Campbell-Walsh-Wein
UROLOGY

Campbell-Walsh-Wein UROLOGY

Editor-in-Chief

Alan W. Partin, MD, PhD

The Jakurski Family Director
Urologist-in-Chief
Chairman, Department of Urology
Professor, Departments of Urology, Oncology and Pathology
Johns Hopkins Medical Institutions
Baltimore, Maryland

Editors

Roger R. Dmochowski,
MD, MMHC, FACS

Professor, Urologic Surgery,
Surgery and Gynecology
Program Director, Female Pelvic
Medicine and Reconstructive Surgery
Vice Chair for Faculty Affairs and
Professionalism
Section of Surgical Sciences
Associate Surgeon-in-Chief
Vanderbilt University Medical Center
Nashville, Tennessee

Louis R. Kavoussi,
MD, MBA

Professor and Chair
Department of Urology
Zucker School of Medicine
at Hofstra/Northwell
Hempstead, New York;
Chairman of Urology
The Arthur Smith
Institute for Urology
Lake Success, New York

Craig A. Peters,
MD

Chief, Pediatric Urology
Children's Health System Texas;
Professor of Urology
University of Texas Southwestern
Medical Center
Dallas, Texas

TWELFTH EDITION

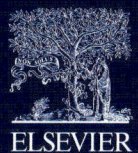

Elsevier
1600 John F. Kennedy Blvd.
Ste 1600
Philadelphia, PA 19103-2899

CAMPBELL-WALSH-WEIN UROLOGY, TWELFTH EDITION

ISBN: 978-0-323-54642-3
Volume I ISBN: 978-0-323-76066-9
Volume II ISBN: 978-0-323-76067-6
Volume III ISBN: 978-0-323-76068-3

INTERNATIONAL EDITION

ISBN: 978-0-323-67226-9
Volume I ISBN: 978-0-323-76005-8
Volume II ISBN: 978-0-323-76006-5
Volume III ISBN: 978-0-323-76007-2

Copyright © 2021 by Elsevier, Inc. All rights reserved.

No part of this publication may be reproduced or transmitted in any form or by any means, electronic or mechanical, including photocopying, recording, or any information storage and retrieval system, without permission in writing from the publisher. Details on how to seek permission, further information about the Publisher's permissions policies and our arrangements with organizations such as the Copyright Clearance Center and the Copyright Licensing Agency, can be found at our website: www.elsevier.com/permissions.

This book and the individual contributions contained in it are protected under copyright by the Publisher (other than as may be noted herein).

Notice

Practitioners and researchers must always rely on their own experience and knowledge in evaluating and using any information, methods, compounds or experiments described herein. Because of rapid advances in the medical sciences, in particular, independent verification of diagnoses and drug dosages should be made. To the fullest extent of the law, no responsibility is assumed by Elsevier, authors, editors or contributors for any injury and/or damage to persons or property as a matter of products liability, negligence or otherwise, or from any use or operation of any methods, products, instructions, or ideas contained in the material herein.

Previous editions copyrighted 2016, 2012, 2007, 2002, 1998, 1992, 1986, 1978, 1970, 1963, and 1954.

ISBN: 978-0-323-54642-3

Senior Content Strategist: Belinda Kuhn
Senior Content Development Specialist: Jennifer Ehlers
Publishing Services Manager: Catherine Jackson
Senior Project Manager: Kate Mannix
Design Direction: Amy Buxton

Printed in Canada

Last digit is the print number: 9 8 7 6 5 4 3 2 1

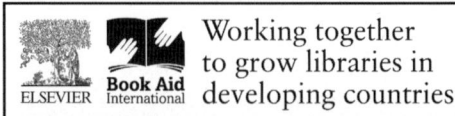

Dedicated to my wife, family, residents, and faculty, all of whom have supported me in this work in various and important ways and helped make this edition of Campbell-Walsh-Wein *possible.*

AP

For this edition of Campbell's *I would like to thank my spouse and my children for their unbelievable support during my career in urology. I would also like to thank my past and present residents and fellows for all that they have taught me about the importance of listening. I would like to recognize a few mentors who have taught me a great deal about the specialty and humanity: Dr. Herb Seybold, Dr. Marty Resnick, Dr. Joe Segura, Dr. Joseph Corriere, Dr. George Benson, Dr. Gerald Jordan, and Dr. Jay Smith.*

RD

To my mentors, whose reassuring voices forever guide me: Bill Catalona, Ralph Clayman, Alan Retik, and Pat Walsh.

LK

The privilege of compiling and editing this book makes us reflect on the vast body of knowledge and experience that makes up the field of urology, and the efforts and dedication of our predecessors and mentors, to whom I dedicate this work. Without the examples, teaching, and inspiration (with not infrequent cajoling and correction), none of us would have been able to grow into who we are or participate in this textbook. For myself, these mentors have been many and varied, guiding me to this day in areas of clinical care, teaching, research, and mentoring. Some are no longer with us but they all continue to inspire.
I also include my wife and children, who inspire, teach, and support me in so many ways. Their commitment has meant the world to me.

CP

PREFACE

Continuing in a great tradition of publishers, editors, and authors, we proudly present to you, our readers, the twelfth edition of the "Bible of Urology"—*Campbell-Walsh-Wein Urology*. Started in 1954 as *Campbell's Urology* and retitled *Campbell-Walsh Urology* in 2012, the present editors felt it was appropriate to honor Alan J. Wein, MD, PhD (Hon) for his many years of dedication to this text by adding his name to the previous chief editors. During his time as chief editor, Dr. Wein was responsible for keeping the textbook in pace with a rapidly growing field in medicine—for this diligence and dedication we are grateful.

As with previous editions, the twelfth edition presents many exciting advances in our use and understanding of technology, physiology, pharmacology, epidemiology, and pathophysiology while maintaining our basic classical urological knowledge.

We are dedicated to keeping the content of this textbook fresh and on the cutting edge of care. *CWW-12* adds 10 novel chapters and more than 150 first-time authors, including several new authors from international sites. *CWW-12* has 3 volumes, 162 chapters, 3706 pages, and more than 3000 illustrations.

The format continues to include color images, Key Points, Suggested Readings, boldfaced important text, and online linkable references to streamline the access and usefulness of the material. Additionally, as in previous editions, a companion Review book with questions and answers for each chapter is available separately under the leadership of Drs. Alan Wein and Thomas F. Kolon.

Volume I (54 chapters) covers basic urological evaluation, imaging and principles and fundamentals of surgery, endourology, and laparoscopy. Also in Volume I is a completely revamped and updated evaluation, the exstrophy-epispadias complex, pediatric stone disease, hypospadias, disorders of sexual development, and many more topics.

Volume II (50 chapters) covers infections within the urinary tract, sexually transmitted diseases, male reproduction, male infertility, erectile dysfunction, neoplasms/management of the testes and penis, medical/surgical management of urological stone disease, and many more topics.

Volume III (58 chapters) covers anatomy, physiology, pharmacology, pathophysiology, oncology, and surgery of the adrenal glands; all chapters covering diagnosis, physiology, and pathophysiology of female and male lower urinary tract disorders; all oncologic aspects (imaging, diagnosis, staging, treatment, and outcomes) of the bladder and prostate; urinary diversion; and physiology, diagnosis, and medical and surgical treatment of benign prostatic hyperplasia.

We all remain extremely proud once again to present you with this textbook and are especially thankful for our spouses and families who have put up with us during the months of review, editing, and proofing. We also give special thanks to the hundreds of authors whose time, expertise, and effort have made all of this possible. We would also like to thank our editorial support staff from Elsevier: Jennifer S. Ehlers (Senior Content Development Specialist) and Belinda Kuhn (Senior Content Strategist), who helped us to coordinate *CWW-12*.

We truly hope you will enjoy reading this textbook.

From the Editors
Alan W. Partin
Roger R. Dmochowski
Louis R. Kavoussi
Craig A. Peters

CONTRIBUTORS

Robert Abouassaly, MD, MS
Assistant Professor, Urology
University Hospitals Case Medical Center
Cleveland, Ohio

Ömer Acar, MD
Department of Urology
College of Medicine
University of Illinois at Chicago
Chicago, Illinois

Mark C. Adams, MD, FAAP
Professor of Urology and Pediatrics
Vanderbilt University
Nashville, Tennessee

Riyad Taher Al-Mousa, MBBS, SSCU, FEBU, MSHA
Consultant Urologist/Neuro-urologist
Urology Department
King Fahad Specialist Hospital–Dammam
Dammam, Saudi Arabia

Mohamad E. Allaf, MD
Vice Chairman and Professor of Urology, Oncology, and Biomedical Engineering
Director of Minimally Invasive and Robotic Surgery
Department of Urology
Brady Urological Institute
Johns Hopkins University School of Medicine
Baltimore, Maryland

Christopher L. Amling, MD, FACS
John Barry Professor and Chair
Department of Urology
Oregon Health & Science University
Portland, Oregon

Christopher B. Anderson, MD, MPH
Assistant Professor, Urology
Columbia University Medical Center
New York, New York

Karl-Erik Andersson, MD, PhD
Professor
Aarhus Institute for Advanced Studies
Aarhus University
Aarhus, Jutland, Denmark;
Professor
Wake Forest Institute for Regenerative Medicine
Wake Forest University School of Medicine
Winston-Salem, North Carolina

Sero Andonian, MD, MSc, FRCS(C), FACS
Associate Professor
Department of Urology
McGill University
Montreal, Canada

Emmanuel S. Antonarakis, MD
Professor of Oncology and Urology
Johns Hopkins Sidney Kimmel Comprehensive Cancer Center
Baltimore, Maryland

Jodi A. Antonelli, MD
Assistant Professor
Department of Urology
University of Texas Southwestern Medical Center
Dallas, Texas

Joshua Augustine, MD
Associate Professor of Medicine
Cleveland Clinic Lerner College of Medicine
Cleveland Clinic
Cleveland, Ohio

Paul F. Austin, MD
Professor
Division of Urologic Surgery
Washington University School of Medicine
St. Louis, Missouri

Timothy D. Averch, MD
Professor and Vice Chair for Quality
University of Pittsburgh Medical Center
Pittsburgh, Pennsylvania

Gina M. Badalato, MD
Assistant Professor, Urology
Columbia University Medical Center
New York, New York

Daniel A. Barocas, MD, MPH, FACS
Associate Professor, Urologic Surgery
Vanderbilt University Medical Center
Nashville, Tennessee

Julia Spencer Barthold, MD
Principal Research Scientist
Nemours Biomedical Research/Division of Urology
Alfred I. duPont Hospital for Children
Wilmington, Delaware;
Professor
Urology and Pediatrics
Thomas Jefferson University
Philadelphia, Pennsylvania

Laurence S. Baskin, MD
Chief of Pediatric Urology
University of California–San Francisco Benioff Children's Hospital
San Francisco, California

Stuart B. Bauer, MD
Professor of Surgery (Urology)
Harvard Medical School;
Senior Associate in Urology
Department of Urology
Boston Children's Hospital
Boston, Massachusetts

Mitchell C. Benson, MD
Herbert and Florence Irving Professor and Chairman Emeritus
Department of Urology
Columbia University;
Attending Physician
Department of Urology
New York Presbyterian Hospital–Columbia
New York, New York

Sara L. Best, MD
Associate Professor
Department of Urology
University of Wisconsin School of Medicine and Public Health
Madison, Wisconsin

Lori A. Birder, PhD
Professor of Medicine and Pharmacology
Medicine–Renal Electrolyte Division
University of Pittsburgh School of Medicine
Pittsburgh, Pennsylvania

Jay T. Bishoff, MD
Director, Intermountain Urological Institute
Intermountain Health Care
Salt Lake City, Utah

Trinity J. Bivalacqua, MD, PhD
R. Christian Evenson Professor of Urology
Johns Hopkins University
Baltimore, Maryland

Marc A. Bjurlin, DO, MSc
Assistant Professor, Urology
New York University
New York, New York

Brian G. Blackburn, MD
Clinical Associate Professor
Internal Medicine/Infectious Diseases and Geographic Medicine
Stanford University School of Medicine
Stanford, California

ix

Bertil Blok, MD, PhD
Department of Urology
Erasmus Medical Center
Rotterdam, Netherlands

Michael L. Blute, MD
Chief, Department of Urology
Walter S. Kerr, Jr., Professor of Urology
Massachusetts General Hospital
Harvard Medical School
Boston, Massachusetts

Timothy B. Boone, MD, PhD
Chairman, Urology
Houston Methodist Hospital;
Professor and Associate Dean
Weill Cornell Medical College
Houston, Texas

Stephen A. Boorjian, MD, FACS
Carl Rosen Professor of Urology
Mayo Clinic
Rochester, Minnesota

Kristy McKiernan Borawski, MD
Clinical Assistant Professor of Urology
Department of Urology
University of North Carolina–Chapel Hill
Chapel Hill, North Carolina

Michael S. Borofsky, MD
Assistant Professor, Urology
University of Minnesota
Minneapolis, Minnesota

Steven B. Brandes, MD
Department of Urology
Columbia University Medical Center
New York, New York

Michael C. Braun, MD
Chief of Renal Service
Texas Children's Hospital;
Professor
Renal Section Chief
Department of Pediatrics
Program Director, Pediatric Nephrology
 Fellowship Program
Baylor College of Medicine
Houston, Texas

Gregory A. Broderick, MD
Professor of Urology
Department of Urology
Mayo Clinic College of Medicine;
Program Director
Urology Residency Program
Mayo Clinic
Jacksonville, Florida

Elizabeth Timbrook Brown, MD, MPH
Assistant Professor, Urology
MedStar Georgetown University Hospital
Washington, DC

Benjamin M. Brucker, MD
Assistant Professor, Urology
New York University
New York, New York

Kathryn L. Burgio, PhD
Professor of Medicine
Department of Medicine
Division of Gerontology, Geriatrics, and
 Palliative Care
University of Alabama at Birmingham;
Associate Director for Research
Birmingham/Atlanta Geriatric Research,
 Education, and Clinical Center
Birmingham VA Medical Center
Birmingham, Alabama

Arthur L. Burnett II, MD, MBA
Patrick C. Walsh Distinguished Professor
 of Urology
Department of Urology
Johns Hopkins School of Medicine
Baltimore, Maryland

Jeffrey A. Cadeddu, MD
Professor of Urology and Radiology
University of Texas Southwestern Medical
 Center
Dallas, Texas

Anne P. Cameron, MD, FRCSC, FPMRS
Associate Professor, Urology
University of Michigan
Ann Arbor, Michigan

Steven C. Campbell, MD, PhD
Professor of Surgery
Department of Urology
Cleveland Clinic
Cleveland, Ohio

Douglas A. Canning, MD
Professor of Surgery (Urology)
Perelman School of Medicine
University of Pennsylvania;
Chief, Division of Urology
Children's Hospital of Philadelphia
Philadelphia, Pennsylvania

Paolo Capogrosso, MD
Department of Urology
Vita-Salute San Raffaele University
Milan, Italy

Michael A. Carducci, MD
AEGON Professor in Prostate Cancer
 Research
Sidney Kimmel Comprehensive Cancer
 Center at Johns Hopkins
Johns Hopkins University School of
 Medicine
Baltimore, Maryland

Maude Carmel, MD
Assistant Professor
Department of Urology at University of
 Texas Southwestern Medical Center
Dallas, Texas

Peter R. Carroll, MD, MPH
Professor and Chair, Urology
University of California, San Francisco
San Francisco, California

K. Clint Cary, MD, MPH
Assistant Professor
Department of Urology
Indiana University
Indianapolis, Indiana

Erik P. Castle, MD
Professor of Urology
Mayo Clinic Arizona
Phoenix, Arizona

Toby C. Chai, MD
Professor and Chair, Department of
 Urology
Boston University School of Medicine;
Chief of Urology
Boston Medical Center
Boston, Massachusetts

Charbel Chalouhy, MD
Assistant Professor of Urology
Campus des Sciences Médicales
St. Joseph University
Beirut, Lebanon

Alicia H. Chang, MD, MS
Instructor
Department of Internal Medicine/
 Infectious Diseases and Geographic
 Medicine
Stanford University School of Medicine
Stanford, California;
Medical Consultant
Los Angeles County Tuberculosis Control
 Program
Los Angeles County Department of Public
 Health
Los Angeles, California

**Christopher R. Chapple, MD, FRCS
(Urol)**
Professor and Consultant Urologist
Department of Urology
The Royal Hallamshire Hospital, Sheffield
 Teaching Hospitals
Sheffield, South Yorkshire, United Kingdom

Thomas Chi, MD
Associate Professor
Associate Chair for Clinical Affairs
Department of Urology
University of California–San Francisco
San Francisco, California

John P. Christodouleas, MD, MPH
Professor of Radiation Oncology
Urologic Cancer Program
Penn Medicine
Philadelphia, Pennsylvania

Peter E. Clark, MD
Professor and Chairman, Urology
Atrium Health;
Chair, Urologic Oncology
Levine Cancer Institute
Charlotte, North Carolina

Douglass B. Clayton, MD, FAAP
Assistant Professor
Urologic Surgery
Vanderbilt University
Nashville, Tennessee

Joshua A. Cohn, MD
Assistant Professor of Urology
Department of Urology
Einstein Healthcare Network;
Assistant Professor of Urology
Department of Surgery, Division of Urologic Oncology
Fox Chase Cancer Center
Philadelphia, Pennsylvania

Michael Joseph Conlin, MD, MCR
Professor, Urology
Portland VA Medical Center;
Professor, Urology
Oregon Health & Sciences University
Portland, Oregon

Christopher S. Cooper, MD, FAAP, FACS
Professor
Department of Urology
University of Iowa;
Associate Dean, Student Affairs and Curriculum
University of Iowa Carver College of Medicine
Iowa City, Iowa

Kimberly L. Cooper, MD
Associate Professor of Urology
Columbia University Medical Center
New York, New York

Lawrence A. Copelovitch, MD
Assistant Professor of Pediatrics
Department of Nephrology
The Children's Hospital of Philadelphia
Philadelphia, Pennsylvania

Hillary L. Copp, MD
Associate Professor, Pediatric Urology
University of California–San Francisco
San Francisco, California

Nicholas G. Cost, MD
Assistant Professor
Department of Surgery
Division of Urology
University of Colorado School of Medicine
Aurora, Colorado

Anthony J. Costello, FRACS, MD
Professor, Urology
Royal Melbourne Hospital, Parkville Victoria
Victoria, Australia

Lindsey Cox, MD
Assistant Professor of Urology
Medical University of South Carolina
Charleston, South Carolina

Paul L. Crispen, MD
Associate Professor
Department of Urology
University of Florida
Gainesville, Florida

Juanita M. Crook, MD, FRCPC
Professor, Radiation Oncology
University of British Columbia;
Radiation Oncologist
Center for the Southern Interior
British Columbia Cancer Agency
Kelowna, British Columbia, Canada

Gerald Cunha, PhD
Professor Emeritus, Urology
School of Medicine
University of California, San Francisco
San Francisco, California

Douglas M. Dahl, MD, FACS
Associate Professor of Surgery
Harvard Medical School;
Chief, Division of Urologic Oncology
Department of Urology
Massachusetts General Hospital
Boston, Massachusetts

Siamak Daneshmand, MD
Associate Professor of Urology (Clinical Scholar)
Institute of Urology
University of Southern California, Los Angeles
Los Angeles, California

Casey A. Dauw, MD
Assistant Professor, Urology
University of Michigan
Ann Arbor, Michigan

Shubha K. De, MD, FRCSC
Assistant Professor
Department of Surgery
Division of Urology
University of Alberta
Edmonton, Alberta, Canada

Guarionex Joel DeCastro, MD, MPH
Assistant Professor, Urology
Columbia University Medical Center;
Department of Urology
New York Presbyterian Hospital/ Columbia University
New York, New York

Jean J.M.C.H. de la Rosette, MD, PhD
Professor, Urology
AMC University Hospital
Amsterdam, Netherlands

Francisco T. Dénes, MD, PhD
Associate Professor, Division of Urology
Chief, Pediatric Urology
University of São Paulo Medical School;
Hospital das Clínicas
São Paulo, Brazil

Dirk J.M.K. De Ridder, MD, PhD, FEBU
Professor, Urology
University Hospitals KU Leuven
Leuven, Belgium

Mahesh R. Desai, MS, FRCS
Chief Urologist and Managing Trustee
Department of Urology
Muljibhai Patel Urological Hospital, Nadiad
Gujarat, India

David Andrew Diamond, MD
Urologist-in-Chief
Department of Urology
Boston Children's Hospital;
Professor of Surgery (Urology)
Harvard Medical School
Boston, Massachusetts

Heather N. Di Carlo, MD
Director, Pediatric Urology Research
Assistant Professor of Urology
Johns Hopkins Medicine
Baltimore, Maryland

Colin P.N. Dinney, MD
Chairman and Professor
Department of Urology
The University of Texas MD Anderson Cancer Center
Houston, Texas

Roger R. Dmochowski, MD, MMHC, FACS
Professor, Urologic Surgery, Surgery and Gynecology
Program Director, Female Pelvic Medicine and Reconstructive Surgery
Vice Chair for Faculty Affairs and Professionalism
Section of Surgical Sciences
Associate Surgeon-in-Chief
Vanderbilt University Medical Center
Nashville, Tennessee

Charles G. Drake, MD, PhD
Associate Professor of Oncology, Immunology, and Urology
James Buchanan Brady Urological Institute
Johns Hopkins University;
Attending Physician
Department of Oncology
Johns Hopkins Kimmel Cancer Center
Baltimore, Maryland

Brian Duty, MD
Associate Professor, Urology
Oregon Health & Science University
Portland, Oregon

James A. Eastham, MD
Chief, Urology Service
Department of Surgery
Memorial Sloan-Kettering Cancer Center;
Professor, Urology
Weill Cornell Medical Center
New York, New York

Scott Eggener, MD
Professor, Surgery
University of Chicago
Chicago, Illinois

Mohamed Aly Elkoushy, MD, MSc, PhD
Professor, Urology
Faculty of Medicine
Suez Canal University
Ismailia, Egypt

Jonathan Scott Ellison, MD
Assistant Professor of Urology
Medical College of Wisconsin
Children's Hospital of Wisconsin
Milwaukee, Wisconsin

Sammy E. Elsamra, MD
Assistant Professor of Surgery (Urology)
Department of Urology
Rutgers Robert Wood Johnson Medical School;
Director of Robotic Surgical Services
Robert Wood Johnson University Hospital
RWJ-Barnabas Health
New Brunswick, New Jersey

Jonathan I. Epstein, MD
Professor of Pathology, Urology, Oncology
The Reinhard Professor of Urological Pathology
Director of Surgical Pathology
The Johns Hopkins Medical Institutions
Baltimore, Maryland

Carlos R. Estrada, MD, MBA
Associate Professor, Surgery
Harvard Medical School;
Associate in Urology
Boston Children's Hospital
Boston, Massachusetts

Jairam R. Eswara, MD
Assistant Surgeon
Division of Urology
Brigham and Women's Hospital
Boston, Massachusetts

Fernando A. Ferrer, MD, FACS, FAAP
Professor of Urology
Department of Urology
Mount Sinai School of Medicine
New York, New York

Neil Fleshner, MD, MPH, FRCSC
Professor of Surgery and Martin Barkin Chair
Department of Urology
University of Toronto;
Surgeon, Uro-Oncology
University Health Network
Toronto, Ontario, Canada

Bryan Foster, MD
Associate Professor
Department of Radiology
Oregon Health & Science University
Portland, Oregon

Richard S. Foster, MD
Professor, Department of Urology
Indiana University
Indianapolis, Indiana

Pat F. Fulgham, MD
Director of Surgical Oncology
Department of Urology
Texas Health Presbyterian Dallas
Dallas, Texas

Arvind P. Ganpule, MS, DNB
Department of Urology
Muljibhai Patel Urological Hospital
Nadiad, Gujarat, India

Kris Gaston, MD
Carolinas Medical Center
Charlotte, North Carolina

John P. Gearhart, MD
The James Buchanan Brady Urological Institute
Johns Hopkins Medical Institutions
Baltimore, Maryland

Matthew T. Gettman, MD
Professor and Vice-Chair, Urology
Mayo Clinic
Rochester, Minnesota

Reza Ghavamian, MD
Eastern Regional Director of Urology
Department of Urology
Northwell Health
Greenlawn, New York;
Professor of Urology
Zucker School of Medicine at Hofstra Northwell
New Hyde Park, New York

Bruce R. Gilbert, MD, PhD
Professor of Urology
The Smith Institute for Urology
Zucker School of Medicine of Hofstra/ Northwell
New Hyde Park, New York

Timothy D. Gilligan, MD, MS, FASCO
Associate Professor of Medicine
Solid Tumor Oncology
Cleveland Clinic Lerner College of Medicine;
Program Director, Hematology/Oncology Fellowship
Taussig Cancer Institute
Cleveland Clinic
Cleveland, Ohio

David A. Goldfarb, MD
Professor of Surgery, CCLCM
Glickman Urological and Kidney Institute
Cleveland Clinic
Cleveland, Ohio

Marc Goldstein, MD, DSc (hon), FACS
Matthew P. Hardy Distinguished Professor of Urology and Male Reproductive Medicine
Department of Urology and Institute for Reproductive Medicine
Weill Medical College of Cornell University;
Surgeon-in-Chief, Male Reproductive Medicine, and Surgery
Department of Urology and Institute for Reproductive Medicine
New York Presbyterian Hospital–Weill Cornell Medical Center
New York, New York

Leonard G. Gomella, MD, FACS
Professor and Chair
Department of Urology
Thomas Jefferson University
Philadelphia, Pennsylvania

Alex Gomelsky, MD
B.E. Trichel Professor and Chairman
Department of Urology
Louisiana State University Health–Shreveport
Shreveport, Louisiana

Mark L. Gonzalgo, MD, PhD
Professor and Vice Chairman, Urology
University of Miami Miller School of Medicine
Miami, Florida

Michael A. Gorin, MD
Assistant Professor
Department of Urology
Johns Hopkins University School of Medicine
Baltimore, Maryland

Tamsin Greenwell, MD, PhD
Consultant Urological Surgeon
University College London Hospitals
London, United Kingdom

Tomas L. Griebling, MD, MPH
John P. Wolf 33-Degree Masonic Distinguished Professor of Urology
Department of Urology
The Landon Center on Aging
The University of Kansas
Kansas City, Kansas

Khurshid A. Guru, MD
Chair, Department of Urology
Director of Robotic Surgery
Robert P. Huben Endowed Professor of Urologic Oncology
Roswell Park Comprehensive Cancer Center
Buffalo, New York

Thomas J. Guzzo, MD, MPH
Assistant Professor of Urology
The Hospital of the University of Pennsylvania
University of Pennsylvania
Philadelphia, Pennsylvania

Jennifer A. Hagerty, DO
Attending Physician
Departments of Surgery/Urology
Nemours/Alfred I. duPont Hospital for Children
Wilmington, Delaware;
Assistant Professor
Departments of Urology and Pediatrics
Sidney Kimmel Medical College of Thomas Jefferson University
Philadelphia, Pennsylvania

Simon J. Hall, MD
Professor
Smith Institute for Urology
Hofstra Northwell School of Medicine
Lake Success, New York

Barry Hallner, MD
Associate Program Director, Female Pelvic Medicine & Reconstructive Surgery
Assistant Professor
Departments of OB/GYN and Urology
Louisiana State University Health New Orleans School of Medicine
New Orleans, Louisiana

Ethan J. Halpern, MD, MSCE
Professor of Radiology and Urology
Department of Radiology
Thomas Jefferson University
Philadelphia, Pennsylvania

Misop Han, MD, MS
Professor, Urology and Oncology
Johns Hopkins Medicine
Baltimore, Maryland

Philip M. Hanno, MD, MPH
Clinical Professor, Urology
Stanford University School of Medicine
Palo Alto, California

Siobhan M. Hartigan, MD
Female Pelvic Medicine and Reconstructive Surgery Fellow
Department of Urology
Vanderbilt University Medical Center
Nashville, Tennessee

Christopher J. Hartman, MD
Assistant Professor of Urology
The Smith Institute for Urology
Northwell Health System
Long Island City, New York

Hashim Hashim, MBBS, MRCS (Eng), MD, FEBU, FRCS (Urol)
Consultant Urological Surgeon
Honorary Professor
Director of the Urodynamics Unit
Bristol Urological Institute
Southmead Hospital
Bristol, United Kingdom

Dorota J. Hawksworth, MD, MBA
Director of Andrology and Male Sexual Health
Department of Urology
Walter Reed National Military Medical Center
Bethesda, Maryland

Sarah Hazell, MD
Radiation Oncology Resident
Department of Radiation Oncology and Molecular Radiation Sciences
Johns Hopkins University School of Medicine
Baltimore, Maryland

John P.F.A. Heesakkers, MD, PhD
Urologist
Radboudumc
Nijmegen, Netherlands

Sevann Helo, MD
Southern Illinois University School of Medicine
Division of Urology
Springfield, Illinois

Amin S. Herati, MD
Assistant Professor of Urology
Department of Urology
The James Buchanan Brady Urological Institute
Johns Hopkins University School of Medicine;
Assistant Professor
Gynecology and Obstetrics
Johns Hopkins University School of Medicine
Baltimore, Maryland

C.D. Anthony Herndon, MD, FAAP, FACS
Professor of Surgery
Director of Pediatric Urology
Surgeon-in-Chief, Children's Hospital of Richmond
Department of Urology
Virginia Commonwealth University
Richmond, Virginia

Piet Hoebeke, MD, PhD
Professor, Urology
Dean, Faculty of Medicine and Health Sciences
Ghent University
Ghent, Belgium

David M. Hoenig, MD
Professor and Chief
North Shore University Hospital
Smith Institute for Urology
North Shore-LIJ-Hofstra University
Lake Success, New York

Michael Hsieh, MD, PhD
Stirewalt Endowed Director
Biomedical Research Institute
Rockville, Maryland;
Associate Professor, Urology
George Washington University
Washington, DC

Valerio Iacovelli, MD
Urology Unit
University of Rome Tor Vergata
San Carlo di Nancy General Hospital
GVM Care and Research
Rome, Italy

Stephen V. Jackman, MD
Professor, Urology
University of Pittsburgh
Pittsburgh, Pennsylvania

Joseph M. Jacob, MD, MCR
Assistant Professor, Urology
SUNY Upstate Medical Center
Syracuse, New York

Micah A. Jacobs, MD, MPH
Department of Urology
University of Texas Southwestern Medical School
Dallas, Texas

Thomas W. Jarrett, MD
Professor and Chairman, Urology
George Washington University
Washington, DC

Gerald H. Jordan, MD, FACS, FAAP (Hon), FRCS (Hon)
Associate Professor, Urology
Eastern Virginia Medical School
Norfolk, Virginia

Martin Kaefer, MD
Professor, Urology
Indiana University School of Medicine
Indianapolis, Indiana

Kamaljot S. Kaler, MD
Clinical Assistant Professor
Section of Urology
Department of Surgery
University of Calgary
Calgary, Alberta, Canada

Panagiotis Kallidonis, MD, MSc, PhD, FEBU
Consultant Urological Surgeon
Department of Urology
University of Patras
Patras, Greece

Steven Kaplan, MD
Professor and Director
The Men's Health Program
Department of Urology
Icahn School of Medicine at Mount Sinai
New York, New York

Max Kates, MD
Assistant Professor, Urology
Johns Hopkins Medical Institutions
Baltimore, Maryland

Melissa R. Kaufman, MD, PhD
Associate Professor, Urologic Surgery
Vanderbilt University
Nashville, Tennessee

Louis R. Kavoussi, MD, MBA
Professor and Chair
Department of Urology
Zucker School of Medicine at Hofstra/
    Northwell
Hempstead, New York;
Chairman of Urology
The Arthur Smith Institute for Urology
Lake Success, New York

Parviz K. Kavoussi, MD, FACS
Reproductive Urologist
Department of Urology
Austin Fertility and Reproductive
    Medicine;
Adjunct Assistant Professor
Psychology: Neuroendocrinology and
    Motivation
University of Texas at Austin
Austin, Texas

Miran Kenk, PhD
University Health Network
Toronto, Canada

Mohit Khera, MD, MBA, MPH
Professor of Urology
Scott Department of Urology
Baylor College of Medicine
Houston, Texas

Antoine E. Khoury, MD, FRCSC, FAAP
Walter R. Schmid Professor of Pediatric
    Urology
Head of Pediatric Urology
Children's Hospital of Orange County
Orange, California

Eric A. Klein, MD
Chairman, Glickman Urological and
    Kidney Institute
Cleveland Clinic
Cleveland, Ohio

Laurence Klotz, MD, FRCSC
Professor, Surgery
University of Toronto;
Urologist
Sunnybrook Health Sciences Centre
Toronto, Ontario, Canada

Bodo Egon Knudsen, MD, FRCSC
Associate Professor
Vice Chair Clinical Operations
Department of Urology
Wexner Medical Center
The Ohio State University
Columbus, Ohio

Kathleen C. Kobashi, MD
Section Head, Urology and Renal
    Transplantation
Virginia Mason Medical Center
Seattle, Washington

Chester J. Koh, MD
Associate Professor of Urology (Pediatric)
TCH Department of Surgery
Scott Department of Urology
Baylor College of Medicine
Texas Children's Hospital
Houston, Texas

Ervin Kocjancic, MD
Professor of Urology
Department of Urology
University of Illinois Health and Science
Chicago, Illinois

Badrinath R. Konety, MD, MBA
Professor and Chair, Dougherty Family
    Chair in UroOncology
Associate Director for Clinical Affairs and
    Clinical Research
Masonic Cancer Center;
Department of Urology
University of Minnesota
Minneapolis, Minnesota

Casey E. Kowalik, MD
Department of Urologic Surgery
Vanderbilt University
Nashville, Tennessee

Martin A. Koyle, MD, FAAP, FACS, FRCSC, FRCS (Eng)
Division Head, Pediatric Urology
Women's Auxiliary Chair in Urology and
    Regenerative Medicine
Hospital for Sick Children;
Professor of Surgery
University of Toronto
Toronto, Ontario, Canada

Amy E. Krambeck, MD
Michael O. Koch Professor of Urology
Indiana University
Indianapolis, Indiana

Jessica E. Kreshover, MD, MS
Assistant Professor
Arthur Smith Institute for Urology
Donald and Barbara Zucker School of
    Medicine at Hofstra-Northwell
Lake Success, New York

Venkatesh Krishnamurthi, MD
Director, Kidney/Pancreas Transplant
    Program
Glickman Urological and Kidney
    Institute, Transplant Center
Cleveland Clinic Foundation
Cleveland, Ohio

Ryan M. Krlin, MD
Assistant Professor of Urology
Department of Urology
Louisiana State University
New Orleans, Louisiana

Alexander Kutikov, MD, FACS
Professor and Chief, Urologic Oncology
Fox Chase Cancer Center
Philadelphia, Pennsylvania

Jaime Landman, MD
Professor of Urology and Radiology
Chairman, Department of Urology
University of California Irvine
Orange, California

Brian R. Lane, MD, PhD
Chief, Urology
Spectrum Health;
Associate Professor
Michigan State University College of
    Human Medicine
Grand Rapids, Michigan

David A. Leavitt, MD
Assistant Professor, Urology
Vattikuti Urology Institute
Henry Ford Health System
Detroit, Michigan

Eugene K. Lee, MD
Assistant Professor, Urology
University of Kansas Medical Center
Kansas City, Kansas

Gary E. Lemack, MD
Professor of Urology and Neurology
University of Texas Southwestern Medical
    Center
Dallas, Texas

Thomas Sean Lendvay, MD, FACS
Professor, Urology
University of Washington;
Professor, Pediatric Urology
Seattle Children's Hospital
Seattle, Washington

Herbert Lepor, MD
Professor and Martin Spatz Chairman
Department of Urology
NYU School of Medicine;
Chief, Urology
NYU Langine Health System
New York, New York

Evangelos Liatsikos, MD, PhD
Professor, Urology
University of Patras
Patras, Greece

Sey Kiat Lim, MBBS, MRCS (Edinburgh), MMed (Surgery), FAMS (Urology)
Associate Consultant, Urology
Changi General Hospital
Singapore

W. Marston Linehan, MD
Chief, Urologic Oncology Branch
National Cancer Institute
National Institutes of Health
Bethesda, Maryland

Richard Edward Link, MD, PhD
Carlton-Smith Chair in Urologic Education
Associate Professor of Urology
Director, Division of Endourology and Minimally Invasive Surgery
Scott Department of Urology
Baylor College of Medicine
Houston, Texas

Jen-Jane Liu, MD
Director of Urologic Oncology
Assistant Professor
Department of Urology
Oregon Health & Science University
Portland, Oregon

Stacy Loeb, MD, MSc
Assistant Professor, Urology and Population Health
New York University and Manhattan Veterans Affairs
New York, New York

Christopher J. Long, MD
Assistant Professor of Urology
Department of Surgery
Division of Urology
Children's Hospital of Philadelphia
Philadelphia, Pennsylvania

Roberto Iglesias Lopes, MD, PhD
Assistant Professor
Division of Urology
Department of Surgery
University of São Paulo Medical School
São Paulo, Brazil

Armando J. Lorenzo, MD, MSc, FRCSC, FAAP, FACS
Staff Paediatric Urologist
Department of Surgery
Division of Urology
Hospital for Sick Children;
Associate Professor
Department of Surgery
Division of Urology
University of Toronto
Toronto, Ontario, Canada

Yair Lotan, MD
Professor
Department of Urology
University of Texas Southwestern Medical Center
Dallas, Texas

Alvaro Lucioni, MD
Department of Urology
Virginia Mason Medical Center
Seattle, Washington

Tom F. Lue, MD, ScD (Hon), FACS
Professor of Urology
University of California–San Francisco
San Francisco, California

Nicolas Lumen, MD, PhD
Professor, Urology
Ghent University Hospital
Ghent, Belgium

Marcos Tobias Machado, MD, PhD
Head, Urologic Oncology Section
Department of Urology
Faculdade de Medicina do ABC, Santo André
São Paulo, Brazil

Stephen D. Marshall, MD
Attending Physician
Laconia Clinic Department of Urology
Lakes Region General Hospital
Laconia, New Hampshire

Aaron D. Martin, MD, MPH
Associate Professor
Department of Urology
Louisiana State University Health Sciences Center;
Pediatric Urology
Children's Hospital New Orleans
New Orleans, Louisiana

Laura M. Martinez, MD
Instructor in Clinical Urology
Houston Methodist
Houston, Texas

Timothy A. Masterson, MD
Associate Professor, Urology
Indiana University Medical Center
Indianapolis, Indiana

Surena F. Matin, MD
Professor
Department of Urology
The University of Texas M.D. Anderson Cancer Center;
Medical Director
Minimally Invasive New Technology in Oncologic Surgery (MINTOS)
The University of Texas M.D. Anderson Cancer Center
Houston, Texas

Brian R. Matlaga, MD, MPH
Professor
James Buchanan Brady Urological Institute
Johns Hopkins Medical Institutions
Baltimore, Maryland

Kurt A. McCammon, MD, FACS
Devine Chair in Genitourinary Reconstructive Surgery
Chairman and Program Director
Professor
Department of Urology
Eastern Virginia Medical School
Norfolk, Virginia

James M. McKiernan, MD
Chairman and Professor, Urology
Columbia University Medical Center/NYPH
New York, New York

Chris G. McMahon, MBBS, FAChSHP
Director
Australian Centre for Sexual Health
Sydney, New South Wales, Australia

Kevin T. McVary, MD, FACS
Professor and Chairman
Division of Urology
Department of Surgery
Southern Illinois University School of Medicine
Springfield, Illinois

Luis G. Medina, MD
Medical Doctor and Researcher
Department of Urology
University of Southern California
Los Angeles, California

Kirstan K. Meldrum, MD
Professor
Department of Surgery
Central Michigan University
Saginaw, Michigan

Matthew J. Mellon, MD, FACS
Associate Professor, Urology
Indiana University
Indianapolis, Indiana

Maxwell V. Meng, MD
Professor, Urology
Chief, Urologic Oncology
University of California–San Francisco
San Francisco, California

David Mikhail, MD, FRCSC
Endourology Fellow
Department of Urology
Arthur Smith Institute for Urology/Northwell Health
New Hyde Park, New York

Nicole L. Miller, MD
Associate Professor
Department of Urologic Surgery
Vanderbilt University Medical Center
Nashville, Tennessee

Alireza Moinzadeh, MD
Director of Robotic Surgery
Institute of Urology
Lahey Hospital & Medical Center
Burlington, Massachusetts;
Assistant Professor, Urology
Tufts University School of Medicine
Boston, Massachusetts

Robert M. Moldwin, MD
Professor of Urology
The Arthur Smith Institute for Urology
Hofstra Northwell School of Medicine
Lake Success, New York

Manoj Monga, MD, FACS
Director, Stevan Streem Center for Endourology & Stone Disease
Department of Urology
Cleveland Clinic
Cleveland, Ohio

Francesco Montorsi, MD, FRCS (Hon)
Professor and Chairman, Urology
Vita-Salute San Raffaele University
Milan, Italy

Daniel M. Moreira, MD, MHS
Assistant Professor, Urology
University of Illinois at Chicago
Chicago, Illinois

Allen F. Morey, MD, FACS
Professor, Urology
University of Texas Southwestern Medical Center
Dallas, Texas

Todd M. Morgan, MD
Associate Professor
Department of Urology
University of Michigan
Ann Arbor, Michigan

John J. Mulcahy, MD, PhD, FACS
Clinical Professor, Urology
University of Alabama
Birmingham, Alabama

Ravi Munver, MD, FACS
Vice Chairman
Department of Urology
Hackensack University Medical Center;
Professor of Surgery (Urology)
Department of Urology
Seton Hall-Hackensack Meridian School of Medicine
Hackensack, New Jersey

Stephen Y. Nakada, MD, FACS, FRCS (Glasg.)
Professor and Chairman, The David T. Uehling Chair of Urology
Department of Urology
University of Wisconsin School of Medicine and Public Health;
Professor and Chairman
Department of Urology
University of Wisconsin Hospital and Clinics
Madison, Wisconsin

Neema Navai, MD
Assistant Professor, Urology
The University of Texas MD Anderson Cancer Center
Houston, Texas

Diane K. Newman, DNP, ANP-BC, FAAN
Adjunct Professor of Urology in Surgery
Division of Urology
Perelman School of Medicine;
Research Investigator Senior
Perelman School of Medicine
University of Pennsylvania
Philadelphia, Pennsylvania

Craig Stuart Niederberger, MD, FACS
Clarence C. Saelhof Professor and Head
Department of Urology
University of Illinois at Chicago College of Medicine;
Professor, Bioengineering
University of Illinois at Chicago College of Engineering
Chicago, Illinois

Victor W. Nitti, MD
Professor of Urology and Obstetrics & Gynecology
Shlomo Raz Chair in Urology
Chief, Division of Female Pelvic Medicine and Reconstructive Surgery
David Geffen School of Medicine at UCLA
Los Angeles, California

Samuel John Ohlander, MD
Assistant Professor, Urology
University of Illinois at Chicago
Chicago, Illinois

L. Henning Olsen, MD, DMSc
Professor, Urology
Section of Pediatric Urology
Aarhus University Hospital
Skejby, Denmark;
Professor
Institute of Clinical Medicine
Aarhus University
Aarhus, Denmark

Aria F. Olumi, MD
Professor of Surgery/Urology
Department of Urologic Surgery
Beth Israel Deaconess Medical Center
Harvard Medical School
Boston, Massachusetts

Nadir I. Osman, MBChB (Hons), MRCS
Department of Urology
Royal Hallmashire Hospital
Sheffield, South Yorkshire, United Kingdom

Brandon J. Otto, MD
Assistant Professor, Urology
University of Florida
Gainesville, Florida

Priya Padmanabhan, MD, MPH
Assistant Professor, Pelvic Reconstruction and Voiding Dysfunction
The University of Kansas
Kansas City, Kansas

Rodrigo Lessi Pagani, MD
Assistant Professor, Urology
University of Illinois at Chicago
Chicago, Illinois

Lance C. Pagliaro, MD
Professor
Department of Genitourinary Medical Oncology
The University of Texas MD Anderson Cancer Center
Houston, Texas

Ganesh S. Palapattu, MD
Chief of Urologic Oncology
Associate Professor, Urology
University of Michigan
Ann Arbor, Michigan

Drew A. Palmer, MD
Endourology Fellow
Department of Urology
University of North Carolina at Chapel Hill
Chapel Hill, North Carolina

Jeffrey S. Palmer, MD, FACS, FAAP
Director, Pediatric and Adolescent Urology Institute
Cleveland, Ohio

Lane S. Palmer, MD, FACS
Professor and Chief, Pediatric Urology
Cohen Children's Medical Center of New York
Zucker School of Medicine of Hofstra/Northwell
Long Island, New York

Meyeon Park, MD, MAS
Assistant Professor in Residence, Medicine
University of California–San Francisco
San Francisco, California

William P. Parker, MD
Department of Urology
University of Kansas Health System
Kansas City, Kansas

Alan W. Partin, MD, PhD
The Jakurski Family Director
Urologist-in-Chief
Chairman, Department of Urology
Professor, Departments of Urology, Oncology and Pathology
Johns Hopkins Medical Institutions
Baltimore, Maryland

Roshan M. Patel, MD
Clinical Instructor
Department of Urology
University of California–Irvine
Orange, California

Margaret S. Pearle, MD, PhD
Professor, Urology, Internal Medicine
University of Texas Southwestern Medical Center
Dallas, Texas

David F. Penson, MD, MPH
Professor and Chair, Urologic Surgery
Vanderbilt University;
Director
Center for Surgical Quality and Outcomes Research
Vanderbilt Institute for Medicine and Public Health
Nashville, Tennessee

Craig A. Peters, MD
Chief, Pediatric Urology
Children's Health System Texas;
Professor of Urology
University of Texas Southwestern Medical Center
Dallas, Texas

Curtis A. Pettaway, Sr., MD
Professor
Department of Urology
University of Texas M.D. Anderson Cancer Center
Houston, Texas

Janey R. Phelps, MD
Department of Anesthesia
University of North Carolina School of Medicine
Chapel Hill, North Carolina

Ryan Phillips, MD, PhD
Resident Physician
Radiation Oncology and Molecular Radiation Sciences
Johns Hopkins University School of Medicine
Baltimore, Maryland

Phillip M. Pierorazio, MD
Associate Professor
Urology and Oncology
Brady Urological Institute and Department of Urology
Johns Hopkins University
Baltimore, Maryland

Hans G. Pohl, MD, FAAP
Associate Professor, Urology and Pediatrics
Children's National Medical Center
Washington, DC

Thomas J. Polascik, MD
Professor, Urologic Surgery
Duke Comprehensive Cancer Center
Duke Cancer Institute
Durham, North Carolina

Michel Pontari, MD
Professor and Vice-Chair, Urology
Lewis Katz School of Medicine at Temple University
Philadelphia, Pennsylvania

John C. Pope IV, MD
Professor, Urologic Surgery and Pediatrics
Vanderbilt University Medical Center
Nashville, Tennessee

Jay D. Raman, MD, FACS
Professor and Chief, Urology
Penn State Health Milton S. Hershey Medical Center
Hershey, Pennsylvania

Ranjith Ramasamy, MD
Director, Reproductive Urology
Department of Urology
University of Miami
Miami, Florida

Ardeshir R. Rastinehad, DO, FACOS
Director, Focal Therapy and Interventional Urology
Associate Professor of Radiology and Urology
Icahn School of Medicine at Mount Sinai
New York, New York

Yazan F.H. Rawashdeh, MD, PhD
Consultant Pediatric Urologist
Section of Pediatric Urology
Aarhus University Hospital
Aarhus, Denmark

Pramod P. Reddy, MD
The Curtis Sheldon and Jeffrey Wacksman Chair of Pediatric Urology
Division of Pediatric Urology
Cincinnati Children's Hospital Medical Center;
Professor of Surgery
Division of Urology
University of Cincinnati College of Medicine
Cincinnati, Ohio

W. Stuart Reynolds, MD, MPH
Assistant Professor, Urologic Surgery
Vanderbilt University
Nashville, Tennessee

Koon Ho Rha, MD, PhD, FACS
Professor
Department of Urology
Urological Science Institute
Yonsei University College of Medicine
Seoul, Republic of Korea

Lee Richstone, MD
Chief, Urology
Long Island Jewish Medical Center
Lake Success, New York;
System Vice Chairman, Urology
Northwell Health
New York, New York

Stephen Riggs, MD
Urologic Oncology
Levine Cancer Institute
Charlotte, North Carolina

Richard C. Rink, MD, FAAP, FACS
Emeritus Professor, Pediatric Urology
Riley Hospital for Children Indiana University School of Medicine;
Faculty, Pediatric Urology
Peyton Manning Children's Hospital St. Vincent
Indianapolis, Indiana

Michael L. Ritchey, MD
Professor, Urology
Mayo Clinic College of Medicine
Phoenix, Arizona

Claus G. Roehrborn, MD
Professor and Chairman, Urology
University of Texas Southwestern Medical Center
Dallas, Texas

Ashley Evan Ross, MD, PhD
Assistant Professor, Urology
Johns Hopkins Brady Urological Institute
Baltimore, Maryland

Sherry S. Ross, MD
Department of Anesthesia
The University of North Carolina at Chapel Hill
Chapel Hill, North Carolina

Christopher C. Roth, MD
Associate Professor of Urology
Louisiana State University Health Sciences Center;
Pediatric Urology
Childrens Hospital New Orleans
New Orleans, Louisiana

Kyle O. Rove, MD
Urologist
St. Louis Children's Hospital
Washington University
St. Louis, Missouri

Eric S. Rovner, MD
Professor
Department of Urology
Medical University of South Carolina
Charleston, South Carolina

Steven P. Rowe, MD
Assistant Professor
Department of Radiology
Johns Hopkins University
Baltimore, Maryland

Matthew P. Rutman, MD
Associate Professor, Urology
Columbia University College of Physicians and Surgeons
New York, New York

Simpa S. Salami, MD, MPH
Assistant Professor
Department of Urology
University of Michigan
Ann Arbor, Michigan

Andrea Salonia, MD, PhD
Director, Urological Research Institute
Milan, Italy

Edward M. Schaeffer, MD, PhD
Professor and Chair, Urology
Northwestern University
Chicago, Illinois

Bruce J. Schlomer, MD
Assistant Professor, Urology
University of Texas Southwestern Medical Center
Dallas, Texas

Michael J. Schwartz, MD, FACS
Associate Professor of Urology
The Smith Institute for Urology
Hofstra Northwell School of Medicine
New Hyde Park, New York

Allen D. Seftel, MD
Professor of Urology
Department of Surgery
Cooper Medical School of Rowan University;
Chief, Division of Urology
Cooper University Health Care
Camden, New Jersey

Rachel Selekman, MD, MAS
Instructor, Surgery
Division of Pediatric Urology
Children's National Medical Center
Washington, DC

Abhishek Seth, MD
Assistant Professor, Urology
Baylor College of Medicine
Houston, Texas

Karen S. Sfanos, PhD
Assistant Professor, Pathology
Johns Hopkins University School of Medicine
Baltimore, Maryland

Paras H. Shah, MD
Urologic Oncology
Department of Urology
Mayo Clinic
Rochester, Minnesota

Mohammed Shahait, MBBS
Clinical Instructor of Urology
University of Pittsburgh Medical Center
Pittsburgh, Pennsylvania

Robert C. Shamberger, MD
Chief of Surgery
Boston Children's Hospital;
Robert E. Gross Professor of Surgery
Harvard Medical School
Boston, Massachusetts

Alan W. Shindel, MD, MAS
Associate Professor, Urology
University of California, San Francisco
San Francisco, California

Aseem Ravindra Shukla, MD
Director of Minimally Invasive Surgery
Department of Pediatric Urology
Children's Hospital of Philadelphia
Philadelphia, Pennsylvania

Jay Simhan, MD, FACS
Vice Chairman, Department of Urology
Einstein Healthcare Network;
Associate Professor of Urology
Temple Health/Fox Chase Cancer Center
Philadelphia, Pennsylvania

Brian Wesley Simons, DVM, PhD
Assistant Professor, Urology
Johns Hopkins University School of Medicine
Baltimore, Maryland

Eila C. Skinner, MD
Professor and Chair, Urology
Stanford University
Stanford, California

Armine K. Smith, MD
Assistant Professor
Brady Urological Institute
Johns Hopkins University;
Assistant Professor, Urology
George Washington University
Washington, DC

Daniel Y. Song, MD
Associate Professor, Radiation Oncology and Molecular Radiation Sciences
Johns Hopkins University School of Medicine
Baltimore, Maryland

Rene Sotelo, MD
Physician, Surgeon, Urologist
Minimally Invasive and Robotic Surgery Center
Instituto Medico La Floresta, Caracas
Miranda, Venezuela

Michael W. Sourial, MD, FRCSC
Assistant Professor, Urology
Wexner Medical Center
The Ohio State University
Columbus, Ohio

Anne-Françoise Spinoit, MD, PhD
Pediatric and Reconstructive Urologist
Department of Urology
Ghent University Hospital
Ghent, Belgium

Arun K. Srinivasan, MD
Pediatric Urologist
Children's Hospital of Philadelphia
Philadelphia, Pennsylvania

Ramaprasad Srinivasan, MD, PhD
Head, Molecular Cancer Section
Urologic Oncology Branch
Center for Cancer Research
National Cancer Institute
National Institutes of Health
Bethesda, Maryland

Irina Stanasel, MD
Assistant Professor, Urology
University of Texas Southwestern Medical Center/Children's Health
Dallas, Texas

Andrew J. Stephenson, MD, MBA, FRCSC, FACS
Associate Professor of Surgery
Department of Urology
Cleveland Clinic Lerner College of Medicine
Case Western Reserve University;
Director, Urologic Oncology
Glickman Urological and Kidney Institute
Cleveland Clinic
Cleveland, Ohio

Julie N. Stewart, MD
Assistant Professor
Department of Urology
Houston Methodist Hospital
Houston, Texas

John Stites, MD
Minimally Invasive and Robotic Urologic Surgery
Hackensack University Medical Center
Hackensack, New Jersey

Douglas W. Storm, MD, FAAP
Assistant Professor
Department of Urology
University of Iowa Hospitals and Clinics
Iowa City, Iowa

Douglas William Strand, PhD
Assistant Professor, Urology
University of Texas Southwestern Medical Center
Dallas, Texas

Li-Ming Su, MD
David A. Cofrin Professor of Urologic Oncology
Chairman, Department of Urology
University of Florida College of Medicine
Gainesville, Florida

Chandru P. Sundaram, MD, FACS, FRCS (Eng)
Professor, Urology
Indiana University School of Medicine;
Program Director and Director of Minimally Invasive Surgery
Department of Urology
Indiana University School of Medicine
Indianapolis, Indiana

Samir S. Taneja, MD
James M. and Janet Riha Neissa Professor of Urologic Oncology
Departments of Urology and Radiology
NYU Langone Medical Center
New York, New York

Nikki Tang, MD
Assistant Professor, Dermatology
Johns Hopkins University
Baltimore, Maryland

Gregory E. Tasian, MD, MSc, MSCE
Assistant Professor, Urology and
  Epidemiology
University of Pennsylvania–Perelman
  School of Medicine;
Attending Physician, Urology
The Children's Hospital of Philadelphia
Philadelphia, Pennsylvania

**Kae Jack Tay, MBBS, MRCS (Ed), MMed
(Surgery), MCI, FAMS (Urology)**
Consultant
Department of Urology
Singapore General Hospital
SingHealth Duke-NUS Academic Medical
  Center
Singapore

John C. Thomas, MD, FAAP, FACS
Associate Professor of Urologic Surgery
Division of Pediatric Urology
Monroe Carell Jr. Children's Hospital at
  Vanderbilt
Nashville, Tennessee

J. Brantley Thrasher, MD, FACS
William L Valk Distinguished Professor
Department of Urology
University of Kansas Medical Center
Kansas City, Kansas

Edouard J. Trabulsi, MD, FACS
Professor
Department of Urology
Kimmel Cancer Center
Sidney Kimmel Medical College
Thomas Jefferson University
Philadelphia, Pennsylvania

Chad R. Tracy, MD
Assistant Professor, Urology
University of Iowa
Iowa City, Iowa

Paul J. Turek, MD, FACS, FRSM
Director
The Turek Clinic
San Francisco, California

Mark D. Tyson, MD, MPH
Department of Urology
Mayo Clinic College of Medicine and
  Science
Phoenix, Arizona

Robert G. Uzzo, MD, FACS
Professor and Chairman
Department of Surgery
The G. Willing "Wing" Pepper Professor
  in Cancer Research
Adjunct Professor of Bioengineering
Temple University College of Engineering
Fox Chase Cancer Center–Temple
  University Health System
Lewis Katz School of Medicine
Philadelphia, Pennsylvania

Brian A. VanderBrink, MD
Urologist
Division of Urology
Cincinnati Children's Hospital
Cincinnati, Ohio

Alex J. Vanni, MD, FACS
Associate Professor
Department of Urology
Lahey Hospital and Medical Center
Burlington, Massachusetts

David J. Vaughn, MD
Professor of Medicine
Division of Hematology/Oncology
Department of Medicine
Abramsom Cancer Center at the
  University of Pennsylvania
Philadelphia, Pennsylvania

Vijaya M. Vemulakonda, MD, JD
Associate Professor of Pediatric Urology
Division of Urology
Department of Surgery
University of Colorado School of
  Medicine
Aurora, Colorado

Manish A. Vira, MD
Vice Chair of Urologic Research
Smith Institute for Urology
Northwell Health
Lake Success, New York;
Associate Professor of Urology
Zucker School of Medicine of Hofstra/
  Northwell
Hempstead, New York

Ramón Virasoro, MD
Associate Professor, Urology
Eastern Virginia Medical School
Norfolk, Virginia;
Fellowship Director, Urology
Universidad Autonoma de Santo
  Domingo
Santo Domingo, Dominican Republic

Alvin C. Wee, MD
Surgical Director, Kidney Transplantation
Glickman Urological and Kidney Institute
Cleveland Clinic
Cleveland, Ohio

Elias Wehbi, MD, FRCSC
Assistant Professor
Department of Urology–Division of
  Pediatric Urology
University of California Irvine
Orange, California

Alan J. Wein, MD, PhD (Hon), FACS
Founders Professor and Emeritus Chief of
  Urology
Co-Director, Urologic Oncology Program
Co-Director, Voiding Function and
  Dysfunction Program
Division of Urology
Penn Medicine, Perelman School of
  Medicine
Philadelphia, Pennsylvania

Dana A. Weiss, MD
Assistant Professor, Urology
University of Pennsylvania;
Attending Physician, Urology
The Childrens Hospital of Philadelphia
Philadelphia, Pennsylvania

Jeffrey P. Weiss, MD, FACS
Professor and Chair
Department of Urology
SUNY Downstate College of Medicine
Brooklyn, New York

Robert M. Weiss, MD
Donald Guthrie Professor of Surgery/
  Urology
Yale University School of Medicine
New Haven, Connecticut

Charles Welliver, Jr., MD
Assistant Professor
Division of Urology
Albany Medical College
Albany, New York

Hunter Wessells, MD, FACS
Professor and Nelson Chair
Department of Urology
Affiliate Member
Harborview Injury Prevention and
  Research Center
University of Washington
Seattle, Washington

Duncan T. Wilcox, MD, MBBS
Surgeon-in-Chief
Ponzio Family Chair of Pediatric Urology
Department of Pediatric Urology
Children's Hospital Colorado
Aurora, Colorado

Jack Christian Winters, MD, FACS
Professor and Chairman, Urology
Louisiana State University Health Sciences
  Center
New Orleans, Louisiana

Anton Wintner, MD
Instructor in Surgery
Harvard Medical School;
Assistant in Urology
Massachusetts General Hospital
Boston, Massachusetts

J. Stuart Wolf, Jr., MD, FACS
Professor and Associate Chair for Clinical
  Integration and Operations
Departments of Surgery and Perioperative
  Care
Dell Medical School
The University of Texas at Austin
Austin, Texas

Christopher E. Wolter, MD
Assistant Professor, Urology
Mayo Clinic Arizona
Phoenix, Arizona

Dan Wood, PhD
Consultant Urologist in Adolescent and
 Reconstructive Surgery
The University College Hospitals
London, United Kingdom

Michael E. Woods, MD
Associate Professor, Urology
University of North Carolina
Chapel Hill, North Carolina

Hailiu Yang, MD
Department of Urology
Cooper Health
New York, New York

Richard Nithiphaisal Yu, MD, PhD
Pediatric Urology Attending
Department of Urology
Boston Children's Hospital
Boston, Massachusetts

Joseph Zabell, MD
Assistant Professor
Department of Urology
University of Minnesota
Minneapolis, Minnesota

Mark R. Zaontz, MD
Professor of Clinical Urology in Surgery
Perelman School of Medicine
University of Pennsylvania;
Attending Physician, Urology
Children's Hospital of Philadelphia
Philadelphia, Pennsylvania

Rebecca S. Zee, MD, PhD
Chief Resident of Urology
University of Virginia School of Medicine
Charlottesville, Virginia

CONTENTS

VOLUME I

PART I Clinical Decision Making

1. Evaluation of the Urologic Patient: History and Physical Examination, 1
   Sammy E. Elsamra, MD

2. Evaluation of the Urologic Patient: Testing and Imaging, 14
   Erik P. Castle, MD, Christopher E. Wolter, MD, and Michael E. Woods, MD

3. Urinary Tract Imaging: Basic Principles of CT, MRI, and Plain Film Imaging, 28
   Jay T. Bishoff, MD, and Ardeshir R. Rastinehad, DO, FACOS

4. Urinary Tract Imaging: Basic Principles of Urologic Ultrasonography, 68
   Bruce R. Gilbert, MD, PhD, and Pat F. Fulgham, MD

5. Urinary Tract Imaging: Basic Principles of Nuclear Medicine, 91
   Michael A. Gorin, MD, and Steven P. Rowe, MD

6. Assessment of Urologic and Surgical Outcomes, 101
   David F. Penson, MD, MPH, and Mark D. Tyson, MD, MPH

7. Ethics and Informed Consent, 115
   Vijaya M. Vemulakonda, MD, JD

PART II Basics of Urologic Surgery

8. Principles of Urologic Surgery: Perioperative Care, 119
   Simpa S. Salami, MD, MPH

9. Principles of Urologic Surgery: Incisions and Access, 135
   David Mikhail, MD, FRCSC, and Simon J. Hall, MD

10. Principles of Urologic Surgery: Intraoperative Technical Decisions, 145
    Manish A. Vira, MD, and Christopher J. Hartman, MD

11. Lower Urinary Tract Catheterization, 152
    Joseph M. Jacob, MD, MCR, and Chandru P. Sundaram, MD, FACS, FRCS (Eng)

12. Fundamentals of Upper Urinary Tract Drainage, 160
    Casey A. Dauw, MD, and J. Stuart Wolf, Jr., MD, FACS

13. Principles of Urologic Endoscopy, 185
    Brian Duty, MD, and Michael Joseph Conlin, MD, MCR

14. Fundamentals of Laparoscopic and Robotic Urologic Surgery, 203
    Roshan M. Patel, MD, Kamaljot S. Kaler, MD, and Jaime Landman, MD

15. Basic Energy Modalities in Urologic Surgery, 235
    Michael W. Sourial, MD, FRCSC, Shubha K. De, MD, FRCSC, Manoj Monga, MD, FACS, and Bodo Egon Knudsen, MD, FRCSC

16. Evaluation and Management of Hematuria, 247
    Stephen A. Boorjian, MD, Jay D. Raman, MD, FACS, and Daniel A. Barocas, MD, MPH, FACS

17. Complications of Urologic Surgery, 260
    Reza Ghavamian, MD, and Charbel Chalouhy, MD

18. Urologic Considerations in Pregnancy, 282
    Melissa R. Kaufman, MD, PhD

19. Intraoperative Consultation, 296
    Michael J. Schwartz, MD, FACS, and Jessica E. Kreshover, MD, MS

PART III Pediatric Urology

SECTION A Development and Prenatal Urology, 305

20. Embryology of the Genitourinary Tract, 305
    Laurence S. Baskin, MD, and Gerald Cunha, PhD

21. Urologic Aspects of Pediatric Nephrology, 341
    Michael C. Braun, MD, and Chester J. Koh, MD

22. Perinatal Urology, 358
    C.D. Anthony Herndon, MD, FAAP, FACS, and Rebecca S. Zee, MD, PhD

SECTION B Basic Principles, 388

23. Urologic Evaluation of the Child, 388
    Rachel Selekman, MD, MAS, and Hillary L. Copp, MD, MS

24. Pediatric Urogenital Imaging, 403
    Hans G. Pohl, MD, FAAP

25. Infection and Inflammation of the Pediatric Genitourinary Tract, 426
    Christopher S. Cooper, MD, FAAP, FACS, and Douglas W. Storm, MD, FAAP

26. Core Principles of Perioperative Management in Children, 447
    Sherry S. Ross, MD, and Janey R. Phelps, MD

27. Principles of Laparoscopic and Robotic Surgery in Children, 458
    Thomas Sean Lendvay, MD, FACS, and Jonathan Scott Ellison, MD

SECTION C Lower Urinary Tract Conditions, 473

28. Clinical and Urodynamic Evaluation of Lower Urinary Tract Dysfunction in Children, 473
    Duncan T. Wilcox, MD, MBBS, and Kyle O. Rove, MD

29. Management Strategies for Vesicoureteral Reflux, 489
    Antoine E. Khoury, MD, FRCSC, FAAP, and Elias Wehbi, MD, FRCSC

30. Bladder Anomalies in Children, 518
    Aaron D. Martin, MD, MPH, and Christopher C. Roth, MD

31. Exstrophy-Epispadias Complex, 528
    John P. Gearhart, MD, and Heather N. Di Carlo, MD

xxi

32 Prune-Belly Syndrome, 581
Francisco Tibor Dénes, MD, PhD, and Roberto Iglesias Lopes, MD, PhD

33 Posterior Urethral Valves, 602
Aseem Ravindra Shukla, MD, and Arun K. Srinivasan, MD

34 Neuromuscular Dysfunction of the Lower Urinary Tract in Children, 624
Carlos R. Estrada, MD, MBA, and Stuart B. Bauer, MD

35 Functional Disorders of the Lower Urinary Tract in Children, 652
Paul F. Austin, MD, and Abhishek Seth, MD

36 Management of Defecation Disorders, 667
Martin A. Koyle, MD, FAAP, FACS, FRCSC, FRCS (Eng), and Armando J. Lorenzo, MD, MSc, FRCSC, FAAP, FACS

37 Lower Urinary Tract Reconstruction in Children, 680
John C. Thomas, MD, FAAP, FACS, Douglass B. Clayton, MD, FAAP, and Mark C. Adams, MD, FAAP

SECTION D Upper Urinary Tract Conditions, 714

38 Anomalies of the Upper Urinary Tract, 714
Brian A. VanderBrink, MD, and Pramod P. Reddy, MD

39 Renal Dysgenesis and Cystic Disease of the Kidney, 741
John C. Pope IV, MD

40 Pathophysiology of Urinary Tract Obstruction, 776
Craig A. Peters, MD, and Kirstan K. Meldrum, MD

41 Ectopic Ureter, Ureterocele, and Ureteral Anomalies, 798
Irina Stanasel, MD, and Craig A. Peters, MD

42 Surgery of the Ureter in Children: Ureteropelvic Junction, Megaureter, and Vesicoureteral Reflux, 826
L. Henning Olsen, MD, DMSC, and Yazan F.H. Rawashdeh, MD, PhD

43 Management of Pediatric Kidney Stone Disease, 853
Gregory E. Tasian, MD, MSc, MSCE, and Lawrence A. Copelovitch, MD

SECTION E Genitalia, 871

44 Management of Abnormalities of the External Genitalia in Boys, 871
Lane S. Palmer, MD, FACS, and Jeffrey S. Palmer, MD, FACS, FAAP

45 Hypospadias, 905
Christopher J. Long, MD, Mark R. Zaontz, MD, and Douglas A. Canning, MD

46 Etiology, Diagnosis, and Management of the Undescended Testis, 949
Julia Spencer Barthold, MD, and Jennifer A. Hagerty, DO

47 Management of Abnormalities of the Genitalia in Girls, 973
Martin Kaefer, MD

48 Disorders of Sexual Development: Etiology, Evaluation, and Medical Management, 990
Richard Nithiphaisal Yu, MD, PhD, and David Andrew Diamond, MD

SECTION F Reconstruction and Trauma, 1019

49 Surgical Management of Differences of Sexual Differentiation and Cloacal and Anorectal Malformations, 1019
Richard C. Rink, MD, FAAP, FACS

50 Adolescent and Transitional Urology, 1043
Dan Wood, PhD

51 Urologic Considerations in Pediatric Renal Transplantation, 1054
Craig A. Peters, MD, and Armando J. Lorenzo, MD, MSc, FRCSC, FAAP, FACS

52 Pediatric Genitourinary Trauma, 1065
Bruce J. Schlomer, MD, and Micah A. Jacobs, MD, MPH

SECTION G Oncology, 1087

53 Pediatric Urologic Oncology: Renal and Adrenal, 1087
Michael L. Ritchey, MD, Nicholas G. Cost, MD, and Robert C. Shamberger, MD

54 Pediatric Urologic Oncology: Bladder and Testis, 1111
Fernando A. Ferrer, MD, FACS, FAAP

VOLUME II

PART IV Infections and Inflammation

55 Infections of the Urinary Tract, 1129
Kimberly L. Cooper, MD, Gina M. Badalato, MD, and Matthew P. Rutman, MD

56 Inflammatory and Pain Conditions of the Male Genitourinary Tract: Prostatitis and Related Pain Conditions, Orchitis, and Epididymitis, 1202
Michel Pontari, MD

57 Interstitial Cystitis/Bladder Pain Syndrome and Related Disorders, 1224
Robert M. Moldwin, MD, and Philip M. Hanno, MD, MPH

58 Sexually Transmitted Diseases, 1251
Kristy McKiernan Borawski, MD

59 Cutaneous Diseases of the External Genitalia, 1273
Richard Edward Link, MD, PhD, and Nikki Tang, MD

60 Tuberculosis and Parasitic Infections of the Genitourinary Tract, 1307
Alicia H. Chang, MD, MS, Brian G. Blackburn, MD, and Michael Hsieh, MD, PhD

PART V Molecular and Cellular Biology

61 Basic Principles of Immunology and Immunotherapy in Urologic Oncology, 1333
Charles G. Drake, MD, PhD

62 Molecular Genetics and Cancer Biology, 1346
Karen S. Sfanos, PhD, and Mark L. Gonzalgo, MD, PhD

PART VI Reproductive and Sexual Function

63 Surgical, Radiographic, and Endoscopic Anatomy of the Male Reproductive System, 1370
Parviz K. Kavoussi, MD, FACS

64 Male Reproductive Physiology, 1390
Paul J. Turek, MD, FACS, FRSM

65 Integrated Men's Health: Androgen Deficiency, Cardiovascular Risk, and Metabolic Syndrome, 1411
Neil Fleshner, MD, MPH, FRCSC, Miran Kenk, PhD, and Steven Kaplan, MD

66 Male Infertility, 1428
Craig Stuart Niederberger, MD, FACS, Samuel John Ohlander, MD, and Rodrigo Lessi Pagani, MD

67 Surgical Management of Male Infertility, 1453
Marc Goldstein, MD, DSc (hon), FACS

68 Physiology of Penile Erection and Pathophysiology of Erectile Dysfunction, 1485
Alan W. Shindel, MD, MAS, and Tom F. Lue, MD, ScD (Hon), FACS

69 Evaluation and Management of Erectile Dysfunction, 1513
Arthur L. Burnett II, MD, MBA, and Ranjith Ramasamy, MD

70 Priapism, 1539
Gregory A. Broderick, MD

71 Disorders of Male Orgasm and Ejaculation, 1564
Chris G. McMahon, MBBS, FAChSHP

72 Surgery for Erectile Dysfunction, 1582
Matthew J. Mellon, MD, FACS, and John J. Mulcahy, MD, PhD, FACS

73 Diagnosis and Management of Peyronie's Disease, 1599
Allen D. Seftel, MD, and Hailiu Yang, MD

74 Sexual Function and Dysfunction in the Female, 1627
Ervin Kocjancic, MD, Valerio Iacovelli, MD, and Ömer Acar, MD

PART VII Male Genitalia

75 Surgical, Radiographic, and Endoscopic Anatomy of the Retroperitoneum, 1658
Drew A. Palmer, MD, and Alireza Moinzadeh, MD

76 Neoplasms of the Testis, 1680
Andrew J. Stephenson, MD, MBA, FRCSC, FACS, and Timothy D. Gilligan, MD, MS, FASCO

77 Surgery of Testicular Tumors, 1711
Stephen Riggs, MD, Kris Gaston, MD, and Peter E. Clark, MD

78 Laparoscopic and Robotic-Assisted Retroperitoneal Lymphadenectomy for Testicular Tumors, 1734
Mohamad E. Allaf, MD, and Louis R. Kavoussi, MD, MBA

79 Tumors of the Penis, 1742
Curtis A. Pettaway, Sr., MD, Juanita M. Crook, MD, FRCPC, and Lance C. Pagliaro, MD

80 Tumors of the Urethra, 1776
Christopher B. Anderson, MD, MPH, and James M. McKiernan, MD

81 Inguinal Node Dissection, 1790
Rene Sotelo, MD, Luis G. Medina, MD, and Marcos Tobias Machado, MD, PhD

82 Surgery for Benign Disorders of the Penis and Urethra, 1804
Ramon Virasoro, MD, Gerald H. Jordan, MD, FACS, FAAP (Hon), FRCS (Hon), and Kurt A. McCammon, MD, FACS

83 Surgery of the Scrotum and Seminal Vesicles, 1843
Dorota J. Hawksworth, MD, MBA, Mohit Khera, MD, MBA, MPH, and Amin S. Herati, MD

PART VIII Renal Physiology and Pathophysiology

84 Surgical, Radiologic, and Endoscopic Anatomy of the Kidney and Ureter, 1865
Mohamed Aly Elkoushy, MD, MSc, PhD, and Sero Andonian, MD, MSc, FRCS(C), FACS

85 Physiology and Pharmacology of the Renal Pelvis and Ureter, 1877
Dana A. Weiss, MD, and Robert M. Weiss, MD

86 Renal Physiology and Pathophysiology Including Renovascular Hypertension, 1905
Thomas Chi, MD, and Meyeon Park, MD, MAS

87 Renal Insufficiency and Ischemic Nephropathy, 1921
Joshua Augustine, MD, Alvin C. Wee, MD, Venkatesh Krishnamurthi, MD, and David A. Goldfarb, MD

88 Urologic Complications of Renal Transplantation, 1936
Mohammed Shahait, MBBS, Stephen V. Jackman, MD, and Timothy D. Averch, MD

PART IX Upper Urinary Tract Obstruction and Trauma

89 Management of Upper Urinary Tract Obstruction, 1942
Stephen Y. Nakada, MD, FACS, FRCS(Glasg.), and Sara L. Best, MD

90 Upper Urinary Tract Trauma, 1982
Steven B. Brandes, MD, and Jairam R. Eswara, MD

PART X Urinary Lithiasis and Endourology

91 Urinary Lithiasis: Etiology, Epidemiology, and Pathogenesis, 2005
Margaret S. Pearle, MD, PhD, Jodi A. Antonelli, MD, and Yair Lotan, MD

92 Evaluation and Medical Management of Urinary Lithiasis, 2036
Nicole L. Miller, MD, and Michael S. Borofsky, MD

93 Strategies for Nonmedical Management of Upper Urinary Tract Calculi, 2069
David A. Leavitt, MD, Jean J.M.C.H. de la Rosette, MD, PhD, and David M. Hoenig, MD

94 Surgical Management for Upper Urinary Tract Calculi, 2094
Brian R. Matlaga, MD, MPH, and Amy E. Krambeck, MD

95 Lower Urinary Tract Calculi, 2114
Arvind P. Ganpule, MS, DNB, and Mahesh R. Desai, MS, FRCS

PART XI Neoplasms of the Upper Urinary Tract

96 Benign Renal Tumors, 2121
William P. Parker, MD, and Matthew T. Gettman, MD

97 Malignant Renal Tumors, 2133
Steven C. Campbell, MD, PhD, Brian R. Lane, MD, PhD, and Phillip M. Pierorazio, MD

98 Urothelial Tumors of the Upper Urinary Tract and Ureter, 2185
Panagiotis Kallidonis, MD, MSc, PhD, FEBU, and Evangelos Liatsikos, MD, PhD

99 Surgical Management of Upper Urinary Tract Urothelial Tumors, 2199
Thomas W. Jarrett, MD, Surena F. Matin, MD, and Armine K. Smith, MD

100 Retroperitoneal Tumors, 2226
Timothy A. Masterson, MD, K. Clint Cary, MD, MPH, and Richard S. Foster, MD

101 Open Surgery of the Kidney, 2248
Aria F. Olumi, MD, and Michael L. Blute, MD

102 Laparoscopic and Robotic Surgery of the Kidney, 2279
Daniel M. Moreira, MD, MHS, and Louis R. Kavoussi, MD, MBA

103 Nonsurgical Focal Therapy for Renal Tumors, 2309
Chad R. Tracy, MD, and Jeffrey A. Cadeddu, MD

104 Treatment of Advanced Renal Cell Carcinoma, 2324
Ramaprasad Srinivasan, MD, PhD, and W. Marston Linehan, MD

VOLUME III

PART XII The Adrenals

105 Surgical and Radiographic Anatomy of the Adrenals, 2345
Ravi Munver, MD, FACS, and John Stites, MD

106 Pathophysiology, Evaluation, and Medical Management of Adrenal Disorders, 2354
Alexander Kutikov, MD, FACS, Paul L. Crispen, MD, and Robert G. Uzzo, MD, FACS

107 Surgery of the Adrenal Glands, 2405
Sey Kiat Lim, MBBS, MRCS (Edinburgh), MMed (Surgery), FAMS (Urology), and Koon Ho Rha, MD, PhD, FACS

PART XIII Urine Transport, Storage, and Emptying

108 Surgical, Radiographic, and Endoscopic Anatomy of the Female Pelvis, 2427
Priya Padmanabhan, MD, MPH

109 Surgical, Radiographic, and Endoscopic Anatomy of the Male Pelvis, 2444
Jen-Jane Liu, MD, Bryan Foster, MD, and Christopher L. Amling, MD, FACS

110 Physiology and Pharmacology of the Bladder and Urethra, 2461
Toby C. Chai, MD, and Lori A. Birder, PhD

111 Pathophysiology and Classification of Lower Urinary Tract Dysfunction: Overview, 2514
Elizabeth Timbrook Brown, MD, MPH, Alan J. Wein, MD, PhD (Hon), FACS, and Roger R. Dmochowski, MD, MMHC, FACS

112 Evaluation and Management of Women With Urinary Incontinence and Pelvic Prolapse, 2525
Alvaro Lucioni, MD, and Kathleen C. Kobashi, MD

113 Evaluation and Management of Men With Urinary Incontinence, 2539
Riyad Tasher Al-Mousa, MBBS, SSCU, FEBU, MSHA, and Hashim Hashim, MBBS, MRCS (Eng), MD, FEBU, FRCS (Urol)

114 Urodynamic and Video-Urodynamic Evaluation of the Lower Urinary Tract, 2550
Benjamin M. Brucker, MD, and Victor W. Nitti, MD

115 Urinary Incontinence and Pelvic Prolapse: Epidemiology and Pathophysiology, 2580
Gary E. Lemack, MD, and Maude Carmel, MD

116 Neuromuscular Dysfunction of the Lower Urinary Tract, 2600
Casey CG. Kowalik, MD, Alan J. Wein, MD, PhD (Hon), FACS, and Roger R. Dmochowski, MD, MMHC, FACS

117 Overactive Bladder, 2637
W. Stuart Reynolds, MD, MPH, and Joshua A. Cohn, MD

118 The Underactive Detrusor, 2650
Christopher R. Chapple, MD, FRCS (Urol), and Nadir I. Osman, MBChB (Hon), MRCS

119 Nocturia, 2664
Stephen D. Marshall, MD, and Jeffrey P. Weiss, MD, FACS

120 Pharmacologic Management of Lower Urinary Tract Storage and Emptying Failure, 2679
Karl-Erik Andersson, MD, PhD

121 Conservative Management of Urinary Incontinence: Behavioral and Pelvic Floor Therapy, Urethral and Pelvic Devices, 2722
Diane K. Newman, DNP, ANP-BC, FAAN, and Kathryn L. Burgio, PhD

122 Electrical Stimulation and Neuromodulation in Storage and Emptying Failure, 2739
John P.F.A. Heesakkers, MD, PhD, and Bertil Blok, MD, PhD

123 Retropubic Suspension Surgery for Incontinence in Women, 2756
Siobhan M. Hartigan, MD, Christopher R. Chapple, MD, FRCS (Urol), and Roger R. Dmochowski, MD, MMHC, FACS

124 Vaginal and Abdominal Reconstructive Surgery for Pelvic Organ Prolapse, 2776
Jack Christian Winters, MD, FACS, Ryan M. Krlin, MD, and Barry Hallner, MD

125 Slings: Autologous, Biologic, Synthetic, and Mid-urethral, 2830
Alex Gomelsky, MD, and Roger R. Dmochowski, MD, MMHC, FACS

126 Complications Related to the Use of Mesh and Their Repair, 2877
Anne P. Cameron, MD, FRCSC, FPMRS

127 Additional Therapies for Storage and Emptying Failure, 2889
Timothy B. Boone, MD, PhD, Julie N. Stewart, MD, and Laura M. Martinez, MD

128 Aging and Geriatric Urology, 2905
Tomas L. Griebling, MD, MPH

129 Urinary Tract Fistulae, 2924
Dirk J.M.K. De Ridder, MD, PhD, FEBU, and Tamsin Greenwell, MD, PhD

130 Bladder and Female Urethral Diverticula, 2964
Lindsey Cox, MD, and Eric S. Rovner, MD

131 Surgical Procedures for Sphincteric Incontinence in the Male, 2993
Hunter Wessells, MD, FACS, and Alex J. Vanni, MD, FACS

PART XIV Benign and Malignant Bladder Disorders

132 Bladder Surgery for Benign Disease, 3010
Paras H. Shah, MD, and Lee Richstone, MD

133 Genital and Lower Urinary Tract Trauma, 3048
Allen F. Morey, MD, FACS, and Jay Simhan, MD, FACS

134 Special Urologic Considerations in Transgender Individuals, 3062
Nicolas Lumen, MD, PhD, Anne-Françoise Spinoit, MD, PhD, and Piet Hoebeke, MD, PhD

135 Tumors of the Bladder, 3073
Max Kates, MD, and Trinity J. Bivalacqua, MD, PhD

136 Management Strategies for Non–Muscle-Invasive Bladder Cancer (Ta, T1, and CIS), 3091
Joseph Zabell, MD, and Badrinath R. Konety, MD, MBA

137 Management of Muscle-Invasive and Metastatic Bladder Cancer, 3112
Thomas J. Guzzo, MD, MPH, John P. Christodouleas, MD, MPH, and David J. Vaughn, MD

138 Surgical Management of Bladder Cancer: Transurethral, Open, and Robotic, 3133
Neema Navai, MD, and Colin P.N. Dinney, MD

139 Use of Intestinal Segments in Urinary Diversion, 3160
Anton Wintner, MD, and Douglas M. Dahl, MD, FACS

140 Cutaneous Continent Urinary Diversion, 3206
Guarionex Joel DeCastro, MD, MPH, James M. McKiernan, MD, and Mitchell C. Benson, MD

141 Orthotopic Urinary Diversion, 3233
Eila C. Skinner, MD, and Siamak Daneshmand, MD

142 Minimally Invasive Urinary Diversion, 3258
Khurshid A. Guru, MD

PART XV The Prostate

143 Development, Molecular Biology, and Physiology of the Prostate, 3274
Brian Wesley Simons, DVM, PhD, and Ashley Evan Ross, MD, PhD

144 Benign Prostatic Hyperplasia: Etiology, Pathophysiology, Epidemiology, and Natural History, 3305
Claus G. Roehrborn, MD, and Douglas William Strand, PhD

145 Evaluation and Nonsurgical Management of Benign Prostatic Hyperplasia, 3343
Paolo Capogrosso, MD, Andrea Salonia, MD, PhD, and Francesco Montorsi, MD, FRCS (Hon)

146 Minimally Invasive and Endoscopic Management of Benign Prostatic Hyperplasia, 3403
Sevann Helo, MD, R. Charles Welliver, Jr., MD, and Kevin T. McVary, MD, FACS

147 Simple Prostatectomy: Open and Robotic-Assisted Laparoscopic Approaches, 3449
Misop Han, MD, MS, and Alan W. Partin, MD, PhD

148 Epidemiology, Etiology, and Prevention of Prostate Cancer, 3457
Andrew J. Stephenson, MD, MBA, FRCSC, FACS, Robert Abouassaly, MD, MS, and Eric A. Klein, MD

149 Prostate Cancer Biomarkers, 3478
Simpa S. Salami, MD, MPH, Ganesh S. Palapattu, MD, Alan W. Partin, MD, PhD, and Todd M. Morgan, MD

150 Prostate Biopsy: Techniques and Imaging, 3490
Edouard J. Trabulsi, MD, FACS, Ethan J. Halpern, MD, MSCE, and Leonard G. Gomella, MD, FACS

151 Pathology of Prostatic Neoplasia, 3506
Jonathan I. Epstein, MD

152 Diagnosis and Staging of Prostate Cancer, 3514
Stacy Loeb, MD, MSc, and James A. Eastham, MD

153 Active Management Strategies for Localized Prostate Cancer, 3522
Samir S. Taneja, MD, and Marc A. Bjurlin, DO, MSc

154 Active Surveillance of Prostate Cancer, 3537
Laurence Klotz, MD, FRCSC

155 Open Radical Prostatectomy, 3548
Edward M. Schaeffer, MD, PhD, Alan W. Partin, MD, PhD, and Herbert Lepor, MD

156 Laparoscopic and Robotic-Assisted Laparoscopic Radical Prostatectomy and Pelvic Lymphadenectomy, 3566
Li-Ming Su, MD, Brandon J. Otto, MD, and Anthony J. Costello, FRACS, MD

157 Radiation Therapy for Prostate Cancer, 3587
Ryan Phillips, MD, PhD, Sarah Hazell, MD, and Daniel Y. Song, MD

158 Focal Therapy for Prostate Cancer, 3616
Kae Jack Tay, MBBS, MRCS(Ed), MMed(Surgery), MCI, FAMS (Urology), and Thomas J. Polascik, MD

159 Treatment of Locally Advanced Prostate Cancer, 3640
Maxwell V. Meng, MD, and Peter R. Carroll, MD, MPH

160 Management Strategies for Biochemical Recurrence of Prostate Cancer, 3659
Eugene K. Lee, MD, and J. Brantley Thrasher, MD, FACS

161 Hormonal Therapy for Prostate Cancer, 3671
Scott Eggener, MD

162 Treatment of Castration-Resistant Prostate Cancer, 3687
Emmanuel S. Antonarakis, MD, and Michael A. Carducci, MD

Index, I-1

VIDEO CONTENTS

PART I Clinical Decision Making

Chapter 4 Urinary Tract Imaging: Basic Principles of Urologic Ultrasonography

Video 4.1 Importance of survey scans. *Courtesy Bruce R. Gilbert and Pat F. Fulgham*
Video 4.2 Perineal ultrasound. *Courtesy Bruce R. Gilbert and Pat F. Fulgham*

PART II Basics of Urologic Surgery

Chapter 11 Lower Urinary Tract Catheterization

Video 11.1 Female urethral catheterization. *Courtesy Jay Sulek and Chandru Sundaram*
Video 11.2 Male urethral catheterization. *Courtesy Jay Sulek and Chandru P. Sundaram*

Chapter 12 Fundamentals of Upper Urinary Tract Drainage

Video 12.1 "Eye-of-the-needle" fluoroscopically guided antegrade access into the upper urinary tract collecting system. *Courtesy J. Stuart Wolf, Jr.*

Chapter 13 Principles of Urologic Endoscopy

Video 13.1 Ureteroscopy and retrograde ureteral access. *Courtesy Ben H. Chew and John D. Denstedt*

PART III Pediatric Urology

SECTION A Development and Prenatal Urology

Chapter 22 Perinatal Urology

Video 22.1 Prenatal urinary tract dilation of the fetal kidneys. *Courtesy C.D. Anthony Herndon and Rebecca S. Zee*
Video 22.2 Fetal measurement of amniotic fluid index. *Courtesy C.D. Anthony Herndon and Rebecca S. Zee*
Video 22.3 Fetal ultrasound documenting multicystic dysplastic kidney. *Courtesy C.D. Anthony Herndon and Rebecca S. Zee*

SECTION B Basic Principles

Chapter 23 Urologic Evaluation of the Child

Video 23.1 Male examination. *Courtesy Rachel Selekman and Hillary Copp*
Video 23.2 Female examination. *Courtesy Rachel Selekman and Hillary Copp*

Chapter 27 Principles of Laparoscopic and Robotic Surgery in Children

Video 27.1 Robotic-assisted ureteral reimplantation. *Courtesy Thomas Sean Lendvay and Jonathan Ellison*
Video 27.2 Robotic-assisted ureteroureterostomy. *Courtesy Thomas Sean Lendvay and Jonathan Ellison*
Video 27.3 Robotic-assisted buccal graft pyeloureteroplasty with omental quilting. *Courtesy Thomas Sean Lendvay and Jonathan Ellison*
Video 27.4 Robotic-assisted ureteral polyp resection. *Courtesy Thomas Sean Lendvay and Jonathan Ellison*

SECTION C Lower Urinary Tract Conditions

Chapter 32 Prune-Belly Syndrome

Video 32.1 Abdominoplasty in prune-belly syndrome. *Courtesy Francisco T. Dénes and Roberto Iglesias Lopes*

Chapter 33 Posterior Urethral Valves

Video 33.1 Cystoscopic incision and ablation of posterior urethral valve. *Courtesy Drs. Long, Shukla, and Srinivasan*
Video 33.2 Repair of Y-configuration urethral duplication. *Courtesy Drs. Srinivasan and Bowen*

Chapter 37 Lower Urinary Tract Reconstruction in Children

Video 37.1 Implanting catheterizable channel into bladder. *Courtesy John C. Thomas and Mark C. Adams*
Video 37.2 Catheterizable channel (Monti). *Courtesy John C. Thomas and Mark C. Adams*
Video 37.3 Laparoscopic-assisted MACE in children. *Courtesy Steven G. Docimo*

SECTION E Genitalia

Chapter 45 Hypospadias

Video 45.1 First stage proximal hypospadias repair with dermal patch graft correction of ventral penile curvature
Video 45.2 First stage hypospadias repair with dermal graft correction of ventral chordee and free inner preputial graft glansplasty
Video 45.3 Reverse pedicle barrier flap for circumcised boys with hypospadias
Video 45.4 Belman flap
Video 45.5 Meatal advancement glansplasty (MAGPI)
Video 45.6 M inverted V plasty (MIV)
Video 45.7 Thiersch-Duplay
Video 45.8 Thiersch-Duplay without meatoplasty
Video 45.9 Duckett tube
Video 45.10 Second stage urethroplasty with tunica vaginalis coverage
Video 45.11 First stage repair of perineal hypospadias with penoscrotal transposition
Video 45.12 Buccal graft interposition for complex hypospadias reconstruction
Video 45.13 Closure of urethrocutaneous fistula
Video 45.14 Repeat Thiersch-Duplay for coronal urethrocutaneous fistula
Video 45.15 Buccal mucosa graft inlay
Video 45.16 Urethral diverticulum closure

Chapter 46 Etiology, Diagnosis, and Management of Undescended Testis

Video 46.1 Inguinal orchidopexy
Video 46.2 Transscrotal orchidopexy
Video 46.3 Laparoscopic orchiopexy

PART VI Reproductive and Sexual Function

Chapter 67 Surgical Management of Male Infertility

Video 67.1 General preparation for vasovasostomy. *Courtesy Marc Goldstein*
Video 67.2 Surgical techniques for vasovasostomy. *Courtesy Marc Goldstein*
Video 67.3 Microsurgical vasovasostomy (microdot suture placements). *Courtesy Marc Goldstein*
Video 67.4 General preparation for vasoepididymostomy. *Courtesy Marc Goldstein*

Video Contents

Video 67.5 Preparation for anastomosis in vasoepididymostomy. *Courtesy Marc Goldstein*
Video 67.6 Varicocelectomy. *Courtesy Marc Goldstein*
Video 67.7 Vasography. *Courtesy Marc Goldstein*
Video 67.8 Vasography and transurethral resection of the ejaculatory ducts. *Courtesy Marc Goldstein*

Chapter 72 Surgery for Erectile Dysfunction
Video 72.1 Implantation of AMS 700 LGX inflatable penile prosthesis. *Courtesy Drogo K. Montague*
Video 72.2 Prosthetic surgery for erectile dysfunction. *Courtesy Drogo K. Montague*

Chapter 73 Diagnosis and Management of Peyronie's Disease
Video 73.1 Reconstruction for Peyronie's disease: incision and grafting. *Courtesy Gerald H. Jordan*

PART VII Male Genitalia

Chapter 75 Surgical, Radiographic, and Endoscopic Anatomy of the Retroperitoneum
Video 75.1 Interaortal caval region. *Courtesy James Kyle Anderson*
Video 75.2 Right retroperitoneum. *Courtesy James Kyle Anderson*
Video 75.3 Left lumbar vein. *Courtesy James Kyle Anderson*
Video 75.4 Lumbar artery. *Courtesy James Kyle Anderson*

Chapter 77 Surgery of Testicular Tumors
Video 77.1 Retroperitoneal lymph node dissection: the split and roll technique. *Courtesy Kevin R. Rice, K. Clint Cary, Timothy A. Masterson, and Richard S. Foster*

Chapter 78 Laparoscopic and Robotic-Assisted Retroperitoneal Lymphadenectomy for Testicular Tumors
Video 78.1 Laparoscopic retroperitoneal lymph node dissection: patient 1. *Courtesy Frederico R. Romero, Soroush Rais-Bahrami, and Louis R. Kavoussi*

Chapter 79 Tumors of the Penis
Video 79.1 Partial penectomy. *Courtesy Curtis A. Pettaway, Juanita M. Crook, Lance C. Pagliaro*
Video 79.2 Low dose rate brachytherapy. *Courtesy Curtis A. Pettaway, Juanita M. Crook, Lance C. Pagliaro*

Chapter 80 Tumors of the Urethra
Video 80.1 Male total urethrectomy. *Courtesy Hadley M. Wood and Kenneth W. Angermeier*

PART VIII Renal Physiology and Pathophysiology

Chapter 84 Surgical, Radiologic, and Endoscopic Anatomy of the Kidney and Ureter
Video 84.1 Left gonadal vein. *Courtesy James Kyle Anderson*
Video 84.2 Left renal hilum. *Courtesy James Kyle Anderson*
Video 84.3 Right kidney before dissection. *Courtesy James Kyle Anderson*
Video 84.4 Left lower pole crossing vessel. *Courtesy James Kyle Anderson*
Video 84.5 Digital nephroscopy: the next step. *Reproduced with permission from Andonian S, Okeke Z, Anijar M, et al. Digital nephroscopy: the next step. J Endourol Part B Videourology 24, 2010a.*
Video 84.6 Digial ureteroscopy: the next step. *Reproduced with permission from Andonian S, Okeke Z, Smith AD: Digital ureteroscopy: the next step. J Endourol Part B Videourology 24, 2010b.*

Chapter 88 Urological Complications of Renal Transplantation
Video 88.1 Technique of laparoscopic live donor nephrectomy. *Courtesy Michael Joseph Conlin and John Maynard Barry*
Video 88.2 Laparoscopic live donor nephrectomy. *Louis R. Kavoussi*

PART IX Upper Urinary Tract Obstruction and Trauma

Chapter 89 Management of Upper Urinary Tract Obstruction
Video 89.1 Laparoscopic pyeloplasty. *Courtesy Frederico R. Romero, Soroush Rais-Bahrami, and Louis R. Kavoussi*
Video 89.2 Robotic-assisted laparoscopic pyeloplasty. *Courtesy Sutchin R. Patel and Sean P. Hedican*

PART X Urinary Lithiasis and Endourology

Chapter 94 Surgical Management for Upper Urinary Tract Calculi
Video 94.1 Blast wave lithotripsy. *Courtesy Brian R. Matlaga and Amy E. Krambeck*
Video 94.2 Shock wave lithotripsy. *Courtesy Brian R. Matlaga and Amy E. Krambeck*
Video 94.3 Shockpulse lithotripsy. *Courtesy Brian R. Matlaga and Amy E. Krambeck*
Video 94.4 Venturi effect. *Courtesy Brian R. Matlaga and Amy E. Krambeck*

PART XI Neoplasms of the Upper Urinary Tract

Chapter 101 Open Surgery of the Kidney
Video 101.1 Patient case study. *Courtesy Aria F. Olumi and Michael L. Blute*
Video 101.2 Global ischemia. *Courtesy Aria F. Olumi and Michael L. Blute*
Video 101.3 Regional ischemia. *Courtesy Aria F. Olumi and Michael L. Blute*
Video 101.4 Vena cava tumor thrombectomy. *Courtesy Aria F. Olumi and Michael L. Blute*

Chapter 102 Laparoscopic and Robotic Surgery of the Kidney
Video 102.1 Laparoscopic partial nephrectomy. *Courtesy Frederico R. Romero, Soroush Rais-Bahrami, and Louis R. Kavoussi*

Chapter 103 Nonsurgical Focal Therapy for Renal Tumors
Video 103.1 Percutaneous renal cryoablation. *Courtesy Arvin K. George, Zhamshid Okhunov, Soroush Rais-Bahrami, Sylvia Montag, Igor Lobko, and Louis R. Kavoussi*

PART XII The Adrenals

Chapter 105 Surgical and Radiographic Anatomy of the Adrenals
Video 105.1 Left adrenal vein. *Courtesy James Kyle Anderson*
Video 105.2 Right adrenal vein. *Courtesy James Kyle Anderson*

Chapter 107 Surgery of the Adrenal Glands
Video 107.1 Laparoscopic adrenalectomy. *Courtesy Frederico R. Romero, Soroush Rais-Bahrami, and Louis R. Kavoussi*

PART XIII Urine Transport, Storage, and Emptying

Chapter 110 Physiology and Pharmacology of the Bladder and Urethra
Video 110.1 Urothelial cells responding to carbachol, a nonspecific muscarinic agonist. *Courtesy Toby C. Chai, University of Maryland School of Medicine*

Video Contents **xxix**

Video 110.2 Actin-myosin cross bridge cycling. *Courtesy Toby C. Chai, Yale School of Medicine*
Video 110.3 Digital calcium fluorescent microscopy of a muscle myocyte contraction. *Courtesy George J. Christ, David Burmeister, and Josh Tan, Wake Forest University School of Medicine*
Video 110.4 Calcium spark development in myocyte. *Courtesy Toby C. Chai, Yale School of Medicine*

Chapter **112** Evaluation and Management of Women With Urinary Incontinence and Pelvic Prolapse
Video 112.1 Discussion of normal lower urinary tract function. *Courtesy Roger Dmochowski*
Video 112.2 Live interview of a patient with pelvic floor disorders. *Courtesy Roger Dmochowski*
Video 112.3 Case study of a patient with mixed urinary incontinence. *Courtesy Roger Dmochowski*
Video 112.4 Examination of a patient with significant anterior vaginal wall prolapse. *Courtesy Roger Dmochowski*
Video 112.5 Case study of a patient with symptomatic prolapse and incontinence. *Courtesy Roger Dmochowski*
Video 112.6 Demonstration of "eyeball" filling study in a patient with incontinence and prolapse. *Courtesy Roger Dmochowski*
Video 112.7 Q-tip test in a patient with minimal urethral mobility. *Courtesy Roger Dmochowski*

Chapter **114** Urodynamic and Video-Urodynamic Evaluation of the Lower Urinary Tract
Video 114.1 Overview of urodynamic studies in female pelvic floor dysfunction. *Courtesy Alan J. Wein, Louis R. Kavoussi, Alan W. Partin, and Craig A. Peters*

Chapter **115** Urinary Incontinence and Pelvic Prolapse: Epidemiology and Pathophysiology
Video 115.1 The Pelvic Organ Prolapse Quantification (POPQ) system. *Courtesy Jennifer T. Anger and Gary E. Lemack*

Chapter **125** Slings: Autologous, Biologic, Synthetic, and Midurethral
Video 125.1 Distal urethral polypropylene sling. *Courtesy Shlomo Raz and Larissa Rodriguez*
Video 125.2 Rectus fascia pubovaginal sling procedure. *Courtesy Alan J. Wein, Louis R. Kavoussi, Alan W. Partin, and Craig A. Peters*
Video 125.3 Top-down retropubic mid-urethral sling: SPARC. *Courtesy Alan J. Wein, Louis R. Kavoussi, Alan W. Partin, and Craig A. Peters*
Video 125.4 Outside-in transobturator mid-urethral sling: MONARC. *Courtesy Alan J. Wein, Louis R. Kavoussi, Alan W. Partin, and Craig A. Peters*
Video 125.5 MiniArc single-incision sling system. *Courtesy Alan J. Wein, Louis R. Kavoussi, Alan W. Partin, and Craig A. Peters*

Chapter **129** Urinary Tract Fistulae
Video 129.1 Robotic-assisted laparoscopic repair of complex vesicovaginal fistula in a patient with failed open surgical and vaginal repair. *Courtesy Ashok K. Hemal and Gopal H. Badlani*
Video 129.2 Martius flap. *Courtesy Shlomo Raz and Larissa Rodriguez*
Video 129.3 Transvaginal repair of a vesicovaginal fistula using a peritoneal flap. *Courtesy Shlomo Raz and Larissa Rodriguez*
Video 129.4 Transvaginal bladder neck closure with posterior urethral flap. *Courtesy Brett D. Lebed, J. Nathaniel Hamilton, and Eric S. Rovner*

Chapter **131** Surgical Procedures for Sphincteric Incontinence in the Male
Video 131.1 Surgical treatment of the male sphincteric urinary incontinence: the male perineal sling and artificial urinary sphincter. *Courtesy David R. Staskin and Craig V. Comitor*
Video 131.2 Male sling. *Courtesy Hunter Wessells*

PART XIV Benign and Malignant Bladder Disorders

Chapter **133** Genital and Lower Urinary Tract Trauma
Video 133.1 Technique demonstrating protection of phallus during removal of penile strangulation device. *Courtesy Allen F. Morey and Jay Simhan*

Chapter **134** Special Urologic Considerations in Transgender Individuals
Video 134.1 Creation of the neo-urethra
Video 134.2 Creation of the neoscrotum
Video 134.3 Procedure for implantation of erectile device

Chapter **135** Tumors of the Bladder
Video 135.1 Patient case studies using blue light cystoscopy (BLC). *Courtesy Max Kates and Trinity J. Bivalacqua*

Chapter **136** Management Strategies for Non–Muscle-Invasive Bladder Cancer (Ta, T1, and CIS)
Video 136.1 Demonstration of the technique of en bloc resection of bladder tumor completed cystoscopically with a resectoscope and bipolar cutting loop. *Courtesy Giulia Lane*

Chapter **140** Cutaneous Continent Urinary Diversion
Video 140.1 Stapled right colon reservoir with appendiceal stoma. *Courtesy Mitchell C. Benson*

Chapter **141** Orthotopic Urinary Diversion
Video 141.1 T-pouch ileal neobladder. *Courtesy Eila C. Skinner, Donald G. Skinner, and Hugh B. Perkin*
Video 141.2 The modified Studer ileal neobladder. *Courtesy Siamak Daneshmand*

PART XV The Prostate

Chapter **146** Minimally Invasive and Endoscopic Management of Benign Prostatic Hyperplasia
Video 146.1 Holmium laser enucleation of the prostate (HoLEP). *Courtesy Mitra R. de Cógáin and Amy E. Krambeck*

Chapter **147** Simple Prostatectomy: Open and Robot-Assisted Laparoscopic Approaches
Video 147.1 Robot-assisted laparoscopic simple prostatectomy. *Courtesy Misop Han*

Chapter **151** Prostate Biopsy: Techniques and Imaging
Video 151.1 Images from a transrectal prostate biopsy. *Courtesy Leonard G. Gomella, Ethan J. Halpern, and Edouard J. Trabulsi*
Video 151.2 Ultrasonography and biopsy of the prostate. *Courtesy Daniel D. Sackett, Ethan J. Halpern, Steve Dong, Leonard G. Gomella, and Edouard J. Trabulsi*

Chapter **155** Open Radical Prostatectomy
Video 155.1 Radical retropubic prostatectomy. *Courtesy Herbert Lepor and Dmitry Volkin*
Video 155.2 High release of the neurovascular bundle. *Courtesy Patrick C. Walsh*
Video 155.3 Incision on the endopelvic fascia and division of puboprostatic ligaments. *Courtesy Patrick C. Walsh*

Video 155.4 Control of the dorsal vein complex. *Courtesy Patrick C. Walsh*
Video 155.5 Division of the urethra and placement of the urethral sutures. *Courtesy Patrick C. Walsh*
Video 155.6 Division of the posterior striated sphincter. *Courtesy Patrick C. Walsh*
Video 155.7 Preservation of the neurovascular bundle. *Courtesy Patrick C. Walsh*
Video 155.8 Use of the Babcock clamp during release of the neurovascular bundle. *Courtesy Patrick C. Walsh*
Video 155.9 Wide excision of the neurovascular bundle. *Courtesy Patrick C. Walsh*
Video 155.10 Reconstruction of the bladder neck and vesicourethral anastomosis. *Courtesy Patrick C. Walsh*
Video 155.11 Use of the Babcock clamp during vesicourethral anastomosis. *Courtesy Patrick C. Walsh*

Chapter 156 Laparoscopic and Robotic-Assisted Radical Prostatectomy and Pelvic Lymphadenectomy

Video 156.1 Operating room setup. *Courtesy Li-Ming Su and Jason P. Joseph*
Video 156.2 Vas and seminal vesicle dissection. *Courtesy Li-Ming Su and Jason P. Joseph*
Video 156.3 Posterior dissection. *Courtesy Li-Ming Su and Jason P. Joseph*
Video 156.4 Entering retropubic space. *Courtesy Li-Ming Su and Jason P. Joseph*
Video 156.5 Endopelvic fascia and puboprostatics. *Courtesy Li-Ming Su and Jason P. Joseph*
Video 156.6 Dorsal venous complex ligation. *Courtesy Li-Ming Su and Jason P. Joseph*
Video 156.7 Anterior bladder neck transection. *Courtesy Li-Ming Su and Jason P. Joseph*
Video 156.8 Posterior bladder neck transection. *Courtesy Li-Ming Su and Jason P. Joseph*
Video 156.9 Bladder neck dissection: anterior approach. *Courtesy Li-Ming Su and Jason P. Joseph*
Video 156.10 Neurovascular bundle dissection. *Courtesy Li-Ming Su and Jason P. Joseph*
Video 156.11 Division of dorsal venous complex and apical dissection. *Courtesy Li-Ming Su and Jason P. Joseph*
Video 156.12 Pelvic lymph node dissection. *Courtesy Li-Ming Su and Jason P. Joseph*
Video 156.13 Entrapment of prostate and lymph nodes. *Courtesy Li-Ming Su and Jason P. Joseph*
Video 156.14 Posterior reconstruction. *Courtesy Li-Ming Su and Jason P. Joseph*
Video 156.15 Vesicourethral anastomosis. *Courtesy Li-Ming Su and Jason P. Joseph*
Video 156.16 Extraction of specimen. *Courtesy Li-Ming Su and Jason P. Joseph*

PART IV: Infections and Inflammation

55 — Infections of the Urinary Tract

Kimberly L. Cooper, MD, Gina M. Badalato, MD, and Matthew P. Rutman, MD

Urinary tract infections (UTIs) are common, affect men and women of all ages, vary dramatically in their presentation and sequelae, and are one of the most frequent reasons for prescribing antibiotics. The overwhelming majority of UTIs contribute to varying levels of morbidity yet rarely progress to life-threatening emergencies. In certain populations, however, UTIs can contribute to significant mortality if undiagnosed and untreated. When bacterial virulence increases or host defense mechanisms decrease, bacterial inoculation, colonization, and infection of the urinary tract occur. Careful diagnosis and treatment result in successful resolution of infections in most instances. A better understanding of the pathogenesis of UTIs and the role of host and bacterial factors has improved the ability to identify patients at risk and prevent or minimize sequelae. Recent evidence has proven that urine is not sterile; indeed, in many cases bacteriuria is protective against the development of UTIs. In this era of widespread multidrug-resistant (MDR) bacteria it is crucial that we do not overdiagnose UTIs and expose patients to unnecessary antibiotics. The appropriate management of UTIs includes implementation of antibiotic stewardship, which undoubtedly will have a beneficial impact on global public health. Clinical presentation, in conjunction with analysis of urine samples that are collected in a proper fashion, must be critically determined before recommending antibiotics for bacteriuria and UTIs. Guidelines should be incorporated into clinical practice to improve the use of antibiotics in terms of choice of and duration of therapy. Education of practitioners and patients regarding best practices related to bacteriuria and UTIs is paramount.

DEFINITIONS

UTI is an inflammatory response of the urothelium to bacterial invasion that is usually associated with bacteriuria and pyuria.

Bacteriuria is the presence of bacteria in the urine. It has been assumed to be a valid indicator of either bacterial colonization or infection of the urinary tract. Although this is usually true, studies in animals (Hultgren et al., 1985; Mulvey et al., 1998) and humans (Elliott et al., 1985) have indicated that bacteria may be in the urothelium in the absence of bacteriuria. Alternatively, bacteriuria may represent bacterial contamination of an abacteriuric specimen during collection.

Pyuria, the presence of white blood cells (WBCs) in the urine, is generally indicative of infection and/or an inflammatory response of the urothelium to bacteria, stones, an indwelling foreign body, or other conditions that can contribute to pyuria. Bacteriuria without pyuria is generally indicative of bacterial colonization without overt infection of the urinary tract. Pyuria without bacteriuria, or sterile pyuria, warrants further evaluation (see the discussion of pyuria in the section on urinalysis).

Infections are often defined clinically by their presumed site of origin. *Cystitis* describes a clinical syndrome of dysuria, frequency, urgency, and occasionally suprapubic pain. These symptoms, although generally indicative of bacterial cystitis, may also be associated with infection of the urethra or vagina or noninfectious conditions such as interstitial cystitis/ painful bladder syndrome, bladder carcinoma, or calculi.

Acute pyelonephritis **is a clinical syndrome of chills, fever, and flank pain that is accompanied by bacteriuria and pyuria, a combination that is reasonably specific for an acute bacterial infection of the kidney.** Often there are no associated lower urinary symptoms. The term should not be used if flank pain is absent. It may have no morphologic or functional components detectable by routine clinical modalities. There may be significant difficulties in diagnosing spinal cord–injured and elderly patients who may be unable to localize the site of their discomfort.

Chronic pyelonephritis describes a shrunken, fibrosed kidney, diagnosed by morphologic, radiologic, or functional evidence of renal disease that may be postinfectious but is frequently not associated with current (active) UTI. Bacterial infection of the kidney may cause a *focal, coarse scar* in the renal cortex overlying a calyx, almost always accompanied by some calyceal distortion (Fig. 55.1), which can be detected radiographically or by gross examination of the kidney. These radiographic changes are identical to those that may be produced by vesicoureteral reflux (VUR) or calyceal stone disease. Less commonly, renal scarring from infection can result in atrophic pyelonephritis or generalized thinning of the renal cortex, with a small kidney appearing radiographically similar to one with postobstructive atrophy (Fig. 55.2). Xanthogranulomatous pyelonephritis (XGP) is a rare form of chronic pyelonephritis often associated with stone disease and characterized by destructive replacement of normal renal parenchyma with granulomatous inflammation; it is associated with ipsilateral loss of renal function (see the section on XGP).

UTIs may also be described in terms of the anatomic or functional status of the urinary tract and the health of the host.

Uncomplicated **describes an infection in a healthy patient with a structurally and functionally normal urinary tract; this often specifically refers to the absence of obstruction to any part of the urinary tract.** The majority of these patients are women with isolated or recurrent bacterial cystitis or acute pyelonephritis, and the infecting pathogens are usually susceptible to and eradicated by a short course of oral antimicrobial therapy.

A *complicated* infection is associated with factors that increase the chance of acquiring bacteria and decrease the efficacy of therapy (Box 55.1). **The urinary tract is structurally or functionally abnormal, the host is compromised, and/or the bacteria have increased virulence or antimicrobial resistance.**

Renal diseases that reduce the concentrating ability of the kidney or voiding dysfunction that alter bladder-emptying capabilities are commonly encountered functional abnormalities. Examples of renal diseases, which mainly affect the tubulointerstitial compartment, include postobstructive nephropathy, sickle cell nephropathy, lithium nephropathy, chronic tubulointerstitial nephritis, and inherited diseases such as medullary cystic kidney disease. Examples of anatomic abnormalities include enlargement of the prostate or congenital or

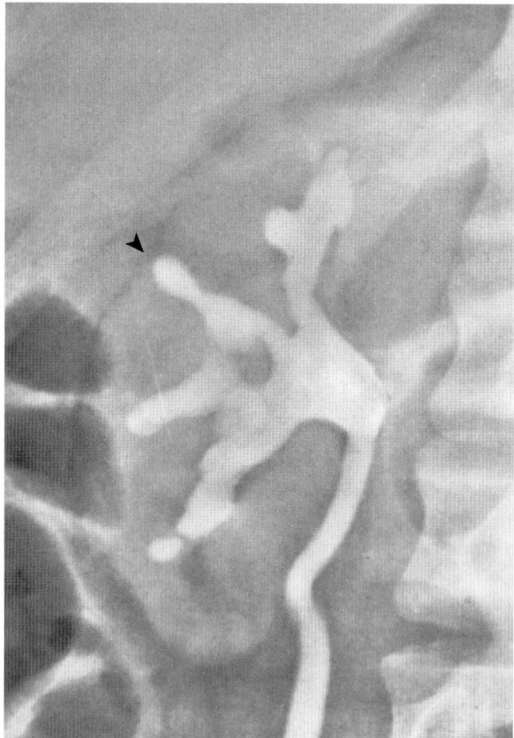

Fig. 55.1. Excretory urogram demonstrates focal, coarse scarring in the right kidney of an 18-year-old girl with a history of many recurrent fevers between 2 months and 2 years of age. A cystogram when the patient was 2 years old established an atrophic left kidney with marked reflux up to the left kidney and slight reflux up to the right kidney. Excretory urography at the age of 6 years established severe atrophy of the left kidney. She had no infections between the ages of 6 and 15 years. Several reinfections occurred at the age of 15 years, and they ceased with prophylactic therapy. Her blood pressure has remained normal, and her serum creatinine level was 0.9 mg/dL at the age of 18 years. At 21 years of age she stopped antimicrobial prophylaxis for 18 months without infections or introital colonization with Enterobacteriaceae. Note that all calyces are blunted and that one extends to the capsule *(arrowhead)* because of atrophy of the overlying cortex.

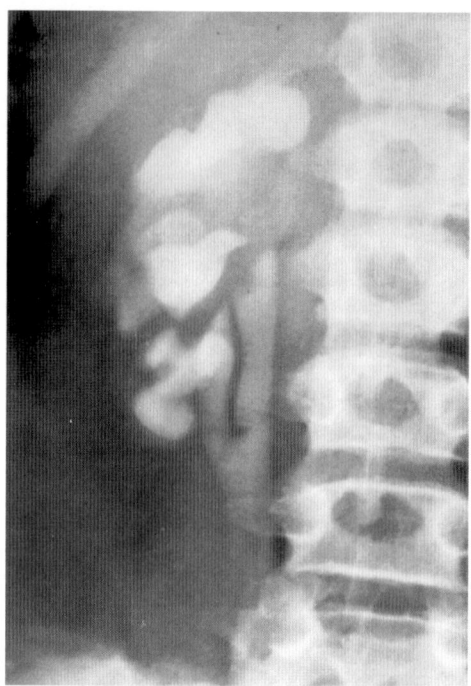

Fig. 55.2. Pyelonephritic atrophy, suggestive of postobstructive atrophy, in a 20-year-old woman with spina bifida, neurogenic bladder, and many episodes of fever and bacteriuria in early childhood. Observe the uniform, regular atrophy of the renal cortex that suggests reflux of bacteria simultaneously into virtually all nephrons. This type of pyelonephritic atrophy is uncommon and is characteristic of obstruction with superimposed infection.

BOX 55.1	**Factors That Suggest a Complicated Urinary Tract Infection**

Functional or anatomic abnormality of urinary tract
Male gender
Pregnancy
Elderly patient
Diabetes
Immunosuppression
Childhood urinary tract infection
Recent antimicrobial agent use
Indwelling urinary catheter
Urinary tract instrumentation
Hospital-acquired infection
Symptoms for more than 7 days at presentation

Data from Schaeffer AJ: Urinary tract infections. In Gillenwater JY, Grayhack JT, Howards SS, et al., editors: *Adult and pediatric urology*, Philadelphia, 2002, Lippincott Williams & Wilkins, p 212.

---

acquired sites of residual urine, such as calyceal or urethral or bladder diverticula. Bladder outlet obstruction, neurogenic bladder, and detrusor underactivity also contribute to functional abnormalities. A complicated infection is frequently caused by multidrug-resistant bacteria.

Chronic, although implying long time frames, is a poor term that should be avoided in the context of UTIs, except for chronic pyelonephritis or bacterial prostatitis, because the duration of the infection is not defined.

UTIs may also be defined by their relationship to other UTIs:
- A *first* or *isolated* infection is one that occurs in an individual who has never had a UTI or has one remote infection from a previous UTI.
- An **unresolved** infection is one that has not responded to antimicrobial therapy and is documented to be the same organism with a similar resistance profile.
- A *recurrent* infection is one that occurs after documented, successful resolution of an antecedent infection. Consider these two different types of recurrent infection:
  1. *Reinfection* describes a new event associated with reintroduction of bacteria into the urinary tract.
  2. *Bacterial persistence* refers to a recurrent UTI caused by the same bacteria reemerging from a focus within the urinary tract, such as an infectious stone or the prostate. *Relapse* is frequently used interchangeably. These definitions require careful clinical and bacteriologic assessment and are important because they influence the type and extent of the patient's evaluation and treatment.

Antimicrobial prophylaxis (AP) is the attempted prevention of reinfections of the urinary tract by the administration of antimicrobial drugs. If the term is used correctly in reference to the urinary tract, it can be assumed that bacteria have been eliminated before prophylaxis is begun. **Surgical AP entails administration of an antimicrobial agent before and for a *limited* time after a procedure to prevent local or systemic postprocedural infections** (see the later section on American Urological Association (AUA) guidelines for prophylaxis).

Antimicrobial suppression is the attempted prevention of growth of a focus of bacterial persistence that cannot be eradicated.

Domiciliary or *outpatient UTIs* occur in patients who are not hospitalized or institutionalized at the time they become infected.

Nosocomial or *health care–associated UTIs* occur in patients who are hospitalized or institutionalized.

Catheter-associated UTIs (CAUTIs) occur within that population of patients with indwelling bladder drainage catheters. They are cumulatively the most common cause of secondary bacteremia and are associated with increased morbidity and mortality (Flores-Mireles et al., 2015). Prolonged catheterization, female gender, advanced age, and diabetes represent risk factors for developing a CAUTI (Chenoweth et al., 2014) (see the later section on CAUTIs).

> **KEY POINTS: DEFINITIONS**
>
> - Bacteriuria and pyuria are not synonymous with a UTI.
> - UTIs are classified based on their presumed site of origin.
> - UTIs can be uncomplicated (occurring in healthy patients with normal urinary tracts) or complicated (associated with factors that increase the likelihood of bacteriuria and decrease the efficacy of therapy).

INCIDENCE AND EPIDEMIOLOGY

UTI-related complaints are among the most common primary diagnoses for women visiting the emergency department in the United States (Foxman, 2014; Niska et al., 2010). **In 2007 in the United States alone, there were an estimated 10.5 million office visits for UTI-related complaints (accounting for a total of 0.9% of all ambulatory visits), and 2 to 3 million visits to the emergency room** (Schappert, 2011). **Nearly 30% of women have had a symptomatic UTI requiring antimicrobial therapy by age 24, and almost half of all women experience a UTI during their lifetime** (Foxman, 2002). Moreover, 11% of women over the age of 18 have one UTI annually.

Given the frequency of this problem, the associated **financial impact is staggering.** In the United States the direct and indirect costs for the treatment of UTIs annually was estimated to be $2.3 billion in 2010 (Foxman, 2010). For each of these infections, the cost in treating an antimicrobial-resistant organism is greater than treating susceptible bacterial counterparts (Neidell et al., 2012). Furthermore, as it pertains to acute pyelonephritis, the direct and indirect costs were estimated at $2.14 billion in 2000, which is projected to be $2.9 billion in 2013 (Brown et al., 2005).

The incidence of bacteriuria increases with institutionalization or hospitalization and concurrent conditions (Sourander et al., 1966). CAUTIs are the most common nosocomial infection, constituting more than 80% of nosocomial UTIs (Foxman, 2002; Sedor, 1999). **The incidence of UTIs is also elevated during pregnancy and in patients with spinal cord injury (SCI), diabetes, multiple sclerosis, organ transplant recipients, and human immunodeficiency virus (HIV) infection/acquired immunodeficiency syndrome (AIDS).**

Once a patient has an infection, he or she is likely to develop subsequent infections. In fact, historical data by Mabeck originally established that the probability of recurrent UTIs increases with the number of previous infections (Mabeck, 1972). More recent cohort analyses have verified this trend among diverse populations (Foxman, 2014). First, the risk of recurrence is particularly high among young, sexually active women. In a prospective trial following 285 college women after their first UTI, the risk of a second infection was 24% within the 6-month follow-up period (Foxman et al., 2000). In another study examining a group of 796 women starting a new method of contraception, subset analysis showed that those women with a history of 2 or more previous UTIs had 2 to 5 times the risk of recurrence at 1 year compared with counterparts who only had 1 or no previous infections (Hooton et al., 1996). Postmenopausal women with a history of UTIs are similarly at increased risk of recurrence. A 2012 double-bind, non-inferiority study by Beerepoot et al. compared daily trimethoprim-sulfamethoxazole (TMP-SMX) versus lactobacilli prophylaxis among 252 postmenopausal women with approximately 7 symptomatic UTIs in the preceding year. At 12 months, a total of 69.3% recurred in the antibiotic arm compared with 79.1% in the probiotics group, with the mean number of recurrences in the 12-month follow-up period being 2.9 and 3.3, respectively (Beerepoot et al., 2012). Last, among men treated in an ambulatory setting for a UTI within the Veteran Affairs system, the risk of recurrence at 30 days was 4.1% in one retrospective study (Drekonja et al., 2013). Overall, these data examining different demographic groupings underscore the finding that populations with a track record of UTIs do have predisposition to recur.

Further information on this topic is available online at Expert Consult.com.

The sequelae of complicated UTIs are substantial. It is well established in the presence of obstruction, infection stones, diabetes mellitus, and other risk factors that UTIs in adults can lead to progressive renal damage (Freedman, 1975). **The long-term effects of uncomplicated recurrent UTIs are not completely known, but, so far, no association between recurrent infections and renal scarring, hypertension, or progressive renal azotemia has been established** (Asscher et al., 1973; Freedman, 1975).

> **KEY POINTS: INCIDENCE AND EPIDEMIOLOGY**
>
> - UTIs are the most common bacterial infection and, as such, make a significant impact on health care costs.
> - The incidence of bacteriuria increases with institutionalization/hospitalization as well as with pregnancy and certain comorbidities that alter lower urinary tract function or cause immunosuppression.
> - No clear association has been described between recurrent uncomplicated UTIs and renal sequelae such as scarring, hypertension, or progressive renal insufficiency.

PATHOGENESIS

UTIs occur as a result of interactions between the uropathogen and the host. **Successful infection of the urinary tract is determined in part by the virulence factors of the bacteria, the inoculum size, and the inadequacy of host defense mechanisms.** These factors also play a role in determining the ultimate level of colonization and damage to the urinary tract. Whereas increased bacterial virulence appears to be necessary to overcome strong host resistance, bacteria with minimal virulence factors are able to infect patients who are significantly compromised.

Routes of Infection

Ascending Route

Most bacteria enter the urinary tract from the bowel and skin reservoir via ascent through the urethra into the bladder. Adherence of pathogens to the introital and urothelial mucosa plays a significant role in ascending infections. This route is further enhanced in individuals with significant soilage of the perineum with feces, women who use spermicidal agents (Foxman, 2002; Handley et al., 2002; Hooton et al., 1996), and patients with intermittent or indwelling catheters.

Most episodes of pyelonephritis are caused by retrograde ascent of bacteria from the bladder through the ureter to the renal pelvis and parenchyma. Although reflux of urine is probably not required for ascending infections, edema associated with cystitis may cause sufficient changes in the ureterovesical junction to permit reflux (Fig. 55.3). Once the bacteria are introduced into the ureter, they may ascend to the kidney unaided. **However, this ascent would be greatly increased by any process that interferes with the normal ureteral peristaltic function. Gram-negative bacteria and their endotoxins, as well as pregnancy, ureteral obstruction, and high lower tract pressures have a significant antiperistaltic effect.**

Bacteria that reach the renal pelvis can enter the renal parenchyma by means of the collecting ducts at the papillary tips and then ascend upward within the collecting tubules. This process is hastened and exacerbated by increased intrapelvic pressure from ureteral obstruction or VUR, particularly when it is associated with intrarenal reflux.

Further information about routes of infection is available online at ExpertConsult.com.

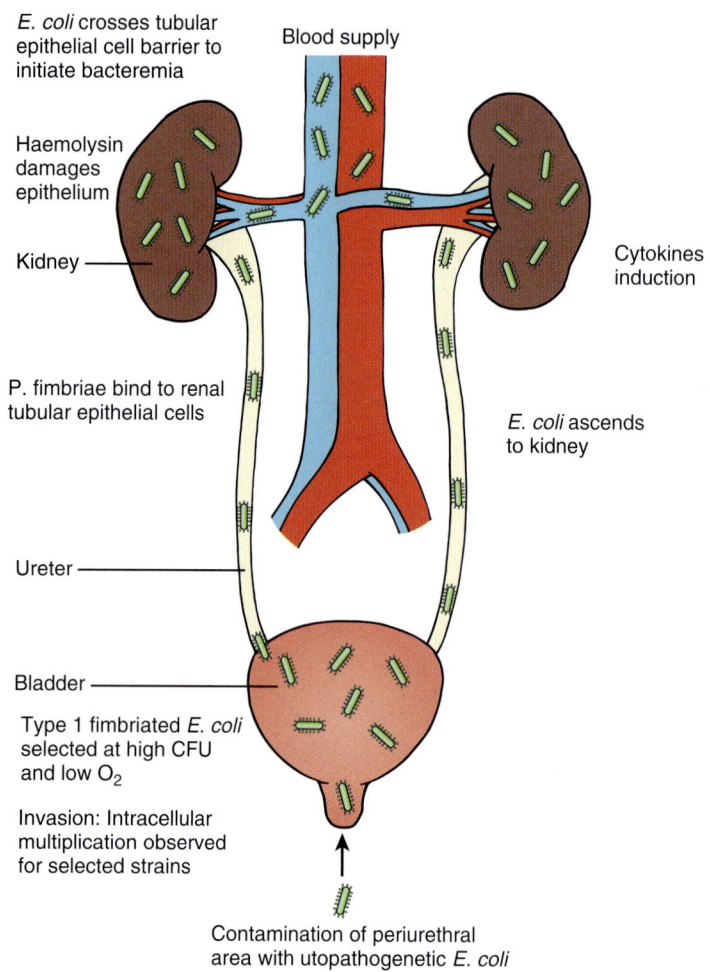

Fig. 55.3. Bacterial adherence in ascending urinary tract infections. (Modified from Glover M, Moreira CG, Sperandio V, et al.: Recurrent urinary tract infections in healthy and nonpregnant women. *Urological Sci* 25:1, 2014, pp 1–8.)

Urinary Pathogens

Most UTIs are caused by facultative anaerobes usually originating from the bowel flora. Uropathogens such as *Staphylococcus epidermidis* and *Candida albicans* originate from the flora of the vagina or perineal skin (Fig. 55.4).

E. coli is by far the most common cause of UTIs, accounting for 85% of community-acquired and 50% of hospital-acquired infections. Other gram-negative Enterobacteriaceae, including *Proteus* and *Klebsiella*, and gram-positive *Enterococcus faecalis* and *Staphylococcus saprophyticus* are responsible for the remainder of most community-acquired infections. **Nosocomial infections** are caused by *E. coli*, *Klebsiella*, *Enterobacter*, *Citrobacter*, *Serratia*, *Pseudomonas aeruginosa*, *Providencia*, *E. faecalis*, and *Staphylococcus epidermidis* (Kennedy et al., 1965). Less common organisms such as *Gardnerella vaginalis*, *Mycoplasma* species, and *Ureaplasma urealyticum* may infect patients, some of whom have intermittent or indwelling catheters (Fairley, 1989; Josephson et al., 1988). *U. urealyticum* and *M. hominis* have been identified in the urine of women with chronic urinary symptoms but negative standard urine cultures; antibiotic treatment targeted at these organisms has resulted in improvement in symptoms (Baka et al., 2009; Potts et al., 2000). Within the intensive care unit, where virtually all patients who develop a UTI have indwelling catheters, the most frequent pathogens include *Escherichia coli*, *Pseudomonas aeruginosa*, enterococci, and *Candida albicans*, with species distribution and resistance patterns differing considerably among institutions and regions (Bagshaw, 2006).

With the development of more sophisticated urine culture techniques and the identification of the urinary microbiome (see the section on microbiome), several emerging uropathogens have been identified. Although some may suggest these organisms are part of the microbiome, patients who have these emerging pathogens may be symptomatic and require treatment. *Aerococcus urinae* is a rare pathogen that causes UTIs in older adults with significant comorbidities, including some urologic malignancies (Higgins, 2017). *A. urinae* is often mistaken for *Staphylococcus*, *Streptococcus*, and *Enterococcus* spp. Another emerging pathogen, *Raoultella planticola*, is a gram-negative rod that has been associated with UTIs in immunocompromised patients (Skelton et al., 2017). *Myroides odoratimimus*, a gram-negative rod commonly found in environmental sources such as soil, has been identified as the causative agent in UTIs in immunocompromised patients and is particularly dangerous because of its extensive drug resistance (Licker et al., 2018).

E. coli strains mediating extraintestinal infections are typically grouped into broad phylogenetic classes by multiplex polymerase chain reaction (Clermont et al., 2000), where 70% of uropathogenic *E. coli* (UPEC) isolates fall into the B2 group (Johnson et al., 2001). More recent studies have used multilocus sequence typing to further define and characterize *E. coli* strains mediating UTI and other infections at the level of "sequence type." *E. coli* **sequence type ST131 (serotype O25b:H4) merits special attention as a rapidly emerging cause of multidrug-resistant infections, including UTI** (Johnson et al., 2010; Kudinha et al., 2013). Although first noted for extended-spectrum β-lactamases (ESBLs), fluoroquinolone resistance is a hallmark phenotype among ST131 isolates. **The prevalence of infecting organisms is influenced by the patient's age.** For example, *S. saprophyticus* is recognized as causing approximately 10% of symptomatic lower UTIs in young, sexually active females (Latham et al., 1983), whereas it rarely causes infection in males and elderly individuals.

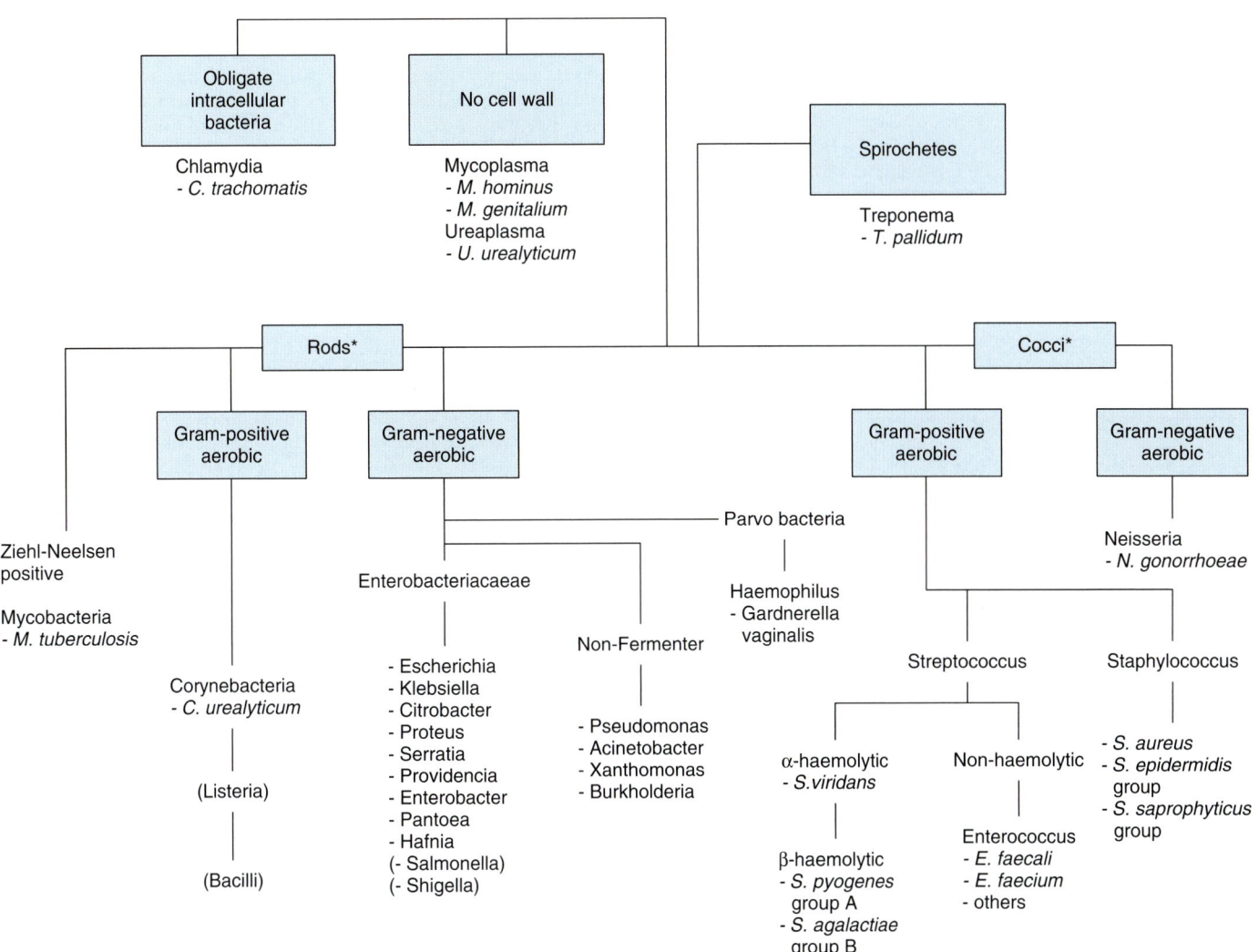

Fig. 55.4. Relevant bacteria for urological infections. *Anaerobic bacteria not considered (see Grabe et al., 2015, p. 60 for clarification). (From Grabe M, Bartoletti R, Bjerklund Johansen TE, et al: *Guidelines on urological infections*, 2015 (website): https://uroweb.org/wp-content/uploads/19-Urological-infections_LR2.pdf.)

Fastidious Organisms

Anaerobes in the Urinary Tract

Symptomatic anaerobic infections of the urinary tract are uncommon. However, the distal urethra, perineum, and vagina are normally colonized by anaerobes. Whereas 1% to 10% of voided urine specimens are positive for anaerobic organisms (Finegold, 1977), anaerobic organisms found in suprapubic aspirates are much more unusual (Gorbach and Bartlett, 1974). Clinically symptomatic UTIs in which only anaerobic organisms are cultured are rare, although they may frequently be a contaminant in midstream urine cultures (Hooton et al., 2013). Nevertheless, **these organisms must be suspected as causative when a patient with persistent bladder irritative symptoms has cocci or gram-negative rods seen on microscopic examination of the centrifuged urine** (catheterized, suprapubic aspirated, or voided midstream urine) **and routine quantitative aerobic cultures fail to grow organisms** (Ribot et al., 1981).

Anaerobic organisms are frequently found in cases of enteric fistualization with the urinary tract or in **suppurative infections of the genitourinary (GU) system**. In one study of suppurative GU infections in males, 88% of scrotal, prostatic, and perinephric abscesses included anaerobes among the infecting organisms (Bartlett and Gorbach, 1981). The organisms found are usually *Bacteroides* species, including *B. fragilis*, *Fusobacterium* species, anaerobic cocci, and *Clostridium perfringens* (Finegold, 1977). The growth of clostridia may be associated with cystitis emphysematosa (Bromberg et al., 1982).

Mycobacterium tuberculosis and Other Nontuberculous Mycobacteria

Mycobacterium tuberculosis and other nontuberculous mycobacteria may be found in the urinary tract (Brooker and Aufderheide, 1980; Thomas et al., 1980). Urinary tuberculosis (UTB) most commonly occurs with hematuria (either gross hematuria, microhematuria, and/or sterile pyuria), storage symptoms, and/or dysuria, with or without systemic symptoms such as fever and weakness. Diagnosis and subsequent treatment are often delayed because of nonspecific symptoms, potentially contributing to impaired renal function and eventual renal failure. Polymerase chain reaction for *M. tuberculosis* has replaced acid-fast staining as the ideal method of diagnosis (Altiparmak et al., 2015; Figueiredo and Lucon, 2008; Ghaleb et al., 2013).

Chlamydia

Chlamydiae are not routinely grown in aerobic culture but have been implicated in GU infections.

Bacterial Virulence Factors

Virulence characteristics play a role in determining if an organism will invade the urinary tract and the subsequent level of infection within the urinary tract. It is generally believed that uropathogenic strains resident in the bowel flora, such as UPEC, can infect the urinary tract not only by chance but also by the expression of virulence factors that enable them to adhere to and colonize the perineum and urethra and migrate to the urinary tract, where they establish an inflammatory response in the urothelium (Moreno et al., 2008; Schaeffer et al., 1981; Schlager et al., 2002; Yamamoto et al., 1997). The same virulence factors can be found on bacterial strains that cause recurrent UTI in patients (Foxman et al., 1995). Some of these virulence determinants are located on 1 of approximately 20 UPEC-specific pathogenicity-associated islands (PAIs) ranging in size from 30 to 170 kb. These PAIs collectively increase the size of the pathogen genome by about 20% over a commensal strain. UPEC phylogroups (A, B1, B2, and D) have been defined based on the presence of genomic PAIs and the expression of associated virulence factors such as adhesions, toxins, surface polysaccharides, flagella, and iron-acquisition systems (Bien et al., 2012).

Early Events in Uropathogenic *E. coli* Pathogenesis

The steps of UPEC pathogenesis include (1) UPEC colonization of the periurethral and vaginal tissue as well as the urethra; (2) ascending infection into the bladder lumen and within the urine; (3) adherence to the surface urothelium and interaction with the bladder epithelial cell defense mechanism; (4) biofilm elaboration; (5) invasion and replication by forming bladder Intracellular Bacterial Communities (IBCs), in which quiescent intracellular reservoirs (QIRs) can form and stay dormant in the underlying urothelium; (6) and, in some cases, renal colonization and host tissue damage with high risk for sepsis (Terlizzi et al., 2017; Fig. 55.5).

Bacterial Adherence

Bacterial adherence to vaginal and urothelial epithelial cells is an essential step in the initiation of UTIs. This interaction is influenced by the adhesive characteristics of the bacteria, the receptive characteristics of the epithelial surface, and the fluid bathing both surfaces. Bacterial adherence is a specific interaction that plays a role in determining the organism, the host, and the site of infection. Portions of this section on bacterial adherence have been published elsewhere (Schaeffer et al., 1981).

Bacterial Adhesins. UPEC expresses a number of adhesins that allow it to attach to urinary tract tissues (Mulvey, 2002). These adhesins are classified as either **fimbrial** or **afimbrial**, depending on whether the adhesin is displayed as part of a rigid fimbria or pilus. Bacteria may produce a number of antigenically and functionally different pili on the same cell; others produce a single type; in some, no pili are seen (Klemm, 1985). A typical piliated cell may contain 100 to 400 pili. The pilus is usually 5 to 10 nm in diameter, is up to 2 μm long, and appears to be composed primarily of subunits known as *pilin* (Klemm, 1985). Pili are defined functionally by their ability to mediate hemagglutination of specific types of erythrocytes. The most well-described pili are types 1, P, and S.

Type 1 (Mannose-Sensitive) Pili. Type 1 pili are commonly expressed on nonpathogenic and pathogenic *E. coli*. Type 1 pili consist of a helical rod composed of repeating FimA subunits joined to a 3-nm–wide distal tip structure containing the adhesin FimH (Jones et al., 1995). These pili mediate hemagglutination of guinea pig erythrocytes (Duguid et al., 1966). The reaction is inhibited by the addition of mannose; thus type 1 pili are termed *mannose-sensitive hemagglutination* (MSHA) (Reid and Sobel, 1987; Svenson et al., 1984).

The role of type 1 pili as a virulence factor in UTIs has been established. This evidence has been obtained (1) from the analysis of bacteria isolated from the urine of patients with UTIs, which were found to express mannose-sensitive (MS) adhesins (Ljungh and Wadstrom, 1983); (2) from studies with animal models (Fader and Davis, 1982, Hagberg et al., 1983a,b; Hultgren et al., 1985; Iwahi et al., 1983) in which inoculation of type 1 piliated organisms into the bladder resulted in significantly more colonization of the urinary tract than inoculation of nonpiliated organisms; and (3) from the observation that anti–type 1 pili antibodies and competitive inhibitors such as methyl-α-D-mannopyranoside protected mice from contracting UTIs (Aronson et al., 1979; Hultgren et al., 1985). **Studies have demonstrated that interactions between FimH and receptors expressed on the luminal surface of the bladder epithelium are critical for the ability of many UPEC strains to colonize the bladder and cause disease** (Connell et al., 1996; Langermann et al., 1997; Mulvey et al., 1998; Thankavel et al., 1997).

P (Mannose-Resistant) Pili. P pili confer tropism to the kidney; the designation "P" stands for pyelonephritis (Mulvey, 2002). P pili, which are found in most pyelonephritogenic strains of UPEC, mediate hemagglutination of human erythrocytes that is not altered by mannose and is thus termed *mannose-resistant hemagglutination* (MRHA) (Kallenius et al., 1979). The adhesin PapG, at the tip of the pilus, recognizes the α-D-galactopyranosyl-(1-4)-β-D-galactopyranoside moiety present in the globoseries of glycolipids (Kallenius et al., 1980; Leffler and Svanborg-Eden, 1980), which are found on P blood group antigens and on uroepithelium (Svenson et al., 1983). The *fm* operon of UPEC encodes the type 1 pili and the *pap* operon encodes the P- or Pap-pili. Clinical isolates of UPEC have demonstrated

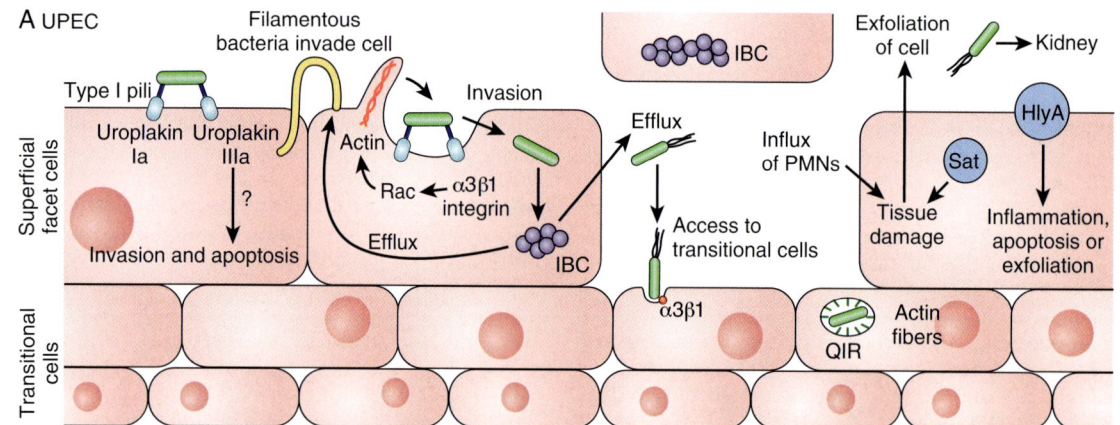

Fig. 55.5. Uropathogenic *E. coli* (UPEC). UPEC attaches to the uroepithelium through type 1 pili, which bind the receptors uroplakin Ia and IIIa; this binding stimulates unknown signalling pathways (indicated by the question mark) that mediate invasion and apoptosis. Binding of type 1 pili to α3β1 integrins also mediates internalization of the bacteria into superficial facet cells to form intracellular bacterial communities (IBCs) or pods. Exfoliation of the uroepithelium exposes the underlying transition cells for further UPEC invasion, and the bacteria can reside in these cells as quiescent intracellular reservoirs (QIRs) that may be involved in recurrent infections. (Modified from Croxen MA, Finlay BB. Molecular mechanisms of *Escherichia coli* pathogenicity. *Nat Rev Microbiol* 8:26–38, 2010.)

that the fm operon is constitutive and the pap component is part of a PAI that contains other virulence factors (Terlizzi et al., 2017).

Svanborg-Eden and Svennerholm (1978) were the first to report a correlation between bacterial adherence and severity of UTIs. They showed that UPEC strains from girls with acute pyelonephritis had high adhesive ability, whereas strains causing asymptomatic bacteriuria or from the feces of healthy girls had low bacterial adherence. Between 70% and 80% of the pyelonephritic strains, but only 10% of the bowel isolates, had adhesive capacity. Furthermore, P pili were present in 91% of urinary strains causing pyelonephritis, 19% of strains causing cystitis, and 14% of strains causing asymptomatic bacteriuria but only 7% of bowel isolates from healthy children, highlighting the correlation between bacterial adherence and UTIs (Kallenius et al., 1981).

Whereas P pili are strongly associated with pyelonephritis, these virulence factors are not associated with renal scarring and reflux caused by bacterial infection (Vaisanen et al., 1981). Studies suggest minimal correlation between P-piliated *E. coli* strains and recurrent pyelonephritis with gross reflux in girls (Lomberg et al., 1983). Thus it would appear that P pili in acute pyelonephritis are important mainly in nonrefluxing or minimally refluxing children.

Other Adhesins. Although pili are important in the initial attachment of UPEC to urothelium, UPEC also expresses a group of afimbrial adhesins (AFA) that are responsible for maintaining this connection (Vigil et al., 2011). One common adhesion TosA was found to be expressed during UTI and was found in 30% of urinary tract samples. Another example includes the iron-regulated adhesion Iha, which mediated adherence to bladder epithelial cells (Johnson et al., 2005).

Catch Bonds. Not surprisingly, UPEC adhesins have evolved to meet the physical dynamics of the urinary tract, and this is best understood for FimH. Using hemagglutination assays and flow cell approaches, **the affinity of *E. coli* expressing specific FimH alleles for erythrocytes was found to be enhanced by shear stress,** and mutations that abolished FimH-erythrocyte interactions in static conditions did not affect dynamic affinities (Thomas et al., 2002). Conversely, static conditions reduced FimH-erythrocyte interactions. Known as *catch bonds*, this fingertrap-like mechanism is mediated by shear-altered interactions between the FimH pili and mannose-binding domains that result in force-induced tightening of the mannose-binding pocket (Le Trong et al., 2010). Similar shear-enhanced binding now appears widespread in biology and includes *E. coli* P-fimbriae (reviewed in Sokurenko et al., 2008). The implications of catch bonds for UPEC adherence and UTI pathogenesis are obvious. **Enhanced adherence in the presence of shear would promote UPEC retention in the urethra and bladder during voiding and in the ureters against peristalsis. In the absence of shear, reduced FimH affinity would facilitate diffusion and thereby promote ascending infection.**

Information on phase variation in vivo is available online at ExpertConsult.com.

Epithelial Cell Receptivity

Vaginal Cells

The significance of epithelial cell receptivity in the pathogenesis of ascending UTI has been studied initially by examining adherence of *E. coli* to vaginal epithelial cells and uroepithelial cells collected from voided urine specimens. Fowler et al. (1977) established that certain indigenous microorganisms (e.g., lactobacilli, *S. epidermidis*) avidly attached themselves to washed epithelial cells in large numbers. When vaginal epithelial cells were collected from patients susceptible to reinfection and compared with such cells obtained from controls resistant to UTI, the *E. coli* strains that cause cystitis adhered much more avidly to the epithelial cells from the susceptible women. **These studies established increased adherence of pathogenic bacteria to vaginal epithelial cells as the first demonstrable biologic difference that could be shown in women susceptible to UTI.**

Subsequently, Schaeffer et al. (1981) **confirmed these vaginal differences in women, but in addition they observed that the increased bacterial adherence was also characteristic of buccal epithelial cells.** As can be seen in Fig. 55.7, there is a striking similarity in the ability of both cell types to bind to the same *E. coli* strain. In

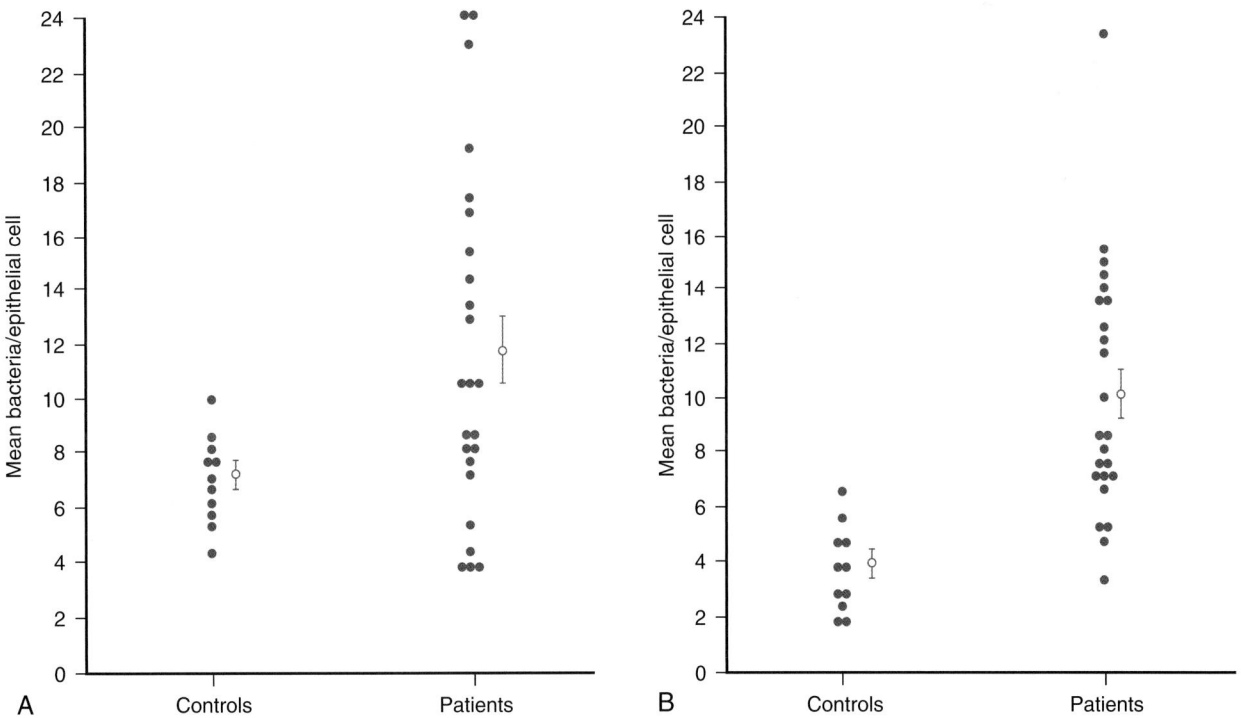

Fig. 55.7. In vitro adherence of *Escherichia coli* to vaginal (A) and buccal (B) cells from healthy controls and patients with recurrent urinary tract infections. Values represent an average of 14 (A) and 11 (B) determinations in each individual. The *open circles* and *bars* represent the means + standard error of the mean. (Data from Schaeffer AJ, Jones JM, Dunn JK: Association of in vitro *Escherichia coli* adherence to vaginal and buccal epithelial cells with susceptibility of women to recurrent urinary tract infections. *N Engl J Med* 304:1062–1066, 1981.)

addition, there was a significant relationship between vaginal cell and buccal cell receptivity. Seventy-seven different *E. coli* strains were tested for their ability to bind to vaginal and buccal epithelial cells. A direct nonlinear relationship between buccal and vaginal adherence in controls and patients was confirmed for urinary, vaginal, and anal isolates. Thus high vaginal cell receptivity was associated with high buccal cell receptivity.

These observations emphasize that the increase in receptor sites for UPEC on epithelial cells from women with recurrent UTIs is not limited to the vagina and thus suggest that a genotypic trait for epithelial cell receptivity may be a major susceptibility factor in UTIs. This concept was extended by examining the human leukocyte antigens (HLAs), which are the major histocompatibility complex in humans and have been associated statistically with many diseases (Schaeffer et al., 1994). The A3 antigen was identified in 12 (34%) of the patients, which is significantly higher than the 8% frequency observed in healthy controls. Thus HLA-A3 may be associated with increased risk of recurrent UTIs.

Variation in Receptivity. A small variation in vaginal cell and buccal cell receptivity may be observed from day to day in healthy controls. Adherence ranges from 1 to 17 bacteria per cell and appears to be cyclic and repetitive. When adherence was correlated with the days of a woman's menstrual cycle, higher values were noted in the early phase, diminishing shortly after the time of expected ovulation (day 14). The number of bacteria per epithelial cell often correlated with the value obtained on the same day of the menstrual cycle 1 or 2 months previously. Premenopausal women are particularly susceptible to attachment of UPEC and nonpathogenic lactobacilli at certain times during the menstrual cycle and to *E. coli* during the early stages of pregnancy. **The importance of such hormones as estrogens in the pathogenesis of UTI is therefore a matter of great interest, especially because the clinical urologist may see women who have recurrent cystitis at regular intervals, possibly in response to these hormonal changes.**

Reid and Sobel (1987) found that uropathogens attached in larger numbers to uroepithelial cells from women older than 65 years of age than to cells from premenopausal women 18 to 40 years of age. Raz and Stamm (1993) noted that **susceptibility to recurrent UTI was increased by the lowered estrogen levels found in the postmenopausal women and that estrogen replacement decreased uropathogenic bacterial colonization and the incidence of UTI.**

Blood group antigens and carbohydrate structures bound to membrane lipids or proteins also constitute an important part of the uroepithelial cell membrane. The **presence or absence of blood group determinants on the surface of uroepithelial cells may influence an individual's susceptibility to a UTI.** Sheinfeld et al. (1989) determined the blood group phenotypes in women with recurrent UTI and compared them with those of age-matched women controls. There is a higher frequency of Lewis nonsecretor Le(a+b−) and recessive Le(a−b−) phenotypes among women with recurrent UTIs. The nonsecretor status has also been associated with female acute uncomplicated pyelonephritis, especially in premenopausal women (Ishitoya et al., 2002). Stapleton et al. (1995) have shown that unique *E. coli*–binding glycerides are found in vaginal epithelial cells from nonsecretors but not from secretors. **These studies individually and collectively support the concept that there is an increased epithelial receptivity for *E. coli* on the introital, urethral, and buccal mucosa that is characteristic of women susceptible to recurrent UTIs and may be a genotypic trait.**

The possibility that vaginal mucus may influence bacterial receptivity was investigated by Schaeffer et al. (1994). Type 1 piliated *E. coli* bound to all of the vaginal fluid specimens (Venegas et al., 1995). The binding capacity of vaginal fluid from women colonized with *E. coli* in vivo was greater than that from noncolonized women (Schaeffer and Stuppy, 1999). The importance of vaginal fluid in bacteria/epithelial cell interactions was investigated in an in vitro model that measured the effect of vaginal fluid on the binding of bacteria to an epithelial cell line (Gaffney et al., 1995). Vaginal fluid from colonized women enhanced binding of bacteria to epithelial cells. Conversely, vaginal fluid from noncolonized women inhibited adherence. Thus the **vaginal fluid appears to influence adherence to cells** and, presumably, vaginal mucosal colonization. Subsequent studies demonstrated that secretory IgA is the primary glycoprotein responsible for vaginal fluid receptivity (Rajan et al., 1999).

Bladder Cells

FimH binds mannosylated residues on the uroplakin molecules covering bladder superficial epithelial cells. The luminal surface of the bladder is lined by umbrella cells. The apical surfaces of umbrella cells appear as a quasi-crystalline array of hexagonal complexes composed of four integral membrane proteins known as *uroplakins* (Sun, 1996). In vitro binding assays have shown that two of the uroplakins, UPIa and UPIb, can specifically bind UPEC expressing type 1 pili (Wu et al., 1996). High-resolution freeze-fracture electron microscopy has shown that the tips of these pili, including the adhesins, are buried in the central cavity of the uroplakin hexameric rings (Mulvey et al., 2000; Fig. 55.8). **Thus FimH-mediated binding to the bladder epithelium is the initial step in the intricate cascade of events leading to UTIs.** Immediate urothelial responses to UPEC may be triggered by uroplakins because FimH binding to UPIb was shown to result in phosphorylation of UPIII and subsequent UPIII-mediated increases in intracellular calcium (Thumbikat et al., 2009).

Uropathogenic *E. coli* Persistence in the Bladder. Soon after attachment to the epithelium, UPEC is quickly internalized into the bladder superficial cells (Anderson et al., 2004a,b; Martinez and Hultgren, 2002; Fig. 55.9). Invasion into the superficial epithelium of the bladder allows UPEC to establish a new niche in an effort to protect itself from the host innate immune response (Anderson et al., 2004a,b).

Once intracellular, the UPEC organisms rapidly grow and divide within the cell cytosol, forming small clusters of bacteria termed *early intracellular bacterial communities* (IBCs) (Anderson et al., 2004a,b; Justice et al., 2004). As they grow, the bacteria maintain their typical rod shape of approximately 3 μm and form a loosely organized cluster, with microorganisms randomly oriented in the cell cytoplasm. Between 6 and 8 hours after inoculation, early IBCs show a drop in bacterial growth rate, resulting in doubling times greater than 60 minutes, a significant shortening of the bacterial morphology to an average of 0.7 μm, and a phenotypic switch into a biofilm-like community (Justice et al., 2004) Similar bacteria-engorged urothelial cells have been identified in 22% of voided urine specimens from patients with UTI with *E. coli* (Rosen et al., 2007). Importantly, **UPEC isolated from the human IBC-like cells were capable of infecting mice and recapitulating IBCs** (Garofalo et al., 2007).

Biofilms shield bacteria from environmental challenges such as antimicrobial agents and the host immune response (Donlan and Costerton, 2002). **Characteristics of the biofilm that increase protection include the slower growth rate of the bacteria with associated physiologic changes, expression of factors that inhibit antimicrobial activity, and the inability of the antimicrobial agent to penetrate the biofilm matrix** (Anderson et al., 2004a,b). The biofilm also protects the bacteria from neutrophils because they are unable to effectively penetrate the IBC and engulf the bacteria. In animal models, bacteria on the edge of IBCs eventually detach, differentiate to typical rod morphology, become motile, and then escape the host cell into the bladder lumen in a process called *fluxing* (Mulvey et al., 2001). These bacteria may become highly filamentous, reaching up to 70 μm or greater in length. This process occurs by approximately 24 hours after inoculation (Justice et al., 2004). It is possible that the filaments may help the bacteria evade the immunologic response. Moreover, a large majority of UPEC isolated from women with acute, asymptomatic, or recurrent UTIs have shown the presence of flagellum-mediated movement, which may play an important role in adherence and dispersal during biofilm elaboration (Nakamura et al., 2016; Wright et al., 2005).

The escaped bacteria re-adhere and reinvade superficial cells to lead to second IBC formation. In subsequent rounds, further IBC formation occurs. After a few days, the invasive bacteria become more quiescent. In animal models, the bacteria can persist in this dormant reservoir state for some time before reemerging to cause recurrent UTIs (Anderson et al., 2004a,b). Indeed, in murine UTI, individuals with sterile urine nonetheless may contain thousands of viable UPEC within bladder tissue (Mulvey et al., 2001), suggesting that IBCs may be a transient intermediate in the establishment of stable UPEC reservoirs

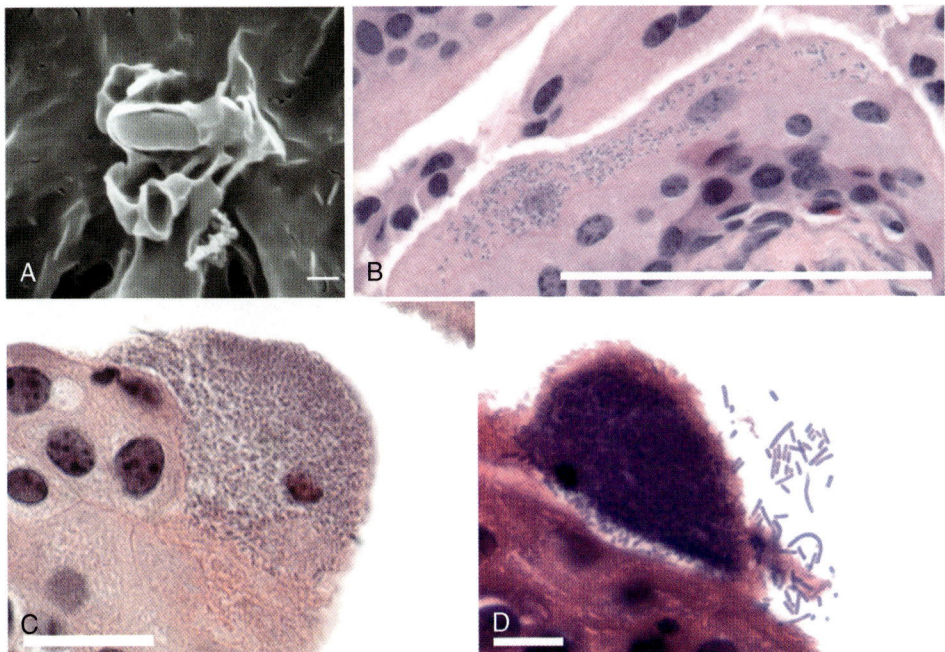

Fig. 55.8. Uropathogenic *Escherichia coli* (UPEC) binds, invades, and multiplies inside the superficial cells of the bladder epithelium. (A) Scanning electron microscopy shows a single UPEC bound to the surface of a bladder cell. Type 1 pilus–mediated contact between bacterium and host cell initiates signaling cascades in the bladder cell, leading to localized actin rearrangements and membrane protrusions around the bacterium. Scale bar, 0.5 μm. (B) Once inside the bladder superficial cells, UPEC rapidly multiplies to form disordered bacterial clusters in the host cell cytoplasm, called an early intracellular bacterial community (IBC). Bacteria are visible as dark-staining rods inside the cell in this hematoxylin and eosin (H&E)-stained thin bladder section. Scale bar, 100 μm. (C) H&E-stained thin bladder section reveals a middle IBC, wherein the constituent bacteria have organized themselves into a biofilm-like state within the bladder cell. Scale bar, 20 μm. (D) A late IBC, visible by H&E staining, is typified by detachment of peripheral bacteria and fluxing of these organisms into the bladder lumen. Scale bar, 10 μm. (From Anderson GG, Martin SM, Hultgren SJ: Host subversion by formation of intracellular bacterial communities in the urinary tract. *Microbes Infect* 6:1094–1101, 2004.)

within the bladder. Exfoliation of superficial urothelial cells (see later) exposes underlying transitional cells. In contrast to the cytosolic UPEC aggregates characteristic of IBCs, UPEC invasion of transitional cells results in membrane-bound bacteria limited to two to four bacteria per cell (Justice et al., 2004). These intracellular UPEC remain quiescent, and thus such transitional cells are referred to as *quiescent intracellular reservoirs* (QIRs) (Mysorekar and Hultgren, 2006). However, chemically perturbing the urothelium to evoke urothelial differentiation caused reemergence of UPEC from QIR marked by significant bacterial proliferation. **Together, these findings suggest that bladder reservoirs of intracellular UPEC may contribute to recurrent UTI in susceptible individuals as the transitional cells undergo differentiation.**

Natural Defenses of the Urinary Tract

Periurethral and Urethral Region

The normal flora of the vaginal introitus, the periurethral area, and the urethra usually contain microorganisms such as lactobacilli, coagulase-negative staphylococci, corynebacteria, and streptococci that form a barrier against uropathogenic colonization (Fair et al., 1970; Marrie et al., 1978; Pfau and Sacks, 1977). Changes in the vaginal environment related to estrogen, cervical IgA (Stamey et al., 1978), and low vaginal pH (Stamey and Timothy, 1975) may alter the ability of these bacteria to colonize. More commonly, however, acute changes in colonization have been associated with use of antimicrobial agents and spermicidal agents that alter the normal flora and increase the receptivity of the epithelium for uropathogens.

Little is known about the factors that predispose patients to urethral colonization with uropathogens. The proximity of the urethral meatus to the vulvar and perianal areas suggests that contamination occurs frequently. The nature of urethral defense mechanisms other than flow of urine is largely unknown. Bacterial multiplication in the normal urethra may be inhibited by the indigenous flora (Chan et al., 1984). Although colonization of the periurethral and urethral regions is prerequisite to most infections, the ability of the organisms to overcome the normal defense mechanisms of the urine and the bladder is clearly pivotal.

Urine

In general, fastidious organisms that normally colonize the urethra will not multiply in urine and rarely cause UTIs (Cattell et al., 1973). In contrast, urine usually supports the growth of nonfastidious bacteria (Asscher, et al. 1973). **Urine from normal individuals may be inhibitory, especially when the inoculum is small** (Kaye, 1968). **The most inhibitory factors are the osmolality, urea concentration, organic acid concentration, and pH. Bacterial growth is inhibited by either very dilute urine or a high osmolality when associated with a low pH.** Much of the antimicrobial activity of urine is related to a high urea and organic acid content (Solomon et al., 1983). From a clinical perspective, however, these conditions do not appear to significantly distinguish between patients who are susceptible or resistant to infection.

Uromodulin (Tamm-Horsfall protein), a kidney-derived mannosylated protein that is present in an extraordinarily high concentration in the urine (>100 mg/mL), **may play a defensive role by saturating all the mannose-binding sites of the type 1 pili, thus potentially blocking bacterial binding to the uroplakin receptors of the urothelium** (Duncan, 1988; Kumar and Muchmore, 1990).

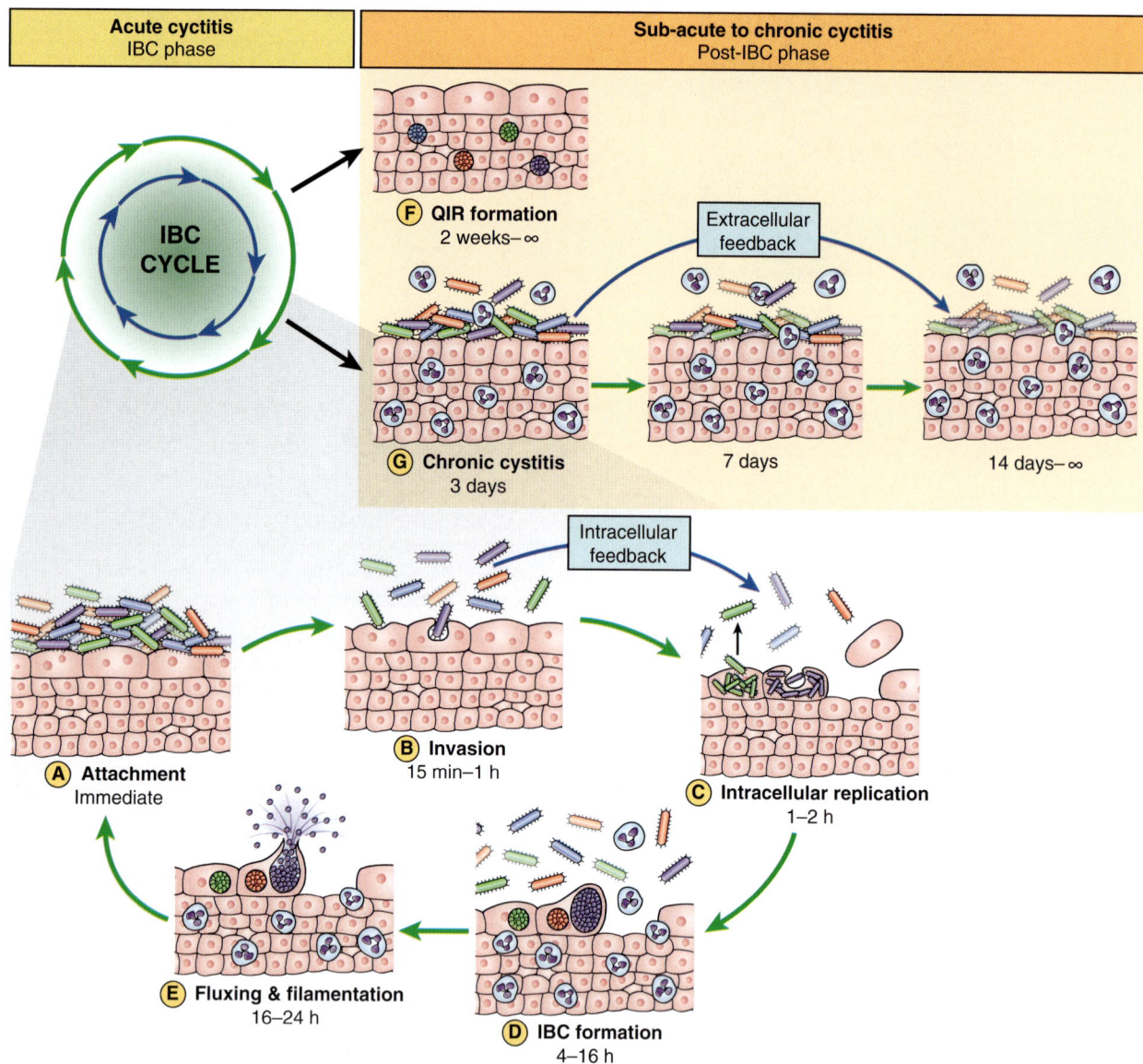

Fig. 55.9. Uropathogenic *Escherichia coli* model for acute cystitis, chronic cystitis, and quiescent intracellular reservoir formation: intracellular bacterial community (IBC) formation starts when bacteria attach onto the apical transitional epithelium of the bladder via type 1 pili. These bacteria are then enveloped and invade the epithelium, replicating and forming IBCs. As a host response to infection, the urothelium typically exfoliates, resulting in IBC liberation and IBC recreation in a clonal fashion. IBCs may also progress to quiescent intracellular reservoirs, which are not metabolically active and do not produce a measurable inflammatory response. (Modified from Hannan TJ, Totsika M, Mansfield KJ, et al.: Host-pathogen checkpoints and population bottlenecks in persistent and intracellular uropathogenic *Escherichia coli* bladder infection. *FEMS Microbiol Rev* 3:616e48, 2012.)

Bladder

Bacteria presumably make their way into the bladder frequently. Whether small inocula of bacteria persist, multiply, and infect the host depends in part on the ability of the bladder to empty (Cox and Hinman, 1961). Additional factors responsible for defense involve innate and adaptive immunity and exfoliation of epithelial cells.

Immune Response

Pathogen Recognition. The host recognition of the pathogen is mediated by a series of pathogen-associated molecular pattern receptors (PAMPs), such as Toll-like receptors (TLRs) (Anderson et al., 2004a,b), which provide the link between recognition of invading organisms and development of the innate immune response. TLRs recognize molecular patterns that are conserved among many species of pathogens, such as lipopolysaccharide (LPS) and peptidoglycan (PG), and activate signaling pathways that initiate immune and inflammatory responses to kill pathogens. Superficial bladder epithelial cells express TLR4 on their membranes, which, along with CD14, recognize LPS from the bacteria and activate the innate immune response (Anderson et al., 2004a,b). The newly identified TLR11, which recognizes UPEC and protects the kidneys from ascending infection, is also expressed on uroepithelial cells, as well as renal cells (Zhang et al., 2004).

The innate system response to an infection in the bladder or kidneys is primarily local inflammation. **The innate immune response occurs more rapidly than the adaptive response and involves a variety of cell types, including polymorphonuclear leukocytes, neutrophils, macrophages, eosinophils, natural killer cells, mast cells, and dendritic cells.** In addition, increased transcription of inducible nitric oxide synthase by polymorphonuclear leukocytes results in high levels of nitric oxide and related breakdown products that also have toxic effects on the bacteria (Poljakovic and Persson 2003; Poljakovic et al., 2001). Adaptive immunity involves the specific recognition of pathogens by T and B lymphocytes and production of high-affinity antibodies, a process that occurs 7 to 10 days after infection.

For additional data regarding the immunologic response to UTI, the idea of immunization, and the roles of lipopolysaccharide, see ExpertConsult.com.

Alterations in Host Defense Mechanisms

Obstruction

Obstruction to urine flow at all anatomic levels, whether secondary to anatomic abnormalities or elevated storage pressure, is a key factor in increasing host susceptibility to UTI. Obstruction inhibits the normal flow of urine, and the resulting stasis compromises bladder and renal defense mechanisms. **Stasis also contributes to the growth of bacteria in the urine and their ability to adhere to the urothelial cells.** In the animal model of experimental hematogenous pyelonephritis, the kidney is relatively resistant to infection unless a ureter is ligated. Under these circumstances, only the obstructed kidney becomes infected (Beeson and Guze, 1956). Clinical observations support the role of obstruction in pathogenesis of UTI and in increasing severity of infection. **Minimal episodes of cystitis or pyelonephritis can become life threatening when obstruction to urine flow becomes present.** Although obstruction clearly increases the severity of infection, it need not be a predisposing factor. For example, men with large residual urine may remain uninfected for years.

Vesicoureteral Reflux

Hodson and Edwards (1960) first described the association of VUR, UTI, and renal clubbing and scarring. **Children with high-grade reflux and UTIs usually develop progressive renal damage manifested by renal scarring, proteinuria, and renal failure. Those with a lesser degree of reflux usually improve or completely recover spontaneously or after treatment of the UTI. In adults, the presence of reflux does not appear to decrease renal function unless there is high storage pressure or stasis and concurrent UTIs.**

Underlying Disease

There is a high incidence of renal scarring in patients with underlying conditions that cause chronic interstitial nephritis, almost all of which produce primary renal papillary damage. These conditions include diabetes mellitus, sickle cell disorders, adult nephrocalcinosis, hyperphosphatemia, hypokalemia, analgesic abuse, sulfonamide nephropathy, gout, heavy-metal poisoning, and aging (Freedman, 1979).

Diabetes Mellitus

An increased incidence of asymptomatic bacteriuria and symptomatic UTIs appears to occur in women with diabetes mellitus, but there is no substantial increase among men with diabetes (Forland et al., 1977; Meiland et al., 2002; Ooi et al., 1974; Vejlsgaard, 1973). Some contributory factors to the increased incidence include incomplete bladder emptying, poor glucose control, and impaired immune response (Boyko et al., 2005)

Diabetes appears to predispose the patient to more severe infections. Frequent courses of antibiotics for asymptomatic bacteriuria and symptomatic UTIs in patients with diabetes result in a higher incidence of resistant pathogens (ESBL-positive Enterobacteriaceae, carbapenem-resistant Enterobacteriaceae, and vancomycin-resistant enterococci [VRE]). Multiple studies have investigated the relationship between risk of UTI and glycosuria, but there is no evidence to support this relationship (Johnsson et al., 2013; Rizzi and Trevisan, 2016). One study using antibody-coated bacteria techniques to localize the site of infection showed the upper urinary tract to be involved in nearly 80% of patients with diabetes and UTIs (Forland et al., 1977). This evidence of increasing immunologic response in patients with diabetes who acquire bacteriuria suggests renal parenchymal involvement and a potential increase in morbidity.

Infections are frequently caused by atypical organisms such as yeast and result in upper tract infections and significant sequelae

---

BOX 55.2 Conditions Associated With Renal Papillary Necrosis

Diabetes mellitus
Pyelonephritis
Urinary tract obstruction
Analgesic abuse
Sickle cell hemoglobinopathies
Renal transplant rejection
Cirrhosis of the liver
Dehydration, hypoxia, and jaundice of infants
Miscellaneous: renal vein thrombosis, cryoglobulinemia, renal candidiasis, contrast media injection, amyloidosis, calyceal arteritis, necrotizing angiitis, rapidly progressive glomerulonephritis, hypotensive shock, acute pancreatitis

Data from Eknoyan G, Qunibi WY, Grissom RT, et al.: Renal papillary necrosis: an update. *Medicine* 61:55, 1982.

---

such as emphysematous pyelonephritis, papillary necrosis, perinephric abscess, or metastatic infection (Stapleton, 2002; Wheat, 1980).

Renal Papillary Necrosis

The role of infection in the development and progression of renal papillary necrosis (RPN) is controversial. **Multiple predisposing conditions have been associated with the development of RPN, particularly diabetes, analgesic abuse, sickle cell hemoglobinopathy, and obstruction** (Box 55.2).

Clinically, RPN is a spectrum of disease. Patients may have an acute fulminating illness with rapid progression or may have a chronic disease that is incidentally discovered. Some patients may chronically pass necrotic tissue in their urine (Hernandez et al., 1975), whereas some may never experience papilla loss in the urine (Lindvall, 1978). Retained necrotic papillae may calcify, especially in association with infection. Furthermore, this necrotic tissue may form the nidus for chronic infection. Opportunistic fungal infections have been reported (Juhasz et al., 1980; Madge and Lombardias, 1973; Tomashefski and Abramowsky, 1981; Vordermark et al., 1980). Renal sonography may be useful to diagnose RPN (Buonocore et al., 1980; Hoffman et al., 1982).

The early diagnosis of RPN is important to improve prognosis and reduce morbidity. In addition to chronic infection, patients with analgesic abuse–associated papillary necrosis may have an increased incidence of urothelial tumors; routine urinary cytologic examinations may be helpful to diagnose these tumors early (Jackson et al., 1978). In patients who have analgesic abuse–induced RPN, the disease stabilizes if the analgesic intake is stopped (Gower, 1976). Furthermore, adequate antimicrobial therapy to control infection and early recognition and treatment of ureteral obstruction caused by sloughed necrotic tissue can minimize a decline in renal function. **A patient who suffers from an acute ureteral obstruction caused by a sloughed papilla and who has a concomitant UTI has a urologic emergency.** In this case, immediate removal of the obstructing papilla by stone basket (Jameson and Heal, 1973) or acute drainage of the kidney by ureteral catheter or percutaneous nephrostomy is necessary.

In the case of sickle cell disease, it is particularly important that patients engage with nephrology early to prevent the progression of sickle cell nephropathy, which includes glomerular disease in addition to papillary necrosis. Preventive measures include ensuring adequate fluid intake, blood pressure control, and the use of angiotensin-converting enzyme (ACE) inhibitors or angiotensin II receptor blockers (ARBs) in patients who have microalbuminuria and/or proteinuria (Gebreselassie et al., 2015).

Other conditions that may increase the susceptibility of the kidney to infection include hypertension and vascular obstruction (Freedman, 1979). The association of renal infection with several other renal diseases, including glomerulonephritis, atherosclerosis, and tubular necrosis, which are not associated with papillary necrosis, does not lead to pyelonephritis and scarring.

Human Immunodeficiency Virus

UTIs are fivefold more prevalent in HIV-positive individuals than in control subjects (Schonwald et al., 1999). The pathologic bacteria include higher rates of *Acinetobacter* and *Salmonella* species in HIV-positive patients. Patients with AIDS (defined by either an AIDS-defining illness and/or CD4 count <200 cells/mm^3) are at higher risk for atypical infections including fungal (*Candida* spp., *Aspergillus* spp., *Cryptococcus neoformans*, and other endemic fungi such as *Histoplasma*), mycobacterial (tuberculosis and nontuberculous mycobacteria), and viral (cytomegalovirus and adenoviruses) infections. Patients with a CD4 count below 200 cells/mm^3 are typically placed on *Pneumocystis* pneumonia prophylaxis; often TMP-SMX (which decreases UTI risk), unless the patient has a sulfa allergy or G6PD deficiency.

Other Conditions That Increase Risk of Urinary Tract Infections

Renal Transplantation

UTIs are among the most common infection sustained by renal transplant recipients, with more than one-third of renal transplant recipients sustaining at least one infection after surgery; they also remain a potential risk factor for poorer graft outcomes (Golebiewska et al., 2011). Transplant recipients are noted to have a higher incidence of infections with bacteria-harboring antibiotic resistance capability and are prone to recurrent episodes of symptomatic infection, likely related to colonization within their urinary tract (Hollyer and Ison, 2017). Exposure to intensified immunosuppression resulting from acute rejection episodes, female gender, advanced age of the recipients, long catheter duration, and cadaveric donor remains the risk factor for recurrent UTIs (Wu et al., 2016).

Menopause

UTIs among women increase in frequency after menopause; the rationale and treatment strategies for this are discussed in subsequent sections.

Pregnancy

See the section entitled *Bacteriuria in Pregnancy* for a complete discussion of this topic.

Spinal Cord Injury With High-Pressure Bladders

Of all patients with bacteriuria, no group compares in severity and morbidity with those who have SCI. Nearly all these patients require catheterization early after their injuries because of bladder overactivity or flaccidity, and significant numbers develop ureterectasis, hydronephrosis, reflux, and renal calculi. Bacteriologic and urodynamic advances in the management of these patients have greatly reduced their morbidity and mortality. Special problems associated with SCI are presented in a later section.

> **KEY POINTS: PATHOGENESIS**
>
> - Most UTIs are caused by bacteria, usually originating from the bowel and skin flora.
> - Bacterial virulence factors, including adhesin, play a role in determining which bacteria invade and the extent of infection.
> - Increased epithelial cell receptivity predisposes patients to recurrent UTIs and is a genotypic trait.
> - Obstruction to urine flow is a key factor in increasing host susceptibility to UTIs.

EVALUATION

Diagnosis of a UTI must involve a thorough history with a specific focus on signs and symptoms of the urinary complaints as well as investigating risk factors for infection. Physical exam, although necessary, is often unrevealing. Diagnosis of UTI is dependent on a properly collected urine sample. Additional testing is sometimes warranted, depending on the history.

Signs and Symptoms

Cystitis is typically associated with symptoms of dysuria, frequency, and/or urgency. Suprapubic pain, hematuria, and fever may also be present. Pyelonephritis is classically associated with fever, chills, flank pain, and costovertebral-angle tenderness. Nausea, vomiting, and malaise may be present. Urinary symptoms may or may not be present. Complicated UTIs can occur with other signs and symptoms. If patients complain of pneumaturia or fecaluria, a vesicoenteric or vesicovaginal fistula should be suspected. Renal or perirenal abscess may cause indolent fever and flank mass and tenderness. Patients with indwelling catheters often have asymptomatic bacteriuria, but fever associated with bacteremia may occur rapidly and become life threatening. Diagnosing a UTI in the geriatric population presents unique challenges (see the section on UTIs in the elderly).

In addition to focusing on presenting symptoms, **other relevant information that must be ascertained includes recent infections (urologic and nonurologic) and/or antibiotic use, significant comorbidities that may predispose to infections, recent hospitalizations, presence of pediatric voiding dysfunction, sexual and reproductive history, known urologic anatomic abnormalities, prior surgery of the urinary tract, reproductive organs or spine, family history, and current medications** (Box 55.3).

In the differential diagnosis of UTIs clinicians should consider **voiding dysfunction that is not secondary to bacterial factors and will not improve with antibiotics targeted at a UTI** (see chapters on interstitial cystitis/painful bladder syndrome, hematuria evaluation, STDs, VUR). For example, the symptoms associated with painful bladder syndrome may mimic a UTI, and, unfortunately, many patients who suffer from this syndrome are often treated with many courses of antibiotics despite the absence of documented positive cultures.

Furthermore, vaginitis is characterized by irritative voiding associated with vaginal irritation and is subacute in onset. A history of vaginal discharge or odor and multiple or new sexual partners is common. Frequency, urgency, hematuria, and suprapubic pain are not present. Physical examination reveals a vaginal discharge, and examination of vaginal fluid demonstrates inflammatory cells. Differential diagnosis includes herpes simplex virus, gonorrhea, *Chlamydia*, trichomoniasis, yeast, and bacterial vaginosis.

Last, urethritis causes dysuria that is usually subacute in onset and is associated with a history of discharge and new or multiple sexual partners. Frequency and urgency of urination may be present but are less pronounced than in patients with cystitis, and fever and chills are absent. Urethral discharge with inflammatory cells or initial pyuria in the male is characteristic. The common causes of urethritis include

---

> **BOX 55.3** Important Information in Evaluation of Urinary Tract Infection
>
> - Recent infections/antibiotic use
> - Recent hospitalizations
> - Comorbidities
> - History of pediatric voiding dysfunction
> - Sexual and reproductive history
> - Anatomic urologic abnormalities
> - Prior surgery of genitourinary tract, reproductive organs, spine
> - Family history
> - Current medications

Neisseria gonorrhoeae, Chlamydia, herpes simplex virus, and trichomoniasis. Appropriate cultures and immunologic tests are indicated. Urethral injury associated with sexual intercourse, chemical irritants, or allergy may also cause dysuria. A history of trauma or exposure to irritants and a lack of discharge or pyuria are characteristic.

As a general rule, **painless gross hematuria, or microhematuria in the absence of a positive culture, should always raise the suspicion for urologic malignancy, and a hematuria evaluation must be initiated.**

Physical examination should focus on the abdominal and pelvic regions. On examination of the suprapubic area, bladder distention may be palpated, often an indicator of an elevated postvoid residual. The presence or absence of costovertebral-angle tenderness should be assessed, particularly if the suspicion for pyelonephritis is high. During pelvic examination in a woman the presence of vaginal discharge should be noted. Inspection and palpation of the urethral area may identify the presence of a urethral diverticulum or Skene gland infection. If either of these are present, a cystic-appearing structure may be palpable or visualized. Fluid may be expressed on palpation of the area and tenderness may be elicited when palpating the cystic structure directly. In postmenopausal women careful attention should be focused on assessing the quality of the vaginal epithelium, specifically noting the degree of vaginal atrophy; atrophic vaginal tissue is an indicator of a hypoestrogenic state, which is a known risk factor for the development of UTIs. Pelvic organ prolapse may be identified as well; prolapse can contribute to incomplete emptying, which can be associated with a UTI. In men a rectal exam should be performed to assess the prostate. A focused neurologic exam on the pelvic area should be performed to assess whether sensation is intact.

Diagnosis by Urine Testing

Urine Collection

The diagnosis of a UTI is dependent on obtaining a properly collected urine sample with subsequent analysis of urine (urinalysis) and urine culture. Diagnostic accuracy and decreased rates of false-positive urinalysis and culture can be improved by reducing bacterial contamination during collection. Although studies have not demonstrated a clear benefit to cleansing the meatus before giving a midstream voided sample, it is a commonly accepted practice that is endorsed universally.

Before sample collection in circumcised men, the glans should be cleansed with a 2% castile soap towelette. For those uncircumcised, the foreskin should be retracted and the glans cleansed with the towelette before specimen collection. A midstream specimen should be obtained by collecting it in a sterile cup.

In women, contamination of a midstream urine specimen with introital bacteria and WBCs is common, particularly when the woman has difficulty maintaining separation of the labia. Women should therefore be instructed to spread the labia, wash and cleanse the periurethral area with a 2% castile soap towelette, and then collect a midstream urine specimen. The voided specimen is contaminated if it shows evidence of vaginal epithelial cells and lactobacilli on urinalysis. **Increased BMI, significant vaginal atrophy, decreased manual dexterity, and the inability to bear weight are factors that contribute to difficulty obtaining an adequate clean-catch midstream sample in women. The presence of an intravaginal pessary also increases the likelihood of obtaining a contaminated sample; if a woman has an indwelling pessary, analysis of a catheterized sample is preferable** (Box 55.4).

The collection receptacle also can affect the reliability of the sample. In some cases, voided urine samples, not collected via a midstream clean-catch sample, are collected from a bedpan or a nonsterile paper cup, rather than a sterile cup. This may occur in an emergency room setting or when a urine sample is requested during a well visit with a general practitioner or gynecologist. Analysis of these samples should be disregarded, but unfortunately patients are often treated based on abnormal findings in such erroneous samples, irrespective of symptoms. **If a patient has an indwelling Foley catheter and there is suspicion of a UTI, the catheter should be removed and a new catheter should be placed under sterile conditions to obtain a sample that reflects microbes in the urine, as opposed to microbes that may be colonizing the catheter or drainage bag.** Likewise, samples should not be taken from an ostomy appliance; rather they should be obtained via intubation of the stoma.

BOX 55.4 Factors That Affect Ability to Provide Adequate Midstream Clean-Catch Sample

- Increased body mass index
- Vaginal atrophy
- Poor manual dexterity
- Inability to bear weight
- Intravaginal pessary
- Nonsterile collection receptacle

Catheterization with collection of a mid-catheterized specimen is more accurate than a voided specimen; however, because of its invasive nature it is only used in certain circumstances. Situations in which a catheterized sample should be considered include when the voided sample shows clear evidence of contamination (i.e., many squamous epithelial cells), a patient has a pessary, the patient is unable to provide an adequate clean-catch sample, or the patient cannot provide any sample at all. Although time intensive, the risk of iatrogenic infection is low and catheterization is critical to obtain the best quality samples, particularly if the symptoms of a UTI are equivocal. Indeed, a recent study evaluating the utility of catheterized samples in patients with symptoms not strongly suggestive of a UTI revealed obtaining a catheterized sample decreased the percent of patients who would have been treated with an antibiotic based on a positive voided sample by slightly more than 50% (Aisen et al., 2018).

Suprapubic aspiration is highly accurate, but because it is associated with some morbidity, there is limited clinical usefulness except for a patient who cannot urinate on command, such as patients with SCI. However, even in those populations, catheterized samples are preferred over suprapubic aspiration. A single aspirated specimen reveals the bacteriologic status of the bladder urine without introducing urethral bacteria.

Further information on this topic is available online at Expert Consult.com.

Key Issues in Analysis of Urine Samples. Certain components of a urine sample are highly suggestive of a UTI. Leukocyte esterase is produced by the breakdown of WBCs in the urine. Its presence is an indication of pyuria, but not bacteria specifically. As mentioned previously, the presence of WBCs and therefore leukocyte esterase is not uncommon in women with vaginal contamination. Nitrites are present when bacteria reduce dietary nitrates, via bacterial nitrate reductase activity. Not all bacteria produce nitrites, though, so the absence of nitrites does not mean bacteria are not present. **All Enterobacteriaceae produce nitrites, including *E. coli, Klebsiella, Enterobacter, Proteus, Citrobacter, Morganella,* and *Salmonella* spp. Non–nitrite-producing bacteria include all gram positives and Pseudomonads (e.g., Pseudomonas and Acinetobacter).** In addition, patients who adhere to low-nitrate diets may have false-negative results. The presence of nitrites has a high specificity but much lower sensitivity. The presence of leukocyte esterase and nitrites is more reliable when bacterial counts are more than 100,000 colony-forming units (CFUs) per milliliter. Cloudy urine may occur because of pyuria but it can also occur because of precipitated phosphate crystals in alkaline or concentrated urine.

Ideally a sample is analyzed in proximity to the time at which it was received. If a sample is left standing too long, it may become alkaline and subsequently may contain bacteria or lysed red cells. If the sample will not be analyzed within a few hours, it must be refrigerated, especially if not in a specimen cup that contains preservatives. Hydration can also dilute the concentration of certain constituents.

Urine Dipsticks. Dipsticks, or chemically impregnated reagent strips, are often used in urgicares or medical clinics, or by patients at home when they develop symptoms of a UTI. **Although dipsticks are most helpful in ruling out a UTI, each parameter has false positives and negatives, which make it less reliable in determining whether**

a patient has a UTI. However, in a patient who has symptoms strongly suggestive of a UTI, a positive dipstick can be helpful in determining whether to initiate antibiotics. A positive nitrite is the independent variable most likely to rule in a UTI, when analyzed in conjunction with symptoms (Meister et al., 2013). Analysis of several of the components of a dipstick increases the diagnostic abilities compared with just one component. **Positive nitrites or positive leukocyte esterase and blood on a dipstick most accurately diagnose a UTI** (Little et al., 2009; Marques et al., 2017).

However, the borderline sensitivity of dipsticks, especially among patients with less characteristic symptoms of UTIs, does not allow these inexpensive tests to replace careful microscopic urinalysis in symptomatic patients (Semeniuk and Church, 1999). In addition, results of a dipstick can be inaccurate if the test strips are expired or improperly stored. Some of the dipstick reagents, like nitrites, are sensitive to air exposure, so if a container of strips is not closed as soon as one is used, the other strips are more likely to give false-positive results in the future. The leukocyte reaction takes up to 5 minutes to occur, so if a strip is not observed for the appropriate duration, a patient may display a false-negative result.

Urinalysis. Automated urinalysis allows for more sensitive detection of hematuria and bacteria in the urine as compared with dipsticks. Preferred collection tubes for urinalysis are those that have non-mercuric preservatives, such as a combination of chlorhexidine, ethylparaben, and sodium propionate. Such preservatives ensure the quality of the sample for up to 72 hours without refrigeration, therefore preventing bacterial overgrowth. Approximately 6 to 8 mL of urine is centrifuged at 1800 to 2000 RPM for 4 minutes, then examined. Microscopic analysis reports on the number of RBCs, WBCs, squamous epithelial cells, bacteria, crystals, and casts. The number of squamous cells is an indicator of the sample quality.

Abnormal results of any one urinary constituent is usually not pathognomonic of a UTI; thus several constituents must be evaluated together. **Multiple aspects of the urinalysis may indicate an acute inflammatory response, particularly pyuria (the presence of at least 5 to 10 leukocytes per high-power field) and hematuria. This information is valuable in conjunction with culture results given that bacteriuria may represent chronic colonization** versus acute infection. In addition, cultures typically require 48 to 72 hours to result; thus urinalysis provides for quick analysis. Ideally a sample is sent for analysis soon after the sample is given, with attention paid to proper sample collection. The strongest predictors of a UTI, in the correct clinical context, include moderate bacteriuria, moderate pyuria, and nitrites (Meister et al., 2013).

Pyuria can be found in several conditions other than UTIs, so the mere presence of WBCs in the urine is not diagnostic. Increasing numbers of WBCs present in a symptomatic patient, however, do support a UTI diagnosis. Indeed, it has been suggested that moderate pyuria, defined as WBC count greater than 50, in conjunction with symptoms suggestive of a UTI, justifies treatment with antibiotics (Meister et al., 2013). Other conditions known to cause pyuria include GU tuberculosis, urolithiasis, injury to the urothelium (including chlamydial urethritis), and interstitial nephritis. Depending on the level of hydration, the intensity of the tissue reaction producing the cells, and the method of urine collection, any number of WBCs can be seen in the microscopic sediment in the presence of an uninfected urinary tract. **The absence of pyuria should cause the diagnosis of UTI to be questioned until urine culture results are available. If a culture is positive yet no pyuria is demonstrated on urinalysis, clinicians should consider obtaining a catheterized sample.**

Bacteria may be present on initial urinalysis even though the final culture is negative, thus rendering the bacteria found on urinalysis a false-positive result. This is most likely to occur when vaginal bacteria, such as lactobacilli and corynebacteria, are present in a voided sample from a female patient.

Automated urinalysis can reliably rule out a UTI and preclude the need to order a urine culture (Kayalp et al., 2013). However, ruling in a UTI based on a urinalysis is not as straightforward, because urinalyses may have abnormal parameters even in healthy, asymptomatic women, using preferred collection techniques (Frazee et al., 2015). Thus **relying on results of urinalyses alone can lead to overdiagnosis of UTIs. It is critically important that results of urinalyses are interpreted in conjunction with the clinical presentation and eventually correlation with a urine culture.**

Urine Culture. Standard urine culture is the gold standard for identifying the presence of bacteriuria, which supports a diagnosis of UTI in the symptomatic patient. The technique was originally described in the 1950s. Ideally, urine is collected via a midstream clean-catch sample or catheterized sample and is placed in a vacutainer tube that contains freeze-dried preservatives, which practically eliminate false-positive results. The sample is then placed on blood agar and MacConkey culture plates.

Historically, a colony count of at least 10^5 CFU/mL of urine was used to diagnose a UTI. Initially, this colony count confirmed a diagnosis of pyelonephritis (Kass, 1956) but has subsequently been employed to make a diagnosis of cystitis as well. However, many studies have demonstrated that women with dysuria may have lower bacterial colony counts. Indeed, 20% to 40% of women with symptomatic UTIs have bacteria counts of 10^2 to 10^4 CFU/mL of urine (Kraft and Stamey, 1977; Kunz et al., 1975; Stamey et al., 1965), probably because of the slow doubling time of bacteria in urine (every 30 to 45 minutes) combined with frequent bladder emptying (every 15 to 30 minutes) from irritation. **Thus, in dysuric patients, an appropriate threshold value for defining significant bacteriuria is 10^2 CFU/mL of a known pathogen** (Stamm and Hooton, 1993).

Urine culture results are reported as negative, commensal flora, or positive. Commensal flora includes coagulase-negative staphylococci, alpha and non-hemolytic streptococci, diphtheroids, nonpathogenic *Neisseria* spp., and yeasts. Results of positive urine cultures are reported with antibiotic sensitivities for each pathogen: S (sensitive), I (indeterminate), and R (resistant), with the minimum inhibitory concentration (MIC) following the sensitivities. **The MIC is the lowest concentration of an antibiotic that inhibits growth of an organism.** If an antibiotic is listed as sensitive, it suggests that growth of an organism is inhibited by the serum concentration of the medication that is achieved using the recommended dose. If listed as indeterminate, the antibiotic still may be effective in locations where the medication is physiologically concentrated or a higher-than-recommended dose can be used. Resistant organisms are those that are resistant to standard achievable serum drug levels (Fig. 55.10). **Efficacy of the antimicrobial therapy is critically dependent on the antimicrobial levels in the urine and the duration that this level remains above the minimal inhibitory concentration of the infecting organism** (Hooton and Stamm, 1991). **Resolution of infection is closely associated with the susceptibility of the bacteria to the concentration of the antimicrobial agent achieved in the urine** (McCabe and Jackson, 1965; Stamey et al., 1965, 1974). The concentration of useful antimicrobial agents in the serum and urine of healthy adults is shown in eTable 55.1, which demonstrates that the **urinary levels are often several hundred times greater than the serum levels.** Inhibitory concentrations in urine are achieved after oral administration of all commonly used antimicrobial agents, except for the macrolides (erythromycin).

Factors other than the MIC should be taken into account when selecting an antibiotic, such as anatomic location of the infection and fluid type that is harboring infection (i.e., urine vs. blood). The lowest MIC is not always the most effective option. Route of administration should also be considered when determining which antibiotic to choose. This is particularly important in the outpatient setting when patients demonstrate the presence of multidrug-resistant organisms.

The specific pathogen identified in the culture is also a critical factor in evaluating the need to proceed with treatment, particularly if symptoms are equivocal. Although there is consensus regarding the benefit of treating a symptomatic patient who has gram-negative rods in the urine, the significance of gram-positive organisms in women is more controversial. In many cases a gram-positive organism may represent a periurethral contaminant. In a study comparing the presence of uropathogens in voided samples versus catheterized samples in symptomatic premenopausal women, the presence of *E. coli* in midstream samples had a high positive predictive value (93%) of bladder bacteriuria,

ORDERER PROCEDURE	Urine culture	
Source	Clean Catch	
Body site		
FINAL REPORT	>100,000 CFU/mL	Escherichia coli
Organism	Positive	Escherichia coli
SUSCEPTIBILITY METHOD	Microscan Minimun	Inhibitory Concentrations
Organism	Positive	Escherichia coli µg/mL
AMIKACIN	Susceptible	<=4 µg/mL
AMPICILLIN	Resistant	>16 µg/mL
AMPICILLIN-SULBACTAM	Intermediate	16/8 µg/mL
AZTREONAM	Susceptible	<=2 µg/mL
CEFAZOLIN	Susceptible	<=2 µg/mL
CEFEPIME	Susceptible	<=2 µg/mL
CEFOXITIN	Susceptible	<=2 µg/mL
CEFTAZIDIME	Susceptible	<=2 µg/mL
CEFTRIAXONE	Susceptible	<=1 µg/mL
ERTAPENEM	Susceptible	<=0.5 µg/mL
GENTAMICIN	Susceptible	<=1 µg/mL
LEVOFLOXACIN	Susceptible	<=0.5 µg/mL
MEROPENEM	Susceptible	<=1 µg/mL
NITROFURANTOIN	Susceptible	<=32 µg/mL
PIPERACILLIN-TAZOBACTAM	Susceptible	<=8 µg/mL
TETRACYCLINE	Resistant	>8 µg/mL
TOBRAMYCIN	Susceptible	2 µg/mL
TRIMETHOPRIM-SULFAMETHOXAZOLE	Resistant	>2/32 µg/mL

Fig. 55.10. Minimum inhibitory concentration for *E. coli* urinary tract infection, demonstrating sensitivity to most antibiotics except ampicillin, ampicillin-sulbactam, tetracycline, and trimethoprim-sulfamethoxazole.

even at low colony counts, whereas the presence of enterococci and group B streptococci were not predictive of bladder bacteriuria at any colony count (Hooton et al., 2013). In women who grew enterococci and/or group B streptococci in a voided sample, *E coli* grew from a catheterized sample in 61% of these subjects. The authors concluded that gram-positive organisms rarely cause acute cystitis in isolation.

In some cases, despite symptoms and a UA that are suggestive of a UTI, a standard urine culture may be negative. In this scenario a culture should be sent specifically looking for atypical organisms such as *Ureaplasma urealyticum* or *Mycoplasma hominis*.

Recently, more sensitive culture techniques have been described, known as the Expanded Quantitative Urine Culture (EQUC) (see the section on microbiome). Although the EQUC is not widely used yet, its ability to detect more organisms in the urine challenges traditional thinking about cutoff thresholds for the diagnosis of UTIs as well as the concept that polymicrobial presence should be discounted as a contaminant. Some have argued that the standard urine culture should no longer be considered the gold standard for detecting uropathogens (Price et al., 2018). **With more sophisticated techniques available to detect microbes, clinical judgment is paramount to prevent overtreatment of bacteriuria.**

> **KEY POINTS: EVALUATION**
>
> - Clinical presentation is critical in considering diagnosis; results of urine testing cannot be analyzed without knowledge of signs and symptoms.
> - Urine must be collected in a manner that minimizes contamination.
> - Formal urinalysis is preferred over dipstick testing.
> - Urine culture results provide information regarding bacterial sensitivities.

LOCALIZATION

Ureteral Catheterization

In cases of bacterial persistence it is useful to try to identify the source. Ureteral catheterization allows separation of not only bacterial persistence into upper and lower urinary tracts but also the infection between one kidney and the other, and even localization of infection to ectopic ureters or to nonrefluxing ureteral stumps (by using saline solution irrigation) (Stamey, 1980). Attempts to identify one or both kidneys as a source of infection are particularly important in patients with fever, flank pain, and/or costovertebral angle tenderness. This modality of diagnostics is also particularly important for the patient with renal transplant in determining if the native kidneys are harboring infection contributing to a UTI (see eTable 55.1).

Stone Cultures

It is clinically useful to culture stones removed from the urinary tract to identify the bacteria—and their sensitivities—that reside within their interstices. Urinary and stone cultures must be analyzed separately because results may be discordant. UTIs are the most common complication after stone removal procedures. Manipulation of infected stones, and possible release of endotoxins into the bloodstream, can lead to systemic inflammatory response syndrome (SIRS) or potentially fatal urosepsis. Studies have shown that stone cultures, rather than periprocedure urine cultures, are a better predictor of postoperative sepsis and SIRS (Korets et al., 2011; Mariappan et al., 2005).

IMAGING

Imaging studies are not required in most cases of UTI because clinical and laboratory findings are sufficient for correct diagnosis, initiation of treatment, and adequate management of most patients. However, infections in most men, compromised hosts, febrile infections, signs or symptoms of urinary tract obstruction, failure to respond to appropriate therapy, and a pattern of recurrent infections suggesting bacterial persistence within the urinary tract warrant imaging for identification of underlying abnormalities that require modification of medical management or percutaneous or surgical intervention (Box 55.5).

A UTI associated with possible urinary tract obstruction must be urgently evaluated. This refers to patients with calculi, especially

> **BOX 55.5 Indications for Radiologic Investigation in Acute Clinical Pyelonephritis**
>
> Potential ureteral obstruction (e.g., caused by stone, ureteral stricture, tumor)
> History of calculi, especially infection (struvite) stones
> Potential papillary necrosis (e.g., patients with sickle cell anemia, severe diabetes mellitus, analgesic abuse)
> History of genitourinary surgery that predisposes to obstruction, such as ureteral reimplantation or ureteral diversion
> Poor response to appropriate antimicrobial agents after 5 to 6 days of treatment
> Diabetes mellitus
> Polycystic kidneys in patients in dialysis or with severe renal insufficiency
> Neuropathic bladder
> Unusual infecting organisms, such as tuberculosis, fungus, or urea-splitting organisms (e.g., *Proteus*)

> **BOX 55.6 Correctable Urologic Abnormalities That Cause Bacterial Persistence**
>
> - Infection stones
> - Chronic bacterial prostatitis
> - Unilateral infected atrophic kidneys
> - Ureteral duplication and ectopic ureters
> - Foreign bodies
> - Urethral diverticula and infected periurethral glands
> - Unilateral medullary sponge kidneys
> - Nonrefluxing, normal-appearing, infected ureteral stumps after nephrectomy
> - Infected urachal cysts
> - Infected communicating cysts of the renal calyces
> - Papillary necrosis
> - Perivesical abscess with fistula to bladder

infection (struvite) stones; ureteral tumors; ureteral strictures; congenital obstructions; or previous GU surgery, such as ureteral reimplantation or urinary diversion procedures that may have caused obstruction. Patients with **diabetes mellitus** can develop special complications from UTIs; they may acquire emphysematous pyelonephritis or papillary necrosis. **Impacted necrotic papillae** may cause acute ureteral obstruction. Patients with **polycystic kidney disease who are on dialysis** are particularly prone to developing perinephric abscesses.

Urologic imaging is indicated in patients whose symptoms of acute clinical pyelonephritis persist after several days of appropriate antimicrobial therapy; they may manifest perinephric or renal abscesses. In addition, **patients with unusual organisms,** including urea-splitting organisms (e.g., *Proteus* species), should be examined for abnormalities within the urinary tract, such as obstructing stones, strictures, or fungus aggregates.

The second reason for radiologic evaluation is to diagnose a focus of bacterial persistence. **In patients whose bacteriuria fails to resolve after appropriate antimicrobial therapy or who have rapid recurrence of infection, abnormalities that allow bacterial persistence should be sought.** Although uncommon, it is important to identify causes of persistence because they may represent surgically correctable urologic abnormalities. Acquired or congenital urologic abnormalities that can cause unresolved or recurrent UTIs are listed in Box 55.6.

Ultrasonography

Renal and bladder ultrasound (RBUS) is an important imaging technique because it is noninvasive, easy and rapid to perform, and offers no radiation or contrast agent risk to the patient. Ultrasound is particularly useful in identifying calculi and hydronephrosis, pyonephrosis, and perirenal abscesses. Although with the known pitfalls of limited sensitivity, a single radiograph for calculi could accompany ultrasonography. Ultrasonography is also useful for diagnosing postvoid residual urine. A disadvantage is that the study is dependent on the interpretative and performance skills of the examiner. Furthermore, the study may be technically poor in patients who are obese or have other anatomic challenges, or who have dressings, drainage tubes, or open wounds overlying the area of interest. **The sensitivity of ultrasound for demonstrating renal parenchymal abnormalities in acute pyelonephritis is lower than that of CT and MRI; it is lower than that of CT for detecting small renal stones and most ureteral stones and is less accurate than CT in detecting ureteral obstruction.**

Computed Tomography and Magnetic Resonance Imaging

The radiologic modalities that offer the best anatomic detail for evaluation of UTI are CT and MRI. These studies are more sensitive than excretory urography or ultrasonography in the diagnosis of acute focal bacterial nephritis, renal and perirenal abscesses, and radiolucent calculi (Kuhn and Berger, 1981; Mauro et al., 1982; Soler et al., 1997; Soulen et al., 1989; Wadsworth et al., 1982). When used to localize renal and perirenal abscesses, CT improves the approach to surgical drainage and permits percutaneous approaches. MRI has not supplanted CT in the evaluation of renal inflammation, but it has provided some advantages in delineating extrarenal extension of inflammation. Pelvic MRI is the most useful imaging modality for detecting a urethral diverticulum.

Voiding Cystourethrogram

The voiding cystourethrogram is an important examination in assessing VUR. In women with a history of febrile UTIs, known VUR as a child, or recurrent pyelonephritis as an adult, a voiding cystourethrogram (VCUG) should be performed. VCUG should also be considered in patients with a history of recurrent UTIs and hydronephrosis detected on upper tract imaging. Historically VCUG with a double-balloon catheter was recommended if there was suspicion of a urethral diverticulum; however, the current standard of care used is pelvic MRI.

Information about radionuclide studies is available online at ExpertConsult.com.

MICROBIOME

Contrary to traditional thought, urine is not sterile. In recent years, 16S ribosomal RNA sequencing analysis has been used to help determine that many bacterial species inhabit the urinary tract of healthy men and women who do not have symptoms of a UTI (Lewis et al., 2013; Nelson et al., 2010; Wolfe et al., 2012). Standard culture techniques readily identify fast-growing bacteria that thrive in an oxygen-rich environment. However, many bacteria require special nutrients or are anaerobic and thus will not grow in standard culture preparations. This initial work involving the urinary microbiome has since revolutionized our thought process when it comes to identifying bacteria in the urinary tract. Although bacteria in the urine were traditionally thought of as categorically pathological, it is now established that bacteria are present in the urine of symptomatic as well as asymptomatic men and women.

Once the female urinary microbiome was identified, researchers started investigating whether modifying standard culture techniques would enable detection of bacteria that previously would have been missed. Indeed, using an expanded quantitative urine culture (EQUC) protocol, many bacteria were identified that would have been missed using standard culture preparations (Hilt et al., 2014). The EQUC specifically analyzed a larger volume of urine, which was subject to different atmospheric conditions and longer incubation times. Hilt et al. then compared standard culture protocols to the EQUC protocol in 65 samples from patients with or without overactive bladder symptoms. They found that 52/65 samples grew bacteria in the EQUC protocol group, yet 48 of these 52 were negative in standard culture cohort. Beyond typical bacteria often cultured in urine, 35 different genera and 85 different species were identified. This discovery further supported the notion that the female urinary microbiome exists and contains many different nonpathogenic microbiota (Table 55.2).

Now that we are aware of the existence of the female urinary microbiome, we face the "challenge of interpretation": we must determine when and how to treat bacteria in the urinary tract with the acknowledgment that we will never, nor should we strive to, eradicate all bacteria (Brubaker and Wolfe, 2017). Indeed, many bacteria within the microbiome are considered protective (Brubaker et al., 2014; Pearce et al., 2014). Ongoing research seeks to determine if disruptions in the established microbiota are seen in certain forms

TABLE 55.2 List of Bacterial Species Cultured in Different Conditions

ORGANISM	AEROBIC 35°	AEROBIC 30°	CO$_2$ 35°	ANAEROBIC 35°	CAMPY (6% O$_2$, 10% CO$_2$) 35°
Actinobaculum schaalii (7)	+		+	+	+
Actinobaculum urinale (1)				+	
Actinomyces europaeus (2)			+		
Actinomyces graevenitzii (1)					+
Actinomyces naeslundii (1)		+			
Actinomyces neuii (5)	+		+	+	
Actinomyces odontolyticus (2)	+		+	+	
Actinomyces oris (1)			+		
Actinomyces turicensis (3)	+	+	+	+	
Actinomyces urogenitalis (3)	+	+			
Aerococcus sanguinicola (3)	HD	HD	+		
Aerococcus urinae (9)	+	+	+	+	+
Aerococcus viridans (1)			+		
Alloscardovia omnicolens (4)	+		+	+	
Arthrobacter cumminsii (4)	+	+	+	+	
Bacillus subtilis (1)	HD	+			
Bifidobacterium bifidum (1)			+	+	
Bifidobacterium breve (6)			+	+	+
Bifidobacterium dentum (1)			+	+	
Bifidobacterium longum (1)				+	
Brevibacterium ravenspurgense (2)			+	+	
Campylobacter ureolyticus (1)	HD			+	
Candida glabrata (2)	+		+	+	
Corynebacterium afermentans (2)	+			+	
Corynebacterium amycolatum (3)		+	+	+	+
Corynebacterium aurimucosum (3)	+	+	+	+	
Corynebacterium coyleae (7)	+	+	+	+	+
Corynebacterium freneyi (2)	+		+	+	
Corynebacterium imitans (2)	+	+	+		
Corynebacterium lipophile-group F1 (4)	+	+	+	+	+
Corynebacteirum matruchotii (1)			+		
Corynebacterium minutissium (1)		+		+	
Corynebacterium riegelii (4)	+	+	+	+	
Corynebacterium tuberculostearicum (2)	+				
Corynebacterium tuscaniense (3)	+		+		
Corynebacterium urealyticum (3)	+		+		
Enterobacter aerogenes (1)	+	+	+	+	+
Enterococcus faecalis (7)	+	+	+	+	+
Escherichia coli (3)	+	+	+	+	+
Facklamia hominis (5)	+	+		+	
Fingoldia magna (1)	HD			+	
Fusobacterium nucleatum (1)	HD			+	
Gardnerella vaginalis (10)	+	+	+	+	
Gardnerella sp. (3)	+		+	+	+
Gemella haemolysans (1)		+			
Gemella sanguinis (1)		+			
Klebsiella pneumoniae (1)	+	+	+	+	+
Kocuria rhizophila (1)		+			
Lactobacillus crispatus (6)			+	+	
Lactobacillus delbrueckii (1)			+	+	

Continued

TABLE 55.2 List of Bacterial Species Cultured in Different Conditions—cont'd

ORGANISM	AEROBIC 35°	AEROBIC 30°	CO$_2$ 35°	ANAEROBIC 35°	CAMPY (6% O$_2$, 10% CO$_2$) 35°
Lactobacillus fermentum (1)					+
Lactobacillus gasseri (12)	+	+	+	+	+
Lactobacillus iners (6)	+		+	+	+
Lactobacillus jensenii (10)	+		+	+	+
Lactobacillus johnsonii (1)			+		
Lactobacillus rhamnosus (2)			+	+	
Micrococcus luteus (9)	+	+	+		+
Micrococcus lylae (1)	+		+		
Neisseria perflava (1)			+		
Oligella urethralis (5)					+
Peptoniphilus harei (3)				+	
Prevotella bivia (1)				+	+
Propionibacterium avidum (1)				+	
Propionimicrobium lymphophilum (1)				+	
Pseudomonas aeruginosa (1)			+		
Rothia dentocariosa (1)	+		+		
Rothia mucilaginosa (2)	+		+		+
Slackia exigua (1)				+	
Staphylococcus capitis (1)	+		+	+	
Staphylococcus epidermidis (7)	+	+	+	+	+
Staphylococcus haemolyticus (2)	+		+		
Staphylococcus hominis (2)	+		+		
Staphylococcus lugdunesis (2)	+	+	+	+	+
Staphylococcus simulans (2)	+			+	+
Staphylococcus warneri (2)	+				+
Streptococcus agalactiae (1)	+	+		+	+
Streptococcus anginosus (15)	+	+	+	+	+
Streptococcus gallolyticus (1)	+	+	+	+	+
Streptococcus gordonii (1)		+	+	+	
Streptococcus parasanguinis (1)	+				
Streptococcus pneumonia/mitis/oralis (6)	+	+	+	+	+
Streptococcus salivarius (3)				+	
Streptococcus sanguinis (2)			+		
Streptococcus vestibularis (1)	HD		+	+	
Trueperella bernardiae (3)	+		+		
Unclassified#1 (1)	+	+			
Unclassified#2 (1)	+	+			+
Unclassified#3 (1)			+		
Unclassified#4 (1)	+	+			
Unclassified#5 (1)				+	
Unclassified#6 (1)	+		+		
Unclassified#7 (1)	+				
Unclassified#8 (1)	+			+	+

The "+" symbol designates the environmental conditions from which the organism was isolated and identified. The "HD" symbol indicates that only high-dilution (1 μL) urine was plated for that condition and that no growth was observed. A blank space designates no growth in that condition for that particular organism using a low-dilution (100 μL) inoculum. The (#) next to the organism name designates the number of times the organism has been isolated.
Data from Hilt EE, McKinley K, Pearce MM, et al.: Urine is not sterile: use of enhanced urine culture techniques to detect resident bacterial flora in the adult female bladder. *J Clin Microbiol.* 52(3):871–876, 2014.

of lower urinary tract pathology, focusing particularly on determining whether the microbiome differs in women with conditions such as urge incontinence or painful bladder syndrome (Nickel et al., 2016; Thomas-White et al., 2016).

In line with this understanding of a dynamic urinary microbiome that affects bladder physiology, emerging scientific theories continue to develop and explore the concept that urine has a role beyond purely functioning as a vehicle for excretory waste. First, the Urinology Think Tank, a group supported by the National Institute of Diabetes and Digestive and Kidney Disease, is investigating the notion that properties intrinsic to urine, including the microbiotia, exfoliated cells, exosomes, pH, metabolites, protein, and specific gravity, may interact with the urothelium to influence bladder function and homeostasis (Urinology Think Tank Writing, 2018). Furthermore, emerging basic science work continues to explore the possibility that the constituents of urine, including donor-derived urine stem cells, can be used for human cell therapy and autologous repair (Pavathuparambil Abdul Manaph et al., 2018).

> **KEY POINTS: MICROBIOME**
>
> - Urine is not sterile.
> - The female urinary microbiome has been identified using RNA sequencing techniques, and knowledge of these microbiota should inform UTI management and interpretation of novel culture techniques such as the EQUC protocol.

ASYMPTOMATIC BACTERIURIA

The management of asymptomatic bacteriuria has evolved with time, even before the identification of the urinary microbiome, which essentially renders the term "asymptomatic bacteriuria" obsolete. Nonetheless, for the purposes of this chapter, we will continue to use this term and review its significance.

The term *asymptomatic bacteriuria* is appropriately used when a person has no signs or symptoms of a UTI, yet bacteria are identified in a noncontaminated urine sample. In women, the term *asymptomatic bacteriuria* is used when the same bacteria is identified in quantitative counts of greater than or equal to 100,000 CFUs in two consecutive voided samples that are obtained in a fashion that minimizes contamination. In men, only one clean-catch voided sample that identifies one bacterial species in quantitative counts greater than or equal to 100,000 CFUs is necessary to use the term *asymptomatic bacteriuria* appropriately. Alternatively, in men or women, one catheterized sample that identifies a single bacterial species in a quantitative count of greater than or equal to 100 can make the diagnosis of asymptomatic bacteriuria (Nicolle, et al., 2005; Box 55.7).

The prevalence of asymptomatic bacteriuria varies based on age, sex, and comorbid conditions. First, the prevalence of asymptomatic bacteriuria increases with age: it has been identified in approximately 1% of school-age girls but is present in greater than 20% of healthy women older than 80 years of age who are community dwellers (Nicolle, 2003). It also correlates with sexual activity; in fact population studies have identified a prevalence in premenopausal, married women of 4.6%, whereas in age-matched nuns the prevalence is only 0.7% (Kunin and McCormack, 1968). Menopause is also a risk factor for asymptomatic bacteriuria with a prevalence estimated as 1% to 5% in healthy premenopausal women and 2.8% to 8.6% in postmenopausal women between the ages of 50 and 70 (Nicolle, 2003). In younger men, asymptomatic bacteriuria is uncommon (Lipsky, 1989). As men age, the prevalence increases; in elderly (>75 years old) community dwellers it has been quoted as 6% to 15% (Nicolle, 2003). The overall prevalence is increased in both sexes living in long-term care facilities: it has been reported in 25% to 50% of women and 15% to 40% of men in facilities (Nicolle, 1997). Asymptomatic bacteriuria is more common in female patients with diabetes as compared with males (9%–27% vs. 0.7%–11%) (Zhanel et al., 1991a,b). The presence of asymptomatic bacteriuria is also strongly associated with duration of disease as well as comorbidities associated with poorly controlled diabetes (Zhanel et al., 1995). In patients with SCI who perform clean intermittent catheterization (CIC), the prevalence is 23% to 89% (Bakke and Digranes, 1991). Finally, the prevalence in patients with long-term indwelling catheters is 100% (Warren et al., 1982). **As demonstrated by all of these statistics, risk factors for asymptomatic bacteriuria include advanced age, female gender, institutionalization, comorbid conditions such as diabetes, and catheterization/presence of an indwelling Foley catheter** (Colgan et al., 2006; Table 55.3).

In older women living in the community, *E. coli* is the predominant pathogen isolated in asymptomatic women; it was found in 51.4% of samples in one study. Other species of bacteria were found in fewer than 10% of samples and included *Klebsiella pneumoniae*, *Proteus mirabilis*, and *Enterococcus faecalis* (Linhares et al., 2013). The *E. coli* strains identified in women with asymptomatic bacteriuria have less virulence factors than other strains that cause symptomatic urinary infections (Svanborg, 1997). Molecular studies have shown that

> **BOX 55.7** Diagnosis of Asymptomatic Bacteriuria
>
> - Lack of signs and symptoms of UTI
> - Diagnosis based on urine specimen collected in a manner that minimizes contamination
> - For asymptomatic women: 2 consecutive voided urine specimens with isolation of same bacterial strain in quantitative counts ≥100,000 CFUs/mL
> - For asymptomatic men: single voided urine specimen with one bacterial species isolated in quantitative count ≥100,000 CFUs/mL
> - For women or men: single catheterized urine specimen with one bacterial species isolated quantitative count ≥100 CFUs/mL

CFUs, Colony-forming units; *UTI*, urinary tract infection.
Data from Nicolle LE, Bradley S, Colgan R, et al.: Infectious Diseases Society of America guidelines for the diagnosis and treatment of asymptomatic bacteriuria in adults. *Clin Infect Dis* 40(5):643–654, 2005. Based on ISDA guidelines.

TABLE 55.3 Prevalence of Asymptomatic Bacteriuria in Selected Populations

POPULATION	PREVALENCE (%)	REFERENCE
Healthy, premenopausal women	1.0–5.0	Nicolle, 2003
Pregnant women	1.9–9.5	Nicolle, 2003
Postmenopausal women aged 50–70 years	2.8–8.6	Nicolle, 2003
Patients with diabetes		
Women	9.0–27	Zhanel et al., 1991a
Men	0.7–11	Zhanel et al., 1991a
Elderly persons in the community		
Women	10.8–16	Nicolle, 2003
Men	3.6–19	Nicolle, 2003
Elderly persons in a long-term care facility		
Women	25–50	Nicolle, 1997
Men	14–50	Nicolle, 1997
Patients with spinal cord injuries		
Intermittent catheter use	23–89	Bakke and Digranes, 1991
Sphincterotomy and condom catheter in place	57	Waites et al., 1993b
Patients undergoing hemodialysis	28	Chaudhry, 1993
Patients with indwelling catheter use		
Short-term	9–23	Stamm, 1991
Long-term	100	Warren, 1982

Data from Nicolle LE, Bradley S, Colgan R, et al.: Infectious Diseases Society of America guidelines for the diagnosis and treatment of asymptomatic bacteriuria in adults. *Clin Infect Dis* 40:643–654, 2005.

some *E. coli* strains are actually commensal strains, whereas others may have initially been virulent but transitioned into commensal strains (Klemm et al., 2007; Zdziarski et al., 2008). In men, gram-negative bacilli, enterococci, and coagulase-negative staphylococci are common pathogens identified in the urine (Lipsky et al., 1984; Mims et al., 1990). The bacterial isolates vary in institutionalized patients or those with indwelling catheters, as compared with community dwellers. In this former population, polymicrobial bacteriuria is frequent; common bacteria found in these populations include *Pseudomonas aeruginosa*, *Morganella morganii*, and *Providencia stuartii* (Nicolle, 1993, Nicolle et al., 2005).

Historically there was concern that untreated asymptomatic bacteriuria may be a risk factor for recurrent UTIs and long-term sequelae such as hypertension, renal insufficiency, or development of urinary tract cancer. However, studies have shown that this is not the case (Bengtsson et al., 1998; Tencer, 1988). **On the contrary, more recent work establishes that treating asymptomatic bacteriuria in all groups is potentially deleterious** (Cai et al., 2012, 2015). Indeed, treatment can lead to an increased risk of subsequent symptomatic UTIs, increased costs associated with treatment of bacteriuria, and potential adverse effects of antibiotics.

To promote a universal approach to the diagnosis and management of asymptomatic bacteriuria in adult populations greater than 18 years old, the **Infectious Disease Society of America (IDSA) published guidelines in 2005 (that are endorsed by the AUA)** (Nicolle et al., 2005). **These guidelines clearly stipulate that, in the majority of patients, asymptomatic bacteriuria should not be treated.** Specifically, it should not be treated in the following populations: premenopausal, non-pregnant women; women with diabetes; older community dwellers; elderly institutionalized patients; patients with SCI; and patients with indwelling catheters. On the contrary, it should always be treated in pregnant women and in patients who are undergoing procedures in which transmucosal bleeding is anticipated. Pyuria, which in isolation often triggers many practitioners to recommend antimicrobial therapy, is not an indication to treat even if it is found in conjunction with asymptomatic bacteriuria. No recommendation was made for whether to treat asymptomatic bacteriuria in renal transplant patients or other immunocompromised hosts (Box 55.8). The IDSA published an update to this guideline in 2019. This update included populations not addressed in the 2005 guideline, specifically children and patients with solid organ transplants or neutropenia (Nicolle et al., 2019).

The **US Preventive Services Task Force (USPSTF) concurred with the IDSA, and in 2008 published a statement urging people not to indiscriminately screen for asymptomatic bacteriuria** (Lin et al., 2008). This task force looked at several different types of studies that included pregnant and non-pregnant women as well as men. The Taskforce concluded that women who are pregnant are the only group who should be screened for asymptomatic bacteriuria.

Likewise, a Cochrane review published in 2015 also concluded that treatment of asymptomatic bacteriuria is not recommended (Zalmanovici Trestioreanu et al., 2015). This review included nine randomized or "quasi" randomized controlled studies, which included a total of 1614 subjects. Studies were not included in this review if they contained any of the following subjects: pregnant women, subjects who either had indwelling catheters or performed CIC, subjects who had indwelling stents or nephrostomy tubes, transplant recipients, subjects who had bacteriuria related to recent urologic procedures, patients with SCI, or hospitalized patients. The review found that symptomatic UTI, complications, and death were similar between the subjects who were treated with antibiotics and those who were not. Although bacteriuria was eradicated more often in those treated, more adverse effects were also noted in this population. No decline in renal function was identified in those not treated.

One of the studies included in the Cochrane review looked at young sexually active women who were seen in a sexually transmitted disease clinic in Italy for recurrent UTIs between 2005 and 2009 (Cai et al., 2012). Subjects were included in the study if they had at least one symptomatic UTI in the 12 months before enrollment and had documented asymptomatic bacteriuria at the onset of the study. The participants were then randomized into two groups: in group A, asymptomatic bacteriuria was observed, whereas in group B, it was treated. At periodic intervals (3, 6, 12 months), their urine samples were analyzed for the presence of bacteriuria. A total of 673 women between the ages of 18 and 40 were studied. The data showed that those in group B had a higher rate of symptomatic UTI over 1 year, as compared with the untreated women in group A. Multivariate analysis showed that antibiotic use was an independent risk factor ($P < 0.001$; hazard ratio, 3.09; 95% CI) for the development of a symptomatic UTI. The majority of subjects who had not had a symptomatic UTI did have asymptomatic *E. faecalis* present in their urine with late follow-up. The investigators concluded that treatment of asymptomatic bacteriuria may remove the protective benefit of an asymptomatic strain.

With extended follow-up of this study population (albeit a smaller total population of 550 subjects because of dropout during extended follow-up), the difference in recurrence rates for symptomatic UTIs was statistically significant ($P < 0.001$) at a mean of 38.8 months (Cai et al., 2015). In group A, 97 (37.7%) subjects recurred, while in group B, 204 (69.6%) recurred. In addition to demonstrating higher recurrence rates in the treated group, the *E. coli* isolated in group B showed higher resistance to several antibiotics, including amoxicillin-clavulanic acid, TMP-SMX, and ciprofloxacin as compared with *E. coli* isolates from group A. The increased resistance rates were not seen until at least 2 years of follow-up. The authors concluded that use of antibiotics in women with asymptomatic bacteriuria and a history of recurrent UTIs must be discouraged. These findings overall further corroborate the IDSA guidelines.

Despite the extensive data available that argue against treating asymptomatic bacteriuria, unfortunately inappropriate antibiotic treatment is still a widespread problem. Ferroni et al. cite several translational barriers to the adoption of IDSA principles among all practitioners; these include a lack of awareness, confusion regarding the guidelines, and continued fear about adverse outcomes associated with not prescribing an antibiotic (Ferroni and Taylor, 2015; James et al., 1998; Wolfe et al., 2004). Indeed a study by Ditkoff et al. (2018) showed that more than 50% of practitioners from a variety of specialties including family practice, internal medicine, gynecology, urology, and emergency medicine were not aware of IDSA guidelines for management of asymptomatic bacteriuria or acute cystitis. Cumulatively, these data suggest that there is more work to be done to normalize the standards of care, because the sequelae of in appropriate antibiotic use remains a growing concern from the standpoint of individual patient care and from a public health perspective.

Further information about this topic is available online at ExpertConsult.com.

The management of asymptomatic bacteriuria before nonurologic surgery is another topic that lacks a universal approach. Perhaps this question has best been studied as it pertains to the management of asymptomatic bacteriuria before joint replacement surgery. Recent data challenge the traditional dogma that asymptomatic bacteriuria should be treated before joint surgery to reduce the risk of developing a septic joint. One multicenter, multinational study by Sousa et al. (2014) specifically looked at the incidence of postoperative joint infections in 2497 patients with and without asymptomatic bacteriuria who underwent knee or hip arthroplasties. A total of 12.1% ($n = 303$) of

---

BOX 55.8 Treat or Not Treat Asymptomatic Bacteriuria

Do Not Treat: premenopausal, non-pregnant women, women with diabetes, older community dwellers, elderly institutionalized patients, patients with spinal cord injury, patients with indwelling catheters, pyuria with asymptomatic bacteriuria

Treat: pregnant women, patients undergoing procedures in which transmucosal bleeding is anticipated

Data from Nicolle LE, Bradley S, Colgan R, et al.: Infectious Diseases Society of America guidelines for the diagnosis and treatment of asymptomatic bacteriuria in adults. *Clin Infect Dis* 40(5):643–654, 2005. Based on ISDA guidelines.

these patients had asymptomatic bacteriuria preoperatively, and 154 patients in this cohort were pretreated before surgery. The postoperative joint infection rate within the entire population was 1.7%. In patients with asymptomatic bacteriuria, the joint infection rate was significantly higher than in the group who were not bacteriuric (4.3% vs. 1.4%; OR 3.23; 95% CI). However, treatment of asymptomatic bacteriuria did not significantly affect the development of postoperative joint infections. In those treated, which was a decision made by the individual physician and was not randomized, the rate of infections was 3.9%, whereas in the untreated group it was 4.7%, which was not a statistically significant difference. Interestingly, although the bacteriuric patients had a higher incidence of gram-negative prosthetic infections, the organism cultured from the urine was not the same as the organism cultured from the joint. The authors concluded that the presence of asymptomatic bacteriuria is a surrogate marker for increased risk of infection overall, but preoperative treatment of the bacteriuria did not modulate the likelihood of remaining infection free in the joint. Therefore **treatment of asymptomatic bacteriuria before orthopedic surgery is not recommended.**

A more recent study by Lamb et al. (2017) concluded that obtaining preoperative urine cultures before joint replacement surgery is not necessary because the presence of asymptomatic bacteriuria does not correlate with the incidence of prosthetic joint infections. They compared the incidence of joint infections during a period when preoperative urine cultures were routinely obtained to the incidence after the adoption of a policy that eliminated urine cultures from preoperative order sets. Although the joint infection rate was no different, the financial impact to the health care system was drastic: without the cost of processing urine cultures the savings were approximately $20,000 per year. This study thus introduces another added consideration, in the form of cost savings, when advocating for restraint in the screening and treatment of asymptomatic bacteriuria.

KEY POINTS: ASYMPTOMATIC BACTERIURIA

- The prevalence of asymptomatic bacteriuria varies with age, sex, and comorbid conditions.
- Untreated asymptomatic bacteriuria is not associated with hypertension or renal insufficiency.
- Several guidelines recommend not screening for or treating asymptomatic bacteriuria except in specific patient populations.
- Asymptomatic bacteriuria should be screened for and treated in pregnant women and in patients who are undergoing urologic procedures in which mucosal bleeding is anticipated.
- Treatment of asymptomatic bacteriuria contributes to development of multidrug-resistant symptomatic UTIs.

PRINCIPLES OF ANTIMICROBIAL THERAPY

Antibiotics have been the mainstay of therapy for UTIs. A decision regarding the antimicrobial selection and the duration of therapy must consider the spectrum of activity of the drug against the known pathogen or the most probable pathogen based on the presumed source of acquisition of infection, whether the infection is judged to be uncomplicated or complicated, potential adverse effects, and cost. The concentration of the antimicrobial agent achieved in blood is not important in treatment of uncomplicated UTIs. However, blood levels are critical in patients with bacteremia and febrile urinary infections consistent with parenchymal involvement of the kidney and prostate.

In patients with renal insufficiency, dosage modifications are necessary for agents that are cleared primarily by the kidneys and cannot be cleared by another mechanism. In renal failure, the kidneys may not be able to concentrate an antimicrobial agent in the urine; therefore difficulty in eradicating bacteria may occur. Urinary tract obstruction may also reduce concentration of antimicrobial agents within the urine.

An often underemphasized but important characteristic is the drug's impact on the bowel and vaginal flora and the hospital bacterial environment. Bacterial susceptibility varies dramatically in patients exposed to antimicrobial agents and in individuals in inpatient and outpatient settings. Each clinician must keep abreast of changes that affect antimicrobial use and susceptibility patterns.

Most important, the decision to initiate antibiotic therapy should not be based on treating a positive urine culture alone; rather clinical presentation, in conjunction with urine testing, should be considered, and we must assess the likelihood that the patient will benefit from or be harmed by antibiosis. As stated by Thomas Hooton in 2012, **"Acute uncomplicated cystitis rarely progresses to severe disease, even if untreated; thus, the primary goal of treatment is to ameliorate symptoms."** In an era when we are witnessing the increasing resistance of bacterial strains as well as managing the sequelae of inappropriate antibiotic use, decisive clinical judgment and antibiotic stewardship are imperative. As Thomas Finucane wrote, **"Clinicians considering intervention should not ask whether the individual has a real 'UTI' but should ask instead whether there is evidence that antibiotic treatment directed at standard bacteriuria is more likely to benefit than harm this individual"** (Finucane, 2017). It is the firm belief of the authors that these considerations should guide management of UTIs in the contemporary era.

Urinary analgesics are an invaluable adjunct to antibiotic management and may not only reduce symptoms but also shorten the course of antibiotics (Finucane, 2017). In fact a randomized trial involving 500 women younger than 65 years of age compared immediate fosfomycin treatment to ibuprofen alone for the treatment of acute cystitis (Gagyor et al., 2015). At 28 days, the fosfomycin group had received 283 total courses of antibiotics as compared with 94 in the ibuprofen group, corresponding to a significant incidence in the reduction of antibiotic use by 66.5%. An effective urinary analgesic may thus be an important advance in curtailing antibiotic use.

Ecologic Impact and Collateral Damage

Collateral damage refers to the ecologic adverse events associated with antibiotics such as bacterial resistance and selection and/or colonization with multidrug-resistant organisms, which have been associated with the use of broad-spectrum cephalosporins and quinolones (Gupta et al., 2011; Paterson, 2004; Ramphal and Ambrose, 2006). **It is particularly important to consider the collateral impact of antibiotics with respect to uncomplicated cystitis, because (1) there is minimal risk of progression to tissue invasion and sepsis, and (2) this problem is one of the most common sources of antibiotic exposure in otherwise healthy populations, thus potentially magnifying the impact of adverse events when they do occur** (Gupta et al., 2001a,b). **In the past several years, the frequency and spectrum of antimicrobial-resistant UTIs have increased in the hospital and community.** The increasing frequency of drug resistance has been attributed to combinations of microbial characteristics, bacterial selection pressure caused by antimicrobial use, and societal and technologic changes that enhance the transmission of drug resistance (Shepherd and Pottinger, 2013). Resistance patterns have been shown to vary by geographic location (Manges et al., 2001).

Bacterial resistance may occur because of intrinsic chromosomal-mediated resistance or by acquired chromosomal- or extrachromosomal (plasmid)-mediated resistance caused by exposure of an organism to antimicrobial agents.

Intrinsic chromosomal resistance exists in a bacterial species because of the absence of the proper mechanism on which the antimicrobial agent can act.

Acquired chromosomal resistance occurs during therapy for UTIs. The bacteria susceptible to the administered antimicrobial agent will be eradicated by therapy, but within 24 to 48 hours a repeat urine culture will show high bacterial counts of some resistant mutants. In essence, the antimicrobial therapy has selected the resistant mutant. This phenomenon is most likely to occur when the antimicrobial level in the urine is close to or below the minimal inhibitory concentration of the drug. **Selection of resistant clones in the course of therapy for a previously sensitive bacteriuric population occurs between 5% and 10% of the time, clearly not an insignificant factor.** Underdosing and noncompliance, as well as diuresis induced by increased fluid intake, can contribute to this process. Therefore, when the decision is made that a patient would benefit from antibiotics, the clinician should select an antimicrobial agent with a urinary concentration that exceeds the minimal inhibitory concentration, avoid underdosing, and emphasize patient compliance.

Extrachromosomal-mediated resistance may be acquired and transferable via plasmids, which contain the genetic material for the resistance. **This mechanism of resistance occurs in the bowel flora and is much more common than selection of preexisting mutants in the urinary tract. All antimicrobial classes are capable of causing plasmid-mediated resistance.** In addition, the plasmids carrying the resistant genetic material are transferable within species and across genera. Thus, for example, a patient receiving tetracycline may harbor several bowel strains that are resistant to tetracycline, ampicillin, sulfonamides, and TMP. Because the bowel flora is the major reservoir for bacteria that ultimately colonize the urinary tract, infections that occur after antimicrobial therapy and that can cause plasmid-mediated resistance are commonly caused by organisms with multidrug resistance.

Several bacteria have evolved to develop specific resistance genes to different classes of antibiotics. In 1983 the first report of plasmid-mediated β-lactamases capable of hydrolyzing extended-spectrum cephalosporins was made. They have since been characterized as extended-spectrum β-lactamases (ESBLs) and confer resistance to most β-lactam antibiotics, including third-generation cephalosporins; also, ESBL *E. coli* can have co-resistance to other classes of antibiotics, including fluoroquinolones and aminoglycosides (Pitout and Laupland, 2008; Prakash et al., 2009). In a similar vein, AmpC β-lactamases are cephalosporinases encoded on chromosomes of many Enterobacteriaceae and a few other organisms that confer resistance to broad-spectrum cephalosporins; transmissible plasmids with the AmpC enzyme genes can now appear in bacteria such as *E. coli* that had poor chromosomal expression of this gene (Jacoby, 2009). In 2001 the first *K. pneumoniae* carbapenemase (KPC)–producing bacteria, a group of highly drug-resistant gram-negative bacilli, was isolated. It has since become the most prevalent mechanism of carbapenem resistance in the United States at the time of this writing (Lee et al., 2009). Although *K. pneumoniae* remains the most relevant bacterial species carrying KPCs, the enzyme has been identified in other gram-negative bacilli (Kitchel et al., 2009).

Antimicrobial resistance is influenced by the duration and amount of antimicrobial agent used. For example, documented increased use of fluoroquinolones in the hospital setting has been directly associated with increased resistance of bacteria (particularly *Pseudomonas* spp.) to the fluoroquinolones. Resistance tends to increase the longer the agent is used. Conversely, reduction in duration of therapy and in the amount of the drug used may lead to reemergence of more susceptible strains.

The inappropriate and excessive use of fluoroquinolones for UTIs and other infections has contributed to the growing problem of quinolone resistance among uropathogens (Chen et al., 2012). According to the European Center for Disease Prevention and Control 2015 report, fluroquinolone resistance was noted among 22.8% of *E. coli* strains and 29.7% *K. pneumoniae* isolates (European Centre for Disease Prevention and Control, 2017.)

In institutionalized settings, such as intensive care units or nursing homes, extended-spectrum β-lactamase–producing *E. coli* and *K. pneumoniae* isolates have a reported 40% to 45% resistance rate to quinolones (Itokazu, et al., 1996; Wiener et al., 1999). Furthermore, specific to a transplant unit, where fluoroquinolones are commonly administered prophylactically, *E. coli* resistance can be up to 80%. **Previous use of fluoroquinolones and the presence of underlying urologic diseases were the strongest determinants for UTIs caused by resistant strains** (Ena et al., 1995). **Last, fluoroquinolone resistance is associated with more frequent multidrug-resistant bacterial strains** and may thus serve as a harbinger of increased individual risk of resistance to first-line antibiotics (Karlowsky et al., 2006).

In fact, many of the adverse events related to antibiotics are also related to a perturbation in commensal microbiomes, such as in the gut and vagina (MacDonald et al., 1993; Vollaard and Clasener, 1994). Antibiotic-related disruption to the intestinal microbiota has been associated with the development of *Clostridium difficile* and colonization with vancomycin-resistant bacteria (Khoruts et al., 2010; Ubeda et al., 2010). Studies in animal models have demonstrated that changes to the intestinal flora after antibiotics can then result in an increased susceptibility to subsequent enteric infection (Sekirov et al., 2008). As far as the implications for the vaginal microbiome, there is a clear association between the risk for vaginal candidiasis and previous treatment with antibiotics (MacDonald et al., 1993). The likelihood of vaginal candidiasis appears directly related to the duration of antibacterial use, particularly with broad-spectrum agents, as well as those who have had repeated episodes of *Candida* infection (Spinillo et al., 1999). Narrowing the spectrum of antibiotic choice and limiting treatment course, particularly in cases of uncomplicated UTIs, are thus instrumental measures in mitigating the systemic implications of treatment.

Antimicrobial Formulary

The mechanism of action, reliable coverage, and common adverse reactions, precautions, and contraindications for antimicrobial agents used in the treatment of UTIs are indicated in Tables 55.4 through 55.7. Bactericidal antibiotics refer to those that cause irreversible death of bacteria, whereas bacteriostatic agents inhibit bacterial replication without killing the organisms (i.e., reversible stoppage).

Nitrofurantoin

Nitrofurantoin is effective against most common uropathogens. It is rapidly excreted from the urine but does not obtain therapeutic levels in most body tissues, including the gastrointestinal (GI) tract. Therefore it is not useful for upper tract, complicated infections, or blood-borne infections (Wilhelm and Edson, 1987). **It has minimal effects on the resident bowel and vaginal flora.** Acquired bacterial resistance to this drug is exceedingly low. Nitrofurantoin can cause GI upset and rare pulmonary issues, such as pulmonary fibrosis, when used chronically. Nitrofurantoin should also be avoided in patients with suspicion of or known glucose-6-phosphate dehydrogenase (G6PD) deficiency because it can lead to hemolytic anemia. It had always been recommended that nitrofurantoin be avoided in patients with chronic renal insufficiency, defined as a CrCl less than 60 mL/min, because of lack of efficacy from poor renal concentrating ability. However, in the 2015 American Geriatric Society Beers Criteria, this threshold was reduced to 30 mL/min because of new data regarding its effectiveness in certain populations with renal impairment. Despite this revision, it remains prudent to use nitrofurantoin with caution in patients with significant renal impairment, particularly for long courses. In fact, Geerts, et al. (2013) found that in a cohort of 21,317 women treated with 3 to 10 days of nitrofurantoin for UTI, renal impairment (defined as CrCl 30–50 mL/min) was not significantly associated with treatment ineffectiveness; nevertheless, a significant association was noted

TABLE 55.4 Bacteriostatic Versus Bactericidal Agents

BACTERIOSTATIC	BACTERICIDIAL
Chloramphenicol	Aminoglycosides
Clindamycin	Quinolones
Macrolides (e.g., azithromycin, erythromycin)	β-lactams
Sulfonamides	Vancomycin
Tetracycline	
Trimethoprim	

Nitrofurantoin is generally bacteriostatic, but it can be bactericidal in high doses and against certain organisms.

TABLE 55.5 Mechanism of Action of Common Antimicrobials Used in the Treatment of Urinary Tract Infections

DRUG OR DRUG CLASS	MECHANISM OF ACTION	MECHANISMS OF DRUG RESISTANCE
β-Lactams (penicillins, cephalosporins, aztreonam)	Inhibition of bacterial cell wall synthesis	Production of β-lactamase Alteration in binding site of penicillin-binding protein Changes in cell wall porin size (decreased penetration)
Aminoglycosides	Inhibition of ribosomal protein synthesis	Downregulation of drug uptake into bacteria Bacterial production of aminoglycoside-modifying enzymes
Quinolones	Inhibition of bacterial DNA gyrase	Mutation in DNA gyrase-binding site Changes in cell wall porin size (decreased penetration) Active efflux
Fosfomycin	Inhibition of bacterial cell wall synthesis	Novel amino acid substitutions or the loss of function of transporters
Nitrofurantoin	Inhibition of several bacterial enzyme systems	Not fully elucidated—develops slowly with prolonged exposure
Trimethoprim-sulfamethoxazole	Antagonism of bacterial folate metabolism	Draws folate from environment (enterococci)
Vancomycin	Inhibition of bacterial cell wall synthesis (at β-lactams)	Enzymatic alteration of peptidoglycan at different point than target

TABLE 55.6 Reliable Coverage of Antimicrobials Used in the Treatment of Urinary Tract Infections of Commonly Encountered Pathogens[a]

ANTIMICROBIAL AGENT OR CLASS	GRAM-POSITIVE PATHOGENS	GRAM-NEGATIVE PATHOGENS
Amoxicillin or ampicillin	*Streptococcus* Enterococci	*Proteus mirabilis*
Amoxicillin with clavulanate	*Streptococcus* Enterococci	*P. mirabilis* *Klebsiella* species
Ampicillin with sulbactam	*Staphylococcus* (not MRSA) Enterococci	*P. mirabilis* *Haemophilus influenzae, Klebsiella* species
Antistaphylococcal penicillins	*Streptococcus* *Staphylococcus* (not MRSA)	None
Antipseudomonal penicillins	*Streptococcus* Enterococci	Most, including *Pseudomonas aeruginosa*
First-generation cephalosporins	*Streptococcus* *Staphylococcus* (not MRSA)	*Escherichia coli* *P. mirabilis* *Klebsiella* species
Second-generation cephalosporins (cefamandole, cefuroxime, cefaclor)	*Streptococcus* *Staphylococcus* (not MRSA)	*E. coli, P. mirabilis* *H. influenzae, Klebsiella* species
Second-generation cephalosporins (cefoxitin, cefotetan)	*Streptococcus*	*E. coli, Proteus* species (including indole-positive) *H. influenzae, Klebsiella* species
Third-generation cephalosporins (ceftriaxone)	*Streptococcus* *Staphylococcus* (not MRSA)	Most, excluding *P. aeruginosa*
Third-generation cephalosporins (ceftazidime)	*Streptococcus*	Most, including *P. aeruginosa*
Aztreonam	None	Most, including *P. aeruginosa*
Aminoglycosides	*Staphylococcus* (urine)	Most, including *P. aeruginosa*
Fluoroquinolones	*Streptococcus*[a]	Most, including *P. aeruginosa*
Nitrofurantoin	*Staphylococcus* (not MRSA) Enterococci	Many Enterobacteriaceae (not *Providencia, Serratia, Acinetobacter*) *Klebsiella* species
Fosfomycin	Enterococci	Most Enterobacteriaceae (not *P. aeruginosa*)
Pivmecillinam	None	Most, excluding *P. aeruginosa*
Trimethoprim-sulfamethoxazole	*Streptococcus* *Staphylococcus*	Most Enterobacteriaceae (not *P. aeruginosa*)
Vancomycin	All, including MRSA	None

[a]Depends on the antimicrobial agent.
MRSA, Methicillin-resistant *Staphylococcus aureus*.

TABLE 55.7 Common Adverse Reactions, Precautions, and Contraindications for Antimicrobial Agents Used in Treatment of Urinary Tract Infection

DRUG OR DRUG CLASS	COMMON ADVERSE REACTIONS	PRECAUTIONS AND CONTRAINDICATIONS
Amoxicillin or ampicillin	Hypersensitivity (immediate or delayed) Diarrhea (especially with ampicillin), GI upset AAPMC Maculopapular rash (not hypersensitivity) Decreased platelet aggregation	Increased risk of rash with concomitant viral disease, allopurinol therapy
Amoxicillin with clavulanic acid	Increased diarrhea, GI upset with amoxicillin/clavulanic acid	
Ampicillin with sulbactam	Same as with amoxicillin/ampicillin	
Antistaphylococcal penicillins	Same as with amoxicillin/ampicillin GI upset (with oral agents) Acute interstitial nephritis (especially with methicillin)	
Antipseudomonal penicillins	Same as with amoxicillin/ampicillin Hypernatremia (these drugs are given as sodium salt; especially carbenicillin, ticarcillin) Local injection site reactions	Use with caution in patients very sensitive to sodium loading.
Cephalosporins	Hypersensitivity (less than with penicillins) GI upset (with oral agents) Local injection site reactions AAPMC Positive Coombs test Decreased platelet aggregation (especially with cefotetan, cefamandole, cefoperazone)	Should not be used in patients with immediate hypersensitivity to penicillins; may use with caution in patients with delayed hypersensitivity reactions
Aztreonam	Hypersensitivity (less than with penicillins)	Less than 1% incidence of cross-reactivity in penicillin- or cephalosporin-allergic patients; may be used with caution in these patients
Aminoglycosides	Ototoxicity: vestibular and auditory components Nephrotoxicity: nonoliguric azotemia Neuromuscular blockade with high levels	Avoid in pregnant patients, except in pyelonephritis. Avoid if possible in patients with severely impaired renal function, diabetes, or hepatic failure. Use with caution in myasthenia gravis patients (because of potential for neuromuscular blockade). Use with caution with other potentially ototoxic and nephrotoxic drugs.
Fluoroquinolones	Mild GI effects; dizziness, lightheadedness; photosensitivity Central nervous system effects, including dizziness, tremors, confusion, mood disorder, hallucinations Tendon rupture	Avoid in children or pregnant patients because of arthropathic effects. Concomitant antacid, iron, zinc, or sucralfate use dramatically decreases oral absorption; use another antimicrobial agent or discontinue sucralfate use while taking quinolones. Space administration of quinolones from antacids, iron, or zinc products by at least 2 h to ensure adequate absorption. Ensure adequate patient hydration. These agents can significantly increase theophylline plasma levels (ciprofloxacin and enoxacin seem to have a greater effect than norfloxacin or ofloxacin); avoid quinolones or monitor theophylline levels closely. These agents can lower seizure threshold; avoid in patients with epilepsy and in patients with other risk factors (medications or illness) that may lower the seizure threshold. Monitor glucose levels in patients taking antidiabetic agents because hypoglycemia and hyperglycemia have been reported in patients treated concurrently with fluoroquinolones and antidiabetic agents. These agents can enhance warfarin effects; closely monitor coagulation tests.

TABLE 55.7 Common Adverse Reactions, Precautions, and Contraindications for Antimicrobial Agents Used in Treatment of Urinary Tract Infection—cont'd

DRUG OR DRUG CLASS	COMMON ADVERSE REACTIONS	PRECAUTIONS AND CONTRAINDICATIONS
Fosfomycin	Headache GI upset Vaginitis	Hypersensitivity to fosfomycin or any component of the formulation
Pivmecillinam	Rash GI upset	Use with caution in patients with penicillin hypersensitivity.
Nitrofurantoin	GI upset Peripheral polyneuropathy (especially in patients with impaired renal function, anemia, diabetes, electrolyte imbalance, vitamin B deficiency, and debilitated) Hemolysis in patients with G6PD deficiency Pulmonary hypersensitivity reactions can range from acute to chronic and include cough, dyspnea, fever, and interstitial changes.	Do not use in patients with low creatinine clearance (<50 mL/min) because adequate urine concentrations will not be achieved. Monitor long-term patients closely. Avoid concomitant probenecid use, which blocks renal excretion of nitrofurantoin. Avoid concomitant magnesium or quinolones, which are antagonistic to nitrofurantoin.
Trimethoprim-sulfamethoxazole	Hypersensitivity, rash GI upset Photosensitivity Hematologic toxicity (AIDS patients)	Higher incidence of all adverse reactions occurs in AIDS patients and in the elderly. Avoid in pregnant patients. Avoid in patients receiving warfarin; concomitant use can significantly elevate prothrombin time.
Vancomycin	"Red-man syndrome": flushing, fever, chills, rash, hypotension (histaminic effect) Nephrotoxicity and/or ototoxicity when combined with other nephrotoxic and/or ototoxic drugs Local injection site reactions	Use with caution with other potentially ototoxic and nephrotoxic drugs.

AAPMC, Antimicrobial-associated pseudomembranous colitis; *AIDS*, acquired immunodeficiency syndrome; *GI*, gastrointestinal; *G6PD*, glucose-6-phosphate dehydrogenase.
Data from McEvoy GK, editor: *American Hospital Formulary Service drug information*, Bethesda, MD, 1995, American Society of Health-System Pharmacists.

between renal impairment (CrCl < 50 mL/min) and pulmonary adverse events leading to hospitalization.

The Beers Criteria strongly recommend against the *long-term* use of nitrofurantoin for the purposes of antibiotic suppression, founded on the potential adverse events described earlier; nevertheless, **there is no specific recommendation against the *short-term* use of these agents within a carefully selected geriatric population, specifically those with normal renal function.** It is the authors' shared opinion that this agent can still remain a first-line treatment option for the acute management of uncomplicated cystitis within select elderly populations, although the categorical recommendation against long-term usage has created insurance coverage barriers to prescribing nitrofurantoin even for limited courses in these patients.

Trimethoprim-Sulfamethoxazole

The combination of TMP-SMX has been one of the most widely used antimicrobial agents for the treatment of acute UTIs. TMP-SMX attains therapeutic levels in most tissues and is effective against most common uropathogens, with the notable exception of *Enterococcus* and *Pseudomonas* spp. TMP-SMX is inexpensive and has minimal adverse effects on the bowel flora. Disadvantages are relatively common adverse effects, consisting primarily of rashes and GI complaints (Cockerill and Edson, 1991). Stevens-Johnson syndrome and toxic epidermal necrolysis are rare and potentially life-threatening, blistering skin reactions that have been associated with TMP-SMX. In fact, one contemporary Canadian retrospective review analyzing the inciting agent for the 64 documented cases seen at their regional hospital between 2001 and 2011 identified TMP-SMX as the antibiotic most often associated with this reaction; it was implicated in 4 of the 64 patients reviewed (6%) (Miliszewski et al., 2016).

Fosfomycin

Fosfomycin, an oral bactericidal antimicrobial agent similar to phosphonic acid in chemical structure, is active against most uropathogens. Its major benefit is its limited cross-resistance between most other common antibacterial agents, as well as its efficacy against the majority of gram-negative organisms and vancomycin-resistant *Enterococcus* (VRE). Further, it has been shown to be effective as a single-dose agent when used as an empirical treatment for uncomplicated cystitis. It is an excellent oral option for MDR bacteria that would otherwise necessitate treatment with intravenous antibiotics. It is generally well tolerated with low incidences of GI upset and headache and very rare adverse events seen in multiple trials (Patel et al., 1997). Fosfomycin should not be used in the setting of urosepsis/blood-borne infections. Currently, in the United States a 3-g sachet of fosfomycin costs $70 to $90 or more, depending on the insurance coverage; this expense may preclude its use in some patients.

Fluoroquinolones

Fluoroquinolones share a common predecessor in nalidixic acid and inhibit DNA gyrase, a bacterial enzyme integral to replication. The fluoroquinolones have a broad spectrum of activity that makes them ideal for the empirical treatment of UTIs. **They are effective against Enterobacteriaceae and *P. aeruginosa*. Activity is also high against *S. aureus* and *S. saprophyticus*, but, in general, antistreptococcal coverage is marginal.** Most anaerobic bacteria are resistant to these drugs; therefore the normal vaginal and bowel flora are not altered (Wright et al., 1993). **Bacterial resistance initially appeared to be uncommon but has increased because of indiscriminate use of these agents** (Vromen et al., 1999; Wright et al., 1993).

These drugs are not nephrotoxic, but renal insufficiency prolongs the serum half-life, requiring adjusted dosing in patients with creatinine clearances of less than 30 mL/min. Among the adverse reactions reported for fluoroquinolones, GI disturbances are the most common, and this is likely related to the collateral damage to commensal microbiota in the gut (Stewardson et al., 2015). Hypersensitivity, skin reactions, central and peripheral nervous system reactions, and even acute renal failure have been reported (Hootkins et al., 1989). In addition, serious central nervous system side effects, anxiety/depression, hallucinations, confusion, and suicidal thoughts have been cited (FDA Drug Safety Communication, 2016).

In 2008 the US Food and Drug Administration (FDA) announced a black box warning of tendon ruptures associated with fluoroquinolones. In 2013 it added a risk of irreversible nerve damage to the warning. In 2015 the FDA acknowledged the existence of fluoroquinolone-associated disability (FQAD) in 178 patients, with chronic pain reported as the most common symptom. Although it does not affect the majority of patients, FQAD may be "underappreciated" (Tennyson and Averch, 2017). Some have speculated that mitochondrial damage is responsible for the serious adverse effects, but there is no consensus about this theory (Marchant, 2018).

Achilles tendon disorders, including rupture, have been estimated to occur in 20 cases per 100,000 and therefore fluoroquinolone use should be discontinued at the first sign of tendon pain (Greene, 2002). Drug-induced tendinopathy is listed as a class effect of fluoroquinolones; indeed, there is a 3.8-fold increased risk of Achilles tendinopathy compared with use of other antibiotics (Chhajed et al., 2002). A recent study determined that factors that contribute to an increased risk of sustaining an Achilles tendon disorder while taking a fluoroquinolone include advanced age, chronic renal failure, male gender, normal body mass index (BMI), and concurrent use of corticosteroids (Godoy-Santos et al., 2018). The mechanism of tendon rupture is unclear, but ciprofloxacin stimulates matrix-degrading protease activity from fibroblasts and exerts an inhibitory effect on fibroblast metabolism and synthesis of matrix ground substance, factors that may contribute to tendinopathy (Williams, et al., 2000). Other soft tissue and peripheral nervous system side effects reported with fluoroquinolones include paresthesias, myalgias, and arthralgias (2016). Administration of the fluoroquinolones to immature animals has caused damage to the developing cartilage; therefore they are currently contraindicated in children, adolescents, and pregnant or nursing women (Christ et al., 1988). More research is needed to better characterize side effects associated with fluoroquinolone usage and understand why certain people are susceptible to these adverse results (Marchant, 2018).

Because of the disabling and potentially irreversible side effects of these drugs on soft tissue and the nervous system, in 2016 the FDA revised the boxed warning on these products to reflect the fact these agents should be prescribed sparingly. According to this warning, "fluoroquinolones should be reserved for use in patients who have no other treatment options for...uncomplicated urinary tract infections because the risk of these serious side effects generally outweighs the benefits in these patients." A new FDA warning issued in 2018 warns against the development of mental health side effects, specifically agitation, disorientation, delirium, memory impairment, nervousness, and problems with attention. In addition, the FDA expressed concerns about blood sugar disturbances associated with fluoroquinolone use (FDA, 2018b). Later in 2018 the FDA issued a warning about an increased risk of aortic dissection associated with fluoroquinolone use (FDA, 2018a).

There are important drug interactions associated with the fluoroquinolones. The World Health Organization (WHO) warns of rare increases in the anticoagulant effects of Coumadin when taken with fluoroquinolones. Antacids containing magnesium or aluminum interfere with absorption of fluoroquinolones (Davies et al., 1972). Certain fluoroquinolones (enoxacin and ciprofloxacin) elevate plasma levels of theophylline and prolong its half-life (Wright et al., 1993).

Cephalosporins

Three generations of cephalosporins have been used for the treatment of acute UTIs (Wilhelm and Edson, 1987). In general, as a group, activity is high against Enterobacteriaceae and poor against enterococci. First-generation cephalosporins have greater activity against gram-positive organisms, as well as common uropathogens such as *E. coli* and *K. pneumoniae*, whereas second-generation cephalosporins have activity against anaerobes. Third-generation cephalosporins are more reliably active against community-acquired and nosocomial gram-negative organisms than other β-lactam antimicrobials. First-generation cephalosporins such as cephalexin can be prescribed in doses that range from 500 mg twice daily to three or four times daily for 3 to 7 days for uncomplicated cystitis; dosing is highly variable depending on the source. Fourth- and fifth-generation cephalosporins can be used for complicated UTIs.

Aminopenicillins

Ampicillin and amoxicillin have been used often in the past for the treatment of UTIs, but the emergence of resistance in 40% to 60% of common urinary isolates has lessened the usefulness of these drugs (Gupta et al., 2011; Hooton and Stamm, 1991). The effects of these agents on the normal bowel and vaginal flora can predispose patients to reinfection with resistant strains and often lead to candidal vaginitis (Iravani, 1991). The addition of the β-lactamase inhibitor clavulanate to amoxicillin greatly improves activity against β-lactamase–producing bacteria resistant to amoxicillin alone. However, its high cost and frequent GI side effects limit its usefulness. The extended-spectrum penicillin derivatives (e.g., pivmecillinam, piperacillin, mezlocillin, azlocillin) retain ampicillin's activity against enterococci and offer activity against many ampicillin-resistant gram-negative bacilli. **This makes them attractive agents for use in patients with nosocomially acquired UTIs and as the initial parenteral treatment of acute uncomplicated pyelonephritis acquired outside of the hospital, although less-expensive agents are equally effective.**

Aminoglycosides

When combined with TMP-SMX or ampicillin, aminoglycosides are the first drugs of choice for febrile UTIs. Their nephrotoxicity and ototoxicity are well recognized; therefore careful monitoring of patients for renal and auditory impairment associated with infection is indicated. Once-daily aminoglycoside regimens have been instituted to maximize bacterial killing by optimizing the peak concentration-to-minimal inhibitory concentration ratio and reduce the potential for toxicity (Fig. 55.11; Nicolau et al., 1995). Administering an aminoglycoside as a single daily dose can take advantage not only of its concentration-dependent killing ability but also of two other important characteristics: time-dependent toxicity and a more prolonged postantimicrobial effect (Gilbert, 1991; Zhanel et al., 1991a,b). The regimen consists of a fixed 5 to 7-mg/kg dose of gentamicin or 5 to 7 mg/kg tobramycin. Subsequent interval adjustments are made by using a single concentration in serum and a nomogram designed for monitoring of once-daily therapy (Fig. 55.12). Antimicrobial doses are given at the interval determined by the drug concentration of a sample obtained after the start of the initial infusion. For example, if the serum concentration was 7 mg/mL 10 hours after the start of the infusion, subsequent 7-mg/kg doses would be given every 36 hours. This regimen is clinically effective, reduces the incidence of nephrotoxicity, and provides a cost-effective method for administering aminoglycosides by reducing ancillary service times and serum aminoglycoside determinations.

Aztreonam

Aztreonam has a similar spectrum of activity as the aminoglycosides, and as with all β-lactams, it is not nephrotoxic. However, its spectrum

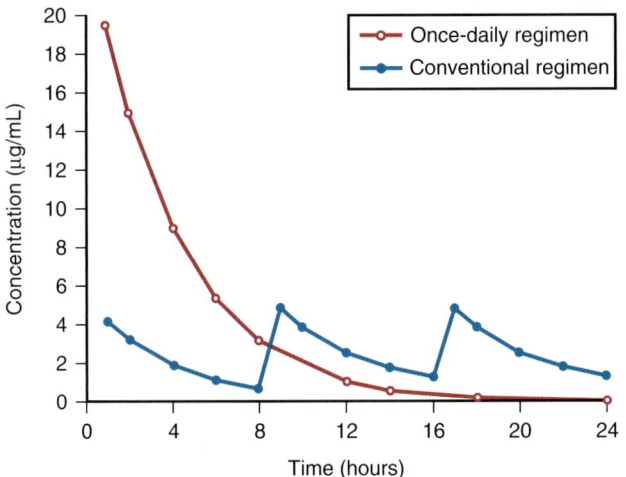

Fig. 55.11. Simulated concentration-versus-time profile of once-daily (7 mg/kg/24 h) and conventional (1.5 mg/kg/8 h) regimens for patients with normal renal function. (From Nicolau DP, Freeman CD, Belliveau PP, et al.: Experience with a once-daily aminoglycoside program administered to 2,184 adult patients. *Antimicrob Agents Chemother* 39:650–655, 1995.)

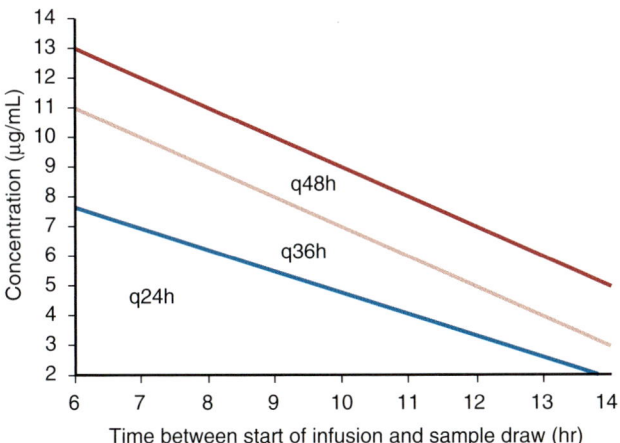

Fig. 55.12. Once-daily aminoglycoside nomogram for gentamicin and tobramycin at 7 mg/kg. (From Nicolau DP, Freeman CD, Belliveau PP, et al.: Experience with a once-daily aminoglycoside program administered to 2,184 adult patients. *Antimicrob Agents Chemother* 39:650–655, 1995.)

of activity is less broad than the third-generation cephalosporins. **It should be used primarily in patients who have penicillin allergies.**

Pivmecillinam

Pivmecillinam is a penicillin-like β-lactam antibiotic that is the prodrug of mecillinam. It has high activity against gram-negative organisms and is primarily used in Nordic countries for empirical treatment of uncomplicated cystitis. **It is not currently available in the United States,** but it has been shown to have low resistance patterns (roughly 2% of *E. coli*) as well as being safe and effective (Grainger et al., 1982).

Choice of Antimicrobial Agents

Many antimicrobial agents have been shown to be effective in the treatment of UTIs. **Factors important in aiding selection of empirical therapy include whether the infection is complicated or uncomplicated; the spectrum of activity of the drug against the probable pathogen; a history of hypersensitivity; potential side effects, including renal and hepatic toxicity; the ecologic impact of antibiotic choice; and cost.** The bacterial susceptibility and cost of the drug vary dramatically among inpatient and outpatient settings throughout the country. Therefore it is imperative that each clinician keep abreast of changes in bacterial susceptibility via regional antibiograms as well as cost patterns and use current information when choosing antimicrobial agents.

As mentioned earlier, antibiotic-related disruption to the intestinal microbiota can result in GI side effects, specifically diarrhea. *C. difficile* infections (CDIs) are particularly concerning. In recent years CDIs have become more common and more resistant to treatment. In 2011 453,000 CDIs were diagnosed, resulting in 29,000 deaths in the United States (Lessa et al., 2015). Antibiotics most likely to cause CDI include cephalosporins, clindamycin, carbapenems, trimethoprim/sulfamethoxazole, fluoroquinolones, and penicillin combinations. Macrolides, tetracyclines, and aminoglycosides are not associated with CDI (Slimings, 2014). The diagnosis of CDI requires the presence of diarrhea (diagnosed as greater than or equal to 3 unformed stools in 24 hours) or radiologic evidence of ileus or toxic megacolon and a stool test that is positive for toxigenic *C. difficile* or its toxins or histopathologic or colonoscopic evidence of pseudomembranous colitis. Treatment of CDI should be guided by the severity of illness and the risk of recurrence or complications. Metronidazole and vancomycin are the treatment of choice for CDI; recent data reveal higher treatment failure rates associated with metronidazole with increasing disease severity. Thus, with more mild cases metronidazole is the preferred treatment of choice, whereas with more severe cases vancomycin is recommended (Bagdasarian et al., 2015).

Duration of Therapy

The duration of therapy needed to cure a UTI appears to be related to a number of variables, including the extent and duration of tissue invasion, the bacterial concentration in urine, the achievable urine concentration of the antimicrobial agent, and risk factors (see later) that impair the host and natural defense mechanisms.

> **KEY POINTS: PRINCIPLES OF ANTIMICROBIAL THERAPY**
>
> - Antimicrobial resistance is increasing because of excessive use.
> - Antimicrobial selection should be influenced by efficacy, safety, cost, and compliance.
> - The choice of the agent as well as the duration of therapy are critical in preventing the perpetuation of antimicrobial resistance as well as adverse events related to treatment.

BLADDER INFECTIONS

Uncomplicated Cystitis

The overwhelming majority of infections encountered in urology are acute uncomplicated cystitis. Often these infections are treated by practitioners other than urologists. **Most cases of uncomplicated cystitis occur in women. Each year, approximately 10% of women report having had a UTI, and more than 50% of all women have at least one such infection in their lifetime** (Foxman et al., 2000). Uncomplicated cystitis occasionally occurs in prepubertal girls, but it increases greatly in incidence in late adolescence and during the second and fourth decades of life. Twenty-five to 30 percent of women 20 to 40 years of age have a history of UTIs (Kunin, 1961). **Although it is much less common, young men may also experience acute cystitis without underlying structural or functional abnormalities of the urinary tract** (Krieger et al., 1993). Risk factors (Box 55.9) include sexual intercourse and use of spermicides (Foxman, 2002; Handley et al., 2002; Hooton et al., 1996). Sexual transmission of uropathogens has been suggested by demonstrating identical *E. coli* in the bowel and urinary flora of sex partners (Johnson and Stamm, 1989).

> **BOX 55.9** Risk Factors for Urinary Tract Infections
>
> **REDUCED URINE FLOW**
> Outflow obstruction, prostatic hyperplasia, prostatic carcinoma, urethral stricture, foreign body (calculus)
> Neurogenic bladder
> Inadequate fluid uptake (dehydration)
>
> **PROMOTE COLONIZATION**
> Sexual activity—increased inoculation
> Spermicide—increased binding
> Estrogen depletion—increased binding
> Antimicrobial agents—decreased indigenous flora
>
> **FACILITATE ASCENT**
> Catheterization
> Urinary incontinence
> Fecal incontinence
> Residual urine with ischemia of bladder wall

E. coli is the causative organism in 75% to 90% of cases of acute cystitis in young women (Latham et al., 1985; Ronald, 2002). *S. saprophyticus*, a commensal organism of the skin, is the second most common cause of acute cystitis in young women, accounting for 10% to 20% of these infections (Jordan et al., 1980). Other organisms less commonly involved include *Klebsiella*, *Proteus*, and *Enterococcus* spp. In men, *E. coli* and other Enterobacteriaceae are the most commonly identified organisms.

Clinical Presentation

The validated UTI Symptom Assessment questionnaire includes seven symptoms that are most likely reported in association with a UTI: frequency, urgency, painful urination, incomplete emptying, suprapubic pain/pressure, low back pain, and hematuria. In addition to identifying the presence or absence of individual patient-reported symptoms, the degree of severity and bother are also assessed with this questionnaire (Clayson et al., 2005). Cystitis is a superficial infection of the bladder mucosa, so fever, chills, and other signs of dissemination are usually not present.

Although many patients complain of foul-smelling or cloudy urine when requesting treatment for a UTI, studies have not identified these symptoms as reliable indicators of the presence of a UTI, particularly in the absence of specific urinary symptoms. If patients have one or both of these symptoms, yet none of the earlier-mentioned classic symptoms, they should be encouraged to hydrate vigorously and then reassess.

Studies suggest that having more than one symptom raises the likelihood of being diagnosed with a UTI. However, dysuria alone is the most reliable indicator of UTI; when present it contributes to higher severity and bother scores compared with other typical UTI symptoms (Dune et al., 2017). Diagnosis of a UTI can be challenging because many patients complain of symptoms such as frequency, urgency, or incontinence at baseline associated with other lower urinary tract pathology. Thus, when critically evaluating a patient with symptoms suggestive of UTI, clinicians must establish whether the symptoms are different from their baseline voiding dysfunction symptoms. In addition, patients often complain of "burning," which may be burning associated with urination (dysuria), or burning in the vaginal or pelvic area that is present irrespective of voiding. If patients complain of "burning," it is important to have them articulate their complaint beyond just "burning."

A review of nine studies (published between 1965 and 2001) investigating the accuracy of history and physical examination in properly detecting acute uncomplicated UTI determined that **in the absence of vaginal discharge or irritation, the combination of symptoms of dysuria and frequency can predict the presence of a UTI in more than 90%. Overall, the probability of having a UTI is increased when a patient experiences frequency, dysuria, hematuria, and back pain, along with demonstrating CVAT on exam** (Bent et al., 2002).

Similarly, a recent meta-analysis compiled 16 studies encompassing 3711 patients in an effort to ascertain the diagnostic accuracy of individual symptoms by correlating them to urine culture results. In this investigation, the presence of frequency, dysuria, hematuria, nocturia, and urgency increased the probability of having a UTI, whereas the presence of vaginal discharge decreased the likelihood of having a UTI. When hematuria was associated with nitrites on a dipstick, the probability of having a UTI was at least 90% (Giesen et al., 2010).

Overall, acute onset of dysuria and acute change in baseline voiding symptoms are most consistent with a diagnosis of acute uncomplicated cystitis.

Laboratory Diagnosis

See prior discussion of urine testing in the evaluation section.

Management

Antimicrobial Selection. Oral antimicrobial agents for treatment of acute uncomplicated cystitis are outlined in Fig. 55.13. The recommendations set forth for the management of uncomplicated cystitis in women, described herein, are based on the IDSA and European Society of Microbiology and Infectious Diseases guidelines statement (Gupta et al., 2011). In general, these treatment algorithms should inform management, and the ultimate choice of agent should be individualized based on allergy status, projected compliance, local antibiograms/practice patterns, availability, and cost.

Nitrofurantoin has maintained an excellent level of activity over 4 decades and is well tolerated. Nitrofurantoin (100 mg twice daily for 5 days) is an appropriate choice for first-line therapy because of minimal resistance and propensity for ecologic adverse side effects; its efficacy is comparable with 3 days of TMP-SMX.

TMP and TMP-SMX (DS twice daily for 3 days) are effective and inexpensive agents for empirical therapy, resulting in bacteriologic cure (i.e., eradication of the pathogen from the urine) within 7 days after the start of treatment in approximately 94% of women (Warren et al., 1999). **They are recommended in areas where the prevalence of resistance to these drugs among *E. coli* strains causing cystitis is less than 20%** (Gupta et al., 2011). When used alone, TMP is as efficacious as TMP-SMX and is associated with fewer side effects, presumably because of the absence of the sulfa component (Harbord and Gruneberg, 1981). It can be prescribed to patients who are allergic to sulfa. However, TMP can cause hypersensitivity and rashes that may be erroneously attributed to sulfa (Alonso et al., 1992).

Fosfomycin trometamol (3 g in a single dose) is an appropriate choice for therapy where it is available because of minimal resistance and propensity for collateral damage, but it may have inferior efficacy compared with standard short-course regimens according to data submitted to the FDA and summarized in the Medical Letter (1997; Gupta et al., 2011).

Pivmecillinam (400 mg twice daily for 3 to 7 days) is an appropriate choice for therapy in regions where it is available (availability limited to some European countries; not licensed and/or available for use in North America) because of minimal resistance and propensity for collateral damage, but it may have inferior efficacy compared with other available therapies (A-I; Gupta et al., 2011).

The **fluoroquinolones** have been used in the management of uncomplicated cystitis in the past, and they are effective in 3-day regimens (Gupta et al., 2011). **They have a high propensity for collateral damage (i.e., ecological adverse effects, such as drug resistance) and should be reserved as antimicrobials of last resort for acute cystitis; indeed this is in agreement with the FDA warning mentioned in an earlier section** (2016; Gupta et al., 2011).

β-lactam agents (such as amoxicillin-clavulanate, cefdinir, cefaclor, and cefpodoxime-proxetil) remain second-line treatment options

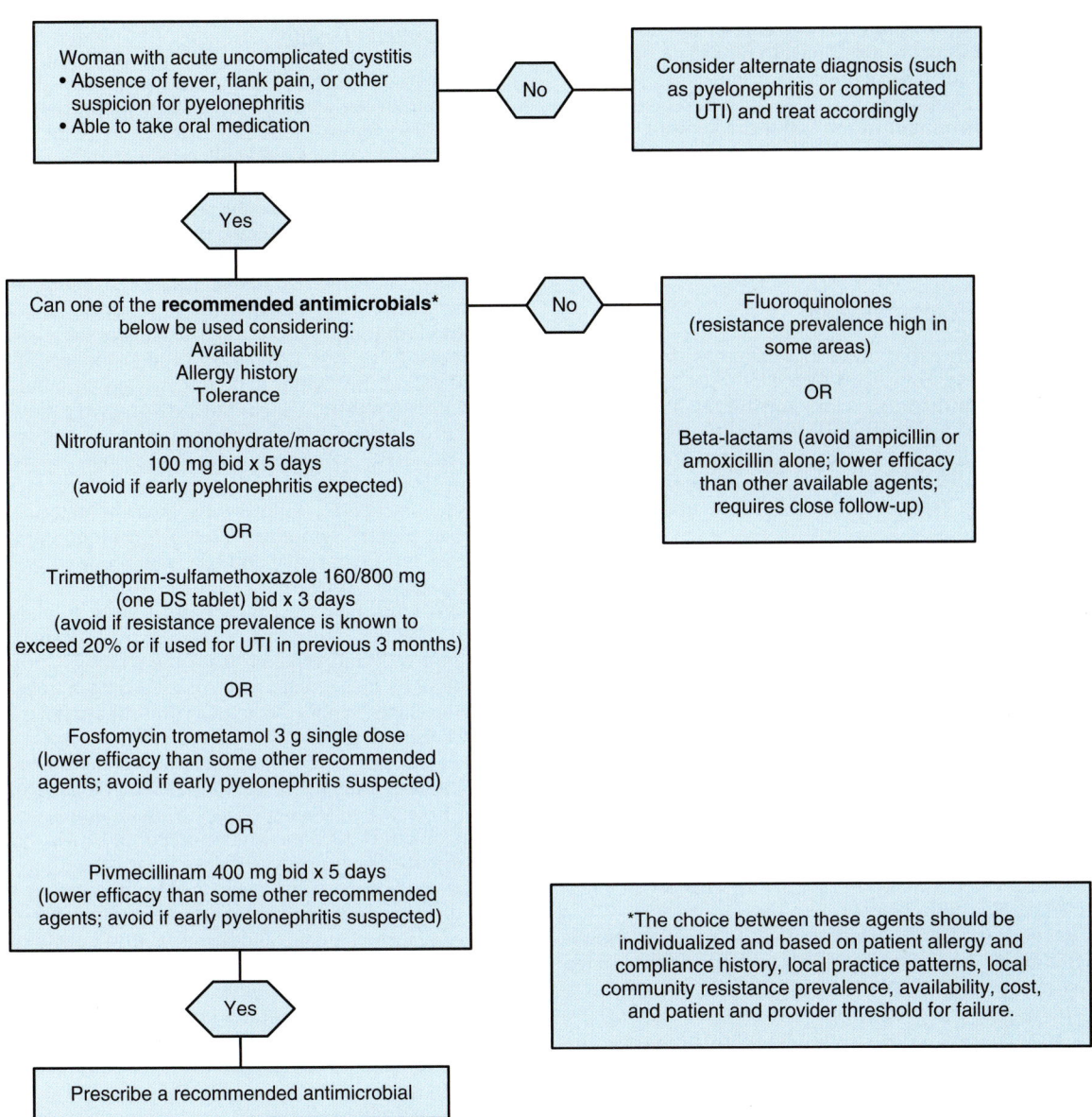

Fig. 55.13. IDSA-recommended treatment of acute uncomplicated cystitis.

for uncomplicated cystitis and can be used in 3- to 7-day regimens (Gupta et al., 2011).

Duration of Therapy. Three-day therapy is the preferred regimen for uncomplicated cystitis in women (Norrby, 1990; Warren et al., 1999). In an excellent review of more than 300 separate clinical trials of single-dose, 3-day, or 7-day treatment with TMP, TMP-SMX, fluoroquinolones, and β-lactam antimicrobial therapies, it was concluded that, irrespective of the antimicrobial used, 3-day therapy is more effective than single-dose therapy. Three-day therapy with TMP-SMX and TMP has been associated with cure rates similar to longer courses of therapy and an incidence of adverse effects about as low as that seen with single-dose therapy and lower than seen with longer courses of therapy (Charlton et al., 1976; Kunin, 1985; McCue, 1986; Warren et al., 1999). Because 7-day therapy often causes more adverse effects, it is recommended only for women with symptoms of 1 week or more, men, and individuals with possible complicating factors. Other durational variations include nitrofurantoin 5-day therapy and fosfomycin single-dose therapy.

Seven-day therapy is the preferred regimen for cystitis in men.

Cost of Therapy. The cost of treating a UTI involves not only the initial evaluation and cost of the drug but also what occurs subsequently. The most important prediction of high cost-effectiveness is high efficacy against the most common urinary pathogen, *E. coli*. The lower the effectiveness against this bacterium, the greater the number of revisits, cases of progression to pyelonephritis, and follow-up costs. Antimicrobial cost is a poor prediction of cost-effectiveness (Rosenberg, 1999).

Follow-Up

Approximately 90% of women are asymptomatic within 72 hours after initiating antimicrobial therapy (Fihn et al., 1985). **A follow-up visit or culture is not required in women who are asymptomatic after therapy. Further urologic evaluation is unnecessary in women who respond to therapy** (Abarbanel et al., 2003; Lipsky, 1989). **However, UTIs in most men should be considered complicated until proven otherwise.** Andrews et al. (2002) showed that approximately 50% of men with UTIs have a significant abnormality. Furthermore, if a patient does not respond to therapy, appropriate microbiologic urologic evaluations should be undertaken for the causes of unresolved and complicated UTIs.

Compliance With Recommended Agents. Despite the compelling argument for the purposeful and selective use of antibiotic therapy with respect to the treatment of uncomplicated cystitis, practice patterns within the prescribing community as a whole have yet to change. In a recent questionnaire distributed to physicians, including non-urologists, more than half of the 260 respondents were not familiar with the IDSA guidelines, and 30% did not recommend a first-line agent for the treatment of uncomplicated cystitis (Ditkoff et al., 2017). This suggests that further education and outreach efforts are critical to ensure all practitioners managing patients with uncomplicated cystitis are practicing the standard of care; only this way can the negative ecologic impact of inappropriate antibiotic use be mitigated on a population level.

Complicated Urinary Tract Infections

Complicated UTIs are those that occur in a patient with a compromised urinary tract or that are caused by a very resistant pathogen (Table 55.8). **These complicating factors may be readily apparent from the severity of the presenting illness or the past medical history. However, they may not be obvious at first and may only become evident from subsequent failure of the patient to respond to appropriate therapy** (see later discussion on unresolved or recurrent UTIs).

The clinical spectrum ranges from mild cystitis to life-threatening kidney infections and urosepsis (kidney infections and urosepsis are discussed subsequently). These infections can be caused by a broad range of bacteria with resistance to multiple antimicrobial agents. Therefore urine cultures are mandatory to identify the bacteria and its antimicrobial susceptibility.

Because of the wide range of host conditions and pathogens and a lack of adequate controlled trials, guidelines for empirical therapy are limited. For patients with mild to moderate illness who can be treated as an outpatient with oral therapy, 10 to 14 days of fluoroquinolones have traditionally been recommended because of their concentration in the urine and good tissue penetration (Stamm and Hooton, 1993); however, emerging resistance patterns to this class of antibiotics as well as concerns about side effects will likely change prior practice patterns.

For patients requiring hospitalization, IV antimicrobials should be administered based on the susceptibility patterns of the known uropathogens at that institution.

Because therapy will be compromised without addressing complicating factors, every effort should be made to correct any underlying urinary tract abnormalities, such as obstruction, and treat host factors that exacerbate the infection.

Therapy is usually continued for 10 to 14 days on culture-specific antibiotics and switched from parenteral to oral therapy when the patient is afebrile and clinically stable. Repeat urine cultures should be performed if the patient fails to respond to therapy.

Emphysematous Cystitis

Emphysematous cystitis is a rare and potentially life-threatening form of complicated cystitis that is associated with a mortality rate of up to 7% (Amano and Shimizu, 2014). Early medical therapy is important in achieving a favorable outcome and avoiding the need for surgical intervention. The pathognomonic finding of this disease process is gas noted within the wall on cross-sectional imaging. Emphysematous cystitis is typically observed in elderly women (60–70 years of age) with poorly controlled diabetes; additional risk factors include any condition that may predispose to incomplete emptying and lower urinary stasis, such as neurogenic bladder and bladder outlet obstruction. Although various microorganisms have been associated with this disease process, *E. coli* (60%) and *K. pneumoniae* (10%–20%) are most commonly implicated (Amano and Shimizu, 2014).

Clinical Presentation. The clinical signs and symptoms are variable, ranging from asymptomatic (reported in up to 7%) to overt sepsis (Kuo et al., 2009; Wortmann and Fleckenstein, 1998). The most common symptom in these patients is abdominal pain (80%) (Grupper et al., 2007) followed by gross hematuria (60%), and obstructive urinary symptoms (10%) (Yoshida et al., 2010). The presence of fever is variable and has been reported in 30% to 50% of these patients (Amano and Shimizu, 2014).

Radiologic Findings. The characteristic feature on plain radiograph involves curvilinear areas of increased radiolucency delineating the bladder wall and separate from the rectal gas posteriorly; the distribution of the air has been described as a cobblestoned or "beaded necklace" appearance, reflecting the irregular submucosal blebs (Grayson et al., 2002). A CT scan of the pelvis will also show air pocketed diffusely within the bladder wall, and possibly intraluminally; a CT scan is necessary to make the diagnosis and exclude other sources of pelvic air such as a fistula, trauma, or gangrene of adjacent structures (Amano and Shimizu, 2014; Fig. 55.14).

Management. The majority (90%) of these patients are treated with medical therapy alone, which consists of antibiotics (often parenteral), bladder drainage, and treatment of comorbid conditions such as poorly controlled diabetes (Amano and Shimizu, 2014). Antibiotic treatment regimens include agents that offer broad gram-negative coverage that can then be narrowed based on culture sensitivities and clinical response; if an initial Gram stain identifies gram-positive cocci, ampicillin or amoxicillin should be incorporated into the treatment regimen for better enterococcal coverage. The need for surgical intervention is rare and is reserved for those cases that respond poorly to initial medical management or severe necrotizing infections. The severity of the condition determines the nature of the surgical intervention,

TABLE 55.8 Host Factors Classifying a Urinary Tract Infection as Complicated

COMPLICATION	EXAMPLES
Anatomic abnormality	Cystocele, fistula, diverticulum
Iatrogenic	Nosocomial infection, surgery, indwelling catheter
Urinary tract obstruction	Bladder outlet obstruction, ureteropelvic junction obstruction, ureteral stricture
Voiding dysfunction	Neurologic disease, pelvic floor dysfunction, vesicoureteral reflux, incontinence, high postvoid residual
Other	Pregnancy, urolithiasis, diabetes, other immunosuppression

Data from Dason S, Dason J, Kappor A, et al.: Guidelines for the diagnosis and management of recurrent urinary tract infections in women. *Can Urol Assoc J* 5(5):316–322, 2011.

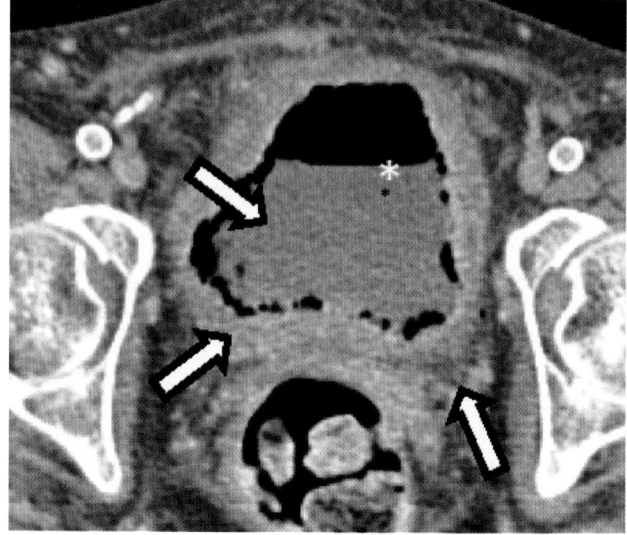

Fig. 55.14. Computed tomography of emphysematous cystitis. *Arrows* indicate intramural gas; there is also air in the bladder lumen (*).

but case reports have described debridement, partial cystectomy, and total cystectomy in advanced cases (Thomas et al., 2007).

Unresolved Urinary Tract Infections

Clinical Presentation

Unresolved infection indicates that initial therapy has been inadequate in eliminating symptoms and/or pathologic bacterial growth in the urinary tract. If the symptoms of UTI do not resolve by the end of treatment or if symptoms recur shortly after therapy, a urinalysis and urine culture with susceptibility testing should be obtained. If the patient's symptoms are significant and cannot be alleviated with urinary analgesics, broad-spectrum antibiotics may be initiated as empirical therapy pending the availability of the culture and susceptibility testing.

The causes of unresolved bacteriuria during antimicrobial therapy are shown in Box 55.10. **Most commonly, the bacteria are resistant to the antimicrobial agent selected to treat the infection.** Typically, the patient has received the antimicrobial therapy in the recent past and developed bowel colonization with resistant bacteria. β-lactams, tetracycline, and sulfonamides are notorious for causing plasmid-mediated R factors that simultaneously carry resistance to multiple antimicrobial agents. **The second most common cause is development of resistance in a previously susceptible population of bacteria during the course of treatment of UTIs.** This problem occurs in approximately 5% of the patients receiving antimicrobial therapy. It is easy to recognize clinically because the culture on therapy shows that the previous susceptible population has been replaced by resistant bacteria of the same species. It can be shown that resistant organisms were actually present before contact with the initial antimicrobial agent, but they were present in such low numbers that it was impossible to detect by in vitro susceptibility studies before therapy. When the antimicrobial concentration in the urine is insufficient to kill all the bacteria present, the more resistant forms will emerge. This characteristically is seen in patients who are underdosed or who are poorly compliant and hence have inadequate dose regimens. **The third cause is the presence of an unsuspected, second pathogen that was present initially and is resistant to the antimicrobial therapy chosen.** Treatment of the dominant organism unmasks the presence of the second strain. **The fourth cause is rapid reintroduction of a new resistant species while the patient is undergoing initial therapy.** Rapid reinfection that mimics unresolved bacteriuria should alert the clinician to the possibility of an enterovesical fistula.

If the culture obtained on therapy shows that the initial species is still present and susceptible to the antimicrobial chosen to treat the infection, the unresolved infection must be caused by inability to deliver an adequate concentration of antimicrobial agents into the urinary tract, an excessive number of bacteria that "override" the antimicrobial activity, or noncompliance with the regimen.

> **BOX 55.10** Causes of Unresolved Bacteriuria, in Descending Order of Importance
>
> Bacterial resistance to the drug selected for treatment
> Development of resistance from initially susceptible bacteria
> Bacteriuria caused by two different bacterial species with mutually exclusive susceptibilities
> Rapid reinfection with a new, resistant species during initial therapy for the original susceptible organism
> Azotemia
> Papillary necrosis from analgesic abuse
> Giant staghorn calculi in which the "critical mass" of susceptible bacteria is too great for antimicrobial inhibition
> Self-inflicted infections or deception in taking antimicrobial drugs (a variant of Munchausen syndrome)

In patients with azotemia, a determination of urinary antimicrobial concentrations usually shows that the level of the drug is below the minimal inhibitory concentration of the infecting organism.

In patients with papillary necrosis, severe defects in the medullary concentrating ability dilute the antimicrobial agent. A large mass of bacteria within the urinary tract is most commonly associated with a giant staghorn calculus. Even though adequate urinary levels of bactericidal drugs are present, the concentration is inadequate to sterilize the urine. This occurs because even susceptible bacteria cannot be inhibited once they reach a certain critical density, particularly if attached to a foreign body.

The last cause of unresolved bacteriuria occurs in those patients who have variants of Munchausen syndrome. These patients secretly inoculate their bladders with uropathogens or omit their oral antimicrobial agents while steadfastly asserting that they never miss a dose. The patient with Munchausen syndrome has an inconsistent clinical history and invariably a normal urinary tract on urologic imaging. Careful bacteriologic observations usually indicate the implausibility of the clinical picture.

Laboratory Diagnosis

Urinalysis and urine culture are mandatory to determine the cause of unresolved bacteriuria. The first four causes associated with resistant bacteria require no further evaluation. However, if reculture shows that the bacteria are sensitive to the antimicrobial agent the patient is taking, renal function and radiologic evaluation should be performed to identify renal or urinary tract abnormalities.

Management

If the patient's symptoms are significant, initial broad-spectrum empirical antimicrobial treatment may be initiated, and selection should be based on the assumption that the bacteria are resistant. Therefore an antimicrobial agent different from the original agent should be selected.

Recurrent Urinary Tract Infections

A recurrent UTI is defined as two UTIs in a 6-month period or three or more UTIs in a 12-month period. Recurrent UTIs are common in otherwise healthy women. Indeed, in healthy college-age women, 20% had at least one culture-documented UTI within 6 months of an index UTI (Foxman et al., 2000). Other studies have reported a 20% to 30% recurrence rate in women (Albert et al., 2004; Gupta et al., 2001a,b). It is well established that one of the most significant risk factors for development of a UTI is a prior recent UTI. Recurrent infections are hypothesized to be secondary to either bacterial persistence within the urinary tract or, more commonly, novel reinfection. Persistence, caused by the same bacterial strain, usually leads to recurrent infections in a short time frame, whereas reinfections generally occur over a more remote period. Reinfections are caused by either the same organism more than 2 weeks after treatment or a different organism. Reinfection is likely secondary to ascent of uropathogens from fecal flora into the urinary tract or from reemergence of bacteria from uroepithelial intracellular colonies. In men, reinfections raise suspicion for the presence of anatomic abnormalities.

Evaluation

In evaluation of a woman with recurrent UTIs, the clinical focus should be on preventing recurrence by identifying risk factors for, and altering behaviors that contribute to, recurrent infections. The history and physical exam should eliminate overt external anatomic or obvious functional abnormalities of the urinary tract that predispose to recurrent UTIs. If any of these factors are identified, the UTIs are classified as complicated.

Obtaining a thorough medical history is imperative. Emphasis should be on ascertaining the prior number of infections and

BOX 55.11 Risk Factors for Recurrent Urinary Tract Infections

- Sexual activity
- New sexual partner within past year
- Family history of urinary tract infection (UTI) in first-degree female relative
- Recent antimicrobial use
- Spermicide use
- History of UTI before menopause
- Menopause
- Incontinence, elevated postvoid residual, cystocele (in postmenopausal women)

TABLE 55.9 Indications for Further Investigation of Recurrent Urinary Tract Infection

Previous urinary tract trauma or surgery
Previous bladder or renal calculi
Gross hematuria after resolution of infection
Obstructive symptoms, low uroflowmetry, or high postvoid residual
Urea-splitting bacteria on culture
Previous abdominopelvic malignancy
Bacterial persistence after sensitivity-based therapy
Diabetes or other immune compromise
Pneumaturia, fecaluria, anaerobic bacteria, or history of diverticulitis
Repeated pyelonephritis
Asymptomatic microhematuria after resolution of infection should be evaluated

Data from Dason S, Dason J, Kappor A, et al.: Guidelines for the diagnosis and management of recurrent urinary tract infections in women. *Can Urol Assoc J* 5(5):316–322, 2011.

their frequency, culture results, associated symptoms, and identifiable triggers or risk factors. Symptoms such as pneumaturia, fecaluria, obstipation, as well as prior history of diverticulitis, prior pelvic surgery, or radiation should raise suspicion for vesicoenteric or vesicovaginal fistula. Description of any concomitant bowel symptoms, such as chronic constipation, diarrhea, and fecal incontinence may provide additional information to identify reversible contributing factors. Prior treatment strategies and patient response should be carefully investigated. **Significant risk factors for recurrence in women include sexual activity, a new sexual partner within the past year, menopause, spermicidal use, family history of UTI in a first-degree female relative, and recent antimicrobial use** (Dielubanza and Schaeffer, 2011; Hooton et al., 1996; Scholes et al., 2000, 2010). **In postmenopausal women, risk factors for recurrent UTIs include incontinence, elevated postvoid residual, and presence of a cystocele. A history of a UTI before menopause has also been identified as a risk factor** (Raz et al., 2000) (Box 55.11).

On physical examination, palpating the suprapubic area and performing a pelvic examination are important. One may identify a distended bladder; a significant postvoid residual contributes to bacteriuria. On pelvic examination the appearance of vaginal epithelium, particularly in postmenopausal women, should be characterized. The presence of pelvic organ prolapse or a urethral diverticulum could help establish the cause of recurrent UTIs.

Obtaining laboratory data, specifically urinalysis and urine culture, is imperative in patients with recurrent UTIs. Many of these patients are treated based on symptoms that overlap significantly with irritative storage symptoms and may in fact be inappropriately treated for UTIs. It is important in this population to establish that their symptoms are secondary to bacteriuria. In addition, quantification of the bacterial burden, species, and degree of resistance, if present, is also important information. Obtaining a urine culture in women with uncomplicated recurrent UTIs resulted in decreased hospitalization for treatment of UTI and decreased intravenous antibiotic usage (Suskind et al., 2016).

In many patients obtaining a postvoid residual and uroflow measurement provides important information. **In patients with emptying symptoms or a distended bladder on physical examination, documentation of a postvoid residual is critical.** In postmenopausal women with recurrent UTIs, higher postvoid residual and decreased urine flow were associated with uncomplicated recurrent UTIs (Raz et al., 2000). In fact, elevated PVR or decreased flow rates are often considered parameters that contribute to complicated UTIs; thus identification of abnormal values is important if the suspicion is high.

Imaging and cystoscopic evaluation are not warranted in all women with recurrent UTIs. Indeed, the yield of imaging in women without suspected complicated UTI is low and is not recommended by the American College of Radiology, the Canadian Urological Association Guidelines, or the European Association of Urology (EAU) Guidelines (Dason et al., 2011; EAU Guidelines, 2015; Segal et al., 2000). However, **in women with risk factors for a complicated UTI the evaluation should include imaging and cystoscopy.** These diagnostic tests may reveal kidney or bladder stones, neoplasms, fistulae, anatomic renal anomalies including scarring or papillary necrosis, or many other possible abnormalities (Table 55.9). Preferred imaging includes renal and bladder ultrasound with possible plain radiograph of the abdomen. In some cases, a CT scan is recommended as well, especially if there is a high index of suspicion for a complicated infection with no abnormality demonstrated on prior imaging. In patients with stones or obstruction, a CT scan is particularly useful in providing structural detail. In premenopausal women with a functional uterus, it is imperative to ask whether they may be pregnant; if they are uncertain, a pregnancy test should be obtained before any imaging that confers radiation (Fairchild et al., 1982).

Many providers perform cystoscopy for the evaluation of all women with recurrent UTIs; however, several studies substantiate the fact that cystoscopy does not confer any added value beyond imaging, particularly in uncomplicated UTIs (Lawrentschuk et al., 2006; Pagano et al., 2017; van Haarst et al., 2001). These data demonstrate that, if imaging has been performed, an invasive diagnostic procedure should not be considered in the uncomplicated setting. There is utility for cystoscopic evaluation in patients with complicated UTIs.

Bacterial Persistence

For culture-documented infections with acute symptoms, if patients fail to respond to an appropriate course of antibiotics, then bacterial persistence may be present. **The incidence of bacterial persistence in the recurrent UTI population is very small, but, when present, it is critical to diagnose the source of persistence. In such cases of bacterial persistence, cystoscopic evaluation and imaging studies are necessary.** With persistence there are usually correctable urologic abnormalities that may be reversible (see Box 55.6). Such abnormalities create persistence often immune from treatment because of the inability of antibiotics to penetrate or eliminate the nidus of infection. In select instances, surgical removal of the source of infection has been shown to eradicate the infections (Stamey, 1980).

Proper evaluation for bacterial persistence includes endoscopic evaluation of the urinary tract as well as radiologic studies. Cystoscopy, ultrasonography, and CT scan may be useful in identifying the source. VCUG is useful when there is suspicion of VUR or the presence of a nonrefluxing ureteral stump. Pelvic MRI is standard of care to identify a urethral diverticulum. Retrograde urethrogram should be considered in men with suspected urethral stricture disease.

One of the most common causes of bacterial persistence are struvite renal calculi. Urea-splitting organisms, such as *P. mirabilis*, contribute to such infection stones (see Chapter 91, Table 91.3). Urease-splitting organisms cause alkalinization of urine with precipitation of calcium, magnesium, ammonium, and phosphate salts. These minerals contribute to formation of branched struvite stones. The bacteria in these stones often persist despite antibiotic treatment; urine cultures may show no growth after treatment, but this is misleading because the bacteria remain sheltered within these stones. Oxalate and apatite stones that become secondarily colonized also may contribute to bacterial persistence. Risk factors for the development of infection stones include chronic indwelling catheters, urinary diversions, or other urinary tract abnormalities that affect stasis. To eradicate bacteriuria thought to be related to stone disease, surgical treatment of the infection stones is recommended in all patients safe for intervention, per the AUA Guidelines: Medical Management of Kidney Stones (American Urological Association, 2014). In those patients with residual or recurrent struvite stones who are not surgical candidates, acetohydroxamic acid in conjunction with antibiotic suppression may be offered (American Urological Association, 2014).

Management of nonobstructing stones in recurrent UTIs is controversial. One study identified certain patient characteristics that increase the likelihood of recurrent UTIs despite complete stone extraction, including type 2 diabetes mellitus, hypertension, and black ethnicity (Omar et al., 2015). In this cohort of 120 patients 50% remained infection free 1 year after surgical extraction of the stone. Further research is necessary to determine whether eradicating small, nonobstructing stones has a beneficial effect on reducing the incidence of recurrent UTIs.

Management

The majority of women with recurrent infections do not have identifiable and/or correctible anatomic abnormalities. Options for minimizing recurrent infections include behavioral modifications, use of non-antibiotic therapies, and, as a last resort, antibiotic treatment and prophylaxis.

In this era of widespread antibiotic overuse and the prevalence of alarming numbers of multidrug-resistant bacteria, judicious use of antibiotics is imperative.

The development of multidrug-resistant bacteria is associated with increased and prolonged hospitalization rates and significant adverse effects, including death. The Centers for Disease Control and Prevention (CDC) has reported that antibiotic resistance is one of the most serious health threats we encounter. More than 2 million people annually are infected with an antibiotic-resistant infection, which results in more than 20,000 deaths (CDC, 2014).

To minimize overuse of antibiotics and preserve their effectiveness, antibiotic stewardship programs have been developed. These programs have been efficacious at improving antibiotic prescribing patterns, improving patient outcomes, decreasing adverse effects, and improving rates of susceptibilities to particular agents (Barlam et al., 2016). Indeed, a recent Cochrane review demonstrated that stewardship programs have improved compliance with antibiotic guideline recommendations and have helped decrease the duration of antibiotic courses (Davey et al., 2017). **The management of UTIs must adhere to antibiotic stewardship efforts (Fig. 55.15).**

Behavioral Modification. It is a clinically accepted principle that employing behavioral modification is a reasonable strategy to minimize recurrent UTIs, despite the lack of scientific evidence in support of several aspects of this approach. Such behavioral modifications carry minimal to no risks and enhance overall bladder health. Many women prone to UTIs acknowledge that they drink insufficient quantities of water and/or have a tendency to hold urine for extended periods despite feeling urges to void. Hydration is recommended to augment innate immunity by sloughing of urothelial cells and flushing of adherent bacteria. A recent study found that in premenopausal

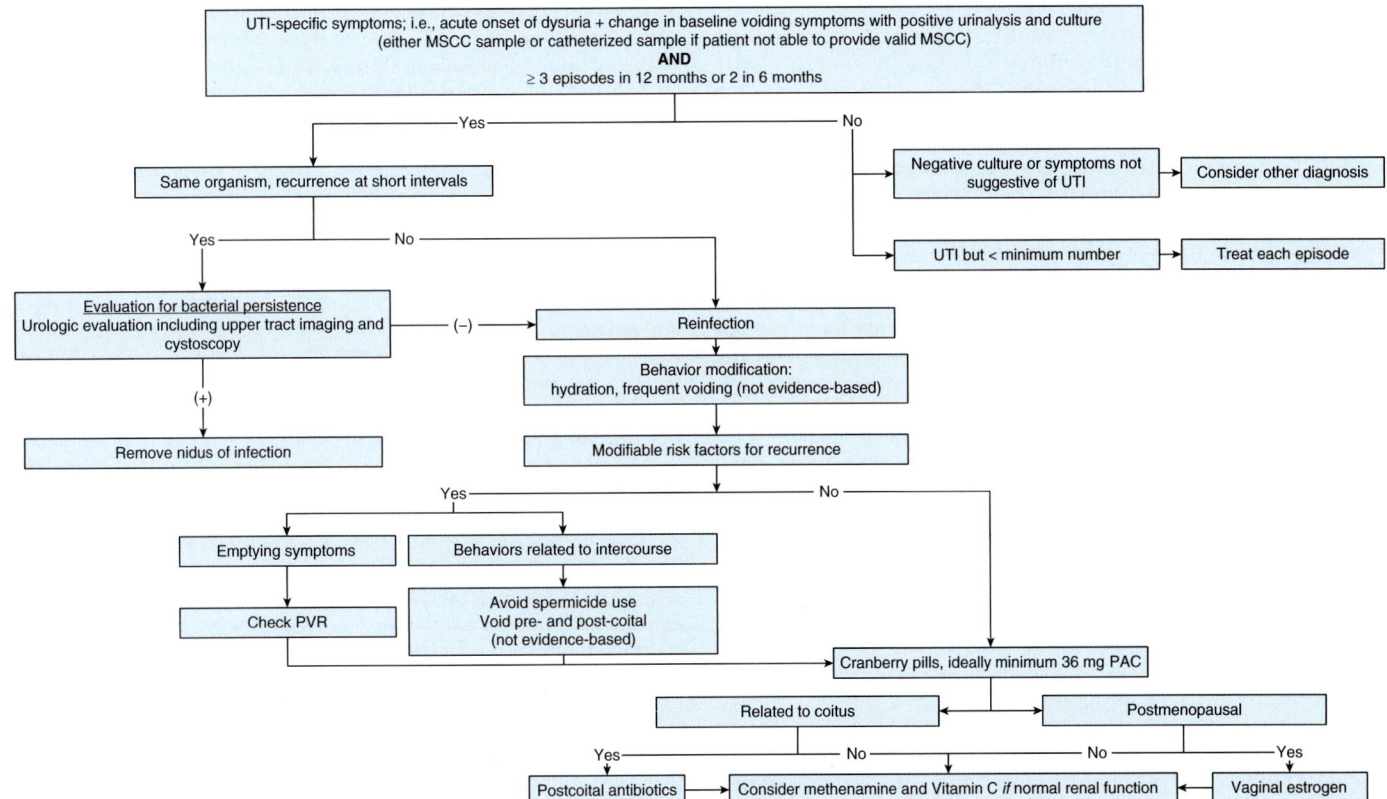

Fig. 55.15. Algorithm for management of recurrent urinary tract infections. *MSCC*, Midstream clean-catch sample; *PAC*, proanthocyanidin; *PVR*, postvoid residual; *UTI*, urinary tract infection.

women with a history of recurrent UTIs, increasing water intake by 1.5 L daily led to a significant decrease in the number of cystitis episodes (Hooton et al., 2018). Likewise, frequent voiding helps to continually empty the bladder, which is particularly important if women have a tendency to hold urine for extended periods or do not empty their bladders adequately when they do void. Sexual activity is a known risk factor for UTIs because it transiently increases bacteriuria. Therefore emptying the bladder after intercourse should help minimize the likelihood that the transient bacteriuria will progress to clinical symptomatology of a UTI. By this same logic that has been favored for managing patients with a history of UTIs, voiding pre-intercourse, when possible, may also be beneficial. Spermicides (nonoxynol-9) have been associated with an increased risk of developing a UTI because they contribute to decreased population of normal vaginal flora and subsequently alter the vaginal pH, making the environment more hospitable for uropathogenic bacteria to thrive (Fihn et al., 1985,1996; Handley et al., 2002). Clinicians have speculated that shaving pubic hair and wearing thong underwear may contribute to recurrent UTIs; however, scientific data confirming this do not exist.

Self-Start Therapy. One widespread practice that has been favored for managing patients who suspect they have a UTI involves allowing reliable patients to start antimicrobial therapy with onset of their typical UTI symptoms, sometimes without providing a urine sample or consulting their health care provider. Although this practice empowers the appropriate patient with the ability to self-diagnose and allows for instant access to antibiotics, it countermands the principles of antibiotic stewardship and the meaningful use of culture-specific antibiotics described in previous sections. Historical literature provided justification of this practice, with older studies suggesting patients have excellent diagnostic skills and will appropriately treat only when necessary (Gupta et al., 2001a,b; Schaeffer and Stuppy, 1999). Initially this approach depended on patients providing urine samples and following up for culture results after initiating antimicrobial therapy. With time, however, the expectation of providing samples has dissipated, and, in the current era, most patients begin antibiotics without making an effort to confirm the presence of a UTI, much less the causative organism and sensitivities.

Historically, patients were encouraged to rely on broad-spectrum antibiotics to treat their symptoms, and fluoroquinolones were considered "ideal" agents for self-start therapy. However, although this approach is endorsed by many practitioners, partially because of ease of patient management, this strategy only perpetuates antibiotic overuse by relying on self-diagnosis. Many patients with a history of UTIs have anxiety because of fear of when the next UTI will appear. These patients may prematurely and incorrectly initiate treatment if they notice any change in their typical urinary habits; often patients are quick to assume they have another UTI if they have a slight increase in urgency, or mild discomfort with urination. **Our anecdotal clinical experience suggests that patients are not always adequate diagnosticians when it comes to UTIs, and the risks outweigh the benefits of self-start therapy. A practice that allows patients to self-medicate, often with extended courses of broad-spectrum antibiotics, is not a sustainable strategy.**

In the management algorithm for recurrent infections, many experienced clinicians encourage patients to medicate with urinary analgesics with the onset of symptoms to provide some relief, provide a urine sample, and continue observation unless they display significant symptoms. For persistent issues despite analgesics, prescription of IDSA-recommended antibiotics, in consultation with local antibiograms, may be administered and tailored once culture results are available. In many cases patient symptoms are transient and unrelated to bacterial infection and thus are self-limiting; this approach spares a course of unnecessary antibiotics.

Low-Dose Continuous Prophylaxis. Another widely advocated management option for recurrent UTIs is daily prophylaxis with low-dose antibiotics. Conceptually, this strategy has been promoted because particular antimicrobial agents eradicate pathogenic bacteria from introital and bowel reservoirs without fostering bacterial resistance. Many papers were published in the late 20th century endorsing the use of TMP-SMX, TMP alone, nitrofurantoin, cephalexin (low dose) and fluoroquinolones, as well as several other antibiotics no longer in use (Bailey et al., 1971; Martinez et al., 1985; Nicolle, et al., 1989; Raz and Boger, 1991; Stamm et al., 1980a). In these studies, some of which were placebo controlled, patients who received daily prophylaxis, generally for 6 months to a year, demonstrated lower rates of UTIs (compared with placebo or with the patients' prior experiences as controls). Although these studies concluded that daily antibiotic use was safe and effective, some did mention an increased incidence of non-*E.coli* UTIs after such prophylaxis.

A 2004 Cochrane review of AP against recurrent UTIs in non-pregnant women concluded that **women with uncomplicated recurrent UTIs are less likely to have an infection if they take prophylactic antibiotics for 6 to 12 months** (Albert et al., 2004). This review included 19 randomized controlled studies, involving 1120 women. Study designs of these 19 studies included comparing antibiotics with placebo, the same antibiotic with different regimens (i.e., daily vs. weekly vs. monthly vs. postcoital), different antibiotics, or antibiotics versus non-antibiotic pharmacologic interventions. The majority of these studies evaluated 6 months of prophylaxis; only one studied subjects for 1 year of treatment. The most recently published study included was published in 1995. The studies reported on the number of recurrences while subjects were on prophylaxis as well as after prophylaxis was discontinued. Adverse effects of antibiotic use were also investigated. The authors concluded that continuous antibiotic use did decrease the clinical and microbiologic recurrence rate; however, there were more adverse effects attributed to the antibiotics.

Only two studies performed follow-up 6 months beyond the prophylactic period (Schaeffer et al., 1982; Stamm et al., 1980). In these two studies, once prophylaxis was discontinued, the recurrence rate was comparable between those treated and the placebo group. Therefore, **although prophylaxis was deemed an effective strategy in the short term, in the long term patients who were treated prophylactically demonstrated the same risk of recurrence as those not treated.** Two of the studies assessed postcoital antibiotic use; one compared it with placebo, the other compared it with daily antibiotics use. Both studies found that postcoital antibiotic use, in women with recurrent UTIs secondary to intercourse, is an effective strategy and is preferable to daily antibiotic use.

Although many practitioners advocate prophylactic antibiotics, at least in part because of the conclusions of this Cochrane review, several points must be emphasized. The authors of the Cochrane review questioned the quality of the clinical trials reviewed, specifically citing concerns regarding inconsistent definitions of recurrent UTIs, outcomes analyzed, analysis of antibiotic side effects, and follow-up of subjects. Although continuous antibiotics were effective, no consensus existed related to how long to continue suppression. The studies analyzed in this review are several decades old, performed at a time when antibiotic resistance rates were much lower than those encountered today. Clearly long-term suppressive antibiotics pose a major risk to society because this practice undoubtedly will contribute to perpetuation of multidrug-resistant organisms. **Because of the risk of adverse effects of exposure to antibiotics, long-term treatment with daily prophylaxis is not an appropriate contemporary approach.** Indeed, the European Association of Urology (EAU) guidelines for urologic infections state that recent concerns highlight the "need for reconsidering long-term antibiotic prophylaxis in recurrent UTI and assess in each individual case effective alternative preventive measures" (Grabe et al., 2015). If patients desire indefinite daily prophylaxis they should be educated that no long-term data exist in support of this strategy and that they are exposing themselves to potentially severe side effects and development of multidrug-resistant organisms.

Postcoital antibiotic use is an acceptable strategy in patients with a clear-cut causal relationship between intercourse and onset of UTIs when other management options have not been effective. Ideally, prior cultures with sensitivities should be taken into consideration when choosing an antibiotic, in addition to a patient's allergies as well as local resistance patterns and ecologic effects of the chosen agent.

Nitrofurantoin remains a popular choice for prophylaxis because it concentrates in urine, is efficacious against many uropathogens, and does not promote widespread resistance. However, nitrofurantoin is associated with significant adverse effects, particularly with long-term use. Unfortunately, providers do not routinely address the risk of pulmonary fibrosis or renal and neurotoxicity, and many patients are encouraged to take it daily, indefinitely, lacking appropriate counseling detailing the potential harm they may encounter in the future. A recent systematic review and meta-analysis of common antibiotics used for prophylaxis in women concluded that nitrofurantoin was equally as effective, in terms of clinical and microbiologic cure, as norfloxacin, trimethoprim, sulfamethoxazole/trimethoprim, cefaclor, estriol, or methenamine hippurate. However, it was also associated with increased risk of adverse effects, mostly related to the GI tract (Price et al., 2016).

Non-Antibiotic Management. Although it has been historically acceptable to recommend AP, a review of the literature from the last 10 years suggests that the majority of recent research has focused on non-antibiotic strategies to prevent UTIs. Contemporary research corroborates that, although AP may be effective, increasing rates of antibiotic resistance and subsequent adverse ecologic effects associated with AP make this strategy less desirable. **It is imperative that we develop alternatives to antibiotics for minimizing UTIs without further contributing to the alarming rates of antibiotic resistance; as stated earlier more than two million illnesses and more than 20,000 deaths occur yearly because of antibiotic resistance.**

Recent articles have reviewed several forms of non-AP; one included a systematic review and meta-analysis of available randomized controlled trials (RCTs). The authors found that the oral immunostimulant OM-89, the vaginal vaccine Urovac, vaginal estrogen, cranberry, and acupuncture had varying degrees of success in lowering the risk of recurrent UTIs; however, oral estrogens and lactobacilli were not effective (Beerepoot et al., 2013). Another review article examined the efficacy of vitamin C, cranberry, estrogen, lactobacilli, methenamine, OM-89, and Urovac (Geerlings et al., 2014). Use of vitamin C was not deemed effective in reducing the incidence of UTIs, whereas the others had varying degrees of success. Researchers acknowledge that further studies must be undertaken, particularly comparisons between specific products and the gold-standard AP, before strong recommendations can be made in support of non-antibiotic strategies. In addition, standardized doses and products should be used in all studies to make the conclusions more powerful.

Cranberry. Cranberry products for UTI prophylaxis have been investigated for years in the scientific and lay press. **One of the active ingredients in cranberry is the polyphenol type A proanthocyanidin (PAC), which prevents the P fimbriae of *E. coli* from adhering to uroepithelial cells** (Howell et al., 2010). Studies have investigated various formulations of cranberry, including juice/concentrate, capsules, tablets and extract, in comparison with placebo or no treatment (Barbosa-Cesnik et al., 2011; Kontiokari et al., 2001; Stothers, 2002). Other studies have examined the efficacy of cranberry versus AP (Beerepoot et al., 2011; McMurdo et al., 2009).

Some of the earlier studies were analyzed in a **Cochrane review from 2008** (Jepson and Craig, 2008). This review included 10 studies (1049 subjects) that investigated cranberry supplementation in patients with recurrent UTIs. Most of these studies (seven) evaluated use of juice, whereas tablet formulations were evaluated in four studies. One study investigated juice and tablets. Investigators concluded that cranberry was effective in reducing the incidence of recurrent UTIs in women as compared with older men or women, or people who required catheterization (either indwelling catheters or who performed CIC). Indeed, **in women with recurrent UTIs cranberry significantly reduced the incidence of UTIs at 1 year** (RR 0.65; 95% CI 0.46–0.90). As discussed by investigators who conducted this review, an obstacle in drawing conclusions about the efficacy of cranberry is that there was significant heterogeneity of products available and routes of administration, thus making the dosage of cranberry in each study population variable. Although side effects were minimal, there was a large dropout rate, particularly in those who ingested the juice.

A more recent Cochrane review added 14 more studies to the original review; thus a total of 24 studies (4473 subjects) were included (Jepson et al., 2012). In these investigations various cranberry formulations were evaluated and compared with placebo, water, antibiotics, methenamine, lactobacillus, or no treatment. In contrast to the earlier meta-analysis, these data reported that cranberry supplementation did not significantly reduce the symptomatic UTI rate overall, in comparison with water, placebo, or no treatment (RR 0.86; 95% CI 0.71–1.04). **In subgroup analysis, cranberry did not significantly reduce the recurrence rate of UTIs in any group, including in women with a history of recurrent UTIs (RR 0.74; 95% CI 0.42–1.31), a contradictory finding compared with the prior Cochrane review.** Interestingly, two of the studies compared cranberry capsules or syrup with AP in women with recurrent UTIs and found that cranberry was equally as effective as antibiotic in reducing the risk of recurrent UTIs (RR 1.31; 95% CI 0.85–2.02).

Although GI adverse effects were no higher in those who took cranberry products compared with placebo or no treatment, many studies did report low compliance rates/high dropout rates, which were attributed to tolerability of the products, particularly juice intake. **The authors of the review did acknowledge that most studies did not report on how much active ingredient, or PAC, the products had, and thus the products may not have been potent enough to achieve desired results. Based on this more recent review, cranberry juice cannot be recommended for prevention of recurrent UTIs; however, the efficacy of other cranberry products must be further examined and must include standardization of the preparation and confirmation of the presence of active ingredient. Based on prior research, 36 mg of PAC equivalents/day has been shown to be effective, but 72 mg may be even more effective** (Howell et al., 2010; Fig. 55.16). In addition, because the anti-adhesion effect is not long acting, the product should be taken twice a day.

Administering 72 mg of PAC daily to women in nursing homes was ineffective in decreasing the rates of bacteriuria plus pyuria, or of developing a symptomatic UTI, over a 1-year period (Juthani-Mehta et al., 2016). However, the majority of these women did not have bacteriuria plus pyuria or recurrent symptomatic UTIs before the study period, so the benefit of PAC may not have been as apparent as it may have been in a different cohort, namely those who were prone to UTIs. In addition, samples were obtained via midstream clean-catch samples, rather than catheterized samples, despite that these women were most likely atrophic and may have had comorbidities that made providing appropriate voided samples more challenging. Furthermore, postvoid residual volumes or degree of incontinence were not characterized; these are two known risk factors for bacteriuria in the elderly population. Although this study had significant limitations, some argued that these data confirm that "it is time to move on from cranberries" (Nicolle, 2016). However, challenging the efficacy of cranberry in preventing recurrent UTIs in all women based on results from a nursing home cohort does not seem wise.

The most recent systematic review and meta-analysis of cranberry products included 28 studies (4947 subjects) and concluded that ingestion of cranberry products confer a significant reduction in the risk of recurrent UTIs (Luis et al., 2017). A subgroup analysis determined that subjects with a history of recurrent UTIs and those who had undergone gynecologic surgery benefitted the most from cranberry products.

Although research has determined that a minimum quantity of 36 mg of PAC is most important in achieving efficacy against recurrent UTIs, few products report on the PAC content. In addition the cost of those products that report on PAC dosage may make them prohibitively expensive for some.

A pre-existing FDA warning to avoid cranberries and cranberry products when taking warfarin was removed in 2011. The concern about adverse interactions, specifically that cranberry elevates the INR and thus increases bleeding diathesis, has not been substantiated in scientific studies (Ansell et al., 2009; Mellen et al., 2010; Zikria et al., 2010). **Practitioners should feel comfortable recommending cranberry products even if their patient is taking warfarin.**

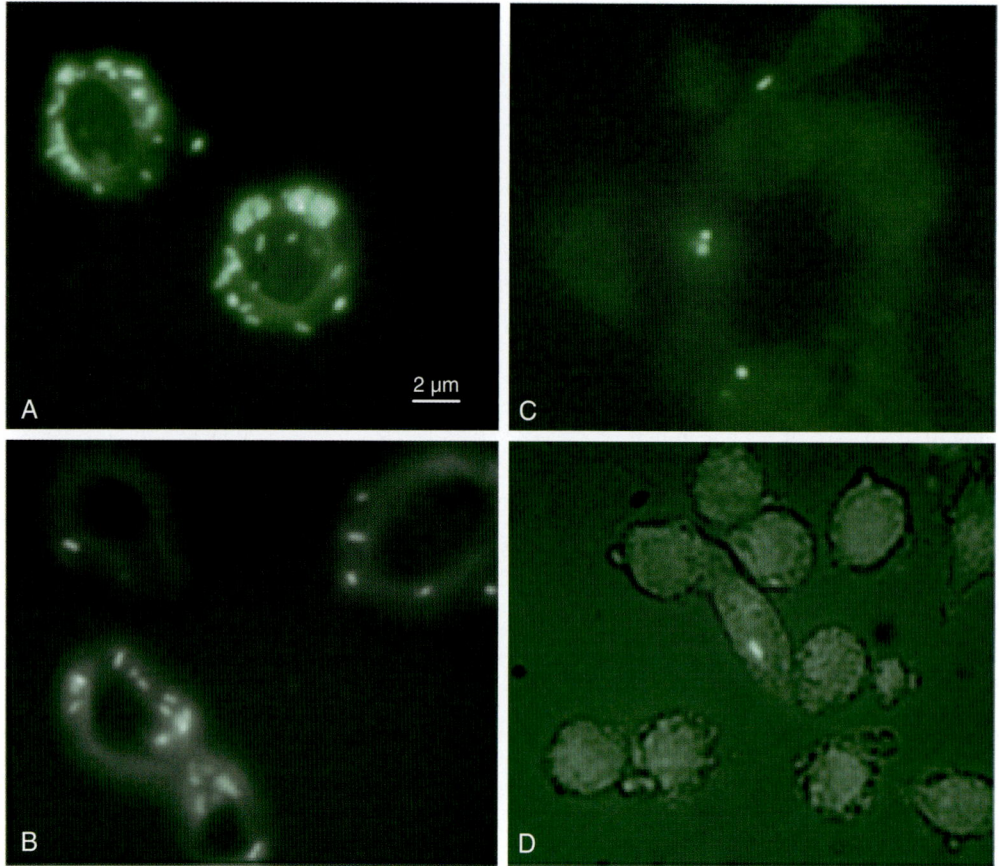

Fig. 55.16. *Escherichia coli* and effect of proanthocyanidin (PAC). (A) *E. coli* cultured in urines collected after placebo consumption. (B) *E. coli* cultured in urines collected 6 hours after consumption of cranberry powder containing 18-mg PAC. (C) *E. coli* cultured in urines collected 6 hours after consumption of cranberry powder containing 36-mg PAC. (D) *E. coli* cultured in urines collected 6 hours after consumption of cranberry powder containing 72-mg PAC.

As evidenced by the contradictory conclusions of the Cochrane reviews, as well as various other articles reviewed, the efficacy of cranberry supplements in minimizing recurrent UTIs is controversial at best and remains an area ripe for more investigation. The authors do recommend cranberry supplements, ideally those with a minimum of 36 mg of PAC, based on our successful anecdotal experience.

Estrogen. Postmenopausal women may have frequent reinfections (Hooton and Stamm, 1991; Raz and Stamm, 1993). Such infections are **sometimes attributable to residual urine** after voiding, which is often associated with bladder or uterine prolapse. **In addition,** decreased estrogen levels contribute to the transformation to atrophic vaginal epithelium and increased vaginal pH, which creates a more hospitable environment for bacteria to thrive. Indeed, **the lack of estrogen causes marked changes in the vaginal microflora,** including a loss of lactobacilli and increased colonization by *E. coli* (Raz and Stamm, 1993). An early placebo-controlled study with 93 women showed that the use of vaginal estriol reduced the number of UTIs as compared with placebo (RR 0.25; 95% CI 0.13–0.50) (Raz, 1993). The UTI rate was significantly lower in the group that received the vaginal estriol (0.5 vs. 5.9 episodes per patient-year, $P < 0.001$) (Fig. 55.17). The efficacy was attributed to the reemergence of vaginal lactobacilli and the decrease in vaginal pH in those who received vaginal estrogen. Adverse effects were minimal, although there was a 28% dropout rate in the estrogen group as compared with 17% in the placebo group; the most common reason for dropout was bothersome local adverse reactions to estriol including vaginal burning, itching, or irritation. Another study compared the use of an estradiol-releasing vaginal ring to no estrogen administration and found that the use of vaginal estrogen lowered the likelihood

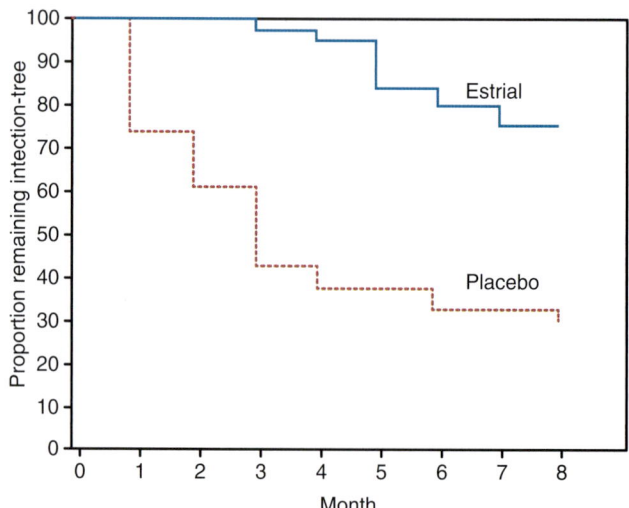

Fig. 55.17. Kaplan-Meier analysis showing the cumulative proportions of women remaining free of urinary tract infections in the Estriol and placebo groups ($P < 0.001$ by the Log-Rank Test). (Data from Raz R, Stamm WE: A controlled trial of intravaginal estriol in postmenopausal women with recurrent urinary tract infections, *N Engl J Med* 329(11):753–756, 1993.)

of developing a UTI in postmenopausal women with a history of recurrent UTIs (RR 0.64; 95% CI 0.47–0.86; Eriksen, 1999).

This literature was included in a **Cochrane review** that investigated the efficacy of oral and vaginal estrogen in preventing recurrent UTIs in postmenopausal women (Perrotta et al., 2008). A total of nine studies that included 3345 women were analyzed. Oral estrogens compared with placebo, analyzed in four studies, were not effective in preventing a UTI. Some of the studies comparing oral antibiotics to vaginal estrogen showed significant heterogeneity and results could not be pooled. Based on the two studies discussed earlier, the authors concluded that **vaginal estrogen is effective in preventing recurrent UTIs in postmenopausal women. The beneficial effect from vaginal estrogen use can take at least 12 weeks to manifest.** Adverse effects included breast tenderness, nonphysiologic discharge, and vaginal bleeding/spotting, irritation, itching and burning. Investigators encouraged the performance of future studies that investigated the optimal administration of vaginal estrogen.

A recent review of various forms of vaginal estrogen was performed and found that all forms (estrogen cream, tablets, and ring) improved symptoms of vaginal atrophy, but the impact on UTIs specifically was not analyzed (Lethaby et al., 2016).

Package inserts for vaginal estrogen preparations include warnings about potential systemic effects of estrogen administration, which likely contributes to some patients' reluctance to initiate vaginal estrogen therapy. However, the boxed warnings refer to all forms of estrogen administration, regardless of route of administration, and concerns about the risks of *vaginal* estrogen have not been supported by scientific studies. Although estrogen is detectable in plasma after vaginal administration, the levels are lower compared with those achieved with oral administration of low-dose conjugated estrogens. Daily administration of low-dose vaginal estrogen resulted in steady-state estrogen concentrations that were noted to be within or slightly above the normal reference range for postmenopausal women (Dorr et al., 2010). Indeed, all low-dose vaginal estrogen preparations result in minimal systemic absorption that results in levels that do not exceed normal postmenopausal levels (Santen, 2015).

RCTs of vaginal estrogen use have not been designed to analyze outcomes such as cancer or cardiovascular disease. However, observational studies have found no increased risk of fracture or breast cancer in women who used vaginal estrogen (Lyytinen et al., 2006; Michaelsson et al., 2002). Analysis of data from subjects in the Women's Health Initiative Observational Study confirmed that vaginal estrogen preparations do not confer an increased risk of cancer or cardiovascular disease (Crandall et al., 2018).

Vaginal estrogen use in breast cancer survivors has been studied. An increased risk of breast cancer recurrence was not demonstrated (Dew et al., 2003; Le Ray et al., 2012), including in those who were taking tamoxifen. The safety of vaginal estrogen use in survivors who are taking aromatase inhibitors has not been clearly demonstrated (Wills et al., 2012). All of these studies focused on vaginal estrogen use for amelioration of symptoms secondary to vulvovaginal atrophy. Despite the lack of data demonstrating an increased risk of recurrence, vaginal estrogen use is generally discouraged in this population (Santen et al., 2017). However, for these women who are suffering from recurrent UTIs vaginal estrogen can be prescribed after endorsement from their oncologist. As discussed, data *do not* demonstrate an increased risk of cancer recurrence but *do* demonstrate a decreased risk of recurrent UTIs.

Laser therapy to treat symptoms associated with vulvovaginal atrophy has become popular in recent years as an alternative to hormonal therapies. The MonaLisa Touch laser is a fractional CO_2 laser designed for the vaginal mucosa. It stimulates the production of new collagen. Scientific data supporting this modality to decrease the risk of recurrent UTIs do not exist.

Probiotics. Certain strains of lactobacilli can interfere with the presence of uropathogenic bacteria in the urogenital epithelium. The maintenance of normal urogenital flora may be enhanced by strains that produce antibacterial substances such as hydrogen peroxide (Falagas et al., 2006). Initial studies evaluated various strains for prevention of recurrent UTIs, including a *Lactobacillus* GC drink and the vaginal suppository *L. casei v rhamnosus* (Baerheim et al., 1994; Kontiokari et al., 2001). However, neither product proved effective in reducing the UTI recurrence rates. More recent studies using *L. crispatus* vaginal suppositories and *L. rhamnosus GR-1* and *L. reuteri RC-14* oral capsules showed more promising results (Beerepoot et al., 2012; Stapleton et al., 2011).

A Cochrane review published in 2015 examined the efficacy of probiotic use in women and children (Schwenger et al., 2015). This review included 9 studies; study design compared probiotics with placebo, no treatment, or antibiotics. Many forms and dosages of probiotics and duration of treatment were used in the studies reviewed. This review concluded that **probiotics cannot be recommended as an effective strategy for prevention of recurrent UTIs.** However, the authors acknowledge the studies reviewed were small and had design flaws. More investigation into the efficacy of probiotics is necessary before they become part of the urologist's treatment algorithm.

Methenamine. Methenamine salts, which have been used for urinary indications for approximately 100 years, are 70% to 90% renally excreted and are converted to ammonia and formaldehyde in an acidic environment (pH < 6) (Lo et al., 2014). Formaldehyde is either bactericidal or bacteriostatic in urine depending on its concentration. To achieve acidification of the urine when these oral tablets are taken, high doses of ascorbic acid (vitamin C) (1–4 g) can be ingested in conjunction with the methenamine (recommended dose is 1 g twice daily). Two formulations of methenamine are FDA approved, methenamine hippurate and methenamine mandelate. Two early randomized placebo-controlled trials conducted in otherwise healthy women demonstrated a 56% to 75% reduction in recurrent UTIs with the use of methenamine mandelate 500 mg four times daily with ascorbic acid 500 mg four times daily, and methenamine hippurate 1 g twice daily without the addition of vitamin C (Cronberg et al., 1987; Harding, 1974). The acid salts, mandelate and hippurate, have nonspecific bacteriostatic properties and are therefore not effective against urease-producing bacteria. Methenamine is contraindicated if the creatinine clearance is less than 50 cc/min or in patients with severe liver disease or hypersensitivity to the drug or its components. It must also be avoided in patients who are also taking sulfonamides, antacids, and carbonic anhydrase inhibitors (Table 55.10).

A Cochrane Review published in 2012 included 13 studies (2032 subjects) of methenamine hippurate (Lee et al., 2012). Various doses were investigated in these studies, ranging from 1 to 4 g per day. Acidification agents were combined with methenamine in only two of the studies. Researchers concluded that there was significant heterogeneity in the studies reviewed; thus definitive conclusions could not be made. However, methenamine showed some benefit in patients with normal urinary tracts (symptomatic UTI: RR 0.24; 95% CI 0.07–0.89; bacteriuria: RR 0.56; 95% CI 0.37–0.83), but not in patients with anatomic abnormalities (symptomatic UTI: RR 1.54; 95% CI 0.38–6.20; bacteriuria: RR 1.29; 95% CI 0.54–3.07). **In patients who had normal urinary tracts and did not have indwelling catheters, short-term (≤7 days) therapy contributed to a significant reduction in symptomatic infections (RR 0.14; 95% CI 0.05–0.38).** Methenamine hippurate was not effective in patients

TABLE 55.10 Methenamine Drug Interactions

Antacids: may diminish therapeutic effect
Carbonic anhydrase inhibitors: may diminish therapeutic effect
Sodium picosulfate: therapeutic effect may be diminished by concomitant methenamine use
Foods/diets that alkanize urine (pH >5.5)[a]: may diminish therapeutic effect

[a]Almonds; chestnuts; flax, pumpkin, and sunflower seeds; berries; cherries; grapes; citrus; cantaloupe; figs; kiwi.
Data from Lo TS, Hammer KD, Zegarra M, Cho WC: Methenamine: a forgotten drug for preventing recurrent urinary tract infection in a multidrug resistance era. *Expert Rev Anti Infect Ther* 12(5):549–554, 2014.

with known urinary tract abnormalities. Adverse effects were infrequent; nausea and diarrhea were most frequently encountered.

Concern has been raised about the use of a product that gets converted to formaldehyde, which is listed as a carcinogen in the 2011 National Toxicology Program Report on Carcinogens. However, in this report, formaldehyde has been associated with nasopharyngeal cancer, sinonasal cancer, and lymphohematopoietic cancers. Formaldehyde was not listed as being associated with urothelial cancers. The risk of developing bladder cancer secondary to the use of methenamine thus appears to be theoretical (Geerlings et al., 2014).

D-Mannose. D-mannose is a simple sugar that has shown some promise recently in preventing bacterial adhesion to the urothelium. It binds and blocks Fim H, an adhesin protein located at the tip of type 1 pili of enteric bacteria, therefore functioning as a competitive inhibitor of bacterial adhesion mechanisms. Historically it has been used for treating UTIs in some animals (Altarac and Papes, 2014). Recent studies have found that D-mannose was equally as efficacious as nitrofurantoin in reducing the risk of recurrent UTIs and demonstrated a significantly lower risk of adverse effects. D-mannose was also effective in reducing symptoms associated with acute cystitis as well as preventing recurrent UTIs (Domenici et al., 2016; Kranjcec et al., 2014). More studies must be performed to draw more definitive conclusions about the efficacy of D-mannose. Optimal dosing for D-mannose formulations remains unknown.

Immunoactive Prophylaxis. Bacterial extracts have been investigated as potential prophylactic agents against UTIs. Oral and vaginal products exist and have been studied.

The oral immunostimulant OM-89 (Uro-Vaxum) is an extract that contains 18 serotypes of heat-killed uropathogenic *E. coli*. The different serotypes increase neutrophils and macrophage phagocytosis, thereby stimulating the host immune system to target uropathogenic *E. coli*. Several studies have investigated the efficacy of OM-89 in women with recurrent UTIs (Bauer et al., 2005; Magasi et al., 1994; Schulman et al., 1993; Tammen, 1990). A meta-analysis of these studies included 891 patients who took 1 capsule a day of OM-89 or placebo (Beerepoot et al., 2013). In the treated group the risk ratio of developing at least one UTI was significantly lower in the OM-89–treated group (RR 0.61; 95% CI 0.48–0.78). The mean number of UTIs was also about 50% lower in the treated group, as compared with placebo. Adverse effects were equally common in the treated and placebo groups, with headaches and GI complaints reported most frequently. The manufacturer of OM-89 funded some of the studies, so results must account for potential funding bias. A more recently conducted meta-analysis of existing studies of OM-89 identified 15 double-blind randomized controlled studies but only included 5 in their analysis because of methodologic flaws with the other 10 studies (Taha Neto et al., 2016). Although analysis of the literature demonstrated a benefit in favor of OM-89, the authors concluded that the studies were of variable quality, demonstrated potential reporting bias, and had short follow-up. They emphasized the need for future high-quality studies with longer follow-up before endorsement of OM-89 for use in prophylaxis is justified.

A vaginal vaccine (Urovac) that works via stimulating IgA and IgG in the urinary tract and subsequently decreasing potential colonization of uropathogens has also been studied (Hopkins et al., 2007). The vaccine contains 10 heat-killed uropathogenic bacterial species, including six serotypes of uropathogenic *E. coli*, *Proteus vulgaris*, *K. pneumoniae*, *Morganella morganii*, and *E. faecalis*. Three trials that included 220 women total were conducted by the same group of investigators. In one trial, primary immunization (three vaginal vaccine suppositories at weekly intervals) was compared with placebo (Uehling et al., 1997); in the other two trials booster immunizations (three additional suppositories at monthly intervals) followed initial primary immunization (Hopkins et al., 2007; Uehling et al., 2003). Women who received the boosters were less likely to develop a UTI. A meta-analysis of these three studies concluded that Urovac slightly reduced recurrent UTI rates (RR 0.81; 95% CI 0.68–0.96) (Beerepoot et al., 2013). More studies with much larger numbers of subjects must be conducted before robust conclusions can be made about Urovac.

In 2019 the AUA released a guideline on evaluation and management of recurrent uncomplicated UTIs in women (American Urological Association, 2019).

> **KEY POINTS: RECURRENT URINARY TRACT INFECTIONS**
>
> - Obtaining a thorough history is critical, with emphasis on prior symptoms, urinalysis and culture results, and triggers for infections.
> - Sources of possible bacterial persistence must be identified and eradicated.
> - Imaging and cystoscopy are NOT recommended for recurrent uncomplicated UTIs.
> - Prevention of recurrence should focus on nonantibiotic interventions.

KIDNEY INFECTIONS

Renal Infection (Bacterial Nephritis)

Although renal infection is less prevalent than bladder infection, it often is a more difficult problem for the patient and his or her physician because of its often varied and morbid presentation and course, the difficulty in establishing a firm microbiologic and pathologic diagnosis, and its potential for significantly impairing renal function. **Although the classic symptoms of acute onset of fever, chills, and flank pain are usually indicative of renal infection, some patients with these symptoms do not have renal infection. Conversely, significant renal infection may be associated with an insidious onset of nonspecific local or systemic symptoms, or it may be entirely asymptomatic.** Therefore a high clinical index of suspicion and appropriate radiologic and laboratory studies are required to establish the diagnosis of renal infection.

Unfortunately, **the relationship between laboratory findings and the presence of renal infection often is poor. Bacteriuria and pyuria, the hallmarks of UTI, are not predictive of renal infection. Conversely, patients with significant renal infection may have sterile urine if the ureter draining the kidney is obstructed or the infection is outside of the collecting system.**

The pathologic and radiologic criteria for diagnosing renal infection may also be misleading. Interstitial renal inflammation, once thought to be caused predominantly by bacterial infection, is now recognized as a nonspecific histopathologic change associated with a variety of immunologic, congenital, or chemical lesions that usually develop in the absence of bacterial infection. Infectious granulomatous diseases of the kidney often have either radiologic or pathologic characteristics that mimic renal cystic disease, neoplasia, or other renal inflammatory disease.

The effect of renal infection on renal function is varied. Acute or chronic pyelonephritis may transiently or permanently alter renal function, but nonobstructive pyelonephritis is no longer recognized as a major cause of renal failure (Baldassarre and Kaye, 1991; Fraser et al., 1995). However, pyelonephritis, when associated with urinary tract obstruction or granulomatous renal infection, may lead rapidly to significant inflammatory complications, renal failure, or even death.

Pathology

The opportunity for pathologic confirmation of **acute bacterial nephritis** is rare. The kidney may be edematous. Focal acute suppurative bacterial nephritis caused by hematogenous dissemination of bacteria to the renal cortex is characterized by multiple focal areas of suppuration on the surface of the kidney (Fig. 55.18). Histologic examination of the renal cortex shows focal suppurative destruction of glomeruli and tubules. Adjacent cortical structures and the medulla are not involved in the inflammatory reaction. **Acute ascending pyelonephritis** is characterized by linear bands of inflammation extending from the medulla to the renal capsule (Fig. 55.19). Histologic examination usually reveals a focal wedge-shaped area of acute interstitial inflammation with the apex of the wedge in the renal medulla. Polymorphonuclear leukocytes or a predominantly lymphocytic and plasma cell response are seen. Bacteria also may be present.

Chapter 55 Infections of the Urinary Tract **1167**

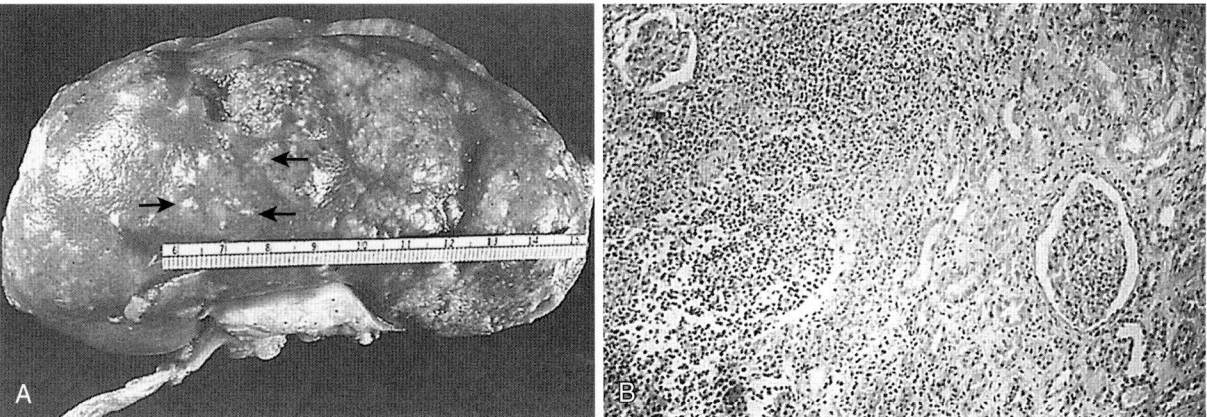

Fig. 55.18. Acute focal suppurative bacterial nephritis. (A) Surface of kidney. *Arrows* indicate focal areas of suppuration. (B) Renal cortex showing focal suppuration destruction of glomeruli and tubules. (From Schaeffer AJ: Urinary tract infections. In Gillenwater JY, Grayhack JT, Howards SS, et al., editors: *Adult and pediatric urology*, Philadelphia, 2002, Lippincott Williams & Wilkins, pp 211–272.)

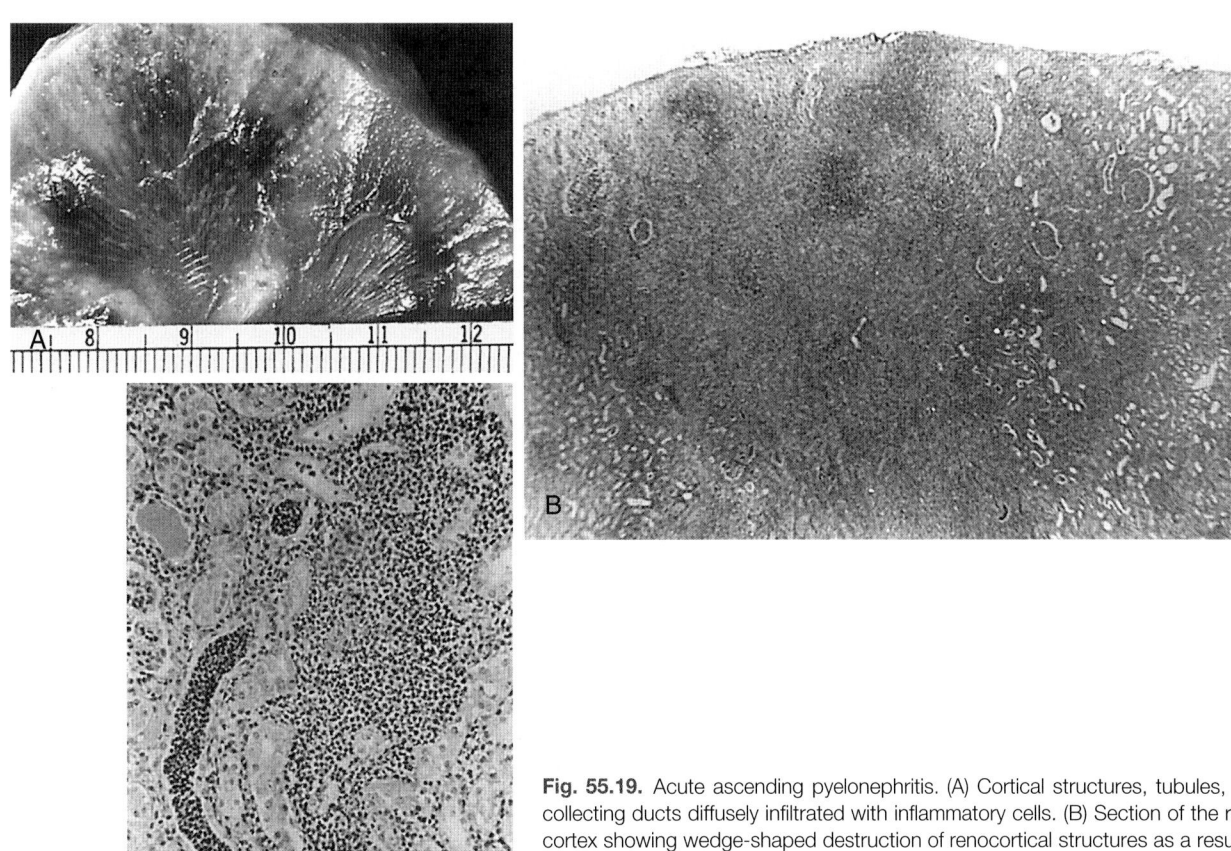

Fig. 55.19. Acute ascending pyelonephritis. (A) Cortical structures, tubules, and collecting ducts diffusely infiltrated with inflammatory cells. (B) Section of the renal cortex showing wedge-shaped destruction of renocortical structures as a result of ascending infiltration with inflammatory cells. (C) Thickened and inflamed tissue surrounding the collecting ducts in the medulla. A polymorphonuclear cast of segmented neutrophils is clearly visible. (From Schaeffer AJ: Urinary tract infections. In Gillenwater JY, Grayhack JT, Howards SS, et al., editors: *Adult and pediatric urology*, Philadelphia, 2002, Lippincott Williams & Wilkins, pp 211–272.)

The changes that appear to be most specific for **chronic pyelonephritis** are evident on careful gross examination of the kidney and consist of a cortical scar associated with retraction of the corresponding renal papilla (Freedman, 1979; Heptinstall, 1974; Hodson, 1965; Hodson and Wilson, 1965). The kidney shows evidence of patchy involvement with numerous chronic inflammatory foci mainly confined to the cortex but also involving the medulla (Fig. 55.20).

The scars may be separated by intervening zones of normal parenchyma, causing a grossly irregular renal outline. The microscopic appearance, as with most chronic interstitial disease, includes the presence of lymphocytes and plasma cells. Although glomeruli within scars may be surrounded by a cuff of fibrosis or be partially or completely hyalinized, glomeruli outside these severely scarred zones are relatively normal. Vascular involvement is variable, but in patients with hypertension, nephrosclerosis may be found. Papillary abnormalities include deformity, sclerosis, and sometimes necrosis. Studies in animals have clearly indicated the critical role of the papilla in the initiation of pyelonephritis (Freedman and Beeson, 1958). However,

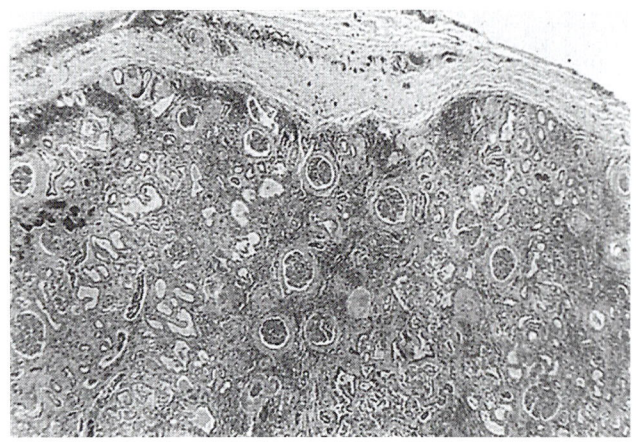

Fig. 55.20. Chronic pyelonephritis. The renal cortex shows thickened fibrous capsule and focal retracted scar on surface of kidney. Focal destruction of tubules in center of picture is accompanied by periglomerular fibrosis and scarring. (From Schaeffer AJ: Urinary tract infections. In Gillenwater JY, Grayhack JT, Howards SS, et al., editors: *Adult and pediatric urology*, Philadelphia, 2002, Lippincott Williams & Wilkins, pp 211–272.)

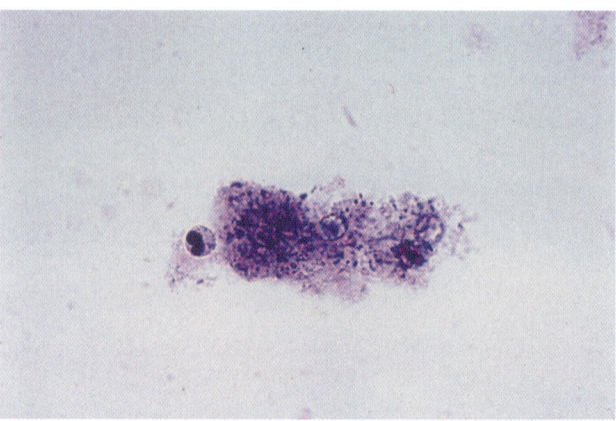

Fig. 55.21. Brightfield micrograph of a mixed bacterial leukocyte cast from patient with acute pyelonephritis. Only the bacteria and the nucleus of a leukocyte stain strongly. Many bacteria are clearly demonstrated by through-focusing (toluidine blue O stain, magnification ×640). (Modified from Lindner LE, Jones RN, Haber MH: A specific urinary cast in acute pyelonephritis. *Am J Clin Pathol* 73:809–811, 1980.)

these changes are not necessarily specific for bacterial infection and may occur in the absence of infection as a result of other disorders such as analgesic abuse, diabetes, and sickle cell disease.

Acute Pyelonephritis

Although pyelonephritis is defined as inflammation of the kidney and renal pelvis, the diagnosis is clinical. True infection of the "upper urinary tract" can be proved by catheterization tests (ureteral catheterization or bladder washout) as described in this chapter, but these are impractical and unnecessary in most patients with acute pyelonephritis. None of the noninvasive tests that have been developed to determine infection in the kidney or bladder are totally reliable.

Clinical Presentation. The clinical spectrum ranges from gram-negative sepsis to cystitis with mild flank pain (Stamm and Hooton, 1993). **The classic presentation is an abrupt onset of chills, fever (100.3°F or greater), and unilateral or bilateral flank or costovertebral angle pain and/or tenderness. These so-called upper tract signs are sometimes accompanied by dysuria, increased urinary frequency, and urgency, but in many cases lower urinary symptoms are not present.**

Although some authors regard loin pain and fever in combination with significant bacteriuria as diagnostic of acute pyelonephritis, it is clear from localization studies using ureteral catheterization (Stamey and Pfau, 1963) or the bladder washout technique (Fairley et al., 1967) that **clinical symptoms correlate poorly with the site of infection** (Eykyn et al., 1972; Fairley, 1972; Smeets and Gower, 1973; Stamey et al., 1965).

On physical examination, there often is tenderness to deep palpation in the costovertebral angle. Variations of this clinical presentation have been recognized. Acute pyelonephritis may also simulate GI tract abnormalities with abdominal pain, nausea, vomiting, and diarrhea. Asymptomatic progression of acute pyelonephritis to chronic pyelonephritis, particularly in compromised hosts, may occur in the absence of overt symptoms. Acute renal failure may be present in the rare case (Olsson et al., 1980; Richet and Mayaud, 1978).

Laboratory Diagnosis. The patient may have leukocytosis with a predominance of neutrophils. **Urinalysis usually reveals numerous WBCs, often in clumps, and bacterial rods or chains of cocci. The presence of large amounts of granular or leukocyte casts in the urinary sediment is suggestive of acute pyelonephritis.** A specific type of urinary cast characterized by the presence of bacteria in its matrix has been demonstrated in the urine of patients who have had acute pyelonephritis (Fig. 55.21; Lindner et al., 1980). Blood tests may show leukocytosis with a predominance of neutrophils, increased erythrocyte sedimentation rate, elevated C-reactive protein levels, and elevated creatinine levels if renal failure is present. In addition, creatinine clearance may be decreased. Blood cultures may be positive.

Bacteriology. Urine cultures are positive, but about 20% of patients have urine cultures with fewer than 10^5 CFU/mL and therefore negative results on Gram staining of the urine (Rubin et al., 1992).

E. coli, **which constitutes a unique subgroup that possesses special virulence factors, accounts for 80% of cases.** If VUR is absent, a patient bearing the P blood group phenotype may have special susceptibility to recurrent pyelonephritis caused by *E. coli* that have P pili and bind to the P blood group antigen receptors (Lomberg et al., 1983). Bacterial K antigens and endotoxins also may contribute to pathogenicity (Kaijser et al., 1977). Many cases of community-acquired pyelonephritis are caused by a limited number of multiantimicrobial-resistant clonal groups (Manges et al., 2004).

More resistant species, such as *Proteus, Klebsiella, Pseudomonas, Serratia, Enterobacter,* or *Citrobacter,* should be suspected in patients who have recurrent UTIs, are hospitalized, or have indwelling catheters, as well as in those who required recent urinary tract instrumentation. Except for *E. faecalis, S. epidermidis,* and *S. aureus,* gram-positive bacteria rarely cause pyelonephritis.

Blood cultures are positive in about 25% of cases of uncomplicated pyelonephritis in women, and the majority replicate the urine culture and do not influence decisions regarding therapy. Therefore blood cultures should not be routinely obtained for the evaluation of uncomplicated pyelonephritis in women. **However, they should be performed in men and women with systemic toxicity or in those requiring hospitalization or with risk factors such as pregnancy** (Velasco et al., 2003).

Renal Ultrasonography, Computed Tomography, and Magnetic Resonance Imaging. Ultrasound may show focal parenchymal swelling and regions of increased or decreased echogenicity (Fig. 55.22). CT and MRI also may show focal swelling and diminished and inhomogeneous parenchymal contrast enhancement (Fig. 55.23). Without contrast, CT may show diminished density of affected areas and MRI may show regions of restricted diffusion. Acute pyelonephritis may cause chronic renal scarring; however, radiographic changes usually resolve; therefore future renal imaging will show a normal-appearing kidney.

Differential Diagnosis. **Acute appendicitis, diverticulitis, and pancreatitis can cause a similar degree of pain, but the location of the pain often is different.** Results of the urine examination are usually normal. Herpes zoster can cause superficial pain in the region of the kidney but is not associated with symptoms of UTI; the diagnosis will be apparent when shingles appear.

Management

Initial Management. Infection in patients with acute pyelonephritis can be subdivided into (1) uncomplicated infection that does not warrant hospitalization, (2) uncomplicated infection in patients with normal urinary tracts who are ill enough to warrant hospitalization for parenteral therapy, and (3) complicated infection associated with hospitalization, catheterization, urologic surgery, or urinary tract abnormalities (Fig. 55.24).

It is critical to determine whether the patient has an uncomplicated or complicated UTI because significant abnormalities have been found in 16% of patients with acute pyelonephritis (Shen and Brown, 2004). In patients with presumed uncomplicated pyelonephritis who will be managed as outpatients, initial radiologic evaluation can usually be deferred. However, if there is any reason to suspect a problem or if the patient will not have reasonable access to imaging if there should be no change in condition, we prefer renal ultrasonography to rule out stones or obstruction. In patients with known or suspected complicated pyelonephritis, CT provides excellent assessment of the status of the urinary tract and the severity and extent of the infection.

Oral ciprofloxacin (500 mg twice daily) for 7 days is an appropriate first-line therapy in patients not requiring hospitalization where the prevalence of uropathogen resistance to quinolones in the community does not exceed 10%, as per the IDSA guidelines on management

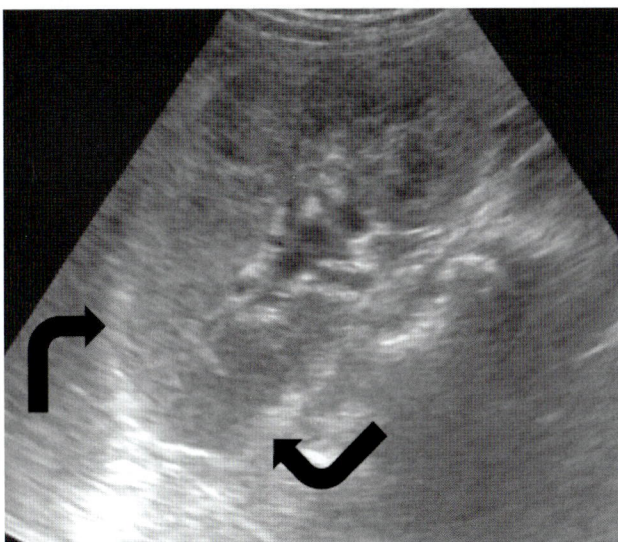

Fig. 55.22. Ultrasound of acute pyelonephritis. *Arrows* show abnormally echogenic and swollen upper pole.

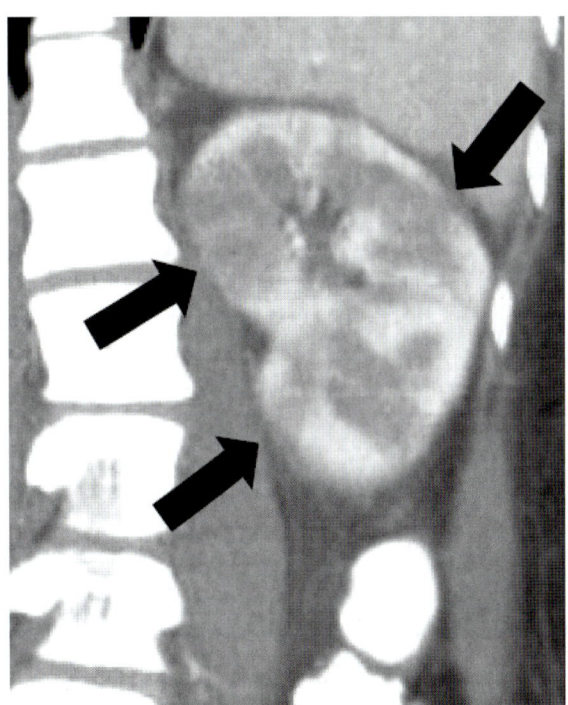

Fig. 55.23. Computed tomography of focal pyelonephritis. *Arrows* show patchy regions of diminished heterogeneous enhancement and swelling.

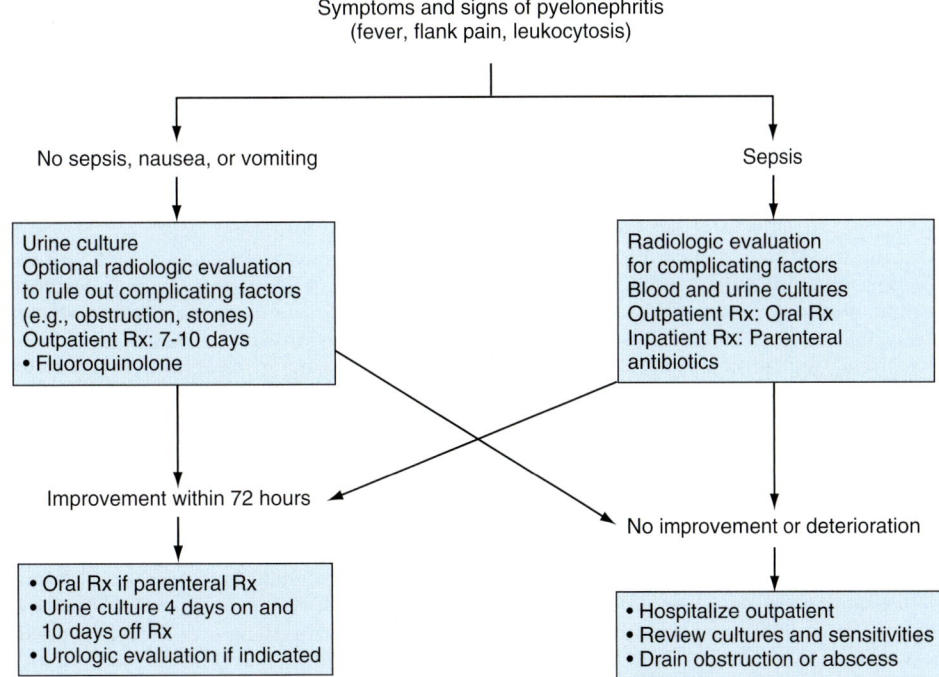

Fig. 55.24. Management of acute pyelonephritis.

TABLE 55.11 Treatment Regimens for Acute Complicated and Uncomplicated Pyelonephritis in Women

CIRCUMSTANCES	ROUTE	DRUG	DOSAGE[e]	FREQUENCY PER DOSE	DURATION (DAYS)
Outpatient—moderately ill, no nausea or vomiting	Oral[a]	TMP-SMX DS[b]	160–800 mg	q12h	14
		Ciprofloxacin[c]	500 mg	q12h	7
		Ciprofloxacin[c] (extended release)	1000 mg	q24h	7
		Levofloxacin[c]	750 mg	q24h	5
Inpatient—severely ill, possible sepsis	Parenteral[d]	Ampicillin and gentamicin	1–2 g 1–1.5 mg/kg	q6h q8h	10–14
		Levofloxacin[c]	500–750 mg	q24h	10–14
		Ceftriaxone	1 g	q24h	10–14
		Carbapenem	(dosage varies)		10–14
Pregnant	Parenteral[d]	Ampicillin and gentamicin	1–2 g 1–1.5 mg/kg	q6h q8h	10–14
		Aztreonam	1 g	q8h	10–14
	Oral	Cephalexin	500 mg	q6h	

DS, Double strength; TMP-SMX, trimethoprim-sulfamethoxazole.
[a]May be given with an initial 1-time intravenous dose of a long-acting parenteral antimicrobial such as 1 g of ceftriaxone or a consolidated 24-hour dose of an aminoglycoside. See IDSA recommendations.
[b]Appropriate choice if uropathogen is known to be susceptible. If susceptibility is unknown, an initial dose of long-acting parenteral antimicrobial such as 1 g of ceftriaxone or a consolidated 24-hour dose of an aminoglycoside is recommended.
[c]May be used in areas where the prevalence of resistance of community uropathogens to fluoroquinolones is not known to exceed 10%.
[d]For parenteral agents, take until afebrile then transition to oral agents according to sensitivities.
[e]All dosages should be adjusted for renal function.

of acute pyelonephritis (Gupta et al., 2011). If an initial one-time parenteral dose of antibiosis is chosen, a long-acting agent such as 1 g of ceftriaxone or a consolidated 24-hour dose of an aminoglycoside can be used as an alternative to an intravenous fluoroquinolone (Gupta et al., 2011). Once-daily oral fluoroquinolones, such as ciprofloxacin 1000 mg extended release for 7 days or levofloxacin 750 mg for 5 days, are also reasonable alternatives in non-hospitalized patients in whom resistance patterns in the community are low (Gupta et al., 2011). Oral TMP-SMX (160/800 mg [1 double-strength tablet] twice daily for 14 days) is an appropriate agent if the organism is known to be sensitive; if the susceptibility is unknown, an initial intravenous dose of a long-acting parenteral antibiotic, such as 1 g ceftriaxone or a consolidated 24-hour dose of an aminoglycoside is recommended (Gupta et al., 2011; Talan et al., 2000) (Table 55.11). As mentioned in previous sections, with the emerging resistance and potential for collateral damage associated with quinolones, future guidelines will likely need to address the role of cephalosporins for outpatient treatment of pyelonephritis.

If a patient has an uncomplicated infection but is sufficiently ill to require hospitalization (high fever, high WBC count, vomiting, dehydration, evidence of sepsis), has complicated pyelonephritis, or fails to improve during the initial outpatient treatment period, a parenteral antibiotic is recommended. In women with pyelonephritis requiring hospital admission, recent IDSA guidelines recommend an intravenous regimen such as a fluoroquinolone, an aminoglycoside with or without ampicillin, an extended-spectrum cephalosporin with or without an aminoglycoside, or a carbapenem (Gupta et al., 2011; Warren et al., 1999). If gram-positive cocci are causative, ampicillin/sulbactam with or without an aminoglycoside is recommended.

Hospitalization, IV fluids, and antipyretics are required.
Overall kidney function is not affected in the presence of unilateral obstruction. **However, a solitary obstructed kidney causes acute renal failure; antimicrobial agents are dosed based on the GFR. Any substantial obstruction must be relieved expediently by the safest and simplest means, such as ureteral stent or percutaneous nephrostomy tube placement.**

A Gram stain of the urine sediment is helpful to guide the selection of the initial empirical antimicrobial therapy. In all cases, antimicrobial therapy should be active against potential uropathogens and achieve antimicrobial levels in renal tissue and urine.

Subsequent Management. Even though the urine usually becomes sterile within a few hours of starting antimicrobial therapy, patients with acute uncomplicated pyelonephritis may continue to have fever, chills, and flank pain for several more days after initiation of successful antimicrobial therapy (Behr et al., 1996). They should be observed.

Alterations in antimicrobial therapy may be made depending on the patient's clinical response and the results of the culture and susceptibility tests. Susceptibility tests should also be used to replace potentially toxic drugs, such as aminoglycosides, with less toxic drugs, such as aztreonam and cephalosporins.

Patients with complicated pyelonephritis and positive blood cultures should be treated with parenteral therapy until clinically stable. If blood cultures are negative, 2- to 3-day parenteral therapy is sufficient. After parenteral therapy, an appropriate oral antimicrobial drug (fluoroquinolone, TMP, TMP-SMX, or amoxicillin or amoxicillin/clavulanic acid for gram-positive organisms) should be continued in full dosage for an additional 10 to 14 days.

Unfavorable Response to Therapy. When the response to therapy is slow or the urine continues to show infection, an immediate reevaluation is mandatory. Urine and blood cultures must be repeated and appropriate alterations in antimicrobial therapy made on the basis of susceptibility testing. CT is indicated to attempt to identify unsuspected obstructive uropathy, abscess formation, urolithiasis, or underlying anatomic abnormalities that may have predisposed the patient to infection, prevented a rapid therapeutic response, or caused complications of the infectious process, such as renal or perinephric abscess. **In patients with fever lasting longer than 72 hours, CT is most helpful for ruling out obstruction and identifying renal and perirenal infections** (Soulen et al., 1989). Radionuclide imaging may be useful to demonstrate functional changes associated with acute pyelonephritis (decrease in renal blood flow, delay in peak function, and delay in excretion of the radionuclide) (Fischman and Roberts, 1982) and cortical defects associated with VUR.

Follow-Up. Depending on the clinical presentation and response and initial urologic evaluation, some patients may require additional evaluation (e.g., VCUG, cystoscopy, bacterial localization studies) and correction of an underlying abnormality of the urinary tract. Raz et al. (2003) evaluated the long-term impact of acute pyelonephritis in women. Scanning with ^{99m}Tc-dimercaptosuccinic acid (^{99m}Tc-DMSA) 10 to 20 years after acute pyelonephritis revealed scars in approximately 50% of the patients, but changes in renal function were minimal and not associated with renal scarring.

Information on bacterial nephritis is available online at Expert Consult.com.

Emphysematous Pyelonephritis

Emphysematous pyelonephritis is a urologic emergency characterized by an acute necrotizing parenchymal and perirenal infection caused by gas-forming uropathogens. The pathogenesis is poorly understood. Because the condition usually occurs in patients with diabetes, it has been postulated that the high tissue glucose levels provide the substrate for microorganisms such as *E. coli*, which are able to produce carbon dioxide by the fermentation of sugar (Schainuck et al., 1968). Although glucose fermentation may be a factor, the explanation does not account for the rarity of emphysematous pyelonephritis despite the high frequency of gram-negative UTI in patients with diabetes, nor does it explain the rare occurrence of the condition in nondiabetic patients.

In addition to diabetes, many patients have urinary tract obstruction associated with urinary calculi or papillary necrosis and significant renal functional impairment. The overall mortality rate has been reported to be between 19% (Huang and Tseng, 2000) and 43% (Freiha et al., 1979).

Clinical Presentation. Nearly all of the documented cases of emphysematous pyelonephritis have occurred in adults (Hawes et al., 1983). Juvenile patients with diabetes do not appear to be at risk. Women are affected more often than men.

The usual clinical presentation is severe, acute pyelonephritis, although in some instances a chronic infection precedes the acute attack. Almost all patients display the classic triad of fever, vomiting, and flank pain (Schainuck et al., 1968). Emphysematous pyelonephritis affects predominantly female patients with diabetes and can occur in insulin-dependent and non–insulin-dependent patients in the absence of ureteral obstruction. Patients without diabetes can also develop this form of pyelonephritis but often have ureteric obstruction and do not seem to develop extensive disease (Pontin and Barnes, 2009). Pneumaturia is absent unless the infection involves the collecting system. Results of urine cultures are invariably positive. *E. coli* is most commonly identified. *Klebsiella* and *Proteus* spp. are less common.

Radiologic Findings. The diagnosis is established radiographically. Tissue gas that is distributed in the parenchyma may appear on abdominal radiographs as mottled gas shadows over the involved kidney (Fig. 55.26). This finding is often mistaken for bowel gas. A crescentic collection of gas over the upper pole of the kidney is more distinctive. As the infection progresses, gas extends to the perinephric space and retroperitoneum. This distribution of gas should not be confused with cases of emphysematous pyelitis in which air is in the collecting system of the kidney. Emphysematous pyelitis is secondary to a gas-forming bacterial UTI, often occurs in patients without diabetes, is less serious, and usually responds to antimicrobial therapy.

Ultrasonography usually demonstrates strong focal echoes suggesting the presence of intraparenchymal gas (Brenbridge et al., 1979; Conrad et al., 1979). **CT is the imaging procedure of choice in defining the extent of the emphysematous process and guiding management** (Fig. 55.27). **An absence of fluid in CT images or the presence of streaky or mottled gas with or without bubbly and loculated gas appears to be associated with rapid destruction of renal parenchyma and a 50% to 60% mortality rate** (Best et al., 1999; Wan et al., 1996). The presence of renal or perirenal fluid, the presence of bubbly or loculated gas or gas in the collecting system, and the absence of streaky or mottled gas patterns are associated with a less than 20% mortality rate.

In line with these observations, in 2000, Huang and Tseng developed a radiologic classification system based on the extent of gas involvement in the renal tissue on CT scan that has been used to help guide management; the system uses a four-category system that grades

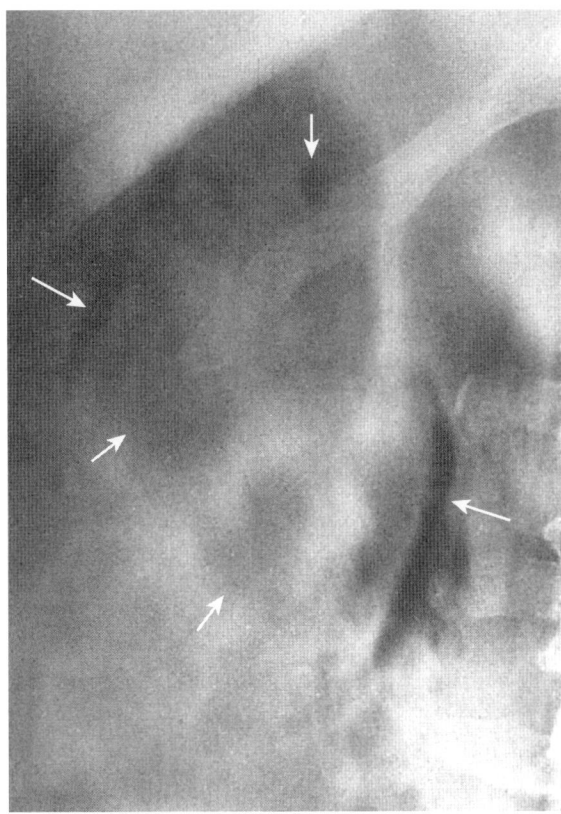

Fig. 55.26. Emphysematous pyelonephritis; plain film. Extensive perinephric *(long arrows)* and intraparenchymal *(short arrows)* gas secondary to acute bacterial pyelonephritis. (From Schaeffer AJ: Urinary tract infections. In Gillenwater JY, Grayhack JT, Howards SS, et al., editors: *Adult and pediatric urology*, Philadelphia, 2002, Lippincott William & Wilkins, pp 211–272.)

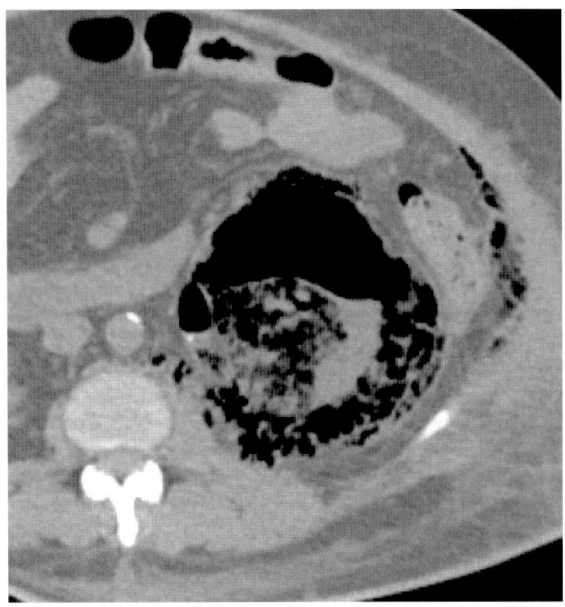

Fig. 55.27. Computed tomography of emphysematous pyelonephritis. There is air within and surrounding the left kidney.

progressively more gas involvement with the renal and adjacent renal tissue with ascension through the classes (Huang, 2000).

Obstruction is demonstrated in approximately 25% of the cases. A nuclear renal scan should be performed to assess the degree of renal function impairment in the involved kidney and the status of the contralateral kidney.

Management. Emphysematous pyelonephritis is a urologic emergency. Most patients are septic, and fluid resuscitation, glucose and electrolyte management, and broad-spectrum antimicrobial therapy are essential. Ureteral obstruction, if present, is alleviated by a percutaneous nephrostomy tube or a stent (Pontin and Barnes, 2009). Hypoalbuminemia, shock at initial presentation, bacteremia, indications for hemodialysis, thrombocytopenia, altered mental status, and polymicrobial infection are among various prognostic risk factors that have been associated with increased mortality in different outcomes studies involving emphysematous pyelonephritis patients (Huang and Tseng, 2000; Lu et al., 2014). Treatment has evolved over the years from nephrectomy to more conservative management with percutaneous catheter drainage or the use of a double-J ureteral stent depending on the severity of presentation. Until the late 1980s, management involved emergency nephrectomy with or without open surgical drainage and antibiosis, although this management was still associated with a mortality rate of 40% to 50% (Ahlering et al., 1985; Michaeli et al., 1984). Since this time, the overall mortality rate has decreased with advancements in medicine, and **definitive management is by percutaneous drainage, except in cases of extensive diffuse gas with renal destruction; in this latter scenario, nephrectomy is advised** (Huang and Tseng, 2000; Pontin and Barnes, 2009). Early diagnosis and treatment of patients with diabetes and urinary infection is important to potentially avoid progression of this disease process and in turn nephrectomy (Pontin and Barnes, 2009).

Renal Abscess

Renal abscess or carbuncle is a collection of purulent material confined to the renal parenchyma. Before the antimicrobial era, 80% of renal abscesses were attributed to hematogenous seeding by staphylococci (Campbell, 1930). In addition, historically, patients with abscesses were young men with no prior renal disease. Although experimental and clinical data document the facility for abscess formation in normal kidneys after hematogenous inoculation with staphylococci, widespread use of antimicrobial agents since about 1950 appears to have diminished the propensity for gram-positive abscess formation (Cotran, 1969; DeNavasquez, 1950). The current index patient typically has a history of renal disease or obstruction, no gender predominance, and no laterality, and the infection is typically with a gram-negative organism.

Since about 1970, gram-negative organisms have been implicated in the majority of adults with renal abscesses. The most common organisms include *E. coli, Klebsiella, Proteus,* and *Pseudomonas* spp. (Fowler and Perkins, 1994; Shu et al., 2004). Hematogenous renal seeding by gram-negative organisms may occur, but this is not likely to be the primary pathway for gram-negative abscess formation. Clinically, there is no evidence that gram-negative septicemia antedates most lesions. Further, gram-negative hematogenous pyelonephritis is almost impossible to produce in animals unless the kidney is traumatized or completely obstructed (Cotran, 1969; Timmons and Perlmutter, 1976). Like the normal kidney, the partially obstructed kidney rejects blood-borne gram-negative inocula. Thus ascending infection associated with tubular obstruction from prior infections or calculi appears to be the primary pathway for the establishment of gram-negative abscesses. Two-thirds of gram-negative abscesses in adults are associated with renal calculi or damaged kidneys (Salvatierra et al., 1967; Siegel et al., 1996). Although the association of pyelonephritis with VUR is well established, the association of renal abscess with VUR has been infrequently noted (Segura and Kelalis, 1973). Case reports in the pediatric literature exist, but literature within the adult population is sparse. More recent observations, however, indicate that reflux is frequently associated with renal abscesses and persists long after sterilization of the urinary tract (Anderson and McAninch, 1980; Timmons and Perlmutter, 1976). Renal abscesses are also associated with IV drug abuse.

Clinical Presentation. The patient may present with fever, chills, abdominal or flank pain, and occasionally weight loss and malaise. Symptoms of cystitis may occur. Occasionally, these symptoms may be vague and delay diagnosis until surgical exploration or, in more severe cases, autopsy (Anderson and McAninch, 1980). A thorough history may reveal a gram-positive source of infection 1 to 8 weeks before the onset of urinary tract symptoms or symptoms consistent with UTI or pyelonephritis in the weeks prior (Hung et al., 2007). **The infection may have occurred in any area of the body.** Multiple skin carbuncles and IV drug abuse introduce gram-positive organisms into the bloodstream. Other common sites are the mouth, lungs, and bladder (Lyons et al., 1972). Complicated UTIs associated with stasis, calculi, pregnancy, neurogenic bladder, and diabetes mellitus also appear to predispose the patient to abscess formation (Anderson and McAninch, 1980).

Shu et al. (2004) published their experience with 26 cases of renal/perirenal abscesses with anatomically normal GU tracts, and no stones or prior urologic manipulation. In 24 of the 26 cases, the patients had at least 1 predisposing factor (diabetes mellitus, HIV, steroid use, IV drug abuse, liver disease, UTI, pregnancy). Diabetes mellitus is noted to be a very significant risk factor for development of renal abscesses, as is increased length of hospitalization (Ko et al., 2011, 2013).

Laboratory Diagnosis. The patient typically has marked leukocytosis. In a series by Siegel et al. (1996) of 52 patients, blood cultures were positive 28% of the time, whereas Yen et al. (1999) published a series of 78 patients, 25 of which (32%) had positive blood cultures. In comparison of positive cultures in all three types of fluids (abscess, blood, urine) only 1 patient of the 78 had identical isolates in all three. Urine and abscess culture had a 15% identical culture rate, whereas blood and abscess had a 13% identical culture rate (Yen et al., 1999). Pyuria and bacteriuria may not be evident unless the abscess communicates with the collecting system. **Because gram-positive organisms are most commonly blood-borne, urine cultures in these cases typically show no growth or a microorganism different from that isolated from the abscess.** Another study showed not only a bacteremia rate of 26% but also that positive urine cultures were only present in roughly 30% of patients (Shu et al., 2004).

Ultrasonography and CT distinguish abscess from other inflammatory renal diseases. **Ultrasonography is the quickest and least expensive method to demonstrate a renal abscess. An echo-free or low-echodensity space-occupying lesion with increased transmission is found on the ultrasound image** (Fig. 55.28). The margins of an abscess are indistinguishable in the acute phase, but the structure contains a few echoes and the surrounding renal parenchyma is edematous (Fiegler, 1983). Subsequently, the appearance tends to be that of a well-defined mass. The internal appearance, however, may vary from a virtually solid lucent mass to one with large numbers of low-level internal echoes (Schneider et al., 1976). The number of echoes depends on the amount of cellular debris within the abscess. The presence of air results in a strong echo with a shadow.

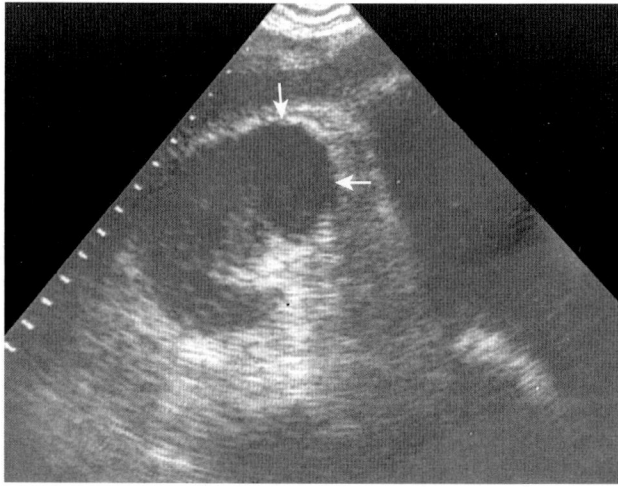

Fig. 55.28. Acute renal abscess. Transverse ultrasound image of the right kidney demonstrates a poorly marginated rounded focal hypoechoic mass *(arrows)* in the anterior portion of the kidney.

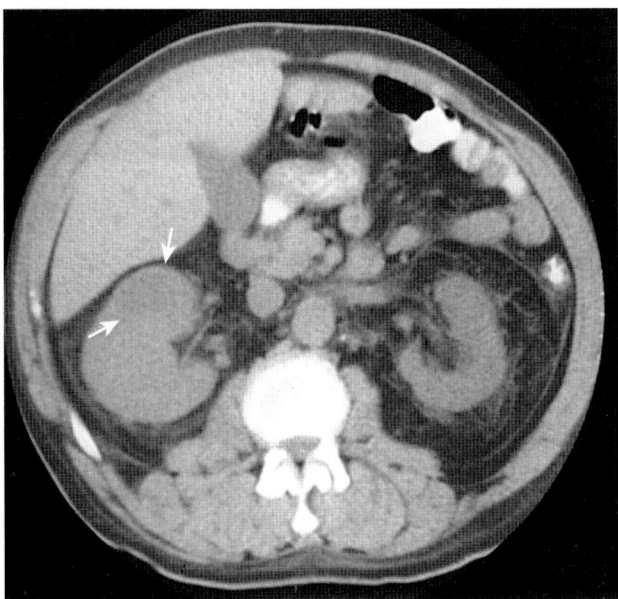

Fig. 55.29. Acute renal abscess. Nonenhanced computed tomography scan through the mid pole of the right kidney demonstrates right renal enlargement and an area of decreased attenuation *(arrows)*. After antimicrobial therapy, a follow-up scan showed complete regression of these findings.

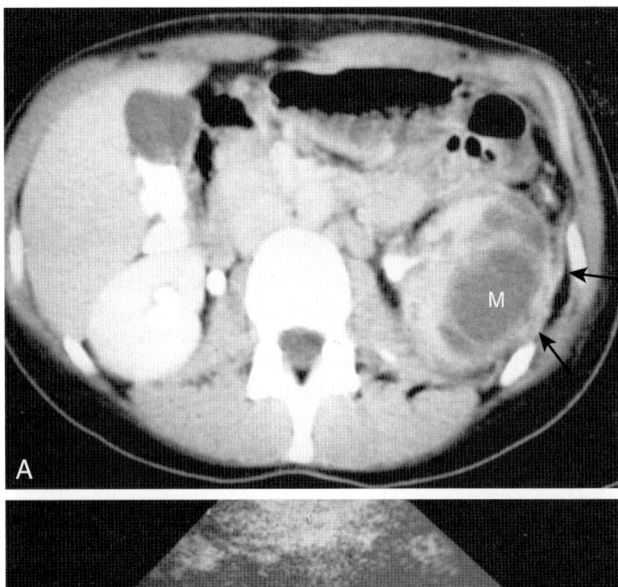

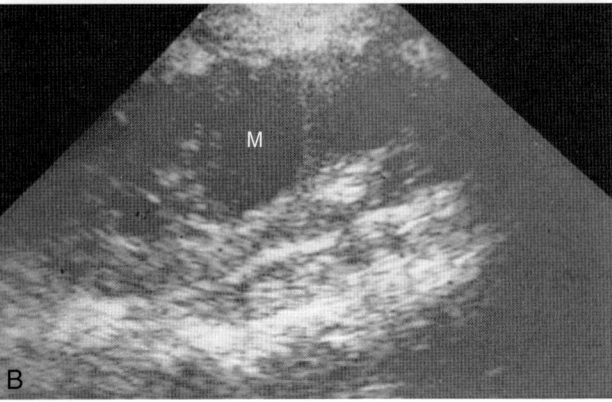

Fig. 55.30. Chronic renal abscess. (A) Enhanced computed tomography scan shows an irregular septated low-density mass *(M)* extensively involving the left kidney. Note thickening of perinephric fascia *(arrows)* and extensive compression of the renal collecting system. Findings are typical of renal abscess. (B) Ultrasound longitudinal image demonstrates a septated hypoechoic mass *(M)* occupying much of the renal parenchymal volume.

Differentiation between an abscess and a tumor is impossible in many cases. Arteriography is used infrequently to demonstrate abscesses. The center of the mass tends to be hypervascular or avascular, with increased vascularity at the cortical margins and lack of vascular displacement and neovascularity.

CT appears to be the diagnostic procedure of choice for renal abscesses because it provides excellent delineation of the tissue. On CT, abscesses are characteristically well defined before and after contrast agent enhancement. The findings depend in part on the age and severity of the abscess (Baumgarten and Baumgartner, 1997). Initially, CT shows renal enlargement and focal, rounded areas of decreased attenuation (Fig. 55.29). After several days of the onset of the infection, a thick fibrotic wall begins to form around the abscess. An echo-free or slightly echogenic mass caused by the presence of necrotic debris is seen. CT of a chronic abscess shows obliteration of adjacent tissue planes, thickening of the Gerota fascia, a round or oval parenchymal mass of low attenuation, and a surrounding inflammatory wall of slightly higher attenuation that forms a ring when the scan is enhanced with contrast material (Fig. 55.30). The ring sign is caused by the increased vascularity of the abscess wall (Callen, 1979; Gerzof and Gale, 1982).

Radionuclide imaging with gallium or indium is sometimes useful in evaluating patients with renal abscesses (see previous sections).

Management. Although the classic treatment for an abscess has been percutaneous or open incision and drainage, there is good evidence that use of IV antimicrobial agents and careful observation of a small abscess less than 3 cm or even 5 cm in a clinically stable patient is appropriate. Antibiotics, if begun early enough in the course of the process, may obviate surgical procedures (Hoverman et al., 1980; Levin et al., 1984; Shu et al., 2004). CT- or ultrasound-guided needle aspiration may be necessary to differentiate an abscess from a hypervascular tumor. Aspirated material should be cultured and appropriate antimicrobial therapy instituted on the basis of the findings.

All patients should be immediately started on IV antibiotic therapy. The selection of empirical antimicrobial therapy is dependent on the presumed source of the infection and the resistance patterns within the hospital. When hematogenous dissemination is suspected, the pathogenic organism most frequently is penicillin-resistant *Staphylococcus,* and the antimicrobial of choice therefore is a penicillinase-resistant penicillin (Schiff et al., 1977). If a history of penicillin hypersensitivity is present, the recommended drug is vancomycin. Cortical abscesses that occur in the abnormal urinary tract are associated with more typical gram-negative pathogens secondary to ascending infection and should be treated empirically with IV third-generation cephalosporins, antipseudomonal penicillins, or aminoglycosides until specific therapy can be instituted. Patients should have serial examinations with ultrasonography or CT until the abscess resolves. The radiographic evolution or resolution of the abscesses typically further dictates clinical management. The suspicion of misdiagnosis or an uncontrolled infection with the development of perinephric abscess or infection with an organism resistant to the antimicrobial agents used in therapy should be suspected with worsening clinical picture.

After patients are started on IV antibiotic therapy and there is radiographic confirmation of abscess, the size of the abscess typically dictates management. Abscesses 3 cm or less can be managed with antibiotics alone (Lee et al., 2010; Shu et al., 2004; Siegel et al., 1996). In a series from South Korea of 49 patients with normal urinary tracts and abscesses smaller than 5 cm, there was 100% resolution of abscesses confirmed with CT scan with antibiotics alone (Lee et al., 2010).

Although fewer data exist for patients with obstruction or anomalous urinary tracts, **abscesses 3 to 5 cm in diameter should be conservatively managed initially in the setting of stable clinical parameters.** We suggest following the clinical course and size of the abscess radiographically to assess for improvement. Should the patient progress, percutaneous drainage should be considered. Abscesses of all sizes in immunocompromised hosts or those that do not respond to antimicrobial therapy should be drained percutaneously (Fernandez et al., 1985; Fowler and Perkins, 1994; Siegel et al., 1996). **However, percutaneous drainage remains the first-line procedure of choice for most renal abscesses larger than 5 cm in diameter.** Typically, abscesses of this size require multiple drains, multiple drain manipulations, or eventual surgical washout and potential nephrectomy (Siegel et al., 1996).

Infected Hydronephrosis and Pyonephrosis

Infected hydronephrosis is bacterial infection in a hydronephrotic kidney. The term *pyonephrosis* refers to infected hydronephrosis associated with suppurative destruction of the parenchyma of the kidney, in which there is total or nearly total loss of renal function (Fig. 55.31). Where infected hydronephrosis ends and pyonephrosis begins is difficult to determine clinically. Rapid diagnosis and treatment of pyonephrosis are essential to avoid permanent loss of renal function and to prevent sepsis.

Clinical Presentation. The patient is usually very ill, with high fever, chills, flank pain, and tenderness. Occasionally, however, a patient may have only an elevated temperature and a complaint of vague gastrointestinal discomfort. A previous history of urinary tract calculi, infection, or surgery is common. **Bacteriuria may not be present if the ureter is completely obstructed.**

Radiologic Findings. The ultrasonographic diagnosis of infected hydronephrosis depends on demonstration of internal echoes within the dependent portion of a dilated pyelocalyceal system. CT is nonspecific but may show thickening of the renal pelvis, stranding of the perirenal fat, and a striated nephrogram. Ultrasonography demonstrates hydronephrosis and fluid debris levels within the dilated collecting system (Corriere and Sandler, 1982; Fig. 55.32A). The diagnosis of pyonephrosis is suggested if focal areas of decreased echogenicity are seen within the hydronephrotic parenchyma.

Management. Once the diagnosis of pyonephrosis is made, the treatment is initiated with appropriate antimicrobial drugs and drainage of the infected pelvis. A ureteral catheter can be passed to drain the kidney, but if the obstruction prevents this, a percutaneous nephrostomy tube should be placed (Camunez et al., 1989; Fig. 55.32B). When the patient becomes hemodynamically stable, other procedures are usually needed to identify and treat the source of the obstruction.

Perinephric Abscess

A perinephric abscess extends beyond the renal capsule but is contained by Gerota fascia and **usually results from rupture of an acute cortical abscess into the perinephric space,** extravasated infected urine from obstruction, **or from hematogenous seeding from sites of infection.** Patients with pyonephrosis, particularly when a calculus is present in the kidney, are susceptible to perinephric abscess formation. **Diabetes mellitus is present in approximately one-third of patients with perinephric abscess** (Edelstein and McCabe, 1988; Meng et al., 2002). **In about one-third of the cases, perinephric abscess is caused by hematogenous spread, usually from sites of skin infection** (Gardiner et al., 2011). A perirenal

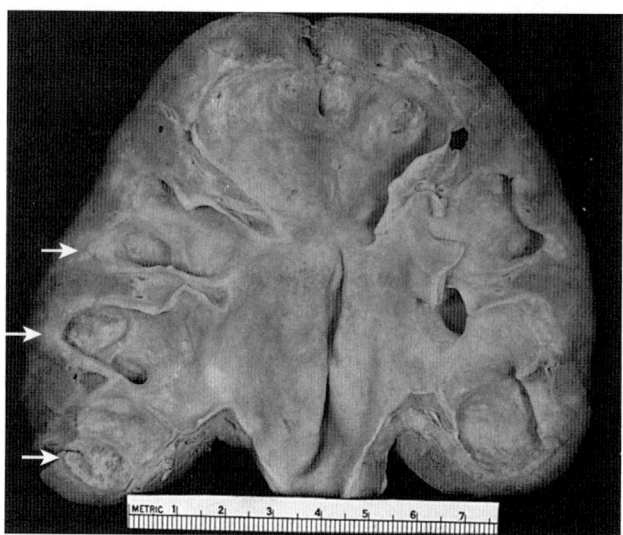

Fig. 55.31. Pyonephrosis: gross specimen. The kidney shows marked thinning of the renal cortex and medulla, suppurative destruction of the parenchyma *(arrows)*, and distention of the pelvis and calyces. Previous incision released a large quantity of purulent material. The ureter showed obstruction distal to the point of section.

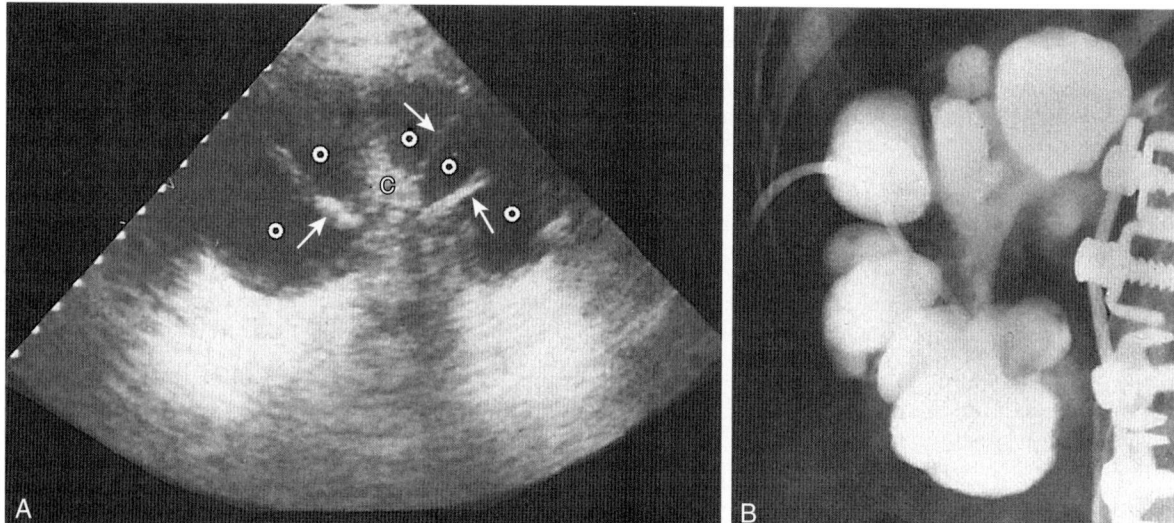

Fig. 55.32. Pyonephrosis. (A) Longitudinal ultrasound image of the right kidney demonstrates echogenic central collecting complex (C) with radiating echogenic septa *(arrows)* and thinned hypoechoic parenchyma. Multiple dilated calyces *(o)* with diffuse low-level echoes are seen. (B) Antegrade pyelogram performed through a percutaneous nephrostomy catheter correlates well with the ultrasound image. Dilated pus-filled calyces are demonstrated. The renal pelvis is obliterated by chronic scarring and stone disease. The kidney did not regain function. (From Schaeffer AJ: Urinary tract infections. In Gillenwater JY, et al., editors: *Adult and pediatric urology*, Philadelphia, 2002, Lippincott Williams & Wilkins, pp 211–272.)

hematoma can become secondarily infected by the hematogenous route or by direct extension of a primary renal infection. When a perinephric infection ruptures through the Gerota fascia into the pararenal space, the abscess becomes paranephric. Paranephric abscesses may also result from infectious disorders of the bowel, pancreas, or pleural cavity. Conversely, perinephric or psoas abscess may be the result of bowel perforation, Crohn disease, or spread of osteomyelitis from the thoracolumbar spine. *E. coli*, *Proteus*, and *S. aureus* account for most infections.

Clinical Presentation. The onset of symptoms is typically insidious. Symptoms are present for more than 5 days in most patients with perinephric abscess compared with only about 10% of patients with pyelonephritis. The clinical presentation may be similar to that of pyelonephritis; however, more than one-third of patients may be afebrile. An abdominal or flank mass can be felt in about half of the cases; costovertebral angle tenderness is typically present. Psoas abscess should be suspected if the patient has a limp and flexion and external rotation of the ipsilateral hip. Laboratory features include leukocytosis, elevated levels of serum creatinine, and pyuria in more than 75% of cases. Edelstein (1988) showed that results of urine cultures predicted perinephric abscess isolates in only 37% of cases; a blood culture, particularly with multiple organisms, was often indicative of perinephric abscess but identified all organisms in only 42% of cases. Meng et al. (2002) showed that roughly 75% of patients had a positive culture. Urine was statistically significantly more sensitive than blood and abscess fluid collection in their study. Therefore caution should be exercised when choosing therapy based on the results of urine and blood cultures because data may sometimes be inadequate. Pyelonephritis usually responds within 4 to 5 days of appropriate antimicrobial therapy; perinephric abscess does not. Thus perinephric abscess should be suspected in a patient with UTI and abdominal or flank mass or persistent fever after 4 days of antimicrobial therapy. Perinephric abscesses are commonly seen concomitantly with renal abscesses.

CT is particularly valuable for demonstrating the primary abscess. In some cases, the abscess is confined to the perinephric space; however, extension to the flank or psoas muscle may occur (Fig. 55.33). CT is able to show with exquisite anatomic detail the route of spread of infection into the surrounding tissues and will demonstrate any obstruction that may be present (Fig. 55.34). This information may be helpful in planning the approach for surgical drainage. Ultrasonography demonstrates a diverse appearance ranging from a nearly anechoic mass displacing the kidney to an echogenic collection that tends to blend with normally echogenic fat within the Gerota fascia (Corriere, 1982). Occasionally, a retroperitoneal or subdiaphragmatic infection may spread to the paranephric fat that is outside this fascia. The clinical symptoms of insidious onset of fever, flank mass, and tenderness are indistinguishable from those associated with perinephric abscess. UTI, however, is absent. Ultrasonography and CT can usually delineate the abscess outside the Gerota fascia.

Improved imaging techniques have decreased the mortality rate of 40% to 50% in early series to roughly 12%, but there is still an average of 3.4 days' lag time before appropriate diagnosis in a contemporary series (Meng et al., 2002). Only 35% of patients were correctly diagnosed on presentation in the Meng series, and this lag time contributed to mortality in nearly all patients in that series. Having an appropriate threshold for imaging will continue to improve the rate of correct diagnoses.

Management. Antimicrobial agents should be immediately started upon diagnosis of perinephric abscess. Gram stain identifies the pathogenesis and guides antimicrobial therapy. An aminoglycoside together with an antistaphylococcal agent, such as methicillin or oxacillin, should be started immediately. If the patient has a penicillin hypersensitivity, cephalothin or vancomycin may be used.

In addition to controlling sepsis and preventing further spread of infection, Meng et al.'s series of 25 patients suggests that, for small perinephric abscesses (<3 cm), antibiotics alone can appropriately treat immune-competent patients (Meng et al., 2002). Eight out of the 10 patients treated with antibiotics alone had full resolution after a mean of 10 days in the hospital. The average size of abscess treated was 1.8 cm. Siegel et al. (1996) also showed good resolution of perinephric abscesses less than 3 cm, with cure seen in all five patients in their series.

For larger collections or those not responsive to initial antibiotic therapy, intervention is the next step in treatment. **Surgical drainage, or nephrectomy if the kidney is nonfunctioning or severely infected, was the classic treatment for perinephric abscesses. However, with the advent of the field of interventional radiology and improvements in percutaneous drainage techniques, renal ultrasonography and CT- or ultrasound-guided percutaneous aspiration and drainage of perirenal collections is now a good option for therapy.** In Meng's study, 11 of the 25 patients had percutaneous drainage in addition to antibiotics (Meng et al., 2002). The mean abscess size was 11 cm and the mean time to resolution was 25 days. Four of

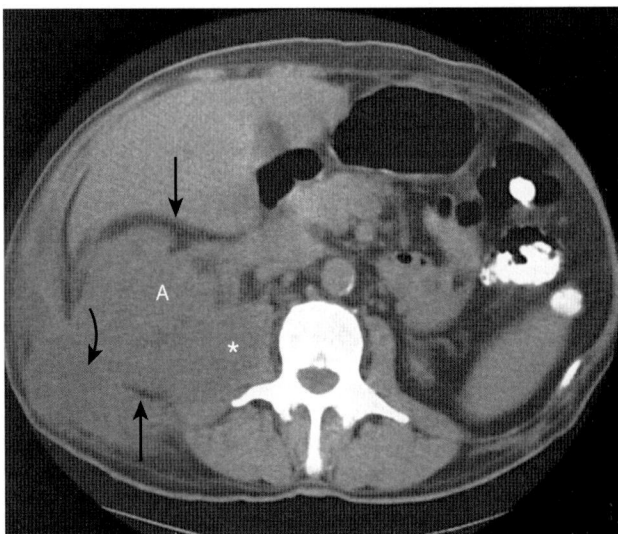

Fig. 55.33. Nonenhanced computed tomography scan through the lower pole of the right kidney (previous left nephrectomy) shows extensive perinephric abscess. Extensive abscess (A) distorts and enlarges the renal contour, infiltrates perinephric fat *(straight arrows)*, and extends into the psoas muscle *(asterisk)* and the soft tissues of the flank *(curved arrow)*. Also note that normal renal collecting system fat has been obliterated by the process.

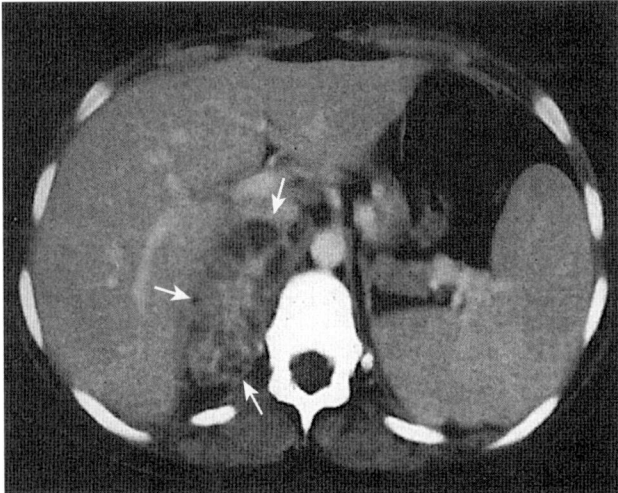

Fig. 55.34. Perinephric abscess involving the right adrenal gland. Computed tomography scan shows large right pararenal mass *(arrows)* with multiple low-density areas within. At surgery, a large pararenal abscess with extensive involvement of the right adrenal was found. (From Schaeffer AJ: Urinary tract infections. In Gillenwater JY, Grayhack JT, Howards SS, et al., editors: *Adult and pediatric urology*, Philadelphia, 2002, Lippincott Williams & Wilkins, pp 211–272.)

these patients eventually required open surgical exploration and drainage. All removed kidneys demonstrated hallmarks of minimal function. **Unlike in renal abscesses, early drainage of abscesses greater than 3 cm in diameter is recommended.**

Once the perinephric abscess has been drained, the underlying problem must be addressed. Some conditions such as renal cortical abscess or enteric communication require prompt attention. Nephrectomy for pyonephrosis may be performed concurrent with drainage of the perinephric abscess if the patient's condition is good. In other instances it is best to drain the perinephric abscess first and correct the underlying problem or perform a nephrectomy when the patient's condition has improved. Meng's series of 11 patients with abscesses greater than 11 cm had a roughly 33% need for nephrectomy (Meng et al., 2002). Although this is a high number in patients who are likely diabetic, whereas the nephron-sparing approach is ideal, it is decidedly lower than the historical nephrectomy rate, likely secondary to more successful percutaneous drainage rates. In three of their patients with small perinephric abscesses and hydronephrosis, antibiotics and drainage of the obstructed urinary system led to cure.

Perinephric Abscess Versus Acute Pyelonephritis. Once again, the greatest obstacle to the treatment of perinephric abscess is the delay in diagnosis. **In the series by Thorley et al. (1974), a common misdiagnosis was acute pyelonephritis;** Meng's study showed a similar delay of roughly 3 to 4 days in appropriate diagnosis in a modern study (Meng et al., 2002). **Thorley's study found that two factors differentiated perinephric abscess and acute pyelonephritis: (1) most patients with uncomplicated pyelonephritis were symptomatic for less than 5 days before hospitalization, whereas most with perinephric abscesses were symptomatic for longer than 5 days; and (2) no patient with acute pyelonephritis remained febrile for longer than 4 days once appropriate antimicrobial agents were started. All patients with perinephric abscesses had a fever for at least 5 days, with a median of 7 days.** Similar results were noted by Fowler and Perkins (1994).

Patients with polycystic renal disease who undergo hemodialysis may be particularly susceptible to the progression from acute UTIs to perinephric abscess. Of 445 patients undergoing chronic hemodialysis at the Regional Kidney Disease Program in Minneapolis, 5.4% had polycystic kidney disease and 33.3% developed symptomatic UTIs (Sweet and Keane, 1979). Eight (62.5%) developed perinephric abscesses, and three of these patients died. According to the investigators, all UTIs, even those that progressed to perinephric abscesses, were promptly treated with appropriate antimicrobial agents, and all patients in this group became afebrile and asymptomatic when the agents were stopped. However, later, after various times, symptoms attributable to perinephric abscess developed in eight of the patients. The mechanism of this process is not clear, but the limited bioavailability of some antimicrobial agents in cysts is variable and could contribute to the progression of renal infection.

Chronic Pyelonephritis

In patients without underlying renal or urinary tract disease, chronic pyelonephritis secondary to UTI is a rare disease and an even more rare cause of chronic renal failure. In patients with underlying functional or structural urinary tract abnormalities, however, chronic renal infection can cause significant renal impairment. Thus it is essential that appropriate studies be used to diagnose, localize, and treat chronic renal infection.

The prevalence of chronic pyelonephritis has also been assessed in patients undergoing dialysis for end-stage renal disease. Despite a 2% to 5% prevalence of bacteriuria in women, pyelonephritis uncomplicated by obstruction or urinary tract malformation does not cause end-stage renal disease. Schechter et al. (1971) analyzed the cause for renal failure in 170 patients referred to them for dialysis. Chronic pyelonephritis was the primary cause of end-stage renal disease in 22 (13%) but was usually associated with an underlying structural defect. Unequivocal nonobstructive chronic pyelonephritis was not found. Symptomatic infections tended to occur before the onset of azotemia in most patients with chronic pyelonephritis. Similarly, Huland and Busch (1982) evaluated 161 patients with end-stage renal disease and found that 42 had chronic pyelonephritis. However, in addition to a history of UTIs, these 42 patients had complicating defects, such as VUR, analgesic abuse, nephrolithiasis, or obstruction. Nonobstructive uncomplicated UTI alone was never found to be the cause of renal insufficiency. Thus, using end-stage renal disease seen at autopsy or at the dialysis clinic as an indicator, the occurrence of uncomplicated chronic bacterial pyelonephritis is rare.

In addition, the role of bacterial infection in development of chronic renal disease can be assessed in patients with renal interstitial and tubular damage similar to that which has classically been called chronic pyelonephritis. The frequency with which various potential causes of interstitial damage are operative in patients with interstitial nephritis was assessed by Murray and Goldberg (1975). These investigators not only concluded that UTI is rarely the sole cause of chronic renal disease in the adult but also observed that 89% of their azotemic patients had a readily identifiable primary cause of their interstitial nephritis. Thus, when patients with a clinical diagnosis of chronic interstitial nephritis are selected as the starting point, it is easy to associate many factors with this disease, but UTI does not seem to be one of them.

Clinical Presentation. **There are no symptoms of chronic pyelonephritis until it produces renal insufficiency, and then the symptoms are similar to those of any other form of chronic renal failure.** If a patient's chronic pyelonephritis is thought to be a result of many episodes of acute pyelonephritis, a history of intermittent symptoms of fever, flank pain, and dysuria may be elicited. Similarly, urinary findings and the presence of renal infection correlate poorly. Bacteriuria and pyuria, the hallmarks of UTI, are not predictive of renal infection. Conversely, patients with significant renal infection may have sterile urine if the ureter draining the kidney is obstructed or the infection is outside of the collecting system.

The pathologic and radiologic criteria for diagnosing renal infection may also be misleading. Asscher (1980) has tabulated eight long-term follow-up studies from the literature on kidneys of adults with UTIs. The data from these reports on 901 patients show that bacteriuria present in otherwise healthy adults for long periods may be associated with nonexistent or extremely minimal evidence of kidney damage. Conversely, patients who have chronic pyelonephritis may have negative urine cultures.

Radiologic Findings. **The diagnosis of chronic pyelonephritis can be made with the greatest confidence on the basis of pyelographic findings. The essential features are asymmetry and irregularity of the kidney outlines, blunting and dilation of one or more calyces, and cortical scars at the corresponding site** (Fig. 55.35). In addition to stones, obstruction, tuberculosis, and analgesic nephritis with papillary necrosis (which can be readily excluded by history), chronic pyelonephritis can also produce a localized scar over a deformed calyx. In advanced pyelonephritis, calyceal distortion and irregularity together with cortical scars complete the picture. Calyceal stones and reflux nephropathy may produce a scarred kidney that is indistinguishable from post-pyelonephritis findings. Regardless of the cause of chronic pyelonephritis, CT findings will be consistent with atrophy, cortical/parenchymal thinning, calyceal clubbing, and possible hypertrophy of residual normal tissue and asymmetry (Craig et al., 2008). Fig. 55.36 (D'Souza et al., 1995) showed a linear relationship between renal parenchymal volume loss and function decline as assessed by DMSA scan. Hodson and Wilson (1965) pointed out that renal infarction, an extremely rare condition, may closely resemble pyelonephritic scars but that the renal pyramid remains with renal infarction in contradistinction to pyelonephritis.

Pathology. **In chronic pyelonephritis, the gross kidney is often diffusely contracted, scarred, and pitted.** The scars are Y-shaped, flat, broad-based depressions with red-brown granular bases. The scarring is often polar with underlying calyceal blunting. The parenchyma is thin, and the corticomedullary demarcation is lost. **Histologic changes are patchy.** There is usually an interstitial infiltrate of lymphocytes, plasma cells, and occasional polymorphonuclear cells. Portions of the parenchyma may be replaced by fibrosis, and, although glomeruli may be preserved, periglomerular fibrosis is often seen. In some affected areas, glomeruli may be completely fibrosed and tubules atrophied. Leukocyte and hyaline casts are sometimes present in the tubules; the

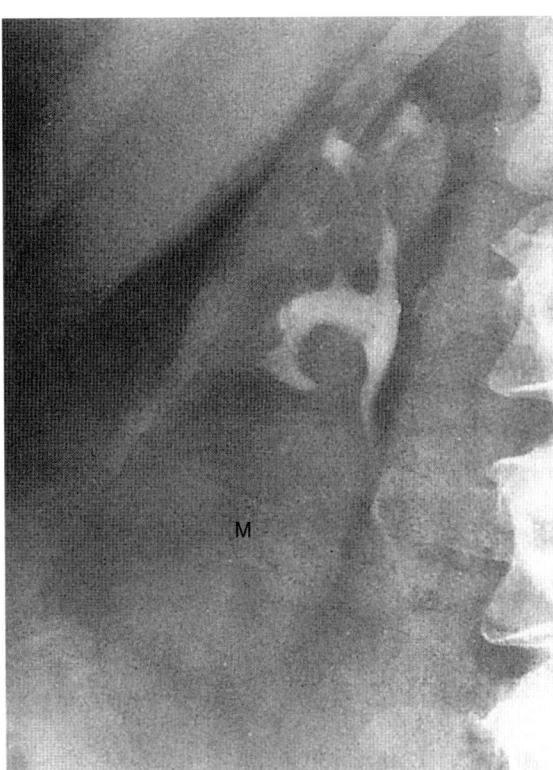

Fig. 55.35. Chronic pyelonephritis. Ten-minute excretory urogram demonstrates irregular renal outline with upper pole parenchymal atrophy. Note significant loss of renal cortical thickness over blunted and dilated calyces. Lower pole mass (M) is a simple cyst. (From Schaeffer AJ: Urinary tract infections. In Gillenwater JY, Grayhack JT, Howards SS, et al., editors: *Adult and pediatric urology*, Philadelphia, 2002, Lippincott Williams & Wilkins, pp 211–272.)

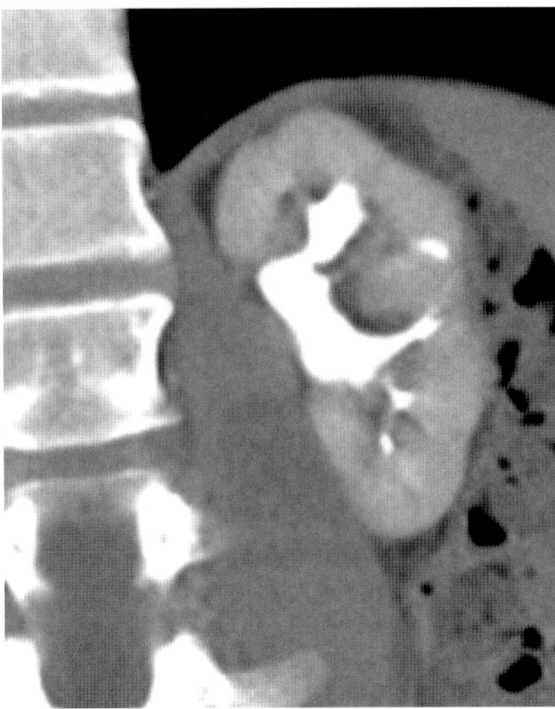

Fig. 55.36. Computed tomography of chronic pyelonephritis. There are cortical scars and blunted calyces.

latter may cause resemblance to the thyroid colloid, hence the description *renal thyroidization* (Braude, 1973). In general, the changes are nonspecific; they also may be seen in toxic exposures, postobstructive atrophy, hematologic disorders, postirradiation nephritis, ischemic renal disease, and nephrosclerosis. **The pathology of stone-induced scars and reflux-induced scars may be identical.**

Management. Management of radiographic evidence of pyelonephritis should be directed at treating infection if present, preventing future infections, and monitoring and preserving renal function. The treatment of existing infection must be based on careful antimicrobial susceptibility tests and selection of drugs that can achieve bactericidal concentrations in the urine and yet are not nephrotoxic. Achievement of acceptable bactericidal levels of a drug in the urine of a patient with chronic pyelonephritis may be difficult because the diminished concentrating ability of pyelonephritis may impair excretion and concentration of the antimicrobial agent. The duration of antimicrobial therapy is often prolonged to maximize the chance of cure. With patients in whom renal damage develops or progresses in the presence of UTI, the working hypothesis should be that there is an underlying renal, usually papillary, lesion or underlying urologic condition, such as obstruction or calculus, which has increased susceptibility to renal damage. Appropriate nephrologic and urologic evaluation should be undertaken to identify and, if possible, correct these abnormalities.

Information about bacterial relapse is available online at Expert Consult.com.

Infectious Granulomatous Nephritis

Xanthogranulomatous Pyelonephritis

Xanthogranulomatous pyelonephritis (XGP) is a rare, severe, chronic renal infection typically resulting in diffuse renal destruction. Most cases are unilateral and result in a nonfunctioning, enlarged kidney associated with obstructive uropathy secondary to nephrolithiasis. XGP is characterized by accumulation of lipid-laden foamy macrophages. It begins within the pelvis and calyces and subsequently extends into and destroys renal parenchymal and adjacent tissues. It has been known to imitate almost every other inflammatory disease of the kidney, as well as renal cell carcinoma, on radiographic examination (Malek and Elder, 1978; Tolia et al., 1980). In addition, the microscopic appearance of XGP has been confused with clear cell adenocarcinoma of the kidney on frozen section and has led to radical nephrectomy (Anhalt et al., 1971; Flynn et al., 1979; Lorentzen and Nielsen, 1980; Malek and Elder, 1978; Tolia et al., 1980). The entity is uncommon and is found in only about 0.6% (Malek et al., 1972) to 1.4% (Ghosh, 1955) of patients with renal inflammation who are evaluated pathologically.

Pathogenesis. The primary factors involved in the pathogenesis of XGP are nephrolithiasis, obstruction, and infection (Gregg et al., 1999). Nephrolithiasis has been noted in as many as 83% of the patients in various series; approximately half of the renal stones have been of the staghorn type (Chuang et al., 1992; Nataluk et al., 1995; Parsons et al., 1983). It has been proposed clinically and demonstrated experimentally that primary obstruction followed by infection with *E. coli* can lead to tissue destruction and collections of lipid material by macrophages (Povysil and Konickova, 1972). These macrophages (xanthoma cells) are distributed in sheets around parenchymal abscesses and calyces and are intermixed with lymphocytes, giant cells, and plasma cells. The bacteria appear to be of low virulence because spontaneous bacteremia has rarely been described. Other possible interrelated factors include venous occlusion and hemorrhage, abnormal lipid metabolism, lymphatic blockage, failure of antimicrobial therapy in UTI, altered immunologic competence, and renal ischemia (Friedenberg and Spjut, 1963; Goodman et al., 1979; McDonald, 1981; Mering et al., 1973; Tolia et al., 1981). The concept that XGP is related to incomplete bacterial degradation and altered host response has received mixed support (Khalyl-Mawad et al., 1982; Nielsen and Lorentzen, 1981). Thus it appears that there is probably no single factor instrumental in the pathogenesis of this disease. Rather, there is an inadequate host acute inflammatory response within an obstructed, ischemic, or necrotic kidney.

Pathology. The kidney is usually massively enlarged and has a normal contour. XGP may be diffuse, as in approximately 80% of

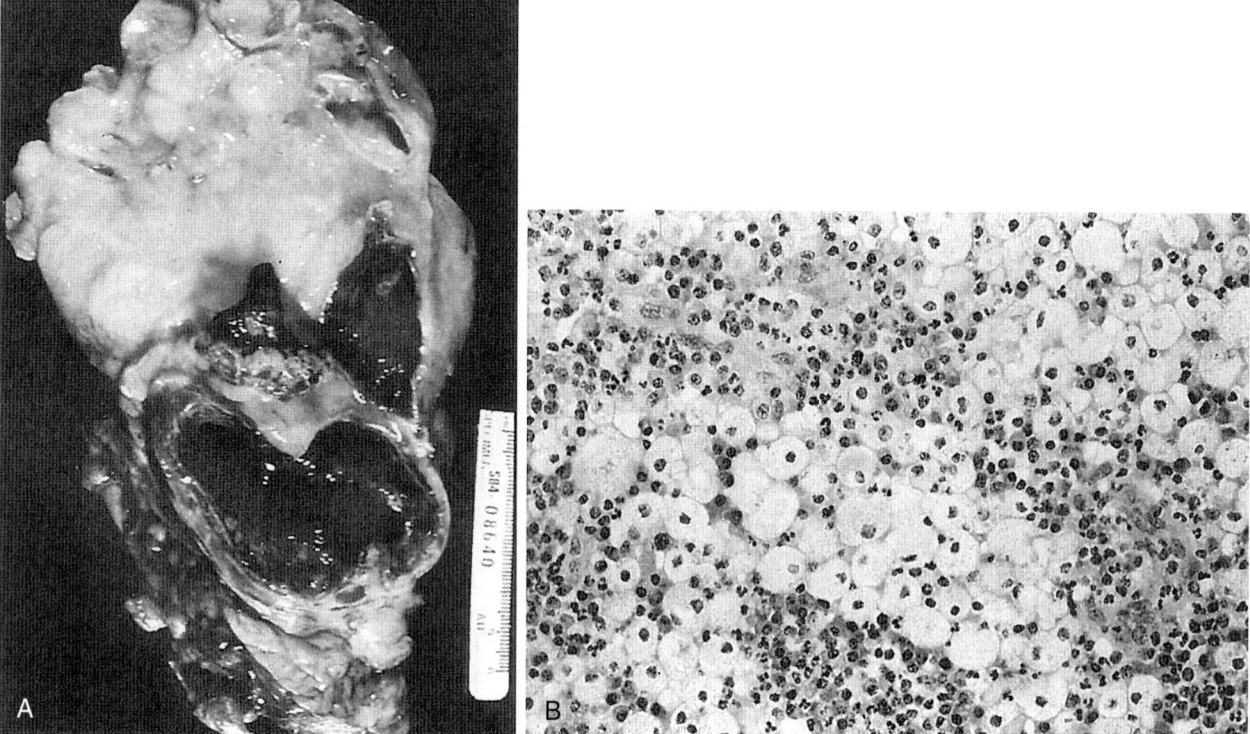

Fig. 55.37. Xanthogranulomatous pyelonephritis. (A) Gross specimen. Kidney is massively enlarged, measuring 23 × 12 cm; the normal architecture is replaced by a shaggy yellow upper pole mass corresponding to xanthogranulomatous inflammation and numerous distorted and dilated calyces. (B) Microscopically, the shaggy yellow tissue is composed primarily of lipid-laden histiocytes mixed with other inflammatory cells. (From Schaeffer AJ: Urinary tract infections. In Gillenwater JY, Grayhack JT, Howards SS, et al., editors: *Adult and pediatric urology*, Philadelphia, 2002, Lippincott Williams & Wilkins, pp 211–272.)

the patients, or segmental. In the diffuse form of the disease, the entire kidney is involved, whereas in segmental XGP, only the parenchyma surrounding one or more calyces or one pole of a duplicated collecting system is involved. On sectioning, the kidney usually demonstrates nephrolithiasis and peripelvic fibrosis. The calyces are dilated and filled with purulent material, but fibrosis surrounding the pelvis usually prevents dilation. The papillae are often destroyed by papillary necrosis (Goodman et al., 1979). In advanced stages of the disease, multiple parenchymal abscesses are filled with viscous pus and lined by yellowish tissue (Fig. 55.37A). The cortex is often thin and replaced by xanthogranulomatous tissue. The capsule is often thickened, and extension of the inflammatory process into the perinephric or paranephric space is common (Goodman et al., 1979; Gregg et al., 1999; McDonald, 1981).

On microscopic examination, the yellowish nodules that line the calyces and surround the parenchymal abscesses contain dark sheets of lipid-laden macrophages (foamy histiocytes with small, dark nuclei and clear cytoplasm) intermixed with lymphocytes, giant cells, and plasma cells (Fig. 55.37B). Xanthogranulomatous cells are not specific to XGP but may be present anywhere inflammation or obstruction coexists. The origin of the fatty substance is disputed. Cholesterol esters that make up a part of the lipid may be derived from lysis of erythrocytes after hemorrhage (Saeed and Fine, 1963).

Clinical Presentation. XGP should be suspected in patients with UTIs and a unilateral enlarged nonfunctioning or poorly functioning kidney with a stone or a mass lesion indistinguishable from malignant tumor. Most patients experience flank pain (69%), fever and chills (69%), and persistent bacteriuria (46%) (Malek and Elder, 1978). Additional vague symptoms, such as malaise, may be present. On physical examination, 62% of the patients had a flank mass and 35% had previous calculi (Malek and Elder, 1978). Less commonly, hypertension, hematuria, or hepatomegaly is the presenting complaint. The medical history is often positive

for UTIs and urologic instrumentation (Eastham et al., 1994; Flynn et al., 1979; Goodman et al., 1979; Grainger et al., 1982; Malek and Elder, 1978; Nataluk et al., 1995; Petronic et al., 1989; Yazaki et al., 1982). People with diabetes also appear to be at greater risk of developing the disease (Eastham et al., 1994). Although it may occur at any age, the peak incidence of XGP is in the fifth to the seventh decade. Women are more commonly affected than men. There is no predilection for either kidney.

Bacteriology and Laboratory Diagnosis. Although review of the literature shows *Proteus* to be the most common organism involved with XGP (Anhalt et al., 1971; Tolia et al., 1981), *E. coli* is also common. The prevalence of *Proteus* organisms may reflect their association with stone formation and subsequent chronic obstruction and irritation. Malek and Elder (1978), in their analysis of 26 cases, found that renal tissue cultures grew bacteria in 22 of 23 cases. Anaerobes also have been cultured (Malek and Elder, 1978).

Approximately 10% of patients have mixed cultures. About one-third of patients have no growth in their urine, probably because many patients have recently taken or are taking antimicrobial agents when cultures are obtained. The infecting organism may be revealed only by tissue cultures obtained during surgery. Urinalysis usually shows pus and protein. In addition, blood tests often reveal anemia and may show hepatic dysfunction in up to 50% of the patients (Malek and Elder, 1978).

XGP is almost always unilateral; therefore azotemia or frank renal failure is uncommon (Goodman, et al. 1979; Gregg et al., 1999).

CT is probably the most useful radiologic technique in evaluating patients with XGP (Fig. 55.38). Fifty to eighty percent of patients show the classic triad of unilateral renal enlargement with little or no function and a large calculus in the renal pelvis (Elder, 1984). CT usually demonstrates a large, reniform mass with the renal pelvis tightly surrounding a central calcification but without pelvic dilatation (Goldman et al., 1984; Hartman, 1985;

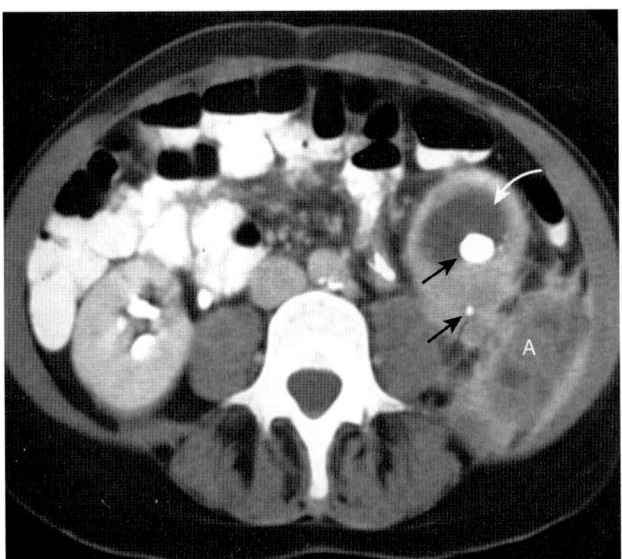

Fig. 55.38. Xanthogranulomatous pyelonephritis. Enhanced computed tomography scan shows collecting system and parenchymal calculi *(straight black arrows)* with lower pole pyonephrosis *(curved white arrow)* and an irregular, predominantly low-density perinephric abscess *(A)* extending into the soft tissues of the flank.

Solomon et al., 1983). Renal parenchyma is replaced by multiple water-density masses representing dilated calyces and abscess cavities filled with varied amounts of pus and debris. On enhanced scans, the walls of these cavities demonstrate a prominent blush because of the abundant vascularity within the granulation tissue. The cavities themselves, however, fail to enhance, whereas tumors and other inflammatory lesions usually do. The CT scan is particularly helpful in demonstrating the extent of renal involvement and may indicate whether adjacent organs or the abdominal wall are involved by XGP (Eastham et al., 1994; Kaplan et al., 1997).

Ultrasonography usually demonstrates global enlargement of the kidney (Merenich and Popky, 1991). The normal renal architecture is replaced by multiple hypoechoic fluid-filled masses that correspond to debris-filled, dilated calyces or foci of parenchymal destruction (Fagerholm, 1983; Hartman et al., 1984). With focal involvement, a solid mass involving a segment of the kidney is sometimes called tumefactive xanthogranulomatous pyelonephritis. There may or may not be an associated calculus in the collecting system or ureter. Renal cell carcinoma and other solid renal lesions must be considered in the differential diagnosis (Elder, 1984).

Radionuclide renal scanning using ^{99m}Tc-DMSA is used to confirm and quantify the differential lack of function in the involved kidney (Gregg et al., 1999). MRI has not yet superseded CT in the evaluation of renal inflammation, but it provides some advantages in delineating extrarenal extension of inflammation (Soler et al., 1997). Lesions of XGP may appear as cystic foci of intermediate intensity signal on T1-weighted images and hyperintensity on T2-weighted images. Arteriography shows hypervascular areas, but there may be some hypovascular areas (Malek and Elder, 1978, Tolia et al., 1981; Van Kirk et al., 1980). Therefore radiologic studies, although distinctive, often cannot be used to differentiate between XGP and renal cell carcinoma.

Differential Diagnosis. Diagnosis of segmental XGP without calculi may be difficult. XGP in association with massive pelvic dilation cannot be distinguished from pyonephrosis. When XGP occurs within a small contracted kidney, the radiographic findings are nonspecific and nondiagnostic. Renal parenchymal malacoplakia may show renal enlargement and multiple inflammatory masses replacing the normal renal parenchyma, but calculi are usually not present. Renal lymphoma may be associated with multiple hypoechoic masses surrounding the contracted, nondilated pelvis, but lymphoma is usually clinically obvious, and renal involvement is usually bilateral and not associated with calculi (Hartman et al., 1984).

Management. The primary obstacle to the correct treatment of XGP is incorrect diagnosis. Today with CT technology, the diagnosis of XGP is made preoperatively nearly 90% of the time (Eastham et al., 1994; Nataluk et al., 1995). Antimicrobial therapy may be necessary to stabilize the patient preoperatively, and, occasionally, **long-term antimicrobial therapy will eradicate the infection and restore renal function** (Mollier et al., 1995). Because the renal abnormality may be diagnosed preoperatively as a renal tumor and/or is diffuse, **nephrectomy is usually performed.** If localized XGP is diagnosed preoperatively or at exploration, it is amenable to partial nephrectomy (Malek and Elder, 1978; Osca et al., 1997; Tolia et al., 1980).

The lipid-laden macrophages associated with XGP, however, closely resemble clear cell adenocarcinoma and may be difficult to distinguish solely on the basis of frozen section. Furthermore, XGP has been associated with renal cell carcinoma, papillary transitional cell carcinoma of the pelvis or bladder, and infiltrating squamous cell carcinoma of the pelvis (Pitts et al., 1981; Schoborg et al., 1980; Tolia et al., 1981); thus, if malignant renal tumor cannot be excluded, nephrectomy should be performed. When diffuse and extensive disease into the retroperitoneum exists, removal of the kidney and perinephric fat may be needed. Under these circumstances, the surgery may be difficult and may involve dissection of granulomatous tissue from the diaphragm, great vessels, and bowel (Flynn et al., 1979; Malek and Elder, 1978). It is important to remove the entire inflammatory mass because in nearly three-fourths of patients, xanthogranulomatous tissue is infected. If incision and drainage alone are performed rather than nephrectomy, the patient may continue to suffer from protracted debilitating illness and may develop a renal cutaneous fistula; an even more difficult nephrectomy will then be necessary. One early case-matched series of laparoscopic nephrectomies performed for XGP concluded that the benefits of laparoscopic surgery do not extend to the treatment of this disease (Bercowsky et al., 1999); however, a larger review of a modern XGP experience suggests that laparoscopic nephrectomy is a reasonable treatment approach (Guzzo et al., 2009; Kapoor et al., 2006; Vanderbrink et al., 2007). Some studies suggest a retroperitoneal approach laparoscopically and, if transperitoneal, the use of a hand-assist port (Tobias-Machado et al., 2005). Although feasible, removal of an XGP kidney is difficult, and high conversion rates were seen across multiple studies (Korkes et al., 2008).

Malacoplakia

Malacoplakia, from the Greek word meaning "soft plaque," is an unusual inflammatory disease originally described to affect the bladder but has been found to affect the GU and GI tracts, skin, lungs, bones, and mesenteric lymph nodes. It is an inflammatory lesion described originally by Michaelis and Gutmann (1902). It was characterized by von Hansemann (1903) as soft, yellow-brown plaques with granulomatous lesions in which the histiocytes contain distinct basophilic lysosomal inclusion bodies or Michaelis-Gutmann bodies. Although its exact pathogenesis is unknown, malacoplakia probably results from abnormal macrophage function in response to a bacterial infection, which is most often *E. coli*.

Pathogenesis. The pathogenesis is unknown, but several theories are popular. In 93 patients who had cultures of urine, diseased tissue, or blood, 89.4% had coliform infections (Stanton and Maxted, 1981). Moreover, 40% of the patients in this review had an immunodeficiency syndrome, autoimmune disease, carcinoma, or another systemic disorder. **This association of coliform infections and compromised health status in patients with malacoplakia is well recognized.**

It is hypothesized that bacteria or bacterial fragments form the nidus for the calcium phosphate crystals that laminate the Michaelis-Gutmann bodies. Most investigations into the pathogenesis of this disease support theories that a defect in intraphagosomal bacterial digestion accounts for the unusual immunologic response that causes malacoplakia.

Pathology. The diagnosis is made by biopsy. The lesion is characterized by large histiocytes, known as *von Hansemann cells*, and small basophilic, extracytoplasmic, or intracytoplasmic calculospherules called *Michaelis-Gutmann bodies*, which are pathognomonic

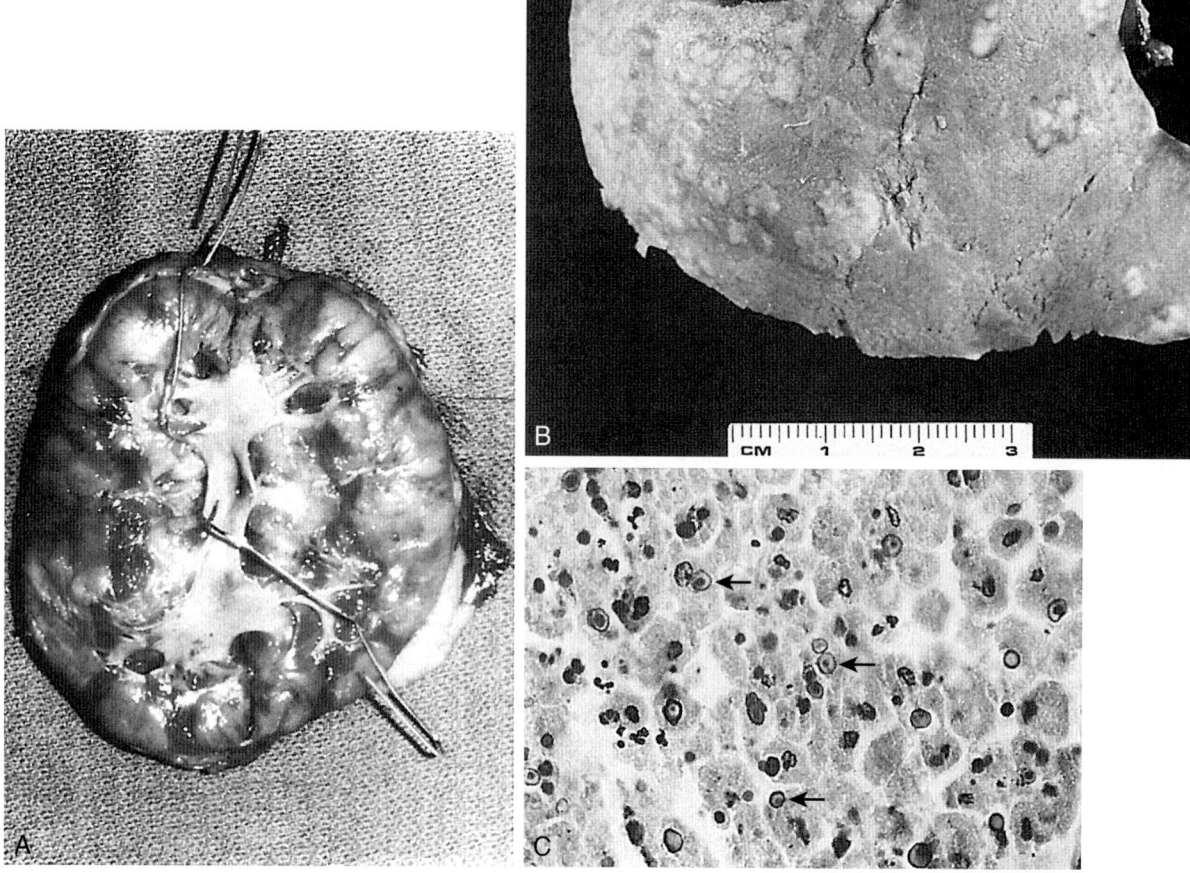

Fig. 55.39. Renal parenchymal malacoplakia. (A) Cut surface demonstrates extensive cortical and upper medullary replacement by multifocal, confluent, tumorlike masses. (B) Cortical surface exhibits multiple, firm, plaquelike lesions. (C) Hallmark of malacoplakia is demonstration of the Michaelis-Gutmann body *(arrows)*, which represents incompletely destroyed bacteria surrounded by lipoprotein membrane (hematoxylin and eosin stain). (From Hartman DS: Radiologic pathologic correlation of the infectious granulomatous diseases of the kidney: I and II. *Monogr Urol* 6:3, 1985.)

(Fig. 55.39). Electron microscopy has revealed intact coliform bacteria and bacterial fragments within phagolysosomes of the foamy-appearing malacoplakic histiocytes (Lewin et al., 1976; Stanton and Maxted, 1981). In their review of the subject, Stanton and Maxted (1981) and Esparza et al. (1989) emphasized that, although pathognomonic for the disease, Michaelis-Gutmann bodies may be absent in early malacoplakia and are not necessary for the diagnosis.

It has been shown that macrophages in malacoplakia involving the kidney and bladder contain large amounts of immunoreactive α_1-antitrypsin (Callea et al., 1982). The amount of α_1-antitrypsin remains unchanged during the morphogenetic stages of the pathologic process. Macrophages from other pathologic processes, closely resembling malacoplakia but without Michaelis-Gutmann bodies, do not contain α_1-antitrypsin except for a few macrophages in tuberculosis and XGP. **Therefore immunohistochemical staining for α_1-antitrypsin may be a useful test for an early and accurate differential diagnosis of malacoplakia.**

Clinical Presentation. Most patients are older than 50 years. **The ratio of females to males with malacoplakia within the urinary tract is 4:1, but this disparity does not occur in other body tissues** (Stanton and Maxted, 1981). **The patients often are debilitated and immunosuppressed and have other chronic diseases. In fact, malakoplakia is increasingly described after solid organ transplantation, particularly renal transplant recipients** (Nieto-Rios et al., 2017). The symptoms of bladder malacoplakia are bladder irritability and hematuria. Cystoscopy reveals mucosal plaques or nodules. As these lesions progress, they may become fungating, firm, sessile masses that cause filling defects of the bladder, ureter, or pelvis on excretory urograms. The distal ureter may become strictured or stenotic and cause subsequent renal obstruction or nonfunction (Sexton et al., 1982). A typical patient with renal parenchymal disease may have one or more radiographic masses and chronic *E. coli* infections. Renal parenchymal malacoplakia may be complicated by renal vein thrombosis and inferior vena cava thrombosis (McClure, 1983). When malacoplakia involves the testis, epididymo-orchitis is present. Malacoplakia of the prostate is rare, but, when it occurs, it may be confused with carcinoma clinically (Shimizu et al., 2005). Mortality can exceed 50%, and the morbidity can be substantial (Stanton and Maxted, 1981).

Radiologic Findings. **Multifocal malacoplakia on excretory urography typically is seen as enlarged kidneys with multiple filling defects.** Renal calcification, lithiasis, and hydronephrosis are absent. The multifocal nature is best appreciated by using ultrasonography, CT, or arteriography. Ultrasound examination may demonstrate renal enlargement and distortion of the central echo complex. The masses are often confluent, resulting in an overall increase in the echogenicity of the renal parenchyma (Hartman et al., 1980). On CT, the foci of malacoplakia are less dense than the surrounding enhanced parenchyma (Hartman, 1985). Arteriography typically reveals a hypovascular mass without peripheral neovascularity (Cavins and Goldstein, 1977; Trillo et al., 1977).

Unifocal malacoplakia on excretory urography appears as a noncalcified mass that is indistinguishable from other inflammatory

or neoplastic lesions. Ultrasonography and CT may demonstrate a solid or cystic structure, depending on the degree of internal necrosis. Angiography may demonstrate neovascularity (Trillo et al., 1977). Extension beyond the kidney, which can occur with either multifocal or uniform malacoplakia, is best demonstrated by CT.

Differential Diagnosis. The differential diagnosis includes renal cystic disease, neoplasia, and renal inflammatory disease (Hartman, 1985). **Malacoplakia should be considered when one or more renal masses are observed, particularly in female patients with recurrent UTIs with *E. coli*, altered immune response syndromes, or cystoscopic evidence of malacoplakia or filling defects in the collecting system** (Charboneau, 1980). **Malacoplakia should also be suspected when these radiographic findings occur in a renal transplant patient who has persistent UTI despite appropriate antimicrobial therapy.** Cystic disease generally can be excluded by careful sonographic and CT evaluations. Renal involvement with metastatic disease or lymphomas usually occurs late in the course of the disease, which is well established. Multifocal renal cell carcinoma is most often seen in the context of von Hippel-Lindau disease with its other clinical manifestations. Patients with XGP usually have signs and symptoms of UTI. As with malacoplakia, the involved kidney is enlarged but renal calculi and obstruction are common. Multiple renal abscesses are often associated with hematogenous dissemination resulting from cardiac disease.

Management. Management of malacoplakia should be directed at control of the UTIs, which should stabilize the disease process. This subject is well reviewed by Stanton and Maxted (1981). Although multiple long-term antimicrobial agents, including many antituberculosis agents, have been used, the sulfonamides, rifampin, doxycycline, and TMP are thought to be especially useful because of their intracellular bactericidal activity (Maderazo et al., 1979). Fluoroquinolones are taken up by macrophages directly and have also proven effective in the management of malacoplakia (Vallorosi et al., 1999). Other investigators have used ascorbic acid and cholinergic agents such as bethanechol in conjunction with antimicrobial therapy and have reported good results (Abdou et al., 1977; Stanton et al., 1983; Zornow et al., 1979). Both agents are thought to increase intracellular cyclic guanosine monophosphate levels, which have been postulated as the biologic defect causing macrophage dysfunction. Surgical intervention, however, may be necessary if the disease progresses in spite of antimicrobial treatment. Nephrectomy is usually performed for the treatment of symptomatic unilateral renal lesions.

The long-term prognosis appears to be related to the extent of the disease. When parenchymal renal malacoplakia is bilateral or occurs in the transplanted kidney, death usually occurs within 6 months (Bowers and Cathey, 1971; Deridder et al., 1977). Patients with unilateral disease usually have a long-term survival after nephrectomy.

Information on renal echinococcosis is available online at ExpertConsult.com.

OTHER INFECTIONS
Fournier Gangrene

Fournier gangrene is a potentially life-threatening form of necrotizing fasciitis involving the male genitalia. It is also known as idiopathic gangrene of the scrotum, streptococcal scrotal gangrene, perineal phlegmon, and spontaneous fulminant gangrene of the scrotum (Fournier, 1883, 1884). As originally reported by Baurienne in 1764, then by Fournier in 1883, it was characterized by an abrupt onset of a rapidly fulminating genital gangrene of idiopathic origin in previously healthy young patients that resulted in gangrenous destruction of the genitalia. The disease now differs from these descriptions in that it involves a broader age range, including older patients (Bejanga, 1979; Wolach et al., 1989), follows a more indolent course, and has a less abrupt onset; and, in approximately 95% of the cases, a source can now be identified (Burpee and Edwards, 1972; Jamieson et al., 1984; Kearney and Carling, 1983; Macrea, 1945; Spirnak et al., 1984).

Infection most commonly arises from the skin, urethra, or rectal regions. An association between urethral obstruction associated with strictures and extravasation and instrumentation has been well documented. **Predisposing factors include diabetes mellitus, local trauma, paraphimosis, periurethral extravasation of urine, perirectal or perianal infections, and surgery such as circumcision or herniorrhaphy. In cases originating in the genitalia, specifically as a result of urethral obstruction, the infecting bacteria probably pass through Buck fascia of the penis and spread along the Dartos fascia of the scrotum and penis, Colles fascia of the perineum, and Scarpa fascia of the anterior abdominal wall.** In view of the typical foul odor associated with this condition, a major role for anaerobic bacteria is likely. **Wound cultures generally yield multiple organisms, implicating anaerobic-aerobic synergy** (Cohen, 1986; Meleney, 1933; Miller, 1983). Mixed cultures containing facultative organisms (*E. coli*, *Klebsiella*, enterococci) along with anaerobes (*Bacteroides*, *Fusobacterium*, *Clostridium*, microaerophilic streptococci) have been obtained from the lesions.

Clinical Presentation

Patients frequently have a history of recent perineal trauma, instrumentation, urethral stricture associated with sexually transmitted disease, or urethral cutaneous fistula. Pain, rectal bleeding, and a history of anal fissures suggest a rectal source of infection. Dermal sources are suggested by history of acute and chronic infections of the scrotum and spreading recurrent hidradenitis suppurativa or balanitis.

The infection commonly starts as cellulitis adjacent to the portal of entry. Early on, the involved area is swollen, erythematous, and tender as the infection begins to involve the deep fascia. Pain is prominent, and fever and systemic toxicity are marked (Paty and Smith, 1992). The swelling and crepitus of the scrotum quickly increase, and dark purple areas develop and progress to extensive gangrene. If the abdominal wall becomes involved in an obese patient with diabetes, the process can spread very rapidly. Specific GU symptoms associated with the condition include dysuria, urethral discharge, and obstructed voiding. Alterations in mental status, tachypnea, tachycardia, and temperature greater than 38.3°C (101°F) or less than 35.6°C (96°F) suggest gram-negative sepsis.

Laboratory Diagnosis and Radiologic Findings

Anemia occurs secondary to a decreased functioning erythrocyte mass caused by thrombosis and ecchymosis coupled with decreased production secondary to sepsis (Miller, 1983). Elevated serum

---

> **KEY POINTS: KIDNEY INFECTIONS**
>
> - Acute pyelonephritis classically is seen as the abrupt onset of chills, fever, and flank or costovertebral angle tenderness but can involve symptoms as mild as cystitis or as severe as sepsis.
> - Emphysematous pyelonephritis is a life-threatening infection diagnosed radiographically by the presence of gas in the parenchyma or collecting system and can be managed via percutaneous drainage or surgically.
> - Renal abscesses are well delineated by CT and are classically managed with IV antimicrobial agents and drainage. Smaller abscesses may be amenable to conservative treatment with medical management.
> - Pyonephrosis is a bacterial infection in a hydronephrotic kidney. Prompt diagnosis is critical; treatment entails intravenous antimicrobial agents and drainage of the obstructed renal unit.
> - XGP is a chronic renal infection that is often found in poorly functioning renal units obstructed secondary to nephrolithiasis. XGP can be mistaken for renal tumors.
> - Malacoplakia is an unusual inflammatory disease thought to result from abnormal macrophage function. Michaelis-Gutmann bodies are lysosomal inclusion bodies that characterize this disease microscopically.

creatinine levels, hyponatremia, and hypocalcemia are common. Hypocalcemia is believed to be secondary to bacterial lipases that destroy triglycerides and release free fatty acids that chelate calcium in its ionized form.

Because crepitus (subcutaneous gas) is often an early finding, a plain film of the abdomen may be helpful in identifying air. Scrotal ultrasonography is also useful in this regard. Biopsy of the base of an ulcer is characterized by superficially intact epidermis, dermal necrosis, vascular thrombosis, and polymorphonuclear leukocyte invasion with subcutaneous tissue necrosis. Stamenkovic and Lew (1984) noted that the use of frozen sections within 21 hours after the onset of symptoms could confirm a diagnosis earlier and lead to early institution of appropriate treatment.

Management

Prompt diagnosis is critical because of the rapidity with which the process can progress. The clinical differentiation of necrotizing fasciitis from cellulitis may be difficult because the initial signs including pain, edema, and erythema are not distinctive. However, **the presence of marked systemic toxicity out of proportion to the local finding should alert the clinician.** Intravenous hydration and antimicrobial therapy are indicated in preparation for surgical debridement. Antimicrobial regimens include broad-spectrum antibiotics (β-lactam plus β-lactamase inhibitor) such as piperacillin-tazobactam (especially if *Pseudomonas* is suspected), ampicillin plus sulbactam, or vancomycin or carbapenems plus clindamycin or metronidazole (Morpurgo and Galandiuk, 2002).

Immediate debridement is essential. In the patient in whom diagnosis is clearly suspected on clinical grounds (deep pain with patchy areas of surface hypoesthesia or crepitation, or bullae and skin necrosis), direct operative intervention is indicated. **Extensive incision should be made through the skin and subcutaneous tissues, going beyond the areas of involvement until normal fascia is found. Necrotic fat and fascia should be excised, and the wound should be left open. A second procedure 24 to 48 hours later is indicated if there is any question about the adequacy of initial debridement. Orchiectomy is almost never required** because the testes have their own blood supply independent of the compromised fascial and cutaneous circulation to the scrotum. **Suprapubic diversion should be performed in cases in which urethral trauma or extravasation is suspected. Colostomy should be performed if there is colonic or rectal perforation.** Hyperbaric oxygen therapy has shown some promise in shortening hospital stays, increasing wound healing, and decreasing the gangrenous spread when used in conjunction with debridement and antimicrobials (Paty and Smith, 1992). Once wound healing is complete, reconstruction (e.g., using myocutaneous flaps) improves cosmetic results.

Outcome

The mortality rate averages approximately 20% (Baskin et al., 1990; Clayton et al., 1990; Cohen, 1986) but ranges from 7% to 75%. Higher mortality rates are found in patients with diabetes, alcoholics, and those with colorectal sources of infection who often have a less typical presentation, greater delay in diagnosis, and more widespread extension. Regardless of the presentation, **Fournier gangrene is a true urologic emergency that demands early recognition, aggressive treatment with antimicrobial agents, and surgical debridement to reduce morbidity and mortality.**

Periurethral Abscess

Periurethral abscess is a life-threatening infection of the male urethra and periurethral tissues. Initially, the area of involvement can be small and localized by Buck fascia. However, when Buck fascia is penetrated, there can be extensive necrosis of the subcutaneous tissue and fascia. Fasciitis can spread as far as the buttocks posteriorly and the clavicle superiorly. Rapid diagnosis and treatment are essential to reduce the morbidity and high mortality historically associated with this disease.

Pathogenesis

Periurethral abscess is frequently a sequela of gonorrhea, urethral stricture disease, or urethral catheterization. Frequent instrumentation is also associated with periurethral abscess formation. The source of the infecting organism is the urine. Gram-negative rods, enterococci, and anaerobes are most frequently identified. The presence of multiple organisms is common. Anaerobes, normal residents of the male urethra, are also frequently found in wound cultures.

Clinical Presentation

Presenting signs and symptoms include scrotal swelling in 94% of patients, fever (70%), acute urinary retention (19%), spontaneously drained abscess (11%), and dysuria or urethral discharge (5% to 8%). The average interval between initial symptoms and presentation is 21 days. Urinalysis of the first glass specimen reveals pyuria and bacteriuria.

Management

Treatment consists of immediate suprapubic urinary drainage and wide debridement. Antimicrobial therapy with an aminoglycoside and a cephalosporin is usually adequate for empirical coverage. More selective antimicrobial therapy can be instituted when the antimicrobial susceptibility of the organisms is available. Perineal urethrostomy or chronic suprapubic diversion occasionally has been helpful to prevent recurrences, and it should be considered in patients with diffuse stricture disease. The presence of a malignancy is unusual, but biopsy is important.

> **KEY POINTS: OTHER INFECTIONS**
>
> - Fournier gangrene is necrotizing fasciitis arising from the perineal skin, scrotum, urethra, or rectum.
> - Emergent surgical debridement and broad-spectrum antimicrobial agents are the essentials of treatment of Fournier gangrene.
> - Periurethral abscess can occur secondarily to urethral stricture or catheterization; treatment entails surgical debridement, suprapubic urinary drainage, and antimicrobial agents.

BACTEREMIA, SEPSIS, AND SEPTIC SHOCK

Sepsis is a clinical syndrome characterized by extremes of body temperature, heart rate, respiratory rate, and WBC count that occurs in response to an infection. A detailed list of potential characteristics can be found in Box 55.12. Severe sepsis and septic shock are extensions of the sepsis spectrum and involve acute organ dysfunction and life-threatening hypotension not responsive to fluid resuscitation (Dellinger et al., 2008). A typical host response to infection involves localized containment and elimination of bacteria and repair of damaged tissue. This process is facilitated by macrophages and dendritic cells and orchestrated by $CD4^+$ T helper cells via the release of proinflammatory and anti-inflammatory molecules (cytokines, chemokines, interferons). Sepsis occurs when a local infectious process becomes an uncontrolled systemic blood-borne inflammatory response resulting in damage to tissues or organs remote from the initial site of infection or injury. The extremes of the spectrum are lethal in one in four patients, and there are an estimated 750,000 cases (3 cases per 1000 population) of sepsis or septic shock in the United States each year (Dellinger et al., 2008; Rivers et al., 2001). Much like other medical emergencies, including polytrauma, acute myocardial infarction, and stroke, early recognition and appropriate treatment significantly influence outcome; these are commonly known as "the golden hours."

> **BOX 55.12   Potential Characteristics of Sepsis Spectrum**
>
> **GENERAL**
> Fever (core temperature >38.3°C)
> Hypothermia (core temperature <36°C)
> Heart rate >90 min, 1 or 2 SD above the normal value for age
> Tachypnea
> Altered mental status
> Significant edema or positive fluid balance (20 mL/kg/24 h)
> Hyperglycemia (plasma glucose >120 mg/dL or 7.7 mmol/L) in the absence of diabetes
>
> **INFLAMMATORY**
> Leukocytosis (WBC count >12,000/μL)
> Leukopenia (WBC count <4000/μL)
> Normal WBC count with >10% immature forms
>
> **ORGAN DYSFUNCTION**
> Arterial hypoxemia (PaO$_2$/FiO$_2$ >300)
> Acute oliguria (urine output 0.5 mL/kg in 1 h for at least 2 h)
> Creatinine increase of 0.5 mg/dL
> Coagulation abnormalities (INR 1.5 or aPTT >60 sec)
> Ileus (absent bowel sounds)
> Thrombocytopenia (platelet count <100,000/μL)
> Hyperbilirubinemia (plasma total bilirubin >4 mg/dL or 70 mmol/L)
>
> **TISSUE PERFUSION**
> Hyperlactatemia (>1 mmol/L)
> Decreased capillary refill or mottling

aPTT, Activated partial thromboplastin time; *INR*, international normalized ratio; *SD*, standard deviation; *WBC*, white blood cell.
Data from Levy MM, Fink MP, Marshall JC, et al.: 2001 SCCM/ESICM/ACCP/ATS/SIS International Sepsis Definitions Conference. *Crit Care Med* 31:1250–1256, 2003.

Definitions

- **Bacteremia:** the presence of viable bacteria in the blood
- **Systemic inflammatory response syndrome (SIRS):** a clinical syndrome characterized by the 2001 International Sepsis Definitions Conference (Levy et al., 2003) as extremes of body temperature, heart rate, ventilation, and immune response. SIRS can occur in response to multiple insults, including systemic infection, trauma, thermal injury, or a sterile inflammation.
- **Sepsis:** SIRS and infection either documented or strongly suspected
- **Severe sepsis:** sepsis plus sepsis-induced organ dysfunction or tissue hypoperfusion, typically systolic blood pressure (SBP) less than 90 mm Hg or mean arterial pressure (MAP) less than 70 mm Hg
- **Septic shock:** an extreme form of sepsis with sepsis-induced hypotension persisting despite adequate fluid resuscitation; findings may include elevated lactic acid or oliguria

Pathophysiology

Initial studies of pathophysiologic features of septic shock concentrated on the interactions of lipopolysaccharides (LPS) from the gram-negative bacterial cell wall with various innate immune system pathways. More recent investigations now focus on understanding the activation and regulation of the innate and acquired immune systems and the array of cytokines that are released during localized and systemic inflammatory responses.

Bacterial Cell Wall Components in Septic Shock

The exotoxins produced by some bacteria (e.g., exotoxin A produced by *P. aeruginosa*) can initiate septic shock. **However, the bacteria themselves, and in particular their cell wall components, are primarily responsible for the development of septic shock. These components activate numerous innate immunologic pathways, including macrophages, neutrophils, and dendritic cells and the complement system. The prime initiator of gram-negative bacterial septic shock is endotoxin, an LPS component of the bacterial outer membrane.** Endotoxin can directly activate the coagulation, complement, and fibrinolytic systems, leading to the release of small molecules that cause vasodilation and increased endothelial permeability (Tapper and Herwald, 2000).

Cytokine Network

Monocytic cells appear to have a pivotal role in mediation of the biologic effects of SIRS and septic shock. Monocytes can remove and detoxify LPS and be beneficial to the host. However, LPS-stimulated monocytes produce cytokines such as tumor necrosis factor (TNF) and interleukin (IL)-1. The intravascular activation of inflammatory systems involved in septic shock is mainly the consequence of an overproduction of these and other cytokines. Production of these cytokines is modulated by CD4$^+$ T helper cells. Type I CD4$^+$ T helper cells release proinflammatory cytokines including TNF-α, interferon-γ, and IL-2. These cytokines are also produced by macrophages, endothelial cells, and other cells stimulated by microbial products. The systemic release of large amounts of the cytokine TNF is associated with death from septic shock in humans (Calandra et al., 1988; Girardin et al., 1988; Waage, 1987). However, despite the fact that TNF is classically regarded as a central mediator of pathophysiologic changes associated with sepsis, the role of attenuation of this and other proinflammatory cytokines remains unclear. For example, in one animal model of peritonitis, survival was worsened by the administration of antibodies blocking TNF (Eskandari et al., 1992). Also, patients suffering from rheumatoid arthritis treated with TNF-α agents remain susceptible to the development of septic shock. Last, a meta-analysis of clinical trials using anti-inflammatory agents in sepsis suggested these agents were generally harmful in all but a small subset of patients (Hotchkiss and Karl, 2003). More recently, anti-inflammatory cytokines, including IL-4 and IL-10, released by type II CD4$^+$ T helper cells, have also been noted to be elevated in sepsis, further illustrating the complex regulation of proinflammatory and anti-inflammatory cytokines in a septic patient. In summary, proinflammatory and anti-inflammatory cytokines are elements of early sepsis; however, the role of cytokine modulation in the treatment of sepsis remains unclear.

Clinical Presentation and Diagnosis

Early signs of systemic inflammatory response syndrome include **temperature extremes (>38°C [100.4°F] or <36°C [96.8°F]), tachycardia (heart rate >90 beats/min), tachypnea, and altered mental status.** The classic bedside findings differentiating septic shock from other types of shock include a warm patient, brisk capillary refill, and a bounding pulse reflecting pyrexia, peripheral vasodilation, and decreased systemic vascular resistance. Other diagnostic criteria include evidence of **organ dysfunction** such as hypotension, oliguria, or ileus and **laboratory abnormalities** including leukocytosis or leukopenia, hyperbilirubinemia, hyperlactatemia, hyperglycemia, coagulation abnormalities, and elevated C-reactive protein and procalcitonin (see Box 55.12). The classic clinical presentation of fever and chills followed by hypotension is manifest only in about 30% of patients with gram-negative bacteremia (McClure, 1983). Even before temperature extremes and the onset of chills, bacteremic patients often begin to hyperventilate. Thus the **earliest metabolic change in septicemia is a resultant respiratory alkalosis.** In critically ill patients, the sudden onset of hyperventilation should lead to blood drawing for culture and careful evaluation of the patient. **Changes in mental status can also be important clinical** clues. Although the most common pattern is lethargy or obtundation, an occasional patient may become excited, agitated, or combative. Cutaneous manifestations such as the bull's-eye lesion associated with *P. aeruginosa* may be identified.

Metastatic infections secondary to GU tract bacteremia have been described (Siroky et al., 1976). In this review of 137 patients who developed metastatic infections from bacteremia with a GU source, 79% had undergone prior urologic instrumentation, 59% developed skeletal infections, mainly of the spine, and 29% developed endocarditis, most commonly caused by *E. faecalis*.

Bacteriology

In classic studies of sepsis syndrome and septic shock, gram-negative bacteria were predominant organisms isolated in 30% to 80% of cases and gram-positive bacteria in 5% to 24% (Bone, 1991; Calandra et al., 1988; Ispahani et al., 1987). Although *E. coli* is the most common organism causing gram-negative bacteremia, many nosocomial catheter-associated infections are caused by highly resistant gram-negative organisms: *P. aeruginosa*, *Proteus*, *Providencia*, and *Serratia* spp. *Acinetobacter* and *Enterobacter* spp. are also emerging as important nosocomial pathogens. In a large series, *E. coli* caused about one-third of the cases; the *Klebsiella-Enterobacter-Serratia* family, approximately 20%; and *Pseudomonas*, *Proteus*, *Providencia*, and anaerobic species, approximately 10% each (Kreger et al., 1980). Anaerobic organisms may cause bacteremia when the source is a postsurgical intra-abdominal abscess or transrectal prostatic biopsy. **More recent studies suggest the incidence of sepsis caused by gram-positive bacterial and fungal organisms is increasing** (Martin et al., 2003) **and reinforce the need for initial broad-spectrum antimicrobial coverage.**

Management

The principles of management of sepsis include resuscitation, supportive care, monitoring, administration of broad-spectrum antimicrobial agents, and drainage or elimination of infection (Dellinger et al., 2008; Sessler et al., 2004). Although the identification and early intervention of sepsis by the urologist is important, the use of expert consultants is also recommended because management of sepsis and the critically ill patient is complex and always evolving. Early goal-directed therapy remains the standard approach since it was shown to be significantly beneficial in a 263-patient study by Rivers et al. (2001).

Principles of resuscitation include support of the airway and breathing and optimization of perfusion with the use of invasive pressure monitoring with central access (Rivers et al., 2001). Intubation and mechanical ventilation may be required in patients who are obtunded and unable to protect their airway. Supplemental oxygen may be instituted, but supranormal oxygen delivery is no longer considered a goal of therapy (Dellinger et al., 2008). **Tissue perfusion should first be optimized** with fluid resuscitation to restore mean circulating filling pressures; this may include crystalloid and or colloid/blood products. If additional blood pressure support is needed, vasoactive agents including phenylephrine, norepinephrine, vasopressin, and dopamine can be instituted; however, low-dose dopamine administration for renal protection is no longer recommended by critical care experts. Other principles of resuscitation and supportive care include optimization of oxygen delivery, correction of coagulopathies if clinically significant, maintenance of blood glucose levels below 110 mg/dL with intensive insulin therapy (van den Berghe et al., 2001), and implementation of hemofiltration as needed (Schiffl et al., 2002). The use of hydrocortisone therapy in septic shock patients did not show a survival or disease-specific benefit in patients in a large study (Sprung et al., 2008).

Identification of the presumptive source of infection and cultures from corresponding fluids and blood should be obtained before the initiation of antimicrobial therapy. Multiple blood cultures for aerobic and anaerobic organisms should be obtained. In addition, all potential sources of bacteremia must be cultured (i.e., urine, sputum, and wounds). Careful attempts to identify the source of infection should be made because the choice of appropriate antimicrobial coverage depends on the organisms that are thought most likely to cause the infection. The severity of the underlying disease and the possibility of synergistic interactions are also important considerations. **If the urinary tract is the most likely portal of entry, a broad-spectrum antimicrobial either alone or in combination with an aminoglycoside should be administered. Three clinical factors have been predictive of the subsequent isolation of a resistant pathogen: (1) the use of an antimicrobial drug in the last month, (2) advanced age, and (3) male sex** (Leibovici et al., 1992). If the infection is hospital acquired, or if the patient has had multiple infections or is immunocompromised or severely ill, an aminoglycoside and anti-*Pseudomonas* β-lactam or a third-generation cephalosporin should be used. When identification and drug susceptibilities of the offending organism are known, antimicrobial therapy should be changed to use the lowest cost, least toxic antimicrobial with the narrowest antimicrobial coverage. Antimicrobial treatment should be continued until the patient has been afebrile for 3 to 4 days and is clinically stable. Local infections that may have provided the focus for the bacteremia should be treated individually as appropriate. The surviving sepsis campaign suggests the initiation of broad-spectrum antibiotics within 1 hour of diagnosis of septic shock (Dellinger et al., 2008).

> **KEY POINTS: BACTEREMIA, SEPSIS, AND SEPTIC SHOCK**
>
> - Sepsis is a clinical syndrome characterized by extremes of body temperature, heart rate, respiratory rate, and WBC count that occurs in response to an infection.
> - The principles of management of sepsis include resuscitation, supportive care, monitoring, administration of broad-spectrum antimicrobial agents, and drainage or elimination of infection.
> - The surviving sepsis campaign and early goal-directed therapy have been shown to improve outcomes in critically ill patients.

Bacteriuria in Pregnancy

Pregnancy

The prevalence of bacteriuria in pregnant women varies from 4% to 7%, and the incidence of acute clinical pyelonephritis ranges from 25% to 35% in untreated bacteriuric women (Stamey, 1980). This is probably the result of dilation of the ureters and pelvis of the kidney secondary to pregnancy-related hormonal alterations. In addition, urine obtained from a pregnant woman at any gestational stage exhibits a more suitable pH for growth of *E. coli* (Asscher et al., 1973). **It is not surprising that untreated bacteriuria in the first trimester is accompanied by a substantial increase in the incidence of acute pyelonephritis because half of these women have upper tract bacteriuria** (Fairley et al., 1966).

Untreated bacteriuria involving these dilated upper tracts could be expected to cause a significant number of abnormalities that should be radiologically apparent. Kincaid-Smith and Bullen (1965) performed a culture on 4000 women at their first antenatal visit. Out of 240 bacteriuric women, 148 returned for excretory urography 6 weeks after delivery. Approximately 40% of these patients had radiologic abnormalities consistent with pyelonephritis or analgesic nephritis. Brumfitt et al. (1967) showed that the incidence of radiologic abnormalities in bacteriuria of pregnancy was proportional to the difficulty in clearing the infection. Patients who responded promptly to a single course of therapy had a 23% incidence of radiologic abnormalities, but those who remained bacteriuric despite repeated therapeutic efforts had a 65% incidence of radiologic changes. Thus prolonged bacteriuria and pyelonephritis of pregnancy appear to be **associated** with significant radiologic abnormalities. However, there is little evidence to suggest that bacteriuria of pregnancy or acute pyelonephritis of pregnancy **causes** these renal radiologic abnormalities.

Recurrent UTIs are common in pregnant women and can result in preterm labor and low-birth-weight babies. All pregnant women should routinely be screened for bacteriuria. Aggressive management of the bacteriuria is necessary: as stated earlier, pregnant women are one of the few categories of patients who require treatment of asymptomatic bacteriuria, per the IDSA guidelines. **Screening with urine culture is recommended at the initial visit by the American College of Obstetricians and Gynecologists (ACOG). Treatment of asymptomatic bacteriuria has been shown to reduce morbidity and complications. Asymptomatic bacteriuria is one of the most common infectious issues encountered during pregnancy. The prevalence of asymptomatic bacteriuria does not change with the occurrence of pregnancy and ranges from 2% to 7%** (Hooton et al., 2000). The risk of acquiring bacteriuria during pregnancy increases with lower socioeconomic class, multiparity, and sickle cell traits (Patterson and Andriole, 1987; Stenqvist et al., 1989).

The site of bacteriuria in pregnant female patients probably also reflects the situation before conception. In two studies that localized the origin of the bacteriuria, one using the Stamey ureteral catheterization technique and the other the Fairley bladder washout, upper tract infections were found in 44% and 24.5% of pregnant female patients, respectively (Fairley et al., 1966; Heineman and Lee, 1973). In non-pregnant females with recurrent bacteriuria, Stamey (1980) has reported about a 50% probability that the origin is in the upper tract. With other techniques, which may reflect the severity of tissue infection rather than the location of infection, the results are similar; approximately 50% of women with screening bacteriuria of pregnancy are fluorescent antibody-positive (Fa$^+$) and thus have evidence of upper tract infection (Harrison et al., 1974). Fairley and his group (1973) found that the site of infection is unrelated to the likelihood that pyelonephritis will develop during pregnancy.

Spontaneous resolution of bacteriuria detected by standard urine culture in pregnant women is unlikely unless it is treated. Non-pregnant patients often clear their asymptomatic bacteriuria (Hooton et al., 2000), **but pregnant women become symptomatic more frequently and tend to remain bacteriuric** (Elder et al., 1971).

Pyelonephritis develops in 1% to 4% of all pregnant women (Sweet, 1977) **and in 15% to 45% of pregnant women with untreated bacteriuria** (Pedler and Bint, 1987; Wright et al., 1993). **Of the women who develop pyelonephritis during pregnancy, 60% to 75% acquire it during the third trimester** (Cunningham et al., 1973), **when hydronephrosis and stasis in the urinary tract are most pronounced. As many as 10% to 20% of pregnant women who get pyelonephritis develop it again before or just after delivery** (Cunningham et al., 1973; Gilstrap et al., 1981). Moreover, a third of pregnant women who develop pyelonephritis have a documented prior history of pyelonephritis (Gilstrap et al., 1981). **The increased likelihood that bacteriuria may progress to acute pyelonephritis during pregnancy alters the morbidity of bacteriuria for this group. Treatment of screening bacteriuria of pregnancy decreases the incidence of acute pyelonephritis during pregnancy from a range of 13.5% to 65% to a range of 0 to 5.3%** (Sweet, 1977).

Pathogenesis

The anatomic and physiologic changes induced by the gravid state significantly alter the natural history of bacteriuria (Patterson and Andriole, 1987). **These changes may cause pregnant women to be more susceptible to pyelonephritis and may require alteration of therapy.** These changes have been well summarized in several reviews (Davidson and Talner, 1978; Waltzer, 1981).

Anatomic and Physiologic Changes During Pregnancy

Increase in Renal Size

Renal length increases approximately 1 cm during normal pregnancy. It is thought that this does not represent true hypertrophy but is the result of increased renal vascular and interstitial volume. No histologic changes have been identified in renal biopsies (Waltzer, 1981).

Smooth Muscle Atony of the Collecting System and Bladder

The collecting system, especially the ureters, undergoes decreased peristalsis during pregnancy, and most women in their third trimester show significant ureteral dilation (Davison and Lindheimer, 1978; Kincaid-Smith, 1978; Waltzer, 1981; Fig. 55.41). **This hydroureter has been attributed to the muscle-relaxing effects of increased progesterone during pregnancy and to mechanical obstruction of the ureters by the enlarging uterus at the pelvic brim.** Progesterone-induced smooth muscle relaxation also may cause an increased bladder capacity (Waltzer, 1981). Later in pregnancy, the dilation may be the result of the obstructive effect of the enlarging uterus (Poole and Thorsen, 1999).

Bladder Changes

The enlarging uterus displaces the bladder superiorly and anteriorly. The bladder becomes hyperemic and may appear congested when viewed endoscopically (Waltzer, 1981). Estrogen stimulation probably causes bladder hypertrophy, as well as squamous changes of the urethra (Waltzer, 1981).

Augmented Renal Function

The transient increases in glomerular filtration rate and renal plasma flow during pregnancy have been well summarized by several authors, and are probably secondary to the increase in cardiac output (Davison and Lindheimer, 1978; Kincaid-Smith, 1978; Waltzer, 1981; Zacur and Mitch, 1977). **Glomerular filtration increases by 30% to 50%, and urinary protein excretion increases. The significance of these physiologic changes is apparent when the normal serum creatinine and urea nitrogen values for pregnant women are surveyed** (Table 55.12). **Values considered normal in non-pregnant women may represent renal insufficiency during pregnancy.**

Davison and Lindheimer (1978) recommend that pregnant patients with serum creatinine levels greater than 0.8 mg/dL or urea nitrogen levels greater than 13 mg/dL undergo further evaluation of renal function. Similarly, **urinary protein in pregnancy is not considered abnormal until more than 300 mg of protein in 24 hours is excreted.**

These significant physiologic changes in pregnancy, which may develop as early as the first trimester, lead to urinary stasis and mild hydroureteronephrosis, and contribute to development of pyelonephritis.

Recent studies of *E. coli* adhesins and their respective specific tissue receptors have established an adhesin-based mechanism for pyelonephritis-induced pre-term birth and low birth weight in mice (Kaul et al., 1999). There is a higher incidence of *E. coli*–bearing Dr adhesins during the third trimester of pregnancy in women with gestational pyelonephritis (Nowicki et al., 1994) and an upregulation of Dr adhesin in the kidney, endometrium, and placenta during the third trimester of pregnancy (Martens et al., 1993). When infected intravesically with *E. coli*–bearing Dr adhesin, nearly 90% of mice that were hyporesponsive to bacterial lipopolysaccharide and that had a deficient immune response delivered pre-term. However, only 10% of mice infected with *E. coli* without Dr adhesion delivered pre-term. Also, there was a significant reduction in fetal birth weight

TABLE 55.12 Average Values for Serum Creatinine and Urea Nitrogen

	NON-PREGNANT FEMALES (mg/dL)	PREGNANT FEMALES (mg/dL)
Serum creatinine	0.7	0.5
Urea nitrogen	13.0	9.0

Data from Davison JM, Lindheimer MD: Renal disease in pregnant women. *Clin Obstet Gynecol* 21:411, 1978.

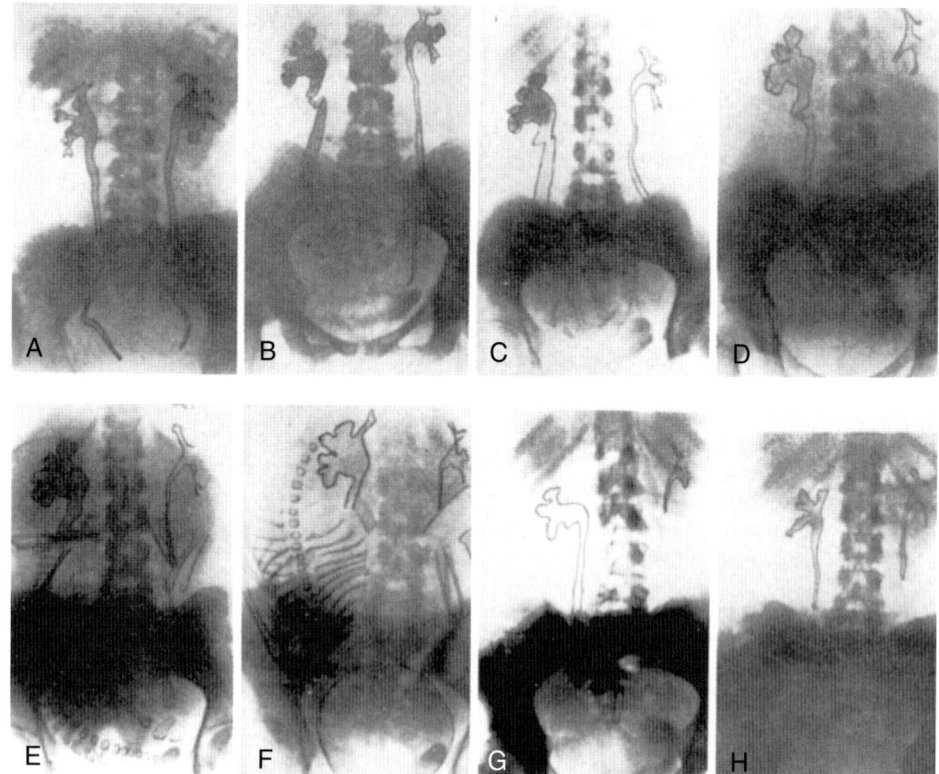

Fig. 55.41. Progressive hydroureter and hydronephrosis observed on intravenous pyelogram during a normal pregnancy. (A) 15 weeks; (B) 18 weeks; (C) 22 weeks; (D) 26 weeks; (E) 34 weeks; (F) 39 weeks; (G) 1 week postpartum; (H) 6 weeks postpartum. Bilateral hydroureter and hydronephrosis are shown as early as 15 weeks (A). (B to H) Successive urograms are from one patient during a normal pregnancy. Dilation occurs mainly on the right side, and both urinary tracts are normal by 6 weeks after delivery. (From Hundley JM, Walton HJ, Hibbits JT, et al.: Physiologic changes occurring in the urinary tract during pregnancy. *Am J Obstet Gynecol* 30:625–649, 1935.)

in the Dr adhesin–infected group. Bacterial tissue culture showed systemic spread of the *E. coli*–bearing Dr adhesins to the placentae and fetuses.

Complications Associated With Bacteriuria During Pregnancy

Prematurity and Prenatal Mortality

In the pre-antimicrobial era, pregnant women with symptomatic UTIs and bacterial pyelonephritis were reported to have a high incidence of prematurity, low birth weight, and death (Gilstrap et al., 1981). The relationship between asymptomatic bacteriuria and prematurity is less clear. Gilstrap et al. (1981) found no difference in prematurity rates between pregnant patients treated for asymptomatic bacteriuria and non-bacteriuric controls. However, Cunnington's review suggests that ascending GU tract infections may contribute to up to 50% of premature deliveries, especially when they occur before 30 weeks' gestation (Cunnington et al., 2013). **Pregnant women with asymptomatic bacteriuria are at higher risk for developing symptomatic UTIs that result in adverse fetal outcomes, pyelonephritis, and possible maternal sequelae such as sepsis. Therefore all pregnant women with asymptomatic bacteriuria should be treated** (Smaill, 2001).

Information on maternal anemia is available online at Expert Consult.com.

Laboratory Diagnosis

Significant false-negative rates occur if screening is conducted by urinalysis or reagent strip testing (McNair et al., 2000; Preston et al., 1999). **Therefore an initial screening culture should be performed in all pregnant women during the first trimester** (Stenqvist et al., 1989). The US Preventive Services Task Force (USPSTF) recommends screening for asymptomatic bacteriuria with urine culture in pregnant women at 12 to 16 weeks' gestation or at the first prenatal visit, if later (Lin et al., 2008). If the culture shows no growth, repeat cultures are generally unnecessary because **patients who have no growth in their urine early in their pregnancy are unlikely to develop bacteriuria later** (McFadyen et al., 1973; Norden and Kass, 1968). Pregnant women with a history of recurrent UTI or VUR may benefit from AP (Bukowski et al., 1998).

Management

Selection of an antimicrobial agent to treat the bacteriuria must be made, however, with special considerations given to maternal and fetal toxicity. The physiologic changes of pregnancy such as maternal expanded fluid volume, the distribution of the drug to the fetus, increased renal blood flow, and increased glomerular filtration may decrease the serum drug concentration. **If the culture is positive, special consideration must be given to the selection of antimicrobial agents chosen to treat infection and prevent fetal toxicity.** The pathogens are similar to those seen in non-pregnant women (MacDonald et al., 1983). Table 55.13 lists the antimicrobial agents and dosing for use in pregnancy. The **aminopenicillins and cephalosporins are considered safe and generally effective throughout pregnancy. In patients with penicillin allergy, nitrofurantoin is a reasonable alternative. It may be used safely during the first two trimesters in patients without glucose-6-phosphate dehydrogenase deficiency.** Nitrofurantoin is often used **because fluoroquinolones and TMP-SMX are contraindicated in pregnancy.**

TABLE 55.13 Oral Antimicrobial Agents Used in Pregnancy

DRUG	DOSAGE	COMMENTS
AGENTS CONSIDERED SAFE		
Penicillins		
Ampicillin	500 mg four times daily	Extensively used
Amoxicillin	250 mg three times daily	Safe and effective
Penicillin V	500 mg four times daily	Used less frequently but achieves excellent urinary levels
Cephalosporins		
Cephalexin	500 mg four times daily	Extensively used
Cefaclor	500 mg four times daily	Somewhat more effective against gram-negative organisms
Nitrofurantoin	100 mg four times daily	May be used during the first two trimesters; may result in hemolytic anemia in patients with G6PD deficiency
AGENTS THAT SHOULD BE AVOIDED		
Fluoroquinolones		Possible damage to immature cartilage
Chloramphenicol		Associated with "gray baby" syndrome
Trimethoprim		Inhibits folic acid metabolism and is thus teratogenic especially with respect to neural tube defects
Erythromycin		Associated with maternal cholestatic jaundice
Tetracyclines		May cause acute liver decompensation in the mother and inhibition of new bone growth in the fetus

G6PD, Glucose-6-phosphate dehydrogenase.
Modified from Schaeffer AJ: Urinary tract infections. In Gillenwater JY, Grayhack JT, Howards SS, et al., editors: *Adult and pediatric urology*, Philadelphia, 2002, Lippincott Williams & Wilkins, pp 211–272.

If nitrofurantoin is used, however, this is discontinued at 35 weeks of gestation because of an increased risk of hemolytic anemia in the neonate. If a pregnant woman has a single episode of pyelonephritis or two episodes of cystitis, daily suppression with either nitrofurantoin or cephalexin should be considered until delivery. It is prudent to prescribe a full 3- to 7-day course of therapy in pregnant women.

In 2011 a Cochrane Review completed by Widmer et al. showed that antibiotic treatment of asymptomatic bacteriuria in pregnant women significantly decreases the risk of pyelonephritis and preterm delivery. However, there was not adequate evidence at that time to suggest that a single-dose treatment was as effective as standard conventional treatment (Widmer et al., 2011). A more recent Cochrane review published in 2015 looked at the duration of treatment for asymptomatic bacteriuria (Widmer et al., 2015). The authors looked at 13 studies that included 1622 women and compared single-dose treatment with 4- to 7-day course (short) treatment. The review found that a 7-day regimen was more effective than a 1-day course, especially for preventing a low-birth-weight outcome, but this was based on only one study. There were no differences for other review outcomes such as pyelonephritis and preterm birth. The authors concluded by saying although more trials were needed, women with asymptomatic bacteriuria in pregnancy should be treated with a standard time regimen of antibiotics.

Follow-up cultures should be obtained to document absence of infection. If the culture is positive, the cause of bacteriuria must be determined to be lack of resolution, bacterial persistence, or reinfection. If the infection is unresolved, proper selection and administration of another drug will likely solve the problem. If the problem is bacterial persistence or rapid reinfection, antimicrobial suppression of infection or prophylaxis (Pfau and Sacks, 1992) throughout the remainder of the pregnancy should be considered.

Pregnant women with acute pyelonephritis should be hospitalized and initially treated with parenteral antimicrobial agents until clinical improvement is noted. There is no strong evidence to recommend a specific treatment regimen in pregnant women. β-Lactam antibiotics are commonly used because they are considered relatively safe for the fetus. Carbapenems are generally used in select severe cases including those caused by multidrug-resistant bacteria (Matuszkiewicz-Rowinska et al., 2015). However, older series reported that more than 95% of these patients respond within 24 hours using ampicillin and an aminoglycoside (Cunningham et al., 1973) or cephalosporins (Sanchez-Ramos et al., 1995). Despite known toxicities, a recent study concluded that aminoglycosides, specifically gentamicin, are still used often in pregnant women with UTIs, thus subjecting them unnecessarily to ototoxicity (Kushner et al., 2016). Parenteral treatment should be tailored on the basis of culture sensitivities before transitioning to oral antibiotics. If improvement is not seen within 72 hours of the commencement of antibiotics, a renal ultrasound should be performed to assess for stone, obstruction, or abscess. If there is a strong suspicion of a urologic stone that cannot be seen with ultrasound, a plain radiograph of the abdomen or a low-dose spiral CT should be considered in urgent cases.

A Cochrane review published in 2015 looked at interventions for preventing recurrent UTI during pregnancy. The authors concluded that close surveillance alone was as effective as a daily dose of nitrofurantoin and close surveillance together to prevent recurrent UTIs, although the evidence was low quality. They also found there was a significant reduction in asymptomatic bacteriuria in women who had a high clinic attendance rate and had received nitrofurantoin and close surveillance (Schneeberger et al., 2015).

Medications that are relatively contraindicated during pregnancy include the fluoroquinolones, TMP, chloramphenicol, erythromycin, tetracycline, sulfonamides, and sometimes nitrofurantoin (Nicolle, 1987). Fluoroquinolones are contraindicated because of their effects on immature cartilage. TMP may have teratogenic effects and should be avoided, especially in the first trimester. The "gray baby" syndrome is a toxic effect of chloramphenicol on neonates resulting from the inability of the infant to metabolize or excrete the drug. Erythromycin may cause cholestatic jaundice in the mother. Tetracycline may cause fetal malformations and maternal liver decompensation. Sulfonamides may cause kernicterus and neonatal hyperbilirubinemia and should be avoided in the third trimester. As mentioned earlier, nitrofurantoin can cause hemolytic anemia in mother and child when glucose-6-phosphate dehydrogenase deficiency is present (Nicolle, 1987).

Information about pregnancy in women with renal insufficiency is available online at ExpertConsult.com.

> **KEY POINTS: BACTERIURIA IN PREGNANCY**
> - Screening for bacteriuria via urine culture should be performed in all pregnant women during the first trimester.
> - The prevalence of bacteriuria does not change with the occurrence of pregnancy; however, unlike in non-pregnant women, spontaneous resolution of bacteriuria in pregnant women is unlikely.
> - All pregnant women with bacteriuria should be treated.
> - Bacteriuria more commonly progresses to acute pyelonephritis during pregnancy.

BACTERIURIA AND URINARY TRACT INFECTIONS IN THE ELDERLY

As the average life expectancy increases, the diagnosis, treatment, and morbidity and mortality of UTIs in the geriatric population will continue to be of utmost importance. In 2012 there were 43.1 million Americans older than 65 years of age (Ortman et al., 2014). By the year 2050, however, the population aged 65 and over in the United States is projected to be 83.7 million. Certainly, this trajectory in population dynamics within the US alone highlights the public health issue inherent to this topic.

Epidemiology

At least 20% of women and 10% of men older than 65 years have bacteriuria that is detected by standard urine culture (Boscia and Kaye, 1987). In contrast to young adults, in whom bacteriuria is 30 times more prevalent in women than in men, this ratio in the elderly progressively decreases to 2:1. Most elderly patients with bacteriuria are asymptomatic.

The prevalence of bacteriuria in the elderly increases with age (Brocklehurst et al., 1968; Sourander, 1966) and concurrent disease and may exceed 50% in selective groups (Boscia and Kaye, 1987; Schaeffer, 1991). Bacteriuria is present in greater than 20% of healthy community-dwelling women older than 80 years of age and in 6% to 15% of community-dwelling men who are older than 75 years of age (Nicolle, 2003). Estimates of bacteriuria in those living in long-term care facilities range from 25% to 50% of women and 15% to 40% of men (Nicolle, 1997). Risk factors can be compounded. In a study of 373 women and 150 men older than 68 years of age, 24% of functionally impaired nursing home residents had bacteriuria compared with 12% of healthy domiciliary subjects (Boscia et al., 1986).

Screening for Bacteriuria

Screening for asymptomatic bacteriuria in elderly residents in the community or long-term care facilities is not recommended (Abrutyn et al., 1994; Boscia et al., 1987; Nicolle et al., 1983, 2005; Nordenstam et al., 1986). There is no documented relationship between asymptomatic bacteriuria and uncomplicated UTIs and worsening renal function. The treatment of asymptomatic bacteriuria to improve incontinence has not been justified (Baldassarre and Kaye, 1991; Ouslander et al., 1995). Although studies have demonstrated decreased survival in bacteriuric patients compared with non-bacteriuric control subjects, it is unclear whether increased mortality rates and bacteriuria are causally related (Abrutyn et al., 1994; Baldassarre and Kaye, 1991).

Pathogenesis

The pathophysiology of increased susceptibility to bacteriuria/UTIs is multifactorial and poorly understood. **Age-related changes include a decline in cell-mediated immunity, incomplete bladder emptying, neurogenic bladder dysfunction, increased perineal soiling as a result of fecal and urinary incontinence, increased incidence of urethral catheter placement, and, in women, changes in the vaginal environment associated with estrogen depletion** (Arnold et al., 2016; Raz and Stamm, 1993; Schaeffer, 1991).

Bacteriologic characteristics of infection in the elderly differ from those in younger patients (Baldassarre and Kaye, 1991). *E. coli* **remains the most common uropathogen overall, causing 50% to 75% of these infections** (Nicolle, 2001). However, there is a **significant increase in the incidence of *Proteus*, *Klebsiella*, *Enterobacter*, *Serratia*, and *Pseudomonas* spp., as well as enterococci**. One study found that in community-dwelling older women, organisms responsible for asymptomatic bacteriuria include *E. coli* (51.4%), *K. pneumoniae* (4.1%), *Proteus mirabilis* (3.3%), and *Enterococcus faecalis* (2.5%) (Linhares et al., 2013). Enterococci in the elderly tend to resolve without treatment; this is felt to represent colonization (Das et al., 2009). Bacteriuria caused by gram-positive bacteria is much more common in elderly men than in elderly women (Jackson et al., 1962); however, *S. saprophyticus* is not seen in this population. Polymicrobial bacteriuria is also more common among the geriatric population (Nicolle et al., 1987). Cumulatively, the shift in the pattern of uropathogens, the high frequency of polymicrobial infections, and antimicrobial resistance in the elderly are due in large part to an increase in institutionalization and hospitalization, catheterization, and overall antimicrobial usage (Routh et al., 2009).

Diagnosis

In the elderly, UTI symptoms may be more subtle, such as generalized abdominal discomfort or delirium. **Even severe upper tract infections may not be associated with fever or leukocytosis** (Baldassarre and Kaye, 1991). **However, new signs or symptoms localized to the lower urinary tract, specifically dysuria, remain the most important UTI criteria, even in the elderly.** Traditionally, altered mental status has often been attributed to a UTI in the elderly. However, because bacteriuria is more common with age, the mere presence of a positive urine culture in a patient with altered mental status is not tantamount with a UTI. This dilemma makes diagnosing a UTI, particularly in a patient who cannot reliably report symptoms, challenging. **Although it has been common practice to treat elderly bacteriuric patients with antibiotics because of confusion, no data demonstrate treatment improves a patient's condition** (Finucane, 2017).

Because new signs or symptoms localized to the GU tract are most important even in the geriatric population, dizziness and confusion, in the absence of urinary symptoms, should not be attributed to a UTI. Therefore it is not recommended to send urine cultures on patients for nonspecific symptoms or chronic urinary symptoms such as incontinence and frequency, nor for asymptomatic patients (Mody and Juthani-Mehta, 2014; Nicolle, 2002). Sending urine studies in patients with dementia or other impaired mental status (when defining dysuria is difficult) may be of clinical benefit when not responsive to other interventions (i.e., hydration). **If elderly patients experience mental status changes yet no urinary complaints, they should be hydrated then reassessed. If altered mental status and/or change in character of urine persists despite fluid resuscitation, then urine testing should be considered** (see figure at https://www.ncbi.nlm.nih.gov/pmc/articles/PMC4194886/) (Mody and Juthani-Mehta, 2014). Finally, obtaining a culture to document clearance of bacteria is never recommended (Mody and Juthani-Mehta, 2014).

A high index of suspicion is warranted when evaluating geriatric patients; therefore diagnosis should rely on the results of a carefully obtained urinalysis and culture. **The presence of greater than 10^5 CFU/mL of urine remains the standard for diagnosis** in patients with clinical signs and symptoms of UTI. However, **counts of 10^2 or more bacteria are clinically significant in catheterized specimens** (Kunin, 1987; Nicolle et al., 2005).

The use of laboratory testing in the diagnosis of UTI in the elderly also poses some challenges. Urinary dipstick testing for leukocyte esterase, nitrites, or both has a different specificity and sensitivity depending on the clinical population. Sensitivity and specificity for a positive dipstick test in older adults is 82% (95% CI 74%–92%) and 71% (95% CI 55%–71%), making the urine dipstick a more valuable test to rule out UTI than diagnosing its presence

(Deville et al., 2004; Kunin, 1994). These data are linked to the fact that, unlike in younger adults, pyuria and in turn the presence of leukocyte esterase, has been shown to be an inaccurate predictor of bacteriuria in the elderly. **Pyuria is common in elderly patients, and pyuria alone is not a good predictor of bacteriuria nor an indication for antimicrobial treatment in the elderly population** (Nicolle et al., 2005; Ouslander et al., 1996). Accordingly, Boscia et al. (1989) reported that more than 60% of women with pyuria of 10 WBCs/mm^3 or greater (noted in midstream specimens) did not have a concurrent bacteriuria. However, **the absence of pyuria was a good predictor of the absence of bacteriuria**, and this accounts for the high specificity associated with dipstick testing.

Finally, declining functional and mental status in elderly adults, as well as a potentially difficult body habitus, often makes obtaining a true midstream clean-catch urine specimen extremely challenging. In institutionalized elderly patients and those with limited dexterity, a catheterized specimen may be the only way to obtain an uncontaminated urine specimen (Nicolle, 2002; Nicolle et al., 2005).

Because urinary tract abnormalities can predispose to and complicate the management and sequela of bacteriuria in the elderly, a thorough urologic evaluation is warranted. Renal dysfunction, calculi, hydronephrosis, urinary retention, neurogenic bladder dysfunction, and other abnormalities should be identified by serum creatinine measurement, CT, ultrasonography, urodynamics (UDS), and/or cystoscopy. The timing and sequence of these tests should be dictated by the clinical setting.

Bacteriuria that leads to UTIs in elderly subjects in the presence of underlying structural urinary tract abnormalities (e.g., obstruction with hydronephrosis) or systemic conditions (e.g., severe diabetes mellitus) are clinically significant, can lead to renal failure, and require prompt therapy. In addition, UTIs caused by urea-splitting bacteria, such as *Proteus* or *Klebsiella* species that cause formation of infection stones, may also lead to severe renal damage.

Sepsis and its sequelae (sepsis syndrome and septic shock) are increasingly common in the elderly. Risk factors include the aggressive use of catheters (Kunin et al., 1992) and other invasive equipment, implantation of prosthetic devices, and the administration of chemotherapy to cancer patients or corticosteroids in other immunosuppressed patients. In addition, modern medical care has given longer life spans to the elderly and other populations of patients with metabolic, neoplastic, or immunodeficiency disorders who remain at increased risk for infection.

Management

Prospective randomized comparative trials of antimicrobial or no therapy in elderly male and female nursing home residents with asymptomatic bacteriuria consistently document no benefit of antimicrobial therapy. On the contrary, treatment with antimicrobial therapy increases the occurrence of adverse drug effects and reinfection with resistant organisms and increases the cost of treatment. **Therefore asymptomatic bacteriuria in elderly residents of long-term care facilities should not be treated with antimicrobial agents.**

The McGeer infection surveillance definitions provide standardized criteria for infections that commonly occur in residents of aged-care homes. The criteria to be diagnosed with a UTI include a combination of clinical signs and microbiology (Stone et al., 2012). The criteria required vary, depending on whether the patient has an indwelling catheter or not. Critics of the McGeer criteria point out that the ability to interpret the clinical signs in those who are cognitively impaired is limited (Ryan et al., 2018; Table 55.14).

If patients have lower tract symptoms and symptoms are mild, it is prudent to wait for urine culture before treatment. For those elderly patients who require immediate treatment, empirical antibiotics should be started. Traditionally, 7 days of therapy has been recommended. However, a recent Cochrane review of the antibiotic duration

TABLE 55.14 Surveillance Definitions for Urinary Tract Infections

CRITERIA
A. For residents without an indwelling catheter (both criteria 1 and 2 must be present)
 1. At least 1 of the following sign or symptom subcriteria
    a. Acute dysuria or acute pain, swelling, or tenderness of the testes, epididymis, or prostrate
    b. Fever or leukocytosis and at least 1 of the following localizing urinary tract subcriteria
       i. Acute costovertebral angle pain or tenderness
       ii. Suprapubic pain
       iii. Gross hematuria
       iv. New or marked increase in incontinence, urgency, or frequency
    c. In the absence of fever or leukocytosis, then 2 or more of the following localizing urinary tract subcriteria
       i. Suprapubic pain
       ii. Gross hematuria
       iii. New or marked increase in incontinence
       iv. New or marked increase in urgency
       v. New or marked increase in frequency
 2. One of the following microbiologic subcriteria
    a. At least 10^5 CFU/mL of no more than 2 species of microorganisms in a voided urine sample
    b. At least 10^2 CFU/mL of any number of organisms in a specimen collected by in-and-out catheter[5]
B. For residents with an indwelling catheter (both criteria 1 and 2 must be present)
 1. At least 1 of the following sign or symptom subcriteria
    a. Fever, rigors, or new-onset hypotension, with no alternate site of infection
    b. Either acute change in mental status or acute functional decline, with no alternate diagnosis and leukocytosis
    c. New-onset suprapubic pain or costovertebral angle pain or tenderness
    d. Purulent discharge from around the catheter or acute pain, swelling or tenderness of the testes, epididymis, or prostate
 2. Urinary catheter specimen culture with at least 10^5 CFU/mL of any organism(s)

Comment: A diagnosis of UTI can be made without localizing symptoms if a blood culture isolate is the same as the organism isolated from the urine and there is no alternate site of infection.

From Stone ND et al.: Surveillance definitions of infections in long-term care facilities: revisiting the McGeer criteria. *Infect Control Hosp Epidemiol* 33(10):965–977, 2012. Reprinted with permission © Cambridge University Press & The Society for Healthcare Epidemiology of America.
From McGeer Criteria, p68, Ryan, Gillespie et al. 2018.

for treating uncomplicated symptomatic UTIs in the elderly included 15 studies totaling 1644 women and showed no difference in short-term clinical failure between short-course (3–6 days) and long-course (7–14 days) oral antibiotic regimens. The rate of persistent UTI was lower with short-term therapy compared with single-dose (Lutters and Vogt-Ferrier, 2008). For individuals with fever or more severe systemic infection, 10 to 14 days of therapy was recommended. The goal in this population was to eliminate symptoms but not sterilize the urine (McMurdo and Gillespie, 2000).

The elderly population is more susceptible than young patients to the toxic and adverse effects of antimicrobial agents (Boscia et al., 1986; Carty et al., 1981; Grieco, 1980). The metabolism and excretion of antimicrobial agents may be impaired, and the resulting increased serum levels can further damage renal function. Interactions with other medications can occur (Stahlmann and Lode, 2003). The safety margin between therapeutic and toxic doses is significantly narrowed. Therefore antimicrobial agents must be used judiciously, and dosing and drug levels should be carefully monitored. **The recent black box warning pertaining to fluoroquinolones urges caution in patients older than 60, in whom the risk of tendon rupture is greatest.** See the Management section for further discussion of antibiotic prescribing regimens/considerations for complicated and uncomplicated infections.

> **KEY POINTS: BACTERIURIA IN THE ELDERLY**
> - Screening for bacteriuria is not recommended in elderly patients because there is no relationship between asymptomatic bacteriuria and uncomplicated UTIs and deteriorating renal function; asymptomatic bacteriuria should not be treated.
> - Infections of the urinary tract may present as subtle signs, and a high index of suspicion is often required for diagnosis.
> - Treatment of symptomatic UTI requires modifications for physiologic and pathophysiologic conditions of the elderly.
> - Obtaining a urine culture to document clearance of bacteriuria is not recommended.

CATHETER-ASSOCIATED URINARY TRACT INFECTION

Guidelines from the CDC define a CAUTI as a UTI after placement of an indwelling urinary catheter for more than 2 days (Centers for Disease Control and Prevention: Urinary Tract Infection, 2015). To be diagnosed with a CAUTI, patients must have one symptom of a UTI (suprapubic tenderness, CVA tenderness, urinary frequency/urgency/dysuria, or fever >100.4°F) and a urine culture with a single organism more than 100,000 CFU/mL.

Catheter-associated bacteriuria is widely recognized as the most common hospital-acquired infection. The development of bacteriuria in the presence of an indwelling catheter is inevitable and occurs at an incidence of approximately 10% per day of catheterization. Sterile and clean intermittent catheterization has been associated with rates of bacteriuria ranging from 1% to 3% per catheterization (Warren, 1997). **The most important risk factors associated with increased likelihood of developing catheter-associated bacteriuria are duration of catheterization, female gender, absence of systemic antimicrobial agents, and catheter-care violations** (Stamm, 1991). **Most patients with catheter-associated bacteriuria are asymptomatic.** In patients with short-term catheter placement, only 10% to 30% of bacteriuric episodes produce typical symptoms of acute infection (Haley et al., 1981; Hartstein et al., 1981). Similarly, although patients with long-term catheters are bacteriuric, the incidence of febrile episodes occurs at a rate of only 1 per 100 days of catheterization (Warren, 1991).

Each CAUTI is estimated to cost between $589 and $758 (Anderson et al., 2007; Tambyah et al., 2002). In patients requiring intensive care, the cost is roughly $2000 per nosocomial UTI (Chen et al., 2009). The nosocomial costs for *E. coli* infections with relatively susceptible strains are considerably lower than for those caused by resistant gram-negative bacteria, which often require expensive parenteral antimicrobial therapy (Tambyah et al., 2002).

In 2008 the Center for Medicare and Medicaid Services (CMS) announced that it will no longer reimburse hospitals for the extra costs resulting from CAUTIs. Judicious use of indwelling Foley catheters in perioperative patients helps to prevent CAUTI. Current recommendations for perioperative use of an indwelling urinary catheter include intraoperative urine output monitoring, prolonged surgeries, and urologic surgeries (Gould, 2009). Limiting the duration of indwelling catheters in these patients is critical. Large nationwide hospital initiatives have helped to reduce the CAUTI rates. The Mayo Clinic reported a 70% decrease in their CAUTI rate over 1 year. They described their protocol as the bundled 6-C CAUTI approach: consider (appropriate placement and daily need for indwelling catheter), connect, clean (catheter care), closed (maintain closed system), call (irrigation when necessary) and culture (only for indication) (Sampathkumar et al., 2016).

Pathogenesis

Bacteria enter the urinary tract of a catheterized patient by several routes. **Bacteria can be introduced at the time of initial catheter placement** by either mechanical inoculation of urethral bacteria or contamination from poor technique. **Subsequently, the bacteria most commonly gain access via a periurethral or intraluminal route** (Stamm, 1991). In women, periurethral entry is the most prevalent. Daifuku and Stamm (1984) found that among 18 women who developed catheter-associated bacteriuria, 12 had antecedent urethral colonization with the infecting strain. **Bacteria may also enter the drainage bag and follow the intraluminal route to the bladder.** This route is particularly common in patients who are clustered among other patients with indwelling catheters (Maizels and Schaeffer, 1980; Tambyah et al., 1999).

The urinary catheter system provides a unique environment that allows for two distinct populations of bacteria: those that grow within the urine and those that grow on the catheter surface. A bacterial **biofilm** represents a microbial environment of microorganisms embedded in an extracellular matrix of bacterial products and host components that often lead to catheter encrustation (Bonadio et al., 2001; Stamm, 1991). The bacterial biofilm prevents antibiotic contact with the bacteria and can result in CAUTI and antibiotic resistance (Chenoweth and Saint, 2016). Certain bacteria, particularly of the *Pseudomonas* and *Proteus* species, are adept at biofilm growth, which may explain their higher incidence in this clinical setting (Mobley and Warren, 1987). The uropathogens isolated from the catheterized urinary tract often differ from those found in uncatheterized ambulatory patients. *E. coli* is still the most common organism isolated, but *Pseudomonas, Proteus,* and *Enterococcus* spp. are prevalent (Warren, 1991). In patients with long-term catheterization (more than 30 days), the bacteriuria is usually polymicrobial, and the presence of four or five pathogens is not uncommon (Warren et al., 1982). Although certain species may persist for long periods, the bacterial populations in these patients tend to be dynamic.

Clinical Presentation

Most patients are asymptomatic. Suprapubic discomfort and development of fever, chills, or flank pain may indicate a symptomatic UTI.

Laboratory Diagnosis

Significant bacteriuria in patients with catheters is present when greater than 100 CFU/mL is present, because even this low level progresses to greater than 10^5 CFU/mL in almost all patients (Maizels and Schaeffer, 1980; Stark and Maki, 1984). Pyuria is not a discriminate indicator of infection in this population.

Management

**Careful aseptic insertion of the catheter and maintenance of a closed dependent drainage system are essential to minimize development of bacteriuria. The catheter-meatal junction should be cleaned daily with water, but antimicrobial agents should be avoided because they lead to colonization with resistant pathogens, such as *Pseudomonas*.

Incorporation of silver oxide (Schaeffer et al., 1988) or silver alloy (Saint et al., 1998) into the catheter and hydrogen peroxide into the drainage bag has been reported to decrease the incidence of bacteriuria in some studies (Schaeffer et al., 1988), but not in other populations (Stamm, 1991). **The major benefit of silver alloy is that it decreases the likelihood of bacteriuria in hospitalized adults catheterized for the short term** (Brosnahan et al., 2004; Newton et al., 2002; Saint et al., 2000).

If an asymptomatic catheterized patient has had an indwelling catheter for 3 or more days and will have the catheter removed, a dipstick test can be used to rule out bacteriuria (Tissot et al., 2001). Concurrent administration of systemic antimicrobial agents transiently decreases the incidence of bacteriuria associated with short-term catheterization, but after 3 to 4 days the incidence of bacteriuria is similar to the rate in catheterized patients not taking systemic antimicrobials agents, and the prevalence of resistant bacteria and side effects is substantial. **Therefore this practice is not recommended.** The concept of instilling nonvirulent bacteria into the bladder to completely block colonization and infection by pathogens has been tested in patients with SCI (Hull et al., 2000). Patients successfully colonized with the nonvirulent strain had reduced symptomatic UTI and a subjective improvement in quality of life.

Patients with indwelling catheters should be treated only if they become symptomatic (e.g., febrile). Urine cultures should be performed before initiating antimicrobial therapy. The antimicrobial agent should be discontinued within 48 hours of resolution of the infection. Because the catheter has been indwelling, encrustation may shelter bacteria from the antimicrobial agent; therefore the catheter should be changed.

KEY POINTS: CATHETER-ASSOCIATED BACTERIURIA

- Careful aseptic insertion of the catheter and maintenance of a closed, dependent drainage system are essential to minimize development of bacteriuria.
- The development of catheter-associated bacteriuria is inevitable.
- Only symptomatic CAUTIs require treatment.

MANAGEMENT OF URINARY TRACT INFECTIONS IN PATIENTS WITH SPINAL CORD INJURY

Patients with SCI have unique characteristics that affect the risk, diagnosis, and management of UTIs, all of which are considered complicated. **Of all patients with bacteriuria, no group compares in severity and morbidity with those who have SCI.** Nearly all these patients require catheterization early after their injuries because of bladder overactivity or flaccidity, and significant numbers develop ureterectasis, hydronephrosis, VUR, and renal calculi. Bacteriologic and urodynamic advances in the management of these patients have greatly reduced their morbidity and mortality.

Epidemiology

Before the advent of CIC and modern antibiotics, UTI and renal failure accounted for the great majority of deaths in the SCI population (Barber and Cross, 1952). The National Spinal Cord Injury Statistical Center published a report in 2012 stating that GU infections account for only 3% of deaths in the SCI population, the 11th most common cause of deaths; the advent of CIC and antibiotics has clearly decreased the morbidity attributed to UTIs and renal failure, as compared with mid–20th century statistics.

UTIs are among the most common urologic complications of SCI. It has been estimated that approximately 33% of patients with SCI have bacteriuria at any time (Stover et al., 1989) and that eventually almost all patients with SCI will become bacteriuric; many will suffer significant morbidity and mortality. One prospective study of patients on intermittent catheterization or condom catheterization reported an incidence of significant bacteriuria (18 episodes per person per year) and an annual incidence of febrile UTIs of 1.8 per person per year (Waites et al., 1993a). In addition, **UTI is the most common cause of fever in the patient with SCI** (Beraldo et al., 1993). The 1992 National Institute on Disability and Rehabilitation Research Consensus Conference examined the problems associated with UTIs in patients with SCI (National Institute on Disability and Rehabilitation Research, 1993). **Among the risk factors identified were impaired voiding, overdistention of the bladder, elevated intravesical pressure, increased risk of urinary obstruction, VUR, urinary tract instrumentation, and presence of stones. Other factors that have been implicated are decreased fluid intake, poor hygiene, perineal colonization, decubiti, and other evidence of local tissue trauma, as well as reduced host defense associated with chronic illness** (Gilmore et al., 1992; Waites et al., 1993a).

Pathogenesis

The method of bladder management has a profound impact on the incidence of UTI. The National Institute on Disability and Rehabilitation Research Consensus Conference noted that indwelling catheters were most likely to lead to UTI and that the majority of patients with an indwelling catheter for 30 days are bacteriuric (National Institute on Disability and Rehabilitation Research, 1993). Suprapubic catheters and indwelling urethral catheters eventually have an equivalent infection rate (Biering-Sorensen, 2002; Kunin et al., 1987; Tambyah and Maki, 2000). However, the onset of bacteriuria may be delayed using a suprapubic catheter compared with a urethral catheter. During a 2-year period, 170 patients with SCI were evaluated regarding type of urinary drainage and infection (Warren et al., 1982). In patients using indwelling urethral catheters, all urine cultures were positive. The corresponding values for the suprapubic catheter group were 44%. Condom drainage systems are also associated with an incidence of bacteriuria from 63% (Dukes, 1928) to almost 100% (Pyrah et al., 1955).

Since its introduction by Lapides et al. (1972), clean (but not sterile) intermittent catheterization (CIC) has dramatically changed the management of patients with SCI. **Although never rigorously compared with indwelling urethral catheterization, CIC has been shown to decrease lower urinary tract complications by maintaining low intravesical pressure and by reducing the incidence of stones** (Stover et al., 1989). CIC also appears to reduce complications associated with an indwelling catheter, such as UTI, fever, bacteremia, and local infections such as epididymitis and prostatitis. Weld and Dmochowski (2000) followed 316 patients with SCI (who had received different bladder management) for a mean of 18.3 years and recorded all complications. The CIC group had statistically significantly lower complication rates compared with the urethral catheterization group and no significantly higher complication rates relative to all other management methods for each type of complication studied. Thus it is generally agreed that **CIC places patients with SCI at the lowest risk for significant long-term urinary tract complications** (Stamm, 1975).

There is conflicting evidence over the value of sterile versus nonsterile or "no touch" methods of CIC. Some studies have reported a lower incidence of infection in patients treated with sterile techniques (Foley, 1929), whereas others have not (Nyren et al., 1981; Pyrah et al., 1955). Bennett et al. (1997) reported on a sterile method of CIC that uses an introducer tip to bypass the distal 1.5 cm of the urethra and showed a significant decrease in UTI. Different types of catheters have been used for CIC. The low-friction catheters may be less traumatic for the urethra (Casewell and Phillips, 1977; Garibaldi et al., 1980), but their impact on bacteriuria and UTI has yet to be proven. Cardenas et al. (2011) looked at the time to first UTI in SCI patients using hydrophilic catheters compared with standard nonhydrophilic catheters. They reported that half of each group experienced symptomatic UTI within a 20-day period, although the hydrophilic group had a longer time before UTI.

Clinical Presentation

The majority of patients with SCI with bacteriuria are asymptomatic. Many are managed with CIC, suprapubic catheters, and indwelling Foley catheters, which can lead to asymptomatic bacteriuria. Asymptomatic bacteriuria should not be treated in the patient with SCI (Nicolle et al., 2005; Vigil and Hickling, 2016). Furthermore, asymptomatic patients with SCI who use indwelling, condom, or intermittent catheters should not be screened with urinalysis or urine culture. There is no standard definition for UTI in patients with SCI. Because of a loss of sensation, patients usually do not experience frequency, urgency, or dysuria, making the diagnosis of UTI a challenge in this population. More often, they complain of flank, back, or abdominal discomfort, leakage between catheterizations, increased spasticity, malaise, lethargy, and/or cloudy, malodorous urine. As noted earlier, UTI is the most common cause of fever in this population.

Bacteriology and Laboratory Diagnosis

Urinalysis will show bacteriuria and pyuria. Pyuria is not diagnostic of infections because it may occur from the irritative effects of the catheter. The National Institute on Disability and Rehabilitation Research Consensus Statement recommended criteria for the diagnosis of significant bacteriuria in spinal cord–injured patients (National Institute on Disability and Rehabilitation Research, 1993). Any detectable bacteria from indwelling or suprapubic catheter aspirates was considered significant because the majority of patients with an indwelling catheter and low-level bacteriuria showed an increase to greater than 10^5 CFU/mL within a short period of time (Cardenas and Hooton, 1995). For patients on CIC, greater than or equal to 10^2 CFU/mL was considered significant. For catheter-free males, a clean voided specimen showing greater than or equal to 10^4 CFU/mL was considered significant.

Bacteriuria in patients with SCI differs from that in patients with intact spinal cords with regard to cause, complexity, and antimicrobial susceptibility and is influenced by the type and duration of catheterization. *E. coli* is isolated in approximately 20% of patients. Enterococci, *P. mirabilis*, and *Pseudomonas* spp. are more common in patients with SCI than in patients with intact spinal cords. Other common organisms are *Klebsiella* spp., *Serratia* spp., *Staphylococcus*, and *Candida* spp. Most bacteriuria in short-term catheterization is single-organism, whereas patients catheterized for longer than a month usually demonstrate a polymicrobial flora caused by a wide range of gram-negative and gram-positive bacterial species (Edwards et al., 1983).

Management

As a result of the diverse flora and high probability of bacterial resistance, a urine culture must be obtained before initiating empirical therapy. For afebrile patients, β-lactams, TMP-SMX, and nitrofurantoin can be used while awaiting culture results. An oral fluoroquinolone may considered as second-line option, given the concerns about resistance patterns and side effects with this class of antibiotics (Cardenas and Hooton, 1995). An indwelling catheter should be changed to ensure maximal drainage and eliminate bacterial foci in catheter encrustations. **Patients with SCI and fever or chills are usually admitted and treated with a parenteral aminoglycoside and either a penicillin or a third-generation cephalosporin** (Cardenas and Hooton, 1995). In this patient population consultation with a physician with expertise in antimicrobial management may be necessary, especially in a patient with recurrent infections.

If clinical improvement does not occur within 24 to 48 hours, repeat culture and adjustment of antimicrobial therapy based on the initial culture and susceptibility should be performed. Imaging studies should be obtained to rule out obstruction, stones, and abscess. Post-therapy cultures are usually not necessary because asymptomatic recolonization is common and not clinically significant. However, if a urea-splitting bacterium is identified, a follow-up culture should be obtained to ensure its eradication. Bladder irrigation with saline or antibiotic solutions (Waites et al., 2006) has not traditionally been recommended because the rates of catheter-associated bacteriuria and UTI were not reduced with such methods. However, Cox et al. reported in 2017 on 22 patients (cause of NGB was 63.6% SCI) who underwent gentamicin bladder installations. Patients had fewer symptomatic UTIs and underwent fewer courses of oral antibiotics after initiating gentamicin irrigations. In addition, the proportion of multidrug-resistant organisms in urine cultures decreased (Cox et al., 2017).

AP is not supported for patients who have neurogenic bladder caused by SCI (Morton et al., 2002; Vigil and Hickling, 2016). AP did not significantly decrease symptomatic UTIs and resulted in an approximately twofold increase in antimicrobial-resistant bacteria (Nicolle et al., 2019).

Patients with SCI with recurrent symptomatic UTIs should undergo urinary tract imaging and urodynamic testing and a review of their bladder management program. Particular attention should be given to catheter drainage, intermittent catheterization techniques, and frequency of intermittent catheterization or voiding schedule (Cardenas and Hooton, 1995). **Recurrent UTIs may be associated with high storage pressures, and intervention to lower storage pressure may decrease the incidence of symptomatic UTI. Evidence from studies in patients with SCI suggests that bladder catheterization for longer than 10 years is associated with an increased risk of carcinoma of the bladder.** West et al. (1999) examined two databases with more than 33,000 patients with SCI, and over a 5-year period identified 130 patients with bladder cancer (0.4%). Several risk factors for bladder cancer have been proposed. Vereczky et al. (cited in Weyrauch and Bassett, 1951) tested different risk factors based on the outcome of 153 patients with SCI, of which 7 were diagnosed with bladder cancer. Upon identification of 31 possible predictors, only duration of catheterization was significant. **Chronic infection and inflammation of the bladder mucosa could be the carcinogenic stimulus in these patients** (Pyrah et al., 1955). **Nitrosamines produced in infected urine have also been implicated** (Najenson et al., 1969).

KEY POINTS: MANAGEMENT OF URINARY TRACT INFECTION IN PATIENTS WITH SPINAL CORD INJURY

- The majority of patients with SCI with bacteriuria are asymptomatic. Only symptomatic patients require therapy.
- Patients with SCI and UTI commonly experience fever; flank, back, or abdominal discomfort; leakage between catheterizations; increased spasticity; malaise; lethargy; and/or cloudy, malodorous urine.
- Urine culture before the initiation of empirical therapy is essential because patients with SCI often have evidence of diverse flora with a high probability of bacterial resistance.
- CIC places patients with SCI at the lowest risk for significant long-term urinary tract complications.
- Chronic infection can be carcinogenic.

KIDNEY TRANSPLANT RECIPIENTS

There is no current consensus on the role of antibiotics in renal transplant patients with asymptomatic bacteriuria. The IDSA guideline published in 2005 made no recommendation because of insufficient evidence (Nicolle et al., 2005). In the update to this guideline published in 2019, the recommendation is not to screen or treat asymptomatic bacteriuria if the transplant occured more than 1 month prior (Nicolle et al., 2019). In 2013 The American Society of Transplantation Infectious Diseases Community of Practice recommended not treating asymptomatic bacteriuria after 3 months post-transplantation, except in those patients who had a rise in serum creatinine. If the kidney donor has asymptomatic bacteriuria at the time of transplantation, the recipient should be treated. Also, transplant recipients usually receive TMP-SMX for PCP prophylaxis, which can reduce the chance of UTIs (Parasuraman et al., 2013).

In 2018 a Cochrane Review looked at antibiotics for asymptomatic bacteriuria in kidney transplant recipients (Coussement et al., 2018). Asymptomatic bacteriuria occurs in 17% to 51% of kidney transplant recipients and is thought to increase the risk for eventual UTI. The data only included two studies, totaling 212 patients, and excluded those patients with indwelling urethral catheters or ureteral stents. Because of the limited data in the Cochrane Review, the authors concluded there was insufficient evidence to support routine antibiotic treatment of asymptomatic bacteriuria in renal transplant patients. Furthermore, they stated it is unclear if screening for asymptomatic bacteriuria with urine cultures should be performed.

Whether to treat asymptomatic bacteriuria in renal transplant patients remains controversial.

Because of the immunosuppressed state of a kidney transplant recipient, particularly early in the first few months, recognition and treatment of UTI in this population is paramount and may be critical for graft survival. **Transplant recipients are at higher risk for VUR. Risk factors for infection include female gender, diabetes, cadaveric graft, two episodes of asymptomatic bacteriuria, and prolonged hemodialysis before transplantation** (Castaneda et al., 2013). Treatment duration, particularly in the early post-transplantation period (6 months), is usually 14 days for uncomplicated UTIs and 21 to 28 days for complicated UTIs (Säemann and Hörl, 2008).

ANTIMICROBIAL PROPHYLAXIS FOR COMMON UROLOGIC PROCEDURES

Principles of Surgical Antimicrobial Prophylaxis

The prior urologic best practice statement (BPS) was written in 2008 and validated in 2011. There has been a great deal of effort placed on examining AP over the last decade and the latest BPS published in 2019 should update the practicing urologist. Surgical AP entails treatment with an antimicrobial agent before and for a *limited* time after a procedure to prevent local or systemic postprocedural infections. This is in contrast to antimicrobial treatment, which uses an antimicrobial agent to eradicate a suspected or documented infection.

The 2019 BPS recommends consideration of periprocedural AP for all urologic procedures in which a tissue barrier break will occur. For most procedures, prophylaxis should be initiated within 60 minutes of the procedure (Bratzler et al., 2004). When used as AP, vancomycin and fluoroquinolones should be initiated within 120 minutes of the procedure. Single-dose AP is most appropriate in the majority of uncomplicated urologic surgery. **Efficacious levels should be maintained for the duration of the procedure and, in only special circumstances, a limited time (24 hours, at most) after the procedure** (Bratzler and Houck, 2004). Although prospective studies addressing prophylaxis for urologic procedures exist, most focus on only a narrow spectrum of procedures. However, application of the principles of these studies with additional consideration of the patient and the type of procedure provides a framework for determining when and what type of AP may be indicated. The AP agent chosen should target the likely local organisms and be supported by sensitivities reflected in local antibiograms; cost and safety should be part of the decision-making process. An additional, nontraditional type of prophylaxis in urology entails periprocedural treatment of the urinary tract with an antimicrobial agent to prevent local or systemic sequelae from the manipulation of colonized hardware such as stents or urethral catheters.

A wide array of patients undergo invasive procedures in urology. Two important considerations when assessing the need for AP are the ability of a host to respond to bacteriuria or bacteremia and the sequelae of a possible infection. Additional considerations include the likelihood of bacterial invasion at the surgical site and possible sequelae. Factors that affect the host's ability to respond to infection include advanced age, anatomic anomalies, poor nutritional status, smoking, chronic corticosteroid use, other concurrent medication use, and immunodeficiency, such as untreated HIV infection (Box 55.13). In addition, chronic indwelling hardware, infected endogenous material such as stones, distant infectious sites, and prolonged hospitalizations also increase the risk of infectious complications, by increasing the local bacterial concentration and/or altering the spectrum of bacterial flora.

BOX 55.13 Host Factors That Increase the Risk of Infection

Advanced age
Anatomic anomalies
Poor nutritional status
Smoking
Chronic corticosteroid use
Immunodeficiency
Chronic indwelling hardware
Infected endogenous/exogenous material
Distant coexistent infection
Prolonged hospitalization

Data from Cruse PJ: Surgical wound infection. In Wonsiewicz MJ, editor: *Infectious disease*, Philadelphia, 1992, WB Saunders, pp 758–764; Mangram AJ, Horan TC, Pearson ML, et al.: Guideline for prevention of surgical site infection, 1999. Hospital Infection Control Practices Advisory Committee. *Infect Control Hosp Epidemiol* 20:250–278; quiz 279–280, 1999.

The type of procedure will also help direct the timing, duration, and spectrum of AP needed (see Table 55.15 for a summary of AP recommendations). Consideration should be given to the extent of the local tissue injury incurred and the anticipated type of flora at the site. The choice of AP agent should consider the patient's comorbidities, allergies, and the specific AP risk. As stated earlier in the chapter, the FDA issued a black box warning for quinolones because of serious side effects and specifically discouraged their use in treating uncomplicated cystitis; this must be kept in mind while considering use of fluoroquinolones for AP.

AP is not without morbidity because drug reactions and allergic complications, although rare, may result in minor reactions such as rashes or gastric disturbances, or significant sequelae such as allergic nephritis, or anaphylaxis.

The new BPS on Urologic Procedures and Antimicrobial Prophylaxis includes some key updated recommendations, specifically regarding asymptomatic bacteriuria and funguria. Asymptomatic bacteriuria and asymptomatic funguria do not require treatment before a surgical procedure that does not violate the urothelium. The orthopedic literature has shown that there is no benefit to treating asymptomatic bacteriuria even in the setting of a total knee or hip prosthetic replacement (Sousa et al., 2014). The same is true of patients undergoing open heart surgeries (Soltanzadeh and Ebadi, 2013). Repeat urinalysis to demonstrate clearing of asymptomatic bacteriuria is also not recommended (Ramos et al., 2016).

The EAU infection guidelines published in 2017 concluded that before urologic surgery, in diagnostic and therapeutic procedures not entering the urinary tract, asymptomatic bacteriuria is not generally considered a risk factor, and screening and treatment are not considered necessary. However, the EAU guideline states that in procedures entering the urinary tract and breaching the mucosa, particularly in endoscopic urologic surgery, bacteriuria is a definite risk factor. In these patients, a urine culture must be taken before interventions and in case of asymptomatic bacteriuria, preoperative treatment is recommended (Bonkat et al., 2019). The EAU guideline also reports the treatment of asymptomatic bacteriuria is not recommended before arthroplasty surgery.

In addition, low-risk patients with asymptomatic bacteriuria and/or funguria may not require prophylaxis before a urologic surgical procedure that does not violate the urothelium with the exception of pregnant females. However, the statement does recommend single-dose antifungal prophylaxis for patients undergoing endoscopic, robotic, or open surgery on the urinary tract.

The IDSA 2016 clinical practice guidelines for management of candidiasis strongly recommended all patients with candiduria who are undergoing any urologic procedure be treated with either oral fluconazole or intravenous amphotericin B for several days before

TABLE 55.15 Recommended Antimicrobial Prophylaxis for Urologic Procedures

PROCEDURE	LIKELY ORGANISMS	PROPHYLAXIS INDICATED	ANTIMICROBIAL(S) OF CHOICE	ALTERNATIVE ANTIMICROBIAL(S), IF REQUIRED	DURATION OF THERAPY[¶]
LOWER TRACT INSTRUMENTATION					
Cystourethroscopy with minor manipulation, break in mucosal barriers, biopsy, fulguration, etc.; clean-contaminated	GNR, rarely enterococci[†]	Uncertain[§]; consider host-related risk factors. Increasing invasiveness increases risk of SSI	TMP-SMX, Amoxicillin/Clavulanate	1st/2nd generation Cephalosporin + Aminoglycoside (Aztreonam[¥]) ± Ampicillin	Single dose
Transurethral cases: e.g. TURP, TURBT, laser enucleative and ablative procedures, etc.; clean-contaminated[l]	GNR, rarely enterococci	All cases	Cefazolin, TMP-SMX	Amoxicillin/Clavulanate, Aminoglycoside (Aztreonam[¥]) ± Ampicillin	Single dose
Prostate brachytherapy or cryotherapy; clean-contaminated	S. aureus, skin; GNR	All cases	Cefazolin	Clindamycin**	Single dose
Transrectal prostate biopsy; contaminated	GNR, anaerobes[††]; consider MDR coverage, if risks of systemic antibiotics within 6 months, international travel, healthcare worker	All cases	Fluoroquinolone, 1st/2nd/3rd gen. Cephalosporin (ceftriaxone commonly used) + Aminoglycoside	Aztreonam May need to consider ID consultation	Single dose
UPPER TRACT INSTRUMENTATION					
Percutaneous renal surgery; e.g. PCNL; clean-contaminated	GNR, rarely enterococci, and skin[‡‡], S. aureus	All cases	1st/2nd gen. Cephalosporin, Aminoglycoside (Aztreonam[¥]) + Metronidazole, or Clindamycin	Ampicillin/Sulbactam	≤24 hours
Ureteroscopy, all indications; clean-contaminated	GNR, rarely enterococci	All cases; of undetermined benefit for uncomplicated diagnostic only procedures	TMP-SMX, 1st/2nd gen. Cephalosporin	Aminoglycoside (Aztreonam[¥]) ± Ampicillin, 1st/2nd gen. Cephalosporin, Amoxicillin/Clavulanate	Single dose
OPEN, LAPAROSCOPIC OR ROBOTIC SURGERY					
Without entering urinary tract, e.g. adrenalectomy, lymphadenectomy, retroperitoneal or pelvic; clean	S. aureus, skin	Consider in all cases; may not be required	Cefazolin	Clindamycin	Single dose
Penile surgery, e.g. circumcision, penile biopsy, etc.; clean-contaminated	S. aureus	Likely not required			

TABLE 55.15 Recommended Antimicrobial Prophylaxis for Urologic Procedures—cont'd

PROCEDURE	LIKELY ORGANISMS	PROPHYLAXIS INDICATED	ANTIMICROBIAL(S) OF CHOICE	ALTERNATIVE ANTIMICROBIAL(S), IF REQUIRED	DURATION OF THERAPY[¶]
Urethroplasty; reconstruction anterior urethra, stricture repair, including urethrectomy; clean; contaminated; controlled entry into the urinary tract	GNR, rarely enterococci, S. aureus	Likely required	Cefazolin	Cefoxitin, Cefotetan, Ampicillin/Sulbactam	Single dose
Involving controlled entry into urinary tract e.g. renal surgery, nephrectomy, partial or otherwise, ureterectomy pyeloplasty, radical prostatectomy; partial cystectomy, etc.; clean-contaminated	GNR (E. coli), rarely enterococci	All cases	Cefazolin, TMP-SMX	Ampicillin/Sulbactam, Aminoglycoside (Aztreonam[ψ]) + Metronidazole, or Clindamycin	Single dose
Involving small bowel (i.e. urinary diversions), cystectomy with small bowel conduit, other GU procedures; uretero-pelvic junction repair, partial cystectomy, etc.; clean-contaminated	Skin, S. aureus, GNR, rarely enterococci	All cases	Cefazolin	Clindamycin and aminoglycoside Cefuroxime (2nd generation cephalosporin), Aminopenicillin combined with a β-lactamase inhibitor + Metronidazole	Single dose
Involving large bowel[§§]; colon conduits; clean-contaminated	GNR, anaerobes	All cases	Cefazolin + Metronidazole, Cefoxitin, Cefotetan, or Ceftriaxone + Metronidazole, Ertapenem NB: these IV agents are used along with mechanical bowel preparation and oral antimicrobial (neomycin sulfate + erythromycin base or neomycin sulfate + metronidazole)	Ampicillin/Sulbactam Ticarcillin/Clavulanate Pipercillin/ Tazobactam	Single parenteral dose
Implanted prosthetic devices: AUS, IPP, sacral neuromodulators; clean	GNR, S. aureus, with increasing reports of anaerobic, and fungal organisms	All cases	Aminoglycoside (Aztreonam[ψ]) + 1st/2nd gen. Cephalosporin or Vancomycin[χ]	Aminopenicillin β-lactamase inhibitor, including Ampicillin/ Sulbactam Ticarcillin, or Tazobactam;	≤24 hours
Inguinal and scrotal cases; e.g. radical orchiectomy, vasectomy, reversals, varicocelectomy, hydrocelectomy, etc.; clean	GNR, S. aureus	Of increased risk; all cases	Cefazolin	Ampicillin/Sulbactam	Single dose

Continued

TABLE 55.15 Recommended Antimicrobial Prophylaxis for Urologic Procedures—cont'd

PROCEDURE	LIKELY ORGANISMS	PROPHYLAXIS INDICATED	ANTIMICROBIAL(S) OF CHOICE	ALTERNATIVE ANTIMICROBIAL(S), IF REQUIRED	DURATION OF THERAPY[¶]
Vaginal surgery, female incontinence, e.g. urethral sling procedures, fistulae repair, urethral diverticulectomy, etc.; clean-contaminated	S. aureus, streptococci, enterococci, vaginal anaerobes; skin	All	2nd gen. Cephalosporin (Cefoxitin, Cefotetan) provides better anaerobic coverage than 1st gen. cephaloporins; however, Cefazolin is equivalent coverage for the vaginal anaerobes in sling procedures	Ampicillin/Sulbactam; + Aminoglycoside Aztreonam[¥]) + Metronidazole, or Clindamycin	Single dose
OTHER Shock-wave lithotripsy; clean	GNR, rarely enterococci; GU pathogens	Only if risk factors	If risks, consider TMP-SMX, 1st gen. Cephalosporin (Cefazolin), 2nd gen. Cephalosporin (Cefuroxime), Aminopenicillin combined with a β-lactamase inhibitor + Metronidazole	1st/2nd gen. Cephalosporin, Amoxicillin/ Clavulanate Ampicillin + Aminoglycoside (Aztreonam[¥]), Clindamycin	Single dose

[†]GU GNR: Common urinary tract organisms are *E. coli*, *Proteus* spp, *Klebsiella* spp, and GPC *Enterococcus*.
[§]If urine culture shows no growth prior to the procedure, antimicrobial prophylaxis is not necessary.
[¶]Or full course of culture-directed antimicrobials for documented infection (which is treatment, not prophylaxis).
[¥]Aztreonam can be substituted for aminoglycosides in patients with renal insufficiency.
[ǀ]Includes transurethral resection of bladder tumor and prostate, and any biopsy, resection, fulguration, foreign body removal, urethral dilation or urethrotomy, or ureteral instrumentation including catheterization or stent placement/removal.
[**]Clindamycin, or aminoglycoside + metronidazole or clindamycin, are general alternatives to penicillins and cephalosporins in patients with penicillin allergy, even when not specifically listed.
[††]Intestine: Common intestinal organisms include aerobes and anaerobes: *E. coli*, *Klebsiella* spp, *Enterobacter*, *Serratia* spp, *Proteus* spp, *Enterococcus*, and *Anaerobes*.
[‡‡]Skin: Common skin organisms are *S. aureus*, coagulase negative *Staphylococcus* spp, Group A *Streptococcus* spp.
[§§]For surgery involving the colorectum, bowel preparation with oral neomycin plus either erythromycin base or metronidazole are added to systemic agents.
[χ]Routine administration of vancomycin for AP is not recommended.[43] The antimicrobial spectrum of Vancomycin is less effective against methicillin-sensitive strains of *S. aureus*.
From Lightner DJ, Wymer K, Sanchez J, et al: *Urologic procedures and antimicrobial prophylaxis*, 2019 (website): https://www.auanet.org/Documents/Guidelines/PDF/Antimicrobial%20Prophylaxis%20Table%20V.pdf.

and after intervention (Pappas et al., 2016). The AUA BPS disagrees with this recommendation and states that antifungal prophylaxis should be used in patients undergoing specific endoscopic procedures in which high pressure irrigants are used (transurethral resection of bladder tumor [TURBT], transurethral resection of the prostate (TURP), ablative outlet procedures, therapeutic URS, and entry into urinary tract). Full antifungal treatment is recommended for patients with symptomatic fungal UTIs at the time of stent or drainage tube change. Neutropenic patients with funguria and a urinary tract obstruction require a longer course of periprocedural antifungal treatment. Those patients undergoing treatment of fungal balls (mycetoma) should have preoperative fungal cultures and periprocedural antifungal treatment for 5 to 7 days.

The panel recommended considering AP at the time of select procedures, including voiding trials, and catheter, drain, stent, or nephrostomy tube removals, particularly if other risk factors are present. A recent meta-analysis published in 2013 revealed a significantly lower prevalence of symptomatic UTIs with AP at the time of catheter removal in surgical and medical patients (Marschall et al., 2013).

The BPS specifically looked at the use of single-dose AP for each category of skin incision. The statement suggests that single-dose AP is not necessary in Class 1/Clean Procedures (uninfected, no GU or GI tract entry) except in groin or perineal incisions. The BPS recommends AP for those patients undergoing Class II/clean-contaminated GU procedures, which includes prostate biopsy. For transurethral procedures and therapeutic upper endoscopic procedures, single-dose AP (including first- or second-generation cephalosporins or trimethoprim/sulfamethoxazole) covering enterococci and gram-negative pathogens is recommended. For patients undergoing Class

III/contaminated procedures, AP is strongly recommended because the risk of a surgical site infection (SSI) or systemic infection is high. The BPS recommends coverage of aerobic and anaerobic organisms for those undergoing colorectal surgical procedures (first-generation cephalosporin and metronidazole). The BPS does not discuss GU prosthetic antimicrobial coverage. However, it does comment that generally, AP that covers skin flora (coagulase-negative staphylococci and gram-negative bacilli) is recommended. Finally, class IV wounds are infected, and empirical antibiotics are initiated until final culture results are available.

Urethral Catheterization and Removal

The indications for the routine use of prophylactic antimicrobial agents before urethral catheterization vary and depend on the health, sex, and specific living circumstances of the individual patient, as well as the indication for catheterization (Schaeffer, 2006). The risk of infection after one-time urethral catheterization is 1% to 2% in healthy domiciliary women; however, this risk rises significantly in hospitalized patients (Thiel and Spuhler, 1965; Turck et al., 1962). Thus, for patients with risk factors for infection (see Box 55.13), AP with an oral agent such as TMP-SMX should decrease the risk of postprocedural infection (see Table 55.15).

A recent Cochrane review published in 2013 looking at AP for short-term catheter (defined as ≤14 days) bladder drainage in adults found that surgical patients who received AP (3-day duration postop or from postop day 2 to catheter removal) had a reduced rate of bacteriuria and other signs of infection, including pyuria, fevers, and gram-negative urine cultures (Lusardi et al., 2013). Importantly, the authors did conclude that because of the limited evidence and allergic reactions or side effects from the AP, the results should be interpreted with caution. Patients who require long-term intermittent catheterization should not be on routine prophylaxis, because the rates of UTI are comparable and the overall risk of infection is low (Clarke et al., 2005; Duffy et al., 1995).

Prolonged use of an indwelling urethral catheter is common in hospitalized patients and is associated with an increased risk of bacterial colonization, with a 5% to 10% incidence of bacteriuria per catheter day for each day the catheter is in place (Saint and Lipsky, 1999; Sedor and Mulholland 1999; van der Wall et al., 1992). **Prophylactic administration of antimicrobial agents during catheterization is not generally recommended** because bacterial resistance can develop rapidly and complicate subsequent necessary antimicrobial treatment (Clarke et al., 2005). This is supported by the Cochrane Database of Systematic Reviews that concluded that antimicrobials given postprocedurally until catheter removal or for the first 3 postoperative days did not reduce rates of bacteriuria or infection (Niël-weise and van den Broek, 2005).

The natural history of bacteriuria after catheter removal has not been comprehensively studied. Harding et al. (1991) reported that in asymptomatic bacteriuric women who had been catheterized for 4 to 6 days, 25% developed a UTI within 14 days of catheter removal. In this study, 1-day treatment with TMP-SMX was as effective as a 10-day course in resolving infections. Similar studies on the natural history of post-catheterization bacteriuria have not been performed in male patients.

Data from Polastri et al. (1990) suggest that AP for chronic indwelling catheter changes is not indicated. In their study of 46 catheter changes, bacteremia occurred 4% of the time and, when noted, was associated with very low concentrations of bacteria in the cultures. Systemic sequelae were not noted.

Urodynamics

Urodynamics (UDS), like cystoscopy, is a minimally traumatic procedure with limited urothelial injury that poses a small risk of local infection in hosts with normal anatomy and immune response. Several recent studies support this notion. According to the AUA Best Practice Policy on Urologic Surgery Antimicrobial Prophylaxis, prophylactic antibiotics are not indicated before UDS for patients without UTI risk factors ("index patients") (Wolf et al., 2008).

A large systematic review published in 2008 including 8 RCTs with 995 (mostly female) patients undergoing UDS compared prophylactic antibiotics with placebo or no treatment. The authors concluded there was a 40% reduction in the risk of bacteriuria and that 13 patients would need to be given prophylactic antibiotics to prevent one episode of bacteriuria (Latthe et al., 2008). This review did not assess the occurrence of symptomatic UTI, but it has been estimated that only 8% of women develop a symptomatic UTI within 1 week of a diagnosis of asymptomatic bacteriuria (Hooton et al., 2000). **In 2012 a Cochrane review evaluated the role of prophylactic antibiotics to reduce the risk of UTIs after UDS** (Foon et al., 2012). The review included 9 RCTs with 973 patients (76% female). Patients receiving prophylaxis had fewer UTIs (20% vs. 28%), but there was no statistically significant difference. **The authors concluded there was not enough evidence that prophylaxis reduced symptomatic UTIs.**

In 2017 the Society of Urodynamics, Female Pelvic Medicine, and Urogenital Reconstruction (SUFU) published a Best Practice Policy Statement on UDS AP in the non-index patient (Cameron et al., 2017). **The statement recommends that all patients be screened for symptoms of UTI and undergo dipstick urinalysis. If the provider suspects a UTI, the UDS should be postponed until the UTI has been treated. Patients undergoing UDS who do NOT require AP include those with no known GU anomalies, patients with diabetes, those with prior GU surgery or a history of prior UTI, postmenopausal women, recently hospitalized patients, and patients with cardiac valvular disease, nutritional deficiencies, or obesity. The panel does recommend periprocedural antibiotics in those patients with increased risk factors for UTI after UDS: relevant neurogenic LUT dysfunction, elevated postvoid residual, asymptomatic bacteriuria, immunosuppression (including renal transplant patients), age over 70, and an indwelling catheter, external collection device, or intermittent catheterization. The majority of these recommendations are based on Level IV (low level) evidence because of the lack of well-done studies. As always, clinical judgment of each individual scenario should supersede these recommendations, which, as stated, are not based on high-level evidence.** The authors strongly recommend careful and judicious use of AP until better evidence reveals the true need. Finally, the panel did recommend AP for patients undergoing UDS who have had an orthopedic total joint implant within the prior 2 years or who are considered at increased risk of developing joint infections from bacteremia (see Table 3 of Cameron et al. 2017, p 924). The first choice for prophylaxis is a single oral dose of TMP-SMX before UDS. Acceptable alternatives include first- and second-generation cephalosporins, amoxicillin/clavulanate, fluoroquinolones, and parenteral aminoglycoside plus ampicillin. The panel only found one study that used a 1-day AP course of nitrofurantoin in patients undergoing UDS and cystoscopy. They demonstrated no improvement in bacteriuria with nitrofurantoin AP (Cundiff et al., 1999). In light of the black box warning on quinolones and the lack of well-done studies, the authors currently use nitrofurantoin as an alternative to TMP-SMX.

Transrectal Ultrasound-Guided Prostate Biopsy

Infectious complications after prostate biopsy have increased in recent years, with reported rates from 0.1% to 7.0% and sepsis rates from 0.3% to 3.1% (Loeb et al., 2011; Nam et al., 2010). **The most common cause for infection after transrectal prostate biopsy is fluoroquinolone-resistant *E. coli*** (Liss et al., 2015). **The most common risk factor is exposure to antimicrobials within 6 months of the biopsy. The use of prophylactic antimicrobials for transrectal ultrasound-guided prostate biopsy (TRUS-Bx) reduces postprocedural fever and UTI in most studies.** The class and duration of antimicrobial treatment are more varied and controversial. AP with fluoroquinolones has been shown to significantly reduce the rate of infectious complications compared with placebo (8% vs. 25%) (Kapoor et al., 1998; Shandera et al., 1998; Sieber et al., 1997; Tal et al., 2003; Taylor and Bingham, 1997a,b; Zani et al., 2011).

However, **several recent studies have highlighted an increasing trend of infectious complications caused by fluoroquinolone-resistant** organisms among men undergoing TRUS-Bx (Binsaleh et al., 2004; Feliciano et al., 2008; Han et al., 2005; Lange et al., 2009; Ng and Chan, 2008; Young et al., 2009; Zaytoun et al., 2011). Prevalence rates for colonization with fluoroquinolone-resistant organisms in this patient population have been reported to be as high as 22% (Liss et al., 2011). Nevertheless, more than 90% of urologists continue to use fluoroquinolones empirically for AP before TRUS-Bx (Antsupova et al., 2014; Shandera et al., 1998). The increasing prevalence of infectious complications with fluoroquinolone-resistant bacteria in men undergoing TRUS-Bx suggests that this approach may not be judicious for some patients (Taylor et al., 2012). Indeed, of fluoroquinolone-resistant strains obtained (by rectal swabs) from men before prostate biopsy, 70% had an enhanced virulence profile (Liss et al., 2013).

Empirical augmented prophylaxis with a typical combination of aminoglycosides and fluoroquinolones has been effective in recent studies (Ho et al., 2009; Kehinde et al., 2013). A recent meta-analysis of 3 RCTs showed the superiority of augmented prophylaxis in reducing UTIs and hospitalizations after prostate biopsy (Yang et al., 2015); however, it is inevitable that bacterial resistance will evolve to challenge even these regimens.

Rectal swab culture obtained before TRUS-Bx allows for the isolation and identification of fluoroquinolone-resistant organisms from a patient's native intestinal flora. Targeted prophylaxis has been extensively studied. A meta-analysis published in 2014 included 8 studies comparing targeted prophylaxis with empirical fluoroquinolone prophylaxis. The study reported that targeted prophylaxis was more efficacious in reducing infectious complications (Roberts et al., 2014). A more recent study by Liss et al. (2015) found no significant difference (between empirical and targeted prophylaxis) in sepsis rates in 5355 patients at Kaiser Permanente centers in the United States. In a study using targeted prophylaxis based on bacterial sensitivities of rectal swabs before TRUS-Bx, 19.6% of men had fluoroquinolone-resistant organisms. There were no infectious complications in the men who received targeted prophylaxis, whereas there were infectious complications, including sepsis, in 2.6% on empirical prophylaxis (Taylor et al., 2012). Cost-effectiveness analysis revealed that targeted prophylaxis yielded a cost savings of $4499 per post–TRUS-Bx infectious complication averted. Per estimation, 38 men would need to undergo rectal swab before TRUS-Bx to prevent 1 infectious complication. **Thus screening before TRUS-Bx and targeted prophylaxis should be considered as a thoughtful, predictable alternative to empirical prophylaxis.** That being said, there are a number of issues related to the actual process of targeted prophylaxis including costs, time of extra visits, special culture media, and lab requirements. There have been recent data to suggest that fosfomycin is as effective as fluoroquinolone in UTIs after TRUS-Bx (Noreikaite et al., 2018; Ongun et al., 2012; Roberts et al., 2018).

Recent studies suggest that a single-dose/day of fluoroquinolones is as effective as 3 days of treatment (Sabbagh et al., 2004). Together these data suggest that a minimum of 1 day of an antimicrobial agent is indicated for transrectal ultrasound-guided prostate biopsies. **In 2017 an Update of the AUA White Paper on the prevention and treatment of the more common complications related to prostate biopsy was published** (Liss et al., 2017). **The authors made several key recommendations including preoperative assessment of risk factors for resistant bacteria, and urine culture and treatment of infections in men with lower urinary tract symptoms. The White Paper recommends fluoroquinolone AP within 1 hour of the prostate biopsy. If a rectal swab culture is done, culture-specific antibiotics should be administered (gentamicin and ceftriaxone are most common agents). Local antibiograms can help identify resistance patterns and the authors advocate alternative antibiotics if *E. coli* has more than 20% fluoroquinolone resistance. The EAU guideline recommends the use of AP in men before transrectal prostate biopsy as well as rectal cleansing with povidone-iodine in men before transrectal prostate biopsy.**

Shock-Wave Lithotripsy

The AUA Guidelines on Surgical Management of Stones suggest that noninvasive procedures such as shock-wave lithotripsy do not require AP if the preoperative urine microscopy is benign (Assimos et al., 2016). A meta-analysis of nine RCTs examined the efficacy of AP for shock-wave lithotripsy and demonstrated no statistically significant benefit in reducing postoperative bacteriuria, fevers, or UTIs (Lu et al., 2012). In addition, a prospective study published in 2013 evaluating 526 shock-wave patients, of whom just 10 received AP, revealed very low rates of asymptomatic bacteriuria (0.8%) and UTI (0.2%) (Honey et al., 2013). **Prophylaxis for shock-wave lithotripsy is not recommended based on the low rates of bacteriuria and UTI; however, a history of a recent UTI or of infection stones should warrant a full treatment course of antimicrobial agents before shock-wave lithotripsy.**

Endoscopic Procedures: Lower Urinary Tract

Simple Cystoscopy (Without Manipulation)

Cystoscopy is a minimally traumatic procedure with limited urothelial injury performed on a diverse spectrum of patients, including young healthy women and older men. Several prospective trials (Burke et al., 2002; Clark and Higgs, 1990; Manson, 1988) of patients with preprocedure sterile urine report culture-proven rates of UTI between 2.2% and 7.8% after cystoscopy without AP. In Clark's report the risk of infection was higher in patients with a previous history of UTI. In a similarly designed study, Rane et al. (2001) reported a significantly higher postprocedure culture-proven infection rate of 21% without AP. Johnson et al. (2007) reported results of a randomized controlled trial of more than 2000 patients demonstrating reductions in bacteriuria with administration of single-dose trimethoprim or ciprofloxacin. In all the studies, single doses of antimicrobial agents reduced infections to between 1% and 5%. None of these studies had significant systemic infections reported after the cystoscopic procedures.

More recently, several studies have concluded that AP is not necessary before diagnostic cystoscopy. A retrospective review of more than 2000 patients who did not receive AP reported that only 1.9% of subjects developed a febrile UTI less than 30 days after a cystoscopy and all of the UTIs responded quickly to oral antibiotics; no patients required hospitalization for sepsis (Herr, 2014). This cohort included patients who had negative cultures before the cystoscopy (76%) as well as patients with asymptomatic bacteriuria (24%). A recent systematic review and meta-analysis published in 2015 showed no significant differences in post-cystoscopy UTIs when comparing patients who received AP with those who did not (Garcia-Perdomo et al., 2015). Arrabal-Polo et al. (2017) recently looked at the effect of AP in patients undergoing flexible cystoscopy and concluded that the use of ciprofloxacin or fosfomycin as prophylaxis does not appear to be indicated in flexible cystoscopy. Recent antibiotic use or hospitalization have been identified as risk factors that increase the likelihood of developing a UTI post-cystoscopy (Gregg JR et al., 2015). In a subsequent study these same investigators found that incorporating infection risks in conjunction with analysis of an antibiogram decreased the use of AP before cystoscopy without increasing the rate of post-procedure UTIs (Gregg et al., 2018).

Based on recent evidence, AP is not necessary for the overwhelming majority of diagnostic cystouroscopic procedures. The EAU 2017 guideline on infections states "given the low absolute risk of post-procedural UTI in well-resourced countries, the high number of procedures being performed, and the high risk of contributing to increasing antimicrobial resistance the panel consensus was to strongly recommend not to use antibiotic prophylaxis in patients undergoing urethrocystocopy (flexible or rigid)" (Bonkat et al., 2019).

Transurethral Resection of the Prostate and Bladder (Cystourethroscopy With Manipulation)

Therapeutic transurethral lower urinary tract procedures increase the risk of localized infections compared with simple diagnostic cystoscopy. Although not delineated in any prospective studies, several risk factors likely increase infectious complications, including trauma to the mucosa, increased duration and/or degree of difficulty of the procedure, pressurized irrigants, and manipulation or resection of infected material. The most well-studied lower urinary tract procedure is **transurethral resection of the prostate (TURP).** In a meta-analysis of 32 studies comprising 4260 patients, a risk reduction was noted in bacteriuria from 26% to 9.1% on postoperative urine cultures obtained 2 to 5 days after the procedure for patients treated with prophylactic antimicrobial agents (Berry and Barratt, 2002). Similarly, septicemia (defined as rigors, persistently elevated temperature [>38.5°C], and an elevated C-reactive protein level) decreased from 4.4% to 0.7% with AP. The most effective antimicrobial classes included fluoroquinolones, aminoglycosides, cephalosporins, and TMP-SMX. **Single doses of antimicrobial agents did lower the relative risk of bacteriuria, but not as significantly as antimicrobial agents administered for short courses (2 to 5 days) while the urethral catheter remained in place.** Although continuation of antimicrobial therapy while the catheter is in place is not truly prophylaxis, continuation of the initial prophylactic antimicrobial agent for an anticipated short period of time (with catheter in place) does not increase the risk of developing antimicrobial-resistant organisms. In a randomized controlled trial of 243 patients undergoing transurethral resection of bladder tumors (TURBTs), three perioperative doses of cephadrine (compared with no antimicrobial) reduced the rate of bacteriuria (MacDermott et al., 1988). No recent trials have otherwise investigated prophylaxis for **TURBT**; however, **evidence from TURP procedures suggests that prophylaxis would reduce bacteriuria in these procedures. However, the EAU guidelines based on a systematic review of two RCTs found no benefit for AP in patients undergoing TURBT and recommends AP prophylaxis to reduce infectious complications in only high-risk patients undergoing transurethral resection of the bladder.**

Other cystoscopic procedures with manipulation (e.g., laser prostatectomy, bladder biopsies) have not been well studied. However, the similarity in terms of tissue trauma and invasiveness would suggest that the data regarding TURP and TURBT can be extrapolated. Nevertheless, a recent publication looked at the utility of preoperative antibiotics before bladder biopsy and showed that there was no difference in the rate of UTI or febrile UTI in those patients undergoing bladder biopsy in the office setting (without prophylaxis) versus the operating room (with prophylaxis) (Lipsky et al., 2017). **This is a challenge as the current Center for Medicare and Medicaid Services (CMS) mandates require AP before cystoscopy and biopsy in the OR. IDSA and the AUA guidelines concur with the CMS mandate.** The IDSA guidelines on surgical prophylaxis in urology recommend AP with a fluoroquinolone, trimethoprim-sulfamethoxazole, or cefazolin for lower tract instrumentation in patients with risk factors for infection. However, although CMS and the IDSA and AUA guidelines recommend AP before bladder biopsy, the recent study lends support to the notion that AP in all patients undergoing biopsy may not be necessary.

Patient risk factors associated with increased infectious risk include obesity, diabetes, smoking, immunosuppression, and malnutrition (Bratzler et al., 2013). **In addition, the authors mention urologic-specific risk factors, including urinary tract anatomic anomalies, urinary obstruction, stones, and indwelling or externalized catheters.** In 2009 Yokoyama et al. evaluated the possibility of discarding AP in patients undergoing TURBT. Their prospective study of 162 patients concluded that AP in patients undergoing TURBT did not provide benefit (symptomatic UTI rate of 3.4% in control group vs. 2.3% in the prophylaxis group, as well as no sepsis episodes in either) (Yokoyama et al., 2009).

Patients who are known preoperatively to have UTIs should have the infections eradicated before the procedure is started; therefore, in these patients, preoperative antimicrobial agents are therapeutic and not prophylactic. Failure to eradicate bacteriuria results in bacteremia in 50% of patients (Morris et al., 1976).

Diagnostic and therapeutic upper tract studies that are performed with pressurized irrigants may induce urothelial injury. **Prophylaxis with antimicrobial agents that cover uropathogens is indicated.**

Endoscopic Procedures: Upper Urinary Tract

Ureteroscopy

Diagnostic and therapeutic upper tract endoscopic procedures have an increased risk of localized infections compared with simple diagnostic cystoscopy because of several factors, including increased trauma to the mucosa, increased duration and/or degree of difficulty of most ureteroscopic procedures, increased pressure of irrigants, and (when applicable) manipulation or resection of infected material. **The use of AP is supported** by a randomized trial involving 113 patients undergoing ureteroscopy in which prophylactic fluoroquinolone administration significantly reduced postprocedure bacteriuria (13% vs. 2%) in a healthy population of individuals with ureteral stones and uninfected preoperative urine (Knopf et al., 2003). If an infection or infectious material is suspected, culture and a full treatment course of an appropriate antimicrobial are recommended before the procedure. Some urologists advocate for medical diuresis with furosemide during the procedure.

A recent systematic review and meta-analysis looked at a total of 11 studies with more than 4500 patients undergoing ureteroscopic lithotripsy. Deng et al. (2018) found no significant difference in risk of postoperative febrile urinary tract infections between those patients with and those without AP. However, those patients receiving a single dose of preoperative antibiotics had a significantly lower risk of bacteriuria and pyuria (Deng et al., 2018). The authors concluded by recommending a single dose of oral preoperative AP for patients undergoing ureteroscopic lithotripsy.

Ureteral Stenting

AP should be administered at the time of stent removal. If the patient has significant risk factors, stent culture should be performed at this time to help direct potential antimicrobial treatment if infection occurs. The rates of colonization of the urine range from 0 to 29% without the use of AP (Kehinde et al., 2004; Lojanapiwat, 2006; Riedl et al., 1999). Rates of stent colonization in the same series were significantly higher, ranging from 42% to 70%. Dwell time of the stent was the most significant factor influencing stent colonization, and this was not reduced by prophylaxis. Urine culture correctly identified the colonizing organism (stent culture) in only 15% of the cases.

Percutaneous Renal Surgery (Prophylaxis Indicated in All Patients)

Percutaneous renal surgery is commonly performed for large renal stones, ureteropelvic junction obstruction, and transitional cell carcinoma surveillance. Pyrexia and bacteremia occur frequently and likely stem from a combination of renal parenchymal injury, pressurized irrigation, and, in some cases, manipulation of infectious stones. There are no RCTs confirming the need for prophylaxis, but several studies demonstrated a relationship between the risk of postoperative infectious complications (including bacteriuria and sepsis) and the duration of the procedure, and amount of irrigant used (Dogan et al., 2002). **If preoperative urine cultures are positive, treatment of the infection should occur before surgery. Conversely, if preoperative cultures are negative, AP covering common urinary pathogens should be instituted** (Wolf et al., 2008) (see Table 55.6).

Open, Laparoscopic, and Robotic Surgery

Open surgical procedures can be classified as clean, clean contaminated, contaminated, and dirty (Table 55.16). **AP is indicated for clean-contaminated and contaminated wounds, whereas antimicrobial treatment with an appropriate agent should be instituted for dirty-infected wounds.** No large studies have evaluated the risk of surgical site infections for different laparoscopic urologic procedures. However, data in the general surgery literature suggest that the laparoscopic approach lowers the risk of surgical

TABLE 55.16 Wound Classifications

Class I/clean	Uninfected operative wound without entry into pulmonary, GI or GU systems	Inguinal and scrotal procedures for noninfectious indications, RPLND.
Class II/clean-contaminated	Entry into pulmonary, GI or GU under controlled conditions; no other contamination	Opening into urinary tract, as in nephrectomy, cystectomy, prostatectomy, endoscopic procedures.
Class III/contaminated	Infected stone procedures, use of bowel segments	PCNL on struvite stones, infected stones. TRUS prostate biopsy.
Class IV/dirty	Open trauma, abscesses	Debridement; implication that the offending organisms were present prior to the index procedure.
Prosthesis Implantation	IPP, AUS	Antibiotic prophylaxis should cover likely skin organisms; increasing resistance, MRSA colonization has led many surgeons to use vancomycin perioperatively.

Modified from Mangram, AJ, Horan, TC, Pearson, ML, et al: Guideline for prevention of surgical site infection. *Am J Infect Control* 27:97, 1999.
AUS, Artificial genitourinary sphincter; *GI*, gastrointestinal; *GU*, genitourinary; *IPP*, implantable penile prosthesis; *MRSA*, methicillin-resistant *Staphylococcus aureus*; *PCNL*, percutaneous nephrolithotomy; *RPLND*, retroperitoneal lymph node dissection; *TRUS*, transrectal ultrasound guided.

site infections (Kluytmans, 1997). Clean surgeries in urology include radical nephrectomy if the urinary tract is not entered. **All urologic procedures in which the urinary tract is opened electively are considered clean-contaminated procedures (Class II), whereas entry into an infected urinary tract is considered a contaminated procedure (Class III)** and carries a higher rate of surgical site infection (Cruse, 1992). **Antimicrobial agents should be active against the most likely infecting organism, should be administered within 1 hour of the procedure, and discontinued 24 hours after**, because several studies have failed to demonstrate beneficial effects of long courses of prophylaxis (Conte et al., 1972; Goldmann et al., 1977).

In the United States, first-generation cephalosporins are commonly used for prophylaxis of clean-contaminated procedures because they have low incidences of allergic reactions, long half-lives, and low cost. For patients with a β-lactam allergy, the 2004 National Surgical Infection Prevention Project (NSIPP) guidelines recommend either vancomycin or clindamycin. Prophylaxis for urinary reconstruction with intestine requires increased anaerobic coverage, so the use of first-generation cephalosporins and anaerobic coverage with metronidazole is recommended. When use of the colon or appendix is anticipated for urologic reconstruction, the 2004 NSIPP and WHO recommendations include orally administered antimicrobial bowel preparation (neomycin plus erythromycin or neomycin plus metronidazole) 18 to 24 hours before surgery, and parenteral cefotetan or cefoxitin 30 to 60 minutes before incision (Bratzler and Houck, 2004). Recommendations for patients with a β-lactam allergy include clindamycin plus gentamicin, aztreonam, or ciprofloxacin. Dirty wounds in urology include all abscesses and traumatic perforations of the GU tract. Treatment of a dirty wound should begin with broad coverage of anticipated organisms and intraoperative wound cultures. Subsequent therapy and treatment duration depends on the sensitivities of the cultured organism.

Skin Preparation for Surgery

Although AP plays an important role in minimizing the risk of a surgical site infection, additional considerations are important to lessen the risk of introducing pathogens into the operative site. Pre-hospital bathing, mechanical bowel prep, hair removal, and perioperative skin preparation play a role in preventing infections. See AUA BPS for more information.

Vaginal Surgery

RCTs have not been reported for vaginal urologic surgery, but there is a large body of evidence for vaginal hysterectomy. An old meta-analysis demonstrated a dramatic decrease in incidence of pelvic infections when AP was used (Duff and Park, 1980). Chang et al. (2005) reported the results of a RCT showing that a course of antimicrobials of less than 24 hours was as effective as a long course in patients undergoing laparoscopic assisted vaginal hysterectomy. The AUA AP BPS recommended AP for all vaginal procedures including midurethral sling (MUS) surgery in 2010 and again in 2019. This recommendation is based on expert opinion. Several studies have looked to see if AP is necessary in MUS surgery. One study looked at 174 patients undergoing MUS without AP. The lack of AP was not found to lead to any higher risk of infections, although there was no control arm in this study (Harmanli et al., 2012). An RCT with and without prophylactic antibiotics for MUS was ended early because of lower-than-predicted infectious complications in both groups (Harmanli et al., 2011). Shepherd et al. (2014) performed a decision analysis looking at the necessity of AP before MUS surgery for SUI and concluded that since infectious complications are rare, AP may not be necessary.

Special Considerations

Patients With Risk of Endocarditis

The risk of infectious endocarditis (IE) after urologic procedures is low. Previous guidelines from the American Heart Association (AHA) had recommended routine prophylaxis, but the current recommendation is that the use of prophylactic antibiotics solely to prevent IE is **not recommended** (Wilson et al., 2007). However, these guidelines do acknowledge that instrumentation of the GU tract may result in transient enterococcal bacteremia. Since 2007 the AHA recommends that AP during GU procedures is not an effective strategy for the sole prevention of IE (Wilson et al., 2007).

The latest American College of Cardiology (ACC)/AHA guidelines state that administration of antibiotics is not beneficial for patients undergoing urologic procedures (Nishimura et al., 2017). The guideline states that IE is more likely to result from random bacteremia than from a GU procedure and that prophylaxis may prevent a very small number of cases, if any. The AHA does not recommend antimicrobial treatment even for high-risk patients (prosthetic cardiac valves, previous infectious endocarditis, or cardiac transplant patients with valve disease) undergoing instrumentation of the GU tract.

Regardless, the guidelines do state that **for patients with certain concomitant conditions (prosthetic cardiac valve, previous IE, congenital heart disease, cardiac transplantation) and an active infection or colonization who are to undergo GU tract manipulation, including elective cystoscopy, antibiotic therapy to sterilize the urine may be reasonable (Class IIb evidence).** Amoxicillin or ampicillin is suggested as a first-line agent for enterococci, vancomycin for those who cannot tolerate ampicillin, or culture-directed agents when possible (Wilson et al., 2007).

Patients With Indwelling Orthopedic Hardware

In 2003 a joint commission of the AUA, American Academy of Orthopedic Surgeons (AAOS), and infectious disease specialists released an advisory statement on AP for urologic patients with total joint replacement. The commission did not advise AP for urologic patients with joint replacements, pins, plates, or screws that were at least 2 years old. However, if the prosthetic joint or implant was inserted within 2 years, prophylaxis was recommended with either an oral quinolone or 2 g of ampicillin intravenously and 1.5 mg/kg of gentamicin (vancomycin if ampicillin allergy) intravenously 30 to 60 minutes before the procedure. The AAOS's most recent statement in 2009 recommends that clinicians consider AP for all total joint replacements prior to any invasive procedure that may cause bacteremia. The impetus for this recommendation was the combination of the significant cost of treating infected joint replacements and the potential adverse outcomes. In addition, the recent AUA BPS statement from 2019 does recommend AP for the prevention of prosthetic hip or knee prostheses, particularly for urologic procedures at high risk of bacteremia, those patients within 2 years of joint replacement, and high-risk patient populations. Although the risk for infection with urologic procedures is weak, the panel recommended AP because of the potential of catastrophic harm with a joint infection (Table 55.17).

Prophylaxis on the basis of potential seeding of a prosthetic joint should be instituted for procedures including stone manipulation, transmural incision of the urinary tract, upper tract endoscopic procedures, procedures involving bowel segments, and transrectal prostate biopsy. In addition, patients with recent prosthetic joints or compromised host factors and urinary diversions, indwelling stents or catheters, a recent history of urinary retention, or UTIs should receive AP before urinary tract procedures.

ACKNOWLEDGMENTS

The authors thank Justin Matulay, MD, and Michael Lipsky, MD, for their assistance with the compilation of references and creation of a new flow sheet for management of rUTIs, and they also thank Jeffrey Newhouse, MD, for his expert review of radiologic information and for providing images for the chapter.

TABLE 55.17 Antimicrobial Regimens for Patients With Indwelling Orthopedic Hardware

PATIENT TYPE	ANTIMICROBIAL RECOMMENDATION
Total joint inserted >2 yr ago, pins, plates, screws + no host risk factors	Not recommended empirically
Total joint inserted <2 yr ago or aberrant host factor(s)	Oral quinolone or ampicillin, 2 g IV + gentamicin, 1.5 mg/kg IV, 30–60 min before procedure Substitute vancomycin, 1 g IV, over 1–2 h before procedure if ampicillin allergy

From American Urological Association and American Academy of Orthopaedic Surgeons: Antibiotic prophylaxis for urological patients with total joint replacements. *J Urol* 169:1796–1797, 2003.

KEY POINTS: ANTIMICROBIAL PROPHYLAXIS FOR COMMON UROLOGIC PROCEDURES

- AP entails treatment with an antimicrobial agent before and for a limited time after a procedure to prevent local or systemic postprocedural infections.
- The type of procedure and competency of the host defenses determine the need for AP.
- Special considerations for AP include patients undergoing TRUS-Bx, those with a risk of endocarditis and bacteriuria, and patients with indwelling orthopedic hardware.

REFERENCES

The complete reference list is available online at ExpertConsult.com.

56 Inflammatory and Pain Conditions of the Male Genitourinary Tract: Prostatitis and Related Pain Conditions, Orchitis, and Epididymitis

Michel Pontari, MD

PROSTATITIS

Historical Perspective

In a presentation to the 1929 American Urological Association held in Seattle, Dr. Franklin Farman of Los Angeles gave a brief history of prostatitis and proposed a classification. He noted that knowledge of the prostate dates back to mentions by Herophilus in 350 BCE, and that Nicola Massa, a Venetian physician living the 16th century, is accredited with discovering and describing the prostate. The first description of prostatitis dates to 1838 by Verdies. Treatment by prostate massage was described by Posner of Berlin in 1893. Before this therapy, diseases of the prostate were treated by "applications to the perineum in the form of counter-irritation, heat, cupping, leeches and the like." He proposed a classification of prostatitis divided into two groups based on bacterial cause: the specific or gonorrheal type and the nonspecific or secondary focal type. The gonococcal was divided into three types: simple catarrhal or follicular prostatitis from acute infection and spread from the posterior urethra, true chronic parenchymous prostatitis from repeated infections, and a final category of atrophic or atonic prostatitis. This latter category, he asserted, also includes symptoms of premature ejaculation and impotency but has other causative factors, "a discussion of which involves the field of neuro and psycho-pathology." The second category of prostatitis was thought to come about from hematologic seeding from other infections.

The clinical course of infectious prostatitis was changed significantly with the development of antibiotics (Nickel, 2000). Krieger and Weidner (2003) contend that the contemporary history of prostatitis began with a letter to the editor published in the *Journal of Urology* in 1978 by George Drach et al. (1978). This is described as the first scientific recommendations for a systematic classification of patients with symptoms of prostatitis. The diagnosis was based on the microscopic examination and quantitative cultures of segmented urogenital tract specimens described by Meares and Stamey (1968) and four categories presented: (1) acute bacterial prostatitis with acute infection, (2) chronic bacterial prostatitis with recurrent episodes of bacteriuria by the same organism, (3) chronic bacterial prostatitis in which patients had symptoms of prostatitis, negative cultures, and inflammatory cells, and (4) prostatodynia, with symptoms of prostatitis including "prostatic discomfort" but no recognizable infection or inflammation.

Current Classification of Prostatitis

The current classification of prostatitis was developed at consensus conferences in 1995 and 1998; the National Institutes of Health (NIH) classification was published in 1999 (Krieger et al., 1999).

NIH Classification

I. Acute bacterial prostatitis
II. Chronic bacterial prostatitis
IIIA. Chronic prostatitis/pelvic pain syndrome, inflammatory
IIIB. Chronic prostatitis/pelvic pain syndrome, noninflammatory
IV. Asymptomatic inflammatory prostatitis

Categories I and II are similar to the Drach classification (Drach et al., 1978). Bacterial prostatitis accounts for 5% to 10% of cases. The categories of nonbacterial prostatitis and prostatodynia were transformed into category III chronic prostatitis/chronic pelvic pain syndrome (CP/CPPS). Category III is subdivided as category IIIA, inflammatory, with the presence of white blood cells in expressed prostatic secretions (EPS), post–prostate massage urine (VB3) or seminal plasma, or category IIIB, noninflammatory, without the inflammatory cells. This mirrors the distinction between nonbacterial prostatitis and prostatodynia. There have been no clinically significant differences demonstrated between these two subclasses.

The term *prostatitis* for category III may be confusing. Historically, the pain was thought to come from the prostate, from infection, or from inflammation. However, we now recognize that the prostate may not be the source of the pelvic pain in these men, and the term *chronic pelvic pain syndrome* was adopted to reflect this understanding. Although categorized as prostatitis, the pain of CP/CPPS may have nothing to do with inflammation or the prostate in some men. Type IV is asymptomatic inflammatory prostatitis and is diagnosed in men with no genitourinary pain complaints. Thus type IV is most commonly found in the evaluation of other genitourinary tract issues, such as in biopsy looking for prostate cancer or on semen analysis for evaluation for infertility.

The NIH definition of category III CP/CPPS as adopted by the Chronic Prostatitis Research Network is that of symptoms of pain or discomfort in the pelvis for at least 3 of the previous 6 months (Schaeffer et al., 2002b). Several exclusion criteria are also included, such as demonstration of uropathogenic bacteria detected by standard microbiologic methods, urogenital cancer, prior radiation or chemotherapy, urethral stricture, or neurologic disease affecting the bladder (Schaeffer et al., 2002b). Similar inclusion and exclusion criteria are being used in the ongoing NIH study on the multidisciplinary approach to pelvic pain (MAPP) (Landis et al., 2014).

Histopathology

Histology

The term *prostatitis* can refer to the presence of inflammation on a histology examination of the prostate or is also used to describe clinical syndromes manifest by genitourinary discomfort or pain described in the NIH classification. The relationship is certainly not completely clear, and use of the terms can be confusing. The classification also contains category IV, which is prostatic inflammation, including prostate-specific specimens such as EPS, VB3, seminal plasma, and biopsies. Asymptomatic in this classification is the absence of pain. Histologic inflammation is commonly found in specimens resected for benign prostatic hyperplasia (BPH) (Nickel et al., 1999) and in biopsies done looking for prostate cancer. In a study by McNeal, prostatic inflammation was found in 44% of sampled adult prostates (McNeal, 1968). More contemporary series have found that more than 70% of men at autopsy to have chronic inflammation (Zlotta et al., 2014). Increased numbers of intraepithelial lymphocytes in areas of category IV prostatitis compared with areas of normal prostate suggest that it may be immune or autoimmune in origin (Dikov et al., 2015).

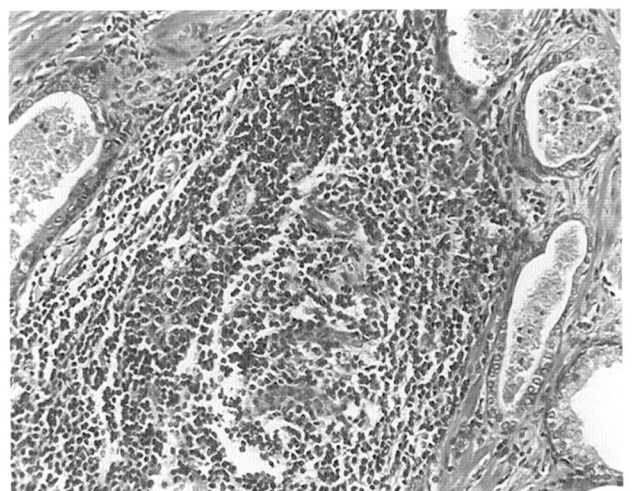

Fig. 56.1. Histologic preparation of a prostate specimen demonstrating areas of glandular, periglandular, and stromal inflammation (×400). (Courtesy Dr. Alexander Boag.)

A classification system proposed by Nickel et al. recommended reporting inflammation in prostatitis by its anatomic location in the prostate, either glandular (within a duct/gland epithelium or lumen), periglandular (lies within stroma but centered around ducts and glands and approaches 50 μm or less), or stromal (in the stroma and >50 μm from a gland). Extent of inflammation is defined as focal (<10%), multifocal (10%–50%), or diffuse (> 50%). Grade is 1, or mild (individual inflammatory cells separated by distinct spaces, <100 cells); 2, or moderate (confluent sheets of cell with no tissue destruction or lymphoid follicles, 100–300 cells); and 3, or severe (confluent sheets of inflammatory cells with tissue destruction or nodule formation, 100–500 cells) (Nickel et al., 2001). Fig. 56.1 shows a representative section illustrating the three locations of prostatic inflammation.

Associated entities include corpora amylacea, which form from the deposition of prostatic secretions around sloughed epithelial cells; they do not usually cause inflammation unless they cause obstruction (Morales et al., 2005). Prostate calculi may contribute to inflammation by causing local obstruction or by providing a nidus for bacterial growth. The chemical composition of many stones suggest they may be caused by chronic infection (Dessombz et al., 2012). The presence of stones has been correlated to the symptoms of men with CP/CPPS (Shoskes et al., 2007). Occasionally they grow large enough to cause urethral obstruction and warrant surgical removal (Goyal et al., 2013).

Specific Cases of Prostatic Inflammation

Granulomatous Prostatitis

Granulomatous prostatitis is diagnosed by the histologic finding of epithelioid granulomas with or without other inflammatory cells (Uzoh et al., 2007). It is commonly found on specimens from transurethral resections and prostate biopsies. The most widely accepted grading system categorizes granulomatous prostatitis as specific, nonspecific, after transurethral resection of the prostate (TURP), and allergic granulomatous prostatitis (Epstein and Hutchins, 1984). It is commonly seen after intravesical Bacillus Calmette-Guerin (BCG) therapy for bladder cancer and can cause transient elevated levels of prostate-specific antigen (PSA) (Leibovici et al., 2000). Tuberculosis can also cause granulomatous prostatitis (Kulchavenya et al., 2012).

Immunoglobulin G Subclass 4 (IgG4)

Prostatitis has been described from IgG4-related disease (IgG4-RD). IgG4-RD is a recently described fibroinflammatory disease with multiorgan involvement. The first case of histologically confirmed IgG4 prostatitis was in 2006 (Yoshimura et al., 2006). IgG4-related disease is a fibroinflammatory condition characterized by several features: tendency to form tumorlike lesions at multiple sites, dense infiltrate of lymphocytes and IgG4 +plasma cells, characteristic pattern of fibrosis, and often, but not always, elevated levels of serum IgG4 (Deshpande et al., 2012). First described in autoimmune pancreatitis, multiple previously described disorders including Ormond disease (retroperitoneal fibrosis) are now considered to fall within this category (Stone et al., 2012). One of the characteristics of IgG4 disease is a dramatic response to corticosteroids. Patients with lower urinary tract symptoms from IgG4 disease have responded to corticosteroids with improvement in symptoms (Hart et al., 2013). There is as yet no characteristic presentation that would allow for identification of men with IgG4 prostatitis to allow for selection for treatment with steroids instead of surgery or standard BPH medications (Pontari, 2014). An obvious but perhaps small group is those men with concomitant autoimmune pancreatitis or sclerosing cholangitis and lower urinary tract symptoms (LUTS; Buijs et al., 2014). The diagnosis could be considered if histologic findings at the time of prostate biopsy for elevated PSA or a nodule suggest the diagnosis.

Category I Prostatitis: Acute Bacterial Prostatitis

Acute bacterial prostatitis (ABP) generally affects men age 20 to 40 years but also has a second peak of incadence in men over the age of 60 (Krieger et al., 2011; Roberts et al., 1998). The causes of acute bacterial prostatitis are many. One is from ascending urethral infection. Characterization of virulence factors in the bacteria of men diagnosed with acute prostatitis indicated similar organisms in the urine specimens and rectal swab of the patient or sexual partner as the causative organism of the prostatitis in 6 of 9 men tested, indicating an ascending route of infection (Terai et al., 2000). Direct seeding from a prostate biopsy is a common cause. Other causes include intraprostatic reflux of infected urine that enters the ejaculatory and prostatic ducts of the posterior prostatic urethra and rarely spreads from the rectum via the lymphatic system. Hematogenous dissemination in the setting of bacterial sepsis or other blood-borne infections such as tuberculosis can occur (Brede and Shoskes, 2011).

Risk factors for the development of acute prostatitis include unprotected sexual intercourse, specifically insertive anal intercourse, phimosis, condom catheter use, indwelling urethral catheters, and urinary tract instrumentation, including endoscopic procedures and prostate biopsy (Dielubanza et al., 2014). Dysfunctional voiding and disorders causing urinary stasis, including distal urethral stricture and BPH, also put men at risk of developing prostatitis (Heyns, 2012). Acute prostatitis can occur after an episode of bacterial cystitis or epididymo-orchitis (Brede and Shoskes, 2011). A review of complications of clean intermittent catheterization showed that prostatitis occurs in up to 33% of these patients (Wyndaele, 2002).

The presentation of category I prostatitis is acute symptoms of a urinary tract infection (UTI), characteristically including urinary frequency and dysuria. Some patients have symptoms suggestive of systemic infection, such as malaise, fever, and myalgias (Krieger et al., 1999). Because of the UTI, pain can also be present in the lower abdomen and perineum. Urinary retention may be present because of acute swelling of the prostate, pain, or spasm of the bladder neck. In severe cases, patients can experience symptoms of sepsis: high fevers and chills, cardiovascular instability, and mental status changes (Brede and Shoskes, 2011). The presentation can vary by the cause of the prostatitis. As compared with spontaneous acute prostatitis as seen in younger men, patients who develop acute prostatitis after lower urinary tract manipulation or biopsy tend to be older and have a greater likelihood of septicemia (Kim et al., 2015; Millan-Rodriguez et al., 2006). Patients with Extended spectrum beta–lactamase (ESBL) positive bacteria also have significantly higher rates of septicemia (Kim et al., 2015). **Acute prostatitis should be considered in any man who presents with a febrile UTI. Febrile UTI in men can be from pyelonephritis, acute cystitis, or prostatitis. In a prospective study of 70 men with febrile UTI** (Ulleryd et al., 1999), **more than 90% had increases in PSA and/or prostate volume.** In this cohort one-third had flank pain. This indicates that the prostate is likely involved even if the patient has signs of pyelonephritis.

Microbiology. The most common causative organism is *Escherichia coli*, implicated in 65% to 80% of cases (Millan-Rodriguez et al., 2006). Other common gram-negative organisms include *Pseudomonas aeruginosa*, *Proteus mirabilis*, and *Klebsiella* and *Serratia* spp. (Etienne et al., 2008; Kim et al., 2014; Yoon et al., 2012). *Enterococcus* spp. account for up to 10% of cases of acute prostatitis (Kravchick et al., 2004; Schneider et al., 2003a). *Neisseria gonorrhoeae* should be considered as a possible cause in sexually active young men. Rare causes of bacterial prostatitis include obligate anaerobes and gram-positive bacteria other than *Enterococcus* spp. *Mycobacterium tuberculosis* is a rare cause of prostatitis and is usually associated with immunodeficiency. Prostate involvement is seen in approximately 10% of cases of genitourinary tuberculosis (TB). Common symptoms in these patients include perineal pain and dysuria (Kulchavenya, 2013; Kulchavenya et al., 2013). In tuberculous prostatitis, abscess cavities can form in the prostate, which can connect with sinuses to the perineum and result in fistula formation. In patients with impaired immunity such as HIV, other infecting organisms can cause prostatitis, including *Staphylococcus aureus*, *Klebsiella pneumonia*, *Pseudomonas aeruginosa*, *Serratia marcescens*, *Salmonella typhi*, *M. tuberculosis*, and *Mycobacterium avium intracellulare* (Weinberger et al., 1988).

There are multiple virulence factors associated with the bacteria found in men with acute prostatitis. A contemporary study of previously healthy men aged 17 to 40 years old with acute prostatitis demonstrated 26 virulence genes from the cultured *E. coli* representing 5 virulence factors, including adhesins, toxins, and siderophores in addition to the expression of α-hemolysin, aerobactin, cytotoxic necrotizing factor-1 (CNF1), cytolethal distending toxin type 1 (CDT-1), and colicins. The isolates averaged 12.5 virulence genes (Krieger et al., 2011). URIs are uncommon in young healthy men, and this study demonstrates that bacterial virulence has a significant contribution to the development of acute prostatitis in this population (Krieger and Thumbikat, 2016). Another virulence factor that occurs in the bacteria causing acute prostatitis is the production of biofilms. Biofilms are a group of bacteria together in one area protected by a polysaccharide matrix. This makes the penetration of antibiotics more difficult. In a study of uropathogenic *E. coli* causing infection, biofilm formation was found more often in bacteria recovered from men with acute prostatitis (63%) as compared with cystitis (43%) and pyelonephritis (40%) (Soto et al., 2007), consistent with other studies (Kanamaru et al., 2006).

An important concept that has emerged is the difference in bacterial cause of prostatitis and antibiotic susceptibility depending on the cause. There are differences in organisms, depending on whether the acute prostatitis developed in the community or was nosocomial. A review indicated that community-acquired infections were three times more common than nosocomial infections. *E. coli* was the predominant organism, but nosocomial cases were more often caused by *P. aeruginosa*, enterococci, or *S. aureus* and had greater antimicrobial resistance and clinical failures (Etienne et al., 2008). Further distinctions are noted, depending on whether the acute prostatitis is spontaneous or occurs after lower urinary tract instrumentation or prostate biopsy. Patients with spontaneous acute prostatitis have predominantly *E. coli* (Millan-Rodriguez et al., 2006). Patients with acute prostatitis after manipulation also have predominantly *E. coli* but have a much higher prevalence of *Pseudomonas* spp. (20%) and have a higher risk of prostate abscess (Ha et al., 2008). Acute prostatitis after transrectal biopsy also has predominantly *E. coli*, but these bacteria are more resistant to fluoroquinolones (Kim et al., 2014), more likely to have ESBL-producing bacteria, and more likely to have positive blood cultures (Kim et al., 2015). **Thus the antibiotic selection for acute prostatitis must take into consideration the route of infection.**

Evaluation. Patient history is important given the differences in the cause of the infection. The determination should be made if the patient has spontaneous acute prostatitis or has had lower urinary tract manipulation or a recent transrectal prostate biopsy. LUTS such as frequency urgency and dysuria are common. Associated signs of bacteremia and sepsis can be present, including fever, chills, and sweats (Brede and Shoskes, 2011). The history should assess for possible complicating factors such as diabetes, HIV, neurologic disease, and recent antibiotic use (Dielubanza et al., 2014). A palpable bladder may indicate urinary retention. **Acute prostatitis is the one situation in which one may palpate a truly "boggy" prostate from edema from inflammation. The prostate is tender and swollen in 60% to 90% of cases** (Etienne et al., 2008; Millan-Rodriguez et al., 2006). **Caution should be used to avoid aggressive palpation that could lead to bacterial dissemination and sepsis.**

Laboratory tests include a CBC, urinalysis, and midstream urine culture. Urine culture is positive in 60% to 85% of cases (Etienne et al., 2010). In a series of 347 patients with acute prostatitis, positive blood cultures were associated with a fever of more than 101.1°F, and although they generally grew organisms similar to the urine culture, contributed to the microbiologic diagnosis in 5% of cases (Etienne et al., 2010). Blood cultures should be drawn for patients with fever or chills before fever who have not yet received antibiotics. Prostate massage for prostate fluid should not be performed in the acute setting. Urinalysis can show white and red blood cells consistent with an infection. If the patient has a urethral discharge, urine can be sent for nuclear amplification tests for gonorrhea or chlamydia, but the prevalence of sexually transmitted infections in the setting of acute bacterial prostatitis is approximately 2% (Etienne et al., 2008). Renal function should be assessed to help guide antibiotic therapy. An assessment of postvoid residual urine should be made to rule out urinary retention, preferably noninvasively with an ultrasound. PSA testing is not recommended because the level is expected to be high during the acute phase (Game et al., 2003) and must be followed to ensure resolution back to normal levels. This may take up to 6 months to normalize and must be followed if elevated to make sure there is no elevation from an underlying prostate cancer (Zackrisson et al., 2003). Imaging studies are generally not indicated unless a prostate abscess is suspected. A transrectal ultrasound or CT scan can be used in this setting (Horcajada et al., 2003). There is no role for prostate biopsy for acute prostatitis.

Treatment. It is important to fully treat acute prostatitis not only for the sake of the acute illness but also to prevent progression to a chronic infection as category II prostatitis (10.2%) or category III (9.6%) (Yoon et al., 2012). Infection with ESBL bacteria after a transrectal prostate biopsy is also a risk factor for progression to chronic prostatitis, reported as 25% of those with ESBL bacteria (Oh et al., 2013). Patients with systemic signs of infection need admission for IV antibiotics, hydration, and monitoring of laboratory studies. Some patients can be treated as an outpatient if they have no signs of systemic illness, can tolerate oral intake, and do not have urinary retention (Brede and Shoskes, 2011).

Antibiotics are the mainstay of therapy for acute bacterial prostatitis. The most recent European Association of Urology (EAU) guidelines on treating UTIs recommend the parenteral administration of high-dose bactericidal antibiotics such as a broad-spectrum penicillin, third-generation cephalosporin, or a fluoroquinolone. In initial therapy, any of these can be combined with an aminoglycoside (Grabe et al., 2015). One problem with this recommendation is the issue of men presenting with acute prostatitis after transrectal prostate biopsy. **Given the rates of resistance to quinolones and the incidence of ESBL bacteria seen in these cases, a strong argument can be made to use a carbapenem antibiotic in men presenting with fever and prostatitis after a transrectal prostate biopsy** (Dielubanza et al., 2014). **This concern is reflected in the Update of the American Urological Association White Paper on the prevention and treatment of complications after prostate biopsy** (Liss et al., 2017), **which states patients who have a fever after prostate biopsy should:**

- Not be offered fluoroquinolones or trimethoprim-sulfamethoxazole (TMP-SMX)
- Be managed with aggressive resuscitation and broad-spectrum antibiotic coverage: carbapenems, amikacin, or second- and third-generation cephalosporins (after urine and blood cultures)

Once the fever has subsided, or as initial treatment in patients who can be safely discharged, an oral fluoroquinolone, provided the bacteria is susceptible, is a good choice of therapy. Ciprofloxacin 500 mg twice daily or levofloxacin 500 mg daily can be used (Brede and Shoskes, 2011). It is recommended to reculture the urine after

1 week to make sure the bacteria has been cleared (Dielubanza et al., 2014). The traditional recommendation for antibiotic therapy for acute prostatitis to prevent chronic infection has been 4 weeks. However, 2 weeks of ciprofloxacin in men with a febrile UTI has been shown to produce a similar bacterial cure rate compared with 4 weeks of therapy (89% vs. 97%) and clinical cure rates at 1 year (72% vs. 82%). Thus 2 weeks is likely sufficient for duration of oral antibiotics (Ulleryd and Sandberg, 2003). Treatment for tuberculous prostatitis is with anti-TB chemotherapy for at least 6 months (Kulchavenya et al., 2016).

Adjuncts to Antibiotic Therapy. The use of nonsteroidal anti-inflammatory medications can help with pain and inflammation. Patients may also benefit from the use of alpha-blockers if they have LUTS. For patients in urinary retention requiring drainage, traditional thinking has been to place a suprapubic catheter to avoid irritation of the prostate and possible bacteremia. For short-term care, straight catheterization or a brief period of urethral catheterization may be attempted (Brede and Shoskes, 2011). Not every author agrees with this, however (Dielubanza et al., 2014), but for long-term bladder drainage, a suprapubic catheter is recommended.

Prostatic Abscess

Prostatic abscess should be suspected in men with high fever or a history of immunosuppression such as diabetes or HIV or who do not respond to initial therapy after 48 hours (Ha et al., 2008). Risk factors for development of abscess include history of prior catheter use, history of genitourinary surgery, increasing age and increased medical co-morbidities, indwelling catheter, instrumentation of the lower urinary tract, bladder outlet obstruction, acute and chronic bacterial prostatitis, chronic renal failure, hemodialysis, biopsy of the prostate, diabetes, cirrhosis, and HIV (Abdelmoteleb et al., 2017; Weinberger et al., 1988).

Imaging should be performed to look for a prostatic abscess. Methods recommended are transrectal ultrasound or CT scan. Ultrasound will show a hypoechoic area. CT offers the advantage of clarity of location and preoperative planning, as well as identification of any spread beyond the prostate (Vaccaro et al., 1986). Smaller lesions less than 1 to 2 cm may be treated conservatively with antibiotics (Abdelmoteleb et al., 2017). In a recent series, patients with an abscess smaller than 2 cm could be cured by medical therapy alone, but those who underwent surgical drainage required a shorter duration of antibiotic treatment than those treated conservatively (Lee et al., 2016). In men with progression of symptoms, treatment is indicated. Localized lesions, or those that are very peripheral, can be treated by percutaneous drainage under ultrasound guidance (Varkarakis et al., 2004). The recurrence rate after aspiration ranges from 15% to 33% (Ackerman et al., 2018). Lesions that do not respond to initial percutaneous drainage or lesions too large to adequately drain percutaneously should be taken for TURP to unroof the abscess (Fig. 56.2). A maneuver that has proven helpful is palpation and massage of the prostate after unroofing to help fully drain the abscess cavity. Rare cases of abscess that extend beyond the prostate may require open surgical treatment (Ludwig et al., 1999).

> **KEY POINTS**
> - Men with category I acute prostatitis experience acute symptoms of dysuria, frequency, and possibly fever.
> - The most common causative organism is *E. coli.*
> - Types of bacteria and antibiotic sensitivities differ by cause: spontaneous, after transurethral procedure, or after transrectal biopsy.
> - Men with acute prostatitis after transrectal biopsy should be treated with carbapenems, amikacin, or second- and third-generation cephalosporins.
> - A suprapubic tube should be used if long-term drainage is needed.
> - Failure to respond to therapy should prompt imaging to look for a prostatic abscess.

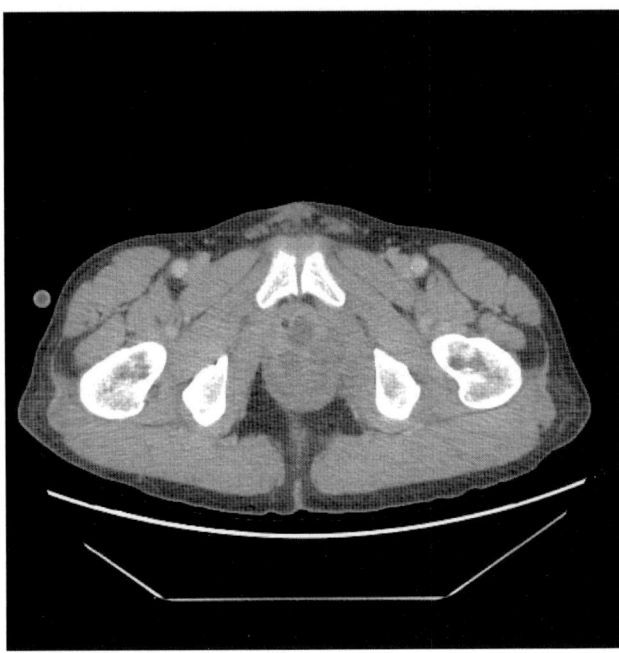

Fig. 56.2. Large prostate abscess in patient with dysuria and fever. Abscess was treated by transurethral unroofing.

Category II: Chronic Bacterial Prostatitis

Chronic bacterial prostatitis is characterized by recurrent urinary tract infections with the same organism (Krieger et al., 1999). This suggests a persistent prostatic source. This category accounts for 5% to 10% of cases of prostatitis (Krieger and Egan, 1991). **The symptoms of dysuria and pain generally respond to antibiotic treatment, and, unlike men with category III CP/CPPS, they are then relatively asymptomatic between episodes.**

Bacteria-Causing Category II Prostatitis. Causative organisms for causing acute bacterial prostatitis, in most cases, are *E. coli, Pseudomonas, Proteus, Klebsiella,* and *Enterobacter* spp. (Gill and Shoskes, 2016). The role of enterococcus in causing chronic bacterial prostatitis is generally accepted. Of 6211 patients attending an Italian prostatitis clinic between 1997 and 2008, *Enterococcus faecalis* was found in 2745, or 44% (Cai et al., 2011). The significance of other gram-positive bacteria such as staphylococci and streptococci is debated. Microorganisms also considered to be of debatable significance include *Corynebacterium, Ureaplasma urealyticum,* and *Mycoplasma hominis.* Fastidious organisms that may require different culture techniques include *Mycoplasma tuberculosis* and *Candida* spp. (Schneider et al., 2003b). Similar to bacteria causing category I prostatitis, bacteria causing chronic bacterial prostatitis also are likely to form biofilms, which make them less likely to respond to treatment (Bartoletti et al., 2014).

Role of Chlamydia in Prostatitis? The role of chlamydia as a cause of chronic bacterial prostatitis is still controversial. *Chlamydia* is an obligate intracellular gram-negative bacterium. It is surrounded by a rigid cell wall and needs other living cells to multiply because it cannot synthesize some essential nutrients (Mackern-Oberti et al., 2013). *Chlamydia* spp. can cause prostatic infection by an ascending route after urethral inoculation in animal models (Pal et al., 2004). The main argument is the difficulty of attributing the findings of *Chlamydia* spp. in the expressed prostatic secretions or semen to prostate infection alone given the possibility of urethral contamination, as *Chlamydia* spp. are a common cause of urethritis (Weidner et al., 2002). Studies of prostate tissue show *Chlamydia* spp. in 3% to 30%; however, the possibility of contamination from the prostatic urethra exists in tissue from TURP, transrectal biopsies, or open surgery and is eliminated only by perineal biopsy from the lateral lobes. Two studies of biopsies from the lateral lobes of the prostate have not detected *Chlamydia* spp. (Doble et al., 1989b; Weidner et al., 1991b).

However, a growing body of literature on the possible role of *Chlamydia* spp. in prostate infection suggests some involvement. In a study looking for *Chlamydia* spp. in men with prostatitis compared with controls, *Chlamydia* spp. were identified by plasmid DNA found in the ejaculate of 35 of 78 patients but in none of 20 controls. Antichlamydial mucosal IgA was found in 69.2% of patients, with none found in the controls. The IgA levels correlated with symptoms and levels of IL-8 (Mazzoli et al., 2007). The presence of *Chlamydia* spp. has been linked to premature ejaculation (PE). In men with chronic prostatitis attributed to *Chlamydia* spp., 118 of 317 had PE (37.2%) as compared with 73 of 639 (11.5%) men with chronic prostatitis from common uropathogenic bacteria ($P < 0.0002$) (Cai et al., 2014). More compelling evidence was the report of a reduction in serum PSA in men with EPS or VB3 positive for *Chlamydia* spp. but negative VB1 treated with 4 weeks of a combination of levofloxacin and azithromycin; the resultant eradication of *Chlamydia* spp. and PSA response was also accompanied by a decrease in symptoms. This strongly suggests prostate involvement. Despite ongoing concerns (Benelli et al., 2017), some evidence supports a causative role for *Chlamydia* spp. in chronic bacterial prostatitis.

Diagnosis and Evaluation. The diagnosis is currently made by the pre-massage and post-massage test (or two-glass test). The VB3 specimen gives information as to a persistent prostatic source of bacteria. The patient provides a midstream pre-massage urine specimen and a urine specimen (initial 10 mL) after prostatic massage to obtain expressed prostatic secretions (EPS) (Nickel et al., 2006). These specimens are then sent for culture. The previous method was the "four-glass test" as described by Meares and Stamey, which includes the first voided urine looking for urethral bacteria (VB1), the midstream urine (VB2), post-massage urine for EPS (VB3), and collection of the prostate fluid itself for culture (Meares and Stamey, 1968). The two-glass pre-massage and post-massage test is a simpler method and yields similar results. A study from the NIH Chronic Prostatitis Collaborative Research Network (CPCRN) examined a cohort of 353 men with CP/CPPS with complete four-glass data and noted that the two-glass test predicted a positive four-glass result with clinically acceptable accuracy (more than 95% of men would have had the same diagnosis if the four-glass test were performed) (Nickel et al., 2006). In men with human immunodeficiency virus (HIV), cultures should be sent not only for the usual bacteria but also for more atypical organisms, including anaerobes, anaerobes, fungi, and TB (Heyns and Fisher, 2005). There are no recommended diagnostic cutoff points for bacterial counts between the two specimens obtained, but some clinics use a 10-fold increase in the post-massage urine as being diagnostic of CP II (Benelli et al., 2017). Semen cultures are not recommended because of limited detection of causative bacteria (Weidner and Anderson, 2008) and decreased specificity resulting from skin contamination (Gill and Shoskes, 2016).

Urine should be assessed for hematuria. If present in the setting of infection, it should be rechecked 4 to 6 weeks after resolution of infection to look for resolution of the hematuria. Persistent hematuria should prompt an evaluation. Physical examination should evaluate for fever. Abdominal examination is necessary to rule out other causes of abdominal/suprapubic pain. Scrotal examination is needed to evaluate for any associated areas of inflammation and possible infection such as the epididymis and testis. A digital rectal examination is indicated to look for prostate size and any abnormalities to suggest prostate cancer. It is important to assess for bladder outlet obstruction and urinary retention. Retention of urine may predispose to recurrent urinary tract infection. A postvoid residual urine of more than 180 mL has been correlated with increased risk of infection (Truzzi et al., 2008). Urinary retention also increases the pathogenicity of bacteria (Johnson et al., 1993).

Not all patients with chronic bacterial prostatitis need imaging. In men younger than 45 years old with a first event of acute UTI, imaging showed no abnormalities. It is recommended, however, in this group to rule out urethral stricture. Men with a flow rate of more than 15 mL/min should be further evaluated (Abarbanel et al., 2003). Urethral strictures can occur with a UTI in up to 41% of cases (Santucci et al., 2007). Imaging is recommended for men with a UTI and history of diabetes, chronic kidney disease, stones, voiding difficulties, neurologic disease, poor response to antibiotics, infection with urea-splitting bacteria, or hematuria more than 1 month after the infection (Heyns, 2012).

Treatment of Chronic Bacterial Prostatitis (Category II). The treatment of category II prostatitis is limited to antibiotics that can penetrate the prostate and achieve therapeutic levels. The prostate capillary bed lacks active transport mechanisms for antibiotics (Stamey et al., 1970). Penetration into the prostate, therefore, is dependent on passive transport, and the factors that influence this transport are drug concentration, lipid solubility, degree of ionization or charge, degree of protein binding, and size and shape of the molecule (Wagenlehner et al., 2013). Quinolones have excellent prostate penetration because of their configuration, including positively and negatively charged groups, also called a zwitterion. The fluid of chronic bacterial prostatitis is alkaline and contributes to concentration of the quinolones (Wagenlehner et al., 2005). These molecules also have high lipid solubility (Perletti et al., 2009). Other antimicrobial agents that have good to excellent penetration into prostatic fluid and tissue include tetracyclines because of their lipid solubility, macrolides because of their pKa values, and trimethoprim, which is a lipid-soluble base with a favorable pKa (Charalabopoulos et al., 2003b).

There are no American Urological Association (AUA) guidelines for antibiotic treatment of chronic bacterial prostatitis/category II, but the EAU has guidelines for this condition (Grabe et al., 2015). Fluoroquinolones such as ciprofloxacin and levofloxacin are the antibiotics of choice not only because of their tissue penetration but also because of their spectrum of coverage, which includes gram-negatives, including *Pseudomonas*, gram-positives, and atypical pathogens such as *Chlamydia* spp. and genital *Mycoplasma* spp. Duration of treatment is based on expert opinion; the recommendation is 4 to 6 weeks. This is in agreement with recent guidelines published by the Prostatitis Expert Reference Group from the UK (Rees et al., 2015b). Because of their ability to penetrate biofilms, the addition of a macrolide may be beneficial. In a trial by Magri et al., the combination of azithromycin 500 mg three times per week added to ciprofloxacin 750 mg per day for 4 weeks increased bacterial eradication rates compared with azithromycin and ciprofloxacin at the more standard regimen of 500 mg per day for 6 weeks (Magri et al., 2011).

Overall it is estimated that 60% to 80% of patients with *E. coli* and other gram-negative Enterobacteriaceae can be cured by the quinolone regimen (Wagenlehner et al., 2013). This is in comparison with only 30% to 50% with a 12-week course of Bactrim (timethoprim-sulfamethoxazole [TMP-SMX]) (Kurzer and Kaplan, 2002). However, in cases in which the bacteria are resistant to fluoroquinolones but susceptible to TMP-SMX, a 3-month course of TMP-SMX can be given. There are no evidence-based recommendations for treatment if the bacteria are resistant to both agents. A 2013 Cochrane review examined the treatment of chronic prostatitis (Perletti et al., 2013). For traditional bacterial prostatitis, there was no difference among the oral fluoroquinolones. No conclusion could be drawn regarding the optimal treatment duration; treatment ranged from 4 to 12 weeks. For chlamydial prostatitis, azithromycin was superior to Cipro and equivalent to clarithromycin.

CP II in HIV/Immunocompromised Patients. In men with HIV, consideration should be made for low antimicrobial suppression for some time to reduce the risk of recurrence (Santillo and Lowe, 2006). In patients who are already treated with highly active antiretroviral therapy (HAART) and are still persistently immunocompromised, lifetime suppressive antimicrobials have been recommended to risk progression to prostatic abscess (Lee et al., 2001).

Beyond Quinolones. In the setting of increasing quinolone resistance and trimethoprim resistance, other alternatives are needed. Alternatives that have data for use in chronic bacterial prostatitis include netilmicin, an aminoglycoside (no longer available in the US; Magri et al., 2016) and cefoxitin (Demonchy et al., 2018). Piperacillin-tazobactam achieves prostatic levels that would be adequate to treat infections from *E. coli, Klebsiella,* and *Proteus* but not adequate levels to treat *Pseudomonas* (Kobayashi et al., 2015). Fosfomycin has in vitro activity against *E. coli* with antimicrobial resistance, including

ESBL strains (Karlowsky et al., 2014). It also has good penetration into the prostate (Gardiner et al., 2014). A dosage of 3 g every 48 to 72 hours was used in 15 patients with bacterial eradication in 8 and clinical cure in 7 (Los-Arcos et al., 2015).

Adjunct treatments for refractory chronic bacterial prostatitis include alternate regimens of antibiotics and surgery. When antibiotic therapy fails to eradicate infection, the patient can be started on a daily dose of an antibiotic targeting an identified bacterial isolate. Duration is approximately 6 months, after which it should be titrated down to maintain the lowest dose that results in symptom relief (Dielubanza et al., 2014). A trial of the medicine near 6 months may also be advisable to see if the antibiotic is still necessary. In self-start therapies, men send urine cultures when they have a recurrence of symptoms and start the antimicrobials at the start of symptoms (Dielubanza et al., 2014). For patients whose symptoms are refractory to medical therapy, TURP has been used with results of 52% to 67% of patients responding to TURP down to the surgical capsule (Barnes et al., 1982; Decaestecker and Oosterlinck, 2015).

KEY POINTS

- Chronic bacterial prostatitis is characterized by recurrent urinary tract infections with the same organism.
- Unlike men with category III prostatitis/chronic pelvic pain syndrome, men with category II are relatively asymptomatic between episodes.
- Urinary retention as a cause of recurrent UTI must be ruled out.
- Men younger than 45 years old do not need imaging but need assessment for a urethral stricture.
- Treatment is with antibiotics that achieve adequate prostate concentrations.
- For refractory cases daily suppressive antibiotics or TURP can be used.

Etiology

Despite a concerted research effort in the past 20 years, the cause and much of the pathogenesis of CP/CPPS remain unknown. However, there is evidence to support a possible role for infection, neurologic causes, and inflammatory/autoimmune, endocrine, and psychological factors. It is likely the interplay between all of these that contributes to the creation and continuation of pelvic pain (Pontari, 2013). One hypothesis is that an insult such as infection, stress, or trauma in a genetically susceptible individual leads to neurogenic inflammation, which is maintained by these other factors (Fig. 56.3).

Infection

The symptoms of CP/CPPS are similar to that of a true prostatic infection. Therefore infection has been commonly assumed by patients and clinicians to be the cause of the symptoms. A history of prior sexually transmitted disease (STD) increases the odds of prostatitis by 1.8 times (Collins et al., 2002). Although a history of STD seems to lead to greater risk of CP/CPPS, there is no evidence of an active STD in these men (Weidner et al., 1991a). There is no difference in the routine cultures of men with CP/CPPS and asymptomatic controls from urine, prostatic fluid, and post-prostate massage urine or seminal plasma (Nickel et al., 2003). Eight percent of men had uropathogenic bacteria, and roughly 70% had some form of bacteria in each group. This indicates that some asymptomatic men appear to routinely have bacteria in the prostate but may not by themselves produce disease or symptoms.

Molecular techniques that can identify bacteria without culture include polymerase chain reaction, which has failed to show a clear organism emerging as the source of CP/CPPS (Badalyan, 2003; Hochreiter et al., 2000; Krieger et al., 2000; Leskinen et al., 2003; Riley et al., 1998; Shoskes and Shahed, 2000; Takahashi et al., 2003; Xiao et al., 2013). A newer technique involves using a specific set of primers that amplifies bacterial DNA, and then algorithms can match the resultant sequences to specific organisms. This technique can identify all bacterial species present at more than 1% to 3% of the biome (Ecker et al., 2008). Using this technique, Nickel et al. reported the only significant difference was found in the initial stream (VB1) samples, with the organism *Burkholderia cenocepacia* overrepresented in the CP/CPPS patients ($P = 0.002$) compared with controls (Nickel et al., 2015). This organism is an opportunistic pathogen in patients with cystic fibrosis and is known to be able to form biofilms (Fazli et al., 2014; Ganesan and Sajjan, 2011). Organisms of this genus have been described in acute prostatitis (Arzola et al., 2007). In an animal model, a strain of bacteria called CP1, isolated from a man with CP/CPPS, induced and sustained chronic pelvic pain that persisted after bacterial clearance from the genitourinary tract (Rudick et al., 2011). Thus possibly certain bacteria produce pelvic pain. Recent studies also have found alterations in the microbiome of men with CP/CPPS compared with controls. Men with CP/CPPS have increased diversity of bacteria in the urinary tract at the phylogenic level that exhibit more varied clustering than men without symptoms (Shoskes et al., 2016). A parallel study showed less diversity in the gut microbiome in the CP/CPPS patients compared with controls (Shoskes et al., 2016).

Inflammation

The term *prostatitis* implies inflammation of the prostate gland. However only about one-third of men with clinical CPPS have been found to have prostatic inflammation on biopsy (True et al., 1999). **In those with inflammation in VB3, EPS, or seminal plasma, the degree of inflammation does not correlate with symptoms** (Schaeffer et al., 2002a). Data looking at individual cytokines vary widely and are not conclusive. The possibility of an autoimmune response in some men is supported by reports that some men with CP/CPPS have an increased lymphoproliferative response to prostate antigens (Motrich et al., 2007) compared with controls. These include a region of the prostatic acid phosphatase molecule, PSA (Kouiavskaia et al., 2009), and human seminal vesicle secretory protein 2 (SVS2) (Hou et al., 2012). Levels of the chemokines monocyte chemoattractant protein-1 and macrophage inflammatory protein-1-α are significantly elevated in patients with CP/CPPS compared with those without urologic disease or BPH, and elevated MIP-1-α levels showed positive correlation with not only absolute NIH-CPSI scores, but with pain components of the NIH-CPSI as well (Desireddi et al., 2008). Levels of IL-17 are elevated in men with CP/CPPS and correlate with patient symptoms (Murphy et al., 2015).

Neurologic Causes

The cardinal symptom in CP/CPPS is pain, which is mediated through the nervous system. In addition to the increased self-report of neurologic disease in men with CP/CPPS compared with controls (Pontari et al., 2005), there is evidence for differences in the autonomic nerve function of men with CP/CPPS. **There is evidence for central sensitization in the afferent and efferent nervous system in men with CP/CPPS** (Yang et al., 2003; Yilmaz U et al., 2007). Central sensitization is characterized by continued nerve activity in the absence of stimulation or which requires a very low level of nociceptive stimulation to continue (Woolf, 1983). There are no differences in sensory perception thresholds in these patients, indicating that there is no peripheral neuropathy (Yilmaz et al., 2010). Changes in brain structure and function have been seen on neuroimaging. Farmer et al. (2011) studied spontaneous pelvic pain, with men lying in the fMRI scanner for 10 minutes and rating their fluctuations in brain activity in the absence of any external stimulus. Pain perception was localized to the anterior insula and correlated with the intensity of self-reported pain (Fig. 56.4). There were also differences in the relationship of gray and white matter in men with CPPS compared with controls (Farmer et al., 2011). The findings in men with CPPS differ from those in other pain conditions, including low back pain (Baliki et al., 2011). Other imaging studies have indicated UCCPS patients have lower white matter tract density in areas of perception, integration of sensory information

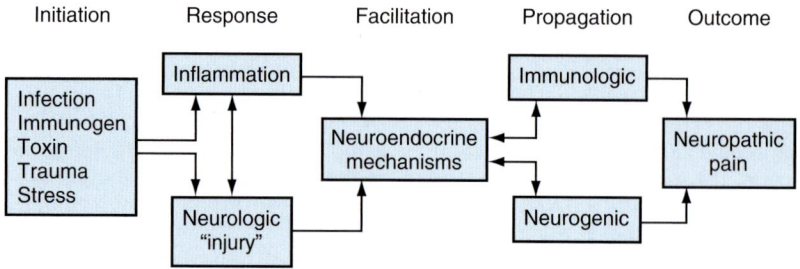

Fig. 56.3. Proposed cascade of initiation of chronic prostatitis and chronic pelvic pain syndrome (CPPS). Initial insult such as infection, immune response, toxin, trauma, or stress in genetically susceptible host leads to neurogenic inflammatory response. This is then facilitated and propagated by psychological, immune, neurologic, and endocrine mechanisms to produce the final outcome of the phenotype of CPPS.

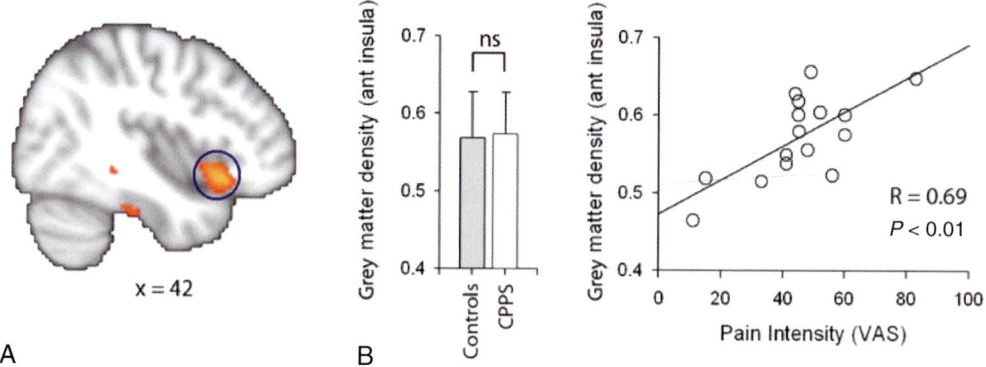

Fig. 56.4. Anterior insula activity is related to chronic prostatitis and chronic pelvic pain syndrome (CP/CPPS) pain intensity. (A) Peak activity from anterior insula *(blue circle)* identified from pain. The visual contrast shows significantly larger activity in pain task versus visual task *(bar graph)*, and shows significant positive relationship between activity and CP/CPPS pain intensity (each symbol is individual subject in scatterplot). (B) Correlation of peak activity from anterior insula with clinical parameters of CP/CPPS. In addition to spontaneous pain intensity MPQ exhibited significant correlation with insular activity. (From Farmer MA: Brain functional and anatomical changes in chronic prostatitis/chronic pelvic pain syndrome. *J Urol.* 186[1]:117–124, Fig 3.)

and pain modulation (Woodworth et al., 2015). Men with CP/CPPS have decreased connectivity between motor areas involved in pelvic floor control and the right posterior insula, an area involved in pain processing and sympathetic autonomic control. The greater pain was associated with less connectivity between the areas (Kutch et al., 2015).

Pelvic Floor Dysfunction

Neurologic abnormalities are postulated to also cause spasm in the pelvic floor. Patients with CP/CPPS have pathological tenderness of the striated pelvic floor muscle and poor to absent function in ability to relax the pelvic floor efficiently with a single or repetitive effort (Zermann et al., 1999). An electromyogram (EMG) study of the pelvic floor in these patients showed that compared with controls, men with CP/CPPS had (1) greater preliminary resting hypertonicity and instability and (2) lowered voluntary endurance contraction amplitude (Hetrick et al., 2006). A study by the CPCRN found that on physical examination, 14% of patients with CP/CPPS had tenderness of the internal pelvic floor, 13% had external pelvic floor tenderness, and neither was found in controls (Shoskes et al., 2008). On transabdominal ultrasound measurement of pelvic floor muscle mobility, compared with controls, men with CPPS have on average lower pelvic floor mobility resulting from increased tension (Khorasani et al., 2012).

Psychosocial Factors

Greater perceived stress is associated with greater pain intensity ($P = 0.03$) and disability ($P = 0.003$) in men with CP/CPPS (Ullrich et al., 2005). **Helplessness and catastrophizing predict overall pain along with urinary symptoms and depression** (Tripp et al., 2006). This was confirmed by a systematic review of 69 research articles looking at psychosocial influences (Riegel et al., 2014) that found an association of pain intensity with catastrophizing, perceived stress, and low satisfaction with relationships including sexual functioning. In the Boston Area Community Health (BACH) Survey, men who reported experiencing sexual, emotional, or physical abuse were at increased risk for symptoms of CP/CPPS (OR 1.7–3.3; Hu et al., 2007).

Endocrine Abnormalities

One of the common findings in chronic pain conditions is alterations of the hypothalamic-pituitary-adrenal axis; similar findings have been reported in CP/CPPS. On awakening, serum cortisol levels rise; there is a significantly greater cortisol rise in men with CPPS compared with controls. **Men with CPPS also have a lower baseline adrenocorticotropic hormone (ACTH) level and blunted ACTH rise in response to stress than men without symptoms** (Anderson et al., 2008).

Genetics

A twin study from the University of Washington compared self-reported lifetime physician diagnosis of CP/CPPS with so-called chronic overlapping pain conditions (COPC), including fibromyalgia, chronic fatigue syndrome, irritable bowel syndrome (IBS), temporomandibular disorder, tension headaches, and migraine headaches. Compared with their non-CP/CPPS twin, those with CP/CPPS were

6 to 30 times more likely to report a COPC. The conclusion is that familial factors, either shared environmental factors or genetic factors, play a large role in the relationship between CP/CPPS and COPC (Gasperi et al., 2017).

Biomarkers

There have been few biomarkers that correlate with symptoms in CP/CPPS. One of these markers is nerve growth factor (NGF), a neuropeptide that plays a role in nociception (Miller et al., 2002). NGF is reported to also decrease in men with CPPS who respond to treatment but not in those who do not respond (Watanabe et al., 2011). In the MAPP study, in men with UCCPS, pain severity was significantly positively associated with concentrations of matrix metallopeptidase 9 (MMP-9) and MMP-9/NGAL (neutrophil gelatinase-associated lipocalin) complex, and urinary severity was significantly positively associated with MMP-9, MMP-9/NGAL complex, and VEGF-R1 (vascular endothelial growth factor receptor 1) (Dagher et al., 2017). VEGF and MMP-9 are known to play a role in neuropathic pain (Ji et al., 2009; Selvaraj et al., 2015), although MMP/NGAL may be a marker of infection or inflammation (Chen et al., 2007).

Abnormal Sensory Processing

One of the hallmarks of patients with centralized chronic pain is generalized or global abnormality of sensory processing (Jensen et al., 2009; Kosek et al., 1996). In the MAPP study, this was tested using quantitative sensory testing (QST), in which a quantifiable pain stimulus, a computer-controlled pressure stimulus, is applied to the thumbnail. Patients with UCCPS (49% male) had significantly increased pain sensitivity compared with healthy controls (41% males). However, they were less sensitive to a mixed pain comparison group of patients with fibromyalgia, chronic fatigue syndrome, and irritable bowel syndrome (Clemens et al., 2018).

KEY POINTS

- Men with CP/CPPS have amounts of bacteria in urine, prostate fluid, and seminal plasma equal to that in men without pain.
- There is evidence of central sensitization of the central nervous system (CNS) in afferent and efferent nerves.
- In those with inflammation in VB3, EPS, or seminal plasma, the degree of inflammation does not correlate with symptoms.
- Helplessness and catastrophizing predict overall pain along with urinary symptoms and depression.
- Men with CPPS also have a lower baseline ACTH level and blunted ACTH rise in response to stress than men without symptoms.
- Men with CP/CPPS have increased pain sensitivity compared with controls.

Symptoms in Chronic Prostatitis and Chronic Pelvic Pain Syndrome

The symptom that distinguishes category III prostatitis CP/CPPS from other conditions such as BPH is pain. One of the early attempts to catalog the symptoms of CP/CPPS was an Internet survey by Alexander and Tressel that surveyed of 163 men with prostatitis and reported that the most frequently reported and most severe symptom was pain in the pelvic region, followed by urinary frequency and obstructive voiding symptoms. The most frequent site of pain was the perineum (Alexander and Trissel, 1996).

In 1999 the NIH set out to develop a symptom score that could be used as an outcome measure for clinical trials (Litwin et al., 1999). It also has proved useful to help categorize the symptoms of CPPS. The development included focus groups of patients judged to have CP/CPPS, generally pelvic pain in the absence of infection. The resulting index included three domains: pain, urinary symptoms, and quality of life. Pain domains include pain in the perineum, lower abdomen/suprapubic area, testes, penis, pain with ejaculation, and dysuria. The other two sections include voiding symptoms and interference/quality of life. It has been validated (Litwin, 2002), and the pain and quality of life subscales are sensitive to change (Propert et al., 2006).

Prevalence of Individual Symptoms in Men With Chronic Prostatitis and Chronic Pelvic Pain Syndrome

A large study of 1563 men with CP/CPPS in Europe and North America looked at symptoms reported on the NIH-CPSI (Wagenlehner et al., 2013). The mean NIH-CPSI score in the group was 20.4. The most common location of pain was in the perineum 63.3%, testicular 57.6%, tip of penis 32.4%, suprapubic area 42.3%, dysuria 43.3%, and pain with ejaculation 47.7%. Patients with dysuria were significantly more likely to have ejaculatory pain ($P < 0.001$). Patients with a greater number of pain locations also had greater severity of pain, voiding symptoms, and worse quality-of-life scores. Frequency and intensity of pain had the highest impact on overall quality of life; urinary symptoms did not correlate with changes in quality of life. Overall, using the total pain domain score as a measure, 32% had mild pain, 52% moderate pain, and 16% severe pain.

Summary of Findings From the Multidisciplinary Approach to Pelvic Pain Study

The NIH-sponsored MAPP study recruited men as part of a large phenotyping study. A large battery of urologic and psychological questions was administered. Some of the important findings to date are the following:

1. Patients who have pain beyond the pelvis have more severe symptoms than those with pelvic pain only.

   The MAPP project used a whole body map to record sites of pain (Lai et al., 2017). Forty-five sites are designated on the body map divided into seven zones. The severity of the nonpelvic pain increased with the number of regions reported. Patients with a greater number of pain sites also reported significantly greater sleep disturbance, depression and anxiety, psychological stress, somatic symptom burden, and negative affect. They also had more symptoms consistent with IBS, fibromyalgia, and migraine headaches.

2. Men with COPC have more severe symptoms than those with only urologic symptoms.

   In the MAPP study, 31% of men with pelvic pain enrolled have one or more of these so-called COPCs, the most common being IBS; patients with COPC also report more severe urologic symptoms and more frequent depression and anxiety compared with those without COPC (Krieger et al., 2015).

3. Patients with bladder-focused symptoms (bladder pain with filling and painful urgency) report more severe symptoms than those who do not have bladder symptoms.

   Of 191 men enrolled in the first MAPP study, 75% were found to have either painful urgency (i.e., urgency to urinate because of pain pressure or discomfort and not because of fear of leaking) or pain that was made worse with bladder filling (Lai et al., 2015). Compared with men with pelvic pain only, men with painful urgency or bladder pain had more flares and higher levels of catastrophizing and more frequently reported having IBS. They also had more severe symptoms of pain, frequency, and urgency. These symptoms are usually thought to be associated with interstitial cystitis/bladder pain syndrome, in which older studies have reported a 10:1 female-to-male ratio (Clemens, 2015; Hanno et al., 2011; Lai et al., 2015). In the RAND Interstitial Cystitis Epidemiology male study, there was a 17% overlap between men who met the high specificity IC/BPS definition and the case definition for CP/CPPS (Suskind et al., 2013). Thus there is considerable symptom overlap between CP/CPPS and IC/BPS as currently defined.

4. Pain and urinary symptoms should not be measured together as part of a composite score.

Principal components and exploratory factor analysis were used to examine questionnaire items that had been administered to participants in the MAPP study (Griffith et al., 2016). Exploratory factor analysis is used to identify a small number of factors that can explain a correlation matrix among a set of questionnaire items. The analysis suggested that two separate factors drove the correlations for the questionnaires, the first being pelvic pain and the second urinary symptoms. An association with depression was predicted by pain but not by urinary symptoms, indicating these symptoms vary in their impact on patients. The conclusion of this study was that it is important to assess pain and urinary symptoms separately rather than combined as in the present symptom questionnaires, the NIH-CPSI (Litwin et al., 1999) and the GUPI (Clemens et al., 2009). The implication for treatment trials is that if they used a combined score, as has been done for the majority of trials in CP/CPPS since 1999, then there may be significant effects on either pain or urinary symptoms that were not seen because the overall change in score was not clinically significant.

Fluctuations in Symptom Severity

In the MAPP study of 424 participants with urologic pelvic pain syndrome, of whom 191 were male, symptoms were assessed every 2 weeks for 1 year (Stephens-Shields et al., 2016). The percentage of patients who improved was 24.8% for pain symptoms and 15% for urinary symptoms. The percentages for those whose symptoms became worse were 9.4% for the pain and 6.1% for the urinary symptoms. Factors that were predictive of worsening symptoms at 1 year were the extent of widespread pain, the presence of nonurologic symptoms (COPC), and poorer overall health. Pain catastrophizing and self-reported stress were predictive of just worsening pain scores. There was no contribution of anxiety, depression, and general mental health to symptom worsening (Naliboff et al., 2017).

Significant exacerbations of symptoms have been termed *flares* (Sutcliffe et al., 2012). Many factors have been postulated to cause flares. In a case crossover study from the MAPP network, 79 reported no flare at baseline or at any time thereafter in the 1 year follow-up. In a group of 292 (69%) patients with at least one flare, 116 were men. Only recent sexual activity and UTI-like symptoms were predictive of flare. Issues that did not predict a flare included diet, physical activity or sedentary behavior, stress, and constipation (Sutcliffe et al., 2018).

Sexual Dysfunction

The prevalence of ED in men with CP/CPPS is reported at 15% to 40% (Tran and Shoskes, 2013). In addition, a case control study of a large Taiwanese health database showed that men with a diagnosis of ED were more likely to have been previously diagnosed with CP/CPPS, 8.6%, compared with 2.5% of randomly selected controls ($P < 0.001$) (Chung et al., 2012). Other symptoms of sexual dysfunction are ejaculatory dysfunction/pain and premature ejaculation. From the CPCRN cohort, 74% of the men had ejaculatory pain at some point (Shoskes et al., 2004). Similar levels of premature ejaculation have been reported (Tran and Shoskes, 2013).

Anxiety and Depression

In the original CPCRN cohort study, men with CP/CPPS were twice as likely to report anxiety and depression as age-matched controls (Pontari et al., 2005). Similar findings were reported in the subsequent MAPP study, as compared with age- and education-matched controls, males with pelvic pain showed greater levels of current and lifetime stress, poor illness coping, and increased self-report of cognitive deficits (Naliboff et al., 2015). A large database study from Taiwan found that men with CP/CPPS were significantly more likely to have a diagnosis of anxiety disorder than men without the diagnosis. The odds ratio (OR) was 2.10 (95% confidence interval [CI] 1.92–2.29, $P < 0.001$). The association held for all age groups and was particularly strong in men aged 40 to 59 years old in which the OR was 2.53 (Chung and Lin, 2013).

Association With Other Medical Diseases

Cardiovascular Disease. In the CPCRN study that compared cases with age-matched controls, men with CP/CPPS were six times more likely to self-report a history of cardiovascular disease, most commonly hypertension. A follow-up study by Shoskes et al. found greater arterial stiffness in men with CPPS compared with controls (Shoskes et al., 2011). The association of hypertension and CP/CPPS was also examined in the Health Professionals follow-up study, which found no association on multivariate analysis with hypertension overall, but there was in men with a BPH/LUTS history (OR 1.36) (Zhang et al., 2015). Other studies have been mixed, reporting no correlation for hypertension as part of metabolic syndrome in men with CP/CPPS (Wang et al., 2013) or a significantly higher rate of hypertension in men with CP/CPPS than controls (Chung and Lin, 2013).

Neurologic Disease. Men with CP/CPPS were 5 times more likely to self-report a history of nervous system disease compared with asymptomatic age-matched controls in the CPCRN study (Pontari et al., 2005). In the NIH cohort, the symptom that most contributed to the difference in neurologic disease was numbness and tingling in the limbs. Also significant was a history of vertebral disk disease/surgery. Migraine headaches were common in the cases, but they were not significantly different than controls.

Phenotypic Approach to Symptoms and Symptom Clustering: UPOINT

The phenotype of patients meeting the criteria for CP/CPPS is variable and can include multiple different types of symptoms. This has been well outlined by Shoskes et al. in the UPOINT classification (Shoskes et al., 2009). This includes the categories of urinary, psychosocial, organ-specific, infection, neurologic/systemic, and tenderness of skeletal muscle (Fig. 56.5). The impetus for the classification was in part the recognition of the failure of monotherapies in clinical trials in men with CP/CPPS (Nickel et al., 2004). With this classification, therapy can be targeted to specific domains of symptoms. The clinical description of the UPOINT classification includes several factors under each domain, and descriptions of the compilation of symptoms have been published (Nickel and Shoskes, 2010). The percentage of men who fall in to each domain has been strikingly similar across multiple studies; the largest domain has been organ-specific and urinary, and the smallest domain

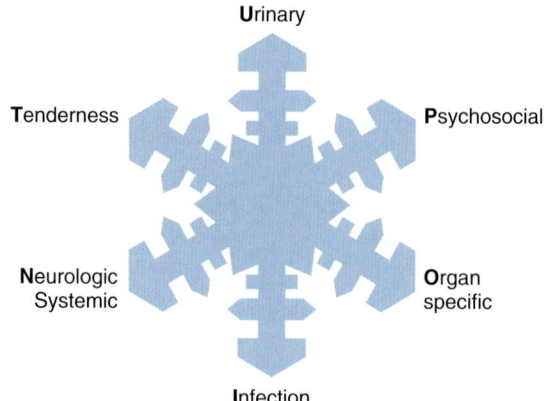

Fig. 56.5. The UPOINT classification has six clinically defined domains: urinary, psychological, organ-specific, infection, neurologic/systemic, and tenderness. Each individual patient has a unique phenotype, thus the idea of the "snowflake hypothesis." (Data from M. Pontari: *Common features and dissimilarities of urologic and other chronic pain syndromes: CP/CPPS, NIH meeting on phenotyping patients with pelvic pain*, Baltimore, MD, June 2008.)

has been the infectious category. Men with CP/CPPS generally are characterized by multiple domains. In an early description, only one in five men were positive for only one domain, one-third of men were characterized by two domains, and the rest by three or more domains (Shoskes et al., 2009). There is a strong correlation between the number of domains of UPOINT and severity of symptoms (Shoskes et al., 2009; Shoskes et al., 2010; Shoskes and Nickel, 2013).

Evaluation of Chronic Prostatitis and Chronic Pelvic Pain Syndrome

CP/CPPS is a diagnosis of exclusion, and the evaluation must rule out identifiable causes of pelvic pain. To meet the NIH consensus definition, patients should not have active urethritis, urogenital cancer, urinary tract disease, functionally significant urethral stricture, or neurologic disease affecting the bladder (Krieger et al., 1999). A list of inclusion and exclusion and deferral criteria for diagnosis of CP/CPPS that have been used in NIH studies and trials were published by the CPCRN research network (Schaeffer et al., 2002).

Many other medical problems may be present in men with CPPS. One challenge for the urologist is that these include areas outside of the usual scope of urology, including neurologic, immunologic, and psychological factors that influence the disease process.

Two recent guidelines from the UK Prostatitis Expert Reference group (Rees et al., 2015a) and the International Consultation on Urologic Disease (Nickel et al., 2013) have published a description and recommendations for evaluation. The recommendations of these reports are incorporated into this description of the evaluation of CP/CPPS.

History

Given the wide variety of possible causes of CP/CPPS, information on possible cause can be obtained by a detailed history of the circumstances at the onset. Patients with onset associated with significant stress or psychological trauma may be more likely to have pelvic floor dysfunction. A history of trauma could indicate problems based on neurologic damage or musculoskeletal abnormalities. Some patients seek medical attention after a urinary tract infection or STD and should be assessed for persistence of infection.

Assessment

Pain. The National Institutes of Health Chronic Prostatitis Symptom Index (NIH-CPSI) includes sections on pain including location, frequency and severity of pain, voiding symptoms, and interference/quality of life (Litwin et al., 1999). One limitation of the NIH-CPSI is that it does not have questions about pain thought to be related to the bladder. In the NIH-sponsored MAPP study, 42% of males enrolled at baseline met criteria for a diagnosis of IC/PBS (Krieger et al., 2015). A modification of the NIH-CPSI called the Genitourinary Pain Index (GUPI) (Fig. 56.6) contains two questions related to pain with bladder filling or emptying and better captures bladder symptoms (Clemens et al., 2009). The clinical importance is to remember to assess for symptoms of bladder pain in men with pelvic pain because this can prompt using bladder-specific treatments that are not useful in men with no bladder pain.

Other Urologic Symptoms
Voiding: The NIH-CPSI and GUPI list only two questions on voiding dysfunction. The AUA symptom index can be useful to assess these other voiding symptoms (Barry et al., 1992).
Sexual function: The history should include an assessment including a history of erectile dysfunction, libido, and ejaculatory problems. The Sexual Health Inventory for Men (SHIM) instrument can be used to quantify the erectile dysfunction-reference (Cappelleri and Rosen, 2005). This is a shortened version of the International Index of Erectile Function (IIEF) (Rosen et al., 2002).

Review of Symptoms

Neurologic: Given the prevalence of neurologic disease in men in the CPCRN cohort, patients should be evaluated for concomitant neurologic disease (Pontari et al., 2005). A complaint of back pain with numbness or pain radiating down the legs should suggest lumbar-sacral disk disease. A history of migraine headache should be obtained. Changes in vision in a young male could suggest multiple sclerosis. Sensitivity to auditory, visual, or olfactory stimuli could also indicate underlying neurologic disease (Geisser et al., 2008).
GI: Men with CP/CPPS are more likely to have IBS (Rodriguez et al., 2009). There is overlapping innervation of the bowel and bladder such that irritation of the colon in experimental models results in inflammation of the bladder (Christianson et al., 2007). Irritation of one organ in experimental models results in inflammation of the other (Pezzone et al., 2005). The evaluation therefore of men with CP/CPPS must assess problems such as constipation, diarrhea, and the relation of discomfort to bowel movements. In the MAPP study, 31% of men had an associated chronic overlapping pain condition, the vast majority of which were IBS (Krieger et al., 2015). Men with GI symptoms can benefit from referral to a gastroenterologist, preferably one experienced in treating IBS. Thus asking about symptoms of IBS such as constipation, diarrhea, or both is important to help direct the patient to a GI specialist for treatment.
Rheumatologic: Men with CP/CPPS are at higher risk for systemic chronic pain syndromes such as fibromyalgia and chronic fatigue syndrome, although not nearly as increased a risk as IBS (Krieger et al., 2015). Fibromyalgia manifests as pain in many areas of the body. Pain with significant fatigue may indicate chronic fatigue syndrome. These conditions should be further evaluated by a rheumatologist.
Psychological symptoms: There are no published criteria for the psychological evaluation of men with CP/CPPS. However, men should be queried about significant anxiety, depression, and symptoms of obsessive compulsive behavior. Given the association of panic attacks with thyroid disease and interstitial cystitis, an assessment for panic attacks can be helpful (Weissman et al., 2004). A questionnaire that may be useful is the pain catastrophizing scale (Osman et al., 1997). Guidelines from the UK (Rees et al., 2015a) suggest using the Patient Health Questionnaire-9 (PHQ-9) (Moriarty et al., 2015) or a shortened version called the PHQ-2 and/or the Generalized Anxiety Disorder Screener-7 (GAD-7) (Lowe et al., 2008). They also offer several simple questions for initial assessment:
Anxiety: In the past month, how often have you been bothered by feeling nervous, anxious, or on edge, or by not being able to stop or control worrying?
Depression: In the last month, how often have you been bothered by feeling down, depressed, or hopeless? Having little interest or pleasure in doing things?

Physical Examination

Neurologic examination: Screening examination for abnormalities
Abdominal examination: To look for other causes of abdominal and/or suprapubic pain
Genitourinary examination: An examination for hernia, hydrocele, testicular masses, penile lesions, or other findings of the genitalia should be performed. A rectal and prostate examination should be performed. Rectal masses or hemorrhoids should be assessed. On rectal examination the prostate is tender in less than half of men (Shoskes et al., 2008); severe tenderness suggests acute prostatitis. Nodularity should not be attributed to inflammation and should prompt a consideration of prostate cancer.
Muscle tenderness: During rectal examination, palpation of the muscles lateral to the prostate and extending to the coccyx can identify myofascial trigger points and identify patients that may benefit from pelvic floor physical therapy and relaxation techniques (Berger et al., 2007). During palpation of the pelvic floor, having the patient abduct the leg on either side can make it easier to examine the muscles. An extended genitourinary pelvic floor examination has been evaluated with the MAPP study and detected pelvic floor tenderness in 47% of men with CP/CPPS compared

Male Genitourinary Pain Index

1. In the last week, have you experienced any pain or discomfort in the following areas?

   a. Area between rectum and testicles (perineum)   ☐₁ Yes   ☐₀ No
   b. Testicles   ☐₁ Yes   ☐₀ No
   c. Tip of penis (not related to urination)   ☐₁ Yes   ☐₀ No
   d. Below your waist, in your pubic or bladder area   ☐₁ Yes   ☐₀ No

2. In the last week, have you experienced:

   a. Pain or burning during urination?   ☐₁ Yes   ☐₀ No
   b. Pain or discomfort during or after sexual climax (ejaculation)?   ☐₁ Yes   ☐₀ No
   c. Pain or discomfort as your bladder fills?   ☐₁ Yes   ☐₀ No
   d. Pain or discomfort relieved by voiding?   ☐₁ Yes   ☐₀ No

3. How often have you had pain or discomfort in any of these areas over the last week?

   ☐₀ Never   ☐₁ Rarely   ☐₂ Sometimes   ☐₃ Often   ☐₄ Usually   ☐₅ Always

4. Which number best describes your AVERAGE pain or discomfort on the days you had it, over the last week?

   ☐ 0   ☐ 1   ☐ 2   ☐ 3   ☐ 4   ☐ 5   ☐ 6   ☐ 7   ☐ 8   ☐ 9   ☐ 10

   No Pain   Pain as bad as you can imagine

5. How often have you had a sensation of not emptying your bladder completely after you finished urinating, over the last week?

   ☐₀ Not at all   ☐₁ Less than 1 time in 5   ☐₂ Less than half the time   ☐₃ About half the time   ☐₄ More than half the time   ☐₅ Almost always

6. How often have you had to urinate again less than two hours after you finished urinating, over the last week?

   ☐₀ Not at all   ☐₁ Less than 1 time in 5   ☐₂ Less than half the time   ☐₃ About half the time   ☐₄ More than half the time   ☐₅ Almost always

7. How often have your symptoms kept you from doing the kinds of things you would usually do, over the last week?

   ☐₀ None   ☐₁ Only a little   ☐₂ Some   ☐₃ A lot

8. How much did you think about your symptoms, over the last week?

   ☐₀ None   ☐₁ Only a little   ☐₂ Some   ☐₃ A lot

9. If you were to spend the rest of your life with your symptoms just the way they have been during the last week, how would you feel about that?

   ☐₀ Delighted
   ☐₁ Pleased
   ☐₂ Mostly satisfied
   ☐₃ Mixed (about equally satisfied and dissatisfied)
   ☐₄ Mostly dissatisfied
   ☐₅ Unhappy
   ☐₆ Terrible

Fig. 56.6. Genitourinary Problem Index (GUPI): Modification of the National Institutes of Health Chronic Prostatitis Symptom Index with addition of questions on bladder pain (with permission from Validation of a modified National Institutes of Health chronic prostatitis symptom index to assess genitourinary pain in men and women. (From Clemens JQ; Calhoun EA; Litwin MS; McNaughton-Collins M; Kusek JW; Crowley EM; Landis JR; Urologic Pelvic Pain Collaborative Research Network. *Urology*. 74[5]:983–987, quiz 987.e1-3, 2009 Nov.)

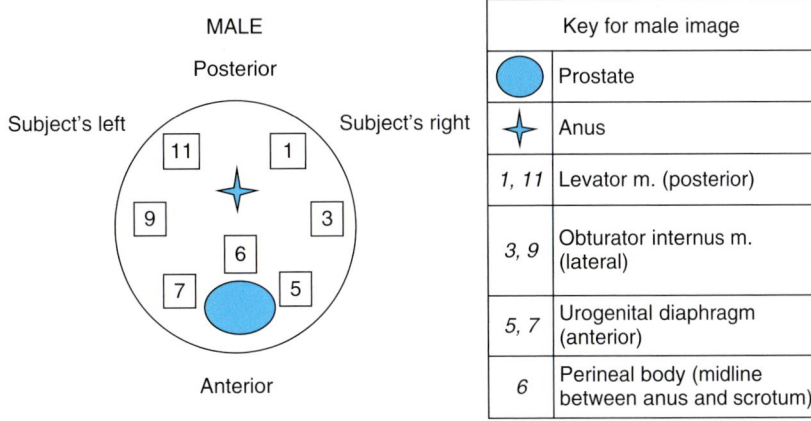

Fig. 56.7. Diagram for male pelvic muscle examination. Sites of palpation, performed through the rectum, with subject's anterior surface facing down relative to examiner. Numbers correspond to clock-face positions. (From Yang CC et al.: Physical examination for men and women with urological chronic pelvic pain syndromes: a MAPP network study. *Urology.* 116:23–29, 2018.)

with 6% of healthy controls. Prostatic tenderness was found in 22 of the cases and none of the controls (Yang et al., 2018). The importance of an extended examination is to maximize detection of pelvic floor tenderness, which can be amenable to pelvic floor physical therapy and targeted muscle relaxation treatments. The examination includes the perineal body, levator, obturator, and urogenital diaphragm muscles. The perineum was palpated midway between the anus and inferior edge of the scrotum. The pelvic floor muscles were palpated through the rectum: the urogenital diaphragm muscles were palpated anteriorly at the prostate apex; the obturator muscles were palpated anteriorly and laterally; the levator muscles were palpated posteriorly. The figure from the study is helpful as a roadmap to examination (Fig. 56.7).

Laboratory/Office Studies

Urinalysis: Men should have a urinalysis to look for unevaluated hematuria. A positive urine dip must be confirmed by finding 3 or more RBC per high-power field on a microscopic evaluation of the urine (Davis et al., 2012). Microscopy of the post-prostate massage urine (VB3) or expressed prostatic secretions have been used in the past to categorize men as category IIIA or IIIB; however, given the absence of clinical utility in making this distinction, this is not recommended.

Assessment for infection: A midstream urine sample for culture is recommended. If there is no documentation of culture results available, then a urinalysis and culture should be obtained at the time of symptom recurrence (Schaeffer, 2006). Optional in the UK guidelines but recommended by the International Consultation on Urological Diseases (ICUD) is the two-glass test, using the VB2 and VB3 specimens (Nickel et al., 2006). This is a standard diagnostic method in men with recurrent UTIs. Those men with a positive midstream urine culture, however, would be diagnosed with category II prostatitis, chronic bacterial and not category III CP/CPPS. The significance of a positive VB3 with a negative VB2 is unclear. This previously was considered to be a diagnosis of chronic bacterial prostatitis in older classification systems (Nickel and Moon, 2005). Asymptomatic men with no pelvic pain can be found to have positive localization cultures (Nickel et al., 2003). A positive VB3 has been used to classify as infectious in the UPOINT classification (Shoskes et al., 2009) and can be an indication for treatment with antibiotics (Shoskes et al., 2010).

Urine assessment for nontraditional organisms: It is not recommended to routinely send urine for culture for atypical organisms. However, in men who have a concomitant urethral discharge, nuclear amplification test should be performed for gonorrhea and chlamydia.

Semen cultures are not recommended.

Urine cytology: This is optional but indicated in men with irritative voiding symptoms such as frequency, dysuria, or hematuria. Carcinoma in situ of the bladder has been diagnosed in men presenting for evaluation of CP/CPPS, and hematuria is not always present (Nickel et al., 2002).

Postvoid residual: This should be checked by catheterization or ultrasound to rule out urinary retention as a cause of symptoms.

Blood tests: APSA test is not indicated. If, however, a PSA is measured and found to be elevated, the elevation should not be ascribed to CP/CPPS but should be further evaluated as in any patient (Nadler et al., 2006).

Imaging studies are optional and may be appropriate in some patients:

CT scan of abdomen and pelvis: Patients with concomitant abdominal pain may require imaging with CT to exclude an intra-abdominal process such as chronic appendicitis or diverticulitis.

Scrotal ultrasound: Testicular pain should be evaluated with a scrotal ultrasound.

Prostate ultrasound: Transrectal ultrasound has limited utility in men with CP/CPPS (Nickel et al., 2013).

MRI of lumbar and sacral spine: Patients with signs and symptoms of lumbar radiculopathy should be considered for MRI.

Uroflowmetry: This is an optional study in the evaluation of CP/CPPS. It may be helpful in a young male with complaints of decreased force of stream as an investigation into stricture disease.

Urodynamics and cystoscopy: Urodynamics are optional studies used in men with CPPS. They should be used in those who fail medical therapy and have significant voiding symptoms, decreased uroflowmetry, and or elevated postvoid residual urine (Hruz et al., 2003). In addition to bladder outlet obstruction, urodynamics can also diagnose men with pseudodyssynergy, which is retained electrical activity of the external sphincter during voiding in the absence of abdominal straining; brief and intermittent closing of the membranous urethra during voiding detected by electromyography; or fluoroscopy in videourodynamics (Gonzalez and Te, 2006). These men are considered to have pelvic floor dysfunction.

Cystoscopy can be used in men with decreased uroflow and/or elevated postvoid residual urine to evaluate for urethral stricture. Cystocopy should also be used in men who give a history of pain with bladder emptying and/or relieved by bladder emptying, suggestive of IC/BPS because in a small set of these patients a Hunner's ulcer is present, which responds to fulguration or intralesional injections (Gonzalez and Te, 2006; Hanno et al., 2011).

Prostate biopsy is not recommended for the diagnosis of CP/CPPS alone.

Clinical phenotyping tool: UPOINT

The phenotype of patients meeting the criteria for CPPS is variable and can include several different types of symptoms. This has been well outlined by Shoskes et al. in the UPOINT classification (Shoskes et al., 2009). This includes the categories of urinary, psychosocial, organ-specific, infection, neurologic/systemic, and tenderness of skeletal muscle. This classification is a convenient way to remember the assessment and is also available online. The UK guidelines (Rees et al., 2015a) and ICUD summary (Nickel et al., 2013) recommend the use of UPOINT (or equivalent) as a means to phenotype symptoms and ultimately aid in directing therapy.

An outline of recommended tests sorted into mandatory, recommended, and optional categories is provided in Box 56.1.

KEY POINTS

- CP/CPPS is a diagnosis of exclusion and should be made only after a thorough search for other causes of pelvic pain.
- CP/CPPS has potential issues outside of the pelvis (and usual scope of urology) such as psychological issues and neurologic problems.
- Patients with CP/CPPS must be assessed for other chronic pain syndrome such as irritable bowel syndrome, fibromyalgia, and chronic fatigue syndrome.
- Patients with tenderness on pelvis examination may benefit from pelvic floor physical therapy/myofascial release.
- Therapy for CPPS is best done in a multimodal fashion; the symptom classification UPOINT can be helpful in directing evaluation and subsequently therapy.

BOX 56.1 Evaluation for Men With Chronic Pain and Chronic Pelvic Pain Syndrome

MANDATORY

History
- Pelvic pain: pain in penis, testes, suprapubic area, perineum; pain with bladder filling and/or relieved by bladder emptying; pain with ejaculation, dysuria, voiding symptoms
- Review of symptoms
  - Neurologic problems: changes in vision, back pain, numbness in legs or pelvis/perineum, migraine
  - GI problems: constipation or diarrhea, pain relieved by bowel movement
  - Rheumatologic: excessive fatigue, pain in many areas throughout body
  - Psychological: significant anxiety, depression, history of traumatic experience, pain worse with stress

Physical Examination
- GU examination for hernia, hydrocele, penile lesions
- Prostate nodules or tenderness
- Pelvic floor examination
- Abdominal examination for other sources of pain

Laboratory Studies
- Urinalysis to rule out hematuria reflex to formal urinalysis
- Urine culture

RECOMMENDED
- Symptom inventory: Use NIH-CPSI or GUPI
- Sexual function assessment
- Two-glass urine VB2 and VB3
- Flow rate
- Urine cytology for dysuria or gross hematuria
- Bladder ultrasound for postvoid residual urine

NOT RECOMMENDED FOR INITIAL EVALUATION IN ALL PATIENTS; OPTIONAL IN SELECT PATIENTS
- Evaluation for STD with nuclear amplification (urine)
- Imaging studies
  - Scrotal US for testicular pain or lesions
  - CT of abdomen/pelvis for abdominal pain
  - Transrectal ultrasound
  - MRI of lumbar/sacral spine for symptoms suggestive of disk herniation
- Other
- Urodynamics/flow rate and cystoscopy: for refractory voiding symptoms, elevated residual urine volume
- PSA: for prostate cancer screening

GI, Gastrointestinal; *GU*, genitourinary; *GUPI*, Genitourinary Pain Index; *PSA*, prostate-specific antigen; *STD*, sexually transmitted disease; *US*, ultrasound; *VB2*, midstream urine; *VB3*, post-massage urine.

Treatment of Chronic Prostatitis and Chronic Pelvic Pain Syndrome

Pharmacologic Treatment

Antibiotic Treatment. Small, uncontrolled studies have lent credence to the efficacy of antibiotic therapy in ameliorating patients' symptoms, but large randomized, placebo-controlled studies have failed to consistently show meaningful benefit. Studies without a placebo control that have shown a benefit include 500 mg of tetracycline combined with a nutraceutical and an ethylenediaminetetraacetic acid suppository for 3 months (Shoskes et al., 2005); 90 days of therapy with 200 mg levofloxacin or 200 mg levofloxacin plus 0.2 mg of tamsulosin in a study of 105 men with CP/CPPS (Ye et al., 2008); 6 weeks of levofloxacin 100 mg twice daily and combination with doxazosin 4 mg at bedtime (Jeong et al., 2008); the combination of ciprofloxacin 500 mg twice daily plus tamsulosin 0.2 mg (Kim et al., 2008); and a 6-week course of levofloxacin 200 mg twice per day or in combination with terazosin 2 mg before sleep (Wang et al., 2016).

There are relatively few placebo-controlled studies of antibiotics in the treatment of CP/CPPS. Only one of these showed a benefit. A randomized trial of levofloxacin 500 mg daily in 80 men with a diagnosis consistent with CP/CPPS found that NIH-CPSI symptom scores were not significantly improved after 6 weeks of therapy (Nickel et al., 2003). An NIH-sponsored trial randomized men with CP/CPPS and an NIH-CPSI score of at least 15 to ciprofloxacin 500 mg twice daily or placebo. The trial found that NIH-CPSI symptom scores were not significantly improved after 6 weeks of therapy (change in symptom score from baseline −5.4 versus −3.9 with placebo); additional changes 6 weeks later were minimal (Alexander et al., 2004). A third trial that showed a benefit looked at tetracycline HCL 500 mg orally per day combined with 0.4 g/day of vitamin C and 0.2 g/day of co-vitamin B compared with vitamin B used as a placebo. The premise of the trial was that the antibiotic plus vitamins would be effective against nanobacterial infection (Zhou, 2008).

Several questions arise in the use of antibiotics in CP/CPPS. One is whether there is a difference based on duration of a patient's symptoms and/or prior antibiotic exposure. Trials of antibiotics in men with shorter duration of symptoms have shown greater symptom benefit (Nickel and Xiang, 2008) than those in men with longer duration of symptoms (Alexander et al., 2004). Another question with using antibiotics in men with a clinical diagnosis of CP/CPPS is why they would work in this group of patients in whom the diagnosis requires UTI to be excluded by definition. Several factors have been proposed. One is that antibiotics, especially fluoroquinolones, have anti-inflammatory properties. Ciprofloxacin decreases IL-6 and tumor necrosis factor-alpha (TNF-α) production in cell lines, animal models, and in semen and postmasturbation urine samples in men with CP/CPPS (Ogino et al., 2009; Stancik et al., 2008). Another factor could be the effect of antibiotics on bacteria that are localized to the prostate fluid (VB3 or EPS) but not resulting in a positive midstream urine culture. These men are currently classified as category III; in older classifications such as the 1978 classification of Drach et al. they would have been classified as category II or chronic bacterial prostatitis (Nickel and Moon, 2005).

Several meta-analysis and systemic review studies have been published on the treatment of men with CP/CPPS. The data indicated that the greatest decrease in symptom score was seen in the combination of antibiotics and alpha-blockers, with a decrease in total NIH-CPSI of 13.8 points compared with placebo (Anothaisintawee et al., 2011). A follow-up analysis by the same group included some of the studies that used a comparator but not a lone placebo and reached a similar conclusion (Thakkinstian et al., 2012). Another meta-analysis included only the two controlled trials using fluoroquinolone antibiotics (Alexander et al., 2004; Nickel et al., 2003) and concluded that antibiotics failed to show statistically significant or clinically significant reduction in NIH-CPSI scores (Cohen et al., 2012). A meta-analysis that included all the trials listed above use a random effects model to account for the heterogeneity of the studies and concluded that antibiotics are not effective in the treatment of CP/CPPS (Zhu et al., 2014).

Fluoroquinolones have been the most widely studies antibiotics for this condition. The rationale for their use is originally based on their spectrum of activity as well as their pharmacokinetic properties allowing for high prostatic concentration (Charalabopoulos et al., 2003a). In patients with fluoroquinolone-resistant bacteria, trimethoprim alone (TMP), or in combination with sulfamethoxazole can be used. Other second-line agents include tetracycline, doxycycline, and macrolides (Nickel and Moon, 2005; Perletti et al., 2013).

Summary of Treatment Recommendations. At the time of this writing, there were no AUA guidelines on the treatment of CP/CPPS. There are recommendations from the European Association of Urology (Engeler et al., 2013), which were antimicrobial therapy (quinolones or tetracyclines) over a minimum of 6 weeks in treatment-naïve patients with a duration of CPPS less than 1 year. The group convened by Prostate Cancer UK (Rees et al., 2015a) adds that a repeated course of antibiotic therapy (4 to 6 weeks) should be offered if a bacterial source is confirmed or if there is a partial response to the first course. Repeated courses of antibiotics in the absence of a positive urine culture is not accepted therapy.

Alpha-Blocker Treatment. Alpha-blockers have long been used for treating CP/CPPS. The rationale includes the idea that some cases of CP/CPPS come from dysfunctional voiding (Lee et al., 2007). The α receptors in the central nervous system have also been shown to be active in long-term pain syndromes (Teasell and Arnold, 2004). Earlier randomized trials of alpha-blockers in men with CP/CPPS showed positive results, including those that used the NIH-CPSI score and those that predated its use. These include studies of terazosin (Cheah et al., 2003; Gul et al., 2001), doxazosin (Evliyaoglu and Burgut, 2002; Tugcu et al., 2007), alfuzosin (Mehik et al., 2003), tamsulosin (Chen et al., 2011; Nickel et al., 2004), and silodosin (Nickel et al., 2011).

Two large NIH-sponsored trials failed to show a benefit for alpha-blockers. Alexander found no benefit with tamsulosin in men who were treated for 6 weeks compared with placebo (Alexander et al., 2004). Men in this study were not necessarily alpha-blocker naive. A study of alfuzosin in men with shorter duration of symptoms and who were alpha-blocker naive did not show any benefit compared with placebo after 12 weeks (Nickel et al., 2008). Several meta-analyses have been published examining the use of treatments including alpha-blockers to show that there is no benefit (Cohen et al., 2012) or likely a benefit to using alpha-blockers, and the best results were in combination with antibiotics (Anothaisintawee et al., 2011) or with antibiotics and anti-inflammatory medications (Thakkinstian et al., 2012). **The ICUD study recommends alpha-blockers for newly diagnosed, alpha-blocker–naive patients who have voiding symptoms** (Nickel et al., 2013). **The EAU guidelines recommend use of alpha-blockers for patients with a duration of PPS less than 1 year** (Engeler et al., 2013).

Anti-Inflammatory Therapy. The term *prostatitis* implies inflammation although only one-third of men with symptoms of CP/CPPS have inflammation on prostate biopsy (True et al., 1999). A randomized placebo trial of a cyclooxygenase (COX)-2 inhibitor, rofecoxib, which is no longer available because of cardiac side effects, showed the total and subscale NIH-CPSI scores significantly decreased from baseline in all groups, and no statistically significant difference was found. Patient global assessment of pain, a secondary outcome, favored rofecoxib over placebo (Nickel et al., 2003). A study of another COX-2 inhibitor, celecoxib, in a study of men with IIIA prostatitis showed significant reduction in total NIH-CPSI score, pain, and quality-of-life subscores, but not the urinary subscore (Zhao et al., 2009).

Other forms of anti-inflammatory medication have been tried. A small trial of 17 patients compared a leukotriene inhibitor, zafirlukast, to placebo in a study in which all patients also received doxycycline and found no difference (Goldmeier et al., 2005). A trial similar in size compared placebo with a 4-week course of prednisone with a dose reduction from 20 mg to 5 mg once per day over a 4-week period. No significant change in symptom scores was seen (Bates et al., 2007). A different approach to anti-inflammatory treatment was investigated in an observational study of beclomethasone dipropionate suppositories, a rectal form of corticosteroid. Clinically significant improvement in pain and voiding symptoms were seen in 162 of the 180 patients. No significant adverse effects were reported (Bozzini et al., 2016).

Results from meta-analyses indicate that anti-inflammatory medications are considered to have beneficial effects for some patients (Thakkinstian et al., 2012). They are likely ineffective if used alone but useful in combination therapy with an alpha-blocker and a muscle relaxant that also has anti-inflammatory properties (Cohen et al., 2012). The pooled RR for studies of anti-inflammatory medications for CP/CPPS was 1.8 (95% CI 1.2–2.6) compared with placebo (Anothaisintawee et al., 2011). **In conclusion, anti-inflammatory monotherapy is not recommended but can be used as part of multimodal therapy** (Nickel et al., 2013), **but long-term side effects have to be considered** (Engeler et al., 2013).

Reductase Inhibitors. A significant improvement with finasteride compared with placebo in the Prostatitis Symptom Severity Scale, a precursor to the NIH-CPSI, but not in pain was seen demonstrated in a small 12-month pilot study from Finland (Leskinen et al., 1999). A 6-month trial comparing finasteride with placebo in patients with category IIIA (defined as any inflammation in the EPS or VB3 specimen) at 4 academic centers showed improvement in symptoms compared with placebo but did not reach statistical significance (Nickel JC et al., 2004). Dutasteride at 0.5 mg was studied in the REDUCE trial, a 4-year, randomized, double-blind, placebo-controlled study of prostate cancer risk reduction. The NIH-CPSI survey was used to measure baseline and change in symptom severity. After 48 months, the dutasteride group noted a significant decrease of 6 points or greater in CPSI total score compared with placebo (49% vs. 37%, $P = 0.0033$) (Nickel et al., 2011).

Overall, 5α-reductase inhibitor (5ARI) medications appear to be effective in some patients. This is demonstrated when the previous trials are subjected to a meta-analysis, with significant reduction in NIH-CPSI scores compared with placebo (−4.6, 95% CI −8.7 to −0.5) (Anothaisintawee et al., 2011). The decision in whom to use 5ARI medications must also be made in the context of side effects, including reduced volume of ejaculate, erectile dysfunction, and decrease in libido (Thompson et al., 2003). This indicates that they may be best used in older patients with CP/CPPS who also have voiding symptoms from BPH (Rees et al., 2015a).

Medications for Neuropathic Pain. Given the data to support a possible neuropathic basis for CP/CPPS, it is logical that medications used to treat neuropathic pain are commonly used for treatment. A randomized placebo-controlled trial of the anticonvulsant pregabalin in men with CPPS showed an effect that approached significance but did not reach the primary endpoint ($P = 0.07$) (Pontari et al., 2010). However, several secondary endpoints were significantly improved. This suggests that in a subset of men with CPPS, pregabalin may be effective (Berger, 2011). Patients with suspected neuropathic pain are commonly started on tricyclic antidepressants. Non–placebo-controlled studies have shown a beneficial effect of duloxetine when combined with tamsulosin and saw palmetto (Giannantoni et al., 2014) or with the alpha-blocker doxazosin (Zhang et al., 2017). Amitriptyline has been widely used in women with interstitial cystitis, but data in men with CPPS are lacking. In the IC/PBS studies, a better response was seen if the dose was increased up to 50 mg (Foster et al., 2010).

A phase IIa proof of concept clinical trial using tenazumab, a monoclonal antibody against nerve growth factor, in men with CPPS showed at week 6 there was marginal improvement in average daily pain and urgency frequency compared with placebo, with no difference in overall NIH-CPSI score (Nickel et al., 2012). A trial of an inhibitor of fatty acid amide hydrolase (FAAH), a synaptic membrane enzyme responsible for the breakdown of endogenous cannabinoids (eCBs), showed no improvement in pain reduction compared with placebo. However, there was greater improvement in voiding frequency compared with placebo in all groups tested (Wagenlehner et al., 2017).

Phototherapy. Wagenlehner et al. compared treatment with the pollen extract Cernilton for 12 weeks to placebo and found significant improvement in total NIH-CPSI scores, as well as pain and quality-of-life domains (Wagenlehner et al., 2009). Similar results in a controlled trial were reported using another pollen extract product for 6 months, showing significant reduction in pain, voiding symptoms, and sexual function in the treatment group (Elist, 2006). The mechanism of action of pollen extract is unknown but is thought to induce smooth muscle relaxation and anti-inflammatory effects (Wagenlehner et al., 2011). Quercetin, a plant-derived bioflavonoid, showed a significant improvement in symptoms after 4 weeks compared with placebo in a small trial and also has been used in IC/PBS (Shoskes et al., 1999).

Bladder Specific: Pentosan Polysulfate. Pentosan polysulfate (PPS) is a medication used to treat symptoms of interstitial cystitis, thought to work by augmenting the bladder's layer of glycosaminoglycans, which acts as a protective barrier. Use of PPS in men with CP/CPPS has shown modest improvement compared with placebo, with no significant changes in Clinical Global Improvement (CGI) scores but significant improvement in the NIH-CPSI quality-of-life scores (Nickel et al., 2005). It is recommended by the EAU guidelines but with a strength rating of weak (Engeler et al., 2013). For men with painful bladder filling relieved by emptying, consideration should be made to use treatments outlined in the AUA guidelines for treating interstitial cystitis (Hanno et al., 2011).

Other Medications

Allopurinol. It was theorized that the intraprostatic ductal reflux of urine increases the concentration of metabolites containing purine and pyrimidine bases in the prostatic ducts, causing inflammation (Persson and Ronquist, 1996). Therefore allopurinol was compared with placebo in a randomized, double-blind controlled study in 54 men. The allopurinol groups had lower levels of serum urate, urine urate, and EPS urate and xanthine (Persson et al., 1996). However, re-review of the data and statistical methods showed that the changes in the urine and prostatic secretion of purine and pyrimidine bases resulted in significant amelioration of symptoms (Nickel et al., 1996). A follow-up randomized clinical trial further showed no advantage of allopurinol compared with placebo (Ziaee et al., 2006).

Mepartricin. This is a mediation that reduces serum estrogen levels and prostatic estrogen receptors in animal models. One small trial indicated beneficial effects on total NIH-CPSI scores in men with CP/CPPS (De Rose et al., 2004).

PDE5 Inhibitors. PDE5 inhibitors are useful to treat erectile dysfunction in men with CPPS at any age. Tadalafil can treat lower urinary tract symptoms, erectile dysfunction, and possibly the symptoms of CP/CPPS (Grimsley et al., 2007; Oelke et al., 2012). This may be of benefit in men with concomitant erectile dysfunction.

Other Treatments for Chronic Prostatitis and Chronic Pelvic Pain Syndrome

Conservative

Lifestyle Changes: Diet and Exercise. In a survey of 62 patients with CPPS, 47% reported having sensitivity to some foods. The most common were spicy foods, coffee, tea, chili, and alcoholic beverages. Items that improved symptoms included docusate, psyllium (dietary fiber), water, herbal teas, and polycarbophil (fiber laxative) (Herati and Moldwin, 2013). There are no specific dietary recommendations for all patients with CP/CPPS, and they should be individualized based on the patient's food sensitivities. A study in men with CPPS demonstrated significant improvement in pain scores, quality of life, and overall NIH-CPSI scores in men in an aerobic exercise group compared with placebo/stretching after 18 weeks (Giubilei et al., 2007).

Stress Management/Psychological Treatments. Of 134 men with chronic prostatitis treated with stress reduction alone, 110 (86%) reported that they were better, much better, or "cured" (Miller, 1988). Options for our patients with these psychological factors include traditional therapy with a psychologist or psychiatrist. A feasibility trial of cognitive therapy showed significant reduction in pain, disability, and catastrophizing in a small cohort of patients who completed an 8-week program (Tripp et al., 2011). Although not yet widely available, these types of program provide a promising future method of treatment, including using these treatments via the Internet (Perry et al., 2017).

Acupuncture. The mechanism of the improvement in CPPS symptoms after acupuncture is unknown but can be postulated to have an ameliorating effect on neuropathic pain. Acupuncture for CP/CPPS is typically performed using 4 to 6 needle points (Herati and Moldwin, 2013). Controlled trials using sham needles placed at sites away from the true acupuncture sites have also shown a significant improvement over sham including increase in β-endorphin and leucine encephalin levels (Lee et al., 2011). The use of electrical stimulation in addition to needle placement has been used and shown to be superior to sham and advice and exercise alone in men with CPPS (Lee and Lee, 2009). A systematic review of trials of acupuncture in the treatment of CPPS identified 9 clinical trials involving 890 patients that met criteria for inclusion and concluded that the evidence for the efficacy of acupuncture for treating CPPS was encouraging, but the quantity and quality of the available evidence precluded making firm conclusions in favor of acupuncture (Posadzki et al., 2012). In clinical practice, given the relatively few side effects of acupuncture, it can be suggested to individuals who do not respond to first-line medical therapy or to those who would prefer to not take medications for their discomfort.

Minimally Invasive Therapies

Pelvic Floor Physical Therapy and Skeletal Muscle Relaxants. Studies of noninvasive techniques to treat pelvic floor dysfunction include biofeedback and pelvic floor retraining, or learning to selectively contract and then relax the pelvic muscles. Reports of small series of this technique have shown significant improvement (Clemens et al., 2000; Cornel et al., 2005; Nadler, 2002). Results of pretreatment urodynamics and sphincter EMG were not predictive of outcomes (Clemens et al., 2000). Biofeedback and pelvic floor therapy are also effective in patients who have pseudodyssynergy on urodynamics (Kaplan et al., 1997).

A series of uncontrolled studies from Stanford have reproducibly shown a benefit to combining myofascial trigger point release and paradoxic relaxation training, essentially biofeedback training (Anderson et al., 2005). In addition to pain and urinary symptoms, improvements in sexual function including ejaculatory pain, decreased libido, or erectile dysfunction are also noted (Anderson et al., 2005; Anderson et al., 2006). A shorter 6-day course of myofascial release and trigger point manipulation has been described and produced a 6-point or greater decrease in total NIH-CPSI score at 6 months in 70 of 116 patients (60%) completing the course (Anderson et al., 2011).

One of the difficulties in assessing the effects of pelvic floor physical therapy (PT) is how to control the study. A study from the NIH-sponsored Urological Pelvic Pain Collaborative Research Network (UPPCRN) group showed the feasibility of using global massage as a control for patients undergoing myofascial physical therapy (Fitzgerald et al., 2013). Although not powered or designed to be a definitive outcome study, patients undergoing myofascial therapy had a significantly greater response on global assessment response than the therapeutic massage group, 57% to 21% (P = 0.03). **Referral to a physical therapist who is familiar with pelvic floor PT techniques, if possible, is recommended as the improvement after pelvic floor PT appears to be better after therapy received from specialized centers** (Polackwich et al., 2015b).

Adjuncts to Pelvic Floor Physical Therapy. For refractory cases of pelvic floor spasm, needling of the area, either as dry needling or with the injection of local anesthesia, can be used (Moldwin and Fariello, 2013). The use of perineal injection of *Botulinum* toxin has also been reported to relax tender muscle/trigger points (Gottsch et al., 2011). Other described methods to relax the pelvic floor include the use of extracorporeal shock wave therapy (ESWT). Early studies appeared promising (Zimmermann et al., 2008; Zimmermann et al., 2009), but a study looking at long-term results of ESWT in CP/CPPS patients demonstrated no benefit compared with sham control at 24 weeks as a follow-up to the same patient cohort that showed significant results at 12 weeks (Moayedinia et al., 2014).

Prostate Massage. Prostate massage may help break up areas of ductal obstruction and help with flow and antibiotic penetrance into the prostate. Given the transrectal approach, it could also potentially have some effect on the pelvic floor. Uncontrolled studies (Nickel et al., 1999; Shoskes and Zeitlin, 1999) found clinical benefits in one-third to two-thirds of patients treated with repetitive prostatic massage (2 to 3 times per week) for 4 to 6 weeks along with antibiotic therapy. Other studies did not show a benefit when combined with antibiotics, in patients with either category II or III prostatitis (Ateya et al., 2006). **A subsequent systematic review of the literature concluded that evidence for a role of repetitive prostatic massage as an adjunct in the management of CP is, at most, "soft" but that the practice could be considered as part of multimodal therapy in selected patients** (Mishra et al., 2008).

Circumcision. A study looked at the additive effect of circumcision to a regimen of antibiotic, anti-inflammatory, and alpha-blocker medications. A control group received medication only. A total of 774 men were randomized, and 713 completed the trial. At the end of 3 months, the percentage of men in each group with at least a 4-point drop in the NIH-CPSI score was 84.6% in the circumcision group and 68.5% in the control group (P < 0.001). Significant changes were seen in all three domains of the NIH-CPSI compared with the control group (P < 0.001) (Zhao et al., 2015). These data must be replicated, and the therapy is obviously limited to men who are not already circumcised but present an interesting adjunct to therapy.

Prostate-Specific Treatments

Local Hyperthermia and Needle Ablation. In a series of 105 patients, those treated with transrectal radiofrequency hyperthermia with or without antibiotics for 6 weeks had a significant improvement in the domains of the NIH-CPSI compared with patients treated with antibiotics alone (Gao et al., 2012). Older studies have used microwave thermotherapy for CP/CPPS (Kastner et al., 2004; Michielsen et al., 1995; Suzuki et al., 1995). Few controlled trials are reported. Nickel and Sorensen reported that, at 3 months' follow-up, the transurethral microwave thermotherapy–treated patients had significantly improved symptom scores compared with sham-treated patients; 7 of 10 men treated with transurethral microwave thermotherapy had a favorable result compared with 1 of 10 men treated with a sham therapy (Nickel and Sorensen, 1996). Thermotherapy is not currently recommended for CP/CPPS but could be used in men with concomitant BPH. Transurethral need ablation (TUNA) has been used in men with CP/CPPS with mixed results (Chiang and Chiang, 2004; Chiang et al., 1997; Leskinen et al., 2002) and is not recommended for treatment.

Intraprostatic Injection of Onabotulinumtoxin A. Recent studies have reported on intraprostatic injection of onabotulinumtoxin A (Botox). This has been used in the past for BPH. One small, uncontrolled study indicated that Botox worked better via a transrectal route than transurethral and in smaller glands (El-enen et al., 2015). Two controlled studies used the transurethral route. At a dose of 100 to 200 U there was significant benefit to the Botox injection compared with saline (Falahatkar et al., 2015) or cystoscopy without injection (Abdel-Maguid et al., 2018). Side effects included exacerbation of dysuria in almost half of patients, hematuria in 3% to 17%, and hematospermia in 7% to 14% (El-enen et al., 2015; Falahatkar et al., 2015).

Surgical Therapy for Chronic Prostatitis and Chronic Pelvic Pain Syndrome

Surgical Therapy for Bladder Neck Hypertrophy. Based on the possibility of centralization and lack of evidence of the prostate as a primary pain source in men with CPPS, transurethral resection is not expected to improve pain. One entity that may be important in a subset of patients is bladder neck hypertrophy. There are no pathognomonic diagnostic criteria. This should be suspected in men with chronic pelvic pain who also have significant obstructive voiding symptoms. Pressure flow urodynamics are expected to show increased voiding pressure and decreased flow, with a relative narrowing of the bladder neck (Hruz et al., 2003). It is important to rule out pseudodyssynergy, which would show inappropriate relaxation of the external urethral sphincter on EMG (Huckabay and Nitti, 2005). Te and Kaplan reported significant improvement in 31 of 32 men with bladder neck hypertrophy and symptoms of chronic prostatitis treated with bladder neck incision (Kaplan et al., 1994).

Neurostimulation. Sacral nerve stimulation (SNS) and percutaneous tibial nerve stimulation (PTNS) are FDA approved for urinary symptoms but not specifically for pelvic pain. Most studies have looked at SNS in patients with interstitial cystitis/bladder pain syndrome and are case series. The implantation rate after test stimulation (>50% reduction in symptoms) ranges from 56% to 68%; of those implanted and followed for up to 5 years, 64% to 72% can achieve a durable, significant improvement (Yang, 2013). In a study of 89 patients with CP/CPPS randomized to PTNS or sham, there was significant reduction in pain, urgency, and NIH-CPSI score in the treatment group compared with the sham at 12 weeks (Kabay et al., 2009). An open trial of transcutaneous electrical nerve stimulation (TENS) was successful after 12 weeks of treatment in 29 (48%) patients, and a positive effect was sustained during a mean follow-up of 43.6 months in 21 patients (Schneider et al., 2013). At this time, it appears reasonable to offer PTNS as therapy in patients with CPPS and SNS in those with pelvic pain who also have urinary frequency and urgency.

Electromagnetic Stimulation. In an open-label trial of electromagnetic stimulation, patients sat on a chair with electromagnetic energy for 30 minutes twice weekly for 6 weeks; 22 of 37 men demonstrated a greater than 6-point drop in NIH-CPSI compared with baseline at 24 weeks. Mean total and pain subscales were significantly improved at 24 weeks compared with baseline. International Prostate Symptom Score (IPSS) scores were also significantly improved compared with baseline (Kim et al., 2013). A previous study by Rowe showed a significant improvement in mean symptoms scores at 3 months and 1 year compared with the sham control group (P < 0.05) at 1 year (Rowe et al., 2005).

Cystoscopy and Fulguration of Hunner's Ulcer. Men with pain thought to be of bladder origin (i.e., pain with bladder filling and/or relieved by bladder emptying) should have a cystoscopy to look for a Hunner ulcer. Although not commonly found, fulguration of these areas can provide symptom relief (Gonzalez and Te, 2006; Hanno et al., 2011).

Not Recommended: Radical Prostatectomy. Not recommended is surgical removal of painful structures in the setting of pain elsewhere in the pelvis. Certainly **radical prostatectomy is not recommended in the absence of treatment for prostate carcinoma** (McLoughlin et al., 2014). A concern for pain relief is the possibility of neural centralization and that the prostate is not the isolated source of pain in these patients

Cochrane Review of Nonpharmacological Interventions for Treating Chronic Prostatitis and Chronic Pelvic Pain Syndrome

A 2018 Cochrane Database review examined the evidence for acupuncture, circumcision, electromagnetic chair, lifestyle modifications, physical activity, prostate massage, extracorporeal shockwave lithotripsy, and transrectal thermotherapy (compared with medical therapy). They did not find adequate information on psychological therapy or prostatic surgery. Their conclusion was that "some of the interventions can decrease prostatitis symptoms in an appreciable number without a greater incidence of adverse events. The quality of evidence was mostly low." They encouraged future clinical trials with more detailed report of the methods, including sample size, masking, and outcomes including adverse events (Franco et al., 2018).

Treatment: Summary and Approach

A significant limitation to treatment of CP/CPPS is that there are no positive clinical trials for monotherapy in men with CP/CPPS (Nickel et al., 2013). Certainly therapy should start with the most conservative treatments possible, including lifestyle changes. Further therapy is best directed at simultaneous multimodal therapy based on the patient's individual phenotype (Shoskes et al., 2010). The UPOINT classification offers a convenient framework in which to plan treatment(s) and is recommended in current guidelines for treatment by the EAU (Engeler et al., 2013) and ICUD (Nickel et al., 2013). Finally, many if not most patients need to see more than one type of specialist. This often involves neurology, gastroenterology, psychiatry/psychology, physical medicine, and rehabilitation in addition to urology. Referral to a pain clinic, especially one with a multimodal approach may also be helpful (Baranowski et al., 2013). A referral to pain management specialists is also recommended if a patient requires the use of opioids.

> **KEY POINTS**
> - Repeated courses of antibiotics in the absence of a positive urine culture are not indicated.
> - The best treatment combination from meta-analyses is antibiotics plus alpha-blockers.
> - Men with bladder pain should be considered for bladder-specific therapies.
> - Men with tenderness on pelvic floor examination should be referred for pelvic floor physical therapy.
> - Sacral neuromodulation can be used in men with pain who also have frequency and urgency.
> - Treatment is best undertaken as simultaneous multimodal therapy addressing all aspects of the patients symptoms.

ACUTE AND CHRONIC ORCHITIS AND ORCHIALGIA
Acute Orchitis

The incidence of acute orchitis is not known. In a recent review of 669 cases of acute scrotum in an emergency room over a 10-month period, patients were diagnosed with orchitis in 10.3% of cases and orchid-epididymitis in 28.7%; isolated epididymitis was diagnosed in 28.4% of the patients. The mean age of those in the orchitis group was 44.6 years old and for those in the orchidoepididymitis group, the mean age was 46.5 years old (Lorenzo et al., 2016).

Etiology

Acute orchitis can be divided into specific orchitis and viral orchitis. Specific orchitis can be caused by a wide variety of infectious diseases including by a hematogenous route. In a large series examining evaluation of the acute scrotum, men with orchitis and epidymo-orchitis over the age of 35 most commonly have bacterial infection with predominantly gram-negative bacteria, *E. coli* and *Pseudomonas*, similar to the distribution of age and infection in acute epididymitis (Kaver et al., 1990). Other reported infectious agents include *Treponema pallidum* (Chu et al., 2016), *M. tuberculosis* (Yadav et al., 2017), and many others that are not common in the United States, including *Brucella* (Savasci et al., 2014) and *Filariasis* spp. (Richens, 2004). Candiduria can lead to epididymoorchitis (Kauffman et al., 2011).

Viral orchitis is most commonly caused by the mumps virus (Ludwig, 2008). Despite vaccination that almost eliminated this disease by 2001, sporadic outbreaks have occurred since, involving a high percentage of persons with a history of vaccination (Cortese et al., 2011; Dayan and Rubin, 2008). The usual clinical scenario in Mumps is a prodrome of headache, malaise, and myalgias followed by parotitis developing 2 to 3 weeks after exposure and lasting for 2 or 3 days (Rubin et al., 2015). Orchitis is usually associated with epididymitis and fever, resolving within 1 week. Atrophy of the testis occurs in half the cases and can be associated with oligospermia and decreased fertility but usually not complete infertility (Dejucq and Jegou, 2001). Another virus that is associated with orchitis is the human immunodeficiency virus type 1 (HIV-1). This is the result of direct infection of the virus in the testis and as a consequence of immunosuppression from the infection (De Paepe et al., 1989). Orchitis is a symptom of infectious mononucleosis, indicating that the Epstein-Barr virus may have a direct effect on the testes (Cheung et al., 1993; Dejucq and Jegou, 2001). HSV-2 has been detected in the testes (DeTure et al., 1976). Many other viruses have been reported to infect the testes including dengue, smallpox, and chickenpox (Riggs and Sanford, 1962).

Autoimmune orchitis is defined as an autoimmune aggression of the testes characterized by the presence of anti-sperm antibodies (ASA). Conditions that produce symptomatic orchitis are classified as secondary autoimmune orchitis, as opposed to primary autoimmune orchitis, which is characterized by the presence of ASA, no associated systemic disease, and they are asymptomatic (Silva et al., 2014). Primary autoimmune orchitis is primarily a problem in the evaluation of male infertility. The main causes of secondary autoimmune orchitis are usually associated with a primary vasculitis, particularly Behçet's disease, polyarteritis nodosa, and Schönlein-Henloch purpura (Pannek and Haupt, 1997). The testis is an immune-privileged site, but in autoimmune orchitis the blood testis barrier is altered by a T cell–mediated inflammatory response with an increased production of proinflammatory cytokines such as IFN-g, IL-1, IL-6, IL-12, IL-17, and IL-23 and the resultant production of anti-sperm antibodies (Jacobo et al., 2011a; Jacobo et al., 2011b).

Evaluation

Medical history should include circumstances of onset, including sexual history, recent instrumentation or surgery, and prior episodes. A history of trauma should be elicited. The duration of pain is important given that one of the prime differential diagnoses is testicular torsion. A history of symptoms of upper respiratory symptoms and/or parotitis consistent with mumps should be established. Fever, sweats, headache, and back pain are common in infection with brucellosis (Street et al., 2017). Inquiry should also be made about a history of the multiple conditions that can cause secondary autoimmune orchitis. Physical examination should include assessment for signs of systemic involvement including fever and tachycardia. Examination of the scrotum usually reveals a tender testis and spermatic cord.

Urine culture should be obtained in all patients. Urine culture has been reported to be positive in 38.5% of patients diagnosed with isolated orchitis and 37.5% of those diagnosed with orchido-epididymitis (Lorenzo et al., 2016). In sexually active patients, especially with epididymal involvement, testing for STD should be performed. Imaging with scrotal US can help to distinguish testicular torsion from orchitis and identify testicular tumors and abscess (Altinkilic et al., 2013).

Treatment

In patients with signs of infectious orchitis, antibiotics to treat gram-negative uropathogens should be started and treatment adjusted based on the result of urine culture. In patients with suspicion of STD, especially younger patients with concomitant epididymitis, treatment for STD should be started (Centers for Disease Control and Prevention, 2015). Mumps orchitis can be treated by interferon but does not always prevent testicular atrophy (Ku et al., 1999). Secondary autoimmune orchitis may be treated with systemic medications, including corticosteroids, immunosuppressive medications such as azathioprine, or IV cyclophosphamide, and intravenous immunoglobulin (Silva et al., 2014). In men with HIV, treatment requires initial antibiotic treatment followed by a period of maintenance suppression, particularly if salmonella is identified as the causative organism (Shindel et al., 2011). Patients with orchitis need to be followed up, especially those whose symptoms do not resolve to rule out missed torsion or testicular tumor. Patients should also be counseled that, although the acute pain can resolve in 1 to 3 days, the ensuing inflammation can last 2 to 4 weeks before completely resolving (Trojian et al., 2009).

Chronic Scrotal Pain Syndrome: Orchialgia

Orchialgia is defined as scrotal pain, intermittent or constant, lasting at least 3 months, and can be unilateral or bilateral (Kavoussi and Costabile, 2013). **One of the first considerations in assessing orchialgia is to determine if the pain is limited to the testis/scrotum or if it is part of a larger pelvic pain problem including other pain sites consistent with CP/CPPS** (Clemens JQ et al., 2009; Litwin et al., 1999).

Epidemiology

In Europe, orchialgia accounts for 2.5% to 4.8% of clinic visits (Ciftci et al., 2010; Strebel et al., 2005). The prevalence in the United States is not known, but Zermann et al. reported in one series that almost 40% of chronic pelvic pain localizes to the scrotum (1999). Approximately 100,000 cases per year are estimated in the United States. The breakdown of known causes reported are 6% to 12% after vasectomy, 18% after inguinal hernia repair, up to 5% after scrotal surgery, and 1% to 2% after abdominal or groin surgery (Parekattil et al., 2013). The most common age for presentation is 20 to 30 years old (Calixte et al., 2017).

Cause of Chronic Orchialgia

There are multiple identifiable causes of chronic scrotal pain. Short-term scrotal pain, which lasts a few weeks, can occur in 30% of men undergoing a vasectomy, whereas developing into long-term chronic pain that causes men to seek treatment is reported in anywhere from 1 in 1000 men (up to 15%) (Kavoussi and Costabile, 2013; Tandon and Sabanegh, 2008). Other causes include iatrogenic injury after hernia repair in up to 14% of cases or laparoscopic surgery, and inguinal hernia repair in 18% of patients, with a greater risk in patients who undergo surgery for a recurrent hernia or in which mesh was used (Dickinson et al., 2008; Massaron et al., 2007). Orchialgia can also occur after varicocele or varicocele surgery, referred pain from a mid or distal ureteral stone, indirect hernia, aortic or iliac artery aneurysm, trauma, and/or perineural fibrosis (Sigalos and Pastuszak, 2017). Another more recent finding has been that of pelvic floor dysfunction. In a series of men with chronic orchialgia, 93% had at least one symptom of pelvic floor dysfunction, and 88% were found to have increased resting pelvic floor muscle tone (Planken et al., 2010). Approximately 18% to 25% of chronic orchialgia is considered idiopathic (Quallich and Arslanian-Engoren, 2013).

The importance of alterations in nerve function may be very important in the pathophysiology and subsequent management of chronic orchialgia. Parekattil et al. (2013) reported on the finding of Wallerian degeneration (WD) on nerve biopsy in a significantly greater proportion of patients with pain (84%) than controls (20%) ($P = 0.0008$). Also, the degeneration appeared to be in reproducible patterns, involving the cremasteric muscle layer, perivasal tissues, and posterior periarterial/lipotamous tissues, the so-called "trifecta nerve complex." WD is a well-coordinated response of a nerve to injury, including proliferation of Schwann cells, changes in the local extracellular matrix, and recruitment of neurotrophin and cytokines, to facilitate axonal regeneration (Dubovy, 2011). The subsequent neuroinflammation can also lead to neuropathic pain. However, because 20% of the asymptomatic control group also had degeneration, this is not always the case (Parekattil et al., 2013). Staining with calcitonin gene-related peptide (CGRP), which is a marker of sensory nociceptors (Greco et al., 2008), has found increased levels of CGRP-positive nerves in spermatic cords of patients with pain compared with those with no testicular pain (Oka et al., 2016).

Granulomatous orchitis is marked by the presence of granulomatous inflammation in the testis and has multiple causes, including tuberculosis, brucellosis, actinomycosis, syphilis, leprosy, and sarcoidosis (Akinci et al., 2006; Roy et al., 2011). Idiopathic granulomatous orchitis is a rare inflammatory condition of unknown cause characterized by nonspecific granulomatous inflammation with multinucleated giants cells without caseation (Roy et al., 2011). Diagnosis is usually made after orchiectomy for suspected malignancy as the presentation is similar on ultrasound. Patients may have chronic pain but may also present with painless testicular enlargement (Dhand and Casalino, 2011). Just as has been described in the prostate, IG4-related inflammation has emerged as the cause of scrotal content pain, affecting the testis cells (de Buy Wenniger et al., 2013) and perivasal tissue-causing fibrosis (Najari et al., 2014). IG4-positive cells have also been reported in specimens of idiopathic granulomatous orchitis in men with no history of systemic IG4 disease (Karram et al., 2014). Another inflammatory condition that can cause orchitis is malakoplakia. The distinction from granulomatous orchitis is a dense infiltrate of histiocytes, and pathognomonic Michaelis-Gutmann bodies (Roy et al., 2011).

Evaluation

The diagnosis is directed at ruling out the other causes of chronic orchalgia. A history should evaluate for signs and symptoms of intermittent torsion and for infection with history of prior testicular or epididymal infection. On review of systems, the presence of symptoms of bowel dysfunction with constipation or diarrhea that may be indicative of IBS should be asked (Ciftci et al., 2010). Also important are symptoms of lower back pain and vertebral disk disease, because orchalgia can be referred pain from back problems (Rowell and Rylander, 2012). LUTS could indicate a history of voiding dysfunction, which could lead to UTIs. Cui and Terlecki reported that on screening for low testosterone or B12 levels in men with chronic orchialgia, 125 of 154 were found to be deficient in either or both compounds (Cui and Terlecki, 2016). A thorough examination of the genitalia including testes, epididymis, prostate, and pelvic floor is mandatory. Inguinal hernias should be ruled out. Laboratory studies include a urinalysis. **A duplex Doppler ultrasound should be performed to assess for anatomic or congenital abnormality, or mass** (Costabile et al., 1991b). If a ureteral stone is suspected, a CT scan can be performed.

Therapy for Idiopathic Orchialgia and Chronic Scrotal Pain Syndrome

Medical Therapies. Much like CP/CPPS, antibiotics are commonly used but rarely indicated (Strebel et al., 2005). Doxycycline and quinolones are recommended because of their penetration into the scrotal structures and because they can be used for up to 4 weeks (Levine, 2010). Anti-inflammatory medications are commonly used for the analgesic effects. There is little supporting evidence however for a specific therapeutic target (Starke and Costible, 2017). Given that CSPS is a chronic pain condition, medications used for neuropathic pain are prescribed. These include tricyclic antidepressants and gabapentin (Costabile et al., 1991a).

Spermatic Cord Block. When the initial evaluation does not show a discrete treatable cause and conservative medical management does not improve symptoms, a reasonable next step is spermatic cord block with bupivacaine. If positive, this can help confirm the diagnosis of orchialgia (Sigalos and Pastuszak, 2017). It may also help predict if spermatic cord denervation will be effective as a treatment. In a series of 74 patients, a positive response to a spermatic cord block with more than 50% temporary reduction in pain was an independent predictor of pain response to microsurgical denervation of the spermatic cord (MDSC) (Benson et al., 2013).

Surgical therapy: see the following for nonpharmacologic treatment of chronic scrotal pain.

Acute and Chronic Epididymitis (Epididymalgia)

Acute Epididymitis. Acute epididymitis is defined as pain, swelling, and inflammation of the epididymis that lasts more than 6 weeks. Epididymitis is a common condition. The incidence rates range from 25 to 65 per 10,000 person years and accounts for up to 600,000 cases per year in the outpatient setting in the United States (Cek et al., 2017). The average age of acute epididymitis is variable and affects pediatric and adult populations.

Etiology. The widely accepted route of infection is the ascent of microorganisms from the urethra, as reported by Campbell in 1927 in cases of gonococcal urethritis and subsequent epididymitis (Centers for Disease Control and Prevention, 2015). This was confirmed in later studies that compared isolates from the urine/urethra and simultaneously epididymitis and identified concurrence between the areas of approximately 80% (Berger et al., 1987; Doble et al., 1989a; Melekos and Asbach, 1987).

The causative organisms depend on the age of the patient. The classic teaching has been that men over the age of 35, as well as in children, the organisms are similar to those causing a urinary tract infection, such as *E. coli*. In men under 35 who are sexually active, *Chlamydia trachomatis* and *Neisseria gonorrhoeae* are more common (Holmes et al., 1979). Risk factors in the older men without sexually transmitted epididymitis include history of prostate infections or UTIs, recent surgical intervention in the urinary tract, bladder outlet obstruction such as BPH or stricture, uncircumcised penis or congenital deformity of the urinary tract, and immunosuppression (Ryan et al., 2018).

An updated examination of the causes of epididymitis was recently undertaken by a German group, using updated diagnostic methods for bacteria and viruses (Pilatz et al., 2015). A bacterial pathogen was found in 130/150 patients (87%), the most common was *Escherichia* (56%). The most common sexually transmitted infection was *Chlamydia* followed by *Mycoplasma* and *N. gonorrhoeae*. The sexual history did not always match the diagnosis, and men under 35 had enteric organisms in 42% of cases. **The conclusions from this very well-executed study are the following:**

1. **The age cutoffs of younger than 35 for a sexually transmitted infection (STI) as cause of acute epididymitis and older than age 35 to have an enteric bacterial pathogen are not strict rules.**
2. **A sexual history suggests that STI is not predictive of STI and that men with STI may not have a convincing history. Therefore all sexually active men with acute epididymitis should be screened for an STI.**
3. **Viruses were not a significant contributing factor to acute epididymitis, and mumps were not detected.**
4. **13% of cases still had no identifiable microbial cause.**

Clinical Evaluation. The signs and symptoms of acute epididymitis include pain and swelling. Swelling usually starts at the cauda of the epididymis and then ascends to reach the rest of the epididymis and then to the testis. Presentation is unilateral in 96% of cases (Cek et al., 2017). In the large series of Pilatz et al., 26% of patients presented with a fever defined as greater than 38°C, whereas 6.7% presented with an epididymal abscess (Pilatz et al., 2015). Dysuria is reported in one-third of patients (Kaver et al., 1990; Pearson et al., 1988).

Medical history should include circumstances of onset, including sexual history, recent instrumentation or surgery, and prior episodes. Physical examination should include assessment for signs of systemic involvement, including fever and tachycardia. Examination of the scrotum usually reveals a tender epididymis and spermatic cord. Induration of the cauda or whole epididymis is frequently present, and orchitis is noted in half of cases (Kaver et al., 1990).

Diagnostic evaluation should include laboratory studies to assess for white blood cell count, urine for routine urine culture and susceptibility, assessment of inflammation by leukocyte esterase on first-void urine or microscopic examination of sediment from a spun first-void urine (Centers for Disease Control and Prevention, 2015). In older men with acute epididymitis, an assessment of postvoid residual urine should be made to rule out urinary retention as a cause of UTI and subsequent epididymitis.

The differential diagnosis of acute scrotal pain such as seen with acute epididymitis includes testicular torsion, torsion of the appendix testis, inguinal hernia, testicular carcinoma, pain from varicocele, scrotal or testicular abscess, acute orchitis, and/or testicular trauma (Cek et al., 2017). Imaging studies include scrotal ultrasound. Common ultrasound features include hydrocele, epididymal enlargement, hyperperfusion, and testicular involvement (Pilatz et al., 2013). This is an important tool to confirm the diagnosis and to rule out testicular torsion as a cause of the acute scrotal pain (Altinkilic et al., 2013).

Treatment. For symptom relief, the traditional recommendations are bed rest, elevation of the scrotum, and local cooling. Nonsteroidal anti-inflammatory medications can also be useful. Most patients can be managed on an outpatient basis, but those with elevated white blood cell counts and fever should likely be admitted. Antimicrobial therapy depends on the most likely pathogen. The CDC guidelines divide this into three groups: acute epididymitis likely caused by STD, likely caused by STD and enteric organism (men who practice insertive anal sex), and likely only caused by enteric organisms. For the first group, the recommendation is ceftriaxone 250 mg in single IM dose plus doxycycline 100 mg orally twice per day for 10 days; for the second group levofloxacin 500 mg PO daily (or ofloxacin 300 mg PO twice per day) for 10 days is substituted for doxycycline, and for the third group levofloxacin (or ofloxacin) alone is recommended. Men with confirmed chlamydia or gonorrhea should also be tested for other STDs including HIV, and their sex partners should also be referred for evaluation and presumptive treatment (Centers for Disease Control and Prevention, 2015).

Follow-Up. It is recommended that men whose symptoms do not resolve within 72 hours be re-evaluated. Follow-up ultrasound may be needed in patients who are not clinically responding to rule out progression of an infection to an abscess or testicular infarction, which would require surgical treatment. Close follow-up of urine cultures for susceptibility is also important given the increasing rates of fluoroquinolone-resistant bacteria (Ryan et al., 2018).

Chronic Epididymitis. The definition of chronic epididymitis is similar to that for orchalgia (i.e., symptoms of discomfort and/or pain for at least 3 months' duration), localized to 1 or both epididymis (Nickel et al., 2002). In a survey of Canadian urologists over a 2-week period, of 6037 male patients seen, 57 or 0.9% had chronic epididymitis with a mean duration of 2.5 years and an average age of 41.1 years (Nickel et al., 2002).

Etiology. Nickel et al. recommended a classification of chronic epididymitis as being one of three categories: inflammatory, postobstructive, and chronic epididymyalgia, implying no clear cause (Nickel et al., 2002). Causes in the inflammatory group include infective from chlamydia, postinfective after acute bacterial epididymitis, granulomatous from tuberculosis, drug-induced from amiodarone, and idiopathic inflammatory. Patients with AIDS are also prone to develop tuberculous epididymitis (Heyns et al., 2009). The postobstructive group includes pain associated with congenital, acquired, or iatrogenic obstruction, such as postinfective or postsurgical, including postvasectomy.

Evaluation. Medical history should include any history of treatment for acute epididymitis. A Chronic Epididymitis Symptom Index has been published (Nickel et al., 2002). In the Canadian classification of epididymitis, the inflammatory chronic epididymitis is associated with abnormal swelling or induration. The obstructive may have induration, and in the idiopathic group or epididymalgia, the epididymis is palpably normal (Nickel et al., 2002). Patients may also experience testicular pain. Specific to tuberculous epididymitis, the onset is described as subacute, with swelling of the epididymis that may not be painful. Systemic signs of TB, along with scrotal thickening and a characteristic fistula, may be present. A scrotal mass may be present. Although TB often commonly involves the testis, the epididymis is solely infected in 45% of cases (Yadav et al., 2017). Laboratory tests include a urinalysis and midstream urine for culture. Patients with a urethral discharge should be evaluated with testing for an STD. Imaging studies including scrotal ultrasound are helpful to look for epididymal and testicular tumors. Patients should be assessed for neurologic problems that contribute to the pain, especially back pain indicating disk disease (Calixte et al., 2018).

Treatment. Conservative measures are recommended to start. Ruling out a malignancy allows for counseling the patient on the benign nature of the condition and observation if symptoms are mild. Scrotal support and warm compresses may be beneficial. Medical treatments lack evidence-based studies. Many types of medications have been used including antibiotics, anti-inflammatories, phytotherapy, and anxiolytics (Cek et al., 2017). Approximately one-quarter of patients receive pain medications (Nickel, 2003).

Tubercular Epididymitis

The EAU has published guidelines for the treatment of genitourinary TB (Kulchavenya et al., 2016). Medical treatment is with anti-TB regimens of antibiotics. The usual regimen is 4 anti-TB drugs simultaneously for a minimum of 6 months. Five different regimens of chemotherapy are used depending on the form of urogenital TB. Surgery to drain an abscess may be needed, or removal of a chronically infected epididymis or testis may be necessary. All surgical procedures should be performed while on anti-TB medications. The treatment duration is then judged based on the histology of the removed tissue. **An indication for surgery is failure of a scrotal mass to respond or increases in size after 3 weeks of antitubercular chemotherapy; the mass should be explored by an inguinal incision to rule out testicular or epididymal malignancy** (Cek et al., 2005).

Nonmedical Therapy for Chronic Scrotal Pain: Chronic Orchitis (Orchalgia) and Chronic Epididymitis (Epididymalgia)

Minimally Invasive Treatments

Pelvic Floor Physical Therapy. Given the results of a study of 41 men with chronic testicular pain showing increased resting pelvic floor tone (Planken et al., 2010), **pelvic floor PT should be considered in men with orchlgia and abnormal tone on digital rectal examination.** A series of 30 patients with chronic orchalgia treated with pelvic floor physical therapy reported that after 12 sessions, pain improved in 50% of men, and complete resolution of pain occurred in 13% (Farrell et al., 2016).

Botox. Local cord denervation with onabotulinumtoxin A (Botox) has been used for chronic scrotal pain. Khambatil et al. reported on 18 patients with chronic scrotal pain with a cord injection of Botox. All patients had experienced temporary relief from a cord block of 0.5% Marcaine and 2% xylocaine. One hundred units of Botox were injected 1 to 2 cm distal to the external ring, targeting the branches of the genitofemoral and ilioinguinal nerves. At 1 month follow-up pain was reduced in 72% of patients, and at 3 months in 56%. Most men had return of pain and tenderness by 6 months (Khambati et al., 2014).

Pulsed Radiofrequency of the Spermatic Cord. Pulsed radiofrequency has been performed for chronic back pain and sciatica, as well as for chronic visceral pelvic pain. Five patients with chronic scrotal pain (one bilateral) who responded to local anesthetic cord block were treated with pulsed radiofrequency (PRF) denervation of the spermatic cord. The treatment time was 3 minutes at 42 °C. At a mean follow-up of 25 weeks, the mean visual analog scores for pain decreased from 9 to 1. No complications such as testicular atrophy or decreased sensation of the scrotal or penile skin were reported (Basal et al., 2012). There are no long-term results available with this technique.

Nonradical Surgical Treatments

Neuromodulation

A sacral nerve stimulation trial that entered the caudal epidural space resulted in an 80% decrease in pain at 4 months in a male with recurrent epididymitis (McJunkin et al., 2009). Although the stimulator works on the S2-S4 area, the result with the testis was attributed to recent re-evaluation of dermatomes that reports that dermatomes are larger than described in most textbooks (Lee et al., 2008) and that based on cadaver studies, 25% of pudendal nerves receive a contribution from S1 (Shafik et al., 1995). Spinal cord stimulation in the epidural space to the level of T10 and T11 has been reported to help chronic scrotal pain (Nouri and Brish, 2011) as has cutaneous stimulation of the cutaneous branch of the ilioinguinal and genital branch of the genitofemoral nerves (Rosendal et al., 2013).

Surgical Therapy

Surgical Therapy for Orchalgia in Patients With Identifiable Intrascrotal Lesions

Patients can present with pain that appears to be localized to specific lesions (i.e., a varicocele or spermatocele). Patients can also have surgery for intermittent torsion. The results of surgery for pain resulting from hydrocelectomy, spermatocelectomy, and orchidopexy for intermittent torsion are reported as 100%, 94%, and 89%, respectively (Gray et al., 2001). The most common surgery for a specific target is spermatic vein ligation for treatment of a painful varicocele with a complete resolution rate of 85% by primary microsurgical and 72% for nonmicrosurgical repair; for laparoscopic repair the mean complete resolution rate is 81% with a recurrence rate of 6.8% (Shridharani et al., 2012). Percutaneous embolization can be effective for painful varicocele, but recurrence rates are generally higher than for microsurgical repair. The rate of success for microsurgical repair as a salvage procedure for recurrent or persistent varicocele after varicocelectomy has been reported at 90% (Chawla et al., 2005). Predictors of response to varicocelectomy include greater number of veins ligated (>7), greater preoperative pain score (>6), and longer duration of pain (>9 months) (Chen, 2012).

Vasovasostomy or Vasoepididymostomy for Treatment of Postvasectomy Pain

An option unique to patients with postvasectomy pain syndrome is to reverse the vasectomy and restore patency of the vas. Complete response rates are 34% to 50%, and overall improvement is 82% to 93% (Horovitz et al., 2012; Lee et al., 2014; Myers et al., 1997; Nangia et al., 2000; Polackwich et al., 2015a). A 20% reoperation rate from 1 to 9 years was reported by Polackwich et al. (2015a). Pain relief may take 3 months or more after the procedure, an important point in counseling patients and managing expectations (Horovitz et al., 2012). Given the relatively minimal morbidity, this is an attractive option for patients who have persistent long-term pain after vasectomy in the absence of other identifiable causes.

Microsurgical Denervation of the Spermatic Cord

Microsurgical denervation of the spermatic cord (MDSC) was first described by Devine and Schellhammer in two patients in 1978 (Devine and Schellhammer, 1978). This procedure involves transecting the nerves in the spermatic cord, while preserving the blood supply and lymphatics to prevent formation of a hydrocele (Tan and Levine, 2016). The internal spermatic veins are ligated, and the cremaster muscle and spermatic cord fascia are preserved (Strom and Levine, 2008). **Three areas identified by Parekatil et al. that had the highest areas of WD were the cremasteric muscle fibers, the perivasal sheath, and the posterior lipomatous tissue; these areas were called the trifecta nerve complex, which is thought to form the anatomic basis for relief from the denervation procedure** (Parekattil et al.,

2013). This approach has led to a more targeted MDSC approach in which the inner spermatic sheath is completely spared and only 5% to 10% of the spermatic cord is ligated, minimizing risk to the testicular and vasal arteries. A biowrap is also placed around the cord to minimize scarring and neuroma formation (Calixte et al., 2018).

Numerous studies on the efficacy of MDSC have been published (Benson et al., 2013; Larsen et al., 2013; Oomen et al., 2014; Parekattil et al., 2013; Strom and Levine, 2008) and report cure rates of 50% to 70%. By far the largest series is from Calixte et al., who report on 860 cases of robot-assisted microsurgical denervation. At a median follow-up of 24 months, complete resolution of pain was achieved by 49% of their patients, and 34% had a greater than 50% reduction in pain. The improvement in pain continued to progress with higher rates reported at 4 years than 6 months postoperatively (Calixte et al., 2018). Two studies have reported on specifically the results in men with postvasectomy pain syndrome, one from 1997 in which 13 of 17 reported complete relief of pain at the first follow-up visit and the other 4 had improvement (Ahmed et al., 1997). A much more recent report of overall success was achieved in 20/27 units. Patients with involvement of multiple structures in the scrotum (i.e., testis, epididymis, spermatic cord) had a success rate of 81% and were more likely to have a successful surgery ($P < 0.001$) (Tan et al., 2018). Men who have had a prior attempt at surgical repair at pain relief respond in a similar fashion to men who have not had any prior attempts at surgical therapy for chronic scrotal pain (Larsen et al., 2013; Tan et al., 2018).

Positive response to spermatic cord block predicts success with MSDC. The amount of pain relief obtained after cord block correlates with pain relief after undergoing MSDC, and those with a good response are likely to have durable and complete resolution of their pain (Benson et al., 2013). Some men may experience more pain relief with MSDC than cord block. The recommendation by Jonas et al. is to consider MSDC in men who have at least a 50% reduction in pain on spermatic cord block with 20 mL of 0.25% bupivacaine injected at the level of the pubic tubercle (Benson et al., 2013). Discussion of the risks and benefits are important because although the majority of results are good and there are few reported complications, one of those complications is testicular atrophy (Strom and Levine, 2008).

Epididymectomy for Chronic Pain

In the series of Davis of 10 patients who underwent epididymectomy, only 1 had significant pain relief and 9 subsequently underwent subsequent orchiectomy as definitive treatment (Davis et al., 1990). However, other series have reported better results. These range from 32% cure rate (Sweeney et al., 2008) up to 100% (Selikowitz and Schned, 1985). Most series report complete improvement in 50% to 75% of patients and improvement in another 15% to 21% (Chen and Ball, 1991; Hori et al., 2009; Lee et al., 2014; Padmore et al., 1996; Siu et al., 2007). Results are better in patients with a palpable area of tenderness, area of abnormality on ultrasound, or a cyst (Calleary et al., 2009; Padmore et al., 1996). Results for specifically postvasectomy pain are mixed and range from 12% to 80% cure rates (Hori et al., 2009; Lee et al., 2011; Lee et al., 2014; Siu et al., 2007; Sweeney et al., 2008). **Better rates are reported in cases with incorporation of the distal portion of the vasectomy site with the epididymectomy specimen** (Hori et al., 2009). This removes perineural inflammation, sperm extravasation, and fibrosis that may contribute to ongoing pain (Nariculam et al., 2007a). The rate for progression to orchiectomy after epididymectomy resulting from persistent pain is reported at 22% (Sweeney et al., 2008) up to 90% (Davis et al., 1990).

Orchiectomy for Chronic Scrotal Pain

The results for orchiectomy for chronic scrotal pain vary from 0 to 75% pain relief and partial improvement in 20% to 43% (Costabile et al., 1991b; Davis et al., 1990; Nariculam et al., 2007b; Yamamoto et al., 1995). Better results for an inguinal approach were noted by Davis than using a scrotal approach, 75% versus 55% complete response (Davis et al., 1990). In 17 patients after inguinal hernia repair, 65% were pain free at an average follow-up of 7 years. Of these, 6 patients were operated on for testicular ischemia. Patients operated on for nociceptive pain resulting from testicular injury such as ischemia have a better response than those operated for neuropathic pain from testicular nerve injury (Ronka et al., 2015).

Orchiectomy performed for persistent pain an average of 13.8 months after microsurgical resulted in a complete pain response in 70% and 30% still on pain medications. Men with bilateral scrotal content pain were at higher risk to develop pain after MDSC (Lipscomb and Williams IV, 2016). Although orchiectomy may be considered the last resort for treatment of scrotal pain, pain may persist, called a phantom pain (Puhse et al., 2010). Treatment of pain that persists after orchiectomy is handled in a manner similar to that described for treating persistent testicular pain after inguinal hernia repair. The genital branch of the genitofemoral nerve at the external ring is identified and neuroma is resected, and the proximal end of the nerve is placed in the pelvis. This has resulted in excellent relief in 8 out of 10 men treated for residual pain after prior orchiectomy at a mean of 17.5 months' follow-up. The remaining two men reported a good result (Dellon et al., 2014).

An algorithm for the progression of surgical therapy in men with chronic scrotal pain is shown in Fig. 56.8.

> **KEY POINTS**
>
> - Viral orchitis is most commonly caused by the mumps virus.
> - For scrotal pain a duplex Doppler ultrasound should be performed to assess for anatomic or congenital abnormality, torsion, or mass.
> - Pelvic floor physical therapy should be considered in men with orchalgia and abnormal tone on digital rectal examination.
> - Acute epididymitis is more commonly caused by an STD in men younger than 35 and enteric organism in men older than 35.
> - For MDSC, three areas that should be addressed are the cremasteric muscle fibers, the perivasal sheath, and the posterior lipomatous tissue.
> - The distal vas deferens should be incorporated into the surgical specimen during an epididymectomy for postvasectomy pain syndrome.

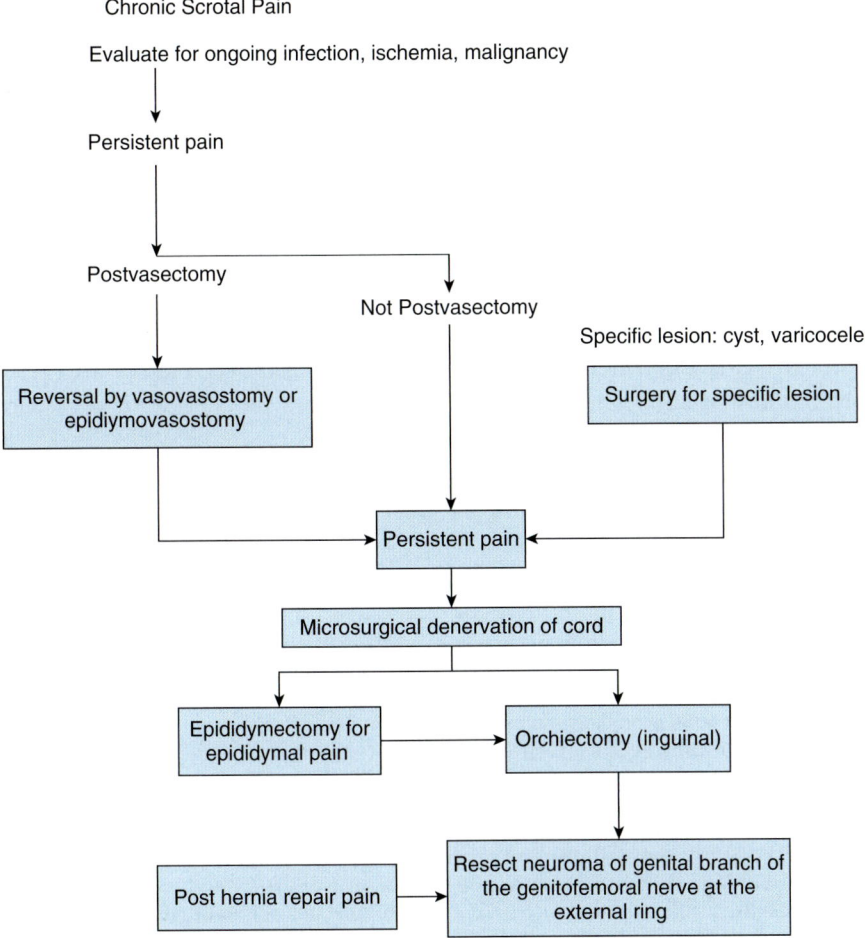

Fig. 56.8. Algorithm for progression of surgical therapy for men with chronic scrotal pain.

REFERENCES

The complete reference list is available online at ExpertConsult.com.

57

Interstitial Cystitis/Bladder Pain Syndrome and Related Disorders

Robert M. Moldwin, MD, and Philip M. Hanno, MD, MPH

A BRIEF HISTORY AND OVERVIEW

Our current understanding of interstitial cystitis/bladder pain syndrome (IC/BPS) has evolved much from 1876, when Dr. Samuel Gross coined the term *interstitial cystitis*, describing a condition of chronic bladder inflammation of unknown etiology (Gross, 1876). In 1918, Dr. Guy Hunner extended this work in his report of "classical" interstitial cystitis; rare patients presented with bladder pain on filling and the cystoscopic finding of inflamed areas of the bladder wall (Hunner, 1915, 1918). This was later termed *Hunner lesions (HLs)*. Clinical experience over the next 50 years revealed that the vast majority of patients who presented with bladder pain had no evidence of bladder wall abnormality on routine cystoscopic examination. A 1987 National Institutes of Health/National Institute of Diabetes and Digestive and Kidney Diseases (NIH/NIDDK) meeting of "experts" produced a definition of IC with the objective to provide a homogenous population of patients for clinical trials (Gillenwater and Wein, 1988). Many clinicians incorporated these criteria into their practices only to find that they excluded approximately 60% of individuals who would otherwise have been clinically diagnosed with the condition (Hanno et al., 1999). Clearly, our definition needed to broaden, and this needed to be reflected in its nomenclature. Although controversy remains, the term *bladder pain syndrome (BPS)* is currently most commonly used and was selected to meet standards of medical pain taxonomy (Baranowski, et al., 2008). Today, IC/BPS may be defined clinically as **"an unpleasant sensation (pain, pressure, discomfort) perceived to be related to the urinary bladder, associated with lower urinary tract symptoms (LUTS) of more than six weeks duration, in the absence of infection or other identifiable causes"** (Hanno and Dmochowski, 2009). This definition is based on what we now believe to be a heterogeneous syndrome, a form of chronic pelvic pain that spans the gamut of patients to include not only those who present with gross inflammatory disease of the bladder wall but also those who have no visible inflammation but endorse bladder pain and often have multiple nonurologic complaints of pain (Nickel and Moldwin, 2018; Tripp et al., 2012) (Fig. 57.1).

Difficulties encountered with the development of treatment strategies may be confounded by this heterogeneity, prompting many investigators to suggest that better phenotyping of the patient population may result in better clinical outcomes (Nickel and Moldwin, 2018). As our definition of the condition has broadened, prevalence estimates have increased dramatically. Current population-based studies conservatively estimate 2.1 million men (Suskind, et al., 2013) and 3.3 million women (Berry et al., 2011) in the United States having symptoms consistent with IC/BPS.

DEFINITION, NOMENCLATURE, AND TAXONOMY

> "The beginning of wisdom is the definition of terms." —Socrates (Nails, 2018)

How we define and what we name a medical condition may have an enormous impact on its diagnosis, its epidemiology, the protocol of clinical trials, recognition by the medical community, the names of patient support groups, and (in many countries) patient insurance coverage and physician reimbursement. Even subtle changes in definition, whether it be the character of pain, the location, its association with voiding or not, or its duration may have a profound effect on many of these parameters. A simple example is that of the International Continence Society's definition of *painful bladder syndrome (PBS)* as "the complaint of suprapubic pain related to bladder filling, accompanied by other symptoms such as increased daytime and night-time frequency, in the absence of proven urinary infection or other obvious pathology" (Abrams et al., 2002). Simply requiring pain to be suprapubic and linked to bladder filling eliminated 34% of patients who were clinically diagnosed with IC/PBS (Warren et al., 2006). Another example is the study by Berry et al. in which a minor change in definition (high sensitivity vs. high specificity definitions) resulted in a difference of 4.3 million estimated to have symptoms suggestive of the condition (Berry et al. 2011)!

The reader may note that current literature is replete with varied terms including *hypersensitive bladder* (Homma et al., 2009), *painful bladder syndrome/interstitial cystitis (PBS/IC)* (Hanno et al., 2005a), *interstitial cystitis/painful bladder syndrome (IC/PBS)* (Hanno et al., 2005b), and *bladder pain syndrome/interstitial cystitis (BPS/IC)* (Fall et al., 2010). **For purposes of clarity and in accordance with the guidelines of the American Urological Association (AUA), this chapter will default to the terminology of the International Consultation on Incontinence (ICI)—*bladder pain syndrome*—but keeps the term *interstitial cystitis* to facilitate recognition and understanding.**

Mounting evidence suggests that BPS is indeed a syndrome and distinct from those patients presenting with HLs (Abrams et al., 2018; Akiyama et al., 2018; Fall and Peeker, 2013; Han et al., 2018; Hanno et al., 2011, 2013) (see Fig. 57.1). This was a topic highlighted at a recent U.S. Food and Drug Administration (FDA) Bone, Reproductive, and Urologic Drugs Advisory Committee (BRUDAC) meeting. The primary question discussed was whether patients with IC and BPS should be combined in future clinical trials. The question itself implied that IC and BPS are two clinically and pathologically separate conditions. Ultimately by unanimous decision, the committee chose to study the two conditions together primarily *based on symptoms* that are indistinguishable from one another (Nickel and Moldwin, 2018).

Interstitial Cystitis/Bladder Pain Syndrome Research Criteria and Their Influence on Clinical Practice

In an effort to define IC so that patients in different geographic areas and under the care of different physicians could be compared, the NIDDK held a workshop in August 1987 at which consensus criteria were established for the diagnosis of IC (Gillenwater and Wein, 1988). **These criteria were not meant to define the disease, but rather to ensure that groups of patients included in basic and clinical research studies would be relatively comparable.** After pilot studies were carried out to test the criteria, they were revised at another NIDDK workshop 1 year later (Wein et al., 1990) (Box 57.1).

HISTORICAL PERSPECTIVE OF INTERSTITIAL CYSTITIS/BLADDER PAIN SYNDROME: EARLY 1800S TO 1970S

A detailed historical perspective for IC/BPS from the 1800s to 1970s and an evolution of definitions for IC/BPS can be found online at ExpertConsult.com.

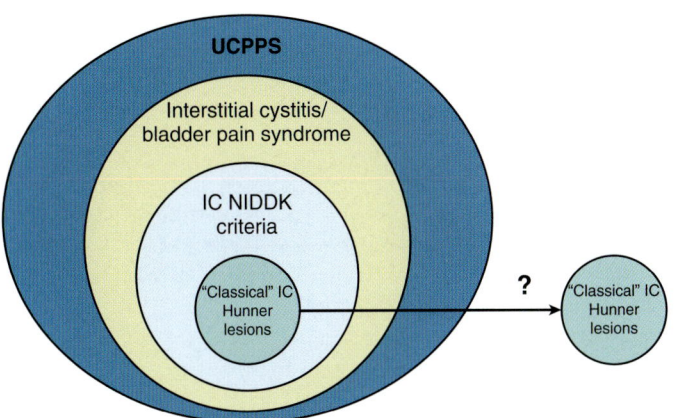

Fig. 57.1. Evolving nomenclature/taxonomy and definitions are associated with a larger and more diverse patient population, all with a similar clinical presentation. The "?" denotes mounting interest to separate "classical IC" (as a disease typified by easily identifiable bladder wall inflammation) from the remainder of "syndromic" patients. *UCPPS*, Urologic chronic pelvic pain syndrome. (Modified from Nickel JC, Moldwin R. FDA BRUDAC 2018 Criteria for Interstitial Cystitis/Bladder Pain Syndrome Clinical Trials: Future Direction for Research. *J Urol* 200[1]:39–42, 2018.)

Unexpectedly, the medical community began to use the NIDDK research criteria to establish a diagnosis in their clinical practice, leading to concerns of underdiagnosing the condition. The specificity of the finding of bladder glomerulations before or after distention came into question (Erickson, 1995; Tomaszewski et al., 2001; Waxman et al., 1998). Many patients who presented with IC symptoms had no evidence of glomerulations under anesthesia (Al Hadithi et al., 2002; Awad et al., 1992). Even the consistency of finding glomerulations at varying time points had been called to question (Shear and Mayer, 2006).

The multicenter Interstitial Cystitis Data Base (ICDB) study conducted through the NIDDK accumulated data on 424 patients with IC, enrolling patients from May 1993 to December 1995. Entry criteria were much more symptom driven than those promulgated for research studies (Simon et al., 1997). Notably, no evidence of HLs or glomerulations was needed for study participation. In an analysis of the defining criteria (Hanno et al., 1999), it appeared the NIDDK research criteria fulfilled their mission. **Fully 90% of expert clinicians agreed that patients diagnosed with IC by those criteria in the ICDB indeed had the disorder. However, 60% of patients deemed to have IC by these experienced clinicians would not have met NIDDK research criteria.** With this dilemma in mind, the European Society for the Study of Interstitial Cystitis (ESSIC) (recently renamed the International Society for the Study of BPS) developed a definition by which patients would be required to meet less stringent criteria: pelvic pain for longer than 6 months; pressure or discomfort perceived to be related to the urinary bladder accompanied by at least one other urinary symptom such as persistent urge to void or frequency; and the exclusion of confusable diseases as the cause of the symptoms (van de Merwe et al., 2008). The broader definition facilitated the diagnosis and treatment in many patients who would otherwise remain undiagnosed (Proaño et al., 2013). Although not mandated, cystoscopy with hydrodistention (CHD) and biopsy was suggested to allow subtyping.

IC/BPS is now viewed not only through the paradigm of a chronic pain syndrome that manifests through bladder-related symptoms, but as a syndrome that may not be a true disease of the bladder alone in many patients (Hanno, 2008). This paradigm is reflected in the ongoing Multi-Disciplinary Approach to the Study of Chronic Pelvic Pain (MAPP) Research Network (https://www.mappnetwork.org/), where the breadth of pelvic pain studied extends to IC/BPS and men afflicted with chronic prostatitis/chronic pelvic pain syndrome, collectively termed *urologic chronic pelvic pain syndrome (UCPPS)*. UCPPS is characterized by chronic pain in the pelvic region or genitalia, often accompanied by urinary frequency and urgency (Clemens et al., 2019; Landis et al., 2014).

BOX 57.1 National Institute of Diabetes and Digestive and Kidney Diseases Diagnostic Criteria for Interstitial Cystitis

To be diagnosed with interstitial cystitis, patients must have either glomerulations on cystoscopic examination or a classic Hunner ulcer, and they must have either pain associated with the bladder or urinary urgency. An examination for glomerulations should be undertaken after distention of the bladder under anesthesia to 80 to 100 cm H_2O for 1 to 2 minutes. The bladder may be distended up to two times before evaluation. The glomerulations must be diffuse—present in at least three quadrants of the bladder—and there must be at least 10 glomerulations per quadrant. The glomerulations must not be along the path of the cystoscope (to eliminate artifact from contact instrumentation). The presence of any one of the following excludes a diagnosis of interstitial cystitis:

1. Bladder capacity of greater than 350 mL on awake cystometry using either a gas or liquid filling medium
2. Absence of an intense urge to void with the bladder filled to 100 mL of gas or 150 mL of liquid filling medium
3. The demonstration of phasic involuntary bladder contractions on cystometry using the fill rate just described
4. Duration of symptoms less than 9 months
5. Absence of nocturia
6. Symptoms relieved by antimicrobial agents, urinary antiseptic agents, anticholinergic agents, or antispasmodic agents
7. A frequency of urination while awake of fewer than eight times per day
8. A diagnosis of bacterial cystitis or prostatitis within a 3-month period
9. Bladder or ureteral calculi
10. Active genital herpes
11. Uterine, cervical, vaginal, or urethral cancer
12. Urethral diverticulum
13. Cyclophosphamide or any type of chemical cystitis
14. Tuberculous cystitis
15. Radiation cystitis
16. Benign or malignant bladder tumors
17. Vaginitis
18. Age younger than 18 years

From Wein AJ, Hanno PM, Gillenwater JY. Interstitial cystitis: an introduction to the problem. In: Hanno PM, Staskin DR, Krane RJ, et al., eds. *Interstitial cystitis*. London: Springer-Verlag; 1990:13–15.

VOIDING SYMPTOMS AND INTERSTITIAL CYSTITIS/BLADDER PAIN SYNDROME

Although bladder pain is the central symptom of IC/BPS and the most frequent reason for seeking health care (Clemens et al., 2018), urinary urgency is also commonly described. The ICS definition of urgency as "*a sudden* compelling desire to pass urine, which is difficult to defer" (Abrams et al., 2002) has been useful for the diagnosis of overactive bladder (OAB), and its presence in the IC/BPS patient has prompted suggestions that IC/BPS and OAB syndrome may represent a spectrum of bladder hypersensitivity (Homma, 2008; Lai et al., 2014). Nevertheless, qualitative differences in urgency usually exist between OAB and IC/BPS. **As compared with the OAB patient who fears urine loss, IC/BPS patients often describe a compelling need to void centered on mounting (not sudden) pain, pressure, or pelvic discomfort that occurs with filling.**

Urgency is not a symptom that defines IC/BPS. It is a term often poorly defined and comprehended by patients and cannot be used to clearly discriminate between IC/BPS and OAB (Clemens et al.,

KEY POINTS: BLADDER PAIN SYNDROME AND INTERSTITIAL CYSTITIS

- *Bladder pain syndrome* is a term developed to meet current standards of pain taxonomy. BPS encompasses patients with pain perceived to be bladder-based associated with urinary urgency or frequency in the absence of other identified causes of symptoms. BPS includes subgroups such as those meeting NIDDK criteria and the smaller subgroup of patients with "classical disease" (HLs).
- The term *interstitial cystitis* is currently wrapped in controversy, as it is not a modern histologic description of the condition, even for those patients who manifest gross inflammatory disease of the bladder. Nevertheless, the term remains beside BPS (as IC/BPS) to facilitate patient care and to acknowledge patient support groups such as the Interstitial Cystitis Association (ICA; www.ichelp.org). Whether the older term *interstitial cystitis* should refer to a distinct subgroup of BPS (i.e., those with HLs) is, as yet, unclear.
- The HL (formerly termed *Hunner ulcer*) is the pathognomonic finding for the "classical form" of IC and represents a minority of the IC/BPS population. HLs are easily identified during office cystoscopy, although bladder distention beyond functional capacity and other imaging strategies have been used to enhance identification (Ueda et al., 2008). There is a lack of consensus as to which pathologic findings, if any, are required for, or even suggestive of, a tissue diagnosis (Hanno et al., 2005a; Tomaszewski et al., 1999, 2001).

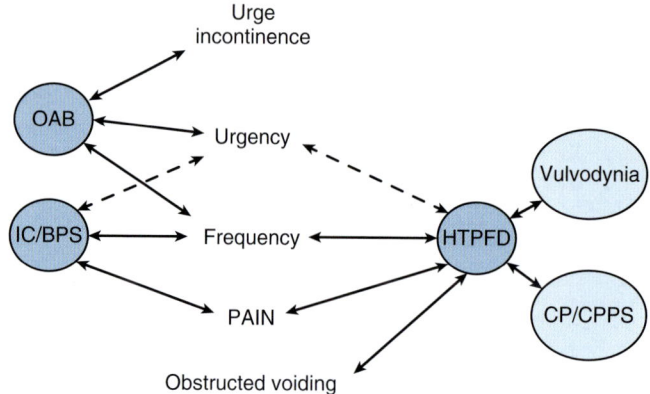

Fig. 57.2. Urinary complaints shared by commonly encountered urological conditions, adding to the complexity of diagnosis. Note that the varied constellation of symptoms associated with pelvic floor dysfunction/spasm may be remarkably similar to those of IC/BPS and OAB. HTPFD may also be associated with other pain syndromes that have been associated with IC/BPS. *CP/CPPS*, Chronic prostatitis/chronic pelvic pain syndrome; *HTPFD*, high-tone pelvic floor dysfunction; *IC/BPS*, interstitial cystitis/bladder pain syndrome; *OAB*, overactive bladder. (Modified from Abrams P, Hanno P, Wein A. Overactive bladder and painful bladder syndrome: there need not be confusion. *Neurourol Urodyn* 24[2]:149–150, 2005.)

KEY POINTS: LOWER URINARY TRACT SYMPTOMS AND THE PATIENT WITH INTERSTITIAL CYSTITIS/BLADDER PAIN SYNDROME

- Urgency has been defined as the complaint of a sudden compelling desire to pass urine that is difficult to defer. Fear of incontinence is more consistent with OAB, whereas pressure, pain, or discomfort suggests IC/BPS.
- As compared with the relatively uncommon finding of OAB, HTPFD is present in the majority of IC/BPS patients. This functional disorder may pose a diagnostic challenge as associated LUTS and pelvic pain overlap with IC/BPS.

2011). Studies through the MAPP Network also demonstrate that descriptions of urgency vary independently from pain (Lai et al., 2015), suggesting that these symptoms should be monitored separately. Making matters more complex, the diagnosis of IC/BPS does not preclude coexisting detrusor overactivity (DO). In studies through the NIDDK database, Nigro et al. (1997a) found a 14% incidence of urodynamic DO in the IC/BPS patients, a prevalence probably close to what one might expect in the general population if studied urodynamically (Salavatore et al., 2003).

The downstream effect of urinary urgency would, of course, be low-volume urinary frequency (Abrams, 2005). **Although BPS patients may have significantly higher voiding frequencies, smaller voided volumes, and narrower ranges of voided volume compared with OAB patients** (Kim et al., 2014), **one cannot distinguish between the two syndromes based on a voiding diary.**

High-tone pelvic floor dysfunction (HTPFD; often termed *hypertonicity of the pelvic floor musculature, nonrelaxing pelvic floor dysfunction, pelvic floor spasm*, or *myalgia of the pelvic floor*) may produce irritative and/or obstructive voiding symptoms and/or pelvic pain (Kuo et al., 2015). **HTPFD has been identified in 70% to 94% of IC/BPS patients either on the basis of urodynamically proven voiding dysfunction** (Butrick et al., 2009) **or reproduction of pelvic pain on examination of the pelvic floor musculature** (Peters et al., 2007, 2008). The clinical diagnostic dilemmas generated by the presence of HTPFD include its ability to generate pain alone or in association with IC/BPS, and the overlap of symptoms between these conditions. The associated irritative symptoms may be confused for OAB. HTPFD may also be responsible for complaints associated with other pain syndromes such as chronic prostatitis/chronic pelvic pain syndrome (CP/CPPS) (Shoskes et al., 2008) and vulvodynia (Bornstein et al., 2016) (Fig. 57.2).

EPIDEMIOLOGY OF INTERSTITIAL CYSTITIS/BLADDER PAIN SYNDROME

Since initial population-based studies of the 1970s to early 1990s, we have seen a significant increase in IC/BPS prevalence estimates, likely a result of a more liberalized definition, one without any specific physical findings needed or biochemical markers available (Nickel, 2018) (Table 57.1). Methodologic differences may also account for much of the variability in prevalence noted among investigations.

The relatively low prevalence of IC/BPS reported by Bade et al. (1995) of 8 to 16 of 100,000 might be expected as data were derived from questionnaires completed by urologists, 80% of whom used elevated mast cell counts on bladder biopsy to make the diagnosis. Two symptom-based questionnaire studies by Parsons et al. (2002a) demonstrated the other side of the prevalence spectrum. One survey queried female health care professionals or their spouses attending a lecture by the author, and the other focused on third-year American female medical students (Parsons and Tatsis, 2004). Both studies suggested that IC/BPS prevalence might be as high as 20,000 per 100,000 of the female population. Assessment of male IC/BPS prevalence has been particularly challenging because of clinical similarities between IC/BPS and CP/CPPS (Arora and Shoskes, 2015).

The most sophisticated large-scale, population-based IC/BPS prevalence study to date was conducted by the RAND Corporation and termed the RICE (RAND Interstitial Cystitis Epidemiology) study. With use of a case definition with an 83% specificity, a random sample of 146,231 households was contacted by telephone, and 12,752 women completed the questionnaire; 2.7% met the high-specificity definition of BPS. **The figures correspond to 3.3 million women in the United States 18 years of age or older with symptoms compatible with the diagnosis** (Berry et al., 2011). Prevalence increased with age from 2.21% for 18 to 29 years of age to a high

TABLE 57.1 Population-Based Prevalence Studies for Interstitial Cystitis/Bladder Pain Syndrome

AUTHOR	DATE OF PUBLICATION	COUNTRY	STUDY DESIGN	IC/BPS PREVALENCE (PER 100,000) F/M
Oravisto	1975	Finland	Physician Dx	18.1/–
Held et al.	1990	USA	Physician Dx	30.0/–
Bade et al.	1995	Netherlands	Physician Dx	8–16/–
Jones/Nyberg	1997	USA	Patient report	865/–
Curhan et al. (NHS I/II)	1999	USA	Physician Dx / Patient report	52/– (I) / 67/– (II)
Ito et al.	2000	Japan	Physician Dx	4.5/–
Parsons et al.	2002a	USA	Questionnaire	20,000/–
Leppilahti et al.	2002 / 2005	Finland / Finland	Questionnaire / Questionnaire	450/– / 300–680/–
Roberts et al.	2003	USA (Olmstead County, MN)	Physician Dx	114/69.7
Parsons and Tatsis	2004	USA	Questionnaire	20,000/–
Clemens et al.	2005	USA (Kaiser)	Physician Dx	197/41
Temml et al.	2007	Austria	Questionnaire	306/–
Inoue et al.	2009	Japan	Questionnaire	265/–
Song et al.	2009	China	Questionnaire	100/–
Choe et al.	2011	S Korea	Questionnaire	261/–
Berry et al.	2011	USA	Questionnaire	2700–6300/–
Suskind et al.	2013	USA	Questionnaire	–/2000–4200

Dx, Diagnosis; *F/M*, female/male; *IC/BPS*, interstitial cystitis/bladder pain syndrome.

of 3.41% for 50 to 59 years of age and then decreased to 1.70% for 70 to 75 years of age. Of note is that less than 10% of these women had a clinical diagnosis of IC/BPS. When the same methodology was applied to men, the **findings suggested that 1.9% (2.1 million) of adult US males have symptoms of IC/BPS**, higher than the weighted prevalence of chronic prostatitis and CPPS (Suskind et al., 2013). Although these prevalence studies suggest that a high percentage of IC/BPS patients are male, one must note that they were based on symptoms rather than diagnoses. **Investigations based on diagnoses in clinical practice suggest a female-to-male ratio of 5:1** (Clemens et al., 2005).

Interstitial Cystitis/Bladder Pain Syndrome in Children

No studies exist that detail the prevalence of IC/BPS in childhood; however, the condition is considered to be uncommon. On the other hand, children with voiding dysfunction, often associated with disturbances of bowel and pelvic floor behavior, are commonly evaluated in pediatric urology practices (Aguiar and Franco, 2018; Santos et al., 2017). Many of these patients present with varied complaints of pelvic and/or urethral pain that easily can be confused with those of IC/BPS. A recall-based study suggested that adult female IC/BPS patients have a higher prevalence of urinary urgency and recurrent urinary tract infections during childhood than an asymptomatic cohort (Peters et al., 2009). In a recent recall survey, Doiron et al. (2017) also detected a link back to childhood bladder and bowel dysfunction. They found that IC/BPS patients with irritable bowel syndrome (IBS)–like symptoms frequently complained of the need to push for a bowel movement, voided only once or twice daily, and had painful urination during childhood. This coupled with the known high prevalence of HTPFD in the IC/BPS population merits concerns that adult IC/BPS patients may have linked bladder-bowel-pelvic floor dysfunction dating back to childhood (Costantini et al., 2018).

There is a small cohort of children with chronic symptoms of bladder pain, urinary frequency, and sensory urgency in the absence of infection who have been evaluated with urodynamics, cystoscopy, and bladder distention and have findings consistent with the diagnosis of IC/BPS. In a review of 20 such children by Close et al., the median age of **onset was younger than 5 years, and the vast majority of patients had long-term remissions with bladder distention** (Close et al., 1996). This group also emphasized the need to differentiate these patients from those with dysfunctional voiding.

THE EPIDEMIOLOGY OF HUNNER LESIONS

One might expect epidemiologic studies related to the classical form of IC/BPS to be straightforward, given that this is a diagnosis primarily based on physical findings. Unfortunately, this has not been the case. The relative rarity of these lesions has hampered patient accrual for the development of longitudinal data. Medical coding strategies often do not distinguish HL patients from those without lesions, thus making even retrospective studies difficult to perform. Most patient populations related to HLs have been derived from tertiary care centers and are, therefore, unlikely to truly reflect general population demographics. Despite these limitations, common epidemiologic threads among studies do exist.

Data regarding the prevalence of HLs in practice range from 3.5% to 56% (Table 57.2), generating an average prevalence among studies of approximately 20%. The vast majority of these data come from clinical practices within tertiary care centers. This selection bias and other concerns, previously detailed, suggest that extrapolation of prevalence data to the general IC/BPS population should be done with caution.

Patients with HLs tend to be older than those without HLs (Table 57.3). This finding was first identified by Hand (1949), who evaluated 223 IC/BPS patients and found that 13% had grade 3 lesions, a description that is consistent with most current HL definitions. He found that these patients were older at symptom onset than those without lesions (average age 41 years vs. 35.5 years, respectively). Female HL patients had a longer interval between symptom onset and diagnosis than non-HL patients (11.5 years vs. 7.5 years, respectively).

Koziol et al. (1993) evaluated 374 IC/BPS patients and found that 20.1% had HLs. HL patients had similar age of symptom onset, age of diagnosis, and duration of symptoms to non-HL patients. A subsequent study by the same lead author (1996) evaluating 565 IC/BPS patients (111 with and 454 without HL), however, found the average age of symptom onset to be older in the HL group (46.9 years) than in the non-HL group (40.9 years).

Peeker et al. (2000b) compared 130 HL patients to 101 non-HL patients. They found that HL patients had a higher mean age at symptom onset (55 vs. 30 years of age) and at the time diagnosis (62 vs. 38 years of age).

Rais-Bahrami et al. (2012) analyzed patient demographics, disease characteristics, and symptoms of 268 patients with IC/BPS seen at a tertiary care center between 1990 and 2008 across three age cohorts (<30 years of age, 30 to 60 years of age, and >60 years of age. They found HL in all cohorts, however, there were more HL patients in the older age cohorts (12.0%, 42.0%, and 39.8%, respectively).

The prevalence of HL in young IC/BPS patients is not well established. Hammett et al. (2013) published a case study of a 13-year-old girl with documented HL.

Heredity and Interstitial Cystitis/Bladder Pain Syndrome

In a pioneering study, Warren et al. (2004) suggested a hereditary aspect to incidence. They found that **adult female first-degree relatives of patients with IC/BPS may have a prevalence of IC/BPS 17 times that found in the general population.** This, together with previously reported evidence showing a greater concordance of IC/BPS among monozygotic than dizygotic twins, suggests but does not prove a genetic susceptibility to IC/BPS that could partially explain the discord in prevalence rates in different populations (Warren et al., 2001, 2004). A recent study using genetic linkage analysis suggested that a genetic variant on chromosome 3 and possibly on chromosomes 1, 4, 9, and 14 contribute to an IC/BPS predisposition (Allen-Brady et al., 2018). The same group examined familial clustering of IC/BPS with 21 associated medical conditions. Diagnoses of myalgia and myositis/unspecified (fibromyalgia syndrome [FMS]) and constipation were found in significant excess in the IC/BPS patients and their first-degree and second-degree relatives. Although environmental factors may account for some of this effect, the excess clustering in more distant relatives suggests that shared genetic factors may account for the coexistence of these conditions (Allen-Brady et al., 2015). Familial clustering has also been reported between IC/BPS and CP/CPPS (Dimitrakov, 2001), a finding not surprising given the clinical overlap between these conditions (Arora and Shoskes, 2015; Moldwin, 2002).

Natural History, Effects on Quality of Life, and Economic Burden

The natural history of IC/BPS has primarily been assessed through patient recall. Rais-Bahrami et al. found that patients diagnosed at

TABLE 57.2 Percentage of Hunner Lesion Patients Within Varied IC/BPS Studies

YEAR	AUTHOR	HL PREVALENCE/ TOTAL NUMBER OF IC/BPS PATIENTS
1949	Hand	13%/223
1987a	Holm-Bentzen et al.	3.5%/115
1987	Parsons and Mulholland	28%/75
1993	Koziol et al.	20%/374
1996	Koziol et al.	19.6%/565
1997a	Nigro et al.[a]	11.3%/113
1997	Simon et al.[a]	10.5%/190
1997	Messing et al.[a]	11.3%/150
2001	Forrest et al.[b]	10%/52
2002	Peeker and Fall	56%/231
2004	Forrest and Schmidt[b]	10%/92
2008	Braunstein, et al.	39%/223
2011	Peters et al.	17%/214
2012	Logadottir et al.	55%/393
2013	Killinger et al.	17%/214

[a]Interstitial Cystitis Data Base data. HL prevalence varied from 5.3% to 33.3% between referral centers.
[b]Forrest et al. evaluated only male patients.
HL, Hunner lesion; IC/BPS, interstitial cystitis/bladder pain syndrome.

TABLE 57.3 Age Difference: Hunner Lesion (HL) Patients Versus Non-HL Patients

		HL		NON-HL		
YEAR	AUTHOR	MEAN AGE OF SYMPTOM ONSET	MEAN AGE OF DIAGNOSIS OR AT TIME OF STUDY*	MEAN AGE OF SYMPTOM ONSET	MEAN AGE OF DIAGNOSIS OR AT TIME OF STUDY[a]	COMMENTS
1949	Hand	41	53.5	35.5	43	No males were noted to have HL
1977	DeJuana and Everett		58[a]			Female predominant; HL was inclusion criteria for study
1993	Koziol	43.6	57.1[a]	42	52[a]	
1996	Koziol	46.9		40.9		
2002	Peeker and Fall	55	62	30	38	
2008	Braunstein et al.		60[a]		47[a]	Female predominant in HL and non-HL patients
2011	Peters et al.		62[a]		55[a]	
2012	Logadottir et al.		62		42	Female predominant in HL and non-HL patients
2013	Killinger et al.		62[a]		55[a]	

[a]Study did not report the age at diagnosis; rather it only supplied information about the ages of patients at the time of the study.

> **KEY POINT: PREVALENCE OF INTERSTITIAL CYSTITIS/ BLADDER PAIN SYNDROME**
>
> - Prevalence studies for IC/BPS show wide variation with a general upsurge over time likely related to a more "liberalized" definition of the condition.
> - IC/BPS is uncommon in children, but when present may occur with or without HLs.
> - Dysfunctional voiding with bowel and pelvic floor dysfunction may give rise to symptoms similar to IC/BPS and should be considered in the differential diagnosis.
> - HL may be identified in approximately 20% of IC/BPS patients in clinical practice.
> - Patients with HL are generally older than those without HL.
> - Studies, although limited in number, suggest genetic transmission of IC/BPS in some patients.

the youngest ages experienced significantly more urinary urgency, frequency, dysuria, dyspareunia, and genital pain. Older patients had a higher incidence of nocturia, urinary incontinence, and HLs (Rais-Bahrami et al., 2012). Patients with mild symptoms at onset appear to show symptom stability at 3 years, whereas those with concomitant chronic fatigue syndrome at symptom onset tend to show symptom progression of IC/BPS over time (Warren et al., 2013). **Prodromal symptoms related to pelvic pain and irritative voiding are often experienced decades before a formal diagnosis.** Urinary frequency without pain was identified in 42% of those patients with prodromal symptoms (Warren et al., 2018). These patients are more likely to have nonbladder syndromes (e.g., FMS) and a poorer prognosis. These findings are consistent with the previously discussed increase in childhood voiding complaints recalled by adult female IC/BPS patients.

Longitudinal studies will often show symptom improvement over the first few weeks simply based on a regression to the mean and an intervention effect (improvement based on the increased follow-up and care) (Propert et al., 2000). This phenomenon was also described by the MAPP Network with the most significant symptom reduction identified between baseline and week 2. A smaller reduction was noted between weeks 2 and 4. This phenomenon reinforces the need for randomized controlled trials (RCTs) and a possible pre-enrollment interval (Stephens-Shields et al., 2016).

Two distinct pain phenotypes have been identified in the IC/BPS patient: those with pelvic pain only and those with "pelvic pain and beyond." Nickel et al. (2015) found that 81% of female IC/BPS patients were afflicted with pain beyond the pelvis and had notably higher levels of sensory type pain, a poorer physical QoL, greater somatic depression, and more sleep disturbance than those with the sole complaint of pelvic pain. Pelvic pain and beyond was also identified in approximately 75% of the MAPP Network's UCPPS patients, a population that also included male CPPS and IC/BPS patients (Clemens et al., 2019). Krieger et al. (2015) reported that 38% of UCPPS patients had at least one nonurologic-associated somatic syndrome (IBS, chronic fatigue syndrome, or FMS). This cohort had more severe symptoms, symptoms of longer duration, and higher rates of depression and anxiety than those with UCPPS only. Collectively, these studies suggest that a significant proportion of IC/BPS patients may have widespread and possibly "centralized" pain that may not respond adequately when only local therapies are applied. The findings also support a role for phenotyping strategies such as UPOINT (Urinary, Psychosocial, Organ specific, Infection, Neurologic/Systemic, Tenderness) for clinical and future research (Nickel et al., 2009b).

Information detailing symptom remission is difficult to capture as the lack of complaints usually obviates the need for office evaluation. The IC database study detailed 35% of IC/BPS patients as having at least one occurrence of symptom remission for greater than 3 months, with 38% of that group having remission for at least 6 months (Simon et al., 1997). **A MAPP Network two-site study found that symptom "flares" occurred in 98% of female UCPPS patients (100% who met IC/BPS criteria).** Flares varied widely in terms of duration (seconds to months), frequency (multiple times per day to once per year or less), symptom type (pain vs. urinary symptoms), and intensity. The most common length of flare was multiple days (87%), with increasing duration of flare associated with greater pelvic pain, urologic symptoms, disruption to participants' activities, and bother (Sutcliffe et al., 2014). A subsequent case-crossover study found sexual activity to be the only consistent factor associated with flare onset. Subpopulations appeared to be triggered by various dietary factors and abdominal exercises (Sutcliffe et al., 2018). These findings support the role to intervene if a trigger for flares is identified, but a rigid plan for flare prevention is not recommended.

As with all forms of chronic pain, IC/BPS is often associated with a decline in mental and physical quality of life (QoL), poor coping skills, anxiety, and depression (Hanno et al., 2005a; Michael et al., 2000; Rothrock et al., 2002, 2003; Vasudevan and Moldwin, 2017). Symptom severity in female IC/BPS patients was an independent predictor of a poorer QoL (body pain, general health, and mental health). A "married" status was associated with both lower symptom severity and improvement in multiple QoL domains (El Khoudary et al., 2009). Furthermore, spousal distraction techniques appear to blunt the effect of pain on the mental QoL.

Sexual dysfunction in female IC/BPS patients may have a profound effect on their physical and mental QoL, underscoring the importance of identifying and ultimately treating this problem when present (Nickel et al., 2007). Catastrophic thinking (defined as believing that the worst may happen and the individual would not be able to tolerate it) was common and associated with greater impairments in various domains, including depressive symptoms, general mental health, social functioning, vitality, and pain (Rothrock et al., 2003). Disability may be partially explained by the impact of negative affect and catastrophizing (Katz et al., 2013). Cognitive behavior therapy approaches that address catastrophizing and mood may serve an important role (Muere et al., 2018).

The symptoms of IC/BPS may affect the patient's ability to adequately function or to function at all in the workplace. IC/BPS patients are six times more likely than individuals in the general population to cut down on work time because of health problems but only half as likely to do so as patients with arthritis (Shea-O'Malley and Sant, 1999). Data collected from the RICE study demonstrated that the *impact* of bladder symptoms on life activities was the most consistent predictor of work outcomes. This suggests an important role for behavioral therapies devoted to improve coping skills and self-management strategies (Beckett et al., 2014).

Abuse and Symptoms

The Boston Area Community Health Survey (BACH) found emotional, sexual, and physical abuse to be a risk factors for symptoms suggestive of IC/BPS (Link and Lutfey, 2007), and this has been borne out in other studies. A Michigan study compared a control group of 464 women with 215 IC/BPS patients and found that 22% of the control group had experienced abuse versus 37% of the patient group (Peters et al., 2007b). A study performed through the Kaiser Permanente database found a 3.8% prevalence of child abuse versus 0.4% in a control population (Clemens et al., 2008b). Those with a history of sexual abuse may have more pain and fewer voiding symptoms (Seth and Teichman, 2008). How reliable these data are is not clear, and it would be wrong to jump to any conclusions about abuse in an individual patient. However, practitioners need to have sensitivity to the possibility of an abusive relationship history in all pain patients, and BPS patients in particular. When patients are found to have multiple diagnoses, the rate of previous abuse also increases, and these patients may need referral for further counseling at a traumatic stress center (Fenton et al., 2008).

Medical Costs

Costs of the disorder are not insignificant and can range from $4000 to $7000 per year, not including lost wages, costs preceding diagnosis, costs of alternative therapies, and costs attributable to misdiagnosis

(Clemens et al., 2008a, 2009b). A recent large-scale US-based study was conducted to describe and compare health care utilization, direct costs, and comorbidities for patients with and without IC/BPS during the first year after diagnosis. A diagnosis of IC/BPS was associated with $7223 higher total health care costs than not having IC/BPS, with outpatient costs contributing to 71% of the difference. HL patients used more health care resources as reflected by total health care costs $6895 higher than patients without HL (Tung et al., 2017).

KEY POINTS: NATURAL HISTORY, EFFECTS ON QUALITY OF LIFE, AND ECONOMIC BURDEN

- Symptoms tend to fluctuate, with the majority of patients showing no long-term deterioration.
- Two distinct pain phenotypes have been identified in the IC/BPS patient: those with pelvic pain only and those with "pelvic pain and beyond," with the latter group representing over 75% of patients.
- Symptom flares are common and are most commonly experienced for several days. Triggers for flares vary widely among patients.
- Prodromal symptoms related to pelvic pain and irritative voiding are often experienced decades before a formal diagnosis.
- QoL in almost all domains is significantly affected.
- The ability to function effectively or at all in the workplace is affected to a significant degree by coping skills.

Associated Disorders

Multiple medical ailments are associated with IC/BPS. Many of these conditions such as FMS, chronic fatigue syndrome, temporomandibular disorder, and irritable bowel syndrome (IBS) are functional pain disorders that may account for some portion of the 75% to 80% of IC/BPS patients who endorse pain beyond the bladder. Other pain disorders of the pelvis such as HTPFD and vulvodynia are often associated with IC/BPS. Symptoms produced by these other "pain generators" may overlap with those of the bladder, further worsen pain, and complicate management strategies. The association of IC/BPS and other disorders may give clues to underlying etiology and aid in the development of phenotyping strategies.

Based on data developed by the Interstitial Cystitis Association (ICA), a large-scale survey of 6783 individuals diagnosed by their physicians as having IC/BPS studied the prevalence of associated diseases (Alagiri et al., 1997). Data from this group was combined with two smaller studies evaluating the presence of autoimmune disease. These data are compared with a more recent albeit smaller multi-institutional study (205 IC/BPS and 117 age-matched controls) (Nickel et al., 2010b) and presented in Table 57.4. Of note, among studies is the high prevalence of pain syndromes that are believed to have a centralized pain component, that is, FMS, chronic fatigue syndrome, and IBS. **IBS was the most commonly identified associated condition, afflicting over 30% of IC/BPS patients and having the highest prevalence relative to the general population of any functional somatic pain syndrome.** Altered visceral sensation has been implicated in IBS in that these patients experience intestinal pain at intestinal gas volumes that are lower than those that cause pain in healthy persons (Lynn and Friedman, 1993), strikingly similar to the pain on bladder distention in IC. Visceral organ crosstalk presumably mediated through the convergence of sensory neural pathways in the dorsal root ganglion, spinal cord, and/or brain could be responsible for some of this association (Greenwood-Van Meerveld et al., 2015).

FMS was also overrepresented in the IC/BPS population. This is a painful nonarticular condition predominantly involving muscles; it is the most common cause of chronic, widespread musculoskeletal pain. FMS is typically associated with persistent fatigue, nonrefreshing sleep, and generalized stiffness. Females were once thought to be afflicted ten times more commonly than men (Jacobsen et al., 1993). Paralleling the path of IC/BPS, current epidemiologic findings for FMS suggest that males compose 60% of the population (Wolfe et al., 2018). The association between FMS and IC/BPS is intriguing because both conditions have similar demographic features, modulating factors, associated symptoms, and response to tricyclic compounds (Chelimsky et al., 2012; Clauw et al., 1997).

Sexual pain and dysfunction are commonly encountered in the female IC/BPS patient (Bogart et al., 2011; Rubin and Malphrus,

TABLE 57.4 Diagnoses Frequently Reported in Interstitial Cystitis/Bladder Pain Syndrome (IC/BPS) Patients

DIAGNOSIS	Van de Merwe, 2003, 2007; Alagiri et al., 1997; Peeker et al., 2003 — PREVALENCE BASED UPON SYMPTOMS (%)	PREVALENCE OF CONDITION IN IC/BPS/PREVALENCE OF CONDITION IN GENERAL POPULATION	Nickel et al., 2010 — SELF-REPORTED DIAGNOSIS (%) IC/BPS VS. CONTROL SIGNIFICANT STATISTICAL DIFFERENCES IDENTIFIED FOR ALL DIAGNOSES
Allergy	44	2	
Irritable bowel syndrome	34.3	12	38.6/5.2
Sensitive skin	26.5	2.4	
Vulvodynia	25	3.1[a]	17/0.9
Fibromyalgia	25	7.8	17.7/2.6
Chronic fatigue syndrome	13	1.5	9.5/1.7
Migraine	22.4	1	29.9/11.2
Asthma	9.8	1.6	
Inflammatory bowel disease	8.2	117	
Systemic lupus erythematosus	2.3	46	
Rheumatoid arthritis	4–13	10	
Sjögren syndrome	8.0	15	
Temporomandibular disorder			12/5.2
Low back pain			46.6/18.8

[a]Estimated prevalence for vulvodynia in the general population at the time of study was 15%. A current prevalence estimate is 8% (Harlow et al., 2014). Ratio shown is consistent with updated information.

2018). Some of this pain may be related to **vulvodynia,** a condition defined as vulvar pain of at least 3 months duration without clear identifiable cause, which may have potential associated factors (Bornstein et al., 2016). Studies of vulvodynia prevalence in the IC/BPS patient vary widely from 17% (Nickel et al., 2010b) to almost all patients being affected (Gardella et al., 2011). Furthermore, vulvodynia and IC/BPS share common comorbid conditions including IBS, FMS, and orofacial pain (Nguyen et al., 2013; Reed et al., 2012). The concordance of these noninfectious inflammatory syndromes involving the tissues derived from the embryonic urogenital sinus and the overlap of coexisting functional syndromes argue for a common cause (Fariello and Moldwin, 2015; Fitzpatrick et al., 1993).

Well-defined inflammatory diseases such as Crohn disease, **systemic lupus erythematosus (SLE), Sjögren syndrome (SS),** and rheumatoid arthritis are infrequently seen in the IC/BPS patient, but their relative occurrence (in the few studies available) in this population is astoundingly high. The most frequently encountered of these conditions is IBS/Crohn disease in which prevalence in the IC/BPS population varies between 104 and 117 higher than in the general population (Alagiri et al., 1997). This finding has not been corroborated yet by other investigators.

Several publications have noted an association between IC/BPS and SLE (Boye et al., 1979; de la Serna and Alarcon-Segovia, 1981; Fister, 1938; Meulders et al., 1992; Weisman et al., 1981). Alagiri et al. (1997) suggested a 34 to 46 times higher prevalence of SLE in IC/BPS patients compared with the general population. Complicating studies is the common presentation of bladder symptoms predating an SLE diagnosis (Liberski et al., 2018). The question has always been whether the bladder symptoms represent an association of these two disease processes or rather are a manifestation of lupus involvement of the bladder (Yukawa et al., 2008). This is an important distinction to make as unlike IC/BPS, lupus cystitis may have a much more virulent clinical course with the development of gross inflammatory changes, bladder wall fibrosis, and hydroureteronephrosis (Abelha-Aleixo et al., 2015). Bladder symptoms may also be a consequence of myelopathy with involvement of the sacral cord in a small group of these patients (Sakakibara et al., 2003).

An association has been reported between IC/BPS and SS, an autoimmune exocrinopathy with a female preponderance manifested by dry eyes, dry mouth, and arthritis, but which can also include fever, dryness, and gastrointestinal and lung problems. Van de Merwe et al. (1993) investigated 10 IC patients for the presence of SS. Two patients had both keratoconjunctivitis sicca and focal lymphocytic sialoadenitis, allowing a primary diagnosis of SS. Only two patients had neither finding. He later reported an incidence of 28% of SS in patients with IC (van de Merwe et al., 2003). The incidence of symptoms of IC/BPS in patients with SS has been estimated to be up to 5% (Leppilahti et al., 2003). Patients with SS may have bladder symptoms from DO, and each patient requires careful individual evaluation before a diagnosis of IC/BPS is made (Lee et al., 2011).

HTPFD as identified by tender and hypertonic pelvic floor and associated musculature can be found in approximately 80% of IC/BPS patients (Bassaly et al., 2011). Its clinical importance stems from symptoms that may extensively overlap with IC/BPS, making diagnosis of both conditions more challenging (see Fig. 57.2). The etiology of HTPFD is unknown, but may date back to childhood voiding dysfunction (Doiron et al., 2017). Other etiologic considerations include its development as guarding behavior related to bladder pain. Some authors suggest that cross-talk through viscerosomatic and viscerovisceral neural pathways may play a bidirectional role in the development of IC/BPS and HTPFD (Pezzone et al., 2005). Interestingly, resting state functional MRI demonstrated altered activity and connectivity of pelvic floor sensorimotor cortical control regions in women with IC/BPS (Kilpatrick et al., 2014).

Nickel et al. (2010b) proposed that distinct phenotypes begin to emerge when one examines the epidemiology of IC/BPS and associated medical conditions (Fig. 57.3). The smallest group comprises individuals who only endorse bladder symptoms. Other groups comprise individuals in whom pain is derived from either regional or widespread pain syndromes. More complexity is added, as multiple forms of regional and widespread pain may be present in the IC/BPS patient.

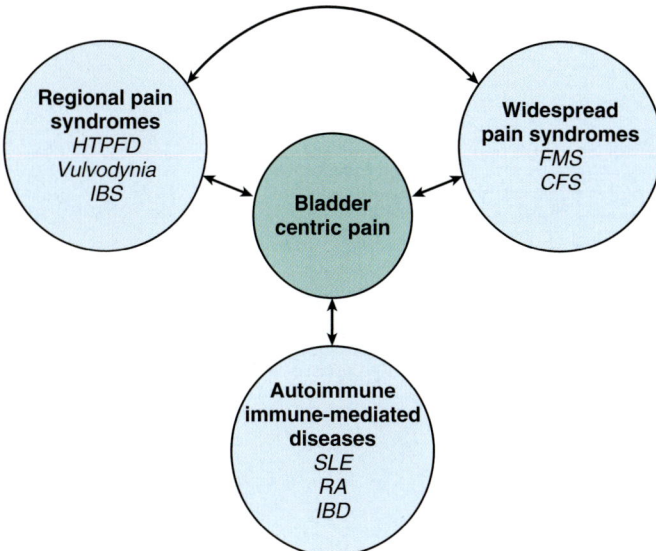

Fig. 57.3. Broad categories of illnesses associated with interstitial cystitis/bladder pain syndrome. *CFS,* Chronic fatigue syndrome; *FMS,* fibromyalgia syndrome; *HTPFD,* high-tone pelvic floor dysfunction; *IBD,* inflammatory bowel disease; *IBS,* irritable bowel syndrome; *RA,* rheumatoid arthritis; *SLE,* systemic lupus erythematosus. (Modified from Nickel JC, Tripp DA, Pontari M, et al. Interstitial cystitis/painful bladder syndrome and associated medical conditions with an emphasis on irritable bowel syndrome, fibromyalgia and chronic fatigue syndrome. *J Urol* 184(4):1358–1363, 2010b.)

Data derived from prior prevalence studies suggest that autoimmune and/or immune-mediated pain may represent another distinct group associated with IC/BPS. Further epidemiologic studies are warranted, because the epidemiology of this disorder may ultimately yield as many clues into cause and treatment as other avenues of research. The heterogeneity of causes and symptoms of IC/BPS suggests that proper clinical phenotyping could foster the development of better treatments for individual phenotypes and more successful treatments for all affected patients (Baranowski et al., 2008; Shoskes et al., 2009).

> **KEY POINTS: ASSOCIATED DISORDERS**
>
> - The bladder-centric patient with IC/BPS is uncommon.
> - Regional pain syndromes such as HTPFD, vulvodynia, and IBS may worsen pain. They may also complicate diagnosis because of overlapping symptoms.
> - The presence of distinct groups of medical conditions associated with IC/BPS underscores the heterogeneity of the condition, but also suggests that individualized strategies of care will ultimately benefit patients.

ETIOLOGY

It is likely that IC/BPS has a multifactorial cause that may act predominantly through one or more pathways, resulting in the typical symptoms (Clemens et al., 2019, Hanno et al., 2013; Nordling et al., 2017; Patnaik et al., 2017) (Fig. 57.4). There is an abundance of theories regarding its pathogenesis, but confirmatory evidence gleaned from clinical practice has proven sparse. Among numerous proposals that have been explored are "leaky epithelium," mast cell activation, and neurogenic inflammation, or some combination of these and other factors leading to a self-perpetuating process resulting in chronic bladder pain and voiding dysfunction (Elbadawi, 1997). IBS, FMS, chronic fatigue syndrome, and various other chronic pain disorders may precede or follow the development of IC/BPS in some patients (Kim and Chang, 2012), but development of associated syndromes is not inevitable by any means, and their relationship to the cause is currently unknown (Warren et al., 2009). It has been postulated

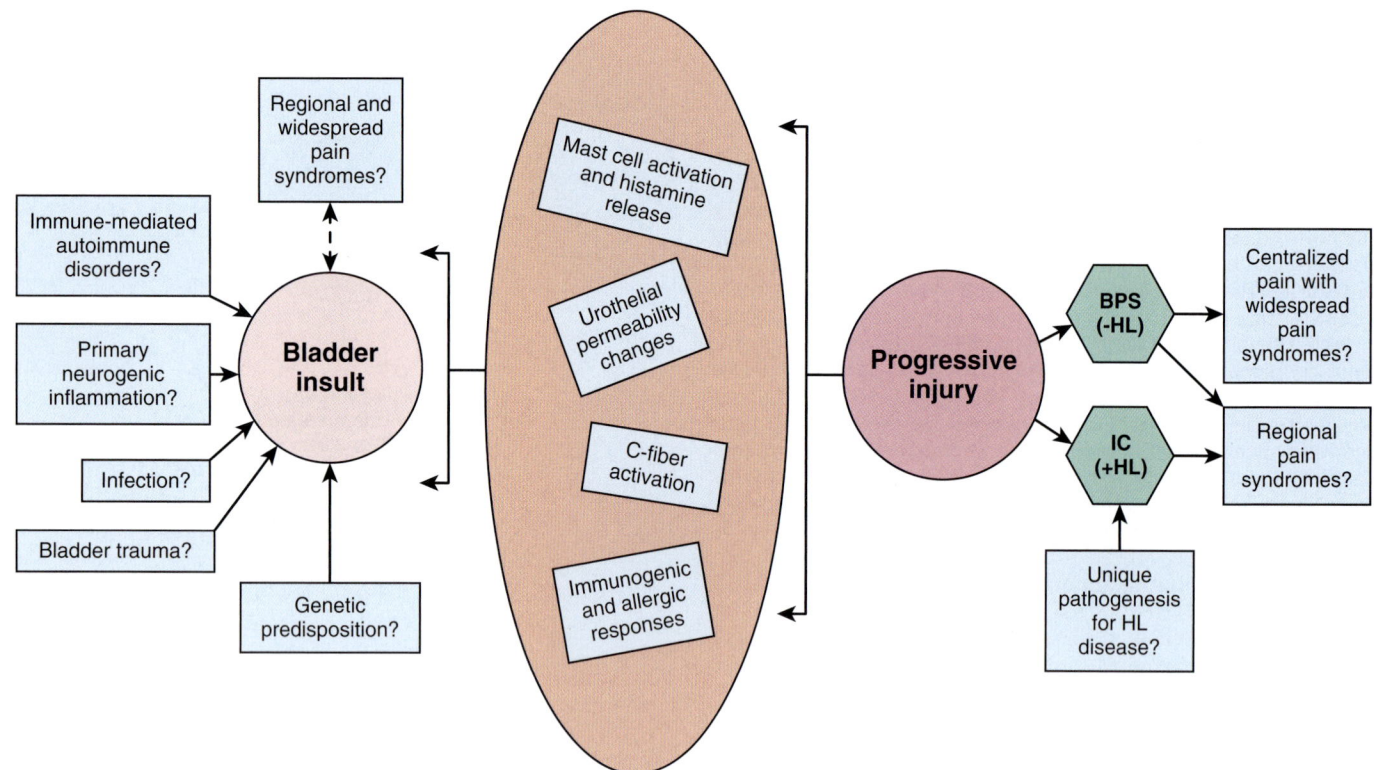

Fig. 57.4. Multiple etiologic factors may play a role in the development of interstitial cystitis *(IC)*/bladder pain syndrome *(BPS)* symptoms. Current concepts of pathogenesis include its common association with pain beyond the bladder, (regional and widespread). Note the proposed distinction between patients with Hunner lesions (+HL), designated as *IC*, and those without Hunner lesions (–HL), designated as *BPS*.

that neural cross-talk in the dorsal root ganglia, in the spinal cord, and at the level of the brain might play a role in the development of chronic pain disorders and their clinical associations through central sensitization (Furuta et al., 2012). This phenomenon may explain the lack of physical findings in many IC/BPS patients and their non-response to local therapies.

A discussion of animal models and the possible role of infection, autoimmunity, inflammation, mast cells, histamine, epithelial permeability, antiproliferative factor (APF), neurogenic factors, cross-sensitization, urine abnormalities, genetic factors, stress, and pelvic floor dysfunction can be found online at ExpertConsult.com.

PATHOLOGY

There is no histology pathognomonic of IC/BPS. This is not surprising given a medical condition that is primarily based on the complaint of visceral pain; and this reinforces the need for accurate phenotyping. Other factors that may obfuscate histologic studies include: duration of disease, recent trauma (e.g., hydrodistention), history of bacterial cystitis, and even the location or type of biopsy. These factors align with the great variation in the reported histologic appearance of biopsy specimens from IC/BPS patients, and even the microscopic variation among biopsies taken from the same patients over time (Gillenwater and Wein, 1988).

Histologic features of IC/BPS can be remarkably bland. On the other hand, inflammatory features can be seen in 24% to 76% of patients without a visible HL (Erickson et al., 2008b). Rosamilia presented data comparing light microscopic changes of IC/BPS bladder biopsies to controls (Hanno et al., 2005a; Rosamilia et al., 2003). Although epithelial denudation, submucosal edema, congestion and ectasia, and inflammatory infiltrate were increased in the IC/BPS group, histologic parameters were normal and indistinguishable from control subjects in 55% of IC/BPS specimens. Method of biopsy can be important in interpreting findings, because transurethral resection biopsy specimens tend to show mucosal ruptures, submucosal hemorrhage, and mild inflammation (Johansson and Fall, 1990), whereas histology is normal approximately half the time with cold-cup forceps biopsy specimens (Lynes et al., 1990a; Mattila, 1982; Rosamilia et al., 2003).

Striking differences in histopathology, primarily based on severity of inflammatory events, distinguish IC/BPS with HLs (IC/BPS+HL) and IC/BPS without HLs (IC/BPS-HL). This point, along with little data to support transition from IC/BPS-HL to IC/BPS+HL (Fall et al., 1987), **argues that these conditions may be completely separate disorders.** Johansson and Fall (1990) evaluated 64 patients with IC/BPS+HL and 44 with IC/BPS–HL. The former group had mucosal ulceration and hemorrhage, granulation tissue, intense inflammatory infiltrate (predominantly plasma cells and lymphocytes), elevated mast cell counts, and perineural infiltrates. The IC/BPS–HL group, despite having the same severe symptoms, had a relatively unaltered mucosa with a sparse inflammatory response, the main feature being multiple, small mucosal ruptures and suburothelial hemorrhages that were noted in a high proportion of patients. As these specimens were almost all taken immediately after hydrodistention, how much of the admittedly minimal findings in the IC/BPS–HL group was purely iatrogenic is a matter of speculation. The same group later reported the frequent finding of completely normal biopsy specimens in IC/BPS–HL patients (Johansson and Fall, 1994). Furthering these results, Maeda et al. (2015) found a severe lymphoplasmocytic infiltrate in 93% of IC/BPS+HL biopsies versus only 8% of IC/BPS–HL biopsies. They identified epithelial denudation to be a distinct feature of IC/BPS+HL that is not confined to the HL, and suggests a fieldlike change to the bladder surface. Although most studies report few inflammatory events associated with IC/BPS–HL (Akiyama et al., 2019), a recent study described more severe bladder wall fibrosis and increased mast cell infiltration in these patients (Kim et al., 2017). Several studies have suggested that a severely abnormal pathology may be associated with a poor prognosis (McDougald and Landon, 2003; Nordling et al., 2004); this is not necessarily the case (MacDermott et al., 1991a).

Mast cell proliferation, activation, and degranulation may play a role in the pathogenesis of IC/BPS (Theoharides and Stewart, 2017). Mast cells trigger inflammation that is associated with local pain, but the mechanisms mediating pain are unclear. In a murine model of neurogenic cystitis, Rudick et al. (2008) demonstrated that mast cells promote cystitis pain and bladder pathophysiology through the separable actions of histamine and TNF, respectively. Mast cell density has been repeatedly studied as a potential marker for IC/BPS, but results have been disparate (Gamper et al., 2015; Holm-Bentzen et al., 1987a; Larsen et al., 2008; Moore et al., 1992; Regauer et al., 2017) partially because of methodologic differences. A recent study employing immunohistochemical localization of mast cells with anti–mast cell tryptase found increased subepithelial and detrusor mast cell density in patients with IC/BPS+HL, but this finding was of low predictive value. Furthermore, there were no differences in mast cell density between IC/BPS–HL and specimens from patients with OAB (Gamper et al., 2015). Another study using digital quantitative analysis detailed the similarities of mast cell density between IC/BPS+HL and specimens with "chronic cystitis" and between IC/BPS–HL and normal controls. As one might expect, mast cell density correlated to general lymphoplasmocytic cell density (Akiyama et al., 2017). **Collectively, these findings suggest that mast cell counts, although perhaps relevant to pathogenesis, have no role in the diagnosis of IC/BPS.**

Specialized preparation of specimens may yield insights into pathophysiology and aid in diagnosis. Immunohistochemical staining techniques were used to identify nerve fibers, B-lymphocytes, the NGF receptor (p75^{NTR}), and mast cells performed on biopsy specimens from IC/BPS–HL, IC/BPS+HL, OAB, and normal control individuals. Sensory hyperinnervation, basal urothelial p75^{NTR} staining, and an assessment of B-lymphocyte and tissue integrity enabled the differentiation of both IC/BPS+HL and IC/BPS–HL from OAB and normal control specimens (Regauer et al., 2017).

At this time, the role of histopathology in the diagnosis of IC/BPS is limited to those patients with HLs in whom one must rule out carcinoma and carcinoma in situ, eosinophilic cystitis, tuberculous cystitis, and any other entities with a specific tissue diagnosis (Hellstrom et al., 1979; Johansson and Fall, 1990; Tsiriopoulos et al., 2006).

KEY POINTS: PATHOLOGY

- The role of histopathology is primarily to exclude other possible diagnoses that might be responsible for the symptoms.
- There is no histology pathognomonic of IC/BPS, and one cannot make the diagnosis on pathology alone in the absence of the cardinal symptoms.
- Completely normal-appearing bladder biopsy specimens in symptomatic patients are common.

Diagnosis

Current diagnostic strategies for IC/BPS are primarily based on its definition rather than strict research criteria established about 30 years ago. The definition—chronic pain, pressure, or discomfort associated with the bladder, usually accompanied by urinary frequency in the absence of any other identifiable cause (Hanno et al., 2005a, 2005b)—has been carefully crafted to incorporate noxious terms beyond "pain" that are commonly voiced by patients. The definition incorporates "urinary frequency" (that is often driven by the pain) but intentionally omits "urgency," a term that is poorly understood by patients and clinicians alike and generally aligns with a diagnosis of OAB syndrome.

Perhaps the most challenging aspect to accurately diagnose IC/BPS is excluding other identifiable causes of symptoms. In the authors' experience, failure to diagnose other causes of pelvic pain that may occur with or without IC/BPS is one of the most common reasons for therapeutic failure.

Table 57.5 summarizes confusable diseases related to IC/BPS and their mode of exclusion based on diagnostic proposals and procedures modified from the ESSIC group (van de Merwe et al., 2008). **It is of utmost importance for the clinician to identify and treat all pelvic pain generators (usually in a stepwise fashion) for optimal success, and this is stressed in a suggested diagnostic algorithm modified from AUA guidelines (Fig. 57.5).**

A detailed history, physical examination, and urine studies will, in almost all circumstances, give the clinician enough clues to exclude common well-described sources of pelvic pain that might be confused with IC/BPS (Box 57.2). As described in guidelines suggested by the American Urological Association, basic urine studies including a urinalysis and urine culture are needed. The urine culture is suggested to exclude low counts of bacteria that might produce symptoms in the face of a negative urinalysis (Duldulao et al., 1997; Hanno et al., 2011). The value of urine cytology needs to be weighed against the emotional distress that could result from the frequently encountered false-positive result (Davis et al., 2012). Nevertheless, the examination should be considered in the face of clinical factors such as smoking history, age over 40 years, and irritative voiding symptoms.

Difficulties of diagnosis are multiplied by the overlap of other visceral pain syndromes such as male CPPS (Forrest and Schmidt, 2004; Hakenberg and Wirth, 2002). As mentioned earlier in this chapter, similarities between these groups of patients are so striking that they are currently being studied collectively under the rubric of UCPPS by the MAPP Network (Clemens et al., 2015).

Although a table of common confusable disorders is provided (see Table 57.5), two confusable conditions bear special mention as they are likely to be encountered more frequently by the urologic community over the next several years.

Ketamine Cystitis

Ketamine, an NMDA receptor antagonist, is an anesthetic agent and newly popularized treatment for depression that when used recreationally may produce a clinical picture indistinguishable from IC/BPS (Chen et al., 2018; Gauney et al., 2016). Ketamine's rise in popularity as a recreational "club" drug (with street names including "special K," "super K," "super acid," "kate," "cat valium," "ket," "keller," and "vitamin K") includes its rapid onset and short duration of action (Smith et al., 2002). Ketamine also produces a "dissociative anesthesia" that may be characterized as an unconscious, trancelike state with profound analgesia (Sinner and Graf, 2008). Although ketamine's recreational use appears to have initially blossomed in Asia, abuse has since spread internationally. In 2015, an estimated 2.3 million people in the United States older than 12 years of age were reported to have abused ketamine, with 200,000 having used it within the previous year (National Institute on Drug Abuse, 2015). In a survey of 1900 New York City club-frequenting adults 18 to 29 years of age, 21% admitted to ketamine use, with slightly higher usage by men (Kelly et al., 2006). Mounting evidence suggests ketamine and/or its urine metabolites (e.g., hydroquinone), may be responsible for many of the pathologic and clinical manifestations of this condition (Baker et al., 2016; Misra, 2018). Specific pathologies that have been identified include bladder barrier dysfunction, neurogenic inflammation, immunoglobulin-E–mediated inflammation, overexpression of carcinogenic genes, enhanced apoptosis, and nitric oxide synthase–mediated inflammation (Jhang et al., 2015). The severity of ketamine cystitis' inflammatory effects appear to be related to the duration of abuse (Gauney et al., 2016; Mak et al., 2011). Early presentation may manifest as only LUTS. Progression of disease is typified by additional complaints including dysuria, worsening frequency, gross hematuria, and pelvic pain. Further ketamine use may produce gross inflammatory changes similar in appearance but usually more widespread than HLs. These inflammatory changes, left unchecked, may result in irreversible bladder wall fibrosis, upper urinary tract changes, and renal dysfunction (Chen et al., 2011; Middela and Pearce, 2011). Successful management of ketamine cystitis begins with early identification and the cessation of ketamine abuse, the latter being the most important and challenging part of care. Hence, we cannot stress enough the importance of rehabilitation

TABLE 57.5 Disorders That May Be Mistaken for IC/BPS

CONFUSABLE DISORDER	EXCLUDED OR DIAGNOSED BY
Carcinoma and carcinoma in situ	Cystoscopy, biopsy
Infection with:	
Common intestinal bacteria	Routine bacterial culture
Chlamydia trachomatis, Ureaplasma urealyticum, Mycoplasma hominis, Mycoplasma genitalium, Corynebacterium urealyticum, Candida species, *Mycobacterium tuberculosis*	Special cultures Dipstick; if "sterile" pyuria, culture for *M. tuberculosis*
Herpes simplex, herpes zoster	Medical history, physical examination
Radiation	Medical history
Chemotherapy, including immunotherapy with cyclophosphamide	Medical history
Anti-inflammatory therapy with tiaprofenic acid	Medical history
Ketamine cystitis	Medical history
Bladder neck obstruction and neurogenic outlet obstruction	Medical history, urodynamic evaluation
Bladder stone; lower ureteral stone	Imaging or cystoscopy, CT
Urethral diverticulum	Medical history, physical examination, MRI
Colon cancer, diverticulitis, irritable bowel syndrome; inflammatory bowel disease	Medical history, physical examination, colonoscopy
Urogenital prolapse	Medical history, physical examination
Endometriosis, adenomyosis	Medical history, physical examination, imaging studies (i.e., MRI/pelvic ultrasonography) as appropriate
Pelvic congestion syndrome	Medical history, pelvic ultrasonography
Vaginal candidiasis	Medical history, physical examination, vaginal cultures as appropriate
Cervical, uterine, and ovarian cancer	Physical examination, pelvic ultrasonography
Vulvodynia	Medical history and physical examination
Incomplete bladder emptying (retention)	Postvoid residual urine volume measured by ultrasound evaluation
Overactive bladder	Medical history; urodynamic evaluation as appropriate
Prostate cancer	Physical examination, serum PSA
Benign prostatic obstruction	Medical history, physical examination, uroflowmetry and pressure-flow studies in selected cases
Chronic bacterial prostatitis	Medical history, physical examination, culture
Chronic nonbacterial prostatitis	Medical history, physical examination, culture
Pudendal nerve entrapment	Medical history, physical examination, nerve block may prove diagnosis
Abdominal wall hernia	Medical history, physical examination
Pelvic floor muscle–related pain	Medical history, physical examination

CT, Computed tomography; *MRI,* magnetic resonance imaging; *PSA,* prostate-specific antigen.
Modified from van de Merwe JP, Nordling J, Bouchelouche P, et al. Diagnostic criteria, classification, and nomenclature for painful bladder syndrome/interstitial cystitis: an ESSIC proposal. *Eur Urol* 53(1):60–67, 2008.

in this patient population. **Although ketamine abuse may be seen at any age, the clinician should be especially wary of the young patient who presents with a clinical picture of IC/BPS with visible inflammation of the bladder wall.**

High-Tone Pelvic Floor Dysfunction

HTPFD is commonly identified in patients with urologic, gynecologic, and colorectal pain syndromes (Kuo et al., 2015). Symptoms associated with HTPFD often include pelvic pressure, persistent urgency, the sensation of incomplete bladder emptying (in severe cases, poor bladder emptying is identified), urinary hesitancy, constipation, dyspareunia (pain often experienced the next day), and perineal, penile, and ejaculatory pain (Srinivasan et al., 2007). Although not essential for diagnosis, video-urodynamic evaluation suggests that poor relaxation of the external sphincter is common in IC/BPS (Kuo and Kuo, 2018). Examination of the pelvic floor has identified a myofascial trigger point in approximately 78% of IC/BPS patients, with multiple trigger points identified in 68% of individuals (Bassaly et al., 2011).

HTPFD often magnifies the pain of IC/BPS, or it may be the sole cause of symptoms. In either case, it has been our observation that failure to diagnose HTPFD in the presumed IC/BPS patient will commonly lead to a suboptimal response, as treatment strategies differ between the two conditions. **Hallmarks of HTPFD include the presence of hypertonic pelvic and nearby accessory musculature, muscle banding, and myofascial trigger points, the latter being described as tender "knots" in taut muscle band that produce pain** (Bron and Dommerholt, 2012). One should be particularly concerned about the presence of HTPFD in the patient who endorses a history of dysfunctional voiding, bowel disturbances, and sexual pain; the bowel

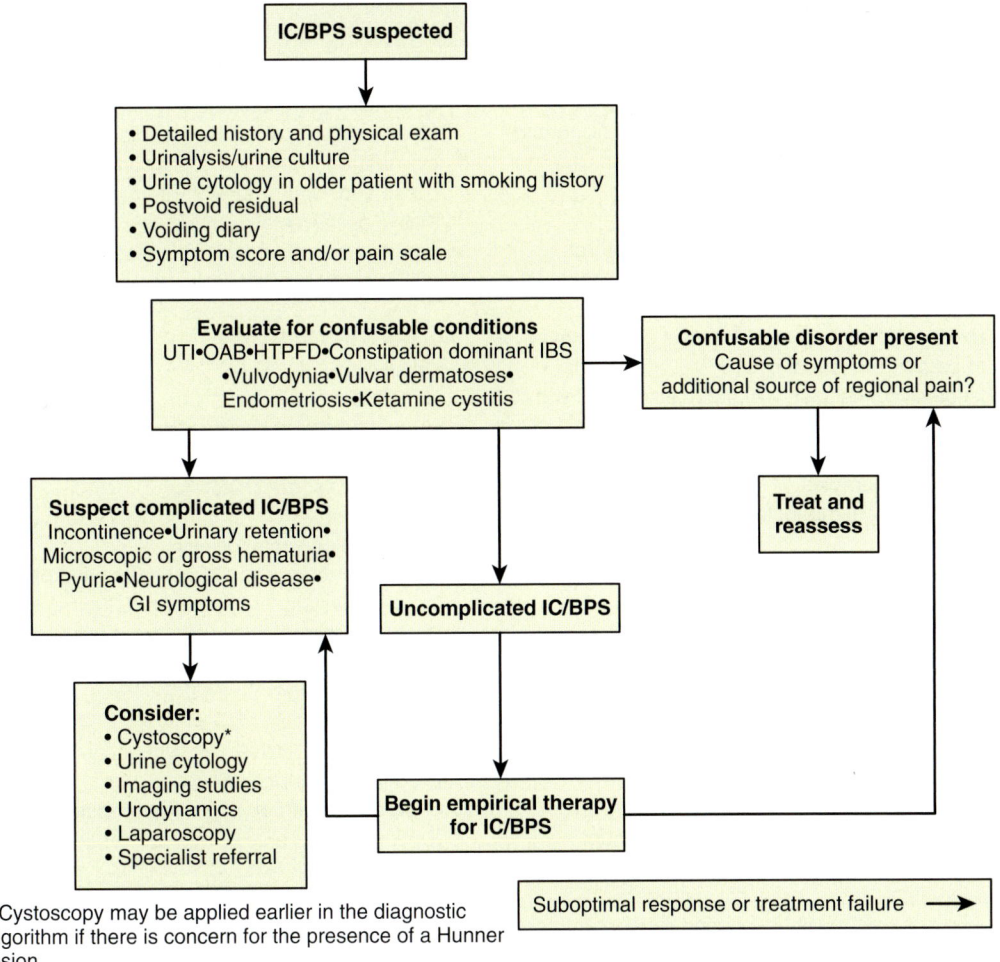

Fig. 57.5. Proposed diagnostic algorithm for evaluation of interstitial cystitis/bladder pain syndrome (IC/BPS). *GI*, Gastrointestinal; *HTPFD*, high-tone pelvic floor dysfunction; *IBS*, irritable bowel syndrome; *OAB*, overactive bladder; *UTI*, urinary tract infection. Modified from Hanno PM, Burks DA, Clemens JQ, et al. AUA guideline for the diagnosis and treatment of interstitial cystitis/bladder pain syndrome. *J Urol* 185(6):2162–2170, 2011.

and bladder disturbances often date back to childhood (Doiron et al., 2017). Physical examination should include a detailed palpation of the pelvic floor musculature and adjacent musculature. If HTPFD is suspected, physical therapy evaluation by a pelvic floor specialist is suggested (Polackwich et al., 2015). A multimodal program consisting of physical therapy, behavior modification (avoidance of straining maneuvers, "reverse Kegels," stress reduction), topical heat application, skeletal muscle relaxants, control of constipation, and even anesthetic or botulinum neurotoxin type A (BTX-A) injections (myofascial trigger point injections) to affected muscles may be helpful to ameliorate symptoms (Moldwin and Fariello, 2013; Halder et al., 2017).

BEYOND THE HISTORY, PHYSICAL EXAMINATION, AND URINE STUDIES

The Voiding Diary

Baseline information regarding urinary frequency and volumes voided are helpful for diagnostic purposes and to follow patient progress. One 24-hour period with time of void and volume is usually all that is needed (Mazurick and Landis, 2000). Mounting pelvic discomfort with filling typically drives *low-volume urinary frequency*. The voiding pattern may be indistinguishable from other conditions including OAB or other forms of voiding dysfunction. On the other hand, the finding of frequent but high-volume voids that solely occur during the daytime may suggest other diagnoses.

The use of Symptom Scales for Clinical Assessment and Research is described online at ExpertConsult.com.

Urodynamic Evaluation

The primary value of urodynamic studies in the evaluation of IC/BPS is limited to the identification of other functional bladder pathology(ies) that may confound diagnosis and hinder therapeutic progress.

Cystometry in IC/BPS patients typically demonstrates normal detrusor function but a decreased bladder capacity and hypersensitivity. Bladder compliance is normal, as hypersensitivity would prevent the bladder from filling to the point of noncompliance (Siroky, 1994). Pain on bladder filling that reproduces the patient's symptoms is very suggestive of the diagnosis.

Many dispute the need for urodynamic study noting that most patients can be treated successfully based on the clinical presentation. Bladder outlet obstruction is a common occurrence in the female IC/BPS patient, presumably related to pelvic floor dysfunction (Cameron and Gajewski, 2009). The authors suggested that typical symptoms of voiding dysfunction should prompt a course of dedicated therapy and that urodynamic evaluation adds little information to change the course of care.

DO and IC/BPS may coexist in 15% to 19% of patients (Gajewski et al., 1997, Kirkemo et al., 1997). The case for urodynamics to exclude concomitant DO as a cause for irritative voiding symptoms

BOX 57.2 Highlights of Clinical Evaluation for the Pelvic Pain Patient

HISTORY
General thorough medical history emphasizing the following:
1. Location of pelvic pain and relationship to bladder filling and emptying
2. Presence/absence of initiating event for pain
3. Duration, quality, and radiation of pain
4. Presence/absence of regional pain (i.e., penile, urethral [dysuria?], vulvar, perineal, perianal, testicular, inguinal, coccygeal)
5. Presence or absence of voiding and/or bowel dysfunction
6. Relationship of pain to menstrual cycle
7. Presence/absence of sexual pain (i.e., pain associated with ejaculation, orgasm, entry, and/or deep dyspareunia)
8. Factors that trigger or decrease pain
9. Response to previous therapies
10. History of urologic/gastroenterologic, gynecologic/neurologic/rheumatic disease
11. Previous bladder/pelvic surgery
12. Previous urinary tract infection
13. Previous pelvic irradiation
14. Autoimmune diseases
15. Associated syndromes (irritable bowel, fibromyalgia, chronic fatigue)

PHYSICAL EXAMINATION
Physical examination emphasizing the following:
1. Abdominal examination: identification of tender anterior abdominal wall musculature, hernias, abdominal distention (tympany), bladder distention, suprapubic tenderness
2. Females: vaginal examination with inspection for abnormal discharge, vulvar dermatoses (i.e., introital mucosal atrophy, lichen sclerosus); pain mapping of vulvar region with Q-tip; one-digit vaginal palpation to identify tenderness or other abnormalities of the bladder, bladder neck, and/or urethra; evaluation for tenderness, hypertonicity, or trigger points of pelvic floor and obturator internus muscles

   Males: digital rectal examination with pain mapping of the scrotal-anal region; evaluation for tenderness, hypertonicity, or trigger points of anal sphincter, pelvic floor, and obturator internus muscles

LABORATORY TESTING
1. Urinalysis
2. Urine culture
3. Urine cytology in risk groups

SYMPTOM EVALUATION
1. Voiding diary
2. Visual analog scale for pain
3. Symptom score (i.e., O'Leary-Sant symptom and problem index, University of Wisconsin IC Scale, Pelvic Pain and Urgency/Frequency questionnaire [PUF], Genitourinary Pain Index [GUPI], male or female version, Bladder Pain/Interstitial Cystitis Symptom Score [BPIC-SS])

OTHER EVALUATIONS
1. Urodynamics (optional)
2. Cystoscopy with or without hydrodistention under anesthesia (Optional. The value of hydrodistention is controversial as indicated in the text.)
3. Bladder biopsy if bladder lesion identified

Modified from Hanno P, Lin AT, Nordling J, et al. Bladder pain syndrome. In: Abrams P, Cardozo L, Khoury S, et al., eds. *Incontinence.* Paris: Health Publications Limited; 2009:1459–1518.

(not pain) is debatable, as empirical therapy can easily be justified as a first-line maneuver. Additionally, medications such as amitriptyline, often used early in the course of care, have anticholinergic properties, which may resolve the issue. Of course, urodynamic evaluation would likely provide useful information for those patients who fail empirical therapy or those who present with a confusing clinical picture (e.g., pain, urgency frequency, and urinary retention). Complex cases may benefit from full video-urodynamic studies (Carlson et al., 2001).

Office Cystoscopy

Current guidelines established by the American Urological Association do not require cystoscopic evaluation in the *routine* management of IC/BPS as visual findings are generally unrevealing. We favor early endoscopy as the finding of a Hunner lesion would direct management in a different (usually more aggressive) direction. **Although the extent of HLs has been correlated to symptom severity and bladder capacity** (Akiyama et al., 2018), **they cannot be reliably identified on the basis of clinical presentation or urine studies** (Braunstein et al., 2008; Doiron et al., 2016). Experimental data suggest that measurement of increased nitric oxide levels in the bladder can accurately identify those with inflammatory disease, but this has not folded over to routine clinical care (Logadottir et al., 2004). Flexible cystoscopy in the office setting can be accomplished with minimal discomfort and often provides the patient with immediate relief from concerns of bladder cancer. HLs can be identified (Fig. 57.6). Narrow-band imaging may enhance the identification of subtle lesions during the office procedure (Kajiwara et al., 2014).

Although perhaps not as sophisticated as standard urodynamic evaluation, bladder filling during the examination allows an assessment of bladder capacity (best obtained with the voiding diary) and reproduction of pain with bladder filling. Specific sites of hyperalgesia such as the bladder neck can also be identified using the tip of the cystoscope as an examining finger. On a final note, office cystoscopy offers an opportunity to drain the bladder, then to introduce an anesthetic (i.e., alkalinized) lidocaine. Significant relief of pain after this "anesthetic challenge" suggests a bladder origin to pain. Lack of response does not exclude a diagnosis of IC/BPS (Cox et al., 2016).

Cystoscopy With Hydrodistention and Biopsy

Long before it was considered a diagnostic tool, cystoscopy with hydrodistention (CHD) was used as a therapeutic modality for IC/BPS (Bumpus, 1930). **CHD under anesthesia allows for sufficient distention of the bladder to afford visualization of submucosal pinpoint petechial hemorrhages, termed *glomerulations* (Fig. 57.7). After filling to 80 cm of water pressure for 1 to 2 minutes, the bladder is drained and refilled. The terminal portion of the effluent is often blood-tinged. Reinspection will reveal the glomerulations that develop throughout the bladder after distention and** are not usually seen during examination without anesthesia (Nigro et al., 1997b).

Glomerulations are not specific for IC/BPS (Erickson, 1995; Waxman et al., 1998), and only when seen in conjunction with the clinical criteria of pain and frequency can the finding of glomerulations be viewed as potentially significant. **Glomerulations can be seen after radiation therapy, in patients with carcinoma, after exposure to

Chapter 57 Interstitial Cystitis/Bladder Pain Syndrome and Related Disorders

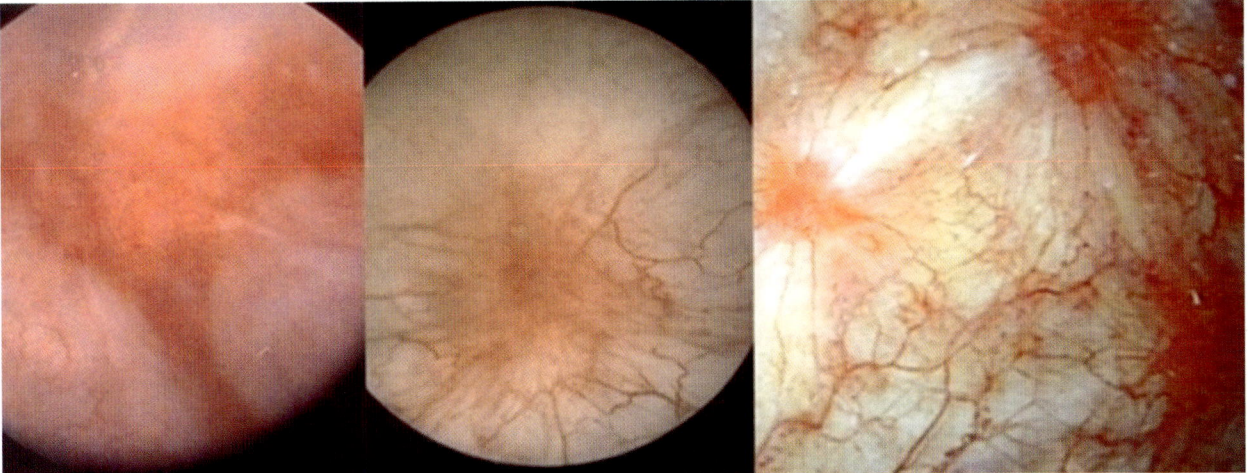

Fig. 57.6. Varied appearances of Hunner lesions identified on routine cystoscopic examination. Note the stellate appearance. Bleeding and disruption of the lesions usually occurs centrally with bladder distention. Fibrous bridging between lesions may occur, which further restricts bladder capacity.

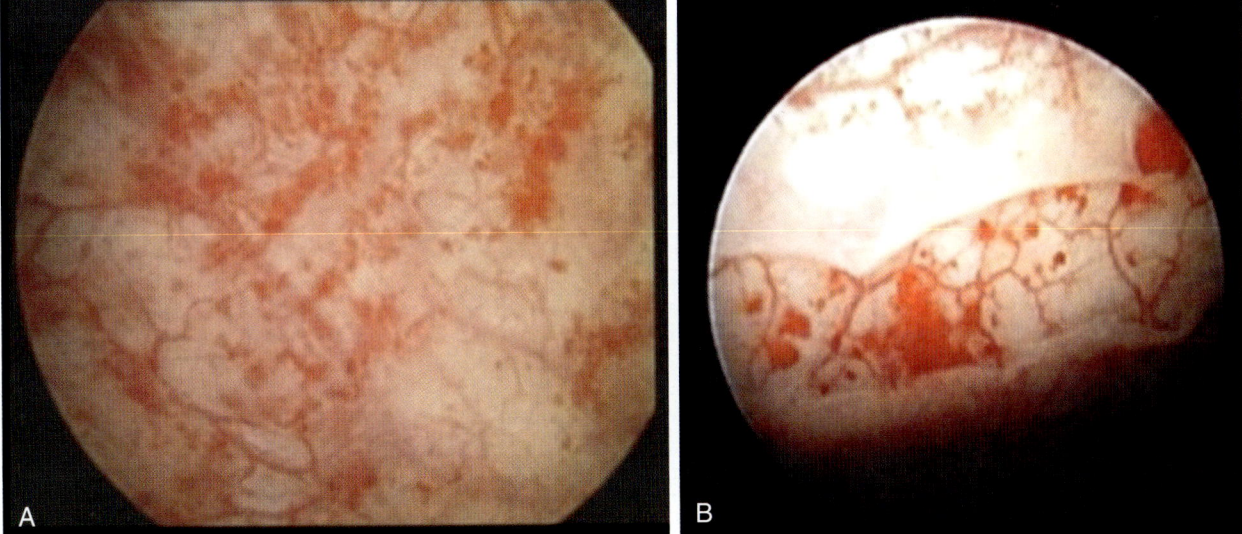

Fig. 57.7. (A) Typical appearance of glomerulations after bladder distention in a patient with interstitial cystitis/bladder pain syndrome without a Hunner lesion. (B) Mucosal tears that frequently develop during hydrodistention, often near the bladder neck (note the submucosal glomerulations).

toxic chemicals or chemotherapeutic agents, and often in patients on dialysis or after urinary diversion when the bladder has not filled for prolonged periods. They have been reported in the majority of men with prostate pain syndromes, begging the question as to whether CPPS in men is closely linked with IC (Berger et al., 1998). They are observed in up to 20% of men undergoing transurethral prostatectomy for LUTS (Furuya et al., 2007). We have speculated that they may simply reflect the response of the bladder to distention after a prolonged period of chronic underfilling because of sensory urgency, rather than resulting from a primary pathologic process.

Further confusion arises when the patient demonstrates the symptoms of IC/BPS but the cystoscopic findings under anesthesia are completely normal. This occurred in 8.7% of patients undergoing CHD entered into the IC database (Messing et al., 1997). Awad et al. recognized this entity soon after the NIDDK research criteria had been described. They reported on a series of patients in whom the symptomatology, urodynamic evaluation findings, histology, and response to therapy were identical to IC/BPS but in whom findings on CHD were normal. It was termed *idiopathic reduced bladder storage* (Awad et al., 1992). Clinical, urodynamic, and cystoscopic data strongly suggest that the presence of glomerulations is not selecting out a meaningful difference in patients with symptoms of IC/BPS (Al Hadithi et al., 2002; Wennevik et al., 2016).

The presence of glomerulations on cystoscopy with hydrodistention may identify a group of patients with worse daytime frequency and nocturia, lower mean voiding volumes, and lower bladder capacity under anesthesia, but does not have any relationship to biopsy findings, bladder pain, or urgency (Boudry et al., 2013; Erickson et al., 2005). **A low bladder capacity at the time of hydrodistention (anesthetic bladder capacity) may represent a distinct clinical phenotype, having higher symptom scores and fewer reports of depression and IBS, essentially a more bladder-centric patient picture** (Walker et al., 2017).

Although hydrodistention has been commonly employed to provoke the appearance of an HL, this practice has been recently questioned (Nickel and Moldwin, 2018). As noted in the preceding section, office cystoscopy can easily identify these lesions. Furthermore, the finding of a focal bladder lesion that can only be identified on the basis of distention of the bladder well beyond its normal functional capacity suggests that this group may represent a different place in the spectrum of disease or a different phenotype altogether.

Despite a possible role to phenotype patients, the value of cystoscopy with hydrodistention for diagnosis appears to be clinically limited. Bladder biopsy is indicated only if necessary to rule out other disorders that might be suggested by the

cystoscopic appearance. One common indication for biopsy is to differentiate an HL from carcinoma in situ.

The Search for a Marker

Development of a specific marker for a symptom complex that may coexist with other regional or widespread pain syndromes is daunting and probably unrealistic. Rather, we hope that biomarker development will help stratify patients into phenotypic subgroups that may share similar pathology and response to therapy. The markers themselves may also represent therapeutic targets for future drug development. Markers that have been studied fall into groups including: inflammatory mediators, proteoglycans, urinary hexosamines and GAG, proliferative factors, nitric oxide, urothelial proinflammatory gene expression, and viruses (Grigorescu et al., 2016).

One of the earliest studied markers for diagnosis of IC/BPS was the mast cell count. Biopsies were routinely obtained (at the time of hydrodistention) and analyzed in a standardized fashion with greater than 27 mast cells per cubic millimeter being indicative of mastocytosis (Larsen et al., 2008). Studies regarding the mast cell count's role for IC/BPS diagnosis were conflicting, and no study to date has associated mast cell counts with response to therapy (e.g., antihistamines). Given these factors, the use of mast cell criteria is not recommended outside the realm of research (Christmas and Rode, 1991; Dundore et al., 1996; Feltis et al., 1987; Hanno et al., 1991; Holm-Bentzen et al., 1987a; Kastrup et al., 1983; Lynes et al., 1987; Moore et al., 1992). Methylhistamine, a histamine metabolite found in the urine and thought to reflect mast cell activation, was not associated with symptom scores, response to bladder distention, cystoscopic findings, or bladder biopsy features including mast cell determination by tryptase staining (Erickson et al., 2004).

Multiple urinary markers have been investigated (Erickson, 2001, Erickson et al., 2002), including eosinophil cationic protein (Lose et al., 1987), GAG excretion (Hurst et al., 1993), and urinary histamine and methylhistamine (El Mansoury et al., 1994). Proposals for measuring smooth muscle isoactin expression (Rivas et al., 1997) and urinary levels of neurotrophin-3, nerve growth factor, glial cell line–derived neurotrophic factor, and tryptase (Okragly et al., 1999) have been suggested. Low levels of GP51, a urinary glycoprotein with a molecular weight of 5 kDa, have been documented in IC patients compared with normal controls and patients with other urinary tract disease (Byrne et al., 1999), suggesting surface mucin aberrations.

The measurement of elevated nitric oxide levels in air instilled and incubated in the bladder has been proposed for office screening (Ehrén et al., 1999; Lundberg et al., 1996). Increased levels of endogenously formed nitric oxide in patients with IC correspond to increased iNOS mRNA expression and protein levels in these patients. Furthermore, iNOS was found to be localized to the urothelium, but it was also found in macrophages in the bladder mucosa (Koskela et al., 2008). The simple technique allows for discrimination of ulcer from non-HL disease (Logadottir et al., 2004) and may provide an objective measure of treatment response (Hosseini et al., 2004).

Urinary macrophage inhibitory factor (MIF) levels in female patients with IC/BPS and HLs are approximately fivefold higher than MIF levels in female non-IC/BPS patients or IC/BPS patients without HLs. Urinary MIF was also elevated in males with other forms of bladder inflammation (bacterial and radiation cystitis), indicating that, although a good marker to detect inflammation, MIF was not specific for the presence of IC/BPS with HLs. Nevertheless, the assay may better select out those patients who would benefit from early cystoscopic evaluation, and it may pose as a target for future therapies for IC/BPS and other inflammation-based bladder diseases (Vera et al., 2018).

Patients with HLs were found to have a 5-fold to 20-fold increase in the chemokines CXCL-10 and CXCL-1, interleukin-6, and nerve growth factor when compared with BPS patients without HLs (Tyagi et al., 2012). Different expression patterns of the genes involved in pronociceptive inflammatory reactions suggest distinct pathophysiologies for HL patients compared with patients with IC/BPS without HLs (Homma et al., 2013).

Of all biomarkers analyzed for the diagnosis of IC/BPS to date, none has shown higher sensitivity (95%) and specificity (95%) to differentiate IC/BPS from healthy controls than urinary antiproliferative factor (APF), a "frizzled 8 protein" that belongs to a family of proteins that appear to have a role in the development of nerve tissues, skin, and the lining of organs (Keay et al., 2004b). APF is known to inhibit the proliferation of urothelial cells in vitro and is associated with decreased production of heparin-binding epidermal growth factor–like growth factor (HB-EGF) (Keay et al., 2000). APF activity was related to increased production of epidermal growth factor (EGF), insulin-like growth factor-1, and insulin-like growth factor–binding protein-3 by the bladder cells from IC/BPS patients but not by the cells from healthy bladders. Studies of IC/BPS patients and asymptomatic controls showed **urine levels of APF, HB-EGF, and EGF to reliably separate IC/BPS from controls** (Erickson et al., 2002; Keay et al., 2001b). Despite current concepts of overlapping pathologies between men with IC/BPS and CP/CPPS, APF levels in the urine were found to discriminate between men with IC/BPS versus those with CPPS or nonbacterial prostatitis (Keay et al., 2004a). Data regarding the reproducibility of APF and any practical clinical uses are lacking.

Uroplakin III-delta 4 is a potential marker for identifying IC/BPS with HLs (Zeng et al., 2007). The feasibility of diagnosing IC/BPS in humans and domestic cats from the spectra of dried serum films (DSFs) using infrared microspectroscopy has been reported (Rubio-Diaz et al., 2009).

Recent studies through the MAPP Network have shown female IC/BPS patients to exhibit a heightened inflammatory response compared with healthy controls as identified through stimulation of Toll-like receptor 2 (TLR2) and TLR4 in patient-derived peripheral blood mononuclear cells (PBMCs). A TLR4 inflammation score correlated strongest for pain frequency and intensity (Schrepf et al., 2014). A one standard deviation increase in TLR4 inflammatory response was associated with a 1.59 greater likelihood of extrapelvic pain. Furthermore, patients with comorbid syndromes had higher inflammatory responses to TLR4 stimulation in PBMCs. The TLR4 response was also associated with low-pressure pain thresholds (Schrepf et al., 2015). TLR7 is associated with SLE and SS, two inflammatory conditions that are more frequently identified in the IC/BPS population. Ichihara et al. identified increased *TLR7* gene expression and TLR7 immunoreactive cells in the bladder biopsies of IC/BPS patients with HLs compared with control specimens, further suggesting that these conditions may represent two different pathologic states (Ichihara et al., 2017). Differentiation of IC/BPS with HLs from other forms of cystitis is crucial for future investigations.

Potassium Chloride Test

The intravesical KCl challenge has been described as an aid to diagnose IC/BPS (Parsons et al., 1998). The test essentially compares the sensory nerve provocative ability of sodium versus potassium using a 0.4-M KCl solution. Pain and provocation of symptoms constitutes a positive test result. Whether the results indicate abnormal epithelial permeability in the subgroup of positive patients or hypersensitivity of the sensory nerves is unclear. When first described, the KCl test was thought to help identify the IC/BPS patient without the need for cystoscopy and hydrodistention under anesthesia. Of course, as our diagnostic paradigm has shifted to one that is symptom-based, the need for a provocative test, one that can result in a great deal of patient discomfort, has waned. Accordingly, **used as a diagnostic test for IC/BPS, the KCl test is not recommended.** Interestingly, a negative KCl test will be seen in up to 25% of patients meeting strict NIDDK research criteria (suggesting a lack of sensitivity in a group of patients that would more likely respond). Specificity has also been of concern as a 36% false-positive rate was identified in asymptomatic men (Yilmaz et al., 2004) and a 33% positive rate in a fixed population of Turkish textile workers (Sahinkanat et al., 2008). Sensitivity to the KCl solution may also be present in 25% of patients with OAB. Virtually all patients with irritative symptoms from radiation cystitis and urinary tract infection test positive (Parsons et al., 1994b, 1998). The results with chronic prostatitis and CPPS in men are variable, but 50% to 84% of men have been reported to test positive (Parsons and Albo, 2002; Parsons et al., 2005; Yilmaz et al., 2004). In women with pelvic pain, the results are similar (Parsons et al., 2002b), and, based on these findings, Parsons has expressed the view that IC/BPS may affect over 20% of the female population of the United States (Parsons et al., 2002a). Another way to interpret the findings would be that the KCl test is very nonspecific, missing a significant number of IC/BPS patients and overdiagnosing much of the population.

> **KEY POINTS: DIAGNOSIS**
>
> - IC/BPS remains a diagnosis of exclusion in patients who meet the symptomatic criteria for diagnosis.
> - The identification of confusable conditions that may mimic bladder-based pain or present as additional pain generators (e.g., HTPFD) is essential for a successful therapeutic outcome.
> - Although cystoscopy is not mandatory for diagnosis, a flexible office cystoscopy may be considered early in the course of care to exclude the presence of HLs.
> - Cystoscopy and upper tract imaging are mandatory in patients with hematuria who have not been previously evaluated for this finding.
> - Urodynamics are optional and usually reserved for complex cases.
> - There are no commonly available laboratory markers that substantially contribute to diagnosis.

TREATMENT OF INTERSTITIAL CYSTITIS/BLADDER PAIN SYNDROME

Before embarking on therapy for the IC/BPS patient, the clinician must first be cognizant that there is no "home run" therapy available that will apply to all patients, most certainly a result of heterogeneity of the population. This leaves a trial-and-error approach to treatment that can quickly breed frustration for the patient. Much of this frustration and perhaps secondary depression can be mitigated to a significant degree by establishing treatment goals and realistic expectations, moving forward as partners in management.

As in all disciplines of medicine, improved outcomes are often derived from factors that cannot be acquired from medical textbooks or videos. This is particularly apropos to IC/BPS, where management remains somewhat of an art form. (See Box 57.4, an algorithm with six tiers of therapeutic intervention.) This may sound straightforward, but can you use therapies of different tiers together? If so, which would be the best ones, and for which patients? Why should you choose one therapy over another? And what about those other pain generators? The answers to these questions are as diverse as the IC/BPS population. They are honed from routinely caring for afflicted patients; performing detailed, unhurried evaluations; making educated decisions regarding therapy based on multiple clinical factors (as diverse as difficulties with transportation to poor sleep quality to sexual dysfunction) along with known benefits and risks of the interventions; and then simply observing the therapeutic responses, good or bad.

General Principles of Therapy

As a general medical principle, conservative treatment strategies are recommended with progression to more aggressive care in the setting of poor symptom control and an unacceptable QoL (see Box 57.4). Re-evaluation to identify other sources of pain should also be considered in those patients who are not improving. Initial aggressive (higher-tier) care may be indicated for patients who present with severe symptomatology that, in the clinician's opinion, is unlikely to have an adequate response to more conservative measures. Although not formally studied, clinical experience suggests that concomitant treatments may yield the benefit of addressing different aspects of the patient's symptom profile and may reduce the need for higher-tier care. Placebo effect and regression to the mean is common in this population and needs to be taken into consideration during the first 3 to 4 weeks of therapy (Stephens-Shields et al., 2016). Clinicians and patients should discuss discontinuance (if only

BOX 57.4 Tiered Therapy for IC/BPS per AUA Guidelines[a]

FIRST-LINE TREATMENTS
- General relaxation/stress management
- Patient education
- Self-care/behavior modification
- Pain management

SECOND-LINE TREATMENTS
- Specialized manual physical therapy
- Oral agents: amitriptyline, hydroxyzine, cimetidine, PPS
- Intravesical therapy: DMSO, heparin, lidocaine
- Pain management

THIRD-LINE TREATMENTS
- Cystoscopy under anesthesia with hydrodistention
- Treatment of Hunner lesions, if found
- Pain management

FOURTH-LINE TREATMENTS
- Intradetrusor botulinum A toxin
- Neuromodulation
- Pain management

FIFTH-LINE TREATMENTS
- Cyclosporine A
- Pain management

SIXTH-LINE TREATMENTS
- Urinary diversion (with or without cystectomy)
- Substitution cystoplasty
- Pain management

[a]Note exceptions for sequential management in text.
Modified from Hanno PM, Erickson D, Moldwin R, et al. Diagnosis and treatment of interstitial cystitis/bladder pain syndrome: AUA Guideline Amendment. *J Urol* 193(5):1545–1553, 2015.

on a temporary basis) of longstanding therapy that has been of questionable benefit.

IC/BPS is a multifaceted condition that may require the talents of other practitioners to achieve an adequate reduction in symptoms. For example, cognitive behavior therapy applied by experienced mental health professionals may be helpful to address often-encountered catastrophic thinking (Tripp et al., 2017). If pudendal neuralgia is thought to be present, pudendal nerve blocks applied by trained clinicians may be helpful therapy and can also aid in diagnosis (Gupta et al., 2015; Singh et al., 2017). Anesthetic or BTX-A (non-FDA approved for this purpose) trigger-point injections to the pelvic floor musculature may reduce pain associated with HTPFD when more conservative methods such as directed physical therapy have reached a therapeutic plateau (Moldwin and Fariello, 2013). Chronic opioid therapy, with its well-known and recently highly publicized risks, is not routinely recommended for the IC/BPS patient (Engeler et al., 2013). Nevertheless, benefit may be had for carefully selected patients treated by pain management specialists familiar with "universal precautions" (Atkinson and Fudin, 2017). Gynecologic, gastroenterologic, and rheumatologic consultation, among others, should be sought early on in care, as appropriate.

Conservative Therapies

Stress reduction, exercise, warm tub baths, and efforts by the patient to maintain a normal lifestyle all contribute to overall QoL (Whitmore, 1994). In a large patient survey, dietary changes, application of heat or cold, and stress reduction all had positive response rates in more than 80% of responders (O'Hare et al., 2013). In a controlled study of 45 IC/BPS patients and 31 healthy controls, higher levels of stress were related to greater pain and urgency in patients with IC but not in the control group (Rothrock et al., 2001). Maladaptive strategies for coping with stress may adversely affect symptoms (Rothrock et al., 2003). Catastrophic thinking, the irrational, consuming fear of a disastrous outcome, appears to enhance the perception of pain, but may be modified with cognitive behavior therapy (Tripp et al., 2017).

Biofeedback, soft-tissue massage, and other physical therapies may aid in muscle relaxation of the pelvic floor (Holzberg et al., 2001; Lukban, et al., 2001; Markwell, 2001; Meadows, 1999; Mendelowitz et al., 1997). This is a reasonable intervention, given the strong association of HTPFD and IC/BPS (Bassaly et al., 2011; Peters et al., 2007a). A preliminary NIDDK trial demonstrated the feasibility of such a study and strongly suggested the efficacy of physical therapy when compared with global therapeutic massage (FitzGerald et al., 2009). This was confirmed in an RCT comparing 10 scheduled treatments of myofascial physical therapy versus global therapeutic massage at 11 North American clinical centers. The Global Response Assessment (GRA) response rate was 26% in the global therapeutic massage group and 59% in the myofascial physical therapy group ($P = .0012$) (FitzGerald et al., 2012).

Mendelowitz et al. had a 69% success rate in 16 patients treated with electromyographic biofeedback (Mendelowitz et al., 1997), but treatment response did not correlate to changes in muscle identification, and the placebo effect may have been considerable. **Acupuncture has been used for IC/BPS and many other chronic pain syndromes.** IC/BPS results with acupuncture have been disappointing, with most studies showing it to be no more effective than placebo, sham acupuncture, or standard care (Ezzo et al., 2000; Geirsson et al., 1993). Conversely, a more recent albeit open-label study showed significant improvement in multiple clinical parameters after 5 weeks of treatment (two sessions per week) that lasted 3 months. A progressive worsening of symptoms back to baseline was identified at 1-year follow-up. No doubt, further sham or placebo-controlled trials with perhaps standardization of methodology for needle placement are needed (Sönmez and Kozanhan, 2017).

Diet

Dietary triggers are endorsed by an estimated 53% to 93% of IC/BPS patients, based on patient surveys (Interstitial Cystitis Association, 2005; Koziol et al., 1993; Shorter et al., 2007). All are hampered by methodologic difficulties; however, they are remarkably consistent with regard to the specific items that are felt to trigger symptoms. Often these include caffeine, alcohol, artificial sweeteners, hot peppers, and acidic beverages such as cranberry juice (Shorter et al., 2007).

One placebo-controlled dietary study, although small, failed to demonstrate a relationship between diet and symptoms (Fisher et al., 1993). Contrary to that study, a recent controlled clinical trial from Japan investigated the effect of "intensive dietary manipulation" on 40 IC/BPS patients (30 receiving intensive and 10 receiving nonintensive manipulation) using parameters including O'Leary-Sant Symptom and Problem indices, urgency visual analog scale score, bladder or pelvic pain visual analog scale score, and numerical patient-reported QoL index. Foods/beverages that were removed or restricted included tomatoes, tomato products, soybean, tofu, spices, excessive potassium, citrus, high-acidity–inducing substances, and others. Statistically significant improvement was identified in the "intensive" group versus the "nonintensive" group at all time points up to 1 year (Oh-oka, 2017).

Urine pH has been thought to be a factor that might trigger symptoms. Indeed, several acid-sensing ion channel subunits are expressed in human bladder, and the upregulation of some of these channels in IC/BPS patients suggests involvement in increased pain and hyperalgesia (Sanchez-Freire et al., 2011). This hypothesis was somewhat dispelled by Nguan et al., who performed a prospective, double-blind, crossover study consisting of crossover instillations of urine at physiologic pH (5.0) and neutral buffered pH (7.5) (Nguan et al., 2005). There was no statistically significant difference in subjective pain scores, suggesting that adjusting urine pH with diet or dietary supplements may have little influence on symptomatology. Orange and grapefruit juices, rich in potassium and citrate, tend to *increase* urinary pH (Wabner and Pak, 1993) but are avoided by many IC patients based on "IC diet" recommendations and their personal experience with food-related flares. The discrepancy between patients' descriptions of symptom flares based on the ingestion of acidic products and these research findings suggests that either there is very frequent misinterpretation of these agents as triggers or that some other process(es) (e.g., bladder bowel cross-talk) might be involved. Alkalinizing the urine may still be worth trying, but supporting studies are lacking. Some patients have had benefit with calcium glycerophosphate, an over-the-counter food acid–reducing agent (Hill et al., 2008; O'Hare et al., 2013), but, once again, controlled trials are lacking.

A stepwise method to determine dietary sensitivities such as an elimination diet may play an important role in patient management. This strategy requires patients to keep diaries of food intake, voiding, and pain. They begin with a bland diet using foods and beverages often chosen from food lists compiled by prior questionnaire-based studies (Box 57.5). They then slowly

---

BOX 57.5 Foods/Beverages Identified as Most and Least Bothersome to Patients With Interstitial Cystitis/Bladder Pain Syndrome

MOST BOTHERSOME	LEAST BOTHERSOME
Coffee (caffeinated)	Water
Coffee (decaffeinated)	Milk, low-fat
Tea (caffeinated)	Milk, whole
Cola carbonated beverage	Bananas
Non-cola carbonated beverage	Blueberries
	Honeydew melon
Diet carbonated beverage	Pears
Caffeine-free carbonated beverage	Raisins
	Watermelon
Beer	Broccoli
Red wine	Brussels sprouts
White wine	Cabbage
Champagne	Carrots
Grapefruit	Cauliflower
Lemon	Celery
Orange	Cucumber
Pineapple	Mushrooms
Cranberry juice	Peas
Grapefruit juice	Radishes
Orange juice	Squash
Pineapple juice	Zucchini
Tomato	White potatoes
Tomato products	Sweet potatoes/yams
Hot peppers	Eggs
Spicy foods	Turkey
Chili	Beef
Horseradish	Pork
Vinegar	Lamb
Monosodium glutamate	Shrimp
NutraSweet	Tuna fish
Sweet'N Low	Salmon
Equal (sweetener)	Chicken
Saccharin	Oats
Mexican food	Rice
Thai food	Pretzels
Indian food	Popcorn

Modified from Friedlander JI, Shorter B, Moldwin RM. Diet and its role in interstitial cystitis/bladder pain syndrome (IC/BPS) and comorbid conditions. *BJU Int* 109(11):1584–1591, 2012.

add potentially "offensive" items back into their diet and record results. The value of this approach rests with its ability to detect and avoid foods that appear to trigger symptoms. It also prevents patients from eliminating more foods than necessary, so that they continue to meet their nutritional requirements (Friedlander et al., 2012). Baseline data regarding diet sensitivities may be collected on a short, validated questionnaire (Shorter et al., 2014).

In a large National Institutes of Health study, patients with newly diagnosed IC/BPS were treated with a focus on four targeted areas: (1) controlling or managing symptoms, (2) controlling fluid intake, (3) changing the diet to one that might improve symptoms, and (4) bladder training and urge suppression. A behavioral approach to stress and pain management was also used to help patients learn skills to reduce stress in their lives. Of 135 patients randomized to this approach without additional medication, 45% were moderately or markedly improved at the 12-week end point (Foster et al., 2010). In another trial, hydrodistention followed by bladder training produced a statistically significant better response at 24 weeks postprocedure than hydrodistention alone (Hsieh et al., 2012).

The Role of Patient Support Groups

Several support groups exist to serve IC/BPS patients, providing up-to-date education and on-line support. The Interstitial Cystitis Association (ICA) (www.ichelp.org), a not-for-profit organization, has been in existence for 34 years, providing educational services for physicians and patients, sponsoring national patient symposia and charity walks, promoting research in the field, and even running their own pilot research program for young investigators. Other excellent resources for patients include the Interstitial Cystitis Network (ICN) (www.ic-network.com) and another not-for-profit group, The International Painful Bladder Foundation (IBPF) (painful-bladder.org).

Oral Therapies (Table 57.6)

Amitriptyline

Amitriptyline, a tricyclic antidepressant (TCA), has become a staple of oral treatment for IC/BPS. The tricyclics possess varying degrees of at least three major pharmacologic actions: (1) They have central and peripheral anticholinergic actions at some but not all sites, (2) they block the active transport system in the presynaptic nerve ending that is responsible for the reuptake of the released amine neurotransmitters serotonin and noradrenaline, and (3) they are sedatives, an action that occurs presumably on a central basis but perhaps is related to their antihistaminic properties. Amitriptyline, in fact, is one of the most potent tricyclic antidepressants in terms of blocking H_1-histaminergic receptors (Baldessarini, 1985). It may also stimulate β-adrenergic receptors in bladder body smooth musculature, an action that would further facilitate urine storage by decreasing the excitability of smooth muscle in that area (Barrett et al., 1987).

Hanno and Wein first reported a therapeutic response in IC/BPS after noting a "serendipitous" response to amitriptyline in one of their patients concurrently being treated for depression (Hanno and Wein, 1987). Reasoning that a drug used successfully at relatively low doses for many types of chronic pain syndromes, that would also have anticholinergic properties, β-adrenergic bladder effects, sedative characteristics, and strong H_1-antihistaminic activity, would seem to be ideal for IC, the first clinical trials with doses ranging from 25 to 75 mg were carried out with promising results (Hanno, 1994; Hanno et al., 1989); however, drop-out rates were high. Sedation was the most common complaint. Other uncontrolled studies followed, all demonstrating success (Kirkemo et al., 1990; Pranikoff and Constantino, 1998) along with another TCA, desipramine (Renshaw, 1988).

In a 4-month intent-to-treat, placebo-controlled, double-blind trial of 50 patients, 63% on amitriptyline at doses of 25 to 75 mg (dose as tolerated) before bed reported good or excellent satisfaction versus 4% on placebo (van Ophoven et al., 2004a). At 19-month follow-up, there was little tachyphylaxis, and good response rates were observed in the entire spectrum of IC/BPS symptoms (van Ophoven and Hertle, 2005).

TABLE 57.6 Grade and Level of Evidence According to Oxford System for Oral and Intravesical Therapies

TREATMENT	ICI[a]	EAU[b]	GIANNANTONI[c]
ORAL THERAPIES			
Amitriptyline	B: 2	A: 1	A: 1
Analgesics	C: 4	C: 2	
Hydroxyzine	D: 1	A: 1	
PPS	D: 1	A: 1	C: 1
Cyclosporine	C: 3	A: 1	A: 1
l-Arginine	–A: 1		A: 1
Antibiotics regimens	D: 4		
Azathioprine	D: 4		
Benzydamine	D: 3		
Chloroquine derivatives	D: 4		
Cimetidine	C: 3		
Doxycycline	D: 4		
Duloxetine	–C: 4		
Gabapentin	C: 4		
Methotrexate	D: 4		
Misoprostol	D: 4		
Montelukast	D: 4		
Nalmefene	–A: 1		
Nifedipine	D: 4		
Quercetin	D: 4		
Tanezumab	D: 1		
Suplatast tosilate	D: 3		
Vitamin E	D: 4		
INTRAVESICAL THERAPIES			
Lidocaine	C: 2		
DMSO	B: 2	A: 1	
Heparin	C: 3		
Hyaluronic acid	D: 1	B: 2	
Chondroitin sulfate	D: 4	B: 2	A: 1
PPS	D: 4	A: 1	
Oxybutynin	D: 4		
BTX (intramural)	A: 1		A: 1

[a]Hanno P, Dinis P, Lin A, et al. Bladder pain syndrome. In: Abrams P, Cardozo L, Khoury S, et al., eds. *Incontinence*. Paris: International Consultation on Urological Diseases/European Association of Urology; 2013:1583–1649.
[b]Fall M, Baranowski AP, Elneil S, et al. EAU guidelines on chronic pelvic pain. *Eur Urol* 57(1):35–48, 2010.
[c]Giannantoni A, Bini V, Dmochowski R, et al. Contemporary management of the painful bladder: a systematic review. *Eur Urol* 61:29–53, 2012.
BTX, Botulinum toxin; DMSO, dimethyl sulfoxide; EAU, European Association of Urology; ICI, International Consultation on Incontinence; PPS, pentosan polysulfate.
From Committee on Bladder Pain Syndrome. *Fifth International Consultation on Incontinence*. Paris, France; 2012.

The large, double-blind, RCT by the NIDDK comparing education and behavioral modification with and without oral amitriptyline showed no significant differences in symptom improvement between the groups at 12 weeks. However, reanalysis of these data selecting out patients who could tolerate doses of 50 mg or higher, did show efficacy beyond control, 77% versus 53%, respectively (Foster et al., 2010).

Amitriptyline appears to have efficacy that is unrelated to the presence or absence of an HL, and cystoscopy shows no predictive value for treatment outcome (Sun et al., 2014). It may also be beneficial in the treatment of other pain disorders that often accompany IC/BPS, (e.g., vulvodynia) (Ventolini, 2013).

Amitriptyline has proven analgesic efficacy with a **median preferred dose of 50 mg in a range of 25 to 150 mg daily.** Patients should be cautioned about fatigue, constipation, dry mouth, increased appetite (with weight gain), and dizziness. **Slowly titrating the dose on a weekly basis, beginning at 10 mg in the evening and increasing by 10 mg weekly to a maximum tolerated dose of 50 mg before bed seems to minimize side effects.** Despite the findings of research trials, long-term clinical benefits may be seen at doses lower than 50 mg. The clinician should be cautious when contemplating amitriptyline's use in the IC/BPS patient who complains of obstructive voiding symptoms or those patients who suffer from chronic constipation as the drug can easily worsen these conditions. Delayed ejaculation, anorgasmia, and decreased libido are common side effects of all TCAs (Shankar, 2015).

Tricyclic antidepressants are contraindicated in patients with long QT syndrome or significant conduction system disease (bifascicular or trifascicular block) after recent myocardial infarction (within 6 months), unstable angina, congestive heart failure, frequent premature ventricular contractions, or a history of sustained ventricular arrhythmias. They should be used with caution in patients with orthostatic hypotension (Low and Dotson, 1998). Doses greater than 100 mg are associated with increased relative risk for sudden cardiac death (Ray et al., 2004).

Antihistamines

Theoharides postulated that the unique piperazine H_1-receptor antagonist *hydroxyzine*, a first-generation antihistamine, would block neuronal activation of mast cells, and thereby mitigate IC/BPS symptoms (Minogiannis et al., 1998; Simons, 2004; Theoharides, 1994). In 40 patients treated with 25 mg before bed increasing over 2 weeks (if sedation was not a problem) to 50 mg at night and 25 mg in the morning, virtually every symptom evaluated improved by 30%. Only three patients had absolutely no response. As with many IC drug reports, these responses were evaluated subjectively and without blinding or placebo control. A subsequent study suggested improved efficacy in patients with documented allergies and/or evidence of bladder mast cell activation (Theoharides and Sant, 1997; Theoharides et al., 1997). **No significant response to hydroxyzine was found in an NIDDK placebo-controlled trial** (Sant et al., 2003). **Nevertheless, a good safety profile along with its ability to improve sleep (often in conjunction with amitriptyline) and commonly reported allergy symptoms, makes hydroxyzine a useful medication in selected patients.**

Why an H_2-antagonist would be effective is unclear, but uncontrolled studies show improvement of symptoms in two-thirds of patients taking cimetidine in divided doses totaling 600 mg (Lewi, 1996; Seshadri et al., 1994). It proved effective in a double-blind, placebo-controlled trial with 400-mg twice-daily dosing (Thilagarajah et al., 2001), but histologic studies show the bladder mucosa to be unchanged before and after treatment, and the mechanism of any efficacy remains unexplained (Dasgupta et al., 2001). Cimetidine is a common treatment in the United Kingdom, where over one-third of patients reported having used it (Tincello and Walker, 2005).

Montelukast

Mast cell triggering releases two types of proinflammatory mediators, including granule stored preformed types such as heparin and histamine and newly synthesized prostaglandins and leukotrienes B_4 and C_4. Classic antagonists, such as montelukast, zafirlukast, and pranlukast, block cysteinyl leukotriene-1 receptors. In a pilot study, 10 women with IC and detrusor mastocytosis received 10 mg of montelukast daily for 2 months (Bouchelouche et al., 2001b). Frequency, nocturia, and pain improved dramatically in 8 of the patients. Further study would seem to be warranted, especially in patients with detrusor mastocytosis, defined as more than 28/mm^2 (Traut et al., 2011).

Pentosan Polysulfate Sodium

Pentosan polysulfate (PPS; brand name Elmiron) was approved in the United States for the "relief of bladder pain or discomfort associated with interstitial cystitis" in 1996 under the FDA's orphan products program. It remains the only FDA oral medication approved for this indication. PPS is a synthetic sulfated polysaccharide, similar in structure to glycosaminoglycans (GAG) of the bladder surface. Taken orally, 3% to 6% of PPS is excreted into the urine (Barrington and Stephenson, 1997) and purportedly improves symptoms by correction of GAG defects that produce a dysfunctional, "leaky" bladder epithelium. Another hypothesis proposed by Parsons is the drug's ability to sequester "toxic cations" (Parsons, 2017).

Initial studies reported encouraging results (Parsons et al., 1983). Fourteen subsequent trials have been disparate. Trials have been plagued with methodologic differences and problems inherent to all IC/BPS clinical trials, the heterogeneity of the population (Moldwin, 2017). Small studies suggest that it may be of value in the management of radiation cystitis (Hampson and Woodhouse, 1994; Parsons, 1986) and cyclophosphamide cystitis (Toren and Norman, 2005).

An industry-sponsored trial showed no dose-related efficacy response in the range of 300 to 900 mg daily; however, adverse events *were* dose related (Nickel et al., 2005). A phase IV, randomized, double-blind, placebo-controlled trial evaluating the efficacy of PPS for IC/BPS found no statistically significant difference for the primary end point, defined as a 30% or greater reduction from the baseline Interstitial Cystitis Symptom Index (ICSI) total score between two different doses of PPS (100 mg once a day and 100 mg three times a day) and a placebo group. In this well-constructed study that included intent-to-treat analysis, the investigators used a less rigorous definition of IC/BPS for enrollment (although sub-stratification for patients meeting NIDDK criteria was also performed). They did not exclude patients with comorbid conditions such as IBS, pelvic floor dysfunction, or depression. Likewise, patients were not excluded if they had already used PPS in their clinical care. Hence, these and other factors (such as drop-out for reasons other than nonresponse to therapy and adverse events) may have had an effect on outcome (Nickel et al., 2015).

Adverse events with PPS occurred in less than 4% of patients at the dose of 100 mg three times daily and included reversible alopecia, diarrhea, nausea, and rash (Hanno, 1997). Rare bleeding problems have been reported (Rice et al., 1998). Of recent concern is a report of a **pigmentary maculopathy**, manifest by "difficulty reading," developing in 6 patients after long-term PPS use (Pearce et al., 2018). This finding merits follow-up investigation. Caution has been suggested when using PPS in groups with high risk for breast cancer and premenopausal women as the drug promotes cellular proliferation in vitro in the MCF-7 breast cancer cell line (Zaslau et al., 2004).

Despite efficacy and safety concerns, clinical practice suggests that PPS can produce clinical responses in a subset of patients (Al-Zahrani and Gajewski, 2011), and tachyphylaxis seems to be uncommon in these individuals. Hence, along with amitriptyline, hydroxyzine, and cimetidine, this agent has been recommended as a second-tier agent for IC/BPS (Hanno et al., 2015). Clinical usefulness is hampered by the inability to select patients most likely to benefit. This is magnified by high cost and a clinical response that may take 3 months (and on rare occasions, up to 6 months) to occur. Its use remains controversial among practicing clinicians.

Immunomodulator Drugs

Cyclosporine A. Cyclosporine A (CyA), a widely used immunosuppressive drug in organ transplantation, was the subject of a novel IC/BPS trial (Forsell et al., 1996). Eleven patients received cyclosporine for 3 to 6 months at an initial dose of 2.5 to 5 mg/kg daily and a maintenance dose of 1.5 to 3 mg/kg daily. Micturition frequency decreased, and mean and maximum voided volumes increased significantly. Bladder pain decreased or disappeared in 10 patients. After cessation of treatment, symptoms recurred in the majority of patients.

In a longer-term follow-up study, 20 of 23 refractory IC patients on CyA followed for a mean of 60.8 months became free from bladder pain. Bladder capacity more than doubled. Eleven patients subsequently stopped therapy, and in 9, symptoms recurred within months but responded to reinitiating CyA (Sairanen et al., 2004). Sairanen et al. (2005) further found that cyclosporine A was far superior to sodium PPS in all clinical outcome parameters measured at 6 months. Patients who responded to cyclosporine A had a significant reduction of urinary levels of EGF (Sairanen et al., 2008). Retrospective data from three centers in the United States reported success in 23 of 34 patients with HLs, but in only 3 of 10 patients without HLs (Forrest et al., 2012), suggesting that the HL phenotype might be the best group to target with CyA therapy. A 3- to 4-month trial was suggested to gauge treatment success. Similar results were seen in a recent open-label study of patients who failed at least two prior therapies (Crescenze et al., 2017).

Measurement of luminal nitric oxide has correlated lower levels with treatment response to cyclosporine (Ehrén et al., 2013). A case report highlighted success in a patient with primary SS and IC/BPS (Emmungil et al., 2012). **CyA is a recommended fifth-tier therapy as its side effects do not warrant early use in most patients.** Its association with renal dysfunction, hypertension, heightened risk for infection and lymphoma, development of gum hyperplasia, alopecia, tremor, among others, along with multiple drug and food interactions make this a medication that requires close initial and subsequent patient follow-up. Doses that have been described are usually 1 to 3 mg/kg/day, lower than those used in the setting of renal transplant (Crescenze et al., 2017; Forrest et al., 2012; Forsell et al., 1996; Sairanen et al., 2004). Protocols for follow-up vary among centers, all focusing on monitoring for hypertension and serum studies (including estimated glomerular filtration rate [eGFR]). Crescenze et al. (2017) found a CyA serum level drawn 2 hours after dose administration to be helpful for monitoring and allowed for dose reduction in about 40% of patients.

Other Immunoregulating Agents. Soucy and Grégoire studied the value of **prednisone** (25 mg/day, followed by dose tapering) in patients with refractory ulcerative IC, noting a 22% reduction in symptom scores and a 69% improvement in pain (Soucy and Grégoire, 2005). **With a lack of follow-up trials and concerns for long-term safety, chronic steroid therapy is not currently recommended in the treatment algorithm.** In a single report in 1976, Oravisto et al. used **azathioprine or chloroquine derivatives** for IC/BPS patients not responding to other treatments (Oravisto and Alfthan, 1976). About 50% of patients responded. Low-dose oral **methotrexate** significantly improved bladder pain in four of nine women with IC/BPS but did not change urinary frequency, maximum voided volume, or mean voided volume (Moran et al., 1999). No placebo-controlled RCT has been done with this agent. Immunoregulating medications that have been studied but failed to show efficacy for IC/BPS include suplatast tosilate (Ueda, 2000), mycophenolate mofetil (Yang et al., 2011), and adalimumab (Bosch, 2014).

Miscellaneous Agents

L-Arginine. Foster and Weiss were the original proponents of L-arginine in the therapy of IC (Foster et al., 1997). Eight patients with IC were given 500 mg of L-arginine three times daily. After 1 month, urinary NOS activity increased eightfold, and 7 of the 8 patients noticed improvement in symptoms. An open-label study of 11 patients showed improvement in all 10 of the patients who remained on L-arginine for 6 months (Smith et al., 1997). Further open-label studies (Ehrén et al., 1998) and RCTs (Cartledge et al., 2000; Korting et al., 1999) have shown no clinically significant improvement for IC/BPS. L-Arginine is therefore not a recommended therapy.

Quercetin. Quercetin, a bioflavonoid available in many over-the-counter products, may have the anti-inflammatory effects of other members of this class of compounds found in fruits, vegetables, and some spices. Katske et al. (2001) administered 500 mg twice daily to 22 IC/BPS patients for 4 weeks. All but one patient had some improvement in the O'Leary-Sant symptom and problem scores and in a global assessment score. Further larger studies with placebo controls are necessary to determine efficacy.

Antibiotics. Exclusion of a urinary tract infection is part and parcel of the IC/BPS diagnosis. No study to date has identified any organism by any technology that can be consistently identified as the cause for symptoms. Nevertheless, some studies indirectly suggest that the topic may need further study. Warren et al. (2000) randomized 50 patients to receive 18 weeks of placebo or antibiotics including rifampin plus a sequence of doxycycline, erythromycin, metronidazole, clindamycin, amoxicillin, and ciprofloxacin for 3 weeks each. Intent-to-treat analysis demonstrated that 12 of 25 patients in the antibiotic group and 6 of 25 patients in the placebo group reported overall improvement, whereas 10 and 5 patients, respectively, noticed improvement in pain and urgency. The study was complicated by the fact that 16 of the patients in the antibiotic group underwent new IC/BPS therapy during the study, as did 13 of the placebo patients. There was no statistical significance reached. What was statistically significant was the occurrence of adverse events in 80% of participants who received antibiotics compared with 40% in the placebo group. Nausea and/or vomiting and diarrhea were the predominant side effects. Most patients on antibiotics correctly guessed what treatment arm they were in, and those who guessed correctly were significantly more likely to note improvement after the study. No duration in improvement after completion of the trial of antibiotics was reported.

Burkhard et al. (2004) recorded a 71% success rate in 103 women with a history of urinary urgency and frequency and chronic urethral and/or pelvic pain often associated with dyspareunia and/or a history of recurrent urinary tract infection. This was a large, inclusive group and one that is probably broader than the IC/BPS on which we are focusing. Nevertheless, Burkhard recommended empirical doxycycline in this group. The overwhelming majority of IC/BPS patients have been treated with empirical antibiotics before diagnosis.

At this time, there is no evidence to suggest that antibiotics have a place in the therapy of IC/BPS in the absence of a culture-documented infection (Maskell, 1995). It is unlikely that the baseline symptoms of IC/BPS will respond to the incidental finding of bacteriuria without the presence of a symptom flare (Nickel et al., 2010a). Nevertheless, it would not be unreasonable to treat patients with *one* empirical course of antibiotic, if they have never been on an antibiotic for their urinary symptoms. In the event of a symptom flare thought to be caused by infection, a urinalysis and urine culture would be mandatory. An additional practical note: Some IC/BPS patients will develop recurring, uncomplicated bacterial cystitis. These episodes may trigger significant symptom flares that last for extended intervals. In these instances, the clinician should consider the use of antibiotic prophylactic protocols to "side table" these events.

Nifedipine. The calcium channel antagonist nifedipine inhibits smooth muscle contraction and cell-mediated immunity. In a pilot study, 30 mg of an extended-release preparation was administered to 10 female patients and titrated to 60 mg daily in 4 of the patients who did not get symptom relief (Fleischmann, 1994). Within 4 months, 5 patients showed at least a 50% decrease in symptom scores, and 3 of the 5 were asymptomatic. No further studies have been reported.

Misoprostol. The oral prostaglandin analogue misoprostol was studied in 25 patients at a dose of 600 µg daily (Kelly et al., 1998). At 3 months 14 patients were significantly improved, and at 6 months 12 patients still had a response. A cytoprotective action in the urinary bladder was postulated.

Dextroamphetamine. A single anecdotal series of six patients reported benefit from use of 30 mg of dextroamphetamine sulfate daily, with return of symptoms on discontinuation of medication (Check et al., 2013).

Phosphodiesterase Inhibitors. The use of phosphodiesterase type 5 inhibitors (PDE5Is) for IC/BPS has long been considered. PDE5Is are hypothesized to relax smooth muscle or structures involved in afferent signaling and suppress smooth muscle spontaneous activity (Chen et al., 2014; Hanna-Mitchell and Birder, 2011; Truss et al., 2001). Trials using them for BPS are underway.

Gabapentin. Gabapentin, introduced in 1994 as an anticonvulsant, has found efficacy in neuropathic pain disorders including diabetic neuropathy (Backonja et al., 1998) and postherpetic neuralgia (Rowbotham et al., 1998). It demonstrates synergism with morphine in neuropathic pain (Gilron et al., 2005). It may give some benefit in CPPS and IC/BPS (Sasaki et al., 2001). Pregabalin is also reported to be effective for neuropathic pain and the pain of FMS (Agarwal and Elsi Sy, 2017; Arnold et al., 2008; Freynhagen et al., 2005).

> **KEY POINTS: ORAL THERAPIES**
> - Few of the oral therapies commonly used for the treatment of IC/BPS have unequivocal evidence of efficacy in large, multicenter, clinical RCTs.
> - There is little evidence that any of these therapies change the natural history of the disease, although many seem effective in individual patients.
> - Consider "drug holidays" to periodically check drug effectiveness.
> - Consider multidrug therapy as needed to maximize clinical improvement and avoid adverse events of single high-dose medications.

Intravesical Therapies

Intravesical therapy (see Table 57.6) has the appeal of treating the bladder directly and may be an excellent choice for the patient with limited tolerance to oral agents or simply to further treat symptoms when the effects of oral medications and other conservative measures appear to have plateaued. The downside of therapy is that pain produced centrally or from other pelvic pain generators will be left untreated. Furthermore, response to an intravesical agent may be limited by poor adherence and/or poor absorption through the urothelial surface. Caustic medications that have been described as treatment options (e.g., silver nitrate, oxychlorosene sodium [Clorpactin]) are rarely used today. Many of the current commonly used agents can be self-instilled, thus enhancing patient empowerment and limiting their need for frequent trips to the medical office. Intravesical instillation therapy is suggested to be used as second-line treatment in the management of IC/BPS by the AUA (Hanno et al., 2011).

The use of silver nitrate and Clorpactin is described online at ExpertConsult.com.

Dimethyl Sulfoxide

A mainstay for the treatment of IC/BPS is the intravesical instillation of 50% dimethyl sulfoxide (DMSO) (Sant, 1987). DMSO is sometimes administered in a solution with sodium bicarbonate, heparin, and/or steroid, but its only FDA-approved use is as a stand-alone treatment (Gafni-Kane et al., 2013; Stav et al., 2012). DMSO is a byproduct of the wood pulp industry and a derivative of lignin. It has exceptional solvent properties and is freely miscible with water, lipids, and organic agents. One must be cognizant of systemic absorption of coadministered agents. Pharmacologic properties include membrane penetration, enhanced drug absorption, anti-inflammatory action (Kim et al., 2011), analgesic effects, collagen dissolution, muscle relaxation, and mast cell histamine release. In vitro effects on bladder function belie its positive effects in vivo (Freedman et al., 1989), where histamine release has not been demonstrated after treatment (Stout et al., 1995). It has been suggested that DMSO actually desensitizes nociceptive pathways in the lower urinary tract (Birder et al., 1997). Tests for DMSO for treatment of human illness began in the 1960s in the areas of musculoskeletal inflammation and the cutaneous manifestations of scleroderma.

Stewart et al. are credited for popularizing intravesical DMSO for IC/BPS (Stewart et al., 1967). Further reports by this group confirmed safety and efficacy (Shirley et al., 1978; Stewart and Shirley, 1976; Stewart et al., 1971, 1972) with symptom-free intervals of 1 to 3 months in 73% of patients. Ek et al. (1978) reported a 70% success rate but found that most patients ultimately required retreatment or further therapy with other modalities. Prospective series of Fowler (1981) and Barker et al. (1987) revealed symptomatic success rates higher than 80%, although relapse was not uncommon. Fowler noted only minimal improvements in functional bladder capacity and attributed the beneficial effects of DMSO to a direct effect on the sensory nerves of the bladder. Perez-Marrero et al. (1988) compared DMSO with saline and showed a 93% objective improvement and 53% subjective improvement compared with 35% and 18%, respectively, for saline. Patients with bladder instability do not respond (Emerson and Feltis, 1986). Stav et al. (2012) and Hung et al. (2012) reported 60% success rates and recommended it be considered a first-line therapy. Tomoe (2015) reported better efficacy in patients with HLs.

With its ease of administration (Biggers, 1986), **low morbidity, and reasonable efficacy, DMSO certainly merits its place as a useful treatment for IC/BPS.** In vivo studies on rat bladder strips exposed to various concentrations of DMSO for 7 minutes showed absence of electrical field stimulation contraction at 40% concentration and diminished compliance at 30% concentration (Melchior et al., 2003). Concentrations of 25% or less had negligible effects in this model. How it relates to use of DMSO in humans is unknown. A rare case of eosinophilic cystitis has been reported after DMSO instillation (Abramov et al., 2004). Patients should be informed that they might experience severe urgency and frequency with the first several instillations. Patients will typically have a garlic-like odor to their breath caused by partial pulmonary excretion, making blinded clinical trials impossible to carry out.

DMSO is often administered as part of an "intravesical cocktail" (50 mL Rimso-50 + 10 mg triamcinolone + 44 mEq sodium bicarbonate + 20,000 to 40,000 units intravesical heparin) weekly for 6 weeks. If there is a good clinical response, maintenance therapy consisting of administration of the cocktail monthly for 6 months has been employed. Other combinations of agents used in DMSO cocktails have been described, but none has shown clear superiority (Rawls, et al., 2017).

Glycosaminoglycans

Exogenous glycosaminoglycans (GAGs) have been shown to be effective in providing an epithelial permeability barrier in bladders in which the epithelium has been injured with protamine (Nickel et al., 1998). Heparin, which can mimic the activity of the bladder's own mucopolysaccharide lining (Hanno et al., 1978b), has anti-inflammatory effects and actions that inhibit fibroblast proliferation, angiogenesis, and smooth muscle cell proliferation. Given intravesically, there is virtually no systemic absorption, even in an inflamed bladder (Caulfield et al., 1995). Ten thousand units can be administered intravesically in sterile water either alone or with DMSO at varying intervals with favorable results reported (Parsons et al., 1994a; Perez-Marrero et al., 1993). Kuo reported a 50% or greater improvement in the International Prostate Symptom Score in 29 of 40 women with IC treated with 25,000 units intravesically twice weekly for 3 months (Kuo, 2001).

Parsons used daily intravesical doses of 40,000 units of heparin in 20 mL of sterile water administered by the patient daily and held for 30 to 60 minutes. "Reasonable improvement of symptoms" can be expected between 6 months and 2 years after initiation of therapy (Parsons, 2000). Adding alkalinized lidocaine to the heparin instillation provides better pain relief (Parsons, 2005). The addition of 8 mL of 2% lidocaine and 4 mL of 8.4% sodium bicarbonate may improve results (Welk and Teichman, 2008). In fact, a combination of 200 mg of lidocaine alkalinized with the sequential instillation of 8.4% sodium bicarbonate (10 mL total solution) *without* heparin showed a 30% response rate 3 days after completion of daily intravesical administration for 5 days and was statistically superior to a placebo cocktail (Nickel et al., 2009b). A Japanese study reported high success rates with weekly intravesical instillation of 20,000 units of heparin with 5 mL of 4% lidocaine and 25 mL of 7% sodium bicarbonate for 12 weeks (Nomiya et al., 2013). Intravesical administration of a solution of lidocaine and heparin has been proposed as a treatment for symptom flare (Parsons et al., 2012).

Another GAG analogue, pentosan polysulfate sodium (PPS), administered intravesically (300 mg twice weekly in 50 mL of normal saline) showed some modest benefit in a small trial (Bade et al., 1997). A 41-patient trial comparing oral PPS with oral and intravesical administration showed that the 24% reduction in O'Leary-Sant scores with oral therapy alone rose to a 46% reduction in the group that also received intravesical PPS (Davis et al., 2008).

The nonsulfated GAG hyaluronic acid has also been used intravesically. Trials using 40 mg dissolved in 46 mL of normal saline weekly for 4 to 6 weeks and then monthly treatments thereafter have had response rates varying from 71% (Morales et al., 1996) to 30% (Porru et al., 1997). In the summer of 2003, Bioniche Life Sciences and in the spring of 2004 Seikagaku Corporation reported double-blind, placebo-controlled, multicenter clinical studies of their hyaluronic acid preparations (40 mg or 200 mg/mL, respectively), and neither showed significant efficacy of sodium hyaluronate compared with placebo. These negative studies have not been published in peer-reviewed literature. Neither preparation has been approved for use for IC/BPS in the United States. An Austrian open-label study showed that 13 of 27 patients with IC/BPS and a positive potassium test result responded to intravesical hyaluronic acid 40 mg weekly for 10 weeks, though initial nonresponders at 5 weeks also were treated with intravesical PPS 200 mg three times weekly for the remaining 5 weeks (Daha et al., 2008). The best results for hyaluronic acid come from Riedl, who studied 126 patients with a positive modified potassium test result who could hold the solution for 2 hours, using 40 mg weekly for a minimum 10 weeks; 84% had significant improvement (Riedl et al., 2008). Treatment-resistant cases have been managed with a combination of sequential bladder distention under anesthesia accompanied by a hyaluronic acid instillation every 1 to 3 months depending on response, with a 74% success rate in 23 patients (Ahmad et al., 2008). Although hyaluronic acid has been seemingly efficacious in uncontrolled trials (Engelhardt et al., 2011; Figueiredo et al., 2011; Lai et al., 2013; Lv et al., 2012; Van Agt et al., 2011), **the efficacy of hyaluronic acid for IC/BPS remains unproven in controlled and blinded trials** (Iavazzo et al., 2007). It remains unapproved for IC/BPS in the United States.

Chondroitin sulfate plays an important role for bladder barrier function (Janssen et al., 2013). Hurst showed by immunohistochemistry a deficit of chondroitin sulfate from the luminal bladder surface in IC patients (Hurst, 2003). Intravesical chondroitin sulfate inhibited recruitment of inflammatory cells in an experimental "leaky bladder" model of cystitis (Engles et al., 2012). Small, uncontrolled studies using intravesical chondroitin sulfate showed success rates of 33% to 75% (Sorensen, 2003; Steinhoff et al., 2002; Tornero et al., 2013). A multicenter, open-label study using a 2% solution of sodium chondroitin sulfate weekly for 6 weeks and then monthly for 4 months had a 60% response rate with no safety issues (Nickel et al., 2009a). A larger follow-up study failed to demonstrate significant efficacy (Nickel et al., 2012; Thakkinstian and Nickel, 2013). A large open-label experience using the device for all forms of "chronic cystitis" concluded that it was effective in improving urgency, voided volumes, and nocturia, and well tolerated when administered weekly for a maximum of eight instillations (Nordling and van Ophoven, 2008).

The GAGs have been combined for instillation with favorable results reported in uncontrolled studies (Cervigni, 2015; Cervigni et al., 2008, 2012; Giberti et al., 2013; Porru et al., 2012). A recent study of combined hyaluronic acid and chondroitin sulfate demonstrated similar pain reduction and fewer associated adverse events compared with 50% DMSO when the intent-to-treat population was examined (Cervigni et al., 2016).

A large analysis of GAG layer replenishment therapy with intravesical GAGs concluded that despite the fact that GAG intravesical therapy has been in use for over two decades, most of the studies have been uncontrolled, have been poorly done, and have had a small number of patients. Large-scale RCTs are urgently needed to underline the benefit of this type of therapy. Distinct patient groups (well phenotyped) need to be confirmed by definite diagnostic findings (Madersbacher et al., 2013).

Other Intravesical Therapies

Sodium Channel Blocking Anesthetics (Lidocaine). Intravesical instillations of anesthetics agents (most commonly used with other medications in cocktail solutions) have the advantage of observing almost immediate results, making this form of care potentially helpful for symptom flares or for maintenance therapy. Its value also rests with its ability to help discern the source of pain, with many centers using a positive response to alkalinized lidocaine preparations as evidence for a bladder-centric phenotype (Henry et al., 2015). The most common agent used has been lidocaine, a sodium channel blocker that also has anti-inflammatory and antimicrobial properties (Cassuto et al., 2006). Lidocaine has a short half-life in serum and is not absorbed to a significant degree through the urothelial surface unless in an alkaline environment. Hence, most instillations are buffered in a sodium bicarbonate. Nickel et al. (2009) explored the role of alkalinized intravesical lidocaine in an RCT that showed moderate or marked improvement 3 days after completing the 5-day course of treatment (30% and 9.6%, respectively, for patients treated with lidocaine and placebo; $P = 0.012$). The 30% response for lidocaine underscores the high percentage of patients whose pain may be derived from extravesical sources. Long-acting local anesthetics such as bupivacaine have been suggested in combination with or replacing lidocaine; however, no controlled trails have been performed for assessment. The clinician should note that lidocaine and similar preparations are associated with a tachyphylaxis. As such, patients should be monitored for decreasing efficacy of therapy over time.

> **KEY POINTS: INTRAVESICAL THERAPIES**
>
> - The potential for high efficacy combined with safety and a low side-effect profile that is gained by applying a treatment directly to the bladder lining has made research into new methods of intravesical therapy a high priority of researchers and pharmaceutical companies.
> - Patients in whom pain and other symptoms are not related directly to bladder pathology would not be expected to respond well to this type of organ-directed therapy.
> - Although intravesical therapy may be helpful to control symptoms of IC/BPS, the frequency and duration of therapy and the value of maintenance therapy have not been well studied.

Intradetrusor Therapy

Onabotulinum Toxin-A (BTX-A). Intradetrusor BTX-A is approved by the FDA for the treatment of refractory neurogenic bladder and OAB. BTX-A has been used effectively for years in different conditions associated with muscular hypercontractions and has been described for treatment of HTPFD and other associated pain syndromes (e.g., vulvodynia) with promising results (Bertolasi et al., 2009; Moldwin and Fariello, 2013; Morrissey et al., 2015). The drug is not FDA approved for use in IC/BPS, and, although results between studies have been inconsistent (Rahnama'i et al., 2018), mounting evidence suggests efficacy and low risk in selected cases and has prompted the suggestion that BTX-A be considered as fourth line therapy for IC/BPS (Hanno et al., 2015). Consideration for earlier-stage management may occur when dosing and templates for injection become more refined. As with intravesical instillations, this therapy is probably best suited to patients with what the clinician believes to be a bladder-centric phenotype.

The therapeutic potential of BTX-A for IC/BPS is related to factors beyond its known ability to temporarily inhibit the release of acetylcholine and other neurotransmitters. BTX-A also has analgesic properties (Rajkumar and Conn, 2004). Initially this effect was thought to be a result of relief of muscle spasm. However, botulinum has been shown to reduce peripheral sensitization by inhibiting the release of several neuronal signaling markers, including glutamate and substance P, and reducing *c-Fos* gene expression. It may affect the sensory feedback loop to the central nervous system by decreased input from the muscle tissue, possibly by inhibiting acetylcholine release from gamma motor neurons innervating intrafusal fibers of the muscle spindle (Rosales et al., 1996). It inhibits the release of sensory neurotransmitters from isolated bladder preparations in rat bladder models of both acute injury and chronic inflammation

(Lucioni et al., 2008). Chronic inflammation and apoptosis is significantly reduced after repeated BTX-A injections in patients with IC/BPS (Shie et al., 2013). Intravesical BTX-A administration blocks the acetic acid–induced calcitonin gene–related peptide (CGRP) release from afferent nerve terminals in the bladder mucosal layer in rats (Chuang et al., 2004). In an animal model of bladder permeability barrier disruption, intravesical BTX-A minimized bladder irritability and restored afferent neural responses to baseline levels (Vemulakonda et al., 2005).

Two early RCTs showed no significant improvement from BTX-A above placebo; however, these results may have been related to injection sites that differ from other groups (e.g., periurethral) (Gottsch et al., 2010) or were performed with abobotulinum toxin A rather than onobotulinum toxin A in conjunction with therapies that have known potential benefit (e.g., bladder hydrodistention) (Manning et al., 2014). These studies were included in a meta-analysis of five RCTs, ultimately demonstrating a statistically significant improvement in subjective indices including visual analog scores for pain (Shim et al., 2016). A 1-year follow-up in 15 patients treated with 200 units of BTX-A in 20 mL of normal saline showed that the success rate fell from 86.6% at 3 months to 26.6% at 5 months and was 0 at 12 months (Giannantoni et al., 2008). Bladder biopsy 2 weeks after BTX-A intradetrusor injection showed that nerve growth factor production levels fell to those of controls in patients who responded (Liu et al., 2009).

Pinto et al. (2010) championed limiting injections to 100 units divided into 10 injection sites, all in the trigone. More than 50% of patients experienced efficacy with a duration of 9 months, and no voiding dysfunction was noted. There appears to be little tachyphylaxis associated with the treatment. Repeated injections at regular intervals, or when symptoms recur, remain effective (Kuo, 2013; Pinto et al., 2013). A recent RCT using 100 units trigonal BTX-A injections versus saline demonstrated a greater than 50% reduction in pain in 60% of BTX-A patients, versus 22% for placebo (Pinto et al., 2018). One downside of BTX-A is its inability to traverse the urothelial surface; hence the need for injection-based therapy. An innovative approach using instillation of liposome-encapsulated BTX-A to enhance its surface effect unfortunately did not show benefit above placebo (Chuang and Kuo, 2017). **Intradetrusor injection of onabotulinum toxin A appears to be a reasonable treatment for IC/BPS that is refractory to standard conservative, oral, and intravesical treatment** (Mangera et al., 2011; Yokoyama et al., 2012), **meriting its incorporation to AUA guidelines as a fourth-line consideration** (Hanno et al., 2015). When injected into the trigone in 10-unit aliquots (100 units total), the risk for impaired bladder emptying seems to be minimized. Nevertheless, BTX-A should be used with caution in patients who present with symptoms and/or signs of incomplete bladder emptying.

Neuromodulation

The International Neuromodulation Society defines therapeutic neuromodulation as "the alteration of nerve activity through targeted delivery of a stimulus, such as electrical stimulation or chemical agents, to specific neurological sites in the body" (https://www.neuromodulation.com). This has appeal in the field of pelvic pain by its possible effect on transport or perception of pain-related information. Furthermore, its effects on pelvic floor behavior may mitigate symptoms from associated HTPFD.

Perhaps the simplest form of neuromodulation is **transcutaneous electrical nerve stimulation (TENS)**, a simple and safe cutaneous method for pain relief of a variety of painful conditions (Fall, 1987). The mechanism by which conventional TENS presumably lessens pain is through the selective activation of large-diameter non-noxious afferents (Aβ fibers), thus affecting pain gate control. Another described mechanism is the release of endorphins and their precursors into the cerebrospinal fluid (Coutaux, 2017). As a secondary effect, urinary frequency may also be reduced.

Fall et al. (1980) were first to use electrical stimulation in IC/BPS, reporting on 14 women treated successfully with long-term intravaginal nerve stimulation or TENS. Subsequently, McGuire et al. (1983) noted improvement in 5 of 6 patients treated with electrical stimulation. In the most complete review of the subject (Fall and Lindstrom, 1994), 33 patients with IC/BPS with HLs and 27 patients without HLs were treated by means of suprapubic TENS. Favorable results or remission was described in 26% of patients without HLs and a surprising 54% of patients with HLs. Fall and Lindstrom (1994) caution that the experience is based on open studies, relatively few patients, and the knowledge of a significant placebo effect with peripheral pain stimulation. One of the major values of TENS is that it can easily be applied by patients in conjunction with other conservative management strategies. Further study with RCTs will be needed to determine efficacy. The best locations for electrode placement and stimulation settings still need to be determined (Fall, 2017).

Acupuncture's controversial role in the treatment of IC/BPS is discussed in the Conservative Therapies section earlier in this chapter.

Posterior tibial nerve stimulation (PTNS) was successful in 60% of 37 patients with symptoms of bladder overactivity in an uncontrolled Dutch study (van Balken et al., 2001). An Australian double-blind placebo-controlled study of transdermal posterior tibial nerve laser therapy showed no benefit in 56 patients when comparing active with placebo arms, but the placebo effect was remarkably strong, indicating the importance of such trials in evaluation of invasive therapies (O'Reilly et al., 2004). A Chinese study of PTNS twice weekly for 5 weeks in IC/BPS patients failed to show improvement in pain scores, and none of the 18 patients thought the treatment had a significant effect (Zhao et al., 2008). A more recent study of PTNS in 20 female IC/BPS patients with 12-weekly sessions found no clinically relevant improvements (Ragab et al., 2015). Taken as a whole, **there is little evidence to recommend PTNS for the pain associated with IC/BPS. An exception would be the patient who presents with symptoms of DO.**

Sacral neuromodulation (SNM) for IC/BPS, usually entailing electrical stimulation of the S3 sacral nerve, was developed through the basic and clinical research of Fandel and Tanagho (2005) and Schmidt (1993). Its current FDA-approved use in urology is for the treatment of nonobstructive urinary retention and the symptoms of OAB, including urinary urge incontinence and significant symptoms of urgency-frequency alone or in combination, in patients who have failed or could not tolerate more conservative treatments. SNM has also received FDA approval for the treatment of fecal incontinence. The device is not FDA approved for the treatment of IC/BPS; however, treatment results in this population have been encouraging (Peters, 2017). Treatment benefits for IC/BPS may be related to effects on pain gate regulation at the spinal segmental and higher levels, endorphin release, and modulation of pelvic floor muscle behavior (Rahnama'i, et al., 2018). In fact, many have observed that patients who do best with this treatment are those who have identifiable pain *and* HTPFD (Aboseif et al., 2002; Everaert et al., 2001; Siegel et al., 2001). Patients reporting pelvic pain in the absence of demonstrable pelvic floor dysfunction and levator tenderness did poorly (Schmidt, 2001). Decreases in urinary chemokines (most notably MCP-1) have been associated with favorable treatment responses (Peters et al., 2015). A successful test stimulation produced a decrease in antiproliferative activity and normalization of HB-EGF levels (Chai et al., 2000a).

A staged approach to device implantation (usually 1 to 4 weeks), as compared with a 3- to 4-day temporary electrode placement appears to improve final implantation rates (Baxter and Kim, 2010; Peters et al., 2003). Long-term efficacy related to these differences in technique is unknown.

Studies on the therapeutic potential of electrical stimulation for IC/BPS began in the late 1990s (van Kerrebroeck, 1999) followed by the use of SNM for intractable pelvic pain in 10 patients. This study showed improvement in 6 patients at a median of 19 months (Siegel et al., 2001). Peters et al. (2003) reported success in two-thirds of IC/BPS patients with sacral nerve stimulation. A single-blind, randomized crossover trial of sacral versus pudendal nerve stimulation suggested that direct stimulation of the pudendal nerve might achieve higher success rates (Peters et al., 2007). **Several studies, albeit largely uncontrolled, now attest to the benefits of sacral neuromodulation for IC/BPS** (Comiter, 2003; Ghazwani et al., 2011; Lavano et al., 2006;

Marinkovic et al., 2011; Tirlapur et al., 2013b; Vaarala et al., 2011). Evaluation of long term outcomes show a mean reduction of visual analog pain scores varying from 41% to 63% (Elhilali et al., 2005; Gajewski et al., 2011; Ghazwani et al., 2011; Marinkovic et al., 2011; Powell and Kreder, 2010; Rahnama'i et al., 2018). **These reports and expert opinion have placed SNM as suggested fourth-line therapy in AUA guidelines, now recommended alongside BTX-A and pain management interventions.**

Unilateral stimulation should be performed before bilateral sacral stimulation is considered (Oerlemans and van Kerrebroeck, 2008). A bilateral test stimulation could be indicated when a unilateral test fails (Steinberg et al., 2007). The only prospective randomized crossover trial to compare the unilateral with bilateral sacral nerve stimulation found no significant differences comparing the results (Scheepens et al., 2002). The presence of pain is a predictor of adverse events (White et al., 2009), and although sacral neuromodulation is effective in 56% of patients with urgency and frequency, when pain is the major complaint, caution is indicated.

Although sacral neuromodulation can significantly decrease opioid requirements in refractory IC/BPS, the majority of patients taking chronic opioids for pain will likely continue to use them for pain relief even after implantation (Peters and Konstandt, 2004). Treatment results do not appear to be age dependent (Peters et al., 2013). Sexual functioning in women may improve as well (Yih et al., 2013). The presence of urgency may be a positive predictor of long-term success (Gajewski and Al-Zahrani, 2011). When used for IC/BPS symptoms, frequent reprogramming is often required (Maxwell et al., 2008). Dorsal root ganglion, spinal cord, and deep brain stimulation are procedures that may have a role in the treatment of pelvic pain syndromes in the future. Literature is scarce and mainly limited to case studies of pelvic pain unrelated to IC/BPS (Roy et al., 2018).

> **KEY POINTS: NEUROMODULATION**
>
> - Multiple forms of neuromodulation may improve symptoms of IC/BPS. TENS is probably underutilized by practitioners and may serve a role as conservative self-therapy.
> - Although PTNS has shown efficacy for LUTS, its role in the management of pelvic pain is questionable.
> - BTX-A and SNM are recommended as fourth-line options for IC/BPS. The clinician might favor SNM over BTX-A in those patients with obstructive voiding symptoms and/or pain related to HTPFD.

Surgical Therapy

Hydrodistention

Hydrodistention of the bladder under anesthesia has been used as a treatment for IC/BPS since its original description in 1922 by Frontz. Since that time, varied methods have been explored with a technical focus on duration of distention and intravesical pressure applied. Reports of hydrodistention with systolic pressures as end points and durations of up to 3 hours showed good symptomatic results but unacceptable adverse events such as bladder rupture (Dunn et al., 1977). A more recent similar study using a balloon distention technique had equivalent results (Glemain et al., 2002). These initial observations made clinicians keenly aware that the bladder in IC patients can be very thin. **The possibility of perforation or rupture during any hydrodistention must always be kept in mind and discussed with the patient** (Badenoch, 1971; Hamer et al., 1992). Further observations suggested that **prolonged distention probably has little or no benefit over a short-term distention measured in minutes** (McCahy and Styles, 1995; Taub and Stein, 1994). **AUA guidelines suggest that short-duration (1- to 3-minute), low-pressure (60- to 80-cm H_2O) bladder hydrodistention be considered as a third-line treatment option** (Hanno et al., 2015).

Our method is to perform an initial cystoscopic examination (the findings of which are usually unremarkable), and distend the bladder for 1 to 2 minutes at a pressure of 80 cm H_2O. The bladder should be inspected throughout the procedure as tears of the mucosa or deeper can occur rapidly. Digital compression of the urethra against the cystoscope may be needed if urine leakage occurs during filling. The bladder is emptied and then refilled to allow observation for glomerulations. A therapeutic hydraulic distention follows for another several minutes. Biopsy is rarely necessary in the setting of therapeutic hydrodistention, but, if needed, it should be done *after* the hydrodistention is completed to avoid perforation. Patients should be counseled that a postprocedural flare in symptoms is a common occurrence often necessitating short-course therapy using agents as varied as urinary anesthetics and opioids. Placement of an intravesical anesthetic may improve postprocedural discomfort. Hoke et al. (2016) retrospectively reviewed their experience using a transvaginal trigonal nerve block to improve the response to hydrodistention. Although the block did not appear to have any effect as compared with hydrodistention patients not receiving the block, the postoperative improvements in pain were impressive, with a 51% to 64% reduction in pain scores 1 month after the procedure. Therapeutic responses in patients with a bladder capacity under anesthesia of less than 600 mL showed 26% with excellent results and 29% with fair results compared with 12% with excellent results and 43% with fair results in patients with larger bladder capacities (Hanno and Wein, 1991). Most favorable responses were extremely brief. The rare patient experiencing long-term improvement (>6 months) would be a candidate for repeat therapeutic distention. Favorable results were reported combining hydrodistention and BTX-A for IC/BPS (Kuo and Chancellor, 2009), ketamine cystitis (Zeng et al., 2017), and GAG therapy (Shao et al., 2010).

Hydrodistention has no benefits for patients with DO (McCahy and Styles, 1995; Taub and Stein, 1994). Over one-half of men with "prostate pain" and without bacteriuria may have glomerulations. Symptoms in this group have been reported to improve with hydrodistention (Berger et al., 1998), yet another example of the pathophysiologic crossover between these conditions.

A review of cystodistention by Olson et al. (2018) was condemning, citing that the "quality of available evidence falls below the level that would be expected of a new intervention before widespread usage, particularly in the context of evidence-based medicine." They advocated for its use to be restricted to those enrolled in an RCT or as part of a standardized national/international protocol with uniform technique and PROMs. Despite these admonitions, acute hydrodistention does not appear to result in any long-term bladder dysfunction (Kang et al., 1992; Lasanen et al., 1992) or decrease in capacity (Kirk et al., 2018), and clinical experience has been generally favorable. Nevertheless, further RCTs assessing the efficacy of hydrodistention are needed if the procedure is to remain as a viable third-line option.

Surgical Considerations

Nowhere in the treatment of IC/BPS does the caveat *primum non nocere* bear more relevance than when considering surgical options. **Although the high success rate/low complication rate for cystoscopy with fulguration of HLs merits its place as a third-line treatment option, major reconstructive procedures (sixth-line care) should be entertained only when all trials of conservative treatment have failed.** One worst-case scenario is the patient who develops significant postoperative complications and is still in pain, a situation that highlights the difficulties entailed with patient selection. Conversely, suicides have been attributed to unremitting pain where more aggressive intervention was withheld. When moving forward with a major surgical procedure, the clinician must feel that the patient has realistic expectations regarding risks and outcomes. If this is not felt to be the case, further counseling will be needed. Surgery should be reserved for the motivated and well-informed patient who falls into the category of having extremely severe, unresponsive disease, a group that comprises less than 10% of patients (Irwin and Galloway, 1994; Parsons, 2000).

Historical Procedures

Many surgical approaches have been employed for IC, and it is worth mentioning a few for historical perspective alone. Sympathectomy and intraspinal alcohol injections have been used to treat pelvic pain (Greenhill, 1947). Differential sacral neurotomy was reported in three patients with favorable results (Meirowsky, 1969), but like most deinnervation procedures never gained popularity because of subsequent poor results. Transvesical infiltration of the pelvic plexuses with phenol failed in 5 of 5 patients with IC (Blackford et al., 1984). With a significant complication rate of 17% (McInerney et al., 1991), it is rarely if ever currently used for sensory urgency disorders or detrusor hyperreflexia. There are several reports on cystolysis going back to Richer in 1929 (Bourque, 1951). Worth and Turner-Warwick reported some short-term benefit, but unpredictable long-term results (Worth, 1980; Worth and Turner-Warwick, 1973). Freiha and Stamey (1979) used cystolysis in six IC patients with favorable results in four. Albers and Geyer (1988) reported long-term follow-up in 11 IC patients and only 1 success. Denervation procedures have a notoriously high late-failure rate, and the procedure is not justified for IC/BPS (Stone, 1991; Walsh, 1985). In fact, Rogers (2003) concluded that there are no convincing clinical studies to recommend surgical procedures to interrupt visceral nerve pathways in women with any type of chronic pelvic pain.

Surgery for Hunner Lesion

Transurethral resection of an HL as initially reported by Kerr (1971), can provide symptomatic relief. Fall resected ulcerated lesions in 30 patients, resulting in initial disappearance of pain in all and a decrease in urinary frequency in 21 (Fall, 1985). Similar results have been attained with the neodymium: yttrium-aluminum-garnet (YAG) laser (Rofeim et al., 2001; Shanberg et al., 1985, 1989). Extreme caution is critical with use of a laser in the IC/BPS bladder, because forward scatter through these thin bladders with resulting bowel injury is an ever-present danger. As fulguration appears to be a relatively safe and effective technique, there would seem to be little justification to use laser for the treatment of HLs. Applying energy of any sort to glomerulations or to tissue having normal appearance is unlikely to benefit the patient (Shanberg et al., 1997).

Fulguration with low energy settings usually entails the use of a rollerball or bugbee electrode. Rapid development of surrounding hyperemia and edema is a hallmark finding seen during HL fulguration; these effects likely secondary to release of vasoactive substances from the inflamed tissue. The majority of patients require repeat fulguration as recurrence of the lesions and symptoms is to be expected over ensuing months to years (Hillelsohn et al., 2012). The use of an injectable steroid has the theoretical advantage of treating a focal inflammatory disease (although field changes have been noted) and preventing the development of bladder wall fibrosis and decrease in bladder capacity. Submucosal injection of 10 mL of 40 mg/mL **triamcinolone acetonide** injected in 0.5-mL aliquots was used for the treatment of HLs in 30 patients (Cox et al., 2009). Seventy percent of patients were very much improved, and duration of improvement was estimated to be 7 to 12 months. Similar benefits were derived from lower (66 mg) triamcinolone dosing (Funaro et al., 2018). The surgeon should be aware that injection of an HL is not as benign a process as BTX-A injection in the office. These are vascular lesions that often bleed when injected, often necessitating some fulguration.

Major Surgical Procedures

Proper patient selection and education is crucial when contemplating a major surgical procedure for the IC/BPS patient as risks include potentially devastating surgical complications and the suboptimal control of pain. On the other hand, every practitioner in this field knows the pure joy expressed by the patient whose chronic, life-altering symptoms are no longer present. As one might imagine, the patient most likely to respond to urinary diversion/substitution with or without cystectomy is one whose symptoms are generated solely or at least primarily by the bladder. It is therefore of great importance to identify and treat any other pain generators of the pelvis that might be present. As noted earlier in this chapter, HTPFD is the most common finding, but it is important to keep in mind that myalgia of the pelvic floor may be a consequence of bladder pain. Other factors that often clue the clinician to a bladder source of pain are the reproduction of the pain with bladder filling/palpation and urinary frequency that is driven by that pain. A profound reduction in bladder pain with the intravesical instillation of an anesthetic may also reflect a bladder source of pain. Brookoff and Sant (1997) proposed trying a differential spinal anesthetic block before considering cystectomy. If the patient continues to perceive bladder pain after a spinal anesthetic at the T10 level, it can be taken as an indicator that the pain signal is being generated at a higher level in the spinal cord and that surgery on the bladder will not result in pain relief. Some patients with intractable urinary frequency will opt for simple conduit urinary diversion alone, feeling that their QoL will be improved independent of the pain piece of the puzzle. Of course, treatment outcomes would be much more predictable in the patient with a poor QoL in the setting of HLs and a small, contracted, "end-stage" bladder unresponsive to conservative measures.

"Less Is More"

Bladder diversion, replacement, or augmentation is an attractive alternative to the standard ileal conduit and cystectomy for the young, otherwise healthy patient. Apart from carrying higher immediate and delayed postoperative risks, many can produce further difficulties for the patient, including pain, that will be discussed later. These factors must be kept in mind when considering anything but the simplest form of diversion possible.

Urinary diversion with or without cystourethrectomy is the ultimate surgical answer to the dilemma of IC/BPS, akin to cutting the "Gordian knot." Most patients will have relief from pain with or without simple cystectomy, suggesting that it is bladder distention or the contact with agents in urine that drive the pain (Nordling and Blaivas, 2014; Redmond and Flood, 2017). Leaving the bladder in situ is clearly associated with lower morbidity, but the potential for future problems including pyocystis, hemorrhage, severe pain, and unremitting feelings of incomplete emptying and spasm (Adeyoju et al., 1996; Eigner and Freiha 1990). Bladder carcinoma has also been reported after urinary diversion but is not specifically associated with IC/BPS (Hanno and Tomaszewski, 1982). Theoretically, conduit diversion seems to be reasonable if one is concerned about disease occurring in any continent storage type of reconstruction. Although the simplest approach, urinary diversion is not without risk. A Finnish group noted failure in 2 of 4 patients treated with cystectomy and conduit diversion because of persistent pain (Lilius et al., 1973). Baskin and Tanagho (1992) also cautioned about persistence of pelvic pain after cystectomy and continent diversion, discussing three such patients, and this has been the basis for discussion of HTPFD as a confusable source of pelvic pain. A similar report followed (Irwin and Galloway, 1992).

Supratrigonal cystectomy and the formation of an enterovesical anastomosis with bowel segments (substitution cystoplasty) has been a popular surgical procedure for intractable IC/BPS. The diseased bladder is resected in its entirety, sparing only a 1-cm cuff around the trigone to which the bowel segment is anastomosed (Irwin and Galloway, 1994; Worth et al., 1972). Although it is not always clear in the literature how much bladder has been resected, the results reported using these procedures for IC/BPS have been mixed at best. Badenoch operated on 9 patients, with 4 becoming much worse and 3 ultimately undergoing urinary diversion (Badenoch, 1971). Flood et al. (1995) reviewed 122 augmentation procedures, 21 of which were done for IC/BPS. Patients with IC/BPS had the most unfavorable results of any group, with only 10 having an "excellent" outcome. Wallack et al. (1975) reported 2 successes; Seddon et al. (1977) had success in 7 of 9 patients; and Freiha et al. (1980) ended up performing formal urinary diversion in 2 of 6 patients treated with augmentation cecocystoplasty. Weiss et al. (1984) had success in 3 of 7 patients treated with sigmoidocystoplasty, and Lunghi et al. (1984) had no excellent results in 2 patients with IC/BPS. Webster and Maggio (1989) reviewed their data in 19 patients and concluded that only patients with bladder capacities under anesthesia less than 350 mL should undergo substitution cystoplasty. Hughes et al. (1995) lowered the threshold to less than 250 mL.

More recent series on subtotal cystectomy plus augmentation have been somewhat more positive (Chesa et al., 2001; Costello et al., 2000). Peeker et al. (1998) had favorable results in all 10 patients with ulcerative IC/BPS but unfavorable results in the 3 patients operated on without HLs. He no longer performs the procedure in the latter group. Linn et al. (1998) had success in 20 of 23 patients (only 2 with IC/BPS with HLs) treated with subtotal cystectomy and orthotopic bladder substitution with an ileocecal pouch. He recommends a supratrigonal cystectomy. A Spanish series reported success in 13 of 17 procedures with a mean follow-up of 94 months (Rodriguez Villamil et al., 1999). The University of Alabama group reported long-term success in 1 of 4 patients with orthotopic neobladders and 1 of 3 with augmentation cystoplasty (Lloyd, 1999). A German report on substitution cystoplasty sparing the trigone was quite enthusiastic, detailing a 78% pain-free rate in 18 patients treated with ileocecal augmentation (10) or ileal substitution (8) at a mean follow-up of 57 months (van Ophoven et al., 2002). Two patients failed to get any pain relief, and 4 required either long-term intermittent catheterization or suprapubic drainage to empty the neobladder. The results of standard bladder augmentation are significantly worse than seen with supratrigonal resection and bowel augmentation. Enterocystoplasty performed for 7 IC/BPS patients showed failure in all patients, and 67 of 69 patients treated for other benign diagnoses were either cured or improved (Blaivas et al., 2005).

From a purely conceptual perspective, a **supratrigonal cystectomy with augmentation cystoplasty** would seem to be the perfect procedure: one that can remove the pain-producing tissue, maintain urethral voiding, and avoid "the bag." Unfortunately, even in patients with HLs, any remnant of tissue left above the trigone may become inflamed and produce further pain. Patients with preexisting urethral pain would be poor candidates for this approach, as upwards of 30% of patients will need to self-catheterize because of poor emptying. Many will also need to perform intermittent bladder irrigations to remove collected mucus. These factors along with the previously described reports of suboptimal benefit need to be considered when choosing this approach.

Bejany and Politano reported excellent results in 5 patients treated with total bladder replacement and recommended **neobladder reconstruction** (Bejany and Politano, 1995). A Thai experience using cystectomy and ileal neobladder in women in whom conservative therapy failed reported favorable results in all 35 patients treated (Kochakarn et al., 2007). Spontaneous voiding with minimal residual urine was found in 33 patients, and the remaining 2 patients had spontaneous voiding with residual urine requiring clean intermittent catheterization.

Keselman et al. (1995) had 2 failures in 11 patients treated with **continent diversion** and attributed this to surgical complications. Webster et al. (1992) had 10 failures in 14 patients treated with urinary diversion and cystectourethrectomy. Ten patients had persistent pelvic pain, and 4 of them also complained of pouch pain with only 2 patients noting symptom resolution. An English study of 27 patients who underwent cystectomy and bladder replacement with a Kock pouch noted successful treatment of pain in all patients, but follow-up was limited (Christmas et al., 1996). Parsons (2000) suggests that pouch pain will occur in 40% to 50% of patients within 6 to 36 months of surgery. In the event of neobladder pain after subtotal cystectomy and enterocystoplasty or continent diversion, it appears safe to retubularize a previously used bowel segment to form a urinary conduit for a straightforward urinary diversion without significant risk for conduit pain (Elzawahri et al., 2004).

Rössberger et al. (2007) shared their experience with 47 IC/BPS patients subjected to reconstructive or extirpative surgery, 34 of whom had classic HLs. Surgeries for the entire group included 23 substitution cystoplasties, 12 conduit diversions, and 10 Kock pouches. Twenty-eight of these 34 patients with HLs had complete symptom resolution from the initial surgical procedure. Four of the remaining 6 required urinary diversion, cystectomy, or HL resection in a trigonal remnant, but ultimately did well. Only 3 of 13 patients with non-Hunner IC/BPS had successful symptom resolution after reconstructive surgery, 2 of whom required conduit diversion. These results make one wonder whether an ileal conduit with cystectomy would have been a better initial approach for many of these patients.

> **KEY POINTS: SURGICAL THERAPY**
>
> - Major surgery for IC/BPS is a reasonable alternative for patients with severe symptoms in whom standard attempts at treatment have failed and when the disease course suggests that spontaneous remission of symptoms is unlikely.
> - Patients with a small bladder capacity under anesthesia are less likely to respond to conservative attempts at therapy.
> - Patients with HLs may have the best results with major surgery.
> - Although pain is usually the dominant feature of IC/BPS, unremitting urinary frequency refractory to conservative therapies may be an indication to proceed with urinary diversion.
> - Diversion, and even cystectomy with diversion, cannot guarantee a pain-free result, and it is critical for the patient to factor this into the decision about this often irrevocable step.
> - A simple ileal conduit or continent diversion without cystectomy can be an acceptable treatment choice with favorable clinical results.
> - Subtotal cystectomy with bladder augmentation may fail to give pain relief in more than one-third of patients (Andersen et al., 2012).

FINAL THOUGHTS

While a urology fellow, I (RM) listened to Phil Hanno lecturing about IC (as nomenclature directed at that time), likening the condition to a hole in the air…a vagueness that was hard to see or grasp from every clinical direction. Now, more than ever before, this metaphor holds true for a condition defined by a set of symptoms. The well-known heterogeneity of IC/BPS has confounded all clinical research, and, unfortunately, no animal model to date can reproduce the complexities of the IC/BPS universe.

What is essential moving forward is further work in the realm of phenotyping, both on a clinical and bench-top level. One major development stressed in this chapter is the growing acceptance of IC/BPS with HLs as a group that distinguishes itself demographically, pathologically, and, most importantly, in terms of clinical response to varied therapies from those without these lesions. Could patients with HLs represent a group with enough pathologic consistency to be ideal for future therapeutic trials? Work underway by the MAPP Network has already begun to find clusters of patients that may have differential responses to therapies. In the end, the development of biomarkers may not be helpful at defining the IC/BPS patient. Rather, the hope is that they will help guide the clinician toward therapies that will be of most benefit. Clinical phenotyping strategies have already been scrutinized to help clinicians establish the source(s) of pelvic pain in rapid fashion and to help foster better therapeutic outcomes.

A phenotypic approach to patient care is all well and good, and we are getting there, but the look of concern and fearfulness that we see from so many of our patients needs to be addressed by taking time to listen, to educate, and to work with them as partners in care. I am certain that these simple "human things" that clinicians do can improve the quality of a patient's life more than many of the therapies discussed in our chapter.

SUGGESTED READINGS

Berry SH, Elliott MN, Suttorp M, et al: Prevalence of symptoms of bladder pain syndrome/interstitial cystitis among adult females in the United States, J Urol 186(2):540–544, 2011.

Clemens JQ, Mullins C, Ackerman AL, et al: Urologic chronic pelvic pain syndrome: insights from the MAPP Research Network, Nat Rev Urol 16(3):187–200, 2019.

FitzGerald MP, Payne CK, Lukacz ES, et al: Randomized multicenter clinical trial of myofascial physical therapy in women with interstitial cystitis/painful bladder syndrome and pelvic floor tenderness, J Urol 187(6):2113–2118, 2012.

Grigorescu B, Powers K, Lazarou G: Update on urinary tract markers in interstitial cystitis/bladder pain syndrome, *Female Pelvic Med Reconstr Surg* 22(1):16–23, 2016.

Hanno PM, Burks DA, Clemens JQ, et al: AUA guideline for the diagnosis and treatment of interstitial cystitis/bladder pain syndrome, *J Urol* 185(6):2162–2170, 2011.

Hanno PM, Erickson D, Moldwin R, et al: Diagnosis and treatment of interstitial cystitis/bladder pain syndrome: AUA Guideline Amendment, *J Urol* 193(5):1545–1553, 2015.

Henry RA, Morales A, Cahill CM: Female urology beyond a simple anesthetic effect: lidocaine in the diagnosis and treatment of interstitial cystitis/bladder pain syndrome, *Urology* 85(5):1025–1033, 2015.

Kuo TL, Ng LG, Chapple CR: Pelvic floor spasm as a cause of voiding dysfunction, *Curr Opin Urol* 25(4):311–316, 2015.

Lai HH, Krieger JN, Pontari MA, et al: Painful bladder filling and painful urgency are distinct characteristics in men and women with urological chronic pelvic pain syndromes: a MAPP Research Network Study, *J Urol* 194(6):1634–1641, 2015.

Nickel JC, Moldwin R: FDA BRUDAC 2018 criteria for interstitial cystitis/bladder pain syndrome clinical trials: future direction for research, *J Urol* 200(1):39–42, 2018.

Nickel JC, Tripp DA, Pontari M, et al: Interstitial cystitis/painful bladder syndrome and associated medical conditions with an emphasis on irritable bowel syndrome, fibromyalgia and chronic fatigue syndrome, *J Urol* 184(4):1358–1363, 2010b.

Nordling J, Anjum FH, Bade JJ, et al: Primary evaluation of patients suspected of having interstitial cystitis (IC), *Eur Urol* 45(5):662–669, 2004.

Norus T, Fode M, Nordling J: Ileal conduit without cystectomy may be an appropriate option in the treatment of intractable bladder pain syndrome/interstitial cystitis, *Scand J Urol* 48(2):210–215, 2014.

Parsons JK, Parsons CL: The historical origins of interstitial cystitis, *J Urol* 171(1):20–22, 2004.

Sairanen J, Forsell T, Ruutu M: Long-term outcome of patients with interstitial cystitis treated with low dose cyclosporine A, *J Urol* 171:2138–2141, 2004.

Suskind AM, Berry SH, Ewing BA, et al: The prevalence and overlap of interstitial cystitis/bladder pain syndrome and chronic prostatitis/chronic pelvic pain syndrome in men: results of the RAND Interstitial Cystitis Epidemiology male study, *J Urol* 189(1):141–145, 2013.

Tam J, Loeb C, Grajower D, et al: Neuromodulation for chronic pelvic pain, *Curr Urol Rep* 19(5):32, 2018.

Tung A, Hepp Z, Bansal A, et al: Characterizing health care utilization, direct costs, and comorbidities associated with interstitial cystitis: a retrospective claims analysis, *J Manag Care Spec Pharm* 23(4):474–482, 2017.

REFERENCES

The complete reference list is available online at ExpertConsult.com.

58. Sexually Transmitted Diseases

Kristy McKiernan Borawski, MD

EPIDEMIOLOGY OF SEXUALLY TRANSMITTED DISEASES

A 1997 Institute of Medicine (IOM) report described sexually transmitted diseases (STDs) as, "hidden epidemics of tremendous health and economic consequence in the United States," and stated that the "scope, impact, and consequences of STDs are under recognized by the public and healthcare professionals" (Institute of Medicine Committee on Prevention and Control of Sexually Transmitted Diseases et al., 1997). Unfortunately, this still holds true two decades later, and we are now seeing the resurgence of various STDs such as syphilis and gonorrhea that had previously seen a decline in reported cases. Data from the 2016 Centers for Disease Control and Prevention (CDC) report are summarized in Table 58.1 (CDC, 2016a). Nearly 20 million new STD cases occur every year, with one-half occurring among people 15 to 24 years of age (Satterwhite et al., 2013). The direct cost of treating STDs in the United States is nearly $16 billion annually (Owusu-Edusei et al., 2013).

Clinical Prevention Guidance

Five major strategies should be used to guide prevention and control of STDs (Frieden et al., 2015). They are as follows:
- Accurate risk assessment, education, and counseling of persons at risk in prevention strategies
- Pre-exposure vaccination of persons at risk for vaccine-preventable STDs
- Identification of symptomatic or asymptomatic persons infected with STDs
- Effective diagnosis, treatment, counseling, and follow-up of infected persons
- Evaluation, treatment, and counseling of sex partners of infected persons

The first step in prevention is identifying the at-risk population. Risk factors include higher numbers of lifetime sexual partners, unprotected sex without a condom, substance abuse, and risky sexual partners. Men who have sex with men (MSM) are at an increased risk for STDs. Although the incidence of human immunodeficiency virus (HIV) and bacterial STDs had been decreasing in this group in the mid-1990s, there has now been increasing rates of syphilis, gonorrhea, and chlamydial infections. In fact, approximately two-thirds of primary and secondary syphilis cases in the United States are in MSM (Chesson et al., 2010; Kerani et al., 2007; Patton et al., 2014).

Screening Recommendations

In 2014, a multi-organization report was released that recommended clinical and nonclinical providers assess an individual's behavior and biologic risk for acquiring and transmitting STDs and/or HIV and tailor risk-reduction counseling and screening based on those risk factors (CDC, 2014).

Screening recommendations are also tailored to an individual's risk. The 2015 CDC screening guidelines are listed in the following sections. (Please note that these recommendations summarize federal agency and medical professional organizations' clinical guidelines) (Workowski, 2015).

Young or at-Risk Women

Young or at-risk women should be screened for the following:
- Routine screening for *Chlamydia trachomatis* on an annual basis for all sexually active women younger than 25 years of age (LeFevre, 2014)
- Routine screening for *Neisseria gonorrhoeae* on an annual basis for all sexually active women younger than 25 years of age (LeFevre, 2014)
- Annual screening for *C. trachomatis* and *N. gonorrhoeae* in women with risk factors

Pregnant Women

- All pregnant women in the United States should be screened for HIV infection at the first prenatal visit, even if they have been previously tested (Chou et al., 2012; Moyer, 2013).
- A serologic test for syphilis should be performed for all pregnant women at the first prenatal visit (US Preventive Services Task Force, 2009).
- All pregnant women younger than 25 years of age and older women at increased risk for infection should be screened for *C. trachomatis* and *N. gonorrhoeae* at the first prenatal visit (LeFevre, 2014).
- All pregnant women at risk for hepatitis C should be screened at the first prenatal visit.

Persons in Correctional Facilities

- Women younger than 35 years of age and men younger than 30 years of age in correctional facilities should be screened for *C. trachomatis* and *N. gonorrhoeae*.
- Universal screening should be conducted on the basis of local area and institutional prevalence of early infectious syphilis.

Men Who Have Sex With Men

Screening recommendations for MSM are as follows:
- HIV serology test if HIV status is unknown or negative and the patient or his partner has had more than one sex partner since the most recent HIV test.
- Syphilis serology test to establish whether patients with reactive tests have untreated syphilis, have partially treated syphilis, are manifesting a slow serologic response to appropriate prior therapy, or are serofast.
- Test for urethral infection regardless of condom use during exposure for *C. trachomatis* and *N. gonorrhoeae* in men who have had insertive intercourse during the preceding year.
- Test for rectal infection regardless of condom use during exposure for *C. trachomatis* and *N. gonorrhoeae* in men who have had receptive intercourse during the preceding year.
- Test for pharyngeal infection regardless of condom use during exposure for *N. gonorrhoeae* in men who have had receptive oral intercourse during the preceding year.

---

*The Centers for Disease Control and Prevention (CDC) provides national guidelines on the diagnosis and treatment of sexually transmitted diseases. The 2015 guidelines were used at the time this chapter was written (Workowski KA, Bolan GA; Centers for Disease Control and Prevention. Sexually transmitted diseases treatment guidelines, 2015. *MMWR Recomm Rep.* 2015;64[RR-03]:1–137. As these guidelines are periodically updated based on review of the most recent literature, readers are encouraged to check for updates from the CDC before treating patients with STDs.

TABLE 58.1 Sexually Transmitted Disease Cases 2016

	CASES REPORTED	RATE PER 100,000 PEOPLE	CHANGE FROM 2015
Chlamydia	1,598,354	497.3	4.7% increase
Gonorrhea	468,514	145.8	18.5% increase
Syphilis (primary and secondary)	27,814	8.7	17.6% increase

Centers for Disease Control and Prevention. Sexually transmitted disease surveillance; 2016a. Available at: https://www.cdc.gov/std/stats16/default.htm.

Transgender Men and Women

- Assess STD and HIV-related risk based on current anatomy and sexual behaviors.

Reporting Sexually Transmitted Disease

There are six mandated reportable diseases in every state: syphilis (including congenital), gonorrhea, chlamydia, chancroid, HIV infection, and acquire immunodeficiency syndrome (AIDS). The requirements for reporting other STDs vary by state. State and local health department resources are useful to identify reportable STDs in your area.

Prevention Methods

There are several methods available for the prevention of STDs. These include pre-exposure vaccination, abstinence and reduction in the number of sex partners, condoms (both male and female), cervical diaphragms, and topical microbicides and spermicide.

When used correctly, male condoms are highly effective in preventing the transmission of HIV. In heterosexual serodiscordant relationships (i.e., one infected and one uninfected) in which condoms were consistently used, HIV-negative partners were 80% less likely to become infected with HIV compared with serodiscordant relationships in which condoms were not used. Condom use decreases the risk for other STDs and, by limiting lower genital tract inflammation, may reduce the risk for pelvic inflammatory disease. When the infected area or site of potential exposure is covered, condoms can also reduce the risk for HPV, genital herpes, syphilis, and chancroid transmission.

Because they are regulated as medical devices, condoms are subject to random sampling by the US Food and Drug Administration (FDA). Breakage rates are approximately 2 per 100 used in the United States with slightly higher rates of breakage with anal intercourse.

Alternatives to latex condoms include polyurethane or other synthetic condoms and natural membrane condoms. **Polyurethane male condoms provide comparable protection against STDs/HIV and pregnancy to that of latex condoms.** Polyurethane condoms are compatible with the use of both oil-based and water-based lubricants. The effectiveness of other synthetic condoms to prevent STDs had not been extensively studied. **Natural membrane condoms ("lambskin" condoms) are made from the lamb cecum and can have pores up to 1500 nm in diameter, and, although they prevent passage of sperm, the large pore size allows passage of HIV and hepatitis B virus** (Workowski, 2015).

URETHRITIS

STDs can cause urethritis, or urethral inflammation. Typical symptoms include urethral discharge, dysuria, urethral stinging/itching, and penile tip irritation, however, urethritis is often asymptomatic (Moi et al., 2015; Horner et al., 2016).

Etiology

There are an estimated 2.8 million cases of urethritis each year that can be associated with complications including acute epididymitis, orchitis, and prostatitis (Brill, 2010). Several organisms can cause infectious urethritis. *N. gonorrhoeae* is presumed the cause of urethritis in the presence of gram-negative intracellular diplococci. Nongonococcal urethritis (NGU) is caused by *C. trachomatis* in 15% to 40% of cases (Bradshaw et al., 2006; Frieden et al., 2015). *Mycoplasma genitalium* has emerged as the second most common cause of NGU accounting for 15% to 25% of all cases (Taylor-Robinson et al., 2004; Ross and Jensen, 2006; Manhart et al., 2007). Less common causes of NGU include *Trichomonas vaginalis*, herpes simplex virus (HSV), *Haemophilus vaginalis*, and adenovirus.

Diagnosis

Previously, urethritis was diagnosed by examination of the purulent discharge with Gram stain showing greater than or equal to 5 white blood cells (WBCs) per high-power field (hpf) (Workowski, Berman, 2010). The sensitivity of the urethral Gram stain is highly dependent on the experience of the provider and the method of collection (i.e., swab vs. loop vs. spatula [increasing yield in the same order]) (Frieden et al., 2015). Several studies demonstrated that utilizing a threshold of greater than or equal to 5 WBC/hpf could miss a significant proportion of individuals with *Chlamydia trachomonatis*, *N. gonorrhoeae*, and *M. genitalium* (Couldwell et al., 2010; Rietmeijer and Mettenbrenk, 2012, 2017; Bachmann et al., 2015). **In light of these studies, the current CDC guidelines recommend using a threshold of greater than or equal to 2 WBCs per oil immersion field for the diagnosis of urethritis** (Frieden et al., 2015). The diagnosis of urethritis can be documented on the basis of any of the following signs or tests (Frieden et al., 2015):
- Mucoid, mucopurulent, or purulent discharge on examination
- Gram stain of urethral secretions demonstrating greater than or equal to 2 WBCs per oil immersion field
- Positive leukocyte esterase from a first-void urine
- Greater than 10 WBCs/hpf from a first-void urine

If point-of-care diagnostic tests (Gram stain microscopy) are not available, all men should have a nucleic acid amplification test (NAAT). In males, urine is the preferred specimen for NAATs. NAATs are also recommended in the presence of greater than or equal to 2 WBCs per oil immersion field and no intracellular gram-negative or purple diplococci (Papp et al., 2014; Frieden et al., 2015).

Gonococcal Urethritis

In 2016, there were 468,514 cases of gonorrhea reported, a significant increase over previous years (CDC, 2016a). Screening for *N. gonorrhoeae* is covered earlier in this chapter. *N. gonorrhoeae* is a gram-negative dipplococcus that has an incubation period of 3 to 14 days. Men will usually have symptoms that prompt treatment such as urethritis, epididymitis, prostatitis, or proctitis and rarely disseminated gonococcal infection. Women are usually asymptomatic and may present with sequela of the disease, pelvic inflammatory disease (PID), tubal scarring, infertility, ectopic pregnancy, and chronic pelvic pain (Hook et al., 2008).

Diagnosis of Gonococcal Urethritis

A positive Gram stain of a male urethral specimen that demonstrates polymorphonuclear leukocytes with intracellular gram-negative diplococci can be considered diagnostic for *N. gonorrhoeae* in symptomatic men. Because of its low sensitivity, a negative Gram stain does not rule out infection with *N. gonorrhoeae*. Cultures and NAATs are available for the detection of genitourinary *N. gonorrhoeae* infections. Cultures for *N. gonorrhoeae* require urethral swabs, whereas NAATs can be performed on first-catch urine and urethral swabs (Papp et al., 2014). As an aside, NAATs are not FDA-cleared for diagnosing rectal, oropharyngeal, and conjunctival infections; culture is the preferred option in these instances. As of 2014, there were five commercially available NAAT assays available for detection of both *N. gonorrhoeae* and *C. trachomatis*. **Because of their higher sensitivity, NAATs are now the preferred method for detecting *N. gonorrhoeae* and *C. trachomatis*.** In certain circumstances, however, culture for *N. gonorrhoeae* is recommended, such as in cases of sexual assault of prepubescent boys, to evaluate suspected gonorrhea treatment failures, and to monitor developing resistance to current treatment regimens. If multiple specimens are being collected from an anatomic site (e.g., urethral swab), *N. gonorrhoeae* cultures should be obtained first to maximize the sample and increase the likelihood of a successful culture (Elias and Vogel, 2011).

Treatment of Gonococcal Urethritis

Treatment of *N. gonorrhoeae* has become more complex given the evolution of antimicrobial resistance to the antibiotics historically used to treat gonorrhea and the decreased use of culture given the widespread availability and ease of NAATs (Kirkcaldy et al., 2016). In 1986, the CDC established the Gonococcal Isolate Surveillance Project (GISP) to monitor antimicrobial susceptibilities in the United States (Schwarcz et al., 1990). **Currently, the CDC recommends that gonococcal infections be treated with a single dose of both ceftriaxone 250 mg (intramuscularly) and azithromycin 1 g orally** (Workowski, 2015; Kirkcaldy et al., 2016). **If ceftriaxone is not available, alternative regimens are cefixime 400 mg orally in a single dose plus Azithromycin 1 g orally in a single dose** (Workowski, 2015). The use of ceftriaxone is contraindicated in patients with allergies to cephalosporins and in those with an IgE-mediated penicillin allergy (Pichichero and Casey, 2007; Ahmed et al., 2012). **Patients in whom the use of cephalosporins is contraindicated should be treated with azithromycin 2 g orally in a single dose plus either gemifloxacin 320 mg orally or intramuscular gentamicin 240 mg** (Kirkcaldy et al., 2014, 2016; Workowski, 2015).

Increasing antibiotic resistance has been noted among *N. gonorrhoeae* isolates. In 2014, 25% of isolates were resistant to tetracycline, 19.2% were resistant to ciprofloxacin, and 16.2% were resistant to penicillin. There was also an increase in the percentage of isolates demonstrating reduced susceptibility to azithromycin (0.6% in 2013 to 2.5% in 2014). Reduced susceptibility to cefixime and ceftriaxone remained low in 2014 (0.8% and 0.1%, respectively) but followed similar increasing trends of resistance (Kirkcaldy et al., 2016).

Treatment failures, defined as lack of symptom resolution within 3 to 5 days and no sexual contact during this period and/or a patient with a positive test of cure when no sexual contact is reported, should be evaluated with a culture along with antimicrobial susceptibility testing (Kidd and Ye, 2012; Workowski, 2015).

All patients who are diagnosed with gonorrhea should be tested for other STDs, namely chlamydia, syphilis, and HIV. Patients who are diagnosed with gonorrhea should be instructed to abstain from sexual activity for 7 days after treatment and until all sex partners have been adequately treated. All sex partners with whom they have had sexual contact within the 60 days preceding the onset of symptoms should be referred for evaluation, testing, and presumptive treatment. Because of high rates of reinfection, a follow-up test is recommended in 3 to 4 months (Workowski, 2015).

Nongonococcal Urethritis

Five percent to 20% of urethritis cases are caused by gonorrhea. The remaining NGU cases are caused by a variety of organisms, the most common of which is *C. trachomatis*, which accounts for approximately 15% to 40% of NGU cases and is more common in younger men (Wetmore et al., 2011). Many men diagnosed with urethritis will have no definitive diagnosis (Bradshaw et al., 2006; Schwebke et al., 2011). The second most common identifiable cause of NGU, *M. genitalium*, is found in 15% to 25% of men with symptomatic NGU (Taylor-Robinson and Jensen, 2011; Manhart et al., 2013; Horner and Martin, 2017). *Ureaplasma urealyticum* has been weakly associated with NGU, specifically among young men with few sexual partners. It should, however, be considered in men with no other identifiable pathogens (Frølund et al., 2011; Bachmann et al., 2015). *Trichomonas vaginalis* rates vary greatly by age and geography and should be considered in areas of high prevalence (Bachmann et al., 2015; Workowski, 2015). Other causes of NGU include herpes simplex virus (HSV)-1, HSV-2, and adenovirus (Bradshaw et al., 2002; Frølund et al., 2011).

Chlamydia

Chlamydia, caused by *C. trachomatis*, is the most frequently reported infectious disease in the United States, with the highest prevalence in persons younger than 24 years of age (CDC, 2016a). It has an incubation period of 3 to 14 days. Other sequela of *C. trachomatis* include epididymitis and Reiter syndrome. Diagnosis and treatment is also aimed to prevent transmission to their female partners as ascending chlamydial infections in women can lead to scarring of the fallopian tubes, pelvic inflammatory disease, pelvic pain, and infertility (Gottlieb et al., 2013; Lanjouw et al., 2016). As with gonorrhea, detecting *C. trachomatis* in men can be done both through urethral swab and NAATs. **NAATs using first-catch urine are the most sensitive test for detecting *C. trachomatis* infections in men and, as such, are the recommended test** (Papp et al., 2014; Workowski, 2015).

The recommended treatment for *C. trachomatis* is **azithromycin 1 g orally in a single dose OR doxycycline 100 mg orally twice daily for 7 days** (Workowski, 2015; Lanjouw et al., 2016). Alternative regimens include erythromycin base 500 mg orally four times daily for 7 days, erythromycin ethylsuccinate 800 mg orally four times a day for 7 days, levofloxacin 500 mg orally once daily for 7 days, or ofloxacin 300 mg orally twice a day for 7 days (Workowski, 2015). HIV status does not affect treatment recommendations.

Like in gonorrhea, persons testing positive for chlamydia should be advised to abstain from intercourse for 7 days after single-dose treatment or until completion of all 7 days of treatment with resolution of symptoms. **Concurrent testing for gonorrhea, HIV, and syphilis should be performed with any chlamydia diagnosis.** Although a test of cure is not advised for persons completing the advised treatment regimens (and, if retested within 3 weeks, the test may not be valid because of residual pathogen-derived nucleic acids), a 3-month retest is recommended (Fung et al., 2007; Hosenfeld et al., 2009; O'Connell and Ferone, 2016). All sex partners with whom the patient has had sexual contact within the 60 days preceding the onset of symptoms should be referred for evaluation, testing, and presumptive treatment.

Mycoplasma Genitalium

M. genitalium, first identified in the early 1980s, is responsible for 15% to 20% of NGU cases, 20% to 25% of nonchlamydial NGU cases, and approximately 30% of persistent or recurrent urethritis cases (Taylor-Robinson and Jensen, 2011; Workowski, 2015). Transmission is primarily by direct genital-genital mucosal contact. It has been detected in anorectal samples and as such, transmission from penile-anal sexual contact has been identified. Oral-genital transmission is less likely given decreased concentration of *M. genitalium* in the oro-pharynx (Jensen et al., 2016).

Cultures for *M. genitalium* can take up to 6 months, and, as such, few laboratories can recover clinical isolates (Workowski, 2015). As *M. genitalium* lacks a cell wall, it cannot be Gram stained. NAATs identifying *M. genitalium*–specific nucleic acid (DNA or RNA) are the only clinically useful methods for diagnosis. Unfortunately, although NAAT assays are commercially available, none have been approved by the FDA for diagnostic use (Horner and Martin, 2017; Sethi et al., 2017). **Because of the lack of approved diagnostic tests, *M. genitalium* should be suspected in cases of persistent or recurrent urethritis.**[*]

Antimicrobial resistance has become quite prevalent for *M. genitalium*. Doxycycline, a first-line treatment option for NGU, has only

---

[*]2016 European guidelines on *M. genitalium* recommend the use of NAATs for the diagnosis of *M. genitalium*. The authors also strongly recommend that all positive NAATs be followed up with an assay capable of detecting macrolide resistance–mediating mutations.

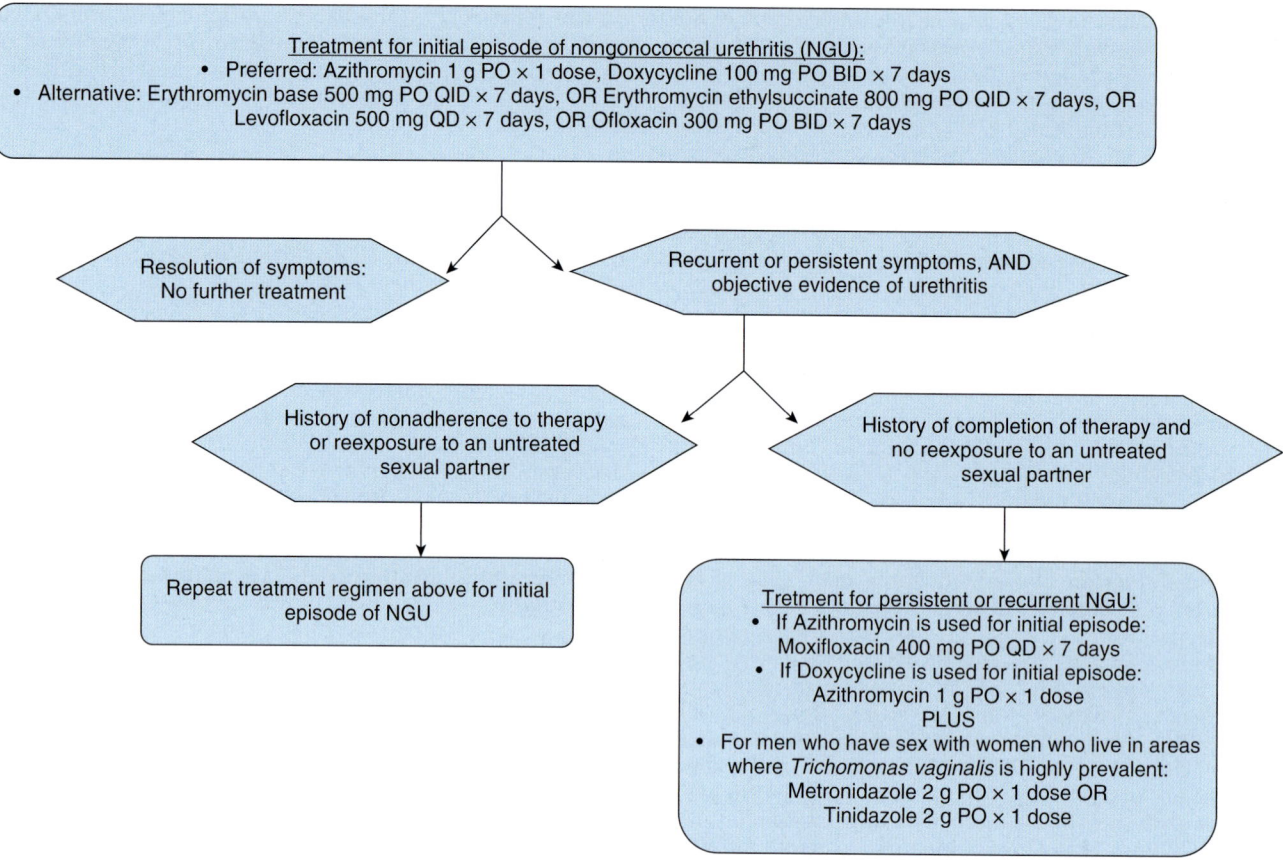

Fig. 58.1. Treatment algorithm for nongonococcal urethritis (NGU). *BID,* Twice daily; *PO,* per os (orally); *QD,* once daily; *QID,* four times daily. (Data from Bachmann LH, Manhart LE, Martin DH, et al. Advances in the understanding and treatment of male urethritis. *Clin Infect Dis.* 2015;61(Suppl 8):S763–S769.).

a 31% median cure rate (Schwebke et al., 2011). Currently, the CDC recommends a single dose of 1 g of azithromycin (Workowski, 2015). Historically, this regimen had a median cure rate of 85%, however this has dropped to 40% in a recent study (Manhart et al., 2013). Because of the treatment failures associated with the single-dose azithromycin regimen, a longer course of azithromycin was considered (500 mg initial dose followed by 250 mg daily for 4 days). Although considered, the CDC still recommends a single 1-g azithromycin dose for first-line therapy. The European guidelines differ in treatment recommendations (Jensen et al., 2016).* Treatment failures should then receive moxifloxacin 400 mg daily for 7, 10, or 14 days. Moxifloxacin appears promising in early reports, with 100% cure rates. Treatment recommendations are not affected by HIV status.

Patients testing positive for *M. genitalium* should be advised to abstain from intercourse until they have completed treatments and symptoms have resolved. Sex partners should be managed according to guidelines for patients with NGU (Workowski, 2015; Horner and Martin, 2017). **Patients with *M. genitalium* infections should be screened for other STDs including *C. trachomatis*, *N. gonorrhoeae*, syphilis, HIV, and *T. vaginalis* when appropriate** (Jensen et al., 2016). All sex partners with whom the patient has had sexual contact within the 60 days preceding the onset of symptoms should be referred for evaluation, testing, and presumptive treatment.

Trichomaonas Vaginalis

T. vaginalis is a flagellated parasite that preferentially infects the urethra in men and women and the vaginal and vulvar area in women (Muzny and Schwebke, 2013; Meites et al., 2015). Occurrence rates of *T. vaginalis* vary by age and geography with ranges from 2% to 13% (Bachmann et al., 2011, 2015). NAATs, although not FDA-approved for use in males, are replacing wet mounts of cultures for diagnosing *T. vaginalis*. The low prevalence of *T. vaginalis* in NGU does not warrant using these tests in the initial workup, although they should be considered for male sexual partners to women with trichomoniasis and for other male populations in high prevalence areas of the country. The recommended treatment for *T. vaginalis* is metronidazole 2 g orally once or tinidazole 2 g orally once (Bachmann et al., 2015).

Persistent or Recurrent Nongonoccal Urethritis

Persistence or recurrence can be a result of resistance to the completed treatment course, noncompliance with the initial treatment regimen, or re-exposure to an untreated sex partner. Consideration should be given to resistant *M. genitalium* and/or infection with *T. vaginalis*. A urine specimen can be sent for testing. A treatment algorithm for NGU can be found in Fig. 58.1. In men with persistent symptoms, urologic evaluation does not usually identify a specific cause for the urethritis. One consideration is to make sure there is no pain elsewhere in the pelvis that could indicate chronic pelvic pain syndrome as opposed to localized urethritis (Nickel et al., 2003).

---

*The 2016 European guidelines on *Mycoplasma genitalium* treatment differ from the CDC recommendations. For uncomplicated *M. genitalium* infections in the absence of macrolide resistance, the recommended treatment is azithromycin 500 mg on day 1 then 250 mg on days 2 to 5 OR josamycin 500 mg three times daily for 10 days. Uncomplicated *M. genitalium* macrolide-resistant infections should be treated with moxifloxacin 400 mg orally for 7 to 10 days. Second-line treatment for uncomplicated persistent *M. genitalium* infections is moxifloxacin 400 mg orally for 7 to 10 days. Please note that these guidelines also recommend a test of cure no earlier than 3 weeks after the start of treatment.

TABLE 58.2 Genital Ulcer Disease

DISEASE	LESIONS	LYMPHADENOPATHY	SYSTEMIC SYMPTOMS
Primary syphilis	Painless, indurated, with a clean base, usually singular	Nontender, rubbery, nonsuppurative bilateral lymphadenopathy	None
Genital herpes	Painful vesicles, shallow, usually multiple	Tender, bilateral inguinal adenopathy	Present during primary infection
Chancroid	Tender papule, then painful, undermined purulent ulcer, single or multiple	Tender, regional, painful, suppurative nodes	None
Lymphogranuloma	Small, painless vesicle or papule progresses to an ulcer	Painful, matted, large nodes with fistulous tracts	Present after genital lesion heals

EPIDIDYMITIS

Acute epididymitis is characterized by pain, swelling, and inflammation of the epididymis that lasts less than 6 weeks (Tracy et al., 2008; Workowski, 2015). The testis may be involved (epididymo-orchitis). Given the often similar presentation, one should maintain a high index of suspicion for testicular torsion. Although concurrent urethritis is often present, it is often asymptomatic. In men younger than 35 years of age, epididymitis is often caused by *C. trachomatis* or *N. gonorrhoeae*. Enteric organisms (*Escherichia coli, Pseudomonas*) may be present among men who are the insertive partner during anal intercourse (Workowski, 2015). In men older than 35 years of age who do not report insertive anal intercourse, epididymitis is often caused by uropathogenic organisms (*E. coli*) resulting from bladder outlet obstruction, urinary tract surgery, or instrumentation (Street et al., 2017). Chronic epididymitis is characterized by a history of symptoms of discomfort in the scrotum, testicle, or epididymis for 6 weeks or longer. There are both infectious (most commonly from *Mycobacterium tuberculosis*) and noninfectious causes of chronic epididymitis.

Diagnosis of Epididymitis

Acute epididymitis routinely presents as unilateral testicular pain and tenderness with a reactive hydrocele and palpable swelling of the epididymis. **Ultrasonography should not be used to diagnose acute epididymitis as a negative ultrasound in the setting of the appropriate clinical context would not alter clinical management.** Ultrasonography can be helpful if torsion is suspected. The diagnosis of epididymitis should include one of the following (Workowski, 2015):
- Gram stain or methylene blue stain of urethral secretion demonstrating greater than or equal to 2 WBCs per oil immersion field
- Positive leukocyte esterase on first-void urine
- Greater than or equal to 10 WBCs per high-power field on spun first-void urine

All suspected cases of acute epididymitis should be tested for *C. trachomatis* and *N. gonorrhoeae* with NAATs. Urine bacterial cultures should be obtained in men with sexually transmitted enteric infections and in older men with epididymitis caused by genitourinary bacteriuria (Workowski, 2015).

Treatment of Epididymitis

Empiric therapy should be started before laboratory results are available. **For acute epididymitis likely caused by an STD, the CDC recommends ceftriaxone 250 mg* intramuscularly in a single dose PLUS doxycycline 100 mg orally twice daily for 10 days. For acute epididymitis most likely caused by STD and enteric organisms (MSM), the recommended treatment is ceftriaxone 250 mg intramuscularly in a single dose PLUS levofloxacin 500 mg orally once daily for 10 days OR ofloxacin 300 mg orally twice daily for 10 days. For acute epididymitis likely caused by enteric organisms and if gonorrhea has been ruled out, treatment can be either levofloxacin or ofloxacin using the same dose/duration.** Similar to other infections caused by *C. trachomatis* and *N. gonorrhoeae*, if positive for these pathogens, patients should be counseled to abstain from sexual intercourse until they and their partners have been treated and symptoms have resolved. Testing for other STDs and HIV should proceed as mentioned in previous sections (Workowski, 2015; Street et al., 2017)

GENITAL, ANAL, AND PERIANAL ULCERS

Most young sexually active patients with genital ulcers in the United States have either genital herpes (more common) or syphilis or less commonly chancroid and donovanosis (Table 58.2). Noninfectious causes include carcinoma, yeast, trauma, psoriasis, and fixed drug eruption. Because of the inaccuracies with history and physical examination alone, all patients with genital, anal, or perianal ulcers need serologic testing, darkfield examination of polymerase chain reaction (PCR) testing if available for syphilis, culture or PCR for genital herpes, and serologic testing for type-specific herpes simplex virus (HSV) antibody. In endemic areas, a test for *Haemophilus ducreyi* should also be performed. HIV testing should be done in patients without known HIV status. Despite evaluation, 25% of patients with genital ulcers will have no specific diagnosis, and ulcers that do not respond to initial therapy or appear unusual should be sent for biopsy (Workowski, 2015).

Genital Herpes Simplex Virus Infections

Herpes simplex virus (HSV) type 1 and HSV-2 are double-stranded DNA viruses. Most cases of genital herpes are caused by HSV-2. In the United States, approximately 16% of adults are HSV-2 seropositive, but only 10% to 25% of persons with HSV-2 infections will have recognized genital herpes (Tronstein et al., 2011). **HSV-1 is now the leading cause of first-episode genital herpes in high-income countries, particularly in women and MSM younger than 25 years of age** (Johnston and Corey, 2016; Ryder et al., 2009). Although many persons may have mild or unrecognized infections, the virus is shed intermittently in the anogenital area. Shedding has been shown to occur on 10% of days, even among persons with asymptomatic HSV-2 infection (Tronstein et al., 2011). Transmission risk appears to be greatest during lesional recurrences or prodrome (Patel et al., 2017). All patients with genital herpes should be tested for HIV infection.

Pathophysiology of Genital Herpes

During primary infection, HSV-2 infects epithelial cells and then nerve endings followed by retrograde axonal transport to establish

---
*2016 European guidelines on the management of epididymo-orchitis recommends the same antibiotic choices with these notable dose differences: ceftriaxone 500 mg rather than 250 mg (CDC); ofloxacin 200 mg twice daily for 14 days rather than 300 mg twice daily for 10 days (CDC).

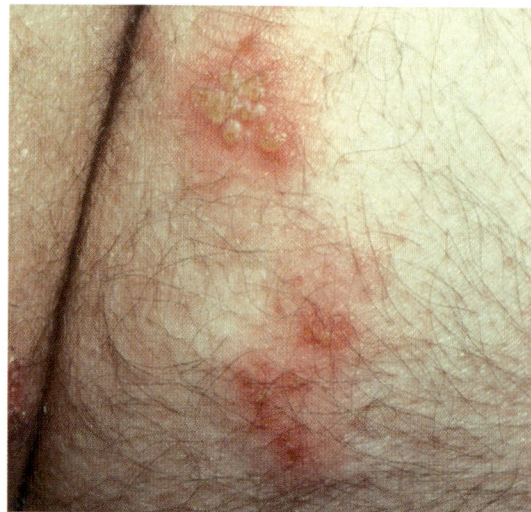

Fig. 58.2. Typical vesicular eruptions of herpes simplex virus.

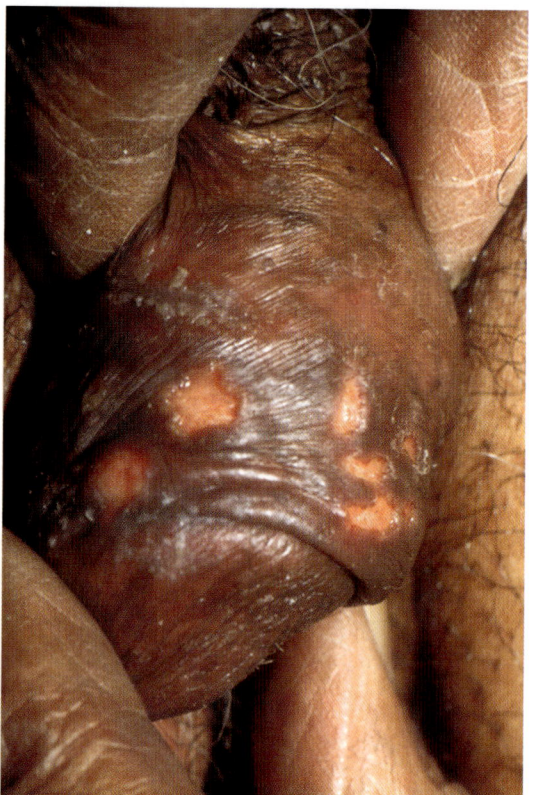

Fig. 58.3. Herpes simplex virus infection on the penis.

persistent infections in the sacral ganglia entering into a latent state. During reactivation, the virus travels down the axon to skin and mucosal surfaces, where viral shedding may be associated with genital ulcers, or more commonly, is asymptomatic (Johnston and Corey, 2016). **Periodic recurrence of genital, anal, or perianal ulcers are a hallmark of genital HSV infection, with a median of five recurrences in the first year after primary infection with genital HSV-2 and a median of one recurrence after infection with genital HSV-1** (Benedetti et al., 1999). After the first year of infection, the recurrence rate for HSV-2 decreases by a median of 2 recurrences per year, although recurrence rates may be highly variable (Johnston and Corey, 2016). Events that trigger HSV reactivation include local trauma such as surgery or ultraviolet light, immunosuppression, or fever (Gupta et al., 2007).

Presentation of Genital Herpes

Classic genital herpes can be recognized by the presence of a typical painful papular lesion progressing to vesicle (Fig. 58.2) and ulcer (Fig. 58.3) formation with local adenitis (Patel et al., 2017) that arises 4 to 7 days after exposure. Many herpetic lesions do not have the classic appearance and can look like fissures and furuncles, and they can manifest as vulvar erythema in women (Koutsky et al., 1992). Primary genital HSV-1 cannot be distinguished from HSV-2 and requires serologic testing. Possible complications include aseptic meningitis and autonomic dysfunction that can lead to urinary retention (Corey et al., 1983). Recurrent cases are usually preceded by a prodromal lesion but then can have similar presentations as mentioned earlier.

Diagnosis of Genital Herpes

Because the prognosis and the types of counseling needed depend on the type of genital herpes (HSV-1 or HSV-2), the clinical diagnosis of genital herpes should be confirmed by type-specific laboratory testing (Workowski, 2015). Cell culture and PCR are the preferred HSV testing and can be acquired from swabs from the base of genital ulcers. If needed, vesicles should be unroofed with a needle or scalpel blade (Gupta et al., 2007; Patel et al., 2017). Failure to detect HSC by culture or PCR, especially in the absence of active lesions, does not indicate an absence of HSV infection because viral shedding is intermittent (Workowski, 2015). Type-specific HSP serologic assays are useful in the following situations: (1) recurrent genital symptoms or atypical symptoms with negative HSV PCR or culture; (2) clinical diagnosis of herpes without laboratory confirmation; (3) a patient whose partner has genital herpes (Workowski, 2015). Type-specific HSV serologic assays are based on the HS-specific glycoprotein GS2 (HSV-2) and glycoprotein GS1 (HSV-1) (Song et al., 2004). Repeat testing is indicated if recent acquisition of genital herpes is suspected (Workowski, 2015).

Treatment of Genital Herpes

Because of the potential for developing severe or prolonged symptoms, all patients with symptomatic first-episode genital herpes should receive antiviral therapy (Table 58.3) (Workowski, 2015).

Almost all persons with symptomatic first-episode genital HSV-2 infections will have recurrent episodes of genital lesions; recurrences are less frequent with HSV-1. Antiviral therapy for recurrent genital herpes can be administered either as suppressive therapy to reduce the frequency or recurrences or episodically to ameliorate the duration of lesions (Workowski, 2015). Suppressive therapy can also decrease the risk for genital HSV-2 transmission to susceptible partners (Romanowski et al., 2003; Corey et al., 2004). The 2015 CDC

TABLE 58.3 Recommended Treatment Regimens for First Clinical Episode of Genital Herpes[a]

Acyclovir 400 mg orally three times a day for 7–10 days
OR
Acyclovir 200 mg orally five times a day for 7–10 days
OR
Valacyclovir 1 g orally twice a day for 7–10 days
OR
Famciclovir 250 mg orally three times a day for 7–10 days

[a]Treatment can be extended if healing is incomplete after 10 days of therapy.
Data from Workowski KA, Bolan GA; Centers for Disease Control and Prevention. Sexually transmitted diseases treatment guidelines, 2015. *MMWR Recomm Rep.* 2015;64(RR-03):1–137.

guideline recommendations for suppressive therapy for recurrent genital herpes can be found in Table 58.4, and recommendations for episodic therapy for recurrent genital herpes are in Table 58.5. Effective episodic treatment requires the initiation of therapy within 1 day of lesion onset or during the prodrome that precedes some outbreaks.

Counseling of infected persons and their sex partners is important in the management of genital herpes. A complete list of recommended topics can be found in the 2015 CDC guidelines (Workowski, 2015).

Syphilis

Syphilis is a systemic disease caused by *Treponema pallidum*, a coiled spiral spirochete bacterium, and is classified as acquired or congenital. The global burden of syphilis is high, with an estimated 10.6 million incident cases occurring annually (Stoltey and Cohen, 2015). **Syphilis rates are rising among MSM in the USA** (CDC, 2017). Acquired syphilis is usually caused by exposure during sexual contact (vaginal, anogenital, and orogenital) but rarely can be acquired through blood products, organ donation, and occupational exposures (Chambers et al., 1969; Perkins and Busch, 2010; Owusu-Ofori et al., 2011; Stoltey and Cohen, 2015). It is estimated that 50% to 60% of sexual contacts of individuals with early syphilis will acquire syphilis (Schober et al., 1983).

TABLE 58.4 Recommended Suppressive Treatment Regimens for Recurrent Genital Herpes

Acyclovir 400 mg orally twice a day
OR
Valacyclovir 500 mg orally once a day[a]
OR
Valacyclovir 1 g orally once a day
OR
Famciclovir 250 mg orally twice a day for 7–10 days

[a]Valacyclovir 500 mg once a day might be less effective than other valacyclovir or acyclovir regiments in patients who have frequent recurrences (≥10 per year).
Data from Workowski KA, Bolan GA; Centers for Disease Control and Prevention. Sexually transmitted diseases treatment guidelines, 2015. *MMWR Recomm Rep*. 2015;64(RR-03):1–137.

TABLE 58.5 Recommended Episodic Treatment Regimens for Recurrent Genital Herpes

Acyclovir 400 mg orally three times a day for 5 days
OR
Acyclovir 800 mg orally twice a day for 5 days
OR
Acyclovir 800 mg orally three times a day for 2 days
OR
Valacyclovir 500 mg orally twice a day for 3 days
OR
Valacyclovir 1 g orally once a day for 5 days
OR
Famciclovir 125 mg orally twice a day for 5 days
OR
Famciclovir 1 gram orally twice daily for 1 day
OR
Famciclovir 500 mg orally once followed by 250 mg twice daily for 2 days

Data from Workowski KA, Bolan GA; Centers for Disease Control and Prevention. Sexually transmitted diseases treatment guidelines, 2015. *MMWR Recomm Rep*. 2015;64(RR-03):1–137.

All patients who test positive for either primary or secondary syphilis should be tested for HIV infection. The incidence rate for syphilis in the HIV population has been reported as 77 times greater than that of the general population (Chesson et al., 2005). Syphilis is associated with HIV shedding in blood plasma (HIV concentrations can increase as much as 0.22 log values before syphilis treatment) and the genital tract (Kalichman et al., 2011, Workowski, 2015). Rarely, an unusual serologic response has been observed among patients with HIV infection who have syphilis. When clinical findings are suggestive or syphilis but serologic tests are nonreactive or unclear, alternative tests (biopsy, darkfield examination) can be considered (Workowski, 2015).

Primary Syphilis

The incubation period between contact and the development of a chancre is usually between 10 and 90 days. Primary syphilis is characterized by the development of an ulcer (chancre) usually with regional lymphadenopathy. **The chancre is usually painless, single, and indurated with a clean base discharging clear serum** (Figs. 58.4 and 58.5). Lesions are often atypical in appearance and may be multiple, deep, and indistinguishable from herpes (Rompalo et al., 2001a, 2001b; Hope-Rapp et al. 2010; Janier et al., 2014). Untreated lesions heal spontaneously in 3 to 8 weeks (Ho and Lukehart, 2011).

Secondary Syphilis

Secondary syphilis arises from the development of bacteremia that usually occurs 3 to 5 months after the initial infection. **It is characterized by a maculopapular rash (Fig. 58.6) involving the palms of the hands and soles of the feet (usually does not itch) and mucous membrane lesions involving the vagina or anus.** The rash can ulcerate and lead to condyloma lata (large, raised gray or white lesions). Additional symptoms include fever, lymphadenopathy, alopecia, and weight loss (CDC, 2017a). There is also a broad vasculitis that, in approximately 10% of patients, may lead to manifestations such as hepatitis, iritis, nephritis, and neurologic problems including headache and cranial nerve involvement (VIII, auditory) (Mindel et al., 1989). The neurologic sequelae should be individualized as early neurosyphilis (Janier et al., 2014).

Latent Syphilis

Latent syphilis is defined as seroreactivity with no clinical evidence of disease and is broken up into early versus late latent syphilis. Early latent syphilis includes patients with a positive serologic test for syphilis, preceded by a negative serology test within 1 year or recent contact with an infected person. All other cases of latent

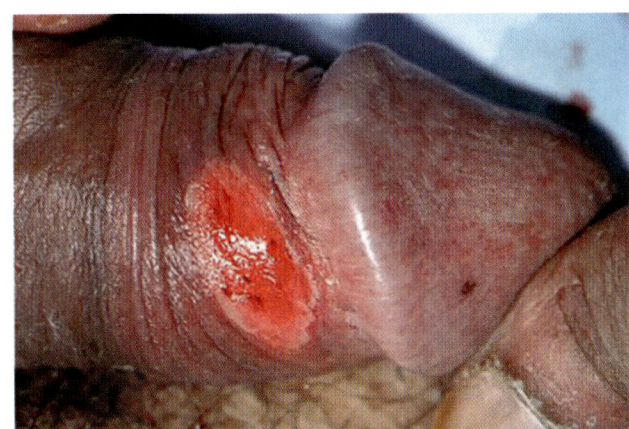

Fig. 58.4. Syphilis with penile chancre. (From James WD, Berger TG, Elston DM. Syphilis, yaws, bejel and pinta. In: *Andrews' diseases of the skin: clinical dermatology*, 12th ed. Philadelphia, PA: Elsevier; 2016:345).

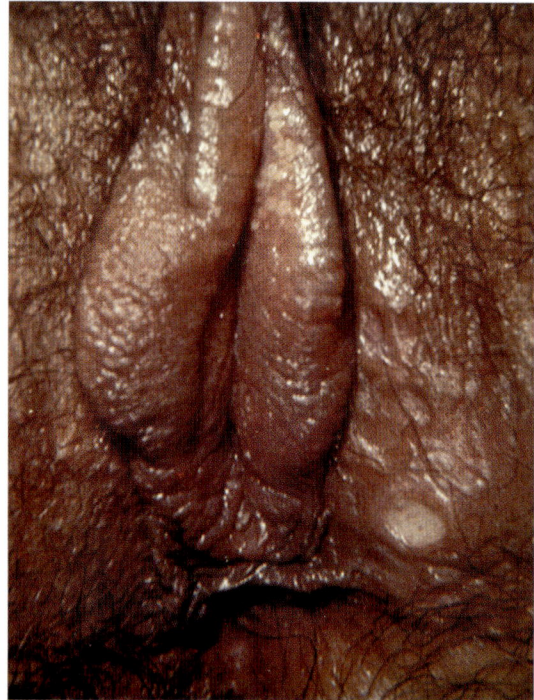

Fig. 58.5. Syphilis with vulvar chancre.

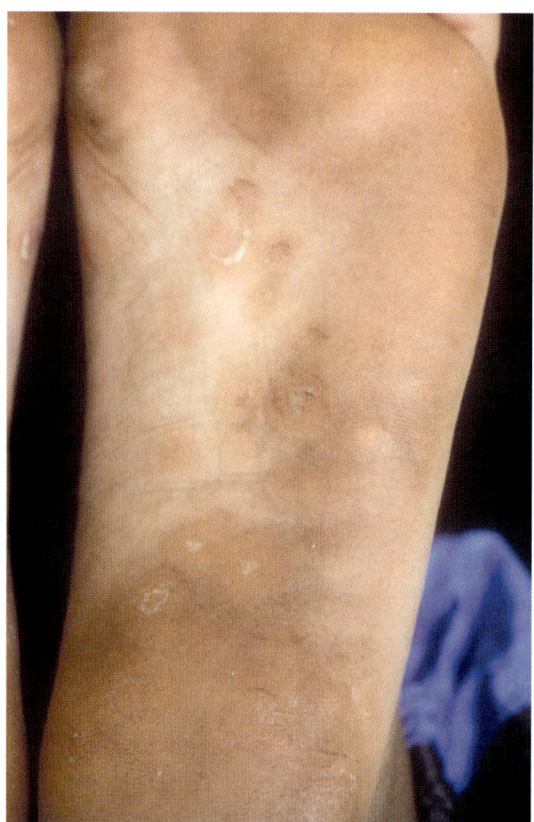

Fig. 58.6. Secondary syphilis affecting the soles of the feet.

syphilis is defined as late latent syphilis or syphilis of unknown duration (Workowski, 2015).

Tertiary Syphilis

About 35% of individuals with late latent syphilis will develop the late manifestations of syphilis, which include neurosyphilis, cardiovascular syphilis, and gummatous syphilis. These are rare outside of developing countries. Neurosyphilis can be seen in secondary syphilis, and meningovascular syphilis also occurs in tertiary syphilis. The incubation period is usually 5 to 12 years. After 10 to 20 years, the spinal column and brain can also be involved. The spinal cord syndrome is called *tabes dorsalis,* and the brain syndrome is called *general paralysis of the insane* (Danielsen et al., 2004; French, 2007). Cardiovascular syphilis occurs 15 to 30 years after infection and may occur in any large vessel (French, 2007).

Diagnosis of Syphilis

Darkfield Examination

Cultures for *T. pallidum* are not possible in vitro. A darkfield examination to detect *T. pallidum* directly from lesion exudate or tissue is the definitive method for diagnosing early syphilis. It is very cumbersome and is not widely utilized (Workowski, 2015).

Serology

A presumptive diagnosis of syphilis requires the use of two tests: a nontreponemal test and a treponemal test. Use of only one serology test is insufficient as it can result in false-negative results in patients tested during primary syphilis and false-positive results in patients without syphilis.

Nontreponemal Tests

Nontreponemal tests (NTTs) identify nontreponemal antibodies that bind lipids that have bound to the treponeme and become antigenic (Lafond and Lukehart, 2006). NTTs become positive 10 to 15 days after the beginning of the primary chancre. Nontreponemal tests include Venereal Disease Research Laboratory (VDRL) or rapid plasma reagin (RPR) (Janier et al., 2014). False-positive NTT results can be caused by other infections (HIV), autoimmune conditions, immunizations, pregnancy, drug use, and old age. **All persons with a reactive NTT should always receive a confirmatory treponemal test** (Workowski, 2015).

Nontreponemal test antibody titers might correlate with disease activity and can be used to follow treatment response. A fourfold change in titer, equivalent to a change of two dilutions (e.g., from 1:16 to 1:4 or from 1:8 to 1:32) is required to demonstrate a clinically significant difference between two NTTs. Sequential serologic tests in individual patients should be performed using the same NTT (Workowski, 2015). NTT titers usually decline after treatment and may become nonreactive with time. Some treponemal antibodies can persist for a long period (serofast) (Workowski, 2015).

Treponemal Tests

Treponemal antibodies are detected by immunofluorescence in the fluorescent treponemal antibody absorption test (FTA-ABS), the *T. pallidum* particle agglutination test (TP-PA), various enzyme immunoassays (EIAs), chemiluminescence immunoassays, immunoblots, or rapid treponemal assays (Workowski, 2015). False-positive results are uncommon but can occur in patients with collagen disease, lupus, and other infections (Hart, 1986). **Most patients who have a reactive treponemal test (TT) will have reactive tests for the remainder of their lives regardless of treatment or disease activity.** Fifteen percent to 25% of patients treated in the primary stage revert to nonreactive after 2 to 3 years (Romanowski et al., 1991; Workowski, 2015). Rapid syphilis tests including the enzyme-linked immunosorbent assay (ELISA) are available and approved by the FDA. These can give results in 5 to 10 minutes but cannot distinguish between active and treated syphilis. A reverse screening algorithm utilizes this rapid test as a screen and if positive, a reflexive NTT is performed. If the NTT is negative, a second TT should be performed (preferably one based on different antigens than the original). If the second TT is positive, persons with a history of previous treatment need no further management unless sexual history suggests re-exposure. In this instance, a repeat

NTT is recommended in 2 to 4 weeks. Those without a history of treatment and a positive second TT should be offered treatment for latent syphilis. If the second TT is negative and risk factors are low, further evaluation is not indicated (Workowski, 2015).

Treatment for Syphilis

Intravenous penicillin G is the preferred drug for treating all stages of syphilis. The preparation used, dosage, and duration of treatment will depend on the stage and clinical manifestation of the disease. Treatment guidelines from the CDC for adults with syphilis are detailed in Table 58.6 (Workowski, 2015). **Combinations of different penicillin G preparations are not appropriate for the treatment of syphilis.** Patients should be informed of the possibility for a Jarisch-Herxheimer reaction with the first 24 hours after initiation of treatment. This is an acute febrile reaction accompanied by headache, myalgia, and other symptoms that most commonly happens among persons who have early syphilis, presumably because of higher bacterial burdens. Patients should be counseled that this is not an allergic reaction to penicillin but a reaction to the treatment of treponemes. Treatment is conservative with nonsteroidal anti-inflammatory drugs (Workowski, 2015).

Clinical and serologic evaluation should be performed at 6 and 12 months. **Patients who have signs or symptoms that persist or recur and those with at least a fourfold increase in nontreponemal test titer persisting for longer than 2 weeks likely are either treatment failures or were reinfected.** These patients should be retreated and re-evaluated for HIV, and CSF examination can be considered. Retreatment consists of weekly injections of benzathine penicillin G 2.4 million units IM for 3 weeks unless neurosyphilis is diagnosed (Workowski, 2015).

Chancroid

Chancroid is caused by the gram-negative bacillis *Haemophilus ducreyi* (Albritton, 1989). *H. ducreyi* is usually spread through sexual intercourse, and it is believed that microabrasions are required to be present before infection can be established in the genital epithelium and underlying tissue (Morse, 1989; Lewis, 2003). Currently in the United States, chancroid is restricted to rare sporadic cases, although it remains endemic in North India and Malawi (Gonzalez-Beiras et al., 2016; Lautenschlager et al., 2017). Chancroid is more prevalent among individuals from lower socioeconomic groups, female commercial sex workers and their male partners, and uncircumcised men. Chancroid is a risk factor for HIV transmission (Lewis, 2003).

Chancroid initially starts as tender erythematous papules, most often on the prepuce and frenulum in men and on the vulva, cervix, and perianal area in women. The papules quickly progress into pustules that rupture after a few days and develop into superficial ulcers with ragged and undetermined edges (Fig. 58.7). The incubation period is usually 3 to 7 days. Inguinal lymphadenitis, usually unilateral and painful, develops in approximately 50% of patients, which may progress into fluctuant buboes that may spontaneously rupture (Lautenschlager et al., 2017).

TABLE 58.6 Treatment of Syphilis

STAGE OF SYPHILIS	PENICILLIN TREATMENT	PENICILLIN-ALLERGIC PATIENTS
Primary, secondary, and early latent syphilis with no neurologic involvement	Benzathine penicillin G 2.4 million units IM, single dose	Doxycycline 100 mg PO bid for 14 days Tetracycline 500 mg PO qid for 14 days
Late latent or latent syphilis of unknown duration with no neurologic involvement	Benzathine penicillin G 2.4 million units IM once a week for 3 weeks	Doxycycline 100 mg PO bid for 28 days Tetracycline 500 mg PO qid for 28 days
Tertiary (late) syphilis with no neurologic involvement	Benzathine penicillin G 2.4 million units IM once per week for 3 weeks	Consult infectious disease specialist
Neurosyphilis Alternative regimen	Aqueous crystalline penicillin G 3–4 million units IV q4h or continuous IV infusion for total 18–24 million units per day, both for 10–14 days Procaine penicillin 2.4 million units IM daily plus probenecid 500 mg PO qid, both for 10–14 days	

bid, Twice daily; *IM*, intramuscular; *IV*, intravenously; *PO*, per os (orally); *q4h*, every 4 hours; *qid*, four times daily.
From Workowski KA, Bolan GA; Centers for Disease Control and Prevention. Sexually transmitted diseases treatment guidelines, 2015. *MMWR Recomm Rep.* 2015;64(RR-03):1–137.

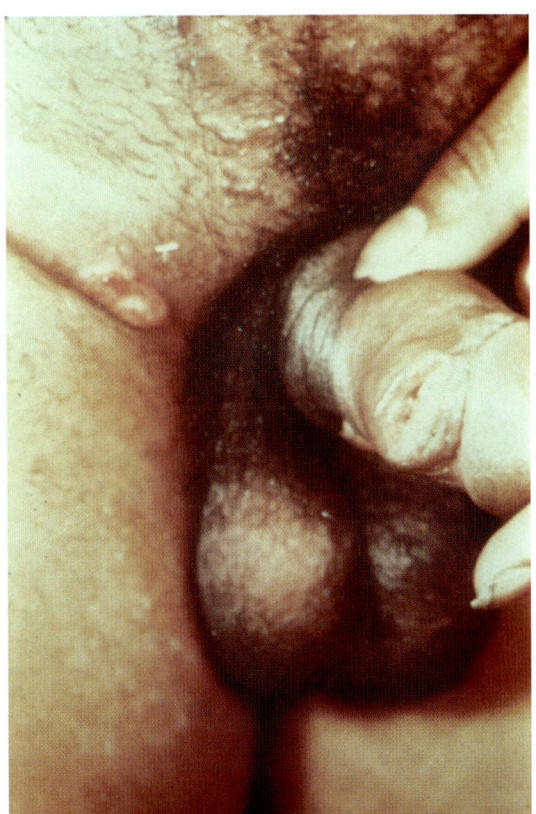

Fig. 58.7. Chancroid with regional lymphadenopathy.

A definitive diagnosis of chancroid requires identification of *H. ducreyi* on a special culture medium that is not widely available. Although no FDA-cleared PCA test for *H. ducreyi* is available in the United States, testing can be performed by laboratories that have developed their own PCR test and have conducted clinical laboratory improvement amendments (CLIA) verification studies (Workowski, 2015). For both clinical and surveillance purposes, the diagnosis of chancroid can be made if the following criteria are met: (1) the patient has one or more painful genital ulcers; (2) the clinical presentation, appearance of genital ulcers and, if present, regional lymphadenopathy are typical for chancroid; (3) the patient has no evidence for *T. pallidum* infection by either darkfield examination of ulcer exudate or serologic testing for syphilis performed at least 7 days after onset of ulcers; and (4) an HSV PCR test or HSV culture performed on the ulcer exudate is negative (Workowski, 2015).

Treatment is with any *one* of the following options: azithromycin 1 g orally in a single dose, ceftriaxone 250 mg intramuscularly in a single dose, ciprofloxacin 500 mg orally twice a day for 3 days, or erythromycin base 500 mg orally three times a day for 7 days. Patients should be tested for HIV at the time of diagnosis and if negative, testing for syphilis and HIV should be repeated in 3 months. Patients with HIV or those who are uncircumcised do not respond as well to treatment and may require a prolonged course (Workowski, 2015). Patients with fluctuant buboes may require treatment in the form of either needle aspiration or incision and drainage (Lautenschlager et al., 2017).

Granuloma Inguinale (Donovanosis)

Granuloma inguinale is a genital ulcerative disease caused by the intracellular gram-negative bacterium *Klebsiella granulomatis* (formerly *Calymmatobacterium granulomatis*) (Carter et al., 1999). It occurs rarely in the United States, although cases are still reported from Papua New Guinea, South Africa, India, Brazil, and Australia (Velho et al., 2008; O'Farrell and Moi, 2016). The incubation period is approximately 50 days, after which papules develop into ulcers that gradually increase in size. These are usually painless, slowly progressive ulcerative lesions on the genitals or perineum without regional lymphadenopathy. Despite the name, only 10% of cases involve the inguinal region. The lesions are highly vascular (beefy red appearance) and tend to bleed easily (Fig. 58.8) (Workowski, 2015). The most common site of extragenital spread is the mouth, but it can also occur in the pelvis, intra-abdominal organs, and other bones (Velho et al., 2008). All patients who receive a diagnosis of granuloma inguinale should be tested for HIV (Workowski, 2015).

There are no FDA-cleared molecular tests for the detection of *K. granulomatis*. Diagnosis requires visualization of dark-staining Donovan bodies on tissue crush preparation of biopsy (Workowski, 2015). The recommended treatment is azithromycin 1 g orally weekly or 500 mg daily for at least 3 weeks and until all lesions are completely healed. Alternative agents may be found in the CDC guidelines (Workowski, 2015). Squamous cell carcinoma of the penis may mimic granuloma inguinale and, as such, a biopsy should be done if antibiotics fail to resolve ulcers (O'Farrell and Moi, 2016).

Lymphogranuloma Venereum

C. trachomatis is an obligate intercellular pathogen. It's fifteen serovars can be classified into three groups based on type of infection; trachoma (serovars A, B, Ba, and C), anogenital infections (serovars D and K), and lymphogranuloma venereum (LGV; serovars L1, L2, and L3) (Schachter et al., 2008; Stamm, 2008). In Western countries, the incidence of LGV has been increasing since 2003, primarily among HIV men who have sex with men (Ronn et al., 2014). LGV symptoms are classically divided into three stages: local infection (primary stage), regional dissemination (second stage), and progressive tissue damage (tertiary stage). Although often asymptomatic, a self-limited genital ulcer or papule develops about 3 to 30 days after inoculation. Direct rectal inoculation can result in proctitis with rectal bleeding, rectal pain, tenesmus, constipation, or hemopurulent rectal discharge (Workowski, 2015; O'Byrne et al., 2016). About 2 to 6 weeks after the primary lesion appears, regional tissue invasion occurs with constitutional symptoms (i.e., fever, chills, malaise, myalgia). With penile, urethral, or vulvar inoculation, inguinal syndrome occurs characterized by unilateral, painful inguinal or femoral lymphadenopathy known as buboes (Fig. 58.9) (O'Byrne et al., 2016). Inguinal nodes are more common in men because the lymph drainage of the cervix and vagina are to the retroperitoneal rather than inguinal nodes (Mabey and Peeling, 2002). If left untreated, LGV can lead to irreversible tissue destruction and scarring resulting in regional lymphedema and genital elephantiasis. In cases of rectal involvement, perirectal abscesses, anal fissures, and strictures can form (Workowski, 2015; O'Byrne et al., 2016). LGV does not appear to occur more frequently or with more virulence in HIV-positive individuals (Jebbari et al., 2007).

Diagnosis is based on clinical suspicion, epidemiologic information, and the exclusion of other etiologies. Genital lesions, rectal specimens, and lymph node specimens can be tested for *C. trachomatis* by culture, direct immunofluorescence, or NAAT. Although NAATs for *C. trachomatis* detection from a rectal sample are not FDA-cleared for this purpose, many laboratories have performed CLIA validation studies needed and as such NAAT performed on rectal specimens is the preferred approach for testing. Chlamydia serology (complement fixation titers greater than or equal to 1:64 or microimmunofluorescence

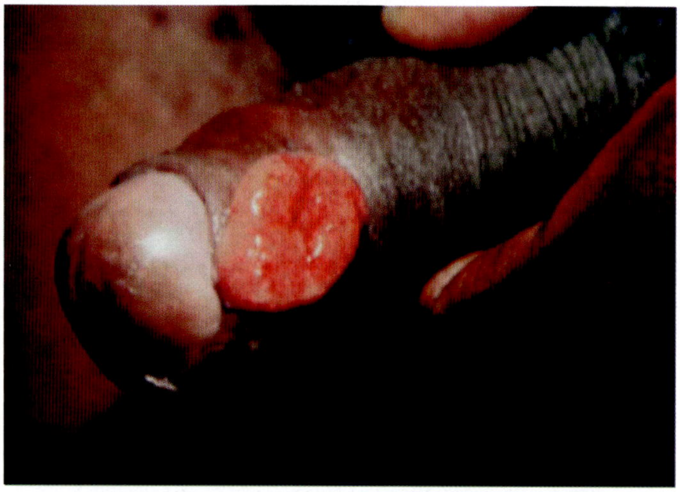

Fig. 58.8. Lymphogranuloma venereum (donovanosis) lesion on the penis. (From O'Farrell N. Donovanosis. *Sex Transm Infect.* 2002;78:452–457.).

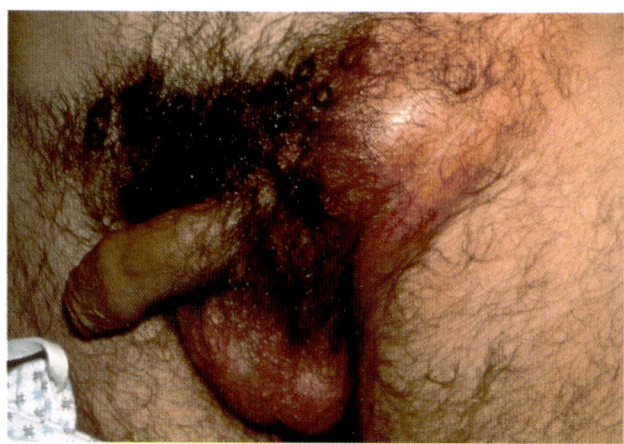

Fig. 58.9. Lymphogranuloma venereum with inguinal adenopathy.

titers >1:256) might support the diagnosis of LGV in the appropriate clinical context (Workowski, 2015).

Recommended treatment is doxycycline 100 mg orally twice a day for 21 days. An alternative regimen is erythromycin base 500 mg orally four times a day for 21 days (Workowski, 2015). Recently, studies have evaluated the use of a 7-day course of doxycycline with excellent cure rates (Simons et al., 2018). As of now, however, the CDC guidelines still recommend a 21-day course of doxycycline. Patients who test positive for LGV should be screened for other STDs, especially HIV, gonorrhea, and syphilis.

Molluscum Contagiosum

Molluscum infection is a benign epidermal eruption of the skin caused by molluscum contagiosum, a large double-stranded DNA virus (Myskowski, 1997). Four serotypes of molluscum contagiosum have been identified, molluscum contagiosum virus (MCV)-1 followed by MCV-2. MCV-2 appears relatively common in the setting of immunocompromise and HIV (Fernando et al., 2015). **As an STD, molluscum infection usually affects young adults and appears to be increasing in frequency** (Villa et al., 2010). Sexually transmitted molluscum lesions usually affect the genitals, pubic region, lower abdomen, upper thigh, and/or buttocks.

Molluscum lesions present as smooth-surfaced, firm, dome-shaped papules with central umbilication. Lesions are usually 2 to 5 mm, and patients commonly have 1 to 30 lesions that are usually asymptomatic (Fig. 58.10). **Molluscum infection will usually spontaneously regress in 6 to 12 months in the immunocompetent individual with no sequelae** (Villa et al., 2010). Infections can be much more severe and extensive in immunocompromised patients, namely those with HIV. Molluscom infection in immunocompromised persons can be much more aggressive and widespread, presenting with 100 or more lesions and progressive as confluent, coalescing

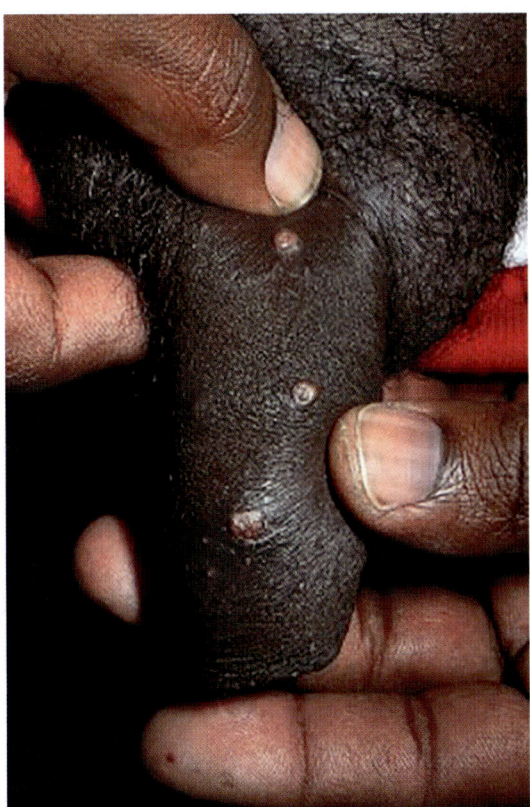

Fig. 58.10. Molluscum contagiosum on the penis. (From James WD, Berger TG, Elston DM. Viral diseases. In: *Andrews' diseases of the skin: clinical dermatology*, 12th ed. Philadelphia, PA: Elsevier; 2016:389).

large lesions (Schwartz and Myskowski, 1992; Brown et al., 2000; Trope and Lenzi, 2005; Nakamura-Wakatsuki et al., 2011).

Diagnosis is predominantly clinical on the basis of characteristic lesions. Biopsy is indicated in cases of atypical presentations in which malignancy must be excluded (Trope and Lenzi, 2005).

Expectant management (no treatment) is an option for immunocompetent patients. Patients should be warned of the risk for autoinoculation and advised against shaving or waxing the genitals to prevent further spread. Towels, bed linen, clothes, and so on should not be shared when active lesions are present (Fernando et al., 2015). For those seeking treatment, multiple options exist including cryotherapy, curettage, light emitting, and pulse dye lasers. Topical therapies include 0.5% podophyllotoxin (avoid in pregnancy), 5% imiquimod cream (avoid in pregnancy), and multiple other chemical preparations. For patients with HIV, the first treatment should be HAART as a low CD4 count is inversely proportional with the number of molluscum lesions, and lesions have been shown to regress after initiation of HAART in some cases (Myskowski 1997; Fernando et al., 2015).

ANOGENITAL WARTS
Human Papillomavirus

Human papillomaviruses (HPVs) are a small group of nonenveloped, double-stranded DNA viruses belonging to the *Papillomaviridae* family. To date, more than 170 types of HPV have been identified, one-half of which affect the genital tract (Boda et al., 2018). **High-risk mucosal HPV types, predominantly 16, 18, 31, 33, and 35, have been associated with most cervical, penile, vulvar, vaginal, anal, and oropharyngeal cancers and precancers.** HPV 16 and 18 are the most common high-risk types and are considered to be responsible for greater than 70% of all cervical cancer cases (Clifford et al., 2003; Boda et al., 2018). **HSV 6 and 11 are nononcogenic and are responsible for about 90% or anogenital warts** (Garland et al., 2009). HPV infections are often asymptomatic and unrecognized, and the majority of sexually active persons become infected with HPV at least once in their lifetime (Myers et al., 2000). Oncogenic high-risk HPV strains have the strongest contribution to the occurrences of precancerous and cancerous lesions (Stokley et al., 2014). In 2009, there were an estimated 34,788 new HPV-associated cancers and 355,000 new cases of anogenital warts (Chesson et al., 2012; Jemal et al., 2013; Patel et al., 2013).

Presentation and Diagnostic Considerations

Anogenital warts (condylomata acuminatum) are usually asymptomatic, but depending on the size and location, they can be painful or pruritic. The warts are usually flat, papular, or pedunculated growths (Fig. 58.11). They occur commonly at certain anatomic sites, including the vaginal introitus, under the foreskin of an uncircumcised penis, and on the shaft of a circumcised penis, although they may be seen at multiple sites in the anogenital epithelium or within the anogenital tract, such as the cervix, vagina, urethra (Fig. 58.12), perineum, perianal skin, anus, and scrotum (Workowski, 2015). Bowenoid papulosis is characterized by flat, often hyperpigmented papules a few millimeters to several centimeters in diameter. These occur singly or, more often, may be found in multiples on the penis, near the vulva, or perianally. Bowenoid papulosis is now called HSIL (high-grade squamous intraepithelial lesion) and is usually caused by HPV-16. Giant condyloma acuminatum is a rare, aggressive, wartlike growth that is a verrucous carcinoma. Unlike other HPV-induced genital carcinomas, this tumor is usually caused by HPV-6. It occurs most often on the glans or prepuce of an uncircumcised male; less often, it may occur on perianal skin or the vulva. Despite its bland histologic picture, it may invade deeply, and infrequently it may metastasize to regional lymph nodes (James and Elston, 2016).

The diagnosis of anogenital warts is usually made by clinical examination. Although HPV tests are available to detect oncogenic types of HPV, the tests should not be used for male partners of women with HPV or women younger than 25 years of age for diagnosis

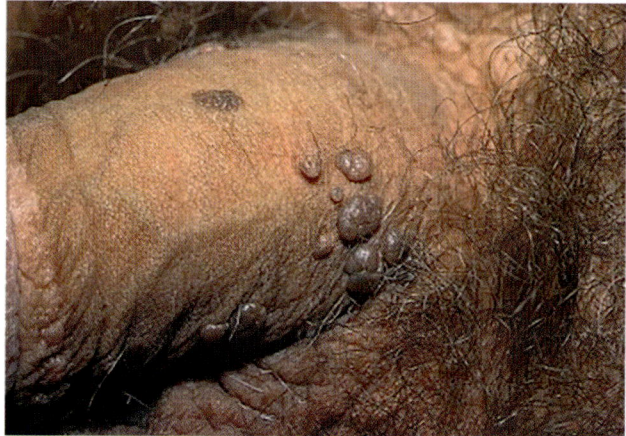

Fig. 58.11. Penile warts (Condylomata acuminata) caused by human papillomavirus. (From James WD, Berger TG, Elston DM. Viral diseases. In: *Andrews' diseases of the skin: clinical dermatology*, 12th ed. Philadelphia, PA: Elsevier; 2016:405).

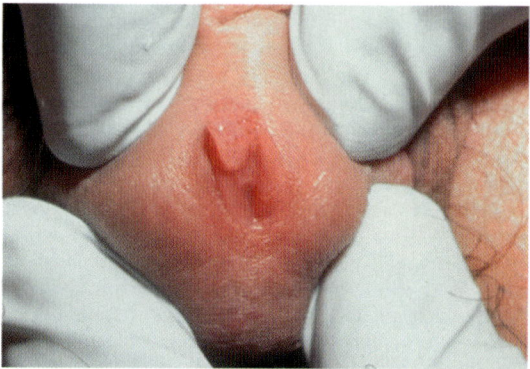

Fig. 58.12. Meatal wart caused by human papillomavirus.

of genital warts or as a general STD test (Workowski, 2015). The use of 3% to 5% acetic acid to visualize potentially affected areas is not recommended. **Biopsy may be indicated in the following conditions: (1) the diagnosis is uncertain; (2) the lesions do not respond to standard therapy; (3) the disease worsens during therapy; (4) the patient is immunocompromised; (5) the warts are pigmented, indurated, or affixed to underlying tissue; or (6) there is persistent ulceration or bleeding** (Workowski, 2015).

Treatment of Anogenital Warts

The main goal of treatment is removal of the wart and improvement in associated symptoms. Some warts may spontaneously resolve within 1 year, and, as such, some patients may opt for observation. **Wart size, number, anatomic location, patient preference, cost, and potential adverse effects should guide treatment.** Treatment regimens are divided into patient-applied and provider-applied options (Workowski, 2015).

Patient-applied treatments for HPV are as follows:
- Imiquimod cream 3.75% applied once daily at bedtime for up to 16 weeks; should be washed off 6 to 10 hours after application
- Imiquimod cream 5% applied daily at bedtime three times a week for up to 16 weeks; should be washed off 6 to 10 hours after application
- Podofilox 0.5% solution or gel up to 0.5 mL/day, applied twice a day for 3 days, then no therapy for 4 days, up to four cycles. Total wart area should not exceed 10 cm^2.
- Sinecatechins 15% ointment three times per day for up to 16 weeks. This should not be washed off after application.

Provider-administered treatments for HPV are as follows:
- Cryotherapy such as liquid nitrogen, which induces cytolysis. Application can be repeated every 1 to 2 weeks. Large warts may need local anesthesia because of possible pain with application.
- Surgical therapy including direct excision with scissors, tangential shave excision, curettage, or laser therapy using a CO$_2$ laser. Consider collaboration with a plastic surgeon for large lesions that require large areas of excision, especially on the penis or in the groin creases. Should be performed in an appropriately ventilated room using standard precautions and local exhaust ventilation (CDC, 1999; Siegel et al., 2007, updated 2017).
- Trichloroacetic acid (TCA) or bichloroacetic acid (BCA) 80% to 90%; these acids destroy warts by chemical coagulation of wart proteins. Apply to wart, and allow to dry before patient stands up; if intense pain ensues after administration, neutralize the acid with soap and water or sodium bicarbonate. Can be repeated weekly.

Imiquimod stimulates production of interferon and other cytokines, and, as a result, its use can result in local inflammatory reactions (redness, irritation, induration, ulceration, or vesicle formation) and hypopigmentation (Mashiah and Brenner, 2008; Workowski, 2015). There are limited data on the use of imiquimod in pregnancy, although animal data suggests that it may pose low risk (Ciavattini et al., 2012; Workowski, 2015). **Both the 3.75% and 5% imiquimod cream can weaken condoms and vaginal diaphragms.**

Podofilox (podophyllotoxin) is an antimitotic drug that causes wart necrosis. It is recommended that providers apply the initial treatment to demonstrate proper application technique. **Podofilox use is contraindicated in pregnancy** (Workowski, 2015).

Sinecatechins contains the green tea extract catechins, which exhibit specific antioxidant, antiviral, antitumor, and immunostimulatory properties (Tzellos et al., 2011). Genital, anal, and oral sexual contact should be avoided while using this ointment. Side effects include erythema pruritus, burning, pain, ulceration, edema, induration, and rash. This treatment is not recommended for immunocompromised or pregnant patients as its safety and efficacy has not been established. Sinecatechins may weaken condoms and vaginal diaphragms.

Most anogenital warts respond to treatment within 3 months. If significant improvement is not noted, another treatment modality should be used. As mentioned earlier, biopsy may be considered for lesions that do not respond to treatment.

Patients with anogenital warts should be screened for other STDs. Patients should be counseled that even with treatment of warts, HPV can still be transmitted to partners. **Because HPV can infect areas not covered by condoms, the routine use of condoms, although it can decrease the risk for transmission, does not eliminate its possibility** (Workowski, 2015).

Human Papillomavirus Vaccine

Abstaining from sexual activity is the most reliable method for preventing genital HPV infections. Other risk-reducing behaviors include correct condom use and limiting the number of sex partners (Boda et al., 2018). In 2006, a quadrivalent HPV vaccine (Gardasil) was introduced that prevents infection with HPV types 6, 11, 16, and 18. Initially, it was approved in 2006 for use in females 9 to 26 years of age. Later, in 2009, it was approved for use in males 9 to 26 years of age. There are currently two other HPV vaccines available in the United States: a bivalent vaccine (Cervarix) that covers HPV 16 and 18 and a 9-valent vaccine (Gardasil 9) that covers HPV 6, 11, 16, 18, 31, 33, 45, 52, and 58 (Nicol et al., 2015; Boda et al., 2018). All vaccines are given in a two- or three-dose series (depending on age of initiation) of intramuscular injections over a 6-month period. All vaccines offer coverage for HPV types 16 and 18, which account for 66% of all cervical cancers. The quadrivalent vaccines offers additional protection against HPV type 6 and 11, which accounts for 90% of anogenital warts. The 9-valent vaccine covers five additional HPV types (31, 33, 45, 52, and 58), which account for 15% of all cervical cancer cases (Workowski, 2015; Boda et al., 2018). **As of the end of 2016, only the 9-valent HPV vaccine will be available in the United States** (CDC, 2018c).

Currently, the 9-valent vaccine is recommended for males and females 11 to 12 years of age (can start at 9 years) and for females 13 to 26 years of age and males 13 to 21 years of age who were not adequately vaccinated previously. Vaccination is also recommended for gay, bisexual, and other MSM; transgendered persons; and persons 22 to 26 years of age with certain immunocompromising conditions who were not adequately vaccinated when they were younger (CDC, 2018c).

HPV vaccines were previously administered as a three-dose regimen. This has been updated and, currently, **if the first dose of any HPV vaccine is given before the 15th birthday, vaccination should be completed according to a two-dose schedule.** In this regimen, the second dose is recommended 6 to 12 months after the first dose, with a minimum of 5 months between the first and second dose (if a shorter interval, the third vaccine dose is given at a minimum of 12 weeks after the second dose and a maximum of 5 months after the second dose). If the first dose of any HPV vaccine is given after the 15th birthday, a three-dose series schedule should be used. In this series, the second dose is recommended 1 to 2 months after the first dose, and the third dose is recommended 6 months after the first dose (CDC, 2018c). All immunocompromised patients should receive the three-dose regimen.

Multiple studies have demonstrated the safety of HPV vaccines. One of the largest was released in 2013 that included over 300,000 young girls who had received nearly 700,000 doses of the HPV vaccine (quadrivalent). The study noted no increased number of cases of autoimmune disease, neurologic problems, or venous thromboembolic adverse effects in the girls who received the HPV vaccine compared with controls (Arnheim-Dahlstrom et al., 2013, Nicol et al., 2015). HPV vaccines have not been associated with earlier initiation of sexual activity, increased risky sexual behaviors, or perceptions about sexually transmitted infections (Workowski, 2015; Madhivanan et al., 2016). Rates of HPV vaccination are increasing; in 2016, more than 60% of adolescents 13 to 17 years of age have received at least one dose (Walker et al., 2017).

ZIKA VIRUS

Zika virus is a flavivirus related to dengue, yellow fever, and West Nile virus that was first isolated in 1947 in Uganda. Transmission by *Aedes aegypti* to laboratory animals was reported in 1956, and the first human infection was reported in 1964 (Petersen et al., 2016b; Wikan and Smith, 2017). The first large outbreak of Zika virus occurred in 2007 on the island of Yap in Micronesia followed by a second outbreak in French Polynesia during 2013 to 2014. It was during the French-Polynesian outbreak that the link between Zika virus and Guillain-Barré syndrome (GBS) was first reported (Stassen et al., 2018). In 2016, because of the rapid expansion of Zika virus and the suspected causal relationship between the virus and microcephaly in Brazil, the World Health Organization declared Zika virus a public health emergency of international concern (Hennessey et al., 2016; Stassen et al., 2018). By July 2017, more than 700,000 confirmed and suspected mosquito-borne cases of Zika virus had been reported to the Pan American Health Organization from 48 countries and territories in the Americas (Petersen et al., 2016b; Pan American Health Organization, 2017).

Transmission of Zika Virus

Like other flaviviruses, Zika virus is mainly transmitted by female mosquito vectors. Other modes of transmission include maternal-fetal transmission, blood donation, and sexual transmission (male to female, male to male, and female to male). The first suspected case of Zika sexual transmission occurred in 2008 (Foy et al., 2011; Magalhaes et al., 2018; Mead et al., 2018). Transmission has been reported for condomless vaginal and anal intercourse (Magalhaes et al., 2018).

Zika virus RNA has been detected in blood samples, male and female reproductive tract samples, urine, saliva, breast milk, and conjunctival and other body fluids. Infectious virus has been recovered from most of these body fluids but to a much lesser extent (Magalhaes et al., 2018; Uraki et al., 2017). The median time to Zika virus RNA clearance post–symptom onset from infected patients' urine and semen is 8.2 days (6.4 to 10.0) and 34.4 days (27.9 to 40.8), respectively (Paz-Bailey et al., 2017). Zika virus RNA has been detected as late as 188 days after symptom onset. The longest recorded time for Zika virus viability (infectious virus in cell culture) was 69 days after symptom onset (Moreira et al., 2017; Mead et al., 2018). Of note, Zika virus has been detected in the ejaculate of at least two vasectomized men (Magalhaes et al., 2018).

Symptoms

Symptoms of Zika virus can be highly variable. Most people (up to 80%) are asymptomatic. Symptoms, when present, tend to be mild and nonspecific and can include mild fever, conjunctivitis, maculopapular rash, myalgia, and headache (Rabaan et al., 2017; Mead et al., 2018). In Zika virus–infected men, prostatitis, hematospermia, and microhematospermia have been reported (Stassen et al., 2018). Although it is unknown what cells or tissues are affected with Zika virus, the presence of hematospermia in some patients suggests one or more tissues of accessary genital tract (seminal vesicles, prostate and bulbourethral gland) are likely infected (Magalhaes et al., 2018).

Zika virus infections have been associated with severe neurologic manifestations such as microcephaly and Guillain-Barré syndrome (Koppolu and Shantha Raju, 2018). In Brazil, an average of 163 cases of microcephaly were recorded annually between 2001 and 2014, however in the year leading up to January 30, 2016, 4783 microcephaly and/or CNS malformation cases had already been recorded (Rabaan et al., 2017). Zika virus infections have also been linked to other neurologic manifestations such as meningoencephalitis, fetal cerebral calcifications, central nervous system alterations, and myelitis. Although the ocular manifestations in adults are usually mild (conjunctivitis and uveitis), they can be much more severe in infants. Zika virus ocular manifestations in infants can include blindness, optic neuritis, chorioretinal atrophy, bilateral iris coloboma, and intraretinal hemorrhage (Koppolu and Shantha Raju, 2018).

Diagnosis

The CDC currently recommends Zika virus testing for anyone with possible Zika virus exposure (defined as living in, traveling to, or having unprotected intercourse with someone who lives in or traveled to an area with risk for Zika virus) who has recently experienced symptoms of Zika. Testing is recommended for symptomatic pregnant women with possible Zika exposure, asymptomatic pregnant women with ongoing possible Zika exposure, and pregnant women with possible Zika exposure who have a fetus with prenatal ultrasound findings consistent with congenital Zika virus infection. Testing may be considered for asymptomatic pregnant women with recent possible but no ongoing Zika exposure. Zika virus testing is not recommended for nonpregnant asymptomatic individuals or for preconception counseling (CDC, 2018e).

Nonpregnant symptomatic individuals with possible Zika virus exposure should receive testing of serum and urine by Zika virus ribonucleic acid (RNA) NAAT and Zika virus and/or dengue virus IgM testing of serum. NAAT testing is dependent on the timing of specimen collection and should be performed only on specimens collected less than 14 days after symptom onset. Zika virus and dengue virus IgM serology testing should be performed on all NAAT-negative samples collected less than 14 days from symptom onset and on all samples collected 14 days or longer from symptom onset (CDC, 2018e).

Preconception Counseling and Prevention of Sexual Transmission of Zika Virus

Because of the range of time after symptom onset that Zika virus RNA has been detected in the semen of symptomatic men, the CDC recommends that men with possible Zika exposure, regardless of symptom status, wait at least 6 months from symptom onset (if symptomatic) or last possible exposure before attempting conception with their partner. Women with possible Zika virus exposure are recommended to wait to conceive until at least 8 weeks after symptom onset of last possible exposure. Couples who want to conceive in which one or both partners live in areas with active Zika virus transmission should be tested for Zika virus if they are symptomatic. Men with positive results should wait 6 months from onset of symptoms, and women should wait 8 weeks from symptom onset to attempt conception. If testing is negative, a discussion with a health care provider should be had regarding the timing of conception in the setting of ongoing risk for potential exposure. Couples with possible Zika exposure who are not pregnant and do not plan to become pregnant and who want to minimize their risk for sexual transmission of Zika virus should be advised to abstain from intercourse or use condoms for the same period mentioned earlier (men 6 months and women 8 weeks) (Petersen et al., 2016a).

Treatment for Zika Virus Infections

To date, there are no approved vaccine or antiviral therapies to treat Zika infection. Therefore, the best approach to control Zika virus infections relies on preventing transmission of the virus (both from the vector *A. aegypti* and sexual transmission). Avoiding travel to Zika-endemic areas (found at https://wwwnc.cdc.gov/travel/page/zika-information), utilizing insect repellent with DEET, treating clothes with permethrin, and eliminating standing water to prevent mosquito egg laying and larval development are recommended choices to prevent infection (Koppolu and Shantha Raju, 2018).

HUMAN IMMUNODEFICIENCY VIRUS (HIV) AND ACQUIRED IMMUNODEFICIENCY SYNDROME (AIDS)

Since AIDS was first described in 1981 and HIV identified in 1986, the HIV pandemic has affected millions of people worldwide (Heyns et al., 2013). As of 2016, there were 36.7 million people living with HIV worldwide (1.1 million in the United States as of 2015), with 1.8 million new cases of HIV diagnosed in 2016. Worldwide, 1 million people died from AIDS-related illnesses in 2016. In 2016, 39,782 people in the United States were diagnosed with HIV, a 5% decrease from 2011 to 2015, with MSM accounting for 67% (26,570) of the newly diagnosed cases. Heterosexual contact accounted for 24% (9578 cases), IV drug use accounted for 6% (2224 cases), and a combination of MSM and IV drug use accounted for 3% of newly diagnosed cases (1201 cases). African-Americans had the highest rate of newly diagnosed HIV (44%, or 17,528 cases) followed by Caucasians (26% or 10,345 cases) and Hispanic/Latinos (25%, or 9766 cases). Only 15%, or 1 in 7 people, know that they are infected with HIV (https://www.cdc.gov/hiv/basics/statistics.html).

HIV is a retrovirus that infects T cells and dendritic cells. HIV is spread through blood, semen, vaginal fluid, or breast milk. Immunosuppression occurs with the progressive loss of CD4 T-lymphocytes. There are two types of HIV: HIV-1 and HIV-2. Although HIV-1 accounts for the majority of infections in the United States, HIV-2 infections should be suspected in persons with an unusual clinical presentation or with risk factors including having lived in an endemic area or having sex with a partner from an endemic area (West Africa, Portugal), having a sex partner with known HIV-2, or having a blood transfusion or nonsterile injection in an endemic area (Workowski, 2015). There are three recognized stages of HIV infection. **Stage 1 (acute stage) occurs 2 to 4 weeks after infection and presents as flulike symptoms. Because of high viral load during this stage, patients are at an increased risk for transmitting the virus.** Unfortunately, routine tests for HIV antibodies are often negative during this phase. **Stage 2 (clinical latency, asymptomatic HIV infection or chronic HIV infection) is marked by slow viral replication that can last years to decades depending on treatment.** Patients are often asymptomatic during this phase. **Stage 3 (AIDS) is diagnosed when the CD4 count is less than 200 cells/mm^3 or if the patient acquires an AIDS-defining condition** (CDC, 2018a).

Diagnosis of Human Immunodeficiency Virus

The CDC currently recommends HIV screening for patients 13 to 64 years of age in a health care setting. Patients should be counseled and notified that testing will be performed and given the option to decline. **All persons who seek evaluation and treatment for STDs should be screened for HIV infection.**

HIV infection can be diagnosed by serologic tests that detect antibodies against HIV-1 and HIV-2 and by virologic tests that detect HIV antigens or RNA. Testing usually begins with a sensitive screening test, usually antigen/antibody combination or antibody immunoassay. Available serologic tests are highly sensitive and specific and can detect all known subtypes of HIV-1, and most can also detect HIV-2 and uncommon variants of HIV-1. These are rapid tests, but these rapid assays often become reactive later than conventional laboratory-based antibody or combination antigen/antibody serologic assays. This can result in a negative result in a recently infected person. The recommended algorithm for HIV infections consists of laboratory-based immunoassay which, if repeatedly reactive, is followed by a supplemental test (e.g., HIV-1/HIV-2 antibody differentiation assay, Western blot, or indirect immunofluorescence assay). A positive supplemental test confirms the diagnosis. Because laboratory antigen/antibody immunoassays detect HIV infection earlier than the supplemental tests, during very early infection, discordant HIV tests have been reported as negative (i.e., reactive immunoassay with negative supplemental test). To minimize this, a combination of HIV-1/HIV-2 antigen-antibody immunoassay, which, if reactive, is followed by an HIV-1/HIV-2 antibody differentiation assay. This allows for an additional advantage of detecting HIV-2 antibodies, which if present, carry different monitoring and treatment protocols. Discordant tests should be conformed with RNA testing to determine if the discordance is caused by acute HIV infection (Workowski, 2015).

Once diagnosed, persons with HIV infection should be encouraged to notify their partners and to refer them for counseling and testing. Partner notification services are usually available through the health department. Partners who have been reached and are not known to have HIV exposure should be offered postexposure prophylaxis (PEP) with combination retrovirals medications if they were exposed to genital secretions or blood of a partner with HIV infection.

Decreasing the Transmission Risk

Male Circumcision

Three randomized, controlled studies performed in sub-Saharan Africa demonstrated that circumcision decreased the risk for HIV infection by 50% to 60% (Auvert et al., 2005; Bailey et al., 2007; Gray et al., 2007). Similar reductions were also noted for STDs such as high-risk HPV and genital herpes. Several mechanisms have been shown to potentially account for the reduced risk for HIV acquisition with circumcision. Numerous HIV target cells are present under the dermis of the foreskin. The inner surface of the foreskin is poorly keratinized and potentially prone to lacerations, which can act as a site for HIV entry. Lastly, infection of the prepuce with anaerobic bacteria can lead to the infiltration Langerhans cells, which the HIV virus targets (Heyns et al., 2013). Circumcision has not been shown to reduce the risk for HIV transmission in a man who already has HIV (Wawer et al., 2009). Circumcision has not been shown to reduce the risk for HIV transmission in MSM, although limited data suggest it may be beneficial in MSM who were the insertive partner only in anal intercourse (Heyns et al., 2013; Workowski, 2015). The World Health Organization and the Joint United National Programme on HIV/AIDS (UNAIDS) have recommended that male circumcision efforts be scaled up as an effective intervention for the prevention of heterosexually acquired HIV infection.

Postexposure Prophylaxis

A case-controlled study demonstrating an 81% reduction in the odds of HIV transmission among health care workers (HCWs) with percutaneous exposure to HIV who received zidovudine prophylaxis was the first to describe the efficacy of PEP (Cardo et al., 1997). Because of ethical and operational challenges, no randomized controlled trials have been conducted to test the efficacy of non–occupational postexposure prophylaxis (nPEP) directly, and as such, this trial reports the strongest evidence of benefit of antiretroviral prophylaxis initiated after HIV exposure among humans (CDC, 2016b). **The current guidelines recommend that persons should be evaluated for nPEP when they present less than 72 hours after a potential nonoccupational HIV exposure that poses a substantial risk for HIV acquisition (source of body fluid is known to be HIV-positive, and the reported exposure presents a substantial risk for transmission).** Evaluation includes determination of HIV status, and if this is either negative or results are unavailable, nPEP should be initiated without delay. nPEP is not recommended for exposures with no substantial risk for HIV transmission or if care is sought more than 72 hours after potential exposure. **All persons offered nPEP should be prescribed a 28-day course of a three-drug antiretroviral regimen.** The regimen consists of tenofovir disoproxil fumarate 300 mg with emtricitabine 200 mg daily PLUS raltegravir 400 mg twice daily OR dolutegravir 50 mg daily. HIV status should be monitored at 6 weeks, 3 months, and again at 6 months after exposure (CDC, 2016b).

Pre-Exposure Prophylaxis

Daily oral pre-exposure prophylaxis (PrEP) with the fixed-dose combination of tenofovir disoproxil fumarate (TDF) 300 mg and emtricitabine (FTC) 200 mg has been shown to be safe and effective in reducing the risk for sexual HIV acquisition in adults. PrEP is recommended in the following populations: as one prevention option for sexually active adult MSM who are at substantial risk for HIV acquisition; adult heterosexually active men and women who are at substantial risk for HIV acquisition; adult persons who inject drugs (PWID; also called injection drug users [IDU]) at substantial risk for HIV acquisition; and heterosexually active women and men whose partners are known to have HIV infection (i.e., HIV-discordant couples) as one of several options to protect the uninfected partner during conception and pregnancy so that an informed decision can be made in awareness of what is known and unknown about benefits and risks of PrEP for the mother and fetus (CDC, 2017c).

Urologic Manifestations of HIV/AIDS

HIV and Other STDs

Testing for HIV is recommended for anyone who is diagnosed with an STD or is at risk for an STD (Workowski, 2015). In many populations, the pattern of HIV infection mirrors that of other STDs (Quinn et al., 1988). Genital herpes, syphilis, and chancroid have all been associated with an increased risk for HIV transmission and acquisition. Several factors contribute to this finding including bleeding from irritated genital ulcers and the presence of HIV in ulcer exudate. In HIV-negative patients, genital ulcerations can increase the risk for acquisition of HIV by interrupting the mucosal integrity and recruiting HIV-positive immune cells to the site of the ulcer (Magro et al., 1996). HSV shedding is increased in persons with HIV, and HSV-2 is thought to affect 50% to 90% of HIV-positive patients (Strick et al., 2006). Coinfection with syphilis increases the viral load and decreases the CD4 count leading to rapid progression and immunosuppression (Heyns et al., 2013).

Nonulcerating Skin Infections

Cellulitis of the perineum is more common in men with HIV, and empiric coverage should cover the potential for methicillin-resistant *Staphylococcus auerus* (MRSA) (Shindel et al., 2011). Necrotizing fasciitis, although rare, occurs more commonly in HIV patients. Tuberculosis might involve the scrotal skin or penis resulting in sinuses, nodular lesions, or ulcerative lesions (Heyns et al., 2013).

Genital warts are present in 20% of HIV patients and are most commonly caused by HPV 6 and 11. These lesions can also be quite extensive in HIV/AIDS patients forming giant condyloma (Fig. 58.13). Molluscum contagiousum is found in 5% to 18% of HIV patients. Although it is usually self-limited in healthy individuals, the lesions may not regress in HIV-positive patients and can serve as a nidus for secondary bacterial infections (Shindel et al., 2011).

Urinary Tract Infections

Patients who have HIV experience a greater risk for urinary tract infection (UTI) when their CD4 count is less than 500/mm^3 (Lee et al., 2001; Lebovitch and Mydlo, 2008). The risk for UTI is even higher among those with a CD4 count less than 200/mm^3 or those with a high viral load. Thirty percent of patients with a CD4 count less than 200/mm^3 have bacteriuria compared with 11% with CD4 counts between 200/mm^3 and 500/mm^3 and 0% for counts greater than 500/mm^3 (Hoepelman et al., 1992; Nicolle, 2014). Although immunosuppression is the principal driving factor behind the increased incidence of UTI, voiding dysfunction may also predispose to UTI development. Typical pathogens include the *E. coli, Enterobacter, Proteus, Klebsiella,* and other gram-negative bacteria (Hoepelman et al., 1992; Lebovitch and Mydlo, 2008). *Pseudomonas aeruginosa* can be found in up to 30% of HIV-infected patients with a UTI (Hyun and Lowe, 2003). ***Salmonella* UTI is of particular concern given its increased potential for fatal recurrence and as such, should be aggressively managed with lifelong prophylaxis** (Reddy et al., 2010; Shindel et al., 2011). Urine culture is recommended before initiation of empiric treatment because of the resistance patterns seen within this group (Vignesh et al., 2008).

HIV-infected patients who do not respond after a few days of empiric antibiotics and those with a CD4 count less than

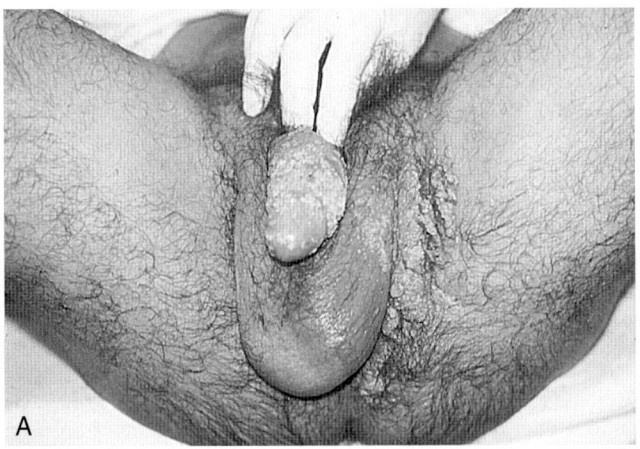
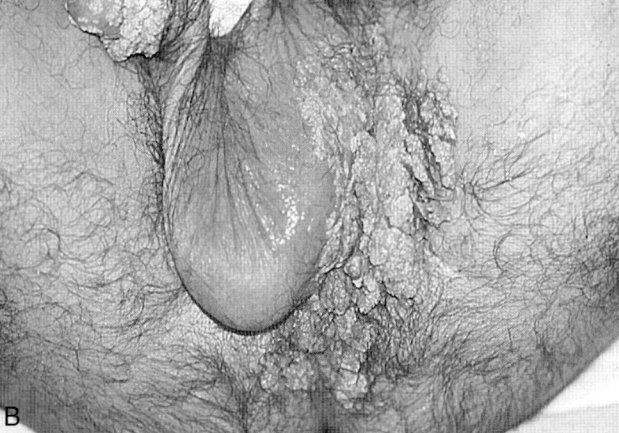

Fig. 58.13. (A and B) Acquired immunodeficiency syndrome patient with extensive genital condyloma.

500/mm³ (especially <250/mm³) should be screened for atypical and opportunistic infections. Organisms of concern include fungi such as *Candida, Aspergillus, Blastomyces, Cryptococcus, Cryptosporidia,* and *Histoplasma*; parasites such as *Toxoplasma* and *Pneumocystis*; *M. tuberculosis,* and viruses such as cytomegalovirus (CMV) and adenovirus (Lee et al., 2001; Shindel et al., 2011; Heyns et al., 2013). The diagnosis of viral UTI can be confirmed with molecular techniques such as PCR, and treatment consists of cidofovir (Paduch, 2007; Heyns et al., 2013).

Renal Infections

Gram-negative bacteria are the most common cause of pyelonephritis in the HIV population. Opportunistic renal pathogens include *Pneumocystis carinii, Mycobacterium* spp., *Candida,* and *Histoplasmosis.* Renal mycobacterial infections have been detected at autopsy in 6% to 23% of AIDS patients, most of whom had not experienced any symptoms of infection before death (Shindel et al., 2011). The most common mycobacterial organism is *M. tuberculosis* followed by *Mycobacterium avium* and *Mycobacterium intracellulare.* **Mycobacterial infection of the urinary tract usually occurs in a descending fashion, and it can remain latent for many years after the initial infection until reactivation.** Diagnosis of renal tuberculosis (TB) is made by a positive Ziehl-Nielsen stain of urine; urine culture for acid-fast bacilli, which requires three to six early morning cultures and may take up to 6 weeks to grow; or PCR, which, although it can produce quick results (48 hours), it is not widely available because of technical difficulties (Heyns et al., 2013). TB can also present as an iliopsoas abscess. Approximately 10% of iliopsoas abscesses are caused by *M. tuberculosis,* and approximately 25% of these are associated with HIV (Navarro Lopez et al., 2009). If treatment includes rifampin, HIV drug levels should be monitored as rifampin induces cytochrome p450, which can lower the concentration of protease inhibitors (PIs) and nonnucleoside reverse transcriptase inhibitors. **Because of the increased risk for relapse, HIV patients with treated renal TB should have an annual urine culture for acid-fast bacilli up to 10 years after treatment to screen for recurrence** (Shindel et al., 2011).

Prostatitis

Although relatively uncommon in the general population (1% to 2%), prostatitis is diagnosed in 3% of men with HIV and 14% of those with AIDS, although these numbers predate HAART treatment (Leport et al., 1989; Lebovitch and Mydlo, 2008). Common symptoms include chronic pelvic/perineal pain, dysuria, urgency frequency, and other lower urinary tract symptoms (LUTS). Prostatitis is usually caused by *E. coli,* but other organisms including *S. aureus, Klebsiella pneumonia, Pseudomonas aruginosa, Serratia marcescens, Salmonella typhi, M. tuberculosis, M. avium,* and *M. intracellulare* can also cause prostatitis in the HIV/AIDS population. Fungal infections can cause prostatitis, especially with CD4 counts less than 200/mm³. These organisms include *Candida albicans, Aspergillus fumigatus, Cryptococcus neogormans,* and *Histoplasma capsulatum* (Weinberger et al., 1988; Benson and Smith, 1992; Santillo and Lowe, 2006). **The risk for developing a prostatic abscess or urosepsis is greater than in the general population because of the atypical pathogens that may be present.** Prolonged treatment with antimicrobial or antifungal therapy is needed (Leport et al., 1989; Hyun and Lowe, 2003). Despite prolonged therapy, up to 70% of HIV-infected patients have relapsing symptoms (Leport et al., 1989; Kwan and Lowe, 1992; Shindel et al., 2011; Heyns et al., 2013). Special consideration should be given to cryptococcal prostatitis, which may persist after treatment in up to 29% of cases and may serve as a reservoir for relapsing meningitis; as such, these patients may require long-term or even lifelong antifungals depending on their immune status (Lee et al., 2001; Shindel et al., 2011).

Testis, Epididymis, and Seminal Vesicles

Infection of the epididymis and/or testicle is a common finding in men with HIV and tends to be recurrent and chronic (Coburn, 1998). Changes have been found within the tubular structures of the epididymis in AIDS patients. These changes are likely caused by persistent inflammation and predispose patients to recurrent infections because of inadequate clearance of secretions (Dalton and Harcourt-Webster, 1991). Autopsy studies of AIDS patients who have succumbed to opportunistic infections have shown that 25% to 39% of men have the identical organism harvested from their testes, suggesting that the testes and epididymis may be a reservoir for delayed opportunistic infections. The most common organisms harvested from the testes in these cases were *Gonococcus, Salmonella,* CMV, *M. avium, M. intracellulare, Toxoplasma, Histoplasma,* and *Candida* (De Paepe and Waxman, 1989; Heyns et al., 2013). Treatment requires a period of initial antibiotics followed by maintenance suppression, particularly if *Salmonella* is present (Shindel et al., 2011).

Testicular atrophy is a frequent autopsy finding in HIV-infected patients. The etiology is likely multifactorial including fever, chronic illness, opportunistic infections, cachexia, activation of cytokines, and the cytotoxic effect of the HIV virus itself. Patients with an extremely low body mass index (BMI) (<20) were 3.5 times more likely to have testicular atrophy than those with a BMI greater than or equal to 20. An association between disseminated CMV infection and testicular atrophy has been noted. HIV-infected patients with CMV end-organ infection had a fivefold increased incidence of pronounced testicular atrophy (Mhawech et al., 2001).

Nephrolithiasis

Historically, PIs (indinavir specifically) have been implicated as a cause of nephrolithiasis in up to 22% of HIV-infected patients, and autopsy studies have demonstrated urinary stones in up to 40% of HIV-infected patients (Shindel et al., 2011; Raheem et al., 2012). Risk factors for nephrolithiasis in the HIV-infected population include hepatitis coinfection and exposure to PIs (Lin et al., 2015). Twenty percent of indinavir is not metabolized and is excreted by the kidneys within 24 hours. Indinavir is most soluble at a pH less than 5, and, as such, tends to precipitate in alkaline urine forming radiolucent stones (Raheem et al., 2012). Indinavir as a stone component is only seen in 29% of calculi, and the remaining stone components are calcium oxalate, ammonium acid urate, and uric acid (Lebovitch and Mydlo, 2008). Indinavir is used less often currently, although the newer PIs, such as lopinavir, atanaznavir, amprinavir, and belfinavir, have also been associated with the development of nephrolithiasis, although at much lower rates relative to indinavir (Shindel et al., 2011).

Other factors that may contribute to nephrolithiasis in HIV-infected patients include malnutrition, diarrhea, dehydration, urinary acidification, hypocitraturia, and hyperuricosuria secondary to cell lysis after chemotherapy for AIDS-associated lymphoma (Heyns et al., 2013). **Once diagnosed, patients should undergo a complete metabolic evaluation including stone analysis if possible, 24-hour urine collection, and serum studies (creatinine, uric acid, and calcium)** (Lebovitch and Mydlo, 2008). In patients with protease stones and in whom conservative management is possible, first-line treatment involving discontinuation of the drug and hydration has been successful in up to 70% of cases (Kohan et al., 1999).

Renal Dysfunction

Despite HAART, kidney disease and renal failure are still common causes of death in HIV-positive patients (Croxford et al., 2017). Renal disease can be a consequence of both HIV infection and its treatments. Potential causes of renal dysfunction in persons with HIV or AIDS include the depletion of intravascular volume owing to diarrhea and vomiting, sepsis, metabolic dysfunction, nephrotoxic medications, intrinsic diseases such as HIV-associated nephropathy (HIVAN), and ureteric obstruction caused by urolithiasis, blood clots, retroperitoneal lymphoma, fungal collections, or fibrosis (Lebovitch and Mydlo, 2008; Heyns et al., 2013). Drugs that can cause acute kidney injury in HIV-infected patients include antibiotics, antifungal agents (amphotericin B and pentamidine), antiviral agents, and antiretroviral drugs (indinavir, atazanavir, abacavir, and tenofovir) (Kalyesubula and Perazella, 2011).

As life expectancy for HIV-infected patients has increased since the introduction of HAART, the risk for developing chronic kidney disease has also increased. Untreated HIV or AIDS increases the risk for acute kidney injury. With the initiation of HAART, renal failure persists but life expectancy increases (Heyns et al., 2013). Additionally, with increased life expectancy comes an increased risk for age-related risk factors such as hypertension and diabetes. HIV-infected men on HAART have a fourfold higher incidence of diabetes than HIV-negative men (Kalyesubula and Perazella, 2011; Heyns et al., 2013).

HIVAN is characterized by an elevated serum creatinine and nephrotic-range proteinuria (>3.5g/day), although edema and hypertension are frequently absent. HIVAN typically occurs with CD4 counts less than 200 cells/mm^3 and a blood load of greater than 1000 copies/mL, and it affects 7% to 32% of HIV-positive patients. It has a 12:1 greater incidence in black patients compared with white patients and has become the third leading cause of end-stage renal disease among black patients 20 to 64 years of age. The diagnosis is made by biopsy that demonstrates a collapsing variant of focal segmental glomerulosclerosis, proliferation of renal tubular and visceral cells, tubular microcystic formation, edema, interstitial fibrosis, and infiltration of the interstitium with leukocytes. Patients progress rapidly to end-stage renal disease with dialysis requirement occurring within 10 months of diagnosis. **Treatment includes HAART if the patient is not already on HIV medications and angiotensin-converting enzyme inhibitors.** Despite treatment, 1-year mortality reaches 50% (Lebovitch and Mydlo, 2008; Shindel et al., 2011; Heyns et al., 2013; Ekrikpo et al., 2018).

Voiding Dysfunction

LUTS can be a common source of morbidity in the HIV-infected population and tends to worsen as the disease progresses. **In an Internet survey of MSM, HIV status was an independent risk factor for bothersome LUTS, and a history of AIDS was a risk factor for severe disease** (Breyer et al., 2011). With acute HIV infections, LUTS, including acute retention and sacral loss, may be the sentinel event that presages HIV conversion (Zeman and Donaghy, 1991; Lee et al., 2001; Shindel et al., 2011; Heyns et al., 2013). With disease progression, symptoms can worsen, possibly related to recurrent or chronic UTI, central nervous system disturbances (i.e., HIV encephalitis, cerebral toxoplasmosis, HIV demyelination disorders, CMV polyradiculopathy, central nervous system neoplasms, and HIV-related dementia), peripheral neurologic deficits, and side effects of HAART or other medications (Lebovitch and Mydlo, 2008; Shindel et al., 2011). Awareness of CMV infection is important in the HIV-positive population because there is a greater than 40% rate of virus reactivation with subsequent risk for bladder end-organ damage and life-threatening infection. Combined bladder dysfunction, bowel dysfunction, and back or sciatic pain should prompt consideration for CMV polyradiculopathy. Diagnosis is made by lumbar puncture, and prompt treatment may improve symptoms (Collier et al., 1987; Shindel et al., 2011).

Erectile Dysfunction

In a study comparing the prevalence of erectile dysfunction (ED) in HIV-infected men compared with HIV-negative men, the prevalence of ED (mild, moderate, and severe) was shown to be higher in HIV-infected men in all decades of age, and on multivariate analysis HIV infection was the strongest predictor of ED (Zona et al., 2012). A larger meta-analysis confirmed the finding of increased prevalence of ED in HIV-infected men (Luo et al., 2017). ED is common in HIV-infected men younger than 50 years of age, reported as 50% of infected men younger than 30 years of age, 48% of those 31 to 40 years of age, and 53% of those 41 to 50 years of age (Zona et al., 2012). Sexual dysfunction may be caused by HIV-associated organic comorbidities affecting the neurologic, vascular, and hormonal systems; psychological stress; depression; hypogonadism; age; and BMI (Lebovitch and Mydlo, 2008; Heyns et al., 2013; Luo et al., 2017). Several studies have found that antiretroviral therapy, especially PIs, is associated with an increased prevalence of ED. Indinavir and ritonavir have been reported to worsen ED. HAART contributes to increased body weight circulating lipids, glycemia, and decrease in serum testosterone levels, which can lead to a metabolic pattern that promotes endothelial dysfunction (Luo et al., 2017). Sexual dysfunction is also a complex condition that not only includes ED, but disorders of ejaculation, sexual desire, orgasm, and satisfaction during intercourse. The prevalence of ejaculation disorders is higher in men with HIV infection (Jones et al., 1994). Libido has been shown to be lower in HIV-infected patients and even more so in those taking HAART (2% without HIV, 26% with HIV and no HAART, and 48% with HIV and HAART) (Lamba et al., 2004).

Treatment with PDE-5 may interact with PIs. PIs can block the CYP3A enzyme leading to a threefold to 10-fold increase in serum concentrations of sildenafil. Sildenafil should be started at a lower dose in the setting of PIs (Lebovitch and Mydlo, 2008; Heyns et al., 2013).

Malignancy

Malignancy is more common in the HIV-positive individual than in age-matched HIV-negative individuals. Possible mechanisms for this include decreased immune surveillance, a direct effect of viral proteins, or cytokine dysregulation. Other factors that can contribute to the increased risk include high-risk behaviors such as tobacco use, which is two to three times more prevalent in the HIV-infected patient (Albini et al., 2013). AIDS-defining cancers (ADCs) are Kaposi sarcoma (associated with the DNA viruses Kaposi sarcoma–associated herpesvirus (HHV 8), Epstein Barr virus (EBV), and HPV), non-Hodgkin lymphoma, cervical carcinoma, and anal carcinoma (Heyns et al., 2013). HAART has reduced the incidence and mortality for KS and NHL but not for cervical or anal cancer. Since the widespread use of HAART, there has been a threefold increase in non-ADCs including prostate cancer; carcinomas of the anus, lung, breast, skin, conjunctiva, head and neck, liver, and testis; Hodgkin lymphoma; plasma-cell neoplasia; multiple myeloma; leukemia; melanoma; and leiomyosarcoma. Currently these non-ADCs comprise 70% of all cancers diagnosed in HIV-infected people on HAART compared with 20% in the pre-HAART era (Crum-Cianflone et al., 2009; Heyns et al., 2013).

Kaposi Sarcoma

KS was first described in 1872 by a Hungarian dermatologist, Moritz Kaposi. It was the simultaneous occurrence of KS with *Pneumocystis* pneumonias in young MSM in 1981 that led to the first description of AIDS (Hoffmann et al., 2017). Measured at 5 years after AIDS onset, the cumulative incidence of KS in the United States has decreased from 14.3% in 1980 to 1989 to 6.7% in 1990 to 1995 and to 1.8% in 1996 to 2006 (Simard et al., 2011). KS is characterized by abnormal neoangiogenesis, inflammation, and the proliferation of tumor cells. KS is induced by infection with herpes virus 8 (HHV-8) also known as KS-associated herpesvirus (Hoffmann et al., 2017). HHV-8 is now considered a necessary condition for the development of KS, although not all persons with HHV-8 will develop KS. Transmission of HHV-8 occurs predominantly via saliva but also sexually, vertically, and via blood products (Haq et al., 2016).

KS can begin in any area of the skin but may also appear on oral, genital, or ocular mucous membranes. It typically manifests as a few asymptomatic purple macules or nodules usually along skin tension lines. The tumors can remain unchanged for a prolonged period or grow rapidly within a few weeks. Rapid growth can lead to localized pain and eventually develop central necrosis and ulceration. The prognosis depends on the extent of the tumor, immune status, and the presence of systemic illness.

Large randomized trials have shown the protective effect of HAART against the development of KS (Silverberg et al., 2007; Borges et al., 2016; Hoffmann et al., 2017). If KS is diagnosed in an HIV-infected patient naïve to HAART, HAART should be initiated. In patients on HAART without complete suppression of HIV plasma viremia, the regimen should be optimized. With decreasing plasma viremia and immune reconstitution, many KS lesions stabilize or even resolve without any KS-specific treatment. Treatment can be local or systemic. Local treatments include cryosurgery, intralesional injections, radiation, or imiquimod (Hoffmann et al., 2017). In patients with rapidly progressive disease, KS-related symptoms, or visceral disease or lymphedema, HAART should be combined with cytotoxic chemotherapy. Prognosis is favorable, even in advanced disease, with an 85% 5-year survival rate (Bower et al., 2014a). KS may dramatically flare after initiation of HAART in what is called *immune reconstitution inflammatory syndrome (IRIS)*, which is seen in HIV-positive patients with initial low CD4 counts and high viral load. IRIS can be seen as early as 3 weeks with a mean onset of 5 weeks, and the syndrome can be fatal (Hoffmann et al., 2017).

Non–AIDS-Defining Urologic Malignancies

Testicular Tumors

HIV-infected men are at a slightly greater risk for testis cancer then HIV-negative men. In particular, seminoma and extragonadal germ cell cancer (GCC) occur more frequently in HIV-infected patients, and the risk for nonseminoma is not, or only marginally, increased (Hentrich and Pfister, 2017). The occurrence of GCC appears to be unrelated to CD4 count and duration of HIV/AIDS. Limited data are available on survival differences between HIV-positive and HIV-negative patients in the post-HAART era. Primary treatment should be the same as in HIV-negative patients. Three cycles of cisplatin, etoposide, and bleomycin (BEP) suppresses the CD4 count by 25% to 50%, and it is probable that one to two cycles of BEP will also be suppressive. Therefore, low-risk nonseminoma patients should be offered surveillance, and adjuvant therapy should only be considered for high-risk nonseminoma patients (Bower et al., 2014b).

Prostate Cancer

The risk for prostate cancer is not increased in the setting of HIV, with several studies showing a slightly lower risk for HIV-positive men compared with HIV-negative men, although its relevance in the HIV-positive population is increasing as life expectancy increases (Hentrich and Pfister, 2017). **The indications for prostate-specific antigen testing in the HIV-positive patient should be the same as in the general population.** Morbidity after prostate biopsy or prostate cancer treatment is not increased in HIV-positive patients compared with HIV-negative men. An increase in infectious complications with radical prostatectomy may be seen in patients with a lower CD4 count and higher viral loads, but no other adverse perioperative outcomes were noted (Lebovitch and Mydlo, 2008; Shindel et al., 2011; Heyns et al., 2013).

Renal Cell Carcinoma

The risk for renal cell carcinoma (RCC) appears modestly elevated in subjects infected with HIV. In the D:A:D study, 1.4% of all non-ADCs were reported to be RCC (Worm et al., 2013). There does not seem to be an association between CD4 count at AIDS onset and the risk for RCC (Hentrich and Pfister, 2017). Based on data from the two largest case series on HIV-related RCC, there does not seem to be a difference in clinical presentation, pathology, stage distribution, and outcomes between HIV-infected and uninfected patients (Gaughan et al., 2008; Ong et al., 2016).

Bladder Cancer

There does not appear to be an increased risk for bladder cancer in HIV-infected patients, and the risk may actually be lower compared with the general population. The age of onset, however, may be lower in the HIV-infected population (Chawki et al., 2015). The outcome of HIV-infected patients with bladder cancer seems to be similar to that for HIV-negative patients. Patients with HIV should be managed according to the standard guidelines for HIV-negative patients (Hentrich and Pfister, 2017). One possible difference in treatment of HIV-positive patients is to use caution in deciding to use intravesical bacillus Calmette-Guérin (BCG) therapy. Intravesical BCG is dependent on a functioning immune system to exert its local effects. There is a theoretical risk for disseminated infection, with one case report of documented bilateral interstitial pneumonitis in an HIV-positive patient after intravesical BCG therapy. Additionally, because of the decrease in CD4+ cells, BCG may not be able to sufficiently stimulate the host immune system to create the necessary antitumor activity in the HIV-infected patient. **Given the risk for disseminated infection and potential suboptimal response to this therapy in HIV-infected patients, BCG therapy should probably be used with caution in the HIV-infected patient** (Gaughan et al., 2009).

Penile Cancer

Penile cancers and precursor lesions, such as Bowen disease and penile carcinoma in situ (CIS), are more common in HIV-positive men. Squamous cell carcinoma and verrucous carcinoma are more common and typically follow a more aggressive course in HIV patients. Part of the increased susceptibility to these cancers may be related to the generally increased risk for STDs in HIV-positive individuals, including infection with HPV 16 and 18 (Shindel et al., 2011). The diagnosis and management of penile cancer is the same for HIV-infected men as for the general population (Shindel et al., 2011).

VIRAL HEPATITIS

Hepatitis B

Hepatitis B virus (HBV) infection remains to be a major public health burden. Approximately 240 million people worldwide are chronically infected with HBV, which contributes to about 30% of cirrhosis cases and 45% of hepatocellular carcinoma (HCC) cases (Wu and Ning, 2017). Hepatitis B is caused by infection with the HBV, with an incubation period that can span 6 weeks to 6 months. Increased concentrations of the HBV are found in blood, with lower concentrations in other body fluids such as wound exudate, semen, vaginal fluid, and saliva. Hepatitis B infections are more stable in the environment than other blood-borne pathogens (HIV, hepatitis C virus), and, as such, they are more infectious. **The primary risk factors associated with infection among adolescents and adults are unprotected sex with an infected partner, multiple partners, MSM, history of other STDs, and IDU** (Frieden et al., 2015).

HBV infections can be self-limited or chronic. If present, symptoms of acute HBV infection can include constitutional symptoms such as fever, fatigue, and loss of appetite. Gastrointestinal symptoms such as abdominal pain, jaundice, nausea, and vomiting may be present. Discoloration of stool and urine may also be noted. **The risk for developing chronic HBV infections is inversely related to the age of acquisition, with 90% of infected infants developing chronic HBV infections verses 2% to 6% of infected adults** (Hyams, 1995). The risk for premature death from cirrhosis or HCC is 15% to 25% among those with chronic HBV (Frieden et al., 2015).

Diagnosis

The diagnosis of HBV infection requires serologic testing. Serologic testing allows for differentiation among those susceptible to HBV infections, those with either resolved HBV infection or vaccine-induced immunity, and those with either acute or chronic HBV infection. Table 58.7 details the interpretation of these serologic tests (CDC, 2018d).

Screening

The American Association for the Study of Liver Diseases (AASLD) 2017 practice guidelines recommends screening with HBsAg and anti-HBs. **Screening is recommended in all persons born in counties**

TABLE 58.7 Interpretation of Serologic Tests for HBV Infection

SEROLOGIC TEST	SUSCEPTIBLE	IMMUNE DUE TO NATURAL INFECTION	IMMUNE DUE TO HBV VACCINE	ACUTELY INFECTED	CHRONICALLY INFECTED	UNCLEAR
HBsAg	Negative	Negative	Negative	Positive	Positive	Negative
Anti-HBc	Negative	Positive	Negative	Positive	Positive	Positive
Anti-HBs	Negative	Positive	Positive	Positive	Negative	Negative
IgM anti-HBc				Positive	Negative	

HBsAg, Hepatitis B surface antigen; *anti-HBc*, antibody to hepatitis B core antigen; *anti-HBs*, antibody to hepatitis B surface antigen; *IgM anti-HBc*, IgM antibody to hepatitis B core antigen; *HBV*, hepatitis B virus.
From Centers for Disease Control and Prevention. Interpretation of hepatitis B serologic test results. 2018; Available at: https://www.cdc.gov/hepatitis/hbv/pdfs/SerologicChartv8.pdf.

with an HBsAg seroprevalence of greater than or equal to 2%, US-born persons not vaccinated as infants whose parents were born in regions with high HBV endemicity (8%), pregnant women, persons needing immunosuppression, and at-risk groups. All anti-HBs–negative screened persons should be vaccinated. Screening for anti-HBc to determine prior exposure is not routinely recommended (Terrault et al., 2018).

Treatment

The goal of anti-HBV therapy is to prevent the progression of disease to cirrhosis, end-stage liver disease, and HCC and to improve the survival of patients with chronic hepatitis B (Wu and Ning, 2017). Patients with HBV infections should be referred to providers who are familiar with recent updates in HBV infection. Although out of the scope of this chapter, the AASLD guidelines outline the management, including necessary surveillance and antiviral treatments, for HBV infection (Terrault et al., 2018).

Prevention

Prevention is a two-tier approach including decreasing the risk for transmission among HBV-infected individuals and vaccinating at-risk populations to prevent infection with HBV.

Counseling Patients Who Are HBsAg Positive

Counseling patients who are HBsAg positive is focused on preventing transmission of the HBV and maximizing overall health. These patients should be counseled on ways to reduce transmission, such as the following:
- Have household and sexual contacts vaccinated
- Use barrier protection during sexual intercourse if partner is not vaccinated or naturally immune
- Do not share toothbrush or razors
- Do not share injection equipment/glucose testing equipment
- Clean open cuts and scratches
- Clean blood spills with bleach solution
- Do not donate blood, organs, or sperm

Children with HBsAg should not be excluded from activities, day care, or school participation. **HCWs should not be excluded from training or practice because they have HBV infection. Those HCWs whose job requires performance of exposure-prone procedures should seek advice from their institution.** The AASLD states that HCWs should not perform exposure-prone procedures if their serum HBV DNA levels exceed 1000 IU/mL but may resume these procedures once levels are lower and maintained at less than 1000 IU/mL (Terrault et al., 2018).

The CDC recommends screening of all pregnant women for HBsAg and HBV DNA testing for women who are HBsAg positive. If HBV DNA is greater than 200,000 IU/mL, antiviral treatment is suggested to decrease the perinatal transmission risk (Schillie, 2018b).

Vaccination

The CDC recommends HBV vaccination for the following (Schillie, 2018b):
- Prophylaxis for infants born to HBsAG-positive women (also include hepatitis B immunoglobulin [HBIG])
- Universal vaccination of all infants beginning at birth as a safeguard for infants born to HBV-infected mothers not identified prenatally
- Routine vaccination of all previously unvaccinated children younger than 19 years of age
- Vaccination of adults at risk for HBV infection, including those requesting protection from HBV without acknowledgment of a specific risk factor

Both single-antigen HepB vaccines and combination vaccines are available. The two single-antigen vaccines recommended for use in the United States, Engerix-B (GlaxoSmithKline Biologicals, Rixensart, Belgium) and Recombivax HB (Merck & Co., Inc., Whitehouse Station, New Jersey), are used for vaccination of persons starting at birth. Combination vaccines are Pediarix (GlaxoSmithKline Biologicals, Rixensart, Belgium), which contains recombinant HBsAg, diphtheria, and tetanus toxoids, acellular pertussis adsorbed, and inactivated poliovirus and is used for persons 6 weeks to 6 years of age, and Twinrix (GlaxoSmithKline Biologicals, Rixensart, Belgium), which contains recombinant HBsAg and inactivated hepatitis A virus and is used for persons 18 years of age and older (Schillie, 2018b). On November 9, 2017, Heplisav-B (HepB-CpG), a single-antigen HepB vaccine with a novel immunostimulatory sequence adjuvant, was approved by the FDA for prevention of HBV in persons 18 years of age and older. The vaccine is administered as 2 doses, 1 month apart (Schillie, 2018a). Vaccine schedules are determined on the basis of immunogenicity data, and the need for additional/concurrent immunizations. Updated vaccine schedules can be found in the CDC's Recommendations of the Advisory Committee on Immunization Practices (Schillie, 2018b).

Postvaccination Serologic Testing for Response

Postvaccination serologic testing for response is generally not indicated. Testing is recommended for those in whom knowledge of their immune status is needed (e.g., HCWs or public safety workers at high risk for continuous percutaneous or mucosal exposure to blood/bodily fluids). It is also recommended for persons with HIV infections and other immunocompromised persons to determine the need for revaccination. It is also recommended for sex partners and needle-sharing partners of HBsAg-positive persons to determine the need for revaccination and other methods to protect themselves from HBV infection (Frieden et al., 2015). Booster doses or revaccination is not recommended unless anti-HBs remains less than 10 mIU/mL, after initial vaccination of infants born to HBsAg-positive mothers, in HCWs, in hemodialysis patients, and in other immunocompromised individuals (Terrault et al., 2018).

Postexposure Prophylaxis

For those who are exposed to HBV through an identifiable exposure to blood or body fluids, all wounds and skin sites that have come into contact with potentially infected fluids should be washed with soap and water. Mucous membranes should be flushed with water. Applying caustic agents (e.g., bleach) or injection of antiseptics into the wound is not recommended (Schillie, 2018b).

Postexposure in a Previously Vaccinated Health Care Worker

Recommendations for postexposure in a previously vaccinated HCW are as follows:

- If anti-HBs is known to be greater than 10 mIU/mL, no testing of the source patient for HBV is indicated, and no postexposure prophylaxis is indicated.
- If anti-HBs is unknown, the HCW should be tested for anti-HBs levels, and the source patient should be tested for HBsAg.
- If anti-HBs is less than 10 mIU/mL and it is not known if the source patient is HBsAg-positive, the HCW should get one dose of HBIG and be revaccinated with two doses.
  - Check anti-HBs 1 to 2 months after the second vaccine dose.
- If anti-HBs is less than 10 mIU/mL and the source patient is HBsAg-negative, the HCW should receive one vaccine dose.
  - Check anti-HBs 1 to 2 months after vaccine dose.
- If anti-HBs is greater than 10 mIU/mL, no hepatitis B immunoglobulin (HBIG) or additional vaccine is indicated.
- For vaccinated HCWs with anti-HBs less than 10 mIU/mL after two vaccine series, the source patient should be tested as soon as possible.
- If source patient is positive, two doses of HBIG are indicated, one at the time of exposure and an additional dose 1 month later.
- No additional vaccine is indicated.

Postexposure in an Unvaccinated or Incompletely Vaccinated Health Care Worker

The source patient should be tested as soon as possible. If the source patient is HBsAg-positive or unknown, the dose regimen is as follows:
- HCW should receive one dose of HBIG and one vaccine dose.
  - Complete remainder of vaccine series
  - Anti-HBs 1 to 2 months after last vaccine dose (at least 6 months from HBIG dose)

If the source patient is HBsAg-negative, the dose regimen is as follows:
- HCW should complete vaccine schedule
  - Anti-HBs 1 to 2 months after last vaccine doses

Clinical Management of the Health Care Worker Exposed to HBV

In HCWs with anti-HBs less than 10 mIU/mL or unvaccinated/incompletely vaccinated HCWs with exposure to an HBsAg-positive or unknown status, testing for total anti-HBc should be done immediately followed by HBsAg and total anti-HBc 6 months later. **The exposed HCW should refrain from donating blood, plasma, organs, or semen. Sexual practices do not need to be modified, and exposed HCWs do not need to refrain from pregnancy. Breastfeeding does not have to discontinue based on exposure.** No modification of HCW patient-care responsibilities is necessary to prevent transmission to patients (Schillie, 2018b).

Hepatitis C

Approximately 2.7 to 3.9 million individuals are currently living with chronic hepatitis C virus (HCV) infection, with approximately 41,200 new cases of HCV in 2016 (CDC, 2018b). Approximately 50% of those infected are unaware they have HCV. HCV is transmitted primarily through percutaneous exposure that can result from intravenous drug use, needle-stick injuries, and inadequate infection control in health care settings. Injection drug use now accounts for 60% of acute HCV infections (American Association for the Study of Liver Diseases–Infectious Diseases Society of America [AASLD-IDSA], 2018; Tohme, 2010). Less commonly, HCV transmission occurs among HIV-positive individuals who have had sexual contact with an HCV-infected partner (especially among MSM), individuals who have received tattoos in an unregulated environment, and infants born to HCV-infected mothers (Tohme, 2010; CDC, 2018b).

Diagnosis

One-time testing is indicated for those born between 1945 and 1965 and for all persons with behaviors, exposures, or conditions/circumstances associated with increased risk for HCV infection. These other factors are listed as follows (AASLD-IDSA, 2018):

- Behaviors: any history of injection drug use or intranasal illicit drug use
- Risk exposures: long-term hemodialysis; percutaneous/parental exposure in an unregulated setting; HCW or public safety worker after needle-stick, sharps, or mucosal exposure to HCV-infected blood; children born to HCV-infected women; persons who received a transfusion of blood or blood component or underwent an organ transplant before July 1992; those who received clotting factor concentrates produced before 1987; and those who were incarcerated.
- Other conditions/circumstances: HIV infection, sexually active persons about to start pre-exposure prophylaxis for HIV, unexplained chronic liver disease, solid organ donors

Annual testing is recommended for persons who inject drugs and for HIV-infected MSM. Periodic testing should be offered to those with ongoing risk factors for HCV exposure (AASLD-IDSA, 2018).

HCV antibody testing is recommended for the initial diagnosis of HCV infection. A positive HCV antibody test indicates current infection (acute or chronic), resolved prior infection, or a false-positive result. Any positive HCV antibody test should be followed by a HCV nucleic acid test to detect HCV viremia. HCV RNA testing should be done in those with a negative HCV antibody test who are immunocompromised or who may have been exposed within 6 months of the test.

Occupational HCV Exposure in the Health Care Worker

The risk for HCV transmission after exposure to an HCV-positive needle stick or sharps exposure is 0.1% (Egro et al., 2017; CDC, 2018b). If known, the source should be tested for HCV RNA. If the source HCV RNA is negative, no further testing is indicated for the HCW. If the source HCV RNA is positive or unknown, the HCW should have an anti-HCV test within 48 hours. If positive, a reflexive HCV RNA should be sent and the HCW should be referred for treatment of a pre-existing HCV infection. If it is negative, follow-up testing should include an HCV RNA test 3 weeks or longer postexposure. If positive, refer for care. If negative, an optional anti-HCV test can be performed at 6 months postexposure.

As with HBV exposure, HCW who are exposed to an HCV-positive or unknown source should refrain from donating blood, plasma, organs, or semen. Sexual practices do not need to be modified, and exposed HCWs do not need to refrain from pregnancy. Breastfeeding does not have to discontinue based on exposure (CDC, 2001).

Treatment

The goal of treatment of HCV-infected persons is to reduce mortality and liver-related health conditions including end-stage liver disease and hepatocellular carcinoma (AASLD-IDSA, 2018). Since the approval of highly effective HCV protease inhibitor therapies in 2011, the treatment for HCV infections has evolved significantly. Current therapies can achieve a sustained virologic response (absence of detectable virus 12 weeks after treatment), indicative of a cure, in greater than 90% of HCV patients regardless of HCV genotype. Currently, the AASLD-IDSA recommend treatment for all individuals with chronic HCV infections except those with a short life expectancy who cannot be improved with HCV therapy, liver transplantation, or another directed therapy (AASLD-IDSA, 2018).

Treatment is driven by genotype and the presence and degree of cirrhosis. A complete list of treatment recommendations based on genotype and presence/absence and degree of cirrhosis is detailed in the joint AASLD-IDSA HCV guidelines (AASLD-IDSA, 2018).

ECTOPARASITIC INFECTIONS

Pediculosis Pubis (Phthirus Pubis): *Pubic or Crab Louse*

Pediculosis pubis is an infectious disease caused by the infestation with the parasite *Phthirus pubis*. The infection is transmitted by sexual contact, close body contact, or, less commonly, contact with objects. *Phthirus pubis* infects the terminal hairs of the pubic and perianal areas (Salavastru et al., 2017). The lifetime of the adult parasite is less than 1 month during which the female lays eggs that need 1 week to hatch (Galiczynski and Elston, 2008). The incubation period is usually less than 1 month but may be longer (Salavastru et al., 2017). Transmission is not prevented with the use of condoms. **The presence of pubic lice in children does not imply definite sexual contact as they can be acquired by contact with an infected person** (Chosidow, 2000). Patients with pediculosis pubis should be evaluated for other STDs including HIV (Workowski, 2015).

The main complaint is usually itching in the genital area. On examination, visible nits and/or lice are attached to hairs. Initial exposure can result in symptoms in 2 to 6 weeks, but subsequent exposures are associated with quicker onset of symptoms. Because empty egg shells can remain on the hair for many months, the diagnosis is only by identifying live lice or visible eggs (Chosidow, 2000). **Recommended treatments include permethrin 1% cream rinse (applied to affected areas and washed off after 10 minutes) or pyrethrins with piperonyl butoxide applied in the same manner** (Workowski, 2015). Reported resistance to perimethrin and pyrethrins has been increasing and becoming more widespread (Meinking et al., 2002; Yoon et al., 2003). Malathion 0.5% lotion (applied to affected areas and washed off after 8 to 12 hours) can be used when treatment failure is thought to be caused by resistance (Workowski, 2015).

Bedding and clothing should be machine washed (at 50°C), dry-cleaned, or sealed and stored in a plastic bag for 3 days (Workowski, 2015; Salavastru et al., 2017). Fumigation of living areas is not needed. Sex partners within the previous month should be treated. Follow-up evaluation should be done in 1 week, and if lice or eggs are found, retreatment may be necessary. If no clinical response was noted with the use of a recommended regimen, retreatment with an alternative regimen is recommended (Workowski, 2015).

Scabies

Scabies is an infectious disease caused by infestation with the parasite *Sarcoptes scabiei* var. *hominis*. The infection occurs by skin-to-skin contact including sexual intercourse, or less commonly, contact with infected fomites (e.g., clothing) (Salavastru et al., 2017). *S. scabiei* mites burrow into the epidermis in which the female parasite lays eggs that hatch and develop into adults in 2 weeks. Adult parasites die outside their human host within 24 to 36 hours (Arlian et al., 1984). The mites and mite products (feces, eggs, and dead parasites) generate an immediate or delayed (type IV) hypersensitivity reaction such that scabies symptoms usually start 3 to 6 weeks after primary infestation and then 1 to 3 days after reinfestation (Chosidow, 2006; Walton and Oprescu, 2013; Salavastru et al., 2017).

The most common presentations are skin rash and itching, especially at night. **Female scabies mites can burrow under the skin, producing tiny raised and serpiginous lines on the skin** (Salavastru et al., 2017). Scratching can lead to secondary infection with *S. aureus* or β-hemolytic streptococci, and these secondary infections have been associated with poststreptococcal glomerulonephritis (Svartman et al., 1972). A more concentrated area of mites can form a crust and is called *crusted* scabies (Norwegian scabies). This is an aggressive infestation that usually occurs in immunodeficient, debilitated, or malnourished individuals. Diagnosis is suspected based on the characteristics of itch, clinical findings, and suggestive history (e.g., exposure). **Definitive diagnosis is made by microscopic examination of skin scrapings, which identifies mites, eggs, or fecal pellets.** In sexually active patients, STD screening including HIV is recommended (Salavastru et al., 2017).

Recommended treatments include permethrin 5% cream or ivermectin 200 µg/kg orally, repeated in 2 weeks. Topical treatment should be applied at night to all skin regions, including the scalp, groin, navel, external genitalia, finger and toe web spaces, and the skin beneath the ends of nails, and is left in place for 8 to 12 hours. An alternative therapy is lindane 1%, however, because of its toxicity, it should only be used in patients >10 years of age who cannot tolerate the recommended therapies or if the therapies have failed (Mounsey et al., 2008, 2009, 2013; Workowski, 2015). Substantial treatment failures will likely happen with these treatment regimens in the management of crusted scabies. Combination treatment recommendations for crusted scabies consisting of a topical scabicide (25% topical benzyl benzoate or 5% permethrin cream) in a full body application repeated for 7 days and then twice weekly until cured) and oral ivermectin 200 µg/kg on days 1, 2, 8, 9, and 15 (additional treatment on days 22 and 29 for severe cases). Lindane should not be used for crusted scabies (Workowski, 2015). **Bedding and clothing should be machine washed (at 50°C), dry-cleaned, or sealed and stored in a plastic bag for 3 days.** Persons who have had sexual, close personal, or household contact with the patient within the preceding month should be examined, and those found to be infested should be treated.

Scabies epidemics frequently occur in nursing homes, hospitals, residential facilities, and other communities (Bouvresse and Chosidow, 2010). Ivermectin can be considered in this setting, although specialty consultation is recommended (Workowski, 2015).

VAGINITIS

Vaginitis is characterized by vaginal symptoms including discharge, odor, itching, irritation, and burning. Most women have at least one episode of vaginitis in their lives. The most common forms of vaginitis are bacterial vaginosis (BV), vulvovaginal candidiasis, and trichomoniasis. BV accounts for 40% to 50% of cases in which a cause is identified, vulvovaginal candidiasis accounts for 20% to 25% of cases, and trichomoniasis accounts for 15% to 20% of cases. BV and trichomoniasis are sexually transmitted. **The diagnosis can be made by Amsel's criteria: pH, KOH test (potassium hydroxide preparation), and microscopic examination of fresh discharge samples** (Table 58.8) (Paladine and Desai, 2018).

Bacterial Vaginosis

BV is a polymicrobial syndrome resulting from replacement of the normal hydrogen peroxide–producing *Lactobacillus* sp. in the vagina with high concentrations of anaerobic bacteria (i.e., *Prevotella* sp. and *Mobiluncus* sp.), *G. vaginalis*, Ureaplasma, Mycoplasma, and numerous fastidious or uncultivated anaerobes. Although BV is the most common diagnosis in women seeking care for vaginal symptoms, most women with BV are asymptomatic. BV is associated with having multiple male or female partners, douching, lack of condom use, and lack of vaginal lactobacilli. Women with BV are at an increased risk for STDs, complications after gynecologic surgery, pregnancy complications, and recurrence of BV. BV increases the risk for HIV transmission to the male partner. The gold standard for diagnosing BV is a Gram stain used to determine the relative concentration of lactobacilli, gram-negative and gram-variable rods and cocci, and curved gram-negative rods characteristic of BV. **Clinical diagnosis requires three of the following symptoms or signs: (1) homogeneous, thin, white discharge that smoothly coats the vaginal walls; (2) clue cells (vaginal epithelial cells studded with bacteria); (3) vaginal fluid pH greater than 4.5; or (4) fishy odor of vaginal discharge before or after addition of 10% KOH. Treatment is recommended for symptomatic women and consists of metronidazole 500 mg orally twice daily for 7 days or metronidazole gel 0.75%**

TABLE 58.8 Differential Diagnosis of Vaginitis in Women

	VAGINAL DISCHARGE	pH	WHITE BLOOD CELLS	MICROSCOPY	SYMPTOMS
Normal	White, thick, smooth	≤4.5	Absent	Lactobacilli	None
Candidiasis	White, thick, curdlike	≤4.5	Absent	Mycelia	Vulvar pruritus, external or superficial dysuria
Trichomoniasis	Frothy or purulent	≥4.5	Present	Mobile trichomonads present Amine odor	Vulvar erythema and edema, punctate strawberry lesions on cervix
Bacterial vaginosis	Thin, white homogeneous	≥4.5	Absent	Paucity of lactobacilli (75% of patients) Amine odor Clue cells	Fishy odor and increased vaginal discharge

(one full applicator: 5 g) intravaginally once daily for 5 days. An alternative option is clindamycin 2% cream (5 g) intravaginally at bedtime for 7 days. Importantly, clindamycin cream can weaken latex condoms and diaphragms for 5 days after use. **Routine treatment of sex partners is not recommended** (Workowski, 2015).

Trichomoniasis

Trichomoniasis, caused by the protozoan *T. vaginalis*, is the most prevalent nonviral sexually transmitted infection in the United States, affecting 3.7 million people. Although most patients are asymptomatic, symptoms can include diffuse, malodorous, yellow-green discharge with or without vulvar irritation. *T. vaginalis* infection is associated with twofold to threefold increased risk for HIV acquisition, preterm birth, and other pregnancy-related complications. **NAAT is highly sensitive in detecting *T. vaginalis* infections and can be used on vaginal, endocervical, or urine specimens from women.** Culture is available, but NAAT is more sensitive. Microscopic evaluation of wet preparations of genital secretions is common because of low cost. The sensitivity is quite low, however (51% to 65%). If used, slides should be evaluated immediately because sensitivity decreases by up to 20% within 1 hour after collection. **Recommended treatment is a single oral dose of 2 g of metronidazole or 2 g of tinidazole. Because of poor cure rates with a single dose of metronidazole in women with HIV, the CDC recommends metronidazole 500 mg orally twice daily for 7 days for trichomoniasis treatment in HIV-infected women.** Alcohol consumption should be avoided for 24 hours after completion of metronidazole or 72 hours after completion of tinidazole. Because of the high rate of reinfection for trichomoniasis, retesting for *T. vaginalis* is recommended for all sexually active women within 3 months after initial treatment. **All sex partners should be referred for presumptive therapy to avoid reinfection** (Workowski, 2015).

Candidiasis

Vulvovaginal candidiasis (VVC) is usually caused by *C. albicans* but occasionally by other species of *Candida* or yeasts. Seventy-five percent of women will have at least one episode of VVC. Vaginal candidiasis is classified as complicated or uncomplicated based on clinical criteria. Uncomplicated cases involve infections that are sporadic or infrequent, produce mild to moderate symptoms, and are likely to be caused by *C. albicans*, and they occur in immunocompetent women. Complicated cases involve recurrent candidiasis (four or more episodes of symptomatic vulvovaginal candidiasis in 1 year), severe infection, and non–*C. albicans* causes, and they occur in women with uncontrolled diabetes, debilitation, or immunocompromising conditions. Approximately 10% to 20% of cases of vulvovaginal candidiasis will be complicated. **Vaginal cultures should be obtained in patients with recurrent vulvovaginal candidiasis because conventional antimycotic treatments are not as effective against atypical species such as *Candida glabrata*.** The diagnosis is made via wet prep with saline or KOH; a Gram stain of vaginal discharge that demonstrates yeast, hyphae, or pseudohyphae; or a culture that shows *Candida* or other yeast species. Wet mounts should first be done for all patients and culture used for those with symptoms with negative wet mounts. Treatment is not recommended for an asymptomatic patient with a positive culture as 10% to 20% of women are colonized with *Candida* sp. and other yeasts in the vagina.

Treatment for uncomplicated vulvovaginal candidiasis includes numerous over-the-counter intravaginal agents including clotrimazole creams, miconazole as a cream or intravaginal suppository, or tioconazole ointment. Prescription treatment formulations include butoconazole cream, terconazole cream or vaginal suppository, nystatin vaginal suppository, or one oral dose of fluconazole 150 mg. A woman who has persistent symptoms or a recurrence 2 months after having used an over-the-counter treatment should be evaluated. In cases of recurrence, a longer duration of therapy such as 7 to 14 days of topical therapy or a dose of fluconazole every third day for a total of three doses is recommended. Treatment for non–*C. albicans* vulvovaginal candidiasis is not standardized (Workowski, 2015).

KEY POINTS

- Patients with urethritis need to be treated for both gonorrhea and chlamydia. Because of higher sensitivity, NAATs are now the preferred method for detecting *N. gonorrhoeae* and *C. trachomatis*. Urethral swab is no longer indicated.
- Most genital ulcers in the United States are either herpes (most common) or syphilis. Chancroid occurs in some parts of the United States, but granuloma inguinale usually does not. LGV is increasing in incidence in MSM.
- Men with possible Zika exposure, regardless of symptom status, should wait at least 6 months from symptom onset (if symptomatic) or from last possible exposure before attempting conception with their partner. Women with possible Zika virus exposure are recommended to wait to conceive until at least 8 weeks after symptom onset of last possible exposure.
- Vaccines to prevent HPV-associated diseases are available and recommended for men and women younger than 26 years of age, preferably to start before the onset of sexual activity.
- Testing for HIV is recommended for anyone with an STD or at risk for acquiring an STD.
- HIV is becoming a chronic disease, and many of the associated problems are from aging and chronic disease instead of immunosuppression.

REFERENCES

The complete reference list is available online at ExpertConsult.com.

59 Cutaneous Diseases of the External Genitalia

Richard Edward Link, MD, PhD, and Nikki Tang, MD

The diagnosis and treatment of cutaneous diseases of the external genitalia remain important elements of urologic practice. Often overlooked during formal urology residency training, this topic lies at the interface of multiple specialties, including urology, diagnosis of infectious diseases, rheumatology, allergy-immunology, and dermatology.

INTRODUCTION TO BASIC DERMATOLOGY

Dermatology is the clinical discipline focused on the normal biology and pathogenesis of diseases and disorders of the skin. The diagnosis of skin disease depends critically on the history and physical examination, with laboratory testing often relegated to a peripheral and confirmatory role. In many cases, visual inspection alone suffices to narrow the diagnosis significantly. On the other hand, the skin has a limited repertoire of morphologic expression. Therefore the urologist should not hesitate to perform a skin biopsy, when indicated, or to order a variety of laboratory investigations when needed to distinguish between two or more clinical mimics.

The skin is divided into three layers: the epidermis, dermis, and hypodermis (subcutaneous tissue; Fig. 59.1). The epidermis, composed of stratified squamous epithelia, can vary in thickness from 0.05 to 1.5 mm depending on location. Melanocytes (pigment-producing cells) populate the lower layers of the epidermis. The dermis, composed of collagen, elastin, and reticular fibers, can be divided into two layers: the thin superficial layer (papillary dermis) and the thicker deeper layer (reticular dermis). Located within the dermis are mesenchymal structures, such as blood vessels and nerves. The bottom layer of the skin, known as the hypodermis or subcutaneous tissue, is composed largely of fat.

Literally hundreds of cutaneous diseases exist that may involve the external genitalia. In addition, within each disease there may be significant variation in appearance and symptoms as the process for each condition evolves. For this reason, a methodical and systematic approach is essential to reach a rational diagnosis. The dermatologic history should focus on the duration, rate of onset, location, associated symptoms, family history, allergies, occupation, and previous treatment of the condition (Habif, 2004). Common symptoms include pruritus (itching), burning, stinging, and pain. The *lack* of symptoms, such as pain, can also be important in arriving at the correct diagnosis and should therefore be noted.

The physical examination should address the distribution of primary and secondary skin lesions. **It is important to perform a thorough skin survey and not to focus solely on the area of affected genital skin.** For example, the presence of red silvery-scaled plaques on the genital skin of a patient who has similar lesions on their extensor body surfaces may guide the physician toward adding psoriasis to the differential diagnosis.

Most skin conditions begin with a characteristic primary lesion that is an important key to diagnosis. A precise description of this lesion includes documenting its color (red, brown, black, yellow, white, blue, or green) and morphology (macule, papule, plaque, nodule, pustule, vesicle, bulla, or wheal; Table 59.1) (Habif, 2004). Because of the mucosal nature of genital skin, papular and macular lesions may present as erosions in this area (Margolis, 2002). Secondary skin lesions develop as the skin condition evolves or are caused by scratching, rubbing, or superinfection. A secondary lesion should also be classified morphologically as a scale, crust, erosion, ulcer, atrophy, thickening, or scar (Table 59.2).

After gross morphology is determined, laboratory testing may confirm the diagnosis. To identify cutaneous fungi such as dermatophytes and *Candida* species, potassium hydroxide (KOH) or periodic acid–Schiff staining may be applied to scraped or touched skin specimens. KOH dissolves keratin, leaving fungal hyphal walls prominently visible under the microscope. Likewise, mineral oil drops may help visualize mites or eggs, and Tzanck preparations may aid in identifying viral agents such as herpes simplex, varicella zoster, and molluscum contagiosum.

For difficult cases or those in which malignancy is suspected, skin biopsy may be indicated. A variety of techniques exist for this purpose, including curettage, punch, shave, and incisional and complete excisional biopsies. For small scrotal or phallic shaft lesions, these techniques can usually be performed in the office setting under local anesthesia. For larger lesions or those involving the urethral meatus, biopsy in the operating room is recommended. It is often possible to determine the correct diagnosis with a very small (2- to 3-mm) punch biopsy. The resultant defect can easily be closed with one or two 6-0 or 7-0 nylon sutures or even be left open to heal secondarily.

Additional diagnostic maneuvers that may prove invaluable in select situations include serologic testing (e.g., serologic tests for syphilis), culture (e.g., culture for *Pseudomonas aeruginosa*), Wood's ultraviolet lamp (e.g., skin fluorescence of skin affected by vitiligo or erythrasma), and immunohistochemistry stains of biopsy specimens (e.g., examination for specific types of cytokeratins associated with different variants of lichen sclerosus).

DERMATOLOGIC THERAPY

Medical therapy for dermatologic conditions consists of a broad range of topical and systemic compounds.

For systemic therapy, useful drug classes include antibiotics, antifungals, antivirals, anti-inflammatories, and antipruritics. Less commonly used agents, including chemotherapeutic and biologic drugs (e.g., methotrexate, cyclophosphamide, adalimumab, etanercept, infliximab, and ustekinumab), immunosuppressants (e.g., azathioprine, cyclosporine, tacrolimus), and hydroxyurea, are discussed within the specific disease entities.

A lack of familiarity with cutaneous diseases affecting the genitalia may lower the threshold of urologists in prescribing systemic antibiotics for these conditions. Unfortunately, these agents carry significantly greater risks than topical preparations, including promotion of resistant organisms, interaction with other medications, and disruption of the normal bowel and vaginal flora. Alterations in bacterial flora or in their antimicrobial susceptibility patterns may persist for protracted periods, thus emphasizing the need for truly appropriate antibiotic use (Jernberg et al., 2010). Similar caveats apply to systemic antifungal agents such as fluconazole, ketoconazole, and terbinafine. Superficial dermatophytes, such as those causing tinea cruris, generally respond well to diligent application of topical antifungal preparations. **Systemic antifungals are indicated only for very extensive cutaneous dermatophytosis, endemic mycoses with skin involvement, deep infection involving the hair follicles (Majocchi granuloma), or fungal infections in severely immunocompromised individuals** (Lesher and McConnell, 2003). In some cases, even in immunocompetent individuals, systemic antifungals are necessary to treat infections resistant to local therapy (Lesher, 1999). On the other hand, warnings have emphasized the need to

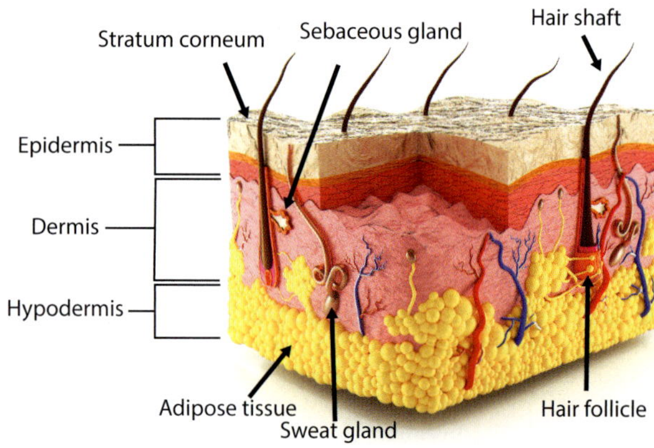

Fig. 59.1. Anatomy of hair-bearing human skin. (Used and modified under license, Anton Nalivayko/Shutterstock.com.)

TABLE 59.1 Primary Cutaneous Lesions

PRIMARY LESION	DESCRIPTION
FLAT	
Macule	A circumscribed, **flat** discoloration that may be brown, blue, red, or hypopigmented
ELEVATED, SOLID	
Papule	An **elevated, solid** lesion up to 0.5 cm in diameter of variable color. Papules may become confluent to become plaques
Nodule	A circumscribed, **elevated solid** lesion >0.5 cm in diameter
Plaque	A circumscribed, **elevated**, superficial, **solid** lesion >0.5 cm in diameter
FLUID-FILLED	
Vesicle	A circumscribed **collection of free fluid** ≤0.5 cm in diameter
Bulla	A circumscribed **collection of free fluid** >0.5 cm in diameter
Pustule	A circumscribed collection of leukocytes and free fluid (**pus**)
Wheal (hive)	A firm **erythematous plaque** resulting from **infiltration** of the dermis with fluid (may be transient)

From Habif TP: *Clinical dermatology: a color guide to diagnosis and therapy*, Edinburgh, 2004, Mosby.

TABLE 59.2 Secondary Cutaneous Lesions

SECONDARY LESION	DESCRIPTION
Scale	Excess dead epidermal cells that are produced by abnormal keratinization and shedding
Crust	A collection of dried serum and cellular debris (a scab)
Erosion	A focal loss of epidermis. Erosions do not penetrate below the dermoepidermal junction and they heal without scarring
Ulcer	A focal loss of epidermis and dermis, which heals with scarring
Fissure	A linear loss of epidermis and dermis with sharply defined, vertical walls
Atrophy	A depression in the skin resulting from thinning of the epidermis or dermis
Scar	An abnormal formation of connective tissue implying dermal damage

From Habif TP: *Clinical dermatology: a color guide to diagnosis and therapy*, Edinburgh, 2004, Mosby.

avoid the routine use of some systemic antifungal medications (such as ketoconazole) for superficial cutaneous infections because of the unpredictable risk of life-threatening hepatotoxicity and adrenal insufficiency (FDA, 2013). Systemic anti-inflammatory agents, in particular the glucocorticosteroids (GCS), deserve additional attention. Oral GCS are absorbed in the jejunum with peak plasma concentrations occurring in 30 to 90 minutes (Lester, 1989). Despite short plasma half-lives of 1 to 5 hours, the duration of effect of GCS lasts between 8 and 48 hours, depending on the agent (Nesbitt, 2003). These drugs have widespread anti-inflammatory effects. They release neutrophils from bone marrow, but they inhibit their movement to sites of inflammation in tissue. They also impair T-cell activation and antigen presentation by dendritic cells (Nesbitt, 2003). **For short-term (≤3 weeks) treatment of dermatologic conditions such as allergic contact dermatitis** (Feldman, 1992), **a single morning dose of GCS is administered to minimize suppression of the hypothalamic-pituitary-adrenal axis** (Myles, 1971). Prednisone is generally the GCS of choice because of its low cost, intermediate duration of action, and variety of dosage forms, although methylprednisolone may be substituted to reduce the mineralocorticoid effects (Wolverton, 2001). **Longer-term treatment with systemic GCS may lead to a wide variety of adverse effects, including osteoporosis, cataract formation, hypertension, obesity, hyperglycemia, aseptic necrosis of the femoral head, immunosuppression, and psychiatric changes** (Nesbitt, 2003). For this reason, the use of topical steroids (see following) is preferable to reliance on systemic GCS whenever clinically feasible. Systemic antipruritic therapies include oral antihistamines such as hydroxyzine and diphenhydramine, and tricyclic agents such as doxepin and selective serotonin reuptake inhibitors (SSRIs).

Topical preparations are the mainstay of therapy for a wide range of cutaneous diseases affecting the genitalia. Urologists tend to be less familiar with the use of these medications than are dermatologists. **Topical medications can be broken down into five general classes: emollients, anti-inflammatories, antibiotics, antifungals, and chemotherapeutic agents.**

Topical preparations include active ingredients that also include a vehicle that determines the rate at which the active ingredients are absorbed by the skin. Emollients restore water and lipids to the epidermis and are useful for dry-skin diseases. Emollients should be applied to moist skin for maximal effect, such as after bathing. Ointments are generally preferred because they less often cause irritation or burning associated with creams (Edwards and Lynch, 2018). Preparations containing urea (e.g., Carmol, vanadine) or lactic acid (Lac-Hydrin, AmLactin) may be particularly potent hydrating agents (Habif, 2004). Ceramides (combinations of a fatty acid and a sphingoid base), the main natural intercellular lipids in the outermost layer of skin, are critical for maintaining normal cutaneous hydration and barrier function (Weber et al., 2012). For this reason, new formulations containing ceramides (CeraVe) may also be particularly useful for skin conditions characterized by xerosis (dryness). Topical corticosteroids are potent anti-inflammatory agents available in a myriad of preparations and strengths. A detailed review of the use and dosing of topical corticosteroids is beyond the scope of this chapter, and the reader is directed to several excellent dermatology textbooks for more detail (Bologna et al., 2018; Edwards and Lynch, 2018; Habif, 2004). **Topical corticosteroids can include significant adverse effects from systemic absorption and from the results of local application. Local effects include epidermal atrophy and the development of striae on the upper portion of the inner thigh, dermal changes (telangiectasias, hypopigmentation), allergic reactions, and negative alterations in the usual course of skin infections and infestations** (Burry, 1973). Special care must be taken when applying corticosteroids to the skin of the male genitalia, which is at a higher risk for steroid atrophy because of its thin dermal depth. In most cases, atrophy is a reversible process that can be expected to resolve during the course of several months but can also be permanent (Sneddon, 1976). Atrophy is particularly troublesome if corticosteroids are applied under the foreskin, which can serve as an occlusive "dressing" and can enhance penetration of the drug (Fig. 59.2; Goldman and Kitzmiller, 1973).

A variety of physical modalities have also been applied to treat dermatologic problems, including ultraviolet light therapy, photodynamic therapy, laser therapy, and cryosurgery. Ultraviolet light therapy, with broadband and narrow-band ultraviolet B (UVB), has been used to treat atopic dermatitis, psoriasis, seborrheic dermatitis, and vitiligo (Honigsmann and Schwarz, 2003). There are now several convenient single-wavelength UVB (308 nm) laser units with small spot sizes, which are particularly useful for treating vexing localized areas of genital psoriasis or vitiligo; such narrow-spectrum machines are believed not to carry the risk of inducing the nonmelanoma skin cancer that is associated with broadband full-body light boxes. Psoralens, when combined with long-wave ultraviolet A radiation (psoralen ultraviolet A [PUVA] therapy), generate a phototoxic effect that is beneficial for treating psoriasis (Honigsmann, 2001; Stern, 2007), vitiligo (Honigsmann and Schwarz, 2003), atopic dermatitis (Morison, 1992), and lichen planus (Honigsmann and Schwarz, 2003). In general, the narrow-band UVB boxes and lasers have supplanted PUVA therapy, as the latter carries a substantial risk of squamous cell carcinoma (SCC) when performed throughout a prolonged period (Stern and Study, 2012). One significant downside to these particular treatments is the inconvenience patients face in attending weekly or biweekly laser sessions. Photodynamic therapy involves the use of cytotoxic oxygen radicals generated from photoactivated molecules to achieve a therapeutic response (Braathen et al., 2007; Tope and Shaffer, 2003).

Photodynamic therapy is useful in treating a variety of inflammatory, malignant, and infectious skin conditions. Studies have shown its success as monotherapy and in combination with cryosurgery, CO_2 laser ablation, and curettage in the management of large or resistant condyloma acuminata or in genital warts occurring during pregnancy (Scheinfeld, 2013a). The downside to this promising modality is that there is not yet an established optimum regimen for off-label use, including for genital warts. Lasers so far play a smaller role in the management of genital lesions, although some lasers (CO_2, pulsed dye) have been used effectively to manage genital condyloma acuminata (Veitch et al., 2017). Overall, cryosurgery is more widely used than laser therapy to treat genital and suprapubic molluscum contagiosum.

ALLERGIC DERMATITIS

Allergic contact or "eczematous" dermatitis (ACD) consists of a group of allergy-mediated processes leading to pruritic skin lesions (Box 59.1).

Atopic Dermatitis (Eczema)

Atopic dermatitis (AD) is a chronic relapsing dermatitis with a predilection for skin flexures that is associated with intense pruritus and damage to the epidermis (Williams, 2005). **The characteristic lesions are erythematous papules and thin plaques with secondary excoriations** (Fig. 59.3; Kang et al., 2003). In general, the lesions do not have a precise border as is common for papulosquamous disorders (Margolis, 2002). Although any age can be affected, 90% of AD patients manifest their condition before the age of 5 years (Rajka, 1989). AD is associated with susceptibility to a wide variety of substances that act as irritants (e.g., fragrances, preservatives, and various proteins). Patients suffering from AD also have a propensity to develop asthma and allergic rhinitis.

The genetic susceptibility to AD has been extensively explored. In a study of 372 AD patients, 73% had a positive family history for atopy. Likewise, twin concordance studies have demonstrated an AD risk of 0.86 for monozygotic twins compared with only 0.21 for dizygotic twins. These findings have spurred an intense search for genes involved in atopy and AD (Wollenberg and Bieber, 2000). Although no single gene has been found to be a unique marker for the disease, at least 11 genetic foci seem to be closely associated with AD (Ellinghaus et al., 2013; Kang et al., 2003). The most important genetic defects confer an inability to synthesize functional filaggrin properly. This structural

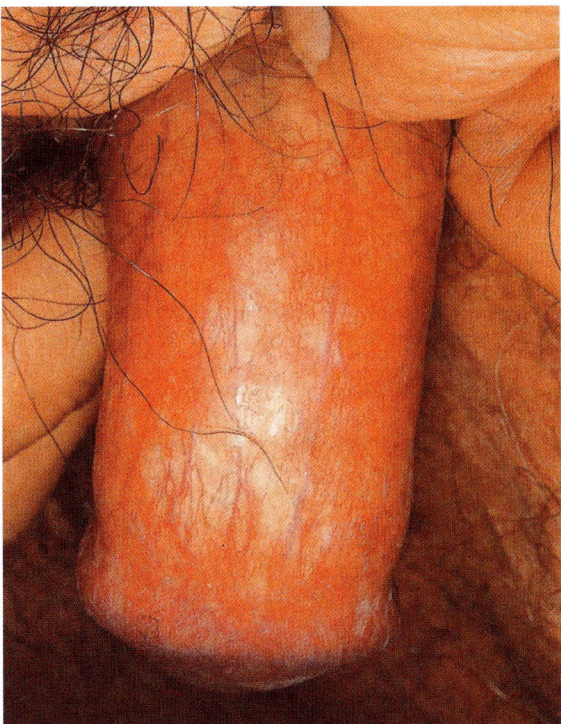

Fig. 59.2. Steroid atrophy of penile shaft skin after application of corticosteroid under the foreskin for 8 weeks. (From Habif TP: *Clinical dermatology*, Edinburgh, 2004, Mosby; 2004, p 36.)

BOX 59.1 Differential Diagnosis of Allergic Dermatitis
Eczema
Allergic dermatitis
Seborrheic dermatitis
Intertrigo
Contact dermatitis
Irritant dermatitis
Balanoposthitis
Zoon balanitis
Candidal-related illness
Impetigo
Herpes simplex
Herpes zoster
Drug reaction

From Margolis DJ: Cutaneous disease of the male external genitalia. In Walsh PC, ed: *Campbell's urology*, Philadelphia, 2002, Saunders.

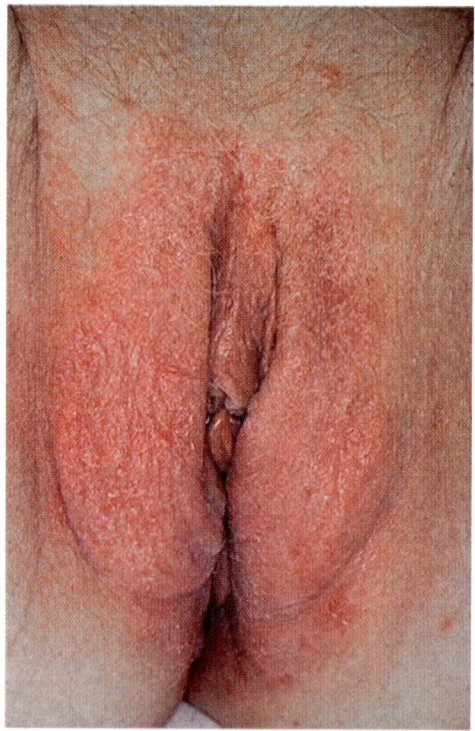

Fig. 59.3. Eczema involving the vulva. (From Simpson R, Nunns D: Skin diseases affecting the vulva. *Obstetrics, Gynaecology, and Reproductive Medicine* 27(3): 77–85, 2017. Fig. 2.)

abnormality results in a "leaky" epithelial barrier and chronic immune activation, which contribute to the pathophysiology of this common skin disease (Heimall and Spergel, 2012).

Intense pruritus is the hallmark of AD, and controlling the patient's urge to scratch is critical for successful treatment (Przybilla et al., 1994). Itching is often worse during evening hours and can be exacerbated by sweating, occlusive undergarments, or wool clothing (Kang et al., 2003). Scratching of lesions may contribute to the clinical complications of AD, including superinfection with *Staphylococcus aureus* species (Ogawa et al., 1994). There is growing evidence that bacterial toxins may serve as superantigens that drive an inflammatory cascade that sustains AD (Skov and Baadsgaard, 2000; Skov et al., 2000).

Clinically, there is no pathognomonic laboratory test, biopsy result, or single clinical feature that allows the definitive diagnosis of AD. The association with a personal or family history of atopy is a critical clue to the diagnosis (Kang et al., 2003). For patients with genital findings, extragenital involvement is commonplace.

A variety of "trigger factors" have been implicated in the exacerbation of AD, including chemicals, detergents, and household dust mites. Removal of these factors from the environment may be beneficial on an individualized basis. Dust mite exposure, in particular, has received significant attention in the literature. Although several studies have demonstrated modest improvement in AD with mite reduction (Kubota et al., 1992; Tan et al., 1996), others report that reduction is associated with no significant clinical benefit (Colloff et al., 1989; Gutgesell et al., 2001).

Treatments for AD include gentle cleaning with nonalkali soaps or soap substitutes (e.g., Cetaphil, Aquanil) and the frequent use of emollients. Evaporation of liquid from the skin may trigger AD (Kang et al., 2003), so frequent bathing especially with hot water is not encouraged. Soaking may help during episodes of bacterial superinfection but should be discontinued after the infection has resolved (Margolis, 2002). Topical corticosteroids may be needed to control pruritus but should be used only for short courses with a rapid taper to avoid local complications of skin atrophy and dyschromia. Topical immunomodulatory agents such as the calcineurin inhibitors tacrolimus and pimecrolimus have shown efficacy in the treatment of AD (Leung et al., 2009; Luger and Paul, 2007; Meagher et al., 2002; Nghiem et al., 2002), and these agents may decrease the need for corticosteroids during long-term therapy (Zuberbier et al., 2007). Antihistamines such as diphenhydramine or a variety of nonsedating agents, such as cetirizine, loratadine, and analogues of these, may be helpful in breaking the "itch-scratch cycle" in AD, particularly when administered before bedtime (Kang et al., 2003). Oral antistaphylococcal drugs have not been shown to significantly improve AD in a randomized, double-blind trial (Ewing et al., 1998). Systemic treatment with azathioprine, corticosteroids, cyclosporine, methotrexate, or mycophenolate mofetil may rarely be indicated for severe, widely disseminated cases (Cooper, 1993; Denby and Beck, 2012; Salek et al., 1993). The newest systemic treatment for moderate to severe AD is dupilumab (Dupixent), the first monoclonal antibody injection approved by the U.S. Food and Drug Administration (FDA) to effectively treat AD by targeting the Th2 pathway (Simpson et al., 2016).

Contact Dermatitis

Contact dermatitis can be broken down into two distinct entities: irritant contact dermatitis (ICD) and ACD. Although the mechanisms differ significantly, the clinical presentation of ICD and ACD may be similar. Most notably, the affected area is usually sharply limited to an area of skin exposure to true allergen or irritating chemical. The primary mode of treatment is to identify and reduce exposure to the offending agent.

ICD results from a direct cytotoxic effect of an irritant chemical touching the skin and is responsible for approximately 80% of contact dermatitis cases (Marks et al., 2002). Examples of offending agents include soaps, solvents, metal salts, and acid- or alkali-containing compounds. Occupational ICD is a serious public health problem and contributes to costs on the scale of $1 billion annually in the United States (Cohen, 2000). The clinical manifestations of ICD depend on the identity of the irritating substance as well as the duration of contact, concentration, temperature, pH, and location of exposure. Acute ICD, such as may result from an occupational accident, generally peaks within minutes to hours after exposure and then begins to heal. Symptoms of burning, stinging, and soreness may be accompanied by erythema, edema, bullae, or frank necrosis in a sharply defined area corresponding to the exposed skin (Cohen and Bassiri-Tehrani, 2003). There are also a variety of subacute forms of ICD that result from repeated subthreshold skin insults. Pruritus is much more common in these more chronic conditions, and the skin lesions are not as well demarcated. The mainstay of treatment for ICD lies in avoiding skin contact with the causative irritants through the use of protective clothing, safe occupational practices, and the use of skin barrier preparations such as ointments, emollient creams, or protective foams. Some commercially available barrier products include Atopiclair, Biafine, EpiCeram, MimyX, Neosalus Foam, and PruMyx (Berndt et al., 2000; Draelos, 2012).

In contrast, ACD represents a local type IV hypersensitivity reaction to a skin allergen to which an individual has been previously exposed and sensitized. Although ACD is a common reason for outpatient dermatology visits, involvement of the genital skin is rare (2.4%) (Bhate et al., 2010). The typical appearance is a well-demarcated pruritic eruption, which may manifest blistering or weeping in the acute phase or the development of scaly plaques more chronically (Mowad and Marks, 2003). In 2003 and 2009 the North American Contact Dermatitis Group (NACDG) reported a long list of common allergens implicated in ACD based on patch testing results (Zug et al., 2009). Similar lists that were produced subsequently contain the same set of allergens, with only a few exceptions. Patch testing is a simple technique of exposing an area of skin to a variety of potential allergens at a known concentration in a grid template (Fig. 59.4). Generally performed by dermatologists, patch testing can help to confirm the diagnosis of ACD and the allergen involved. The most common sensitizing allergen identified by the NACDG was nickel sulfate (Zug et al., 2009), which is a common component of costume jewelry and belt buckles (Fig. 59.5). Although traditionally a cause of earlobe dermatitis from pierced earrings, nickel sensitivity may

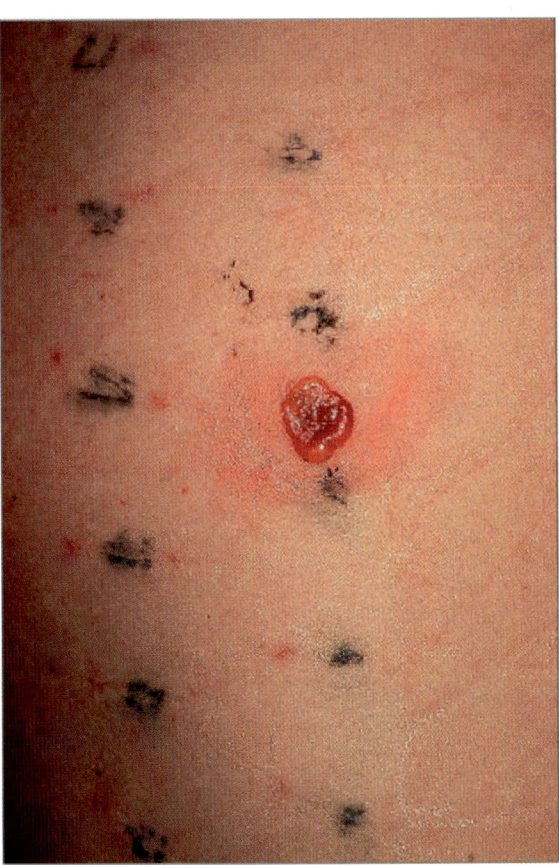

Fig. 59.4. An example of patch testing with a positive response to nickel. (From Bolognia JL, Jorizzo JL, Rapini RP: *Dermatology*, Edinburgh, 2003, Mosby, p 233.)

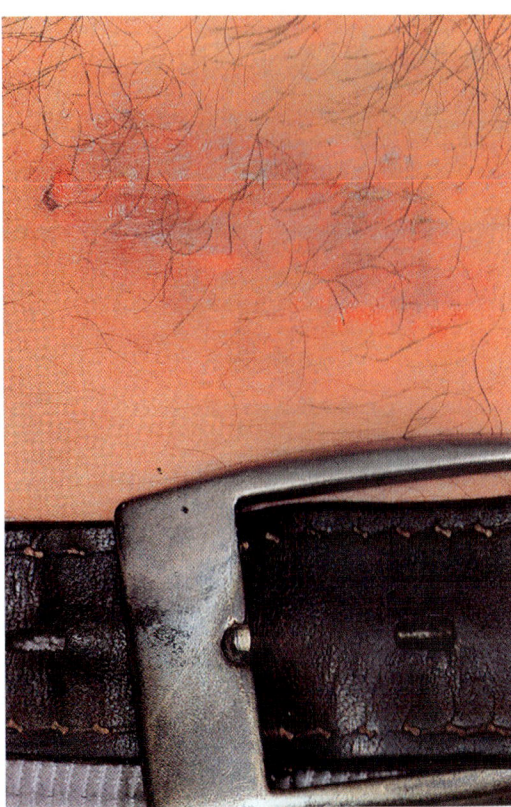

Fig. 59.5. Contact dermatitis caused by a nickel allergy from a belt buckle. (From Habif TP: *Clinical dermatology*, Edinburgh, 2004, Mosby, p 94.)

be a potential cause of genital ACD resulting from the increasing prevalence of genital piercing. Other important allergens include textile dyes, topical antibiotics (neomycin, bacitracin), perfumes and other fragrance materials, formaldehyde-releasing preservatives, the latex in condoms, and topical corticosteroids. When ACD is suspected, the urologist always should inquire about the use of over-the-counter products such as genital moisturizers, spermicides, antiyeast and anti-itch preparations, and lubricants used during sexual intercourse. Oral antihistamines may be helpful for the symptomatic control of ACD in combination with the removal of the inciting allergen. Severe ACD should *not* be treated with a short course of systemic steroids but rather with a 3-week tapering dose of prednisone.

Erythema Multiforme and Stevens-Johnson Syndrome

Erythema multiforme (EM) is a generalized skin disease that may involve the genitalia. **EM can be subdivided into minor and major forms.**

EM minor was first described in 1860 by an Austrian dermatologist, Ferdinand von Hebra (von Hebra, 1860). **This condition is an acute, self-limited skin disease characterized by the abrupt onset of symmetrical fixed red papules that may evolve into target lesions** (Weston, 1996). EM is a clinical rather than a histologic diagnosis. Papules and target lesions are usually grouped and can be present anywhere on the body, including the genitalia (Fig. 59.6A). There is also a predilection for involvement of the oral mucous membranes, as well as the palms and soles.

The majority of cases of recurrent EM minor are precipitated by human herpesvirus 1 and 2 (Nikkels and Pierard, 2002; Schofield et al., 1993), **with herpetic lesions usually preceding the development of target lesions by 10 to 14 days** (Lemak et al., 1986). Although continuous suppressive acyclovir may prevent EM episodes in patients with herpes infection (Tatnall et al., 1995), administration of the drug after development of target lesions is of no benefit (Huff, 1988). The natural history of EM minor is spontaneous resolution after several weeks without sequelae (Schofield et al., 1993), although recurrences are common (Huff and Weston, 1989). Oral antihistamines may provide symptomatic relief. For immunosuppressed patients, the time course of EM minor outbreaks may be longer, and the frequency of recurrence may be greater (Schofield et al., 1993).

The major form of EM has been called Stevens-Johnson syndrome (SJS) in the past, although there remains some controversy as to whether EM major and SJS are distinct entities or are part of a spectrum of disease (Bachot and Roujeau, 2003; Williams and Conklin, 2005). SJS is a much more serious illness than EM minor, and it includes features similar to extensive skin burns (Parrillo, 2007). In its more severe forms, SJS may mimic life-threatening toxic epidermal necrolysis. Admission to the intensive care unit or burn unit may significantly reduce the morbidity and mortality of this condition (Wolf et al., 2005). **Most patients with SJS exhibit a prodromal upper respiratory illness (fever, cough, rhinitis, sore throat, and headache), which progresses after 1 to 14 days to the abrupt development of red macules with blister formation and areas of epidermal necrosis. Genital involvement includes erythema and erosions of the labia** (Fig. 59.7), **penis, and perianal region.**

A vast array of inciting factors has been implicated in the development of SJS, with drug exposures being the most commonly identified. Among the most common offending agents are nonsteroidal anti-inflammatory agents, sulfonamides (particularly cotrimoxazole), tetracycline and doxycycline, penicillin and cephalosporins, and a wide range of anticonvulsants (Chan et al., 1990). In contrast to EM minor, there is rarely an association with an infectious agent (Weston, 2003). SJS generally follows a protracted course of 4 to 6 weeks and may include a mortality rate approaching 30%. **Severe scarring of denuded skin may result in a range of complications, including joint contractures, labial synechia, vaginal stenosis, urethral meatal stenosis, and anal strictures** (Brice et al., 1990; Weston, 2003). Treatment involves immediate removal of the offending drug and

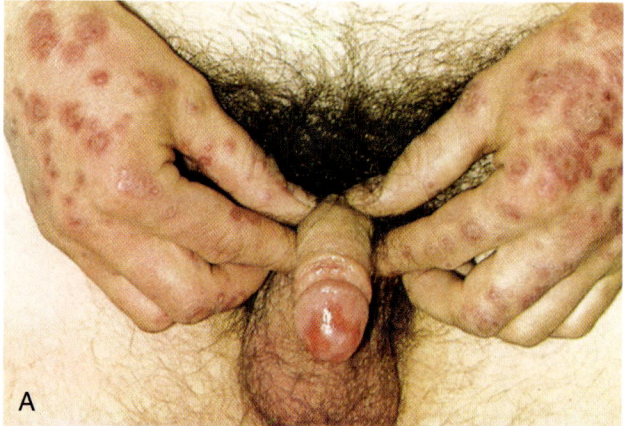

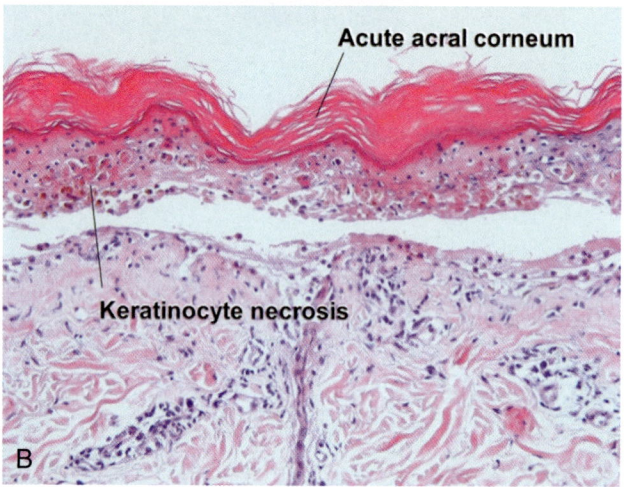

Fig. 59.6. Erythema multiforme (EM). (A) Targetoid lesions of the hands and penis. (B) Typical microscopic picture of EM with a normal stratum corneum, necrotic keratinocytes in the epidermis, and a lymphoid infiltrate. (A, From Korting GW: *Practical dermatology of the genital region*, Philadelphia, 1981, Saunders, p 16. B, From Elston DM, Ferringer T: *Dermatopathology*, Edinburgh, 2009, Saunders, p 147.)

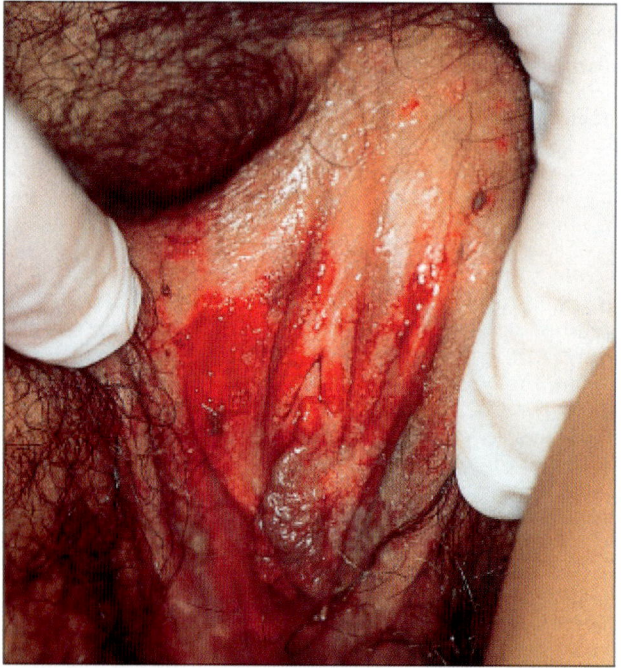

Fig. 59.7. Labial erosions in a case of Stevens-Johnson syndrome. (Courtesy of Yale Dermatology Residents' Slide Collection. From Bolognia JL, Jorizzo JL, Rapini RP. *Dermatology*. Edinburgh: Mosby; 2003.)

supportive care similar to the management of severe burns. There is currently no strong evidence for any specific medical therapy for SJS (Weston, 2003), and the role of systemic corticosteroids in treating SJS remains controversial (Rasmussen, 1976; Tripathi et al., 2000; Weston, 2003). Newer modalities that have had limited randomized controlled studies include cyclosporine (3 to 5 mg/kg/day), tumor necrosis factor (TNF)-α inhibitors, plasmapheresis, and, especially noted, intravenous immunoglobulin (Mockenhaupt, 2011; Paradisi et al., 2014; Worswick and Cotliar, 2011). Care of the SJS patient is best accomplished via a multispecialty team approach.

PAPULOSQUAMOUS DISORDERS

Papulosquamous disorders are a disparate group of diseases that share a common primary lesion: scaly papules and plaques (Box 59.2).

Psoriasis

Psoriasis is a common disease affecting up to 2% of the population (Christophers, 2001; Nestle et al., 2009). For patients with a predisposition, which is likely polygenic in nature, triggering factors such as trauma, infection (streptococcal disease), psychological stress, or new medications can elicit a flare in the psoriatic phenotype. One-third of affected patients have a family history of psoriasis (Hensler and Christophers, 1985; Margolis, 2002; Melski and Stern, 1981).

The characteristic lesion is a sharply demarcated erythematous plaque with silvery-white scales and results from rapid proliferation of the epidermis (van de Kerkhof, 2003). Its pattern can be limited to the elbows or knees or can be distributed on the entire surface of the skin. Although psoriasis can appear at any age, two peaks of onset have been identified: 20 to 30 and 50 to 60 years of age. Patients complain of a significant impairment in their quality of life as a result of pruritus and bleeding, as well as the cosmetic and psychosocial impact of these visible plaques.

Psoriatic involvement of the genitalia is relatively common, although it is usually within the context of a generalized cutaneous disorder. **Patients may present with concerns for malignancy or sexually transmitted disease (STD) when psoriatic lesions are present on the genitalia.** Genital psoriasis leads to impaired self-esteem and reduced sexual self-image, thereby interfering with normal intimate relationships, particularly in women (Magin et al., 2010; Meeuwis et al., 2011). The presence of characteristic lesions on the elbows, knees, buttocks, nails, scalp, and umbilicus may help direct the diagnosis (Fig. 59.8A) (Margolis, 2002). When lesions are present in the inguinal folds and intergluteal cleft, scaling may

---

BOX 59.2 Differential Diagnosis of Papulosquamous Lesions

Psoriasis
Seborrheic dermatitis
Dermatophyte infection
Erythrasma
Secondary syphilis
Pityriasis rosea
Discoid lupus
Mycosis fungoides
Lichen planus
Fixed drug eruption
Reactive arthritis
Pityriasis versicolor
Bowen disease
Extramammary Paget disease

From Margolis DJ: Cutaneous disease of the male external genitalia. In Walsh PC, ed: *Campbell's urology*, Philadelphia, 2002, Saunders.

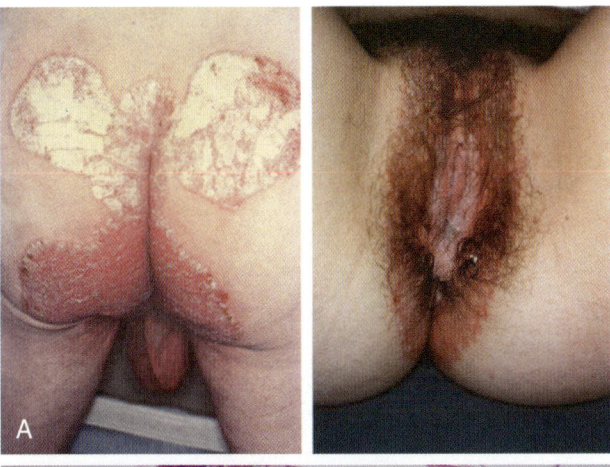

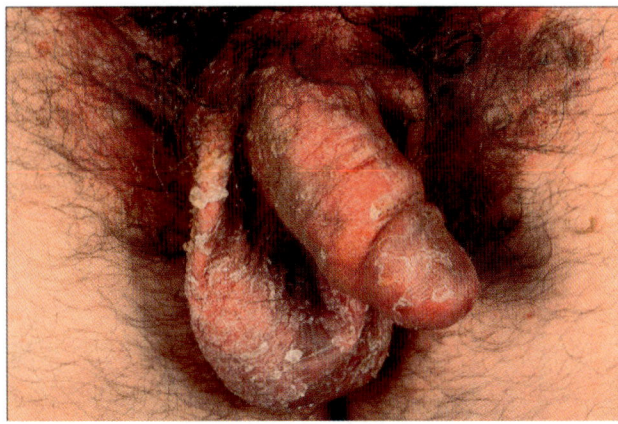

Fig. 59.9. Psoriasis involving the entire penis and scrotum. (Courtesy of Peter CM van de Kerkhof, MD. From Bolognia JL, Jorizzo JL, Rapini RP. *Dermatology*. Edinburgh: Mosby; 2003.)

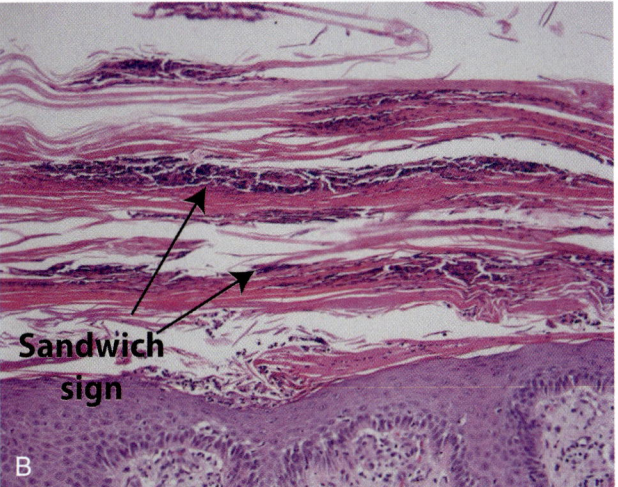

Fig. 59.8. Psoriasis. (A) Silver scales on an erythematous base. (B) Alternating neutrophils and parakeratosis in the stratum corneum of plaque psoriasis (sandwich sign). (A, From Callen JP, Greer DE, Hood AF, et al.: *Color atlas of dermatology*, Philadelphia, 1993, Saunders, p 320. B, From Elston DM, Ferringer T: *Dermatopathology*, Edinburgh, 2009, Saunders p 152.)

be absent (so-called inverse psoriasis) (Goldman, 2000). When evaluating nonscaling erythematous plaques in the inguinal folds, the diagnosis of fungal involvement (i.e., tinea or *Candida*) should be considered and ruled out by KOH preparation or fungal culture. In circumcised men, psoriatic plaques are often present on the glans and corona, whereas in uncircumcised men, lesions are commonly hidden under the preputial skin (Buechner, 2002). In some cases, however, psoriasis involves the entire penis and scrotum (Fig. 59.9).

Psoriasis is a chronic disease with a relapsing and remitting course. A variety of topical and systemic therapies have been developed and are applied to this difficult problem. Despite the variety of therapy, however, as many as 40% of psoriasis patients express frustration at the ineffectiveness of current treatments (Krueger et al., 2001). **For genital psoriasis, the mainstay of therapy is the use of low-potency topical corticosteroid creams for short courses** (Kalb et al., 2009). Examples include a preparation of 3% liquor carbonis detergens (a tar derivative) in 1% hydrocortisone cream or hydrocortisone butyrate 0.1% (Fisher and Margesson, 1998). These preparations should not be used for more than 2 weeks continuously on thin genital skin or in areas occluded by skin folds (Margolis, 2002). If the psoriatic plaque is very thick, a stronger topical corticosteroid such as triamcinolone 0.1% may be used initially. Other topical therapies for psoriasis include vitamin D_3 analogues (calcitriol, calcipotriene), topical calcineurin inhibitors (pimecrolimus cream and tacrolimus ointment), and low-potency retinoids, although these agents are sometimes too irritating or not sufficiently effective. Photochemotherapy combining an ingested PUVA has been used extensively to treat psoriasis (Stern, 2007). However, a dose-dependent increase in the risk of genital SCC has been associated with high-dose PUVA therapy for psoriasis elsewhere on the body (Stern, 1990; Stern et al., 2002). Genital shielding during PUVA therapy is strongly recommended; therefore this modality is contraindicated for treating psoriatic lesions localized to genital skin. For patients with extensive psoriasis, systemic therapy with methotrexate, cyclosporine, retinoids, phosphodiesterase 4 (PDE4) inhibitor (apremilast), or one of the approved TNF-α inhibitors (adalimumab, etanercept, infliximab), interleukin (IL)-17 inhibitor (ixekizumab) or IL-12/23 inhibitors (ustekinumab) may be appropriate. The 308-nm excimer laser (Gerber et al., 2003) is now approved for psoriasis treatment. Experimental therapies that have shown promise in treating psoriasis include vitamin D receptor ligands (Bos and Spuls, 2008) and antibodies or antisense oligonucleotides against T-lymphocyte surface molecules (Gottlieb et al., 2000), TNF (Bos and Spuls, 2008; Chaudhari et al., 2001), or intracellular adhesion molecules (Gottlieb et al., 2000).

Reactive Arthritis (Formerly Reiter Syndrome)

Reactive arthritis (formerly Reiter syndrome) is composed of urethritis, arthritis, ocular findings, oral ulcers, and skin lesions. Only about one-third of all patients with this disorder demonstrate all of the manifestations. The skin findings, particularly when present on the genitalia, may be mistaken for psoriatic lesions (Fig. 59.10). Reactive arthritis is more common in men than in women and is rarely diagnosed in children. **Reactive arthritis is generally preceded by an episode of either urethritis (*Chlamydia*, *Gonococcus*) or gastrointestinal infection (*Yersinia*, *Salmonella*, *Shigella*, *Campylobacter*, *Neisseria*, or *Ureaplasma* species) and is more common in human immunodeficiency virus (HIV)-positive patients** (Margolis, 2002; Rahman et al., 1992; Wu and Schwartz, 2008). **There is a strong genetic association with the human leukocyte antigen (HLA)-B27 haplotype.** Whether or not cross-reactivity between bacterial antigens and HLA-B27 leads to autoimmunity in reactive arthritis remains controversial (Ringrose, 1999; Yu and Kuipers, 2003).

Conjunctivitis is the most common ocular manifestation, although iritis, uveitis, glaucoma, and keratitis may occur. Polyarthritis and sacroiliitis are the most common orthopedic complaints and may lead to chronic disability in a small minority of cases (van de Kerkhof, 2003). Scaly, erythematous psoriaform skin lesions appearing on the penis are referred to as *balanitis circinata* (Fig. 59.11), and similar lesions on the soles are referred to as *keratoderma blennorrhagicum*. **These lesions may be difficult to distinguish from psoriasis, and histologic analysis of biopsy specimens cannot consistently differentiate the two conditions** (Margolis, 2002). Other disease entities that should be excluded include pustular psoriasis, gonococcal infection, and Behçet syndrome. The course of reactive arthritis involving the genitalia is usually self-limited, lasting a few weeks to

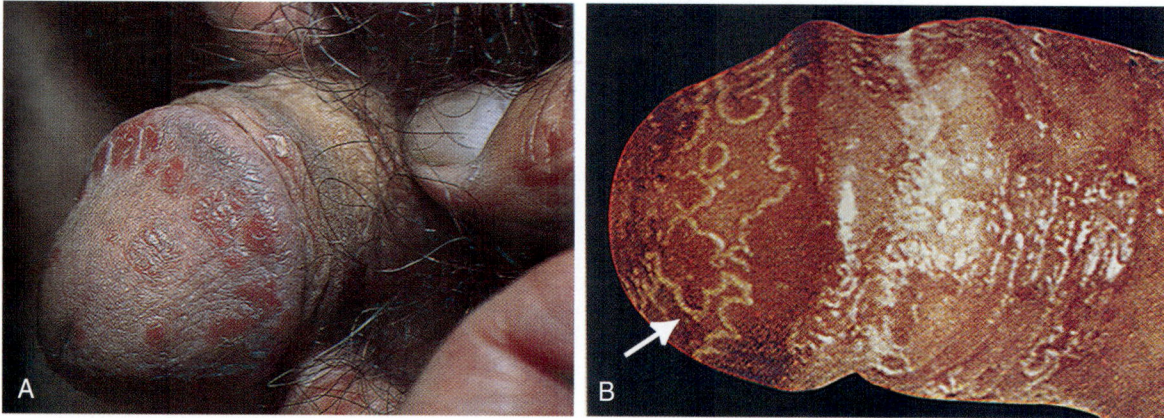

Fig. 59.10. Comparison of psoriasis (A) and reactive arthritis (B) (balanitis circinata) involving the glans penis. Note the highly characteristic coalescence of lesions in this case of reactive arthritis forming a wavy pattern *(arrow)*. (From Habif TP: *Clinical dermatology*, Edinburgh, 2004, Mosby, p 217.)

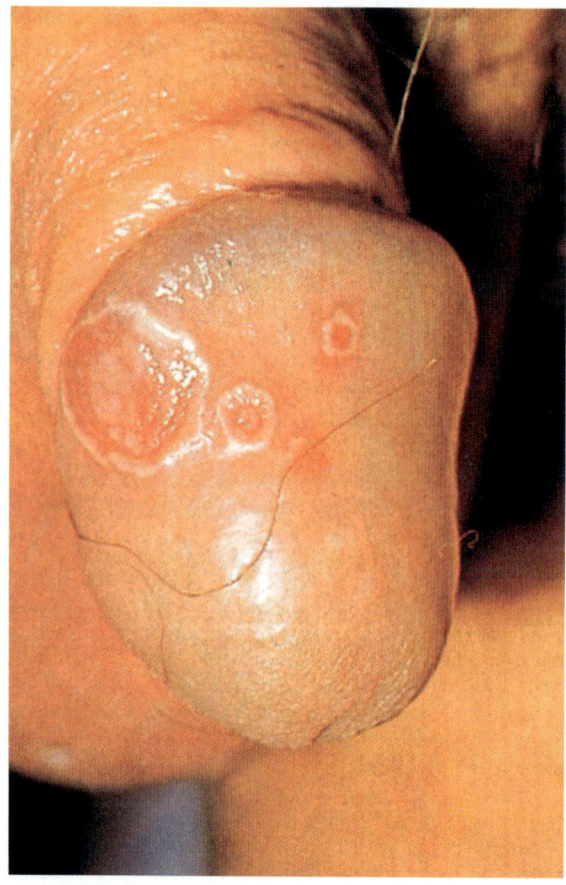

Fig. 59.11. Erosive psoriaform lesions of the glans penis (reactive arthritis; balanitis circinata) may also lack the wavy pattern, making them difficult to differentiate from genital psoriasis. (From Callen JP, Greer DE, Hood AF, et al.: *Color atlas of dermatology*, Philadelphia, 1993, Saunders, p 160.)

months. Lesions may respond to low-potency topical corticosteroids, and systemic therapy is rarely required. Lesions on soles, however, are more persistent; these respond well to the application of potent topical retinoids such as tazarotene or systemic retinoids such as acitretin (Lewis et al., 2000).

Lichen Planus

Lichen planus (LP), the prototype of the lichenoid dermatoses, is an idiopathic inflammatory disease of the skin and mucous membranes. The characteristic "lichenoid tissue reaction" is characterized by epidermal basal cell damage that is associated with a massive infiltration of mononuclear cells in the papillary dermis (Shiohara and Kano, 2003). Cutaneous LP may affect up to 1% of the adult population (Boyd and Neldner, 1991) and oral lesions may be present in as many as 4% (Scully et al., 1998). The pathogenesis of LP appears related to an autoimmune reaction against basal keratinocytes, which express altered self-antigens on their surfaces (Morhenn, 1986).

The primary lesion of LP is a small, polygonal-shaped, violaceous, flat-topped papule. These lesions may be widely separated or may coalesce into larger plaques that may ulcerate, particularly on mucosal surfaces. LP commonly involves the flexor surfaces of the extremities, the trunk, the lumbosacral area, the oral mucosa, and the glans penis (Margolis, 2002). **On the male genitalia, the clinical presentation of LP can vary and includes isolated or grouped papules, a white reticular pattern, or an annular (ringlike) arrangement with or without ulceration** (Fig. 59.12). In some cases, the lesions appear to form linear patterns related to skin trauma (the so-called Koebner phenomenon, which is also seen with psoriasis). On the female genitalia, painful erosion of erythematous plaques is common; in long-standing LP of the vulva, some areas of hyperhydrated hyperkeratosis (manifesting as white plaques) may surround shallow erosions. In women more than in men, concomitant oral LP may be found on the buccal mucosa or tongue (Santegoets et al., 2010). The differential diagnosis of LP includes invasive and in situ SCC, Zoon balanitis, psoriasis, secondary syphilis, herpes and extramammary Paget disease, and lupus erythematosus. Biopsy may be necessary to establish the diagnosis, particularly when the lesions are small, multiple, and ulcerated (Shiohara and Kano, 2003). Lichenoid reactions can also occur in response to ingested drugs and contact allergens, and a careful search for potential offending agents is appropriate.

The natural history of papular LP is benign, and the spontaneous resolution of cutaneous lesions has been observed in up to two-thirds of cases after 1 year (Shiohara and Kano, 2003). **However, the oral and erosive forms may persist significantly longer, and isolated cases of SCC arising within chronic genital LP have been reported**, warranting regular skin checks throughout the course of the disease (Mignogna et al., 2000). Although bothersome pruritus (more often in men) or pain/burning (more often in women) is common with LP, asymptomatic lesions on the genitalia do not require treatment. Care should be taken with LP of the vagina because erosive disease can cause adhesions and permanent damage (Edwards and Lynch, 2018). The primary modality of treatment for symptomatic genital LP is the application of an ultrapotent topical corticosteroid (such as clobetasol 0.05% or halobetasol 0.05%). There is also a role for topical calcineurin inhibitors (pimecrolimus cream, tacrolimus ointment) in the management of genital LP (Luger and Paul, 2007). For severe cases, systemic corticosteroids (15 to 20 mg/day; 2- to

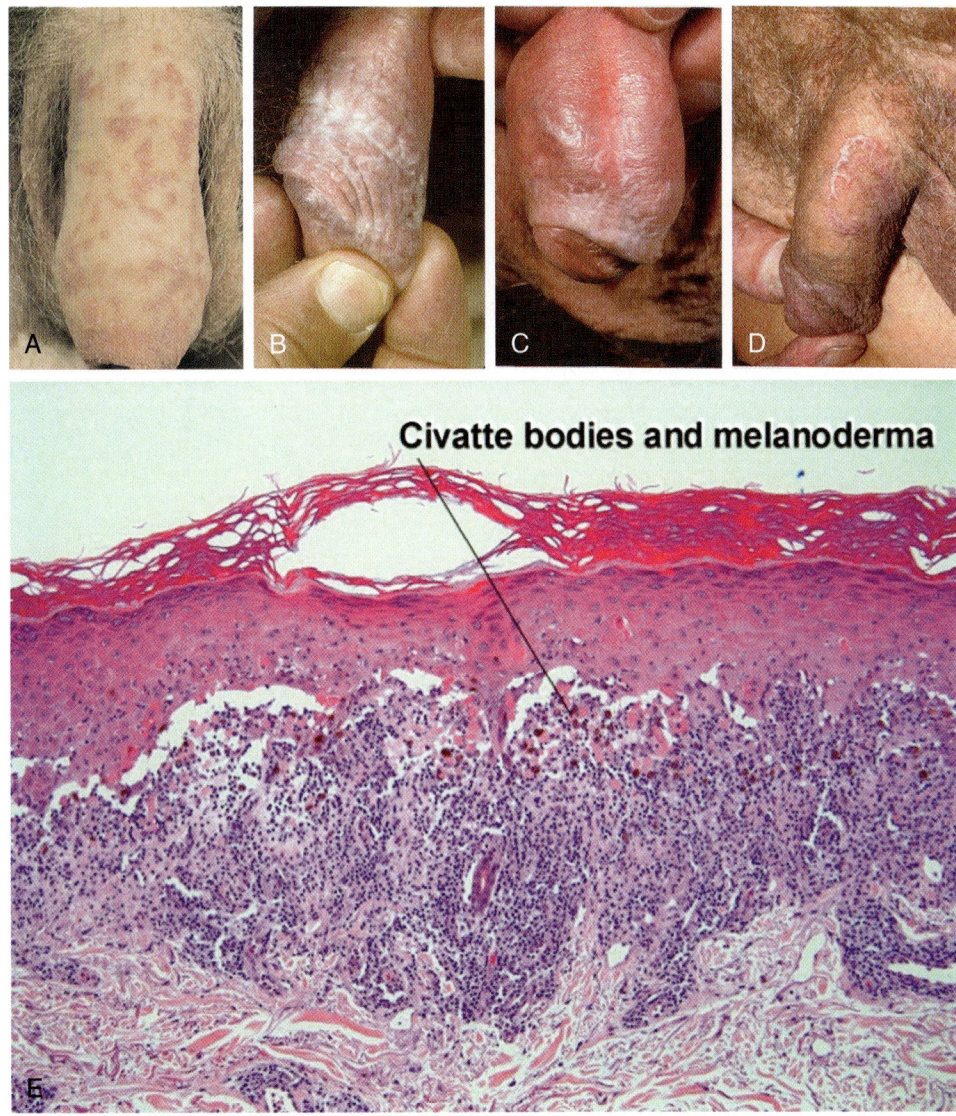

Fig. 59.12. Lichen planus (LP). Various presentations of LP on the male genitalia. (A and B) Individual and grouped purple papules on the penile shaft, some oriented in a linear pattern. (C) A white reticular pattern sometimes seen in LP. (D) An annular (ringlike) arrangement with a shiny surface. (E) Histologically, LP is characterized by destruction of the basal layer, a sawtooth rete ridge pattern, the presence of Civatte bodies and dermal melanocytes, and the absence of parakeratosis or eosinophils. (A, From Korting GW: *Practical dermatology of the genital region*, Philadelphia, 1981, Saunders, p 29. B, C, and D, From du Vivier A: *Atlas of clinical dermatology*, London, 2002, Churchill Livingstone, p 100. E, From Elston DM, Ferringer T: *Dermatopathology*, Edinburgh, 2009, Saunders p 137.)

6-week course) (Boyd and Neldner, 1991) have been shown to shorten the time course to clearance of LP lesions from 29 weeks to 18 weeks (Cribier et al., 1998). Other systemic therapies for severe LP include cyclosporine, tacrolimus, griseofulvin, metronidazole, and acitretin (Boyd and Neldner, 1991; Buyuk and Kavala, 2000; Cribier et al., 1998; Ho et al., 1990; Madan and Griffiths, 2007), although randomized trials demonstrating efficacy are generally lacking. In fact, as pointed out in an exhaustive meta-analysis, there is no overwhelmingly reliable evidence for the efficacy of *any* single treatment for erosive mucosal LP, including application of an ultrapotent topical steroid, which is the widely accepted first-line therapy (Cheng et al., 2012).

Lichen Nitidus

Lichen nitidus (LN) is an unusual inflammatory eruption characterized by tiny, discrete, flesh-colored papules arranged in large clusters. Although there is some debate as to whether LN may represent a variant of LP (Aram, 1988), the two entities are histologically distinct.

LN has a dense, well-circumscribed, lymphohistiocytic infiltrate that is closely apposed to the epidermis (Shiohara and Kano, 2003). Commonly involved sites include the flexor aspects of the upper extremities, the genitalia, the trunk, and the dorsal aspects of the hands. Nail involvement is common. Similar to LP, the natural history of LN is one of spontaneous resolution, with the majority of patients (69%) manifesting the disease for less than 1 year (Lapins et al., 1978). Patients should be reassured that these genital lesions are not infectious and should resolve with time. For symptomatic pruritus, genital lesions usually respond to mid- to low-potency topical corticosteroids and oral antihistamines (Shiohara and Kano, 2003).

Lichen Sclerosus

Lichen sclerosus et atrophicus (LS) is a chronic inflammatory disease of unknown cause with a predilection for the external genitalia. LS is 6 to 10 times more prevalent in women than in men, generally occurring either around the time of menopause or in the prepubertal

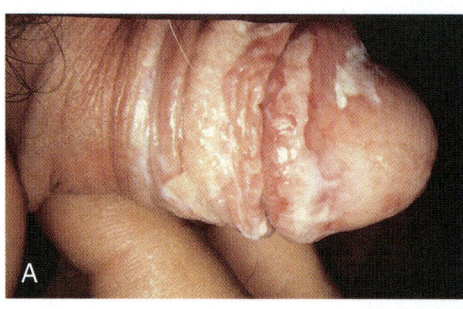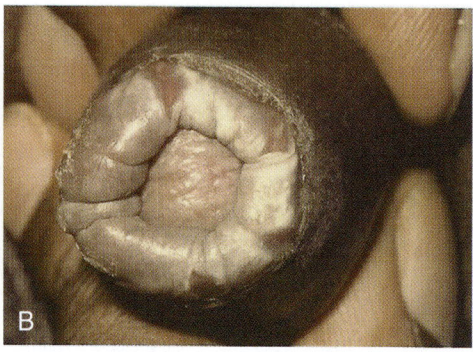

Fig. 59.13. (A and B) Lichen sclerosus et atrophicus (balanitis xerotica obliterans) of the penis. Note the erythematous and white plaques involving the penile shaft, preputial skin, and glans. (A, From Callen JP, Greer DE, Hood AF, et al.: *Color atlas of dermatology*, Philadelphia, 1993, Saunders p 327. B, Courtesy of Ron Rapini, MD. From Bolognia JL, Jorizzo JL, Rapini RP. *Dermatology*. Edinburgh: Mosby; 2003.)

years (Wojnarowska and Cooper, 2003). It tends to affect older men (>60 years of age) (Ledwig and Weigand, 1989) and can be associated with pain during voiding or erection (Margolis, 2002). There is a strong familial predisposition for this disorder, suggesting a genetic contribution (Sherman et al., 2010). For patients with genital LS, 15% to 20% experience extragenital disease (Powell and Wojnarowska, 1999). LS is ultimately a scarring disorder characterized by tissue pallor, loss of architecture resulting from fibrosis, and hyperkeratosis (Fig. 59.13). Some cases of LS may demonstrate prominent purpura and fissuring; the former may be so severe as to obscure the typical "white" color of the disease. The glans penis and foreskin are usually affected, and in contrast to women, perianal involvement in men is usually absent. Preputial scarring from LS can lead to phimosis, and circumcision is usually curative, although recurrence in the circumcision scar may occur. The late stage of this disease is called *balanitis xerotica obliterans*, which can involve the penile urethra and result in troublesome urethral strictures. In women, the disease can eventually lead to vulvar adhesions, labial fusion, clitoral phimosis, and vaginal obstruction. LS can also be the cause of considerable genital itching, burning, pain, and dyspareunia in women.

Despite the similarities in name, LS shares little in common with LP and LN other than pruritus and a predilection for the genital region. **Another critical distinction is that LS has been associated with SCC of the penis and vulva, particularly those variants not associated with human papillomavirus (HPV), and LS may represent a premalignant condition** (Bleeker et al., 2009; van de Nieuwenhof et al., 2011; Velazquez and Cubilla, 2003). LS includes specific histologic features, including basal cell vacuolation, epidermal atrophy, marked dermal edema, collagen homogenization, focal perivascular infiltrate of the papillary dermis, and plugging of the ostia of follicular and eccrine structures (Margolis, 2002). Biopsy is worthwhile to confirm the diagnosis and to exclude malignant change (Powell and Wojnarowska, 1999). The differential diagnosis includes erosive LP, vulvar eczema, lichen simplex chronicus, child sexual abuse, morphea, and mucous membrane pemphigoid. It has been suggested that the expression of selected cellular markers (such as p53, survivin, telomerase, Ki-67, and cyclin D1) can help distinguish between indolent LS and LS with true malignant potential (Carlson et al., 2013). In the future, biopsy specimens may routinely be investigated for these (and other) protein markers to determine prognosis.

From a management standpoint, long-term follow-up of patients with LS is important because of the association with SCC. Fissures, ulcers, papules, or nodules that are nonhealing should be carefully monitored. The application of potent topical steroids (such as clobetasol propionate 0.05% or halobetasol 0.05%) for long courses (3 months) followed by tapering and limited (twice weekly) application to maintain remission is well established as a treatment for LS in women and may improve symptoms and reverse the disease process (Dalziel et al., 1991). This regimen is contrary to the usual policy of avoiding long courses of steroid application to genital skin. The efficacy of similar approaches has not been definitively confirmed in adult men, although benefits have been demonstrated in the pediatric age group (Kiss et al., 2001). Several studies show calcineurin inhibitors to have some positive effect on symptoms, but trials comparing calcineurin inhibitors to topical steroids demonstrate greater efficacy for topical steroids (Funaro et al., 2014). The application of topical and administration of systemic retinoids, as well as photodynamic therapy, may be therapeutic options in rare cases refractory to standard therapeutic interventions. Because of a high rate of recurrence (40% to 50%) after seemingly successful initial therapy, some experts suggest the routine use of proactive (prophylactic) maintenance therapy with either midpotency topical steroids (such as mometasone furoate 0.1%) or topical calcineurin inhibitors (Goldstein et al., 2011; Hengge et al., 2006; Virgili et al., 2013).

Fixed Drug Eruption

A fixed drug eruption is one of the most common types of cutaneous drug reactions and occurs in response to oral medications, usually 1 to 2 weeks after the first exposure. It typically involves the lips, face, hands, feet, and genitalia, particularly the glans penis (Fig. 59.14). After subsequent re-exposure to the drug, the reaction occurs in the exact same location, usually within 24 hours (hence the term "fixed"). The most common medications causing this reaction are sulfonamides, nonsteroidal anti-inflammatory agents, barbiturates, tetracyclines, carbamazepine, phenolphthalein, oral contraceptives, and salicylates (Kauppinen and Stubb, 1985; Stubb et al., 1989; Thankappan and Zachariah, 1991). There have been isolated reports of fixed drug eruption associated with urologic drugs, such as finasteride, tadalafil, and fluconazole (administered for vulvovaginal candidiasis).

When present on the penile shaft or glans, these lesions usually appear as an asymptomatic, solitary, violaceous-colored, well-defined patch or plaque surrounded by an erythematous halo, and they may become bullous, pruritic, erosive, and painful (Margolis, 2002). On the genitalia, the differential diagnosis includes herpes simplex infection or an insect bite. Removing the offending agent usually results in resolution of the lesion, although a postinflammatory brown pigmentation may remain. There should be no long-lasting residual functional defect from this process.

Seborrheic Dermatitis

Seborrheic dermatitis (SD) is a common skin disease characterized by the presence of sharply demarcated pink-yellow to red-brown plaques covered with an adherent flaky scale. It shares a variety of features in common with eczematous dermatitis and could easily be grouped in that category. Common dandruff is a mild form of SD localized to the scalp. It has a predilection for areas rich in sebaceous glands and is generally present only during the first few

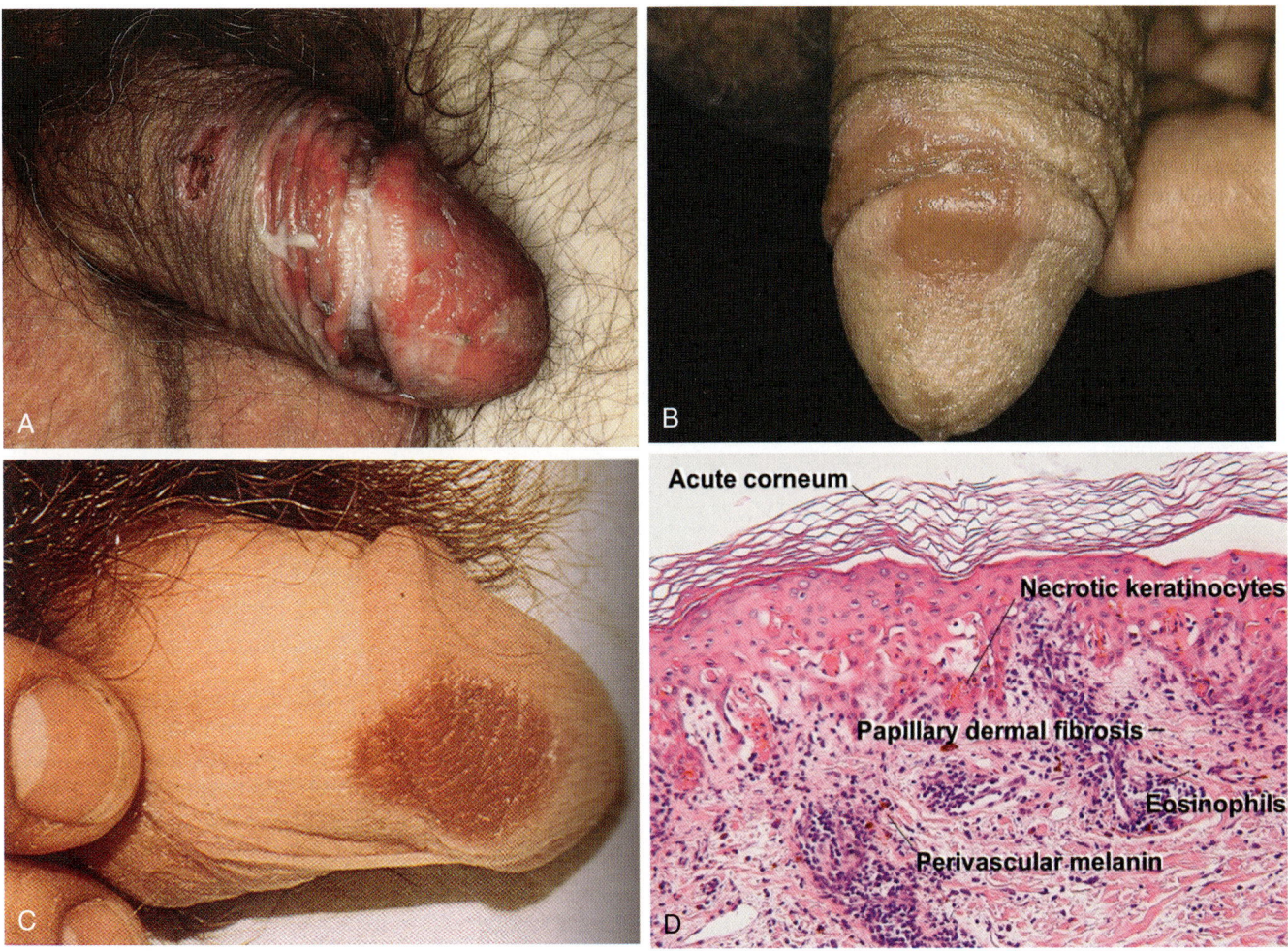

Fig. 59.14. Fixed drug eruptions. (A to C) Involvement of the penis. (D) Histologic features include a normal stratum corneum with chronic changes in the superficial dermis including an eosinophilic infiltrate. (A, From Callen JP, Greer DE, Hood AF, et al.: *Color atlas of dermatology,* Philadelphia, 1993, Saunders, p 160; B, Courtesy of Kalman Watsky, MD. From Bolognia JL, Jorizzo JL, Rapini RP. *Dermatology.* Edinburgh: Mosby; 2003. C, From Habif TP: *Clinical dermatology,* Edinburgh, 2004, Mosby, p 492, D, From Elston DM, Ferringer T: *Dermatopathology,* Edinburgh, 2009, Saunders, p 149.)

months of life or postpuberty, when sebaceous glands are active. Commonly affected areas include the scalp, eyebrows, nasolabial folds, ears, and chest, although the anus, glans penis, and pubic areas may also be involved (Margolis, 2002). Circumcision may be somewhat protective against the development of SD. In one study of 357 patients, the risk of developing penile SD was 2.5 times greater in the uncircumcised state (Mallon et al., 2000).

Adult SD includes a chronic relapsing course (Webster, 1991). **This condition is particularly common in patients with Parkinson disease, and up to 83% of acquired immunodeficiency syndrome (AIDS) patients may manifest SD** (Froschl et al., 1990; Gupta and Bluhm, 2004). Particularly in immunosuppressed individuals, SD may involve a significant proportion of the body surface area. **Extensive and/or severe SD should raise concerns for possible underlying HIV infection** (Fritsch and Reider, 2003). SD may be pruritic, and differentiation from psoriasis may occasionally be problematic. Unlike psoriasis, however, SD rarely involves the nails and tends to have a thinner associated scale.

Controversy concerning the etiology of SD revolves around a possible autoimmune response to a component of normal skin flora, the yeast *Malassezia furfur (Pityrosporum ovale).* Although *M. furfur* can be isolated from the lesions of SD, the number of organisms is only about twice that observed in normal control skin (Nenoff et al., 2001). Likewise, severely SD-affected HIV patients do not harbor more organisms than HIV patients who do not manifest SD (Pechere et al., 1999). Another factor potentially linked to SD is an elevated level of triglycerides and cholesterol at the skin surface (Fritsch and Reider, 2003).

Creams or foams containing topical antifungals (i.e., ketoconazole) are the mainstay of SD treatment on the body and include a 75% to 90% response rate (Elewski et al., 2007; Faergemann, 2000; Fritsch and Reider, 2003). For hair-bearing areas, "antidandruff" shampoos containing zinc, salicylic acid, selenium sulfide, tar, ciclopirox olamine, or 1% to 2% ketoconazole are effective (Margolis, 2002; Squire and Goode, 2002). Because of the chronic and relapsing nature of SD, treatment often must be repetitive and prolonged. Low-potency topical corticosteroids such as 2.5% hydrocortisone may play a role during the initial treatment of severe cases, but they should not be the primary mode of treatment for this condition because of the potential for local steroid side effects.

VESICOBULLOUS DISORDERS

Vesicobullous disorders are uncommon conditions often characterized by autoimmune damage to the epidermis or basement membrane (Box 59.3). Although intact blisters may be found on the groin and suprapubic skin per se, the rupture of vesicles and bullae on the genitalia may only leave behind residual erosions (Margolis, 2002).

> **BOX 59.3** Differential Diagnosis of Vesicobullous Disorders
>
> Bullous pemphigoid
> Pemphigus vulgaris
> Pemphigus foliaceus
> Zoon balanitis
> Behçet syndrome
> Contact dermatitis
> Dermatitis herpetiformis
> Porphyria cutanea tarda
> Herpes zoster
> Herpes simplex
> Lymphangioma circumscriptum
> Impetigo
> Fixed drug eruption
> Factitial
> Innocent trauma
> Benign familial pemphigoid (Hailey-Hailey disease)

From Margolis DJ: Cutaneous disease of the male external genitalia. In Walsh PC, ed: *Campbell's urology*, Philadelphia, 2002, Saunders.

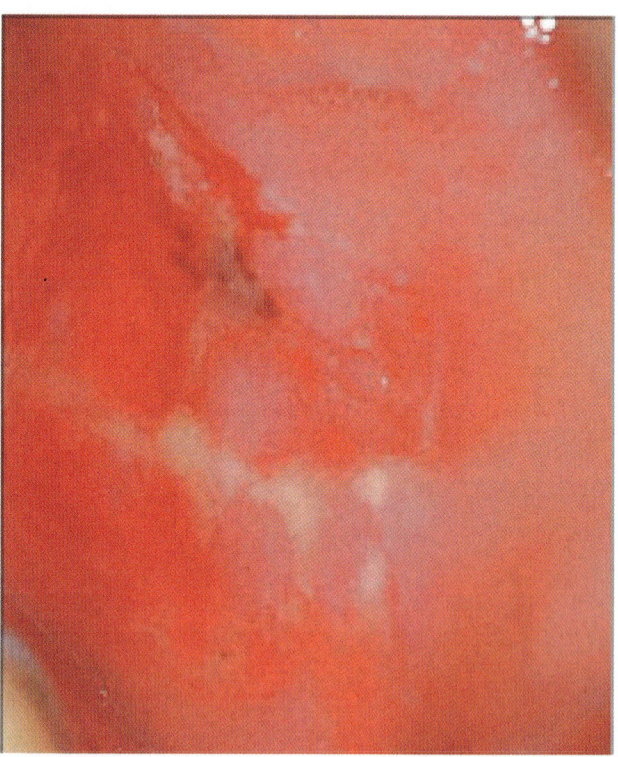

Fig. 59.15. Characteristic painful oral mucosal erosions in pemphigus vulgaris. (Courtesy of Masayuki Amagai. From Bolognia JL, Jorizzo JL, Rapini RP. *Dermatology.* Edinburgh: Mosby; 2003.)

Pemphigus Vulgaris

Pemphigus is a family of autoimmune blistering diseases characterized by intraepidermal blisters resulting from the loss of keratinocyte cell-cell adhesion (Martel and Joly, 2001). These blisters are located in the deep epidermis close to the basal cell layer. The proposed immunopathology includes the development of autoantibodies directed against keratinocyte cell surface markers and desmosomes, which show characteristic histologic changes on biopsies for routine H&E staining and direct immunofluorescence (Amagai et al., 1996; Joly et al., 2000; Zhou et al., 1997).

Almost all pemphigus patients exhibit painful oral mucosal erosions, and more than half experience cutaneous blisters that may involve the genitalia. Characteristic oral lesions are therefore an important clue to the diagnosis (Fig. 59.15). The cutaneous blisters are thin-walled and easily broken so that the presenting morphology is often a collection of nonspecific nonscarring erosions. The loss of epidermal cohesion seen in pemphigus leads to the characteristic Asboe-Hansen or indirect Nikolsky sign: spreading of fluid under the adjacent normal-appearing skin away from the direction of pressure on the blister (Amagai, 2003). **In severe cases without appropriate treatment, pemphigus may lead to fatal septicemia as a result of the loss of the epidermal barrier function of large areas of affected skin.** Treatment for pemphigus traditionally depends on systemic corticosteroids, although minimization of steroid dose is an important goal to limit side effects. The addition of immunosuppressive agents such as azathioprine, cyclophosphamide, and mycophenolate mofetil may be beneficial because of their corticosteroid-sparing effect (Amagai, 2003). In recent years, the use of rituximab as monotherapy (1000 mg administered intravenously on days 1 and 15; repeated in 1 month if necessary) has gained considerable support because of high efficacy rates (>70% with a single cycle) and low relapse rates (22% at 8 to 12 months) (Leshem et al., 2013). The infusion of intravenous immunoglobulin with or without rituximab may also prove effective and presents an inherent advantage of lowering infectious complication rates (Ruocco et al., 2013). The management of pemphigus is difficult and should always be performed in concert with a dermatologist or a rheumatologist who has experience with this disease.

Bullous Pemphigoid

Bullous pemphigoid (BP) is a subepidermal blistering disease that is more common in men and generally afflicts patients older than 60 years of age (Rzany and Weller, 2001). There is enrichment for specific HLA class II alleles in patients with BP as compared with normal controls (Delgado et al., 1996), supporting an autoimmune mechanism of pathogenesis. In BP autoantibodies against specific proteins involved in cell-cell adhesion (BP180, BP230) are present. These proteins are components of hemidesmosomes, which are structures that mediate epidermal-stromal adhesion. Binding of autoantibodies to these structures leads to complement activation and a cascade of events resulting in tissue damage, epidermal-dermal separation, and blister formation (Kitajima et al., 1994; Lin et al., 1997). Drugs such as furosemide, penicillins, ibuprofen, psoralens and angiotensin-converting enzyme inhibitors have been associated with BP (Stavropoulos et al., 2014).

The clinical presentation of BP can be highly variable. It generally begins with a nonbullous phase characterized by severe itching and nonspecific skin findings, including erythematous plaques that mimic urticaria. If the disease progresses into the bullous phase, vesicles and tense blisters filled with wheat-colored or hemorraghic fluid appear on normal skin. Skin involvement can be limited or extensive, tend to form on flexor surfaces, and favor the inner thighs and genitalia (Fig. 59.16A). Mucous membranes may also be involved, although this is less common than in pemphigus. **The diagnosis is made by a combination of clinical, histologic, and, often most importantly, immunohistochemical features such as the deposition of IgG antibodies along the basement membrane** (see Fig. 59.16B; De Jong et al., 1996). Treatment of BP in the United States is traditionally similar to that described for pemphigus, with systemic corticosteroids and various immunosuppressives playing primary roles (Kirtschig and Khumalo, 2004). However, based on the results of several randomized comparative studies, the Europeans favor the use of superpotent topical steroids for the management even of extensive pemphigoid (Joly et al., 2002; Joly et al., 2009). Certainly, treatment of limited-extent pemphigoid should rely heavily on topical, rather than systemic, corticosteroids. For treatment-resistant cases, oral methotrexate, intravenous immunoglobulin, plasmapheresis, or intravenous rituximab may be beneficial (Hatano et al., 2003;

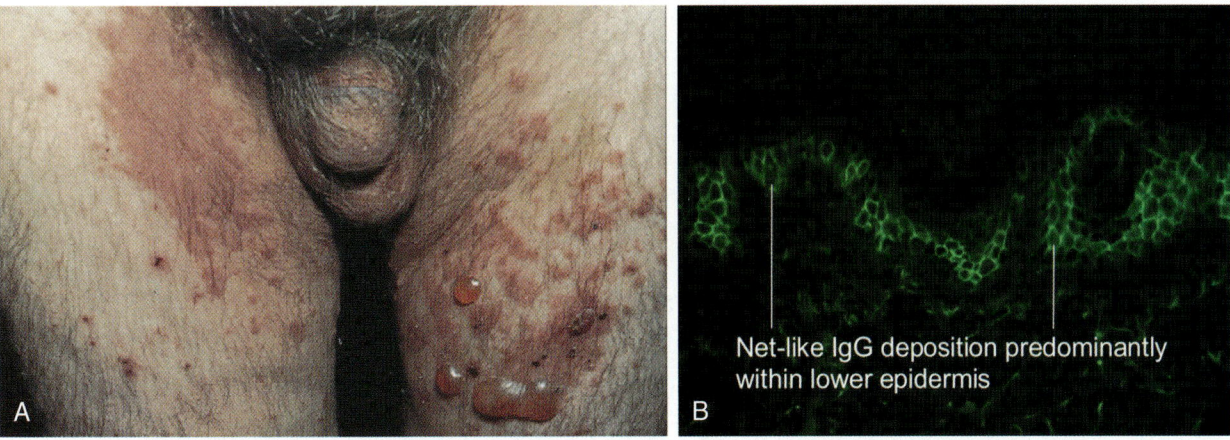

Fig. 59.16. Bullous pemphigoid (BP). (A) Involvement of the inner thighs. Note the confluent plaques and tense blisters in the inguinal area. (B) Direct immunofluorescence of BP showing deposition of autoantibodies (IgG) at the dermoepidermal junction. (A, Courtesy of Luca Borradori, MD, and Philippe Bernard, MD. From Bolognia JL, Jorizzo JL, Rapini RP. *Dermatology*. Edinburgh: Mosby; 2003. B, From Elston DM, Ferringer T: *Dermatopathology*, Edinburgh, 2009, Saunders, p 169.)

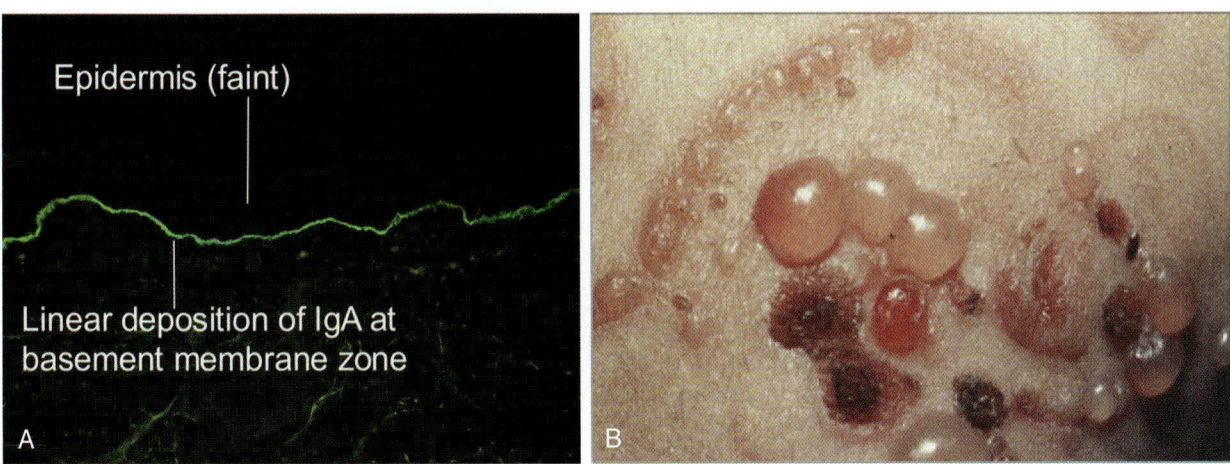

Fig. 59.17. Linear IgA bullous dermatosis. (A) Direct immunofluorescence showing linear deposition of IgA along the dermoepidermal junction. (B) Typical circumferential and linear patterns of vesicles. (A, From Elston DM, Ferringer T: *Dermatopathology*, Edinburgh, 2009, Saunders, p 170. B, Courtesy of Mark D Herron, MD, and John J Zone, MD. From Bolognia JL, Jorizzo JL, Rapini RP. *Dermatology*. Edinburgh: Mosby; 2003.)

Lee et al., 2003; Ruetter and Luger, 2004; Shetty and Ahmed, 2013; Wetter et al., 2005).

Dermatitis Herpetiformis and Linear IgA Bullous Dermatosis

Both of these entities are blistering autoimmune skin diseases associated with the deposition of IgA antibodies at the basement membrane.

Dermatitis herpetiformis (DH) is a cutaneous manifestation of celiac disease and is generally associated with gluten sensitivity (Karpati, 2004). It is most common in people of northern European origin. There is a close association of dermatitis herpetiformis with certain HLA class II DQ2 alleles (DQA1*0501, DQB1*02) (Reunala, 1998). Epidermal transglutaminase is the autoantigen in DH. Pruritic plaques, papules, and vesicles in a symmetrical distribution characterize this disease. These vesicles may form "herpetiform" groups on an erythematous base. Patients may also complain of pain and burning over the lesions. Diagnosis can be confirmed by biopsy and direct immunofluorescence, which shows a granular pattern of IgA deposition at the basement membrane. Treatment includes the use of dapsone and a strict gluten-restricted diet (Andersson and Mobacken, 1992; Frodin et al., 1981).

Linear IgA bullous dermatosis (LABD), in contrast, is not associated with celiac disease. As the name implies, a linear pattern of antibody deposition at the basement membrane is found on immunohistochemistry in LABD (Fig. 59.17). Characteristic clinical features include vesicles and bullae arranged in a combination of circumferential and linear orientations. Treatment with either sulfapyridine or dapsone is usually effective in controlling LABD, and long-term spontaneous remission rates of 30% to 60% have been described (Wojnarowska et al., 1988). In contrast to pemphigus and BP, neither dermatitis herpetiformis nor LABD commonly affects genital or perigenital skin.

Hailey-Hailey Disease

Hailey-Hailey disease, also known as benign familial pemphigus, is a rare autosomal dominant blistering dermatosis related to various mutations in the *ATP2C1* gene. The *ATP2C1* gene encodes the protein product hSPCA1, which is a Ca^{2+}/Mn^{2+} transporter.

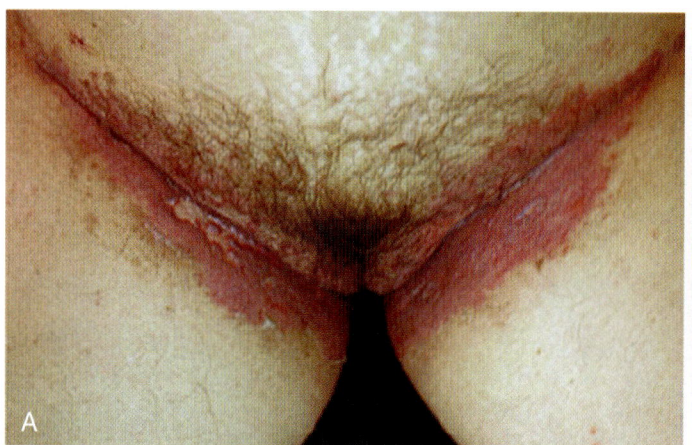
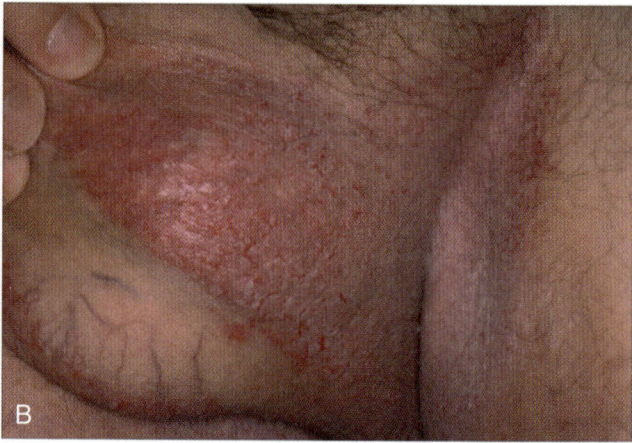

Fig. 59.18. Genital presentations of Hailey-Hailey disease. (A) The vulva and groin are covered in a vesicular eruption that has become confluent and macerated. (B) Erythematous plaque with maceration of the inguinal canal and scrotum. (**A,** From Zhao QF, Hasegawa T, Komiyama E, et al: Hailey-Hailey disease: a review of clinical features in 26 cases with special reference to the secondary infections and their control. *Dermatologica Sinica* 35(1): 7–11, 2016. Fig. 1A. B, Courtesy of Daniel Hohl, Theodora Maura, Jean Phillipe Görög. From Bolognia JL, Jorizzo JL, Rapini RP. *Dermatology.* Edinburgh: Mosby; 2003.)

This protein is responsible for calcium homeostasis in the Golgi apparatus required for the post-translational processing of junctional proteins involved in proper epidermal cell-cell adhesion. Hailey-Hailey disease usually develops within the second or third decade of life (Burge, 1992). It has a characteristic predilection for the intertriginous areas including the neck, axillae, groin, and perianal region (Fig. 59.18). In women, disease in the inframammary folds is common although vulvar disease is unusual (Wieselthier and Pincus, 1993). Symptoms include an unfortunate combination of pruritus, pain, and a foul odor. As heat and sweating exacerbate the condition, Hailey-Hailey disease tends to worsen dramatically during the summer months (Burge, 1992). Skin findings include confluent areas of fragile white skin with small linear fissures, exudate, vesicles, and pustules that form as a result of the aberrant keratinocyte cell adhesion. Mucous membrane involvement does not occur. Lesions may be confined to the axilla or groin, and superinfection with yeast, bacteria, or herpes simplex virus may compound the problem. Histologic examination may be helpful in differentiating Hailey-Hailey disease from impetigo, pemphigus, intertrigo, and Darier disease (Margolis, 2002). Treatment includes wearing lightweight, breathable clothing to avoid friction and sweating. Lesions may respond to topical or intralesional corticosteroids, with the caveats mentioned previously about the use of these agents on intertriginous skin. For disease that is resistant to medical therapy, wide excision and skin grafting have been effective, as have local ablative techniques such as dermabrasion, photodynamic therapy, electron beam radiotherapy, glycopyrrolate, afamelanotide, and CO_2 or erbium-YAG laser vaporization (Alsahli et al., 2017; Christian and Moy, 1999; Farahnik et al., 2017; Hamm et al., 1994; Hohl et al., 2003). An innovative approach to this disorder is to inject infected areas with botulinum toxin type A; this therapy greatly reduces sweating and thereby reduces disease severity (Bessa et al., 2010).

NONINFECTIOUS ULCERS

Genital ulcers can be a result of infectious and noninfectious causes (Box 59.4).

Aphthous Ulcers and Behçet Disease

Aphthous ulcers are small, painful erosions that commonly involve the oral cavity (so-called canker sores), but they can occasionally

---

BOX 59.4 Differential Diagnosis of Ulcers

Syphilis
Chancroid
Herpes simplex
Crohn disease
Aphthous ulcer
Behçet disease
Granuloma inguinale
Genital bite wound
Lymphogranuloma venereum
Factitial dermatitis
Wegener granulomatosis
Leukocytoclastic vasculitis
Pyoderma gangrenosum

From Margolis DJ: Cutaneous disease of the male external genitalia. In Walsh PC, ed: *Campbell's urology*, Philadelphia, 2002, Saunders; 2002.

---

be present on the genitalia. When oral and genital aphthous ulcers coexist, the clinician should seriously consider the diagnosis of Behçet disease (BD). BD is a generalized relapsing and remitting ulcerative mucocutaneous disease that likely involves a genetic predisposition and an autoimmune mode of pathogenesis (Mendes et al., 2009; Sakane, 1997). Although many genetic loci have been implicated, perhaps the strongest association is with *HLA B51*. Oxidative stress related to the overproduction of superoxide radicals by neutrophils has also been implicated in the development of this condition (Freitas et al., 1998; Najim et al., 2007). However, a large number of other etiopathogenetic mechanisms have been proposed and supported by experimental findings (such as IL-10 gene mutations) (Remmers et al., 2010). The notable variability in efficacy for any of the therapeutic interventions enumerated later suggests that pathways of inflammation in BD are unlikely to be uniform. BD has a high prevalence in Turkey (80 per 100,000), Israel (15 per 100,000), and Japan (10 to 12 per 100,000), but it is rare in the United States (0.12 to 5.0 per 100,000) (Arbesfeld and Kurban, 1988; Calamia et al., 2009). Affected individuals may also suffer from epididymitis, thrombophlebitis, aneurysms (particularly of the pulmonary artery), and gastrointestinal, neurologic, and arthritic problems (Aykutlu

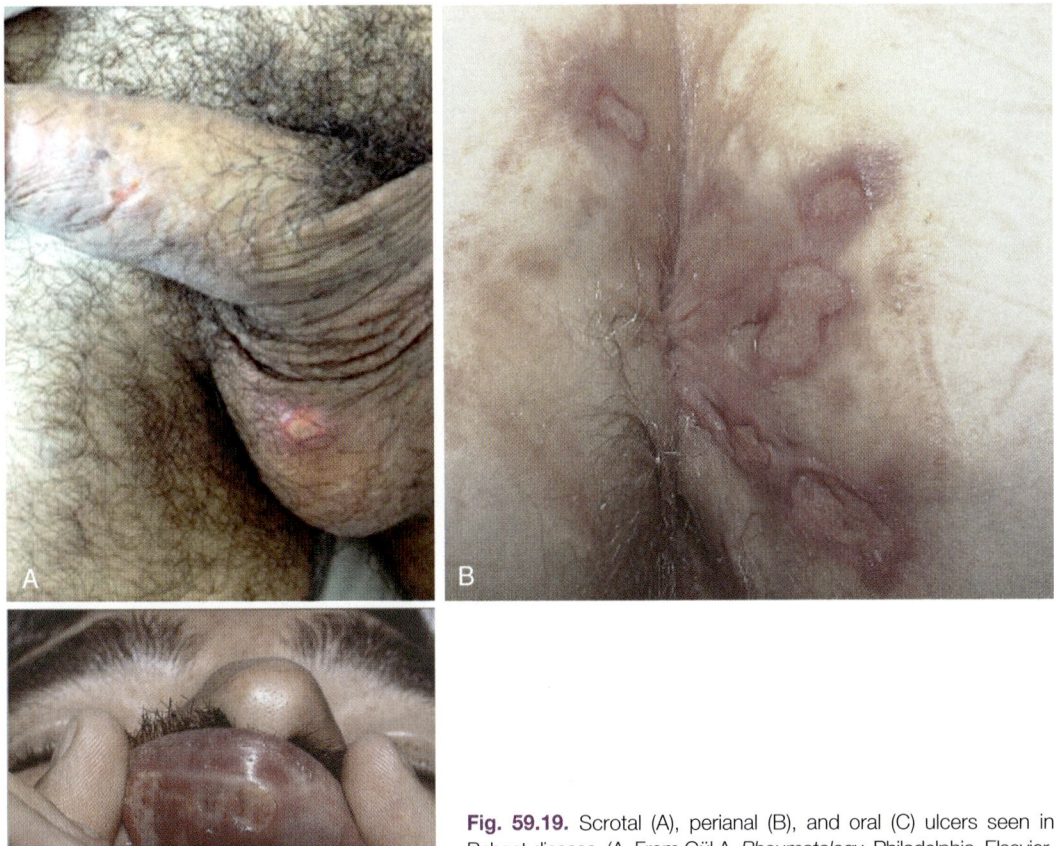

Fig. 59.19. Scrotal (A), perianal (B), and oral (C) ulcers seen in Behçet disease. (A, From Gül A. *Rheumatology*. Philadelphia, Elsevier, 2019. Fig. 167-1; B and C, Courtesy of Samuel L Moschella, MD. From Bolognia JL, Jorizzo JL, Rapini RP. *Dermatology*. Edinburgh: Mosby; 2003.)

et al., 2002; Cetinel et al., 1998; Koc et al., 1992; Krause et al., 1999; Margolis, 2002; Tuzun et al., 1997). BD occurs with roughly similar frequency among males and females, although men typically experience a more severe course.

Mucocutaneous lesions of the oral cavity and genitalia (Fig. 59.19) and ocular involvement (uveitis) form a triad of clinical features in BD. The genital lesions are larger and generally more painful than the oral lesions. Optic involvement occurs in 90% of cases and may lead to blindness (Moschella, 2003). It is now considered a multisystem disease, with new criteria classifying a patient as having BD if they score at least 4 points in the following: 2 points each (ocular lesions, oral aphthosis, and genital aphthosis) and 1 point each (skin lesions, central nervous system involvement, and vascular manifestations) (International Team for the Revision of the International Criteria for Behçet's Disease, 2014). Other causes for genital ulceration, however, including simple or complex aphthous ulcers, primary syphilis, herpes simplex, and chancroid, must be considered before a diagnosis of BD is made (Margolis, 2002). In the context of these accepted criteria, oral ulceration is the most sensitive lesion and genital ulceration is the most specific lesion. The latter therefore is the most clinically useful lesion in diagnosing BD according to this schema. Nonetheless the diagnosis of BD depends exclusively on the aggregate clinical findings, because there are no specific laboratory, radiologic, genetic, or histologic findings that conclusively confirm this diagnosis (Hatemi et al., 2013).

The clinical course of BD is protean, and randomized controlled trials in support of specific therapy are currently limited (Kaklamani and Kaklamanis, 2001). A wide range of topical and systemic agents has been applied to treat BD with variable success, including corticosteroids, dapsone, colchicine, immunosuppressants, 5-aminosalicylic acid (5-ASA) derivatives, cyclosporine A, and TNF-α inhibitors (especially infliximab and adalimumab) (Kose et al., 2009; Moschella, 2003). It has become clear that earlier and more aggressive treatment of BD-associated significant organ involvement with immunosuppressives and biologics has improved the overall outcome. Rheumatologic consultation is advised when this diagnosis is suspected.

Pyoderma Gangrenosum

Pyoderma gangrenosum (PG) is a rare ulcerative neutrophilic skin disease associated with systemic illnesses including inflammatory bowel disease, arthritis, collagen vascular disease, chronic active hepatitis, HIV infection, and myeloproliferative disorders (Moschella, 2003). **It most commonly affects women between the second and fifth decade of life and likely has an autoimmune pathogenesis given its association with other autoimmune diseases.** Between 20% and 50% of cases, however, are idiopathic. The annual incidence of PG in the United States is about 1 case per 100,000 individuals.

The classic morphologic presentation of PG is painful cutaneous and mucous membrane ulceration, often with extensive loss of tissue and a purulent base (Fig. 59.20). The classic appearance is a rapidly developing ulcer on the lower legs with an overhanging, undermined violaceous border that developed at a site of trauma. Although unusual, PG can involve the penis, scrotum, vulva, and peristomal sites (Cairns et al., 1994). As was the case in BD, no specific diagnostic laboratory test or histopathologic feature is pathognomonic for PG, although a history of an underlying systemic disease may raise suspicion. Biopsy should be performed 5 to 10 mm from the edge of the ulcer, where a dense neutrophilic infiltrate will be present (Edwards and Lynch, 2018). Aside from ulcerative STDs, the differential diagnosis of penile PG includes calciphylaxis, BD, necrotizing fasciitis, cutaneous metastatic Crohn disease, deep fungal infection, pemphigus vegetans,

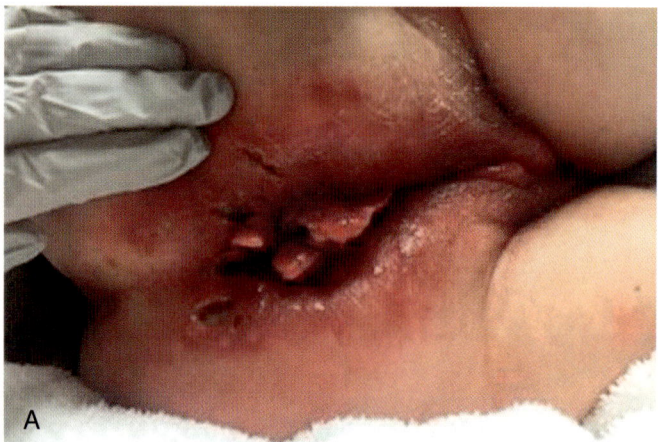
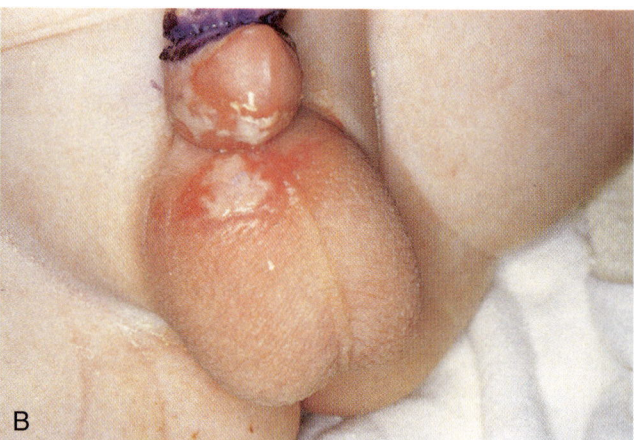

Fig. 59.20. Pyoderma gangrenosum involving the genitals of a woman with rheumatoid arthritis (A) and the penis and scrotum (B). (A, From Pinard J, Chiang DY, Mostaghimi A, et al: Wounds that would not heal: pyoderma gangrenosum. *Am J Med* 131(4): 377–379, 2018, Fig 1B; B, from Callen JP, Greer DE, Hood AF, et al. *Color atlas of dermatology*. Philadelphia: Saunders; 1993, p. 330.)

Fournier gangrene, neoplastic conditions, erosive LP, trauma, and factitious damage (Badgwell and Rosen, 2006). Treatment includes a combination of local and systemic corticosteroid therapy with or without adjunctive immunosuppressants (i.e., cyclosporine, TNF-α inhibitors, and intravenous immunoglobulin) (Chow and Ho, 1996; Feldman et al., 2018; Song et al., 2018). Minocycline, sulfasalazine, and thalidomide have been used in combination with corticosteroids in a small number of cases. Genital PG may also be amenable to topical treatment with calcineurin inhibitors (Lally et al., 2005).

Traumatic Causes

Cutaneous lesions of the genitalia, including ulceration, can be caused by local trauma, which should be included in the differential diagnosis. **This can be either accidental ("innocent trauma") or self-inflicted ("factitial dermatitis/dermatitis artefacta," and "psychogenic neurotic excoriation").** Accidental injuries may be a result of trauma during sexual practices (including genital bite wounds), ornamentation (i.e., piercing), or unusual hygiene practices (i.e., cleaning) (Margolis, 2002). **Factitial dermatitis is a psychocutaneous disorder in which the individual self-inflicts cutaneous lesions usually for an unconscious motive or because of an underlying mental illness. Factitial lesions are occasionally produced deliberately with the hope of some secondary gain (such as product liability litigation).** An association between factitial dermatitis and borderline personality disorder appears to exist (Koblenzer, 2000). Other disorders to be considered include Munchausen syndrome by proxy, body dysmorphic disorder, and malingering, if secondary-gain issues exist. **Psychogenic excoriations are seen in patients with underlying psychological dysfunction, namely depression, bipolar disorder, delusional disorder, or obsessive-compulsive disorder** (Fig. 59.21; Ehsani et al., 2009; Mutasim and Adams, 2009). Although rare, factitial dermatitis or neurotic excoriations should always be considered in the differential diagnosis of unusual genital lesions, including oddly configured angulated erosions and ulcerations (Verma et al., 2012).

INFECTIONS AND INFESTATIONS

Sexually Transmitted Diseases

STDs with genital cutaneous manifestations include lymphogranuloma venereum, granuloma inguinale, herpes simplex, chancroid, molluscum contagiosum, HPV, and syphilis (Fig. 59.22). These conditions are discussed in detail in Chapter 15.

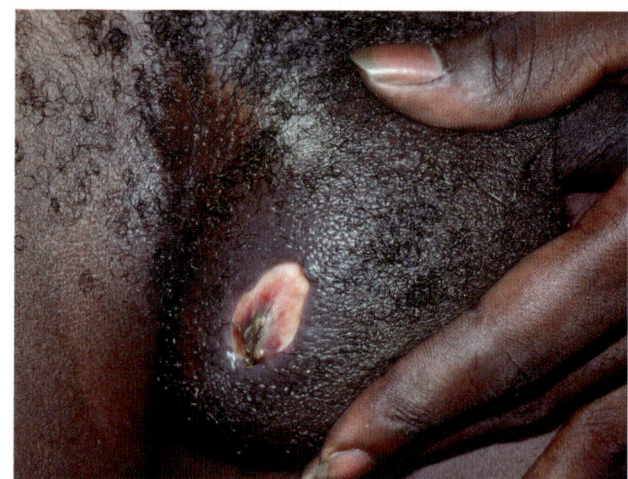

Fig. 59.21. Factitial ulcer of the scrotum caused by repeated picking at the scrotal skin.

Balanitis and Balanoposthitis

Balanitis is an inflammatory disorder of the glans penis. When the process involves the preputial skin in uncircumcised men, it is termed *balanoposthitis*. In children, bacterial infections are the predominant cause. In adult men, the cause may be intertrigo, ICD, local trauma, or candidal and bacterial infections (Fig. 59.23). Treatment includes removal of irritating agents, improved hygiene, topical antibiotics and antifungals, and occasionally short courses of low-potency topical corticosteroids (Margolis, 2002). When treatment fails, the differential should include neoplastic diseases, Zoon balanitis, psoriasis, and alternative infectious agents such as HPV (Wikstrom et al., 1994). Balanoposthitis tends to occur in patients with phimosis, and circumcision may be curative in select recurrent cases. Balanoposthitis may also result from bacterial superinfection in the setting of poor hygiene and neutropenia (Manian and Alford, 1987).

Cellulitis and Erysipelas

Cellulitis is an infection of the deep dermis and subcutaneous tissues most commonly caused by gram-positive organisms (*Streptococcus pyogenes* and *S. aureus*) (Lewis, 1998). In immunocompetent individuals, organisms usually gain entry to the site of

Chapter 59 Cutaneous Diseases of the External Genitalia **1289**

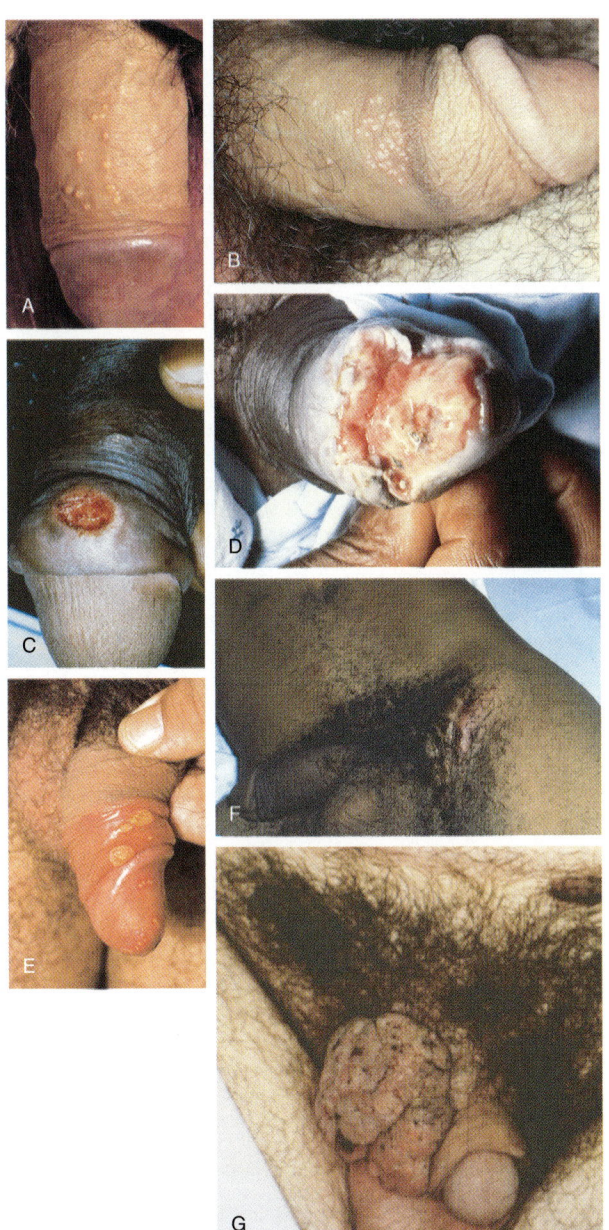

Fig. 59.22. Genital lesions associated with sexually transmitted diseases. (A) Herpes simplex virus. (B) Molluscum contagiosum. (C) Syphilitic chancre. (D) Granuloma inguinale. (E) Chancroid. (F) Lymphogranuloma venereum. (G) Condyloma accuminata. (From Callen JP, Greer DE, Hood AF, et al.: *Color atlas of dermatology*, Philadelphia, 1993, Saunders.)

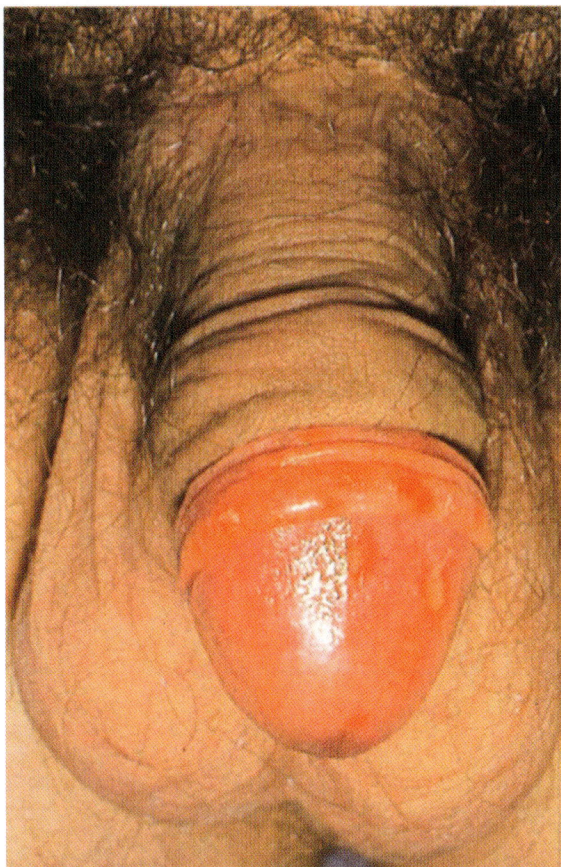

Fig. 59.23. Candidal balanoposthitis. (From Korting GW: *Practical dermatology of the genital region*, Philadelphia, 1981, Saunders, p 159.)

infection through a break in the skin barrier. In immunocompromised patients, a blood-borne route of infection is more common. Systemic signs of illness include fever, chills, and general malaise. Local signs include erythema (rubor), warmth (calor), pain (dolor), and swelling (tumor) at the site with indistinct borders (Fig. 59.24). Treatment includes systemic antibiotics with activity against *S. pyogenes* and *S. aureus* species. The clinician may be forced to rely on known local antimicrobial sensitivity patterns because obtaining satisfactory material for culture may be difficult. In cases associated with diabetes, mixed flora may be present and antibiotic coverage should be broadened. Marking the zone of cellulitis at the onset of therapy is an important step to allow progression and resolution of cellulites to be monitored during therapy.

Erysipelas is a superficial bacterial skin infection limited to the dermis with lymphatic involvement. This disease commonly occurs at the extremes of age and often involves the face. In contrast to the cutaneous lesion of cellulitis, erysipelas generally exhibits a raised and distinct border at the interface with normal skin. The causative organism is usually *S. pyogenes*.

Fournier Gangrene (Necrotizing Fasciitis of the Perineum)

Fournier gangrene (FG) is a potentially life-threatening progressive infection of the perineum and genitalia (Morpurgo and Galandiuk, 2002). In the genital region, most cases of FG are caused by mixed bacterial flora, which include gram-positive, gram-negative, and anaerobic bacteria. *Escherichia coli*, *Bacteroides* spp., *S. pyogenes*, and *S. aureus* are common etiologic pathogens. Risk factors for developing FG include underlying alcoholism, diabetes, cancer and malnutrition, advanced age, recent urogenital or colorectal instrumentation or trauma, and preexisting peripheral vascular disease. However, group A streptococcal necrotizing fasciitis can occur in healthy immunocompetent individuals.

The hallmark of FG is a rapid progression from the signs and symptoms of cellulitis (erythema, swelling, and pain) to blister formation, to clinically visible ischemia, and ultimately to foul-smelling necrotic lesions (Fig. 59.25). **Infection may spread along fascial planes; therefore the exterior skin findings may represent only a small proportion of the underlying infected and necrotic tissue. The diagnosis of FG is a surgical emergency because progression from genitalia to perineum to abdominal wall may occur extremely rapidly (often within hours). Spread of tissue infection is accompanied by an ever-increasing risk of bacterial septicemia, usually the eventual cause of death. The exclusion of FG therefore should be a priority during every consultation for soft-tissue infection of the genitalia.** Pain out of proportion to the visible extent of infection should raise suspicion for FG. The skin may also exhibit a grayish cast or fetid odor uncharacteristic of uncomplicated genital cellulitis. Imaging of the genitalia with plain radiographs, computed tomography, and/or bedside ultrasonography (Amendola et al., 1994; Avery and Scheinfeld, 2013) may demonstrate gas bubbles within the tissue, although the delay associated with imaging should not postpone surgical intervention in obvious cases.

Treatment involves a combination of broad-spectrum antibiotics and extensive surgical debridement to margins of healthy bleeding tissue. These patients often require a second-look operation after 24 to 48 hours to exclude further disease progression (Gurdal et al., 2003). During surgical debridement for scrotal FG, the testicles and other structures within the tunica vaginalis can almost always be spared, although loss of tissue in the abdominal wall may be extensive because of bacterial spread along fascial planes. The indications for adjunctive hyperbaric oxygen therapy in FG remain controversial, although several groups have reported favorable results (Dahm et al., 2000; Eke, 2000; Jallali et al., 2005). There may also be potential benefit to the use of vacuum-assisted closure devices in FG (Czymek et al., 2009). However, despite aggressive modern management, the mortality of FG may be as high as 16% to 40% (Blume et al., 2003; Dahm et al., 2000; Eke, 2000; Sorensen et al., 2009; Yeniyol et al., 2004). A number of different numeric scoring scales have been applied to FG in an attempt to predict proactively the patients who are at the highest risk for mortality and who should receive the most aggressive intervention. These include the FG Severity Index and the Uludag FG Severity Index, as well as the more general Age-Adjusted Charlson Comorbidity Index (ACCI) and the recently introduced surgical Apgar score (sAPGAR). A study verified that *all* of these scoring systems are valid methods for assessing patients in the setting of FG, and adoption of one may assist the clinician in making therapeutic decisions (Vyas et al., 2013).

Among patients who survive an episode of FG, there most likely will be ongoing disability and reduced functionality for months to years. Sexual dysfunction is common (~65%) (Czymek et al., 2013). Therefore FG survivors should expect to receive long-term care from a variety of specialists.

Folliculitis

Folliculitis is a common disorder characterized by perifollicular pustules on an erythematous base (Kelly, 2003). It occurs most frequently in heavily hair-bearing areas such as the scalp, beard, axilla, groin, and buttocks and can be exacerbated by local trauma from prolonged occlusion (e.g., truck drivers), shaving, rubbing, or clothing irritation (Margolis, 2002). Patients may complain of pruritus or pain over the area; conversely, symptoms may be entirely absent. Cultures are generally negative, and diagnosis is usually made clinically, although a variety of infectious organisms have been associated with folliculitis, including *S. aureus*, *Pseudomonas* spp., fungi, and herpes simplex virus. Folliculitis has also been associated with the use of contaminated hot tubs and swimming pools, with the offending organism usually *P. aeruginosa* (Fig. 59.26; Gregory and Schaffner, 1987; Rolston and Bodey, 1992). Treatment for folliculitis

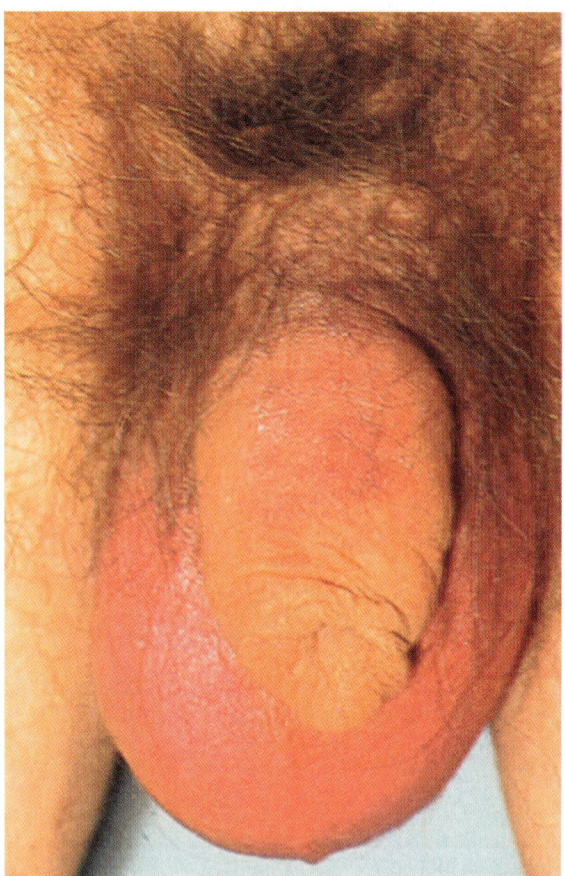

Fig. 59.24. Penoscrotal cellulitis. (From Korting GW: *Practical dermatology of the genital region*, Philadelphia, 1981, Saunders, p 37.)

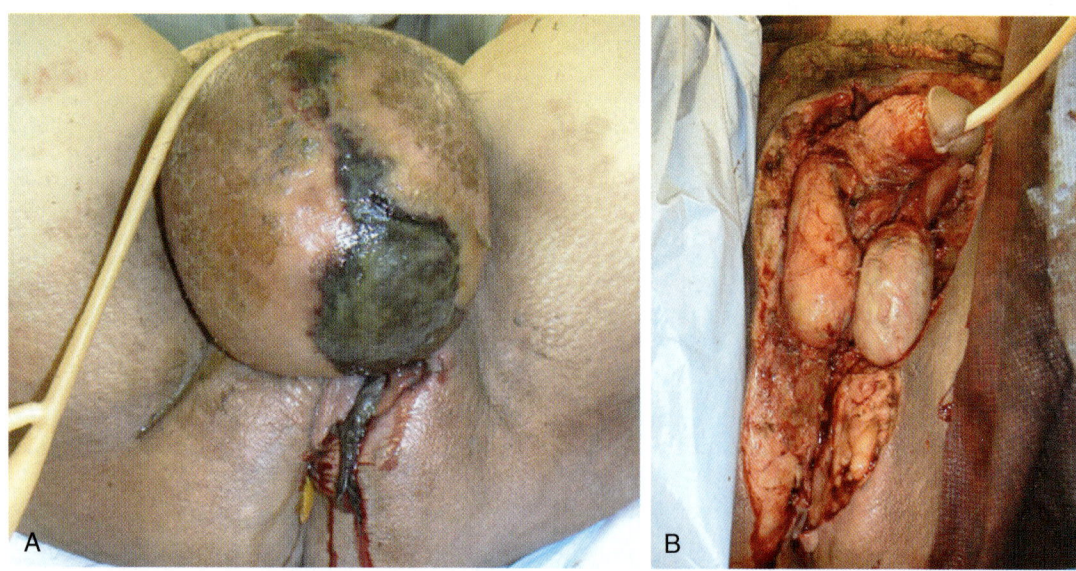

Fig. 59.25. Fournier gangrene of the scrotum. (A) Surface appearance of scrotum and perineum showing area of frank necrosis. (B) Extent of soft tissue debridement required to achieve margins of viable tissue. Note that the testes within their tunica vaginalis compartment are spared.

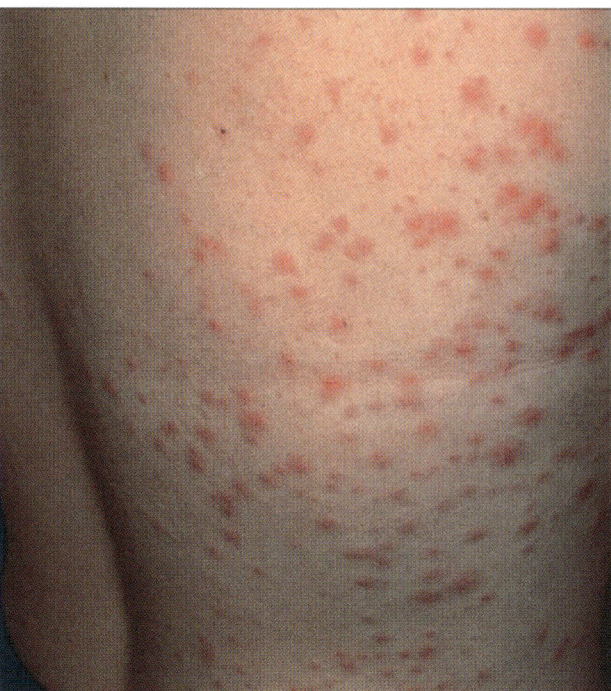

Fig. 59.26. Pseudomonal folliculitis caused by the use of a hot tub. (Courtesy of Yale Dermatology Residents' Slide Collection. From Bolognia JL, Jorizzo JL, Rapini RP. *Dermatology*. Edinburgh: Mosby; 2003.)

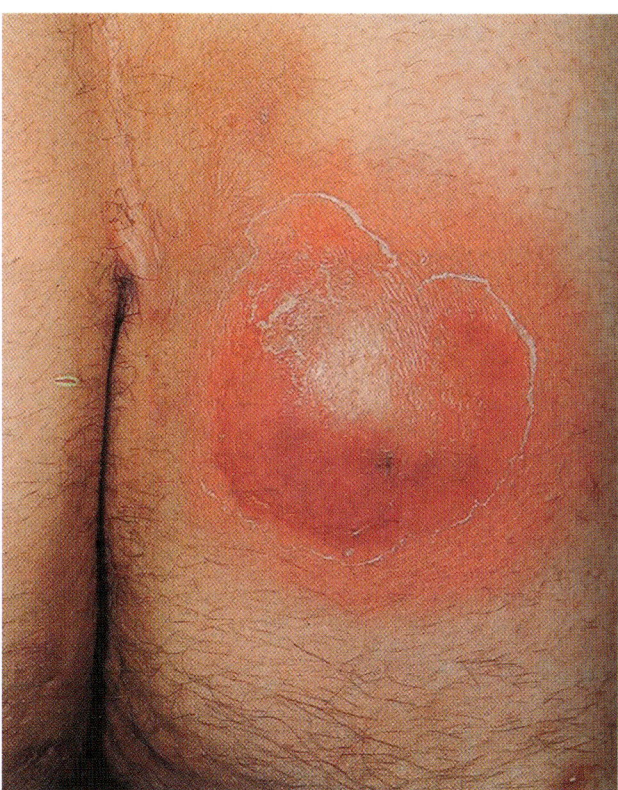

Fig. 59.27. A large furuncle located on the buttocks. (From Habif TP: *Clinical dermatology*, Edinburgh, 2004, Mosby, p 284.)

includes good hygiene, removal of offending irritants, and appropriate topical or systemic antiviral, antibiotic, or antifungal agents. However, recurrence is common. The results of a surveillance study indicate that 96% of *P. aeruginosa* isolates tested from swimming pools and hot tubs were multidrug resistant (Lutz and Lee, 2011). These results may have important implications for immune-suppressed individuals, where infection with multidrug-resistant *P. aeruginosa* has a greater potential impact. Failure to respond to conservative measures should lead to lesion culture with concomitant antimicrobial susceptibility testing.

Furunculosis

Furuncles and abscesses are walled-off collections of pus. **Although abscesses can occur anywhere on the body, a furuncle is by definition associated with a hair follicle.** Although inflammation of the superficial portion of the hair follicle is present in folliculitis, furunculosis is characterized by involvement of the deeper follicle leading to a red and tender "boil" (Edwards and Lynch, 2018). Furuncles tend to occur in areas prone to minor trauma including the groin and buttocks (Fig. 59.27). *S. aureus* is the most common causative organism, although anaerobes may be present. Risk factors include diabetes mellitus, obesity, poor hygiene, and immunosuppression (Brook and Finegold, 1981). Warm compresses may be beneficial, and larger lesions may require incision and drainage, as for any abscess. Other lesions in the differential include an epidermal cyst or Bartholin's gland duct cyst. When there is associated cellulitis, a systemic antibiotic with activity against staphylococci should be administered. In today's environment of methicillin-resistant staphylococci, coverage for such organisms is advisable if they are prevalent within the clinician's community. To reduce recurrence, mupirocin ointment to the nares may also be applied to eliminate carrier status.

Hidradenitis Suppurativa (Acne Inversa)

Hidradenitis suppurativa (HS) is a chronic disease of apocrine gland-bearing skin with a predilection for the axillae and anogenital regions (Alikhan et al., 2009; Kelly, 2003). **The condition generally begins after puberty and a familial form with an autosomal dominant pattern of inheritance has been described** (Von Der Werth et al., 2000). Originally believed to be a disease of apocrine glands, HS is now thought to be an epithelial disorder of hair follicles (Jansen et al., 2001). HS is more common in women and patients of African-American descent. Although superinfection of HS lesions may occur, bacterial infection does not appear to be the primary initiator. During the pathogenesis of HS, hair follicles become plugged and swollen. **Rupture of follicular contents (including bacteria and keratin) into the surrounding dermis initiates a marked inflammatory response with the formation of abscesses and sinus tracts** (Slade et al., 2003).

The clinical features of HS include painful inflammatory nodules and sterile abscesses developing in the axillae, groin, perianal, and inframammary areas (Fig. 59.28; Kelly, 2003). With time, draining sinus tracts and hypertrophic scars develop. Serious complications of HS can occur, including hypoproteinemia, secondary amyloidosis, the development of fistulae to the urethra (Gronau and Pannek, 2002), bladder, peritoneum, and rectum (Nadgir et al., 2001), and SCC in areas of heavy scarring (Altunay et al., 2002; Rosenzweig et al., 2005).

Treatment of HS includes smoking cessation, improvement in hygiene, weight reduction, management of metabolic syndrome or underlying hormone-related disorders, and efforts to minimize friction and moisture in affected areas (i.e., loose undergarments, absorbent powder) (Kelly, 2003; Kohorst et al., 2015). No single therapeutic intervention is universally effective. Topical clindamycin or the combination of oral clindamycin or minocycline with oral rifampicin may be beneficial for some patients (Gener et al., 2009). In a double-blind randomized trial, systemic therapy with tetracycline was no more effective than topical clindamycin in HS (Jemec and Wendelboe, 1998). Other oral agents that sometimes prove beneficial include dapsone (50 to 200 mg/day), zinc (40 to 80 mg/day elemental zinc), retinoids (acitretin 25 to 50 mg/day or isotretinoin 1 mg/kg/day), cyclosporine (4 mg/kg/day), and hormone blockers (spironolactone and oral contraceptives in women and finasteride and dutasteride in men) (Scheinfeld, 2013b). Systemic corticosteroids may improve HS, but relapse is the rule after cessation of therapy (Slade et al., 2003). Lithium may exacerbate HS or limit its response to conventional medical therapy (Gupta et al., 1995). Although recurrent incision

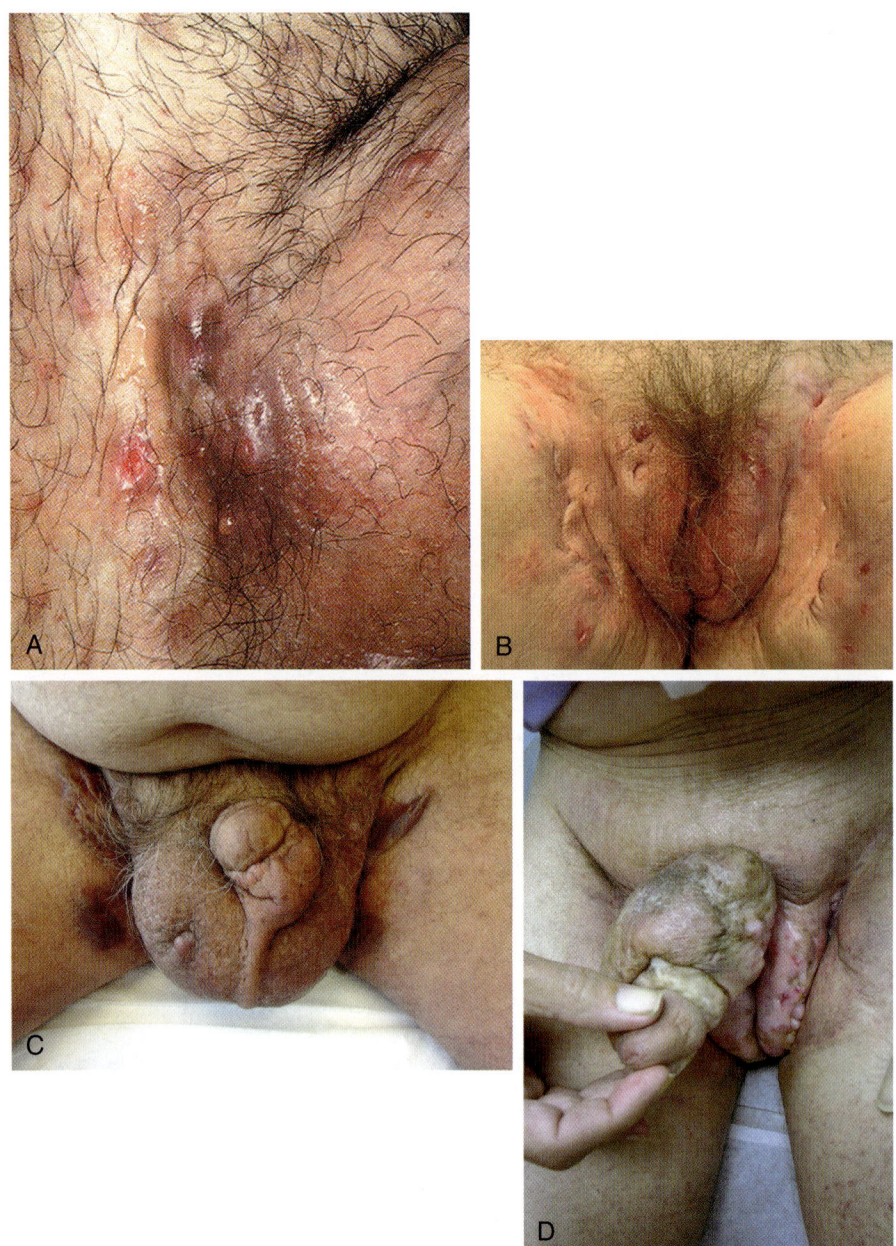

Fig. 59.28. Hidradenitis suppurativa. (A) Characteristic painful papules and draining sinus tracts. (B) Histology shows follicular plugging and connection to a dilated apocrine duct. (C and D) Examples of severe genital involvement of hidradenitis, which would make surgical management difficult. (A, From Danby FW, Margesson LJ: Hidradenitis suppurativa. *Dermatologic Clinics* 28(4): 779–793, 2010, Fig. 2. B, Courtesy of Yale Dermatology Residents' Slide Collection. From Bolognia JL, Jorizzo JL, Rapini RP. *Dermatology*. Edinburgh: Mosby; 2003.)

and drainage of HS lesions are discouraged, wide and deep excision with skin grafting has been effective (Bocchini et al., 2003; Rompel and Petres, 2000). A variety of new approaches, including the use of the CO_2 and Nd:YAG lasers to treat HS, are under investigation (Lapins et al., 1994; Madan et al., 2008; Tierney et al., 2009). Off-label administration of newer biologic agents such as TNF-α blockers (particularly subcutaneous adalimumab, 40 mg/week) has proven variably effective in the management of HS in select patients when surgery is simply not feasible (Shuja et al., 2010).

Corynebacterial Infection (Trichomycosis Axillaris and Erythrasma)

Trichomycosis axillaris is a superficial bacterial infection of axillary and pubic hair caused by corynebacteria. Yellow, red, or black nodules are visible on the hair shafts (Fig. 59.29) and there is frequently a characteristic odor (Blume et al., 2003). There is an association with hyperhidrosis (Margolis, 2002). The differential diagnosis includes infestation with pediculosis pubis or fungal infection (piedra) (Avram et al., 1987), although examination with magnification can generally distinguish trichomycosis axillaris from these conditions. Shaving can provide immediate improvement, and antibacterial soaps may prevent further infection (Blume et al., 2003). For pubic trichomycosis axillaris, clindamycin gel, bacitracin, and oral erythromycin have also proven effective (Bargman, 1984; Blume et al., 2003).

Erythrasma is a *Corynebacterium minutissimum* infection of the skin that results in sharply bordered, light red to dark brown, scaling patches in moist areas, particularly the groin and axilla. These lesions may be pruritic or asymptomatic and may be confused with dermatophyte infection (tinea cruris) (Sindhuphak et al., 1985). Under a Wood

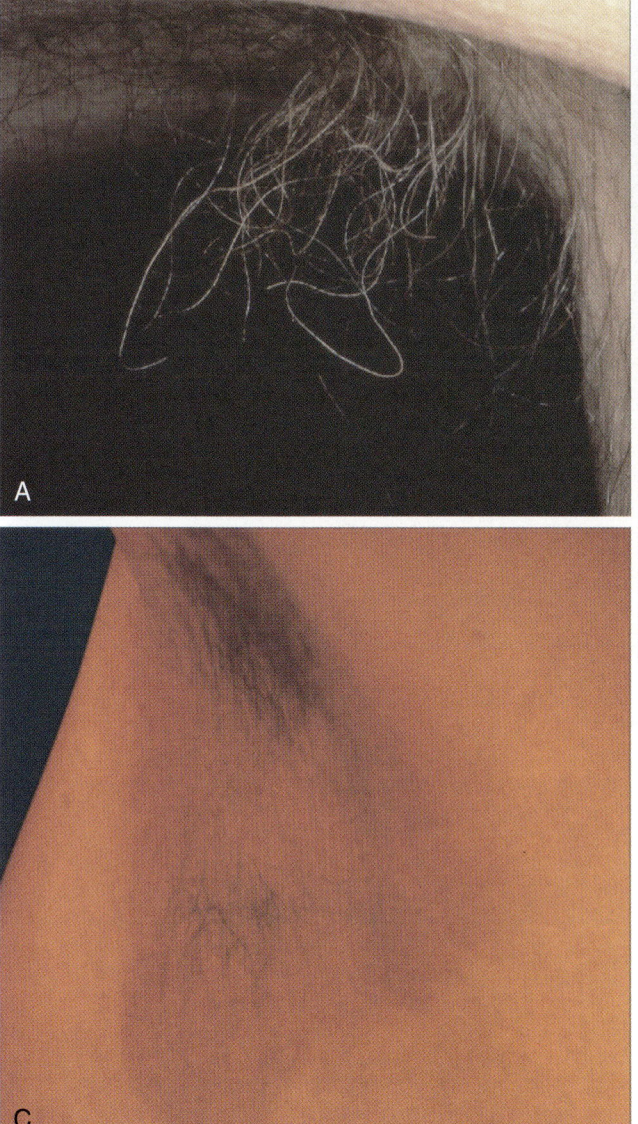
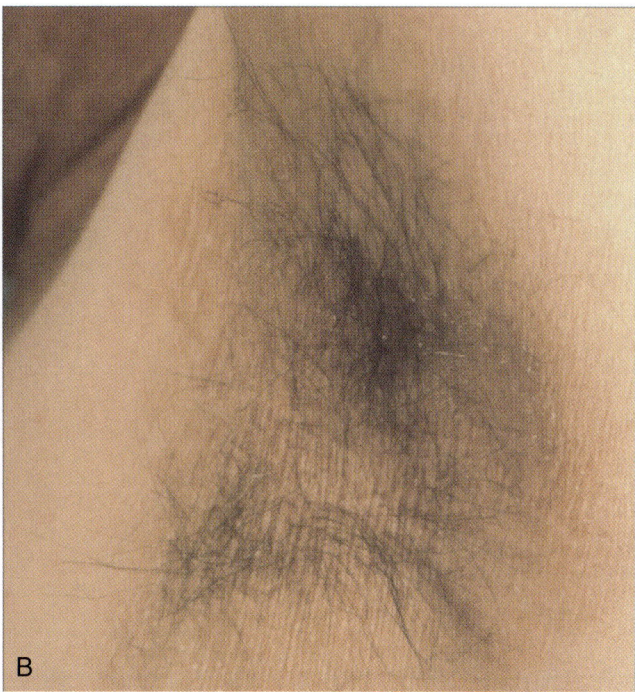

Fig. 59.29. Corynebacterial infections of the skin. (A) Trichomycosis axillaris. (B and C) Erythrasma under white light (B) and Wood lamp (C) showing coral-red fluorescence. (From Bolognia JL, Jorizzo JL, Rapini RP: *Dermatology*, Edinburgh, 2003, Mosby.)

light, the lesions show a characteristic bright coral-red fluorescence (see Fig. 59.29) (Halprin, 1967). Effective treatments include antibacterial soaps, topical aluminum chloride, topical clindamycin 1% solution or gel, miconazole 1% cream, and oral erythromycin (500 to 1000 mg/day) (Cochran et al., 1981; Holdiness, 2002).

Ecthyma Gangrenosum

Ecthyma gangrenosum is a rare cutaneous manifestation of pseudomonal septicemia that presents most commonly on the anogenital area in debilitated, immunosuppressed, or neutropenic patients. The lesions of ecthyma gangrenosum are tender grouped erythematous macules that may progress to form bullae or rupture to produce a gangrenous ulcer covered by a thick, black eschar (Fig. 59.30; Blume et al., 2003). On histologic examination, necrotizing vasculitis and gram-negative organisms are present. The differential diagnosis includes PG, necrotizing vasculitis, cryoglobulinemia, and septic emboli containing other organisms, including *Candida*, *Aspergillus*, *Citrobacter*, *E. coli*, *Aeromonas hydrophila*, and *Fusarium* (Altwegg and Geiss, 1989; Gucluer et al., 1999; Martino et al., 1994; Reich et al., 2004). Consistent with the underlying sepsis, ecthyma gangrenosum carries a poor prognosis, and immediate treatment with intravenous antipseudomonal antibiotics is indicated. Wound debridement may also be necessary (Collini et al., 1986).

Genital Bite Wounds

After deliberate or accidental bite wounds to the genitalia, a normal component of the human oral flora, *Eikenella corrodens*, may be implanted into genital skin. This results in the rapid development of extremely painful, necrotic ulcerations at the bite site(s) (Fig. 59.31) (Rosen, 2005; Rosen and Conrad, 1999). The rapidity of ulceration, extraordinary degree of discomfort, and a history of traumatic orogenital contact help distinguish this type of infection from the more common STDs and other genital ulcers. The treatment is high-dose oral amoxicillin-clavulanate (1500 mg/day) until healing occurs.

Candidal Intertrigo

Fungal infection of macerated skin folds can occur with candidal species and involve the finger webs and intertriginous areas. Affected pruritic skin is reddened and characteristic satellite lesions may be present (Fig. 59.32). The differential diagnosis includes dermatophyte infection (tinea cruris), pemphigoid, psoriasis, SD, and contact dermatitis (Margolis, 2002). Fungal forms (round yeast cells as well as elongate pseudohyphae) can be seen in scraped skin preparations after treatment with KOH, and culture is usually unnecessary. Daily topical treatment with any imidazole antifungal agent for at least 2

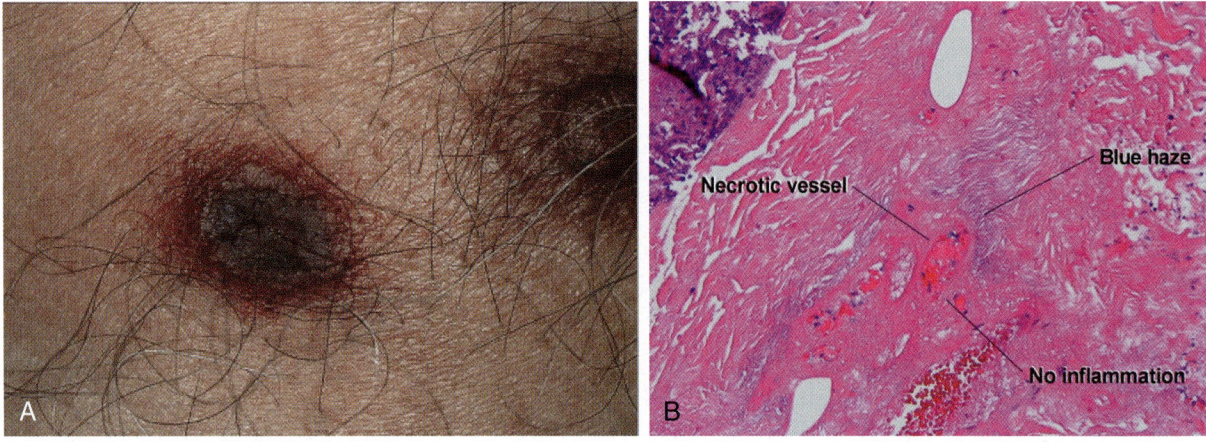

Fig. 59.30. Ecthyma gangrenosum. (A) Involvement on the chest wall. Note the necrotic center and erythematous border around the lesion. (B) Histologically, necrotic vessels surrounded by a "blue haze" of organisms characterize ecthyma gangrenosum. (A, Courtesy, Yale Residents' Slide Collection. From Bolognia JL, Jorizzo JL, Rapini RP. *Dermatology*. Edinburgh: Mosby; 2003. B, From Elston DM, Ferringer T: *Dermatopathology*, Edinburgh, 2009, Saunders, p 263.)

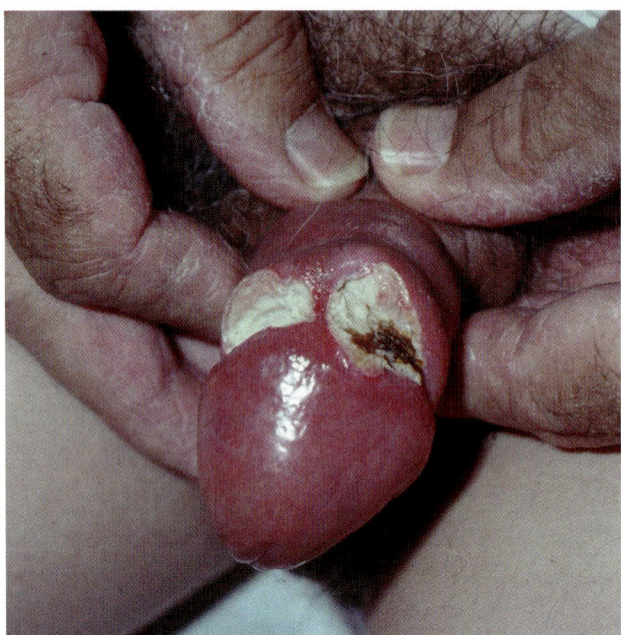

Fig. 59.31. Ulceration after a human bite wound to the penile shaft.

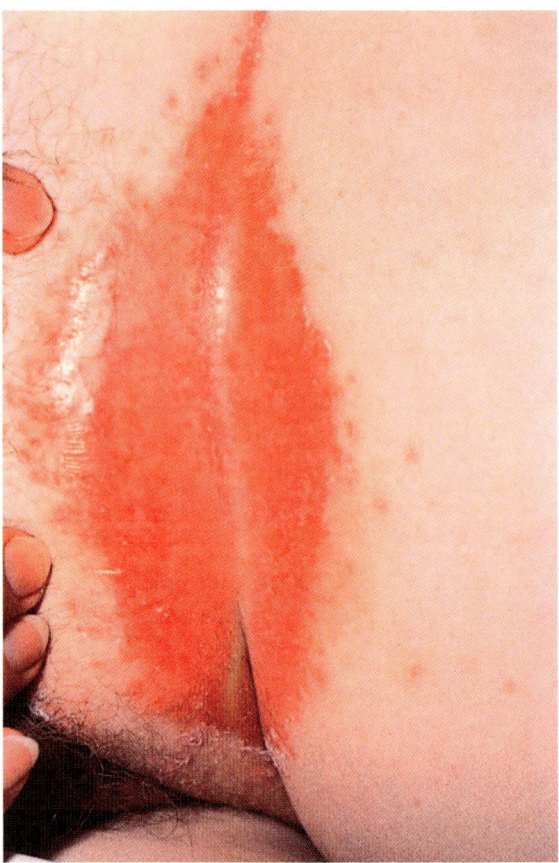

Fig. 59.32. Candidal intertrigo with erythema, areas of tissue maceration, and satellite lesions. (From Callen JP, Greer DE, Hood AF, et al.: *Color atlas of dermatology*, Philadelphia, 1993, Saunders, p 318.)

weeks is usually necessary for intertrigo, and oral antifungals (such as fluconazole 150 mg/day) are occasionally required (Cullin, 1977). Maneuvers to decrease moisture and skin maceration, such as the use of drying powders and loose clothing, may also help prevent relapse. Candida intertrigo may be a presenting sign of diabetes, and appropriate laboratory testing should be performed to rule this out as a predisposing condition.

Dermatophyte Infection

Dermatophytes are fungi of three genera *(Trichophyton, Microsporum, Epidermophyton)* that have the propensity to invade and grow within keratinized tissues such as the skin, hair, and nails. These fungi produce keratinases, which break down keratin and facilitate invasion (Viani et al., 2001). In addition, mannans in the cell wall of some dermatophytes produce immunoinhibitory effects (Dahl, 1994).

Tinea cruris is the term applied to dermatophyte infection of the groin and genital area and is commonly known as "jock itch." More common in males than females, this condition is favored by hot, humid environments and concomitant dermatophyte infection of the feet *(tinea pedis)*. Obesity may also be a significant risk factor (Scheinfeld, 2004). The inner thighs and inguinal region are the most commonly affected areas, and the scrotum and penis are usually spared in men. However, isolated penile dermatophytosis has been well described (Pielop and Rosen, 2001). **Conversely, significant**

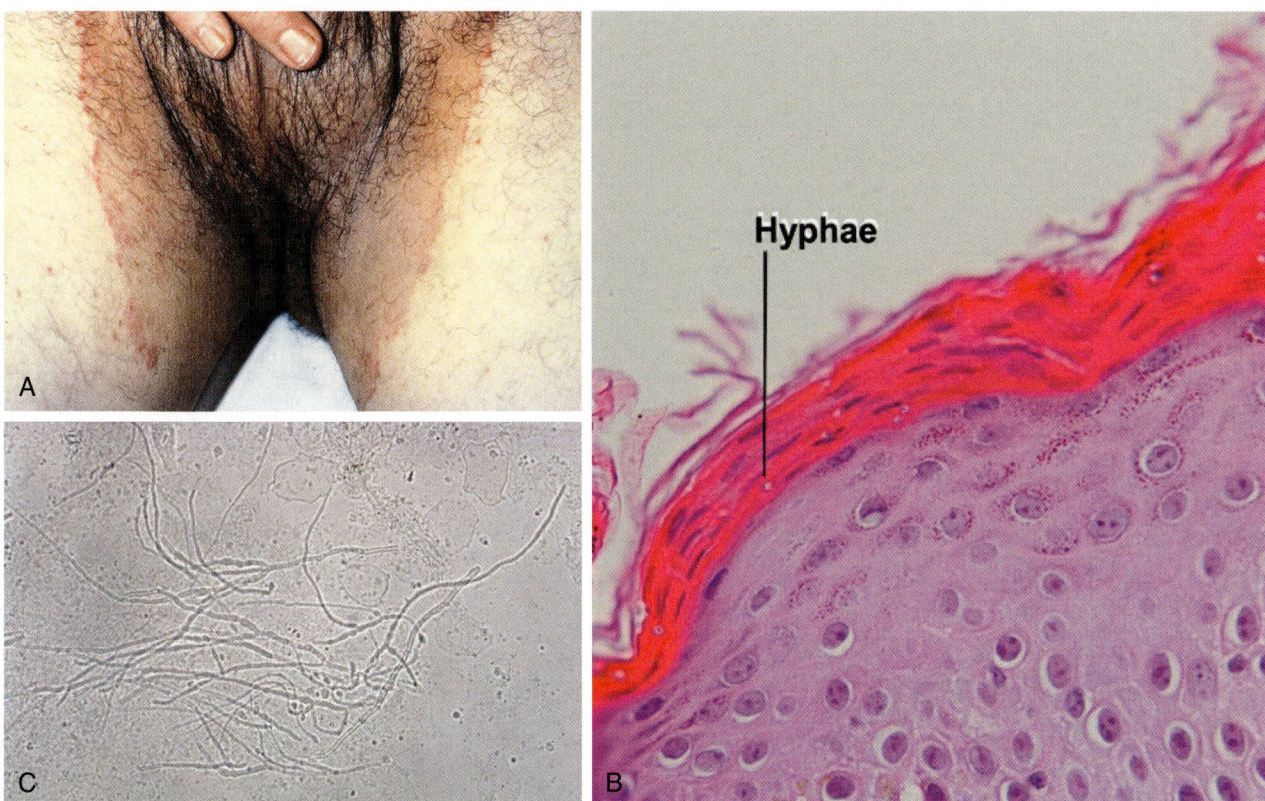

Fig. 59.33. Dermatophyte infection. (A) *Tinea cruris* showing areas of postinflammatory hyperpigmentation and active infection at the border of the lesions. (B) Histologically, fungal hyphae are localized within a compact stratum corneum layer. (C) Potassium hydroxide preparation from a scraping showing fungal forms. (A, From Callen JP, Greer DE, Hood AF, et al.: *Color atlas of dermatology*, Philadelphia, 1993, Saunders, p 318. B and C, From Elston DM, Ferringer T: Dermatopathology, Edinburgh, 2009, Saunders, p 275.)

scrotal involvement should raise suspicion for cutaneous candidiasis as an alternative diagnosis (Sobera and Elewski, 2003). Characteristic lesions in tinea cruris are sharply demarcated erythematous plaques with a raised scaly border (Fig. 59.33), and they may be intensely pruritic. A variety of disorders can mimic dermatophytes infection, including SD, psoriasis, contact dermatitis, and erythrasma. The diagnosis of fungal infection can be confirmed with skin scrapings and a KOH preparation. Culture is rarely required, because organisms are easily visualized microscopically.

Good hygienic practices can be beneficial in preventing recurrent disease, including wearing loose clothing, cleaning of contaminated garments, weight reduction, and the use of topical powders to keep the intertriginous areas dry (Sobera and Elewski, 2003). Topical antifungal preparations are the primary agents for treatment; the powdered forms have the added benefit of drying moist areas. Azoles have sufficient coverage against yeast as well as tinea-causing dermatophytes, whereas the allylamines terbinafine and naftifine are not as effective against yeast (Edwards and Lynch, 2018). Furthermore, although nystatin is effective to treat candidiasis, it is not effective against dermatophytes. **Care should be taken to treat only active disease and not the postinflammatory hyperpigmentation that can occur with recurrent chronic dermatophyte infection** (Margolis, 2002). Systemic antifungals are rarely necessary to treat groin infection with dermatophytes. However, should this prove necessary, as is sometimes the case when tinea infection has follicular involvement too deep for topical therapy to penetrate, the current drug of choice is terbinafine in a dosage of 250 mg/day for 1 week (Farag et al., 1994).

Infestation

Pediculosis pubis and scabies *(Sarcoptes scabiei)* are the most common infestations involving the genital region.

Infestation with the crab louse *(Phthirus pubis)* causes pediculosis pubis, a pruritic disorder of the genitalia, which may coexist with other STDs (Opaneye et al., 1993; Varela et al., 2003). In one study of adolescent males, patients with pediculosis pubis showed a risk of concomitant gonorrhea or chlamydial infection more than twofold higher than normal controls (Pierzchalski et al., 2002). Louse infestation is not limited to the genitals and may involve other hair-bearing areas such as the eyelashes, beard, and axillae (Meinking, 1999). The diagnosis is confirmed by identification of crab lice attached to hairs (Fig. 59.34), often with associated perifollicular erythema. **Transmission of pediculosis pubis is usually through sexual contact, although contaminated clothing, bedding, and towels have also been implicated in some cases** (Meinking, 1999). **The standard treatment is the application of 5% permethrin cream overnight to all affected hair-bearing areas with a repeat application 1 week later** (Meinking, 1999). Note that the second application of permethrin is important, because the rate of treatment success with a single application may be as low as 57% (Kalter et al., 1987). For rare cases refractory to topical therapy or those involving the eyelashes *(tinea palpebrarum)*, the addition of oral ivermectin may be curative (Burkhart and Burkhart, 2000). Interestingly, because of the adoption of the widespread removal of pubic hair among young adults of both genders ("Brazilian waxing"), the incidence of pubic louse infestation in industrialized countries has fallen dramatically in recent years.

Another important infestation involving the genitalia is scabies, caused by the female itch mite *S. scabiei*. **Scabies is a worldwide problem, and factors such as overcrowding, delayed treatment of primary cases, and poor public awareness encourage spread** (Meinking et al., 2003). Transmission is common between close contacts and family members (Burkhart et al., 2000). The number of mites living on an immunocompetent host is usually small (<100) (Arlian et al., 1988), although far greater numbers may be recovered

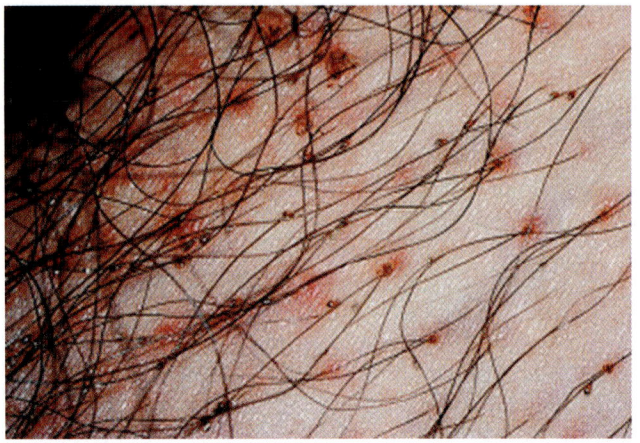

Fig. 59.34. Pediculosis pubis. Several crab lice are visible. (From Buttaravoli P, Leffler SM: *Minor Emergencies*. Philadelphia, Elsevier, 2012, Fig. 174-5.)

in cases of immunosuppression (so-called crusted or Norwegian scabies). The incubation period before symptoms develop after infestation can vary from days to months in duration but is most typically about 6 weeks.

Severe pruritus is the hallmark of scabies, often accentuated at night or after bathing (Meinking et al., 2003). In both genders, the genital areas are commonly affected. Small erythematous and pruritic papules are present, and excoriations with secondary bacterial infection may occur (Fig. 59.35). **Thin, gray or white burrows may be visible and are pathognomonic for scabies infestation. Crusted scabies affecting genital skin presents as it does in other anatomic sites: with thickly crusted plaque(s)** (Perna et al., 2004). In the absence of visible burrows, a broad differential must be considered, including AD, pyoderma, psoriasis, and other insect bites. As in the case of pediculosis pubis, the treatment of choice for scabies is 5% permethrin cream applied to the entire body overnight with a second application 1 week later. An alternative topical scabicide, lindane, is not favored because of central nervous system toxicity in children and a rising rate of resistance among mites (Boix et al., 1997; Elgart, 1996; Purvis and Tyring, 1991). Oral ivermectin (200 μg/kg/dose, 2 doses administered 2 weeks apart) is an alternate regimen that has been successfully used to treat scabies (Chouela et al., 2002; Heukelbach et al., 2004; Karthikeyan, 2005). A randomized comparative trial showed that permethrin was slightly more effective than ivermectin when the latter is only provided as a single dose (Goldust et al., 2012). **Note that pruritus may persist for several weeks despite successful treatment and that all intimate contacts should also be treated to prevent reinfestation.** Even with effective treatment, itchy nodules may remain on the glans penis; intralesional injections of minute amounts of dilute triamcinolone acetonide (2 to 3 mg/mL) may facilitate resolution of these postscabies nodules.

NEOPLASTIC CONDITIONS
Squamous Cell Carcinoma in Situ

Squamous cell carcinoma in situ (SCCis) is a full thickness intraepidermal carcinoma (Miller and Moresi, 2003). Bowen originally described this condition in 1912, hence the term "Bowen disease" (Bowen, 1912). On extragenital sites, there is a strong association between SCCis and ultraviolet light exposure (Reizner et al., 1994). **Commonly presenting in the seventh decade of life with a slight female predominance** (Arlette, 2003; Hemminki and Dong, 2000), **SCCis usually has an indolent clinical course and rarely progresses to invasive disease. When it occurs on mucosal surfaces of the male genitalia, most notably the glans penis of uncircumcised men, this entity is referred to as erythroplasia of Queyrat** (Fig. 59.36). Yet another name for this entity is penile intraepithelial neoplasia. In the female, the comparable SCCis on the vulva would be called vulvar intraepithelial neoplasia. In these locations, coinfection with HPV types 8, 16 (70%), and other serotypes (30%) has been identified (Wieland et al., 2000). Other risk factors for SCCis include ionizing radiation, immunosuppression, thermal injury, arsenic exposure, chronic dermatoses (such as long-standing LP), and LS of the glans penis (Arlette, 2003; Centeno et al., 2002; Euvrard et al., 1995; Nasca et al., 1999; Powell et al., 2001).

SCCis lesions are sharply demarcated, solitary, pink to red scaly plaques that may be confused with basal cell carcinoma, eczema, seborrhea, or psoriasis. SCCis on or near the vulva may be heavily pigmented and resemble melanoma and external genital warts. When localized to the penile shaft, SCCis may have a more thickened, verrucoid appearance. Although usually asymptomatic, these lesions may also be pruritic or painful. The diagnosis is confirmed by histologic evaluation, and several areas should be sampled to exclude the presence of dermal invasion (Margolis, 2002).

Primary treatment of SCCis involves either surgical excision or tissue ablation. For accessible areas, such as the scrotum, simple excision with a 5-mm margin is favored (Bissada, 1992; Margolis, 2002). For areas where tissue preservation is more critical, Mohs microsurgery, laser therapy, and cryoablation may play a role (Leibovitch et al., 2005; Sonnex et al., 1982b; van Bezooijen et al., 2001). Topical treatment with either 5-fluorouracil or imiquimod 5% can be effective for management of selected cases of SCCis involving the genitalia, although response is variable and the risk of recurrence is higher than with surgical treatment (Arlette, 2003; Deen and Burdon-Jones, 2017; Gerber, 1994; Micali et al., 2003; Orengo et al., 2002).

Bowenoid Papulosis

Bowenoid papulosis is an uncommon condition found on the penis and vulva of sexually active adults, with a peak incidence in the third decade of life (Schwartz and Janniger, 1991). **It histologically resembles Bowen disease except that the abnormal keratinocytes are spread discontinuously throughout the epidermis** (Margolis, 2002). Typical lesions are multiple small erythematous papules that may coalesce to form plaques with a verrucous surface similar to a genital wart (Fig. 59.37). There is a clear association with HPV type 16. **Female partners of men with bowenoid papulosis have an increased risk of cervical neoplasia and should receive close cervical follow-up** (Rosemberg et al., 1991). In men, however, bowenoid papulosis generally has a benign course and spontaneous regression may occur (Eisen et al., 1983; Feng et al., 2013; Giam and Ong, 1986). Therefore, in a young and reliable patient, observation alone may be justified. If treatment is desired, conservative local therapy with topical agents (0.5% 5-fluorouracil, 0.5% tazarotene cream, or imiquimod 5%) or ablative measures (electrodessication, liquid nitrogen cryotherapy, laser ablation) is usually appropriate (Margolis, 2002).

Squamous Cell Carcinoma

Invasive SCC involving the genitalia (Fig. 59.38) is covered in detail in Chapter 37.

Verrucous Carcinoma (Buschke-Lowenstein Tumor)

Verrucous carcinoma is a locally aggressive, exophytic, low-grade variant of SCC that has little metastatic potential (Habif, 2004). **The Buschke-Lowenstein tumor is a verrucous carcinoma of the anogenital mucosal surface and may represent up to 24% of all penile tumors** (Schwartz, 1995). It most commonly occurs in uncircumcised men on the glans or prepuce, although similar lesions can be found on the vulva, vagina cervix, or anus. Verrucous carcinoma has been associated with HPV types 6 and 11 infection but not with the more classically oncogenic types 16 and 18 (Ahmed et al., 2006; Chan et al., 1994; Margolis, 2002; Yasunaga et al., 1993).

Verrucous carcinoma lesions have a warty appearance and are often large and fungating when presenting on the genitalia (Fig. 59.39). Aside from genital sites, these lesions can also present within the oral and nasal cavities and plantar surfaces of the feet. They are

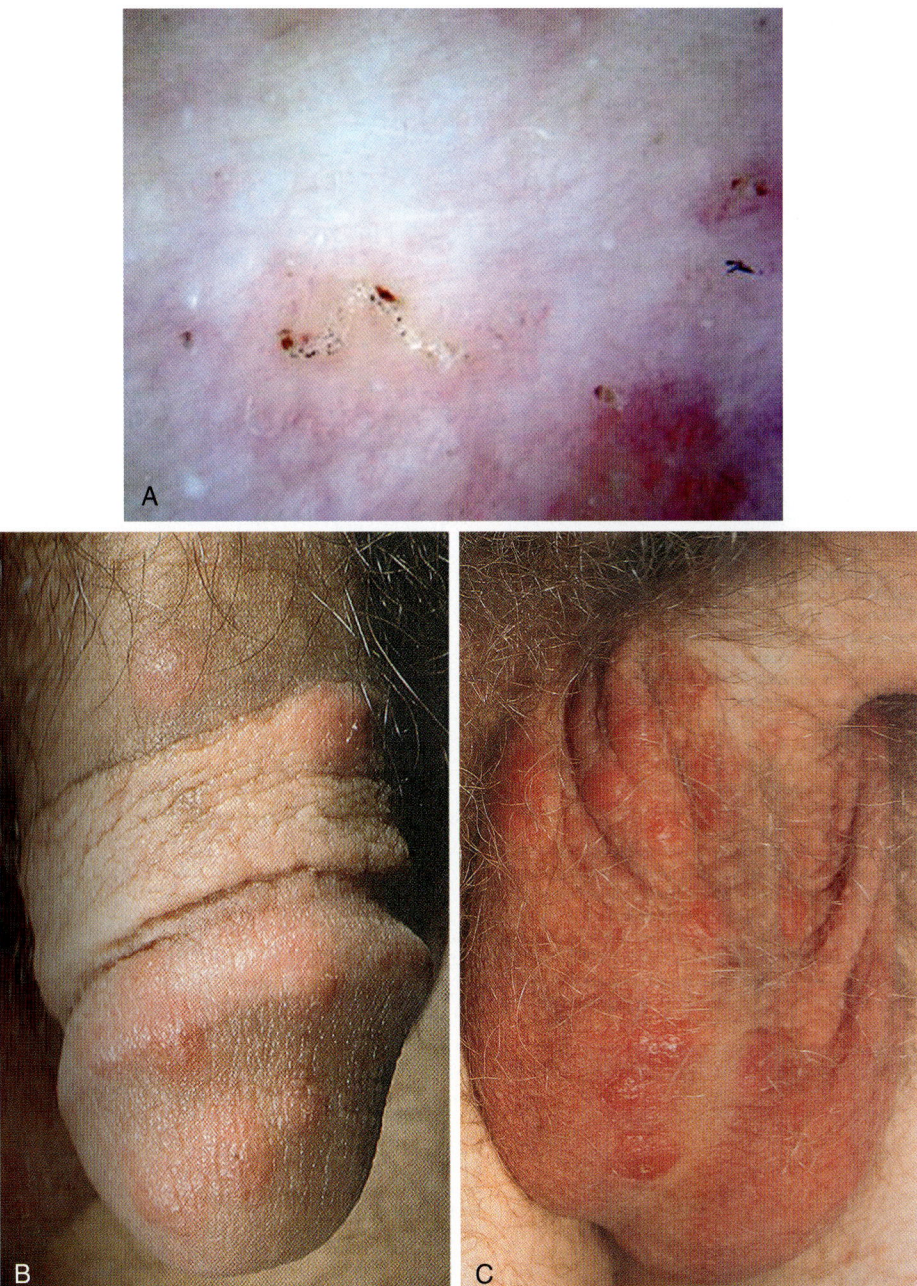

Fig. 59.35. Scabies. (A) A papular eruption with a visible characteristic burrow. (B and C) Classic established genital scabies with eroded papules on the glans penis and scrotum. (A, From Panuganti B, Tarbox M: Evaluation and management of pruritis and scabies in the elderly population. *Clinics in Geriatric Medicine* 29(2): 479–499, 2013, Fig. 3. B and C, From Habif TP. *Clinical dermatology*. Edinburgh: Mosby; 2004, p. 501.)

slow growing and locally destructive, often extending deeply into underlying tissue. Preferred treatment is by local excision. Mohs micrographic surgery may be helpful in tracing out the tumor and minimizing tissue loss. **Primary radiotherapy is relatively contraindicated because of the potential for anaplastic transformation with a subsequent increase in metastatic potential** (Andersen and Sorensen, 1988; Fukunaga et al., 1994; Stehman et al., 1980; Vandeweyer et al., 2001).

Basal Cell Carcinoma

Basal cell carcinoma (BCC) is the most common cutaneous neoplasm overall, arising most often on areas of chronically sun-exposed skin such as the head and neck. Genital BCC has also been described as a very rare entity, most commonly involving the scrotal skin in the male and the vulva in the female (Benedet et al., 1997; Esquivias Gomez et al., 1999; Kinoshita et al., 2005; Nahass et al., 1992). In the world medical literature, fewer than 100 total cases of BCC have been described involving all the potential genital sites (penis, scrotum, vulva). Several subtypes of BCC have been defined including nodular, superficial, micronodular morpheaform, and infiltrating. The nodular variant accounts for 60% of extragenital BCCs and almost all genital BCCs, and this variant presents as a pearly, skin-toned papule or plaque often with telangiectasias overlying the tumor (Fig. 59.40; Miller and Moresi, 2003). These lesions may ulcerate centrally and manifest a very low metastatic potential. Treatment is by local excision. Because preservation of genital skin is important, both for form and function, the use of Mohs micrographic surgery may be advisable for the rare genital BCC. In patients with metastatic, locally advanced, and/or unresectable BCC, vismodegib and sonidegib are Hedgehog signaling pathway inhibitors that were approved by the FDA in 2012 and 2015, respectively.

Kaposi Sarcoma

Kaposi sarcoma (KS) is a disease of endothelial cell origin. Whether KS is a neoplastic or hyperplastic process remains controversial, and evidence exists for and against clonal expansion (Gill et al., 1998; Rabkin et al., 1997). Before the onset of the AIDS epidemic, KS was considered a chronic disease afflicting elderly men of Jewish, Mediterranean, or Eastern European descent ("classic KS") (Safai, 1987). However, infection with HIV-1 has increased the incidence of KS by more than 7000-fold (Margolis, 2002; Miles, 1994). KS generally affects HIV-infected patients with advanced immune impairment (CD4+ T-cell counts of <500 cells/mm) (Tappero et al., 1993). Approximately 40% of homosexual men with AIDS have developed KS as compared with less than 5% in other risk groups (North et al., 2003; Rogers et al., 1987), although the prevalence in this population has decreased since the widespread use of highly active antiretroviral therapy. There is also a clear association between infection with human herpesvirus 8 and the development of KS (Boshoff and Weiss, 1997; Weiss et al., 1998). In this regard, the other group at risk for development of KS associated with human herpesvirus 8 infection includes recipients of solid organ transplants (Riva et al., 2012).

Classic KS in immunocompetent individuals presents as slowly growing, blue-red to overtly violaceous pigmented macules on the lower extremities. Although oral and gastrointestinal lesions may occur, the genitalia are seldom involved. This is in contrast to the case with AIDS ("epidemic KS"), in which a solitary genital lesion may be the first manifestation of KS (Lowe et al., 1989). **The clinical features of KS in AIDS patients and solid organ transplant recipients are diverse, ranging from a single lesion to disseminated cutaneous and visceral disease** (Fig. 59.41). Lesions may coalesce to cover large areas of skin and may result in lymphatic or venous blockage leading to local edema (Margolis, 2002). When these lesions involve the glans penis, they can cause obstruction at the urethral meatus or fossa navicularis (Swierzewski et al., 1993). However, penile KS is still rare, even among those infected with HIV-1; only about 3% of AIDS patients will ever develop KS of the genitalia (Rosen et al., 1999).

Treatment must be tailored to the individual clinical case, and complete cure may be an unrealistic goal. No treatment is necessary for solitary lesions. However, if treatment is desired, local therapies such as surgical excision, laser ablation, cryotherapy, topical imiquimod 5%, or intralesional injection of chemotherapeutic agents (i.e., vinblastine) may be beneficial (Chun et al., 1999; Heyns and Fisher, 2005; Rosen, 2006; Schwartz, 2004). For extensive locoregional disease, radiotherapy (15 to 30 Gy) has an objective response rate of greater than 90% (Cattelan et al., 2002; Kirova et al., 1998). For widely disseminated KS, systemic chemotherapy with vincristine, doxorubicin, and bleomycin is the treatment of choice (Aversa et al., 1999). For KS associated with organ transplantation,

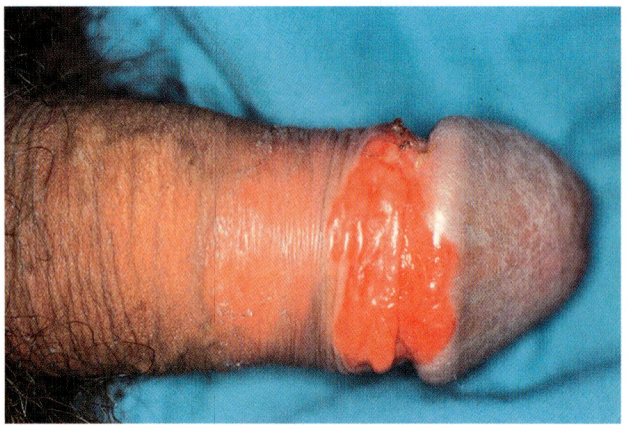

Fig. 59.36. Erythroplasia of Queyrat. Squamous cell carcinoma involving the glans penis. (From Callen JP, Greer DE, Hood AF, et al.: *Color atlas of dermatology*, Philadelphia, 1993, Saunders, p 330.)

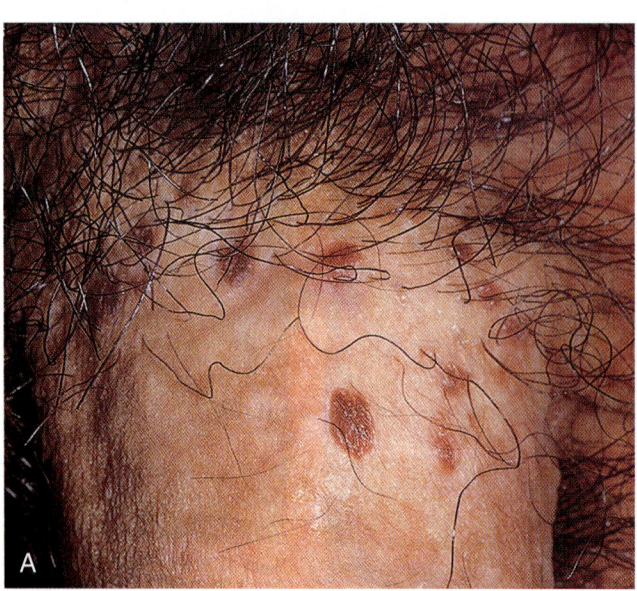
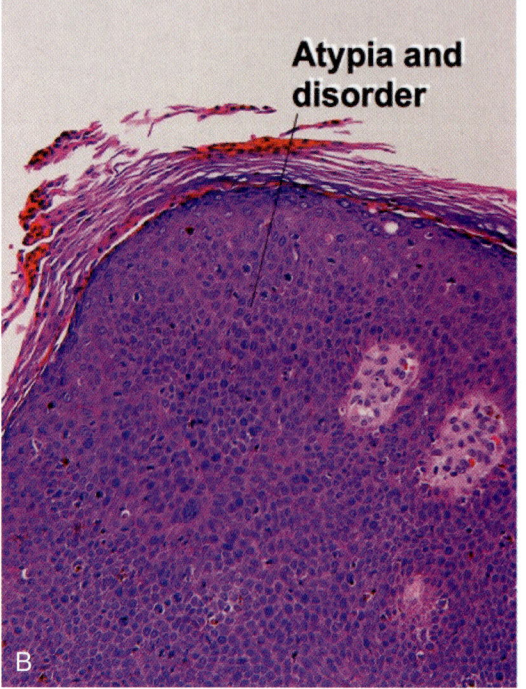

Fig. 59.37. Bowenoid papulosis. (A) Involvement of the penile shaft. Note multiple brown verrucous papules on the penile shaft. (B) Characteristic full thickness atypia, which may be mistaken for Bowen disease. (A, From Habif TP: *Clinical dermatology*, Edinburgh, 2004, Mosby, p 343. B, From Elston DM, Ferringer T: *Dermatopathology*, Edinburgh, 2009, Saunders, p 293.)

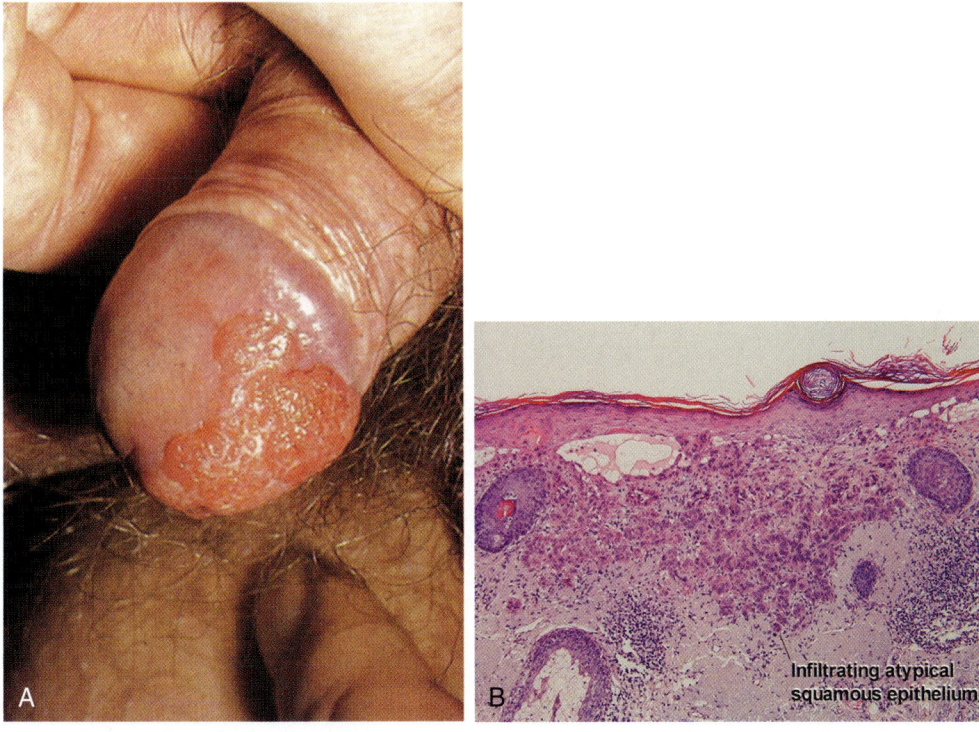

Fig. 59.38. Squamous cell carcinoma (SCC). (A) Exophytic erosive lesion on the glans with evident keratinization. (B) Atypical keratinocytes invading the dermis in SCC. (A, From Callen JP, Greer DE, Hood AF, et al.: *Color atlas of dermatology,* Philadelphia, 1993, Saunders, p 129. B, From Elston DM, Ferringer T: *Dermatopathology,* Edinburgh, 2009, Saunders, p 57.)

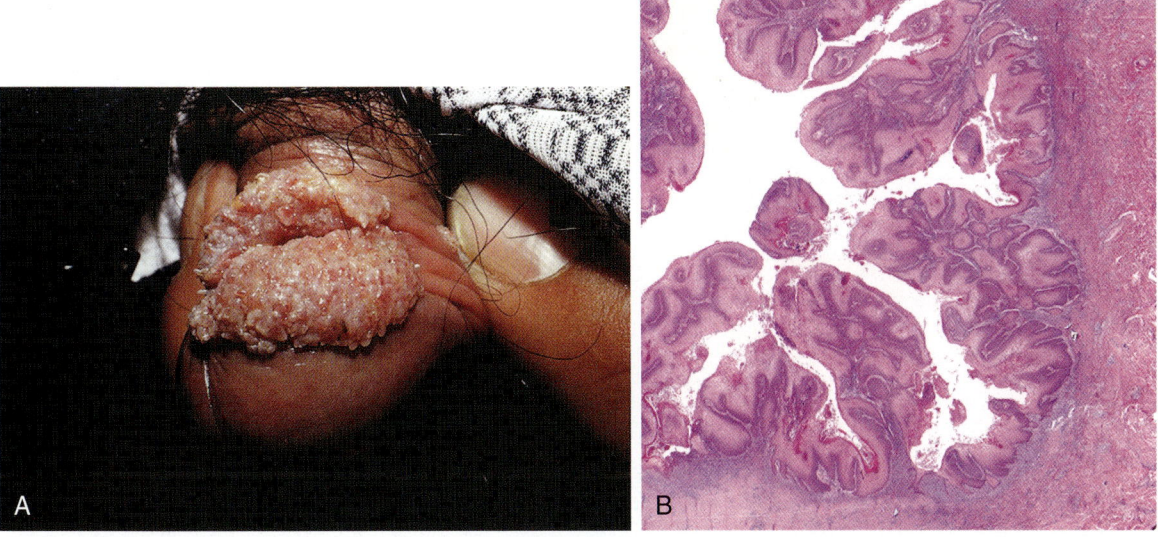

Fig. 59.39. Verrucous carcinoma of the penis (Buschke-Lowenstein tumor). (A) Note the exophytic and wartlike appearance. (B) Histologic features of verrucous carcinoma. (A, From Callen JP, Greer DE, Hood AF, et al.: *Color atlas of dermatology,* Philadelphia, 1993, Saunders, p 330, B, From Elston DM, Ferringer T: *Dermatopathology,* Edinburgh, 2009, Saunders, p 58.)

reduction in the degree of postoperative immunosuppression or switching from a calcineurin inhibitor to an mTOR inhibitor may lead to KS resolution without any additional intervention (Riva et al., 2012).

Pseudoepitheliomatous, Keratotic, and Micaceous Balanitis

Pseudoepitheliomatous, keratotic, and micaceous balanitis (PEKMB) is a rare entity characterized by the development of a thick, hyperkeratotic plaque on the glans penis of older men (Fig. 59.42). The term *micaceous* refers to the white, scaly appearance of the lesions (Child et al., 2000). PEKMB was originally thought to be a purely benign process, although several case reports have documented the presence of concurrent verrucous carcinomas associated with this lesion (Child et al., 2000). Controversy remains as to whether PEKMB is a premalignant condition (Beljaards et al., 1987; Jenkins and Jakubovic, 1988; Read and Abell, 1981). Histologic examination is essential to exclude the presence of SCC and verrucous carcinoma

(Margolis, 2002). PEKMB is characterized on histology by a hyperplastic epidermis with ridges extending deeply into the dermis (Jenkins and Jakubovic, 1988). These lesions should be treated locally either by surgical excision or ablative techniques, and close follow-up is essential (Bargman, 1985; Read and Abell, 1981). There are also anecdotal reports of successful treatment using topical 5-fluorouracil cream (Bargman, 1985; Choo et al., 2017; Krunic et al., 1996).

Melanoma

Malignant melanoma is a neoplasm arising from melanocytes. The incidence of melanoma has risen 3% to 7% during the past several decades (Nestle and Kerl, 2003). Risk factors for development of

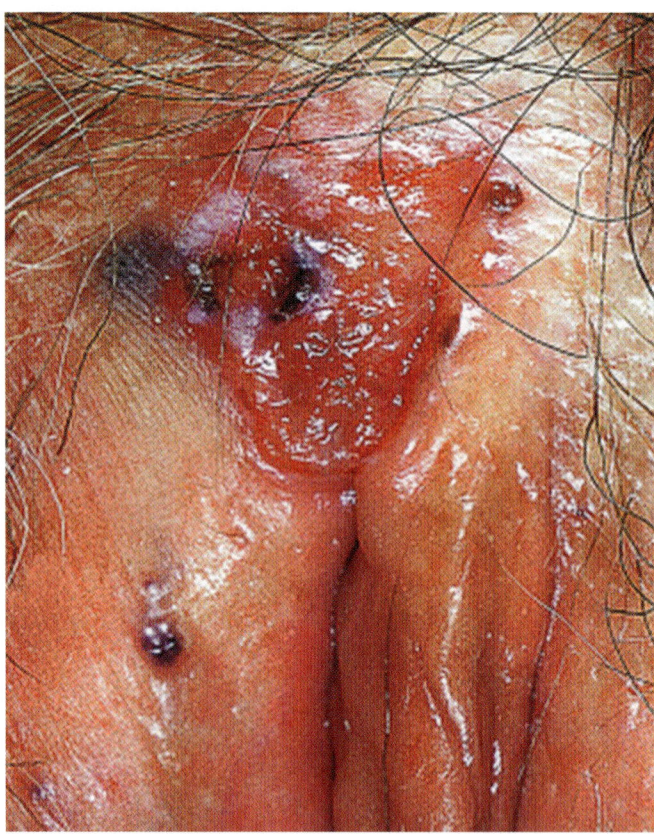

Fig. 59.40. Basal cell carcinoma involving the vulva. (From Chapman MS: *Skin disease: diagnosis and treatment*. Philadelphia, Elsevier, 2018. Fig. 17-11.)

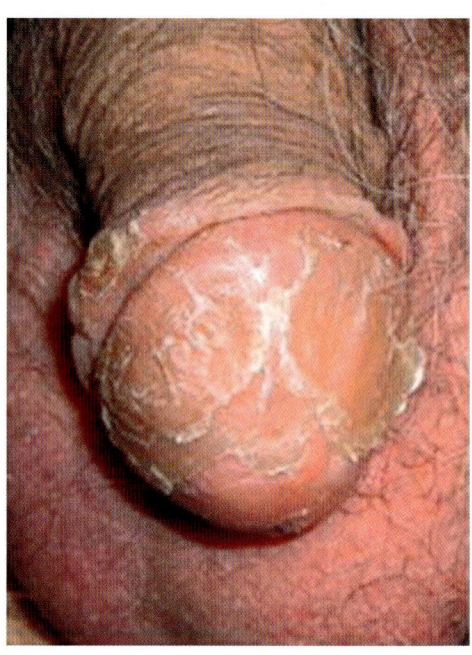

Fig. 59.42. Pseudoepitheliomatous, keratotic, and micaceous balanitis. The glans becomes covered with mica (asbestos-like) scales and horny crusts. (From Ferràndiz-Pulido C, de Torres I, García-Patos V: Penile squamous cell carcinoma. *Dermatology* 103(6): 478–487, 2012, Fig. 1A.)

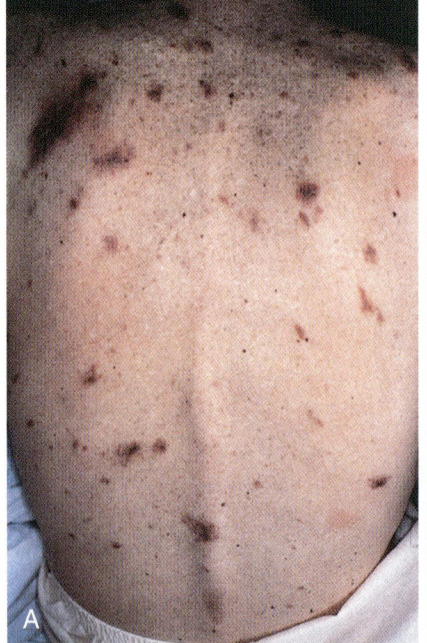
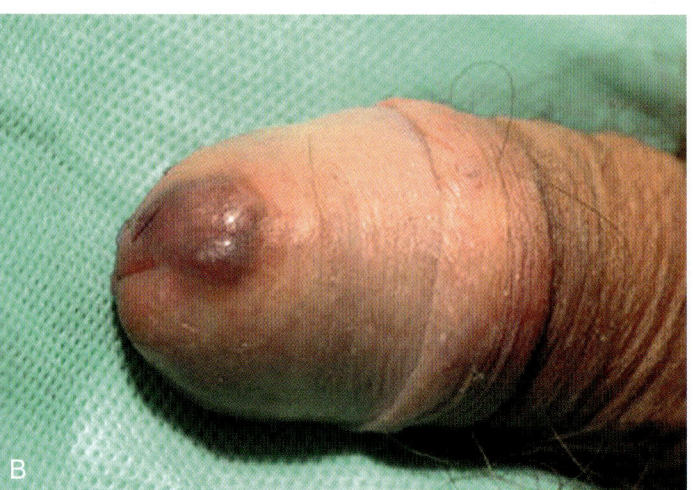

Fig. 59.41. Kaposi sarcoma. Classic macular lesions seen on the back (A) and glans penis **(B)**. (A, From Callen JP, Greer DE, Hood AF, et al. *Color atlas of dermatology*. Philadelphia: Saunders; 1993, p. 220; B, From Imko-Walczuk B, Kielbowicz M, Malyszko J, et al: Kaposi sarcoma in the genital area in a kidney-transplant patient: a case report and literature review. *Transplant Proc* 48(5):1843–1848, 2016, Fig. 1.)

the disease include family history, certain genetic markers, fair skin, light eye color, and a history of excessive ultraviolet radiation exposure (especially multiple blistering sunburns as a child or adolescent). Primary melanoma of the male genitalia is an uncommon entity with only approximately 100 cases reported in the literature (Sanchez-Ortiz et al., 2005), and melanoma of the male urethra is even more rare (Oliva et al., 2000). The same cannot be said for females, as melanoma makes up about 7% to 10% of all vulvar malignancies and remains the second most common such lesion after SCC (Suwandinata et al., 2007). Although vulvar melanoma is more common among Caucasian women, the prognosis is worse among African-American women (Mert et al., 2013).

Genital melanoma usually presents as a pigmented macule or papule with an irregular border, although unpigmented lesions and ulceration may also be present (Margolis, 2002). **Early diagnosis is critical because local treatment of superficial lesions with wide local excision or partial penectomy can provide excellent disease control** (Sanchez-Ortiz et al., 2005; Stillwell et al., 1988). **The same caveats are true in female patients.** In contrast, patients with biopsy-proven metastatic disease have traditionally had a universally poor prognosis despite aggressive surgical management and multiagent cytotoxic chemotherapy. In the last several years, however, several drugs have gained regulatory approval for the treatment of metastatic and unresectable melanoma as a result of an increase of knowledge in melanoma-specific molecular biology and immunology. The efficacy of small-molecule BRAF (e.g., vemurafenib, dabrafenib, trametinib) and MAP-ERK kinase (MEK) inhibitors, as well as the immune checkpoint inhibitors (e.g., ipilimumab and the anti-PD1/PDL1 antibodies lambrolizumab and nivolumab), have transformed the treatment of advanced melanoma.

Extramammary Paget Disease

Extramammary Paget disease (EPD) is an uncommon intraepithelial adenocarcinoma of sites bearing apocrine glands (Zollo and Zeitouni, 2000). The majority of patients with EPD are elderly Caucasian females, and involvement of the male penis and scrotum is exceedingly rare (Park et al., 2001; van Randenborgh et al., 2002). The vulva is the most commonly involved genital site in women followed by the perianal region in men (Wojnarowska and Cooper, 2003). **There is an important association between EPD and another underlying malignancy in at least 10% to 30% of cases** (Margolis, 2002; Ng et al., 2001; Payne and Wells, 1994). An investigation in a cancer specialty hospital suggested that this association may be even stronger in men than previously appreciated (Hegarty et al., 2011). In the male, associations between urethral, prostate, bladder, rectal, and apocrine malignancies with EPD have been described (Hayes et al., 1997; Hegarty et al., 2011; Salamanca et al., 2004). **It is critical, therefore, to perform a systematic evaluation for underlying carcinoma in all cases of EPD.**

The lesion in EPD is usually an erythematous plaque with a sharp border between normal and involved skin (Fig. 59.43). It may be asymptomatic, pruritic, or associated with burning pain. The diagnosis is confirmed histologically by the presence of vacuolated Paget cells in the epidermis that stain for glandular cytokeratins, epithelial membrane antigen, and carcinoembryonic antigen (Wojnarowska

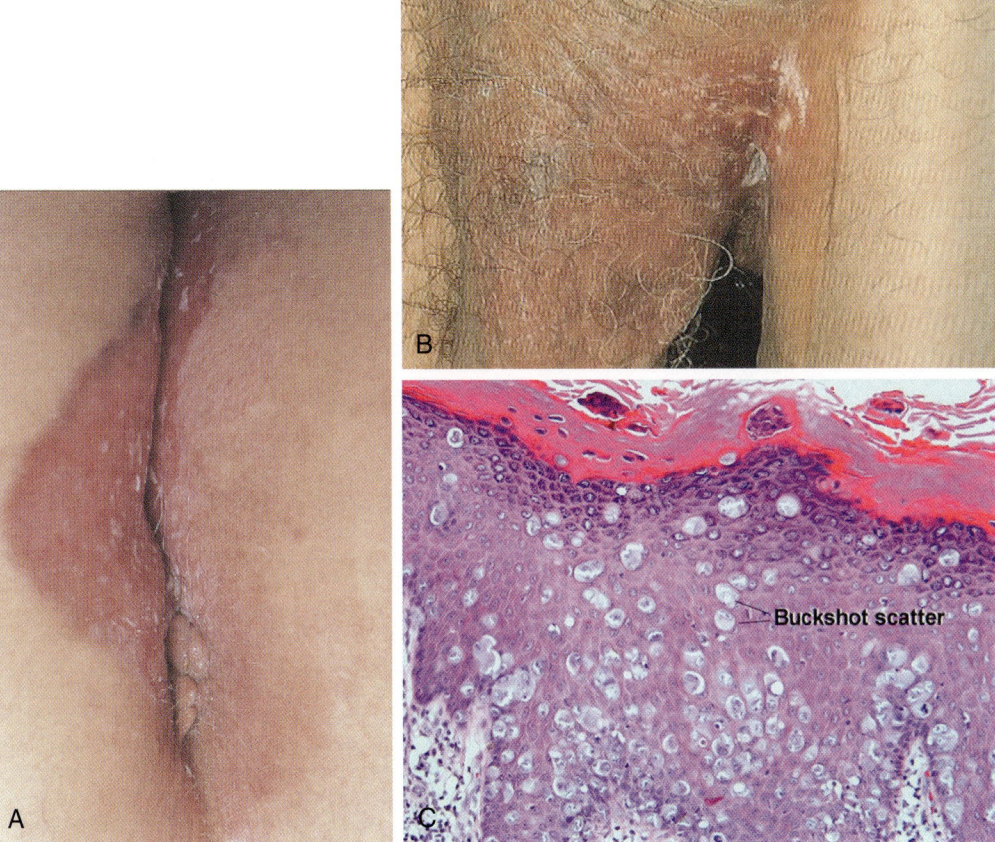

Fig. 59.43. Extramammary Paget disease involving the vulva (A) and base of scrotum (B). Note the well-demarcated border between the lesion and normal adjacent skin. (C) Tumor cells distributed throughout the epidermis ("buckshot scatter"). (A, Courtesy of Fenella Wojnarowska, MD, and Susan M. Cooper, MD. From Bolognia JL, Jorizzo JL, Rapini RP. *Dermatology*. Edinburgh: Mosby; 2003. B, From Bolognia JL, Jorizzo JL, Rapini RP: *Dermatology*, Edinburgh, 2003, Mosby, p 1108. C, From Elston DM, Ferringer T: *Dermatopathology*, Edinburgh, 2009, Saunders, p 66.)

and Cooper, 2003). Treatment generally involves surgical excision or Mohs micrographic surgery, although radiotherapy, photodynamic therapy, and topical imiquimod 5% or 5-fluorouracil have also been used successfully (Bewley et al., 1994; Brown et al., 2000; Guerrieri and Back, 2002; Lee et al., 2009; Moreno-Arias et al., 2003; Qian et al., 2003; Sillman et al., 1985).

Cutaneous T-Cell Lymphoma

Cutaneous T-cell lymphoma (CTCL) represents a group of related neoplasms derived from T cells that home to the skin. CTCL includes a variety of conditions including mycosis fungoides, Sézary syndrome, lymphoid papulosis, and pagetoid reticulosis (Willemze, 2003). There is an increased risk of CTCL associated with HIV infection (Biggar et al., 2001). Although these disorders may involve the genitalia of both genders, extragenital disease is usually also present. CTCL accounts for the majority of primary cutaneous lymphomas with B-cell–derived lymphomas accounting for only 20% to 25% (Willemze et al., 1997; Willemze et al., 2005). Definitive diagnosis depends on biopsy histopathology.

CTCL generally presents initially as pruritic patches that must be differentiated from a variety of benign dermatoses including psoriasis, eczema, superficial fungal infections, and drug reactions. **The initial lesions of CTCL have a strong predilection in both sexes to occur on suprapubic and/or buttock skin.** Patients may subsequently develop hematologic involvement (Sézary syndrome) and cutaneous plaques, erosions, ulcers, or frank skin tumors (Fig. 59.44) (Margolis, 2002). CTCL is a chronic condition that may progress throughout many years. Topical treatments include application of ultrapotent corticosteroids, nitrogen mustard, and carmustine with complete remission rates of approximately 60% (Vonderheid et al., 1989; Zackheim et al., 1998). Other treatments include radiotherapy (including total body electron beam treatment), phototherapy (PUVA or Narrowband Ultraviolet B), and systemic treatment with chemotherapy, interferons, or retinoids (Diederen et al., 2003; Hoppe et al., 1990; Olsen and Bunn, 1995; Querfeld et al., 2005).

BENIGN CUTANEOUS DISORDERS SPECIFIC TO THE MALE GENITALIA

Angiokeratoma of Fordyce

Angiokeratomas of Fordyce are vascular ectasias of dermal blood vessels that may be visible on the penis and scrotum of adult men (Bechara et al., 2002). These lesions appear as 1- to 2-mm red or purple papules (Fig. 59.45A), and associated generalized scrotal redness may exist (Miller and James, 2002). This is usually a benign condition without systemic manifestations, although it may rarely be a source of troublesome scrotal bleeding (Hoekx and Wyndaele, 1998; Taniguchi et al., 1994). Similar lesions can be observed in Fabry disease (Fig. 59.45B), which is a rare glycogen storage deficiency. Although treatment is usually unnecessary for angiokeratoma of Fordyce, several authors have reported success using erbium:YAG, Nd:YAG, KTP, and Argon laser photocoagulation in select cases (Bechara et al., 2004; Occella et al., 1995; Ozdemir et al., 2009).

Pearly Penile Papules

Pearly penile papules are white, dome shaped or filiform, closely spaced small papules located on the glans penis (Fig. 59.45C). They are often arranged circumferentially at the corona. Pearly penile papules are common lesions found in up to 14% to 48% of young postpubertal adults, particularly if the penis is not circumcised (Khoo and Cheong, 1995; Rehbein, 1977; Sonnex and Dockerty, 1999). **Although pearly penile papules may occasionally be misdiagnosed as condyloma, the available evidence does not support a role for HPV in causing pearly penile papules, and no association with cervical intraepithelial neoplasia in female partners has been demonstrated** (Hogewoning et al., 2003). Patients should be reassured that this is a benign condition or normal variant that does not usually require treatment. If treatment is desired because of cosmetic concerns, local destruction with either the CO_2 laser or cryotherapy has been applied successfully (Lane et al., 2002; Ocampo-Candiani and Cueva-Rodriguez, 1996). **Histologically, these lesions are angiofibromas similar to the lesions seen on the face in tuberous sclerosis.**

Zoon Balanitis

Zoon balanitis, also called plasma cell balanitis and balanitis plasmacellularis, occurs in uncircumcised men from the third decade onward and has an unknown cause (Pastar et al., 2004). Smooth, moist, erythematous, well-circumscribed papules and plaques on the glans penis characterize the disease (see Fig. 59.14D). Shallow erosions are often present (Yoganathan et al., 1994), and the lesions can be large (up to 2 cm in diameter) (Margolis, 2002). Lesions may be asymptomatic or exhibit mild pruritus or tenderness. SCC and EPD must be excluded, typically by biopsy. Circumcision appears to be proof against development of the disease and can be performed to cure the majority of cases (Ferrandiz and Ribera, 1984; Sonnex et al., 1982a). For patients averse to circumcision, topical corticosteroids may provide symptomatic relief, and topical calcineurin inhibitors (tacrolimus or pimecrolimus), topical retinoids, and laser therapy may also play a role in alleviation (Albertini et al., 2002; Baldwin and Geronemus, 1989; Rallis et al., 2007; Retamar et al., 2003; Tang et al., 2001; Wojnarowska and Cooper, 2003).

Sclerosing Lymphangitis

Nonvenereal sclerosing lymphangitis is a rare penile lesion consisting of an indurated, slightly tender cord involving the coronal sulcus

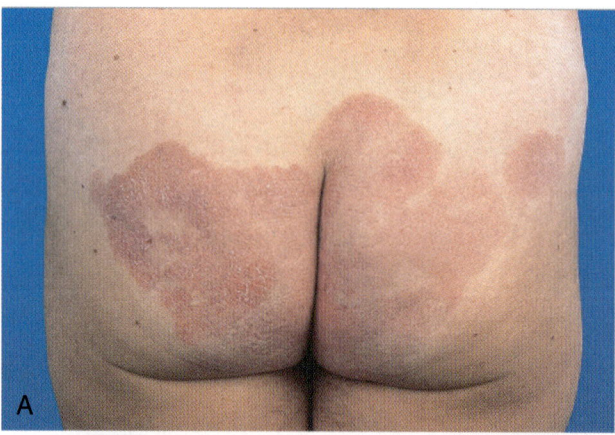
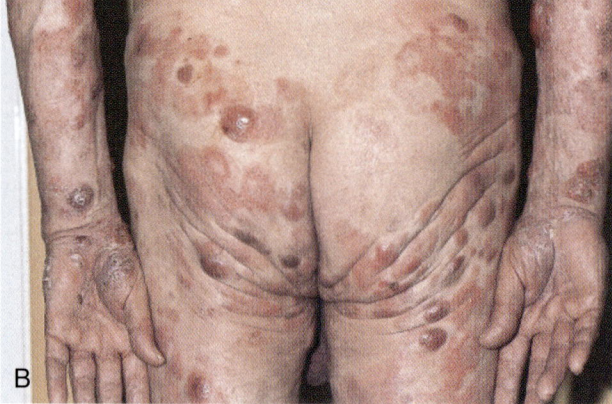

Fig. 59.44. Mycosis fungoides (a cutaneous T-cell lymphoma) involving the buttocks. (A) The limited plaque stage. (B) A more advanced case with plaques, patches, and tumors present. (From Bolognia JL, Jorizzo JL, Rapini RP: *Dermatology*, Edinburgh, 2003, Mosby.)

Chapter 59 Cutaneous Diseases of the External Genitalia 1303

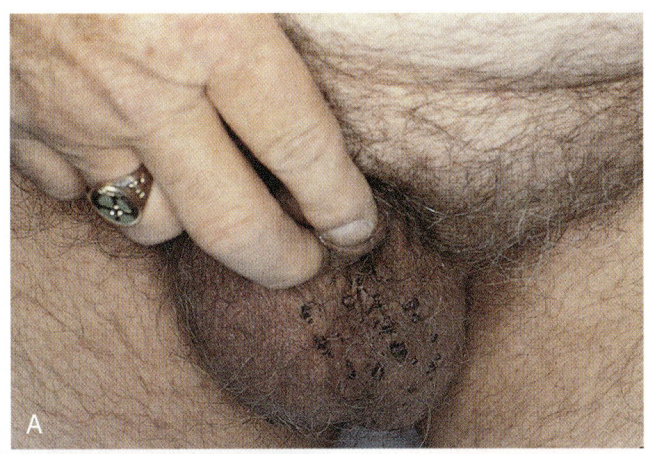
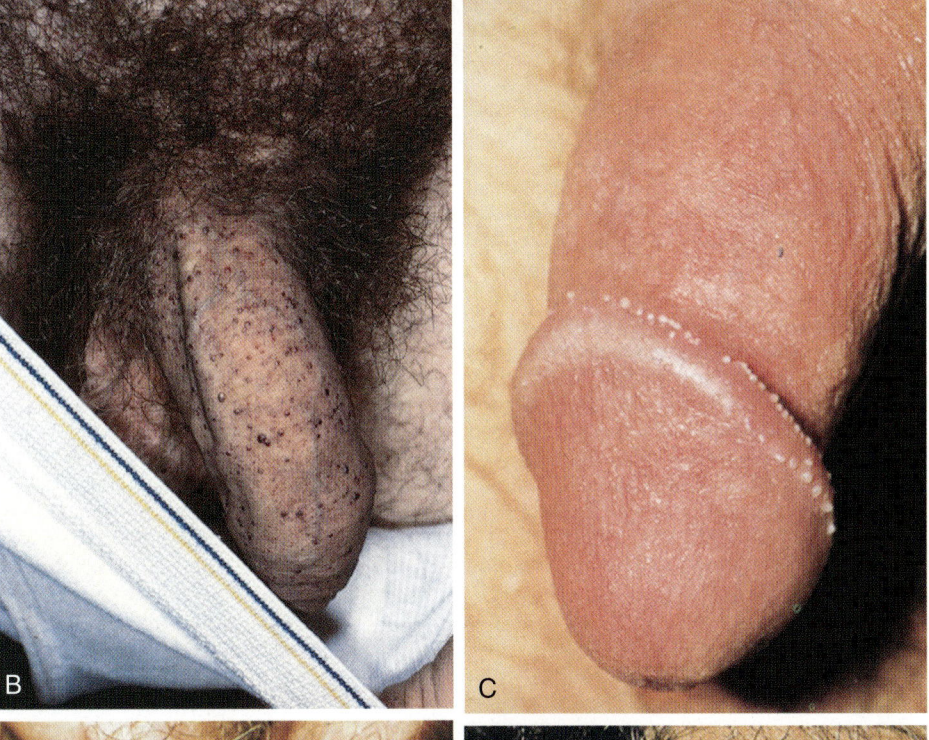
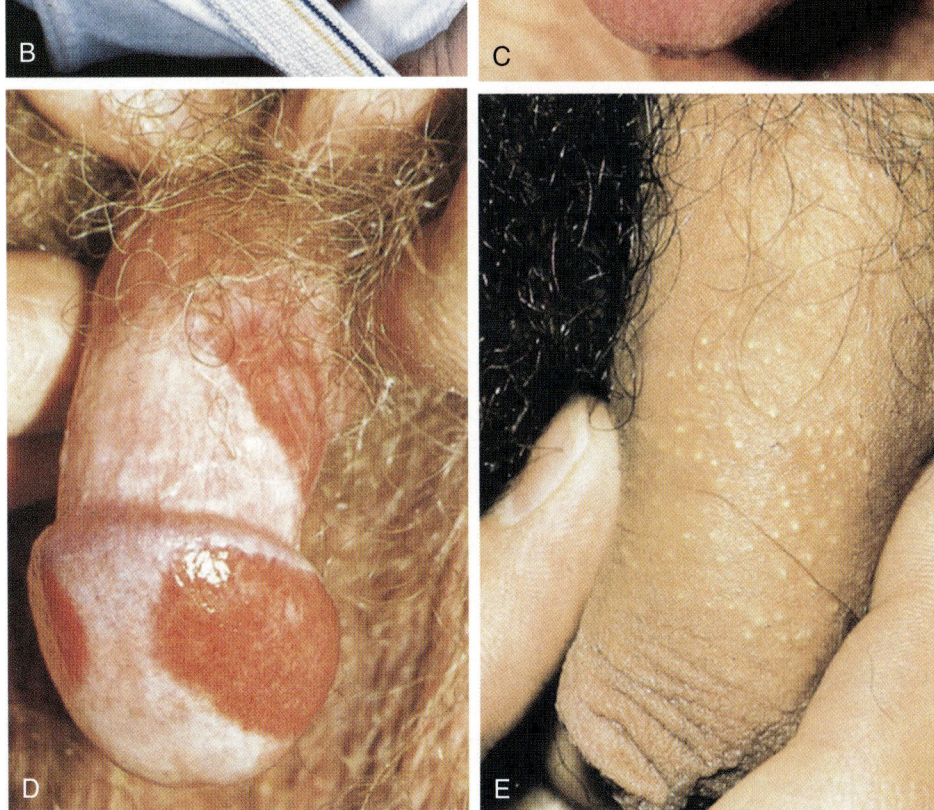

Fig. 59.45. Benign cutaneous disorders specific to the male genitalia. (A) Angiokeratoma of Fordyce showing purple scrotal vascular malformations. (B) Fabry disease: a glycogen storage deficiency with associated purple vascular malformations on the penile shaft. (C) Pearly penile papules located on the corona of the glans penis. (D) Zoon balanitis of the glans penis. (E) Ectopic sebaceous glands on the penile shaft. (A, B, and E, From Callen JP, Greer DE, Hood AF, et al.: *Color atlas of dermatology,* Philadelphia, 1993, Saunders. C and D, From Korting GW: *Practical dermatology of the genital region,* Philadelphia, 1981, Saunders.)

and adjacent penile skin (Gharpuray and Tolat, 1991; Rosen and Hwong, 2003). It is usually flesh colored but may occasionally be red. A mechanism related to thrombosis of lymphatic vessels has been proposed. There is an association with vigorous sexual activity, and resolution usually occurs within several weeks (Margolis, 2002; Sieunarine, 1987). Although somewhat controversial, a search for concomitant gonococcal and nongonococcal urethritis may be advisable in these cases.

Median Raphe Cysts

Median raphe cysts occur in young men on the ventral aspect of the penis, most commonly near the glans (Stone, 2003). Although these cysts are believed to develop from aberrant urethral epithelium, they do not communicate with the urethra (Asarch et al., 1979). Treatment is accomplished by surgical removal.

Ectopic Sebaceous Glands

Ectopic sebaceous glands on the penile shaft may be visible as pin-sized, flesh-colored papular lesions that may be mistaken for verruca (see Fig. 59.45E) (Margolis and Wein, 2002). There is no indication for treating these asymptomatic benign lesions and patient reassurance is sufficient.

COMMON MISCELLANEOUS CUTANEOUS DISORDERS

Skin Tag

Skin tags (acrochordons, fibroepithelial polyps) are soft, skin-colored, pedunculated lesions that can be present anywhere on the body but have a clear predilection for the neck, axillae, and inguinal folds. Although usually asymptomatic, these lesions may become painful secondary to local trauma or as a result of torsion and infarction in rare cases. These are common lesions, and up to 50% of all individuals may have at least one skin tag (Banik and Lubach, 1987). **It is important to distinguish these lesions from the hamartomatous skin lesions (multiple fibrofolliculomas) associated with Birt-Hogg-Dube syndrome, which are histologically distinct from common skin tags** (De la Torre et al., 1999). When skin tags cause either discomfort or cosmetic distress, they can easily be removed by snip excision and light electrocautery or chemical cautery with aluminum chloride applied to the base to achieve hemostasis. When a large number of skin tags appear at a relatively young age (<40), there may be an association with benign and malignant lower gastrointestinal tract polyposis, and gastroenterologic referral for endoscopy should be considered (Piette et al., 1988).

Epidermoid Cysts

Epidermoid or epidermal-inclusion cysts are the most common cutaneous cysts, and these lesions can be found anywhere on the body, including the genitalia. They are particularly common on the scrotum (see Fig. 59.46E). **The term "sebaceous cyst" should be avoided because the contents of these cysts are not sebaceous in origin** (Stone, 2003). Although not painful at baseline, rupture of the cyst wall can lead to a severe inflammatory reaction that is extremely painful. Definitive treatment requires surgical excision of the entire cyst wall to prevent cyst recurrence. Inflamed or superinfected epidermoid cysts may require incision and drainage and antibiotic therapy if there is adjacent cellulitis. Dystrophic calcification of scrotal epidermoid cysts may be a cause of scrotal calcinosis (Dare and Axelsen, 1988; Michl et al., 1994).

Seborrheic Keratosis

Seborrheic keratoses are very common beige to dark brown macules, plaques, and papules affecting individuals older than 30 years, and the incidence increases in frequency with advancing age. They are most common on the face, neck, and trunk although any body site except the palms, soles, and mucous membranes may be affected. The degree of pigmentation can vary significantly, and darker lesions may be confused with melanoma (Pierson et al., 2003). **These lesions have a waxy, "stuck-on" appearance (see Fig. 59.46D) and patients may note that they drop off spontaneously and then regrow** (Margolis, 2002). Treatment by shave excision or destruction with liquid nitrogen is usually performed for cosmetic reasons. **An abrupt increase in the size and number of multiple seborrheic keratoses has been termed the "Sign of Leser-Trelat" and has been implicated as a cutaneous marker of occult internal malignancy** (Chiba et al., 1996; Ginarte et al., 2001; Heaphy et al., 2000; Vielhauer et al., 2000).

Lentigo Simplex

Lentigo simplex is a condition characterized by the presence of brown-pigmented macules unrelated to sunlight exposure (Fig. 59.46A). These lesions can be found anywhere on the body, including the mucous membranes and nail beds. In the genital area (benign genital lentiginosis), these lesions present commonly on the labia, vaginal introitus, perineum, and glans penis (penile melanosis). The lesions of lentigo simplex are usually smaller than those seen in melanocytic nevi. Although usually benign, the lesions of lentigo simplex may deserve biopsy evaluation in cases demonstrating atypical shape or coloration. When present in a discontinuous manner at multiple sites, the diagnosis of genital melanoma becomes less likely compared with the probability of benign genital lentiginosis. **Finally, the combination of multiple pigmented lesions associated with intestinal polyposis should raise suspicion for Peutz-Jeghers syndrome.**

Mole (Nevus)

A mole or nevus of the skin is composed of slightly altered melanocytes called "nevus cells" arranged in a cluster. The location of the cluster determines the type of nevus. Junctional nevi are located between the epidermis and dermis and are usually flat, tan to black, small (<5 mm), and sharply bordered (Margolis, 2002). Intradermal nevi have clusters within the dermis and are usually small (<5 mm) and lighter in coloration, with sharp borders. Compound nevi have clusters in both locations and are usually darker and raised as a papule (Fig. 59.46B). As is the case for any pigmented lesion, marked irregularity in coloration or border and rapid morphologic change with time are indications for excisional biopsy to rule out dysplastic nevus or melanoma.

Dermatofibroma

Dermatofibromas are small hyperpigmented nodules that occur most commonly on the lower extremities and occasionally on the genitalia (see Fig. 59.46C). Pinching of these lesions causes a downward movement of the tumor (the so-called dimple sign) (Kamino and Pui, 2003). These are benign lesions with a characteristic histologic pattern of spindle-shaped fibroblasts and myofibroblasts arranged in fascicles. Treatment by surgical excision is usually unnecessary and may leave a scar that is cosmetically inferior to the original lesion (Kamino and Pui, 2003).

Neurofibroma

Neurofibromas are common tumors composed of neuromesenchymal tissue with residual nerve axons. They can be present anywhere on the body including the labia and scrotum (Kantarci et al., 2005; Mishra et al., 2002; Singh et al., 1992; Yoshimura et al., 1990). They are usually skin-colored, soft or rubbery nodules that may be pedunculated (Fig. 59.46F). **Digital pressure on the lesion causes invagination or so-called button-holing** (Habif, 2004). These can be solitary lesions or multiple, which should raise suspicion for neurofibromatosis or von Recklinghausen disease.

Capillary Hemangioma

Capillary hemangiomas are proliferations of blood vessels that are either present at birth or develop rapidly during the neonatal period.

Chapter 59 Cutaneous Diseases of the External Genitalia 1305

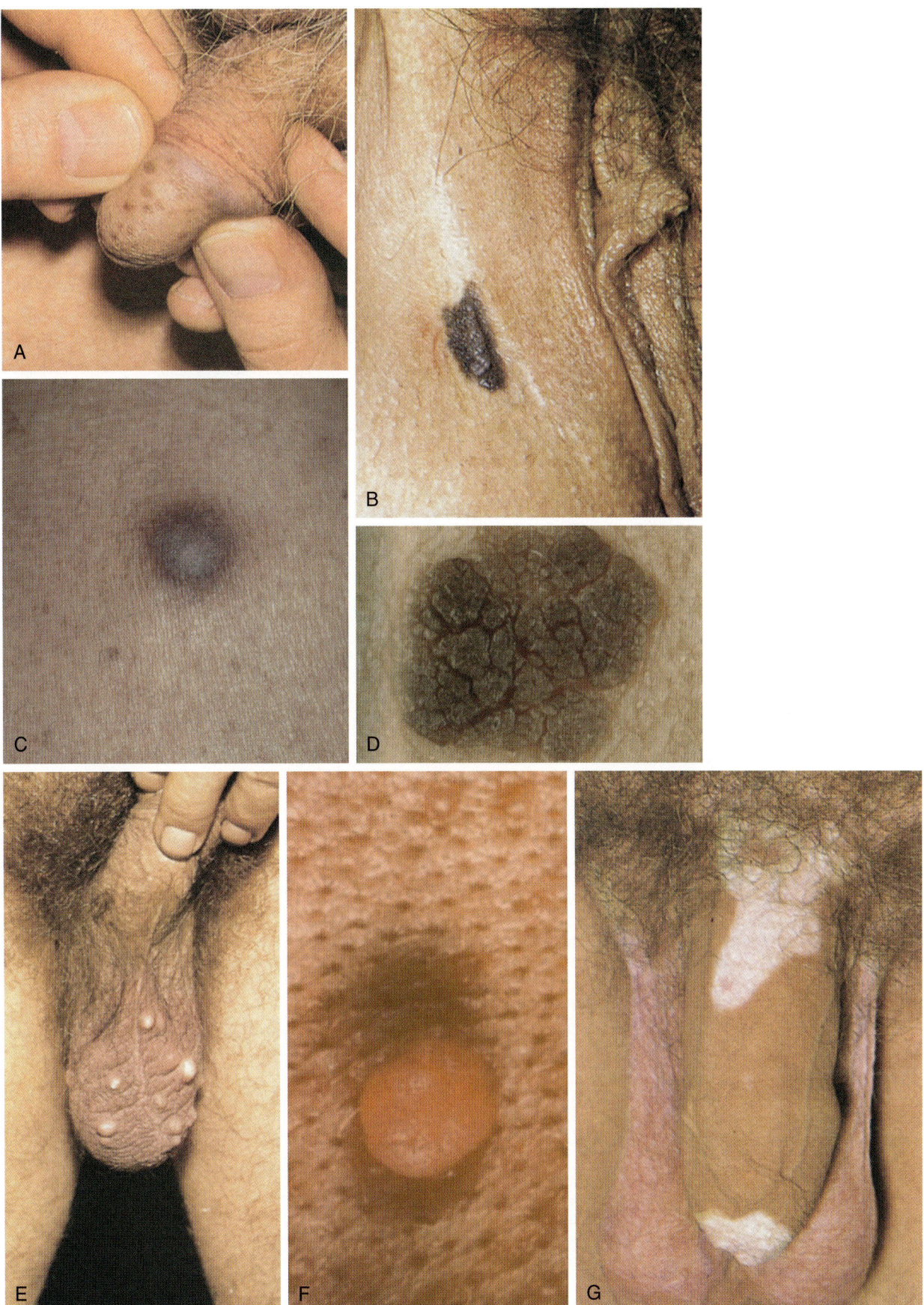

Fig. 59.46. Miscellaneous cutaneous disorders. (A) Lentigo simplex involving the glans penis (penile melanosis). (B) A compound melanocytic nevus in the inguinal crease. (C) A dermatofibroma on the lower extremity. (D) A characteristic seborrheic keratosis showing the "stuck-on" waxy appearance. (E) Epidermoid cysts of the scrotum. (F) Pedunculated neurofibroma. (G) Vitiligo involving the penile shaft. (A, B, E, and G, From Korting GW: *Practical dermatology of the genital region,* Philadelphia, 1981, Saunders. C, From Bolognia JL, Jorizzo JL, Rapini RP: *Dermatology,* Edinburgh, 2003, Mosby. D, From Habif TP: *Clinical dermatology,* Edinburgh, 2004, Mosby.)

These lesions can involve the anogenital region, can lead to bleeding, or can cause obstruction of the urethra, vagina, or anus (Roberts and Devine, 1983; Sharma et al., 1981). The majority will involute during childhood or early adolescence (Margolis, 2002). An innovation in the treatment of very large, persistent, and/or obstructive hemangiomas is the systemic administration of propranolol; because this treatment is not without some risk, it should be initiated and supervised by a clinician experienced with this modality (Izadpanah et al., 2013). Topical timolol therapy has also shown to be efficacious (Zheng and Li, 2018).

Vitiligo

Vitiligo is an acquired autoimmune disorder of the skin, leading to depigmentation, affecting 0.5% to 2% of the global population (Ortonne, 2003). It may occur at any age, and the precise pathogenesis of vitiligo remains a topic of intense research effort. Large patches of skin become completely amelanotic. Although the skin appears white, it is otherwise completely normal. The borders with unaffected skin are usually sharp and well defined (Fig. 59.46G). This condition is particularly noticeable in darker-skinned individuals and on body sites that are normally hyperpigmented. Vitiligo limited to the genitalia has been observed in less than 0.3% of the male population (Moss and Stevenson, 1981). Lesions have a tendency to enlarge circumferentially with time and may develop at sites of local trauma (Koebner phenomenon). Genital vitiligo must be differentiated from LS and postinflammatory hypopigmentation (Margolis, 2002). Wood's light can be used to accentuate vitiliginous areas. Treatments include temporary repigmentation with topical cosmetics, topical corticosteroids, topical calcipotriol (Vitamin D analogue), calcineurin inhibitor (pimecrolimus), ultraviolet light, PUVA therapy, and skin grafting. Use of the excimer laser to induce melanin production is particularly suited to the genitalia. **The diagnosis of vitiligo should prompt a screening for autoimmune thyroid disease.**

> ### KEY POINTS
> - The diagnosis of cutaneous diseases of the external genitalia depends critically on a thorough history and physical examination. Extragenital findings may provide the key to diagnosis. The urologist should perform a thorough skin survey and should not focus solely on the area of affected genital skin.
> - The side effects of topical corticosteroids are significant from systemic absorption and locally. Adverse effects may be worsened if these agents are applied under the foreskin, which may serve as an occlusive dressing. In general, when applied to genital skin, only low-potency topical corticosteroids should be used for short treatment courses.
> - Cutaneous disorders of the external genitalia can be broken down into the general categories of allergic, papulosquamous, vesicobullous, ulcerative, infectious, neoplastic, and miscellaneous diseases.
> - Histopathologic analysis of biopsy specimens plays an important role in differentiating cutaneous diseases with similar clinical features and in excluding malignancy.
> - Local treatment modalities including the use of laser energy, photodynamic therapy, ultraviolet radiation, and cryotherapy are being applied successfully to a variety of genital cutaneous disorders and offer an alternative to surgical excision in some cases.

SUGGESTED READINGS

Bhate K, Landeck L, Gonzalez E, et al: Genital contact dermatitis: a retrospective analysis, *Dermatitis* 21(6):317–320, 2010.
Bhattacharya M, Kaur I, Kumar B: Lichen planus: a clinical and epidemiological study, *J Dermatol* 27:576–582, 2000.
Bolognia JL, Schaffer JV, Cerroni L: *Dermatology*, 4th ed, Edinburgh, 2018, Elsevier.
Criteria for diagnosis of Behçet's disease. International Study Group for Behçet's Disease, *Lancet* 335:1078–1080, 1990.
Czymek R, Kujath P, Bruch HP, et al: Treatment, outcome and quality of life after Fournier's gangrene: a multicentre study, *Colorectal Dis* 15:1529–1536, 2013.
Denby KS, Beck LA: Update on systemic therapies for atopic dermatitis, *Curr Opin Allergy Clin Immunol* 12:421–426, 2012.
Eke N: Fournier's gangrene: a review of 1726 cases, *Br J Surg* 87:718–728, 2000.
Ellinghaus D, Baurecht H, Esparza-Gordillo J, et al: High-density genotyping study identifies four new susceptibility loci for atopic dermatitis, *Nat Genet* 45:808–812, 2013.
Hatemi G, Yazici Y, Yazici H: Behçet's syndrome, *Rheum Dis Clin North Am* 39:245–261, 2013.
Krueger G, Koo J, Lebwohl M, et al: The impact of psoriasis on quality of life: results of a 1998 National Psoriasis Foundation patient-membership survey, *Arch Dermatol* 137:280–284, 2001.
Leibovitch I, Huilgol SC, Selva D, et al: Cutaneous squamous carcinoma in situ (Bowen's disease): treatment with Mohs micrographic surgery, *J Am Acad Dermatol* 52:997–1002, 2005.
Mallon E, Hawkins D, Dinneen M, et al: Circumcision and genital dermatoses, *Arch Dermatol* 136:350–354, 2000.
Morpurgo E, Galandiuk S: Fournier's gangrene, *Surg Clin North Am* 82:1213–1224, 2002.
Rompel R, Petres J: Long-term results of wide surgical excision in 106 patients with hidradenitis suppurativa, *Dermatol Surg* 26:638–643, 2000.
Ruocco E, Wolf R, Ruocco V, et al: Pemphigus: associations and management guidelines: facts and controversies, *Clin Dermatol* 31:382–390, 2013.
Sanchez-Ortiz R, Huang SF, Tamboli P, et al: Melanoma of the penis, scrotum and male urethra: a 40-year single institution experience, *J Urol* 173:1958–1965, 2005.
Scheinfeld N: Hidradenitis suppurativa: a practical review of possible medical treatments based on over 350 hidradenitis patients, *Dermatol Online J* 19:1, 2013.
Stern RS, PUVA Follow-Up Study: The risk of squamous cell and basal cell cancer associated with psoralen and ultraviolet A therapy: a 30-year prospective study, *J Am Acad Dermatol* 66:553–562, 2012.
Wolf R, Orion E, Marcos B, et al: Life-threatening acute adverse cutaneous drug reactions, *Clin Dermatol* 23:171–181, 2005.
Wollenberg A, Bieber T: Atopic dermatitis: from the genes to skin lesions, *Allergy* 55:205–213, 2000.
Worswick S, Cotliar J: Stevens-Johnson syndrome and toxic epidermal necrolysis: a review of treatment options, *Dermatol Ther* 24:207–218, 2011.

REFERENCES

The complete reference list is available online at ExpertConsult.com.

60

Tuberculosis and Parasitic Infections of the Genitourinary Tract

Alicia H. Chang, MD, MS, Brian G. Blackburn, MD, and Michael Hsieh, MD, PhD

GENITOURINARY TUBERCULOSIS

Tuberculosis (TB) can affect any organ system of the body, including the genitourinary (GU) tract. **Untreated, GU TB can lead to irreparable tissue damage with serious consequences such as renal failure and infertility, making it critical for clinicians to consider TB in the differential diagnosis of GU disorders.** Described as the second "great imitator" (after syphilis; Sievers, 1961), TB can mimic many other diseases and complicate the correct diagnosis and treatment of infected patients. As TB becomes less common in industrialized nations, the diagnosis of GU TB increasingly relies on clinical recognition and a high index of suspicion.

History

Genomic analyses suggest that *Mycobacterium tuberculosis* coevolved with humans. Its early progenitor, *Mycobacterium prototuberculosis*, possibly infected early hominids more than 3 million years ago (Gutierrez et al., 2005). Bony lesions consistent with TB have been detected in a 500,000-year-old *Homo erectus* skeleton (Kappelman et al., 2008). The oldest microbiologic confirmation of *M. tuberculosis* infection in humans dates back to the Neolithic Period with use of DNA isolated from 9000-year-old skeletons of a woman and child found in a prehistoric site in the eastern Mediterranean (Hershkovitz et al., 2008). Microscopic and molecular findings of tubercle bacilli have been documented in Egyptian mummies from circa 3000 BCE (Nerlich et al., 1997; Zimmerman, 1979). Descriptions of TB can be found in written records of old civilizations from ancient East Asia, to New World cultures in the Americas, to Western hemisphere societies such as the Greeks and Romans, and continuing into modern history (Daniel, 2006). It was not until the 18th and 19th centuries, however, that TB reached epidemic proportions and ravaged Europe and North America. "Consumption," as it was known, was responsible for as many as 25% of deaths during the Industrial Age (Chalke, 1959). The turning point in the history of TB came on March 24, 1882, when Robert Koch famously presented to the scientific community the first successful isolation and identification of the tubercle bacillus (Sakula, 1982). In honor of Dr. Koch, March 24 has become World Tuberculosis Day.

Microbiology

TB is caused by a group of closely related acid-fast bacteria referred to as the *Mycobacterium tuberculosis* complex (MTBC). The complex includes species known to cause disease in only humans: *M. tuberculosis* and *Mycobacterium africanum*; species that cause disease in humans and other mammals: *Mycobacterium bovis*, *Mycobacterium canettii*, *Mycobacterium microti*, *Mycobacterium caprae*, *Mycobacterium orygis*, and *Mycobacterium pinnipedii*; and species that thus far have only been identified in animals: *Mycobacterium mungi* and *Mycobacterium suricattae* (Alexander et al., 2010; Coscolla et al., 2013; Parsons et al., 2013). **By far, the most frequently isolated species in human TB worldwide is *M. tuberculosis*, followed by *M. bovis*.** Local geographic differences exist, however, such as in West Africa, where *M. africanum* causes up to 40% of human TB cases (Yeboah-Manu et al., 2017). The species *M. tuberculosis*, however, has become synonymous with TB and is often inaccurately used to represent the entire complex. The species in the complex that infect humans cause clinically indistinguishable disease, but drug susceptibility patterns may differ among them. *M. bovis*, for example, has innate resistance to pyrazinamide, which is one of the first-line agents against *M. tuberculosis*.

Epidemiology

The World Health Organization (WHO) 2013 estimates that one-quarter of the world's population is infected with MTBC in its latent form. In 2016 there were 10.4 million new cases of active TB disease and 1.7 million deaths from TB worldwide, a continued decline since the year 2000. TB mortality has fallen by 45% since 1990 (WHO, 2016). However, different obstacles in TB control remain. These include medical conditions that promote resurgence of TB such as the human immunodeficiency virus (HIV) epidemic in sub-Saharan Africa and the rapid increase in obesity and diabetes worldwide. The increase of multidrug and extensive drug resistance also compromises TB control.

In the United States, there were 9272 reported cases of active TB in 2016 (2.9 per 100,000 persons). TB incidence in the United States has been steadily declining since its resurgence in the 1980s and its peak in 1992. In the United States, TB disproportionately affects non–US-born persons. In 2016 the incidence among non–US-born individuals was 14 times higher than among US-born persons (Centers for Disease Control and Prevention [CDC], 2017).

The frequency of GU involvement among patients who develop TB varies significantly depending on the population studied. **More than 90% of GU TB cases occur in developing countries, where the frequency approaches 15% to 20% of patients with pulmonary TB. In contrast, the frequency of GU TB in developed countries is 2% to 10% of patients with pulmonary TB** (Figueiredo and Lucon, 2008). In the developing world, the GU tract is the second most common extrapulmonary site after lymph nodes (Wong et al., 2013). **In the United States, GU TB is the third most common form after pleural and lymphatic TB and is found in 27% of extrapulmonary** cases (Daher et al., 2013). Approximately two-thirds of those affected are men. GU TB is generally a disease of adults, although it has been reported in children as young as 2 years of age (Merchant et al., 2013).

Infection, Host Immune Response, and Transmission

The initial mode of entry of MTBC into the host is via inhalation of cough-generated infectious aerosols, although there are reported cases of direct inoculation of MTBC into soft tissues (Angus et al., 2001). Once the bacilli reach the alveoli, they are phagocytosed by alveolar macrophages. In some persons, MTBC organisms are killed by the macrophages at this point and effectively cleared from the body. These persons do not develop infection nor an adaptive immune response (Walzl et al., 2011). In others, MTBC bacilli escape killing, begin to replicate within macrophages, and establish infection. Up to 12 weeks may pass before a cellular immune response is detectable (Dannenberg, 1994), and before this development, the tubercle bacilli can spread through the lymphatics to the hilar lymph nodes and ultimately through the bloodstream to seed distant organs.

The host attempts to contain MTBC infection by forming granulomas. Infected macrophages secrete inflammatory cytokines, such as interleukin-6 (IL-6), IL-12, IL-1β, and tumor necrosis factor-α (TNF-α) and recruit a variety of immune cells to surround them. Foamy macrophages, epithelioid cells, and multinucleated giant cells (Langhans cells) cluster to the center of the granuloma and are surrounded by a cuff of lymphocytes (Silva et al., 2012). Antigen processing and presentation lead to T-cell activation and the mounting of an adaptive cellular response against MTBC (Schluger R et al., 1998). T cells secrete cytokines such as IL-2, TNF-α, and most important, interferon-γ (IFN-γ) to maintain the granuloma and to induce killing of the infected macrophages and the infectious bacilli. When killing is not achieved, the granuloma can still successfully sequester viable tubercle bacilli, which stop replicating and become dormant. In 90% to 95% of persons, TB is controlled at this point and enters what has historically been considered as latency (Boom et al., 2003). Latent TB is marked by cicatrization and granuloma calcification. In fewer than 5% of infected persons the initial infection fails to be controlled and progresses within the year to active TB disease (primary progression). After latency is established, MTBC can resurface years later to cause reactivation TB. The process of reactivation is not well understood. The development of some conditions such as old age, renal failure, diabetes mellitus, malnutrition, HIV infection, and other causes of immune suppression shifts the balance between host and pathogen in favor of the pathogen. A series of events then occur that lead to renewed bacillary replication and release, granuloma caseation (the characteristic lesion of TB), and reactivation. **The lifetime risk of reactivation TB is estimated at 5% to 15%, although the risk is higher in patients with the medical comorbidities mentioned previously.** Once TB reactivates, the patient can then generate infectious respiratory aerosols that are breathed in by close contacts. In general, those with exclusively extrapulmonary disease, such as GU TB, are not considered infectious, although transmission by direct skin inoculation or other aerosol producing procedures from infected fluids and tissues can occur. **The two forms of TB described—latent TB infection and active TB disease—represent a simplification of what is now understood to be a spectrum; a dynamic continuum between contained TB infection, subclinical TB disease, and progressively infectious TB disease.** An individual who has acquired TB can move forward and backward along this spectrum through his or her lifetime, depending on changes in host immunity such as imparted by medical comorbidities or changes in the bacilli such as imparted by treatment for latent TB infection (Pai et al., 2016).

Development of Genitourinary Disease

There are four means by which GU TB develops. The principal route is via hematogenous spread of MTBC. Clinical disease may occur soon after bacilli reach the GU system, or they may enter a period of latency before becoming clinically active (Figueiredo and Lucon, 2008; Patterson et al., 2012). Typically, GU TB becomes evident after a prolonged latency, ranging up to 46 years (Christensen, 1974; Narayana, 1982). Hematogenous seeding may localize to only the GU tract or widely disseminate to multiple organ systems. The typical sites for GU seeding are the kidneys and epididymis. Other organs of the GU tract become infected via contiguous spread from these initial landing sites.

Ascending or retrograde infection through the urinary system is the second route of infection, albeit significantly less common than hematogenous spread. This is the case in GU TB after bladder irrigation with bacille Calmette-Guérin (BCG) for the treatment of bladder cancer. BCG is a live, attenuated vaccine derived from *M. bovis*, a member of the *M. tuberculosis* complex. Although rare, GU TB complicates 0.9% of patients receiving BCG irrigation (Lamm et al., 1992). Cases described include pyelonephritis, renal abscesses, ureteric obstruction, cystitis, prostatitis, and epididymo-orchitis (Demers and Pelsser, 2012; Parker and Kommu, 2013; Squires et al., 1999).

Rarely, TB can also reach the GU system via contiguous spread from other organ systems or direct inoculation. TB is one of the few infectious diseases that does not respect anatomic boundaries. Extension of TB from the spine, psoas, and to the kidneys has been described (Kothari et al., 2001). Similarly, gastrointestinal (GI) TB can extend into the GU tract to form enterorenal and enterovesical fistulae (Merchant, et al., 2013; Ney and Friedenberg, 1981). Direct inoculation is exceedingly rare. Cases include autoinoculation of external genitalia from infected stool or urine, and person-to-person genital inoculation after contact with infected genital or oral lesions (Angus et al., 2001).

Clinical Manifestations and Pathologic Features

Symptoms and signs of GU TB are often nonspecific. Patients are often treated for other bacterial infections (sometimes repeatedly) or are evaluated for possible malignancy before GU TB is entertained. Symptoms correlate with the severity and location of disease. Renal TB, for example, can be progressive and destructive but symptomatically silent until it extends into the bladder. In developed countries, where patients with TB tend to seek medical attention earlier in the disease process, 8.4% of GU TB patients are asymptomatic (Figueiredo and Lucon, 2008). **The typical TB constitutional symptoms of fever, weight loss, night sweats, and malaise are present in fewer than 20% of patients** (Simon et al., 1977). Up to 50% of patients with GU TB have only dysuria on presentation, 50% have storage symptoms, and 33% have hematuria and flank pain (Figueiredo and Lucon, 2008). Renal colic occurs in fewer than 10% of patients, and corresponds to the passage of necrotic papillary tissue, clots, stones, and caseous phlegmon in patients with severe pyelonephritis (Eastwood et al., 2001; Simon et al., 1977). Typical laboratory findings include sterile pyuria and/or hematuria. **This combination is found in more than 90% of GU TB patients in developing countries.**

Kidney

Eighty percent of GU TB occurs in the kidney (Wong et al., 2013; Yadav et al., 2017). Renal infection is progressive and highly destructive over time. The pathological findings in the kidney vary greatly depending on disease severity.

The most insidious lesions are found in patients with pulmonary TB and renal failure, with or without pyuria, who have no changes visible on imaging of the GU tract. In these patients, kidney biopsies reveal TB-induced granulomatous interstitial nephritis (Ram et al., 2011). Renal histology shows granulomas, which are sometimes caseating. In some patients, treatment reverses the associated renal insufficiency (Eastwood et al., 2001). Other microscopic changes in the kidney include glomerulonephritis from immune complex deposition or amyloidosis secondary to TB (Sun et al., 2012). In these cases, the kidneys are collateral damage of pulmonary or systemic disease.

When renal infection is the outcome of widely disseminated TB in multiple organ systems, hematogenous spread of high number of bacilli leads to innumerable small (3-mm), pale clumps of granulomas that look like scattered millet seeds on gross pathological examination of the kidney. This form of disseminated TB is known as *miliary TB* and carries a high mortality. In the kidney, the "milia" can be found studding the renal cortex and medulla and do not usually affect renal function (Eastwood et al., 2001).

In more localized infection of the kidney, tubercle bacilli become lodged first in the periglomerular capillaries. Granulomas form in the renal parenchyma and coalesce. When they caseate, cavities with necrotic material form. These can result in frank abscesses, chronic pyelonephritis, and parenchymal and papillary necrosis. Sinus tracts may emerge along the flanks (Bhatt and Lodha, 2012; Patterson et al., 2012). Examination findings at this stage can include costovertebral angle tenderness (Gokce et al., 2002). As infection advances, the calyces become inflamed and eventually calcify, resulting in calyceal distortion, dilation, and stenosis (Merchant et al., 2013a).

With enough disease progression, the kidney becomes nonfunctional, a process called *autonephrectomy* (Teo and Wee, 2011). This complication is present in up to 33% of patients with GU TB. There are two types of autonephrectomy. The first is the caseocavernous type, in which viable tissue is replaced with granulomas and cavities filled with inflammatory exudate. This type of autonephrectomy occurs with and without calcification. The second type is fibrotic, with severe scarring and calcification resulting in a shrunken kidney (Fischmann, 1951).

End-stage renal failure develops in approximately 7% of cases (Figueiredo and Lucon, 2008). Chronic inflammation may lead to squamous metaplasia in the renal pelvis that persists after treatment, posing a risk for squamous cell carcinoma (Byrd et al., 1976).

Ureter

TB in the ureters occurs via descent of infection from the kidneys. As bacilli pass in the urine through the ureter, granulomas can form along the walls. Infected calculi can also descend and lodge in the ureters. The ensuing inflammation leads to scarring and strictures, commonly in the distal end of the ureter at the vesicoureteral junction (Patterson et al., 2012). Strictures can also occur throughout the ureter in a "pan-ureteral" fashion, leading to a "beaded corkscrew" appearance (Wong et al., 2013). When ureters are distorted from scarring, obstruction and urinary reflux can develop (Eastwood et al., 2001). **Urinary obstruction resulting from strictures is an important cause of renal failure in GU TB** (Carl and Stark, 1997).

Bladder

Descending infection to the bladder usually begins near the ureteral orifices and spreads along the lymphatics to other areas. Similar to TB in the ureters, bacilli implant in the urothelium and cause a patchy cystitis. Ulcerations may develop in areas where large granulomas coalesce. The dome of the bladder is the most affected, whereas the trigone and neck usually remain normal. Mucosal inflammation, friability, and hematuria follow (Wong et al., 2013). After approximately a year of chronic inflammation and mucosal scarring, bladder contracture develops (Singh et al., 2013). Urinary frequency, urgency, pain, and dysuria become prominent when bladder capacity shrinks to less than 100 mL. The severely contracted "thimble" bladder typically has a capacity of less than 20 mL. Bladder contraction is a late complication of GU TB and is more common in the developing world (12% vs. 4% of GU cases in developed countries), where diagnosis occurs after disease is more advanced (Figueiredo and Lucon, 2008).

Epididymis, Vas Deferens, Testes, and Scrotum

The epididymis, the second most common GU site of hematogenous seeding after the kidney, is involved in 10% to 55% of GU TB patients. Infection is bilateral in 34%. The disease initially affects the more vascular globus minor. Granulomas in the epididymal epithelium elicit chronic inflammation leading to fibrous narrowing and obliteration of the lumen. With disease progression, large caseous granulomas result in a nodular epididymis. On examination, the epididymis may appear swollen or hardened (Fraietta et al., 2003). Granulomas may adhere to the overlying skin, ulcerate, and in up to 50% of patients, a tuberculous sinus tract develops on the posterior surface of the scrotum (Ferreira et al., 2011). After the infection spreads to the vas deferens, it becomes thickened and beaded on examination as a result of nodular scarring (Kulchavenya et al., 2012).

Isolated epididymis or testicular infections are rare but have been described (Kho and Chan 2012; Shenoy et al., 2012). More commonly, epididymal TB extends into the testes. Granulomas form within the seminiferous tubular epithelium as well as in the connective tissue of the testis. Eventually, normal tissue becomes replaced with granulomatous tissue and fibrosis. The hardened masses that develop mimic testicular tumors. Approximately 5% of patients develop hydrocele.

Prostate and Seminal Vesicles

The prostate is infected via either hematogenous spread or urinary contamination and is involved in 22% to 49% of GU TB patients (Yadav et al., 2017). With hematogenous spread, prostatic lesions can be found in the periphery with sparing of the urethra. Disease then remains asymptomatic and progresses to calcification and gland hardening. Infection via the urinary route often involves the urethra and manifests more like bacterial prostatitis. Prostatic nodules or fluctuation may be palpated on examination. **TB should be suspected in patients with chronic prostatitis that persists despite antibiotics. Quinolones used to treat routine bacterial prostatitis are also active against MTBC. However, the shorter courses used for bacterial prostatitis are not sufficient for TB prostatitis, and the symptoms will not resolve or will quickly recur.** Prostatic abscesses are rare but do occur, particularly in acquired immunodeficiency syndrome (AIDS) patients (Figueiredo and Lucon, 2008).

TB of the seminal vesicles may cause infertility, which can be the first symptom of GU TB (Lubbe et al., 1996). The bacilli reach the seminal vesicles through the vas deferens in cases of TB of the testis or epididymis or through the urethra and ejaculatory ducts in cases of TB of the kidneys, bladder, or prostate. Granulomas develop in the walls of the seminal vesicles, and the lumen may be filled by caseation. Eventually calcification ensues. Patients may have low-volume ejaculate, oligospermia, azoospermia, or hemospermia. TB can rarely cause seminal vesicle abscesses (Eastham et al., 1999). Physical examination may reveal enlarged seminal vesicles in early disease or hardened nodules in advanced disease.

Urethra and Penis

The urethra appears somewhat resistant to TB infection and is involved in only 1.9% to 4.5% of GU TB cases. It is typically associated with prostate infection and can occur with urethroscrotal fistulae. Isolated urethral TB is very rare but has been reported (Bouchikhi et al., 2013). Similarly, primary TB in the penis is exceedingly rare. Penile lesions begin on the skin as an inflamed papule or a keratotic plaque (also known as lupus vulgaris). The lesions then ulcerate and spread to the cavernous tissue. Pea-sized nodules can be felt in the cavernous bodies and urethra corresponding to coalescing granulomas. These nodules can be painless and hard or appear as a fungating mass. Both presentations can mimic malignancy. When fibrosis develops, the penis can become distorted or the patient can experience erectile dysfunction (Angus et al., 2001; Gupta et al., 2008; Kar and Kar, 2012; Yadav et al., 2017).

Orificial TB, a rapidly necrotic form of penile TB, has also been reported (Ramesh and Vasanthi, 1989). It has been described in immunocompromised or severely debilitated patients. It arises from autoinoculation of the penile skin with infected stool or urine from the patient or rarely from hematogenous or lymphatic spread (Wilkinson et al., 2010). Painful ulcers coated with pseudomembrane appear and can erode into deeper structures (Chen et al., 2000). Orificial TB is a presentation of very advanced and severe TB elsewhere in the GU or GI tract and carries a poor prognosis.

An exceedingly rare form of penile TB is papulonecrotic tuberculid (PNT) (Dandale et al., 2013). This is a cutaneous manifestation of TB on the glans penis and can occur in other skin areas as well. PNT of the penis has been described in Japan, South Africa, and India. The tuberculids are red papules that erupt on the skin, ulcerate, and undergo varioliform scarring. Unlike primary TB of the penis, these ulcers can be painless and do not contain tubercle bacilli. The tuberculids are hypersensitivity reactions to MTBC antigens that were disseminated to the skin from other infectious foci, and as such they are culture negative and typically polymerase chain reaction (PCR) negative. Histology is often inconclusive; mature granulomas are not always seen. The recurrent lesions are easily confused with syphilis, Behçet disease, recurrent herpes simplex, balanitis, and squamous cell carcinoma. Recognizing this entity is the first step in diagnosis, and response to empirical TB treatment despite negative cultures confirms it.

Diagnosis

In developed countries, the primary goal of the diagnostic workup is isolation of MTBC in culture for drug susceptibility testing. In the right clinical context, tissue samples demonstrating caseating granulomas can support a diagnosis of TB when cultures or DNA tests are negative. Absent those, diagnosis of patients with GU TB relies on the constellation of consistent clinical findings in a patient with probable exposure and response to empirical medical

treatment. Because up to 20% of GU TB occurs concurrently with pulmonary TB (Figueiredo and Lucon, 2008), **it is useful to also assess for the presence of pulmonary disease.**

Culture

The current gold standard for the diagnosis of GU TB is urine acid-fast bacilli (AFB) culture. First-void urine is the best sample because urine is the most concentrated at that time. Three to five urine samples on consecutive days should be collected for maximum yield. These should be cultured immediately after collection because prolonged exposure to urine acidity can retard mycobacterial growth (American Thoracic Society, 2000). The sensitivity of urine AFB cultures is as high as 80% to 90% when done in this manner (Lewinsohn et al., 2017). Real-world practice, however, compounded by sporadic shedding of bacilli into urine, leads to sensitivity as low as 10% (Abbara and Davidson, 2011). Ziehl-Neelsen stains can be done on the urine as well, but the sensitivity is less than 50%. In addition, any tissue obtained from biopsy or surgery should also be cultured.

M. tuberculosis complex has traditionally been cultured on solid, egg-based, Lowenstein-Jensen (LJ) medium. This method is laborious and time consuming; usually 4 to 6 weeks are required before growth of MTBC can be detected. LJ remains the medium of choice in developing countries because it is the least expensive and requires no specialized equipment. In developed countries, urine is cultured on more expensive, agar-based, transparent, solid media such as Middlebrook 7H10. With this medium, colonies can be visualized approximately 1 week earlier than with LJ media. Liquid-based detection systems such as the BACTEC Mycobacteria Growth Indicator Tube (MGIT) are also used in the developed world. The MGIT is a fully automated system that uses fluorescence quenching to detect mycobacterial growth in as little as 10 days. Current guidelines recommend culturing on at least one solid medium concurrently with the liquid system to maximize yield (American Thoracic Society, 2000). Other available detection methods include semiautomated systems that use radiometric liquid culture. Antibiotic susceptibility can be tested using any of the culture methods described earlier. Typically, susceptibility to first-line TB drugs is tested "in house" using the MGIT instrument. Susceptibility testing for second-line TB drugs is generally performed only at reference laboratories.

Nucleic Acid Amplification Tests

Several nucleic acid amplification tests (NAATs) have been developed to speed the detection of MTBC, providing results within 1 to 2 days. NAATs can aid detection of MTBC in patients with low bacillary load, in whom culture may fail to isolate the organisms. However, nonrespiratory specimens such as urine contain natural inhibitors that interfere with the DNA or RNA amplification process, potentially lowering test sensitivity (Chawla et al., 2012; Mehta et al., 2012; Moussa et al., 2000). The sensitivity of PCR tests for GU TB depends on the type of specimen tested, the sequence amplification used, and the specific amplification protocol. Assays using the MTBC repetitive IS6110 insertion sequence and those using nested PCR techniques perform better than those amplifying 16S-rRNA (Moussa et al., 2000). Differences in test performance exist between NAAT assays that are commercially developed, automated, or in-house "home-brew" tests.

Since 2010, the newest commercial NAAT assay on the market, the GeneXpert MTB/RIF also provides molecular detection of rifampin drug resistance simultaneously with MTBC detection. The system is self-contained and automates sputum processing, DNA extraction, and amplification. Because more than 90% of rifampin-resistant strains are also isoniazid-resistant, rifampin resistance serves as a surrogate marker for multidrug-resistant TB (MDR-TB), defined as resistance to isoniazid and rifampin (Ioannidis et al., 2011).

Systematic review of the use of various NAATs in urinary tract TB patients indicate sensitivity ranging from 70% to 100%, although studies were small and heterogeneous and produced estimates with wide confidence intervals. The pooled sensitivity of GeneXpert MTB/RIF in urine samples ranged from 83% to 95% and specificity of 79% to 99% when compared with urine AFB culture (Altez-Fernandez et al., 2017). Sensitivity of NAAT on epididymal biopsy tissue was 87.5% in one study (Chawla et al., 2012).

In the United States, NAATs are recommended as an adjunct in the evaluation of GU TB but should not replace culture for diagnosis. They should also not be used to exclude extrapulmonary TB because there are insufficient high-quality studies to confirm sensitivity of the assays (Lewinsohn et al., 2017). In developing countries, the cost of NAATs and the need for expensive equipment have been obstacles, although the WHO recommends GeneXpert MTB/RIF as part of the initial workup of all patients with TB (2013). Unlike cultures, NAATs cannot be used to monitor response to treatment because nucleic acids are shed from dead organisms and tests can remain positive despite adequate treatment (American Thoracic Society, 2000).

Histopathology

Because urine AFB cultures in GU TB are sometimes negative, tissue biopsy can help establish a diagnosis of GU TB (Kulchavenya et al., 2013). Although mycobacteria are often not seen in the tissue, the finding of caseating granulomas and the appropriate clinical context can help establish a diagnosis of GU TB. Histopathology shows findings consistent with TB in 38.3% of GU TB cases in developed countries and 21.9% of cases globally. In patients with epididymal nodules, fine-needle aspiration cytology can provide a diagnosis in 67.5%. Adding a TB NAAT can further augment diagnostic sensitivity to tissue specimens (Yadav et al., 2017).

Screening Tests

The tuberculin skin test (TST) and interferon-gamma release assays (IGRAs) do not differentiate between latent infection and active TB disease. They have limited utility in the diagnosis of active disease, although they are widely used and approved by the US Food and Drug Administration (FDA) for this purpose. A positive test cannot rule in TB disease, and a negative test cannot rule it out. The ideal use for these tests is in the screening of individuals for the presence of TB infection. **Of the two types of tests, IGRAs are currently recommended as the preferred method to screen persons 5 years or older born in TB-endemic countries, although TST is still an acceptable alternative** (Lewinsohn et al., 2017).

Tuberculin Skin Test, Purified Protein Derivative, Mantoux Test. The TST evaluates the presence of an existing cellular immune response to MTBC antigens, which should be present in persons who have been infected. Tuberculin is a sterile suspension of protein extracted from cultures of *M. tuberculosis* and is injected intradermally into the volar aspect of the forearm. After 48 to 72 hours, delayed-type hypersensitivity will cause induration at the site of injection in those with prior immune priming. The CDC guidelines for interpretation of a positive test depend on the risk factors of the patient. Three distinct cut-points for positivity have been defined according to risk. For persons with recent contact with a patient with TB, with fibrotic changes on chest radiograph that are consistent with prior TB, or who are immunosuppressed, 5 mm or more of induration is positive. For immigrants from high prevalence countries, residents of or workers in high-risk institutions, injection drug users, and persons with medical comorbidities that increase risk of active TB, 10 mm or more of induration is positive. For the general public, 15 mm or more is positive (Table 60.1; Lewinsohn et al., 2017).

Although initial training of personnel in test placement and interpretation is necessary, the TST has some advantages. It is cheap, does not require a laboratory, and is easy to perform. The main disadvantage is that the TST is not specific for MTBC. Vaccination with BCG and infection with nontuberculous mycobacteria may elicit a positive reaction. In addition, the TST requires a second visit from the patient for test reading, which can be difficult to ensure. False-negative results can occur in 10% to 25% of persons with active TB (Huebner et al., 1993). In one study, the TST result was positive in 85% to 95% of patients with GU TB (Figueiredo and Lucon, 2008).

TABLE 60.1 Guidelines for Determining a Positive Tuberculin Skin Test Reaction

INDURATION ≥5 mm	INDURATION ≥10 mm	INDURATION >15 mm
• HIV-positive persons • Silicosis • Fibrotic changes on chest radiograph consistent with old TB • Patients with organ transplants • Immunosuppressed therapy (receiving the equivalent of > 15 mg/d prednisone for ≥ 1 month, or TNF-α antagonists) • Recent contacts of person with TB disease • Children < 5 years of age	• Immigrants from high-prevalence countries (TB incidence >20/100,000) • Residents and employees[a] of high-risk congregate settings: prisons and jails, nursing homes and other health care facilities, residential facilities for AIDS patients, and homeless shelters • Mycobacteriology laboratory personnel • Persons with clinical conditions that make them high risk: silicosis diabetes mellitus, chronic renal failure, some hematologic disorders (e.g., leukemias and lymphomas), other specific malignancies (e.g., carcinoma of the head or neck and lung), weight loss of >10% of ideal body weight, gastrectomy, jejunoileal bypass • Injection drug users	• Persons with no risk factors for TB

[a]For persons who are otherwise at low risk and are tested at entry into employment, a reaction of >15 mm induration is considered positive.
From Lewinsohn DM, Leonard MK, LoBue PA, et al.: Official American Thoracic Society/Infectious Diseases Society of America/Centers for Disease Control and Prevention clinical practice guidelines: diagnosis of tuberculosis in adults and children. *Clin Infect Dis.* 64(2): 111-115, 2017.
AIDS, Acquired immunodeficiency syndrome; *HIV,* Human immunodeficiency virus; *TB,* tuerculosis; *TNF-α,* tumor necrosis factor-alpha.

Interferon-Gamma Release Assays. IGRAs are blood tests that measure the level of IFN-α (a surrogate of cellular immune reactivity) produced in response to MTBC-specific antigens, akin to an in vitro MTBC-specific TST. Persons infected with MTBC have circulating T cells that quickly recognize MTBC antigens and secrete IFN-α upon re-exposure. The antigens used in IGRAs are absent from all BCG strains and most nontuberculous mycobacteria, and thus exposure to these organisms does not result in a positive IGRA. Results are available after 24 hours.

There are two IGRAs available in the United States, the Quanti-FERON (QFT) and the. The QFT assay has undergone several iterations and in 2017, the fourth-generation assay T-SPOT.TB test was introduced to the market, the QFT-Plus. In the QFT-Plus, whole blood is collected in four specialized test tubes: one containing the MTBC antigens ESAT-6, CFP-10; one containing proprietary MTBC antigens that activate CD8 T cells; and two controls (negative and positive). The blood is incubated directly in the collection tubes for 16 to 24 hours. Plasma is then separated and IFN-α is measured using enzyme-linked immunosorbent assay (ELISA). Test results are read as positive, negative, or indeterminate, based on the level of IFN-α produced in relation to the negative and positive controls.

In the T-SPOT.TB assay, peripheral blood mononuclear cells (PBMCs) are separated from whole blood and then incubated with ESAT-6 and CFP-10 in wells coated with antibodies that capture IFN-α. Enzyme-linked immunospot (ELISPOT) assay is used to detect an increase in the number of cells (appearing as spots in each test well) that secrete IFN-α in relation to a negative control. Spots are manually counted, and the test is read as positive, negative, or borderline. Despite the increased difficulty of performing T-SPOT.TB over QFT, it is the more sensitive test. Pooled studies estimate a sensitivity of 83% for third-generation QFT and 91% for T-SPOT.TB, versus 89% for TST in cases of for culture-confirmed TB (Mazurek et al., 2010). Pooled studies of the fourth-generation QFT are currently being undertaken.

Radiography

GU TB generates a wide spectrum of imaging findings. The test of choice depends on disease location and should be driven by symptoms and other clinical data. Imaging is often the first test that indicates TB is the cause of a GU disorder.

Plain Radiography. The kidney-ureter-bladder (KUB) radiograph frequently demonstrates calcifications caused by TB, which are present

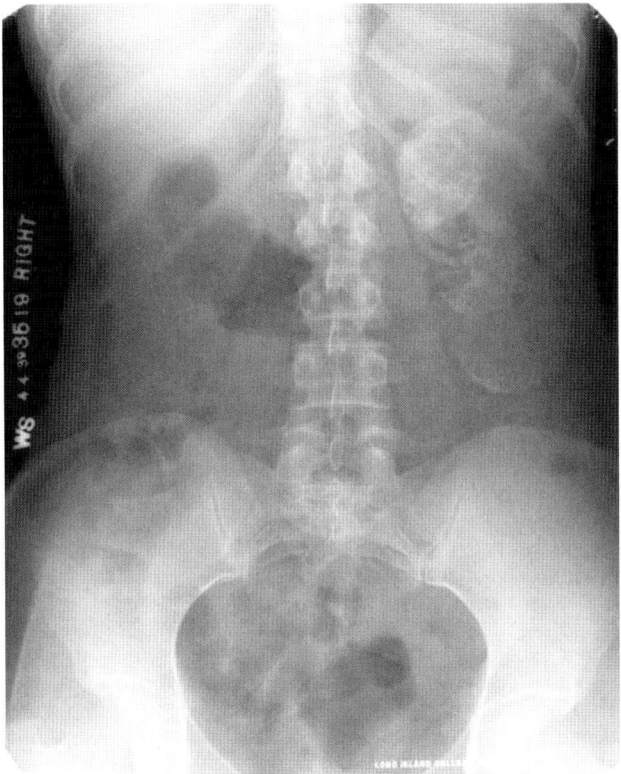

Fig. 60.1. Kidney-ureter-bladder radiographic view in a patient with left renal tuberculosis with associated calcifications.

in more than 50% of patients (Merchant et al., 2013a). Initial renal lesions may appear as faint punctate calcifications within the parenchyma. As TB progresses, the KUB film may show globular calcifications that correspond to a tubercular mass (Fig. 60.1). Papillary necrosis appears as triangular ringlike calcifications in the collecting system. With fibrotic autonephrectomy, the KUB film shows a small, shrunken, calcified "cement" or "putty" kidney, in which calcific rims outline the individual renal lobes; this lobar pattern is pathognomonic for end-stage renal TB.

A plain radiograph can also demonstrate renal and ureteral TB-infected calculi. Stones may take strange shapes as they form in a deformed and fibrosed renal pelvis. A stone in the shape of an upward arrowhead may indicate a renal pelvis that has been "hiked up" by contraction from scarring.

The KUB film can also show ureteral calcifications, which are characteristically intraluminal as opposed to the mural calcifications of schistosomiasis. Bladder wall calcifications are not very common except in late cases of bladder contraction. Calcifications of the prostate and seminal vesicles are seen in 10% of patients. Plain film findings suggestive of TB may be seen in surrounding tissues as well, appearing as erosions of the vertebral bodies or calcifications in cold abscesses of the psoas muscle (Merchant et al., 2013a; Teo and Wee, 2011).

All patients being evaluated for GU TB should also have a chest x-ray to exclude concomitant infectious pulmonary TB (American Thoracic Society, 2000).

Intravenous Urography. Intravenous urography (IVU) is the gold standard for imaging early renal TB. Initial erosive changes of the urothelium appear as loss of sharpness and edge irregularities (Figueiredo and Lucon, 2008). Calyceal erosions have a "moth-eaten" appearance (Patterson et al., 2012). Filling defects may be seen, caused by tuberculomas rupturing into the calyx or by papillary necrosis. IVU can demonstrate medullary cavities that communicate with the collecting system. When a calyx or infundibulum is stenosed, contrast excretion by the renal parenchyma may fail, creating a "phantom calyx" in the location where the calyx should be visible (Eastwood et al., 2001). Ureteral TB can manifest as a rigid, calcified, straightened, pipestem ureter that is tubular and lacks normal peristaltic activity on IVU. The ureter may also take on the appearance of a beaded corkscrew as a result of nodular fibrosis along the entire ureter. The pipestem and corkscrew findings are highly suggestive of TB, particularly when seen concurrently with either kidney or bladder abnormalities. IVU can also detect nonfunctional kidneys because of autonephrectomy, as well as a fibrosed, contracted bladder (Fig. 60.2). On occasion, perinephric abscess may be suggested, particularly if there is restriction of renal movement with breathing or ureteral displacement on IVU.

The most common findings on IVU, however, are obstructive changes resulting from scarring and distortion of the collecting system: calyceal obliteration, infundibular narrowing, hydrocalycosis, segmental or total hydronephrosis, and hydroureter (Figs. 60.3 and 60.4). Calyceal dilation and distortion present a typical cloverleaf pattern on film (Carl and Stark, 1997). Ureterovesical junction obstruction is caused by tuberculous cystitis or strictures of the distal third of the ureter (Fig. 60.5). The finding of a "hiked-up" renal pelvis, with sharp angulation of the ureteropelvic junction (UPJ), is known as "Kerr's kink" (Merchant et al., 2013a).

Computed Tomography With Urography. Computed tomography (CT) with urography is the most frequently used modality for imaging TB in developed countries, where it has largely replaced IVU (Merchant et al., 2013b). High-end multi-detector scanners can detect lesions as small as 3 to 4 mm. With the administration of intravenous contrast, CT can assess kidney function during different phases of excretion. Similar to KUB and IVU, CT reveals calcifications, scarring, and signs of obstruction (Fig. 60.6). CT is more sensitive than KUB in detecting calcifications and thickening of the collecting ducts. It is particularly useful in the evaluation of patients with complicated and extensive TB. Perinephric and psoas abscesses can be seen, as well as any pathology in lymph nodes, vertebrae, spleen, or liver. Pathology in the prostate and seminal vesicles can also be visualized, including enlargement, necrosis, cavitations and abscesses, as well as calcifications.

CT does have disadvantages. CT is less sensitive for detecting the minimal urothelial thickening, subtle papillary necrosis, and other changes of early renal TB, for which IVU is still the preferred study. In addition, CT imparts a higher radiation dose than IVU.

Retrograde Pyelography and Antegrade Pyelography. Both retrograde and antegrade pyelography, with either percutaneously or endoscopically administered contrast, have been replaced by CT urography. However, when IVU or CT cannot be done because of

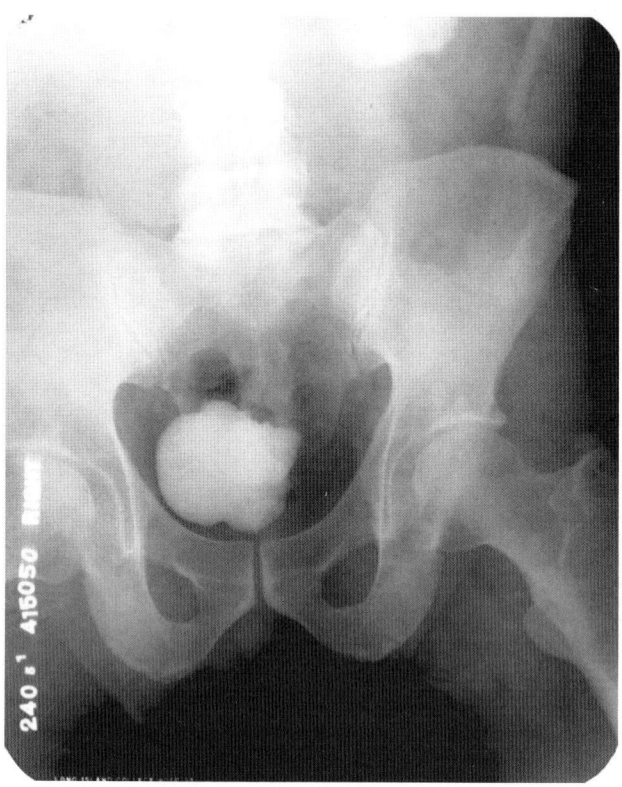

Fig. 60.2. The cystogram portion of an intravenous pyelogram in a patient with left renal tuberculosis. Note the contracted left side of the bladder that is secondary to fibrosis from the tuberculosis.

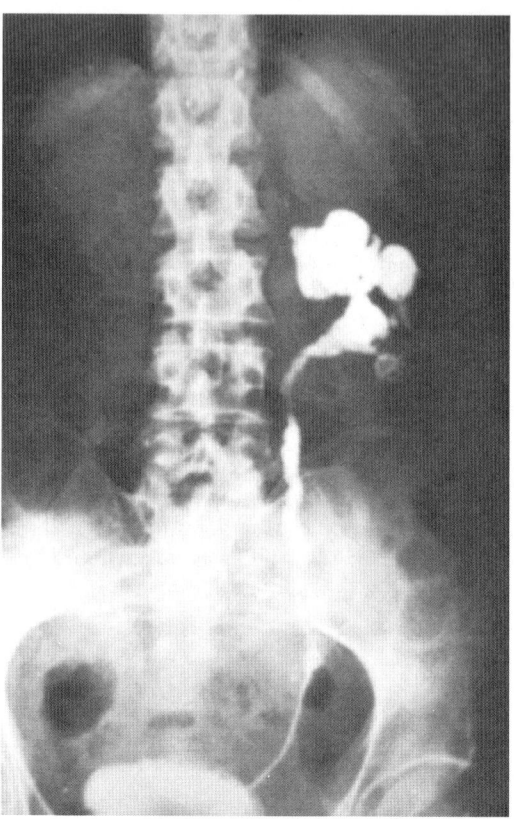

Fig. 60.3. Occluded calyx.

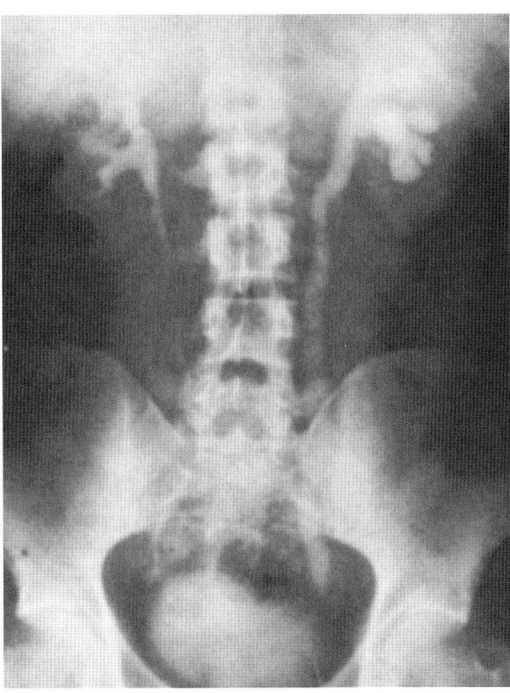

Fig. 60.4. Severe calyceal and parenchymal destruction.

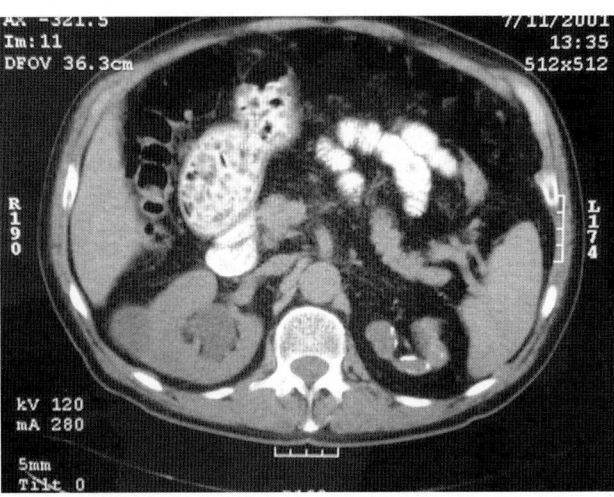

Fig. 60.6. CT after oral contrast medium in a patient with bilateral tuberculosis. The right kidney is hydronephrotic secondary to infundibular stenosis but has retained good function. The left kidney is an end-stage nonfunctioning atrophic kidney with calcification.

Ultrasonography

Ultrasonography (US) has a limited role in the diagnosis of GU TB because findings are generally nonspecific, and visualization is not as clear as with CT. It is useful in pediatric or pregnant patients because of the lack of radiation exposure. US is also less expensive than CT. US is used to evaluate the testes, epididymis, and, with transrectal US, the prostate and seminal vesicles, which appear thickened. US can also locate abscesses or cavities in the kidney. Cystic lesions with septations suggest chronic infection (Wong et al., 2013). Focal calcifications appear as highly echogenic areas with distal shadowing. Restriction of renal movement during breathing suggests a perinephric or psoas abscess. Like CT, US can provide concurrent information about the abdomen, such as the presence of ascites, lymphadenopathy, or omental caking. A primary use of US in GU TB is to follow hydronephrosis in patients who are receiving medical treatment because fibrosis during healing can worsen urinary obstruction.

Magnetic Resonance Imaging

Magnetic resonance imaging (MRI) is not commonly used in the workup of GU TB because of the many other imaging modalities available (Merchant et al., 2013b). Like ultrasound, it can be useful in pediatric or pregnant patients to avoid exposure to radiation. MRI can detect a single granuloma. Small lesions are hypointense on T1 and T2 images. Larger lesions have central hyperintensity on T2 images because of the increased cellularity at the center of the granuloma. Larger TB lesions can mimic malignancy, and it is not always possible to differentiate the two.

A magnetic resonance urogram (MRU) can be more sensitive than IVU in showing urothelial thickening and caliectasis. The addition of diffusion-weighted imaging (DWI) can help distinguish hydronephrosis from pyonephrosis. Various techniques have been explored with MRI to study TB, including cineMRU and dynamic MRU, which can evaluate ureteral peristalsis. MRI with DWI can be used to monitor renal fibrosis. Apparent diffusion coefficients (ADCs) decrease with fibrosis and can be used to gauge the stage of TB, including the effect of treatment. Caution should be used when using gadolinium in renal failure patients because of the risk of developing nephrogenic systemic fibrosis.

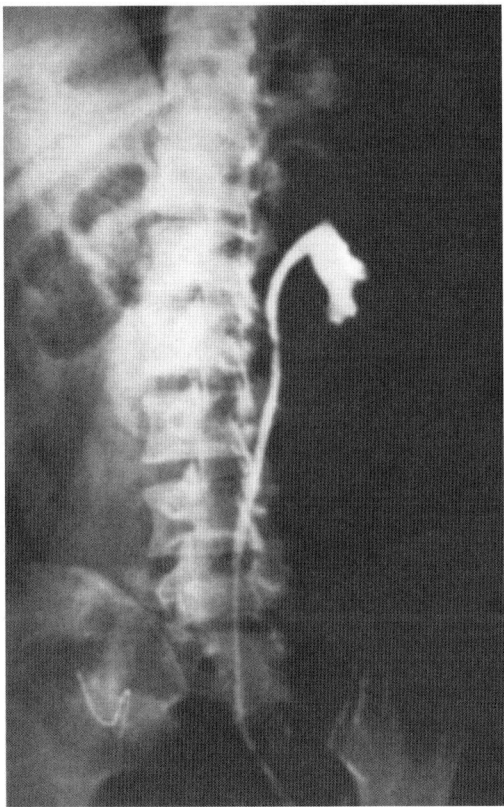

Fig. 60.5. Stricture at the distal left ureter.

renal insufficiency or contrast allergy, these modalities can be helpful in delineating the distortions in GU anatomy. In addition, these tests can be used in conjunction with IVU to determine whether cavitations are obstructive or nonobstructive, and whether they are in communication with the urinary collecting system or not (Merchant et al., 2013b).

Cystoscopy and Ureteroscopy

Endoscopy plays a limited role in the diagnosis of TB. Although it allows direct visualization of lesions, findings can be nonspecific.

They include local hyperemia, mucosal erosion, ulceration, granulomatous masses, and irregularity of the ureteral orifices. Ulcerative lesions may mimic malignancy. A "golf-hole" ureteric orifice is suggestive of TB, and, when found, upper tract imaging or endoscopy should be obtained (Fig. 60.7). Biopsies should be performed when possible, especially if malignancy is a possibility. Although a positive urine culture for MTBC is sufficient for diagnosis, results may not be available quickly enough. Furthermore, in those with negative urine cultures, bladder biopsy can be 19% to 52% sensitive for TB (Figueiredo and Lucon, 2008).

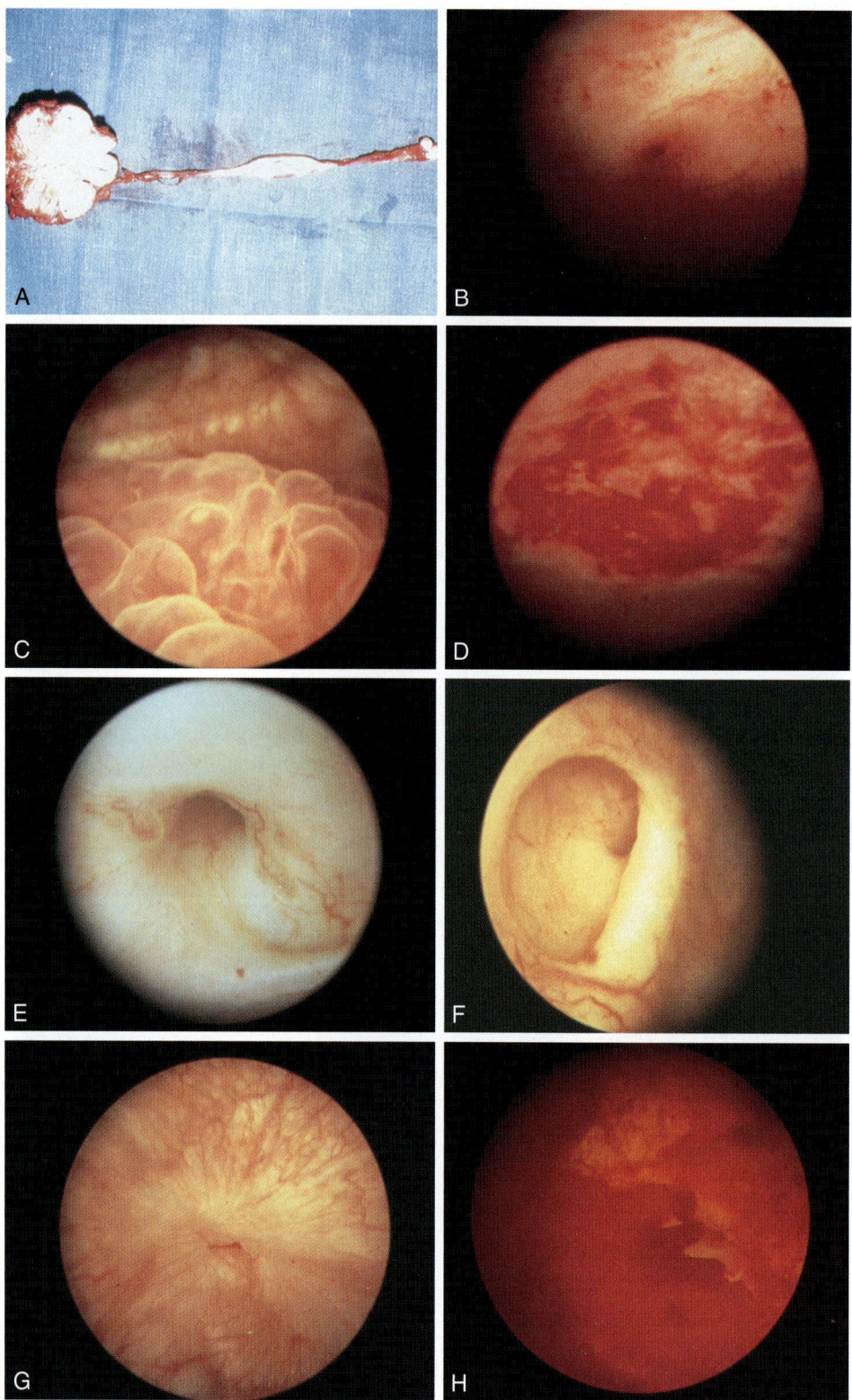

Fig. 60.7. (A) Extensive tuberculosis of the kidney and ureter with calcification and stricture formation. (B) Acutely inflamed ureteric orifice. (C) Tuberculous bullous granulations. (D) Acute tuberculous ulcer. (E) Tuberculous golf-hole ureter. (F) Tuberculous golf-hole ureter, severely withdrawn. (G) Healed tuberculous lesion. (H) Acute tuberculous cystitis with ulceration.

TABLE 60.2 First-Line Antituberculous Drugs

DRUG/FORMULATION	ADULT DOSAGE (DAILY)[a]	ADULT DOSAGE (INTERMITTENT)[b]	MAIN ADVERSE EFFECTS
Isoniazid[c] 50-, 100-, 300-mg tablet 50 mg/5 mL syrup 100 mg/mL injection	5 mg/kg (typically 300 mg)	3 times/week 15 mg/kg (typically 900 mg)	Hepatic toxicity, peripheral neuropathy
Rifampin[d] 150-, 300-mg capsule 600-mg injection powder	10 mg/kg (typically 600 mg)	3 times/week 10 mg/kg (typically 600 mg)	Hepatic toxicity, flulike syndrome, pruritus, drug interactions
Rifabutin[e] 150-mg capsule	5 mg/kg (typically 300 mg)	Not recommended	Hepatic toxicity, flulike syndrome, uveitis, neutropenia, drug interactions
Rifapentine[f] 150-mg tablet		Once weekly 10–20 mg/kg/week PO (600 mg and higher) in continuation phase only in very select patients	Similar to rifampin
Pyrazinamide 500-mg tablet	40–55 kg: 1000 mg 56–75 kg: 1500 mg 76–90 kg[g]: 2000 mg	3 times/week: 40–55 kg: 1500 mg 56–75 kg: 2500 mg 76–90 kg: 3000 mg	Arthralgias, hepatic toxicity, pruritus, rash, hyperuricemia, gastrointestinal upset
Ethambutol 100-, 400-mg tablet	40–55 kg: 800 mg 56–75 kg: 1200 mg 76–90 kg[g]: 1600 mg	3 times/week: 40–55 kg: 1200 mg 56–75 kg: 2000 mg 76–90 kg: 2400 mg	Decreased red-green color discrimination, decreased visual acuity, optic neuritis

[a]Or 5 times/week daily observed therapy (DOT).
[b]Daily therapy is preferred. Intermittent therapy (administered by DOT) only during the continuation phase of therapy. The World Health Organization and CDC no longer recommend dosing intervals less frequent than 3 times/week.
[c]Pyridoxine 25–50 mg should be given to prevent neuropathy in malnourished or pregnant patients and those with HIV infection, renal failure, thyroid disease, alcoholism or diabetes.
[d]In general, cannot be taken by HIV-infected persons taking protease inhibitors or certain NNRTIs.
[e]When taken with efavirenz, the rifabutin dose is increased to 450 mg/day or 600 mg 3 times/week. When taken with fosamprenavir, nelfinavir or indinavir, the rifabutin dose is 150 mg/day or 300 mg 3 times/week. With lopinavir/ritonavir (Kaletra), ritonavir alone, atazanavir alone or ritonavir combined with other protease inhibitors, the rifabutin dose is 150 mg every other day or 3 times/week; some experts believe this dose to be subtherapeutic and recommend 150 mg daily or 300 mg 3 times/week with close monitoring for rifabutin toxicity, particularly uveitis.
[f]Rifapentine is contraindicated in HIV+ persons, in persons with cavitary pulmonary disease, or persons with extrapulmonary tuberculosis. Use of once weekly rifapentine is not advocated by WHO.
[g]In patients >90 kg, dosing is recommended based on lean body weight.
From The Medical Letter. Drugs for tuberculosis. *Treat Guidel Med Lett* 10(116): 29–36, 2012; Modified from CDC: Treatment of tuberculosis, American Thoracic Society, CDC, and Infectious Diseases Society of America. *MMWR Recomm Rep.* 52(No. RR-11):1–77, 2003.

Treatment

Before the development of antimicrobials, treatment of TB relied primarily on rest and nourishment in sanatoria; and in those with severe GU disease, extirpative surgery was the best hope for cure. With the development of streptomycin in 1944, followed by isoniazid in 1952 and the rifamycins in 1957, medical treatment with antituberculous drugs replaced sanatoria and surgical procedures (Daniel, 2006). **Today, most TB patients can be treated medically and in the ambulatory setting, even those with MDR-TB. Surgery primarily establishes a diagnosis or is an adjunct to antibiotics in advanced cases** (Abbara and Davidson, 2011).

Medical Therapy

Successful medical treatment of TB requires multiple drugs for several reasons (CDC, 2003). First, the tubercle bacilli exist in different microenvironments within the host. These apply different pressures on the organism and cause it to exhibit different metabolic needs and replication speeds. The drugs vary in their activity against MTBC; some are bactericidal, whereas others are only bacteriostatic. Some drugs work best on rapidly replicating bacteria, whereas others are more effective against less metabolically active bacilli. The drugs also penetrate differently into various tissues and perform optimally at different pHs. In addition, multiple drug therapy prevents the emergence of drug-resistant strains.

Combination therapy with first-line antituberculous drugs achieves the best cure rates in the shortest timeframe (Table 60.2). Treatment should start with these—namely, isoniazid (INH), rifampin, pyrazinamide, and ethambutol. Before the start of treatment, baseline measurements should include platelet count and liver and kidney function tests. Patients should also be tested for HIV, and, when appropriate, for hepatitis B and C and diabetes. Medical therapy should be tailored according to drug susceptibility data when available. Directly observed treatment (DOT) should be employed to ensure medication adherence and minimize the likelihood of developing drug-resistant strains (Nahid et al., 2016).

Second-line agents are reserved for patients who experience side effects from first-line agents, whose MTBC organisms exhibit drug resistance or in whom first-line agents fail. Second-line agents vary in tolerability and ease of administration (Table 60.3). Recent drugs added to the second-line agents are the fluoroquinolones and linezolid (Lee et al., 2012), both of which were developed to treat other bacterial infections, and bedaquiline, the first new drug in 40 years specifically developed for TB (CDC, 2013).

TABLE 60.3 Second-Line Antituberculous Drugs

DRUG/FORMULATION	ADULT DOSAGE (DAILY)[a]	MAIN ADVERSE EFFECTS
Streptomycin[b]	15 mg/kg IM, IV (max 1 g)	Vestibular and auditory toxicity, renal damage
Capreomycin[b]	15 mg/kg IM, IV (max 1 g)	Vestibular and auditory toxicity, renal damage, electrolyte imbalance
Amikacin/kanamycin[b]	15 mg/kg IM, IV daily	Ototoxicity, renal damage
Cycloserine[c]	10–15 mg/kg in two doses (250–500 mg bid) PO	Psychiatric symptoms, seizures
Ethionamide	15–20 mg/kg in 1 or 2 doses (250–500 mg qd or bid) PO	Gastrointestinal and hepatic toxicity, hypothyroidism, optic neuritis, neurotoxicity
Levofloxacin	500–1000 mg PO, IV	Gastrointestinal toxicity, central nervous system effects, rash, dysglycemia, QT prolongation, tendonitis/tendon rupture
Moxifloxacin	400 mg PO, IV	Gastrointestinal toxicity, central nervous system effects, rash, dysglycemia, QT prolongation, tendonitis/tendon rupture
Para-aminosalicylic acid	8–12 g split into 2–3 doses PO	Gastrointestinal disturbance, hepatitis, hypothyroidism
Linezolid	600 mg PO	Bone marrow suppression, peripheral and optic neuropathy, hepatic toxicity
Bedaquiline[d]	400 mg PO × 2 weeks, then 200 mg PO thrice-weekly	Headache, nausea, arthralgias, QT prolongation, hepatic toxicity

[a]Dosage may need to be adjusted for renal impairment.
[b]Generally given 5–7 times/week (15 mg/kg, or a maximum of 1 g per dose) for an initial 2 to 4 months, and then (if needed) 3 times/week (20 to 30 mg/kg, or a maximum of 1.5 g per dose). Dosing less frequently than 3 times/week is no longer recommended. For patients >59 years old, dosage is reduced to 10 mg/kg (max 750 mg per dose). Dosage should be decreased if renal function is diminished.
[c]Some authorities recommend pyridoxine 50 mg for every 250 mg of cycloserine to decrease the incidence of adverse neurologic effects.
[d]Bedaquiline is given at 400 mg orally with food, daily for 2 weeks, then 200 mg orally three times/week.
Modified from Lewinsohn DM, Leonard MK, LoBue PA, et al.: Official American Thoracic Society/Infectious Diseases Society of America/Centers for Disease Control and Prevention Clinical Practice Guidelines: diagnosis of tuberculosis in adults and children. *Clin Infect Dis* 64(2):111–115, 2017; Lee M, Lee J, Carroll MW, et al.: Linezolid for treatment of chronic extensively drug-resistant tuberculosis. *N Engl J Med* 367(16):1508–1518, 2012; Centers for Disease Control and Infection (CDC): Provisional CDC guidelines for the use and safety monitoring of bedaquiline fumarate (Sirturo) for the treatment of multidrug-resistant tuberculosis. *MMWR Recomm Rep.* 62(RR-09):1–12, 2013.
bid, Twice daily; *IM*, intramuscularly; *IV*, intravenously; *PO*, per os (orally); *qd*, every day.

GU TB can be successfully treated with the standard short-course regimen of 6 months of first-line antituberculous drugs (Nahid et al., 2016). Treatment begins with an intensive phase of 2 months of daily INH, rifampin, and pyrazinamide, followed by a continuation phase of 4 months of INH and rifampin given daily or alternatively, thrice weekly. Twice-weekly administration during the continuation phase is no longer recommended (WHO, 2010). Pyridoxine (vitamin B_6) administration minimizes the risk of INH-induced peripheral neuropathy. Ethambutol is added at the beginning of treatment pending drug susceptibilities and is discontinued if the strain is found to be susceptible to the other first-line drugs. First-line drugs reach high concentrations in the urine and work well in acidic environments. The intensive phase of treatment targets rapidly multiplying bacteria, whereas the continuation phase attempts to eradicate slow, sporadic multipliers and persistent bacteria.

Although 6 months is the duration of standard short-course therapy, clinical scenarios regularly arise that require prolongation of treatment. The type of clinical disease present and the antituberculous drugs used affect duration of treatment (Nahid et al., 2016). For example, at least 9 months of treatment is recommended for extensive pockets of infection, concurrent smear-positive cavitary pulmonary disease, central nervous system involvement, or delay in positive cultures converting to negative. If the patient is unable to take pyrazinamide for at least 2 months, either because of side effects or drug resistance, therapy should also last 9 months or longer. Some clinicians recommend 12 months of therapy for GU TB because of high relapse rates of up to 22% when therapy is given for only 6 months (Gokalp et al., 1990). Because of the complexities that often arise with regimen choice, drug interactions, and side effects, any deviation from standard short-course therapy should be discussed with specialists experienced in treating TB.

During therapy, liver enzymes should be monitored monthly in those with preexisting liver disease because all first-line agents except ethambutol can cause hepatic toxicity that can be reversed with drug discontinuation. Patients should be advised to abstain from alcohol and other hepatotoxic drugs. Although treatment is, in general, well tolerated, severe hepatic injury has occurred. Visual acuity and red-green color perception also should be monitored while on ethambutol. Close follow-up of patients is necessary, not only to monitor for side effects, but also because renal lesions may worsen with drug treatment. **The healing process is sometimes accompanied with new fibrosis, which can worsen urinary obstruction and bladder contraction** (Psihramis and Donahoe, 1986). **Steroids may help in the management of these patients (see following). Surgical intervention to relieve worsening or newly developed obstruction may be necessary.**

Corticosteroids. The role of adjunctive corticosteroids for the treatment of TB disease still must be fully elucidated. The antiinflammatory effects of corticosteroids are thought to prevent an unchecked host immune response from causing excessive tissue destruction and scarring. Steroids provide a mortality benefit in TB meningitis and are strongly recommended in that setting. Although not routinely recommended, steroids are sometimes used in patients with severe pulmonary TB, when antibiotic treatment leads to a paradoxic worsening of symptoms (Breen et al., 2004), and in some patients with TB pericarditis to prevent constrictive pericarditis (Nahid et al., 2016). Steroids have also been used in a few cases of GU TB to prevent ureteral strictures and bladder contraction, but these cases are anecdotal, and no clinical trials have been conducted. A recent review and meta-analysis of published clinical trials of corticosteroid use in pulmonary, meningeal, pleural, pericardial, and peritoneal TB showed that, regardless of which organ system was affected, steroids reduced mortality by 17% (Critchley et al., 2013).

Surgical Therapy

About 55% of patients with GU TB require surgical management during their course of disease (Wong et al., 2013). Intervention is more frequent as disease advances. **Surgical procedures are performed to relieve urinary obstruction and drain infected material, to remove nonworking infected kidneys in cases resisting cure, to improve medically resistant hypertension secondary to a functionally excluded kidney, or to reconstruct the urinary tract.** Abscesses that do not respond to therapy may require aspiration or percutaneous or open drainage. Currently, more than half of operations performed for TB are reconstructive (Gupta et al., 2008). The optimal timing of surgery is 4 to 6 weeks after the initiation medical therapy. This delay allows active inflammation to subside, the bacillary load to decrease, and lesions to stabilize.

Procedures to Relieve Obstruction. Prompt relief of obstruction is emergently required in cases of uremia or sepsis. Bilateral obstruction or unilateral obstruction of a functionally solitary kidney is often the cause of renal failure. Early ureteral stenting or percutaneous nephrostomy (PCN) for tuberculous ureteral strictures limits the loss of renal function and increases the opportunity for later reconstructive surgery (Shin et al., 2002). Temporary and immediate drainage of obstruction is recommended, preferably by retrograde ureteric stenting. An indwelling double-J stent can be placed until the patient's condition has been optimized. Retrograde placement is successful in 41% of cases (Ramanathan et al., 1998). When this is not technically feasible, an antegrade, internalized or externalized ureteral stent is placed via percutaneous puncture of the obstructed kidney. If that also fails, a PCN is left in place until definitive management. Because strictures and fibrous scars may be present, more than one PCN may be necessary (Carl and Stark, 1997). PCN must be followed by correction of the cause of obstruction. A tuberculous cutaneous fistula can develop if the PCN is simply removed, although this is less likely to develop with effective concurrent medical therapy. If the kidney is unsalvageable, a nephrectomy may become necessary. High-contrast injection pressures during stent and PCN placement should be avoided to prevent possible dissemination of infection (Salem, 2008).

Nephrectomy. Organ preservation is the fundamental goal in surgical management of GU TB. However, total nephrectomy is considered in two settings. The first is the patient with a nonfunctional kidney and recalcitrant or recurrent TB despite optimal medical therapy. After nephrectomy of the infected kidney, relapse rates of less than 1% have been reported after short-course medical treatment (Figueiredo and Lucon, 2008). The second setting in which a nephrectomy is considered is the patient with a nonfunctional kidney and medically resistant hypertension. Nephrectomy improves hypertension in 65% of cases (Flechner and Gow, 1980). Overall, nephrectomy is performed in 27% of GU TB patients, and the frequency is similar between developed and developing countries (Figueiredo and Lucon, 2008).

Because of the extensive fibrosis often present, the traditional approach to the kidney is through an oblique retroperitoneal incision that can be extended dorsally or ventrally as needed. In rare patients the perinephric fat may appear to have granulomatous masses or caseous cavities. These should be removed with the specimen. Individual ligation of the renal artery and vein is preferred to limit risk of late arteriovenous fistula. The ureters are usually not taken out concurrently. Care must be taken to minimize disruption of the surrounding lymphatics and to avoid entering the pleural or peritoneal space during the procedure.

More recently, laparoscopic nephrectomy has gained popularity (Hemal, 2011; Lee et al., 2002) despite concerns that extensive fibrosis associated with TB would render a laparoscopic approach suboptimal. Several investigators have reported good outcomes and suggest that it should be the preferred approach because of decreased blood loss and more rapid patient recovery (Chibber et al., 2005; Gupta et al., 2008; Zhang et al., 2005). In experienced hands, laparoscopic nephrectomy for renal TB is a somewhat longer procedure than when it is done for other reasons, but in one study the procedure took only half an hour longer on average (Lee et al., 2002).

Ureteropelvic and Ureteral Surgery. Strictures of the ureteropelvic junction (UPJ) and ureter may be temporarily stented to allow improvement of renal function before definitive management. Upper and midureteric strictures are rare and may be amenable to endourologic treatment. Lower ureteric strictures are more common and often require open surgical intervention. The length and degree of the stricture, whether it can be passed by a guidewire or not, vascular supply to the lesion, and renal function are important factors to be considered in the management of patients (Kim et al., 1993).

Endoscopic Management. Tuberculous ureteric strictures are characterized by mucosal ischemia and dense fibrosis. Therefore success rates of endoscopic management of strictures resulting from other causes may not necessarily apply to TB strictures. In general, short strictures with residual lumens in patients with good renal function yield the best outcome. Strictures forming during medical treatment and managed by early stenting (double-J placement) can stabilize and require no further treatment (Shin et al., 2002). Balloon dilation by retrograde or antegrade access has been described for TB strictures of the ureter, UPJ, ureterovesical junction, and calyceal infundibula (Kim et al. 1993; Murphy et al., 1982). A stent is often placed after dilation. Because of high failure rates, repeat procedures are often needed.

Follow-up imaging (US or IVU) of all patients with ureteric strictures is needed, especially those managed endoscopically, because some strictures worsen during the healing process as a result of fibrosis and cicatrization. Corticosteroids may be added if deterioration is detected. Failure to improve or progression after 6 weeks of medical treatment is an indication for open surgical management.

Open Surgical Options. Long, complex strictures require open surgical repair. Because of fibrosis, loss of elasticity, and reduced vascularity, mobilization of structures may be difficult. Repair of UPJ scarring is more challenging in TB cases than for congenital stenosis. Dismembered pyeloplasty is feasible for extrarenal pelves with short segment scarring. Nondismembered (flap) pyeloplasty is preferred for longer strictures but may not be feasible because of excessive scarring of the pelvis. When anatomic reconstruction is not possible, ureterocalicostomy (anastomosis of the ureter to the lower pole calyx) is an option. The renal capsule should be preserved to cover the lower pole of the kidney. If not enough capsule is available, omentum can be used to avoid stenosis at the calicoureteral anastomosis (Carl and Stark, 1997).

Upper and middle ureteric strictures can be managed by excision of the diseased segment, and, with adequate mobilization, a primary tension-free ureteroureterostomy can be performed. Alternatively, lysis of adhesions and intubation (Davis intubated ureterotomy) may be done. Lower ureter strictures requiring surgery are best managed by complete excision of the entire affected ureteric segment back to healthy ureteric mucosa that has good blood supply. The resultant gap is bridged with a tension-free, well-vascularized anastomosis to healthy bladder (ureteroneocystostomy). Various procedures exist to bring the bladder closer to the ureteric end. Simple mobilization of the lateral attachments of the bladder on the contralateral side, accompanied by dividing the superior vesical artery, may provide 2 to 3 cm of length to bridge a small gap. In patients with good bladder capacity, a psoas hitch may also be performed. Care must be taken to avoid the genitofemoral and femoral nerves when placing these sutures. A well-performed psoas hitch can bridge a gap of up to 5 cm. A Boari flap is another method of bridging a longer gap of 10 to 15 cm and may be performed in combination with a psoas hitch (Sankari, 2007). A poorly executed Boari flap can compromise bladder capacity. Contracted bladders from TB cystitis may not have sufficient surface area and elasticity to allow flap creation. Finally, ileal interposition (ileal ureteric replacement) can be done in cases of multiple or recurrent strictures in which the native ureter is no longer an adequate conduit (Goel and Dalela, 2008).

Bladder Surgery. Augmentation cystoplasty and bladder substitution are options in the management of the tuberculous contracted bladder. First described in the 19th century for a tuberculous contracted bladder, augmentation is indicated when frequency, nocturia, urgency, pain, and hematuria, become intolerable—typically when bladder capacity is less than 100 mL (Gupta et al., 2008). For severely contracted bladders, ileocecum or sigmoid segments are most suitable. When only half the bladder is diseased, ileum is often used. Other segments used in augmentation include stomach and cecum. The general rules of incorporating the bowel into the urinary tract apply, such as thoroughly evaluating renal function, reconfiguring a low-pressure reservoir (de Figueiredo et al., 2006), providing patient education, and conducting long-term follow-up. Thimble bladders with capacity less than 20 mL are best managed by orthotopic bladder substitution (Hemal and Aron, 1999). Complications of either bladder augmentation or substitution include mucus production, electrolyte derangements, and secondary bacterial infection.

Urethral Procedures. Bladder neck contracture is best managed endoscopically by transurethral incision of the contracture. Urethral strictures are also managed endoscopically and often require repeated procedures. Tuberculous urethral fistulae are treated by initiation of medical therapy and suprapubic bladder drainage. Delayed reconstruction is preferred. Drainage of a seminal vesicle tuberculous cavity into the bladder by cold knife incision has been reported (Dewani et al., 2006).

Genital Surgery. Extirpative surgery for genital TB is considered only for patients in whom medical therapy has failed. When the epididymis is infected with sparing of the testis, every effort should be made to perform an epididymectomy alone without orchiectomy. Preserving testicular blood supply is important during dissection of the epididymis. Initiating dissection at the globus minor after ligation of the vas facilitates excision. If the testes are infected, a scrotal orchiectomy can be done. Involvement of the vas deferens by TB is usually distal to the external ring and ligation of at the level of the ring is possible and sufficient.

Monitoring for Tuberculosis Relapse

Even with optimized treatment, as with any infection, TB can relapse in 2% to 6% of pulmonary TB patients, particularly within the first year after treatment (CDC, 2003). A second, longer, or different drug course is then required. GU TB patients may relapse at a higher rate than pulmonary TB patients, in 6.3% to 22% of cases, even after 12 months of medical therapy (Figueiredo and Lucon, 2008). The extensively diseased kidney can contain innumerable foci of tubercle bacilli. Difficulty in achieving complete sterilization of all foci with antituberculous drugs may be the reason for the higher relapse rate. Viable bacilli have been identified in the kidneys even after 9 months of treatment (Figueiredo and Lucon, 2008). In all cases of recurrent TB, extra effort should be exerted to isolate the organism for drug susceptibility testing. Pulmonary TB patients are usually followed for 2 years after completing treatment; for GU TB patients, some investigators have recommended 10 years of follow-up, as the average time of relapse was 5.3 years (Gokce et al., 2002).

Management of Genitourinary Tuberculosis in Special Situations

Each of the special situations below requires careful selection of the antituberculous regimen because of side effects, interactions, and drug toxicities. Expert advice should be sought from infectious diseases specialists or physicians experienced in the treatment of TB.

Multidrug-Resistant and Extensively Drug-Resistant Tuberculosis

Persons with MTBC strains that are resistant to both INH and rifampin (the two most important first-line agents) have MDR-TB by definition. Worldwide, approximately 3.3% of newly diagnosed patients and 20% of previously treated patients have MDR-TB (WHO, 2016). In the United States, 1.4% of TB cases were MDR-TB. The percentage of drug-resistant TB has remained stable in the United States for the last 20 years (CDC, 2017). Treatment is complicated by the need to use regimens typically longer than 18 months. The cure rate is 50% to 60% compared with 94% to 97% in patients with drug-susceptible TB (CDC, 2009). Among MDR-TB cases, 9.7% have additional drug resistance (WHO, 2016). Extensively drug-resistant TB (XDR-TB) is defined by resistance to INH, rifampin, any fluoroquinolone, and at least one of the injectable second-line aminoglycosides (amikacin, kanamycin, or capreomycin). XDR-TB is exceedingly difficult to cure, with complicated patient drug regimens involving 5 to 6 drugs for 2 years or more. As a result, the cure rate of patients with XDR-TB is only 30% to 50% (CDC, 2013)

Pregnancy and Lactation

Women of childbearing age should be advised to avoid pregnancy while being treated for active TB. If the diagnosis is discovered during pregnancy, prompt therapy should be initiated because the risk to the fetus from TB outweighs the risk of adverse drug effects. Treatment consists of INH, ethambutol, rifampin, and pyridoxine for 9 months. The use of pyrazinamide is controversial in the United States because drug effects on the fetus are not well established and because of the perceived increased risk for hepatotoxicity in the pregnant patient. However, the WHO recommends using pyrazinamide in pregnant women as part of the standard first-line treatment. Postpartum women may breastfeed their infants once noninfectious because drug concentrations in breastmilk are too low to cause toxicity (Nahid et al., 2016).

Human Immunodeficiency Virus Infection

HIV infection increases the risk of active TB 30-fold. With HIV and TB coinfection, each disease accelerates the other. All TB patients should be tested for HIV. Among HIV-positive persons in the world, almost 25% of deaths are due to TB (WHO, 2016). This is reminiscent of TB mortality rates in 18th- and 19th-century Europe.

Extrapulmonary, and consequently, GU TB may be more common in HIV-positive patients. In a small study in India, GU TB was found postmortem in 49% of AIDS patients (Lanjewar et al., 1999). In HIV-positive patients, GU TB can be more disseminated, with more lymph node enlargement and bilateral renal disease. There is usually less caseation, necrosis, and fibrosis because a competent immune system is necessary for the vigorous inflammatory process that leads to fibrosis and scarring. As a result, among patients with GU TB, stenosis of the collecting system occurs less frequently (12.5% vs. 93.8% in HIV-negative persons), and there is a lower incidence of bladder contracture (12.5% vs. 65.3% in HIV-negative persons with GU TB) (Figueiredo et al., 2009). Despite the lower incidence of obstructive cicatricial lesions, GU TB in HIV-positive persons is associated with high mortality.

Treatment in HIV-positive patients with GU TB should not be delayed. Treatment guidelines are similar to those for persons without HIV infection. Short-course chemotherapy for 6 months is effective, and 9 months of treatment is no longer routinely recommended. Instead, duration of treatment is determined by the usual factors: disease location and severity, drugs tolerated, response, and also importantly, whether the patient is on effective antiretrovirals. If the HIV-infected patient is not on consistent and effective antiretrovirals, TB treatment for 9 months is recommended. Daily instead of intermittent treatment is recommended and preferred for HIV-positive patients (Nahid et al., 2016). Drug interactions with antiretrovirals can be complex and must be considered. The rifamycins (rifampin and, to a lesser degree, rifabutin) may decrease serum levels of antivirals to suboptimal levels. Dose increases may be needed as a result (Kaplan et al., 2009).

Renal Transplant Recipients

Renal allograft TB is rare. Infection usually presents in kidney transplant patients within 6 months of transplantation but can occur as late as 7 years after. The shorter interval may be a result of the immunosuppression required for the graft or of pre-existing TB in the donor kidney. Because patients are seen very early in the disease process, no changes are usually visible on imaging. Furthermore, the immunosuppression prevents much of the pathology that is part of the natural course of GU TB. Diagnosis is difficult because many of the symptoms and findings of GU TB are absent. Fever is the usual presenting symptom. Urinary symptoms are present in only 20% of cases (el-Agroudy et al., 2003). Chest x-ray findings are abnormal but not specific in 55% of patients. Regardless of chest x-ray findings, 56% have positive sputum cultures. In one study, urine AFB culture was positive in 100% of patients (Dowdy et al., 2001). Many patients are diagnosed after graft nephrectomy with histopathology (Lorimer et al., 1999).

Treatment is complicated by drug interactions between the rifamycins and the immunosuppressive drugs, necessitating frequent monitoring of serum drug levels and dosing adjustments. Rifamycin-free regimens are possible but lengthen the duration of treatment to at least 18 months. Complications in transplant patients include graft rejection, disseminated TB, and death in up to 36% of patients (Dowdy et al., 2001).

> **KEY POINTS: TUBERCULOSIS**
> - Untreated genitourinary TB can lead to irreparable tissue damage with serious consequences such as renal failure and infertility, making it critical for clinicians to consider TB in the differential diagnosis of GU disorders.
> - Genitourinary tuberculosis is associated with nonspecific symptoms and can be indolent; typical constitutional symptoms of TB are infrequent. A high index of suspicion is necessary for correct diagnosis.
> - The gold standard for diagnosis of genitourinary tuberculosis is a positive AFB culture from urine or tissue biopsy. However, often a diagnosis can be made using alternate methods such as with NAAT or the finding of granulomas on histopathology examination of tissue.
> - The optimal timing of surgery is 4 to 6 weeks after the initiation medical therapy. This delay allows active inflammation to subside, the bacillary load to decrease, and lesions to stabilize.
> - Monitoring for relapse is important after treatment of genitourinary TB because it can occur in up to 22% of cases.

PARASITIC INFECTIONS OF THE UROGENITAL TRACT

A number of parasitic infections affect the urogenital tract. Although urologists practicing in nonendemic areas may encounter patients with urogenital parasitic infections only rarely, it is nevertheless critical for physicians to understand these diseases to facilitate appropriate diagnosis and therapy of affected individuals. Parasitic infections relevant to urology include urogenital schistosomiasis, filariasis, amebiasis, enterobiasis, and echinococcosis.

Schistosomiasis

More than 200 million people globally are infected by *Schistosoma* species. The three species of primary medical importance are *Schistosoma mansoni* (found primarily in Africa, the Arabian Peninsula, and South America), *Schistosoma japonicum* (China and Southeast Asia), and *Schistosoma haematobium* (Africa and the Arabian Peninsula). Whereas *S. mansoni* and *S. japonicum* affect primarily the liver and gastrointestinal tract, *S. haematobium* infection affects primarily the genitourinary tract and is the focus of this chapter. Urogenital schistosomiasis is a disease featuring a complex parasite life cycle, multifaceted human disease, and close ecological links to the environment. *S. haematobium* likely has coevolved with humans and nonhuman primates for millennia; as a result, even ancient civilizations realized the constellation of signs and symptoms associated with urogenital schistosomiasis.

History

The presence of schistosome antigens in Egyptian mummies (circa 3500 BCE), including more recent mummies with confirmed *S. haematobium* eggs in tissues (Deelder et al., 1990), confirms that urogenital schistosomiasis has been with *Homo sapiens* for millennia. Indeed, the Egyptians recognized this infection and named it "A-a-a disease", which was depicted hieroglyphically by a penis dripping with bloody urine (Hanafy et al., 1974; Shokeir et al., 1999). Later, the German pathologist Theodore Bilharz, performing autopsies in Cairo in 1852, found worms in mesenteric veins and linked them to eggs found in human urine and stool.

Biology and Life Cycle

Human infection is initiated by the penetration of *S. haematobium* cercariae through (even intact) skin that is in contact with infested fresh water (Fig. 60.8). The average lifespan of cercariae is 1 day. Penetration success rates fall off quickly within hours of cercarial shedding from the intermediate snail host (King, 2006).

After penetration, schistosomes transform from free-living cercariae into obligate parasites called *schistosomulae* by first shedding their tails over approximately 90 to 120 minutes and then undergoing a series of structural changes (Melo and Pereira, 1985). The transformed schistosomulae migrate to the lungs via the bloodstream or lymphatics and then the liver via the venous circulation (Wilson, 2009). Migration out of the skin and into the lungs takes several weeks (Rheinberg et al., 1998; Wilson, 2009).

The juvenile schistosomes then arrive at the liver sinusoids via the venous circulation, where they begin blood feeding. Soon thereafter, the now-mature worms preferentially migrate to the venous plexus of the bladder and other pelvic organs, where they live an average of 3 to 5 years. The developmental period from cercaria to adult worm ranges from 80 to 110 days. After worm pairing, males clasp the females in a ventral groove termed the "gynecophoric" canal, using their muscular bodies to help females pump host blood into their mouths and secreting chemical signals to stimulate oviposition (Gupta and Basch, 1987).

Eggs are laid by adult female worms in the pelvic venous circulation. Human schistosomes are very fecund, with egg-laying rates of hundreds to thousands of eggs per female per day. *S. haematobium* eggs are ovoid, measuring approximately 140 microns long and featuring a terminal spine (Loker, 1983; Ratard and Greer, 1991; Fig. 60.9). Eggs must penetrate the endothelium to reach the lumen of bladder to exit in the urinary stream, reach fresh water, and hatch to become miracidia. Some *S. haematobium* eggs are also excreted into the feces after expulsion from the intestinal wall. It is estimated that less than half of the eggs produced are successfully excreted in urine. The rest are retained in the body where the immune response causes significant pathology.

Eggs can survive approximately 20 days as long as they remain wet. Upon contact with fresh water and light, the eggs hatch, releasing miracidia, which are the larval stage of the parasite. The ciliated miracidia of *S. haematobium* infect intermediate host snails of the *Bulinus* genus. *Bulinus* snails prefer slow-flowing fresh-water habitats and are able to withstand low oxygen conditions.

The typical life span of a miracidium is 6 hours. If during this brief period a *Bulinus* snail is encountered, the miracidia will penetrate the snail tissue and form a primary sporocyst. After several days, 20 to 40 daughter sporocysts are generated by the primary sporocyst. These eventually mature into 200 to 400 cercariae (per sporocyst) that are released back into water. The prepatent period (the time between initial penetration of the snail by a miracidium and release of the first cercariae) varies with water temperature, and at temperatures below 15°C or greater than 35°C, no cercariae are shed (Pflüger et al., 1984).

Epidemiology

The geographic distribution of urogenital schistosomiasis is dependent on the tropical conditions required by *S. haematobium* and its specific snail hosts. Consequently, *S. haematobium* is endemic throughout much of sub-Saharan Africa and in portions of North Africa and the Middle East. However, in 2013, 120 schistosomiasis cases were diagnosed on the French island of Corsica, representing the first

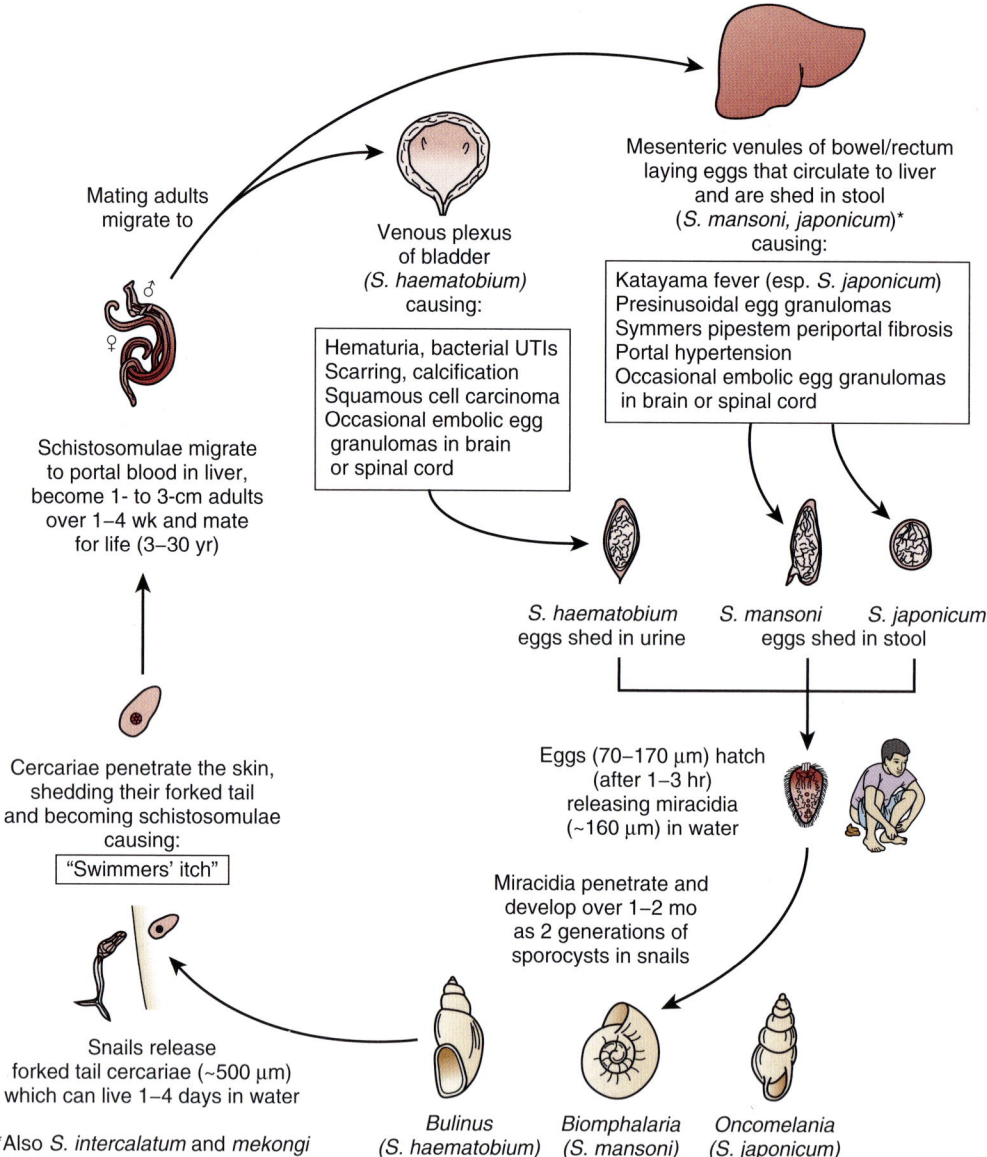

Fig. 60.8. Life cycle of a schistosome. *UTIs,* Urinary tract infections. (From King CH: Schistosomiasis. In Guerrant RL, Walker DH, Weller PF, editors: *Tropical infectious diseases, principles, pathogens, and practice,* ed 2, Philadelphia, 2006, Elsevier Churchill Livingstone, pp 1341–1348.)

time autochthonously transmitted schistosomiasis had been detected in Europe for more than a century (Holtfreter et al., 2014). The subsequent finding of additional cases there in 2015 suggests that this may now be an endemic focus of schistosomiasis (Berry et al., 2016). Interestingly, some of these infections may have been caused by *Schistosoma bovis* (typically a bovine-specific schistosome) or *S. haematobium-S. bovis* hybrids. Older calculations have estimated that most of the more than 200 million people worldwide with schistosomiasis have the urogenital form of infection (van der Werf et al., 2003). Newer estimates suggest that the number of people with schistosomiasis may be more than 440 million, including *S. haematobium*-induced infection (Colley et al., 2014). Up to 150,000 people die annually from *S. haematobium*-induced obstructive renal failure alone (van der Werf et al., 2003). It has been calculated that in a 2-week period in 2003, 70 million and 32 million individuals in sub-Saharan Africa experienced *S. haematobium*-induced hematuria and dysuria (respectively) and that major bladder wall pathology and major hydronephrosis were present in 18 and 10 million people, respectively (van der Werf et al., 2003).

For individuals, the risk of contracting urogenital schistosomiasis is driven primarily by the nature and length of contact with contaminated fresh water. Rural women and children can be exposed during domestic chores when they use *S. haematobium*-infested ponds, rivers, and lakes as their water supply (e.g., for laundry and dishwashing). Children may also be infected while playing and swimming in infested water. Men and women can be exposed during freshwater fishing, washing cars, and working in agricultural areas with high water-intensity crops such as rice and sugar cane (Hunter et al., 1993). In endemic areas, schistosomiasis prevalence is usually highly focal because of the localized nature of water-dependent transmission.

On a regional level, land-use patterns and ecological changes can lead to a higher burden of schistosomiasis in some areas, sometimes even resulting in outbreaks. For instance, it has been recognized for at least a century that building dams and irrigation schemes can increase schistosomiasis transmission by creating year-round, slow-flowing, fresh water habitats for the intermediate snail hosts and by promoting increased human population density associated with expanded agriculture. Accordingly, data from Africa consistently show that populations living near dams and irrigation schemes have a greater risk of contracting schistosomiasis compared with populations living distantly from these schemes (Steinmann et al., 2006).

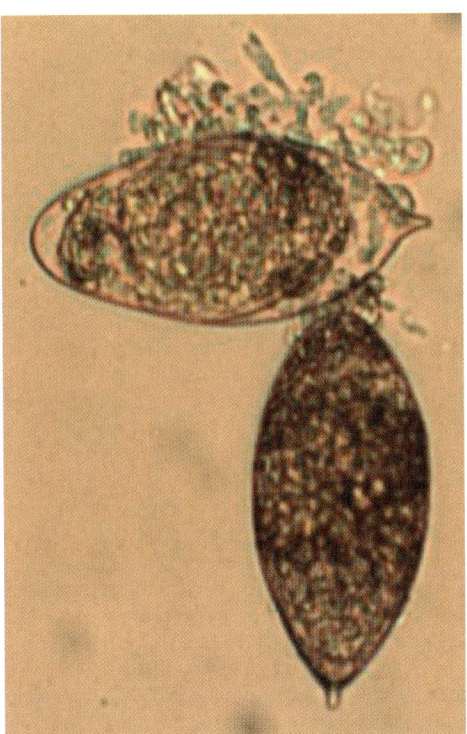

Fig. 60.9. Micrographs of *Schisosoma haematobium* eggs. Note the characteristic terminal spines of the eggs. (From Ray et al., 2012.)

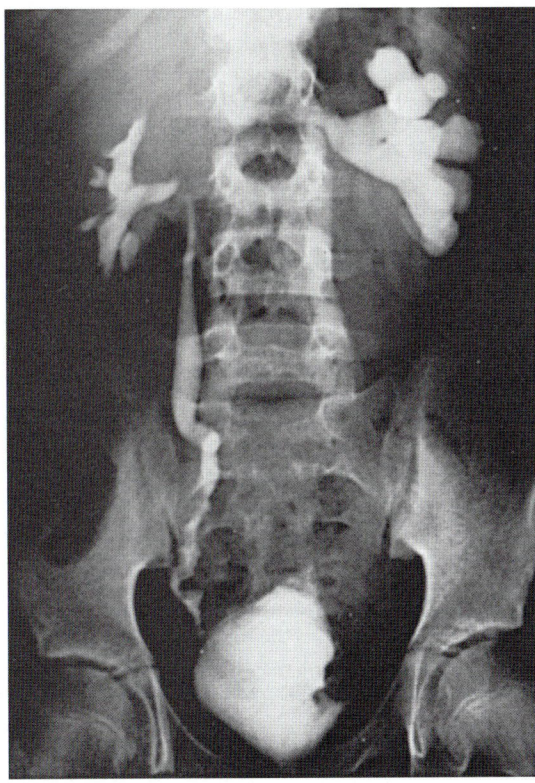

Fig. 60.10. Intravenous urogram in an Egyptian boy shows scalloping of the bladder and right lower ureter by schistosomal polypoid lesions.

In the 1930s, after the construction of the Aswan Low Dam in Egypt that led to a conversion from ancient, flood-based irrigation to perennial irrigation, the prevalence of schistosomiasis increased from less than 11% to more than 75% in some regions (Hunter et al., 1993). A similar series of events occurred after the construction of the Aswan High Dam in Egypt during the 1960s (Malek, 1975) and the Diama Dam in West Africa during the 1980s (Malek, 1975; Talla et al., 1990).

Communities in endemic areas with poor sanitary conditions and especially those without clean, running water generally have the highest prevalence rates of schistosomiasis (WHO, 2014a). Children are disproportionately affected, with the highest parasite burden occurring in those aged 5 to 15 (Anderson et al., 1992). It is unclear whether this age distribution results from higher exposure among children or a higher inherent susceptibility (Woolhouse et al., 1991).

Schistosomiasis is associated with poverty for a number of reasons. First, the aquatic snails that harbor the larval forms of schistosomes are distributed within tropical and subtropical developing countries, whereas they are not present in developed nations in temperate zones. Second, inadequate sanitation facilitates *Schistosoma* transmission because the schistosome life cycle requires an influx of eggs from human excreta into surface fresh waters. Moreover, prolonged contact with surface fresh water is promoted by lack of safe water supplies, leading to a higher risk of infection (Soares et al., 2011). Finally, schistosomiasis contributes to the perpetuation of poverty. Chronic infection adversely affects childhood growth, development, and learning, as well as worker productivity (Bonds et al., 2010).

Pathogenesis and Pathology

Cercarial skin penetration is facilitated by secreted molecules such as proteases, which initiate the cellular and humoral responses to schistosome infection (Curwen et al., 2006). However, likely as a result of the parasite strategy of modulating the host immune response from the moment of first contact, brief cercarial penetration does not typically induce an immune response beyond localized skin inflammation (Jenkins et al., 2005). Regardless, repeated exposure to schistosomulae can lead to hypersensitization and the development of a maculopapular rash.

During subsequent maturation into adult worms, schistosomulae begin to generate a double lipid bilayer outer surface (the tegument) that allows them to evade an immunopathologic response and remain in the host for years, facilitating chronic infection. As the survival of the worm within the host depends significantly on the tegument, numerous mechanisms are employed for immune evasion, including host antigenic mimicry, continual membrane turnover, immunomodulatory proteins and proteases, host-evading biophysical properties of the tegument, and modulation of expression of surface antigens (Abath and Werkhauser, 1996).

Because it is difficult to study the natural pathogenesis of egg-associated disease in humans, much of our knowledge stems from autopsy studies and animal models. In contrast to the relatively silent immune response to worms, the main immunopathologic responses raised against *S. haematobium* are triggered by oviposition in the walls of the bladder and other pelvic organs. With heavy worm burdens, egg deposition in the pelvic organs leads to granuloma development and eventual fibrosis, often obstructing the flow of blood or urine. Granulomas are characterized by a mixed leukocytic infiltration, including eosinophils, plasma cells, and lymphocytes. Because of continuous oviposition, all stages of granulomas are simultaneously present in individuals with chronic infection. Composite, coalescing granulomas are common, secondary to *S. haematobium* egg deposition in clusters. Grossly, granulomatous inflammation can form bulky, hyperemic, and polypoid masses projecting into the bladder lumen (Fig. 60.10). Other factors that have been shown to influence the host immune response and resulting disease severity include host genetics, in utero sensitization to parasitic antigens, and co-infection by other microbes/parasites (Pearce and MacDonald, 2002). *S. haematobium* eggs appear to rapidly induce bladder expression of type 2 inflammation–associated genes and suppress transcription of urothelial barrier function-related genes (Fu et al., 2012; Ray et al., 2012). These findings suggest that the parasite and human host may share the goal of expelling eggs from the bladder wall, across a temporarily lowered urothelial barrier, and out into the urinary stream.

Although *S. haematobium* has tropism for the pelvic organs, some oviposition occurs in the portal tract. As a result, portal hypertension can occur if a large burden of eggs are swept into the liver, clog pre-sinusoidal capillaries, induce granuloma formation, and consequently block the hepatic vasculature. Alternatively, embolized eggs can cause granulomatous and fibrotic portal areas and the dilation of collateral porto-systemic shunts, permitting the lodging of eggs in these vessels and the formation of pipe-stem fibrosis (Symmer's fibrosis) (Aubry et al., 1980). Hepatosplenomegaly is one clinical manifestation of Symmer's fibrosis, although susceptibility to its development depends largely on the variability of individual immune responses. Besides portal involvement, migration of worm pairs to the pulmonary vessels can result in oviposition in the lungs. Generally, pulmonary schistosomiasis develops only in very severe cases of infection and when pathogenesis in other organs (i.e., pelvic) has already occurred (Borgstein, 1964). When pulmonary oviposition occurs, eggs may obstruct the lung vasculature and lead to pulmonary fibrosis, pulmonary hypertension, and/or cor pulmonale (Bedford et al., 1946).

Naturally acquired immunity to urogenital schistosomiasis exists: some individuals maintain negative urine egg counts for at least 5 years despite never receiving anthelmintics in the face of continual exposure to *S. haematobium* (McManus and Loukas, 2008). The resistance of these individuals to reinfection has been attributed to the involvement of a T-helper type 1 (Th1) and a Th2-type cytokine response, whereas chronically infected individuals exclusively mount a Th2 response (McManus and Loukas, 2008). In some individuals, the activity of potentially protective IgE antibodies may be blocked by IgG4 antibodies generated against worm and egg antigens, possibly hampering the development of protective immunity to schistosomiasis (Hagan et al., 1991).

Because levels of IgE antibodies to worm antigens have been observed to increase with age (Roberts et al., 1993), many workers have suggested an immune-mediated development of resistance. This age-dependent trend, however, could be due to either behavioral or immunologic changes, because studies in endemic communities have ascertained a general decline in contact with infected water with increasing age (Dalton and Pole, 1978). Nevertheless, recent analyses suggest that even when exposure to infected water is controlled, age may play a role in the development of resistance.

Eggs that are not promptly expelled from pelvic organs calcify, including those in the bladder and ureters. The accumulation of eggs results in decreased compliance of the urinary tract and increases upper tract pressures. In turn, this promotes the development of urinary stasis, hydronephrosis, and hydroureter (Cheever et al., 1975). The extent of organ calcification can often be identified through radiologic imaging and is roughly correlated with the tissue burden of calcified eggs (Cheever et al., 1975). The anatomic level of obstruction involves the ureteral meatus (1%), interstitial ureter (10% to 30%), juxtavesical ureter (20% to 60%), lower third of the ureter (15% to 50%), or a contiguous combination of these areas (30% to 60%) (Al-Shukri and Alwan 1983; Gelfand, 1948; Smith et al., 1977). Three patterns of hydroureter are associated with urogenital schistosomiasis: segmental (i.e., cylindrical or fusiform), tonic, and atonic (Smith et al., 1977). About one-quarter of obstructive uropathy cases involve segmental ureteral dilation; 80% of those cases occur in the lower ureter. The dilations occur above areas of concentric ureteral muscular replacement by fibrosis and sandy patches. It is unusual for segmental lesions to cause significant hydronephrosis. Up to 30% of obstructive uropathy is caused by tonic hydroureter. This is characterized by dilated, tortuous, thick-walled, and trabeculated ureters with marked ureteral muscular hypertrophy and impaired peristalsis. Typically, the entire ureter proximal to an obstructive lesion is involved, generating a functional stenosis. This is often accompanied by significant hydronephrosis, which is reversible if the obstruction is relieved (Smith et al., 1977). Atonic hydroureters are found in the remaining patients with obstructive uropathy. These ureters are markedly dilated, very tortuous and thin-walled, lack peristalsis, and are associated with atrophic, fibrotic ureteral muscle.

Schistosomal hydroureter typically precedes hydronephrosis (Cheever et al., 1978; Lehman et al., 1973). Left untreated, schistosomal hydronephrosis progresses from worsening renal pelvic dilation to medullary atrophy to medullary effacement and cortical atrophy (Smith et al., 1974; Smith et al., 1977). This pathophysiological sequence accounts for the abrogation of tubular function (especially concentrating ability) before compromise of glomerular function (Lehman et al., 1971; Lehman et al., 1973).

Patients with chronic *S. haematobium* are at increased risk of bacterial urinary tract superinfections (Adeyeba and Ojeaga, 2002; Laughlin et al., 1978; Uneke, 2009), possibly because the bacteria can affix to the tegument of adult worms, or secondary to urinary stasis or immunomodulation. Patients infected with *S. haematobium* are also at higher risk for bladder cancer, especially squamous cell carcinoma. The relationship between *S. haematobium* and bladder cancer is perhaps the strongest of any helminthic infection-cancer association. This association is supported by epidemiologic studies (particularly in Egypt) and experimental models (Mostafa et al., 1999). Rates of bladder cancer are linked with duration and severity of infection and are associated with a mortality rate as high as 10.8 per 100,000 males in Egypt (Mustacchi, 2003).

Female genital schistosomiasis (FGS) remains poorly understood. Sequestration of eggs in the female reproductive tract results in the formation of fibrotic nodules, or "sandy patches," in the uterus, cervix, and lower genital tract (Badawy, 1962) (Fig. 60.11). Little is known about the mechanism through which *S. haematobium* generates female genital disease aside from the increased vascularization of the female genital mucosa that occurs due to the presence of eggs (Jourdan et al., 2011).

Other bladder sequelae of long-term *S. haematobium* infection include the development of urothelial hyperplasia, squamous metaplasia, urothelial dysplasia, and eventually urothelial or squamous cell carcinoma. Bladder cancer is the final pathological sequela of schistosomiasis. Schistosomal bladder cancer features an early onset (40 to 50 years) and is often squamous cell carcinoma (60%–90%) or adenocarcinoma (5%–15%) (Al-Shukri et al., 1987; Bedwani et al., 1998; Cheever et al., 1978; Lucas, 1982; Thomas et al., 1990). More than 40% of schistosomiasis-associated bladder squamous cell carcinomas are well differentiated and verrucous and feature an overall good prognosis. Tumors are found on the posterior wall about half of the time and on the lateral wall approximately 30% of the time. Exophytic neoplasms account for roughly two-thirds of schistosomal bladder cancers, whereas the remainder are ulcerative endophytic tumors. Mass drug administration (MDA) campaigns in Egypt have been associated with an overall reduction of bladder neoplasms from 28% to 12% and a shift from squamous cell carcinomas to transitional cell carcinomas (Gouda et al., 2007). Although transitional cell carcinomas of the bladder are less frequently associated with *S. haematobium* infection (Michaud, 2007), some epidemiologists believe that the relatively high rate of smoking in schistosomiasis-endemic regions may further increase the risk of bladder cancer, possibly synergistically with *S. haematobium* infection (Bedwani et al., 1998). However, some unselected autopsy series from the same regions have reported similar frequencies of bladder cancers in patients without schistosomiasis (Cheever et al., 1978; Smith et al., 1977).

Egg deposition into the bladder wall has been implicated as a major factor in carcinogenesis, and *S. haematobium* has recently been classified as a "Class I" agent ("carcinogenic to humans") by the International Agency for Research on Cancer within the World Health Organization (Working Group, 2011). Vascular endothelial growth factor (VEGF) is increased in the bladder early after *S. haematobium* egg exposure (Fu et al., 2012; Ray et al., 2012; Salem et al., 2012). VEGF may promote tumor vasculogenesis and facilitate carcinogenesis and/or cancer progression. One potential pathway of schistosomal bladder oncogenesis may be initiated when papillomas merge with the basal transitional epithelium, forming benign fibro-epithelial papillary growths. After successive episodes of inflammation and fibrosis, some of the urothelial cells may sequester together (or expand clonally) and form potentially precancerous lesions, including squamous metaplasia (Mustacchi, 2003). Molecular profiling of the

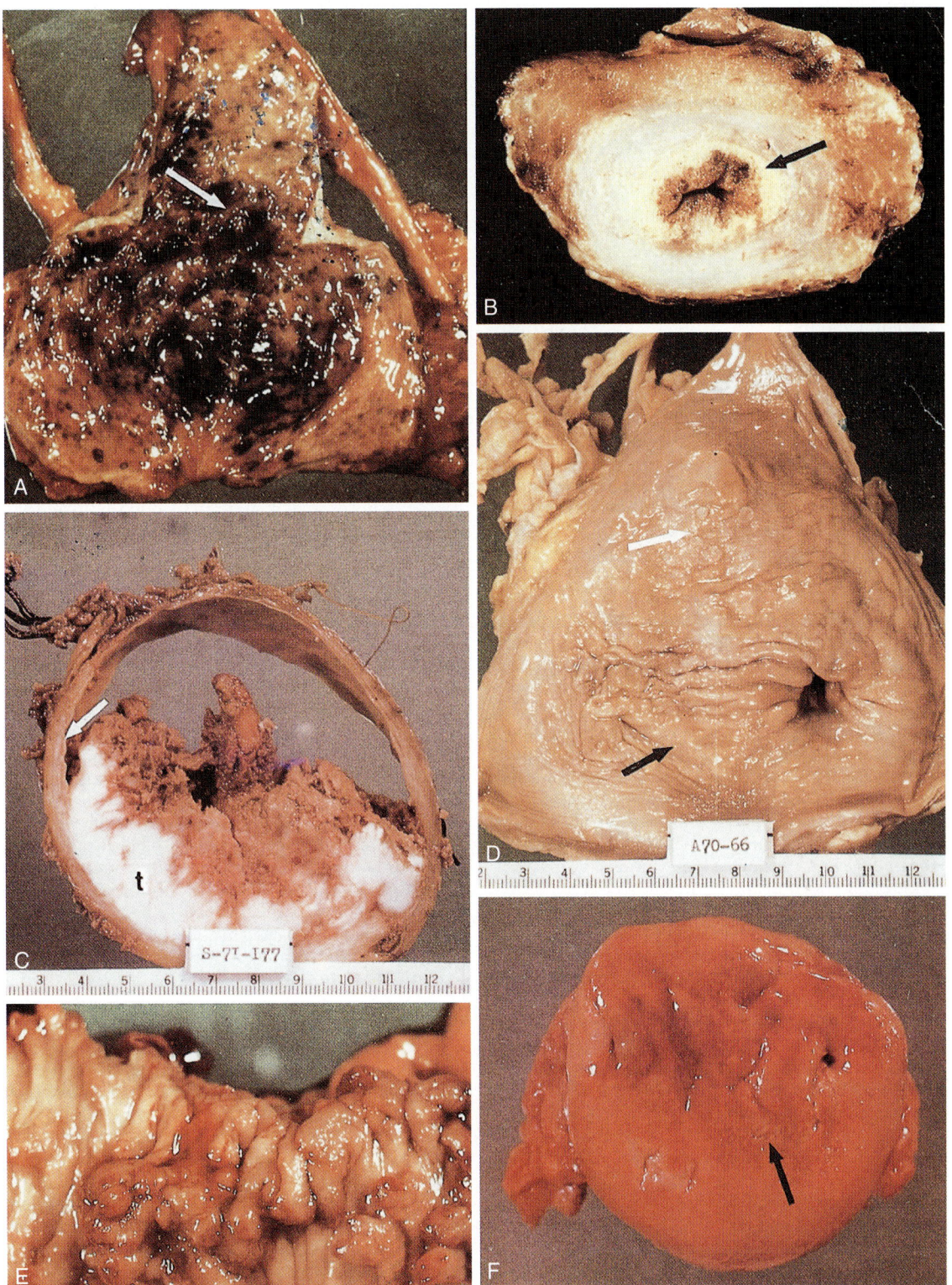

Fig. 60.11. Macroscopic appearance of human urinary schistosomiasis. (A) Urinary bladder opened with an anterior Y incision. The posterior and apical walls have many erythematous, granular, sessile, and pedunculated polyps *(arrow)* characteristic of the early active stage of urinary schistosomiasis. (B) Coronal section through the apex of a formalin-fixed urinary bladder. The lamina propria has been expanded and is replaced by a yellow-tan, finely granular, sandy patch *(arrow)*, which is characteristic of chronic inactive foci. Small, sandy patches are sprinkled through the fibrotic, atrophic detrusor muscle, even in perivesical fat. The more superficial erythematous portion of the lamina propria contains some viable eggs with granulomatous response (chronic active stage of urinary schistosomiasis). (C) Coronal section through the middle of a urinary bladder after formalin inflation and fixation. The lamina propria *(arrow)* has been replaced by a concentric sandy patch, most prominent at the margin of the exophytic, moderately differentiated squamous cell carcinoma. The bladder wall is attenuated except for the tumor (t). No evidence of recent oviposition was found in the lower urinary tract (chronic inactive stage of urinary schistosomiasis, usually found with the bilharzial bladder cancer syndrome). (D) Urinary bladder opened with anterior Y incision shows several features of severe chronic inactive urinary schistosomiasis. The entire lamina propria has been replaced by a sandy patch. Foci of epidermization are seen at or near the *white arrow*. The left ureteral orifice (right) is markedly dilated (the so-called golf-hole ureter of schistosomal uropathy). The right ureteral orifice *(point of black arrow)* is markedly stenotic. (E) Rectosigmoid colon with polyposis. Numerous sessile and pedunculated polyps are seen. Many are erythematous, indicative of active oviposition with granuloma formation. Some have necrotic hemorrhagic tips. (F) Mucosal surface of partial cystectomy specimen (4- to 5-cm ellipse) from a patient with the chronic inactive stage of the disease. There is a stellate chronic schistosomal ulcer. Despite the inactivity of the disease, these ulcers may bleed profusely. Pale mucoid flecks at the margin of the ulcer *(arrow)* are areas of adenoid (goblet cell) metaplasia.

mouse bladder indicates that S. *haematobium* egg exposure induces transcriptional alterations in bladder carcinogenesis-related signaling pathways (Ray et al., 2012). Bacterial urinary tract co-infections may also contribute to S. *haematobium*-associated bladder carcinoma, given that S. *haematobium* increases the ability of bacteria to reduce nitrates to nitrosamines, which can alkylate proteins and nucleic acids (Grisham and Yamada, 1992). Resulting mutations in oncogenes (i.e., p53) may then contribute to neoplasia (Mustacchi, 2003).

Clinical Manifestations

Acute schistosomiasis encompasses the transient human responses to cercarial penetration and the longer-lasting responses to schistosome tissue migration and maturation. Chronic schistosomiasis results from the immune response to protracted oviposition, often lasting for years and leading to organ damage. As a result, clinically apparent chronic schistosomiasis is limited to long-term residents of endemic areas, who are continually re-infected, have long-term, high worm burdens, and are re-exposed to eggs. As with most human helminths, *Schistosoma* spp. cannot complete their life cycle nor replicate in the human host. Thus, in tourists or short-term visitors who are exposed once to the parasite, even in the absence of efficacious chemotherapy, adult worms die of senescence within 3 to 5 years, limiting subsequent pathology.

Acute Schistosomiasis. The first clinical manifestation of schistosomiasis is often an itchy maculopapular rash (cercarial dermatitis), usually within 1 to 2 days of cercarial penetration. The rash usually resolves before travelers have returned from endemic areas, making the diagnosis more difficult (Stuiver, 1984).

Between 2 and 8 weeks later, acute schistosomiasis is seen in some patients during their primary infection (although it is silent in many). The well-known eponym for acute schistosomiasis, "Katayama fever," is named after early descriptions of the syndrome in the Katayama Valley in Japan; it occurs most commonly with heavy primary *S. japonicum* infections, less commonly with *S. mansoni*, and rarely with *S. haematobium*. The initial signs and symptoms of Katayama fever include fever, dry cough, fatigue, headache, diarrhea, eosinophilia, neck pain, and urticaria (Jauréguiberry et al., 2010). Acute schistosomiasis is seen rarely among people living in endemic areas (Meltzer et al., 2006). Because the signs and symptoms of acute schistosomiasis are nonspecific, cases often remain undiagnosed or confused with other endemic diseases such as malaria or enteric fever (Jensen et al., 1995).

Because acute schistosomiasis may be clinically silent, all individuals with exposure to potentially infested water should be aware of the possibility of infection, with considerations for accurate diagnosis and treatment based on these factors (Jauréguiberry et al., 2010).

Chronic Schistosomiasis. Adult *S. haematobium* worm pairs shed eggs into the bladder wall beginning about 8 to 12 weeks after infection. This is sometimes heralded by painless, recurrent hematuria, dysuria, or urinary frequency (Mahmoud, 2001). In some highly endemic cultures, hematuria in males is seen as a sign of puberty, and can be sufficiently severe as to result in anemia (Wilkins et al., 1985). Proteinuria is also often associated with urogenital schistosomiasis. Hematuria is a consistent and specific enough sign of infection that it is used as a primary diagnostic technique in endemic areas. However, given the many other possible causes of hematuria, urogenital schistosomiasis is often unsuspected and misdiagnosed in infected travelers returning to their nonendemic, home countries (Raglio et al., 1995).

Long-term urogenital schistosomiasis results in fibrosis that may obstruct urinary drainage and result in organ dysfunction. Egg deposition in the ureters and subsequent granuloma, polyp, and ulcer formation increases the risk of hydronephrosis and hydroureter because of impaired peristalsis of the walls of the renal pelvis and ureter, which in turn can result in obstruction and vesicoureteral reflux. Recovery of renal function may be achieved through anthelminthic therapy in shorter term infections, although surgical repair of the ureter or urinary diversion may be necessary during late stage or more severe disease (Mahmoud, 2001).

Female genital schistosomiasis (FGS) is another form of chronic schistosomiasis that occurs in 33% to 75% of females with S. *haematobium* infection as a result of eggs deposition into the Fallopian tubes, cervix, vagina, vulva, ovaries, and/or uterus (Kjetland et al., 2012). Friable mucosal lesions ("sandy patches") can result, which often bleed on contact during pelvic examinations or sexual intercourse (Hotez and Fenwick, 2009). Dyspareunia, pelvic and abdominal pain, vaginal bleeding and discharge, urinary frequency, and infertility are common, but resemble urinary tract infections and sexually transmitted diseases of other etiologies, so FGS is often misdiagnosed and left untreated (Hotez and Fenwick, 2009).

Men can carry high numbers of *S. haematobium* eggs in the ejaculatory ducts and seminal vesicles, and blood and/or schistosome eggs may be present in the ejaculate before they are detectable in the urine. Patients with involvement of these urogenital structures often present with a testicular mass or scrotal pain. Egg burdens of the epididymis, ovaries, and fallopian tubes are generally higher than those of the testes, uterus, and vagina (Cheever et al., 1977; Cheever et al., 1978; Helling-Giese et al., 1996).

As infection progresses, a late, chronic, active stage develops when tissue egg burdens peak. Chronic suprapubic and pelvic pain with associated urinary urgency, frequency, and incontinence are classic for the "schistosomal contracted bladder" (Duvie, 1986). Frequently the trigone appears normal or somewhat hyperemic and edematous, whereas the remainder of the detrusor muscle is thickened and indurated, as is the entire bladder wall. Functional bladder capacity can be as low as 50 mL in adults.

Over years, active infection becomes more quiescent, oviposition and egg excretion occur at a lower rate, and symptoms are dampened. More than 30% of light infections become asymptomatic in some endemic regions (Rutasitara and Chimbe, 1985). In spite of this, clinically silent obstructive uropathy may evolve throughout this period as fibrosis replaces polypoid lesions and the bladder and ureters undergo sometimes irreversible damage. As a result, severe hydroureteronephrosis can develop insidiously.

Infected individuals can enter a chronic inactive phase, in which viable eggs are no longer detected in urine or tissues. Signs and symptoms at this stage are caused by sequelae and complications of the immune reaction to the calcified, dead eggs rather than the schistosomal infection itself. Unfortunately, among patients with schistosomal obstructive uropathy, 40% to 60% see urologists at this end stage (Smith and Christie, 1986). In heavily endemic regions, poorly or nonfunctioning kidneys are common in patients who are asymptomatic. About half of patients develop bacterial urinary tract co-infections superimposed on their schistosomal obstructive uropathy. The bacteria associated with urogenital schistosomiasis are the same organisms that cause UTIs in patients without schistosomiasis. Some series have noted an association of chronic or recurring urinary tract infections caused by *Salmonella*, often associated with intermittent bacteremia in some patients with urogenital schistosomiasis (King, 2001). The latter association suggests that *Salmonella* bacteriuria in this setting may actually be "spillover" of bacteremia into the urinary stream. *Salmonella* organisms reside in the apical invaginations of the schistosome tegument, where they are sheltered from host defenses and antibiotics. Awareness of this association can lead to treatment of both infections with good response. Antibiotics alone do not fully resolve this process.

Another manifestation of urogenital schistosomiasis is the development of bladder urothelial ulcers (Smith et al., 1977). Acute schistosomal ulcers rarely are seen in the active stage, when necrotic polyps slough into the urine leaving behind a urothelial ulcer. The more common chronic bladder ulcer is a late sequela of heavy infection. This lesion is associated with a constant "burning" and intense suprapubic and pelvic pain. The majority of these patients exhibit gross hematuria and pyuria.

Eosinophilia is very common during acute schistosomiasis and is seen even during chronic infection. During chronic infection, the eosinophilia is usually low grade, and although neither sensitive nor specific for schistosomiasis, its presence can be a clue that a parasitic infection such as schistosomiasis may be present. Exceptions to this usual sequence of acute and chronic infection may occur and sometimes manifest in the form of ectopic pulmonary schistosomiasis, neuroschistosomiasis, and female genital schistosomiasis.

Diagnosis

Finding *S. haematobium* eggs in urine or stool remains the gold standard for diagnosis of active infection, although eggs do not appear until oviposition begins 8 to 12 weeks after initial infection. As maximal egg shedding in the urine peaks at noon, urine samples should be ideally collected between 9 AM and 3 PM for examination (Doehring et al., 1983; Doehring et al. 1985). Urine samples can be concentrated to increase sensitivity and detect low-intensity infections. If eggs are not found in the urine or stool but clinical suspicion remains high and serology is consistent with exposure, tissue biopsy can be considered. A rectal snip biopsy should be performed before a bladder biopsy, because eggs are common in the rectal mucosa and the risk of a bladder biopsy-related complication (i.e., infection, perforation) is avoided. A squash preparation of the biopsy specimen between glass slides is superior to histopathologic analysis, because it is more sensitive and allows determination of egg viability. In potential cases of female genital schistosomiasis, microscopic inspection of biopsies of lesions on the vulva, vagina, or cervix may result in egg identification and diagnosis (Helling-Giese et al., 1996). Visual- and dipstick-based detection of gross or microscopic hematuria and urine turbidity are also used to indirectly diagnose urogenital schistosomiasis, although these methods are less sensitive and specific and best combined with already-established diagnostic tools; they are most commonly used in the developing world as part of control and elimination campaigns (Adesola et al., 2012).

Serologic tests that combine a FAST-ELISA followed by Western blot analysis are available at the Centers for Disease Control and Prevention (CDC) (Al-Sherbiny et al., 1999; CDC, 2014; Wilson et al., 1995). Together, the assays are more than 90% sensitive and specific for *S. haematobium* infection. In cases in which the diagnosis is suspected but eggs are not present, serology can be useful but does not distinguish between acute and chronic infection because antibody titers remain positive even after curative chemotherapy. Other serologic assays are also available at commercial laboratories. Patients generally first become antibody positive about 4 to 6 weeks after infection (Schwartz et al., 2005).

Ultrasonography can also be useful and may demonstrate bladder or ureteral wall thickening, polypoid lesions, hydroureter, hydronephrosis, urinary tract calcifications, and even bladder carcinoma (Kardorff and Döhring, 2001). Plain abdominal radiographs may reveal urinary tract calcifications; a calcified bladder, which may resemble a fetal head in the pelvis, is characteristic of chronic urogenital schistosomiasis (Fig. 60.12). The prostate, seminal vesicles, posterior urethra, distal ureters, and, occasionally, colon may also demonstrate calcifications.

The earliest radiographic changes on intravenous urography appear to be striations in the ureters and renal pelvis (Hugosson, 1987). Ureteral calcification is typically intramural, and the ureters are dilated. This differs from the calcifications seen in tuberculosis, which form casts of nondilated ureters. Other findings on intravenous urography include hydronephrosis, hydroureter, nonfunctioning kidney, ureteral stenosis, and bladder and ureteral filling defects caused by polypoid lesions. Similar lesions can also be identified through ultrasonography. With intravenous urography, delayed films are often necessary in the presence of severe obstructive uropathy to discern distended ureters and kidneys. Postvoid views may reveal bladder neck obstruction with retention. Combining intravenous urography with fluoroscopy can differentiate between tonic and atonic ureters (Abdel-Halim et al., 1985) and identify nonstenotic, immobile ureters.

CT can detect obstructive uropathy and calcified lesions in the colon and urinary tract (Jorulf and Linstedt, 1985), a potential advantage over intravenous urography. MRI does not yet seem to provide enough diagnostic superiority to warrant widespread use (Kohno et al., 2008). Fluoroscopic voiding cystourethrography can detect vesicoureteral reflux, which occurs in 25% of infected ureters. Cystoureterscopy may reveal mucosal lesions in the bladder (Fig. 60.13). Retrograde fluoroscopic pyelography during cystoureterscopy may reveal important details regarding ureteral anatomy and drainage.

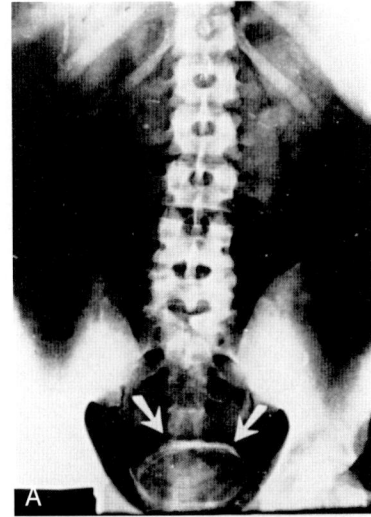
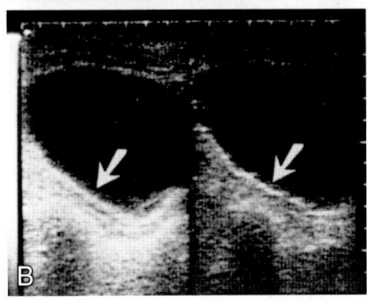

Fig. 60.12. Bladder calcification in a 30-year-old Egyptian farmer. (A) Plain x-ray film of the abdomen shows a rim of calcification surrounding the urinary bladder *(arrows)*. (B) Abdominal ultrasound study shows a bright line surrounding the bladder with a definite dark rim behind it *(arrows)*. (A and B, Courtesy G. Thomas Strickland, MD. From Abdel-Wahab MF, Ramzy I, Esmat G, et al.: Ultrasonography for detecting Schistosoma haematobium urinary tract complications: comparison with radiographic procedures. *J Urol.* 148:346, 1992.)

Antigen detection or PCR may be a more sensitive means of diagnosis. Serum or urine samples from infected individuals can be tested for the presence of circulating anodic and circulating cathodic schistosome antigens (CAA and CCA). CAA and CCA are specific for active infection because they are only released by viable adult worms and have the added benefit of producing quantitative measurements useful for determining infection severity (Agnew et al., 1995; Kremsner et al., 1994). Moreover, the development of an ELISA reagent strip test for urine samples has allowed for point-of-care detection of CCA that is more user friendly and field applicable (Midzi et al., 2009; van Dam et al., 2004). However, in some hands the CCA test completely failed to detect *S. haematobium* infection (versus >80% sensitivity and specificity for detection of *S. mansoni* infection) (Stothard et al., 2006) and is relatively expensive for widescale use in the developing world.

By far the most sensitive method for diagnosing urogenital schistosomiasis from urine or even stool samples is PCR (Obeng et al., 2008; ten Hove et al., 2008). PCR is also highly sensitive and specific for diagnosing female genital schistosomiasis from vaginal lavage samples, although detection may vary based on patient age and length of infection (Kjetland et al., 2009). Unfortunately, PCR is difficult to use in the developing world and in the field because it requires highly trained technicians and the use of organic solvents and commercial kits. Still, in the context of transmission control and disease surveillance, especially in settings of low-intensity transmission, PCR is a useful option.

Globally, many cases of urogenital schistosomiasis remain undetected and untreated because most are diagnosed only through direct egg detection rather than more sensitive methods. The need

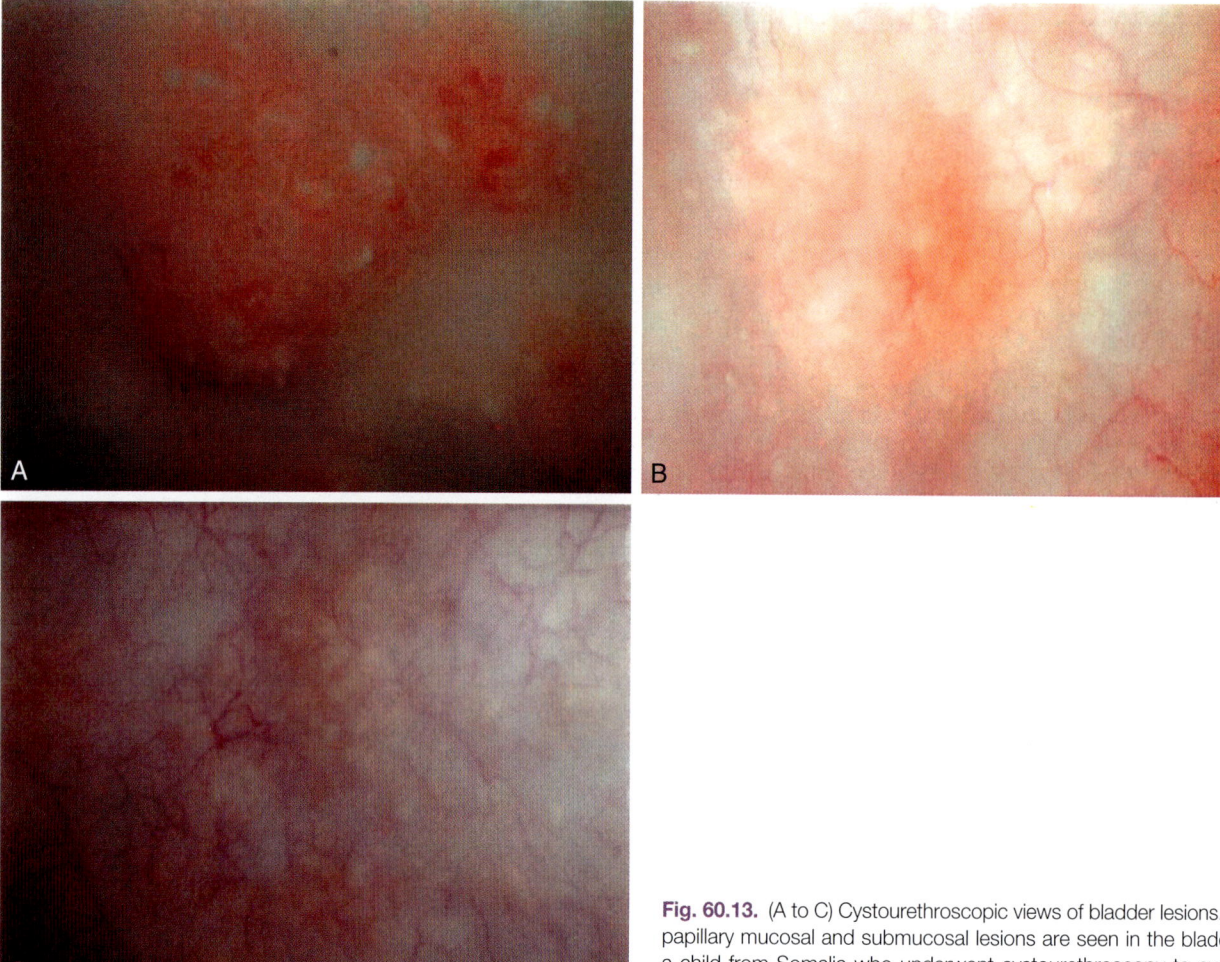

Fig. 60.13. (A to C) Cystourethroscopic views of bladder lesions. Both papillary mucosal and submucosal lesions are seen in the bladder of a child from Somalia who underwent cystourethroscopy to evaluate intermittent hematuria and dysuria. (Courtesy Craig Peters, MD.)

for more reliable and accessible diagnostic tools is thus particularly important for the development of more effective schistosomiasis control strategies in the developing world.

Treatment

Medical Management. Praziquantel (PZQ) is currently the only WHO-recommended drug for schistosomiasis (WHO, 2014b) and has replaced metrifonate and oxamniquine as the main therapeutic agent. Although dependence on a single drug increases the potential for parasitic resistance, PZQ's efficacy, widespread availability, and low toxicity are favorable factors, and there has been little incentive for the development of alternative drugs. Two 20-mg/kg oral doses of PZQ are given on the same day, 6 to 8 hours apart (or alternatively, one 40-mg/kg dose) for S. haematobium infections. Corticosteroids are often added for the treatment of acute schistosomiasis (Katayama fever).

As measured by egg reduction and cure rate, PZQ's efficacy is 60% to 90% (Danso-Appiah et al., 2008; Doenhoff, et al., 2008). Even in those not cured, the worm burden is likely substantially reduced, which significantly decreases the chances of developing further infectious sequelae. After a patient is treated with PZQ, it is reasonable to monitor egg counts in urine and stool specimens and to perform serial ultrasonographic studies of the urogenital tract to assess response to drug therapy. Repeat PZQ courses can be given if there is a concern for persistent infection.

PZQ has a favorable pharmacokinetic and side effect profile. The most common side effects (abdominal pain, nausea, headache, and dizziness) are typically mild, generally occur within 3 to 4 hours postadministration, and resolve spontaneously. Most patients experience few or no side effects (N'Goran et al., 2003). However, PZQ pills are large and bitter tasting, making oral administration difficult to tolerate, especially for children (Meyer et al., 2009). A pediatric formulation of PZQ is in development. Perhaps because of its FDA classification as a Pregnancy Category B drug (deemed safe in lactating and pregnant women based only on animal studies), many chemotherapy programs exclude pregnant and lactating women. However, there are few reports of adverse effects resulting from PZQ among the millions of pregnant women treated with praziquantel (Olds, 2003).

PZQ is less efficacious against schistosomulae than adult worms, which may partly explain the lower cure rates in areas with high rates of schistosomiasis transmission and reinfection. In addition, it means that PZQ cannot be used to abort infection shortly after exposure. Multiple PZQ doses administered several weeks apart can ensure that juvenile schistosomes missed by the first administration are eradicated after maturation (Doenhoff et al., 2008).

Whether schistosomes are developing resistance to PZQ is debatable. Most large studies conducted on S. haematobium–infected individuals suggest little drug resistance in endemic areas (Guidi et al., 2010; King et al., 2000). However, there have been reports of PZQ failures in the treatment of travelers or military personnel returning from endemic areas (Doenhoff et al., 2008). Even if resistance to PZQ is not already evolving, it could occur in the future. Hopefully, use of alternative drugs and combining drug treatment programs with environmental control programs (snail control and sanitation improvement) may lower transmission and reduce the use of PZQ enough to prevent this.

Artemisinin and its analogues (artemether and artesunate, currently in use as antimalarials) are chemoprophylactic alternatives to

PZQ because they specifically target the schistosomular stage of *S. haematobium*. Artemether or artesunate are 90% to 97% efficacious in preventing schistosomiasis but are poor treatments for established infections. Combined administration of PZQ and artemisinin derivatives results in lower infection rates than PZQ alone and thus offers a valuable tool for mass drug administration programs, especially in areas of high transmission and reinfection rates. However, a major concern regarding the use of artemesinins in this manner is the induction of malaria resistance to artemisinin derivatives. Because of this, widespread PZQ-artemisinin derivative combination therapy should not be used in schistosomiasis-malaria co-endemic areas (Liu et al., 2011).

Surgical Management. The efficacy and ease of PZQ therapy for urogenital schistosomiasis, together with the possible reversibility of early stage disease (Richter et al., 1996; Richter, 2000) mean that, in most cases, trials of medical therapy should be undertaken before elective surgical approaches (Cioli, 1995). Generally, surgery is reserved for complications that have not responded to adequate medical treatment within a reasonable follow-up period or for those settings where immediate surgical intervention is necessary. For example, severe bladder hemorrhage is one common cause for urgent surgical intervention.

Prostatitis and prostatic enlargement are uncommon in schistosomiasis. Accordingly, numerous autopsy studies have failed to demonstrate evidence of anatomic bladder outlet obstruction (Cheever et al., 1977; Cheever et al., 1978; Smith et al., 1974). However, clinical studies consistently report cystoscopic (FAM, 1964), urodynamic (Sabha and Nilsson, 1988), and elevated postvoid residual urine volumes, which are evidence of functional bladder outlet obstruction that occasionally requires surgical intervention in patients with severe inactive urinary schistosomiasis (Abdel-Halim et al., 1985). *S. haematobium* infection–associated scrotal induration, pain, and enlargement associated with epididymitis can lead to surgery for the suspicion of a testicular tumor.

Surgery is indicated for irreversibly contracted bladders; procedures include vesical denervation, urinary diversion, ileocystoplasty, or hydrodistention. Any treatment, however, must be performed in conjunction with medical chemotherapy. Chronic, deep bladder ulcers may necessitate a partial cystectomy, because fulguration rarely produces either symptomatic relief or ulcer healing. Urothelial hyperplasia is strongly associated with severe urogenital schistosomiasis, whereas urothelial dysplasia and metaplasia commonly accompany schistosomal bladder cancer (Khafagy et al., 1972). Treatment of bladder cancer secondary to schistosomiasis is typically surgical and discussed elsewhere (see Chapters 92 through 96).

The most frequent sequelae of urinary schistosomiasis result from ureteral involvement causing obstructive uropathy (Cheever et al., 1978; Lehman et al., 1973; Smith and Christie, 1986; Smith et al., 1974). Hydroureter and hydronephrosis are linked to the intensity of *S. haematobium* infection. **Because ureteral obstruction observed during schistosomiasis is most often caused by concentric or hemiconcentric polypoid lesions that "girdle" the ureteral muscle in the intramural and adjacent extravesical ureter, it often responds well to medical management alone.** Complete resolution of deteriorated renal function because of active infection–associated obstructive uropathy responds within 1 to 2 months of PZQ chemotherapy (Lehman et al., 1973). Chemotherapy not only reverses schistosomal obstructive uropathy but also can prevent it, even in persons who are continually reinfected (Subramanian et al., 1999). However, in late, chronic, active and inactive urinary schistosomiasis, anatomic obstruction may be less amenable to chemotherapeutic cure.

Anatomic ureteral stenosis, with or without calculi, has been identified in up to 80% of patients with ureteral obstruction (Al-Shukri and Alwan, 1983; El-Nahas et al., 2003; Lehman et al., 1973; Smith et al., 1977). **When residual ureteral stenosis persists after chemotherapy, it is usually amenable to surgical intervention. Depending on the location and extent of the stricture, procedures involving dilation or excision have been employed.** Balloon dilation is efficacious with anatomic stenosis (Jacobsson et al., 1987), but mechanical dilation is frequently plagued by recurrent stenosis (Wishahi, 1987). When the ureteral meatus, intramural ureter, ureterovesical junction, or distal ureter is involved, options to reconstruct a functional valve include a variety of plastic operations. Most of these procedures are variants of the Politano-Leadbetter operation (Leadbetter and Leadbetter, 1961; Politano and Leadbetter, 1958). Although highly efficacious for some patients (Al-Shukri and Alwan, 1983; Smith et al., 1977), other authors have noted that restenosis can occur (Umerah, 1981).

In long or multifocal lesions of the ureter, excision of the affected portion may leave an inadequate residual ureter for reimplantation or simple ureteroureterostomy. In these cases, surgeons have successfully employed the Boari flap, ileal conduit, suprapubic intravesical ureterostomy (in which the obstructed ureteral segment is bypassed using a peritoneal dialysis catheter and drained into the bladder), and replacement of the ureter with ileal segments, taking care to maintain an isoperistaltic direction of the ileal segment (Abdel-Halim, 1980; Abdel-Halim, 1984; Abu-Aisha et al., 1985; Al-Shukri and Alwan, 1983). Isolated meatal stenosis of the ureter may be amenable to simple meatoplasty (Al-Shukri and Alwan, 1983). When a ureter is hopelessly obstructed and cannot be reconstructed, long-term nephrostomy drainage is another option.

Prognosis. **Most patients with urogenital schistosomiasis have mild infections and a good prognosis. The morbidity and mortality of urogenital schistosomiasis is determined by the overall intensity of infection and genetic polymorphisms for relevant immune response genes** (He et al., 2008; Isnard et al., 2011; Isnard and Chevillard, 2008; Kouriba et al., 2005; Ouf et al., 2012). In regions of low *S. haematobium* prevalence, such as Nigeria, essentially no urogenital schistosomiasis-related mortality is observed and the frequency and severity of schistosomal obstructive uropathy is low. In contrast, when Egypt had a prevalence of 50%, schistosomiasis contributed to mortality in 10% of *S. haematobium*-infected individuals (Cheever et al., 1978; Smith et al., 1974). Among patients with severe disease, mortality approached 50% in 2 to 5 years (Lehman et al., 1970). **Patients who die of schistosomal obstructive uropathy (bilateral end-stage hydronephrosis, or unilateral hydronephrosis with contralateral non-schistosomal end-stage renal disease) are typically in their 20s and have heavy total egg burdens.** Patients who develop the complications of pyelonephritis and urothelial cancer are commonly older than age 40, consistent with time- and intensity-related pathology (Christie et al., 1986; Smith and Christie, 1986).

The prognosis for patients with urinary tract lesions has dramatically improved with PZQ therapy. In children with obstructive polyps, the uropathy usually completely resolves within 2 to 6 weeks of treatment. For patients with chronic obstructive uropathy resulting from sandy patches and fibrosis, the prognosis is less clear. Some individuals tolerate advanced obstructive uropathy with little, if any, deterioration in renal function. **Schistosomal obstructive uropathy, urolithiasis, bladder outlet obstruction, and bacterial cystitis all predispose to pyelonephritis.** Bacterial superinfection can be life-threatening and should be treated aggressively and promptly. Finally, for **those who develop a bladder malignancy, their prognosis is dependent on the aggressiveness of their tumor.**

Prevention and Control

Travelers to endemic areas should be advised to avoid contact with potentially infested fresh water (streams, rivers, ponds, and lakes). Fast-flowing water can still harbor *S. haematobium*. **Heating water to more than 125°F for 5 minutes kills the cercariae, as does chlorination and allowing the water to stand for more than 2 days in a setting free of snails.** Since the advent of PZQ in the late 1970s and its subsequent mass distribution beginning in the 1980s and 1990s, schistosomiasis has become relatively simple and affordable to treat but remains difficult to control. For the past 3 to 4 decades, control efforts have focused heavily on reducing morbidity using periodic, typically annual targeted mass drug treatments with PZQ, a strategy advocated by the WHO. However, when access to safe water is not available, rural poor communities are subject to vicious cycles of infection, treatment, and reinfection, making more frequent PZQ administration necessary. Sanitation improvements, health education, and snail control are approaches used to break the cycle of transmission by slowing or halting the influx of eggs into the aquatic habitat, decreasing individual exposure, and reducing the availability of snail intermediate hosts, respectively. Although PZQ is inexpensive, the cost effectiveness of chemotherapy fluctuates widely among MDA settings because of variations in the number of doses of PZQ given per person, variability in transportation and delivery costs, and the potential to take advantage of pre-existing public health control programs or other infrastructure (Brooker et al., 2008). The per-person cost in control campaigns is typically under $0.50, although even this modest cost, at sufficient scale, may exceed the available resources of many endemic countries (Hotez et al., 2009). Fortunately, a number of pharmaceutical companies and foundations are donating PZQ for use in MDA campaigns.

Because asexual reproduction in the snail host allows the parasite to amplify rapidly, sanitation programs and drug treatment campaigns must reduce egg input into the environment by nearly 90% before a substantial decrease in transmission can be achieved (Woolhouse, 1992). Reductions in snail populations, in contrast, can theoretically effect proportional decreases in disease transmission risk; some experts feel snail control may be the best means of schistosomiasis control (Sokolow et al., 2016; Woolhouse, 1992). However, considering that adult worms can live for years in the human host, without concurrent mass treatment, snail population control alone would have to persist for many years to eliminate transmission. Thus integrated campaigns focusing on three aims (treating human cases, reducing contact of humans and their wastes with infested water, and controlling snails) offer the most promise (Sokolow et al., 2016; Sokolow et al., 2018).

Other control efforts include molluscicides (Knopp et al., 2011; Knopp et al., 2012; Zhang and Jiang, 2011), biologic control using snail predators or competitors (Allen and Victory, 2003; Coelho et al., 2004; Mkoji et al., 1999; Pointier and Jourdane, 2000; Roberts and Kuris, 1990; Sokolow et al., 2013), and vaccine development (although an efficacious vaccine currently remains out of reach) (Bethony et al., 2008; Gray et al., 2010). Water, sanitation, and hygiene ("WASH") programs are also, once again, taking center stage, and feature many additional benefits beyond potential schistosomiasis reduction (Giné Garriga and Pérez Foguet, 2013; Soares et al., 2011).

In contrast to the outcomes seen with attempts at elimination and control of other parasitic infections (e.g., malaria, lymphatic filariasis, onchocerciasis), the mass drug administration and other control programs aimed at schistosomiasis have not resulted in a reduction in the worldwide prevalence of this infection in recent years. At the same time, schistosomiasis has been eliminated in 10 countries to date (Iran, Japan, Lebanon, Malaysia, Martinique, Montserrat, Morocco, Thailand, Tunisia, and Turkey) (Amarir et al., 2011; Rollinson et al., 2012). At the 65th WHO World Health Assembly (May 2012), resolution WHA65.21 was passed, calling on the global community to "make available the necessary and sufficient means and resources…to intensify control programs in most disease-endemic countries and initiate elimination campaigns, where appropriate" (WHO, 2014). Representing a shift from morbidity control to a new focus on elimination, this marks an exciting and hopeful milestone in the global fight against schistosomiasis.

> **KEY POINTS: SCHISTOSOMIASIS**
> - *S. haematobium* worms can survive in human hosts for years to decades. A careful travel and social history is crucial to identify potential exposures, correlate them with urogenital symptoms, and determine the need to perform specific diagnostic assays.
> - Praziquantel therapy of early stage urogenital schistosomiasis can reverse inflammatory lesions, including fibrosis of the urinary tract caused by the host response to eggs deposited in tissues.
> - The gold standard for diagnosis of active urogenital schistosomiasis is the identification of eggs in urine, stool, or bladder or rectal biopsies. Serological and PCR-based assays are highly sensitive but may not distinguish between active versus resolved infection and are impractical in endemic regions.

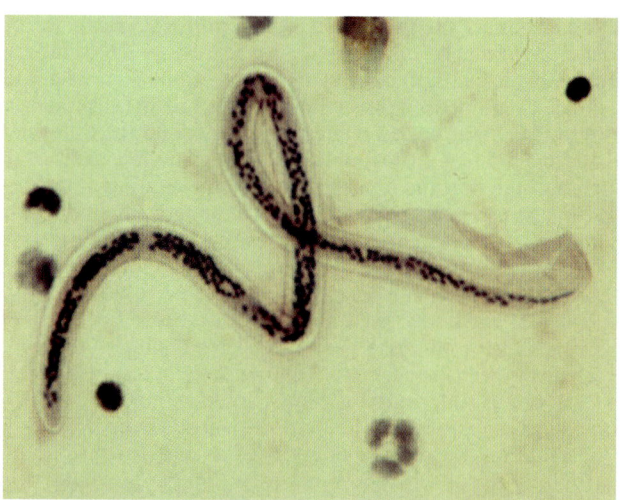

Fig. 60.14. Microfilaria of *Wuchereria bancrofti* in peripheral blood. (Courtesy Division of Parasitic Diseases and Malaria, Centers for Disease Control and Prevention.)

Filariasis

The filariae are vector-borne tissue nematodes. Human pathogens in this group include the agents of **lymphatic filariasis** (LF), *Onchocerca volvulus*, and *Loa loa*.

LF is caused by the mosquito-borne helminths *Wuchereria bancrofti*, *Brugia malayi*, and *Brugia timori*. The symptoms of LF range from acute lymphatic inflammation to chronic lymphatic dilation with hydrocele, lymphedema, and elephantiasis of the limbs.

Organisms

W. bancrofti, *B. malayi*, and *B. timori* are threadlike nematodes. Infective (third-stage) larvae are transmitted to humans by mosquito bites. After entering humans, larvae migrate to central lymphatic vessels and eventually mature (over 6 to 9 months) into adult male or female worms. Adults (approximately 20 to 100 mm × 0.2 mm) are considerably larger than microfilariae (approximately 200 μm × 10 μm) (Fig. 60.14). Adult worms live primarily in the afferent lymphatics, especially in the lower extremities (inguinal, iliac, and periaortic lymphatics) and (for *W. bancrofti* only) male genitalia (epididymis, spermatic cord, testicles). The natural lifespan of adult worms is approximately 5 to 7 years.

After mating with males, female worms release large numbers of microfilariae. In most endemic areas, *W. bancrofti* and *Brugia* microfilaremia peak in the middle of the night as an adaptation to facilitate transmission, coinciding with peak local mosquito vector activity. In some parts of the Pacific, the periodicity of *W. bancrofti* is diurnal rather than nocturnal. After mosquito ingestion, microfilariae mature over 10 to 14 days into infective third-stage larvae.

W. bancrofti and *Brugia* species harbor an obligate rickettsia-like endosymbiont (*Wolbachia*). These endosymbionts are involved in embryogenesis, and antimicrobial therapy (e.g., doxycycline) kills them, resulting in decreased microfilariae release and suppressed larval molting (Hoerauf et al., 2001).

Epidemiology

Worldwide, millions of people are infected with LF, many of whom experience significant morbidity. Recent estimates place the global prevalence of LF at approximately 68 million, a substantial decline compared with the early 2000s (Ramaiah and Ottesen, 2014). More than 90% of infections are caused by *W. bancrofti*, mostly in sub-Saharan Africa, South and Southeast Asia, and the western Pacific. In the Americas, *W. bancrofti* is endemic only to Haiti, the Dominican Republic, Guyana, and Brazil. Infection with *B. malayi* is limited to Asia and several Pacific islands (e.g., Indonesia and the Philippines).

B. timori infection occurs only in southeastern Indonesia. Within a given geographic area, the distribution of LF is often heterogeneous. Several genera of mosquitoes are capable of transmission, including *Anopheles* (rural Africa and the Pacific), *Culex* (urban areas, especially India), *Aedes aegypti* in some Pacific islands, and others.

Although varying among different locales and mosquito vectors, transmission of LF is relatively inefficient, and obstructive lymphatic disease is generally seen only in persons repeatedly infected over many years (i.e., usually long-term residents of endemic areas). In endemic communities, prevalence increases from childhood through the third or fourth decade of life, after which it remains fairly constant (because of the gradual accumulation of adult-stage worms in the population over time). Lymphedema and genital disease are rare before age 10 but increase in prevalence with age. Overall, about one-third of infected persons have clinically overt disease. The likelihood of developing clinical manifestations is particularly high in India, Papua New Guinea, and Africa, whereas it is lower in the Americas (Kazura et al., 1997).

Pathology and Clinical Manifestations

The initial immune response to infective larvae and early adult worms is mostly proinflammatory (involving Th1 and Th2 T-cell responses). The contribution of humoral immunity includes an increase in filaria-specific IgE titers. Eosinophil-mediated killing of microfilariae also likely plays a role. With the onset of microfilaremia, T-cell responses decrease, mediated by IL-10, IgG4-blocking antibodies, and antigen-specific suppressor T cells. Whether protective immunity develops has been difficult to determine, but groups of individuals have remained infection free despite long-term exposure in highly endemic settings (Steel et al., 1996).

Clinical manifestations in infected patients vary greatly, ranging from subclinical infection to severe disfigurement of the limbs and genitalia. Damage from established infection is cumulative because of progressive scarring and lymphatic obstruction over time. Medical therapy does not readily reverse such damage but can prevent further progression in patients with active LF infection. Although rarely fatal, LF can cause severe disability and among parasitic infections is responsible for the third-highest number of disability-adjusted life years (DALYs) lost globally.

The mechanisms leading to lymphedema have been poorly established. However, parasite-derived factors are at least partly responsible for initial lymphatic dilation, with subsequent contributions from secondary bacterial infections and inflammatory responses to dying or dead parasites. *Wolbachia* endosymbionts also appear to drive a proinflammatory response. Lesions vary from nodular inflammation to suppuration, histologically appearing as granulomas around worms, sometimes with tissue eosinophils (Fig. 60.15). A vicious cycle can result, with acute attacks worsening lymphedema, predisposing to more secondary infections, worsening lymphedema, and so on; episodic filarial inflammation eventually abates, leaving obliterated lymphatics surrounded by scar tissue. Elephantiasis or hydrocele is then the end stage in some patients.

Subclinical Infection. Most LF-infected persons have few overt clinical manifestations, even with high-grade microfilaremia. However, though the infection is clinically asymptomatic, virtually all persons with patent *W. bancrofti* or *B. malayi* infection have at least some subclinical disease (e.g., dilated lymphatics, scrotal lymphangiectasia, microscopic hematuria, or proteinuria). Eosinophilia is also very common with most forms of LF.

Acute Adenolymphangitis. Acute adenolymphangitis (ADL) is often the first clinical manifestation of LF, consisting of fever, lymphadenitis, lymphangitis, and edema that usually lasts days to a week. The lymphangitis is retrograde (extending peripherally), which distinguishes it from bacterial lymphangitis. Although all four extremities can be involved in bancroftian and brugian filariasis, the genital lymphatics are affected almost exclusively by *W. bancrofti* infection. This can result in funiculitis, epididymitis, scrotal pain, tenderness, and lymph scrotum (ruptured lymphatic vesicles on the scrotal skin that yield a whitish discharge and secondary bacterial infections).

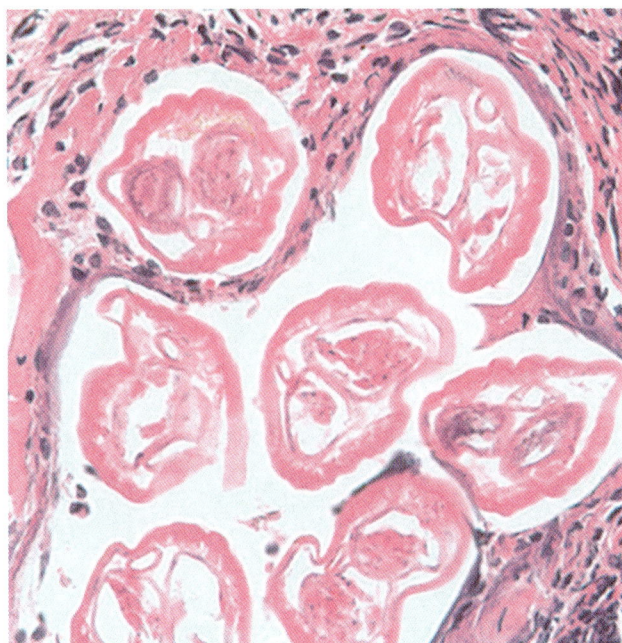

Fig. 60.15. Section of an adult *Brugia* organism in a lymph node. (Courtesy Division of Parasitic Diseases and Malaria, Centers for Disease Control and Prevention.)

Another acute manifestation, **dermatolymphangioadenitis** (DLA), is characterized by fever, chills, myalgias, and headache. Edematous inflammatory plaques occur, as well as hyperpigmentation, vesicles, and ulcers, often at the site of an inciting skin injury. Inflammation progresses proximally and is thought to be secondary to bacterial infections.

Lymphedema. Lower or upper extremity edema is the most common chronic manifestation of LF, with lower extremity edema being the more prevalent. Bancroftian filariasis typically involves the entire limb, whereas brugian filariasis usually involves only the leg below the knee. Although both lower extremities are often affected, asymmetrical involvement is most common. The overlying skin may exude serous fluid. Breast involvement can also occur in females.

Genitourinary Manifestations. Male genital involvement is very common with bancroftian filariasis but uncommon with *Brugia* infection. The prevalence of female genital involvement has not been well established, although anecdotal evidence suggests that it is uncommon (Nutman and Kazura, 2011). Genital disease is not usually experienced until at least the teenage years. Acute painful episodes of (usually unilateral) epididymitis or funiculitis accompanied by fever and malaise can last several days and are one of the most common consequences of bancroftian filariasis.

Funiculoepididymitis. Funiculoepididymitis is characterized by palpable cordlike swellings and edema. Although the condition is usually self-limited, recurrences and the subsequent development of chronic lymphedema are common. Filarial funiculitis rarely results in sterility or orchitis, because the spermatic cord usually remains uninvolved. This manifestation is often mistaken for malignancy, and many patients undergo surgery as a result (including orchiectomy). Varicocele may complicate inflammation, increasing pain and swelling. Bacterial superinfection is a rare but severe complication, with exquisite pain and septic thrombophlebitis often present.

Hydroceles. Chronic disease of the male genitals often results in hydroceles, which can be very large (Fig. 60.16). In endemic areas, differentiation of filarial from nonfilarial hydrocele is difficult, and parasites are rarely detected in the hydrocele fluid. Hydrocele accompanied by nodules in the cord or epididymis and a history of travel to or residence in an endemic area suggests LF. A thick, fibrous tunica, especially with cholesterol or calcium deposits, also suggests LF.

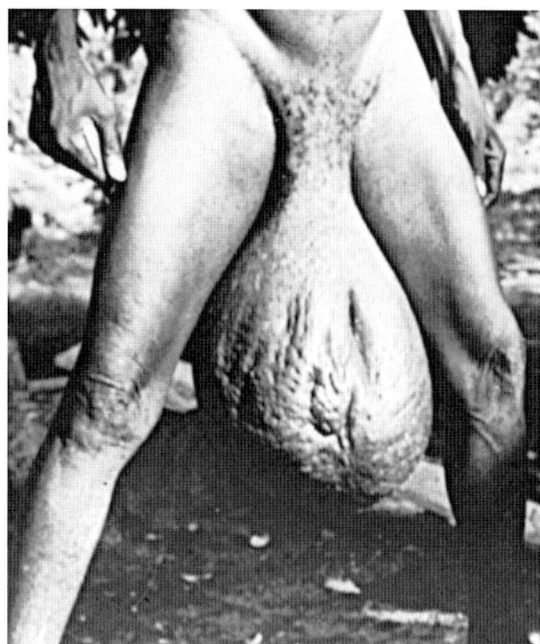

Fig. 60.16. Huge hydrocele and scrotal elephantiasis. (Courtesy Dr. B. H. Kean. From Zaiman H: A pictorial presentation of parasites, Valley City, ND.)

Hydroceles are usually painless unless complicated by acute epididymitis or funiculitis. The scrotal skin may also be thickened and brawny as a result of lymphedema, with oozing lymph. Patients with filarial hydrocele rarely experience bacterial superinfection, although those with elephantiasis and lymph scrotum are often superinfected.

Scrotal and Penile Elephantiasis. Mild scrotal edema is not unusual during early infection or with established hydrocele. Conversely, penile edema is unusual, and massive enlargement of the scrotum or penis occurs late, largely in individuals with poor access to medical care. Genital elephantiasis rarely arises from causes other than LF.

Chyluria. Chyluria occurs when GU tract lymphatics are damaged, resulting in lymph passage into the urine and massive fat and protein loss. Although rare, this can result in serious nutritional consequences. It usually occurs earlier in the natural history of filariasis than genital elephantiasis. Chyluria is usually intermittent and may spontaneously remit.

Tropical Pulmonary Eosinophilia. Tropical pulmonary eosinophilia (TPE) is a syndrome characterized by paroxysmal cough and wheezing (usually nocturnal), fever, adenopathy, high-grade eosinophilia, and elevated IgE levels. It is caused by an allergic response to microfilarial antigens and is seen most commonly in South and Southeast Asia. Chest radiographs range from normal to diffuse reticulonodular infiltrates, and pulmonary function tests show restrictive (and sometimes obstructive) defects. If done, lung biopsy reveals an eosinophilic interstitial pneumonitis. Microfilaremia is usually absent.

Diagnosis

In residents of endemic areas, lymphedema or male genital disease is epidemiologically more likely a result of LF than a similar presentation in the developed world (assuming no other cause of secondary edema is present). Still, tuberculosis, *S. haematobium* infection (urogenital schistosomiasis), and gonorrhea may also produce funiculoepididymitis and are in the differential diagnosis. In addition, nonfilarial hydrocele is common in tropical and nontropical areas. However, hydrocele occurs at an earlier age and with greater frequency in filariasis-endemic areas.

For parasitologic confirmation, it is difficult to visualize adult worms directly because they are localized in the lymphatics; they are usually seen only via histologic examination of surgical or biopsy specimens (in which visualizing adult worms is diagnostically definitive but insensitive). However, ultrasound examination of lymphatics has at least 80% sensitivity in some settings, in part because live adult worms have a distinctive pattern of movement (the **"filaria dance sign"**) (Amaral et al., 1994). Online examples can be found at https://www.youtube.com/watch?v=ER1BFx4_qGc and http://www.filariajournal.com/content/2/1/3/figure/F1?highres=y. Plain radiographs may reveal calcifications, which are also suggestive of LF in the appropriate clinical setting.

Microfilariae can be found in blood and occasionally in other body fluids; they are best detected by a Giemsa-stained blood smear. The timing of blood collection should be based on the periodicity of the microfilariae in the geographic location involved (highest during the night in most cases). Microfilaremia is found in only a minority of infected persons, and definitive diagnosis in amicrofilaremic cases can be more difficult. Detection of circulating *W. bancrofti* antigens is one means to detect such infections, and this can be done with an ELISA and a point-of-care immunochromatographic card test (ICT). Recently, a new ICT (the Alere Filariasis Test Strip) has shown better sensitivity in field conditions than the BinaxNOW Filariasis ICT, which has been in use for the past 10 to 20 years (Weil et al., 2013). There are currently no tests for circulating antigens in brugian filariasis. PCR-based assays for *W. bancrofti* and *B. malayi* in blood are very sensitive but are not yet widely available.

Antibody-based assays for diagnosing LF have traditionally suffered from poor specificity. IgG4 antibodies are less cross-reactive to nonfilarial helminth antigens and thus are more specific. Specificity has also been improved with species-specific antigens for brugian and bancroftian infection. A dipstick antibody test has been developed for brugian filariasis (Weil et al., 2011).

Patients with so-called burned-out infections (e.g., those who have received antiparasitic therapy or who departed endemic areas years previously and in whom the worms have died) often have lasting damage (i.e., lymphedema, genital disease, and other clinical manifestations). In these patients, negative testing for microfilaremia and circulating antigens does not exclude the possibility that their lesions could be a result of LF. However, such patients are usually LF antibody positive.

Radionuclide lymphoscintigraphic imaging reliably demonstrates lymphatic abnormalities in patients with LF. Although helpful in documenting the degree of damage associated with infection, this is not useful for differentiating LF from other causes of lymphatic disease.

Treatment

Because most patients with microfilaremia have at least subclinical disease, treatment is recommended for symptomatic and asymptomatic individuals with microfilaremia. Diethylcarbamazine (DEC, 2 mg/kg orally three times a day) is the treatment of choice for active LF (microfilaremia, antigen positivity, or live adult worms on ultrasound). A 1-day course seems as effective as the traditional 12-day regimen for most patients (CDC, 2013a), although those with TPE should receive a 2- to 3-week course. DEC kills microfilariae but has only modest activity against adult worms and in the United States is available only through the CDC (phone: 404-639-3670; website: https://www.cdc.gov/parasites/health_professionals.htm). DEC should not be given to persons from areas co-endemic for onchocerciasis or *L. loa* (e.g., West and Central Africa) unless these infections have been excluded because of potentially serious side effects related to the killing of these parasites by DEC. Alternatives for LF include albendazole and ivermectin. Albendazole (400 mg orally twice daily for 21 days) has microfilaricidal and macrofilaricidal activity, but the activity of ivermectin (150 to 400 µg/kg orally once) is limited mostly to microfilariae.

Side effects of DEC include fever, chills, arthralgias/myalgias, headaches, nausea, and vomiting. In heavily infected patients, painful skin nodules, lymphadenitis, and epididymitis may occur as a reaction to dying parasites or *Wolbachia* endosymbionts, usually days to weeks after initiation of therapy. Ivermectin has a side effect profile similar to DEC when used for LF; it also must be used with caution if co-infection with *L. loa* is possible (see below). Albendazole (when used in single-dose regimens; see later) has relatively few side effects when used for LF.

Doxycycline (200 mg daily) augments the suppression of microfilaremia induced by antifilarial drugs and has some macrofilaricidal activity. Prolonged courses (4 to 8 weeks) render adult worms sterile (Kappagoda et al., 2011). Individuals treated with doxycycline can experience substantial improvements in lymphedema and hydrocele. These benefits are seen even in patients with lymphedema who do not have active infection, suggesting that the benefit of doxycycline extends beyond the macrofilaricidal and anti-*Wolbachia* activity of this drug (Mand et al., 2012). The prolonged course is problematic for administration in the developing world, and doxycycline cannot be given to pregnant women or young children. However, in the United States a 6-week treatment course of this drug is a reasonable consideration in properly selected patients.

In persons with chronic lymphedema, prevention of secondary bacterial infections, good hygiene, elastic stockings, elevation, and physiotherapy are important for morbidity control. Antiparasitic therapy in these patients should be reserved for those with active infection. Surgical correction is challenging and often unnecessary. Lymphatic-venous and nodal-venous anastomoses for elephantiasis have been somewhat successful in decreasing leg swelling as has reconstructive surgery for genital involvement. The long-term effects of these intensive surgical techniques have not been determined.

Genital elephantiasis is rarely amenable to surgery, and lymphadenectomy may further compromise lymph drainage and worsen symptoms. In some cases of funiculoepididymitis, surgery, such as decompression or excision of filarial nodules, may be indicated to preserve the testis and spermatic cord. When funiculoepididymitis is recurrent, painful, and deforming or complicated by blood vessel involvement, more radical surgery is warranted. Drainage of hydroceles provides immediate relief, although recurrence is common in the absence of medical and definitive surgical therapy. Hydrocelectomy is often indicated for large or symptomatic hydroceles. Excision of the intact hydrocele sac is the procedure of choice; alternatively, inversion with partial excision can be considered. When identified, leaking or dilated lymphatic vessels should be sutured or excised. Small hydroceles that do not enlarge usually do not require surgery. Reconstruction of the scrotum or vulva, with removal of redundant tissue, can also provide symptomatic relief to selected patients.

Prevention and Control

Individual protection against LF infection involves avoidance of infected mosquitoes through personal protective measures and long-lasting insecticide-treated bednets (LLINs); LLINs have been shown to be a valuable tool for the control and elimination of LF (Reimer et al., 2013). Elimination of microfilariae within communities can interrupt transmission because patent microfilaremia is necessary for mosquitoes to transmit the infection from person to person. However, because chemotherapy does not kill all of the adult worms, it is necessary to continue intermittent administration of antiparasitic drugs for many years, until the adult worms die of senescence. This strategy can be effective for *W. bancrofti* elimination (Molyneux, 2009) but is more challenging in *Brugia*-endemic areas because animals also serve as reservoirs of infection for the latter. MDA campaigns (involving distribution of single annual doses of albendazole plus either DEC or ivermectin, which have a sustained microfilaricidal effect to most of the population) are the mainstay of control programs in Africa (albendazole/ivermectin) and elsewhere (albendazole/DEC). These campaigns have been successful in control and elimination of LF with many areas nearing elimination and are the primary reason for the decrease in global LF prevalence described previously. These programs have also prevented 19 million hydrocele cases globally since 2000, decreasing by half the number of hydroceles because of LF over that time period (Ramaiah and Ottesen, 2014). Encouragingly, recent small studies suggest that triple antiparasitic therapy (DEC + albendazole + ivermectin) reduces microfilaremia more profoundly and for a more prolonged time than dual antiparasitic therapy, with no additional serious adverse effects (Thomsen et al., 2016). If confirmed at a larger scale, this may herald a major advance for MDA programs in areas where all three drugs can be used together.

Onchocerciasis, also known as **river blindness**, is a filarial infection usually caused by *Onchocerciasis volvulus*. The infection is transmitted by *Simulium* black flies; 99% of onchocerciasis cases are found in Africa, with limited foci in Latin America (within Brazil and Venezuela) and the Arabian Peninsula (Yemen). About 17 million people are infected globally (WHO, 2017), which represents a 55% decrease in prevalence compared with 2000, largely because of successful MDA programs. As with LF, transmission is inefficient and highly focal. Adult worms live for up to 15 years in subcutaneous nodules (mean natural life span, 9 to 10 years) and release microfilariae that travel through the skin (and eye). *O. volvulus* adults also harbor *Wolbachia* endosymbionts. Infection classically causes dermatitis/pruritis, keratitis, and chorioretinitis, with blindness as an end result after many years, from corneal scarring. Diagnosis is confirmed by microscopically examining skin snips for microfilariae, finding adult worms in subcutaneous nodules, or seeing microfilariae in the anterior chamber of the eye via slit lamp. Antibody and antigen detection tests are less well developed than for LF.

In late stages, *Onchocerca* infection may produce "hanging groin" or scrotal elephantiasis as a result of recurrent lymphadenitis and loss of skin elasticity. Histology demonstrates atrophy and fibrosis of inguinal lymph nodes with subcutaneous edema and fibrosis. Onchocerciasis is also occasionally accompanied by massive inguinal lymphadenopathy. Recently, *Onchocerca lupi* (a parasite of canines) has been recognized as a rare cause of human disease, with infections in six US residents reported since 2013 (five of whom were children); all lived in the southwestern United States, and developed nodules that contained adult *O. lupi* worms (three in the spine, two in the skin/soft tissues, and one in the extraocular muscles) (Cantey et al., 2016).

Ivermectin is the treatment of choice (150 µg/kg orally once, repeated every 6 to 12 months until patients are asymptomatic) for onchocerciasis. Although the activity of ivermectin is primarily against microfilariae, emerging data suggest that it has at least some activity against adult worms and that macrofilariae life spans may be shortened 50% to 70% by multiple doses of ivermectin (Walker et al., 2017). As noted later, ivermectin must be used with caution if coinfection with *L. loa* is possible. Adverse effects include fever, rash, dizziness, pruritus, myalgias, arthralgias, and lymphadenopathy, mostly caused by dying filariae and *Wolbachia*. After ivermectin treatment, 6 weeks of doxycycline (200 mg/day orally) therapy kills or reduces the life span of most adult female *Onchocerca* worms and sterilizes most of the remainder, greatly reducing or clearing microfilaremia in most treated individuals (Debrah et al., 2014; Hoerauf, 2011; Walker et al., 2015). DEC should not be administered to persons infected with onchocerciasis because blindness and systemic toxicity can result from the resulting ocular and systemic inflammatory responses related to the dying parasites.

Loaiasis is caused by *L. loa*, a filarial infection that is limited to Central and West Africa and transmitted by *Chrysops* flies. Adult worms migrate in subcutaneous tissues, and microfilariae circulate diurnally in the blood. *L. loa* adults do not harbor *Wolbachia*. Most infected persons have asymptomatic eosinophilia; some have urticaria, migratory subcutaneous lesions, and visible worms migrating across the conjunctivae *(eye worms)*. Hematuria and proteinuria occur in 30% of patients; lymphadenitis and hydrocele also rarely occur. DEC (2 to 3 mg/kg orally three times a day for 14 to 21 days) is effective against loaiasis, although multiple courses may be necessary (Klion and Nutman, 2011). Treatment can cause pruritus, arthralgias, migratory swellings, fever, eye worms, diarrhea, and renal failure. Patients with detectable microfilaremia (particularly more than 2500 to 8000 microfilariae per milliliter of blood) are at risk of treatment-associated encephalopathy (especially if they receive ivermectin), which may be ameliorated by pretreatment apheresis. Albendazole (200 mg orally twice daily for 3 weeks) is associated with a lower risk of encephalopathy than DEC and may be safer in patients with high-grade parasitemia (Kappagoda et al., 2011).

Other Nonfilarial Genitourinary Parasites

Echinococcosis

Echinococcus granulosus is a cestode (tapeworm) that causes cystic echinococcosis. Infection results from ingestion of food or water contaminated with *Echinococcus* eggs or contact with infected dogs. Prevalence is high in pastoral communities, particularly in South America, the Mediterranean littoral, Eastern Europe, the Middle East, East Africa, Central Asia, China, Russia, and Australia. After infection the parasites encyst, usually in the liver or (less commonly) in the lungs. Although rare, cysts can grow ectopically in almost any organ in the body, with the kidneys being the third most common organ affected after the liver and lungs (<2% to 3% of cases) (Moscatelli et al., 2013). Initially, cysts are asymptomatic, but over time they enlarge (1–2 cm/yr) and eventually cause pain or a palpable abdominal mass; hydatiduria and renal colic occur in a minority of patients. Renal function is usually unaffected. Imaging shows a thick-walled, fluid-filled spheric cyst, often with a calcified wall; the appearance helps define the stage of the disease and, in turn, management strategies. Serologic testing is adjunctive for diagnosis, with a sensitivity of only 60% to 90%. Although use of percutaneous puncture, aspiration, injection, and reaspiration (PAIR) is a good therapeutic option for liver cysts, this is not done for lung or renal cysts, for which the only options are surgical resection or antiparasitic chemotherapy. Albendazole (400 mg orally twice per day for 1 to 6 months) is the recommended medical therapy (Kappagoda et al., 2011). Surgical excision is indicated in some patients because of the size or location of the lesions. Cyst rupture can cause anaphylaxis. Some evidence suggests that PZQ plus albendazole preoperatively and postoperatively may minimize secondary seeding and metastatic infection (Bygott and Chiodini, 2009).

Enterobiasis

Enterobius vermicularis (pinworm) causes enterobiasis, which occurs worldwide (common in both temperate and tropical countries). The worms live in the proximal colon and migrate to the perianal region to lay eggs, which become infectious after 6 hours. Transmission is mainly person-to-person, often via fecal-oral contamination of hands or fomites. Although most infections are asymptomatic, perianal pruritus can be severe. Rarely, pinworms can also migrate ectopically, including through the vagina, uterus, and fallopian tubes and into the peritoneal cavity of females. Dead worms and eggs incite granulomas and adhesions. Vulvar and cervical granulomas, salpingitis, oophoritis, tubo-ovarian abscess, appendicitis, and peritonitis can result. Epididymal involvement and inguinal hernias have been rarely reported in men (Moore and McCarthy, 2011).

Treatment with single-dose albendazole (400 mg orally) or mebendazole (100 mg orally) is highly effective. Alternatives include ivermectin (200 μg/kg orally once). Household and other close contacts should be treated, and treatment should be repeated after 2 weeks because of frequent reinfection and autoinfection (Kappagoda et al., 2011).

Amebiasis

Entamoeba histolytica, a protozoan transmitted by the fecal-oral route, is most common in tropical regions. Most infected persons remain asymptomatic, but 10% develop symptoms in other organs, including (rarely) the kidneys. Cutaneous amebiasis can also occur, with painful ulcers often involving the perianal area and genitals (Peterson et al., 2011). Treatment is with tinidazole (2 g orally per day for 3 to 5 days) or metronidazole (750 mg orally three times a day for 10 days), followed by paromomycin (8 to 12 mg/kg orally three times a day for 7 days) or iodoquinol (650 mg orally three times a day for 20 days) (Kappagoda et al., 2011).

Trichomoniasis

Trichomonas vaginalis is a common sexually transmitted protozoan. See Chapter 58 for details.

> **KEY POINTS: LYMPHATIC FILARIASIS**
>
> - Lymphatic filariasis is caused by three species of tissue nematodes that are transmitted to humans by mosquito vectors.
> - LF is endemic to much of the tropics but is transmitted inefficiently, and clinically apparent LF is usually seen only in long-term residents of endemic countries.
> - LF is diagnosed by blood smears, antibody/antigen assays, and radiologic and clinical means.
> - Antiparasitic treatment for active LF is with diethylcarbamazine (DEC); ivermectin and albendazole also have activity, and all three drugs are used in mass chemotherapy control programs. Doxycycline also results in a clinical benefit in many patients.

SUGGESTED READINGS

A Rev. Hum. Carcinog. Biol. Agents (Working Group of the International Agency for Research on Cancer, W. H. O.) 100B, 377–390 (World Health Organization, 2011).

Doenhoff MJ, Cioli D, Utzinger J: Praziquantel: mechanisms of action, resistance and new derivatives for schistosomiasis, *Curr Opin Infect Dis* 21:659–667, 2008.

Drugs for Parasitic Infections, 2013, The Medical Letter, Inc (website): http://secure.medicalletter.org/TG-article-132b.

Elliott DE: Schistosomiasis: pathophysiology, diagnosis, and treatment, *Gastroenterol Clin North Am* 25:599–625, 1996.

Figueiredo AÉÉ, Lucon AÉÉ: Urogenital tuberculosis: update and review of 8961 cases from the world literature, *Rev Urol* 10(3):207–217, 2008.

Fu C-L, Odegaard JI, Herbert DR, et al: A novel mouse model of schistosoma haematobium egg-induced immunopathology, *PLoS Pathog* 8:e1002605, 2012.

Goel A, Dalela D: Options in the management of tuberculous ureteric stricture, *Indian J Urol* 24(3):376–381, 2008.

Gryseels B, Polman K, Clerinx J, et al: Human schistosomiasis, *Lancet* 368:1106–1118, 2006.

Gupta NP, Kumar A, Sharma S, et al: Reconstructive bladder surgery in genitourinary tuberculosis, *Indian J Urol* 24(3):382–387, 2008.

Hemal AK: Laparoscopic retroperitoneal extirpative and reconstructive renal surgery, *J Endourol* 25(2):209–216, 2011.

IARC Working Group on the Evaluation of Carcinogenic Risks to Humans: Biological agents. Volume 100 B. A review of human carcinogens, *IARC Monogr Eval Carcinog Risks to Humans* 100:1–441, 2012.

Kappagoda S, Singh U, Blackburn BG: Antiparasitic therapy, *Mayo Clin Proc* 86:561–583, 2011.

King C: Schistosomiasis. In Guerrant R, Walker D, Weller P, editors: *Tropical infectious diseases: principles, pathogens, and practice*, London, 2006, Elsevier Churchill Livingstone, pp 1341–1348.

Mahmoud AAF: *Schistosomiasis*, London, 2001, Imperial College Press, p 524.

Meltzer E, Artom G, Marva E, et al: Schistosomiasis among travelers: new aspects of an old disease, *Emerg Infect Dis* 12:1696–1700, 2006.

Merchant S, Bharati A, Merchant N: Tuberculosis of the genitourinary system—urinary tract tuberculosis: renal tuberculosis—Part I, *Indian J Radiol Imaging* 23(1):46–63, 2013.

Mustacchi P In Kufe D, Pollack R, and Wischselbaum R: *Cancer Med.* (BC Decker, 2003).

Nahid P, Dorman S, Alipanah N, et al: Executive summary: official American thoracic Society/Centers for disease control and Prevention/Infectious diseases society of America clinical practice guidelines: treatment of drug-susceptible tuberculosis, *Clin Infect Dis* 63(7):853–867, 2016.

Pai M, Behr MA, Dowdy D, et al: Tuberculosis, *Nat Rev Dis Primers* 2:1–23, 2016.

Ray D, Nelson T, Fu C-L, et al: Transcriptional profiling of the bladder in urogenital schistosomiasis reveals pathways of inflammatory fibrosis and urothelial compromise, *PLoS Negl Trop Dis* 6:e1912, 2012.

Sakula A: Robert Koch: centenary of the discovery of the tubercle bacillus, 1882, *Thorax* 37(4):246–251, 1982.

Shokeir AA, Hussein M: The urology of Pharaonic Egypt, *BJU Int* 84:755–761, 1999.

Stuiver PC: Acute schistosomiasis (Katayama fever), *Br Med J (Clin Res Ed)* 288:221–222, 1984.

van der Werf MJ, et al: Quantification of clinical morbidity associated with schistosome infection in sub-Saharan Africa, *Acta Trop* 86:125–139, 2003.

REFERENCES

The complete reference list is available online at ExpertConsult.com.

PART V
Molecular and Cellular Biology

61
Basic Principles of Immunology and Immunotherapy in Urologic Oncology

Charles G. Drake MD, PhD

Immunotherapy is an important treatment modality for multiple tumor types, including bladder cancer, kidney cancer, melanoma, and lung cancer (Drake et al., 2014; LaFleur et al., 2018). What is often underappreciated as the field advances is the prominent role that immunotherapy has long played in bladder cancer (Brandau and Suttmann, 2007). In fact, the use of bacille Calmette-Guérin (BCG) in bladder cancer provides an ideal framework through which to understand immunotherapy for genitourinary (GU) cancers, although there are still many unanswered questions regarding BCG's mechanism of action. In addition to BGC, which is a relatively nonspecific agent, immunotherapy for GU cancers has also involved the concept of inducing a specific anticancer immune response via a cancer vaccine. Vaccine approaches for prostate cancer and kidney cancer are discussed; more detailed clinical information is included in specific chapters dedicated to treatment. Perhaps most clinically relevant is the concept of immune checkpoint blockade (ICB); it is now clear that antigen-specific immune responses to cancer are restrained by a specific set of molecules expressed on CD4 and CD8 tumor-infiltrating lymphocytes (TILs) (LaFleur et al., 2018). These "checkpoint" molecules, typified by PD-1 and PD-L1, are critical in restraining an antitumor immune response so that treatment with monoclonal antibodies blocking immune checkpoint interactions can lead to objective clinical responses (i.e., tumor shrinkage) in approximately 20% of patients with kidney cancer or bladder cancer. The immunologic mechanisms underlying the efficacy of ICB are discussed, and key clinical data are highlighted. ICB is more effective when combined with other treatment modalities, and immune-based combination therapy will likely become standard of care in the future. Potential combination partners include conventional chemotherapy (in bladder cancer), vascular endothelial growth factor (VEGF) inhibition (in kidney cancer), and androgen-deprivation therapy (in prostate cancer). Finally, anti-CTLA-4, which likely targets suppressive CD4 populations, is an important component in combination approaches and is discussed as well.

INNATE IMMUNE SYSTEM

For didactic purposes, the immune system is often divided into two subsystems, the **innate** and the **adaptive**. Evolutionarily, the innate immune system is the older of the two, and it is present in all vertebrate organisms. Functionally, the innate system recognizes its targets through repeated patterns associated with pathogens. These pathogen-associated molecular patterns (or PAMPs) are recognized by a series of receptors related to Toll molecules in drosophila and are known as Toll-like receptors, or TLRs (Medzhitov and Janeway, 2000). The binding of PAMPs to TLRs is a fundamental immunologic mechanism though which an organism recognizes "danger." Urologists who treat bladder cancer with intravesical BCG employ these innate immune immunologic mechanisms clinically; peptidoglycans in the BCG cell wall are canonical PAMPs, which bind to TLR2 on innate immune cells resident in the bladder wall, activating them and initiating a multi-step immune response (Brandau and Suttmann, 2007).

The initial immune cell that responds to an invading pathogen (or to instilled BCG) is most likely a tissue resident macrophage (Table 61.1). Their names are derived from the Greek *makros* (large) and *phagos* (to eat), thus macrophages are large cells that evolved to engulf and destroy pathogens. Recognition of PAMPs by tissue-resident macrophages leads to their activation, and subsequent secretion of chemical messengers are known as cytokines and chemokines (see following), which in turn recruit and activate additional immune cells important in controlling a local infection. Again, BCG therapy for bladder cancer provides an excellent example: recognition by macrophages and the adherence of bacteria to urothelial cells lining the bladder result in the secretion of a series of chemokines and cytokines (Fig. 61.1). Some of these secreted cytokines attract a second cell type of major importance in the innate immune system, the neutrophil (also known as a polymorphonuclear neutrophil, or PMN). PMNs are the most abundant immune cell in the peripheral circulation, comprising approximately 60% of the white cells in the blood. These cells have a half-life measured in hours in the peripheral blood but can survive for days in the tissue at a site of infection or inflammation. In that sense, PMNs are the major cellular constituent of pus and the hallmark of acute inflammation. One remarkable feature of neutrophil biology is the neutrophils' ability to emigrate from the circulation into tissues; this occurs when they squeeze between cells in the vascular endothelium as they follow a chemokine concentration gradient toward an area of infection within tissues. The hypersegmented configuration of their nucleus likely helps in this process by presenting a less formidable structural barrier to deformation. Like macrophages, neutrophils synthesize a variety of secretory granules, which are released upon PAMP recognition and facilitate destruction of an invading pathogen.

Cytokines and Chemokines

Cytokines and chemokines are small molecule chemical messengers through which epithelial cells communicate with key cells in the immune system and through which cells in the immune system communicate with each other. There are a large number of such molecules, and their nomenclature can be confusing. However, these molecules play a critical role in acute and chronic inflammation, the innate immune response, and the adaptive immune response to cancer, so understanding a few key members is important.

In that regard, the term *cytokine* is a rather general one, referring to any small immunologically relevant molecule secreted by a cell. Because many (but not all) of these molecules are involved in the migration of cells, the name derives from *cyto* (cell), and *kinesis* (movement). Typical cytokines include the type I interferons (IFN-α and IFN-β), which are produced by virally infected or otherwise stressed epithelial cells. Immunologically, type I interferons render epithelial cells more sensitive to immunologic attack by increasing their recognition by cells of the adaptive immune system and by directly facilitating epithelial cell death. As is discussed later, intravesical instillation of IFN-α has been evaluated in a number of clinical trials in bladder cancer, with encouraging but somewhat mixed results (Askeland et al., 2012).

TABLE 61.1 Selected Cell Types Involved in the Immune Response to Genitourinary Cancers

CELL TYPE	IMMUNOLOGIC ROLE
Epithelial/urothelial cell	Secrete type I interferons as well as chemokines in response to stress, inflammation, viral infection, or danger signals mediated by pathogen-associated molecular patterns (PAMPs)
Macrophage	An innate immune cell that engulfs pathogens and dead/dying cells and secretes cytokines and chemokines to amplify or initiate an immune response
Neutrophil (PMN)	The most numerous of all innate immune cells in the peripheral blood, critically important in controlling bacterial infections. A collection of neutrophils (pus) is a characteristic of acute inflammation
Dendritic cell	The cell type that bridges the innate and adaptive immune systems by presenting antigens (peptides) from dead/dying cells or debris to T cells in the lymph node. Like macrophages, dendritic cells are activated by "danger" signals transmitted through PAMPs or by cytokines in the microenvironment
CD4 T cell	A "helper" T cell that can either help CD8 T cells to kill or B cells to secrete antibodies
CD8 T cell	A "killer" T cell that, once activated, serially lyses specific targets
Regulatory T cell (Treg)	A subset of CD4 T cells characterized by expression of the transcription factor FoxP3. Major role is to down-regulate an ongoing immune response. In cancer, this is generally a detrimental function

The term *chemokine* refers to a subset of cytokines whose primary function is to induce the migration of immune cells along a chemical concentration gradient. The prototypical example is CXCL8, which can be secreted by most epithelial cell types, including bladder urothelium, in response to inflammatory signals. CXCL8 is a powerful chemoattractant for neutrophils and is likely important in the immune response to BCG in bladder cancer patients. The final subset of cytokines worthy of discussion are a series of molecules originally described as facilitating communication between leukocytes, the interleukins. Interleukins were numbered in the order of their discovery, leading to an unfortunately complex situation in which an interleukin's designation usually has very little to do with its functional role or cell of origin. Interleukin-1 (IL-1), for example, is really more of an innate cytokine than an interleukin; it is secreted from stressed epithelial cells, attracts a variety of immune cells, and in the systemic circulation is one of the primary mediators of an elevated temperature in response to infection. More generally, though, there are two discrete sets of cytokines associated with a broad polarization in the adaptive (T cell–mediated) immune response. These are termed the Th1 and Th2 families of cytokines (Table 61.2 and Fig. 61.2). These cytokines are secreted by CD4 (helper) T cells in response to various stimuli and are critically important in polarizing the immune system in one of several broad directions (Weaver et al., 2006).

In bladder cancer, these patterns of response are especially important because a Th1 response is associated with a successful response to BCG treatment, whereas a Th2 response is associated with BCG failure (de Reijke et al., 1996; Saint et al., 2001; Saint et al., 2002; Thalmann et al., 2000). Mechanistically, this skewing occurs as naive CD4 helper cells are activated (see Fig. 61.2). In an environment rich in IL-12, CD4 T cells differentiate into Th1 cells and in turn secrete interleukin 2 (IL-2), tumor necrosis factor-α (TNF-α) and interferon gamma (IFN-γ). These Th1 cytokines help to activate CD8 (killer) T cells and are important in a successful antitumor response. Conversely, when naive CD4 T cells recognize their targets in the context of interleukin 4 (IL-4), they differentiate into Th2 cells, which are associated with chronic inflammation and antibody production, and secrete IL-4, IL-5, IL-10, and IL-13. In bladder cancer these cytokines can be detected **systemically** after BCG treatment, so elevated serum IL-2 post-treatment is associated with a favorable outcome. These are important data, showing that the immune effects of BCG are not solely local and illustrating the point that activation of the immune system in one organ site can have detectable effects throughout the entire organism.

ADAPTIVE IMMUNE SYSTEM

The adaptive immune system includes CD4 (helper) T cells, CD8 (killer) T cells, and B cells. These cells are recruited to an immune response in response to activation of the innate immune system and are vital to two key facets of the immune response: its specificity and its ability to "remember" prior antigen encounters and respond more robustly when that antigen is encountered again in the future. Before expounding on those properties, it is important to understand how information from the innate immune system is transferred to the adaptive immune system. This transfer depends on a unique cell type known as the dendritic cell, which serves as a bridge between an innate and an adaptive immune response. Dendritic cells (DCs) get their name from their long and fine cytoplasmic projections, which microscopically resemble nerve cells. Functionally, dendritic cells are scattered throughout the peripheral tissues, as exemplified by Langherhans cells in the skin. DCs spend the majority of their lifespan at rest, continually sampling their microenvironment, taking in fluid and protein antigens through the process of pinocytosis. In the absence of an activating or "danger" signal, DCs remain quiescent and sessile. A danger signal can come in the form of cytokines, such as TNF-α secreted from innate immune cells such as macrophages, or through direct contact with bacterial products through pattern receptors (TLRs) on DCs. When DCs are activated, a remarkable transition takes place. First, they cease taking in antigens because their

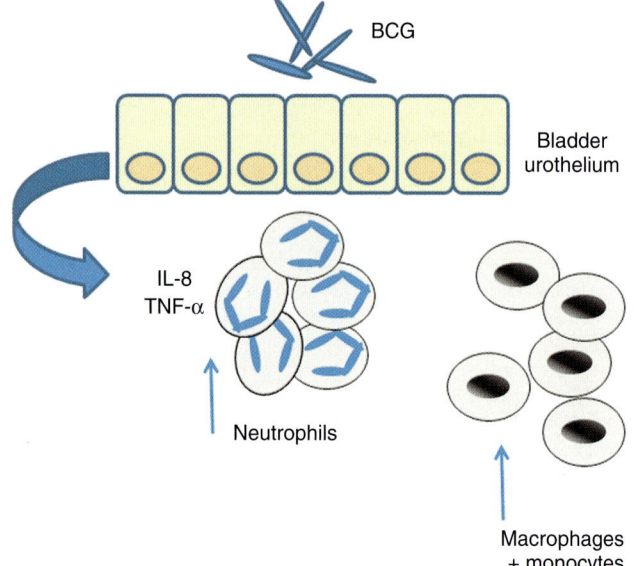

Fig. 61.1. Activation of the innate immune system by bacille Calmette-Guérin (BCG). *IL-8*, Interleukin-8; *TNF-α*, tumor necrosis factor-α. (Modified from Brandau S, Suttmann H: Thirty years of BCG immunotherapy for non-muscle invasive bladder cancer: a success story with room for improvement. *Biomed Pharmacother* 61:299–305, 2007.)

TABLE 61.2 Selected Cytokines, Chemokines, and Interleukins Involved in the Immune Response to Genitourinary Cancers

CYTOKINE	CELL OF ORIGIN	ROLE
TYPE 1 INTERFERONS		
Interferon-α	Urothelial cells, epithelial cells Macrophages	A type 1 interferon typically secreted by a virally infected cells, or cells sensing "danger" through Toll-like receptor (TLR) engagement. Up-regulates class I MHC and antigen processing, rendering cells more susceptible to immunologic attack
Interferon-β	Urothelial cells, epithelial cells Macrophages	Similar to IFN-α, another type 1 interferon
CHEMOKINES		
CXCL8	Urothelial cells Epithelial cells	A chemokine that is a powerful chemoattractant for neutrophils
IL-1	Epithelial cells Macrophages	Like IL-8, also attracts other immune cells such as monocytes from the circulation
SLC	Stromal cells in lymph nodes	Also known as CXCL21, SLC attracts activated dendritic cells and T cells into the lymph nodes. It is sensed by the receptor CCR-7
INTERLEUKINS AND TH1/TH2 POLARIZATION		
IL-12	Dendritic cells	A Th1-inducing cytokine, when naive CD4 T cells are activated in the presence of IL-12, they differentiate into Th1 cells
IL-4	Dendritic cells, natural killer T cells	A Th2 cytokine, when naive CD4 T cells are activated in the presence of IL-4, they differentiate into Th2 cells
IL-2, TNF-α and IFN-γ	Th1 cells (CD4 T cells)	Canonical cytokines secreted by Th1 cells, and which are associated with a favorable response to BCG in bladder cancer. These cytokines are also associated with inducing CD8 (killer) T-cell function
IL-4, IL-5, IL-10, IL-13	Th2 cells (CD4 T cells)	Canonical cytokines secreted by Th2 cells, and which are associated with an unfavorable response to BCG in bladder cancer. These cytokines are also associated with the induction of antibody production

BCG, Bacille-Calmette-Guérin; *IL,* interleukin; *MHC,* major histocompatibility complex.

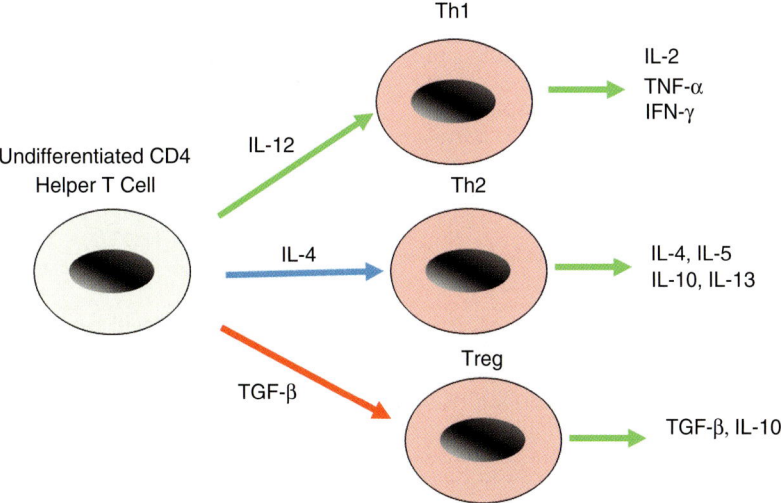

Fig. 61.2. CD4 T-cell polarization and the Th1 and Th2 families of cytokines. *IFN,* Interferon; *IL,* interleukin; *TGF,* transforming growth factor; *TNF,* tumor necrosis factor. (Modified from Weaver CT, Harrington LE, Mangan PR, et al.: Th17: an effector CD4 T cell lineage with T-cell ties. *Immunity* 24:677–688, 2006.)

new role is to present the antigens they have already taken up to T and B cells. Thus their dendrites are retracted and the cells develop a more compact morphology. Second, they upregulate cell surface molecules important for presenting the antigens they have engulfed to T cells. Key cell surface molecules include major histocompatibility molecules, which bind 9 to 12 amino acid peptide antigens in their grooves for interacting with specific receptors on T cells (TCRs), as well as a set of molecules designed to optimally stimulate T cells; these are called co-stimulatory molecules and include B7-1, B7-2, and others. Finally, DCs must solve a spatial problem: resting lymphocytes (T cells and B cells) reside in the secondary lymphoid structures (i.e., in the lymph nodes), while resting DCs are situated in the tissues. Thus DCs must migrate into the lymphatic system and enter into the lymph nodes (LNs) through afferent lymphatic vessels. This is accomplished via chemotaxis; activated DCs follow a gradient of secondary lymphoid chemokine (SLC) using a receptor known as CCR7 to traffic to the LN. Once in the lymph nodes, DCs interact with (and activate) specific CD4, CD8, and B lymphocytes, completing the transfer of information from the innate immune system to the adaptive.

A naive CD4 T cell is activated when an antigen-presenting DC presents its cognate (specific) peptide antigen (usually 11 AA long) in the context of a Class II major histocompatibility complex (MHC). CD4 T cells are helper cells, they either help CD8 T cells to become fully activated and exert their lytic function or assist B cells in making antibodies. As described earlier, CD4 T-cell responses fall into several basic categories, including a Th1 response, which fully activates CD8 (killer cells) and a Th2 response, which helps B cells to mature into antibody-secreting plasma cells. An additional CD4 T cell subtype of interest is the regulatory T cell (Treg) (Chao and Savage, 2018; Sakaguchi et al., 2008). These cells suppress adaptive immune responses and appear to play a role in preventing a successful adaptive Th1/CD8–driven anticancer response. The origin of Treg is complex; a population of "natural" Treg arises de novo in the course of T-cell development in the thymus, while a second population is "induced" when naive CD4 T cells recognize their antigen in a microenvironment that is low in proinflammatory signals and rich in transforming growth factor beta (TGF-β) (see Fig. 61.2). The relative contribution of these two types of Treg to the progression of GU cancers in humans is unclear; however, recent laboratory data point to a critical role for natural, thymus-derived Treg (Savage et al., 2013).

Perhaps the most fascinating adaptive immune cell is the CD8 T cell. These cells recognize their specific cognate antigen as 9 amino acid peptides; these peptides are recognized when bound in the groove of Class I MHC molecules. Class I MHC molecules are present on almost all cell types and are upregulated in the context of inflammation and on virally infected cells. When a specific CD8 T cell recognizes its target, it secretes a series of molecules, which results in destruction of that cell type. This killing process is remarkably specific; in the autoimmune disease type 1 diabetes, CD8 T cells can lyse beta cells in the pancreas while leaving immediately adjacent alpha cells completely intact. The mechanism of killing itself is also exquisite; CD8 T cells employ multiple molecular mechanisms to induce their target cells to commit suicide (i.e., to undergo programmed cell death or apoptosis; Martinez-Lostao et al., 2015). Finally, CD8 T cells are serial killers, able to lyse multiple specific targets in a sequential manner. CD8 T cells can be specifically activated by cancer vaccines, as will be discussed later; blocking immune checkpoint molecules is an important clinical modality for augmenting the activity of CD8 T cells specific for cancer antigens.

IMMUNE EDITING HYPOTHESIS

Before moving forward with a discussion of how the immune system may be manipulated to treat GU cancers, it is worthwhile considering the immune system's baseline role in either the promotion or the elimination of cancer. With the exception of certain virally mediated tumors that occur most commonly in immunocompromised individuals, human cancers develop in immunologically intact hosts. As tumorigenesis proceeds from low-grade/localized disease to distant metastases, an interaction between the host immune system and the evolving tumor occurs. This process has been well characterized in a number of animal models and can be divided into three distinct stages (Dunn et al., 2004). In the first stage of the process, early tumors are recognized by the immune system in a productive, proactive way, leading to **elimination** of small, clinically undetectable masses. Elimination is most likely mediated by a concerted effort between the innate (macrophages and dendritic cells) and the adaptive immune systems. As tumors progress, they acquire genetic, epigenetic, and stromal alterations that render an antitumor immune response less efficacious. Thus, in the next phase of tumor/immune system interactions, tumors are able to exist in a dynamic **equilibrium** with the host immune response, with progression slowed by an ongoing immune response, but in which tumors can no longer be successfully eliminated. Equilibrium may persist for a significant period of time, and some tumors may remain in the equilibrium stage for the life of the host. Eventually, though, many tumors proceed to **escape** the host immune response and become clinically apparent. The molecular mechanisms involved in the escape phase are multiple and include down-regulation of tumor antigens against which a host response is directed, down-regulation of MHC molecules, and the induction or expansion of regulatory T cells (Treg) that actively inhibit an immune response (Drake et al., 2006). Together, the three phases of tumor/host interactions (elimination, equilibrium, and escape) collectively form the "immune editing hypothesis," which serves as a valuable framework through which to understand the immune response to cancer. Indeed, subversion of a productive host antitumor response is now designated as one of the hallmarks of cancer (Hanahan and Weinberg, 2011).

> **KEY POINTS: BASIC IMMUNOLOGY**
> - An immune response begins with an innate response, which is rapid but relatively nonspecific, then progresses to include the adaptive immune system, which is characterized by specificity and memory.
> - For an antitumor immune response, a Th1 response dominated by IFN-γ, IL-2, and TNF-α is desired.
> - CD4+ regulatory T cells (Treg) inhibit an adaptive immune response.
> - The immune editing hypothesis explains how early tumors can be recognized and eliminated by the immune system, whereas clinically evident tumors must escape immune recognition to evolve.

CHRONIC INFLAMMATION AND THE ENDOGENOUS IMMUNE RESPONSE TO GENITOURINARY CANCERS

Although the immune editing hypothesis suggests that antitumor immune responses are generally beneficial, those data must be considered along with a great deal of apparently contradictory data suggesting that inflammation can promote tumor progression (Balkwill et al., 2005; de Visser et al., 2006). Human and animal studies showed that inflammation has a clear role in the development of bladder cancer (Michaud, 2007) and likely plays a role in the development of prostate cancer (PC) as well (De Marzo et al., 2007).

CHRONIC INFLAMMATION AND THE IMMUNE RESPONSE TO BLADDER CANCER

Among GU malignancies, bladder cancer provides the strongest evidence for a link between chronic inflammation and carcinogenesis. The evidence linking inflammatory schistosomiasis infections to bladder cancer is particularly robust, and *Schistosoma haematobium* has been classified as a known carcinogen by the International Agency for Research on Cancer. Epidemiologically, countries with high rates of endemic infection have high rates of bladder cancer, and elevated levels of infestation are associated with a squamous cell phenotype (Mostafa et al., 1999). Other sources of bladder inflammation that have been linked to carcinogenesis include chronic urinary tract infections (Kantor et al., 1984), chronic indwelling catheters (Groah et al., 2002), and cystitis induced by cyclophosphamide treatment (Talar-Williams et al., 1996). The cellular and molecular mechanisms by which chronic bladder infection leads to cancer have not been fully elucidated; they likely involve mechanisms similar to those described in other cancers (Mantovani et al., 2008), that is, dysfunctional (M2) macrophages that produce immune suppressive cytokines, a subset of myeloid cells that suppress an active immune response (myeloid-derived suppressor cells, MDSCs; Gabrilovich, 2017), and a polarization of the adaptive immune response toward a Th2 and Treg phenotype.

Once bladder tumors develop, the immune editing hypothesis (Fig. 61.3) would suggest that early tumors may be recognized by the immune system and eliminated. That hypothesis is supported by data showing that CD8 T-cell infiltration correlates with outcome in patients with muscle-invasive bladder cancer (Sharma et al., 2007). Obviously a successful CD8-mediated antitumor response does not occur in all cases, and recent data describe an important mechanism by which bladder tumors, kidney cancer, and other tumor types "escape" immune recognition (Drake et al., 2014; LaFleur et al., 2018). This occurs through the interaction between immune checkpoint molecules expressed on cancer-specific T cells and their ligands, expressed on either tumor cells or tumor-associated macrophages (Fig. 61.4). This interaction is profoundly inhibitory to T cell activity, attenuating proliferation as well as effector function. In this regard, several tissue-based studies showed that the epithelial cells in bladder cancer express the immune checkpoint ligand PD-L1. In one early study, PD-L1 expression was noted in approximately 15% to 35% of cases, and expression was associated with increased tumor grade (Nakanishi et al., 2007). Interestingly, in these patients, PD-L1 expression was more closely associated with prognosis than was World Health Organization grade, pointing to a functional role for the PD-1/PD-L1 interaction in bladder cancer progression. A second related study confirmed the relationship between PD-L1 expression and high-grade tumors and further demonstrated that PD-L1 expression was associated with tumor infiltration by immune cells (Inman et al., 2007). Interestingly, this group also showed that PD-L1 was highly expressed in BGG-induced granulomas in patients progressing on therapy, suggesting a possible escape mechanism. Mechanistically, these data support a model known as "adaptive immune resistance" (Fig. 61.5), which explains how PD-L1 expression is a critical mechanism by which tumors evade the immune response (Taube et al., 2012). In this model, mutations arising as a tumor progresses lead to an adaptive immune response defined by CD8 T cell recognition. These CD8 T cells migrate to the tumor, as a consequence of acquiring effector function secrete the cytokine IFN-γ. IFN-γ is a powerful inducer of PD-L1 expression in tumor cells and myeloid cells and epithelial cells, and it is these induced PD-L1 molecules on tumor cells that interact with PD-1 on the infiltrating CD8 T cells to effectively curtail their antitumor effector function

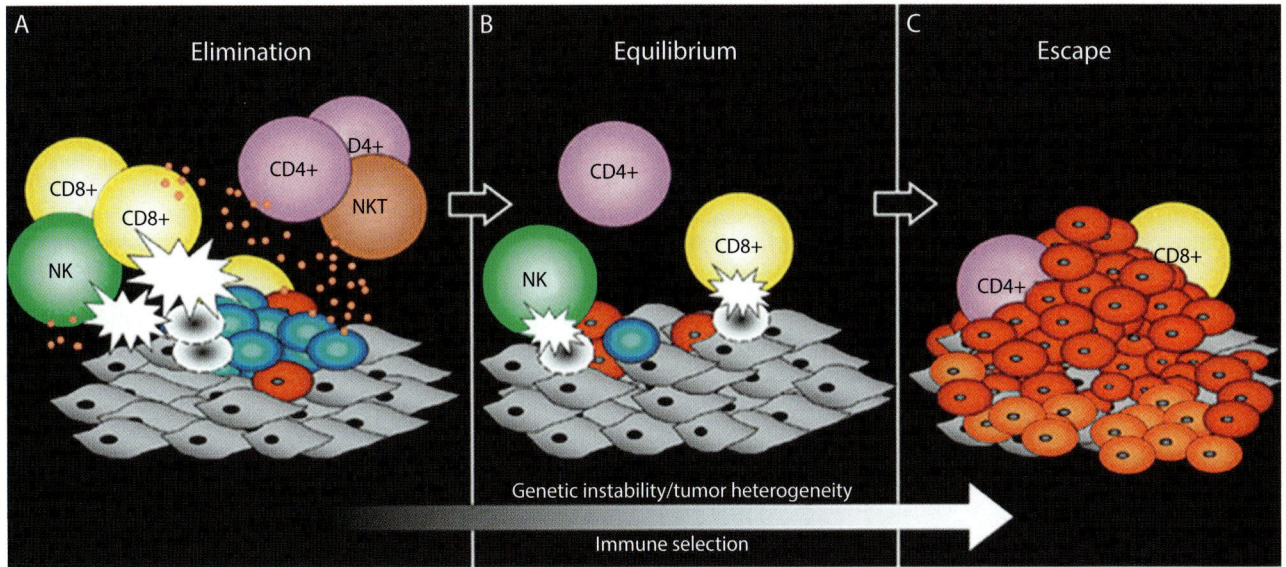

Fig. 61.3. The immune editing hypothesis. *NK*, Natural killer cell; *NKT*, natural killer T cell. (From Dunn GP, Old LJ, Schreiber RD: The immunobiology of cancer immunosurveillance and immunoediting. *Immunity* 21:137–148, 2004.)

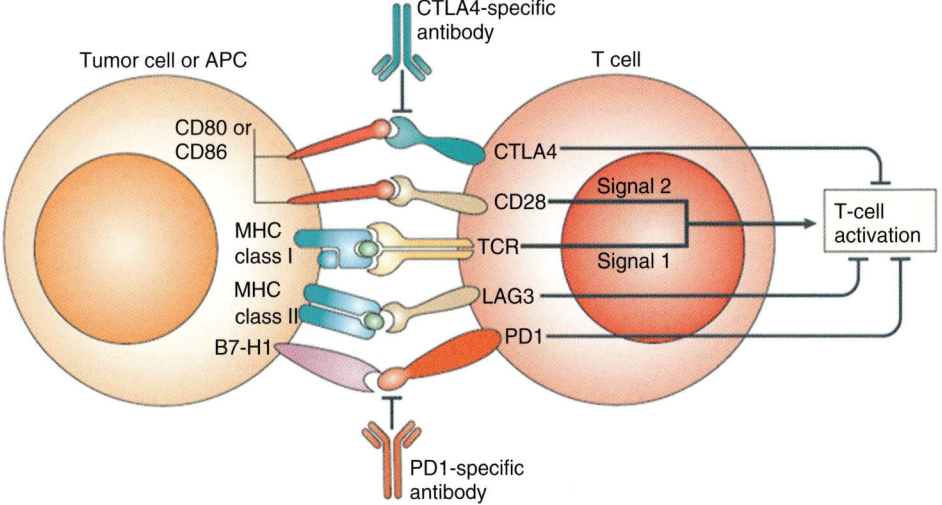

Fig. 61.4. Immune checkpoint molecules. *APC*, Antigen-presenting cell; *MHC*, major histocompatibility complex. (From Drake CG: Prostate cancer as a model for tumour immunotherapy. *Nat Rev Immunol* 10:580–593, 2010.)

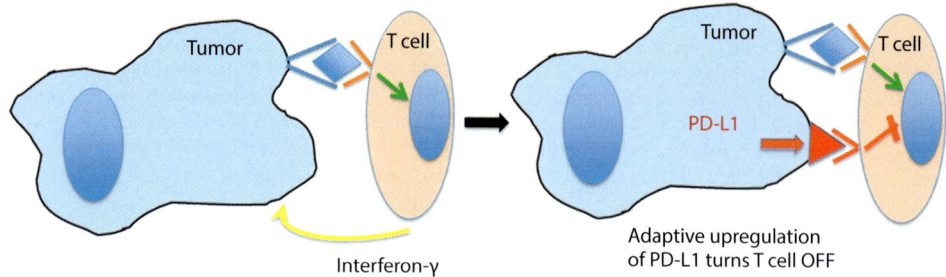

Fig. 61.5. Adaptive immune resistance.

(Taube et al., 2012). Those data would suggest that a monoclonal antibody that blocks either PD-1 or PD-L1 could potentially lead to objective tumor responses in patients with bladder cancer, a hypothesis strongly confirmed by phase II and III studies in bladder and kidney cancer (see following).

IMMUNE MICROENVIRONMENT IN KIDNEY CANCER

Unlike bladder and prostate cancer, a link between chronic inflammation and kidney cancer is less clear and is only weakly suggested by the associations of kidney cancer with proinflammatory risk factors such as smoking or obesity (Chow et al., 2010). Several lines of evidence suggest that the tumor microenvironment (TME) of kidney cancer may be different from that of other tumor types. One important difference is the influence of tumor-infiltrating CD8 T cells; in most other cancers, increasing CD8 T cell density is associated with improved prognosis (Fridman et al., 2012). In kidney cancer, older (Nakano et al., 2001) and more contemporary (Giraldo et al., 2015) data show that an increased CD8 T cell density is associated with a **less favorable** outcome. This relationship holds for metastatic lesions and primary tumors (Remark et al., 2013). Unfortunately, the mechanisms underlying this paradoxic relationship are unknown. In terms of prognosis, one study identified a group of patients with elevated CD8 T cell infiltration, increased expression of immune checkpoint molecules such as PD-1 and lymphocyte activation gene–3 (LAG-3). That subgroup also had relatively few functional antigen presenting cells and showed a particularly poor outcome (Giraldo et al., 2015). To more fully understand the tumor microenvironment in kidney cancer, one group used an advanced flow cytometry method to deeply profile the immune landscape in a substantial number (>70) of biopsies from primary tumors (Chevrier et al., 2017). Those data revealed an impressive complexity; clustering analyses of the infiltrating immune cells showed a total of 17 macrophage subsets and 22 T cell subsets. PD-1 was broadly expressed on infiltrating lymphocytes, whereas other immune checkpoint molecules such as LAG-3 and TIM-3 were more narrowly expressed. In terms of potential future trials, these data identified a macrophage population highly that expressed the cell surface marker CD38, and which was associated with the presence of PD-1 expressing T cells. Clinically, these data suggest that CD38 blockade may be a reasonable target for combination therapies; this is important because several anti-CD38 antibodies are either FDA approved (Mateos et al., 2018) or are in clinical development.

CHRONIC INFLAMMATION AND THE IMMUNE RESPONSE TO PROSTATE CANCER

The prostate microenvironment is infiltrated by several types of inflammatory cells, including innate cells such as macrophages and adaptive cells such as T and B cells even in the absence of symptoms or cancer. This baseline inflammation is likely tumor promoting, and accumulating data from several groups support a model in which chronic prostatic inflammation drives the development of cancer (De Marzo et al., 2007). Multiple lines of evidence link chronic inflammation to prostate cancer tumorigenesis. First, chronic inflammation in the prostate gland is frequently focused in the peripheral zone, the region in which more than 90% of tumors arise (McNeal et al., 1988). Second, epidemiologic studies show that western nations, in which chronic prostatic inflammation is endemic, have a significantly increased incidence in prostate cancer as compared with Asian populations, in which inflammation is less prevalent (Sfanos and De Marzo, 2012). Finally, and perhaps most convincing, are data surrounding a prostatic lesion known as prostatic inflammatory atrophy (PIA), a lesion characterized by flattened, but proliferating, epithelial cells and associated inflammatory cells (De Marzo et al., 1999). Morphologic studies showed that regions of PIA are located geographically proximal to high-grade prostatic intraepithelial neoplasia (PIN) lesions (Putzi and De Marzo, 2000), suggesting a possible causative link between PIA and the eventual development of cancer.

The adaptive T cell environment of prostate cancer is dominated by regulatory T cells (Treg), which have been described in the gland itself as well as in neoplastic lesions (Fox et al., 2007; Miller et al., 2006; Sfanos et al., 2008). A role for Treg likely extends to metastatic lesions; studies showed an increased prevalence of functional Treg in the bone marrow of patients with prostate cancer (Zhao et al., 2012). In keeping with the notion of immunosuppression in prostate cancer, data from humans (Kiniwa et al., 2007) and animals (Shafer-Weaver et al., 2009) suggest that, in prostate cancer, CD8 T cells can also have a suppressive, protumor phenotype. In perhaps the most convincing of these studies, one group showed that regulatory CD8 T cells in the peripheral blood were sufficiently suppressive as to mask an antigen-specific T cell response driven (Olson and McNeel, 2007). Finally, as in other GU cancers, there is some evidence that the PD-1/PD-L1 axis may restrain an adaptive T cell response to prostate cancer, because the CD8 T cells that infiltrate the prostate gland are clearly PD-1 positive (Sfanos et al., 2009) as well as clonally restricted. Taken together, these data suggest that prostate cancer develops in an environment characterized by chronic inflammation, as well as a nonproductive adaptive CD4 and CD8 T cell response (Bronte et al., 2005; Gannon et al., 2009).

> **KEY POINTS: CHRONIC INFLAMMATION AND THE ENDOGENOUS IMMUNE RESPONSE TO GU CANCERS**
>
> - Bladder cancer is promoted by chronic inflammation initiated by infection or other stimuli.
> - In kidney cancer, there is good evidence for an ongoing adaptive, CD8 T-cell–mediated response, but paradoxically, an increased CD8 density is associated with a worse prognosis.
> - Prostate cancer may also be driven by chronic inflammation.
> - Expression of immune checkpoint molecules on TILs attenuates the adaptive immune response to GU tumors.

IMMUNOTHERAPY FOR GENITOURINARY CANCERS

Bacille Calmette-Guérin in Bladder Cancer

The mechanism of action of BCG provides an excellent framework through which to understand the course of an induced immune

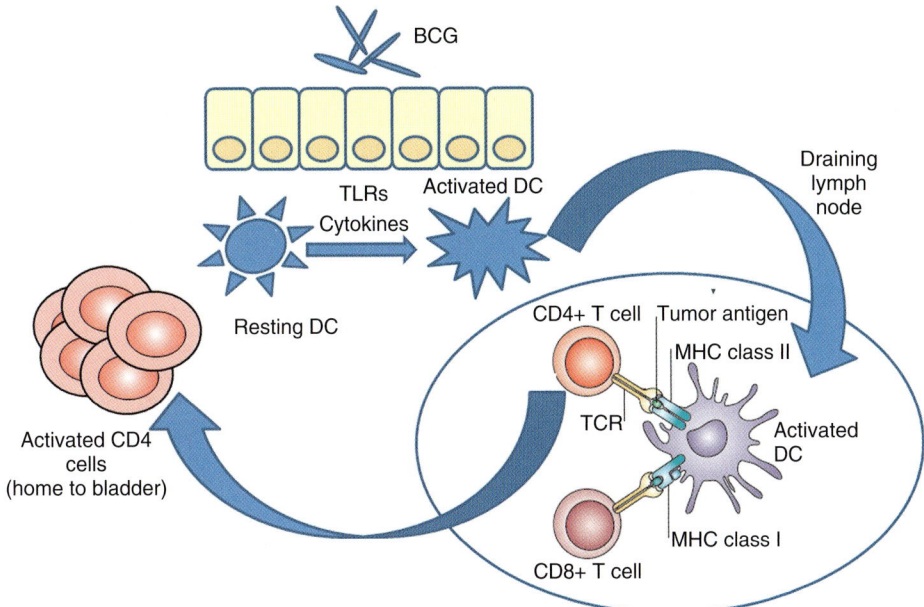

Fig. 61.6. Bacille Calmette-Guérin (BCG) and an adaptive immune response. *DC*, Dendritic cell; *MHC*, major histocompatibility complex; *TCR*, T-cell receptor; *TLRs*, Toll-like receptors. (Modified from Brandau S, Suttmann H: Thirty years of BCG immunotherapy for non-muscle invasive bladder cancer: a success story with room for improvement. *Biomed Pharmacother* 61:299–305, 2007; Drake CG: Prostate cancer as a model for tumour immunotherapy. *Nat Rev Immunol* 10:580–593, 2010.)

response, an understanding that will be useful in appreciating the mechanisms of other immunotherapy modalities described in this chapter (Brandau and Suttmann, 2007; see Fig. 61.6). The process begins with the instillation of 1 to 5×10^8 viable mycobacteria into the bladder. Most of these will be washed out with the first postinstillation void, but a significant fraction will adhere to the urothelial cells lining the bladder via a fibronectin attachment protein (Kavoussi et al., 1990). Repeated patterns (PAMPs) on the bacterial cell wall stimulate urothelial cells to secrete cytokines, acting through the toll-like receptors TLR-2 and TLR-4. Direct activation of resident macrophages and dendritic cells by BCG components is also likely but has been less well described. The BCG-stimulated urothelial cells initiate a stepwise immune response by secreting the chemokine IL-8 (among many others); IL-8 is a powerful neutrophil attractant. TNF-α is also secreted, and this setting, this Th1 family cytokine recruits and activates macrophages. A few hours after BCG installation, a sizable wave of neutrophils migrates into bladder wall (de Boer et al., 1991). This influx of neutrophils is characteristic of acute inflammation, and the recruited neutrophils clear residual bacilli by secreting cytotoxic granules in addition to releasing a series of cytokines that help activate dendritic cells to potentiate the eventual involvement of the adaptive immune system. The next step in this inflammatory cascade occurs over several weeks as an adaptive immune response, primarily CD4 T cell driven, is recruited to the bladder (Kates et al., 2017). Although the precise mechanisms through which CD4 T cells are recruited have not been well documented, this most likely occurs in the same manner as it does in other immune responses: dendritic cells are activated by neutrophil and urothelial cell-derived cytokines (in addition to bacterial products) and traffic to the draining lymph nodes, where they present antigens to CD4 T cells to activate specific lymphocytes. The antigenic targets of CD4 T cells during BCG therapy for bladder cancer have not been well described, but likely include bacterial antigens as well as tissue-/tumor-specific antigens. Nevertheless, an adaptive immune response has been demonstrated to be required for successful BCG therapy of bladder cancer in laboratory studies (Ratliff et al., 1987), and the identification of CD4 T cell–rich granulomas in BCG-treated patients provides evidence that this is likely to be the case in humans as well (Prescott et al., 1992). As described earlier, the adaptive immune response is capable of generating long-lived memory T cells, which may persist for the life of a vaccinated patient. The generation of memory CD4 cells by BGC treatment of bladder cancer has not been well studied in patients, but their induction is strongly suggested by the significant fraction (approximately 50%) of patients whose non-muscle invasive disease remains in remission for years after BGG therapy. In summary, successful BCG immunotherapy for bladder cancer represents a typical immune response, initially characterized by activation and involvement of the innate immune system (neutrophils and macrophages), which then evolves toward an adaptive immune response driven by CD4 T cells polarized to secrete Th1 cytokines (IL-2, TNF-α, and IFN-γ), followed by consolidation in the form of long-lived T cell memory.

Cancer Vaccines

Like BCG, a "cancer vaccine" aims to raise a T-cell response against cancer (Fig. 61.7). When a "vaccine" is injected into the skin, the components of the vaccine known as PAMPs (Medzhitov and Janeway, 2000) activate resting dendritic cells and program them to migrate to a local lymph node. Thus a vaccine necessarily includes some component(s) intended to activate dendritic cells, although the precise substances employed vary between different vaccines. Another common term for these activating components is "adjuvant," because they "add" immunogenicity to the protein or peptide components of a vaccine. The other key component of a vaccine is a target protein or proteins that are expected to be relatively overexpressed in a tumor relative to normal tissue. The choice of vaccine antigen(s) is somewhat empiric and, like adjuvant choice, varies widely between approaches. Once a resting dendritic cell has been loaded with antigen, activated, and has migrated to a lymph node, it then displays fragments of antigen in the form of small peptides. Cellular recognition of these small peptide fragments (antigens) is complex; as introduced earlier, these peptides are not presented alone but instead are recognized when bound to a genetically diverse set of host molecules collectively encoded by a set of genes within the major histocompatibility complex (MHC). Specific receptors (TCRs) on CD4 and CD8 T cells recognize a structure composed of MHC molecules and a specific peptide. Simple recognition (a good fit) is insufficient for full T cell activation; T cells must also receive additional co-stimulatory signals provided by mature DCs to proliferate and acquire effector

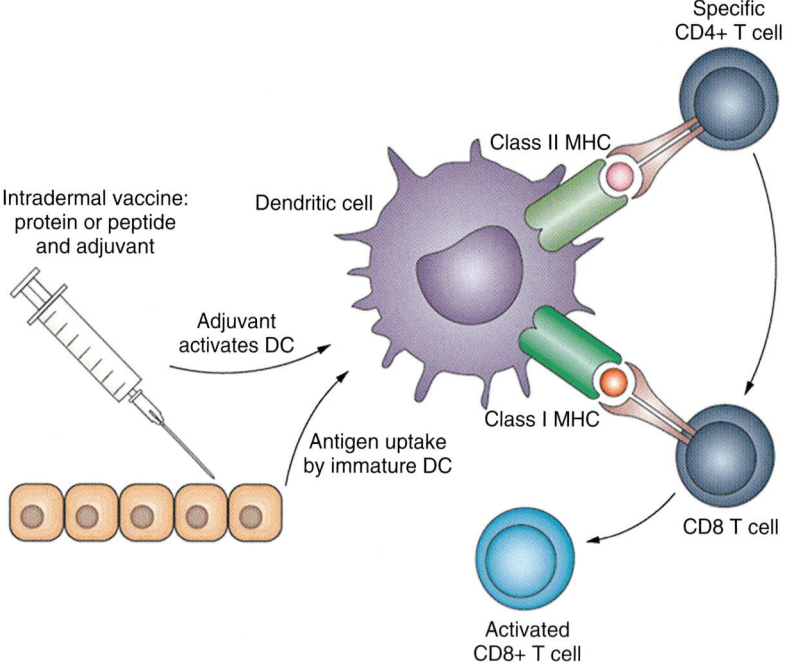

Fig. 61.7. Cancer vaccines. *DC*, Dendritic cell; *MHC*, major histocompatibility complex. (From Drake CG, Lipson EJ, Brahmer JR: Breathing new life into immunotherapy: review of melanoma, lung and kidney cancer. *Nat Rev Clin Oncol* 11:24–37, 2014b.)

function. In the case of CD8 T cells, the principal desired effector function is the ability to lyse target cells expressing the same MHC/peptide complex that activated them (i.e., their target antigen). For CD4 T cells, a Th1 response is desired. Once fully activated, CD8 T cells leave the lymph node and traffic widely through the host in search of their targets.

Vaccines for Kidney Cancer

Although an in-depth discussion of all the cancer vaccine approaches in GU cancers is beyond the scope of this chapter, several vaccines are highlighted. The examples chosen illustrate key immunologic principles, as well as the challenges inherent in developing vaccine-based immunotherapy. In that regard, one interesting vaccine approach for kidney cancer focused on targeting multiple carefully selected antigens with a fairly simple adjuvant. To select relevant antigens, resected kidney tumors from a series of patients expressing the common class I MHC allele HLA-A2 were isolated, and the cell surface peptides residing in class I MHC molecules eluted and analyzed using mass spectrometry (Walter et al., 2012). This approach identified a set of tumor-associated peptides, which were used to design a vaccine incorporating granulocyte-macrophage colony-stimulating factor (GM-CSF) as an adjuvant. GM-CSF is a strong inducer of DC migration, but perhaps less robust than the TLR agonists in terms of inducing DC activation. In the phase I study of this agent (IMA901), 28 patients with renal cell carcinoma (RCC) were enrolled; because the peptides in the vaccine are only presented by the MHC class I allele HLA-A2, patients were required to be A2 positive. These patients received up to eight multi-peptide vaccinations, each preceded by GM-CSF as an adjuvant. The vaccine was well tolerated, with no grade 3 or 4 adverse events reported. At a 3-month follow-up point, a single patient showed a partial response, 16 patients had disease progression, and 11 had stable disease. Immune responses to the targeted peptides were detected in several of the treated patients (Walter et al., 2012). To improve the relatively sparse clinical activity noted, investigators made use of data showing that low doses of the alkylating agent cyclophosphamide have vaccine-potentiating immune effects (North, 1982), these effects are at least partially mediated by the depletion of the regulatory T cells (Treg) that turn off an immune response (Machiels et al., 2001; Wada et al., 2009). In a randomized phase II trial, 68 HLA-A2 positive patients with RCC were randomly assigned to either vaccine, or to vaccine preceded by a single immunomodulatory dose of intravenous cyclophosphamide (300 mg/m^2). Objective tumor regressions were rare, with a single confirmed partial response among 64 patients. Subsequent immunologic analyses showed an increased T-cell response to the targeted peptides, and verified that low-dose cyclophosphamide depletes regulatory T cells in humans. Despite these phase II results, a randomized phase III trial comparing standard of care first-line sunitinib to the combination of sunitinib + vaccine was initiated (NCT01265901). With a median follow-up of approximately 3 years, overall survival was not improved by the addition of vaccine to TKI, with a nonsignificant trend toward improved survival **in the nonvaccinated group** (HR 1.34, $P = 0.087$). These data are consistent with the data described earlier, suggesting that CD8 T cell infiltration in RCC may be associated with a less favorable outcome (Giraldo et al., 2015).

A second illustrative vaccine approach in kidney cancer involved autologous vaccines, in which antigens are derived from a patient's individual tumor lysate or whole cells. Such vaccines were tested in RCC and lung cancer (Eager and Nemunaitis, 2005; Simons et al., 1997); autologous vaccine approaches are complicated by the complexity in generating a vaccine from variable amounts of patient material. To overcome these challenges, a novel approach was developed, whereby a vaccine is generated using RNA extracted from patient-derived tumor material, rather than tumor lysate or cells (Figlin et al., 2012). With this approach (AGS-003), substantial quantities of vaccine can be manufactured using a relatively small amount of resected tumor. Rather than relying on the patient's endogenous DCs (which are often defective or dysfunctional [Gabrilovich et al., 1997]), the AGS-003 vaccine uses autologous DCs generated ex vivo, through maturation of immature monocytes in the presence of the cytokines IL-4 and GM-CSF (Palucka et al., 2005). So, to manufacture AGS-003, patients undergo leukopheresis, and DCs are cultured. Simultaneously, tumor RNA is prepared from a resected mass and is used to transfect those autologous DCs to generate a mature, cell-based vaccine, which is then frozen and stored for repeated intranodal injections.

A phase III trial of AGS-003 randomly assigned approximately 600 patients with metastatic high-risk RCC to receive either ongoing treatment with the standard-of-care tyrosine kinase inhibitor sunitinib or one cycle of sunitinib followed by AGS-003 co-administered along with sunitinib (NCT01582672). The primary end point of the study was progression-free survival; unfortunately that study phase III also failed to meet its primary endpoint, although follow-up continues.

Vaccines for Prostate Cancer

As outlined earlier, one approach to overcoming DC dysfunction is to generate new DC outside of the patient's tolerogenic environment. In PC, this approach is exemplified by Sipuleucel-T, which was the first cancer vaccine approved by the FDA for the treatment of patients with a solid tumor (Kantoff et al., 2010a). Sipuleucel T is individually manufactured for each patient with PC in a process that includes multiple steps. Briefly, patients undergo leukopheresis and peripheral blood mononuclear cells (PBMCs) are extracted and then incubated with PAP2024, a fusion protein that links the target antigen prostatic acid phosphatase (PAP) to GM-CSF. After approximately 36 hours of incubation, cells are prepared for reinfusion. In this approach, GM-CSF serves as the adjuvant that helps to activate dendritic cells. Of interest, the final Sipuleucel-T product is heterogeneous and includes mature antigen-presenting cells (APCs) as well as other cell types, including T cells, B cells, and natural killer cells (Sonpavde et al., 2012). Once infused, the autologous ex vivo-activated APC prime PAP-specific CD4+ and CD8+ T cells (Antonarakis et al., 2018) in a manner similar to a classical vaccine-mediated prime-boost regimen, in which the first infusion primes the immune system and subsequent infusions boost the response.

A second prostate cancer vaccine that reached late stages of clinical development is ProstVac VF (Bavarian Nordic, USA; Madan et al., 2009). This vaccine approach is different from the peptide or cell-based vaccines discussed earlier and relies on the incorporation of a target antigen into a virus to specifically activate the immune system (Fig. 61.8). The antigen chosen here was prostate-specific antigen (PSA), and the viral backbone comes from poxviruses, which are related to the vaccine used in the campaign that led to the successful worldwide eradication of smallpox.

This technology has been honed over several decades, and the iteration in the phase III trial includes a number of important modifications designed to optimize immunogenicity. First, the vaccine involves a heterologous prime boost regimen, in which the initial vaccine is based on a modified vaccinia Ankara (MVA) backbone, followed by a series of booster vaccines with a fowlpox backbone. This is necessary because the humoral (antibody-mediated) immune response to the MVA backbone is robust, such that boosting with an identical vaccine is limited by the host's immune antibody response to the viral backbone itself. To further increase immunogenicity, the vaccine was engineered to incorporate a triad of co-stimulatory molecules designed to generate dendritic cells with an enhanced potential for T-cell activation (Hodge et al., 1999). Finally, similar to IMA901 in RCC, administration of GM-CSF at the vaccination site is used to help recruit local DCs and enhance antigen presentation. In patients, poxvirus vectors most likely infect epithelial cells, a proportion of which undergo cell death. Cellular debris, including encoded antigens, are then taken up by nearby immature DC, which, when appropriately activated, can present these antigens to CD4+ and CD8+ T cells in a proinflammatory context (Drake, 2010). Direct infection of DC, particularly the Langerhans cells in the skin, is another mechanism by which poxvirus vectors may prime an immune response. The end result of ProstVac treatment is postulated to be activation and proliferation of PSA-specific CD8 and CD4 T cells, which was demonstrated in early correlative studies. In contrast to Sipuleucel-T (GuhaThakurta et al., 2015), ProstVac-VF does not appear to prime an extensive antibody response; indeed antibodies specific for PSA are extremely rare with this agent. Based on a potential survival benefit shown in a randomized phase II trial (Kantoff et al., 2010b), an international randomized phase III of ProstVac VF was initiated (NCT01322490). This trial enrolled 1200 patients with metastatic castration-resistant prostate cancer and randomized them to placebo, ProstVac-VF plus subcutaneous GM-CSF, or to ProstVac-VF alone. The primary endpoint of the trial was overall survival. Unfortunately as was the case for the two RCC vaccine trials mentioned earlier, the phase III trial of ProstVac VF was closed by the data safety monitoring committee because it was deemed unlikely to meet its primary endpoint of an improved overall survival.

> **KEY POINTS: IMMUNOTHERAPY FOR GENITOURINARY CANCERS**
>
> - BCG therapy for bladder cancer stimulates the innate and adaptive immune systems and is a prototype for successful cancer immunotherapy.
> - Cancer vaccines have been evaluated in kidney and prostate cancer, and a single vaccine (Sipuleucel-T) is FDA approved for metastatic prostate cancer.
> - Several other vaccine approaches failed in phase III trials in kidney and prostate cancer.

PD-1/PD-L1 Blockade in Genitourinary Cancers

As introduced earlier, most tumors involve multiple mechanisms to evade immune-mediated destruction (Drake et al., 2006). The most

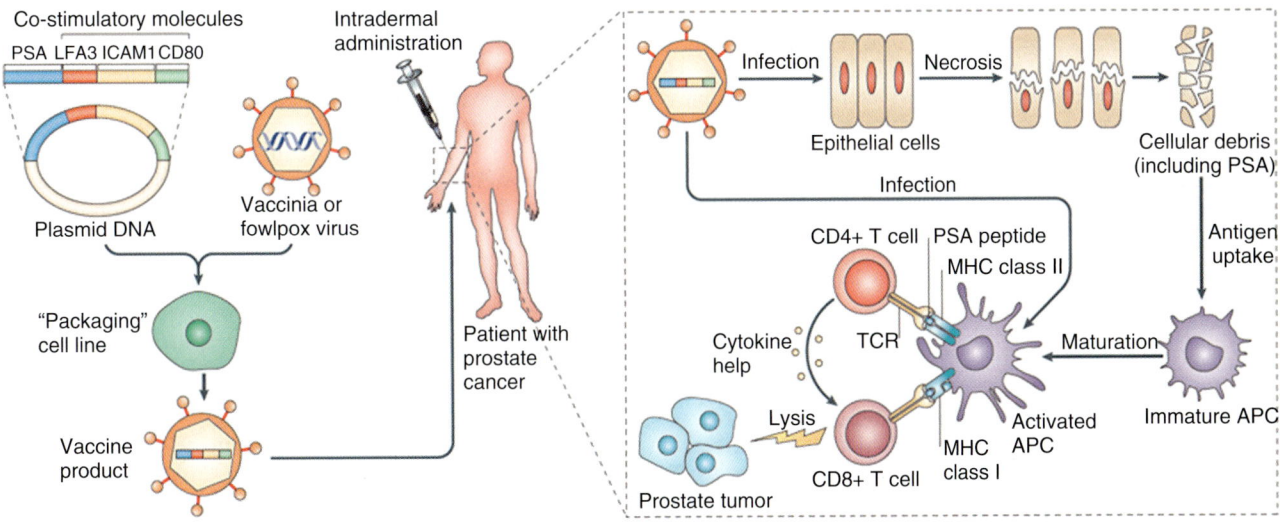

Fig. 61.8. Virus-based cancer vaccines (ProstVac VF). *APC*, Antigen-presenting cell; *MHC*, major histocompatibility complex; *PSA*, prostate-specific antigen; *TCR*, T-cell receptor. (From Drake CG: Prostate cancer as a model for tumour immunotherapy. *Nat Rev Immunol* 10:580–593, 2010.)

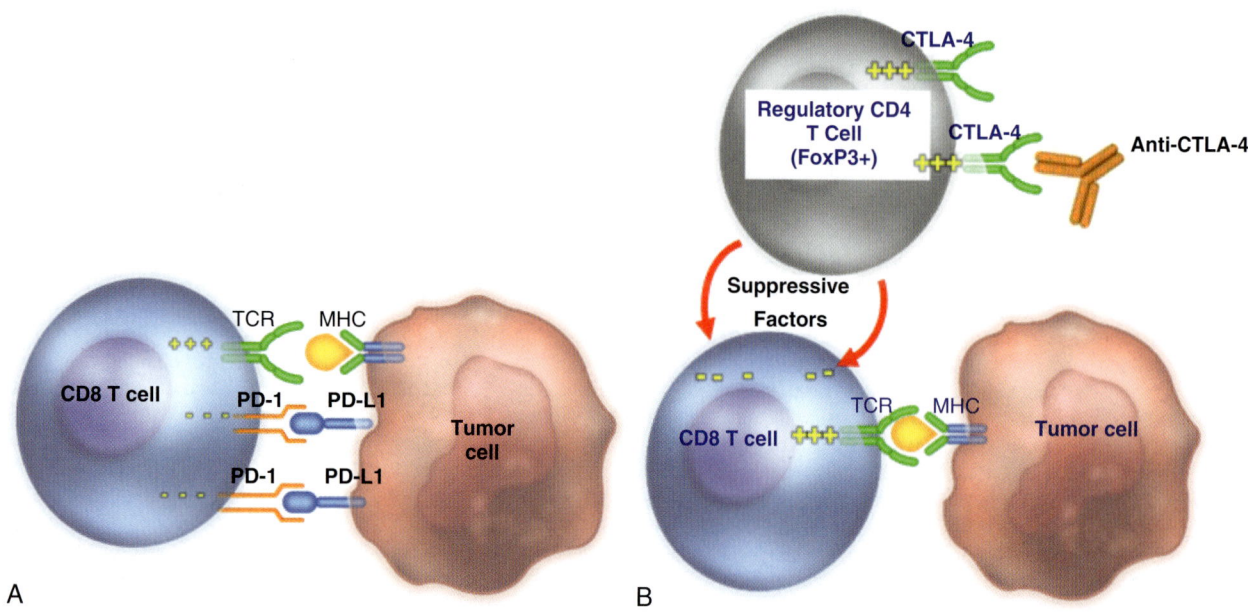

Fig. 61.9. Immune checkpoint blockade. (A) PD-1/PD-L1 blockade. (B) CTLA-4 blockade.

important of these mechanisms involves T-cell expression of one PD-1, which binds to its ligand PD-L1 to effectively limit T-cell proliferation and killing capacity (Drake et al., 2014; LaFleur et al., 2018; Fig. 61.9A).

PD-1/PD-L1 Blockade in Second-Line Bladder Cancer

Because bladder cancer frequently expresses PD-L1, blocking PD-1 and/or PD-L1 in that disease would seem a logical approach; at this time five anti-PD-1/PD-L1 agents are FDA approved for *second-line* treatment of metastatic bladder cancer. All five have objective response rates (ORRs) between 15% and 23% in unselected patients in the second-line setting. The majority were approved based on single-arm studies comparing median overall survival (OS) and ORR with historical controls. These include the following:

1. **Atezolizumab**, a humanized anti-PD-L1 IgG1 antibody engineered to minimize binding to Fc receptors; this was the first immune checkpoint therapy granted approval by the FDA for urothelial bladder cancer (UBC). Approval was based on the IMvigor 210 study (Rosenberg et al., 2016), a single-arm phase II trial in which second-line bladder cancer patients were treated with 1200 mg of atezolizumab every 3 weeks. The ORR was 14.8% (CI 11.1–19.3) and based on a prespecified response rate of 10% in historical controls, approval was granted for patients who progress after platinum-based therapy or who have progressed within 1 year of neoadjuvant or adjuvant therapy with a platinum-containing regimen.
2. **Nivolumab**, a fully human IgG4 anti-PD1 antibody hinge-modified to improve half-life, received accelerated approval from the FDA for second-line therapy in bladder cancer patients previously treated with a platinum-containing regimen. This approval was based on data from a single-arm phase II study that enrolled 270 patients to receive nivolumab at 3 mg/kg every 2 weeks (Sharma et al., 2017) and had an overall response rate of 19.6%.
3. **Pembrolizumab**, a hinge-stabilized, humanized IgG4 anti-PD1 antibody that, like nivolumab, disrupts the engagement of PD-1 with its ligands PD-L1 and PD-L2. Of the FDA-approved antibodies blocking the PD-1/PD-L1 interaction, pembrolizumab is the only agent approved based on data from a randomized, phase III study (Bellmunt et al., 2017). Accelerated approval was granted by the FDA based on that open-label study, which randomly assigned 542 patients who had recurred or progressed after platinum-based therapy to investigator's choice chemotherapy (paclitaxel, docetaxel, or vinflunine) versus pembrolizumab at 200 mg every 3 weeks. The median overall survival in the pembrolizumab arm was improved as compared with the chemotherapy arm (10.3 months vs. 7.4 months, $P = 0.002$), and the ORR for the pembrolizumab treated patients was significantly greater than that in the chemotherapy group (21.1% vs. 11.4%, $P = 0.001$).
4. **Durvalumab**, a fully human anti-PD-L1 antibody, was approved based on a single-arm phase I/II study evaluating 61 patients with platinum-treated advanced urothelial cancer (UC) (Massard et al., 2016). Patients were eligible if they had disease relapse within 1 year of neoadjuvant or first-line chemotherapy. In PD-L1 selected patients, the overall response rate was 31.0%. A follow-up analysis reporting on 191 unselected patients treated with durvalumab reported an ORR of 17.8% (Powles et al., 2017).
5. **Avelumab**, an IgG1 anti-PD-L1 antibody that blocks the interaction between PD-1 and PD-L1 but not PD-1 and PD-L2 evaluated in a phase Ib study of unselected patients with platinum refractory bladder cancer; the ORR was 18.2% with a reported median OS of 13.7 months (Apolo et al., 2017). A second pooled analysis of an additional cohort of 241 patients with platinum refractory UC demonstrated a confirmed ORR of 17.6%, with a median overall survival for the pooled cohort of approximately 7.0 months (CI 5.6–11.1) (Patel et al., 2018).

PD-1/PD-L1 Blockade in First-Line Bladder Cancer

With the idea that the immune system may be more intact in chemotherapy-naive patients, the anti-PD-L1 antibody atezolizumab was evaluated in the first-line setting in cisplatin-ineligible patients in one arm of the ImVigor 210 study. The majority of those patients suffered from renal impairment that prohibited cisplatin-based therapy (70%). The ORR for first-line cisplatin-ineligible patients was approximately 23%, with an overall survival of 15.9 months (95% CI 10.4 m. – not estimable). Based on those data, atezolizumab was approved for treating cisplatin-ineligible patients with metastatic urothelial carcinoma. Pembrolizumab was also approved for use as first-line therapy in cisplatin-ineligible patients in mUC based on data from an single-armed phase II study (Bajorin et al., 2015).

Selecting Bladder Cancer Patients for PD-1/PD-L1–Based Immunotherapy

Although blocking the PD-1/PD-L1 interaction has clinical activity in patients with metastatic bladder cancer, it is clear that not all patients benefit. This is particularly important in the first-line setting, where cisplatin-ineligible patients can be treated either with a carboplatin-based regimen or with first-line anti-PD-1 (pembrolizumab) or first-line anti-PD-L1 (atezolizumab). Based on the notion that PD-L1 expression identifies tumors in which an adaptive immune response is engaged, it makes sense that PD-L1 expression, quantified by immunohistochemistry, could serve as a reasonable predictive biomarker to select patients for immunotherapy (Aggen and Drake, 2017). Indeed, the majority of the trials outlined earlier tested the predictive properties of PD-L1 expression, with the general finding that PD-L1 expression enriches for patients likely to respond to anti-PD-1/PD-L1 monotherapy. As a predictive biomarker, PD-L1 expression is far from perfect, with several factors limiting its capabilities. Perhaps the most obvious of those is sampling error; PD-L1 expression is expressed heterogeneously throughout a tumor nodule, so results may be critically dependent on the lesion interrogated by biopsy (McLaughlin et al., 2016). Complicating sampling error is the factor that at least five different immunohistochemical (IHC) assays have been developed, each with different staining protocols and antibodies. Although these may generally give concordant results (Hirsch et al., 2017), cutoffs for "positivity" vary between assays. Finally, in most of these studies objective responses, even complete responses, have been observed in patients whose tumors were completely negative for PD-L1 expression by IHC. Taken together, those data suggest that PD-L1 expression is at best a weak biomarker in bladder cancer.

PD-1/PD-L1 Blockade in Kidney Cancer

Because RCC is usually considered to be an immune-sensitive tumor type, the observation of single-agent objective responses in RCC patients treated with single-agent anti-PD-1 in phase I trials was not completely unexpected. Indeed, one patient with advanced RCC showed a stable partial response for more than 4 years in the first-in-man dose-escalation study (Brahmer et al., 2010). Perhaps more noteworthy, this sustained partial response eventually evolved into a documented complete response, and the patient has remained off treatment for more than 10 years at last follow-up (Lipson et al., 2013). This initial observation of clinical activity for PD-1 blockade in RCC was supported by data from a more dose-intense phase Ib trial; here, the objective response rate was 30% to 35%, with an additional 10% of patients showing stable disease (McDermott et al., 2015). Based on the activity seen in phase I trials, several phase I and II studies of PD-1 blockade using nivolumab in RCC were initiated. One interesting trial was a dose-ranging study (NCT01354431); this trial enrolled a total of 150 patients, randomized into treatment cohorts at doses of 0.3 mg/kg, 2 mg/kg, and 10 mg/kg, treated every 3 weeks (in contrast to the once-every-2-week dosing in the phase Ib study). The results of that trial showed surprisingly equivalent activity and toxicity for each of the three doses tested (i.e., in RCC there is not a clear dose-response relationship for anti-PD-1 treatment using nivolumab). These findings led to a pivotal phase III trial (Checkmate 025) comparing 3 mg/kg of nivolumab to the mTOR inhibitor everolimus in patients with metastatic RCC (mRCC) after progression on TKI therapy; the primary endpoint of this trial was of OS (Motzer et al., 2015). With 821 patients randomized, median OS was 25.0 months with nivolumab versus 19.6 months with everolimus. The ORR was 24% with nivolumab versus 5% with everolimus. Similar to pembrolizumab in UC, there was no difference in progression-free survival (PFS). Unlike UBC, there is a single anti-PD-1/PD-L1 agent FDA approved for second-line RCC.

PD-1/PD-L1 Blockade in Prostate Cancer

PD-1 blockade was evaluated in a small number of patients with metastatic castrate-resistant prostate cancer, the majority of whom were heavily pretreated (Topalian et al., 2012). These data were generally disappointing; no objective responses were noted in approximately 20 men. Biologically, the lack of response to PD-1 blockade in prostate cancer may be explained by the notion that prostate cancer cells generally do not appear to express PD-L1 (Haffner et al., 2018), although the majority of CD8 T cells that infiltrate the gland do express PD-1 (Sfanos et al., 2009). Based on the observation that PD-L1 expression is increased after treatment with the second-generation androgen receptor inhibitor enzalutamide (Bishop et al., 2015), a single-armed study added PD-1 blockade to enzalutamide in patients progressing on enzalutamide. Early data from that trial were encouraging, with 3 out of the initial 10 treated patients showing PSA and/or objective responses (Graff et al., 2016). Those data are important because they suggest that, at least under certain circumstances, prostate cancer patients may respond to blockade of the PD-1/PD-L1 axis.

Taken together, the results mentioned earlier show that ICB will clearly play an important role in treating RCC and bladder cancer, but additional combinatorial efforts will almost certainly be required to achieve objective responses in men with prostate cancer.

> **KEY POINTS: IMMUNOTHERAPY FOR GENITOURINARY CANCERS**
>
> - BCG therapy for bladder cancer stimulates the innate and adaptive immune systems and is a prototype for successful cancer immunotherapy.
> - Cancer vaccines have been evaluated in kidney and prostate cancer.
> - A single vaccine (Sipuleucel-T) is FDA approved for metastatic prostate cancer.
> - Cancer vaccines are generally well tolerated but result in few objective clinical responses.
> - Blocking the PD-1/PD-L1 interaction is effective in second-line bladder cancer and has activity in first-line patients who are cisplatin ineligible.
> - PD-L1 expression may distinguish bladder cancer patients more likely to respond to anti-PD-1/anti-PD-L1 therapy.
> - Anti-PD-1 is effective in second-line kidney cancer.
> - Anti-PD-1/PD-L1 has not shown robust monotherapy activity in metastatic prostate cancer.

Combination Immunotherapy Regimens in Genitourinary Cancers

CTLA-4 Blockade in Prostate and Kidney Cancer

Cytotoxic T lymphocyte antigen-4 (CTLA-4) is an immune checkpoint molecule expressed on T cells within the tumor microenvironment. Its expression patterns are different than PD-1; CTLA-4 appears to be relatively overexpressed on the population of FoxP3+ CD4 T cells that down-regulate immune responses, regulatory T cells (Treg) (Peggs et al., 2009; Simpson et al., 2013) (see Fig. 61.9). Thus blockade of CTLA-4 likely attenuates the function of Treg, enabling the CD8 tumor infiltrating lymphocytes to exert antitumor activity (Fig. 61.9B).

ICB using anti-CTLA-4 (ipilimumab) monotherapy was evaluated in a number of early phase studies in men with prostate cancer. These data show that treatment is associated with a PSA response rate of approximately 15% to 20%, but with few objective (radiographic) responses (Slovin et al., 2013). In several of these studies, a low dose of radiation therapy was included in an effort to release antigen and potentiate an immune response. However, in those published data, there was no evidence for such an effect; for example, the PSA response rate in patients treated with a dose of 10 mg/kg of ipilimumab was 12% in the presence of radiation therapy (RT) versus 25% without.

Despite this relatively low PSA response rate, and little evidence that low-dose RT applied to a single lesion in men with metastatic disease improved the PSA response rate to ipilimumab, a phase III trial combining RT and ipilimumab, was launched in men with mCRPC who had progressed on or after treatment with docetaxel chemotherapy. This trial enrolled approximately 800 men and randomized them to a single low-dose treatment of RT alone versus RT followed by ipilimumab at a dose of 10 mg/kg every 3 weeks × 4 weeks, with every 3-month maintenance for men who were not progressing. The trial did not meet its primary endpoint (overall survival) with a median OS of 11.2 months in the ipilimumab arm versus 10.0 months for placebo (Kwon et al., 2014). The prespecified secondary endpoint was met, with a PFS of 4.0 months in the ipilimumab group versus 3.1 months in the placebo group (HR = .070, $P < 0.001$). These data provide evidence that ipilimumab may have clinical activity in prostate cancer but were insufficient for regulatory approval. Retrospective analyses of the phase III data showed that men with more favorable disease characteristics (no visceral metastases, normal alkaline phosphatase, normal hemoglobin) appeared to benefit from treatment. One fascinating finding of those post-hoc analyses was that men with visceral disease appeared to derive absolutely no benefit from ipilimumab treatment, whereas in men with bone-only disease there was a clear suggestion of clinical benefit. The precise mechanisms underlying this dichotomy are unclear but may reflect a different immune microenvironment in bone versus soft-tissue metastases in prostate cancer (Drake, 2014). Relevant to those findings, a second phase III trial in the pre-chemotherapy setting has completed enrollment; that trial specifically excluded men with soft-tissue disease; unfortunately that study also failed to meet its primary overall survival endpoint (Beer et al., 2017). Taken together, these phase III data showed that anti-CTLA-4 monotherapy is not an effective treatment for metastatic castration resistant prostate cancer.

If PD-1 is largely expressed on CD8 (killer) T cells that infiltrate tumors, and CTLA-4 is predominantly expressed on CD4 regulatory T cells (Treg), then combined blockade of both pathways could lead to therapeutic synergy. This was true in animal models; combined PD-1/CTLA-4 blockade was the first immune checkpoint combination to show synergistic effects in animals (Curran et al., 2010). Based on preclinical data, the combination of PD-1 and CTLA-4 inhibition has been tested in multiple tumor types, most notably in RCC. In a phase 1b study (CheckMate 016), patients with mRCC had a response rate of approximately 40% to combination therapy, an impressive result that should perhaps be tempered by the rate of grade III/IV immune-related adverse events, which was also in the 40% range (Hammers et al., 2014). Those data led to a phase III front-line trial (Checkmate 214), comparing the combination of anti-PD-1 and anti-CTLA-4 to standard of care sunitinib in front-line RCC patients. Phase III results were similar to the phase 1b data, with combined treatment reaching its combined endpoints of overall response rate (i.e., the ORR for ipilimumab plus nivolumab was 41.6% vs. 26.5% with sunitinib) (Motzer et al., 2018). Based on these data, combination immunotherapy is an FDA-approved first-line treatment option for patients with metastatic RCC.

Combining PD-1/PD-L1 Blockade With Androgen Deprivation Therapy in Prostate Cancer

In general, androgen-deprivation therapy (ADT) has proinflammatory effects. Some of these involve the thymus, which is an organ important for T cell ontogeny. In younger mammals, the thymus is sizable and functional, resulting in the ongoing output of naive T cells. As the organism ages, the thymus involutes so that the daily output of new naive T cells decreases progressively. In aged mice (and presumptively in humans as well), androgen ablation restores the size and cellularity of the thymus, resulting in an increased T-cell output (Sutherland et al., 2005). Consistent with those data, androgen ablation before prostate cancer surgery results in the infiltration of CD4+ T cells into the gland; these cells have an activated phenotype (Mercader et al., 2001). Also supporting a proimmunogenic role for androgen ablation are data demonstrating the induction of novel antibody specificities in treated patients (Nesslinger et al., 2007).

The FDA-approved prostate cancer vaccine was evaluated in combination with intermittent androgen ablation; the results of that study showed that administration of the vaccine before androgen ablation increased CD8 T cell responses to the target antigen, with a handful of patients maintaining low PSA levels even after recovery of testosterone (Antonarakis et al., 2017). Androgen ablation has been combined with immune checkpoint blockade, a phase III trial randomized patients progressing on the next-generation androgen synthesis inhibitor abiraterone acetate to either enzalutamide or the combination of enzalutamide plus anti-PD-L1 (atezolizumab). This trial (NCT03016312) has a primary endpoint of overall survival; the readout is expected in 2020.

Combining PD-1/PD-L1 Blockade With Chemotherapy in Bladder Cancer

Although chemotherapy is often thought of as antagonistic to the immune system, studies showed that some chemotherapy agents, particularly the alkylating agent cyclophosphamide, could in fact enhance a vaccine-directed immune response (Machiels et al., 2001; Wada et al., 2009). In-depth explorations of chemotherapy/immunotherapy combinations showed that additive effects were dependent on several factors. First among those is the chemotherapy agent under study; certain chemotherapy agents are more immunogenic than others in animal models (Galluzzi et al., 2015). This disparity even exists among agents in the same class, for example, among the platinum-based compounds, oxaliplatin appears to be more immunogenic than its sister agents carboplatin or cisplatin. Mechanistically, immunologically favorable chemotherapy agents appear to induce "immunogenic cell death" (Fig. 61.10), in which tumor cells are killed in a manner that facilitates antigen uptake by resting dendritic cells, followed by subsequent trafficking to the draining lymph node and presentation to tumor-antigen–specific T cells. In addition to the type of agent employed, the schedule seemed to be critically important, with small differences being crucial to a proimmune effect. The dose is also critical, with animal studies (Machiels et al., 2001; Wada et al., 2009) and human studies (Emens et al., 2009) showing that a lower dose of chemotherapy is generally required for optimal combinatorial activity. The majority of those data were generated using vaccine-based regimens; in humans, full-dose platinum-doublet–based chemotherapy clearly adds efficacy to anti-PD-1–based immunotherapy (Rizvi et al., 2016), and the combination of PD-1 blockade plus full-dose standard therapy is a standard-of-care treatment regimen for patients with non–small-cell lung cancer (Gandhi et al., 2018). Based to some degree on those data, there are currently a number of ongoing phase III trials in bladder cancer, adding PD-1 or PD-L1 blockade to standard first-line gemcitabine/cisplatin regimen. Those are important trials; if successful they will transform first-line bladder cancer to a disease treated with a chemotherapy/immunotherapy combination. Such a result could provide patient benefit but would leave in question an optimal second-line treatment for progressing or nonresponsive patients.

Combining PD-1/PD-L1 Blockade With VEGF Inhibition in Kidney Cancer

Antiangiogenic therapy is the mainstay of therapy for metastatic RCC; by inhibiting the formation of new blood vessels, tumor progression can be diminished. In general, the blood vessels within tumors are abnormal, with increased tortuosity and permeability to soluble molecules (Jain, 2001). That permeability does not apply to T lymphocytes; the blood vessels in tumors generally inhibit T cell migration. Treatment with either small molecule agents that inhibit VEGF tyrosine kinase signaling or with antibodies that bind to VEGF promotes the normalization of tumor vasculature, promoting the emigration of T cells from the circulation into the tumor. This process was demonstrated in animal models and in cancer patients (Hegde et al., 2017). In one especially relevant example, a phase 1 trial combining anti-CTLA-4 (ipilimumab) with anti-VEGF (bevacizumab) in patients with metastatic melanoma (Hodi et al., 2014) showed a clear increase in the CD8 T cell infiltrate in the tumor bed. In RCC, combining bevacizumab with the anti-PD-L1 antibody atezolizumab also showed an increase in intratumoral CD8 T cell infiltration (Wallin et al., 2016), and clinical results from that trial drove a randomized phase III trial of the bevacizumab/atezolizumab combination regimen in the first-line setting in RCC patients. An additional notable aspect of VEGF biology is that the molecule itself is immunosuppressive (Kandalaft et al., 2011). Thus VEGF signaling promotes a tolerogenic phenotype in APCs, inducing them to mediate T cell suppression rather than activation. Inhibition of VEGF signaling reverses this process, restoring APC phenotype and function. It is also significant that VEGF TKIs are associated with objective responses in RCC, and in many models the level of cancer-driven immunosuppression correlates with tumor burden. Thus there are three major mechanisms by which VEGF inhibition may facilitate an antitumor

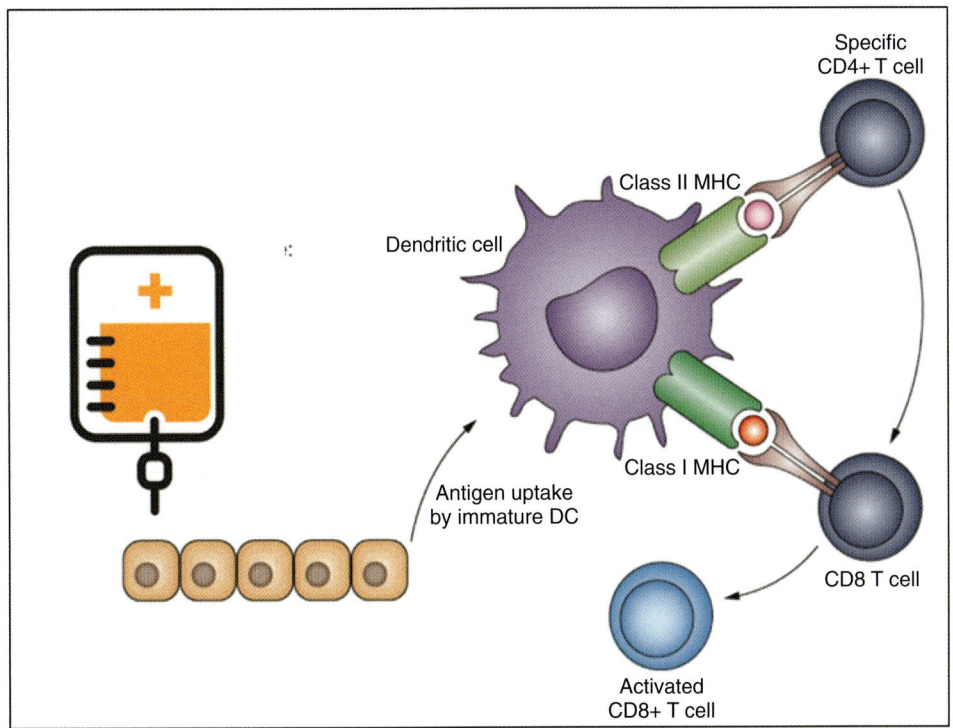

Fig. 61.10. Immunogenic cell death. *DC*, Dendritic cell; *MHC*, major histocompatibility complex.

immune response in RCC: (1) normalizing the tumor vasculature, enabling T cell infiltration; (2) reversing a suppressive effect on APCs; and (3) driving tumor regression, thus minimizing a tolerogenic tumor burden. A single-armed phase II study combining PD-1 blockade with VEGF-TKI treatment reported an overall response rate of 73%, supporting the notion that VEGF/immunotherapy combinations have clinical activity. Similar combinations are the subject of a number of first-line, randomized phase III trials in RCC.

CONCLUSIONS

Cancer immunotherapy is a rapidly advancing field, and progress in this area has been particularly strong in the case of GU cancers. A more robust understanding of basic immunology and immune resistance to tumors has driven recent progress, and there are a large number of ongoing trials. BCG immunotherapy for bladder cancer was one of the first immune-based treatments to enter into routine clinical practice in any cancer type. As discussed in other chapters, the future of immunotherapy will most likely involve combination approaches: the combination of PD-1 blockade with CTLA-4 blockade is now FDA approved in first-line RCC treatment. Other combinations of interest include ADT in prostate cancer, VEGF inhibition in RCC, and chemotherapy plus immunotherapy combinations in bladder cancer. Although these combinations hold considerable promise, it is unlikely that most patients will benefit; in the future it will be important to understand mechanisms of resistance to combined therapy in preclinical models as well as in patients.

SUGGESTED READINGS

Balkwill F, Charles KA, Mantovani A: Smoldering and polarized inflammation in the initiation and promotion of malignant disease, *Cancer Cell* 7:211–217, 2005.
Brandau S, Suttmann H: Thirty years of BCG immunotherapy for non-muscle invasive bladder cancer: a success story with room for improvement, *Biomed Pharmacother* 61:299–305, 2007.
De Marzo AM, Platz EA, Sutcliffe S, et al: Inflammation in prostate carcinogenesis, *Nat Rev Cancer* 7:256–269, 2007.
Drake CG, Jaffee E, Pardoll DM: Mechanisms of immune evasion by tumors, *Adv Immunol* 90:51–81, 2006.
Drake CG: Prostate cancer as a model for tumour immunotherapy, *Nat Rev Immunol* 10:580–593, 2010.
Dunn GP, Old LJ, Schreiber RD: The immunobiology of cancer immunosurveillance and immunoediting, *Immunity* 21:137–148, 2004.
Gabrilovich D: Mechanisms and functional significance of tumour-induced dendritic-cell defects, *Nat Rev Immunol* 4:941–952, 2004.
Gannon PO, Poisson AO, Delvoye N, et al: Characterization of the intraprostatic immune cell infiltration in androgen-deprived prostate cancer patients, *J Immunol Methods* 348:9–17, 2009.
Hanahan D, Weinberg RA: Hallmarks of cancer: the next generation, *Cell* 144:646–674, 2011.
Hodi FS, O'Day SJ, McDermott DF, et al: Improved survival with ipilimumab in patients with metastatic melanoma, *N Engl J Med* 363:711–723, 2010.
Kantoff PW, Higano CS, Shore ND, et al: Sipuleucel-T immunotherapy for castration-resistant prostate cancer, *N Engl J Med* 363:411–422, 2010a.
Kantoff PW, Schuetz TJ, Blumenstein BA, et al: Overall survival analysis of a phase II randomized controlled trial of a Poxviral-based PSA-targeted immunotherapy in metastatic castration-resistant prostate cancer, *J Clin Oncol* 28:1099–1105, 2010b.
Madan RA, Arlen PM, Mohebtash M, et al: Prostvac-VF: a vector-based vaccine targeting PSA in prostate cancer, *Expert Opin Investig Drugs* 18:1001–1011, 2009.
Medzhitov R, Janeway C Jr: Innate immune recognition: mechanisms and pathways, *Immunol Rev* 173:89–97, 2000.
Michaud DS: Chronic inflammation and bladder cancer, *Urol Oncol* 25:260–268, 2007.
Ostrand-Rosenberg S, Sinha P: Myeloid-derived suppressor cells: linking inflammation and cancer, *J Immunol* 182:4499–4506, 2009.
Palucka AK, Laupeze B, Aspord C, et al: Immunotherapy via dendritic cells, *Adv Exp Med Biol* 560:105–114, 2005.
Pardoll DM: The blockade of immune checkpoints in cancer immunotherapy, *Nat Rev Cancer* 12:252–264, 2012.
Ribas A: Tumor immunotherapy directed at PD-1, *N Engl J Med* 366:2517–2519, 2012.
Savage PA, Malchow S, Leventhal DS: Basic principles of tumor-associated regulatory T cell biology, *Trends Immunol* 34:33–40, 2013.
Slovin SF, Higano CS, Hamid O, et al: Ipilimumab alone or in combination with radiotherapy in metastatic castration-resistant prostate cancer: results from an open-label, multicenter phase I/II study, *Ann Oncol* 2013.
Topalian SL, Hodi FS, Brahmer JR, et al: Safety, activity, and immune correlates of anti-PD-1 antibody in cancer, *N Engl J Med* 366:2443–2454, 2012b.

REFERENCES

The complete reference list is available online at ExpertConsult.com.

62

Molecular Genetics and Cancer Biology

Karen S. Sfanos, PhD, and Mark L. Gonzalgo, MD, PhD

Despite decades of intensive biomedical research, cancer remains a significant cause of morbidity and mortality worldwide. In part, this is due to the complexity inherent in this disease, which is, in fact, not truly a single disease at all. It involves more than 100 separate subtypes, all grouped together under the single term, *cancer*.

In the United States cancer strikes more than half a million victims annually and is the second leading cause of death; it is poised to become the leading cause of death in the near future, should recent trends continue. Genitourinary (GU) malignancies make up 25% (440,560) of all estimated cancer cases in 2018 in the United States (basal and squamous skin cancers excluded) and 16% (96,460) of all cancer deaths (Siegel et al., 2018). However, significant advances in the diagnosis and treatment of certain GU cancers have been made. For example, the cure rate for testicular cancer now approaches 100% (Einhorn, 2002; Horwich et al., 2006). Unfortunately, this cancer is unusual in its responsiveness to therapy and is relatively uncommon. We have had less success with the more prevalent GU malignancies in men, such as prostate, bladder, and renal cancers; the first, fourth, and sixth most common cancers in men, respectively (Siegel et al., 2018). It is encouraging, however, that mortality figures for these malignancies have shown a slow but steady decline over the past decade, and there is every reason to believe that these trends will continue and even accelerate in the future.

Much of our current understanding of cancer is the direct result of the molecular biology revolution that developed rapidly after the elucidation of the molecular structure of DNA by Watson and Crick in 1953 (Watson and Crick, 1953). In subsequent years, the field of molecular genetics has complemented and greatly expanded upon knowledge gleaned by other disciplines, such as biochemistry and cell biology, providing important insights, at the molecular level, regarding the abnormalities present in cancer cells. Recent years have seen a tremendous expansion in the tools available for studying the genetic basis of human cancer. This includes whole genome and whole "exome" (the coding regions of the genome) sequencing efforts that have become relatively affordable and routine. Thus a great deal is now known concerning the numerous molecular signaling pathways that provide positive and negative regulatory signals that, in normal cells, stringently control cell proliferation so that any losses in cell number are precisely counterbalanced, thereby maintaining tissue and organ homeostasis, processes that go awry in cancer cells. Renegade populations of autonomously proliferating cells represent a serious threat to survival of the organism, particularly to large, long-lived species such as ourselves; therefore we have evolved multiple barriers to prevent such outbreaks from occurring. Notably, this means **that incipient cancer cells must overcome several hurdles on the way to becoming fully malignant, a multi-step process that takes many years or even decades to complete.** Consequently, it has been recognized that **cancer cells must acquire at least eight key attributes to make the transition from a normal cell to a malignant one. These attributes include (1) genetic instability and mutation, (2) autonomous growth, (3) insensitivity to internal and external antiproliferative signals, (4) resistance to apoptosis and other forms of induced cell suicide, (5) unlimited cell division potential, (6) the ability to induce new blood vessel formation (angiogenesis), (7) locally invasive behavior that uniquely distinguishes malignant from benign neoplasms, and (8) evasion of the immune system.** In addition, cancer cells must deal with various cellular stresses that are byproducts of their abnormal physiology as well as increase their energy metabolism required to fuel autonomous growth and unlimited replication. It is also currently recognized that tumor-associated inflammation may drive the development of early preneoplastic lesions into invasive cancers and/or promote tumor progression. **Finally, many cancers develop an additional, lethal attribute: the ability to leave the site of the primary tumor to colonize and thrive in distant organs or tissues as metastases** (Hanahan and Weinberg, 2000; Hanahan and Weinberg, 2011; Luo et al., 2009; Solimini et al., 2007).

This chapter outlines fundamental concepts of molecular genetics that are directly related to human cancer in general, with an emphasis on GU malignancies in particular. Spurred by recent technologic advances such as high-throughput DNA and RNA sequencing, our knowledge of the molecular genetics of cancer is rapidly expanding, providing new insights for use in novel diagnostic, prognostic, and therapeutic applications.

TUMOR SUPPRESSOR GENES AND ONCOGENES

For a detailed description of basic molecular genetics (DNA, RNA, and transcription, protein synthesis, chromosomes, and gene structure), see ExpertConsult.com.

Tumor Suppressor Genes

Tumor suppressor genes negatively regulate cellular growth and play a critical role in the normal processes of the cell cycle. These genes are also important for DNA repair and cell signaling. The absence of tumor suppressor gene function may lead to dysregulation of normal growth control and malignancy. **Loss of function of both copies (alleles) of a tumor suppressor gene is typically required for carcinogenesis. This functional loss can occur via (1) homozygous gene deletion, (2) loss of one allele and mutational inactivation of the second allele, (3) mutational events involving both alleles, or (4) loss of one allele and epigenetic inactivation of the second allele, often involving DNA methylation, which suppresses expression of the gene.** Classic tumor suppressor genes discussed later in this chapter are the retinoblastoma gene *(RB1)* and the *TP53* gene (see Cell Cycle Deregulation).

The "two-hit" hypothesis was first proposed in cases of retinoblastoma, which required mutations in both alleles for disease manifestation (Knudson, 1971). This is due to the fact that if just one allele is inactivated, the remaining allele could produce sufficient amounts of the correct protein to maintain the normal state (Fig. 62.6). However, specific types of mutations in certain genes may not follow this two-hit rule and can function in a dominant negative capacity when mutated, inhibiting the function of the normal protein from the unaltered allele. An example is when two or more of the same protein molecules act together (such as dimerization), as is the case for TP53 (Baker et al., 1990). Alternatively, deletion or mutation of a single allele may result in insufficient protein production (haploinsufficiency), resulting in an increased carcinogen susceptibility as in the case of the *CDKN1B* (p27Kip1) gene (Fero et al., 1998).

Oncogenes

Oncogenes are positively associated with cellular proliferation and are the mutated form of normal genes (proto-oncogenes). Two

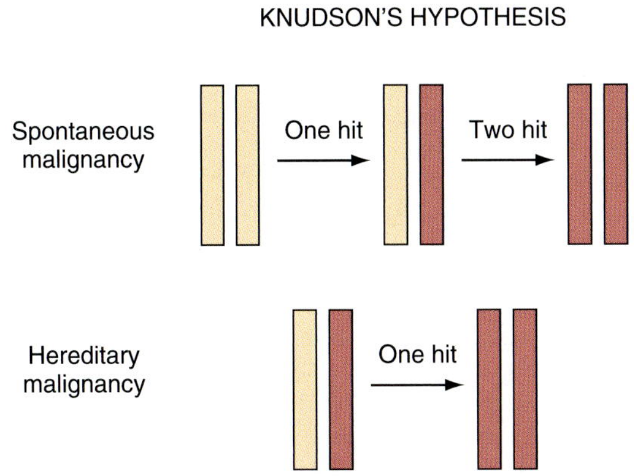

Fig. 62.6. Knudson's hypothesis was that inactivation of the same gene was responsible for sporadic and hereditary malignancies. Patients with sporadic tumors had two normal copies of the gene, and therefore the sporadic tumors required inactivation of both copies of the gene. Patients with hereditary tumor syndromes were born with only one functioning copy of the gene of interest, and therefore the hereditary tumors required inactivation of only one copy.

KEY POINTS: TUMOR SUPPRESSOR GENES AND ONCOGENES

- Mutations in DNA can lead to changes in protein function or expression that increase the potential for cancer initiation, progression, or metastasis.
- Tumor suppressor genes normally negatively regulate and control cellular growth. Oncogenes normally promote cell growth.
- Loss of tumor suppressor gene function can occur primarily by (1) homozygous deletion, (2) loss of one allele and mutational inactivation of the second allele, (3) mutational events involving both alleles, and (4) loss of one allele and epigenetic inactivation of the second allele.
- Certain tumor suppressor genes do not follow the "two-hit" hypothesis and may be inactivated via dominant negative mutations or haploinsufficiency.
- Proto-oncogenes can be converted to oncogenes by (1) mutation of the proto-oncogene resulting in an activated form of the gene, (2) gene amplification, and (3) chromosomal rearrangement.

---

oncogenes that have been found to be overexpressed in a variety of cancers include *MYC* and *MET* (Bottaro et al., 1991; Wong et al., 1986). The proto-oncogene, *MYC*, encodes an early response gene product that is a transcription factor responsible for regulating cellular proliferation. Amplification of *MYC* is a frequent event in prostate cancer, and expression of MYC in human prostate epithelial cells has been associated with immortalization (Gil et al., 2005).

Hepatocyte growth factor acts through a receptor encoded by the proto-oncogene *MET* (Bottaro et al., 1991). Increased expression of *MET* has been reported in renal cell carcinoma and is also more frequent in higher grade cancers (Pisters et al., 1997). Missense mutations of the *MET* proto-oncogene may also result in constitutive activation of the MET protein in tumors associated with hereditary renal cell carcinoma (Schmidt et al., 1997).

Mechanisms by which a proto-oncogene can be converted to an activated oncogene are via (1) mutation of the proto-oncogene resulting in an active form of the gene product, (2) gene amplification, and (3) chromosomal rearrangement. A mutation occurring within the protein coding sequence of a gene can lead to a continuous proliferation signal from the mutant protein. For example, mutation of the proto-oncogene *ERBB*, which encodes for the epidermal growth factor receptor (EGFR), results in expression of a receptor that is constitutively active (Downward et al., 1984). Errors that occur during chromosomal replication may result in gene amplification and aneuploidy. Such an increase in gene copy number often results in an increased number of mRNA transcripts and overproduction of the corresponding protein. For instance, certain types of bladder cancer overexpress *MYC* by this mechanism (Christoph et al., 1999). Immunohistochemical staining of bladder cancer specimens has demonstrated overexpression of MYC protein in more than half of papillary and invasive tumors (Schmitz-Drager et al., 1997). Finally, chromosomal structural rearrangements such as translocation events can result in the formation of an oncogene; for example, genetic rearrangement leading to the fusion of a portion of the *TMPRSS2* gene and the *ERG* oncogene in a large proportion of prostate cancers (Tomlins et al., 2005).

CELL CYCLE DEREGULATION

Apart from development and growth, **cell division is tightly regulated so that the production of new cells precisely balances those lost during normal wear and tear, thus maintaining tissue and organ homeostasis.** Unlike single-celled eukaryotes, individual human cells are not allowed to make autonomous decisions regarding their proliferation. Rather, **a complex series of external growth inhibitory and growth stimulatory signals are integrated by the cell, resulting in either cell division or quiescence. In cancer, activated oncogenes and inactivated tumor suppressor genes alter the balance between these signals so that net proliferation is continuously favored.**

Quiescent cells are considered to be out of cycle in a reversible state known as "G_0," which is the default state for most cells. When signaled to proliferate, cells activate their **cell cycle** machinery, initiating **an orderly, unidirectional, series of events resulting in (a) duplication of the cell's genome during the DNA synthetic phase (S phase), followed by (b) segregation of each genomic complement to each of two resulting daughter cells, a process referred to as mitosis (M phase).** These two critical phases are **separated by two so-called "Gap" phases (G_1 and G_2).** Throughout the cell cycle, which takes approximately 24 hours to complete, each step is dependent upon completion of the prior step before progressing further (Hartwell et al., 1974). In addition, **checkpoint mechanisms closely monitor DNA integrity as well as certain critical cell cycle events. If problems are detected (e.g., DNA damage), the cell cycle will be paused to allow for repair** (Hartwell and Weinert, 1989). **If repair is not possible, normal cells often then commit cellular suicide through an active process termed *apoptosis.* Many oncogenes and tumor suppressors exert their effects by interfering with cell cycle checkpoints and apoptotic pathways, allowing cancer cells to divide continuously and accumulate. Loss of ability to respond appropriately to damaged DNA is particularly dangerous because it fosters genetic instability, a key attribute of cancer cells. Loss of DNA damage checkpoint controls results in an increased mutation rate, accelerating the mutation of cancer-associated genes, thus contributing to carcinogenesis and disease progression** (Bartek et al., 1999).

Additional details of the eukaryotic cell cycle (cyclin-dependent kinases and cyclins, cell cycle entry, the retinoblastoma protein and the restriction point, S-phase, mitosis, and cell cycle checkpoints) can be found online at ExpertConsult.com.

Retinoblastoma Protein and Genitourinary Malignancies

The retinoblastoma susceptibility protein, RB1 (formerly pRb), plays a central role in controlling the R-point, a decision point in late G_1 beyond which an irreversible commitment to divide is made. The inappropriate, continuous proliferation of cancer cells is largely due to a loss of R-point control, typically the result of functional inactivation of the RB1 pathway (Pardee, 1989). *RB1* gene mutations have been identified in approximately one-third of bladder tumors (Horowitz et al., 1990), and reintroduction of the *RB1* gene into bladder carcinoma cell lines has been found to inhibit cell growth in vitro and tumor formation in vivo (Takahashi et al., 1991). Altered expression of RB1 protein has been also identified in approximately one-third of bladder carcinomas (Logothetis et al., 1992), and altered expression has been correlated with higher stage disease and decreased patient survival (Cordon-Cardo et al., 1992).

Prostate carcinoma has not been as strongly linked to *RB1*. Although *RB1* mutations are present in 10% to 30% of prostate cancer specimens (Bookstein et al., 1990; Kubota et al., 1995), decreased expression is not consistently identified with high-risk patients or recurrent disease (Kibel and Isaacs, 2000). In other studies, no correlation was found between expression and grade or stage (Ittmann and Wieczorek, 1996), but Theodorescu et al. (1997) reported that low RB1 protein expression correlated with decreased disease-specific survival in univariate and multivariate analysis.

Renal carcinoma has not been clearly linked to *RB1*. *RB1* is rarely inactivated in renal carcinoma cell lines or tumors (Ishikawa et al., 1991), and analysis of clinical specimens has not demonstrated a clear association between prognosis and *RB1* expression (Lipponen et al., 1995).

Cyclin-Dependent Kinase Inhibitors

The temporal sequencing of events occurring throughout the cell cycle is affected by a highly conserved set of protein kinases termed cyclin-dependent kinases, or CDKs (Meyerson et al., 1992). CDKs phosphorylate specific protein substrates involved in executing the phase-specific activities of the cell cycle. The enzymatic activities of the CDKs are dependent upon a class of regulatory proteins called cyclins, so named because their abundances are tightly linked to specific phases of the cell cycle, during which they physically associate with and activate the CDK enzymatic activity (De Bondt et al., 1993; Jeffrey et al., 1995) (see eFig. 62.7). Another group of proteins termed *cyclin-dependent kinase inhibitors (CDKIs)* bind to and directly inhibit CDK activity or their activating phosphorylations (Peter and Herskowitz, 1994; Sherr and Roberts, 1995). Thus, although cyclins play major regulatory roles in orchestrating CDK activities, CDKs are subject to additional levels of control, and these processes are commonly altered in cancer cells. CDKIs belong to either of two different classes, the Cip/Kip family, which includes the proteins CDKN1A (p21), CDKN1B (p27) and CDKN1C (p57); and the INK4 (*in*hibit CD*K4*) family, which includes INK4B (p15), INK4A (p16), INK4C (p18), and INK4D (p19). The Cip/Kip proteins are broadly acting, able to inhibit multiple cyclin-CDK complexes throughout the cell cycle (Clurman and Porter, 1998), whereas the INK4 group are more restricted in their activities, inhibiting CDK4 and CDK6-containing complexes; thus they are critical regulators of the R-point and the G_1/S transition because they can block RB1 phosphorylation (see eFig. 62.8). **Increased expression and accumulation of CDKIs is used by the cell as a means of halting the cell cycle in response to various stresses.** For example, p21 expression is increased in response to DNA damage (el-Deiry et al., 1993). CDKIs function in nonstress situations as well. For example, p27 levels are high in quiescent cells, and all of the Cip/Kip proteins appear to play some role in maintenance of the G_0 state in terminally differentiated cells (Halevy et al., 1995; Matsuoka et al., 1995; Parker et al., 1995).

Among the INK4 family, **inactivating mutations and abnormal gene promoter methylation of p15 and p16 have been strongly implicated in cancer in general** (Hirama and Koeffler, 1995; Kamb et al., 1994) and specifically in genitourinary malignancies (Cairns et al., 1995; Herman et al., 1995). The best studied of the INK4 proteins is p16. The p16 protein binds to cyclin-dependent kinases 4 and 6 and inhibits their interaction with cyclin D1 that normally mediates passage through G_1 phase of the cell cycle by phosphorylation of the RB1 protein (Serrano et al., 1993). The *INK4A* gene encoding p16 was initially found to be mutated and deleted in a wide variety of tumors including bladder and kidney (Kamb et al., 1994). Subsequent analysis has demonstrated that **inactivation often occurs by DNA hypermethylation at the *INK4A* promoter**—an alternative, epigenetic method of gene inactivation (Merlo et al., 1995).

The *INK4A* gene is frequently inactivated by deletion in bladder carcinomas (Cairns et al., 1995; Williamson et al., 1995). Importantly, despite its proximity, the *INK4B* gene was ruled out as the primary tumor suppressor at this site because it was not within the deletion interval. A study by Orlow et al. (1999) found that deletion and methylation of the *p16* gene occurred frequently in superficial bladder carcinoma, but only those deletions that affect both the *p16* and *p14* genes, which are located at the same locus, correlated with a decrease in disease-free survival. In contrast to bladder cancer, mutational inactivation of INK4 family members appears to be rare in prostate carcinoma. However, inactivation of *INK4A* by promoter hypermethylation has been implicated in prostate cancer. Herman et al. (1995, 1996) demonstrated *INK4A* hypermethylation in 60% of prostate cancer cell lines, whereas *INK4B* was rarely inactivated. However, these results are tempered by the fact that silencing of the *INK4A* gene by promoter hypermethylation often occurs during the establishment of cell lines in vitro.

Surprisingly, despite the critical role that Cip/Kip family members play in G1S cell cycle arrest, they are rarely mutated in a wide variety of malignancies, including genitourinary tumors, and there are only rare reports of promoter hypermethylation (Kawamata et al., 1995; Shiohara et al., 1994). However, expression of this family of CDK inhibitors plays an important role in cancer in general (Catzavelos et al., 1997; Loda et al., 1997; Yatabe et al., 1998) and in genitourinary carcinomas in particular. Stein et al. (1998) found increased expression of *CDKN1A* (p21) in 64% of bladder tumors and found that increased expression was associated with a decreased probability of tumor recurrence and improved patient survival. Decreased *CDKN1B* (p27) expression has also been linked to increasing tumor grade, pathologic stage, and poor survival in bladder carcinoma (Del Pizzo et al., 1999).

The expression of *CDKN1A* in prostate cancer has not demonstrated a clear correlation with advanced disease or poor outcome (Kibel and Isaacs, 2000). However, specific genetic polymorphisms in *CDKN1A* and *CDKN1B* have been associated with advanced disease (Kibel et al., 2003), and altered expression of *CDKN1B* has been implicated in aggressive disease in multiple studies. Cordon-Cardo et al. (1998) examined radical prostatectomy specimens and found that absent or low CDKN1B production by immunohistochemistry was an independent risk factor for decreased disease-free survival by multivariate analysis. Cote et al. (1998) found that decreased CDKN1B nuclear staining correlated with not only decreased disease-free survival but also overall survival in radical prostatectomy patients, whereas Freedland et al. (2003) found that CDKN1B-positive cells in the prostate needle biopsy specimen had a 2.5-fold increased risk of biochemical recurrence (PSA relapse).

The relevance of *CDKN1B* to prostate cancer is also supported by studies of mouse models. For example, mice deficient in *CDKN1B* develop prostate hyperplasia, confirming the potential importance of this gene in prostate tissue homeostasis (Cordon-Cardo et al., 1998). More excitingly, studies have shown that mice deficient in both CDKN1B and PTEN have a high incidence of prostate cancer (Di Cristofano et al., 2001).

TP53 Tumor Suppressor

The TP53 tumor suppressor protein is a key player in cell cycle checkpoints, responding to DNA damage by signaling cell cycle arrest and repair of the damage (see eFig. 62.9). If the DNA damage cannot be repaired, TP53 may trigger cell death (apoptosis). *TP53* is the most commonly mutated gene in cancer and plays a prominent role in GU malignancies. *TP53* was also recently found to be the most commonly mutated gene in the mutational landscape of metastatic cancer across a screen of 62 principal tumor types (Zehir et al., 2017). Alterations to *TP53* in regard to genitourinary cancers is discussed in detail in the following sections.

DNA METHYLATION

The covalent modification of the C-5 position of cytosine by a methyl group is mediated by DNA methyltransferase, resulting in the formation of 5-methylcytosine; an epigenetic modification of DNA that

KEY POINTS: CELL CYCLE DEREGULATION

- The cell cycle consists of an ordered, unidirectional series of events, the main goal of which is to replicate the cell's genome and partition one copy into each of two resulting daughter cells.
- The cell cycle is divided up into four phases; G1, S, G2, and M. The transition from G1 into S is critically dependent on phosphorylation of the RB1 tumor suppressor protein. Mutations in *RB1* are common in urologic malignancies.
- Phase-specific phosphorylation of substrate proteins by cyclin-dependent kinases (CDKs) orchestrates progression through the cycle.
- The activities of CDKs depend upon their association with specific cyclin proteins. Cyclins accumulate and are rapidly degraded in a phase-specific manner, thus ensuring the proper sequencing and irreversibility of key events throughout the cell cycle.
- Primary points of cell cycle control are the G1S and G2M checkpoints. Checkpoints employ cyclin-dependent kinase inhibitor proteins (CDKIs) to pause the cell cycle in response to a variety of signals, including DNA damage, cell-cell contact, cytokine release, and hypoxia.
- The TP53 tumor suppressor protein is a key player in cell cycle checkpoints, responding to DNA damage by signaling cell cycle arrest and repair of the DNA damage. If the DNA damage cannot be repaired, TP53 may trigger cell death (apoptosis).
- *TP53* is the most commonly mutated gene in cancer and plays a prominent role in GU malignancies.
- Defects in cell cycle checkpoints lead to unregulated cell proliferation and genetic instability.

occurs in vertebrates and is essential for normal embryonic development (Bird, 1992; Jones, 1986). Methylation of cytosine occurs primarily at the CpG palindrome in DNA. The presence of 5-methylcytosine at CpG dinucleotides has resulted in a significant depletion of this sequence from the genome during the course of vertebrate evolution (Schorderet and Gartler, 1992). This reduction in frequency of CpG dinucleotides in the genome is the result of spontaneous deamination of 5-methylcytosine to thymine (Rideout et al., 1990; Sved and Bird, 1990). Notably, certain areas of the genome do not show a depletion of the CpG dinucleotides and contain the expected frequency of this sequence. These regions are referred to as CpG islands and make up approximately 1% of vertebrate genomes yet account for approximately 15% of the total number of CpG dinucleotides in DNA (Bird, 1986; Gardiner-Garden and Frommer, 1987). CpG islands are typically located upstream of many ubiquitous housekeeping and tissue-specific genes. CpG island methylation affects the levels of gene transcription (Cedar, 1988). Hypermethylation of CpG islands usually results in transcriptional downregulation, whereas hypomethylation of these regions may increase gene expression.

CpG islands located in the promoter regions of tumor suppressor genes are normally unmethylated. Abnormal methylation of these regions may result in a progressive reduction in gene expression, thus altering normal cellular growth control in favor of proliferation. Methylation of CpG islands may lead to decreased gene expression by mechanisms including changes in local chromatin structure, inhibition of transcription factor binding, or exclusion of transcriptional machinery from methylated promoter DNA (Bird and Wolffe, 1999). The epigenetic properties of methylation may therefore affect gene activity without altering the DNA sequence and represents an alternative means of gene inactivation apart from gene mutation or deletion.

Changes in global levels and regional patterns of DNA methylation are among the earliest and most frequent events known to occur in human cancer (Jones and Baylin, 2002). Alterations in DNA methylation have a direct impact on mutational and epigenetic components that may contribute neoplastic transformation. **Three major pathways by which DNA methylation may result in genetic dysregulation in human cancer include (1) inherent mutational effects of 5-methylcytosine, (2) epigenetic effects of promoter methylation on gene transcription, and (3) potential gene activation and induction of chromosomal instability by DNA hypomethylation** (Gonzalgo and Jones, 1997; Jones and Gonzalgo, 1997).

DNA Methylation and Prostate Cancer

Glutathione S-transferases belong to a superfamily of enzymes responsible for detoxification of a wide range of xenobiotics. These enzymes catalyze the nucleophilic attack of reduced glutathione on potentially damaging electrophilic compounds. **Aberrant methylation of the CpG island at the Glutathione S-transferase Pi-1 *(GSTP1)* locus is the most frequent somatic genome alteration reported in prostate cancer** (Jerónimo et al., 2001; Lee et al., 1994). Methylation of *GSTP1* has been detected in more than 90% of prostate carcinomas and approximately 70% of prostatic intraepithelial neoplasia (PIN) lesions but is not present in normal prostate tissue or benign prostatic hyperplasia (Lee et al., 1994). In normal prostate tissue, expression of *GSTP1* is limited to basal cells, but it can be upregulated in columnar epithelial cells exposed to oxidative stress. Increased levels of DNA methylation have also been associated with worse clinical outcomes in patients with prostate cancer (Maruyama et al., 2002).

The ras association domain family protein 1, isoform A *(RASSF1A)* gene is located on chromosome 3p21. *RASSF1A* is a tumor suppressor gene that is frequently altered in a variety of human cancers. Abnormal methylation of *RASSF1A* has been reported to occur in 60% to 70% of prostate carcinomas (Kuzmin et al., 2002). Loss of heterozygosity (LOH) of the 3p21 region is associated with methylation and silencing of the remaining *RASSF1A* allele during tumorigenesis. Methylation *RASSF1A* has been observed more frequently in higher-grade prostate cancers compared with less aggressive tumors (Liu et al., 2002).

Genome-wide methylation analyses have been conducted in prostate cancer, with the results indicating that there are widespread changes in methylation patterns (hypermethylation and hypomethylation) that occur in gene-associated and conserved intergenic regions. Interestingly, although interindividual heterogeneity in DNA methylation patterns was observed among prostate cancer patients, within individuals with metastatic prostate cancer, DNA methylation alterations were highly conserved across all of their metastases, suggesting that DNA methylation alterations undergo clonal selection (Aryee et al., 2013; Yegnasubramanian et al., 2011).

Role of DNA Methylation in Bladder Cancer

Mutations of the *TP53* gene are present in more than half of all human malignancies. Many of the mutational hotspots found in the *TP53* gene occur at CpG dinucleotides that are normally methylated, thus implicating 5-methylcytosine as an endogenous mutagen in the genome (Greenblatt et al., 1994; Rideout et al., 1990; Tornaletti and Pfeifer, 1995). Mutational inactivation of *TP53* is a frequent event in urothelial dysplasia, carcinoma in situ (CIS), and invasive bladder cancer (Spruck et al., 1994).

The contribution of DNA methylation to these mutational events varies depending upon the type of bladder cancer and the etiologic agent believed to be responsible for tumor formation (Jones et al., 1998). Urothelial carcinomas in western countries and Japan have relatively few mutations at CpG sites, suggesting that DNA methylation may not play a major role in inducing these changes. In contrast, a higher frequency of mutations at CpG dinucleotides consistent with 5-methylcytosine deamination is observed in patients with squamous cell carcinoma and urothelial carcinoma with a history of exposure to phenacetin or arsenic (Jones et al., 1998). These observations highlight the potential mutagenic effects of DNA methylation upon the genome and the contribution of methylation to *TP53* inactivation during bladder carcinogenesis.

INK4A (p16) Methylation in Bladder Cancer

Inactivation of the *INK4A* gene may occur by a variety of mechanisms including deletion, mutation, and promoter methylation (Gonzalez-Zulueta et al., 1995; Herman et al., 1995; Spruck et al., 1994). Mutation or deletion of one *INK4A* allele and concurrent methylation of the remaining allele results in complete loss of functional activity. Methylation of *INK4A* has been reported in 27% to 60% of primary urothelial carcinomas (Chan et al., 2002; Chang et al., 2003). Such epigenetic changes are among the earliest molecular events associated with transformation and may therefore precede morphologic alterations in cellular architecture.

The first detailed study investigating the effects of *INK4A* promoter methylation on transcriptional activity was performed in bladder cancer cells, where a reduction in *INK4A* expression was associated with higher levels of methylation in the upstream promoter region methylation of specific CpG sites in the *INK4A* promoter was shown to significantly downregulate transcriptional activity of the gene (Gonzalgo et al., 1998). Administration of the demethylating agent 5-aza-2′-deoxycytidine (5-Aza-CdR) was capable of reactivating *INK4A* expression in bladder cancer cells that were previously shown to contain methylated alleles of the gene. Methylation in exon 2 of the *INK4A* gene is also a frequent occurrence in a variety of cancers and is an excellent marker for transformation, although the presence of methylation in this region of the *INK4A* gene does not affect *INK4A* transcription in bladder cancer cells (Gonzalgo et al., 1998).

Hypermethylation of Other Genes in Bladder Cancer

The E-cadherin *(CDH1)* gene encodes a transmembrane glycoprotein that modulates calcium-dependent intercellular adhesion in epithelial tissues. Methylation of the CpG island located in the *CDH1* promoter is associated with decreased gene expression in high-grade urothelial carcinoma, including disease-associated with carcinoma in situ (Graff et al., 1995; Horikawa et al., 2003). *CDH1* methylation has also been reported in histologically normal urothelium; however, many of these cases were from patients older than 70 years of age and may be related to a potential link between methylation and aging (Ahuja and Issa, 2000; Bornman et al., 2001). Lower levels of CDH1 expression may increase β-catenin/TCF signaling activity and proliferation in urothelial carcinomas (Maruyama et al., 2002; Thievessen et al., 2003).

Methylation of *RASSF1A* has been reported in up to 97% of primary bladder tumors, suggesting that epigenetic inactivation of this gene may play an important role in bladder carcinogenesis (Lee et al., 2001). High tumor grade, nonpapillary growth pattern, and muscle invasive disease are associated with *RASSF1A* promoter methylation in bladder cancer (Maruyama et al., 2001).

Hypomethylation in Bladder Cancer

Global DNA hypomethylation is also a frequent event in tumorigenesis (Jones and Baylin, 2002). **Hypomethylation may result in genomic instability via alterations in chromatin structure, increased genetic recombination between repetitive elements, or derepression of retrotransposons** (Baylin et al., 2001). Methylation of CpG sites is usually maintained by the enzymatic activities of DNA methyltransferase 1 *(DNMT1)*, whereas de novo methylation of CpG sites is mediated by DNA methyltransferases 3A and 3B *(DNMT3A* and *DNMT3B)* (Jones and Baylin, 2002). **One important role for methylation is genomic imprinting, which results in monoallelic gene expression without altering the genetic sequence.** Loss of imprinting (LOI) is a reduction in the methylation of the normally methylated allele, which can lead to activation of the normally silent copy of a growth-promoting gene (Feinberg and Tycko, 2004). This phenomenon has been reported for the human insulin-like growth factor-2 gene *(IGF2)* in a variety of cancers (Sakatani et al., 2005; Woodson et al., 2004).

Methylation of long interspersed nuclear element (L1 LINE) sequences is reduced in bladder cancer cell lines and primary tumors compared with normal bladder mucosa (Jürgens et al., 1996). DNA methyltransferase expression, however, did not correlate with methylation status of cell lines, and methyltransferase activity was reduced in quiescent cells, suggesting that aberrant expression of DNMT1 does not account for the altered methylation patterns found in urothelial carcinoma (Jürgens et al., 1996). Decreased DNMT1 expression and induction of DNMT3A and DNMT3B in bladder cancer has also been reported (Kimura et al., 2003). These data suggest that downregulation of DNMT1 expression may be at least partly responsible for hypomethylation of repetitive elements in bladder cancer.

KEY POINTS: DNA METHYLATION

- Methylation occurs specifically at CpG dinucleotides in the genome. The presence of 5-methylcytosine in DNA can result in spontaneous deamination to thymine and therefore the formation of C→T transition mutations.
- DNA methylation can affect gene function by subsequent mutational events or epigenetic mechanisms. Methylation of CpG islands associated with the promoter region of genes may result in suppression of gene expression.
- Loss of promoter methylation of normally methylated genes can lead to inappropriate gene expression (e.g., expression of oncogenes).

DNA DAMAGE AND REPAIR

Cancer is fundamentally a genetic disease. Alterations in numerous genes provide the malignant cell the means to activate cancer-associated pathways and inactivate tumor suppressive barriers, making possible the acquisition of the key set of attributes associated with the cancer phenotype. **The intrinsic accuracy of DNA polymerase coupled with associated error-correction mechanisms keeps the error rate during DNA replication to an astonishingly low estimated value of approximately 3 incorrect bases per cell division; this in a genome of more than 3 billion bases! These processes are not perfect, however, and cancer-causing changes do occur in oncogenes and tumor suppressor genes via epigenetic, mutational, and copy number alterations, in addition to epigenetic abnormalities.** Many of these genetic changes are thought to result from a variety of endogenous (e.g., mitochondrial respiratory byproducts) and exogenous (e.g., chemicals, radiation) DNA damaging agents that constantly assault the genome (Ames and Gold, 1991, 1998). To counter these threats, our cells employ a plethora of defensive mechanisms, including free-radical scavengers such as α-tocopherol, vitamin C, carotenoids, bilirubin, and urate, as well as protective enzymes such as superoxide dismutases, glutathione peroxidases, and glutathione transferases, which detoxify a wide range of carcinogens (Finkel and Holbrook, 2000; Mates and Sanchez-Jimenez, 1999). Loss of expression, because of promoter hypermethylation, of the glutathione S-transferase pi enzyme encoded by the *GSTP1* gene is observed in the vast majority of prostate cancer cases (Lee et al., 1994; Lin et al., 2001), and recent studies have found associations between genetic polymorphisms in GSTs and the risk of biochemical recurrence in prostate cancer patients (Nock et al., 2009). Epidemiologic and retrospective studies on prostate cancer risk have found a protective effect for selenium, which is used as a co-factor by glutathione peroxidases (Colli and Amling, 2009; Lowe and Frazee, 2006), raising hope that dietary intervention may be protective against prostate cancer. However, a recent large clinical trial showed no benefit for dietary supplementation with selenium (Hatfield and Gladyshev, 2009), and it now appears that selenium's observed protective effects may be limited to men with low baseline selenium levels. Results from other clinical chemoprevention trials in prostate cancer have, unfortunately, been similarly disappointing (Gaziano et al., 2009).

In addition to DNA damage prevention, the cell employs a host of DNA repair systems. The set of pathways dealing with DNA damage recognition and repair is **referred to as the DNA damage**

response, or DDR, and encompasses a plethora of genes. The DDR includes the replication machinery (with its associated proofreading capability), as well as the many components of specific DNA repair systems such as base-excision repair, nucleotide-excision repair, double-strand break repair, and mismatch repair described in detail later (Loeb, 1998; Schmutte and Fishel, 1999).

As previously mentioned, **the cell cycle and the DDR are closely integrated. In response to DNA damage, the first step is to arrest the cell cycle so that the DNA can be repaired. It is therefore not surprising that there is substantial overlap between the initiators of DNA repair and cell cycle arrest** (Kastan and Bartek, 2004). For example, ATM and ATR kinases are activated in response to DNA damage, and both activate TP53, CHK1, and other proteins critical to cell cycle arrest (Bartek and Lukas, 2003).

Considering the number of genetic changes calculated to be required for cancer development, the large number of changes actually observed in cancer cells, and the extraordinarily low spontaneous mutation rates in normal human cells, Loeb was led to conclude that the spontaneous mutation rate is insufficient to explain the number of mutations observed in the majority of human cancers. Loeb hypothesized that, early in the process of tumorigenesis, preneoplastic cells may develop defects in one or more of the genes responsible for the fidelity of DNA replication (Cheng and Loeb, 1993; Loeb et al., 1974; Loeb, 1991). Such a defect would then lead to an increased mutation rate resulting in a so-called "mutator phenotype." This hypothesis gains further support from the fact that most cells in proliferating tissues, such as epithelial tissues (the source of the vast majority of human cancers), are relatively short lived, being eliminated either by cell shedding or apoptosis. Thus the target population of cells at risk for becoming cancerous is far less than the total number of cells in the body, yet cancers are certainly not uncommon. In addition, cells with a "hypermutable" phenotype are often more difficult to treat because the selection pressure of therapy may rapidly select tumor cells with mutations conferring resistance (Tlsty et al., 1989).

The term *mutator phenotype* was originally used to refer to defects in the DNA replication and repair proteins, resulting in relatively small-scale errors in the DNA sequence, such as single base substitutions, deletions, and duplications. **Despite (or perhaps because of?) the many potential targets for mutator genes, few such genes have been found to be consistently mutated in significant proportions of common human cancers**, a notable exception being the mismatch repair pathway. Mismatch repair defects are the underlying cause of hereditary nonpolyposis colorectal cancer (HNPCC) (Aaltonen et al., 1993) and have been reported in as many as 15% of sporadic colon cancers (Liu et al., 1995).

Although defects in DNA repair genes in sporadic malignancies, including genitourinary tumors, have been identified, Loeb's concept of the mutator phenotype, as originally stated, has yet to be fully evaluated. It currently appears that it may not be a major player in the development of the majority of common sporadic human cancers. **If, however, the mutator concept is broadened to include systems involved in *chromosomal* stability, then it may become widely applicable. At any rate, the current consensus is that genetic instability of *some* sort is required for cancer development.**

Additional information on DNA repair mechanisms (nucleotide excision repair, base excision repair, mismatch repair, DNA double-strand break repair, nonhomologous end joining) can be found online at ExpertConsult.com.

GENOMIC ALTERATIONS

Research by many different groups on several different tumor types has strongly implicated genetic instability as an important determinant of tumorigenesis, although the ultimate source of genetic instability in cancer is still not entirely clear (Hartwell, 1992; Loeb, 1991). As mentioned previously, although certainly important in specific instances such as inherited cancer susceptibility syndromes, deficiencies in genes involved in the replication, maintenance, and repair of DNA have not yet been shown to play a major

> **KEY POINTS: DNA DAMAGE AND REPAIR**
> - DNA damage does not often lead to malignancy because the cell possesses multiple repair mechanisms.
> - Defects in DNA repair facilitate the accumulation of the mutations critical for tumor formation and progression.
> - NER is a major defense against DNA damage caused by ultraviolet radiation and chemical exposure.
> - BER repairs damage caused by spontaneous deamination of bases, radiation, oxidative stress, alkylating agents, and replication errors.
> - Mismatch repair removes nucleotides mispaired by DNA polymerase.
> - DSB repair is a major defense against DNA damage caused by ionizing radiation, free radicals, and chemicals.
> - Many syndromes involve inherited defects in DNA repair exhibit marked increases in cancer susceptibility; strongly linking genomic instability and cancer.

direct role in the genesis of most sporadic human cancers. **Recent studies on a number of human cancers found that the genomes of each cancer have numerous mutations (on average 33 to 66 somatic mutations in solid tumors) in gene coding sequences that are predicted to significantly alter the corresponding protein products** (Vogelstein et al., 2013). **Comprehensive sequencing efforts coupled with statistical methods to predict the effects of individual mutations have revealed that approximately 140 genes, when mutated, can "drive" tumorigenesis (e.g., "driver" genes). Most tumors only contain two to eight such driver mutations, whereas the remaining mutations in any particular cancer case are considered "passengers" that do not confer a selective growth advantage** (Sjoblom et al., 2006; Vogelstein et al., 2013; Wood et al., 2007).

Apart from the sequence alterations predicted to arise from the original mutator phenotype concept, *chromosomal* instability leads to gross changes in chromosome number and/or structure. The spectrum and severity of such chromosomal alterations may differ for different tumor types. For instance, **hematologic malignancies often are seen with simple diploid or near-diploid karyotypes with only one or very few detectable, often balanced, chromosomal rearrangements**. However, as a class these cancers only account for about 10% of all human cancers. **In stark contrast, the presence of large variations in chromosome numbers and complex structural rearrangements, as well as intratumoral variation in these aberrations, are hallmarks of most human solid tumors**, which represent the bulk of human malignancies. Important exceptions include certain tumors deficient in mismatch repair. **In prostate cancer, as well as most human tumor types and transplantable tumor models, the extent of chromosomal abnormalities correlates with disease severity and aggressiveness**, pointing to a role for these changes in cancer progression and spanning from premalignant lesions to localized primary tumors, and, finally, to metastatic disease to which patients typically succumb (Bostwick et al., 1996; Brothman et al., 1990; Isaacs et al., 1995; Lundgren et al., 1992; Sandberg, 1992). For example, in a study that used a computational method to infer aneuploidy based on gene expression data of genes that are located in adjacent chromosomal regions, greater levels of aneuploidy were found to confer worse survival rates (Carter et al., 2006). Likewise, a recent study in prostate cancer performed unsupervised hierarchical clustering of copy-number alterations (CNAs) in 218 tumor samples and found that tumors with the highest number of genome-wide CNAs had a significantly accelerated time to biochemical recurrence (Taylor et al., 2010).

The chromosomal changes seen in solid tumors can be broken down into two main classes: changes in the number of whole chromosomes and changes in chromosomal structure. Numerical chromosomal alterations can be further subdivided into changes in the numbers of specific individual chromosomes (aneusomies; e.g., monosomies and trisomies) and changes in the number of

> **BOX 62.2 Gross Chromosomal Abnormalities Frequently Observed in Cancer**
>
> **NUMERICAL ABNORMALITIES**
> Aneuploidies
>   Abnormal numbers of whole chromosome complement (e.g., triploidy, tetraploidy)
>   Losses or gains of single chromosomes (e.g., monosomy, trisomy)
>
> **STRUCTURAL ABNORMALITIES**
> Rearrangements
>   Inversions
>   Translocations (either balanced or unbalanced)
>   Chromothripsis
> Chromosomal fusions
>   End-to-end fusion = dicentric chromosome
>   Intra-chromosomal fusion = ring chromosome
> Deletions (from small segments up to entire chromosome arms)
> Duplications, amplifications
> Double minutes (often containing amplified sequences)
> Isochromosomes (loss of one chromosomal arm, replaced by duplication of the remaining arm)
> Complex (a variety of combinations of the previously mentioned abnormalities)

copies of the entire diploid set of chromosomes (ploidy changes; e.g., tetraploidy, octaploidy). Possible mechanisms responsible for such numerical changes include nondisjunction, endoreduplication (an abrupt doubling of the chromosome complement without cell division) cytokinesis defects, and cell fusion events. Likewise, structural changes can be subdivided into several distinct types of chromosomal aberrations as listed in Box 62.2. An additional mechanism for genomic rearrangement, termed chromothripsis (literally meaning "chromosome shattering"), has been described that was initially extrapolated from genomic sequencing studies on cancer cells (Stephens et al., 2011). Chromothripsis is evidenced by a large number (possibly hundreds) of chromosomal rearrangements in confined chromosomal regions that have occurred after apparent shattering and rejoining of a chromosomal region in a sometimes disordered fashion.

As previously mentioned, cancer-associated chromosomal changes were recognized as early as the 1900s by Boveri, who proposed that such abnormalities may be involved in cancer causation. Much later, Klein put forth the idea that chromosomal rearrangements affect the expression of cancer-related genes located near the observed chromosomal breakpoints (Klein, 1981). This hypothesis has been validated over the ensuing years, in large part because of studies on what were observed to be consistent chromosomal changes found in hematologic malignancies and soft-tissue sarcomas, eventually leading to the isolation and cloning of the resident genes involved (Nowell, 1994). Over the years, painstaking dissection of chromosomal regions that are repeatedly found to undergo alteration in specific tumor types or subtypes has led to the discovery of hundreds of individual cancer-associated genes. Typically, genomic loci that are frequently lost tend to harbor tumor suppressor genes, whereas those loci exhibiting copy number gains (e.g., gene amplification) point toward oncogenes (Snijders et al., 2005). Examples of genes frequently amplified in cancers include members of the *MYC*, *RAS*, *EGFR*, and *FGF* gene families, as well as cell cycle regulatory genes such as *CCND1* (cyclin D gene), *CDK4*, and *HDM2*. **Gene amplifications in cancer are usually seen either as multiple small extrachromosomal copies called double minutes, or as amplified regions within chromosomes, so-called homogeneously staining regions (HSRs)** (Cowell, 1982).

Specific Chromosomal Rearrangements in Genitourinary Malignancies

Recurrent Gene Rearrangements in Prostate Cancer

Although they are much less frequently observed in common adult solid tumors, recurrent translocations do occur, often amid the backdrop of countless chromosomal abnormalities (Sandberg, 1985). **One of the most exciting recent findings in prostate cancer research has been the discovery of recurrent structural rearrangements in the majority of prostate cancer cases, primarily involving oncogenic ETS transcription factor family members.** The initial report by Tomlins et al. in 2005 described the use a novel bioinformatic approach that led to the identification of recurrent gene fusions between the upstream regulatory region of the androgen-regulated gene *TMPRSS2* and *ERG*, an ETS family member previously known to be involved in Ewing sarcoma and various leukemias (Tomlins et al., 2005). These two genes reside 3 Mb apart on chromosome 21 (*TMPRSS2*, 21q22.3; *ERG* 21q22.2), and detailed molecular analysis revealed that in the majority of rearranged cases (approximately 2/3), the gene fusion occurs via deletion of the intervening sequence, with the remaining fusions resulting from more complex, translocation-type of rearrangements (Perner et al., 2007; Tomlins et al., 2005). In either case, **the net result is to place a known oncogenic transcription factor under the control of an androgen-regulated promoter, resulting in androgen-driven expression of the fusion transcript** (Wang et al., 2008a). As expected, increased *ERG* transcription and ERG protein expression is positively correlated with presence of the gene fusion. In addition to a variety of splice variants, there are multiple forms of the genomic rearrangement, the most common one being a fusion between exon 1 of *TMPRSS2* to exon 4 of *ERG*. **These gene rearrangements can be readily detected, either by assaying for the presence of the fusion transcripts by reverse transcriptase polymerase chain reaction (RT-PCR) or by assaying for the rearrangement directly by multiprobe, multi-color fluorescence in situ hybridization (FISH), and such approaches are currently being evaluated for potential use in noninvasive diagnostic applications** (e.g., in urine or blood). More recently, detection of ERG protein expression by immunostaining has been shown to be an excellent surrogate marker for chromosomal rearrangements involving the ERG gene, thus providing a simpler method for their detection (Chaux et al., 2011; Falzarano et al., 2011; Park et al., 2010).

Since the publication of the initial report by Tomlins et al. (2005), several large retrospective studies have been performed assessing these fusions in localized prostate cancers in PSA-screened cohorts. These studies confirmed the initial finding and found the prevalence of the *TMPRSS2-ERG* fusion in prostate cancer to be in the range of 40% to 60%, making this one of the most common somatic genetic alterations in prostate cancer (Gopalan et al., 2009b; Mehra et al., 2007; Mosquera et al., 2009; Nam et al., 2007; Perner et al., 2007; Tu et al., 2007; Wang et al., 2008a). One intriguing anatomic exception is cancer originating in the transition zone of the prostate, which appears to completely lack *TMPRSS2-ERG* gene rearrangements (Guo et al., 2009a).

As assessed by FISH in tissue sections, the *TMPRSS2-ERG* fusion has not been observed in benign prostate epithelial or stromal cells, although it has been reported to be present in high-grade prostatic intraepithelial neoplasia (HGPIN), the presumptive precursor lesion for prostate adenocarcinoma, at frequencies between 15% and 20%, which is about one-half the frequency observed in localized PSA-detected cancers (Cerveira et al., 2006; Han et al., 2009; Mosquera et al., 2008; Perner et al., 2007). This finding implies that, at least in a subset of cases, the rearrangement may be an early event in prostate tumorigenesis. **With the important exceptions of transition zone cancers and HGPIN, the prevalence and high degree of specificity of the *TMPRSS2-ERG* fusion for prostate cancer makes this a potentially useful biomarker for diagnosis and disease monitoring, one that could be used in conjunction with current markers such as serum PSA, which have limited specificity.** Indeed, the detection of *TMPRSS2-ERG* fusion-driven

ERG overexpression in prostate biopsies from men found only to have HGPIN was shown to be predictive of cancer diagnosis on subsequent biopsy (Park et al., 2013), and multiple studies have demonstrated the utility of *TMPRSS2-ERG* detection in the blood or urine either alone or in combination with the non–protein-coding RNA prostate cancer antigen 3 (PCA3) in enhancing the sensitivity of prostate cancer diagnosis (Hessels et al., 2007; Leyten et al., 2012; Tomlins et al., 2011).

Apart from its promising potential as a diagnostic prostate cancer marker, it is as of yet unclear if additional clinical information may be provided by determining a patient's *TMPRSS2-ERG* gene fusion status. As such, **the prognostic significance of fusion status in prostate cancer remains uncertain.** Although several studies have reported associations between *TMPRSS2-ERG* rearrangement and various indicators of disease aggressiveness, including higher stage, presence of metastases, and disease-specific death (Attard et al., 2008a; Barwick et al., 2010; Cheville et al., 2008; Demichelis et al., 2007; Leyten et al., 2012; Mehra et al., 2007; Nam et al., 2007; Perner et al., 2007; Rajput et al., 2007), several other published studies failed to observe such associations (Albadine et al., 2009; Dai et al., 2008; Darnel et al., 2009; Fine et al., 2010; Gopalan et al., 2009b; Lapointe et al., 2007; Lotan et al., 2009; Rouzier et al., 2008; Tu et al., 2007; Yoshimoto et al., 2006). A large prospective study of 1180 men treated by radical prostatectomy found that the presence of the *TMPRSS2-ERG* rearrangement was not predictive of recurrence or mortality but was associated with tumor stage (Pettersson et al., 2012). Studies examining the prognostic capabilities of *TMPRSS2-ERG* positivity in predicting treatment outcomes to androgen deprivation (Leinonen et al., 2010), abiraterone (Danila et al., 2011), or radiotherapy (Dal Pra et al., 2013) show no association. In addition, one study reported a link between gene fusion and *favorable* prognosis (Saramaki et al., 2008), and Petrovics et al. reported that higher levels of *ERG* mRNA expression appeared to be positively associated with disease-free survival (Petrovics et al., 2005). Another study reported that *ERG* gene copy number gain without the presence of the gene fusion is prognostic for recurrence after radical prostatectomy (Toubaji et al., 2011). The precise reasons for these conflicting results are not apparent. A number of variables differ between many of these studies, including the nature of the study cohort, sample size, method of cancer detection, manner in which the tissues were obtained, intratumoral heterogeneity in the presence of the fusion (Minner et al., 2012), manner in which the gene fusions were detected (e.g., PCR or FISH), length of patient follow-up, and the clinical end points assessed. Further research in this area is clearly warranted to better resolve these issues.

After the report of *TMPRSS2-ERG* rearrangements, further study revealed additional gene fusions in prostate cancer. Thus the *TMPRSS2* gene can fuse to other ETS family member genes, including *ETV1*, *ETV4*, and *ETV5* (Helgeson et al., 2008; Tomlins et al., 2005; Tomlins et al., 2006). These additional translocations are much rarer than the *TMPRSS2-ERG* rearrangement, which is estimated to represent more than 90% of all fusions involving ETS genes in prostate cancer (Kumar-Sinha et al., 2008). In addition, fusions involving upstream fusion partners other than *TMPRSS2* have also been found, including the fusions *SLC45A3-ETV5*, *SLC45A3-ERG*, *HNRPA2B1-ETV5*, and *SLC45A3-ELK4*; however, these are also relatively rare (Attard et al., 2008a; Attard et al., 2008b; Hermans et al., 2008; Maher et al., 2009; Rickman et al., 2009; Tomlins et al., 2007). Whereas the fusion events in prostate cancer are typically driven by genomic rearrangements, the SLC45A3-ELK4 fusion was later found to be due to RNA cis-splicing events between these two genes (which are located adjacent to each other on chromosome 1 band q32) with no alterations to the DNA sequence (Zhang et al., 2012). Additional low frequency gene fusions have been identified in prostate cancer that involve non-ETS family members such as *CDKN1A*, *CD9*, *IKBKB*, the oncogene *PIGU*, the tumor suppressor *RSRC2*, and members of the RAF pathway (*BRAF, RAF1*) (Palanisamy et al., 2010; Pflueger et al., 2011; Ren et al., 2012). These studies have been facilitated by next-generation RNA sequencing (RNA-seq or whole "transcriptome" shotgun sequencing) technologies that unbiasedly sequence all RNA species in a sample with an analysis that is not limited to "annotated" sequences. The results of RNA-seq studies indicate that some of the fusion events that occur in prostate cancer may be "private events" (e.g., only occurring in one patient), implying that the frequency and range of fusion events in prostate cancer may be far greater than what is currently understood (Pflueger et al., 2011).

Recurrent Gene Rearrangements in Renal Cancer

A novel subtype of renal cell carcinoma, microphthalmia transcription factor (MiTF)/TFE family translocation carcinomas, has been described that features chromosomal translocations involving one of two members of the MiTF family (Argani and Ladanyi, 2005; Hemesath et al., 1994). The first involves the *TFE3* gene on chromosome Xp11.2, which translocates to one of several partner genes including *PRCC* (1q21), *ASPL* (17q25), *PSF* (1p34), *NonO* (Xq12; rearranged via inversion), and an unknown gene at 3q23 (Argani et al., 2001a; Argani et al., 2001b; Argani and Ladanyi, 2005; Argani et al., 2005; Martignoni et al., 2009; Sidhar et al., 1996; Weterman et al., 1996). These translocations place the *TFE3* gene under the control of strong promoters that then drive inappropriate expression of *TFE3* (or a *TFE3*-containing fusion protein). In these cancers, TFE3 protein is readily detectable in the nucleus by immunohistochemical (IHC) staining with anti-*TFE3* antibody, thus aiding in diagnosis. TFE3 renal cell carcinomas are found primarily in children and adolescents and account for the majority of pediatric renal cell carcinoma (RCC) cases (Argani and Ladanyi, 2005). It has recently been reported that activation of the *MET* proto-oncogene may play a role with *TFE3* in these tumors (Tsuda et al., 2007), which is of interest because these tumors display papillary histologic architecture, and mutations in the *MET* gene are the underlying cause of hereditary papillary renal cell carcinoma (Jeffers et al., 1997).

A second class of MiTF/TFE family translocation carcinomas contains a specific translocation between the *TFEB* gene on 6p21 and the *ALPHA* gene on 11q12 (Argani et al., 2005). Like the Xp11 translocation RCCs, this entity is also most commonly found in children and adolescents and shares many other features with the TFE3 translocation tumors. In addition to IHC staining for TFE3 and TFEB proteins, it was recently demonstrated that these tumors are also marked by staining for the protein cathepsin K, a shared transcriptional target gene of these transcription factors (Martignoni et al., 2009). The use of such markers or PCR to detect these specific gene fusions may have clinical importance because, as the cathepsin K example shows, these tumors likely are controlled by a different transcriptional program than conventional RCC, thus therapeutic targets used against these cancers may not be effective against translocation RCCs.

Recurrent Gene Rearrangements in Testicular Cancer

In testicular germ cell tumors (TGCTs), gain of the short arm of chromosome 12 is a nearly universal finding, with the notable exception of the rare spermatocytic seminoma subtype (Atkin and Baker, 1982; Rodriguez et al., 1993; Rosenberg et al., 1998; Verdorfer et al., 2004). In the majority of cases (approximately 80%) this occurs through a structural rearrangement producing an isochromosome 12p, that is, a version of chromosome 12 consisting of 2 p-arms and no q (long) arm. In the remainder of cases 12p material is gained through more complex chromosomal rearrangements (Looijenga et al., 2007; Ottesen et al., 2003; Rosenberg et al., 2000). More detailed analyses have revealed amplification of specific regions on 12p, including the area 12p11-12p13. One common region of amplification at 12p11.2-12p12.1 contains 22 potential genes, including *KRAS*, a promising candidate TGCT gene, which also undergoes activating mutations in TGCTs (Goddard et al., 2007; Moul et al., 1992; Olie et al., 1995; Rodriguez et al., 2003; Zafarana et al., 2003). An additional region of interest lies at 12p13.31, where the so-called "stem cell cluster region" resides. This region contains several stem cell–related genes, including *CD9*, *EDR1*, *GDF3*, *SCNN1A*, *NANOG*, and *STELLAR*, which exhibit coordinate overexpression (Clark et al., 2004; Korkola et al., 2006).

Other Genomic Alterations in Genitourinary Malignancies

Apart from chromosomal translocations, which are primarily specific changes in the spatial organization of the genome, an overall derangement of the chromosomal complement is nearly universal in human cancer, particularly in carcinomas; cancers that originate from epithelial cells and represent the majority of adult GU malignancies. Such abnormalities are wide ranging, affecting the genome at multiple scales, including losses and gains of entire chromosomes or chromosomal arms, as well as deletions and amplifications of chromosomal regions large and small. **These changes are generically referred to as CNAs.** In addition to mutations, structural rearrangements, and epigenetic changes, CNAs are yet another reflection of the underlying genomic instability in cancer cells, resulting in the large number of genetic changes required for malignant transformation. This instability generates a great degree of genetic heterogeneity. For instance, when metaphase chromosomes of tumor cells are examined during karyotypic analysis, a bewildering array of chromosomal aberrations is typically observed, such that no two karyotypes within a given cancer cell population are exactly the same. However, within this seemingly random assortment of alterations there are some changes that are seen in multiple different cells and multiple tumor samples, providing a strong indication that a gene or genes located in the region undergoing recurrent alteration is involved in the pathogenesis of the disease. Over the past several decades, using ever more sophisticated and higher-resolution molecular methods, many such changes have been catalogued and candidate cancer genes identified. Two general approaches are used here. In the first, inherited (germline) defects in genes that cause hereditary cancer predisposition syndromes are sought, often by performing genetic linkage analysis in affected and nonaffected family members in an attempt to find genetic loci that track in a Mendelian fashion with disease status. Several familial cancer predisposition syndromes are now understood in significant detail, some featuring GU malignancies, others not (Tables 62.1 and 62.2). In the second approach, a variety of techniques are employed to discover disease-associated genes in sporadic cancers that lack a strong familial component (caused by somatic rather than germline genetic alterations). **The detection of copy number alterations in a particular gene (or region containing the gene) coupled with mutations in the other allele is persuasive evidence for that gene functioning as a disease-relevant oncogene (with activating mutations) or tumor suppressor gene (featuring inactivating mutations or promoter methylation).** In the case of cancer-related genes identified in hereditary predisposition syndromes, hopefully alterations of genes discovered in familial forms of the disease are also relevant to their more common sporadic counterparts. In a number of instances this has been found to be true: for example, gene abnormalities linked to certain familial forms of kidney cancer are also involved in sporadic forms of the disease. In the following sections we describe some of the recurrent genetic changes identified in familial and sporadic forms of genitourinary malignancies.

Hereditary Prostate Cancer

Family history is one of the strongest prostate cancer risk factors (Steinberg et al., 1990), and criteria defining a hereditary form of the disease have been established (Carter et al., 1993). Twin studies have estimated a heritable risk for prostate cancer of approximately 50% (Lichtenstein et al., 2000; Page et al., 1997). Traditional linkage analysis is well suited to identify highly penetrant genetic alterations (Fig. 62.12). **The overall low yield and irreproducibility seen in hereditary prostate cancer (HPC) linkage studies have led to the conclusion that rather than being caused by a few high-impact genes, HPC is instead likely to depend upon alterations in many genes, each of which has only a modest effect** (Easton et al., 2003; Schaid, 2004).

Initial genome-wide searches in HPC families uncovered evidence for susceptibility loci on chromosome 1q, 4q, 5p, 7p, 13q, and Xq (Smith et al., 1996). The first strong candidate locus, HPC1, was localized to the region 1q24.25 (Gronberg et al., 1997) and a gene, *RNASEL*, was later identified at this locus (Carpten et al., 2002; Rokman et al., 2002). Although this linkage was replicated in some studies, it was not confirmed in others (Bergthorsson et al., 2000; Cooney et al., 1997; Eeles et al., 1998; McIndoe et al., 1997). Similarly, a failure to consistently confirm linkage has plagued other candidate HPC loci/genes as well, highlighting the difficulty in conducting such studies. Because prostate cancer is a relatively common disease, HPC families are contaminated with sporadic cases ("phenocopies"). Furthermore, it has become apparent that familial prostate cancer may lack the type of high-risk susceptibility genes such as *BRCA1* or *BRCA2* that are clearly linked to hereditary forms of breast and ovarian cancers (Simard et al., 2003). Among other considerations, these facts underline the need for large, well-defined HPC cohorts,

TABLE 62.1 Tumor Syndromes Associated With Genitourinary Malignancies

SYNDROME	TUMOR	CHROMOSOME(S)	GENE(S)	(FUNCTION)
Wilms' tumor	Wilms' tumor	11p13	WT1	(Transcriptional repressor)
Beckwith-Wiedemann	Wilms' tumor	11p15	CDKN1C	(Cell cycle regulator)
Von Hippel-Lindau	Clear cell renal cell carcinoma Pheochromocytoma	3p25	VHL	(Transcriptional elongation and ubiquitination)
Hereditary papillary renal cancer	Papillary renal cell carcinoma	7q31	MET	(Receptor tyrosine kinase)
Birt-Hogg-Dubé	Papillary renal cell carcinoma Oncocytoma	17p11.2	FLCN	(Unknown function)
Multiple endocrine neoplasia type II	Pheochromocytoma	10q11	RET	(Receptor tyrosine kinase)
Hereditary nonpolyposis colorectal cancer	Upper tract transitional cell carcinoma	2p22, 3p21.3, 2p18, 2q31-q33, 7p22, 14q24.3	MSH2, MLH1, MSH6, PMS1, PMS2, MLH3	(DNA mismatch repair)
Hereditary prostate cancer	Prostate cancer	1q24-25, 1p36, 1q42-43, 8p22-23, 17p11, 20q13, Xq27-28	RNASEL, MSR1, ELAC2	(Endoribonuclease, macrophage specific receptor, cell cycle regulator)

TABLE 62.2 Selected Tumor Syndromes Not Strongly Associated With Genitourinary Malignancies

SYNDROME	PRIMARY TUMOR	CHROMOSOME(S)	GENE(S)	(FUNCTION)
Familial retinoblastoma	Retinoblastoma	13q14	RB	(Transcriptional regulation)
Li-Fraumeni	Sarcoma, breast carcinoma	17p13	TP53	(Transcription factor, serine kinase)
	22q12	hCHK2		
Familial adenomatous polyposis	Colorectal carcinoma	5q21	APC	(Regulates β-catenin activity)
Familial breast carcinoma	Breast carcinoma	17q21, 13q12	BRCA1, BRCA2	(DNA double-strand break repair)
Cowden's disease	Breast carcinoma	10q23	PTEN	(Phosphatase; PI3K antagonist)
Multiple endocrine neoplasia type I	Pancreatic islet cell carcinoma	11q13	MEN1	(Transcription factor)

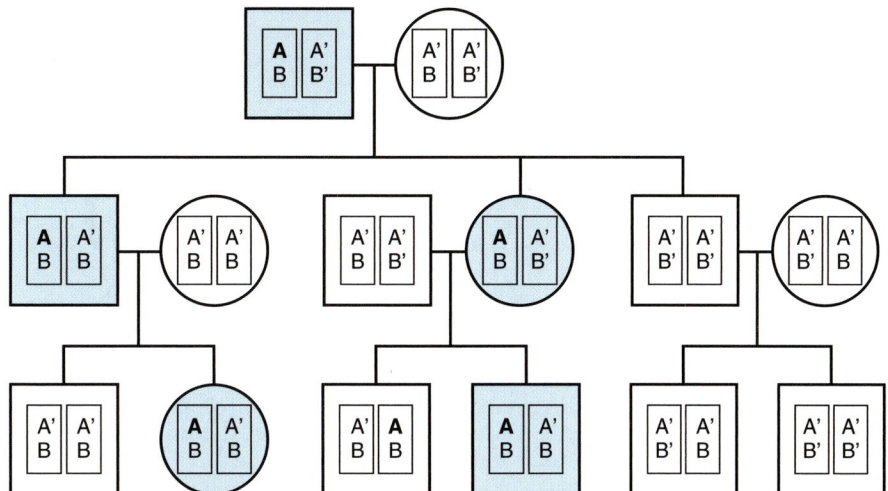

Fig. 62.12. The familial tumor syndrome is passed from generation to generation. Genotyping demonstrates that the polymorphic marker A *(marked in bold)* is passed also from generation to generation in concert with the phenotypic disease. Presumably a gene responsible for the syndrome is located near marker A. Linkage analysis is complicated by incomplete penetrance (not all members of the family with the allele get the disease), phenocopies (family members who have sporadic disease), inability to get DNA from all family members, and the large number of markers being simultaneously analyzed.

making genetic studies difficult to perform. One large HPC cohort of 175 pedigrees identified a region in chromosome 17q21-22 near BRCA1 with linkage to prostate cancer susceptibility (Lange et al., 2003). This region has subsequently become one of the most intensively investigated regions of the genome for HPC susceptibility. Furthermore, germline mutations in BRCA2 have subsequently been found to not only increase the risk of developing prostate cancer but also confer worse prognosis and have implications in the management of the disease, such as the use of platinum and taxane chemotherapy and PARP inhibitors (Castro and Eeles, 2012).

Targeted next-generation sequencing of exons in 202 genes on chromosome 17q21-22 from germline DNA of unrelated patients with prostate cancer from families that were selected for linkage to the 17q22-22 region identified a variant in the HOXB13 gene (HOXB13 G84E) that significantly increased the risk of HPC (Ewing et al., 2012). The carrier frequency of the G84E allele was found in 0.1% of men without prostate cancer and 1.4% of men with prostate cancer. Furthermore, the frequency of the allele was much higher in men with early-onset, familial prostate cancer (3.1%) versus men with late-onset, nonfamilial prostate cancer (0.6%) (Ewing et al., 2012). Although the carrier rate of the G84E allele is rare, the strong linkage to prostate cancer risk may warrant genetic testing for the variant, much like is currently performed for BRCA1 or BRCA2 in hereditary breast and ovarian cancers. Other candidate HPC susceptibility genes include ELAC2 (HPC2), macrophage scavenger receptor-1 (MSR-1) and PODXL (Casey et al., 2006; Nupponen et al., 2004; Tavtigian et al., 2001; Xu et al., 2002a). It is intriguing that two of the HPC candidates, RNASEL and MSR-1, are associated with functions of the immune response, because inflammation is currently considered a likely contributor to the pathogenesis of prostate cancer (De Marzo et al., 2007; Sfanos and De Marzo, 2012).

Sporadic Prostate Cancer

In sporadic prostate cancer, initial studies found recurrent changes involving losses of genetic material at 6q, 7q, 8p, 10q, 13q, 16q, 17p, 17q, and 18q; however, in most cases the precise genes involved have yet to be identified (Karan et al., 2003). **Changes in chromosome 8, typically loss of the p-arm and gain of the q-arm, or portions of these arms, are the most frequently observed genetic alterations.** At least two or three separate regions are deleted on 8p, implying the existence of multiple tumor suppressor genes (TSG). Chromosome **8p22 is commonly deleted, with frequencies of 32% to 65% reported in primary tumors and 65% to 100% in metastases. MSR-1 lies in this region** and sequence variants in MSR-1 have been found to be associated with increased disease risk; however, mutations in MSR-1 have not been reported in sporadic prostate cancers (Nupponen et al., 2004; Wiklund et al., 2009; Xu et al., 2002a). **Another promising candidate TSG on 8p is the prostate-restricted homeobox gene NKX3.1 at 8p21** (He et al., 1997). Mice engineered with a loss of a single allele of NKX3.1 develop prostate hyperplasia and PIN, an example of haploinsufficiency, wherein a phenotypic effect is observed because of the loss of a single allele (Abdulkadir et al., 2002; Bhatia-Gaur et al., 1999).

8q gain, often involving the entire chromosomal arm leading to isochromosome 8q formation, is the most common chromosomal abnormality found in advanced prostate cancer (e.g., hormone-refractory lymph node metastases) and is correlated with disease progression and resistance to hormone deprivation or blockade (Alers et al., 2000; Isaacs, 2002; van Dekken et al., 2003). **The proto-oncogene MYC at 8q24 is a likely candidate gene on 8q,** but the observed gains are large and more work is required to properly assess this possibility. Elevated expression of another gene in this region, *EIF3S3*, has been documented in cancer compared with benign prostatic hyperplasia (Savinainen et al., 2004). Mouse models lend support for a linkage to *MYC* because transgenic mice with forced prostate-specific expression of human *MYC* develop PIN and invasive adenocarcinomas (Ellwood-Yen et al., 2003). Furthermore, amplification at the *MYC* locus has been reported in some human prostate cancers and is associated with a poor prognosis (Jenkins et al., 1997; Sato et al., 1999).

Chromosome 7 abnormalities are also frequently observed in prostate cancer. Aneusomy of the entire chromosome (trisomy 7) has been reported in PIN and cancer and has been associated with advanced stage and a poor prognosis (Alcaraz et al., 1994; Arps et al., 1993; Macoska et al., 1993; Qian et al., 1995; Zitzelsberger et al., 1994). Apart from whole chromosome gains, losses involving 7q31.1 have been documented, suggesting a tumor suppressor resides here (Takahashi et al., 1995; Zenklusen et al., 1994). A potential candidate TSG in this region is caveolin *(CAV1)*, whose expression is reportedly decreased in cancer (Bender et al., 2000; Wiechen et al., 2001). On the other hand, positive IHC staining for caveolin has been associated with *poor* prognosis; thus its role in prostate cancer remains unclear (Tahir et al., 2001; Yang et al., 1999). Another attractive candidate gene in this region is *EZH2*, which codes for a histone methyl-transferase involved in gene silencing. In microarray analyses, *EZH2* has been found to be overexpressed in prostate cancer metastases and its expression in primary tumors is associated with disease (PSA) recurrence (Lapointe et al., 2004; Rhodes et al., 2003; Varambally et al., 2002).

Chromosome 10 also undergoes alteration in prostate cancer, with deletions observed at 10p11.2 and 10q23-q24 (Ittmann, 1996; Trybus et al., 1996). The tumor suppressor gene *PTEN*, a PI3 kinase antagonist, maps to this second region and has been linked to human prostate cancer in a number of studies (Ayala et al., 2004; Li et al., 1997a). *PTEN* undergoes homozygous (both copies) deletion, loss of heterozygosity (LOH), and promoter hypermethylation and is also mutated in prostate cancer. **Overall, PTEN is more frequently altered in advanced disease** (reported rates of 60% to 100%) compared with primary tumors (Cairns et al., 1997; Han et al., 2009; Pesche et al., 1998; Sarker et al., 2009; Whang et al., 1998). Interestingly, the frequency of *PTEN* LOH greatly exceeds *PTEN* mutation; therefore it is suggested that another gene or genes may be targeted for deletion in this region of chromosome 10. One possibility is the *MXI1* gene, whose protein product binds to and antagonizes *MYC*. In the mouse, *PTEN* deficiency exhibits synergy when combined with other mouse models of prostate cancer (Carver et al., 2009; Chen et al., 2006; Di Cristofano et al., 2001; Kim et al., 2002; King et al., 2009).

LOH on 13q has been reported in greater than 50% of prostate cancer cases examined. Three separate regions of loss have been identified, containing the potential cancer genes *BRCA2*, *RB1*, *EDNRB*, and *KLF5* (Chen et al., 2003; Cooney et al., 1996b; Hyytinen et al., 1999). High rates of *RB1* loss (up to 80%) have been reported in advanced cancers (Cher et al., 1996); however, the *RB1* mutation rate is relatively low, and RB1 expression is not well correlated with the gene dosage or disease status (Bookstein et al., 1990; Ittmann and Wieczorek, 1996; Kibel and Isaacs, 2000; Kubota et al., 1995). However, Theodorescu et al. reported that low RB1 protein expression was correlated with decreased disease-specific survival in univariate and multivariate analysis (Theodorescu et al., 1997).

Losses on 16q have been observed with reported frequencies ranging from 30% to 56% of prostate cancer cases, more commonly seen in advanced cancer and associated with a poor prognosis (Bergerheim et al., 1991; Carter et al., 1990; Elo et al., 1997; Li et al., 1999; Suzuki et al., 1996). A common region of loss at 16q22-q24 contains two likely candidate genes, the *CDH1* gene at 16q22.1 that codes for the calcium-dependent cell-cell adhesion protein E-cadherin (Morton et al., 1993; Murant et al., 2000; Rubin et al., 2001; Umbas et al., 1994) and the *ATBF1* gene at 16q22, coding for an AT-sequence binding transcription factor (Sun et al., 2005). Loss of *CDH1* has been associated with metastatic prostate cancer; however, IHC staining studies have produced mixed results and reports of mutation or LOH of E-cadherin are lacking; therefore *CDH1* may not be the primary target of the 16q deletion. The *ATBF1* gene, on the other hand, has been reported to be mutated in 40% of prostate cancers (Sun et al., 2005).

Reports of LOH on 6q range from 30% to 50%, with a minimal region of loss at 6q14-q22, although no strong candidate gene has been identified in this region (Cooney et al., 1996a; Hyytinen et al., 2002).

Allelic losses of a region on 17p that includes the *TP53* gene have been documented but are relatively infrequent in primary prostate cancer compared with more advanced disease (Brooks et al., 1996). This matches findings of mutational analyses in which TP53 mutations are rarely found in primary tumors but are reported in up to 40% of advanced disease (Bookstein et al., 1993; Navone et al., 1993; Visakorpi et al., 1992). A recurrent region of loss on 17q is located near the *BRCA1* gene at 17q21; however, the identified common area of loss does not include this critical tumor suppressor gene (Brothman et al., 1995; Williams et al., 1996).

Deletions on 18q are mainly observed in advanced prostate cancer, with a common region of deletion encompassing the known cancer-related genes *DCC*, *SMAD2*, and *SMAD4* (Ueda et al., 1997; Yin et al., 2001).

Loss of the cell cycle regulatory gene *CDKN2A* on 9p21, which encodes the cyclin-dependent kinase inhibitor p16, has been reported in 20% of prostate cancers and at twice this frequency in advanced disease (Cairns et al., 1995; Jarrard et al., 1997). As discussed previously, this locus also contains the p14 and p15 genes as well, making it difficult to pinpoint the exact target(s) of genetic loss in this region. Reduced expression and LOH of another *CDKI* gene, *CDKN1B* on 12p13.1-p12, which encodes the p27 protein, are also found in prostate cancer and are associated with more advanced disease (Guo et al., 1997; Kibel et al., 1998; Yang et al., 1998).

One additional locus that has particular relevance for prostate cancer is the androgen receptor *(AR)* gene located on Xq12. **The region Xq11-q13 containing *AR* is amplified in up to 30% of cases of advanced disease failing hormonal ablation therapy, in stark contrast with untreated (hormonally naive) cases that do not show *AR* amplification** (Chen et al., 2004; Linja and Visakorpi, 2004; Mellado et al., 2009; Visakorpi et al., 1995a). *AR* mutations, which often act to broaden the receptor's ligand specificity or otherwise provide a gain of function, occur in advanced as well as lower stage cancer, although they are rarely found in cases untreated by androgen deprivation therapy (Culig et al., 2001; Gottlieb et al., 2004; Hara et al., 2003; Newmark et al., 1992; Taplin et al., 1995; Tilley et al., 1996). Even in the absence of gene amplification, AR protein levels have been seen to be elevated in prostate cancer (Latil et al., 2001; Linja et al., 2001), further emphasizing the importance of AR hyperactivation in this disease. In addition to mutation, alternatively spliced versions of the *AR* lacking the androgen ligand-binding domain have been identified in prostate cancer cells (Dehm et al., 2008; Guo et al., 2009b; Hu et al., 2009). Such *AR* splice variants are active in the absence of bound ligand and therefore may contribute to the emergence of prostate cancer refractory to androgen ablative therapies.

Subsequent studies using the comparative genomic hybridization (CGH) technique, in which competitive reactions between differentially labeled tumor-derived versus normal-derived genomic DNA highlight regions lost or gained in the tumor sample, have largely confirmed and also extended the genomic alterations previously uncovered using LOH analysis. These CGH studies indicate that the number of different alterations is increased in advanced disease and that losses are more frequent than gains in early stages of the disease, with gains and genetic amplifications more commonly seen in advanced hormone-refractory disease (Cher et al., 1996; Nupponen and Visakorpi, 2000; Visakorpi et al., 1995b). Sun et al. reviewed all published prostate cancer CGH studies (Sun et al., 2007) and found that, overall, 13 regions were found to be altered in at least 10% of prostate cancer cases, with 8 regions showing deletion and 5 regions showing copy number gain. An additional 6 regions (3 with gains, 3 with losses) were found to be altered in more than 10% of advanced cancers. In agreement with earlier studies, 8p was the most frequent region of genomic loss (with a peak at 8p21.3), being observed in one-third of all cases and one-half of advanced disease. Likewise, 8q was gained most often (bimodal peaks at 8q22.2 and 8q24.13), being observed in one quarter and one half of all cases and in advanced disease, respectively (Sun et al., 2007). The other regions commonly lost, in decreasing order of frequency, included 13q21.31, 6q14.1-q21, 16q13-q24.3, and 18q12.1-q23, while regions exhibiting gain included 7q11.21-q32.3, Xq11.1-q23, 17q24.1-q25.3, and 3q26.23-q33. Also in keeping with the general observation that more aggressive and advanced cancers typically harbor more genetic abnormalities than their lower grade and lower stage counterparts, advanced prostate cancers displayed 2- to 3-fold more copy number alterations.

The application of modern high-resolution methods for assessing CNA, such as representational oligonucleotide microarray analysis and single nucleotide polymorphism (SNP) mapping arrays, will vastly improve our ability to detect CNA, particularly smaller alterations below the resolution limit of CGH, as well as aid in the identification of the resident oncogenes and tumor suppressor genes (Liu et al., 2006; Lucito et al., 2003; Sebat et al., 2004; Slater et al., 2005; Zhao et al., 2005).

High-density SNP microarrays have been used in genome-wide association studies (GWASs); high-resolution association studies between common DNA sequence variants (SNPs) and prostate cancer risk. Unlike the more traditional linkage analyses of the past, the platform is amenable to very large cohorts and is better able to detect genetic variations with small to moderate effects on disease risk (Jorgenson and Witte, 2007; Manolio, 2010; Risch and Merikangas, 1996). Several GWASs have been published on prostate cancer, resulting in the identification of more than 70 germline variants (SNPs) that are associated with the risk of developing prostate cancer (Amundadottir et al., 2006; Breyer et al., 2009; Duggan et al., 2007; Eeles et al., 2008; Eeles et al., 2009; Eeles et al., 2013; Gudmundsson et al., 2007; Gudmundsson et al., 2008; Haiman et al., 2007; Nakagawa et al., 2012; Thomas et al., 2008; Witte, 2007; Yeager et al., 2009). With larger meta-analyses being conducted worldwide, the number of prostate cancer SNPs is expected to increase to more than 100 in the near future (Nakagawa, 2013).

Interestingly, most of the SNPs are not located in or even near genes previously shown to be involved in prostate cancer pathogenesis. Notably, three independent loci were identified on 8q24, all contained within 1 Mb of the DNA segment; however, no genes have yet been identified to account for these risk alleles (Cheng et al., 2008). Systematic review of replication studies in prostate cancer susceptibility loci identified from GWASs finds that the 8q24 region continues to be the most implicated in prostate cancer risk and among different racial cohorts (Ishak and Giri, 2011). Although the MYC gene is in this vicinity, it is still 200 Kb away from the nearest SNP, thus its relevance, if any, remains uncertain. Importantly, unlike the loci identified in earlier linkage studies in HPC families, the risk alleles identified in these GWASs have been independently confirmed. As predicted, the risk attributable to each locus is small to modest, yet, because of the large cohorts studied, each association is highly statistically significant and each has been shown to confer risk independent of the other loci, thus these risk alleles act in a fairly additive fashion (Kote-Jarai et al., 2008; Sun et al., 2008; Witte, 2009; Zheng et al., 2008).

The clinical utility of using SNP "panels" for prostate cancer risk assessment is currently being investigated (Chatterjee et al., 2013; Nam et al., 2009; Zheng et al., 2009). However, **although men in the top decile in terms of number of combined risk alleles have a two- to fourfold increased risk for prostate cancer compared with the bottom decile, the numbers of men harboring such large numbers of risk alleles is small, thus these SNPs are unlikely to have utility for population screening purposes.** An important facet to these studies is that so far most of these prostate cancer risk alleles do not appear to be associated specifically with risk for aggressive disease (Kader et al., 2009; Wiklund et al., 2009). This is unfortunate because the lack of strong prognostic markers is a key shortcoming in the field that must be resolved. **The majority of current GWASs used case-control designs; therefore it will likely require new case-case studies, comparing aggressive versus nonaggressive disease, to uncover new SNPs informative for disease aggressiveness. It is thought that the recently identified SNPs are therefore more likely related to prostate cancer initiation rather than progression.** One such study that compared SNP frequencies among prostate cancer patients who were defined as having aggressive versus nonaggressive disease identified a region of 17p12 (TT genotype of SNP rs4054823) that was consistently higher among patients with more aggressive disease (Xu et al., 2010). The SNP in 17p12 resides in a region that does not contain any known genes; therefore, at present, the molecular mechanism by which it is associated with aggressive disease remains unknown. **Another approach that has had some early success in other cancers is to use gene expression array data to develop "gene signatures" able to predict aggressive behavior** (Cheville et al., 2008; Mucci et al., 2008; Setlur et al., 2008).

Recent rapid advances in next-generation sequencing technologies, allowing for whole-genome sequencing and whole-exome sequencing of multiple tumor samples at a time, have enabled comprehensive analyses of the complete landscape of genomic alterations (e.g., SNPs, CNAs, chromosomal rearrangements) present in human prostate cancer. One such study that conducted massively parallel sequencing of tumor and matched genomic DNA from seven patients with Gleason grade 7 or higher tumors identified a median of 3866 putative somatic base mutations (range 3192–5865) covering approximately 80% of the genome per tumor with a 10-fold higher mutation rate in CpG dinucleotides than all other genomic positions (Berger et al., 2011). Of the somatic mutations identified, a median of 20 mutations per tumor that cause a change in amino acid sequence were found to occur within protein-coding genes. Specific genes found to be mutated in multiple tumors included the scaffold protein SPTA1, a modulator of the transcriptional regulator DAXX called SPOP, chromatin modifiers CHD1, CHD5, and HDAC9, and members of the heat shock protein (HSP) stress response complex HSPA2, HSPA5, and HSP90AB1. In addition to somatic mutations, a median of 90 chromosomal rearrangements were identified per tumor genome (range 43–213), all of which produced balanced translocations without genomic loss and with the generation of "chimeric" chromosomes. Additional genes found to be specifically targeted by mutation and/or rearrangements were the tumor suppressor PTEN and the PTEN-interacting protein MAGI2. In a separate study of whole exome sequencing of 112 prostate tumor and normal pairs, mutations in SPOP were again detected, and this was found to be the most frequently mutated gene (Barbieri et al., 2012). Interestingly, Barbieri et al. found that SPOP mutations occurred in the tumors that lacked ETS family gene rearrangements, possibly defining a new molecular subtype of prostate cancer. Additional recurrent mutations were identified in the forkhead transcription factor gene FOXA1 and MED12, a protein involved in transcription initiation. As exome sequencing becomes more and more routine, attention has turned to the possibility of performing rapid high-throughput sequencing of patient samples that can inform therapeutic decisions on men newly diagnosed with advanced prostate cancer (Roychowdhury et al., 2011).

In addition to novel gene fusions that have been identified via RNA-seq analyses, a number of novel noncoding RNA (ncRNA) species have been identified in prostate cancer samples. Much of the focus of ncRNAs in prostate cancer has been on microRNA (miRNA) species, which are small, approximately 22 nucleotide molecules that function in gene silencing and may be linked to prostate cancer aggressivenss, promote the development of castration resistance, or may serve as markers of prostate cancer stem cells (reviewed in Bolton et al., 2013). Recently, this also includes the discovery of multiple novel long noncoding RNA (lncRNA) transcripts that may play a functional role in prostate carcinogenesis (Lu et al., 2017). lncRNAs are distinguished from small ncRNA species (such as microRNAs, siRNAs, and small nucleolar RNAs) in that they are typically more than 200 nucleotides in length. Although they do not encode for functional peptides, lncRNAs do play a role in gene regulation and other cellular processes (Ulitsky and Bartel, 2013). One of the most clinically advanced biomarkers of prostate cancer, *PCA3* (also known as DD3), in fact happens to be an lncRNA (Bussemakers et al., 1999). RNA-seq performed on a cohort of 102 prostate tissues and cell lines identified 106 unannotated intergenic RNAs that were differentially expressed between prostate cancer and benign prostate samples (Prensner et al., 2011). One of the top upregulated transcripts, an lncRNA called *PCAT-1*, was markedly upregulated in metastases and was found to act as a target of the polycomb repressive complex 2 (PRC2). Interestingly, *PCAT-1* is located on chromosome 8q24, discussed previously in regard to susceptibility loci in prostate cancer, and is approximately 725 kb upstream of the *c-MYC* oncogene. Another lncRNA identified in this study, *SChLAP1*, was found in follow-up studies to antagonize chromatin remodeling complex activity and serve as a prognostic indicator of poor prostate cancer outcome (Mehra et al., 2016; Prensner et al., 2013).

Renal Cancer

Renal cell carcinomas (RCC) include a spectrum of subtypes and can be subdivided into at least five different categories: clear cell RCC (ccRCC), which account for the majority (70% to 80%) of adult cases; papillary RCC, which accounts for most of the remaining 10% to 20%; chromophobe RCC, collecting duct RCC, and the MiTF/TFE family translocation carcinomas described earlier. In addition, there are more than four inherited forms of RCC. **Importantly, the genes discovered to have germline mutations that cause these familial forms of the disease have also been found to play important roles in sporadic RCC as well** (Coleman, 2008).

Patients with Von Hippel-Lindau (VHL) syndrome are predisposed to a number of tumor types, notably ccRCC (Coleman, 2008). The finding of consistent losses of 3p in this disease led to the identification of the von Hippel-Lindau *(VHL)* gene located at 3p25-p26, germline mutation of which causes VHL disease (Latif et al., 1993; Stolle et al., 1998; Tory et al., 1989; Zbar et al., 1987). **Once the *VHL* gene was identified, its status was assessed in sporadic (nonfamilial) RCC, where it was found to be mutated in more than half of sporadic ccRCC cases** (Gnarra et al., 1994; Shuin et al., 1994). More than 300 different *VHL* mutations have been catalogued and ccRCC cases not harboring *VHL* mutations often undergo LOH (deletion) or silencing of the gene by promoter hypermethylation; thus altogether, the vast majority of ccRCC have compromised *VHL*. **The VHL protein normally functions as part of a multiprotein complex with elonginB, elonginC, Cul-2 (cullin-2), and Rbx1 (ring box-1), which exhibits E3 ubiquitin ligase activity and targets subunits of the hypoxia-inducible factor-1 (HIF-1) transcription factor for ubiquitination and subsequent proteasomal destruction** (Iliopoulos et al., 1996; Kaelin, 2002; Kamura et al., 1999; Kibel et al., 1995; Pause et al., 1997). **HIF-1 functions as a master regulator of the cellular response to low oxygen levels.** Under normal conditions, specific proline amino acid residues in the two HIF-1 subunits, HIF-1α and HIF-1β, are hydroxylated by the oxygen-dependent proline hydroxylase enzymes *EGLN1-3*. This oxygen-dependent modification signals HIF-1's ubiquitination and thus HIF-1 is rapidly turned over (Bruick and McKnight, 2001; Ivan et al., 2001; Jaakkola et al., 2001; Maxwell et al., 1999). **Under conditions of oxygen deprivation (hypoxia) the prolyl hydroxylases fail to act; thus HIF-1 is spared and accumulates, allowing its translocation to the nucleus, where it activates a number of target genes**, including the glucose transporter *GLUT-1*, the proangiogenic growth factors *PDGF* and *VEGF*, the chemokine *CXCL-1* and its receptor *CXCL4*, TGFα and the HGF receptor, MET (Hu et al., 2003; Igarashi et al., 2002; Linehan et al., 2007; Staller et al., 2003; Wykoff et al., 2001). That the HIF-1 pathway is activated in ccRCC is supported by the highly vascular nature of these tumors and the fact that expression of HIF-1 target genes are found to be elevated. Thus, **in ccRCC, the loss of VHL function leads to a state of "pseudohypoxia," in which the cells respond as if they are being starved for oxygen.**

Several of the genes activated by HIF-1 have been singled out for therapeutic targeting, and positive results in clinical trials have led to FDA approval of some of these agents (Hansel and Rini, 2008; Linehan, 2002). For example, the monoclonal antivascular endothelial growth factor (VEGF) antibody bevacizumab and the small molecule kinase inhibitors sunitinib and sorafenib, which inhibit VEGF and PDGF, have shown improvements in progression-free survival in clinical trials for metastatic RCC, leading in the latter two cases to FDA approval (Hansel and Rini, 2008).

The VHL/sporadic ccRCC example epitomizes the potential for translational application of cancer molecular genetics, beginning with studies on a familial cancer that were then translated to the sporadic form of the disease, culminating in the rational design of therapeutic agents against revealed molecular targets having a positive impact in the clinic.

A second familial form of RCC is hereditary papillary renal carcinoma, the cause of which has been pinpointed to activation of the proto-oncogene tyrosine kinase c-Met, which is the cell surface receptor for the growth factor HGF (Jeffers et al., 1997). *MET* is located at 7q31-q34, which is notable because the vast majority of sporadic papillary RCC cases show trisomy of chromosome 7 (Kovacs, 1993). In addition, activating mutations, typically affecting the tyrosine kinase domain, leading to a constitutively active receptor, have also been found in sporadic cases (Schmidt et al., 1997).

A third type of hereditary RCC predisposition is Birt-Hogg-Dube (BHD) syndrome. Individuals with BHD most commonly develop chromophobe RCC, but other forms such as clear cell RCC, papillary RCC, and benign oncocytomas are also observed (Pavlovich et al., 2002; Pavlovich et al., 2005). The *BHD* gene underlying the disease is located at 17p11.12 and codes for the protein folliculin (Schmidt et al., 2001). A spectrum of disruptive mutations and gene deletions support a tumor suppressor gene function for folliculin (Khoo et al., 2002; Nickerson et al., 2002; Schmidt et al., 2005; Vocke et al., 2005); however, the precise function of this protein has not been elucidated, although evidence indicates it affects the ERK and Akt/mTOR signaling pathways (Baba et al., 2008).

A fourth familial RCC subtype, albeit rare, is hereditary leiomyomatosis RCC (HLRCC), featuring an aggressive form of papillary RCC (Kiuru and Launonen, 2004; Merino et al., 2007; Sudarshan et al., 2007). The cause of HLRCC has been traced to the fumarate hydratase gene at 1q42.3-q43, whose protein product converts fumarate to malate in the Krebs cycle. Once again, the HIF-1 pathway is implicated in RCC tumorigenesis, as the resulting accumulation of fumarate acts as a competitive inhibitor of the prolyl hydroxylases *EGLIN1-3*, preventing modification of HIF-1 subunits, prolonging their half-lives and leading to a pseudohypoxic state, as was the case for mutated *VHL*. In support of this pathogenetic scheme, increased expression of VEGF and a high microvessel density has been found in HLRCC tumors (Isaacs et al., 2005; Pollard et al., 2005).

In 2011 a germline missense substitution was discovered in microphthalmia-associated transcription factor (*MITF*, another member of the MiTF family discussed earlier in regard to MiTF/TFE family translocation carcinomas) that conferred a greater than fivefold increase in risk of developing RCC, melanoma, or both types of cancer (Bertolotto et al., 2011). The germline substitution in codon 318 (E318K) was found to impair SUMOylation of MITF, leading to transcriptional activation of genes that function in the hypoxia pathway *(HIF1A, CCR7, HMOX1)*, the importance of which in RCC has already been discussed.

Bladder Cancer

Although first-degree relatives of patients with bladder cancer are at increased risk of developing the disease, high-risk families are very rare and lack clear Mendelian inheritance patterns, precluding classical linkage analysis. Bladder cancer is therefore not considered a familial disease. Instead, it has been proposed that there likely exist many susceptibility genes with small to moderate effects on disease risk (Aben et al., 2006; Kiemeney, 2008). Recent attention has therefore turned to the use of GWAS, which are better suited to the discovery of low penetrance susceptibility loci. The first such studies that have been published and reported susceptibility loci include 8q24.21, near the MYC proto-oncogene, 3q28, associated with the TP53 relative TP63, and at 5p15.33, which is near the HTERT gene coding for the cancer-associated telomere maintenance enzyme telomerase (Kiemeney et al., 2008; Kiemeney et al., 2009; Rafnar et al., 2009; Wang et al., 2009a). Notably, gain of 5p15.33 had previously been identified as being associated with bladder cancer progression (Yamamoto et al., 2007), and reduced or absent TP63 expression has been associated with disease progression and poor prognosis (Koga et al., 2003; Urist et al., 2002). An additional GWAS reported by Wu et al. found a missense variant in the prostate stem cell antigen (PSCA) gene to be associated with bladder cancer risk in Caucasians (Wu et al., 2009b) and was subsequently shown in a GWAS by Wang et al. to be associated with bladder cancer risk in a Chinese population (Wang et al., 2010). Interestingly, the rs2294008 variant of PSCA has also been shown to be significantly associated with gastric cancer in Japan and China (Matsuo et al., 2009; Sakamoto et al., 2008; Wu et al., 2009a). This mutation is predicted to result in truncation of the first 9 amino acids of the PSCA protein. Earlier studies reported that PSCA mRNA and protein levels are increased in bladder cancer compared with normal urothelium, with mRNA expression serving as an independent predictor of recurrence in superficial bladder cancer (Amara et al., 2001; Elsamman et al., 2006; Wang et al., 2010). Recent years have seen an explosion in large-scale GWASs in Europe and the United States that have now accounted for at least 11 extensively replicated urinary bladder cancer susceptibility loci: 1p13.3 (GSTM1), 2q37.1 (UGT1A cluster), 3q28 (TP63), 4p16.3 (TMEM129 and TACC3-FGFR3), 5p15.33 (HTERT-CLPTM1L), 8p22 (NAT2), 8q24.21 (MYC), 8q24.3 (PSCA), 18q12.3 (SLC14A1), 19q12 (CCNE1), and 22q13.1 (CBX6, APOBEC3A) (García-Closas et al., 2011; García-Closas et al., 2005; Kiemeney et al., 2008; Kiemeney et al., 2010; Moore et al., 2011; Rafnar et al., 2009; Rothman et al., 2010; Tang et al., 2012; Thorunn Rafnar et al., 2011; Wu et al., 2009b) with additional loci recently reported on 3q26.2 and 11p15.5 and two suggested regions on 20p12.2 and 6q22.3 as well (Figueroa et al., 2014). Pathway analysis of 5 GWASs conducted on bladder cancer cases and controls of European background found that the genetic variants associated with bladder cancer to belong to three fundamental cellular processes: metabolic detoxification, mitosis, and clathrin-mediated vesicles (Menashe et al., 2012).

The majority (75% to 85%) of bladder cancer and cancer-associated lesions seen in the clinic are of superficial type (stages pTa, pTis, pT1). Recurrences after therapy are frequent, requiring diligent surveillance by urine cytology and cystoscopy resulting in frequent resections. In addition, the risk of progression is likewise high. Accurate assessment of risk for recurrence and progression to muscle-invasive disease are critical needs for which current predictive schemes based on histopathologic features are suboptimal. Hopefully the information at the molecular level will help improve current methods of risk stratification.

Much work has been done to identify genetic alterations in bladder cancer. In general, changes observed fall into two groups: those that are mostly unrelated to clinical subtype (e.g., changes in chromosome 9 and RAS mutations), and those that are related to specific grades and/or stages of the disease (e.g., FGFR3 mutations in low-grade noninvasive papillary urothelial bladder cancer; TP53 and RB1 alterations in muscle-invasive disease) (Knowles, 2008). In 2014 work by The Cancer Genome Atlas (TCGA) Research Network identified several additional mutated genes that had not been previously reported as significantly mutated in bladder cancer (TCGA Research Network, 2014). These genes included genes involved in cell cycle regulation (CDKN1A), nucleotide excision repair (ERCC2), and retinoic acid-mediated gene activation (RXRA).

More than half of urothelial cell carcinomas of all grades show chromosome 9 alterations; commonly these are losses of the entire chromosome or entire chromosomal arms, whereas LOH events of more restricted regions are also seen, leading to the current consensus that there are multiple tumor suppressor genes located on both chromosomal arms (Cairns et al., 1993; Linnenbach et al., 1993; Tsai et al., 1990). In otherwise near-diploid tumors, complete loss of one copy (monosomy 9) is the only karyotypic abnormality seen (Fadl-Elmula et al., 2000; Gibas et al., 1984). The region at 9p21 containing the genes for the CDKI proteins INK4B (p15) and INK4A (p16), which suppress the RB1 pathway, as well as harboring the TP53-stabilizing gene p14ARF, is a strong candidate bladder cancer TSG locus. This region commonly undergoes LOH or homozygous deletion in bladder cancers, including low-grade and low-stage tumors (Berggren et al., 2003; Devlin et al., 1994; Orlow et al., 1995; Williamson et al., 1995), and mutations have been associated with high-grade disease and tumor progression (Orlow et al., 1999).

At least three different regions of loss have been mapped on 9q. Candidate bladder cancer TSGs have been proposed, including the patched gene, PTCH, at 9q22, which shows mutations and LOH in up to 40% of cancers (Aboulkassim et al., 2003; McGarvey et al., 1998); the region termed DBC1 at 9q32-q33, which exhibits deletion and silencing in approximately 50% of cases (Habuchi et al., 1998; Nishiyama et al., 1999); and 9q34, which exhibits LOH and contains the gene TSC1 (tuberous sclerosis gene 1), a strong candidate bladder TSG resulting from the finding of TSC1 mutations in conjunction with LOH (Adachi et al., 2003; Hornigold et al., 1999; Knowles et al., 2003). The TSC1 gene encodes the protein hamartin, which is a phosphorylation target of Akt and functions in negative regulation of mTOR (mammalian target of rapamycin), a downstream target of the PI3K pathway, which is also dysregulated in bladder cancer via inactivation of the PI3K antagonist PTEN, as well as mutational activation of the p110 catalytic subunit of PI3 kinase; PIK3CA (Aveyard et al., 1999; Cairns et al., 1998; Wang et al., 2000).

Noninvasive (superficial, pTa) papillary UCC represents a major bladder cancer subgroup at diagnosis. Apart from changes involving chromosome 9, these tumors appear relatively stable with respect to chromosomal structural changes, with losses and gains reported for approximately a dozen different chromosomal locations, most in 20% or fewer of cases examined (Knowles, 2008; Koed et al., 2005). More subtle genetic alterations in oncogenes and tumor suppressor genes also occur with varying frequencies. As recently reviewed by Knowles (2008), activating mutations in the RAS family of proto-oncogenes (H-, K-, and N-RAS) have been reported in up to 15% of cases, mutations in PIK3CA in 16% of cases, and amplification/overexpression of CCND1 and HDM2 in 10% to 20% and approximately 30% of cases, respectively.

In addition to oncogene activation, inactivation of several tumor suppressor genes by either deletion or promoter hypermethylation has been reported in superficial papillary UCC. These genes include several genes on chromosome 9 such as CDKN2A (p16) affected in 30% to 60% of cases; PTCH, the DBC1 locus and TSC1, all reportedly affected in 60% of cases (Knowles, 2008).

The most frequently altered TSG in superficial Ta disease is the fibroblast growth factor receptor 3 (FGFR3), with mutation frequencies approaching 90% of cases reported (Billerey et al., 2001; Cappellen et al., 1999; Sibley et al., 2001; Tomlinson et al., 2007). The most common FGFR3 mutation is a serine-to-cysteine mutation at amino acid 249, which has been shown to cause constitutive ligand-independent receptor activation because of induced receptor dimerization via intermolecular Cys-Cys disulfide bonding (Li et al., 2006). **The frequency of FGFR3 mutations is much lower in higher stage, invasive bladder cancers, and mutations are lacking in the superficial Tis stage (CIS), which has a high propensity for recurrence and progression to invasive disease.** In addition, in Ta disease there is a strong inverse correlation between mutation and tumor grade (Billerey et al., 2001). The high preferential prevalence of FGFR3 mutations in Ta disease suggests an association with low-risk bladder cancer (Tomlinson et al., 2007). FGFR3 mutations are also associated with benign tumors of the skin (seborrheic keratoses) (Hafner et al., 2006; Logie et al., 2005). In a recent prospective study, Hernandez et al. (2006) concluded that FGFR3 mutations are associated with a subgroup of tumors having good prognosis, and Burger et al. reported FGFR3 status is useful in risk stratification for patients with high-grade non–muscle-invasive UCC. Finally, there are indications that FGFR3 mutations and RAS family mutations are mutually exclusive (Hafner et al., 2006; Jebar et al., 2005; Logie et al., 2005). These findings may be rationalized by considering that FGFR3 is known to activate the RAS/RAF/MEK/ERK pathway (Choi et al., 2001). Likewise, reports of mutational exclusivity have been made regarding FGFR3 and TP53, which are mutated in only about 5% of pTa cases and are associated with higher grade disease (Bakkar et al., 2003; Zieger et al., 2005). Interestingly, in pT1 disease, the frequency of FGFR3 mutations is lower, TP53 mutation frequency is higher, and unlike pTa disease, these mutations are not necessarily mutually exclusive (Bakkar et al., 2003; Tomlinson et al., 2007; van Rhijn et al., 2004).

Although the frequency of chromosome 9 alterations and RAS family mutations are comparable across all grades and stages of bladder cancer, **muscle-invasive urothelial carcinomas (stage pT2 and higher) exhibit more genetic alterations (qualitatively and quantitatively) than lower stage disease; in keeping with the general observation that more aggressive cancers tend to exhibit evidence of greater genetic instability than their less aggressive counterparts.** Invasive bladder tumors exhibit a wide range of copy number alterations across virtually every chromosome, although the gene targets of these changes are largely unknown at present (Koed et al., 2005). In a similar vein, Blaveri et al. used cluster analysis of array CGH (aCGH) data to successfully separate bladder tumors of differing stages and grades from one another. In addition, a quantitative measure of the fraction of genome altered (FGA) was shown to be inversely related to patient survival time in cases with muscle-invasive cancer (Blaveri et al., 2005). Ploidy, another reflection of genomic instability, has been found to be associated with progression from noninvasive to invasive bladder cancer (Holmang et al., 2001). Mutational inactivation of TP53 is seen in greater than 40% of invasive pT2 tumors, in sharp contrast to the low mutational rate seen in pTa disease, where TP53 mutation is associated with risk for progression (Fujimoto et al., 1992; George et al., 2007; Spruck et al., 1994; Uchida et al., 1995). Likewise, inactivation of RB1, either by LOH or through INK4A inactivation, is common in invasive bladder cancer but is infrequent in pTa tumors (Benedict et al., 1999; Cairns et al., 1991; Chatterjee et al., 2004; Shariat et al., 2004). Loss of the region of 10q harboring the PTEN tumor suppressor gene is also more frequent in muscle-invasive bladder cancer than in lower stage pTa tumors (Aveyard et al., 1999; Cappellen et al., 1997; Kagan et al., 1998).

Intrinsic Subtypes of High-Grade Bladder Cancer

At least two intrinsic subtypes of high-grade bladder cancer have been identified (Choi et al., 2014; Damrauer et al., 2014). Luminal and basal-like subtypes, which have characteristics of different stages of urothelial differentiation, have been correlated with patient outcomes. These subtypes are also similar to molecular changes that have been identified in breast cancer. Distinct genomic alterations such as FGFR3 and TSC1 mutations are commonly found in the luminal subtype, whereas alterations in the RB1 pathway are enriched in basal-like bladder cancer (Damrauer et al., 2014).

Low-grade papillary tumors are found to have frequent FGFR3, RAS, and receptor tyrosine kinase alterations, whereas high-grade tumors are characterized by loss of tumor suppressor genes, such as PTEN, TP53, and RB1 pathway alterations. A model of bladder cancer initiation and progression that incorporates data related to these distinct molecular subtypes suggests that low-grade tumors that progress are high-grade papillary tumors of the luminal molecular subtype, and high-grade tumors that originate de novo are more consistent with the basal-like expression subtype (Damrauer et al., 2014).

Using whole genome mRNA expression profiling, three molecular subtypes of muscle-invasive bladder cancer that resembled molecular subtypes of breast cancer have been identified (Choi et al., 2014). Basal-type bladder cancers are characterized by p63 activation, squamous differentiation, and more aggressive disease at presentation. Luminal-type bladder cancers had active PPARg and estrogen receptor transcription and are enriched with activating FGFR3 mutations. The p53-like bladder cancers are frequently resistant to neoadjuvant methotrexate, vinblastine, doxorubicin, and cisplatin chemotherapy, and all chemoresistant tumors were found to have a p53-like phenotype after therapy (Choi et al., 2014). These data suggest that the level of "p53-ness" plays an important role in bladder cancer chemoresistance.

Genetic Alterations in Bladder Pre-Neoplasia

Urothelial hyperplasias with flat or papillary histomorphology have been proposed to be precursors of low-grade bladder cancers, although this concept is somewhat controversial (Chow et al., 2000). In support, Hartman et al. reported that, when present, genetic alterations (assayed at 9q21, 9q22, and 17p13) in hyperplasias were also found in superficial papillary tumors from the same patient (Hartmann et al., 1999). Genetic studies on hyperplasias have reported moderate to high frequencies of chromosome 9 alterations, whereas other genetic changes that are associated with aggressive forms of bladder cancer are reportedly infrequent (Chow et al., 2000). Dysplastic urothelial lesions have been found to be have frequent changes of chromosome 9 and frequent aneuploidy, and approximately half are TP53 mutated (Hartmann et al., 2002; Mallofre et al., 2003). The prevalence of changes seen in low-grade intraurothelial neoplasia was lower than that observed in high-grade (CIS) lesions (Hartmann et al., 2002). CIS lesions (pTis) are aggressive, high-grade precursor lesions, exhibiting high rates of recurrence and progression to invasive disease. In contrast with superficial papillary lesions, CIS exhibits frequent (50%–70% range) genetic alterations (LOH) of 4q, 8p, 11p, 13q, and 14q, in addition to several other chromosomal alterations observed at lower but still significant frequencies (Rosin et al., 1995). CIS lesions may be subdivided into primary lesions, which are isolated without associated cancer and cancer-associated secondary lesions. It has been reported that chromosome 9 changes are infrequent in primary lesions, whereas the majority of secondary lesions exhibit deletions on chromosome 9 (Billerey et al., 2001; Hartmann et al., 2002; Hopman et al., 2002; Spruck et al., 1994).

As expected, given their aggressive nature, FGFR3 mutation rates are low in CIS, whereas the TP53 pathway shows frequent alterations. TP53 mutation occurs in more than half of CIS lesions and is correlated with strong nuclear TP53 staining by IHC (Hartmann et al., 2002; Hopman et al., 2002). Nuclear TP53 expression in TCC has been associated with increased risk of recurrence and death, independent of tumor grade, stage, and lymph node status in TCC patients (Esrig et al., 1994; Lipponen, 1993; Sarkis et al., 1993).

Genetic Alterations in Normal and Benign Bladder Urothelium

Given bladder cancer's propensity to recur, plus the fact that it is often multifocal, it has been proposed that there may be genetic changes in broad areas of the urothelium. Such a hypothesis would be in keeping with the "field cancerization" concept (also known as "field effect"), first devised by Slaughter et al. in 1953 to help explain the multifocal nature and high local recurrence rates of cancers of the oral cavity, as well as the finding of histologically abnormal epithelium in areas adjacent to cancer. Slaughter et al. proposed that multiple cancer foci arose within a wider field of abnormal epithelium that had been preconditioned by some prior carcinogenic insult(s). Genetic changes have been detected in samples of histologically normal-appearing urothelium obtained from surgical samples from cancer patients. For example, Muto et al. (2000) found shared instances of LOH as well as promoter hypermethylation of the INK4A gene between normal-appearing and tumor areas from the same case. Likewise, Stoehr et al. (2005) performed LOH analyses on a large number of cases in which normal-appearing epithelium was isolated by laser capture microdissection. They also reported cancer-associated genetic changes in the normal-appearing urothelium, which, in some cases, matched the changes found in concurrent cancers in the same case. However, caution is warranted when assessing such results, given the possibility of contamination of the normal areas sampled by small multifocal cancer lesions or by pagetoid spread of tumor cells (Junker et al., 2003). On the other hand, a study by Obermann et al. using interphase FISH in tissue sections detected losses involving chromosome 9 in normal-appearing cells, which, from a technical standpoint, should be effective at excluding possible confounding microscopic foci of cancer cells (Obermann et al., 2004).

Inverted papillomas of the urinary bladder are considered benign entities. In keeping with this, they exhibit infrequent LOH at cancer-associated chromosomal loci, as well as infrequent (less than 10%) mutations of *FGFR3* (Eiber et al., 2007; Sung et al., 2006). In contrast to inverted papillomas, papillary urothelial neoplasia of low malignant potential (PUN-LMP) exhibit high rates (85%) of *FGFR3* mutation (van Rhijn et al., 2002), a genetic alteration that, as described previously, is strongly associated with bladder tumors of low stage and low grade. However, a study by Cheng et al. found frequent LOH at several loci that typically undergo LOH in advanced bladder carcinoma (greater than or equal to pT2) (Cheng et al., 2004).

Molecular Genetic-Based Assays for Bladder Cancer Detection and Surveillance

The large amount of data concerning common genetic alterations in bladder cancer have been exploited to aid in detecting the presence of bladder cancer. One widely used test termed Urovysion (Abbott Molecular/Vysis) is a multiplex, multicolor FISH-based assay that features a cocktail of 4 hybridization probes that assess the status of 4 chromosomes (Bubendorf et al., 2001; Halling, 2003). Probes specific for the centromeres of chromosomes 3, 7, and 17 provide information on cancer-associated gains of these chromosomes, whereas the fourth probe is specific for 9p21, which harbors the p14 and p16 genes often deleted in bladder cancers. This test, approved by the US FDA in 2005, is used in conjunction with standard urine cytology in diagnosing suspected cases as well as monitoring for local recurrence in patients previously diagnosed and treated (Hajdinjak, 2008; Halling et al., 2000). In addition, the test may have utility in monitoring response in patients with superficial bladder cancer treated with intravesical bacille Calmette-Guérin (BCG) therapy (Kipp et al., 2005) and may be useful in distinguishing inverted papillomas from urothelial carcinoma with inverted growth pattern (Jones et al., 2007).

Currently there are 6 FDA-approved urine-based molecular tests for bladder cancer focused on either genetic or immunochemical targets, and many other potential markers are under development (Herman et al., 2008; Sullivan et al., 2009; van Rhijn et al., 2005; Zwarthoff, 2008). **However, although these tests improve upon standard urine cytology, they do not supplant it.**

Finally, a recent study by Wang et al. (2009b) reported the development of a quantitative-PCR (Q-PCR) gene signature for predicting progression in cases of non–muscle-invasive bladder cancer.

Testicular Cancer

Testicular germ cell tumors (TGCTs) are a fascinating set of malignancies possessing many unique features (Oosterhuis and Looijenga, 2005). These cancers appear to originate from totipotent stem cells, with evidence strongly supporting TGCT initiation in utero, whereby abnormal primordial germ cells (PGCs) or gonocytes are blocked in their differentiation, remaining dormant until puberty. This is supported by expression in TGCTs of markers closely associated with PGCs, including placental alkaline phosphatase (PLAP), the stem cell factor tyrosine kinase receptor KIT (c-kit), and the transcription factors POU5F1 (Oct3/4) and NANOG that are involved in maintenance of pluripotency or "stemness." The presumptive common precursor to TGCTs is the intratubular germ cell neoplasia unclassified (ITGCNU), which closely resembles PGCs, sharing many of the same markers (PLAP, KIT, POU5F1) (Skakkebaek et al., 1987). ITGCNU, also traditionally referred to as CIS (carcinoma in situ), although this nomenclature is technically inaccurate, has a very high rate of progression to invasive disease, estimated to be almost 100% if allowed sufficient time (Linke et al., 2005).

TGCTs are classified into two main categories: seminomas and the nonseminomas. A third type, the so-called spermatocytic seminomas, are extremely rare and are not discussed here (Ulbright, 1993). **Like the TGCT precursor ITGCNU, seminomas closely resemble PGC/gonocytes, morphologically and in their expression of molecular markers** (positive expression of PLAP, KIT, POU5F1, NANOG, STELLAR, SOX17) (de Jong et al., 2008; Sperger et al., 2003). **Nonseminomatous TGCTs resemble embryonic and extra-embryonic tissues that have undergone varying extents of differentiation.** The nonseminomas include four subtypes. Embryonal carcinoma (EC) are similar in many respects to embryonic stem cells, or perhaps primitive ectoderm, and express POU5F1, NANOG, and STELLAR, as well as SOX2 (Gopalan et al., 2009a). Extraembryonic differentiation is apparent in the yolk sac tumors (YSTs) and choriocarcinoma (CC), whereas somatic tissue differentiation is found in the teratomas.

Besides their unique pathogenesis, TGCTs are also unique in their responsiveness to treatment modalities that induce DNA damage (e.g., ionizing radiation and cisplatin-based chemotherapy). Thus the majority of patients are currently curable, even those with advanced disseminated disease (Einhorn, 2002). This extreme sensitivity to DNA damage is thought to be related to the origins of TGCT; their normal stem cell counterparts are poised to undergo apoptosis in response to DNA damage, and the fact that **most TGCTs maintain wild type TP53 and apparently intact DDR** (Bartkova et al., 2007; Gorgoulis et al., 2005; Kersemaekers et al., 2002). Interestingly, responsiveness to therapy in TGCT is inverse that seen in most other cancers, that is, sensitivity decreases with increasing differentiation state, such that ITGCNU are eliminated with low-dose radiation, whereas teratomas exhibit resistance to radiation and chemotherapy.

Family history is a strong risk factor for the development of TGCT, stronger than that found in most other cancers (Czene et al., 2002; Forman et al., 1992; Mai et al., 2009; Westergaard et al., 1996). Despite this fact, initial reports of an association between specific losses on Yq and risk were not later confirmed (Krausz and Looijenga, 2008). Genetic polymorphisms in CAG tract length, which codes for polyglutamine repeats in the androgen receptor, were assessed but were not found to be associated with disease risk (Garolla et al., 2005; Giwercman et al., 2004; Rajpert-De Meyts et al., 2002). Furthermore, **linkage and more recent GWASs have not revealed evidence for major TGCT-related genetic loci, implying instead the existence of multiple loci having modest influence** (Crockford et al., 2006; Lutke Holzik et al., 2005; Rapley, 2007). **However, in two recent GWASs, Kanetsky et al. and Rapley et al. reported that common genetic variants at 5q31.3 near sprouty 4 (*SPRY4*, an inhibitor of the MAPK signaling pathway) and in the *KITLG* gene region (c-KIT ligand, also known as stem cell factor or steel factor) on 12q22 are significantly associated with TGCT risk**, including seminomas and nonseminomas (Kanetsky et al., 2009; Rapley et al., 2009). In addition, Rapley et al. (2009) identified a susceptibility locus on chromosome 6 in an intron of *BAK1*, a gene that promotes apoptosis.

Spontaneous (as opposed to inherited) genetic alterations have been catalogued in TGCTs. Apart from aneuploidy, there are relatively few genetic changes or gene mutations found in TGCTs, giving an overall picture of a relatively low level of genetic instability, which may be in large part the result of the aforementioned intact DDR and predominately wild type *TP53* status in these cancers (Bignell et al., 2006; Greenman et al., 2007). One recurrent nearly universal genetic alteration in TGCT (excluding the rare spermatocytic seminomas) is the previously described gain of 12p, which may involve the *KRAS* gene or genes such as *NANOG* and *STELLAR* located in the stem cell cluster region at 12p13.31. Additional evidence for *KRAS* involvement in TGCT includes reports of activating mutations in up to 40% of cases, as well as increases in expression in concert with increased gene copy number. Interestingly, *BRAF* mutations have also been identified in TGCT but are seen to be mutually exclusive to K-Ras overexpression (McIntyre et al., 2005b; Sommerer et al., 2005).

Other changes that have been reported in sporadic TGCT include gains of material on chromosomes 1, 5, 7, and X; and losses on chromosome 18 in ITGCNU and invasive cancer; and losses from chromosomes 4 and 13, plus gain of 2p, which were more restricted to invasive cancers (Summersgill et al., 2001).

In seminomas, recurrent gains of 4q12, 16p13, and Xq22 plus losses of 3q29, 11q12.1, and 14q13.2 have been reported (Goddard et al., 2007). The *KIT* gene, whose protein product is a receptor tyrosine kinase also known as CD117, is located at 4q12. *KIT* amplifications have been reported in 24% of seminomas and gene-specific amplifications in 17%, but these changes were lacking in nonseminomas and ITGCNU (McIntyre et al., 2005a). Also, mutations in c-kit represent the most common somatic mutations found in seminomas (25% of cases) but are rarely found in nonseminomas (Coffey et al., 2008; Forbes et al., 2006). Despite the apparent lack of c-kit gene amplifications in ITGCNU, activating mutations in *KIT* have been reported, and IHC staining is positive for this entity as well as seminomas, although it not seen in nonseminomas or spermatocytic seminomas (Goddard et al., 2007; Kemmer et al., 2004; Looijenga et al., 2003; Przygodzki et al., 2002; Tian et al., 1999).

Gains of 17q11.2-q21 have been reported in TGCT, and this region contains the *ERBB2* receptor tyrosine kinase gene as well as the *GRB7* adaptor protein gene. *ERBB2* ties into the RAS pathway, whereas GRB7 binds to and likely regulates KIT, ERBB2, and RAS and is reportedly overexpressed in TGCT and their ITGCNU precursor (Kraggerud et al., 2002; Skotheim et al., 2003).

The previously mentioned results create an emerging picture of derangement of growth stimulatory protein kinase signaling pathways in TGCT, including activations in the RAS and KIT pathways in most seminomas and nonseminomas (Kemmer et al., 2004; Sommerer et al., 2005). In keeping with the fact that **RAS and KIT activate the PI3K/AKT pathway,** activated Akt has also been observed (Kemmer et al., 2004). In addition, **the PI3K antagonist PTEN is reported to be frequently inactivated by either mutation or deletion in seminomas and nonseminomas,** further suggesting an important role for activated PI3K/AKT pathway in TGCT (Di Vizio et al., 2005; Teng et al., 1997).

Normal PGCs undergo programmed erasure of DNA CpG methylation marks and thus a loss of imprinting. Recent IHC studies using an anti-5-methyl cytosine antibody to assess global methylation status in situ have confirmed and extended prior reports focusing on specific loci. These new studies found very low to absent 5-methyl cytosine in the majority of ITGCNU and seminoma compared with robust detection of 5-methyl cytosine in nonseminomas (Netto et al., 2008; Peltomaki, 1991; Smiraglia et al., 2002; Zhang et al., 2005). These results are supportive of a model for TGCT pathogenesis, in which ITGCNU is derived from retained abnormal PGC, which have matured to the point of 5-methyl cytosine erasure but before the point in normal PGC development at which epigenetic marks are re-established via de novo DNA methylation. Such observed changes in global methylation do not necessarily rule out the existence of hypermethylation at specific gene promoters. For instance, epigenetic silencing of specific genes such as the tumor suppressor *RASSF1A* has been reported in seminoma (Honorio et al., 2003; Koul et al., 2002).

TELOMERES AND TELOMERASE

As we have seen, **cancer cells exhibit marked genetic, morphologic, and behavioral heterogeneity, a reflection of their underlying genetic complexity and instability.** In addition, **most cancers display a strong positive association with increasing age.** As discussed previously, it has been persuasively argued that an increase over the extremely low baseline mutation rate (a mutator phenotype) is needed for accrual of sufficient mutations to bring about malignant transformation (Loeb, 1991).

Cancer genomes exhibit clear evidence of genetic instability; however, defective DNA maintenance and repair genes do not appear to be major contributors to the development of most sporadic cancers, thus the source of the genetic instability involved in the majority of cancers has been unclear. This has been particularly true of chromosomal instability, a nearly ubiquitous feature of carcinomas. Although alterations in chromosome number may arise via defects in centrosomes or the mitotic spindle checkpoint, little information exists regarding the origins of structural chromosomal abnormalities (Pihan et al., 2003; Roh et al., 2003). **An attractive candidate for the source of chromosomal instability in cancer is telomere dysfunction. Telomeres may provide a common link between genetic instability, cellular proliferation, and aging** (DePinho, 2000; Shay, 1997).

Telomeres and Chromosomal Instability

Telomeres are structures composed of specialized repetitive DNA complexed with telomere-specific binding proteins, located at the ends of every human chromosome, where they stabilize and protect the ends (Blackburn, 1991). Telomeric DNA is noncoding and consists of tandem repeats of the six base pair sequence TTAGGG (Meyne et al., 1989; Moyzis et al., 1988). In normal human cells, telomere lengths typically range from 6 to 12 kilobases per chromosome. **Telomeres that are too short are dysfunctional ("uncapped"), causing chromosomal destabilization** (Karlseder, 2003; Saldanha et al., 2003).

Importantly, telomeres are dynamic; shortening by approximately 100 base pairs each time a cell divides because of inability of DNA polymerases to completely replicate terminal DNA sequences (Harley et al., 1990; Lindsey et al., 1991). **Thus telomere length is inversely correlated with the number of times a cell has divided** (Hastie et al., 1990; Levy et al., 1992). Telomere shortening may also occur because of unrepaired single-strand breaks caused by oxidative damage to telomeric DNA (Kruk et al., 1995; von Zglinicki et al., 2000). Conversely, telomeres may be elongated through the action of the telomere synthetic enzyme telomerase or, uncommonly, via a telomerase-independent genetic recombination mechanism termed ALT (Greider and Blackburn, 1985; Heaphy et al., 2011; Reddel et al., 2001).

Chromosomes with short, dysfunctional telomeres are prone to fusion, leading to the formation of dicentric chromosomes that missegregate or break in mitosis during anaphase. The newly generated chromosomal breaks are fusogenic, thus perpetuating a cycle of chromosome fusion and breakage (Lo et al., 2002; McClintock, 1941). It is in this way that critically short telomeres initiate chromosomal instability (Artandi and DePinho, 2000; Feldser et al., 2003; Vukovic et al., 2007). **Numerous studies support the link between telomere dysfunction and chromosomal instability in human cancers.** For example, in head and neck tumors, chromosomes bearing severely short telomeres are associated with chromosomal fusions, rearrangements, anaphase bridges, and multipolar mitoses (Gisselsson et al., 2000).

> **KEY POINTS: GENOMIC ALTERATIONS**
>
> - Large variations in chromosome numbers and complex structural rearrangements, as well as intratumoral variation in these aberrations, are hallmarks of most human solid tumors.
> - The extent of chromosomal abnormalities typically correlates with disease severity and aggressiveness.
> - Recurrent structural rearrangements occur in prostate (ETS gene fusions), renal (MiTF/TFE family translocation carcinomas), and testicular cancers (isochromosome 12p).
> - Copy number alterations in a particular gene, coupled with changes in the other allele, are evidence for gene functioning as a disease-relevant oncogene or tumor suppressor gene.
> - Genes discovered to have germline mutations that cause familial forms of cancer may also be involved in the sporadic form of the disease (e.g., VHL in ccRCC).
> - High-density SNP microarrays have been used in GWAS to identify DNA sequence variants associated with cancer risk.
> - Low-grade bladder cancers that progress are typically high-grade papillary tumors of the luminal molecular subtype, and high-grade bladder cancers that originate de novo are more consistent with basal-like expression.

Telomere Shortening Acts as a Tumor Suppressive Mechanism in Normal Cells

Normal cells closely monitor their telomere lengths. Moderate telomere shortening either signals entry into an irreversible cell cycle arrest termed *replicative senescence* or initiates programmed cell death, responses thought to have evolved as tumor suppressive barriers against abnormal clonal expansion and the development of excessive telomere shortening that would accompany further cell division, were it to be allowed to continue (Wright and Shay, 2001). Thus **progressive telomere shortening acts as a "mitotic clock," counting down cell divisions and signaling cell cycle exit once one or more telomeres reaches a threshold length** (Harley et al., 1990).

Forced expression of the enzyme telomerase in presenescent cells counteracts telomere shortening, thus preventing replicative senescence and endowing the cells with unlimited cell division potential or "immortalization" (Bodnar et al., 1998; Vaziri and Benchimol, 1998). In normal somatic human cells, telomerase activity is stringently repressed, thus telomere length will decrease in proliferating cells and can be used as a signal to halt further expansion. **Although the precise mechanism(s) by which short telomeres trigger senescence and apoptosis are still under study, evidence implicates the tumor suppressors TP53 and RB1 as being involved in the response to shortened telomeres** (Vaziri and Benchimol, 1999). Importantly, abrogation of this telomere length checkpoint allows continued cell division and, in the absence of telomerase, severe telomere shortening, beyond the minimum length required for proper telomere function, therefore causing telomere uncapping and chromosomal destabilization (Counter et al., 1992).

In summary, **telomere shortening presents two important barriers to incipient cancer cells. First, moderate shortening instigates the senescence cell cycle exit or apoptosis. Second, extreme telomere shortening causes chromosomal instability, which, although it increases, the mutation rate will also tend to result in genetic abnormalities lethal to the cell** (Fig. 62.13).

Cancers and Premalignant Lesions Possess Abnormally Short Telomeres

The majority of human cancer tissues and cancer-derived cell lines examined have been found to contain abnormally short telomeres (Furugori et al., 2000; Hastie et al., 1990; Mehle et al., 1996; Remes et al., 2000; Takagi et al., 1999). For example, using a Southern blot technique for bulk telomere length assessment, Sommerfeld et al. and Konenman et al. observed substantial telomere shortening in primary prostate cancer tissues compared with matched adjacent normal-appearing and benign prostatic hyperplasia (BPH) areas in radical prostatectomy specimens (Koeneman et al., 1998; Sommerfeld et al., 1996). Likewise, results from direct telomere length assessment in archival tissue samples using telomere-specific FISH reveal significantly shorter telomeres in prostate cancer cells, when compared with their normal epithelial cell counterparts within the same tissue samples (Meeker et al., 2002a).

When examined using high-resolution telomere-specific FISH, it has been found that **premalignant lesions, including those of bladder and prostate cancer, tend to have abnormally short telomeres** (Hansel et al., 2006; Kawai et al., 2007; Meeker and Argani, 2004; Meeker et al., 2004; van Heek et al., 2002). This finding indicates that **telomere loss occurs early in the disease process**, at the IEN stage, **strongly implying a causal role for telomere shortening in carcinogenesis through the initiation of chromosomal instability** (O'Shaughnessy et al., 2002). In the prostate, the premalignant precursor is high-grade prostatic intraepithelial neoplasia (HGPIN) (Bostwick and Cheng, 2012). **A new regulatory motif in cell-cycle control causing specific inhibition of cyclin D/CDK4, the majority of which (93%) were found to harbor abnormally short telomeres by FISH (Meeker et al., 2002b). Notably, in this study, telomere shortening in HGPIN foci was restricted to the *luminal* secretory epithelial cells only, whereas the underlying basal epithelial cells and surrounding stromal cells displayed normal telomere lengths. In a separate study, Vukovic et al. reported significant telomere

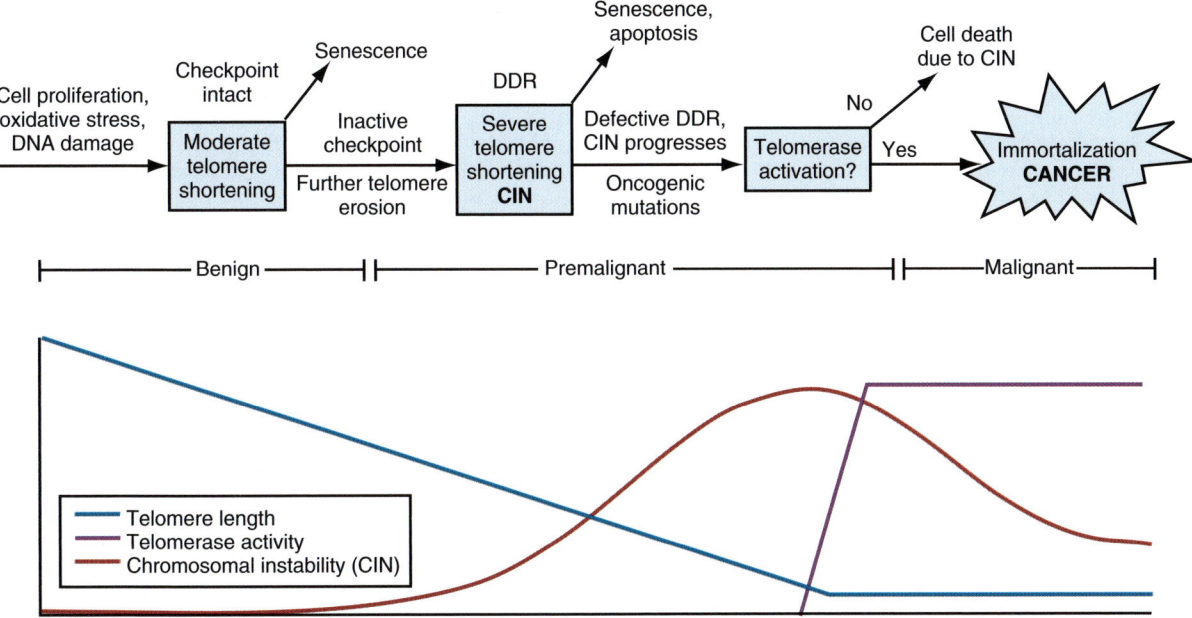

Fig. 62.13. Contributions of telomere loss and telomerase activation to oncogenesis. Bypass of the normal telomere length-sensitive cell senescence checkpoint allows severe telomere loss which initiates chromosomal instability (CIN). Defective DNA damage response (DDR) allows CIN to continue, generating potentially oncogenic mutations but also producing intolerable levels of genomic damage. Transformed cells may proceed through this second barrier by activating telomerase, which stabilizes the telomeres and also provides an unlimited proliferative potential ("immortalization").

shortening in 63% of HGPIN, with a higher rate of telomere shortening (80%) reported for foci situated near (within 2 mm) adenocarcinoma within the same tissue sample (Vukovic et al., 2003). Studying a cohort of men with a diagnosis exclusively of HGPIN in prostate needle biopsies, Joshua et al. (2007) reported an association between short telomeres in the PIN lesions or surrounding stromal cells and eventual diagnosis of prostate cancer, as well as time to diagnosis.

Because the majority of PIN lesions are not thought to progress to invasive cancers, intact telomere-based replicative senescence or apoptosis checkpoints may represent a critical bottleneck restraining the outgrowth of most PIN lesions. Even if incipient cancer cells manage to abrogate these checkpoints, as described later, they would still have to activate telomerase to avoid intolerable levels of genetic instability and provide an immortalized phenotype.

Telomerase Activity Restabilizing Chromosomes and Allowing Unlimited Cellular Replication

Although dysfunctional telomeres may help initiate cancer formation, if left unchecked, continued telomere shortening in premalignant lesions and cancers would cause increasing levels of genetic instability, ultimately becoming lethal to the tumor. Cancer cells overcome this problem by restabilizing their telomeres, primarily through activation of the enzyme telomerase, a specialized reverse transcriptase that adds back telomere DNA repeats to chromosome ends (Greider and Blackburn, 1987). Telomerase provides at least two critical functions to the tumor cell; namely, quelling chromosomal instability and supplying the capacity for unlimited replication ("immortalization") (Greider, 1998; Shay and Wright, 1996). Research has revealed that telomere length maintenance appears to be a necessary step for human cells to become malignant; confirming the long-held belief that cellular immortalization is a key attribute of cancer cells (Elenbaas et al., 2001; Hahn et al., 1999). Although telomerase activity appears to be the preferred way cancer cells stabilize their telomeres, 10% to 15% of human cancer cases lack detectable telomerase activity. At least a subset of these, particularly certain CNS tumors and some cancers of mesenchymal origin, maintain their telomeres via a telomerase-independent genetic recombination pathway known as *alternative lengthening of telomeres (ALTs)* (Heaphy et al., 2011; Reddel, 2003). With the exceptions of nonseminomatous testicular germ cell tumors (15%), chromophobe renal cell carcinoma (9%) and small cell carcinoma of the bladder (23%), ALT is rarely if ever observed in common GU malignancies (Heaphy et al., 2011). However, almost all tissue samples assayed for ALT thus far have been from primary tumors. Interestingly, despite a lack of ALT in more than 1000 primary prostate cancers examined, ALT was found in all distant metastases assayed in a single patient with lethal prostate cancer. In this case, detailed genomic analysis indicated that ALT was acquired during the transition from local to disseminated growth, raising the intriguing possibility that ALT may play a role in advanced disease (Haffner et al., 2013).

Several studies have reported on telomerase activity in clinical prostate samples with positivity ranging from 47% to 100%, whereas normal and BPH tissues taken from prostates without evidence of cancer are typically negative for telomerase activity (Caldarera et al., 2000; Engelhardt et al., 1997; Kallakury et al., 1997; Kamradt et al., 2003; Kim et al., 1994; Koeneman et al., 1998; Lin et al., 1997; Sommerfeld et al., 1996; Wullich et al., 1999; Zhang et al., 1998). Although two of these studies found a positive correlation between either the presence or level of telomerase activity and tumor grade, four other studies found no correlation with grade, stage, or preoperative PSA levels. However, the number of cases in many of these studies was small.

Telomerase Activity as a Potential Diagnostic Marker

The high prevalence and relatively strong activity found in prostate cancers compared with normal tissue plus the very high sensitivity of the standard telomerase activity assay have led to evaluation of the telomerase activity assay as a potential diagnostic marker for cancer. Unfortunately, the potential utility of aiding cancer diagnosis appears limited, primarily because of problems with false-negative and false-positive results seen with the technically demanding telomerase activity assay. False-negative results may occur as a result of inactivation of the labile enzyme during isolation, whereas false-positive results may stem from the presence of inflammatory cells in the sample (Meeker and Coffey, 1997). In addition, other molecular cancer biomarkers often outperform telomerase. For example, the detection of telomerase components by RT-PCR in urine provides some improvement in the sensitivity and specificity over urine cytology in bladder cancer detection, particularly in low-grade disease (Eissa et al., 2007). However, a review of the literature on urinary molecular markers for bladder cancer detection concluded that other markers (e.g., microsatellites, FISH, and Cytokeratin 20) outperform telomerase (van Rhijn et al., 2005).

In an intriguing study, Wu et al. (2003) found that shorter **telomeres in peripheral blood leukocytes (PBLs), as measured with telomere-specific Q-PCR, were associated with increased risk for a number of cancers, including bladder and renal cancer.** Similar associations between short telomeres and bladder cancer risk were observed when comparing telomere lengths measured in buccal cells and PBL (Broberg et al., 2005; McGrath et al., 2007). **In contrast, no association was observed between PBL telomere length and prostate cancer risk in a recent study** (Mirabello et al., 2009). The variations in the PBL telomere lengths measured in these studies are thought to be due to inherited interindividual differences in telomere lengths modified by changes occurring postnatally, perhaps because of diet and lifestyle factors.

Potential Prognostic Value of Telomere Length in Prostate Cancer

Telomere shortening is predictive of poor prognosis in several cancers, including those of the lung, endometrium, and breast and neuroblastoma (Bisoffi et al., 2006; Griffith et al., 1999; Hiyama et al., 1995a; Hiyama et al., 1995b; Smith and Yeh, 1992). A potential link between telomere length and prostate cancer prognosis was first reported by Donaldson et al. In this retrospective case-control study, biochemical recurrence and overall survival were significantly correlated with tumor telomere content, a surrogate for telomere length. Specifically, all 7 prostatectomy patients whose tumor telomeric DNA contents were less than that of control samples (placental DNA) showed evidence of biochemical recurrence (elevated PSA) within 10 years after surgery (Donaldson et al., 1999). Of the 9 patients in this study with short tumor telomeres, 7 died within 10 years, in contrast to 100% 10-year survival for patients with normal-to-long tumor telomeres. In addition, these patients also showed no evidence of biochemical recurrence. Potential drawbacks of this study include a small sample size (18 cases; only 7 of 9 men in the short telomere category underwent surgery), and the fact that it was not known whether the deaths observed were due specifically to prostate cancer.

In a more recent retrospective study using 77 prostatectomy samples and a more sensitive chemiluminescent slot blot assay, Fordyce et al. (2002) reported that less-than-normal telomere content in primary prostate cancers was associated with recurrence, independent of patient age, grade (Gleason sum), and regional lymph node status (Fordyce et al., 2005). The magnitude of the relative hazard for disease recurrence associated with low telomere content (RH = 5.02) was on par with that of Gleason grade and nodal status. Interestingly, a positive correlation was found between telomere content of the tumor and that of the surrounding normal-appearing prostate tissue within the same prostatectomy samples. An association was also found between telomere content of these normal-appearing prostate tissues and 72-month recurrence-free survival. The authors postulated that telomere loss in morphologically normal tissue represents areas at heightened risk of experiencing genetic instability. This is reminiscent of the so-called "field effect" phenomenon that has long been discussed in the cancer literature (Bostwick et al., 1998; Crissman et al., 1993; Foster et al., 2000; Yu et al., 2004). The authors further proposed that cancers arising in such areas may show greater genotypic and phenotypic heterogeneity and thus be more prone to behave aggressively because of a greater level of chromosomal instability caused by short telomeres (Fordyce et al., 2005; Heaphy et al., 2013). Finally, in a recent prospective population-based study of prostate cancer using telomere-specific FISH, it was found that short telomeres in tumor-associated stroma cells as well as greater cell-to-cell variability in telomere length among cancer cells were associated with higher risk of death resulting from prostate cancer. These associations were found to be largely independent of other traditional poor prognostic indicators and the risk associations were essentially additive, such that men with the shortest stromal telomeres and most variable cancer telomeres had a 14-fold increased risk of dying from their cancer compared with men with the longest stromal telomeres and the least variable cancer cell telomeres (Heaphy et al., 2013).

Telomerase-Based Opportunities for Therapy

Given that the majority of human tumors rely on telomerase for immortalization and genomic stabilization, this enzyme is an attractive target for anticancer therapy. There are two overall strategic paradigms for therapeutic targeting of telomerase in cancer. The first involves taking advantage of the tumor's dependence on telomerase enzymatic activity for survival. This strategy includes approaches aimed at directly inhibiting telomerase enzymatic activity or blocking its expression. The second approach attempts to exploit the fact that the telomerase gene *(HTERT)* promoter is selectively active in cancer cells, for example, by using the telomerase promoter to drive oncolytic virus or gene therapy vectors to limit their replication or expression to tumor cells or by directing immunotherapy against cells expressing hTERT protein.

Many of these approaches have undergone preclinical testing using prostate cancer cell lines and xenografts, and some are currently in early clinical trials. One point of concern with antitelomerase therapies has to do with the question of selectivity of action against tumor cells over normal telomerase-positive cells, such as the stem cells of the hematopoietic system and those within tissues with high turnover rates. This is of particular importance for those approaches in which telomerase-positive cells are actively targeted for destruction, including immunotherapy, gene therapy, and oncolytic viral therapies. Encouragingly, work to date describing the treatment of human tumor xenografts in mice have, in general, not produced major toxicity in normal tissues.

KEY POINTS: TELOMERES AND TELOMERASE

- Telomeres contain stretches of terminal, noncoding, repetitive DNA that cap the ends of each chromosome, thereby stabilizing them.
- Telomere DNA repeats are progressively lost as cells divide and as a result of oxidative DNA damage at the telomeres.
- Normal cells monitor their telomere lengths and permanently exit the cell cycle (cellular senescence) or commit suicide (apoptosis) in tumor suppressive responses to telomere shortening. This telomere length checkpoint involves TP53 and RB1.
- Loss of telomere length checkpoints leads to critical telomere shortening, which initiates chromosomal instability contributing to cancer initiation.
- Most cancers and premalignant lesions have abnormally short telomeres.
- Most cancers express the enzyme telomerase that restabilizes the telomeres and allows unlimited cell division potential (immortalization); thus telomerase represents an attractive therapeutic target.

APOPTOSIS

Apoptosis, also known as programmed cell death, is a tightly regulated process used by multicellular organisms to eliminate **unwanted cells.** For example, apoptosis is used in tissue remodeling during development and in the immune system to eliminate self-reactive T cells (Ashkenazi and Dixit, 1998; Kerr et al., 1972). **Apoptosis contrasts sharply with necrosis, a nonprogrammed form of cell death** in which cells that are acutely injured (e.g., by physical trauma) swell and burst, abruptly releasing their contents, and act as potent inducers of the inflammatory response. **Apoptosis is a more orderly, energy-requiring process in which the dying cell's contents are degraded and neatly packaged into so-called apoptotic bodies, which are then engulfed by neighboring cells or macrophages; a process that does not elicit a strong inflammatory response** (Fadok et al., 1992).

Apoptosis and Cancer

Unlike unicellular organisms, cancer poses a risk to multicellular life forms; thus a variety of potentially tumorigenic abnormalities can signal a cell to eliminate itself as a potential threat via apoptosis. For example, if a cell suffers DNA damage (potentially mutagenic) but fails to make repairs, it will be eliminated and replaced from the organism's pool of undamaged cells. Therefore it is not surprising that aberrations of apoptosis can be detrimental and that failure of dividing cells to initiate apoptosis contributes to cancer (Ashkenazi and Dixit, 1998).

Abnormalities in the apoptotic machinery have implications for malignancy beyond an individual cell's ability to respond appropriately to cell physiologic stresses such as DNA damage. First, **the apoptosis cascade is critical to the immune system's ability to eliminate cancer cells by inducing them to undergo apoptosis** (Nagata, 1997). This has clear implications for the organism's intrinsic immune surveillance for malignancy and the tumor's response to extrinsic immunotherapy. Second, because cytotoxic cancer therapies also depend in large part on inducing apoptosis, **defects in the apoptotic cascade can profoundly influence tumor responses to chemotherapy and radiotherapy** (Minn et al., 1995; Thornberry and Lazebnik, 1998; Walton et al., 1993).

Apoptosis, an Evolutionarily Conserved Process

Apoptosis is tightly regulated by an evolutionarily conserved system of positive and negative signals, the balance of which determines whether the cell will undergo apoptosis. These signals ultimately converge upon an important family of proteases called caspases ("cysteine proteases with aspartic acid specificity"), key components of the apoptotic machinery (Thornberry, 1998). Caspases, of which there are at least 13, are **broadly categorized as either initiator caspases (e.g., caspases-8, 9 and 10) or executioner caspases (e.g., caspases-3, 6, and 7). Caspases are synthesized as larger, inactive forms called procaspases, which require specific proteolytic cleavage to become active proteases themselves.** Often a procaspase is activated by another caspase, setting in motion a sequential, amplifying, proteolytic cascade. **Initiator caspases begin the cascade that ultimately leads to activation of executioner caspases downstream. Once activated, the executioner caspases attack several intracellular protein targets.** Executioner caspases cleave antiapoptotic proteins, such as Bcl-2 and Bcl-XL, which not only destroy their anti-apoptotic function but also actually release proapoptotic carboxyl-terminal fragments, further stimulating cell death (Wolf and Green, 1999). Executioner caspases then target proteins critical to cell survival. Cleavage of DNA repair and replication proteins, such as DNA-PKcs and replication factor C, leads to nuclear dysregulation. Nuclear structural proteins, such as lamins NuMa and SAF-A, are fragmented, contributing to dissolution of the nucleus and nuclear condensation, a hallmark of apoptosing cells. Proteolysis of cytoskeletal proteins such as keratin and actin lead to destruction of the internal structural integrity of the cell. Last, cleavage of proteins critical to cell-cell interaction, such as beta-catenin and focal adhesion kinase, precipitates the specific and irreversible phenotypic changes associated with apoptosis (Orth et al., 1996; Wen et al., 1997; Wolf and Green, 1999). **The end result is a stereotypical death in which the cytoplasm shrinks, the cell membrane blebs, and the nuclear chromatin condenses.**

The entire apoptotic process can be completed in just 60 minutes (Thornberry and Lazebnik, 1998).

Additional details of the intrinsic and extrinsic apoptotic pathways can be found online at ExpertConsult.com.

Role of TP53 in Apoptosis

In addition to the key roles played by TP53 in cell cycle arrest and DNA damage repair, TP53 can also induce apoptosis (May and May, 1999). TP53-induced apoptosis is mediated through the Bcl-2 family, via the intrinsic pathway, and dysregulation of this apoptotic pathway has direct relevance to the cause of cancer. TP53-induced apoptosis is mediated by transcriptional activation of genes that initiate the apoptotic cascade and inhibition of genes that block the cascade (Miyashita et al., 1994; Miyashita and Reed, 1995; Oda et al., 2000). TP53-induced apoptosis is dependent on the Apaf-1/caspase-9 activation pathway (Soengas et al., 1999). Whereas the Bcl-2 family member Bax has been implicated as the primary factor responsible for TP53 induction of this cascade (Miyashita and Reed, 1995), Bax is not essential for TP53-dependent apoptosis (Knudson et al., 1995). It is possible that inhibition of Bcl-2 (Miyashita et al., 1994) or upregulation of the proapoptotic Bcl-2 family member noxa may allow cells lacking Bax to still undergo TP53-dependent apoptosis (Oda et al., 2000).

Considering TP53's role in multiple tumor-suppressive pathways (DNA damage response, cellular senescence, and apoptosis), it is not surprising that it is so frequently mutated in cancer.

Apoptosis and Genitourinary Malignancies

Because a tumor cell's inability to undergo apoptosis is a hallmark of malignancy, multiple groups have attempted to characterize the apoptotic response of genitourinary malignancies. Because cells undergoing apoptosis exhibit a stereotypical death, global analysis of apoptosis is possible using assays designed to detect key hallmarks of the apoptotic process, such as the fragmentation of DNA characteristic of the process, as well as assays designed to detect abnormalities in specific apoptotic proteins.

Global Defects in Apoptosis

HGPIN and prostate carcinoma actually have significantly higher levels of apoptosis than normal prostatic epithelium. The level of apoptotic activity is relatively low compared with other malignancies and is opposed by increased replication. Importantly, many prostate cancer cells can be induced to undergo apoptosis in response to androgen withdrawal, which represents a front-line therapy for patients with advanced disease (Denmeade and Isaacs, 1996; Isaacs, 1994; Kyprianou et al., 1990; Tu et al., 1996). Unfortunately, clearly not all of a patient's cancer cells succumb, as recurrences inevitably arise. As the tumor progresses to androgen independence, it is unclear if the androgen-resistant cells have an increased or decreased rate of apoptosis, because studies have demonstrated both in hormone-refractory disease (Berges et al., 1995; Koivisto et al., 1997). The conflicting data may reflect the tumor's dynamics and the effect of therapy. There is a clear survival advantage for the advanced cancer cell that can protect itself from apoptosis. However, **a rapidly growing, infiltrative, advanced tumor, which is outgrowing its blood supply and mutating its DNA, may have a high apoptotic rate in spite of protective mechanisms the tumor's cells have acquired.**

Studies of apoptosis in bladder carcinoma have demonstrated an association with aggressive high-grade advanced disease but not with decreased disease-free survival (King et al., 1996; Lipponen and Aaltomaa, 1994). External-beam radiation therapy has been associated with a modest improvement in survival for tumors with high apoptotic rates. This may reflect the fact that external-beam radiation therapy requires an intact apoptotic mechanism to be effective (Rodel et al., 2000).

As previously mentioned, **most testicular germ cell tumors maintain intact DDR and wild type TP53, thus display high cure rates in response to therapies that induce DNA damage** (Bartkova et al., 2007; Einhorn, 2002; Gorgoulis et al., 2005; Kersemaekers et al., 2002).

Individual members of the apoptotic machinery have been frequently studied. However, all studies are unable to assay all elements of the apoptotic machinery simultaneously and therefore to globally assess the tumor's ability to undergo programmed cell death.

TP53 mutations and abnormalities in expression are among the most frequent in cancer and have been identified in prostate, bladder, and renal cancers (Hollstein et al., 1991; Reiter et al., 1993; Sidransky et al., 1991). Abnormalities in TP53 cause dysregulation of the cell cycle and DNA repair mechanisms in addition to apoptosis and are covered in more detail in the section Cell Cycle.

Bcl-2 family members have been studied in genitourinary malignancies. **Elevated levels of Bcl-2 have been identified in the majority of hormone-refractory prostate tumors, reflecting the tumor's relative resistance to apoptosis in the advanced state** (Colombel et al., 1993; McDonnell et al., 1992). Increased and decreased levels of Bcl-2 have been identified in localized prostate tumors, and few studies have found a correlation with grade, stage, and progression (Byrne et al., 1997; Lipponen and Vesalainen, 1997; Theodorescu et al., 1997). Other antiapoptotic members of the Bcl-2 gene family, Bcl-X_L and Mcl1, may also be linked to prostate carcinoma (Krajewska et al., 1996). Analysis of bladder carcinoma has demonstrated similar results. Bcl-2 levels are higher in more aggressive bladder carcinoma, but expression of Bcl-2 had no effect on treatment outcome (King et al., 1996; Rodel et al., 2000). As noted earlier, phosphorylation of Bad by Akt can also tilt the scales toward cell survival, especially in concert with elevated levels of Bcl-2. Akt activation is commonly seen in many urologic malignancies and can result from loss of the tumor suppressor PTEN, mutation and constitutive activation of PI3 kinase, and/or activation of tyrosine kinase receptors such as HER2/NEU, EGFR, and the insulin-like growth factor receptor (IGFR).

Other Bcl-2 family members have not been as well studied. Loss of Bax expression is apparently not a common mechanism for the development of prostate carcinoma (Johnson and Hamdy, 1998; Krajewska et al., 1996) but may play a role in progression of localized bladder carcinoma (Ye et al., 1998).

In summary, deficiencies in signal transduction pathways leading to apoptosis clearly play a role in the initiation and progression of malignancy. It is unclear if expression analysis of the apoptotic machinery will provide additional prognostic information from traditional histochemical analysis. However, it is clear that effective chemotherapy and radiation therapy is in large part dependent on apoptosis. In addition, in the future the apoptotic machinery may be manipulated using novel ligands that bind to death receptors and promote TP53-independent cancer cell death.

Alternative Regulators of Apoptosis in Genitourinary Malignancies

In addition to the classic regulators of apoptosis, a number of other pathways for cell survival and death have been uncovered that play key roles in urologic cancer. Some of these pathways are being actively explored as targets for cancer therapy. The Vancouver group has mapped out a detailed gene profile of prostate tumors treated with neoadjuvant hormonal ablation therapy to identify key regulators of cell death and survival after castration. In addition to Bcl-2, which is upregulated in surviving cancer cells, they have also reported on clusterin and Hsp27. **Clusterin, or testosterone-repressed prostate message-2, is upregulated in patient samples after hormone ablation as well as in the Shionogi and CWR-22 xenograft models of hormone-sensitive tumors. Although its precise function is not known, a large body of evidence suggests that clusterin is induced by stress and functions to stabilize the cell during periods of stress** (Miyake et al., 2000). In this model, clusterin is believed to act like HSPs, whose role as a protein chaperone is also to stabilize client proteins. Clusterin is activated by heat shock protein 1 (HSP1). Functional evidence of clusterin's role comes from studies in which clusterin is either overexpressed or knocked down using antisense strategies. In the first scenario, clusterin expression promotes hormone-refractory cell growth and prevents androgen withdrawal–induced apoptosis. In the second scenario, treatment of hormone-refractory cells with antisense clusterin promotes apoptosis (Gleave and Miyake, 2005; July et al., 2002; Miyake et al., 2004). This same group of investigators has also reported that the heat shock protein HSP27 is also frequently overexpressed in hormone-refractory prostate cancers. Similar experiments using overexpression and antisense strategies have suggested that targeting HSP27 may influence the course of hormone-refractory cancers, in particular in combination with cytotoxic chemotherapies (Rocchi et al., 2004).

Another family of cellular signaling molecules that play a role in the regulation of cell survival and apoptosis is the sphingolipids. Sphingolipids are one of three major constituents of the cell membrane, along with phospholipids and cholesterol. **Sphingolipid generation is regulated by a large cast of enzymes, notably the sphingomyelinases, ceramide synthase, and the ceramidases.** Ceramide is produced from sphingomyelin by sphingomyelinase and from sphinganine by ceramide synthase. Ceramidases, on the other hand, degrade ceramide and lead to formation of sphingosine and sphingosine-1-phosphate. Ceramide is a potent proapoptotic molecule that can promote apoptosis through the classical mitochondrial activation of caspases or through a nonclassical caspase-independent form of apoptosis (Kolesnick and Fuks, 2003). Sphingosine-1-phosphate, in contrast, is a powerful antiapoptotic molecule that may modulate the degree of apoptosis like a rheostat (Maceyka et al., 2002).

The importance of ceramide to genitourinary tumors is that it appears to be a key modulator of radiation-induced tissue damage and apoptosis. As with clusterin and other heat shock proteins, ceramide appears to be a critical mediator of stress response in cells, in this case promoting apoptosis as opposed to cell survival. Studies supporting ceramide's role in radiation-induced apoptosis are manifold, including studies demonstrating the direct cell death signal induced by exogenous treatment of cells with ceramide, studies of radiation response in mouse knockout models, and studies of radiation response in the presence and absence of inhibitors of sphingolipid metabolism. It is hoped that therapeutics that increase ceramide production and promote apoptosis can be developed. The role of sphingolipid-1-phosphate has also emerged from these studies, and recent work suggests that this molecule is a promising target for cancer therapy (Gulbins and Kolesnick, 2003; Kester and Kolesnick, 2003; Perry and Kolesnick, 2003).

STEM CELLS AND CANCER

Stem cells are found in multicellular organisms and are characterized by the ability of self-renewal through mitotic cell division and differentiation into a diverse range of specialized cell types. **Common properties of stem cells include the ability of self-renewal, generation of cellular progeny, localization within specialized niches, and the ability to give rise to all cell types within an organ.** For example, human prostate stem cells are believed to be localized within the basal epithelium and give rise to a hierarchy of progenitor cells that may differentiate into secretory or neuroendocrine cells (Burger et al., 2005; Xin et al., 2005).

Recent studies suggest that neoplastic cells mimic normal tissue development and may arise from and are dependent on a small population of stem cells. **The cancer stem cell hypothesis argues that cancers arise from transformation of stem or progenitor cells that are capable of multilineage differentiation.** Cancer stem cells may account for only a small percentage of any tumor, but this small population of cells is critical for tumor survival. The most readily accepted experimental demonstration of cancer stem cells relies on serial transplantation of tumor cell populations isolated based on one or numerous putative cancer stem cell markers into immune deficient mice or 3D culture systems and recapitulation of the heterogeneous primary tumor. Using this experimental strategy, initial evidence to support the cancer stem cell hypothesis was discovered in leukemia, breast, and neurologic cancers. For example, a CD44+/CD24low/- population of cells in primary breast tumors were specifically capable of new tumor formation when engrafted into nude mice (Al-Hajj et al., 2003; Dontu et al., 2003). Similar reports in glioblastoma suggest that a CD133 positive population as the putative stem cell (Dirks, 2005; Singh et al., 2003). One challenge to the field of cancer stem cell research is the lack of any one marker that is exclusively expressed by cancer stem cells. For any given tumor type, typically many different markers can be identified that confer a cancer stem cell phenotype, and absence of the marker does not always imply that a cell is not a cancer stem cell. For example, in glioblastoma, CD133+ and CD133- cell populations have been shown to possess cancer stem cell-like properties (Beier et al., 2007).

A tumor-initiating cell (T-IC) subpopulation has also been identified in human bladder cancer. This group of cells was found to express CD44+/CK5+/CK20- markers similar to normal bladder basal cells (Chan et al., 2009). The bladder T-IC subpopulation was also capable of forming xenograft tumors in vivo that recapitulated characteristics of the original tumor. Furthermore, CD47 was highly expressed in this group of cells and blockade of CD47 resulted in macrophage engulfment of bladder cancer stem cells in vitro. This finding suggests a potential role for therapeutic targeting of CD47 and the T-IC subpopulation in bladder cancer (Chan et al., 2009). A number of other putative cancer stem cell populations have been identified in bladder cancer, including CK17+/67LR+/CAECAM- cells, embryonic stem cell marker *POU5F1+* cells, and high aldehyde dehydrogenase activity (ALDH^{hi}) cells (reviewed in van der Horst et al., 2012).

CHECKPOINT INHIBITION

Programmed cell death protein 1 (PD-1 or CD279) is a cell surface receptor involved with downregulation of the immune system and

KEY POINTS: APOPTOSIS

- Apoptosis is a rapid, orderly programmed form of cell death that is used by multicellular organisms to eliminate unwanted cells.
- Apoptosis is believed to play an important role in tumor suppression because many of the signals that induce apoptosis arise from potentially tumorigenic cell stresses such as DNA damage.
- Cancer is characterized by interruptions in the normal process of apoptosis, resulting in inappropriate cell survival.
- Apoptosis is mediated by a conserved family of proteases known as caspases. Initiator caspases start caspase proteolytic cascades terminating in the activation of executioner caspases which target several cellular proteins.
- Two main apoptotic pathways have been identified. In the intrinsic pathway, Bcl-2 family members modulate the release of cytochrome c from the mitochondria, which participates in the activation of initiator caspases. The extrinsic pathway activates caspases in response to signals from extracellular "death receptors."
- In addition to its functions in cell cycle arrest and DNA repair, TP53 plays a key role in apoptosis.
- Bcl-2 is a classic inhibitor of the mitochondrial pathway of apoptosis and is overexpressed in some genitourinary malignancies.
- Therapeutic response is often dependent upon the integrity of apoptotic pathways in the cancer cells. Most TGCTs retain intact DDR, wild type TP53 and apoptotic responses, providing high cure rates with DNA damaging agents.
- Novel agonists and antagonists of apoptosis, such as ceramide and clusterin, may successfully be controlled to combat cancer.

> **KEY POINTS: STEM CELLS AND CANCER**
>
> - Stem cells are defined by their ability to differentiate along multiple lineages and their immortality.
> - Cancer is believed to be a stem cell disease in which a small population of cancer stem cells maintains the larger tumor.
> - Cancer may ultimately be eradicated by targeting only the cancer stem cell.

promotes self-tolerance by suppressing T-cell inflammatory activity (Pardoll, 2012). **The PD-1 pathway limits immune activity, resulting in decreased autoimmunity and cytokine secretion.** The 2 ligands for PD-1, PD-L1, and PD-L2 are cell surface glycoproteins within the B7 family of costimulatory and coinhibitory molecules. In the PD-1 pathway, antigen is typically presented to T cells by tumor cells or antigen-presenting cells (APCs) via expression of MHC molecules. PD-1 receptor is expressed on the T-cell surface in response to activation of the T-cell receptor complex. The T-cell mediated immune response is inhibited by the interaction of PD-L1 and PD-L2 ligands on APCs and tumor cells with PD-1 receptors.

PD-L1 is highly expressed in several cancer types, and the PD-1/PD-L1 pathway may be exploited by cancer cells to evade the immune system. Expression of PD-L1 by cancer cells is associated with an immunosuppressive phenotype that allows for tumor evasion. **Inhibition of the interaction between PD-1 and PD-L1 can enhance T-cell response and mediate antitumor activity. This is phenomenon is known as immune checkpoint blockade.** Blockade of the PD-1/PD-L1 interaction has been used for various malignancies, including metastatic urothelial carcinoma with significant response rates.

The utility of PD-1/PD-L1 blockade for treatment of bladder cancer has been investigated in several clinical trials. In an open-label, phase 3 trial of 542 patients with advanced urothelial cancer that recurred or progressed after platinum-based chemotherapy, treatment with pembrolizumab (antibody against PD-1) was associated with a median overall survival of 10.3 months compared with 7.4 months for patients treated with chemotherapy (Bellmunt et al., 2017). No significant difference was observed between groups with respect to progression-free survival or among patients who had a tumor PD-L1 combined positive score of ≥ 10%. Fewer treatment-related adverse events were observed among patients treated with pembrolizumab compared with patients treated with chemotherapy.

A multicenter, phase 2 study evaluated atezolizumab (anti PD-L1 antibody) as first-line therapy in a cohort of previously untreated patients with locally advanced or metastatic urothelial carcinoma who were cisplatin ineligible (Balar et al., 2017). Objective and complete response rates of 23% and 9% were observed among 119 patients treated with atezolizumab in the first-line setting, respectively. Median progression-free and overall survival was 2.7 and 15.9 months, respectively. **Atezolizumab shows potential as a first-line treatment option for patients who are not able to receive cisplatin-based chemotherapy.** Biomarker data was also validated in this study linking intrinsic TCGA subtypes and mutational load with immunotherapy response.

Expression of PD-L1 has also been evaluated as a prognostic marker for bladder cancer with mixed results. Increased expression of glycoprotein B7-H3 in bladder cancer may be an early event in upregulation of PD-1 (Boorjian et al., 2008). Expression of T-cell coregulators B7-H1, B7-H3, and PD-1 were evaluated in paraffin-embedded sections from 318 consecutive patients with urothelial carcinoma who underwent radical cystectomy. Expression of B7-H3 was significantly increased compared with adjacent, nontumor urothelium. Increased B7-H3 expression was independent of tumor stage and expression of B7-H1 by tumors and PD-1 by tumor infiltrating lymphocytes was significantly associated with increased pathologic stage.

The utility of checkpoint inhibitor therapy has also been investigated in RCC. Nivolumab is a fully human IgG4 programmed death 1 (PD-1) immune checkpoint inhibitor antibody that selectively blocks interaction between PD-1 and PD-L1 (and PD-L2). Previous studies have shown that PD-L1 expression is associated with a poor prognosis in RCC (Thompson et al., 2004). **A randomized, open-label, phase 3 study comparing nivolumab with everolimus in patients with RCC who received previous treatment demonstrated improved overall survival and fewer severe adverse events with nivolumab therapy** (Motzer et al., 2015). Whole exome sequencing of metastatic clear cell RCC has also been performed to identify genomic alterations that correlate with response to anti-PD-1 therapy. **In a cohort of 35 patients, loss-of-function mutations in PBRM1 were associated with clinical benefit** (Miao et al., 2018). This observation was confirmed in a validation cohort of 63 patients with clear cell RCC treated with PD-L1 blockade.

> **KEY POINTS: CHECKPOINT INHIBITION**
>
> - The PD-1 pathway limits immune activity resulting in decreased autoimmunity and cytokine.
> - Inhibition of the interaction between PD-1 and PD-L1 can enhance T-cell response and mediate antitumor activity.
> - PD-1/PD-L1 blockade for treatment of advanced or metastatic bladder cancer has demonstrated efficacy as first-line treatment for cisplatin-ineligible patients.
> - Nivolumab has been shown to improve overall survival with fewer adverse events compared with everolimus in patients with RCC who received previous treatment.
> - Loss-of-function mutations in PBRM1 were associated with clinical benefit among patients with metastatic clear cell RCC who received anti-PD-1 therapy.

MICROBIOME AND CANCER: THE METAGENOME

Modern sequencing tools have allowed for a greater understanding of the molecular genetics of a previously less well recognized part of the human body that may nevertheless greatly influence cancer development, progression, and response to therapy: **the metagenome** (the genetic material comprising the human-associated microbiota). **Recent years have seen an explosion of studies aimed at characterizing the human microbiome (the environment, including the microbiota, any proteins or metabolites they make, their metagenome, as well as host proteins and metabolites in this environment) in health and disease.** One area of particular interest is the effect that the microbiome has on cancer. This effect may be through direct interactions at the site of cancer development in cancers with a known microbial cause (such as gastric and cervical cancer), as well as indirect interactions such as regulation of the immune system, effects on metabolism, and effects on cancer therapies. In many cases, direct and indirect interactions with the microbiome are in play.

Direct interactions of the microbiome with cancer include the induction of chronic inflammation by pathogenic microbes that drives cellular proliferation and DNA damage responses, direct genotoxicity (e.g., by bacteria-produced genotoxins [Balskus, 2015]), and the introduction of oncogenes (such as virally encoded oncogenes). **Of keen interest to the study of GU cancers is the recent discovery of a urinary microbiome.** Recent evidence has challenged the long-held clinical dogma that urine is "sterile" and found that urine contains microorganisms (e.g., bacterial, viral, fungal, protozoan) that are representative of a distinct flora in the urinary tract, including the urethra and the bladder (Whiteside et al., 2015). The urinary microbiome has been overlooked in the past partially because of reliance on standard urine culture and clinical microbiology practices that are not suitable for culturing most urinary microbiota. Slight changes to culture conditions, such as using anaerobic and aerobic culture and extending the length of culture time, increases the efficacy of detecting resident bacterial flora in the urine (Hilt et al., 2014). Although the urinary tract shares species with adjacent niches such as the skin and vaginal flora, the evidence suggests that the urinary microbiome is distinct to the other sites of the human body that harbor microbiota. There is not yet definitive evidence linking the urinary microbiome to the development and/or progression of genitourinary cancers; however, this is currently an area of active study in bladder cancer, prostate cancer, and other cancers (Alfano et al., 2016, Shrestha et al., 2018).

Indirect effects of the microbiome (e.g., the effects of the gastrointestinal [GI] microbiota on cancer at a distant anatomic site) on tumorigenesis are less understood and could include modulation of antitumor immune responses and effects on host metabolism (Schwabe and Jobin, 2013). Importantly, evidence is also emerging to indicate that the GI microbiota can exert a profound influence on the efficacy of certain cancer treatments, including chemotherapy and immunotherapy (Jobin, 2018). As with direct interactions, there are only a few published studies examining indirect interactions between the microbiome and genitourinary cancers; however, several compelling studies are emerging in the field of kidney cancer. One recent study demonstrated that the **GI microbiota composition, and specifically the presence of the mucin degrading bacterium *Akkermansia muciniphila*, predicts response to anti-PD-1 targeted immunotherapy in RCC** and other epithelial tumors (Routy et al., 2018). **Importantly, Routy et al. also demonstrated that T-cell activation stimulated by *Akkermansia* was related to patient response to anti-PD-1 treatment.** Studies in RCC have also shown a relationship between the GI microbiota and the symptoms of diarrhea after receiving vascular endothelial growth factor (VEGF)-tyrosine kinase inhibitors (Pal et al., 2015). Finally, **there is also recent evidence that antibiotic use (that would alter/abolish the GI flora) diminishes the effectiveness of immunotherapy in RCC** (Routy et al., 2018).

KEY POINTS: MICROBIOME AND CANCER

- The clinical dogma that urine is sterile has been challenged by studies describing distinct microbiota present in urine that are representative of species residing within the urinary tract. These microorganisms would have previously been under- or unrecognized using standard clinical microbiology culture techniques.
- Direct interactions between the urinary microbiome and genitourinary cancer development or progression is now an area of active study.
- Indirect interactions between the microbiome, such as the GI microbiota, and genitourinary cancers is also an area of active research. The GI microbiota may have a strong influence on treatment response and/or related toxicities to cancer therapies.

SUGGESTED READINGS

Ames BN, Gold LS: The causes and prevention of cancer: the role of environment, *Biotherapy* 11:205–220, 1998.
Blackburn EH: Telomeres, *Trends Biochem Sci* 16:378–381, 1991.
DePinho RA: The age of cancer, *Nature* 408:248–254, 2000.
Fearon ER: Human cancer syndromes: clues to the origin and nature of cancer, *Science* 278:1043–1050, 1997.
Feinberg AP: The epigenetics of cancer etiology, *Semin Cancer Biol* 14:427–432, 2004.
Greider CW: Telomerase activity, cell proliferation, and cancer, *Proc Natl Acad Sci USA* 95:90–92, 1998.
Guttmacher AE, Collins FS: Genomic medicine—a primer, *N Engl J Med* 347:1512–1520, 2002.
Hahn WC, Counter CM, Lundberg AS, et al: Creation of human tumour cells with defined genetic elements, *Nature* 400:464–468, 1999.
Hanahan D, Weinberg RA: The hallmarks of cancer, *Cell* 100:57–70, 2000.
Hanahan D, Weinberg RA: Hallmarks of cancer: the next generation, *Cell* 144:646–674, 2011.
Hartwell L, Weinert T, Kadyk L, et al: Cell cycle checkpoints, genomic integrity, and cancer, *Cold Spring Harb Symp Quant Biol* 59:259–263, 1994.
Jones PA, Baylin SB: The fundamental role of epigenetic events in cancer, *Nat Rev Genet* 3:415–428, 2004.
Jones PA, Baylin SB: The epigenomics of cancer, *Cell* 128:683–692, 2007.
Kaelin WG Jr: Molecular basis of the VHL hereditary cancer syndrome, *Nat Rev Cancer* 2:673–682, 2002.
Kastan MB, Bartek J: Cell-cycle checkpoints and cancer, *Nature* 432:316–323, 2004.
Massague J: G1 cell-cycle control and cancer, *Nature* 432:298–306, 2004.
Rebbeck TR, Spitz M, Wu X: Assessing the function of genetic variants in candidate gene association studies, *Nat Rev Genet* 5:589–597, 2004.
Reya T, Morrison SJ, Clarke MF, et al: Stem cells, cancer, and cancer stem cells, *Nature* 414:105–111, 2001.
Sancar A, Lindsey-Boltz LA, Unsal-Kacmaz K, et al: Molecular mechanisms of mammalian DNA repair and the DNA damage checkpoints, *Annu Rev Biochem* 73:39–85, 2004.
Sjoblom T, Jones S, Wood LD, et al: The consensus coding sequences of human breast and colorectal cancers, *Science* 314:268–274, 2006.
Vogelstein B, Papadopoulos N, Velculescu VE, et al: Cancer genome landscapes, *Science* 339:1546–1558, 2013.
Watson J, Crick F: Molecular structure of nucleic acids: a structure for deoxyribose nucleic acid, *Nature* 171:737–738, 1953.

REFERENCES

The complete reference list is available online at ExpertConsult.com.

PART VI Reproductive and Sexual Function

63 Surgical, Radiographic, and Endoscopic Anatomy of the Male Reproductive System

Parviz K. Kavoussi, MD, FACS

A fundamental comprehension of male genital anatomy is necessary for understanding normal reproduction as well as pathology and treatment options. This chapter provides a general anatomic framework of the surgical, radiographic, and endoscopic anatomy of the normal male reproductive system. Because this chapter is dedicated solely to the anatomy of the male reproductive system, please refer to Chapter 109 for further description of pelvic anatomy, including bones, soft tissue, circulation, and innervation of the pelvis not directly related to reproduction.

TESTIS

Gross Structure

The testicles are paired organs within the scrotum that have reproductive and endocrine functions. It is common for the right testis to hang lower than the left in approximately 85% of men. **The dimensions of the normal testis include a length of 4 to 5 cm, a width of 3 cm, and a depth of 2.5 cm; the testis normally has a volume of 15 to 25 mL.** The organ is ovoid and white (Prader, 1966; Tishler, 1971). There is a small, pedunculated or sessile body at the upper pole of the testis, which is known as the appendix testis. A tough capsule envelops the testis, composed from external to internal of the visceral tunica vaginalis, the tunica albuginea, and the tunica vasculosa, before reaching the parenchyma of the testis. The tunica albuginea is composed of smooth muscle cells that pass through collagenous tissue (Langford and Heller, 1973). It is believed that these smooth muscle cells provide the testicular capsule with some ability to contract and may affect arterial flow into the testis. They may also promote the flow of seminiferous tubule fluid on its way out of the testis (Davis and Horowitz, 1978; Rikmaru and Shirai, 1972; Schweitzer, 1929). The testis attaches to the epididymis on the posterolateral aspect of the testis (Figs. 63.1 and 63.2).

Microanatomic Architecture

The tunica albuginea invaginates into the testis to form the mediastinum testis, where vessels and ducts traverse the testicular capsule. The mediastinum testis sends septa that attach to the inner surface of the tunica albuginea to form 200 to 300 cone-shaped lobules, each of which contains one or more convoluted seminiferous tubules. Each lobule contains a centrifugal artery. Seminiferous tubules are coiled and long, with both ends typically ending in the rete testis. The seminiferous tubules contain germ cells and supporting cells, including Sertoli cells, fibrocytes, and myoid cells of the basement membrane. Each seminiferous tubule is U-shaped, but if a seminiferous tubule were stretched out from its convoluted form, each would measure nearly 1 m in length. **Each seminiferous tubule in the normal testis contains developing germ cells. The testosterone-producing Leydig cells are interdispersed in the loose tissue around the seminiferous tubules.** The interstitial tissue includes Leydig cells, mast cells, macrophages, nerves, blood vessels, and lymphatic vessels. This interstitial tissue makes up a total of 20% to 30% of the testicular volume (Setchell and Brooks, 1988). Sertoli cells line the seminiferous tubules and rest on the tubular basement membrane. The cellular characteristics of Sertoli cells include a low mitotic index, prominent nucleoli, and nuclei with irregular shapes. There are strong, tight junctions between the Sertoli cells, which compartmentalize the seminiferous tubular space into adluminal and basal spaces (Fig. 63.3). The seminiferous tubules straighten and become tubuli recti toward the apex of each lobule, where they enter the mediastinum testis and anastomose with a network of tubules lined by flattened epithelia. This tubular network is the rete testis and forms 12 to 20 efferent ductules that anastomose into the caput of the epididymis. At this point, the efferent ductules convolute, enlarge, and form conical lobules. Each lobule produces a duct that drains into a single epididymal duct. The epididymal duct would be approximately 6 m in length if it were stretched out. It winds within the epididymis to form the body and the tail of the epididymis, all of which are surrounded by a fibrous sheath. The thickening and straightening of the duct forms the vas deferens as it reaches the tail of the epididymis (Figs. 63.4 and 63.5).

Arterial Supply

There are three arterial supplies to the testis: the testicular (internal spermatic) artery, the artery of the vas deferens (deferential artery), and the cremasteric (external spermatic) artery (Harrison and Barclay, 1948). **The testicular artery is the main blood supply to the testis, and its diameter is greater than the deferential and cremasteric arteries combined** (Raman and Goldstein, 2004). The testicular artery arises from the abdominal aorta and descends in the intermediate stratum of the retroperitoneum to enter the internal inguinal ring. From its aortic origin, it crosses the psoas muscle and the ureter to reach the inguinal ring to enter the spermatic cord. As the testicular artery descends toward the testis, it branches into an internal artery and an inferior testicular artery and into a capital artery to the caput epididymis. There may be variation at the level of this branching, which has been found to occur within the inguinal canal in 31% to 88% of cases (Beck et al., 1992; Jarow et al., 1992). In 56% of cases, a single artery enters the testis. In 31% of cases, there are two branches, and in 13% there are three or more branches of this artery (Kormano and Suoranta, 1971). Arterial anastomosis occurs at the head of the epididymis, allowing for a rich blood supply between the testicular and capital arteries. At the tail of the epididymis, arterial anastomoses are formed between the testicular, epididymal, cremasteric, and vasal arteries. The testicular arteries pass into the mediastinum testis and supply the tunica vasculosa in the anterior portion of the upper pole of the testis and the anterior, medial, and lateral portions of the lower pole of the testis. Therefore care must be taken not to devascularize the testis by passing a traction suture through the lower pole, as well as by performing testis biopsies in the medial or lateral surfaces of the upper pole to minimize the risk of vascular injury. The middle of the testis has fewer vessels than the upper or lower poles. The deferential artery derives from the internal iliac artery or from the superior vesical artery. The cremasteric artery

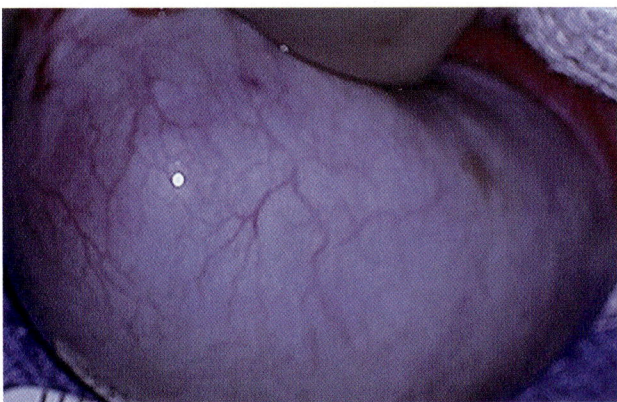

Fig. 63.1. The appearance of the testis with its shiny tunica albuginea layer.

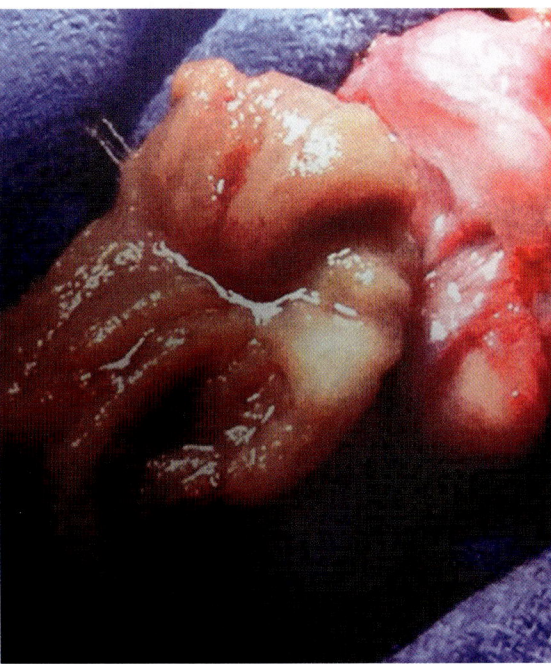

Fig. 63.2. The appearance of the testicular parenchyma when bivalved. The white nodule at the right inferior margin represents a sarcoid nodule.

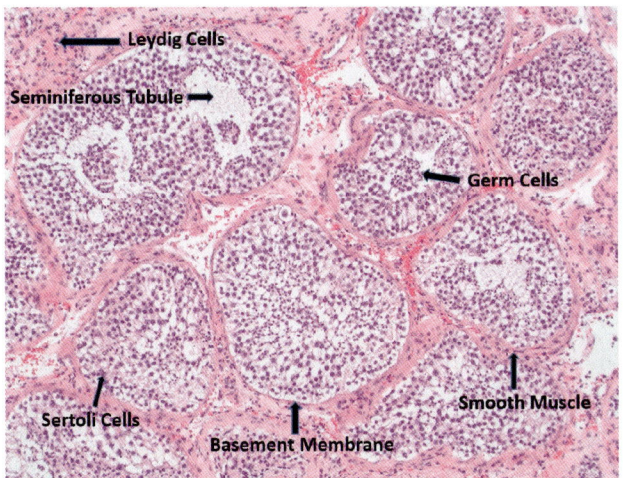

Fig. 63.3. Testicular microanatomic architecture with Leydig cells, seminiferous tubules, germ cells, Sertoli cells, basement membrane, and smooth muscle labeled at 10× magnification. (Courtesy Xiao Yun Wang, MD.)

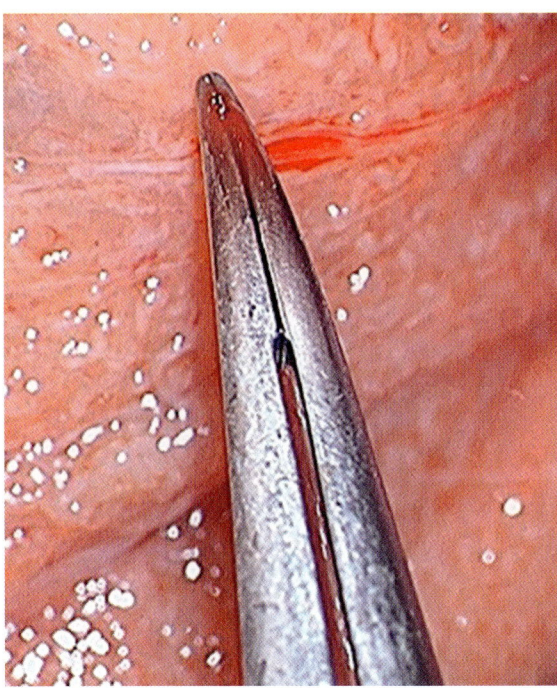

Fig. 63.4. Appearance of the seminiferous tubules under magnification.

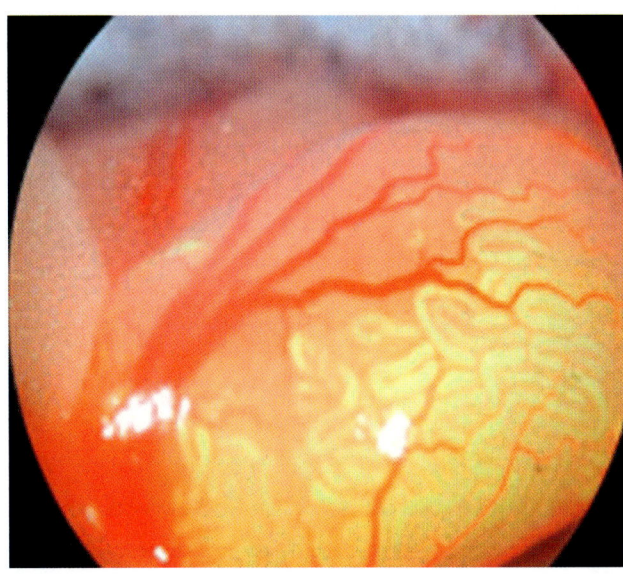

Fig. 63.5. Microbeads injected retrograde through the rete testis into the seminiferous tubules demonstrating the tubular structure. This is a mouse testis that has very similar architecture to the human testis. (Courtesy Jeffrey Lysiak, PhD.)

derives from the inferior epigastric artery and primarily supplies the tunica vaginalis, but it has branches going to the testis. Centrifugal arteries, which are the individual arteries supplying the seminiferous tubules, pass within the septa containing the seminiferous tubules and branch into arterioles that ultimately become intertubular and peritubular capillaries (Muller, 1957). Although in the case of testicular artery ligation, the deferential and cremasteric arteries can potentially provide adequate blood supply to the testis, atrophy and/or azoospermia has resulted from testicular artery ligation in adults and children. Men who have undergone vasectomy deserve special attention in preserving the testicular artery in future surgeries such as varicocelectomy because of the risk of having had the deferential artery compromised at the time of vasectomy (Lee et al., 2007; Figs. 63.6 and 63.7).

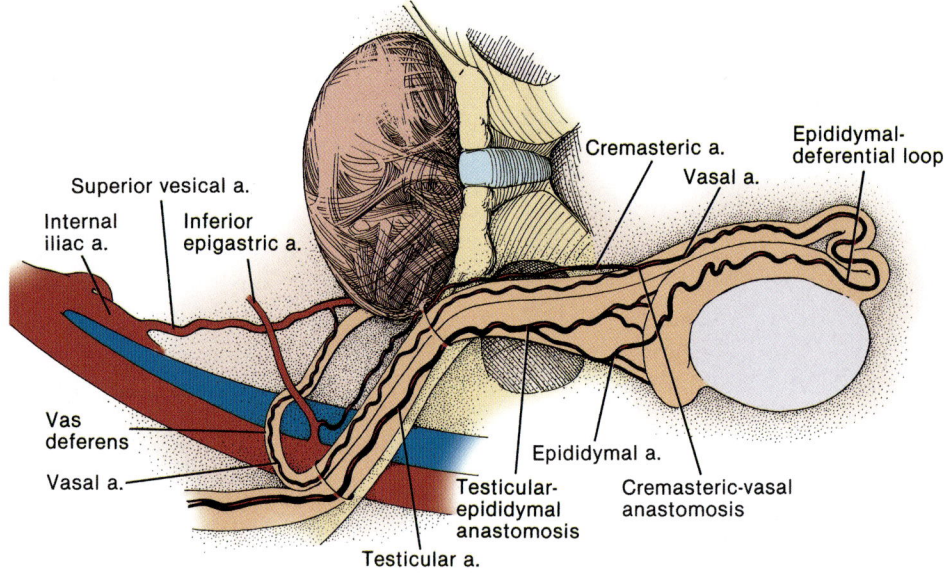

Fig. 63.6. Collateral arterial circulation to the testis. (From Hinman F Jr: *Atlas of urosurgical anatomy*, Philadelphia, 1993, Saunders, p 497.)

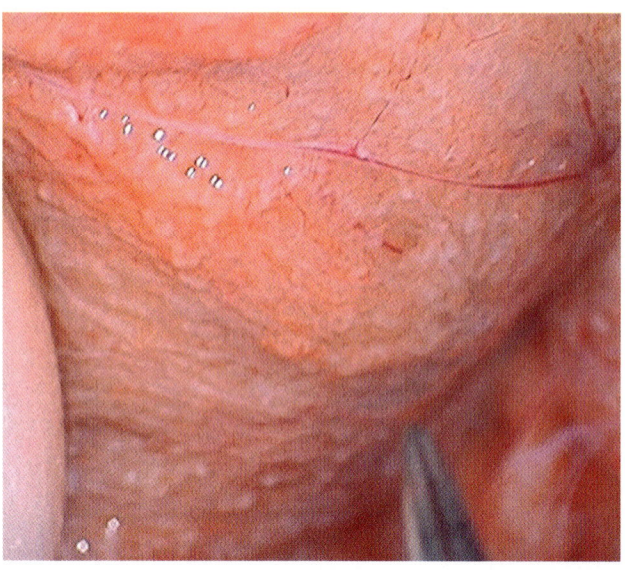

Fig. 63.7. Microsurgical view of arterial supply to the testicular parenchyma.

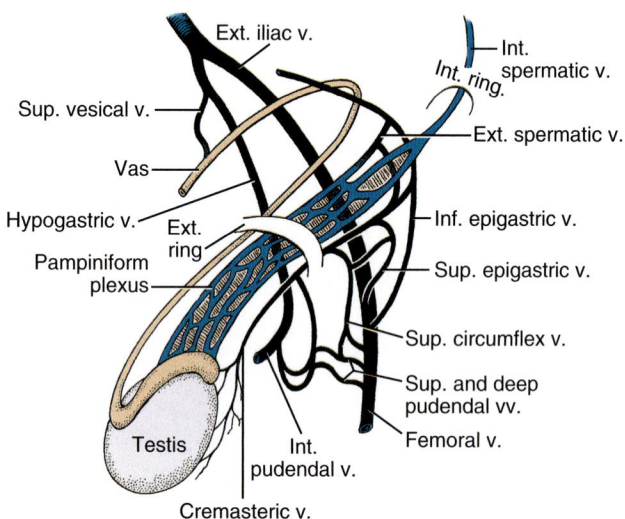

Fig. 63.8. Venous drainage of the testis and epididymis. Note connections between the pampiniform plexus and the saphenous, internal iliac, and external iliac veins.

Venous Drainage

Unlike most other venous patterns in the human body, veins within the testis do not travel with their corresponding arteries. Small parenchymal veins drain into either a group of veins near the mediastinum testis or veins on the surface of the testis (Setchell and Brooks, 1988). These two groups of veins anastomose with each other and the deferential veins to form the pampiniform plexus. The pampiniform plexus is a network of testicular veins that anastomose as they ascend surrounding the testicular artery. This allows for a countercurrent heat exchange that cools the blood flow within the testicular artery. Ultimately, these veins join to form two or three veins at the level of the inguinal canal, and then they form one vein that ascends to drain into the inferior vena cava on the right and into the renal vein on the left side. There may be variations where the testicular veins can anastomose with the external pudendal, cremasteric, and vasal veins; this can allow varicocele ablations to result in recurrence (Figs. 63.8 and 63.9).

Lymphatic Drainage

Lymphatic channels from the testis drain into the para-aortic and interaortocaval lymph nodes. These lymphatic channels ascend within the spermatic cord after leaving the testis (Hundeiker, 1969; Fig. 63.10).

Nerve Supply

Visceral innervation to the testis and epididymis arise in the renal and aortic plexuses and course alongside the gonadal vessels. This is autonomic innervation; the testis does not have any known somatic innervation (Mitchell, 1935). The pelvic plexus, in association with the vas deferens, offers additional gonadal afferent and efferent nerves (Rauchenwald et al., 1995). Three distinct anatomic distributions of nerves have been isolated within the spermatic cord and are thought to be the primary contributors in men with chronic orchialgia. These include a perivasal complex, posterior periarterial/

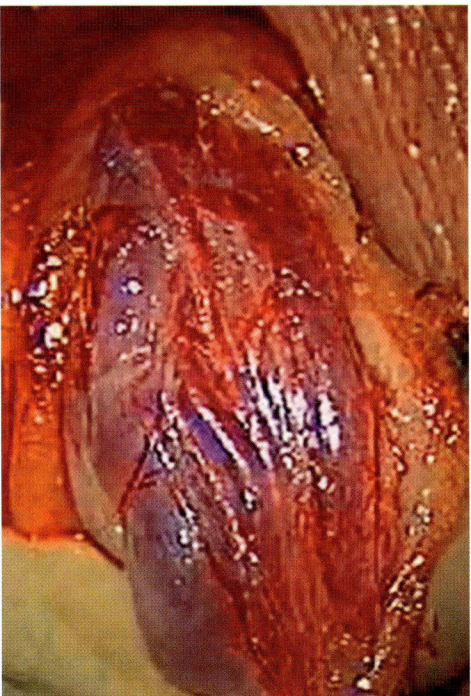

Fig. 63.9. Microsurgical view of the veins of the pampiniform plexus during varicocele ligation through a subinguinal approach.

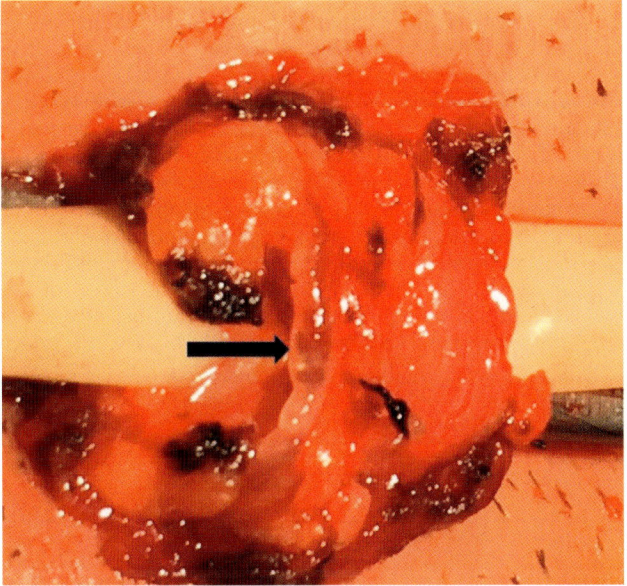

Fig. 63.10. Microsurgical view of a lymphatic channel *(arrow)* as it travels through the spermatic cord as identified during a subinguinal microsurgical varicocele repair.

lipomatous complex, and intracremasteric complex (Parekattil et al., 2013). Some afferent and efferent nerves cross over to the contralateral pelvic plexus (Taguchi et al., 1999). This may account for pathology in one testis affecting the function of the contralateral testis, which has been reported with varicoceles and testicular tumors. **The genital branch of the genitofemoral nerve primarily supplies sensation to the parietal and visceral tunica vaginalis and the overlying scrotum.** These nerves travel along the testicular artery to reach the testis. These nerves ramify within the tunica albuginea but do not enter the seminiferous tubules. Nerves are absent from the seminiferous epithelium.

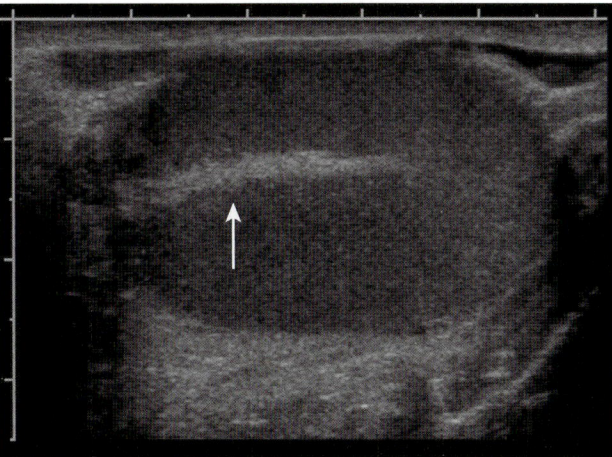

Fig. 63.11. Testis ultrasound image demonstrating rete testis *(arrow)*.

Blood-Testis Barrier

The fluid passing from the seminiferous tubules and exiting from the testis has been found to have a substantially different fluid composition than that of blood plasma or lymphatics. This suggests that compounds do not freely diffuse to and from the tubules, indicating that a barrier exists, which is known as the blood-testis barrier (Setchell and Waites, 1975). There are extremely strong, tight junctions between Sertoli cells, which provide an intracellular barrier that allows for spermatogenesis in an immune privileged site. This is the barrier known as the blood-testis barrier (Ewing et al., 1980). This accounts for the anatomic component of the blood-testis barrier. The functional component is further discussed in Chapter 64.

Ultrasonography

Ultrasonography is the primary imaging modality used to interrogate the scrotum and its contents. Scrotal ultrasound uses high-frequency transducers (7.5 to 10 MHz), gray-scale real-time techniques, as well as color flow and power Doppler. The patient is placed in the supine position and a coupling gel is used with the transducer probe on the scrotal skin. The normal scrotal wall is 3 to 4 mm thick and is hypoechoic. An anechoic area between the echogenic scrotal wall and testicle is commonly visualized, which represents a small amount of physiologic fluid between the visceral and parietal layers of the tunica vaginalis. The mediastinum testis is visualized posteriorly as an echogenic band parallel to the epididymis. It may have variable lengths and thicknesses dependent on each patient's physiology (Dogra et al., 2003). **The echo pattern of the normal testis is fine, uniform, with a medium-level echo pattern.** Sonographically, the normal testis measures approximately 5 cm × 3 cm × 2 cm (Dogra et al., 2001). Color Doppler can identify testicular vessels in the majority of patients (Spirnak and Resnick, 2002). Waveforms from intratesticular arteries and testicular capsular arteries demonstrate consistently low-impedance patterns with high levels of diastolic flow. This represents the lower vascular resistance of the testis. Supratesticular arteries are also sonographically identifiable and show low-impedance waveforms from the testicular, deferential, and cremasteric arteries (Middleton et al., 1989; Figs. 63.11 and 63.12).

Magnetic Resonance Imaging

Ultrasonography is the primary imaging modality of the testis; however, magnetic resonance imaging (MRI) can be used to image the testis as a secondary imaging modality. The normal structures of the scrotum can be depicted clearly and the tunica albuginea can be easily differentiated from the testis parenchyma and the epididymis. MRI can distinguish intratesticular from extratesticular lesions and differentiate between solid and cystic lesions. Complicated and simple fluid collections can be differentiated (Rholl et al., 1987). Delineation of normal and pathologic structures greater than 1 mm is possible. An advantage of MRI is the ability to image both hemiscrota in one imaging plane as well as the inguinal region (Hajek, 1987). Magnetic resonance angiography (MRA) has also been performed for the evaluation of the nonpalpable testis and has identified inguinal testicular nubbin tissue (Eggener et al., 2005).

> **KEY POINTS: TESTIS**
>
> - The seminiferous tubules contain developing germ cells.
> - The Leydig cells produce testosterone.
> - There are three arterial supplies to the testis, including the testicular artery, deferential artery, and cremasteric artery.
> - Lymphatic channels from the testis drain into the para-aortic and interaortocaval lymph nodes.
> - The nerves contributing to chronic orchialgia include a perivasal complex, posterior periarterial/lipomatous complex, and intracremasteric complex.
> - Tight junctions between Sertoli cells make up the anatomic component of the blood-testis barrier.
> - Ultrasonography is the primary imaging modality for intrascrotal content.

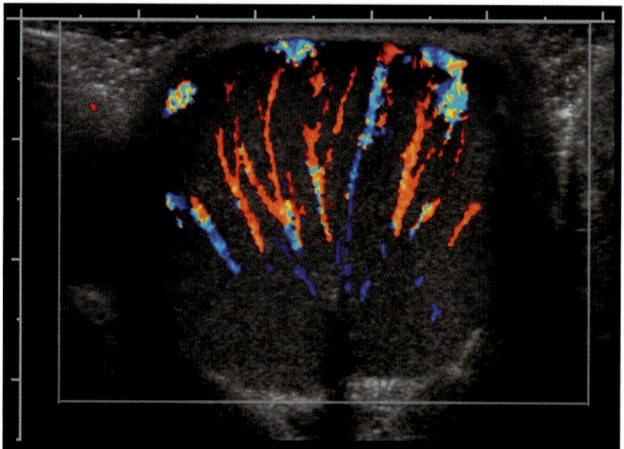

Fig. 63.12. Doppler ultrasound image of testis demonstrating spokelike radiation of testicular vessels originating from the mediastinum testis.

EPIDIDYMIS

Gross Structure

The epididymis is a duct or tubule that is attached to the posterolateral aspect of the testis and is nearest to the testis at its upper pole. Its lower pole is connected to the testis with fibrous tissue. The epididymis is comma shaped. The epididymis is tightly coiled and encapsulated within the tunica vaginalis sheath and would measure 3 to 4 m in length if stretched out (Turner et al., 1978; Von Lanz and Neuhaeuser, 1964). Septa form by extensions of the tunica vaginalis sheath into interductal spaces that divide the duct into histologically characteristic areas (Kormano and Reijonen, 1976). The three areas are characterized as the caput (head), the corpus (body), and the cauda (tail) of the epididymis. Eight to 12 ductuli efferentes from the testis make up the caput epididymis. The caput epididymis is connected to the testis by multiple efferent ducts. The tightly coiled duct, which makes up the epididymis, is continuous with the vas deferens at the most distal portion of the cauda epididymis. Adjacent to the testis, this duct is irregularly shaped and comparatively large. The duct becomes more narrow and concentric near the junction with the ductus epididymis. The duct diameter remains unchanged throughout the corpus epididymis. The diameter of the duct enlarges and becomes irregular in shape in the cauda epididymis. The duct then progresses distally to form the vas deferens. A cystic body on the upper pole of the caput epididymis, which may be pedunculated or sessile, is known as the appendix of the epididymis (Figs. 63.13 through 63.15).

Microanatomic Architecture

There are two primary types of cells throughout the epididymis: principal cells and basal cells (Holstein, 1969; Vendrely, 1981). From caput to cauda, the height of the epithelium decreases, whereas the diameter of the ductus and lumen increases. There are stereocilia that shorten progressively from the proximal to the distal epididymis. In the proximal epididymis, these stereocilia measure 120 μm in height and decrease to 50 μm in the distal epididymis. The principal cells contain elongated nuclei that are commonly clefted, and they contain one or two nucleoli. As the principal cells have absorptive and secretive functions, the apex of each of these cells contains multiple coated pits, membranous vesicles, multivesicular bodies, micropinocytic vesicles, and an extensive Golgi apparatus (Vendrely and Dadoune, 1988). There is a much larger number of principal cells in the epididymal epithelium than the number of basal cells that exist there. The basal cells are interdispersed between the principal

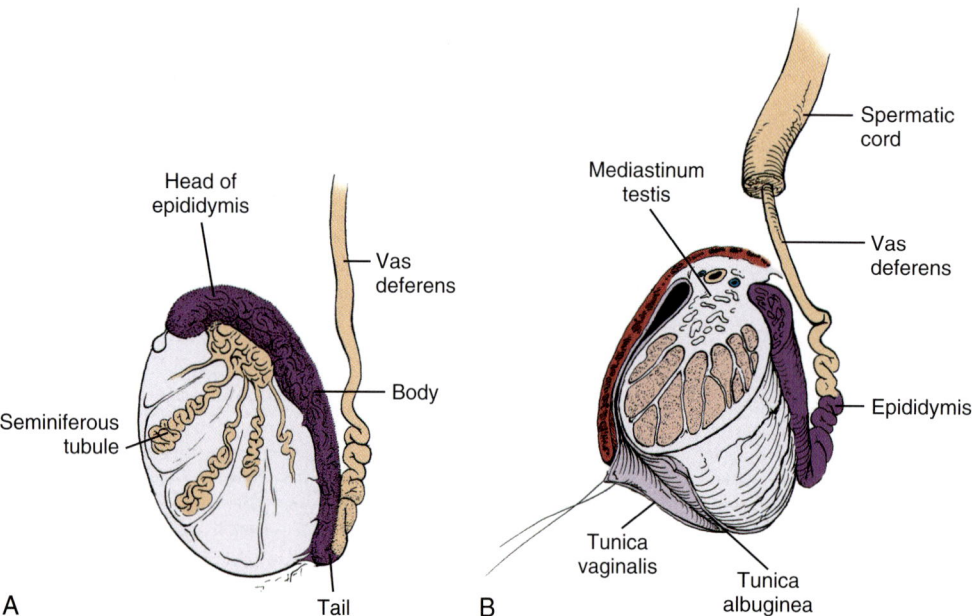

Fig. 63.13. Testis and epididymis. (A) One to three seminiferous tubules fill each compartment and drain into the rete testis in the mediastinum. Twelve to 20 efferent ductules become convoluted in the head of the epididymis and drain into a single coiled duct of the epididymis. The vas is convoluted in its first portion. (B) Cross section of the testis, showing the mediastinum and septations continuous with the tunica albuginea. The parietal and visceral tunica vaginalis are confluent where the vessels and nerves enter the posterior aspect of the testis.

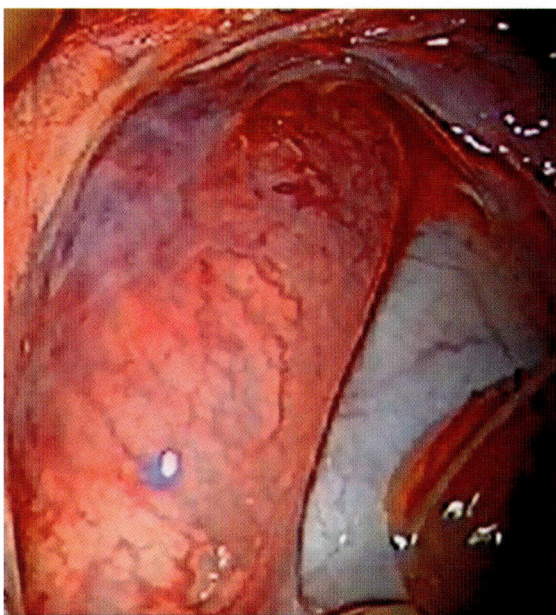

Fig. 63.14. Gross microsurgical appearance of the epididymal caput and corpus.

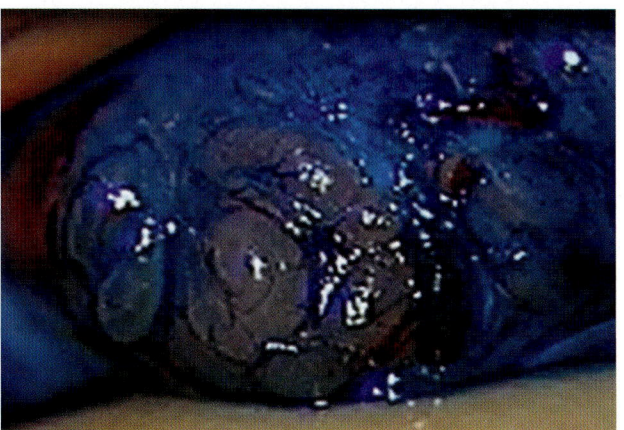

Fig. 63.15. Microsurgical appearance of the epididymal duct after being stained with methylene blue.

cells. The basal cells are tear-shaped. They are positioned on the basal lamina and are 25 µm in length as they reach up toward the lumen. As opposed to the morphology of the principal cells, which varies throughout the epididymis, the basal cells' shape remains relatively consistent throughout the entirety of the epididymis. The basal cells are believed to be derived from macrophages and to be precursors of principal cells. There is a fair amount of variability in the nature of the epithelium of the epididymis, which is dependent on the region. There is a clear transition from a low to a high cuboidal epithelium where the rete testis and ductuli efferentes meet. The ductuli efferentes contain ciliated and nonciliated cells and the epithelium appears uneven (Holstein, 1969). The epithelium of the proximal ductuli efferentes primarily consists of nonciliated cells with extending apices thought to be for secretory function. The ciliated cells conduct sperm cells from the efferent duct to the epididymis, and they are widely dispersed throughout the epithelium (Vendrely, 1981). Junctional complexes join ciliated and nonciliated cells together at their apices, suggesting a blood-epididymis barrier (Hoffer and Hinton, 1984; Suzuki and Nagano, 1978; Turner, 1979). In the ductuli efferentes, the proximal corpus epididymis, and the distal caput epididymis there are contractile cells around the tubule in a loose, two- to four-cell–deep layer (Baumgarten et al., 1971). Nexus-like junctions connect these contractile cells, and each cell contains myofilaments. These cells are larger and appear like thin smooth muscle cells in the distal corpus epididymis, where they have fewer intracellular junctions. Thick smooth muscle cells are found in the cauda epididymis. The smooth muscle cells are organized in three layers. The cells have a longitudinal orientation in the two outer layers and a circular orientation in the central layer. The thickness of the distal contractile layer progressively increases as it forms the vas deferens.

Arterial Supply

A branch of the testicular artery supplies the caput and corpus epididymis. This arterial branch then further divides to supply the superior and inferior epididymal branches (Macmillan, 1954). **The deferential artery also provides vascular supply to the epididymis.** Branches from the deferential artery supply the cauda epididymis. As with the testis, the deferential and cremasteric arteries also supply the epididymis and can compensate for a ligated testicular artery. The connective tissue sheaths forming septa in the epididymis are the entry points for arterial supply within the epididymis. The coiled vessels ultimately straighten to form the microvascular bed within the epididymis (Kormano and Reijonen, 1976). The density of the microvasculature decreases progressively, with the caput containing the highest density of microvasculature and the more distal segments containing lower density (Clavert et al., 1981).

Venous Drainage

The corpus and cauda epididymis have their venous drainage through the vena marginalis of Haberer, draining into the pampiniform plexus via the vena marginalis testis, or through deferential or cremasteric veins (Macmillan, 1954).

Lymphatic Drainage

Similar to that of the testis, the caput and corpus epididymis have their lymphatic drainage through channels that travel with the internal spermatic vein, draining to the preaortic nodes. Lymphatic channels from the cauda epididymis join those leaving the vas deferens to drain ultimately into the external iliac nodes.

Nerve Supply

The superior portion of the hypogastric plexus and the pelvic plexus yield the intermediate and inferior spermatic nerves, respectively, which innervate the epididymis (Mitchell, 1935). Fibers from the sympathetic nervous system sparsely innervate the proximal portion of the epididymis as well as the ductuli efferentes (Baumgarten and Holstein, 1967; Baumgarten et al., 1971). These fibers form a peritubular plexus that is adjacent to the vasculature. The corpus epididymis includes sparse numbers of nerve fibers, and the density of nerve fibers increases progressively traveling toward the cauda epididymis. The density of fibers begins to increase at the midcorpus of the epididymis and the progressive increase in fibers is associated with the progressive proliferation of smooth muscle cells (Baumgarten et al., 1971).

Ultrasonography

The epididymis can be visualized ultrasonographically in its posterolateral position to the testis. **The epididymis appears either hyperechoic or isoechoic in comparison with the testis** (Spirnak and Resnick, 2002). Compared with the testis, the caput epididymis is typically isoechoic, the corpus epididymis is hypoechoic, and the vas deferens is anechoic (Puttemans et al., 2006). The epididymis is typically homogeneous, with well-defined echoes surrounding the epididymis that represent the fascial lining (Black and Patel, 1996). By sonographic measurement, the normal caput epididymis diameter measures between 10 mm and 12 mm, and the normal corpus

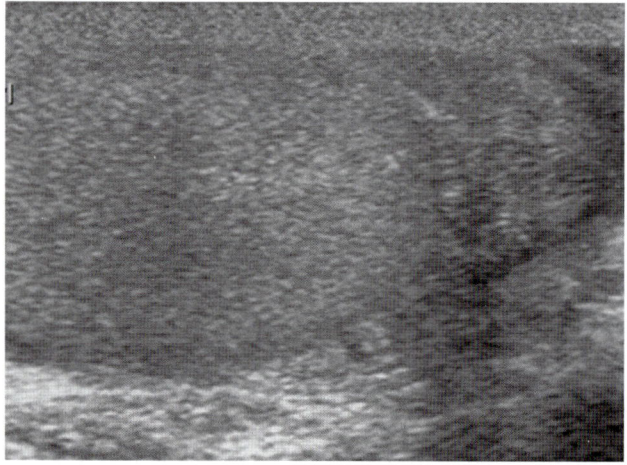

Fig. 63.16. Ultrasound imaging of the caput epididymis, which appears hyperechoic to the testis and is at the right of the testis on this image.

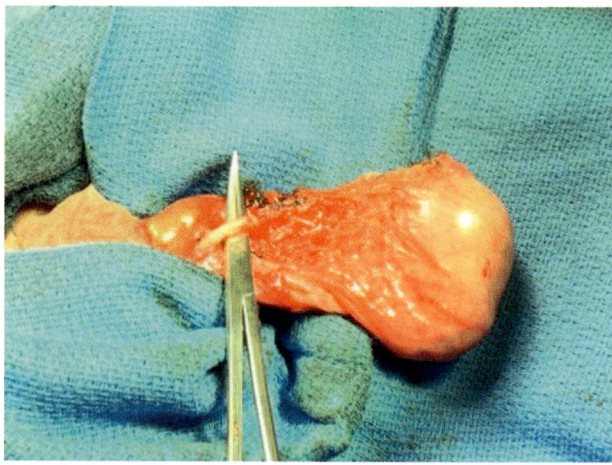

Fig. 63.17. Gross appearance of the vas deferens positioned in the posterior spermatic cord.

epididymis measures between 2 mm and 5 mm (Pezzella et al., 2013). In 98% of men, the caput epididymis is above the upper pole of the testis, with the corpus epididymis typically lateral to the testis. The corpus epididymis is posterior to the body of the testis in 6% of men. The epididymis is inverted with the caput epididymis inferior to the lower pole of the testis in 2.4% of men (Puttemans et al., 2006). The appendix epididymis can be identified as an isoechoic structure attached to the caput epididymis (Black and Patel, 1996). Vascular flow is detectable with pulsed Doppler and color Doppler in all regions of the epididymis in nonpathologic states. The mean resistive index throughout the normal epididymis is approximately 0.55 (Keener et al., 1997; Fig. 63.16).

Magnetic Resonance Imaging

Ultrasonography is the primary modality of imaging of the epididymis, but MRI can be used as an adjunct to image the epididymis. Differences in signal intensity allow for clear delineation of the epididymis with high-resolution MRI (Baker et al., 1987).

> **KEY POINTS: EPIDIDYMIS**
> - The two primary cell types throughout the epididymis are principal cells and basal cells.
> - The arterial supply to the caput and corpus epididymis is from a branch of the testicular artery and the cauda is supplied from deferential arterial branches.

VAS DEFERENS

Gross Structure

The vas deferens, also known as the ductus deferens, extends from the distal end of the cauda epididymis. It is tubular and its embryologic origin is the mesonephric (wolffian) duct. The vas deferens is tortuous for 2 to 3 cm as it leaves the epididymis (the convoluted vas deferens), after which it becomes the straight vas deferens. From the cauda epididymis to its termination at the ejaculatory duct, the vas deferens measures between 30 and 35 cm in length. **The vas deferens travels posteriorly along the spermatic cord, behind the vessels in the cord. The vas deferens passes through the inguinal canal and enters the pelvis lateral to the epigastric vessels** (Fig. 63.17). On entering the pelvis, after passing through the internal inguinal ring, the vas deferens separates from the testicular vessels. The vas deferens ultimately reaches the posterior base of the prostate after traveling

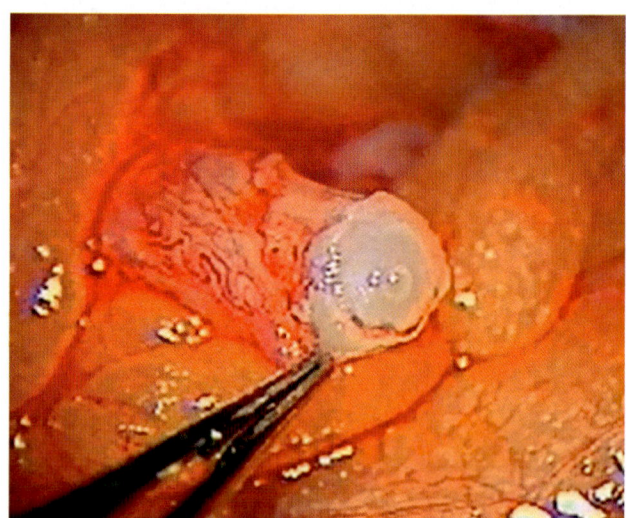

Fig. 63.18. Microsurgical appearance of the transected vas deferens at the time of vasovasostomy.

medial to the pelvic sidewall. The vas deferens is compartmentalized into five different regions. The first is the epididymal segment within the tunica vaginalis, which does not have a sheath. The second is the segment within the scrotum. The third segment is that within the inguinal canal. The fourth is the retroperitoneal segment, and the fifth is the ampulla of the vas deferens (Lich et al., 1978). **The lumen of the vas deferens ranges between 0.2 and 0.7 mm in diameter, depending on the segment.** The outer diameter of the vas deferens ranges between 1.5 and 2.7 mm (Middleton et al, 2009; Figs. 63.18 and 63.19).

Microanatomic Architecture

There is an outer adventitial connective tissue layer surrounding the vas deferens that contains blood vessels and small nerves. Within this connective tissue layer, smooth muscle cells compose the thick wall of the vas deferens. These smooth muscle cells are organized as an inner and outer longitudinal layer, a middle circular layer, and a pseudostratified columnar epithelial layer with nonmotile stereocilia as the inner lining, known as its mucosa (Neaves, 1975; Paniagua et al., 1981). The epithelial cell height decreases progressively throughout the length of the vas deferens from the testis to the seminal vesicle. There are three types of tall, thin columnar cells, as well as basal

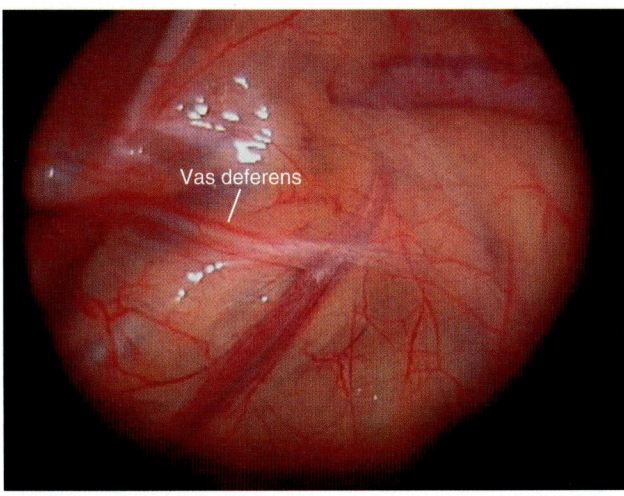

Fig. 63.19. Laparoscopic visualization of the vas deferens.

> **KEY POINTS: VAS DEFERENS**
> - The lumen of the vas deferens ranges between 0.2 and 0.7 mm in diameter, depending on the segment.
> - The superior vesical artery gives off the deferential artery, which supplies the vas deferens.
> - A vasogram should be performed only in conjunction with reconstructive surgery.

cells, making up the pseudostratified epithelium of the vas deferens (Hoffer, 1976; Paniagua et al., 1981). Principal cells, pencil cells, and mitochondria-rich cells make up the columnar cells that extend from the epithelial base to the lumen. The columnar cells have irregularly shaped convoluted nuclei and have stereocilia. In the proximal vas deferens, principal cells are the predominant cell type. Traveling more distally throughout the vas deferens, more pencil cells and mitochondria-rich cells are present. The muscular layer of the vas deferens progressively decreases from proximal to distal.

Arterial Supply

The superior vesical artery gives off the deferential artery, which supplies the vas deferens (Sjostrand, 1965).

Venous Drainage

The venous drainage of the scrotal vas deferens is via the deferential vein, which drains into the pampiniform plexus. The pelvic vas deferens' venous drainage is to the pelvic venous plexus.

Lymphatic Drainage

Lymphatic drainage from the vas deferens travels to the external and internal iliac nodes.

Nerve Supply

The vas deferens receives sympathetic and parasympathetic innervation (Sjostrand, 1965). The sympathetic adrenergic nerves travel via the presacral nerve from the hypogastric nerve (Batra and Lardner, 1976; McConnell et al., 1982). All three layers of the vas deferens tunica muscularis contain adrenergic fibers, but the greatest density of these nerve fibers is found in the outer longitudinal layer (McConnell et al., 1982). Other types of neurotransmitters have been identified within neurons, such as somatostatin, galanin, enkephalin, neuropeptide Y, vasoactive intestinal peptide, and nitric oxide. The function of these neurotransmitters in the vas deferens is not well understood (Dixon et al., 1998).

Vasogram

The vasogram was previously considered to be the radiographic test of choice to evaluate the prostate, ejaculatory duct, and seminal vesicles in the infertile male. The vasogram has been replaced by transrectal ultrasonography for the most part, and the vasogram is used only in conjunction with reconstructive surgery (Honig, 1994).

SEMINAL VESICLES AND EJACULATORY DUCTS

Gross Structure

The seminal vesicles are paired, viscous organs that are positioned posterior to the bladder and prostate. The seminal vesicle is a lateral outpouching of the vas deferens. It has the capacity for 3 to 4 mL of volume, and the nonobstructed seminal vesicle typically measures 5 to 7 cm in length and 1.5 cm in width. The seminal vesicle is a single tube that is highly coiled, and it forms several outpouchings and would measure 15 cm in length if stretched out. The joining of the seminal vesicle with the vas deferens creates the ejaculatory duct. The smooth muscle sheaths from the seminal vesicle and the vas deferens combine with the capsule of the prostate at the prostatic base. The seminal vesicles' excretory duct joins the duct of the ampullary vas deferens as it enters the prostate.

The ejaculatory ducts are positioned at the junction of the vas deferens and the seminal vesicle. The ejaculatory ducts are paired visceral organs. **They ultimately empty through the verumontanum into the prostatic urethra.** The ejaculatory duct is divided into three distinct anatomic regions. These include the extraprostatic region (proximal), intraprostatic region (mid), and the distal region, which joins the lateral aspect of the verumontanum to empty into the prostatic urethra (Nguyen et al., 1996). In contrast to the first two regions, the third distal region is not surrounded by an outer muscular layer and does not form an anatomic sphincter at the ejaculatory duct orifice at the verumontanum (Nguyen et al., 1996).

Microanatomic Architecture

The seminal vesicle has a columnar epithelium with goblet cells. The seminal vesicle tube is surrounded by a thin layer of smooth muscle cells, which is enveloped by a loose adventitia. The three layers composing the tubule of the seminal vesicle include an inner mucous membrane, a collagenous middle layer, and the outer circular and longitudinal muscle layers. The muscle layers account for 80% of the thickness of the wall of the seminal vesicle (Nguyen et al., 1996). The thin, folded mucosa of the seminal vesicle comprises nonciliated, pseudostratified cuboidal or columnar cells. The ejaculatory ducts have similar microanatomic architecture to the seminal vesicles, but they do not have the outer circular muscle layer that is found in the seminal vesicle (Nguyen et al., 1996). The inner epithelial layer of the ejaculatory duct is composed of simple and pseudostratified columnar cells in a folded pattern.

Arterial Supply

The arterial supply to the seminal vesicle originates from the superior vesical artery, which branches into the vesiculodeferential artery. The vesiculodeferential artery supplies the anterior surface of the seminal vesicle in proximity to its tip. The internal iliac artery and inferior vesical artery provide additional arterial supply to the seminal vesicle via the prostatovesicular branch (Clegg, 1955). Variations of arterial supply include the prostatovesicular branch originating from the pudendal artery or the superior vesical artery. Arterial supply to the ejaculatory duct arises from branches of the inferior vesical artery.

Venous Drainage

The venous drainage of the seminal vesicle follows the arterial supply draining through the vesiculodeferential veins and the inferior vesical plexus to the pelvic venous plexus.

Lymphatic Drainage

The lymphatic drainage from the seminal vesicle is to the internal iliac nodes (Mawhinney and Tarry, 1991).

Nerve Supply

Seminal vesicle parasympathetic innervation originates from the pelvic plexus with the sympathetic nervous system contributing fibers from the hypogastric nerves and the superior lumbar nerves (Kolbeck and Steers, 1993). The pelvic plexus innervates the ejaculatory ducts.

Transrectal Ultrasonography

The seminal vesicles can be imaged by transrectal ultrasonography, because they are positioned posteriorly at the base of the prostate. The seminal vesicles appear hypoechoic, compared with the prostate, and are crescent shaped, paired, and symmetrical. The normal seminal vesicle measures 2 cm in width and 4.5 to 5.5 cm in length. They can be visualized as oriented horizontally in the transverse plane. Hypoechoic fatty tissue can be seen separating the seminal vesicles from the base of the prostate. The ejaculatory ducts may occasionally be seen by transrectal ultrasonography, and they appear hypoechoic as they enter the prostate posteriorly.

Computed Tomography

Computed tomography (CT) can image the seminal vesicles. The mean measurements by CT of the seminal vesicles are 3 cm in length and 1.5 cm in width. No significant change is seen by CT in seminal vesicle length on the basis of age. However, the width of the seminal vesicle is smaller in men of increasing age. The pudendal venous plexus can be identified by CT as small punctuate densities along the lateral aspect of the seminal vesicle (Silverman et al., 1985).

Magnetic Resonance Imaging

MRI of the normal seminal vesicles demonstrates signal intensity similar to that of the bladder or muscle on T1 imaging. The seminal vesicles demonstrate a higher signal intensity than the surrounding fat on T2 imaging (King et al., 1989; Secaf et al., 1991; Fig. 63.20; also see Fig. 63.19).

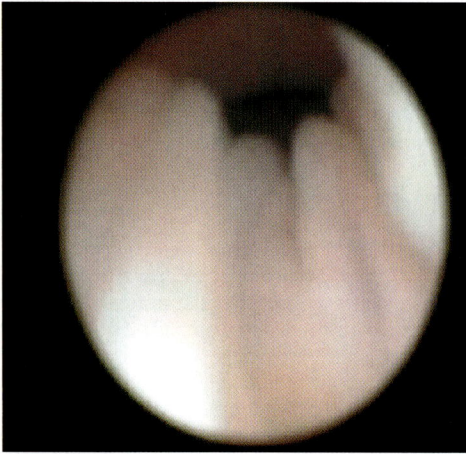

Fig. 63.20. Endoscopic view into the os of the ejaculatory duct transurethrally.

> ### KEY POINTS: SEMINAL VESICLES AND EJACULATORY DUCTS
>
> - The nonobstructed seminal vesicle typically measures 5 to 7 cm in length and 1.5 cm in width.
> - The ejaculatory ducts empty through the verumontanum into the prostatic urethra.
> - Transrectal ultrasound, CT, and MRI can image the seminal vesicles.

PROSTATE

Gross Structure

The normal prostate gland is ovoid and measures 3 cm in length, 4 cm in width, and 2 cm in depth; it has a weight of 18 to 20 g. It is homologous to the Skene glands in females. The prostate is composed of glandular elements and fibromuscular stroma. The prostate is positioned just inferior to the bladder. The prostatic urethra travels through the prostate gland. **The base of the prostate is at the bladder-prostate junction, and the narrowed apex is the most inferior portion of the prostate gland, reaching the urogenital diaphragm.** The prostate is palpable approximately 4 cm from the anus on digital rectal examination. **The apex of the prostate is continuous with the striated urethral sphincter.** The prostate comprises an anterior surface, a posterior surface, and lateral surfaces, and these are in relationship to the prostatic urethra traversing the prostate. A collagen, elastin, and smooth muscle capsule envelops the prostate. The capsule measures 0.5 mm in thickness posteriorly and laterally on average. There is no true prostatic capsule at the apex of the prostate, where normal prostate glands are seen blending into the striated muscle of the urethral sphincter. Similarly, there is no true capsule at the base separating the prostate from the bladder, where the detrusor muscle's outer longitudinal fibers fuse with the fibromuscular capsule of the prostate (Epstein, 1989). The prostate capsule blends with the continuation of the endopelvic fascia on the anterior and anterolateral aspects of the prostate. The prostate is fixed to the pubic bone anteriorly by the puboprostatic ligaments near the apex of the prostate. The superficial branch of the dorsal vein is positioned in the retropubic fat outside the prostatic fascia. It drains into the dorsal vein complex. The levator ani's pubococcygeal portion hugs the lateral aspects of the prostate and is related to its overlying endopelvic fascia. The prostate capsule and the pelvic fascia separate below the parietal and visceral endopelvic fascia juncture (arcus tendineus fascia pelvis). Fatty areolar tissue and the lateral branches of the dorsal vein complex take up the space of this separation between the prostate capsule and the pelvic fascia. **The cavernosal nerves travel within the parietal pelvic fascia, also known as the lateral prostatic fascia, posterolateral to the prostate.** As more anatomic attention has been taken with higher-magnification robotic techniques at the time of radical prostatectomy, the lateral prostatic fascia has been defined in greater detail in an effort to preserve the cavernosal nerves. Nerve bundles have been identified traveling along the prostate laterally and anterior to the previously defined neurovascular bundle (Eichelberg et al., 2007; Raychaudhuri and Cahill, 2008; Fig. 63.21).

The prostate has been divided into distinct anatomic zones. These zones can be identified with transrectal ultrasonography. The transition zone is the smallest of the zones of the prostate. The ducts of the transition zone begin at the angle dividing the preprostatic and the prostatic urethra, and they travel beneath the preprostatic sphincter to course along its lateral and posterior sides. The transition zone makes up 5% to 10% of the glandular tissue of the normal prostate. The transition zone is separated from the rest of the glandular compartments of the prostate by a distinct fibromuscular band. Benign prostatic hyperplasia most commonly occurs in the transition zone. The central zone ducts are positioned circumferentially, surrounding the openings of the ejaculatory ducts. This zone expands toward the base of the bladder, surrounding the ejaculatory ducts, in the shape of a cone. The central zone makes up 25% of the glandular tissue of the prostate. The glands of the central zone are thought to be of wolffian duct origin; they differ immunohistochemically and structurally from the other glands of the prostate (McNeal, 1988). **The peripheral zone of the prostate is the largest zone.**

Seventy percent of the glandular tissue of the prostate is made up of the peripheral zone. The peripheral zone makes up the posterior and lateral aspects of the prostate gland. The ducts of the peripheral zone drain into the prostatic sinus along the entire length of the postsphincteric prostatic urethra. Seventy percent of prostate cancers are found in the peripheral zone. The nonglandular anterior fibromuscular stroma is found extending from the bladder neck to the striated sphincter, and it may make up to one-third of the mass of the prostate. It is composed of collagen, smooth and striated muscle, and elastin. It is anatomically continuous with the anterior visceral fascia, the anterior preprostatic sphincter, and the prostatic capsule.

The prostate is also compartmentalized clinically, based on digital rectal examination and cystoscopic appearance. A central sulcus divides the two lateral lobes of the prostate and a middle lobe. The middle lobe may become hyperplastic and may extend into the bladder neck with age (Fig. 63.22).

Microanatomic Architecture

Seventy percent of the prostate's composition is glandular elements, whereas 30% is made up of fibromuscular stroma. The epithelial cells of the prostate glands are cuboidal or columnar. These secretory epithelial cells are terminally differentiated, have a low proliferative index, and measure 10 to 20 μm in height (De Marzo et al., 1998). These epithelial cells have abundant secretory granules and are organized in rows with their apices projecting into the lumen and their bases attached to a basement membrane (Knox et al., 1994). The nuclei of the cells are at their base, below the Golgi apparatus. The luminal apices have microvilli. The epithelial cells line the periphery of the acinus and secrete into the acinus, which drains into ducts to the urethra ultimately. The tubuloalveolar glands have simple branching patterns. Flattened, undifferentiated basal cells line each acinus beneath the epithelial cells. A thin layer of connective tissue and stromal smooth muscle surrounds each acinus. The secretory cells have scattered, terminally differentiated, nonproliferating neuroendocrine cells between them. Two types of neuroendocrine cells have been identified in the prostate. One is a closed cell with dendrite-like processes that extend toward epithelial cells and basal cells in its proximity. The other type of neuroendocrine

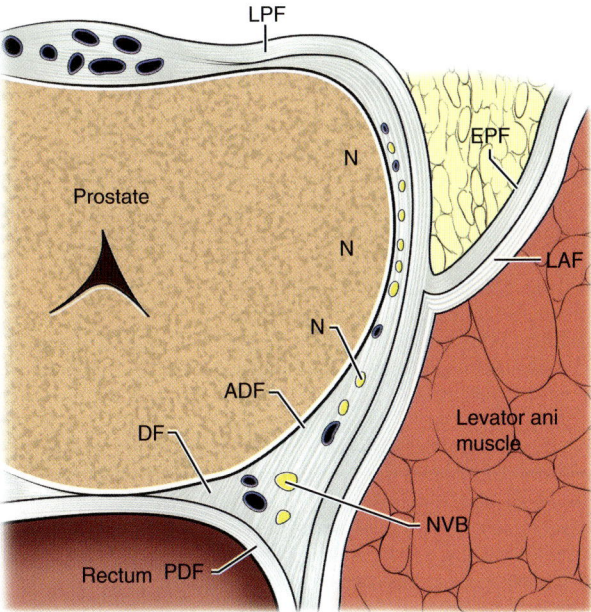

Fig. 63.21. Cross section of prostate with prostatic fascial layers outlined, including the lateral prostatic fascia (*LPF*), endopelvic fascia (*EPF*), levator ani fascia (*LAF*), Denonvilliers fascia (*DF*), anterior lamina of Denonvilliers fascia (*ADF*), posterior lamina of Denonvilliers fascia (*PDF*), neurovascular bundle (*NVB*), and lateral nerves (*N*). (From Walz J, Graefen M, Huland H: Basic principles of anatomy for optimal surgical treatment of prostate cancer. *World J Urol* 25:31–38, 2007.)

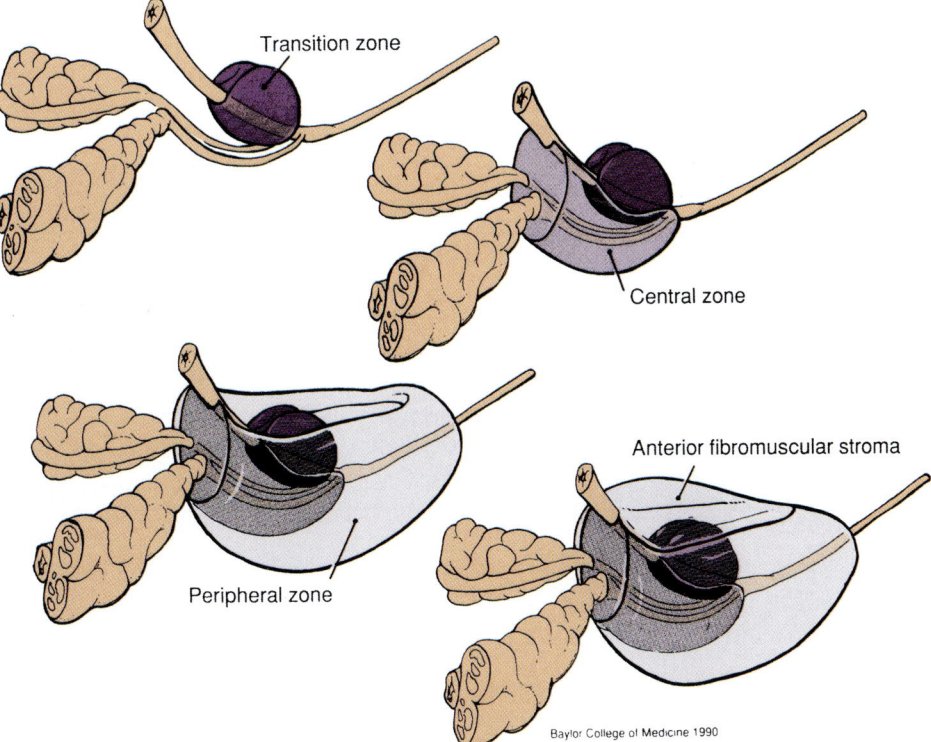

Fig. 63.22. Zonal anatomy of the prostate as described by McNeal (1988). The transition zone surrounds the urethra proximal to the ejaculatory ducts. The central zone surrounds the ejaculatory ducts and projects under the bladder base. The peripheral zone constitutes the bulk of the apical, posterior, and lateral aspects of the prostate. The anterior fibromuscular stroma extends from the bladder neck to the striated urethral sphincter. (Copyright 1990, Baylor College of Medicine.)

cell type seen is an open one with microvilli extending into the lumen (Abrahamsson, 1999; di Sant'Agnese and De Mesy Jensen, 1984; Vashchenko and Abrahamsson, 2005). The stroma is composed of smooth muscle, which is rich in α-actin, myosin, and desmin, and it is also composed of collagen and is continuous with the prostatic capsule. At the junction of the prostate gland, the prostatic urethra, the transitional cells of the prostatic urethra's epithelium, may extend into prostatic ducts. The preprostatic (internal urethral) sphincter encloses the small periurethral prostatic glands without periglandular smooth muscle, and these glands are positioned between fibers of longitudinal smooth muscle. Posterior to the prostate, microscopic smooth muscle bands fuse with Denonvilliers fascia after extending from the posterior aspect of the prostatic capsule. There is a plane of loose, areolar tissue between Denonvilliers fascia and the rectum.

Arterial Supply

The inferior vesical artery is the typical arterial supply to the prostate. The inferior vesical artery branches into urethral arteries that enter the prostatovesical junction posterolaterally and course in a perpendicular route to the urethra. They travel toward the bladder neck with the largest branches posteriorly, approaching the bladder neck in the one o'clock to five o'clock positions and the seven o'clock to eleven o'clock positions. They then supply the urethra after making a caudal turn to run parallel to the urethra. These branches supply the urethra, the periurethral glands, and the transition zone of the prostate (Flocks, 1937). The inferior vesical artery also branches into the capsular artery. The capsular artery yields small branches that supply the anterior prostatic capsule. The capsular branches enter the prostate at 90-degree angles and provide arterial supply to the glandular tissues, coursing along the reticular bands of the stroma. The majority of the inferior vesical artery travels posterolateral to the prostate to form the neurovascular bundles coursing with the cavernous nerves, terminating at the pelvic diaphragm. Branches from the internal pudendal artery and the middle rectal (hemorrhoidal) artery also contribute a supply to the prostate (Fig. 63.23).

Venous Drainage

The prostate includes abundant venous drainage through the periprostatic plexus. **The periprostatic plexus anastomoses with the deep dorsal vein of the penis and the internal iliac (hypogastric) veins.**

Lymphatic Drainage

The obturator and internal iliac nodes are the primary sites of lymphatic drainage from the prostate. The presacral group or, infrequently, the external iliac nodes may receive a small portion of the initial lymphatic drainage.

Nerve Supply

The cavernous nerves provide sympathetic and parasympathetic innervation to the prostate from the pelvic plexus. Innervations to the glandular and stromal elements of the prostate are found traveling with branches of the capsular artery. Sympathetic fibers innervate the smooth muscle of the capsule and stroma for contraction. The parasympathetic nerves promote secretory function by terminating in the acini. Prostate smooth muscle relaxation may be affected by peptidergic and nitric oxide synthase–containing neurons that have been identified in the prostate (Burnett, 1995). The pelvic plexuses carry afferent neurons from the prostate to the pelvic and thoracolumbar spinal centers.

Transrectal Ultrasonography of the Prostate

Transrectal ultrasonography of the prostate provides multiple diagnostic utilities, including assessing prostate volume, locating focal abnormalities, assessing patients with infertility with suspicion of obstruction, and guiding prostate biopsies. The prostate is imaged with biplane, multiplane, and end-fire endorectal transducer probes with a frequency ranging from 6 to 8 MHz. The patient should be positioned either in the lateral decubitus or the dorsal lithotomy position, and a well-lubricated transrectal probe is gently passed into rectum above the anal verge. The prostate and seminal vesicles should be systematically examined in the longitudinal and transverse orientations. Pertinent images should be recorded and labeled (Terris et al., 1992). **The normal prostate has a stipple grey echogenicity and appears homogeneous.** The capsule appears echogenic, continuous, and well defined. **The zonal compartments can be identified.** A distinct layer of echogenic fibrous tissue separates the zones. The prostate presents a semilunar shape and appears symmetrical in the transverse orientation. The peripheral zone has a homogeneous, fine echo pattern. The periurethral tissue is centrally positioned and appears hypoechoic. The relation of the prostate to the surrounding structures, such as the seminal vesicles, bladder neck, and prostatic urethra, can be identified in the longitudinal orientation. The urethra will appear curved within the central portion of the prostate.

The prostate volume can be measured using transrectal ultrasonography with an accuracy of within 5% of its true weight (Hastak et al., 1982). Transverse and longitudinal orientations are used to measure the length, width, and height of the prostate. An ellipsoid formula is then used to estimate the volume of the prostate: Volume = $\frac{4}{3}\pi \times length \times width \times height$ (Roehrborn et al., 1986; Fig. 63.24).

Magnetic Resonance Imaging of the Prostate

MRI of the prostate has been used to provide high-quality, clear images. MRI's direct multiplanar imaging has allowed for detailed

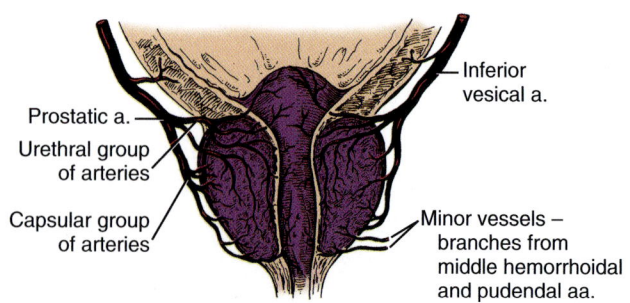

Fig. 63.23. Arterial supply of the prostate. (Modified from Flocks RH: The arterial distribution within the prostate gland: its role in transurethral prostatic resection. *J Urol* 37:527, 1937.)

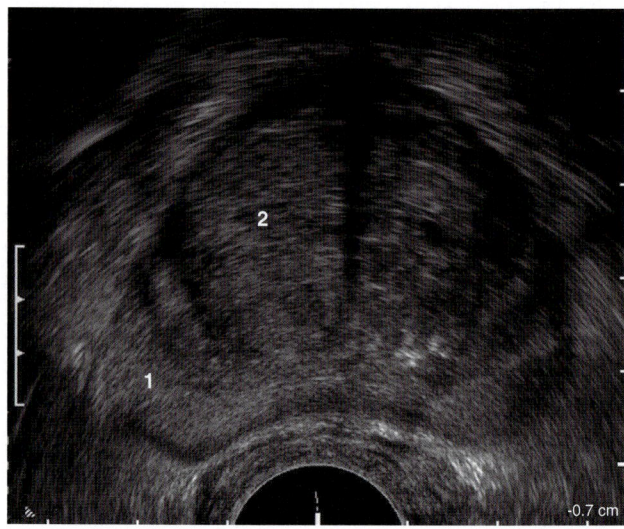

Fig. 63.24. Transrectal ultrasound of the prostate demonstrating the peripheral zone (*1*) and the transition zone (*2*).

demonstration of prostate anatomy (Dooms and Hricak, 1986). Zonal anatomy can be more clearly demonstrated by MRI using 0.5-cm slices. The peripheral zone showed higher signal intensity than the other zones and can be well visualized in the coronal, sagittal, and transverse planes. The central zone was well visualized in the coronal and sagittal planes and was of low signal intensity. The transition zone showed similar MR parameters to the central zone (Hricak et al., 1987). **Zonal anatomy is best demonstrated by T2-weighted images** (Gevenois et al., 1990). Using a specific pulse sequence, the periprostatic venous plexus can be imaged (Poon et al., 1985). The endorectal surface coil has been used to enhance resolution (Schnall and Pollack, 1990). The use of MRI of the prostate has become more frequent for use with pathologic processes (Fig. 63.25).

URETHRA

The urethra is contained within the vascular corpus spongiosum and the glans penis. **The normal urethral diameter is 8 to 9 mm.** Anatomists have organized the urethra into multiple different segmental divisions. It has been categorized in two broad segments: the anterior urethra and the posterior urethra. **The anterior urethra begins at the perineal membrane and continues distally to the urethral meatus. The posterior urethra begins distal to the bladder neck and the transition to the anterior urethra is made at the perineal membrane.** The segments have been further divided to characterize urethral anatomy more precisely. **The urethral epithelium is transitional until the urethral epithelium becomes squamous where it traverses the glans penis.** The submucosa contains smooth muscle, connective tissue, and elastic tissue. The glands of Littre are in the submucosa and their ducts empty into the urethral lumen. **The arterial supply to the urethra is from the internal pudendal artery whose bulbourethral branches supply the urethra, the corpus spongiosum, as well as the glans penis.** The venous drainage from the urethra drains to the pudendal plexus, which drains into the internal pudendal vein. The lymphatics from the urethra drain to the internal iliac (hypogastric) and common iliac nodes (Fig. 63.26).

> **KEY POINTS: PROSTATE**
> - The normal prostate gland measures 3 cm in length, 4 cm in width, and 2 cm in depth, and it has a weight of 18 to 20 g.
> - There is no true prostatic capsule at the apex of the prostate.
> - The cavernosal nerves travel within the lateral prostatic fascia, posterolateral to the prostate.
> - Benign prostatic hyperplasia most commonly occurs in the transition zone of the prostate.
> - A total of 70% of the glandular tissue of the prostate is composed of the peripheral zone, and 70% of prostate cancers are found in the peripheral zone.
> - Seventy percent of the prostate's composition includes glandular elements, whereas 30% is made up of fibromuscular stroma.
> - The inferior vesical artery is the typical arterial supply to the prostate.
> - The periprostatic plexus anastomoses with the deep dorsal vein of the penis and the internal iliac (hypogastric) veins.
> - The obturator and internal iliac nodes are the primary sites of lymphatic drainage from the prostate.
> - Transrectal ultrasonography of the prostate is useful for assessing prostate volume, locating focal abnormalities, assessing patients with infertility with suspicion of obstruction, and guiding prostate biopsies.

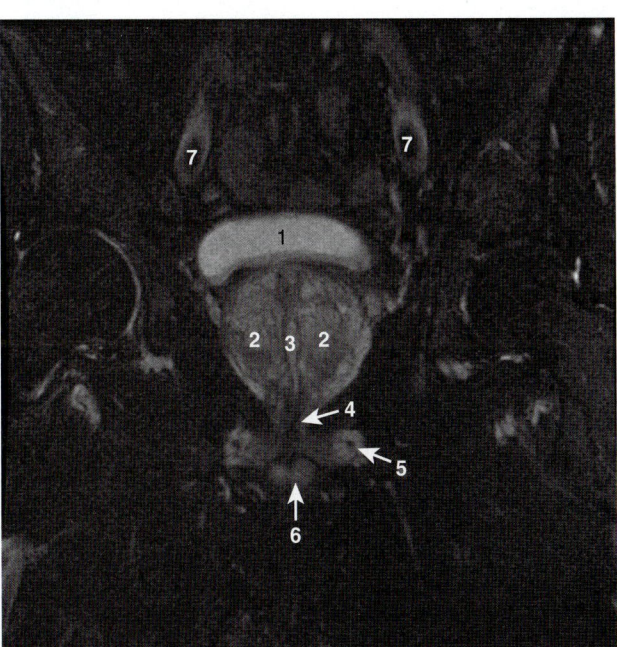

Fig. 63.25. Axial T2-weighted magnetic resonance image of the male pelvis through the prostate gland and adjacent structures. *1*, Urinary bladder; *2*, lateral lobes of prostate; *3*, verumontanum; *4*, striated urethral sphincter; *5*, inferior pubic ramus; *6*, corpus spongiosum in cross section; *7*, external iliac artery.

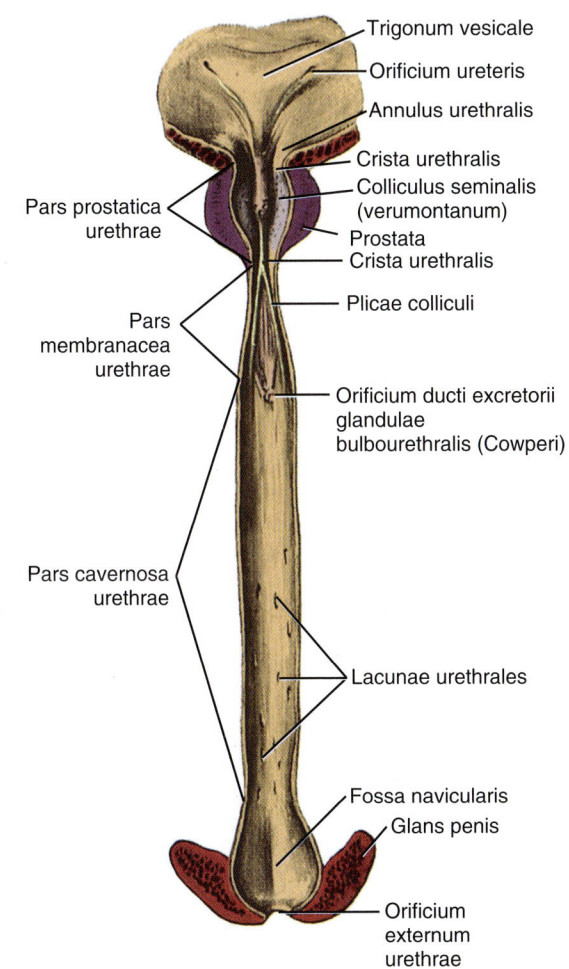

Fig. 63.26. Posterior wall of the male urethra. (From Anson BJ, McVay CB: *Surgical anatomy*, ed 6, Philadelphia, 1984, Saunders, p 833.)

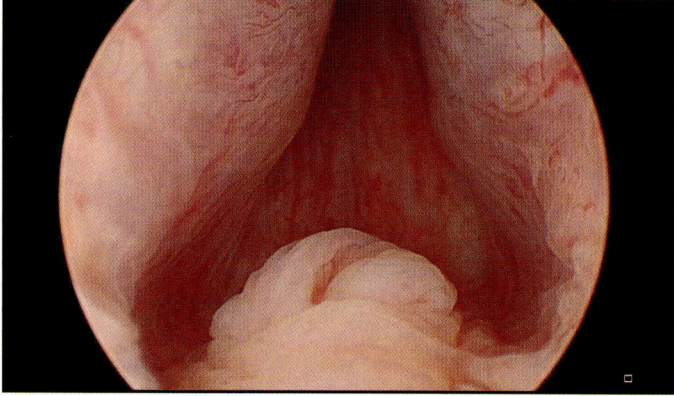

Fig. 63.27. Cystoscopic appearance of the verumontanum. (Courtesy David Leavitt, MD.)

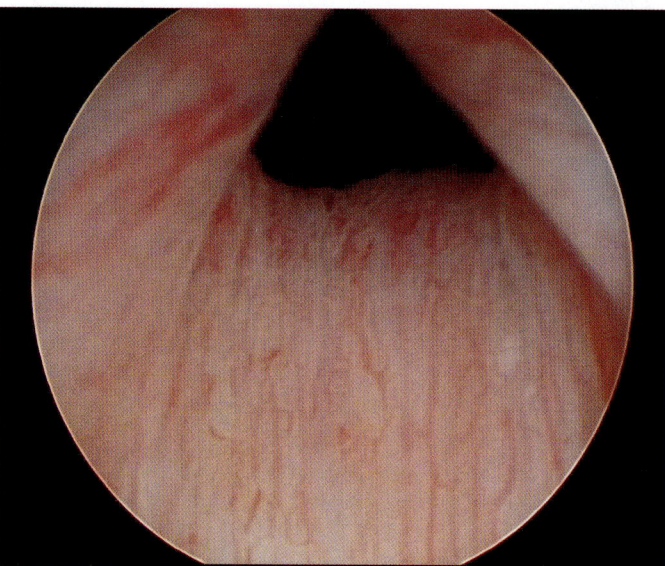

Fig. 63.28. Cystoscopic appearance of the bladder neck. (Courtesy David Leavitt, MD.)

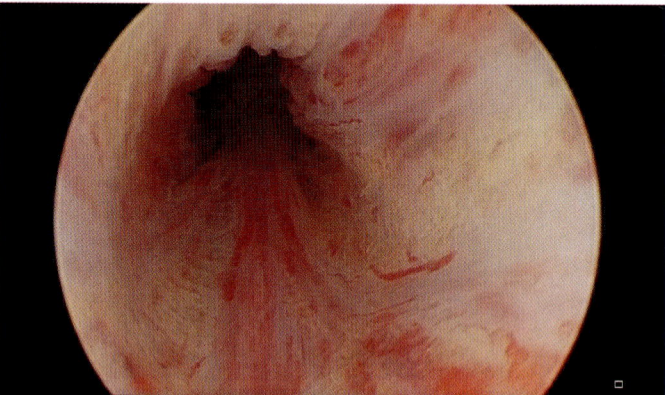

Fig. 63.29. Cystoscopic appearance of the striated sphincter. (Courtesy David Leavitt, MD.)

Prostatic Urethra

The prostatic urethra travels the length of the prostate and is in greater proximity to the anterior surface of the prostate. A urethral crest extends inward from the posterior midline of the prostatic urethra and is present throughout the length of the prostatic urethra. This urethral crest is no longer present at the level of the striated sphincter. All glandular elements of the prostate drain into prostatic sinuses, which are positioned on either side of the urethral crest (McNeal, 1972). The urothelium of the prostatic urethra is made up of transitional epithelial cells. This transitional urothelium may extend into prostatic ducts. An angle at the midpoint of the prostatic urethra turns 35 degrees anteriorly and separates the prostatic urethra into anatomically and functionally distinct segments. These are termed the preprostatic (proximal) and prostatic (distal) segments of the prostatic urethra. This angle may range from zero to 90 degrees depending on variable anatomy (McNeal, 1972, 1988). All glandular elements of the prostate open into the prostatic urethra past the urethral angle. **The verumontanum is formed by the widening and protrusion of the urethral crest from the posterior wall. The prostatic utricles orifice appears like a slit at the apex of the verumontanum.** The utricle's orifice is cystoscopically visible and measures 6 mm. **The prostatic utricle is a müllerian remnant.** The two small openings of the ejaculatory ducts are located on either side of the utricular orifice. After forming at the juncture of the vas deferens and seminal vesicles, the ejaculatory ducts travel approximately 2 cm through the prostate surrounded by circular smooth muscle, until they finally open into the distal prostatic urethra. The preprostatic sphincter is made up of thickened circular smooth muscle, synonymous with the internal urethral sphincter in the proximal segment. The prostatic segment is innervated by motor somatic fibers with an absence of any autonomic innervation (Figs. 63.27 and 63.28).

Membranous Urethra

On average the membranous urethra measures 2 to 2.5 cm in length and spans between the prostatic apex and the perineal membrane (Myers, 1991). A thin, smooth muscle layer spans across the membranous urethra. An outer layer of circularly arranged striated muscle in the shape of a horseshoe near the prostatic apex is found on the anterior surface of the urethra. The striated muscle reaches from the base of the bladder and the anterior aspect of the prostate extending the complete length of the membranous urethra. This signet ring–shaped striated sphincter is broad based and narrows as it courses through the urogenital hiatus of the levator ani to reach the prostatic apex. The posterior portion of the striated sphincter inserts into the perineal body throughout its length (Strasser et al., 1998). The striated sphincter is anterior to the dorsal vein complex and lateral to the levator ani. The band of fibrous tissue that suspends the urethra from the pubis anteriorly and that forms the suspensory ligament of the penis posteriorly, is made up of connective tissue from deep within the anterior and lateral walls. The striated sphincter's lumen consists of a pseudostratified columnar epithelium. There is a vascular submucosa that is surrounded by the longitudinal and circular urethral smooth muscle, which is the instrinsic component of the external sphincter (Raz et al., 1972). The pudendal nerve supplies innervation to the striated sphincter (Tanagho et al., 1982). A branch of the sacral plexus that travels along the surface of the levator ani provides another source of somatic innervation to the sphincter (Hollabaugh et al., 1997). The cavernous nerves are believed to supply autonomic innervation to the intrinsic smooth muscle of the membranous urethra (Steiner et al., 1991). The urethral stroma contains longitudinally organized collagen fibers and elastin fibers (Hickey et al., 1982). Lymphatic drainage from the membranous urethra travels in front of the prostate to join lymphatic channels draining the anteroinferior bladder. These channels terminate in the anterior or medial retrofemoral nodes and the middle node of the medial group of the external iliac nodes. Innervation is solely by motor somatic fibers without autonomic innervation. The ventral root of S3, with some contribution from S2, provides the somatic supply. The supply branches to the pelvic (splanchnic) nerve and passes to the pelvic (inferior hypogastric) plexus. Sensory innervation from the striated sphincter travels through the pudendal nerves via S2, and to a lesser extent S3, to travel to the node of Onuf centrally (Fig. 63.29).

Penile Urethra

The penile urethra, also known as the pendulous urethra and the spongy urethra, as it is surrounded by the corpus spongiosum, makes up the urethra distal to the membranous urethra. The urethra is often subdivided even further at the junction of the membranous and penile urethra and is termed the bulbomembranous urethra. This region comprises a 2-cm length of urethra within the urogenital diaphragm as well as being within the striated urethral sphincter and the first few proximal centimeters of the bulbous urethra, just distal to the sphincter within the penile bulb. The bulbospongy urethra begins a few centimeters distal to the membranous urethra and extends distally to the level of the suspensory ligament. The lumen widens to form the urethral bulb. The bulbourethral glands, also known as Cowper glands, empty into this region at the three o'clock and nine o'clock positions. The bulbourethral glands are located more proximally on either side of the membranous urethra. The penile urethra measures approximately 15 cm in length in its entirety from the suspensory ligament to the meatus. It is positioned more dorsally than ventrally within the corpus spongiosum. The bulb and the fossa navicularis are the two segments of urethral lumen widening; otherwise the luminal diameter is relatively consistent throughout. The mucosa of the penile urethra includes a transitional epithelium until it reaches the fossa navicularis. The muscle layer is made up of an inner longitudinal, a middle circular, and an inconsistently characterized outer longitudinal stratum. The glands of Littre are composed of small, mucus-secreting cells that lubricate the urethra before ejaculation, and they empty into orifices on the posterior wall of the penile urethra. The glands of Littre are rich in goblet cells and enter the spongy tissue between the vascular spaces and the trabeculae. **The penile urethra receives arterial supply from a branch of the internal pudendal artery, which enters at the level of the penile bulb, and is known as the bulbourethral artery.** Venous drainage of the bulbar urethra is by bulbar veins that drain into the prostatic plexus, which is the internal pudendal vein. The penile urethral lymphatics drain through a lymphatic network that is associated with the mucous membrane. These lymphatic channels course longitudinally but anastomose transversely and obliquely. The lymphatic channels drain proximally into trunks at the bulbomembranous urethra. The bulbomembranous lymphatic drainage may be variable. Some lymphatic drainage travels along the urethral artery or artery of the bulb, whereas others drain to the medial retrofemoral node after traveling behind the symphysis pubis. The penile urethral sensory innervation runs through submucosal axons that pass centrally through the dorsal nerve of the penis (Fig. 63.30).

Fossa Navicularis

The glanular portion of the urethra is known as the fossa navicularis, where its caliber dilates when compared with the urethra proximal to the fossa navicularis. It narrows again at the urethral meatus. **Unlike the transitional epithelium of the remainder of the urethra, the urethral mucosa that traverses the glans penis is a squamous epithelium.** These cells become keratinized near the meatus. The epithelium is separated from the smooth muscle of the spongy tissue by loose connective tissue, and a muscularis mucosa is absent. There are multiple pockets on the dorsal and lateral surfaces of the fossa navicularis. The lacuna magna (Morgagni) is a large pocket opening on the roof of the fossa navicularis (Figs. 63.31 through 63.33).

PENIS

Structure

The gross structures of the penis can be divided into distinct anatomic compartments. **The paired corpora cavernosa, which are the erectile bodies, prolongate proximally as the crus and attach to the pubic arch. The urethra travels through the corpus spongiosum, with its proximal segment known as the bulb. The glans penis is an expansion of the corpus spongiosum.** The superior surface of the penis during erection is known as the dorsum and the inferior surface during erection, containing the urethra, is known as the ventrum. The major portion of the body of the penis is formed by the corpora cavernosa as they join beneath the pubis (penile hilum). **A septum**

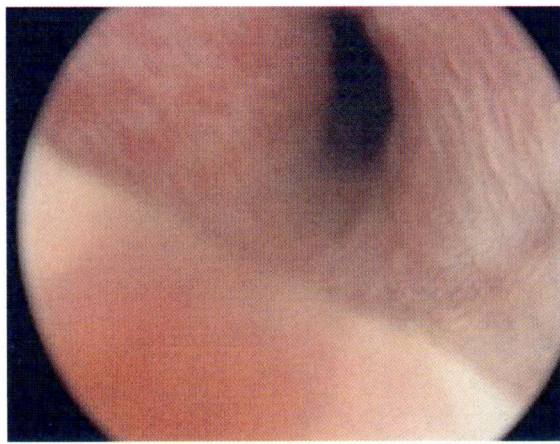

Fig. 63.31. Cystoscopic appearance of the fossa navicularis.

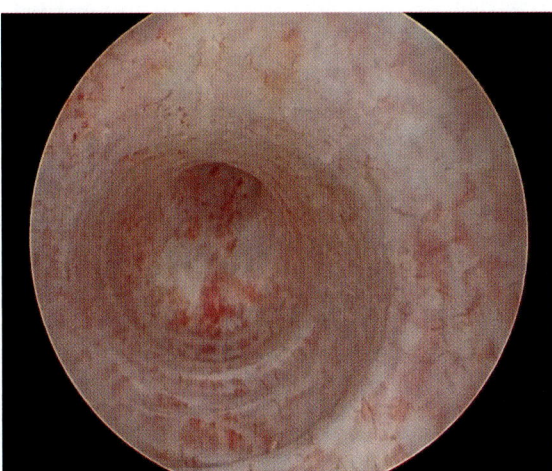

Fig. 63.30. Cystoscopic appearance of the bulbar urethra. (Courtesy David Leavitt, MD.)

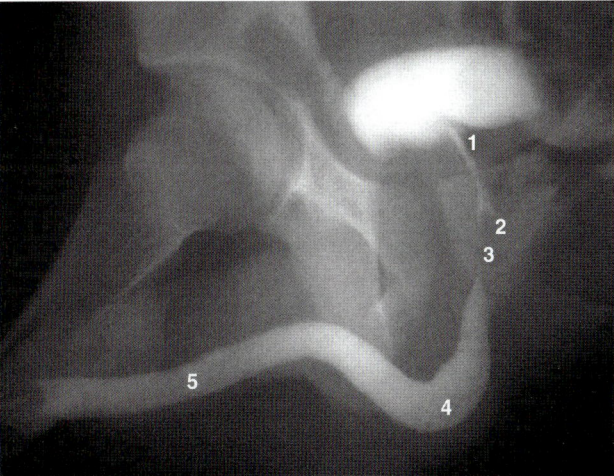

Fig. 63.32. Retrograde urethrogram of the male urethra demonstrating urethral anatomy. *1*, Prostatic urethra; *2*, verumontanum, into which enter the ejaculatory ducts; *3*, membranous urethra, note physiologic narrowing of urethral luminal diameter resulting from external striated sphincter; *4*, bulbar urethra; *5*, pendulous urethra.

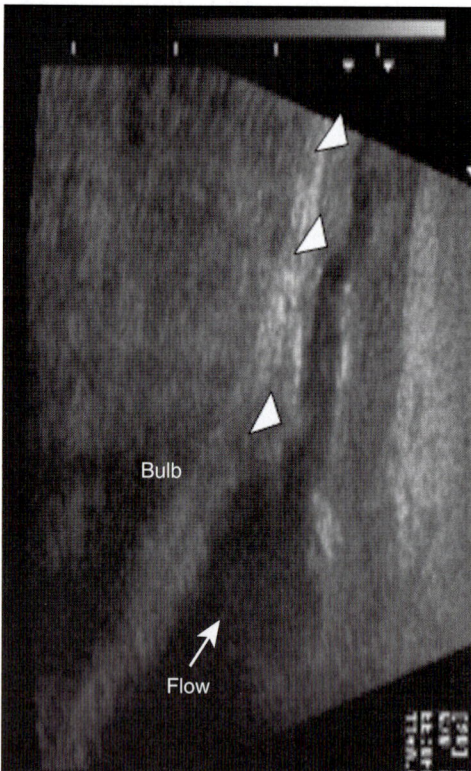

Fig. 63.33. Urethral ultrasonography has been used to assist in assessing the urethra in a noninvasive fashion. The *arrowheads* indicate the direction of urine flow during voiding in a normal urethra without stricture. (Courtesy Jonathan Rhee, MD.)

> **KEY POINTS: URETHRA**
>
> - The urethra is contained within the corpus spongiosum and the glans penis.
> - The anterior urethra begins at the perineal membrane and continues distally to the urethral meatus.
> - The posterior urethra begins distal to the bladder neck and the transition to anterior urethra is made at the perineal membrane.
> - The urethral epithelium is transitional in type until the urethral epithelium becomes squamous where it traverses the glans penis at the fossa navicularis.
> - The arterial supply to the urethra is from the internal pudendal artery whose bulbourethral branches supply the urethra, the corpus spongiosum, and glans penis.
> - The verumontanum is formed by the widening and protrusion of the urethral crest from the posterior wall.
> - The prostatic utricles (müllerian remnants) orifice appears like a slit at the apex of the verumontanum.

---

separates the corpora cavernosa but is permeable distally to allow for free communication between their vascular spaces. This incomplete septum allows the two corporal bodies to function physiologically and pharmacologically as a single unit. The tunica albuginea is the tough connective tissue layer that envelops the corpora cavernosa and is primarily collagenous with a mean thickness of 2 to 3 mm. The tunica albuginea is composed of elastic fibers, which form a tough irregular lattice that is predominantly collagenous with type I and type III fibers. The tunica albuginea becomes thicker ventrally to form a groove to accommodate the corpus spongiosum. The tunica albuginea is bilayered with an inner layer with circularly oriented bundles, which support and contain the cavernous tissue.

Intercavenosal pillars radiate from the inner layer into the corpora, acting as struts supporting the erectile tissue. The outer layer is composed longitudinally, extending from the glans penis to the proximal crura, finally inserting on the inferior pubic ramus. With erection, the outer longitudinal layers and inner circular fibers of the tunica albuginea are tightly stretched, and in the flaccid state they form an undulating meshwork (Goldstein et al., 1982).

The cavernosal structure provides the penis with flexibility, strength, and rigidity. Smooth muscle bundles consisting mainly of collagen (types I, IV, and in lesser amounts type III), elastin, and fibroblasts traversing the corpora cavernosa form endothelial-lined cavernous sinuses. Smooth muscle makes up 45% of the corpora cavernosal volume. Smooth muscle cells in the corpora are thin, thick, and intermediate filamentous structures. Thin filaments, light chains, are composed mainly of actin, thick filaments of myosin, and the intermediate filaments of desmin or vimentin. Myoendothelial junctions, which are cellular extensions through the internal elastic lamina, have been identified as connecting the vascular smooth muscle cells to the endothelial cells. Gap junctions have been identified at the point of cell-to-cell contact in the myoendothelial junction (Kavoussi et al., 2015). Endothelial nitric oxide synthase (eNOS) is expressed in the endothelium of corporal tissue and is recognized to have a major function in the maintenance of erection (Musicki and Burnett, 2007; Fig. 63.34). The corpus spongiosum tapers and travels ventrally to the corpora cavernosa, distal to the bulb. The glans penis is the most distal expansion of the corpus spongiosum. The shaft of the penis and the base of the glans are separated by the corona. The corpora cavernosa are surrounded by Buck fascia dorsally. Buck fascia splits to surround the corpus spongiosum ventrally. The fundiform ligament of the penis is composed of collagenous and elastic fibers from the rectus sheath blending with and surrounding Buck fascia. The suspensory ligament of the penis is made up of deeper fibers from the pubis. Deep to the muscles of the corpora cavernosa, the tunica albuginea and the Buck fascia fuse (Uhlenhuth et al., 1949). Buck fascia joins the base of the glans at the corona distally. The penile shaft skin is very elastic and its only glandular elements are the smegma-producing glands, located at the base of the corona. The penile skin is very mobile as its dartos fascia backing is very loosely attached to Buck fascia. In uncircumcised men, the prepuce (foreskin) is the penile skin as it folds over the glans and attaches below the corona. The glans penis skin is immobile as it is attached to the tunica albuginea below it (Figs. 63.35 and 63.36).

Arterial Supply

There is a superficial arterial system supplying the penis, which originates from the external pudendal arteries, and a deep arterial system that arises from each side from the internal pudendal arteries. The pudendal artery branches into a deep artery, supplying the corpora cavernosa, a dorsal artery, and the bulbourethral artery. Above the perineal membrane, the common penile artery travels in the Alcock canal, and it supplies the corpora cavernosa via three branches. The bulbourethral artery penetrates the perineal membrane, where it enters the corpus spongiosum from above at its posterolateral border. This provides arterial supply to the corpus spongiosum, glans, and urethra. The cavernosal artery penetrates the corpus cavernosum in the penile hilum to nearly the center of the erectile tissue. It provides straight and helicine arteries that supply the cavernous sinuses. After it travels between the crus and the pubis, the dorsal artery of the penis supplies the dorsal surfaces of the corporeal bodies. The dorsal artery travels between the dorsal vein and the dorsal penile nerve, and they all attach to the underside of Buck fascia. The dorsal artery travels distally toward the glans and supplies cavernous branches and circumferential branches to the urethra and the corpus spongiosum (Devine and Angermeier, 1994). There can be a great deal of variability in penile arteries (Bare et al., 1994). A single cavernosal artery may supply both corpora cavernosa or it may be completely absent. In some cases, an accessory pudendal artery may supplement or completely take the place of branches of the common penile artery (Breza et al., 1989). The arterial supply to the penile skin is from the external pudendal branches of the femoral vessels. These

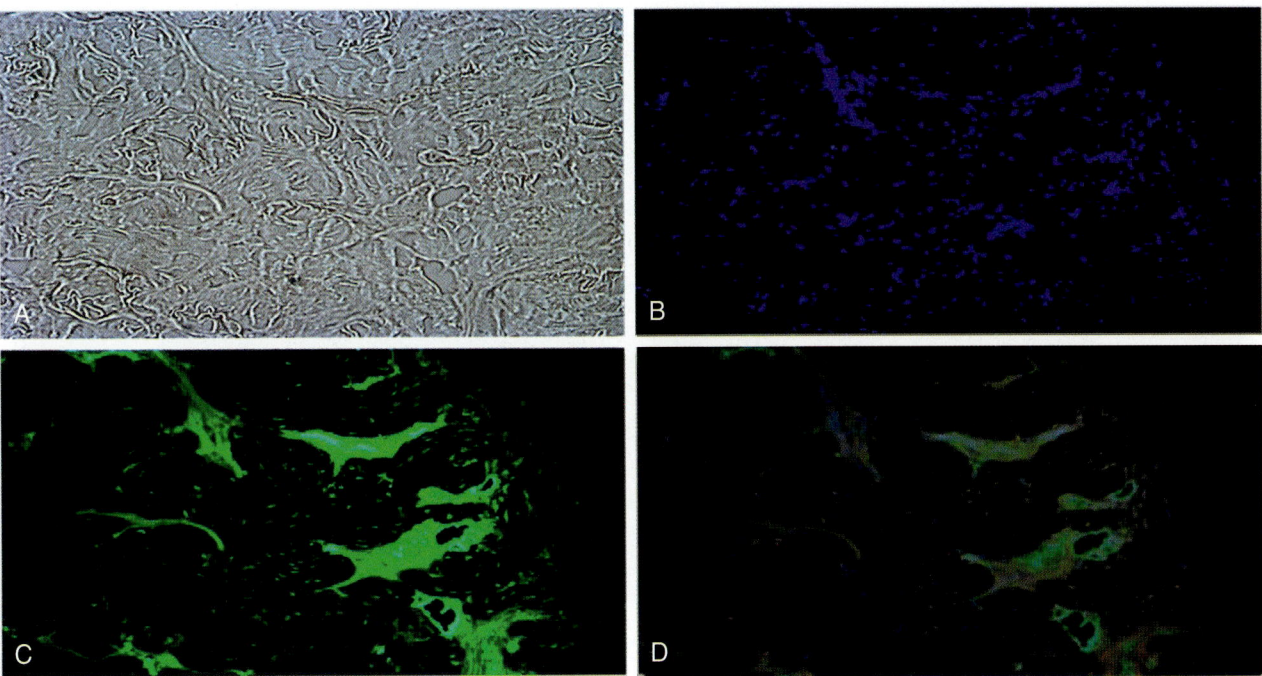

Fig. 63.34. Immunofluorescence of human corpus cavernosum. (A) Phase contrast. (B) DAPI identifying nuclei. (C) eNOS identifying endothelium. (D) DAPI and eNOS overlapped.

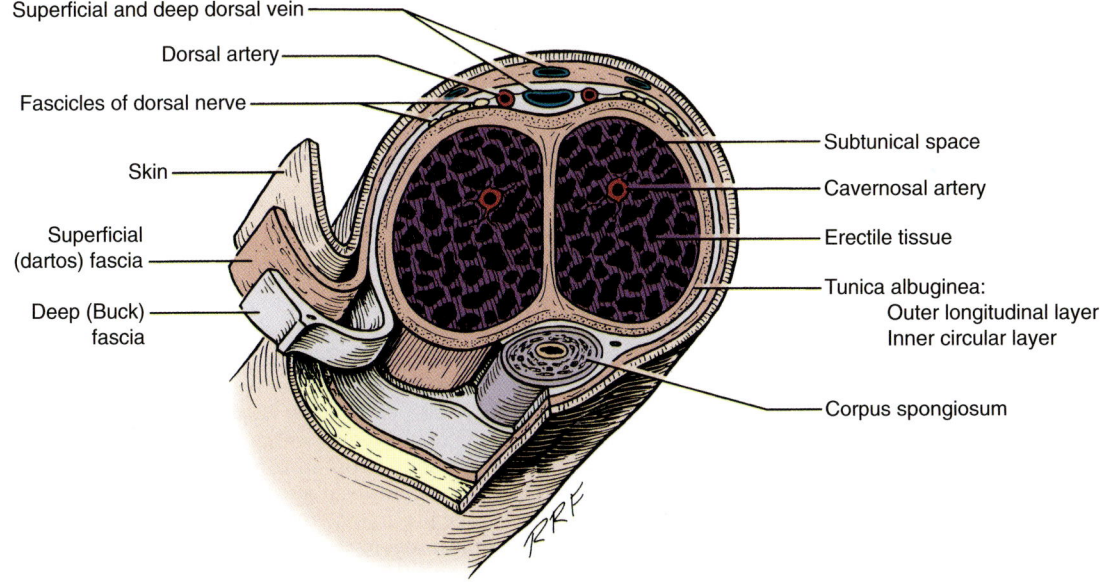

Fig. 63.35. Cross section of the penis, demonstrating the relationship between the corporal bodies, penile fascia, vessels, and nerves. (From Devine CJ Jr, Angermeier KW: Anatomy of the penis and male perineum, *AUA Update Series* 13:10–23, 1994.)

vessels run longitudinally in the dartos fascia layer and provide a rich blood supply after entering the base of the penis (Fig. 63.37).

Venous Drainage

The superficial dorsal vein lies external to Buck fascia, whereas the deep dorsal vein is beneath Buck fascia and runs between dorsal arteries. A number of venous channels anastomose at the base of the glans to form the dorsal vein of the penis. **The dorsal vein travels between the corporal bodies, in a groove, and drains into the preprostatic plexus.** In the distal two-thirds of the penile shaft, the circumflex veins from the corpus spongiosum course around the corpora cavernosa to enter the deep dorsal vein perpendicularly. There are typically 3 to 10 circumflex veins. The cavernous sinuses form intermediary venules that empty into the subtunical capillary plexus. Emissary veins from these plexuses travel obliquely between the layers of the tunica and drain into the circumflex veins dorsolaterally. Emissary veins form two to five cavernous veins in the proximal third of the penis, joining on the dorsomedial surface of the corpora cavernosa. These veins travel between the bulb and crura at the hilum of the penis. They receive branches from the bulb and the crura and empty into the internal pudendal veins.

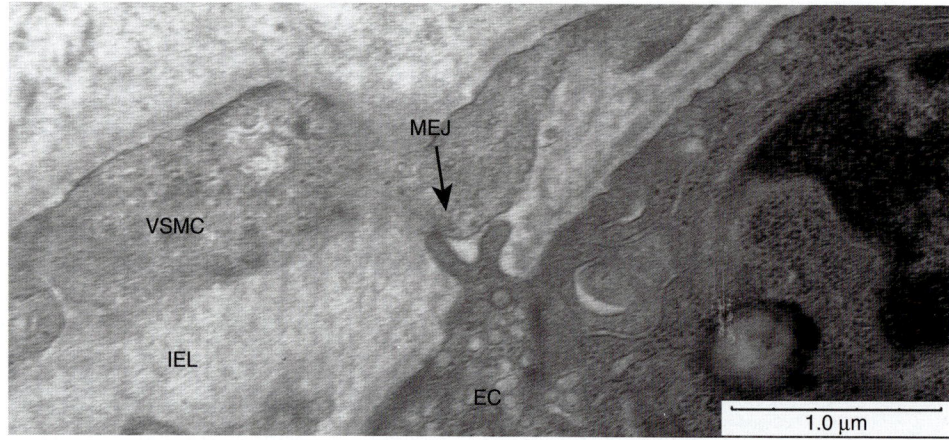

Fig. 63.36. Electron microscopy of a myoendothelial junction (*MEJ*) in human corpus cavernosal tissue. The MEJ is extending from the endothelial cell (*EC*) through the internal elastic lamina (*IEL*) to communicate with the vascular smooth muscle cell (*VSMC*).

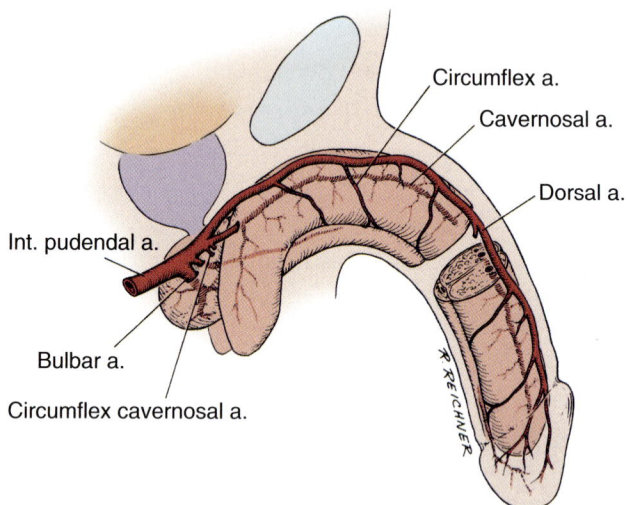

Fig. 63.37. Arterial supply of the penis.

Lymphatic Drainage

Lymphatics from the skin of the penis drain to the superficial inguinal and subinguinal lymph nodes. **Penile shaft lymphatics converge on the dorsum and ramify to both sides of the groin to drain into inguinal lymph nodes.** Lymphatics from the glans run deep to Buck fascia dorsally to drain to the superficial and deep inguinal nodes bilaterally. Some studies have suggested direct lymphatic channels from the glans to pelvic nodes as well as studies proposing lymphatic drainage through sentinel nodes positioned medial to the superficial epigastric veins. These models have been challenged (Catalona, 1988).

Nerve Supply

Sensory innervation of the penis is through the dorsal nerves. These nerves richly supply the glans. The dorsal nerves travel alongside the dorsal arteries. Small branches of the perineal nerve supply the ventrum of the penis as distally as the glans (Uchio et al., 1999). The somatic nerve supply originates from spinal nerves S2, S3, and S4 via the pudendal nerve. The pudendal nerve passes through the Alcock canal and continues as the dorsal nerve of the penis. The cavernous nerves supply sympathetic and parasympathetic innervation from the pelvic plexus to the corporeal bodies after penetrating them to ramify in the erectile tissue (Fig. 63.38).

Cavernosogram

Cavernosograms historically were used primarily to assist in the diagnosis of venous leak erectile dysfunction. Radiopaque contrast is injected into the corporal body with plain film imaging. This is not a commonly used diagnostic test any longer, but it is occasionally used at the time of penile fracture repair (Fitzpatrick and Cooper, 1975; Mydlo et al., 1998; Fig. 63.39).

Doppler Ultrasound of the Penis

Doppler penile ultrasound was first described in the 1970s and has been used over the years for assessment for erectile dysfunction, Peyronie disease, arteriocorporal fistulas (Fig. 63.40), and other penile pathologic processes (Malvar et al., 1973). High-resolution (7.5–12 MHz) real-time ultrasonography and color-pulsed Doppler can visualize the dorsal and cavernous arteries and can perform hemodynamic blood-flow analysis (Lue et al., 1989; Sikka et al., 2013). The entire length of the penis from the crura in the pelvis to the tip of the glans penis can be imaged. Color duplex demonstrates the direction of blood flow within the vessels, with blood flow toward the probe transducer appearing red and blood flow away from the probe transducer appearing blue (Broderick and Arger, 1993; Herbener et al., 1994). Penile arterial and venous flow velocities can be measured. The tunica alguinea can be assessed in cases of Peyronie disease (Chou et al., 1987).

Magnetic Resonance Imaging

Normal anatomy and pathologic anatomy of the penis can be evaluated with MRI. Anatomic detail and morphologic characteristics of the corpora cavernosa and corpus spongiosum can be demonstrated. Pathology such as congenital anomalies, penile prostheses, malignancies, hematoma, or fibrous tissue as a result of trauma, penile fractures, and fibrous plaques in men with Peyronie disease can be clearly visualized by MRI (Boudghene et al., 1992; Hricak et al., 1988). Complete morphologic analysis of the penis with fine anatomic detail can be obtained with combined evaluation of T1 and T2 images. Fine differentiation of penile tissues is possible with MRI, including penile skin, dartos fascia, hypodermal connective tissue, vascular characterization of corporus cavernosa and spongious tissue, the urethral lumen, deep penile arteries, superficial dorsal veins, and the tunica albuginea with high resolution (Satragno et al., 1989; Fig. 63.41).

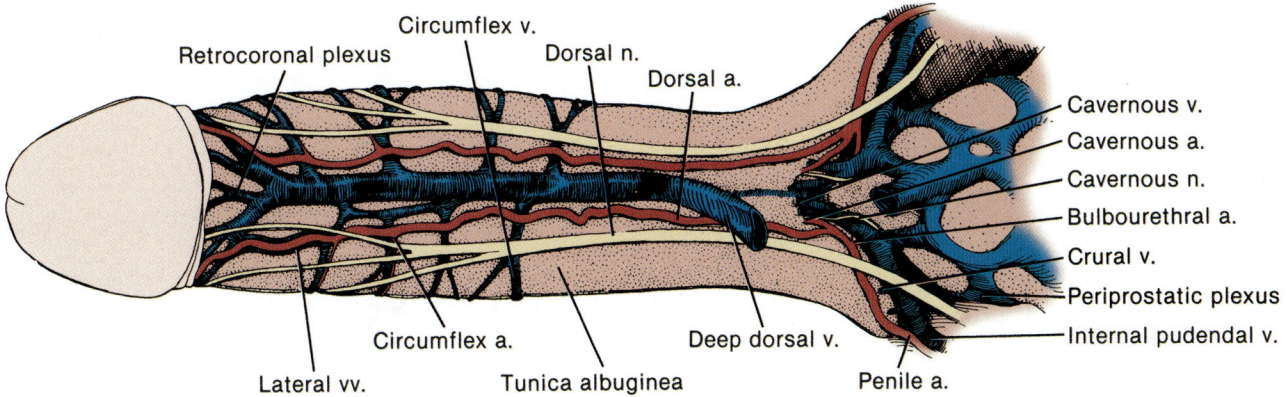

Fig. 63.38. Dorsal penile arteries, veins, and nerves. (From Hinman F Jr: *Atlas of urosurgical anatomy*, Philadelphia, 1993, Saunders, p 445.)

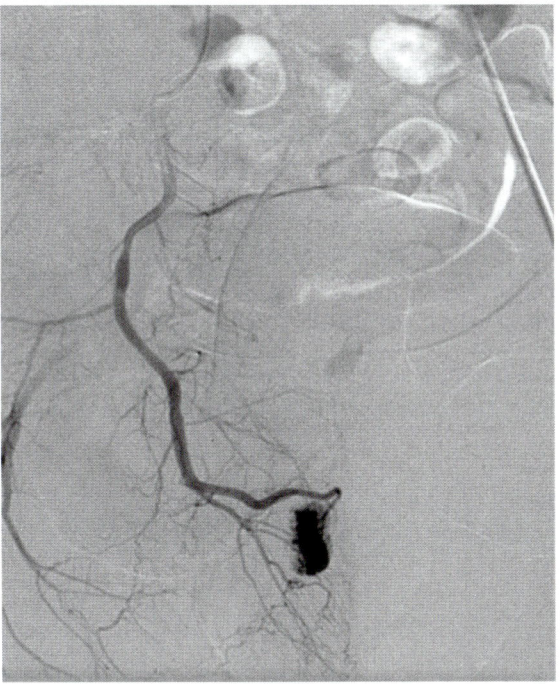

Fig. 63.39. Angiogram of arteriocorporeal fistula in patient with nonischemic priapism showing filling of the right corpus cavernosum.

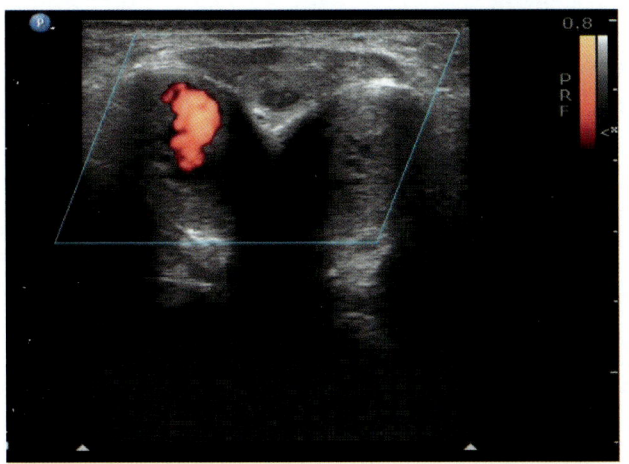

Fig. 63.40. Penile Doppler ultrasound of arteriocorporal fistula in patient with nonischemic priapism showing arterial flow into right corpus cavernosum *(red)*.

> **KEY POINTS: PENIS**
>
> - The paired erectile bodies are known as the corpora cavernosa.
> - The glans penis is an expansion of the corpus spongiosum.
> - A permeable septum separates the corpora cavernosa for free communication between their vascular spaces.
> - The superficial arterial system to the penis originates from the external pudendal arteries, and a deep arterial system arises from the internal pudendal arteries.
> - The dorsal vein runs between the corporeal bodies and drains into the preprostatic plexus.
> - Penile shaft lymphatics converge on the dorsum and ramify to both sides of the groin to drain into inguinal lymph nodes.
> - Sensory innervation of the penis is through the dorsal nerves, and the somatic nerve supply originates from spinal nerves S2, S3, and S4 via the pudendal nerve.

SCROTUM

Gross Structure

The scrotal skin is hair bearing, pigmented, with abundant sebaceous and sweat glands, and has an absence of fat. It is variable and may be folded with transverse rugae or it may appear loose and shiny. Its appearance depends on the tone of the underlying dartos smooth muscle. The median raphe runs longitudinally in the midline from the urethral meatus to the anus. Deep to the raphe, the scrotum is divided by a septum into two compartments, each containing a testis. The smooth muscle of the dartos fascia underlying the skin is continuous with Colles, Scarpa, and the dartos fascia of the penis. The spermatic fasciae are layers of the abdominal wall that extend to form parts of the scrotal wall. The external oblique extends to form the external spermatic fascia, which attaches to the borders of the external inguinal ring. The internal oblique extends to form the cremaster muscle and fascia, which attach to the inguinal ligament laterally, to the iliopsoas laterally, and to the pubic tubercle medially. The transversalis fascia continues to become the internal spermatic fascia in the scrotum. A peritoneal derivative known as the parietal and visceral tunica vaginalis surrounds the testis with a mesothelium-lined pouch. The tunica vaginalis is continuous with the testis posterolaterally at its mesentery, where it is attached to the scrotal wall. The gubernaculum fixes the testis at its inferior pole (Fig. 63.42).

Arterial Supply

The external pudendal arteries supply the anterior wall of the scrotum. **The arteries run parallel to the rugae and do not cross the median**

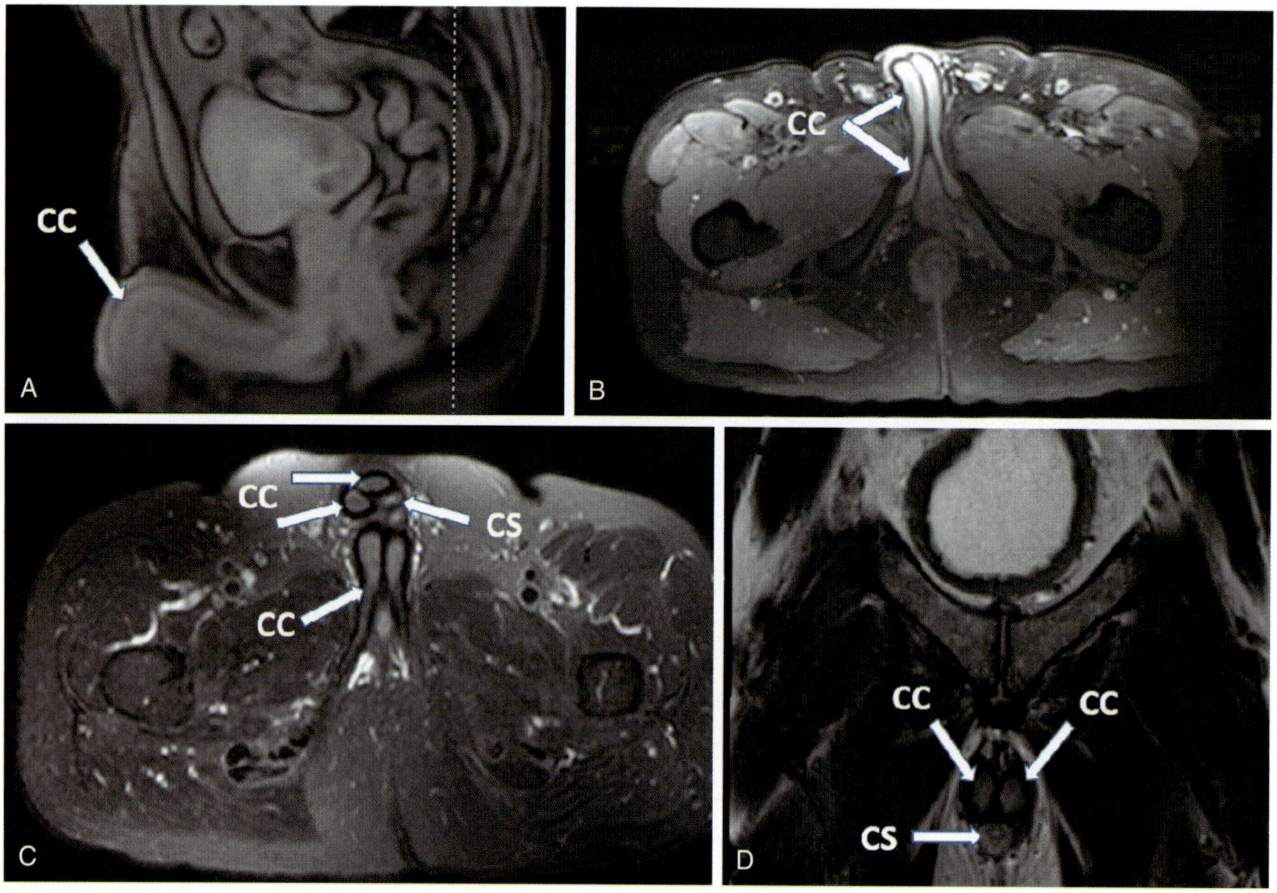

Fig. 63.41. MRI of the penis. *CC*, Corpus cavernosum; *CS*, corpus spongiosum. (A) T2 sagittal image of the penis. (B) T2 axial image of the corporal bodies with *arrows* showing them paired adjacent to each other and diverging at the crus. (C) T1 axial image of the penis in the deep pelvis as well as a cross-sectional view of the corporal bodies. (D) T2 coronal image demonstrating the corpora cavernosa and the corpus spongiosum in cross section.

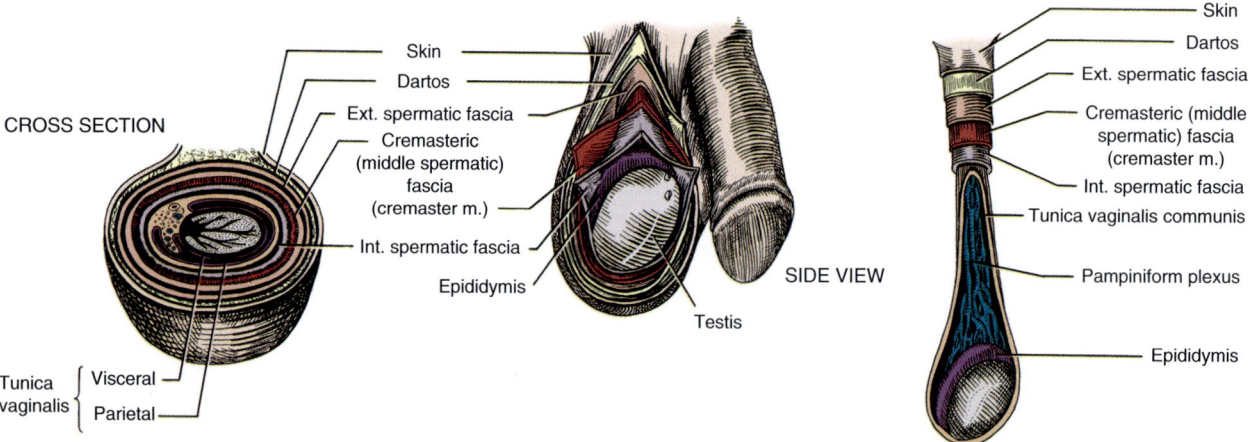

Fig. 63.42. Scrotum and its layers. (From Pansky B: *Review of gross anatomy,* ed 6, New York, 1987, McGraw-Hill.)

raphe. The posterior aspect of the scrotum has arterial supply from perineal branches. Arterial supply to the spermatic fascia is from the cremasteric, testicular, and deferential branches.

Venous Drainage

The external pudendal veins drain the anterior scrotal wall. The veins run parallel to the rugae and do not cross the median raphe.

Lymphatic Drainage

Scrotal lymphatics do not cross the median raphe and drain into the superficial inguinal nodes on the ipsilateral side.

Nerve Supply

Branches of the ilioinguinal and genitofemoral nerves innervate the anterior scrotal wall. The nerves run parallel to the rugae and do not cross the median raphe. The posterior aspect of the scrotum receives innervation from scrotal branches of perineal nerves as well as from branches of the posterior femoral cutaneous nerve (S3).

> **KEY POINTS: SCROTUM**
> - The smooth muscle of the dartos fascia underlying the scrotal skin is continuous with Colles, Scarpa, and the dartos fascia of the penis.
> - The scrotal wall arteries run parallel to the rugae and do not cross over the median raphe.
> - Branches of the ilioinguinal and genitofemoral nerves innervate the anterior scrotal wall.

SUGGESTED READINGS

Breza J, Aboseif SR, Orvis BR, et al: Detailed anatomy of penile neurovascular structures: surgical significance, *J Urol* 141(2):437–443, 1989.
Clegg EJ: The arterial supply of the human prostate and seminal vesicles, *J Anat* 89(2):209–216, 1955.
Devine CJ Jr, Angermeier KW: Anatomy of the penis and male perineum, *AUA Update Series* 13:10–23, 1994.
Dogra VS, Gottlieb RH, Oka M, et al: Sonography of the scrotum, *Radiology* 227(1):18–36, 2003.
Epstein J: *The prostate and seminal vesicles*, New York, 1989, Raven.
McNeal JE: The prostate and prostatic urethra: a morphologic synthesis, *J Urol* 107(6):1008–1016, 1972.
Setchell BP, Brooks DI: *Anatomy, vasculature, innervation and fluids of the male reproductive tract*, New York, 1988, Raven Press.

REFERENCES

The complete reference list is available online at ExpertConsult.com.

64 Male Reproductive Physiology

Paul J. Turek, MD, FACS, FRSM

The male reproductive axis of hormones and organs is a well-orchestrated and precisely managed biologic system that has evolved over millions of years. It is responsible for reproductive tract formation and development, fertility potential at puberty, and the maintenance of adult maleness. This chapter explores our current understanding of this complex system by defining its anatomy and physiology, including the hypothalamic-pituitary-gonadal (HPG) hormonal axis, spermatogenesis, and androgen production within the testicle and maturation and transport of sperm in the ductal system. In addition, new concepts in genetic and epigenetic infertility, stem cell science, and ejaculatory physiology are explained. Through such rigorous intellectual dissection, the true beauty and sophistication of the reproductive process is appreciated.

HYPOTHALAMIC-PITUITARY-GONADAL AXIS

The HPG axis plays a critical role during development and adulthood in four physiologic processes: (1) **phenotypic gender** development during embryogenesis, (2) **sexual maturation** at puberty, (3) testis endocrine function—**testosterone production**, and (4) testis exocrine function—**sperm production**.

Basic Endocrine Concepts

Two types of hormones mediate communication in the reproductive axis: peptide and steroid. **Peptide hormones are small, secretory proteins that act through cell surface receptors.** Hormone signals are transduced by one of several second-messenger pathways (Fig. 64.1). Most peptide hormones induce phosphorylation of proteins that alter cell function. Examples of peptide hormones are luteinizing hormone (LH) and follicle-stimulating hormone (FSH). In contrast, **steroid hormones are derived from cholesterol. They are not stored in secretory granules; consequently, steroid secretion directly reflects rates of hormone production.** In plasma, these hormones are usually bound to carrier proteins, and because they are lipophilic, steroid hormones are cell membrane permeable. After binding to intracellular receptors, steroids are translocated to nuclear DNA recognition sites and regulate target gene transcription. Examples of reproductive axis steroid hormones are testosterone and estradiol.

Hormonal signaling within the HPG axis is hierarchically governed by a free-running pulse generator within the hypothalamus. The amplitude and frequency with which hormone secretions occur within the reproductive axis determine downstream organ responsiveness. Feedback control is the principal mechanism through which hormonal regulation occurs (Fig. 64.2). With feedback control, a hormone can regulate the synthesis and action of itself or of another hormone. **In the HPG axis, negative feedback activity is primarily responsible for minimizing perturbations and maintaining homeostasis.**

Components of the Reproductive Axis

Hypothalamus

As the integrative center of the HPG axis, the hypothalamus receives neuronal input from the amygdala, thalamus, pons, retina, olfactory cortex, and many other areas (see Fig. 64.2). The pulse generator for the cyclic secretion of pituitary hormones, **the hypothalamus is anatomically linked to the pituitary gland by a portal vascular system and neuronal pathways.** By avoiding the systemic circulation, the portal vascular system allows direct delivery of hypothalamic hormones to the anterior pituitary.

The most important hypothalamic hormone for reproduction is **gonadotropin-releasing hormone (GnRH)**, a 10–amino acid peptide generated in the neuronal cell bodies in the preoptic and arcuate nuclei. **Currently, the only known function of GnRH is to stimulate the secretion of LH and FSH from the anterior pituitary.** GnRH has a plasma half-life of approximately 5 to 7 minutes and is almost entirely removed on the first pass through the pituitary either by receptor internalization or enzymatic degradation. GnRH secretion results from integrated input of stress, exercise, and diet from higher brain centers, gonadotropins secreted from the pituitary, and circulating gonadal hormones. Substances known to regulate GnRH secretion are listed in Table 64.1. In **Kallman syndrome,** characterized by congenital hypogonadotropic hypogonadism, the GnRH precursor neurons fail to migrate normally, with a subsequent absence of hypothalamic GnRH secretion (Bick et al., 1992; Dode et al., 2003). Affected individuals have delayed puberty or infertility because of lack of testosterone production.

GnRH output exhibits several types of rhythmicity: seasonal, on a time scale of months and peaking in the spring; circadian, resulting in higher testosterone levels during the early morning hours; and pulsatile, with GnRH peaks occurring every 90 to 120 minutes on average. The importance of pulsatile GnRH secretions in normal HPG axis function is aptly demonstrated by the ability of exogenous GnRH agonists (e.g., leuprolide acetate) to stop testicular testosterone production by changing pituitary exposure to GnRH from a cyclic to a constant pattern.

Anterior Pituitary

Located within the bony sella turcica of the skull, the pituitary has two lobes: posterior and anterior. The posterior lobe, or neurohypophysis, secretes two hormones, oxytocin and vasopressin, and is driven by neural stimuli. In contrast, **the anterior pituitary, or adenohypophysis, is regulated by blood-borne factors and is the site of action of GnRH** (see Fig. 64.2). GnRH stimulates the production and release of FSH and LH by a calcium flux–dependent mechanism. The sensitivity of pituitary gonadotrophs for GnRH varies with an individual's age and hormonal status. **LH and FSH are the primary pituitary hormones that regulate testis function.** They are glycoproteins composed of two polypeptide chain subunits, termed α and β, each coded by a separate gene. The α subunit of each hormone is identical and is similar to that of all other pituitary hormones; biologic and immunologic activities are conferred by the unique β subunit. Both subunits are required for endocrine activity. Sugars linked to these peptide subunits, consisting of oligosaccharides with sialic acid residues, differ in content between FSH and LH and likely account for differences in their plasma clearance rates. Secretory pulses of LH vary in frequency from 8 to 16 pulses in 24 hours and vary in amplitude by onefold to threefold. These pulse patterns closely reflect GnRH release. **Androgens and estrogens regulate LH secretion through negative feedback.** On average, FSH pulses occur every 1.5 hours and vary in amplitude by 25%. The FSH response to GnRH is more difficult to assess than that of LH for two reasons: (1) FSH has a smaller amplitude response and a longer serum half-life and (2) **the gonadal proteins inhibin and activin may affect FSH secretion and are thought to account for the relative secretory independence of FSH from GnRH secretion.**

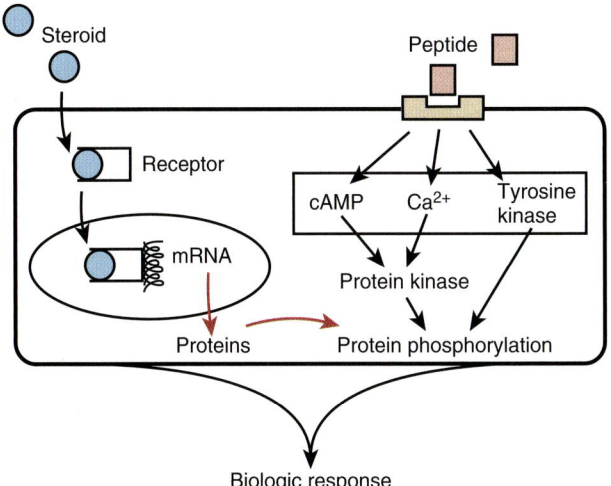

Fig. 64.1. Two kinds of hormone classes mediate intercellular communication in the reproductive hormone axis: peptide and steroid. (Modified from Turek PJ: Male infertility. In Tanagho EA, McAninch JC, editors: *Smith's urology*, ed 16, Stamford, CT, 2008, Appleton & Lange.)

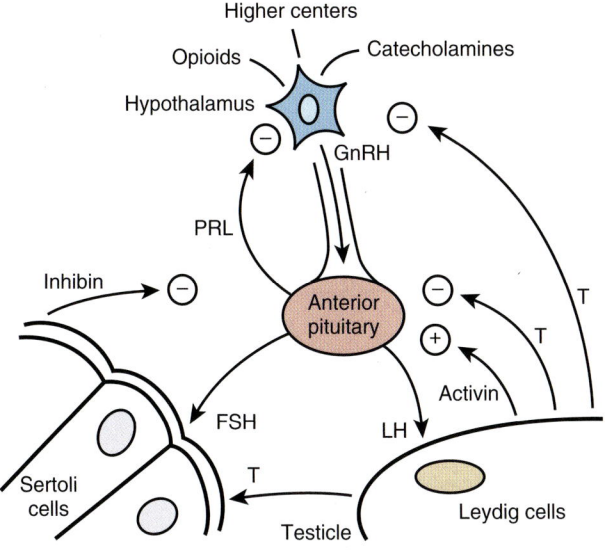

Fig. 64.2. Diagram of the hypothalamic-pituitary-testis hormonal axis. +, Positive feedback; −, negative feedback; *FSH*, follicle-stimulating hormone; *GnRH*, gonadotropin-releasing hormone; *LH*, luteinizing hormone; *PRL*, prolactin; *T*, testosterone. (Modified from Turek PJ: Male infertility. In Tanagho EA, McAninch JC, editors: *Smith's urology*, ed 16, Stamford, CT, 2008, Appleton & Lange.)

TABLE 64.1 Substances That Modulate Gonadotropin-Releasing Hormone (GnRH) Secretion

GnRH MODULATOR	TYPE OF FEEDBACK	EXAMPLES
Opioids	Negative	β-Endorphin
Catecholamines	Variable	Dopamine
Peptide hormones	Negative	FSH, LH
Sex steroids	Negative	Testosterone
Prostaglandins	Positive	PGE$_2$
Insulin	Positive	Insulin
Kisspeptins	Positive	Kisspeptin (puberty)
Leptins	Positive	Leptin

FSH, Follicle-stimulating hormone; *LH*, luteinizing hormone; *PGE$_2$*, prostaglandin E$_2$.

FSH and LH are only known to act in the gonads. They activate adenylate cyclase, which leads to increases in intracellular cyclic adenosine monophosphate (cAMP). In the testis, LH stimulates steroidogenesis within Leydig cells by inducing the mitochondrial conversion of cholesterol to pregnenolone and testosterone. **FSH binds to Sertoli cells and spermatogonial membranes within the testis and is the major stimulator of seminiferous tubule growth during development. FSH is essential for the initiation of spermatogenesis at puberty.** In the adult, the major physiologic role of FSH is to stimulate **quantitatively normal** levels of spermatogenesis (Tapanainen et al., 1997).

A third anterior pituitary hormone, prolactin, can also affect the HPG axis and fertility. Prolactin is a large, globular protein of 199 amino acids (23 kD) that is responsible for milk synthesis during pregnancy and lactation in women. No human mutations have been found in either the human prolactin gene or its receptor (Goffin et al., 2002). **The role of prolactin in men is less clear, but it may increase the concentration of LH receptors on Leydig cells and sustain normal, high intratesticular testosterone levels. It may also potentiate the effects of androgens on the growth and secretions of the male accessory sex glands** (Steger et al., 1998; Wennbo et al., 1997). Normal prolactin levels may be important to maintain libido. Although low prolactin levels are not necessarily pathologic, hyperprolactinemia abolishes gonadotropin pulsatility by interfering with episodic GnRH release. In addition, the anterior pituitary contains cells that secrete other glycoprotein hormones: adrenocorticotropic hormone (ACTH), growth hormone (GH), and thyroid-stimulating hormone (TSH). These glycoprotein hormones can also have significant effects on male reproduction.

Testis

Normal male virility and fertility require the collaboration of the exocrine and endocrine testis (see Fig. 64.2). The interstitial compartment, composed mainly of Leydig cells, is responsible for steroidogenesis. The seminiferous tubules produce spermatozoa.

Normal testosterone production in men is approximately 5 g/day, and secretion occurs in a damped, irregular, pulsatile manner (nyctohemeral). Testosterone is metabolized into two major active metabolites in target tissue: (1) the major androgen **dihydrotestosterone (DHT)** from the action of **5α-reductase,** and (2) the estrogen **estradiol** through the action of **aromatases.** DHT is a much more potent androgen than is testosterone. In most peripheral target tissues, testosterone reduction to DHT is required for androgen action, but in the testis and skeletal muscle, conversion to DHT is not essential for hormonal activity.

The primary site of FSH action is on Sertoli cells within seminiferous tubules. In response to FSH, Sertoli cells produce androgen-binding protein (ABP), transferrin, lactate, ceruloplasmin, clusterin, plasminogen activator, prostaglandins, and growth factors. Through these FSH-mediated factors, seminiferous tubule growth is stimulated during development, and sperm production is initiated during puberty. Mice FSH knockout studies suggest that FSH is not essential for spermatogenesis; indeed, affected mice can be fertile (Levallet et al., 1999).

The testis also produces the protein hormones inhibin and activin (Itman et al., 2006). Inhibin is a 32-kD protein made by Sertoli cells that inhibits FSH release from the pituitary. Within the testis, **inhibin production is stimulated by FSH and acts by negative feedback at the pituitary or hypothalamus.** Activin, a testis protein with close structural homology to transforming growth factor-β (TGF-β), exerts a stimulatory effect on FSH secretion. Activin receptors are found in a host of extragonadal tissues, suggesting that this hormone may have growth factor or regulatory roles in the body.

Negative feedback suppression of GnRH release by testosterone occurs through androgen receptors (ARs) in hypothalamic neurons and in the pituitary. **In studies of genetic mutations, it is clear that testosterone and estrogen participate in negative feedback** (Shupnik and Schreihofer, 1997). Steroid negative feedback results mainly from AR binding to testosterone, with a smaller contribution from estradiol binding. **Testosterone feedback occurs mainly at the hypothalamus, whereas estrogen feedback is mainly in the pituitary** (Santen, 1975). It also appears that although testosterone is the primary regulator of LH secretion, estradiol (along with inhibin from Sertoli cells) is the predominant regulator of FSH secretion (Hayes et al., 2001).

Development of the Hypothalamic-Pituitary-Gonadal Axis

Sex determination is genetic in humans. **A critical gene for sex determination is *SRY* (sex-determining region Y gene) on the short arm of the Y chromosome.** The *SRY* gene product is a protein with a high mobility group (HMG) box sequence, a highly conserved DNA-binding motif that kinks DNA. This DNA bending effect alters gene expression, leading to testis formation and subsequently to the male phenotype. However, the *SRY* gene does not act in isolation to determine human sex. *DAX1*, a nuclear hormone receptor gene, can alter *SRY* activity during development by suppressing genes downstream to *SRY* that would normally induce testis differentiation. A second gene, *WNT4*, largely confined to the adult ovary, may also serve as an "antitestis" gene. The discovery of these genes has significantly altered theories of sex determination. In the past, the female genotype was considered the "default," *SRY*-negative, developmental pathway. **It is now clear that genes such as *WNT4* and *DAX1* can proactively induce female gonadal development, even in the presence of *SRY*** (DiNapoli and Capel, 2008).

Once gonadal sex is determined, Leydig cells make **testosterone**, which induces development of the **internal genitalia** (Fig. 64.3). Leydig cells also synthesize **insulin-like growth factor-3** to promote **transabdominal testis migration** into the scrotum. DHT masculinizes the genital anlage to form the **external genitalia** (see Fig. 64.3). In addition, Sertoli cells within the developing testis synthesize **müllerian-inhibiting substance (MIS, or antimüllerian hormone [AMH])**, which **prevents the müllerian duct from developing into uterus and fallopian tubes and keeps the early germ cells quiescent in the testis** (Fig. 64.4). In general, deficiencies in these developmental pathways result in either birth defects or intersex disorders.

The hormonal feedback relationships within the HPG axis become established during gestation. **The expression of kisspeptin protein is in part responsible for activating GnRH neurons and triggering GnRH release.** In addition, SF-1, an orphan nuclear receptor, is secreted by developing Sertoli cells and contributes to HPG axis development (Val et al., 2003). After the withdrawal of placental steroids at birth, there is a period of high gonadotropin secretion in the neonate. Subsequently, as axis sensitivity to gonadotropins increases, FSH and LH secretions fall to the low levels characteristic of childhood. Puberty begins with GnRH pulsing, leading gonadotropins to increase to adult levels and subsequently to increase sex hormones. **The hypothalamic capacity to generate GnRH pulses arises at puberty, usually starting around the 12th year in males. Puberty begins at critical growth, weight, and nutritional rates for boys and girls and is likely initiated by kisspeptin, melatonin, and leptin** (Clement et al., 1998). The adipocyte hormone leptin is the body's regulatory signal governing the size of the fat stores, and there is increasing evidence that leptin modulates hypothalamic and pituitary activity (Caprio et al., 1999; Kiess et al., 1999; Quinton et al., 1999).

Aging and the Hypothalamic-Pituitary-Gonadal Axis

A progressive decline in testosterone and sperm production occurs with age, such that men in the seventh decade have mean plasma testosterone levels 35% lower than young men (Vermeulen et al., 1995). The consequence of this is a phenomenon that has been variously termed **male menopause, male climacteric, andropause, or, more appropriately, partial androgen deficiency in the aging male (PADAM)**. The changes to the seminiferous epithelium with age include decreases in seminiferous tubule volume and length. **An age-related decrease in sperm production in older testes appears to stem from decreased germ cell proliferation rather than increased cellular degeneration.** Correspondingly, FSH levels also increase with age, with mean values threefold higher in older than younger men. The cause of the age-related decline in HPG axis function is multifactorial. Testosterone production is reduced because of fewer Leydig cells and more testosterone-binding proteins. Diurnal variation of testosterone secretion is also lost in elderly men. With age, there is also evidence for a blunted HPG feedback response to low testosterone (despite generally high levels of gonadotropins) and to GnRH stimulation. Finally, normal pulsatile GnRH release is replaced by irregular pulses that are less effective in stimulating gonadotropin release (Mulligan et al., 1997). A combination of these effects is likely responsible for diminished HPG axis function with age.

Testis

Gross Architecture

The testis is a white, ovoid organ that is normally 15 to 25 mL in volume (Prader, 1966) and has a length of 4.5 to 5.1 cm (Tishler, 1971; Winter and Faiman, 1972). The tunica albuginea has smooth muscle cells that course through collagenous tissue (Langford and

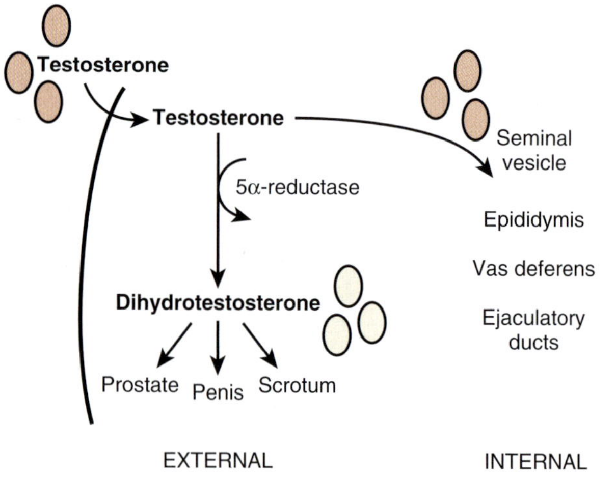

Fig. 64.3. Diagram of internal and external genitalia development. Testosterone is the main androgenic steroid responsible for the developing male internal genitalia, whereas dihydrotestosterone is the main androgen responsible for development of male external genitalia.

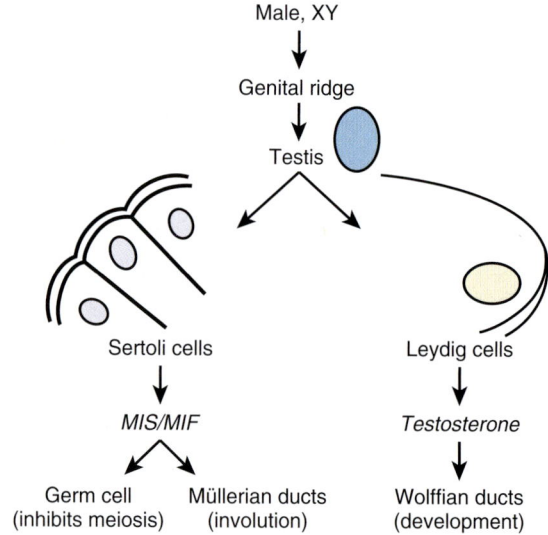

Fig. 64.4. Early differentiation pathway of the male. *MIS/MIF,* Müllerian inhibiting substance/factor. (Modified from Turek PJ. Male infertility. In Tanagho EA, McAninch JC, editors: *Smith's urology,* ed 16, Stamford, CT, 2008, Appleton & Lange.)

KEY POINTS: HYPOTHALAMIC-PITUITARY-GONADAL AXIS

- Normal testosterone and sperm production depends on the pulsatile secretion of hypothalamic GnRH and LH and FSH from the anterior pituitary gland.
- Regulation of HPG axis hormones occurs primarily through negative feedback.
- The determination of maleness is derived from the *SRY* gene on the Y chromosome. However, developmental genes such as *WNT4* and *DAX1* are considered antitestis genes and can proactively induce female gonadal development.
- Changes to the HPG axis with paternal age include lower testosterone levels, blunted axis feedback, and irregular hormone pulsatility.

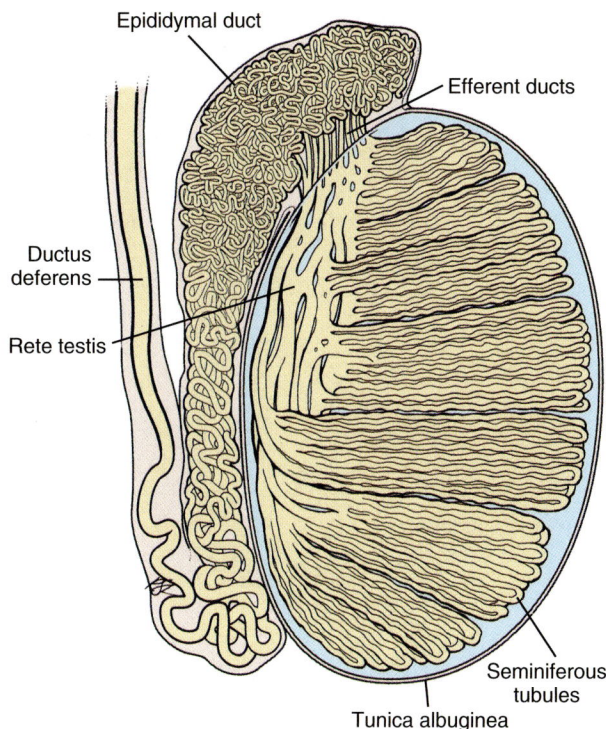

Fig. 64.6. Drawing of the human testis showing the seminiferous tubules (250 m in length), epididymis (3 to 4 m in length), and vas deferens. (Based on Hirsh AV: The anatomical preparations of the human testis and epididymis in the Glasgow Hunterian Collection. *Hum Reprod Update* 1:515–521, 1995.)

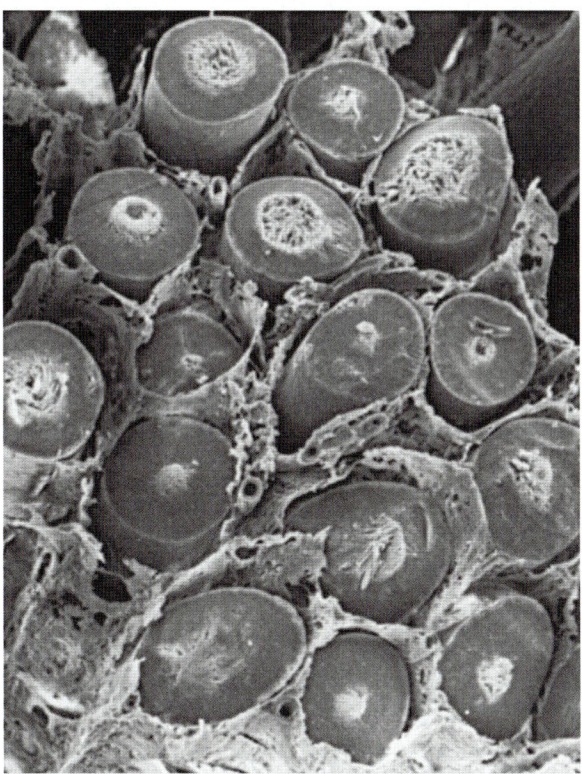

Fig. 64.5. Scanning electron micrograph of the cut surface of the human testis. Note the relationship of interstitial tissue to seminiferous tubules. (From Christensen AK. Leydig cells. In Greep RO, Astwood EB, editors: *Handbook of physiology*, Washington, DC, 1975, American Physiology Society, pp 57–94.)

Heller, 1973). Smooth muscle cells may impart contractile capability to the capsule (Rikmaru and Shirai, 1972), may affect blood flow into the testis (Schweitzer, 1929), and promote the flow of seminiferous tubule fluid from the testis (Davis and Horowitz, 1978).

The testis parenchyma is divided into compartments by septa. Each septum divides seminiferous tubules into lobes that each contain a centrifugal artery. **Individual seminiferous tubules harbor developing germ cells. Interstitial tissue is composed of Leydig cells, mast cells, macrophages, nerves, and blood and lymph vessels. In humans, interstitial tissue makes up 20% to 30% of total testicular volume** (Setchell and Brooks, 1988). The relationship between seminiferous tubules and interstitial tissue anatomy is demonstrated in Fig. 64.5. Seminiferous tubules are long, highly coiled, and looped. Both ends terminate in the rete testis. **The combined length of the 600 to 1200 tubules in the human testis is estimated to be 250 m** (Lennox

and Ahmad, 1970; Fig. 64.6). The "hub" of the testis, also termed the **rete testis,** coalesces to form 6 to 12 **ductuli efferentes** that carry testicular fluid and spermatozoa into the **caput epididymis** (see Fig. 64.6).

The arterial supply to the testis and epididymis is derived from three sources: the internal spermatic artery, the deferential (vasal) artery, and the external spermatic (or cremasteric) artery (Harrison and Barclay, 1948). The internal spermatic artery arises from the abdominal aorta and is intimately associated with the pampiniform plexus of veins. The vascular arrangement within the pampiniform plexus, with counterflowing artery and veins, facilitates the exchange of heat and small molecules. For example, testosterone passively diffuses from veins to the artery in a concentration-limited manner (Bayard et al., 1975). **The countercurrent heat exchange supplies arterial blood to the testis that is 2°C to 4°C lower than the rectal temperature in normal men** (Agger, 1971). A loss of the temperature differential is associated with testicular dysfunction in men with varicocele (Goldstein and Eid, 1989) and cryptorchidism (Marshall and Edler, 1982). As the spermatic cord is commonly dissected during varicocele repair, it is surgically relevant to know that a single artery is observed in 50% of spermatic cords, with two arteries in 30% and three arteries in 20% of cases (Beck et al., 1992).

Inferior to the scrotal pampiniform plexus and near the mediastinal testis, the spermatic artery is highly coiled and branches before entering the testis. Extensive interconnections, especially between the internal spermatic and deferential arteries, allow maintenance of testis viability even after division of the internal spermatic artery (Fig. 64.7). From angiographic studies, a single artery enters the testis in 56% of cases; two branches in 31% of cases, and three or more branches in 13% of testes (Kormano and Suoranta, 1971). In men with a single testicular artery, its interruption can result in testicular atrophy (Silber, 1979). The testicular arteries penetrate the tunica albuginea and travel inferiorly along the posterior surface of the testis within the parenchyma. Branching arteries pass anteriorly over the testicular parenchyma. Major testicular artery branches also

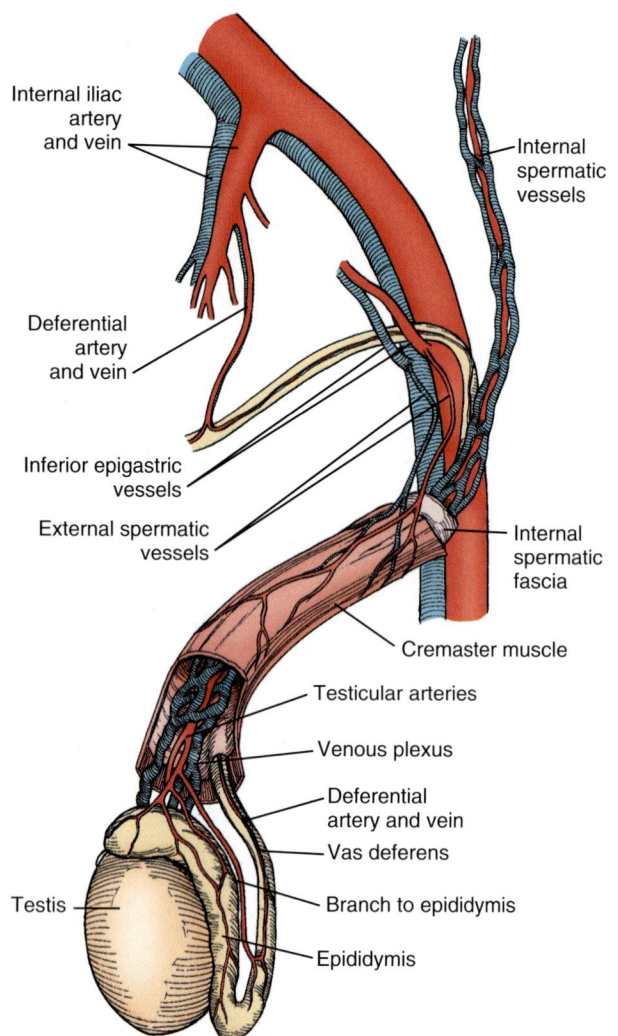

Fig. 64.7. Schematic illustration of interconnections between internal spermatic, external spermatic (cremasteric), and deferential vessels in the peritesticular region and spermatic cord.

travel over the inferior pole of the testis, pass anteriorly, and branch out over the surface of the testis. The location of these vessels is clinically important, because they may be injured during orchiopexy, testis biopsy, or sperm retrieval procedures (Jarow, 1991; Schlegel and Su, 1997). **The midsection of the testis has relatively fewer vessels compared with superior or inferior areas.** Individual arteries to the seminiferous tubules, termed **centrifugal arteries**, travel within the septa. Centrifugal artery branches give rise to arterioles that supply individual intertubular and peritubular capillaries (Muller, 1957). The intertubular capillaries are located within the columns of interstitial tissue, whereas the ladder-like capillaries running near the seminiferous tubule are called **peritubular capillaries.** Through this vascular complex, the human testis is provided with 9 mL of blood per 100 g of tissue per minute (Pettersson et al., 1973).

Veins within the testis are unusual in that they do not run with the corresponding intratesticular arteries. Small parenchymal veins empty either into the veins on the testis surface or into a group of veins near the mediastinum testis that travels along the rete testis (Setchell and Brooks, 1988). These two sets of veins join together with deferential veins to form the pampiniform plexus as they ascend into the scrotum. Pampiniform plexus veins are thin walled, which likely contributes to the effective diffusion of testosterone and heat with the closely associated spermatic artery.

The testis has no known somatic innervation. It receives autonomic innervation primarily from the intermesenteric nerves and renal plexus (Mitchell, 1935). These nerves run along the testicular artery into the testis. It appears that testicular adrenergic innervation is restricted primarily to small blood vessels that supply Leydig cell clusters that may regulate Leydig cell steroidogenesis (Baumgarten et al., 1968; Turnbull and Rivier, 1997). It is thought that vascular tone in the testis is regulated at several levels (Linzell and Setchell, 1969), including autoregulation of capsular arteries (Davis et al., 1990), and regional variation is based on local metabolic need and governed by peptides such as atrial natriuretic peptide (Collin et al., 1997) and assisted transport of molecules such as LH across the vascular endothelium (Milgrom et al., 1997). Indeed, these observations suggest a highly specialized function for the microvasculature of the testis (see review by Desjardins [1989]).

Prominent lymphatics can be observed within the spermatic cord (Hundeiker, 1971). Obstruction of these ducts results in dilation of the testis interstitium but not the seminiferous tubules, suggesting that the interstitial space is drained by lymphatics.. **Lymphatic obstruction can also result in hydrocele formation, a known complication of varicocelectomy and herniorrhaphy procedures.** The sperm-containing intratubular fluid that bathes Sertoli cells flows from the seminiferous tubules into the rete testis and subsequently into the caput epididymis. This fluid, isosmotic with plasma, is thought to be mainly of seminiferous tubule origin (Setchell and Brooks, 1988). **Reabsorption of this fluid within the rete testis and efferent ductules is regulated by estrogens** (Lee et al., 2000). Tubular fluid composition is markedly different from blood plasma or lymphatics, suggesting that substances are not freely diffusible into and out of the tubules (Setchell and Waites, 1975). This has led to the concept of a "blood-testis barrier" to be discussed later.

Testis Cytoarchitecture

Interstitium

Leydig Cells. The testis interstitium contains blood vessels, lymphatics, fibroblasts, macrophages, mast cells, and Leydig cells (Fig. 64.8). **Leydig cells are responsible for the bulk of testicular steroid production. Leydig cells differentiate from mesenchymal precursor cells by the seventh week of gestation.** The activation of Leydig cell steroidogenesis correlates with the onset of androgen-dependent differentiation of the male reproductive system. Leydig cells differentiate from stem cell precursors under the influence of LH and placental-derived human chorionic gonadotropin (hCG) and from the effect of local paracrine factors such as insulin-like growth factor-1 (IGF-1) (Huhtaniemi and Pelliniemi, 1992; Le Roy et al., 1999; Teerds and Dorrington, 1993). **By 3 months after birth, a second wave of Leydig cell differentiation occurs in response to pituitary LH production, briefly elevating testosterone levels.** Androgen produced during the early male neonate's life is thought to hormonally imprint the hypothalamus, liver, and prostate such that they respond appropriately to androgen stimulation later in life. **After reactivation of the HPG axis at puberty, stereologic analysis has revealed that a single testis from a young adult contains approximately 700 million Leydig cells** (Kaler and Neaves, 1978).

Testosterone. Testosterone, synthesized from cholesterol, is the principal steroid produced by the testis (Lipsett, 1974). Numerous C18, C19, and C21 steroids are also produced (Ewing and Brown, 1977; Lipsett, 1974). Cholesterol is transported into Leydig cell mitochondria, where the cholesterol side-chain cleavage enzyme converts it to pregnenolone. Maintenance of cholesterol stores is part of normal Leydig cell function; LH stimulation evokes cholesterol mobilization through cholesterol esterase activity. Pregnenolone is transported out of the mitochondrial membrane into the smooth endoplasmic reticulum, where it is converted into testosterone. Testosterone diffuses across the cell membrane and is trapped within the extracellular fluid and blood plasma by steroid-binding proteins.

Cholesterol transport to the inner membrane of the mitochondrion is regulated by two transport proteins: steroidogenic acute regulatory (StAR) protein and peripheral benzodiazepine receptor (PBR). LH binding elicits StAR synthesis in the Leydig cell, which then threads through the outer mitochondrial membrane to

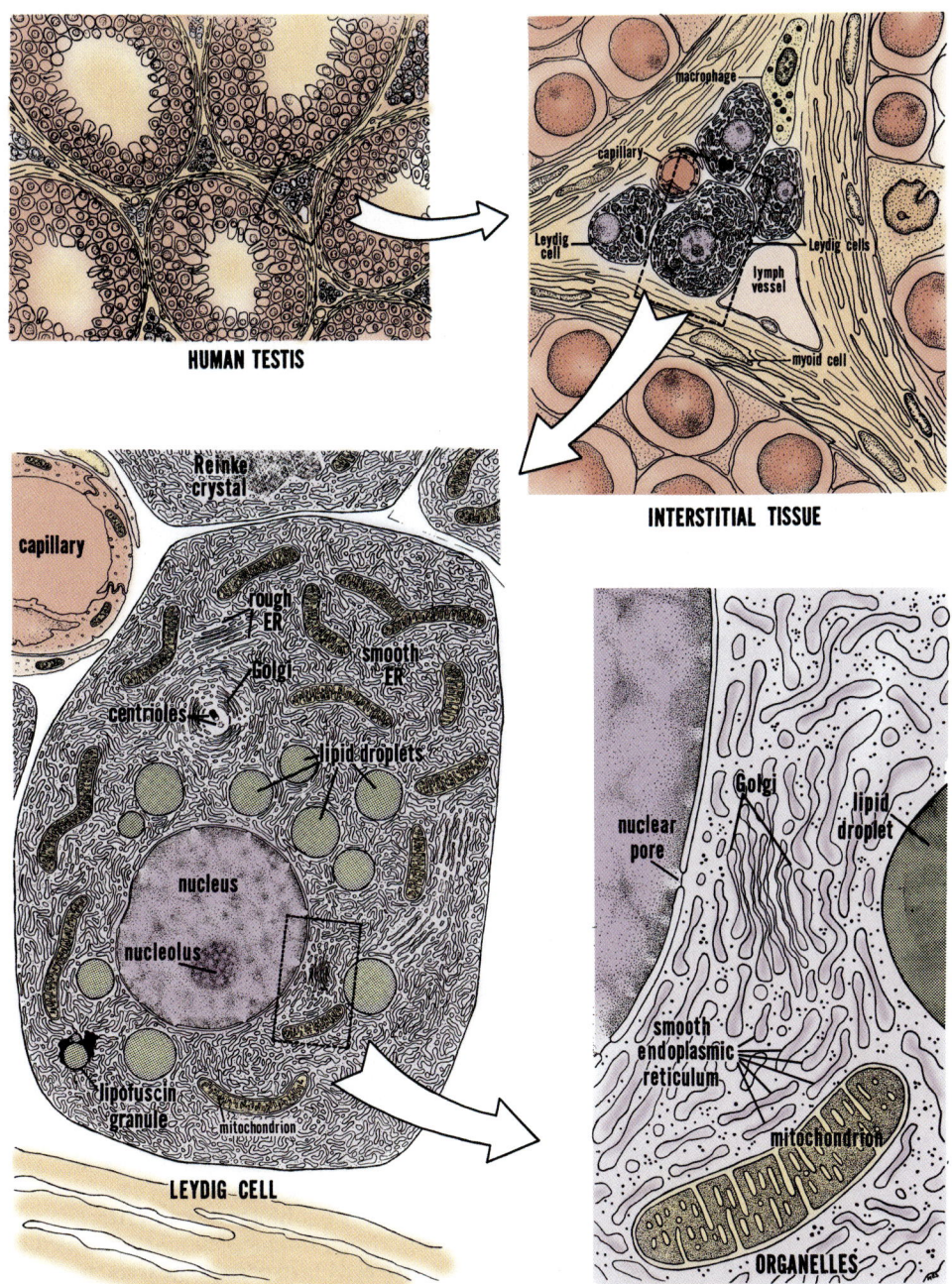

Fig. 64.8. Fine structure of human Leydig cells. Leydig cells occur in clusters in the interstitium between seminiferous tubules *(upper left)*. Interstitial tissue *(upper right)* contains macrophages and fibroblasts and capillaries and lymph vessels. The most abundant organelle within the Leydig cell cytoplasm is the smooth endoplasmic reticulum *([ER], lower left)*. Organelles seen in greater detail *(lower right)*. (From Christensen AK: Leydig cells. In Greep RO, Astwood WB, editors: *Handbook of physiology*, Baltimore, 1975, Williams & Wilkins. Copyright 1975, American Physiological Society, Bethesda, MD.)

facilitate cholesterol transport (Stocco, 2000). PBR forms a channel for cholesterol in the mitochondrial membrane (Culty et al., 1999), but it is not clear whether PBR functionally interacts with StAR (West et al., 2001).

The four major enzymes participating in testosterone biosynthesis from pregnenolone are cholesterol side-chain cleavage enzyme, 3β-hydroxysteroid dehydrogenase, cytochrome P450 17α-hydroxylase/C17-20-lyase, and 17β-hydroxysteroid dehydrogenase. The enzymology, chromosomal locations, and molecular genetics of these enzymes are well described (Payne and Hales, 2004). Mutations in the genes encoding these enzymes have been described, and the resulting disorders of androgen biosynthesis are a relatively rare cause of sexual ambiguity in chromosomally normal males (Miller, 2002).

Control of Testosterone Synthesis. The control of Leydig cell steroidogenesis is complex and involves pituitary and nonpituitary factors (Payne and Youngblood, 1995). **The most important regulator of testosterone production is LH.** After binding LH, through the second messenger cAMP, Leydig cells initiate transport of cholesterol into mitochondria. Pituitary peptides other than LH (e.g., FSH and prolactin) modify the response to LH (Ewing, 1983). Other, nonpituitary factors capable of modifying steroid production by Leydig cells include **GnRH** (Sharpe, 1984); **inhibin** and **activin** (Bardin et al., 1989); **epidermal growth factor (EGF), IGF-1, and TGF-β** (Ascoli and Segaloff, 1989; Saez et al., 1991); prostaglandins (Eik-Nes, 1975); and adrenergic stimulation (Eik-Nes, 1975). Moreover, direct inhibition of Leydig cell steroidogenesis may

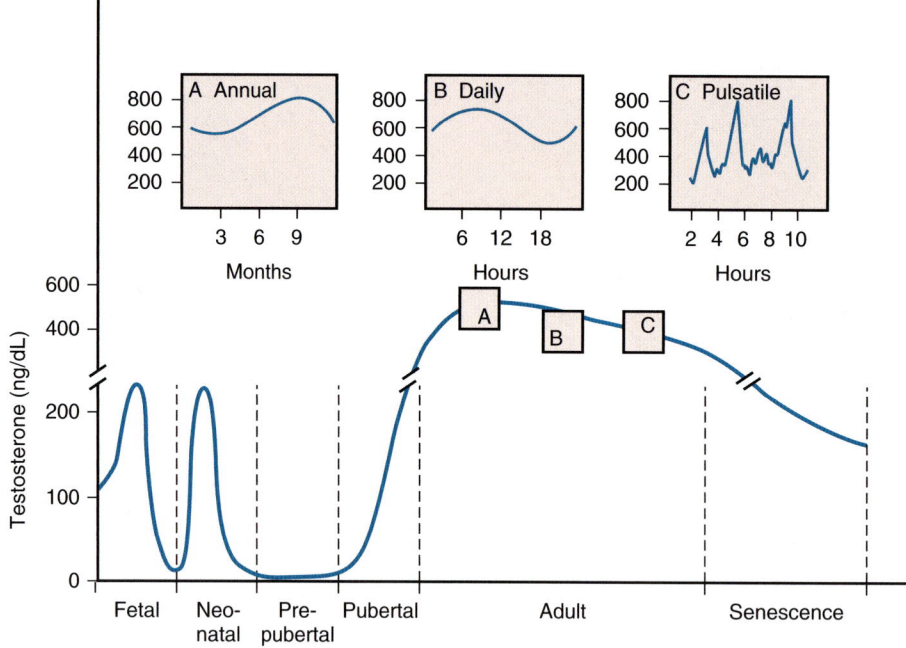

Fig. 64.9. Peripheral blood testosterone levels in the human male during the life cycle. The fetal testosterone peak occurs at 12 to 18 weeks' gestation *(lower left corner; gestational age not shown)*. The neonatal peak occurs at approximately 2 months of age. Testosterone declines to low levels during the prepubertal period. The pubertal increase in testosterone occurs at 12 to 17 years of age. Testosterone concentration in the adult reaches its maximum during the second or third decade of life and then declines slowly. Testosterone declines dramatically during senescence. *Inset A* shows the annual rhythm in testosterone concentration in the human male. The peak and nadir occur in the fall and spring, respectively. *Inset B* shows the daily rhythm in testosterone concentration. The peak and nadir occur in the morning and evening, respectively. *Inset C* shows the frequent and irregular fluctuations in testosterone concentration. (From Ewing LL, Davis JC, Zirkin BR: Regulation of testicular function: a spatial and temporal view. In Greep RO, editor: *International review of physiology*, Baltimore, 1980, University Park Press, p 41.)

also occur through **estrogens and androgens** (Darney et al., 1996; Ewing, 1983).

Testosterone Cycles. Testosterone blood levels change dramatically during human fetal, neonatal, and adult life. Fig. 64.9 shows that a testosterone peak occurs in the human fetus at 12 to 18 weeks of gestation. Another testosterone peak occurs at approximately 2 months of age. A third testosterone peak occurs during the second decade of life. After this, there is a plateau, and then a slow decline with age. Superimposed on this, there are annual and daily rhythms of testosterone production (see Fig. 64.9, insets A and B) and irregular daily fluctuations in testosterone (see Fig. 64.9, inset C). These temporal changes in testosterone production reflect a complex and continuous interaction between the pituitary gland and testis. The testosterone peaks correspond temporally to four developmental events: (1) the development of the fetal reproductive tract, (2) the neonatal "imprinting" of androgen-dependent target tissues, (3) masculinization at puberty, and (4) the maintenance of growth and function of androgen-dependent organs in the adult. This topic has been reviewed thoroughly by Swerdloff and Heber (1981).

Seminiferous Tubules

The seminiferous tubules consist of germ cells and supporting cells and are a unique environment for gamete production. Support cells include Sertoli cells and fibrocyte and myoid cells of the basement membrane. The germ cells include a slowly dividing stem cell population, more rapidly proliferating spermatogonia and spermatocytes, and metamorphosing spermatids.

Sertoli Cells. The seminiferous tubules are lined with Sertoli cells that rest on the tubular basement membrane and extend cytoplasmic ramifications into its lumen (Fig. 64.10). The ultrastructural features of Sertoli cells are well described (Bardin et al., 1994). They have irregularly shaped nuclei, prominent nucleoli, and a low mitotic index and exhibit unique **tight junctional complexes** between adjacent Sertoli cells. **These tight junctions are the strongest intercellular barriers in the body. They divide the seminiferous tubule space into basal (basement membrane) and adluminal (lumen) compartments** (see Fig. 64.10). This anatomic arrangement forms the basis for the **blood-testis barrier** and allows spermatogenesis to occur in an immunologically privileged site. **Sertoli cells serve as nurse cells for spermatogenesis, nourishing developing germ cells within and between Sertoli cell cytoplasmic projections.** The undifferentiated **spermatogonia** are near the basement membrane of the tubule, whereas the more advanced **spermatocytes and spermatids** are near the luminal surface. Thus the Sertoli cell is a polarized epithelium in which the base approximates the plasma environment, and its apex harbors an environment unique to the seminiferous tubule (Ewing et al., 1980).

Sertoli cells nurture germ cell development by (1) providing a specialized adluminal microenvironment, (2) supporting germ cells through gap junctions between Sertoli and germ cells, and (3) allowing migration of developing germ cells within the tubule (see Fig. 64.10). The tight junctions between Sertoli cells are constantly remodeled to allow "opening" and "closing" necessary for germ cell interaction and migration (Mruk and Cheng, 2004). Ligand-receptor complexes, such as c-kit and kit ligand, are likely involved in mediating communication between germ and Sertoli cells. Sertoli cells also participate in germ cell phagocytosis and produce and secrete fluid and important effector molecules. Androgen-binding protein (ABP) is one of earliest described Sertoli cell secretory products (Hansson and Djoseland, 1972). ABP is an intracellular carrier of androgen within the Sertoli cell. **By binding testosterone, ABP maintains high levels of androgen (50-fold higher than serum) within the seminiferous tubules.** Testosterone also plays an important role in

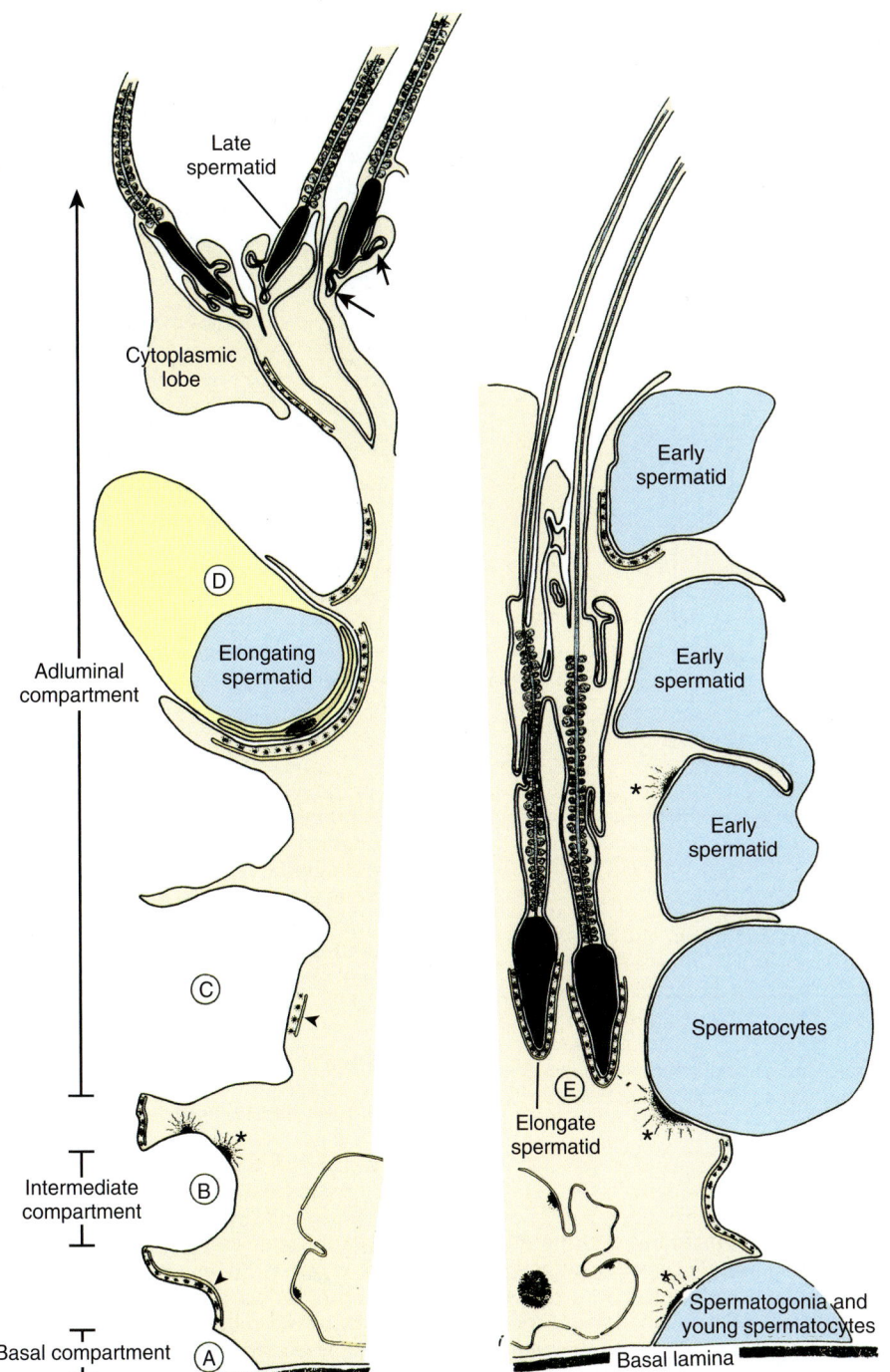

Fig. 64.10. Representation of the tree-shaped Sertoli cell with a thickened central portion, or "trunk," and more delicate processes, or "limbs." Note the basal, intermediate, and adluminal compartments of the seminiferous epithelium. *(A)* Spermatogonia and early spermatocytes share positions on the basal lamina and are enveloped by adjacent Sertoli cells that join to form tight junctional complexes (site of blood-testis barrier). *(B)* Sertoli cells form junctional complexes above and below leptotene-zygotene spermatocytes as they translocate from the basal to adluminal compartments. *(C)* The spermatocytes enter the adluminal compartment when Sertoli tight junctions dissociate. *(D)* The elongating spermatid is situated within a narrow recess of the Sertoli cell trunk. *(E)* As the spermatid elongates further, the cell becomes lodged within the body of the Sertoli cell. The advanced spermatid moves toward the lumen of the epithelium in preparation for spermiation. Only the sperm head remains in intimate contact with the Sertoli cell. Specialized cell-to-cell contacts: *asterisks,* desmosome-gap junction complex; *arrowheads,* ectoplasmic specializations; *isolated arrows,* tubulobulbar complexes. (From Russell L: Sertoli-germ cell interactions: a review. *Gamete Res.* 3:179, 1980.)

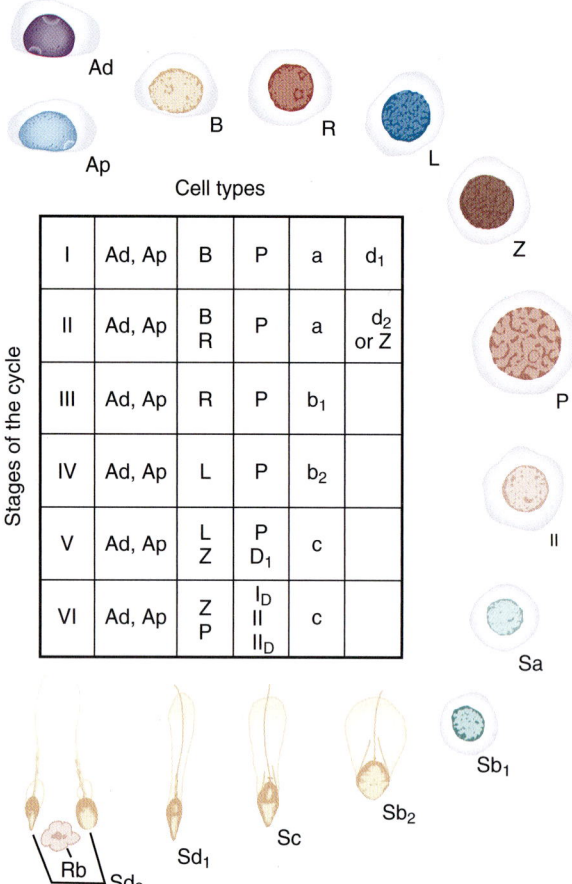

Fig. 64.11. The steps of spermatogenesis in man. *Ad*, Dark type A spermatogonium; *Ap*, pale type A spermatogonium; *B*, type B spermatogonium; *II*, secondary spermatocyte; *L*, leptotene spermatocyte; *P*, pachytene spermatocyte; *R*, resting or preleptotene primary spermatocyte; *Rb*, residual body; $Sa(a)$, Sb_1 (b_1), Sb_2 (b_2), Sc (c), Sd_1 (d_1), Sd_2 (d_2), spermatids; *Z*, zygotene spermatocyte. The table shows cells that make up the six stages of the "cycle" of the seminiferous epithelium (I to VI): D_1, diakinesis; ID and IID, first and second maturation divisions of spermatocytes. (Modified from Clermont Y: Renewal of spermatogonia in man. *Am J Anat.* 118:509, 1966.)

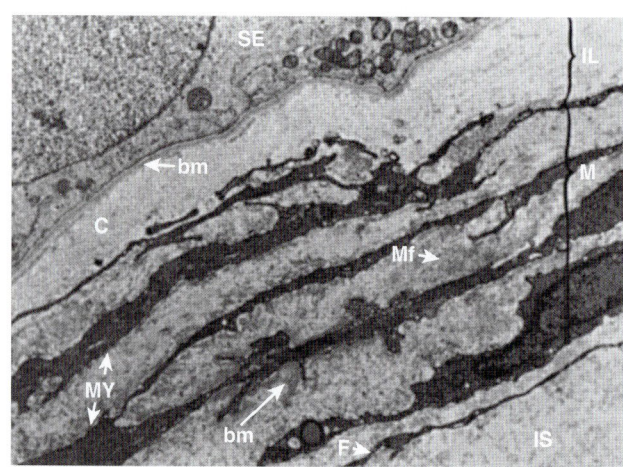

Fig. 64.12. Low-power electron micrograph of human peritubular testis tissue. Peritubular tissue lies between the basement membrane *(bm)* of the seminiferous epithelium *(SE)* and the interstitial tissue *(IS)*. Peritubular tissue has three zones: the inner lamella *(IL)*; the myoid layer *(M)*, containing myoid cells *(MY)* with abundant microfibrils *(Mf)*; and an adventitial layer containing fibroblasts *(F)*. (From Hermo L, Lalli M, Clermont Y: Arrangement of connective tissue elements in the walls of seminiferous tubules of man and monkey. *Am J Anat.* 148:433–446, 1977.)

the regulation of Sertoli cell function, including ABP production (Griswold et al., 1988). **Inhibin is Sertoli cell derived** and plays an important regulatory role in the negative feedback loop of FSH secretion. Inhibin B is an important endocrine marker of Sertoli cell function in the male infertility evaluation (Pierik et al., 1998).

As keepers of the testis immunologic sanctuary, Sertoli cells maintain a germ cell microenvironment entirely distinct from that of plasma. As such, Sertoli cells secrete numerous other products, including extracellular matrix components (lamin, collagen type IV, and collagen type I) and proteins such as ceruloplasmin, transferrin, glycoprotein 2, plasminogen activator, somatomedin-like substances, T proteins, H-Y antigen, clusterin, cyclic proteins, growth factors, and somatomedin (Mruk and Cheng, 2004). Dihydrotestosterone, testosterone, androstenediols, 17β-estradiol, and other C21 steroids are also produced by Sertoli cells (Ewing et al., 1980; Mather et al., 1983), although the roles they play in Sertoli cell function are largely unknown.

Germ Cells. Within the human seminiferous tubule, germ cells give rise to approximately 123×10^6 (range, 21 to 374×10^6) spermatozoa daily (Amann and Howards, 1980). This equates to the production of about 1000 sperm per heartbeat. Within the seminiferous tubule, germ cells are arranged in a highly ordered sequence from the basement membrane to the lumen. **Morphologic analysis of the various germ cells reveals at least 13 recognizable germ cell types in the human testis** (Clermont, 1963; Heller and Clermont, 1964; Fig. 64.11). Each cell type is thought to represent a different step in the spermatogenic process. Proceeding from the least to the most differentiated, based on morphologic appearance, they have been named **dark type A spermatogonia (Ad); pale type A (Ap) spermatogonia; type B spermatogonia (B); preleptotene (R), leptotene (L), zygotene (Z), and pachytene (P) primary spermatocytes; secondary spermatocytes (II); and Sa, Sb, Sc, Sd_1, and Sd_2 spermatids.** Sertoli cell tight junctions maintain spermatogonia and early spermatocytes within the basal compartment and all subsequent germ cells in the adluminal compartment.

Peritubular Structure

The human seminiferous tubule is surrounded by several layers of peritubular tissue (Hermo et al., 1977; Fig. 64.12). The outer adventitial layer consists of fibrocytes. In the middle layer are myoid cells interspersed with connective tissue lamellae. The inner layer consists of a collagen matrix. The peritubular myoid cells are thought to have contractile function (Toyama, 1977). Myoid cells also actively secrete extracellular matrix components fibronectin and collagen type I and produce the inner collagenous layer (Tung et al., 1984). Notably, myoid cells are known to associate with Sertoli cells in a precise mesenchymal-epithelial interaction. Skinner et al. (1988) isolated a myoid-derived paracrine factor produced, P-Mod-S (peritubular modifies Sertoli), that profoundly affects Sertoli cell synthetic functions in vitro.

Blood-Testis Barrier

Dyes and other substances, when injected into the bloodstream of animals, rapidly appear throughout all body tissues but fail to penetrate regions of the brain and testis. This led to the concept of the existence of a blood-testis barrier. **More appropriately termed the "blood–seminiferous tubule barrier," it has two components: an anatomic or mechanical element and functional elements.** The mechanical barrier is created, in part, by muscle-like myoid cells that surround seminiferous tubules (Dym and Fawcett, 1970; Fawcett et al., 1970). Regulation of molecular traffic also occurs at the level of capillary endothelial cells. However, the most important component of this barrier is the synaptic tight junctions between Sertoli cells that preclude the passage of large molecules and lymphocytes. These anatomic elements are necessary but not sufficient for maintaining the immunologic "sanctuary" status within the tubule, because they are not observed in other protected areas of the reproductive tract (Brown et al., 1972; Tung et al., 1971).

Thus, although the mechanical barrier contributes to the isolation of the testis, other "functional" components must also exist to suppress the normal immune response. Several mechanisms likely work in concert to protect sperm from destruction. First, the types and number of lymphocytes are restricted in anatomically vulnerable regions in the germinal epithelium (Anderson and Hill, 1988; el-Demiry et al., 1985; Mahi-Brown et al., 1988). There is also evidence to suggest that immunologic tolerance plays a role in the functional blood-testis barrier. The leading theory proposes that within the anatomically weaker areas (rete testis, efferent tubule, epididymis) of the barrier, there is a small, continuous leak of sperm antigens (Tung, 1980). This leak generates T-suppressor cells and immune tolerance, similar to desensitization protocols for common environmental allergens. However, with larger antigenic challenges, a true immune response results (Turek, 1997). Contributing to this tolerance, it is now clear that Sertoli cells express various mediators that act locally to generate an immunosuppressive environment within the testis (Filippini et al., 2001). These include the "master immune regulator" molecule galectin 1 (Chui et al., 2011) as well as the cytokines interferon-γ, soluble Fc receptor, and TGF-β (Ben-Rafael and Orvieto, 1992; Perussia et al., 1987; Turek, 1997), and androgens (Diemer et al., 2003).

Why does the blood-testis barrier exist? Because it develops at spermarche (Kormano, 1967), it is likely important for meiosis, because it may immunologically isolate developing male gametes that are not recognized as self by the adult male immune system. In this sense, **the value of a blood-testis barrier is fully realized after puberty, because foreign "antigens" on postmeiotic germ cells exist only after spermarche. A testicular insult such as biopsy, torsion, or trauma will not induce antisperm antibodies if it occurs before puberty.** After puberty, however, immunologic infertility is a known risk (Turek, 1997). Clinically, the blood-testis barrier may also limit chemotherapy access to cancer cells sequestered behind it and result in isolated cancer recurrence within the testis.

Spermatogenesis

Spermatogenesis is a remarkably complex and specialized process of DNA reduction and germ cell metamorphosis. Older studies have estimated that the entire process in humans requires approximately 64 days (Clermont, 1972). However, an in vivo kinetic study in healthy men revealed that **the total time to produce an ejaculated sperm ranges from 42 to 76 days,** suggesting that the duration of spermatogenesis can vary widely among individuals (Misell et al., 2006; Fig. 64.13). Spermatogenesis involves (1) **a proliferative phase** as spermatogonia divide to replace their number (self-renewal) or differentiate into daughter cells that become mature gametes; (2) **a meiotic phase** when germ cells undergo a reduction division, resulting in haploid (half the normal DNA complement) spermatids; and (3) **a spermiogenesis phase** in which spermatids undergo a profound metamorphosis to become mature spermatozoa. (For excellent reviews, see Steinberger [1976] and de Kretser and Kerr [1988].)

A **cycle of spermatogenesis** involves the division of primitive spermatogonial stem cells into subsequent germ cells. Several cycles of spermatogenesis coexist within the germinal epithelium, and they are described morphologically as **stages.** If spermatogenesis is viewed from a single fixed point within a seminiferous tubule, six recognizable cellular associations or stages are predictably observed in humans (Heller and Clermont, 1964) (see Fig. 64.11). In addition, there is also a specific organization of spermatogenic cycles within the tubular space, termed **spermatogenic waves.** The best evidence suggests that human spermatogenesis exists in a spiral or helical cellular arrangement that ensures sperm production is a continuous and not a pulsatile process (Schulze, 1989; Fig. 64.14).

Testis Stem Cell Migration, Renewal, and Proliferation

Testis Stem Cell Migration. During early prenatal development, **primordial germ cells** migrate to the gonadal ridge and associate with Sertoli cells to form primitive testicular cords (Witschi, 1948).

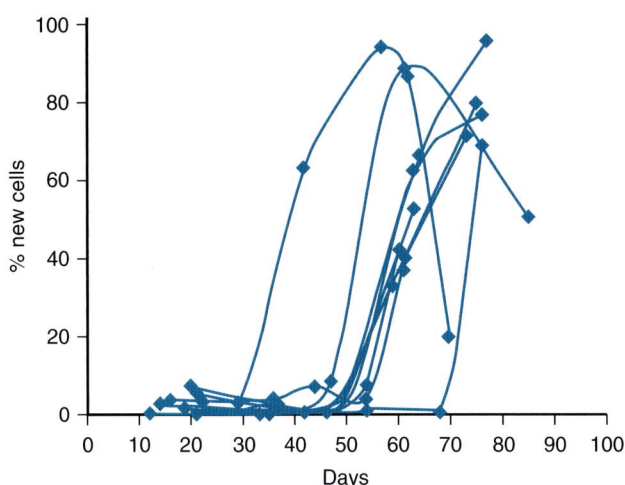

Fig. 64.13. Time to make and ejaculate human sperm. Combined spermatocyte labeling curves for 11 individuals with normal semen quality who ingested 50 mL of ^2H_2O twice daily for 3 weeks. New ejaculated sperm was found as early as 42 days after ingestion of label, and there was considerable interindividual variation in the time to make and ejaculate sperm. (From Misell LM, Holochwost D, Boban D, et al.: A stable isotope/mass spectrometric method for measuring the kinetics of human spermatogenesis in vivo. *J Urol.* 175:242–246, 2006.)

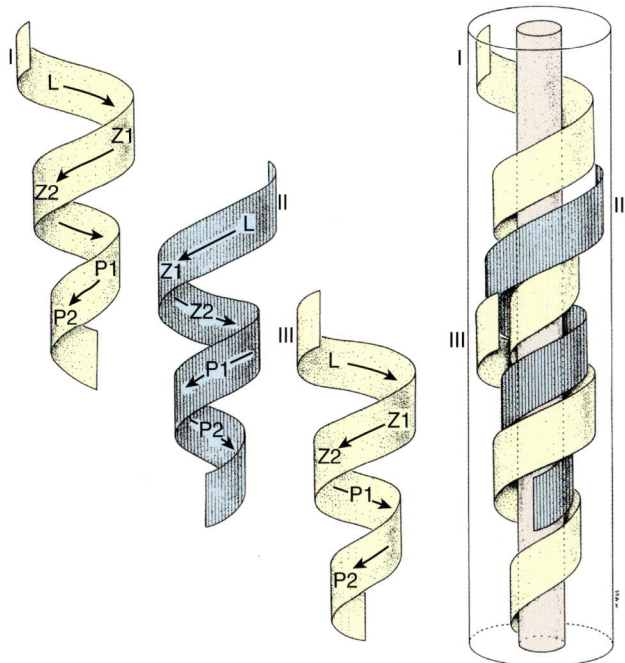

Fig. 64.14. Helical configuration of seminiferous tubule epithelial cycles in man, forming overlapping waves of spermatogenesis that keep sperm production constant. (From Schulze W, Rehder U: Organization and morphogenesis of the human seminiferous epithelium. *Cell Tissue Res.* 237:395–407, 1984.)

These primitive germline stem cells are termed **gonocytes** after the gonad differentiates into a testis by forming seminiferous cords. They are called **spermatogonia** after migration to the periphery of the tubule (Gondos and Hobel, 1971). **These early migrating germ cells have properties similar to embryonic stem cells and are likely the source of adult germ cell tumors** (Ezeh et al., 2005). The failure of germ cells to migrate into the primitive testicle is also thought to be a cause of **extragonadal germ cells tumors** and adult infertility resulting from **azoospermia** with Sertoli cell–only testicular histology (Nikolic et al., 2016).

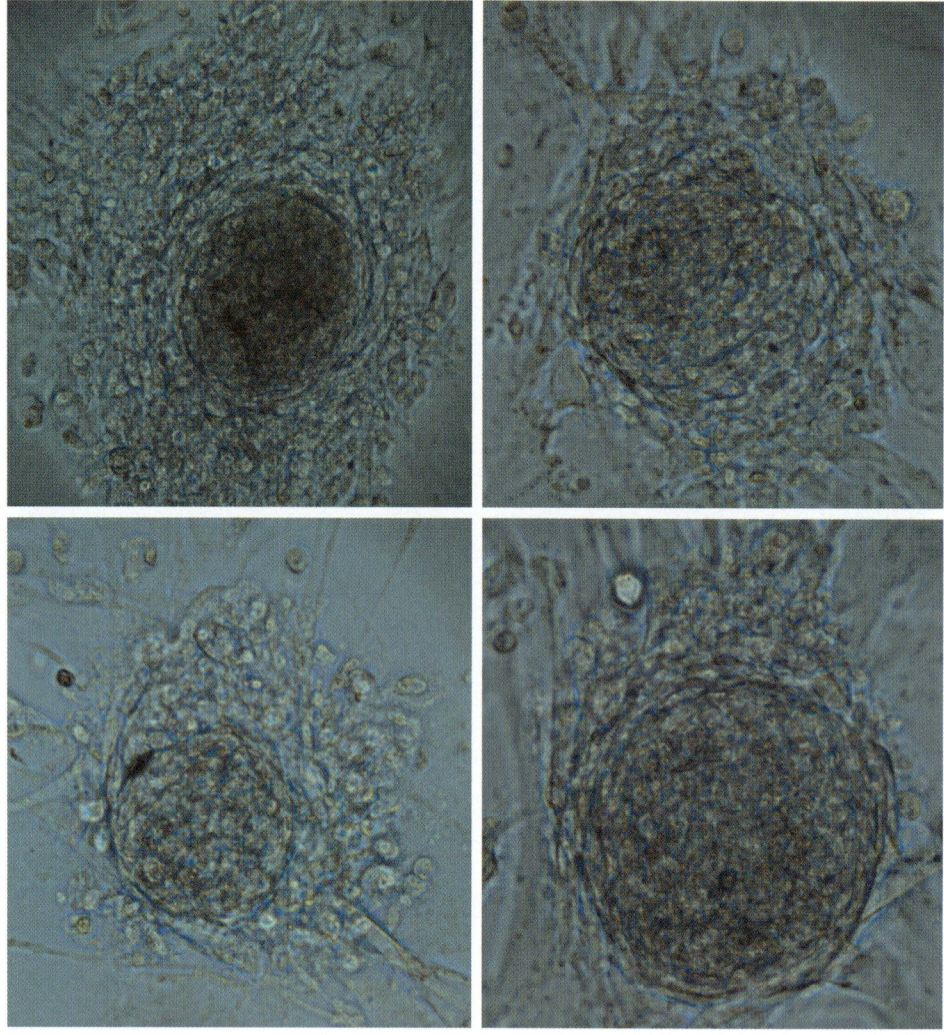

Fig. 64.15. Microphotograph of four different colonies of adult testis spermatogonial-derived stem cells. Cell clusters are the result of reprogramming of adult spermatogonia in culture conditions used for human embryonic stem cells (HESCs). They exhibit the typical cobblestone appearance of HESCs and are functionally multipotent.

Testis Stem Cell Renewal. Spermatogonia within the testis stem cell niche are replenished in a process termed **stem cell renewal**. The growth factor receptor kit ligand/c-kit receptor system and the niche factor glial cell line–derived neurotrophic factor (GDNF) appear involved in this process (Oatley and Brinster, 2008). **Recent studies have also shown that human spermatogonial stem cells can be reprogrammed in vitro to become embryonic-like stem cells** (Conrad et al., 2008; Kossack et al., 2009; Fig. 64.15). Obtained from adult testis biopsies, the embryonic-like cells express distinct markers of pluripotency *(OCT-4, SOX-2, STELLAR, GDF-3)*, can form all three germ layers, maintain a normal karyotype, form teratomas, and express appropriate levels of epigenetic markers and telomerase (Kossack et al., 2009). This finding suggests that in the future the testis may be a source of patient-specific stem cells for cell-based therapy.

Testis Stem Cell Proliferation. In the human, pale type A (Ap) spermatogonia in the basal stem cell niche of the seminiferous tubule divide at 16-day intervals (Clermont, 1972) to form B spermatogonia. B spermatogonia are committed to become spermatocytes, but the cytoplasm between spermatogonial daughter cells remains conjoined after mitosis, forming cytoplasmic bridges between adjacent cells. These **cytoplasmic bridges are observed between germ cells of all classes throughout spermatogenesis** (Ewing et al., 1980). These bridges could be important for synchronized cellular proliferation and differentiation and for regulation of gene expression.

Meiosis

Somatic cells replicate by mitosis, in which genetically identical daughter cells are formed. **Germ cells replicate by meiosis, in which the genetic material is halved to allow reproduction.** Meiosis generates genetic diversity, providing a richer source of material on which natural selection can act. Cell replication by mitosis is a precise, well-orchestrated sequence of events involving duplication of the genetic material (chromosomes), breakdown of the nuclear envelope, and equal division of the chromosomes and cytoplasm into daughter cells. **The essential difference between mitotic and meiotic replication is that a single DNA duplication step is followed by only one cell division in mitosis but two cell divisions in meiosis (four daughter cells).** Consequently, daughter cells contain only half of the chromosome content of parent cells. Thus a diploid ($2n$) parent cell becomes a haploid (n) gamete. Other major differences between mitosis and meiosis are outlined in Table 64.2. Research has shown that small RNA molecules (small RNAs), including small interfering RNAs (siRNAs), microRNAs (miRNAs), and piwi-interacting RNAs (piRNAs), are important regulators of gene germ cell expression at the post-transcriptional or translation level (He et al., 2009; Tolia and Joshua-Tor, 2007).

Spermatogenesis begins with type B spermatogonia dividing mitotically to form primary spermatocytes within the adluminal compartment. **Primary spermatocytes are the first germ cells to**

TABLE 64.2 Essential Differences: Mitosis and Meiosis

MITOSIS	MEIOSIS
Occurs in somatic cells	Occurs in sexual cells
One cell division, two daughter cells	Two cell divisions, four daughter cells
Chromosome number maintained	Chromosome number halved
No pairing, chromosome homologs	Synapse of homologs, prophase I
No crossovers	More than one crossover per homolog pair
Centromeres divide, anaphase	Centromeres divide, anaphase II
Identical daughter genotype	Genetic variation in daughter cells

undergo meiosis (Kerr and de Kretser, 1981). In this process, a meiotic division is followed by a typical mitotic reduction division, resulting in daughter cells with a haploid chromosome complement. In addition, as a consequence of chromosomal recombination, each daughter cell contains different genetic information. The resultant cell is the Sa spermatid (see Fig. 64.11).

Chromosomal recombination, the defining feature of mammalian meiosis, ensures that haploid gametes differ genetically from their adult precursors and is the real engine of genetic diversity and evolution. During meiotic prophase, formation of a synaptonemal complex with pairing of homologous (maternal and paternal) chromosomes occurs, along with physical interaction and exchange of DNA through reciprocal sites of crossing over **(chiasmata)** between homologs. Recent research has shown that defects in the fidelity of recombination within human male germ cells can cause azoospermia and male infertility (Walsh et al., 2009). **In one study, 10% of nonobstructive azoospermic men had significant defects in recombination compared with men with normal spermatogenesis** (Gonsalves et al., 2004). In addition, among men with maturation arrest pattern on testis biopsy, faulty recombination was observed in about half of cases, providing evidence that faulty recombination is linked to poor sperm production (Gonsalves et al., 2004). Variations in recombination also have implications for sperm aneuploidy, because alterations in crossover position are risk factors for chromosomal nondisjunction. **Indeed, evidence suggests that the correlation of faulty recombination and sperm aneuploidy in azoospermic men is strong enough to explain the higher rate of chromosomal abnormalities in offspring conceived with in vitro fertilization (IVF) and intracytoplasmic sperm injection (ICSI)** (Sun et al., 2008).

Spermiogenesis

During spermiogenesis, round Sa spermatids mature into spermatozoa (see Fig. 64.11). During this maturation sequence, cell division does not occur, but there are extensive changes to the spermatid nucleus and cytoplasm. **These include the loss of cytoplasm, migration of cytoplasmic organelles, formation of the acrosome from the Golgi apparatus, formation of the flagellum from the centriole, nuclear compaction to about 10% of former size, and reorganization of mitochondria around the sperm midpiece** (Kerr and de Kretser, 1981). The nucleus of the round spermatid changes from spheric to asymmetrical as chromatin condenses. Many cellular elements contribute to the reshaping process, including chromosome structure, associated chromosomal proteins, the perinuclear cytoskeletal theca layer, the manchette of nuclear microtubules, subacrosomal actin, and Sertoli cell interactions. With completion of spermatid elongation, the Sertoli cell cytoplasm retracts around the developing sperm, stripping it of all unnecessary cytoplasm and extruding it into the tubule lumen.

The mature sperm has remarkably little cytoplasm and is produced in massive quantities—up to 300 per gram of testis per second.

Sertoli Cell–Germ Cell Interaction

A complex network of cell-cell interactions exists within the testis between Leydig cells and Sertoli cells, between Leydig cells and peritubular cells, between Sertoli and peritubular cells, and between Sertoli cells and germ cells. Several Sertoli cell–germ cell associations in mammalian testes are illustrated in Fig. 64.10 (Romrell and Ross, 1979; Russell and Clermont, 1976; Skinner, 1995). In addition, there are factors that can reversibly disrupt the blood-testis barrier, including TGF-β3 and tumor necrosis factor-α (TNF-α). These substances act by reducing the levels of occludin and zonula occludens-1 (ZO-1) in the barrier through a p38 mitogen-activated protein (MAP) kinase signaling pathway (Xia et al., 2009). This represents only a piece of the remarkably complex and highly interactive process that characterizes spermatogenesis.

Genetics

Genetic causes of abnormal spermatogenesis have been identified as point mutations in single genes inherited in Mendelian fashion (e.g., cystic fibrosis), and as chromosomal disorders in which segments of (or entire) chromosomes have structural or numerical abnormalities. The reader is referred to Turek and Reijo Pera (2002) for a comprehensive review of such disorders. The postulation that deletions in the long arm of the Y chromosome cause azoospermia was made over three decades ago (Tiepolo et al., 1976). Based on cytogenetic analysis, this theoretic region was termed the *azoospermia factor (AZF)*. **Currently, the positional patterns of deletions (termed *microdeletions*) in the AZF region are used to subdivide this region into AZFa, AZFb, and AZFc subregions** (Vogt et al., 1996). **Regional deletions of the Y chromosome, termed *Yq microdeletions*, occur in 6% to 8% of severely oligospermic men and in 15% of azoospermic men** (Reijo et al., 1996). Taken together, such deletions are the most commonly defined molecular cause of male infertility (Kostiner et al., 1998).

There is emerging literature addressing the prognostic value of AZF deletions. In contrast to partial and complete AZFc-deletion patients, in whom sperm is often found on semen analysis or testis biopsy, finding ejaculated or testis sperm in men with complete AZFa or AZFb deletions is highly unlikely (Hopps et al., 2003; Park et al., 2013). Complete AZFa deletions are associated with germ cell aplasia or Sertoli cell–only histology. In general, complete AZFb deletions are associated with maturation arrest at the primary spermatocyte (early) or spermatid (late) stages, but ejaculated sperm has also been reported in isolated cases (Park et al., 2013). AZFc deletions are associated with hypospermatogenesis or a Sertoli cell–only pattern with foci of spermatogenesis. Sperm have been detected in ejaculates of men with presumed and confirmed *partial* AZFa and AZFb deletions (Foresta et al., 2001). Similarly, ejaculated sperm in men with AZFa + b, and AZFb + c deletions (presumably partial deletions) has also been reported (Park et al., 2013), but the finding of AZFa – c deletions has been associated with azoospermia and no sperm on testis biopsy.

More recently, it has become clear that the **X chromosome** is also important for spermatogenesis. In 2001 Wang et al. reported on a systematic search for genes expressed exclusively in mouse spermatogonia and found that 10 were localized to the X chromosome (Wang et al., 2001). Further studies of X-linked genes in male infertility patients have identified the *SOX3* gene (sex determining region Y box 3) and the *FATE* gene as two potential candidate fertility genes (Olesen et al., 2003; Raverot et al., 2004), confirming the concept that X chromosome genes may contribute significantly to currently unexplained cases of male infertility (Mueller et al., 2013).

Genetics and Paternal Age

Age-Related Sperm Chromosomal Anomalies. The chromosomal status of sperm was first investigated because of concern that advanced paternal age was associated with increased cases of trisomy, especially trisomy 21 or Down syndrome, in offspring. With fluorescence in situ hybridization (FISH) technology, subtle paternal-age effects on sperm aneuploidy are now evident. **The paternal age effect appears to increase the fraction of sperm with sex chromosomal aneuploidies** (Wyrobek et al., 1996). However, there is **little evidence to support a paternal age–related increase in aneuploid births, except for possibly trisomy 21 and disomy 1 (very rare).** Examining sperm chromosome structural abnormalities, Martin and Rademaker (1987) described a significant linear relationship between paternal age and the frequency of structural anomalies in sperm ($r = 0.63$). One explanation for this association may be that **continued cell division during spermatogenesis places germ cells at risk for chromosomal injury, especially with advanced paternal age.** Except for reciprocal translocations, however, there is little evidence to indicate that this association leads to an increased frequency of offspring with de novo structural chromosomal anomalies.

Age-Related Sperm Genetic Mutations. Single gene defects in sperm result from errors in DNA replication. Although it has been difficult to assess the presence or absence of such defects in sperm, the effect of advanced paternal age on conditions in offspring associated with single-gene mutations is clear. These disorders are listed in Box 64.1 and consist of autosomal dominant diseases that have known associations with advanced paternal age. They are termed *sentinel phenotypes* because they are disorders of significant frequency and low fitness and stem from highly penetrant mutations. **One mechanism for the development of new single-gene mutations with age implicates the characteristic and continuous process of spermatogonial cell division.** By puberty, 30 cell divisions of spermatogonia have occurred; however, after puberty, 23 divisions occur per year in these cells. **The simple fact that the spermatogonia of older men have undergone numerous cell divisions may increase the chance of errors in DNA transcription, the source of single-gene defects.** Formal risk estimates exist for the contribution of advanced paternal age to autosomal dominant mutations. In men younger than 29 years, the risk of a mutation occurring in offspring is 0.22 per 1000 births. This risk doubles (0.45 per 1000) at paternal ages 40 to 44, and then climbs to 3.7 per 1000 births at ages older than 45 (Friedman, 1981).

Age-Related Sperm Epigenetic Changes. There is also emerging evidence that DNA methylation marks in sperm that control gene expression, termed epigenetics, are altered with paternal age (Jenkins et al., 2014). Sperm appear to accumulate hundreds of DNA methylation defects with age that localize to specific genomic sites, many of which control genes associated with neurodevelopment (e.g., schizophrenia, bipolar disease, autism, mood disorders). In a study of sperm donated twice by men, once when young and again when older, the rate of epigenetic change in sperm doubled that estimated for other body tissues (Jenkins et al., 2014). Even more intriguing, the epigenetics changes that occurred in sperm as men age tended to cluster in genes associated with schizophrenia and bipolar disorder, diseases known to occur more in offspring as paternal age increases. Thus at least a subset of paternal age-related disorders in offspring may be a consequence of epigenetic alterations transmitted in sperm (Yatsenko and Turek, 2018).

KEY POINTS: TESTIS

- The testis contains 250 m of seminiferous tubules and 700 million Leydig cells in the young adult.
- Spermatogenesis occurs in stages, cycles, and waves to ensure constant sperm production.
- Genes on the X, as well as the Y, chromosome govern spermatogenesis and contribute to male infertility.
- With paternal age, there are increases in sperm structural chromosomal abnormalities, autosomal-dominant mutations, and epigenetic alterations leading to disease in offspring.

EPIDIDYMIS

Gross Architecture

The epididymis is a comma-shaped organ located along the posterolateral surface of the testis. **Passage through the epididymis induces many changes to newly formed sperm, including gains in functional motility, and alterations in surface charge, membrane proteins, immunoreactivity, phospholipids, fatty acid content, and adenylate cyclase activity. These changes improve cell membrane structural integrity, improve motility and sperm chemotaxis, and increase fertilization ability.** Spermatozoa within the testis have very poor or no motility. They become progressively motile and functional only after traversing the epididymis.

The epididymis is a tubule or duct 3 to 4 m in length and tightly coiled and encapsulated within the sheath of connective tissue of the tunica vaginalis (Lanz and Neuhauser, 1964; Turner et al., 1978). Extensions from the sheath enter interductal spaces and form septa that divide the duct into histologically characteristic regions (Kormano and Reijonen, 1976). Anatomically, these are classically divided into caput or head, corpus or body, and cauda or tail (Fig. 64.16). The caput epididymis consists of 8 to 12 ductuli efferentes from the testis. The lumen of the ductuli efferentes is large and somewhat irregular in shape near the testis, becoming narrow and oval near the junction with the ductus epididymis. Distal to this junction, the duct diameter increases slightly and thereafter remains constant in the corpus epididymis. In the bulky cauda epididymis, the tubule diameter enlarges substantially and acquires an irregular shape. Progressing distally, the tubule gradually assumes the characteristic appearance of the vas deferens.

Vascular and Lymph Supply

In humans, the caput and the corpus epididymis receive arterial blood from a branch of the testicular artery (see Fig. 64.7). It subsequently divides into superior and inferior epididymal branches (MacMillan, 1954). The epididymis also receives blood from branches of the deferential arteries (artery of the vas deferens), and collateral

---

BOX 64.1 Genetic Disorders in Offspring Associated With Advanced Paternal Age

Achondroplasias
Aniridia
Apert syndrome
Bilateral retinoblastoma
Crouzon syndrome
Fibrodysplasia ossificans
Hemophilia A
Lesch-Nyhan syndrome
Marfan syndrome
Neurofibromatosis
Oculodentodigital syndrome
Polycystic kidney disease
Polyposis coli
Progeria
Treacher Collins syndrome
Tuberous sclerosis
Waardenburg syndrome
Schizophrenia
Bipolar disorder
Autism
Attention deficit disorders
Alzheimer disease (postulated)

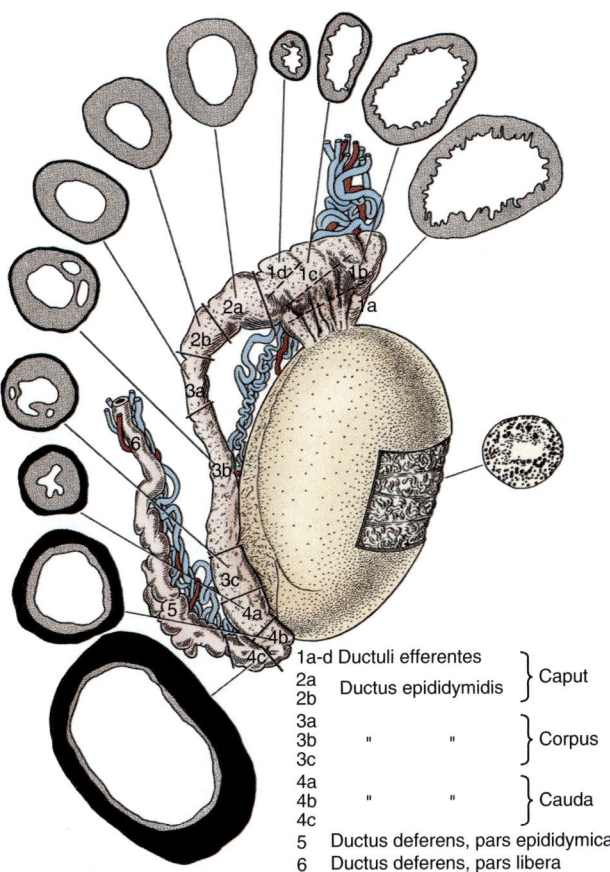

Fig. 64.16. Drawing of the human epididymis showing regionalization of the ductal epithelium and muscle layer. Epididymal segment locations are shown in cross section and are identified by number. (From Baumgarten HG, Holstein AF, Rosengren E: Arrangement, ultrastructure, and adrenergic innervation of smooth musculature of the ductal efferentes, ductus epididymidis, and ductus deferens in man. *Z Zellforsch Mikrosk Anat.* 120:37, 1971.)

1a-d Ductuli efferentes
2a
2b   Ductus epididymidis   } Caput
3a
3b   "   "   } Corpus
3c
4a
4b   "   "   } Cauda
4c
5   Ductus deferens, pars epididymica
6   Ductus deferens, pars libera

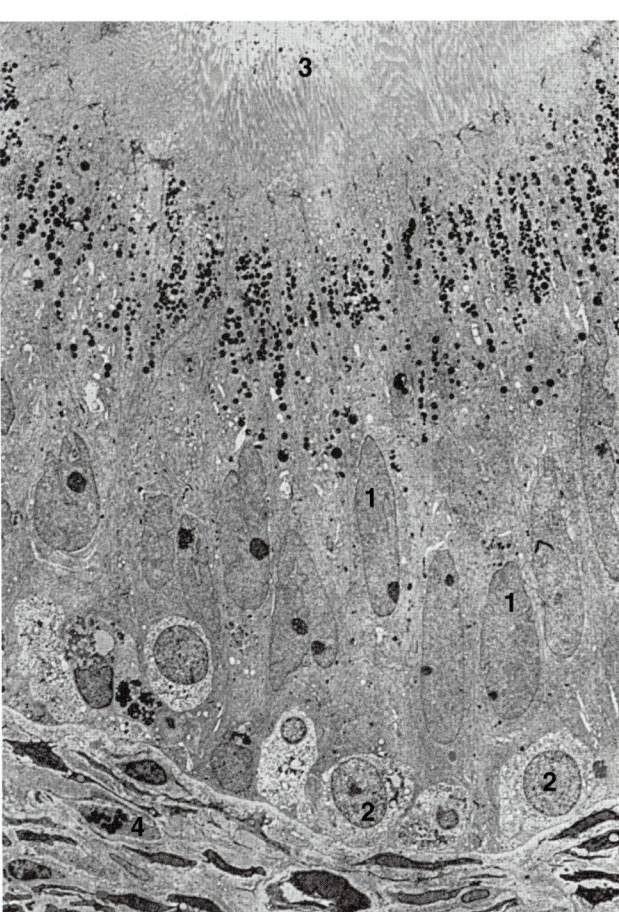

Fig. 64.17. Electron micrograph of a human epididymis in cross section. Major components of the luminal epithelium are principal cells *(1)*, basal cells *(2)*, stereocilia *(3)*, and myofilaments *(4)*. Magnification approximately ×1800. (From Holstein AF: In Hafez ESE, editor: *Human semen and fertility regulation in men*, St. Louis, 1976, Mosby.)

vessels connect the deferential artery to the testicular blood supply. The cauda epididymis is supplied by branches of the deferential artery. **The deferential and cremasteric arteries serve as collateral sources to the epididymis, when the main testicular artery is obstructed or ligated.** The arterial branches within the epididymis enter along septa formed from the connective tissue sheath. These vessels coil extensively before transforming into the straight vessels of the microvascular bed (Kormano and Reijonen, 1976). Microvascularization density varies significantly along the length of the epididymis, with the proximal caput containing the densest subepithelial capillary network and the more distal segments harboring less dense vascularization. From animal studies, the epididymal capillary network is under hormonal control. For example, in rabbits, bilateral hormonal castration results in progressive deterioration and eventual disappearance of the epididymal capillary network (Clavert et al., 1981). It is not clear whether vascularization in the human epididymis is similarly controlled.

According to MacMillan (1954), venous drainage from the corpus and cauda epididymis joins to form the vena marginalis epididymis of Haberer. These veins drain into the pampiniform plexus through the vena marginalis testis or through the cremasteric or deferential veins. Lymphatic drainage of the epididymis occurs through two routes (Wenzel and Kellermann, 1966). Lymph from the caput and corpus epididymis are removed through the same route as that described for the testis. These vessels course beside the internal spermatic vein and ultimately terminate in the preaortic nodes. Lymph vessels from the cauda epididymis join those draining the vas deferens and terminate in the external iliac nodes.

Innervation

The innervation of the human epididymis is derived primarily from the intermediate and inferior spermatic nerves that arise from the superior portion of the hypogastric plexus and pelvic plexus, respectively (Mitchell, 1935). The ductuli efferentes and the proximal segments of the epididymis are sparsely innervated by sympathetic fibers (Baumgarten et al., 1968; Baumgarten and Holstein, 1967). In these regions, the fibers are principally associated with blood vessels. Many more fibers are observed in the midcorpus epididymis, and their density increases progressively with progression along the epididymis, coincident with the appearance and proliferation of smooth muscle cells in these areas (Baumgarten et al., 1971). The distribution of contractile cells and sympathetic nerves within the epididymis may explain the rhythmic peristaltic movements of the ductuli efferentes and initial epididymal segments, as well as the intermittent contractile activity of the cauda epididymis and the vas deferens during emission (Risely, 1963). These physiologic contractions are critical to the movement of sperm through the epididymis.

Cytoarchitecture

Epididymal Epithelium

The histology of the human epididymis has been reviewed by Holstein (1969) and Vendrely (1981). It consists of two main cell types: **principal cells and basal cells** (seen at low ultrastructural magnification in Fig. 64.17). Principal cells vary in height along the length of the epididymis because of the length of stereocilia (microvilli, not cilia). In general, tall stereocilia (120 μm) are found in the proximal epididymis, and smaller or shorter stereocilia (50 μm) are observed in more distal regions. The nuclei in principal cells are elongated and often possess large clefts and one or two nucleoli. Consistent with the idea that principal cells carry out absorptive and secretive processes, their cellular apices have numerous coated pits, micropinocytotic vesicles, multivesicular bodies, irregularly shaped membranous vesicles, and an extensive Golgi apparatus. Because these cytologic features vary along the length of the epididymis, it suggests that there is varying absorptive and secretory capacity along the length of the duct (Vendrely and Dadoune, 1988).

There are far fewer basal cells than principal cells lining the epididymal epithelium. Tear-shaped basal cells rest on the basal lamina and extend toward the lumen, their apices forming threads between adjacent principal cells. They are thought to be derived from macrophages and may in fact be the precursors of principal cells. Unlike the principal cells, the morphology of basal cells remains relatively constant throughout the epididymal duct.

The epithelium of the epididymis exhibits regional differences along its length. Within the epididymis proper, the epithelium is pseudostratified and consists of principal and basal cells as described earlier. Proximally, at the junction of the rete testis and ductuli efferentes, there is a distinct transition from a low to a high cuboidal epithelium. The epithelium in the ductuli efferentes consists of ciliated and nonciliated cells (Holstein, 1969). The ciliated cells conduct sperm from the efferent ducts into the epididymis. The nonciliated cells with protruding apices are likely secretory in nature and predominate in the proximal ductuli efferentes (Vendrely, 1981). Other nonciliated cells have microvilli suggestive of resorptive activity and predominate in the distal ductuli efferentes. Nonciliated and ciliated cells are joined apically through junctional complexes. This suggests the existence of a blood-epididymis barrier analogous to the blood-testis barrier (Hoffer and Hinton, 1984; Suzuki and Nagano, 1978). **Although not as dense as the blood-testis barrier, the blood-epididymis barrier extends from the caput to the cauda epididymis and may play an important role in influencing the composition of fluid within the epididymal lumen of its differing segments** (Turner, 1979).

Epididymal Contractile Tissue. Peripheral to the basal lamina of the ductuli efferentes are various contractile cells (Baumgarten et al., 1971) (see Fig. 64.17). In the ductuli efferentes (distal regions of the caput and the proximal corpus epididymis), the contractile cells form a loose layer, two to four cells deep, around the tubule. These cells contain myofilaments and are connected by numerous nexus-like junctions. In the corpus epididymis, there are larger contractile cells with fewer nexus-like intracellular junctions that resemble smooth muscle cells. In the cauda epididymis, the thin contractile cells are replaced by thick smooth muscle cells that form three layers—the outer two layers oriented longitudinally and the central layer circularly. This distal contractile layer increases in thickness as it forms the vas deferens. The contractile tissue throughout the epididymis is likely involved in sperm transport.

Epididymal Function

Described variations in the anatomy and histology of the epididymal tubule from the caput to cauda regions suggest that the epididymis actually consists of several different functional tissues (Vendrely, 1981). It is clear that sperm transport and storage, fertilizing ability, and motility maturation are several consequences of epididymal passage. This is addressed more fully in reviews by Robaire and Hermo (1988) and Moore and Smith (1988).

Sperm Transport

Sperm transport through the human epididymis has been calculated to take from 2 to 12 days (Johnson and Varner, 1988). Sperm transit time through the caput-corpus epididymis is roughly similar to the transit time through the cauda epididymis and is more likely related to daily testicular sperm production rather than a man's age or the frequency of ejaculation (Amann, 1981; Johnson and Varner, 1988). In one study, sperm epididymal transit time averaged 2 days in men with a high daily rate of sperm production, compared with 6 days in men with low daily sperm production (Johnson and Varner, 1988). Although the frequency of sexual activity does not affect sperm transit time through the caput and corpus epididymis, "recent emissions" can reduce transit time through the cauda epididymis by 68% (Amann, 1981).

Because normal human testicular sperm are immotile as they enter the epididymis and remain relatively immotile within the caput, **mechanisms other than sperm motility must exist to transport sperm through the epididymis**. Animal studies have been very revealing in this regard (Bedford, 1975; Courot, 1981; Hamilton, 1977; Jaakkola, 1983; Jaakkola and Talo, 1982). Initially, sperm are carried into the ductuli efferentes by rete testis fluid, and **fluid flow is facilitated by fluid resorption by ductal epithelial cells mediated by the estrogen receptor**. Motile cilia and myoid cell contractions within the ductuli efferentes also assist with sperm movement. **Within the epididymis proper, the principal mechanism responsible for sperm transport is likely the spontaneous, rhythmic contraction of the contractile cells surrounding the epididymal duct.**

Sperm Storage

After migrating through the caput and corpus epididymis, sperm are retained in the cauda epididymis for varying lengths of time, depending on the frequency of sexual activity. In men 21 to 55 years of age, **an average of 155 to 209 million sperm are present in each epididymis** (Amann, 1981; Johnson and Varner, 1988), **and approximately half are stored in the caudal region**.

Spermatozoa stored in the cauda epididymis, unlike testicular sperm, are capable of progressive motility and are able to fertilize eggs. The exact amount of time that sperm can remain fertile within the epididymis is unclear, but animal studies have shown that sperm can remain viable for several weeks after vas deferens ligation (Hammond and Asdell, 1926; Young, 1929). However, it is also clear that sperm fertility measured in vivo diminishes when sperm are maintained in the epididymis for prolonged periods of time (Cooper and Orgebin-Crist, 1977; Cuasnicu and Bedford, 1989). In humans, sperm aging as a result of extended epididymal transit time and prolonged storage may contribute to reduced fertility (Johnson and Varner, 1988).

The exact fate of unejaculated epididymal sperm is unknown. In animals, sperm are lost through spontaneous seminal discharge, through oral self-cleaning (Martan, 1969), in urine (Lino et al., 1967), or by epididymal reabsorption (Amann and Almquist, 1961). Phagocytosis of spermatozoa by macrophages (spermiophages) within the epididymal lumen has been observed in humans after ligation of the vas deferens (Alexander, 1972). However, whether this mechanism can remove large numbers of spermatozoa from the epididymis of unvasectomized men is unclear.

Sperm Maturation

Sperm Motility. **Sperm gain the capacity for motility with migration through the epididymis. This is observed as a change in the pattern of motility and as an increase in the proportion of sperm exhibiting "mature" motility patterns.** Bedford et al. (1973) first observed that most sperm from the ductuli efferentes, when placed in culture medium, are immotile or show only weak, twitching movement or "immature" tail movements characterized by "thrashing" beats in wide arcs that result in little forward progression. Within the initial epididymal segment, this immature motility pattern persisted. However, in the corpus region, there was an increase in the fraction of sperm with a "mature" motility pattern characterized by high-frequency, low-amplitude beats that result in progressive motility (Fig. 64.18). Within the cauda epididymis, the majority of sperm had a mature motility pattern.

The relative importance of epididymal contact time versus region-specific maturation to gains in sperm motility patterns is unknown. Animal studies indicate that motility maturation may, in part, be

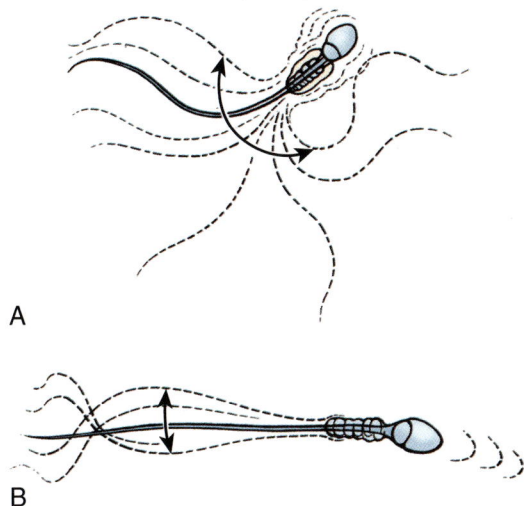

Fig. 64.18. Patterns of tail movement of human epididymal sperm. (A) The pattern shown by sperm taken from the proximal epididymis is characterized by high-amplitude, low-frequency beats producing little forward movement. (B) In contrast, tail movement in a large proportion of sperm from the cauda epididymis is characterized by low-amplitude, rapid beats with forward progression. (From Bedford JM, Calvin HI, Cooper GW: The maturation of spermatozoa in the human epididymis. *J Reprod Fertil.* 18:199–213, 1973.)

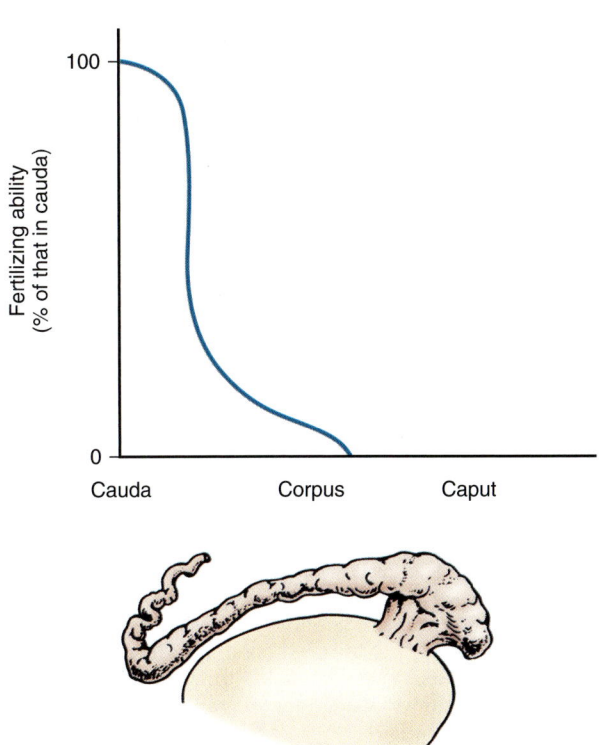

Fig. 64.19. Sperm fertility maturation in the human epididymis. Sperm fertilizing ability was assessed using zona pellucida–free hamster eggs and by changes in motility. (From Bedford JM: The bearing of epididymal function in strategies for in vitro fertilization and gamete intrafallopian transfer. *Ann N Y Acad Sci.* 541:284–291, 1988.)

an intrinsic process that occurs independent of epididymal interactions (Horan and Bedford, 1972; Orgebin-Crist, 1969). Human studies in obstructed patients with congenital absence of the vas deferens or epididymal obstruction also frequently report poor motility in spermatozoa aspirated from the distal epididymis and better sperm motility in the proximal epididymis (Matthews et al., 1995; Silber, 1989). When combined, **these observations suggest that spermatozoa are able to develop motility based on contact time with the proximal epididymal epithelium.** However, this maturation process may not be identical to that which occurs through sperm interaction with the epididymis during migration through all ductal regions.

Sperm Fertility. Testicular sperm are incapable of fertilizing eggs unless injected into them with micromanipulation (Bedford, 1974; Orgebin-Crist, 1969; Yanagimachi, 2005). In most animals, the ability of sperm to fertilize eggs is acquired gradually as the sperm pass through the epididymis (Fig. 64.19). Indeed, it has been shown in rabbits that sperm from the caput, corpus, and cauda epididymis can fertilize 1%, 63%, and 92% of rabbit eggs, respectively (Orgebin-Crist, 1969). Human in vitro experiments using zona pellucida–free hamster eggs have corroborated these findings (Moore et al., 1988). In a study that assessed the fertilizing capacity of human epididymal sperm, Hinrichsen and Blaquier (1980) demonstrated that, although sperm from the proximal epididymis are able to bind to zona-free eggs, only sperm from the cauda epididymis can actually penetrate eggs. **Thus sperm fertility maturation is, for the most part, achieved at the level of the late corpus or early cauda epididymis.**

Recent clinical observations, however, challenge the idea that fertility maturation requires sperm migration through the entire epididymis. Indeed, patients with epididymal obstruction or congenital absence of the vas deferens can achieve natural pregnancies after vasoepididymostomy at the level of the ductuli efferentes (Schoysman and Bedford, 1986; Silber, 1989). This suggests that obstruction induces proximal skewing of the maturation sequence along the epididymal duct or that there may be a reduced flow of sperm through the epididymis after such bypass procedures, allowing more contact and sperm maturation time (Orgebin-Crist, 1969; Turner and Roddy, 1990). Despite this observation, **it is generally believed that the likelihood of fertility is greater as the surgical anastomosis is performed more distally in the epididymis** (Thomas, 1987). Additional findings from the reversal of older vasectomies (>15 years of obstruction) suggest that, although postoperative ejaculated sperm concentrations are maintained after reversals with prolonged obstructive intervals, sperm motility is significantly decreased. This indicates that acquired epididymal dysfunction resulting from prolonged blockage may play an important role in the fertility potential of men after vasectomy reversal (Mui et al., 2014).

Sperm Biochemical Changes. Sperm undergo many biochemical changes with passage through the epididymis (Brooks, 1983). **Epididymal sperm transit induces a net negative surface membrane charge** (Bedford et al., 1973), **and sperm membrane sulfhydryl groups oxidize to disulfide bonds, improving sperm structural rigidity necessary for progressive motility and egg penetration** (Bedford et al., 1973; Reyes et al., 1976). Other post-testicular modifications of sperm membranes include changes in sperm lectin-binding properties (Courtens and Fournier-Delpech, 1979; Olson and Danzo, 1981), phospholipid and lipid content (Nikolopoulou et al., 1985), glycoprotein composition (Brown et al., 1983), immunoreactivity (Tezón et al., 1985), and iodination characteristics (Olson and Danzo, 1981). **Overall, these membrane modifications during epididymal passage may enhance sperm adherence to the egg zona pellucida** (Blobel et al., 1990; Orgebin-Crist and Fournier-Delpech, 1982). Sperm also undergo numerous metabolic changes during epididymal transit (Dacheux and Paquignon, 1980). These include an increased capacity for glycolysis (Hoskins et al., 1975), changes in intracellular pH and calcium content, modification of adenylate cyclase activity (Casillas et al., 1980), and alterations in cellular phospholipid and phospholipid-like fatty acid content (Voglmayr, 1975).

Regulation of Epididymal Function

Sperm changes within the epididymis are likely influenced by fluids and secretions within the epididymal lumen (Blaquier et al., 1989; Robaire and Hermo, 1988). The biochemical composition of epididymal fluid differs from that of serum and also shows regional differences in osmolarity, electrolyte content, and protein composition (Robaire and Hermo, 1988). These differences are likely the consequence of variations in vascularization, blood-epididymis barrier activity, and selective absorption and secretion of substances such as glycerylphosphorylcholine (GPC), carnitine, and sialic acids along the epididymal duct. Proteins within epididymal fluid that are known to have physiologic effects on sperm in vitro include forward motility protein (Brandt et al., 1978), sperm survival factor (Morton et al., 1978), progressive motility sustaining factor (Sheth et al., 1981), sperm motility-inhibiting factor (Turner and Giles, 1982), acidic epididymal glycoprotein (Pholpramool et al., 1983), and the EP2-EP3 proteins that induce sperm binding to zona pellucida (Cuasnicu et al., 1984; Blaquier et al., 1988). Thus variations in epididymal tubule fluid characteristics play an important role in sperm maturation during epididymal transit. It is not surprising, then, that the epididymis is a potentially important source of sperm dysfunction and male infertility.

Epididymal function is hormonally regulated. Testosterone and DHT are found in very high concentrations within the epididymis (Leinonen et al., 1980). This suggests the importance of androgens for epididymal function (Brooks and Tiver, 1983). In animals, castration results not only in the loss of androgen-dependent epididymal proteins but also in losses in epididymal weight, changes in luminal histology, and alterations in the synthesis and secretion of epididymal fluid GPC, carnitine, and sialic acid. Ultimately, the castrated epididymis loses the ability to sustain sperm motility, fertility maturation, and sperm storage capacities, processes that are reversed with androgen replacement.

Compared with other accessory sex glands, the epididymis requires relatively higher levels of androgen to maintain its structure and function (Prasad and Rajalakshmi, 1976). **Androgen effects on the epididymis are mediated mainly through DHT, the primary androgen in epididymal tissue** (Pujol et al., 1976), and/or 5α-androstane-3α, 17β-diol (3α-diol) (Orgebin-Crist et al., 1975). Indeed, this is corroborated by the fact that the enzymes Δ4-5α-reductase (catalyzes DHT formation from testosterone) and 3α-hydroxysteroid dehydrogenase (converts DHT to 3α-diol), which produce testosterone metabolites, are also found in the human epididymis (Kinoshita et al., 1980; Larminat et al., 1980). It may also help to explain the recent observation that the clinical use of 5α-reductase inhibitors is associated with impaired semen quality (Amory et al., 2007).

Epididymal function is also influenced by temperature (Foldesy and Bedford, 1982; Wong et al., 1982). Chronic exposure of the epididymis to elevated temperatures, for example, by placing them within the abdomen, results in the loss of sperm storage and electrolyte transport functions. The effect of temperature on epididymal function may help explain how varicocele and cryptorchidism affect male infertility. Abnormalities in epididymal myoid cell contractility may also influence epididymal function. In the rat, partial surgical denervation of the epididymis results in an abnormal accumulation of sperm within the cauda epididymis and a decrease in the swimming speed of sperm (Billups et al., 1990). These findings have implications for infertility from neuropathic causes such as spinal cord injury and diabetes mellitus.

> **KEY POINTS: EPIDIDYMIS**
>
> - The epididymis consists of principal cells with absorptive and secretory function, basal cells derived from macrophages, and contractile cells that facilitate sperm transport.
> - During epididymal passage, sperm mature by gaining progressive motility and the ability to bind to and penetrate the egg zona pellucida.
> - Epididymal function is temperature and androgen (mainly DHT) dependent, important considerations for cryptorchidism, varicocele, and 5α-reductase use.

DUCTUS (VAS) DEFERENS

Gross Architecture

The vas deferens is a tubular organ derived from the mesonephric (wolffian) duct. In humans, the vas deferens is 30 to 35 cm long, beginning at the cauda epididymis and terminating in the ejaculatory duct, medial to the seminal vesicle and posterior to the prostate. It is classically divided into five regions: (1) the sheathless epididymal segment contained within the tunica vaginalis, (2) the scrotal segment, (3) the inguinal segment, (4) the retroperitoneal or pelvic portion, and (5) the ampulla (Lich et al., 1978). In cross section, the vas deferens consists of an outer adventitial connective tissue sheet containing blood vessels and small nerves, a muscular coat that consists of a middle circular layer surrounded by inner and outer longitudinal muscle layers, and an inner mucosal layer with an epithelial lining (Neaves, 1975). The outer diameter of the vas deferens varies from 1.5 to 3 mm, and the lumen of the unobstructed vas deferens varies from 200 to 700 μm in diameter (Middleton et al., 2009).

The vas deferens receives its blood supply from the deferential artery, a branch of the superior vesical artery. Venous drainage corresponds to arterial supply. The vas deferens receives innervation from the sympathetic and the parasympathetic nervous systems (Sjostrand, 1965). The cholinergic supply does not appear important for motor activity of the vas deferens (Baumgarten et al., 1975). There is a rich supply of sympathetic adrenergic nerves derived from hypogastric nerve coursing via the presacral nerve (Batra and Lardner, 1976; McConnell et al., 1982). Adrenergic nerve fibers have been observed in all three layers of the vas muscularis, with the greatest concentration in the outer longitudinal layer (McConnell et al., 1982). The vas deferens also receives a short adrenergic nerve (Sjostrand, 1965) and has an abundance of purinergic receptors in its smooth muscle membranes, suggesting sympathetic and purinergic cotransmission in sperm transport and ejaculation (Gur et al., 2007). Neurons containing other neurotransmitters, including neuropeptide Y, enkephalin, galanin, somatostatin, vasoactive intestinal polypeptide, and nitric oxide, have also been identified; however, their role in vas deferens function is unknown (Dixon et al., 1998). Notably, human vas deferens specimens obtained at vasovasostomy after vasectomy show a marked reduction in the density of muscular noradrenergic and subepithelial secretomotor nerves in testicular compared with abdominal segments. These changes may influence subsequent sperm transport in the vas deferens and therefore procedural success after vasectomy reversal (Dixon et al., 1998).

Cytoarchitecture

The human vas deferens is lined by pseudostratified epithelium (Paniagua et al., 1981). The height of the epithelium decreases along the length of the vas deferens from the testis to the seminal vesicle. In addition, the longitudinal epithelial folds are simpler near the testis and become more complex distally. The pseudostratified epithelium vasal lining is composed of basal cells and three types of tall, thin columnar cells (Hoffer, 1976; Paniagua et al., 1981). The columnar cells, extending from the epithelial base to the lumen, include principal cells, pencil cells, and mitochondria-rich cells. All columnar cells exhibit stereocilia and irregular convoluted nuclei. Principal cells are the most frequent columnar cell type in the proximal vas deferens, whereas pencil cells and mitochondria-rich cells increase in density distally. The thickness of the total muscle layer gradually decreases along the length of the vas deferens. This complex cytoarchitecture strongly suggests that the vas deferens is more than simply a passive conduit for sperm transport.

Vas Deferens Function

Sperm Transport

Sperm transport through the vas deferens is influenced by several physiologic processes. First, **the human vas deferens exhibits spontaneous motility** (Ventura et al., 1973). **It also has the capacity** to respond when stretched (Bruschini et al., 1977). **Finally, fluid within the vas deferens can be propelled into the urethra by strong peristaltic contractions elicited either by electrical stimulation of the hypogastric nerve** (Bruschini et al., 1977) **or by adrenergic neurotransmitters** (Bruschini et al., 1977; Lipshultz et al., 1981). This suggests that immediately before emission, with sympathetic stimulation, sperm is rapidly transported from the distal epididymis through the vas deferens to the ejaculatory duct. **This rapid transport is consistent with the vas deferens having the highest muscle-to-lumen ratio (approximately 10:1) of any hollow viscus in the body.**

Sperm reserves in the vas deferens have been estimated at approximately 130 million, suggesting that a significant proportion of human ejaculated sperm is stored in the vas deferens (Amann and Howards, 1980). In addition, vasal sperm quality, as assessed from fertile men at the time of vasectomy, is very similar to that of the ejaculate, with 71% motility and 91% viability (Bachtell et al., 1999). In the rabbit, it has been shown that during sexual rest, epididymal sperm are transported through the vas deferens and leak into the urethra in small amounts (Prins and Zaneveld, 1979, 1980a, 1980b). This suggests that the vas deferens is involved in ridding the epididymis of excess, stored sperm. On sexual stimulation, rabbit sperm are transported through the vas deferens similar to humans. **After sexual stimulation, however, the vas deferens contents are propelled proximally toward the epididymis because the distal vas deferens contracts with greater amplitude, frequency, and duration than the proximal segment** (Prins and Zaneveld, 1980a). Notably, with prolonged sexual rest, excess epididymal sperm are once again transported distally, supporting the idea that the vas deferens is important for sperm transport and for maintenance of epididymal sperm reserves.

Absorption and Secretion

Based on its cytoarchitecture, the human vas deferens likely has absorptive and secretory functions (Hoffer, 1976; Paniagua et al., 1981). The principal cells are typical of cells that synthesize and secrete glycoproteins (Bennett et al., 1974; Gupta et al., 1974). The stereocilia, apical blebbing, and primary and secondary lysosomes within principal cells are also characteristic of cells involved in absorptive function (Friend and Farquhar, 1967; Murakami et al., 1988). Last, spermiophagy by epithelial cells in the ampullary vas deferens has been observed with scanning electron microscopy in men and monkeys (Murakami et al., 1988). **Normal vas deferens function is likely to be androgen dependent because the vas deferens actively converts testosterone to DHT** (Dupuy et al., 1979). Castration causes atrophy of—and testosterone treatment, restoration of—monkey vas cytoarchitecture (Dinakar et al., 1977), and spontaneous and α- and β-adrenergic–stimulated contractions of the rat vas deferens are altered by castration (Borda et al., 1981). Thus, although once thought to be a simple muscular conduit for sperm, the vas deferens is now viewed as a complex reproductive organ.

SEMINAL VESICLE AND EJACULATORY DUCTS

Gross Architecture and Cytoarchitecture

Seminal Vesicle

In the adult, the seminal vesicles are paired, elongated, hollow viscous organs located posterior to the prostate and bladder. Each seminal vesicle is 5 to 7 cm long and up to 1.5 cm wide. Each seminal vesicle actually consists of a tubule that is 15 cm long and highly coiled and convoluted. **The tubule is composed of three layers: the inner lining is a moist and folded mucous membrane; the middle layer is largely collagenous; and the outer layer consists of circular and longitudinal muscle layers that constitute 80% of the wall thickness** (Nguyen et al., 1996). The mucosa of the seminal vesicle, mainly nonciliated, pseudostratified columnar or cuboidal cells, is notable for many thin, complicated folds that produce numerous crypts. The excretory duct of the seminal vesicle opens into the ampullary vas deferens as it enters the prostate gland.

The blood supply to the seminal vesicle arises from the internal iliac artery and inferior vesicular artery through the prostatovesicular branch (Clegg, 1955). The prostatovesicular artery can also arise from the superior vesicular artery or from the pudendal artery. Most commonly, the prostatovesicular artery has anterior and posterior branches that supply the respective surfaces of the seminal vesicle. The lymphatic drainage of the seminal vesicle is through the internal iliac lymph nodes. The seminal vesicles are innervated through sympathetic nerves from the superior lumbar and hypogastric nerves. Parasympathetic innervation occurs through the pelvic plexus.

Ejaculatory Ducts

The ejaculatory ducts are paired, collagenous, tubular structures that commence at the junction of the vas deferens and seminal vesicle, course through the prostate, and empty into the prostatic urethra at the verumontanum. Histologically, the ejaculatory ducts are a continuation of the seminal vesicle, except that the outer circular muscle layer does not extend into the ducts (Nguyen et al., 1996). There are three distinct anatomic regions to the ejaculatory duct: the proximal, extraprostatic portion; the middle intraprostatic segment; and a short distal segment incorporating the lateral aspect of the verumontanum in the urethra (Nguyen et al., 1996; Fig. 64.20). Although the ejaculatory duct contains an outer muscular layer in its extraprostatic and intraprostatic segments, as the duct courses distally the outer muscular layer dissipates, and **there is no valvelike, muscular "sphincter" at the ejaculatory duct orifice,** as was once thought (Nguyen et al., 1996; Fig. 64.21). Instead, urinary reflux is prevented and ejaculatory continence is maintained by the acute angle of duct insertion into the urethra. The inner epithelial layer of the ejaculatory ducts is also complex and folded and consists of simple and pseudostratified columnar cells. The ejaculatory ducts receive their blood supply from branches of the inferior vesical artery and are innervated through the pelvic plexus.

Seminal Vesicle and Ejaculatory Duct–Unit Function

Animal studies suggest that **the seminal vesicle and ejaculatory duct relationship is functionally similar to that of the bladder and urethra** (Turek et al., 1998). **The seminal vesicle is a contractile, compliant, smooth muscular organ with dynamic properties analogous to those of the bladder, and the ejaculatory duct serves as a urethra-like conduit.** This theory allows the classification of ejaculatory duct obstruction into **two types of disorders, analogous to bladder outlet obstruction: (1) obstruction resulting from physical blockage of the ducts, similar to bladder outlet obstruction and (2) "functional" obstruction of the seminal vesicle, similar to voiding dysfunction caused by bladder myopathy.** In addition, this has implications for the diagnosis of ejaculatory duct disorders because "static" anatomic imaging, such as transrectal ultrasonography, may not be sufficient to differentiate between these disorders, and medications and conditions (such as diabetes) may predispose the system to seminal vesicle dysfunction (Smith et al., 2008).

Seminal Vesicle Function

The seminal vesicles secrete a significant proportion (80%) of the seminal fluid, and these secretions are found in later fractions of the ejaculate, after the sperm-rich epididymal and prostatic secretions. After ejaculation, sperm pass into and through the female cervical mucus and subsequently the uterus to enter the oviduct, where fertilization occurs. During residence in the female reproductive tract, sperm must undergo capacitation before oocyte fertilization. During capacitation, the acrosome reaction and development of hyperactivated motility occurs (Yanagimachi, 1994). It is not clear if prostatic or seminal vesicle secretions contribute to capacitation.

In fact, the exact physiologic role of seminal vesicle fluid is not clear, although in rodents it functions as a plug or barrier that reduces the chances for sperm from a subsequent male to fertilize the oocyte. Before ejaculation, semen is a liquid, and after all components mix with the seminal vesicle secretions, it coagulates.

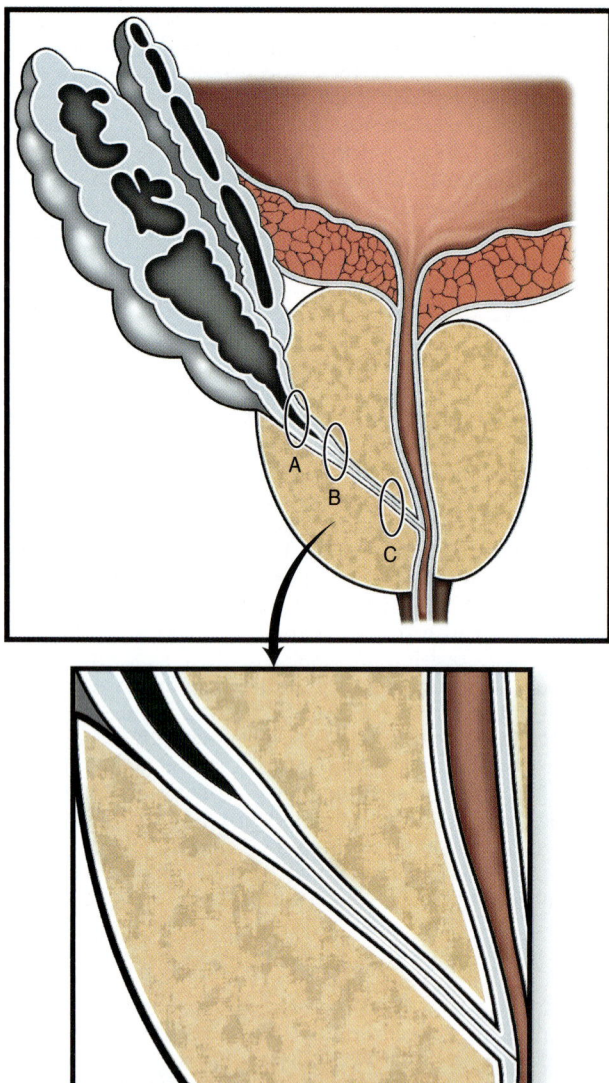

Fig. 64.20. Schematic anatomy of the human ejaculatory duct complex. (A) Proximal; (B) intraprostatic or middle; and (C) distal ejaculatory duct regions. The *inset* shows how the muscle layer thins out in the middle segment. (From Nguyen HT, Etzell J, Turek PJ, et al.: Normal human ejaculatory duct anatomy: a study of cadaveric and surgical specimens. *J Urol.* 155:1639–1642, 1996.)

The major component of the coagulum is **semenogelin I, a 52-kD protein expressed exclusively in the seminal vesicles** (Robert et al., 1999). **Through coagulating semen, seminal vesicle secretions may promote sperm motility, increase stability of sperm chromatin, and suppress immune activity in the female reproductive tract.** The best-elucidated function of **human semen** is its ability to **provide antioxidative protection to sperm.** Semen is rich in antioxidant enzymes, including glutathione peroxidase, superoxide dismutase, and catalase (Yeung et al., 1998). In addition, the antioxidant molecules taurine, hypotaurine, and tyrosine are present in high concentrations (van Overveld et al., 2000). Lipofuscin granules from dead epithelial cells give seminal vesicle secretions a yellow-white color. In addition, seminal vesicle secretions are alkaline and contain fructose, mucus, vitamin C, flavins, phosphoryl choline, and prostaglandins. High fructose levels provide nutrient energy for sperm. The mixing of seminal vesicle with prostatic secretions results in human semen having a mildly alkaline pH. **Acidic ejaculate (pH <7.2) is associated with blockage or absence of seminal vesicles** (Turek, 2005).

> **KEY POINTS: VAS DEFERENS, SEMINAL VESICLE, AND EJACULATORY DUCTS**
>
> - The vas deferens is of wolffian (mesonephric) duct origin and transports sperm from the cauda epididymis to the ejaculatory duct during seminal emission.
> - The seminal vesicle and ejaculatory duct unit is analogous to the bladder and urethra and is subject to physical blockage and functional disorders that result in infertility.

SPERMATOZOA

Anatomy and Physiology

The human spermatozoon is approximately 60 μm in length and is divided into three morphologic sections: head, neck, and tail (Fig. 64.22). The oval **sperm head**, about 4.5 μm long and 3 μm wide, contains a nucleus with highly compacted **chromatin** and an **acrosome**, a membrane-bound organelle that harbors enzymes required for penetration of the outer vestments of the egg before fertilization (Yanagimachi, 1978). The **sperm neck** maintains the connection between the sperm head and tail. It consists of the **connecting piece** and **proximal centriole**. The **axonemal complex** extends from the proximal centriole through the sperm tail. The **tail** harbors the **midpiece, principal piece, and endpiece** (Zamboni, 1992). The midpiece is 7 to 8 μm long and is the most proximal

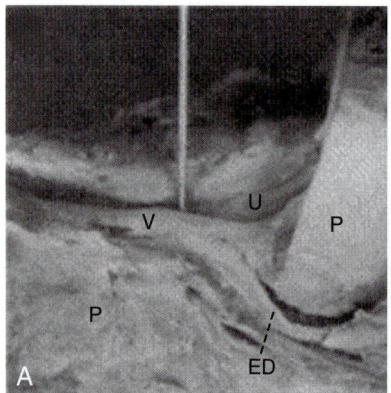 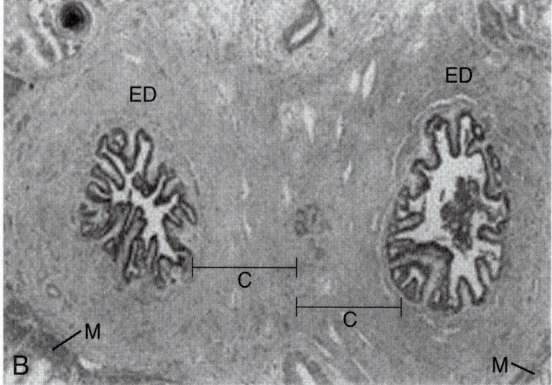

Fig. 64.21. Human ejaculatory duct gross and microscopic anatomy from cadaver specimens. (A) Sagittal section through the midline with pin in ejaculatory duct orifice and ejaculatory duct *(ED)* and veru *(V)*, urethra *(U)*, and prostate *(P)* visible. (B) Microphotograph of the paired ejaculatory ducts in the middle intraprostatic segment showing the thick collagenous layer *(C)* surrounding the mucosa with a thin, outer muscular layer *(M)*. (From Nguyen HT, Etzell J, Turek PJ, et al.: Normal human ejaculatory duct anatomy: a study of cadaveric and surgical specimens. *J Urol.* 155:1639–1642, 1996.)

segment of the tail, terminating in the annulus. It contains **the axoneme**, with its characteristic microtubule arrangement and surrounding **outer dense fibers** (Fig. 64.23). It also contains the **mitochondrial sheath,** which is helically arranged around the outer dense fibers. The outer dense fibers, rich in disulfide bonds, are not contractile proteins but are thought to provide the sperm tail with the elastic rigidity necessary for progressive motility (Oko and Clermont, 1990). Similar in structure to the midpiece, the principal piece has several columns of outer dense fibers that are replaced by the fibrous sheath. The fibrous sheath consists of **longitudinal columns** and **transverse ribs**. The sperm terminates in the endpiece, the most distal segment of the sperm tail, and contains axonemal structures and the fibrous sheath. Except for the endpiece region, the sperm is enveloped by a highly specialized plasma membrane that regulates the transmembrane movement of ions and other molecules (Friend, 1989).

The spermatozoon is a remarkably complex metabolic and genetic machine. The 75 sperm mitochondria that surround the axoneme contain enzymes required for oxidative metabolism and produce adenosine triphosphate (ATP), the primary energy molecule for the cell. Mitochondria are organelles that produce cellular energy and can also cause apoptotic cell death through the release of cytochrome *c*. Mitochondria are composed of outer and inner membranes. The inner membrane forms deep folds into the matrix, called the cristae, which make the surface area of the inner membrane larger than that of the outer membrane. Five distinct respiratory chain complexes span the width of the inner membrane and are necessary for oxidative phosphorylation: nicotinamide adenosine diphosphate (NADPH) dehydrogenase, succinate dehydrogenase, cytochrome *bc1*, cytochrome *c* oxidase, and ATP synthase complexes. Contained within the matrix are citric acid cycle, fatty acid, and amino acid oxidative enzymes; newly made ATP; mitochondrial DNA (mtDNA); and ribosomes.

Human mitochondria contain DNA (mtDNA) that is distinct from sperm nuclear DNA. mtDNA consists of a circular, histone-free chromosome of 16,569 base pairs of DNA arranged in a single heavy and single light strand and **encodes respiratory-chain–complex subunit proteins, mitochondrial rRNAs, and tRNAs used for protein synthesis.** These genes have no introns. mtDNA is also far more susceptible to mutations than is nuclear DNA (estimated 40 to 100 times higher). Reasons for this may include the fact that mitochondria are near respiratory-chain complexes and may be easily attacked by reactive oxygen species. **In addition, mtDNA is not coated with protective histones, and mitochondria have very limited DNA repair mechanisms** (Hirata et al., 2002). **The fact that mitochondria rapidly accumulate mutations suggests the necessity of degrading all paternal mtDNA in the fertilized egg.** This degradation is likely mediated by the small proteolytic polypeptide ubiquitin, which regulates proteolysis in many tissues (Sutovsky et al., 1999).

From animal studies, it is clear that the plasma membrane covering the sperm-head region harbors specialized proteins that participate in sperm-egg interaction (Saling, 1989). Indeed, carbohydrate-binding proteins on the sperm membrane interact with the species-specific ZP3 protein in the egg zona pellucida, resulting first in sperm binding to the zona and subsequently to induction of the acrosome reaction

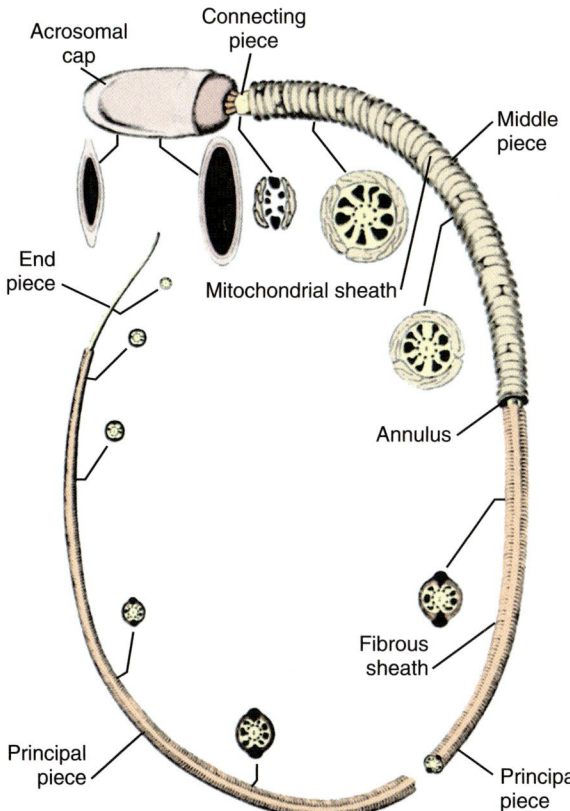

Fig. 64.22. Diagram of a typical mammalian spermatozoon. The plasma membrane is omitted to illustrate the major cellular components. Cross-sectional insets show the orientation of the internal cell structures. (From Fawcett DW: The mammalian spermatozoon. *Dev Biol.* 44:394–436, 1975.)

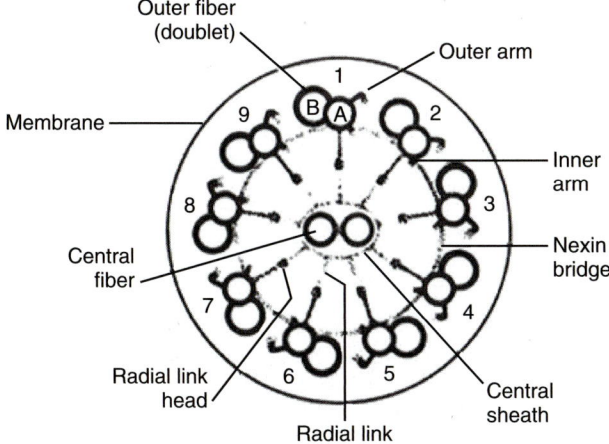
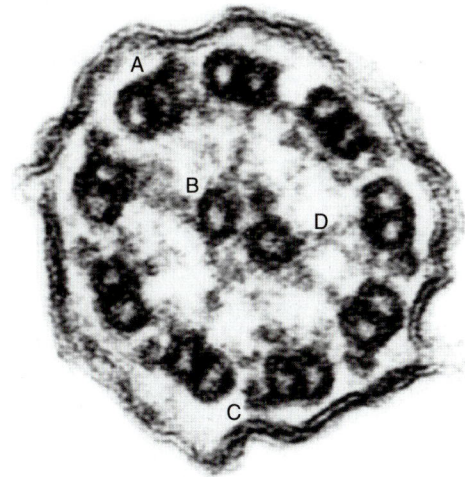

Fig. 64.23. The "9 + 2" sperm axonemal structure. *Left,* Schematic cross section of axoneme, demonstrating microtubule arrangement. *Right,* Electron micrograph of axoneme. *(A)* Outer doublet; *(B)* inner central doublet; *(C)* outer dynein arm; *(D)* radial link.

(Shabanowitz, 1990). Another sperm membrane protein, PH30, is present on testicular sperm, is modified during sperm migration through the epididymis, and functions as a fusion protein between the sperm and egg membranes at fertilization (Blobel et al., 1990; Primakoff et al., 1987).

Physiologically, the axoneme is the true motor assembly and requires 200 to 300 proteins for proper function. Among these, the "9 + 2" pattern of outer and inner doublets of microtubules is the best-understood component (see Fig. 64.23). The dynein proteins extend from one microtubule doublet to the adjacent doublet and form the inner and outer arms of the axoneme. **The sperm axoneme contains the enzymes and structural proteins necessary for the chemical transduction of ATP into mechanical movement and motility.** Dynein is a large (2000 kD), Mg^{2+}-stimulated ATPase responsible for ATP-generated microtubule sliding that causes axonemal bending and, ultimately, sperm flagellar movement. The dynein structure has two or three globular, outer (heavy) chain heads (500 kD) joined to a common stem. The heads control movement along the microtubules. The inner (light) chain arms (14 to 120 kD) are the primary effectors of movement and are associated with the radial spokes of the dynein assembly. Sperm with outer arm mutants have reduced motility, and those with inner arm mutants have no motility. Radial links or spokes connect a microtubule of each doublet to the central inner doublet and consist of a complex of proteins. The central inner doublet is surrounded by a ringlike helical sheath to which the radial links from the outer doublets are attached. Tektins are proteins associated with the outer microtubular doublets, and nexin links are proteins that connect the outer doublets to one another and maintain the cylindric axonemal shape.

The phenotype of defective sperm structure has been recognized as ciliary dyskinesia. Although infertility is the rule with ciliary dyskinesias, ejaculated sperm can be motile and sperm concentrations can be normal. With ICSI, clinical pregnancies and live births have been reported after use of affected sperm (Cayan et al., 2001). Because the inheritance is usually recessive, normal offspring are likely. In general, patients suspected of harboring sperm structural defects exhibit severely compromised sperm motility (<10%). Sperm electron microscopy can reveal ultrastructural or functional sperm abnormalities. Sperm structural abnormalities are currently categorized by Chemes (2000) as follows:

1. **Nonspecific flagellar anomalies.** This is the most frequent flagellar anomaly underlying severely low motility and shows a structural phenotype of random, heterogeneous, microtubular alterations. These anomalies can arise from correctable disorders such as varicocele, reactive oxygen species, and gonadotoxin exposure. There is no evidence of familial occurrence.
2. **Dysplasia of the fibrous sheath.** This condition is a systematic sperm abnormality, usually associated with near-complete or total immotility. It has a more homogenous and distinctive phenotype characterized by sperm fibrous sheath, axonemal, and periaxonemal distortions. A subset of these patients exhibit the classic **ciliary dyskinesia** (formerly **immotile cilia syndrome**) in which sperm immotility is associated with respiratory disease and dextrocardia. There is a strong familial incidence, suggesting that such conditions are genetic.

SUMMARY

Spermatogenesis is a remarkably intricate and complex process that is driven by precisely regulated secretions of GnRH, LH, and FSH from the HPG axis. Perturbations in this hormonal milieu are common causes of male infertility. Sperm production in the testis functions optimally at 2°C to 4°C below body temperature and generates mature human sperm in 64 days. Well-integrated cycles and waves of spermatogenesis ensure that human sperm production is constant at about 1200 sperm per second. Spermatogenesis is an androgen-dependent process that occurs with very high intratesticular testosterone levels. The product of spermatogenesis, the spermatozoa, leave the testis as immotile cells with limited capacity to fertilize oocytes. After epididymal transit, sperm are typically motile and capable of fertilization. During ejaculation, sperm are rapidly transported through the ejaculatory ducts into the urethra from the distal epididymis. The ejaculate supports sperm metabolism and motility, serves as an antioxidant, and acts as a barrier to exclude subsequent gamete deposits from gaining access to the egg.

SUGGESTED READINGS

Akre O, Richiardi L: Does a testicular dysgenesis syndrome exist?, *Hum Reprod* 24:2053–2060, 2009.
Carrell DT: Epigenetics of the male gamete, *Fert Steril* 97:267–292, 2012.
Cornwall GA: New insights into epididymal biology and function, *Hum Reprod Update* 15:213–227, 2009.
De Jonge CJ, Barratt CL, editors: *The sperm cell: production, maturation, fertilization, regeneration*, New York, 2006, Cambridge University Press.
DiNapoli L, Capel B: SRY and the standoff in sex determination, *Mol Endocrinol* 22:1–9, 2008.
Itman C, Mendis S, Barakat B, et al: All in the family: TGF-beta family action in testis development, *Reproduction* 132:233–246, 2006.
Masters V, Turek PJ: Ejaculatory physiology and dysfunction, *Urol Clin North Am* 28:363, 2001.
Payne AH, Hales DB: Overview of steroidogenic enzymes in the pathway from cholesterol to active steroid hormones, *Endocr Rev* 25:947–970, 2004.
Robaire B, Hinton BT, editors: *The epididymis: from molecules to clinical practice: a comprehensive survey of the efferent ducts, the epididymis and vas deferens*, New York, 2002, Kluwer Academic and Plenum.
Skinner MK, Griswold MD, editors: *Sertoli cell biology*, San Diego, 2005, Elsevier.
Smith JF, Turek PJ: Ejaculatory duct obstruction, *Urol Clin North Am* 35:221–227, 2008.
Turek PJ: Male infertility. In Tanagho EA, McAninch JC, editors: *Smith's urology*, ed 17, Stamford (CT), 2007, Lange Clinical Medicine.
Turek PJ, Reijo Pera RA: Current and future genetic screening for male infertility, *Urol Clin North Am* 29:767–792, 2002.
Walker WH: Molecular mechanisms of testosterone action in spermatogenesis, *Steroids* 74:602, 2009.

REFERENCES

The complete reference list is available online at ExpertConsult.com.

KEY POINTS: SPERM

- Sperm are ciliated cells that possess a "9 + 2" axonemal structure that allows motility.
- It is estimated that 200 to 300 genes regulate sperm motility.
- Sperm motility defects, termed *ciliary dyskinesias*, are common and can be either correctable (nonspecific flagellar anomalies) or genetic (dysplasia of the fibrous sheath).
- Human sperm mtDNA is a circular, histone- and intron-free DNA ring that encodes for respiratory-chain–complex proteins and is very susceptible to mutations.

65 Integrated Men's Health: Androgen Deficiency, Cardiovascular Risk, and Metabolic Syndrome

Neil Fleshner, MD, MPH, FRCSC, Miran Kenk, PhD, and Steven Kaplan, MD

RATIONALE FOR INTEGRATIVE MEN'S HEALTH

Introduction to the Problem

In almost every corner of our planet, health outcomes among boys and men are significantly inferior to those among girls and women. Despite these differences, attention from health policy leadership and local, national, and supranational entities toward addressing this issue has remained scant. Efforts to reduce gender inequality in health are desperately needed and require a substantial adjustment in multiple facets of life, including workplace safety, global peace, sociology, psychology, and lifestyle.

Gender Longevity Gap

Human longevity continues to increase on a global scale (Fries, 1980; Oeppen and Vaupel, 2002). Emphasis on perinatal care, labor and delivery, childhood vaccinations, smoking cessation, and healthier lifestyles in terms of diet and exercise have made a true impact on extending human life span around the world (Mathers and Loncar, 2006; Oeppen and Vaupel, 2002). Interestingly, one peculiar statistic seems to stand out from the general progress: the gap in longevity between male and female humans. **On average, men throughout the world live shorter lives than women.** Average life expectancy in the United States is currently 79.3 years (World Health Organization [WHO], 2016b). However, when one breaks this statistic out by gender, women live on average 81.6 years, whereas men live only 76.9; a difference of 4.7 years. Table 65.1 presents global data on life expectancy, demonstrating the differences in longevity between men and women. The gap exists across the globe and across all strata of industrial development; eastern Europe demonstrates the largest gap, approximately 7 years. Even in sub-Saharan Africa, the region with the shortest life expectancy in the world, men are living on average 5.3 years less than women (Jamison et al., 2013). In fact, there is not one part of the world where men on average outlive women.

In addition to the discrepancy present in current statistics, trends recorded over the past 50 years do not demonstrate a narrowing of the longevity gap. The Global Burden of Disease Study (Wang et al., 2016) demonstrated not only that, between 1970 and 2010, women had a higher life expectancy than men, but also that the gains in longevity over this period were more pronounced among women than men. Average gain in life duration for men was 11.1 years, compared with 12.1 for women. Thus, **although the average longevity of men and women is improving, it tends to be improving more among women than among men** (Klenk et al., 2016; Fig. 65.1).

Health and Wellness Gap by Gender

Men live not only shorter lives than women but also sicker lives. Men fall ill younger and are more prone to major chronic diseases such as cancer, hypertension, and cardiovascular disease. Table 65.2 lists the major causes of death among Americans, along with the ratios of their prevalence in males and females. The 10 conditions listed are responsible for 75% of all deaths in the United States. As is evident from this table (Murphy et al., 2017), **6 of the 10 most common causes of death are more prevalent among males.** The discordance between genders is glaringly obvious in cancer, heart disease, accidents, diabetes, and suicide. Similar trends are reported around the world and are even more disparate, not surprisingly, in nations with a larger gender longevity gap (WHO, 2016a). In addition to the total life duration, differences in healthy-life expectancy (HLE) are commonly observed between genders. HLE is a metric that corrects the mean life expectancy by weighted disability factors to derive the number of years on average that a particular country's citizens are free from chronic illness (GBD 2015 DALYs and HALE Collaborators, 2016). Between 2008 and 2010 HLE for males at birth in the United Kingdom was 63.5 years, equivalent to more than 81% of total life expectancy spent in very good or good general health. For women in the United Kingdom, HLE at birth was more than 2 years higher in the same period, at 65.7 years (Tokudome et al., 2016; UK Office for National Statistics, 2012; Van Oyen et al., 2013).

Explanation of the Poorer Health of Men

In most societies men possess more power, opportunity, and wealth than women; yet these privileges do not seem to translate into an advantage or parity between the genders in regard to health and comorbidity. **A series of factors have been identified that place men at higher risk of death and disease. These include increased exposure to physical and environmental harm in the workplace, propensity for risk-taking behaviors, and masculinity-defined norms of health behavior that may negatively affect acute and chronic illness-related outcomes.**

Propensity for Risk-Taking Behavior

Men are more likely to engage in risk-taking behaviors than women. This has been demonstrated across cultures and is a recognized world-wide phenomenon (Byrnes et al., 1999). Hazardous pursuits such as alcohol use, smoking, and risky sexual practices are more prevalent among men (Creighton and Oliffe, 2010; Dolan, 2011; Stergiou-Kita et al., 2015). Men tend to consume more alcohol than women and are more likely to binge drink. In a study by Wilsnack et al. (2009), global samples of individuals of various ages were questioned about their drinking habits. As expected, ratios of drinking rates between males and females were greater than 1.0 in 98 of 104 evaluated countries. Furthermore, lifetime abstainers from alcohol were far more likely to be female. High-volume alcohol consumption was also more prevalent among men. Other studies have demonstrated similar findings (Balabanova and McKee, 1999; Hao et al., 2004; Lim et al., 2007; Parry et al., 2005; Popova et al., 2007; Slone et al., 2006; Van Gundy et al., 2005; Wilsnack et al., 2000). It was estimated that in 2010, 3.14 million men, as opposed to 1.72 million women, died from causes linked to excessive alcohol use (Lim et al., 2012).

In most of the world being male is one of the greatest predictors of tobacco use. Global consumption of tobacco is fourfold higher among men than among women (48% vs. 12%) (WHO, 2015). Although the differences are smaller in the United States (with approximately 1 in 4 Americans using tobacco), tobacco use is, according to the 2016 National Survey on Drug Use and Health (NSDUH) more prevalent among men (Substance Abuse and Mental Health Services Administration, 2017). In a recent study, 16.7% of men and 13.6% of adult women in the United States used cigarettes on a regular basis (Jamal et al., 2018; Ng et al., 2014; Preston and Wang, 2006; Syamlal et al., 2017).

There are three major reasons underlying this difference in tobacco use: cultural, behavioral, and physiologic. Of particular interest are

TABLE 65.1 Gender Longevity Gap

COUNTRY	POPULATION (000s)	MALE	FEMALE	OVERALL	GENDER GAP (YEARS)
Afghanistan	32,527	59.3	61.9	60.5	2.6
Albania	2897	75.1	80.7	77.8	5.6
Algeria	39,667	73.8	77.5	75.6	3.7
Angola	25,022	50.9	54.0	52.4	3.1
Antigua and Barbuda	92	74.1	78.6	76.4	4.5
Argentina	43,417	72.7	79.9	76.3	7.2
Armenia	3018	71.6	77.7	74.8	6.1
Australia	23,969	80.9	84.8	82.8	3.9
Austria	8545	79.0	83.9	81.5	4.9
Azerbaijan	9754	69.6	75.8	72.7	6.2
Bahamas	388	72.9	79.1	76.1	6.2
Bahrain	1377	76.2	77.9	76.9	1.7
Bangladesh	160,996	70.6	73.1	71.8	2.5
Barbados	284	73.1	77.9	75.5	4.8
Belarus	9496	66.5	78.0	72.3	11.5
Belgium	11,299	78.6	83.5	81.1	4.9
Belize	359	67.5	73.1	70.1	5.6
Benin	10,880	58.8	61.1	60.0	2.3
Bhutan	775	69.5	70.1	69.8	0.6
Bolivia (Plurinational State of)	10,725	68.2	73.3	70.7	5.1
Bosnia and Herzegovina	3810	75.0	79.7	77.4	4.7
Botswana	2262	63.3	68.1	65.7	4.8
Brazil	207,848	71.4	78.7	75.0	7.3
Brunei Darussalam	423	76.3	79.2	77.7	2.9
Bulgaria	7150	71.1	78.0	74.5	6.9
Burkina Faso	18,106	59.1	60.5	59.9	1.4
Burundi	11,179	57.7	61.6	59.6	3.9
Cabo Verde	521	71.3	75.0	73.3	3.7
Cambodia	15,578	66.6	70.7	68.7	4.1
Cameroon	23,344	55.9	58.6	57.3	2.7
Canada	35,940	80.2	84.1	82.2	3.9
Central African Republic	4900	50.9	54.1	52.5	3.2
Chad	14,037	51.7	54.5	53.1	2.8
Chile	17,948	77.4	83.4	80.5	6
China	1,383,925	74.6	77.6	76.1	3
Colombia	48,229	71.2	78.4	74.8	7.2
Comoros	788	61.9	65.2	63.5	3.3
Congo	4620	63.2	66.3	64.7	3.1
Costa Rica	4808	77.1	82.2	79.6	5.1
Côte d'Ivoire	22,702	52.3	54.4	53.3	2.1
Croatia	4240	74.7	81.2	78.0	6.5
Cuba	11,390	76.9	81.4	79.1	4.5
Cyprus	1165	78.3	82.7	80.5	4.4
Czechia	10,543	75.9	81.7	78.8	5.8
Democratic People's Republic of Korea	25,155	67.0	74.0	70.6	7
Democratic Republic of the Congo	77,267	58.3	61.5	59.8	3.2
Denmark	5669	78.6	82.5	80.6	3.9
Djibouti	888	61.8	65.3	63.5	3.5
Dominican Republic	10,528	70.9	77.1	73.9	6.2
Ecuador	16,144	73.5	79.0	76.2	5.5
Egypt	91,508	68.8	73.2	70.9	4.4
El Salvador	6127	68.8	77.9	73.5	9.1
Equatorial Guinea	845	56.6	60.0	58.2	3.4
Eritrea	5228	62.4	67.0	64.7	4.6
Estonia	1313	72.7	82.0	77.6	9.3
Ethiopia	99,391	62.8	66.8	64.8	4
Fiji	892	67.0	73.1	69.9	6.1
Finland	5503	78.3	83.8	81.1	5.5
France	64,395	79.4	85.4	82.4	6
Gabon	1725	64.7	67.2	66.0	2.5
Gambia	1991	59.8	62.5	61.1	2.7

TABLE 65.1 Gender Longevity Gap—cont'd

COUNTRY	POPULATION (000s)	MALE	FEMALE	OVERALL	GENDER GAP (YEARS)
Georgia	4000	70.3	78.3	74.4	8
Germany	80,689	78.7	83.4	81.0	4.7
Ghana	27,410	61.0	63.9	62.4	2.9
Greece	10,955	78.3	83.6	81.0	5.3
Grenada	107	71.2	76.1	73.6	4.9
Guatemala	16,343	68.5	75.2	71.9	6.7
Guinea	12,609	58.2	59.8	59.0	1.6
Guinea-Bissau	1844	57.2	60.5	58.9	3.3
Guyana	767	63.9	68.5	66.2	4.6
Haiti	10,711	61.5	65.5	63.5	4
Honduras	8075	72.3	77.0	74.6	4.7
Hungary	9855	72.3	79.1	75.9	6.8
Iceland	329	81.2	84.1	82.7	2.9
India	1,311,051	66.9	69.9	68.3	3
Indonesia	257,564	67.1	71.2	69.1	4.1
Iran (Islamic Republic of)	79,109	74.5	76.6	75.5	2.1
Iraq	36,423	66.2	71.8	68.9	5.6
Ireland	4688	79.4	83.4	81.4	4
Israel	8064	80.6	84.3	82.5	3.7
Italy	59,798	80.5	84.8	82.7	4.3
Jamaica	2793	73.9	78.6	76.2	4.7
Japan	126,573	80.5	86.8	83.7	6.3
Jordan	7595	72.5	75.9	74.1	3.4
Kazakhstan	17,625	65.7	74.7	70.2	9
Kenya	46,050	61.1	65.8	63.4	4.7
Kiribati	112	63.7	68.8	66.3	5.1
Kuwait	3892	73.7	76.0	74.7	2.3
Kyrgyzstan	5940	67.2	75.1	71.1	7.9
Lao People's Democratic Republic	6802	64.1	67.2	65.7	3.1
Latvia	1971	69.6	79.2	74.6	9.6
Lebanon	5851	73.5	76.5	74.9	3
Lesotho	2135	51.7	55.4	53.7	3.7
Liberia	4503	59.8	62.9	61.4	3.1
Libya	6278	70.1	75.6	72.7	5.5
Lithuania	2878	68.1	79.1	73.6	11
Luxembourg	567	79.8	84.0	82.0	4.2
Madagascar	24,235	63.9	67.0	65.5	3.1
Malawi	17,215	56.7	59.9	58.3	3.2
Malaysia	30,331	72.7	77.3	75.0	4.6
Maldives	364	76.9	80.2	78.5	3.3
Mali	17,600	58.2	58.3	58.2	0.1
Malta	419	79.7	83.7	81.7	4
Mauritania	4068	61.6	64.6	63.1	3
Mauritius	1273	71.4	77.8	74.6	6.4
Mexico	127,017	73.9	79.5	76.7	5.6
Micronesia (Federated States of)	104	68.1	70.6	69.4	2.5
Mongolia	2959	64.7	73.2	68.8	8.5
Montenegro	626	74.1	78.1	76.1	4
Morocco	34,378	73.3	75.4	74.3	2.1
Mozambique	27,978	55.7	59.4	57.6	3.7
Myanmar	53,897	64.6	68.5	66.6	3.9
Namibia	2459	63.1	68.3	65.8	5.2
Nepal	28,514	67.7	70.8	69.2	3.1
Netherlands	16,925	80.0	83.6	81.9	3.6
New Zealand	4529	80.0	83.3	81.6	3.3
Nicaragua	6082	71.5	77.9	74.8	6.4
Niger	19,899	60.9	62.8	61.8	1.9
Nigeria	182,202	53.4	55.6	54.5	2.2
Norway	5211	79.8	83.7	81.8	3.9
Oman	4491	75.0	79.2	76.6	4.2

Continued

TABLE 65.1 Gender Longevity Gap—cont'd

COUNTRY	POPULATION (000s)	MALE	FEMALE	OVERALL	GENDER GAP (YEARS)
Pakistan	188,925	65.5	67.5	66.4	2
Panama	3929	74.7	81.1	77.8	6.4
Papua New Guinea	7619	60.6	65.4	62.9	4.8
Paraguay	6639	72.2	76.0	74.0	3.8
Peru	31,377	73.1	78.0	75.5	4.9
Philippines	100,699	65.3	72.0	68.5	6.7
Poland	38,612	73.6	81.3	77.5	7.7
Portugal	10,350	78.2	83.9	81.1	5.7
Qatar	2235	77.4	80.0	78.2	2.6
Republic of Korea	50,293	78.8	85.5	82.3	6.7
Republic of Moldova	4069	67.9	76.2	72.1	8.3
Romania	19,511	71.4	78.8	75.0	7.4
Russian Federation	143,457	64.7	76.3	70.5	11.6
Rwanda	11,610	61.9	67.4	64.8	5.5
Saint Lucia	185	72.6	77.9	75.2	5.3
Saint Vincent and the Grenadines	109	71.3	75.2	73.2	3.9
Samoa	193	70.9	77.5	74.0	6.6
Sao Tome and Principe	190	65.6	69.4	67.5	3.8
Saudi Arabia	31,540	73.2	76.0	74.5	2.8
Senegal	15,129	64.6	68.6	66.7	4
Serbia	8851	72.9	78.4	75.6	5.5
Seychelles	96	69.1	78.0	73.2	8.9
Sierra Leone	6453	49.3	50.8	50.1	1.5
Singapore	5604	80.0	86.1	83.1	6.1
Slovakia	5426	72.9	80.2	76.7	7.3
Slovenia	2068	77.9	83.7	80.8	5.8
Solomon Islands	584	67.9	70.8	69.2	2.9
Somalia	10,787	53.5	56.6	55.0	3.1
South Africa	54,490	59.3	66.2	62.9	6.9
South Sudan	12,340	56.1	58.6	57.3	2.5
Spain	46,122	80.1	85.5	82.8	5.4
Sri Lanka	20,715	71.6	78.3	74.9	6.7
Sudan	40,235	62.4	65.9	64.1	3.5
Suriname	543	68.6	74.7	71.6	6.1
Swaziland	1287	56.6	61.1	58.9	4.5
Sweden	9779	80.7	84.0	82.4	3.3
Switzerland	8299	81.3	85.3	83.4	4
Syrian Arab Republic	18,502	59.9	69.9	64.5	10
Tajikistan	8482	66.6	73.6	69.7	7
Thailand	67,959	71.9	78.0	74.9	6.1
The former Yugoslav Republic of Macedonia	2078	73.5	77.8	75.7	4.3
Timor-Leste	1185	66.6	70.1	68.3	3.5
Togo	7305	58.6	61.1	59.9	2.5
Tonga	106	70.6	76.4	73.5	5.8
Trinidad and Tobago	1360	67.9	74.8	71.2	6.9
Tunisia	11,254	73.0	77.8	75.3	4.8
Turkey	78,666	72.6	78.9	75.8	6.3
Turkmenistan	5374	62.2	70.5	66.3	8.3
Uganda	39,032	60.3	64.3	62.3	4
Ukraine	44,824	66.3	76.1	71.3	9.8
United Arab Emirates	9157	76.4	78.6	77.1	2.2
United Kingdom	64,716	79.4	83.0	81.2	3.6
United Republic of Tanzania	53,470	59.9	63.8	61.8	3.9
United States of America	321,774	76.9	81.6	79.3	4.7
Uruguay	3432	73.3	80.4	77.0	7.1
Uzbekistan	29,893	66.1	72.7	69.4	6.6
Vanuatu	265	70.1	74.0	72.0	3.9
Venezuela (Bolivarian Republic of)	31,108	70.0	78.5	74.1	8.5
Viet Nam	93,448	71.3	80.7	76.0	9.4
Yemen	26,832	64.3	67.2	65.7	2.9

Chapter 65 Integrated Men's Health: Androgen Deficiency, Cardiovascular Risk, and Metabolic Syndrome

TABLE 65.1 Gender Longevity Gap—cont'd

COUNTRY	POPULATION (000s)	MALE	FEMALE	OVERALL	GENDER GAP (YEARS)
Zambia	16,212	59.0	64.7	61.8	5.7
Zimbabwe	15,603	59.0	62.3	60.7	3.3
WHO Region					
African Region	989,173	58.2	61.7	60.0	3.5
Region of the Americas	986,705	74.0	79.9	77.0	5.9
South-East Asia Region	1,928,174	67.3	70.7	68.9	3.4
European Region	910,053	73.2	80.2	76.8	7
Eastern Mediterranean Region	643,784	67.4	70.4	68.8	3
Western Pacific Region	1,855,126	74.5	78.7	76.6	4.2
Global	7,313,015	69.1	73.7	71.4	4.6

From World Health Organization, 2015.

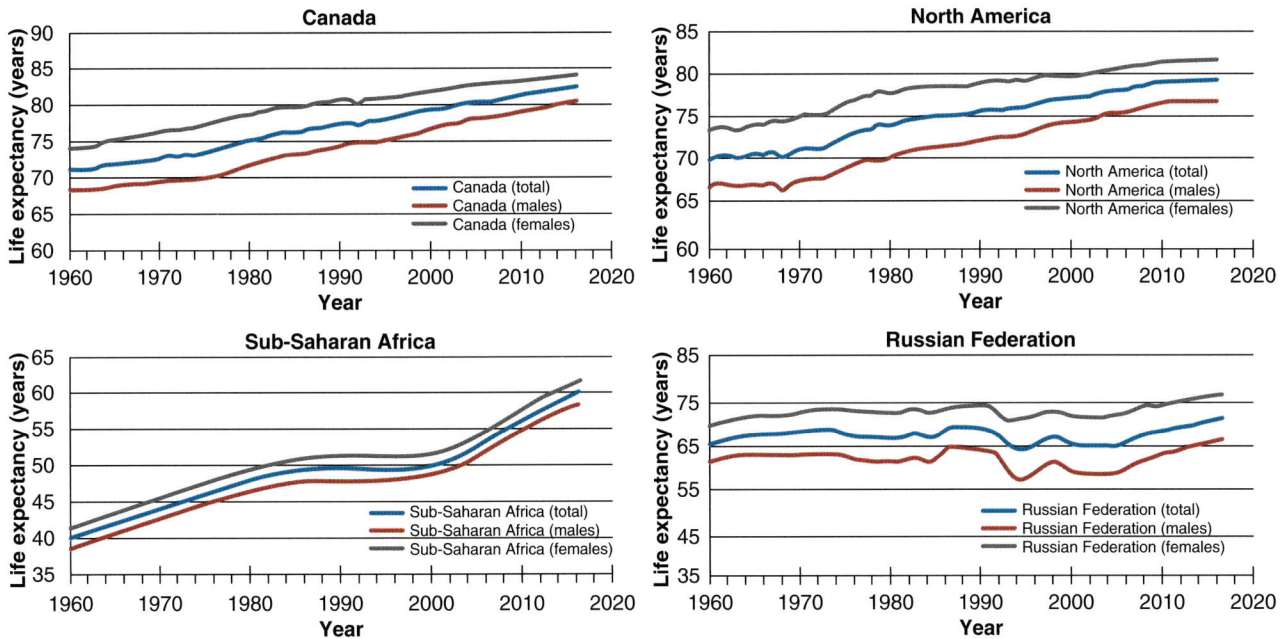

Fig. 65.1. Life expectancy at birth over recent decades, demonstrating improvements in longevity for males and females. (Data from The World Bank.)

TABLE 65.2 Major Causes of Death, United States 2016

CAUSE OF DEATH	ANNUAL NO. OF DEATHS	MALE-TO-FEMALE INCIDENCE RATIO
Heart disease	633,842	1.12
Cancer	595,930	1.11
Chronic obstructive lung disease	155,041	0.88
Accidents	146,571	1.73
Stroke	140,323	0.71
Dementia	110,561	0.44
Diabetes	79,535	1.18
Influenza/pneumonia	57,062	0.89
Nephrological conditions	49,959	1.03
Suicide	44,193	3.33

From Centre for Disease Control and Prevention/National Center for Health Statistics (CDC/NCHS): *National vital statistics system, mortality 2017*, Atlanta 2017, US Department of Health and Human Services.

recent neuropsychologic studies suggesting that exposure to tobacco products stimulates different parts of the brain in men compared with women (Birge et al., 2017). This neurophysiologic difference between genders may explain why women are less likely to quit smoking than men. The ill effects of tobacco exposure are well known, accounting for almost 25% of all cardiovascular disease. Importantly, a recent study has demonstrated that almost 50% of deaths associated with 12 different cancer types were related to smoking, including liver, colon and rectum, lung, oral cavity and throat, esophagus, larynx, stomach, pancreas, bladder, kidney, and cervical cancer, as well as acute myeloid leukemia (Abdel-Rahman et al., 2017; Botteri et al., 2008; Gandini et al., 2008; Haverkos et al., 2003; International Collaboration of Epidemiological Studies of Cervical Cancer et al., 2006; Iodice et al., 2008; Lee et al., 2016; Ugai et al., 2018).

Unhealthy sexual practices are also more prevalent among men than among women. Sexual promiscuity and high-risk sexual practices affect health in many separate domains. Sexually transmitted diseases such as human immunodeficiency virus (HIV), syphilis, and hepatitis are associated with ill health and early death (McElligott, 2014). Multiple studies from almost every country in the world have demonstrated that men are more apt to engage in higher-risk sexual practices and less likely to use protection such as condoms or antiretroviral therapies as compared with women (Dir et al., 2014; Lan et al., 2017; Vagenas et al., 2013; Ward-Peterson et al., 2018).

On a neurohormonal level, studies have observed more intense changes in dopaminergic activity (Spear, 2000) and higher levels of sensation seeking and risk taking (Bongers et al., 2003; Eysenck et al., 1984) in young males, whereas higher levels of negative urgency were found in females (d'Acremont and Van der Linden, 2005). In the domain of sexual activity, males start having sex at a younger age compared with females, report greater number of sexual partners over their lifetimes, and tend to engage in multiple risky sexual behaviors (Grunbaum et al., 2002; Kotchick et al., 2001; Newman and Zimmerman, 2000; Romer and Hennessy, 2007).

Aside from the mentioned three hazardous practices, men across different cultures tend to engage in higher risk activities, such as drag racing, parachuting, and extreme sports more frequently than women.

Masculinity Defined Norms of Behavior and Attitudes Toward Health

No dissertation on men's health can omit the concept of "masculinity," its attributes and its influence on the perception of health and disease. Men throughout the globe are more likely than women to adopt beliefs and behaviors that increase the risks to their health and safety and are less likely to engage in behaviors that are linked with preservation or improvement of health and longevity. Gender is constructed from cultural and subjective meanings that constantly shift and vary, depending on the time and geographic location (Kimmel, 1996). Stereotypes used by society in the construction of gender are composed of characteristics generally believed to be typical either of women or of men. There is widespread agreement in western society about what are considered to be typically feminine and typically masculine characteristics (Golombok and Fivush, 1994; Street et al., 1995; Williams and Best, 1982). People of both genders are encouraged to adhere to stereotypic beliefs and behaviors and commonly do conform to and adopt the dominant norms of femininity and masculinity present in their culture (Bohan, 1993; Deaux, 1984; Eagly, 1983).

Research indicates that men and boys experience relatively more social pressure than females to endorse gender stereotypes such as the health-related beliefs that men are independent, self-reliant, strong, robust, and tough (Golombok and Fivush, 1994; Martin, 1995; Williams and Best, 1982). It is therefore not surprising that male behaviors tend to be more stereotypic than those of women and girls (Katz and Ksansnak, 1994; Levant et al., 1998; Rice and Coates, 1995; Street et al., 1995).

In most parts of the world, the resources used by males to construct their masculinity are largely not conducive to preservation of health (Courtenay, 2000). Men construct their gender in part by dismissing their health care needs. They boast about not visiting physicians, refuse to take time off work when ill, and idolize high tolerance to alcohol (e.g., by boasting that drinking alcohol does not impair their driving skills). As a result, global masculinity has evolved, in part, into a construct that predisposes men to early death and disability. There are many examples of how this plays out in the practical world. Men, for instance, do not visit primary care doctors as often as women do. Although women may have a reproductive bias in favor of more visits, even when maternity-related visits are accounted for, women in the United States visit their practitioners one-third more times than men (Centers for Disease Control and Prevention [CDC], 2015). Similar studies in Europe, Australia, United Kingdom, Lithuania, and Canada have corroborated this observation (Galdas et al., 2005; UCL Institute of Health Equity, 2013), which is particularly pronounced at ages between 20 and 44 (Hippisley-Cox and Vinogradova, 2009).

Men are less likely to be compliant with prescribed medications (Berg et al., 2004; Hadji et al., 2016; Monane et al., 1996), although a few exceptions have been noted (Li and Froelicher, 2007; Manteuffel et al., 2014). Men are also less likely to adhere to physician care plans than women and are less likely to undergo recommended screening services (Henry J. Kaiser Family Foundation [KFF], 2015).

Physical and Chemical Exposure in the Workplace

One of the most obvious domains of risk to men's health is the workplace. Throughout the globe, men are more likely to die from work-related injuries than women. In the United States, Australia, and Canada, 92%, 96%, and 97% of all risk fatalities were among men, respectively (Bilsker et al., 2010). Significant work-associated health care and workers' compensation costs are prevalent throughout the developed world (Safe Work Australia, 2016; US Bureau of Labor Statistics, 2016). For example, in the United States it is estimated that more than $1 billion per week (US Department of Labor, 2018) was spent for expenses related to workplace injury and illness in 2012. The costs of workplace injuries and illnesses include direct and indirect costs. Direct costs include workers' compensation stipends, medical charges, and legal outlays. Indirect costs include training for replacement workers, accident inquiry, lost productivity, equipment and property damage repairs, and charges linked to diminished worker morale and absenteeism.

A host of reasons explain why the male gender is at higher risk of work-related illness and injury. First is the largely gender-segregated and specific aspects of either occupations themselves or the subdivision of labor within certain job categories. Male employees are statistically represented in greater numbers in certain industries, including mining, military, farming, protective services (fire/police), and fishing (Arcury et al., 2014; Curtis Breslin et al., 2007; Desmond, 2006; Ibanez and Narocki, 2011; Lawson, 2010; Messing et al., 2003; Phakathi, 2013; Power and Baqee, 2010; Power, 2008). Furthermore, even within many of the more gender-balanced industries, heavy, "physical" work tasks are disproportionately performed by male workers (Arcury et al., 2014; Desmond, 2006). Men are thus overexposed to high-risk workplaces and associated hazards and injuries.

Targets and Effective Interventions

Improving men's health on the epidemiologic scale requires innovative solutions creatively implemented to reverse the aforementioned causes of the gender gap in life expectancy and health outcomes. The health of people in local communities is linked to global systems. The world economy and labor markets, for example, can have a powerful effect on men's health outcomes. As industrial production expands, workers face a range of occupational health and safety hazards, particularly in relatively economically disadvantaged countries. The social structural relationships that organize men's work life and their health are not simply imposed on men by global forces; these relationships are local, global, and reciprocal. Any positive change in these relationships requires us not only to improve overall health and longevity but also to ideally position men's health on par with that of their female counterparts. To do this, the major change must come in the form of a social movement, one that undoes the risk factors for early demise and reduces the risk or prevalence of high-risk activities in which men tend to engage. Such a change would, specifically, work toward improving the work environment and creating a gender balance, minimizing high-risk behaviors, and, last, altering the construct of masculinity to one that encourages healthy lifestyles, facilitates open communication among peers, and engages men to interact more frequently with the health care systems (particularly between the ages of 18 and 40). Urologists can have a major impact in this regard: many men re-enter the health care systems by way of a urologist's office complaining of lower urinary tract symptoms resulting from benign prostatic hyperplasia (BPH) or erectile dysfunction (ED) or seeking a vasectomy. Indeed, the urologist should develop training to recognize and even intervene among his or her male patients who demonstrate adverse risk factors for chronic disease or death, such as smoking, excess alcohol usage, and metabolic syndrome. It is clear that simple public health messaging about healthy choices and lifestyle have limited results. Despite intensive education campaign, much of the developed world has a problem with increasing body weight (Swinburn et al., 2011), especially in North America, where obesity prevalence is approaching 40% in the United States (Hales et al., 2017), 32.4% in Mexico, and 26.7% in Canada (Organization of Economic Co-operation and Development [OECD], 2017).

In recent decades, research has been devoted to improving health outcomes of vulnerable men, with findings suggesting novel directions to move forward. Innovative programs designed to reach out to men through their preferred sport activities have been shown to be promising (Bottorff et al., 2015). The interest of men in soccer in Europe (Gray et al., 2013; Hunt et al., 2014) and hockey in Canada (Blunt et al., 2017; Petrella et al., 2017) demonstrate particular effectiveness and potential for affecting health perspectives on health. Public health campaigns featuring prominent athletes and celebrities targeting the 18- to 40-year-old demographic have begun to emerge (Canadian Men's Health Foundation, 2018; Movember Foundation, 2011), although it is too early to conclusively measure their outcomes. Societal change does not happen overnight, and thoughtful change in men's lifestyle choices requires a sustained and innovative effort, which is unlikely to pay off for decades. On a more microepidemiologic level, clinicians must strive to counsel their patients on healthier lifestyle choices.

Global Men's Health Movement

The awareness of men's health as a unique need in the medical, psychological, and sociologic fields has taken root. A host of national and international organizations have sprung forward to aid in this regard. The WHO has recognized that decreasing the gender health gap is required for achieving the stated goal of global health equity (Baker et al., 2014). Fundraising organizations such as Movember have also fueled these efforts via grassroots funding campaigns seeking to augment governmental supports (Movember Foundation, 2018; Ontario gov).

Clearly, one of the major challenges in these efforts is reaching men living in societies with the greatest discrepancies, such as the countries in sub-Saharan Africa and Eastern Europe. In addition to the efforts by the supranational organizations, most major national urologic associations have their own efforts. A number of countries have published, or are developing, national men's health programs such as those put forward by Ireland, Australia, and Brazil. These programs are seeking to address the specific health care needs of men by improving their engagement with the medical practice, standardizing the approaches to addressing men's health, and researching best practices that would lead to improving health outcomes in men.

> **KEY POINTS: RATIONALE FOR INTEGRATIVE MEN'S HEALTH**
>
> - Men throughout the world live shorter lives then women throughout the world.
> - The gender gap persists despite improvements in overall life expectancy at birth.
> - Men live not only shorter lives than women but also sicker lives.
> - Gender differences in illness-related outcomes reflect social, environmental, and physiologic factors.
> - Innovative and coordinated programs targeting men are required to promote social and behavioral changes that would improve men's health.

METABOLIC SYNDROME AND MEN'S HEALTH

Introduction, History, and Definitions

Metabolic syndrome is defined as a series of interconnected biochemical, physiologic, metabolic, and clinical factors that increase the individual's risk of type 2 diabetes mellitus (T2DM), heart disease, and early mortality. The syndrome was first conceived in 1920 when a Swedish investigator (Kylin, 1923) noted an association between hypertension, gout, and elevated blood glucose levels. In 1947 the concept was further refined when Vague (1947) noted that visceral organ fatty deposits were linked with cardiovascular disease and type 2 diabetes mellitus. In 1988 Reaven (Reaven, 1988; Reaven, 1993) described an aggregate of risk factors for cardiovascular disease and diabetes that he named Syndrome X. Syndrome X was renamed the deadly quartet in 1989, incorporating glucose intolerance, hypertriglyceridemia, hypertension, and upper body obesity (Kaplan, 1989). Finally, the term metabolic syndrome was coined in 1998 by the World Health Organization (Alberti and Zimmet, 1998; WHO, 1999). Since then, other subspecialty societies concerned with this condition have released their own definitions and criteria (Fig. 65.2). Table 65.3 lists the criteria set out by major organizations for the diagnosis of metabolic syndrome.

Although the listed definitions possess a number of common criteria, the WHO, American Association of Clinical Endocrinologists (AACE), and the European Group for the Study of Insulin Resistance

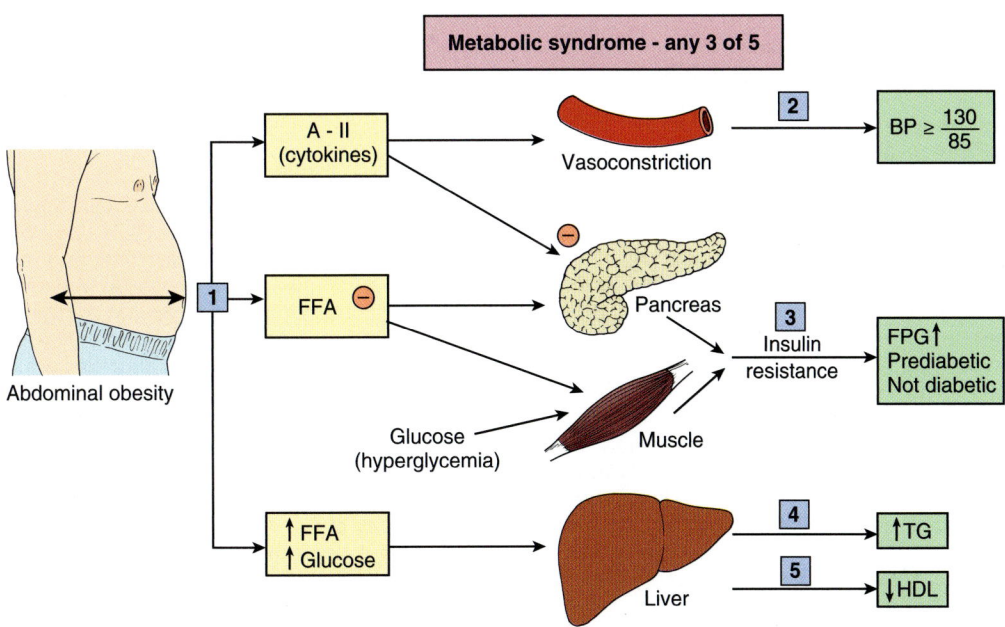

Fig. 65.2. Diagnosis of metabolic syndrome requires a tape measure, an accurate eye, and fasting lipogram, plasma glucose measurements, and blood pressure measurements. (Adapted from Lionel H. *Circulation* 115-e32-e35, 2007.)

TABLE 65.3 Metabolic Syndrome Definitions and Criteria

CLINICAL PARAMETER	WHO (1999)	EGIR (Balkau and Charles, 1999)	ATP III (NCEP, 2001)	AACE (Einhorn et al., 2003)	IDF (Alberti et al., 2005)
Obesity/body fat distribution	Waist/hip ratio >0.90 in men, >0.85 in women; or BMI >30 kg/m²	Waist circumference ≥94 cm in men, ≥80 cm in women	Waist circumference >102 cm in men, >88 cm in women	BMI ≥25 kg/m²	Waist circumference ≥94 cm in men, ≥80 cm in women
Insulin resistance/hyperglycemia	IGT, IFG, T2DM, or other evidence of insulin resistance	Hyperinsulinemia (plasma insulin >75th percentile)	Fasting glucose ≥110 mg/dL	Fasting glucose ≥110 mg/dL	Fasting glucose ≥100 mg/dL, T2DM
Triglyceridemia	≥150 mg/dL	≥177 mg/dL	≥150 mg/dL	>150 mg/dL	>150 mg/dL or on treatment
Cholesterol	HDL-C <35 mg/dL in men or <39 mg/dL in women	HDL-C <39 mg/dL	HDL-C <40 mg/dL in men; <50 mg/dL in women	HDL-C <40 mg/dL in men; <50 mg/dL in women	HDL-C <40 mg/dL in men; <50 mg/dL in women; or on treatment
Blood Pressure	≥140/90 mm Hg	≥140/90 mm Hg or on treatment	>130/85 mm Hg	≥130/85 mm Hg	>130/85 mm Hg or on treatment
Other	Microalbuminuria[a]			Other features of insulin resistance[b]	

AACE, American Association of Clinical Endocrinologists; *ATP III*, National Cholesterol Education Program Adult Treatment Panel III Report; *BMI*, body mass index; *EGIR*, European Group for the Study of Insulin Resistance; *HDL-C*, high-density lipoprotein cholesterol; *IDF*, International Diabetes Federation; *IFG*, impaired fasting glucose; *IGT*, impaired glucose tolerance; *T2DM*, type II diabetes mellitus; *WHO*, World Health Organization.
[a]Microalbuminuria defined as urinary albumin excretion ≥70 μg/min or albumin/creatine ratio ≥30 mg/g.
[b]Family history of T2DM, hypertension, or CVD; polycystic ovary syndrome; sedentary lifestyle; advancing age; ethnic groups having high risk for T2DM or CVD.

criteria emphasize insulin resistance, which requires a cumbersome oral glucose tolerance test to be ascertained. The Adult Treatment Panel III criteria were developed to use readily available anthropometric measures and clinical laboratory tests, thereby facilitating epidemiologic research. Defining obesity cutoffs for specific ethnic groups also remains problematic, which is why the International Diabetes Federation (IDF) have further adjusted their specific criteria to provide cutoff points that are specific for different racial/ethnic populations (Ritchie and Connell, 2007).

Prevalence and Predictors of Metabolic Syndrome

Metabolic syndrome is a prevalent condition across the world. Depending on the ethnic, gender, racial, and geographic makeup of the studied group, prevalence of metabolic syndrome ranges between 10% and 84% of the population. Choice of definition used can lead to significant differences in the estimates of prevalence. In a paper by Morote et al., the range of patients with a diagnosis of prostate cancer before commencing androgen deprivation therapy afflicted by metabolic syndrome ranged between 9.4% by the WHO definition and 50% by International Diabetes Federation definition within the same cohort (Morote et al., 2015). The IDF estimates that about one-fourth of adults in the world meet the criteria for metabolic syndrome.

Risk factors for metabolic syndrome include sedentary lifestyle, excess caloric intake, and higher socioeconomic status. It is interesting to ponder that, for the first time in human history, we are witnessing the emergence of medical syndromes that arise from overconsumption and sedentary lifestyle; this would have been unimaginable 100 years ago. In the National Health and Nutrition Examination Survey (NHANES) advancing age and advancing weight were associated with metabolic syndrome. As an example, 5% of subjects with normal weight had metabolic syndrome compared with 60% of obese individuals. Similarly, 10% of individuals aged 20 to 29 had metabolic syndrome compared with 45% of those 60 to 69 years old (Ford et al., 2002).

Physiology of Metabolic Syndrome

Although the physiologic alterations associated with metabolic syndrome have not been fully elucidated, recent research has greatly expanded our understanding of the condition. In general, **it is believed that genetic risk factors interact with lifestyle exposure (physical inactivity, smoking, caloric excess, psychological stress) to create a positive energy imbalance.** This in turn leads to adiposity with concomitant alteration in fatty acid metabolism and increased release of adipokines (Fig. 65.3). Ultimately, this leads to endothelial dysfunction, atherogenic dyslipidemia, insulin resistance, hypertension, hypercoagulability, and low-grade inflammation.

Abdominal Obesity

Obesity is largely driven by excess consumption of calorie-dense foods and diminished physical activity. Adipose tissue is composed of adipocytes, stromal preadipocytes, immune cells, and endothelium. It responds rapidly and dynamically to excess caloric intake with adipocyte hypertrophy and hyperplasia (Halberg et al., 2008). With obesity and progressive adipocyte enlargement, adipocyte hypoxia ensues (Cinti et al., 2005), leading to necrosis and macrophage infiltration into adipose tissue. This progressive process is accompanied by the release of biologically active metabolites known as adipokines, which include glycerol, free fatty acids (FFAs), proinflammatory mediators (such as tumor necrosis factor-α and interleukin-6 [IL-6]), plasminogen activator inhibitor-1 (PAI-1), and C-reactive protein [CRP]) (Lau et al., 2005). This localized inflammatory process in the adipose tissue propagates an overall systemic inflammation, which is associated with the development of comorbidities (Trayhurn and Wood, 2004). Adipokines integrate the endocrine, autocrine, and paracrine signals to mediate multiple processes, including insulin sensitivity (Saleem et al., 2009), oxidative stress (Tsimikas et al., 2009), energy metabolism, blood coagulation, and inflammatory responses (Jacobs et al., 2009). Combined, these physiologic changes

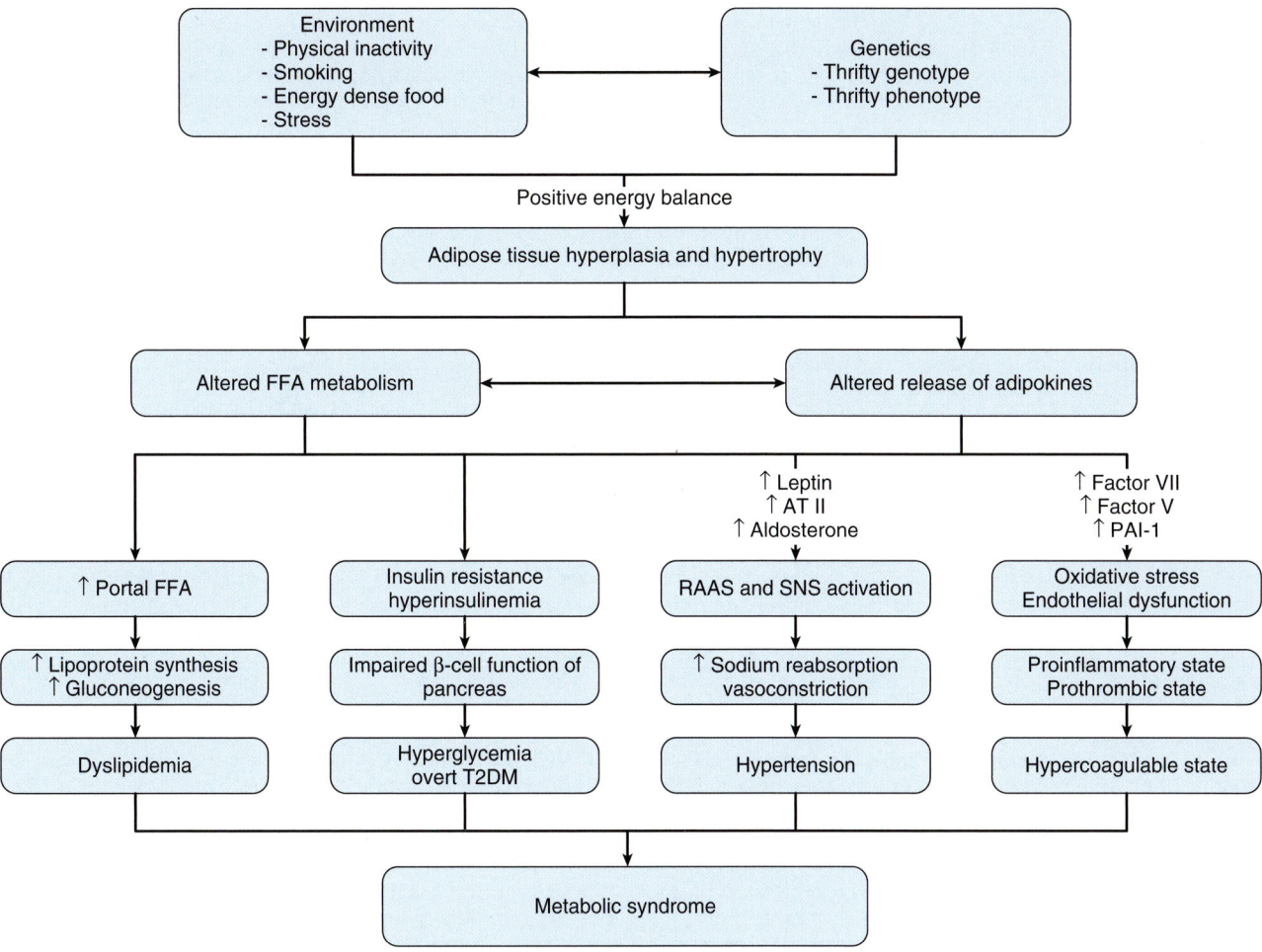

Fig. 65.3. Schematic presentation of metabolic syndrome. *AT II*, Angiotensin II; *FFA*, free fatty acids; *PAI-1*, plasminogen activator inhibitor 1; *RAAS*, renin-angiotensin-aldosterone system; *SNS*, sympathetic nervous system; *T2DM*, type 2 diabetes mellitus.

accelerate atherosclerosis, plaque rupture, and atherothrombosis. Thus the adipose tissue no longer only acts to store excess energy as lipids but rather evolves into an endocrine organ, releasing numerous cytokines and eliciting systemic physiologic alterations.

Insulin Resistance

Insulin-resistant individuals exhibit impaired glucose metabolism and tolerance, which manifests as an abnormal response to a glucose challenge, elevated blood fasting glucose levels, and/or overt hyperglycemia, or a reduction in the effect of insulin after its intravenous administration. Insulin resistance is defined as a pathophysiologic condition in which normal insulin concentration fails to induce normal responses in target tissues, such as adipose, muscle, and liver. Under this abnormal condition, pancreatic beta cells are stimulated to secrete more insulin (thereby inducing hyperinsulinemia) to overcome the hyperglycemia. Although hyperinsulinemia may compensate for insulin resistance in regard to some of its biologic effects, including maintenance of normoglycemia, it can result in exaggerated insulin effects in normally sensitive tissues. This accentuation of a subset of insulin actions, coupled with a resistance to its other actions, results in the clinical manifestations of metabolic syndrome (Gill et al., 2005). An inability of the pancreatic beta cells over time to produce sufficient amounts of insulin to correct the worsening insulin resistance in target tissues leads to hyperglycemia and overt type 2 diabetes mellitus (Petersen and Shulman, 2006).

Dyslipidemia

Dyslipidemia in metabolic syndrome is characterized by a host of lipid anomalies reflecting disturbances in the structure, metabolism, and activity of atherogenic lipoproteins and antiatherogenic high-density lipoprotein cholesterol. Insulin resistance leads to atherogenic dyslipidemia through multiple processes. First, because insulin normally inhibits lipolysis in adipocytes, impaired insulin signaling increases lipid breakdown and increases circulating FFA levels. In the hepatic tissue, FFAs serve as substrates for triglyceride formation. Second, insulin resistance directly increases very low-density lipoprotein (VLDL) production. Third, insulin regulates the activity of enzyme lipoprotein lipase, the rate-limiting enzyme and a major mediator of VLDL clearance. Hypertriglyceridemia in insulin resistance is therefore the result of an increase in VLDL production and a decrease in VLDL clearance. VLDL is metabolized to remnant lipoproteins and small, dense low-density lipoproteins (LDL), both of which can promote the formation of atherosclerotic deposits. On balance, it is believed that the dyslipidemia associated with insulin resistance is a direct consequence of increased VLDL secretion from the liver (Ginsberg et al., 2005). These anomalies are closely associated with increased oxidative stress and endothelial dysfunction, thereby reinforcing the proinflammatory phenotype of atherosclerotic disease.

Hypertension

Essential hypertension is frequently associated with several metabolic abnormalities, of which obesity, glucose impairment, and dyslipidemia are the most prevalent (Ferrannini and Natali, 1991). Studies suggest that hyperglycemia and hyperinsulinemia activate the renin-angiotensin system (RAS). There is also evidence that insulin resistance and hyperinsulinemia lead to sympathetic nervous system hyperactivation, which increases renal sodium reabsorption, persistently increases cardiac output, and causes arterial vasoconstriction, resulting in hypertension (Morse et al., 2005). Evidence also suggests that adipocytes produce aldosterone in response to the stimulation of angiotensin ATII receptors (Briones et al., 2012).

Genetics

Increasing evidence suggests that genetics plays a major role in the cause of metabolic syndrome (Ordovas, 2007). Some individuals who are not obese by traditional measures develop insulin resistance and exhibit metabolic risk factors. This occurrence is particularly frequently encountered in individuals who have a family history of T2DM, with either both parents or one parent and a first- or second-degree relative suffering from the disease (Perseghin et al., 1997). A similar paradigm also is found more frequently in people of South Asian heritage (Abate et al., 2004; Martin et al., 2003). It is probable that the expression of each metabolic risk factor falls partially under its own genetic control, which then influences the individual's response to environmental exposures. This is exemplified by data suggesting that polymorphisms in genes affecting lipoprotein metabolism are associated with the worsening of dyslipidemia among obese people (Laakso, 2004; Poulsen et al., 2005).

Neel et al. (1962) proposed the *thrifty genotype hypothesis*, postulating that **persons living in a calorically depleted environment would maximize their probability of survival if they could maximize storage of surplus energy**. Genetic selection would thus favor the energy-conserving genotypes in such environments. However, these same selected genetic variations may become unfavorable when the nutrition improved and high-calorie food becomes abundant. This may explain why certain immigrant populations are at highest risk for metabolic syndrome in the United States and other countries (Banerjee and Shah, 2018; Berkowitz et al., 2016; Ogden et al., 2014). This hypothesis assumes that the common genetic variants of thrifty genes predispose to metabolic syndrome. Hales and Barker in 1992 hypothesized that babies who experienced a fetal caloric deprivation in utero adapted to a poor nutritional environment by reducing energy expenditure and becoming "thrifty." Support for this postulated construct is found in the association between diminished birth weight and risk of adult-onset insulin resistance and T2DM (Hales et al., 1997).

Endothelial Dysfunction

Metabolic syndrome is characterized by impaired endothelium-dependent vasodilation, reduced arterial compliance, and accelerated atherosclerosis (Kraemer-Aguiar et al., 2008). Mediators of these anomalies include elevated levels of oxidative stress reactants, hyperglycemia, advanced glycation products, FFAs, inflammatory cytokines, and adipokines.

Hypercoagulable State

Metabolic syndrome induces a proinflammatory state characterized by elevated circulating cytokines and acute-phase reactants (e.g., CRP). In addition, anomalies in the procoagulant factors fibrinogen, factors VII and VIII, and the antifibrinolytic factor plasminogen activator inhibitor-1 (PAI-1) have been demonstrated. Grundy (2004) has shown that fibrinogen is an acute-phase reactant protein. Therefore prothrombotic and proinflammatory states appear to be linked metabolically.

Dietary Factors

Numerous studies (Aljada et al., 2004) have shown that diets high in fat and processed foods are associated with the generation of reactive oxygen species and an activation of the proinflammatory transcription factor nuclear factor-κB (NF-κB) (Aljada et al., 2004). In contrast, a diet rich in fruits and fiber tends not to induce these changes.

Glucocorticoid and Stress-Response Mediators

Chronic hypersecretion of stress mediators, such as the stress hormone cortisol, may lead to the accumulation of visceral fat in the body. Low levels of growth hormone and low testosterone may also potentiate the interaction between stress and metabolism (Charmandari et al., 2005). Stress steroids also increase the activity of enzymes involved in fatty acid synthesis, promote the secretion of lipoproteins (Wang et al., 1995), induce hepatic gluconeogenesis (Argaud et al., 1996), induce the differentiation of preadipocytes to adipocytes (which may promote increased body fat mass) (Hauner et al., 1989), and increase lipolysis, which leads to peripheral insulin resistance (Guillaume-Gentil et al., 1993). Investigators have demonstrated associations between blood cortisol levels and a number of features of metabolic syndrome, including visceral obesity and sarcopenia, which are known to lead to dyslipidemia, hypertension, and T2DM (Chrousos, 2009).

Obstructive Sleep Apnea

Increasing evidence points to linkages between obstructive sleep apnea (OSA) and metabolic syndrome. OSA is estimated to affect 4% of male and 2% of female adults in the United States (Young et al., 1993). The results of the Sleep Heart Health Study demonstrate that increased degree of sleep-disordered breathing is associated with metabolic syndrome components, including high body mass index (BMI), waist-to-hip ratio, hypertension, diabetes, and blood lipid levels. The presence of alterations in sympathetic activity and hypothalamic-pituitary-adrenal axis in OSA could suggest a possible mechanistic linkage between the two disorders (Calvin et al., 2009).

Metabolic Syndrome and Urologic Disorders

Although metabolic syndrome was classically associated with elevated risk of cardiovascular disease, diabetes, and stroke, it in fact has a broader range of manifestations. Certainly, cancers common in developed nations, such as colorectal and breast cancers, may be linked to metabolic syndrome (Bhandari et al., 2014; Esposito et al., 2012; Esposito et al., 2013a; Esposito et al., 2013b; Jinjuvadia et al., 2013). **Urologic conditions are recognized to be highly prevalent among aging men, especially those with metabolic syndrome.** Awareness of metabolic syndrome and its constituent conditions is important for urologists in terms of counseling and diagnostic suspicion.

Renal Conditions

Metabolic syndrome and frank T2DM have a significant impact on renal physiology, as described earlier in this chapter. The three major renal conditions associated with metabolic syndrome are renal insufficiency, urolithiasis, and renal cell carcinoma (RCC).

Renal Insufficiency. Renal disorders are a major cause of death and disability in the developed world (see the earlier section on men's health). It is estimated that 1 in 10 residents of the United States suffers from chronic kidney disease (De Nicola and Zoccali, 2016). Rates of renal replacement therapy, transplantation and dialysis, are growing (Tonelli et al., 2011; Tonelli et al., 2018) as populations age and risk factors for renal disease become more prevalent. Furthermore, even patients with chronic kidney failure who do not require renal replacement therapy appear to have accelerated rates of death, largely from cardiovascular disease (Go et al., 2004). Hypertension and diabetes (Kastarinen et al., 2010), obesity (Bruck et al., 2018), and perhaps nontraditional risk factors such as anemia, hyperphosphatemia, high plasma C reactive protein and fibrinogen, high sympathetic activity, and accumulation of endogenous inhibitors of nitric oxide synthase (Salem, 2002) appear to be the main drivers of chronic kidney disease at the population level. These processes are consequences of metabolic syndrome.

Stones. Urolithiasis is more frequently found among patients exhibiting features of metabolic syndrome. In the study by Chou et al. (2011), calcium oxalate and uric acid stones were more prevalent among patients with obesity. Okomoto et al. used a murine model fed a diet including 1% ethylene glycol to study metabolic syndrome and potential for urolithiasis. The study showed an increased formation of calcium oxalate crystals as well as higher calcium deposits within the renal tissue (Okamoto et al., 2010). Several mechanisms have been suggested to explain these associations, including lipase activity, mitochondrial dysfunction, and lipid peroxidation, factors known to cause cellular damage and result in debris, which in turn leads to nucleation phenomenon (Jonassen et al., 2005) and hypercalciuria (Baggio and Budakovic, 2005).

Hypercalciuria is associated with components of metabolic syndrome (Conen et al., 2004; Nakagawa et al., 2006; Schachter, 2005), such as obesity, dyslipidemia, hyperglycemia, and hypertension. The burden of elevated uric acid levels is further worsened by the fact that patients with metabolic syndrome tend to excrete slightly acidic urine. A defect in the production of ammonia in the proximal tubule at the mitochondrial level has been identified as the primary source of aciduria, as reinforced by studies demonstrating that obesity and urinary pH are inversely associated (Powell et al., 2000). Drugs used to manage hypertension among patients with metabolic syndrome may also influence renal stone formation (Alexander et al., 2017).

Tumors. Demonstrating an association between metabolic syndrome and RCC is a challenging epidemiologic exercise. Diagnostic bias exists: patients with hypertension and glucose intolerance are more frequently exposed to renal imaging than the general population, resulting in discovery of small renal masses. Emerging evidence, however, does suggest an association with components of the metabolic syndrome. Obesity, for example, is a well-established risk factor for RCC among women, although emerging data suggest that frank T2DM is also associated with higher rate of the disease. A systematic review conducted by Larsson and Wolk (2011) demonstrated that a history of T2DM is associated with a 26% increase in risk of RCC in men (relative risk [RR] 1.26, 95% confidence interval [CI] 1.06–1.49). These results were subsequently confirmed by Bao et al. (2013) and Tseng et al. (2015). In addition, T2DM may lead to a worse prognosis in RCC and worse overall survival in these patients (hazard ratio [HR] 1.56, $P < 0.001$) (Chen et al., 2015).

Bladder Cancers

Only a small number of studies have examined the association between metabolic syndrome and bladder cancer. In a prospective cohort study of 580,000 subjects, Haggstrom et al. (2011) showed that metabolic syndrome was associated with a significantly increased risk of bladder cancer in men (RR 1.10, 95% CI 1.01–1.18) but not in women. Russo et al., using a different study design to evaluate medication-exposed cohorts, showed a similar association limited to men (2008). In the meta-analysis by Esposito et al., metabolic syndrome was significantly associated with bladder cancer (RR 1.10, 95% CI 1.02–1.18) (2012). Certainly the well-accepted association with tobacco exposure and of both bladder cancer and metabolic syndrome remains a confounder difficult to disentangle from an etiologic perspective. Several epidemiologic studies have demonstrated a positive association between obesity and an increased risk of bladder cancer (Holick et al., 2007; Koebnick et al., 2008), whereas others did not observe this relationship (Haggstrom et al., 2011; Larsson et al., 2008). Qin et al. (2013) published a meta-analysis of 11 cohort studies, showing an overall significant correlation between obesity and an increased risk of bladder cancer (RR 1.10, 95% CI 1.06–1.16).

Obesity has been examined as a risk factor in terms of prognosis of superficial bladder cancer. Kluth et al. (2013), in a retrospective cohort study, showed that obese patients experienced worse outcomes than those who were nonobese, with an increased risk of disease recurrence (HR 2.66, 95% CI 2.12–3.32), disease progression (HR 1.49, 95% CI 1.00–2.21), cancer-specific mortality (HR 3.15, 95% CI 1.74–5.67), and any cause of mortality (HR 1.42, 95% CI 1.06–1.92). Similarly, Wyszynski et al. (2014), in a US population-based study of 726 patients with superficial bladder cancer, reported that high BMI at diagnosis was modestly associated with an increased risk of recurrence (HR 1.33, 95% CI 0.94–1.89). Taken together, these observations suggest further clinical studies are required to elucidate this possible relationship.

Overactive Bladder

There is increasing evidence for a link between overactive bladder (OAB) and metabolic syndrome. Because it is often difficult to uncouple the effects of OAB and BPH on lower urinary tract symptoms (LUTS), the best evidence for a link between OAB and metabolic syndrome is obtained by studying female populations (Bunn et al., 2015). From a pathophysiologic point of view, there are a host of reasons why women with metabolic syndrome may be at greater risk of developing OAB. These include sympathetic hyperactivity, proinflammatory status, endothelial dysfunction leading to ischemic damage during bladder distention, and diminished bladder perfusion. As discussed previously, insulin resistance resulting from obesity is a significant component of metabolic syndrome, and it is argued that the proinflammatory state, increased FFAs, hypercoagulability, and cellular oxidative stress combined lead to premature vascular disease (Gallagher et al., 2011). A positive correlation between serum insulin levels and OAB has been reported in women. In addition, circulating HDL cholesterol levels were shown to be lower in patients with OAB (Uzun et al., 2012) compared with healthy controls. Bunn et al. recently conducted a literature review of published studies on this topic (2015), noting that many of the studies were limited by methodologic challenges, as well as by being focused on the individual components (e.g., obesity or hyperlipidemia) as opposed to metabolic syndrome as an aggregate construct. Pertinent findings include the fact that all studies examining the postulated linkage between metabolic syndrome and OAB were positive (i.e., suggesting a correlation between the two entities), but the evidence was deemed to be of modest quality. Similarly, the majority of studies that examined connections between obesity and OAB were positive. Overall, these data support an association between OAB and obesity at the very least, and likely metabolic syndrome as well. Further work in this area is encouraged.

Lower Urinary Tract Symptoms

Epidemiologic data suggest that LUTS may be associated with metabolic syndrome. Inflammation has been proposed as a common mechanistic link between these clinical entities. Several studies have demonstrated that components of metabolic syndrome such as hyperinsulinemia, T2DM, dyslipidemia, and hypertension directly correlate with a proinflammatory and fibrotic state (Devaraj et al., 2009; Fagerberg et al., 2008; Fibbi et al., 2010; Greenfield and Campbell, 2006; Powell, 2007). One cause may be the presence of inflamed adipose tissue (Devaraj et al., 2009; Kalyani and Dobs, 2007). IL-8 is a proinflammatory chemokine that contributes to inflammation by acting with IL-1β and IL-6. IL-8 seems to be the most reliable and predictive surrogate marker of prostatitis (Fibbi et al., 2010; Kalyani and Dobs, 2007; Penna et al., 2007), and elevated IL-8 levels have been reported in the expressed prostatic secretions of subjects with BPH (Hochreiter et al., 2000; Liu et al., 2009). IL-8 has been shown to be actively involved in BPH-associated chronic inflammation and mediates epithelial and stromal cell proliferation (Lotti et al., 2014; Lotti et al., 2015; Penna et al., 2009).

Further evidence suggests that IL-8 may stimulate prostatic growth (Lotti and Maggi, 2013; Penna et al., 2007). The majority of observational clinical studies suggest that inflammation is linked to the development of BPH and LUTS. These observations around prostatic inflammation may explain why men with metabolic syndrome are more likely to have larger prostates than men without and why LUTS symptomatology is more adverse even with comparable prostate volumes among men with metabolic syndrome than those without (Bhindi et al., 2014). Not surprisingly, the degree of inflammation has been directly correlated with prostatic volume and IPSS scores (He et al., 2016).

Prostate Cancer

The inflammatory and cytokine-induced mitogenic environment associated with metabolic syndrome is also highly carcinogenic. Pivotal work by Bhindi et al. demonstrated that **men with metabolic syndrome are more likely to have cancer and to exhibit high-risk features among a cohort of men presenting for prostate biopsy** (Bhindi et al., 2014, 2015, 2016). Importantly, combinations of individual components of metabolic syndrome increased the risk of aggressive disease in a "dose-response" relationship. Obese men who undergo active surveillance were also found to be at higher risk for disease progression (Bhindi et al., 2016). A recent meta-analysis (Gacci et al., 2017) of more than 24 studies examined the published literature regarding this potential association. The authors concluded that the risk of prostate cancer per se was only minimally increased (odds ratio [OR] 1.17, 95% CI 1.00–1.36) but that the risk of advanced/high-grade features such as high Gleason score, adverse pathologic stage, and biochemical recurrence was increased, with the rates of biochemical failure almost doubled. An important consideration in these studies is that many men, particularly in the developed world, receive therapy that abrogates metabolic syndrome pathways such as statins or antidiabetic agents, which have been linked with protection from these adverse features (Hamilton, 2017; Hamilton and Freedland, 2008a; Hamilton and Freedland, 2008b; Hamilton et al., 2008; Margel, 2014; Margel et al., 2013a, 2013b). It thus remains possible that the strength of these associations is actually larger than those reported in the epidemiologic literature.

Low Testosterone and Erectile Dysfunction

A number of epidemiologic studies support the associations between obesity (Bajos et al., 2010; Larsen et al., 2007), the metabolic syndrome, (Bal et al., 2007; Kupelian et al., 2006), T2DM (Malavige and Levy, 2009), and low serum testosterone (Wu et al., 2010) with sexual dysfunction, including ED (Diaz-Arjonilla et al., 2009). These studies highlight the complex and often multidirectional relationships between obesity, metabolic status, low testosterone levels, and ED in men. Cohort and case-control studies support a bidirectional association between low serum testosterone concentration and metabolic syndrome. Low serum total testosterone is associated with the development of central obesity and intra-abdominal adiposity (Allan and McLachlan, 2010; Brand et al., 2011; MacDonald et al., 2010). In addition, lower androgen axis measures such as total and free testosterone and sex hormone binding globulin (SHBG) levels are associated with an increased risk of metabolic syndrome (Allan and McLachlan, 2010; Brand et al., 2011; MacDonald et al., 2010). Castration therapy among older men with prostate cancer induces metabolic syndrome (Faris and Smith, 2010; Morote et al., 2015) and elevated risk of cardiovascular disease and type 2 diabetes (Alibhai et al., 2009; Keating et al., 2006). From the opposite point of view, high BMI, central adiposity, and the metabolic syndrome are also associated with low androgen axis parameters (Allan and McLachlan, 2010; Brand et al., 2011; Laaksonen et al., 2005; MacDonald et al., 2010). **It therefore appears that the association between these two clinical entities is bidirectional. ED is also associated with metabolic syndrome, given its interaction with hypertension, diabetes (extreme of glucose intolerance), obesity, vasculopathy, and generalized inflammation** (Wang et al., 2011).

Targeting Metabolic Syndrome as a Novel Strategy in Disease Etiology

Despite the growing recognition of the myriad of associations between metabolic syndrome and numerous chronic urologic disorders, the extent to which reversing the constituent features (e.g., obesity, insulin resistance) either via lifestyle adjustment or pharmacologic means can alter the natural history of the disease remains debatable.

Diet and Exercise

Extensive physiologic studies have been conducted in lean and obese men evaluating the effects of exercise on the androgen axis parameters. Blood concentrations of testosterone and cortisol were found to increase after exercise: testosterone levels increase immediately after exercise, whereas the cortisol response tends to be slightly delayed into recovery, depending on the exercise protocol. For these endocrine changes to occur, an exercise protocol must be of sufficient length and intensity. Obese men require more vigorous exercise (Moradi, 2015).

Statins

Statins inhibit the HMG-CoA reductase enzyme of the mevalonate pathway. This group of drugs is approved for the management of hypercholesterolemia and prevention of secondary cardiac events among at-risk men. A high proportion of patients prescribed statins exhibit at least a subset of the components of metabolic syndrome, if not the disorder. **Although significant epidemiologic literature suggests that statins may provide protection from the progression of prostate cancer** (Hamilton and Freedland, 2008b), **the only evidence has come from association studies.** Randomized intervention trials, such as the Canadian LIGAND trial examining atorvastatin in patients with biochemical failure, are currently underway (Clinicaltrials.gov, 2018).

Metformin

Metformin is a biguanide drug that has recently received attention in the epidemiologic literature (Sayyid and Fleshner, 2016), as well as the lay press. Metformin has been used to treat T2DM for decades and is an inexpensive (because of being available in generic formulations) drug with a well-established safety profile. Metformin exhibits many newly discovered properties but essentially elicits its metabolism-modifying effects by generating energetic stress in the liver through inhibition of oxidative phosphorylation (Fleshner and Bhindi, 2014). These properties are of particular interest in the context of early stage prostate cancer, which predominantly uses the oxidative phosphorylation pathway for energy generation. **Numerous epidemiologic studies suggest that men with diabetes treated with metformin have lower risk of incidence and death from a number of cancers, including prostate** (Margel et al., 2013b) **and potentially bladder carcinoma** (Richard et al., 2018). Most studies using metformin are association studies. In one small interventional trial, metformin was administered to nondiabetic men before radical prostatectomy and elicited a reduction in cancer cell proliferation and perturbation of the PTEN/PI3K-AKT pathway (a major cancer progression pathway) (Joshua et al., 2014). Although positive randomized trials are lacking to date, a number of studies are currently underway, including the Canadian MAST trial (Clinicaltrials.gov), which aims to accrue 408 active surveillance patients and randomize them between metformin and placebo. This study was modeled after the REDEEM study (Fleshner et al., 2012).

Testosterone Therapy

As previously stated, although metabolic syndrome is associated with low testosterone levels, treatment with exogenous testosterone may partially reverse individual aspects of metabolic syndrome, such as facilitating weight loss, reducing lipolysis, and potentially providing additional benefits that are covered elsewhere in this book (Anaissie et al., 2017; Shigehara et al., 2018).

Metabolic Syndrome in Integrative Men's Health

Integrative men's health engenders the need for urologists and their associates to be facile and comfortable when discussing nutrition and exercise. Given the association of obesity with various urologic conditions such as BPH, sexual dysfunction, hypogonadism, and urologic cancer, a more holistic approach is a valuable addition in providing quality care. **Obesity, defined as a BMI of at least 30 kg/m^2 in adults by the National Institutes of Health, has been associated with a myriad of conditions, including various aspects of metabolic dysfunction such as dyslipidemia, T2DM, hypertension, cardiovascular disease, and stroke** (Chu et al., 2015). Downstream consequences of obesity include increased risk of falls and fractures and increased rates of orthopedic surgery on weight-bearing joints (Derman et al., 2014). Between 1980 and 2008 mean global BMI increased by 0.4 to 0.5 kg/m^2 per decade in men and women. In 2008 an estimated 1.46 billion adults worldwide had a BMI of 25 kg/m^2 or greater, and of these, 205 million men and 297 million women were obese (Finucane et al., 2011).

As with many cancers, numerous risk factors are related to prostate cancer, including age, race, and hormonal and genetic factors. However, there are several modifiable risk factors, such as diet and physical fitness, which may affect incidence and outcomes in men with prostate cancer on numerous levels. Dietary or lifestyle modifications may improve outcomes in many of these urologic diseases. Research has demonstrated that frequent physical exercise reduces the risk of chronic diseases, including T2DM, CVD, and cancers, by a number of mechanisms. First, exercise is well known to increase insulin-mediated glucose uptake. Exercise also decreases inflammation by reducing levels of insulin-like growth factor-1 (IGF-1). A recent study of 26 men with prostate cancer treated with androgen deprivation therapy (ADT) found that IGF-1 levels were reduced ($P = 0.019$) at month 3 but not month 6 in those who competed in a 24-week home-based aerobic or resistance-based exercise training program versus controls. Modifications in outcomes, including weight and BMI, were also directly correlated with changes in biomarkers, demonstrating physiologic benefit of exercise (Santa Mina et al., 2013).

Exercise is also a universally known practice that helps people reduce excess weight or prevent weight gain; therefore obesity and exercise are interconnected. **There is a growing body of data linking obesity, inactivity, and prostate cancer with regard to risk and outcomes such as biochemical recurrence (BR).** A large meta-analysis has demonstrated that physical exercise imparts a small benefit with regard to reducing prostate cancer risk. The authors scrutinized 43 articles that met the inclusion criteria and included 19 cohort and 24 case-controlled studies in their analysis (Liu et al., 2011). They confirmed that there was a statistically significant 10% reduction in risk of prostate cancer between men with the highest versus lowest levels of activity (RR 0.90, 95% CI 0.84–0.95, $P = 0.001$) (Liu et al., 2011). Studies examining the impact of high BMI (25–29 overweight, >30 obese) on prostate cancer risk have also been performed, with a recent meta-analysis incorporating 12 and 13 studies of localized and advanced prostate cancer, respectively. The analysis found an inverse linear relationship between BMI and localized prostate cancer ($P_{trend} < 0.001$, RR 0.94, 95% CI 0.91–0.97 for every 5 kg/m^2 increase) and a direct relationship between BMI and advanced prostate cancer ($P_{trend} = 0.001$, RR 1.09, 95% CI 1.02–1.16 for every 5 kg/m^2 increase) (D'Amico et al., 2002). This study strongly suggests a twofold effect of adiposity on the development of prostate cancer; however, the cause of this correlation is still unclear. Interestingly, a number of studies have demonstrated the association between low circulating concentrations of free testosterone and aggressive prostate cancer (Dai et al., 2012; Severi et al., 2006), although other studies have showed no relationship between testosterone levels and aggressive prostate cancer (Sher et al., 2009).

The consequences of obesity on surgical outcomes in prostate cancer have also been established. Robotic-assisted radical prostatectomy, although safe in the hands of experienced surgeons, is known to be more technically demanding in obese patients. **Moreover, numerous studies linking the effects of obesity on disease outcomes and biochemical recurrence have been suggested.** A recent study demonstrated that metabolic syndrome and specifically obesity and hypertension were risk factors for biochemical recurrence in 1428 men after radical prostatectomy (adjusted hazard ratio [aHR] = 1.37, 95% CI 0.92–2.09) (Asmar et al., 2013). A retrospective analysis of 1038 patients treated with radical prostatectomy demonstrated that elevated BMI (mean BMI 28.5 kg/m^2) was associated with increased risk of biochemical recurrence (HR 1.06, $P = 0.007$), noting that adjusting for PSA nadir attenuated, but did not eliminate, the association (HR 1.04, $P = 0.043$) (Ho et al., 2012b). Another recent study comprising 1734 men who underwent radical prostatectomy or radiation therapy demonstrated that men with elevated blood glucose (serum glucose closest to the date of diagnosis, ≥100 mg/dL) had a 50% increased risk of recurrence (HR 1.5, 95% CI 1.1–2.0) compared with those with normal glucose levels (<100 mg/dL) in men who underwent either radical prostatectomy (HR 1.9, 95% CI 1.0–3.6) or radiation therapy, respectively (HR 1.4, 95% CI 1.0–2.0) (Wright et al., 2013).

A few prospective studies have evaluated exercise interventions in men with prostate cancer, with one study demonstrating that physical activity had a significant and positive association with improved sexual functioning in men who had received external beam radiation therapy ($P < 0.001$) (Dahn et al., 2005) However a more recent study demonstrated that an aerobic training program was safe and feasible but did not improve ED in men after radical prostatectomy (Jones et al., 2014).

In addition, studies have shown that supervised exercise training for prostate cancer survivors benefits cardiorespiratory fitness and physical function and strength in comparison with patients who received educational material alone (Galvao et al., 2014). **A recent meta-analysis of studies examining exercise interventions in men with advanced prostate cancer have indicated that various types of programs, including aerobic and resistance type training, improve many quality-of-life factors** (Gardner et al., 2014).

Finally, one compelling prospective study supporting the impact of exercise in prostate cancer was a recent analysis of the effect of exercise on gene expression. This study examined the association between self-reported physical activity and gene expression patterns in the prostate tissue of 71 men with low-risk PCa undergoing surveillance. Results revealed that 25 gene sets were upregulated in men who engaged in more than 3 hours per week of vigorous physical activity compared with those who did not. **Upregulated gene sets included many that regulate cell and DNA repair pathways.** Twelve gene sets associated with obesity and steroid hormone metabolism were also upregulated in men who were overweight or obese versus men with a normal BMI (Magbanua et al., 2014).

There are other global risk factors associated with metabolic dysfunction and urologic conditions. However, there have been few studies examining the effects of cardiovascular risk factor modification on urologic conditions such as ED (Kalka et al., 2013). **A number of studies suggest that dietary change, weight loss, and exercise may result in improvement of ED in some patients** (DeLay et al., 2016; Gupta et al., 2011). Few studies have evaluated whether cardiovascular risk factor modification can have ameliorative effects on ED. Shared risk factors include modification of tobacco use, hyperlipidemia, and dietary change/weight loss/exercise in targeted patients, each of which can result in improvement in ED (DeLay et al., 2016; Kalka et al., 2013; Kostis and Dobrzynski, 2014). Esposito et al. conducted a randomized single-blind study of 110 obese men aged between 35 and 55 years without diabetes, hypertension, or hyperlipidemia, who had an International Index of Erectile Function (IIEF) score of 21 or less, examining the effects of weight loss and increased physical activity on erectile and endothelial function. At 2 years, BMI decreased more in the intervention group compared with control patients, as did serum concentrations of interleukin-6 and C-reactive protein (Esposito et al., 2004). **These data suggest that aggressive risk modification for ED and CVD may alter the arc of progression.**

Ultimately, how can we translate the conclusions of these studies to meaningful recommendations for the urologist? What does this mean to our patients? **The challenge is less in instructing a patient to eat better and exercise, but more in promoting long-term, standardized, working strategies for every type of patient.** Among the key steps needed for implementing treatment plans that will meaningfully affect these modifiable risk factors for patients is more high-quality research. The implementation of safe and effective programs that prioritize the importance of exercise in the general health care setting and our own urology departments is a priority. **Our shared aim should be directed at creating optimal and individualized interventional approaches that address the dietary and physical activity needs for all urologic conditions and improve men's health overall.**

Conclusion

Metabolic syndrome is a complex pathophysiologic disorder with far-reaching implications for integrative men's health, public health, and healthy aging. Much has been learned about the cause of this condition in recent years. In the next decade, interventional trials should confirm whether targeting metabolic syndrome or its components can provide tangible benefits to patients with cancer and other chronic conditions apart from those already known to the medical community (e.g., heart disease).

> **KEY POINTS: METABOLIC SYNDROME AND MEN'S HEALTH**
>
> - Metabolic syndrome, defined as a combination of dyslipidemia, glucose insensitivity, and obesity, is increasingly prevalent around the world.
> - In addition to its association with increased CVD risks, metabolic syndrome is linked with pelvic health issues, including LUTS, ED, and hypogonadism, as well as genitourinary tumors (kidney, bladder, prostate).
> - Dietary or lifestyle modifications may improve outcomes in many of these urologic diseases, with clinical trials currently testing metabolic modulators statins and metformin.
> - Exercise-based interventions in men with advanced prostate cancer improve quality of life.
> - Dietary change, weight loss, and exercise may improve erectile function.
> - Men's health should include individualized and precision-based intervention programs to alter the arc of pelvic conditions.

TESTOSTERONE THERAPY AND CARDIOVASCULAR RISK: ADVANCES AND CONTROVERSIES

Introduction and Historical Context

Perhaps no topic in the field of men's health is currently more controversial than the indications, efficacy, and potential adverse effects associated with testosterone replacement therapy. Testosterone was initially isolated in 1935 by Brown-Sequard, with synthetic forms commercially available since the 1950s (Brinkmann, 2011). Testosterone formulations were approved and made available for treatment of frankly hypogonadal males, including men with testicular trauma and those with rare bilateral tumors. The benefits and safety profile of exogenous testosterone administration have not been established for the treatment of low testosterone levels that occur as part of aging, even if a man's symptoms appear to reflect a deficiency in this hormone. Indeed, large-scale, placebo-controlled, decades-long trials (ideal in the setting of a possible long-term commitment to prolonged testosterone supplementation) have not been completed at this time.

Despite the lack of conclusive clinical trial data, use of testosterone supplements has increased significantly over the past decade. Handelsman (2013) demonstrated that global trends of testosterone prescribing increased in 37 of 41 studied countries between 2001 and 2011. In the United Kingdom, prescriptions almost doubled over the period in question (Gan et al., 2013). Perhaps in no jurisdiction did prescriptions for testosterone replacement therapy increase more than in the United States (Gabrielsen et al., 2016; Rao et al., 2017). The value of annual testosterone prescriptions filled in the United States have increased from $18 million in 1988 to $70 million in 2000, and to more than $2 billion in 2013, with most of these sales oriented toward middle-aged and older men without frank hypogonadism (Bhasin, 2016).

Testosterone replacement therapy has been studied for potential benefits in a host of medical conditions, including depression, dementia, cardiac failure, osteopenia, chronic obstructive pulmonary disease, rheumatoid arthritis, ED, and anemia (Amanatkar et al., 2014; Katznelson et al., 1996; Snyder et al., 2016). Testosterone is also taken by some to abate the general effects of aging and to improve athletic performance (Page et al., 2005). There are many forms of testosterone supplementation currently available, including oral, intramuscular, transdermal, sublingual, subdermal, or transnasal routes (Bassil et al., 2009).

In light of the increased use of testosterone replacement therapy and lack of long-term well-conducted randomized clinical trials, it remains important to understand the risks and benefits associated with testosterone supplementation. Lack of clear understanding of the physiologic effects of low testosterone levels may be particularly relevant for estimating the patient's risk of developing cardiovascular disease, which is a major cause of death in aging men. Potential clinically relevant interactions between cardiovascular risks and circulating testosterone levels were brought to the forefront by the FDA with a warning issued regarding this connection in January of 2014 (Nguyen et al., 2015).

Clinical Trials: Evidence of Effectiveness

Recent larger-scale (albeit short-term) placebo-controlled randomized trials have been conducted to evaluate the benefits of testosterone replacement therapy in aging men with symptomatic hypogonadism. Snyder et al. (2016) randomized 790 patients to receive either testosterone or placebo gel for 1 year in the context of an overall program assessing testosterone supplementation (Testosterone Trials). Despite the fact that the study was a combination of seven coordinated clinical trials, three specific domains of aging were recently reported: sexual function, vitality, and physical functioning. In terms of *sexual function substudy*, testosterone replacement therapy was associated with significantly improved sexual performance, as well as increased sexual desire and erectile function. In terms of *physical functioning substudy*, no significant differences were observed between the groups in the proportion of men whose 6-minute walking distance significantly improved (primary trial outcome). In addition, no change was detected in 6-minute walking distance or the percentage of men whose physical functioning subscore of the 36-Item Short Form Health Survey (SF36) increased by at least 8 points. However, significant differences were reported between treatment groups in the change from baseline in physical functioning scores (mean difference, 2.75 points; $P = 0.03$). When the populations of all three trials were pooled, improvements in physical functioning were noted in testosterone-treated participants. In addition, men who received testosterone were more likely than those who received placebo to perceive an improvement in their walking ability since the beginning of the trial ($P = 0.002$). Taken together, these data suggest a modest impact on physical functioning associated with testosterone replacement therapy. In terms of the *vitality t substudy*, testosterone replacement elicited no significant benefit with respect to vitality, as assessed by the Functional Assessment of Chronic Illness Therapy (FACIT)–Fatigue scale. Once again, when study populations of all three trials were combined, testosterone was associated with small but significant benefits with respect to mood and depression symptoms. Men in the testosterone-treated group were more likely to report improved energy levels. A smaller Asian study confirmed these findings (Tong et al., 2012).

Meta-analyses have been performed to summarize the accumulated trial information and assess the risks and benefits associated with testosterone replacement therapy (Amanatkar et al., 2014; Bolona et al., 2007; Calof et al., 2005; Corona et al., 2014; Elliott et al., 2017; Fernandez-Balsells et al., 2010; Guo et al., 2016; Haddad et al., 2007; Xu et al., 2013; Zarrouf et al., 2009). These pooled analyses, although not perfect, provide a method of overcoming power deficiencies of many smaller or shorter-term randomized clinical trials (Higgins et al., 2008). Although there are a number of differences in terms of these analyses, credible evidence suggests that, among healthy aging males with symptomatic hypogonadism, testosterone replacement therapy does improve a number of factors, including overall quality of life, depression symptoms, libido, and erectile function. Taken together, these data do provide credible evidence of benefit of testosterone replacement among appropriately selected men with age-related symptomatic hypogonadism.

Cardiovascular Risk

Credibly assessing cardiac risk associated with testosterone replacement is methodologically challenging. Men who exhibit signs of hypogonadism disproportionately exhibit comorbidities such as obesity, hypertension, and glucose intolerance, risk factors that by themselves place them at elevated risk of cardiovascular events. It is therefore difficult to disentangle the adverse events associated with drug exposure from the risk associated with the disease unless randomized data are available. Randomized trials in this space, however, are limited by short- or intermediate-term drug exposure (i.e., there are no studies with 10- to 20-year exposure data) and are often insufficiently powered to analyze rare events such as cardiovascular conditions. Publication biases are also potentially relevant (Xu et al., 2013). Among the published randomized clinical trials that have assessed the risk of mortality resulting from cardiovascular factors, 19 trials reported on these risks (Ho et al., 2012a; Hoyos et al., 2012; Jones et al., 2011; Kalinchenko et al., 2010; Kaufman and Vermeulen, 2005; Srinivas-Shankar et al., 2010; Xu et al., 2013), with a total of 4 deaths reported among 1851 placebo-treated men and 9 among 2088 men receiving testosterone replacement therapy (OR 2.15, $P > 0.05$).

Nonfatal cardiac events, however, were shown in some studies to be more prevalent among testosterone users in randomized trials. In 2010 Basaria et al. conducted a relatively small randomized study (n = 209) that demonstrated an almost fivefold higher incidence of cardiovascular events among testosterone-treated men (23 in testosterone replacement therapy group vs. 5 in placebo). Xu et al. subsequently assessed adverse event rates in a meta-analysis and estimated a 54% increase in the risk of cardiovascular events associated with testosterone therapy (Xu et al., 2013). Interestingly, trials sponsored by pharmaceutical companies demonstrated no increased risk, whereas those that were not funded by the industry demonstrated a twofold increase in risk (OR 2.06, $P < 0.05$), suggestive of a publication bias.

As alluded to earlier, retrospective cohort analyses and health record linkage studies are sometimes the only way to assess risk with longer-term exposures when such data are not available from randomized clinical trials. Although these analyses suffer from biases mentioned earlier, studies by Finkle et al. (2014) and Vigen et al. (2013) demonstrated increased risk with testosterone therapy. In the study by Vigen et al., men in the Veterans' Affairs system who underwent coronary angiography were included in the study analysis. Men who had hypogonadism and were on testosterone replacement therapy exhibited a 1.29-fold increase in cardiac events, corresponding to a 5.8% increase in absolute risk. Finkle et al. evaluated a cohort of almost 56,000 men, assessing the risk of myocardial infarction following testosterone-replacement therapy institution (Finkle et al., 2014). An excess risk was noted among older men and younger men with pre-existing cardiovascular disease. The results of these trials led the FDA, as well as other jurisdictional agencies (Health Canada, WHO, etc.) to issue a warning regarding the potential association between cardiac events and testosterone supplementation (Nguyen et al., 2015).

Investigators eagerly await the results of the cardiovascular trial substudy of the Testosterone Trials (Alamir). In this substudy, atherosclerotic plaque progression will be measured using computed tomography (CT) angiography, with results hopefully available by the end of 2018. These trials will, however, not represent the final word on this controversy because, even if plaque progression is not worsened by testosterone replacement therapy, other cardiovascular events such as plaque rupture or arrhythmia could, in theory, be affected. Indeed, electrocardiographs conducted in testosterone-treated patients demonstrated a prolongation in the QT interval in one pooled analysis of data from two separate randomized control trials (Gagliano-Juca et al., 2017).

What Is a Clinician to Do?

The scope of current knowledge regarding testosterone replacement therapy, like most other medical conundrums, requires the practicing clinician to understand the controversies and be able to communicate them to his or her patients. Professional guidelines can also help. The Endocrine Society in 2018 updated their guidelines regarding testosterone replacement therapy (Bhasin et al., 2018). The main points outlined in their document include (1) limiting the diagnosis of testosterone deficiency to symptomatic males with unequivocally low testosterone levels; (2) recommending against testosterone replacement therapy in men planning fertility in the near term, in men with breast or prostate cancer, or in those with significant prostate cancer risk, elevated hematocrit, untreated severe obstructive sleep apnea, severe lower urinary tract symptoms, uncontrolled heart failure, myocardial infarction or stroke within the last 6 months, or thrombophilia; and (3) discussing the potential risks of therapy associated with testosterone replacement therapy, clarifying that there are currently insufficient data to establish a causal association between cardiovascular disease and testosterone supplementation.

> **KEY POINTS: TESTOSTERONE REPLACEMENT THERAPY**
>
> - The use of testosterone replacement therapy in countering low testosterone levels that occur as part of the aging process is controversial because of inadequately elucidated effectiveness and safety profile.
> - Recent large-scale randomized trials demonstrated some improvements in sexual and physical function and vitality.
> - Limited clinical trial evidence and retrospective cohort analyses suggest that testosterone replacement therapy increases the risk of cardiovascular events.
> - Practicing urologists should keep current with the recently updated guidelines and current research on testosterone replacement therapy to be able to discuss the risks and benefits for individual patients.

ASSOCIATION BETWEEN CARDIOVASCULAR DISEASE AND ERECTILE DYSFUNCTION

Predisposing Factors

There are a host of predisposing risk factors and underlying pathophysiologic processes for CVD and ED. These include, but are not limited to dyslipidemia, smoking, hypertension, and T2DM. The underlying mechanisms of CVD and ED include inflammation, atherosclerosis, and endothelial dysfunction (Vlachopoulos et al., 2013). There is emerging consensus that ED and CVD are independent risk factors for each other. The Princeton Consensus Conference (Nehra et al., 2012) identified ED as a substantial independent risk factor for CVD, and the QRISK group published one of the first risk scores to incorporate ED as an independent risk factor into their updated 10-year CVD risk model, calculating a 25% increased risk for average middle-aged men with ED (Hippisley-Cox et al., 2017).

Erectile Dysfunction and Subclinical Cardiovascular Disease

The temporal relationship between ED and subclinical CVD progression is less clear. Is ED a precursor to CVD, or does underlying CVD first manifest as ED? Available data come from either cross-sectional studies correlating symptoms of ED and overt CVD or highly limited prospective cohort studies correlating ED incidence and severity with incident CV events (Banks et al., 2013; Chew et al., 2010; Fung et al., 2004; Montorsi et al., 2006). The data suggest that there is a 2- to 3-year time interval between the onset of ED and CVD symptoms (Montorsi et al., 2006), whereas more recent studies have examined the interrelationships between subclinical CVD (i.e., early atherosclerosis), ED, and overt CVD (myocardial infarction [MI] or major adverse cardiac events [MACEs]; Chew et al., 2010; Inman et al., 2009). A landmark study, the Multi-Ethnic Study of Atherosclerosis (MESA; Feldman et al., 2016) demonstrated that subclinical CVD is a predictor of ED and potentially of ensuing MACEs. **Among the key findings in the study was that the coronary artery calcium (CAC) score can serve as a "disease score" and surrogate marker of accelerated atherosclerosis process in arteries, including penile arteries and vascular ED** (Jackson et al., 2010).

About 50% of men with sudden CVD events may have had no previous symptoms of CAD, and between 70% and 89% of sudden cardiac events occur in men (Fox et al., 2004; Ni et al., 2009; Podrid and Myerburg, 2005). **More importantly, ED may be the single warning of the elevated risk of sudden CVD events** (Gandaglia et al., 2014). Finally, severity and duration of ED has been correlated with the magnitude of coronary disease, with the presence of ED being independently associated with CVD events (Gandaglia et al., 2014; Shin et al., 2011).

It appears that development of ED may occur during the progression of baseline subclinical vascular disease to more clinically manifest CVD. In the MESA study, there was a strong association between baseline subclinical disease, as assessed by CAC and carotid plaque burden, and subsequent ED. This further suggests the value of atherosclerosis testing (i.e., CAC scoring and measurement of carotid plaque burden) in predicting ED and overt CVD (Feldman et al., 2016). More important, given the strengths of ED as a predictor of future vascular events, it may be prudent to implement increased evaluation of subclinical CVD in at-risk patients before and after the onset of ED (Detrano et al., 2008; Gibson et al., 2014).

> **KEY POINTS: CARDIOVASCULAR DISEASE AND ERECTILE DYSFUNCTION**
>
> - There are a number of overlapping risk factors for CVD and ED.
> - The temporal relationship between ED and subclinical CVD remains to be determined.
> - CAC score can serve as a "disease score" and a surrogate for accelerated atherosclerosis process in arteries, including penile arteries, with implications for vascular ED.

MENTAL HEALTH AND OPIOID ABUSE IN MEN

Mental Illness in Men

Mental illnesses, including anxiety, depression, and suicide, are becoming increasingly prevalent in men, while concomitantly being underdiagnosed. Any mental illness (AMI), defined as a mental, behavioral, or emotional disorder, occurs in 14.5% of men and in 14.5% of men age 50 or older in the United States (National Institute of Mental Health, 2018; Substance Abuse and Mental Health Services Administration [SAMHSA], 2017). Among men with AMI, 33.9% received treatment, including 46.8% of men aged 50 or over. The prevalence in US adults of serious mental illness (SMI), defined as AMI that substantially interferes with or limits one or more major life activities, is 4.2% (5.3% in women and 3.0% in men). In 2016, among the 10.4 million adults with SMI, 6.7 million received treatment (68.8% in women and 57.4% in men) (Substance Abuse and Mental Health Services Administration [SAMHSA], 2017).

More specifically, more than 6 million men suffer from depression, including symptoms such as fatigue, irritability, and loss of interest in work or hobbies. It has been estimated that 3,020,000 men in the United States suffer from panic disorder and a myriad of phobias. An equal number of men and women (total: 2.3 million) develop bipolar disorder, and 90% of people who are diagnosed with schizophrenia by age 30 are men (NIMH, 2018; Substance Abuse and Mental Health Services Administration [SAMHSA], 2017; http://www.cdc.gov/msmhealth/mental-health.htm). These high rates of AMI and SMI have led to a significant increase in incidences of suicide and substance abuse. More than 44,000 people in the United States in 2015 committed suicide, defined as ending one's own life, according to the CDC, making it the 10th leading cause of death overall. Although many suicide prevention programs focus on helping teenagers, the highest number of suicides in the United States in 2015 occurred among people ages 45 to 54. Men are especially at risk, with a suicide rate approximately four times higher than that of women. There are a host of underlying risk and predisposing factors, including a significant decline in traditional male industries such as manufacturing, forestry, and fisheries, with subsequent unemployment. About 76% of suicides in the United Kingdom are in men, and suicide is the most common cause of death for men under the age of 35 (UK Office of National Statistics, 2012). A review by the Samaritans in 2012 noted that men who are predisposed to suicide include those who are middle aged and of lower socioeconomic class (Wyllie et al., 2012). Six key themes identified in this group were personality traits, sense of masculinity, relationship breakdowns, challenges of midlife, emotional illiteracy, and socioeconomic factors.

Consequences of Opioid Abuse

In recent years the emotional and economic consequences of opioid misuse on public health has increased dramatically and is now understood as a major source of morbidity and mortality in the United States. Despite a decrease in the number of total opioids prescribed in the United States from a peak in 2012, some 33,000 people died of opioid overdoses in 2015 (including 15,000 from prescription sources), and currently more than 115 Americans die daily after overdosing on opioids (Centers for Disease Control and Prevention/National Center for Health Statistics [CDC/NCHS], 2017).

From a men's health perspective, understanding the magnitude of this crisis and in particular how urologists will interact with patients will be a very important part of our training in the future. Efforts to decrease the supply of opioids will require increasing commitment from all prescribers, including surgeons. As drug monitoring programs seek to offer greater scrutiny, urologists are tasked with improving their understanding of how opioids are dispensed to patients and how best to reduce overprescription. Moreover, there are direct endocrine consequences of opioid use, including hypogonadism, that adversely affect men's health (Leapman and Kaplan, 2017).

The opioid epidemic is notable for the expansiveness of the problem in the United States, spanning divisions of gender, race, age, and income level. Although greater increases in prescription pain reliever opioid deaths were seen between 1999 and 2010 among women (400%) compared with men (273%), men are still significantly more likely to misuse, overdose, and die from opioids.

Opioid Prescriptions

There appears to be a high degree of variability in the dispensing of pain medications after surgery and there are some who routinely dispense above recommended safety thresholds. Not only do these overprescribed doses represent potential dangers for the patients receiving the prescriptions, but they also are a source of risk for those in the individual's family and community. The potential supply of opioids is vast given that most patients report using far less than is prescribed by their surgeons (Hill et al., 2017; Kumar et al., 2017). This is magnified by the fact that most patients who are prescribed opioids after surgery report they store unused opioids in unsecured locations (Bartels et al., 2016).

The risks of new-onset opioid use or overdose after general and urologic surgery is also increasing and should be a concern to trainees and prescribers in those specialties (Brummett et al., 2017; Shah et al., 2017). There are particular verticals that are predisposed to increased pain and the potential for opioid overprescribing, including cancer surgery and stone disease. **In a publication examining nearly 70,000 patients undergoing cancer surgery with curative intent, the risk of new persistent opioid use was 10.4% and more common in patients receiving adjuvant chemotherapy** (Lee et al., 2017).

Gonadal Dysfunction

Male gonadal function is affected by opioid use and abuse. By disrupting the pulsatile release of gonadotropin-releasing hormone (GnRH), opioids suppress the hypothalamic-pituitary-gonadal axis and result in hypogonadism (Ceccarelli et al., 2006). Sustained gonadal suppression is commonly noted in chronic opioid users and may impair male sexual health, with manifestations including low libido, fatigue, depression, anxiety, osteoporosis, and loss of muscle mass (Aloisi et al., 2009; Reddy et al., 2010).

For some individuals, the identification of opioid-related endocrine dysfunction can serve as an opportunity to seek formal treatment. **In light of the growing prevalence of opioid use, clinicians who treat hypogonadism should continue to take note of the potential contributions of chronic opioid use as a causative agent for symptomatic hypogonadism.** Nevertheless, with a growing population of opioid users—including those receiving chronic opioid substitution therapies such as methadone—there is a potential role to consider exogenous androgen supplementation. For example, in a randomized, double-blind, placebo-controlled trial of testosterone replacement in men with opioid-induced androgen deficiency, patients receiving testosterone supplementation experienced greater improvements in pain sensitivity, sexual desire, body composition, and overall quality of life (Basaria et al., 2015). These findings suggest that in selected patients who do have nonmodifiable opioid use, consideration of supplementation may be warranted.

Role of Urology

As part of an expanding integrative men's health program, there will be a need for urologists to foster greater awareness of the potential harms associated with even short courses of opioids (Leapman and Kaplan, 2017). Those prescribing are encouraged to adopt responsible prescribing practices, such as **initially prescribing the *lowest effective dose*** and offering repeat assessments as needed, rather than upfront high-dose therapy. In addition to direct consequences of overdose and dependence, opioids can adversely affect men's health by resulting in hypogonadism, and a urology consult should be regarded as a potential opportunity to primarily address chronic use.

> **KEY POINTS: MENTAL HEALTH**
>
> - Mental health issues, including anxiety, depression, and suicide, are increasingly prevalent in men and are concomitantly being underdiagnosed.
> - More than 6 million men in the United States suffer from depression, including symptoms such as fatigue, irritability, and loss of interest in work or hobbies.
> - Men are at higher risk for suicide, with a rate approximately four times higher than that of women.
> - Opioid abuse is now a leading health care crisis, with significant morbidity and mortality.
> - The opioid epidemic is notable for the expansiveness of the problem in the United States, spanning divisions of gender, race, age, and income level.
> - Clinicians who treat hypogonadism should be cognizant of the relationship between chronic opioid and symptomatic hypogonadism.

BUILDING AN INTEGRATIVE MEN'S HEALTH CENTER

Components

Inherent to the delivery of more efficient men's health care is an understanding of why men seem to lag women in entering the health care space. Concurrently, identifying how men do or do not seek health care, and, more importantly, how men interpret and deal with acute and chronic health conditions will help elucidate a more comprehensive and successful approach. Urologic and cardiac conditions make up a significant portion of men's health issues, but a broader approach based on age and geographic location will provide a more sustainable program for diagnoses and therapy. Moreover, attention toward exercise, nutrition, and complementary and alternative solutions will provide a more robust approach. Finally, health care providers need to be adequately trained to care for men who have sex with men, transgender patients, and complex geriatric men.

Curriculum

Miner et al. (2018) developed a comprehensive and sensible approach to integrative men's health. The four general categories are the following:
1. Conditions that are unique to men (e.g., prostate cancer, prostate disease, and ED)
2. Diseases or illnesses more prevalent in men compared with women (e.g., CVD, stroke, and renal disease)
3. Health issues for which risk factors and adverse outcomes are different in men (e.g., obesity)
4. Health issues for which different interventions to achieve improvements in health and well-being at the individual or population level are required for men (e.g., access to care)

A men's health curriculum must be rooted in the deep understanding of the impact of masculinity factors on health care engagement and outcomes. Various psychosocial stressors, including employment, culture, and geographic location, can directly and indirectly contribute to high rates of unhealthy behaviors, chronic disease diagnoses, and premature mortality among men. These underlying factors should be considered in a multi-specialty and tiered approach to improving receipt of appropriate health care services (Miner et al., 2018).

Future Business Plan

Before a business plan is developed for an integrative men's health center (IMHC), it has to be decided what and whom it will encompass, organization, revenue versus expenses, sustainability, and opportunities for growth. From a ground-level perspective and in building a pathway to sustainable success, there must be a buy-in from leadership (in either an academic or private practice setting) as well as a host of medical specialties, including partnerships with various subspecialists in cardiology, endocrinology, psychiatry, orthopedics, and dermatology. All these partners should be vested in the need for integration of thought, goals, and vision.

In the past, many IMHCs have focused on aging, sexual health, and the administration of testosterone (Miner et al., 2018). There is a rapidly evolving health care landscape, wherein there is an increased stress on the medical system and health care providers. This includes the need for adaptation of a patient-centered medical home model, electronic medical records, and increasing scrutiny of testing and outcomes dovetailing with patient satisfaction metrics, which add to the burden of clinical management of male patients.

The future of men's health will be predicated on improving more efficient entry pathways to enhance the patient journey and experience. This includes a more holistic and integrated approach including proper education and testing and careful shared decision making between the patient and provider.

REFERENCES

The complete reference list is available online at ExpertConsult.com.

66

Male Infertility

Craig Stuart Niederberger, MD, FACS, Samuel John Ohlander, MD, and Rodrigo Lessi Pagani, MD

EPIDEMIOLOGY

The disease of infertility affects approximately 15% of couples, rendering nearly one of six childless (World Health Organization [WHO], 1991). Multiple sources of bias historically have distorted assessment of the contribution of each gender to infertility, but we can reasonably expect men and women to contribute an equal number of faulty gametes (Tielemans et al., 2002). Therefore accurate evaluation and treatment of males is of great importance in addressing this significant health care issue.

Unfortunately, much of infertility care for men is delivered outside of well-established reimbursement systems, compromising accurate calculation of epidemiologic metrics (Meacham et al., 2007). Fortunately, the American Society for Reproductive Medicine's professional group, the Society for Assisted Reproductive Technologies (SART), compels in vitro fertilization (IVF) clinics to report outcomes in a systematic fashion, allowing limited evaluation of the impact of male infertility. However, this assessment is through the lens of women seeking the most evolved technology for female reproductive care and necessarily skews the appraisal of the incidence and prevalence of the male contribution to the disease. Recent data compiled from the National Survey of Family Growth (NSFG) found that 18% to 27% of men within infertile couples were never evaluated, further supporting the likely underreporting of male factor infertility (Eisenberg et al., 2013). Based upon the NSFG data, approximately 7.5% of sexually active men seek care at some point in their lifetime for difficulty conceiving, of which 18% of men reported a clinician-diagnosed male reproductive problem (Anderson et al., 2009).

The Urologic Diseases in America (UDA) Project included collection of male reproductive epidemiologic data from a variety of sources, which, albeit sparse, allowed for some limited analysis of the parameters of the disease of male infertility (Meacham et al., 2007). Considering ambulatory surgery for conditions associated with male infertility, it is unsurprising that men aged 25 to 34 years had higher usage with an average rate of 126 per 100,000 compared with men aged 35 to 44 with 83 per 100,000 and those aged 45 and older at 20 per 100,000 (Meacham et al., 2007). Thus younger men represent more than half of male infertility cases, and nearly 1 in 11 cases occurs in men in the 5th decade and older (Meacham et al., 2007). Considering geographic distribution in the United States, men living in the west had lower use of ambulatory surgery compared with those in the northeast and midwest (29 per 100,000, 104 per 100,000, and 72 per 100,000, respectively) (Meacham et al., 2007).

From an economic perspective, the UDA Project estimated total expenditures for treating primary male infertility at $17 million dollars in 2000, clearly an underestimate because of the delivered care absent from traditional databases (Meacham et al., 2007). Because a significant amount of male reproductive medical care delivery involves assisted technologies for the female partner, accounting for this care, the assessed total cost is a sizable $18 billion (Meacham et al., 2007). A cost questionnaire completed by men pursuing fertility care demonstrated that patients spent 16% to 20% of their annual income on infertility-related expenses (Elliott et al., 2016).

Complicating epidemiologic assessment is the fact that the primary assay for male infertility, the semen analysis, is a poor predictor with a low receiver operating characteristic (ROC) curve area for all available parameters (Guzick et al., 2001). Consequently, men with some presence of sperm on semen analysis may be inaccurately judged to be fertile and omitted from accurate accrual in a tabulation of insufficient reproductive potential.

HISTORY

The production and delivery of the male gamete requires orchestration among endocrine, immune, and neural systems, passage through intricately constructed anatomy, complex orchestrated sequences of gene expression and chromosomal structural events, and the proper embryologic and postnatal development of all systems. It is consequently unsurprising that myriad disparate conditions contribute to male reproductive dysfunction. Table 66.1 enumerates percentages of final diagnoses made in one infertility clinic (Sigman et al., 2009). As will become clear in this chapter, the percentages in Table 66.1 for each condition are highly variable depending on how the individual conditions are assessed in published studies, and the data contained within the table are an indictment of how poorly male reproductive information is systematically collected. However, the table does demonstrate the wide variety of diagnoses associated with male infertility. To address all potential possibilities, the practitioner must approach inquiring about past history in a methodical fashion. For the sake of efficiency, the patient may complete a form at home or in the waiting area before the physician encounter.

Reproductive health is an unusual aspect of medicine: two patients are required for a positive outcome. Several consequences arise from this unique circumstance, the first being that a probabilistic approach to diagnosing infertility is necessary. In the best circumstances, with intercourse timed to menstruation and a rigorous calculation of optimal timing, including assessment of quality of cervical mucus and measurement of basal body temperature, cumulative pregnancy rates for all tracked subjects in one well-conducted study were 38% at one cycle, 68% at three cycles, 81% at six cycles, and 92% at 12 cycles (Gnoth et al., 2003). For those who ultimately became pregnant, the cumulative pregnancy rates were 42% at one cycle, 75% at three cycles, 88% at six cycles, and 98% at 12 cycles (Gnoth et al., 2003). Therefore a couple seeking treatment for infertility a month or two after discontinuing contraceptive measures should be counseled to continue to try for a few more months unless other significant conditions exist. **A minority of couples who have not conceived after 6 cycles may still do so. It is reasonable to initiate an evaluation after 6 months with the understanding that some couples will still conceive shortly afterward.** It is useful to communicate to patients the probabilistic nature of reproduction by describing each month of trying as rolling a die or flipping a coin.

An important question to ask is how often the couple is having intercourse. In general, semen parameters peak after 1 or 2 days of abstinence and then decline (Levitas et al., 2005). Often in an attempt to accumulate sperm, men wait long periods before attempting to impregnate their partners. Data suggest that not only is this practice unhelpful, it actually results in poorer sperm quality (Levitas et al., 2005). **For an optimal characterization of semen, a man should be instructed to wait 1 or 2 days after an ejaculation to submit a specimen for semen analysis** (Levitas et al., 2005). **However, for increasing the probability of conception and pregnancy, intercourse every day around the time of ovulation is likely the best strategy** (Scarpa et al., 2007).

TABLE 66.1 Distribution of Final Diagnoses From a Male Infertility Clinic

CATEGORY	NUMBER	%
Immunologic	121	2.6%
Idiopathic	1535	32.6%
Varicocele	1253	26.6%
Obstruction	720	15.3%
Normal female factor	503	10.7%
Cryptorchidism	129	2.7%
Ejaculatory failure	95	2.0%
Endocrinologic	70	1.5%
Drug or radiation	64	1.4%
Genetic	56	1.2%
Testicular failure	52	1.1%
Sexual dysfunction	32	0.7%
Pyospermia	25	0.5%
Cancer	20	0.4%
Systemic disease	15	0.3%
Infection	10	0.2%
Torsion	5	0.1%
Ultrastructural	5	0.1%
TOTAL	4710	100.0%

From Sigman M, Lipshultz LI, Howards SS: Office evaluation of the subfertile male. In Lipshultz LI, Howards SS, Niederberger CS, editors: *Infertility in the male*, ed 4, New York, 2009, Cambridge University Press, p 153–176.

Another consequence of the fact that two patients are required for a positive outcome in this unique area of medicine is that consideration of the female partner's age is a critical component in judging reproductive potential and planning therapeutic strategies. Whereas the effects of male age on reproductive potential remain to be fully elucidated, advancing male age appears to affect bulk seminal parameters and sperm DNA packaging to only a limited degree, allowing a male to father children well into his later years (Cocuzza et al., 2008a; Colin et al., 2010; Hellstrom et al., 2006; Henkel et al., 2005; Moskovtsev et al., 2006; Schmid et al., 2007; Silva et al., 2012; Sloter et al., 2007; Yang et al., 2007). For the woman, age is a critical predictor of reproductive potential, especially when artificial reproductive technologies are used (Balasch and Gratacós, 2012; te Velde and Pearson, 2002). **On average, female fecundity declines precipitously after age 35** (Balasch and Gratacós, 2012). In some geographic regions, female fertility appears to decline more rapidly than others (Zargar et al., 1997). Therefore determining the female partner's age and assessing it in the context of her locale are essential aspects of the reproductive history.

An important general question to ask is whether the man and his partner have previously conceived children, or if each has with other partners, and the age or ages of the offspring. Proven fertility at some point in time demonstrates a functioning reproductive system after puberty, which eliminates a number of concerns regarding congenital issues.

The typical enumeration of systemic diseases and past surgeries in taking the reproductive history reveals a number of conditions associated with reproductive dysfunction. Diabetes mellitus and multiple sclerosis interfere with normal coordinated ejaculatory function, as does spinal cord injury (Kafetsoulis et al., 2006; Tepavcevic et al., 2008; Vinik et al., 2003). **Even before spermatotoxic chemotherapy, cancer appears to negatively affect spermatogenesis, especially if the cancer is of testicular origin** (de Bruin et al., 2009). Azoospermia may reveal cancer, and the physician considering a man with no sperm on semen analysis should regard testis cancer as a possible cause (Mancini et al., 2007). Surgeries such as transurethral resection of the prostate and minimally invasive therapies for prostatic enlargement are associated with ejaculatory dysfunction (Elshal et al., 2012; Jaidane et al., 2010). As discussed elsewhere in this text, retrograde ejaculation of varying degrees may occur after retroperitoneal lymph node dissection for testis cancer, depending on the type of dissection and the clinical context within which the dissection occurs.

Herniorrhaphy may result in obstruction of the vas deferens (Hallén et al., 2011, 2012; Shin et al., 2005; Tekatli et al., 2012). Mesh in particular appears to incite a dense foreign body inflammatory response that may entrap the vas deferens even if the placement of mesh is not immediately adjacent to the vas (Hallén et al., 2011, 2012; Maciel et al., 2007; Tekatli et al., 2012). If vasal occlusion is the sole cause of infertility, then both vasa must be occluded, an expectedly infrequent event. However, occlusion of one vasa from herniorrhaphy with contralateral spermatogenic dysfunction of another source may cause infertility in the male.

Aside from the typical questions regarding medical and surgical history, answers to a number of questions specifically related to male reproduction may elucidate causes of infertility. If the practitioner is not using a history form, a helpful mnemonic is *TICS*, as if one is ticking off items on a list. T stands for toxins, I for infectious/inflammatory disease, C for childhood history, and S for sexual history.

Spermatotoxicity

In the *TICS* mnemonic, *T* is for toxins. A variety of substances interfere with spermatogenesis, mature sperm function, and sperm delivery. Many common medications, prescribed and over the counter, can be associated with male reproductive dysfunction.

Endocrine Modulators

Medications may affect the ratio of estrogen to androgen through a variety of mechanisms, including a molecular similarity to estrogen, increased estrogen synthesis, increased aromatase activity, dissociation of steroids from sex hormone–binding globulin (SHBG), decreased testosterone synthesis, competitive and noncompetitive binding to steroid receptors, decreased synthesis of adrenal steroids, and induction of hyperprolactinemia (Bowman et al., 2012). **Some of the more commonly encountered agents warranting inquiry include the antiandrogens bicalutamide, flutamide, and nilutamide; the antihypertensive spironolactone; the antiretroviral protease inhibitors such as indinavir; the nucleoside reverse transcriptase inhibitors such as stavudine; corticosteroids, especially in adolescence; and exogenous estrogen** (Bowman et al., 2012).

Although a source of debate, the 5α-reductase inhibitors finasteride and dutasteride appear to have only limited spermatogenic suppressive effects if at all (Amory et al., 2007; Overstreet et al., 1999). Occasional anecdotal case reports and a prospective database review suggest that sperm parameters dramatically improve in an individual man after discontinuation of a 5α-reductase inhibitor, including the low dose for androgenic alopecia, but the substantial interassay variability of semen parameters calls into question whether these effects could simply be the result of chance (Chiba et al., 2011; Samplaski et al., 2013).

Primarily through conversion to estradiol by aromatase and consequent inhibition of luteinizing hormone (LH) secretion by the pituitary, exogenous testosterone acts to decrease intratesticular testosterone synthesis and reduce spermatogenesis (Grimes et al., 2012). Agents with androgenic properties similarly diminish sperm production (de Souza and Hallak, 2011). In fact, investigators have studied testosterone and androgenic steroids as potential targets for male contraception since the 1970s (Grimes et al., 2012; Gu et al., 2009; Ilani et al., 2012; WHO Task Force, 1990). In general, these studies have a duration of 2 years or less of application of testosterone or androgenic steroid and demonstrate reversibility with return to sperm in the ejaculate after approximately 4 months or more of discontinuation of the contraceptive agent (Grimes et al., 2012; Gu et al., 2009; Ilani et al., 2012; WHO Task Force, 1990). However, whether and when spermatogenesis returns after longer periods of use are unknown.

Recreational Drugs

Although data are conflicting, most studies suggest that cannabis decreases plasma testosterone in a dose-dependent and duration-dependent manner (Gorzalka et al., 2010). Recent data identified a nonlinear decrease in semen concentration and total sperm count with frequency of cannabis use and suggested a threshold effect at use of more than once per week (Gundersen et al., 2015). More robust data associate chronic alcohol intake with decreases in androgens and sperm parameters (Pasqualotto et al., 2004; Villalta et al., 1997). Heavy chronic alcohol intake also appears to increase aromatization of testosterone to estradiol (Purohit, 2000). Investigators have observed that more moderate use of alcohol may decrease intracytoplasmic sperm injection (ICSI) outcomes (Braga et al., 2012).

Early studies suggested worsening of bulk seminal parameters with cigarette smoking (Stillman et al., 1986). Although the results of subsequent studies associating smoking and bulk parameters were conflicting, more recent cross-sectional analysis has supported deterioration of seminal parameters in a dose-dependent manner, arguing more strongly that cigarette smoking impairs male reproductive potential (Ramlau-Hansen et al., 2007). Investigators observed that cigarette smoking increased seminal oxidative stress parameters and decreased metrics of sperm DNA quality (Pasqualotto et al., 2008b; Sharma et al., 2016; Taha et al., 2012). An abnormal ratio of protamines 1 and 2 was observed in smokers with evidence of atypical protamine 2 expression, pointing to DNA packaging as directly compromised by tobacco use (Hammadeh et al., 2010). The negative effects of cigarette smoking on sperm bulk parameters and DNA quality appear to be especially acute in the presence of a clinical varicocele, suggesting the possibility of additive toxicity (Fariello et al., 2012b). Researchers studied effects of an aryl hydrocarbon receptor ligand present in cigarette smoke and found that it induced apoptosis in the fetal testis in a manner that was preventable with an aryl hydrocarbon receptor antagonist, providing evidence that maternal smoking may affect the reproductive potential of male offspring (Coutts et al., 2007). Consistent with these laboratory findings, epidemiologic data associated maternal cigarette smoking to smaller testes, lower sperm counts, and alterations in sex hormones in the adult male offspring (Jensen et al., 2005; Ravnborg et al., 2011). Epidemiologic evidence supports that the secondary sex ratio, the ratio of boys to girls born, is altered in mothers who smoke (Beratis et al., 2008). One explanation is that cigarette smoking alters circulating testosterone concentrations in pregnant women (James, 2002).

Electronic cigarettes that aerosolize with typically a nicotine-containing solvent are becoming increasingly popular, although there remains of paucity of data related to potential health consequences. There are reports of lower levels for carcinogens and toxicants compared with smokers, although no long-term data exist (Goniewicz et al., 2017; Hecht et al., 2015; McRobbie et al., 2015). At this time, no data exist related to impact on androgens or semen parameters.

Antihypertensives

Further details about this topic are available online at Expert Consult.com.

Antipsychotics

The most common mechanism of action for antipsychotic drugs is antagonism of dopamine, which causes loss of libido as a side effect in the majority of patients (Stimmel and Gutierrez, 2006). Another proposed reason for diminished libido with use of antipsychotics is elevation of prolactin levels, which appears to be most acute for risperidone and to a lesser extent olanzapine (Melkersson, 2005). As discussed elsewhere in this text, selective serotonin reuptake inhibitors (SSRIs) are commonly associated with anorgasmia and delayed or absent ejaculation (Clayton and Montejo, 2006; Stimmel and Gutierrez, 2006).

Opioids

Opioid analgesics suppress LH release primarily through hypothalamic-mediated mechanisms and consequently reduce testosterone synthesis (Subirán et al., 2011). Experimental evidence in animals demonstrates endogenous opioid peptides, their precursors, and their receptors in various testis cell types (Subirán et al., 2011). Endogenous opioid peptides are primarily synthesized by Leydig and Sertoli cells and inhibit Sertoli cell function via autocrine and paracrine mechanisms (Subirán et al., 2011). Therefore opioids not only can induce the hypogonadotropic hypogonadism commonly observed in chronic use but may also diminish spermatogenesis directly in the testis (Brennan, 2013; Subirán et al., 2011). Evidence suggests that discontinuation of opioid analgesics may be associated with rapid return of androgen, perhaps as early as within 1 month (Brennan, 2013). **With the widespread prescribing of opioid analgesics and the epidemic of opioid abuse, their use as a cause of hypogonadotropic hypogonadism should be suspected in all such hypoandrogenic men.**

Antibiotics

Further details about this topic are available online at Expert Consult.com.

Cytotoxic Chemotherapeutics

Because chemotherapeutic agents are most effectively applied to suppress a briskly proliferating population of cells, and the pathway of male gamete development primarily involves a rapidly dividing stem cell cohort, it is unsurprising that medical therapies directed toward cancers impair spermatogenesis. Alkylating agents such as the nitrogen mustard cyclophosphamide have been long identified to impair sperm production (Vaisheva et al., 2007). These spermatogenic suppressive effects were noted to be dose and time dependent, with lower doses and shorter durations of therapy leading to reversible dysfunction but ultimate return to male fertility potential, and higher doses and longer durations of therapies resulting in permanently impaired fertility (Vaisheva et al., 2007). Other chemotherapeutic agents commonly used in conjunction with cyclophosphamide to treat non-Hodgkin lymphoma, including doxorubicin, vincristine, and prednisone, have been reported to impair spermatogenesis as individual agents (Vaisheva et al., 2007). Likewise, investigators reported that cisplatin, etoposide, and bleomycin were associated with diminished sperm parameters in a dose- and time-dependent manner (Gandini et al., 2006).

One concern of patients and physicians is how much chemotherapy damages the DNA of sperm (Delbes et al., 2007; O'Flaherty et al., 2008, 2010; Robbins, 1996; Smit et al., 2010; Spermon et al., 2006; Stahl et al., 2006; Tempest et al., 2008). Evidence suggests that sperm DNA damage can be detected at least up to 2 years after chemotherapy, arguing that cryopreservation of sperm before treatment with cytotoxic chemotherapeutic agents is preferable to awaiting the return of sperm after chemotherapy (Tempest et al., 2008). The question is whether sperm is "safe" to use after a discrete amount of time after the induction of chemotherapeutic agents that may mutate cellular DNA in a way that may be translated through the germ line into offspring. An informed answer to that question based on well-conducted clinical trials is not yet available.

This lack of knowledge frustrates male reproductive specialists who counsel patients on whether their own biologic material or donor sperm would be the best choice after cytotoxic chemotherapy. **Questions about sperm DNA integrity and mutagenicity after chemotherapy serve as a second reason to encourage men undergoing such oncologic therapy to cryopreserve sperm before induction, because cryopreservation presents a well-established means for fertility preservation in the setting of cancer** (Anger et al., 2003; Crha et al., 2009; Meseguer et al., 2006). Proper cryopreservation of sperm results in long-term potential for reproductive success, and patients may be assured that should they store sperm in this way, it will be available when they need it (Rofeim and Gilbert, 2005).

Although many patients may recover sperm in the ejaculate after cytotoxic chemotherapy, and it is very possible that, after a period as yet to be determined, ejaculated sperm after chemotherapy will be safe for conception, many men do not develop sufficient ejaculated sperm for fertility. These men do use cryopreserved sperm if available to successfully father offspring (Meseguer et al., 2006).

Systemic application of antitumor medication is not necessarily the only form of chemotherapy that may alter fertility potential. Investigators noted in a small series of young men that local instillation of bacille Calmette-Guérin into the bladder for superficial transitional cell carcinoma resulted in a significant decrease in sperm concentration and motility (Raviv et al., 2005).

A special case arises in peripubertal boys undergoing cytotoxic chemotherapy for cancer. Oncologists are often in a rush to apply lifesaving therapy, and parents may be uncomfortable discussing topics such as masturbation for semen collection with their children. However, if oncologic therapy is successful, it is precisely these patients with a potentially long life expectancy who would benefit from sperm cryopreservation as an option for future fertility. Peripubertal boys are capable of producing semen samples suitable for cryopreservation, and it is entirely feasible to obtain an ejaculate suitable for storage (Menon et al., 2009; van Casteren et al., 2008). The urologist must simply be comfortable enough to discuss the advantages of fertility preservation and the methods to achieve it.

Anti-Inflammatory Agents

Further details about this topic are available online at Expert Consult.com.

Phosphodiesterase V Inhibitors

Further details about this topic are available online at Expert Consult.com.

Environmental Toxicants

Further details about this topic are available online at Expert Consult.com.

Thermal Toxicity

For reasons not entirely clear but engendering much speculation, mammals evolved so that the scrotal container of the testis was housed outside the body cavity, keeping its contents at a temperature considerably cooler than that of the internal organs (Setchell, 1998; Thonneau et al., 1998). **Scrotal temperature in humans is maintained to be 2°C to 4°C below core body temperature by mechanisms including a countercurrent heat exchange between a central set of linear arteries directing blood toward the testis and a plexus of veins surrounding the arteries draining blood back toward the vena cava** (Setchell, 1998; Thonneau et al., 1998). Many investigators have exhaustively studied the effects of heat on spermatogenesis in animals, observing depopulation of germ cells, perturbations in the various spermatogenic cell types, and apoptosis within specific cell types (Absalan et al., 2010; Setchell, 1998). Cryptorchidism provides a model by which the effects of heat can be studied on sperm production: increasing testis temperature to that of the abdominal cavity significantly impairs spermatogenesis (Setchell, 1998).

The degree to which scrotal temperature can be raised without affecting male fertility remains an open question. Clothing, physical activity, and body posture (e.g., whether the legs are crossed or not in a sitting position) change scrotal temperature to an incremental degree, but whether that translates to alterations in spermatogenesis is purely speculative (Jung et al., 2005; Mieusset et al., 2007). Researchers observed an increase in scrotal temperature on the order of a half a degree Celsius with prolonged sitting on heated car seats and speculated that such an effect may be additive to the intrascrotal temperature rise that occurs when sitting (Jung et al., 2008). One study observed that when a man was naked, mean scrotal temperature was significantly lower on the left than on the right, but when he was clothed, the temperature was significantly higher on the left than on the right (Bengoudifa and Mieusset, 2007). Clothing may thus confer a greater differential increase in left scrotal temperature than right scrotal temperature (Bengoudifa and Mieusset, 2007).

A number of studies associate occupational exposure resulting in a significant increase in intrascrotal temperature with detrimental effects on sperm (De Fleurian et al., 2009; Thonneau et al., 1998). However, other researchers have observed no significant negative effects on sperm in fertile men exposed to high heat at work and postulated that in the normal state, compensatory mechanisms protect the testis when a prolonged rise in ambient temperature occurs (Momen et al., 2010).

Laptop computers radiate heat, and researchers have studied the effects of these devices on scrotal temperature. In one study, under controlled conditions, having a laptop computer resting on the lap for 1 hour raised the scrotal temperature an average 2.6°C on the left and 2.8°C on the right side (Sheynkin et al., 2005). However, simply sitting without a laptop raised the scrotal temperature an average of 2.1°C (Sheynkin et al., 2005). Whether the extra approximately half-degree Celsius imparts significant damage to spermatogenesis remains an open question. However, investigators have observed that a man sitting with his legs apart and for shorter periods of time experiences less of an increase in scrotal temperature (Sheynkin et al., 2011).

Radiation

Testes directly exposed to ionizing radiation suffer germ cell loss and Leydig cell dysfunction (Bahadur and Ralph, 1999; Castillo et al., 1990; Clermont, 1972; Gandini et al., 2006; Green et al., 2010). In one survey of boys with acute lymphoblastic leukemia who underwent testicular irradiation at 12, 15, and 24 Gray (Gy), all became azoospermic, but those receiving less than 24 Gy had normal testosterone production (Castillo et al., 1990). The investigators observed elevated gonadotropins and noted that this finding indicated the possibility of subclinical Leydig cell damage (Castillo et al., 1990). **In a survey of childhood cancer survivors, chances of having future offspring were lessened by radiation doses to the testes of 7.5 Gy and above** (Green et al., 2010). The testis need not be directly irradiated for spermatogenic impairment to occur; if the radiation field is proximal to the testis and the dose is sufficient, sperm production may be diminished even if the testis is shielded (Gandini et al., 2006).

With widespread use of radiofrequency devices for telecommunications and wireless networks, investigators have questioned the effects of this band of the electromagnetic spectrum on sperm (Agarwal et al., 2008b; Agarwal et al., 2009; Avendano et al., 2012; Baste et al., 2008; Erogul et al., 2006; Falzone et al, 2008). Researchers observed negative effects on sperm motility parameters, viability, and reactive oxygen species (ROS) generation after electromagnetic radiation generated by 850- and 900-MHz cell phone transmission systems in vitro (Agarwal et al., 2009; Erogul et al., 2006; Falzone et al., 2008). A similar analysis was performed in vitro by exposing aliquots of semen to 4 hours under a wireless Internet-connected laptop computer, emitting 7 to 15 times more radiofrequency electromagnetic waves compared with unexposed controls (Avendano et al., 2012). The authors identified a significant decrease in motility and an increase in DNA fragmentation of the exposed aliquot (Avendano et al., 2012). However, in vitro exposure of sperm to electromagnetic radiation does not account for the distance and material, including biologic tissues, that separate a cell phone transceiver or laptop computer and sperm during common use. To address a more typical usage scenario, investigators have used epidemiologic data to gauge potential in vivo effects. In one questionnaire-based study of Norwegian sailors exposed to high-power electromagnetic fields in a military environment, researchers noted a significant linear relationship between increasing exposure and reported infertility (Baste et al., 2008). The offspring's sex ratio at birth also revealed a linear relationship, with a decreasing ratio of boys to girls with higher degrees of exposure to electromagnetic radiation (Baste et al., 2008). Researchers in another epidemiologic study divided men into four groups based on cell phone talking time: no use; less than 2 hours per day; 2 to 4 hours per day; and more than 4 hours per day (Agarwal et al., 2008b). The investigators observed that semen analyses in the four groups of increasing cell phone use revealed a linear decrease in sperm count, motility, viability, and normal morphology (Agarwal et al., 2008b).

Infections and Inflammation

In the *TICS* mnemonic, *I* stands for infectious and inflammatory disease leading to male reproductive dysfunction. Infections of the testis, epididymis, prostate, and urethra may lead to male infertility through anatomic and functional means (Kasturi et al., 2009). Common organisms affecting the prostate include *Escherichia coli*, *Pseudomonas aeruginosa*, and *Klebsiella*, *Proteus*, and *Enterococcus* species (Kasturi et al., 2009). Typical epididymal organisms include *Neisseria gonorrhoeae*, *Chlamydia trachomatis*, and *E. coli* (Kasturi et al., 2009). Infectious urethral organisms in the context of impaired male reproduction include *N. gonorrhoeae*, *C. trachomatis*, *Mycoplasma* species, and *Trichomonas vaginalis* (Kasturi et al., 2009). Although relatively infrequently encountered, infections of the testis may include the Rubulavirus mumps, coxsackievirus B, *N. gonorrhoeae*, *C. trachomatis*, *E. coli*, *P. aeruginosa*, and *Klebsiella*, *Staphylococcus*, and *Streptococcus* species (Kasturi et al., 2009). Mumps orchitis is typically so painful and bizarre to the person so affected that, even at a very young age, a boy whose case of mumps travels into his testis is unlikely to forget the event. Infrequently encountered in modern industrialized nations, *Mycobacterium tuberculosis* may affect any reproductive organ and cause scarring of the vas deferens and epididymis (Niederberger, 2011).

Infectious consequences may be anatomic, such as urethral infection leading to stricture, or functional, impairing sperm (Kasturi et al., 2009). Functional alterations may derive from direct effects of the infectious organism on sperm or through induction of immunologic responses in any male reproductive organ, leading to sperm dysfunction (La Vignera et al., 2011). As an example of direct effects, investigators observed that incubating sperm with increasing concentrations of *C. trachomatis* serovar E elementary bodies was associated with degradation of sperm DNA in a time-dependent manner (Satta et al., 2005). **Although in vitro laboratory experiments have also demonstrated a negative effect of *E. coli* on sperm, the majority of bacteria including *E. coli* have limited or no effects on sperm motility in vivo** (Diemer et al., 2003; Lackner et al., 2006). Whereas bacteria may coexist with sperm without significant pathologic consequence, sexually transmitted organisms may play a more virulent role (Bezold et al., 2007). The differential effects on sperm of common bacteria and sexually transmitted infectious agents remain far from clear.

Viruses proffer a potentially unique negative direct effect on sperm by integration into a man's genome and vertical transmission through his germ line (La Vignera et al., 2011). **Although viral nucleic material appears to be present in the seminal plasma, neither hepatitis C nor human immunodeficiency virus appear to be correlated with a direct negative effect on sperm function** (Garrido et al., 2005). Human papillomavirus was associated with impairment of bulk seminal parameters, and in vitro treatment of sperm in the laboratory with heparinase III appeared to diminish viral load without significantly altering functional semen parameters (Garolla et al., 2012).

Researchers have studied a wide variety of indirect negative effects of infection on sperm, including through leukocytosis, ROSs, interleukins 1, 6, and 8, interferon-γ, macrophage migration inhibitory factor, tumor necrosis factor-α, epididymal macrophages, and dendritic cells (La Vignera et al., 2011). It is logical that any part of the immune system may lose self-recognition of sperm or, in the presence of an active infection, overwhelm sperm defenses.

Evidence suggests that noninfectious or postinfectious inflammatory processes of the prostate may lead to sperm alterations and male infertility, but the degree to which inflammation alters male reproductive potential beyond what infection imparts remains unknown (Ausmees et al., 2013; Schoor, 2002; Wagenlehner et al., 2008). One putative mechanism by which nonbacterial prostatitis may lead to male infertility is through seminal leukocytosis or pyospermia and the release of ROSs resulting in sperm damage (Schoor, 2002). Other possible means of sperm dysfunction via prostatic inflammation include generation of antisperm antibodies and biochemical alterations in prostatic ions such as zinc, magnesium, calcium, or selenium (Schoor, 2002). Prostatitis may damage sperm by inducing ROSs without leukocytosis as an intermediary (Pasqualotto et al., 2000; Schoor, 2002).

Childhood Diseases

The *C* in *TICS* stands for childhood diseases. Maladies of early development include anatomic maldevelopment leading to obstruction or misdirection of the male gamete as it traverses the journey from the testis to the female reproductive tract and disorders that lead to disturbed sperm production or to conditions that damage mature sperm.

Pediatric Surgery

Hydroceles and hernias repaired during childhood are associated with a low but discrete incidence of complications causing vasal obstruction (Lao et al., 2012). In one large series, the rate of testis atrophy after pediatric inguinal hernia was 0.3% (Ein et al., 2006). As hernias repaired during adolescence often include surgical mesh, vasal occlusion as a result of inflammation associated with this material should be considered in an infertile man with such a procedure in his surgical history (Hallén et al., 2011, 2012; Lao et al., 2012; Shin et al., 2005; Tekatli et al., 2012). Other surgical procedures during childhood may also affect future reproductive status. In earlier series, investigators associated scarring from posterior urethral valve ablation with male reproductive dysfunction, but in more recent series, fertility complications with urethral valve surgery are rarely observed (Caione and Nappo, 2011). Older procedures for restoring bladder neck anatomy in children were associated with retrograde ejaculation, but these surgeries are rarely performed today (Sigman et al., 2009).

Testis Torsion

For males 25 years old and younger, testis torsion is more than three times more common than testis cancer, with an estimated incidence of 4.5 cases per 100,000 per year (Mansbach et al., 2005; Mellick, 2012). Contralateral testicular biopsy findings are abnormal in 57% to 88% of males when torsion occurs, which suggests either that unnoticed torsion is damaging the testis before torsion becomes clinically evident or that some underlying pathology is present that manifests as abnormal scrotal anatomy and as spermatogenic dysfunction (Visser and Heyns, 2003). **Approximately half of men with torsion develop adverse spermatogenic effects** (Visser and Heyns, 2003). Overall after torsion, 36% to 39% of men will have sperm concentrations below 20 million/mL (Visser and Heyns, 2003). Because torsion is a traumatic event that disrupts intratesticular architecture, including the tight junctions between the Sertoli cells that make up the blood-testis barrier, it is unsurprising that up to 11% of men develop antisperm antibodies after torsion (Visser and Heyns, 2003).

Cryptorchidism

As described elsewhere in this text, during the fifth week of gestation, cells destined to become gonads arise in the posterior abdominal wall of the developing embryo (Lewis and Kaplan, 2009). A complex set of highly orchestrated sequenced events occurs, including differentiation of the various testis cell types, organization into what will ultimately become histologic compartments within the testicle, and development of the outer container of the testis and its connection to the distal organs where sperm ultimately will be routed (Lewis and Kaplan, 2009). The most overt anatomic change is migration of germ cells from the posterior abdominal wall toward the nascent inguinal canals and eventually into the scrotum, resulting in an extra-abdominal localization of the male gonads (Lewis and Kaplan, 2009). This process does not conclude until the third trimester (Lewis and Kaplan, 2009). Researchers have identified multiple regulatory triggers in animal models that direct descent of the testis, including the insulin-like 3 (*INSL3*) gene, the relaxin/insulin-like family peptide receptor 2 (*LGRF8*) gene, antimüllerian hormone (AMH), and members of the *HOX* gene family such as *HOX10* (Hughes and Acerini, 2008; Lewis and Kaplan, 2009). Dysfunction of certain of these genes may result primarily in arresting the mechanical journey of the germ cells, whereas aberrant expression of others may be involved in the processes of spermatogenesis and descent, causing infertility in ways beyond the thermal toxicity to which undescended testes are subject in later reproductive life. **Androgens are required to induce regression of the cranial suspensory ligament during the fourth month of gestation to allow descent of the testis** (Hughes and Acerini, 2008; Lewis and Kaplan, 2009). Failure of any of these processes impedes descent of the testis into the scrotum, resulting in cryptorchidism, which is widely known to be associated with impaired reproductive potential in later life (Sigman et al., 2009).

Undescended testes occur in up to 4% of newborn boys at term (Barthold and González, 2003). The prevalence of cryptorchid testes decreases to less than 1.5% by 1 year of age (Barthold and González, 2003; Chung and Brock, 2011). Cryptorchidism concordance analysis in twins and siblings indicates a pattern of maternal inheritance but also suggests that the intrauterine environment plays an important role (Jensen et al., 2010). In most series, the incidence of unilateral cryptorchidism is usually around twice that of bilateral undescended testes (Barthold and González, 2003). The distinction is important, because prognosis is related to whether cryptorchidism is unilateral or bilateral. The reproductive prognosis in later life is similar in men with no history of cryptorchidism and in those with a unilateral undescended testis who underwent orchidopexy as a child, regardless of age at surgery or the size of the undescended testis (Lee et al., 2001; Miller et al., 2001). **In one large epidemiologic study of men who had orchidopexy during childhood, successful rates for those attempting paternity with a history of surgically treated unilateral cryptorchidism were 96% compared with a control population, but only 70% for those who had bilateral cryptorchidism** (Lee, 2005). In that study, men with bilateral cryptorchidism had levels of the Sertoli cell product and marker of spermatogenesis inhibin B that were nearly one-third of the levels in controls compared with men with unilateral undescended testes repaired in childhood who had inhibin B levels approximately two-thirds of controls (Lee, 2005). Differences in testosterone concentrations were less than those of inhibin B, arguing that fertility impairment caused by cryptorchidism is less based in Leydig cell steroidogenesis than in dysfunction of the seminiferous epithelium (Lee, 2005). Congruent with the identified differences in inhibin B between men with neither, one, or both testes undescended, researchers observed that sperm density on semen analysis is lower in men who had surgical repair of bilateral cryptorchidism than in those with a unilateral undescended testis, which in turn is lower than in men with normally descended testes (Lee, 1993; Lee and Coughlin, 2001; Moretti et al., 2007). With transmission electron microscopy, investigators also found a greater number of ultrastructural defects in men who had cryptorchidism surgically treated as a child compared with controls, and sperm from men with bilateral undescended testes had more defects than from those with unilateral disease (Moretti et al., 2007).

Conclusive data associating the timing of orchidopexy with reproductive outcomes in later life remain elusive. It is widely recognized that surgical correction of undescended testes after puberty likely has minimal effect on bulk semen analysis parameters (Grasso et al., 1991). However, the age before puberty at which orchidopexy results in optimal effect in reproductive potential has not been definitively established. Regression analysis demonstrated that serum testosterone concentrations in men were negatively correlated to increasing age at orchidopexy, indicating that Leydig cell function is better spared by earlier age of surgical correction for cryptorchidism (Lee, 2005). Conventional wisdom contended that full germ cell development is arrested and remains quiescent before puberty, implying that orchidopexy performed at any earlier age would have similar outcomes. However, maturational alterations may occur in the hypothalamic, pituitary, and testicular endocrine axis much earlier than adolescence (Hadziselimovic, 2002). Likewise, a transition from the spermatogonial cell types of the fetal germ cell reservoir to that of the adult occurs at a very early age (Hadziselimovic, 2002).

Studies of men undergoing testis sperm extraction with the intent for use in ICSI and who had cryptorchidism and orchidopexy at an earlier time offer some information about the optimal timing of surgical correction of undescended testes, although results are conflicting. In an early study of 30 azoospermic men who had bilateral cryptorchidism, no correlation was found between the age at bilateral orchidopexy and the rate of successful surgical sperm retrieval, which was 73% overall (Negri et al., 2003). In a later study of 42 azoospermic men in whom all but two had bilateral cryptorchidism, no significant differences in surgical sperm retrieval rate were observed comparing men who had orchidopexy up to 10 years of age (61.9%) and men whose testes were brought into the scrotum after 10 years of age (57.1%) (Wiser et al., 2009). However, in an early study of 38 azoospermic men with 30 having had bilateral cryptorchidism, the successful surgical retrieval of sperm in 94% for men who had orchidopexy before 11 years old, 43% from 11 to 20 years old, and 44% after age 20 years was statistically different at the selected threshold of 10 years ($P < 0.01$) (Raman and Schlegel, 2003). Congruent with these results, in 79 azoospermic men, 62% having had bilateral orchidopexy and 20.3% having had unilateral orchidopexy (with 17.7% unknown), ROC curve analysis revealed age at orchidopexy to have the second greatest area under the curve (AUC) after testosterone in discriminating successful surgical sperm retrieval (Vernaeve et al., 2004). **It consequently appears prudent to recommend orchidopexy before 10 years of age from a reproductive perspective, recognizing that cryptorchid boys who pass that threshold still may have sperm surgically retrieved for use in ICSI later in life.**

Testes that change in position after descent and those that are nearly but not fully descended present special challenges in assessing potential alterations in reproductive potential. Numerous reports clearly document testes as being descended that are later observed to have ascended to varying degrees (Barthold and González, 2003; Gracia et al., 1997). Whereas most appear to ascend to a location distal to the inguinal canal, clinicians have reported ascent as high as to an intra-abdominal position (Barthold and González, 2003; Gracia et al., 1997). Unfortunately, the fertility potential for these patients has not yet been systematically studied, and their reproductive prognosis must be considered unknown at present. For men with retractile testes, limited data suggest that although sperm are often observed in the ejaculate in a man, sperm density is lower than would be expected in a man with normal fertility, approaching that of men with a history of cryptorchidism (Caroppo et al., 2005).

Testicular Dysgenesis Hypothesis

Further details on this topic are available online at Expert Consult.com.

Genetics

Current knowledge of the genetic basis of male infertility is discussed systematically later in this chapter. A good reproductive history should include whether any blood relatives experienced difficulty conceiving offspring. The evaluating physician should also inquire as to the presence in the patient's family of genetic syndromes known to be related to reproductive dysfunction such as cystic fibrosis and other entities detailed in the latter part of this chapter (Anguiano et al., 1992).

Sexual History

The *S* in *TICS* is for the sexual history. Although it may seem intuitive that a couple would engage in a sufficient frequency of intercourse when attempting to conceive, lifestyle or proclivities may intervene and interfere. As discussed previously in this chapter, optimum timing for intercourse appears to be daily around the time of ovulation (Scarpa et al., 2007). Some women accurately predict the periovulatory period by symptoms, the so-called mittelschmerz

(O'Herlihy et al., 1980). However, many women mistake bodily sensations as ovulation, and symptoms alone cannot reliably be used to assess optimal timing for intercourse. **Because ovulation is detectable by basal body temperature or home hormonal kits *after* it has occurred, a couple should be encouraged if possible to record the day of ovulation for two or three menstrual cycles and begin daily intercourse several days before the earliest recorded day.** Such a method is impractical for women with advanced age, because it delays potential reproductive therapies. In the setting of advanced maternal age, more aggressive strategies in collaboration with the female fertility specialist should be considered.

Lubricants commonly used during sexual activity such as K-Y Jelly, Keri Lotion, Astroglide, and others are associated with impaired sperm motility (Sigman et al., 2009). Saliva should also be considered toxic to sperm (Sigman et al., 2009). Researchers incubated a variety of lubricants with sperm and observed that the isotonic preparation Pre-Seed did not result in a significant decrease in sperm motility or chromatin integrity as assessed by an acridine orange–based sperm chromatin structure assay (Agarwal et al., 2008a). In that study, FemGlide, Replens, and Astroglide lubricants resulted in a significant decrease in motility, and FemGlide and K-Y Jelly resulted in a significant decline in sperm chromatin quality (Agarwal et al., 2008a). Laboratory investigators have also provided evidence that use of Pre-Seed during semen collection for analysis does not affect assessment of bulk seminal parameters, sperm membrane functional integrity, levels of ROSs, total antioxidant capacity (TAC), and DNA integrity (Agarwal et al., 2013).

The urologist should inquire about erectile function, because obviously if intercourse is impeded or impossible, sperm will not be deposited successfully in the vaginal vault near the cervical os. The physiology, evaluation, and treatment of erectile dysfunction are discussed extensively elsewhere in this text.

The psychological weight of having a diagnosis of infertility and the stress of therapy are significant (Schanz et al., 2005; Volgsten et al., 2008). One metric of whether infertility is exerting an adverse psychological effect on the male is frequency of intercourse, which may be altered in up to half of men being treated for infertility and is associated with libido and sexual satisfaction (Ramezanzadeh et al., 2006). A revealing question for a man undergoing male reproductive evaluation is whether the frequency of coitus has changed during the process.

Men and women adapt to the stress of infertility in different ways with different coping mechanisms (Peterson et al., 2006). Men tend to distance themselves and problem solve, whereas women are more likely to seek social support (Peterson et al., 2006). Men and women may consequently interpret their partner's natural adaptive strategy as problematic, when in fact it is simply a different means of coping. **A common misconception is that men conflate fertility with masculinity, which in fact happens only infrequently** (Fisher et al., 2010).

Stress may impair semen quality, creating a vicious circle for men experiencing infertility and its related psychological distress (Gollenberg et al., 2010). Fortunately, evidence suggests that once men have entered into reproductive medical therapy including IVF with their partners, the diagnosis of male infertility does not disturb psychological well-being and well-adjusted relationships (Holter et al., 2007). The clinician treating male reproductive dysfunction should consider referral to a qualified psychologist to ease the transition from the fearsome diagnosis of infertility to the many effective therapies that are available. If the discussion is couched in terms of problem solving, many men are very willing to engage in psychological counseling.

> **KEY POINTS: MALE REPRODUCTIVE HISTORY**
>
> - The most important determinant of a couple's reproductive potential is maternal age.
> - Many conditions may affect male reproductive function. The examining physician may organize the male reproductive history into toxicants, infectious processes, childhood conditions, and sexual history.

PHYSICAL EXAMINATION

General Physical Examination

Because male infertility may be related to many systemic and genetic conditions, the general physical examination often yields clues as to the source of reproductive dysfunction. Male and female faces are morphologically distinct, and female facial characteristics alert the examining physician to potential sex chromosomal and androgenization disorders (Velemínská et al., 2012). Alterations in secondary sexual characteristics such as facial, truncal, axillary, and pubic hair suggest inadequate androgenization (Sigman et al., 2009). If androgenization is significantly impaired through puberty, a high-pitched voice may result (Sokol, 2009). An overabundance of endogenous or therapeutically induced estradiol may lead to gynecomastia (Sigman et al., 2009). If testosterone production during puberty is so low that closure of the epiphyses of the long bones of the extremities fails to occur, typical body morphology will include an arm span 5 cm longer than the patient's height and a lower body segment as defined by pubic-to-heel distance more than 5 cm longer than the upper body segment as measured from the crown to the pubis (Sokol, 2009).

With the lack of virilization at the anticipated time of puberty, Klinefelter syndrome is classically detailed in textbooks as resulting in gynecomastia, an eunuchoid appearance, and tall height for age (Oates and Lamb, 2009). However, it should be noted that many men with a 47,XXY karyotype do not display the typical body morphology and habitus so described.

Obesity should be noted because substantial evidence associates it with male reproductive dysfunction. **It is well established that obese men have elevated estradiol as a result of peripheral conversion from testosterone by an overabundance of adipose cells that contain the enzyme aromatase** (Aggerholm et al., 2008; Chavarro et al., 2010; Hammoud et al., 2006; Hammoud et al., 2010b; Hofny et al., 2010). A TTTA aromatase polymorphism appears to be particularly related to increasing estradiol with increasing body mass, and those with the polymorphism are most likely to experience decreasing estradiol when they lose weight (Hammoud et al., 2010b). **Serum testosterone is also well known to be lower in obese men** (Hammoud et al., 2006). Four main causes are hypothesized: negative feedback of estradiol on the hypothalamic-pituitary axis resulting in decreased LH release; increased leptin; insulin resistance; and sleep apnea (Hammoud et al., 2006; Hofny et al., 2010). Although some studies correlate increasing obesity with decreased LH, others do not, and the mechanism of reduced testosterone in obese men may be unrelated to gonadotropins (Aggerholm et al., 2008; Hammoud et al., 2006; Hofny et al., 2010; Paasch et al., 2010; Pauli et al., 2008; Teerds et al., 2011).

SHBG is typically reduced in obese men, in general ascribed to increased circulating insulin in obesity (Hammoud et al., 2006; 2008; Pauli et al., 2008; Teerds et al., 2011). The consequence of lowered SHBG is that bioavailable testosterone may be greater than what total testosterone predicts, and an obese man may be more androgenized than expected on superficial laboratory assessment.

Researchers observed an inverse correlation between serum inhibin B concentrations and body mass index (BMI) in men but not prepubertal boys (Winters et al., 2006). The association between decreasing inhibin B and increasing obesity in men potentially indicates decreased Sertoli cell number, and the fact that the relationship is not seen before puberty suggests that obesity exerts its negative effect on Sertoli cells during puberty (Winters et al., 2006).

Although these kinds of studies have associated obesity with altered male hormones that consequently result in infertility through an endocrine effect, researchers have also implicated increased BMI with decreased paternity in investigations that suggest that the adverse effects of obesity on male reproduction may be independent of the endocrine system (Pauli et al., 2008; Stewart et al., 2009). Some evidence suggests that only extreme obesity negatively affects male fertility through an endocrine pathway (Chavarro et al., 2010). Other published studies have observed a relationship only between sperm motility and BMI but not an association with sperm concentration, suggesting that obesity may interfere primarily with epididymal function that imparts motility to sperm (Martini et al., 2010). Some studies indicate that obesity may degrade sperm DNA integrity and mitochondrial activity, whether through the final common pathway of the endocrine system or another hormonal-independent mechanism (Fariello et al., 2012a). Although this evidence suggests that the endocrine system is a probable target for impairment of reproductive effects in the male, it is likely that the full elucidation of the means by which excess adiposity exerts its effects on male reproduction is beyond such a singular process.

Male Reproductive Physical Examination

Fortunately for the examining physician, much of the male reproductive system is located outside of the body cavity, where it can be easily palpated. Because much of the male reproductive physical examination is most effectively performed with the patient standing, it is important to put the patient at ease and before a low examining table or chair, because some men develop syncope during palpation of the scrotum. Asking a man about his work often distracts him from the male genital examination (Niederberger, 2011).

If the partner of the patient is present during the history, she may relate valuable information. However, the patient may also feel reluctant to divulge specific facts of reproductive significance before his partner, and the physical examination presents an opportunity to tactfully ask her to leave the room to allow the man time to discuss issues with his physician privately (Niederberger, 2011).

Examining the Scrotum

Visual observation of the scrotum may be revealing. One or both sides may be hypoplastic, indicating an absence of the scrotal contents since birth (Niederberger, 2011). One side may be substantially larger than the other, suggesting a reactive hydrocele or tumor. A varicocele may be so large as to be visible. Finally, proximity to the thighs in a large or obese male may indicate an insufficient difference between intrascrotal and body temperature.

Examining the Testis and Epididymis

The examiner first palpates the testis and epididymis through the scrotum, noting any abnormalities. The epididymis is typically difficult to appreciate; if it is easily palpated, it is likely engorged, which suggests obstruction. Segmentation of the epididymis is also worthwhile to note: if the portion near the upper pole is easy to discern but the lower pole is not, wolffian ductal development may have been incomplete (Lewis and Kaplan, 2009).

Testis size correlates with sperm production and is consequently an important assessment in the physical examination of the infertile male (Bujan et al., 1989; Takihara et al., 1987). The size of the testis may be assessed by calipers often referred to as the *Seager orchidometer* (Fig. 66.1; Niederberger, 2011). **The long axis of the testis is gently grasped between the jaws of the calipers, and a measurement of 4.6 cm or less is associated with spermatogenic impairment** (Schoor et al., 2001). A second method to ascertain testis size is to compare the examiner's palpation findings with a string of ellipsoids of increasing size with marked volumes as shown in Fig. 66.2 (Niederberger, 2011). **A volume of 20 mL or less is considered low** (Sigman et al., 2009). Finally, testis volume may be more directly measured by ultrasonography of the scrotum (Abdulwahed et al., 2013; Sakamoto et al., 2007a, 2007b). However, it is unclear the degree to which the incremental increase in accuracy that testis ultrasound adds to that obtained by the caliper or Prader orchidometer translates to clinically useful information (Sakamoto et al., 2007a).

Examining the Spermatic Cord

Palpation of the spermatic cord yields two features of reproductive significance: whether the vas deferens is palpable, and whether a varicocele is present. The vas is a firm, cordlike structure differentiated from vasculature within the spermatic cord by the compressibility

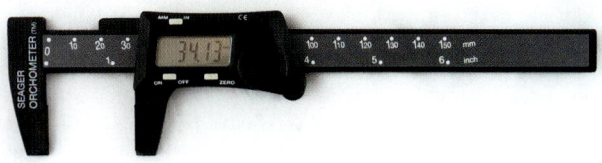

Fig. 66.1. Caliper (Seager) orchidometer.

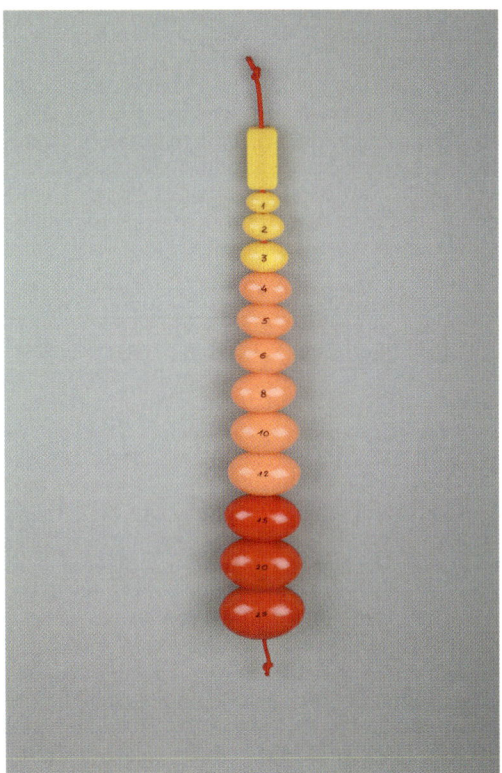

Fig. 66.2. Prader orchidometer. (Courtesy Erler Zimmer GmbH and Co. KG, Germany.)

of the vessels. Because the veins within the cord may be mistaken for the vas on manual examination of the upper scrotum, absence of the vas can be a difficult physical sign to identify. **For the clinician with experience in vasectomy, one useful method of identifying whether the structure is absent is to search for the vas as if performing the first step of a vasectomy, bringing it to the surface of the skin.** If what is presumed to be the vas disappears from the examiner's fingers three times, the clinician can be confident that the vas is absent. This pearl is referred to as *Meacham's maxim* after Randall Meacham, who described the technique (Niederberger, 2011).

Unilateral absence of the vas deferens suggests the possibility of a complete lack of wolffian ductal development on that side, including renal agenesis. In such patients, a renal ultrasound may be considered to investigate whether the patient has a solitary kidney (Niederberger, 2011). **If both vasa are absent, the man has a high likelihood of a cystic fibrosis gene mutation** (Anguiano et al., 1992). In such patients, laboratory genetic assessment of the cystic fibrosis transmembrane conductance regulator gene sequence is indicated (Bombieri et al., 2011; Lyon and Miller, 2003). As investigators observed renal agenesis in 11% of men with congenital bilateral absence of the vas deferens (CBAVD), renal ultrasound may also be considered to investigate whether a solitary kidney is present (Schlegel et al., 1996).

In addition to assessing the presence, absence, and continuity of the vas deferens, the clinician examining the upper scrotum views its surface to determine if a plexus of varicose veins arising from the spermatic cord is visible and then gently palpates to identify whether a varicocele may be felt. Although sporadic reports before 1955 described cases in which surgery on varicocele yielded evidence of improved reproductive potential, W. Selby Tulloch was the first to systematically report a series of cases of infertile men undergoing high ligation of a varicocele and subsequent improvement in sperm counts (Tulloch, 1955). Lawrence Dubin and Richard Amelar studied varicocele and its treatment in larger series and broadly educated urologic surgeons on its pathology and the merits of therapy (Dubin and Amelar, 1975; Nagler and Grotas, 2009).

The varicocele is the most commonly encountered nonductal surgically addressable pathologic entity potentially affecting male reproductive potential (Nagler and Grotas, 2009). **In general, incidence estimates in the general population range from one-fifth to one-sixth, whereas most studies suggest the incidence of varicocele in infertile males to be between one-third and one-half** (Fretz and Sandlow, 2002; Nagler and Grotas, 2009; Pryor and Howards, 1987). That not all men with varicocele are infertile remains one of the most perplexing problems in male reproductive medicine; the choice of therapy for a particular man with a varicocele is challenging.

Clinical studies of varicocele have used multiple grading systems to describe the severity of the entity, further complicating the task of the evaluating physician (Nagler and Grotas, 2009; Williams, 2011). Most systems use three or four grades; the first usually is a varicocele that cannot be palpated but can be detected only by radiographic evaluation, typically ultrasound (Dubin and Amelar, 1970; Nagler and Grotas, 2009; Williams, 2011). Some systems differentiate varicoceles that can be palpated only during the Valsalva maneuver (Dubin and Amelar, 1970; Nagler and Grotas, 2009). Because the majority of studies concur that treatment of subclinical varicoceles does not significantly improve male reproductive potential, a sensible grading system would include these entities, which are best left untreated, to differentiate them from those that ought to be addressed with therapy (Niederberger, 2011). Likewise, the difference between varicoceles that can be seen and those that can only be felt is clinically obvious, and a reasonable grading system would differentiate the two (Niederberger, 2011). **Therefore the modern evidence-based clinical grading varicocele system includes subclinical, which is not palpable or visible and can only be detected by radiographic evaluation such as Doppler ultrasound; grade I, which is palpable only with the patient standing and performing a Valsalva maneuver; grade II, which is palpable but not visible; and grade III, a varicocele that is so large as to be visible by the examining physician through the rugae of the scrotum** (Dubin and Amelar, 1970; Nagler and Grotas, 2009; Practice Committee of the American Society for Reproductive Medicine, 2014).

Examining the Phallus

In the typical setting of intercourse, semen must be deposited proximal to the cervical os for optimal chance of reproduction. Consequently, any abnormality of the phallus that may prevent placement of the semen at that locale should be noted by the examining physician. These abnormalities include phimosis, meatal displacement in hypospadias or epispadias, and significant penile curvature (Niederberger, 2011).

Examining the Prostate and Seminal Vesicles

In general, examination of the prostate and seminal vesicles does not add a significant amount of information to the evaluation of the infertile male. If the patient is sufficiently apprehensive about digital rectal examination, it may be prudently omitted. Should rectal examination be performed, the clinician notes the size of the prostate, because it may be aplastic or hypoplastic in cases of congenital malformation or significant hypoandrogenism (Niederberger, 2011). **The seminal vesicles cannot typically be palpated; if they are palpable, it is an abnormal finding suggesting engorgement and possible ejaculatory ductal obstruction** (Niederberger, 2011).

> **KEY POINTS: MALE REPRODUCTIVE PHYSICAL EXAMINATION**
>
> - Obesity impairs male reproductive potential by endocrine-dependent and endocrine-independent mechanisms.
> - Testis size directly reflects spermatogenic mass.
> - Unilateral absence of the vas deferens suggests a wolffian ductal anomaly; bilateral absence is associated with mutations in the gene responsible for cystic fibrosis. In both, renal agenesis may result.

LABORATORY EVALUATION OF MALE INFERTILITY

Like other aspects of urology, much can be learned about the condition of male infertility from blood tests, in this case, primarily of the endocrine system. Also similar to other urologic fields, genomic assessment of male reproductive function is a burgeoning area of research and increasing clinical usefulness. However, the laboratory inquiry into male infertility also includes a way of directly appraising the severity of the condition by observing the male gametes in the semen analysis. These three general laboratory assessments make up the laboratory evaluation of male infertility: the endocrine evaluation, analysis of semen, and genomic assessment.

Endocrine Evaluation

Because spermatogenesis is highly dependent on intratesticular testosterone synthesis, it is unsurprising that hypoandrogenism is associated with male infertility. Testosterone levels in men vary widely, and most investigators use either 280 ng/dL or 300 ng/dL as a threshold for adequate androgenization in a man (Petak et al., 2002; Sokol, 2009). Approximately 45% of men with azoospermia caused by spermatogenic dysfunction are observed to have testosterone levels less than 300 ng/dL. Serum testosterone below that threshold is found in 43% of men with oligospermia and 35% of men in an infertility clinic with sperm density greater than the threshold of 20 million/mL specified in the fourth edition of the WHO laboratory manual for the examination and processing of human semen (Sussman et al., 2008). Because 90% of men with sperm density of 22 million/mL or less will not have conceived with their partners within 1 year, many with sperm density less than that value are expected to have pathologic reproductive dysfunction; consequently in approximately one-third, it is likely related to endocrinopathy (WHO, 2010). **Androgenization should therefore be assessed by laboratory evaluation in all men presenting for infertility, including those in whom sperm density is greater than 20 million/mL.** An upper limit of sperm density has not been established above which endocrine dysfunction is unlikely to be discovered. Clinicians may reasonably use the 50th percentile value in the 5th edition of the WHO manual of 73 million/mL with time to pregnancy within 1 year as a guide, suggesting that a full endocrine evaluation is not necessary (WHO, 2010).

Testosterone circulates in three main forms: tightly bound to SHBG; loosely bound to protein, primarily albumin; and unbound or free (Matsumoto and Bremner, 2011). The forms inducing cellular activity are free and loosely bound together, comprising what is referred to as *bioavailable testosterone* (Matsumoto and Bremner, 2011). In the healthy man, 30% to 44% of circulating testosterone is bound to SHBG, 54% to 68% is loosely bound to albumin, and 0.5% to 3.0% is unbound (Matsumoto and Bremner, 2011). **Using a threshold of 300 ng/dL for testosterone and the lower limit of 54.5% for percent bioavailable testosterone, a reasonable lower limit for the concentration of bioavailable testosterone would consequently be 164 ng/dL.**

SHBG is altered in a variety of medical conditions and states such as obesity and aging (Box 66.1; Bhasin et al., 2010). The clinician

> **BOX 66.1** Conditions Associated With Altered Sex Hormone–Binding Globulin (SHBG) Concentrations
>
> **CONDITIONS ASSOCIATED WITH DECREASED SHBG**
> Obesity
> Nephrotic syndrome
> Hypothyroidism
> Glucocorticoids, progestins, and androgenic steroid therapy
> Acromegaly
> Diabetes mellitus
>
> **CONDITIONS ASSOCIATED WITH INCREASED SHBG**
> Aging
> Hepatic cirrhosis and hepatitis
> Hyperthyroidism
> Anticonvulsant therapy
> Estrogen therapy
> Human immunodeficiency virus disease

Modified from Bhasin S, Cunningham GR, Hayes FJ, et al.: Testosterone therapy in men with androgen deficiency syndromes: an Endocrine Society clinical practice guideline. *J Clin Endocrinol Metab* 95:2536–2559, 2010.

cannot rely on total testosterone to gauge bioavailable testosterone. Because obtaining an accurate laboratory assessment of free testosterone can be difficult, a practical method of determining bioavailable testosterone is to calculate it from total testosterone, SHBG, and albumin (Vermeulen et al., 1999). Internet-based and smartphone calculators are available; as of this writing, the International Society for the Study of the Aging Male hosts a calculator at www.issam.ch/freetesto.htm, and a calculator for iOS devices may be found at http://itunes.apple.com/us/app/bioavailable-testosterone/id308770722.

In young, healthy men, total serum testosterone exhibits a circadian rhythm, with a peak in the early morning and trough levels in the late afternoon (Plymate et al., 1989). SHBG displays an opposing circadian rhythm in men of all ages, with a peak in the late afternoon and a trough in the early morning (Plymate et al., 1989). **Consequently, bioavailable testosterone demonstrates a marked circadian rhythm in young, healthy men, with a peak in the early morning and trough in the late afternoon** (Plymate et al., 1989). In older men, total testosterone and its circadian rhythm are attenuated, and the circadian rhythm and concentration of bioavailable testosterone are substantially diminished (Plymate et al., 1989). To standardize sampling of total and bioavailable testosterone in all men, assays are typically performed in the morning, although the necessity of such timing is more important in younger men.

In the case of hypoandrogenism, a pituitary or testicular source is identified by assessing LH (Niederberger, 2011). If testicular Leydig cell dysfunction is the cause, LH is elevated to varying degrees (Niederberger, 2011). In the case of pituitary dysfunction, LH is decreased (Niederberger, 2011). The clinician may assess LH after total or bioavailable testosterone returns with a low value, or, for efficiency, both assays may be performed simultaneously. Because testosterone and LH are released in a pulsatile fashion, borderline results may be investigated further by obtaining three morning samples at 20-minute intervals (Sokol, 2009). Historically, clinicians pooled these samples for a single measure, but three separate assay results may be determined and arithmetically averaged.

The Sertoli cell products inhibin B and activin regulate pituitary follicle-stimulating hormone (FSH) by respectively inhibiting and stimulating its release (Caroppo, 2011). Because the Sertoli cells are regulated by robust paracrine interaction with germ cells, with depopulation of the latter, inhibin levels decrease and FSH consequently increases (Niederberger, 2011). Clinicians have consequently used FSH as an indirect assessment of germ cell mass; higher concentrations of FSH indicate increasing germ cell dysfunction and depopulation (Niederberger, 2011). **Combined with testis size as measured by a caliper orchidometer, FSH is an accurate predictor of whether azoospermia is a result of obstruction or spermatogenic dysfunction: 96% of men with obstructive azoospermia had FSH assay values of 7.6 IU/L or less and testis long axis greater than 4.6 cm, whereas 89% of men with azoospermia caused by spermatogenic dysfunction had FSH values greater than 7.6 IU/L and testis long axis 4.6 cm or less** (Schoor et al., 2001). In the case of male reproductive dysfunction in which sperm is present in the ejaculate, the odds ratio of abnormal sperm concentration increased markedly at an FSH value of 4.5 IU/L, suggesting another threshold that the clinician may use to assess male reproductive dysfunction (Gordetsky et al., 2011).

Assays of inhibin B are clinically available, and investigators have investigated whether measuring inhibin B directly is a more accurate assessment of spermatogenic function than the indirect assay of FSH (Grunewald et al., 2013; Jørgensen et al., 2010; Kumanov et al, 2006; Muttukrishna et al., 2007; Myers et al., 2009; van Beek et al., 2007). In general, these studies include analyses of correlation between inhibin B or FSH and sperm parameters or testis parameters measured by physical examination. Many studies observe greater accuracy with measuring inhibin B than with FSH in these correlations, and some data suggest that lower ranges of inhibin B allow improved correlation (Grunewald et al., 2013; Kumanov et al., 2006; Myers et al., 2009; van Beek et al., 2007). **However, the incremental improvement in accuracy is typically small, and inhibin and FSH provide clinically useful markers of spermatogenic function** (Myers et al., 2009). The clinician may consequently use either marker based on cost and availability.

Like inhibin B, AMH is a member of the transforming growth factor-β (TGF-β) family synthesized by Sertoli cells, and investigators have studied its use as an assay in assessing spermatogenic function (Fénichel et al., 1999; Fujisawa et al., 2002; Muttukrishna et al., 2007). Although results from pilot studies are encouraging, reported data sets remain small, and use of AMH is considered primarily experimental.

Aromatase enzymes convert cholesterol-based molecules such as testosterone to estrogens and are found in many organ systems including testis, adipose tissue, liver, and brain (Kim et al., 2013). Estradiol is consequently measurable in men, and investigators have proposed that elevated estradiol adversely affects male reproductive potential (Gregoriou et al., 2012; Raman and Schlegel, 2002; Schlegel, 2012). **A ratio of total testosterone to estradiol below 10:1 is suggested to indicate reproductive dysfunction** (Gregoriou et al., 2012; Raman and Schlegel, 2002; Schlegel, 2012). Unfortunately, the full scope of the role of estradiol is unknown, but low levels may adversely affect male reproductive potential as well (Schulster et al., 2016). Although there is a primarily inhibitory effect in somatic cells, and, subsequently, spermatogenesis, there is a stimulatory effect in germ cells. It has been shown that estradiol has a dose-dependent, nonadditive effect in germ cell proliferation. Lack of functional aromatase also leads to dysfunctional spermatogenesis (Carreau et al., 2002; Robertson et al., 1999).

The pituitary hormone prolactin is known to inhibit gonadotropins and suppress testosterone production in men; prolactin levels may be elevated in pituitary hyperplasia, adenoma, or tumors (Sokol, 2009). Clinically significant disease of the pituitary is typically associated with symptoms such as visual field changes, headache, or erectile dysfunction (Niederberger, 2011). Prolactin assay should be considered when these symptoms accompany male infertility, especially if total or bioavailable testosterone is low. However, the incidence of clinically significant prolactinoma is very low in infertile males, with only four detected in 1035 men in one large screening study, and prolactin need not be routinely included in the initial endocrine evaluation of an infertile man (Sigman and Jarow, 1997). Prolactin is commonly a labile assay; if its levels are elevated, repetition of the test is warranted (Niederberger, 2011). Assessment of other pituitary hormones such as thyroid-stimulating hormone, adrenocorticotropic hormone, or growth hormone is indicated if a space-occupying pituitary lesion is suspected or found on imaging examination (Sokol, 2009). Likewise, should signs of other endocrine disease such as exophthalmos, striations, moon facies, or facial bony changes be observed, thyroid hormone, cortisol, or growth hormone assays may be entertained. However, they need not be included in the initial screening evaluation of an infertile man. **A reasonable initial laboratory screen to assess an endocrine basis for male reproductive dysfunction should be performed in the morning and includes total testosterone, SHBG, and albumin to calculate bioavailable testosterone; LH and FSH to gauge pituitary function; and estradiol to evaluate aromatization.**

Men with a history of congenital adrenal hyperplasia (CAH) may develop testicular adrenal rest tumors and infertility later in life (Aycan et al., 2013; Pierre et al., 2012). In these patients, serum 17-hydroxyprogesterone, Δ4-androstenedione, renin, and testosterone can be used to assess response to therapy (Pierre et al., 2012).

Evaluation of Semen

Reproduction is a probabilistic system: the more viable sperm that begin their journey in the female reproductive tract, the greater the chance that one will penetrate and fertilize the ovum. In this sense, there is only one definitive result of a semen analysis, and that is the condition in which no sperm are present; only in that case can a man be absolutely considered sterile.

In 1951 the physiologist John MacLeod published the first stringent statistical assessment comparing what could be observed under the light microscope in semen from men who had successfully impregnated their partners versus semen of men who had not done so (MacLeod, 1951). MacLeod applied a descriptive statistical approach, computing cumulative probability histograms for each observable parameter and determining quartiles for each of the two groups of men (MacLeod, 1951). Basic parameters studied included the concentration of sperm, their movement, and their shape (MacLeod, 1951). What is immediately evident from MacLeod's seminal publication is that the histograms for sperm parameters from fertile and infertile men are largely overlapping, meaning that a substantial range of values for any parameter does not discriminate between male fertility and infertility (MacLeod, 1951). MacLeod sensibly approached this problem by considering lower sperm parameter values to be more appropriate thresholds for suggesting male infertility; however, values above these lower thresholds do not confirm fertility (MacLeod, 1951). This was difficult to grasp in clinical implementation. The field of reproductive medicine is rife with the incorrect assumption that should a parameter be above a threshold—for example, sperm concentration greater than 20 million/mL—then the man is considered fertile. The only conclusion that may be drawn from such a comparison is that if the parameter is lower than the threshold, the man is likely to be infertile; the converse is not necessarily true.

One general approach to the problem of an assay for which the values representing disease and health are overly coincident is to establish two thresholds, beyond which health or disease is probable, and within which no predictive statement can be made. In one study to develop two such sets of thresholds for semen analysis, investigators applied the computational method classification and regression tree (CART) analysis to semen analyses from fertile men and those whose wives were undergoing intrauterine insemination (IUI) and for whom female infertility had been largely excluded (Guzick et al., 2001). **As an example, for sperm concentration, 13.5 million/mL was found to be the lower parameter, and 48.0 million/mL was identified as the upper parameter** (Guzick et al., 2001). Using these parameters, the clinician would counsel a man whose sperm concentration was less than 13.5 million/mL that he was likely infertile, and one with a concentration greater than 48.0 million/mL that he was likely fertile. Should the man's concentration be greater than 13.5 million/mL and less than 48.0 million/mL, no assessment of fertility potential could be accurately made.

Bulk Semen Parameters and the World Health Organization Criteria

Building on the original work by MacLeod and deriving consensus from a group of experts, WHO established criteria for semen analysis parameters in its laboratory manual for the examination and processing of human semen (Cooper et al., 2010; Niederberger, 2011; Murray et al., 2012; WHO, 2010). For the first four editions of the manual, criteria were set by both expert panel and survey data and included such thresholds as sperm density of 20 million/mL, which would be judged as a reasonable number below which a man should be considered likely infertile (Cooper et al., 2010; Murray et al, 2012; Niederberger, 2011; WHO, 2010). The problems with such a set of criteria are evident: the sperm density of fertile men may be found below the thresholds and that of infertile men above.

The 5th edition of the WHO laboratory manual departed from the previous four by emphasizing the statistical description of the population of men on which it was based (Cooper et al., 2010; WHO, 2010). Values for percentiles of semen parameters from men whose partners became pregnant within 1 year of discontinuation of contraceptives are tabulated, allowing the clinician to compare an infertile patient's results with a fertile cohort (Table 66.2; Cooper et al, 2010; WHO, 2010). Two limitations of such an approach are clear: first, the data are derived from a fertile population and not an infertile one, and second, the clinician cannot rely on descriptive statistics to predict outcomes. Nonetheless, the manual's tables offer the physician useful comparative information that would be otherwise unavailable in evaluating and treating infertile men.

Somewhat confusingly, the 5th edition of the manual published alongside the full percentile table a separate list of the 5th percentiles and their 95% confidence intervals (CIs) (Cooper et al., 2010; WHO, 2010). For example, the 5th percentile value for sperm density is 15 million/mL with a 95% CI range of 12 to 16 million/mL (Cooper et al., 2010; WHO, 2010). Although the authors of the companion publication to the manual very clearly describe the problems inherent in using thresholds derived from descriptive statistics of a fertile male population, the enumeration of the 5th percentile values has appeared to spur their use as new thresholds. The best use of the tables in the 5th edition of the manual would be for the urologist

TABLE 66.2 Bulk Semen Analysis Parameter Percentiles

PERCENTILE	2.5	95% CI	5	95% CI	10	25	50	75	90	95	97.5
Semen volume (mL)	1.2	(1.0–1.3)	1.5	(1.4–1.7)	2	2.7	3.7	4.8	6	6.8	7
Sperm concentration (million/mL)	9	(8–11)	15	(12–16)	22	41	73	116	169	213	259
Total number (million/ejaculate)	23	(18–29)	39	(33–46)	69	142	255	422	647	802	928
Total motility (%)	34	(33–37)	40	(38–42)	45	53	61	69	75	78	81
Progressive motility (%)	28	(25–29)	32	(31–34)	39	47	55	62	69	72	75
Normal forms (%)	3	(2.0–3.0)	4	(3.0–4.0)	5.5	9	15	24.5	36	44	48
Vitality (%)	53	(48–56)	58	(55–63)	64	72	79	84	88	91	92

CI, Confidence interval.
Modified from Cooper TG, Noonan E, von Eckardstein S, et al.: World Health Organization reference values for human semen characteristics. *Hum Reprod Update* 16(3):231–245, 2010.

to present to a man alongside the patient's own parameters as a reference for an ultimately fertile population, but clinical reality dictates that physicians and patients are interested in defining what represents infertility to consider when medical or surgical therapy is appropriately invoked. Communicating the 5th percentile value as one that likely represents infertility and the 50th percentile as typical for a man conceiving with his wife within 1 year is reasonable practice for clinical urology. As an example, sperm density lower than 15 million/mL would suggest infertility, and 73 million/mL would be considered typical (Cooper et al., 2010; WHO, 2010).

To complicate matters, semen analysis parameters are highly variable, and investigators typically recommend a minimum of two analyses separated by 2 to 3 weeks for assessment (Centola, 2011). Although data exist to the contrary, most investigators observe a decline in bulk seminal parameters with increasing days of abstinence, and variability in abstinence may be responsible for variability in semen analysis results (Elzanaty, 2008; Levitas et al., 2005; Keel, 2006; Keihani et al., 2017). Consequently, the physician evaluating a man for his reproductive potential should ensure that the duration of abstinence before an ejaculated specimen is as constant as possible. **Historically, men were instructed to wait 2 to 5 days after an ejaculation to submit a sample for semen analysis** (Centola, 2011; WHO, 2010). **More recent studies suggest that a single day of abstinence is optimal for assessing bulk seminal parameters** (Elzanaty, 2008; Levitas et al., 2005).

A nontoxic wide-mouthed glass or plastic cup is used to collect the semen sample (WHO, 2010). In the case of religious or cultural stipulations that do not allow collection by masturbation, a special nontoxic condom may be used (WHO, 2010).

The physical and chemical characteristics of a semen sample are first assessed before microscopic examination. Ejaculated semen first forms a coagulum, and the sample is allowed to liquefy for 30 minutes before evaluation (Centola, 2011). Viscosity is assessed by aspiration into a pipette and measuring the length of the drop that forms, which should be no longer than 2 cm (Centola, 2011; WHO, 2010). The sample is then inspected visually for coloration. A normal ejaculate is white or light gray; a yellow or green hue may indicate infection, jaundice, or vitamins or medication; brown is often observed in spinal cord–injured men; and red suggests blood (Centola, 2011; WHO, 2010).

Historically, semen pH was reported, but its measurement is no longer recommended because environmental conditions may alter it, and the original intent of using pH to gauge whether obstruction exists is hampered by the vast difference in size between a hydrogen ion and sperm head (Centola, 2011). For bulk seminal parameters describing microscopic features, a specialized slide with a compartment with defined volume such as a hemocytometer or Makler counting chamber is typically used (Centola, 2011).

Semen Volume. Often unreported by laboratories infrequently performing semen analysis, semen volume is clinically important (Niederberger, 2011). Conditions causing seminal hypovolemia include anatomic factors, such as ejaculatory ductal obstruction or hypoplasia of the prostate and seminal vesicles as may occur in severe androgen deficiency or CBAVD; functional issues, such as in retrograde ejaculation; neurologic conditions, such as in spinal cord injury, diabetes mellitus, or multiple sclerosis; and pharmacologic factors, which may occur in men prescribed α-adrenergic blocking agents such as tamsulosin (Niederberger, 2011; Sigman et al., 2009). The 5th percentile for volume according to the 5th edition of the WHO laboratory manual is 1.5 mL with a 95% CI of 1.4 to 1.7 mL, and the 2.5th percentile is 1.2 mL with a 95% CI of 1.0 to 1.3 mL (WHO, 2010). **For practical purposes, the most frequently used threshold value for volume is 1.0 mL to initiate evaluation for seminal hypovolemia** (Niederberger, 2011).

Aspermia, dry ejaculate, and *anejaculation* refer to the condition in which no fluid is discharged from the urethra during male orgasm (Sigman et al., 2009). It is caused by the same conditions associated with seminal hypovolemia (Niederberger, 2011; Sigman et al., 2009). **If aspermia or seminal hypovolemia is observed, a postejaculatory urinalysis is performed to identify retrograde ejaculation, and some form of investigation such as transrectal ultrasonography (TRUS) is conducted to evaluate whether ejaculatory ductal obstruction may be present** (Niederberger, 2011; Sigman et al., 2009). For postejaculatory urinalysis, the patient is instructed to void before ejaculation for a semen analysis and then to urinate after collection of the semen sample into separate containers (Sigman et al., 2009). The urine is reconstituted by centrifugation, and the number of sperm in the pellet is counted (Sigman et al., 2009). A small number of sperm in the urine is of little consequence if the number of sperm in the antegrade sample is large. In general, if the number of sperm in the urine nears or exceeds that in the antegrade specimen, retrograde ejaculation is considered clinically significant (Sigman et al., 2009).

Seminal hypervolemia with an ejaculate volume exceeding 5 mL is a rare condition (Sigman et al., 2009). It is proposed to interfere with male reproduction by diluting sperm (Sigman et al., 2009). If a too-large seminal volume is of concern, the sperm may be reconstituted by processing into a smaller volume and IUI performed (Centola, 2011; Sigman et al., 2009).

Sperm Density. Sperm density or concentration is typically recorded in millions per milliliter. The term *oligospermia* or *oligozoospermia* refers to low sperm density, and *cryptozoospermia* denotes sperm so few as to be difficult to reliably measure (Niederberger, 2011). The 5th percentile for sperm density according to the 5th edition of the WHO laboratory manual is 15 million/mL with a 95% CI of 12 to 16 million/mL, and the 50th percentile is 73 million/mL (Cooper et al., 2010; WHO, 2010). Previous editions of the WHO laboratory manual included a threshold for sperm density of 20 million/mL, and it was common in the past for practitioners to define oligospermia as lower than that value. With the descriptive tabulation of sperm parameters in the 5th edition of the WHO manual, oligospermia is more appropriately defined in a clinical context: a man with a single semen sample demonstrating 10 million/mL who has had no difficulty impregnating his wife may not be oligospermic, whereas one with small testes, an elevated FSH, and densities on several semen analyses ranging from 20 to 25 million/mL may be reasonably considered oligospermic. **As mentioned previously, a large CART analysis revealed 13.5 million/mL to be a lower parameter for sperm density and 48.0 million/mL to be an upper parameter** (Guzick et al., 2001). In CART analysis, the ROC AUC for sperm density was 0.60, indicating relatively poor discriminating ability between fertile and subfertile subgroups (Guzick et al., 2001).

Total sperm count or number is calculated by multiplying semen volume and sperm density and is typically recorded in millions (Niederberger, 2011). The 5th percentile for total sperm number according to the 5th edition of the WHO laboratory manual is 39 million with a 95% CI of 33 to 46 million, and the 50th percentile is 255 million (Cooper et al., 2010; WHO, 2010).

Sperm Motility. Sperm motility is assessed optimally within 30 minutes of liquefaction and refers to a percentage of sperm observed with defined motion (WHO, 2010). Low motility is termed *asthenospermia* or *asthenozoospermia* (Niederberger, 2011). The 5th edition of the WHO manual classifies motility into three categories—progressive, nonprogressive, and immotility—replacing the four categories of older grading systems (a through d, where a and b indicated "rapid" and "slow" progressive motility; WHO, 2010). *Progressive motility* is defined as sperm "moving actively, either linearly or in a large circle, regardless of speed," and nonprogressive motility is defined as "all other patterns of motility with an absence of progression" (WHO, 2010). The 5th percentile for progressive motility according to the 5th edition of the WHO laboratory manual is 32% with a 95% CI of 31% to 34%, and the 50th percentile is 55% (Cooper et al., 2010; WHO, 2010). **CART analysis revealed 32% to be a lower parameter for sperm motility and 63% to be an upper parameter** (Guzick et al., 2001). In CART analysis, the ROC AUC for sperm motility was 0.59, revealing low discriminating ability for this parameter (Guzick et al., 2001).

Sperm Morphology. Human sperm is highly pleomorphic with more bizarrely shaped sperm in any man's ejaculate than those with configuration anticipated to successfully penetrate and fertilize an ovum (Niederberger, 2011). An overabundance of abnormal forms is termed *teratospermia* or *teratozoospermia* (Niederberger, 2011). Earlier editions of the WHO manual described fairly generous criteria as characterizing an acceptably shaped sperm, and even then, the majority of sperm were classified as misshapen in a normal semen analysis (Niederberger, 2011). **In an attempt to improve the predictive capability of sperm morphology, Kruger proposed a grading system in which several aspects of sperm were assessed, and if any one was out of range, the sperm was counted as abnormal** (Kruger et al., 1987; van der Merwe et al., 2005). This system is variably referred to as "strict" morphology, "Kruger" morphology, and "Tygerberg" morphology, and as a result of the more stringent criteria defining a normal sperm, thresholds in the range of 5% typically characterize a normal ejaculate (van der Merwe et al., 2005). The 5th edition of the WHO manual adopted strict morphology as its assessment of sperm shape (WHO, 2010). The 5th percentile for normal morphologic forms according to the 5th edition is 4% with a 95% CI of 3.0% to 4.0%, and the 50th percentile is 15% (Cooper et al., 2010; WHO, 2010). CART analysis revealed 9% to be a lower parameter for strict morphology and 12% to be an upper parameter (Guzick et al., 2001). In CART analysis, the ROC AUC for sperm motility was 0.66, with the bulk parameters of density and motility revealing low discriminating capacity (Guzick et al., 2001).

The clinical predictive value of strict morphology is questionable. Although limited data suggest that the parameter may be associated with embryo formation, the majority of studies support that strict morphology is unassociated with sperm nuclear integrity and that it does not predict natural conception, IUI, or IVF outcomes (Avendaño et al., 2009; Dayal et al., 2010; Dubey et al., 2008; French et al., 2010; Keegan et al., 2007; Lockwood et al., 2015; Morbeck et al., 2011; Sripada et al., 2010). To complicate matters, evidence suggests that as laboratory technicians have learned to inspect each sperm more closely for eccentricities of shape, an increasing number of men are described as having lower percentages of sperm with normal morphology (Morbeck et al., 2011). The practical implication of this trend is that currently many men who seek evaluation are identified as having isolated teratozoospermia and are likely to have adequate reproductive potential.

Conditions exist in which specific biologic defects are associated with the majority of sperm. For example, should the acrosome fail to form, the preponderance of sperm will have small, round heads, a disorder referred to as *globozoospermia* (WHO, 2010). During spermiation, if the basal plate does not attach to the nucleus opposite the acrosome, the heads are absorbed (WHO, 2010). This defect results in only tails observed and is termed *pinhead sperm* (WHO, 2010). Undoubtedly, these relatively uncommon specific morphologic conditions affect male reproductive potential.

Further details on this topic are available online at Expert Consult.com.

Sperm Vitality. *Vitality* refers to the portion of sperm that are metabolically active living cells (Niederberger, 2011; WHO, 2010). *Necrospermia* or *necrozoospermia* is the condition describing a large number of nonliving sperm (Niederberger, 2011). **The assessment of whether sperm are living is essential if near or total asthenospermia is observed to discriminate whether the lack of motility is a result of cell death or of dysfunction of molecular processes involved in sperm motion** (Niederberger, 2011; WHO, 2010). If the test is purely diagnostic and the sperm are not to be used in IVF, it is performed by staining with eosin Y and with or without nigrosin (Niederberger, 2011; WHO, 2010). A metabolically active sperm excludes the eosin Y dye, whereas a dead one cannot and absorbs the pigment (Niederberger, 2011; WHO, 2010). Nigrosin darkens the background and increases the contrast between it and the live sperm heads, allowing them to be identified more easily (WHO, 2010). The 5th percentile for sperm vitality according to the 5th edition of the WHO laboratory manual is 58% with a 95% CI of 55% to 63%, and the 50th percentile is 79% (Cooper et al., 2010; WHO, 2010).

A method of assessing sperm vitality in a nondestructive manner amenable to subsequent use in IVF is the hypo-osmotic swelling (HOS) test (Jeyendran et al., 1984). When incubated in hypo-osmotic medium, the tails of live sperm with unimpaired membranes swell within 5 minutes, allowing for identification of viable gametes (WHO, 2010).

Further details on this topic are available online at Expert Consult.com.

Secondary Semen Assays

The haploid male gamete expresses different surface antigens than the remainder of diploid cells in the male body and consequently must be protected from the immune system by tight junctions between Sertoli cells (Walsh and Turek, 2009). If this "blood-testis barrier" is disrupted, sperm exposed to the immune system may incite an immune response of varying severity involving secretory and humoral immunoglobulins and affecting multiple regions of the surface of the sperm cell (Walsh and Turek, 2009). **Conditions observed to be associated with antisperm antibody formation include vasectomy, testis trauma, orchitis, cryptorchidism, testis cancer, and varicocele** (Walsh and Turek, 2009).

Leukocytes may be harmful to sperm, with evidence suggesting that production of ROSs may be the destructive mechanism (Agarwal et al., 2006; Aktan et al., 2013; Desai et al., 2009; Domes et al., 2012; Lackner et al., 2006; Pasqualotto et al., 2000). Moderate levels of leukocytes in semen may be physiologic and may even be beneficial for sperm function (Barraud-Lange et al., 2011).

Use of an assay for antisperm antibodies should be entertained if agglutination of sperm is observed or if sperm motility is decreased, especially if conditions associated with antisperm antibodies exist (Brannigan, 2011; Niederberger, 2011; Walsh and Turek, 2009; WHO, 2010). Two types of assays for antisperm antibodies are available: those that test for immunoglobulins on the surface of sperm are referred to as *direct* tests, and those that measure antibodies in fluid such as seminal plasma or serum are *indirect* assays (Brannigan, 2011; WHO, 2010). **Direct assays are preferred for clinical relevance, because antibodies in plasma or serum may not correlate to sperm surface binding** (Brannigan, 2011; Niederberger, 2011; Walsh and Turek, 2009). Because of its large size, immunoglobulin M (IgM) is present in very low quantities if at all in semen, and consequently IgG and IgA are the primary assay targets (Brannigan, 2011; Niederberger, 2011; Walsh and Turek, 2009).

Two direct assays are available: the mixed antiglobulin reaction (MAR) test and the immunobead assay (Brannigan, 2011; WHO, 2010). The MAR test uses latex beads coated with an anti-IgG or anti-IgA "bridging" antibody incubated with sperm, whereas the direct immunobead test involves polyacrylamide beads coated with rabbit immunoglobulins against human IgG or IgA (Brannigan, 2011; WHO, 2010). **In both cases, after incubation the technician identifies the presence of antisperm antibodies by association of moving particles proximal to motile sperm, and thus some amount of sperm motion is essential for these assays; complete asthenospermia renders direct antisperm antibody assays unable to be performed** (Brannigan, 2011; Niederberger, 2011; WHO, 2010). The direct immunobead test is more laborious than the MAR assay but yields more precise information (WHO, 2010).

The WHO laboratory manual loosely specifies 50% as a threshold for the MAR and immunobead tests and notes that reference values are not established, leaving the interpretation of these assays to the physician considering the degree and localization of antisperm antibody binding and the clinical context (WHO, 2010). Sperm head binding is considered to be of greater clinical significance than tail binding (Niederberger, 2011).

Pyospermia Assays. Under phase contrast microscopy without staining, leukocytes and immature germ cells are indistinguishable (Brannigan, 2011). Consequently, when faced with a report indicating an abundance of cells resembling leukocytes observed only with phase contrast microscopy, the evaluating physician cannot accurately diagnose pyospermia (Brannigan, 2011). Fortunately, laboratory testing to evaluate the presence of leukocytes is not difficult. The Papanicolaou stain may be used to differentiate leukocytes from immature germ cells based on nuclear morphology (WHO, 2010). **The current consensus threshold for leukocytes according to the WHO laboratory manual is 1 million/mL** (WHO, 2010). Semen cultures are generally unhelpful because positive results in asymptomatic men have not been shown to have clinical significance

(Moretti et al., 2009; Shalika et al., 1996). If a patient is symptomatic, the prostatitis algorithm found elsewhere in this book may be followed. If pyospermia is excluded, the patient can be reassured that the presence of immature germ cells is common and not of pathologic significance (Brannigan, 2011).

Tertiary and Investigational Sperm Assays

The limitations of bulk seminal parameters spawned myriad additional means to assess sperm structure and function in hopes of better diagnosing male reproductive dysfunction, applying therapies, and predicting outcomes in techniques such as IVF. Most are promising, but few are even close to proven. Many provide insight into the biologic processes involved in reproduction, but similarly designed studies report conflicting results when these assays are applied to clinical problems. Emphasizing a lack of consensus on how they are to be used clinically, the 5th edition of the WHO manual details these assays in its "research procedures" chapter (WHO, 2010). The prudent practitioner will continue to follow the literature as it evolves and use these assays clinically should a clear consensus emerge regarding usefulness.

Sperm DNA Integrity Assays. Sperm DNA molecular and spatial organization is highly specific to cells of the male gamete. Sperm DNA is six times more compact than in somatic cells, and it is arranged with protamines to form tightly linear side-by-side sheets (Ward and Coffey, 1991). Investigators have hypothesized that fragmentation or disturbances in DNA arrangement lead to aberrations in sperm function, fertilization, implantation, and pregnancy (Agarwal et al., 2003; Lewis et al., 2013). Conflicting data and opinions abound in testing this hypothesis, indicating that our understanding of the role of sperm DNA quaternary structure is limited, the assays available are imperfect, or both. Poor sensitivity and specificity of the current testing modalities have prevented widespread acceptance of the utility of DNA integrity testing. The lack of standardized testing protocols and diagnostic thresholds has led to a significant ongoing debate on the applicability and prognostic value of such testing. The current published literature does not provide clear evidence to support routine use.

In general, there are two types of test methods that assess DNA structural integrity (Sakkas and Alvarez, 2010). In one, DNA fragmentation is measured directly (Sakkas and Alvarez, 2010). In general, this type of assessment is preferred by andrology laboratories at present because it appears to more effectively correlate with clinical outcomes (Sakkas and Alvarez, 2010). In the other, DNA is denatured before analysis (Sakkas and Alvarez, 2010). In a comprehensive meta-analysis, higher rates of miscarriage were associated with an overall approximately double risk ratio with increasing sperm DNA fragmentation, but different assays yielded markedly different risk ratios (Robinson et al., 2012).

TUNEL Assay. The terminal deoxynucleotidyl transferase dUTP nick end labeling (TUNEL) assay represents a general method in widespread use in molecular biology to assess DNA fragmentation by labeling the terminal end of nucleic acid strands with a fluorescent marker, and it was adopted in the andrology laboratory with various modifications to detect sperm head DNA fragmentation (Gavrieli et al., 1992; Mitchell et al., 2011). Fig. 66.3 details one method. In panels A and B, a fluorescent stain that binds to DNA regions, rich in adenine and thymine, 4′,6-diamidino-2-phenylindole (DAPI), identifies sperm heads containing packed DNA. Panel A is a brightfield image that allows sperm tails to be seen, confirming that the area under scrutiny is a sperm. Panel B is a fluorescent image, allowing comparison with TUNEL-positive sperm, which are identified in panel C. In general, results are reported as a DNA fragmentation index (DFI), which is calculated as the ratio of TUNEL-positive sperm to all sperm and expressed as a percentage. **TUNEL is considered a direct measure of sperm DNA fragmentation, and in a meta-analysis of miscarriage rates, TUNEL had the highest associated risk ratio at nearly 4** (Robinson et al., 2012; Sakkas and Alvarez, 2010).

Comet Assay. Like the TUNEL assay, the comet assay, also referred to as the *single-cell gel electrophoresis assay*, is widely used in molecular biology laboratories to assess DNA fragmentation and has been

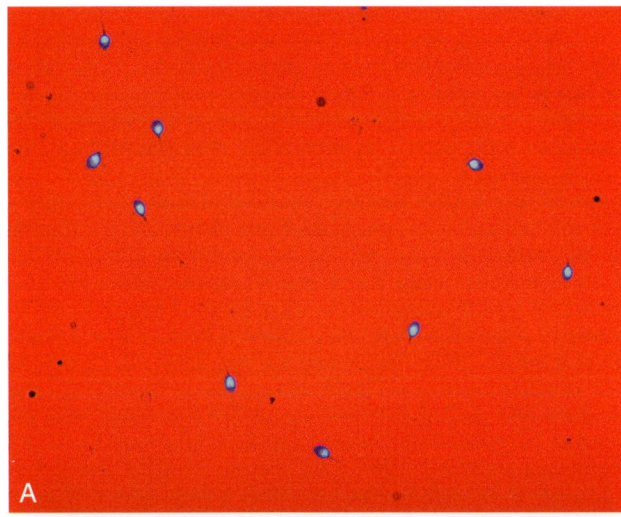
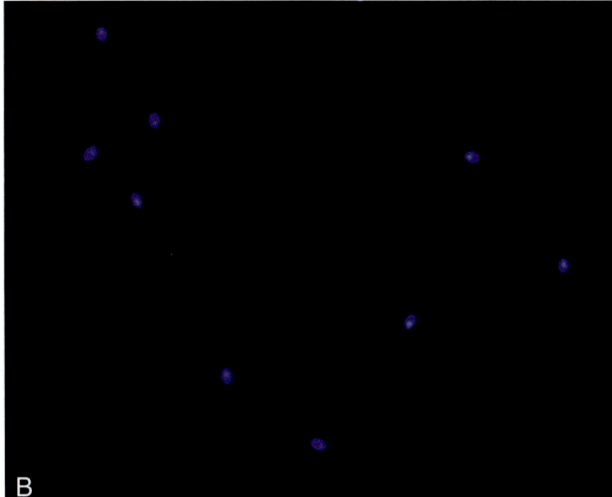
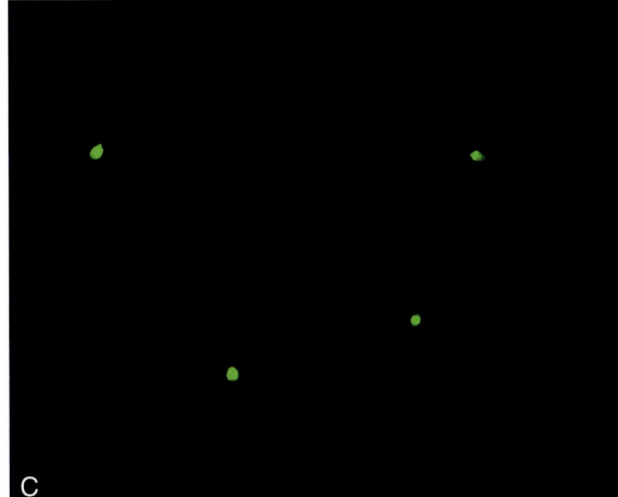

Fig. 66.3. TUNEL assay. (A) Brightfield. (B) Sperm heads by fluorescence are demonstrated. (C) TUNEL-positive sperm.

adopted in the andrology laboratory for sperm (Sakkas and Alvarez, 2010; Tice et al., 2000). It is a simple assay that involves migration of single sperm head DNA in an electrophoretic agarose gel, and the tail, resembling a comet, indicates the degree of fragmentation (Tice et al., 2000). At neutral pH, this assay is considered a direct measure of sperm DNA fragmentation (Sakkas and Alvarez, 2010). Data are conflicting regarding its use as a tool for predicting clinical outcomes (Ribas-Maynou et al., 2012; Robinson et al., 2012;

Simon et al., 2010, 2011). Investigators have used the comet assay in a variety of research settings to understand the effects of various entities on sperm DNA, including varicocele, toxins, male age, and testis cancer (Bertolla et al., 2006; Blumer et al., 2008; Cho et al., 2016; Delbes et al., 2007; Fariello et al., 2012b; Lacerda et al., 2011; Meeker et al., 2004, 2008; O'Flaherty et al., 2008; Schmid et al., 2007; Wu et al., 2009).

Denatured Sperm DNA Assays. A number of assays denature sperm DNA before structural analysis (Sakkas and Alvarez, 2010). The comet assay performed in acidic or alkaline conditions denatures DNA, and like the comet assay, the sperm chromatin dispersion (SCD) assay allows visual identification of individual sperm head DNA structure by dispersion on agarose followed by nucleic acid staining (Fernández et al., 2003; Sakkas and Alvarez, 2010). The most established assay for sperm head DNA structure is the Sperm Chromatin Structure Assay (SCSA) (SCSA Diagnostics, Brookings, SD) (Boe-Hansen et al., 2006; Chohan et al., 2006; Evenson and Jost, 2000; Evenson and Melamed, 1983; Larson et al., 2000). The SCSA does not identify individual sperm but rather a population of cells by flow cytometry after denaturation in acidic conditions followed by staining with acridine orange (Evenson and Jost, 2000; Larson et al., 2000). Graphic analysis of flow cytometric data yields several outcome parameters for SCSA; the DFI and high DNA stainability (HDS) are the two reported in common clinical use (Evenson and Jost, 2000; Larson et al., 2000). Although a number of studies have associated human reproductive outcomes with SCSA reported values, many failed to find statistically valid correlations (Boe-Hansen et al., 2006; Bungum et al., 2007, 2008; Evenson and Jost, 2000; Larson et al., 2000; Lin et al., 2008; Payne et al., 2005). In a meta-analysis of miscarriage rates, SCSA had a risk ratio of 1.47 with a 95% CI of 1.04 to 2.09, indicating a weak likely association.

Reactive Oxygen Species. Naturally occurring chemical reactions generate highly reactive molecules with unpaired electrons termed *free radicals*. Free radicals produced from oxidative reactions are referred to as *reactive oxygen species*. ROS are involved in multiple physiologic processes important to sperm function, but investigators theorize that if present in excess, seminal ROS may cause reproductive dysfunction (Agarwal et al., 2006, 2008c; Desai et al., 2009). TAC may be quantified in seminal fluid, and one popular method of quantifying how ROSs may affect sperm function is calculation of a ROS-TAC score (Rice-Evans and Miller, 1994; Sharma et al., 1999). Researchers have assessed ROS activity in aging, prostatitis, varicocele, lubricants, radiation, smoking, toxins, and obesity (Agarwal et al., 2009, 2013; Cocuzza et al., 2008a, 2008b; Farombi et al., 2008; Hsu et al., 2009; Palmer et al., 2012; Pasqualotto et al., 2000, 2008a; Smith et al., 2005; Taha et al., 2012).

Acrosome Reaction. Further details on this topic are available online at ExpertConsult.com.

Sperm Mucus Interaction. Further details on this topic are available online at ExpertConsult.com.

Sperm Ovum Interaction. Further details on this topic are available online at ExpertConsult.com.

Sperm Ultrastructural Assessment. MSOME involving sperm head morphologic inspection with high-power Nomarski differential interference contrast optics that magnify the field more than 6000× is discussed in the section on sperm morphology in this chapter. Although electron microscopy is widely used in scientific research on the male gamete, it also has a place in the clinical assessment of the infertile male (Chemes and Rawe, 2003). **Sperm motility is dependent on the ultrastructural arrangement of microtubules in the tail with a peripheral array of nine pairs and a central two microtubules connected by dynein arms** (Chemes and Rawe, 2003). This "9 + 2" architecture is shared with cilia, and genetic disorders affecting it can manifest as respiratory pathology associated with **male reproductive dysfunction, referred to as the** *immotile cilia syndrome, primary ciliary dyskinesia* **(PCD), or** *Kartagener syndrome* (Chemes and Rawe, 2003; Eliasson et al., 1977; Guichard et al., 2001). Kartagener syndrome results in sperm that are nearly totally or completely immotile but metabolically active (Peeraer et al., 2004). Semen samples with less than 10% motility and vitality demonstrated by testing may be investigated with electron microscopy to assess tail ultrastructural defects (Zini and Sigman, 2009). Electron microscopy is not available in all andrology laboratories.

Sperm Fluorescence in situ Hybridization. With the introduction of assisted reproductive technologies (ARTs), many males affected by errors occurring during stem cell division are now able to yield offspring with increased risk of aneuploidies, in particular of the sex chromosomes (Hansen et al., 2005; Rimm et al., 2004). Fluorescence in situ hybridization (FISH) employs fluorescent-labeled primers that bind specifically to each chromosome in the sperm, allowing measurement of sperm aneuploidies that are of major clinical importance (Templado et al., 2013). One advantage of FISH is that it offers the ability to investigate the cytogenetics of somatic and germ cells, which may differ beyond the expected halving of chromosomes (Martin, 2008). Unfortunately, sperm that undergo a FISH analysis cannot be used for in vitro fertilization afterward.

Sarrate et al. (2010) have verified that the relationship between sperm count and the overall increased rates of chromosome abnormalities in sperm accurately demonstrates an inverse correlation between these two parameters. In reality, exceptionally high levels of sperm aneuploidy were identified in testicular sperm extraction samples of men with azoospermia resulting from spermatogenic dysfunction (Huang et al., 1999). Currently, it has been used as a diagnostic tool for couples with recurrent pregnancy loss or recurrent implantation failure (Kohn et al., 2016; Ramasamy et al., 2015; Zidi-Jrah et al., 2016).

Genomic Assessment

Ironically, genes passed from parent to male offspring may be responsible for a condition that, if left untreated, would prevent those genes from being passed to future generations; evidence suggests that genetics plays a significant role in male reproductive dysfunction (Oates and Lamb, 2009). Known genetic conditions associated with the male sex are detailed in later sections of this chapter. In this section, clinically available assays are described.

Karyotype

Staining chromosomes with dyes binding to various moieties of the chemical structure of DNA resulting in banding patterns represents the classic means of cytogenetic analysis of chromosomes (Swansbury, 2003). FISH uses fluorescent probes hybridizing to determine sequences on chromosomes, allowing for identification of specific regions or entire chromosomes depending on the specificity of the probe (Swansbury, 2003). Other techniques, such as the spectral karyotype (SKY), use combinatorial methods to visualize all chromosomes in multiple colors (Swansbury, 2003). **The American Urological Association Best Practice Statement on the Optimal Evaluation of the Infertile Male recommends that genetic testing including karyotype be performed in all males with azoospermia caused by spermatogenic dysfunction and in those with severe oligospermia defined as less than 5 million sperm/mL** (Jarow et al., 2010). However, because numerical and structural chromosomal anomalies vary by geographic region, and obtaining a karyotype may represent a significant expense to the patient, the treating physician may judge whether this assay is indicated in his or her patient population.

Y Chromosome Microdeletion Testing

The Y chromosome is one of the smallest in humans at approximately 60 megabase (Mb) pairs (Navarro-Costa, 2012; Tilford et al., 2001). It is the determinant of the male gender and is the only chromosome passed directly from father to son (Navarro-Costa, 2012). It consists of a male-specific region with no homologous chromosomal mate and two pseudoautosomal regions (PAR1 and PAR2) (Graves et al., 1998; Krausz and Casamonti, 2017; Navarro-Costa, 2012; Tilford et al., 2001). In an elegant series of cytogenetic analyses for the time, **Tiepolo and Zuffardi determined in 1976 that a region in the long arm of the Y chromosome was critical to the formation of sperm in man, which became known as the** *azoospermia factor* (Chandley et al., 1989; Tiepolo and Zuffardi, 1976).

The portion of the Y chromosome that does not recombine represents approximately 95% of its sequence (Tilford et al., 2001). About one-third of this nonrecombinant region consists of palindromic inner sequences present at least twice in forward and reverse reading frames referred to as *amplicons* (Tilford et al., 2001). This sequence structure is believed to substitute in part in place of sexual recombination in repair of the Y chromosome but may also engender a particular fragility in increasing the likelihood of the loss of segments, or microdeletions (Oates and Lamb, 2009). Based on the work of Tiepolo and Zuffardi, investigators observed microdeletions of three regions on the Y chromosome to be commonly associated with azoospermia or oligospermia, which were termed *AZFa*, *AZFb*, and *AZFc* (Oates and Lamb, 2009). Once thought to be separate and distinct regions, AZFb and AZFc overlap, whereas AZFa is distant and isolated (Jobling and Tyler-Smith, 2003). The *DAZ* genes, believed to be integrally associated with spermatogenesis, are housed within the AZFc region (Saxena et al., 2000). Investigators have also referred to the proximal portion of AZFc as *AZFd*, but the usefulness of isolating this subregion remains unclear (Müslümanoğlu et al., 2005).

Some microdeletions of AZFc appear to be associated with spermatogenic impairment but not failure (Mulhall et al., 1997; Oates et al., 2002). Likewise, the clinical relevance of analysis of AZFc subregions such as gr/gr is unclear, because sperm may be present in the ejaculate and in the testis (Giachini et al., 2008; Lardone et al., 2007; Stouffs et al., 2008; Visser et al., 2009; Wu et al., 2007). However, evidence strongly suggests that deletion of genes *USP9Y* and *DDX3Y* in the AZFa region and deletion of genes *EIF1AY*, *RPS4Y2*, and *KDM5D* in the AZFb region cause significant pathology of the testis resulting in diminishing low likelihood of sperm retrieval by surgery (Hopps et al., 2003). **It is reasonable practice to recommend Y chromosomal microdeletion assessment to azoospermic men before surgical sperm extraction to counsel them on the likelihood of retrieval** (Jarow et al., 2010). However, it is also reasonable to omit testing based on the relative rarity of AZFa and AZFb microdeletions in clinical practice.

Genomic Sequence Assessment

A variety of technologies such as DNA microarrays allow multiple single nucleotide polymorphisms (SNPs) and mutations associated with known diseases to be screened for and reported (Hunter et al., 2008; Lazarin et al., 2013; Schena et al., 1995). These reports can be used to identify whether parents are carriers for a large number of genetic diseases and the probability of affected offspring. Recessive disorder carrier screening is increasingly used in couples undergoing assisted reproduction, particularly those who suffer from early pregnancy loss and recurrent miscarriages. Whole-genome sequencing as a clinical tool is also under current development (Moorthie et al., 2013). It is used in research and select diagnostic applications but is not widely used in clinical diagnosis. Although these technologies may ultimately be used to diagnose underlying causes of male reproductive dysfunction, use as general screening tools in evaluating male infertility is not yet warranted.

Cystic Fibrosis Transmembrane Conductance Regulator Mutation Assessment

The relationship between alterations in the CFTR and maldevelopment of the vas is discussed in the section on developmental disorders in this chapter. This section describes what testing is available.

The protein encoded by CFTR forms a channel for chloride ions and possibly bicarbonate and may regulate transport of other ions (Hampton and Stanton, 2010). More than 1600 CFTR mutations have been identified, and they may be mild or severe, defined by whether the full cystic fibrosis disease phenotype results from the mutation (Bombieri et al., 2011; Hampton and Stanton, 2010; Oates and Lamb, 2009; Ratbi et al., 2007; Yu et al., 2012). **The most common severe mutation is ΔF508, which results from deletion of three base pairs that consequently remove the amino acid phenylalanine typically at position 508 of the encoded protein** (Hampton and Stanton, 2010). A high incidence of patients harbor more than one mutation; approximately 46% have two (Yu et al., 2012). **A severe mutation such as ΔF508 on each allele will result in a child with cystic fibrosis, making screening imperative for the prospective father and mother for those suspected of harboring genetic alterations in CFTR.**

Currently available CFTR screening panels typically include 25 to 40 of the most common mutations. Because a subset of known mutations is screened for, a negative result still carries a defined risk. Testing is commercially available for all known mutations but is, not surprisingly, more expensive. CFTR mutation prevalence varies by ethnicity and geography (Bombieri et al., 2011; Boyd et al., 2004; Foresta et al., 2005; Hamosh et al., 1998; Havasi et al., 2010; Li et al., 2010; Ratbi et al., 2007; Schulz et al., 2006). Consequently, the clinician should take into account location and ethnicity in interpreting results. Typically, CFTR screening panel reports are stratified by ethnicity.

> **KEY POINTS: LABORATORY EVALUATION OF MALE INFERTILITY**
>
> - Endocrine assessment of male reproductive status includes total testosterone, the portion of testosterone not bound to SHBG, estradiol, and the pituitary gonadotropins LH and FSH.
> - The semen analysis represents a probabilistic assessment of male reproductive potential. Aside from azoospermia, no specific threshold applied to any parameter absolutely discerns infertility from fertility.
> - The differential diagnosis for men with semen volumes less than 1.0 mL includes ejaculatory ductal obstruction, retrograde ejaculation, and vasal and accessory sex gland maldevelopment such as that occurring with CBAVD.
> - Sperm vitality staining differentiates complete asthenospermia from necrospermia. Common laboratory staining methods differentiate pyospermia from immature germ cells.
> - A preponderance of sperm with round heads, a condition referred to as *globozoospermia*, indicates deficient acrosome formation. The treatment is IVF with ICSI.
> - Disruption in the blood-testis barrier formed by tight junctions between Sertoli cells results in antisperm antibodies, which have varying clinical significance depending on the degree of binding to sperm heads.
> - Genetic screening of the CFTR in men with CBAVD and their partners identifies the presence of severe mutations such as ΔF508 that may result in clinically overt cystic fibrosis in offspring.

IMAGING IN THE EVALUATION OF MALE INFERTILITY

Radiographic or ultrasonographic imaging is infrequently needed in the diagnosis of male reproductive dysfunction and should be ordered cautiously. Likely benign conditions such as testicular microlithiasis may be detected, resulting in patient distress and often unnecessary additional testing (Dagash and MacKinnon, 2007). The following descriptions of imaging in the evaluation of male reproductive dysfunction should not be interpreted as indicated in typical screening.

Scrotal Ultrasonography

Evaluation of the infertile male includes a detailed manual examination of the scrotum and its contents. As with the scrotal physical examination for any urologic evaluation, abnormalities may be detected that warrant scrotal ultrasonography for further investigation. Scrotal ultrasonography is performed by using a high-frequency linear array transducer. Transverse and longitudinal ultrasonography of the testes and color flow Doppler ultrasonography of testicular and

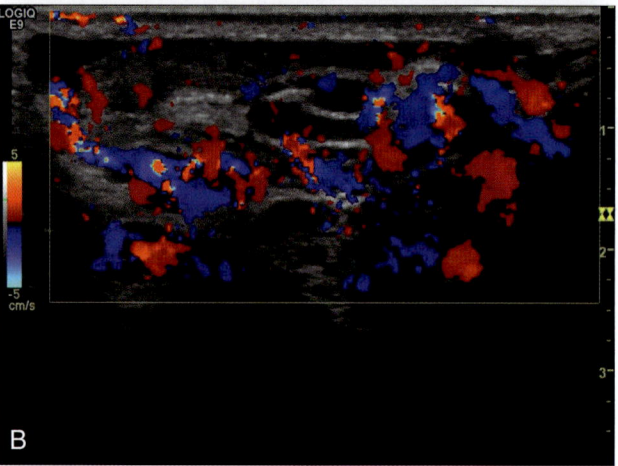

Fig. 66.4. Color duplex Doppler ultrasonography of scrotum demonstrating varicocele. (A) Dilated veins adjacent to the testis. (B) Directional flow in the vessels.

spermatic cord vascularity are performed (Mittal et al., 2017). Testicular volume is calculated as (length × width × anteroposterior diameter) × π/6 and the normal value range is 15 to 20 mL (Ammar et al., 2012). In Fig. 66.4, color duplex Doppler ultrasonography demonstrates a varicocele. Panel A reveals the varicocele to be adjacent to the testis, and the colored areas in panel B demonstrate the direction of flow. The diameter of the largest vein can be measured and reported.

Ultrasonography of the spermatic cord may be indicated if the evaluating physician is uncertain whether a varicocele is present on palpation (Nagler and Grotas, 2009). However, the varicoceles so identified are often so small as to be of questionable clinical significance. Varicoceles become palpable at approximately 2.7 to 3.6 mm in diameter, and surgical treatment of varicoceles smaller than 3.0 mm that are not palpable on physical examination but observed on ultrasound does not result in improved seminal outcomes (Eskew et al., 1993; Hoekstra and Witt, 1995; Jarow et al., 1996; Schiff et al., 2006). **Consequently, the most rational approach based on whether identification of a varicocele is likely to affect treatment outcomes is not to rely on ultrasound as a necessary diagnostic tool.**

Direction of flow may be assessed by color Doppler ultrasound, and investigators have reported that reversal of flow is a positive prognostic sign that surgical treatment of varicocele may result in improved seminal parameters (Hussein, 2006; Schiff et al., 2006). At this time, insufficient numbers of men with nonpalpable varicoceles that are identified with reversal of flow are reported in studies investigating surgical treatment to conclude that color Doppler ultrasound is indicated as a screening modality for infertile men.

In conjunction with TRUS, investigators have observed sensitivity of 75% and specificity of 72% for diagnosing azoospermia caused by spermatogenic dysfunction and sensitivity of 29.8% and specificity of 87% for diagnosing azoospermia caused by obstruction (Abdulwahed et al., 2013). However, given the high accuracy in differentiating azoospermia caused by spermatogenic dysfunction versus obstruction yielded by measuring testis longitudinal axis and assaying serum FSH, it seems more prudent and cost effective not to use ultrasonography in an attempt to diagnose the cause of azoospermia in men with adequate seminal volumes.

Vasography

Contrast vasography in the direction of the abdomen allows determination of patency of the vas deferens from the scrotum to the ejaculatory ducts (Ammar et al., 2012). It is currently rarely performed because image modalities such as TRUS and magnetic resonance imaging (MRI) have superseded it; it is invasive and may result in scar tissue formation in the vasal lumen and obstruction; and injection of saline into the vasal lumen during intended vasal reconstructive procedures with the manual feedback of whether fluid flows easily or backflow occurs offers similar information. **Fluid, contrast or otherwise, should never be injected into the vasal lumen in the direction of the epididymis because it will rupture the delicate epididymal tubules.** Should backflow be identified during intraoperative saline vasography, a monofilament suture such as 4-0 polypropylene may be inserted into the vasal lumen, advanced until resistance is encountered, and then withdrawn and the distance measured to determine the location of the obstruction.

Venography

Further details on this topic are available online at Expert Consult.com.

Transrectal Imaging

The diagnosis of ejaculatory ductal obstruction is considered when azoospermia in conjunction with low seminal volume is encountered (Niederberger, 2011). The earliest and still currently the most prevalent method of investigating whether ejaculatory ductal obstruction in present is TRUS (Jarow, 1996; Niederberger, 2011). **TRUS imaging evidence of ejaculatory duct obstruction includes an anteroposterior seminal vesicle diameter of greater than 1.5 cm with or without a midline prostatic cyst** (Ammar et al., 2012; Jarow, 1996; Niederberger, 2011). Fig. 66.5 demonstrates an intraprostatic cyst, with panel A exhibiting the transverse view and panel B the longitudinal view. Unfortunately, although TRUS is convenient and common, its specificity is low compared with other modalities for identifying whether or not obstruction is present (Purohit et al., 2004). EDO is not always associated with seminal vesicle dilation, and, conversely, normal fertile men can at times have dilated seminal vesicles depending on the duration of sexual abstinence (Mogdil et al., 2016). These other assessments include radiographic imaging after injection of contrast directly into the seminal vesicles, or vesiculography; aspiration of the seminal vesicles to determine whether sperm is present; and injection of diluted indigo carmine or methylene blue dye into the seminal vesicles and observation by cystoscopy of whether the colored dye flows from the ductal orifices at the verumontanum, a technique referred to as *chromotubation* (Purohit et al., 2004). In a small series, vesiculography and chromotubation were more accurate than TRUS by a margin of 25% (Purohit et al., 2004). However, these techniques are more invasive and expensive, and an incremental improvement in diagnostic accuracy compared with TRUS if conclusively demonstrated in larger studies may not justify the additional risk and cost.

Further details on this topic are available online at Expert Consult.com.

Abdominal Imaging

Further details on this topic are available online at Expert Consult.com.

Cranial Imaging

Cranial MRI allows assessment of whether hyperprolactinemia is associated with an anatomic pituitary lesion and is more useful

Chapter 66 Male Infertility

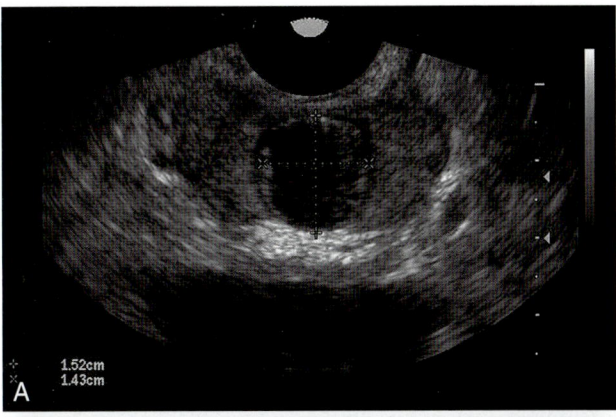

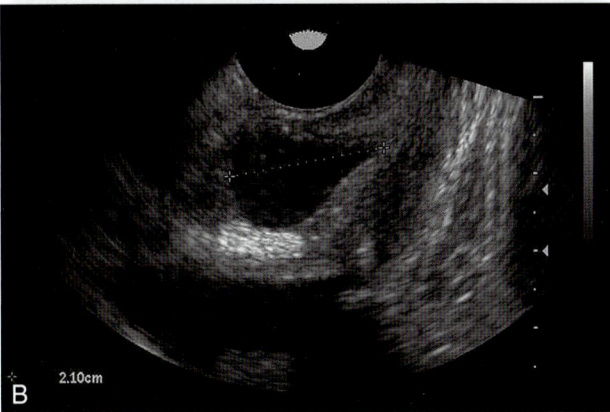

Fig. 66.5. Transrectal ultrasonography revealing an intraprostatic cyst. (A) Transverse. (B) Longitudinal. (Courtesy Marcelo Vieira.)

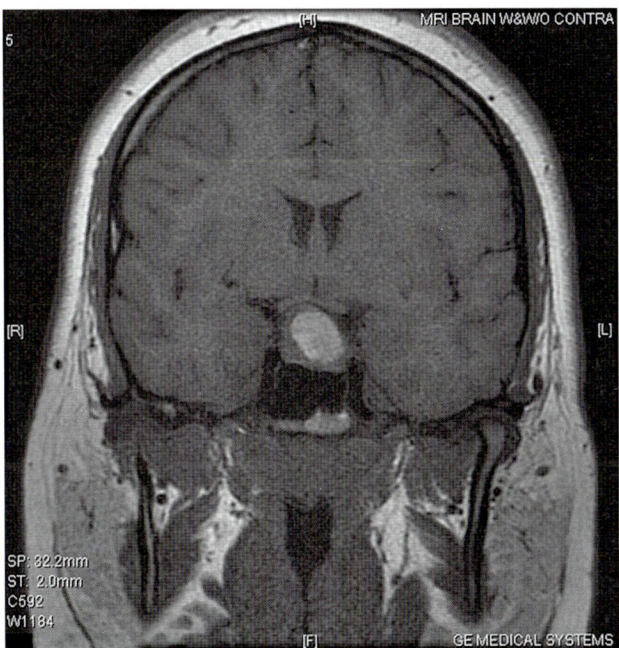

Fig. 66.6. Large pituitary macroadenoma revealed by cranial magnetic resonance imaging.

when prolactin levels are twice the upper limit of normal (Niederberger, 2011; Rhoden et al., 2003). MRI may distinguish between microadenomas and macroadenomas and may assist in judging whether medical or surgical therapy is indicated (Johnsen et al., 1991). Fig. 66.6 demonstrates a cranial MRI revealing a large pituitary macroadenoma.

> **KEY POINT: IMAGING**
>
> - Imaging can reveal sequelae of genetic conditions, such as congenital absence of the vas deferens and renal aplasia, and it can differentiate reasons for seminal hypovolemia, such as ejaculatory ductal obstruction, but it is infrequently necessary to establish diagnoses such as varicocele or spermatogenic dysfunction.

TESTIS HISTOPATHOLOGY

Further details on this topic are available online at Expert Consult.com.

ASSISTED REPRODUCTION

Further details on this topic are available online at Expert Consult.com.

Diagnoses and Therapies

The understanding of the pathophysiology of male reproductive dysfunction has expanded in past years but remains incomplete. The difficulties inherent in the probabilistic nature of reproduction and its assessment pose challenges to the physician evaluating and consequently treating male infertility. However, sufficient information is known for the treating physician to make reasoned assumptions about whether a pathologic explanation involving the man exists, its likely basis, and plausible therapy. This section reviews discrete diagnoses and possible medical therapies.

Genetic Syndromes

With the completion of sequencing of the human genome in 2004, knowledge of how the genes involved in human reproduction conspire to create fully formed and viable sperm will follow (International Human Genome Sequencing Consortium, 2004). As discussed in the section of this chapter describing genomic sequence assessment, broad panels are available that identify carrier risk of known genetic diseases, and whole-genomic sequencing is being used in research. However, current use of broad panels and use of whole-genome sequencing, should it become immediately available, as general screening tools for male reproductive dysfunction are hampered by the lack of an understanding of how the majority of the genetic mechanisms involved in spermatogenesis function in concert to produce viable sperm. A certain number of genetic associations are known to be involved in male infertility, and these are detailed in subsequent sections. In this section, general genetic causes of male fertility involving chromosomal number, structure, and epigenetic mechanisms are discussed.

Chromosomal Numerical Disorders

The presence of a supernumerary X chromosome yielding 47,XXY, or Klinefelter syndrome, is the most commonly identified genetic cause of male infertility (Groth et al., 2013; Oates and Lamb, 2009; Sigman, 2012). A 47,XXY genotype is observed in 1 in 500 to 1000 live births, and in more than 95% of affected adults results in azoospermia, small testes, and elevated gonadotropin levels (Groth et al., 2013; Maiburg et al., 2012). Approximately 75% of children have learning disabilities, and 63% to 85% of men have low testosterone levels (Groth et al., 2013). **Body morphology features such as increased height are observed in only 30% of Klinefelter males, and consequently the condition cannot be excluded by physical examination and physical inspection alone** (Groth et al., 2013). Increased incidence of other disorders related to the testis such as mediastinal germ cell tumors is documented in men with Klinefelter syndrome, suggesting broader testicular effects (Sokol, 2012).

A nonmosaic 47,XXY karyotype is observed in 80% to 90% of men with Klinefelter syndrome (Maiburg et al., 2012). The remainder are mosaic 46,XY/47,XXY or have additional or structurally abnormal X chromosomes (Maiburg et al., 2012). In the man, approximately 8% have sperm in the ejaculate, and the remainder are azoospermic (Oates, 2012). Within the testis, approximately half of men with Klinefelter syndrome have sufficient mature sperm amenable to surgical sperm retrieval for use with IVF and ICSI (Oates, 2012). **Early age at diagnosis appears to offer a more favorable prognosis** (Mehta and Paduch, 2012).

Until recently, fertility management of men with Klinefelter syndrome was limited to diagnosing the condition with karyotype analysis, assessing whether sperm was present in the ejaculate, and attempting to extract sperm from the testis if it was not. Many of these men are identified shortly after puberty with low testosterone levels and prescribed exogenous testosterone alone, suppressing native spermatogenesis if present. Citing the progressive decline in spermatogenesis over time, investigators have argued for aggressive management including surgical extraction of sperm at early to mid puberty before initiation of therapy with exogenous testosterone and aromatase inhibitor (Mehta and Paduch, 2012; Mehta et al., 2013). This approach is primarily investigational at this time.

Structural Chromosomal Anomalies

As discussed in the section detailing Y chromosome microdeletion testing, investigators observed three regions on the Y chromosome, designated AZFa, AZFb, and AZFc, to be associated with azoospermia or oligospermia (Oates and Lamb, 2009). **Microdeletions of AZFc currently have unclear clinical significance, whereas AZFa and AZFb microdeletions are nearly always associated with absence of retrievable sperm from the testis** (Giachini et al., 2008; Hopps et al., 2003; Lardone et al., 2007; Mulhall et al., 1997; Oates et al., 2002; Stouffs et al., 2008; Visser et al., 2009; Wu et al., 2007). **AZFa microdeletions have particular clinical significance because spatially the AZFa region appears to be localized distinctly from AZFb and AZFc, with the latter two overlapping** (Oates and Lamb, 2009). In deletion carriers presenting with oligozoospermia, there is a potential risk of a progressive decrease of sperm concentration over time, and sperm cryopreservation can be considered (Krausz and Casamonti, 2017).

Other structural anomalies of the Y chromosome may be identified by karyotypic analysis (Oates and Lamb, 2009). Two terminal breaks in both chromosome arms and subsequent fusion may lead to a ring Y chromosome, or r(Y), with variable phenotype depending on the amount of chromosomal material lost (Arnedo et al., 2005). Karyotypic anomalies in somatic chromosomes may also be associated with infertility (Mau-Holzmann, 2005).

Epigenetic Anomalies

Not only must the DNA sequence be intact for successful function of the male gamete, but also the DNA must be tightly coiled and packaged (O'Flynn O'Brien et al., 2010). As discussed in the section describing denatured sperm DNA assays, investigators have constructed various methods of interrogating sperm DNA structure with unclear prognostic outcomes at present. Other components of sperm DNA packaging may yield future diagnostic tools; for example, animal studies revealed that premature translation of protamine 1 resulted in postmeiotic maturational arrest in mouse spermatogenesis, and protamine 2 deficiency led to sperm DNA damage and embryo demise (Cho et al., 2003; Lee et al., 1995). In humans, evidence links protamine 2 precursors and the protamine 1–protamine 2 ratio to sperm DNA quality and IVF outcomes (Aoki et al., 2006; de Mateo et al., 2009; Torregrosa et al., 2006). Histones also offer a future target for clinical assessment. They are highly, specifically localized along human sperm DNA, and researchers have observed histone variants to relate to fertility in bulls (de Oliveira et al., 2013; Hammoud et al., 2009). Sonnack et al. (2002) observed that infertile men have significantly decreased levels of histone H4 acetylation associated with impaired spermatogenesis.

DNA methylation allows coordination of gene expression in somatic cell development (Boissonnas et al., 2013). Once thought to be of little consequence in sperm, this epigenetic modification is now considered to play key roles in spermatogenesis and embryogenesis (Boissonnas et al., 2013; Carrell, 2012; Molaro et al., 2011). The pattern of gene promoter methylation is substantially different in somatic and sperm cell DNA and may have future clinical applicability in the assessment of male reproductive potential (Molaro et al., 2011). In addition, multiple RNA species (mRNA, microRNA, Piwi-interacting RNA, etc.) can directly and indirectly affect the sperm's expression profile (Craig et al., 2017).

Testicular Causes

The testis essentially consists of two compartments, the seminiferous tubules that house the developing male gametes and the interstitial spaces between the tubules, inhabited by Leydig cells. Both are required for sperm production, which then must conclude with transit of the male gamete outward. Testicular causes of male reproductive dysfunction may consequently be considered to derive from pathology in the production of sperm in the seminiferous epithelium or in the synthesis of testosterone by Leydig cells, or obstruction in the microductal system transporting sperm toward the ejaculatory ducts.

Spermatogenic Dysfunction

As discussed in the section describing testis histopathology, dysfunction in the seminiferous epithelium may be globally described as hypospermatogenesis, which indicates a decrease in sperm production; maturation arrest, which represents halting of the sequence of steps of the male gamete at some point through premeiotic, meiotic, and postmeiotic development; and Sertoli cell–only syndrome, which denotes a complete depopulation of spermatogonial cells. The molecular mechanisms leading to completion of spermatogenesis are still under investigation, and in the future it is likely that genomic, proteomic, and metabolomic markers will become available for clinical use to diagnose specific causes of spermatogenic dysfunction (Kovac et al., 2013). At present, the primary means of assessing deficiencies in spermatogenesis is histopathologic inspection. As previously described, if azoospermia is present, in 89% of cases spermatogenic dysfunction is identified as the cause with an FSH value greater than 7.6 IU/L and the testis long axis 4.6 cm or less (Schoor et al., 2001).

Another form of spermatogenic pathology arises in the testis and impedes sperm in the ejaculate. In the seminiferous epithelium, Sertoli cell tight junctions protect haploid germ cells from circulating immunologic cells, forming a blood-testis barrier (Brannigan, 2011). **Pathologic conditions that disrupt this blood-testis barrier may expose the immunologically protected spermatids and spermatozoa to antibody formation, which may cause sperm agglutination, impeded sperm motility, and reduced fertilizing potential** (Brannigan, 2011). These conditions include obstruction in the male reproductive tract such as that occurring after vasectomy; inflammation associated with orchitis, prostatitis, or sexually transmitted disease; exposure to heat with varicocele, cryptorchidism, or external sources such as hot tubs; trauma and testis torsion; and genetic associations including thymic maldevelopment and the HLA-B28 haplotype (Walsh and Turek, 2009). Assays for antisperm antibodies are detailed in the section describing the laboratory evaluation of semen.

For treatment of antisperm antibodies, simple measures include use of condoms and washing sperm. Neither has good evidence to substantiate its use (Walsh and Turek, 2009). Washing may remove unbound antibodies, but those that matter remain bound to sperm (Walsh and Turek, 2009). More direct treatments include immunosuppression with corticosteroids and ART. Two controlled trials of corticosteroids offer conflicting results, with one demonstrating improved fertility and the other not (Haas and Manganiello, 1987; Hendry et al., 1990). Whether because of a lack of compelling evidence or because of more direct results, IVF and ICSI have become common treatment for antisperm antibodies.

Steroidogenic Dysfunction

The terms *hypergonadotropic hypogonadism*, *primary hypogonadism*, and *primary hypoandrogenism* refer to impaired testosterone synthesis caused by Leydig cell dysfunction (Sokol, 2009). **This entity is typically identified by elevated LH levels and decreased circulating testosterone** (Sokol, 2009). However, Leydig cell dysfunction may exist concurrently with pituitary insufficiency, and these men will have decreased testosterone concentrations and variable LH levels that do not reflect the typical increase associated with primary Leydig cell insufficiency (Sokol, 2009). Increasing age is a condition associated with decreasing androgen and blunted pituitary response (Feldman et al., 2002; Sokol, 2009).

An absolute requirement for spermatogenesis is intratesticular steroidogenesis, which appears to be especially important for the postmeiotic maturation of sperm (Caroppo, 2011). Men with Klinefelter syndrome often have lower levels of circulating testosterone, but impaired Leydig cell function may not be the only mechanism responsible for a phenotype that resembles those of hypoandrogenic males (Oates, 2012; Sokol, 2009). Investigators have reported evidence of Leydig cell dysfunction in humans associated with mutations in the LH receptor gene and in FSH receptor–deficient mice, and as the genes responsible for steroidogenesis become clinically available for assessment in humans, it is anticipated that more cases of Leydig cell dysfunction with genetic causes will be identified (Baker et al., 2003; Latronico et al., 1996). Other potential clinical causes of Leydig cell dysfunction include orchitis, cytotoxic chemotherapy, and exposure to environmental toxicants (Skakkebaek et al., 2001; Sokol, 2009).

There is currently no accepted therapy for hypoandrogenism caused by Leydig cell insufficiency (Sokol, 2009). Exogenous testosterone is not indicated, because insufficient testicular testosterone concentrations are achieved for spermatogenesis, and pituitary LH release is suppressed (Niederberger, 2011). **Should azoospermia be associated with low testosterone concentrations and significantly elevated LH levels, if the patient desires paternity, the treatment is surgical sperm extraction.**

Microductal Obstruction

Either by congenital or acquired means, the epididymis or scrotal vas deferens may be obstructed. If obstruction is bilateral, azoospermia typically results. As discussed in the section describing the endocrine evaluation, the physician may use the FSH level combined with the testis longitudinal axis as measured by calipers to predict whether azoospermia is associated with obstruction; 96% of men with obstructive azoospermia had FSH concentration of 7.6 IU/L or less and testis long axis greater than 4.6 cm (Schoor et al., 2001). Fig. 66.11 illustrates an algorithm for the evaluation of azoospermia. Microductal obstruction may also be unilateral: in that case, bulk seminal parameters may be reduced or not depending on the function of the contralateral testis. If unilateral obstruction is present with adequate spermatogenesis in the ipsilateral testis and the existence of spermatogenic pathology in the contralateral testis, impaired bulk seminal parameters may result and microductal reconstruction may be indicated.

As discussed in the section describing evaluation of the surgical history of an infertile male, herniorrhaphy especially with mesh may result in obstruction of the vas deferens in the inguinal canal (Hallén et al., 2011, 2012; Maciel et al., 2007; Shin et al., 2005; Tekatli et al., 2012). If both vasa are occluded, azoospermia likely results.

Pituitary Dysfunction

The pituitary hormones LH and FSH regulate spermatogenesis: LH directs Leydig cell steroidogenesis; and FSH controls spermatogenesis via the Sertoli cells (Caroppo, 2011). If by intrinsic dysfunction or external pathology LH, FSH, or both are suppressed, spermatogenesis suffers.

Hypogonadotropic Hypogonadism

Hypogonadotropic hypogonadism refers to the condition of decreased pituitary hormonal secretion. **Kallmann described anosmia associated with decreased pituitary function, and the syndrome bears his name** (Kallmann and Schoenfeld, 1944). The incidence of the syndrome is approximately 1 in 10,000 males, and the mode of inheritance is most frequently autosomal recessive, but autosomal-dominant and X-linked recessive patterns are also observed (Bhagavath et al., 2006; Sokol, 2009). Investigators have identified associations with Kallmann syndrome and the *KAL1* gene encoding anosmin-1 responsible for neurotropic growth factors during embryogenesis, the *GNRHR* gene encoding gonadotropin-releasing hormone (GnRH) receptor, the pituitary-specific transcription factor PIT1, the PIT1-related transcription factor PROP1, the G protein–coupled Kisspeptin receptor GPR54, the homeobox genes *HESX1*, *LEX3*, and *LEX4*, and others (Bhagavath et al., 2006; Dattani et al., 1998; de Roux et al., 2003; Kim et al., 2003; Newbern et al., 2013; Sobrier et al., 2004; Wu et al., 1998). Researchers noted approximately 10% of men with Kallmann syndrome to harbor mutations in either the *GNRHR* or *KAL1* gene (Bhagavath et al., 2006).

Treatment includes replacement of LH with human chorionic gonadotropin (hCG) and replacement of FSH with recombinant

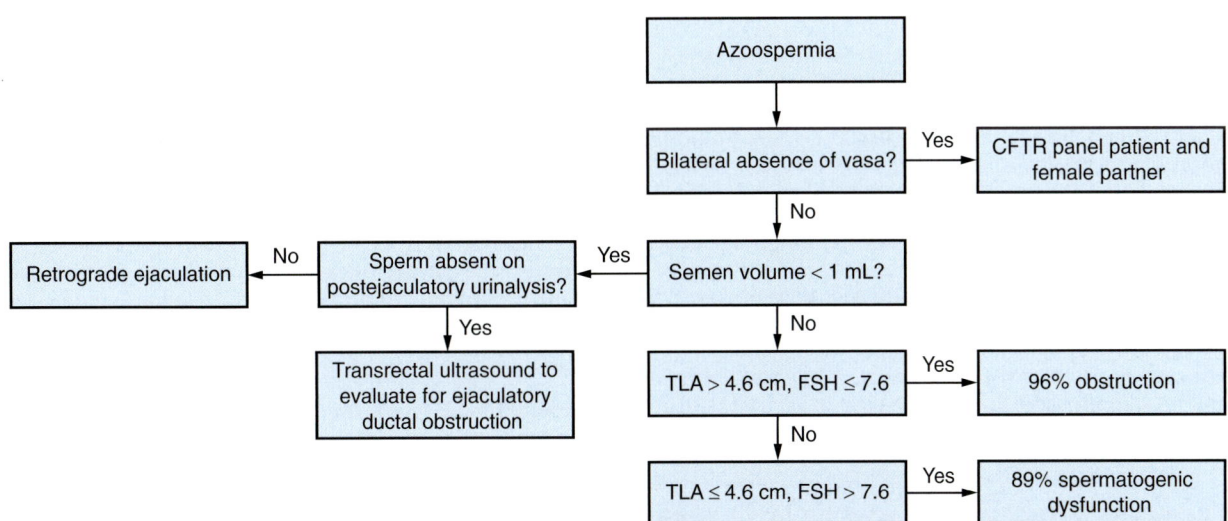

Fig. 66.11. Algorithm for evaluation of azoospermia. *CFTR,* Cystic fibrosis transmembrane conductance regulator; *FSH,* follicle-stimulating hormone; *TLA,* testis longitudinal axis measured by caliper orchidometer.

FSH (rFSH) or hMG, which exhibits LH- and FSH-like activity (Sokol, 2009). Treatment with hCG alone may initiate spermatogenesis; if hMG or rFSH is prescribed, after spermatogenesis returns, these agents may be withdrawn after several months of therapy (Sokol, 2009). Men who are identified as having Kallmann syndrome later in life when reproductive interests occur have often been prescribed exogenous androgen since adolescence. These men may require gonadotropin therapy for 1 to 2 years before sperm becomes evident in the ejaculate. Typical doses for intramuscular or subcutaneous hCG are 1500 to 5000 IU two to three times weekly to a maximum of 10,000 IU/wk and are titrated to serum testosterone results (Hussein et al., 2013; Sokol, 2009). The dose of hMG is 75 IU two to three times weekly, typically administered subcutaneously (Sokol, 2009).

Rarely, men may have isolated decreased secretion of either LH or FSH (Giltay et al., 2004; Sokol, 2009). Isolated LH deficiency was termed the "fertile eunuch syndrome" and characterizes men who have features of hypoandrogenism because of low levels of LH but who produce sperm as a result of adequate FSH (Sokol, 2009). Conversely, men with isolated FSH deficiency have suppressed spermatogenesis but adequate androgenization (Giltay et al., 2004). Treatment of these uncommon conditions includes replacement with the appropriate gonadotropin (Giltay et al., 2004; Sokol, 2009). Men may also infrequently have isolated hypothalamic GnRH deficiency (Nachtigall et al., 1997). Treatment includes GnRH administration by a subcutaneous portable mini-infusion pump every 2 hours, and, as with treatment for Kallmann syndrome, long-term courses of at least 6 months' duration may be required (Nachtigall et al., 1997).

Kallmann and the associated syndromes of hypogonadotropic hypogonadism are the most severe forms of conditions resulting in diminished pituitary hormonal secretion. **Incomplete forms with hypoandrogenism associated with serum LH concentrations above those observed with Kallmann syndrome but lower than expected for the diminished testosterone are common** (Bhagavath et al., 2006). For these men, pituitary stimulation with antiestrogenic agents such as clomiphene or tamoxifen or with aromatase inhibitors such as anastrozole or letrozole may restore testosterone levels and possibly improve spermatogenesis (Hussein et al., 2005, 2013; Ioannidou-Kadis et al., 2006; Katz et al., 2012; Moskovic et al., 2012; Raman and Schlegel, 2002; Roth et al., 2013; Siddiq and Sigman, 2002; Sussman et al., 2008; Whitten et al., 2006). Clomiphene citrate is a selective estrogen receptor modulator that is currently FDA approved for women. It has been used as an off-label treatment for male hypogonadism and infertility for more than 40 years, and it is proven to significantly increase testosterone levels without changes in PSA or hematocrit levels (Chandrapal et al., 2016). The initial dose of clomiphene citrate is typically 25 mg every day or 50 mg every other day and is increased by titrating to serum testosterone to a maximum of 100 mg daily (Hussein et al., 2005, 2013; Sussman et al., 2008). In some studies, the titration target is restoration of normal androgen levels; in others, it is elevated at 600 to 800 ng/dL (Hussein et al., 2005, 2013; Sussman et al., 2008). The typical dosage of anastrozole is 1 mg daily, although there is not a current standardization of dosing given the increasing knowledge of the role of estradiol in male sexual and reproductive health (Raman and Schlegel, 2002).

Prader-Willi syndrome is characterized by failure to thrive in infancy associated with a poor suck reflex followed by loss of satiety in early childhood, which may lead to marked obesity if poorly controlled (Cassidy and Driscoll, 2009). Its incidence is approximately 1 in 15,000 to 30,000 (Cassidy and Driscoll, 2009). Features associated with the syndrome include hypogonadism, small testes, dysmorphic facies, growth hormone deficiency with short stature and small hands and feet, pain insensitivity, and cognitive disorders such as obsessive-compulsive traits (Bervini and Herzog, 2013). Researchers have suspected that the association of growth hormone deficiency and hypogonadism with the syndrome derive from hypothalamic dysfunction, but the precise pathophysiology is still uncertain (Bervini and Herzog, 2013). Prader-Willi syndrome is typically caused by the loss of expression of genes located on human chromosome 15q11-q13 by means of failed imprinting, which is the epigenetic phenomenon that allows genes on only one chromosome to be active (Bervini and Herzog, 2013). **In the healthy state, the genes located on the maternal chromosome 15q11-q13 are silenced, and those on the paternal chromosome are active; in Prader-Willi syndrome, the maternal genes are silenced and the paternal ones inactive** (Bervini and Herzog, 2013).

Pituitary Tumors and Diseases

Space-occupying lesions in the sella turcica such as secretory and nonsecretory tumors and craniopharyngiomas may compress the anterior pituitary and result in varying degrees of LH and FSH suppression (Sokol, 2009). The most common kind of pituitary tumor resulting in male reproductive dysfunction secretes prolactin and is commonly associated with other symptoms such as erectile dysfunction (Sokol, 2009). These tumors are rare; as described in the section discussing the endocrine evaluation, in one series of 1035 men undergoing an infertility evaluation, only 4, or 0.4%, had hyperprolactinemia (Sigman and Jarow, 1997). This finding questions the value of including prolactin as a routine assay in screening infertile men, especially those who are otherwise asymptomatic (Niederberger, 2011; Sigman and Jarow, 1997; Sokol, 2009). **In general, mild elevations of prolactin in the range of 20 to 50 µg/L do not warrant further evaluation; if prolactin is significantly elevated, cranial MRI is indicated** (Niederberger, 2011). The dopamine agonists bromocriptine and cabergoline may be prescribed for prolactin-secreting adenomas for which surgery is not indicated, with cabergoline exhibiting fewer side effects (Klibanski, 2010).

Other Pituitary Lesions

Diseases infiltrating the pituitary may also suppress its secretion of hormones, including granulomata of infection, sarcoidosis, and histiocytosis (Sokol, 2009). Deposition of iron by hemochromatosis or repeated blood transfusions may also invoke hypogonadotropic hypogonadism (Sokol, 2009). Systemic diseases such as morbid obesity, chronic malnutrition, and type 2 diabetes may also be associated with hypogonadotropic hypogonadism (Dhindsa et al., 2004; Sokol, 2009). Treatment of these disorders is aimed at ameliorating the underlying condition.

Extrapituitary Endocrine Modulators

As described in the section discussing the role of investigating endocrine modulators when taking the history of an infertile man, exogenous androgenic agents, especially testosterone, suppress pituitary gonadotropins (Grimes et al., 2012). Also discussed in that section are cannabis, antipsychotics, opioids, and environmental toxicants, which inhibit pituitary function via estrogenic and dopaminergic pathways (Carlsen et al., 1992; Gorzalka et al., 2010; Stimmel and Gutierrez, 2006; Subirán et al., 2011). Treatment is directed toward removing the offending agent when possible. CAH, especially in milder forms that manifest clinically in adolescence or adult life, may be associated with hypogonadotropic hypogonadism (Reisch et al., 2011). A high incidence of testicular adrenal rest tumors adds to the reproductive dysfunction present in these men (Claahsen-van der Grinten et al., 2008; Reisch et al., 2011). Fertility may be restored with corticosteroid therapy (Claahsen-van der Grinten et al., 2007). However, side effects such as weight gain and skin changes from the lengthy application of therapy required to address the long duration of spermatogenesis may prove problematic (Claahsen-van der Grinten et al., 2007).

Extratesticular Endocrine Dysfunction

Because estradiol inhibits gonadotropin release, conditions that increase its concentration may lead to hypogonadotropic hypogonadism. These include the pharmacologic agents described in the section discussing medications that alter the ratio of estrogen to androgen through a variety of means (Bowman et al., 2012). When possible, use of another agent may improve fertility. As described in the section discussing the general physical examination of the infertile male, elevated estradiol is associated with obesity by the mass of adipose cells containing aromatase (Aggerholm et al., 2008; Chavarro et al., 2010; Hammoud et al., 2006, 2010b; Hofny et al., 2010). Multiple factors are suspected to associate obesity with male infertility, and hypogonadotropic hypogonadism may or may not be involved, including "neohormones" leptin and kisspeptin and other comorbidities such as diabetes and sleep apnea (Aggerholm et al., 2008; Craig et al., 2017; George et al., 2010; Hammoud et al., 2006; Hofny et al., 2010; Munzberg et al., 2005; Paasch et al., 2010; Pauli et al., 2008; Teerds et al., 2011). In 2006 a study conducting a group of 20,620 families in Iowa and North Carolina demonstrated a dose-response relationship between BMI and male infertility (Sallmen et al., 2006). These findings were confirmed in other studies around the globe (Nguyen et al., 2007; Ramlau-Hansen et al., 2007). Besides increased aromatization of testosterone to estradiol peripherally, obesity is also responsible for reducing pulse amplitude of the LH secretion from the pituitary as well as decreased response to LH by the testis (Vermeulen et al., 1993). The question remains regarding whether diet, exercise, and weight reduction improve male reproductive potential. Limited animal studies in an obese rodent model suggest that diet and exercise improve sperm parameters, but human studies are sparse and inconclusive (Braga et al., 2012; Luconi et al., 2013; Nguyen et al., 2007; Palmer et al., 2012). In the absence of conclusive data demonstrating a causative effect between weight loss and improved male fertility, it still seems prudent to recommend it in obese men because the ancillary health benefits are certain. Nonetheless, male obesity appears to affect clinical pregnancy, miscarriage, and live birth rates in couples submitted to assisted reproductive technology (Campbell et al., 2015; Provost et al., 2016; Thomsen et al., 2014).

Researchers have investigated the use of aromatase inhibitors such as anastrozole, letrozole, and testolactone for elevated estradiol, demonstrating that for the typical male patient, testosterone levels increase and estradiol levels decline (Gregoriou et al., 2012; Raman and Schlegel, 2002; Schlegel, 2012; Shoshany et al., 2017). Limited data support that sperm parameters may concurrently improve (Gregoriou et al., 2012; Raman and Schlegel, 2002; Schlegel, 2012; Shoshany et al., 2017). As described in the section discussing the endocrine evaluation of male infertility, researchers have proposed that a testosterone-to-estradiol ratio in nanograms per deciliter (ng/dL) to picograms per milliliter (pg/mL) of less than 10 : 1 indicates aromatase overactivity that would benefit from inhibitory therapy (Gregoriou et al., 2012; Raman and Schlegel, 2002; Schlegel, 2012). Prescribers should be cautious in the long-term use of aromatase inhibitors, because bone density in the male may be estradiol dependent, and long-term studies of this class of drug in men are lacking (Khosla et al., 2001; Kim et al., 2013).

Mutations in the androgen receptor *(AR)* gene located on the long arm of the X chromosome at banding region Xq11-12 lead to a spectrum of disorders from complete testicular feminization to male infertility (Davis-Dao et al., 2007; Dowsing et al., 1999; Sokol, 2009). Male reproductive dysfunction appears to be related to a longer cytosine-adenine-guanine (CAG) repeat length in exon one of the *AR* gene (Davis-Dao et al., 2007; Dowsing et al., 1999; Sokol, 2009; Xiao et al., 2016). **Male infertility associated with AR insensitivity is characterized by increased testosterone, estradiol, and LH to variable degrees with typical FSH levels; significantly elevated testosterone in the presence of impaired male fertility should consequently raise the suspicion of AR resistance** (Sokol, 2009). High-dose testosterone therapy may result in improved spermatogenesis, but data on this form of treatment are limited (Tordjman et al., 2014). Pregnancy may be achieved by ICSI with ejaculated sperm or that derived by surgical extraction from the testis (Massin et al., 2012; Tordjman et al., 2014).

Because dihydrotestosterone regulates the anatomic development of external male genitalia, mutations in the gene encoding isozyme 2 of 5α-reductase located on the short arm of chromosome 2 at banding region 2p23 result in a spectrum ranging from a female to a male phenotype (Johnson et al., 1986; Sokol, 2009; Thigpen et al., 1993). Phenotypic females with 5α-reductase 2 mutations may harbor testes with intact spermatogenesis (Johnson et al., 1986; Thigpen et al., 1993). No medical treatment is currently available for this disorder. Pregnancies have been successfully attained with ICSI from sperm from men with 5α-reductase-2 deficiency (Kang et al., 2011; Matsubara et al., 2010).

Developmental Disorders

Anatomic development that results in aberrant genital formation may manifest in later life as male infertility. Main areas of maldevelopment include the testes, the external genitalia, and the reproductive microductal system.

Intersex or Disorders of Sexual Development

Disorders of sex development (DSD) are congenital diseases in which the chromosomal, gonadal, or anatomic sex is abnormal and embraces a wide-ranging spectrum of phenotypes classified in five different groups (Hughes et al., 2006). The first class involves disorders of gonadal differentiation; the second comprehends ovotesticular DSD (formerly known as true hermaphroditism); the third includes 46,XX DSD (formerly known as female pseudohermaphroditism); the fourth encloses 46,XY DSD (formerly known as male pseudohermaphroditism); and the fifth group consists of unclassified forms (Hughes et al., 2006). DSDs are increasingly being understood as the consequence of specific aberrant genes, and the current nomenclature used to describe intersex now includes the karyotype, a clinically descriptive term, and the molecular basis of the disorder if it is known (Ono and Harley, 2013). An example of an intersex description using this nomenclature may be "46,XY DSD complete gonadal dysgenesis with SF1 mutation" (Ono and Harley, 2013). Genes identified to be involved in DSD are too numerous to be listed here, and the reader is referred to Ono and Harley for a current review (Ono and Harley, 2013). In general, the genes involved in DSDs that manifest as male infertility do so by developmental anatomic abnormalities, abnormal or absent spermatogenesis, general endocrinopathy, or encoding for defective endocrine receptors and target complexes (Oates and Lamb, 2009; Ono and Harley, 2013).

Hypospadias and Epispadias

Aberrant anatomic location of the urethra in hypospadias or epispadias may result in deposition of semen too distal in the vaginal vault (Niederberger, 2011). These men may have adequate bulk seminal parameters, and if screening semen analysis is performed before physical examination of the man, the diagnosis may be missed. Hypospadias appears to have genetic and environmental causes, with genetic polymorphisms playing a predominant role rather than isolated gene defects (Macedo et al., 2012). The pathophysiology of epispadias is different from that of hypospadias, and it is typically considered on the spectrum of bladder-exstrophy-epispadias complex (BEEC) disorders (Rasouly and Lu, 2013).

Cryptorchidism

The basis of cryptorchidism and the relationship of the disorder to male reproductive function is detailed in the section of this chapter describing childhood diseases in the reproductive history of the infertile male. The most significant feature related to the prognosis of cryptorchidism is whether the condition is unilateral or bilateral (Lee, 2005; Lee et al., 2001; Miller et al., 2001).

Microductal Aplasia

The vas deferens may fail to develop on one side or both. The distinction is significant, because the pathophysiologic basis of each is different.

Congenital Unilateral Absence of the Vas Deferens. As described in the section detailing the physical examination of the infertile male, unilateral absence of the vas deferens implies that wolffian, or mesonephric, ductal development on the ipsilateral side was aberrant. As these ducts become in embryogenesis the epididymis, vas deferens, and ejaculatory duct, the proximal and distal portions may be malformed or absent as well (Lewis and Kaplan, 2009). The most important consideration if unilateral absence of the vas is observed is that because renal development is coupled with wolffian ductal development, a solitary absent vas deferens may signal renal agenesis (Niederberger, 2011).

Congenital Bilateral Absence of the Vas Deferens. Oates et al. reported in the early 1990s that males with CBAVD had a high frequency of genetic sequence abnormalities associated with cystic fibrosis (Anguiano et al., 1992). **Coupled with the observation that in nearly all men with cystic fibrosis the vasa are absent bilaterally, these findings suggested that CBAVD is frequently a phenotype for a spectrum of disorders involving mutations in the gene responsible for cystic fibrosis** (Anguiano et al., 1992). As described in the section discussing genomic sequence assessment in the laboratory evaluation of the infertile male, that gene encodes a predominantly chloride ion channel termed the *cystic fibrosis transmembrane conductance regulator*, and currently more than 1600 mutations in the gene have been identified, which vary in the severity of the phenotype from CBAVD to cystic fibrosis (Bombieri et al., 2011; Hampton and Stanton, 2010; Oates and Lamb, 2009; Ratbi et al., 2007; Yu et al., 2012).

It is currently believed that two genetic causes of CBAVD exist: one that results from mutations in CFTR and another that results from alterations in as-yet-unidentified other genes involved in mesonephric ductal development (Oates and Lamb, 2009). CFTR mutations represent a spectrum of disease severity; if both alleles harbor severe mutations, cystic fibrosis results, and if one or both alleles contain the milder forms, CBAVD may occur (Bombieri et al., 2011; Hampton and Stanton, 2010; Oates and Lamb, 2009; Ratbi et al., 2007; Yu et al., 2012). As described in the section detailing genomic sequence assessment, the most common mutation is ΔF508, which is severe (Hampton and Stanton, 2010). **The carrier frequency for cystic fibrosis gene mutations is high—approximately 1 in 20 in persons of northern European descent—and it is consequently important to investigate the CFTR status of the female partner of a man identified to have CBAVD in addition to his genetic evaluation** (Oates and Lamb, 2009). Symptoms such as chronic sinus or respiratory infections may be overlooked if mild, and the urologist diagnosing CBAVD may be the first to uncover an indolent form of cystic fibrosis (Oates and Lamb, 2009).

Spermatogenesis in men with CBAVD is typically normal, and ICSI with surgically extracted sperm is typically effective (Kamal et al., 2010). Nevertheless, one study has shown that sperm obtained from men with CFTR mutations and CBAVD were associated with an increased risk of miscarriage and stillbirth after ICSI (Lu et al., 2014). Genetic counseling taking into account the CFTR genetic assessment of the affected man and his female partner allows for the couple to understand the likelihood of cystic fibrosis in offspring and the implications of carrier status, and it may be performed by the urologist or a clinical geneticist.

Varicocele

The diagnosis of varicocele was discussed in the section detailing the physical examination of the infertile man: why imaging such as ultrasound is most rationally not recommended for the screening evaluation of a varicocele is discussed in the section describing imaging.

That most men with varicocele have sperm present on semen analysis has proved to be one of the most confounding aspects of its diagnosis and treatment. As discussed in the section describing the semen analysis, the results of this assay are assessed in a probabilistic context with substantial variability, making analytical statements concerning its effect on male reproductive potential difficult. Taking into account confounding factors involving the female partner that are often opaque and difficult to control in analyses, determining the effect of a varicocele on pregnancy, miscarriage, and birth becomes intractable. However, substantial evidence links varicocele to spermatogenic dysfunction and impaired male reproductive potential.

Because the left internal spermatic vein drains into the left renal vein approximately 8 to 10 cm superior to the entry of the right internal spermatic vein draining into the vena cava, the hydrostatic column of blood on the left predisposes that side to incompetence in its venous valves more so than on the right (Gat et al., 2005; Masson and Brannigan, 2014; Shafik and Bedeir, 1980). **As a result, varicose veins in the pampiniform plexus are more common on the left than on the right** (Gat et al., 2005; Masson and Brannigan, 2014). The incidence of bilateral varicoceles depends on the techniques involved in detection, with more than 80% observed to be bilateral on contact thermography, Doppler sonography, and venography in one series (Gat et al., 2004). Whether these bilateral varicoceles so identified are clinically significant remains an open question. **One clinical consequence of the infrequency of solitary right varicoceles is that should one be identified, renal pathology such as tumor should be considered, especially if the right-sided varicocele is of abrupt onset** (Masson and Brannigan, 2014).

Varicoceles likely arise as most varicose veins do by intravenous valvular incompetence (Gat et al., 2005; Wishahi, 1991). Genetics may predispose to a valvular defect, because investigators have noted an increased incidence of varicoceles in first-degree relatives of men with a known varicocele (Raman et al., 2005).

Substantial evidence correlates the presence of palpable varicoceles to male reproductive dysfunction. Bulk seminal parameters are poorer in men with varicocele than in the fertile population (Al-Ali et al., 2010; WHO, 1992). Testis size, which reflects the mass of spermatogenesis, is smaller in men with varicocele, and investigators have documented progressive atrophy associated with the condition (Lipshultz and Corriere, 1977; Patel and Sigman, 2010; Sakamoto et al., 2008).

Most studies investigating how varicocele exerts deleterious effects on male reproductive function consider the primary event to be an increase in intratesticular temperature secondary to interruption in the countercurrent heat exchange provided in the pampiniform plexus with opposing flow vectors in a central arterial system and surrounding veins (Goldstein and Eid, 1989; Masson and Brannigan, 2014; Zorgniotti and MacLeod, 1973). Varicoceles are also associated with the presence of higher oxidative stress in the semen of patients seeking care for infertility, which in turn can increase DNA fragmentation (Clavijo et al., 2017). Another possible mechanism by which varicocele can affect spermatogenesis is through testicular hypoperfusion and stasis of blood, leading to hypoxia and toxin accumulation (Chakraborty et al., 1985; Gat et al., 2005; Lee et al., 2006). A study conducted by Mostafa et al. (2016) found that men with varicoceles have elevated levels of apoptosis-associated microRNA in seminal fluid. The proposed mechanisms by which male fertility is impaired by this effect mainly include DNA fragmentation and apoptosis, oxidative stress, predisposition to aneuploidy, and intracellular metabolic and ionic changes (Abd-Elmoaty et al., 2010; Agarwal et al., 2008c; Baccetti et al., 2006; Benoff et al., 2004; Bertolla et al., 2006; Blumer et al., 2008; El-Domyati et al., 2010; Enciso et al., 2006; Ghabili et al., 2009; Lima et al., 2006; Pasqualotto et al., 2008a; Shiraishi and Naito, 2007; Smith et al., 2005; Wu et al., 2009; Zucchi et al., 2006).

Varicocele repair can improve semen parameters, pregnancy rates, live birth rates, and sperm DNA fragmentation for most infertile men with clinical varicocele (Baazeem et al., 2011; Kohn et al., 2017; Smit et al., 2013; Wang et al., 2012; Zini et al., 2011). In couples seeking fertility using assisted reproduction techniques, varicocele repair may offer improvement in semen parameters and allow couples to use less invasive forms of treatment (Samplaski et al., 2017).

Ejaculatory Dysfunction

Disorders of ejaculation may be anatomic, functional, or neuropathic in origin, resulting in absence of emission, resistance, or misdirection. The three main categories of ejaculatory dysfunction encountered in a clinical setting include ejaculatory ductal obstruction, retrograde ejaculation, and anejaculation.

Ejaculatory Ductal Obstruction

The ejaculatory ducts are primarily intraprostatic structures that originate at the terminus of the seminal vesicles and serve as their extensions but without their musculature, functioning within the prostate as simple conduits (Nguyen et al., 1996). The ampulla of the vas enters the prostate medially and at an acute angle with the terminating limb of the seminal vesicle (Nguyen et al., 1996). The intraprostatic conduit ends angled at the verumontanum, which contains two layers of longitudinal muscular bundles extending into the urethra (Nguyen et al., 1996).

Obstruction of the ejaculatory ducts is infrequent and is the cause of azoospermia in less than 5% of men without sperm in the ejaculate (Wosnitzer and Goldstein, 2014). Patients with ejaculatory duct obstruction without underlying cause present with 50% prevalence of cystic fibrosis gene *(CFTR)* mutations and should be considered for genetic evaluation (Jarvi et al., 1995). It may occur at any point along the transit of the ducts within the prostate and result from infection, inflammation, prior surgery, or compression by congenital cysts (Wosnitzer and Goldstein, 2014). As detailed in the section discussing the semen analysis, an evaluation for ejaculatory ductal obstruction is indicated when the seminal volume is less than 1.0 mL. Men with partial ejaculatory duct obstruction can have severe oligospermia or azoospermia, decreased motility, and decreased ejaculatory volume (Mogdil et al., 2016). As noted in the section describing imaging to evaluate for ejaculatory ductal obstruction, techniques to investigate it include TRUS, MRI, chromotubation, and hydraulic pressure measurements. TRUS-guided seminal vesicle aspiration can be useful in diagnosing partial ejaculatory duct obstruction. The finding of three or more sperm per high-powered microscopic field (400×) in the aspirate is considered positive and suggestive of obstruction (Jarow, 1996). If clinically significant ejaculatory ductal obstruction is suspected and if the position of the obstruction is amenable to surgery, transurethral resection of the ejaculatory ducts (TURED) is warranted. The level of the resection is guided by synchronous TRUS to avoid inadvertent injury to the rectum (Mogdil et al., 2016). Different studies have shown elimination of painful ejaculation and hematospermia in all patients (Popken et al., 1998; Weintraub et al., 1993), increased ejaculatory volumes (Yurdakul et al., 2008), and improvements in semen quality (Smith et al., 2008).

Retrograde Ejaculation

Ejaculation is a multiphasic event that includes coordinated neural activity and muscular contraction and relaxation (Jefferys et al., 2012; Phillips et al., 2014). Afferent genital stimulation and cognitive ideation initiate the process, which induces emission through sympathetic stimulation of the bladder neck, vasal ampullae, seminal vesicles, and prostate (Jefferys et al., 2012; Phillips et al., 2014). **Essential to antegrade ejaculation, the bladder neck must first close while temporal neural sequencing first causes closure of the external sphincter to create a high pressure compartment that is emptied with its subsequent opening** (Shafik, 1995).

Failure of sufficient resistance at the bladder neck during generation of the high-pressure system within the prostatic urethra may redirect emission into the bladder, causing retrograde ejaculation. Pathologic causes include congenital abnormalities of or surgery to the bladder neck, spinal cord or neural injury during trauma or retroperitoneal lymph node dissection, diabetes mellitus, or idiopathic causes (Jefferys et al., 2012). **Like ejaculatory ductal obstruction, retrograde ejaculation is infrequent and is established as the diagnosis in less than 2% of infertile men** (Jefferys et al., 2012).

As detailed in the section discussing the semen analysis, an evaluation for ejaculatory ductal obstruction is indicated when the seminal volume is less than 1.0 mL and includes a postejaculatory urinalysis, which is considered significant if the number of sperm in the urine nears or exceeds that in the antegrade specimen (Sigman et al., 2009). **Primary treatment modalities include retrieval of retrograde ejaculated sperm and increasing resistance at the bladder neck with sympathomimetic agents.** In both cases, the sperm so obtained is processed for use in IUI or IVF. If retrieval is to be attempted, the urine is typically first alkalinized with oral bicarbonate or diluted by oral fluid intake, and then the voided urine or a catheterized specimen is obtained after masturbation and orgasm (Jefferys et al., 2012). Investigators have also described ejaculation on a full bladder with successful results (Crich and Jequier, 1978; Templeton and Mortimer, 1982). **Clinicians may also use sympathomimetic agents such as synephrine, pseudoephedrine, ephedrine, or phenylpropanolamine, with approximately one in four patients achieving antegrade ejaculation** (Jefferys et al., 2012). Researchers have described other therapy such as anticholinergic agents, acupuncture, and surgery, but these should be considered investigational (Jefferys et al., 2012).

Anejaculation

Anejaculation refers to lack of seminal emission and projectile ejaculation, and it must be distinguished from anorgasmia, in which the absence of an ejaculation has a cerebral cause (Brackett et al., 2009). Conditions that result in anejaculation are primarily neurologic and include retroperitoneal lymph node dissection, pelvic surgery, multiple sclerosis, transverse myelitis, congenital neural tube defects, diabetes mellitus, and spinal cord injury (Brackett et al., 2009; Phillips et al., 2014).

For patients with sufficient peripheral neural function, neurostimulation with penile vibratory devices or application of current with a rectal electrode, or electroejaculation, may result in sufficient sperm for IUI or IVF (Brackett et al., 2009; Phillips et al., 2014). **For men with spinal cord injuries at a level of T6 or above, stimulation may cause autonomic dysreflexia, an uninhibited sympathetic reflex accompanied by headache, diaphoresis, hypertension, bradycardia, and diaphoresis, which may be life threatening.** Autonomic dysreflexia can be addressed before stimulation by treatment with nifedipine and during the procedure with monitoring of cardiac activity and blood pressure (Brackett et al., 2009; Phillips et al., 2014).

The sperm achieved by stimulation in patients with spinal cord injury is typically characterized by adequate count but impaired motility (Brackett et al., 2009). Evidence supports impairment of sexual accessory gland function, a noxious seminal plasma milieu, and immunopathic mechanisms as causative (Brackett et al., 2009).

Stimulation with penile vibratory devices serves as first-line therapy, with electroejaculation used if the former is unsuccessful (Brackett et al., 2009). If electroejaculation does not yield sperm or if other factors prevent its use, surgical extraction is indicated (Brackett et al., 2009).

Structural Sperm Abnormalities

As discussed in the section describing evaluation of sperm morphology, the majority of sperm in fertile men are eccentrically shaped, and associating the typical variation of sperm shape to clinical relevance in a quantifiable manner has proved challenging. Investigators have characterized certain infrequent discrete structural abnormalities with overt clinical manifestations.

Evidence suggests genetic bases and consequences for two rare types of specific sperm head abnormalities, globozoospermia and macrocephaly. In globozoospermia, the majority of the sperm lack acrosomal caps, rendering the heads spheric rather than ovoid. Sperm macrocephaly is characterized by large-headed and multiflagellated spermatozoa (Nistal et al., 1977). Investigators have associated globozoospermia in humans with mutations in the genes *SPATA16* at chromosome band 3q26.32, *PICK1* at 22q12.3-q13.2, and *DPY19L2* at 12q14.2 (Perrin et al., 2013). Both *SPATA16* and *PICK1* localize to proacrosomal granules that are involved in formation of the acrosome during spermatogenesis (Perrin et al., 2013). Sperm macrocephaly can be caused by the occurrence in homozygosity of a 1-bp deletion in the *AURKC* gene, which is essential for correct meiotic chromosomal segregation and cytokinesis (Dietrich et al., 2007). **It is debatable whether higher rates of aneuploidy are present in patients with globozoospermia or teratozoospermia in general; however, for men in whom nearly all sperm have enlarged heads, multiple tails, and abnormal acrosomes, a very high rate of aneuploidy is found** (Machev et al., 2005; Sun et al., 2006). The treatment for globozoospermia is IVF with ICSI as no acrosome reaction can occur to fertilize the egg; owing to the high rate of aneuploidy in sperm associated with macrocephaly and multiple tails, ICSI is not recommended (Machev et al., 2005; Perrin et al., 2013; Sun et al., 2006). Recently, assisted oocyte activation has been proposed as treatment for globozoospermic patients (Kunetz et al., 2013).

As discussed in the section describing the ultrastructural assessment of sperm, *primary ciliary dyskinesia* refers to a rare condition in which the microtubular architecture of cilia is disrupted (Boon et al., 2013). Because structures such as the sperm tail share similar microtubular construction with cilia, conditions that affect this architecture frequently result in a variety of other clinical manifestations such as immotile sperm, congenital heart disease, chronic respiratory and otolaryngologic infections, and laterality defects (Ferkol and Leigh, 2012). PCD occurs in 1 in 15,000 to 30,000 live births and is typically inherited in an autosomal recessive manner, with occasional X-linked inheritance reported (Boon et al., 2013; Ferkol and Leigh, 2012). Investigators have associated numerous genetic mutations with PCD, with mutations in dynein axonemal heavy chain 5 *(DNAH5)* and intermediate chain 1 *(DNAI1)* accounting for 38% of patients with the condition (Boon et al., 2013; Davis and Katsanis, 2012; Ferkol and Leigh, 2012; Hildebrandt et al., 2011; Zariwala et al., 2011). The sperm of infertile male patients with PCD are usually immotile to varying degrees or are even completely static and manifest defective morphology (Sha et al., 2014). ICSI may achieve pregnancy in cases of PCD (Peeraer et al., 2004). The sperm for ICSI could be obtained from ejaculate, epididymis or testis, but it has been demonstrated that fertilization is improved with immotile testicular spermatozoa (Nijs et al., 1996).

Empirical Treatment

Further details on this topic are available online at Expert Consult.com.

> **KEY POINTS: DIAGNOSES AND THERAPIES**
>
> - Klinefelter syndrome, characterized by 47,XXY, is the most commonly identified genetic cause of male infertility. Bodily morphologic features cannot reliably exclude the presence of the condition.
> - The clinical evaluation of a man identified with CBAVD includes CFTR assessment of him and his female partner to determine risk of cystic fibrosis in offspring.
> - Severe hypogonadotropic hypogonadism may be associated with anosmia and is treated with gonadotropin replacement. Less severe forms are more common, and patients may respond to antiestrogenic agents or aromatase inhibitors.

FERTILITY PRESERVATION IN CANCER

Further details on this topic are available online at Expert Consult.com.

SUGGESTED READINGS

Anguiano A, Oates RD, Amos JA, et al: Congenital bilateral absence of the vas deferens. A primarily genital form of cystic fibrosis, *J Am Med Assoc* 267:1794–1797, 1992.

Dubin L, Amelar RD: Varicocelectomy as therapy in male infertility: a study of 504 cases, *Fertil Steril* 26:217–220, 1975.

Dubin L, Amelar RD: Varicocele size and results of varicocelectomy in selected subfertile men with varicocele, *Fertil Steril* 21:606–609, 1970.

Jarow JP, Sigman M, Kolettis PN, et al: *The evaluation of the azoospermic male: AUA best practice statement*, Linthicum, MD, 2011, American Urological Association Education and Research.

Lipshultz LI, Howards SS, Niederberger CS: *Infertility in the male*, 4th ed, New York, 2009, Cambridge University Press.

MacLeod J: Semen quality in 1000 men of known fertility and in 800 cases of infertile marriage, *Fertil Steril* 2:115–139, 1951.

Meacham RB, Joyce GF, Wise M, et al: Male infertility, *J Urol* 177:2058–2066, 2007.

Niederberger CS: *An introduction to male reproductive medicine*, New York, 2011, Cambridge University Press.

Niederberger CS: Current management of male infertility, *Urol Clin North Am* 41(1):2014.

Sigman M: A meta-analysis of meta-analyses, *Fertil Steril* 96:11–14, 2011.

Sigman M, Kolettis PN, McClure RD, et al: *The optimal evaluation of the infertile male: AUA best practice statement*, Linthicum (MD), 2011, American Urological Association Education and Research.

Tilford CA, Kuroda-Kawaguchi T, Skaletsky H, et al: A physical map of the human Y chromosome, *Nature* 409:943–945, 2001.

Vermeulen A, Verdonck L, Kaufman JM: A critical evaluation of simple methods for the estimation of free testosterone in serum, *J Clin Endocrinol Metab* 84:3666–3672, 1999.

World Health Organization (WHO): *World Health Organization laboratory manual for the examination and processing of human semen*, Geneva, 2010, World Health Organization.

REFERENCES

The complete reference list is available online at ExpertConsult.com.

67
Surgical Management of Male Infertility

Marc Goldstein, MD, DSc (hon), FACS

Since the 11th edition of this text was published, the indications for and techniques of surgery for male infertility have been further refined, resulting in substantially increased success in the management of male factor infertility. These advances include (1) increasing use of genetic and molecular biologic markers (see Chapters 64 and 66) to better select patients for surgical treatment; (2) improved techniques for microsurgical reconstruction of obstruction; (3) the use of varicocelectomy for enhancement of spermatogenesis in azoospermic or severely oligospermic men (Kim et al., 1999; Matthews et al., 1998) and for prevention of future infertility and androgen deficiency in young men as well as for treatment of androgen deficiency in men of all ages (Tanrikut et al., 2011); (4) refined microsurgical techniques for sperm retrieval combined with in vitro fertilization (IVF) with intracytoplasmic sperm injection (ICSI) for men with nonobstructive azoospermia. Even men with nonobstructive azoospermia resulting from Klinefelter syndrome and microY deletions, once regarded as hopeless cases, can now father biologic offspring with in vitro fertilization and intracytoplasmic sperm injection (Palermo et al., 1998; Ramasamy et al., 2009; Tournaye et al., 1996).

Experimental use of flow cytometry of semen and testicular tissue has identified viable sperm, whereas conventional microscopy has not (Bolyakov et al., 2016). IVF with ICSI has expanded our ability to treat even the most severe forms of male-factor infertility such as unreconstructable reproductive tract obstruction and nonobstructive azoospermia. However, it is a costly procedure and an intense process for the female partner, with associated risks of complications, including ovarian hyperstimulation, multiple gestations, as well as complications of the procedures for oocyte retrieval. Furthermore, as ICSI bypasses all natural biologic barriers, it raises realistic concerns of passing genetic abnormalities to the offspring (Foresta et al., 2005; Kim et al., 1998) and is associated with an increased incidence of birth defects in resultant children (Davies et al., 2012). On the other hand, recent analyses clearly indicate that **specific treatments for male-factor infertility, such as microsurgical reconstruction for obstructive azoospermia and varicocelectomy for impaired testis function, in properly selected patients, remain the safest and most cost-effective ways of managing infertile men** (Kolettis and Thomas, 1997; Lee et al., 2008; Marmar et al., 2007; Pavlovich and Schlegel, 1997; Smit et al., 2010). **Specific treatment aimed at correcting or enhancing male infertility can upgrade a couple from donor sperm to IVF/ICSI with testicular microdissection to IVF/ICSI with ejaculated sperm or intrauterine insemination or even to naturally conceived pregnancies** (Samplaski et al., 2013).

For men with unreconstructable obstruction as well as men with nonobstructive azoospermia, surgical retrieval of sperm to achieve fertilization, pregnancy, and live birth with IVF/ICSI is a feasible management option. The development and recent refinement of the various techniques of surgical sperm retrieval, from testes, epididymides, or seminal vesicles, with percutaneous or open surgical approaches, have expanded the armamentarium of urologists treating infertile men. In particular, the employment of the operating microscope to evaluate and identify individual seminiferous tubules more likely to contain sperm has significantly improved the success of testicular sperm extraction (Dabaja and Schlegel, 2013; Schlegel, 1999) while minimizing morbidity significantly (Ramasamy et al., 2005; Tsujimura et al., 2002).

The use of microsurgical techniques has also been extended to varicocelectomy. Varicoceles have long been known to be associated with male infertility and have now clearly been shown to result in progressive, duration-dependent testicular injury (Lipshultz and Corriere, 1977; Nagler et al., 1985; Russell, 1957; Sigman and Jarow, 1997). **Furthermore, microsurgical varicocelectomy, previously reserved only for men with oligospermia, has now been applied to men with nonobstructive azoospermia, resulting in induction of spermatogenesis and successful return of sperm to the ejaculate in many cases** (Ishikawa et al., 2008; Kim et al., 1999; Matthews et al., 1998; Pasqualotto et al., 2003, 2006; Youssef et al., 2009). Although varicocelectomy has historically been reserved for the treatment of infertile men as well as varicocele-induced pain, there is an emerging concept of **early repair of varicoceles to prevent future infertility and Leydig cell dysfunction.** Substantial evidence has accumulated suggesting that varicocele adversely affects Leydig cell function, resulting in lower serum testosterone levels when compared with age-matched controls without varicocele (Tanrikut et al., 2011). Varicocelectomy can halt and even partially reverse this decline (Castro-Magana et al., 1989; Cayan et al., 1999; Su et al., 1995; Tanrikut et al., 2011). **In selected men, varicocelectomy may be an effective treatment for symptomatic, age-related androgen deficiency.**

Thus, with safer and more effective microsurgical techniques, early varicocelectomy has expanded the urologist's role from that of salvaging remaining testicular function to that of preventing future infertility and androgen deficiency.

When surgery for male infertility is undertaken, only rarely is the life (or death) of the patient at stake. What is at stake when the surgery described in this chapter is undertaken is new life, with the potential for altering not only the quality of a couple's life but also the future of our species. The responsibilities assumed by the surgeon in these circumstances demand the utmost in judgment and skill. **Many of the procedures described in this chapter are among the most technically demanding in all of urology.** Acquisition of the skills required to perform them demands intensive laboratory training in microsurgery and a thorough knowledge of the anatomy and physiology of the male reproductive system. Attempting such surgery only occasionally and without proper training is a terrible disservice to the patient, the couple, and future humanity.

SURGICAL ANATOMY

The scrotal contents are unique in their accessibility for physical examination, imagining modalities, and surgical intervention. The success of surgery for male infertility and scrotal disorders is predicated upon selection of the correct operation and the most appropriate surgical approach. The details of the history and careful physical examination followed by confirmatory, judiciously selected laboratory and imaging procedures, are presented in Chapter 66. When surgical intervention for diagnostic or therapeutic purposes is indicated, a thorough understanding of the anatomy (see Chapter 63) and physiology (see Chapter 64) of the male reproductive system is requisite for planning and carrying out a surgical procedure with the highest probability of success and lowest morbidity.

The key points of surgical anatomy follow.

Testicular Blood Supply

The main blood supply to the testis is from the testicular (internal spermatic) artery arising directly from the aorta (Table 67.1). A second

TABLE 67.1 Blood Supply to Testis, Epididymis, and Vas Deferens

TESTIS
1. Testicular (internal spermatic) artery from aorta (main blood supply)
2. Deferential artery from internal iliac (hypogastric) artery/superior vesicle artery
3. Cremasteric (external spermatic) artery from inferior epigastric artery

EPIDIDYMIS
1. Superior epididymal artery derived from testicular artery
2. Inferior epididymal artery derived from vassal (deferential) artery

VAS DEFERENS
1. Seminal vesicle end: deferential artery
2. Testicular end: deferential artery and inferior epididymal artery

---

blood supply comes from the artery of the vas deferens (deferential artery), which derives from the hypogastric (internal iliac) artery or the superior vesicle artery (also a branch of the hypogastric). The third blood supply, primarily to the tunica vaginalis but with branches going to the testes, comes from the cremasteric (external spermatic) artery, which derives from the inferior epigastric artery. **The testicular artery is the main blood supply to the testes.** Its diameter exceeds the diameter of the deferential (vasal) artery plus the cremasteric artery combined (Raman and Goldstein, 2004). Although vasal and cremasteric arteries can provide adequate blood supply to the testes in the event that the testicular artery is ligated, especially in children, **atrophy and/or azoospermia has resulted from testicular artery ligation in the adult and in children** (Maluf, 1957; Silber, 1979).

Special attention should be paid to men who have undergone vasectomy, where the vasal artery has likely been compromised. In these men, maintaining the integrity of the testicular artery in any future operations, such as varicocelectomy, is critical (Lee et al., 2007).

Epididymal Blood Supply

The epididymis has a rich blood supply (see Table 67.1). The superior and the medial epididymal arteries derive from the testicular artery. The blood supply to the cauda (inferior pole) of the epididymis derives from the vasal (deferential) artery. The two main blood supplies to the epididymis, running superiorly and inferiorly, form an extensive interconnection such that if the vasal artery is ligated from previous vasectomy, the blood supply to the epididymis from the testicular artery is more than adequate. In addition, in preparation for vasoepididymostomy or vasovasostomy, the epididymis can be intentionally dissected off of the testis and mobilized to the caput (see Fig. 67.13) with the inferior and medial epididymal arteries intentionally ligated without adverse consequence. **As long as the superior epididymal artery remains intact, the blood supply to the epididymis will be adequate.**

Blood Supply of the Vas Deferens

The vas deferens obtains its blood supply from two sources (see Table 67.1). The seminal vesical (abdominal) end of the vas derives its blood supply from the deferential (vasal) artery. The testicular end of the vas receives additional blood supply from the inferior epididymal arterial interconnections, which extend onto the vas deferens. The two blood supplies to the vas deferens freely anastomose with each other. **After vasectomy, if the vasal vessels are ligated, the testicular end of the vas receives all of its blood supply from** branches of the testicular artery and epididymal artery, although the seminal vesical (abdominal) end of the vas receives all of its blood supply from the deferential artery. The vas deferens receives no blood supply from the surrounding cremaster muscle or from any blood vessels from the spermatic cord. Therefore, if the vas deferens is sectioned or obstructed in two different locations, the intervening segment will fibrose because of lack of blood supply. Therefore two simultaneous vasovasostomies cannot be safely performed on the same vas if the vasal vessels have been interrupted in both locations.

Anatomy of the Excurrent Ducts

Sperm and testicular fluid exit the testes through 7 to 11 tiny efferent ducts. These ducts become convoluted when they exit the testes and form the caput of the epididymis (see Chapter 63). At that level, they freely anastomose with each other. They all coalesce at the distal caput to form a single epididymal tubule from the caput-corpus junction all the way to the vas deferens. Therefore, **if the epididymis is accidentally injured or ligated distal to the caput, the entire system on that side will be completely obstructed.** This is an important consideration when performing epididymal surgery or surgery near the epididymis. **Hydrocelectomy** is a common surgical procedure that can result in **iatrogenic injury to the epididymis.** In long-standing large hydroceles, the epididymis is often splayed out and difficult to identify. Use of an operating microscope and transillumination of the hydrocele sac help avoid injury to the epididymis, vas, and testicular blood supply (Dabaja et al., 2013). **Generous margins from the epididymis should be allowed when performing hydrocelectomy** (see Chapter 63). Orchiopexy for torsion can also result in inadvertent injury to the epididymis. **A single stitch through an epididymal tubule in the corpus or cauda will result in complete obstruction** of that side. Because there are multiple lobules at the levels of the caput, **puncture of a single tubule for sperm aspiration can be safely performed at the most proximal region of the caput** without significantly compromising the flow of sperm into the corpus. Multiple punctures of many tubules at the caput or any puncture distal to the caput, however, can cause obstruction (Zhang et al., 2013).

Ejaculatory Ducts

The left and right ejaculatory ducts enter the prostatic urethra at the level of the utricle. Obstruction of ejaculatory ducts can lead to azoospermia. Multiple transrectal prostatic biopsies to diagnose or follow men with prostate cancer can cause stricture or obstruction of the ejaculatory ducts. Those men potentially interested in future fertility, regardless of age, should be encouraged to bank sperm before biopsy. Transurethral resection of the ejaculatory ducts (TURED) can relieve the obstruction. TURED should not be considered a benign procedure because it is occasionally associated with significant morbidity (see later). Normally, the ejaculatory ducts contain a valvelike mechanism that prevents reflux of urine into the ejaculatory duct. **After TURED, a significant percentage of men develop reflux of urine up the excurrent ductal system** (Vazquez-Levin et al., 1994), **causing chemical and/or bacterial epididymitis.**

> **KEY POINTS: SURGICAL ANATOMY**
> - The testicular artery is the main blood supply to the testis.
> - If the epididymis is accidentally injured or ligated distal to the caput, the entire system on that side will be obstructed.

TESTIS BIOPSY

Indications

The indications for testis biopsy are detailed in Chapter 66. Briefly, testis biopsy is indicated in azoospermic men with testis of normal size and consistency, palpable vasa deferentia, normal serum follicle-stimulating hormone (FSH) levels, and a negative serum antisperm antibody assay. Under these circumstances, **biopsy will distinguish obstructive from nonobstructive azoospermia.** In men with **congenital absence of vasa and normal serum FSH levels**, biopsy always reveals spermatogenesis (Goldstein and Schlossberg, 1988), and **biopsy is not necessary** before definitive sperm aspiration and IVF with ICSI. Men with a highly positive serum antisperm antibody test, especially with a history consistent with iatrogenic injury to the vasa (inguinal hernia repair) or epididymides (hydrocelectomy), do not require biopsy before reconstruction because obstruction is almost certain. **Diagnostic biopsy should usually be performed bilaterally irrespective of the size discrepancy of the two testes.** Good spermatogenesis is sometimes found in small, firm testes, whereas biopsies of large, healthy testes may reveal maturation arrest.

The ability to achieve pregnancy with only a single testicular sperm has turned biopsy into a potentially therapeutic, as well as diagnostic, procedure. Even men with markedly elevated serum FSH levels and small, soft testes in whom testicular failure is certain often harbor rare mature sperm in their testes. These sperm can be extracted using techniques described later in this chapter and employed for IVF with intracytoplasmic injection of testicular sperm.

The recently discovered heterogeneity of the testes of men with nonobstructive azoospermia coupled with the ability of testicular sperm to acquire motility (Jow et al., 1993) has resulted in changes in the techniques of testis biopsy. **Examination of fresh, unfixed tissue for the presence of sperm with tails** and possible motility, and examination of multiple samples if sperm are not found initially, is now recommended. Furthermore, optimal care requires the availability, at the time of biopsy, of an andrology laboratory capable of processing and cryopreserving any sperm found at the time of biopsy.

Open Testis Biopsy: Microsurgical Technique

Open biopsy remains the gold standard because it provides an optimal amount of tissue for accurate diagnosis and retrieval of sperm for IVF (Dardashti et al., 2000; Rosenlund et al., 1998; Schlegel, 1999). Open testis biopsy may be performed using either general, spinal, or local anesthetic. Although local anesthesia of just the skin and tunicas without a cord block is uncomfortable, local anesthesia with spermatic cord block can be effective and comfortable. However, there are limitations of the cord block. In animal studies, the incidence of accidental damage to the testicular artery during blind cord block is 5% (Goldstein and Einer-Jensen, 1983). In addition, if there has been previous scrotal surgery with scar or adhesions and more extensive dissection and manipulation may be required, I prefer to use general or spinal anesthetic.

The surgeon's goals when performing a testis biopsy are to provide an optimal tissue sample, avoid trauma to the specimen, and avoid injury to the epididymis or testicular blood supply. Open biopsy under magnification (preferably with an operating microscope) satisfies these requirements.

An assistant stretches the scrotal skin tightly over the anterior surface of the testis and confirms that the epididymis is posterior. Bilateral 1-cm transverse scrotal incisions within the scrotal skinfolds provide good exposure with a minimum of scrotal bleeding. Alternatively, a single vertical incision in the median raphe may be employed. The incision is carried through the skin and dartos muscle, and the tunica vaginalis is opened. **If the anatomy is distorted from previous surgery, the epididymis cannot be clearly palpated posteriorly, or if the tunica albuginea cannot be clearly identified, the incision should be enlarged and the testis delivered.** The edges of the tunica vaginalis are held open with hemostats and any bleeding vessels are cauterized. **Use of loupes or, better yet, the operating microscope allows ready identification of a spot on the tunica albuginea relatively free of visible surface vessels.** The wound should be dry before incising the tunica albuginea to prevent saturation of the biopsy with blood. A 3- to 4-mm incision is made in the tunica albuginea with a 15-degree microknife (Fig. 67.1A). Small crossing vessels are cauterized with bipolar cautery and divided before excising a pea-sized sample of seminiferous tubules with razor-sharp iris scissors (Fig. 67.1B). **When handling testis biopsy material for permanent fixation, avoid tissue handling in any way (including with forceps) because this may traumatize and distort the testicular architecture.** The specimen is then deposited directly into either Bouin's, Zenker's, or collidine-buffered glutaraldehyde solution. **Formalin fixation results in distortion of testicular histology and should not be used for testis biopsy.** A "touch prep" is made by blotting the cut surface of the testis several times with a glass slide (Fig. 67.1C) and adding a drop of saline, lactated Ringer's, or human tubal fluid with IVF medium and a coverslip. Examination under high power using a light microscope with or without phase contrast will reveal the presence of sperm with tails and allow assessment of motility (Fig. 67.1D). If no sperm are found in the touch prep, a second specimen may be cut for a wet "squash prep." In this case, the specimen is placed on a slide, a drop of saline is added, and the specimen is crushed under a coverslip (Jow et al., 1993). If no sperm are found, the tunica is closed with 2 to 3 interrupted sutures of 5-0 vicryl (Fig. 67.1E), and another area is biopsied through the same skin incision. As described later in this chapter, **use of an operating microscope providing 10× to 25× magnification may allow selective sampling of larger seminiferous tubules more likely to contain sperm** (Schlegel, 1999). **If sperm are identified,** the slide as well as additional **tissue removed are sent for cryopreservation** in the andrology laboratory. **The location of the biopsy site where sperm were found is noted, and the tunica albuginea is closed with 2 to 3 interrupted sutures of 6-0 nylon. This facilitates identification of sites of spermatogenesis for future testicular sperm extraction for IVF/ICSI.**

The tunica vaginalis is closed with 5-0 monofilament nonabsorbable suture for hemostasis. Use of a nonabsorbable suture facilitates identification of the biopsy site if sperm were found at that site, and subsequent testicular sperm extraction is required at the time of IVF with ICSI. The testis is returned to the tunica vaginalis, which is closed with a continuous 5-0 Vicryl suture. The skin is closed with a subcuticular 5-0 Monocryl. The wounds are covered with bacitracin ointment and a fluff-type dressing secured with a snug scrotal support. Antibiotics are unnecessary.

Percutaneous Testis Biopsy

Percutaneous testis biopsy using the same 14-gauge biopsy gun employed for prostatic biopsy **is a blind procedure and could result in unintentional injury to either the epididymis or testicular artery. This technique should not be used when previous surgery has resulted in scarring and obliteration of normal anatomy.** Fine-needle aspiration usually yields specimens that contain few tubules with poorly preserved architecture. When performed under local anesthesia, a cord block is necessary to minimize pain. The technique of percutaneous biopsy is described in the section Scrotal Operations. As a therapeutic tool for sperm retrieval, **percutaneous biopsy or aspiration is most useful for fresh sperm retrieval for IVF/ICSI in men with obstructive azoospermia and normal spermatogenesis.**

Percutaneous Testicular Aspiration

Testicular aspiration performed with a 23-gauge needle or angiocath sheath (Marmar et al., 1993) is probably less invasive and less painful than percutaneous biopsy but usually yields few tubules with poorly preserved architecture. Although flow cytometric evaluation of this material can distinguish haploid from diploid cells and therefore confirm the presence or absence of late stages of spermatogenesis (Chan et al., 1984), direct wet examination of the aspirate for sperm and assessment of motility provide the most practical clinical information. Three or four aspirations can be performed until sperm are identified. In cases of obstructive azoospermia, these sperm can be used for IVF with ICSI (Craft et al., 1995) when sperm cannot be retrieved from the epididymis (see later). Fine-needle aspiration has a significantly lower yield of sperm than open micro-TESE in men with nonobstructive azoospermia.

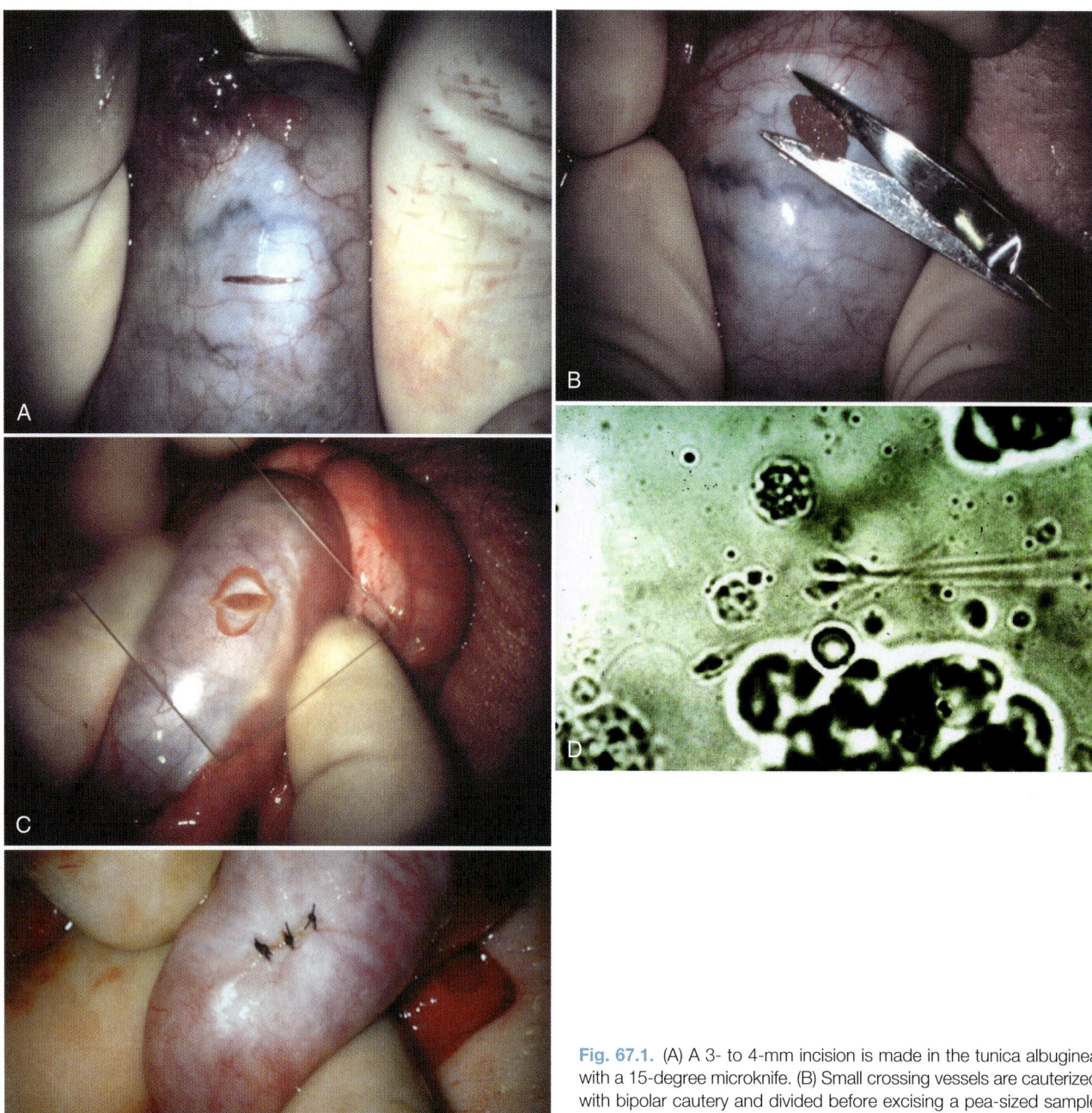

Fig. 67.1. (A) A 3- to 4-mm incision is made in the tunica albuginea with a 15-degree microknife. (B) Small crossing vessels are cauterized with bipolar cautery and divided before excising a pea-sized sample of seminiferous tubules with razor sharp iris scissors. (C) A "touch-prep" is made by blotting the cut surface of the testis several times with a glass slide. (D) Examination under high power using a light microscope with or without phase contrast will reveal the presence of sperm with tails and allow assessment of motility. (E) If no sperm are found, the tunica is closed with 2 to 3 interrupted sutures of 5-0 Vicryl.

Complications of Testis Biopsy

Carefully performed, testis biopsy is associated with few complications (Dardashti et al., 2000; Schlegel and Su, 1997). **The most serious complication associated with testis biopsy is inadvertent biopsy of the epididymis.** If histologic evaluation of the biopsy material reveals epididymis with sperm within the epididymal tubule, obstruction of the epididymis at the site of the biopsy is certain. If, however, there are no sperm within the epididymal tubules, the patient is either obstructed above the level of the epididymal biopsy or has primary seminiferous tubular failure and no harm has been done.

The most common complication of testis biopsy is hematoma. Hematomas can be large and may require drainage. Use of magnification to avoid vessels and a bipolar cautery for hemostasis helps prevent this complication. Proper closure of the well-vascularized tunica vaginalis with a continuous 5-0 suture minimizes bleeding and adhesions.

With the rich blood supply of the scrotum and its contents, wound infection is rare in the absence of hematoma, and antibiotics are unnecessary.

KEY POINTS: TESTIS BIOPSY

- Biopsy is a potentially therapeutic, as well as diagnostic, procedure.

VASOGRAPHY

Indications

The absolute indications for vasography are the following (must include all three):
1. Azoospermia
2. Complete spermatogenesis with many mature spermatids on testis biopsy
3. At least one palpable vas
   Relative indications for vasography are the following:
1. Severe oligospermia with normal testis biopsy
2. High level of sperm-bound antibodies, which indicates unilateral, bilateral, or partial obstruction (Lee et al., 2009)
3. Low semen volume and very poor sperm motility (partial ejaculatory duct obstruction)
   Vasography should answer the following questions:
1. Are there sperm in the vasal fluid?
2. Is the vas obstructed?

If the testis biopsy reveals many sperm, the following are indications:
1. **Absence of sperm in vasal fluid indicates** obstruction on the testicular side of the vasotomy site, most likely an **epididymal obstruction.** Vasography is done in this case with saline or indigo carmine to confirm patency of the seminal vesicle (distal) end of the vas before vasoepididymostomy.
2. **Copious vasal fluid containing many sperm indicates vasal or ejaculatory duct obstruction,** and formal contrast vasography is performed as described later to document the exact location of the obstruction.
3. **Copious thick, white fluid without sperm in a dilated vas indicates secondary epididymal obstruction** in addition to a potential vasal or ejaculatory duct obstruction.

Vasography with radiographic contrast media and intraoperative radiographs are rarely indicated. There is no need to perform vasography at the time of testis biopsy for azoospermia unless immediate reconstruction is planned and the touch/wet-prep biopsy reveals mature sperm with tails. If not meticulously performed, vasography can cause stricture or even obstruction at the vasography site, which can complicate subsequent reconstruction (Howards et al., 1975; Poore et al., 1997). In addition, vasography is of no value in making the diagnosis of epididymal obstruction, and the majority of non–vasectomy-related obstructions are epididymal.

If testis biopsy reveals normal spermatogenesis and the vasa are palpable, vasography, if necessary, should be performed only at the time of definitive repair of obstruction. General anesthesia provides the most flexibility for scrotal exploration, vasography, and repair of obstruction. Although local anesthesia can provide adequate analgesia, patients are often unable to lie still through several hours of microsurgery. Long-acting hypobaric spinal or continuous epidural anesthesia can be satisfactory alternatives.

Technique of Vasography and Interpretation of Findings

Inguinal hernia repair, particularly when performed in childhood, is known to be associated with vasal injury leading to obstruction. If there is no previous inguinal incision and the site of obstruction is unknown, the testis is delivered through a high vertical scrotal incision (see Fig. 67.11). The vas deferens is identified and isolated at the junction of the straight and convoluted portions of the vas deferens. Using an operating microscope and 10× power magnification, the vasal sheath is longitudinally incised and the vasal vessels carefully preserved (Fig. 67.2A).

A clean segment of bare vas is delivered and surrounded with a vessel loop. A straight clamp is placed beneath the vas to act as a platform. Under 25× power magnification, a 15-degree microknife is used to hemitransect the vas until the lumen is revealed (Fig. 67.2B). **Any fluid exuding from the lumen is placed on a slide, mixed with a drop of saline, and sealed with a coverslip for microscopic examination. If the vasal fluid is devoid of sperm with repeated sampling** after milking the epididymis and convoluted vas, **epididymal obstruction is present.** The end of the vas toward the seminal vesicles is then cannulated with a 24-gauge angiocatheter sheath and is injected with 1 mL of Ringer's lactate solution with a 1-mL tuberculin syringe to confirm its patency (Fig. 67.3). If the Ringer's passes easily, formal vasography is not necessary. If further proof of patency of the vas deferens is desired, 1 mL of 50% dilute indigo carmine may be injected and the bladder catheterized. The presence of blue/green dye in the urine confirms patency of the vas. Indigo carmine diluted 50/50 with Ringer's solution is preferred instead of methylene blue because, even at low concentrations, methylene blue kills sperm and renders them useless for cryopreservation or for immediate IVF/ICSI (Chang et al., 1998; Sheynkin et al., 1999a; Wood et al., 2003). **If motile sperm are found in the vas, the testicular end should be gently barbotaged with 0.2 mL of human tubal fluid media, and the fluid processed by the andrology laboratory for sperm cryopreservation for potential future use for ICF/ICSI. This should be done before injection with indigo carmine or x-ray contrast material** (Sheynkin et al., 1999a).

If a large amount of fluid (typically brownish "crank-case oil"–appearing fluid) is found in the vasal lumen and microscopic examination reveals the presence of sperm, the obstruction is toward the seminal vesicle end of the vas. In these cases, the vas is usually markedly dilated. A 2-0 Proline suture can be passed toward the

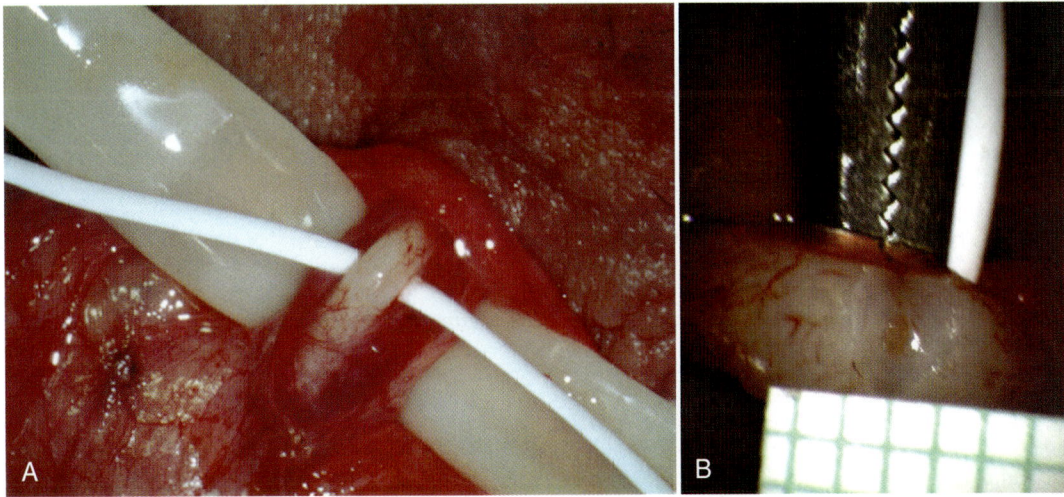

Fig. 67.2. (A) The vasal sheath is longitudinally incised and the vasal vessels carefully preserved. (B) A 15-degree microknife is used to hemitransect the vas until the lumen is revealed.

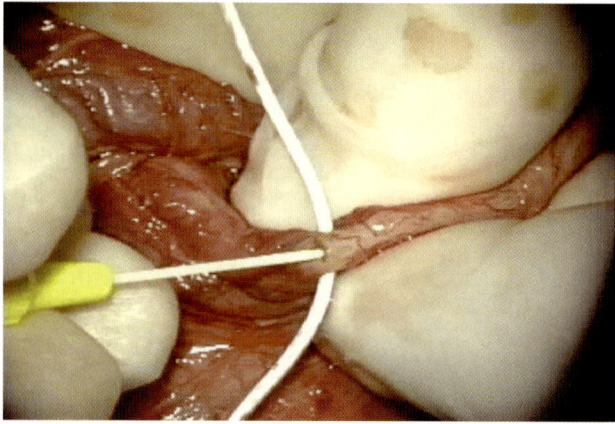

Fig. 67.3. The end of the vas towards the seminal vesicles is cannulated with a 24-gauge angiocatheter sheath and is injected with 1 mL of Ringer's lactate solution with a 1 mL tuberculin syringe to confirm its patency.

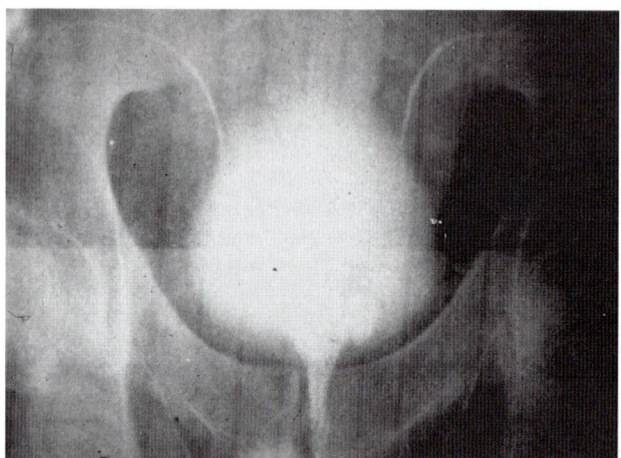

Fig. 67.4. Placing a balloon on gentle traction prior to vasography prevents reflux on contrast into the bladder.

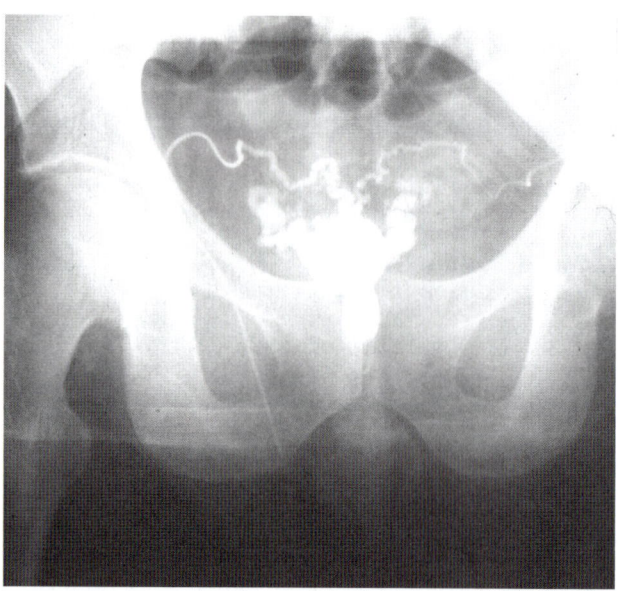

Fig. 67.5. After the vasa have been cannulated, vasograms are performed with the injection of 0.5 mL of water-soluble contrast media.

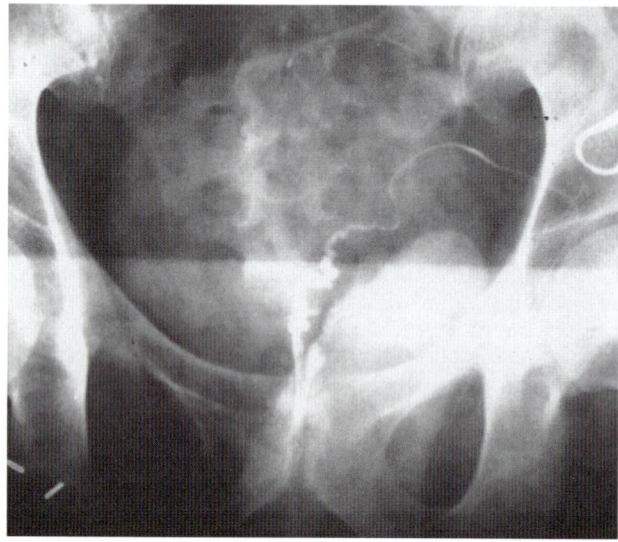

Fig. 67.6. Vasography reveals obstruction at the site of the ejaculatory ducts.

seminal vesicle end of the vas and a clamp placed on the Proline when the suture passes no further. This is particularly useful for delineating the site of inguinal obstruction from prior groin surgery. If the obstruction is proximal to the inguinal scar, formal vasography is performed by passing a No. 3 ureteral catheter toward the seminal vesicle end of the vas. A 16-Fr Foley catheter is placed in the bladder, and the balloon is filled with 5 mL of air. Placing the balloon on gentle traction before vasography prevents reflux of contrast into the bladder, which can obscure detail (Fig. 67.4). The air-filled balloon also identifies the location of the bladder neck relative to any obstruction. After the vasa have been cannulated, vasograms are performed with the injection of 0.5 mL of water-soluble contrast media (Fig. 67.5). **If vasography reveals obstruction at the site of the ejaculatory ducts** (Fig. 67.6), **indigo carmine or, after sperm has been aspirated and cryopreserved, methylene blue is injected in both vasa to facilitate a transurethral resection (TUR) of the ejaculatory ducts** (see the section on electroejaculation indications). If both vasa are visualized after injection of contrast into only one vas (Fig. 67.7), it means both vasa empty into a single cavity, usually a midline ejaculatory duct cyst.

Vasography may reveal the vas deferens ending blindly, far from the ejaculatory ducts (Fig. 67.8). This finding indicates congenital partial absence of the vas deferens, and these patients should be tested for cystic fibrosis mutations (see Chapter 24). If this is found bilaterally (Fig. 67.9), reconstruction is impossible, but vasal or epididymal sperm can be aspirated into standard laboratory pipettes (see Varicocelectomy) and cryopreserved for future IVF with ICSI. If vasography reveals obstruction in the inguinal region (Fig. 67.10), either inguinal vasovasostomy or crossed transseptal vasovasostomy, using the contralateral unobstructed vas (see Fig. 67.24), may be performed. **The hemitransected vasography sites are carefully closed microsurgically** using two or three interrupted 10-0 monofilament nylon sutures for the mucosa and 9-0 for the muscularis and adventitia.

If the vasal fluid reveals no sperm and vasography confirms patency of the seminal vesicle end of the vas, the vas is completely transected, and the seminal vesicle end is prepared for vasoepididymostomy (see Fig. 67.27). If the vasal fluid reveals many sperm and vasography is normal, either retrograde ejaculation, lack of emission, or aperistalsis of the vas (Tiffany and Goldstein, 1985; Tillem and Mellinger, 1999) is the cause of the azoospermia.

Complications of Vasography

Stricture

Multiple attempts at percutaneous vasography using sharp needles can result in stricture or obstruction at the vasography site. Imprecise

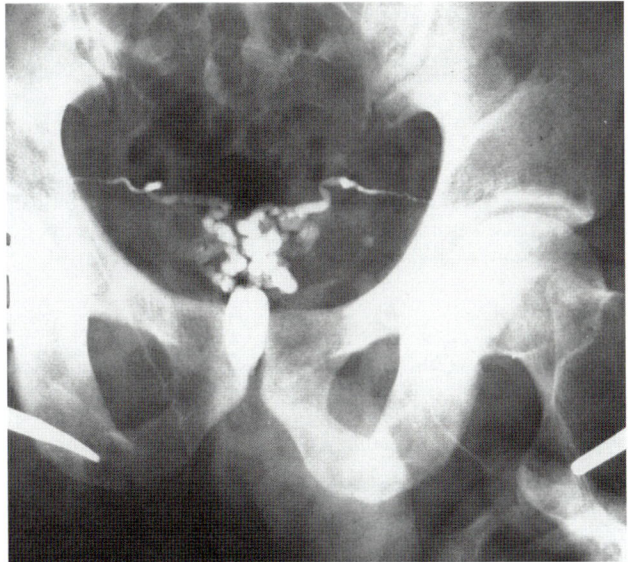

Fig. 67.7. Both vasa are visualized after injection of contrast into only one vas.

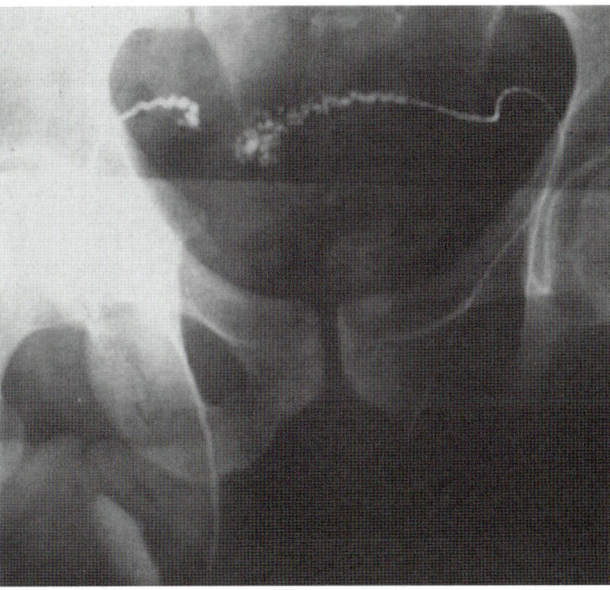

Fig. 67.9. Bilateral congenital partial absence of the vas deferens.

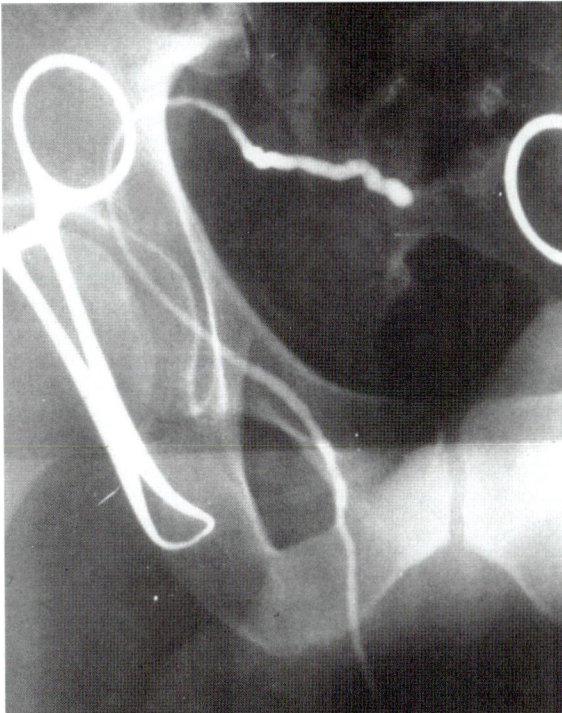

Fig. 67.8. The vas deferens ending blindly, far from the ejaculatory ducts.

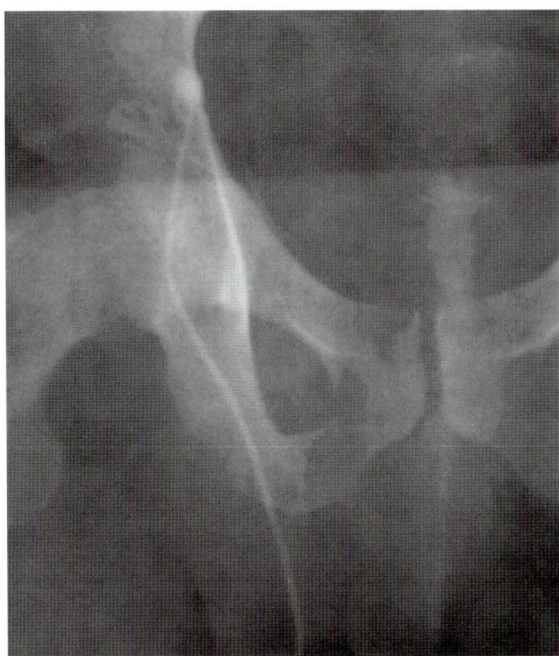

Fig. 67.10. Vasography reveals obstruction in the inguinal region.

closure of a vasotomy can also result in stricture and obstruction (Howards et al., 1975; Poore et al., 1997). Non–water-soluble contrast agents may also result in stricture and should not be employed for vasography.

Injury to the Vasal Blood Supply

If the vasal blood supply is injured at the site of vasography, vasovasostomy proximal to the vasography site may result in ischemia, necrosis, and obstruction of the intervening segment of vas.

Hematoma

A bipolar cautery should be used for meticulous hemostasis to prevent hematoma in the perivasal sheath.

Sperm Granuloma

Leaky closure of a vasography site may lead to the development of a sperm granuloma, which can result in stricture or obstruction of the vas. The microsurgical technique for closure of vasography sites is identical to that employed for vasovasostomy described later in this chapter.

Transrectal Vasography and Seminal Vesiculography

If transrectal ultrasound reveals markedly dilated seminal vesicles and/or a midline müllerian duct cyst in a man with obstructive azoospermia, transrectal aspiration followed by instillation of indigo carmine mixed with radiographic contrast is a useful diagnostic maneuver (Eisenberg et al., 2008; Jarow, 1994; Katz and Nagler, 1994; Riedenklau et al., 1995).

The same bowel prep and antibiotic coverage used for transrectal prostate biopsy is employed. The fine-needle aspirate is examined for sperm. If sperm are present. it means at least one vas and epididymis are patent. Then 0.5 mL of indigo carmine is diluted with 1.5 mL of 50% water-soluble contrast and instilled. If a flat plate reveals a potentially resectable lesion, a TUR of the ejaculatory ducts is performed (see Electroejaculation). Visualization of blue dye effluxing from the ejaculatory ducts or an unroofed cyst aids in determining the adequacy of the resection (Cornel et al., 1999).

This technique obviates the need for formal open scrotal vasography in men with transrectally accessible lesions. If sperm are found in the aspirate, a TUR may immediately be undertaken without violating the scrotum. Sperm-laden aspirates may be frozen for future IVF with ICSI if surgery fails.

If no sperm are found in the aspirated fluid, it suggests that secondary epididymal obstruction exists. Simultaneous TUR of the ejaculatory ducts and vasoepididymostomy is rarely successful. In the face of both ejaculatory duct obstruction and bilateral epididymal obstruction, the best option would be epididymal sperm aspiration for cryopreservation for future IVF/ICSI.

Summary

1. Vasography is performed only if testicular biopsy confirms spermatogenesis consistent with obstructive azoospermia.
2. Vasography is performed only at the time of planned reconstruction.
3. Vasal fluid is always sampled first to allow cryopreservation of motile sperm if found.
4. Indigo carmine is used instead of methylene blue to confirm patency.
5. Formal vasography with x-ray contrast is needed only to locate obstructions proximal to the internal inguinal ring.
6. If transrectal ultrasound reveals dilated seminal vesicles and/or a midline (müllerian duct) cyst, transrectal fine-needle aspiration followed by instillation of contrast and indigo carmine should be performed. If motile sperm are found, they should be cryopreserved.

> **KEY POINTS: VASOGRAPHY**
> - Perform vasography only at the time of planned reconstruction.

VASOVASOSTOMY

The number of American men who undergo vasectomy has remained stable at about 500,000 per year, as has the divorce rate of 50%. Surveys suggest that 2% to 6% of vasectomized men will ultimately seek reversal, and up to 20% express interest in future fertility. Furthermore, obstructive azoospermia can be the result of iatrogenic injuries to the vas deferens, usually from hernia repair, in 6% of azoospermic men (Sheynkin et al., 1998a; Shin et al., 2005).

Preoperative Evaluation

Before attempted surgical reconstruction of the reproductive tract, adequate spermatogenesis should be documented. A prior history of natural fertility prevasectomy is usually adequate.

Physical Examination

1. Testis: Small or soft testes suggest impaired spermatogenesis and predict a poor outcome.
2. Epididymis: An indurated irregular epididymis often predicts secondary epididymal obstruction, necessitating vasoepididymostomy.
3. Sperm granuloma: **A sperm granuloma at the testicular end of the vas suggests that sperm have been leaking at the vasectomy site. This vents the high pressures away from the epididymis and is associated with a better prognosis for restored fertility regardless of the time interval since vasectomy** (Wosnitzer and Goldstein, 2013).
4. Vasal gap: When a very destructive vasectomy has been performed, most of the scrotal straight vas may be absent or fibrotic, and the patient should be advised that inguinal extension of the scrotal incision will be necessary to mobilize adequate length of vas to enable a tension-free anastomosis.
5. Scars from previous surgery: Operative scars in the inguinal or scrotal region should alert the surgeon to the possibility of iatrogenic inguinal (hernia repair) vasal or epididymal obstruction (hydrocelectomy, orchiopexy) (Hopps and Goldstein, 2006; Sheynkin et al., 1998a).

Laboratory Tests

1. Semen analysis with centrifugation and examination of the pellet for sperm should be performed preoperatively. Complete sperm with tails are found in 10% of preoperative pellets a mean of 10 years after vasectomy (Lemack and Goldstein, 1996). Under these circumstances sperm are certain to be found in the vas on at least one side, indicating a favorable prognosis for restored fertility. Men with a low semen volume should have a transrectal ultrasound to ascertain the possibility of an additional ejaculatory duct obstruction.
2. Serum and antisperm antibody studies: The presence of serum antisperm antibodies corroborates the diagnosis of obstruction and the presence of active spermatogenesis (Lee et al., 2009).
3. Serum FSH: Men with small, soft testes should have serum FSH measured. An elevated FSH level predicts impaired spermatogenesis and a poorer prognosis.
4. Prostate specific antigen (PSA): Vasectomy reversal candidates over age 40 should have serum PSA measured.

Anesthesia

General anesthesia is ideal. Slight movements are greatly magnified by the operating microscope and disturb performance of the anastomosis. In cooperative patients regional or even local anesthesia with sedation can be employed if the vasal ends are easily palpable, a sperm granuloma is present, and/or the time interval since vasectomy is short, decreasing the likelihood of secondary epididymal obstruction. When large vasal gaps are present, extensions of the incisions high into the inguinal canal may be necessary. Furthermore, if vasoepididymostomy is necessary, the operating time could exceed 4 or 5 hours. Hypobaric spinal anesthesia with long-acting agents such as Marcaine can provide 4 to 5 hours of anesthesia time and has the advantage of eliminating lower body motion. Epidural anesthesia with an indwelling catheter can be equally effective. Local anesthesia with liposomal bupivacaine and sedation is also workable, especially in men with small vasal gaps and under 10-year interval since vasectomy.

Surgical Approaches: Scrotal

Bilateral high vertical scrotal incisions provide the most direct access to the obstructed site in cases of vasectomy reversal. Length is usually a problem on the abdominal end but not on the testicular end. The location of the external inguinal ring must be marked (Fig. 67.11). **If the vasal gap is large, or the vasectomy site is high, this incision can easily be extended toward the external ring.** If the vasectomy site is low, it is easy to pull up the testicular end. This incision should be made at least 1 cm lateral to the base of the penis. **The testis should be delivered with the tunica vaginalis left intact.** This provides excellent exposure of the entire scrotal vas deferens and, if necessary, the epididymis.

Surgical Approaches: Inguinal

An inguinal incision is the preferred approach in men when obstruction of the inguinal vas deferens from prior herniorrhaphy or orchiopexy is strongly suspected. Incision through the previous scar usually leads directly to the site of obstruction. If the obstruction turns out to be scrotal or epididymal, it is a simple matter to deliver

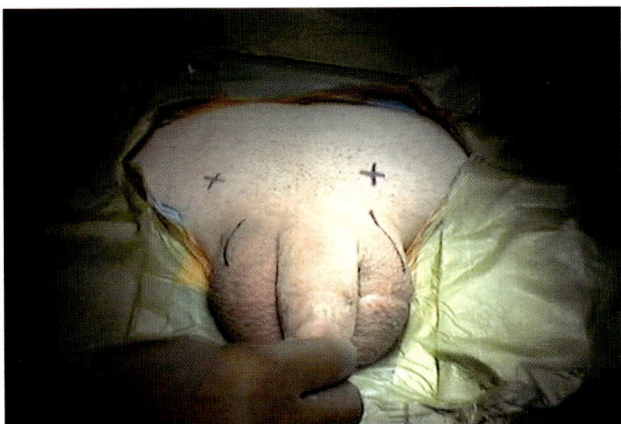

Fig. 67.11. The location of the external inguinal ring is marked.

the testis through the inguinal incision or through a separate scrotal incision to perform the anastomosis.

Preparation of the Vasa

The vas is grasped above and below the site of obstruction with two Babcock clamps. Penrose drains replace the Babcock clamps and facilitate the dissection. The vasal vessels and periadventitial sheath are included. **Transillumination of the periadventitial sheath**, by properly adjusting the operating light, **allows clear visualization of the blood vessels, which facilitates dissection of the periadventitial sheath and prevents damage to the vasal vessels**. The vas is mobilized enough to allow a tension-free anastomosis. To preserve good blood supply **the vas should not be stripped of its sheath**. The obstructed segment and, if present, sperm granuloma at the vasectomy site should be dissected out and excised. By staying right on the vas and/or sperm granuloma during this dissection, the risk of injuring the testicular artery is reduced. **Injury to adjacent cord structures, especially the testicular artery, is likely to result in testicular atrophy because the vasal artery has usually been interrupted at the vasectomy site.**

When large vasal gaps are present, a gauze-wrapped index finger is used to bluntly separate the cord structures from the vas. Blunt finger dissection through the external ring will free the vas to the internal inguinal ring if additional abdominal side length is necessary. These maneuvers leave all the vasal vessels intact. **When the vasal gap is extremely large, additional length can be achieved by dissecting the entire convoluted vas free of its attachments to the epididymal tunica** (Fig. 67.12), allowing the testis to drop upside down. These maneuvers can provide an additional 4 to 6 cm of length. To maintain the integrity of the vasal vessels, this dissection is best performed using magnifying loupes or the operating microscope under low power. If the amount of vas removed is so large that even these measures fail to allow a tension-free anastomosis, the incision can be extended to the internal inguinal ring, the floor of the inguinal canal cut, and the vas rerouted under the floor, as in a difficult orchiopexy. An additional 4 to 6 cm of length can be obtained by dissecting the epididymis off of the testis from the vasoepididymal junction to the caput epididymis (Fig. 67.13A and B). The superior epididymal vessels are left intact and provide adequate blood supply to the testicular end of the vas. With this combination of maneuvers, up to 10-cm gaps can be bridged.

After the vasa have been freed, the testicular end of the vas is cut transversely. An ultrasharp knife drawn through a slotted 2-, 2.5-, or 3-mm diameter nerve-holding clamp (Accurate Surgical and Scientific Instrument Corp., Westbury, NY) yields a perfect 90-degree cut (Fig. 67.14). The cut surface of the testicular end of the vas deferens is inspected using 15× to 25× power magnification. **A healthy white mucosal ring should be seen, which springs back immediately after gentle dilation. The muscularis should appear smooth and soft. A gritty-looking muscularis layer indicates the presence of

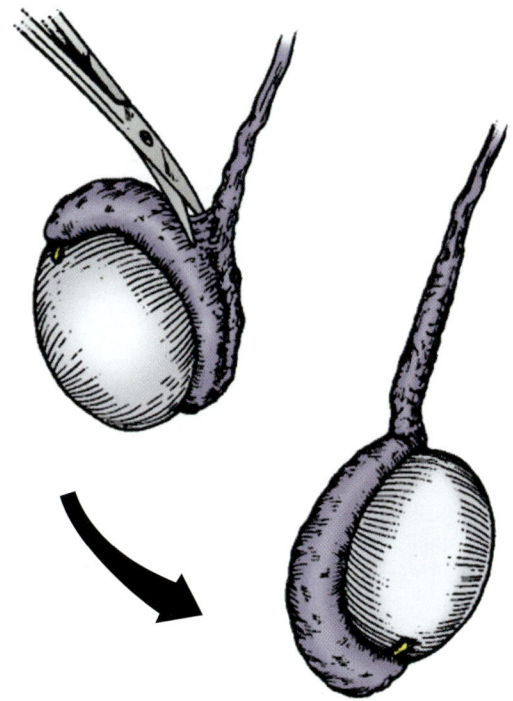

Fig. 67.12. When the vasal gap is extremely large, additional length can be achieved by dissecting the entire convoluted vas free of its attachments to the epididymal tunica.

scar/fibrotic tissues.** The cut surface should look like a bullseye with the three vasal layers distinctly visible. Healthy bleeding should be noted from the cut edge of the mucosa and the surface of the muscularis. If the blood supply is poor or the muscularis is gritty, the vas is recut until healthy tissue is found. The vasal artery and vein are then clamped and ligated with 6-0 nylon. Small bleeders are controlled with a microbipolar forceps set at low power. Once a patent lumen has been established on the testicular end, the vas is milked and a clean glass slide is touched to its surface. The vasal fluid is immediately mixed with a drop or two of saline or Ringer's lactate and preserved under a coverslip for microscopic examination. The abdominal end of the vas deferens is prepared in a similar manner and the lumen gently dilated with a microvessel dilator and cannulated with a 24-gauge angiocatheter sheath. Injection of saline or Ringer's lactate confirms its patency. After Ringer's injection and a test dilation the vas is recut to obtain a fresh surface. **A minimum of instrumentation of the mucosa should be performed.**

After preparation, the ends of the vasa are stabilized with a Microspike approximating clamp (Goldstein, 1985) to remove all tension before the anastomosis is performed. Isolating the field through a slit in a rubber dam prevents microsutures from sticking to the surrounding tissue. A sterile tongue blade covered with a large Penrose drain is placed beneath the ends of the vasa to provide a platform on which to perform the anastomosis.

When to Perform Vasoepididymostomy

The gross appearance of fluid expressed from the testicular end of the vas is usually predictive of findings on microscopic examination (Table 67.2). If microscopic examination of the vasal fluid reveals the presence of sperm with tails, vasovasostomy is performed. If no fluid is found, a 24-gauge angiocatheter sheath is inserted into the lumen of the testicular end of the vas and barbotaged with 0.1 mL of saline while the convoluted vas is vigorously milked. The barbotage fluid is expressed onto a slide and examined. **Men with large sperm granulomas often have virtually no dilation of the testicular end of the vas and little or no fluid initially. However, with barbotage and vigorous milking, invariably sperm can be found in this scant

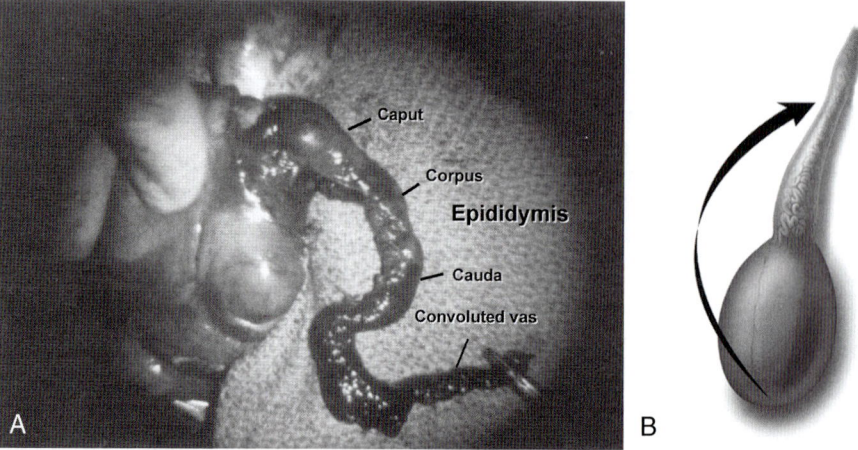

Fig. 67.13. (A and B) An additional 4 to 6 cm of length can be obtained by dissecting the epididymis off of the testis from the vasoepididymal junction to the caput epididymis.

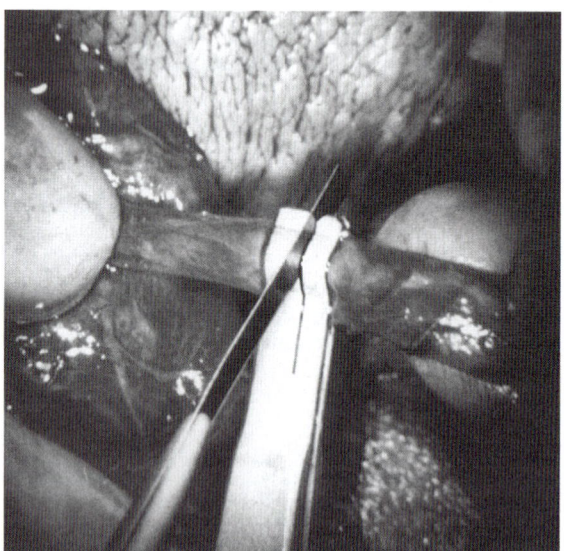

Fig. 67.14. An ultrasharp knife drawn through a slotted nerve holding clamp yields a perfect 90-degree cut.

fluid. If there is no sperm granuloma, and the vas is absolutely dry and spermless after multiple samples are examined, vasoepididymostomy is indicated. If the fluid expressed from the vas is found to be thick, white, water insoluble and toothpaste-like in quality, microscopic examination rarely reveals sperm. Under these circumstances, the tunica vaginalis is opened and the epididymis inspected. If clear evidence of obstruction is found (i.e., an epididymal sperm granuloma with dilated tubules above and collapsed tubules below), vasoepididymostomy is performed. **When in doubt, or if the surgeon is not very experienced with vasoepididymostomy, vasovasostomy should be performed.** However, only 15% of men with bilateral absence of sperm in the vasal fluid after barbotage and an intensive search will have sperm return to the ejaculate after vasovasostomy (Sheynkin et al., 2000).

When copious, crystal clear, waterlike fluid squirts out from the vas and no sperm are found in this fluid, a vasovasostomy is performed because the likelihood is that sperm will return to the ejaculate after vasovasotomy is performed.

Multiple Vasal Obstructions

If saline injection reveals that the abdominal end of the vas deferens is not patent, a 2-0 nylon or polypropylene suture is gently threaded into the vas lumen to determine the site of obstruction. If the obstruction is within 5 cm of the original vasectomy site, the abdominal end of the vas deferens may be dissected to this site and excised. The incision should then be extended inguinally to free the vas up extensively toward the internal inguinal ring. The testicular end then should also be freed up to the vasoepididymal junction. If the site of the second obstruction is so far from the vasectomy site that two vasovasostomies are necessary, a single crossed vasovasostomy should be performed to yield one good system. If this is not possible, vasal or epididymal sperm is aspirated into micropipettes and cryopreserved for future IVF with ICSI. **Simultaneous vasovasostomies at two separate sites will usually lead to devascularization of the intervening segment with fibrosis and necrosis.**

Varicocelectomy and Vasovasostomy

When men presenting for vasovasostomy or vasoepididymostomy are found to have significant varicoceles on physical examination, it is tempting to repair the varicoceles at the same time. **When varicocelectomy is properly performed, all spermatic veins are ligated and the only remaining avenues for testicular venous return are the vasal veins. In men who have had vasectomy and are presenting for reversal, the vasal veins are likely to be compromised from either the original vasectomy or the reversal. Furthermore, the integrity of the vasal artery in those men is also likely to be compromised. Varicocelectomy in such men requires preservation of the testicular artery as the primary remaining testicular blood supply as well as preservation of some avenue for venous return.**

Microscopic varicocelectomy can ensure preservation of the testicular artery in most cases. Deliberate preservation of small cremasteric or perivasal veins provides venous return. In one series of 570 men presenting for vasectomy reversal, 19 had large varicoceles (20 left, 7 bilateral). Microsurgical varicocelectomy was performed at the same time as vasovasostomy. The cremasteric veins and the fine network of veins adherent to the testicular artery were left intact for venous return and to minimize the chances of injury to the testicular artery. Postoperatively 5/26 varicoceles recurred (22%) (Goldstein, 1995). This compares to a recurrence rate of less than 1% in 3500 varicocelectomies performed by the author in nonvasectomized men in whom the vasal vessels were intact and the cremasteric veins and periarterial venous network were ligated. However, Mullhall et al. (1997) performed a series of simultaneous microsurgical vasovasostomies and varicocelectomies without intentionally preserving the cremasteric and periarterial network. They reported a low recurrence rate and no cases of atrophy. Interestingly, the increase in recurrences when the cremasteric veins and periarterial venous network were left intact suggests that these veins contribute to a significant proportion of varicocele recurrences.

TABLE 67.2 Relationship Between Gross Appearance of Vasal Fluid and Microscopic Findings

APPEARANCE OF VASAL FLUID	INTRAOPERATIVE EVALUATION OF ASPIRATE	RECOMMENDED SURGICAL PROCEDURE
Copious, crystal clear, watery	No sperm	Vasovasostomy
Copious, cloudy thin, water soluble	Sperm with tails, including short tails, motile or nonmotile	Vasovasostomy
Copious, creamy yellow, water insoluble	Many sperm heads, often with acrosome visible, scattered throughout the slide	Vasovasostomy
Copious, thick white toothpaste-like, water insoluble	No sperm or sperm heads	Vasoepididymostomy
Scant white thin fluid	No sperm or sperm heads	Vasoepididymostomy
Scant fluid, no granuloma at vasectomy site	No sperm or sperm heads	Vasoepididymostomy
Scant fluid, granuloma present at vasectomy site	Barbotage fluid reveals sperm, usually with tails, often motile	Vasovasostomy
Any fluid	Fluid with occasional grapelike clusters of sperm heads	Vasoepididymostomy

If varicocelectomy is performed at the same time as vasovasostomy or vasoepididymostomy, it is important that a microscope be used and the testicular artery preserved. Another approach, especially when the female partner is young, is to do the vasovasostomy or vasoepididymostomy first. The semen quality is then assessed postoperatively. If necessary, varicocelectomy can be safely performed 6 months or more later when venous and arterial channels have formed across the anastomotic line. This two-stage delayed approach has been completed a dozen times with no atrophy or recurrence.

Anastomotic Techniques: Keys to Success

All successful vasovasostomy techniques depend on adherence to surgical principles that are universally applicable to anastomoses of all tubular structures.

These include the following:

1. **Accurate mucosa-to-mucosa approximation**
   In human vasovasostomy, the lumen on the testicular side is usually dilated, often to diameters 2 to 5 times that of the abdominal side. Techniques that work well with lumina of equal diameters may be less successful when applied to lumina of markedly discrepant diameters.
2. **Leakproof anastomosis**
   Sperm are highly antigenic and provoke an inflammatory reaction when they escape from the normally intact lining of the excurrent ducts of the male reproductive tract. Extravasated sperm adversely influence the success of vasovasostomy (Hagan and Coffey, 1977). Unlike blood vessel anastomoses, in which platelets and clotting factors seal the gaps between sutures, vasal and epididymal fluid contain no platelets or clotting factors, so the water tightness of the anastomosis is entirely dependent on the mucosal sutures.
3. **Tension-free anastomosis**
   When an anastomosis is performed under tension, sperm may appear in the ejaculate for several months after surgery. Ultimately, sperm counts and motility will decrease, and azoospermia may ensue. At re-exploration only a thin fibrotic band is found at the anastomotic site. This can be prevented by adequately freeing up the vasa and placement of re-enforcing sutures in the sheath of the vas.
4. **Good blood supply**
   If the cut vas exhibits poor blood supply, it should be recut until healthy bleeding is encountered. If extensive resection is necessary, additional length should be obtained using the techniques previously described.
5. **Healthy mucosa and muscularis**
   If the mucosa or cut surface of the vas exhibits poor distensibility after dilation, peels away from the underlying muscularis, or shreds easily, then the vas should be cut back until healthy mucosa is found. Surgeons should be aware that if a needle

electrocautery was used in vasectomy, the area of damage to the mucosa and muscularis by the electric current may extend far beyond the tip of the needle cautery. If the muscularis is found to be fibrotic or gritty, the vas must be recut until healthy tissue is found.

6. **Good atraumatic anastomotic technique**
   If multiple surgical errors occur during the procedure, such as inadvertent cutting of the mucosa with the needles when placing sutures, tearing through of sutures, or backwalling of the mucosa, the anastomosis should be resected and redone immediately.

Setup

An operating microscope providing variable magnification from 6× to 32× power is employed. A diploscope providing identical fields for surgeon and assistant is preferred. Foot pedal controls for a motorized zoom and focus leave the surgeon's hands free.

The surgeon and assistant should be comfortably seated on microsurgical chairs that stabilize the chest and arms. This dramatically improves stability and accuracy. An inexpensive alternative is a simple rolling stool with a round bean bag (meditation pillow) taped on top for padding. Two arm boards placed on either side of the surgeon and built up to the appropriate height with folded blankets taped to the board provide excellent arm support. **Right-handed surgeons should sit on the patient's right side** so that their forehand stitch is always on the smaller, more difficult abdominal side lumen.

Microsurgical Multilayer Microdot Method

This method of vasovasostomy can handle lumina of markedly discrepant diameters in the straight or convoluted vas. **The microdot technique ensures precise suture placement by exact mapping of each planned suture. The microdot method separates the planning from the placement** (Dabaja et al., 2013; Goldstein et al., 1998). This allows focus on only one task at a time and results in substantially improved accuracy.

A microtip marking pen (Devon Skin Marker Extra Fine #151) is used to map out planned needle exit points. **Exactly six mucosal sutures are used for every anastomosis** because it is easy to map out and always results in a leakproof closure even when the lumen diameters are markedly discrepant.

Immediately after the cut surface of the testicular end of vas is dried with a Weck-cel sponge, a dot is made at 3 o'clock halfway between the mucosal ring and the outer edge of the muscle layer. A line is extended out from this dot to serve as a reference point. The second dot is made at 9 o'clock, and a line is extended from this dot as well. Additional dots are placed at 11, 1, 5, and 7 o'clock for a total of six. The abdominal end of the vas is marked in the same way to exactly match the testicular end (Fig. 67.15). Monofilament 10-0 nylon sutures are used, double-armed with 70-micron diameter taper-point needles bent into a fish-hook configuration (available from Sharpoint and Ethicon). **Double-armed sutures allow inside-out placement** (Fig. 67.16), **eliminating the need for manipulation of the mucosa and the possibility of back-walling.** If the mucosal rings are not sharply defined, the cut surfaces of the vasal ends are stained with indigo carmine to highlight the mucosa (Sheynkin et al., 1999a). The anastomosis is begun with the placement of three 10-0 mucosal sutures anteriorly (Fig. 67.17). **On the small abdominal side lumen, the lumen is gently and momentarily dilated with a microvessel dilator just before placement of the sutures.** For accurate mucosal approximation only a small amount of mucosa is included but one-third to one-half the muscle wall thickness. **Exactly the same amount of tissue is included in the bites on each side. The needle should exit through the center of each dot.** After placement, the three mucosal sutures are tied. Two 9-0 monofilament nylon deep muscularis sutures are placed exactly in between the previously placed mucosal sutures, just above but not through the mucosa (Fig. 67.18) and then tied. These sutures seal the gaps between the mucosal sutures without trauma to the

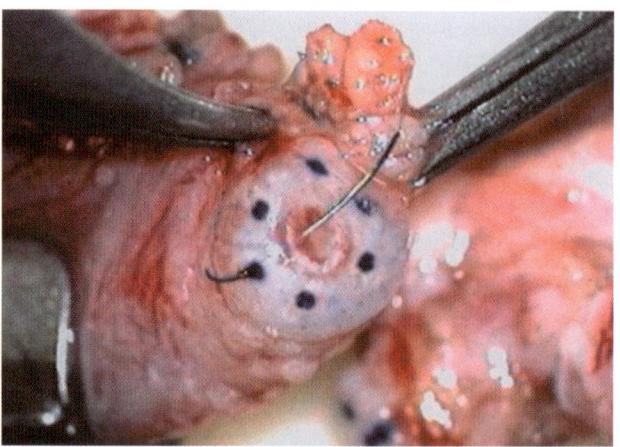

Fig. 67.16. Double-armed sutures allow inside-out placement.

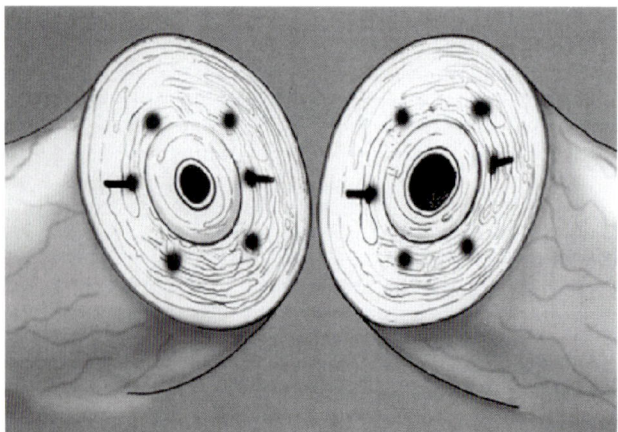

Fig. 67.15. The abdominal end of the vas is marked in the same way to exactly match the testicular end.

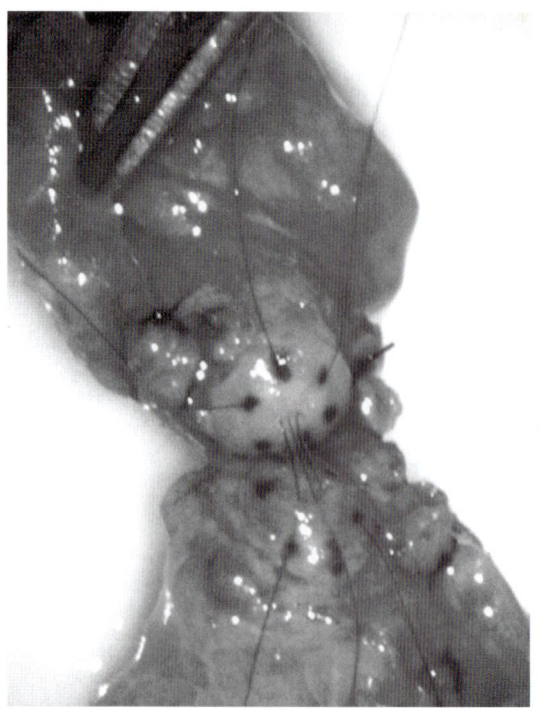

Fig. 67.17. The anastomosis is begun with the placement of three 10-0 mucosal sutures anteriorly.

Chapter 67 Surgical Management of Male Infertility 1465

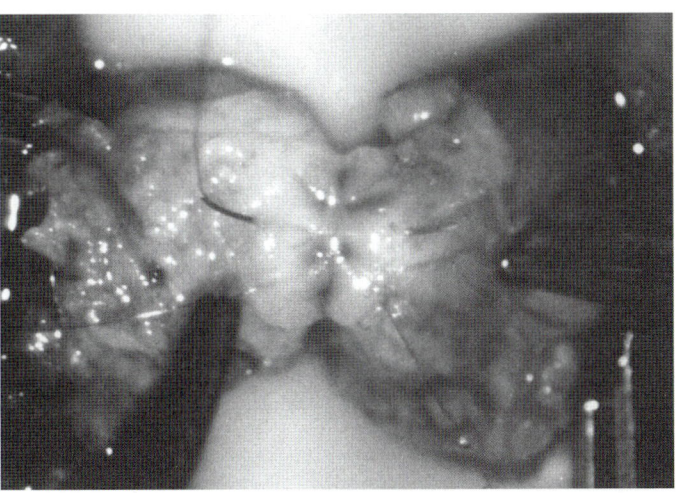

Fig. 67.18. Two 9-0 monofilament nylon deep muscularis sutures are placed exactly in between the previously placed mucosal sutures, just above, but not through the mucosa.

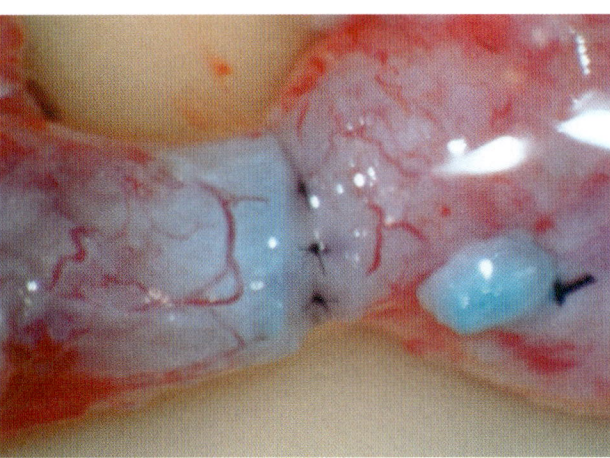

Fig. 67.20. Three additional 10-0 sutures are placed through each microdot and then tied to complete the mucosal portion of the anastomosis.

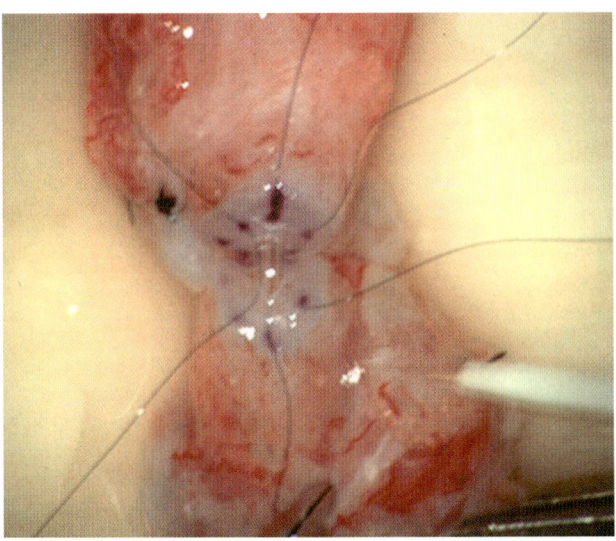

Fig. 67.19. The vas is rotated 180 degrees.

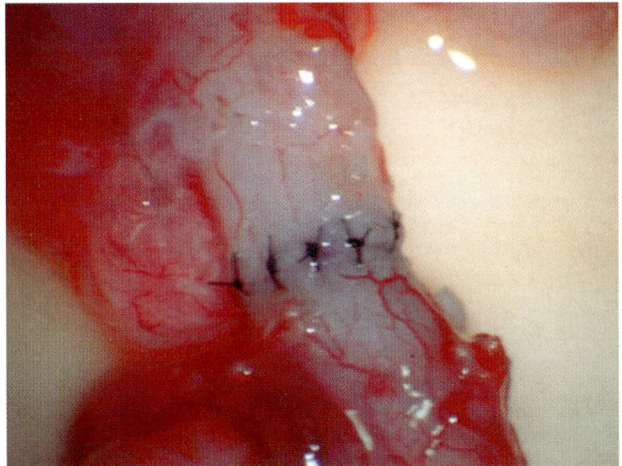

Fig. 67.21. Completion of the mucosal layer.

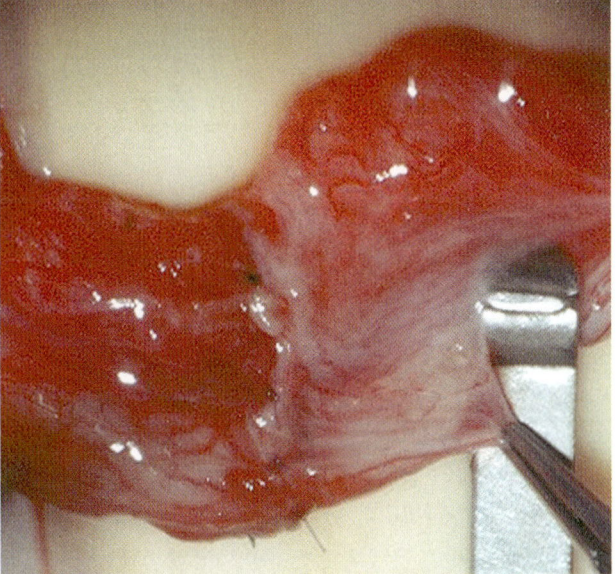

Fig. 67.22. The anastomosis is finished by approximating the vasal sheath with six to eight interrupted sutures of 8-0 nylon completely covering the anastomosis and relieving it of all tension.

mucosa from the larger 100-micron diameter cutting needle required to penetrate the tough vas muscularis and adventitia. The vas is rotated 180 degrees (Fig. 67.19), and three additional 10-0 sutures are placed through each microdot and then tied to complete the mucosal portion of the anastomosis (Fig. 67.20). Just before tying the last mucosal suture, the lumen is irrigated with heparinized Ringer's solution to prevent the formation of clot in the lumen. After completion of the mucosal layer (Fig. 67.21), four more 9-0 deep muscularis sutures are placed exactly in between each mucosal suture, just above but not penetrating the mucosa. Four to six 9-0 nylon interrupted sutures are placed between each muscular suture. This is a purely adventitial later that covers the underlying mucosal suture. The anastomosis is finished by approximating the vasal sheath with six to eight interrupted sutures of 8-0 nylon, completely covering the anastomosis and relieving it of all tension (Fig. 67.22).

Anastomosis in the Convoluted Vas

Vasovasostomy performed in the convoluted portion of the vas deferens is technically more demanding than anastomoses in the straight portion. **Fear of cutting back into the convoluted vas to obtain healthy tissue may lead surgeons to complete an anastomosis in the straight portion when the testicular end of the vas has poor blood**

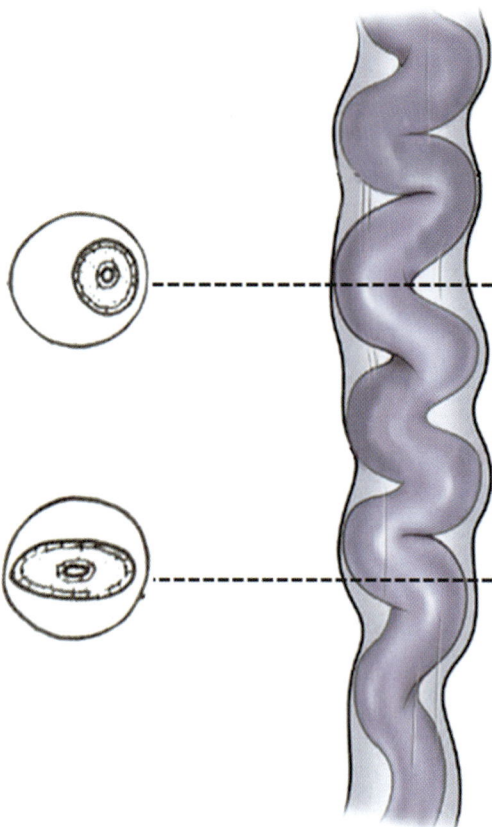

Fig. 67.23. An oblique lumen with a thin flap of muscle and mucosa on one side is not acceptable.

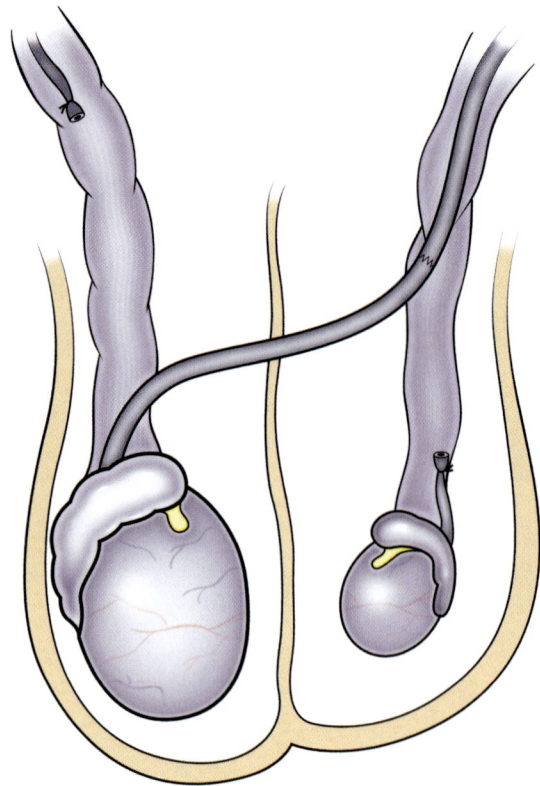

Fig. 67.24. Technique for vasovasostomy or vasoepididymostomy with contralateral testis.

supply, unhealthy or friable mucosa, or gritty fibrotic muscularis. Adherence to the following principles will enable anastomosis in the convoluted vas to succeed as often as those in the straight portion.

1. **A perfect transverse cut yielding a round ring of mucosa and a lumen directed straight down is essential.** A very oblique lumen with a thin flap of muscle and mucosa on one side is not acceptable (Fig. 67.23). The vas should be recut at 0.5-mm intervals until a perfect cut with good blood supply and healthy tissue is obtained. A slotted nerve clamp 2.5 or 3 mm in diameter and ultrasharp knife facilitates this part of the procedure (see Fig. 67.14). Often the vas must be recut 2 or 3 times until a satisfactory cut is obtained.
2. **The convoluted vas should not be unraveled.** This disturbs the blood supply at the anastomotic line.
3. The sheath of the convoluted vas may be carefully dissected free of its attachments to the epididymal tunica (see Fig. 67.12). This minimizes disturbance of its blood supply and provides the necessary length to perform a tension-free anastomosis.
4. Care must be taken to avoid taking large bites of the muscularis and adventitial layers on the convoluted side to prevent inadvertent perforation of adjacent convolutions.
5. Reinforce the anastomosis by approximating the vasal sheath of the straight portion to the sheath of the convoluted portion with six interrupted sutures of 7-0 nylon. This removes all tension from the anastomosis.

Crossed Vasovasostomy

This useful procedure often provides an easy solution for otherwise difficult problems (Hamidinia, 1988; Lizza et al., 1985; Sheynkin et al., 1998a). Crossover is indicated in the following circumstances:

1. Unilateral inguinal obstruction of the vas deferens associated with an atrophic testis on the contralateral side. A crossover vasovasostomy should be performed to connect a healthy testicle to the contralateral unobstructed vas.
2. Obstruction or aplasia of the inguinal vas or ejaculatory duct on one side and epididymal obstruction on the contralateral side

It **is preferable to perform one anastomosis with a high probability of success (vasovasostomy) than two operations with a much lower chance of success** (e.g., unilateral vasoepididymostomy and contralateral TURED).

Technique

The vas attached to the atrophic testis is transected at the junction of its straight and convoluted portion and its patency confirmed with a Ringer's or indigo carmine vasogram (Fig. 67.24). The contralateral vas is dissected with the normal testis toward the inguinal obstruction. It is clamped and transected as high up as possible with a right angle clamp. The testicular end of the vas is crossed through a capacious opening made in the scrotal septum; the surgeon proceeds with vasovasostomy as described earlier. This procedure is much easier than inguinal vasovasostomy, which requires finding both ends of the vas within the dense scar of a previous inguinal operation.

Transposition of the Testis

Occasionally when vasal length is critically short, a tension-free crossed anastomosis can best be accomplished by testicular transposition (Fig. 67.25). The spermatic cord is always longer than the vas. The testes will comfortably cross through a generous opening in the septum and sit nicely in the contralateral scrotal compartment.

Wound Closure

If the vasal dissection was extensive, Penrose drains are brought out the dependent portion of the right and left hemiscrota and fixed in place with sutures and safety pins preferably before the anastomosis is begun. Placement of drains at the end of the procedure

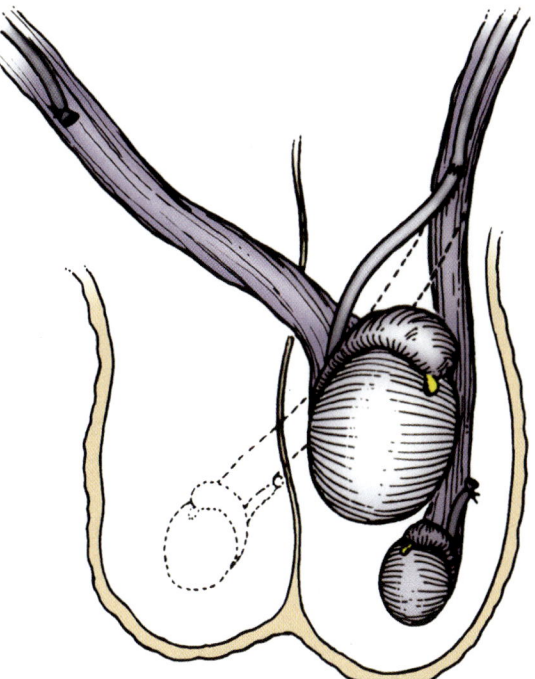

Fig. 67.25. When vasal length is critically short, a tension-free crossed anastomosis can best be accomplished by testicular transposition.

may potentially disturb the anastomosis. The dartos layer is approximated with interrupted 4-0 absorbable sutures and the skin with subcuticular sutures of 5-0 Monocryl. The wound heals with a fine scar. The use of through-and-through skin closures, which give an unacceptable "railroad-track"-looking scar, should be avoided. **Almost all of our procedures are performed on an ambulatory basis.** If drains were placed, the patients are given detailed instructions (with explicit drawings) on how to remove the drains the next morning.

Postoperative Management

Sterile fluffs gauze dressings are held in place with a snug-fitting scrotal supporter. Only perioperative antibiotics are used. Patients are discharged with a prescription for acetaminophen with codeine. They shower 48 hours after surgery. **They wear a scrotal supporter at all times (except in the shower), even when sleeping, for 6 weeks postoperatively. Thereafter, a scrotal supporter is worn during athletic activity, until pregnancy is achieved.** Desk work is resumed in 3 days. No heavy work or sports are allowed for 3 weeks. **No intercourse or ejaculation is allowed for 3 weeks postoperatively.** Semen analyses are obtained at 1, 3, and 6 months postoperatively and every 6 months thereafter. If azoospermia persists at 6 months, a redo vasovasostomy or vasoepididymostomy is necessary.

Postoperative Complications

The most common complication is hematoma. In 2500 operations, 7 small hematomas occurred. None required surgical drainage. Most were walnut sized and perivasal. They take 6 to 12 weeks to resolve. Wound infection did not occur. Late complications include sperm granuloma at the anastomotic site (approximately 5%). This usually is a harbinger of eventual obstruction. Late stricture and obstruction are disappointingly common (see following). **Progressive loss of motility followed by decreasing counts indicates stricture.** Our recent change from Proline to **nylon sutures** (Sheynkin, 1999b), use of the microdot system to prevent leaks, extensive dissection of the vas until healthy mucosa and muscularis is identified, constant attention to the preservation of good blood supply, and generous use of scrotal support until pregnancy is established have reduced the incidence of late obstruction from 12% (Matthews et al., 1995) **to** 5% (Kolettis and Thomas, 1997) **at 18 months after surgery. Because of the risk of late stricture and obstruction, we strongly encourage cryopreservation of semen specimens as soon as motile sperm appear in the ejaculate.**

Long-Term Follow-Up Evaluation After Vasovasostomy

When sperm are found in the vasal fluid on at least one side at the time of surgery, the anastomotic technique described results in appearance of sperm in the ejaculate in 99.5% of men (Dabaja et al., 2013; Goldstein et al., 1998). Pregnancy has occurred in 52% of couples followed for at least 2 years and 63% when female factors are excluded with outcomes dependent on the time since vasectomy and female partner age (Boorjian et al., 2004; Gerrard et al., 2007; Kolettis et al., 2003, 2005; Wosnitzer and Goldstein, 2013).

> **KEY POINTS: VASOVASOSTOMY**
>
> - The presence of serum antisperm antibodies corroborates the diagnosis and presence of active spermatogenesis.
> - The vas deferens should not be stripped of its sheath.
> - When the vasal gap is extremely large, additional length can be achieved by dissecting the convoluted vas free of its attachments to the epididymal tunica. The convoluted vas should not be unraveled.
> - Successful vasovasostomy relies on an accurate mucosa-to-mucosa approximation, a tension-free and leakproof anastomosis, good blood supply, healthy mucosa and muscularis, and good atraumatic anastomotic technique.

SURGERY OF THE EPIDIDYMIS

Detailed knowledge of epididymal anatomy and physiology (presented in Chapters 63 and 64) is essential before undertaking surgery of this delicate but important structure. Sperm motility and fertilizing capacity progressively increase during passage through the 200-micron diameter, 12- to 15-foot long, tightly coiled single tubule. When the epididymis is obstructed and functionally shortened after vasoepididymostomy, even very short lengths of epididymis are able to adapt and allow some sperm to acquire motility and fertilizing capacity (Jow et al., 1993; Silber, 1989). Adaptation may gradually continue up to 2 years after surgical reconstruction, with progressive improvement in the fertility and motility of sperm. Nevertheless, preservation of the greatest possible length of functional epididymis is most likely to result in the best sperm quality after vasoepididymostomy (Schlegel and Goldstein, 1993; Schoysman and Bedford, 1986). Furthermore, because the wall of the epididymis is thinnest in the caput region and gradually thickens and because of the increasing numbers of smooth muscle cells in its more distal (inferior) end, anastomoses are technically easier to perform and more likely to succeed in its distal regions. **Because the corpus and cauda epididymis is a single tubule with a very small diameter, injury or occlusion of a tubule anywhere along its length will lead to total obstruction of outflow at that level.** For these reasons, **magnification, with loupes for macrodissection and with the operating microscope for anastomosis, is essential for performing all epididymal surgery.**

Fortunately, the epididymis is blessed with a rich blood supply derived from the testicular vessels superiorly and the deferential vessels inferiorly (see Testicular Blood Supply and Chapter 21). Because of the extensive interconnections between these branches, either the testicular or deferential branches (but not both) to the epididymis may be divided without compromising epididymal viability.

Conversely, because the epididymal branches of the testicular artery are medial to and separate from the main testicular artery and veins, surgical procedures may be performed on the epididymis without compromise to testicular blood supply.

Vasoepididymostomy

Before the development of microsurgical techniques, accurate approximation of the vasal lumen to that of a specific epididymal tubule was not possible. Vasoepididymostomy was performed by aligning the vas deferens adjacent to a slash made in multiple epididymal tubules and hoping a fistula would form. Results with this primitive technique were poor. Microsurgical approaches allow accurate approximation of the vasal mucosa to that of a single epididymal tubule (Silber, 1978) resulting in marked improvement in the patency and pregnancy rates (Chan et al., 2005; Schlegel, 1993). **However, microsurgical vasoepididymostomy is the most technically demanding procedure in all of microsurgery.** In almost no other operation are results so dependent upon technical perfection. **Microsurgical vasoepididymostomy should be attempted only by experienced microsurgeons who perform the procedure frequently.**

Indications

The indications for vasoepididymostomy at the time of vasectomy reversal were reviewed earlier. For obstructive azoospermia not resulting from vasectomy, **vasoepididymostomy is indicated when complete spermatogenesis in at least one testis is confirmed by either prior biopsy or highly positive serum antisperm antibodies** (Lee et al., 2009), **and scrotal exploration reveals the absence of sperm in the vasal lumen with no vasal or ejaculatory duct obstruction.** The preoperative evaluation is identical to that described for vasovasostomy.

Microsurgical End-to-Side Vasoepididymostomy

End-to-side techniques of vasoepididymostomy have the advantage of being minimally traumatic to the epididymis and relatively bloodless (Table 67.3; Chan et al., 2005; Fogdestam et al., 1986; Krylov and Borovikov, 1984; Schiff et al., 2005; Thomas, 1987; Wagenknecht et al., 1980). The end-to-side technique does not disturb the epididymal blood supply. When the level of epididymal obstruction is clearly demarcated by the presence of markedly dilated tubules proximally and collapsed tubules distally, the site at which the anastomosis should be performed is readily apparent. The end-to-side approach has the advantage of allowing accurate approximation of the muscularis and adventitia of the vas deferens to a precisely tailored opening in the tunica of the epididymis. This is the preferred technique when vasoepididymostomy is performed simultaneously with inguinal vasovasostomy because it is possible to preserve the vasal blood supply deriving from epididymal branches of the testicular artery (Fig. 67.26). This provides blood supply to the segment of vas intervening between the two anastomoses. Maintenance of the deferential artery's contribution to the testicular blood supply is also important in situations in which the integrity of the testicular artery is in doubt because of prior surgery such as orchiopexy, nonmicroscopic varicocelectomy, or hernia repair.

The testis is delivered through a 3- to 4-cm high vertical scrotal incision. The vas deferens is identified, isolated with a Babcock clamp, and then surrounded with a Penrose drain at the junction of the straight and convoluted portions of the vas deferens. Using 8× to 15× power magnification provided by the operating microscope, the vasal sheath is longitudinally incised with a microknife, and a bare segment of vas stripped of its carefully preserved vessels is delivered. The vas is hemitransected with the ultrasharp knife until the lumen is entered (Fig. 67.27). **The vasal fluid is sampled. If microscopic examination of this fluid reveals the absence of sperm, the diagnosis of epididymal obstruction is confirmed.** Patency of the vas and ejaculatory ducts is confirmed by cannulating the abdominal end of the vas with a 24-gauge angiocatheter sheath and gently injecting lactated Ringer's solution with a 1-mL tuberculin syringe (see Fig. 67.3). Further confirmation of patency may be obtained by injecting indigo carmine, catheterizing the bladder, and observing blue-tinged urine. The vas is then completely transected using a 2.5-mm slotted

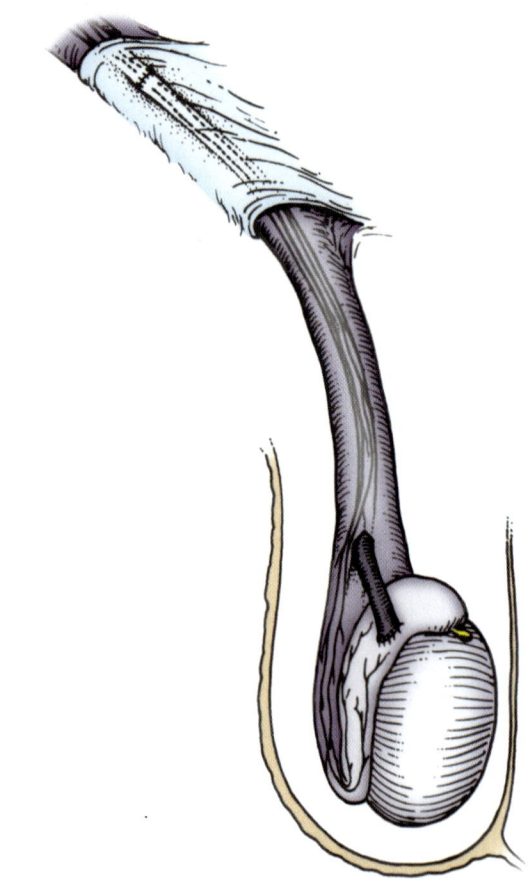

Fig. 67.26. Vasoepididymostomy is performed simultaneously with inguinal vasovasostomy because it is possible to preserve the vasal blood supply deriving from the epididymal branches of the testicular artery.

TABLE 67.3 Comparison of Three Common Techniques for Vasoepididymostomy

TECHNIQUES	ADVANTAGES	DISADVANTAGES
Intussusception (LIVE)	Two sutures placed longitudinally in the dilated epididymal tubule provide four points of fixation Virtually bloodless anastomosis	Cannot assess tubular fluid for sperm before anastomosis setup
End-Side	Virtually bloodless anastomosis Epididymal fluid can be examined before anastomosis	Difficult suture placement to a collapsed tubule
End-End	Epididymal fluid can be examined before anastomosis Easy and rapid identification of the level of obstruction in the epididymis Allows upward mobilization of epididymis to bridge a large vasal gap	Difficult hemostasis on transected epididymis Difficult to identify the proper tubule for anastomosis Difficult outer layer closure Vasal blood supply from inferior epididymal artery is sacrificed

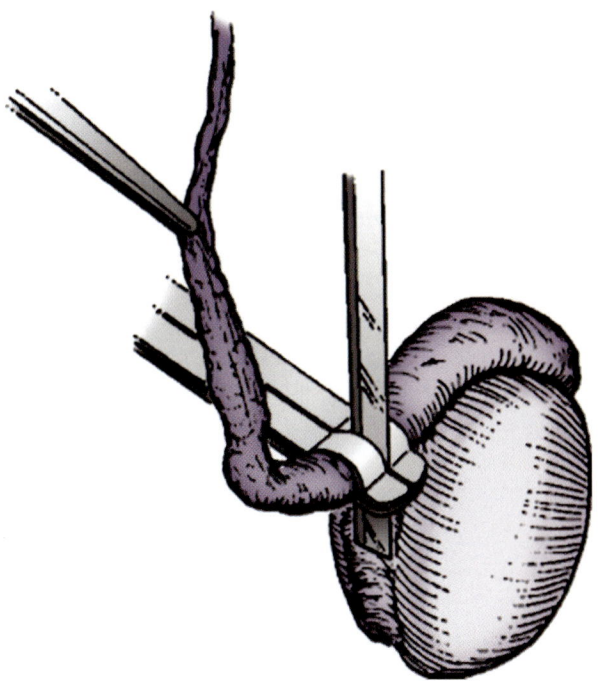

Fig. 67.27. The vas is completely transected using a 2.5-mm slotted nerve clamp.

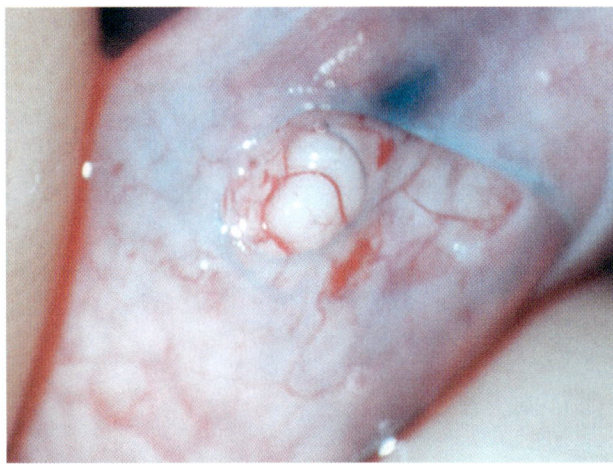

Fig. 67.29. Epididymal tubules are then gently dissected with a combination of sharp and blunt dissection until dilated loops of tubule are clearly exposed.

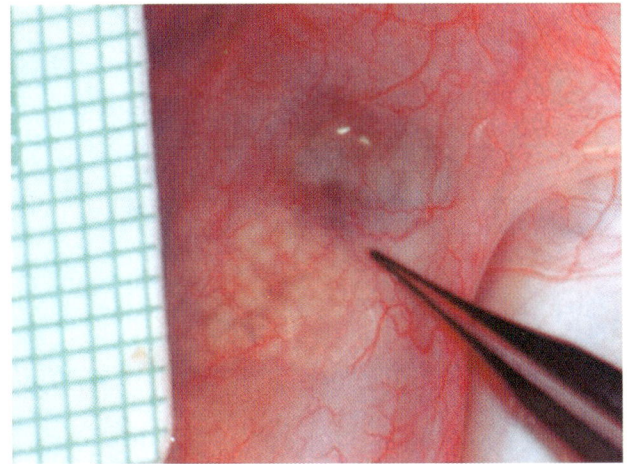

Fig. 67.28. Diluted epididymal tubules are clearly seen beneath the epididymal tunica.

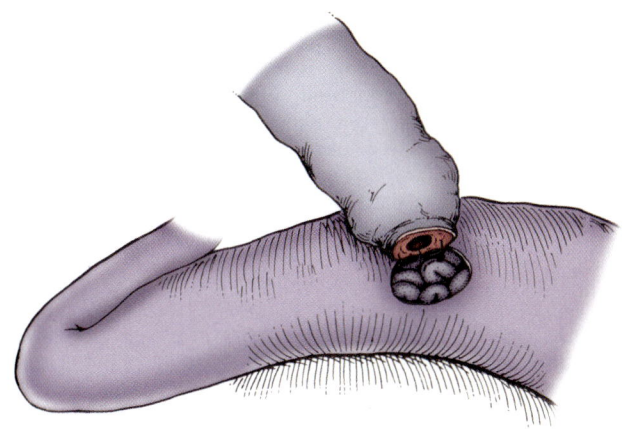

Fig. 67.30. The posterior edge of the epididymal tunica is reapproximated to the posterior edge of the vas muscularis and adventitia with two to three interrupted sutures.

nerve clamp (see Fig. 67.27), and the vas is prepared as for vasovasostomy as described earlier.

After opening the tunica vaginalis, the epididymis is inspected under the operating microscope. An anastomotic site is selected above the area of suspected obstruction, proximal to any visible sperm granulomas, where dilated epididymal tubules are clearly seen beneath the epididymal tunica (Fig. 67.28). A relatively avascular area is grasped with sharp jewelers forceps and the epididymal tunica tented upward. **A 3- to 4-mm buttonhole is made in the tunica with microscissors to create a round opening that matches the outer diameter of the previously prepared vas deferens.** The epididymal tubules are then gently dissected with a combination of sharp and blunt dissections until dilated loops of tubule are clearly exposed (Fig. 67.29). **If the level of obstruction is not clearly delineated, after the buttonhole opening is made in the tunic, a 70-μm diameter tapered needle from the 10-0 nylon microsuture is used to puncture the epididymal tubule beginning as distal as possible and fluid sampled from the puncture site. When sperm are found, the puncture sites are sealed with microbipolar forceps,** a new buttonhole made in the epididymal tunic just proximally, and the tubule prepared as described previously.

The vas deferens is drawn thru an opening in the tunica vaginalis and secured in proximity to the anastomotic site with two to four interrupted sutures of 6-0 polypropylene placed through the vasal adventitia and the tunica vaginalis. **The vasal lumen should reach the opening in the epididymal tunica easily, with length to spare.** The posterior edge of the epididymal tunica is then approximated to the posterior edge of the vas muscularis and adventitia with two to three interrupted sutures of double-armed 9-0 nylon (Fig. 67.30). This is done in such a way as to bring the vasal lumen in close approximation to the epididymal tubule selected for anastomosis.

Intussusception Vasoepididymostomy

Intussusception techniques have supplanted the older end-to-side techniques because they allow needle placement in a dilated tubule. Intussusception also plasters the wall of the epididymis against the inner vasal mucosa, and the normal flow of epididymal fluid from the epididymal tubule to the vas encourages this apposition and makes it more leakproof than older techniques in which the opening in the epididymal tubule was made before needle placement.

The original intussusception technique described by Berger (1998) employed three double-armed 10-0 sutures placed in the epididymal tubule in a triangular fashion and the use of a 9-0 needle to tear an opening in the middle of the triangle. **We now employ a two-stitch longitudinal intussusception (LIVE) technique for all**

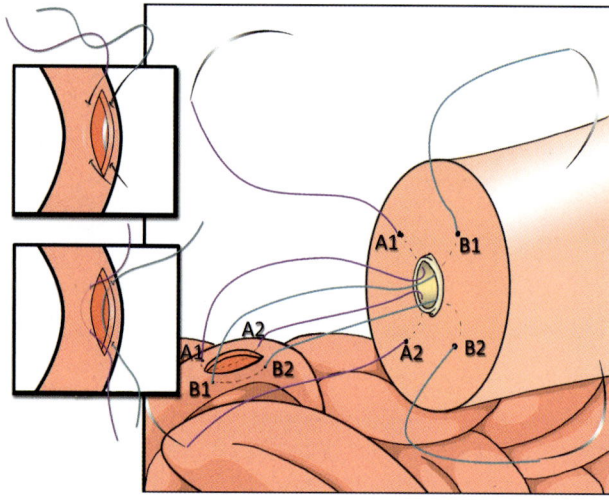

Fig. 67.31. Four microdots are marked on the cut surface of the vas deferens and two parallel sutures are placed in the distended epidiymal tubule longitudinally but not pulled through.

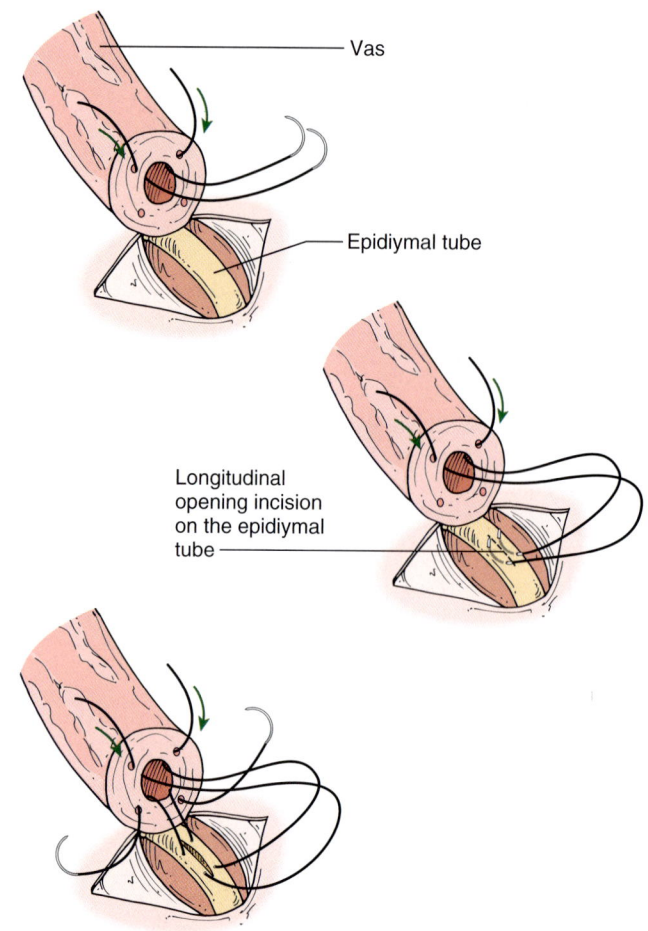

Fig. 67.32. A single-arm technique of vasoepididymostomy is almost as effective as the double-arm technique.

vasoepididymostomies. It is much easier to perform and is even more successful. With this method, four microdots are marked on the cut surface of the vas deferens and two parallel sutures are placed in the distended epididymal tubule longitudinally but not pulled through (Fig. 67.31). Marmar (2000) suggests mounting two needles in the needle holder and placing them simultaneously transversely in the tubule. However, if the needles are not pulled through to avoid leakage of fluid and tubular collapse, they can be placed one at a time with greater control and accuracy (Chan et al., 2005; Schiff et al., 2005). Longitudinal placement also allows a larger opening to be made in the epididymal tubule without risk of completely transecting it. Using a 15-degree microknife, an opening is made exactly between and parallel to the two previously placed sutures. We have also developed a single-arm technique of vasoepididymostomy that is almost as effective as the double-arm technique (Fig. 67.32; Monoski, 2007). This technique may prove valuable when double-arm sutures are not available.

Technique When Vasal Length Is Severely Compromised

When there is inadequate length of the vas deferens to reach the dilated epididymal tubule without tension, the epididymis can be dissected down to the vasoepididymal junction and then dissected off the testes as in the older end-to-end operation.

After the vas has been prepared, the tunica vaginalis is opened and the testis delivered. Inspection of the epididymis under the operating microscope may reveal a clearly delineated site of obstruction. Often a discrete yellow sperm granuloma is noted, above which the epididymis is indurated and the tubules dilated and below which the epididymis is soft and the tubules collapsed. **If the level of obstruction is not clearly delineated, a 70-micron tapered needle from the 10-0 nylon microsuture is used to puncture the epididymal tubule beginning as distal as possible, and fluid is sampled from the puncture site until sperm are found. At that level the puncture is sealed with microbipolar forceps, and the epididymis is ligated just proximal to the puncture site with a 6-0 nylon suture. The epididymis is then dissected off the testis and flipped up to obtain additional length.** To do this, the epididymis is encircled with a small Penrose drain at the level of obstruction and, using 2.5× power loupe magnification, dissected off of the testis for 3 to 5 cm, yielding sufficient length to perform the anastomosis. Usually a nice plane can be found between the epididymis and testis, and injury to the epididymal blood supply can be avoided by staying right on the tunica albuginea of the testis. The inferior and, if necessary, middle epididymal branches of the testicular artery are ligated and divided to free up an adequate length of epididymis. The superior-epididymal branches entering the epididymis at the caput are always preserved and can provide adequate blood supply to the entire epididymis. The tunica vaginalis in then closed over the testis with 5-0 Vicryl. This prevents drying of the testis and thrombosis of the surface testicular vessels during the anastomosis. The dissected epididymis remains outside the tunica vaginalis.

If the epididymis is indurated and dilated throughout its length, the epididymis is dissected to the vasoepididymal (VE) junction. This dissection is often facilitated by first dissecting the convoluted vas to the VE junction from below, and then, after encircling the epididymis with a Penrose drain, dissecting the epididymis to the VE junction from above. In this way the entire VE junction can be freed up. This will allow preservation of maximal epididymal length in cases of distal obstruction near the VE junction. After the epididymis is dissected off of the testis and flipped-up, a two-stitch end-to-side intussusception anastomosis is performed as described earlier.

Varicocelectomy and Vasoepididymostomy

Although varicocelectomy can be simultaneously performed at the time of vasovasostomy (Mulhall et al., 1997), especially if intact deferential veins can be identified going across the anastomosis, I do not recommend doing simultaneous varicocelectomy and vasoepididymostomy. After varicocelectomy, the venous pressure in the epididymal vein is very high and, because vasoepididymostomy is a significantly more delicate and difficult procedure with a lower success rate than vasovasostomy, the increased bleeding at the site of the vasoepididymostomy may negatively affect the success rate. I recommend performing the vasoepididymostomy first, waiting 6 months, and, if sperm quality remains poor, and/or serum testosterone levels are low, then repairing the varicocele microsurgically.

Long-Term Follow-Up Evaluation and Results

Microsurgical vasoepididymostomy in the hands of experienced and skilled microsurgeons results in the appearance of sperm in the ejaculate in 50% to 85% of men. Patency rates with the intussusception technique can exceed 80% (Berger, 1953; Brandell, 1999; Marmar, 2000). With the classic end-to-side or older end-to-end method, the patency rate is about 70%, and 43% of men with sperm will impregnate their wives after a minimum follow-up of 2 years (Pasqualotto et al., 1999; Schlegel and Goldstein, 1993). With the intussception techniques, patency rates are 70% to 90% (Chan et al., 2005; Kolettis and Thomas, 1997; Schiff et al., 2005). Regardless of technique, pregnancy rates are higher the more distal the anastomosis is performed (Silber, 1989). **With the older end-to-end or end-to-side methods, at 14 months after surgery 25% of initially patent anastomoses have shut down** (Matthews et al., 1995). **With intussusception technique, the late shutdown rates appear to be less than 10%,** but long-term follow-up with these techniques have not been reported. **Nevertheless, we recommend banking sperm intraoperatively** (Matthews and Goldstein, 1996) **and as soon as they appear in the ejaculate postoperatively after vasoepididymostomy, regardless of technique employed.** In men with very low counts or poor sperm quality postoperatively and men who remain azoospermic, the sperm intraoperatively can be used for IVF with intracytoplasmic sperm injection. Persistently azoospermic men without cryopreserved sperm can opt for either a redo vasoepididymostomy and/or microscopic epididymal sperm aspiration combined with IVF and intracytoplasmic sperm injection (see Varicocelectomy).

> **KEY POINTS: VASOEPIDIDYMOSTOMY**
>
> - Vasoepididymostomy is the most technically demanding procedure in all of microsurgery and should only be attempted by experienced microsurgeons who perform the procedure frequently.

TRANSURETHRAL RESECTION OF THE EJACULATORY DUCTS

Ejaculatory duct obstruction is usually a congenital anomaly that represents the opposite end of the spectrum of excurrent ductal system anomalies, which begin with congenital complete absence of the vas deferens and most of the epididymis. When the aplastic segment occurs at the terminal end of the vas, where the ejaculatory duct enters the urethra, it is potentially correctable by transurethral resection (TUR; Kadioglu et al., 2001; Ozgok et al., 2001; Paick et al., 2000; Schroeder-Printzen, 2000; Yurdakul et al., 2008). Occasionally ejaculatory duct obstruction results from chronic prostatitis or extrinsic compression of the ejaculatory ducts by prostate or seminal vesical duct cysts (Cornel et al., 1999; Kadioglu et al., 2001; Paick et al., 2000). Higher ejaculatory duct pressures have been directly measured in men with ejaculatory duct obstruction (Eisenberg et al., 2008).

Diagnosis

The workup leading to the diagnosis of probable ejaculatory duct obstruction is covered in Chapter 66. Briefly, **ejaculatory duct obstruction is suspected in azoospermic or severely oligo- and/or asthenospermic men with at least one palpable vas deferens, a low semen volume, acid semen pH, and negative, equivocal, or low semen fructose levels.** If these men have normal serum levels of FSH and testis biopsy reveals normal spermatogenesis, the diagnosis of ejaculatory duct obstruction is entertained.

Digital rectal examination may reveal a midline cystic structure. **Transrectal sonography is key for the diagnosis and treatment of ejaculatory duct obstruction.** A midline cystic lesion or dilated ejaculatory ducts and seminal vesicles can be visualized sonographically. As described earlier in this chapter, **transrectal ultrasound-guided aspiration of the cystic or dilated ejaculatory ducts or seminal vesicles is performed** (Jarow, 1994). **The aspirate is examined microscopically and, if motile sperm are found, they are cryopreserved and 2 to 3 mL indigo carmine diluted with water-soluble radiographic contrast is instilled. If a radiograph confirms a potentially resectable lesion, TUR of the ejaculatory ducts is performed without the need for prior vasography because** the presence of sperm in the seminal vesicles indicates that at least one epididymis is patent and that the cyst or dilated ejaculatory duct communicates with a nonobstructed vas. The instillation of indigo carmine assists in localizing the opening of the ejaculatory duct and confirms when resection has successfully opened the obstructed system. **Transrectal sonography with aspiration should be performed immediately before anticipated surgery and employs the same bowel prep and antibiotic prophylaxis used for transrectal prostate biopsy.**

If no sperm are found in the aspirate, vasography is necessary, as described in Technique of Vasography and Interpretation of Findings. **If no sperm are found in either vas when the vasotomy is made and vasography reveals ejaculatory duct obstruction, it is best to abandon attempts at reconstruction and simply perform microsurgical epididymal sperm aspiration and cryopreservation for future IVF/ICSI. Simultaneous vasoepididymostomy and TUR of the ejaculatory ducts has never worked in my experience.** If ejaculatory duct obstruction is confirmed by vasography employing a 50% water-soluble contrast medium and sperm are present in the vasa, the 3-Fr whistle tip ureteral vasography stents are left in place so that a dilute indigo carmine solution can be injected by the assistant to aid resection.

Technique

Cold knife incision alone almost always leads to reobstruction. The resectoscope, with the 24-Fr cutting loop, is engaged with a finger placed in the rectum, providing anterior displacement of the posterior lobe of the prostate. The ejaculatory ducts course between the bladder neck and the verumontanum and exit at the level of and along the lateral aspect of the verumontanum (Fig. 67.33). **Resection of the veru often reveals the dilated ejaculatory duct orifice or cyst cavity. Resection should be carried out in this region with great care to preserve the bladder neck proximally, the striated sphincter distally, and the rectal mucosa posteriorly.** Efflux of indigo carmine from dilated orifices confirms adequate resection. **Excessive coagulation must be avoided.** If formal vasography was performed, the hemivasotomies are carefully closed, employing microsurgical technique. A Foley catheter is left overnight, and the patient receives an additional 7 days of oral antibiotics.

Complications

Reflux

Reflux of urine into the ejaculatory ducts, vas, and seminal vesicles occurs after a majority of resections. This can be documented by voiding cystourethography or measuring semen creatinine levels (Malkevich and Nagler, 1994). Contamination of semen by urine impairs sperm quality.

Epididymitis

Reflux can lead to acute and chronic epididymitis. Recurrent epididymitis often results in epididymal obstruction. The incidence of epididymitis after TUR is probably underestimated. Symptomatic chemical epididymitis may occur from refluxing urine. **Chronic low-dose antibacterial suppression, such as that employed for vesicoureteral reflux, may be necessary until pregnancy is achieved.** If epididymitis is chronic and recurrent, vasectomy or even epididymectomy may be necessary.

Retrograde Ejaculation

Even when care has been taken to spare the bladder neck, retrograde ejaculation is common after TUR. Pseudoephedrine 60 mg orally,

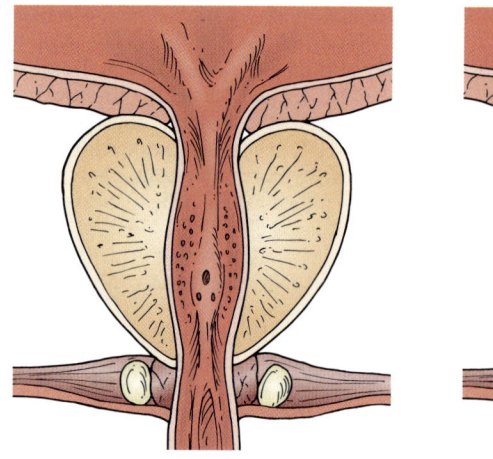
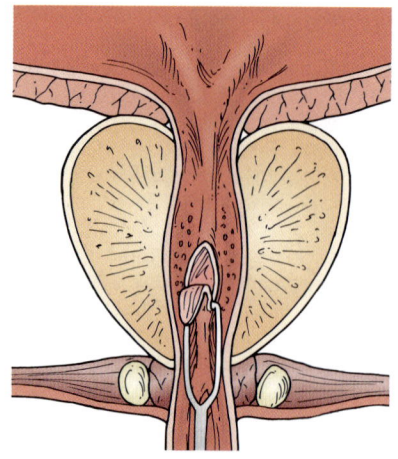

Fig. 67.33. The ejaculatory ducts course between the bladder neck and the verumontanum and exit at the level of and along the lateral aspect of the verumontanum.

90 minutes before ejaculation or Ornade spansules (chlorpheniramine and phenylpropanolamine) twice a day for a week may prevent this. If this is not successful, sperm can be retrieved from alkalinized urine and used for either intrauterine insemination or IVF with ICSI.

Results

TUR of the ejaculatory ducts results in increased semen volume about two-thirds of the time and appearance of sperm in the ejaculate in about half of previously azoospermic men. Pregnancy rates are based on case reports and small series (Fuse et al., 2003; Goldwasser et al., 1985; Ozgok et al., 2001; Paick et al., 2000; Yurdakul et al., 2008). If viable sperm appear in the ejaculate but the quality is poor, IVF with ICSI is recommended, which currently yields delivery rates of up to 38.5% per attempt. Because of the potential for serious complications, **TUR should be performed only in azoospermic men or in severely oligoasthenospermic men and only after the couple has stated they are unwilling to do IVF and have been fully apprised of the risks of TUR.**

ELECTROEJACULATION

Indications

Men with neurologic impairments in sympathetic outflow, such as seen in traumatic spinal cord injury, demyelinating neuropathies (multiple sclerosis), diabetes, or after retroperitoneal lymph node dissection, frequently have abnormalities in or absence of seminal emission. **Ejaculation can be induced in most of these men, especially those with high spinal cord injury, with vibratory stimulation** (Bennett et al., 1987; Brackett et al., 1997; Brindley, 1981; Ohl et al., 1997; Schellan, 1968). **For men who do not respond to vibratory stimulation, electroejaculation has proven to be a safe and effective means of obtaining motile sperm suitable for assisted reproduction techniques (IUI, IVF/ICSI).**

Anesthesia

The procedure is performed under general anesthesia except for in men with a complete spinal cord injury, who do not require anesthesia. **In men with a high thoracic spinal cord lesion (above T6) or in those men with prior history of autonomic dysreflexia, pretreatment with 20 mg of sublingual nifedipine 15 minutes before the procedure is employed.** These men should have intravenous access and their blood pressure and pulse monitored every 2 minutes before, during, and for 20 minutes after electroejaculation. In the event of a sympathetic outflow (autonomic dysreflexia) termination of the procedure should be sufficient to break the response; however, intravenous access allows for delivery of sympatheticolytic agents if they become necessary.

Technique

Before the patient is placed in the lateral decubitus position, the bladder is catheterized and emptied. A 12-Fr or 14-Fr silastic catheter lubricated with a small amount of mineral oil is used because commonly employed lubricants are spermicidal; 10 cc of buffer (HEPES-BSA) is instilled into the bladder. Before the electroejaculation sequence, a digital rectal exam and anoscopy are performed. A rectal probe with 3 large horizontal stripes is well lubricated, inserted with the electrodes facing anteriorly, and applied against the posterior aspect of the prostate and seminal vesicles. The probe is connected to a variable output power source, which simultaneously records probe temperature through a thermistor in the rectal probe. Electrostimulation is started at 3 to 5 volts and increased in 1 volt increments with each stimulation (Ohl et al., 2001). An assistant records probe temperatures and number of stimulations to full erection and ejaculation and collects the ejaculate in a sterile wide-mouth plastic container. The number of stimulations and maximum voltage required are variable and the ejaculate may be retrograde. If probe temperature rises rapidly or above 40°C, stimulation is suspended until the temperature falls below 38°C or probes are changed. At the completion of stimulation, anoscopy is again performed to check for rectal injury. The bladder is recatheterized to obtain any retrograde-ejaculated sperm. The specimens are then delivered to the laboratory for processing. **A second EEJ sequence can be immediately performed under the same anesthetic to obtain additional sperm.**

With use of this technique, sperm can be recovered in greater than 90% of men. Overall pregnancy rates of up to 40% can be achieved after multiple cycles with intrauterine insemination. Use of IVF with ICSI will yield 50% live delivery rates for a single (albeit costly) procedure if motile sperm are obtained.

> **KEY POINTS: ELECTROEJACULATION**
>
> - Indicated in men who do not respond to vibratory stimulation.

SPERM RETRIEVAL TECHNIQUES

Men with congenital absence or bilateral partial aplasia of vas deferens or those with failed or surgically unreconstructable obstructions are treated by using sperm retrieval techniques in conjunction with in vitro fertilization (Table 67.4; Anger et al., 2004; Craft et al., 1995; Janzen et al., 2000; Levine et al., 2003; Qiu et al., 2003; Schlegel et al., 1994; Sheynkin et al., 1998b; Silber et al., 1990; Temple-Smith et al., 1985). These techniques are also useful for intraoperative retrieval of sperm during reconstructive procedures such as vasoepididymostomy, which have significant failure rates. The intraoperatively retrieved sperm

TABLE 67.4 Surgical Techniques for Sperm Retrieval

	ADVANTAGES	DISADVANTAGES
MESA (microsurgical epididymal sperm aspiration)	Microsurgical procedure allows lower complication rate Epididymal sperm has better motility than testicular sperm Large number of sperm can be harvested for cryopreservation of multiple vials in a single procedure	Requires anesthesia and microsurgical skills Not indicated for nonobstructive azoospermia
PESA (percutaneous epididymal sperm aspiration)	No microsurgical skill required Local anesthesia Epididymal sperm has better motility than testicular sperm	Complications include hematoma, pain, and vascular injury to testes and obstruction of the epididymis Variable success in obtaining sperm Small quantity of sperm obtained than with MESA Not indicated in nonobstructive azoospermia
TESA (testicular sperm aspiration)	No microsurgical skill required Local anesthesia Can be used for obstructive azoospermia	Immature or immotile testicular sperm Small quantity of sperm obtained Poor results in nonobstructive azoospermia Complications include hematoma, pain, and vascular injury to testes and epididymis
TESE (testicular sperm extraction)	Low complication rate if performed microsurgically Preferred technique for nonobstructive azoospermia	Requires anesthesia DNA microsurgical skills

may be used immediately if the wife has been prepared for IVF or may be cryopreserved for a future IVF with ICSI cycle in the event the reconstructive surgery is unsuccessful. Sperm obtained from chronically obstructed systems usually have poor motility and decreased fertilizing capacity. **The use of ICSI combined with IVF is essential regardless of the count and motility of the aspirated sperm.**

Microsurgical Epididymal Sperm Aspiration Techniques

Open Tubule Technique

The technique described here can be employed for either intraoperative sperm retrieval at the time of vasoepididymostomy or as an isolated procedure in men with congenital absence of the vas or unreconstructable obstructions (Matthews and Goldstein, 1996; Nudell et al., 1998). A median raphe approach through two small transverse scrotal incisions within the scrotal skinfolds are made. After delivery of the testis, the tunica vaginalis is opened and the epididymis inspected under 16× to 25× magnification using the operating microscope. The epididymal tunica is incised over a dilated tubule as described previously for vasoepididymostomy. Meticulous hemostasis is obtained using the bipolar cautery. A dilated tubule is isolated and incised with a 15-degree microknife. The fluid is touched to a slide, a drop of human tubal fluid media is added, a cover slip is placed, and the fluid is examined. If no sperm are obtained, the epididymal tubule and tunica are closed with 10-0 and 9-0 monofilament nylon sutures, respectively, and an incision is made more proximally in the epididymis or even at the level of the efferent ductules until motile sperm are obtained.

As soon as motile sperm are found, a dry micropipette (5 μL; Drummond Scientific Co., Broomall, PA) is placed adjacent to the effluxing epididymal tubule (Fig. 67.34). A standard hematocrit pipette is less satisfactory but can be used if micropipettes are not available. **Sperm are drawn into the micropipette by simple capillary action.** Negative pressure, as is generated by action of an in-line syringe, should not be applied during sperm recovery because this may disrupt the delicate epididymal mucosa. Two micropipettes may be employed simultaneously to increase speed of sperm recovery.

The highest rate of flow is observed immediately after incision of the tubule. Progressively better quality sperm are often found after the initial washout. **Gentle compression of the testis and epididymis enhances flow from the incised tubule.** With patience, 10 to 20 μL of epididymal fluid can be recovered.

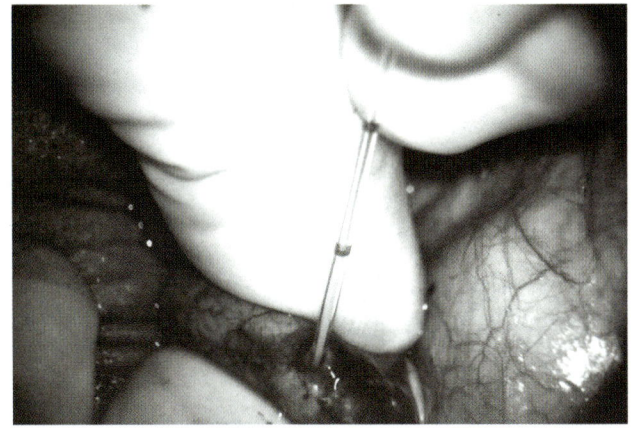

Fig. 67.34. A dry micropipette is placed adjacent to the effluxing epididymal tubule.

The micropipette is connected to a short (3–5 cm) segment of medical grade silicone tubing (American Scientific Products, McGaw Park, IL). Alternatively, the tubing attached to a 25-gauge butterfly needle may be employed. A 20-gauge needle fitted to a Luer-tip syringe is then placed in line. The fluid is flushed with IVF media (0.5–1.0 mL) into a sterile container. Once a micropipette has been used, it is discarded. Residual fluid in the pipette will disrupt capillary action. A typical procedure requires 4 to 12 micropipettes. The sperm bank should be instructed to cryopreserve the aspirate in multiple vials (aliquots) so that several IVF cycles may be attempted if required (Anger et al., 2004; Janzen et al., 2000).

Experience with the technique has revealed that, **paradoxically in obstructed systems, sperm motility is better more proximally in the epididymis with the most motile sperm often found in the efferent ductules** (Fig. 67.35). Interestingly, fertilization rates are highest in men who have the longest length of epididymal tubule available, assuming motile sperm are found at some point in the epididymis. This is likely because the more epididymis present, the more factors are present in the epididymal fluid to promote fertilizing capacity. Even when packed with debris distally, the epididymal tubule may be capable of secreting substances that can diffuse proximally and benefit sperm motility and fertilizing capacity.

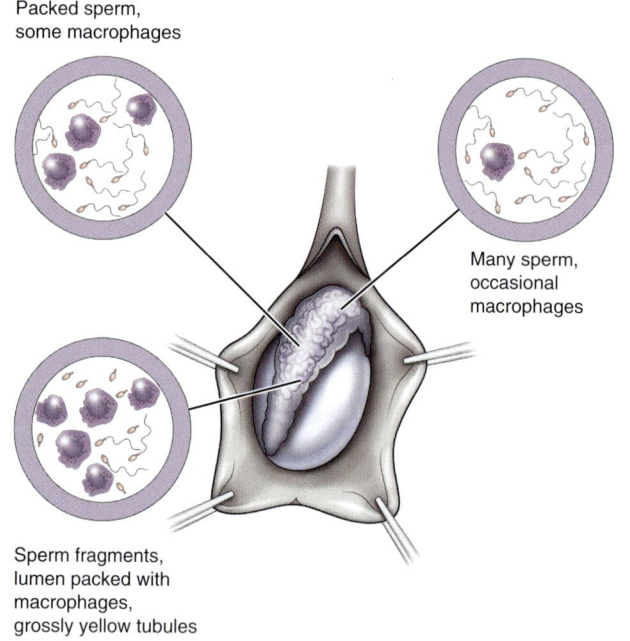

Fig. 67.35. Sperm motility is better more proximally in the epididymis with the most motile sperm often found in the efferent ductules.

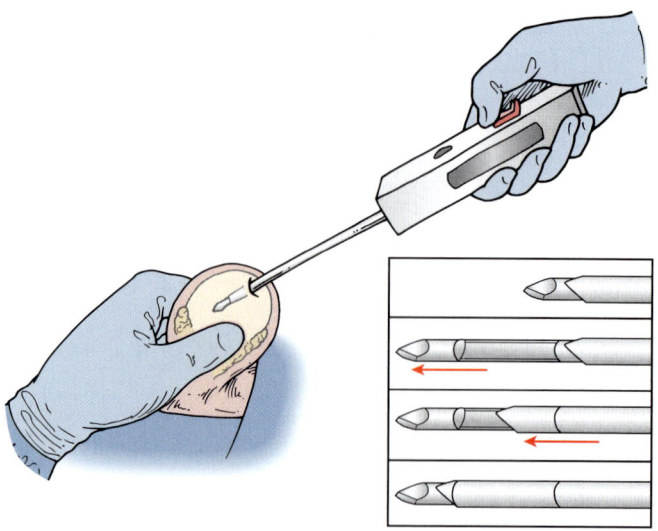

Fig. 67.37. Percutaneous core biopsy using a 14-gauge biopsy gun.

whom future vasoepididymostomy is considered. In view of the enormous costs and effort involved in IVF, epididymal sperm retrieval under direct vision is the preferred technique (Zhang et al., 2013).

> **KEY POINTS: EPIDIDYMAL SPERM ASPIRATION**
> - Puncture of a single tubule for sperm aspiration can be safely performed at the most proximal region of the caput epididymis.
> - In obstructed systems, sperm motility is better more proximally in the epididymis with the most sperm found in the efferent ductules.

Testicular Sperm Extraction

The indications for testicular sperm extraction (TESE) are the following:
1. **Failure to find sperm in the epididymis** in the presence of the spermatogenesis or complete absence of the epididymis
2. **Nonobstructive azoospermia** (Ostad et al., 1998; Schlegel et al., 1997; Su et al., 1999; Tsujimura et al., 2002)

Testicular sperm has been retrieved employing one of three techniques:
1. **Open microsurgical testicular sperm extraction:** preferably employing an operating microscope (micro-TESE) allows retrieval of the largest number of sperm with removal of the smallest amount of testicular tissue; this **is the best technique in men with nonobstructive azoospermia.**
2. Percutaneous core biopsy: uses the same 14-gauge biopsy gun used for prostate biopsy (Fig. 67.37).
3. Percutaneous aspiration (testicular sperm aspiration, TESA) with a high-suction glass syringe and a 23-gauge needle. This is the least invasive but often requires 10 to 20 passes to obtain an adequate yield (Fig. 67.38) (Carpi et al., 2005; Friedler et al., 1997; Harrington et al., 1996; Mercan et al., 2000; Rajfer and Binder, 1989; Sheynkin et al., 1998b).

The percutaneous methods are most appropriate in men with normal spermatogenesis and obstructive azoospermia in whom adequate numbers of sperm can be retrieved in a small amount of tissue (Craft et al., 1995). The pros and cons of these three methods are discussed in Testis Biopsy.

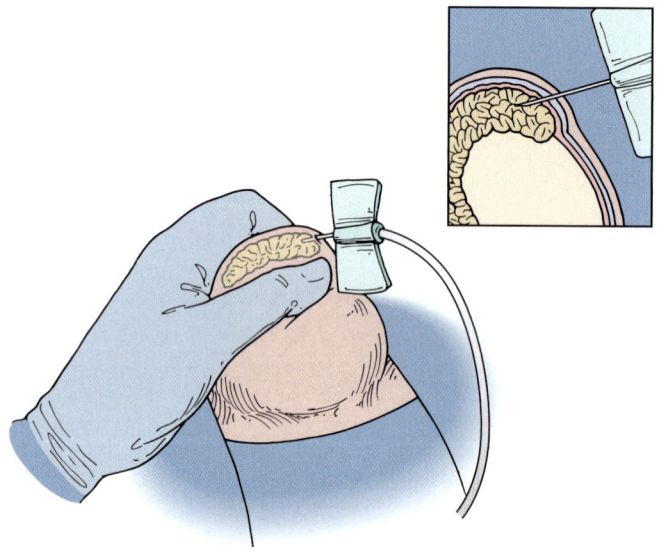

Fig. 67.36. Percutaneous puncture of the epididymis with a fine needle.

With use of ICSI, ongoing pregnancy or delivery rates exceeding 60% have been achieved with this technique using either fresh or cryopreserved epididymal sperm (Nudell et al., 1998; Schlegel et al., 1995). Epididymal sperm aspiration can be done electively, with the cryopreserved sperm used for multiple future IVF cycles (Anger et al., 2004; Janzen et al., 2000).

Percutaneous Epididymal Sperm Aspiration

Percutaneous puncture of the epididymis with a fine needle (Fig. 67.36), or percutaneous epididymal sperm aspiration (PESA), has been successfully employed to obtain sperm and achieve pregnancies (Craft and Tsirigotis, 1995; Levine et al., 2003; Lin et al., 2004; Qiu et al., 2003; Shrivastav et al., 1994). The technique is less reliable than the open retrieval, and the small quantities of sperm obtained are sometimes inadequate for cryopreservation. Reported pregnancy rates are half those achieved with open techniques (Sheynkin et al., 1998b). It can also potentially obstruct the epididymis in men in

Microsurgical Testicular Sperm Extraction

The use of an operating microscope for standard open diagnostic testes biopsy allows identification of an area in the tunica albuginea

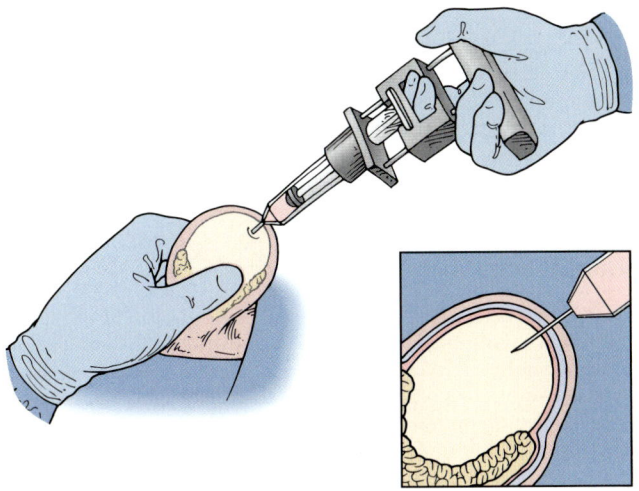

Fig. 67.38. Percutaneous aspiration with a high suction glass syringe and a 23-gauge needle.

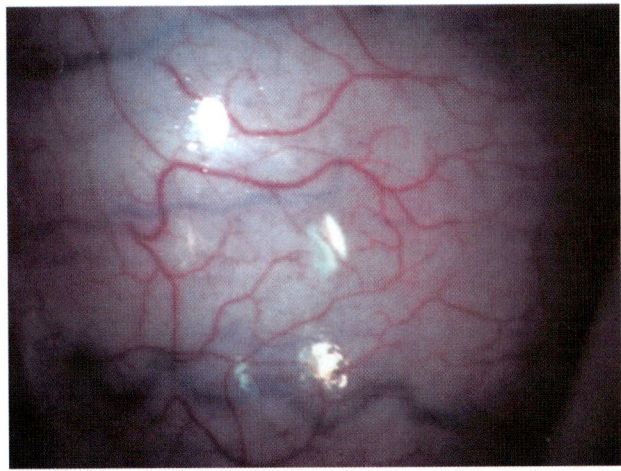

Fig. 67.39. Open diagnostic testis biopsy allows identification of an area in the tunica albuginea free of blood vessels.

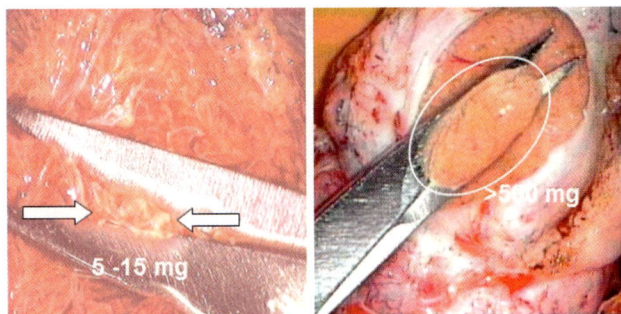

Fig. 67.40. Tubules with spermatogenesis have a considerable larger diameter than tubules that are Sertoli cell-only.

TABLE 67.5 TESE Outcomes by Diagnosis

CONDITION	RETRIEVAL
Klinefelter syndrome	68%
AZFc deletions	70%
Sertoli cell–only	30%
Postchemotherapy	53%
Cryptorchidism (postorchiopexy)	74%
Maturation arrest	40%
AZFa, AZFb deletions	0

TESE, Testicular sperm extraction.
Data from Chan et al., 2001; Hopps et al., 2003; Hung et al., 2007; Raman and Schlegel, 2003; Ramasamy et al., 2009; Ramasamy and Schlegel, 2007.

free of blood vessels (Fig. 67.39), minimizing the risk of injury to testicular blood supply and allowing a relatively blood-free biopsy specimen (Dardashti et al., 2000). Employing the microscope for testis biopsy, Schlegel (1999) discovered that in men with nonobstructive azoospermia, some of the tubules were larger than others. **The larger tubules are more likely to yield sperm.** Previous studies revealed that testicular biopsy in men with nonobstructive azoospermia displays considerable heterogeneity. Examination of permanently fixed biopsy specimens that display heterogeneity reveals that **tubules with spermatogenesis are of considerably larger diameter than tubules that are Sertoli cell–only. This difference can be readily observed under the operating microscope** (Fig. 67.40).

Technique. With the patient under general or regional anesthetic, the testes are exposed through either a single midline median raphe incision or two transverse incisions within the skin lines and between the scrotal blood vessels. The testes is delivered into the wound. The tunica vaginalis is opened and the operating microscope is brought into the field. Using 10× magnification, an avascular plane is identified on the anterior surface of the tunica albuginea. Using a 15-degree microknife, a generous transverse incision is made between the blood vessels through the tunica albuginea. Small blood vessels that are seen coursing across the incision are coagulated with the microbipolar cautery before incising them. This yields a blood-free field. The seminiferous tubules are observed. **Sertoli cell–only tubules tend to be thin, white, and stringy. Tubules with active spermatogenesis are larger, plumper, and somewhat yellow.** Using a micro-needle holder or micro-bipolar forceps, the seminiferous tubules are dissected in an attempt to identify larger tubules. If such a tubule is found, a sharp curved iris scissors is used to selectively excise these tubules. The sample is placed in human tubal fluid media, microdissected with iris scissors, and passed multiple times through a 24-gauge angiocath sheath. This breaks up the tubules and improves the chances of finding sperm (Schlegel, 1999). The processed specimen is then immediately examined by an andrology laboratory technician present in the operating room. After sperm have been found, hemostasis is obtained with the microbipolar cautery. The incision in the tunica albuginea is closed with a 6-0 nylon or Proline suture. The testis is returned to the tunica vaginalis, which is closed with a continuous suture of 5-0 Vicryl. If necessary the opposite testis is explored.

Results. Using the microdissection technique, sperm have been identified in 50% of men explored (Dabaja and Schlegel, 2013; Schlegel, 1999). In those men in whom sperm are found, a pregnancy rate of 45%, with a live delivery rate of almost 40%, has been achieved at Cornell using IVF/ICSI. The spontaneous abortion rate is 19%. The high rate of spontaneous abortion is probably because of the increased incidence of chromosomal abnormalities and DNA damage in the sperm of men with nonobstructive azoospermia (Rucker et al., 1998). Even in severe cases of congenital or acquired testicular failure, as in Sertoli cell–only syndrome (Su et al., 1999), post-chemotherapy azoospermia (Chan et al., 2001), and nonmosaic (47XXY) Klinefelter syndrome (Palermo et al., 1998; Ramasamy et al., 2009), sperm have been found and pregnancy and live births achieved (Table 67.5). An experimental technique using flow cytometry has been able to find sperm, often motile or twitching, in 80% of testicular specimens in which light microscopy by an experienced technician found none (Bolyakov et al., 2016). The technique employs SYTO 17 red fluorescent nucleic acid stain (Invitrogen), which attaches only to sperm. The safety of the dye on human sperm has yet to be proven, but studies on living cells have not demonstrated increased cellular stress (Wlodkowic et al., 2008; Zhao et al., 2009).

> **KEY POINTS: TESTICULAR SPERM EXTRACTION**
>
> - Open microsurgical testicular sperm extraction is the best technique in men with nonobstructive azoospermia.

Postmortem Sperm Retrieval

Postmortem sperm retrieval and cryopreservation (but no pregnancies) were initially reported by Rothman in 1980 and employed removal and mincing of the epididymis. The retrieved sperm can be frozen and subsequently used to achieve pregnancy. Pregnancy has now been achieved with sperm retrieved postmortem using IVF with ICSI (Benshushan and Schenker, 1998; Dostal et al., 2005; Tash et al., 2003).

Retrieval of sperm from the vas can be performed using the technique described for vasectomy (see Vasovasostomy). Once the vas has been delivered, a hemivasotomy is made with a 15-degree microknife (as described in Technique of Vasography and Interpretation of Findings). The testicular end of the vas is cannulated with a 22-gauge angiocatheter and the vas irrigated with a 0.2-mL volume of human tubal fluid medium, while the convoluted vas and epididymis are massaged.

The ethical appropriateness of such retrieval is the most important issue surrounding its use, and current guidelines require the patient to have given permission for sperm retrieval and use before death (Trinkoff and Barone, 2013).

VARICOCELECTOMY

Varicocelectomy is by far the most commonly performed operation for the treatment of male infertility. **Varicocele is found in approximately 15% of the general population: 35% of men with primary infertility and in 75% to 81% of men with secondary infertility.** Animal and human studies have demonstrated that **varicocele is associated with a progressive and duration-dependent decline in testicular function** (Chehval and Purcell, 1992; Gorelick and Goldstein, 1993; Hadziselimovic et al., 1989; Harrison et al., 1986; Kass and Belman, 1987; Lipshultz and Corriere, 1977; Nagler et al., 1985; Russell, 1957; Witt and Lipshultz, 1993).

Repair of varicocele will halt any further damage to testicular function (Gorelick and Goldstein, 1993; Kass and Belman, 1987) and, in a large percentage of men, result in improved spermatogenesis (Dubin and Amelar, 1977; Marmar et al., 2007; Schlegel and Goldstein, 1992), improved live birth rates, and better IVF/ICSI outcomes (Kirby et al., 2016). It also enhances Leydig cell function (Su et al., 1995; Tanrikut et al., 2011). The potentially important role of urologists in preventing future infertility and/or androgen deficiency underscores the importance of utilizing a varicocelectomy technique that minimizes the risk of complications and recurrence. Table 67.6 summarizes the pros and cons of various methods of varicocele repair.

Scrotal Operations

A variety of surgical approaches have been advocated for varicocelectomy. The earliest recorded attempts at repair of varicocele date to antiquity and involved external clamping of the scrotal skin, including the enlarged veins. In the early 1900s an open scrotal approach was employed, involving the mass ligation and excision of the varicosed plexus of veins. At the level of the scrotum, however, the pampiniform plexus of veins are intimately entwined with the coiled testicular artery. Therefore **scrotal operations are to be avoided because damage to the arterial supply of the testis frequently results in testicular atrophy and further impairment of spermatogenesis and fertility.**

Retroperitoneal Operations

Retroperitoneal repair of varicocele involves incision at the level of the internal inguinal ring (Fig. 67.41), splitting of the external and internal oblique muscles and exposure of the internal spermatic artery and vein retroperitoneally near the ureter. This approach has the advantage of isolating the internal spermatic veins proximally, near the point of drainage into the left renal vein. At this level, only one or two large veins are present and, in addition, the testicular artery has not yet branched and is often distinctly separate from the internal spermatic veins. Retroperitoneal approaches involve ligation of the fewest number of veins. This approach is still a commonly employed method for the repair of varicocele, especially in children.

A **disadvantage of a retroperitoneal approach is the high incidence of varicocele recurrence, especially in children and adolescents, when the testicular artery is intentionally preserved.** Recurrence rates after retroperitoneal varicocelectomy are in the range of 15% (Homonnai et al., 1980; Rothman et al., 1981; Watanabe et al., 2005). Failure is usually due to preservation of the periarterial plexus of fine veins (venae comitantes) along with the artery. These veins have been shown to communicate with larger internal spermatic veins. If left intact, they may dilate and cause recurrence. Less commonly, failure is due to the presence of parallel inguinal or retroperitoneal collaterals, which may exit the testis and bypass the ligated retroperitoneal veins rejoining the internal spermatic vein proximal to the site of ligation (Murray et al., 1986; Sayfan et al., 1981). Dilated cremasteric veins (Sayfan et al., 1980) and scrotal collaterals (Kaufman et al., 1983) are also causes of varicocele recurrence and

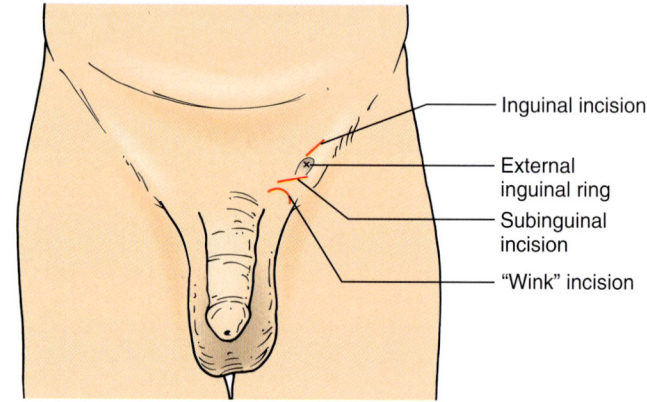

Fig. 67.41. Retroperitoneal repair of varicocele involves incision at the level of the internal inguinal ring.

TABLE 67.6 Techniques of Varicocelectomy

TECHNIQUE	ARTERY PRESERVED	HYDROCELE (%)	FAILURE (%)	POTENTIAL FOR SERIOUS MORBIDITY
Retroperitoneal	No	7	15–25	No
Conventional inguinal	No	3–30	5–15	No
Laparoscopic	Yes	12	3–15	Yes
Radiographic	Yes	0	15–25	Yes
Microscopic inguinal or subinguinal	Yes	0	0.5–1.0	No

cannot be identified with a retroperitoneal approach. Positive identification and preservation of the 1.0- to 1.5-mm testicular artery via the retroperitoneal approach is difficult, especially in children in whom the artery is small. The operation involves working in a deep hole, and, because at this level the internal spermatic vessels cannot be delivered into the wound, they must be dissected and ligated in situ in the retroperitoneum. **In addition, the difficulty in positively identifying and preserving lymphatics using this approach results in postoperative hydrocele formation after 7% to 33% of retroperitoneal operations** (Szabo and Kessler, 1984). The incidence of recurrence appears to be higher in children, with rates reported between 15% and 45% in adolescents (Gorenstein et al., 1986; Levitt et al., 1987; Reitelman et al., 1987). Kass and Marcol (1992) report that **recurrence can be markedly reduced in children and adolescents by intentional ligation of the testicular artery.** This ensures ligation of the periarterial network of fine veins. Although reversal of testicular growth failure has been documented with intentional testicular artery ligation at the time of retroperitoneal repair in children, **the effect of artery ligation on subsequent spermatogenesis is uncertain.** In adults bilateral artery ligation has been documented to occasionally cause azoospermia and testicular atrophy (Silber, 1979). At least **it is inarguable that testicular artery ligation will not enhance testicular function.**

Laparoscopic Varicocelectomy

Laparoscopic repair is in essence a retroperitoneal approach, and many of the advantages and disadvantages are similar to those of the open retroperitoneal approach (Donovan and Winfield, 1992; Enquist et al., 1994; Hagood et al., 1992; Hirsch et al., 1998; Riccabona et al., 2003; Watanabe, 2005).

With use of the laparoscope, the internal spermatic vessels and vas deferens can be clearly visualized through the laparoscope as they course through the internal inguinal ring. **The magnification provided by the laparoscope allows visualization of the testicular artery** (Kobori et al., 2013). **With experience, the lymphatics may be visualized and preserved as well** (Glassberg et al., 2008). With laparoscopic varicocelectomy the internal spermatic veins are ligated at the same level as the retroperitoneal (Palomo) approach. Laparoscopic varicocelectomy should allow preservation of the testicular artery in a majority of cases, as well as preservation of lymphatics. The incidence of varicocele recurrence would be expected to be similar to that associated with the open retroperitoneal operations. These recurrences would be due to collaterals joining the internal spermatic vein near its entrance to the renal vein or entering the renal vein separately.

Currently reported series of laparoscopic varicocelectomy report a recurrence rate of 2.9% to 4.5% in most recent series (Barroso et al., 2009; May et al., 2006; Glassberg et al., 2008) but up to 17% in some (Al-Said et al., 2008). An artery ligation but lymphatic-sparing laparoscopic technique has markedly reduced the incidence of postoperative hydrocele formation in children (Glassberg et al., 2008). The potential complications of laparoscopic varicocelectomy (injury to bowel, vessels, or viscera; air embolism; peritonitis) are significantly more serious than those associated with the open techniques. Furthermore, laparoscopic varicocelectomy requires a general anesthetic. The microsurgical techniques described next can be performed using local or regional anesthesia and employ an incision of 2 to 3 cm for unilateral repair. This is often no greater than the sum of incisions employed for a laparoscopic approach. Postoperative pain and recovery from the laparoscopic technique are the same as those associated with subinguinal varicocelectomy (Hirsch et al., 1998). In the hands of an experienced laparoscopist, the approach is a reasonable alternative for the repair of bilateral varicoceles (Diamond et al., 2009; Donovan and Winfield, 1992; Mendez-Gallart et al., 2009; Tong et al., 2009).

Microsurgical Inguinal and Subinguinal Operations: the Preferred Approaches

Subinguinal microsurgical varicocelectomy is currently the most popular approach. It has the advantage of allowing the spermatic cord structures to be pulled up and out of the wound so that the testicular artery, lymphatics, and small periarterial veins may be more easily identified. In addition, **an inguinal or subinguinal approach allows access to external spermatic and even gubernacular veins** (Kaufman et al., 1983), which may bypass the spermatic cord and result in recurrence if not ligated. Last, an inguinal or subinguinal approach allows access to the testis for biopsy or examination of the epididymis for obstruction or repair of hydrocele (Dabaja et al., 2013).

Traditional approaches to inguinal varicocelectomy involve a 5-cm incision made over the inguinal canal, opening of the external oblique aponeurosis, and encirclement and delivery of the spermatic cord. The cord is then dissected and all the internal spermatic veins are ligated (Dubin and Amelar, 1977). The vas deferens and its vessels are preserved. An attempt is made to identify and preserve the testicular artery and, if possible, the lymphatics. In addition, the cord is elevated, and any external spermatic veins that are running parallel to the spermatic cord or perforating the floor of the inguinal canal are identified and ligated. Compared with retroperitoneal operations, conventional nonmagnified inguinal approaches lower the incidence of varicocele recurrence but do not alter the incidence of either hydrocele formation or testicular artery injury. **Conventional inguinal operations are associated with an incidence of postoperative hydrocele formation varying from 3% to 15% with an average incidence of 7%** (Szabo and Kessler, 1984). Analysis of the hydrocele fluid has clearly indicated that hydrocele formation after varicocelectomy is due to ligation of the lymphatics (Szabo and Kessler, 1984). The incidence of testicular artery injury during nonmagnified inguinal varicocelectomy is unknown. However, case reports suggest that this complication may be more common than realized. It can result in testicular atrophy and, if the operation is performed bilaterally, azoospermia may ensue in a previously oligospermic man. Furthermore, Starzl and his transplant group reported a 14% incidence of testicular atrophy and 70% incidence of hydrocele formation when the spermatic cord was divided and only the vas and vasal vessels preserved (Penn et al., 1972).

The introduction of **microsurgical technique** to varicocelectomy **has resulted in a substantial reduction in the incidence of hydrocele formation** (Cayan et al., 2000; Goldstein et al., 1992; Marmar and Kim, 1994; Matthews et al., 1998). This is **because the lymphatics can be more easily identified and preserved.** Furthermore, the use of **magnification enhances the ability to identify and preserve the 0.5- to 1.5-mm testicular artery, thus avoiding the complications of atrophy or azoospermia.**

Advocates of nonmicrosurgical techniques contend that the deferential (vassal) artery and, if preserved, the cremasteric artery provide adequate blood supply to the testes to prevent atrophy. However, anatomic studies have known that the diameter of the testicular artery is greater than the diameter of the deferential artery and cremasteric artery combined (Raman and Goldstein, 2004). **The testicular artery is the main blood supply to the testis.** Experience with the one-stage Fowler and Steven's orchiopexy, in which the testicular artery is intentionally ligated, reveals that a substantial percentage of such procedures result in an atrophic testis. Also, animal models indicate that artery preservation varicocelectomy results in improved testicular ultrastructure, whereas artery ligation resulted in further deterioration of ultrastructure (Zheng et al., 2008). At the very least, it is inarguable that **ligation of the testicular artery is unlikely to enhance testicular function.**

Anesthesia

If the testis is delivered, as described below, regional or light general anesthesia is preferred. If only the cord is delivered, local anesthesia with a 50-50 combination of 0.25% bupivacaine (preferably liposomal) and 1% lidocaine is satisfactory with adjunctive intravenous sedation. After infiltration of the skin and subcutaneous tissues the cord is infiltrated before delivery. Blind cord block carries with it a small risk of inadvertent testicular artery injury (Goldstein and Einer-Jensen, 1983). A 30-gauge needle should therefore be employed for cord block to minimize the risk of injury and hematoma.

TABLE 67.7 Indications for Inguinal (External Oblique Opened) Versus Subinguinal (Fascia Intact) Varicocelectomy

INGUINAL	SUBINGUINAL
Prepubertal children	Prior inguinal surgery
Solitary testis	Obesity
Tight, low external ring	Lax, capacious external ring
	High external ring
Short cord, high-lying testis	Long cord with low-lying testis
Less experienced with microsurgical repair	Very experienced with microsurgical repair

Inguinal and Subinguinal Approaches

The introduction of the subinguinal approach, just below the external inguinal ring (Marmar et al., 1985) obviates the necessity for opening any fascial layer and is associated with less pain and a rapid recovery. At the subinguinal level, however, significantly more veins are encountered, the artery is more often surrounded by a network of tiny veins that must be ligated, and the testicular artery has often divided into two or three branches, making arterial identification and preservation more difficult (Hopps et al., 2003).

Subinguinally, the arterial pulsations are often dampened by compression on the edge of the external ring, making its identification somewhat more difficult than when the external oblique is opened. Table 67.7 summarizes the criteria for performing the operation inguinally (external oblique opened) versus subinguinally (fascia intact). **In general, it is best to use a subinguinal approach in men with a history of any prior inguinal surgery.** Under these circumstances the cord is usually stuck to the undersurface of the external oblique, and opening the fascia risks injury to the cord. A subinguinal approach is easier in obese men in whom opening and closing the fascia is difficult through a small incision. A subinguinal approach is easier in men with high, lax, capacious external rings and in men with long cords and low-lying testes. In these men the level of the external ring is fairly proximal to the testis, and opening the fascia will not result in a significant diminution in the number of veins to be ligated or in the branching of the testicular artery.

I recommend always opening the external oblique in prepubertal children without prior inguinal surgery. In children the testicular artery is very small and systemic blood pressure is low, making identification of the artery very difficult in a subinguinal approach. The fascia could also be opened in men with a solitary testis in whom preservation of the artery is critical. Exposure of the cord more proximally (at the inguinal level) allows identification of the artery before it has branched, where clear pulsations are more readily observed.

Consider opening the fascia in men with prior failed subinguinal varicocelectomy to dissect proximal to the prior scarred ligation area. The microdissection will be quicker and easier. **A subinguinal operation is significantly more difficult than a high inguinal operation and should only be used by surgeons who perform the operation frequently.** Less experienced microsurgeons should start out doing inguinal operations because they are easier. **An inguinal operation is employed when simultaneous ipsilateral hernia repair is performed** (Schulster et al., 2017).

Before the incision is made, the location of the external inguinal ring is determined by invagination of the scrotal skin and is marked. The size of the incision is determined by the size of the testis when delivery of the testis (see following) is planned. Atrophic testes can be delivered through a 2- to 2.5-cm incision. Larger testes require a 3-cm incision. The incision is made within Langer lines to minimize scarring.

If the decision is made to perform an inguinal operation and thus to open the fascia, the incision is begun at the external ring and extended laterally 2 to 3.5 cm along Langer lines (Fig. 67.42). If the operation is to be performed subinguinally, the incision is placed in the skin lines right over the external ring (Fig. 67.43).

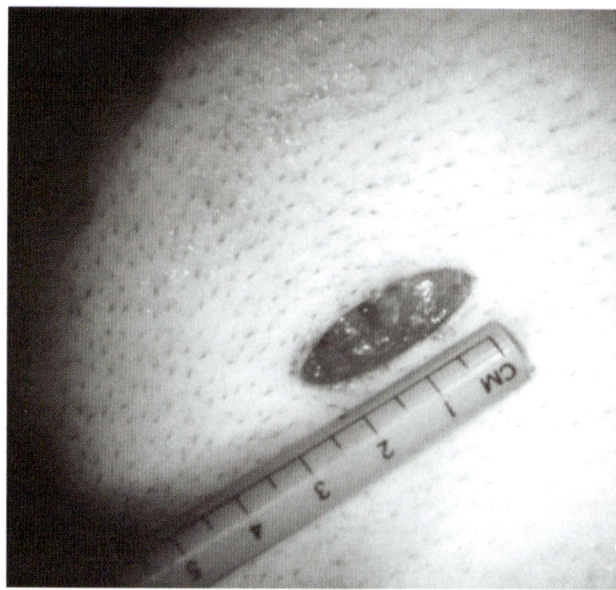

Fig. 67.42. An incision is begun at the external ring and extended laterally 2 to 3.5 cm along Langer lines.

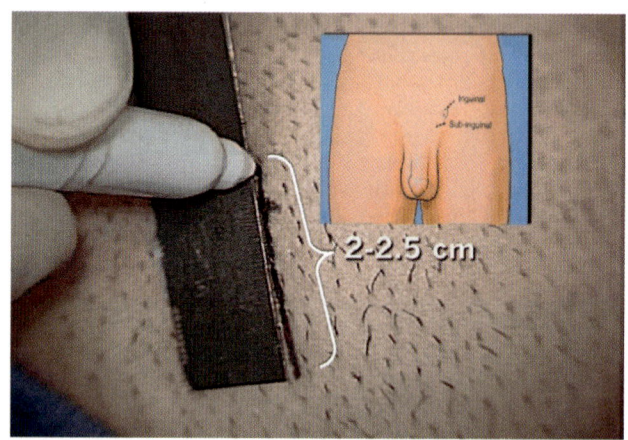

Fig. 67.43. When not performed subinguinally, the incision is placed in the skin lines right over the external ring.

Camper fascia and Scarpa fascia are divided with the electrocautery between the blades of a Crile clamp. The superficial epigastric artery and vein at the superior aspect of the incision and/or the superficial external pudendal artery and vein at the inferior aspect of the incision, if encountered, are retracted or, if in the middle of the incision, may be clamped, divided, and ligated. If an inguinal approach is selected, the external oblique aponeurosis is cleaned and opened the length of the incision to the external inguinal ring in the direction of its fibers. A 3-0 absorbable suture placed at the apex of the opening in the external oblique facilitates later closure.

The spermatic cord is grasped with a Babcock clamp and delivered through the wound. The ilioinguinal and genital branches of the genitofemoral nerve are excluded from the cord, which is then surrounded with a large Penrose drain. If a subinguinal incision was made, Camper and Scarpa fasciae are incised as described earlier. An index finger is introduced into the wound and along the cord into the scrotum. The index finger is then hooked under the external inguinal ring, retracting it cephalad. A small Richardson retractor is slid along the back of the index finger and retracted caudad over the cord toward the scrotum (Fig. 67.44). The spermatic cord will be revealed between the index finger and retractor. The assistant grasps the cord with a Babcock clamp and delivers it through the wound. The cord is surrounded with a large Penrose drain.

Dissection of the Cord

The operating microscope is then brought into the field. Under 6× to 10× power magnification the external spermatic fascia is opened with a Bovie electrocautery in the direction of the cremasteric fibers to avoid injury to the cremasteric arteries. A 5-0 Vicryl suture is placed at the apex of the opening to facilitate later closure. The relatively avascular internal spermatic fascia is opened with scissors as high as possible and held open with the straight mosquito forceps, which are sequentially applied as high as possible while pulling down on the testis (Fig. 67.45A and B). The magnification is increased to 10× to 25× power and, after irrigation with 1% papaverine solution, the cord is inspected for the presence of pulsations revealing the location of the testicular artery.

A micro-Doppler is extremely useful in identifying arteries (Fig. 67.46). **Once the testicular artery is identified, it is dissected free of all surrounding tissue, tiny veins, and lymphatics using a fine-tip nonlocking micro needle holder and microforceps.** The artery is encircled with a vessel loop for positive identification and gentle retraction (Fig. 67.47). The suspected artery is tested by elevating the artery with the tips of the micro needle holder until it is completely occluded and then slowly lowering it until a pulsating blush of blood appears just over the needle holder. The artery is often surrounded by X- or H-like networks of small veins (Fig. 67.48). If the artery is not immediately identified, the cord is carefully dissected beginning with the largest veins. The veins are stripped clean of adherent lymphatics (Fig. 67.49) and the underside of the largest veins inspected for an adherent artery.

In approximately 50% of cases the testicular artery is adherent to the undersurface of a large vein (Beck et al., 1992). All veins within the cord, with the exception of the vasal veins, are doubly ligated with either hemoclips (Fig. 67.50A) or by passing two 4-0 silk ligatures, one black and one white, beneath the vein (Fig. 67.50B). These are then tied and the vein divided. Medium hemoclips are used for veins 5 mm or larger, small auto-hemoclips for veins 1 to 5 mm, and 4-0 silk for veins smaller than 2 mm. The bipolar cautery can be used for veins smaller than 0.5 mm. The vasal veins are preserved, providing venous return. If the vas deferens is accompanied by a dilated vein greater than 2.5 mm in diameter, they are dissected free of the vasal artery and ligated. The vas deferens is always accompanied by two sets of vessels. **As long as at least one set of deferential veins remains intact, venous return will be adequate.**

At the completion of the dissection, the cord is run over the index finger and inspected to verify that all veins have been identified and ligated. Small veins adherent to the testicular artery are dissected free and ligated or, if smaller than 1 mm, cauterized using a bipolar unit with a jeweler's forceps tip and divided. Cremasteric arteries are found (usually between and adherent of two cremasteric veins) and preserved in at least 90% of cases. Recent studies employing power Doppler in men with nonobstructive azoospermia undergoing testicular sperm extraction have found that tubules containing sperm are most likely to be found in areas of the testis with the greatest blood supply. Therefore logic would dictate that preservation of maximum testicular blood supply, including testicular and cremasteric arteries, would be beneficial to testicular function. **At the completion of the dissection, only the testicular arteries, cremasteric arteries,**

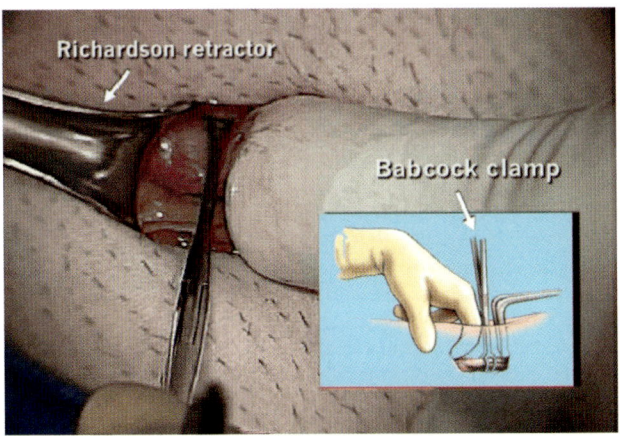

Fig. 67.44. A Richardson retractor is slid along the back of the index finger and retracted caudad over the cord toward the scrotum.

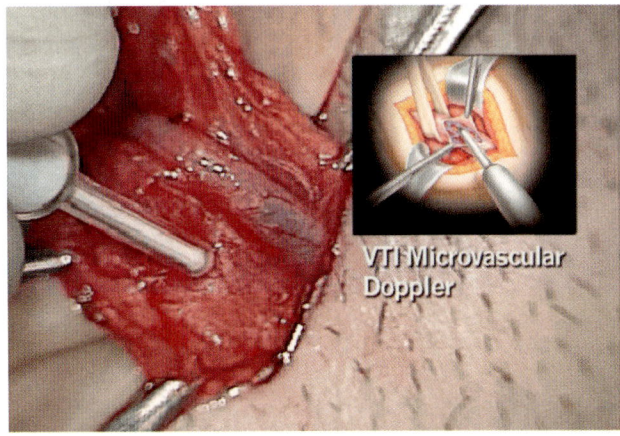

Fig. 67.46. Use of a micro-Doppler to identify arteries.

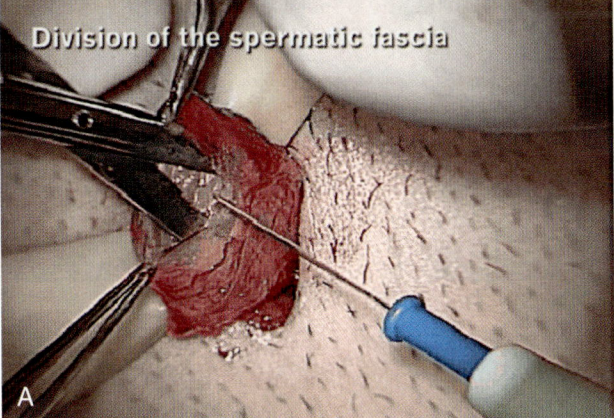
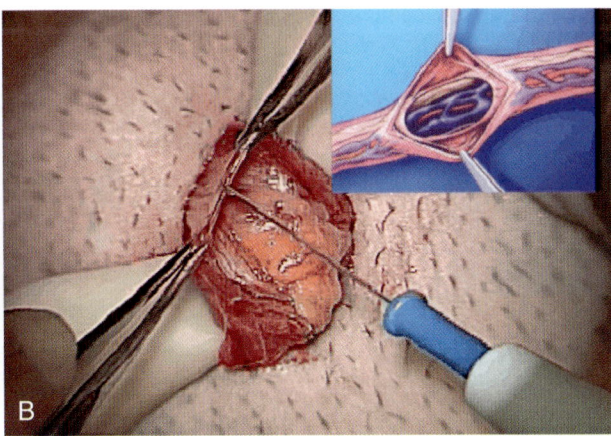

Fig. 67.45. (A and B) The internal spermatic fascia opened with scissors as high as possible (A) and held open with the straight mosquito forceps (B).

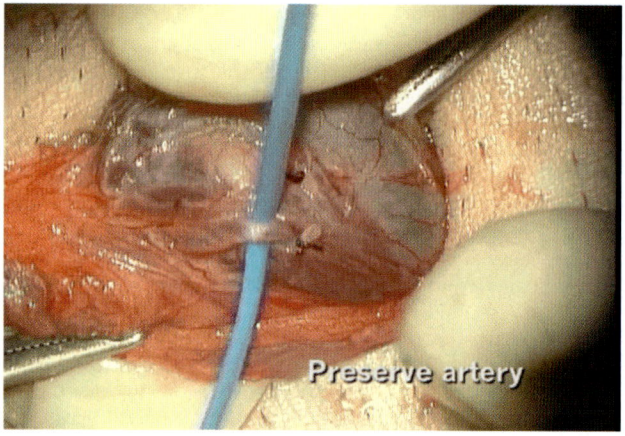

Fig. 67.47. The testicular artery encircled with a vessel loop.

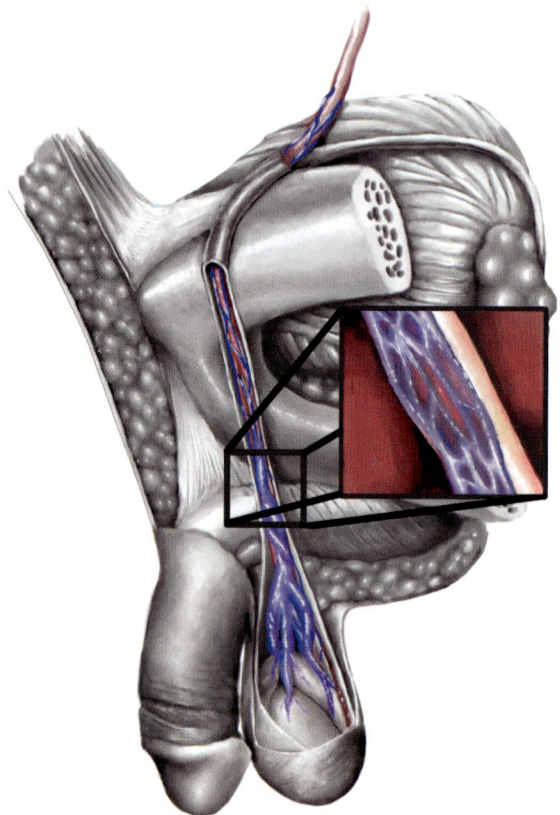

Fig. 67.48. The testicular artery shown surrounded by X- or H-like networks of small veins.

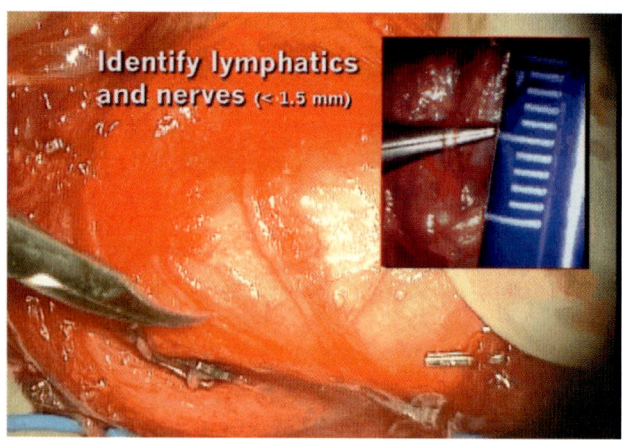

Fig. 67.49. Lymphatics.

lymphatics, and vas deferens with its vessels remain (Fig. 67.51). Dissection is not deemed complete until a run through the cord reveals no additional internal or external spermatic veins. Each time a vein is found and ligated, any remaining veins dilate up.

Delivery of the Testis

Delivery of the testis through a small inguinal or subinguinal incision guarantees direct visual access to all possible avenues of testicular venous drainage. Delivery of only the cord allows access to most external spermatic collaterals but may miss those close to the testis and will not allow access to scrotal or gubernacular collaterals, which have been demonstrated radiographically to be the cause of 10% of recurrent varicoceles (Kaufman et al., 1983).

Orhan et al. retrospectively evaluated these new operative approaches: 82 microsurgical inguinal varicocelectomies and 65 subinguinal cases (Wosnitzer and Roth, 1983). The authors reported no significant difference between the two groups in operative time, semen improvement, or pregnancy rate, although the number of veins and arteries was higher in the subinguinal group. The author delivers the testis to address scrotal collaterals. His rationale for ligating scrotal collaterals is based on the publication of an article by Walsh et al., who found that 10% of failed varicocelectomies were due to scrotal collaterals (Kaufman et al., 1983). Interestingly, Patrick Walsh, the world-renowned urologist at Johns Hopkins who is best known for developing nerve-sparing radical prostatectomy, started out as a male fertility specialist. After completing his urology residency at the University of California, Los Angeles, he did a fellowship in male reproductive endocrinology with Jean Wilson, MD, at the University of Texas, Southwestern. Walsh's original interest in the prostate was on androgen action on the prostate and benign prostatic hypertrophy. He was the first author of the first description of embolization for varicocelectomy published in the *Journal of the American Medical Association* in 1981 (Walsh and White, 1981). The venography images of scrotal collaterals in men with prior failed varicocelectomy in the 1983 article in *Radiology* are very clear (Kaufman et al., 1983), and the authors of the study show that they contribute to the significantly higher failure rate of embolization techniques compared with current microsurgical techniques. Walsh also coauthored a book titled *Male Infertility* with Amelar and Dubin (1977). **It is undeniable that delivery of the testis provides direct visual access to every possible route of venous return,** and in more than 4000 cases done by the author, the failure rate was less than 1% with minimal morbidity (Goldstein et al., 1992; Goldstein, 2016). Finally, open microsurgical varicocelectomy has demonstrated lower recurrence rates and fewer complications compared with a laparoscopic or a high retroperitoneal approach (Goldstein, 2016).

With gentle upward traction on the cord and upward pressure on the testis through the invaginated scrotum, the testis is easily delivered through the wound. All external spermatic veins are identified and doubly ligated with hemoclips and divided (Fig. 67.52). The gubernacula are inspected for the presence for veins exiting from the tunica vaginalis. These are either cauterized or doubly clipped and divided. **When this step is completed, all testicular venous return must be within the Penrose surrounding cord,** which is again run over the index finger, and any remaining internal or external spermatic veins are clipped or ligated. **If the varicocelectomy has been performed successfully, squeezing on the dilated scrotal pampinoform plexus of veins just above the testis will result in transmission of a distinct impulse felt in the biggest veins just on the testicular side of the ligation.** This is similar to transmission of a fluid wave in diagnosing ascites. Absence of a distinct impulse suggests that a significant internal, external, or gubernacular vein has been missed, allowing venous blood to go straight across the area of ligation and warrants rerunning the cord and redelivery of the testis. The reason this "impulse test" works is that it takes time for the testicular venous return to find its way through the deferential veins, so immediately after ligation the venous pressure is high.

The external spermatic fascia is reapproximated with 2 or 3 interrupted sutures of 5-0 Vicryl, facilitated by pulling up on the suture previously placed at the apex of the opening in the external spermatic fascia. This covers up the exposed testicular arteries.

Chapter 67 Surgical Management of Male Infertility 1481

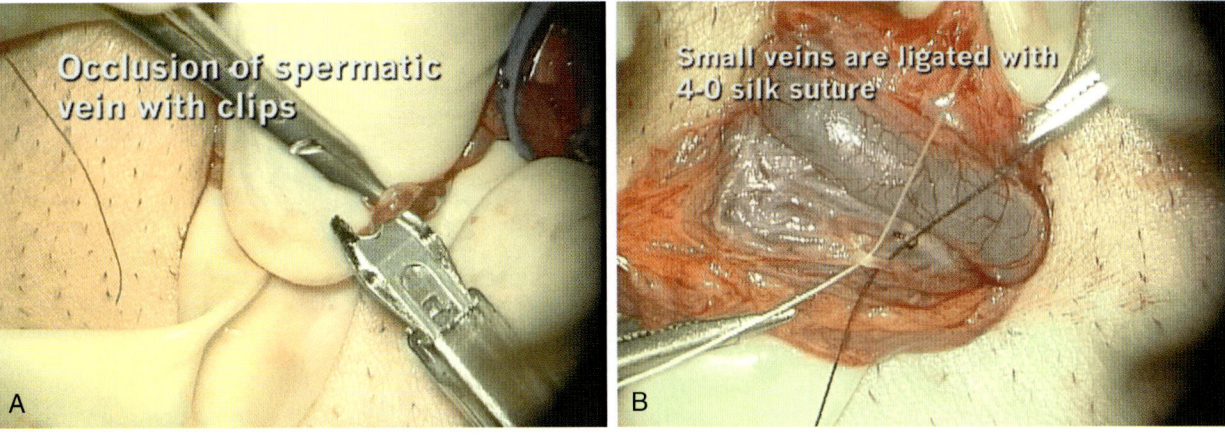

Fig. 67.50. Veins within the cord ligated with hemoclips (A) or by passing two 4-0 silk ligatures, one black and one white, beneath the vein (B).

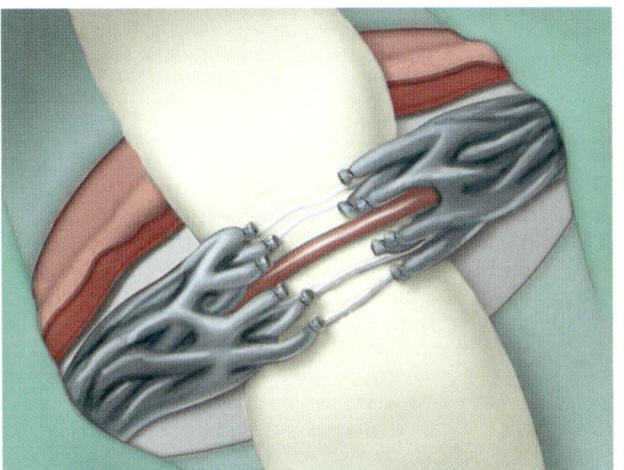

Fig. 67.51. Completed dissection showing the testicular artery, cremasteric arteries, lymphatics, and vas deferens with its vessels remaining.

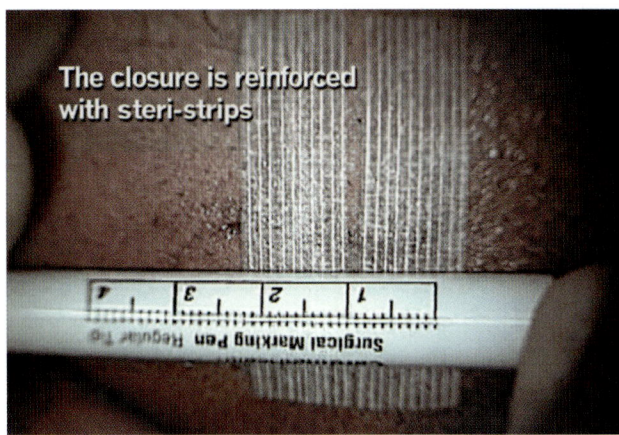

Fig. 67.53. Subcuticular suture reinforced by two to three Steri-Strips.

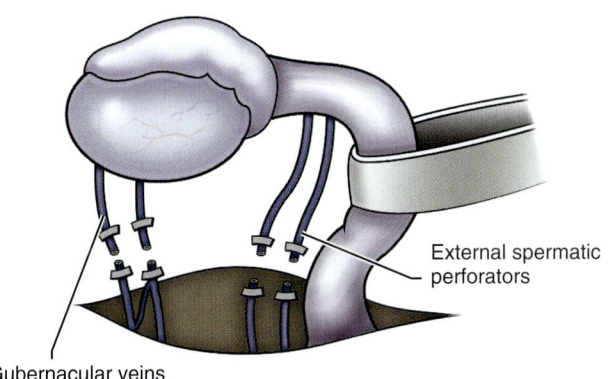

Fig. 67.52. External spermatic and gubernacular veins are doubly ligated with hemoclips and divided.

Hydroceles are found in 15% of testes associated with varicoceles. **As little as 3 cc of hydrocele fluid can significantly alter testicular temperature regulation** (Wysock and Goldstein, 2009). If a hydrocele is noted when the testis is delivered, it is repaired. Small ones may be treated with excision of a segment of the hydrocele sac and cauterization of the edges. Larger hydroceles are treated with either a bottleneck or excision technique. **The temporary high venous pressure immediately after varicocelectomy can make good hemostasis difficult to achieve after excisional hydrocelectomy. Therefore there should be no hesitation to employ a scrotal Penrose drain placed in the dependent portion of the scrotum for 24 hours after combined varicocelectomy and excisional hydrocelectomy.** The testis is then returned to the scrotum and the Penrose drain is left beneath the cord structures.

The external oblique aponeurosis, if opened, is reapproximated with continuous suturing using the previously placed 3-0 suture. Scarpa fascia and Camper fascia are reapproximated with a single or continuous 3-0 plain catgut suture, and the skin is approximated with a 5-0 monofilament absorbable subcuticular suture reinforced by 2 to 3 Steri-Strips (Fig. 67.53). A scrotal supporter is applied and stuffed with fluff type dressings. The patient is discharged on the day of surgery with a prescription for acetaminophen with codeine. The patient is instructed to apply ice to his or her wounds intermittently for 20 minutes for 20 days postoperatively to prevent further swelling and ease discomfort on the effected site. The patient should shower in 48 hours, and light desk work may be resumed in 2 or 3 days. Ejaculation and intercourse may be resumed 1 week postoperatively, light exercise in 2 weeks, and all activities 3 weeks postoperatively.

Radiographic Occlusion Techniques

Radiographic coil occlusion of the internal spermatic veins has been successfully employed for varicoceles (Lima et al., 1978; Walsh and White, 1981; Weissbach et al., 1981). These techniques are performed under a local anesthetic through a small cut-down incision over the femoral vein. The recurrence rate after balloon occlusion was originally 11% and more recently is reportedly as low as 4% (Kaufman et al.,

1983; Matthews et al., 1992; Mitchell et al., 1985; Murray et al., 1986). Failure to successfully cannulate small collaterals and external spermatic veins and scrotal collaterals results in recurrence. **Venographic placement of a balloon or coil in the internal spermatic vein is successfully accomplished in 75% to 90% of attempts** (Morag et al., 1984; Sivanathan and Abernethy, 2003; White et al., 1981; Winkelbauer et al., 1994). **Therefore a significant number of men undergoing attempted radiographic occlusion will ultimately require a surgical approach.** In addition, the radiographic techniques take between 1 and 3 hours to perform compared with 25 to 45 minutes required for surgical repair. Although rare, serious complications of radiographic balloon or coil occlusion have included migration of the balloon or coil into the renal vein, resulting in loss of a kidney, pulmonary embolization of the coil or balloon (Matthews et al., 1992), femoral vein perforation or thrombosis, and anaphylactic reaction to radiographic contrast medium. Antegrade scrotal sclerotherapy via cannulation of a scrotal vein has been employed in Europe (Ficarra et al., 2002; Minucci et al., 2004; Tauber and Johnsen, 1994). The recurrence rate is similar to balloon or coil techniques. Long-term follow-up is not available, and the consequence of escape of the sclerosing agent into the renal vein and vena cava is unknown. In addition, the larger the varicocele, the higher the failure and recurrence rate with this technique. **We have seen many men referred with late (2–5 years) recurrence after radiographic occlusion. They typically present as slow-filling veins that become prominent at the end of the day. Initial cursory physical examination can miss these recurrences. We believe these recurrences are likely due to recanalization through the coils because, unlike in surgical repair, the veins are not ligated and divided.** Although often initially successful, I believe that radiographic occlusion is less durable than microsurgical ligation.

Complications of Varicocelectomy

Hydrocele

Hydrocele formation is the most common complication reported after nonmicroscopic varicocelectomy. The incidence of this complication varies from 3% to 33%, with an average incidence of about 7%. Analysis of the protein concentration of hydrocele fluid indicates that **hydrocele formation after varicocelectomy is due to lymphatic obstruction** (Szabo and Kessler, 1984). At least half of postvaricocelectomy hydroceles grow to a size large enough to warrant surgical excision because of the discomfort and growth of the hydrocele to a large size. The effect of hydrocele formation on sperm function and fertility is uncertain. It is known that men with varicocele have significantly elevated intratesticular temperatures (Goldstein and Eid, 1989; Zorgniotti et al., 1979). This appears to be an important pathophysiologic phenomenon mediating the adverse effects of varicocele on fertility (Saypol et al., 1981). The development of a large hydrocele creates an abnormal insulating layer that surrounds the testis. This may impair the efficiency of the counter-current heat exchange mechanism and therefore obviate some of the benefits of varicocelectomy (Wysock and Goldstein, 2009).

Use of magnification to identify and preserve lymphatics almost eliminates the risk of hydrocele formation after varicocelectomy (Glassberg et al., 2008; Goldstein et al., 1992; Marmar and Kim, 1994). The management of postvaricocelectomy hydrocele is identical to that of other hydroceles (see Chapter 41).

> **KEY POINTS: HYDROCELE**
>
> - A single stitch through an epididymal tubule in the corpus or cauda will result in complete obstruction.

Testicular Artery Injury

The diameter of the testicular artery in humans is 1.0 to 1.5 mm. The testicular artery supplies two-thirds of the testicular blood supply and the vasal and cremasteric arteries the remaining one-third (Raman and Goldstein, 2004). Microdissections of the human spermatic cord have revealed that the testicular artery is closely adherent to a large internal spermatic vein in 40% of men. In another 20% of men the testicular artery is surrounded by a network of tiny veins (Beck et al., 1992). During the course of cord dissection for varicocelectomy, the artery may go into spasm and even in its unconstricted state is often difficult to positively identify and preserve. **Injury or ligation of the testicular artery carries with it the risk of testicular atrophy and/or impaired spermatogenesis.** Starzl's transplant group (Penn et al., 1972) reported a 14% incidence of frank testicular atrophy when the testicular artery was purposely ligated. The actual incidence of testicular artery ligation during varicocelectomy is unknown, but some studies suggest it is common (Wosnitzer and Roth, 1983). Animal studies indicate that the risk of testicular atrophy after testicular artery ligation varies from 20% to 100% (Goldstein and Einer-Jensen, 1983; MacMahon et al., 1976). In humans, atrophy after artery ligation is probably less likely because of the contribution of the cremasteric as well as vasal arterial supply (Raman and Goldstein, 2004). **In children the potential for neovascularization and compensatory hypertrophy of the vasal and cremasteric vessels is probably greater than in adults, making atrophy after testicular artery ligation less likely.** Use of magnifying loupes, or preferably an operating microscope and/or a fine-tip Doppler probe, facilitates identification and preservation of the testicular artery and therefore minimizes the risk of testicular injury. Radiographic balloon or coil occlusion techniques also eliminate this risk.

Varicocele Recurrence

The incidence of varicocele recurrence after surgical repair varies from 0.6% to 45% (Al-Kandari et al., 2007; Barbalias et al., 1998; Cayan et al., 2000; Lemack et al., 1998). Recurrence is more common after repair of pediatric varicoceles. Radiographic studies of recurrent varicoceles visualize periarterial, parallel inguinal, or midretroperitoneal collaterals or, more rarely, trans-scrotal collaterals (Kaufman et al., 1983). **Retroperitoneal operations miss parallel inguinal and scrotal collaterals.** Nonmagnified inguinal operations have a lower incidence of varicocele recurrence but fail to address the issue of scrotal collaterals or small veins surrounding the testicular artery. The microsurgical approach with delivery of the testis lowers the incidence of varicocele recurrence to less than 1% compared with 9% using conventional inguinal techniques (Goldstein et al., 1992; Marmar and Kim, 1994).

Results

Varicocelectomy results in significant improvement in semen analysis in 60% to 80% of men. Reported pregnancy rates after varicocelectomy vary from 20% to 60% (Marmar et al., 2007). A randomized controlled trial of surgery versus no surgery in infertile men with varicoceles revealed a pregnancy rate of 44% at 1 year in the surgery group versus 10% in the control group (Madgar et al., 1995). In our series of 1500 microsurgical operations, 43% of couples were pregnant at 1 year (Goldstein and Tanrikut, 2006) and 69% at 2 years when couples with female factors were excluded. **Microsurgical varicocelectomy results in return of sperm to the ejaculate in up to 50% of azoospermic men with palpable varicoceles** (Ishikawa et al., 2008; Kim et al., 1999; Lee et al., 2007; Matthews et al., 1998; Pasqualotto et al., 2006).

The results of varicocelectomy are also related to the size of the varicocele. **Repair of large varicoceles results in a significantly greater improvement in semen quality than repair of small varicoceles** (Jarow et al., 1996; Steckel et al., 1993). In addition, large varicoceles are associated with greater preoperative impairment in semen quality than small varicoceles, and consequently overall pregnancy rates are similar regardless of varicocele size. Some evidence suggests that the younger the patient is at the time of varicocele repair, the greater the improvement after repair and the more likely the testis is to recover from varicocele-induced injury (Kass et al., 1987). Varicocele recurrence, testicular artery ligation, and postvaricocelectomy hydrocele formation are often associated with poor postoperative results. **In infertile men with low serum testosterone levels, microsurgical varicocelectomy alone results in substantial improvement in serum** testosterone levels (Cayan et al., 1999; Rosoff et al., 2009; Su et al., 1995; Tanrikut et al., 2011; Younes, 2003).

Summary

Varicocele is an extremely common entity, present in 15% of the male population. Varicoceles are found in approximately 35% of men with primary infertility but 75% to 81% of men with secondary infertility. Mounting evidence clearly demonstrates that varicocele causes progressive duration-dependent injury to the testis. Larger varicoceles appear to cause more damage than small varicoceles and, conversely, repair of large varicoceles results in greater improvement of semen quality. **Variocelectomy can halt the progressive duration-dependent decline in semen quality found in men with varicoceles.** The earlier the age at which varicocele is repaired, the more likely is recovery of spermatogenic function. **Variocelectomy can also improve Leydig cell function resulting in increased testosterone levels** (Cayan et al., 1999; Su et al., 1995; Tanrikut et al., 2011; Younes, 2003). **Repair improves live birth rates as well as IVF/ICSI outcomes and increases the chances of finding sperm in men with NOA.**

The most common complications after varicocelectomy are hydrocele formation, testicular artery injury, and varicocele persistence or recurrence. **The incidence of these complications can be reduced by employing microsurgical techniques, inguinal or subinguinal operations, and exposure of the external spermatic and scrotal veins.** Employment of these advanced techniques of varicocelectomy provide a safe, effective approach to elimination of varicocele, preservation of testicular function, and, in a substantial number of men, an increase in semen quality and likelihood of pregnancy, as well as increase in serum testosterone in men with androgen deficiency.

KEY POINTS: VARICOCELECTOMY

- Early repair of varicoceles prevents both future infertility and Leydig cell dysfunction.
- In select men, varicocelectomy may be an effective treatment for symptomatic, age-related androgen deficiency.
- Micro-Doppler is extremely useful in identifying arteries.
- As long as at least one set of deferential veins remains intact, venous return will be adequate.
- At the completion of the dissection, only the testicular arteries, cremasteric arteries, lymphatics, and vas deferens with its vessels remain.
- Ligation of the testicular artery is unlikely to enhance testicular function.
- Microsurgical varicocelectomy results in return of sperm to the ejaculate in approximately 40% of men with nonobstructive azoospermia.

ORCHIOPEXY IN ADULTS

It is well known that cryptorchidism is associated with a high incidence of infertility even when unilateral. Long, hot baths and saunas in humans, on a regular basis, have been shown to impair spermatogenesis. Elevated testicular temperature is also thought to be the primary pathophysiologic feature of varicocele (Goldstein and Eid, 1989; Saypol et al., 1981; Wright et al., 1997; Zorgniotti, 1980). Spermatogenesis is exquisitely temperature sensitive. Animal and human studies have shown that artificial elevation of testicular temperature results in impaired spermatogenesis (Perez-Crespo et al., 2008; Shin et al., 1997; Shiraishi et al., 2009). It will also preserve testicular hormonal function. The technique of orchiopexy in adults is identical to that employed for children. Even with a normal contralateral testis, orchiopexy is worthwhile to bring down a unilateral undescended testis to, if possible, a scrotal location where it can be examined. Leydig cell function in undescended testis can be retained. Orchiopexy in adults with bilateral undescended testes can induce spermatogenesis and allow pregnancy (Shin et al., 1997).

Even **a solitary cryptorchid testis, when properly placed in scrotum, can provide enough testosterone to obviate the need for hormone replacement. When orchiopexy is performed in adults, regular self-examination and yearly sonography is mandatory.**

Retractile or Ectopic Testes in Adults

Retractile testes in boys are usually not surgically repaired if the testes can be manually manipulated to stay down in the scrotum either in the office or under anesthesia. The fate of persistently retractile testis in adults is unknown. A subset of infertile men have retractile testis (Caucci et al., 1997). The semen analyses of these men often demonstrate a typical stressed pattern similar to those of men with varicoceles. These men, however, do not have palpable varicoceles. They all have at least one and frequently both testes that retract out of the scrotum and into the abdomen and remain there for an hour or more a day. In some men these testes remain in the abdomen virtually all the time, except when in a warm shower or under anesthesia. It is likely that these testes will suffer from impaired temperature regulation and impaired spermatogenesis. Scrotal orchiopexy can improve the semen quality and fertility of some of these men. Some men have ectopic testis in which, instead of the testes being side to side, one testis is behind (Fig. 67.54) the other, almost in the perineum. This is also likely to elevate testis temperature.

When scrotal orchiopexy is performed for retractile or ectopic testis in adults, a dartos pouch operation should be performed. Simple suture orchiopexy of the tunica albuginea of the testis to the dartos, such as is performed sometimes to prevent torsion, will not prevent retraction of these testes into the groin. Creation of a dartos pouch keeps the testis well down into the scrotum and permanently prevent retraction. **This is also the most reliable and safest technique for the prevention of testicular torsion** (Redman and Barthold, 1995).

A 3- to 4-cm transverse incision is made in the low scrotal skinfolds overlying the testis. **The incision is kept very superficial, just through**

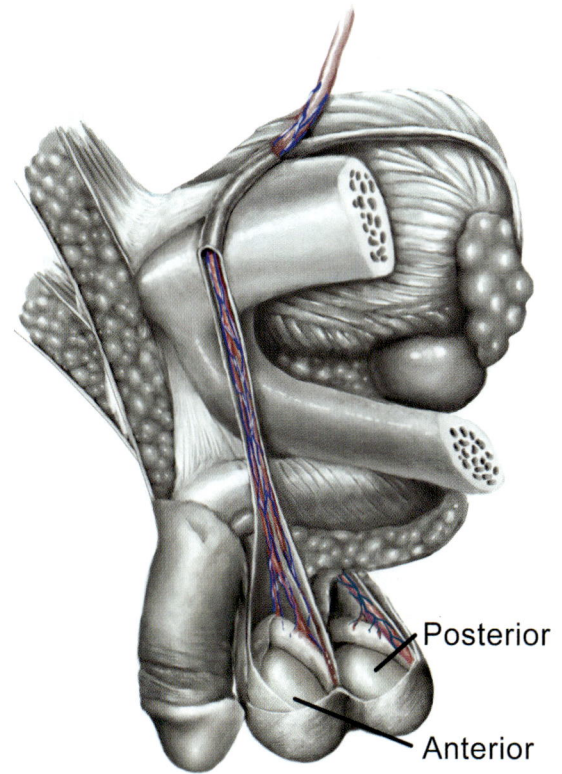

Fig. 67.54. Ectopic testis, where one testis is behind the other, almost in the perineum.

the dermis and not into the dartos. A large pouch must be created to accommodate the adult testis. The place of dissection is above the dartos and just below the skin, which is kept thin.

After a capacious pouch is created, the dartos and underlying tunica vaginalis are vertically incised and the testis delivered. The cremasteric fibers overlying the spermatic cord are divided and ligated to minimize the tendency of the testis to retract. The opening in the dartos is closed around the cord (but not too tightly) to prevent the testis from falling out of the pouch. The cut edge of the everted tunica is approximated to the opening in the dartos with interrupted synthetic monofilament absorbable sutures. This allows placement of the testis in the pouch without the need for fixation sutures in the tunica albuginea (Redman and Barthold, 1995). The skin is closed over the testis with interrupted sutures of 4-0 chromic catgut. This technique obviates the risk of inadvertent injury to and bleeding from the testicular artery, which courses just under the tunica albuginea (Jarow, 1990).

Videos 67.1 to 67-8 show procedures related to this topic.

> **KEY POINTS: ORCHIOPEXY**
>
> - When orchiopexy is performed for retractile or ectopic testis in adults, a dartos pouch should be performed.

ACKNOWLEDGMENTS

I thank Vanessa L. Dudley and Philip Shihua Li, MD, for their immeasurable assistance in the preparation of this manuscript.

REFERENCES

The complete reference list is available online at ExpertConsult.com.

68 Physiology of Penile Erection and Pathophysiology of Erectile Dysfunction

Alan W. Shindel MD, MAS, and Tom F. Lue, MD, ScD (Hon), FACS

"The penis does not obey the order of its master, who tries to erect or shrink it at will. Instead, the penis erects freely while its master is asleep. The penis must be said to have its own mind, by any stretch of the imagination."

Leonardo da Vinci

PHYSIOLOGY OF PENILE ERECTION

Historical Contexts on Our Understanding of Erectile Physiology

The oldest known recorded description of erectile dysfunction (ED) dates from circa 2000 BCE and was set down on Egyptian papyrus. Two types were described: natural ("the man is incapable of accomplishing the sex act") and supernatural (evil charms and spells). Later, Hippocrates reported many cases of ED among the rich inhabitants of Scythia and ascribed it to excessive horseback riding (Brenot, 1994). Aristotle stated that three branches of nerves carry spirit and energy to the penis and that erection is produced by the influx of air (Brenot, 1994). Aristotle's theory was well accepted until Leonardo da Vinci proposed that erection was derived from penile blood flow, based on observations of a large amount of blood in the erect penis of hanged men. These writings were not widely known until the beginning of the 20th century (Brenot, 1994). Although Da Vinci's observation was not widely publicized, in 1585 Ambroise Paré gave a reasonably accurate account of penile anatomy and the concept of blood-derived penile erection. He described the penis as concentric coats of nerves, veins, arteries, two ligaments (corpora cavernosa), a urinary tract, and four muscles. Paré accurately wrote, "When the man becomes inflamed with lust and desire, blood rushes into the male member and causes it to become erect." Dionis elaborated on Paré's theory by stressing the importance of retaining blood in the penis for maintenance of erection (Brenot, 1994). The mechanism of blood retention was thought by Dionis to be related to muscular contraction compressing proximal penile veins. In 1787 Hunter hypothesized that venous spasm prevented the exit of blood from the penis during erection.

Modern investigations of penile hemodynamics began in the 1970s with xenon washout and caversonography studies in human men exposed to audiovisual sexual stimuli. Limitations of these technologies led to conflicting results: Shirai concluded that penile venous flow is increased during erection, but markedly increased arterial flow compensates for this (Shirai et al., 1978). Wagner (1981) advanced the alternative hypothesis that venous drainage is decreased during erection.

Introduction of Doppler ultrasound and improved understanding of molecular biology revolutionized our understanding of erection physiology near the turn of the 20th century (Lue et al., 1985). In the 1980s it was confirmed that increased blood inflow (via arterial vasodilation) and decreased venous outflow (via venous coaptation) were key drivers of penile erection (Lue, 1986; Lue et al., 1983, 1984). In the 1990s nitric oxide (NO) and the enzymes that produce it (endothelial and neuronal nitric oxide synthase, eNOS and nNOS, respectively) were identified as key regulators of penile erection (Rajfer et al., 1992). The antierectile activity of phosphodiesterase type 5 (PDE5) was identified around the same time (Boolell et al., 1996). This understanding led to the development of effective oral pharmacotherapy for ED, which has revolutionized the medical management of sexual dysfunction (Goldstein et al., 1998). Many other molecular determinants of penile erection have been identified, including intracellular gap junctions, potassium, and calcium channels, and alternate molecular pathways such as RHO/Rho-kinase (Matsui et al., 2015). Our understanding of penile tissues has also improved, bettering our understanding of the role of elasticity and fibrosis in penile erection and detumescence (Gonzalez-Cadavid, 2009). Our current understanding of the physiology of erection and pathophysiology of ED is detailed in this chapter.

Functional Anatomy of the Penis

The penis is composed primarily of three cylindric structures. Dorsally, there are paired corpora cavernosa that extend from the pubic rami to the tip of the penis. The ventrally located corpus spongiosum encircles the urethra and is covered by a loose subcutaneous layer and skin. All three corporal bodies contain spongy vascular tissue that has the capacity to expand to contain large volumes of blood (Yiee and Baskin, 2010).

There is wide variability in penile length and girth (Table 68.1; Awwad et al., 2005). The flaccid length and girth of the penis is controlled by content of blood within the corporal bodies, which is in turn controlled by the degree of contraction within the smooth muscles of the spongy erectile tissue. There is marked variability in penile length, and neither age nor the size of the flaccid penis are necessarily accurate predictors of erect penile length (Wessells et al., 1996). There is also a fair degree of variability with respect to congenital penile curvature. Up to 15% of men have a downward penile curvature during erection, and approximately one-quarter have an erect penile angle less than horizontal (Sparling, 1997). Some experts have posited that certain variations in penile anatomy may lead to functional ED (e.g., penile buckling during intercourse) even in the presence of normal arterial and venous function. During attempted penetration, buckling forces from axial load on the penis are dependent not only on intracavernous pressures but also on penile geometry and corporal expandability. Some patients with normal penile hemodynamics may experience sexual difficulty even in the context of full tumescence; in such cases structural causes (i.e., penile curvature from chordee or Peyronie disease) should be considered (Udelson et al., 1998).

Corpora Cavernosa, Corpus Spongiosum, and Glans Penis

The corpora cavernosa are paired, dorsally located cylinders of expansile vascular tissue ensheathed by the tunica albuginea. Their proximal ends, the crura, originate at the undersurface of the puboischial rami as two separate structures but merge under the pubic arch and remain attached up to the glans penis. **Connections are present between the corpora cavernosa in men; in some species (e.g., dogs) a septum completely separates the corporal bodies** (Lue et al., 1983, 1984; Yiee and Baskin, 2010).

Each corpus cavernosum is a conglomeration of vascular sinusoids, larger in the center and smaller in the periphery (Goldstein and Padma-Nathan, 1990). These interconnected sinusoids are separated

TABLE 68.1 Penile Length in Adults

FIRST AUTHOR	YEAR OF REPORT	NO. SUBJECTS	AGE IN YEARS (RANGE)	FLACCID LENGTH (cm)	STRETCHED OR ERECT LENGTH (cm)	COUNTRY
Kinsey	1948	2770	20–59	9.7	15.5 (E)	United States
Bondil	1992	905	17–91	10.7	16.74 (S)	France
Wessells	1996	80	21–82	8.85 +/- 2.38	12.45 +/- 2.71 (S), 12.89 +/- 2.91 (E)	United States
Ponchietti	2001	3300	17–19	9	12.5 (S)	Italy
Ajmani	1985	320	17–23	8.16 +/- 0.94	NA	Nigeria
Schneider	2001	111	18–19	8.6 +/- 1.50	14.48 +/- 1.99 (E)	Germany
		32	40–68	9.22 +/-1.67	14.18 +/- 1.83 (E)	Germany
Awwad	2005	271 (N)	17–83	9.3 +/- 1.9	13.5 +/- 2.3 (S)	Jordan
		109 (ED)	22–68	7.7 +/- 1.3	11.6 +/- 1.4 (S)	Jordan

E, Erect length; *ED*, erectile dysfunction; *N*, normal; *NA*, not available; *S*, stretched length.
Modified from Awwad Z, Abu-Hijleh M, Basri S, et al.: Penile measurements in normal adult Jordanians and in patients with erectile dysfunction. *Int J Impot Res* 17:191–195, 2005.

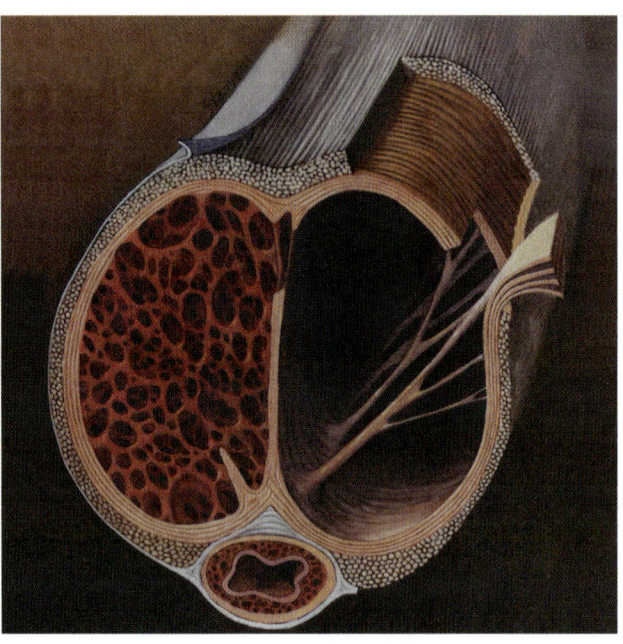

Fig. 68.1. Artist's cross-sectional drawing of the penis, depicting the inner circular and outer longitudinal layers of the tunica albuginea and the intracavernous pillars. The longitudinal layer is absent in the ventral groove housing the corpus spongiosum. (From Lue TF, Akkus E, Kour NW: Physiology of erectile function and dysfunction. *Campbell's Urol Update* 12:1–10, 1994.)

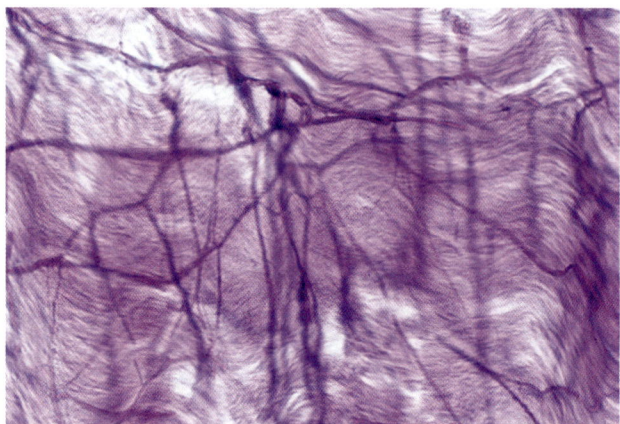

Fig. 68.2. Micrograph of the human tunica albuginea, showing the interwoven elastic fibers and the finer collagen fibers (Hart stain ×100).

by smooth muscle trabeculae surrounded by elastic fibers, collagen, and loose areolar tissue. The structure of the corpus spongiosum and glans is similar to that of the corpora cavernosa except that the sinusoids are larger.

The terminal cavernous nerves and helicine arteries of the phallus are intimately associated with the smooth muscle of the corpora. In the flaccid state, blood slowly diffuses from the central to the peripheral sinusoids, and the blood gas levels are similar to those found in venous blood. During erection, rapid entry of arterial blood to central and peripheral sinusoids enhances oxygen tension and raises pH (Sattar et al., 1995).

Tunica Albuginea

The tunica albuginea are paired, bilayered, fibrous sheaths that cover the corpora cavernosa and afford great flexibility, rigidity, and tissue strength to the penis (Fig. 68.1; Goldstein and Padma-Nathan, 1990). The principle constituent of the tunica is fibrillar collagen (mostly type I but also type III); however, elastic fibers are also present in an irregular, latticed network interwoven with the collagen fibers (Fig. 68.2). Elastin permits the penis to expand during penile erection.

The outer-layer tunica collagen bundles are oriented longitudinally, extending from the glans penis to the proximal crura. Inner-layer collagen bundles support and contain the cavernous tissue and are oriented circularly. Radiating from this inner layer are intracavernous pillars that act as struts to augment the septum between the corpora and to provide essential support to the erectile tissue. These structures insert into the inferior pubic rami but are absent between the 5 o'clock and the 7 o'clock positions. Between the inner and outer tunica layer are oblique-oriented fibers that connect the two main layers.

The detailed histologic composition of the tunica varies with anatomic location and function. The ventral portion of the corporal tunica tends to be thinner (mean thickness 0.8 mm) relative to the dorsal tunica (mean thickness 2.2 mm) because of variations in the outer corporal layer thickness. The absence of intracavernous pillars and thinner tunica layer create an area of relative weakness on the ventrum of the penis that has clinical relevance in cases of penile fracture and implant surgery (Hsu et al., 1994).

The bilayered structure of the tunica is critical to normal erectile function. Emissary veins that drain the corporal bodies run between the inner and outer layers of the tunica for a short distance, often piercing the outer bundles obliquely. These veins are compressed by the expanding corporal sinuses during the early phases of penile erection; this has the effect of obstructing venous outflow and promoting tumescence (Yiee and Baskin, 2010). The cavernous artery and branches of the dorsal artery that supply blood supply to the corpus cavernosum are protected from this compression because they run within the corporal bodies and are surrounded by a periarterial soft-tissue sheath.

The corpus spongiosum is also ensheathed by a tunica layer; however, the spongiosal tunica lacks an outer layer or intracorporeal struts, ensuring a low-pressure system during erection. Furthermore, the tunica of the corpus spongisoum does not extend into the glans penis.

External support of the corpora consists of two ligamentous structures: the fundiform and suspensory ligaments. The fundiform ligament arises from Colles fascia and is lateral, superficial, and not adherent to the tunica albuginea of the corpora cavernosa. The suspensory ligament arises from Buck fascia and consists of two lateral bundles and one median bundle that circumscribe the dorsal vein of the penis. Its main function is to attach the tunica albuginea of the corpora cavernosa to the pubis, and it provides support for the mobile portion of the penis (Hoznek et al., 1998). In patients with congenital deficiency or in whom this ligament has been severed in "penile elongation" surgery, the erect penis may be unstable during attempted penetration.

Arteries

The primary source of penile blood in most men is the paired internal pudendal arteries, which are branches of the internal iliac arteries (Fig. 68.3A). The internal pudendal artery becomes the common penile artery after giving off a branch to the perineum. The three branches of the penile artery are the cavernous, dorsal, and bulbourethral. Distally, they join to form a vascular ring near the glans. The cavernous artery effects tumescence of the corpus cavernosum and enters at the hilum of the penis, where the two crura converge. It gives off many helicine arteries along its course, which supply the trabecular erectile tissue and the sinusoids (Fig. 68.3B). These helicine arteries are contracted and tortuous in the flaccid state and become dilated and straight during erection. The dorsal artery of the penis is responsible for engorgement of the glans during erection; in many men it also supplies branches that penetrate the tunica and merge with the cavernous arteries to supply the distal penis (Diallo et al., 2013). The bulbourethral artery supplies the proximally located penile bulb and corpus spongiosum. The bulbourethral and urethral arteries are situated outside the tunica albuginea of the corpus spongiosum on the lateral and dorsal sides.

In approximately one-third of cases, accessory arteries from the external iliac, obturator, and vesical and femoral arteries also supply the penis; in some men these accessory arteries may be the dominant or only arterial supply to the corpus cavernosum (Breza et al., 1989; Nehra et al., 2008). Penile circulation in approximately 70% of men is thought to be derived from both the internal pudendal and accessory arteries, with circulation entirely from either internal pudendal or accessory arteries in about 15% each (Droupy et al., 1997). Preservation of accessory pudendal arteries is associated with more rapid recovery of sexual function in men after radical prostatectomy (Mulhall et al., 2008).

Veins

The venous drainage from the three corpora originates in tiny venules leading from the peripheral sinusoids immediately beneath the tunica albuginea. These venules travel in the trabeculae between the tunica and the peripheral sinusoids to form the subtunical venous plexus before exiting the inner tunica layer as the emissary veins (Fig. 68.4A). There is wide variability in penile venous circulation (Fig. 68.4B and C; Hsu et al., 2012).

The emissary veins from the corpus cavernosum and spongiosum drain dorsally to the deep dorsal vein, which originates near the coronal sulcus and serves as the primary venous drainage of the glans and distal two-thirds of the corpora (corresponding to the pendulous portion of the penis). The deep dorsal vein runs cephalad and posterior to the symphysis pubis to join the periprostatic venous plexus; occasionally there are two deep dorsal veins. Additional sources of venous drainage include circumflex veins laterally, periurethral veins ventrally, and small venous channels accompanying the paired dorsal artery. Periarterial veins also travel longitudinally to join the dorsal vein or Santorini plexus proximally (Hsu et al., 2003). These become enlarged after the deep dorsal vein is ligated and may be the cause of recurrent leakage in venogenic ED (Chen et al., 2005). Emissary veins from the proximal (infrapubic) penis join to form cavernous and crural veins. These join the periurethral veins from the urethral bulb to form the internal pudendal veins.

The venous drainage of penile skin and subcutaneous tissues is derived from subcutaneous veins that unite near the base of the penis to form a single (or paired) superficial dorsal vein that drains into the saphenous veins. Occasionally, the superficial dorsal vein may also drain a portion of the corpora cavernosa.

Hemodynamics and Mechanism of Erection and Detumescence

Erection involves sinusoidal relaxation, arterial dilation, and venous compression (Lue, 1986). The importance of smooth muscle relaxation has been demonstrated in animal and human studies (Ignarro et al., 1990; Saenz de Tejada et al., 1989, 1991). To summarize

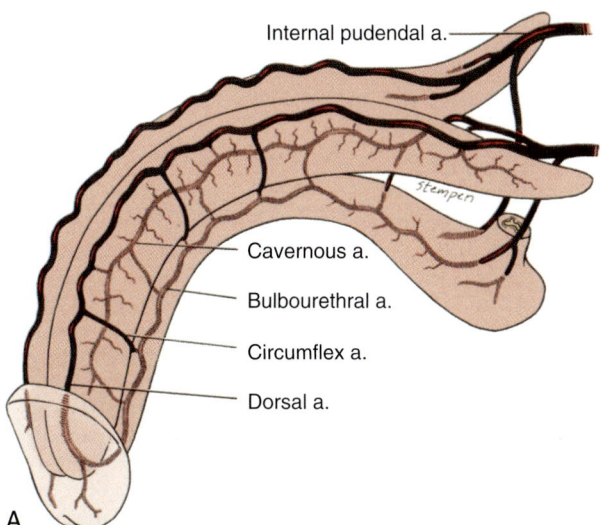
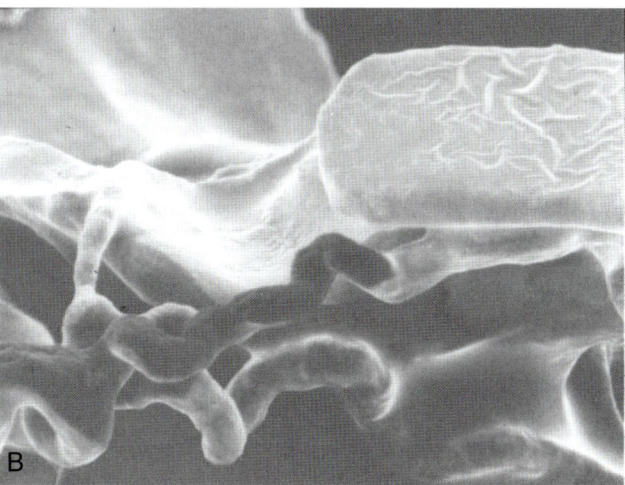

Fig. 68.3. (A) Penile arterial supply. (B) Scanning electron micrograph of a human penile cast showing helicine arteries opening directly into the sinusoids without intervening capillaries. *a*, Artery.

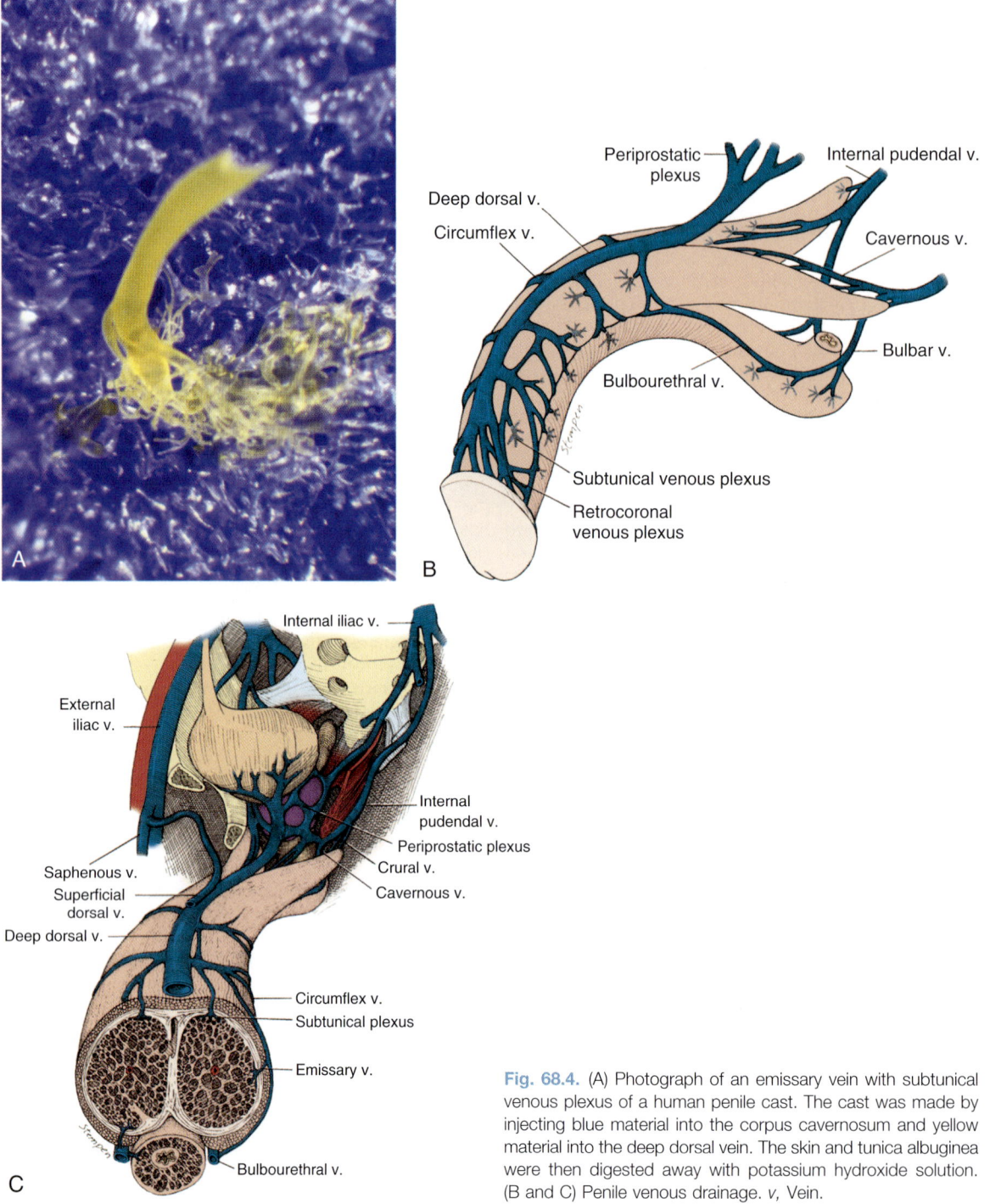

Fig. 68.4. (A) Photograph of an emissary vein with subtunical venous plexus of a human penile cast. The cast was made by injecting blue material into the corpus cavernosum and yellow material into the deep dorsal vein. The skin and tunica albuginea were then digested away with potassium hydroxide solution. (B and C) Penile venous drainage. v, Vein.

the hemodynamic events of erection and detumescence, seven phases have been observed in animal experiments that reflect the changes in and the relationship between penile arterial flow and intracavernous pressure (Fig. 68.5).

Corpora Cavernosa

The penile erectile tissue, specifically the cavernous smooth musculature and the smooth muscles of the arteriolar and arterial walls, plays a key role in the erectile process. In the **flaccid state**, these smooth muscles are tonically contracted, allowing only a small amount of arterial flow into the corpora (Sattar et al., 1995).

Sexual stimulation triggers release of neurotransmitters from the cavernous nerve terminals. This release of neurotransmitters results in relaxation of these smooth muscles, leading to dilation of arterioles and arteries and increased corporal blood flow. The increased corporal blood supply pools in the vascular sinusoids, which expand and compress the subtunical venous plexuses between the tunica albuginea and the peripheral sinusoids, reducing venous outflow during the **latent phase**. As the tunica albuginea expand and are stretched to capacity, the penis enlarges and compresses the emissary veins between the inner circular and outer longitudinal layers; this is the **tumescent phase**. With maximal occlusion of the emissary veins, intracavernous pressure increases to approximately 100 mm Hg, raising the penis from the dependent position to the **full-erection phase**. Intracavernous pressure may be further elevated (up to several hundred millimeters of mercury) with reflex contractions of the ischiocavernosus muscles during maximal sexual arousal (i.e., the **rigid-erection phase**). During rigid erection intracavernosal pressures exceeding systolic blood pressure may **lead to reversal of flow in cavernous arteries** (Fig. 68.6; Lue, 1986).

The angle of the erect penis is determined by its size and attachment to the puboischial rami (the crura) and the anterior surface of the pubic bone (the suspensory and fundiform ligaments). In men with a large penis or a loose suspensory ligament, the penis often points downward even with full rigidity.

After sexual climax or cessation of arousal, the penis detumesces in three overlapping phases. The first (**initial detumescence**) entails a transient intracorporeal pressure increase as arteries vasocontrict and compress vascular sinusoids that are engorged with corporal blood by occlusion of the emissary veins. The second phase consists of a slow pressure decrease as the emissary veins gradually open and permit venous outflow (**slow detumescence**). The final phase involves rapid pressure decrease as venous outflow capacity returns to baseline (**rapid detumescence**) (Bosch et al., 1991).

Corpus Spongiosum and Glans Penis

The hemodynamics of the corpus spongiosum and glans penis differ from those of the corpora cavernosa. **During erection, arterial flow increases, but pressure in the corpus spongiosum and glans is only one-third to one-half of pressure within the corpora cavernosa.** The thin tunica covering of the corpus spongiosum and complete absence of a tunica layer over the glans ensure minimal venous occlusion during tumescence. During the full-erection phase, partial compression of the deep dorsal and circumflex veins between Buck fascia and the engorged corpora cavernosa contributes to glanular tumescence, although the spongiosum and glans essentially function as a large arteriovenous shunt during this phase. In the rigid-erection phase, the ischiocavernosus and bulbocavernosus muscles forcefully compress the spongiosum and penile veins, increasing engorgement and pressure inside the spongiosum and glans (Table 68.2; Lue, 1986).

Neuroanatomy and Neurophysiology of Penile Erection

Spinal Centers and Peripheral Pathways

The innervation of the penis is autonomic (sympathetic and parasympathetic) and somatic (sensory and motor) (Fig. 68.7). From neurons in the spinal cord and peripheral ganglia, the sympathetic and parasympathetic fibers merge to form the cavernous

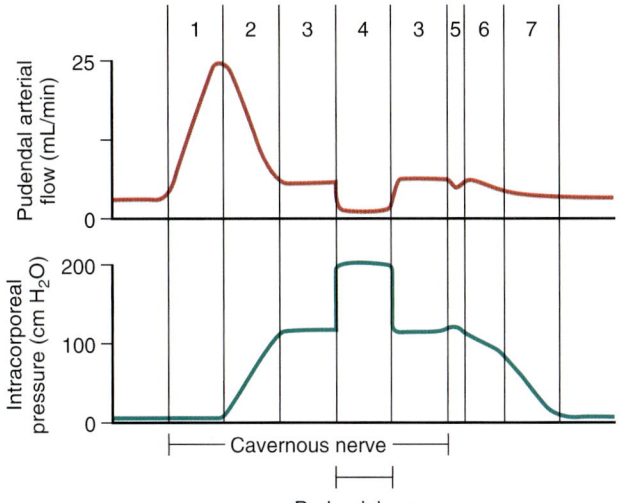

Fig. 68.5. Blood flow and intracavernous pressure changes during the seven phases of penile erection and detumescence: *0,* flaccid; *1,* latent; *2,* tumescence; *3,* full erection; *4,* rigid erection; *5,* initial detumescence; *6,* slow detumescence; *7,* fast detumescence.

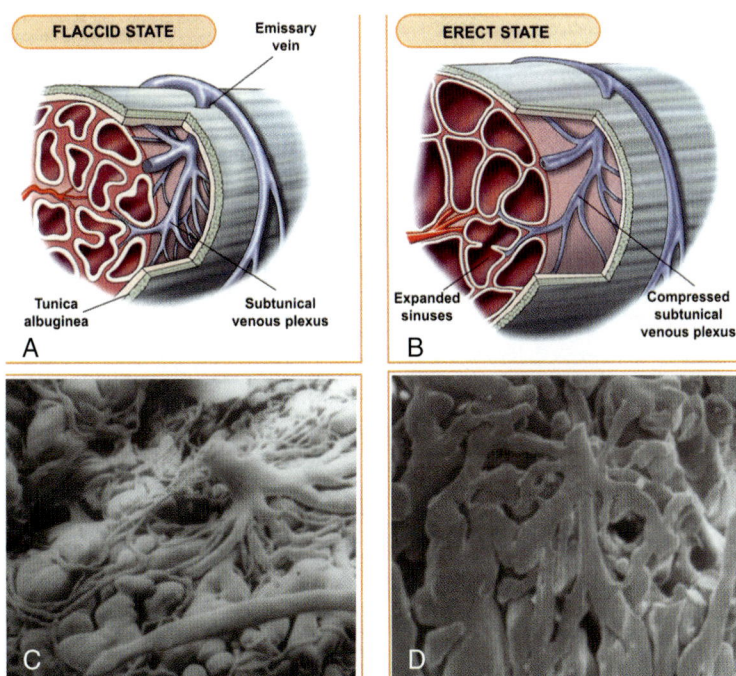

Fig. 68.6. The mechanism of penile erection. (A) In the flaccid state, the arteries, arterioles, and sinusoids are contracted. The intersinusoidal and subtunical venous plexuses are wide open, with free flow to the emissary veins. (B) In the erect state, the muscles of the sinusoidal wall and the arterioles relax, allowing maximal flow to the compliant sinusoidal spaces. Most of the venules are compressed between the expanding sinusoids. The larger venules are sandwiched and flattened between the distended sinusoids and the tunica albuginea. This effectively reduces the venous capacity to a minimum. (C and D) Scanning electron micrographs of casts of a canine subtunical venous plexus in the flaccid (C) and erect (D) states. (A and B, From Lue TF, Giuliano F, Khoury S, et al.: *Clinical manual of sexual medicine: sexual dysfunction in men*, Paris, 2004, Health Publications.)

TABLE 68.2 Comparison of Corpus Spongiosum and Glans Penis

	CORPUS SPONGIOSUM	GLANS PENIS
Tunica albuginea	Thin (circular layer only)	Absent
Main blood supply	Bulbar and spongiosal arteries	Dorsal artery
Venous occlusion during erection	No	No
Compression by skeletal muscle	Yes (ischiocavernosus, bulbocavernosus)	No

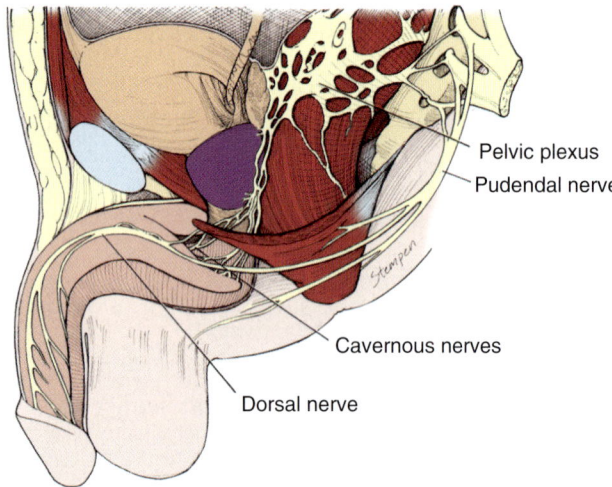

Fig. 68.7. Penile neuroanatomy.

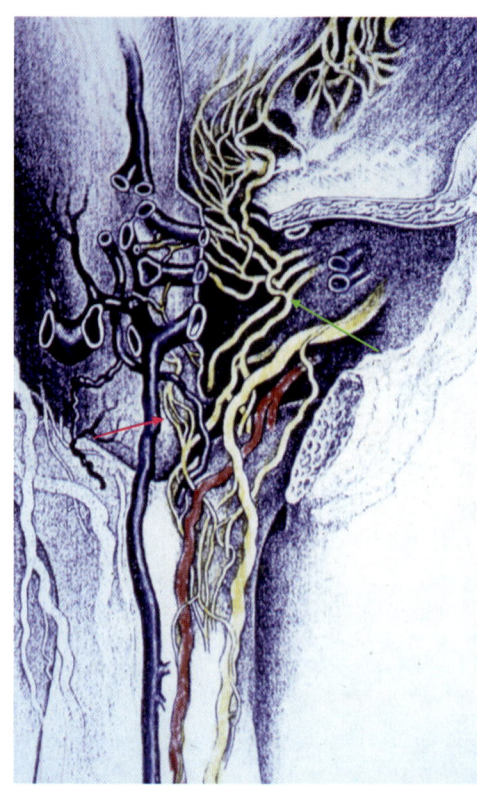

Fig. 68.8. Drawing from a human cadaveric dissection shows the medial (red arrow) and lateral (green arrow) bundles of the cavernous nerve distal to the prostate. (From Paick JS, Donatucci EF, Lue TF: Anatomy of cavernous nerves distal to prostate: microdissection study in adult male cadavers. *Urology* 42:145–149, 1993, with permission from Excerpta Medica, Inc.)

KEY POINTS

- Penile erection is dependent on increased arterial blood flow and coaptation of venous structures.
- The structure of the corporal bodies of the penis is essential to the erectile process.
- There is substantial variability in penile vascular anatomy between patients; this may have functional relevance in case of pelvic surgery.

nerves, which enter the corpora cavernosa and corpus spongiosum. Somatic nerves to the penis are primarily responsible for sensation but also play an important motor function by modulating contraction of the bulbocavernosus and ischiocavernosus muscles during rigid erection and ejaculation (Giuliano, 2011).

Autonomic Pathways. The sympathetic innervation of the penis originates from the 11th thoracic to the 2nd lumbar spinal segments and passes through the white rami to the sympathetic chain ganglia. Some fibers travel through the lumbar splanchnic nerves to the inferior mesenteric and superior hypogastric plexuses, from which fibers travel in the hypogastric nerves to the pelvic plexus. In humans, the T10 to T12 segments are most often the origin of the sympathetic fibers to the penis. Sympathetic chain ganglia cells projecting to the penis are located in the sacral and caudal ganglia (Giuliano, 2011).

The parasympathetic innervation of the penis arises from neurons in the intermediolateral cell columns of the second, third, and fourth sacral spinal cord segments. The preganglionic fibers pass in the pelvic nerves to the pelvic plexus, where they are joined by the sympathetic nerves from the superior hypogastric plexus. **The cavernous nerves are branches of the pelvic plexus that innervate the penis.** Human cadaveric dissection has revealed medial and lateral branches of the cavernous nerves (the former accompanying the urethra and the latter piercing the urogenital diaphragm 4 to 7 mm lateral to the sphincter) and multiple communications between the cavernous and dorsal nerves (Fig. 68.8; Paick et al., 1993). In addition to the cavernous nerve proper, pelvic ganglion cells exist in and along the nerve components and pelvic viscera. These ganglia are localized to the bladder/prostate junction, the dorsal aspect of the seminal vesicles, and along the prostate. There are widespread individual variations in distribution of these extramural ganglion cells in the male pelvis (Takenaka et al., 2005).

Stimulation of the pelvic plexus and the cavernous nerves induces erection, whereas stimulation of the sympathetic trunk causes detumescence. In animal models, removal of the spinal cord below L4 or L5 eliminates reflex erectile response to genital contact. Placement of these animals with a female animal in estrous, electrical stimulation of the medial preoptic area (MPOA), and central administration of the dopamine agonist apomorphine produce erections (Giuliano et al., 1996; Paick and Lee, 1994; Sato and Christ, 2000). Similarly, many men with sacral spinal cord injury retain psychogenic erectile ability even though reflexogenic erection in response to penile stimulation is abolished. These cerebrally elicited erections are found more frequently in patients with lower motor neuron lesions below T12, implying that central inhibition of tonic sympathetic tone is largely responsible for centrally mediated penile erection (Courtois et al., 1999). Further evidence for this relationship is that psychogenic erections do not typically occur in patients with spinal lesions above T9 (Chapelle et al., 1980). Although psychogenic erections may occur in men with spinal cord lesions, the degree of tumescence is often marginal and insufficient for intercourse (Chapelle et al., 1980).

Somatic Pathways. The somatosensory innervation of the penis originates at sensory receptors in the penile skin, glans, and urethra and within the corpus cavernosum. There are numerous afferent terminations in the human glans penis; free nerve endings (sensitive to touch and temperature) are the most common nerve structure and connect to thinly myelinated A_δ and C fibers (Halata and Munger, 1986). Pressure sensitive corpuscular receptors are also present, albeit at a much lower density (Halata and Munger, 1986). Nerve fibers from the various skin receptors converge to form bundles of the dorsal nerve of the penis, which joins other nerves to become the pudendal nerve. The latter enters the spinal cord via the S2-S4 roots to terminate on spinal neurons and interneurons in the central gray region of the lumbosacral segment. Activation of these sensory neurons sends messages of pain, temperature, and touch by means of spinothalamic and spinoreticular pathways to the thalamus and sensory cortex for sensory perception (McKenna, 1998).

The dorsal nerve of the penis is composed of two to six branches. In the majority of men, branches of the dorsal nerve perforate the tunica albuginea and connect to the corpus cavernosum (Kozacioglu et al., 2014). Although largely made up of somatic sensory nerves, the dorsal nerve of the penis in humans and animals also includes nNOS-containing fibers (Burnett et al., 1993; Carrier et al., 1995). These NOS-positive nerve bundles in the dorsal nerve are reduced after damage of the cavernous nerve near the rat prostate (Podlasek et al., 2001). Stimulation of the sympathetic chain at the L4-L5 level elicits an evoked discharge of the dorsal nerve (Giuliano et al., 1993). These findings illustrate that the dorsal nerve has somatic and autonomic components that regulate erectile and ejaculatory functions.

Onuf's nucleus is the center of somatomotor penile innervation and is localized to the second to fourth sacral spinal segments. Somatomotor fibers from this nucleus travel in the sacral nerves to the pudendal nerve to innervate the ischiocavernosus and bulbocavernosus muscles. **Contraction of the ischiocavernosus muscles produces the rigid-erection phase.** Rhythmic contraction and compression of the bulbocavernosus muscle on the proximal corpus is also responsible for the ejection phase of ejaculation (Clement and Giuliano, 2016). Antegrade flow of semen is also dependent on relaxation of the external urinary sphincter and compression of the corpus spongiosum. In animal studies, direct innervation of the sacral spinal motoneurons by brainstem sympathetic centers (A5-catecholaminergic cell group and locus ceruleus) has been identified (Marson and McKenna, 1996). This adrenergic innervation of pudendal motoneurons may be involved in rhythmic contractions of perineal muscles during ejaculation (Chehensse et al., 2017; Facchinetti et al., 2014). Oxytocinergic and serotoninergic innervation of lumbosacral nuclei controlling penile erection and perineal muscles in male rats has also been demonstrated (Tang et al., 1998).

Several spinal reflexes can be elicited by stimulation of the glans penis (Table 68.3). The best known is the bulbocavernosus reflex, which is the basis of genital neurologic examination and electrophysiologic latency testing. The significance of bulbocavernosus reflex testing in assessment of sexual dysfunction assessment is unclear (Giuliano and Rowland, 2013).

Supraspinal Pathways and Centers

Positron emission tomography (PET) and functional magnetic resonance imaging (fMRI) have facilitated a greater understanding of brain activation during sexual arousal in animals and humans (Table 68.4; Hubscher et al., 2010; Tsujimura et al., 2006). Psychogenic ED, premature ejaculation, and orgasmic dysfunction may be associated with alterations in higher brain function. Advanced brain imaging is able to precisely identify brain areas with increased and decreased activity during sexual stimuli (typically induced by exposure to erotic media) and erection relative to activation during nonsexual activities (e.g., exposure to neutral media) (Table 68.5; Chen et al., 2017; Kuhn and Gallinat, 2011; Parada et al., 2016; Tsujimura et al., 2006). These studies are generally well designed but are limited by the complexity and individuality of human emotional and sexual responses.

TABLE 68.3 Spinal Reflexes Involved in Stimulation of Penile Dorsal Nerve

STIMULATION	SPINAL CENTER	EFFERENT	EFFECT
Noxious, abrupt stimulation	Sacral motor neurons	Pudendal nerve (motor)	Bulbocavernous reflex
Low-intensity continuous (e.g., vibratory, manual)	Sacral parasympathetic neurons and interneurons	1. Pelvic nerves 2. Cavernous nerve	1. Detrusor inhibition and closure of bladder neck 2. Penile erection
High-intensity continuous	Sacral motor and parasympathetic Thoracolumbar sympathetic neurons	Pudendal, pelvic, and cavernous nerves	Ejaculation

TABLE 68.4 Brain Centers Involved in Sexual Function

LEVEL	REGION	FUNCTION
Forebrain	Medial amygdala Stria terminalis	Control sexual motivation
	Pyriform cortex	Inhibits sexual drive (hypersexuality when destroyed)
	Hippocampus	Involved in penile erection
	Right insula and inferior frontal cortex Left anterior cingulate cortex	Increased activity during visually evoked sexual stimulation (sexual arousal)
Hypothalamus	Medial preoptic area	Ability to recognize a sexual partner, integration of hormonal and sensory cues
	Lateral preoptic area	Control nocturnal penile tumescence in rats
	Paraventricular nucleus	Facilitates penile erection (via oxytocin neurons to lumbosacral spinal autonomic and somatic efferents)
Brainstem	Nucleus paragigantocellularis	Inhibits penile erection (via serotonin neurons to lumbosacral spinal neurons and interneurons)
	A5-catecholaminergic cell group Locus ceruleus	Major noradrenergic center
Midbrain	Periaqueductal gray	Relay center for sexually relevant stimuli

TABLE 68.5 Common Brain Activation Regions With Visual Sexual Stimuli[a]

BRAIN ACTIVATION REGIONS	FUNCTIONAL ASSOCIATION
Bilateral inferior temporal cortex (right > left)	Visual association area
Right insula	Processes somatosensory information with motivational states
Right inferior frontal cortex	Processes sensory information
Left anterior cingulate cortex	Controls autonomic and neuroendocrine function
Right occipital gyrus	Visual processing
Right hypothalamus	Male copulatory behavior
Left caudate (the striatum)	Processes attention and guides responsiveness to new environmental stimuli

[a]These regions demonstrate activation with visual sexual stimuli in multiple studies.

Integration and processing of afferent inputs (e.g., visual, olfactory, imaginative, genital stimulation) in the supraspinal centers is essential in the initiation and maintenance of penile erection. Spinal transection at the T8 level by revealed neuronal projections from the external genitalia project to the medullary reticular formation via bilateral projections in the dorsal, dorsolateral, and ventrolateral white matter of the spinal cord (Hubscher et al., 2010). In animal studies, the central supraspinal systems controlling sexual arousal are localized predominantly in the limbic system (e.g., olfactory nuclei, MPOA, nucleus accumbens, amygdala, and hippocampus) and hypothalamus (paraventricular and ventromedial nuclei). In particular, the medial amygdala, MPOA, paraventricular nucleus (PVN), periaqueductal gray, and ventral tegmentum are recognized as key structures in the central control of the male sexual response (Andersson, 2011; Melis and Argiolas, 2011). The lateral hypothalamus and anterior part of the middle cingulate cortex show increased blood flow during sexual arousal, whereas the anteroventral hypothalamus and subgenual anterior cingulate cortex show increased flow during penile detumescence after arousal. (Georgiadis et al., 2010). These brain regions are thought to play complementary regulatory roles in the autonomic modulation of sexual response.

In a meta-analysis of fMRI studies of brain activity in response to erotic stimuli, a neural network was identified that appears to constitute a core circuit of male sexual arousal in humans. This neural circuit involves the following components: cognitive (parietal cortex, anterior cingulate gyrus, thalamus, insula), emotional (amygdala, insula), motivational (precentral gyrus, parietal cortex), and physiologic (hypothalamus/thalamus, insula) (Kuhn and Gallinat, 2011). Visual association cortices are also intimately involved in response to erotic stimuli; in sum, the activated regions appear to play roles in cognitive evaluation of external stimuli, modulation of sensory processing, and regulation of urge behavior (Poeppl et al., 2014). Deactivation of the temporal and parietal lobes occurs in men during sexual arousal and/or erection. These areas govern aspects of introspection and self-reflective behaviors, including planning for the future. Inhibition of these regions may play a role in disinhibition before engaging in sexual activity (Poeppl et al., 2014).

Differential brain activation is associated with some discrete sexual issues in men. Men with hypoactive sexual desire retain activity in the left gyrus rectus (within the medial orbitofrontal cortex) during exposure to sexually arousing media; men with normal desire experienced deactivation of this brain region (Stoleru et al., 2003). This region is believed to mediate inhibition of motivated behavior, implying that men with hypoactive sexual desire disorder experience continued inhibition of behavior even with exposure to erotic stimuli. Men with psychogenic ED evidence extended activation of the cingulated gyrus, frontal mesial, and frontal basal cortex during exposure to sexually arousing media. With administration of the dopamine agonist apomorphine activity in these areas became similar to what was observed in healthy controls without ED (Montorsi et al., 2003). Separate studies have suggested that men with psychogenic ED evidence decreased connectivity in the "default mode network" (related to states of wakeful rest and attention to self and other's emotional state and thoughts) and the "salience network" (responsible for processing which environmental cues merit attention). The implication is that psychogenic ED may be related to aberrant appraisal of erotic stimuli and lack of awareness of the self's body state (Cera et al., 2014). Disruption of brain areas responsible for integrating external stimuli and visceral arousal is observed in some patients with ED related to cerebrovascular injury (Winder et al., 2017).

The structures discussed earlier are responsible for the three types of erection: psychogenic, reflexogenic, and nocturnal. Psychogenic erection is a result of audiovisual stimuli or fantasy. Impulses from the brain modulate the spinal erection centers (T11-L2 and S2-S4) to activate the erectile process, primarily by suppression of baseline sympathetic tone that limits penile circulation. Reflexogenic erection is produced by tactile stimulation of the genital organs. The impulses reach the spinal erection centers; some then follow the ascending tract, resulting in sensory perception, whereas others activate the autonomic nuclei to send messages via the cavernous nerves to the penis to induce erection. This type of erection is preserved in patients with upper spinal cord injury (Courtois et al., 2013; Giuliano and Rampin, 2004).

Nocturnal erection occurs mostly during rapid eye movement (REM) sleep (Karacan et al., 1989). PET scanning of humans in REM sleep shows increased activity in the pontine area, the amygdalae, and the anterior cingulate gyrus but decreased activity in the prefrontal and parietal cortex. The mechanism that triggers REM sleep is located in the pontine reticular formation; the cholinergic neurons in the lateral pontine tegmentum are activated, whereas the adrenergic neurons in the locus ceruleus and the serotoninergic neurons in the midbrain raphe are silent. In a brain stimulation study in rats, the sites for eliciting erection during REM sleep were located in the dorsal and intermediate parts of the lateral septum, whereas the ventral part of the lateral septum was the most effective site for eliciting erections during wakefulness (Gulia et al., 2008).

PET has been used to measure increases in regional cerebral blood flow during ejaculation versus sexual stimulation without orgasm in heterosexual volunteers. Primary brain activation was found in the mesodiencephalic transition zone (including the ventral tegmental area), an area frequently activated with "reward" behaviors and with injection of opioids such as heroin. Other activated mesodiencephalic structures included the midbrain lateral central tegmental field; the zona incerta; the subparafascicular nucleus; and the ventroposterior, midline, and intralaminar thalamic nuclei. Increased activation was also observed in the lateral putamen and adjoining parts of the claustrum. Neocortical activity was found in Brodmann areas 7/40, 18, 21, 23, and 47, exclusively on the right side. Conversely, in the amygdala and adjacent entorhinal cortex, a decrease in activation was noted. Remarkably strong increases in blood flow were observed in the cerebellum (Holstege et al., 2003). These findings corroborate the notion that the cerebellum plays an important role in emotional processing.

Although activation of these various brain areas is of great interest, further studies are necessary to better understand the neurobiology of orgasm, ejaculation, and sexual satisfaction in men and to use the results for treatment (Table 68.6; Tsujimura et al., 2006).

Neurotransmitters

Peripheral Neurotransmitters and Endothelium-Derived Factors Facilitating Penile Erection. NO released from nonadrenergic/noncholinergic (NANC, also known as nitrergic) neurons and from the endothelium is thought to be the principal neurotransmitter mediating penile erection. NO activates guanylate cyclase, which increases the production of cyclic guanosine monophosphate (cGMP), which in turn relaxes the cavernous smooth muscle by a

TABLE 68.6 Brain Centers of Orgasm

	BRAIN AREAS	RELEVANCE
Increased activity: primary area	Mesodiencephalic transition zone (including the ventral tegmental area)	"Reward" center also activated by opioid
Increased activity: secondary areas	Midbrain lateral central tegmental field, the zona incerta, subparafascicular nucleus, ventroposterior, midline, and intralaminar thalamic nuclei Lateral putamen and adjoining parts of the claustrum Brodmann areas 7/40, 18, 21, 23, and 47, exclusively on the right side	
Increased activity: other area	Cerebellum	Emotional processing
Decreased activity	Amygdala and adjacent entorhinal cortex	

number of downstream mechanisms (Andersson, 2011). **NO derived from nNOS in NANC nerves is responsible for initiation of corporal smooth muscle relaxation; NO from eNOS is thought to drive maintenance of smooth muscle relaxation and penile erection** (Hurt et al., 2002).

Aside from its role in releasing NO, a number of endothelium-derived substances have also been linked to corporal smooth muscle relaxation. Examples include carbon monoxide (CO), (Decaluwe et al., 2012) hydrogen sulfide (H_2S), (d'Emmanuele di Villa Bianca et al., 2011), endothelium-derived hyperpolarizing factor (EDHF), prostacyclin (PGI_2), and endothelin (which may induce relaxation via activation of endothelin-B receptors) (Saenz de Tejada et al., 1991).

Acetylcholine is released with electrical field stimulation of human erectile tissue, and cholinergic receptors have been localized to the cavernous tissue and endothelium (Blanco et al., 1988; Traish et al., 1990). Although acetylcholine is not the predominant neurotransmitter mediating penile erection, it may contribute indirectly to penile erection by presynaptic inhibition of adrenergic neurons and stimulation of NO release from endothelial cells (Saenz de Tejada et al., 1989). The effect may be minor as inhibition of cholinergic action by intravenous or intracavernous injection of atropine does not abolish erection induced in animals by electrical neurostimulation (Stief et al., 1989).

Peripheral Neurotransmitters and Endothelium-Derived Factors Opposing Penile Erection. Maintenance of intracorporal smooth muscle in a semi-contracted (flaccid) state likely results from three factors: **intrinsic myogenic activity** (Andersson and Wagner, 1995); **adrenergic neurotransmission; and endothelium-derived contracting factors such as angiotensin II, $PGF_{2\alpha}$, and endothelin-1.** Detumescence after erection results from resumption of these factors as well as cessation of NO release, the breakdown of cyclic guanosine monophosphate (cGMP) by phosphodiesterases (PDEs), and/or sympathetic discharge during ejaculation.

Norepinephrine is generally accepted as the principal neurotransmitter mediating penile flaccidity (Andersson, 2011). Both α_1-adrenergic and α_2-adrenergic fibers and receptors have been demonstrated in the corpora cavernosa and surrounding the cavernous arteries (Prieto, 2008). Research findings support a functional predominance of postjunctional α_1-adrenergic receptors for contraction and of prejunctional α_2-adrenergic receptors for downregulating release of norepinephrine and the vasodilator nitric oxide (NO) (Prieto, 2008). Stimulation of adrenergic receptors by norepinephrine produces contraction in penile vessels and the corpora cavernosa; this process is mediated by Ca^{2+} entry into smooth muscle cells via membrane calcium channels. Cellular calcium sensitization mechanisms also contribute and are mediated by protein kinase C (PKC), tyrosine kinases, and Rho-kinase (Andersson, 2011).

Endothelin-1 is a potent vasoconstrictor and mediator of penile detumescence (Holmquist et al., 1990; Saenz de Tejada et al., 1991). Two receptors for endothelin, endothelin-A and endothelin-B_1, mediate the biologic effects of endothelin in vascular endothelial tissue: endothelin-A receptors mediate contraction, whereas endothelin-B_1 receptors induce relaxation. By action on endothelin-A receptors, endothelin induces slow-developing, long-lasting contractions in the corpora cavernosa and cavernosal arteries. Endothelin also potentiates the constrictor effects of catecholamines on trabecular smooth muscle (Christ et al., 1995). Blockade of the endothelin-A receptor ameliorates impaired penile hemodynamics in animal models of obesity (Sanchez et al., 2014).

Several constrictor prostanoids, including prostaglandin I_2 (PGI_2), prostaglandin $F_{2\alpha}$ ($PGF_{2\alpha}$), and thromboxane A_2 (TXA_2), are synthesized by the human cavernous tissue. Prostanoids induce spontaneous contraction in isolated trabecular muscle (Christ et al., 1990) and inhibit the relaxant effects of NO (Azadzoi et al., 1992; Minhas et al., 2001). The contractile effects of prostanoids in corporal tissue appear to be mediated by thromboxane A_2 (TP) receptors (Angulo et al., 2002).

The renin-angiotensin system (RAS) is a well-known mediator of systemic vascular tone, and RAS sensitive receptors have been identified in penile smooth muscle. The RAS consists of two components: a vasoconstrictor/proliferative arm, in which the main mediator is angiotensin II acting on angiotensin (AT1) receptors, and a vasodilator/antiproliferative arm, in which the major effector is angiotensin-(1-7) acting via the G protein–coupled receptor (GPCR) Mas (Fraga-Silva et al., 2013). The opposing functions of the RAS system suggest that this axis may induce pro- and antierectile effects. Administration of angiotensin II with activation of AT1 receptors is associated with increased activity of RhoA/rho-kinase, increased intracellular calcium, and oxidative stress (Fraga-Silva et al., 2013). Administration of angiotensin II in mouse cavernosal cells has also been linked to increased expression of the toll-like receptor 4 (TLR4), a component of the immune system. Inhibition of TLR4 attenuated the enhancement in adrenergic-induced contraction and preserved NOS activity cavernous relaxation (Nunes et al., 2017). The implication is that immune modulation and inflammation (known to be associated with vascular disease) may play a role in alteration of penile hemodynamics (Stallmann-Jorgensen et al., 2015).

Transforming growth factor-beta (TGF-β) is associated with corporal smooth muscle apoptosis, oxidative stress, and reduced smooth muscle-to-collagen ratio (Li et al., 2013). TGF-β appears to be responsible for some of the impaired hemodynamic parameters observed in rat models of diabetes (Li et al., 2013). These effects may be mediated by the Smad2 protein complex, the downstream effectors of TGF-β. Treatment with TGF-β has also been associated with upregulation of the Rho A/Rho-Kinase pathway (Li et al., 2013), increased expression of plasminogen activator inhibitor-1 (PAI-1), and increased activity of the profibrotic Wnt10 pathway (Shin et al., 2014).

Tyrosine kinases induce contraction in rat small penile arteries (Villalba et al., 2010). In a cavernous nerve injury model of ED in rats, treatment with a tyrosine kinase inhibitor led to preservation of NANC nerve fibers and downregulation of sympathetic tyrosine hydroxylase–containing nerve fibers. Also noted in this study was improved smooth muscle-to-collagen ratio and intracorporal pressure response to cavernous nerve stimulation (Lin et al., 2015). These effects may be related to activation of large conductance potassium channels, an effect observed in human cavernous nerve strips exposed to a tyrosine kinase inhibitor in vitro (Gur et al., 2013).

Interactions Among Nerves and Neurotransmitters. There is marked cross-reactivity between pro- and antitumescence pathways and modulation by health conditions in corporal tissue (Angulo et al., 2001; Brave et al., 1993). Numerous factors have been reported to increase NOS activity and NO release, including molecular oxygen, androgen, long-term administration of L-arginine, and repeated intracavernous injection of PGE$_1$ (Escrig et al., 1999; Kim et al., 1993; Marin et al., 1999). Decreased NOS activity has been associated with castration, denervation, hypercholesterolemia, and diabetes mellitus (Alves-Lopes et al., 2017; Lin et al., 2015; Yang et al., 2013). In some cases this may be related to action of adrenergic neurons known to inhibit NO release by binding prejunctional α_2 receptors. NOS isoforms may also regulate the activity of other isoforms. For example, nNOS activity has been shown to decrease expression of inducible nitric oxide synthase (iNOS) after administration of TGF-β1 into the penis (Bivalacqua et al., 2000). NOS isoforms may also be upregulated to compensate for defects in N-production; in nNOS knockout mice, eNOS levels are higher than in control animals, suggesting a possible compensatory mechanism (Burnett et al., 1996).

cAMP-dependent and cGMP-dependent protein kinases can be activated by either cAMP or cGMP, although cross-activation requires an approximately 10-fold higher concentration of the alternate cyclic nucleotide (Walsh, 1994). Although protein kinase A (PKA) and protein kinase G (PKG) may phosphorylate numerous common substrates, several lines of evidence indicate that the activation of PKG by cGMP and cAMP is the predominant mechanism by which cyclic nucleotides decrease intracellular Ca^{2+} to cause vascular smooth muscle relaxation and corporal vasorelaxation (Jiang et al., 1992; Lincoln et al., 1990).

Molecules That Modulate Penile Erection via the Central Nervous System. Major neuropeptides involved in regulation of erectile response include dopamine, oxytocin, NO, norepinephrine, serotonin (5-hydroxytryptamine [5-HT]), and prolactin. **In general, central dopaminergic and adrenergic receptors promote sexual function, and 5-HT receptors inhibit it** (Foreman and Wernicke, 1990). Androgens also play an important role in modulating central nervous system (CNS) control of sexual response.

Dopamine. There are many dopaminergic systems in the brain with ultrashort, intermediate, and long axons. The cell bodies are located primarily in the ventral tegmentum, substantia nigra, and hypothalamus. Five different dopamine receptors have been cloned (D$_1$ to D$_5$), and several of these exist in multiple forms (Ganong, 1999b). Neuroscientists have discovered that specific dopamine receptors (D$_2$, D$_3$, and D$_4$), nNOS, and oxytocin are co-expressed in the cell bodies of oxytocinergic neurons in the PVN and MPOA (Baskerville et al., 2009; Xiao et al., 2005).

In men, the D$_1$ and D$_2$ receptor agonist apomorphine induces erection that is unaccompanied by sexual arousal (Danjou et al., 1988). In male rats, injection of dopaminergic agonists to the PVN stimulates D$_2$, but not D$_3$ or D$_4$, receptors, and increases Ca^{2+} influx in cell bodies of oxytocinergic neurons. The net effect is increased production of NO, which activates oxytocinergic neurotransmission in extrahypothalamic brain areas and spinal cord, leading to penile erection and yawning. Dopamine may also regulate prolactin secretion by actions on the pituitary gland (Ganong, 1999a). The stimulation of D$_4$ receptors increases Ca^{2+} influx and NO production leading to penile erection but not yawning. Nevertheless, D$_4$ receptors are thought to play only a modest role in the proerectile effects of central dopamine (Melis and Argiolas, 2011).

Oxytocin. Oxytocin is a neural hormone secreted by the neurons into the circulation. Oxytocin is localized primarily to the posterior pituitary gland but may also function as a neurotransmitter in neurons projecting from the PVN to the brainstem and spinal cord (Courtois et al., 2013). Serum oxytocin levels are increased during sexual activity in humans and animals. Oxytocin is a potent inducer of penile erection when injected into the central nervous system (CNS). In rats, the most sensitive brain area for the proerectile effect of oxytocin is the PVN of the hypothalamus. Oxytocin release after stimulation of dopamine receptors in the PVN influences the appetitive and reinforcing effects of sexual activity (Succu et al., 2007). PVN neurons contain NOS; interestingly, NOS inhibitors prevent apomorphine-induced and oxytocin-induced erections, implying that NO is a common downstream pathway for dopamine- and oxytocin-mediated erections (Melis and Argiolas, 2011; Vincent and Kimura, 1992).

Nitric Oxide. The NO/cGMP pathway is a critical mediator of erections in the periphery but also plays important roles in the CNS. NO and its downstream effector soluble guanylyl cyclase is localized throughout the human brain, including at the level of the PVN (Melis et al., 1998). Activity of the NO/cGMP pathways in the brain declines with aging (Ibarra et al., 2001) and experimentally induced diabetes (Zheng et al., 2007). Testosterone supplementation has been shown to enhance apomorphine-induced erections and NOS activity in the MPOA; these effects may be mediated by enhanced expression of dopamine-responsive NOS in the MPOA and by NO-induced enhancement of dopamine release in response to external stimuli (Hull et al., 1999).

Serotonin. Neurons containing 5-HT have their cell bodies in the midline raphe nuclei of the brainstem and project to a portion of the hypothalamus, limbic system, neocortex, and spinal cord (Ganong, 1999a). There are numerous 5-HT receptors in the brain, which are classified by type and subtype (Ganong, 1999b). **The general effect of 5-HT in the CNS is inhibitory toward sexual desire and erectile function** (Foreman et al., 1989). However, there is evidence to support a role for 5-HT in facilitating and opposing sexual response, depending on the receptor subtype, the receptor location, and the species investigated (de Groat and Booth, 1993). For instance, activation of the 5-HT$_{1A}$ and 5-HT$_2$ receptors appears to inhibit erectile activity but facilitate ejaculation. Conversely, activation of 5-HT$_{2C}$ receptors facilitates erection in rats (Kimura et al., 2006; Steers and de Groat, 1989). 5-HT$_{2C}$ receptors are localized to the lumbosacral spine and are thought to be potential downstream effectors of the dopamine-oxytocin and melanocortin pathways (Kimura et al., 2008).

Norepinephrine. The cell bodies of norepinephrine-containing neurons are located in the locus ceruleus and the A5-catecholaminergic cell group in the pons and medulla. The axons of these noradrenergic neurons ascend to innervate the paraventricular, supraoptic, and periventricular nuclei of the hypothalamus, thalamus, and neocortex (Courtois et al., 1999). These fibers also descend into the spinal cord and the cerebellum. In contrast to peripheral effects of norepinephrine, **central norepinephrine transmission seems to have a stimulatory effect on sexual function**. In humans and rats, inhibition of norepinephrine release by clonidine, an α_2-adrenergic agonist, is associated with a decrease in sexual behavior. Conversely, yohimbine, an α_2-receptor antagonist, has been shown to increase sexual activity (Clark et al., 1985).

Melanocortins. Melanocortin-4 receptor (MC4R) is expressed in the human and rat CNS, pelvic ganglia, and nerve fibers of the glans penis. This receptor is involved in the control of food intake and energy expenditure and appears to modulate erectile function and sexual behavior. Evidence supporting this notion is based on mouse studies indicating enhanced copulatory behavior and augmentation of erectile response from electrostimulation in mice given an MC4R agonist (Van der Ploeg et al., 2002).

Prolactin. Hyperprolactinemia is known to suppress sexual function in men and experimental animals (Paick et al., 2006; Rehman et al., 2000). **The purported mechanism of action is through inhibition of dopaminergic activity in the MPOA and decreased serum testosterone. Prolactin may also have a direct contractile effect on cavernous smooth muscle** (Table 68.7; Ra et al., 1996).

γ-Aminobutyric Acid. γ-Aminobutyric acid (GABA) activity in the PVN inhibits proerectile signaling. Systemic administration or intrathecal injection at the lumbosacral level of the GABA$_B$ receptor agonist baclofen decreases erection in rats (Bitran and Hull, 1987). At least some of GABA's antierectile effects seem to be mediated by activation of GABA$_A$ receptors, which reduce erectile response to dopamine agonists and oxytocin (Melis and Argiolas, 2002).

Opioids. Endogenous opioids affect sexual function, although the magnitude varies depending on dose and site of administration. Injection of small amounts of morphine into the MPOA induces sexual behavior in rats. However, larger doses of narcotics inhibit penile erection and yawning induced by stimulation of oxytocinergic or dopaminergic pathways (Argiolas, 1992; Melis et al., 1999). Injection of morphine into the PVN of the hypothalamus prevents

TABLE 68.7 Central Neurotransmitters and Their Function

NEUROTRANSMITTER	RECEPTOR AND FUNCTION
Dopamine	D1 and D4 receptor—enhances erection D2 receptor—enhances seminal emission
Serotonin (5-HT)	5-HT—inhibits sex drive and spinal sexual reflex 5-HT1A—inhibits erection, facilitates ejaculation 5-HT2C—enhances erection
Norepinephrine	Enhances sexual function
γ-Aminobutyric acid	Inhibits erectile signals
Opioids	Inhibit penile erection
Cannabinoids	Inhibit sexual function
Oxytocin	Enhances appetitive and reinforcing effects of sexual activity
Nitric oxide	Mediates erection at paraventricular nucleus
Melanocortins	MCR4—enhances erection
Prolactin	Suppresses sexual function

noncontact penile erections and impairs copulation in rats. It is speculated that intracellular NO may be involved in this process (Melis et al., 1999).

Cannabinoids. Cannabinoid CB₁ receptor activation inhibits sexual function by modulating paraventricular oxytocinergic neurons, which mediate erection. Antagonism of CB₁ receptors in the PVN of male rats induces penile erection via the downstream effectors glutamic acid and NO (Melis et al., 2004, 2006).

KEY POINTS: PHYSIOLOGY OF PENILE ERECTION

- Neuronal integrity at the brain, spinal cord, and peripheral level is essential to modulation of penile erections.
- A wide range of neurotransmitters are involved in modulating sexual arousal and penile erection; key examples include dopamine, serotonin, oxytocin, nitric oxide, and norepinephrine.
- Integration of erotic stimuli in the central nervous system is complex; MRI and PET scanning have provided new insight on central mechanisms of sexual arousal in men.

Smooth Muscle Physiology

Cytosolic Calcium and the Calcium Sensitization Pathway

The smooth muscle of the corpora cavernosa are contracted in their normal state. Myosin isoforms in smooth muscle of the corpus cavernosum contain phasic and tonic characteristics (DiSanto et al., 1998). Contractions of the corpus cavernosum smooth muscle may be spontaneous or induced (Yarnitsky et al., 1995). Spontaneous phasic contractions of corpus cavernosum smooth muscle appear to be dependent on an endogenous pacemaker driven by a cytosolic Ca^{2+} oscillator that releases Ca^{2+} from the sarcoplasmic reticulum periodically (Berridge, 2008; Cellek et al., 2002). This cytosolic oscillator can be modulated by neurotransmitters and hormones and may play a role in maintaining corporal smooth muscle function.

Smooth muscle contraction is controlled by two major factors: cytosolic calcium concentration and Rho-kinase signaling (Berridge, 2008). Smooth muscle contraction can occur with or without change in membrane potential (Berridge, 2008; Somlyo and Somlyo, 2000).
Cytosolic Free Calcium. Smooth muscle contraction is regulated by intracellular free calcium (Ca^{2+}) acting through calmodulin. Calcium-bound calmodulin undergoes a conformational change, increasing its affinity for myosin light chain (MLC) kinase. MLC kinase is activated by binding of the calcium-calmodulin complex, leading to phosphorylation of the serine-19 residue of regulatory MLC$_{20}$. In the presence of adenosine triphosphate (ATP), this phosphorylation enables actin to activate the myosin ATPase and initiates cross-bridge cycling. Hydrolysis of ATP by ATPase supplies the energy for the contractile process (Fig. 68.9; Walsh, 1991).

Smooth muscle relaxation requires cessation of MLC kinase activity, which is induced by a decrease of free Ca^{2+} in the sarcoplasm. With decreased intracellular Ca^{2+}, calmodulin dissociates from MLC kinase, inactivating it (Fig. 68.10; Walsh, 1991). MLC$_{20}$ is dephosphorylated (inactivated) by myosin light chain phosphatase (MLCP). MLCP is a holoenzyme consisting of a type 1 phosphatase (PP1c), a myosin-targeting subunit (MYPT1), and a 20-kD subunit of unknown function (Hersch et al., 2004; Ito et al., 2004).
Rho Kinase Signaling Pathway. MLCP inhibition leads to enhanced smooth muscle contraction by preventing inactivation of MLC$_{20}$. The activity of MLCP can be modulated by Rho/Rho-kinase, an important constituent of the *calcium sensitization pathway* that is expressed in penile smooth muscle (Fig. 68.11; Sopko et al., 2014). Agonist activation causes dissociation of RhoA from Rho-guanine dissociation inhibitor; this process leads to activation of Rho-kinase. Rho-kinase phosphorylates the regulatory subunit of MLCP, inhibiting phosphatase activity and enhancing smooth muscle contraction (Hirano, 2007). Tonic contraction of the corporal smooth muscle is thought to be governed primarily by the calcium-sensitizing pathway (Cellek et al., 2002). Tonic contraction of the corporal smooth muscle is also reliant on dephosphorylated myosin remaining bound to actin in the high-affinity state. Calponin may also play a role by simultaneously binding actin and myosin to stabilize cross-bridge interactions and slow the rate of detachment (Szymanski, 2004). These efficiencies have been termed the **latch** state and are critical for sustaining the basal tone of smooth muscle. Evidence from a rat model of cavernous nerve injury also suggests that Rho-kinase activation may contribute to activation of enzymes that drive the transformation of fibroblasts to myofibroblasts, which may contribute to fibrotic changes in tissues (Song et al., 2015).

Molecular Pathways That Directly Modulate Intracellular Free Calcium

Vasoconstrictor agonists such as norepinephrine (α$_1$-adrenergic receptors), endothelin-1 (endothelin-A receptors), angiotensin II (AT1 receptors), prostaglandin F$_{2α}$ (FP receptors), and TXA$_2$ (TP receptors) bind their respective receptors to activate Gq, which stimulates phospholipase C beta. This membrane-bound enzyme hydrolyzes phosphatidylinositol 4,5-bisphosphate to liberate IP$_3$ and 1,2-diacylglycerol. IP$_3$ binds to specific receptors (IP$_3$ receptor) on the smooth endoplasmic reticulum to stimulate the release of Ca^{2+} from intracellular stores. Binding of IP$_3$ to these receptors not only activates Ca^{2+} release but also increases the sensitivity of the IP$_3$ receptor to Ca^{2+} and assists **calcium-induced calcium release**. Increased intracellular Ca^{2+} may also be accomplished by entry of extracellular Ca^{2+} through **receptor-operated channels** without a change in membrane potential (Large, 2002). Norepinephrine, endothelin, vasopressin, and angiotensin II activate Ca^{2+}-permeable, nonselective cation channels, which increase intracellular calcium levels.

Molecular Pathways That Indirectly Modulate Intracellular Free Calcium

Cyclic adenosine monophosphate (cAMP) and cGMP are second messenger molecules involved in smooth muscle relaxation. cAMP-dependent and cGMP-dependent protein kinases phosphorylate proteins and ion channels, the net result of which include

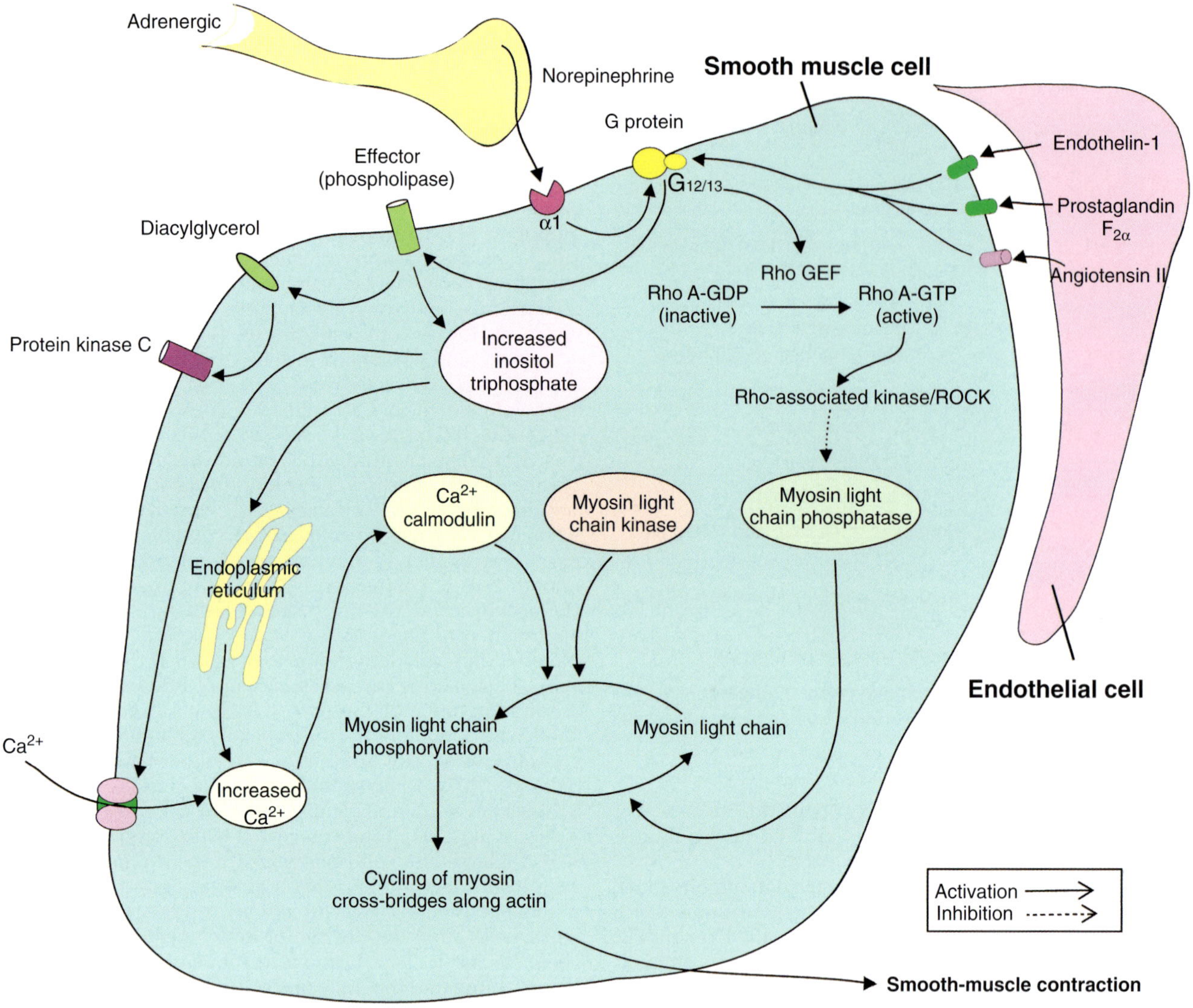

Fig. 68.9. Molecular mechanism of penile smooth muscle contraction. Norepinephrine from sympathetic nerve endings and endothelins, angiotensin II, and prostaglandin F$_{2\alpha}$ from the endothelium activate receptors on smooth muscle cells to initiate the cascade of reactions that eventually result in elevation of intracellular calcium concentrations, activation of Rho-kinase, and smooth muscle contraction. Protein kinase C is a regulatory component of the Ca^{2+}-independent, sustained phase of agonist-induced contractile responses. *GDP*, Guanosine diphosphate; *GEF*, guanine nucleotide exchange factor; *GTP*, guanosine triphosphate.

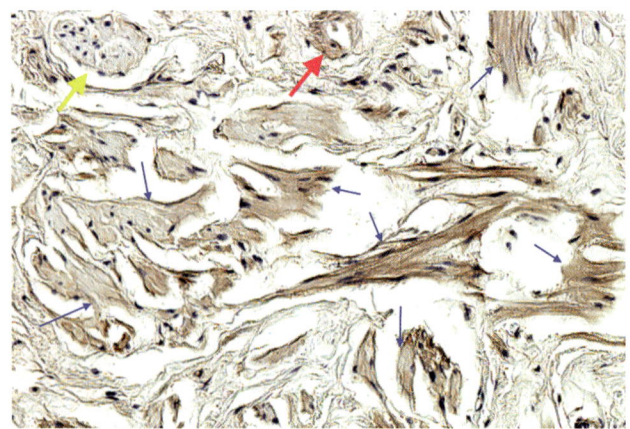

Fig. 68.10. Immunohistochemistry of human penile tissue, showing positive phosphodiesterase type 5 staining of cavernous smooth muscle fibers (*small blue arrows*), nerve (*yellow arrow*), and blood vessel wall (*red arrow*) (×100).

(1) opening of potassium channels and membrane hyperpolarization; (2) sequestration of intracellular calcium by the endoplasmic reticulum; and (3) inhibition of voltage-dependent calcium channels, blocking calcium influx. **The net result is a decrease in cytosolic-free calcium and subsequent smooth muscle relaxation** (Lin et al., 2005).

Modulation of Antitumescence Pathways By Protumescence Pathways

The NO–cGMP–PKG-I pathway suppresses antitumescence pathways by modulating several components of the noradrenergic contractile system; the net impact of these processes is impairment of inositol 1,4,5-triphosphate (IP3) production by phospholipase C (Hirata et al., 1990), IP3 receptor activity (Schlossmann et al., 2000), the RhoA/Rho-kinase pathway (Sauzeau et al., 2000), and the vasoconstrictive activity of endothelin (Mills et al., 2001). Acetylcholine and prostaglandin E1 (PGE$_1$) can also inhibit norepinephrine release, the former by binding to presynaptic receptors on adrenergic neurons (Molderings et al., 1992; Saenz de Tejada et al., 1989).

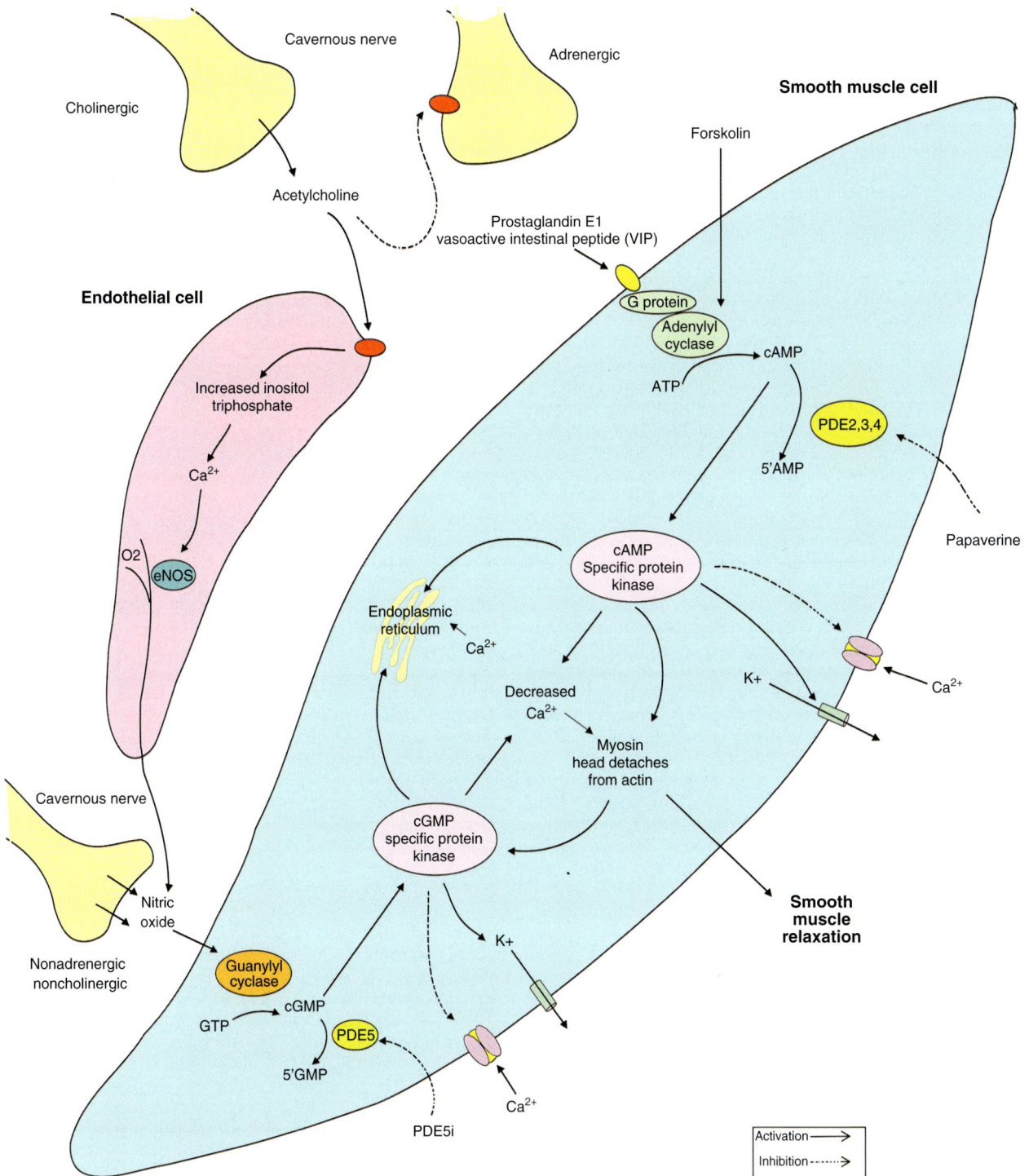

Fig. 68.11. Molecular mechanism of penile smooth muscle relaxation. The intracellular second messengers mediating smooth muscle relaxation, cyclic adenosine monophosphate (cAMP) and cyclic guanosine monophosphate (cGMP), activate their specific protein kinases, which phosphorylate certain proteins to cause opening of potassium channels, closing of calcium channels, and sequestration of intracellular calcium by the endoplasmic reticulum. The resultant decrease in intracellular calcium leads to smooth muscle relaxation. Sildenafil inhibits the action of phosphodiesterase (PDE) type 5 and increases the intracellular concentration of cGMP. Papaverine is a nonspecific phosphodiesterase inhibitor. *ATP*, Adenosine triphosphate; *eNOS*, endothelial nitric oxide synthase; *GTP*, guanosine triphosphate.

Cyclic Guanosine Monophosphate–Signaling Pathway

Nitric Oxide. NO is the best characterized activator of the cGMP pathway. Because of its small size, NO can diffuse inside its target cell, where it interacts with molecules that contain iron in either a heme or an iron-sulfur complex. The most physiologically relevant receptor for NO is soluble guanylate cyclase (sGC), which contains a heme moiety that appears essential for NO-induced vasorelaxation in corporal tissues (Decaluwe et al., 2017). The NO-sGC-cGMP pathway is responsible for the vasorelaxation effect of many endothelium-dependent vasodilators, including histamine, estrogens, insulin, corticotropin-releasing hormone, nitrovasodilators, and acetylcholine (Burnett and Musicki, 2005). **Because of these numerous effects**

NO is believed to be the molecule principally responsible for initiating physiologic penile erection.

Synthesis of NO is catalyzed by NOS, which converts L-arginine and oxygen to L-citrulline and NO. NOS exists as three isoforms in mammals: nNOS and eNOS are preferentially expressed in neurons/nerves and endothelial cells, respectively. iNOS is expressed in almost all cell types. All three NOS isoforms have been identified in the corpus cavernosum, with nNOS and eNOS being considered responsible for initiating and sustaining erection, respectively (Hurt et al., 2002; Musicki et al., 2009). A variant of nNOS (penile nNOS) has been identified as two distinct isoforms in the penis of rats and mice (Magee et al., 1996).

nNOS and eNOS have critical roles in penile erection. The activity and bioavailability of eNOS are regulated by multiple mechanisms, including eNOS phosphorylation, eNOS interaction with regulatory proteins and contractile pathways, and actions of reactive oxygen species. Downregulation of NOS is associated with ED and is identified in the corpus cavernosum of animal models of aging, hypogonadism, and diabetes (Carrier et al., 1997; Penson et al., 1996; Rehman et al., 1997). In human studies single nucleotide polymorphisms of the nNOS (Lacchini et al., 2014) and eNOS genes (Liu et al., 2015) and specific microRNA expression patterns (GamalEl Din et al., 2017) have been associated with greater risk of impaired erectile function and/or differential response to erectogenic medications. An association between microRNA expression and impairment of erectile function in hyperlipidemic (Barbery et al., 2015) and aged rats (Pan et al., 2015, 2016) has also been reported. Interestingly, mice with congenital knockout of nNOS or eNOS often have normal erectile function (Burnett et al., 1996). Compensatory mechanisms, alternative splicing of the disrupted gene (Ferrini et al., 2003), and/or other unknown mechanisms may be involved in the preservation of erectile function in NOS-knockout mice. The NO/cGMP pathway is also known to modulate other relevant pathways in penile erection, including the RhoA/Rho-kinase pathway (Bivalacqua et al., 2007; Chitaley et al., 2001; Priviero et al., 2010).

Carbon Monoxide. CO is a gaseous second messenger that occurs in biologic systems during the oxidative catabolism of heme by the heme oxygenase (HO) enzyme (Wu and Wang, 2005). HO exists in constitutive (HO-2, HO-3) and inducible (HO-1) isoforms and is found in endothelial corporal tissue (Hedlund et al., 2000). CO regulates vascular processes, such as vessel tone, smooth muscle proliferation, and platelet aggregation, and may function as a neurotransmitter (Yetik-Anacak et al., 2015). It is thought to play a potentially important role in penile erection (Abdel Aziz et al., 2009). The neurotransmitter effect of CO may work in part by activation of guanylate cyclase by direct binding to the heme moiety of the enzyme, stimulating the production of cGMP. However, there is also evidence that CO-induced relaxation of corporal tissues may act by non-guanylate cyclase dependent mechanisms (Decaluwe et al., 2012).

Hydrogen Sulfide. H_2S is a gaseous second messenger produced in vascular tissues by breakdown of L-cysteine by the enzyme cystathionine γ-lyase (Zhao and Wang, 2002). Exogenous H_2S or L-cysteine causes relaxation of strips of corpus cavernosum, an effect that is modulated at least in part by membrane potassium channels and appears to work by NOS-dependent and independent pathways (Abd Elmoneim et al., 2017; Meng et al., 2013; Yetik-Anacak et al., 2015). There are species-level differences in precise pathways involved with H_2S-mediated effects (Abd Elmoneim et al., 2017; Meng et al., 2013; Yetik-Anacak et al., 2015). Intracavernosal administration of either H_2S, sodium hydrosulfide (NaHS), or L-cysteine elicits penile erection in rats (d'Emmanuele di Villa Bianca et al., 2011). These observations indicate that a functional L-cysteine/H_2S pathway may be involved in mediating penile erection in men and some mammals, although there appear to be species-level differences in effect.

Natriuretic Peptides. The natriuretic peptide family is involved in the regulation of cardiovascular homeostasis and consists of atrial (ANP), brain (BNP), and C-type (CNP) natriuretic peptides (Matsuo, 2001). ANP and BNP are ligands for the natriuretic peptide receptor NPR-A, whereas CNP is a ligand for the natriuretic peptide receptor NPR-B. Both receptors are members of the guanylyl cyclase family and are called GC-A and GC-B.

CNP increases cGMP and cAMP production in isolated human corporal cells (Rahardjo et al., 2016). CNP appears to be the most potent natriuretic peptide. Whether CNP and NPR-B play a role in physiologic erection has not been determined (Kim et al., 1998; Kuthe et al., 2003; Matsuo, 2001; Sousa et al., 2010).

Guanylyl Cyclase Pathway. In mammals, seven membrane-bound (particulate) guanylyl cyclase isoforms (GC-A to GC-G) and one soluble isoform (sGC) have been identified (Andreopoulos and Papapetropoulos, 2000). Although the membrane-bound guanylyl cyclase system is not known to play a role in physiologic erection, expression of GC-B in human and rat corpus cavernosum and induction of cavernous smooth muscle relaxation by CNP (ligand for GC-B) have been demonstrated (Guidone et al., 2002; Kuthe et al., 2003).

The soluble isoform sGC plays a pivotal role in erectile function because it provides the link between NO and cGMP, the principle extracellular and intracellular signaling molecules, respectively, in physiologic erection (Andersson, 2011). A heterodimeric protein, sGC, consists of α and β subunits, each of which exists in two isoforms ($α_1$, $α_2$, and $β_1$, $β_2$) that are encoded by two separate genes (Andreopoulos and Papapetropoulos, 2000).

Protein Kinase G. PKG, also called cGMP-dependent kinase, is the principal receptor and mediator for cGMP signaling. In mammals, PKG exists in two major forms, PKG-I and PKG-II, which are encoded by two separate genes. In smooth muscle, only PKG-I is expressed and exists as two splice variants (PKG-Iα and PKG-Iβ). **cGMP and/or PKG-I induce smooth muscle relaxation via activation of the plasma membrane Ca^{2+}-ATPase pump, inhibition of IP_3 generation, inhibition of Rho-kinase, stimulation of MLCP, and phosphorylation of heat shock proteins** (Francis et al., 2010). Cavernous smooth muscle strips from PKG-I knockout mice cannot be relaxed by agents that raise cGMP levels, and these mice have a low ability to reproduce, presumably because of ED (Hedlund et al., 2000).

Adenylyl Cyclase Pathway. Signaling molecules in the cAMP pathway bind to and activate specific cytoplasmic membrane receptors that, through their coupled G proteins, activate adenylyl cyclases (Dessauer et al., 2017). Although individual membrane-bound adenylyl cyclases are regulated differently, they all are stimulated by the GTP-bound form of the G_a subunit, and all (except AC9) are stimulated by forskolin in the normal state (Sullivan et al., 1998).

Protein Kinase A. Protein kinase A (PKA), also called cAMP-dependent kinase, is the principal receptor for cAMP, and it mediates most of the cellular effects of cAMP by phosphorylating a wide variety of downstream targets in the cytoplasmic and nuclear compartments (Johnson et al., 2001). In the penis and pelvic ganglion one of these targets is nNOS, which is phosphorylated at serine 1412 by activated PKA (Hurt et al., 2012). PKA is composed of two regulatory (R) and two catalytic (C) subunits that form a tetrameric holoenzyme R_2C_2. Binding of cAMP to the R subunits causes the holoenzyme to dissociate into an $R_2(cAMP)_4$ dimer and two free catalytically active C subunits. The presence of multiple C subunit genes further adds to the diversity and complexity of the various holoenzyme complexes, which differ in biochemical and functional properties as well as patterns of expression and localization. These differences among the isozymes contribute to the broad specificity of PKA in a wide variety of physiologic processes in response to cAMP signaling.

More than 100 different cellular proteins have been identified as physiologic substrates of PKA, with more than 90% (135 of 145) being phosphorylated at serine and the remainder at threonine (Shabb, 2001). The predominant target sequence (>50%) is Arg-Arg-X-Ser, in which Ser is the phosphate acceptor. Three PKA substrate proteins have been identified in penile tissue: phosphodiesterases, cAMP-responsive element-binding protein, and ATP-sensitive potassium (K_{ATP}) channel.

Phosphodiesterase. In each episode of cyclic nucleotide signaling, the increase of intracellular cAMP or cGMP concentration is typically twofold to threefold baseline. Decline occurs rapidly and often during the continued presence of the signaling hormone (Francis et al., 2001). Degradation of cyclic nucleotide signals occurs principally by action of phosphodiesterases (PDE), which catalyze the hydrolysis of cAMP and cGMP to AMP and GMP, respectively. Feedback mechanisms that increase PDE activity and/or expression by the increased cyclic nucleotide level assist cyclic nucleotide degradation (Corbin et al., 2000; Lin et al., 2001a, 2001b).

The superfamily of mammalian PDEs consists of 11 families (PDE1 to PDE11) that are encoded from 21 distinct genes (Lin et al., 2003; Montorsi et al., 2004). Each PDE gene usually encodes more than one isoform; the specific isoform may be determined via alternative splicing or from alternative gene promoters. PDE1, PDE3, PDE4, PDE7, and PDE8 are multigene families, whereas PDE2, PDE5, PDE9, PDE10, and PDE11 are single-gene families. PDE1, PDE2, PDE3, PDE10, and PDE11 hydrolyze cAMP and cGMP; PDE4, PDE7, and PDE8 hydrolyze only cAMP; and PDE5, PDE6, and PDE9 hydrolyze only cGMP.

With the exception of PDE6, which is specifically expressed in photoreceptor cells, all PDEs have been identified in the corpus cavernosum (Kuthe et al., 2001). **PDE5 is the principal PDE for the termination of cavernous cGMP signaling** (Jeremy et al., 1997; Kuthe et al., 2001). Increased expression of PDE5 is noted in serum-starved cultured corporal cells (Carosa et al., 2014) and in mice fed a high-fat diet (Ellati et al., 2013); enhancement of PDE5 activity diminishes erectile response. Inhibition of the cGMP-catalytic activity by PDE5 inhibitors is highly effective in treating ED (Goldstein et al., 1998). Inhibition of PDE5 may also increase cellular levels of cAMP (Stief et al., 2000). This activity is thought to be due to competitive inhibition of PDE3 by cGMP binding, which reduces the ability of PDE3 to break down cAMP (Francis et al., 2001). **Direct inhibition of PDE3 also promotes penile erection** (Kuthe et al., 2002).

Caveolae. Caveolae are invaginated microdomains of plasma membrane that are rich in eNOS and caveolins as well as cholesterol, sphingolipids, and glycosylphosphatidylinositol-linked proteins. Caveolae contain numerous other signaling proteins, such as receptors with seven-transmembrane domains, G proteins, adenylyl cyclase, phospholipase C, protein kinase C, calcium pumps, and calcium channels. Decreased caveolin-1 expression has been reported in the cavernous smooth muscle of aged rats (Bakircioglu et al., 2001). In rodent studies, penile erection appears to require association of sGC in corpus cavernosum with endothelial caveolin-1 (Linder et al., 2006; Shakirova et al., 2009). Decreased caveolin-1 expression has been noted in the corpora of rats after bilateral cavernous nerve injury and in experimentally induced diabetes in mice (Parikh et al., 2017), suggesting that loss of caveolin may contribute to common causes for ED. However, in a rat model of diabetes induced by fructose and streptozotocin, decreased erectile responses were associated with an increase in caveolin-1 expression and decreased eNOS activity (Elcioglu et al., 2010). Caveolae and caveolin are clearly involved in the regulation of erectile function, although the relationship appears complex and may vary based on species and ED cause.

Ion Channels. **Hyperpolarization of smooth muscle cells is associated with smooth muscle relaxation, a process mediated in part by membrane ion channels.** In general, there are four major types of ion channels: (1) external ligand-gated, which open to a specific extracellular molecule (e.g., acetylcholine); (2) internal ligand-gated, which open or close in response to an intracellular molecule (e.g., ATP); (3) voltage-gated, which open in response to a change in membrane potential (e.g., sodium, potassium, and calcium channels); and (4) mechanically gated, which open in response to mechanical pressure (Christ et al., 1993).

Calcium channels play a key role in regulation of corporal smooth muscle. Smooth muscle has neither a T-tubule system nor a well-developed sarcoplasmic reticulum. Extracellular calcium is the primary source of calcium in smooth muscle cells and must cross the plasma membrane via ion channels during an action potential. Three transmembrane proteins are known to specifically regulated calcium inflow and outflow: calcium channels are the major inflow regulators, whereas the calcium-sodium exchanger and calcium-ATPase regulate calcium exit from muscle cells (Christ et al., 1993; Large, 2002).

Calcium permeable channels are known to play an important role in corporal smooth muscle physiology. Although ion channel activity is critical to calcium metabolism in smooth muscle cells, mobilization of intracellular calcium stores also plays a role in induced smooth muscle contraction (Christ et al., 1993).

There are at least four types of potassium channel subtypes in the cavernous smooth muscle: (1) Ca^{2+}-activated K+ channels (e.g., K_{Ca}); (2) ATP-sensitive K+ channels (K_{ATP}); (3) delayed rectifier; and (4) fast transient A current (Christ, 2000; Christ et al., 1993). Activation (opening) of K+ channels leads to movement of positively charged K+ out of the cell, causing hyperpolarization and relaxation of smooth muscle (Andersson, 2011). Hyperpolarization may facilitate smooth muscle relaxation even in the setting of blockade of NO and prostaglandin synthesis (Angulo et al., 2003).

Activation of K_{Ca} channels enhances relaxant response to PDE5I in human diabetic corporal tissue through endothelial mechanisms (Gonzalez-Corrochano et al., 2013). K+ channels appear to be activated by endogenous PKA, PKG, or cGMP. Pharmacologic activation of K_{ATP} channels and large-conductance K_{Ca} channels (i.e., Maxi-K) has been shown to relax corporal smooth muscle in humans (Spektor et al., 2002; Vick et al., 2002). Acetylcholine induces endothelium dependent and independent relaxation of penile arteries, an action that is blocked by inhibition of large conductance K channels. Direct activation of small, medium, and large conductance K channels also produces penile arterial vasodilation (Comerma-Steffensen et al., 2017; Kiraly et al., 2013; Sung et al., 2017); these effects appear to be mediated in part by NO activity but may also have an endothelium independent mechanism of action (Sung et al., 2015).

Calcium-activated chloride channels on the smooth muscle cells of corpus cavernosum are thought to be involved in the maintenance of spontaneous tone and the contractile response to adrenaline and other agonists (Hannigan et al., 2017). The activity of these channels is enhanced in cavernosal tissue from a rabbit model of diabetes-related ED (Lau and Adaikan, 2014).

Additional Cyclic Adenosine Monophosphate–Signaling Pathways

Adenosine. Adenosine is released from various cells as a result of increased metabolic rates and its actions on the vasculature are most prominent when oxygen demand is high (Tabrizchi and Bedi, 2001). The vascular response to adenosine can be either relaxation or constriction, depending on which type of adenosine receptor is activated. Activation of A1 adenosine receptors (coupled to G_i and G_o proteins) and A3 adenosine receptors (coupled to G_i and G_q proteins) results in inhibition of adenylyl cyclase and activation of phospholipase C, both of which lead to vasoconstriction. A2 adenosine receptors are coupled to G_s proteins, and their activation stimulates adenylyl cyclase and subsequent vasorelaxation. The differential distribution of these adenosine receptor subtypes largely determines whether a particular vessel relaxes or contracts as a result of adenosine stimulation (Tabrizchi and Bedi, 2001). Whether adenosine plays a role in physiologic erection is unclear. However, excessive adenosine accumulation in the penis, coupled with increased A_{2B} receptor signaling, contributes to spontaneously prolonged penile erection in adenosine deaminase–deficient mice and sickle cell disease transgenic mice, a well-accepted animal model for priapism (Bivalacqua et al., 2009; Dai et al., 2009) Adenosine receptor deficient mice have reduced erectile response to cavernous nerve stimulation, possibly related to an attenuated reduction in phosphorylated (i.e., activated) myosin light chain during electrostimulation. These animals also manifested higher serum levels of norepinephrine (Ning et al., 2012).

Calcitonin Gene–Related Peptide Family. Calcitonin gene-related peptide (CGRP), amylin, and adrenomedullin are members of the CGRP family. These short-chain peptides are potent vasodilators released from perivascular nerve fibers. They act through the calcitonin receptor–like receptor, which belongs to the G protein-coupled receptor (GPCR) superfamily (Conner et al., 2002).

In rats, CGRP levels in the penis, bladder, kidney, testis, and adrenal gland increase gradually up to maturity and then rapidly decline (Wimalawansa, 1992). Administration of CGRP has been associated with enhanced erectile responses in rats with increased age (Bivalacqua et al., 2001) or diabetes (El-Kamshoushi et al., 2013); the mechanism of erection is thought to involve an increase in corporal cAMP.

Prostaglandins. Prostaglandins are a family of eicosanoids capable of initiating numerous biologic functions. The prime mode of prostaglandin action is through specific prostaglandin receptors that all belong to the GPCR family. There are at least nine known prostaglandin receptor subtypes in mice and humans and several additional splice variants with divergent carboxyl termini (Narumiya and Fitzgerald, 2001). There is variability with respect to ligand specificity and activity between different prostaglandin receptors. "Relaxant" receptors IP, DP1, EP2, and EP4 are coupled to an α_s-containing G protein and are capable of stimulating adenylyl cyclase to increase intracellular cAMP. "Contractile" receptors EP1, FP, and TP are coupled to an α_q-containing G protein, which activates phospholipase C instead of adenylyl cyclase. These contractile receptors do not signal through the cAMP pathway, and their signaling outcome is an increase of intracellular calcium. The EP3 receptor is also a contractile receptor, but it is coupled to an α_i-containing G protein that inhibits adenylyl cyclase to result in a decrease of cAMP formation.

Animal and human corpora cavernosa produce several prostaglandins, including $PGF_{2\alpha}$, PGE_2, PGD_2, PGI_2, and TXA_2 (Moreland et al., 2001). In studies in isolated human penile tissue, different PGs elicit different effects in human corpus cavernosum, corpus spongiosum, and cavernous artery (Hedlund and Andersson, 1985). $PGF_{2\alpha}$, PGI_2, and TXA_2 contract corporal tissue. Conversely, PGE_1 and PGE_2 (but not PGI_2) relax corporal tissue pre-contracted with noradrenaline or $PGF_{2\alpha}$. Although PGI_2 is the predominant vasorelaxant in blood vessels, its action in the erectile tissue is either contractile or neutral. Differences in the action of PGI_2 between blood vessels and the corporal tissue and the variable response to specific prostaglandins in corporal tissue are most likely due to differences in the distribution of prostaglandin receptors (Angulo et al., 2002).

Although the production of prostaglandins and the expression of prostaglandin receptors in the erectile tissue have been clearly demonstrated, their roles in physiologic erection are still undefined. However, **the erectogenic effect of PGE_1 as a pharmaceutical agent for ED has been extensively documented** (Stackl et al., 1988).

Vasoactive Intestinal Peptide. The penis is richly supplied with nerves containing vasoactive intestinal peptide (VIP) and VIP-related peptides such as pituitary adenylate cyclase–activating polypeptide. Most of these nerves also contain immunoreactivity to NOS (Andersson, 2001). Two subtypes of VIP receptors, VPAC1 and VPAC2, belonging to the GPCR family have been cloned from human and rat tissues. VPAC2, but not VPAC1, messenger RNA has been identified in cultured rat cavernous smooth muscle cells (Guidone et al., 2002). In dogs, intracavernous VIP injection induces penile erection (Juenemann et al., 1987). However, in human men the erectile response to VIP as a monotherapy is not robust (Kiely et al., 1989), and VIP release is not essential for neurogenic relaxation of human cavernous smooth muscle (Pickard et al., 1993). The physiologic role of VIP in human penile erection appears minimal (Rahardjo et al., 2016).

Molecular Oxygen as a Modulator of Penile Erection. The PO_2 level of cavernous blood in the flaccid state is similar to that of venous blood (≈35 mm Hg). During erection, influx of arterial blood increases PO_2 to approximately 90 mm Hg (Sattar et al., 1995). Molecular oxygen is a substrate, together with L-arginine, for the synthesis of NO by NOS. In the flaccid state, the low oxygen concentration inhibits NO synthesis; during erection, the higher level of substrate induces NO synthesis. It is estimated that the minimum concentration of oxygen in the cavernous bodies necessary to reach full NOS activity is 50 to 60 mm Hg (Kim et al., 1993).

Similarly, prostaglandin H synthase is also an oxygenase (cyclooxygenase) and uses oxygen as substrate for the synthesis of prostanoids (Lands, 1979; Minhas et al., 2001); low oxygen tension tends to suppress and high oxygen tension tends to facilitate prostaglandin production. Endothelin synthesis is promoted in the setting of low oxygen tension and inhibited when oxygen tension is high (e.g., during erection) (Mills et al., 2001).

Intercellular Communication. Synchronized relaxation and contraction of the corporal smooth muscle requires intercellular communication (Christ et al., 1991). **Gap junctions in the membranes of adjacent smooth muscle cells permit intercellular exchange of ions such as calcium and second-messenger molecules** (Christ et al., 1993). The major component of gap junctions is connexin-43, a membrane-sparing protein of less than 0.25 μm present between smooth muscle cells of human corpus cavernosum (Campos de Carvalho et al., 1993). Cell-to-cell communication through these gap junctions is the most likely explanation for the synchronized responses of corporal smooth muscle to relaxant and contractile stimuli.

Intracavernous Tissue Architecture and Erectile Response

The trabeculae of the corpora cavernosa provide the structural support and regulatory mechanism for the endothelial-lined sinusoidal spaces as well as the conduit for blood vessels and nerves. Relaxation of the trabeculae allows the expansion and filling of the sinusoids by the incoming blood, whereas recoil of the trabeculae expels blood to the emissary veins and returns the penis to a flaccid state. Decreased smooth muscle and elastin content has been associated with impairment of erectile response (Costa et al., 2006).

The complex architecture of the penis is maintained by the dynamic expression and interaction of numerous trophic factors. Sonic hedgehog (SHH) plays a key role in regulating vertebrate organogenesis, cell division, and development of some cancers. **SHH has been identified in the penis; inhibition of SHH in adult rats leads to rapid atrophy and disorganization of the corpus cavernosum** (Podlasek et al., 2003, 2005). In addition, SHH stimulates the expression of vascular endothelial growth factor (VEGF), NOS, and brain-derived neurotrophic factor (BDNF) in the penis (Bond, et al., 2013; Podlasek et al., 2005). Administration of SHH has been linked to improved erectile responses and tissue histology parameters in a number of animal studies (Table 68.8; Choe et al., 2016, 2017).

> **KEY POINTS: SMOOTH MUSCLE PHYSIOLOGY**
> - Relaxation of the cavernous smooth muscle is key to penile erection.
> - NO released by nNOS contained in the terminals of the cavernous nerve initiates the erection process; NO released from eNOS in the endothelium helps maintain erection.
> - NO stimulates the production of cGMP by action on guanylate cyclase.
> - cGMP activates PKG, which opens potassium channels and closes calcium channels.
> - Low cytosolic calcium favors smooth muscle relaxation.
> - Smooth muscle contraction is restored when cGMP is degraded by PDE and intracellular calcium levels return to baseline levels.

PATHOPHYSIOLOGY OF ERECTILE DYSFUNCTION

Just a Water Spout
My nookie days are over, My pilot light is out.
What used to be my sex appeal, Is now my water spout.
Time was when, on its own accord, From my trousers it would spring.
But now I've got a full time job, To find the gosh darn thing.
It used to be embarrassing, The way it would behave.
For every single morning, It would stand and watch me shave.
Now as old age approaches, It sure gives me the blues.
To see it hang its little head, And watch me tie my shoes!!

(Randolph, 1992)

ED is defined as "inability to attain and/or maintain an erection sufficient for satisfactory sexual intercourse" (Montorsi et al., 2010). The term "ED" replaces the antiquated and pejorative term "impotence."

Incidence and Epidemiology

The prevalence of ED increases with advancing age; this relationship was first reported by Kinsey et al. (1948), who reported that ED was present in 2% of men at age 40 but 25% of men by age 65. Contemporary studies using more rigorous definitions have confirmed this relationship between age and ED (Laumann et al.,

TABLE 68.8 Key Molecules Involved in Physiologic Regulation of Cavernous Smooth Muscle

NAME	FUNCTION
CONTRACTION	
High cytosolic calcium	Binds calmodulin to activate MLC kinase
MLC kinase	Converts MLC to active form, MLCP
Phosphorylated MLC (MLCP)	Cycling of myosin cross-bridges along actin results in muscle contraction (vasoconstriction)
MLCP	Dephosphorylates MLCP to inactive form, MLC, reversing vasoconstriction
Rho-kinase (calcium sensitization pathway)	Inhibits MLC phosphatase to maintain muscle contraction and vasoconstriction
RELAXATION	
Nitric oxide	Binds soluble guanylyl cyclase to produce cGMP
cGMP	Activates protein kinase G
Protein kinase G	Opens potassium channels and closes calcium channels
Low cytosolic calcium	Calcium dissociates from calmodulin, muscle relaxation (vasodilation)

cGMP, Cyclic guanosine monophosphate; *MLC*, myosin light chain; *MLCP*, myosin light chain phosphatase.

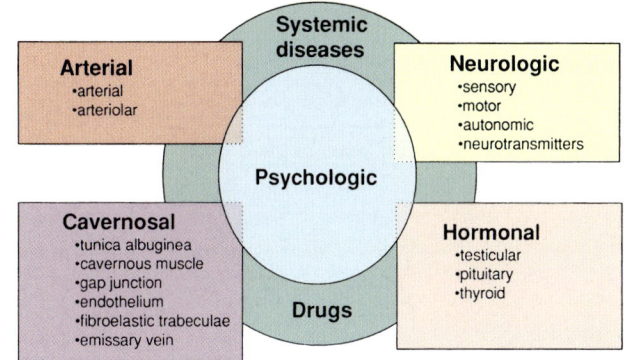

Fig. 68.12. Functional classification of erectile dysfunction. It is unlikely for erectile dysfunction in an individual patient to derive solely from one source. Most cases have a psychogenic component of varying degree, and systemic diseases and pharmacologic effects can be concomitant and causative. (Modified from Carrier S, Brock G, Kour NW, et al.: Pathophysiology of erectile dysfunction. *Urology* 42:468–481, 1993, with permission of Excerpta Medica, Inc.)

2005, 2009; Lewis et al., 2004). However, medical and social conditions often comorbid with aging are significant confounding factors in this epidemiologic trend (Johannes et al., 2000; Laumann et al., 1999).

The National Health and Social Life Survey (**NHSLS**) was a national probability survey of men (N = 1410) and women between the ages of 18 and 59 years living in households in the United States in 1992 and was principally a broad-ranging inquiry into sexual practices and beliefs within that age group (Laumann et al., 1999). The survey collected only limited information on sexual function via single-item questions. **The prevalence of ED (based on a single-item question about attaining/maintain erection) was 7%, 9%, 11%, and 18% for men aged 18 to 29, 30 to 39, 40 to 49, and 50 to 59, respectively.**

The Massachusetts Male Aging Study (MMAS) was the first cross-sectional, community-based, random-sample, prospective epidemiologic survey on ED and its physiologic and psychosocial correlates in men in the United States. A population of 1709 noninstitutionalized men between the ages of 40 and 70 years living in the greater Boston area were surveyed between 1987 and 1989 and resurveyed between 1995 and 1997. Extensive physiologic measures, demographic information, and self-reported ED status (nine items related to erections on a questionnaire) were components of this report (Feldman et al., 1994). **From the incidence rates reported in the MMAS study, per 1000 man-years there were 12.4, 29.8, and 46.4 new cases of ED in men aged 40 to 49, 50 to 59, and 60 to 69, respectively** (Johannes et al., 2000). Similar prevalence rates for ED have been reported from other nations/regions (Moreira Jr., et al., 2003; Schouten et al., 2005). Although the prevalence of ED is higher with advanced age, the degree of subjective bother from ED also tends to decline with age (Gades et al., 2009). Conditions commonly comorbid with age are also strong predictors of incident ED; age-adjusted risk (per 1000 man-years) of ED was higher for men with diabetes mellitus (50.7 cases), treated heart disease (58.3 cases), and treated hypertension (HTN) (42.5 cases).

A large-scale international study of sexual dysfunction in men aged 40 to 80 years of age reported some regional variations in ED prevalence (range 6% to 33%, age standardized). (Laumann et al., 2005; Moreira et al., 2008; Nicolosi, et al., 2005, 2006a, 2006b). Whether these differences represent actual differences in ED prevalence or cultural variability in what constitutes clinically relevant impairment in erectile response is unclear. However, the common risk factors for ED appear to be consistent across geographic regions.

Risk Factors

Conditions commonly associated with ED include poor health status/chronic disease states, vascular and metabolic diseases, conditions of the nervous system, hormonal issues, medication use, psychiatric/psychological disorders, substance abuse, and certain sociodemographic factors (Fig. 68.12). The latter category may relate to comorbid medical conditions (more common in men of lower socioeconomic status), differential expectations of sexual response, or as yet undetermined factors (Kupelian et al., 2008). A unifying theme of most established biologic risk factors for ED is perturbation of vascular and endothelial dysfunction, either directly (as in the case of vascular and metabolic disease) or indirectly (e.g., by effects on neural innervation or hormonal milieu) (Lewis et al., 2004).

Many classification schemes have been proposed for ED cause (Fig. 68.13). Some are based on the cause (diabetic, iatrogenic, traumatic); others are based on the neurovascular mechanism (e.g., failure to initiate [neurogenic], failure to fill [arterial], and failure to store [venous]). One commonly used classification scheme is shown in Box 68.1 (Lizza and Rosen, 1999).

Psychogenic

Previously, psychogenic issues were believed to be the primary cause in up to 90% of men with ED (Masters and Johnson, 1965). Mental health issues (e.g., depression, psychosis) are risk factors for ED (Tan et al., 2012; Zemishlany and Weizman, 2008). The prevalence of ED in men with a range of mental health disorders may be as high as 83% (Mosaku and Ukpong, 2009). Although psychogenic factors are likely to play a role in virtually all cases of ED, most experts now agree that **ED is most often a predominantly functional or physical disorder.**

Sexual behavior and penile erection are controlled by the hypothalamus, limbic system, and cerebral cortex. Stimulatory or inhibitory messages can be relayed to the spinal erection centers to assist or inhibit erection. **Two possible mechanisms have been proposed to explain the inhibition of erection in psychogenic ED: (1) direct inhibition of the spinal erection center by the brain as an exaggeration of the normal suprasacral inhibition**

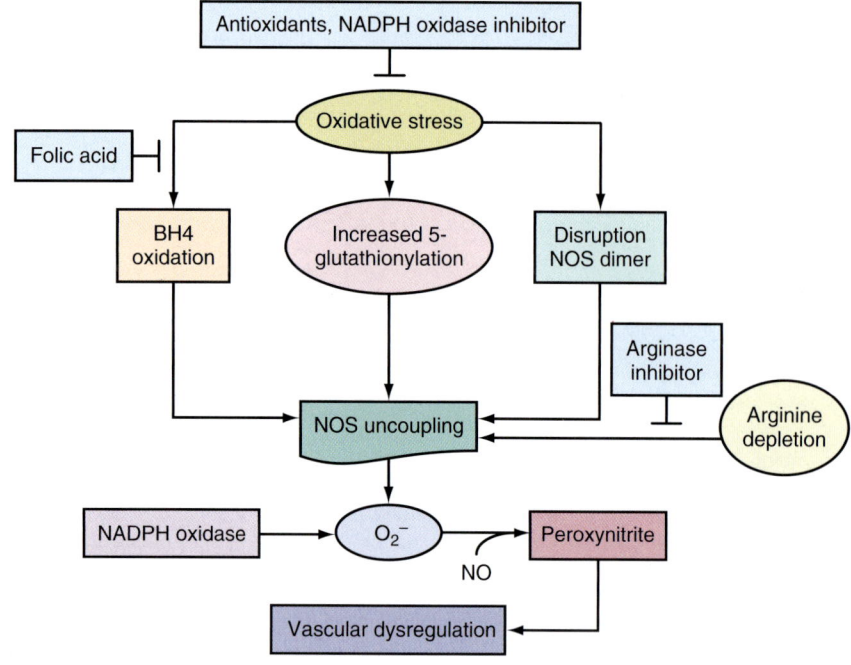

Fig. 68.13. Factors contributing to nitric oxide synthase (NOS) uncoupling and the potential inhibitors. *BH4*, Tetrahydrobiopterin; *NADPH*, reduced nicotinamide adenine dinucleotide phosphate.

BOX 68.1 Classification of Male Erectile Dysfunction

ORGANIC
I. Vasculogenic
   A. Arteriogenic
   B. Cavernosal
   C. Mixed
II. Neurogenic
III. Anatomic
IV. Endocrinologic
V. Medication induced

PSYCHOGENIC
I. Generalized
   A. Generalized unresponsiveness
      1. Primary lack of sexual arousability
      2. Aging-related decline in sexual arousability
   B. Generalized inhibition
      1. Chronic disorder of sexual intimacy
II. Situational
   A. Partner related
      1. Lack of arousability in specific relationship
      2. Lack of arousability because of sexual object preference
      3. High central inhibition because of partner conflict or threat
   B. Performance related
      1. Associated with other sexual dysfunction (e.g., rapid ejaculation)
      2. Situational performance anxiety (e.g., fear of failure)
   C. Psychological distress or adjustment related
      1. Associated with negative mood state (e.g., depression) or major life stress (e.g., death of partner)

(Steers, 2000) and (2) excessive sympathetic nervous system activation and/or elevated peripheral catecholamine levels, which may increase penile smooth muscle tone to prevent relaxation (Kim and Oh, 1992). Animal studies confirm that the stimulation of sympathetic nerves or systemic infusion of epinephrine causes detumescence of the erect penis (Diederichs, et al., 1991a, 1991b). This finding supports the observation that human men with psychogenic ED have higher levels of serum norepinephrine than healthy controls or patients with vasculogenic ED (Kim and Oh, 1992).

Neurogenic

Because erection is a neurovascular event, **any disease, dysfunction, or injury (including surgical) affecting the brain, spinal cord, or peripheral erectogenic nerves (i.e., pudendal and cavernous) can induce ED.** Neurogenic ED may also be comorbid with other diseases that cause ED. The presence of a neurologic disorder or neuropathy does not exclude other causes, and confirming that ED is neurogenic can be challenging.

In the brain the MPOA, PVN, thalamus, and hippocampus are important integration centers for sexual drive and erection (Jeon et al., 2009; McKenna, 1998); lesions of these brain areas are more likely to be associated with ED. Pathologic processes such as **Parkinson disease, stroke, encephalitis, temporal lobe epilepsy tumors, dementias (including Alzheimer disease), multiple system atrophy, and traumatic brain injury (TBI) are often associated with ED.** Insufficiency of dopaminergic and/or oxytocinergic pathways is thought to account for many cases of central neurogenic ED (Chaudhuri and Schapira, 2009). Disruptions of sexual desire are common after CVA and other brain injuries and may contribute to neurogenic ED (Jung et al., 2008).

Spinal lesions, most commonly spinal cord injury but including spina bifida, disk herniation, syringomelia, tumor, and multiple sclerosis, are common causes of ED. The nature, location, and extent of the spinal lesion dictate the effect on erectile function. **Reflexogenic erection (in response to tactile stimulation of the penis) is preserved in approximately 95% of patients with complete upper cord lesions** (Biering-Sorensen and Sonksen, 2001; Chapelle et al.,

1980). Sacral parasympathetic neurons are important in the preservation of these reflexogenic erections, which are typically of short duration and require continuous stimulation for maintenance. **Reflexogenic erections are preserved in approximately 25% of patients with complete lower cord lesions** (Biering-Sorensen and Sonksen, 2001; Chapelle et al., 1980). These patients may experience psychogenic erections (Chapelle et al., 1980); preservation of psychogenic erections in these patients is thought to be mediated by cortically induced inhibition of tonic sympathetic tone from the thoracic spinal cord (Giuliano, 2011). In addition to their impact upon ED, spinal cord lesions may impair the ejaculation reflex; this is particularly apparent in men who have disruption of the emission phase of ejaculation after injury to the sympathetic chain ganglia during retroperitoneal surgery (Dimitropoulos et al., 2016).

Because of the close relationship between the cavernous nerves and the pelvic organs, the incidence of iatrogenic impotence from pelvic surgical procedures (e.g., radical prostatectomy, abdominoperineal resection) is high, ranging up to 100% in some series (Borchers et al., 2006; Walsh and Donker, 1982; Weinstein and Roberts, 1977). **Thorough understanding of the neuroanatomy of the pelvic and cavernous nerves** led to modifications in surgery for cancer of the rectum, bladder, and prostate, which were associated with a lower incidence of iatrogenic ED (Walsh and Donker, 1982). Although nerve-sparing approaches have markedly improved erectile outcomes after pelvis surgery, the majority of men experience at least a temporary decline in erectile function after surgery, and few recover completely to baseline levels. Men with ED at baseline and older than 60 are at greater risk (Nelson et al., 2013).

Animals models indicate that cavernous nerve injury is associated with: (1) upregulation of neurotoxic type M1 macrophages, inflammatory cytokines, RhoA/Rho-kinase signaling, and tyrosine hydroxylase containing neurons; (2) increase in oxidative stress, collagen to smooth muscle ratio, and apoptosis; and (3) downregulation of Sonic hedgehog protein and diminished response to cavernous nerve-induced penile erection (Angeloni et al., 2013; Hannan et al., 2016; Lin et al., 2015; Matsui et al., 2017).

Pelvic fracture can lead to ED secondary to either (or both) cavernous nerve or vascular injury. In men with posterior urethral injury, early realignment has been associated with better potency preservation rate relative to delayed anastomosis (ED rate 34% vs. 42%) (Mouraviev et al., 2005). **Diabetes** may also cause ED via neurogenic or vascular damage, either of which can impair NO release (Saenz de Tejada, et al., 1989). Finally, **age-related declines in penile tactile** sensitivity may contribute to ED by reducing sacral reflexogenic responses (Rowland et al., 1993). Sensory input from the genitalia is essential to achieve and maintain reflexogenic erection and may be particularly important with declines in psychogenic erectile stimuli associated with age or other conditions.

Endocrinologic

Low serum testosterone (T) is a frequent finding in patients with ED. Androgens influence the growth and development of the male reproductive tract and secondary sex characteristics by binding to the androgen receptor (AR) in target tissues; their effects on libido and sexual behavior are well established (Cattabiani et al., 2012; Corona et al., 2016). **In men with low serum T, supplementation (1) enhances sexual interest, (2) increases erectile response, and (3) is linked to improvements in several nonsexual quality-of-life parameters** (Corona et al., 2014; Rosen et al., 2017). The threshold level of T for normal nocturnal erections has been reported at about 200 ng/dL (Granata et al., 1997), although many men experience symptoms (including loss of nocturnal erections) at levels of less than 320 ng/dL (Wu et al., 2010). In a study of patients presenting with ED, reported androgen deficiency symptoms in 47% of men with T levels of less than 200 ng/dL, 33% of men with levels less than 300 ng/dL, 23% of men with levels less than 346 ng/dL, and 7% of men with levels less than 400 ng/dL (Kohler et al., 2008).

Recent investigation has suggested that the number of cytosine-adenine-guanine (CAG) repeats in exon 1 of the AR gene is inversely associated with transcriptional activity of this gene; hypothetically, longer CAG repeats may reduce testosterone/AR activity by limiting the number of available receptors. A weak but significant relationship between CAG repeat length and erectile dysfunction symptoms has been reported but the relationship was significant only for those patients with at least low normal serum T levels (e.g., >330 ng/dL) (Liu et al., 2015; Tirabassi et al., 2016). This effect remains controversial as some studies have not detected a significant relationship between CAG repeats and ED (Andersen et al., 2011).

Low libido is the most common sexual symptom of low T. Older men are at greater risk of symptoms in the context of low T, although whether this relationship is cause or effect is unclear. Importantly, **many men with low T levels are asymptomatic.** Therefore the Endocrine Society recommends that T supplementation be considered only in the context of at least two clearly low morning serum T levels and symptoms clearly referable to low T (Bhasin et al., 2010).

Age, diabetes, high total cholesterol, anemia, increased waist circumference, and obesity (BMI > 30 kg/m^2) are correlated with significantly decreased testosterone levels in men with ED (Hall et al., 2008; Hofstra et al., 2008). In a comprehensive literature review, low serum T predicted elevated fasting insulin, glucose, and hemoglobin A$_{1c}$ values in men who develop diabetes, suggesting that hypogonadism may be a sentinel event in the pathogenesis of diabetes (Traish et al., 2009). **The authors further suggested that androgen deficiency is associated with insulin resistance, type 2 diabetes, metabolic syndrome (MetS), and increased deposition of visceral fat.** Visceral fat may serve as an endocrine organ, producing inflammatory cytokines and promoting endothelial dysfunction and vascular disease (Armani et al., 2017).

Testosterone exerts some effects by regulation of the NO/cGMP pathway and may play a role in RhoA/Rho Kinase signaling, adrenergic tone, and cavernous smooth muscle (Corona et al., 2016). Castration is associated with decreased arterial flow, venous leakage, and reduced erection response to stimulation of the cavernous nerves (Penson et al., 1996; Wang et al., 2015). Castration also increases α-adrenergic responsiveness of smooth muscle (Traish et al., 1999) and decreases smooth muscle and nNOS content in penile tissue (Alves-Lopes et al., 2017). Androgens promote endothelial cell survival, reduce endothelial expression of proinflammatory markers, and inhibit proliferation and intimal migration of vascular smooth muscle cells in in vivo studies. Castration has also been associated with decreased autophagy in cavernous cells in rats; it is speculated that autophagy may help to prevent apoptosis (Wang et al., 2015). At low levels of androgen, increased apoptosis is noted in endothelial cells and smooth muscle cells (Alves-Lopes et al., 2017). Low androgen levels also impairs proliferation, migration, and homing of endothelial progenitor cells as well as myogenic differentiation of mesenchymal progenitor cells (Mirone et al., 2009; Traish and Galoosian, 2013). Clinically, many men receiving long-term androgen ablation therapy for prostate cancer report poor libido and ED (Benedict et al., 2014). Some studies have indicated that testosterone supplementation improves erectile function in men with hypogonadism (Haider et al., 2017; Snyder et al., 2016) but may take sustained treatment for maximal efficacy (Hackett et al., 2016). Other studies have suggested that the benefit of testosterone supplementation relates primarily to sexual desire rather than erectile function (Cunningham et al., 2016).

Any dysfunction of the hypothalamic-pituitary axis can result in low serum T. Hypogonadotropic hypogonadism can be congenital or caused by a tumor or injury of the hypothalamus or pituitary gland. Hypergonadotropic hypogonadism may result from a tumor, injury, testicular surgery, or severe orchitis. In most cases, low serum T is not associated with marked abnormality of gonadotropins (i.e., luteinizing hormone and follicle stimulating hormone) (Kaprara and Huhtaniemi, 2017).

Hyperprolactinemia may occur in the setting of pituitary adenoma or with certain drugs such as antipsychotics (Milano et al., 2017). **High levels of serum prolactin are associated with loss of libido, ED, galactorrhea, gynecomastia, and infertility. Hyperprolactinemia is associated with low serum T, which is thought to be related to inhibition of gonadotropin-releasing hormone secretion at the level of the hypothalamus** (Freeman et al., 2000; Maggi et al., 2013). Although hyperprolactinemia has been clearly linked to sexual issues in men, epidemiologic data have also suggested that low serum prolactin is associated with metabolic syndrome and arteriogenic ED as well as with premature ejaculation and anxiety symptoms (Corona et al., 2009).

ED may also be associated with hyperthyroidism and hypothyroidism. Hyperthyroidism is commonly associated with diminished libido (which may be caused by the increased circulating estrogen levels) and less often with ED. In hypothyroidism, low testosterone secretion and elevated prolactin levels may contribute to ED (Freeman et al., 2000; Maggi et al., 2013).

Arteriogenic

Atherosclerotic or traumatic arterial occlusive disease of the hypogastric-cavernous-helicine arterial tree can decrease the perfusion pressure and arterial flow to the sinusoidal spaces. This has the effect of increasing the time to maximal erection and decreasing rigidity of the erect penis. **In most patients with arteriogenic ED, impaired penile perfusion is a component of a generalized atherosclerotic process. Common health factors associated with penile arterial insufficiency include hypertension, hyperlipidemia, tobacco use, diabetes mellitus, blunt perineal or pelvic trauma, metabolic syndrome, sedentary lifestyle, obesity, and pelvic irradiation** (Bacon et al., 2006; Feldman et al., 1994; Giugliano et al., 2010; Kupelian et al., 2010; Martin-Morales et al., 2001). Abnormalities on penile Doppler examination are associated with vascular disease and greater risk of major cardiac events (Corona et al., 2010). Focal stenosis of the common penile or cavernous artery is most often detected in young patients who have sustained blunt pelvic or perineal trauma (Munarriz et al., 1995). There is a significant relationship between cycling-induced perineal compression leading to vascular, endothelial, and neurogenic dysfunction in men and the development of ED (Sommer et al., 2010). Nevertheless, ED does not commonly occur in men who engage in recreational bicycle riding (Kim et al., 2011). The cardiovascular benefits of routine exercise may mitigate any local effect on the perineal circulation.

Arteriogenic disease is common in men with ED; arteriogenic causes are also potentially amenable to intervention that may yield benefit in terms of erectile function. Men who engage in routine physical activity and maintain healthy body weight are at reduced risk of developing ED (Esposito et al., 2010; Kupelian et al., 2010). Statin-based therapy for hypercholesterolemia has been associated with enhanced erections and improved responsiveness to erectogenic therapy (Cui et al., 2014). Tobacco cessation, weight loss, and exercise have also been associated with improvements in erectile function among men with vascular disease (Meldrum et al., 2012; Verze et al., 2015).

Cardiovascular Diseases. **ED is highly prevalent in men with coronary, cerebral, and peripheral vascular disease** (Bener et al., 2008; Chai et al., 2009; Lahoz et al., 2016; Montorsi et al., 2006). The epidemiologic and mechanistic links between ED and cardiovascular disease include (1) endothelial dysfunction (e.g., eNOS and oxidative stress); (2) smooth muscle defects (e.g., hyperplasia and altered contractility); (3) autonomic dysregulation (e.g., neuropathy and diminished nNOS content); (4) hormonal disruption (e.g., hypogonadism); and (5) metabolic defects (e.g., hyperlipidemia, advanced glycation end products) (Musicki et al., 2015).

Because penile arteries are smaller than coronary arteries, the effect of endothelial dysfunction may be noted in the penis before clinical cardiac disease manifests. In one study of men with CAD, ED preceded CAD in 93% of cases at a mean time interval of 2 years (Montorsi et al., 2006). Microvascular and arterial disease may contribute to the ED phenotype. Reactive hyperemia (a measure of microvascular integrity) had a stronger association with ED than flow-mediated dilation (a measure of larger conduit artery function); the implication is that microvascular disease may play a primary role in the development of ED (Gerber et al., 2015). **ED has thus been promoted by many experts as an early indicator of systemic endothelial dysfunction and an indication for cardiac risk stratification** (Gandaglia et al., 2016; Shah et al., 2016; Vlachopoulos et al., 2013).

Hyperlipidemia. **ED is common in hyperlipidemia** (Roumeguere et al., 2003). Hypercholesterolemia at baseline was a predictor of incident ED over a 25-year study in the Rancho Bernardo Study (Fung et al., 2004). However, a survey of men in the Boston area did not show an association between untreated hyperlipidemia and ED (Hall et al., 2009).

The effect of hypercholesterolemia on erectile function has been studied in various experimental models. Histologic examination of the corpus cavernosum ultrastructure in hyperlipidemia reveals an early atherosclerotic process in the sinusoids (Kim et al., 1994). High levels of oxidized low-density lipoproteins inhibit endothelium-dependent NO-mediated relaxation and enhance corporal smooth muscle contractility (Ahn et al., 1999; Fraga-Silva et al., 2014). Impairment of the NO/cGMP pathway in hyperlipidemia is thought to be due to oxidative stress (Kim et al., 1997), endogenous NOS inhibitors such as NG-monomethyl-L-arginine monoacetate and asymmetrical dimethylarginine (ADMA) (Maas et al., 2005), depletion of the arginine required for production of NO by increased activity of arginase (Fraga-Silva et al., 2014), and production of procontractile factors such as thromboxane and prostaglandin (Azadzoi et al., 1998, 1999). Downregulation of the angiogenic factor VEGF has been detected in rats fed a high-cholesterol diet (Ryu et al., 2006); this has been linked to impairment of endothelium-dependent relaxation (Xie et al., 2005).

Although the eNOS/cGMP pathway is clearly impaired in hyperlipidemic model systems, neuronal vasodilation is not affected (Azadzoi et al., 1998). However, loss of the endothelial layer coupled with a high fat diet has been linked to impaired arterial reactivity and fibrotic changes of the corpora in a rabbit model (Azadzoi et al., 1997; Nehra et al., 1998). This severe phenotype led to impairment of neuronal and endothelial NOS activity (Azadzoi et al., 1999).

Obesity. High body weight, BMI, and total body fat percentage are independently associated with greater prevalence of moderate to severe and complete ED (Esposito et al., 2005; Garimella et al., 2013; Gunduz et al., 2004). Animals models of obesity/metabolic syndrome have demonstrated upregulation of endothelin receptor expression, increased oxidative stress, and decreased reactivity to NO and acetylcholine in cavernous tissues (Sanchez et al., 2014). Visceral fat is an endocrine organ and is thought to produce a number of inflammatory mediators that may promote oxidative stress and insulin resistance in penile and other vascular tissue (Chitaley et al., 2009). Perivascular adipose tissue (PVAT) is another recognized contributor to vascular function. Adipocytes and stromal cells contained within PVAT are sources of molecules with varied paracrine effects on the underlying smooth muscle and endothelial cells, including adipokines, cytokines, reactive oxygen species, and gaseous compounds. In obesity and diabetes, the expanded PVAT and its downstream effects contribute to vascular insulin resistance and atherogenesis. A common denominator of PVAT dysfunction in all these conditions is immune cell infiltration, which triggers the subsequent inflammation, oxidative stress, and hypoxic processes to promote vascular dysfunction (Szasz et al., 2013).

Hypertension. Hypertension (HTN) is an independent risk factor for ED (Feldman et al., 1994; Johannes et al., 2000). In two analyses including more than 270,000 men with ED from a US claims database, the prevalence of hypertension in men with versus without ED was 41.2% versus 19.2%, respectively (Seftel et al., 2004; Sun and Swindle, 2005). Hypertensive damage to end organs (e.g., ischemic heart disease and renal failure) is associated with higher prevalence of ED (Feldman et al., 1994; Johannes et al., 2000; Kaufman et al., 1994). Other determinants of ED in hypertensive men include older age, longer duration of disease, greater severity of hypertension, and the use of antihypertensive medications, some of which may themselves contribute to ED (Doumas et al., 2006).

The cause of HTN-related ED is thought to be related to biochemical and structural changes as opposed to direct effect on vascular walls (Shimizu et al., 2014). Arterial hypertension is characterized by altered vascular tone and increased vascular contractility resulting in high blood pressure. It is accompanied by proliferation, migration of vascular smooth muscle cells, and varying levels of inflammation of the arterial wall. The Rho-kinase pathway plays a crucial role in the regulation of arterial blood pressure (Nunes et al., 2010). Toll-like receptor activation on cells of the vasculature in response to the release of damage-associated molecular patterns and the consequences of this activation on inflammation, vasoreactivity, and vascular remodeling has been proposed as a novel link between inflammation and hypertension (McCarthy et al., 2014). In addition, endoplasmic reticulum stress leading to endothelium-dependent contractile responses in aorta has been proposed as a cause of hypertension in a spontaneously hypertensive rat (SHR) model (Spitler et al., 2013). The RAS pathway, activated in many cases of hypertension, may contribute to reduced nicotinamide adenine dinucleotide phosphate oxidase and subsequent increase in oxidative stress (Jin et al., 2008; Shimizu et al., 2014). Recent evidence from an animal study has also implicated the Rho-kinase pathway in the pathogenesis of hypertension-related ED, with inhibition of Rho-kinase ameliorating the effects of hypertensive state on penile hemodynamics (Zhu et al., 2014).

Mechanism of Vascular Erectile Dysfunction

Arteriogenic ED. In arteriogenic ED, oxygen tension in the corpus cavernosum blood is less than that in psychogenic ED (Tarhan et al., 1997). Formation of PGE_1 and PGE_2 is oxygen dependent, and in rabbit and human corpus cavernosum, increased oxygen tension was associated with elevation of PGE_2 and suppression of TGF-β1-induced collagen synthesis (Moreland et al., 1995; Nehra et al., 1999). Chronic hypoxia leads to decreased smooth muscle content, increased production of TGF-β, and increased production of type I and III collagen in corporal tissue. These effects may be mediated in part by expression of hypoxia inducible factor-1α (HIF-1α) (Lv et al., 2014).

An increased wall/lumen ratio in arteries contributes to increased peripheral vascular resistance in hypertension. Increased resistance has also been detected in the penile vasculature of SHR—an alteration ascribed to structural changes of the arterial and erectile tissue (Arribas et al., 2008; Gradin et al., 2006). Mitochondrial damage (in smooth muscle and endothelial cells), nerve degeneration, oxidative stress, increased contractility in response to adrenergic stimulation, and disruption of NOS expression have also been described in animal models of hypertension (Jiang et al., 2005; Shimizu et al., 2014). These structural changes are mediated in part by action of the RAS pathway, as evidenced by partial prevention from administration of a type 1 angiotensin II receptor blockers (Mazza et al., 2006). Interestingly, comparison arms in these studies using the vasodilator hydralazine or a calcium channel blocker did not show mitigation of penile end organ damage despite lowering systemic blood pressure (Mazza et al., 2006; Shimizu et al., 2014). A similar study comparing the NOS potentiating beta-blocker nebivolol to the calcium channel blocker amlodipine demonstrated that both treatments reduced blood pressure, but only nebivolol mitigated corporal tissue changes (Toblli et al., 2006).

Enhanced Smooth Muscle Contraction and Vasoconstriction. In animal models, increased RhoA/Rho-kinase activity leading to increased contractility of the corporeal smooth muscle has been linked to ED in diabetes (Bivalacqua et al., 2004), hypercholesterolemia (Morikage et al., 2006), hypertension (Fibbi et al., 2008), hypogonadism (Vignozzi et al., 2007), cavernous nerve injury (Martinez-Salamanca et al., 2015), and aging (Jin et al., 2006). Inhibition of Rho-kinase has been associated with decreased pelvic atherosclerosis, improved penile hemodynamics, reduced apoptosis, and preservation of NOS activity in rat models of ED (Hannan et al., 2013; Park et al., 2006). Rho-kinase inhibition has also been linked to relaxation of human corporal cells in vivo (Uvin et al., 2017).

Endothelin-1 levels are elevated in plasma of men with atherosclerosis, hypertension, and hypercholesterolemia. Men with organic ED have higher venous and cavernous blood levels of endothelin-1 as well (El Melegy et al., 2005; Nohria et al., 2003). However, a pilot study using an endothelin-A receptor antagonist as a treatment for men with ED did not produce positive results (Kim et al., 2002).

Angiotensin II may restrict corporal vasodilation by action on the AT1 receptor (Kilarkaje et al., 2013). AT1 receptor antagonists and angiotensin-converting enzyme (ACE) inhibitors have shown promise in the treatment of men with ED and hypertension and men with ED and atherosclerosis, respectively (Baumhakel et al., 2008; Speel et al., 2005).

Defects of maxi-K^+ channel in cells in men with ED are thought to alter hyperpolarization and calcium homeostasis in corporal smooth muscle (Fan et al., 1995). Alterations of intracellular communication between smooth muscle cells via gap junctions (intercellular communication channels) has also been noted in ED (Traish et al., 2013). Specific defects that have been reported include increased collagen content in arteriogenic and obesity-related ED (Tomada et al., 2013) and decreased content of the essential gap junction protein connexin 43 in diabetes and aged animal models of ED (Suadicani et al., 2009; Traish et al., 2013).

High adrenergic tone (related to medical or psychological issues) may lead to insufficient trabecular smooth muscle relaxation (Prieto, 2008). This has the effect of not only reducing arterial inflow but also impairing coaptation of the emissary veins by expanding corporal sinusoids.

Impaired Endothelium-Dependent Smooth Muscle Relaxation. Endothelial dysfunction has been proposed as a common link between cardiovascular disease and ED (Brunner et al., 2005; Musicki et al., 2015). Impairment of endothelium-dependent flow-mediated dilation of the brachial artery has been reported in men with ED; the degree of impairment correlated with the severity of ED (Kovacs et al., 2008). Men with ED related to heart disease, obesity, and low serum testosterone also have fewer circulating endothelial progenitor cells; these regenerative cells are produced in bone marrow and migrate to peripheral vessels to repair endothelial defects (Baumhakel et al., 2006; Esposito et al., 2009; Foresta et al., 2005; Maiorino et al., 2015). Impairment of endothelium-dependent relaxation in hypertensive animal models has been ascribed to angiotensin II (Rajagopalan et al., 1996), thromboxane, superoxide (Cosentino et al., 1998), and direct effects of increased vascular pressure (Paniagua et al., 2000; Table 68.9).

Corporal Structural Defects

Failure to restrict venous outflow from the penis during erection is one of the most common causes of vasculogenic ED (Rajfer et al., 1988). **Veno-occlusive dysfunction may result from various pathophysiologic processes, including degenerative tunica changes, fibroelastic structural alterations, insufficient trabecular smooth muscle relaxation, and venous shunts.**

Degenerative changes (e.g., tissue senescence, diabetes) or traumatic injury to the tunica albuginea (e.g., penile fracture) can impair the compression of the subtunical and emissary veins (Gonzalez-Cadavid, 2009). In Peyronie disease, inelasticity of the tunica albuginea may prevent coaptation of emissary veins (Chiang et al., 1992; Metz et al., 1983). Surgery for correction of Peyronie

TABLE 68.9 Vascular and Structural Changes Leading to Erectile Dysfunction

PENILE STRUCTURE	CHANGES IN ERECTILE DYSFUNCTION
Cavernous artery	Increased vascular resistance, narrow lumen
Smooth muscle	Increased tone (hypertonicity) Decreased smooth muscle content Alteration of potassium channels and gap junctions
Cavernous tissue	Fibrosis (collagen deposition, loss of elastin) Impaired veno-occlusive mechanism
Endothelium	Impaired endothelium-dependent relaxation
Tunica albuginea	Alteration of elastic and collagen fibers
Neurotransmitters	Decreased nNOS, eNOS

eNOS, Endothelial nitric oxide synthase; *nNOS*, neuronal nitric oxide synthase.

disease may also contribute to inadequate corporal veno-occlusion by disruption of the subtunical areolar layer or the tunica (Flores et al., 2011). Acquired venous shunts—the result of operative correction of priapism—may cause persistent glans/cavernosum or cavernosum/spongiosum shunting and venous leakage during erection; however, in these cases ED may also relate to corporal fibrosis from priapism (Pal et al., 2016).

Structural or functional alterations in the fibroelastic components of the trabeculae, cavernous smooth muscle, and endothelium may result in venous leakage. Increased deposition of collagen and decreased elastic fiber content within the corpora has been linked to ED as well as associated disease conditions including diabetes, hypercholesterolemia, vascular disease, and penile injury (Sattar et al., 1994).

Loss of corporal smooth muscle content and functionality is also strongly associated with ED (Mersdorf et al., 1991; Pickard et al., 1993; Saenz de Tejada, et al., 1989). Reductions in smooth muscle content is commonly observed in animal models of vasculogenic and neurogenic ED (Azadzoi et al., 1997; Junemann et al., 1991; Nehra et al., 1998). Interestingly, in a human study penile smooth muscle content was reduced in arteriogenic and venogenic ED but was lowest in men with arterogenic ED (Pickard et al., 1994; Sattar et al., 1996).

Sonic Hedgehog Protein. SHH is one of three proteins in the mammalian hedgehog family, the others being desert hedgehog and Indian hedgehog (Hammerschmidt et al., 1997). SHH plays a key role in regulating neuronal differentiation and axon guidance and appears to play an important role in penile development (Charron et al., 2003; Podlasek et al., 2005). Decreased levels of SHH have been demonstrated after cavernous nerve injury and diabetes; these findings are associated with neve degeneration, corporal apoptosis, and decreased smooth muscle content (Angeloni et al., 2013; Podlasek et al., 2005). Administration of SHH in cavernous nerve injured rats ameliorates many of these findings and improves erectile function (Choe et al., 2017). The mechanism of action may involve brain-derived neurotrophic factor activation (Bond et al., 2013).

Endothelium. **The endothelium is an important source of NO and many other signaling molecules, including EDHF, PGI_2, and hydrogen peroxide.** The endothelium also modulates flow-mediated vasodilation and influences mitogenic activity, platelet aggregation, and neutrophil adhesion; these effects are mediated via transferred chemical mediators (e.g., NO and PGI_2) and/or low-resistance electrical coupling through myoendothelial gap junctions.

Disruption of endothelial function is an early indicator of vascular disease (Triggle et al., 2012). Diabetes and hypercholesterolemia alter the function of endothelium-mediated relaxation of the cavernous muscle and impair erection (Azadzoi and Saenz de Tejada, 1991). Specific mechanisms by which endothelial dysfunction may contribute to ED include decreased endothelial cell density and downregulation of endothelium-specific cell-to-cell junction proteins (e.g., claudin-5, vascular endothelial–cadherin, platelet endothelial cell adhesion molecule 1) (Ryu et al., 2013).

Drug-Induced

Medical therapy is commonly associated with self-reported ED (Razdan et al., 2017). Numerous conditions common in the ED population are themselves risk factors for ED, such as depression, diabetes, and cardiovascular disease (Derby et al., 2001). Medical management of these and other conditions may exacerbate or cause ED. In some cases, sexual symptoms related to medication primarily effect sexual desire, ejaculation, or orgasm; these issues may be reported by patients as "ED" or may lead to secondary issues in erectile response. Self-reported and questionnaire data concerning ED as a side effect of medication should be interpreted with caution.

Antihypertensive Agents. **Almost all antihypertensive drugs have ED listed as a potential side effect.** However, certain antihypertensives carry greater risk of ED than others, and there is evidence that some antihypertensives can be beneficial for erectile function (La Torre et al., 2015). Given the relationship between hypertension and ED, it can be challenging to elucidate the precise cause of ED in men under treatment with antihypertensives; some evidence suggests that the underlying disease process is the principle driver of ED in this population (Kupelian et al., 2013).

Diuretics. Thiazide diuretics are carbonic anhydrase inhibitors that alkalinize cells and cause vasodilation. The predominant activity of thiazide diuretics is to inhibit a directly coupled Na-Cl cotransporter along the distal convoluted tubule of the kidney (Ellison and Loffing, 2009).

Data from a large trial in the United Kingdom showed that twice as many men taking thiazides for mild hypertension reported ED compared with men taking propranolol or placebo (Adverse reactions, 1981). Similar findings were documented from the Treatment of Mild Hypertension Study (TOMHS), in which the prevalence of ED at 2 years in men taking low-dose thiazide was twice that of men taking placebo or alternative agents. After 4 years of treatment, the prevalence of ED in the placebo group approached that of the thiazide group, a finding not fully explained by dropouts (Grimm et al., 1997). A study comparing sexual side effects of thiazide, placebo, or atenolol in hypertensive patients also found a higher rate of ED in the thiazide group, although weight loss was a more powerful mediator of ED resolution (Wassertheil-Smoller et al., 1991). **The mechanism of diuretic-induced ED remains to be elucidated.**

β-Adrenergic Blockers. Receptor studies show that only 10% of adrenoceptors in the penile tissue are of the β type, and their stimulation is thought to mediate smooth muscle relaxation (Andersson and Wagner, 1995). **This response is attenuated in vitro by nonselective drugs such as propranolol, possibly via a prejunctional $β_2$-receptor effect but not by cardiac-selective agents such as practolol** (Srilatha et al., 1999). β antagonists also exert an inhibitory effect within the CNS, perhaps leading to decreased sex hormone levels (Suzuki et al., 1988).

The differential effects of β-adrenoceptor antagonists on erectile function may be explained in part by whether they are general or selective antagonists, and whether they possess vasodilatory properties. **Nonselective β-antagonists such as propranolol are associated with higher prevalence of ED** compared with placebo or ACE inhibitors (Croog et al., 1986). Carvedilol, a general β-adrenoceptor antagonist that also causes vasodilation by blocking $α_1$-adrenoceptors, has been associated with worsening sexual function (Fogari et al., 2001). Selective β-antagonists have a much lower rate of ED that does not significantly differ from what is observed with placebo or ACE inhibitors (Grimm et al., 1997). Some novel $β_1$-adrenoceptor antagonists have vasodilatory effects mediated by release of NO (Reidenbach et al., 2007). In crossover studies using the vasodilating β-antagonist nebivolol versus the selective $β_1$-antagonists metoprolol and atenolol, nebivolol did not decrease sexual intercourse activity in hypertensive men and in some cases had positive effects on erectile function (Boydak et al., 2005; Brixius et al., 2007).

α-Adrenoceptor Blockers. In animal studies, α antagonists (particularly antagonists acting on the $α_1$ receptor) increase and/or prolong the relaxant response of cavernous smooth muscle (Andersson and Wagner, 1995). In addition, prejunctional $α_2$-receptor activation modulates the release of noradrenaline, suggesting a putative relaxant role for $α_2$-antagonists. α-Antagonists used to treat hypertension and/or BPH (e.g., doxazosin) or reduce urinary tract symptoms have not associated with increased prevalence of ED (Flack, 2002; Grimm et al., 1997). Conversely, **$α_2$-receptor agonists (e.g., clonidine) are associated with decreased erectile function thought to relate to peripheral and central mechanisms** (Srilatha et al., 1999). **Methyldopa**, a centrally acting drug, **has also been associated with ED** in controlled trials comparing it with placebo and other antihypertensive agents and is thought to act by antagonizing hypothalamic $α_2$-adrenoceptors (Croog et al., 1988).

Angiotensin-Converting Enzyme Inhibitors. **ACE inhibitors lack any easily appreciated peripheral or central effect that would interfere with sexual function.** Given the relevance of the RAS pathway to ED pathogenesis it is reasonable to hypothesize that these agents may be beneficial in terms of erectile response, an observation that has been confirmed in a number of studies (Toblli et al., 2007). In a rat model of diabetes intracerebroventricular administration of an ACE inhibitor was associated with enhancement of centrally induced erections from sodium nitroprusside or stimulation of the NMDA receptor (Zheng et al., 2013). In the majority of human studies ACE inhibitor use is associated with a neutral to beneficial effect on erectile function (Shindel et al., 2008).

Angiotensin II Type 1 Receptor Antagonists. In studies of hypertensive or aging normotensive animals, AT1 receptor antagonists (e.g., losartan, valsartan, candesartan) reverse structural changes in the penile vasculature and appear to conserve erectile function (Hale et al., 2001, 2002; Hannan et al., 2006; Park et al., 2005; Shindel et al., 2008). In a rat model of diabetes, intracerebroventricular administration of an AT1 receptor antagonist was associated with enhancement of centrally induced erections from sodium nitroprusside or stimulation of the NMDA receptor (Zheng et al., 2013). In human clinical cross-sectional studies, AT1 receptor antagonists, in contrast to other antihypertensive drugs, seem to improve erectile function (Doumas et al., 2006). In a crossover study comparing valsartan with the β-adrenoceptor antagonist carvedilol, valsartan had a beneficial effect on preexisting sexual dysfunction and had no adverse sexual effects during 12 months of treatment (Fogari et al., 2001). Treatment with losartan for 3 months has been associated with improved sexual function (Llisterri et al., 2001).

Calcium Channel Blockers. Clinical studies of calcium channel blockers have demonstrated **no adverse effect on erection** (Cushman et al., 1998; Grimm et al., 1997). However, this class has been linked to ejaculatory complaints, which may be due to decreased force of bulbocavernous muscles (Suzuki et al., 1988).

Aldosterone Receptor Antagonists. Mineralocorticoid receptors have been identified in human corporal tissue (Kishimoto et al., 2013). Spironolactone and eplerenone are mineralocorticoid-blocking agents. Spironolactone is a nonselective mineralocorticoid receptor antagonist with moderate affinity for progesterone and androgen receptors (Corvol et al., 1975). The latter property increases the likelihood of endocrine side effects, including loss of libido, gynecomastia, and ED. Aldosterone has also been linked to adrenergic sensitization in human corporal cells, an effect that tends to promote contraction (Muguruma et al., 2008). However, mineralocorticoids themselves exert inflammatory effects on corporal tissue (including synthesis of tumor necrosis factor-α, nuclear factor-kappa B, and interleukin-6), which may impair erectile responses; treatment of these tissues with spironolactone reduced this effect and thus may theoretically improve peripheral erectile function (Wu et al., 2018). Eplerenone is a next-generation aldosterone receptor antagonist selective for aldosterone receptors alone. It has less affinity for progesterone and androgen receptors (Sica, 2005).

Summary on Antihypertensives. Treatment of mild to moderate hypertension requires agents with an acceptable side-effect profile to minimize noncompliance. Thiazide diuretics and nonselective β-antagonists are associated with higher rates of ED, although this may be reduced by combination therapy and weight loss. α₁-Blockers, ACE inhibitors, and angiotensin II receptor blockers tend to have fewer negative effects on sexual functioning during treatment and may be preferred when starting antihypertensive therapy in men with preexisting ED (Table 68.10).

Psychotropic Medication. Receptor complexity and the convoluted interrelationship of pathways within the CNS make it extremely likely that neurons and ganglia involved in sexual functioning will be affected by psychotropic drugs, leading to functional changes that may be positive and/or negative. For example, nonmedicated patients with schizophrenia are at increased risk of low sexual desire; treatment has been associated with increases in sexual desire but decreased erectile and ejaculatory function (Aizenberg et al., 1995).

Antipsychotics. In a nonrandomized comparative study of antipsychotic medications, the prevalence of sexual dysfunction ranged from 40% to 70% (Wirshing et al., 2002). Newer agents such as clozapine and risperidone are associated with less frequent deficits in sexual desire and erectile function. This class of drugs has many effects on CNS receptors and may act peripherally. The therapeutic effect of antipsychotics is thought to relate to dopaminergic receptor blockade within the limbic and prefrontal areas of the brain. Adverse events with respect to sexual function are thought to be due to β-adrenergic blockade and anticholinergic properties and to antidopaminergic actions within the basal ganglia (Sullivan and Lukoff, 1990).

The occurrence of extrapyramidal effects (i.e., repetitive involuntary muscle movements) differentiates older "typical" antipsychotics (frequent extrapyramidal effects) from newer "atypical" antipsychotics (less common extrapyramidal effects). This variation probably relates to differential affinities for particular classes of receptor or avidity for particular areas of the cerebral cortex (Strange, 2001; Westerink, 2002). An additional effect of dopamine blockade is hyperprolactinemia, which may reduce serum testosterone levels and cerebral dopamine release in permissive cerebral centers. Hyperprolactinemia is more common with older "typical" antipsychotic agents (Smith and Talbert, 1986).

The clinical effect of antipsychotics on sexual function varies according to their affinity for particular receptors. Animal experiments, chiefly in rats, show that D1 receptor activation in the MPOA of the hypothalamus facilitates erection through intermediary oxytocinergic and spinal cholinergic pathways. Activation of D2 receptors in this area may have the opposite effect (Zarrindast et al., 1992). Older agents such as haloperidol and flupenthixol reduce apomorphine-induced erections in experimental animals by means of D1 receptor antagonism (Andersson and Wagner, 1995). However, systemic administration of antipsychotic agents in rabbits produced erection by a local nondopaminergic action, possibly involving antagonism of α₁-adrenoceptors (Naganuma et al., 1993).

Antidepressants. Sexual side effects of antidepressants in men are varied but are important factors governing compliance because these drugs are commonly prescribed to younger and middle-aged adults.

Tricyclics act by inhibiting the reuptake of catecholamines in the CNS. **Their sexual side-effect profile is thought to relate to peripheral anticholinergic and β-adrenergic effects.** It is also possible that they antagonize 5-HT receptors. Controlled clinical studies suggest that **orgasmic disorders in both sexes are frequent,** explaining the use of these drugs as inhibitors of ejaculation (Harrison et al., 1986; Monteiro et al., 1987). *Monoamine oxidase inhibitors* (MAOIs) are associated with **higher rates of orgasmic dysfunction** in controlled trials but the nature of the central or peripheral mechanisms involved is uncertain (Harrison et al., 1986).

TABLE 68.10 Effect of Antihypertensive Agents on Sexual Function

AGENT	EFFECT	MECHANISM
Diuretics	ED (twice as common as placebo)	Unknown
Beta-blocker (nonselective)	ED	Prejunctional α₂-receptor inhibition
α₁-Blocker	Decreases ED rate but may cause alteration of ejaculation	Failure of sympathetic-induced (1) closure of internal sphincter and proximal urethra and (2) failure of seminal emission during ejaculation
α₂-Blocker	ED	Inhibition of central α₂-receptor
Angiotensin-converting enzyme inhibitor	Possible reduction in ED	
Angiotensin II receptor blocker	Possibly reduction in ED	

ED, Erectile dysfunction.

Tricyclics and MAOI are used relatively infrequently in the modern era. *Selective serotonin reuptake inhibitors* (SSRIs) are the class of drug most commonly used to treat depression currently. These drugs inhibit the reuptake of 5-HT into CNS neurons and can produce stimulatory effects on various 5-HT receptors.

It is estimated that **up to 50% of patients taking SSRIs experience a change in sexual function** (Keltner et al., 2002; Rosen et al., 1999). Possible mechanisms include stimulation of 5-HT$_2$ and 5-HT$_3$ receptors, which may inhibit erectogenic pathways within the spinal cord (Tang et al., 1998); decreased dopamine release in the MPOA (Maeda et al., 1994); and alteration of NO metabolism (Angulo et al., 2001). A controlled clinical study suggested that the improvement in sexual function resulting from alleviation of clinical depression with use of SSRIs outweighed any negative effect (Michelson et al., 2001) However, other placebo-controlled randomized studies revealed increased sexual dysfunction, mainly anorgasmia, in the group treated with SSRIs (Croft et al., 1999; Labbate et al., 1998). Further studies have suggested that **these adverse effects can be modified by co-treatment with other drugs such as PDE5 inhibitors** (Fava et al., 2006) or an adjunctive antidepressant agent with dopaminergic activity (e.g., buproprion) (Rudkin et al., 2004) or 5-HT$_{1A}$ activity (e.g., buspirone) (Gitlin et al., 2002).

SSRIs differ in their ability to cause ED. A high incidence of ED has been observed in patients treated with paroxetine (Kennedy et al., 2000), whereas a lesser impact has been reported with citalopram (Mendels et al., 1999). This difference suggests that mechanisms other than inhibition of serotonin reuptake may be involved, which is supported by a report that short-term or long-term administration of paroxetine, but not citalopram, caused ED in rats by inhibiting NO production (Angulo et al., 2001). The inhibitory effects induced by short-term administration of paroxetine on erectile function in the rat can be prevented by inhibition of PDE5 (Angulo et al., 2003).

Other Antidepressants. Animal experiments suggest that stimulation of 5-HT$_{1c}$ receptors within the CNS induces erection (Stancampiano et al., 1994). Newer antidepressants such as mirtazapine and nefazodone tend to have beneficial effects on sexual function, possibly by activating the 5-HT$_{1C}$ receptor, which augments sexual response (Stancampiano et al., 1994), although they may also antagonize the 5-HT$_{2C}$ receptor (Millan et al., 2000). The isolated reports of priapism seen with a prototype agent, trazodone, may be related to the 5-HT$_{1C}$ erectogenic effect seen with its primary metabolite, m-chlorophenylpiperazine, in experimental animals. (Andersson and Wagner, 1995). In a clinical study, trazodone was shown to increase nocturnal erectile activity, despite reducing REM sleep (Ware et al., 1994).

Anxiolytics. Anxiolytics have been implicated in sexual problems (Derby et al., 2001). Benzodiazepines are thought to potentiate the action of GABA in the reticular and limbic system; they may also affect the serotonin and dopaminergic pathways. Experimental studies suggest that GABAergic drugs inhibit erection induced by apomorphine, a dopamine agonist (Zarrindast and Farahvash, 1994). A controlled clinical study demonstrated that a combination of lithium and benzodiazepine was associated with a significantly higher rate of sexual dysfunction than treatment with lithium alone (Ghadirian et al., 1992). More recent anxiolytic agents, such as bupropion, acting mainly by inhibiting dopamine reuptake, and buspirone, acting on 5-HT$_{1A}$ receptors, are less commonly associated with sexual side effects in placebo-controlled trials (Coleman et al., 2001; Gitlin et al., 2002).

Anticonvulsants. Epileptic discharges may affect the function of the hypothalamic-pituitary axis and the level of hormones important for sexual function (Morris and Vanderkolk, 2005). Sexual function, bioavailable testosterone levels, and gonadal efficiency in men with epilepsy who take lamotrigine are comparable with control and untreated values and significantly greater than in men treated with carbamazepine or phenytoin (Herzog et al., 2004). Orgasmic dysfunction is common in patients who receive carbamazepine therapy, and loss of sexual desire is common in men treated with valproate (Kuba et al., 2006). There are reports of improved sexual function and hypersexuality in patients treated with lamotrigine (Gil-Nagel et al., 2006; Grabowska-Grzyb et al., 2006).

Antiandrogens. Androgens are believed to modify sexual behavior by modulating androgen receptors within the CNS. **Antiandrogens cause partial or near-complete blockade of androgen's action by inhibiting production of or antagonizing the androgen receptor.** The effects of androgen deficiency on sexual activity are variable, ranging from complete loss to normal function. Experimental studies in humans suggest that nocturnal erections during REM sleep are androgen dependent, whereas erections in response to visual sexual stimulation are independent (Andersson and Wagner, 1995). An additional peripheral effect has been suggested from animal experiments in which castration decreased NOS activity within the rat corpus cavernosum, leading to reduced erectile activity. Testosterone restored NOS activity, but treatment with finasteride prevented this recovery, suggesting that dihydrotestosterone (DHT) may be the important androgen in penile tissue (Lugg et al., 1995).

The 5α-reductase inhibitors (i.e., finasteride and dutasteride) are antiandrogens with the least effect on circulating testosterone. In randomized placebo-controlled studies of patients given finasteride (5 mg daily) for prostatic symptoms, approximately **5% complained of decreased desire and ED compared with 1% in the placebo group** (Gormley et al., 1992). At the lower dose used to treat male-pattern alopecia (1 mg daily), no sexual dysfunction was seen (Tosti et al., 2001). However, persistent sexual dysfunction for months to years after discontinuation of finasteride for alopecia has been reported. Purported effects include low libido, ED, decreased arousal, and difficulty with orgasm (Irwig and Kolukula, 2011). A rodent study of chronic treatment with a 5α-reductase inhibitor demonstrated decreased erectile response to cavernous nerve electrostimulation, a finding associated with reduced smooth muscle to collagen ratio, depression of eNOS, increased apoptosis, and decreased autophagy (Zhang et al., 2013).

Antagonism at the androgen receptor prevents signal transduction of testosterone and DHT. Nonsteroidal drugs such as flutamide and bicalutamide have relatively pure effects on the androgen receptor. These drugs are used in the palliative treatment of locally advanced and metastatic prostate cancer (Helsen et al., 2014). When used alone, nonsteroidal antiandrogens are associated with an increase in serum testosterone levels. Luteinizing hormone–releasing hormone (LHRH) agonists and antagonists are also frequently used in advanced prostate cancer used to suppress serum testosterone (Clinton et al., 2017; Dellis and Papatsoris, 2017). When a nonsteroidal antiandrogen is used in conjunction with an LHRH agonist or antagonist, the combination reduces testosterone to the castrate range. The main side effect is a reduction of sexual desire, which occurs in up to 70% of patients (Iversen et al., 2001).

In a clinical trial with larger sample size and longer duration, treatment with bicalutamide alone resulted in a smaller decrease in sexual desire than did castration (Iversen et al., 2000). However, in another large controlled trial, treatment with either flutamide or cyproterone resulted in a gradual loss of sexual desire over 2 to 6 years in approximately 80% of patients (Schroder et al., 2000). In a placebo-controlled study, half of patients receiving bicalutamide therapy experienced loss of erectile function, even at a low dose of 50 mg (Eri and Tveter, 1994).

The near-complete androgen deprivation achieved by medical castration with LHRH antagonist (immediate testosterone suppression) or agonists (with an initial surge of testosterone) results in a profound loss of sexual desire, which is usually accompanied by ED (Basaria et al., 2002). In a small study, nocturnal penile tumescence (NPT) monitoring before and after initiation of therapy indicated reductions in nocturnal penile tumescence with medical castration (Marumo et al., 1999).

Miscellaneous Drugs. Many other drugs are purported to induce ED in men. These reports are usually based on anecdotal case reports or post-marketing drug alerts rather than controlled trials.

Digoxin. In an experimental in vitro study with isolated human corpus cavernosum tissue, digoxin attenuated the relaxant response to acetylcholine and intrinsic nerve stimulation; this was linked to findings of reduced penile rigidity not seen in men given a placebo after visual sexual stimulation (Gupta et al., 1998). A randomized clinical study confirmed a negative effect on general sexual functioning linked to a decrease in plasma testosterone (Neri et al., 1987). However, other investigators did not find change in sex and adrenal hormone levels in men taking digoxin (Kley et al., 1984).

Statins. **Statins** are used to reduce lipid levels and are commonly used in men likely to have established risk factors for sexual dysfunction, particularly ED. Several studies have suggested that statins are associated with worsening of ED (Bruckert et al., 1996; Solomon et al., 2006). Although this may relate to drug therapy, it is also plausible that worsening ED in this context may relate to progression of vascular disease in men with hyperlipidemic issues severe enough to warrant medical therapy. Other studies have suggested beneficial erectile effects in men taking statins for ED, including (1) improvement in nocturnal penile activity and mean scores on the Sexual Health Inventory in Men questionnaire from 14.2 to 20.7 in hyperlipidemic patients treated for 4 months (Saltzman et al., 2004); (2) positive effects on ED in men with established penile disease and suboptimal response to PDE inhibitors who were given a statin and an ACE inhibitor (Bank et al., 2006); (3) improvement in the response to sildenafil in men with ED not initially responsive to sildenafil (Herrmann et al., 2006); (4) improvement in erectile function recovery in men who had undergone bilateral nerve-sparing radical prostatectomy and received sildenafil (Hong et al., 2007); and (5) positive effect on International Index of Erectile Function (IIEF) questionnaire scores in patients with hyperlipidemia followed for 12 months (Dogru et al., 2008). A recent meta-analysis of studies concluded that statins are associated with improvements in mean IIEF (Cui et al., 2014).

Histamine H_2 Receptor Antagonists. Cimetidine and ranitidine are widely prescribed for prophylaxis and treatment of peptic ulcer disease. A single in vitro animal study suggested that H_2 receptor stimulation causes cavernous relaxation, possibly via endothelial release of NO (Andersson and Wagner, 1995). Inhibition of this H_2 by these drugs may theoretically contribute to ED.

Opiates. Long-term intrathecal administration of opiates results in hypogonadotropic hypogonadism and associated sexual dysfunction that can be restored with appropriate supplementation (Abs et al., 2000). However, administration of opioid antagonists to older men with ED was not found to improve erectile function measured objectively by nocturnal penile tumescence monitoring (Billington et al., 1990). Opioids have a generalized depressant effect on sexual function when directly administered to the MPOA in rat brain, but treatment with the opioid receptor antagonist naloxone had no sexual effect on healthy male volunteers (Andersson and Wagner, 1995).

Antiretroviral Agents. Hypogonadism and ED appear to be more common among men infected with human immunodeficiency virus (HIV) compared with age-matched men in the general US population (Crum et al., 2005). Sexual dysfunction seems to be a common event after the introduction of antiretroviral therapy (Collazos, 2007). These disturbances seemed to be more common in patients treated with protease inhibitors. Because these patients may have diseases involving several organ systems and may be taking multiple drugs, the precise mechanism of antiretroviral therapy related ED is difficult to determine.

Tobacco. Tobacco use has been clearly linked to ED (Biebel et al., 2016). The Boston Area Community Health (BACH) survey reported a significant dose-response association between smoking and ED with a statistically significant effect observed at 20 or more pack-years of exposure. Passive smoking (i.e., frequent exposure to another individual who is a smoker) was associated with a small, statistically insignificant increase in risk of ED comparable with approximately 10 to 19 pack-years of active smoking (Kupelian et al., 2007).

Nicotine binds to nicotinic receptors and induced contraction of corporal cells in rabbits; inhibition of cyclo-oxygenase, Rho Kinase, and thromboxane A2 synthesis reduces this contractile effect of nicotine (Nguyen et al., 2015). Rats exposed to tobacco smoke have impaired penile hemodynamics in response to cavernous nerve electrostimulation; this is associated with decreased NOS expression and increased oxidative stress and apoptosis in corporal tissues (Huang et al., 2015). Chronic exposure to tobacco extracts has also been linked to impaired NO production from blunted NOS activity, downregulation of nNOS protein, accumulation of endogenous NOS inhibitors, enhanced arginase activity, and upregulation of arginase I protein in cavernous tissue (Imamura et al., 2007).

TABLE 68.11 Drug-Induced Erectile Dysfunction and Suggested Alternatives

CLASS	KNOWN TO CAUSE ERECTILE DYSFUNCTION	SUGGESTED ALTERNATIVES
Antihypertensives	Thiazide diuretics General beta-blockers	**Angiotensin-converting enzyme inhibitors** **Angiotensin II receptor antagonists** **Selective beta-blockers** Alpha-blockers Calcium channel blockers
Psychotropics	Antipsychotics Antidepressants Anxiolytics	Newer anxiolytics (bupropion, buspirone)
Antiandrogen	Androgen receptor antagonists Luteinizing hormone–releasing hormone agonists 5α-Reductase inhibitors	n/a
Recreational drugs	Tobacco Alcohol (large volume)	Tobacco cessation Alcohol in moderate

Alcohol. **Alcohol in small amounts has been associated with improved erection and sexual drive because of its vasodilatory effect and suppression of anxiety. In larger quantities, alcohol can cause central sedation, decreased libido, and transient ED.** In the Western Australia Men's Health Study the age-adjusted odds of ED were lower among current, weekend, and binge drinkers compared with nondrinkers; the odds of ED were higher in ex-drinkers (Chew et al., 2009).

Chronic alcoholism may result in liver dysfunction, decreased testosterone and increased estrogen levels, and alcoholic polyneuropathy, which may also affect penile nerves (Miller and Gold, 1988). In an in vitro study of rabbits given 5% alcohol for 6 weeks, augmented smooth muscle contraction and relaxation to electrical field stimulation and vasoconstrictors such as phenylephrine and potassium chloride was noted. However, there was no increase in relaxation in response to sodium nitroprusside (Saito et al., 1994). Some of the effects of alcohol may be mediated by increased oxidative stress, reactivity to the constrictor effects of endothlin-1, and activation of the RhoA/Rho-kinase pathway (Muniz et al., 2015). Duration of exposure may also play a role; impaired endothelium-dependent relaxation of cavernous smooth muscle and damage of endothelium was reported in mice exposed to subacute ethanol dosing for 14 days; a 7-day exposure group did not manifest significant changes (Table 68.11; Aydinoglu et al., 2008).

Aging, Systemic Disease, and Other Causes

Numerous studies have indicated a progressive decline in sexual function in healthy aging men. **Greater latency to erection, less turgidity, decreased force and volume of ejaculation, a longer refractory period, reduced penile sensitivity, and reduced nocturnal** erections are commonly reported with increasing age (Masters and Johnson, 1977; Rowland et al., 1989; Schiavi and Schreiner-Engel, 1988). **The cause of age-related declines in erectile function in healthy men is incompletely understood but may relate to** heightened cavernous muscle tone (Christ et al., 1990) and age-related decline in serum androgens (Kaiser et al., 1988). Age is also associated with impaired endothelial function through reduced eNOS expression and action, accelerated NO degradation, increased PDE activity, inhibition of NOS activity by endogenous NOS inhibitors, increased arginase activity, increased production of reactive oxygen species, inflammatory reactions, decreased endothelial progenitor cell number and function, and impaired telomerase activity or telomere shortening (Ferrini et al., 2001a, 2001b; Segal et al., 2012; Toda, 2012). Enhanced activity of the RhoA/Rho-kinase (Jin et al., 2006) and RAS pathways (Park et al., 2005) and decreased activity of the relaxant angiotensin-(1-7) pathway (Yousif et al., 2007) have also been associated with aging. At the structural level, age-associated changes in animal models of ED include decreased smooth muscle content and increased caliber of vascular spaces in the corpus cavernosum (Costa and Vendeira, 2008). Additional age-associated changes include decreased gap junction protein connexin 43 content (Suadicani et al., 2009) and increased apoptosis (Ferrini et al., 2001a, 2001b).

Diabetes Mellitus. Diabetes mellitus is a common chronic disease, affecting 0.5% to 2% of the worldwide population. **ED is up to three times more common in men with diabetes (28% vs. 9.6%)** and tends to present at an earlier age (Feldman et al., 1994). The prevalence of ED increases with diabetes of increasing duration (McCulloch et al., 1980; McCulloch et al., 1984). ED among men with diabetes is more frequent in men with coexisting neuropathy and other signs of end-organ damage from diabetes (Fukui et al., 2012). **The presence of ED in a man with diabetes is associated with a greater than 14-fold higher risk of coronary artery disease, and cardiac mortality in men with diabetes** (Gazzaruso et al., 2004). Diabetes mellitus may contribute to ED by disruption of penile arterial circulation (Wang et al., 1993), reduced androgen secretion, peripheral neuropathy, impaired endothelium-dependent relaxation of the corporeal smooth muscle (Saenz de Tejada et al., 1989), loss of smooth muscle structure and activity (Mersdorf et al., 1991), endothelial apoptosis (Condorelli et al., 2013), and oxidative stress (Belba et al., 2016).

Numerous type 1 and type 2 diabetic animal models have been used to study the basic mechanisms of diabetes-induced ED. In these animals, diabetes is associated with endothelial cell dysfunction, incompetent cavernous endothelial cell-cell junctions resulting in an increased prevalence of vascular disease (Ryu et al., 2013). Other effects include decreased nNOS, reduced activity of eNOS, oxidative stress, increased advanced glycation end products, decreased elastin, reduced VEGF, hypercontractility of cavernous erectile tissue, and decreased smooth muscle/collagen ratio leading to impairment of the veno-occlusive mechanism (Yang et al., 2013). Upregulation of the Wnt 10b pathway in corporal cells and fibroblasts of diabetic rats has been associated with fibrotic changes in the penis (Shin et al., 2014). Angiotensin II signaling has also been implicated in diabetes-induced structural changes and oxidative DNA damage in the corpus cavernosum of rats. The mechanisms of angiotensin II–mediated erectile impairment may relate to activation of TGF-β and the RhoA/Rho kinase pathway (Li et al., 2017). Modulation of angiotensin II by captopril, losartan, or angiotensin-(1-7) ameliorated the negative effects of diabetes mellitus (Kilarkaje et al., 2013; Yousif et al., 2014). Activated Rho-kinase mediates diabetes-induced elevation of vascular arginase activation and impairs corpora cavernosa relaxation (Toque et al., 2013). Insulin-like growth factor binding protein 3 (IGFBP3) is increased in animals models of ED; inhibition of IGFBP3 has been associated with improvement in corporal erectile response (Yang et al., 2013). Neuropathy, possibly related to the effect of advanced glycation end products on neuronal microcirculation, may also contribute to diabetes-induced ED (Cellek et al., 2013). Evolving evidence suggests a role for impairment of H_2S metabolism as a potential contributor to the diabetic ED phenotype (Zhang et al., 2016). Summaries of mechanistic studies in humans and animal models, derived from the committee report of the Second International Consultation of Sexual Medicine, are shown in Tables 68.12 and 68.13 (Saenz de Tejada et al., 2005).

Metabolic Syndrome. The metabolic syndrome (MetS) refers to the constellation of glucose intolerance, insulin resistance, dyslipidemia,

TABLE 68.12 Summary Findings of Studies in Patients With Diabetes

FOCUS	FINDING
Anatomic	• Atheromatous lesions in large vessels and stenosis in pudendal and iliac arteries
Functional	• Decreased frequency and rigidity of nocturnal erections • Lower penile rigidity after intracavernous injection of vasodilators • High prevalence of penile arterial insufficiency on Doppler ultrasound
CAVERNOUS TISSUE STUDIES	
Ultrastructural	• Decreased smooth muscle content, increased collagen, thickening of basal lamina, and loss of endothelial cells (more severe in men with diabetes)
Functional	• Reduced eNOS and nNOS-mediated penile smooth muscle relaxation with preservation of NO-donor mediated relaxation • Increased advanced glycation end products in cavernous tissue • Contractile response to α-adrenergic agonist is higher in patients with type 1 but not type 2 diabetes • In human penile arteries, EDHF-mediated endothelium-dependent relaxation is significantly reduced in penile resistance arteries from patients with diabetes • Increased expression of collagen • Increased apoptosis in smooth muscle cells • Expression of tumor necrosis factor-α is also increased • Decreased insulin mediated transport of L-arginine and the essential cofactor NADPH, reducing NOS activity by absence of substrate • Increased expression of inducible arginase (arginase II) while depletes bioavailable L-arginine for NO production

EDHF, Endothelium-derived hyperpolarizing factor; *eNOS*, endothelial nitrous oxide synthase; *NADPH*, reduced nicotinamide adenine dinucleotide phosphate; *nNOS*, neuronal nitrous oxide synthase; *NO*, nitric oxide; *NOS*, nitric oxide synthase.

TABLE 68.13 Summary Findings of Studies in Diabetic Animal Models

MODEL	FINDING
Streptozocin-induced diabetic rats or mice	• NO-dependent selective nitrergic nerve degeneration in diabetes • Decreased endothelial and neurogenic NO-mediated cavernous muscle relaxation • Increased prostacyclin synthesis • Increased cavernous muscle tone owing to upregulation of ET-A receptors • Increased contractile prostaglandins and free oxygen radicals in hyperglycemic state, resulting in reduced response to acetylcholine • Increased glycated hemoglobin, which impairs endothelium-dependent relaxation in aorta and corpus cavernosum from diabetic rats • Impaired responses attributable to EDHF in the vasculature of diabetic animals • Reduced concentration and vascular content of L-arginine
Diabetic rabbit	• Production of cAMP in response to PGE_1 or forskolin is reduced after 6 months • Increased glucose-induced production of PKC mediated by oxidative stress • Oxidative stress interferes with endothelium-dependent relaxation of corpus cavernosum from rabbits

cAMP, Cyclic adenosine monophosphate; *EDHF*, endothelium-derived hyperpolarizing factor; *ET-A*, endothelin-A; *NO*, nitric oxide; PGE_1, prostaglandin E_1; *PKC*, protein kinase C.

and hypertension which are often comorbid and related to visceral adiposity (Kaur, 2014). **MetS is an independent risk factor for ED, and the prevalence of ED increases as the number of metabolic syndrome components increases** (Esposito et al., 2005). MetS is associated with aging and decreased serum testosterone levels (Rodriguez et al., 2007). MetS has also been associated with elevated levels of estrogen, and some of the negative effects of MetS in an animal model (i.e., decreased smooth muscle content and impaired relaxation response to acetylcholine) were mitigated by administration of an estrogen receptor antagonist (Vignozzi et al., 2014). Additional molecular defects that may contribute to ED in MetS include impaired endothelial function and increased systemic inflammation (Esposito et al., 2005; La Vignera et al., 2012). Uncoupling of nNOS and dysfunctional nitrergic vasorelaxation of penile arteries has been reported in an animal model of MetS (see Fig. 68.13) (Sanchez et al., 2012). The various molecular and histologic defects associated with the component elements of MetS also contribute to ED.

Chronic Renal Failure. Decreased sexual desire, ED, and ejaculatory impairment is common in men with chronic renal failure (Lai et al., 2007; Lew-Starowicz and Gellert, 2009). Up to 80% of men with end-stage renal disease manifest evidence of arterial and veno-occlusive ED (Kaufman et al., 1994). Many of the effects of uremia can potentially contribute to the development of ED, including disturbance of the hypothalamic–pituitary–testicular axis, hyperprolactinemia, and accelerated atheromatous disease (Ayub and Fletcher, 2000). Evidence from animal models of chronic uremia suggest that ED in renal failure may also be due to **decreased production and/or reduced bioavailability of endogenous NO, calcification of pudendal arteries, and decreased endothelial reactivity** (Bagcivan et al., 2003; Kielstein and Zoccali, 2005; Maio et al., 2014). Abnormalities of vascular and bulbocavernous reflexes in men with uremia suggest that autonomic neuropathy may also contribute to ED (Campese et al., 1982; Vita et al., 1999). In the setting of uremia nerves are thought to exist in a chronically depolarized state, likely related to serum potassium level. This effect may be mitigated by dialysis and may contribute to ED in this population (Krishnan and Kiernan, 2007). The presence of depressive symptoms is also an independent factor predicting sexual dysfunction in male hemodialysis patients (Peng et al., 2007).

Significant improvement of sexual function may occur after kidney transplantation (Tavallaii et al., 2009). Nevertheless, in a report of 182 men who had undergone kidney transplantation, 49% of men continued to have ED and 18% were sexually inactive (Espinoza et al., 2006).

Hyperuricemia. Elevated serum uric acid has been linked to worse erectile function in men (Aribas et al., 2014), although in one study the effect lost significance after controlling for glomerular filtration rate (Solak et al., 2014). In animal models of hyperuricemia impairment of erectile responses are noted; these findings are associated with decreased expression of NOS isoforms and oxidative stress in the penis (Long et al., 2016).

Other Chronic Medical Conditions. HIV appears to be a direct cause of ED; men with HIV also experience substantial stress (fear of virus transmission, changes in body image, HIV-related comorbidities, infection stigma, obligatory condom use), which may contribute to psychogenic ED (Santi et al., 2014). Other chronic diseases such as hepatitis (Chung et al., 2012), dermatitis (Chung et al., 2012), scleroderma (Rosato et al., 2013), chronic obstructive pulmonary disease (Lauretti et al., 2016), and likely many others are known to be associated with ED.

Primary Erectile Dysfunction

Primary ED refers to a **lifelong inability to initiate and/or maintain erections beginning with the first sexual encounter or masturbation.** Primary psychological ED is often related to anxiety about sexual performance stemming from adverse childhood events, traumatic early sexual experience, or misinformation. Although some cases of primary ED are primarily due to psychological factors and all cases feature psychological components, maldevelopment of the penis or its blood/nerve innervation may also lead to primary ED. Endocrine abnormalities, particularly low testosterone levels, are also implicated in some cases of primary ED, although decreased sex drive is likely to be the main symptom in this situation. Evidence to support these concepts is confined to observational studies with varying numbers of cases (Stief et al., 1989).

Micropenis. Micropenis is defined as symmetrical hypoplasia of the phallus and is often related to urethral developmental abnormalities such as hypospadias and epispadias or endocrine deficiency (Reilly and Woodhouse, 1989). The erectile tissue in such cases often functions normally; sexual dysfunction usually relates to lack of penile length or the degree of chordee, rather than to ED (Woodhouse, 1998).

Vascular Abnormalities. Primary ED in the presence of an externally normal phallus is unusual. Authors have described structural abnormalities of the cavernous tissue, such as absence (Teloken et al., 1993) or replacement by fibrous tissue (Aboseif et al., 1992). Other authors have found vascular abnormalities, including hypoplasia of the cavernous arteries (Montague et al., 1995) or veno-occlusive dysfunction because of aberrant cavernous venous drainage

(Lue, 1999). The underlying cause of these congenital abnormalities is unknown. Treatment in most cases is vascular surgery or implantation of a penile prosthesis; data on outcomes are scant.

> **KEY POINTS: OTHER CAUSES OF ERECTILE DYSFUNCTION**
>
> - Aging is an important contributing factor to ED. The aging process can affect central regulation of erections, hormone levels, neuronal integrity, vascular flow, and penile structures.
> - Diabetes mellitus and metabolic syndrome affect many organ systems and are associated with particularly severe ED phenotypes.
> - ED is associated with a number of chronic health conditions and may be a sentinel event for serious disease.
> - Drugs most commonly associated with ED include antiandrogens, antidepressants, and antihypertensives.
> - Primary ED may be due to psychogenic causes, inexperience, congenital penile anomalies, or defects of penile vascular structures.

PERSPECTIVES

The past two decades have seen a continuing explosion of new information on the physiology of penile erection and the pathophysiology of ED. These new discoveries not only enhance our understanding of the disease process but also provide a solid basis for improving diagnosis and treatment. We can expect that the application of new research tools and information in molecular biology, signal transduction, growth factors, microarrays, and stem cells will improve our understanding of erectile function and ability to help men (and their partners) who are suffering from this condition.

SUGGESTED READINGS

Andersson KE: Mechanisms of penile erection and basis for pharmacological treatment of erectile dysfunction, *Pharmacol Rev* 63:811–859, 2011.
Gandaglia G, Briganti A, Jackson G, et al: A systematic review of the association between erectile dysfunction and cardiovascular disease, *Eur Urol* 65:968–978, 2014.
Gratzke C, Angulo J, Chitaley K, et al: Anatomy, physiology, and pathophysiology of erectile dysfunction, *J Sex Med* 7(1 Pt 2):445–475, 2010.
Montorsi F, Adaikan G, Becher E, et al: Summary of the recommendations on sexual dysfunctions in men, *J Sex Med* 7:3572–3588, 2010.
Musicki B, Bella AJ, Bivalacqua TJ, et al: Basic science evidence for the link between erectile dysfunction and cardiometabolic dysfunction, *J Sex Med* 12:2233–2255, 2015.
Nehra A, Jackson G, Miner M, et al: The Princeton III Consensus recommendations for the management of erectile dysfunction and cardiovascular disease, *Mayo Clin Proc* 87:766–778, 2012.

REFERENCES

The complete reference list is available online at ExpertConsult.com.

69 Evaluation and Management of Erectile Dysfunction

Arthur L. Burnett II, MD, MBA, and Ranjith Ramasamy, MD

HISTORICAL PERSPECTIVE

Sexual medicine has evolved into a mature clinical discipline in the past few decades as a result of steady, considerable progress made in the basic science, epidemiology, clinical investigation, and health services research within this dynamic field. Erectile dysfunction (ED) management, a subcategory of the field addressing specifically difficulty with penile erection/arousal function, has advanced from its well-intended beginnings of psychoanalysis and sex therapy, accompanied by the use of aphrodisiacs, herbal supplements, and hormonal treatments, typifying the knowledge and approach to clinical practice in the 1970s, to an increasingly structured, balanced, and evidence-based process of clinical evaluation and intervention of the contemporary era (Table 69.1).

Well-grounded ED management principles, premised on the highest clinical standards of ethics, quality, safety, and cost effectiveness, are now well accepted by the scientific and clinical community in sexual medicine. These "guidelines" have derived from rigorous and timely review, organization, and reassessments of the constantly evolving body of knowledge in this field performed by assorted consensus bodies representing the spectrum of international and interdisciplinary authorities in sexual medicine. Most notably, the International Consultations on Sexual Medicine (ICSM), cosponsored variously by the World Health Organization, International Consultation on Urological Diseases, American Urological Association (AUA), Société Internationale D'Urologie, and the International Society for Sexual Medicine, have served this role and have published topical proceedings (Hatzimouratidis et al., 2016; Jardin et al., 2000; Lue et al., 2004).

PUBLIC HEALTH SIGNIFICANCE

ED is defined as the inability to attain and/or maintain penile erection sufficient for satisfactory sexual performance (National Institutes of Health [NIH] Consensus Statement, 1992). The definition has been revised over time with recent opinion accepting sufficiency for sexual satisfaction as a valid purpose of this function in the complex human context (McCabe et al., 2016). ED is a medical condition of major health significance, with implications that extend beyond treating the occasional patient who possesses a problem of seemingly non–life-threatening magnitude. **The value of properly assessing and managing ED relates not only to affected individuals and their partners but also to society as a whole, and its scope encompasses physical and mental wellness aspects related to addressing (or failing to address) the sexual dysfunction, concurrent disease management issues, as well as its socioeconomic burden.**

Epidemiology

Epidemiologic investigation, which specifies that study results are readily generalized to the overall male population, has provided powerful information regarding the nature, cause, and prognostic ramifications of ED. **As the most thoroughly studied sexual dysfunction in the context of epidemiologic research, ED is estimated to carry an overall adult male (older than 20 years of age) prevalence rate of 10% to 20% worldwide, with the majority of studies reporting a rate closer to 20%** (Derogatis and Burnett, 2008; Lewis et al., 2010). An age correlation exists for the prevalence of ED, with a worldwide prevalence of 1% to 10% for men younger than the age of 40 years, up to 15% for men age 40 to 49 years, up to 30% for men age 50 to 59 years, up to 40% for men 60 to 69 years, and 50% to 100% for men between 70 and 90 years (Lewis et al., 2010). A cross-sectional study among men seeking first-time medical help for new-onset ED found that one in four men was younger than age 40, and almost 50% of the young men complained of severe ED (Capogrosso et al., 2013). It was estimated that there were more than 152 million men worldwide who experienced ED in 1995, with a projection of the prevalence reaching approximately 322 million men having ED by 2025 (Aytac et al., 1999). This trend is maintained irrespective of racial/ethnic background or geographic region.

Current data have also confirmed that the prevalence of ED mounts with the presence of comorbid medical conditions, which include type 2 diabetes mellitus, obesity, cardiovascular disease, hypertension, dyslipidemia, depression, and prostate disease/benign prostatic hyperplasia (Braun et al., 2000; Laumann et al., 2007; Martin-Morales et al., 2001; Nicolosi et al., 2004; Rosen et al., 2004; Saigal et al., 2006; Seftel et al., 2013). This correlation has supported the premise that ED and comorbid medical conditions share pathophysiologic mechanisms, such as endothelial dysfunction, arterial occlusion, and systemic inflammation (Billups, 2005; Ganz, 2005; Guay, 2007; Kloner, 2005; Montorsi et al., 2004; Solomon et al., 2003).

Novel disease-risk relationships for ED have been described, likely also exhibiting such concomitant pathophysiologic mechanistic associations as endothelial dysfunction and systemic inflammation. These disease relationships include epilepsy (Keller et al., 2012a-e; Pavone et al., 2017), sensorineural hearing loss (Keller et al., 2012a-e), open-angle glaucoma (Chung et al., 2012a-d), urinary calculi (Chung et al., 2011), psoriasis (Cabete et al., 2014; Chung et al., 2012a-d), atopic dermatitis (Chung et al., 2012a-d), chronic periodontitis (Keller et al., 2012a-e), viral hepatitis (Chung et al., 2012a-d), varicocele (Keller et al., 2012a-e), gastric ulcers (Keller et al., 2012a-e), ankylosing spondylitis (Chung et al., 2013a), gout (Gelber, 2015; Schlesinger et al., 2015), inflammatory bowel disease/ulcerative colitis (Kao et al., 2016), interstitial cystitis (Chung et al., 2013b), Parkinson disease (Yang et al., 2017), obstructive sleep apnea (Bozorgmehri et al, 2017; Chung et al., 2016), and premature ejaculation (Brody and Weiss, 2015; Corona et al., 2015).

Although they are few in number, prospectively conducted longitudinal studies have documented the true incidence and disease-risk relationships for ED. In one study, a crude ED incidence rate was 25.9 cases/1000 man-years among men aged 40 to 69 years (Johannes et al., 2000). According to another study, incident ED statistics were 57% at 5 years and 65% at 7 years in men 55 years or older (Thompson et al., 2005). **Such studies have uniquely affirmed predictors for the development of ED, which include age, lower education, diabetes, cardiovascular disease, hypertension, cigarette smoking, cigar smoking, passive exposure to cigarette smoke, and overweight condition** (Buvat et al., 2010; Feldman et al., 2000; Inman et al., 2009; Jackson et al., 2010; Johannes et al., 2000; Salonia et al., 2012b).

However, the strength of the risk association is also gauged from the opposite analytic direction, and incident ED may indeed inform the risk of subsequent disease morbidity and mortality. This relationship has been best demonstrated so far with respect to cardiovascular disease. The placebo arm of the Prostate Cancer Prevention Trial

1513

TABLE 69.1 Evolution in the Management of Erectile Dysfunction

	DIAGNOSTICS	TREATMENTS	GUIDES
Pre-1970	Psychosexual history	Psychosexual therapy Herbal supplements	Studies of Masters and Johnson
1970s	Medical and psychosexual history Nocturnal penile tumescence testing	Penile prosthesis surgery Penile revascularization	International Conferences on Corpus Cavernosum Revascularization
1980s	Physical examination Endocrine evaluation Penile duplex ultrasonography, DICC	Oral medications Intracavernous pharmacotherapy Vacuum device therapy	Goal-directed management
1990s	Combined intracavernous injection and stimulation	Intraurethral pharmacotherapy Oral phosphodiesterase type 5 therapy	NIH Consensus Statement Process of Care Model
2000–Present	Biomarkers of vascular health neuroimaging	? Gene therapy ? Stem cell therapy ? Tissue engineering ? Shock wave therapy	ICUD algorithms (patient-centered approach) AUA Practice Guidelines (evidence-based approach) EAU guidelines

AUA, American Urological Association; *DICC*, dynamic infusion cavernosometry and cavernosography; *EAU*, European Association of Urology; *ICUD*, International Consultation on Urological Diseases; *NIH*, National Institutes of Health.

found that ED is a sentinel for future risk of cardiovascular events, comparable with that of current cigarette smoking or a family history of myocardial infarction (Thompson et al., 2005). This study established that men with ED were 45% more likely than men without ED to experience a cardiac event after 5 years of follow-up (Thompson et al., 2005). In another population-based study of community-dwelling men followed longitudinally, ED was associated with an approximately 80% higher risk of subsequent coronary artery disease at 10 years (Inman et al., 2009). In a long-term follow-up (15 years) of the Massachusetts Male Aging Study (Feldman et al., 1994), ED was found to be positively associated with subsequent all-cause and cardiovascular disease mortality and constituted a risk in this regard similar to that of conventional risk factors, such as increased body mass index, diabetes, and hypertension (Araujo et al., 2009). It is an increasingly recognized and striking observation, made in epidemiologic studies demonstrating the risk association of ED with cardiovascular events, that the development of ED at a younger age heightens this particular risk (Chew et al., 2010; Miner et al., 2012; Vlachopoulos et al., 2014).

Recent meta-analyses of longitudinal studies have supported the findings of earlier reports and have provided relative risk estimates. A meta-analysis of seven prospective cohort studies provided adjusted relative risks for ED subjects compared with healthy subjects, calculating 1.47-fold increased cardiovascular disease events overall and 1.23-fold increased all-cause mortality (Guo et al., 2010). Another meta-analysis of 12 cohort studies calculated overall combined relative risk for men with ED compared with the reference group to be 1.48 with cardiovascular disease, 1.46 for coronary heart disease, 1.35 for stroke, and 1.19 for all-cause mortality (Dong et al., 2011). A further meta-analysis comprising 14 studies documented relative risk of 1.44 for cardiovascular mortality, 1.19 for myocardial infarction, 1.62 for cerebrovascular events, and 1.25 for all-cause mortality for men with ED versus those without ED (Vlachopoulos et al., 2014). A recent study found a significant association between ED severity and overall men's health (measured by the Charlson Comorbidity Index), irrespective of cardiovascular risk factors (Capogrosso et al., 2017).

Besides a predictive relationship of cardiovascular disease based on incident ED, a similar relationship has been suggested with respect to carcinogenesis risk. The Longitudinal Health Insurance Database study in Taiwan showed that cancer risk was 1.42-fold higher in ED patients than in patients without ED during a 5-year follow-up, after adjusting for socioeconomic and comorbid health variables (Chung et al., 2011).

These compelling data regarding occurrence rates and risk factors for ED foster an understanding of the importance of this medical condition. **The subject of ED offers a veritable clinical barometer of overall male health status, and efforts geared toward advancing its management are immediately consequential for disease prevention, health promotion, and survival improvement.**

Health Policy

Sexual dysfunctions and ED specifically have taken on increasing importance with respect to their socioeconomic impact. **In addition to its medical comorbidity associations, ED is recognized to affect adversely quality of life, decrease occupational productivity, and increase the use of health care resources** (Krane et al., 1989; Litwin et al., 1998). Because of the heightened ease of use and availability of effective first-line treatments combined with a growing societal awareness of ED and an acceptance of its treatment, it is understandable that a trend toward increased use of health care services surrounding ED has been observed (Polinski and Kesselheim, 2011; Wessells et al., 2007).

ED can be included among a host of urologic diseases having a substantial burden on the public financially. Total expenditures for outpatient clinical management of ED (exclusive of pharmaceutical costs) in the United States in the year 2000 approximated $330 million, ranking it the ninth most costly among the most frequent urologic diagnoses (Litwin et al., 2005). By contrast, this cost was approximately $185 million in 1994 (Wessells et al., 2007). Individual-level expenditures on an annual basis associated with an ED diagnosis (inclusive of pharmaceutical costs) among affected 18- to 64-year-old males in the United States in 2002 were calculated to be $1107 (Wessells et al., 2007). The Congressional Budget Office estimate of government expense for ED drugs in 2005 was $2 billion for the subsequent 10 years (Polinski and Kesselheim, 2011). These data have enormous implications for governmental as well as nongovernmental agencies in the United States and worldwide, whose work must consider the practical distribution and fiscal allocation of health care services for ED. Some experts have accordingly urged an account of the medical necessity and cost of ED therapy when formulating grounds for insurance coverage (Polinski and Kesselheim, 2011). However, evidence points to rational coverage for ED therapy, and in fact a significantly lower use of this therapy has been shown as compared with ED prevalence (Hornbrook and Holup, 2011). Arguments support the fact that ED is not a frivolous indication for clinical intervention, having quality-of-life and well-being implications as well as importance with respect to health and life preservation.

KEY POINTS: EPIDEMIOLOGY AND HEALTH POLICY

- Approximately 20% of adult men worldwide experience ED.
- Risk factors for ED include increasing age and presence of comorbid medical conditions, such as DM, obesity, CVD, hypertension, depression, and prostate disease.
- Outcomes research has shown that ED merits clinical intervention, having quality-of-life implications and importance regarding health and life preservation.
- ED ranks among the top 10 most costly urologic diagnoses in the United States and must be included in considerations for fiscal allocation of health care services.

TABLE 69.2 Major Erectile Dysfunction Risk Factors

CONDITION	MULTIVARIATE ADJUSTED ODDS RATIO
Diabetes mellitus	2.9
Hypertension	1.6
Cardiovascular disease	1.1
Hypercholesterolemia	1.0
Benign prostate enlargement	1.6
Obstructive urinary symptoms	2.2
Increased body mass index (>30 kg/m^2)	1.5
Physical inactivity	1.5
Current cigarette smoking	1.6
Antidepressant use	9.1
Antihypertensive use	4.0

Data from Francis ME, Kusek JW, Nyberg LM, Eggers PW: The contribution of common medical conditions and drug exposures to erectile dysfunction in adult males. *J Urol* 178:591–596, 2007; and Selvin E, Burnett AL, Platz EA: Prevalence and risk factors for erectile dysfunction in the US. *Am J Med* 120:151–157, 2007.

MANAGEMENT PRINCIPLES

The approach to the evaluation and treatment of ED is most assuredly different from that of many other urologic diseases in several basic respects. The diagnosis of ED customarily involves an acknowledgment of the subjective complaint of erectile inability by the patient (or patient and partner), and extensive diagnostic procedures are generally not required to proffer the diagnosis. In addition, current first-line intervention in the form of effective oral pharmacotherapy is easily prescribed and administered and is frequently successful for the majority of patients. **However, notwithstanding the semblance that the management of ED is fairly uncomplicated, it is a structured process that critically incorporates several clinical practice concepts for bringing the best therapeutic outcomes to patients.**

Early Detection

Epidemiologic and clinical investigation has suggested that many patients with ED retain adverse clinical conditions and also lifestyle factors (e.g., diabetes, cardiovascular disease, prostate disease, overweight condition, current cigarette smoking, and physical inactivity) that potentially compromise erectile function (Laumann et al., 2007; Lewis et al., 2010; Saigal et al., 2006; Selvin et al., 2007). The extent of these risk factors results in an increased global cardiometabolic risk profile in patients with ED (Miner et al., 2012; Nehra et al., 2012). Calculated odds ratios underscore the extent to which various ED risk factors correlate with ED (Table 69.2). **These data support the contention that patients with identifiable ED risk factors likely experience the sexual dysfunction currently or will eventually develop it at some time. Clinical screening of such patients based on these indications is advantageous in allowing opportunities to diagnose and treat ED.**

Growing evidence has also suggested that a patient's genotype influences the risk of developing ED, consistent with proposals that molecular and genetic mechanisms account for the ED phenotype (Andersen et al., 2011; Lippi et al., 2012). This concept fits with the perspective that genetically determined biomarkers will eventually be defined to assess ED risk profile as well as level of responsiveness to a specific ED therapy in the advancing era of precision medicine. Genetic polymorphisms have already been identified among patients with pulmonary hypertension that can predict which patients will benefit most from phosphodiesterase type 5 (PDE5) inhibitors (Hatzimouratidis and Hatzichristou, 2008; Sekine et al., 2014). Precision medicine has the potential not only to optimize treatment but also to guide screening and management of comorbidities. Identifying genes that may link ED and cardiovascular risk would assist in identifying patients in need of further screening and management (Mata et al., 2017).

Medication use has also been associated with ED in up to 25% of presentations (Francis et al., 2007; Keene and Davies, 1999). The most commonly implicated classes of drug include antihypertensive drugs, such as thiazide diuretics and β-adrenoceptor antagonists, and psychotherapeutic drugs, particularly selective serotonin reuptake inhibitor (SSRI) antidepressants. Table 69.3 lists several drug classes commonly associated with ED. It is important to recognize that

TABLE 69.3 Drugs Associated With Erectile Dysfunction

CLASS	SPECIFIC AGENTS
Antihypertensives	Thiazide diuretics, nonselective beta-blockers
Antidepressants	Tricyclics; selective serotonin reuptake inhibitors
Antipsychotics	Phenothiazines
Antiandrogens	Nonsteroidal (flutamide); steroidal; luteinizing hormone–releasing hormone analogues
Antiulcer drugs	Histamine H$_2$ receptor antagonists (cimetidine)
Cytotoxic agents	Cyclophosphamide, methotrexate
Opiates	Morphine

medications may affect other components of the male sexual response cycle, including sexual desire, arousal, and orgasm, which secondarily hamper erectile function. Of additional importance, the assignment of causation of ED for any particular medication is conditional, requiring that an increased prevalence exists in the target population compared with the placebo group after stratification for known risk factors or compared with another drug with an equivalent therapeutic effect, and, further, a credible physiologic mechanism should be established experimentally (Sáenz de Tejada et al., 2005).

Shared Decision Making and Treatment Planning

The therapeutic plan may vary for every patient and couple, and it ultimately depends on a host of factors, including patient considerations and clinical indications and contraindications. **An informed decision-making process should dictate the best therapeutic option.** It follows a balanced and thorough discussion led by the clinician of *all treatment options*, medical and nonmedical, and their expected advantages and disadvantages. Perceived risks and benefits, which may be influenced by the individual clinical situation, should be weighed. The patient may appropriately select a preferred treatment option without necessarily adhering to a strictly prescribed succession of attempted therapies. Patients are supported during the decision-making process to express preferences and values that align with their informed choice (Elwyn et al., 2012). Indeed, the patient may

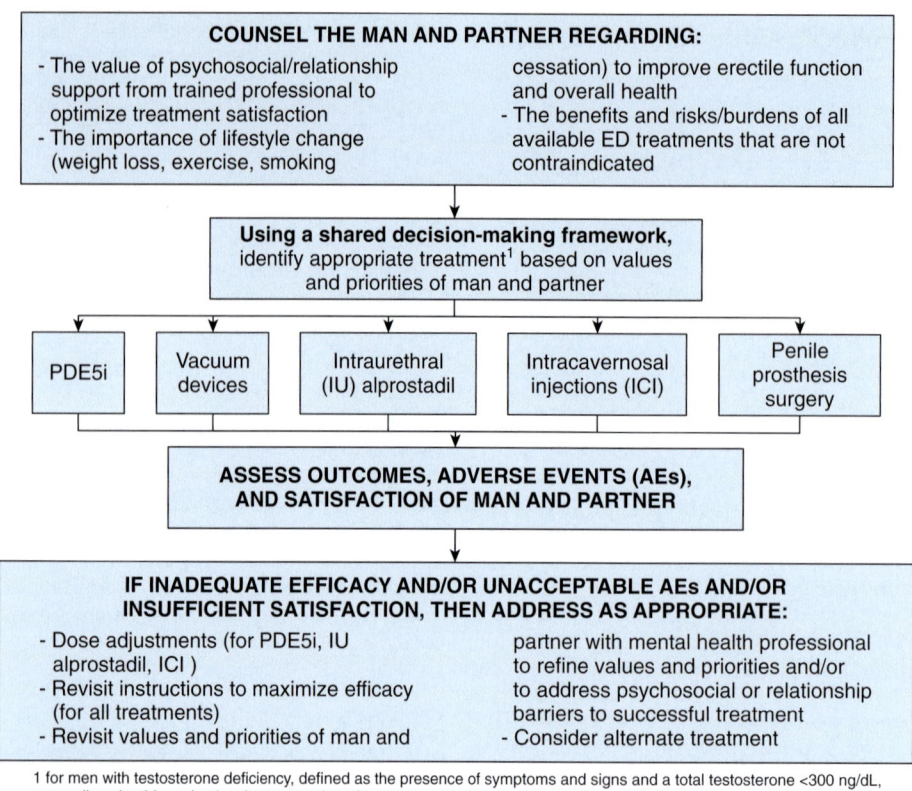

Fig. 69.1. Algorithm for shared decision making and treatment planning. *ED*, Erectile dysfunction; *PDE5i*, phosphodiesterase type 5.

elect to defer treatment altogether. Whatever the patient (or couple) chooses, this option can then be pursued within the boundaries of safety, under the supportive partnership of his clinician. This approach borrows to some extent from the goal-directed ED management approach, which is clearly described by Lue (1990) and fits with the patient-centered framework of managing ED (Hatzichristou et al., 2010). A meta-analysis of randomized clinical trials comparing shared decision making to routine care found that patients participating in shared decision making are more knowledgeable and have higher congruence between the chosen therapy and their values (Stacey et al., 2014). The American Urological Association (AUA) ED guideline panel has endorsed shared decision making as the state of the art in ED management (Burnett et al., 2018; Fig. 69.1).

Step-Care Approach

Practitioners of ED management have always sought a rational approach for implementing diagnostic and therapeutic options. The Process of Care Model for Erectile Dysfunction was proposed as a stepwise methodology, combining processes, actions, and outcomes in the management of the ED patient (Process of Care Consensus Panel, 1999). It specified an algorithm for therapeutic decision making that takes into account patient needs and preferences (goal-directed management), although it was also based on specific criteria such as ease of administration, reversibility, relative invasiveness, and cost of therapies. This algorithm presented a strategy of staged therapy (i.e., first-, second-, and third-line interventions), which ranged from lifestyle modification to surgery. **In concept, the scheme has been borrowed and endorsed by other consensus panels that acknowledged the purpose of patient education and counseling along with medical therapies as initial forms of ED management in common practice** (Hatzichristou et al., 2010; Montague et al., 2005). Although the step-care approach has commonly been used, the contemporary of management of ED emphasize the shared decision-making model (Burnett et al., 2018).

Role of Partner Interview

The partner interview is a critical component in initiating management of ED. Partner interviews have been shown to affect diagnosis and treatment in as many as 58% of cases (Chun and Carson, 2001; Tiefer and Schuetz-Mueller, 1995). **The partner may be the source of important information that guides optimal intervention and response to therapy. The partner may share a new and different perspective on sexual issues affecting the couple, provide insight into the quality of the couple's relationship, and relate his/her role in the sexual dysfunction** (Fisher et al., 2009; Speckens et al., 1995). **The partner's involvement and attitude may also affect the patient's initiation of and adherence to therapy** (Fisher et al., 2005; Jackson and Lue, 1998).

An important additional consideration is that partners' well-being may be affected by the patients' ED conditions. Studies have shown that women partners of men with ED are more likely to have sexual dysfunction or to cease sexual activity entirely (Fisher et al., 2005; Ichikawa et al., 2004; Montorsi and Althof, 2004; Sand and Fisher, 2007). This observation further prompts the facilitatory role of the partner in ED management, which maximizes the success of therapy and inherently the satisfaction of the couple.

In practice, and as necessary, additional office visits, during which the partner accompanies the patient and the patient communicates educational information to the partner, are recommended techniques for involving partners in ED management (Dean et al., 2008).

Cardiac Risk Assessment

The frequent coexistence of ED and cardiovascular disease, as established by clinical epidemiologic study and by basic science research, has steered ED management to include procedures that account for the ED patient's cardiovascular health risks. The Princeton Consensus Conferences, a multidisciplinary forum convened successively on three occasions since the early 2000s, have emphasized

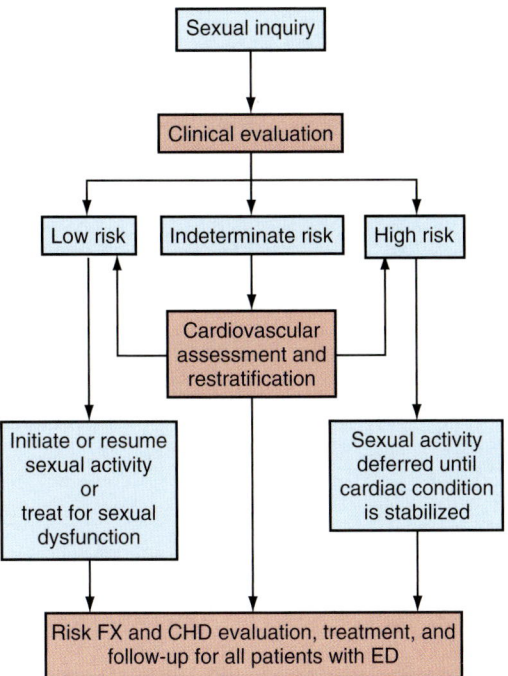

Fig. 69.2. Algorithm for evaluation of the patient with cardiovascular disease recommended by the Second Princeton Panel. *CHD,* Coronary heart disease; *ED,* erectile dysfunction; *FX,* factors.

the link between sexual activity and cardiac risk and have pronounced that all men with ED, even in the absence of manifesting cardiac symptoms, should be regarded as having potential risks for cardiovascular disease (DeBusk et al., 2000; Jackson et al., 2006a,b; Kostis et al., 2005; Nehra et al., 2012). The presence of ED improves the sensitivity of screening asymptomatic cardiovascular disease in men with diabetes (Gazzaruso, 2011; Turek, 2013) and increases the risk of cardiovascular disease, coronary artery disease, and stroke (Dong, 2011; Gandaglia, 2014; Vlachopoulos, 2014).

According to the Princeton Consensus expert panel guidelines, patients with ED are recommended to undergo a full medical assessment with stratification of cardiovascular risk as high, medium, or low (Fig. 69.2). Patients classified as having a high risk would be those with unstable or refractory angina, a recent history of myocardial infarction, certain arrhythmias, or uncontrolled hypertension. For these patients, sexual activity with any particular ED therapy should be deferred until the cardiac condition is stabilized. Such patients should ideally undergo cardiologic referral for cardiovascular stress testing and subsequent risk-reduction therapy. Importantly, even patients at low risk for cardiovascular events should receive the minimum recommendations of cardiovascular disease management. Basic intervention includes counseling for lifestyle modifications such as increased physical activity and improved weight control combined with regular health monitoring by the patient's general practitioner (Kostis et al., 2005). A more comprehensive approach specifies cardiovascular risk reduction and affirmation of exercise tolerance for sexual activity after noninvasive cardiovascular risk assessment that may involve a specialist or collaborative medical team having such expertise (Nehra et al., 2012).

Specialist Referral

The advent of effective oral pharmacotherapy for ED has enabled many primary practitioners to feel comfortable with managing the majority of clinical presentations of ED. At the same time, it is understood that situations arise in which the patient or primary practitioner may request the assistance of a consultant/specialist (e.g., cardiologist, endocrinologist, psychologist, or urologist) for further diagnostic evaluation and treatment beyond the boundaries of initial management (Process of Care Consensus Panel, 1999). Such referrals may be required for individuals with complicated or atypical presentations of ED, representing diagnostic challenges that exceed common clinical practices of nonspecialists. Specialized evaluation and management potentially offer improved therapeutic outcomes for these presentations.

Generally recommended indications for specialized evaluations and associated consultants are failure of initial treatment, referred to a urologist; younger patients with a history of pelvic or perineal trauma, referred to a urologist; patients with significant penile deformity (e.g., Peyronie disease, congenital chordee), referred to a urologist; complicated endocrinopathies (e.g., secondary hypogonadism, pituitary adenoma), referred to an endocrinologist; complicated psychiatric or psychosexual disorders (e.g., refractory depression, hypoactive sexual desire), referred to a psychiatrist; presentations requiring vascular or neurosurgical intervention (e.g., aortic aneurysm, lumbosacral disk disease), referred to a vascular surgeon or neurosurgeon, respectively; and medicolegal reasons (e.g., workers' compensation claims), referred to a urologist.

A caveat is that effort should be made at the time of referral to ensure that patients are fully informed about the rationale, costs, potential risks, and potential outcomes of the referral and possible additional procedures. This recommendation is made in accordance with the principles of patient-centered medicine, by which patients (and partners where possible) should be included in the decision-making process.

Follow-Up Care

Follow-up care is an essential part of ED management and should not be overlooked. The objectives of this action are manifold. A primary basis is to ensure continual success with the therapeutic outcome. It has been shown that treatment discontinuation occurs at high rates among patients who are not reassessed regularly (Albaugh et al., 2002). Additional purposes are to reassess medical and psychosocial conditions adversely affecting ED and success of therapy, evaluate the need for dosage titration or treatment substitution, and monitor adverse drug interactions or drug-interaction effects. As always, follow-up attention offers educational opportunities for patient and partner with regard to addressing sexual health concerns as well as lending guidance for related health care matters.

DIAGNOSTIC EVALUATION

The cornerstone in the evaluation of ED involves a detailed case history, preferably taken from patient and partner, physical examination, and proper laboratory tests (Fig. 69.3). The diagnosis can be submitted based on an individual's report of consistent inability to attain and maintain an erection of the penis sufficient to permit satisfactory sexual intercourse (Lewis et al., 2004; NIH Consensus Statement, 1992). The original National Institutes of Health definition did not specify a parameter for the duration of symptoms to accept the diagnosis. Subsequent organizational statements did apply a 3-month interval as a minimal requirement diagnostically, except for in cases of trauma or surgically induced ED (Lewis et al., 2004).

Sexual, Medical, and Psychosocial History

The comprehensive assessment of any sexual problem begins with the performance of a detailed case history, including sexual, medical, and psychosocial components. The clinician may use brief checklists or questionnaires for the purpose of recognizing the problem and initiating its evaluation, although he or she should routinely perform a detailed interview to understand the nature of the sexual complaint. The sexual history component in particular should be elicited with utmost sensitivity, given the intrapersonal and interpersonal aspects of sexual dysfunction (Althof et al., 2013; Rosen et al., 2004d). Additional emphasis has been directed toward providing

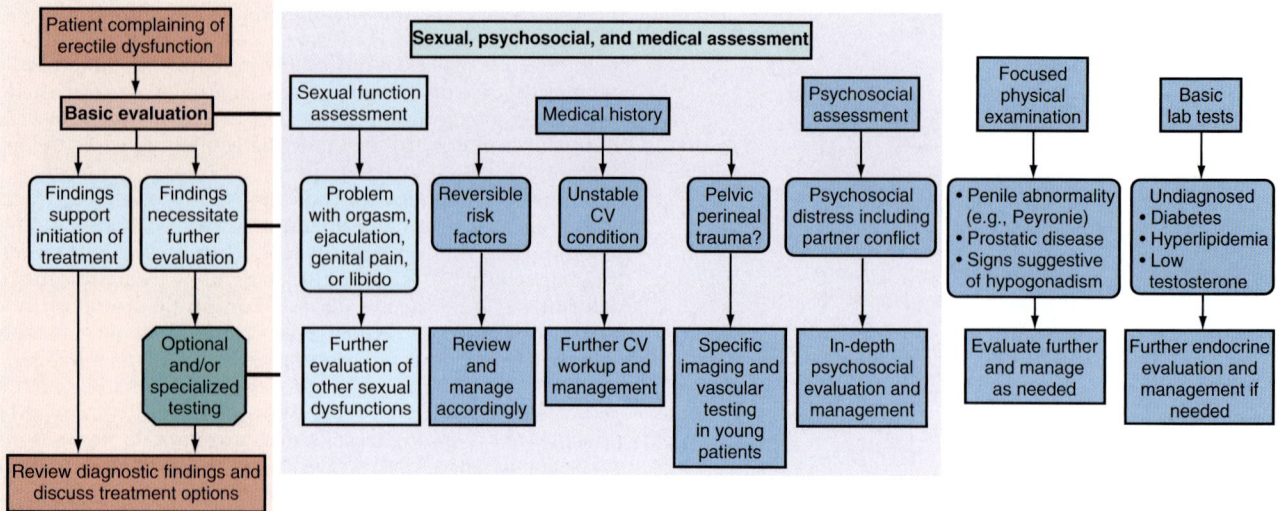

Fig. 69.3. Diagnostic algorithm for erectile dysfunction (ED) recommended by the International Consultations on Sexual Medicine. *CV,* Cardiovascular.

cultural competence when interacting with patients (Hatzichristou et al., 2010). All discussion of sexual matters is done privately and confidentially, and the clinician is required to express trust and concern as well as a nonjudgmental manner that epitomizes the doctor-patient relationship. The clinician should not assume that every patient is involved in a monogamous, heterosexual relationship. However, the situation may be presented in which the partner can be interviewed, and this opportunity may be used, with the approval of the patient, to corroborate aspects of the clinical history and to confirm mutual therapeutic goals.

Sexual History

The sexual history is the central component of the clinical history and can confirm the patient's sexual dysfunction complaint of ED. Objectives of the interview are also to delineate the problem according to such features as its onset, duration, conditions, severity, and cause. The conditions of the problem are often determined by reviewing circumstances that facilitate or hinder erectile function. Circumstances for achievable erections include stimuli used during sexual encounters, erections on awakening, and the role of self-stimulation. Circumstances associated with erectile difficulty include performance anxiety, inability to perform with a designated partner, and motivational factors affecting lovemaking. Other pertinent issues include availability, interest and health of the partner, changes in medical status or other events relating to the onset of ED, and previous attempts to manage the problem by the patient or another caregiver.

The severity of ED can be defined as mild, moderate, or severe/complete, according to increasing degrees of loss of penile rigidity and the associated interference with sexual activity. For instance, mild ED may refer to a minimally decreased ability to attain and/or maintain an erection with intermittent satisfactory sexual performance, moderate ED may refer to a minimally decreased ability to attain and/or maintain an erection with infrequent satisfactory sexual performance, and severe ED may refer to a substantially decreased ability to attain and/or maintain an erection with rare or absent satisfactory performance.

The potential cause of ED is commonly probed and may be categorized as psychogenic, organic, or mixed according to whether there is a presumed psychological or interpersonal determinant (psychogenic), a specific endocrinologic, neurologic, or cardiovascular cause (organic), or the coexistence of psychological or relationship factors and organic causes (mixed) (Table 69.4) (Hatzichristou et al., 2010; Ralph and McNicholas, 2000). Often ED cannot be fully dichotomized into psychogenic and organic categories.

TABLE 69.4 Classification of Erectile Dysfunction

PSYCHOGENIC	ORGANIC
Sudden onset	Gradual onset
Complete immediate loss	Incremental progression
Situational dysfunction	Global dysfunction
Waking erections present	Waking erections poor/absent

Modified from Ralph D, McNicholas T: UK management guidelines for erectile dysfunction. *Br Med J* 321:499–503, 2000.

However, its characterization by a predominant etiologic basis may nonetheless facilitate therapeutic objectives. The interview should also assess whether ED is the primary source of the presenting complaint or secondary to some other aspect of the sexual response cycle (e.g., desire, ejaculation, orgasm) that may also relate to the clinical presentation (Rosen, 2004a). The association of decreased arousal, if present, may be explored as well and evaluated to determine whether it preceded or was incidental to the development of ED.

Medical History

The medical history primarily identifies and evaluates predictors and risk factors associated with ED. **The main objective is to explore the role of possibly related or underlying medical conditions and to ascertain the existence of comorbidities. Recognition of the association between medical conditions and ED may not only lend insight into the possible basis for the ED, which may guide the choice of therapy but also specify reversible or treatable factors associated with ED that may be corrected with an expectation of improving the level of erectile function.**

Medical conditions associated with ED include disease states (e.g., type 2 diabetes mellitus, cardiovascular disease, hypertension, dyslipidemia, neurologic disease, hypogonadism, thyroid disorders), consequences of trauma involving aspects of the body, pelvis, or genitalia (e.g., spinal cord injury, pelvic surgery or radiation, sexual injury), and side effects of medications or recreational substances that disturb biochemical processes of penile erection. Age is recorded in accordance with the well-known association between aging and ED. It is important that comorbidities (e.g., depression, anxiety, anger) are registered because of their bidirectional relationship with ED.

Psychosocial History

The intake of psychosocial history is a necessary part of the clinical history. **The very best sexual performance implies wellness of mind and body acting together, and unstable psychosocial circumstances of intrapersonal and interpersonal contexts may adversely affect sexual function.** Accordingly, the presence and interaction of mental health problems, emotional stressors, and interpersonal relationship difficulties, past and present, should be ascertained. Additional questions may be asked relating to occupational status, financial security, family life, and social support, which may also influence sexual function.

Physical Examination

The physical examination is a highly recommended component of the comprehensive assessment of sexual dysfunctions and complements the clinical case history (Ghanem et al., 2013). It may show possible causes for ED.

This evaluation consists of basic anthropometrics (i.e., height, weight, waist circumference), assessment of body habitus (appearance of secondary sexual characteristics), and examination of relevant body parts pertaining to cardiovascular, neurologic, and genital systems, with a particular focus on the external genitalia. The observation of a classically distinctive body habitus consistent with Kallman or Klinefelter syndrome or obvious physical signs of hypogonadism, such as gynecomastia and general poor masculine development, may suggest an endocrinologic basis for ED.

Findings of obesity, elevated blood pressure, or abnormal femoral or pedal pulses, all signs representative of cardiovascular disease, convey a potential vascular causation. Findings of abnormal genital and perineal sensation or bulbocavernosus reflex (squeezing of the glans penis resulting in contraction of the bulbocavernosus muscle detected by a finger in the anus) may indicate the presence of a peripheral neuropathy in association with a neurologic disorder or diabetes.

Detection of a penile deformity, such as micropenis, congenital chordee, or Peyronie disease–related fibrous plaques in the corpora cavernosa, supports the possibility that a physical impediment accounts for ED. Genital examination findings of abnormal position, size, and consistency of testes may also suggest hypogonadism and indicate that ED exists on endocrinologic grounds.

Questionnaires and Sexual Function Symptom Scores

Self-administered ED questionnaires are extremely useful adjuncts to the case history, and they concur with the patient's self-report in establishing the diagnosis. Questionnaires supplied early in the field were very detailed, such as the Derogatis Sexual Function Inventory (245 items) (Derogatis and Melisaratos, 1979) and the Golombok Rust Inventory of Sexual Satisfaction (GRISS) (28 items) (Rust and Golombok, 1986), and they commonly aimed to differentiate psychogenic and organic ED or to evaluate sexual functioning in the context of the couple. Instruments developed more recently were implemented primarily in clinical trials associated with new drug development, and they particularly captured efficacy end points including sexual interest, performance, and satisfaction. However, as part of pattern shifts of practice that have occurred in ED management in recent years, there has been a growing emphasis on and application of patient self-reported instruments for clinical practice. **These self-report measures have been meant to be brief and practical and to document the presence and severity of ED and the responsiveness of ED to treatment.**

The most widely referenced instruments include the International Index of Erectile Function (IIEF) by Rosen et al. (1997), the Brief Male Sexual Function Inventory (BMSFI) by O'Leary et al. (1995), the Center for Marital and Sexual Health Sexual Functioning Questionnaire by Glick et al. (1997), the Changes in Sexual Functioning Questionnaire by Clayton et al. (1997), and the Erectile Dysfunction Inventory of Treatment Satisfaction (EDITS) by Althof et al. (1999). The IIEF, which contains 15 items that address and quantify five domains (erectile function, orgasmic function, sexual desire, intercourse satisfaction, and overall satisfaction) is the most widely used questionnaire (Fig. 69.4). An abridged five-item version of this instrument, the IIEF-5, has been useful to clinicians in routine clinical practice specifically for the evaluation of ED (Rosen et al., 1999a). The instrument classifies ED severity into five categories: severe (5 to 7), moderate (8 to 11), mild to moderate (12 to 16), mild (17 to 21), and no ED (22 to 25). The Sexual Health Inventory for Men (SHIM) is an abridged version of the IIEF, which also assess the five different sexual function domains. The Male Sexual Health Questionnaire offers another instrument that assesses core components of male sexual function (i.e., desire, erection, ejaculation, satisfaction) and is useful in clinical and research settings (Rosen et al., 2004b). The Sexual Experience Questionnaire is a brief but comprehensive tool for evaluating health-related quality-of-life concepts, and it comprises erection, individual satisfaction, and couple satisfaction domains (Mulhall et al., 2008). A new Visual-Scale Questionnaire has been developed as a quick screening tool for ED (Glavas et al., 2015).

A known limitation of self-administered questionnaires is that they do not distinguish a causative basis for ED; that is, they do not differentiate among the various causes of ED (Blander et al., 1999; Kassouf and Carrier, 2003). **Further, they may not sufficiently indicate the severity of ED that is evidenced on objective grounds** (Tokatli et al., 2006). Although the exact nature of the ED diagnosis arguably is not absolutely necessary to initiate ED treatment today with current management options, it is understood that further clinical evaluation with diagnostic tests may be required to discern the basis and extent of the ED by system (e.g., vascular, neurologic, endocrinologic) and take action that may be most effective and possibly corrective.

Cardiovascular Risk Assessment Tools

A trend in ED assessment is the application of cardiovascular disease-risk prediction models, which are used as scoring instruments to aid in the assessment of any man evaluated for ED (Nehra et al., 2013). **Such models as the Framingham Risk Score or an alternate global risk score, which incorporate such cardiovascular predictive variables as family history of coronary heart disease, body mass index, and metabolic laboratory biomarkers, offer a powerful initial step to characterize and possibly mitigate cardiovascular risk in this clinical setting.**

Laboratory Tests

Appropriate laboratory testing can be considered part of a systematic clinical evaluation for individuals presenting with ED (Ghanem et al., 2013). **Such evaluation may confirm or define etiologic medical conditions associated with the sexual dysfunction. At times, it may identify treatable conditions or previously undetected disease states that may contribute to ED.** A standardized panel of tests can be offered for the man who routinely seeks medical attention for sexual dysfunction including ED. Further laboratory testing can be tailored to the clinical situation. Similarly, specialized endocrinologic assessment can be performed when indicated for select clinical presentations.

Recommended laboratory tests for men with sexual problems typically include serum chemistries, fasting glucose or HbA1c, complete blood count, lipid profile, and serum total testosterone. Total testosterone, measured from a morning-time blood draw, screens androgenic status, and, if abnormally low, serum-free (or bioavailable) testosterone and luteinizing hormone (LH) should be measured. Prolactin measurement may also be done for hormonal assessment. Thyroid function tests may be performed at the clinician's discretion. Serum prostate-specific antigen (PSA) testing is performed as needed if there is a suspicion of prostate pathology that may be promoted by exogenously administered testosterone. Dipstick analysis of urine may show glucosuria, which suggests the diagnosis of diabetes.

SPECIALIZED EVALUATION AND TESTING

The implicit goal of specialized evaluations in medicine in general is to improve diagnostic accuracy and direct successful therapy based

Patient Name: _____ MR#: _____ Date: _____

OVER THE PAST 4 WEEKS

1. How often were you able to get an erection during sexual activity?
   - 0 = No sexual activity
   - 1 = Almost never/never
   - 2 = A few times (much less than half the time)
   - 3 = Sometimes (about half the time)
   - 4 = Most times (much more than half the time)
   - 5 = Almost always/always

2. When you had erections with sexual stimulation, how often were your erections hard enough for penetration?
   - 0 = No sexual activity
   - 1 = Almost never/never
   - 2 = A few times (much less than half the time)
   - 3 = Sometimes (about half the time)
   - 4 = Most times (much more than half the time)
   - 5 = Almost always/always

3. When you attempted sexual intercourse, how often were you able to penetrate (enter)?
   - 0 = Did not attempt intercourse
   - 1 = Almost never/never
   - 2 = A few times (much less than half the time)
   - 3 = Sometimes (about half the time)
   - 4 = Most times (much more than half the time)
   - 5 = Almost always/always

4. During sexual intercourse, how often were you able to maintain your erection after you had penetrated (entered) your partner?
   - 0 = Did not attempt intercourse
   - 1 = Almost never/never
   - 2 = A few times (much less than half the time)
   - 3 = Sometimes (about half the time)
   - 4 = Most times (much more than half the time)
   - 5 = Almost always/always

5. During sexual intercourse, how difficult was it to maintain your erection to complete intercourse?
   - 0 = Did not attempt intercourse
   - 1 = Extremely difficult
   - 2 = Very difficult
   - 3 = Difficult
   - 4 = Slightly difficult
   - 5 = Not difficult

6. How many times have you attempted sexual intercourse?
   - 0 = No attempts
   - 1 = One to two attempts
   - 2 = Three to four attempts
   - 3 = Five to six attempts
   - 4 = Seven to ten attempts
   - 5 = Eleven or more attempts

7. When you attempted sexual intercourse, how often was it satisfactory to you?
   - 0 = Did not attempt intercourse
   - 1 = Almost never/never
   - 2 = A few times (much less than half the time)
   - 3 = Sometimes (about half the time)
   - 4 = Most times (much more than half the time)
   - 5 = Almost always/always

8. How much have you enjoyed sexual intercourse?
   - 0 = No intercourse
   - 1 = No enjoyment
   - 2 = Not very enjoyable
   - 3 = Fairly enjoyable
   - 4 = Highly enjoyable
   - 5 = Very highly enjoyable

9. When you had sexual stimulation or intercourse, how often did you ejaculate?
   - 0 = No sexual stimulation/intercourse
   - 1 = Almost never/never
   - 2 = A few times (much less than half the time)
   - 3 = Sometimes (about half the time)
   - 4 = Most times (much more than half the time)
   - 5 = Almost always/always

10. When you had sexual stimulation or intercourse, how often did you have the feeling of orgasm or climax?
    - 0 = No sexual stimulation/intercourse
    - 1 = Almost never/never
    - 2 = A few times (much less than half the time)
    - 3 = Sometimes (about half the time)
    - 4 = Most times (much more than half the time)
    - 5 = Almost always/always

11. How often have you felt sexual desire?
    - 1 = Almost never/never
    - 2 = A few times (much less than half the time)
    - 3 = Sometimes (about half the time)
    - 4 = Most times (much more than half the time)
    - 5 = Almost always/always

12. How would you rate your level of sexual desire?
    - 1 = Very low/none at all
    - 2 = Low
    - 3 = Moderate
    - 4 = High
    - 5 = Very high

13. How satisfied have you been with your overall sex life?
    - 1 = Very dissatisfied
    - 2 = Moderately dissatisfied
    - 3 = About equally satisfied and dissatisfied
    - 4 = Moderately satisfied
    - 5 = Very satisfied

14. How satisfied have you been with your sexual relationship with your partner?
    - 1 = Very dissatisfied
    - 2 = Moderately dissatisfied
    - 3 = About equally satisfied and dissatisfied
    - 4 = Moderately satisfied
    - 5 = Very satisfied

15. How do you rate your confidence that you could get and keep an erection?
    - 1 = Very low
    - 2 = Low
    - 3 = Moderate
    - 4 = High
    - 5 = Very high

Fig. 69.4. International Index of Erectile Function Questionnaire.

on the specific diagnosis. A similar principle applies to sexual medicine. However, at the present time, despite the availability of various technologies that may specify and define the causation for ED (i.e., vasculogenic, neurogenic, endocrinologic, psychogenic), the treatment plan for this sexual dysfunction can often be formulated without performing extensive diagnostic testing. **Nonetheless, such testing is frequently applied for diagnostic precision, typically by specialists, particularly in settings of complex clinical presentations.** Table 69.5 summarizes the most frequently used evidence-based test procedures for diagnostic evaluations of ED (Rosen et al., 2004d).

TABLE 69.5	Evidence-Based Tests for Organic Erectile Dysfunction and Recommendations

TEST	RECOMMENDATION
VASCULAR	
Dynamic infusion cavernosometry and cavernosography (DICC)	B
Intracavernous injection pharmacotesting (ICI)	B
ICI and color duplex ultrasound	B
Arteriography	C
Computed tomography angiography	D
Magnetic resonance imaging (MRI)	D
Infrared spectrophotometry	D
Radioisotope penography	D
AUDIOVISUAL SEXUAL STIMULATION (AVSS)	
Independent or jointly with vascular testing	C
With or without pharmacologic stimulation (oral, ICI)	C
NEUROPHYSIOLOGIC	
Nocturnal penile tumescence and rigidity (NPTR)	B
Erectiometer/rigidometer	D
Biothesiometry (vibratory thresholds)	C
Dorsal nerve conduction velocity	C
Bulbocavernosus reflex latency	B
Plethysmography/electrobioimpedance	D
Corpus cavernosum electromyography (CC-EMG)	C
MRI or positron emission tomography scanning of brain (during AVSS)	D

Data from Harbour R, Miller J: A new system for grading recommendations in evidence-based guidelines. *Br Med J* 323:334–336, 2001; Rosen RC, Hatzichristou D, Broderick G, et al.: Clinical evaluation and symptom scales: sexual dysfunction assessment in men. In Lue TF, Basson R, Rosen F, et al., editors: *Sexual medicine: sexual dysfunctions in men and women*, Paris, 2004, Health Publications, pp 173–220.

Grades of recommendation:
- A: At least one meta-analysis, systematic review, or randomized controlled trial with a low level of bias and directly applicable to the target population.
- B: A body of evidence including high-quality systematic reviews of case-control or cohort studies directly applicable to the target population and demonstrating overall consistency of results.
- C: A body of evidence including well-conducted case-control or cohort studies with a low risk of confounding, bias, or chance and a moderate probability that the relationship is causal, directly applicable to the target population, with overall consistency of results.
- D: Nonanalytic studies (e.g., case reports, case series, expert opinion).

Vascular Evaluation

The vascular evaluation for ED conceptually connotes surveying the vascular requirements of the sexual organ for the erectile response: arterial blood inflow, blood engorgement, and blood retention within the corporeal structures. **From a diagnostic standpoint, the studies aim to assist in deriving the classic diagnoses of arterial impairment and veno-occlusive dysfunction.** As for all diagnostic testing, hemodynamic tests of the penis require patient counseling regarding the purpose, alternatives, risks, and benefits of any procedure before its implementation.

Combined Intracavernosal Injection and Stimulation

The combined intracavernosal injection and stimulation (CIS) test is a first-line evaluation of penile blood flow because of its very basic manner of administration and assessment. **The test involves the intracavernosal injection of a vasodilatory drug or drugs as a direct pharmacologic stimulus, combined with genital or audiovisual sexual stimulation, and the erectile response is observed and rated by an independent assessor** (Donatucci and Lue, 1992; Katlowitz et al., 1993). **The test is designed to bypass neurologic and hormonal influences involved in the erectile response and allows the clinician to evaluate the vascular status of the penis directly and objectively.**

The clinician may decide the protocol for using vasodilator drugs. Alternative regimens include alprostadil alone (Caverject or Edex, 10 to 20 µg), a combination of papaverine and phentolamine (Bimix, 0.3 mL), or a mixture of all three of these agents (Trimix, 0.3 mL). The procedure requires a syringe with a ¼-inch needle (27- to 29-gauge), which is inserted at the lateral base of the penis directly into the corpus cavernosum for medication delivery. After needle withdrawal, manual compression is applied to the injection site for 5 minutes to prevent local hematoma formation. The assessment is done periodically subsequently with rating of rigidity and duration of response. Repeated dosing may be performed if the initial erectile response is poor. Return to penile flaccidity is required before allowing the patient to leave the office, and if detumescence does not occur spontaneously in approximately an hour after dosing, intracavernosal injection of a diluted phenylephrine solution (500 µg/mL) can be administered every 3 to 5 minutes until flaccidity returns.

A normal CIS test, based on the assessment of a sustainably rigid erection, is understood to signify normal erectile hemodynamics. Alternative diagnoses of psychogenic, neurogenic, or endocrinologic ED may then be considered. However, it is known that false-positive results may occur in as many as 20% of patients with borderline arterial inflow (as defined by the measurement of 25 to 35 cm/s peak cavernous artery systolic flow on duplex ultrasonography) (Pescatori et al., 1994). False-negative results are also possible and occur most commonly because of patient anxiety, needle phobia, or inadequate dosage.

Duplex Ultrasonography (Gray Scale or Color-Coded)

Duplex ultrasound of the penis after pharmacostimulation or CIS represents second-line evaluation of penile blood flow. However, it is the most reliable and least-invasive diagnostic modality for assessing ED. The test adds an imaging dimension and a quantification component to the evaluation of blood flow in the penis distinct from first-line evaluation, which relies solely on the assessor's judgment.

The technique consists of high-resolution (7.5 to 12 MHz) real-time ultrasonography and color-pulsed Doppler, which helps visualize the dorsal and cavernous arteries selectively and perform hemodynamic blood-flow analysis (Lue et al., 1989; Sikka et al., 2013). Scanning is applied to the surface of the penis and may include the entire penis from the crura in the perineum to the tip. Color-coded duplex ultrasonography indicates the direction of blood flow within vessels, with red designating direction toward the probe and blue designating direction away from the probe (Broderick and Arger, 1993; Herbener et al., 1994). Flow velocities are measured at baseline before injection and commonly every 5 minutes afterward up to 20 minutes. Cavernous arterial diameters may also be measured. Vascular anatomic communications between the paired cavernous arteries or between the dorsal and cavernous arteries should be noted (Fig. 69.5). Erection quality should also be simultaneously assessed and rated. An observed poor erection, possibly associated with patient anxiety, should prompt vasodilator redosing as recommended for the CIS test.

A standard pattern of Doppler waveforms occurs with hemodynamic changes in corporeal pressure during progression to normal full erection (Fig. 69.6; Schwartz et al., 1991). In the filling phase when sinusoidal resistance is low (within 5 minutes after vasodilator injection), the waveform increases in size consistent with high forward flow during systole and diastole. As intracavernous pressure increases, diastolic velocities decrease. With full erection, the systolic waveforms sharply peak and may be slightly less than during full tumescence. At maximal rigidity, when intracavernous pressure exceeds systemic diastolic blood pressure, diastolic flow may be zero. The sonographic color pattern of the cavernous artery may demonstrate an impressive shift from red to blue in association with the reversal of diastolic flow.

Normative values have been described for peak systolic velocity (PSV) and diameter of the cavernous arteries during increases in arterial inflow to the penis. Early studies documented that the PSV of the cavernous arteries consistently exceeded 25 cm/s within 5 minutes of vasodilator injection in patients with nonarteriogenic causes of ED (i.e., psychogenic, neurogenic) (Lue et al., 1985; Mueller and Lue, 1988). Investigators subsequently confirmed mean PSV of cavernous arteries after pharmacostimulation to range from 35 cm/s to 47 cm/s in normal subjects (Benson and Vickers, 1989; Shabsigh et al., 1990). A cut point at 25 cm/s included a sensitivity of 100% and a specificity of 95% in patients with abnormal pudendal arteriography (Quam et al., 1989). Diameter changes of the cavernous artery after vasodilator injection were found to increase less than 75% and rarely to exceed 0.7 mm in patients with severe vascular ED (Lue and Tanagho, 1987; Mueller and Lue, 1988). Importantly, unlike PSV changes, a percentage of cavernous arterial vasodilation was not found to correlate well with findings on pudendal arteriography (Jarow et al., 1993).

Vascular arterial anatomic variants may confound the interpretation of duplex ultrasonography (Breza et al., 1989; Jarow et al., 1993). Early cavernous arterial branching or the presence of multiple such branches may affect blood-flow velocity determinations of the main cavernous artery. The presence of distal arterial perforators extending from the dorsal or spongiosal arteries also may alter the measurement of cavernous arterial blood-flow velocity. Accordingly cavernosal artery velocity measurements may vary based on anatomic location (e.g. crus, proximal, and mid-cavernosal) (Pagano and Stahl, 2015). The clinician must recognize these variants as well as anatomic imaging location to avoid making the incorrect diagnosis of arteriogenic ED. On the other hand, asymmetrical blood flow of the cavernous arteries may have diagnostic significance. The findings of dissimilar cavernous artery velocity measurements, which are greater than 10 cm/s between sides, or reversal of flow across a collateral may suggest a significant atherosclerotic lesion (Benson et al., 1993).

Duplex ultrasound measurements are informative for diagnosing vasculogenic ED (Rosen et al., 2004d). **Cavernous arterial insufficiency is suggested when PSV is less than 25 cm/s; a PSV consistently greater than 35 cm/s defines normal cavernous arterial inflow.** Cavernous artery acceleration time (i.e., PSV divided by systolic rise time) greater than 122 ms may also indicate this diagnosis. Cavernous veno-occlusive dysfunction, which refers to failure of erection maintenance despite adequate cavernous arterial inflow, is suggested by assorted sonographic parameters. Generally meaningful at 15 to 20 minutes after stimulatory onset, these parameters include persistent high systolic flow velocities (i.e., PSV >25 cm/s) and high end-diastolic flow velocities (EDV >5 cm/s), accompanied by rapid detumescence, after stimulatory onset. In addition, vascular resistive index (RI), based on the formula written as

$$RI = (PSV - EDV)/PSV$$

has had tremendous diagnostic usefulness in this regard. The parameter is based on the concept that, as penile intracavernous pressure during erection achievement equals or exceeds diastolic pressure, diastolic flow in the corporeal bodies will approach 0 and the value

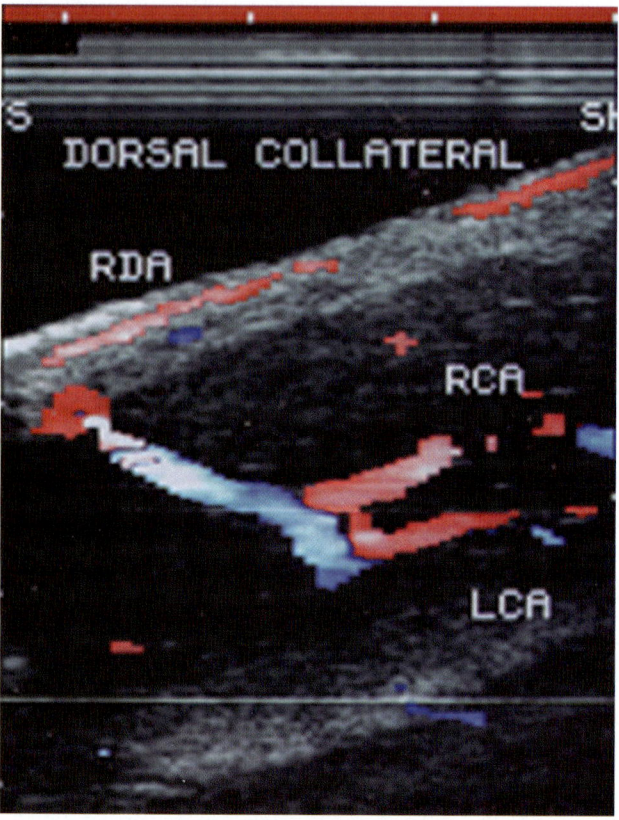

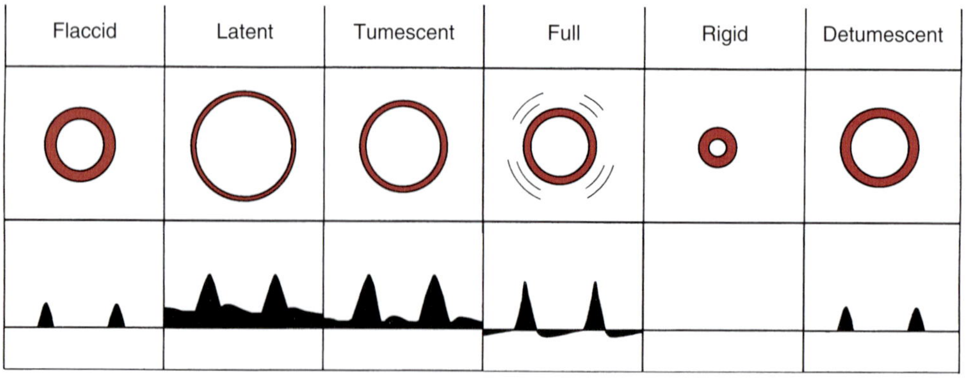

Fig. 69.5. Collateral circulation connecting the right dorsal artery (*RDA*) to the right cavernous artery (*RCA*), and the left cavernous artery (*LCA*) is shown by color duplex ultrasonography in a longitudinal view.

Fig. 69.6. Artist's conception of the changes in diameter and flow waveform in the cavernous arteries induced by intracavernous injection of prostaglandin E_1 in a potent young man as demonstrated by duplex ultrasound. Forceful concentric pulsations are particularly noticeable during full erection.

for RI will approach 1. An RI greater than 0.9 has been associated with normal penile vascular function, and one less than 0.75 is consistent with veno-occlusive dysfunction (Naroda et al., 1996).

Several technical modifications of sonographic evaluation of the penis have been described. A portable Midus-pulsed Doppler unit connected to a laptop computer for in-office testing reliably records the Doppler waveform of the cavernous arteries despite the lack of a real-time ultrasound image (Metro and Broderick, 1999). Power Doppler offers an even more specialized technique to visualize distal ramifications of the main cavernous artery down to the level of arterioles (Golubinski and Sikorski, 2002; Sarteschi et al., 1998). A somewhat more invasive approach that evaluates the integrity of cavernosal arterial flow involves the measurement of the cavernous artery systolic occlusion pressure (CASOP) by a Doppler transducer during saline intracavernosal infusion (Rhee et al., 1995). As a variation on the stimulatory component of penile sonographic testing, a combination of an oral phosphodiesterase type 5 (PDE5) inhibitor in association with visual erotic stimulation has proven an effective, noninvasive method (Baçar et al., 2001; Speel et al., 2001). Sonographically measured postocclusive vasodilation of the cavernous arteries, which is believed to relate to the level of intact endothelial function in the penis, has been found diagnostic for organic ED (Virag et al., 2004). Cavernous artery intima-media thickness as demonstrated by high-resolution echo color Doppler ultrasound has been suggested as being more accurate than PSV in predicting vasculogenic ED (Caretta et al., 2009).

Dynamic Infusion Cavernosometry and Cavernosography

Cavernosometry and cavernosography, precisely referring to functional hemodynamic and radiographic assessments of the corpora cavernosa, represents third-line evaluation of the vascular integrity of the penis. **The testing is indicated for select patients who are suspected of having a site-specific vasculogenic leak resulting from perineal or pelvic trauma or who have had lifelong ED (primary ED).** When used, it generally precedes consideration for corrective penile vascular surgery.

The technique involves two needles inserted into the penis for simultaneous saline infusion and intracavernous pressure monitoring after intracavernosal pharmacologic injection (Glina and Ghanem, 2013). The testing requires complete trabecular smooth muscle relaxation to avoid erroneous results, and repeated and maximal pharmacologic dosing protocols are recommended (Hatzichristou et al., 1995). Measurements of maintenance flow rate, pressure drop, and CASOP are performed to verify complete smooth muscle relaxation (Fig. 69.7).

Dynamic infusion cavernosometry and cavernosography evaluate the penile venous outflow system. **The existence of veno-occlusive dysfunction is indicated by the failure to increase intracavernous pressure to the level of the mean systolic blood pressure with saline infusion or the demonstration of a rapid drop of intracavernous pressure after cessation of saline infusion** (Motiwala, 1993; Puyau and Lewis, 1983; Rudnick et al., 1991; Shabsigh et al., 1991). The flow rate required to maintain erection at an intracavernous pressure of more than 100 mm Hg is normally less than 3 to 5 mL/min, and the pressure decrease in 30 seconds from 150 mm Hg is normally less than 45 mm Hg. Cavernosography follows cavernosometric evaluation and is intended to show the site of venous leakage (Fig. 69.8). With normal veno-occlusive function, there should be opacification of the corpora cavernosa with minimal or no visualization of venous structures or corpus spongiosum. With impaired veno-occlusive function, leakage may be identified into such sites as the glans, corpus spongiosum, superficial dorsal veins, and cavernous and crural veins. More than one site is visualized in the majority of patients (Lue et al., 1986; Rajfer et al., 1988; Shabsigh et al., 1991).

Penile Angiography

Penile angiography is an anatomic study of the arterial vasculature of the penis and represents third-line evaluation of the penile vascular

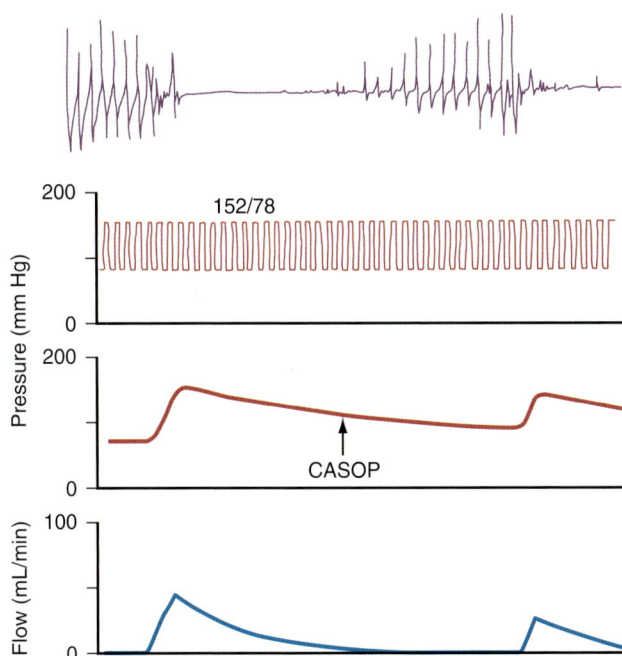

Fig. 69.7. This tracing depicts four simultaneous variables obtained during the third phase of dynamic infusion cavernosometry and cavernosography. *Top to bottom:* Cavernosal artery flow recorded by using a continuous-wave Doppler ultrasound probe; systemic brachial systolic and diastolic arterial blood pressure (150/87 mm Hg); intracavernosal pressure, which varied from 70 to 160 mm Hg in this tracing; and intracavernosal heparinized saline inflow. The intracavernosal pressure at which the cavernosal artery pulsations returned, which is the effective cavernous artery systolic occlusion pressure *(CASOP)*, was 108 mm Hg. The gradient between the brachial and the cavernosal artery systolic occlusion pressures was 150 to 108, or 42 mm Hg, which is abnormal.

system. **It is commonly reserved for the young patient with ED secondary to a traumatic arterial disruption or the patient with a history of penile compression injury who is being considered for penile revascularization surgery** (Sikka et al., 2013).

The procedure involves selective cannulation of the internal pudendal artery and injection of radiographic contrast. The intracavernosal injection of a vasodilating agent is optimally used to induce maximal vasodilation of the penile arterial supply. The anatomy and radiographic appearance of the iliac, internal pudendal, and penile arteries are then evaluated and documented (Fig. 69.9). The inferior epigastric arteries are frequently studied as well to determine their suitability for use in surgical revascularization. Significant variation of the intrapenile arterial anatomy exists, challenging the angiographer to differentiate congenital variations from acquired abnormalities and to establish their clinicopathologic relevance (Bähren et al, 1988; Benson et al., 1993).

Historical and Investigational Studies of Penile Blood Flow

Penile Brachial Pressure Index

The penile brachial pressure index (PBI) test refers to the penile systolic blood pressure divided by the brachial systolic blood pressure. The technique involves applying a small pediatric blood pressure cuff to the base of the flaccid penis and measuring the systolic blood pressure with a continuous-wave Doppler probe. A PBI of 0.7 or less has been used to indicate arteriogenic ED (Metz and Bengtsson, 1981). **The technique has not been found valid because it does not assess the hemodynamic properties of a functionally relevant, induced erection, and thus it is not recommended for use** (Aitchison et al., 1990; Mueller et al., 1990).

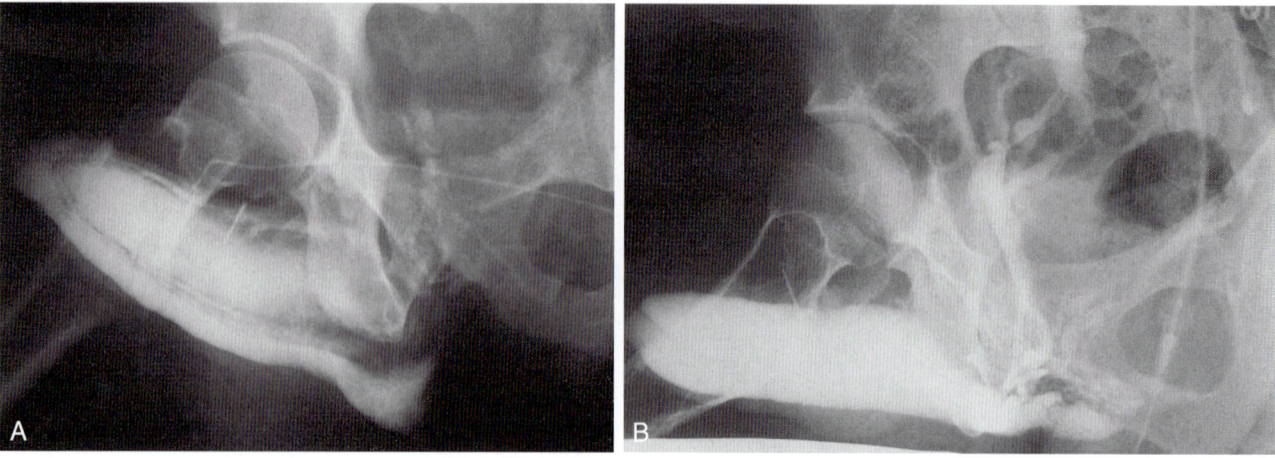

Fig. 69.8. Pharmacologic cavernosography. (A) In a patient 1 year after a penile fracture, a communication between the corpus cavernosum and the spongiosum is seen. (B) In a 27-year-old man with primary impotence, venous leakage from the crura is seen.

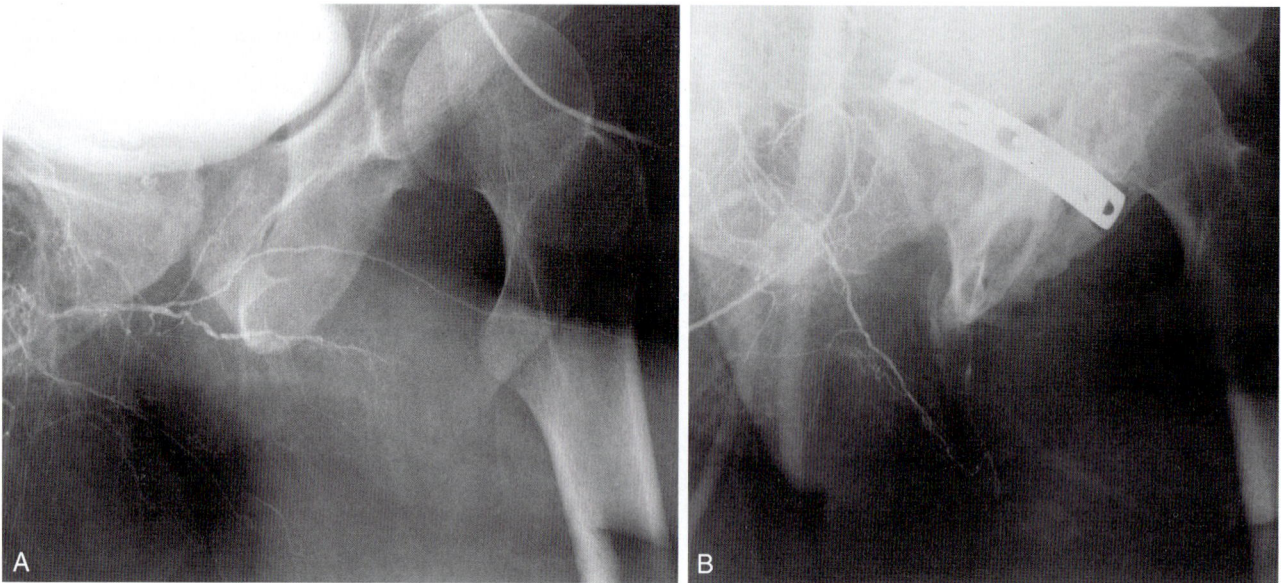

Fig. 69.9. In this patient with a pelvic injury, pharmacologic penile arteriography (after intracavernous injection of 60 mg of papaverine) shows patent common penile, dorsal, and cavernous arteries (A) and nonvisualization of the common penile artery and its branches (B).

Penile Plethysmography (Penile Pulse Volume Recording)

This test evaluates arterial pressure waveforms in the penis with an aggregate of the contributions of all penile vessels (Kedia, 1983). It requires the application of a 2.5- or 3-cm cuff connected to an air plethysmograph applied to the base of the penis, inflating the cuff to a pressure greater than brachial systolic pressure and then decreasing the pressure by 10-mm Hg increments while recording pressure waveform tracings. Abnormal pressure waveforms by diagnostic criteria have been used to indicate vasculogenic ED (Doyle and Yu, 1986). **Because this study is performed in the flaccid penis, as is the PBI, its clinical relevance has been questioned.** Despite this concern, a technical modification that measures postischemic flow-mediated dilation was introduced as being informative regarding penile vascular endothelial function (Dayan et al, 2005; Vardi et al., 2009).

Radioisotopic Penography

This test quantifies changes in penile blood volume after intracavernosal injection of a vasoactive agent using ^{99m}Tc-labeled red blood cells (Shirai et al., 1976). Extremely low flow is understood to mean arteriogenic ED (Smith et al., 1998). An evaluation comparing color duplex ultrasonography and radionuclide penography showed poor correlation (Glass et al., 1996).

Penile Magnetic Resonance Imaging

This test has significant potential applications for the assessment of anatomic details of the penis and penile microcirculation. Angiographic techniques may be combined with this test to evaluate the anatomic condition of the internal iliac and penile vasculature. Magnetic resonance angiography has been shown to correlate well with color duplex ultrasound testing (John et al., 1999; Stehling et al., 1997).

Penile Near Infrared Spectrophotometry

This test provides continuous, quantitative measurements of penile blood flow using a specialized near infrared spectrophotometry instrument (Burnett et al., 2000). It may be applied with an erectile stimulus and documents the hemodynamic phenomena of erection. Penile spectrophotometry has been further investigated in combination with intraurethral pharmacotherapy documenting blood-flow increase to the penis with this erectogenic modality (Padmanabhan and McCullough, 2007). Further investigation of this technique is needed to establish its clinical usefulness.

Cavernous Smooth Muscle Content

This test evaluates the smooth muscle composition of the corporeal tissue by light microscopic and computed morphometric assessment of biopsies of the penis and may serve adjunctively in the diagnosis of vasculogenic ED (Wespes et al., 1992). A reduced proportion of corporeal smooth muscle (and correspondingly increased collagen) has been observed in older men with veno-occlusive dysfunction (19% to 36% smooth muscle) and arteriogenic ED (10% to 25%), compared with that of young, healthy men with normal erections and penile curvature (40% to 52%) (Wespes et al., 1991). In part because of its invasiveness, the test is controversial and thus it remains investigational.

Psychophysiologic Evaluation

The psychophysiologic evaluation of ED seeks to assess the erectile response by applying techniques that directly measure penile tumescence and rigidity. From the historical perspective of ED diagnostics, testing was applied primarily to differentiate psychogenic from organic ED. In general, the documentation of a full erection indicates functional integrity of the neurovascular axis regulating penile erection and thereby raises suspicion of a psychogenic cause.

There are several approaches to perform this evaluation. Importantly, the psychophysiologic evaluation does not currently represent first-line evaluation for ED, largely because of technical and cost limitations associated with current techniques. When considered to undergo any of these tests as part of a diagnostic plan, patients are counseled regarding the expected use, risks, and benefits of the tests.

Penile Tumescence and Rigidity Monitoring

Nocturnal penile tumescence (NPT) monitoring, which describes the study of erections that occur with nighttime sleep, was classically described as a technique offering the assessment of physiologic erectile ability (Wasserman et al., 1980). **As a standard, sleep laboratory nocturnal penile tumescence and rigidity (NPTR) testing applies nocturnal monitoring devices that measure the number of episodes, tumescence (circumference change by strain gauges), maximal penile rigidity, and duration of nocturnal erections** (Kessler, 1988). The conventional approach is to perform monitoring in conjunction with electroencephalography, electro-oculography, and electromyography (EMG), with nasal airflow and oxygen saturation to document rapid eye movement (REM) sleep and the presence or absence of hypoxia (sleep apnea). Documentation of REM sleep is undertaken because of the observation that true erectile phenomena occurring during sleep are associated with the REM sleep phase (Fisher et al., 1965). Sleep movement patterns are also monitored because periodic limb movement disorders are associated with abnormal NPT. Axial rigidity is measured along with photography of the erect penis when awakening the patient at maximal tumescence; a buckling device is applied to the tip of the penis to measure resistance (500 g minimum for vaginal penetration, 1.5 kg suggestive of complete rigidity) (Karacan et al., 1977). NPT traditionally has been performed during two to three nights to overcome the so-called first-night effect when REM sleep is inconsistent. Formal testing, which involves a specially equipped sleep laboratory staffed with trained observers, is costly. The monitoring of diurnal penile tumescence, in reference to monitoring performed during daytime napping, has served alternatively as an in-office evaluation (Morales et al., 1994).

RigiScan (Timm Medical Technologies, Minneapolis, MN) is an automated, portable device used for NPTR, which combines the monitoring of radial rigidity, tumescence, number, and duration of erectile events (Bradley et al., 1985). The device employs two loops, one placed at the base of the penis and the other placed at the

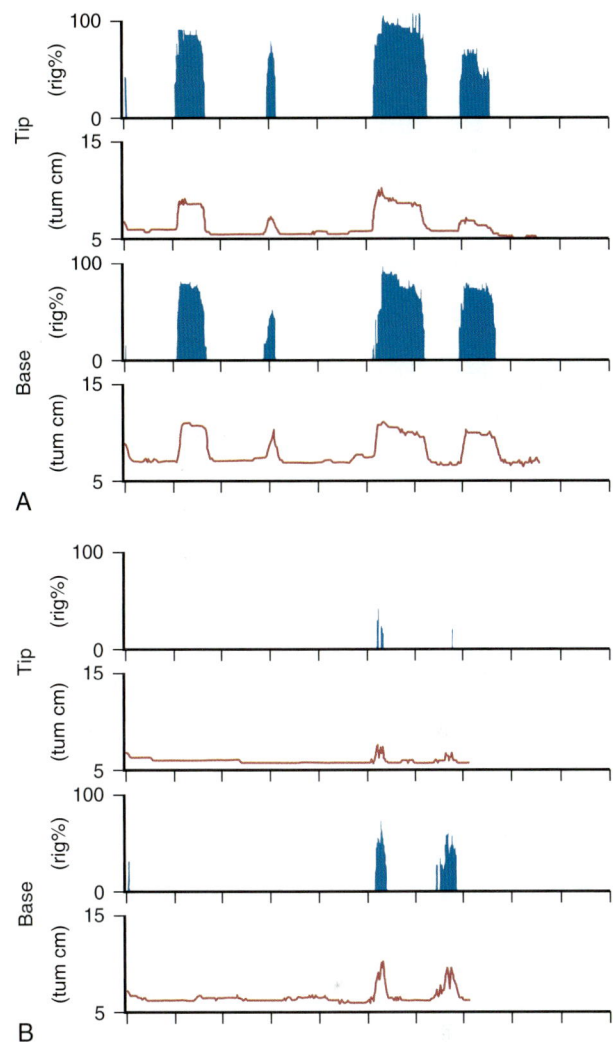

Fig. 69.10. The RigiScan device has been designed to measure penile rigidity during home nocturnal monitoring. (A) A study in a patient with at least two episodes of well-sustained, completely rigid nocturnal erections. (B) A study with two episodes of poorly sustained, poorly rigid nocturnal erections. Such home studies fail to document sleep quality.

coronal sulcus (respectively, base and tip recording sites), and these loops record penile tumescence (circumference) and radial rigidity with timed, standardized constrictions of the loops. A baseline initialization is performed with the patient in the office, and then it is calibrated for home use. At home, registrations of penile rigidity are done every 3 minutes and increased to every 30 seconds when the base loop detects a circumference increase of greater than 10 mm (Fig. 69.10). **Recommended criteria for normal NPTR include four to five normal erectile episodes per night** (Hatzichristou et al., 1998). A computerized program has yielded standardized data measurements according to cumulative distribution of time-intensity measures, defined as tumescence activity units (TAU) and radial rigidity activity units (RAU) (Burris et al., 1989; Levine and Carroll, 1994). A recent study found that RigiScan can accurately predict veno-occlusive dysfunction (Elhanbly and Elkholy, 2012). Potential limitations of RigiScan include the fact that radial rigidity does not accurately predict axial rigidity (Allen et al., 1993; Licht et al., 1995), and considerable variability apparently exists even in normal subjects (Levine and Carroll, 1994). Further, the manner of testing does not allow verification of the presence of REM sleep.

NPT electrobioimpedance (NEVA, American Medical Systems, Minnetonka, MN) is a device introduced more recently that assesses volumetric changes in the penis during nocturnal erections (Knoll and Abrams, 1999). The device consists of three small electrode pads applied to the hip and the penile base and glans and a small recording device attached to the patient's thigh. In operation, an undetectable alternating current is transmitted from the glans electrode to the hip ground, and the penile base electrode measures impedance and changes in penile length. Impedance measures decrease in concert with increases in cross-sectional area of the penis during nocturnal tumescence. Further investigation is needed to establish the relationship of volumetric changes and the rigidity of the penis. Similar to RigiScan, the technique also does not include REM sleep monitoring and correlations.

In summary, NPTR monitoring is an attractive approach for objectively evaluating the somatic basis of erectile ability, theoretically devoid of psychological interference. However, it has several apparent shortcomings that limit its routine use for diagnostic purposes (Jannini et al., 2009). Central issues are that the testing does not indicate the cause and severity of ED and that the results may be poorly reproducible. Another fundamental issue is whether the testing appropriately evaluates wakeful, sexually relevant erections. Indeed, erections observed during NPTR monitoring do not unequivocally equate with erections sufficient for sexual performance, and false-positive results are possible for various clinical situations (e.g., multiple sclerosis). False-negative results may occur in aging patients and in patients with depression or anxiety, which may conditionally affect the physiology of sleep-related erectile phenomena. Nonetheless, NPTR monitoring may be considered in special circumstances such as when the cause of ED is obscure and noninvasive testing is desirable.

Audiovisual and Vibratory Stimulation

Alternative erectogenic methods can be used in conjunction with diagnostic testing of erectile function. **Erotic stimulation by explicit videotape material with monitoring has been used as a reliable as well as a time- and cost-effective alternative to NPTR for differentiating between organic and psychogenic ED presentations** (Bancroft et al., 1991; Sakheim et al., 2007). **It is also considered more physiologic, consistent with erectile behavior when awake.** The testing has potential limitations, with possible false-negative responses occurring in the presence of endocrine abnormalities (Carani et al., 1992; Greenstein et al., 1995) and false-positive responses occurring in psychological situations such as erotic excitement inhibition (Chung and Choi, 1990). As one may infer, these methods can be applied in conjunction with other stimulatory conditions (e.g., pharmacologic erection testing) as well as erectile function assessment approaches (e.g., RigiScan monitoring) (Katlowitz et al., 1993; Martins and Reis, 1997).

Neuroimaging

Diagnostic techniques to evaluate central mechanisms of male sexual arousal have contributed to the psychophysiologic investigation of ED. Positron emission tomography (Miyagawa et al., 2007) and functional magnetic resonance imaging (fMRI; Ferretti et al., 2005; Montorsi et al., 2003; Mouras et al., 2003; Park et al., 2001) have been used in association with video sexual stimulation or an erectogenic pharmacologic stimulus (e.g., oral apomorphine). Studies have documented key brain regions associated with sexual arousal that induce penile erection (i.e., anterior cingulate, insula, amygdala, hypothalamus, and secondary somatosensory cortices). Interestingly, functional abnormalities in the brain have been shown in patients with psychogenic ED, suggesting that this diagnosis may be attributable to an actual biologic basis. More investigation in this area is necessary before determining its clinical role.

Psychological Evaluation

The psychological evaluation of ED addresses psychogenic contributions to clinical presentations, essentially psychological and interpersonal factors interfering with erectile function. These aspects should not be underestimated, and it is well documented in population studies that ED is associated with anxiety, depression, low degrees of self-esteem, negative outlook on life, self-reported emotional stress, and a history of sexual coercion (Feldman et al., 1994; Laumann et al., 2007). The urologist's role in initiating a psychological evaluation is not necessarily complicated, and a basic attempt to use queries about a patient's psychological health is helpful in assessing sexual health (Rowland et al., 2005). A two-question scale may be used in every day clinical practice: "During the past month, have you often been bothered by feeling down, depressed, or hopeless? During the past month, have you often been bothered by little interest or pleasure in doing things?" (Whooley et al., 1997).

The diagnostic interview is central to the psychological evaluation, and this process should be handled in a straightforward manner. Readily discernible causes of sexual dysfunction may be elicited, such as fear of failure, performance anxiety (for widowers, this may include complex interactions of dating, new partners, and unresolved mourning/guilt), insufficient sexual stimulation, loss of attraction for the partner, adjustment to a chronic illness or surgery, and relationship conflicts. In addition, causes that are less immediately discernible may be identified to include unresolved parental attachments, sexual identity issues, history of sexual trauma, occurrence of extramarital affairs, and cultural-religious taboos (Laumann et al., 2007; Leach and Bethune, 1996).

The interviewer should be mindful of the possibility of a primary psychogenic ED presentation (Turnbull and Weinberg, 1983). In the absence of organic risk factors, a primary psychogenic ED causation may be suspected. Further support for the diagnosis may follow the confirmation of noncoital erections (i.e., masturbatory, nocturnal, or when awakening). Clinical subtypes of psychogenic ED may be further identified: (1) generalized versus situational and (2) lifelong (primary) versus acquired (secondary, including substance abuse or major psychiatric illness).

The interviewer should also inquire about relationship factors (Rosen, 2001). Relationship conflicts may be the source of psychogenic ED or otherwise may exacerbate organic ED. A couple's issues include intimacy and trust, status and dominance, loss of sexual attraction, ability to achieve sexual satisfaction without erection, and communication problems. Not only is important information derived from interviewing the patient alone, but also interviews with the couple together and of partners separately may provide insight.

Complex intrapsychic causes of sexual dysfunction are often relevant for the ED presentation and may become evident during the diagnostic interview. The clinical history may show a significant traumatic life experience, cultural or religious strife, compulsive sexual behavior, or neurotic process. It may suggest the presence of serious psychiatric comorbidities, such as substance abuse, depressive symptoms, anxiety disorder, or personality disorder. The urologist may not have the professional background, comfort, or time to address these issues definitively, and a referral to a psychological expert for further attention would be appropriate.

Neurologic Evaluation

The neurologic evaluation of ED is concerned with neurogenic associations with ED presentations. The importance of testing for deficits in the neurologic system relates to the principal regulatory role of this system for governing erectile function. Target sites for evaluation include peripheral, spinal, and supraspinal centers as well as somatic and autonomic pathways involved in this biologic response. In line with this purpose, several diagnostic tests have been introduced. However, thus far they have had limited impact on routine clinical management decisions, and much of the available testing in this realm is reserved for research protocols and medicolegal investigations (Giuliano and Rowland, 2013). In addition, fundamental problems surround the lack of sensitivity, reproducibility, reliability, and validity for many of these tests. This concern is particularly so for autonomic function tests, distinct from somatic function testing, which has been shown to be reproducible and valid. Otherwise, tests that could be most useful for evaluating penile erection, for example, neurotransmitter release, are altogether undeveloped.

Somatic Nervous System

Biothesiometry. This test represents a technique to assess afferent sensory function of the penis (Padma-Nathan, 1988). Testing involves a handheld electromagnetic device placed on the pulp of the index fingers, both sides of the penile shaft, and the glans penis. Measurements of sensory perception threshold are obtained in response to various amplitudes of vibratory stimulation. Investigators have questioned the usefulness of penile glans biothesiometry, which does not accurately portray neurophysiologic function of the dorsal penile nerve because of limitations in recording responses to vibratory stimuli of glanular skin (Bemelmans et al., 1995).

Sacral Evoked Response: Bulbocavernosus Reflex Latency. This test is used to assess the somatosensory reflexogenic mechanism of penile erection. Testing consists of a direct-current stimulator, which delivers square-wave impulses via two stimulating ring electrodes placed around the penis, one secured near the corona and the other secured 3 cm more proximally, and a recorder that gauges responses via concentric needle electrodes placed in the right and left bulbocavernosus muscles. Latency period is measured as the interval from the beginning of each stimulus to the beginning of each response. An abnormal latency time, defined as a value more than three standard deviations above the mean (30 to 40 ms), indicates a high probability of neuropathology (Padma-Nathan, 1988). However, the use of this test has been questioned, and it has been shown that a full battery of electrophysiologic tests evaluating limb nerve function is more sensitive in diagnosing neuropathy than such tests specific to pudendal nerve function alone (Ho et al., 1996; Vodusek et al., 1993).

Dorsal Nerve Conduction Velocity. This test, in concept, extends from pudendal nerve function reflex testing and involves electrophysiologic stimulation with two stimulating electrodes placed at the glans and at the base of the penis for obtaining two bulbocavernosus reflex latency measurements. Conduction velocity of the dorsal nerve is represented by dividing the distance between the two stimulating electrodes by the difference in latency times recorded from both sites. An average conduction velocity of 23.5 m/s with a range of 21.4 to 29.1 m/s is found in normal subjects (Gerstenberg and Bradley, 1983). Abnormal nerve conduction velocities were found to be diagnostic for neurogenic ED in patients with diabetes (Kaneko and Bradley, 1987).

Genitocerebral Evoked Potential. This test is designed to assess afferent sensory mechanisms and stimulus processing at spinal and supraspinal nervous system levels. The testing requires complex electronic equipment for recording the evoked potential waveforms overlying the sacral spinal cord and cerebral cortex in response to dorsal penile nerve electrical stimulation (Spudis et al., 1989). Central conduction time is recorded as the difference between the latency times after stimulation of the first replicated spinal response and the first replicated cerebral response (Padma-Nathan, 1988). The test has been questioned as having poor discriminatory value of response latencies (Pickard et al., 1994). However, it may still serve as an objective tool to define characteristics of afferent penile sensory dysfunction in patients with subtle abnormalities on neurologic examination.

Autonomic Nervous System

Heart Rate Variability and Sympathetic Skin Response. The test of heart rate control (mainly parasympathetic) consists of measuring heart rate variations during quiet breathing, deep breathing, and in response to raising the feet. Normative parameters have been documented. The test of sympathetic skin response involves producing an electrical shock stimulus at a certain location (e.g., median or tibial nerve) and recording the evoked potential elsewhere (e.g., contralateral hand or foot or penis). Recording from the penis is considered to be a potentially useful method of testing penile autonomic innervation (Daffertshofer et al., 1994).

Penile Thermal Sensory Testing. This test assesses the conductance of small sensory nerve fibers that are affected by autonomic disturbances consistent with neuropathy. The testing measures thermal threshold. In studies of the penis, it seems to correlate well with the clinical determination of neurogenic ED (Bleustein et al., 2003; Lefaucheur et al., 2001).

Electrochemical Skin Conductance Testing. Electrochemical skin conductance measured using Sudoscan can be used to assess neurogenic ED. A feasibility study has shown promising results in using Sudoscan in patients with diabetes by measuring electrochemical skin conductance (Lefaucheur, 2017). Diabetic neuropathies can affect penile innervation without causing distal neuropathy, such that penile neuropathy cannot be reliably determined by assessing whether a distal neuropathy has affected the feet. Sudoscan results were more sensitive than sympathetic skin responses in assessing sympathetic innervation impairment. Further studies and clinical trials are needed to determine its diagnostic accuracy.

Corpus Cavernosum Electromyography and Single Potential Analysis of Cavernous Electrical Activity. This test offers a direct recording of cavernous electrical activity, which varies between penile flaccidity and tumescence (Leddy et al., 2012; Wagner et al., 1989). In the normally flaccid penis, electrical activity is described as exhibiting a rhythmic slow wave with intermittent bursts of activity. As penile tumescence occurs (such as in response to visual sexual stimulation or after intracavernosal injection of a smooth muscle relaxant), this activity ceases. During detumescence, the baseline electrical activity returns. Patients with suspected autonomic neuropathy were demonstrated to display a discordant pattern, having continued electrical activity during erectogenic stimuli (Wagner et al., 1989). Recording techniques have been standardized, and normative values have been defined to include maximum peak-to-peak amplitudes between 120 and 500 mV and mean potential durations of 12 seconds (Stief et al., 1994). However, the clinical utility of this test remains in question (Jiang et al., 2003; Kellner et al., 2000).

Hormonal Evaluation

The hormonal evaluation for ED explores an endocrinologic basis for this sexual dysfunction and recognizes accumulating evidence that endocrinopathies potentially affect the physiology of penile erection (Mirone et al., 2009; Traish and Guay, 2006). **Several endocrine conditions are particularly relevant in this regard: testosterone deficiency, formerly termed hypogonadism (decrease or absence of hormonal secretion from the gonads), hyperthyroidism (excessive thyroid hormone release), and diabetes (altered modulation of androgen function** (Maggi et al., 2013; Wang et al., 2011). The diagnostic evaluation may be undertaken in view of their possible influences on erectile function. The clinical history may raise suspicion regarding the diagnosis, although the clinical presentation of an endocrinopathy may be variable. Several questionnaires have been proposed for use in screening, particularly with respect to testosterone deficiency (Daig et al., 2003; Heinemann, 2005; Morley et al., 2000). A new psychometrically validated hypogonadism screener has been developed to identify men with symptoms of testosterone deficiency (Rosen et al., 2011). However, their general lack of specificity for most presentations and the lack of sensitivity for some others has limited their widespread applications (Morales et al., 2007). The central feature of this evaluation involves biochemical testing for serum hormonal levels (Bhasin et al., 2010).

Serum Testosterone Measurements

Much focus in assessing the impact of endocrinopathies on male sexual function has centered on the role of androgens. Androgen deficiency or low testosterone levels are observed in as few as 2% and as many as 33% of men presenting clinically with ED (Citron et al., 1996; Korenman et al., 1990; Soran and Wu, 2005). Differences in patient populations under study likely account for the variation in statistics. In acknowledging that aging may represent a primary cause of declining androgens, thought leaders have variously applied such terms as androgen deficiency of the aging male (ADAM), partial androgen deficiency of the aging male (PADAM), hypoandrogenism, symptomatic late-onset hypogonadism (SLOH), and andropause to designate this association. Adult-onset hypogonadism (AOH) was recently proposed to describe syndromes of testosterone deficiency in men with relationship to adverse adult-onset health conditions rather than aging per se (Khera et al., 2016).

It is important to understand the biology of testosterone production and function to proceed with its laboratory evaluation. **Testosterone circulates in three fractions: free (0.5% to 3%), tightly bound to sex hormone–binding globulin (SHBG) (~30%), and loosely bound to albumin and other serum proteins (~67%)** (Basaria and Dobs, 2001; Freeman et al., 2001). **Free testosterone and albumin-bound portions make up the bioavailable testosterone fraction. The relative concentrations of the carrier proteins (SHBG and albumin) modulate androgen function.** Numerous conditions can alter the SHBG fraction and accordingly affect bioavailable testosterone to some extent even if the total testosterone measurement is unchanged (Bhasin et al., 2010). Decreased SHBG is associated with moderate obesity, nephrotic syndrome, hypothyroidism, and the use of glucocorticoids, progestins, and androgenic steroids, and it produces an elevation in bioavailable testosterone. Increased SHBG is associated with aging, hepatic cirrhosis, hyperthyroidism, human immunodeficiency virus infection, and the use of anticonvulsants and estrogens, and it produces a lowering in bioavailable testosterone. Despite the observation that lower levels of SHBG are associated with insulin resistance (Stellato et al., 2000), variable SHBG levels have been documented in men with diabetes, possibly because of confounding obesity and aging factors, and the diagnosis of hypogonadism in this population should rely on the measurement of a low bioavailable testosterone level (see later) (Kapoor et al., 2007).

Theoretically, the unbound or free fraction measurement of testosterone offers the most relevant determination of testosterone bioavailability. However, commercial assays for free testosterone are known to be inconsistent and have been considered as invalid by some investigators (Field and Wheeler, 2013; Ly et al., 2010; Vermeulen et al., 1999). **The best indicator of androgen status is the calculated bioavailable testosterone (free testosterone and albumin-bound testosterone).** A formula for this calculation is found on the website of the International Society for the Study of the Aging Male (http://www.issam.ch/freetesto.htm), and this formula requires entries for the values of total testosterone and SHBG. In men with serious liver disease or hypoalbuminemia, entry of the serum albumin value may be useful for obtaining the best calculation.

For screening purposes, measurement of total serum testosterone level is generally sufficient. It is recommended that the blood draw be performed between 7:00 AM and 11:00 AM when there is a peak serum testosterone level, accounting for the fact that diurnal variation occurs in younger and middle-aged men (Wang et al., 2009). **The typical reference range for the total testosterone measurement is 280 to 1000 ng/dL.** Because of individual variability, the normal range for testosterone beyond which replacement therapy should be initiated remains unresolved. However, there is a low threshold of testosterone needed to maintain sexual function; the correlation between sexual function and testosterone is weak for levels above 8 nmol/L or 300 ng/dL (Bhasin et al., 2010; Isidori et al., 2014; O'Connor et al., 2011). If the testosterone level is below or at the low limit of normal, blood draw should be repeated for confirmation. On the other hand, a mildly abnormal testosterone level may be found to be normal in 30% of patients on repeat testing (Bhasin et al., 2010). The clinical scenario, such as the presence of conditions that alter testosterone carrier proteins, may prompt further testing and assessment decisions.

Serum Gonadotropin Measurements

With a second total testosterone determination, assessment of LH and prolactin should also be included. Measurement of serum gonadotropins helps to localize the source of the hypogonadism. Testosterone release involves the integrative activity of the hypothalamic-pituitary-gonadal axis and its regulatory feedback mechanisms, and disruption at any level of this axis may account for hypogonadism (Bhasin et al., 2010). A result of low testosterone is decreased negative feedback to the hypothalamus and pituitary, causing increased secretion of LH and follicle-stimulating hormone (FSH). Elevated serum LH and FSH releases are appropriate pituitary responses to low serum testosterone levels, which is consistent with testicular failure (primary hypogonadism). In contrast, normal or low serum LH and FSH releases in the setting of low serum testosterone levels indicate an inappropriate response and suggest a central disorder (secondary hypogonadism).

Serum Prolactin Measurement

Hyperprolactinemia causes hypogonadism by suppression of gonadotropin-releasing hormone from the hypothalamus, which impairs the pulsatile LH secretion required for serum testosterone production by the gonads (Morales et al., 2004). An additional possible mechanism for sexual dysfunction, specifically loss of sexual libido, in patients with hyperprolactinemia independent of the circulating level of testosterone relates to an interference of the peripheral conversion of testosterone to dihydrotestosterone (DHT) (Lobo and Kletzky, 1983). **Suspicion of hyperprolactinemia is raised in the patient with low serum testosterone and low or inappropriately normal LH.** However, controversy surrounds the consideration of routine determinations of prolactin in men with ED, with some indicating the low yield in doing so (Govier et al., 1996; Johnson and Jarow, 1992) and others finding that low serum testosterone or low sexual desire does not always coincide with the diagnosis (Buvat and Lemaire, 1997; Johri et al., 2001). Causes of the condition include various medications such as antipsychotic agents, tricyclic depressants and opiates, prolactin-secreting tumors, hypothyroidism, hypothalamic lesions, renal insufficiency, cirrhosis, and chest wall lesions (Molitch, 2005; Zeitlin and Rajfer, 2000).

Magnetic Resonance Imaging Scans

Cases of central (hypogonadotropic) hypogonadism as well as unexplained hyperprolactinemia prompt central imaging of the pituitary. This evaluation commonly involves magnetic resonance imaging, which can identify structural abnormalities (Citron et al., 1996; Petak et al., 2002; Rhoden et al., 2003). **Generally accepted guidelines provide indications for pituitary imaging: cases of severe central hypogonadism (testosterone <150 ng/dL) and suspicion of pituitary disease (i.e., panhypopituitarism, persistent hyperprolactinemia, or symptoms of tumor mass effect).**

Serum Thyroid Function Tests

Hyperthyroidism is associated with ED, possibly by increasing aromatization of testosterone into estrogen (which raises levels of SHBG) (Morales et al., 2004) **or by increasing adrenergic tone (which causes smooth muscle contractile effects or exerts psychobehavioral effects)** (Carani et al., 2005). Symptoms of hyperthyroidism, such as hyperactivity, irritability, heat intolerance, palpitations, fatigue, and

---

KEY POINTS: DIAGNOSTIC EVALUATION

- The basic evaluation of ED consists of a detailed case history, physical examination, and proper laboratory tests.
- The sexual history should define the characteristics of the ED presentation according to features such as onset, duration, conditions, severity, and cause.
- Cardiac risk assessment and risk reduction interventions are appropriate when necessary for all patients undergoing ED evaluations.
- Hormonal evaluation of ED explores an endocrinologic cause, with special consideration given to testosterone deficiency, hyperthyroidism, and diabetes.
- Questionnaires and other patient self-report measures offer practical help in documenting the presence, severity, and responsiveness to treatment of ED.
- Specialized evaluation and testing may be required for individuals with complicated or atypical presentations of ED.

weight loss, are often reported, and physical signs such as tachycardia, tremor, goiter, and eyelid retraction are often identified. The diagnosis is made biochemically by measurement of high levels of thyroid hormone (total or free thyroxine [T_4] or triiodothyronine [T_3]) with a low-serum thyroid-stimulating hormone level.

TREATMENT CONSIDERATIONS

The treatment of ED axiomatically follows an appropriate diagnostic workup. Although current interventions are etiologically specific and nonspecific, an intervention that is specific for the cause of ED ideally offers the opportunity to treat ED with a corrective purpose in mind. **Current recommendations adhere to a shared decision-making approach to therapy and specify that all therapeutic options are presented to the patient with advantages and disadvantages of each. The perceived risks and benefits based on the patient's clinical situation should be presented and weighed to make an informed decision** (see Fig. 69.1) (Makarov et al., 2016).

Lifestyle Modification

The risk of developing ED is significantly associated with the presence of comorbid health conditions such as diabetes, cardiovascular disease, and metabolic syndromes that are either preventable or to a minimal extent treatable in endeavoring to optimize health status (Kostis et al., 2005). Optimization of these diseases offers opportunities to prevent the development of ED or to ameliorate its extent (Glina et al., 2013).

Epidemiologic studies have shown examinations of potentially modifiable risk factors and in some instances have provided support that risk modification may indeed improve erectile function. For instance, several reports have suggested that the discontinuation of cigarette smoking results in a recovery of functional erection status (Bacon et al., 2006; Feldman et al., 2000; Mannino et al., 1994). A beneficial role of increasing exercise for those with a sedentary lifestyle in men with ED was also evident (Derby et al., 2000; Feldman et al., 1994). In a prospective study, obese men with moderate ED and no overt symptoms of cardiovascular disease showed significant improvements in IIEF scores after exercise and weight control when compared with a control group that followed an educational program alone (Esposito et al., 2004). Significant changes in body mass index, C-reactive protein, and physical activity scores were observed in the intervention group compared with the control group. Mediterranean-style diets and a reduction in caloric intake have been found to improve erectile function in men with metabolic syndrome (Esposito et al., 2006). A change to a no-nose saddle from a conventional saddle was shown to recover erectile function, presumably by alleviating perineal trauma, in a short-term interventional study of men with ED associated with occupational bicycle riding (Schrader et al., 2008).

Reports indicating that ED is potentially ameliorated by lifestyle modifications of risk factors that predispose this sexual dysfunction are most illuminative. The role of lifestyle modifications to prevent or to treat ED has gained support by way of systematic reviews and meta-analysis (Gupta et al., 2011; Kupelian et al., 2010; Porst et al., 2013). The mechanisms of this effect may include reduced cardiovascular risk factors, increased serum testosterone levels, and overall improved mood and self-esteem (Glina et al., 2013; Gupta et al., 2011; Meldrum et al., 2012). **Ongoing clinical and basic science investigation may further affirm the benefits of lifestyle modification and clarify its mechanistic basis.**

Medication Change

It is possible that a certain medication is an offending factor resulting in the clinical presentation of ED. After this inference is made, an appropriate next step would be to change to a different dose or type of medication entirely, considering that this action may reverse ED in some patients (Ralph and McNicholas, 2000). For instance, switching antihypertensive therapies from thiazide diuretics and beta-blockers to calcium channel blockers and renin-angiotensin system inhibitors (i.e., angiotensin-converting enzyme inhibitors and angiotensin receptor blockers) may recover erectile function in men developing ED in this clinical setting. Similarly, in patients suffering adverse sexual dysfunction effects from the use of SSRIs (e.g., ED, retarded ejaculation), treatment strategies such as drug substitution (e.g., bupropion, nefazodone, buspirone, mirtazapine), drug holidays, SSRI dosage reduction, watchful waiting, and administration of PDE5 inhibitors have enabled sexual function recovery (Nurnberg et al., 2001; Rosen et al., 1999b).

Psychosexual Therapy

Because of the frequent interplay of psychological and interpersonal factors in clinical presentations of ED, it is hardly surprising to consider that psychosexual therapy should be included in the therapeutic armamentarium for this sexual dysfunction. A strong limitation in this area is that evidence-based investigation and well-controlled, large-scale outcome research that documents the efficacy of interventions are generally lacking. In practice, psychosexual therapy does represent an ill-defined combination of interventions and interpretations based on behavioral, relational, psychoanalytic, and cognitive psychology concepts. **A variety of interventions are used: systematic anxiety reduction/desensitization, sensate focus, interpersonal therapy, cognitive-behavior therapy, sex education, couples' communication and sexual skills training, and masturbation exercises** (Althof et al., 2005). **Integrated treatments, which combine psychosexual interventions with medical therapies such as oral therapy, intracavernosal injection, or vacuum device therapy, have also proved successful in managing ED presentations, particularly those associated with motivational obstacles** (Althof et al., 2005; Hawton, 1998). The urologist understandably may not feel comfortable or may not possess the necessary training to address complicated psychosocial concerns. However, for mild to moderate psychosocial matters, the urologist may be prepared to proceed with a "biopsychosocial" model that minimally involves awareness of psychosocial issues and preparedness to counsel a patient or couple about normal sexual function and acceptable sexual behaviors (Althof and Needle, 2011). Collaborative efforts with a mental health clinician who has expertise in psychosexual therapy may be necessary to implement intensive therapy techniques.

Hormonal Therapy

A prescription of hormonal therapy is considered for the patient in whom a hormonal disturbance is identified. The urologist's role is appropriate for the treatment of testosterone deficiency and hyperprolactinemia, whereas endocrinologists would be considered as the foremost consultants for other endocrinopathies.

Testosterone Therapy

Androgen replacement directly addresses the clinical complaint associated with testosterone deficiency. As a general principle of sex steroid replacement therapy, serum hormone levels to be achieved daily throughout 24 hours should ideally achieve normal reference values and resemble the normal diurnal pattern. **Evaluating serum testosterone levels before and during treatment is imperative, although the efficacy of testosterone therapy is best judged by clinical response rather than a precise testosterone determination. Current recommendations suggest that a short (e.g., 3-month) therapeutic trial is justified, and, in the absence of a response, testosterone administration should be discontinued** (Bhasin et al., 2010; Wang et al., 2009). Potential adverse effects of androgen therapy (i.e., erythrocytosis, sleep apnea, urinary symptoms, prostate cancer progression risk, gynecomastia, acne) should be recognized (Morales et al., 2004; Wald et al., 2006). The role of testosterone in men's cardiovascular health has been debated; however, a recent meta-analysis of all placebo-controlled randomized controlled trials on how testosterone affects cardiovascular health did not support a causal relationship between testosterone and cardiovascular events

(Corona et al., 2014). **Monitoring of patients on therapy consists of a baseline assessment that includes digital rectal examination and serum PSA testing along with laboratory evaluation (i.e., hemoglobin/hematocrit levels, liver function tests, cholesterol level, and lipid profile) followed by the assessment of treatment efficacy after 3 to 6 months and annually thereafter to ascertain symptom response and any adverse events** (Bhasin et al., 2010; Morales et al., 2004). Short-acting preparations may be preferred in favor of long-acting depot preparations in the initial treatment of patients so that therapy can be discontinued on the occasion of an adverse event (Wang et al., 2009).

For the treatment of testosterone deficiency, several testosterone preparations are offered and can be delivered by various routes: intramuscular, subcutaneous, transdermal (patch and gel), buccal, and oral (Bhasin et al., 2010; Corona et al., 2011; Edelstein et al., 2006; Morgentaler et al., 2008; Wang et al., 2009). A brief description of available therapies follows (see also Table 69.6).

Intramuscular. Testosterone enanthate or cypionate, an injectable depot preparation of testosterone, is delivered by deep intramuscular injection (200 to 250 mg every 2 to 3 weeks). The schedule of therapy results in supraphysiologic levels of testosterone for 72 hours with a steady exponential decline to subphysiologic levels by 10 to 12 days. Alternative dosing of 100 mg every 7 to 10 days can be considered in situations in which patients experience symptomatic mood changes or sexual fluctuations associated with documented early low testosterone level troughs. Another parenteral preparation, testosterone propionate, is also delivered intramuscularly at a dosage of 200 mg every 2 to 3 days because of its shorter half-life, and it may also display serum testosterone fluctuations. Testosterone undecanoate (TU), as a depot formulation consisting of 750- or 1000-mg dosages administered at 10-week dosing intervals, has been used in Europe since 2003, although it is not yet available in the United States.

Subcutaneous. Pellets offer a subcutaneous, long-acting depot formulation of testosterone. Testopel is a pellet containing 75 mg of testosterone. Dosing usually is 2 to 6 pellets (150 to 450 mg testosterone) implanted subcutaneously every 3 to 6 months.

Transdermal. Transdermal delivery options comprise patches and gels, with a delivery approach that intentionally simulates normal circadian levels of testosterone. When patients apply medication in the morning, higher initial absorption mimics normal diurnal variation.

Testoderm was approved initially as a scrotal patch administered daily without adhesive (4 to 6 mg), but its use faltered because of difficulties with its application, the requirement for scrotal shaving, and the finding that it significantly produced high levels of DHT by conversion by 5α-reductase activity that is plentifully present in the scrotal skin. Testoderm TTS represented an alternative formulation avoiding the inconveniences of the scrotal application. Its application is to the arm, back, or buttock as a 5-mg patch. Androderm, an alternative product, delivers 2.5 or 5 mg of testosterone daily. Both patches have been associated with itching, chronic skin irritation, and allergic contact dermatitis. The skin irritation is alleviated by the local application of cortisone cream. Patients are advised to alternate application sites and avoid sun-exposed areas.

AndroGel (testosterone 1% gel) is a topical gel pack that contains 50, 75, or 100 mg of testosterone, with only 10% of the drug being absorbed during a 24-hour period. Testim, also providing 1% testosterone, is an alternative product packaged as a 5-g tube containing 50 mg of testosterone. Both are similarly applied once daily in the morning to clean, dry skin on the shoulders, upper arms, or abdomen, and it is allowed to dry before dressing. Axiron (testosterone 2% solution) is another transdermal product approved by the US Food and Drug Administration (FDA), consisting of 30 mg of testosterone applied to each axilla once daily using a metered applicator. Special considerations for axillary administration include the concealable location and high permeability of the axilla, which has a relatively high level of 5α-reductase activity. Testosterone nasal gel (Natesto) is applied to the nostrils. The recommended dosage of Natesto is 11 mg of testosterone (2 pump actuations; 1 actuation per nostril) administered intranasally two to three times daily for a total daily dose of 22 to 33 mg. The advantages are its quick onset of action, short half-life, and lack of risk of transference. Some of the disadvantages are the possibly irritating nasal route of administration and necessity for administration up to 3 times a day.

Buccal. Striant is a tabletlike, mucoadhesive treatment system (30 mg of testosterone) that continuously delivers medication. It is applied twice daily to the gum tissue above the incisors, allowing testosterone to be absorbed through the buccal mucosa.

Oral. Oral testosterone preparations are limited. Concern is associated with the liver toxicity of testosterone (i.e., hepatitis, cholestatic jaundice, hepatomas, hemorrhagic liver cysts, and hepatocellular carcinoma) related to the large doses necessary to achieve normal serum levels (Bagatell and Bremner, 1996). Large doses (>200 mg/day) are required orally because much of the administration is rendered metabolically inactive during the "first-pass" circulation through the liver. Chemical modifications of oral testosterone have been explored to overcome adverse reactions. Both 17α-methyltestosterone and fluoxymesterone have been formulated, but because of their patient variability of effect with potential liver toxicity risk, they should not be prescribed (Wang et al., 2009). TU, as an oral formulation in oleic acid, is safe by partly escaping hepatic inactivation (Köhn and Schill, 2003). However, it has shown a large individual variability for the time of maximal responses as well as when maximal serum testosterone is attained. Oral TU remains unapproved in the United States. A formulation of TU manufactured by Lipocine, Tlando was reportedly well tolerated in early phase 3 clinical trials and has undergone two additional phase 3 clinical trials with pending results. Lipocine has developed an additional drug with increased solubility and absorption, currently in phase 2 clinical trials.

Alternative Hormone Treatments

Alternative hormonal replacement therapies have been suggested, with certain desirable features and some caveats. DHT as a direct mode of therapy is attractive because of its action as a pure androgen that is not aromatizable to estradiol, and accordingly it has been demonstrated that the hormone does not exert adverse estrogenic effects on prostate growth or lipid profile measurements (Kunelius et al., 2002; Sakhri and Gooren, 2007). A therapeutic DHT gel is available at a dose of 125 to 250 mg/day, yielding plasma DHT levels comparable with physiologic testosterone levels (Kunelius et al., 2002). Dehydroepiandrosterone (DHEA), a hormone supplement with androgen-like and estrogen-like effects, has been used, although limited evidence exists showing it improves sexual function (Baulieu et al., 2000; Morales et al., 2004). The treatment cannot be considered harmless, and the potential exists for DHEA and other nontestosterone androgen precursor preparations (e.g., DHEA-S, androstenediol, androstenedione) to stimulate hormone-sensitive diseases such as breast or prostate cancer. Human chorionic gonadotropin (hCG) has been found to increase total and free testosterone and estradiol 50% above baseline; it would conceivably be of benefit to hypogonadal men in a way similar to the effects of androgen administration. Clinical investigation of hCG has shown some anthropometric effects (i.e., decrease in fat mass, increase in lean body mass) and improvements in serum testosterone concentrations in androgen-deficient men without documented benefits for sexual function (Liu et al., 2002; Tsujimura et al., 2005). Antiestrogens and aromatase inhibitors have been shown to increase endogenous testosterone levels, and selective androgen receptor modulators are under development. Because of insufficient evidence about the therapeutic benefits and adverse effects of alternative replacement therapies in older men with testosterone deficiency, they are not currently recommended for use (Wang et al., 2009).

Hyperprolactinemia Treatments

The treatment of hyperprolactinemia is undertaken with the acknowledgment that testosterone replacement therapy is neither corrective nor sufficient to improve sexual function. The therapeutic objective, rather, is to identify and address the underlying cause, which may then ameliorate ED. Offending drugs, such as estrogens, morphine, sedatives, and neuroleptics, should be discontinued

TABLE 69.6 Testosterone Preparations

FORMULATION	CHEMICAL STRUCTURE	T½	STANDARD DOSAGE	ADVANTAGES	DISADVANTAGES
ORAL AGENTS (NOT FDA APPROVED)					
Testosterone undecanoate	17-α-hydroxyl-ester	4 h	120–240 mg 2–3 times daily	Oral convenience Modifiable dosage	Serum testosterone levels and clinical responses vary Must be taken with meals
Methyltestosterone	17-α-alkylated	3.5 h	20–50 mg 2–3 times daily	Oral convenience Modifiable dosage	Potential hepatotoxicity Treatment considered obsolete
Mesterolone	1-alkylated	8 h	100–150 mg 2–3 times daily	Oral convenience Modifiable dosage	Nonaromatizable to estrogen
INTRAMUSCULAR AGENTS					
Testosterone enanthate	17-α-hydroxyl-ester	4–5 days	250 mg every 2–3 wk	Low cost Modifiable dosage	Wide fluctuations in circulating T levels Multiple injections Relative higher risk of polycythemia
Testosterone cypionate	17-α-hydroxyl-ester	8 days	200 mg every 2–3 wk	Low cost Modifiable dosage	Wide fluctuations in circulating T levels Multiple injections
Testosterone propionate	17-α-hydroxyl-ester	20 h	100 mg every 2 days	Low cost	Wide fluctuations in circulating T levels Multiple injections Relative higher risk of polycythemia
Testosterone undecanoate	17-α-hydroxyl-ester	34 days	1000 mg every 10–14 wk	Testosterone levels maintained within normal range Long lasting Less frequent administration	Pain at injection site
SUBCUTANEOUS AGENTS					
Surgical implants	Native testosterone	—	4 6200-mg implants lasting ≤6 mo	Treatment 3–4×/yr	Placement is invasive Risk of extrusion and site infections
CONTROLLED-RELEASE T-BUCCAL FORMULATION AGENTS					
Testosterone buccal	Native testosterone	12 h	30 mg 2 times daily	Testosterone levels within physiologic range	Possible oral irritation Twice-daily irritation Unpleasant taste
TRANSDERMAL AGENTS					
Testosterone patches	Native testosterone	10 h	5–10 mg/day	Mimics circadian rhythm Simple administration	Skin irritation Daily administration
Testosterone gel 1%–2%	Native testosterone	6 h	5–10 g/day	Testosterone levels maintained within normal range Flexible dose modification Skin irritation less common than with patches	Possible transfer during intimate contact Daily administration
Testosterone nasal gel	Native testosterone	1 h	33 mg/day	Quick onset of action, short half-life, no risk of transference	Two-three times per day administration
Testosterone solution 2%	Native testosterone	NA	60–120 mg/day	Testosterone levels maintained within normal range	Possible transfer during intimate contact Daily administration

NA, Not available; *T*, testosterone; *T½*, drug half-life.
Modified from Corona G, Rastrelli G, Forti G, et al.: Update in testosterone therapy for men. *J Sex Med* 8:639–654, 2011.

(Molitch, 2008). A prolactin-secreting adenoma should be treated medically and, if necessary, surgically. Bromocriptine, a dopamine agonist that lowers prolactin level and restores testosterone to normal, reduces the size of the tumor. Neurosurgical ablation becomes necessary if the therapeutic response to medication does not occur or visual effects are noted in association with optic nerve compression (Gillam et al., 2006). Erection recovery is most evident after treatment of men with significant serum elevations of prolactin (higher than 40 ng/mL) (Netto Júnior and Claro, 1993).

Pharmacologic Therapies

The premise of pharmacologic therapies is that they simulate the biochemical and molecular mechanisms of action naturally governing the erectile response. Conceptually, erectogenic therapies strategically either promote proerectile mechanisms or oppose antierectile mechanisms, at peripheral and central levels of the neurovascular axis responsible for penile erection (Rowland and Burnett, 2000). At a peripheral level, these mechanisms influence corporeal smooth muscle tone. Promotion of proerectile mechanisms is achieved by either inducing corporeal smooth muscle activation through cell-receptor agonists or effectors of tissue relaxant pathways (e.g., stimulating second messenger cyclic nucleotide [cyclic guanosine monophosphate, or cGMP, or cyclic adenosine monophosphate, or cAMP] synthesis) or inhibiting the deactivation of smooth muscle relaxation pathways (e.g., inhibiting phosphodiesterases), whereas opposition of antierectile mechanisms are achieved by decreasing smooth muscle contraction through receptor antagonists of tissue contractile pathways (e.g., α_1-adrenergic inhibitors). At a central nervous system level (i.e., brain or spinal cord), neuronal pathways are affected, and potential opportunities exist to promote proerectile pathways (e.g., agonists of dopaminergic D_2 receptors in the medial hypothalamus) or to oppose antierectile pathways (e.g., antagonists of 5-$HT_{1A/2}$ [serotonergic] receptors in the spinal cord).

Diverse therapies have been touted throughout time, although their efficacy and safety characteristics have not always been clearly defined. Current standards of regulatory agency approval have helped to clarify the qualifications of commercially developed and marketed therapies (Hirsch et al., 2004).

Oral Therapy

Orally administered medication for ED meets many of the attributes of "ideal therapy," which include convenience, simplicity, and noninvasiveness (Morales et al., 1995). Oral therapies are increasingly in demand to meet the therapeutic objective of clinical efficacy as well.

Phosphodiesterase Type 5 Inhibitors. This class of medication was famously inaugurated as an effective ED treatment in the United States after the FDA approval of sildenafil citrate (Viagra, Pfizer, New York, NY) in 1998, vardenafil hydrochloride (Levitra, Bayer Schering Pharma AG, Berlin, Germany), and tadalafil (Cialis, Lilly, Indianapolis, IN) in 2003, and avanafil (Stendra, Vivus, Mountain View, CA) in 2012 (Bruzziches et al., 2013; Porst et al., 2013). **PDE5 inhibitors similarly work to block the catalytic action of the enzyme that degrades cGMP, the downstream effector of the erection mediator nitric oxide, which then facilitates the signal transductional mechanisms of corpus cavernosal smooth muscle relaxation required for penile erection. The medications augment but do not induce the erectile response, and the induction of penile erection requires the release of nitric oxide from penile nerve endings and vascular endothelium under the influence of sexual stimulation** (Burnett, 2005). The high concentration of PDE5 inhibitors in the smooth muscle of the penile corpora cavernosa accounts for the selectivity of their effect.

Despite their similar modes of actions, PDE5 inhibitors differ somewhat in their biochemical properties, pharmacokinetic profiles, and clinical performances (Table 69.7). The chemical structure of PDE5 inhibitors are similar, containing a guaninelike base, a riboselike or desoxyribose-like system, and a phosphate diester-like bond, which confers their ability to bind effectively to the catalytic site of the PDE5 enzyme. The chemical structures of sildenafil and vardenafil are similar, unlike that for tadalafil, and this difference explains some phenomenologic distinctions observed between these agents (Corbin and Francis, 1999). The chemical structure of avanafil differs from the standard model of the other three agents, which may account for some of its selective actions (Kedia et al., 2013). **Distinct from the actions of tadalafil and avanafil, sildenafil and vardenafil cross-react to a greater extent with PDE6, which is expressed in the retina; this difference may explain the complaint of visual disturbances observed with sildenafil and vardenafil use.** Tadalafil minimally cross-reacts with PDE11, unlike the other three PDE5 inhibitors, although the significance of this effect is unclear. The remaining side effects commonly observed with PDE5 inhibitor treatment are associated with inhibition of PDE5 localized in other target tissues, such as vascular and gastrointestinal smooth muscle. Tadalafil possesses a longer half-life of elimination than the other three PDE5 inhibitors. This feature suggests a longer therapeutic window uniquely afforded for tadalafil, which may translate into increased convenience for couples using this agent.

All four PDE5 inhibitors have demonstrated equivalent efficacy and tolerability in clinical trials for the treatment of ED of varying severity and cause (Carson and Lue, 2005; Bruzziches et al., 2013;

TABLE 69.7 Comparison of Four Phosphodiesterase Type 5 Inhibitors Currently Available in the United States

	SILDENAFIL	VARDENAFIL	TADALAFIL	AVANAFIL
Cmax (ng/mL)	450	20.9	378	2153
Tmax (h)	0.8	0.7–0.9	2	0.3–0.5
Onset of action (min)	15–60	15–60	15–120	15–60
Half-life (h)	3–5	4–5	17.5	3–5
Bioavailability	40%	15%	Not tested	30%
Fatty food	Reduced absorption	Reduced absorption	No effect	Reduced absorption
Recommended dosage	25, 50, 100 mg	5, 10, 20 mg	5, 10, 20 mg	50, 100, 200 mg
Side effects:				
Headache, dyspepsia, facial flushing	Yes	Yes	Yes	Yes
Backache, myalgia	Rare	Rare	Yes	Rare
Blurred/blue vision	Yes	Rare	Rare	No
Precaution with antiarrhythmics	No	Yes	No	No
Contraindication with nitrates	Yes	Yes	Yes	Yes

Cmax, Maximal plasma concentration; *half-life*, time required for elimination of one half of the medication from plasma; *Tmax*, time required to attain Cmax.

Giuliano et al., 2010; Hellstrom, 2007; Porst et al., 2013; Yuan et al., 2013). Trial designs for these agents have differed, limiting useful comparisons among them, and superiority cannot be claimed for any particular agent in the absence of directly comparative studies (Carson and Lue, 2005; Khera and Goldstein, 2011). **In general, the agents effectively result in successful sexual intercourse rates of approximately 70%** (Carson and Lue, 2005; Khera and Goldstein, 2011). A somewhat reduced intercourse success rate of 40% to 50% has been reported in patients with diabetes and ED (Fonseca et al., 2004; Safarinejad, 2004) and in patients with ED associated with radical prostatectomy in general (Hatzimouratidis et al., 2009). However, the intercourse success rate for patients after bilateral nerve-sparing radical prostatectomy specifically is somewhat better than for the entire group, and reports have commonly documented rates that approach 60% to 70% for functional erections with therapy.

According to standard dosing recommendations, patients are instructed to take the medications on demand between 30 and 60 minutes before intended sexual activity. This lead-time interval is specified to take advantage of the duration by which the medications achieve peak serum concentrations (i.e., approximately 30 minutes for avanafil, 1 hour for sildenafil and vardenafil, and 2 hours for tadalafil). Although the onset of activity has been documented to occur possibly within 20 minutes for each agent, this characteristic is less important to patients than erection hardness and maintenance of erections with therapy (Claes et al., 2008). A daily dosing regimen has been approved for tadalafil as an alternative treatment schedule to afford patients greater convenience in having sexual intercourse while using this agent (Porst et al., 2006; Shabsigh et al., 2010). **Optimization of effect for all PDE5 inhibitors is also achieved by applying sexual stimulation properly as a prerequisite for nitric oxide release, by reducing food intake, which may delay drug absorption, by escalating drug dosing as needed, and by repeating attempts with the medications several times (up to 9 or 10 attempts affords maximal probability of success)** (Barada, 2003; McCullough et al., 2002; Shindel, 2009). **Correcting or improving adverse health conditions (e.g., glycemic control, hyperlipidemic control, androgen replacement), which affect drug efficacy, has also been demonstrated as potentially beneficial** (Guay, 2003; Sadovsky et al., 2009). As evidence of therapeutic efficacy, patient and partner satisfaction with therapy (as shown for sildenafil) has been well demonstrated (Montorsi and Althof, 2004). Suboptimal acceptance or lack of long-term adherence to therapy (up to 47% of patients) has been reported, which may indicate the influence of psychosocial factors or challenges of a treatment that requires repeated dosing (Al-Shaiji and Brock, 2009; Seftel, 2002). There is controversial evidence that combining testosterone and PDE5 inhibitors may improve response to PDE5 inhibitor therapy (Greco et al., 2006; Spitzer et al., 2012, 2013). A combination of daily doses of 5 mg tadalafil (long-acting) with 50 mg sildenafil (short-acting) may be used in patients with severe ED without increasing side effects (Cui et al., 2015).

Patients using PDE5 inhibitors should be thoroughly counseled regarding precautions (Box 69.1). Cardiovascular safety using this class of compounds has been well demonstrated, although it should be emphasized that given the cardiovascular risks of sexual activity and potential for adverse drug interactions with this therapy, cardiovascular risk assessment and stabilization should be considered for all men before the institution of PDE5 inhibitor therapy. **Controlled and postmarketing studies involving these agents have shown that they do not cause an increase in myocardial infarction or death rates when compared with expected rates in study control populations** (Hellstrom, 2007; Jackson et al., 2006a,b; Nehra, 2009). In addition, patients with known coronary artery disease or heart failure receiving PDE5 inhibitors did not exhibit worsening ischemia, coronary vasoconstriction, or worsening hemodynamics on exercise testing or cardiac catheterization. Caution is advised for the use of PDE5 inhibitors in patients with certain conditions: aortic stenosis, left ventricular outflow obstruction, hypotension, and hypovolemia. The agents have a minimal effect on QTc interval (Morganroth et al., 2004). Vardenafil among PDE5 inhibitors is not recommended in patients who take type 1A antiarrhythmics (e.g., quinidine or procainamide)

BOX 69.1 Warnings and Drug Interactions

The package inserts of all four phosphodiesterase type 5 (PDE5) inhibitors warn against their use in patients with severe cardiovascular diseases and left ventricular outflow obstruction (e.g., aortic stenosis, idiopathic subaortic stenosis), those with severely impaired autonomic control of blood pressure, and patients not studied in clinical trials (US prescribing information of Viagra, Cialis, and Levitra and Stendra, September 2013). These include patients with the following:

- Myocardial infarction, stroke, or life-threatening arrhythmia within the previous 6 months
- New York Heart Association class II or greater heart failure or coronary artery disease causing unstable angina
- Resting hypotension (<90/50 mm Hg) or hypertension (>170/100 mm Hg)
- Known hereditary degenerative retinal disorders, including retinitis pigmentosa
- Severe hepatic impairment (Child-Pugh C) or end-stage renal disease requiring dialysis

Certain drugs such as ketoconazole and itraconazole and protease inhibitors such as ritonavir can impair the metabolic breakdown of PDE5 inhibitors by blocking the CYP3A4 pathway. Such agents may increase blood levels of inhibitors, requiring a PDE5 dose reduction. On the other hand, agents such as rifampin may induce CYP3A4, enhancing the breakdown of inhibitors and requiring higher PDE5 doses. Kidney or hepatic dysfunction may require dose adjustments or warnings.

---

or type 3 antiarrhythmics (e.g., sotalol or amiodarone) or in patients with congenital prolonged QT syndrome.

Nitrate use in any form (e.g., sublingual nitroglycerin, isosorbide dinitrate, other nitrate preparations used to treat angina, amyl nitrite, and amyl nitrate "poppers") represents an absolute contraindication. Past use of nitrates, that is, more than 2 weeks before the use of PDE5 inhibitors, is not considered a contraindication. **If angina occurs during sexual activity when using a PDE5 inhibitor, patients should cease this activity and seek emergency care immediately.** They should inform medical personnel that a PDE5 inhibitor was taken and should avoid nitroglycerin use for a period of 24 hours for sildenafil and vardenafil and 48 hours for tadalafil (Cheitlin et al., 1999). If acute myocardial infarction occurs with the use of PDE5 inhibitors, usual therapies, with the exception of organic nitrates, may be administered. If hypotension results from PDE5 inhibitor use, patients should be placed in the Trendelenburg position and given intravenous fluids along with administration of α-adrenergic agonists (e.g., phenylephrine) as needed. Refractory hypotension warrants intra-aortic balloon counterpulsation, as specified by the American College of Cardiology/American Heart Association guidelines. No pharmacologic antidote to the PDE5 inhibitor/nitrate interaction exists. Caution is advised when PDE5 inhibitors are coadministered with α-adrenergic blockers, because both agents are vasodilators with blood pressure–lowering effects.

Side effects observed with PDE5 inhibitor therapy include headache (7% to 16%), dyspepsia (4% to 10%), flushing (4% to 10%), myalgia/back pain (0 to 3%), nasal congestion (3% to 4%), and visual disturbances (e.g., photophobia, blue vision) (0 to 3%). Randomized controlled trials have documented that flushing and visual side effects are more common in patients receiving sildenafil or vardenafil, whereas back pain/myalgia is more common in patients receiving tadalafil. These events have been found to be mild and to abate with time, and the side effects prompt discontinuation only in few patients (Hellstrom, 2007; Porst et al., 2013).

The concern has been posed with PDE5 inhibitor therapy regarding the development of nonarteritic anterior optic neuropathy (NAION), which can cause blindness, although several systematic reviews of the safety of this class of compounds have not shown an increased risk of NAION or other adverse ocular events associated with their use (Laties, 2009; Porst et al., 2013). Affected patients in postmarketing reports possibly carried risk factors for blindness to include hypertension, diabetes, and hyperlipidemia. At this time, despite the absence of a proven link between PDE5 inhibitor use and serious ocular disorders, physicians should continue to advise patients to stop use of PDE5 inhibitors and to seek immediate medical attention as a safety measure in the event of a sudden loss of vision (Laties, 2009; Porst et al., 2013).

Several investigations have addressed the possible relationship between PDE5 inhibitor use and increased risk for skin cancers, particularly malignant melanoma (Lian Y et al., 2016; Loeb et al., 2015). However, study design flaws and confounders of increased medical surveillance among PDE5 inhibitor users limit any conclusive risk relationship. Similar considerations of a risk relationship for prostate cancer recurrence have also been refuted (Gallina et al., 2015; Loeb et al., 2016).

The interest in extending the use of PDE5 inhibitors beyond an on-demand erectogenic role and rather applying them to recovery or maintenance of the natural vitality of the penis in the face of an ED-associated disease state or condition has been investigated. This proposal has been considered particularly in the clinical context of radical prostatectomy and has been introduced as a therapeutic strategy as "penile rehabilitation," in which the medications are taken in some regularly scheduled fashion to promote the recovery of spontaneous erectile function. Presently, this role remains unclear, because of limited well-designed and conducted (i.e., randomized controlled) clinical trials of PDE5 inhibitor use in this clinical setting (Mulhall et al., 2013). In one supportive trial involving sildenafil treatment of 36 weeks starting 4 weeks after the surgery, 27% of patients using the agent recovered erections defined as "good enough for sexual activity" compared with 4% of patients on placebo at about 1 year after surgery (Padma-Nathan et al., 2008). However, in another trial involving vardenafil treatment of 9 months either on-demand or daily starting 14 days after surgery, erection recovery was no different in patients using vardenafil by either form of administration or placebo at about 1 year after surgery (Montorsi et al., 2008). Another trial randomizing patients to the use of sildenafil nightly or on-demand for 12 months with a 1-month washout showed that erection recovery was not different between patient groups (Pavlovich et al., 2013). By contrast, another study showed that sildenafil administered daily for 6 months improved sexual function among men undergoing radiotherapy; results at 12 months showed that 73% of patients on sildenafil versus 50% of patients on placebo had mild or no ED (Zelefsky et al., 2014). Randomized controlled trials in other ED contexts have failed to show sustained natural erectile function improvement after discontinuing continuous regimens of PDE5 inhibitor therapy (Burnett et al., 2009; Zumbe et al., 2008).

The notion of combining PDE5 inhibitors with other ED therapies such as vasoactive penile pharmacotherapies has been proposed (Lau et al., 2006; McMahon et al., 2006). This strategy is to be considered "off-label," and clinical precautions are advised.

α-Adrenoceptor Antagonists. Phentolamine mesylate is a nonspecific α-adrenergic receptor antagonist with equal affinity for blocking α_1- and α_2-adrenoreceptors. Its mode of action presumably is to produce corporeal smooth muscle relaxation by blocking the (antierectile) postsynaptic α_1-adrenergic receptor (Juenemann et al., 1986). Clinical trials suggested an efficacy rate in men with minimal ED of approximately 40% (Goldstein, 2000). The drug was considered relatively safe; less than 10% of patients using the 40-mg dosage experienced headaches, facial flushing, or nasal congestion. However, further investigation is required before determining whether it will produce erectile responses of sufficient quality for reliable sexual intercourse, particularly in men with more severe ED.

Yohimbine hydrochloride (Yocon), an indolalkylamine alkaloid derived from the bark of the yohimbe tree, reportedly exerts central effects on the mediation of penile erection operating as an α_2-adrenoreceptor antagonist (Clark, 1991; Giuliano and Rampin, 2000). Originally proposed to be an erectogenic and aphrodisiac agent, the drug has been investigated as an authentic ED treatment. It is conventionally prescribed orally at a dosage of 5.4 mg three times daily with observation for improvement throughout at least a month. A meta-analysis of all randomized, placebo-controlled trials involving yohimbine suggested a superior effect for the medication compared to placebo (Ernst and Pittler, 1998). **However, the drug does not appear to enable successful sexual intercourse any better than placebo in men with confirmed organic ED** (Montague et al., 1996; Teloken et al., 1998). Adverse effects appear to be relatively infrequent but include hypertension, anxiety, tachycardia, and headache. Although yohimbine may be well tolerated, its modest results suggest that it may be best limited to men with psychogenic ED (Porst et al., 2013).

Dopaminergic Agonists. Apomorphine (Uprima, TAP Pharmaceutical Products, Lake Forest, IL) is a dopaminergic agent activating D_1 and D_2 receptors at a central level within the paraventricular nucleus of the brain, indicating its particular relevance in the treatment of men with psychogenic ED (Lal et al., 1987). The medication is administered in sublingual form with a dosage range of 2, 4, and 6 mg, and it has no erectile efficacy if it is swallowed (Heaton, 2000). It has a rapid onset of action, with a mean time to erection of 12 minutes. Apomorphine achieves a maximal plasma concentration in 50 minutes, although its window of opportunity extends for approximately 2 hours from administration. In clinical trials involving men with ED of varying severities and causes, the drug achieved a successful sexual intercourse rate of 50.6% at the 4-mg dosage compared with the 33.8% placebo rate (Heaton, 2000). Side effects include nausea (16.9%), dizziness (8.3%), yawning (7.9%), somnolence (5.8%), sweating (5%), and emesis (3.7%). Syncope occurred in 0.6% of patients using the medication at the highest recommended dosage, and this was accompanied by a prodrome consisting of nausea, vomiting, sweating, dizziness, and lightheadedness but no cardiac sequelae. Side effects were minimized when patients were titrated from higher to lower dosages. The drug achieved regulatory approval for commercialization by European authorities in early 2001, but it has not been so approved in the United States.

Melanocortin-Receptor Agonists. Melanocortin analogues (e.g., melanotan II, PT-141) have been studied showing efficacy in inducing erectile responses in early clinical trials (Diamond et al., 2004; Wessells et al., 2000). These drugs operate centrally at melanocortin-4 receptors, which have been implicated in controlling food intake and energy expenditure as well as modulating erectile function and sexual behavior. Flushing and nausea have been reported as side effects. The drugs have not achieved regulatory approval for the treatment of ED.

Serotonin-Receptor Effectors. Trazodone (Desyrel) is an antidepressant that has been associated with priapism, prompting its "off-label" investigation as a possible treatment for ED (Lal et al., 1990). It is purported to work through mechanisms at the spinal-cord level with multiple serotonergic effects (Allard and Giuliano, 2001). The active metabolite of trazodone acts as an agonist of the proerectile 5-HT$_{2C}$ receptor through reuptake inhibition, with some affinity for the 5-HT$_{2A}$ receptor, although it may also operate as an antagonist of antierectile 5-HT$_{1A}$ receptors (Andersson and Wagner, 1995). Rigorous evaluations have not shown clinical efficacy that exceeds placebo responses in eliciting penile erection (Costabile and Spevak, 1999). Given its potential side effects (i.e., drowsiness, nausea, emesis, blood pressure changes, urinary retention, and priapism) and general lack of effect, this medication would appear to have a limited role for ED treatment.

Other Oral Therapies. Additional possibilities for the oral treatment of ED, including l-arginine (the amino acid precursor of nitric oxide), L-dopa (dopamine precursor), limaprost (prostaglandin E$_1$), and naltrexone (opioid antagonist), have been proposed (Burnett, 1999). Each of these agents has a plausible mechanism of action to induce erections. However, they remain insufficiently studied, and their clinical roles remain unclear (Porst et al., 2013).

Intracavernosal Injection

The discovery in 1982 that vasoactive agents, delivered by injection into the penis, induced erections is credited with launching

TABLE 69.8 Intracavernosal Pharmacotherapies

TRADE NAME	DRUG	DOSAGES	EFFICACY (INTERCOURSE)
Caverject	Alprostadil (Prostin VR)	5–40 µg/mL	≈70%
Viradal/Edex	Alprostadil (Prostin VR)	5–40 µg/mL	≈70%
Bimix	Alprostadil + phentolamine	20 µg/mL + 0.5 mg/mL	≈90%
Bimix Androskat (EU)	Papaverine + phentolamine	30 mg/mL + 0.5 mg/mL	≈90%
Trimix	Alprostadil + papaverine + phentolamine	10 µg/mL + 30 mg/mL + 1.0 mg/mL	≈90%
Invicorp	VIP + phentolamine	NA	≈80%

EU, European Union; *NA,* not available; *VIP,* vasoactive intestinal polypeptide.

the movement toward medical therapies for the treatment of ED (Virag, 1982; Zorgniotti, 1985). Since that time, there has been an explosion of basic scientific and clinical research leading to the development and use of various locally administered vasoactive medications having mechanisms of action that result in corporeal smooth muscle relaxation. Although a host of medications have been explored for this purpose, three medications are used regularly in clinical practice: alprostadil, papaverine, and phentolamine (Table 69.8). These have been administered clinically as a single agent (i.e., monotherapy) or in various combinations (e.g., bimix, trimix). Combination therapy offers a synergistic mechanism of the vasoactive agents to elicit maximal erectile responses, particularly among patients who have failed monotherapy (Bennett et al., 1991; Floth and Schramek, 1991; Khera and Goldstein, 2011; Porst et al., 2013; Zorgniotti and Lefleur, 1985). This alternative may also be used to circumvent side effects of a certain agent (e.g., penile pain associated with alprostadil).

A general rule of thumb is to start with a small dose of medication, especially in patients with nonvasculogenic forms of ED. In-office self-injection training and education are recommended before home injection, and this opportunity may also be used to titrate medication toward a dosage that safely yields an erection of sufficient rigidity for sexual intercourse yet lasts no more than an hour (Bénard and Lue, 1990; Fallon, 1995). Comparing empirical and risk-based approaches to intracavernosal injection therapy found no statistically significant differences in patient satisfaction, outcomes, or complications between the two groups (Bernie et al., 2017). The therapy is contraindicated for men with psychological instability, a history or risk for priapism, histories of severe coagulopathy or unstable cardiovascular disease, reduced manual dexterity (although the partner can be trained in the injection technique), and use of monoamine oxidase inhibitors (because of the risk of precipitating a life-threatening hypertensive crisis in the event that an intracavernosal α-adrenergic agonist is used to reverse a priapic episode) (Sharlip, 1998).

Alprostadil. Alprostadil (Prostin VR) is a synthetic form of a naturally occurring fatty acid, prostaglandin E_1, which binds with specific receptors on smooth muscle cells and activates intracellular adenylate cyclase to produce cAMP, which in turn induces tissue relaxation through a second messenger system (Palmer et al., 1994). It currently is the only FDA-approved injectable medication for ED, and it is marketed for this purpose under the trade names Caverject (Pfizer, New York, NY) and Viradel/Edex (Schwarz Pharma, Milwaukee, WI) (Buvat et al., 1998; Linet and Ogrinc, 1996; Porst, 1996). After intracavernosal injection, the medication is locally metabolized by 96% within 60 minutes and does not appreciably enter the peripheral circulation (van Ahlen et al., 1994). At dosages of 10 to 20 µg, alprostadil produces full erections in 70% to 80% of patients with ED (Khera and Goldstein, 2011; Linet and Neff, 1994; Porst et al., 2013). The most common side effects of treatment are pain at the injection site or during erection (in 11% of patients), hematoma/ecchymosis (1.5%), prolonged erection/priapism (1% to 5%), and penile fibrotic lesions (2%) (Linet and Ogrinc, 1996). Perceived advantages of alprostadil for intracavernosal pharmacotherapy relative to other agents are lower incidences of prolonged erection, systemic side effects, and penile fibrosis. Disadvantages include a higher incidence of painful erection and higher cost, and, after reconstitution into liquid from powder, alprostadil has a shortened half-life if not refrigerated.

Papaverine. Papaverine, an alkaloid isolated from the opium poppy, is a nonspecific PDE inhibitor that prevents the degradation of cAMP and cGMP so that these cyclic nucleotides accumulate in smooth muscle cells, thereby increasingly promoting tissue relaxation (Kukovetz et al., 1975). The compound also blocks voltage-dependent calcium channels along the membrane wall, thus impeding calcium influx to the cell, a process known to trigger smooth muscle contraction (Brading et al., 1983; Sunagane et al., 1985). Papaverine is metabolized in the liver, and the plasma half-life is 1 to 2 hours. Its general efficacy in promoting penile erection after intracavernosal administration is approximately 60% (Porst et al., 2013). The drug is inexpensive and stable at room temperature. However, disadvantages include commonly observed liver enzyme elevations, priapism risk (up to 35%), and penile fibrosis risk (1% to 33%), which have led to its abandonment as monotherapy (Fallon, 1995; Lakin et al., 1990; Moemen et al., 2004; Porst, 1996).

Phentolamine. In addition to its purported oral role for ED therapy, phentolamine mesylate is more familiarly applied as an intracavernosal agent. Although its erectogenic effect is mediated by blocking the (antierectile) postsynaptic α_1-adrenergic receptor (Sironi et al., 2000), because of its potential inhibition of the prejunctional α_2-adrenergic receptor, which interferes with norepinephrine reuptake, the drug's tissue relaxant effect for penile erection is believed to be antagonized (Juenemann et al., 1986). This dual effect of the drug probably accounts for its limited success when administered intracavernosally as a sole agent (Blum et al., 1985). It has a short plasma half-life (30 minutes). Common side effects associated with the drug include systemic hypotension, reflex tachycardia, nasal congestion, and gastrointestinal upset.

Vasoactive Intestinal Polypeptide. Vasoactive intestinal polypeptide (VIP), a hormone having 28 amino acids originally isolated from the small intestine, was proposed early on to be the elusive nonadrenergic noncholinergic (NANC) mediator of penile erection because of its potent vasodilatory effects in various tissues (Adaikan et al., 1986). Its mechanism of action in smooth muscle is achieved through specific protein receptor binding and activation of adenylate cyclase, thereby promoting synthesis of cAMP and subsequent tissue relaxation (Anderson and Wagner, 1995). The drug has had disappointing effects when administered alone, although when separately combined with other drugs such as papaverine and phentolamine, erection responses were elicited (Dinsmore and Wyllie, 2008; Kiely et al., 1989). VIP, in combination with phentolamine (Invicorp), is currently being sought for regulatory approval in the United States.

Intraurethral Suppositories

The administration of vasoactive drugs via the urethral channel of the penis was introduced with the hope of affording a less invasive procedure than intracavernosal needle injections to induce penile erection. This technique relies on the absorption of the medication through the mucosal lining into the surrounding corpus spongiosum, with passage via small vascular channels into the main erectile bodies, the corpora cavernosa. The transfer of drug from the urethra to the cavernous tissue varies across men according to anatomic variability. After an initial trial, which demonstrated that prostaglandin E$_2$ was effective in inducing full tumescence in 30% of patients and partial tumescence in 40% of patients (Wolfson et al., 1993), a synthetic formulation of prostaglandin E$_1$ was developed and the FDA approved it in November 1996 as MUSE (Medicated Urethral System for Erection; MEDA Pharmaceuticals, Somerset, NJ) (Hellstrom et al., 1996; Padma-Nathan et al., 1997). MUSE uses a suppository inserted into the urethral opening that dispenses a semisolid pellet (1 × 3 mm) of alprostadil (125-, 250-, 500-, and 1000-µg doses) into the distal urethra (3 cm from the external urethral meatus). Several technical procedures optimize the success of the treatment including properly depositing and manually distributing the medication into the penis and the patient's remaining in the upright position for several minutes after its application. In-office training and monitoring of initial response may afford advantages for optimizing technique and making dosage adjustments before performing the treatment at home.

A calculated final responder rate to MUSE is approximately 50%, and among responders approximately 70% of administrations result in sexual intercourse (Guay et al., 2000; Hellstrom et al, 1996; Khera and Goldstein 2011; Padma-Nathan et al, 1997; Porst et al., 2013). The combined use of an adjustable penile constriction band (ACTIS) was designed and was approved by the FDA to enhance the local retention and effect of the medication (Lewis, 2000). A transurethral bimix consisting of alprostadil and α$_1$-adrenergic antagonist prazosin (ALIBRA) was introduced and in a multicenter trial of nearly 400 patients was shown to increase the at-home responder rate for successful sexual intercourse from 47% with alprostadil alone to 70% with ALIBRA (Qureshi, 2001).

Intraurethral therapy is perceived to have a niche role, associated with its inferior efficacy with regard to PDE5 inhibitors and intracavernosal self-injection therapy (Khera and Goldstein, 2011; Porst et al., 2013). The main indications for this therapy are patients who are nonresponsive to PDE5 inhibitors resulting from damage of the autonomic penile nerve supply (e.g., radical prostatectomy, cystectomy, and trauma) or those who wish to use the therapy in combination with PDE5 inhibitors. Another rare indication for intraurethral therapy is patients complaining about a soft (cold) glans syndrome, which may occur after penile prosthesis implantation or as a clinical entity (Porst et al., 2013).

The most common side effects of MUSE include local urogenital pain (approximately one-third of patients) and minor urethral bleeding (5%) (Guay et al., 2000; Padma-Nathan et al., 1997). Other complications such as hypotension (3%), dizziness (4%), and priapism (0.1%) have been observed as well. MUSE is contraindicated in patients with known hypersensitivity to alprostadil, abnormal penile anatomy, and conditions that increase the risk of priapism. MUSE seems safe for female partners, producing only a 5.8% incidence of vaginal burning or itching, although it should not be used without a condom for intercourse with a pregnant woman.

Transdermal/Topical Pharmacotherapy

The notion to apply vasoactive drugs directly to the surface of the penis is consistent with the general appeal of many transdermal therapies (e.g., gels and creams) in medicine based on their delivery route: convenience, simplicity, and putatively limited systemic adverse effects. Several topical therapies have been explored for ED treatments, although certain obstacles have limited their widespread use. Nitroglycerin, a nitric oxide donor formulated as a 2% paste, was found to produce tumescence but rarely penile rigidity sufficient for sexual intercourse (Owen et al., 1989). This relative inefficacy combined with its headache side effects for patient and partner after absorption and action of the drug as a potent systemic vasodilator have precluded its use in clinical practice. Papaverine, formulated as a gel, was investigated but then abandoned as a topical ED treatment when it was found that its large molecular size (molecular weight 376 Da) interfered with its transdermal absorption (Kim et al., 1995).

Alprostadil has been a more promising prospect, subjected to commercial development for penile glans administration in combination with transdermal delivery enhancers: alprostadil 0.3% in combination with a proprietary permeation enhancer, referred to as Vitaros (Apricus Biosciences, San Diego, CA), and alprostadil combined with NexACT, referred to as Alprox-TD (NexMed, Inc., Robbinsville, NJ). Applied intrameatally, such agents in clinical trials have shown efficacy with rates of vaginal penetration and intercourse success that were small but significantly greater than placebo rates and caused minor side effects of site-specific burning or warmth that were comparable to placebo rates (Goldstein et al., 2001; McMahon, 2002; McVary et al., 1999; Padma-Nathan and Yeager, 2006; Porst et al., 2013; Rooney et al., 2009). Prostaglandin E$_1$ ethyl ester, which is a prodrug of prostaglandin E$_1$, is believed to possess an improved transdermal permeation and less skin irritation than enhancing agents because of its esterification (Schanz et al., 2009). Applied to the shaft of the penis in early clinical trials, this drug achieved significantly higher rigidity scores than placebo. In general, transdermal therapy with alprostadil is likely to meet similar clinical roles as that assigned to transurethral pharmacotherapy. Further clinical trials will be useful to define and establish their place in the treatment of ED.

Medical Device

In patients who do not respond to or who decline oral or local vasoactive pharmacotherapeutic options, vacuum erection device therapy may be alternatively explored. **The principle of vacuum erection device therapy is to mechanically create negative pressure surrounding the penis to engorge it with blood and then restrain blood egress from the organ to maintain the erection-like effect** (Broderick et al., 1992; Nadig et al., 1986). Although the treatment does not produce a truly physiologic erection and the engorged blood predominantly consists of venous blood (Bosshardt et al., 1995), the effect resembles a normal erection and is sufficient for coitus. A particular feature is that the glans penis, and not solely the corpora cavernosa, is engorged with blood by the treatment, such that the treatment is further advantageous for patients experiencing glanular insufficiency (soft glans syndrome).

The standard vacuum erection device consists of a usually clear plastic suction cylinder and vacuum-generating source (manual or battery-operated pump) in one piece. It is placed directly over the flaccid penis and operated, and after the penis is erected an elastic constriction ring or band is positioned at the base of the penis; then the vacuum is released and the device is removed (McMahon, 1997; Montague et al., 1996). **The cylinder has a pressure-release valve designed to prevent penile injury from excessive negative pressure. Sexual intercourse may then ensue, although it is recommended that the ring should not be left in place for longer than 30 minutes. Prescription devices are advised, and metal or other inelastic rings are contraindicated.**

Efficacy rates as high as 90% have been reported for achieving satisfactory erections for ED associated with various severities and causes, but satisfaction rates with the device are lower, ranging commonly from 30% to 70% (Hellstrom et al., 2010; Porst et al., 2013). Attrition is reported to occur and may relate to lack of efficacy with more severe forms of ED, although long-term continuation rates have ranged up to 60% (Porst et al., 2013). Success is limited in patients with severe vascular abnormalities such as proximal venous leakage or arterial insufficiency or fibrosis secondary to priapism or prosthesis infection (Marmar et al., 1988). Patient preferences also dictate long-term success. The device is more acceptable to older men in a steady relationship compared with young, single men. Among basic expectations of the treatment, patients should be informed of possible local discomfort or pain associated with the constriction band, a pivoting effect of the penis because turgidity exists only distal to the band's location, a cyanotic discoloration and coolness of the penis resulting from extracorporeal congestion, and trapping of the ejaculation caused by urethral constriction (Cookson and Nadig, 1993; Sidi et al., 1990; Witherington, 1989). Common complications are minor and include penile pain and numbness, difficult ejaculation, ecchymosis, and petechiae, and major complications (e.g., penile skin necrosis, urethral varicosities, Fournier gangrene) are infrequent. Patients receiving anticoagulant therapy (e.g., aspirin, warfarin) and patients with bleeding disorders should use the device with caution (Limoge et al., 1996). Special uses for this therapy have been sought. It has been successfully combined with oral, intracavernosal, and intraurethral pharmacotherapies to produce erectile responses (Canguven et al., 2009; Chen et al., 1995, 2004; John et al., 1996; Marmar et al., 1988). The device has enhanced erectile effects in the presence of a malfunctioning penile prosthesis (Korenman and Viosca, 1992; Sidi et al., 1990). Further, it may offer a means to preserve the elasticity of penile tissues after priapism or penile prosthesis explantation (Moul and McLeod, 1989; Soderdahl et al., 1997) or after surgical correction of Peyronie disease (Yurkanin et al., 2001), and it has been suggested to facilitate erection recovery after treatments for prostate cancer (Köhler et al., 2007; Raina et al., 2006).

Surgery

Surgical interventions have always served an important role in the armamentarium of ED treatments. **They are often applied in the face of penile injury resulting from genital or pelvic trauma, penile structural deformity occurring in association with Peyronie disease, or possibly cavernosal fibrosis secondary to prolonged ischemic priapism or infection. They are also considered when medical therapy for ED is contraindicated, unsuccessful, or undesirable.**

Penile Prosthesis Surgery

Penile prosthesis or implant surgery is a mechanism for creating penile rigidity that differs from a physiologic or pharmacologically induced erection. Malleable (semirigid) and inflatable (hydraulic) devices are both currently available for this purpose. Details of this treatment option are presented in Chapter 72.

Penile Revascularization Surgery

Based on the requirements of inflow of blood and its retention in the penis for penile erection to occur, vascular surgeries have aggressively been pursued to facilitate or restore these biologic processes.

Arterial Revascularization. In concept, arterial revascularization surgery was designed to create arterial inflow to the corpora cavernosa, in turn addressing the presentation of arteriogenic ED. Several procedures have been described to meet this objective, similarly creating an anastomosis of the inferior epigastric artery either to the corpus cavernosum directly or to vascular conduits of the penis such as the dorsal artery (i.e., revascularization), the deep dorsal vein (i.e., arterialization), or the deep dorsal vein with venous ligation (i.e., arterialization with venous reconstruction) (Hellstrom et al., 2010). Success of these surgeries has been variable and depends on careful patient selection. Penile arteriography is required to establish a penile arterial anatomic defect, and other organic causes of ED (e.g., venous incompetence) that would limit surgical success should be excluded. **According to the current literature, the following inclusion criteria should be met when selecting patients for arterial surgery: age less than 55 years, nonsmoker, nondiabetic, absence of venous leakage, and radiographic confirmation of stenosis of the internal pudendal artery** (Hellstrom et al., 2010; Sohn et al., 2013). **The highest success rates are reported in young men (less than 30 years of age) with isolated arterial stenosis after perineal or pelvic trauma** (Babaei et al., 2009). Complications of arterial revascularization surgery include glans hyperemia (13%), shunt thrombosis (8%), and inguinal hernias (6.5%) (Kawanishi et al., 2004; Manning et al., 1998).

Venous Reconstruction. Venous reconstruction was proposed to prevent the pathologic blood egress from the penis, understandably to correct veno-occlusive ED. Most surgical procedures have centered on ligating or embolizing penile veins (e.g., superficial dorsal vein, deep dorsal vein, crural vein) or surgically compressing the penile crura (e.g., crural plication/ligation, pericavernoplasty) (Hellstrom et al., 2010). **Success with these surgeries has not been affirmed, primarily because of inaccurate or deficient methods for diagnosing and correcting the relevant anatomic defect. The optimal surgical approach remains to be defined, and thus venous reconstructive surgery is presently considered investigational** (Hellstrom et al., 2010; Montague et al., 2005; Sohn et al., 2013). Reported complications of this surgery include glanular hypoanesthesia, skin necrosis, wound infections, penile curvature/shortening, and glans hyperemia.

Combination Therapies

Many patients with ED do not respond acceptably to monotherapy, with nonresponder rates documented in as many as 40% of patients (Porst et al., 2013). Some patients may achieve optimal therapeutic responses by combining treatment options. In addition, it is possible that a dose-limiting adverse effect is associated with ED monotherapy such that combined treatments may then seem advantageous. Multiple combinations may certainly be proposed for ED treatment. The extant literature describes several successful combinations: tadalafil 5 mg daily with 50 mg sildenafil on demand (Cui et al., 2015), oral PDE5 inhibitors with psychosocial counseling (Althof et al., 2005), oral PDE5 inhibitors with testosterone replacement therapy (Greco et al., 2006; Shabsigh et al., 2004; Spitzer et al., 2012, 2013), oral PDE5 inhibitors with transurethral alprostadil (Mydlo et al., 2000; Nehra et al., 2002), oral PDE5 inhibitors and intracavernosal pharmacotherapy (McMahon et al., 1999), oral PDE5 inhibitors and vacuum erection device (Canguven et al., 2009; Chen et al., 2004), intracavernosal pharmacotherapy and vacuum erection device (Chen et al., 1995), transurethral pharmacotherapy and vacuum erection device (John et al., 1996), and transurethral pharmacotherapy and penile prosthesis surgery (Benevides and Carson, 2000). **Caution is advised when initiating combination therapy to observe for potential complications that may be compounded by combined treatments, and in-office evaluations before continuing treatments at home may be considered to offer an additional measure of safety.**

Alternative Therapies

Alternative therapies have long been considered for the treatment of ED, from herbs, ointments, nutraceuticals, and dietary supplements in commercial supply today. The movement toward alternative medicines in this field actually gained momentum during the past decade with the emergence of effective oral therapy in the form of PDE5 inhibitors, which created avenues for producing PDE5 inhibitor-like counterfeit and imitation substances and promoting regulatory agency unapproved products in general. Indeed, the true efficacies of proposed alternative therapies (e.g., ginkgo biloba, L-arginine, Korean red ginseng) remain uncertain in the absence of evidenced benefit in rigorously performed, randomized controlled clinical trials (Khera and Goldstein, 2011; Moyad et al., 2004). The success of these products is ascribed in some measure to the known placebo effect of agents to treat ED, which has been observed to amount to as much as 25% to 50% in properly conducted clinical trials.

Recently, low-intensity extracorporeal shock wave therapy (Li-ESWT), stem cell therapies, and platelet-rich plasma have been proposed as an effective, noninvasive treatment option for ED among men who respond poorly to PDE5 inhibitors. Investigations into the mechanism of action using diabetic animal models treated with Li-ESWT found that erectile function improved by promoting regeneration of nerves, endothelium, and smooth muscle of the penis (Qiu et al., 2013). Studies among men with ED who do not respond to PDE5 inhibitors and after prostatectomy found improved hydrodynamics, endothelial function, and IIEF scores (Frey et al., 2016; Gruenwald et al., 2012, 2013). A meta-analysis of seven randomized clinical trials involving 602 patients with mild to moderate ED showed significant improvement in pooled IIEF-EF scores among men undergoing Li-ESWT compared with placebo (6.40 vs 1.65 points, $P = 0.047$) (Clavijo et al., 2017). The Sexual Medicine Society of North America (SMSNA) released a position statement on restorative and regenerative therapies for erectile dysfunction. Given the current lack of regulatory agency approval for any restorative (regenerative) therapies for the treatment of ED and until such time as approval is granted, SMSNA believes that the use of shock waves, stem cells, or platelet-rich plasma is experimental and requires research protocols in compliance with Institutional Review Board approval. Before the use of alternative therapies can be advocated, further research that demonstrates their mechanisms of action and meaningful efficacy/safety must be performed.

> **KEY POINTS: TREATMENT CONSIDERATIONS**
>
> - Although definitive evidence is necessary, risk modification for preserving erectile health includes recommendation to maintain a healthy and fit lifestyle.
> - Psychosexual therapy offers a role in the integrative management of ED.
> - Various modalities of drug administration including oral, intracavernosal, intraurethral, and transdermal routes are successfully applied or are under study.
> - Vacuum erection device therapy offers an alternative to oral or local vasoactive pharmacotherapeutic options for ED.
> - Surgical intervention (penile prosthesis surgery) are an important treatment when nonsurgical therapy is contraindicated, unsuccessful, or undesirable.
> - Arterial revascularization surgery is offered only to select patients with ED who meet stringent clinical and radiographic criteria for surgical success.

FUTURE DIRECTIONS

Consistent with the ongoing progress in the field of sexual medicine more broadly, advancements in ED management will likely continue. Much has been learned in the physiology and molecular science of penile erection in recent decades, indicative of the amazing scientific discovery occurring in this arena. Science and technology represent the cornerstones for new developments in diagnosis and treatment. In the therapeutic arena, we can expect to see the next generation of pharmacotherapeutics as well as gene, stem cell, and regenerative therapies. Surgical procedures will continue to evolve, including penile reconstructive to prosthetic to tissue replacement surgeries (e.g., penile transplantation). The treatment paradigm will expectedly evolve from treatment based on symptomatic presentation and severity extent of ED to cause-specific ED treatments associated with disease states and genetic factors related to precision medicine. Ongoing progress will likely define the ultimate level of ED management: interventions that restore and maximize natural erectile function.

ACKNOWLEDGMENT

The authors would like to thank Aubrey B. Greer for assisting with updating and editing this chapter.

REFERENCES

The complete reference list is available online at ExpertConsult.com.

70
Priapism
Gregory A. Broderick, MD

Priapism is a persistent erection arising from dysfunction of the mechanisms regulating penile rigidity and detumescence. A correct diagnosis of priapism is a matter of urgency requiring characterization of the underlying hemodynamics.

Scientific organizations have recommended guidelines for the management of priapism, including the American Urological Association (AUA) in 2003 (http://www.auanet.org), the International Society for Sexual Medicine in 2010 (http://www.issm.info), and the European Association of Urology in 2013 (http://www.uroweb.org). Despite the proliferation of guidelines many urologists express a lack of confidence in the assessment and key steps to emergency management of priapism (Bullock et al., 2018). Guidelines committees have promoted uniform definition for priapism and its subtypes but have provided primarily best practice recommendations rather than evidence-based recommendations. Many of these recommendations were first made in prior editions of this book. The literature on priapism is composed mainly of observational reports, many case reports, and small surgical case series. There are few reports of randomized therapeutic trials. Recent case series have included detailed methodologies: duration of priapism, causes of priapism, medicines and procedures employed in managing priapism, and some erectile function outcomes. The epidemiology, cause, pathophysiology of priapism, and clinical research supporting the most effective treatment strategies are summarized in this chapter.

DEFINING PRIAPISM

Priapism is a full or partial erection that continues more than 4 hours beyond sexual stimulation and orgasm or is unrelated to sexual stimulation.

Classifying Priapism

Ischemic Priapism (Veno-occlusive, Low-Flow)

Ischemic priapism is a persistent erection marked by rigidity of the corpora cavernosa (CC) and little or no cavernous arterial inflow. In ischemic priapism there are time-dependent changes in the corporal metabolic environment with progressive hypoxia, hypercarbia, and acidosis. The patient typically reports penile pain after 6 to 8 hours, and the examination reveals a rigid erection. The condition is analogous to a muscle compartment syndrome, with initial occlusion of venous outflow and subsequent cessation of arterial inflows. Well-documented histologic changes occur within the corporal smooth muscle as a consequence of prolonged ischemia. Interventions beyond 36 hours of onset may help relieve erection and pain but have no benefit in preserving potency (Bennett and Mulhall, 2008). Histologically, by 12 hours corporal specimens show interstitial edema, progressing to destruction of sinusoidal endothelium, exposure of the basement membrane, and thrombocyte adherence at 24 hours. After 48 hours thrombus can be found in the sinusoidal spaces, and smooth muscle necrosis with fibroblast-like cell transformation is evident (Spycher and Hauri, 1986). Ischemic priapism is an emergency. When left untreated, resolution may take days to weeks, and severe corporal fibrosis and erectile dysfunction (ED) invariably result (Fig. 70.1).

Stuttering Priapism (Intermittent, Recurrent Ischemic Priapism)

Stuttering priapism is characterized by a pattern of recurrence. The term has historically described recurrent unwanted and painful erections in men with sickle cell disease (SCD) (Serjeant et al., 1985). Patients typically awaken with an erection that persists for several hours. Males with SCD may experience stuttering priapism from childhood; in these patients the pattern of stuttering may increase in frequency and duration, leading to a full episode of unrelenting ischemic priapism. Any patient who has experienced an episode of ischemic priapism is also at risk for stuttering priapism (Hoeh and Levine, 2015).

Nonischemic Priapism (Arterial, High Flow)

Nonischemic priapism is a persistent erection caused by unregulated cavernous arterial inflow. Typically, the corpora are tumescent but not rigid and the penis is not painful. A history of blunt trauma to the perineum or an iatrogenic needle injury is common. Whatever the mechanism of injury, the result is a disruption of the cavernous arterial anatomy creating an arteriolar-sinusoidal fistula. The cavernous environment does not become ischemic and cavernous blood gases do not show hypoxia, hypercarbia, or acidosis. This type of priapism, once properly diagnosed, does not require emergent intervention. Beyond the acute trauma, patients do not report pain. Normal erectile function has been reported after recovery from the initial event, despite persistence of nonsexual partial erection (Fig. 70.2).

PRIAPISM: HISTORICAL PERSPECTIVES

The term *priapism* has its origin in reference to the Greek god Priapus, who was worshipped as a god of fertility and protector of horticulture. Priapus is memorialized in sculptures for his giant phallus. The first recorded account of priapism in English medical literature appears in the *Lancet* and is attributed to Tripe (1845). Historically, the most commonly cited observation on this condition in North American literature is Frank Hinman Sr.'s landmark article describing the natural history of priapism (Hinman, 1914). Subsequently in 1960 his son, Frank Hinman Jr., postulated that venous stasis, increased blood viscosity, and ischemia were responsible for priapism and emphasized that failure to correct these abnormalities in the penile environment was essentially responsible for treatment nonresponse (Hinman, 1960). Advances in our understanding of the physiology of erection and the pathophysiology of ED substantiated early hypotheses that prolonged veno-occlusion within the corporal bodies is analogous to a compartment syndrome. Hauri et al. (1983) first demonstrated the radiologic differences between veno-occlusive and arterial priapism.

Frank Hinman (1914) first described "acute transitory attacks of priapism" as opposed to persistence or rapid recurrence of a single episode. The actual term *stuttering priapism* is attributed to Emond et al. (1980) in observations of patients with SCD in a Jamaican clinic. Stuttering priapism episodes were seen to increase in frequency and length, leading to major, unrelenting occurrence of ischemic priapism. Attempts to manage SCD patients with stuttering ischemic

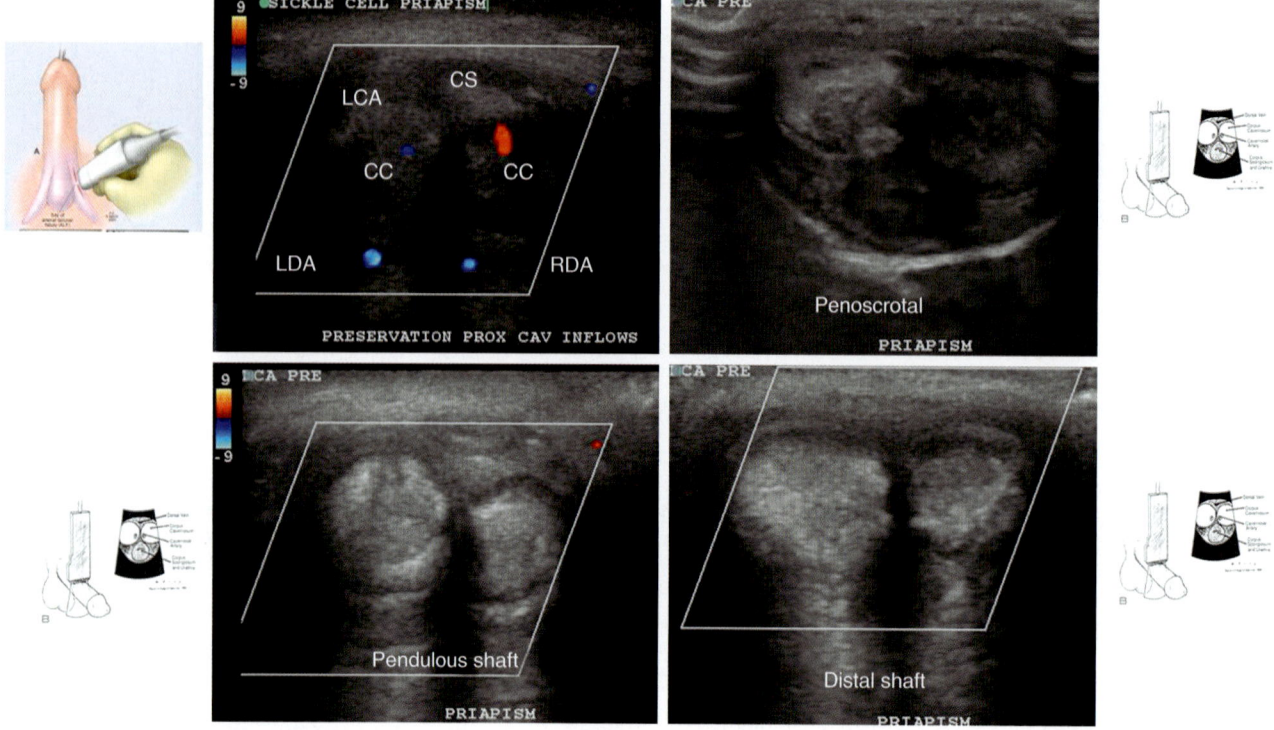

Fig. 70.1. This 21-year-old Nigerian man complained of severe erectile dysfunction after recurrent episodes of sickle cell ischemic priapism. *Top left*, Transperineal imaging with color Doppler shows preservation of cavernous arterial inflow at the crura. *Top right and bottom*, Increasing echogenicity on gray-scale ultrasound of the penile shaft: penoscrotal, pendulous shaft, and distal shaft. These findings are the result of recurring ischemic priapism, which leaves the patient with distal corporal fibrosis. *CC*, Corpus cavernosa; *CS*, corpus spongiosum; *LCA*, left cavernous artery; *LDA*, left dorsal artery; *RDA*, right dorsal artery.

priapism resulted in the early recommendation for hormonal suppression of nocturnal erections and stuttering with estrogen dosing (Serjeant et al., 1985).

Nonischemic priapism is described far less commonly than ischemic priapism in the urologic literature. **Nonischemic priapism is invariably associated with antecedent perineal or penile trauma.** It was first described in the English literature by Burt et al. (1960). After blunt trauma to the perineum, nonischemic (high-flow) priapism (HFP) is associated with disruption of arteriolar-sinusoidal architecture. At this site a region of unregulated arteriolar flow, commonly referred to as a sinusoidal fistula, develops. **Contemporary literature documents that reversal of ischemic priapism may result in conversion to a high-flow state, secondary to either a post-ischemic hyperemia or direct laceration of a cavernous artery and formation of a high-flow fistula at the surgical shunt site** (Bertolotto et al., 2009; Lutz et al., 2012; McMahon, 2002, Rodriguez et al., 2006,).

KEY POINTS: PRIAPISM DEFINITIONS

- Priapism is a full or partial erection that continues more than 4 hours beyond sexual stimulation and orgasm or is unrelated to sexual stimulation.
- Ischemic (low-flow) priapism is a persistent erection marked by rigidity of the CC with little or no cavernous arterial inflow.
- Nonischemic (arterial, high-flow) priapism is a persistent erection caused by unregulated cavernous arterial inflow. The corpora are tumescent but not rigid, and the erection is not painful.
- Stuttering priapism describes a pattern of recurrence. The term has traditionally described recurrent prolonged and painful erections in men with SCD.

EPIDEMIOLOGY OF PRIAPISM

Population-based studies estimate cases per 100,000 person-years (the number of patients with a first episode of priapism divided by the accumulated amount of person-time in the study population). Cases per 100,000 person-years have been calculated in several countries; these data depend on recording of presentations to clinics and hospitals where cases are registered. Kulmala et al. (1995) calculated the cases per 100,000 person-years to be 0.34 to 0.52 from 1975 to 1990 in Finland; Eland et al. (2001) calculated the cases in the Netherlands to be 1.5 per 100,000 person-years; Earle et al. (2003) calculated 0.84 per 100,000 person-years in Australia from 1985 to 2000. These reported incidence rates were significantly affected by the introduction and proliferation of intracavernous vasoactive injections for the management of ED. In Finland during the last 3 years of the study the incidence of priapism doubled to 1.1 cases per 100,000 person-years. These and other reports on the epidemiology and cause of priapism are also greatly influenced by the prevalence of SCD in the populations described. **The lifetime probability of a man with SCD developing ischemic priapism ranges from 29% to 42%** (Emond et al., 1980).

Observation reports in the United States on priapism are evidenced by looking at emergency department data. Two retrospective analyses—the Nationwide Inpatient Sample (NIS) and the Nationwide Emergency Department Sample—provide estimates of the incidence of priapism in the United States. Chrouser et al. (2011) accessed data from the NIS (1998 to 2006). In the sample (4237 hospitalizations), 30% of patients were white, 61.1% were black, and 6.3% were Hispanic; 41.9% of patients had a diagnosis of SCD; and 36.2% of patients required penile surgery. The mean age at time of hospital admission for priapism associated with SCD was 23.8 years and for non-SCD was 40.8 years.

Roghmann et al. (2013) looked at the Nationwide Emergency Department Sample (NEDS). The NEDS includes discharge information

Chapter 70 Priapism **1541**

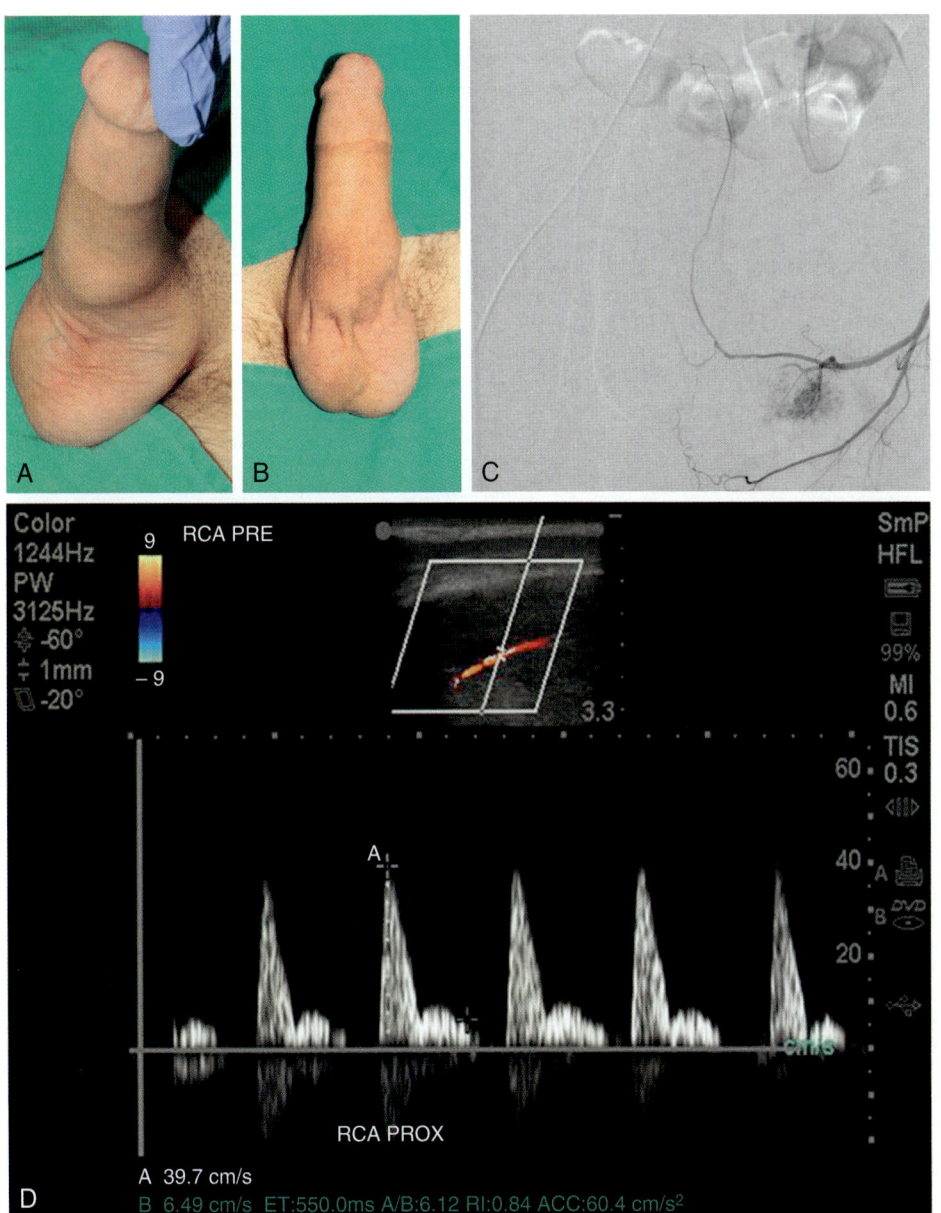

Fig. 70.2. A 21-year-old man with a history of ischemic priapism after binging with alcohol, marijuana, and energy drinks. Patient had a series of penile shunt procedures performed by different urologists in attempts to reverse ischemic priapism: Winter, Al-Ghorab, and subsequently bilateral corpus cavernosum to corpus spongiosum shunts (note bulging at base of pendulous penis). Six months later he sought evaluation for embarrassing persistent nonpainful partial erection. The history and examination were consistent with conversion to high-flow state, likely from an arteriolar sinusoidal fistula. (A) Tumescent shaft with glans scar. (B) Penoscrotal bulging at site of cavernospongiosal shunts. (C) Angiogram of fistula originating at the bulbourethral artery. (D) Doppler evaluation without intracavernous vasoactive injection shows a high-flow state: peak systolic velocity of 39 cm/sec and end diastolic flow of 6 cm/sec and resistive index of 84.

on patients, independent of payers. Data were abstracted for the diagnosis of priapism. Between 2006 and 2009 there were 32,462 emergency department visits for priapism. The incidence of priapism in the United States based on this methodology was 5.34 per 100,000 men per year. The incidence of priapism requiring an emergency room visit was 31.4% higher in summer months; 13% of emergency room visits resulted in hospitalizations; 34% of patients were privately insured; 51% were treated in urban teaching hospitals; 13% of adult patients had SCD; 31% of pediatric patients (<18 years old) had SCD. Sickle cell diagnosis was associated with 57% of pediatric admissions and 20% of adult admissions. **This study** (Roghmann et al., 2013) **and others** (Stein et al., 2013) **suggest that in the United States the incidence of priapism is significantly influenced by the prevalence of SCD in a community and that the majority of contemporary cases are being treated in emergency departments as outpatients rather than requiring hospital admissions and presumably surgery.** Sui et al. (2016) looked at readmissions for priapism in the state of New York; they followed a cohort of patients for 12 months after presenting to emergency departments from 2005 to 2014. They found that 24% of patients were re-admitted in 1 year for another episode of priapism; the majority of patients were readmitted within 60 days. Sickle cell disease and an initial hospital stay for priapism were significant risk factors for readmission.

Etiology of Ischemic Priapism (Veno-occlusive, Low-Flow)

Ischemic priapism accounts for the majority of cases described in the literature. The erection of ischemic priapism may begin with

BOX 70.1 Causes of Priapism

α-Adrenergic Receptor Antagonists
 Prazosin, terazosin, doxazosin, tamsulosin
Antianxiety Agent
 Hydroxyzine
Anticoagulants
 Heparin, warfarin
Antidepressants and Antipsychotics
 Trazodone, bupropion, fluoxetine, sertraline, lithium, clozapine, risperidone, olanzapine, chlorpromazine, thioridazine, phenothiazines
Antihypertensives
 Hydralazine, guanethidine, propranolol
Attention-Deficit/Hyperactivity Disorder Agents
 Methylphenidates (Concerta, Daytrana, Focalin, Metadate, Methylin, Quillivant, Ritalin)
 Atomoxetine (Strattera)
Recreational Drugs
 Alcohol, cocaine (intranasal and topical), crack cocaine, marijuana, synthetic cannabinoids
Genitourinary Conditions
 Straddle injury, coital injury, pelvic trauma, kick to penis or perineum, penile bypass surgery, urinary retention

Hematologic Dyscrasias
 Sickle cell disease, thalassemia, granulocytic leukemia, myeloid leukemia, lymphocytic leukemia, multiple myeloma, hemoglobin Olmsted variant, fat emboli associated with hyperalimentation, hemodialysis, glucose-6-phosphate dehydrogenase deficiency
Hormones
 Gonadotropin-releasing hormone, testosterone
Infectious (Toxin-Mediated) Causes
 Scorpion sting, spider bite, rabies, malaria
Metabolic Conditions
 Amyloidosis, Fabry disease, gout
Neoplastic Causes (Metastatic or Regional Infiltration)
 Prostate, urethra, testis, bladder, rectum, lung, kidney
Neurogenic Conditions
 Syphilis, spinal cord injury, cauda equina compression, autonomic neuropathy, lumbar disk herniation, spinal stenosis, cerebral vascular accident, brain tumor, spinal anesthesia, cauda equina syndrome
Vasoactive Erectile Agents
 Papaverine, phentolamine, prostaglandin E_1, oral phosphodiesterase type 5 inhibitors, combination intracavernous therapy

Modified from Lue TF: Physiology of penile erection and pathophysiology of erectile dysfunction and priapism. In Walsh PC, Retik AB, Vaughan ED, et al., editors: *Campbell's urology*, Philadelphia, 2002, Saunders, pp 1610–1696.

---

sexual stimulation or the administration of pharmacologic agents. **Once an erection persists beyond 4 hours and is not relieved by orgasm or pharmacologic reversal, the pathophysiologic phenomena of ischemic priapism have begun.** Erections lasting up to 4 hours are by consensus defined as "prolonged"; manufacturers of erection-facilitating pharmacotherapies (oral, injectable, and intraurethral) recommend that the patient seek emergent medical consultation for prolonged erection.

Although SCD is a predominant cause of veno-occlusive priapism in the literature, there is a wide variety of reported associations from urinary retention to insect bites (Hoover and Fortenberry, 2004). In 1986 Pohl et al. reported on 230 cases. The cause of priapism was identified as idiopathic in the majority; 21% of cases were associated with alcohol or drug use or abuse, 12% with perineal trauma, and 11% with SCD (Pohl et al., 1986).

Priapism has even been reported after envenomation by arthropods, primarily yellow South American scorpion *Tityus serrulatus* and the Brazilian banana spider, *Phoneutria nigriventer* (Andrade et al., 2008; Nunes et al., 2013; Ravelli et al., 2017; Villanova et al., 2009). The genus *Phoneutria* (from the Greek for "murderess") has eight species. *P. nigriventer* is known to hide in dark and moist places, wander the jungle floor, and stow away within banana shipments. *P. nigriventer* toxin is a neurotoxin; a variety of mechanisms of action have been implicated: calcium channel–blocking properties, inhibiting glutamate release, sodium channel inactivation, and activation of nitric oxide (NO) synthases. Bites cause intense pain, vascular congestion, loss of muscle control—paralysis, breathing problems—asphyxiation, priapism, and death. Two peptides isolated from the venom of *P. nigriventer* have been directly linked with the induction of persistent and painful erections in mammals (Tx2-5 and Tx2-6) (Leite et al., 2012). The protein has been named *eretina* and has been shown to have a highly specific interference at the molecular level with the NO pathway. Penile erection has been induced in vivo with eretina by direct intraperitoneal injection with a minimum effective dose of 0.006 μg/kg (Andrade et al., 2008). The toxin can induce priapism even in mice after cavernous nerve denervations (Ravelli et al., 2017). One pharmacologic review marvels at the potency of arthropod toxins is entitled *"From the stretcher to the pharmacy's shelf"* (Rates et al., 2011).

Hematologic dyscrasias are a major risk factor for ischemic priapism (Box 70.1). Priapism has been described as a complication of SCD, thalassemia, hereditary spherocytosis, paroxysmal nocturnal hemoglobinuria, glucose-6-phosphate dehydrogenase deficiency, glucose-6-phosphate isomerase deficiency, and congenital dyserythropoietic anemia (Burnett, 2005; Kato, 2012). **Thrombotic disease states have also been cited as precipitants of ischemic priapism;** these conditions include asplenia, erythropoietin use, hemodialysis with heparin use, and cessation of Coumadin therapy. Intracavernous heparin given as a therapy for priapism caused by rebound hypercoagulable states has actually worsened the condition (Bschleipfer et al., 2001; Fassbinder et al., 1976). Lue and Garcia (2013) proposed that postoperative recurrence of priapism may be a thromboembolic event like postoperative thrombosis of vascular grafts; they recommend perioperative anticoagulation be administered to patients having shunt procedures for ischemic priapism.

Priapism may occur in patients with excessive white blood cell (WBC) counts. The incidence of priapism in adult male patients with leukemia is 1% to 5% (Chang et al., 2003). Hyperleukocytosis causes priapism in these patients; it is believed that mechanical pressure on abdominal veins secondary to splenomegaly causes congestion of cavernous outflow and sludging of leukemic cells within the CC. When priapism occurs in the oncology setting, evaluation and management of the predisposing condition must accompany interventions directed at the penis. In hematologic malignancies, leukapheresis and cytotoxic therapy (hydroxyurea, cytosine arabinoside) may reduce the numbers of circulating WBCs (Manuel et al., 2007; Ponniah et al., 2004).

Priapism secondary to metastatic infiltrating solid lesions rather than leukemoid reaction is extremely rare. In most case reports of metastatic priapism, the primary malignancy is genitourinary 69% (Cocci et al., 2016). Cocci et al. (2018) noted that the median cancer-specific survival for patients with penile metastasis was 14 months. Other primary cancers have been described in case reports to metastasize to the penis: testis, kidney, and lung. Metastatic infiltration of the penis may proceed with solid replacement or focal nodules within the CC, glans, and CS. Theoretically, metastatic deposits within the corpora could obstruct venous outflow, resulting in ischemic priapism; metastatic deposits could also disrupt sinusoidal architecture and produce a high flow state. Depending on the status of the patient, metastatic lesions may be managed expectantly, with partial or total penectomy, chemotherapy, or irradiation. These cases are too rarely and poorly described to define best practice recommendations (Broderick et al., 2010; Celma Doménech et al., 2008; Chan et al., 1998; Guvel et al., 2003; Robey and Schellhammer, 1984; Fig. 70.3).

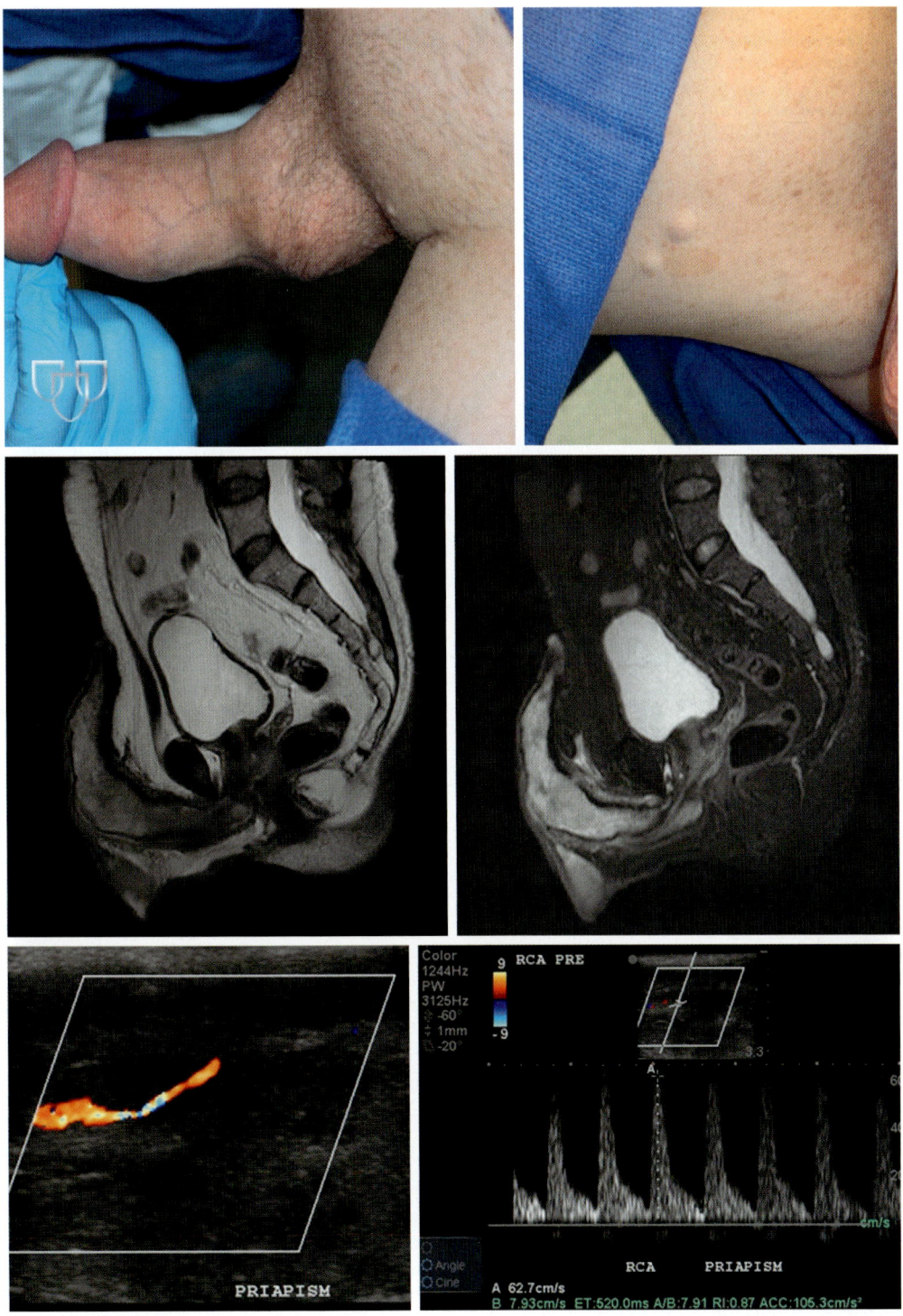

Fig. 70.3. This is a case of biopsy-proven malignant peripheral nerve sheath tumor (neurofibrosarcoma) arising circumferentially around the base of the penis in a 60-year-old man with a known history of neurofibromatosis, type I who presented to the urology clinic with a 4-week history of a continuous erection and 4-cm mass. Physical examination demonstrated a 4-cm nodule deforming the base of penis and partial erection. The patient did have pain with deep palpation. Cutaneous neurofibromas are shown on medial thigh. T1 and T2 coronal MRI images show neurofibrosarcoma replacing corpora cavernosa. Penile color Doppler ultrasound was performed establishing high-flow priapism with elevated peak systolic velocities, elevated end diastolic velocities, but no evidence of an arterial sinusoidal fistula.

Sickle Cell Disease

Blood dyscrasias are a risk factor for ischemic priapism. SCD priapism has traditionally been ascribed to stagnation of blood within the sinusoids of the CC during physiologic erection, secondary to obstruction of venous outflow by sickled erythrocytes (Lue, 2002). Nelson and Winter (1977) described a series of cases in which SCD was the primary cause of ischemic priapism in 23% of adults and 63% of children. **Sickle cell hemoglobinopathy accounts for at least one-third of all cases of priapism,** and, indeed, prevalence of ischemic priapism varies significantly within the population of males in a community with SCD. **From Emond et al.'s 1980 observational study comes the most commonly quoted incidence: among 104 men attending an outpatient sickle cell clinic in Kingston, Jamaica, the incidence of priapism in men with homozygous sickle cell disease (SCD) was 42.** In a US clinical series, Tarry et al. (1987) found that 6.4% of male children in an outpatient sickle cell clinic had a history of priapism. Adeyoju et al. (2002), in an international multicenter observational study of SCD, mailed or interviewed 130 patients attending SCD clinics in the United Kingdom and Nigeria. Respondents ranged in age from 4 to 66 years old, with a mean age of 25. The authors cited mean age of onset of priapism as 15 years, with 75% of patients having their first episode before age 20 and rare first-time presentations by the third decade of life. In the questionnaires a clear distinction was made between acute severe prolonged priapism lasting longer than 24 hours requiring emergency attention and stuttering recurrent priapism of shorter and self-limiting duration. In this population the incidence of acute priapism was 35%; of these patients, 72% gave a history of stuttering priapism. The median frequency of occurrence of stuttering priapism was three times per month; the median duration of each episode was 1.2 hours, with the longest being 8 hours. Precipitating events reported from greatest to least were sexual arousal or intercourse, fever, sleep, cold weather, and dehydration. Self-administered regimens were analgesics, drinking water, and exercise. Twenty-one percent of patients reporting a history of priapism also reported ED. Surprisingly only 7% of young men who had not experienced priapism were even aware that priapism was a potential complication of their SCD. On the basis of the World Health Organization global prevalence map of SCD, Aliyu et al. (2008) estimated that 20 to 25 million individuals worldwide have homozygous SCD: 12 to 15 million in sub-Saharan Africa, 5 to 10 million in India, and 3 million in other world regions. They also found that 70,000 patients with SCD live in the United States (Aliyu et al., 2008).

The sickle cell genetic mutation is the result of a single amino acid substitution in the β-globin subunit of hemoglobin S (HbS). The molecular lesion is a point mutation (GAG substituted for GTG) in exon 1 of the β globin gene; this results in substitution of glutamic acid by valine on the β globin polypeptide chain (Ballas et al., 2012). **Clinical features are seen in homozygous SCD patients: chronic hemolysis, vascular occlusion, tissue ischemia, and end-organ damage.** HbS polymerizes when deoxygenated, injuring the sickle erythrocyte, activating a cascade of hemolysis and vaso-occlusion. Membrane damage results in dense sickling of red cells, causing adhesive interactions among sickle cells, endothelial cells, and leukocytes. Hemolysis releases hemoglobin into the plasma. Free hemoglobin reacts with NO to produce methemoglobin and nitrate. This is a scavenging reaction; the vasodilator NO is oxidized to inert nitrate. Sickled erythrocytes release arginase-I into blood plasma, which converts L-arginine into ornithine, effectively removing substrate for NO synthesis. Oxidant radicals further reduce NO bioavailability. The combined effects of NO scavenging and arginine catabolism result in a state of NO resistance and insufficiency termed *hemolysis-associated endothelial dysfunction* (Aliyu et al., 2008; Kato et al., 2007; Kuypers, 2014; Morris et al., 2005; Rother et al., 2005).

Contemporary science implicates hemolysis and reduced NO in the pathogenesis of pulmonary hypertension, leg ulcers, priapism, and stroke in patients with SCD, whereas increased blood viscosity is believed to be responsible for painful crises, osteonecrosis, and acute chest syndrome (Kato, 2012; Kato et al., 2006). Patients with SCD and priapism have a fivefold greater risk of developing pulmonary hypertension. **SCD priapism is also associated with reduced hemoglobin levels and increased hemolytic markers: reticulocyte count, bilirubin, lactate dehydrogenase (LDH), and aspartate aminotransferase.** Cerebral vascular accidents are more frequent, close to episodes of full-blown priapism; the ASPEN syndrome (association of SCD, priapism, exchange transfusion, and neurologic events) describes cerebral vascular accidents in patients with SCD who have received exchange transfusions (Merritt et al., 2006; Siegel et al., 1993). One series of 136 adult patients with SCD admitted to the intensive care unit (ICU) noted the most common types of crises were severe pain, acute chest syndrome, and infection; 12% of patients were nonsurvivors; thrombocytopenia is more common than thrombocytosis in severe sickle cell crisis (Shome et al., 2018). Sickle cell trait is considered a benign condition; a few complications have been associated with extreme physical exertion. There have been case reports of sickle cell trait as the predisposing factor to ischemic priapism (Birnbaum and Pinzone, 2008; Larocque and Cosgrove, 1974).

Iatrogenic Priapism: Intracavernous Injections

Prolonged erection is more commonly reported than is priapism after therapeutic or diagnostic injection of intracavernous vasoactive medications (Broderick and Lue, 2002; Coombs et al., 2012). Despite the introduction of effective oral medications for ED in 1998, intracavernous injection (ICI) remains an important therapeutic option for men with severe ED in whom a phosphodiesterase type 5 (PDE5) inhibitor fails or who cannot take PDE5 inhibitors because they require nitrates. In many communities patients receiving intracavernous medications for ED will outnumber patients with SCD. **Priapism after ICI is a problem all urologists will encounter and must be prepared to manage.** In a review of worldwide reports on ICI programs, Junemann et al. (1990) noted that diagnostic injection resulted in 5.3% of men getting ischemic priapism, and 0.4% of men reported priapism after injecting at home. In papaverine-based ICI programs, reports of prolonged erections and priapism are poorly distinguished and range from 0 to 35% (Broderick and Lue, 2002). In worldwide clinical trials of the Alprostadil Study Group, prolonged erection (defined as 4 to 6 hours) was described in 5% of patients, and priapism (longer than 6 hours) in 1% (Porst, 1996). In the United States the approved label and package insert for one product (alprostadil [Caverject]) cites the frequency of prolonged erection (4 to 6 hours) as 4% and frequency of priapism as 0.4%. The label recommends that "to minimize chances of prolonged erection or priapism Caverject should be titrated slowly to the lowest effective dosage." Combinations of papaverine/phentolamine/alprostadil commonly referred to as Trimix is the most popular mixture used in ICI programs. In a single-center 5-year retrospective study of 1412 patients, Coombs et al. (2012) noted that 89% of men were using Trimix with significant dropout rates but an overall low rate of priapism (0.5%).

Similar to the clinical trials of Caverject (alprostadil), in clinical trials of Edex (alprostadil) erection lasting longer than 4 hours was reported by 4% of subjects followed for 24 months. Priapism in Edex trials was defined as erection lasting longer than 6 hours; the incidence of priapism was less than 1%. Package inserts approved for marketing Alprostadil injections in the United States contraindicate PGE1 injections for men with sickle cell anemia, sickle cell trait, multiple myeloma, and leukemia.

Injection therapy with alprostadil was first approved in the United States in 1996 and has long since moved out of the spotlight of scientific trials. Neither time nor the introduction of PDE5 inhibitor therapy has completely eclipsed penile injections. Penile injections are the primary alternative offered men who fail or are not satisfied with oral drugs and are the main therapeutic agent offered by men's health clinics. In this author's professional experience the majority of these clinics either fail to do dosage titration in the office or simply "oversell" penile injections, resulting in significantly higher prolonged erection and priapism rates. In a retrospective series from China 214 men were followed for nearly 10 years on alprostadil injections (He et al., 2011). As had been shown in earlier studies dropout rates are significant: 51% of men continue to use treatment for more than 1 year, 6% more than 5 years, 2.9% more than 8 years, and only 1.7% of men were still using penile injectables at 10 years. Major complications identified were pain associated with injection, ecchymosis at injection site, and corporal fibrosis. The authors report that none of the patients in the series required treatment for priapism.

Iatrogenic Priapism: Oral Phosphodiesterase Type 5 Inhibitors, Medications for Attention-Deficit/Hyperactivity Disorder, and Nutritional Supplements for Erectile Dysfunctions

All PDE5 inhibitors have similar side effects related directly to their mode of action, tissue content of substrate, and pharmacologic selectivity for type 5 inhibition versus other phosphodiesterase enzymes. Side effects occurring in 2% or more of patients include headache, flushing, dyspepsia, rhinitis, light sensitivity, and myalgia. Morales et al. (1998) analyzed data from 4274 men who received double-blind treatment with sildenafil or placebo for up to 6 months and 2199 who received long-term open-label sildenafil for up to 1 year. No cases of priapism (erection lasting longer than 4 hours) were reported. No cases of priapism were reported by Montorsi et al. (2004) in a multicenter, open-label, 24-month extension of 8- or 12-week double-blind, placebo-controlled studies assessing the long-term efficacy, safety, and tolerability of tadalafil in 1173 men with ED. Nonetheless, the **indications and usage section of the US Food and Drug Administration (FDA)–approved product labeling (US prescribing information [USPI]) for PDE5 inhibitors** does contain this warning: "There have been rare reports of prolonged erection greater than 4 hours and priapism (painful erections >6 hours duration) for this class of compounds." The USPI and European Summary of Product Characteristics label information contains warning or precautionary language about the use of these agents in men who have conditions predisposing them to priapism. The FDA approved Cialis (tadalafil) as an oral treatment for ED (2.5 mg, 5 mg, 10 mg, and 20 mg) in 2003. Once-daily tadalafil (2.5 mg and 5 mg) was approved for oral treatment of ED in 2008, and subsequently in 2011 tadalafil (2.5 mg and 5 mg) was approved for the signs and symptoms of benign prostatic hyperplasia (BPH) and treatment of ED. Tadalafil 5 mg daily caused no priapism in a phase 2 clinical study of 281 men with history of lower urinary tract symptoms secondary to BPH for 6 weeks, followed by dosage escalation to 20 mg once daily for 6 weeks (McVary et al., 2007). **The 2013 label for the most recently approved PDE5 inhibitor, Stendra (avanafil 50 mg, 100 mg, 200 mg), contains almost identical precautionary wording as prior labels for as-needed (PRN) oral forms of sildenafil, vardenafil, and tadalafil: "There have been rare reports of prolonged erection greater than 4 hours and priapism (painful erections greater than 6 hours)."**

From 1999 to 2007 there were at least nine case-based reports of oral PDE5 inhibitor use and adult priapism and at least one pediatric patient (Aoyagi et al., 1999; Galatti et al., 2005; Goldmeier, 2002; Kassim et al., 2000; King et al., 2005; Kumar et al., 2005; McMahon, 2003; Sur and Kane, 2000; Wilt and Fink, 2004; Wills et al., 2007). **Most case reports detailing priapism after use of a PDE5 inhibitor reveal histories of increased risk for priapism: SCD, SCI, use of a PDE5 inhibitor recreationally, use of a PDE5 inhibitor in combination with ICI, history of penile trauma, use of psychotropic medications, or use of recreational drugs (cocaine).** Wills et al. (2007) described a 19-month-old boy weighing 10 kg who accidentally ingested up to six tablets of sildenafil 50 mg. The child had persistent sinus tachycardia and partial erection for 24 hours; the authors presume this was a high-flow priapism (HFP) because the shaft was neither completely rigid nor painful. Erection in the child subsided spontaneously after overnight intravenous hydration and observation.

In 2013 the FDA issued a warning that methylphenidate medications used in the treatment of attention-deficit/hyperactivity disorder (ADHD) may result in prolonged erection or priapism. The FDA also warns that atomoxetine, another ADHD drug, has been linked to reports of priapism in children, teens, and adults. Drug therapy in ADHD is used in children, adolescents, and adults to increase the ability to pay attention and decrease impulsiveness and hyperactivity. The 2012 Summary Health Statistics for US Children: National Health Interview Survey (Bloom et al., 2013) estimated that more than 6.4 million children ages 4 to 17 have been diagnosed with ADHD; this represents a 41% increase over a decade. The Centers for Disease Control and Prevention (CDC, 2013) further estimate that two-thirds of these children are prescribed methylphenidate medications.

Methylphenidate is a central nervous system stimulant; atomoxetine is a selective norepinephrine reuptake inhibitor. The FDA cautions that physicians may be tempted to switch patients from methylphenidate medications to atomoxetine but that priapism is actually more common in patients taking atomoxetine (US Food and Drug Administration, 2013). **The median age of male patients taking methylphenidate who developed priapism (erection lasting longer than 4 hours) was 12½ years.**

Dietary supplements to enhance erectile function or treat erectile dysfunction have become increasingly popular. These are available over-the-counter and through the Internet. Serial investigations by the Food and Drug Administration have identified that these products may contain prescription levels of the drugs Sildenafil the principal ingredient in Viagra or thiosildenafil, the active ingredient in Cialis. These products are marketed as herbal alternatives that are safe and reliable. There is an emerging trend to seek out nutraceuticals as an alternative to prescription medications. The Center for Drug Evaluation and Research (FDA CDER) has tested more than 300 nutraceuticals for male sexual enhancement finding unlabeled active ingredients (sildenafil or thiosildenafil) at varying dosages. Because of poor quality control active drug concentrations were found to vary from pill to pill in one bottle (Ahmed et al., 2017; ElAmrawy et al., 2016; Nounou et al., 2018, US Food and Drug Administration, 2015).

KEY POINTS: ISCHEMIC PRIAPISM AS A COMPLICATION OF ERECTILE DYSFUNCTION THERAPY

- Prolonged erection is more commonly reported than priapism after therapeutic or diagnostic injection of intracavernous vasoactive medications.
- In worldwide clinical trials of alprostadil, prolonged erection (defined as 4 to 6 hours) occurred in 5% of administrations, and priapism (longer than 6 hours) in 1%.
- In clinical practice, ICI of Trimix (papaverine, phentolamine, and alprostadil) results in prolonged erections in 5% to 35% of administrations.
- Few case reports have documented priapism after PDE5 inhibitor therapy. These reports suggest that men were at increased risk for priapism because of SCD, spinal cord injury, use of a PDE5 inhibitor recreationally, use of a PDE5 inhibitor in combination with ICI, history of penile trauma, use of psychotropic medications, or abuse of narcotics.
- Methylphenidate medications and atomoxetine used in the treatment of ADHD may result in prolonged erection or priapism.

Etiology of Stuttering Priapism (Recurrent Ischemic Priapism)

Stuttering (intermittent) priapism describes a pattern of recurrent priapism. The term has traditionally been used to describe recurrent unwanted and painful erections in men with SCD. **Patients typically awaken with an erection that persists up to 4 hours and becomes progressively painful secondary to ischemia. Patients with SCD may experience stuttering priapism from childhood. Any patient who has experienced ischemic priapism is at risk for stuttering priapism. Patients with stuttering priapism will experience repeated** painful intermittent attacks up to several hours before remission. Affected young men suffer embarrassment, sleep deprivation, and performance anxiety with sexual partners (Chow and Payne, 2008). In a study of 130 patients with SCD, Adeyoju et al. (2002) reported that 46 (35%) had a history of priapism and, of these, 33 (72%) had a history of stuttering priapism. In 75% of patients the first episode of stuttering priapism occurred before the age of 20. Two-thirds of males with SCD ischemic priapism at presentation will describe prior stuttering attacks (Jesus and Dekermacher, 2009). **Commonly reported precipitants of full-blown SCD priapism are stuttering nocturnal or early morning erections, dehydration, fever, and exposure to cold** (Broderick, 2012). Sleep-related erections (SREs) take place during REM sleep. SREs are natural phenomena and appeared to be androgen dependent. The exact duration of nocturnal penile tumescence or normal sleep erections is indeterminate. SREs should occur in men who are eugonadal and have physiologically normal penile blood flow. Several others have noted that SCD patients complain of SREs lasting 3 to 4 hours associated with pain but not necessarily other stigmata of sickle cell crisis (Hoeh and Levine, 2015; Rachid-Filho et al., 2009).

Etiology and Pathophysiology of Nonischemic (Arterial, High-Flow) Priapism

HFP is a persistent erection caused by unregulated cavernous arterial inflow. The epidemiologic data on nonischemic priapism is almost exclusively derived from small case series or individual case reports. **Nonischemic priapism is much rarer than ischemic priapism, and the cause is largely attributed to trauma. Forces may be blunt or penetrating, resulting in laceration of the cavernous artery or one of its branches within the corpora. The cause most commonly reported is a straddle injury to the crura. Other mechanisms include coital trauma, kicks to the penis or perineum, pelvic fractures, birth canal trauma to the newborn male, needle lacerations, complications of penile diagnostics, and vascular erosions complicating metastatic infiltration of the corpora** (Brock et al., 1993; Burgu et al., 2007; Dubocq et al., 1998; Jesus and Dekermacher, 2009; Witt et al., 1990). Although accidental blunt trauma is the most common cause, **HFP has been described after iatrogenic injury from cold-knife urethrotomy, Nesbitt corporoplasty, and deep dorsal vein arterialization** (Liguori et al., 2005; Wolf and Lue, 1992). Any mechanism blunt or penetrating that lacerates a cavernous arteriole can produce unregulated pooling of blood in sinusoidal space with consequent erection. Nonischemic priapism is typically delayed in onset compared with the episode of blunt trauma (Ricciardi et al., 1993). **Sustained partial erection may develop 24 hours after perineal or penile blunt trauma.** It is believed that the hemodynamics of a nocturnal erection disrupts the clot and the damaged artery or arteriole ruptures; the unregulated arterial inflow creates a arteriole-lacunar fistula. As healing progresses with clearing of clot and necrotic smooth muscle tissue, the fistula forms a pseudocapsule. **Formation of a pseudocapsule at the site of fistula may take several weeks to months.**

Contemporary reports suggest that HFP may have a unique subvariety. **Several authors have noted that after either aggressive medical management of ischemic priapism α-adrenergic injection/aspiration protocols or surgical shunting, priapism may rapidly recur with conversion from ischemia to high flow.** HFP has been reported after aspiration and injection of α-adrenergics in the management of ischemic priapism (Bertolotto et al., 2009; McMahon, 2002; Rodriguez et al., 2006). Color Doppler ultrasonography (CDU) has shown formation of an arteriolar-sinusoidal fistula at the site of intervention (needle laceration or shunt site) (see Fig. 70.2). **Secondary HFP should be suspected in patients in whom rapid recurrence, persistence of erection with partial penile rigidity, not associated with pain is evident. Non-fistula type of arterial priapism is the result of dysregulation of cavernous inflows, a post-ischemic hyperemia.** Non-fistula arterial priapism is a rare complication after management of ischemic priapism (Cruz Guerra et al., 2004; Seftel et al., 1998; Wallis et al., 2009). Penile tenderness to palpation is easily confused with the ongoing ache of persistent ischemia. Soft-tissue edema and ecchymosis render the physical examination findings equivocal after medical and surgical maneuvers to alleviate priapism. Dysregulated arterial inflows with or without a fistula can best be distinguished from persistent ischemic priapism by CDU.

> ### KEY POINTS: HIGH-FLOW PRIAPISM
> - Nonischemic priapism is much rarer than ischemic priapism.
> - HFP results from laceration or disruption of a cavernous artery or arteriole.
> - The most common cause is a straddle injury to the crura (bicycle accidents in children).
> - Other mechanisms include coital trauma, kicks to the penis or perineum, pelvic fractures, birth canal trauma to the male newborn, needle lacerations, complications of penile diagnostics, and vascular erosions complicating metastatic infiltration of the corpora.
> - HFP has been described after iatrogenic trauma from cold-knife urethrotomy, corporoplasty, and penile revascularization procedures.

Priapism in Children

Priapism in children and adolescents is most commonly related to SCD. The literature suggests that the incidence of priapism in pediatric sickle cell clinics is 2% to 6% (Jesus and Dekermacher, 2009; Tarry et al., 1987). Adeyoju et al. (2002) conducted a multicenter study of patients with SCD and found that, among 130 males ages 4 to 66, 35% had experienced priapism and more than 70% had experienced stuttering priapism. Donaldson et al. (2014), in a comprehensive review of priapism in children, estimated that SCD is responsible for 65% of cases, leukemia 10%, and trauma 10%.

In the newborn period, fetal hemoglobin predominates, not HbS (Burgu et al., 2007). SCD phenotypes related to ischemic or occlusive crises are unlikely to be evident while fetal hemoglobin persists. Newborn priapism is an extremely rare phenomenon with only limited case reports and rare application of contemporary diagnostic modalities. Erection is frequently elicited in males during the newborn period. In male newborns, simple tactile stimulation such as diaper changing, bathing, and urethral catheterization may result in erection; the erection quickly subsides after cessation of stimuli. Fewer cases of newborn priapism have been reported in the literature and rarely has the cause been defined. Causes have included polycythemia, blood transfusion, and birth canal trauma (Amlie et al., 1977; Karakaya et al., 2016; Leal et al., 1978; Shapiro, 1979; Walker and Casale, 1997). The majority of cases have been conservatively managed with spontaneous resolution reported from hours to days. Minimally invasive diagnostics (CDU) should be performed (Meijer and Bakker, 2003; Pietras et al., 1979). In children who develop priapism after straddle trauma, every effort should be made to localize the arteriolar-sinusoidal fistula. Hatzichristou et al. (2002) reported that identification of the fistula by Doppler ultrasound coupled with direct manual compression softens the high-flow erection and may speed spontaneous resolution. They suggested that this noninvasive therapy likely works in children and not adults because the perineum has considerably less subcutaneous fat and because crural bodies are more easily compressed. **In children HFP is most commonly reported secondary to blunt perineal trauma.** A recent case report of cycling trauma causing arterial priapism identified 12 similar cases in the literature (De Rose et al., 2016). De Rose noted that the delay in presentation may be related to the patient's embarrassment and failure to disclose the primary injury and the subsequent priapism to parents. They describe the efficacy of noninvasive color Doppler ultrasonography (CDU) and magnetic resonance angiography in the assessment of children. **Before proceeding to angiographic embolization of high-flow priapism in children, the urologist should give consideration to the reports that HFP may spontaneous resolve and/or respond to the conservative measure of perineal compression and ice.**

MOLECULAR BASIS OF ISCHEMIC AND STUTTERING PRIAPISM

Advances in our understanding of the molecular basis of priapism have drawn significantly from in vitro and in vivo experimental studies using animal models. Data on the true inciting mechanisms involved in ischemic priapism are emerging. **Ischemic priapism consists of an imbalance of vasoconstrictive and vasorelaxatory mechanisms predisposing the penis to hypoxia and acidosis. In vitro studies have demonstrated that when corporal smooth muscle strips and cultured corporal smooth muscle cells are exposed to hypoxic conditions, α-adrenergic stimulation fails to induce corporal smooth muscle contraction** (Broderick and Harkaway, 1994; Muneer et al., 2005; Saenz de Tejada et al., 1997). Extended periods of severe anoxia significantly impair corporal smooth muscle contractility and cause significant apoptosis of smooth muscle cells and, ultimately, fibrosis of the CC.

In experimental animal models of ischemic priapism, lipid peroxidation, an indicator of injury induced by reactive oxygen species (ROSs), and increased hemo-oxygenase expression occur in the penis during and after ischemic priapism (Jin et al., 2008; Munarriz et al., 2003). Additional pathophysiologic mechanisms involved in the progression of ischemia-induced fibrosis are the upregulation of hypoxia-induced growth factors. Transforming growth factor-β (TGF-β) is a cytokine that is vital to tissue repair. However, excess amounts may induce tissue damage and scarring. Upregulation of TGF-β occurs during hypoxia and in response to oxidative stress (Jin et al., 2008; Moreland et al., 1995). It is hypothesized that TGF-β may be involved in the progression of the corporal smooth muscle to fibrosis (Bivalacqua et al., 2000; Jeong et al., 2004).

Transgenic mouse models of SCD manifest priapism (Beuzard, 1996; Bivalacqua et al., 2009b). There have been two major discoveries in elucidation of the molecular mechanism of ischemic priapism. Mi et al. (2008) have shown that transgenic sickle cell mice CC have enhanced smooth muscle relaxation to electrical field stimulation. Transgenic sickle cell mice and mice lacking endothelial NO synthase (eNOS) gene expression display supraphysiologic erections and spontaneously phasic priapic activity in vivo (Bivalacqua et al., 2006, 2007).

Endothelial cells actively regulate basal vascular tone and vascular reactivity by responding to mechanical forces and neurohumoral mediators with the release of a variety of relaxing and contracting factors. In the penis the vascular endothelium is a source of vasorelaxing factors such as NO and adenosine, as well as vasoconstrictor factors such as RhoA/Rho-kinase. Recent evidence suggests that in states of priapism there may be aberrant NO and adenosine signaling, thus identifying a potential role for NO/cyclic guanosine monophosphate (cGMP), as well as adenosine and RhoA/Rho-kinase signaling in the pathophysiology of ischemic priapism (Bivalacqua et al., 2009a; Champion et al., 2005; Mi et al., 2008).

eNOS knockout mice have an exaggerated erectile response to cavernous nerve stimulation and have phenotypic changes in erectile function consistent with priapism (Bivalacqua et al., 2006; Champion et al., 2005). Mice lacking the *eNOS* gene manifest a priapism phenotype through mechanisms involving defective PDE5 regulatory function in the penis, resulting from altered endothelial NO/cGMP signaling in the organ (Bivalacqua et al., 2006; Lin et al., 2003). Supporting this hypothesis, PDE5 expression is significantly reduced in corpora cavernosa smooth muscle cells (CCSMCs) grown under anoxic and hypoxic cell culture conditions (Lin et al., 2003). **In the context of molecular dysregulation, the cyclic nucleotide cGMP is produced in low steady-state amounts under the influence of priapism-related destruction of the vascular endothelium and thus reduced endothelial NO activity; this situation downregulates the set point of PDE5 function, secondary to altered cGMP-dependent feedback control mechanisms** (Bivalacqua et al., 2006; Burnett and Bivalacqua, 2007; Champion et al., 2005). **When NO is neuronally produced in response to natural erectogenic stimuli or with nocturnal erections, cGMP production surges in a manner that leads to excessive erectile tissue relaxation because of basally insufficient PDE5 enzyme to degrade the cyclic nucleotide.** In addition, reduced Rho-kinase activity (contractile mediator) may contribute to the susceptibility of corporal tissue to excessive relaxation via two distinct molecular mechanisms. **Two distinct molecular mechanisms appear to act in concert to promote stuttering ischemic priapism: enhanced vasorelaxation by uninhibited cGMP and diminished contractile effects of Rho-kinase.** Transgenic sickle cell mice also have significant reductions in penile NO/cGMP signaling leading to deficient PDE5 expression and activity, as well as reduced RhoA/Rho-kinase expression, which causes them to manifest enhanced erectile responses and recurrent priapism (Champion et al., 2005). Another potential cause of enhanced corporal smooth muscle relaxation in SCD-associated priapism is elevated penile adenosine levels, which cause the CC to be in a chronically vasodilated state (Mi et al., 2008). **Taken together, these data suggest that recurrent ischemic priapism results from NO imbalance resulting in aberrant molecular signaling, PDE5 dysregulation, adenosine overproduction, and reductions in Rho-kinase activity, translating into enhanced corporal smooth muscle relaxation and inhibition of vasoconstriction in the penis** (Anele et al., 2015; La Favor et al., 2018).

> **KEY POINTS: SICKLE CELL DISEASE AND PRIAPISM**
> - Sickle cell hemoglobinopathy accounts for at least a third of all cases of ischemic priapism.
> - The sickle cell genetic mutation is the result of a single amino acid substitution in the β-globin subunit of hemoglobin.
> - Clinical features are seen in patients with homozygous SCD: chronic hemolysis, vascular occlusion, tissue ischemia, and end-organ damage.
> - Hemolysis and reduced NO bioavailability are central in the pathogenesis of pulmonary hypertension, leg ulcers, priapism, and stroke in patients with SCD.
> - Increased blood viscosity is responsible for painful crises, osteonecrosis, and acute chest syndrome.
> - SCD patients may experience stuttering priapism from childhood.
> - SCD patients with stuttering priapism will experience repeated painful intermittent attacks up to several hours before remission.
> - Stuttering priapism in SCD is the result of molecular dysregulation with enhanced corporal smooth muscle vasorelaxing forces (secondary to reduced basal levels of PDE5-Inh) and inhibition of vasocontractile forces in the penis.

EVALUATION AND DIAGNOSIS OF PRIAPISM

History

To initiate appropriate management, the physician must determine whether the underlying priapism hemodynamics are ischemic or nonischemic. **Emergency management of ischemic priapism is recommended** (Fig. 70.4). Ischemia should be suspected when the patient has progressive penile pain associated with the duration of erection; has used a known drug associated with priapism; has SCD or another blood dyscrasia; or has a known neurologic condition, especially those affecting the spinal cord. Stuttering priapism history is one of recurrent episodes of prolonged erections, usually nonresolving morning erections. **Nonischemic priapism should be suspected when** there is no pain and the erection duration has not been accompanied by progressive discomfort. There is a history of straddle injury, coital trauma, blunt trauma to the penis or perineum, penile injection, penile surgery, or a diagnostic procedure of the pelvic and penile vessels. The onset of post-traumatic HFP in adults and children may be delayed by hours to several days after the initial injury (Box 70.2).

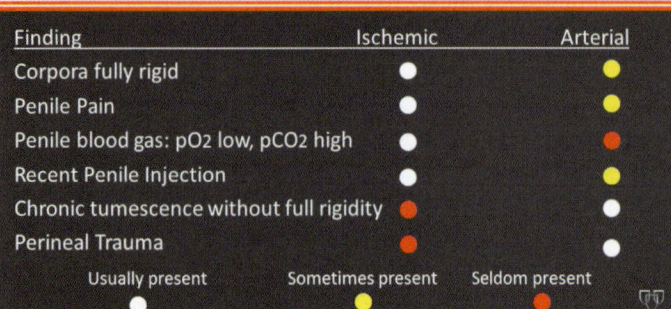
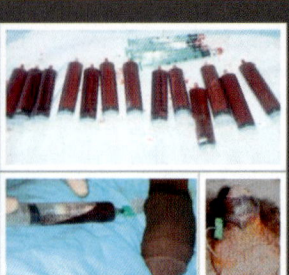
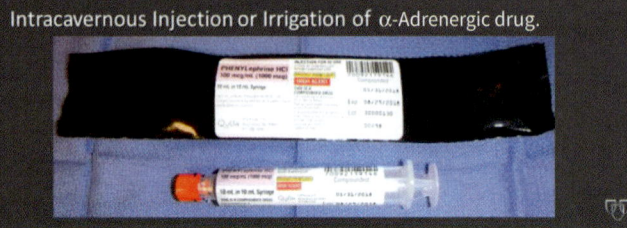

Fig. 70.4. Emergency management of ischemic priapism. (From American Urological Association: Emergency department assessment and management of ischemic priapism: plenary next frontier—panel discussion. *Update on Urologic Emergencies,* San Francisco, 2018, GA Broderick.)

BOX 70.2   Elements in Taking the History of Priapism

Duration of erection
Presence of pain
Previous episodes of priapism and method of treatment
Baseline erectile function
Use of any erectogenic therapies (prescription and nutritional supplements)
Medications and recreational drugs
Sickle cell disease, hemoglobinopathies, hypercoagulable states
Trauma to the pelvis, perineum, or penis

Physical Examination

Inspection and palpation of the penis are recommended to determine the extent and degree of tumescence and rigidity; the involvement of the cavernous bodies; the presence of pain; and the evidence of trauma to the perineum. **In ischemic priapism the corporal bodies will be completely rigid; the glans penis and corpus spongiosum are not.** Although malignancies rarely cause priapism, examination of the abdomen, testicles, perineum, rectum, and prostate may help identify a primary cancer. Malignant infiltration of the penis causes indurated nodules within or replacing corporal tissue. The subtle differences in the penile examination findings may be apparent to the experienced urologist but can be overlooked by emergency personnel (Podolej et al., 2017) on initial evaluation (see Fig. 70.4). If physical examination reveals the penis to be nontender, tumescent, or partially erect, nonischemic priapism should be suspected. **In nonischemic priapism the corpora will be tumescent but not completely rigid.** In children and adults with HFP, depending on the location of trauma and time since the traumatic event, there may be residual bruising at the perineum from straddle injury (Table 70.1).

Laboratory Testing

Evaluation should include a complete blood count (CBC), WBC count with blood cell differential, platelet count, and coagulation profile to assess anemia, rule out infection, detect hematologic abnormalities, and ensure that the patient can safely tolerate surgical interventions should initial medical management fail. In African-Americans, a sickle cell screening should be requested (hemoglobin electrophoresis, reticulocyte count, lactate dehydrogenase). Other hematologic abnormalities may cause priapism, including leukemia, platelet abnormalities, and thalassemia, and these should be sought if the cause is not evident. An elevated reticulocyte count is nonspecific and may be present in priapism caused by SCD and in thalassemia. Urine and serum toxicology panels should be done if recreational narcotic or prescription psychoactive drugs are suspected from the history. A corporal blood gas by aspiration is recommended in the emergency evaluation of priapism. **The corporal blood aspirate differentiates ischemic from nonischemic priapism. Aspiration may be diagnostic and therapeutic.** Visual inspection of the color and consistency of an initial penile aspirate will reveal dark deoxygenated blood with a "crankcase oil" appearance in ischemic priapism. The initial corporal aspirate may be sent for blood gas testing to document pH, Po_2, and Pco_2 (Table 70.2). **CDU should be initiated if the history suggests penile or perineal trauma or if the corporal aspirate reveals well-oxygenated blood** (Fig. 70.5).

Penile Imaging

CDU of the penis and perineum is recommended in the evaluation of priapism. CDU is an adjunct to the corporal aspirate in differentiating ischemic from nonischemic priapism. **Patients with prolonged ischemic priapism will have no blood flow in the cavernous arteries;** the return of the cavernous artery waveform will accompany successful detumescence. **Patients with nonischemic priapism have normal to high blood flow velocities detectable in the cavernous arteries;** an effort should be made to localize the characteristic blush of color emanating from the disrupted cavernous artery or arteriole (Broderick and Lue, 2002). Examination of the entire penile shaft and perineum is recommended; this can be done with the patient supine but frog-legged (see Fig. 70.5). **Penile arteriography should be reserved for the management of HFP, when embolization is planned;** arteriography is too invasive as a diagnostic procedure to differentiate ischemic from nonischemic priapism. The data from penile blood gas assessments become confusing after interventions. CDU should always be considered in the evaluation of a full or partial erection after treatments for ischemic priapism. The differential diagnosis includes resolved ischemia with penile edema, persistent ischemia, and conversion to high-flow state (Burnett, 2004; Lutz et al., 2012, McMahon, 2002; Mistry et al., 2017; Rodriguez et al., 2006). Chiou et al. (2009) have recommended that to accurately categorize presentations as nonischemic or ischemic, careful interpretation of CDU hemodynamics must be done in conjunction with the clinical assessment. They describe eight patients with priapism after ICI (duration ≤7 hours), all of whom showed presence of cavernous arterial inflows with varied peak systolic velocities and end-diastolic velocities. They concluded that most patients with priapism after ICI (and duration <7 hours) have a hemodynamic picture of mixed arteriogenic and veno-occlusive priapism. In their series, men with idiopathic ischemic priapism longer than 20 hours showed no detectable cavernous arterial inflows.

There have recently been reports on the use of magnetic resonance imaging (MRI) in priapism. Kirkham et al. (2008) noted that there

TABLE 70.1 Key Findings in Priapism

FINDINGS	ISCHEMIC PRIAPISM	NONISCHEMIC PRIAPISM
Perineal trauma	Seldom	Usually
Hematologic abnormalities	Usually	Seldom
Recent intracorporal injection	Sometimes	Sometimes
Corpora cavernosa fully rigid	Usually	Seldom
Penile pain	Usually	Seldom
Abnormal penile blood gas	Usually	Seldom
Cavernous inflow (on Doppler)	Seldom	Usually

Modified from Montague DK, Jarow J, Broderick GA, et al.: American Urological Association guideline on the management of priapism. *J Urol* 170:1318–1324, 2003.

TABLE 70.2 Typical Blood Gas Values

SOURCE	Po_2 (mm Hg)	Pco_2 (mm Hg)	PH
Normal arterial blood (room air)	>90	<40	7.40
Normal mixed venous blood (room air)	40	50	7.35
Ischemic priapism (first corporal aspirate)	<30	>60	<7.25

Modified from Montague DK, Jarow J, Broderick GA, et al.: American Urological Association guideline on the management of priapism. *J Urol* 170:1318–1324, 2003.

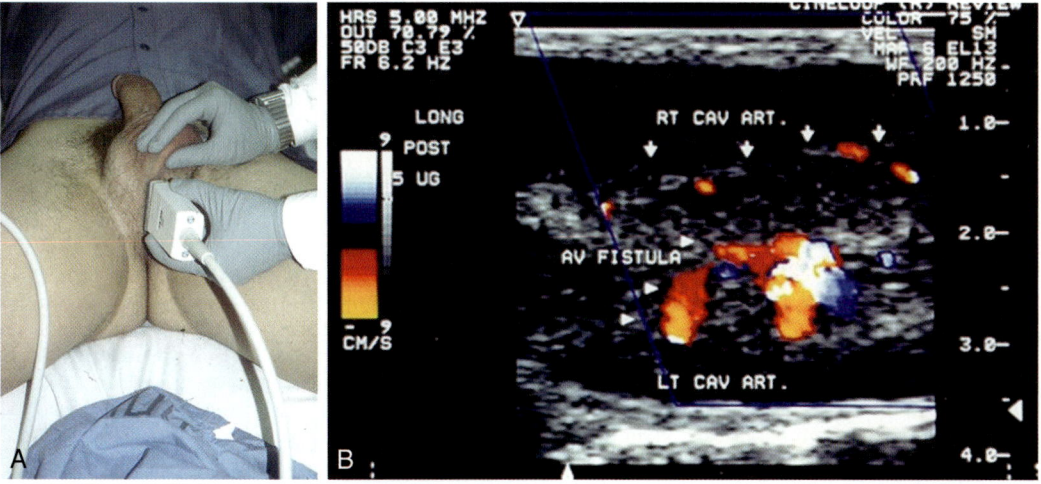

Fig. 70.5. (A) Examination of the crural bodies is required when searching for arterial sinusoidal fistula after straddle injury. (B) Color Doppler image of arterial sinusoidal fistula of left cavernous artery.

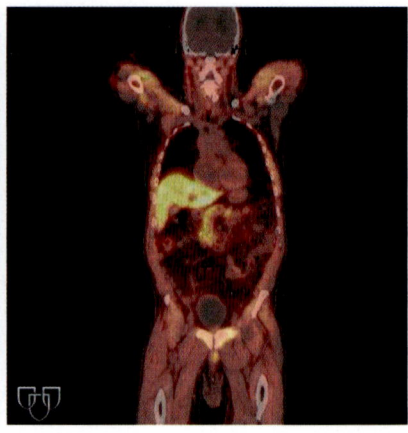

Fig. 70.6. A 76-year-old patient consulted for a penile mass to rule out priapism. His PSA was above 100, and positron emission tomography/computed tomography demonstrated metastatic disease to bone and soft tissue metastasis to the left corpus cavernosum. Metastatic infiltration of the penis must be distinguished from priapism. (Courtesy Dr. Raymond Pak.)

are **three possible roles for MRI** to help in the assessment of priapism; the primary role would be in the **imaging of a well-established arteriolar-sinusoidal fistula**. The authors acknowledge that a limitation of MRI is resolution; MRI cannot demonstrate small vessels as clearly as high-frequency Doppler sonography or angiography. The second role would be in ischemic priapism to **demonstrate the presence and extent of tissue thrombus and corporal smooth muscle infarction.** Ralph et al. (2009) used MRI to assess 50 patients with refractory ischemic priapism. All patients had priapism lasting from 24 to 72 hours, and each had failed medical and surgical interventions. Patients underwent MRI to characterize the extent of smooth muscle necrosis before placement of penile prosthesis. The third role for MRI would be when imaging the penis for **corporal malignancy or metastasis.** MRI may be useful to identify corporal smooth muscle replaced by malignant tissue with or without true ischemic priapism caused by obstruction of venous outflow. In cases in which the history and physical examination are consistent with penile metastasis and not priapism, whole-body surveillance techniques may be confirmatory (Fig. 70.6).

> **KEY POINTS: PRIAPISM IMAGING**
>
> - CDU is an adjunct to the corporal aspirate in differentiating ischemic from nonischemic priapism.
> - CDU imaging should include corporal shaft and transperineal assessment of the crural bodies when there is a history of penile trauma or straddle injury.
> - CDU should always be considered in the evaluation of a persistent or partial erection after treatments for ischemic priapism.
> - Penile arteriography is too invasive as a diagnostic procedure to differentiate ischemic from nonischemic priapism.
> - MRI has three possible roles: imaging of a well-established arteriolar-sinusoidal fistula, identifying corporal thrombus, and identifying corporal metastasis.

MEDICAL TREATMENTS

Ischemic Priapism

Historically, first aid was applied by the patient or recommended by a health practitioner unfamiliar with the hemodynamics of priapism; these interventions included ejaculation, ice packs, cold baths, and cold water enemas. Each of these remedies was thought to end erection by inducing vasoconstriction. Some historical reports advised voiding and exercise. Oral sympathomimetic drugs (etilefrine, pseudoephedrine, phenylpropanolamine, and terbutaline) have been reported to effectively reverse prolonged erection (<4 hours) initiated by ICI therapies with efficacies of 28% to 36% (Lowe and Jarow, 1993). Lowe and Jarow (1993) compared oral terbutaline with pseudoephedrine or placebo in 75 patients with prolonged erection induced by ICI of alprostadil; they reported detumescence in 38% of cases with terbutaline, 28% with pseudoephedrine, and 12% with placebo. In a follow-up study Priyadarshi (2004) specifically investigated the efficacy of oral terbutaline in the management of prolonged erection after ICI (papaverine/chlorpromazine); he administered oral terbutaline 5 mg or placebo to men with persisting erection for more than 2½ hours. Detumescence was achieved in 42% and 15% of cases, respectively, treated with terbutaline or placebo. Terbutaline treatment was unsuccessful in 58% of cases; all of those patients responded to ICI of an α-adrenergic agent.

Every practice administering diagnostic ICI or teaching ICI must be prepared to manage priapism (Fig. 70.7). In my experience, when a vasoactive injection results in a prolonged erection with duration longer than 1 hour but shorter than 4 hours, aspiration may not be necessary. Phenylephrine (200 µg) injected with an ultrafine needle and 1-mL syringe may reverse the erection. Reversing a prolonged erection will spare the patient and the office staff the complexity of treating full-blown ischemic priapism.

Oral agents are not recommended in the management of acute ischemic priapism (>4 hours). The recommended initial treatment of ischemic priapism is the decompression of the CC by aspiration. **Aspiration will immediately soften the erection and relieve pain. Aspiration alone may relieve priapism in 36% of cases.** The AUA Guidelines Panel (2003) advised that there were not sufficient data to conclude that aspiration followed by saline intracorporal irrigation was any more effective than aspiration alone (Montague et al., 2003). Subsequently, Ateyah et al. (2005) reported that a combination of corporal blood aspiration and cold saline irrigation effectively terminated priapism in 66% of cases compared with aspiration alone (24%). **Data to support the efficacy of cold saline are limited. Aspiration should be repeated until no more dark blood can be seen coming out from the corpora and fresh bright red blood is obtained.** This process leads to a marked decrease in the intracavernous pressure, relieves pain, and resuscitates the corporal environment, removing anoxic, acidotic, and hypercarbic blood. A single, large-bore, 19-gauge needle should be inserted at the penoscrotal junction at the 3 or 9 o'clock position to avoid piercing the dorsal neurovascular bundle. The surgeon should compress the penile shaft between the thumb and first digit, just below the 19-gauge needle, aspirating the shaft until it is soft. With the needle left in place, the shaft is permitted to refill. Compression is reapplied and

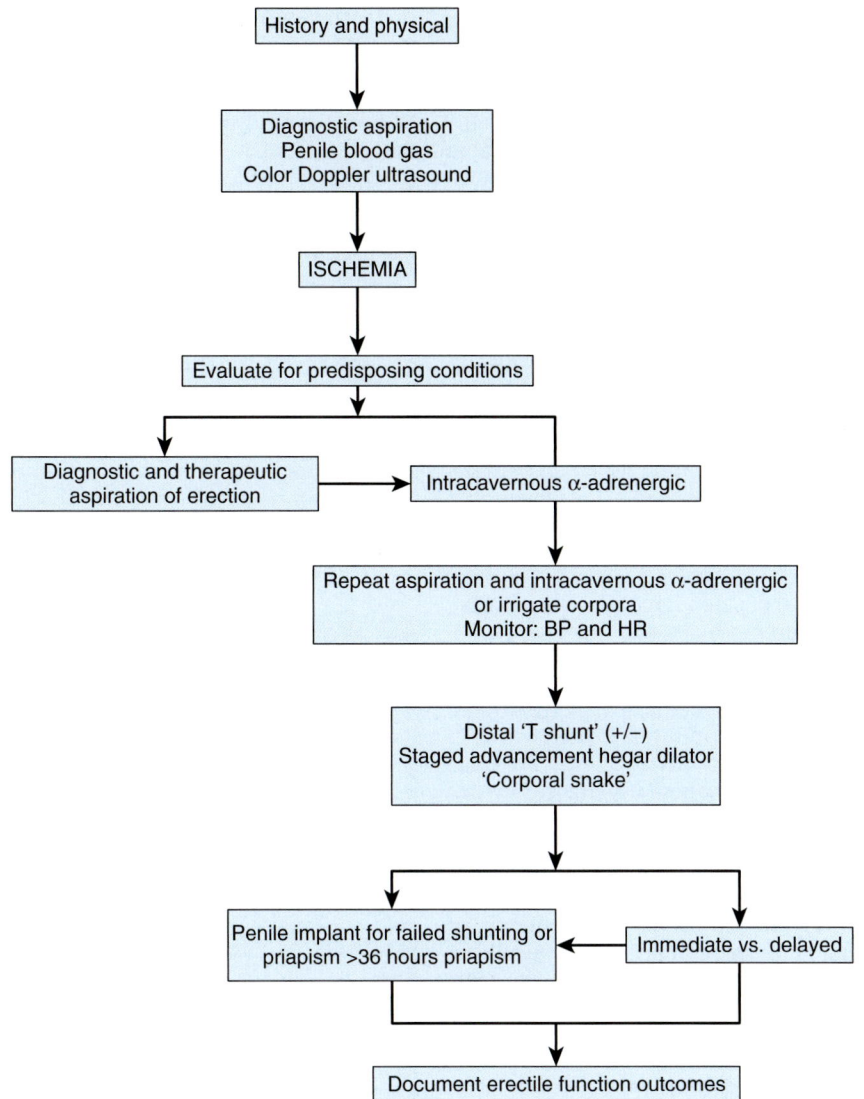

Fig. 70.7. Algorithm for managing ischemic priapism. *BP*, Blood pressure; *ECG*, electrocardiogram; *HR*, heart rate.

aspiration repeated. These maneuvers may have to be serially repeated. Several small, empty syringes should be available (3-mL to 12-mL syringes) (see Fig. 70.4).

Corporal aspiration, if unsuccessful, should be followed by α-adrenergic injection or irrigation. Aspiration followed by the ICI of sympathomimetic drugs was recommended by the AUA Guidelines Panel in 2003 (Broderick et al., 2010; Montague et al., 2003). Sympathomimetic drugs (phenylephrine, etilefrine, ephedrine, epinephrine, norepinephrine, metaraminol) cause cavernous smooth muscle contraction. In the laboratory, normal cavernous smooth muscle preparations from humans, rabbits, and rodents show concentration-dependent contractions on exposure to phenylephrine if the corporal environment is well oxygenated and has a normal pH (Broderick et al., 1994). In patients, time-dependent changes in the corporeal environment begin within 6 hours of persistent erection (Broderick and Harkaway, 1994). Animal models of ischemic priapism have demonstrated impairment in smooth muscle contraction with progressive acidosis, hypoxia, and glucopenia (Broderick et al., 1994; Muneer et al., 2008; Munnarriz et al., 2006; Saenz de Tejada et al., 1997). Corpus cavernosum specimens from patients with prolonged priapism show no contractions to high-dose phenylephrine in vitro.

Phenylephrine is a relatively selective $α_1$-adrenergic receptor agonist with minimal β-mediated ionotropic and chronotropic cardiac effects; it is the agent of choice according to AUA consensus recommendation (2003), the International Consultation on Sexual Medicine (2010), and the European Association of Urology guideline on priapism (2014) (Broderick et al., 2010; Montague et al., 2003; Salonia et al., 2014).

There are no comparative trials of sympathomimetics in the management of priapism, nor are there studies of dosage tolerance to report. In terms of corporal physiology, α-adrenergic agonists are vasoconstrictors of cavernous artery and arterioles. Intracavernous administration of an α-adrenergic agent should contract cavernous smooth muscles, allowing sinusoidal blood to egress from subtunical veins. On the other hand, a β-adrenergic agonist, which would relax cavernous smooth muscle and dilate the cavernous artery and arterioles, could promote oxygenated arteriolar blood to enter the cavernous spaces and wash out deoxygenated blood. Metaraminol is a pure α-adrenergic agent; etilefrine, phenylephrine, and epinephrine are mixed α- and β-adrenergic agonists. Terbutaline is a pure β agonist. Case reports with these agents show varying efficacy from 43% to 81%.

In addition to the specific reversal agent, there is clearly a time-dependent efficacy for pharmacologic reversal of priapism. For acute pharmacologic management of ischemic priapism, the intracavernous administration of dilute solutions of phenylephrine or epinephrine is most commonly described in the United States. In Europe etilefrine is commonly described. Etilefrine is a phenylephrine related β-adrenergic and α-adrenergic agonist. It is available in oral and parenteral formulations internationally (Effortil, ethylandrianol, ethylphenylephrine, phetanol, ethyl noradrianol). Currently, pseudoephedrine, phenylpropanolamine, and ephedrine are the orally active adrenergic agents available in the United States. Pseudoephedrine (Sudafed) is regulated under the Combat Methamphetamine Epidemic Act of 2005, which banned over-the-counter sales of cold medicines containing pseudoephedrine. It is available "behind the counter" without a prescription. Neither Sudafed (pseudoephedrine) nor Sudafed PE (phenylephrine) has been evaluated as an oral agent for the reversal or prevention of priapism in the United States. Phenylephrine is typically diluted in normal saline to a concentration of 100 to 200 µg/mL; it is administered intracavernously as a 1-mL injection every 3 to 5 minutes. Administration should be intermittent over the course of an hour. In my experience, phenylephrine can be concentrated as 200 µg/mL in saline and administered intermittently as 0.5 mL to 1.0 mL every 5 to 10 minutes to a maximum dosage of 1 mg. This will permit up to 10 separate injections of 0.5 mL (100 µg each) or 5 separate injections of 1 mL (200 µg each). The penis is aspirated between successive injections by tightly pinching the shaft at the penoscrotal junction, just below the site of needle insertion. Aspiration should continue until the distal shaft is empty and collapses. This removes deoxygenated acidic blood. Then phenylephrine is injected. Gradually the compression at the penoscrotal junction is released, allowing the shaft to refill with fresh blood. Extremes of age (children vs. elderly), home dosing with pseudoephedrine, and preexisting cardiovascular diseases should be taken into consideration before intracavernous sympathomimetic administration. Serial monitoring of blood pressure and pulse should be performed during and immediately after ICI of sympathomimetic drugs. Potential side effects of intracavernous sympathomimetics include headache, dizziness, hypertension, reflex bradycardia, tachycardia, and irregular cardiac rhythms (Constantine et al., 2017; Sidhu et al., 2018).

Davila et al. (2008) reported subarachnoid hemorrhage in a patient with SCD ischemic priapism. The patient was a 24-year-old African-American man who reported sudden and severe headache immediately after intracorporal administration of phenylephrine 500 µg/mL repeated every 3 minutes for a total of 4 mL (2000 µg = 2 mg). In a retrospective review Ridyard et al. (2016) identified 58 patients presenting to the emergency department with ischemic priapism lasting less than 36 hours. Patients were treated by urology house officers with intracavernous phenylephrine; the protocol resulted in resolution in 86% of patients (Ridyard et al., 2016). Commercially available and compounded phenylephrine HCl (100 mcg/mL) should avoid the risks related to mixing and inadvertently overdosing by emergency personnel (Constantine et al., 2017) (see Fig. 70.4).

SCD and hematologic malignancies are rare but important causes of ischemic priapism. Classically, treatment of SCD-induced ischemic priapism involved analgesics, hydration, oxygen, bicarbonate, and exchange transfusion. Unfortunately, acute neurologic complications may follow exchange transfusions. Hematologists have begun to question the emphasis on intravenous hydration, sodium bicarbonate for alkalinization, and exchange transfusion as first-line therapy for SCD-associated priapism (Kato, 2012). Hydroxycarbamide (hydroxyurea) is a hematologic agent used in the management of vaso-occlusive crises in sickle cell patients (Morrison and Burnett, 2012; Saad et al., 2004). The proposed mechanisms of action are increase in production of hemoglobin F; reduction of leukocytes, platelets, and reticulocytes; and promotion of release of NO. **In the best interests of the patient, the urologist should seek hematologic consultation in the management of boys and men with SCD priapism but remain assertive that hematologic therapy alone is not effective management of SCD priapism** (Ballas, 2017; Rogers, 2005). A 2006 report suggested that transfusion alone has no effective role in the treatment of sickle cell–induced priapism (Merritt et al., 2006).

Reports from hematology centers suggest high success rates with use of penile aspiration, injection, and irrigation with intracavernous sympathomimetics for SCD priapism (Mantadakis et al., 2000). Mantadakis et al. (2000) conducted a prospective trial for the management of children with SCD with prolonged erection, ages 3 to 18 years (no placebo group). For erections lasting longer than 4 hours and less than 12 hours, emergency department interventions were local anesthetic, cavernous aspiration, and irrigation with 10 mL of a 1:1,000,000 solution of epinephrine. If detumescence lasted for 30 minutes, patients were discharged to home. They described 15 patients receiving 39 interventions, of which 37 were successful; 67% required only one aspiration and irrigation treatment. **In the management of SCD pediatric patients with stuttering priapism, several levels of escalating intervention are necessary, with parental and emergency department staff education being the first level.** Gbadoe et al. (2001) described the treatment of 11 patients with SCD (ages 30 months to 15 years) with acute ischemic priapism or stuttering priapism. In their series of cases, if the patient had priapism lasting less than 6 hours, aspiration and injection of 5 mg of etilefrine was given in the emergency department; for stuttering priapism, patients were given oral etilefrine 0.5 mg/kg nightly for 1 month, or 0.25 mg/kg twice daily. Patients (parents) also administered injections at home to reverse painful erection lasting longer than 1 hour. The authors reported no significant hypertension and only one case of "agitation" attributed to daily administration.

> ### KEY POINTS: MEDICAL MANAGEMENT OF ISCHEMIC PRIAPISM
>
> - Oral therapy is not recommended for the treatment of acute ischemic priapism.
> - The initial treatment of ischemic priapism is decompression by aspiration.
> - Aspiration should be repeated until oxygenated blood is seen to refill the corpora.
> - Aspiration should be followed by the ICI (or irrigation) of a diluted α-adrenergic drug.
> - Worldwide availability of adrenergic agents varies; effective reversal of priapism has been documented with dilute injections of ephedrine, epinephrine, etilefrine, metaraminol, or phenylephrine. Phenylephrine is the agent of choice recommended by AUA, International Consultation on Sexual Medicine, and European Association of Urology guidelines.
> - Clinicians are advised to consult their pharmacies and develop clear mixing and dosage protocols for safe administration of adrenergic solutions.
> - Phenylephrine is a sympathomimetic drug with selective α_1-adrenergic receptor actions; it has minimal β-mediated ionotropic and chronotropic cardiac effects.
> - Phenylephrine should be concentrated as 200 µg/mL in normal saline and administered intracavernously as 0.5 mL to 1 mL. Lower concentrations should be used in children and adults with cardiovascular disease. Administration and aspiration may have to be repeated. No recommendations can be made about maximum safe dosage. Hypertensive stroke has been reported as a complication of cumulative administration of 2 mg.
> - Physicians should monitor patients for subjective complaints and objective findings consistent with known undesirable effects: headache, chest discomfort, acute hypertension, reflex bradycardia, tachycardia, palpitations, and cardiac arrhythmia. Patients and parents should be informed about these potential complications.
> - Blood pressure monitoring is recommended with repeated sympathomimetic administration. In patients with significant cardiovascular risks, electrocardiogram monitoring is recommended.
> - Ischemic priapism associated with SCD requires intracavernous treatment. A hematologist may provide concurrent systemic therapies (oxygen, hydration, transfusion), but the best resolution rates are achieved with therapies directed at the penis.

Stuttering Priapism

Various factors must be considered in treating stuttering priapism. **Although an episode may last less than 4 hours, increasing frequency or duration of stuttering episodes may herald a major ischemic priapism.** Multiple frequent visits to the emergency department to resolve the priapism are disruptive to the patient's life and embarrassing. If attacks follow sexual activity, patients may become sexually avoidant (Adeyoju et al., 2002; Chow and Payne, 2008). Safety and efficacy of various treatments are poorly characterized in the literature. The side effects of recommended medications should be understood by the patient. Patients on chronic medical therapy to decrease the frequency of stuttering episodes may significantly benefit from performing a single sympathomimetic intracorporal injection at home as part of a personal treatment algorithm (Teloken et al., 2005; Virag et al., 1996). Multiple treatment options have been described: oral and injectable α-adrenergic agonists, terbutaline, digoxin, the antisickling agent hydroxycarbamide (hydroxyurea), estrogens, gonadotropin-releasing hormone (GnRH) analogues, antiandrogens, baclofen, gabapentin, and recently PDE5 inhibitors (Chow and Payne, 2008).

Etilefrine is available as an oral or injectable treatment in some European countries. The maximum oral dosage is 100 mg in 24 hours, given as 50 mg bid (Okpala et al., 2002). Okpala et al. (2002) followed 18 adults (17 SCD patients and 1 with sickle trait), all with a history of stuttering priapism. Patients were given oral etilefrine in escalating doses from 25 mg at bedtime to a maximum of 100 mg each day. Stuttering episodes were reduced in frequency and duration in 72%. A small series of 6 SCD children were followed with administration twice daily with 0.25 mg of etilefrine per kilogram (Gbadoe et al., 2002). **The experience of multiple investigators using oral α-adrenergics in the management of SCD stuttering ischemic priapism suggests that limited daily administration should be considered in the management of stuttering priapism; drug therapy is typically initiated at bedtime. Oral α-adrenergic administration is a preventative strategy for stuttering priapism.**

Hormonal Therapies

The primary action of systemic hormonal therapy in stuttering priapism is the suppression of the androgenic effects on penile erection. Attempts to treat stuttering priapism with hormones have exploited known regulators of male sexual function by targeting the pituitary gland (GnRH agonists), suppressing pituitary function through feedback inhibition (diethylstilbestrol [DES]), blocking androgen receptors (antiandrogens), and reducing testicular and adrenal synthesis (ketoconazole). The common goal of hormonal therapy in the prevention of stuttering priapism is to reduce serum testosterone to hypogonadal levels or block testosterone's effects on the penis. In the only randomized placebo-controlled trial, a synthetic estrogen, **DES**, caused termination of the stuttering episodes in all patients who received treatment (Chinegwundoh and Anie, 2004). However, in more than 50% of patients (5 of 9) priapism recurred after treatment cessation. Similar results have been described by others in case reports (Gbadoe et al., 2002; Shamloul and el Nashaar, 2005). Long-term estrogen therapy is not recommended because of the potential cardiovascular side effects.

GnRH analogues, goserelin acetate and leuprolide acetate, have been described in case reports (Levine and Guss, 1993; Shamloul and el Nashaar, 2005). Chronic therapy with GnRH analogues in combination with penile injection of α-adrenergics as needed has been reported in the management of ischemic stuttering priapism (Steinberg and Eyre, 1995). Discontinuation of GnRH analogues typically leads to stuttering resumption. **Antiandrogens** including flutamide, bicalutamide, and chlormadinone have been used to interrupt stuttering priapism, and their use has been detailed in case reports. Antiandrogens may have benefit to patients over the GnRH analogues because they are orally administered and because some patients continue having sexually stimulated erections (Costabile, 1998; Dahm et al., 2002; Yamashita et al., 2004). Abern and Levine (2009) used nightly administration of the antifungal agent oral ketoconazole and prednisone to suppress nocturnal erections as a preventive strategy for recurrent ischemic priapism in 8 patients followed for 1½ years. The protocol required titrating dosages and monitoring of nocturnal erections and serum testosterone levels; mean testosterone levels fell from a baseline of 475 ng/dL to 275 ng/dL. The fall in testosterone levels appeared to be a surrogate for efficacy in preventing significant episodes of priapism. Ketoconazole (KTZ) inhibits steroidogenesis in the adrenal and gonadal tissues; it has a half-life of 8 hours. KTZ inhibits cortisol production, necessitating concomitant prednisone administration. In the Abern and Levine protocol, men with recurring ischemic priapism were treated with KTZ 200 mg given orally (PO) every 8 hours and prednisone 5 mg at bedtime for 2 weeks, followed by KTZ nightly without prednisone supplementation. In a follow-up study Hoeh and Levine report on 17 patients with recurrent ischemic priapism and SCD treated with KTZ 200 mg three times daily with prednisone 5 mg daily for 2 weeks and then tapered to KTZ 200 mg nightly for 6 months with no prednisone supplementation. The mean number of emergency department visits for recurrent ischemic episodes lasting more than 4 hours before treatment was 6.5 per patient. Sixteen of seventeen patients had resolution of stuttering during the 6 months of treatment (Hoeh and Levine, 2015).

Rachid-Filho et al. (2009) have described the efficacy of oral **5α-reductase inhibitors** (finasteride) in the management of sickle cell stuttering priapism. They administered finasteride to 35 patients over 120 days in doses that decreased monthly from 5 mg/day to 3 mg/day and then 1 mg/day in the final month. This was not a controlled trial, but careful observation of stuttering episodes was made. They found at the beginning of treatment that the mean number of episodes of stuttering priapism per patient was 22.7, and at the end of 4 months the mean number of episodes per patient was 2.1. The optimal effects were found at 5- and 3-mg daily doses. Six of 35 patients in this study developed painless gynecomastia. Finasteride is a 5α-reductase inhibitor approved in the United States for management of symptomatic BPH (Proscar 5 mg) and male pattern alopecia (Propecia 1 mg); finasteride and dutasteride are type II 5α-reductase inhibitors. This class of drugs reduces conversion of testosterone to dihydrotestosterone, which is believed to be many times more potent at the cellular level. Paradoxically, when measured during clinical trials, serum testosterone levels go up in healthy controls and patients administered finasteride or dutasteride. Neither drug is approved for use in patients with stuttering ischemic priapism.

Baclofen

Studies in rats and humans suggest that baclofen inhibits penile erection and ejaculation, through γ-aminobutyric acid (GABA) receptor activity. In rats, stimulation of $GABA_B$ receptors in the lumbosacral spinal cord inhibits erection (Bitran et al., 1988; Paredes and Agmo, 1995; Vaidyanathan et al., 2004). Denys et al. (1998) reported on nine men with multiple sclerosis or spinal cord injuries who were treated for 44 months with intrathecal baclofen for muscle spasticity; eight of nine reported decreased erectile function, which reversed on cessation of baclofen. Rourke et al. (2002) first reported on the use of oral nightly baclofen 40 mg in the management of recurrent priapism in patients with neurologic lesions. D'Aleo et al. (2009) were the first to report on the use of an intrathecal pump to administer baclofen 180 μg daily for the management of skeletal muscle spasm and recurrent priapism in a patient with spinal cord injury; the patient was refractory to treatment with oral administration of 75 mg/day but responded to a test dose of 25 μg intrathecally. The neurologic literature generally fails to categorize these erectile events as ischemic or nonischemic. Triggering events may be tactile nonsexual stimulation causing repeated reflexogenic erections. Better characterization of these unwanted erections in men with upper motor neural lesions is necessary to appreciate hemodynamics, inciting events, duration, and impact on erectile function. There have been reports to the FDA that men with baclofen infusion pumps experience a withdrawal syndrome when those pumps fail. The withdrawal syndrome has been characterized by return of spasticity, agitation, sleeplessness, and priapism. Advanced symptoms resemble autonomic dysreflexia and may include rhabdomyolysis. The syndrome responds to oral baclofen dosing until intrathecal therapy can be resumed. In non-neurogenic patients, daily administration of baclofen is associated with drowsiness, nausea, complaints of fatigue, and ED. Recurrent reflexogenic erections are clearly an unwanted condition associated with muscle spasticity in men with spinal cord lesions and neurologic disease, but it remains to be demonstrated whether the duration and hemodynamics of such erectile events are similar to ischemic stuttering priapism typical in SCD.

Phosphodiesterase Type 5 Inhibitors in the Management of Stuttering Priapism: A Counterintuitive Treatment Strategy

Bialecki and Bridges (2002) first reported on sildenafil having a paradoxic effect in controlling stuttering priapism in three patients with SCD. Although this proposal would immediately seem illogical on the basis of the understanding that PDE5 inhibitors exert erectogenic effects, there is a scientific basis for using these agents to treat priapism.

In a small case series, Burnett et al. (2006a) showed that daily sildenafil or tadalafil therapy reduces ischemic priapism episodes in men with stuttering priapism. **When used in long-term regimens unassociated with erection stimulatory conditions, PDE5 inhibitor therapy alleviates recurrent priapism episodes in men with SCD-associated priapism without affecting normal erectile capacity** (Bivalacqua et al., 2009a; Burnett et al., 2006b). The working theory is that surges of cGMP go unchecked because of downregulated levels of PDE5; this results in stimuli such as nocturnal erection, which causes unchecked corporal smooth muscle relaxation. In initial series, the short-acting PDE5 inhibitor sildenafil citrate was given at a dose of 25 mg oral daily, with escalation to 50 mg daily. Subsequently these investigators reported on tadalafil at a dose of 5 or 10 mg taken orally three times weekly. Unfortunately a phase 1 placebo controlled trial of sildenafil showed no statistical benefit, with the primary outcome goal of a 50% reduction in biweekly priapism episodes from baseline (Burnett et al., 2014). In the phase 2 (open label) there was a reduction in the primary outcome measure and sildenafil treated patients did have fewer visits to the hospital for priapism episodes. Studies remain ongoing.

SURGICAL MANAGEMENT OF ISCHEMIC PRIAPISM

Surgical management of ischemic priapism is indicated after repeated penile aspirations and injections of sympathomimetics have failed or if such an attempt has resulted in a significant cardiovascular side effect. At present there is a paucity of data regarding the timing of surgical intervention following initiation of medical treatment, although the 2004 International Consultation on Sexual Medicine in Paris recommended corporal aspiration and α-adrenergic agonists for at least 1 hour before consideration of shunting (Pryor et al., 2004). **Early surgical intervention may be preferable in patients with malignant or poorly controlled hypertension or for men who are using monoamine oxidase inhibitor medications contraindicating α-adrenergic therapies.** A comprehensive discussion and documentation that includes baseline erectile function, duration of priapism, risks and benefits of the surgery, and ED should be held with the patient or guardian and an informed consent form signed by the patient or guardian.

Shunting

It is generally accepted that the longer an episode of ischemic priapism lasts, the greater the likelihood of compromised erectile function in the future. Early reviews concluded that priapism lasting longer than 24 hours was associated with a 90% ED rate (Pryor and Hehir, 1982). Kulmala et al. (1996) reported 92% erectile function preservation among patients with ischemic priapism reversed in less than 24 hours, but only 22% preservation of erectile function among men with priapism lasting longer than 7 days. Zacharakis et al. (2014a,b) retrospectively identified 45 patients undergoing distal shunting (2009–2102). Using the operative interventions of simultaneous T shunt and intracavernous tunneling all patients with priapism

> **KEY POINTS: MEDICAL MANAGEMENT OF STUTTERING PRIAPISM**
>
> - The goals of managing a patient with stuttering priapism include prevention of future episodes, preservation of erectile function, and balancing the risks versus benefits of various treatment options.
> - Trials of daily oral α-adrenergic therapy have been in the management of patients (adults and children) with stuttering priapism associated with hemoglobinopathies. Efficacy should be monitored through frequency and duration of stuttering episodes, blood pressure, and normal erectile capacity.
> - Trials of daily oral sildenafil/tadalafil (PDE5 inhibitor), trials of finasteride (5α-reductase inhibitor), and trials of oral ketoconazole/prednisone have been used in the management of adult patients with SCD stuttering priapism. Efficacy should be monitored through frequency and severity of stuttering episodes, side effects, and normal erectile capacity.
> - Trials of GnRH agonists or antiandrogens have been used in the management of adult patients with stuttering priapism. Hormonal agents should not be used in patients who have not achieved full sexual maturation and adult stature. Chronic GnRH or antiandrogen administration in men may affect libido or fertility, cause gynecomastia, cause hot flushes, promote osteoporosis, increase the risks of cardiovascular disease, and worsen sexual function.
> - When administered at home for prolonged morning erections, an injection of an intracavernous α-adrenergic agent may avert a full-blown episode of ischemic priapism. ICI of phenylephrine (by the adult patient or parent) should be considered as an adjunct to daily systemic therapies in patients with stuttering priapism.

duration less than 24 hours were reversed, but only 30% of those lasting more than 48 hours were successfully reversed. Erectile function outcomes at 6 months were significantly reduced and correlated with the duration of priapism.

Recommendations based on well-documented erectile function outcomes are few. One recent study does document erectile function outcomes by contemporary standards. Bennett and Mulhall (2008) carefully documented 39 patients with SCD priapism who came to their emergency department over 8 years; men were routinely interviewed for erectile function status within 4 weeks of priapism using International Index of Erectile Function (IIEF). Of the 39 African-American men followed, 73% acknowledged prior episodes of stuttering, 85% had previously been diagnosed with SCD, but only 5% had been counseled in SCD clinics or were aware that priapism was a complication of SCD. A standard protocol of aspiration and phenylephrine injection was performed; shunting for failure of medical management was performed in 28%. In patients in whom priapism was reversed, spontaneous erections (with or without use of sildenafil) were reported in 100% of men when priapism was reversed by 12 hours; 78% when reversed by 12 to 24 hours; and 44% when reversed by 24 to 36 hours. In this contemporary series of SCD patients, no men reported the return of spontaneous erections after priapism lasting 36 hours or more. **The International Society for Sexual Medicine Standards Committee (expert opinion) stated that shunting is to be considered for ischemic priapism events lasting 72 hours or less. Consideration should be given to foregoing a shunt in priapism events lasting longer, in particular when cavernous thrombosis is evident and no blood can be aspirated from the corporal bodies** (Mulhall, 2006; Pryor et al., 2004).

The objective of shunt surgery is reoxygenation of the cavernous smooth muscle. The shared principle of shunt procedures is to reestablish corporal inflow by relieving venous outflow obstruction; this requires creation of a fistula between the CC and glans penis, CC and corpus spongiosum, or CC and dorsal or saphenous

veins. Shunt procedures are subdivided on the basis of anatomic location on the penis (Lue and Pescatori, 2006; Fig. 70.8).
- Percutaneous distal shunts—Ebbehoj (1974), Winter (1976), or T shunt (Brant et al., 2009)
- Open distal shunt—Al-Ghorab (Borrelli et al., 1983; Hanafy et al., 1976) or corporal snake (Burnett and Pierorazio, 2009)
- Combined T shunt and corporal snake maneuver—Zacharakis et al. (2014b)
- Open proximal shunt—Quackles (1964) or Sacher et al. (1972)
- Saphenous vein—Grayhack et al. (1964)
- Deep dorsal vein shunt—Barry (1976)

A distal cavernoglanular shunt should be the first choice of shunting procedures because it is technically easier to perform than proximal shunting. Percutaneous distal shunting is less invasive than open distal shunting and can be performed with local anesthetic in the emergency department. The most recently described distal shunt (Brant et al., 2009) creates a T-shaped shunt between the CC and glans penis. Brant et al. (2009) describe 13 men with priapism durations longer than 24 hours (in 6 of 13, other distal or proximal shunt procedures had failed). All T shunts were performed after penile anesthetic block; in 12 of 13 patients, the priapism was successfully reversed by initial intervention. In T shunting a No. 10 blade is placed vertically through the glans 4 mm away from the meatus; the blade pierces through the glans to the CC and is rotated 90 degrees away from the urethra and removed (Fig. 70.9). Deoxygenated blood is milked out of the wound. The

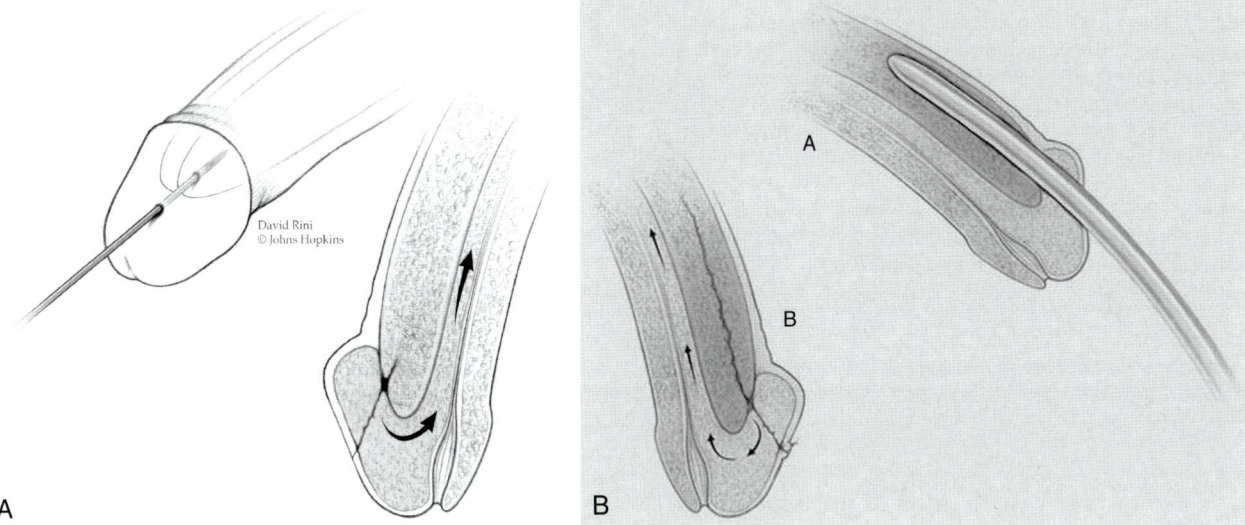

Fig. 70.8. (A) Winter shunt. The distal cavernoglanular shunt procedure is created by transglanular placement of a large-bore needle or angiocatheter into the distal glans and corpus cavernosum. (B) Corporal snake maneuver is a modification of the Al-Ghorab shunt. After excision of a 5-mm circular core of distal tunica albuginea, a 7/8 Hegar dilator is inserted down each corporal body through the tunica window. (B, Copyright Brady Urological Institute. From Burnett AL, Pierorazio PM: Corporal "snake" maneuver: corporoglanular shunt surgical modification for ischemic priapism. *J Sex Med* 6:1171–1176, 2009.)

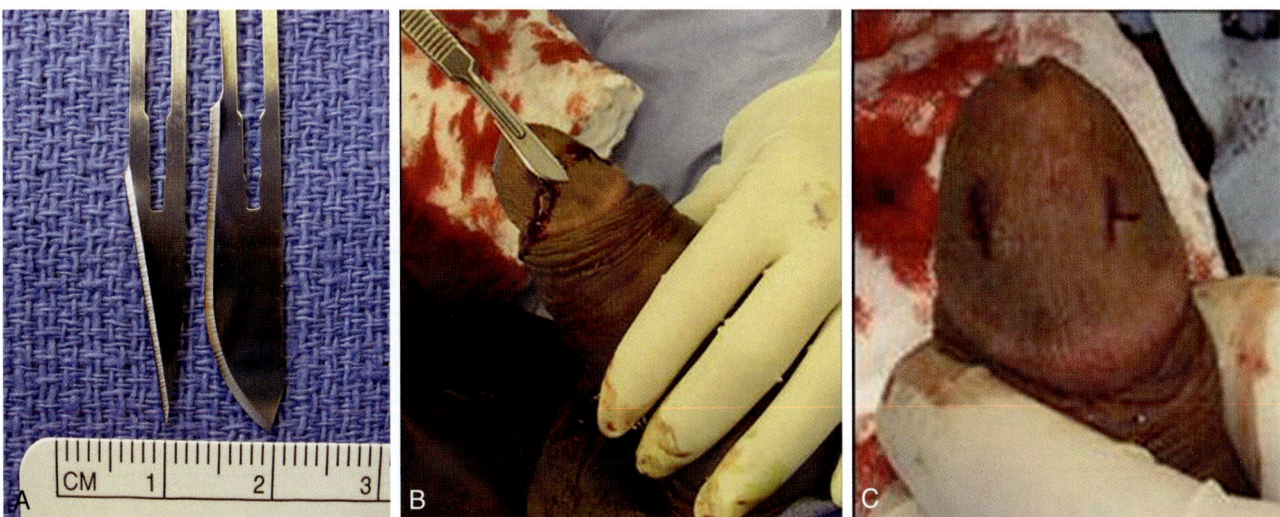

Fig. 70.9. (A) A No. 11 blade is used for an Ebbehoj percutaneous cavernoglanular shunt, and a No. 10 blade is used for a T shunt. (B and C) Note the differences between the Ebbehoj and T shunts. In the Ebbehoj technique the No. 11 blade leaves a straight incision into the glans and corpus cavernosum. In the creation of a T shunt the No. 10 blade is rotated (90 degrees away from the urethra) after insertion and is then withdrawn. In both the percutaneous techniques deoxygenated blood is milked out of the open wounds; once bright red blood is seen, the skin is closed, leaving the deeper incision of the open surgical fistula. In either procedure the maneuver may be repeated on the opposite corpus. (Courtesy Dr. Tom Lue.)

glans is then sutured with absorbable suture. The authors recommend discharge home if the penis remains flaccid for 15 minutes (Brant et al., 2009). If erection returns or persists, a second T shunt is recommended on the opposite side of the meatus. When ischemic priapism has been present for more than 36 hours, immediate placement of bilateral T shunts is recommended, with passage of 20-Fr dilators into the fistula tract and well into the CC down to the crus. This technique is more traumatic and in my experience requires general anesthesia.

Burnett and Pierorazio (2009) have described a similar technique to resolve ischemic priapism refractory to first-line interventions. Their procedure, known as the *corporal snake*, is a modification of the Al-Ghorab corporoglanular shunt (Fig. 70.10). With the patient under general anesthesia, a 2-cm transverse incision is made on the glans; the distal tips of the rigid CC are incised and grasped with 2-0 stay sutures or Kocher clamps. Deoxygenated blood is milked out of the CC, but rather than excising a wedge of tunica and underlying CC muscle, a 7/8 Hegar dilator is advanced through each of the tunica windows proximally several centimeters to release blood and thrombus. The penis is made flaccid by repeated manual compression and release; the glans skin is then approximated with 4-0 chromic sutures; a urethral catheter is placed, and lightly compressive dressing is applied to the genitalia (Fig. 70.11).

Segal et al. (2013) retrospectively reviewed the Johns Hopkins Hospital experience with the corporal snake maneuver. Ten patients with ischemic priapism with a mean duration of 75 hours (range 24 to 288 hours) refractory to medical intervention and simple distal shunting (Winter or Ebbehoj) were treated surgically with the corporal snake maneuver; in 8 the priapism resolved, and they had no postoperative recurrence during 6-month follow-up. In 2 patients the priapism did not respond; they were treated by insertion of inflatable penile implant at time of presentation. Complication rates were significant (20%); complications included wound infection, penile skin necrosis, and urethrocutaneous fistula. The authors documented sexual health function outcomes in these patients treated for refractory priapism lasting 24 to 288 hours; all had significant complaints of ED at 6 months, with 2 of 8 receiving subsequent penile implants (Segal et al., 2013). Zacharakis et al. (2014b) described the efficacy and outcomes of combining the T shunt (Brant et al., 2009) with the corporal snake maneuver in 45 patients. All were refractory to medical reversal of ischemic priapism. The combined distal surgical technique was successful in resolving the acute priapism if duration was less than 24 hours but had limited efficacy in cases of priapism exceeding 48 hours. Corporal needle biopsies were performed in each patient and documented smooth muscle necrosis, worsening as a function of time and uniform in all men with more than 48 hours of ischemia. At 6 months, erectile function outcomes were assessed by the erectile function domain score from the IIEF-5. T shunt with corporal snake tunneling successfully reversed ischemic priapism in all patients with less than 24 hours' duration, but at 6 months ED was reported by 50% of men. Zacharakis et al. (2014b) concluded that the cutoff for reversing ischemic priapism in the hopes of preserving future erectile function is 48 hours. They advise that management of refractory ischemic priapism of longer than 48 hours' duration should include discussion of immediate insertion of a penile implant.

The key factors determining successful surgical reversal of ischemic priapism are evacuation of thrombus, reestablishing cavernous inflow, and patency of shunt. Theoretically, larger open shunt procedures are likely to result in higher shunt patency rates; there are no data comparing percutaneous and open distal shunts. The surgeon must be guided by familiarity with various techniques: percutaneous shunting, open distal shunting, proximal shunting, and vein shunting. Although distal shunting can be performed with penile block and sedation in the emergency department, open shunting, especially that requiring passage of dilators into the CC, will likely require general anesthesia and an operating room suite. At the completion of the shunt, patency can be verified in the operating room and subsequently the recovery room in a number of ways: bright oxygenated blood should be seen emanating from the corporal bodies; intracavernous pressures should fall; the penis should detumesce and refill with sequential compression and release; and CDU should show resumption of cavernous artery inflow (Chiou et al., 2009; Lue, 2002; Nixon et al., 2003; Box 70.3).

Complications of shunting include penile edema, hematoma, infection, conversion of low-flow to high-flow (iatrogenic laceration of a cavernous artery) urethral fistula, penile necrosis, and pulmonary embolism (Mistry et al., 2017). Distal shunt failures may be the consequence of inadequate size and/or formation of a clot at the site. Distal shunt failure invariably leads to further surgical interventions. Shunts cut through the collagen-rich tunica albuginea; collagen-activated platelets and fibrin form as a reaction to surgical injury and will work to seal off the shunt. Premature thrombosis of the site could lead to shunt failure. Three suggestions have

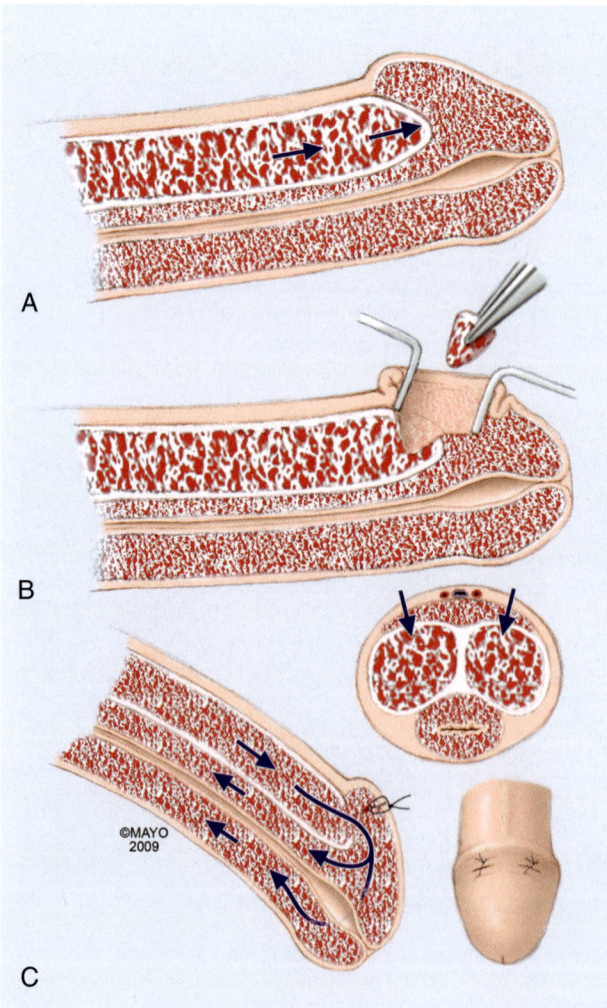

Fig. 70.10. (A to C) The Al-Ghorab shunt requires the excision of circular cone segments of the distal tunica albuginea (5 × 5 mm). (By permission of Mayo Foundation for Medical Education and Research. All rights reserved.)

BOX 70.3	Assessing Corpora Cavernosa Shunt Patency

Visualization of bright red blood in corporal aspirate
Corporal blood gas
Color Doppler ultrasonography
Measurement of intracavernous pressure
Penile compression maneuver (squeeze and release)

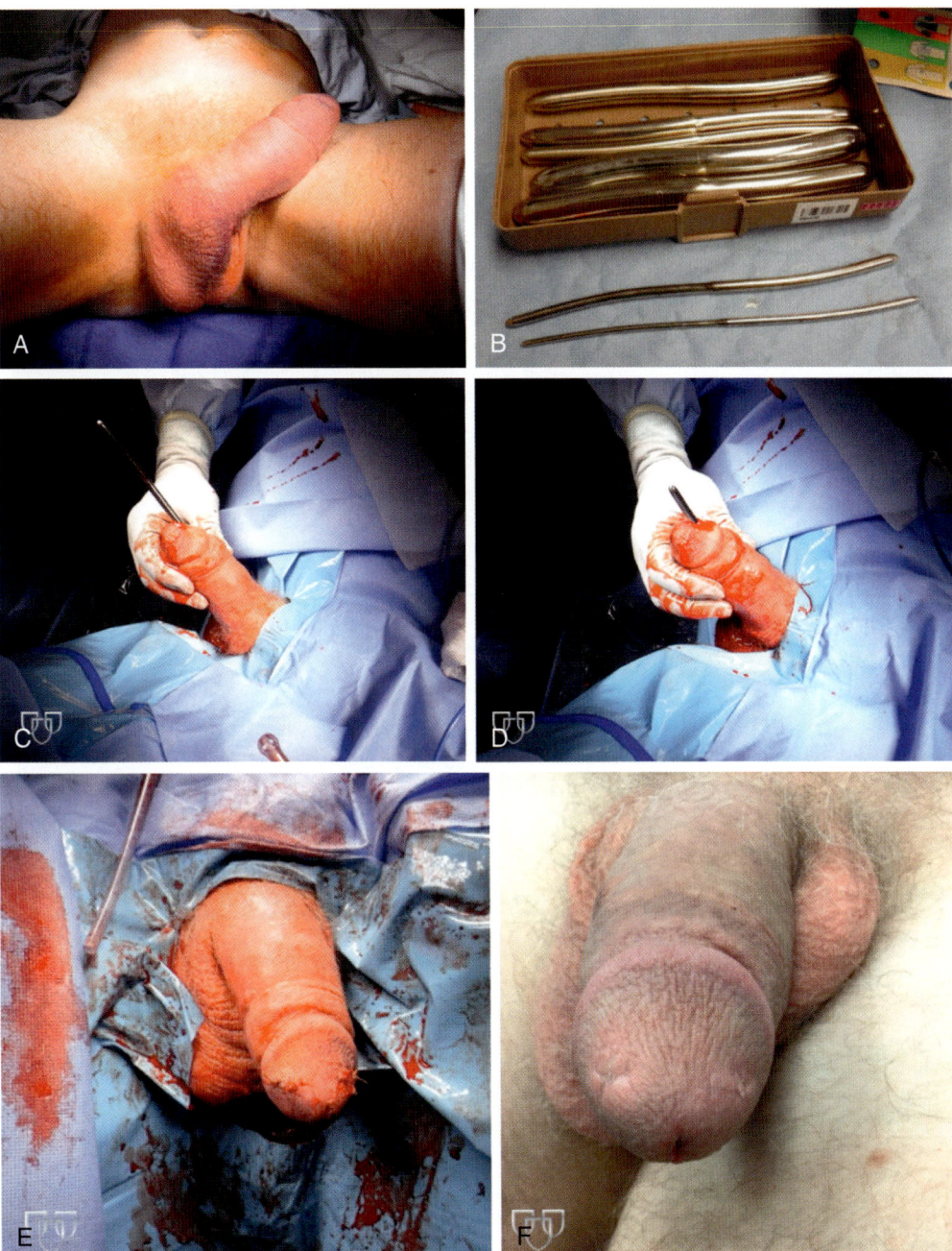

Fig. 70.11. (A) A 54-year-old male who had never been offered a trial of phosphodiesterase type 5 inhibitors before he was started on penile injection therapy by a commercial men's health clinic. He developed priapism after a low-dosage injection of trimix. He failed to respond to prescribed oral Terbutaline and Sudafed. He was treated at 12 to 24 hours in a local emergency department with α-adrenergic irrigations and taken to the operating room (OR) for bilateral distal cavernoglanular shunting with #11 blade. Patient was transferred to Mayo Clinic after more than 48 hours of ischemic priapism, with rigid erection and severe pain. (B) Hegar dilators. (C) Patient was taken to the OR for persistent ischemic priapism and pain. Distal T shunts permitted evacuation of clotting blood, but erection returned while under observation in operating theater. (D) 7/8 French Hegar dilator with staged insertion first distal and then proximal until bright red blood elicited from T shunts. (E) Penis was observed for 5 to 10 minutes in OR with no recurrence of erection; T shunts closed with #3-0 chromic sutures and (F) glans appearance after 3 weeks. The interventions relieved priapism and pain, but patient did develop distal corporal fibrosis and awaits delayed placement of penile prosthesis.

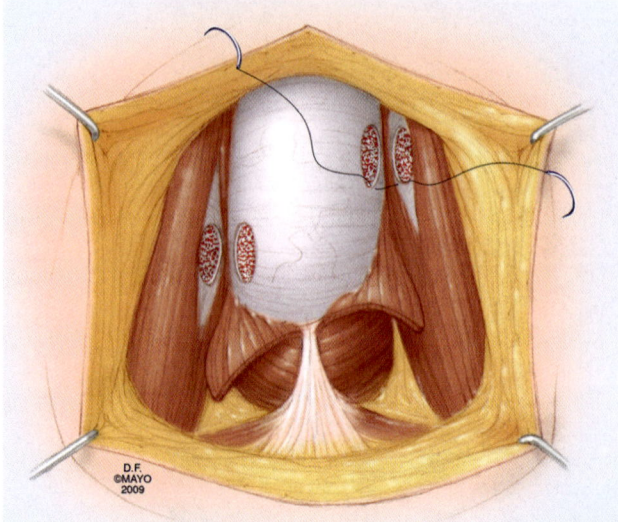

Fig. 70.12. Proximal bilateral shunts are staggered. The right and left sides are separated by a distance of at least 1 cm in an effort to minimize the risk of urethral stricture at the point of corpus cavernosum to corpus spongiosum communication (Sacher et al., 1972). (By permission of Mayo Foundation for Medical Education and Research. All rights reserved.)

been made to prevent shunt obstruction and subsequent failure: (1) compressive penile dressings should be avoided; (2) the patient should periodically squeeze and release the distal penis to "milk" the shunt maintaining patency; and (3) anticoagulation should be considered with shunting. The literature contains only one such recommendation for perioperative anticoagulation for the prevention of premature shunt obstruction in ischemic priapism. That regimen includes preoperative aspirin 325 mg coupled with subcutaneous heparin 5000 units and postoperative aspirin 81 mg daily for 2 weeks (Lue and Garcia, 2013).

A distal shunt combining the T shunt and the "corporal snake" technique of passing dilators has become my treatment of choice. I perform the two techniques in a staged manner in the operating room for priapism refractory to aspiration/α-adrenergic injection. Beginning with bilateral T shunts and milking out of distal corporal clot, I first observe for full evacuation of old blood and appearance of bright red blood. I close the incisions on the glans with 2-0 chromic and wait and observe for maintained detumescence for up to 10 minutes. If the erection resumes I remove the stitches and initiate the corporal snake maneuver with a 7/8 Hegar. The Hegar can be progressively advanced to the proximal shaft, and the size of the Hegar can be progressively increased. This stepwise progression performs a proximal shunt by disruption corporal sinusoidal architecture without the attendant risks of proximal shunting described later. Using the combination of T shunt and intracavernous tunneling Zacharakis et al. (2014a,b) reported on 45 patients with refractory ischemic priapism. The combined technique resolved priapism in less than 24 hours in all patients but in only 30% of men with priapism lasting more than 48 hours. All of these patients with more than 48 hours of ischemia had necrotic cavernous tissue biopsied at time of shunting, and all eventually had penile implants (Zacharakis et al., 2014a,b).

The most commonly described proximal shunt is the unilateral shunt, described by Quackles in 1964 (Fig. 70.12). Proximal corpus cavernosum to corpus spongiosum (CC-CS) shunt procedures require a trans-scrotal or transperineal approach (Quackles, 1964). There are no data comparing bilateral (Sacher et al., 1972) and unilateral CC-CS shunts (Quackles, 1964). Typically, bilateral shunts are staggered; the right side and left side are separated by a distance of at least 1 cm in an effort to minimize the risk of urethral stricture at the point of CC-CS communication. If proximal shunting fails, some

have advocated saphenous vein bypass or deep dorsal vein shunt (Fig. 70.13). A wedge of tunica albuginea is removed, and the vein is anastomosed end to side of CC. There are no comparative trials of vein shunting for ischemic priapism. Authors have described a significant risk of saphenofemoral vein thrombus and pulmonary embolism with vein shunting (Kandel et al., 1968).

> ### KEY POINTS: SURGICAL MANAGEMENT OF ISCHEMIC PRIAPISM
>
> - Shunt surgery should be considered for all patients with ischemic priapism in whom aspiration and ICI of α-adrenergics has failed.
> - Patients should be counseled that erectile function outcomes decline significantly when ischemic priapism has lasted longer than 24 hours and that complete ED is anticipated if ischemic priapism persists for longer than 36 hours.
> - The objective of shunt surgery is reoxygenation of the cavernous smooth muscle.
> - The key factors determining successful surgical reversal of ischemic priapism are evacuation of thrombus, patency of shunt, and resumption of cavernous inflow.
> - A distal cavernoglanular shunt should be the first choice of shunting procedures.
> - Percutaneous distal shunting is less invasive than open distal shunting and may be performed with local anesthetics.
> - There are a number of distal shunting procedures, and the surgeon should be familiar with these procedures and their complications.
> - There are no comparative trials of safety, efficacy, or erectile function outcomes for percutaneous versus open distal shunting techniques. There is increasing evidence to support T shunt in combination with "corporal snake" maneuver as the preferred surgical intervention for refractory ischemic priapism.
> - Proximal shunting establishes a communication between the CC and CS at the base of the penis. The surgeon must be aware of the unique anatomic relationship between the corpus spongiosum and urethra.
> - Shunting may also be accomplished with vein grafting to the CC. Venous shunts have increased the risk of thromboembolism.
> - After medical or surgical reversal of ischemic priapism, penile tumescence rather than complete flaccidity may be evident. A phenomenon of conversion from ischemic priapism to HFP has been described. In cases in which the examination findings may be equivocal, CDU or cavernous blood gas is recommended to demonstrate patency of the shunt and restoration of cavernous inflows.
> - After shunting, the urologist should follow up with the patient regarding erectile function and any subsequent ED therapies.

Immediate Implantation of Penile Prosthesis

Unfortunately, **the natural history of untreated ischemic priapism or priapism refractory to interventions is severe fibrosis, penile length loss, and complete ED** (see Fig. 70.1). Kelami (1985) described the implantation of the Small-Carrion penile prosthesis through an infrapubic incision in the management of postpriapic ED. Bertram et al. (1985) described six postpriapic cases of penile prosthesis; five of the six men had successful implantation of semirigid prostheses. Both groups described extensive corporal fibrosis and

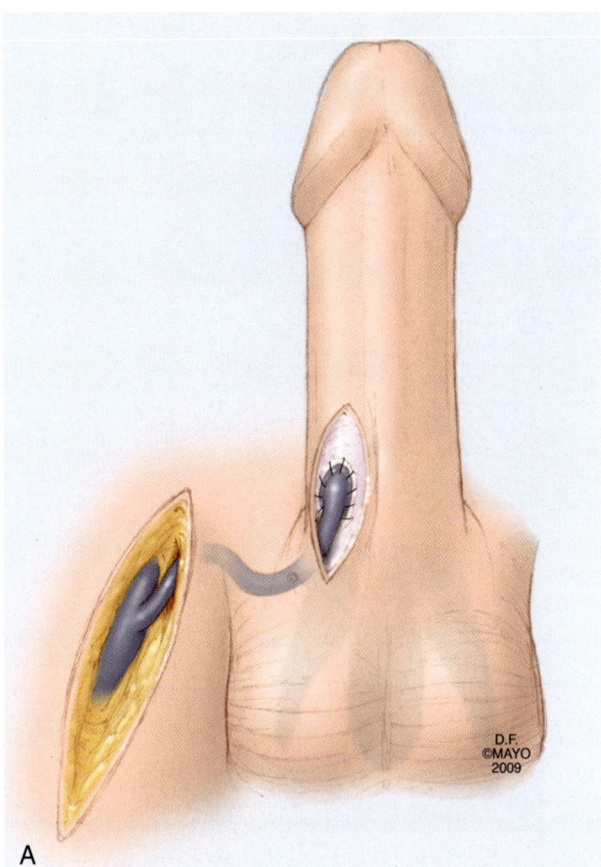 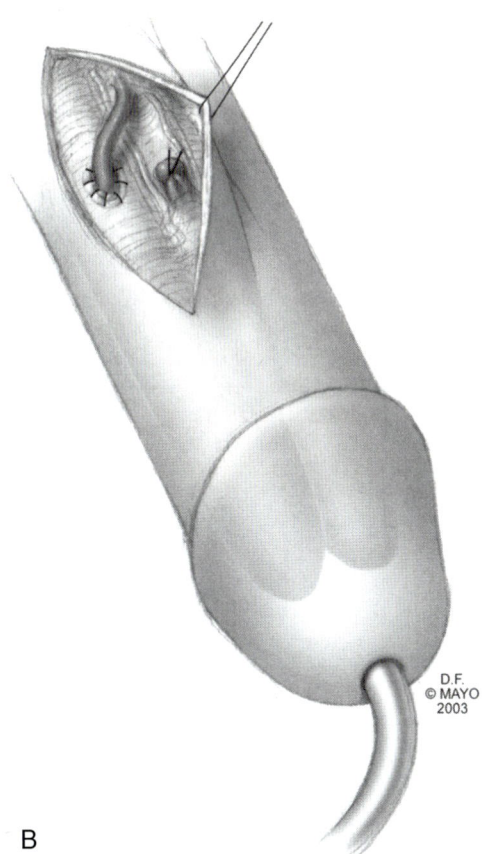

Fig. 70.13. (A) Venous bypass to control ischemic priapism was first described by Grayhack et al. in 1964. The Grayhack shunt mobilizes the saphenous vein below the junction of the femoral vein and anastomoses the vein end to side into the corpus cavernosum. (B) Deep dorsal vein (DDV) shunt with distal ligation of DDV and anastomosis of proximal DDV to corpus cavernosum. A wedge of tunica albuginea is removed. (By permission of Mayo Foundation for Medical Education and Research. All rights reserved.)

suggested that semirigid implants were preferable because inflatable implants would not overcome the corporal fibrosis sufficiently to erect the penis. Douglas et al. (1990) reported on penile prosthesis in five SCD postpriapic men; they described a surgical technique of tunneling and corporal excavation. Inadvertent damage to the tunica albuginea was common, as was subsequent migration of hardware; 11 additional procedures were required after the initial implants. The average time from priapism to implant in Douglas's series was 4 years.

Monga et al. (1996) described implants in young SCD patients (6 patients, average age 26); inflatable implants were placed to treat ED and circumvent ongoing episodes of stuttering priapism. These researchers suggested that potency and recurrent episodes of ischemic priapism could be managed by "early" implantation (Fig. 70.14).

Some have recommended performing an immediate penile prosthesis procedure in the acute management of ischemic priapism in patients in whom sympathomimetic intracavernous therapies and shunting have both failed (Rees et al., 2002). There are two distinct advantages to immediate implantation: corporal fibrosis is not yet established, and penile length may be preserved. **The exact time point at which prosthetic insertion becomes a reasonable option for managing ischemic priapism is unclear** (see Fig. 70.7). Should medical management of ischemic priapism be followed by distal percutaneous shunt, by open distal shunt, and subsequently by proximal shunting before penile implant? Should men with delayed presentation of ischemic priapism and evident corporal thrombus be triaged to an immediate penile implant procedure? What is clear is that any discussion pertaining to early prosthesis insertion should be documented and should include a comprehensive review of the theoretic advantages and actual risks. **Compared with prosthesis insertion in a typical patient with ED, there are significantly higher rates of complications noted in priapism cases: infection, urethral injury, device migration, device erosion, and need for revision surgeries** (Moore et al., 2017; Reddy et al., 2018). The surgeon must be familiar with the additional technical concerns posed by weaknesses in the tunica albuginea in the region of prior shunts.

The advantages of early penile implantation in the acute management of ischemic priapism are preservation of penile length and technically easier implant insertion. Delayed placement of penile prosthesis is technically challenging because of corporal fibrosis (Stember and Mulhall, 2010). Ralph et al. (2009) reported on 50 patients with ischemic priapism. In all patients, conservative management with the instillation of α-adrenergic agents (200 μg phenylephrine repeated to a maximum dose of 1500 μg) failed. Unsuccessful shunts were performed in 13 of 50 cases (Ralph et al., 2009). Mean duration of priapism was 209 hours (range 24 to 720 hours). All patients had evidence of cavernous thrombus and smooth muscle necrosis on MRI, and all 50 underwent insertion of penile prosthesis in the acute setting of refractory ischemic priapism. Revision rates were significantly high, at 24% (12 of 50 patients). The infection rate of 6% was also notably high and likely related to multiple factors including ischemic tissues and preceding penile interventions. The same surgical group recently compared

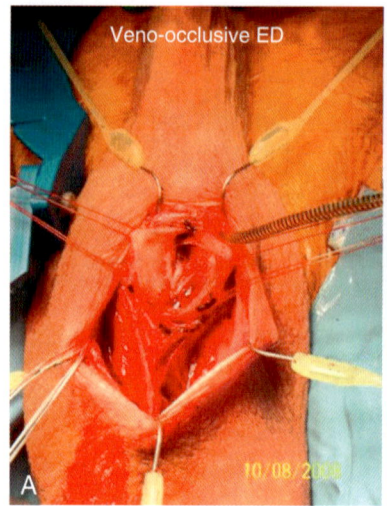 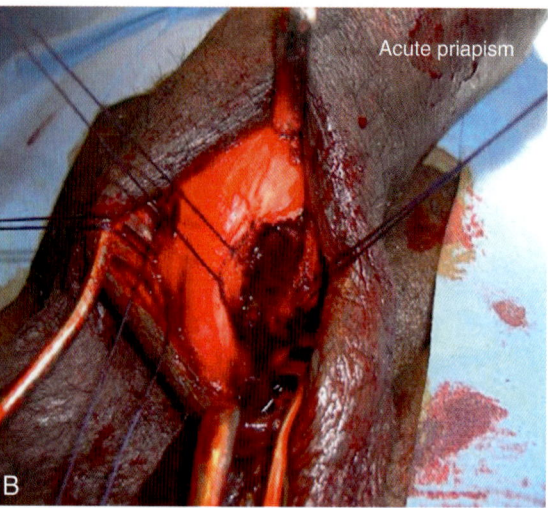

Fig. 70.14. Penoscrotal surgical approach for elective insertion of inflatable penile implant in a white patient with severe veno-occlusive erectile dysfunction (ED) (A) and a patient with sickle cell disease with acute ischemic priapism refractory to pharmacologic interventions and shunting for 48 hours (B). (B, Courtesy David J. Ralph, MD.)

two cohorts of patients undergoing penile implant for refractory ischemic priapism. An early insertion cohort was operated on at a mean of 7 days after onset of priapism, and the delayed cohort was operated on at a mean of 5 months after priapism. In the early insertion group, satisfaction and ability to have intercourse was 96%; in the delayed group, corporal fibrosis made surgery technically more difficult and overall patient satisfaction was 60% (Zacharakis et al., 2014a). The placement of penile implant in the immediate management of refractory ischemic priapism is controversial. There is good evidence that reversing ischemic priapism beyond 36 to 48 hours will have the same long-term outcome as doing no further procedures: corporal fibrosis and complete ED. A successful intervention at 48 hours will certainly spare the patients several weeks of pain and needed analgesia, but it will not result in the recovery of normal if any erections. Some have suggested logistical considerations balance surgical zeal to "fix the problem early." Elective placement of penile implants in the United States requires prior authorization for those surgical services or contracting with the patient for a cash price. Delaying a penile implant to allow some healing of the distal shunt site for 3 weeks allows for prior authorization of the surgical procedure and should theoretically permit operation while there is still unorganized (liquid) clot in the corporal spaces and not dense fibrosis (Tatem and Kovac, 2017).

> **KEY POINTS: SURGICAL MANAGEMENT OF ISCHEMIC PRIAPISM WITH IMMEDIATE PENILE IMPLANT**
>
> - The natural history of untreated ischemic priapism or priapism refractory to interventions is severe fibrosis, penile length loss, and complete ED.
> - The advantages of early penile implantation in the acute management of ischemic priapism are preservation of penile length and easier insertion.
> - The clinician should document baseline erectile function, duration of priapism, history of stuttering, and prior interventions.
> - Penile prosthesis should be considered in the following circumstances:
>   - Aspiration and sympathomimetic ICI have failed.
>   - Distal and proximal shunting procedures have failed.
>   - Ischemia has been present for longer than 36 hours.
> - An MRI before surgery or corporal biopsy at the time of implant should be considered to document corporal smooth muscle necrosis.
> - There are higher rates of revision surgery and complications noted in priapism cases resulting from infection, urethral injury, device migration, and device erosion.

INTERVENTIONAL ANGIOGRAPHY IN THE MANAGEMENT OF ARTERIAL (NONISCHEMIC, HIGH-FLOW) PRIAPISM

Arterial priapism is not an emergency. Spontaneous resolution or response to conservative therapy has been reported in up to 62% of published series (Montague et al., 2003; Pryor et al., 2004). Persistent partial erection from HFP may be evident for months to years without adverse impact on erectile function (Bastuba et al., 1995). Kumar et al. (2006) described a case of HFP in a 24-year-old patient 10 days after straddle injury on a bicycle. The patient had no erection for the first 4 days after injury. Examination revealed a tumescent penis that was compressible. Penile aspiration and blood gas analysis revealed oxygenated corporal blood. CDU of the cavernous artery revealed arteriosinusoidal fistula. Partial erection spontaneously resolved 4 days after diagnostic evaluation, with the patient reporting normal erections 2 weeks later. The authors hypothesized that, in patients with blunt penile and perineal trauma, an arteriolacunar fistula forms; these fistulae, unlike arteriovenous communications, may spontaneously resolve because the less-rigid walls of the lacunae are prone to spontaneous thrombosis. Onset of HFP is typically delayed after injury. The erection is partial, not rigid, and not painful. Although the site of perineal trauma may have hematoma, spreading of the hematoma to the shaft should raise suspicion of rupture of tunica albuginea; this would be highly unusual in blunt perineal (straddle) injury. The pathophysiology of HFP is unregulated arteriolacunar fistula from disruption or crush injury to terminal branches of the cavernous artery. Fistula is typically unilateral. Because there is no restriction of venous outflow, erection is partial and bendable. Patients do report additional engorgement with sexual stimulation with return to partial erection after climax.

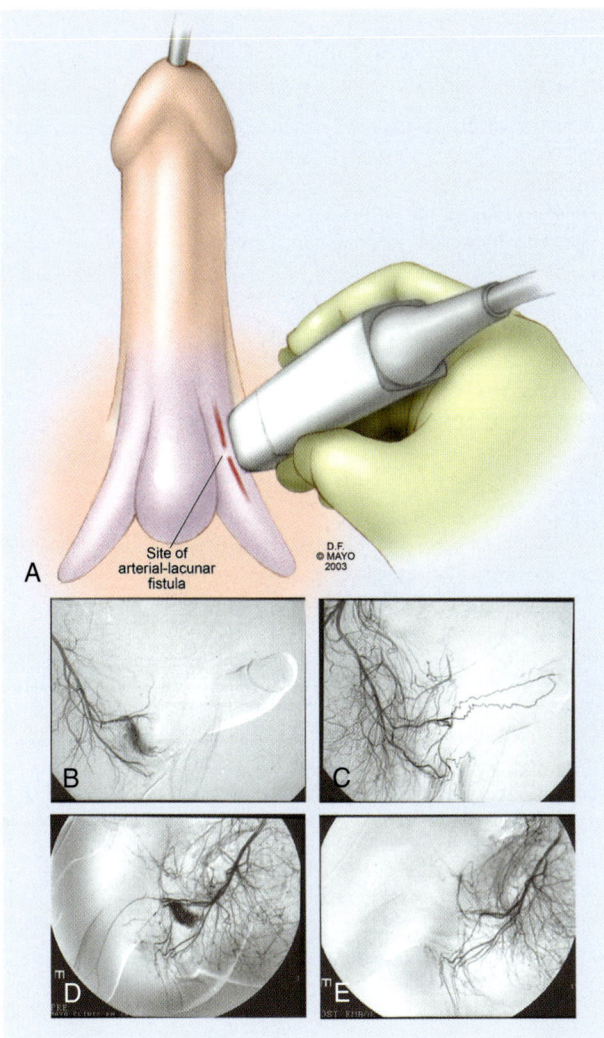

Fig. 70.15. Color Doppler ultrasonography of the penis and perineum is recommended in the evaluation of priapism when the history or examination findings suggest penile trauma (A). Doppler sonography for localization of a fistula correlates well with selective pudendal angiography (B to E); a characteristic fistula blush is shown (B and D), along with normal arteriograms (C and E). (A, By permission of Mayo Foundation for Medical Education and Research. All rights reserved.)

reaction, or antigenicity; it is a temporary occlusive agent and should permit recanalization of the cavernous artery (Park et al., 2001). **The success rates with selective pudendal artery catheterization followed by embolization are high (89% to 100%), regardless of the embolization material used** (Kuefer et al., 2005; Numan et al., 2008). Similar results have been reported by others (Alexander Tønseth et al., 2006; Savoca et al., 2004). **Normal postembolization erectile function has been reported in 75% to 86% of patients** (Cakan et al., 2006; Numan et al., 2008). **A single treatment of embolization carries a recurrence rate of 30% in some series** (Ciampalani et al., 2002; Gandini et al., 2004; Ozturk et al., 2009). **Although ultimately successful, embolization of HFP may require retreatment. The most notable side effect of bilateral arterial embolization is ED.** Recurrence of HPF after embolization may be caused by recanalization of the embolized fistula or unmasking of a fistula in the contralateral cavernous artery. Although it was previously reported that nonpermanent embolization materials cause less ED than permanent ones (5% vs. 39%), reports describing use of the IIEF in evaluation of postembolization erectile function note similar rates of ED—15% and 20% (Alexander Tønseth et al., 2006; Savoca et al., 2004). Older reports show adverse effects including penile gangrene, gluteal ischemia, purulent cavernositis, and abscess of the perineum. These may be due to the less selective embolization techniques (Hakim et al., 1996; Sandock et al., 1996).

Puppo et al. (1985) compared perineal duplex ultrasound and selective internal pudendal arteriography, showing excellent sensitivity of ultrasound in detecting arteriolacunar fistulae that were seen angiographically (12 of 12 cases). Several reports have described combined ultrasound-guided compression with selective arterial embolization to increase success rates in the treatment of nonischemic priapism (Bartsch et al., 2004; Cakan et al., 2006; Hatzichristou et al., 2002). If the follow-up clinical examination is equivocal for recurrence of HFP, a perineal duplex Doppler ultrasound can determine the need for repeat arteriography and embolization (Kim et al., 2007). In a recent series reviewing 16 patients managed at one center with superselective transcatheter artery embolization, 93% of patients responded to a single embolization and 7% required a second embolization for recurrence or persistence of high-flow arteriosinusoidal fistula. All the patients were adults and 70% reported history of trauma; in the majority the onset of HFP was within 10 days of injury. All patients had superselective embolization into the anterior division of the internal iliac artery with advancement of microguidewire and microcatheter (Terumo, Tokyo, Japan) as close to the fistula as possible. Fourteen of 16 patients had unilateral embolization (all with permanent microcoils), and all had preservation of "premorbid erectile function" (Pei et al., 2018).

SURGICAL MANAGEMENT OF ARTERIAL (NONISCHEMIC, HIGH-FLOW) PRIAPISM

Arterial priapism is not a urologic emergency. HFP is painless, and there have been reports of partial erection persisting for years (Nehra, 2006). Any intervention must follow a comprehensive discussion with the patient regarding risks and benefits of any of the procedures advocated by the clinician. **In cases of long-standing arterial priapism in which a pseudocapsule around the fistula has developed, surgical ligation has been reported to be successful. Formation of a pseudocapsule may take weeks to months after trauma. Corporal exploration before the formation of a pseudocapsule** (Fig. 70.16) **may result in ligation of the cavernous artery rather than selective ligation of the fistula.** Currently this intervention is reserved for patients who do not wish to pursue expectant management or who are poor candidates for angioembolization. It is also reserved for patients who refuse the procedure; for patients in places where technology is not available; and for patients in whom angioembolization has failed (Berger et al., 2001; Ji et al., 1994; Mulhall, 2006). The surgical approach is transcorporal. Intraoperative Doppler ultrasound guidance is recommended (Fig. 70.17).

There are no comparative outcome studies of intervention versus conservative management in HFP; there are sufficient case descriptions, especially in children, to recommend initial watchful waiting. Initial observation is recommended for this type of priapism. Conservative measures include ice applied to the perineum and site-specific compression. **Cavernous aspiration has only a diagnostic role in HFP. Repeated aspirations, injection, and irrigation with intracavernous sympathomimetics have no role in the treatment of nonischemic priapism.**

Patients demanding immediate relief can be offered selective arterial embolization. The pathognomonic arteriographic finding is an arteriolacunar fistula; a characteristic intracavernosal cone-shaped blush of contrast is seen at the site of the cavernous artery or arteriole laceration (Fig. 70.15). Selective internal pudendal catheterization and subsequent embolization have been reported with various agents: microcoils, polyvinyl alcohol, N-butylcyanoacrylate, gel-foam, and autologous blood clot (Kuefer et al., 2005). Permanent materials pose a greater theoretic risk of ED; many authors recommend use of autologous blood clot and absorbable gels (Kim et al., 2007; Pryor et al., 2004). Autologous blood clot has a low risk of foreign body

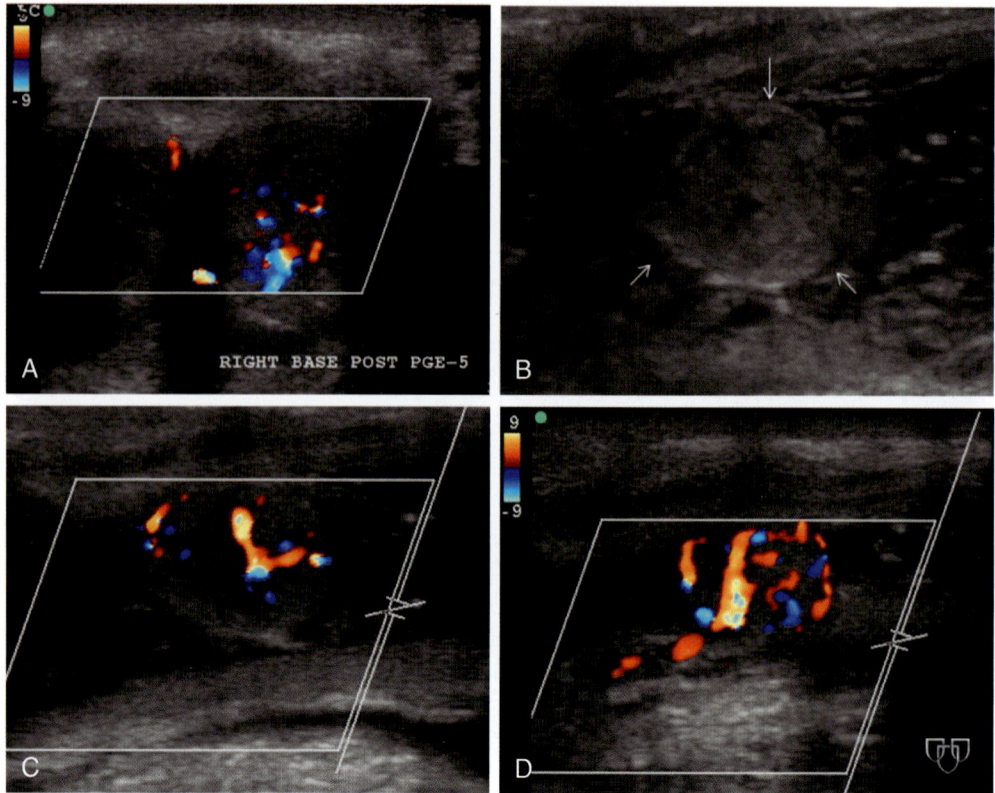

Fig. 70.16. A 60-year-old male presenting more than a year after straddle injury with the complaint of persisting tumescence and no pain. He was unable to achieve rigid erection for sex despite PDE type-5 Inhibitor dosing. (A) Sagittal color Doppler imaging after low dosage alprostadil suggests sinusoidal fistula. (B) Duplex grayscale imaging; *arrows* outline pseudo capsule. (C, D) Coronal images confirm disrupted cavernous arterial and sinusoidal fistula.

KEY POINTS: EVALUATION AND MANAGEMENT OF HIGH-FLOW PRIAPISM

- Arterial priapism is not an emergency and may be managed expectantly.
- Diagnosis of HFP is best made by penile or perineal CDU.
- Penile aspiration and injection of α-adrenergic agents are not recommended for HFP.
- Angioembolization should be preceded by a thorough discussion of chances for spontaneous resolution, risks of treatment-related ED, and lack of significant consequences expected from delaying interventions.
- Overall success rates with embolization are high, although a single treatment carries a variable recurrence rate.
- When angioembolization fails or is contraindicated, surgical ligation is reasonable.
- Formation of a pseudocapsule at the site of a sinusoidal fistula may take weeks to months after trauma.
- CDU guidance is recommended during exploration to locate fistulae.

SUMMARY

Priapism is a full or partial erection that persists more than 4 hours beyond sexual stimulation and orgasm or is unrelated to sexual stimulation. Prompt diagnosis and appropriate management are necessary to spare patients ineffective interventions and optimize erectile function outcomes. Ischemic priapism (veno-occlusive, low-flow) is a persistent painful erection marked by rigidity of the CC. In ischemic priapism there are time-dependent changes in the corpora with progressive hypoxia, hypercarbia, and acidosis. Ischemic priapism is a urologic emergency. Treatment for ischemic priapism is administered in a stepwise manner: decompression of the corpora by needle aspiration, injection and/or irrigation with a dilute sympathomimetic drug (phenylephrine), surgical shunting, and possible consideration of immediate penile implant in refractory cases (see Fig. 70.7). Ischemic priapism is a common pathologic consequence of SCD. Stuttering ischemic priapism describes a pattern of prolonged morning erections that are unwanted and painful in boys and adolescents with SCD. Unfortunately any patient who has experienced an episode of ischemic priapism is also at risk for stuttering priapism. HFP (nonischemic priapism, arterial priapism) is a persistent erection caused by unregulated cavernous arterial inflow. Typically, the corpora are tumescent but not rigid, and the penis is not painful. A history of blunt trauma (a straddle injury) or an iatrogenic needle injury to the penis is common. HFP may follow the primary trauma by several weeks or may be immediate. The cavernous environment in HFP does not become ischemic, and cavernous blood gases do not show hypoxia, hypercarbia, or acidosis. HFP, once properly diagnosed, does not require emergent treatment (see Fig. 70.17).

Urologists intervening to treat priapism should document onset of erection and the presence or absence of pain, trauma, medical history of blood dyscrasias, use of illicit substances, prior prolonged erection events, baseline erectile function, types of interventions, and recovery of erectile function. Physicians should document erectile function outcomes with standardized questionnaires such as Sexual Health Inventory for Men (SHIM) or the International Index of Erectile Function (IIEF). Documenting erectile function outcomes versus the duration of ischemic priapism, time to interventions, and types of interventions will establish evidence-based guidance on how and when to apply those interventions.

Chapter 70 Priapism **1563**

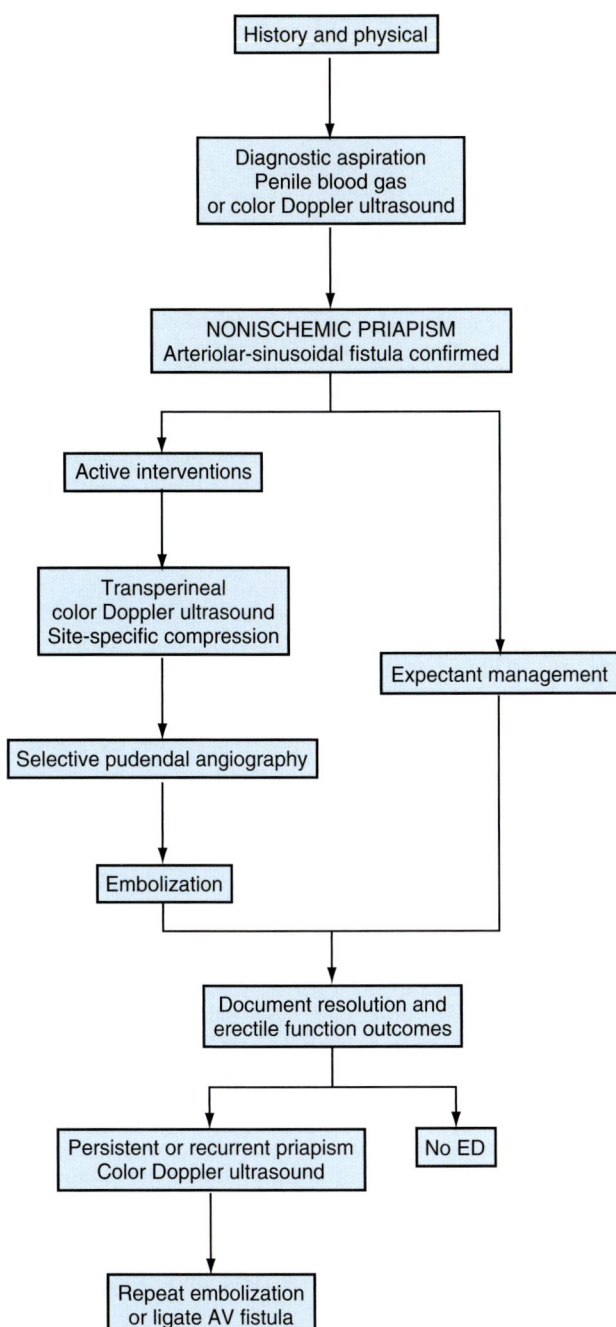

Fig. 70.17. Algorithm for managing high-flow priapism. *AV,* Arteriovenous; *ED,* erectile dysfunction.

SUGGESTED READINGS

Bennett N, Mulhall J: Sickle cell disease status and outcomes of African American men presenting with priapism, *J Sex Med* 5(5):1244–1250, 2008.
Bivalacqua TJ, Champion HC, Mason W, et al: Long-term phosphodiesterase type 5 inhibitor therapy reduces priapic activity in transgenic sickle cell mice, *J Urol* 175:387, 2006.
Brant WO, Garcia MM, Bella AJ, et al: T-shaped shunt and intracavernous tunneling for prolonged ischemic priapism, *J Urol* 181:1699–1705, 2009.
Broderick GA: Priapism and sickle-cell anemia: diagnosis and nonsurgical therapy, *J Sex Med* 9:88–103, 2012.
Broderick GA, Kadioglu A, Bivalacqua TJ, et al: Priapism: pathogenesis, epidemiology, and management, *J Sex Med* 7:476–500, 2010.
Burnett AL, Anele UA, Trueheart IN, et al: Randomized controlled trial of sildenafil for preventing recurrent ischemic priapism in sickle cell disease, *Am J Med* 127(7):664–668, 2014.
Chan PTK, Begin LR, Arnold D, et al: Priapism secondary to penile metastasis: a report of two cases and a review of the literature, *J Surg Oncol* 68(1):51–59, 1998.
Chiou RK, Aggarwal H, Chiou C, et al: Colour Doppler ultrasound hemo-dynamic characteristics of patient with priapism before and after therapeutic interventions, *Can Urol Assoc J* 3(4):304–311, 2009.
Constantine ST, Gopalsami A, Helland G: Recurrent priapism gone wrong: ST-elevation myocardial infarction and cardiogenic shock after penile corporal phenylephrine irrigation, *J Emerg Med* 52(6):859–862, 2017.
Hudnall M, Reed-Maldonado AB, Lue TF: Advances in the understanding of priapism, *Transl Androl Urol* 6(2):199–206, 2017.
Kato GJ: Priapism in sickle-cell disease: a hematologist's perspective, *J Sex Med* 9:70–78, 2012.
La Favor JD, Fu Z, Venkatraman V, et al: Molecular profile of priapism associated with low nitric oxide bioavailability, *J Proteome Res* 17(3):1031–1040, 2018.
Podolej GS, Babcock C: Emergency department management of priapism, *Emerg Med Pract* 19(1):1–16, 2017.
Qi T, Ye L, Chen Z, et al: Efficacy and safety of treatment of high-flow priapism with superselective transcatheter embolization, *Curr Med Sci* 38(1):101–106, 2018.
Ralph DJ, Garaffa G, Muneer A, et al: The immediate insertion of a penile prosthesis for acute ischaemic priapism, *Eur Urol* 56:1033–1038, 2009.
Reed-Maldonado AB, Kim JS, Lue TF: Avoiding complications: surgery for ischemic priapism, *Transl Androl Urol* 6(4):657–665, 2017.
Reddy AG, Alzweri LM, Gabrielson AT, et al: Role of penile prosthesis in priapism: a review, *World J Mens Health* 36(1):4–14, 2018.
Salonia A, Eardley I, Giuliano F, et al: European Association of Urology guidelines on priapism, *Eur Urol* 65:480–489, 2014.
Sidhu AS, Wayne GF, Kim BJ, et al: High-dose intracavernosal phenylephrine for priapism: is it safe?, *J Urol* 197(4 Suppl 1):e1348–e1349, 2017.
Zacharakis E, Raheem AA, Freman A, et al: The efficacy of the T-shunt procedure and intracavernous tunneling (snake maneuver) for refractory ischemic priapism, *J Urol* 191:164–168, 2014b.

REFERENCES

The complete reference list is available online at ExpertConsult.com.

71 Disorders of Male Orgasm and Ejaculation

Chris G. McMahon, MBBS, FAChSHP

Ejaculatory dysfunction (EjD) is one of the most common male sexual disorders. The spectrum of EjD extends from **premature ejaculation (PE)** through delayed ejaculation (DE) to a complete inability to ejaculate (known as anejaculation) and includes retrograde ejaculation (RE), painful ejaculation, ejaculatory anhedonia, and the recently described postorgasmic illness syndrome (POIS).

The sexual response cycle comprises the four interactive stages of **desire, arousal, orgasm, and resolution.** During sexual activity, increasing levels of sexual arousal reach a threshold that triggers the ejaculatory response, which then typically terminates the sexual episode for the male. The perception of the striated muscle contractions and resulting semen expelled during ejaculation, mediated through sensory neurons in the pelvic region, gives rise to the experience of orgasm, a distinct cortical event, experienced phenomenologically, cognitively, and emotionally.

Ejaculatory latency, the time extending from the onset of penile stimulation to the moment of ejaculation, represents a continuum of time that shows variation across men and, within men, across situations. Although the great majority of men appear to reach ejaculation and orgasm after several minutes of penile vaginal stimulation and are, along with their partners, satisfied with the latency of their ejaculatory response, others report dissatisfaction. Specifically, some men ejaculate very rapidly after, or sometimes even before, penetration and do so with minimal stimulation. Others may ejaculate only with great difficulty or not at all, even after prolonged stimulation (McMahon et al., 2013).

ANATOMY AND PHYSIOLOGY OF THE EJACULATORY RESPONSE

The ejaculatory reflex comprises sensory receptors and areas, afferent pathways, cerebral sensory areas, cerebral motor centres, spinal motor centers, and efferent pathways (Fig. 71.1). The brain circuitry controlling ejaculation is part of a more global network controlling other aspects of the sexual response. **Neurochemically, this reflex involves a complex interplay between central serotonergic and dopaminergic neurons, with secondary involvement of cholinergic, adrenergic, oxytocinergic, and γ-aminobutyric acid (GABA) neurons.** The peripheral events leading to ejaculation are controlled by synergistic activation of autonomic (sympathetic and parasympathetic) and somatic divisions of the nervous system. In addition, nonadrenergic noncholinergic (NANC) innervation may contribute to the control of ejaculation through modulation of accessory sex gland activity.

The autonomic and somatic motor efferents originate in five groups of spinal nuclei located in thoracolumbar and lumbosacral segments. Coordinated activation of autonomic and somatic spinal nuclei is controlled by a group of lumbar spinal interneurons (L3-L5) described as the spinal generator of ejaculation. The generator of ejaculation together with the autonomic and somatic spinal nuclei constitutes a spinal network that is under the strong influence of stimulating or inhibiting genital sensory and supraspinal inputs (Clement and Giuliano, 2016).

Several interrelated groups of neurons located in several sensory/integrative, excitatory, and inhibitory areas of the brain form a dedicated neural network for the control of ejaculation. The posteromedial division of the bed nucleus of the stria terminalis, the posterodorsal area of the medial amygdala, the posterodorsal preoptic nucleus, and the parvicellular part of the subparafascicular thalamus contain a group of neurons that are activated during ejaculation (Veening and Coolen, 2014).

Based upon functional, central, and peripheral mediation, the ejaculatory process is typically subdivided into three synchronized phases: **emission, ejection (or penile expulsion), and orgasm.**

Emission consists of contractions of vas deferens, seminal vesicles (SV), and the prostate, with expulsion of sperm and seminal fluid into the posterior urethra and is mediated by synergic activation of sympathetic and parasympathetic pathways (T10-L2) but may also include a cholinergic excitatory mechanism.

Ejection is mediated by somatic nerves (S2 to S4) within the pudendal nerve and involves pulsatile contractions of the bulbospongiosus, ischiocavernosus, and levator ani muscles together with relaxation of the internal urinary sphincter. Ejection also involves a sympathetic spinal cord reflex upon which there is limited voluntary control. The bladder neck (internal urinary sphincter) closes to prevent retrograde flow; the bulbocavernosus, bulbospongiosus, and other pelvic floor muscles contract rhythmically, and the external urinary sphincter relaxes. The external urinary sphincter exhibits intense contractions interrupted by silent periods during ejection of semen.

Orgasm is the result of cerebral processing of pudendal nerve sensory stimuli resulting from increased pressure in the posterior urethra, sensory stimuli arising from the verumontanum, and contraction of the urethral bulb and accessory sexual organs.

Many neurotransmitters are involved in the control of ejaculation, including dopamine, norepinephrine, serotonin, acetylcholine, oxytocin, GABA, and nitric oxide (NO) (McMahon et al., 2004). Of the many studies conducted to investigate the role of the brain in the development and mediation of sexual functioning, dopamine and serotonin have emerged as essential neurochemical factors. **Whereas dopamine promotes seminal emission/ejaculation via D2 receptors, serotonin is inhibitory.** Serotonergic neurons are widely distributed in the brain and spinal cord and are predominantly found in the brainstem, raphe nuclei, and the reticular formation. Currently, multiple serotonin (5-HT) receptors have been characterized (e.g., 5-HT1a, 5-HT1b, 5-HT2a, 5-HT2b) (Peroutka and Snyder, 1979). Stimulation of the 5-HT2c receptor with 5-HT2c agonists results in delay of ejaculation in male rats, whereas stimulation of postsynaptic 5-HT1a receptors results in shortening of ejaculation latency (Ahlenius et al. 1981), leading to the hypothesis that men with PE may have hyposensitivity of 5-HT2c and/or hypersensitivity of the 5-HT1a receptor (Waldinger, 2002; Waldinger and Olivier, 2005).

PREMATURE EJACULATION

Classification of Premature Ejaculation

In 1943 Schapiro proposed classification of PE into two types: types B and A. In 1989 Godpodinoff renamed both types as **lifelong (primary) and acquired (secondary) PE.** Over the years, other attempts to specify subtypes have occurred (e.g., global vs. situational, the effect of a substance).

Lifelong PE is a syndrome characterized by a cluster of core symptoms, including early ejaculation at nearly every intercourse within 30 to 60 seconds in the majority of cases (80%) or between 1 and 2 minutes (20%), with every or nearly every sexual partner and from the first sexual encounters onward (McMahon, 2002; Waldinger et al., 1998).

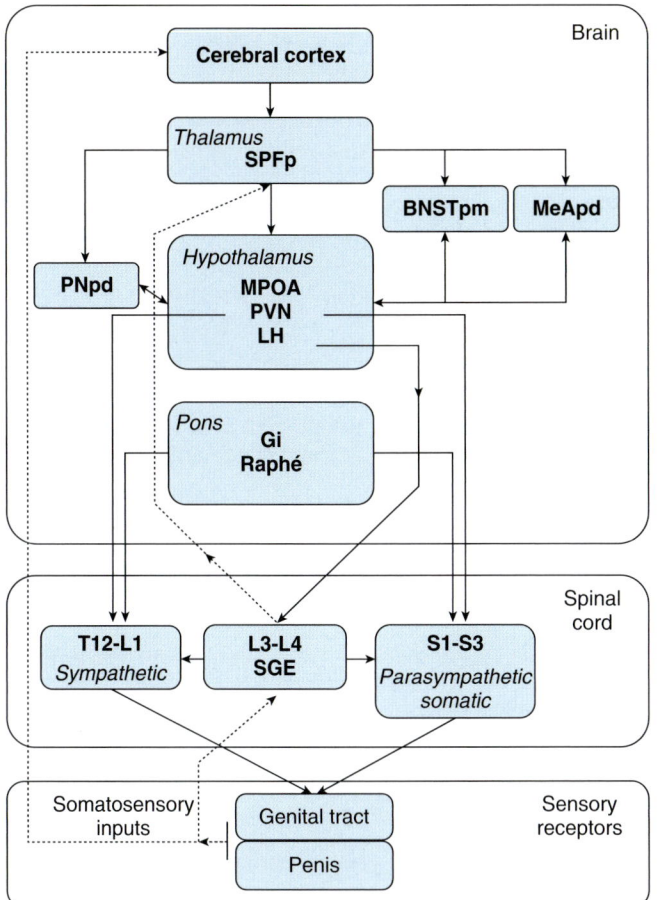

Fig. 71.1. Diagram of the central nervous system network controlling ejaculation. Brain nuclei forming the brain circuitry of ejaculation are indicated with their connections to spinal nuclei involved in the control of ejaculation. Somatosensory afferents originating in genitalia and terminating in the CNS are also presented. *BNSTpm,* Posteromedial part of the bed nucleus of the stria terminalis; *Gi,* gigantocellular nuclei; *LH,* lateral hypothalamus; *MeApd,* posterodorsal part of the medial amygdala; *MPOA,* medial preoptic area; *PNpd,* posterodorsal part of the preoptic nucleus; *PVN,* paraventricular nucleus; *SGE,* spinal generator of ejaculation; *SPFp,* parvicellular part of the subparafascicular nucleus. (Clement P, Giuliano F: Physiology and pharmacology of ejaculation. *Basic Clin Pharmacol Toxicol* 119(Suppl 3):18–25, 2016.)

Acquired PE differs in that sufferers develop early ejaculation at some point in their life, which is often situational, having previously had normal ejaculation experiences. The main distinguishing features between presentations of these two syndromes are the time of onset of symptoms and the reduction in previously normal ejaculatory latency of acquired PE.

Community based normative intravaginal ejaculatory latency time (IELT) research and observational studies of men with PE demonstrated that, although **IELTs of less than 1 minute have a low prevalence of about 2.5% in the general population,** a substantially higher percentage of men with normal IELT complain of PE (Patrick et al., 2005; Waldinger, et al. 2005, 2009). To take account of this diversity, Waldinger and Schweitzer (2006, 2008) proposed a new classification of PE in which **four PE subtypes are distinguished on the basis of the duration of the IELT, frequency of complaints, and course in life. In addition to lifelong PE and acquired PE, this classification includes natural variable PE (or variable PE) and premature-like EjD (or subjective PE).** Men with variable PE occasionally experience an early ejaculation. It should not be regarded as a disorder but as a natural variation of the ejaculation time in men (Waldinger, 2013). On the other hand, men with subjective PE complain of PE while actually having a normal or even extended ejaculation time (Waldinger, 2013). The complaint of PE in these men is probably related to psychological and/or cultural factors. In contrast, the consistent early ejaculations of lifelong PE suggest an underlying neurobiologic functional disturbance, whereas the early ejaculation of acquired PE is more related to underlying medical causes. Serefoglu et al. (2010, 2011) confirmed the existence of these four PE subtypes in a cohort of men in Turkey. Recently, Zhang et al. (2013) and Gao et al. (2013), using a similar methodology, confirmed similar prevalence rates of the four PE subtypes in China to that reported by Serefoglu et al. (2010, 2011). This new classification and continued research into the diverse phenomenology, cause, and pathogenesis of PE is expected to provide a better understanding of the four PE subtypes (Waldinger and Schweitzer, 2008). Although the pathogenesis of lifelong and acquired PE differs, the presence of shared dimensions such as a lack of ejaculatory control and the presence of negative personal consequences suggest a potential for a single unifying definition of lifelong and acquired PE. With continued research into the two other PE subtypes, variable PE and subjective PE, it may be appropriate to expand this unifying definition in the future.

Definition of Premature Ejaculation

Research into the treatment and epidemiology of PE is heavily dependent on how PE is defined. The **medical literature contains several univariate and multivariate operational definitions of PE** (American Psychiatric Association, 1994; Colpi et al., 2004; Jannini et al., 2005; Masters and Johnson, 1970; McMahon et al., 2004, 2008; Metz and McCarthy, 2003; Montague et al., 2004; Waldinger et al., 2005; World Health Organization, 1994; Table 71.1). Each of these definitions characterize men with PE using all or most of the accepted dimensions of this condition: ejaculatory latency, perceived ability to control ejaculation, reduced sexual satisfaction, personal distress, partner distress, and interpersonal or relationship distress. None of these definitions was supported by evidence-based clinical research.

These authority-based definitions are discussed in detail on ExpertConsult.com.

International Society for Sexual Medicine Definition of Premature Ejaculation

In the last decade, substantial progress has been made in the development of evidence-based methodology for PE epidemiologic and drug treatment research using the objective IELT and subjective validated patient-reported outcome (PRO) measures. In October 2007 **the International Society for Sexual Medicine (ISSM) convened an initial meeting of the first Ad Hoc ISSM Committee for the Definition of PE to develop the first contemporary, evidence-based definition of lifelong PE.** Evidence-based definitions seek to limit errors of classification and thereby increase the likelihood that existing and newly developed therapeutic strategies are truly effective in carefully selected dysfunctional populations (Metz and McCarthy, 2003). After critical evaluation of the published data, the committee unanimously agreed that the constructs that are necessary to define lifelong PE are time from penetration to ejaculation, inability to delay ejaculation, and negative personal consequences from PE. They recommended the following definition:

> Lifelong PE is a male sexual dysfunction characterized by the presence of all of these criteria: 1) ejaculation that always or nearly always occurs prior to or within about 1 minute of vaginal penetration; 2) the inability to delay ejaculation on all or nearly all vaginal penetrations; and 3) negative personal consequences such as distress, bother, frustration, and/or the avoidance of sexual intimacy

(McMahon et al., 2008). The committee was, however, unable to identify sufficient published objective data to craft an evidence-based definition of acquired PE. The committee anticipated that future studies would generate sufficient data to develop an evidence-based definition for acquired PE.

In April 2013 the International Society for Sexual Medicine (ISSM) convened a second Ad Hoc ISSM Committee for the Definition of PE in Bangalore, India. The brief of the committee was to evaluate the current published data and attempt to develop a contemporary,

TABLE 71.1 Definitions of Premature Ejaculation (PE)

DEFINITION	SOURCE
PE is a male sexual dysfunction characterized by ejaculation that always or nearly always occurs before or within 1 minute of vaginal penetration (lifelong PE), or, a clinically significant and bothersome reduction in latency time, often to about 3 minutes or less (acquired PE), and the inability to delay ejaculation on all or nearly all vaginal penetrations, and negative personal consequences, such as distress bother, frustration, and/or the avoidance of sexual intimacy	International Society of Sexual Medicine, 2014
Lifelong PE is a male sexual dysfunction characterized by ejaculation that always or nearly always occurs before or within 1 minute of vaginal penetration, and the inability to delay ejaculation on all or nearly all vaginal penetrations, and negative personal consequences, such as distress bother, frustration, and/or the avoidance of sexual intimacy	International Society of Sexual Medicine, 2008 (McMahon et al., 2008)
A persistent or recurrent pattern of ejaculation occurring during partnered sexual activity within approximately 1 minute after vaginal penetration and before the individual wishes it. This symptom must have been present for at least 6 months and must be experienced on almost all or all (approximately 75%–100%) occasions of sexual activity. It causes clinically significant distress in the individual.	DSM-V-TR, 2012 (American Psychiatric Association, 2013)
Persistent or recurrent ejaculation with minimal sexual stimulation before, on, or shortly after penetration and before the person wishes it. The condition must also cause marked distress or interpersonal difficulty and cannot be due exclusively to the direct effects of a substance.	DSM-IV-TR, 2000 (American Psychiatric Association, 2000)
For individuals who meet the general criteria for sexual dysfunction, the inability to control ejaculation sufficiently for both partners to enjoy sexual interaction, manifest as either the occurrence of ejaculation before or very soon after the beginning of intercourse (if a time limit is required, before or within 15 seconds) or the occurrence of ejaculation in the absence of sufficient erection to make intercourse possible. The problem is not the result of prolonged absence from sexual activity.	International Statistical Classification of Disease, 10th Edition (ICD-10) 1994 (World Health Organization, 1994)
The inability to control ejaculation for a "sufficient" length of time before vaginal penetration. It does not involve any impairment of fertility when intravaginal ejaculation occurs.	European Association of Urology, Guidelines on Male Sexual Dysfunction: Erectile Dysfunction and Premature Ejaculation (Hatzimouratidis et al., 2010)
Persistent or recurrent ejaculation with minimal stimulation before, on, or shortly after penetration and before the person wishes it, over which the sufferer has little or no voluntary control, which causes the sufferer and/or his partner bother or distress	International Consultation on Urological Diseases, 2004 (McMahon et al., 2004)
Ejaculation that occurs sooner than desired, either before or shortly after penetration, causing distress to either one or both partners	American Urological Association Guideline on the Pharmacologic Management of PE, 2004 (Montague et al., 2004)
The man does not have voluntary, conscious control or the ability to choose in most encounters when to ejaculate	Metz and McCarthy, 2003 (Metz and McCarthy, 2003)
The Foundation considers a man a premature ejaculator if he cannot control his ejaculatory process for a sufficient length of time during intravaginal containment to satisfy his partner in at least 50% of their coital connections.	Masters and Johnson, 1970 (Masters and Johnson, 1970)
Men with an IELT of less than 1 minute (belonging to the 0.5 percentile) have "definite" PE, whereas men with IELTs between 1 and 1.5 minutes (between 0.5 and 2.5 percentile) have "probable" PE (see Fig. 71.2). In addition, an additional grading of severity of PE should be defined in terms of associated psychological problems. Thus definite and probable PE require further psychological subclassification in asymptomatic, mild, moderate, and severe PE.	Waldinger et al., 2005b (Waldinger et al., 2005)
PE is diagnosed based on the pathologic IELT, as measured by the stopwatch method, with a feeling of loss of voluntary control and/or distress or relational disturbances, as measured by PRO	Jannini, 2005 (Jannini et al., 2005)

IELT, Intravaginal ejaculatory latency time; *PRO*, patient-related outcome (measures).

evidence-based definition of acquired PE and/or a single unifying definition of acquired and lifelong PE. Members unanimously agreed that, although lifelong and acquired PE are distinct and different demographic and etiologic populations, they can be jointly defined, in part, by the constructs of time from penetration to ejaculation, inability to delay ejaculation, and negative personal consequences from PE. The committee agreed that the presence of these mutual constructs was sufficient justification for the development of a single unifying definition of lifelong and acquired PE. Finally, the committee determined that the presence of a clinically significant and bothersome reduction in latency time, often to about 3 minutes or less, was an additional key defining dimension of acquired PE.

The second Ad Hoc ISSM Committee for the Definition of PE (2013) defined PE (lifelong and acquired PE) as a male sexual dysfunction characterized by

- Ejaculation that always or nearly always occurs before or within about 1 minute of vaginal penetration (lifelong PE) or, a clinically significant and bothersome reduction in latency time, often to about 3 minutes or less (acquired PE)
- The inability to delay ejaculation on all or nearly all vaginal penetrations
- Negative personal consequences, such as distress, bother, frustration, and/or the avoidance of sexual intimacy

The unified ISSM definition of lifelong and acquired PE represents the first evidence-based definition for these conditions (Serefoglu et al., 2014). **This definition should form the basis for the office diagnosis of lifelong PE and the design of PE observational and interventional clinical trials. It is limited to men engaging in vaginal intercourse because there are few studies available on PE research in homosexual men or during other forms of sexual expression.** This definition intentionally includes a degree of diagnostic conservatism and flexibility. The 1-minute IELT cutoff point for lifelong PE should not be applied in the most absolute sense because about 10% of men seeking treatment for lifelong PE have IELTs of 1 to 2 minutes. The phrase "within about 1 minute" must be interpreted as giving the clinician sufficient flexibility to diagnose PE also in men who report an IELT as long as 90 seconds. Similarly, a degree of flexible clinical judgement is key to the recognition and interpretation of a bothersome change in ejaculatory latency with reduction of premorbid latency to 3 minutes or less in men with acquired PE. Men who report these ejaculatory latencies but describe adequate control and no personal negative consequences related to their rapid ejaculation do not merit the diagnosis of PE.

The rationale for the ISSM definition of lifelong and acquired PE is fully explored online at ExpertConsult.com.

Diagnostic and Statistical Manual of Mental Disorders Definition of Premature Ejaculation

Based upon the same data that supported the ISSM definition of lifelong PE, **the recently published DSM-5 definition of PE** (American Psychiatric Association, 2013) now includes an objective ejaculatory latency criterion. DSM-5 defines PE as

a persistent or recurrent pattern of ejaculation occurring during partnered sexual activity within approximately 1 minute following vaginal penetration and before the individual wishes it. This symptom must have been present for at least 6 months and must be experienced on almost all or all (approximately 75%–100%) occasions of sexual activity. It causes clinically significant distress in the individual

(American Psychiatric Association, 2013). The DSM-5 definition of PE requires clinicians to specify PE as either lifelong or acquired and as generalized or situational. In addition, the DSM-5 definition of PE distinguishes between mild PE (ejaculation occurring within approximately 30 seconds to 1 minute of vaginal penetration), moderate PE (ejaculation occurring within approximately 15–30 seconds of vaginal penetration), and severe PE (ejaculation occurring before sexual activity, at the start of sexual activity, or within approximately 15 seconds of vaginal penetration).

Prevalence of Premature Ejaculation

Reliable information on the prevalence of lifelong (L-PE) and acquired (A-PE) premature ejaculation in the general male population is lacking. PE has been estimated to occur in 4% to 39% of men in the general community (Grenier and Byers 1997; Laumann et al., 1999; Nathan, 1986; Porst et al., 2007; Reading and Wiest, 1984; Spector and Boyle, 1986; Spector and Carey, 1990) and is often reported as the most common self-reported male sexual disorder (Jannini and Lenzi, 2005). However, **a substantial disparity exists between the incidence of PE in epidemiologic studies, which rely upon either patient self-report of PE and/or inconsistent and poorly validated definitions of PE** (Giuliano et al., 2008; Laumann et al., 1999; Patrick et al., 2005), and that suggested by community-based stopwatch studies of the IELT, the time interval between penetration and ejaculation (Waldinger et al., 2005). The latter demonstrates that the **distribution of the IELT is positively skewed, with a median IELT of 5.4 minutes (range, 0.55–44.1 minutes), decreases with age and varies between countries,** and supports the notion that IELTs of less than 1 minute are statistically abnormal compared with men in the general western population (Fig. 71.2; Waldinger et al., 2005).

Prevalence data derived from patient self-report will be appreciably higher than prevalence estimates based on clinician diagnosis using the more conservative ISSM definition of PE. The following studies demonstrate the varying prevalence estimates ranging from 30% to 3%. Data from the Global Study of Sexual Attitudes and Behaviors (GSSAB), an international survey investigating the attitudes, behaviors,

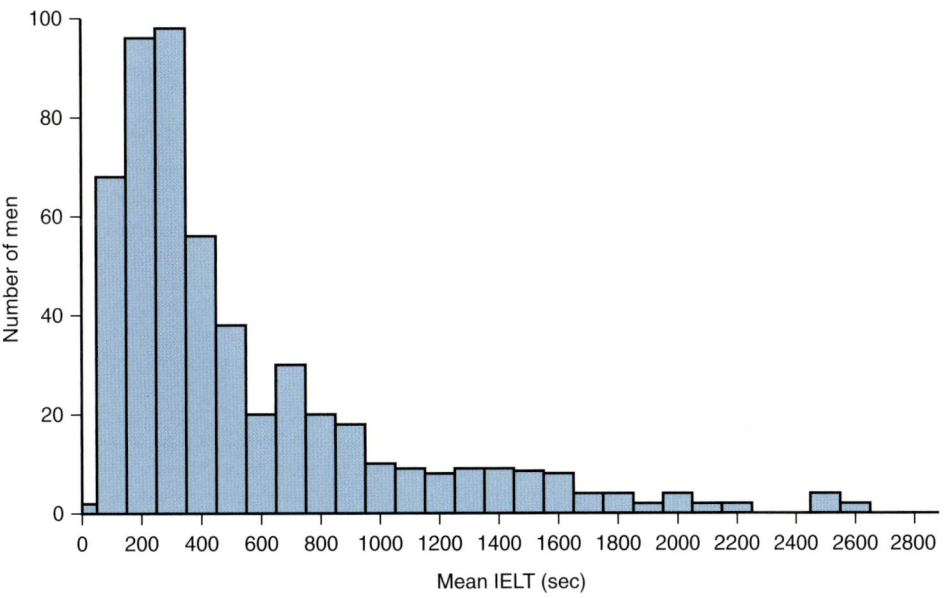

Fig. 71.2. Distribution of intravaginal ejaculatory latency times (IELT) values in a random cohort of 491 men. (Waldinger MD, Quinn P, Dilleen M, et al.: A multinational population survey of intravaginal ejaculation latency time. *J Sex Med* 2[4]:492-497, 2005.)

beliefs, and sexual satisfaction of 27,500 men and women aged 40 to 80 years, reported the global prevalence of PE (based on subject self-report) to be approximately 30% across all age groups (Nicolosi et al., 2004; Laumann et al., 2005). Perception of "normal" ejaculatory latency varied by country and differed when assessed either by the patient or his partner (Montorsi, 2005). A core limitation of the GSSAB survey stems from the fact that the youngest participants were aged 40 years, an age when the incidence of PE may be different from younger males (Jannini and Lenzi, 2005). Contrary to the GSSAB study, the Premature Ejaculation Prevalence and Attitude Survey found the prevalence of PE among men aged 18 to 70 years to be 22.7% (Porst et al., 2007). The real prevalence of PE is difficult to assess in clinical practice (Jannini and Lenzi, 2005).

Fasalo et al. reported that 2658 of 12,558 men (21.2%) attending a free andrological consultation self-diagnosed PE, the majority describing acquired PE (14.8%) and 4.5% describing lifelong PE (Basile Fasolo et al., 2005). In contrast, Serefoglu et al. (2010) reported that the majority of PE treatment-seeking patients described lifelong PE (62.5%) compared with acquired PE (16.1%). Similar findings were reported by Zhang et al., who found that the majority of 1988 Chinese outpatients described lifelong PE (35.6%) or acquired PE (28.07%). These data provide evidence that lifelong and acquired PE patients make up the majority of the patients who seek treatment for the complaint of ejaculating prematurely. In addition, there appears to be a disparity between the incidence of the various PE subtypes in the general community and in men actively seeking treatment for PE.

Consistent with this notion, **Serefoglu et al. (2011) subsequently reported an overall PE prevalence of 19.8% comprising lifelong PE (2.3%), acquired PE (3.9%), variable PE (8.5%), and subjective PE (5.1%).** Using similar research methodology, Gao et al. (2013) reported that 25.80% of 3016 Chinese men complained of PE, with similar prevalence of lifelong PE (3.18%), acquired PE (4.84%), variable PE (11.38%), and subjective PE (6.4%). Of particular interest is the report of Serefoglu et al. (2011) that men with acquired PE are more likely to seek medical treatment than men with lifelong PE (26.53% vs. 12.77%). This finding was confirmed by Gao et al., who demonstrated that acquired PE patients were more likely to seek (17.12% vs. 14.58%) and plan to seek (36.30% vs. 27.08%) treatment for their complaints compared with men with lifelong PE (Gao et al., 2013). These data suggest that the prevalence of acquired PE in the community is approximately around 4% among sexually active adults and that these patients are more likely to seek medical treatment.

Cause of Premature Ejaculation

Historically, attempts to explain the cause of PE have included a diverse range of biologic and psychological theories. Most of these proposed causes are not evidence based and are speculative at best. Although men with lifelong and acquired PE appear to share the dimensions of short ejaculatory latency, reduced or absent perceived ejaculatory control, and the presence of negative personal consequences from PE, they remain distinct and different demographic and etiologic populations (Porst et al., 2010).

Lifelong Premature Ejaculation

Waldinger et al. hypothesized that lifelong early ejaculation in humans may be explained by either a hyposensitivity of the 5-HT2c and/or hypersensitivity of the 5-HT1a receptor (Waldinger, 1998). Recent studies have suggested that **in some men neurobiologic and genetic variations could contribute to the pathophysiology of L-PE,** as defined by the ISSM criteria, and that the condition may be maintained and heightened by psychological/environmental factors (Janssen et al., 2009).

Acquired Premature Ejaculation

Acquired PE is commonly due to **sexual performance anxiety** (Hartmann et al., 2005), psychological or relationship problems (Hartmann et al., 2005), **erectile dysfunction** (ED; Laumann et al., 2005), and occasionally prostatitis (Screponi et al., 2001), hyperthyroidism (Carani et al., 2005), or during withdrawal/detoxification from prescribed (Adson and Kotlyar, 2003) or recreational drugs (Peugh and Belenko, 2001). Consistent with the predominant organic cause of acquired PE, men with this complaint are usually older and have a higher mean BMI and a greater incidence of comorbid disease, including hypertension, sexual desire disorder, diabetes mellitus, chronic prostatitis, and ED compared with lifelong, variable, and subjective PE (Basile Fasolo et al., 2005; Gao et al., 2013; McMahon et al., 2013; Porst et al., 2010; Serefoglu et al., 2010, 2011; Zhang et al., 2013). An increased prevalence of PE has been reported in men with metabolic syndrome (Bolat et al., 2017). Two extensive systematic analyses of reported data report no significant difference in the incidence of PE between circumcised and uncircumcised men (Morris and Krieger, 2013; Tian et al., 2013).

Premature Ejaculation and Sexual Performance Anxiety, and Psychological or Relationship Problems

Anxiety has been reported as a cause of PE by multiple authors and is entrenched in the folklore of sexual medicine as the most likely cause of PE despite scant empirical research evidence to support any causal role (Janssen et al., 2009; Jern et al., 2007). Several authors have suggested that **anxiety activates the sympathetic nervous system and reduces the ejaculatory threshold as a result of an earlier emission phase of ejaculation** (Janssen et al.. 2009).

Hypoactive sexual desire may lead to PE because of an unconscious desire to abbreviate unwanted penetration. Similarly, diminished sexual desire can be a consequence of chronic and frustrating PE.

Female sexual dysfunctions (such as anorgasmia, hypoactive sexual desire, sexual aversion, sexual arousal disorders, and sexual pain disorders such as vaginismus [Bronner et al., 2015; Dogan and Dogan, 2008]) may also be related to acquired PE.

Premature Ejaculation and Comorbid Erectile Dysfunction

Recent data demonstrate that as many as half of subjects with erectile dysfunction (ED) also experience PE (Fasolo et al., 2005; Laumann et al., 2005; Porst et al., 2007). Subjects with ED may either require higher levels of stimulation to achieve an erection or **intentionally "rush" intercourse to prevent early detumescence of a partial erection,** resulting in ejaculation with a brief latency (Jannini et al., 2005). This may be compounded by the presence of high levels of performance anxiety related to their ED, which only worsens their prematurity. However, caution should be exercised in the diagnosis of comorbid ED in men with PE because 33.3% of potent men with PE confuse the ability to maintain erections before ejaculation and after ejaculation, record contradictory response(s) to some/all questions of the SHIM (especially Q3 and Q4), and receive a false-positive SHIM diagnosis of ED (McMahon, 2009).

Premature Ejaculation and Prostate Disease

Acute and chronic lower urogenital infection, prostatodynia, or chronic pelvic pain syndrome (CPPS) is associated with ED, PE, and painful ejaculation (Donatucci, 2006; Rowland et al., 2010; Waldinger et al., 2005; Zohdy, 2009). **Several studies report PE as the main sexual disorder symptom in men with chronic prostatitis or CPPS with a prevalence of 26% to 77%** (Rowland et al., 2010). The exact pathophysiology of the link between chronic prostatitis, ED, and PE is unknown. It has been hypothesized that prostatic inflammation may result in altered sensation and modulation of the ejaculatory reflex, but evidence is lacking (Donatucci, 2006; Shamloul and el-Nashaar, 2006; Sharlip, 2006). It has been reported that antibiotic treatment of microbiologically confirmed bacterial prostatitis in men with acquired PE resulted in a 2.6-fold increase in IELT and improved ejaculatory control in 83.9% of subjects (El-Nashaar and Shamloul, 2007).

Premature Ejaculation and Hyperthyroidism

The majority of patients with thyroid hormone disorders experience sexual dysfunction. Studies suggest a significant correlation between PE and suppressed TSH values in a selected population of andrological and sexological patients. The 50% prevalence of PE in men with hyperthyroidism fell to 15% after treatment with thyroid hormone normalization (Carani et al., 2005). Although occult thyroid disease has been reported in the elderly hospitalized population, it is uncommon in the population who present for treatment of PE and routine **TSH screening is not indicated unless clinically indicated** (Atkinson et al., 1978).

Evaluation of Men Complaining of Premature Ejaculation

Medical History

Men presenting with self-reported PE should be evaluated with a **full medical/sexual history, a focused physical examination, inventory assessment of erectile function, and any investigations suggested by these findings**. Inclusion of the partner in the management process is an important but not a mandatory ingredient for treatment success. Some patients may not understand why the clinician wishes to include the partner, and some partners may be reluctant to join the patient in treatment. However, if partners are not involved in treatment, they may be resistant to changing the sexual interaction (Donahey and Miller, 2000). A cooperative partner can enhance the man's self-confidence, skills, self-esteem, sense of masculinity, and more generally assist the man to develop ejaculatory control (Perelman, 2003). This is, in turn, likely to lead to an improvement in the couple's sexual relationship, as well as the broader aspects of their relationship. There are no controlled studies on the impact of involving partners in treating PE. However, a review of treatment studies for ED demonstrated the important role of including a focus on interpersonal factors on treatment success (Mohr and Bentler, 1990).

Patients expect clinicians to inquire about their sexual health (Schein et al., 1988). Often patients are too embarrassed, shy, and uncertain to mention sexual complaints in the health care professional's (HCP's) office (Humphrey and Nazareth, 2001). Inquiry into sexual health gives patients permission to discuss their sexual concerns and also screens for associated health risks (e.g., cardiovascular risk and ED). Table 71.2 lists recommended and optional questions that patients who complain of PE should be asked (Althof et al., 2010; McMahon et al., 2004). The recommended questions establish the diagnosis and direct treatment considerations and the optional questions gather detail for implementing treatment. Finally, the committee recommends that the HCPs take a medical and psychosocial history.

Diagnosis of Premature Ejaculation

The ISSM definition of PE should form the basis for the diagnosis of PE. A significant population of men with self-reported PE fails to satisfy the criteria of the ISSM definition of PE. This parallels the substantial disparity between the self-reported incidence of PE in epidemiologic studies (Laumann et al., 1999) and that suggested by community-based normative stopwatch IELT studies (Waldinger et al., 2005). This population has recently been categorized as suffering from either variable PE or subjective PE (Waldinger and Schweitzer, 2006, 2008). Men with subjective PE complain of PE but have a normal ejaculatory latency typically of 2 to 6 minutes but on some occasions as long as 25 minutes. It is characterized by a preoccupation with a subjective but false perception of PE with an IELT within the normal range but often with reduced ejaculatory control.

Determination of Intravaginal Ejaculation Latency Time

Self-estimation by the patient and partner of ejaculatory latency should be used to determine IELT in clinical practice. Stopwatch measures of IELT are widely used in clinical trials and observational studies of PE but have not been recommended for use in routine clinical management of PE. Despite the potential advantage of objective measurement, stopwatch measures have the disadvantage of being intrusive and potentially disruptive of sexual pleasure or spontaneity. More recently, studies have indicated that patient or partner self-report of ejaculatory latency correlate relatively well with objective stopwatch latency and may be useful as a proxy measure of IELT (Althof, 1998; McMahon, 2008; Pryor et al., 2005; Rosen et al., 2007). Because patient self-report is the determining factor in treatment seeking and satisfaction, it is recommended that self-estimation by the patient and partner of ejaculatory latency are accepted as the method for determining IELT in clinical practice.

Patient Reported Outcome Measures

Standardized assessment measures such as validated questionnaires and PRO measures can be used as an adjunct to a full medical/sexual history and self-estimation of ejaculatory latency in the evaluation of men presenting with self-reported PE. These measures are all relatively new and were developed primarily for use as research tools. Some have shown good psychometric properties and are potentially valuable adjuncts for clinical screening and assessment.

Several PE measures have been described in the literature (Althof et al., 2006; Arafa and Shamloul, 2007; Patrick et al., 2008; Serefoglu et al., 2009; Symonds et al., 2007; Yuan et al., 2004), although only a small number have undergone extensive psychometric testing and validation. Five validated questionnaires have been developed and published. Currently, there are two questionnaires that have extensive databases and meet most of the criteria for test development and validation: **the Premature Ejaculation Profile (PEP)** and the **Index of Premature Ejaculation (IPE)** (Althof et al., 2006; Patrick et al., 2008). A third brief diagnostic measure, the **premature ejaculation diagnostic tool (PEDT)** has also been developed, has a modest

TABLE 71.2 Recommended and Optional Questions to Establish the Diagnosis of Premature Ejaculation (PE) and Direct Treatment

RECOMMENDED QUESTIONS

What is the time between penetration and ejaculation (coming)?
Can you delay ejaculation?
Do you feel bothered, annoyed and/or frustrated by your PE?

OPTIONAL QUESTIONS

Differentiate lifelong and acquired PE	When did you first experience PE? Have you experienced PE since your first sexual experience on every/almost every attempt and with every partner?
Assess erectile function	Is your erection hard enough to penetrate? Do you have difficulty in maintaining your erection until you ejaculate during intercourse? Do you ever rush intercourse to prevent loss of your erection?
Assess relationship impact	How upset is your partner with your PE? Does your partner avoid sexual intercourse? Is your PE affecting your overall relationship?
Previous treatment	Have you received any treatment for you PE previously?
Impact on quality of life	Do you avoid sexual intercourse because of embarrassment? Do you feel anxious, depressed, or embarrassed because of your PE?

From Althof SE, Abdo CH, Dean J, et al.: International Society for Sexual Medicine's guidelines for the diagnosis and treatment of premature ejaculation. *J Sex Med* 7(9):2947–2969, 2010.

database, and is available for clinical use (Symonds et al., 2007). Two other measures, the Arabic and Chinese PE Questionnaires, have minimal validation or clinical trial data available and are not recommended for clinical use.

Further details of Patient Reported Outcome (PRO) Measures are available online at ExpertConsult.com.

Assessment of Erectile Function

The presence of comorbid ED should be evaluated using a validated instrument such as the International Index of Erectile Function (IIEF) or the IIEF-5 (SHIM). Normal erectile function should be defined as an IIEF EF Domain ≥ 26 or IIEF-5 >21 (Cappelleri et al., 2001; Rosen et al., 1997). Recent data demonstrate that as many as half of subjects with ED also experience PE (Jannini et al., 2005). In the European Premature Ejaculation Prevalence and Attitudes Study, ED present in 31.9% of men with PE compared with 11.8% of non-PE men (Porst et al., 2007). In the Global Study of Sexual Attitudes and Behaviors (GSSAB), the odds ratio for ED in men with PE ranged from was 6.0 in Europe and as high as 11.9 in South America (Laumann et al., 2005). Consistent with this, ED is more prevalent in men with A-PE than L-PE (Basile Fasolo et al., 2005). PE is also more common with increasing severity of ED after adjustment for age (Corona et al., 2004; El-Sakka, 2007; el-Sakka, 2008). Subjects with ED may either require higher levels of stimulation to achieve an erection or intentionally "rush" intercourse to prevent early detumescence of a partial erection, resulting in ejaculation with a brief latency (Jannini et al., 2005). This may be compounded by the presence of high levels of performance anxiety related to their ED, which only worsens their prematurity. However, caution should be exercised in the diagnosis of comorbid ED in men with PE because 33.3% of potent men with PE confuse the ability to maintain erections before ejaculation and after ejaculation, record contradictory response(s) to some or all questions of the SHIM, especially Q3 and Q4, and receive a false-positive SHIM diagnosis of ED (McMahon, 2009).

Physical Examination

Current literature suggests that the diagnosis of L-PE is based purely on the medical history because there are no predictive physical findings or confirmatory investigations (McMahon, 2005). Because differentiation of L-PE and A-PE may be difficult in either young men or men with none or few previous sexual partners and/or limited sexual experience, a physical examination is highly desirable and represents an opportunity for screening for cardiovascular or gender specific diseases. However, **in men with A-PE, a physical examination is mandatory to identify the cause of the PE** and to alleviate its possible cause (Jannini, 2006). The presence of ED should be evaluated either by medical history or with the assistance of a validated instrument. Laboratory or imaging investigations are occasionally required based upon the patient's medical history. A digital prostate examination, routine in an andrological setting for all men over 40, is useful in identifying possible evidence of prostatic inflammation or infection (Jannini, 2006).

Fig. 71.3 is a flow chart for the management of PE (Rowland et al., 2010).

Treatment of Premature Ejaculation

There are **multiple psychosexual and pharmacologic treatments for PE**. Men with L-PE are best managed with PE pharmacotherapy

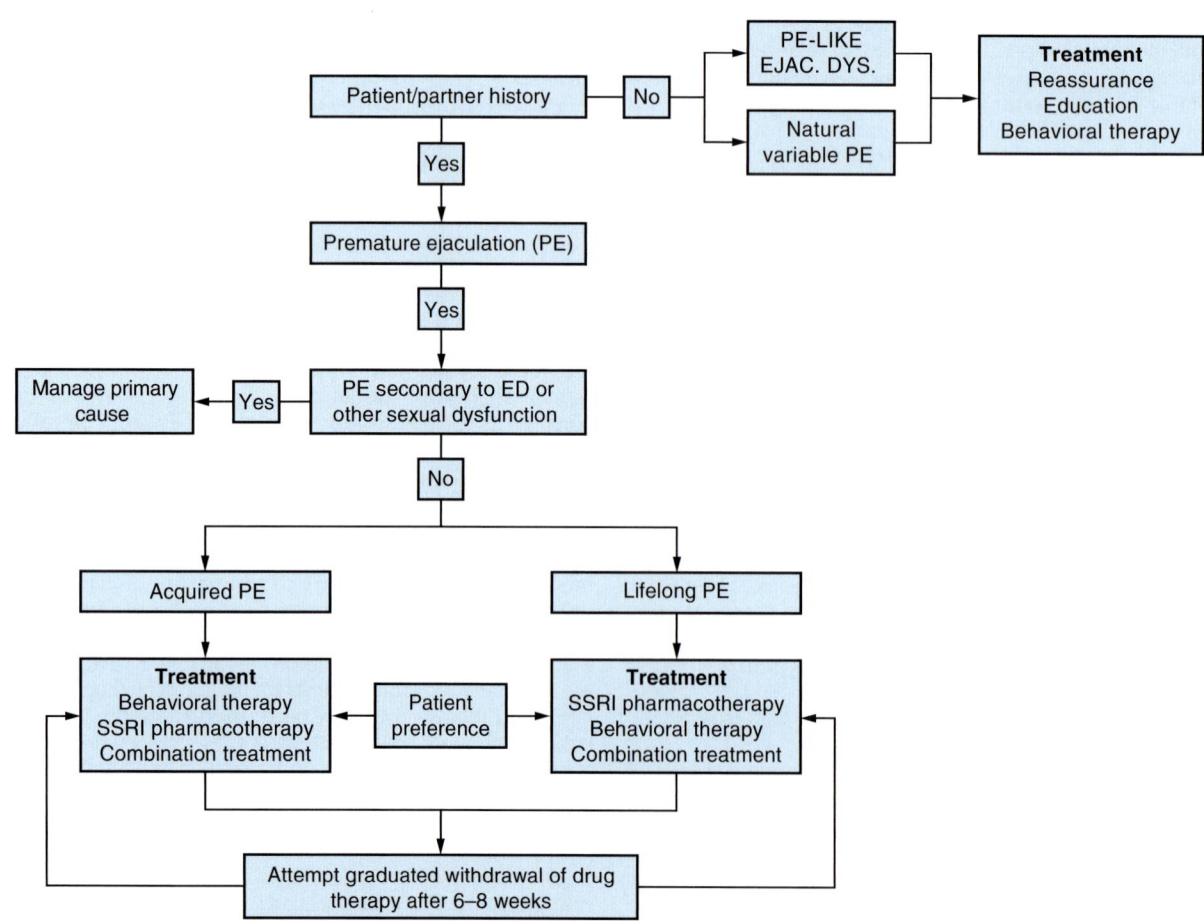

Fig. 71.3. Algorithm for the office management of premature ejaculation. *ED*, Erectile dysfunction; *SSRI*, selective serotonin reuptake inhibitor.

alone or **in combination with graded levels of patient and couple psychosexual therapy.** Men with A-PE should receive cause-specific treatment (e.g., psychosexual counselling or ED pharmacotherapy), alone or in combination with PE pharmacotherapy. Men with natural variable PE or PE-like ejaculatory dysfunction should be primarily treated with psychosexual education and graded patient and couple psychotherapy. Physicians should recognize the association between PE, comorbid ED, metabolic syndrome, sedentary lifestyle, alcohol consumption, and body mass index and counsel patients to exercise more and improve their overall lifestyle (Kilinc et al., 2018; Ventus and Jern, 2016).

Psychosexual Therapy

All men seeking treatment for PE should receive basic psychosexual education or coaching (Althof 2006, 2007; Perelman 2003, 2006). This may include providing information on the prevalence of PE in the general population and the average range of IELT to dispel myths about PE, information on enjoyable sexual activities to extend the man and his partner's sexual repertoire, as well as strategies to address avoidance of sexual activity or unwillingness to discuss sex with his partner. These educational strategies are designed to give the man the confidence to try the medical intervention, reduce performance anxiety, and modify his maladaptive sexual scripts.

Additional information on the role of psychosexual therapy in the management of PE is available online at ExpertConsult.com.

Pharmacologic Treatment

Several forms of pharmacotherapy have been used in the treatment of PE (Giuliano and Clement, 2012). These include the use of **topical local anesthetics, selective serotonin reuptake inhibitors (SSRIs), tramadol, phosphodiesterase type 5 inhibitors (PDE5Is), and α-adrenergic blockers.** The use of topical local anesthetics (LA), such as lidocaine, prilocaine, or benzocaine, alone or in association, to diminish the sensitivity of the glans penis is the oldest known pharmacologic treatment for PE (Schapiro, 1943). The introduction of the selective serotonin reuptake inhibitors—paroxetine, sertraline, fluoxetine, citalopram and the tricyclic antidepressant (TCA) clomipramine—has revolutionized the treatment of PE. These drugs block axonal reuptake of serotonin from the synaptic cleft of central serotonergic neurons by 5-HT transporters, resulting in enhanced 5-HT neurotransmission and stimulation of postsynaptic membrane 5-HT receptors.

Treatment With Selective Serotonin Reuptake Inhibitors and Tricyclic Antidepressants. PE can be treated with **on-demand SSRIs such as dapoxetine or off-label clomipramine, paroxetine, sertraline, and fluoxetine, or with daily dosing of off-label paroxetine, clomipramine, sertraline, fluoxetine, or citalopram.**

Dapoxetine. Dapoxetine has received approval for the treatment of PE in more than 50 countries worldwide. Dapoxetine has not received marketing approval by the US Food and Drug Administration (FDA). It is a **rapid-acting and short half-life SSRI with a pharmacokinetic profile supporting a role as an on-demand treatment for PE** (Pryor et al., 2006). No drug-drug interactions associated with dapoxetine, including phosphodiesterase inhibitor drugs, have been reported. In RCTs, dapoxetine 30 mg or 60 mg taken 1 to 2 hours before intercourse is more effective than placebo from the first dose, resulting in **2.5 and 3.0-fold increases in IELT, increased ejaculatory control, decreased distress, and increased satisfaction.** Dapoxetine was comparably effective in men with L-PE and A-PE (Porst et al., 2010) and was similarly effective and well tolerated in men with PE and comorbid ED treated with PDE5I drugs (McMahon et al., 2013). Treatment-related side effects were uncommon and dose dependent and included nausea, diarrhea, headache, and dizziness (McMahon et al., 2011). They were responsible for study discontinuation in 4% (30 mg) and 10% (60 mg) of subjects. The incidence of treatment-related side effects has been reported to be lower with on-demand dapoxetine compared with daily dosed SSRIs (Verze et al., 2016). There was no indication of an increased risk of suicidal ideation or suicide attempts and little indication of withdrawal symptoms with abrupt dapoxetine cessation (Levine, 2006). Postmarketing experience does, however, report that the discontinuation rate for dapoxetine was high (87% at 12 months) predominantly because of cost and the lack of spontaneity associated with on-demand administration (Park et al., 2017). Jiann et al. reported that 45% of men were satisfied with their response to dapoxetine (30 mg) and that level of satisfaction was closely related to treatment response (Jiann and Huang, 2015).

Off-Label Selective Serotonin Reuptake Inhibitors and Tricyclic Antidepressants. Daily treatment with off-label paroxetine 10 to 40 mg, clomipramine 12.5 to 50 mg, sertraline 50 to 200 mg, fluoxetine 20 to 40 mg, and citalopram 20 to 40 mg is usually effective in delaying ejaculation. A meta-analysis of published data suggests that **paroxetine exerts the strongest ejaculation delay, increasing IELT approximately 8.8-fold over baseline** (Waldinger et al., 2004).

Ejaculation delay usually occurs within 5 to 10 days of starting treatment, but the full therapeutic effect may require 2 to 3 weeks of treatment and is usually sustained during long-term use (McMahon, 2002). Adverse effects are usually minor, start in the first week of treatment, and may gradually disappear within 2 to 3 weeks. They include **fatigue, yawning, mild nausea, diarrhea, or perspiration.** There are anecdotal reports that decreased libido and ED are less frequently seen in nondepressed PE men treated by SSRIs compared with depressed men treated with SSRIs (Waldinger, 2007). Neurocognitive adverse effects include significant **agitation and hypomania in a small number of patients, and treatment with SSRIs should be avoided in men with a history of bipolar depression** (Marangell et al., 2008).

Platelet serotonin release has an important role in hemostasis (Li et al., 1997), and SSRIs, especially with concurrent use of aspirin and nonsteroidal anti-inflammatory drugs, may be associated with **increased risk of upper gastrointestinal bleeding.** Priapism is a rare adverse effect of SSRIs and requires urgent medical treatment. Long-term SSRI use may be associated with **weight gain and an increased risk of type 2 diabetes mellitus** (Fava et al., 2000). In men with normal semen parameters, **paroxetine has been reported to induce abnormal sperm DNA fragmentation in a significant proportion of subjects, without a measurable effect on semen parameters.** The fertility potential of a substantial number of men on paroxetine may be adversely affected by these changes in sperm DNA integrity (Tanrikut et al., 2010).

Systematic analysis of RCTs of antidepressants (SSRIs and other drug classes) in patients with depressive and/or anxiety disorders indicate **a small increase in the risk of suicidal ideation or suicide attempts in youth but not adults.** In contrast, such risk of suicidal ideation has not been found in trials with SSRIs in nondepressed men with PE. Caution is suggested in prescribing SSRIs to young adolescents with PE aged 18 years or less and to men with PE and a comorbid depressive disorder, particularly when associated with suicidal ideation (Khan et al., 2003). Patients should be advised to **avoid sudden cessation or rapid dose reduction of daily dosed SSRIs, which may be associated with an SSRI withdrawal syndrome** (Black et al., 2000).

On-demand administration of clomipramine, paroxetine, sertraline, and fluoxetine 3 to 6 hours before intercourse is modestly efficacious and well tolerated but is associated with substantially less ejaculatory delay than daily treatment in most studies (Kim and Paick, 1999; McMahon and Touma, 1999; Strassberg et al., 1999; Waldinger et al., 2004). On-demand treatment may be combined with either an initial trial of daily treatment or concomitant low-dose daily treatment (McMahon and Touma, 1999).

Patients are often reluctant to begin off-label treatment of PE with SSRIs. Salonia et al. reported that 30% of patients refused to begin treatment (paroxetine 10 mg daily for 21 days followed by 20 mg as needed) and another 30% of those that began treatment discontinued it (Salonia et al., 2009). Similarly, Mondaini et al. reported that, in a clinic population, 90% of subjects either refused to begin or discontinued dapoxetine within 12 months of beginning treatment (McMahon, 2002). Reasons given included not wanting to take an antidepressant, treatment effects below expectations, and cost.

The decision to treat PE with either on-demand dosing of dapoxetine (where available) or daily dosing of off-label SSRIs should be based upon the treating physician's assessment of individual patient requirements. Although many men with PE who engage in sexual intercourse infrequently may prefer on-demand treatment, many men in established relationships may prefer the convenience of daily medication. Well-designed preference trials will provide additional insight into the role of on-demand dosing. In some countries, off-label prescribing may present difficulties for the physician as the regulatory authorities strongly advise against prescribing for indications in which a medication is not licensed or approved. Obviously, this complicates treatment in countries where there is no approved medication and the regulatory authorities advise against off-label prescription.

Topical Local Anesthetics. The use of a topical LA, such as lidocaine and/or prilocaine as a cream, gel, or spray, is well established and is moderately effective in delaying ejaculation. Data suggest that diminishing the glans sensitivity may inhibit the spinal reflex arc responsible for ejaculation (Wieder et al., 2000). Topical anesthetics may be associated with significant penile hypoanesthesia and possible transvaginal absorption, resulting in vaginal numbness and resultant female anorgasmia unless a condom is used (Busato and Galindo, 2004).

PSD502 is a aerosolized eutectic mixture of lidocaine-prilocaine delivered as a metered spray that is designed to optimize tissue penetration and onset of effect (Dinsmore and Wyllie, 2009). The spray only penetrates, and therefore anesthetizes, the mucosa of the glans penis and not the keratinized skin of the shaft. PSD502 has received marketing approval in Europe. The clinical profile of PSD502 is described in one of two double-blind, placebo-controlled, phase III studies.

Dinsmore et al. reported that treatment with PSD502 which is applied to the penis at least 5 minutes before intercourse resulted in a 6.3-fold increase in IELT and associated improvements in PRO measures of control and sexual satisfaction (Dinsmore et al., 2006). In a second prospective multicenter placebo-controlled trial of 256 men with lifelong PE, Carson et al. reported that treatment with PSD502, applied topically to the glans penis 5 minutes before intercourse, increased the geometric mean IELT from a baseline of 0.56 minute and 0.53 minute in the PSD502 and placebo group, respectively, to 2.60 and 0.80 minute (4.6- and 1.5-fold, respectively) (Carson and Wyllie, 2010). There were significantly greater increases in the scores for the IPE domains of ejaculatory control, sexual satisfaction, and distress in the PSD502 group than in the placebo group. There were minimal reports of penile hypoanesthesia and transfer to the partner because of the unique formulation of the compound in both studies.

In 2014 PSD502 (Fortacin) received approval by the European Medicines Agency for the treatment for PE throughout the European Union. The ISSM guidelines for the treatment of PE expert committee identified level 1a evidence to support the efficacy and safety of off-label on-demand label topical anesthetics in the treatment of lifelong PE (Althof et al., 2014). Other topical anesthetics are associated with significant penile hypoanesthesia and possible transvaginal absorption, resulting in vaginal numbness and resultant female anorgasmia unless a condom is used (Busato and Galindo, 2004).

PDE5 Inhibitors. Off-label on-demand or daily dosing of PDE5Is is not recommended for the treatment of L-PE in men with normal erectile function. ED pharmacotherapy alone or in combination with PE pharmacotherapy is recommended for the treatment of L-PE or A-PE in men with comorbid ED. PDE5Is (sildenafil, tadalafil, and vardenafil) are effective treatments for ED. Several authors have reported experience with PDE5Is alone or in combination with SSRIs as a treatment for PE (Abdel-Hamid et al., 2001; Atan et al., 2006; Aversa et al., 2009; Chen et al., 2003; Chia, 2002; Erenpreiss and Zalkalns, 2002; Jannini et al., 2011; Li et al., 2003; Linn et al., 2002; Lozano, 2003; Mathers et al., 2009; Mattos et al., 2008; Mattos and Lucon, 2005; McMahon et al., 2005; Salonia et al., 2002; Sommer et al., 2005; Sun et al., 2007; Tang et al., 2004; Zhang et al., 2005). The putative role of PDE5Is as a treatment for PE is speculative and based only upon the role of the NO/cGMP transduction system as a central and peripheral mediator of inhibitory nonadrenergic, non-cholinergic nitrergic neurotransmission in the urogenital system (Mamas et al., 2003).

Although systematic reviews of studies on the PDE5I drug treatment of PE has failed to provide robust empirical evidence to support a role of PDE5Is in the treatment of PE with the exception of men with PE and comorbid ED (Asimakopoulos et al., 2012; McMahon et al., 2006), recent well-designed studies do support a potential role for these agents, suggesting a need for further evidence-based research (Aversa et al., 2009). In a well-designed study of 42 potent men with L-PE, randomized to receive on-demand vardenafil or placebo, Aversa et al. reported a 7.5-fold increase in geometric mean IELT after treatment with vardenafil (4.5±1.1 vs. 0.6±0.3 minute with placebo; $P < 0.01$) and significant improvements in the IPE domains of ejaculatory control, confidence, overall sexual satisfaction, and distress (Aversa et al., 2009). This study suggests that the role of PDE5Is should be further evaluated in additional well-designed studies. Furthermore, a recent meta-analysis of only RCTs found evidence to suggest that PDE5Is are effective compared with placebo and that a PDE5I combined with an SSRI is more effective than an SSRI alone (Martyn-St James et al., 2017).

The ISSM guidelines for the treatment of PE expert committee identified some evidence to support the efficacy and safety of off-label on-demand or daily dosing of PDE5Is in the treatment of L-PE in men with normal erectile function (LOE4D). However, off-label on-demand or daily dosing of PDE5Is is not recommended for the treatment of L-PE in men with normal erectile function (Althof et al., 2014). ED pharmacotherapy alone or in combination with PE pharmacotherapy is recommended for the treatment of L-PE or A-PE in men with comorbid ED (Althof et al., 2014). Further evidence-based research is encouraged to understand conflicting data (Althof et al., 2014).

Table 71.3 is a summary of recommended pharmacologic treatments for PE.

Treatment of PE with tramadol, α1-adrenoceptor antagonists, intracavernosal injection of vasoactive drugs, emerging investigational drugs, acupuncture, surgical neurotomy, cryoablation, and neuromodulation of the dorsal penile nerve is discussed in detail on ExpertConsult.com.

> **KEY POINTS: PREMATURE EJACULATION**
>
> - PE is a common sexual dysfunction.
> - PE is associated with negative psychological consequences, including distress, bother, and frustration, which may affect quality of life, partner relationships, self-esteem, and self-confidence and can act as an obstacle to single men forming new partner relationships.
> - The evidence-based ISSM definition of lifelong and acquired PE should form the basis of the office diagnosis of lifelong PE.
> - There is limited evidence suggesting that lifelong PE has a genetic basis, and acquired PE is most often due to sexual performance anxiety, psychological or relationship problems, and/or ED.
> - Oral SSRI drugs and topical anesthetic drugs are effective and safe treatments for PE.
> - Psychosexual CBT has a limited role as a first-line treatment for PE but has an important role as an adjunct to pharmacotherapy, especially in men with acquired PE resulting from sexual performance anxiety.
> - Men with acquired PE most secondary to comorbid ED, hyperthyroidism, chronic lower urogenital infection, prostatodynia, or CPPS should receive appropriate cause-specific treatment alone or in combination with an SSRI.

KATE! DELAYED EJACULATION, ANEJACULATION, AND ANORGASMIA

Any psychological or medical disease or surgical procedure that interferes with either central control of ejaculation or the peripheral

TABLE 71.3 Drug Therapy for Premature Ejaculation (PE)

DRUG	DOSE	DOSING INSTRUCTIONS	INDICATION	COMMENTS	LEVEL OF EVIDENCE
Dapoxetine	30–60 mg	On demand, 1–3 hours before intercourse	Lifelong PE Acquired PE	Approved in >50 countries	High
Paroxetine	10–40 mg	Once daily	Lifelong PE Acquired PE		High
Sertraline	50–200 mg	Once daily	Lifelong PE Acquired PE		High
Fluoxetine	20–40 mg	Once daily	Lifelong PE Acquired PE		High
Citalopram	20–40 mg	Once daily	Lifelong PE Acquired PE		High
Clomipramine	12.5–50 µg	Once daily	Lifelong PE Acquired PE		High
	12.5–50 µg	On demand, 3–4 hours before intercourse	Lifelong PE Acquired PE		High
Tramadol	25–50 mg	On demand, 3–4 hours before intercourse	Lifelong PE Acquired PE	Potential risk of opiate addiction	Low
Topical lignocaine/prilocaine	Patient titrated	On demand, 20–30 minutes before intercourse	Lifelong PE Acquired PE		High
Alprostadil	5–20 mcg	Patient administered intracavernosal injection 5 min before intercourse	Lifelong PE Acquired PE	Risk of priapism and corporal fibrosis	Very Low
PDE5 inhibitors	Sildenafil 25–100 mg Tadalafil 10–20 mg Vardenafil 10–20 mg Avanafil 50–200 mg	On demand, 30–50 minutes before intercourse	Lifelong and acquired PE in men with normal erectile function		Low
			Lifelong and acquired PE in men with ED	? Improved efficacy if combined with SSRI	Moderate

ED, Erectile dysfunction; *SSRI*, selective serotonin reuptake inhibitor.

sympathetic nerve supply to the vas and bladder neck, the somatic efferent nerve supply to the pelvic floor, or the somatic afferent nerve supply to the penis can result in delayed ejaculation, anejaculation, RE, and/or anorgasmia. As such, the causes of delayed ejaculation, anejaculation, and anorgasmia are manifold.

Definition, Terminology, and Characteristics of Men With Delayed Ejaculation

Delayed (DE), retarded ejaculation (RE), or inhibited ejaculation (IE) are probably the least common, least studied, least reported, and least understood male sexual dysfunctions. Yet their impact is significant in that it typically results in a lack of sexual fulfilment for both the man and his partner, an effect further compounded when procreation is among the couple's goals of sexual intercourse.

Problems with "difficulty" in ejaculating may range from varying delays in the latency to ejaculation to complete inability to ejaculate (anejaculation). Reductions in the volume, force, and sensation of ejaculation may occur as well. At the extremes are anejaculation (time) and RE (direction), but more commonly encountered is DE. A final disorder, anorgasmia, refers to a perceived absence of the orgasm experience or sexual anhedonia, independent of whether any or all the physiologic concomitants of ejaculation have taken place.

Terminology and Definition

RE, DE, inadequate ejaculation, IE, idiopathic anejaculation, primary impotentia ejaculations, and psychogenic anejaculation have been used synonymously to describe a delay or absence of male orgasmic response. If a distinction is to be made, usually inhibited ejaculation is characterized by the complete absence of ejaculation, although no clear consensus exists. Herein, the preferred terminology DE is meant to describe any and all of the ejaculatory disorders resulting in a delay or absence of ejaculation.

The American Psychiatric Association's DSM-5 defines DE as a marked delay or absence of ejaculation on almost all or all occasions (approximately 75%–100%) of partnered sexual activity and without the individual desiring the delay, which causes clinically significant distress in the individual, is not better explained by a nonsexual mental disorder or as a consequence of severe relationship distress or other significant stressors, and is not attributable to the effects of a substance/medication or another medical condition (American Psychiatric Association, 2013). The disturbance may be either lifelong or acquired, generalized or situational, and mild, moderate, or severe. The DSM-5 definition of "delay" does not have precise boundaries, because there is no consensus as to what constitutes a reasonable time to reach orgasm or what is unacceptably long for most men and their sexual partners. Similarly, the 3rd International Consultation on Sexual Dysfunction defines DE as the persistent or recurrent difficulty, delay in, or absence of attaining orgasm after sufficient sexual stimulation, which causes personal distress (Rowland et al., 2010).

There are no clear criteria as to when a man actually meets the conditions for DE, because operationalized criteria do not exist. Given that most sexually functional men ejaculate within about 4 to 10 minutes after intromission (Patrick et al., 2005), a clinician may assume that men with latencies beyond 25 or 30 minutes (21–23 minutes represents about two standard deviations above the mean) who report distress or men who simply cease sexual activity because of exhaustion or irritation qualify for this diagnosis. Such symptoms, together with the fact that a man and/or his partner decide to seek help for the problem, are usually sufficient for a DE diagnosis.

Epidemiology of Delayed Ejaculation

Although EjD contributes to important patient-related outcomes of procreation, general and performance anxiety, and relationship satisfaction, the prevalence of EjD is unclear (Althof, 2012; Paduch et al., 2015; Rowland et al., 2005). Historically, DE has been reported at low rates in the literature, rarely exceeding 3% (Laumann et al., 1999; Simons and Carey, 2001; Spector and Carey, 1990). However, data from a 2003 multinational survey performed in the United States and Europe showed that approximately 40% of men aged 50 to 79 experienced some form of EjD with prevalence as high as ED (Rosen et al., 2003). Epidemiologic population surveys (Rosen et al., 2003) and cross-sectional observational studies (Corona et al., 2006, 2008; Paduch et al., 2012) have reported various demographic and clinical factors that correlate with EjD. The prevalence of DE appears to be moderately and positively related to age, which is not surprising because ejaculatory function tends to diminish as men age. Lindau et al. reported an incidence of DE of 16.2%, 22.7%, and 33.2% of men aged 57 to 65, 65 to 74, and 75 to 85 years, respectively (Lindau et al., 2007). Furthermore, the prevalence of EjD differs between races (Paduch et al., 2012) and is associated with ED, LUTS, low serum testosterone levels, and hyperlipidemia (Corona et al., 2006, 2008; Paduch et al., 2012; Rosen et al., 2003). However, there is little published literature on the demographic and clinical correlates of EjD in community-dwelling populations, and published observational studies have not subdivided various types of ejaculatory disorders (e.g., delayed vs. absent) or evaluated subjects using psychometrically validated scales of EjD.

Although coital anejaculation is frequently the treatment driver especially for extremely religious individuals referred for fertility problems, men also seek treatment when distressed by their inability to achieve orgasm in response to manual, oral, or vaginal stimulation by their partner. Many men with acquired DE can masturbate to orgasm, whereas others, for multiple reasons, will not or cannot. Loss of masturbatory capacity secondary to emotional or physical trauma is also seen. Approximately 75% of one clinical sample (Perelman, 2004) could reach orgasm through masturbation, whereas the remainder either would not or could not.

Men with DE indicate high levels of relationship distress, sexual dissatisfaction, anxiety about their sexual performance, and general health issues—significantly higher than sexually functional men (Althof, 2012; Corona et al., 2006). In addition, along with other sexually dysfunctional counterparts, men with DE typically report lower frequencies of coital activity (Rowland et al., 2005). A distinguishing characteristic of men with DE is the presence of normal erectile function with some men capable of maintaining erections for prolonged periods of time. However, these men often report low levels of subjective sexual arousal compared with sexually functional men (Rowland et al., 2004).

Cause of Delayed Ejaculation/Anejaculation

Delayed ejaculation/anejaculation may be lifelong or acquired, global, or situational. The pathophysiology of DE is complex, and multiple pathophysiologies have been associated with EjD (Table 71.4). These include congenital disorders as well as ones caused by psychological factors, treatment of male pelvic cancers with surgery or radiotherapy, neurologic disease such as multiple sclerosis and Parkinson disease, hypogonadism, hypothyroidism, infection, and treatment for other disorders such as schizophrenia or mood disorders with major tranquilizers or SSRI antidepressants respectively. Psychological factors include performance anxiety, relationship conflict, poor sexual communication, hypoactive sexual desire, and psychological conflict related to fear of fathering a child, fear of harm to either self or partner, or religious belief–induced

TABLE 71.4 Causes of Retrograde Ejaculation, Delayed Ejaculation, Anejaculation, and Anorgasmia

Aging male	Degeneration of penile afferent nerves
Psychogenic	Inhibited ejaculation
Congenital	Müllerian duct cyst Wolffian duct abnormality Prune-belly syndrome
Anatomic causes	Transurethral resection of prostate Bladder neck incision
Neurogenic causes	Diabetic autonomic neuropathy Multiple sclerosis Spinal cord injury Radical prostatectomy Proctocolectomy Bilateral sympathectomy Abdominal aortic aneurysmectomy Para-aortic lymphadenectomy
Infective	Urethritis Genitourinary tuberculosis Schistosomiasis
Endocrine	Hypogonadism Hypothyroidism
Medication	Alpha-methyldopa Thiazide diuretics Tricyclic and SSRI antidepressants Phenothiazine Alcohol abuse

SSRI, Selective serotonin reuptake inhibitor.

shame (Althof, 2012; Rowland et al., 2005). Some men habitually use an idiosyncratic style of solitary masturbation, which cannot be replicated during coitus and inadvertently condition themselves to DE or anejaculation (Perelman, 2005).

The most common causes of DE seen in clinical practice are psychogenic inhibited ejaculation, degeneration of penile afferent nerves and Pacinian corpuscles in the aging male, hypogonadism, diabetic autonomic neuropathy, treatment with SSRI antidepressants and major tranquilizers, radical prostatectomy or other major pelvic surgery, and radiotherapy.

Psychological Delayed Ejaculation

Psychogenic DE, often described as IE, is usually related to **sexual performance anxiety**, which may draw the man's attention away from erotic cues that normally enhance arousal. Other psychodynamic explanations emphasize psychosexual development issues and have attributed lifelong DE to a wide range of conditions, including fear, anxiety, hostility, orthodoxy of religious belief, and relationship difficulties (Munjack and Kanno, 1979; Waldinger and Schweitzer, 2005). Although some of these factors may contribute to DE in individual men, no well-controlled studies provide broad support, at this point, for any of the various hypotheses for conditions mentioned above (Waldinger and Schweitzer, 2005).

Masters and Johnson were the first to suggest that DE in some men may be associated with **orthodoxy of religious belief** (Masters and Johnson, 1970). Such beliefs may limit the sexual experience necessary for learning to ejaculate or may result in an inhibition of normal function. Many devoutly religious men have masturbated only minimally or not at all, and for some, guilt and anxiety about "spilling seed" may have led to idiosyncratic masturbatory patterns, which, in turn, resulted in DE. Such men often had little contact with women before marriage and, although they may have dated, were less likely than their secular counterparts to experience orgasm with a partner, especially through intercourse.

Idiosyncratic and vigorous masturbation styles that cannot be replicated during intercourse with a partner, or an "auto sexual" orientation in which men derive greater arousal and enjoyment from masturbation than from intercourse, are risk factors for DE (Perelman 2005; Perelman and Rowland, 2006). These men precondition themselves to possible difficulty attaining orgasm with a partner and, as a result, experience acquired DE. These men appear able to achieve erections sufficient for intercourse despite a relative absence of subjective arousal (Apfelbaum, 1989), and their erections are taken as erroneous evidence by the man and his partner that he was ready for sex and capable of achieving orgasm. Disparity between the reality of sex with the partner and the sexual fantasy used during masturbation may inhibit sexual arousal and thus represent another contributor to DE (Perelman, 2001).

Congenital Disorders

Typical congenital problems include müllerian duct obstruction, caused by failure of complete absorption of müllerian duct remnants in the male; wolffian duct abnormalities, which may compromise vas deferens, ejaculatory duct, and seminal vesicle functioning; and prune-belly syndrome.

Infective Disorders

Sexually transmissible infections such as gonorrhea or nonspecific urethritis can produce cicatrization and obstruction anywhere in the male reproductive tract, especially if treatment is delayed. Urinary infection, especially if complicated by epididymitis, can also produce obstruction that may be situated at ejaculatory duct level. Schistosomiasis is endemic in large parts of Africa and is seen with increasing frequency in tourists returning from Africa who have contracted the disease while enjoying water sports. The disease may occur with hematospermia (McKenna et al., 1997), and fibrosis and calcification may lead to genital obstruction. Genitourinary tuberculosis can cause great damage to the male reproductive tracts, and because healing occurs with calcification, the lesions may be irreparable.

Ejaculatory Duct Obstruction

Ejaculatory duct obstruction may be congenital because of müllerian duct cysts or acquired because of prostatitis, STIs such as chlamydia or other pathogens, or duct obstruction by a calculus (Philip et al., 2007). It is the underlying cause for 1% to 5% of male infertility (Pryor and Hendry, 1991). Men with bilateral obstruction suffer from a very low volume, low pH, low-fructose, fluid low-viscosity azoospermic semen or from aspermia, no semen at all. This is due to the absence of the viscous fructose-rich seminal vesicle secretions, which contribute approximately 80% of seminal volume. This low-volume, low-viscosity azoospermic/oligospermic semen distinguishes ejaculatory duct obstruction from the normal volume semen present in bilateral obstruction of vasa deferens. The persistence of pelvic floor muscle contractions and a sensation of orgasm often with postorgasm pelvic pain distinguishes them from most men with anejaculation. Unilateral or partial obstruction may be associated with pelvic pain and oligospermia (Lawler et al., 2006). Diagnosis of ejaculatory duct obstruction by transrectal ultrasound (TRUS), MRI, or transrectal needle-aspiration of the seminal vesicles has relatively low sensitivity (Engin et al., 2009).

Endocrinopathy

Hypothyroidism is commonly strongly associated with DE whereas hyperthyroidism is rarely associated with PE (Carani et al., 2005; Corona et al., 2006) Similarly, **hypogonadism** and low testosterone are associated with DE or anejaculation (Corona et al., 2008, 2011, 2012). In contrast, Morgentaler et al. (2017) reported that linear regression failed to demonstrate an association between IELT and testosterone in men with self-reported DE. The disparity in the results of these studies highlights the complex relationship between testosterone and ejaculatory function and the multifactorial pathogenesis of DE. **Hyperprolactinemia,** via inhibition of hypothalamic GnRH is associated with low testosterone, reduced sexual desire, ED and delayed ejaculation. The effect of prolactin on ejaculation is possibly mediated via its action on the serotonergic system (Corona et al., 2006, 2009).

Iatrogenic Causes

Any prescribed or recreational drug that changes the levels of neurotransmitters, such as serotonin, dopamine, or oxytocin, which are involved in the central or peripheral neural control of ejaculation, may affect ejaculatory latency.

SSRIs are commonly used for the treatment of depression and are associated with a high incidence of sexual dysfunction, with up to 60% reporting some form of treatment-related sexual dysfunction, most commonly ejaculatory dysfunction (Delgado et al., 2005; Madeo et al., 2008; Montejo et al., 2001). Treatment with **antipsychotics,** probably because of either a direct and/or indirect dopamine antagonism (Hull et al., 2004) or increased prolactin levels (Roke et al., 2012), is also commonly associated with DE and retrograde ejaculation (Madhusoodanan and Brenner, 1996; Raja, 1999). Retrograde ejaculation associated with antipsychotics is thought to be due to antagonistic effects on the α-adrenergic system at the level of the bladder neck (Holtmann et al., 2003).

Treatment of Male Pelvic Cancers

Overall QoL and sexual functioning have evolved as key issues in the management of cancer patients. Because of modern surgical techniques, improved quality of drugs for chemotherapy, and modern radiation techniques, more patients can be successfully treated without largely compromising sexual functioning.

Prostate Cancer

Prostate cancer (CaP) has become the most common non-skin malignancy in men in western countries. External-beam radiotherapy (EBRT) and brachytherapy (BT) are, together with the open or robotic radical prostatectomy (RP/RALP), the most common and effective treatments for localized PC. Despite the introduction of very modern radiotherapy (RT) techniques, sexual functioning after CaP treatment remains problematic for many patients. **After RP/RALP, men no longer ejaculate but maintain a sense of orgasm** that can vary from less to more intense than preoperatively and may experience arousal urinary incontinence or climacturia (i.e., urinary incontinence at orgasm).

Ejaculatory disturbances after RT of CaP were reported in as early as the 1980s (Van Heeringen et al., 1988). More recent studies have evaluated the impact of RT on sexual desire, ejaculation, and orgasm. **After EBRT, a decline in sexual desire was reported by 43% of 64 patients and a decreased frequency of orgasm by 57%; all men reported a decrease in ejaculate volume** (Helgason et al., 1995). Using a validated questionnaire, Borghede and Hedelin (1997) reported a decrease in the ability to ejaculate in 56% of the patients. Good prognostic factors for sexual functioning preservation after RT were low age and higher frequency of intercourse.

Early RT studies also assessed sexual functioning. Herr reported already in 1979 on 51 patients treated with retropubic Iodium-125 seeds, with loss of ejaculate experienced by 6% of the patients. In a later study, dry ejaculation was reported by 16% of the patients after BT (Kwong et al., 1984). In both studies, all patients had previously undergone a transurethral resection of the prostate (TURP). For the first time a discomfort with ejaculation was mentioned in two studies (up to 25% of the patients) (Arterbery et al., 1997; Kleinberg et al., 1994). This result is common in clinical practice after BT because of edema of the prostate possibly reducing the elasticity of the urethra and inducing discomfort with ejaculation. In some patients discomfort with ejaculation did not disappear even

18 to 24 months after BT (Beckendorf et al., 1996). Also, decreased interest in sex, sexual desire, and libido was mentioned in up to 50% of the patients evaluated (Arterbery et al., 1997; Beckendorf et al., 1996; Borghede and Hedelin, 1997; Joly et al., 1998).

Several studies on the cause of post-RT decreased libido and ejaculatory disorders have been reported. Daniell et al (2001) studied retrospectively levels of testosterone (TST) and other hormones after RT of PC. TST was found to be low 3 to 8 years after EBRT with lower levels found in older patients. Although testes are very sensitive to radiation, spermatogenesis is more easily affected than androgen productions. The radiation dose calculated in the testes of men irradiated for PC is only 3% to 8% of the dose that could possibly affect androgen production and explain a decrease in TST. A TURP carries a high incidence of RE because it is thought to disrupt the closure mechanism of the vesical neck; this could explain ejaculatory disturbances in most patients after RT with previous TURP.

Rectal Carcinoma

Not much is known about sexual functioning after RT of rectal carcinoma. Preoperative RT for rectal cancer has been associated with a reduction in the rate of local relapse and possibly an advantage in survival. Preoperative RT with the total mesorectal excision (TME) in low-stage rectal cancer has become a common procedure in Europe. **A sharp dissection of the mesorectum associated with visualization and preservation of the pelvic autonomic nerve leads to excellent results regarding erectile and ejaculatory functioning.** Only one study has specifically studied the effects of preoperative RT for rectal carcinoma on male sexual functioning and concluded that it may impair male sexual functioning (Bonnel et al., 2002). However, numbers were too small to draw final conclusion.

Testicular Cancer

Germ cell tumors of the testis are relatively rare, accounting for about 1% of all male cancers. The long-term survival for early disease approaches 100%. Because testicular cancer affects mainly young men in their sexual and fertile life, sexual functioning and ejaculatory disorders are particularly important. The side effects of retroperitoneal lymph node dissection (RPLND) for residual mass after chemotherapy for nonseminomatous cancer are better documented than sexual sequelae of elective abdominal radiotherapy (RT) for seminoma. **Anejaculation occurs in the majority of the patients in non–nerve-sparing techniques.** As a result of careful anatomic studies, the technique of RPLND has been **modified with nerve sparing so that antegrade ejaculation is now maintained in 80% to 100% of patients** (van Basten et al., 1997). Libido and orgasm seem to be normal in these patients.

After RT, deterioration in sexual functioning has been reported by between 1% and 25% of the patients (Caffo and Amichetti, 1999; Incrocci et al., 2002; Jonker-Pool et al., 1997; Schover et al., 1986; Tinkler et al., 1992). Tinkler et al. (1992) reported on 237 patients after orchiectomy and abdominal RT and compared these data with 402 age-matched controls. In almost all parameters studied including erection, ejaculation, and libido, patients scored less than controls (reduction in orgasm, in libido, and interest in sex). Specifically, there was no difference in the ability to ejaculate during sexual activity, but the RT patients reported a noticeable reduction in the amount of semen compared with before treatment (Tinkler et al., 1992). Caffo and Amichetti (1999) evaluated toxicity and QoL of 143 patients treated for early stage testicular cancer: 23% reported a decreased libido, 27% problems with achieving orgasm, and 38% ejaculation disturbances, including PE. A decrease in sexual desire, in orgasm, and volume or semen was negatively correlated with age (Schover et al., 1986). Jonker-Pool et al. (1997) reported on three groups of patients, after RT, wait and see, and chemotherapy. RT patients reported decreased libido in 22% compared with 12% in the wait-and-see group, and 30% in the chemotherapy group. Decrease of absence of ejaculate was reported in 15%, 7%, and 21% in the three groups, respectively; decreased orgasm in 15%, 12%, and 30%, respectively. Although the differences were not statistically significant, in the RT group ejaculation and orgasm disturbances were higher than in the wait-and-see group. Similar results were reported by Arai et al. (1997). PE was reported in up to half of the patients (Arai et al., 1997; Incrocci et al., 2002), but it was the same as recalled before treatment (Incrocci et al., 2002).

The superior hypogastric plexus is responsible for ejaculation, and it is mediated by the sympathetic system; it is a fenestrated network of fibers anterior to the lower abdominal aorta. The hypogastric nerves exit bilaterally at the inferior pole of the superior hypogastric plexus, and have connections with the S1-S2 roots. Normal emission requires integrity of this system. During RPLND these nerves are difficult to recognize and may be damaged, resulting in decreased semen volume or dry ejaculation. Pathways for ejaculation are included in the RT fields for rectal and prostate carcinomas. Damage of the sympathetic nerves could be caused by radiation, but the dose does not seem enough to completely explain the dysfunction. Orgasm is even more complex than ejaculation because it is also affected by cortical input.

Neurologic Disorders

Degeneration of penile fast conducting afferent nerves and Pacinian corpuscles in the **aging male, diabetic autonomic neuropathy, multiple sclerosis, and spinal cord injury** are often associated with delayed ejaculation/anejaculation.

Spinal Cord Injury

The ability to ejaculate is severely impaired by spinal cord injury (SCI). Bors and Comarr highlighted the impact of the level and completeness of SCI on the postinjury erectile and ejaculatory capacity (Table 71.5) (Bors and Comarr, 1960; Comarr, 1970). **Unlike erectile capacity, the ability to ejaculate increases with descending levels of spinal injury. Less than 5% of patients with complete upper motor neuron lesions retain the ability to ejaculate.** Ejaculation rates are higher (15%) in patients with both lower motor neuron lesions and an intact thoracolumbar sympathetic outflow. Approximately 22% of patients with an incomplete upper motor neuron lesion and almost all men with incomplete lower motor neuron lesions retain the ability to ejaculate. In those patients capable of successful ejaculation, the sensation of orgasm may be absent and RE often occurs.

TABLE 71.5 Correlation of Erection, Ejaculation, and Intercourse With Level and Severity of Spinal Cord Injury

CORD LESION		REFLEXOGENIC ERECTIONS (%)	PSYCHOGENIC ERECTIONS (%)	SUCCESSFUL COITUS (%)	EJACULATION (%)
Upper motor neuron	Complete	92	9	66	1
	Incomplete	93	48	86	22
Lower motor neuron	Complete	0	24	33	15
	Incomplete	0	1	100	100

From Comarr AE: Sexual function among patients with spinal cord injury. Urol Int 25(2):134–168, 1970.

Several techniques for obtaining semen from spinal cord injured men with EjD have been reported. **Vibratory stimulation** is successful in obtaining semen in up to 70% of men with spinal cord injury (Brindley, 1984). The use **of electroejaculation** to obtain semen by electrical stimulation of efferent sympathetic fibers of the hypogastric plexus is an effective and safe method of obtaining semen. Brindley et al. (1986) have reported that 71% of men with spinal cord injury who underwent electroejaculation achieved ejaculation. However, both are associated with **a significantly higher risk of autonomic dysreflexia** than electroejaculation. Pretreatment with a fast-acting vasodilator such as nifedipine minimizes the risk of severe hypertension, should autonomic dysreflexia occur with either form of treatment (Steinberger et al., 1990).

Semen collected from men with spinal cord injury is often initially senescent and of poor quality with a low sperm count and reduced sperm motility but may improve with subsequent ejaculations. This poor semen quality may be due to chronic urinary tract infection, dilution of sperm content with urine, chronic use of various medications, elevated scrotal temperature resulting from prolonged sitting, and stasis of prostatic fluid. Testicular biopsies in spinal cord injured men demonstrate a wide range of testicular dysfunction including hypospermatogenesis, maturation arrest, atrophy of seminiferous tubules, germinal cell hypoplasia, interstitial fibrosis, and Leydig cell hyperplasia. In addition, prostatitis secondary to prolonged catheterization, epididymitis, and epididymo-orchitis can precipitate obstructive ductal lesions and testicular damage. Ohl et al. (1989) reported that sperm density and motility were higher in those with incomplete lesions. In a recent collective analysis of 40 paraplegic patients, 22 successfully produced pregnancies by natural insemination or assisted reproductive techniques (Dahlberg et al., 1995).

Evaluation of Men With Delayed Ejaculation

Evaluation of men presenting with DE or anejaculation (aspermia) should include **a full medical/sexual history, a focused physical examination, determination of serum testosterone levels, and any additional investigations suggested by these findings.**

Assessment begins by determining whether DE is lifelong or acquired, global or situational (Table 71.6). Evaluation includes establishment of how often a man can ejaculate during intercourse and the time elapsed between penetration and ejaculation, IELT. If ejaculation fails to occur, the duration of thrusting before suspension of intercourse, the reasons for suspension of intercourse (e.g., fatigue, loss of erection, a sense of ejaculatory futility, or partner request), and whether ejaculation can occur during postcoital self- or partner-assisted masturbation must be determined. The presence or absence of premonitory ejaculatory sensation during intercourse or masturbation suggests achievement of sufficient arousal to almost attain the ejaculation threshold. Variables that improve or worsen performance are noted. The man's ability to relax, sustain, and heighten arousal and the degree to which he can concentrate on sensations are noted.

The presence and extent of patient-, partner-, or interpersonal-related negative psychological consequences such as bother, distress, frustration, or the avoidance of sexual contact should be established. The frequency of intercourse and the identity of the initiator of sexual contacts are useful surrogate measures for these negative psychological consequences. The quality of the nonsexual relationship should also be explored.

In men with acquired DE, previous illness, surgery, medications, or life events/circumstances should be reviewed. The events may include a variety of life stressors and other psychological factors (e.g., after his wife's mastectomy, when the man is afraid of hurting her and therefore is only partially aroused). Societal and religious attitudes that may interfere with excitement are noted, such as the "spilling of seed as a sin."

A focused physical and genital examination to determine whether the testes and epididymes are normal and whether the vasa are present or absent on each side, supported by a screening morning total testosterone level and any other hormonal or imaging investigations indicated by either history or physical examination will identify or exclude organic disease. Digital rectal examination to determine prostate size, anal sphincter tone, and quality of the bulbocavernous reflex (BCR) is indicated in most men except for young men with situational and clear psychogenic inhibited ejaculation. The presence of a neuropathy may require electrophysiologic evaluation of neural pathways controlling

TABLE 71.6 Recommended and Optional Questions to Establish the Diagnosis of Delayed Ejaculation and Direct Treatment

RECOMMENDED QUESTIONS	
For diagnosis	• How often can you ejaculate during sexual intercourse? • During intercourse, how long after penetration does it take for you to either ejaculate or stop intercourse? • When you cannot ejaculate during sexual intercourse, how often do you feel that you are close to ejaculation? • If you cannot ejaculate, why do you stop intercourse? • Do you ever feel that you have ejaculated but fail to release semen? • Do you feel bothered, annoyed, and/or frustrated by your DE? • How often can you ejaculate during masturbation by yourself or with your partner?
OPTIONAL QUESTIONS	
Differentiate lifelong and acquired DE	• When did you first experience DE? • Have you experienced DE since your first sexual experience on every/almost every attempt and with every partner?
Assess erectile function	• Is your erection hard enough to penetrate? • Do you have difficulty in maintaining your erection during intercourse?
Assess relationship impact	• How upset is your partner with your DE? • Do you or your partner avoid sexual intercourse? • Is your DE affecting your overall relationship?
Previous treatment	• Have you received any treatment for you DE previously?
Impact on quality of life	• Do you feel anxious, depressed, or embarrassed because of your DE?

DE, Delayed ejaculation.

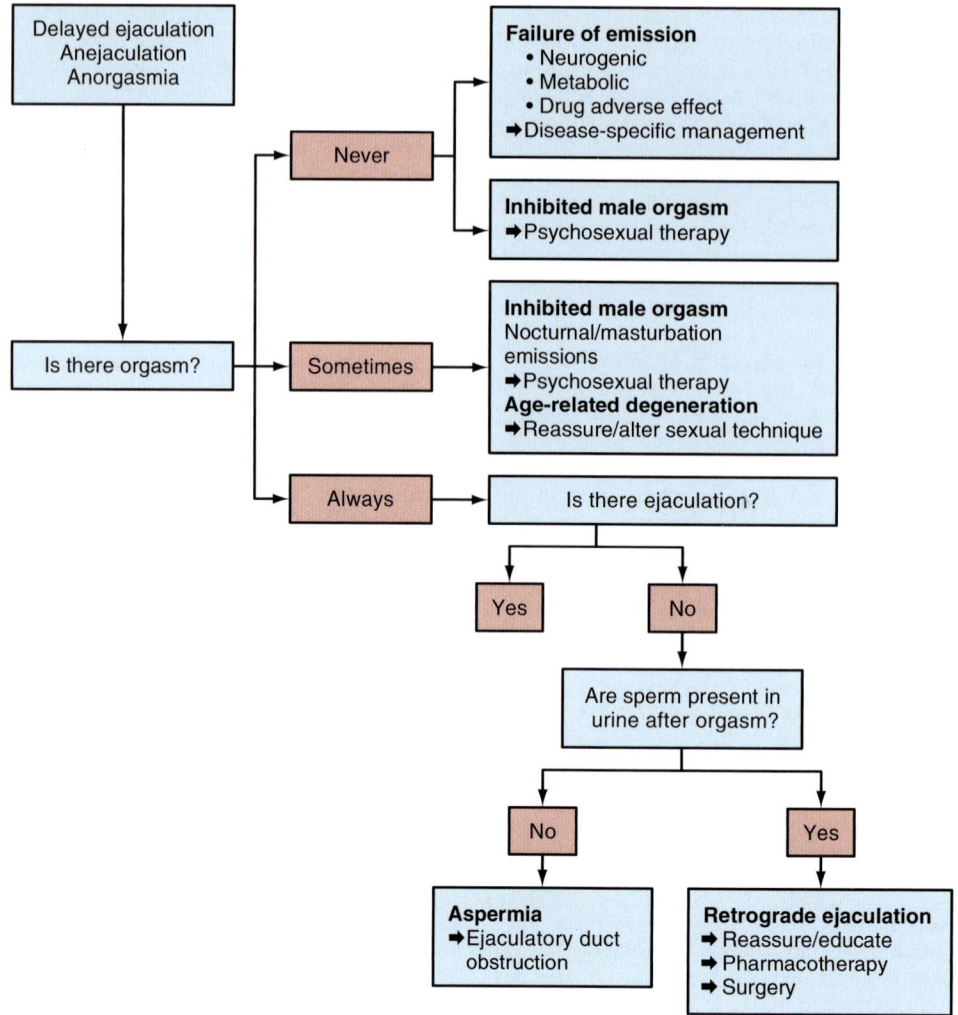

Fig. 71.4. Algorithm for the office management of delayed ejaculation.

ejaculation, pudendal somatosensory and motor-evoked potentials, sacral reflex arc testing, and sympathetic skin responses.

The occurrence of orgasm with either absent or low-volume prograde ejaculation suggests either RE or ejaculatory duct obstruction. The presence of spermatozoa in postmasturbation first-void urine suggests RE, whereas the presence of azoospermia/oligospermic fluid low-viscosity, low-fructose, low-pH semen on semen analysis suggests ejaculatory duct obstruction. If the cause of DE is unclear, culture of expressed prostatic secretion and urine, urine cytology, and serum prostate-specific antigen will exclude prostatitis and bladder and prostatic cancer. Imaging studies such as transrectal ultrasound (TRUS), MRI, or ultrasound of the testicles and epididymes may define any local disease.

Fig. 71.4 is a flow chart for the management of DE (Rowland et al., 2010).

Treatment of Men With Delayed Ejaculation/Anejaculation

Treatment should be cause specific, address the issue of infertility in men of a reproductive age and may include **patient/couple psychoeducation and/or psychosexual therapy, pharmacotherapy, or integrated treatment.** Men/partners of reproductive age undergoing pelvic surgery should be informed of the risk of infertility resulting from anejaculation and the availability of sperm harvesting and assisted reproductive techniques.

Whether a clear pathophysiologic cause is present or absent, patients may be counseled to consider **lifestyle changes, including enjoying more time together to achieve greater intimacy, minimizing alcohol consumption, making love when not tired, and practicing techniques that maximize penile stimulation such as pelvic floor training** (Waldinger and Schweitzer, 2005). Neuropathic DE is usually irreversible and therefore the patient may be counseled to seek alternative methods to achieve mutual sexual satisfaction with his partner.

Psychological Strategies in the Treatment of Delayed Ejaculation

If organic and pharmacologic causes have been eliminated, **referral to an expert psychosexual therapist** is usually indicated to evaluate the causative psychological and behavioral issues. Beneficial effects through psychotherapy depend on the severity of the DE and the individual's receptiveness to engage in counseling and adhere to the counselor's recommendations.

Additional information on the role of psychosexual therapy in the management of DE is available on ExpertConsult.com.

Pharmacotherapy in the Treatment of Delayed Ejaculation

Drug treatment of delayed or inhibited ejaculation has met with **limited success (Table 71.7). These drugs facilitate ejaculation by either a central dopaminergic, antiserotonergic, or oxytocinergic mechanism of action or a peripheral adrenergic mechanism of action.** However, no drugs have been approved by regulatory agencies for this purpose, and most drugs that have been identified for potential use have limited efficacy, impart significant side effects, or are yet considered experimental. **Results are relatively poor in men with psychogenic DE and neuropathic DE.**

TABLE 71.7 Drug Therapy for Delayed Ejaculation and Anejaculation

DRUG	AS NEEDED	DAILY
Cabergoline		0.5–2.0 mg every 3 days
Pramipexole		0.125–0.25 mg
Amantadine	100–400 mg (for two days before coitus)	100–200 mg bid
Bupropion		150 mg daily or bid
Pseudoephedrine		60–120 mg q6h the day before coitus and then twice on the day of coitus
Reboxetine		4–8 mg
Buspirone		5–15 mg bid
Cyproheptadine	4–12 mg (3–4 h before coitus)	
Oxytocin	24 IU intranasal during coitus	

KEY POINTS: DELAYED EJACULATION

- The causes of DE and anejaculation are manifold.
- Failure of ejaculation can be a lifelong problem (25%) or an acquired problem (75%). It may be global and occur in every sexual encounter or be intermittent or situational.
- Treatment of men with DE should be cause-specific and address the issue of infertility in men of reproductive age.
- Drug treatment of men with DE or anejaculation has limited success.

Cabergoline is a central D2 agonist approved for the treatment of hyperprolactinemia that reduces the ejaculatory latency time and facilitates ejaculation (Kruger et al., 2003). Its use has also been described in men with ejaculatory anhedonia or anorgasmia (Wittstock, et al., 2002). The starting dose is 0.5 mg every 3 days and can be escalated to 2 to 3 mg. Adverse effects include nausea, dizziness, and rarely cardiac valvular, pericardial, pulmonary, and retroperitoneal fibroses. Physicians should be cautious with long-term use, and follow-up echocardiography should be performed every 12 months.

α_1-Adrenergic receptor agonists such as on-demand precoital **pseudoephedrine** (120 mg 1–2 h before intercourse) or the **SNRI antidepressant reboxetine** (4–8 mg daily), which inhibits synaptic noradrenaline reuptake, have limited efficacy. The antihistamines **cyproheptadine and loratadine,** a central serotonin antagonist, is anecdotally associated with the reversal of anorgasmia induced by the SSRI antidepressants, but no controlled studies have been reported (Ashton et al., 1997; Aukst-Margetic and Margetic, 2005; McCormick et al., 1990). These studies suggest an effective cyproheptadine dose range of 2 to 16 mg, with administration on a chronic or "on-demand" basis. However, significant dose-related sedative effects are likely to diminish its overall efficacy.

A variety of other pharmacologic agents including **amantadine, apomorphine, bromocriptine, bupropion, and buspirone** have been anecdotally reported as potential DE pharmacotherapy despite an absence of large-population RCTs. Of interest are the recent reports of the **intracoital administration of intranasal oxytocin** in the treatment of anejaculation and anorgasmia (Burri et al., 2008; Ishak et al., 2007; MacDonald and Feifel, 2012; Walch et al., 2001). Although both case reports report reduced ejaculatory latency and/or successful treatment of anorgasmia (Ishak et al., 2007; MacDonald and Feifel, 2012), neither RCT demonstrated statistical superiority to placebo (Burri et al,. 2008; Walch et al., 2001). Furthermore, intranasal oxytocin distribution pharmacokinetics demonstrate that despite achieving supraphysiologic levels of oxytocin in peripheral blood with a Cmax of 15 minutes, very little oxytocin entered the CSF with a substantially longer Cmax of up to 75 minutes (Leng and Ludwig, 2016). In addition, there is no correlation between oxytocin plasma and CSF concentrations (Striepens et al., 2013). In the absence of robust RCT data, no conclusion can be drawn until the efficacy of intranasal OT has been evaluated with formal dose-response studies.

RETROGRADE EJACULATION

Antegrade (normal) ejaculation requires a closed bladder neck (and proximal urethra). **Surgical procedures that compromise the bladder neck closure mechanism may result in RE.** Transurethral incision of the prostate (TUIP) results in RE in 5% (Hedlund and Ek, 1985) to 45% (Kelly et al., 1989) of patients and is probably related to whether one or two incisions are made and whether or not the incision includes primarily the bladder neck or extends to the level of the verumontanum. The importance of contraction of the urethral smooth muscle at the level of the verumontanum has been hypothesized to be important in preventing RE (Reiser, 1961). TURP carries a higher incidence of RE than does TUIP. The reported incidence of RE after TURP ranges from 42% (Edwards and Powell, 1982) to 100% (Quinlan et al., 1991). Although these men may have some antegrade ejaculation and usually experience orgasmic sensation, both events may be reduced as part of the changes that occur in the male sexual response as a man ages. Retrograde ejaculation is more common in DM than in age-matched controls ($P < 0.01$), has been reported in 30% of men with DM, and is not statistically associated with duration of DM, BMI, waist circumference, or HgbA1c or total testosterone levels (Waldinger et al., 2005).

Retrograde ejaculation and failure of emission can be distinguished by examination of a postmasturbatory specimen of urine for the presence of spermatozoa and fructose. The finding of greater than 5 to 10 sperm per high-power field in a postejaculation urine specimen confirms the presence of RE. In patients with low-volume ejaculate, the finding of more sperm in the urine than in the antegrade ejaculate indicates a significant component of RE (Sigman and Howards, 1998).

Treatment

Retrograde ejaculation can be surgically treated with bladder neck reconstruction, but results remain consistently poor (Abrahams et al., 1975; Lipshultz et al., 1981). Drug treatment is the most promising approach. As mentioned earlier, α-adrenergic sympathetic nerves mediate bladder neck closure and emission. Several sympathomimetic amine agents have been described as useful with mixed results (Kedia and Markland, 1975; Proctor and Howards, 1983). These drugs include **pseudoephedrine, ephedrine, midocrine, and phenylpropanolamine.** These agents work by stimulating the release of noradrenaline from the nerve axon terminals but may also directly stimulate α- and β-adrenergic receptors. The most useful is pseudoephedrine, which when administered at a dose of 120 mg every 6 hours on the day before coitus and twice on the day of coitus resulted in prograde ejaculation in 58% of a group of predominantly diabetic men (Shoshany et al., 2017). **The tricyclic antidepressant imipramine, which blocks the reuptake of noradrenaline by the axon from the synaptic cleft, is also occasionally useful** (Ochsenkuhn et al., 1999). The usual dosage is 25 mg twice daily. The current feeling is that long-term treatment with imipramine is likely to be more effective. Preliminary data suggest a potential place for endourethral injection of collagen type 2 in the treatment of RE (Kurbatov et al., 2015).

> **KEY POINTS: RETROGRADE EJACULATION**
>
> - TURP and diabetic autonomic neuropathy are the most common causes of retrograde ejaculation.
> - RE and failure of emission can be distinguished by examination of a postmasturbatory specimen of urine for the presence of spermatozoa and fructose.
> - Pharmacotherapy is associated with variable degrees of success and includes agents such as pseudoephedrine, midocrine, and imipramine.

SPERM RETRIEVAL IN MEN WITH ANEJACULATION PURSUING FERTILITY

Although medical treatment of RE may not always produce normal ejaculation, it may result in some prograde ejaculation. In patients who do not achieve antegrade ejaculation with either surgery or medication, urinary sperm retrieval and artificial insemination using IUI, IVF, or ICSI is an alternative approach with a per-cycle pregnancy rate of 20% to 50% (Nikolettos et al., 1999). The basic method of sperm retrieval involves recovery of previously alkalinized urine by either catheter or voiding after masturbation and then centrifugation and isolation of the sperm.

Penile vibratory stimulation (PVS) and electroejaculation have been used for sperm retrieval in men who are pursuing fertility with psychogenic anejaculation (Wheeler et al., 1988), or EjD secondary to diabetes (Gerig et al., 1997), multiple sclerosis (Previnaire et al., 2014), or SCI (Castle et al., 2014). Application of a medical grade, high-amplitude vibrator to the frenulum activates the afferent nerves of the ejaculatory reflex. In large series, ejaculatory success rate ranged from 65% to 83% (Brackett et al., 1998; Castle et al., 2014; Sonksen et al., 1994). PVS is less effective in SCI below the level of T10, where the nerves of the ejaculatory reflex may be damaged (Sonksen and Ohl, 2002).

Electroejaculation involves the insertion of an electric probe into the rectum adjacent to the prostate gland and delivery of an AC 12- to 24-volt 500 mA current stimulus cycle for 1 to 2 seconds (Denil et al., 1992; Lucas et al., 1991). Ejaculation usually occurs after 2 to 4 stimulus cycles. The stimulus voltage bypasses the reflex arc and applies direct stimulation to the adjacent nerves of the prostate and vas ampulla resulting in contraction of the pelvic floor muscles and ejaculation. Fresh or cryopreserved electroejaculate is subsequently used for IUI, IVF, or ICSI. Ejaculatory success rates range from 80% to 97%, with pregnancy rates ranging from 10% to 12.5% for IUI and 6.3% to 83.3% for IVF or ICSI (Mehta and Sigman, 2015). Electroejaculation pregnancy outcomes appear similar among men with psychogenic anejaculation and men with SCI (Gat et al., 2012), and there appears no significant difference in pregnancy rates with the use of fresh or cryopreserved electroejaculate (Hovav et al., 2002).

It is usually performed under general anesthetic except for men with SCI. It may be associated with rectal mucosal burns with currents more than 500 mA and with autonomic dysreflexia in individuals with a level of spinal cord injury at or above the sixth thoracic vertebral level (T6). Autonomic dysreflexia causes an imbalanced reflex sympathetic discharge, leading to potentially life-threatening hypertension (Sharif and Hou, 2017). Premedication with rapid-acting antihypertensive drugs such as immediate release nifedipine or sublingual or spray nitroglycerine is effective in preventing most AD. Caution should be exercised in older men with coronary artery disease and in men using phosphodiesterase type 5 (PDE5) inhibitors.

EJACULATORY ANHEDONIA

Sexual anhedonia is also known as "ejaculatory anhedonia" or pleasure dissociative orgasm disorder (PDOD). Sufferers may be male or female, are aware of orgasm and ejaculation but experience little or no pleasure. There is little published in peer-reviewed literature, and our understanding of this uncommon disorder is incomplete. Sexual anhedonia may be associated with depression, fatigue, physical illness, hypoactive sexual desire disorder (HSDD), hypogonadism, hyperprolactinemia, spinal cord injury, multiple sclerosis, or during or after cessation of SSRI antidepressants (Csoka et al., 2008) or antipsychotics (Fortier et al., 2003).

Although there is no clear consensus regarding the pathophysiology of PDOD, it is probably a central neurochemical disorder involving multiple neurotransmitters but predominantly dopamine. The dopaminergic neurons of the mesolimbic pathway project into the nucleus accumbens (NAc) and release dopamine in response to reward stimuli including sexual arousal and orgasm. This disorder is probably due to a defect in either the release of dopamine or the interaction between dopamine and the GABAergic neurons of the NAc. This disorder is commonly associated with chronic depression, and the relationship with depression may be bidirectional. As such, there is invariably a psychogenic component driven by the resultant frustration and negativity from the underlying neurochemical disorder.

As part of assessing these men, androgen studies including total and free testosterone, pituitary gonadotropins, and prolactin levels should be performed. If there is evidence of either hyperprolactinemia or secondary hypogonadism, a pituitary MRI should be conducted. The presence of other sexual disorders, including hypoactive sexual desire, opiate addiction, treatment with psychotropic medication (especially major tranquilizers), or genital sensory neuropathy, should be excluded. These men are typically very resistant to the notion that there is a psychogenic cause or contribution to their disorder and as already indicated they may very well be correct. Sufferers are best managed using an integrated approach with pharmacotherapy and psychotherapy. The former may include the use of central dopamine agonists such as for cabergoline at a dose of 0.5 to 3 mg every 3 days.

POST-SSRI SEXUAL DYSFUNCTION

Abrupt cessation, interruption, or dose reduction, antidepressant drugs, particularly selective serotonin re-uptake inhibitors (SSRIs) or serotonin–norepinephrine reuptake inhibitors (SNRIs), can result in an antidepressant withdrawal syndrome (Haddad, 2001). Symptoms are mild and transient and include flulike symptoms and disturbances in sleep, movement, mood, and cognition. Post-SSRI sexual dysfunction (PSSD) is a debilitating condition that adversely affects quality of life, may persist for months to years, yet may spontaneously resolve after prolonged presence (Csoka et al., 2008). The prevalence of persistent sexual side effects after discontinuing SSRIs is unknown, although one study reported a 5% to 15% incidence of PSSD (Bahrick, 2006). The symptoms of PSSD can commence as early as after the first SSRI dose (Csoka et al., 2008) or within days or weeks, persist after discontinuing SSRIs, and include genital anesthesia, HSDD, ED, PE, and ejaculatory anhedonia (Waldinger et al., 2015). It is probable that some subjects thought to have PSSD do in fact have HSDD, ED, and EjD because of underlying depression. The cause of PSSD is unknown, and putative theories include dopamine-serotonin interactions, serotonin neurotoxicity, and downregulation of 5-HT-IA receptor (Bala et al., 2018). Diagnosis of PSSD is challenging and involves review of the patient's drug history, onset and type of symptoms, and the patient's premorbid sexual function. Symptoms must be distinguished from those of the actual mental illness symptoms.

There is no definitive treatment for PSSD, and treatment is limited to specific symptom pharmacotherapy such as PDE5I drugs for ED and/or pharmacotherapy for SSRI-induced sexual dysfunction alone or in combination with individual and couple psychotherapy. Waldinger et al. reported improved penile sensitivity but no improvement in EjD and ED after treatment with low-power laser irradiation or phototherapy of the scrotal and penile shaft skin of a male patient with PSSD (Waldinger et al., 2015).

ORGASMIC HEADACHE

There are multiple single and case series reporting the abrupt onset of a throbbing or a constant headache during sexual activity and at or around the time of orgasm. Lance (1976) reported two variants of sexual headache. The first developed with escalating sexual excitement and had the characteristics of muscle contraction headache. The second was a severe throbbing, vascular-type headache occurring at the time of orgasm. No structural lesions were found in the majority of patients, although the possibility of intracranial vascular or other lesions must be considered. Risk factors included history of migraine, stress, and fatigue.

PAINFUL EJACULATION

Painful ejaculation or odynorgasmia is a poorly characterized syndrome. It may be associated with **urethritis, BPH, acute or chronic prostatitis, chronic pelvic pain syndrome, seminal vesiculitis, seminal vesicular calculi, or ejaculatory duct obstruction** (Corriere, 1997; Kochakarn et al., 2001; Nickel et al., 2005; Weintraub et al., 1993). Often, no obvious etiologic factor can be found. **Painful ejaculation occurs in 17% to 23% of men with LUTS/BPH** (Brookes et al., 2002; Frankel et al., 1998; Tubaro et al., 2001; Vallancien et al., 2003). Men with BPH and painful ejaculation have more severe LUTS and report greater bother. In addition, they report a higher incidence of ED and a reduced ejaculation volume, compared with men with LUTS only (Rosen et al., 2003). Treatment of men with LUTS with α-blocking drugs may be associated with painful ejaculation. A lower incidence of pain has been reported with the uroselective α_1-blocking drug alfuzosin (van Moorselaar et al., 2005). Management should focus on treatment of the underlying cause.

POSTORGASMIC ILLNESS SYNDROME

POIS is a recently described but poorly characterized "orphan" disease comprising a **collection of symptoms, which include severe myalgia and fatigue associated with a flulike state, which occurs within 30 minutes of orgasm.**

Additional information on POIS is available on Expert Consult.com.

CONCLUSION

Recent epidemiologic and observational research has provided new insights into PE and the associated negative psychosocial effects of this dysfunction. The recently developed multivariate evidence-based ISSM definition of lifelong and acquired PE provides the clinician a more discriminating diagnostic tool and should form the basis of the official diagnosis of lifelong PE.

Although there is insufficient empirical evidence to unequivocally identify the cause of PE, there is limited evidence to suggest that lifelong PE may have a genetic basis and acquired PE is most often due to sexual performance anxiety, psychological or relationship problems, and/or ED and to a lesser extent, chronic prostatitis, chronic pelvic pain syndrome, or hyperthyroidism.

Current evidence suggests that psychosexual CBT has a limited role in the contemporary management of PE and confirms the efficacy and safety of oral SSRI drugs and topical anesthetic drugs. It is likely that dapoxetine, despite its modest effect upon ejaculatory latency, has a place in the management of PE, which will eventually be determined by market forces once the challenge of regulatory approval has been met. Treatment with tramadol, intracavernosal injection therapy, or alternate methods of drug delivery cannot be recommended until the results of large well-designed RCTs are published in major international peer-reviewed medical journals.

Delayed ejaculation and anejaculation are more common as men age and have manifold organic and psychogenic causes. They have a significant impact upon sexual fulfilment for the man and his partner and may result in infertility. Treatment of men suffering from DE represents one of the most significant challenges in sexual medicine, and outcome results are often disappointing.

SUGGESTED READINGS

Althof SE, Abdo CH, Dean J, et al: International Society for Sexual Medicine's guidelines for the diagnosis and treatment of premature ejaculation, *J Sex Med* 7(9):2947–2969, 2010.
Corona G, Mannucci E, Petrone L, et al: Psychobiological correlates of delayed ejaculation in male patients with sexual dysfunctions, *J Androl* 27(3):453–458, 2006.
Janssen PK, Bakker SC, Réthelyi J, et al: Serotonin transporter promoter region (5-HTTLPR) polymorphism is associated with the intravaginal ejaculation latency time in Dutch men with lifelong premature ejaculation, *J Sex Med* 6(1):276–284, 2009.
McMahon CG, Altof SE, Waldinger MD, et al: An evidence-based definition of lifelong premature ejaculation: report of the International Society for Sexual Medicine (ISSM) ad hoc committee for the definition of premature ejaculation, *J Sex Med* 5(7):1590–1606, 2008.
McMahon CG, Jannini E, Waldinger M, et al: Standard operating procedures in disorders of orgasm and ejaculation, *J Sex Med* 10(1):204–229, 2013.
Rowland D, McMahon CG, Abdo C, et al: Disorders of orgasm and ejaculation in men, *J Sex Med* 7(4 Pt 2):1668–1686, 2010.
Waldinger MD, McIntosh J, Schweitzer DH: A five-nation survey to assess the distribution of the intravaginal ejaculatory latency time among the general male population, *J Sex Med* 6(10):2888–2895, 2009.

REFERENCES

The complete reference list is available online at ExpertConsult.com.

72 Surgery for Erectile Dysfunction

Matthew J. Mellon, MD, FACS, and John J. Mulcahy, MD, PhD, FACS

Modern penile implants were marketed for the treatment of erectile dysfunction (ED) almost 50 years ago with the introduction of the three-piece inflatable implant by Dr. Scott and the semirigid rod prosthesis by Dr. Small and Dr. Carrion (Scott et al., 1972; Small, 1978). Before that time there were rudimentary penile stiffeners, which gave variable support to the erection but were inconsistently reliable. At that time these devices were the only effective treatment for ED, but as the years progressed, medical therapies in the form of oral medication, intracorporal injections, intraurethral pellets, and vacuum erection devices (VEDs) were marketed with varying success and acceptance. Penile implants have remained a very effective and satisfying treatment of ED, and improvements in design of the product and surgical placement and repair techniques have increased their longevity and functionality. Although satisfaction rates among patients and partners are 80% to 90% and repairs are seen in about 15% of units at 5 years and 30% at 10 years, they remain a secondary treatment of ED (Carson et al., 2000). They tend to be chosen by men who have a strong motivation to continue with sexual activity and who have failed the less-invasive ED treatments or have found them contraindicated or unacceptable. The current goal-directed approach to the patient with ED outlines the treatments available, offers a trial of each therapy as the patient wishes, and settles on that modality that is effective and appealing (Lue, 1990). The need for extensive testing to determine the exact cause of the dysfunction, as had been done in the past, has been proven to be costly and has not changed the therapeutic outcome. It has been reserved for rare and unusual cases.

TYPES OF IMPLANTS AVAILABLE

When penile implants were introduced in the early 1970s, there were two types: the Scott inflatable and the Small–Carrion sponge-filled semirigid rod. As these devices became popular, improvements in design, introduction of competitive models, and the appearance of other vendors to the marketplace fueled the growth of the field. At one point there were five companies selling penile implants. Throughout the 1980s and early 1990s sales of these devices grew almost exponentially each year and reached an apex in 1996 with about 33,000 units sold worldwide in that year. In the same year preliminary data on the effectiveness of sildenafil citrate (Viagra) in restoring fading erections were presented at various medical meetings, and with the resulting publicity implant sales plummeted to a nadir of 12,000 units the following year (Goldstein et al., 1998). The phosphodiesterase type 5 inhibitor (PDEI5) drugs were not universally effective, and implant sales gradually increased over the ensuing years.

Today there are two vendors of penile implants in the United States: Boston Scientific and Coloplast. Other vendors have exited the marketplace because of diminishing sales or corporate acquisition by larger vendors. Worldwide there are currently approximately 50,000 penile implants placed annually, about 24,000 in the United States. Boston Scientific (Marlborough, MA) and Coloplast (Minneapolis, MN) market their products internationally as well. Some foreign vendors do not distribute their products in the United States. Two of the larger foreign vendors are Zephyr Surgical Instruments (Geneva, Switzerland) and Promedon (Cordoba, Argentina).

There are two categories of penile implants, hydraulic and semirigid rod. The hydraulic group comprises the three-piece inflatable and the two-piece inflatable devices. The three-piece inflatable implant is composed of two cylinders with one placed in each corpus cavernosum. These are connected by tubing to a pump located in the scrotum, which, in turn, is connected to an abdominal reservoir. The function of the pump is to transfer fluid between the reservoir and the cylinders. The cylinders function as inner tubes in a bicycle tire and provide very good firmness to the erection when inflated, because they completely fill the interior of the erectile bodies. Because fluid can be totally evacuated from the cylinders, the penis becomes very loose in the flaccid state. **These two features, alternating exceptional rigidity and flaccidity, make the three-piece inflatable group the most popular device among implanting urologists and patients.**

Boston Scientific markets three models of the three-piece inflatable device: (1) the AMS 700 LGX (Video 72.1), which expands in girth and may increase in length up to 25% and (2 and 3) the AMS 700 CX and AMS 700 CXR, which increase in girth only (Fig. 72.1). The CXR is a narrower version of the CX. Coloplast sells two versions of a three-piece inflatable implant, the Titan, and a narrower congener, the Titan narrow, which increase in girth only (Fig. 72.2). The two-piece inflatable implant, the Ambicor of Boston Scientific, comprises a scrotal pump and two cylinders, one placed in each corporal body. Pressing the pump pushes fluid from a reservoir chamber located in the proximal portion of each cylinder to the power chamber, the longer distal part of the cylinder (Fig. 72.3). Bending the penis 65 degrees from the horizontal and holding it in that position for 12 seconds transfers fluid back to the reservoir chamber. Only a small amount of fluid is transferred between the reservoir and power portions of the cylinder when alternating between erect and flaccid states, 6 mL in the larger sizes and 2 mL in the smaller sizes. The device is provided in three fixed girth sizes, and the penile rigidity is determined by the firmness of the cylinders, not the bicycle-tire innertube fit of the three-piece inflatable cylinders. The less the dead space around the cylinders in the corporal body, the greater the penile rigidity is. The rigidity and flaccidity afforded by the Ambicor is inferior to that afforded by the three-piece inflatables. It is chosen when a hydraulic device is desired, but placement of a reservoir in the pelvis is not feasible.

There are currently two types of malleable semirigid rod implants, the Tactra of Boston Scientific and the Genesis of Coloplast. The Tactra is composed of a nickel-titanium alloy (nitinol) core surrounded by a silicone outer coat (Fig. 72.4). The core of the Genesis is individual braided silver wire strands, and it likewise has a silicone outer cover (Fig. 72.5). Each of these rods bends much like a piece of electric wire. The Tactra replaced the recently discontinued Spectra Implant, a mechanical semirigid rod with articulating high molecular weight polyethylene and titanium segments. Both malleable devices are provided in fixed girth sizes. The firmness of the erection depends on the intrinsic rigidity of the cylinders and the amount of dead space in the erectile chambers surrounding the cylinders. Less dead space provides greater rigidity. Placing semirigid rod cylinders slightly shorter than the measured corporal body length gives easier bendability and less recoil to the penis. Mechanical breakage of these implants has been exceedingly rare. The semirigid rods are recommended for patients with limited mental or manual dexterity, or when repairs of a hydraulic device for mechanical problems would be undesirable. Table 72.1 shows the available sizes and components of the penile implants sold in the United States.

INFORMED CONSENT

A thorough explanation of the procedure to the patient and expected results is paramount before the implant is placed. **The greatest**

Chapter 72 Surgery for Erectile Dysfunction **1583**

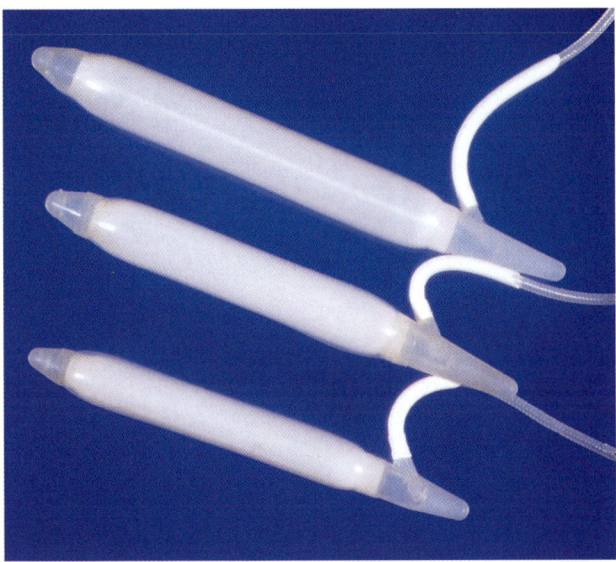

Fig. 72.1. Three AMS 700 18-cm cylinders in full inflation. *Top*, AMS 700 LGX. *Middle*, AMS 700 CX. *Bottom*, AMS 700 CXR.

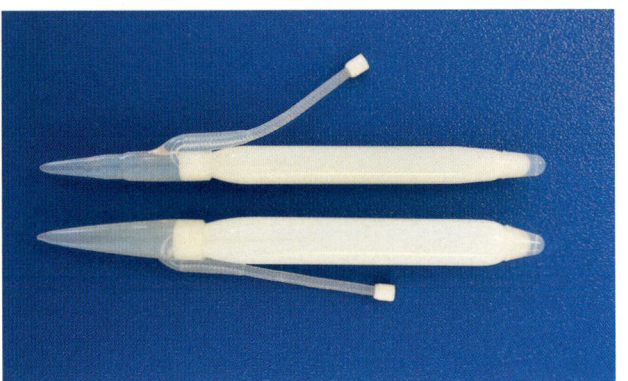

Fig. 72.2. *Top*, Titan Narrow 18-cm inflated cylinder. *Bottom*, Titan 18-cm inflated cylinder.

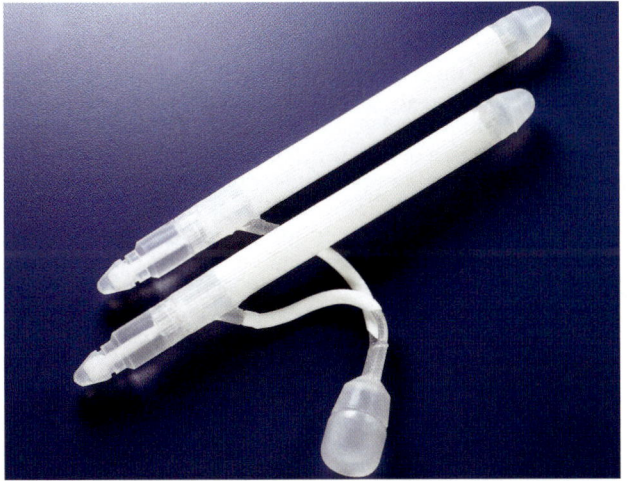

Fig. 72.3. The Ambicor prosthesis.

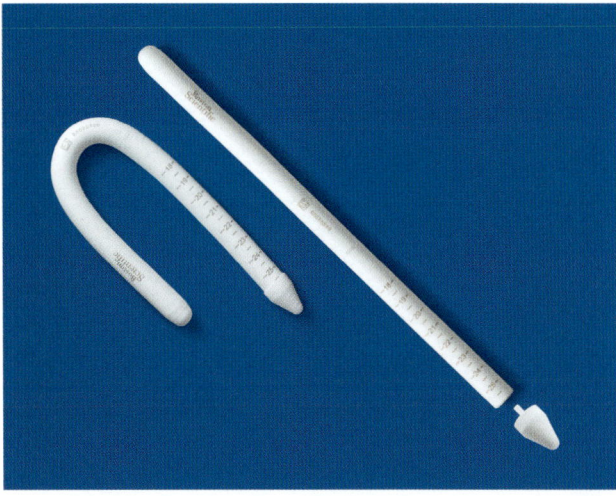

Fig. 72.4. The Tactra malleable semirigid rod implant with trimmable proximal tips and end caps.

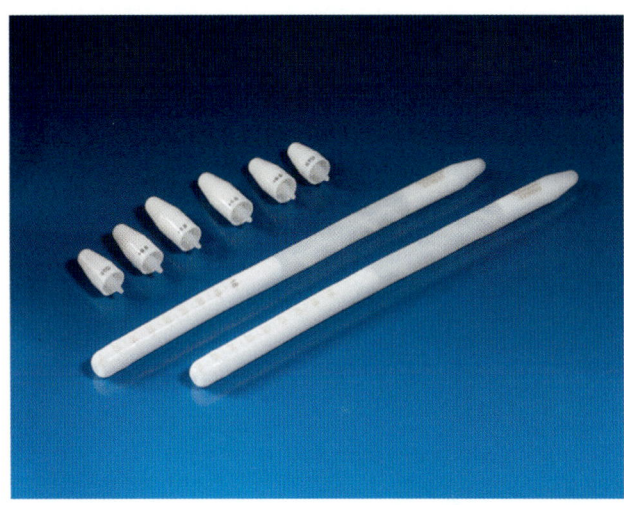

Fig. 72.5. The Genesis malleable semirigid rod implant with trimmable proximal tips and end caps.

disappointment after the surgery is the size of the erection being shorter than what the patient remembers beforehand. This is due to pseudocapsule scar formation covering all parts of the device and limiting expansion of the cylinders. This apparent size reduction seems to be more apparent in patients with Peyronie disease, in which scar tissue is already present in the tunica albuginea, limiting its expansion. This should be stressed to the patient. These devices are mechanically reliable but not indestructible, and repair may be needed in the future. Tissue problems such as pump migration, erosion and extrusion of parts, and infection may also occur, requiring reoperation. Sensation and climax can be affected as well. Alternative ED treatment options, although usually already tried, should be explained and offered. The more experienced the implanter is, the more extensive the informed consent tends to be. Patients who opt for penile implant placement tend to be highly focused on their genitalia. Disappointed and dissatisfied patients can be litigious. **Many patients have unrealistic expectations of the results of penile implant surgery, and the conversation should confirm that the outcome is a firm penis usable for penetrative intercourse not necessarily accompanied by the feelings, desires, and abilities known to the patient previously.**

PREOPERATIVE PREPARATION

Examination of the skin of the genital region and pelvis may reveal conditions such as phimosis, sebaceous lesions, and fungal infections, which should be attended to and eradicated before surgery. Washing the surgical site with a strong soap at home is reinforced. Shaving of pubic hair is done in the preoperative area or in the operating room so that any nicks in the skin will not develop significant bacterial colonization before the surgical skin preparation. In patients with diabetes mellitus the level of blood glucose at the time of surgery

TABLE 72.1 Sizes and Components of Penile Implants Sold in the United States

IMPLANT	CYLINDER LENGTH SIZES AVAILABLE (cm)	CYLINDER DIAMETER SIZES AVAILABLE OR MAXIMUM EXPANSION (mm)	CYLINDER COMPONENTS
BOSTON SCIENTIFIC CORPORATION			
3-Piece Inflatable			
AMS 700 LGX	12, 15, 18, 21	18	Silicone outer
AMS 700 CX	12, 15, 18, 21, 24	18	Polyester/spandex middle
AMS 700 CXR	10, 12, 14, 16, 18	14	Silicone inner
2-Piece Inflatable			
Ambicor	14, 16, 18	12.5	Silicone outer
Ambicor	16, 18, 20	14	Polyester middle
Ambicor	18, 20, 22	15.5	Silicone inner
Malleable Semirigid Rod			
Tactra	14, 23	9.5	Silicone outer
	16, 25	11	Nitinol (nickel titanium alloy) inner core
	18, 27	13	
COLOPLAST CORPORATION			
3-Piece Inflatable			
Titan – Titan Touch	14–28 supplied in even number lengths	19.2–22.1 girth expansion increases with increasing cylinder length	Polyurethane (Bioflex)
Titan Narrow	11, 14, 16, 18	15.2–17.9 girth expansion increases with increasing cylinder length	
Malleable Semirigid Rod			
Genesis	14–23	9.5	Silicone outer covering
	16–25	11	Braided silver wire inner core
	18–27	13	

> **KEY POINTS: INFORMED CONSENT FOR PENILE IMPLANT PLACEMENT**
> - The size of the erect penis after surgery may be shorter and thinner than preoperatively.
> - The goal of implant surgery is to provide a firm penis suitable for intercourse.
> - Penile sensation and ejaculation may both be diminished postoperatively.
> - There will be varying degrees of postoperative pain.
> - Reoperation for a mechanical problem with the implant may be necessary.
> - Tissue problems such as infection may necessitate another surgery.
> - There are other treatments of ED, such as pills, penile inserts and injections, and VEDs.
> - There are a variety of implants, including three-piece and two-piece inflatables and semirigid rods.

should be under 200 mg/dL. If this level is elevated the morning of surgery, an intravenous line may be started and hourly doses of insulin given in 10-unit boluses until the blood glucose is at an acceptable level. Long-term blood glucose control, as manifested by the HbgA1C level, is not as important in the avoidance of implant infection (Ban et al., 2017; Berrios-Torres et al., 2017; Canguven et al., 2018; Wilson et al., 1998). The urine should not be infected, and anticoagulants including low-dose aspirin should be stopped before surgery. The presence of allergies, especially to antibiotics, should be ascertained; these may be used systemically, in irrigating or dipping solutions or coating the surface of the implant. Prior approval from the patient's insurance company is essential because these procedures are very costly, and some insurance policies do not cover treatment of sexual dysfunction. Cash arrangements, frequently with discounts in price, are available, but relatively few patients opt for this approach.

INCISIONS

The original Scott three-piece inflatable implant was placed through an infrapubic incision giving easy access to the dorsal surface of the corporal bodies for cylinder placement and the linea alba for reservoir insertion in the space of Retzius. The incision was vertical from the base of the penis extending up toward the umbilicus. Some implanting surgeons adapted a transverse incision as a variation of this approach. Urologists subsequently adapted the penoscrotal incision, which was first made on the scrotal median raphe. Some surgeons prefer a transverse upper scrotal approach, citing better exposure to the proximal crura and the external inguinal ring for reservoir insertion. Today the majority of urologists use the penoscrotal approach for three-piece inflatable implant placement. A Foley catheter should be placed before the incision to identify the location of the corpus spongiosum. The advantages of the penoscrotal approach are secure placement of the pump in a subdartos pouch and a more cosmetic skin incision. During infrapubic placement care should be taken to identify the dorsal neurovascular bundle and to place the corporotomy stay sutures lateral to this structure at the 10 o'clock and 2 o'clock positions. The nerves coursing through this bundle are sensory to the glans penis and distal penile shaft. The fundiform ligament arising from the mid symphysis pubis is a good guide to the midline when identifying this bundle.

There is a recent report of the three-piece inflatable implant being placed through a subcoronal degloving incision (Weinberg et al., 2016). Using this approach the surgeon can place the cylinders

Chapter 72 Surgery for Erectile Dysfunction **1585**

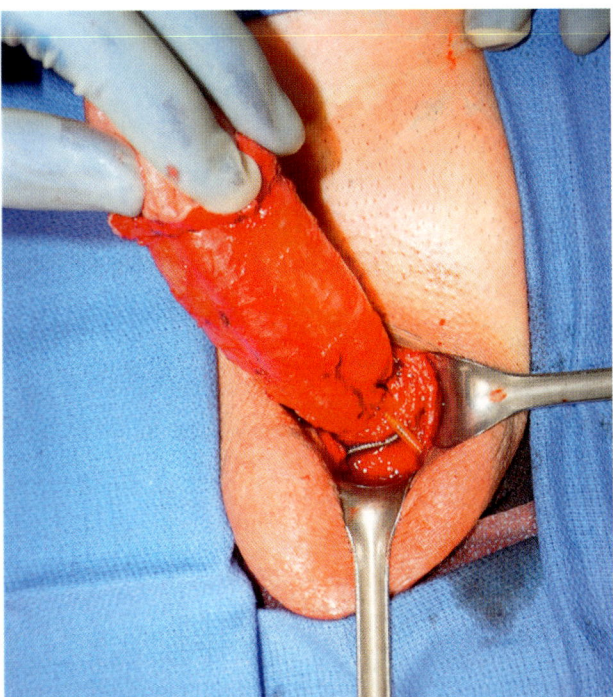

Fig. 72.6. A three-piece inflatable implant placed by the subcoronal approach.

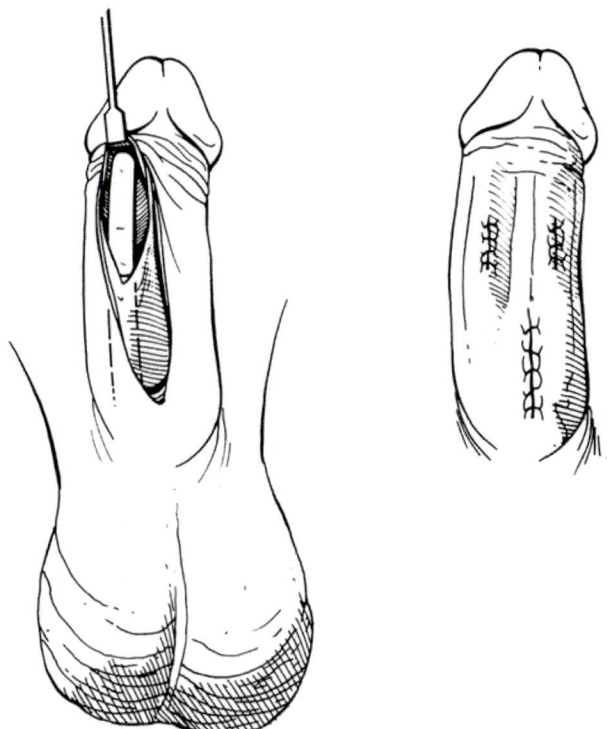

Fig. 72.7. The ventral penile incision for semirigid rod implant placement. The distal end of the corporotomy is lifted over the end of the cylinder with a vein retractor. The midline proximal penile shaft skin incision does not overlap the distal corporotomy incisions.

via penoscrotal or infrapubic corporotomies, and reconstructive procedures on the penile shaft for straightening the erection can be easily performed (Fig. 72.6). The two-piece inflatable implant, the Ambicor, can only be placed through a penoscrotal incision, because it is supplied with short tubing connecting the pump to the cylinders. The semirigid rod implants are usually inserted via a subcoronal incision with corporotomies created laterally. Disadvantages of this approach are a long distance of corporal dilation proximally, which could be challenging in the presence of corporal scarring, and a limited amount of tissue available to close the incision in multiple layers. Circumcision should be performed simultaneously in the uncircumcised patient to avoid maceration of the suture line or lymphedema of the remnant foreskin. An alternative to the subcoronal approach for semirigid rod implant insertion is the ventral penile incision (Wahle and Mulcahy, 1993). A skin incision is made on the proximal penile shaft over the corpus spongiosum. A vein retractor then draws the foreskin distally to expose corporotomy sites at approximately the same location as via the subcoronal approach. The end of the corporotomy is lifted over the end of the rod with the vein retractor during cylinder insertion, thus avoiding the need to bend the cylinder (Fig. 72.7). The proximal penile incision avoids overlapping the corporotomy and skin incisions and allows the uncircumcised patient to retain his foreskin. The perineal incision, originally described for the Small-Carrion implant, is no longer used.

TECHNIQUE OF DEVICE PLACEMENT

Most prosthetic surgeons place patients in the supine position. The bladder is drained with a urinary catheter to ensure safe reservoir placement and avoid inadvertent injury to the urethra. Once the particular surgical approach is selected, the tunica albuginea is exposed and the right and left corporal bodies are skeletonized lateral to the urethra for a penoscrotal approach and lateral to the neurovascular bundles for an infrapubic technique. Two separate 2-0 PDS horizontal mattress sutures are placed approximately 1 cm apart on the respective corporal bodies (Figs. 72.8 and 72.9). These sutures serve as retraction during dilation and also can be used for closure of the incisions once the cylinders are placed. Corporotomies are made between the stay sutures with either electrocautery or a scalpel. These incisions

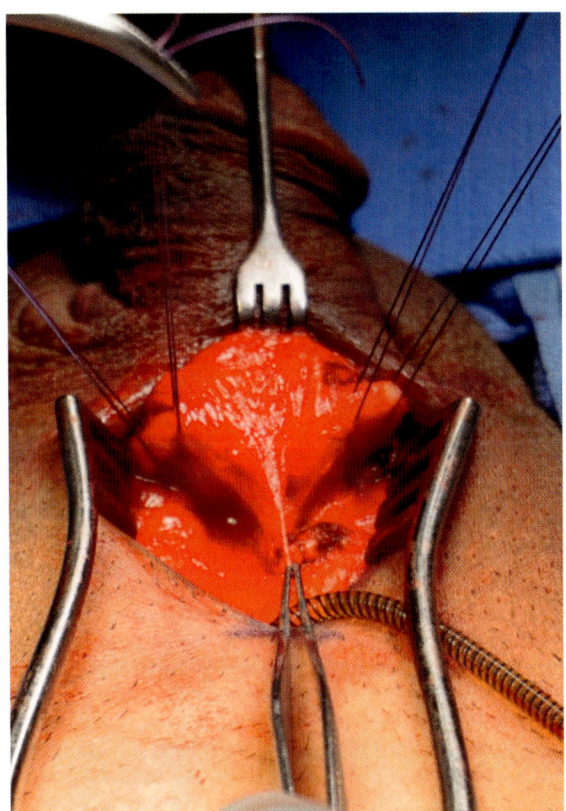

Fig. 72.8. Infrapubic incision for three-piece inflatable implant placement. The corporal stay sutures are placed lateral to the dorsal neurovascular bundle. The Adson forceps is holding the fundiform ligament, a guide to the midline.

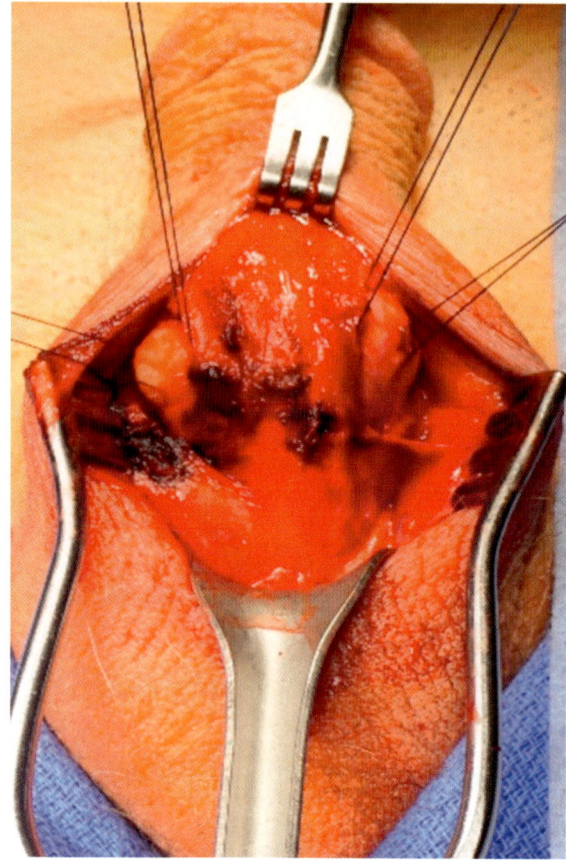

Fig. 72.9. Penoscrotal incision for three-piece inflatable implant placement. Corporal stay sutures are placed lateral to the corpus spongiosum.

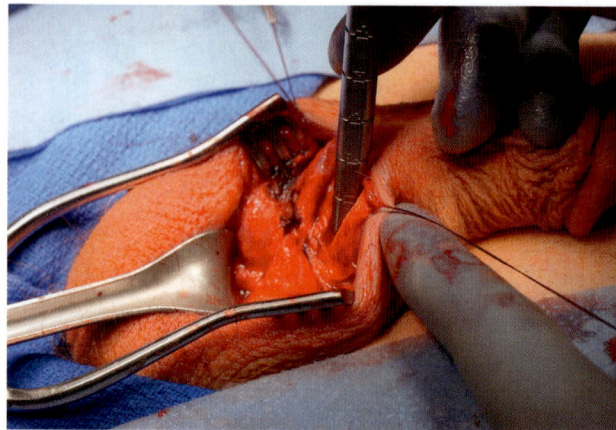

Fig. 72.10. Measuring device indicating an 11-cm proximal corporal measurement. Stay suture used as a reference point.

are longitudinal, parallel to the penile shaft, and can be extended as necessary to facilitate device placement. Dilation begins on the proximal then distal corporal bodies with Metzenbaum scissors followed by Hegar or Brooks dilators, beginning with 7 mm and sequentially moving to 13 mm. The initial corporal tunneling is paramount to avoid corporal crossover, crural perforation, or urethral injury. During proximal advancement, the dilators should be passed gently to the ischial tuberosity to avoid perforation at the point of crural insertion. **Distal passage should progress with the points of the instruments directed laterally, especially as the dilator advances toward the glans to avoid perforation into the urethra or through the midline corporal septum, which is relatively thin.** To assess for these complications, the "goalpost" test is employed by placing dilators simultaneously in the left and right corpora cavernosa first proximally, then distally, and noting their symmetry. Occasionally, fibrosis is encountered, requiring cavernotomes to open or remove the corporal scar tissue, especially in cases of postpriapism ED.

Once adequate dilation is accomplished, the corporal length is measured with a Furlow device. With the stay suture used as a reference point, the proximal and distal measurements are added to determine the total corporal length (Fig. 72.10). A cylinder size equal to or slightly shorter (1 cm) than the measured length is generally recommended to avoid intracorporal buckling and creation of an S-shaped cylinder deformity (Wilson et al., 1996). An inflatable cylinder size is selected and length-adjusted using rear tip extenders. For semirigid rod prosthesis placement, downsizing from the total corporal length measurement 0.5 to 1 cm is recommended. These cylinders generally require a longer corporotomy, if placed through a midcorporal incision, and placement of the proximal crural end first is recommended to facilitate proper seating. A vein retractor or similar instrument can be employed to elevate the distal end of the corporal incision for subcoronal semirigid rod placement. Inflatable cylinders are positioned in the corporal bodies using the Furlow introducer with a Keith needle delivering a traction suture through the glans to pull the cylinders into position distally. Once both cylinders are placed and before corporal closure, a test inflation of the device is performed to evaluate for proper seating, crossover, curvature, or inadvertent perforation. During a primary implant placement, where there is little or no scar tissue in the corpora cavernosa, simply passing the measuring tool to assess corporal length followed by placing the cylinders in the standard fashion without further corporal dilation has resulted in patients noting significantly greater penile length and less postoperative pain compared with those patients in whom the cylinders were placed after standard dilation techniques (Moncada et al., 2010).

The corporal incisions are then closed over the cylinders using the previously placed stay sutures. Alternatively, closure can employ interrupted or running sutures with extreme care taken to avoid puncturing the device with the needles. A small malleable or proximal pushing instrument is useful in protecting the cylinder during needle placement. Placing longitudinal traction on the cylinder with the distal traction suture through the glans aids in minimizing cylinder protrusion and incidental puncture. The surgeon should attempt to keep the input tubing of the cylinders in the most proximal position of the corporotomy. After closure, a second test inflation is performed.

Scrotal pump placement is accomplished by creating a sub-dartos pouch in the most dependent portion of the scrotum on the right or left side. Most patients can operate the pump whether it is placed in the right or left hemiscrotum. This pocket is developed anterior and lateral to the testicle using finger, ring clamp, or nasal speculum dissection. The device pump is then placed in the subcutaneous pouch. Occlusive shodded clamps are employed, and all excessive redundant tubing is removed before the creation of the straight pump to reservoir tubing connection. Once the connection is made, the implant is test-inflated a third time to check for malfunction, displacement, fluid leak, and adequate sizing. The scrotal or infrapubic wound is thoroughly irrigated and closed in standard fashion with two separate subcutaneous layers of 3-0 Vicryl and 4-0 Monocryl skin layer.

The Ambicor and semirigid rod cylinders have fixed girths and are supplied in multiple width sizes. Before the packages containing the implants are opened, it is prudent to determine which width cylinder would be the best fit in the corporal bodies. A useful technique to determine the appropriate size would be to place 2 Hegar dilators parallel to each other simultaneously into the corporal bodies. The urologist should try to touch the thumb to the index finger between the dilators (Fig. 72.11). No separation of the dilators would indicate similar girth cylinders would give a tight fit. Slight separation of the dilators indicates an ideal fit, and touching the thumb to the index finger means a loose fit of comparable size cylinders.

Reservoir Placement

Boston Scientific supplies two versions of the reservoir, a spherical-shaped balloon in volume sizes of 65 mL and 100 mL and a flat,

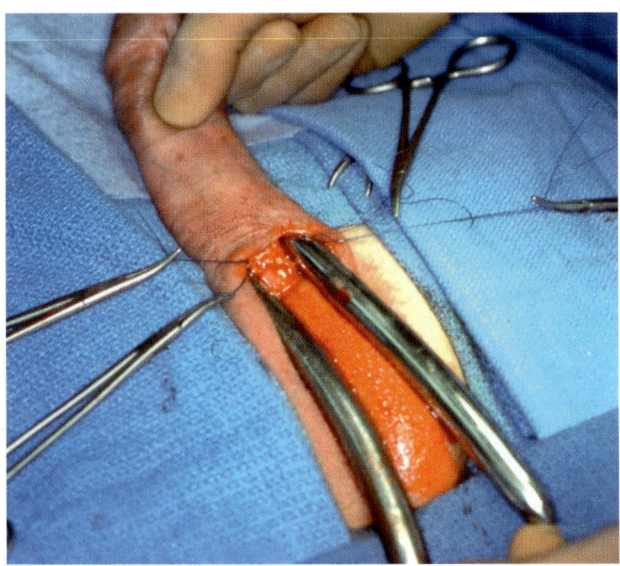

Fig. 72.11. Technique for determining optimal girth size cylinders with Ambicor, Tactra, or Genesis implants.

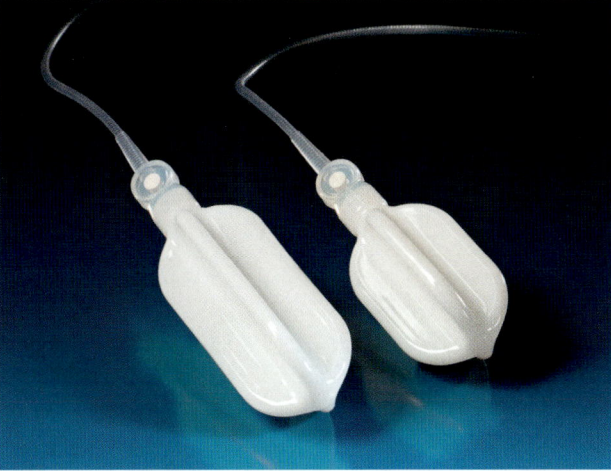

Fig. 72.13. Two sizes of the Coloplast "cloverleaf" reservoir.

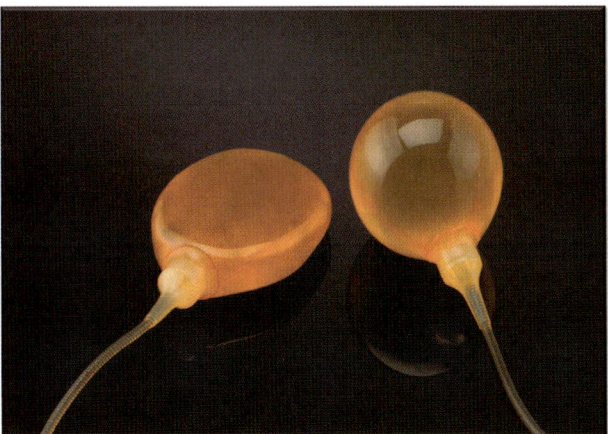

Fig. 72.12. Two types of Boston Scientific reservoirs. *Left,* Disk-shaped "Conceal." *Right,* "Spherical."

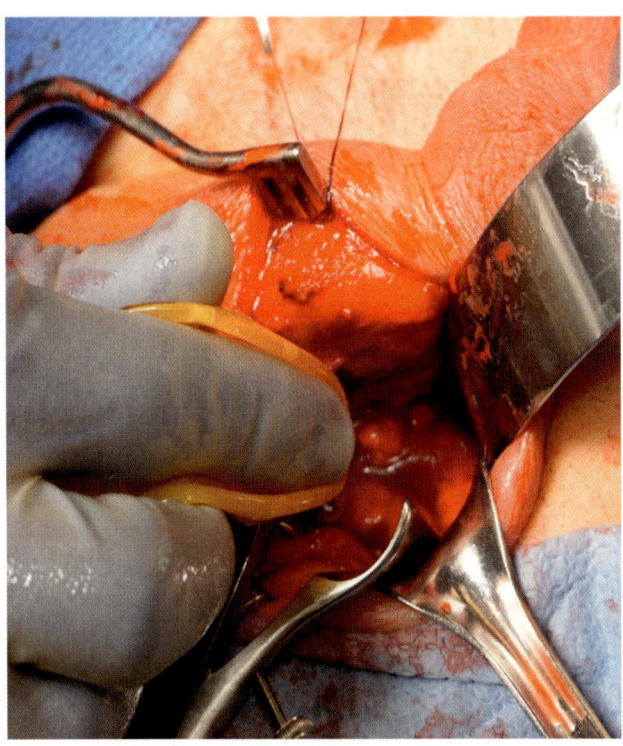

Fig. 72.14. Placing a three-piece inflatable implant reservoir through a long-nosed nasal speculum into the space of Retzius.

disk-shaped balloon called the "Conceal," holding 100 mL of fluid (Fig. 72.12). Coloplast has one shape to the reservoir, resembling a cloverleaf, in two volume sizes, 75 mL and 125 mL (Fig. 72.13). The original reservoirs were placed through the inferior portion of the linea alba, between the rectus muscles in the prevesical space of Retzius. This is still a simple and rapidly accomplished method. With the advent of the penoscrotal incision the reservoirs were advanced via the same incision through the inguinal canal to the side of the bladder. After the bladder is drained and the patient is placed in the Trendelenburg position to reduce the pressure of the bowels on the pelvic structures, a sharp instrument pointing medially pierces the transversalis fascia just above the pubic tubercle, followed by placing the index finger in the fascial defect to ensure location in the space of Retzius. A long nasal speculum is placed beside the finger into the reservoir cavity, the finger is removed, and the reservoir is inserted through the speculum into the space and filled with isotonic saline (Fig. 72.14). The expansion of the reservoir helps to expand the cavity. **The iliac vessels are about 1 inch lateral to the reservoir, and if any resistance is encountered in creating this space, it would be wise to choose another location for placing the reservoir** (Henry et al., 2014). Prior radiation, a previous perivesical urinoma, and previous surgery in the area may generate adhesions that, when disrupted, could damage the vessels. There have been reports of large-capacity reservoirs compressing the iliac vein with resulting leg edema and other untoward sequelae (Da Justa et al., 2003). Today most radical prostatectomy cases are performed robotically. During this approach, the peritoneal reflection over the pelvis is not replaced, and bowel can migrate to the area of the internal inguinal ring, where it can be fixed by adhesions (Sedeghi-Nejad et al., 2011).

Placing the reservoir through the inguinal canal into the space of Retzius in these situations has resulted in bowel being compressed, as the reservoir is inflated, necessitating surgical intervention. Ectopic locations for the reservoir have also been described. The most common is the submuscular suprafascial approach, placing the reservoir between the rectus muscle above and the transversalis fascia below (Morey et al., 2013). A finger is introduced into the inguinal canal, creating a space above the fascia pointing toward the umbilicus. A long nasal speculum is introduced into this space, followed by a long double-hinged clamp or long ring clamp to further develop the cavity about 3 to 4 inches inside the internal inguinal ring (Fig. 72.15). The nipple of the reservoir is grasped with the clamp, driven into the cavity, and held in place while the reservoir is filled with isotonic saline, further expanding the space. Boston Scientific and Coloplast have reservoirs that are flat and will easily rest in this space (Fig. 72.16). The reservoir is under pressure in this location, but both vendors' products have lockout valves preventing fluid from transferring spontaneously from the reservoir to the cylinders. The Boston Scientific lockout valve is located on the pump, whereas the Coloplast lockout valve is positioned at the tubing junction with the reservoir. In the thin patient the reservoir may be visible, and some men report discomfort initially. The location of the reservoir should be checked after placement because these parts have occasionally been found within the peritoneal cavity (Gross et al., 2017).

The tendency is to fill the reservoir to a volume slightly greater than needed to fill the cylinders, which will be more comfortable and less visible in the patient. However, they should be filled almost to capacity, because a smaller volume will allow the reservoir to migrate out of the inguinal canal during cylinder inflation. When replacing the reservoir at a later date, the urologist should inflate the part, make an incision over it, and remove and replace the reservoir through the incision, rather than progressively incising scar tissue around the reservoir tubing to access it. The latter maneuver could destroy a considerable amount of muscle and be accompanied by significant bleeding.

After cystectomy and urinary diversion, implant reservoirs have been successfully placed in the lateral retropubic space through a separate incision medial to the anterior superior iliac spine (Loh-Doyle et al., 2018). To place the reservoir completely out of the pelvis, the epigastric location is a suitable alternative (Riemenschneider, 1981). A left subcostal incision is made, the aponeurosis of the external oblique muscle is incised, the internal oblique and transversus abdominis muscle fibers are separated, and the reservoir is placed in the epigastric space above the omentum. The reservoir tubing is tunneled through the subcutaneous tissue to the scrotum, where the connection to the appropriate pump tubing is made. This approach is seldom used. In the very obese patient the reservoir has been placed successfully in the fat just above the rectus fascia (Garber and Bickell, 2016). These ectopic locations are especially suitable when there is significant intra-abdominal scarring, such as after a cystectomy and urinary diversion or in the presence of a renal transplant.

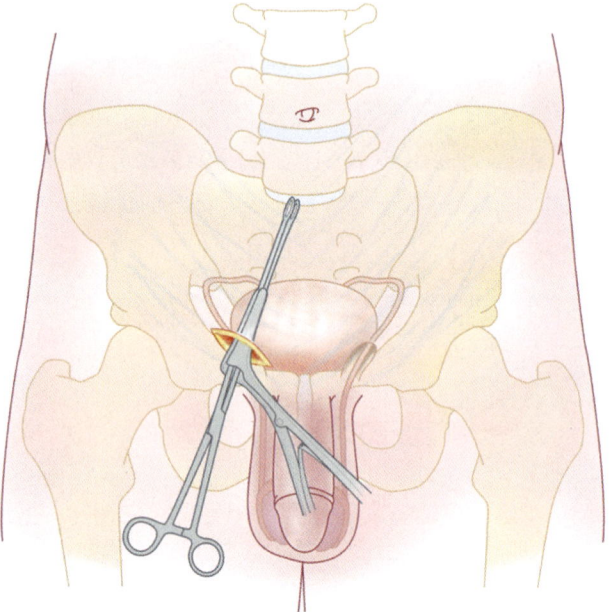

Fig. 72.15. Double-hinged clamp introduced through the inguinal canal pointing toward the umbilicus and developing the submuscular space for reservoir placement.

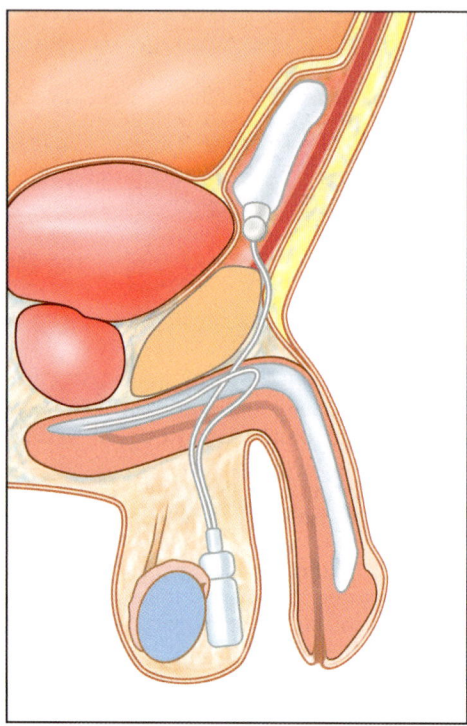

Fig. 72.16. Disk-shaped reservoir positioned below the rectus abdominis muscle and above the transversalis fascia.

> **KEY POINTS: TECHNIQUE OF DEVICE PLACEMENT**
> - The three-piece inflatable implants give the best rigidity and flaccidity and are by far the most popular among patients and urologists.
> - A shorter size to the erection after penile implant placement is the major reason for disappointment after surgery; this should be stressed in the informed consent.
> - Patients with limited dexterity should be encouraged to choose a semirigid rod implant to avoid frustration when trying to manipulate the pump of a hydraulic device.

INTRAOPERATIVE TROUBLESHOOTING

Fibrotic Corpora

Dilation of the corporal bodies is usually straightforward and easily accomplished. Pelvic radiation therapy is commonly used in cases of prostate cancer, and patients with this disease are frequently recipients of a penile implant. There is no greater difficulty in placing a penile implant or in the incidence of postoperative complications after pelvic radiation (Golan et al., 2018; Loh-Doyle et al., 2018). In the presence of scar tissue, such as after an episode of acute ischemic priapism or after cylinders had been previously removed because of infection or erosion, creating cavities for the cylinders can be a challenge. Starting such a dilation with a midshaft corporotomy allows the dilators to pass an equal distance in each direction. If one approach is used for the initial implant placement (i.e., penoscrotal), by using the opposite incision (i.e., infrapubic), the surgeon will encounter less scar tissue. **The dilating instruments should always point dorsolaterally away from the corpus spongiosum, be positioned parallel to the penile shaft, and be seen moving against the lateral wall of the penile shaft.** If scissors are used, they should be passed with a spreading

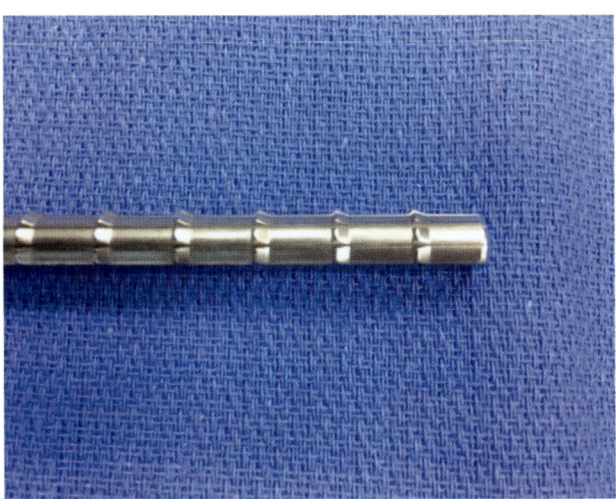

Fig. 72.17. Tip of the Rossello cavernotome showing the raised cups, which shave scarred corporal tissue by pulling the metal rod in and out.

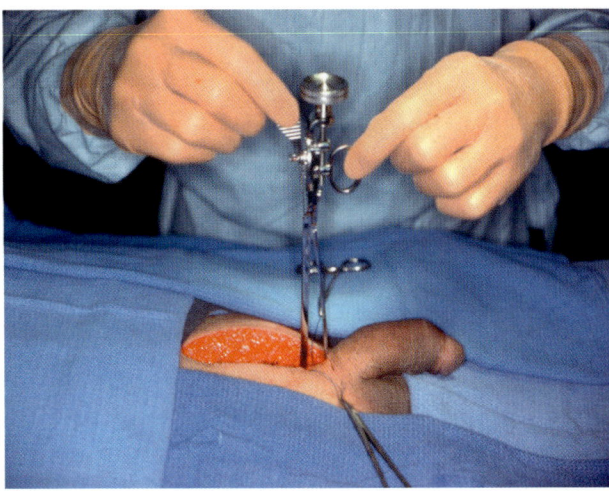

Fig. 72.19. The Otis urethrotome cutting scarred tissue in the proximal crus.

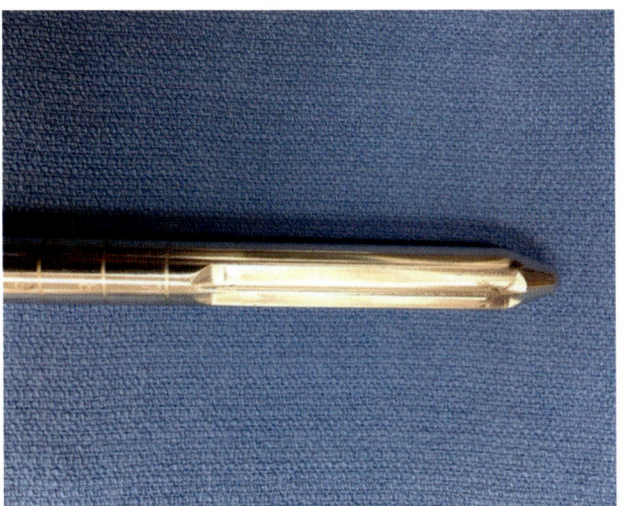

Fig. 72.18. Tip of the Uramix cavernotome showing a raised blade that shaves scarred corporal tissue by moving the blade in a back-and-forth, oscillating motion.

motion, not cutting the tissue. Once a channel is created to the distal subglandular area and to the proximal ischial tuberosity, it can be broadened using the Rossello (Coloplast Corporation) or Uramix (Landsdowne, PA) cavernotomes or the Otis urethrotome. The Rossello cavernotome has raised metal cups, which shave the tissue as a wood rasp shaves wood (Fig. 72.17). The Uramix device has a raised metal blade that shaves tissue as the blade is oscillated from side to side (Fig. 72.18). The Otis urethrotome cuts tissue in one plane, and each cut allows one larger-size dilator to be passed easily (Fig. 72.19). The blade of the Otis urethrotome should be pointed away from the urethra, and this blade should be rotated slightly before a subsequent cut is made to avoid cutting through the tunica albuginea. Excising blocks of corporal scar tissue can also be done using a small, sharp knife blade (Montague and Angermeier, 2006). This is especially useful for exposed scar at the corporotomy site. Both vendors have narrow, inflatable cylinders that will fit more comfortably in a corporal cavity restricted by scar tissue and give comparably good rigidity to the standard-size cylinders because they will completely fill the erection chamber. Use of a single cylinder has been attempted, but the result was suboptimal. The erection appears lopsided, and the rigidity is compromised.

If these measures fail, cavernosal reconstruction can be used. The scarred erectile chamber is incised deeply throughout its length. A cylinder is laid in the cavity and covered by synthetic or natural material as a substitute for native tunica albuginea. **Natural materials used are cadaver pericardium (Tutoplast, Coloplast Corp.)** (Leung-wattanakij et al., 2001) **and porcine small intestinal submucosa (Surgisis, Cook Medical, Bloomington, IN)** (Knoll, 2002). **These grafts are fashioned about 20% larger than the defect to allow for shrinkage and are sewn in place with absorbable suture.** They form a lattice over which the body will form its own scar over a 3-month period. **Synthetic materials used are Dacron (Dupont, Wilmington, DE) and polytetrafluoroethylene (Goretex, Gore Medical, Flagstaff, AZ). A graft the same size as the defect is sewn in place with soft, nonabsorbable sutures.** The natural materials are preferred because they have a lower infection rate. Recently Tachosil (Ethicon, Sommerville, NJ), a hemostatic fibrin sealant and adhesive patch composed of a matrix of equine collagen and marketed for vascular surgery, has been used as a tunical substitute (Patel et al., 2017). This material is fashioned to overlap the tunical edges by about 0.5 cm, applied to the area, and held in place for a short time. No sutures are needed to attach the graft. Cavernosal reconstruction is infrequently used today because urologists have become more proficient at simpler techniques for creating cylinder spaces.

Crural Crossover

The septum between the two erectile chambers is thin and can easily be breached by dilating instruments during cylinder placement. If this occurs and both cylinders wind up on the same side, the erection will look lopsided, the second cylinder will be difficult to place, and corporal length measurements may be significantly different. It is important to recognize and correct this problem during surgery, rather than to have the patient remark at a postoperative visit that the erection looks unusual (Levine and Latchamsetty, 2002). If this problem is identified, both cylinders are removed and a large dilator is placed in the common cavity. The opposite cylinder cavity is redilated with the instruments pointing laterally, and a cylinder is placed into it. The dilator is removed and the second cylinder is placed in the original common cavity. This can be tested by inflating the cylinders and noting that the Foley catheter is in the midline with both inflated cylinders symmetrically located on each side of the catheter. To test for proximal crossover, a dilator is placed in each crus. They should be parallel and of equal height, resembling a football goalpost (Fig. 72.20).

Corporal Perforation

Corporal perforation is unusual and is more commonly seen during secondary cylinder insertion, where corporal scar necessitates aggressive dilation. Proximal perforation through the crus can be suspected if the dilator progresses further inferiorly than its mate and/or corporal measurements differ by more than 1 cm. There is no support, and

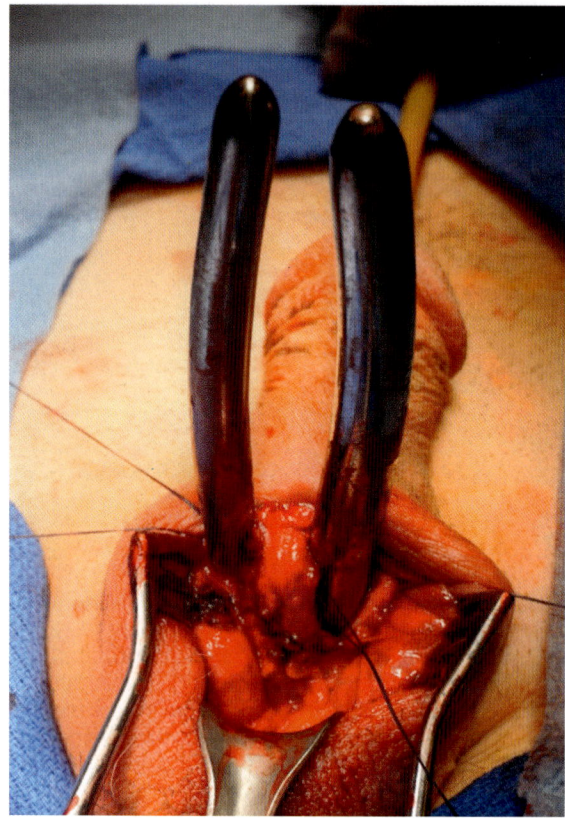

Fig. 72.20. A dilator placed in each proximal crus, parallel and of equal height, indicating no crural crossover or proximal crural perforation, mimicking a football goalpost.

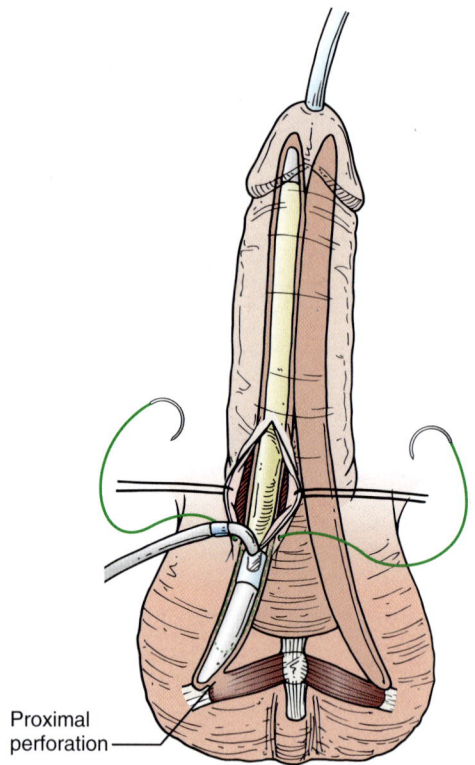

Fig. 72.21. A suture sling of proline placed through the proximal end of an implant cylinder or rear tip extender with each end brought out of the corporal body just distal to the input tube.

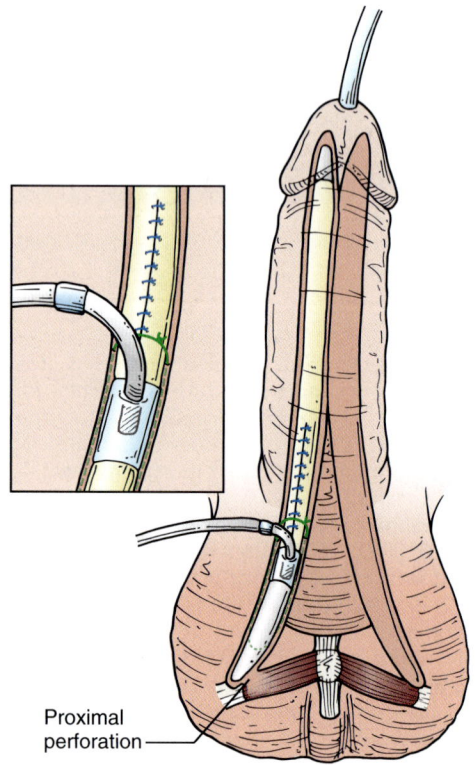

Fig. 72.22. The sling suture (green) tied over the closed corporotomy (blue).

if pushed to the extreme, the metal rod will be palpable 2 inches lateral to the anus. Formerly a windsock of vascular graft material was fashioned into a cup and placed on the cylinder as a rear tip extender (Steidle and Mulcahy, 1987). The cylinder was introduced into the erection chamber and the synthetic cup sewn to the tunica albuginea, preventing proximal cylinder migration. The foreign material was a possible source of infection and difficult to remove during later implant repair because of ingrowth of body tissues into the fabric.

Currently the suture sling is used for this purpose (Wilson, 2010). A nonabsorbable polypropylene stitch with a needle attached to both ends is placed through the proximal end of the cylinder or through the rear tip extender. The cylinder is placed in the corporal body, the distal insertion string is pulled so that the cylinder rests in the corporal body at the same level as its mate, and then the cylinder is partially inflated. The end of each suture is brought out through each side of the tunica just distal to the input tube exit (Fig. 72.21). The corporotomy is closed, the sling suture is tied firmly over the corporotomy closure, and the knot is cut long so that it can be identified and removed at the time of future cylinder replacement (Fig. 72.22). The defect of a perforation or incision into the urethral lumen at the corporotomy site can be closed securely if easily accessible, the wound copiously irrigated, and a cylinder placed (Anele et al., 2014). If there is any question of closure integrity or complexity of repair, the cylinder placement on that side should be aborted, allowing the defect to completely heal. Distal perforation is usually into the fossa navicularis, and the defect is not amenable to closure because of poor exposure. Blood at the urethral meatus, a visible dilator at the meatus, or fluid exiting the urethra after irrigating through the corporotomy is a sign that this has occurred. The cylinder should be left out to allow the defect to heal spontaneously. Placing a urethral catheter is not necessary because the urinary stream will draw tissue fluid into it, and urine will not enter the defect (Bernoulli principle). A cylinder may be placed in the opposite crus to maintain penile length (Sexton et al., 2018). Cylinder placement in the empty erectile chamber can be performed in 5 to 6 months to allow solid scar to form and avoid the dilator entering the original perforation tract. Recently there was a report of 8 cases of distal perforation, in which the urologist created hypospadias, repaired the perforation

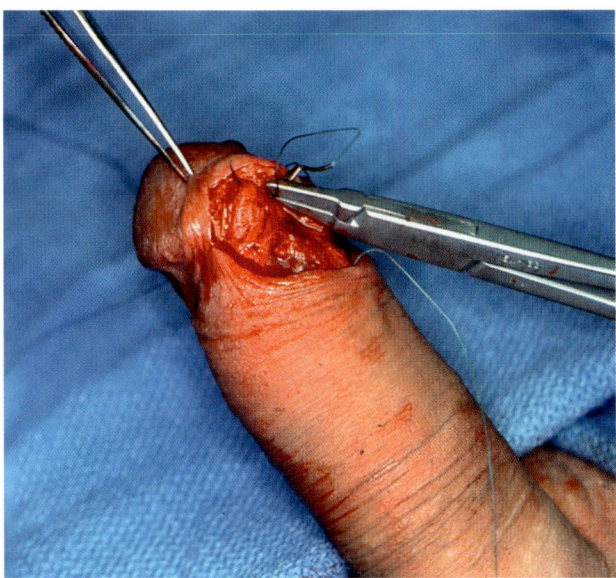

Fig. 72.23. Suture placed through the substance of the glans penis in situation of a hypermobile glans.

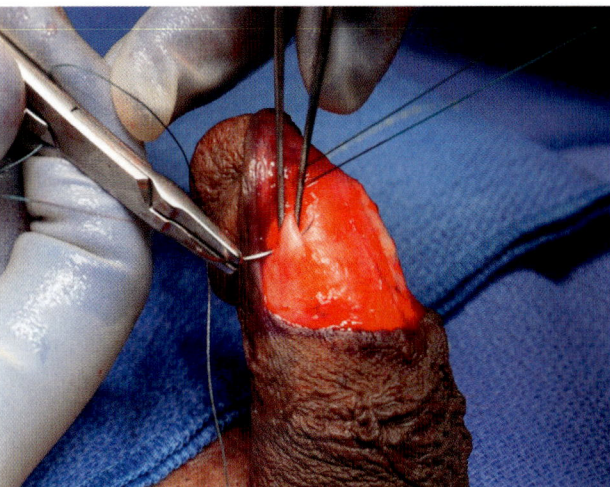

Fig. 72.24. Teeth of an Adson forceps grasping the tunica albuginea over the tip of the underlying implant cylinder as the needle is passed to avoid impaling the cylinder during glans fixation.

defect securely, and placed both cylinders (Perito and Gheiler, 2011). All eight procedures were successful, and four patients requested hypospadias repair at a later date because of spraying of the urinary stream. **It must not be assumed that a urethral injury will heal without closing the defect. Leaving a cylinder in such a situation will likely result in infection.**

Hypermobile Glans Penis

Even though the cylinder tips are positioned in the proper distal location, the glans penis may be excessively mobile or floppy, making penetration during intercourse difficult. The mobility may be dorsal, ventral, or in both directions. This appears to be more common in uncircumcised men. Ventral hypermobility is sometimes called the "SST deformity," mimicking the appearance of the depressed beak of the now-obsolete supersonic transport. If the floppiness is mild, tensing the foreskin toward the scrotum during penetration so that the glans sits more securely on top of the inflated cylinders may be all that is needed. If this is not successful, the problem can be remedied by tacking the glans to the distal tunica albuginea (Ball, 1980; Bickell et al., 2016; Levine and Latchamsetty, 2002). For unidirectional mobility a hemicircumcising incision is made and the glans partially dissected from the distal tunica on either side of the corpus spongiosum or the dorsal neurovascular bundle. A nonabsorbable 3-0 soft suture on an SH needle is driven through the glans substance and then through the tunica albuginea at the level of the inflated cylinder tip (Fig. 72.23). The tunica is grasped in the teeth of an Adson forceps to elevate this tissue from the cylinder and avoid impaling it while placing the needle (Fig. 72.24). The sutures should be placed on both sides before the knot is tied to allow better exposure when placing the second suture. The wound is closed in two layers. Four-quadrant fixation through a complete circumcising incision may be needed for excessive mobility in both directions. **Glans hypermobility and mis-sized cylinders are distinct problems. Cylinders that are too short can be corrected by placing longer cylinders or adding rear tip extenders to the cylinders and should not require glans fixation.**

Curved Erection After Cylinder Placement

Placing and inflating the implant cylinders usually result in a straight erection because the tunica albuginea expands uniformly. However, in the presence of tunical scar from Peyronie disease, a prolonged pharmacologic injection program, or pelvic trauma, areas of the corpora cavernosa will not stretch uniformly. This results in the erection curving in the direction where the scar tissue limits tunical expansion. The semirigid rod implants can usually be bent to overcome the restriction, but when the scar is extensive and thick, straightening the erection with these devices may be difficult, and maneuvers to repair the tunica may be needed. Of the three-piece inflatable cylinders, the AMS 700 CX and the Titan have the best intrinsic rigidity and are better able to correct the curvature than the distally expanding AMS 700 LGX (Kowalczyk and Mulcahy, 1996). Placing and inflating either of these two devices alone will straighten the erection in the majority of cases. An angle of less than 20 degrees of curvature is acceptable and should enable the patient to successfully penetrate for intercourse. The two-piece Ambicor implant does not straighten well and is not recommended when there is significant tunical scarring.

If inflating the cylinders still leaves a significant curve, the modeling maneuver can be employed (Wilson and Delk, 1994). The inflated cylinders are bent forcefully at a right angle away from the direction of the curve and the position held for 90 seconds after the tubing to the pump has been shod-clamped to protect it from back pressure. If initially unsuccessful, the technique can be repeated. Corporotomy disruption and urethral injury have been seen after modeling and should be ascertained. Modeling is less successful in cases of postimplant removal scarring and works best for untreated Peyronie plaques. The penis should be kept partially erect postoperatively for 3 months to allow for pseudocapsule formation with the cylinders straight. If the cylinders are left deflated, a curved erection may return.

Alternatively, a Nesbit procedure/tunical plication or plaque incision and grafting can also be used in recalcitrant cases (Chung et al., 2014; Garafa et al., 2011; Mulcahy and Rowland, 1987). With use of the former technique, the convex surface of the curve is shortened by removing small tunical ellipses followed by closing the defects with absorbable suture or limiting the tunical expansion by placing plication stitches. When incising the tunica over the Titan bioflex material with electrocautery, a setting less than 35 watts should be used to avoid damaging the material (Hakim et al., 1996). The silicone coating of the Boston Scientific products is not affected by the cautery. Incising through the scar on the concave side of the erection allows the force of the cylinder to straighten the erection. The resulting tunical defect can be covered with graft material as described in the section on cavernosal reconstruction.

POSTOPERATIVE COMPLICATIONS

Implant Infection

Numerous precautions to avoid an infection of the implant are taken before, during, and after the surgery. Unfortunately, infections still

> **KEY POINTS: INTRAOPERATIVE TROUBLESHOOTING**
>
> - Injuries between the corpus cavernosum and the exterior should always be closed securely before an implant cylinder is left in place.
> - The AMS 700 CX and Titan implants have the best intrinsic rigidity and are better suited to correct curvature associated with tunica albuginea scarring.
> - Always keep the distal end of scissors or dilating instruments pointing dorsolaterally and parallel to the penile shaft to avoid crural crossover and urethral injury.

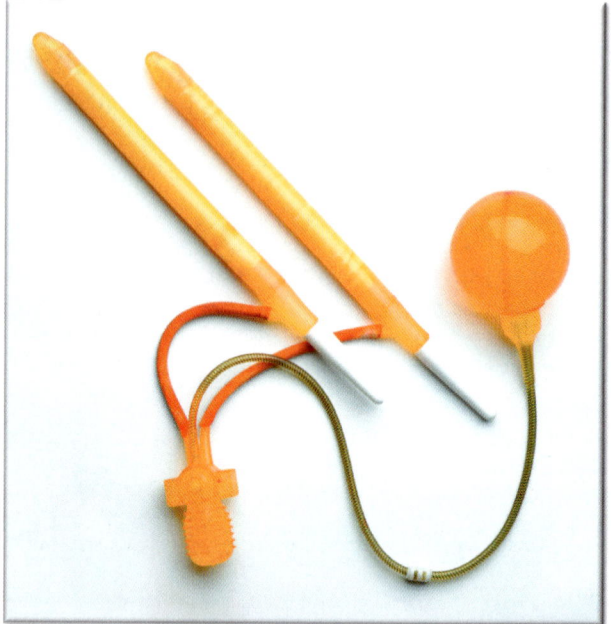

Fig. 72.25. The Inhibizone antibiotic coating of the AMS 700 series implants.

occur, although the incidence is low, in the range of 1% to 3%. Systemic prophylactic antibiotic usage is recommended by American Urological Association guidelines (Wolf et al., 2008). A combination of vancomycin or a third-generation cephalosporin and gentamicin should be started intravenously 1 hour before the incision and continued up to 24 hours postoperatively or until the wound is sealed (De Chiara et al., 2010). **No antibiotics should be needed beyond that point, although most urologists send the patient home on 5 to 14 days of an oral antibacterial** (Darouiche et al., 2013). **It has been shown that the explantation rate for infection is the same whether or not oral postoperative antibiotics are used** (Adamsky et al., 2018).

A recent multi-institutional study assessing the organisms found in 156 infected implants discovered that 86% of the microbes isolated were sensitive to the vancomycin-gentamicin combination (Gross et al., 2017). A three-drug combination of vancomycin, an antifungal such as amphotericin or fluconazole, and piperacillin-tazobactam would neutralize 100% of the organisms found in this series. Use of this three-drug regimen may be prudent prophylactically in patients at high risk for developing an infection and in those with a documented infection before wound culture results are known. Caution regarding the duration of treatment and dosage of the antibiotics should be used because there is increasing evidence of nephrotoxicity with combined vancomycin-piperacillin therapy (Watkins and Deresinski, 2017). Copious irrigation with an antibiotic-containing solution should be used throughout the case, although no particular antiseptic agent is currently recommended. The three-piece inflatable devices of both vendors have antibacterial coatings, and the medications will recede into the tissues over several days. The AMS 700 series is covered with a rifampin-minocycline combination called Inhibizone (Fig. 72.25). These antibiotics were chosen because of low allergic potential and their effectiveness against organisms seen in implant infections. The Titan and the Genesis have a hydrophilic coating that absorbs the liquid into its surface when dipped in the antibiotic solution (Fig. 72.26). The common antibiotics used in the dipping solution are rifampin-gentamicin or sulfamethoxazole-trimethoprim. These new vendor modifications have cut the infection rates in half when compared with using noncoated devices (Carson et al., 2011; Serefoglu et al., 2012).

Dr. Eid (2016) has pioneered the "no-touch technique," in which the skin is completely draped off from the wound and any surgical glove or instrument touching skin is discarded from the operating field. His infection rate in more than 1500 cases was 0.46%. This reinforces the concept that infecting organisms are introduced through the open wound and are not delivered to the surgical site via the bloodstream. A chlorhexidine-alcohol mixture has been shown to be the best preoperative skin prep, showing a 40% lower surgical site infection rate when compared with povidone-iodine (Darouiche et al., 2010).

Twenty-five percent of the population has methicillin-resistant *Staphylococcus aureus* (MRSA) on the skin with greatest concentration in the nasal cavity. Most prosthetic urologists do not screen for MRSA preoperatively. American College of Surgeons Guidelines regarding surgical site infection recommend screening for MRSA in cardiac surgery and orthopedic joint surgery patients. Prosthetic urology patients will likely soon be included among those in whom MRSA screening and decolonization are recommended. If positive MRSA

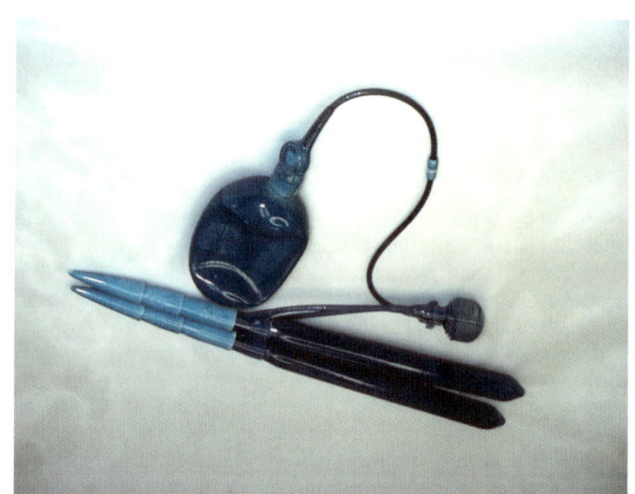

Fig. 72.26. A Titan implant placed in a methylene blue solution showing the solution adhering to the implant surface.

cultures are obtained from the nasal cavity, a decolonization protocol is recommended. This entails chlorhexidine bathing on days 1-3-5 preoperatively and 2% nasal mupirocin (Bactroban) twice a day for 5 days (Ban et al., 2017).

Patients presenting with an infected implant may have the signs and symptoms of fever, chills, and erythema at the incision site, but definitive signs are purulent drainage from the incision, especially when squeezing on the cylinders or pump, visible prosthetic material in the wound, and progressive pain and fixation of the pump to the scrotal wall. **When an infection is present, the incision should be opened and all foreign material removed. Leaving a component behind risks an abscess formation around that part because organisms can migrate along the tubing to remotely located parts of the device.** There are two options after removing the infected device, and these should be thoroughly discussed with the patient before operating. The implant can be left out, irrigation drains placed in each corporal body, and the wound closed (Maatman and Montague, 1984). Solutions containing antibiotics effective against the offending organisms are instilled into each drain every 8 hours for 3 days to eliminate the microbes and prevent a corporal abscess formation. The

BOX 72.1 Antiseptic Washes Used During a Salvage Procedure

- Place dilute povidone–iodine (0.35-3.5%) in implant cavities. Leave in place for 3 minutes.
- Wash out with saline or antibiotic solution.
- Eliminate hydrogen peroxide washes. This substance has no antiseptic advantage over povidone-iodine and can be cytotoxic.
- Chlorhexidine may be more effective than povidone-iodine, but data is insufficient.
- Pressure irrigation is optional.

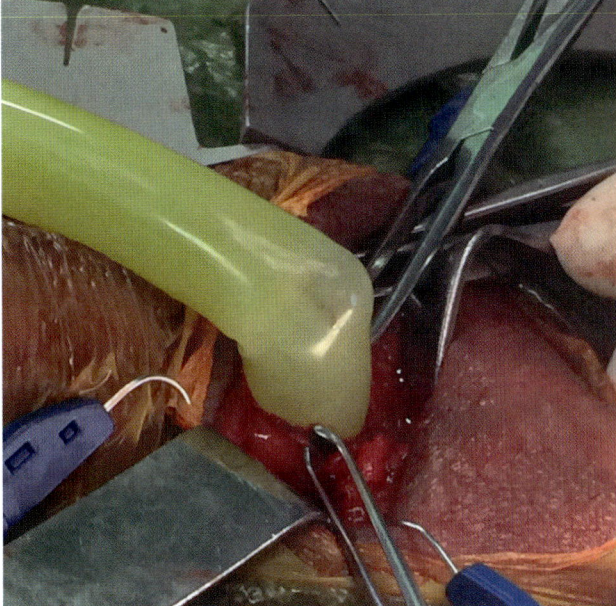

Fig. 72.27. Aneurism of a Titan implant cylinder.

surgeon can return in 2 to 6 months to replace the implant when the infection has cleared. Placing the cylinders will be difficult because of corporal scarring, and the erection will be noticeably shorter. Using a vacuum erection device for 10 minutes daily to stretch the penis while waiting to replace the implant helps minimize this shortening and keeps the erection straight (Canguven et al., 2017).

Another option, termed a "salvage" or "rescue" procedure, entails removing all foreign material, washing the wound thoroughly with a series of antiseptic solutions, changing the wound drapes and in the original protocol, a series of antiseptic solutions including antibiotics, povidone-iodine, and hydrogen peroxide and pressure washing of the implant cavities were employed with a success rate of 84% (Box 72.1; Mulcahy, 2000). The failures were usually associated with onset of infection within 2 months of implant placement, the presence of aggressive organisms, and accompanied by purulence and cellulitis. In a later series four such aggressive infections were successfully cleared by placing the patients on vancomycin and gentamicin systemically, observing receding cellulitis, and performing the salvage procedure after 3 days (Mulcahy, 2015). The original antiseptic irrigating solutions were chosen empirically, and have not been challenged because of their high success rate. Recent evidence from an extensive review of orthopedic joint infection literature suggests a more appropriate content and use of antiseptic irrigating solutions (Pan et al., 2019). A recent series used semirigid rods rather than the patient's original implant type as the replacement cylinders during a salvage procedure with a 94% success rate (Gross et al., 2016). This avoids placing parts in a macerated scrotum or a remote abdominal cavity and takes less time. One-third of these patients requested conversion to a three-piece inflatable implant at a later date. These salvage techniques highlight the goal of corporal length preservation. Delayed reimplantation of a prosthesis after removal for an infection resulted in a total corporal length loss of 3.7 cm in a recent series (Lopategui et al., 2018). Operations to repair a malfunctioning implant that is clinically uninfected have been associated with a high infection rate, in the range of 10% (Henry et al., 2004). Organisms introduced at the time of the original implant placement form a mucopolysaccharide coating called biofilm, which protects them from the body's defense mechanisms (Wilson and Costerton, 2012). The repair procedure disturbs this environment, and bacteria become active, developing a symptomatic infection. **The infection rate in these repair procedures has been reduced to the acceptable 3% range by using a series of antiseptic irrigations in each of the implant cavities after the old parts have been removed and before placing the new implant. This technique has been called a "revision washout" and is recommended for all secondary prosthetic procedures during which old implant parts are removed** (Henry et al., 2005).

Cylinder Aneurysm

A bulge stretching the skin at the base of the penis (Figs. 72.27 and 72.28) may have two causes. In the early postoperative period it is usually a disrupted corporotomy with herniation of the cylinder through the defect. Exploring the wound and repairing the defect at the corporotomy site suffice usually without the need for graft material. Years after implant placement a weakness in the cylinder

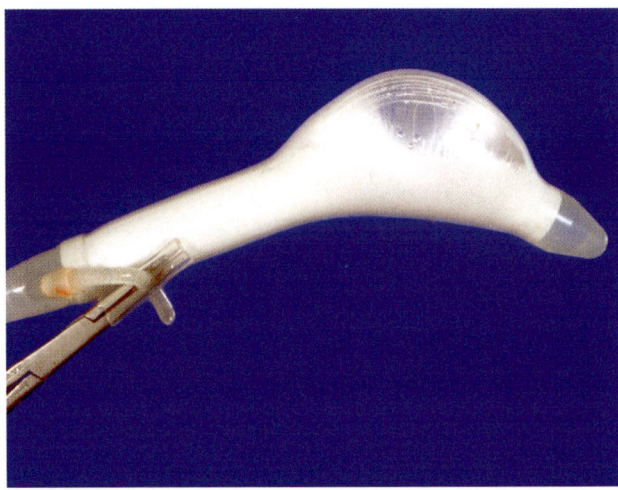

Fig. 72.28. Aneurysm of an AMS 700 cylinder resulting from shredding of the middle fabric layer.

wall may develop as a result of frequent maximal device inflation and aggressive use with resulting bulging of the cylinder wall at the weakened site. If there is a question of an aneurysm, an MRI of the penis will identify the problem, but usually experienced examining fingers can detect the abnormality (Moncada et al., 2004).

The middle fabric layer of the AMS 700 will shred and the polyurethane material of the Titan will deteriorate with excessive wear. Replacing the cylinders corrects this problem. The tunica albuginea may need tapering, but graft material usually is not required.

Cylinder Extrusion

An implant cylinder may extrude through the tunica at the end of the erection chamber and be palpable under the foreskin on the side of the penis (Fig. 72.29) or protrude prominently into the glans, sometimes manifesting as an impending erosion into the urethra at the meatus (Fig. 72.30). Tunical wear from excessive pressure may be due to damage from forceful dilation, placement of oversized cylinders, or aggressive use of the erection over time. Because the prosthetic components are not externally exposed and infection is absent, the cylinder tip can be reseated in a new plane within the

1594 PART VI Reproductive and Sexual Function

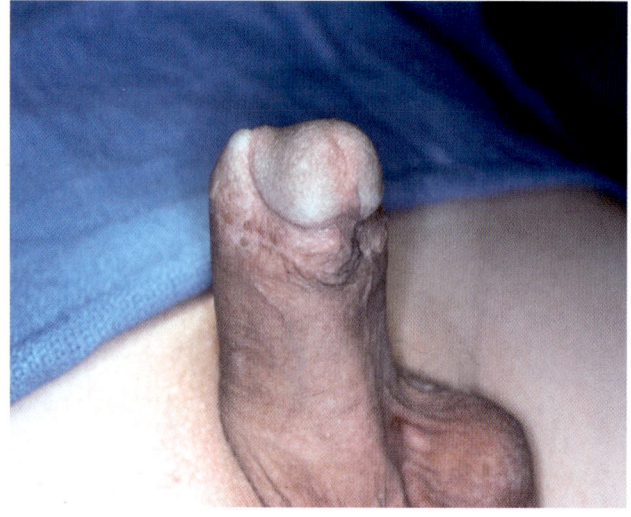

Fig. 72.29. Implant cylinder tip extruding through the distal tunica albuginea.

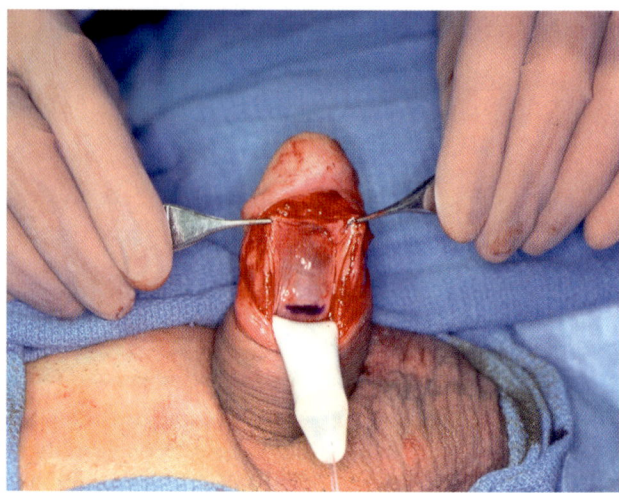

Fig. 72.31. Distal corporoplasty incision into the pseudocapsule surrounding an extruded implant cylinder.

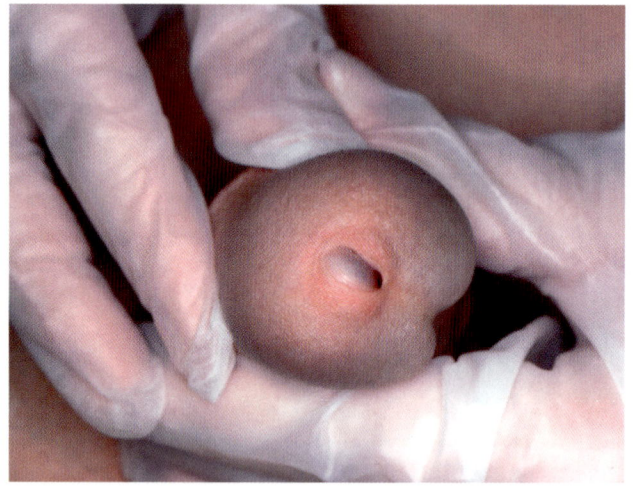

Fig. 72.30. Tip of an implant cylinder protruding into the fossa navicularis.

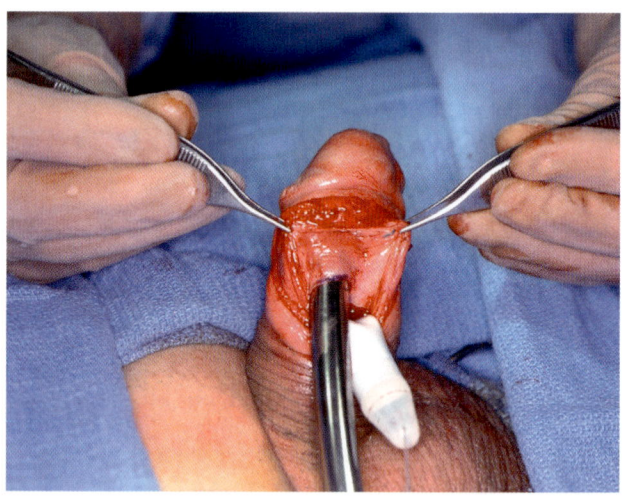

Fig. 72.32. New plane for cylinder placement created behind the pseudocapsule during distal corporoplasty.

corporal cavity, where the distal tunica is intact, a maneuver termed *distal corporoplasty* (Mulcahy, 1999). A hemicircumcising incision followed by a longitudinal corporotomy is made over the extruded cylinder tip. The tip is removed from the cavity and a suture placed through the end to retract the cylinder inferiorly (Fig. 72.31). The back wall of the pseudocapsule is incised, and a dorsomedial plane is developed in the spongy erectile tissue with the scissors and sequential dilators to create a new cylinder cavity (Fig. 72.32). The traction suture at the cylinder tip is used to introduce the cylinder into this new location (Fig. 72.33), and the corporotomy closed. If the problem was associated with an oversized cylinder, replacement with an appropriately downsized device is performed.

Cylinder Erosion

Chronic wear at the cylinder tip over time may cause it to extrude from not only inside the protective tunica albuginea but also through the skin or into the urethra (Fig. 72.34). Protrusion of the cylinder tip may be associated with an underlying device infection, excessive pressure from within the corporal cavity, or external friction of repeated catheterization or instrumentation. Chronic catheterization, either indwelling or intermittent, creates friction against the cylinder tip in the fossa navicularis and has been associated with a high incidence of cylinder erosion into the urethra (Steidle and Mulcahy, 1989). Patients with semirigid rod implants who lack penile sensation,

such as those with a spinal cord injury, are more prone to cylinder erosion (Zermann et al., 2006). The rod tips are hard and cannot be recessed. **Patients with sensory deficits rub the firm penis against undergarments, creating friction against the rod tips. Hydraulic implants should be used in such patients, because they are less prone to erosion.** Urethral erosion sites are inaccessible to repair, and therefore the cylinders and other parts of the implant should be removed and the wound washed with antiseptic solutions. The area is contaminated, and organisms can travel via the tubing to other parts of the device. After the wound is cleansed, a spacer cylinder can be placed in the opposite corporal body to maintain its patency and preserve penile length. A cylinder can be replaced on the side of the erosion after 5 to 6 months, when solid scar has formed and obliterated the original erosion tract. If a cylinder erodes laterally, it should be removed and the wound treated the same way as if it had eroded into the urethra. Placing a new cylinder into the corporal body after an erosion combined with antiseptic irrigations and distal corporoplasty has been tried in such cases but usually proven unsuccessful.

Visceral Erosion of the Reservoir

A very rare occurrence is erosion of the implant reservoir into the urinary bladder or a segment of the bowel. If the reservoir is placed in a restricted perivesical location, the constant pressure of the balloon

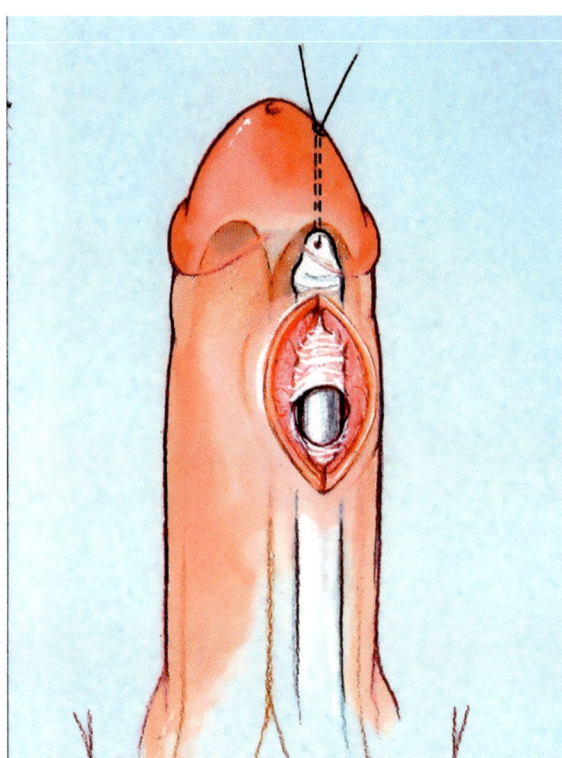

Fig. 72.33. Cylinder placed in new cavity using insertion tool and traction suture during distal corporoplasty.

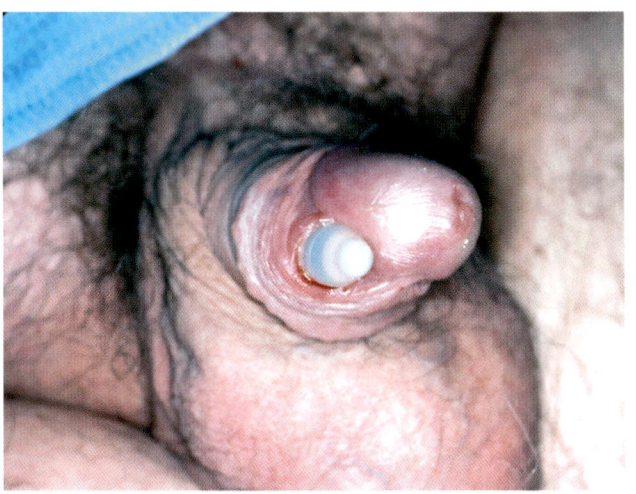

Fig. 72.34. Implant cylinder tip eroding through the skin.

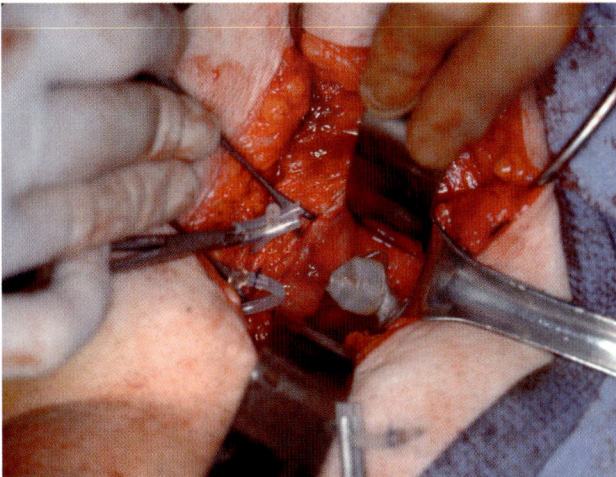

Fig. 72.35. Implant reservoir eroded into the urinary bladder.

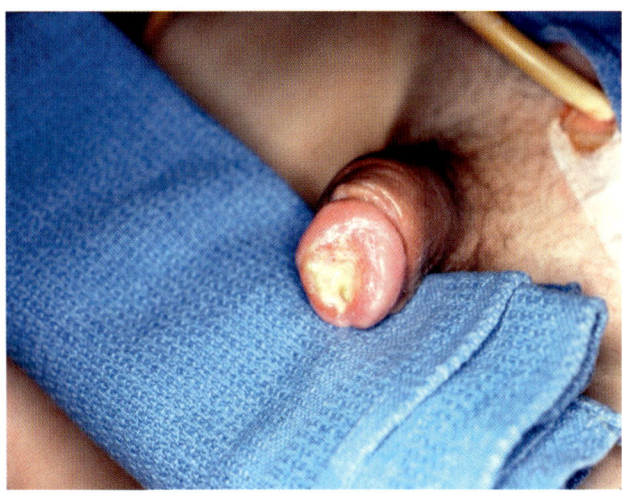

Fig. 72.36. Glans and urethral necrosis after implant placement.

against the bladder wall will cause the latter to break down, and the reservoir will enter the viscus (Fitch and Roddy, 1986). If a reservoir is placed in a very restricted perivesical cavity and expands during filling with isotonic saline, the bladder wall may be torn. The reservoir may enter the bladder, and scar will quickly form in the defect. When the bladder is opened to remove the reservoir, tubing can be seen exiting through a small hole in the bladder wall scar (Fig. 72.35). The wound and the urine are usually sterile and therefore, after the reservoir is removed, a stitch can be placed in the tubing exit site, the bladder closed, and another reservoir placed elsewhere in a capacious cavity. The area should be thoroughly irrigated with antiseptic solutions.

Erosion of the reservoir into the bowel is less common than bladder erosion and occurs when the reservoir is placed adjacent to an immobile bowel segment. Expansion of the reservoir, as it is filled, tears a part of the bowel wall (Singh and Godec, 1992). The problem is quickly noticed as succus entericus invades the tissues and causes significant inflammation. The entire implant should be removed and a general surgeon consulted.

Penile Necrosis After Implant Placement

When placing a penile implant and performing procedures on the tunica albuginea to straighten the erection or better seat the cylinders, the urologist must be mindful that the penis is a digit, and nutrient blood flows in a proximal to distal progression. Ischemia to any part of the penis can result in dry gangrene, and the glans, being the most distal structure, is the most susceptible (Fig. 72.36; Wilson et al., 2017). Longitudinal incisions on the foreskin and tunica albuginea, parallel to the shaft, are less likely to interrupt distal blood supply than transverse incisions. Patients with severe cardiovascular disease, diabetes mellitus, chronic smoking, previous prosthetic implants, and prior pelvic radiation to the area should be considered at risk for this complication, especially when two or more of these comorbidities exist. The distal foreskin may be giving significant glans nourishment, and circumcising incisions may contribute to glans necrosis. Incisions in the tunica albuginea to straighten the erection or rearrange the tunical structure in an attempt to lengthen the erection should be attempted with caution in these high-risk patients. Compressive dressings such as the mummy wrap should be applied without excessive pressure, and the glans should always be left exposed to be certain it has good perfusion. When ischemic necrosis is detected, the cylinders should be removed promptly to take pressure off penile parts and hopefully restore better distal blood flow. Conservative debridement of dead tissue should help with future reconstructive procedures.

> **KEY POINTS: POSTOPERATIVE COMPLICATIONS**
>
> - In the presence of a penile implant infection all foreign material should be removed from the wound because remnant parts may harbor microbes that perpetuate the infection.
> - Patients at risk for reduced penile vascular perfusion should be counseled preoperatively regarding distal penile necrosis. Aggressive reconstructive procedures should be limited or staged in these patients.
> - The implant reservoir should be placed in a capacious cavity to avoid injuring surrounding structures such as bowel or bladder during balloon filling and expansion.

SPECIAL SITUATIONS

Immunosuppressed Patients

Penile implants have been successfully placed in immunosuppressed patients with renal, cardiac, hepatic, and renal/pancreas transplants (Sidi et al., 1987; Sun et al., 2018). An increased incidence of complications in these patients, including implant infection, has not been seen. The immunosuppressive medications are managed by the transplant specialist along with coordination of the prophylactic antibiotics in conjunction with the urologist. Patients who are human immunodeficiency virus positive and are on antiviral regimens with appropriate CD4 counts have often received penile implants without an increased likelihood of an implant infection developing (Davoudzadeh et al., 2016).

Penile Implants in Ischemic Priapism

Acute ischemic priapism of more than a day's duration will result in completely scarred corporal bodies. Months after the episode had subsided the only successful option in restoring the patient's erections is a penile implant. With the significant fibrosis encountered, creating cavities in which to place the cylinders is difficult, and the resulting erection is significantly shorter. The recent trend has been to place the cylinders at the time of the acute episode (Ralph et al., 2009; Yucel et al., 2018). The corporotomy may help relieve the pain of the compartment syndrome. The cavities are edematous, but solid scar has not yet formed, and most of the erectile length will be preserved. Hydraulic or semirigid rod cylinders can be used, and some documentation of spongy tissue necrosis, such as a biopsy, would be prudent to avoid possible future legal ramifications. The patient likely has had distal corporal shunts; these defects should be closed, and placing the distally expanding AMS 700 LGX cylinders should be avoided. Informed consent is paramount, because these are usually young patients with no prior erectile difficulty who are now told that their natural erection will require prosthetic assistance.

Lax Suspensory Ligament

The crural bodies are attached to the symphysis pubis and ischiopubic rami by the suspensory ligament. This structure supports the erection and prevents proximal migration of the penis during the thrusting motions of intercourse. This ligament can infrequently have laxity (Li et al., 2007). The reason for this is not clear and may be congenital or due to trauma during sexual activity. If penile implant cylinders are placed with a proper fit and filling of the corporal bodies, the erection will tend to buckle with a lax supporting ligament. On examining the penis, a gap or cleft can be felt between the crura and the bone, and the penis can be grasped and easily moved side to side (Fig. 72.37). The situation is easily repaired by placing two or three nonabsorbable interrupted sutures securing the tunica

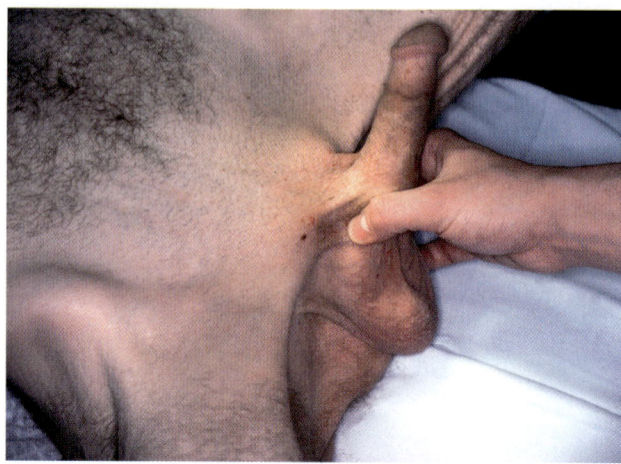

Fig. 72.37. A well-sized penile implant in place providing poor axial rigidity resulting from a lax suspensory ligament. A gap between the crura and the pubic bone is noted, and the crura can easily be moved from side to side.

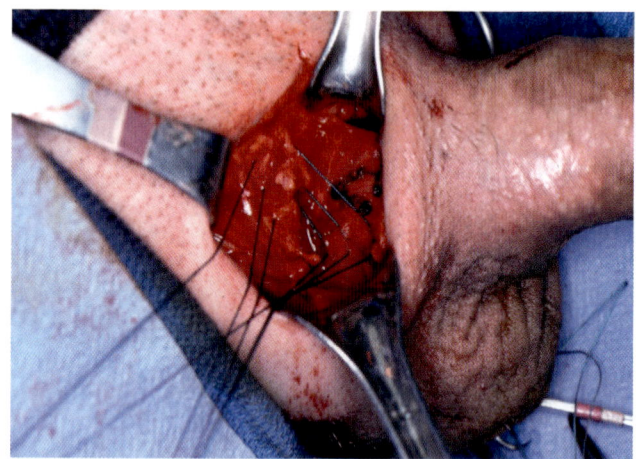

Fig. 72.38. Lax suspensory ligament repaired by three nonabsorbable sutures securing the tunica albuginea to the pubic periosteum bilaterally.

albuginea to the periosteum of the symphysis pubis and the ischiopubic ramus bilaterally (Fig. 72.38).

Long-Distance Bicycle Riding

The crural bodies containing the proximal ends of the implant cylinders or rear tip extenders abut against the anterior projecting horn of the standard bicycle seat. In short-distance recreational bicycle riding this will pose no problem for the patient with a penile implant. In the long-distance frequent rider, however, the firm crura will rub against the seat and may cause pain and/or numbness. This has also been associated with the development of urethral strictures (Awad et al., 2018). Substituting a seat with one that has buttock supports only will solve this problem (Fig. 72.39).

POSTOPERATIVE CARE

After surgery most patients can be discharged home the same day. **During placement of inflatable implants it is recommended that the cylinders be left in a partially erect mode. This allows the recently dilated corporal bodies to heal with scar tissue forming around inflated cylinders and prevents the formation of a contracted pseudocapsule surrounding the cylinders, which could limit their expansion.** A compressive "mummy" wrap can be placed for reduction of postoperative bruising and edema (Henry, 2009).

Chapter 72 Surgery for Erectile Dysfunction 1597

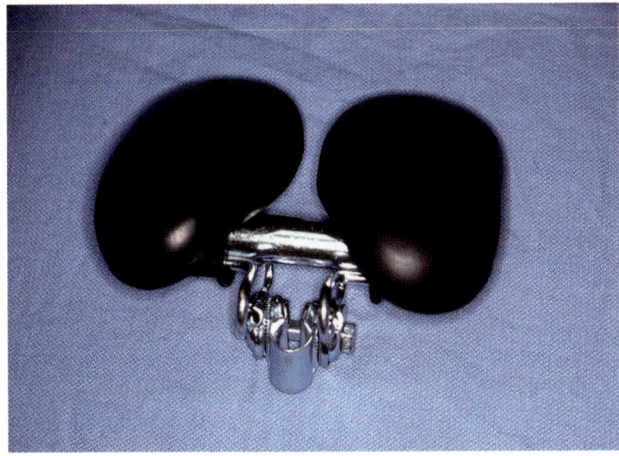

Fig. 72.39. Buttock support bicycle seat used by intense bicycle riders with a penile implant and/or artificial urinary sphincter in place.

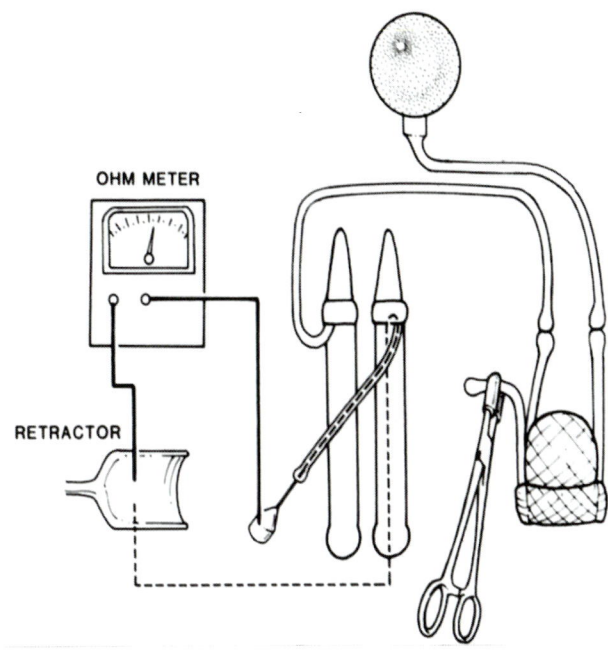

Fig. 72.40. Diagram of ohmmeter testing for leakage in a prosthetic part.

Many surgeons routinely use short-term surgical drains to evacuate scrotal blood and avoid hematoma formation (Kramer et al., 2008). Although safe and not proven to lead to increased infection risk, these drains should be routinely removed within 24 hours. All patients are encouraged to wear compressive underwear for 4 to 6 weeks after the procedure and are instructed to keep the penis pointing upward toward the umbilicus to avoid the inadvertent development of a permanent downward angulation to the erection during healing. In addition, men are encouraged to indirectly apply ice to the scrotum as needed. Most individuals require oral narcotics for a week before transitioning to nonsteroidal anti-inflammatory medication.

Infiltration of the dorsal neurovascular bundle with lidocaine and bupivacaine has reduced postoperative pain and the need for analgesics. Bundle injection with Esparel, a long-acting liposomal suspension of lidocaine and bupivacaine, has been found to reduce the postoperative analgesic pill usage threefold compared with standard lidocaine and bupivacaine bundle injection (Reinstatler et al., 2018). Before formal activation of the device, patients are instructed to retract the pump into a dependent position in the scrotum daily after the infrapubic approach. Using the penoscrotal approach, the pump can be secured in the dartos pouch and daily scrotal manipulation is unnecessary. An office visit is scheduled at 4 to 6 weeks once pain has resolved to begin inflation and deflation of the implant. Ideally, partners attend this session to learn how to use the implant as well as provide assistance for pump manipulation. Men are encouraged to cycle their device daily to passively dilate the cylinders and surrounding corporal bodies as well as gain familiarity with the device operation. Most patients begin using the implant for sexual activity 4 to 6 weeks after surgery.

Mechanical Reliability: Repair for Mechanical Defect

Mechanical malfunction continues to remain the most common complication encountered with penile prosthesis surgery. Semirigid implants are associated with few mechanical failures, and the majority of long-term follow-up data are limited to the three-piece inflatable models. Surgeons may encounter aneurysmal dilation of corporal cylinders, pump malfunction, autoinflation, and tube kinking, although device adaptations by Mentor/Coloplast and American Medical Systems/Boston Scientific have reduced their occurrence. A report on 971 patients who underwent placement of the Mentor Alpha-1 prosthesis after its most recent enhancement in 1992 with more than 5 years of follow-up found that the device survival, free from failure, was 92.6% (Wilson et al., 1999). Alternatively, the AMS 700CX/CXM inflatable penile prosthesis was observed to have long-term reliability of 81.3% with almost 10 years of follow-up in 455 patients (Dhar et al., 2006).

Fluid loss remains the most commonly encountered problem. This may be resolved by replacing the individual leaking component, if identified, and usually occurs late in the device's life span. Implants that have been in place for more than 3 years should be removed and entirely replaced because of wear on parts. If during a repair for mechanical failure the urologist decides to leave parts behind, their hydraulic integrity should be ascertained. Although a leak is found in one part, another part may have a defect as well. The parts may be tested by hydraulic distension of each part and observing for fluid leakage, or more accurately by using an ohmmeter to assess electrical continuity (Fig. 72.40; Mulcahy, 2015). To use this technique, an ohmmeter, set on its most sensitive reading, is placed on a nonsterile Mayo stand adjacent to the operating table. The ends of the ohmmeter cables, which have been previously sterilized, are passed off the operating field and connected to the ohmmeter. A 15-gauge blunt metal needle is inserted into the tubing of the part to be tested, and that part is filled with saline. One cable end is placed on the metal needle; the other cable end is placed on a retractor in another part of the wound. If there is a leak in that part, the sodium and chloride ions will travel through the leak site to the retractor and complete the circuit, giving a positive deflection of the needle. If no leak is present in the tested part, there will be no deflection of the needle. If patients note loss of rigidity with a semirigid implant in place, the surgeon must consider potential fracture of the central cylinder wires. Such an event requires explant and replacement.

PATIENT AND PARTNER SATISFACTION

Although there are many treatment modalities for erectile dysfunction, penile implant placement is associated with high rates of patient satisfaction. A report on 200 patients and 120 sexual partners using AMS 700 three-piece inflatable implants with a mean follow-up of 59 months found that 92% were using the device an average of 1.7 times per week (Montorsi et al., 2000). Ninety-eight percent of patients reported erections as excellent or satisfactory. Importantly, 83% of their partners had similar satisfaction. A more recent study found concurring satisfaction rates, with 97% of patients reporting frequent use of their device (Bettocchi et al., 2010). Only 8% of the 79 patients surveyed were not satisfied with their implant. Complaints of insufficient rigidity and diminished penile length were key drivers of dissatisfaction. In a large series evaluating the satisfaction with the Ambicor implant, 96% of patients and 91% of partners were pleased with the device (Levine et al., 2001). Another large series of 146 men after Ambicor placement reported slightly less satisfaction among patients and partners at 85% and 76%, respectively (Lux et al., 2007).

Another group found that 96% of patients and 85% of their partners had a favorable impression of the Spectra mechanical semirigid rod implant (Akdemir, 2017). In a study comparing the satisfaction of patients with the Spectra and the Genesis, 77% were pleased with the former, whereas 76% found the latter appealing (Casabe, 2016).

These studies highlight a small subset of implant patients who may be dissatisfied with these devices. Complaints regarding perceived penile length, chronic pain or coolness, difficulty with mechanical operation, and decreased sensation of the penis do occur. Preoperative counseling and discussion are paramount. Some patients may benefit from preoperative as well as postprocedure sexual counseling. Surgeons should advise potential candidates that prostheses will not replicate normal erections, but rather provide penile support and rigidity adequate for sexual activity. In addition, ejaculatory dysfunction and penile sensitivity changes may occur and should be discussed with patients before implantation.

Video 72.2 shows prosthetic surgery for erectile dysfunction.

SUGGESTED READINGS

Levine LA, Becher E, Bella A, et al: Penile prosthesis surgery: current recommendations from the international consultation on sexual medicine, *J Sex Med* 13:489–518, 2016.

Pineda M, Burnett AL: Penile prosthesis infections— a review of risk factors, prevention, and treatment, *Sex Med Rev* 4:389–398, 2016.

Video Journal of Prosthetic Urology www.vjpu-issm.info. Contains many videos of penile implant placement and management of complications.

REFERENCES

The complete reference list is available online at ExpertConsult.com.

73

Diagnosis and Management of Peyronie's Disease

Allen D. Seftel, MD, and Hailiu Yang, MD

GENERAL CONSIDERATIONS

Peyronie's disease (PD) was first known as *induratio penis plastica*. It was subsequently named after Francois Gigot de la Peyronie because he was the first to describe and offer treatment for it in a paper published in 1743 (de la Peyronie, 1743). But Guilielmus de Saliceto in the 13th century and Gabriele Falloppio in the 15th century had previously reported on this abnormality of the penis (Musitelli et al., 2008).

PD is currently recognized as a wound-healing disorder of the tunica albuginea (Devine and Horton, 1988) that results in the formation of an exuberant scar, occurring presumably after an injury to the penis activates an abnormal wound-healing response (Greenfield and Levine, 2005; Levine and Burnett, 2013; Ralph et al., 2010; Van de Water, 1997). The resulting scar or plaque is inelastic and therefore results in penile deformity including curvature, indentation, hinge effect, and shortening and is frequently accompanied by erectile dysfunction (ED). One of the most important characteristics of this particular wound-healing disorder is that once the scar has occurred, it does not undergo normal remodeling and therefore the scar and deformity persist (Del Carlo et al., 2008). Progress with treatment of PD has been limited by an incomplete understanding of its pathophysiology, and this lack of understanding has resulted in an inability to prevent the disease from starting and to prevent progression once it has occurred. This, combined with the fact that there is no known reliable treatment to reverse the scarring process, makes PD a challenging disorder to treat.

Multiple misconceptions have been held for decades about PD. Many of these misconceptions have been carried forward and appear to have compromised the proper assessment and early treatment of men with PD (LaRochelle and Levine, 2007). These include that PD is a rare disorder. On the contrary, we now know that the prevalence of PD is somewhere between 3% and 20%, and in certain populations such as those with diabetes mellitus and ED the prevalence may be even higher (Arafa et al., 2007; DiBenedetti et al., 2011; El-Sakka, 2006; La Pera et al., 2001; Lindsay et al., 1991; Mulhall et al., 2004b; Rhoden et al., 2001; Schwarzer et al., 2001; Sommer et al., 2002). Another misconception is that PD has a reasonable likelihood of resolving spontaneously. As a result, men are often told by their physicians that nothing can be done during the acute phase and they should wait 6 months to 1 year before commencing treatment, because there is a "good chance" that the disease process will resolve. We now know from multiple natural history studies that full spontaneous resolution is extremely rare and that it is more likely that within the first 12 to 18 months after presentation, if no treatment is offered, up to 50% of patients will experience worsening of their deformity (Mulhall et al., 2006). Another misconception is that PD is a disorder that occurs only in middle-aged men. Multiple studies have demonstrated that it can occur in teenagers to men in their late 70s (Kadioglu et al., 2002; Levine and Dimitriou, 2000; Tal et al., 2012). Why this process occurs more commonly in middle-aged men is unclear, but theories include that the aging tunica is more apt to be injured in men who are susceptible to the disease, which activates the abnormal wound-healing process (Devine and Horton, 1988; Jarow and Lowe, 1997).

PD is a disorder that appears to go through an active phase during which the scar can grow, resulting in progressive deformity and pain. However, once PD has stabilized, there is usually no further progression (Box 73.1).

NATURAL HISTORY

An understanding of the natural history of PD is critical to counseling patients and selecting treatment options. As noted, there are two phases. The first is the active (acute) phase, which is commonly associated with painful erections and changing deformity of the penis. This is followed by a stable (chronic) phase, which is characterized by stabilization of the deformity and disappearance of painful erections (Devine et al., 1997; Jalkut et al., 2003; Kadioglu et al., 2011a; Ralph et al., 2010). It would seem intuitive that once the scarring process has begun, there would be a progressive increase in deformity; but it has been noted that up to 20% of patients will experience a sudden onset of deformity that can be as great as 90 degrees.

It has been reported that PD can completely resolve in some patients, but this is probably a misconception. It is more likely that some men who traumatize their penises develop curvature secondary to the local inflammatory process. In some of these patients, the inflammation resolves before scarring sets in. Thus, the patient who has resolution of his deformity may not have had PD at all, but rather a slow-healing wound that simply takes longer to undergo the proper remodeling found with normal wound healing. Spontaneous regression has been looked at in several contemporary natural history studies. These data suggest that no more than 13% of patients will have some improvement of their deformity over the first 12 to 18 months after onset of the disease process when not treated (Kadioglu et al., 2002; Hatzimouratidis et al., 2012; Mulhall et al., 2006; O'Brien et al., 2004). Zigelmann et al. (2017) conducted a survey of 126 men undergoing noninjectional and nonsurgical therapy for PD at a single institution as a surrogate for natural disease course. This study found that, although most patients indicated that their penile pain improved (18%) or resolved (64%), only 16% reported that their curvature resolved. The key point to remember is that complete spontaneous resolution of PD is a rare occurrence. Recently, Berookhim et al. (2014) reported on a group of men who elected to have no treatment of their PD. In this study, it appeared that the later in the first year the man sought evaluation after the onset of symptoms, the less likely that he would experience further deformity when left untreated (Berookhim et al., 2014).

EPIDEMIOLOGY

Incidence

The incidence of PD varies widely depending on the population being screened—from 0.39% to 20.3%, with most current estimates of the incidence of PD being between 3% and 9%. The peak age of onset of PD is in the early 50s (Mulhall et al., 2004a; Schwarzer et al., 2001; Stuntz et al., 2016). It was previously held that this was a disorder primarily of white men of northern European descent. It is now recognized that men of every race can develop PD. The variation in recognition of and reporting on this disorder in certain populations may be a result of the interest and presence of physicians

1599

> **BOX 73.1 Peyronie's Disease Caveats**
>
> - Peyronie's disease is not rare.
> - It does not have a high likelihood of spontaneous resolution.
> - It is not a disease of only middle-aged men.
> - It is not a disease of only white men.
> - Trauma to the flaccid and erect penis appears to activate the scarring process in susceptible men.
> - Erectile dysfunction is frequently found in men with Peyronie's disease.
> - Plaque calcification is not an indication of mature, chronic-phase disease.
> - **Peyronie's disease is a disorder that appears to go through an active phase during which the scar can grow, resulting in progressive deformity and pain.**
> - **Once Peyronie's disease has stabilized, there is usually no further progression.**

with expertise in PD, and cultural mores that may make it more or less comfortable for men to share information about changes in their sexual function with a health care provider (Lindsay et al., 1991; Arafa et al., 2007). A recent Japanese study looked at a total of 1090 men undergoing a routine health check and demonstrated the prevalence of PD in healthy men to be quite low at 0.6% (Shiraishi et al., 2012). In a large US web-based survey, 16,000 randomly selected men older than 18 years of age were asked to self-report the symptoms, diagnosis, or treatment of PD. In this study, although only 0.5% to 0.8% of respondents had received a diagnosis of or had been treated for PD, 13% of respondents admitted to having symptoms of PD such as penile deformity or palpable plaque (DiBenedetti et al., 2011). A population-based study of 7711 men in the United States similarly found a 0.7% rate of diagnosed PD, and 11% probably had PD based on symptoms without diagnosis by a physician (Stuntz et al., 2016). Both of these population-based studies demonstrate that although PD is widely prevalent, only a small portion of men with this condition are medically diagnosed. The reasons may include lack of bothersome symptoms and/or reluctance to discuss the signs and symptoms of this embarrassing condition with their physician. Therefore, the prevalence of PD seems to be equivalent to if not greater than other important public diseases such as diabetes and urolithiasis, both established to be present in 3% to 4% of the general population (Sommer et al., 2002).

The incidence of symptomatic PD may be increasing, which is perhaps explained by an increasing tendency to obtain medical help, increasing awareness of people seeking information on the Internet, or increasing use of pharmacologic treatments for ED (e.g., phosphodiesterase inhibitors, intracavernosal injectable agents) (Hellstrom, 2003). Phosphodiesterase inhibitors have not been suggested to directly contribute to the development of PD; rather, their associated use in those with medical conditions such as diabetes that contribute to ED is the likely explanation, because these men now experience erections with deformities they would not have realized were previously present. At this time, there is no suggestion that use of phosphodiesterase type 5 (PDE5) inhibitors should worsen or provoke PD. On the other hand, more recent in vitro and animal model studies have suggested that use of PDE5 inhibitors, as nitric oxide (NO) donors, has an antifibrotic effect that may be beneficial for patients with PD (Valente et al., 2003; Ferrini et al., 2006; Gonzalez-Cadavid and Rajfer, 2009; Chung et al., 2011a). Although treatment for ED, including intracorporeal injection therapy and vacuum devices, has also been implicated as a cause of PD (Carrieri et al., 1998; Jalkut et al., 2003; Bjekic et al., 2006), it seems more likely that these treatments are designed to create a stronger erection, which can then be injured during a sexual encounter, activating the PD disease process in the susceptible individual. Alternatively, as mentioned, these treatments can also unmask unrecognized PD on restoration of erection. To date, there is no evidence that any medicines such as beta-blockers or phenytoin cause PD.

Associated Conditions

Aging

PD is most commonly diagnosed in the fifth decade of life. **A linear increase in prevalence can be seen from 30 to 49 years of age with an exponential increase in prevalence at 50 years of age** upward. (Sommer et al., 2002). Mulhall et al. (2004b) demonstrated an increased PD prevalence of 8.9% in a population being screened for prostate cancer. In this study, the mean patient age was 68 years (Mulhall et al., 2004b). PD may also occur in young men. PD patients younger than 40 years of age tend to present during the acute phase, as there is rapid onset of disease with a penile deformity and pain on erection (Tefekli et al., 2001). Studies have shown that approximately 10% of men with PD are younger than 40 years of age (Levine and Dimitriou, 2000). In addition, Tal et al. (2012) reported on 32 teens diagnosed with PD over a 10-year period with a mean age of 18 (Tal et al., 2012). Sixteen percent reported antecedent trauma, and 37% reported subsequent ED. A high level of distress was reported by 94% of these young men, with 34% seeking treatment for an anxiety or mood disorder (Tal et al., 2012). **The increased prevalence of PD with age is likely a reflection of the increased likelihood of comorbid medical conditions contributing to the development of ED such as hypertension, hyperlipidemia, diabetes, and low testosterone, all of which have been suggested as possible causative factors as the weakened erectile state is associated with PD.** Hypothetically, it could also reflect the reduced tissue elasticity that naturally occurs with aging, predisposing this tissue to stretch-related injury.

Diabetes

One of the more interesting recently studied associations is that of diabetes mellitus and PD. **The prevalence of diabetes in men with PD has been reported to be as high as 33.2%, which is much higher than in the general population** (Bjekic et al., 2006; Cowie et al., 2010; Kadioglu et al., 2002). Further, the prevalence of PD among diabetics has been shown to be increased when compared with the general population, with a reported rate of 8.1% to 20.3% depending on the specific population being screened (Arafa et al., 2007; El-Sakka and Tayeb, 2005; Tefekli et al., 2006). This may reflect particular patient populations, ethnic groups, referral patterns, and expertise of the physicians treating the disorder. Longer duration of diabetes and poor glucose control have also been shown to significantly increase the severity of PD, including duration of PD, deformity, curvature, and erectile function (El-Sakka and Tayeb, 2005; Kendirci et al., 2007). A recent small retrospective study suggested that plaque size and pain may decrease as underlying diabetes is treated (Cavallini and Paulis, 2013).

One theory for the apparent association between PD and diabetes is that men with diabetes are at a higher risk for ED, which may predispose to injury during intercourse because of the less rigid penis pivoting back and forth, potentially resulting in a tissue fatigue–type fracture, activating the scarring disorder (Devine and Horton, 1988) (Fig. 73.1). Another theory suggests that diabetes may lead to decreased compliance of tissues as a result of increased collagen cross-linking (Aronson, 2003). This may make minor injuries less prone to normal remodeling.

Erectile Dysfunction

ED appears to be more common in men with PD than in the general population (Ralph et al., 2010). **The prevalence of ED in men with PD has been reported to be 37% to 58%** (Casabé et al., 2011; Chung et al., 2011b; Kadioglu et al., 2002; Usta et al., 2004). In a duplex ultrasound study of 76 men with PD and ED, 36% had evidence of penile arterial insufficiency, and 59% had veno-occlusive disease as the cause of their ED (Lopez and Jarow, 1993).

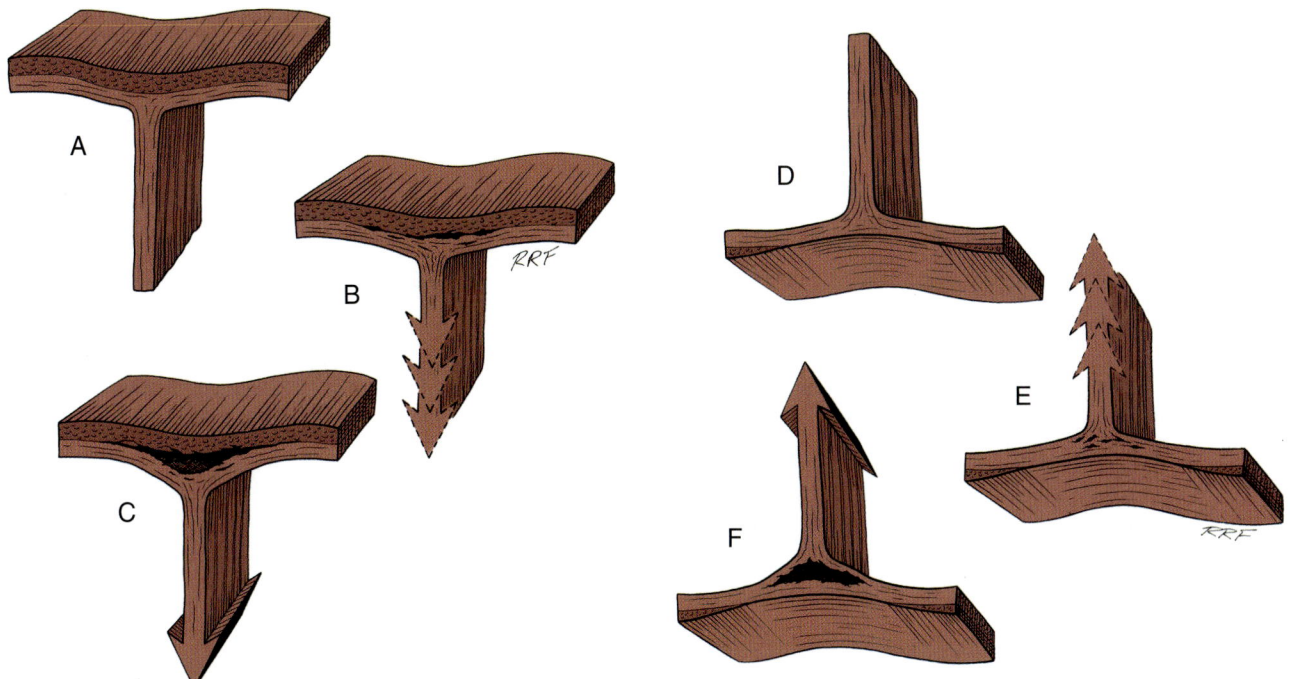

Fig. 73.1. Demonstration of the mechanism of injury during buckling injuries to the penis. (A) Fibers of the septal strands dorsally fan out and are interwoven with the inner circular lamina fibers of the tunica albuginea. The outer lamina consists of longitudinal fibers. (B) In the chronic mechanism of Peyronie's disease, less turgid erections allow flexion of the penis during intercourse, producing elastic tissue fatigue, further reducing elasticity of the tissue and leading to multiple smaller ruptures of the fibers of the tunica with smaller collections of blood, possibly producing multiple scars. (C) In the acute mechanism of Peyronie's disease, bending the erect penis out of column produces tension on the strands of the septum, delaminating the layers of the tunica albuginea. Bleeding occurs, and the space fills with clot. The scar generated by the response of the tissue to this process becomes the Peyronie's disease plaque. (D) Illustration of the situation on the ventrum of the penis, where the bilaminar arrangement of the tunica albuginea becomes thinned, with the midline being monolaminar. The fibers of the septal strands fan out and are interwoven with the inner circular layer. There is no outer circular layer. (E) In the chronic mechanism of Peyronie's disease, less turgid erections allow buckling of the penis as in (B). (F) In the acute mechanism of Peyronie's disease, buckling of the erect penis out of column produces tension on the strands of the septum, causing the septal fibers to tear.

The prevalence of associated comorbidities is higher in patients with PD and ED than in patients with PD and no ED, which may indicate that hypertension, smoking, hypercholesterolemia, diabetes mellitus, and hyperlipidemia are more likely related to ED than to the pathogenesis of PD (Usta et al., 2004). This may be attributable to changes in penile geometry and/or psychological inhibition, which is difficult to determine even in studies in which duplex ultrasound and cavernosometry are used (Kadioglu et al., 2002; Levine and Coogan, 1996).

Psychological Aspects

PD is not only a physically deforming but also a psychologically devastating disorder. Multiple studies have now demonstrated the frequent association of psychological distress in men with PD including diminished self-esteem, shame, embarrassment, self-disgust, anxiety, loss of sexual confidence, and depression, all of which can compromise the man's relationships at home, at work, and in the bedroom (Gelbard et al., 1990; Jones, 1997; Rosen et al., 2008; Smith et al., 2008a). **Penile shortening and the inability to have intercourse are the two most common and consistent risk factors for emotional distress and relationship problems associated with PD** (Rosen et al., 2008; Smith et al., 2008a).

Psychosocial stress is reported by 77% to 94% of men with PD (Gelbard et al., 1990; Nelson and Mulhall, 2013; Tal et al., 2012). Contemporary studies using a validated measure of depression (Center for Epidemiologic Studies Depression Scale [CESD]) have **demonstrated moderate to severe depression in 48% of PD patients, with these rates typically increasing with the duration of PD** (Nelson et al., 2008). PD also commonly affects the patient's sexual partner, causing feelings of helplessness and feelings of personal responsibility for the PD caused by trauma during intercourse, and sadness over loss of intimacy (Rosen et al., 2008).

In an effort to develop a valid outcome measure for assessing psychosocial and sexual consequences of PD, Rosen et al. (2008) conducted a study composed of a series of focus groups with 28 PD patients and identified common concerns. These concerns were grouped into four core domains: (1) physical appearance and self-image, (2) sexual function and performance, (3) PD-related pain and discomfort, and (4) social stigmatization and isolation (Rosen et al., 2008). **With these data, a validated Peyronie's Disease Questionnaire (PDQ) was developed; patient-reported estimates of penile curvature severity correlated with PDQ domains, whereas objective measures of penile curvature did not. For some patients, even a lesser degree of curvature may be highly bothersome or provoke distress** (Hellstrom et al., 2013). This is also evidenced by the fact that self-estimates of penile curvature in men with PD differ from objective measures by an average of 20 degrees, with 54% of patients overestimating their curvature (Bacal et al., 2009). **It is important to remember that despite "successful treatment" that may allow the patient to be sexually functional again, there is often persistent psychological distress, presumably because of residual changes to the patient's pre-PD penile appearance (Gelbard et al., 1990; Jones, 1997). It is critical that the physician recognize these psychological effects, not only to enhance the trust between the patient and physician, but also to identify more advanced indicators of depression, which should initiate referral to a sex therapist, psychologist, or psychiatrist (Levine, 2013).

Radical Prostatectomy

Both prostate cancer and PD are most prevalent in men after their fifth decade of life. The evidence to support or refute a link between radical prostatectomy and PD is limited. In a study of 1011 post–radical prostatectomy patients, Tal et al. (2010) demonstrated an incidence of PD of 15.9% with a mean time to development of disease of 13.9 months (Tal et al., 2010). Although postoperative erectile function was not a predictor of development of PD, younger age at time of prostatectomy and white race were reported risk factors for developing PD after radical prostatectomy. The authors concluded that prospective controlled studies are needed to elucidate the incidence of PD after radical prostatectomy and determine if radical prostatectomy has a causative role in the pathogenesis of PD (Tal et al., 2010).

Ciancio and Kim (2000) also examined the effects of prostatectomy on penile fibrosis and sexual dysfunction. Eleven percent of all patients undergoing prostatectomy developed fibrotic changes in the penis. This fibrosis led to penile curvature in 93%, "waistband" deformity in 24%, and palpable plaques in 69%. Therefore, it does appear that men undergoing radical prostatectomy by an open or robotic approach have a higher risk for developing PD than the general population. The mechanism responsible for this is not known but may include perioperative penile trauma, neurogenic consequences, or via a local release of cytokines that activate the abnormal wound-healing process in men susceptible to PD.

Hypogonadism

The possibility that low serum testosterone may be associated with PD has also been investigated. Results of studies have varied on this topic. Moreno and Morgentaler (2009) demonstrated that severity of curvature was worse in men with low free and total testosterone. Rhoden et al. could not demonstrate this association and concluded in their study that androgen serum levels and sexual dysfunction had no association to PD (Rhoden et al., 2010).

The presence of hypogonadism in patients with PD has been suggested to exaggerate the severity of PD. Nam et al. (2011) showed in a study of 106 patients with PD that curvature, plaque size, ED, and response to medical therapy were worse in patients with testosterone deficiency. Cavallini et al. (2012) investigated whether testosterone replacement in hypogonadal men with PD would affect treatment with intralesional verapamil injection. In these patients, supplementation with testosterone improved the efficacy of intralesional verapamil compared with those who did not receive testosterone replacement. Plaque area and penile curvature were also more severe in hypogonadal men with PD (Cavallini et al., 2012).

Collagen Disorders

There does appear to be an association of PD with other collagen disorders such as Dupuytren disease (DD). DD is believed to be transmitted in an autosomal dominant manner. The prevalence of DD in different geographic locations is extremely variable (0.2% to 56%), and it is not clear whether this is because of genetic or environmental factors. The literature concerning coexisting DD in patients with PD also demonstrates a very large range (0.01% to 58.8%) (Nugteren et al., 2011). As with PD, the prevalence of DD increases with age, from 7.2% among men in the 45- to 49-year-old age group up to 39.5% in those 70 to 74 years of age (Gudmundsson et al., 2000). Other studies have demonstrated DD in 21% to 22.1% of PD patients and in 6.7% who reported having a first-degree relative with DD (Carrieri et al., 1998; Nugteren et al., 2011). Other associated fibrotic conditions are contracture of the plantar fascia (Ledderhose disease) and tympanosclerosis, both of which are uncommon disorders (Box 73.2).

BOX 73.2 Associated Conditions

Aging
Diabetes
Erectile dysfunction
Psychological distress
Radical prostatectomy
Hypogonadism
Collagen disorders

KEY POINTS: EPIDEMIOLOGY

- The incidence of PD varies widely depending on the population being screened and is likely much higher than once thought. Current estimates are between 3% and 9%, and the peak age of onset of PD is the early 50s.
- A linear increase in prevalence can be seen from 30 to 49 years of age, with an exponential increase in prevalence at 50 years of age.
- PDE5 inhibitors have not been suggested to directly contribute to the development of PD; rather, their associated use in those with medical conditions that contribute to ED likely unmasks deformities that would have otherwise gone unrecognized.
- The prevalence of PD among diabetics has been shown to be 8.1% to 20.3% depending on the population screened, which is higher than in the general population. This may reflect particular patient populations, ethnic groups, referral patterns, and expertise of the physicians treating the disorder.
- The prevalence of ED in men with PD has been reported to be 37% to 58%.
- PD is not only a physically deforming but also a psychologically devastating disorder, with 48% of patients showing signs of moderate to severe depression; in general, these rates increase with the duration of PD. Penile shortening and inability to have intercourse are the two most common and consistent risk factors for emotional and relationship problems associated with PD.
- There appears to be an increased incidence of PD in men who have undergone radical prostatectomy, although further prospective studies are required to confirm this association.
- Although hypogonadism may be associated with PD, there is no clear evidence that it is a risk factor. Further study is indicated, and assessment of serum testosterone is recommended.

PENILE ANATOMY AND PEYRONIE'S DISEASE

The exact cause of PD remains to be determined, as noted earlier. Ongoing studies continue to clarify this disorder on the genetic, molecular, and anatomic level. The corpora cavernosa, the erectile bodies of the penis surrounded by the tunica albuginea, possess the ability to become rigid by becoming engorged with blood. **The tunica albuginea is a multilayered structure predominantly composed of type 1 collagen that is oriented with an inner circular and outer longitudinal layer interlaced with elastin fibers separated by an incomplete septum** (Brock et al., 1997; Gentile et al., 1996; Kelly, 2007). This septum is anchored into the inner circular layer and is key to the structural integrity of the tunica; without it, computer models have demonstrated that the stress generated by a full erection of one contiguous corporeal body would be sufficient to rupture the tunica albuginea (Mohamed et al., 2010). **These anchor sites are susceptible to microvascular trauma and tunical delamination, which may be one of the triggers leading to this disease** (Devine

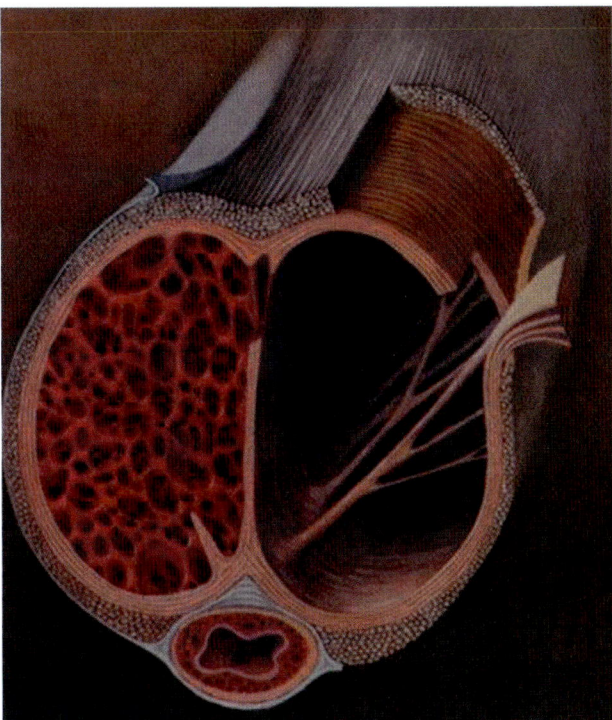

Fig. 73.2. The outer layer bundles, which are coarser and directed in a longitudinal manner, often form an incomplete layer (regions 4 to 5 o'clock, 7 to 8 o'clock, and 11 to 1 o'clock) and condense to form ligament-like structures. Artist's drawing of the penis depicts dorsal and ventral thickening and pillars. (Data from Brock G, Hsu GL, Nunes L, et al. The anatomy of the tunica albuginea in the normal penis and Peyronie's disease. *J Urol* 1997;157:276–81.)

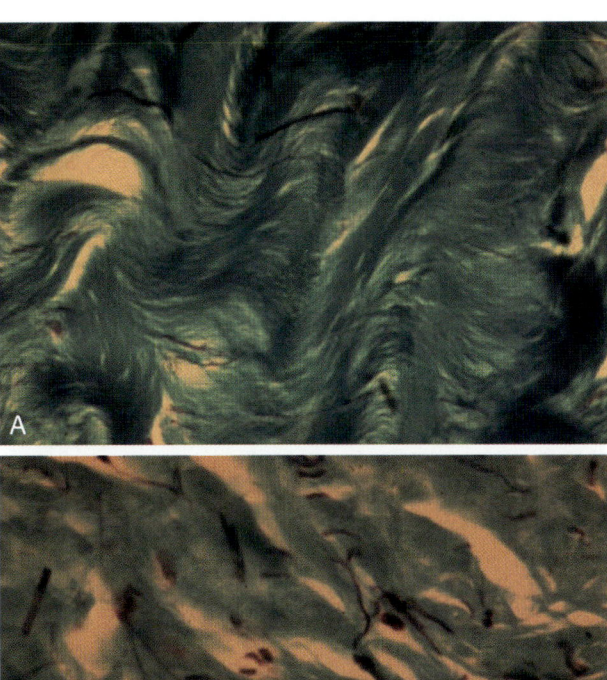
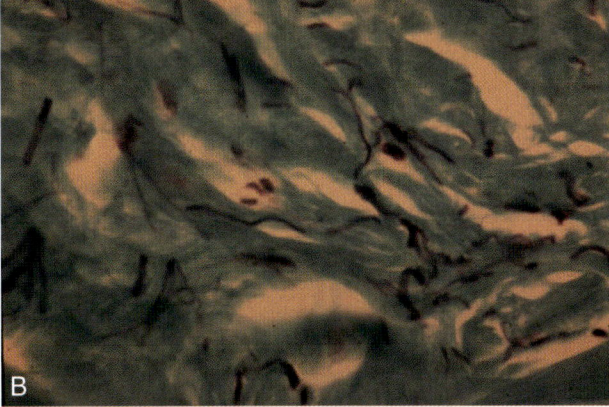

Fig. 73.3. Photomicrographs of the tunica albuginea. (A) Normal tunica albuginea demonstrating the polarized arrangement of collagen. (B) Peyronie's plaque demonstrating the nonpolarized arrangement of collagen and the haphazard arrangement of elastin. Collagen stains green; elastin stains black.

et al., 1997). The structure is further reinforced by intracavernous pillars, which anchor the tunica albuginea across the corpora cavernosa at the 2 to 6 o'clock and 10 to 6 o'clock positions, with finer pillars at the 5 and 7 o'clock positions (Fig. 73.2) (Brock et al., 1997). **It is interesting to note that 60% to 70% of plaques are located on the dorsal aspect of the penis and are usually associated with the septum** (Pryor and Ralph, 2002). It is possible that pressures on the penis during intercourse may cause a delamination between the two layers, activating the abnormal wound-healing process, which is trapped within the tunic, fostering the progressive scarring.

The longitudinal layer of the tunica albuginea is thinnest at the 3 and 9 o'clock positions of the corpora; it is completely absent between the 5 and 7 o'clock positions (Brock et al., 1997). **This may contribute to greater ease of dorsal buckling and may explain why most PD patients exhibit dorsal curvature** (Border and Ruoslahti, 1992; Brock et al., 1997; Devine et al., 1997; Devine and Horton, 1988; Jarow and Lowe, 1997). In normal tunical tissue, each layer appears to be distinct and is able to slide on the adjacent layer. The normal three-dimensional structure of the tunica affords great flexibility, rigidity, and tissue strength to the penis despite the fact that the tunica albuginea is quite thin—1.5 to 3.0 mm, depending on the position around the circumference. **Normal architecture is essentially lost consequent to this disease, resulting in what is known as a Peyronie's "plaque," which, when examined histologically, demonstrates disorganization of collagen fibrils and a decrease in and disorganization of elastin resulting in penile deformity caused by asymmetrical expansion of the corpora (Figs. 73.3 and 73.4)** (Akkus et al., 1997; Brock et al., 1997; Costa et al., 2009; Devine et al., 1997). When expansion is limited at one point along the circumference of the corpora by the inelastic scar of the Peyronie's plaque, deviation to that side occurs; a circumferential plaque may lead to an hourglass deformity (Akkus et al., 1997; Devine et al., 1997).

Impact of Wound Healing on the Development of Peyronie's Disease

In general, PD has been described as a wound-healing disorder of the tunica albuginea. Recent investigations have focused on the mechanisms of wound healing, fibrosis, and scar formation and have correlated the findings with the PD population. Normal wound healing involves three phases: an acute phase, a proliferative phase, and a remodeling phase. These are not to be confused with the acute and chronic phases of PD previously described. By understanding the wound-healing process, one gains a better understanding of PD, targets for drugs used to treat PD, and the animal models that have been developed for the study of PD. In general, during the **acute phase,** blood vessel injury leads to extravasation of blood and aggregation and activation of platelets that release chemotactic agents that act as promoters in the wound-healing cascade by activating and attracting neutrophils during the first 24 hours after clot formation, macrophages after 48 hours, and finally lymphocytes after 72 hours (DiPietro, 1995). Macrophages phagocytose dead or potentially injurious material and destroy bacteria or other foreign cells via oxygen free radical reactions. In addition, macrophages activate keratinocytes, fibroblasts, and endothelial cells by releasing potent tissue growth factors, particularly transforming growth factor-β (TGF-β), and other mediators such as TGF-α, heparin binding epidermal growth factor, fibroblast growth factor (FGF), and collagenase (DiPietro, 1995; Ravanti and Kahari, 2000).

The next phase of normal wound healing is the **proliferative phase,** which marks the shift toward tissue repair beginning at approximately 72 hours after injury and persisting for approximately 2 weeks. It is characterized by fibroblast and myofibroblast migration in response to TGF-β and platelet-derived growth factor (PDGF),

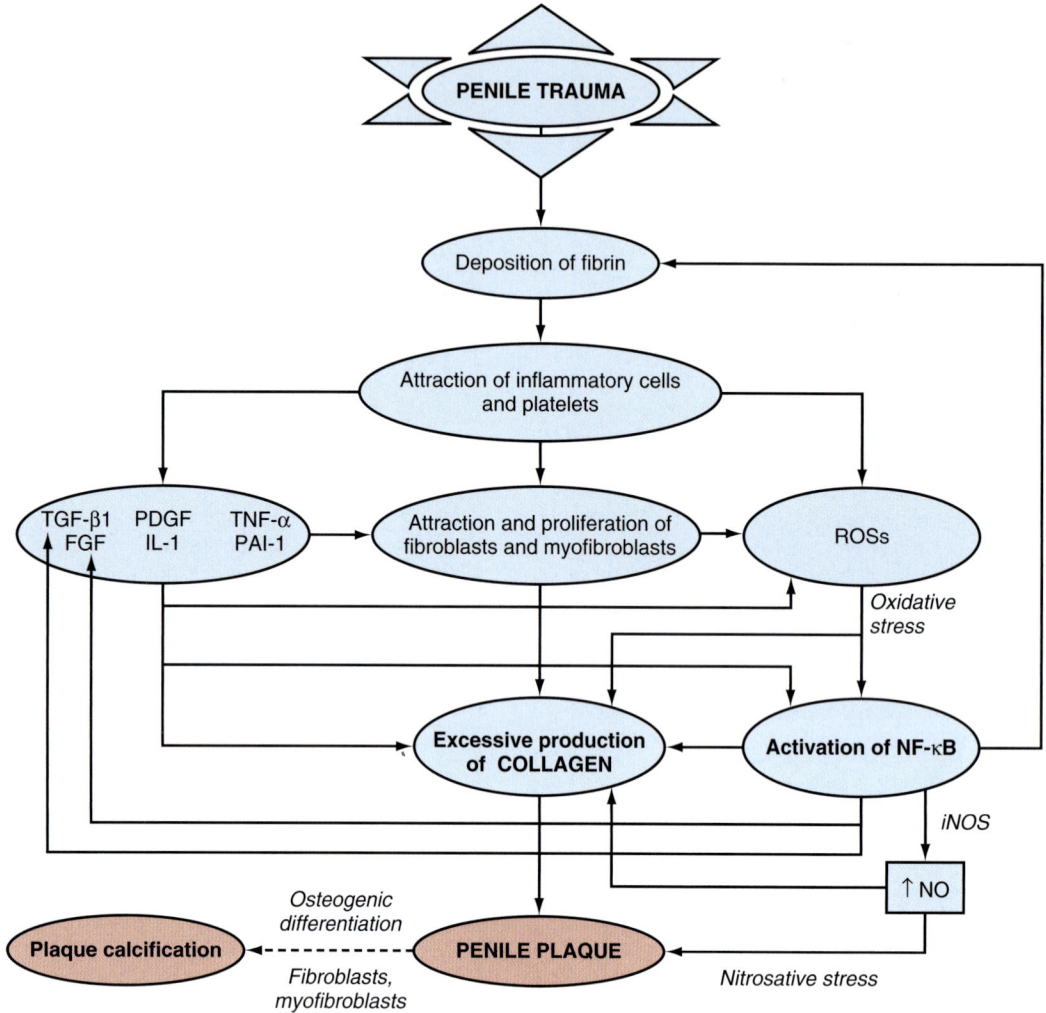

Fig. 73.4. Pathogenetic mechanisms of Peyronie's disease. *FGF*, Fibroblast growth factor; *IL*, interleukin; *iNOS*, inducible nitric oxide synthase; *NF-κB*, nuclear factor-κB; *NO*, nitric oxide; *PAI*, plasminogen activator inhibitor; *PDGF*, platelet-derived growth factor; *ROS*, reactive oxygen species; *TGF*, transforming growth factor; *TNF*, tumor necrosis factor. (Data from Paulis G, Brancato T. Inflammatory mechanisms and oxidative stress in Peyronie's disease: therapeutic "rationale" and related emerging treatment strategies. *Inflamm Allergy Drug Targets* 2012;11:48–57.)

and deposition of newly synthesized extracellular matrix (ECM) composed of type I and type III collagen, hyaluronan, fibronectin, and proteoglycans (Velnar et al., 2009). At this point, fibroblasts are stimulated by TGF-β to change into myofibroblasts, which contain thick actin bundles allowing for wound contraction. TGF-β also signals fibroblasts and myofibroblasts to synthesize types I and III collagen (Tomasek et al., 2002; Gelbard, 2008).

Finally, the **remodeling phase** begins and in the normal situation may last up to 1 or 2 years. The remodeling of an acute wound is tightly regulated by mechanisms that balance the simultaneous degradation and synthesis of collagen and other ECM macromolecules. Any alterations in this process may lead to abnormal wound healing with excessive scarring (Velnar et al., 2009). Matrix metalloproteinases (MMPs) (collagenases), produced by neutrophils, macrophages, and fibroblasts in the wound, are responsible for the degradation of collagen. They are subsequently held in check by inhibitory factors called tissue inhibitors of metalloproteinases (TIMPs). As the activity of TIMPs increases, there is a drop in matrix breakdown by metalloproteinase enzymes, thereby promoting new matrix accumulation (Ravanti and Kahari, 2000). **This balance between TIMPs and MMPs has also been studied in the pathogenesis of PD and is described later in this section.**

Over time, the highly disorganized initial deposition of collagen matrix becomes more oriented and cross-linked during the final stages of the remodeling phase. The process is regulated by a number of factors, with PDGF, TGF-β, and FGF being the most important (Velnar et al., 2009), but also including MMPs, TIMPs, fibrin, or plasminogen activator inhibitor-1 (PAI-1) (Taylor and Levine, 2007; Velnar et al., 2009). **Having accomplished this task, redundant fibroblasts and myofibroblasts are eliminated by apoptosis.** A fundamental understanding of the elements of normal wound healing provides a foundation for understanding which components may go awry in PD. It does appear that most basic science research in this field has focused on the development of the scarring process resulting in the exuberant scar found in men with PD. More recent research has focused on the dysregulation of remodeling that may be responsible for why the fibrosis does not resolve.

ETIOLOGY OF PEYRONIE'S DISEASE

The exact cause of PD has not yet been defined, although most would agree that some injurious stimulus is necessary to trigger the cascade of events that leads to PD in the susceptible individual (Bjekic et al., 2006; Carrieri et al., 1998; Devine et al., 1997; Jalkut et al., 2003; Jarow and Lowe, 1997; Nachtsheim and Rearden, 1996). Trauma may be perceived as a single event experienced by the patient or may take the form of repetitive microtrauma to the penis. Furey (1957) initially suggested that trauma was the primary cause of PD.

The proposed mechanism is that in the erect state, the pressures inside the penis can get quite high and acutely higher when external forces are placed on the penis during intercourse in particular. These pressures may exceed the elasticity and strength of the tunica tissues, resulting in a microfracture. A commonly held misconception is that the trauma to the penis must occur only when it is erect; however, others have noted that trauma to the flaccid penis may also trigger this process. In a recent review of their database of 228 patients (Levine et al., personal communication) who had recognized trauma to the penis shortly before the onset of PD, 16% reported a traumatic event to the flaccid penis (e.g., motor vehicle accident, sports-related injury). As the scar develops, there may also be an inflammatory response, resulting in the pain that can be present in the flaccid penis or when pressure is placed on the penis. Dorsal and ventral sheer stresses occurring during sexual activity may account for the more common dorsal location of plaques (Devine et al., 1997). Investigators have suggested that repetitive microtrauma to the penis leads to delamination of the tunica albuginea and vessels between the layers of the tunica (Somers and Dawson, 1997). This leads to microhemorrhage and initiates the wound-healing cascade described previously.

Carrieri et al. (1998) reported a 16-fold increase in PD in those who had undergone prior invasive procedures and a nearly 3-fold increase in PD in patients who had experienced genital and/or perineal trauma (Carrieri et al., 1998). It is also important to note that although trauma has been considered the most likely trigger activating PD, in our clinical experience no more than 30% of men recall a specific event involving injury to the penis close to the time when the scarring or pain began. Other investigators have reported 16% to 40% of patients having had antecedent trauma (Bjekic et al., 2006; Tal et al., 2012). An injury occurring during sexual activity appears to be the most common recognized event associated with the onset of PD. An association with trauma and position of intercourse has been proposed for some time, based on the assumption that certain positions may be more apt to cause injury. This has not been verified but it does appear from anecdotal experience that the most common sexual position noted to precede the onset of PD is with the partner on top. In this position, a sudden "faux pas de coit" or missed thrust may lead to high intracorporeal pressures (Bitker et al., 1988).

Although trauma undoubtedly plays a pivotal role in the development of disease, it alone cannot explain why some men develop deformity whereas others do not. This is no better illustrated than by a study of 193 penile fracture patients in whom none went on to develop PD (Zargooshi, 2004). Several underlying factors have been considered responsible for PD; genetic predisposition, autoimmune factors, an aberration of localized wound healing, and even infection have been proposed as possible causes (Devine et al., 1991; Jalkut et al., 2003; Mulhall et al., 2002; Ralph et al., 1996; Taylor and Levine, 2007). Therefore, we should be careful about the medicolegal implications of referring to PD as the result of treatment(s) for ED, trauma to the flaccid penis, or catheterization or endoscopy, which are more likely just providing an opportunity for the forces at hand to activate the abnormal wound-healing response in the "genetically" susceptible man rather than being the cause of PD (Carrieri et al., 1998; Levine and Latchamsetty, 2002).

The following discussion focuses on specific research into the pathophysiology of PD.

Role of Oxygen Free Radicals and Oxidative Stress

Oxidative stress has a well-documented role in tissue fibrosis and has been studied in the pathogenesis of PD (Gonzalez-Cadavid and Rajfer, 2005). As stated previously, microvascular trauma leads to extravasation of blood, with thrombus formation that leads to deposition of fibronectin and fibrin. Inflammation ensues with accumulation of inflammatory cells and production of reactive oxygen species (ROS). **During the early phase of PD, an increase in oxidative stress in the form of free radicals induces overexpression of fibrogenic cytokines and augmented transcription and synthesis of collagen.** ROS are increased by TGF-β1, which also directly inhibits collagenase and promotes collagen synthesis (Magee et al., 2002). ROS include superoxide anion, hydrogen peroxide, hydroxyl radical, organic hydroperoxide, alkoxy radicals, and peroxy radicals. Although NO seems to play an antifibrotic role, nitrosative stress and oxidative stress can lead to macromolecular damage, cytotoxic effects, lipid peroxidation, DNA fragmentation, collagen accumulation, and cellular dysfunction (Paulis and Brancato, 2012).

Role of Nitric Oxide in Peyronie's Disease

NO is a small reactive free radical that acts as both an intracellular and an extracellular regulatory molecule. Wound cells, including monocytes, macrophages, and fibroblasts, have been shown to synthesize NO through a nuclear factor-κB (NF-κB)–activated inducible NO synthase (iNOS)–dependent mechanism after injury. The iNOS isoform produces NO; it is usually considered a defense mechanism against infection or cancer, is associated with inflammation, and is significantly increased in human and animal PD plaques (Gonzalez-Cadavid, 2009). NO synthesized by iNOS reacts with ROS, thus reducing ROS levels and presumably inhibiting fibrosis. **The antifibrotic effects of NO may be mediated at least in part by the reduction of myofibroblast abundance and may lead to a reduction in collagen I synthesis** (Vernet et al., 2005). **NO may also play an antifibrotic role by activating guanylyl cyclase, thus producing cyclic guanosine monophosphate (cGMP), which has been suggested to inhibit plaque** formation (Ferrini et al., 2002; Valente et al., 2003).

Role of Myofibroblasts in Peyronie's Disease

The excessive deposition of collagen and ECM accompanied by the loss of functional cells that characterizes tissue fibrosis is caused in some cases by the appearance and accumulation of myofibroblasts (Gonzalez-Cadavid, 2009). Twenty percent of cells cultured from PD tunica albuginea are in fact myofibroblasts, suggesting that they may be one of the primary factors leading to fibrosis in PD (Mulhall et al., 2002). Proposed mechanisms for the presence and persistence of myofibroblasts include a decrease in myofibroblast apoptosis, and stimulation of fibroblast transformation to myofibroblasts by TGF-β and mechanical stress, which has been associated with hypertrophic scarring (Darby and Hewitson, 2007; Gelbard, 2008). **Myofibroblast activation is a key event in the development of fibrosis. Trauma to the tunica albuginea secondary to microscopic delamination increases the adherence of fibroblasts to their surroundings, exposing them to changes in ECM tension, and in the presence of appropriate cytokines initiates their differentiation into myofibroblasts** (Gelbard, 2008). When tension diminishes, myofibroblasts tend to undergo apoptosis. Gelbard postulated that if myofibroblasts are continuously exposed to tension in the form of rigid corpora during erections, they may fail to undergo apoptosis and subsequently contribute to what appears to be a hallmark of PD—inappropriate and persistent stimulation of the wound-healing process (Gelbard, 2008).

Role of Transforming Growth Factor-β1 in the Etiology of Peyronie's Disease

TGF-β1 has been shown to be significantly associated with PD (El-Sakka et al., 1997). **TGF-β is a strong activator of myofibroblasts and is known to be a potent fibrotic growth factor by stimulating the deposition of ECM.** TGF-β binds cell surface receptors and, through a signal transduction cascade, leads to the deposition and remodeling of ECM by stimulating cells to simultaneously **(1) increase the synthesis of most matrix proteins** (Ihn, 2002); **(2) decrease production of matrix-degrading proteases while increasing the production of inhibitors of these proteases** (Knittel et al., 1999); **and (3) modulate the expression of integrins** (Margadant and Sonnenberg, 2010). The action of TGF-β in tissue repair has been shown to involve an initiation of complex sequences of monocyte chemoattraction, induction of angiogenesis, and control of the production of cytokines and other inflammatory mediators (Border and Ruoslahti, 1992). Moreover, TGF-β stimulates the synthesis of individual matrix components including fibronectin, tenascin, collagens, and proteoglycans while simultaneously blocking matrix degradation by decreasing the synthesis of proteases and increasing levels of protease inhibitors (Balza et al., 1988). All of these events can be beneficial in tissue repair; however, the deposition of ECM at a site of tissue injury can lead to scarring and fibrosis. Furthermore, the ability of TGF-β to induce its own production may be the key to the development of scarring and fibrosis (Border and Ruoslahti, 1992). TGF-β1 is not the only member of the large TGF-β superfamily of growth and differentiation factors (GDFs) that have been implicated as fibrotic agents. Myostatin, also known as *GDF-8*, has been proposed not only as an inhibitor of myofiber formation but also as an inducer of fibrosis. Myostatin is expressed in the normal human tunica albuginea (TA) and is overexpressed in PD plaque. Myostatin stimulates myofibroblast generation and collagen deposition in normal tunic and is upregulated by TGF-β1. Myostatin seems to potentiate the effects of TGF-β1 (Cantini et al., 2008).

Fibrotic Gene Expression in Peyronie's Disease

A variety of profibrotic and antifibrotic factors contribute to the development of PD plaque that leads to deformity (Grazziotin et al., 2004). Qian et al. (2004) performed DNA microarray analysis of PD tissue obtained from patients undergoing surgery for PD. The most highly upregulated gene found in the PD plaque, *PTN* or *OSF1*, codes for a secreted heparin-binding protein thought to stimulate mitogenic growth of fibroblasts and osteoblast recruitment, and is possibly related to plaque ossification. Proteins responsible for cell proliferation, cell cycling, and apoptosis were found to be increased, whereas Id-2, an inhibitor of myofibroblast differentiation, was downregulated. The second most upregulated gene, *MCP-1*, is critical to the inflammatory response and ossification (Graves, 1999; Graves et al., 1999). Genes related to myogenic conversion during wound healing and fibroblast differentiation into myofibroblasts were upregulated, whereas collagenase IV, which is critical for collagen degradation and is decreased in fibrosis, was downregulated (Magee et al., 2002). Qian et al. (2004) performed a study comparing gene-expression profiles of PD patients with those of DD patients. A series of 15 genes were upregulated and none were downregulated in the PD plaque versus the normal TA. Of the genes upregulated, the ones most prominently increased were MMPs involved in collagen breakdown, specifically *MMP-2* or *MMP-9* in one-half of the PD plaques, in addition to genes involved in actin-cytoskeleton interactions required for fibroblasts and myofibroblasts to generate contractile forces (Qian et al., 2004). According to the findings of another study, the lower expression of apoptotic genes may cause the persistence of collagen-producing cells that are upregulated, consequently resulting in plaque formation. Similar expression levels of apoptotic genes in both tunica albuginea and Peyronie's plaques may be caused by the generalized physiopathologic alterations in the tunica albuginea that lead to plaque formation at a vulnerable region subjected to recurrent trauma (Zorba et al., 2012).

Del Carlo et al. (2008) investigated the role of MMPs and TIMPs in the pathogenesis of PD by using harvested plaque from patients who had PD. PD tissue samples were found to have diminished or absent levels of MMP-1, MMP-8, and MMP-13 compared with matched perilesional tunica and non-PD controls. PD fibroblasts were cultured with soluble MMPs and TIMPs after treatment with TGF-β or interleukin-1β (IL-1β). They found that IL-1β stimulation increased the production of MMP-1, MMP-2, MMP-8, MMP-9, MMP-10, and MMP-13 in PD fibroblasts, whereas TGF-β increased the production of only MMP-10 and decreased the production of MMP-13, suggesting that PD fibroblasts can be induced to make MMPs (Del Carlo et al., 2008). Baseline aberrant expression of p53, a cell cycle–regulating protein, has been demonstrated in PD fibroblasts and an absent response to sublethal DNA damage. This suggests a role for an aberration in the p53 pathway in the pathogenesis of this condition (Mulhall et al., 2001).

When all of this information is taken together, it is not hard to understand why there are myriad clinical presentations and treatments for this very complex disease. A variety of alterations may be present in a given patient, which may manifest as fibrosis with penile deformity (see Box 73.2). This has been demonstrated by Qian et al., who found **marked heterogeneity in gene expression profiles among men with PD** (Qian et al., 2004). As suggested by the ensuing section on medical therapy, different medical treatments that target different disease mechanisms may not work uniformly among the PD population (see Fig. 73.4).

KEY POINTS: ANATOMY AND ETIOLOGY

- The longitudinal layer of the tunica albuginea is thinnest at the 3 and 9 o'clock positions of the corpora; it is completely absent between the 5 and 7 o'clock positions. This absence of the longitudinal layer ventrally may contribute to greater ease of dorsal buckling and may explain why most PD patients exhibit dorsal curvature.
- Normal architecture is essentially lost consequent to this disease, resulting in what is known as a Peyronie's plaque, which, when examined histologically, demonstrates disorganization of collagen fibrils and a decrease and disorganization of elastin, resulting in penile deformity caused by asymmetric expansion of the corpora.
- Antecedent trauma has been reported in 16% to 40% of patients; most would agree that some injurious stimulus is necessary to trigger a cascade of events that lead to PD in the susceptible individual.
- Oxygen free radicals, oxidative stress, NO, myofibroblasts, TGF-β1, and fibrotic gene expression all play a key role in the development of PD and are key avenues for future research to further elucidate the exact mechanism behind the development of PD.

SYMPTOMS

The most frequent presenting symptoms of patients with PD include penile pain, erect deformity, palpable plaque, and ED (Chung et al., 2011a; Pryor and Ralph, 2002; Smith et al., 2008b). Many men who have PD visit the doctor with a self-misdiagnosis of ED. Not all patients experience pain or are able to palpate a plaque, but the shortening, hinge effect, distal softening, and curvature, when present, are readily recognized. Pain, when present in the acute phase, can occur in the flaccid condition with palpation of the plaque, with erection, or during intercourse. Once the disease process is stable, most pain will resolve, but in some men the pain persists with what has been referred to as "torque" pain associated with a pulling sensation on the plaque when a strong erection occurs (Levine and Larsen, 2013). This should not be confused with the inflammatory pain of the acute phase.

Although curvature can be one of the most recognized and distressing deformities associated with PD, many men are capable of sexual activity with curvature up to 60 degrees, particularly if the curvature is dorsal and more gradual along the shaft. Men with ventral or lateral curvatures may have a more difficult time with intromission because of discomfort. Yet, it is not uncommon to hear that the partner does not complain of discomfort during coitus, regardless of the degree or direction of curvature. Patient estimates of curvature are unreliable. One study demonstrated that 50% of patients overestimated their degree of curvature by an average of 20 degrees (Bacal et al., 2009). Classification by degree of curvature was introduced by Kelami (1983). One center reported on the distribution of curvature by the Kelami classification and found that 39.5% of patients had 30 degrees (mild) or less, 35% had 31 to 60 degrees (moderate), and 13.5% had more than 60 degrees of curvature (severe); 12% had no curvature but did experience an hourglass deformity resulting in an unstable erection (Kadioglu et al., 2011b).

The PD plaque can manifest in a variety of configurations including cords; simple nodules; coinlike, irregular dumbbell shapes; or I-beam plaques. It appears that virtually all plaques have a septal component, which supports the concept of delamination of tunical fibers as a result of axial forces on the septum (Jordan, 2007). Pure septal plaques have also been reported and may result in narrowing, shortening, or no recognized deformity at all (Bella et al., 2007).

The orientation of the plaque usually defines the deformity. Therefore, patients with a simple dorsal plaque are most apt to have dorsal curvature; but if there is transverse or spiraling scarring, which can be partial or circumferential, this could result in varying degrees of indentation including an hourglass deformity, which can result in an unstable penis, or a hinge effect as a result of the inability to tolerate axial forces in the erect condition (Pryor and Ralph, 2002). The distal softening of the shaft beyond the plaque is also difficult to understand, because dynamic infusion cavernosometry and cavernosography (DICC) studies have found that the pressures within the corpora cavernosa are equal, when measured, proximal and distal to the plaque (Jordan and Angermeier, 1993). The cause of distal flaccidity remains speculative and includes local cavernosal fibrosis extending from the involved tunic (Ralph et al., 1992) and site-specific venous leak.

EVALUATION OF THE PATIENT

As with all medical conditions, a detailed history is a critical part of the evaluation of the patient with PD (Levine and Greenfield, 2003). The intake interview should focus on presenting signs and symptoms such as pain, deformity, and palpable plaque. The assessment should also include whether onset was gradual or sudden and the estimated time that symptoms began; it should be determined if there was any inciting event that may have triggered the process, including direct external penile trauma to the flaccid or erect penis or instrumentation. The patient should be asked whether there is any personal or family history of other fibrotic disorders including DD and Ledderhose disease (Fig. 73.5). **Patients should be carefully queried as to their erectile capacity, but ultimately the question is whether the patient is capable of intromission or incapable because of deformity and/or diminished rigidity. A useful question that has been shown to be an effective predictor of postoperative erectile function is "If your penis was straight with the same quality of rigidity that you have now, do you think it would be adequate for penetrative sexual activity?"** (Levine and Greenfield, 2003; Taylor et al., 2012).

Clearly if the patient does not feel his erections would be satisfactory with or without pharmacotherapy, this can help direct the patient to treatment with a penile prosthesis and straightening maneuvers; nonsurgical or other surgical approaches could result in improvement of deformity, but if there is persistent ED, such treatment would likely not give the patient a sexually functional erection.

Further information to be obtained from the sexual history will be whether there are any vascular risk factors for ED, including a history of diabetes, hypertension, elevated cholesterol, and smoking. This is also a useful time to determine if there are issues with premature or delayed ejaculation. A list of medications may also indicate underlying medical conditions that may predispose to ED.

The recently validated PD questionnaire (PDQ) (Rosen et al., 2008; Hellstrom et al., 2013) addresses not only the concerns of the patient regarding structural changes of the penis but also how PD affects his overall psychological condition. The current questionnaire has 15 questions assessing three domains, including (1) Peyronie's psychological and physical symptoms (six items), (2) penile pain (three items), and (3) the effects of PD symptoms (six items). Each domain is intended to be an independent measure, and the scores are not summed for a total instrument score. Higher scores indicate a greater negative impact. With further experience, it may prove to be a useful assessment tool for patients making treatment decisions. The PDQ can be downloaded at http://www.endo.com/File%20Library/Products/Other/PDQ_from_Protocol_1-25.pdf.

The value of a photograph taken at home of the erect penis has been controversial because of the inability to adequately represent and measure a three-dimensional deformity (Bacal et al., 2009; Ohebshalom et al., 2007). At the current time, with the prevalence of smartphones, a photograph can be taken by the patient from above and from the side in the erect state, which can be useful during the initial consultation to get a general impression of the direction and severity of the deformity.

The physical examination should include a general assessment of the femoral pulses, appearance of the flaccid penis, and whether it is circumcised. **To assess the Peyronie's plaque, the penis should be examined on stretch, which allows easier identification of the plaque (Fig. 73.6).** The location of the plaque may be useful to

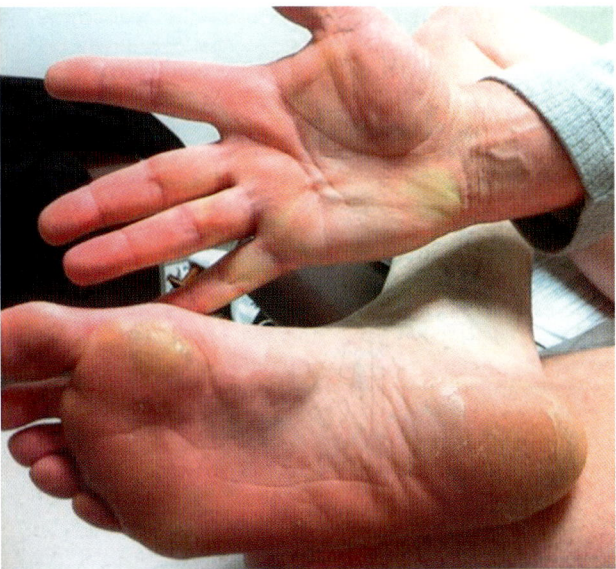

Fig. 73.5. This patient had physical evidence of Dupuytren, Ledderhose, and Peyronie's diseases.

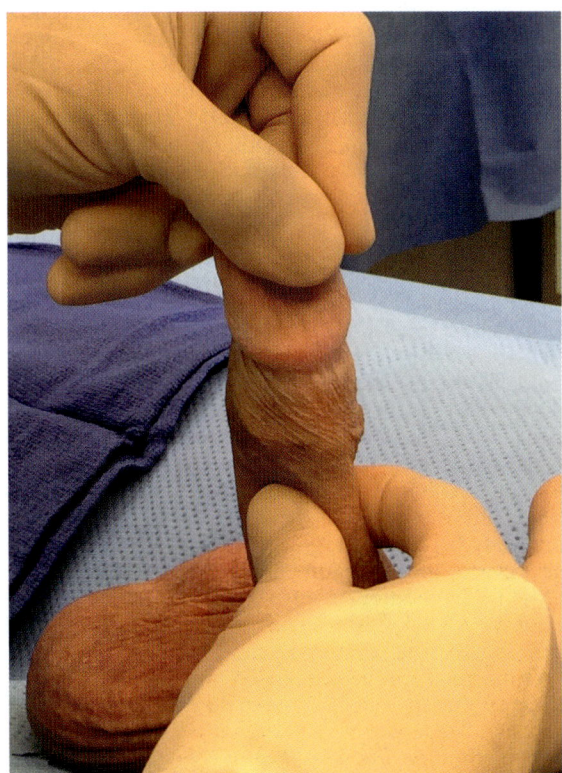

Fig. 73.6. Palpation of the penis on stretch facilitates identification of plaque.

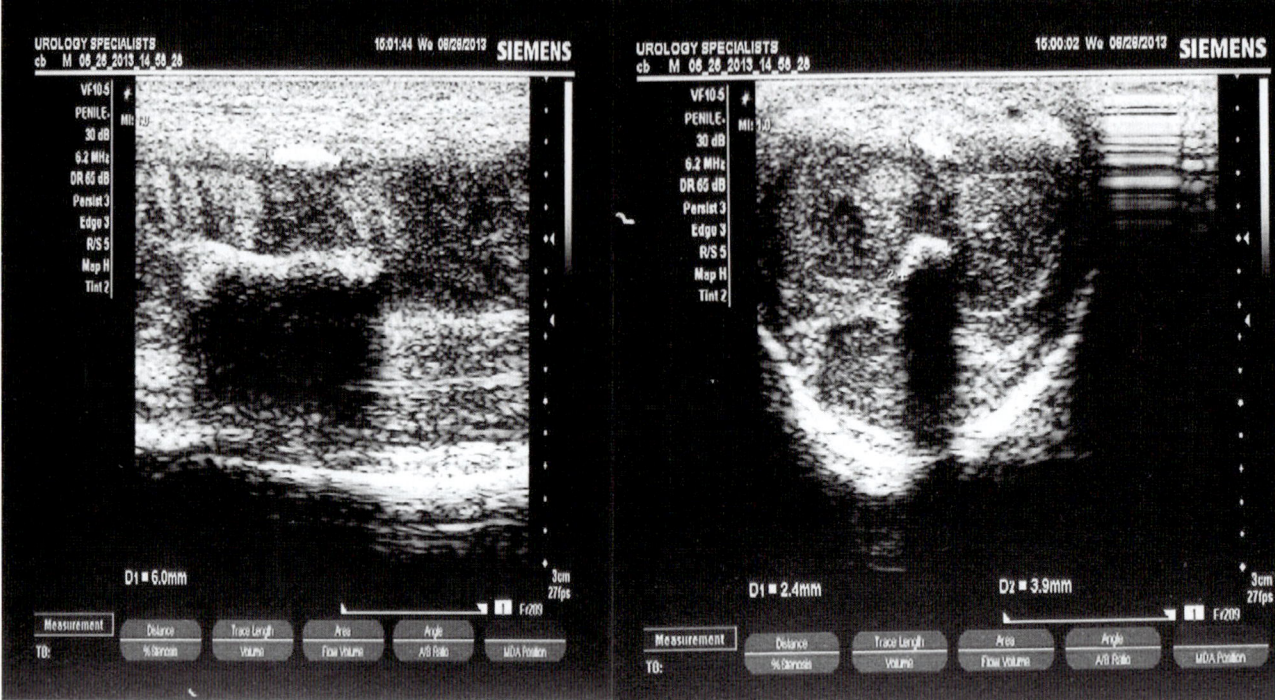

Fig. 73.7. This ultrasound image demonstrates areas of dorsal and ventral calcification. Note shadowing behind calcified plaques.

record, but measurement of the size of the plaque with any modality has been found to be inaccurate because the plaque is rarely a discrete lesion (Bacal et al., 2009; Hatzimouratidis et al., 2012; Levine and Burnett, 2013; Ralph et al., 2010). It has irregular borders and often extends into a septal cord (Levine and Greenfield, 2003; Ralph et al., 2010). **Furthermore, there is no evidence that a reduction in plaque size as a result of treatment is associated with improvement of deformity** (Levine and Burnett, 2013). **The stretched penile length (SPL) is also a critical parameter to measure at the initial consultation. This is performed by placing the penis on stretch by grasping the glans and pulling at a 90-degree angle away from the body** (Wessells et al., 1996). This parameter should be documented, as patient perception of loss of penile length is typically overestimated. It is preferred to measure from the pubis to the corona dorsally, as these are two fixed points and facilitate repeated measurement during the course of treatment and follow-up. The consistency of the plaque may be recorded. A "rock hard" plaque may be an indicator of calcification but will need to be confirmed with some form of imaging, preferably ultrasonography (Fig. 73.7). A calcified plaque is readily identified on ultrasonography because of the hyperdensity of the plaque with shadowing behind it. Computed tomography and magnetic resonance imaging have little value in the evaluation of the patient with PD, but further investigation is ongoing to determine if these modalities can provide prognostic information (Andresen et al., 1998; Hauck et al., 2003).

Only recently has it been recognized that calcification may occur early after the onset of the scarring process, and therefore the previously held notion that calcification is an indication of chronic, severe, and/or mature disease appears untrue (Levine et al., 2013). Calcification is most likely the result of a different genetic subtype of PD in which there is activation of genes involved in osteoblastic activity (Vernet et al., 2005). Why some plaques undergo mineralization and others do not remains unknown, but it does appear that the extent of mineralization may have a bearing on a successful response to nonsurgical therapy; men with more extensive calcification are less likely to benefit from nonsurgical treatment (Chung et al., 2011a). Several investigators have indicated that intralesional injection therapy with verapamil and interferon (IFN) is less likely to be successful in men with significant calcification (Hellstrom et al., 2006; Levine et al., 2002). This is because the drug will not be able to get into or effect change within this mineralized tissue. Furthermore, investigators have also suggested that patients with extensive calcification are more apt to proceed to placement of a penile prosthesis (Breyer et al., 2007; Chung et al., 2012). Recently a calcification grading system was published. The investigators found that patients with grade 3, or the most extensive, calcification (>1.5 cm in any dimension or multiple plaques ≥1.0 cm) were more likely to undergo surgery when they also had satisfactory erectile function. This is in contradistinction to those who had less severe calcification of grade 1 (<0.3 mm) or grade 2 (0.3 to 1.5 cm) or no calcification in whom there was no evidence of an increased likelihood of proceeding to surgery (Levine et al., 2013).

Assessment of penile deformity in the erect state is critical to the evaluation. This has been shown to be most accurately measured after an office vasoactive injection as compared with a home photograph or vacuum-induced erection. As treatment of ED moves toward more invasive treatment, accurate assessment of penile deformity in the erect state is critical. **The AUA 2015 Guideline on Peyronie's Disease now recommends that in-office intracorporeal injection therapy should be performed in every patient before invasive intervention** (Nehra et al., 2015).

The role of vascular testing in the diagnosis of PD has not been clearly defined. In centers that see many patients with this disorder, duplex ultrasound analysis (usually with intracorporeal injection therapy) is routinely performed as part of the initial evaluation, especially for those who are considered surgical candidates (Hatzimouratidis et al., 2012; Levine and Burnett, 2013; Ohebshalom et al., 2007; Ralph et al., 2010). **The benefits of a complete duplex ultrasound assessment include identification of calcification during initial surveillance in the flaccid state, assessment of penile vascular flow parameters after intracavernosal injection of vasoactive agent, observation of the erectile response to the vasoactive injection compared with the patient's sexually induced erection at home, and provision of the best opportunity to objectively assess deformity** (Figs. 73.8 and 73.9; Box 73.3). **These parameters are absolutely critical to the decision process for the patient who is considering surgery** (Fig. 73.10).

Several studies have demonstrated that preoperative erectile function correlates strongly with postoperative surgical results (Jordan and Angermier, 1993; Levine and Greenfield, 2003; Taylor et al., 2012). In an analysis of the relationship of penile deformity to the vascular status of PD, patients with ventral curvature were most likely to have cavernous veno-occlusive dysfunction, which further confirms the concern about postoperative ED after grafting of ventral curves (Kendirci et al., 2005; Lowsley and Boyce, 1950).

Some authors have reported the use of dynamic infusion cavernosometry (DICC) as a tool to assess penile vascular integrity and, in particular, venous leakage before surgery (Alphs et al., 2010; Jordan, 2007). This test appears to add unnecessary invasiveness and expense and provides little value to the diagnostic evaluation over a well-done dynamic penile duplex ultrasonography. Although no standard evaluation for assessment of penile sexual sensitivity has been established, light touch and biothesiometry can be used (Levine and Burnett, 2013). Biothesiometry has been suggested to be an indirect measure of penile sexual sensation. This is controversial because no definitive controlled studies have been reported (Padma-Nathan, 1988). The assumption is that the vibratory nerves travel with the unique sexual nerves of the penis. Therefore, vibratory appreciation with the index fingers used as the positive control and anterior thighs as the negative control can be a surrogate assessment of sexual sensation, which may be compromised by scar infiltration into the sensory nerves or because of other underlying systemic disorders such as diabetes mellitus. In light of the proposed increased prevalence of hypogonadism with ED, a morning serum total testosterone level during the initial evaluation is recommended for men with ED, as per the recently updated AUA ED guideline, but not for men with PD and no ED (Burnett et al., 2018, Moreno and Morgantaler, 2009).

> **BOX 73.3** Value of Penile Duplex Ultrasonography for Peyronie's Disease
>
> - Identification and measurement of plaque calcification
> - Identification of corporeal fibrosis
> - Observation of erectile response to vasoactive intracavernosal injection
> - Measurement of penile vascular parameters (peak systolic velocity, end-diastolic velocity, and resistive index)
> - Optimum objective measurement of erect penile deformity (curvature, girth irregularities, hinge effect)

> **KEY POINTS: EVALUATION**
>
> - Detailed history includes onset of symptoms, vascular risk factors for ED, patient-estimated degree of deformity, and patient assessment of quality of erection with respect to rigidity.
> - Validated questionnaires include the PDQ to document the degree of effect associated with PD.
> - The physical examination focuses on palpability of plaque with the penis on stretch to enhance appreciation of plaque, stretched flaccid penile length, and presence of pain during palpation.
> - Penile deformity should be objectively assessed during a vasoactive drug injection–induced erection, especially if surgery is contemplated.

TREATMENT PROTOCOLS

Multiple treatment protocols have been developed and published. It should be recognized that these algorithms serve only as guidelines and that individualization is key to patient success, which depends on specific findings from the history, physical examination, duplex

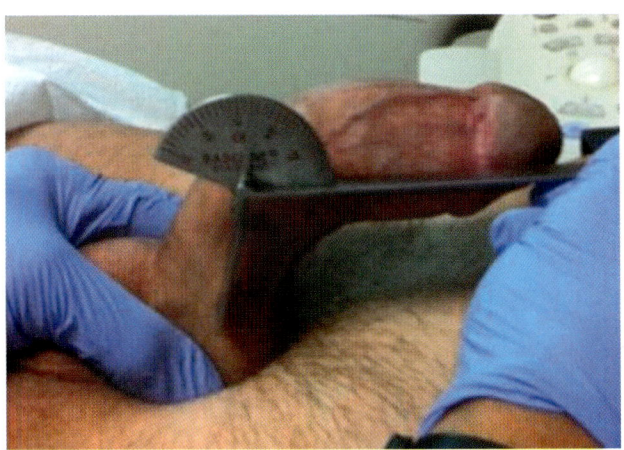

Fig. 73.8. Measurement of curvature with goniometer.

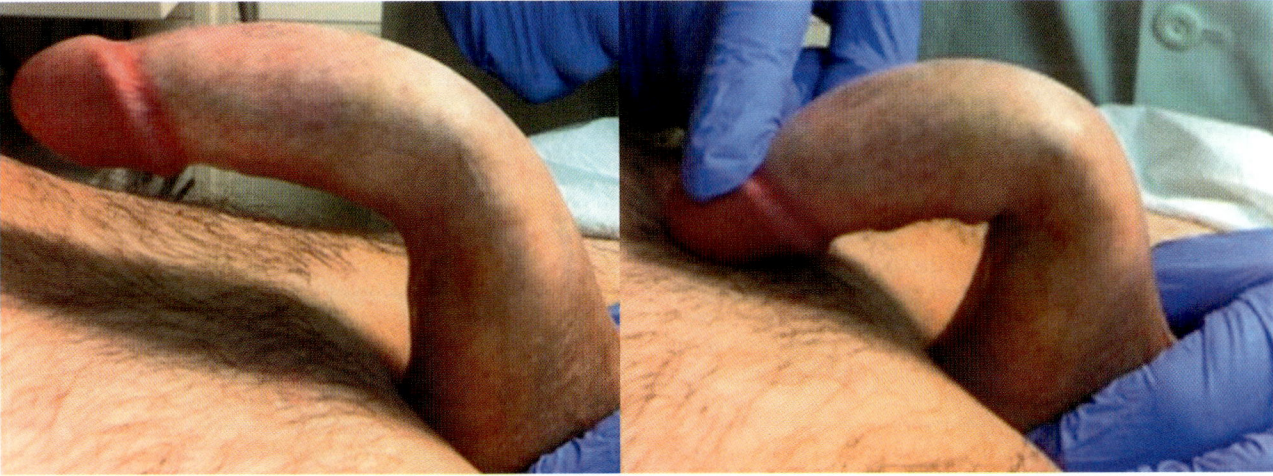

Fig. 73.9. Instability or a hinge effect of the erect penis caused by indentation is demonstrated in this severely dorsally bent penis with application of axial pressure.

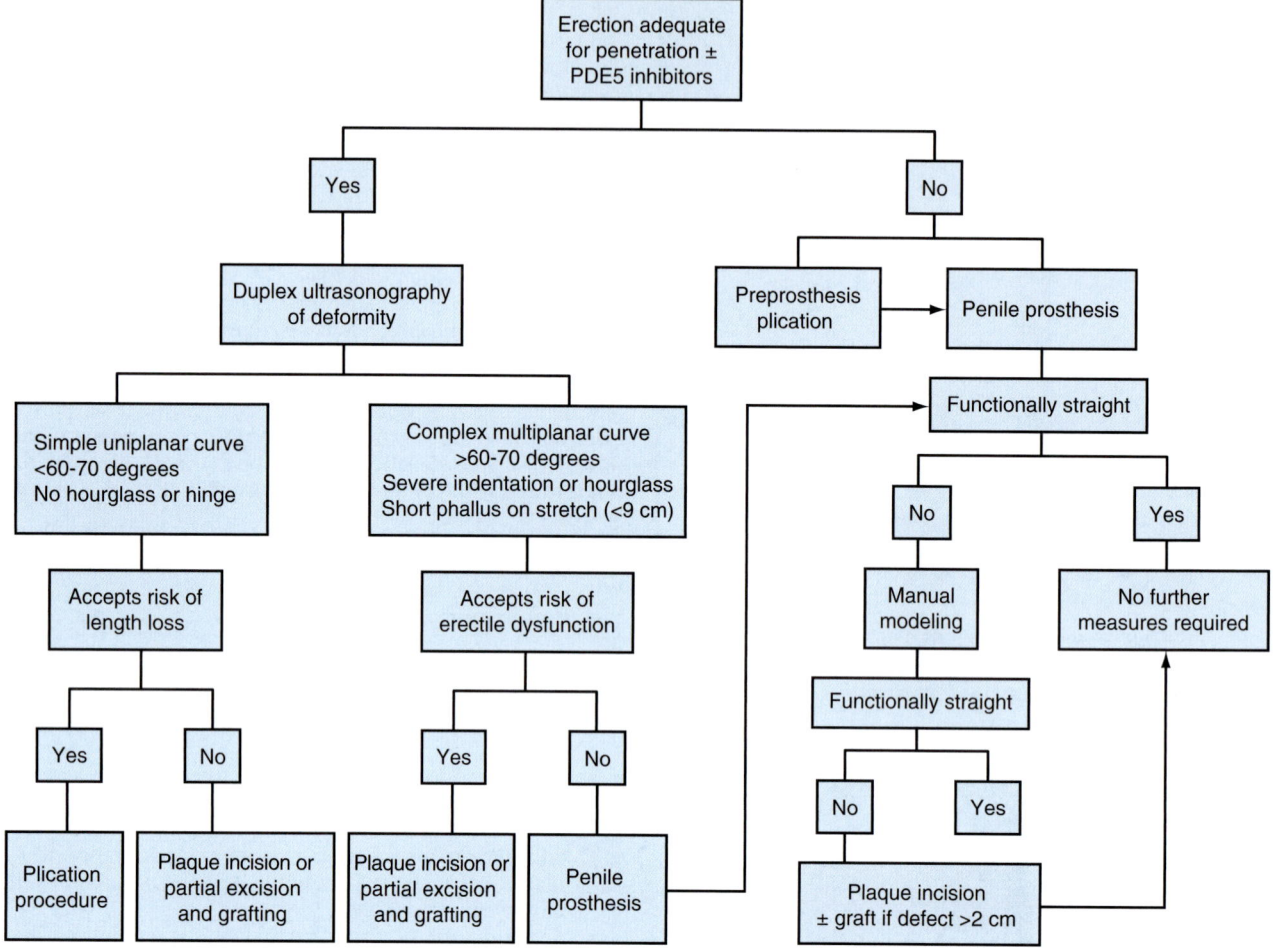

Fig. 73.10. Algorithm for the surgical management of Peyronie's disease. *PDE5*, Phosphodiesterase type 5.

ultrasonography, and patient goals (Bokarica et al., 2005; Hatzimouratidis et al., 2012; Levine and Greenfield, 2003; Levine and Lenting, 1997; Ralph et al., 2010). In an attempt to consolidate guidance to the practicing urologist, the Peyronie's Disease Guideline Panel of the American Urological Association Education and Research was created in 2013. In 2015, the AUA guideline on Peyronie's Disease was published (Nehra et al., 2015).

NONSURGICAL TREATMENT OF PEYRONIE'S DISEASE

Myriad nonsurgical treatments for PD have been offered since the time of de la Peyronie. Medical therapy until very recently has been compromised by suboptimal studies that failed to demonstrate meaningful results because of small numbers of subjects, lack of a control group, lack of randomization, and limited objective measurements (Schaeffer and Burnett, 2012). **In addition, the variety of disease presentations and its poorly understood cause contribute to treatments that have not addressed the underlying pathophysiology of this wound-healing disorder.** As a result, all oral and topical treatments, with the exception of NSAIDs, have been delegated to the "should not offer" status in the 2015 AUA guidelines. In this section, we review the contemporary treatments and focus on placebo-controlled studies when possible.

Some patients require only reassurance, particularly if there is no difficulty or pain for the patient or his partner in accomplishing penetrative sex. Patients should also be reassured that this is not a disorder that will degenerate into a cancer and is therefore not life-threatening.

Oral Medications

Potaba

Potassium para-aminobenzoate (Potaba) is a member of the vitamin B complex. Its mechanism of action has not been studied since 1959, when Zarafonetis and Horrax **demonstrated in fibroblast cell cultures that potassium para-aminobenzoate can reduce the formation of collagen.** According to this in vitro study, it is believed that this drug decreases serotonin levels by increasing monoamine oxidase activity, resulting in enhancement of the endogenous antifibrotic properties of tissues (Zarafonetis and Horrax, 1959).

In a randomized double-blind placebo-controlled trial of 103 treatment-naïve PD patients with noncalcified plaque, 51 patients were assigned to treatment with potassium para-aminobenzoate and 52 to placebo. Mean plaque size decreased in the treatment arm, whereas plaque size remained stable over 12 months of follow-up in the placebo arm. Penile deviation remained stable in those receiving active drug; penile curvature deteriorated significantly in 32.5% of those receiving placebo. No significant differences concerning decrease in pain could be observed between the two groups. The authors concluded, "**Potassium paraaminobenzoate appears to be useful to stabilize the disorder and prevent progression of penile curvature**" (Weidner et al., 2005). No severe adverse events occurred in the study; however, acute hepatitis associated with administration of potassium para-aminobenzoate for PD has been reported (Roy and Carrier, 2008). **Because there is little evidence of benefit with potassium para-aminobenzoate in placebo-controlled trials and it is expensive and difficult to consume (24 tablets daily), the AUA 2015 PD guideline does not recommend its use.**

Vitamin E

Vitamin E is one of the oldest described oral treatments for the treatment of PD (Scardino and Scott, 1949). Vitamin E, a fat-soluble vitamin metabolized in the liver and excreted in bile, is an antioxidant that **is thought to limit oxidative stress of ROS known to be increased during the acute and proliferative phases of wound healing.** Increased free-radical expression and a prolonged inflammatory phase of wound healing have been demonstrated in PD. **Treatment with vitamin E inactivates circulating free radicals that otherwise would inhibit NO from exerting its positive effects on vascular smooth muscle** (Safarinejad et al., 2007).

Several well-designed studies have demonstrated no significant improvement in pain, curvature, and plaque size when compared with placebo (Ralph et al., 2010). Pryor and Farell (1983) conducted a double-blind, placebo-controlled crossover study evaluating vitamin E for the treatment of PD in 40 subjects. No significant improvements were noted in plaque size or penile curvature (Pryor and Farell, 1983). Gelbard et al. compared treatment with vitamin E with the natural history of PD in 97 subjects with disease duration ranging from 3 months to 8 years; no significant differences were found between the two groups in terms of curvature, pain, or the ability to have intercourse (Gelbard et al., 1990). In a randomized double-blind placebo-controlled study of a total of 236 men with PD, vitamin E failed to show benefit with respect to pain, curvature, or plaque size when compared with placebo (Safarinejad et al., 2007). Although there were no significant observed adverse effects reported in this study, there is evidence that vitamin E may increase the risk for cerebrovascular events (Brown et al., 2001). **Vitamin E is the most frequently recommended oral agent in spite of studies showing no benefit over placebo** (LaRochelle and Levine, 2007; Shindel et al., 2008). **The AUA 2015 PD guideline does not recommend its use.**

Tamoxifen

Tamoxifen is a selective estrogen receptor modulator that has both agonist and antagonist effects on target tissues depending on tissue-specific estrogen receptor expression. It has also been demonstrated that tamoxifen can induce the production of TGF-β in an estrogen receptor–independent fashion (Colletta et al., 1990). The use of tamoxifen for the treatment of PD is truly fascinating and underscores how complex the role of TGF-β is in the development of PD. TGF-β released by platelets and activated macrophages plays a central role in the inflammatory response and wound healing. In normal healing, it promotes matrix synthesis by fibroblasts and is self-regulated in an autocrine fashion. However, higher concentrations of TGF-β in the cellular environment inhibit the inflammatory response, causing macrophage deactivation and T-lymphocyte suppression, thus preventing further fibrogenesis (Wahl et al., 1989). This was the initial reasoning for Ralph et al. (1992) to report in a nonrandomized study on the initial use of tamoxifen for the treatment of PD (Ralph et al., 1992).

The initial beneficial effects previously reported were not confirmed in a randomized placebo-controlled trial of 25 patients with PD (Teloken et al., 1999). **The study demonstrated no significant improvement with respect to pain, penile deformity, or plaque size when compared with placebo** (Teloken et al., 1999). **The AUA 2015 PD guideline does not recommend its use.**

Colchicine

Colchicine has been demonstrated to have several different potential mechanisms of action in the treatment of PD. **By binding to tubulin and causing it to depolymerize, colchicine inhibits cell mitosis, mobility, and adhesion of leukocytes; inhibits transcellular movement of collagen; and stimulates the production of collagenase** (Ehrlich and Bornstein, 1972; El-Sakka et al., 1999; Taylor, 1965).

In a randomized double-blind placebo-controlled study to determine the effectiveness and safety of colchicine, 84 PD patients with noncalcified plaque were randomized to colchicine or placebo. Objective measurements did not demonstrate any difference in plaque size or penile curvature. **There were no substantial differences in response to treatment based on duration of disease or within the three Kelami classification groups** (Kelami, 1983). **Significant drug-related adverse effects in the colchicine group included gastrointestinal upset with diarrhea** (Safarinejad, 2004). **The AUA 2015 PD guideline does not recommend its use.**

Carnitine

Carnitine is a trimethylamine molecule that plays a unique role in cell energy metabolism (Reda et al., 2003). **L-Carnitine is hypothesized to act by increasing mitochondrial respiration and decreasing free radical formation** (Bremer, 1983).

In the same double-blind placebo-controlled study mentioned previously, Safarinejad et al. compared the effects of L-carnitine with placebo (Safarinejad et al., 2007). Fifty-nine PD patients were randomized to receive propionyl-L-carnitine, and 59 were randomized to placebo during the 6-month treatment period. **This study again did not show significant improvement in pain, curvature, or plaque size in patients with PD treated with propionyl-L-carnitine as compared with those treated with placebo. The AUA 2015 PD guideline does not recommend its use.**

Pentoxifylline

Pentoxifylline has been shown to block the TGF-β1–mediated pathway of inflammation and to prevent deposition of collagen type I and is a nonspecific phosphodiesterase inhibitor with combined anti-inflammatory and antifibrogenic properties. In an animal model of PD, pentoxifylline reduced the expression of collagen I, α-smooth muscle actin (ASMA), and plaque size by 95% (Valente et al., 2003). Pentoxifylline inhibits tunica albuginea–derived fibroblast proliferation in vitro and attenuates TGF-β–mediated elastogenesis and collagen type I deposition (Shindel et al., 2010). Elastogenesis is inhibited not by decreasing the amount of elastin produced but by inhibiting its deposition through an α_1-antitrypsin–related mechanism (Lin et al., 2010). **Pentoxifylline has also been shown to downregulate TGF-β and increases fibrinolytic activity** (Raetsch et al., 2002; Schandené et al., 1992). Pentoxifylline has been used successfully for the treatment of experimental autoimmune diseases, the presence of which has been suggested as a cause of PD (Ralph et al., 1996). **Pentoxifylline downregulates the release and the production of the profibrotic cytokine tumor necrosis factor (TNF), suppresses the production of platelet-activating factor, and inhibits its action on neutrophils** (Safarinejad et al., 2010).

In a randomized double-blind placebo-controlled study, 114 PD patients were randomized to receive pentoxifylline and 114 were randomized to placebo for 6 months. Of patients in the pentoxifylline group, 12 (11%) had disease progression versus 46 (42%) in the placebo group. **Improvement in penile curvature and plaque volume was significantly greater in patients treated with pentoxifylline than with placebo. The increase in International Index of Erectile Function (IIEF) total score was significantly higher in the pentoxifylline group.** One patient discontinued the medication because of adverse effects. There were no adverse effects in any of the vital signs or in the laboratory data. Pentoxifylline is a peripheral vasodilator and could induce hypotension; consequently, blood pressure should be monitored during treatment with this drug. The most common side effects include nausea, vomiting, dyspepsia, malaise, flushing, dizziness, and headache (Safarinejad et al., 2010). The AUA PD Guidelines Panel judged that some uncertainty remains regarding the efficacy of pentoxifylline given the limited evidence base; replication in a randomized design is needed before pentoxifylline can be recommended as a PD treatment.

Phosphodiesterase Type 5 Inhibitors

PDE5 inhibitors have been shown to be safe and effective in treating ED in patients with PD (Levine and Latchamsetty, 2002). Recently tadalafil was shown to significantly improve IIEF and quality-of-life

(QoL) scores when used in conjunction with penile extracorporeal shock wave therapy (ESWT) as compared with ESWT alone (Palmieri et al., 2012). **There was no advantage with respect to deformity.** (Please note that as per the 2015 AUA PD guideline, clinicians should not use ESWT for the reduction of penile curvature or plaque size).

PDE5 inhibitors have also been suggested as treatment for PD. **By increasing the levels of cGMP, PDE5 inhibitors can inhibit collagen synthesis and induce fibroblast and myofibroblast apoptosis, thus acting as antifibrotic agents by inhibiting scar development** (Gonzalez-Cadavid and Rajfer, 2010; Valente et al., 2003).

In a study by Chung et al., (2011b), **35 men with an isolated septal scar received tadalafil 2.5 mg daily over a 6-month period, after which 24 patients (69%) had resolution of the septal scar. The authors concluded that low-dose daily tadalafil is a safe and effective treatment option in septal scar remodeling** (Chung et al., 2011a). Although oral PDE5 inhibitors are recommended for the treatment of male erectile dysfunction, they are not recommended for the treatment of Peyronie's disease (Nehra et al., 2015).

Intralesional Injection

Verapamil

Calcium channel blockers were originally found to inhibit the incorporation of proline into ECM protein, thus leading to the conclusions that cellular calcium metabolism appears to regulate ECM production and that hypertrophic disorders of wound healing may respond to therapy with calcium channel antagonist drugs (Lee and Ping, 1990).

Verapamil is a calcium channel blocker that has been shown to significantly affect fibroblast function on several levels, including cell proliferation, ECM protein synthesis and secretion, and collagen degradation. In vitro Peyronie's plaque fibroblast proliferation is inhibited by 65% with verapamil at a concentration of 100 to 1000 mg/mL (Anderson et al., 2000). These changes may allow intralesional verapamil to retard, prevent, or possibly reverse plaque formation and progression of PD (Levine and Estrada, 2002). Recently a study demonstrated the mechanism of action of intralesional verapamil injection versus normal saline in a rat model. After verapamil injection, there were histologic changes and reduced plaque size and penile curvature. Verapamil injection also resulted in decreased collagen and elastin fibers, and reduced ASMA, an indicator of myofibroblast activity (Chung et al., 2013b).

Currently, intralesional verapamil is a popular treatment option for the conservative management of PD despite the fact that some studies have not shown as favorable a response (Shindel et al., 2008).

The first reported use of verapamil for the treatment of PD was by Levine et al. and was the first new intralesional treatment since steroid injection was introduced in 1957 (Furey, 1957; Levine et al., 1994). This was a nonrandomized dose-escalating study in 14 men who received biweekly injections of verapamil for 6 months. Subjectively, there was significant improvement in plaque-associated penile narrowing (100%) and curvature (42%). Objectively, a decreased plaque volume of more than 50% was noted in 30% of the subjects. Plaque softening was noted in all patients, and 83% noticed that plaque-related changes in erectile function had arrested or improved. There was no toxicity, nor did symptoms recur when improvement was noted. This preliminary study suggested that intralesional verapamil may be an economical and sensible nonoperative approach to the treatment of PD warranting further study (Levine et al., 1994). In a larger noncontrolled study, verapamil injection resulted in a reduction of pain in 97% of the patients, an improvement in sexual function in 72%, a subjective reduction of deformity in 86%, an improvement in distal rigidity in 93%, and an objective reduction of curvature in 54% (mean curve reduction of 25 degrees) (Levine, 1997).

Rehman et al. (1998) performed a single-blind study on 14 PD patients who were randomly assigned to injection with verapamil or saline. This study demonstrated a significant improvement in plaque size, plaque-associated penile narrowing, and quality of erection in the verapamil-treated men versus the control group. There was no significant difference with respect to penile curvature. There was no local or systemic toxicity except for an occasional ecchymosis or bruise at the injection site (Rehman et al., 1998). Bennett et al. showed in a shorter 3-month trial of 94 patients improvement in curvature in 18%, no change in 60%, and worsening in 22% and concluded that intralesional verapamil can, at a minimum, stabilize penile deformity (Bennett et al., 2007).

In a recent randomized single-blind placebo-controlled trial, Shirazi et al. (2009) randomized 80 patients to receive intralesional verapamil and 40 patients to receive a local saline injection. This study demonstrated no significant difference with respect to plaque size, pain, curvature, plaque softening, or improvement in sexual dysfunction in the active drug and control groups. This study concluded that although some trials have demonstrated intralesional verapamil to be an effective treatment for PD, further larger-scale studies are warranted given these negative findings to assess the effectiveness of intralesional verapamil for the treatment of PD (Shirazi et al., 2009). Drug concentration has also been evaluated, and although 10 mg/10 mL is the most commonly used dose and volume, Cavallini et al. (2007) showed a greater response to injection when 10 mg of verapamil was diluted with 20 mL of injectable saline (Cavallini et al., 2007). These studies highlight the potential for inconsistent results for men with PD, which may vary because of patient selection, presence of calcification, plaque location, drug administration technique, and sample size. Poor candidates for this treatment include those with extensive calcification, curvature of greater than 90 degrees, or ventral curvature, in which it is difficult to adequately infiltrate the plaque (Levine et al., 2002). Predictors of success with intralesional verapamil include younger age (younger than 40 years of age) and curvature greater than 30 degrees (Moskovic et al., 2011). Currently, the AUA PD guideline states that a physician may offer intralesional verapamil for the treatment of patients with Peyronie's disease but should counsel the patients on potential injection site side effects.

Nicardipine

Nicardipine is a dihydropyridine (DHP) type of calcium channel blocker. An in vitro study has suggested that it is more effective than a non-DHP type, verapamil, in reducing glycosaminoglycan biosynthesis and ECM production (Gürdal et al., 1992). Soh et al. (2010) performed the only study on the effectiveness of nicardipine for the treatment of PD. A total of 74 patients were assigned randomly to nicardipine versus saline. Nicardipine demonstrated a significant reduction of pain, improvement in IIEF-5 score, and reduction of plaque size when compared with placebo. Penile curvature was significantly improved in both the active drug and placebo groups without significant difference. There were no severe side effects, such as hypotension or other cardiovascular events (Soh et al., 2010). Nicardipine currently has no recommendations in the AUA 2015 PD guideline.

Interferon Alfa-2b

IFN alfa-2b was first investigated as a treatment for PD in 1991 in the in vitro studies by Duncan et al. (1991). In fibroblasts derived from Peyronie's plaques, the addition of IFN alfa-2b **decreased their rate of proliferation in a dose-dependent fashion, decreased the production of extracellular collagen, and increased the production of collagenase** (Duncan et al., 1991).

In a single-blind, multicenter, placebo-controlled, parallel study to assess the safety and efficacy of intralesional IFN alfa-2b, Hellstrom et al. (2006) randomized a total of 117 consecutive PD patients to IFN alfa-2b or saline. Improvement in penile curvature, plaque size and density, and pain resolution was significantly greater in patients treated with IFN alfa-2b versus placebo. **The treatment group demonstrated a mean decrease in curvature of 27% or 13.5 degrees versus 9% or 4.5 degrees in the placebo group. Although these results were statistically significant, the question arises whether the small difference between the IFN and saline is clinically** significant when taking into account the significant cost of the drug and its side-effect profile, which frequently includes flulike symptoms (fever, chills, and arthralgia) and minor penile swelling with ecchymosis. All of these symptoms were effectively treated with over-the-counter NSAIDs ingested before the injection procedure, and none lasted longer than 36 hours (Hellstrom et al., 2006). **This study was important because it was the first multicenter randomized placebo-controlled trial of intralesional injection for PD. It also was important because it showed that saline injection had little to no effect on penile deformity.**

Per the AUA 2015 PD guidelines, clinicians may administer intralesional interferon α-2b in patients with PD. However, patients should be counseled on the potential adverse events, including sinusitis, flulike symptoms, and minor penile swelling.

Collagenase Clostridium Histolyticum

The first US Food and Drug Administration (FDA)–approved drug for the treatment of PD, collagenase *Clostridium histolyticum* (CCH), is produced by the bacterium *C. histolyticum* and selectively degrades collagen types I and III in connective tissues despite the presence of TIMPs, which have been shown to be elevated in PD and to increase apoptosis of fibroblasts (Del Carlo et al., 2008; Matsushita et al., 2001; Morales et al., 1983; Syed et al., 2012). The recent flurry of investigation on this drug has come many years after the first time it was examined as a treatment for PD by Gelbard et al. (1982), who demonstrated that CCH significantly reduced the size of PD plaques, whereas elastic fibers, vascular smooth muscle, and axonal sheaths were not affected (Gelbard et al., 1982).

In the first prospective, randomized, double-blind, placebo-controlled study of CCH, 49 men with PD were treated with CCH, resulting in significant improvements in plaque size and penile deformity (Gelbard et al., 1993). All patients with a penile bend of 30 degrees or less and/or palpable plaque less than 2 cm responded (N = 3); 36% of patients with a penile bend of 30 to 60 degrees and/or 2 to 4 cm of palpable plaque responded; and 13% of patients with a penile bend of greater than 60 degrees and/or greater than 4 cm of palpable plaque responded. CCH was well tolerated, with no allergic reactions and no significant changes in laboratory parameters (Gelbard et al., 1993). Further investigation was encouraged but took years because of absence of industry support.

In a phase II trial, 25 patients with PD received three intralesional injections of 10,000 units of CCH over 7 to 10 days, with a repeat of treatment at 3 months to assess change from baseline in penile deviation angle and plaque size (Jordan, 2008). A decrease in deviation angle of at least 25% was achieved in 58% of patients, and 95% of patients experienced a reduction in plaque size (Jordan, 2008). More than 50% of patients in this series were considered "very much improved" or "much improved" at all time points in the study; approximately one-third were considered to show minimal improvement or no change, resulting in an investigator's assessment of "worse."

Patients receiving CCH and modeling had a significant change in curvature of penis and decrease in the PD symptom effect score compared to placebo and to CCH without modeling (Gelbard et al., 2012). Patients receiving CCH and modeling had a significant change in curvature of the penis and decrease in the PD symptom effect score compared with placebo (Gelbard et al., 2012).

The phase III IMPRESS (Investigation for Maximal Peyronie's Reduction Efficacy and Safety Studies) I and II trials examined the clinical efficacy and safety of CCH intralesional injections in subjects with PD (Gelbard et al., 2013). A total of 417 and 415 subjects, respectively, went through a maximum of four treatment cycles, each separated by 6 weeks. Men received up to eight injections of 0.58 mg CCH, two injections per cycle separated by approximately 24 to 72 hours with the second injection of each followed 24 to 72 hours later by penile plaque modeling. Men were stratified by baseline penile curvature (30 to 60 degrees versus 61 to 90 degrees) and randomized to CCH or placebo 2 : 1 in favor of active drug. Post hoc meta-analysis of IMPRESS I and II data revealed that **men treated with CCH showed a mean 34% improvement in penile curvature, representing a mean change of −17.0 degrees ± 14.8 degrees per subject, compared with a mean 18.2% improvement in placebo-treated men, representing a mean change of −9.3 ± 13.6 degrees per subject (P < .0001).** The mean change in PD symptom effect score was significantly improved in treated men versus men on placebo (−2.8 ± 3.8 vs. −1.8 ± 3.5, P = .0037). **Patients with extensive calcification, ventral plaques, and disease duration less than 12 months were excluded.** Although serum antibodies to CCH developed in virtually all patients studied, no adverse events were noted as a result. The primary and frequently noted side effect was varying degree of ecchymosis and local penile bruising. Serious adverse events included corporeal rupture in three patients and penile hematoma in three patients. All three corporeal ruptures and one of the three penile hematomas were successfully repaired surgically; another hematoma was successfully drained percutaneously (Gelbard et al., 2013).

The most serious complication of CCH is penile fracture. It is believed that injection weakens the corporal albuginea surrounding the plaque, making it more vulnerable to breaking. The rate of corporal fracture ranges from 0% to 4.9% (Beilan et al., 2018, Jordan 2008, Gelbard et al., 2013, Nguyen et al., 2017). **A pooled analysis of six clinical trials (including the IMPRESS trials) demonstrated that although 85% of patients experienced at least one side effect, most were minor. Only 9 of 1044 patients (0.9%) had a serious side effect, and 4 of 1044 (0.4%) had a penile fracture** (Carson et al., 2015).

There is no consensus treatment protocol for CCH injections. **The current standard of care based on the IMPRESS trials is up to four total treatment sessions consisting of two injections of 0.58 mg of CCH each session (total of 8 injections). However, CCH is expensive, and it is unknown if eight injections are required to achieve an optimal outcome.** There have been several attempts to modify this protocol to achieve maximal benefit while limiting unnecessary treatment. Anaissie et al. (2017) demonstrated that penile curvature improved significantly following the first three cycles but not the fourth cycle. Yang et al. (2016) only administered six 0.58-mg injections over three cycles with an average curvature reduction of 15.4 degrees (32.4%, P < 0.1), which is similar to the IMPRESS trials. Raheem et al. (2017) used a modified CCH protocol to three total treatment sessions of 0.9 mg per treatment over the course of 12 weeks. The mean penile curvature decreased an average of 17 degrees or 31% from baseline of 54 degrees, which is similar to the results of the IMPRESS trials. Although CCH is currently FDA-approved for stable disease, Nguyen et al. (2017) demonstrated in a group of 36 acute-phase patients and 126 stable-phase patients that the mean curvature improvement was comparable: 16.7 degrees for acute-phase patients and 15.6 degrees for chronic-phase patients (P = 0.654). More studies are indicated to justify use of CCH in acute-phase PD.

Further experience will help make CCH injections more cost-effective and predict which patients will benefit the most. This may depend on direction of curve, size of plaque, prevalence of calcification, and duration of disease, among other factors to be determined. A recent presentation did demonstrate that surgical correction with plication or grafting could be successfully performed after CCH injection without added technical difficulty (Larsen and Levine, 2012). CCH received FDA approval for the treatment of PD in December 2013.

The 2015 AUA PD guideline recommends that physicians may administer CCH in patients with a stable curvature greater than 30 degrees and less than 90 degrees with intact erectile dysfunction (with or without use of medications).

As always, the risk and potential side effects of this treatment should be discussed with the patient before initiating treatment.

Topical Drug Application

Several studies have evaluated the effectiveness of topically applied agents for the treatment of PD. Topical application avoids the pain and trauma of intralesional injection therapy. The first study of topical application of a drug, β-aminopropionitrile, showed no benefit with respect to deformity change (Gelbard et al., 1983).

Topically applied liposomal recombinant human superoxide dismutase (lrhSOD) has also been studied in a randomized placebo-controlled trial (Riedl et al., 2005). This substance is proposed to act as an oxygen free radical scavenger, which might interrupt inflammatory cascades and thereby limit further disease progression. Penile curvature was improved by 5 to 30 degrees in 23% of patients, and pain was significantly reduced as well ($P = .017$) compared with placebo after 4 weeks. The authors concluded that lrhSOD is an easily given, safe, and effective local therapeutic for the painful phase of PD (Riedl et al., 2005). A recent randomized controlled trial showed that the H-100 gel, which contains Nicardipine, SOD, and emu oil, applied daily for 6 months resulted significant decrease in mean curvature (40%, $P = 0.0014$) and increase in mean stretched penile length (22.6%, $P = 0.0002$) (Twidwell and Levine, 2016). However, this study was a pilot study with 22 patients, and larger studies are needed to confirm the efficacy of these topical agents before general use.

Fitch et al. (2007) reported on the use of topical verapamil for the treatment of PD (Fitch et al., 2007). Two simultaneous three-armed, double-blind, placebo-controlled studies were conducted in this pilot study. In this study, topical verapamil improved curvature in 14 of 18 patients (77.8%), with a mean curvature improvement of 43.6%. This study also boasted reduction in plaque size in 100% of participants and improvement in erectile function in 72.7%. This study was originally aimed at comparing verapamil to topical trifluoperazine, **but because of the severity of side effects (anxiety, agitation, blurred vision, insomnia, and depression), topical trifluoperazine was discontinued before completion of randomization.** The results of this study have been called into question given the small sample size, lack of a true placebo, and absence of objective measures (Levine, 2007). In addition, simple topical administration of verapamil has been shown to be ineffective in achieving tissue levels within the tunica albuginea sufficient for therapeutic effect (Martin et al., 2002). Favilla et al. (2017), in a prospective double-blind randomized study comparing verapamil and hyaluronic acid in the acute setting showed that although both treatments decreased plaque size, neither resulted in a significant decrease in penile curvature.

At this time, no topically applied agent has been established to be effective in the treatment of PD. The AUA 2015 PD Guidelines Panel identified topical therapy for PD as possibly promising but for which insufficient evidence currently exists to support even a conditional recommendation for its use.

Electromotive Drug Administration

Transdermal drug delivery was proposed to be superior to oral or injection therapy because it bypasses hepatic metabolism and minimizes the pain of injection. Unlike topical verapamil gel, electromotive drug administration (EMDA) with verapamil has been found to deliver detectable levels of the drug to the tunica albuginea (Martin et al., 2002; Levine et al., 2003).

A double-blind, placebo-controlled trial to determine the effectiveness of verapamil delivered through EMDA randomized a total of 42 PD patients to verapamil versus saline. Treatments were performed twice weekly for 3 months. **Both verapamil and saline groups demonstrated essentially equivalent reduction of curvature. The study concluded that further research is necessary to determine whether electric current alone may have a role in the treatment of PD** (Greenfield et al., 2007). Overall, EMDA was well tolerated in each group, and it was noted by all patients to be easy and convenient to perform at home. The only adverse event reported by patients was temporary mild erythema at the treatment site (Greenfield et al., 2007).

In another prospective placebo-controlled study with transdermal EMDA, Di Stasi et al. (2004) randomized patients to receive verapamil and dexamethasone versus placebo. Those receiving active drug demonstrated significant decreases in plaque volume and penile curvature from 43 degrees to 21 degrees, which was significant when compared with placebo. Significant pain relief occurred in both groups, transient in the control group and permanent in the study group. All patients experienced temporary erythema at the electrode site. There were no other side effects (Di Stasi et al., 2004). **Although this approach has limited evidence of benefit, it has not been adopted in most centers. The 2015 AUA PD guideline recommends that clinicians should not offer electromotive therapy with verapamil.**

Extracorporeal Shock Wave Therapy

The mechanism of action involved in ESWT for PD is unclear. However, there are two purported hypotheses: (1) Shock waves cause direct damage to the penile plaque, and (2) ESWT increases the vascularity of the targeted area by generating heat, which leads to the induction of an inflammatory reaction, resulting in lysis of the plaque and removal by macrophages (Gholami et al., 2003).

In the first prospective randomized double-blind placebo-controlled clinical trial evaluating ESWT for the treatment of PD, 100 treatment-naïve PD patients with disease duration less than 12 months were randomly allocated to either ESWT ($n = 50$) or placebo ($n = 50$). For the placebo group, a nonfunctioning transducer was employed. Patients randomized to ESWT demonstrated improvements in pain, IIEF-5 score, and mean QoL score. **Plaque size and penile curvature were not significantly different in the treatment and placebo groups.** After 24 weeks, the mean IIEF-5 score and mean QoL score were stable in the ESWT group, whereas the mean visual analog scale (VAS) score was significantly lower when compared with baseline in both groups. It is interesting to note that after 24 weeks, mean plaque size and mean curvature degree were significantly worse in the placebo group when compared with both baseline and ESWT values. **This difference was less than 3 degrees, which, although statistically significant, is of no clinical significance** (Palmieri et al., 2012).

Recently, a second placebo-controlled, prospective randomized single-blind study was performed in which 102 PD patients were randomly assigned (n = 51) to ESWT or placebo (Hatzichristodoulou et al., 2013b). Pain decreased in 17 of 20 (85%) patients in the ESWT group and in 12 of 25 (48%) patients in the placebo group. Penile deviation was not reduced by ESWT and worsened in 40% and 24.5% of patients in the ESWT and placebo groups, respectively ($P = .133$). Change in sexual function and plaque size reduction was not different between the two groups. In addition, plaque size increased in five patients (10.9%) receiving ESWT only. **The authors concluded that despite some potential benefit of ESWT with regard to pain reduction, it should be emphasized that pain usually resolves spontaneously with time. Given this and the fact that deviation may worsen with ESWT, the treatment cannot be recommended.**

The 2015 AUA PD guideline states that clinicians should not use ESWT for the reduction of penile curvature or plaque size. Clinicians may offer ESWT to improve penile pain.

Penile Traction

Controlled stretching of the penis, or "penile traction," by a device that holds the penis in a cradle and subjects it to tension is indicated for treatment of PD patients as a noninvasive, nonsurgical first-option treatment modality.

Traction has been shown in nonpenile tissue models to induce cellular proliferation by several pathways (Ilizarov, 1989; Sun et al., 1996; Molea et al., 1999; Assoian and Klein, 2008; Bueno and Shah, 2008). It can also trigger scar remodeling; it has been shown that tension applied to tissues leads to a reorientation of collagen fibrils parallel to the axis of stress (Molea et al., 1999; Shapiro, 2008). These changes are the result of a process referred to as *mechanotransduction* whereby mechanical stimuli are converted into chemical responses within the cell (Alenghat and Ingber, 2002). Several signaling cascades are activated by tension on the cytoskeleton, which leads to a proliferative response and activation of various genes (Assoian and Klein, 2008). **An in vitro study to determine the cellular effects of traction on PD cells demonstrated a significant decrease in ASMA in the** strained compared with nonstrained PD cell cultures, whereas an increase in MMPs involved in collagen degradation was observed. In contrast, cytokines and proteins involved in fibroblast replication and inflammation such as ASMA, heat shock protein 47 (HSP47), and TGF-β1 receptor were not upregulated (Chung et al., 2013a). Several studies have been performed examining the clinical effects of traction for the treatment of PD, although none have been controlled trials.

Levine et al. (2008) first demonstrated the use of penile traction for the treatment of PD in a pilot study of 10 men. In nearly all subjects (90%), prior medical therapy had failed. Traction was applied as the only treatment for 2 to 8 hours per day for 6 months. All subjects underwent pretreatment and post-treatment physical examination including measurement of stretched flaccid penile length and biothesiometry. Subjectively, all men noted reduced curvature estimated at 10 to 40 degrees, increased penile length (1 to 2.5 cm), and enhanced girth in areas of indentation or narrowing. **Objective measures demonstrated reduced curvature in all 10 men of up to 45 degrees; average reduction for the group was 33%, from 51 degrees to 34 degrees. SPL increased 0.5 to 2.0 cm, and erect girth increased 0.5 to 1.0 cm with correction of hinge effect in four of four men.** It is important to note that results were maintained at 6 months after completion of therapy. The IIEF erectile function domain score increased from 18.3 to 23.6 for the group. There were no adverse events including skin changes, ulcerations, hypoesthesia, or diminished rigidity (Levine et al., 2008).

Gontero et al. (2009) performed a phase II prospective study on 15 PD patients with a curvature not exceeding 50 degrees with mild or no ED. Penile curvature decreased from an average of 31 degrees to 27 degrees at 6 months, which was not statistically significant. Mean stretched and flaccid penile length increased by 1.3 and 0.83 cm, respectively, at 6 months. Results were maintained at 12 months. Overall treatment results were subjectively scored as acceptable in spite of limited curvature improvements, which varied from "no change" to "mild improvement." **The investigators concluded that the use of a penile extender device provided only minimal improvements in penile curvature but a reasonable level of patient satisfaction, probably attributable to increased penile length. The selection of patients with stabilized disease, many with calcified plaques, and penile curvature not exceeding 50 degrees may have led to outcomes underestimating the potential efficacy of the treatment** (Gontero et al., 2009).

Recently a prospective nonrandomized study was conducted administering traction to PD patients in the acute phase, defined as progressive penile curvature exceeding 15 degrees and/or pain at rest or at erection in the last 12 months (Martínez-Salamanca et al., 2014). A total of 55 patients underwent traction for 6 months and were compared with 41 patients also in the acute phase who did not. Patients were advised to use the device at least 6 hours per day and no more than 9 hours, preventing its use during sleep. Mean duration of use was 4.6 hours per day (3.1 to 9.2 hours). Also, patients were taught to remove the device for at least 30 minutes every 2 hours to prevent glans ischemia. **The mean curvature decreased from 33 degrees at baseline to 15 degrees at 6 months and 13 degrees at 9 months with a mean decrease of 20 degrees in the traction group.** VAS score for **pain decreased from 5.5 to 2.5 after 6 months** ($P < .05$). The percentage of patients who were not able to achieve penetration decreased from 62% to 20% ($P < .03$). Without this intervention, deformity increased significantly, stretched flaccid penile length decreased, VAS score for pain increased, and erection hardness worsened. **Furthermore, the need for surgery was reduced in 40% of patients who would otherwise have been candidates for surgery and simplified the complexity of the surgical procedure (from grafting to plication) in one of three patients.** Treatment-related adverse events included two cases of erythema in the balanopreputial sulcus, which resolved with stopping traction for 24 to 48 hours. Fourteen patients (25.5%) reported some degree of discomfort. Worsening of erectile function over the treatment period was not observed, **and the overall satisfaction rate was 85%** (range 60% to 90%) at 9 months. No case of sensory change after traction was reported (Martínez-Salamanca et al., 2014). **Traction therapy has the potential to be an effective nonsurgical treatment** to recover lost length, reduce curvature, and enhance girth. It is critical that the patient wear the device for 3 or more hours per day to get satisfactory results. There is no recommendation offered by the AUA 2015 PD Guidelines Panel regarding penile traction therapy.

Vacuum Therapy

Application of a penile vacuum device to mechanically straighten the penis has been evaluated in one published noncontrolled study in which subjects wore the vacuum device for 10 minutes twice per day for 12 weeks. This study demonstrated a reduction in the angle of curvature by 5 degrees to 25 degrees in 21 of 31 patients. Three patients' curvature worsened, and in seven the curvature remained unchanged. Fifty-one percent were satisfied with this outcome; the other 49% went on to surgical correction (Raheem et al., 2010). **Although vacuum erection devices are usually considered safe, it would seem that the short-term duration of stretching forces on the penis would not induce the desired physical changes known to occur with mechanotransduction with prolonged stretch therapy.** Several complications such as the development of PD, urethral bleeding, skin necrosis, and penile ecchymosis have been reported with concomitant use of constriction rings and when inappropriately elevated pressures are applied to the penis for an extended period (Kim and Carson, 1993; Ganem et al., 1998).

There is no recommendation offered by the AUA 2015 PD Guidelines Panel regarding vacuum therapy as monotherapy.

Combination Therapy

One study investigated whether a combination of the mechanical effects of penile traction with the chemical effects of intralesional verapamil and oral medications (pentoxifylline and L-arginine) could have a synergistic effect on the tunica albuginea and Peyronie's plaque (Abern et al., 2012). All patients were given oral pentoxifylline and L-arginine, with 39 electing to undergo traction and 35 choosing not to use traction. Both treatment groups had a statistically significant reduction in erect penile curvature. The traction group had a reduction from a mean of 44.4 degrees (standard deviation [SD] 27.5 degrees) at baseline to a mean of 33.4 degrees (SD 25.3 degrees) after the 24-week protocol ($P = .03$). Patients not using traction had a reduction from a mean of 36.6 degrees at baseline (SD 18.5 degrees) to a mean of 21.5 degrees (SD 19.3 degrees) after treatment ($P < .01$). There were no statistically significant differences in curvature outcomes between the two groups. In patients using traction, SPL increased overall by a mean 0.3 cm (SD 0.9 cm) after treatment, which trended toward statistical significance ($P = .06$), whereas the men not using traction lost an average of 0.7 cm (SD 1.1 cm) of length, which was not statistically different ($P = .46$) (Abern et al., 2012). Unfortunately, this study did not control for duration of traction therapy, and some men included in the traction group applied the device for only 1 to 2 hours per week, whereas others wore it for over 50 hours per week. An analysis of traction duration and deformity change demonstrated that wearing the device on average 3 or more hours per day allowed reliable measured deformity improvement, which occurred in a dose-response fashion.

Another combination study examined the effects of combining verapamil injection and verapamil iontophoresis with or without the use of a combination pill that contained vitamin E, potassium para-aminobenzoate, propolis (as galangin), blueberry anthocyanins, soy isoflavones, *Muira puama*, damiana, and *Persea americana*. Intergroup analysis revealed greater plaque size reduction (−30.8% vs. −18.0%) and greater percentage with reduction of curvature (85% vs. 53.5%) with use of the combination pill (Paulis et al., 2013). There is no recommendation offered by the AUA 2015 PD Guidelines Panel regarding combination therapy.

Radiation Therapy

Radiation therapy has been proposed as a treatment for PD since 1964 (Duggan, 1964). **In vitro studies suggest that low-dose** radiation therapy has a potent anti-inflammatory effect, inhibiting leukocyte-endothelium interactions (Arenas et al., 2012). In recent years, radiation therapy has been proposed as a treatment for pain that was thought to be "abnormally persistent." In 1975, a retrospective study examined the use of radiation therapy and found it to be no more effective than no treatment (Incrocci et al., 2000). It is the consensus of multiple experts in the field that radiation should be avoided because of potential risk for malignant change and increase in the risk for ED in aging patients (Hatzimouratidis et al., 2012; Mulhall et al., 2012; Ralph et al., 2010). The 2015 AUA PD guideline recommends that clinicians should not use radiotherapy (RT) to treat Peyronie's disease because of the known risks and uncertain benefits.

Conclusion

It appears that the goal of nonsurgical treatment at a minimum should be to prevent progression of deformity during the acute phase. Reducing deformity to improve sexual function and reduce the effects of the scarring is the ultimate goal of all treatment for PD (Tables 73.1 to 73.3).

SURGICAL MANAGEMENT

Indications

Surgical reconstruction (Video 73.1) is indicated for men with deformity that precludes satisfactory sexual intercourse or causes pain for themselves or their partner during sexual relations or because of distress as a result of the appearance of the erect penis (Kadioglu et al., 2006).

Surgery remains the gold standard treatment to most rapidly and reliably correct the deformity associated with PD; for men who also have ED, placement of a penile prosthesis can provide rigidity for penetrative sexual activity. The indications for surgical correction include stable disease, which is defined as disease that is at least 1 year from onset, and at least 6 months of stable deformity. These indications have not been formally studied but appear to be generally accepted by experts in the field (Jordan, 2007; Levine and Burnett, 2013, Nehra et al., 2015; Ralph et al., 2010). Other indications include a deformity that compromises or makes

KEY POINTS: NONSURGICAL TREATMENT OF PEYRONIE'S DISEASE

- Patients who have no pain or difficulty in accomplishing penetrative sex may require only reassurance, because this is not a disorder that will degenerate into cancer and it is not life-threatening.
- A poor understanding of the cause of this wound-healing disorder contributes to the fact that, to date, conservative treatments often yield inconsistent and clinically insignificant improvements in deformity.
- Currently, no oral agent has been shown in placebo-controlled trials to result in clinically meaningful improvement in curvature. As a result, the only oral medication recommended by the AUA guideline on PD is NSAIDs to reduce pain.
- Topical therapy and ESWT have not been shown to reduce penile deformity.
- Intralesional verapamil and IFN alfa-2b have shown evidence of reduced curvature and improved sexual function. Yet most studies are not controlled trials. These agents at a minimum appear to result in deformity stabilization during the acute phase.
- The first FDA-approved drug for the treatment of PD, CCH (Xiaflex; Endo Pharmaceuticals, Malvern, PA) is produced by the bacterium *C. histolyticum* and selectively degrades collagen types I and III. Mean curvature reduction in the phase III trials in the treatment arm (CCH injection with penile traction) was 34% (17 degrees) versus 18.2% (9.3 degrees) for placebo. The volume of patients seeking treatment for PD may increase over the coming years as public awareness increases with the advent of use of this drug.

impossible the patient's ability to engage in sexual intercourse because of the nature of the deformity and/or inadequate rigidity, and patients in whom conservative therapy has failed (Box 73.4). No single surgical approach is universally defined as the standard of care (Gur et al., 2011; Kendirci and Hellstrom, 2004) because there

TABLE 73.1 Oral Agents for Peyronie's Disease

TREATMENT	MECHANISM OF ACTION	STUDY OUTCOMES	ADVERSE EFFECTS
Potaba	Decreases serotonin levels by increasing monoamine oxidase activity, resulting in enhancement of the antifibrotic properties of tissues	Decreased plaque size, no decrease in curvature	Anorexia, nausea, fever, skin rash, hypoglycemia, acute hepatitis
Vitamin E	Antioxidant, limits oxidative stress of reactive oxygen species shown to be increased in PD	No benefit	Possible cerebrovascular events, nausea, vomiting, diarrhea, headache, dizziness
Tamoxifen	Induces the production of TGF-β in an estrogen receptor–independent fashion, theoretically causing macrophage deactivation and T-lymphocyte suppression, thus preventing further fibrogenesis	No benefit	Alopecia, retinopathy, thromboembolism, pancytopenia
Colchicine	Microtubule depolymerization; inhibits cell mitosis, mobility, adhesion of leukocytes, and transcellular movement of collagen and stimulates the production of collagenase	No benefit	Myelosuppression, diarrhea, nausea, vomiting
Carnitine	Increases mitochondrial respiration; decreases free radical formation	No benefit	Seizures, diarrhea, nausea, abdominal cramps, vomiting
Pentoxifylline	Blocks the TGF-β1–mediated pathway of inflammation; prevents deposition of collagen type I; is a nonspecific phosphodiesterase inhibitor; decreases platelet-activating factor	Decreased curvature in 33% of patients, mean 23 degrees	Nausea, vomiting, dyspepsia, malaise, flushing, dizziness, and headache

TGF, Transforming growth factor.

TABLE 73.2 Intralesional Agents for Peyronie's Disease

Treatment	MECHANISM OF ACTION	STUDY OUTCOMES	ADVERSE EFFECTS
Verapamil	Calcium channel blocker inhibits fibroblast proliferation, extracellular matrix protein synthesis and secretion; increases collagenase activity.	Reduction of curvature and plaque-associated penile narrowing, improvement in quality of erection	Nausea, lightheadedness, penile pain, ecchymoses
Nicardipine	DHP type of calcium channel blocker. In vitro study demonstrated that it is more effective than a non-DHP type, verapamil, in reducing glycosaminoglycan biosynthesis and production of extracellular matrix, such as collagen.	Reduction of pain, improvement in IIEF-5 score, and reduction of plaque size; no benefit in curvature	No severe side effects such as hypotension or other cardiovascular events
Interferon alfa-2b	Decreases plaque fibroblast proliferation in a dose-dependent fashion, decreases production of extracellular collagen, and increases production of collagenase.	Decrease in curvature of 27% (13.5 degrees) vs. 9% (4.5 degrees) in the placebo group	Sinusitis, flulike symptoms (fever, chills, and arthralgia), and minor penile swelling with ecchymosis
Clostridial collagenase	Selectively degrades collagen types I and III in connective tissues despite the presence of TIMPs, which have been shown to be elevated in PD and to increase apoptosis of fibroblasts.	Decrease in penile curvature by 34%, mean decrease of 17 degrees vs. 18%, mean decrease 9.3 degrees in placebo; PD symptom bothersomeness score significantly improved vs. placebo	Contusions, ecchymoses, corporeal rupture

DHP, Dihydropyridine; *IIEF,* International Index of Erectile Function; *PD,* Peyronie's disease; *TIMPs,* tissue inhibitors of metalloproteinases.

TABLE 73.3 External Force Application for Peyronie's Disease

TREATMENT	MECHANISM OF ACTION	STUDY OUTCOMES	ADVERSE EFFECTS
Electromotive drug administration	Bypasses hepatic metabolism, increases concentration of drug to target tissues compared with topical application alone	Verapamil alone: no benefit. Verapamil + dexamethasone: decreases in plaque volume and penile curvature from 43 to 21 degrees	Temporary erythema at the electrode site
Extracorporeal shock wave therapy	Direct damage to the penile plaque; increases vascularity of the targeted area inducing an inflammatory reaction, resulting in lysis of the plaque and removal by macrophages	Improvements in pain, IIEF-5 score, and mean QoL score; no curvature reduction	Local petechiae and ecchymoses
Penile traction	Decreases α-smooth muscle actin, increases matrix metalloproteinases involved in collagen degradation	Length increased 0.5–2.0 cm; girth increased 0.5–1.0 cm; curvature mean decrease of 20 degrees; pain decreased; softening or shrinking of plaque; overall satisfaction 85%	Erythema in the balanopreputial sulcus, discomfort
Vacuum therapy	Unknown; mechanical effects similar to traction have been suggested	Reduction in angle of curvature by 5–25 degrees in 21 of 31 patients	Development of PD, urethral bleeding, skin necrosis, and penile ecchymosis
Radiation therapy	Anti-inflammatory effects via functional modulation of the adhesion of white blood cells to activated endothelial cells and modulation of the induction of nitric oxide synthase in activated macrophages	No clinical benefit	Possible malignant change, increased risk for ED in elderly

ED, Erectile dysfunction; *IIEF,* International Index of Erectile Function; *PD,* Peyronie's disease; *QoL,* quality of life.

> **BOX 73.4** Indications for Surgery
>
> - Stable deformity for at least 6 months from onset of symptoms
> - Inability to engage in satisfactory penetrative sexual intercourse because of deformity and/or inadequate rigidity
> - Failed conservative treatment
> - Desire for most rapid and reliable result

> **BOX 73.5** Preoperative Consent
>
> Set expectations regarding outcome.
> - Persistent or recurrent curvature: The goal is "functionally straight" (curvature <20 degrees)
> - Change in length: The result is more likely shorter with plication than with grafting.
> - Diminished rigidity
>   - ≥5% in all studies—grafting more than plication
>   - ≥30% if suboptimal preoperative rigidity—dependent on preoperative erectile quality
> - Decreased sexual sensation
>   - Typically resolves in 1 to 6 months
>   - Rarely compromises orgasm or ejaculation

are multiple factors to consider, including severity of curvature, direction of curvature, presence of a hinge effect, erection quality, and patient goals. An algorithm for surgical decision making is presented in Fig. 73.10 (Levine and Larsen, 2013).

Preoperative consent is critical because patients with PD are distressed and frequently emotionally devastated. It has been reported that men who have undergone treatment for PD are often not satisfied with their results because of their expectation for recovery of their pre-PD penile appearance (Jones, 1997). **It is therefore important to have a frank discussion with the patient so that he understands the limitations of the operation, and to set appropriate expectations regarding outcomes to optimize patient satisfaction** (Ralph et al., 2010). **The patient should understand that there is a possibility of persistent or recurrent curvature, reduction of penile erect length, diminished rigidity, and decreased sexual sensation (Box 73.5).** Persistent or recurrent curvature is unusual but has been shown in up to 16% of men, the great majority of whom do not require another operation (Ralph et al., 2010; Taylor and Levine, 2007). **The patient should understand that the goal is to make the penis "functionally straight," which expert opinion defines as a residual deformity of 20 degrees or less** (Levine and Burnett, 2013; Ralph et al., 2010). The European Association of Urology (EAU) guidelines committee on PD defines successful curvature correction as 15 degrees or less of residual curvature (Hatzimouratidis et al., 2012). Change (loss) in penile erect length is more likely with plication than with grafting, although all surgical correction procedures have been associated with some length loss. This is extremely important for the patient to understand preoperatively because 70% to 80% of patients initially have loss of length as a result of the fibrotic disease process (Jordan and McCammon, 2007; Pryor and Ralph, 2002; Ralph et al., 2010). Thus, further loss of length can be a major concern. Having stretched flaccid penile length documented preoperatively permits comparison with postoperative length. Diminished rigidity has long been reported after surgery, and studies have demonstrated that up to 50% of men may have some degree of postoperative reduction in rigidity, which may respond to a PDE5 inhibitor. Rigidity will not likely be improved by penile straightening, and therefore in patients who already have significant ED that does not respond to oral medication, placement

of a penile prosthesis should be offered (Ralph et al., 2010; Taylor and Levine, 2007). Men who are considering penile straightening procedures without a penile prosthesis should be carefully evaluated for the quality of their preoperative erections, which does appear to be the most reliable predictor of postoperative ED (Flores et al., 2011; Taylor et al., 2012). In some men with PD and ED, correction of the penile geometry resulted in improved rigidity (Pescatori et al., 2003). **Regardless, it is of critical importance that the patient understand that any operation done on the penis to correct PD may result in diminished rigidity, and that this may subsequently be treated successfully with oral PDE5 inhibitors, injection therapy, or a vacuum device; and those in whom these approaches fail can have a penile prosthesis implanted with little to no additional difficulty** (Chung et al., 2013c; Kendirci and Hellstrom, 2004; Levine et al., 2010). Decreased sexual sensation has been examined and reported on infrequently, but it does appear that approximately 20% of men will describe some reduction in penile sensitivity, rarely interfering with orgasm or ejaculation. During the acute postoperative period, there can be hyperesthesia or hypoesthesia, which tends to resolve and stabilize within 6 to 12 months postoperatively (Taylor and Levine, 2008; Ralph et al., 2010). **The primary determinants for the choice of surgical approach are based on two factors, including quality of the preoperative erection hardness and severity of deformity, including curvature and indentation. In men who have rigidity that is adequate for coital activity with or without pharmacotherapy, tunica plication techniques and plaque incision or partial excision with grafting may be used. Tunica plication techniques are recommended for those who have a simple curvature of less than 70 degrees, those with absence of an hourglass or hinge effect, and those in whom the anticipated loss of length would be less than 20% of the total erect length** (Levine and Lenting, 1997; Mulhall et al., 2005; Ralph and Minhas, 2004). **The estimated penile length loss can be determined during preoperative testing while the penis is erect by measuring the difference in length between the long and short sides of the penis. Grafting procedures are recommended for those with more complex curves of greater than 60 to 70 degrees and/or a destabilizing hourglass resulting in a hinge effect. This hinge effect results in a buckling or unstable penis, which makes penetrative sex difficult. These men must have strong, sexually induced rigidity to reduce the likelihood of postoperative ED** (Flores et al., 2011; Taylor et al., 2012) (Table 73.4). For the man who has PD and ED that is refractory to medical therapy, published algorithms have indicated that penile prosthesis placement is the procedure of choice (Levine and Burnett, 2013; Levine and Dimitriou, 2000; Mulhall et al., 2005; Ralph et al., 2010). This procedure allows for correction of the deformity while also addressing the ED. If curvature is not satisfactorily corrected with the prosthesis inflated during surgery, additional straightening maneuvers may be performed. We recommend manual modeling as the first step as initially reported by Wilson and Delk (1994). If there is residual curvature in excess of 30 degrees after modeling, then a relaxing incision in the tunica albuginea overlying the area of maximum curvature can be made. It is recommended that if the incisional defect is greater than 2 cm, a biograft (i.e., pericardium or small intestine submucosa) should be placed over the defect to prevent cicatrix contracture of the incision or herniation of the prosthesis (Levine and Dimitriou, 2000; Ralph et al., 2010). Plication techniques have been recommended to be performed before placement of the prosthesis to correct curvature in lieu of manual modeling (Dugi and Morey, 2010; Rahman et al., 2004). In this circumstance, if the curvature is dorsal, the erectile deformity can be defined with injection of a vasoactive drug and infusion of saline, then sutures are placed in a Lembert fashion to cause ventral shortening and correction of the curve.

Tunical Shortening Procedures

Penile plication aims to shorten the longer (or convex) side of the tunica albuginea to match the length to the shorter side (Ralph, 2006; Syed et al., 2003). **Advantages to these approaches include shorter surgical time, good cosmetic outcomes, minimal effect**

TABLE 73.4 Outcomes for Plaque Excision or Incision and Grafting

GRAFT MATERIAL	AUTHOR AND DATE	PATIENTS (N)	MEAN FOLLOW-UP (MONTHS)	STRAIGHT AT LATEST FOLLOW-UP (%)	ED (%)	SATISFACTION RATES (%)
Dermal grafts	Wild et al., 1979	10	11	60	6	70
	Levine, 1997	15	11	73	12	70
	Chun et al., 2001	48	19.6	80	25	73
	Kovac and Brock, 2007	50	45	94	NR	NR
	Chung et al., 2011a	6	102	50	NR	35
Saphenous vein grafts	El-Sakka et al., 1998	113	9.72	96	12	92
	Kadioglu et al., 1999	20	13.2	75	5	NR
	Montorsi et al., 2000	50	12	80	6	96
	Akkus et al., 2001	58	16	86	7	92
	Adeniyi et al., 2002	51	32	82	8	88
	Hsu et al., 2003	24	31.2	96	4	100
	Kalsi et al., 2005	113	>60	80	23	60
	Kim et al., 2008	20	>12	85	35	NR
	Wimpissinger et al., 2016	26	156	87	36	73
Buccal mucosa	Shioshvili and Kakonahvili, 2005	26	38	92	8	NR
	Cormio et al., 2009	15	13	100	0	93
	Zucchi et al., 2014	32	43	96.5	3.5	85
Proximal crura	Teloken et al., 2000	7	6	86	0	86
	Schwarzer et al., 2003	31	NR	84	19	94
	Da Ros et al., 2012	27	NR	96	4	70
Tunica vaginalis	Das, 1980	15	4-16	87.5	0	100
	O'Donnell, 1992	25	42.2	88	68	NR
Dura mater	Fallon, 1990	40	12-72	95	25	NR
	Sampaio et al., 2002	40	12-24	95	15	NR
Temporalis fascia	Gelbard and Hayden, 1991	12	NR	100	0	100
Fascia lata	Kalsi et al., 2006	14	31	79	7	93
Small intestinal submucosa (SIS 4-layer)	Breyer et al., 2007	19	15	63	53	Score of 2.7/5.0
	Kovac and Brock, 2007	13	7.8	77	NR	85
	Lee et al., 2008	13	14	100	54	NR
	Staerman et al., 2010	33	14	67	11	79
	Chung et al., 2011b	17	75	77	13	NR
	Valente et al., 2016	28	18	82	17.8	83.2
Bovine pericardium	Egydio et al., 2002	33	19	88	0.0	NR
	Knoll, 2007	162	38	91	21	NR
Tutoplast pericardial graft	Hellstrom and Reddy, 2000	81	58	79	20	78
	Leungwattanakij et al., 2001	19	22	84	16	74
	Usta et al., 2003	11	14	91	NR	NR
	Levine et al., 2003	40	22	98	30	92
	Kovac and Brock, 2007	13	30	100	NR	NR
	Chung et al., 2011a	81	58	91	32	75
	Taylor and Levine, 2008	23	79	87	NR	NR
Acellular dermis	Adamakis et al., 2011	5	6	100	0	100
Synthetic materials	Faerber and Konnak, 1993	9	17.5	100	0	100
TachoSil	Licht and Lewis, 1997	28	22	61	18	30
	Horstmann et al., 2011	43	63	41	9	20
	Yafi et al., 2016	26	20.7	85	0	100
	Hatzichristodoulou, 2018	70	0.2	83.6	NR	NR

ED, Erectile dysfunction; *NR,* not reported.

on rigidity, simple and safe surgery, and effective straightening (Hatzimouratidis et al., 2012; Hudak et al., 2013). **Disadvantages include shortening and failure to correct an hourglass or hinge.** A study of failures with the Nesbit procedure identified three factors associated with an unsatisfactory outcome, including impaired preoperative erectile function, penile shortening of greater than 2 cm, and penile deformity greater than 30 degrees (Andrews et al., 2001). Multiple surgical plication techniques have been offered for PD, beginning with the Nesbit procedure (Nesbit, 1965) (Fig. 73.11). This technique uses excision of an elliptical segment of the tunica on the contralateral side of the curvature. In the setting of a ventral curvature, once Buck's fascia has been elevated, small wedges of the dorsal tunica albuginea are excised and then the defect is closed, typically with permanent suture. Multiple variations on this approach have evolved, including the Yachia procedure, which uses the Heineke-Mikulicz technique (Yachia, 1990, 1993). In the setting of a dorsal curvature, a short (0.5 to 1.5 cm), full-thickness vertical incision is made on the ventral shaft tunic, opposite the area of maximum curvature, which is then closed transversely to shorten the ventral aspect and correct the curvature (Fig. 73.12). This approach must be used carefully so that the length of the incision is not too long, such that transverse closure could result in further narrowing of the shaft, possibly resulting in an unstable erection. Several authors have suggested that this approach has a lower risk for perceived penile shortening (Klevmark et al., 1994; Kümmerling and Schubert, 1995; Nooter et al., 1994; Poulson and Kikeby, 1995; Ralph et al., 1995; Savoca et al., 2000, 2004; Sulaiman and Gingell, 1994).

Imbrication procedures are used to avoid making a full-thickness tunical incision and fold the tunica to correct curvature. The techniques of tunical plication without incision were introduced in 1985 by Essed and Schroeder, who used nonabsorbable sutures placed in a figure-of-eight fashion to enable the knots to be buried (Essed and Schroeder, 1985). Two years later, Ebbehoj and Metz (1987) described their plication technique using multiple rows of sutures to shorten the longer side for congenital curvature (Ebbehoj and Metz, 1987). The 16-dot procedure has become a popular variation of tunical shortening in which there is no incision into the tunic but the tunica albuginea is plicated with permanent suture using an extended Lembert-type suture placement technique (Brant et al., 2007; Gholami and Lue, 2002; Rolle et al., 2005) (Fig. 73.13). Another plication variation is the Levine modification of the Duckett-Baskin tunica albuginea plication (TAP), which was originally used for children with congenital curvature. Here, a partial-thickness incision is made transversely on the contralateral side to the point of maximum curvature (Baskin and Duckett, 1994; Levine, 2006). A pair of transverse parallel incisions 1 to 1.5 cm in length are made through the longitudinal fibers but do not violate the inner circular fibers of the tunic. As a result, the underlying cavernosal tissue is not disturbed, which is thought to reduce the likelihood of postoperative ED. These incisions are separated by 0.5 to 1.0 cm depending on the desired amount of shortening. The longitudinal fibers between the two transverse incisions are excised so as to reduce the bulk of the plication. This procedure is now done with a single central permanent suture (2-0 Tevdek suture, Teleflex Medical, Research Triangle Park, NC, or TiCron suture, Medline, Mundelein, IL) placed in an inverting vertical mattress fashion to bury the knot and then supported with absorbable suture (3-0 polydioxanone [PDS], Ethicon, Somerville, NJ) placed in a Lembert fashion to reduce the palpable nature of the plication and knots (Fig. 73.14).

The key is that all plication procedures shorten the long side of the penis and therefore can result in loss of length on that aspect of the penis. Studies have examined the loss of penile

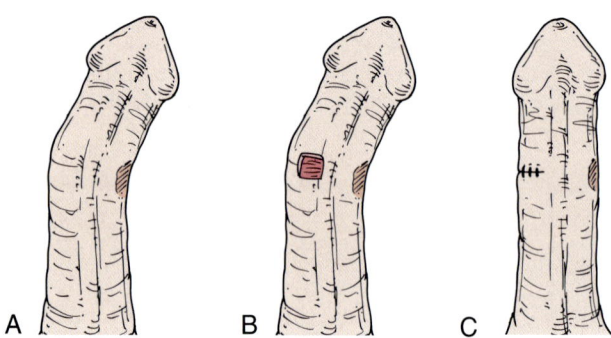

Fig. 73.11. (A) The Nesbit procedure employs a transverse elliptical incision of the tunica albuginea. (B) This is done contralateral to the area of greatest curvature. (C) The defect is closed transversely with permanent suture with or without the addition of absorbable suture.

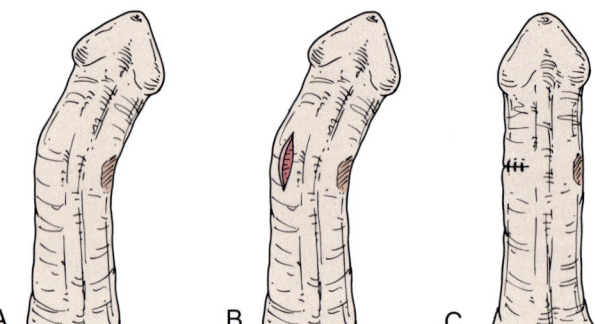

Fig. 73.12. (A) The Yachia procedure employs a full-thickness vertical incision (B) in the tunica albuginea contralateral to the area of greatest curvature and is closed transversely (C) without removal of tunica albuginea.

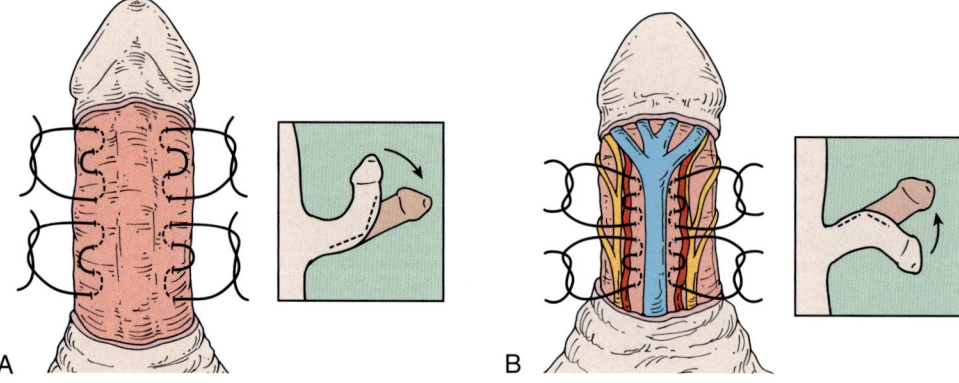

Fig. 73.13. The dot procedure employs no incision. The tunica albuginea is plicated with permanent suture using an extended Lembert-type suture placement following four dots per plication. A, Suture placement for dorsal curve. B, Suture placement for ventral curve.

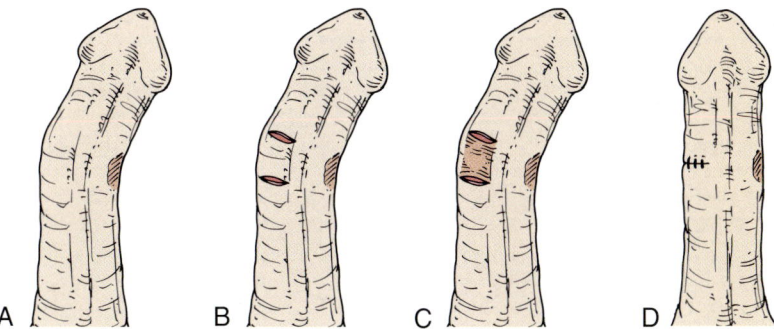

Fig. 73.14. The tunica albuginea plication (TAP) procedure (A) employs a pair of transverse parallel incisions (B) separated by 0.5 to 1.0 cm. The incision is made through the longitudinal fibers but does not violate the inner circular fibers of the tunic. (C) The longitudinal fibers between the two transverse incisions are removed to reduce the bulk of the plication. (D) The defect is then brought together transversely.

length after use of the TAP technique. The expected factors that predicted loss of length included the direction of curvature and the degree of curvature (Greenfield et al., 2006). Greenfield et al. (2006) found that men who had a ventral curvature of greater than 60 degrees tended to have the greatest potential loss of penile length. Preoperative penile length and degree and direction of curvature deformity appear to correlate with postoperative satisfaction (Mulhall et al., 2005; Greenfield et al., 2006).

The drawbacks of any tunica plication procedure for PD are that it does not correct shortening and it potentially may enhance loss of penile shaft length. It does not address hinge or hourglass effect and may exacerbate it, resulting in an unstable penis. The plaque is also left in situ. Penile narrowing or indentation has been reported in up to 17% with these techniques. In addition, there can be pain associated with the knots and suture granulomas (Ralph et al., 2010; Taylor and Levine, 2008; Tornehl and Carson, 2004). Surgical straightening with plication procedures can be expected in 79% to 100% of patients, with a reported satisfaction rate of 65% to 100% (Ding et al., 2010; Larsen and Levine, 2013; Van Der Horst et al., 2004). Recurrence of penile curvature deformity (greater than 30 degrees) has been reported in up to 12% in a limited number of long-term studies (Levine and Burnett, 2013; Taylor and Levine, 2008). The reported risk for new ED ranges from 0% to 38%, and diminished sensation has been reported in 4% to 21% with follow-up of up to 89 months. Other, less common complications include hematoma in up to 9% of patients, urethral injury in less than 2%, and phimosis in up to 5% (Kadioglu et al., 2011b; Larsen and Levine, 2013; Tornehl and Carson, 2004).

A recent International Consultation on Sexual Medicine (ICSM) published recommendations regarding plication procedures in 2010 and reported that there was "no evidence that one surgical approach provides better outcomes over another, but curvature correction can be expected with less risk of new ED" when compared with grafting procedures (Ralph et al., 2010) (Table 73.5 shows a summary of outcomes of tunical shortening procedures).

Clinicians may offer tunical plication surgery to patients whose rigidity is adequate for coitus (with or without pharmacotherapy and/or vacuum device therapy) to improve penile curvature, as per the 2015 AUA PD guideline.

Tunical Lengthening Procedures (Plaque Incision or Partial Excision and Grafting)

Indications for plaque incision and grafting (PIG) or partial plaque excision and grafting (PEG) for surgical correction of PD includes greater complexity of disease with several (or all) of the following: curvature greater than 60 to 70 degrees, shaft narrowing, hinging, and extensive plaque calcification (Kadioglu et al., 2011b; Kendirci and Hellstrom, 2004; Levine and Burnett, 2013; Levine and Lenting, 1997; Ralph et al., 2010; Yafi et al., 2016). **Most important, for the patient to be a candidate for PIG or PEG, he must have strong preoperative erections** (Taylor et al., 2012). This can be determined during the patient interview, when he is asked directly, "If your penis was straight, would the quality of rigidity that you currently have allow penetrative sex?" Should the patient hesitate or note suboptimal-quality erections, a grafting procedure should not be performed unless the patient fully understands the risk for more advanced postoperative ED and the possible need for subsequent prosthesis placement to obtain optimal rigidity. Some men simply reject the idea that they need a prosthesis as a first-line surgical treatment. Others who might be considered candidates for tunica plication reject this approach because of fear of penile length loss. These men may be offered a grafting repair with the understanding that a penile prosthesis can be placed with minimal added difficulty at a later time. The advantage of performing the grafting procedure is that it would likely correct curvature and reestablish more normal shaft caliber while increasing the likelihood of some length recovery in the range of 0.5 to 3.0 cm.

Other factors have been reported in the literature as possible predictors of postoperative ED, including age older than 55 years, evidence of corporeal veno-occlusive dysfunction on duplex ultrasound analysis with a resistance index of less than 0.80, large tunica defect and graft size, ventral curvature, and curvature greater than 60 degrees (Leungwattanakij et al., 2001; Levine et al., 2005; Alphs et al., 2010; Flores et al., 2011). These predictors have been suggested as a result of single-center studies, with a limited number of patients in each cohort. Larger-scale studies indicate that the most critical criterion for any grafting procedure is the quality of preoperative erections (Flores et al., 2011; Taylor et al., 2012). **In fact, Jordan and Angermeier found that there was a linear association between preoperative and postoperative ED** (Jordan and Angermeier, 1993). **Expert opinion has been consistent that patients with ventral deformity do not do well with grafting procedures.** Hellstrom's analysis of the relationship of penile deformity to the vascular status of PD patients showed that men with ventral curvature had the greatest likelihood of having cavernous veno-occlusive dysfunction (Lowsley and Boyce, 1950; Jordan and Angermeier, 1993).

Surgical grafting techniques include PIG and PEG. Historically, total excision of the plaque was practiced to "cut out the disease," resulting in onlays of large grafts with an unacceptably high rate of ED (Kendirci and Hellstrom, 2004; Kadioglu et al., 2006). Therefore, plaque incision was introduced in which a modified-H or double-Y incision is made in the area of maximum curvature (Gelbard, 1995). This allows the tunic to be expanded in this area, thereby correcting the curvature and shaft caliber but minimizing the underlying exposure of the cavernous tissue and thereby reducing the potential fibrosis of the cavernosal tissue and/or interrupting the delicate veno-occlusive mechanism, which has been considered the most likely contributor

TABLE 73.5 Outcomes of Tunical Shortening Procedure for Peyronie's Disease

PROCEDURE	AUTHOR AND DATE	PATIENTS (N)	MEAN FOLLOW-UP (MONTHS)	STRAIGHT AT LATEST FOLLOW-UP (%)	SHORTENING (% OF PATIENTS)	ED (%)	SATISFACTION RATES (%)
Nesbit	Licht and Lewis, 1997	28	22	79	37	4.0	79
	Schneider et al., 2003	48	25	23	44	0	75
	Syed et al., 2003	42	84	91	50	2.0	76
	Savoca et al., 2004	218	89	86.3	17.4	12.9	83.5
	Bokarica et al., 2005	40	81	88	15,[a] 100[b]	5.0	NR
	Ralph, 2006	9	31	NR	NR	NR	67
Plication	Geertsen et al., 1996	28	34	57	NR	3.5	82
	Levine and Lenting, 1997	22	20	91	9	9	NR
	Thiounn et al., 1998	29	34	79	NR	38	81,[a] 62[b]
	Schultheiss et al., 2000	61	39.8	70.5	45.9	3.3	NR
	Chahal et al., 2001	44	49	29	90	36	NR
	Gholami and Lue, 2002	124	31	85	41	6	96
	Van Der Horst et al., 2004	28	30	83	NR	0	67.8
	Paez et al., 2007	76	70	42	NR	60	NR
	Kim et al., 2008	26	≥12	65	69	11	65
	Kadioglu et al., 2008	15	21	87	NR	NR	93
	Taylor and Levine, 2008	61	72	93	18	10	84
	Dugi and Morey, 2010	34	6	98	NR	2.9	93
Yachia	Licht and Lewis, 1997	30	12	100	NR	NR	83
	Rehman et al., 1997	26	32	92	100	7.7	78
	Daitch et al., 1999	14	24.1	93	57	7	79

[a]Patient-perceived shortening.
[b]Objectively measured shortening.
ED, Erectile dysfunction; *NR*, not reported.

to postoperative ED with these grafting procedures (Dalton and Carter, 1991; Hatzimouratidis et al., 2012). Using the modified-H incision allows the correction of the curvature and shaft caliber. Gelbard (1995) has suggested that using multiple incisions and filling them with grafts would result in a smoother correction of curvature and potentially less injury to the underlying cavernosal tissue (Gelbard, 1995).

PEG may be preferable in cases in which the area of maximum deformity is excised, particularly if it is associated with severe indentation. **An increasing number of patients with severe deformity have indentation that if not addressed may result in a straightened penis but with residual narrowing causing instability.** The corners of the defect are darted in a radial fashion to enhance correction of the narrowing in that area (Levine, 2011). Geometric principles have been applied to the grafting technique so as to obtain a properly sized graft with excellent correction of deformity (Egydio et al., 2004). This approach has been considered unnecessarily complex, and there have been reports of a higher rate of postoperative ED when this technique has been used (Flores et al., 2011). **It appears intuitive that to reduce the risk for postoperative ED, the key is to limit trauma to the underlying cavernosal tissue to maintain the veno-occlusive relationship between the cavernosal tissue and the overlying tunica graft.**

Clinicians may offer plaque incision or excision and/or grafting to patients with deformities whose rigidity is adequate for coitus (with or without pharmacotherapy and/or vacuum device therapy) to improve penile curvature, as per the 2015 AUA PD guideline.

Graft Materials

The ideal graft should approximate the strength and elastic characteristics of normal tunica albuginea; should have minimal morbidity and tissue reaction; should be readily available; should not be too thick; should be pliable, easy to size and suture, inexpensive, and resistant to infection; and should preserve erectile capacity (Gur et al., 2011; Kadioglu et al., 2007). Multiple autologous grafts have been used historically, including fat, dermis, tunica vaginalis, dura mater, temporalis fascia, saphenous vein, crura or albuginea, and buccal mucosa (Das, 1980; Devine and Horton, 1974; Hatzichristodoulou et al., 2013a; Kadioglu et al., 2007; Kargi et al., 2004; Leungwattanakij et al., 2003; Liu et al., 2016; Lowsley and Boyce, 1950; Lue and El-Sakka, 1998; Sampaio et al., 2002; Shioshvili and Kakonahvili, 2005; Teloken et al., 2000; Valente et al., 2016; Wimpissinger et al., 2016; Yafi et al., 2016). Although the outcomes of these surgeries are typically good in select patients, they have fallen out of favor because of a need for extended surgery to harvest the graft and a second surgical site, which possesses its own potential complications of healing, scarring, and possible lymphedema. Crural and buccal grafts are compromised by the inability to get enough graft material for large defects (Hatzichristou and Hatzimouratidis, 2002; Schwarzer et al., 2003; Shioshvili and Kakonahvili, 2005). Synthetic polyethylene terephthalate (PETE, Dacron) and polytetrafluoroethylene (PTFE, Teflon) grafts have been used historically and are not recommended now because of the potential risk for infection, localized inflammatory response, and fibrosis (Brannigan et al., 1998; Devine et al., 1997). Finally, "off-the-shelf" allografts and xenografts have emerged, including processed pericardium from a bovine or human source, porcine intestinal submucosa, and porcine skin. The two most common grafts currently used are Tutoplast (Coloplast US, Minneapolis, MN), processed human and bovine pericardium, and porcine small intestinal submucosa (SIS) grafts (Surgisis ES, Cook Urological, Spencer, IN) (Hellstrom, 1994; Hellstrom and Reddy, 2000; Knoll, 2001; Levine and Estrada, 2003, Valente et al., 2016). These packaged processed grafts are being used with increased frequency because of their ease of use and reduction in operating times. The pericardial grafts are thin, are strong, do not contract, and have no reports of infection or rejection. Chun et al. (2001) performed a comparison of dermal and non-Tutoplast processed human cadaveric pericardial grafts in the modified Horton-Devine procedure. Overall, 92% of patients were able to achieve successful coitus with or without assistance. These researchers reported a 33% overall recurrence rate, with 26% of patients who received dermal grafts and 44% of patients who received pericardial grafts experiencing recurrence. However, this study did not report on the severity of recurrence, and all patients were able to achieve erections suitable for coitus. Satisfaction rates were similar, and those who underwent pericardial grafting had shorter operative times and decreased morbidity associated with the absence of a graft donor site (Chun et al., 2001). The SIS grafts have similar advantages to pericardium, except there have been reports of graft contraction, particularly with one-ply grafts, with associated recurrent curvature in the 37% to 75% range (Breyer et al., 2007; Kovac and Brock, 2007; John et al., 2006; Santucci and Barber, 2005; Taylor and Levine, 2008). Other reported postoperative complications with SIS grafts include subgraft hematoma in 26% and an infection rate of 5% (Breyer et al., 2007). However, a contemporary series showed that of 26 patients, there was 82% patient satisfaction and only 1 of 26 patients had a surgical complication (infected hematoma) (Valente et al., 2016).

Tissue-engineered graft materials have been considered more recently and potentially offer the advantage of having a graft seeded with cellular material, which may enhance the take of the graft and potentially reduce local tissue fibrosis with diminished postoperative ED. Adipose tissue–derived stem cell–seeded SIS, human acellular matrix tunica albuginea grafts, and autologous tissue–engineered endothelialized tunica albuginea grafts have been investigated for incision and excision procedures (da Silva et al., 2011; Imbeault et al., 2011; Ferretti et al., 2012; Ma et al., 2012; Schultheiss et al., 2004). Imbeault et al. (2011) demonstrated in vitro creation of artificial tunica albuginea using human dermal fibroblast and human endothelial cells. They concluded that this tissue-engineered endothelialized tubular graft was structurally similar to normal tunic with a high burst pressure and adequate mechanical resistance. Furthermore, the autologous property of this model could represent an advantage compared with other available grafts (Imbeault et al., 2011). Such studies may help elucidate future medical treatments for PD using tissue-engineered grafts for the reconstruction of the tunica albuginea. The biomechanical properties, compatibility with the tunica albuginea, and effective neovascularization of the tissue-engineered grafts need to be investigated further before such basic research can be applied in practice.

More recently, several studies have been published on the efficacy of Tachosil (Baxter Healthcare, Deerfield, IL) to cover the tunica defect from plaque partial excision or incision (Hatzichristodoulou, 2018; Hatzichristodoulou et al., 2013a; Lahme et al., 2002; Yafi et al., 2016). Tachosil is a collagen fleece coated with a tissue sealant that adheres to tissue after several minutes of compression. Because no surgical fixation is required, collagen fleece is easy to administer, and may shorten operating time. Lahme et al. (2002) first reported plaque incision/partial excision using a collagen fleece grafting on 19 patients. At a mean follow-up of 25 months, there were no major complications and recurrence was observed in only 16.7%. Yafi et al. used Tachosil on 26 patients undergoing partial excision and grafting for hourglass deformity with no major complications and an 85% success rate with a mean follow-up of 20 months (Yafi et al., 2016). The 2015 AUA PD guideline offers no opinion on choice of graft material.

Grafting Surgical Technique

Once the patient has achieved satisfactory general anesthesia, it is advised that the patient receive a dose of intravenous antibiotics and that the deep venous thrombosis protection apparatus be applied. The dorsal SPL should be measured. An artificial erection is then created by injecting a vasoactive drug (papaverine, Trimix, prostaglandin E_1) via a 21-gauge butterfly needle placed through the glans into the corpus cavernosum. Saline can be infused to create a full rigid erection, which allows visualization and measurement of the deformity, including curvature and areas of indentation with or without hinge effect. The preferred approach for grafting procedures is a circumcising incision made approximately 1.5 to 2 cm proximal to the corona, or through a previous circumcision site. The penis is degloved down to the Buck fascia, at which point hemostasis is obtained with bipolar cautery. It is advisable for the surgeon to use loupe magnification to reduce the likelihood of injury to neurovascular structures. With the shaft exposed, the erection can again be re-created, demonstrating the area of maximum deformity. In the circumstance of a dorsal or dorsal-lateral curvature, the Buck fascia, with the enclosed neurovascular bundle, is elevated by making a pair of parallel incisions just lateral to the urethral ridge, through the Buck fascia to the tunica albuginea. The Buck fascia is carefully elevated off the tunic. Typically this can be done with delicate, sharp dissection, but occasionally, if there is significant adhesion between the Buck fascia and the tunic, bipolar cautery can be used to elevate this with minimal risk for permanent nerve injury. Once the Buck fascia is elevated off the area of maximum deformity, a full erection is re-created. The area of maximum deformity is marked for incision or partial plaque excision. This allows excision and expansion of areas of severe indentation. It should be noted that even with a pure lateral curvature, the tunic to be excised must traverse through the dorsal septum, because this is the anchor point of the scar and if it is not taken, substantial residual curvature will likely remain (Jordan, 2007). When extensive calcification extends beyond the area of partial plaque excision, the calcified component can be removed, leaving the outer lamina intact because the calcification involves the inner circular fibers. Once the rectangular defect is established, the corners are darted in a radial fashion so as to help to recover normal shaft caliber in the area of indentation. Several authors have simplified the geometric principle technique by ensuring that the lateral sides of the defect are of equal length (Egydio et al., 2004; Levine, 2011). In doing this, we create a uniform-sized square or rectangle, which virtually always allows satisfactory correction of lateral and dorsal curvature. Often the proximal transverse length will be longer than the distal transverse length because of distal tapering of the shaft. The penis can now be measured on stretch again; typically there will be increased dorsal length from 0.5 to 3.0 cm. Stay sutures of 4-0 PDS (Ethicon, Somerville, NJ) are placed in the four corners of the defect and at the midpoint transversely, distally, and proximally. With these stay sutures on stretch, the defect can be measured longitudinally and transversely. Our preference is to use a Tutoplast processed pericardial graft (Coloplast, Minneapolis, MN), because there is usually little graft contraction. The graft should be sized no more than 10% larger than the measured defect on stretch. Porcine SIS grafts (Cook Urological, Spencer, IN) need to be oversized by 25%. Once the graft has been cut to size, it is secured in place with the previously placed stay sutures; then, with 4-0 PDS placed in a running fashion, the graft is secured to the defect. If a large defect is created, it may be advisable to place several interrupted 4-0 PDS sutures in the area of the septum to reduce the volume of blood that can accumulate under the graft. An artificial erection is again reestablished; if there is significant residual curvature, this can be addressed with tunica plication. Authors have found that this is necessary in up to 25% of patients. In patients who have a more prolonged curve or in those who have substantial indentation in one area and a more distal curvature, the grafting should be performed in the area of indentation, and plication is used to address any residual dorsal or lateral curve once grafting has been completed. In this circumstance, a single graft can be used, which has not been shown to have a higher rate of postoperative ED than when multiple grafts are used but does have the advantage of shorter operative time. Once satisfactory deformity correction has been accomplished, the Buck fascia is reapproximated with running 4-0 chromic, and the shaft skin is reapproximated to subcoronal skin with interrupted 4-0 chromic in a horizontal mattress fashion. Of note, for those patients who are uncircumcised and do not have any evidence of phimosis, a circumcision is not necessary (Garaffa et al., 2010); but if there is any question of excessive redundant foreskin and/or phimosis, then circumcision should be performed to reduce the likelihood of postoperative paraphimosis (Garaffa et al., 2010). The penis is dressed with Xeroform gauze (3M, St. Paul, MN) placed over the circumcising incision, and then a Coban wrap (3M, St. Paul, MN) is placed distal to proximal, providing gentle compression. Typically the dressing is left in place for 3 days and then removed, at which point the patient may shower. Submersion of the wound is not advised because this may encourage wound separation.

Postoperative Management

The postoperative rehabilitation period is critical to reduce the risk for postoperative ED and length loss and to optimize straight healing. We find it useful to liken the importance of postoperative rehabilitation after penile surgery to the importance of the rehabilitation needed for successful orthopedic joint replacement. Typically, a patient is seen 2 weeks after surgery, at which point massage and stretch therapy are initiated (Horton et al., 1987). The patient is instructed to grasp the penis by the glans and gently stretch it away from the body and then with his other hand to massage the shaft of the penis for 5 minutes twice per day for 2 to 4 weeks. The massage and stretch can be performed by the patient's partner for the second 2 weeks if possible. This will reinitiate the sexual experience for the couple and hopefully diminish the fear of reinjuring the penis, for which the partner may feel responsible. Investigators have recommended the use of nocturnal PDE5 inhibitors to enhance postoperative vasodilation, which may help support graft take, reduce cicatrix contraction, and theoretically preserve cavernosal tissue, thereby reducing postoperative ED (Levine et al., 2005). Finally, external penile traction devices have been encouraged and have been recently shown to reduce length loss postoperatively and can even enhance length gain after both grafting and plication procedures (Levine et al., 2013). In a recent report, SPL in patients who used postoperative traction therapy was shown to increase after plication and PEG procedures by +0.85 cm and +1.48 cm, respectively, versus length changes of −0.53 cm and +0.24 cm in the plication and PEG groups in which postoperative traction was not used. In fact, 50% of the plication and 89% of the PEG patients using postoperative traction had measured length gain. The reported average daily use was 2.5 hours for 4.5 days per week for an average duration of 3.8 months. There was no patient reported with postoperative length loss among those who used postoperative traction therapy, and although not statistically significant, there was a trend of higher satisfaction for erect length in the groups in which postoperative traction was used. Traction is recommended to be used for 3 or more hours per day, beginning 3 to 4 weeks after surgery, once the wound can tolerate the pressures of the stretching device for 3 months (Rybak et al., 2012).

In a review of published reports on grafting for PD over the past 12 years, satisfactory straightening was found in 74% to 100% of patients, but postoperative ED, which does not have a uniform definition in the literature and may include reduced rigidity, compared with preoperative rigidity to complete loss of rigidity has been reported in 5% to 54% of patients. Diminished sensation after grafting has been reported in a few series with a follow-up of less than 5 years (Taylor and Levine, 2008). In the few single-center surgical outcome reviews with 5 or more years of follow-up, ED has been reported in up to 24%, with recurrent or persistent curvature in the 8% to 12% range (Chung et al., 2011a; Kalsi et al., 2005; Montorsi et al., 2004; Usta et al., 2003). See Table 73.4 for a summary of the outcomes for penile straightening with plaque incision or excision and grafting.

The AUA 2015 PD guideline states that, "Clinicians may offer plaque incision or excision and/or grafting to patients with deformities whose rigidity is adequate for coitus (with or without pharmacotherapy and/or vacuum device therapy) to improve penile curvature. (Moderate Recommendation; Evidence Strength Grade C)."

Penile Prosthesis for Men With Peyronie's Disease

Indications

In men with PD and concurrent ED refractory to PDE5 inhibitors, penile prosthesis placement is the procedure of choice (Kendirci and Hellstrom, 2004; Levine and Dimitriou, 2000; Levine and Lenting, 1997; Mulhall et al., 2005; Ralph and Minhas, 2004). **Additional straightening maneuvers may be necessary, including manual modeling and incising of the tunica albuginea with or without grafting.** Recently, transcorporeal approaches have been used before modeling or relaxing incisions; the plaque is incised or stretched from within the corporeal body (Perito and Wilson, 2013; Shaeer, 2011).

Techniques for Straightening When Placing a Penile Prosthesis for Peyronie's Disease

An inflatable penile prosthesis (IPP) appears to be the preferred surgical implant, as the pressure within the cylinders allows for superior correction of curvature with manual modeling, and improved girth enhancement. Malleable prostheses, when used for PD historically, were associated with narrow, cold, and less than natural erections (Ghanem et al., 1998; Marzi et al., 1997; Montorsi et al., 1993).

Manual modeling via the penoscrotal approach is recommended with a high-pressure inflatable cylinder, but all available three-piece and two-piece devices have been used successfully to correct deformity (Chung et al., 2013c; Levine et al., 2001; Montague et al., 1996; Montorsi et al., 1996; Wilson and Delk, 1994). Our approach is to place the prosthesis cylinders first, followed by closing of the corporotomies. With use of a surrogate reservoir attached to the pump tubing, the prosthesis can be filled to full rigidity, which will allow visualization of the deformity. To protect the pump from the high pressures that may occur during manual modeling, shodded hemostat clamps are applied to the tubing between the pump and the cylinders. The penis is then bent in the contralateral direction to the curvature. It is recommended to try to hold the penis in this position for 60 to 90 seconds, but experience has suggested that approximately 30 seconds may be all that is possible. Once the modeling has been performed, the penis can be reassessed by instilling more fluid, reapplying the hemostats, and then performing the modeling procedure repeatedly until satisfactory curvature correction has been attained. **The modeling technique should be a gradual bending rather than a violent maneuver, because this will reduce the likelihood of inadvertent tearing of the tunic or injury to the overlying neurovascular bundle.** Urethral injuries during performance of this technique as a result of distal extrusion of the prosthetic cylinders at the fossa navicularis have been reported (Wilson and Delk, 1994; Wilson et al., 2001). To reduce the likelihood of this occurring, the bending hand should be placed on the shaft of the penis rather than on the glans, to avoid downward pressure on the tips of the cylinders. The other hand should be grasping the base of the penis with pressure over the corporotomies, which will provide support to this area and reduce the likelihood of disruption of the suture line.

Published reports on the use of modeling have indicated that successful straightening can be expected in 86% to 100% with no higher incidence of device revision; sensory deficit after manual modeling is rare but remains a potential complication that should be discussed with the patient preoperatively (Chung et al., 2013c; Levine et al., 2010; Montague et al., 1996; Wilson and Delk, 1994; Wilson et al., 2001). Although it would appear that for more severe curvature more advanced techniques are necessary, published experience has suggested that manual modeling may be used as first-line therapy for correction of curvature after prosthesis implantation (Chung et al., 2013c; Levine et al., 2010). An alternative to this would be to perform a tunic plication contralateral to the curvature before placement of the prosthesis to correct the curvature (Dugi and Morey, 2010; Rahman et al., 2004). When there is residual curvature of greater than 30 degrees or residual indentation causing the inflated cylinder to buckle, tunical incision is recommended after elevation of the Buck fascia in that area (Levine and Dimitriou, 2000).

The transverse penoscrotal skin incision will allow access to virtually the entire shaft, except when the curvature is distal and dorsal on the shaft, so degloving the penis is not always necessary. The tunical incision is made with the cylinders deflated, using the cautery to release the tunic with an effort to preserve cavernosal tissue over the implant. When Titan cylinders (Coloplast, Minneapolis, MN) are used, the energy should be less than 30 watts to reduce potential cylinder thermal injury (Hakim et al., 1996). Once the incision has been made, the cylinders are reinflated and further modeling can be performed to optimize deformity correction. **Although there is no clearly accepted approach, grafting is recommended when the defect measures greater than 2 cm in any dimension to reduce cicatrix contracture and cylinder herniation** (Carson and Levine, 2014; Levine and Dimitriou, 2000). **Historically, synthetic grafts were used, but currently biografts of pericardium or porcine SIS are recommended. Use of locally harvested dermal grafts is not recommended, because there is a risk for transferring bacteria to the prosthesis.** Collagen fleece spray has also been reported to cover tunical defects in patients undergoing IPP with favorable results (Hatzichristodoulou, 2018; Yafi et al., 2016).

In patients who have suffered debilitating loss of penile length or girth, the "sliding technique" can be used in conjunction with a penile prosthesis to offer some restoration of length and girth (Egydio and Kuehhas, 2015; Rolle et al., 2012). Details regarding this procedure can be found in Rolle et al. (2012). In a large series of 143 patients undergoing this procedure, the average penile length gain was 3.1 cm. There were no prosthesis infections or any major complications at an average follow-up of 9.7 months. Of the 77 patients who had penile curvature, all were corrected and 89.2% of patients were satisfied with their procedure. At this time, experience with this procedure is limited to a single institution, and most patients in this study received a malleable prosthesis.

There have been limited publications looking at the long-term results with regard to outcomes and satisfaction with inflatable penile prostheses in men with PD and ED. Levine et al. (2010) reported on 90 consecutive men undergoing placement of an IPP, with 4% having satisfactory straightening with prosthesis placement alone, 79% having satisfactory curvature correction with prosthesis and modeling, 4% requiring tunical incision, and 12% having incision and pericardial grafting for correction of curvature. There was no evidence that the additional maneuvers increased the rate of mechanical failure or infection with up to 8 years of follow-up. In the nonvalidated questionnaire used in this study, overall patient satisfaction was 84%, whereas only 73% were satisfied with curvature correction. This may indicate a flaw in the design of the questionnaire, but may also reflect the general disappointment and frustration of patients with PD (Levine et al., 2010). Thus, preoperative counseling and setting appropriate expectations as with any prosthesis placement are critical (Akin-Olugbade et al., 2006). It is recommended that preoperative discussion also be focused on the goal of obtaining "functional straightness," in which a residual curvature of 20 degrees or less in any direction would likely not compromise sexual activity and may correct in time as a result of tissue expansion caused by the cylinders. A comparison of outcomes between the two three-piece inflatable devices in North America found no significant advantage with respect to device reliability, infection, or patient satisfaction (Chung et al., 2013c).

By far the most common postoperative complaint heard from men who have undergone penile prosthesis placement is length loss (Montague, 2007). Wang et al. objectively evaluated penile length change after prosthesis implantation and demonstrated decreases of 0.8, 0.75, and 0.74 cm at 6 weeks, 6 months, and 1 year after surgery, respectively (Wang et al., 2009). This is of particular concern in the PD population, who often already have loss of penile length. Any additional length loss as a result of the implant may be distressing to the patient and should be addressed preoperatively. For men who cannot tolerate any further length loss, a recent small pilot study using traction therapy before penile prosthesis placement in men with PD and other disorders causing penile shortening (e.g., prosthesis explants, radical prostatectomy) demonstrated that after 3 to 4 months of daily traction for an average of 3 hours or more per day, there was no further loss of length after prosthesis placement, and the majority had gained some length (0.5 to 2.0 cm) compared with the pretraction SPL (Levine and Rybak, 2011). Postoperative prolonged cylinder inflation has been recommended to maintain penile length and decrease residual curvature; the device is kept inflated for 10 to 30 minutes daily for 3 months starting 6 weeks after surgery. See Table 73.6 for a summary on the outcomes of penile straightening with penile prosthesis placement.

TABLE 73.6 Outcomes of Penile Prosthesis Implantation for Peyronie's Disease

AUTHOR AND DATE	PROSTHESIS TYPE	PATIENTS (N)	MEAN FOLLOW-UP (MONTHS)	ADDITIONAL STRAIGHTENING MANEUVERS (%)	SATISFACTION RATES (%)
Garaffa et al., 2011	Inflatable	129	NR	37	86
	Malleable	80	NR	16	72
Levine et al., 2010	Inflatable	90	49	96	84
DiBlasio et al., 2010	Inflatable	79	20	11	NR
Wilson and Delk, 1994	Inflatable	138	NR	8	NR
Montague, 2007	Inflatable	72	NR	8	67
Chaudhary et al., 2005	Inflatable	46	12	61	93
Rahman et al., 2004	Inflatable	5	22	100	100
Levine and Dimitriou, 2000	Inflatable	46	39	NR	NR
Akin-Olugbade et al., 2006	Inflatable	18	≥6	22.2	60
Usta et al., 2003	Inflatable	42	21 (12–48)	30	84
Wilson et al., 2001	Inflatable	104	60	0	99
Carson et al., 2000	Inflatable	63	NR	NR	88
Morganstern, 1997	Inflatable	309	42	NR	NR
Montorsi et al., 1996	Inflatable	33	17	40	79
Rolle et al., 2012	Both (sliding technique)	3	13	100[a]	100
Antonini et al., 2018	Inflatable	145	NR	NR	NR
Hatzichristodoulou, 2018	Inflatable	15	15.1	100	100
Egydio and Kuehhas, 2015	Both (sliding technique)	143	9.7	100	90.2

[a]Sliding procedure is by definition a straightening maneuver.
NR, Not reported.

KEY POINTS: SURGICAL MANAGEMENT

- Surgical correction of PD with or without penile prosthesis placement remains the gold standard to correct deformity and is indicated when deformity or rigidity compromises or prevents penetrative sexual activity.
- Surgical candidates need to undergo a detailed and comprehensive consent process so that the patient will understand the potential limitations of the surgery and will have appropriate personal expectations, thereby improving postoperative satisfaction.
- For patients with satisfactory preoperative rigidity with curvature less than 60 to 70 degrees without significant indentation, some form of tunica plication is indicated. There does not appear to be any one plication technique that has been demonstrated to be superior to others, as no head-to-head comparative trials have been published.
- Men who have more severe, complex deformity but who have strong preoperative erectile function and no evidence of venous insufficiency on duplex ultrasound analysis should be considered candidates for straightening with plaque incision or PEG.
- Complications associated with all straightening operations include incomplete straightening, recurrent curvature, shaft shortening, diminished penile sexual sensation, and ED.
- It appears that the nature of the graft is less likely the determining factor with respect to postoperative ED. On the other hand, optimum outcomes are most likely a result of proper patient selection with respect to preoperative erectile status and operative technique.
- For men who have inadequate rigidity and PD, penile prosthesis placement with straightening maneuvers as necessary should be considered first-line surgery.
- The AUA 2015 PD guideline recommends the following:
  - Clinicians may offer penile prosthesis surgery to patients with PD with ED and/or penile deformity sufficient to prevent coitus despite pharmacotherapy and/or vacuum device therapy (Moderate Recommendation; Evidence Strength Grade C).
  - Clinicians may perform adjunctive intraoperative procedures, such as modeling, plication, or incision/grafting, when significant penile deformity persists after insertion of the penile prosthesis (Moderate Recommendation; Evidence Strength Grade C).
  - Clinicians should use an inflatable penile prosthesis for the patient undergoing penile prosthetic surgery for treatment of PD.

CONCLUSION

PD is far more common than previously thought and is a growth area in urology not only for clinical practice, but also for basic science research. The mysteries of this wound-healing disorder need to be clarified, and this will likely yield better treatment options and potential strategies to prevent progression. It should be recognized that there are acute and stable phases and that surgery should be offered only after the scarring process has been stable for 3 to 6 months. Patients with PD should be counseled that complete correction of the deformity, including curvature, indentation, and shortening, is not likely and that the goal is to allow the patient to function sexually again. The devastating psychological impact of this disease is important to recognize, and psychological counseling is occasionally indicated and should be offered. For patients in the acute phase, nonsurgical treatment is limited to oral NSAIDs. When surgery is indicated, the goal is to correct the deformity and prevent worsening of ED so that penetrative sexual activity is possible. The patient must understand that recovery of his pre-PD penile appearance is not likely and that surgery carries the risk for incomplete straightening and recurrent curvature, further shaft shortening, change in sexual sensitivity, and, most important, diminished postoperative rigidity. For men with drug-refractory ED and PD, placement of a penile prosthesis with straightening maneuvers is the best approach to address both problems with one operation.

SUGGESTED READINGS

Avant RA, Ziegelmann M, Nehra A, et al: Penile traction therapy and vacuum erection devices in Peyronie's disease, *Sex Med Rev* 2018. [Epub ahead of print]. pii: S2050-0521(18)30019-2.

Eisenberg ML, Smith JF, Shindel AW, et al: Tunica-sparing ossified Peyronie's plaque excision, *BJU Int* 107(4):622–625, 2011.

Goldstein I, Knoll LD, Lipshultz LI, et al: Changes in the effects of Peyronie's disease after treatment with collagenase clostridium histolyticum: male patients and their female partners, *Sex Med* 5(2):e124–e130, 2017.

Gonzalez-Cadavid NF, Rajfer J: Mechanisms of disease: new insights into the cellular and molecular pathology of Peyronie's disease, *Nat Clin Pract Urol* 2:291–297, 2005.

Hatzichristodoulou G, Osmonov D, Kübler H, et al: Contemporary review of grafting techniques for the surgical treatment of Peyronie's disease, *Sex Med Rev* 5(4):544–552, 2017.

Hatzimouratidis K, Eardley I, Giuliano F, et al: European Association of Urology. EAU guidelines on penile curvature, *Eur Urol* 62(3):543–552, 2012.

Levine LA, Burnett AL: Standard operating procedures for Peyronie's disease, *J Sex Med* 10:230–244, 2013.

Lipshultz LI, Goldstein I, Seftel AD, et al: Clinical efficacy of collagenase Clostridium histolyticum in the treatment of Peyronie's disease by subgroup: results from two large, double-blind, randomized, placebo-controlled, phase III studies, *BJU Int* 116(4):650–656, 2015.

Mulhall JP, Schiff J, Guhring P: An analysis of the natural history of Peyronie's disease, *J Urol* 175(6):2115–2118, discussion 2118, 2006.

Nehra A, Alterowitz R, Culkin DJ, et al: Peyronie's disease: AUA guideline, *J Urol* 194(3):745–753, 2015.

Pagano MJ, Weinberg AC, Deibert CM, et al: Penile intracavernosal pillars: lessons from anatomy and potential implications for penile prosthesis placement, *Int J Impot Res* 28(3):114–119, 2016.

Papagiannopoulos D, Yura E, Levine L: Examining postoperative outcomes after employing a surgical algorithm for management of Peyronie's disease: a single-institution retrospective review, *J Sex Med* 12(6):1474–1480, 2015.

Ralph D, Gonzalez-Cadavid N, Mirone V, et al: The management of Peyronie's disease: evidence-based 2010 guidelines, *J Sex Med* 7(7):2359–2374, 2010.

REFERENCES

The complete reference list is available online at ExpertConsult.com.

74

Sexual Function and Dysfunction in the Female

Ervin Kocjancic, MD, Valerio Iacovelli, MD, and Ömer Acar, MD

ANATOMY AND PHYSIOLOGY OF FEMALE SEXUAL ORGANS

Accurate examination of the female external and internal genitalia is mandatory to better understand female sexual function and dysfunction.

The *distal vagina* is the site of female sexual response and it is interrelated with the clitoris and the female urethra. Though in anatomic terms these are distinct structures, the distal vagina, clitoris, and urethra *(clitoral complex)* share blood supply and innervation. During sexual activity, these structures, with their overlying highly vascular skin (the vulva), respond as a unit. Therefore, the vulva can be defined as the wrapping overlying the clitoro-urethro-vaginal complex. The female erectile organs include the clitoris and the vestibular bulbs.

The erectile complex is made of specialized vascular tissues that are sexually responsive and consist of two histologically distinct types of vascular tissue. Trabeculated erectile tissue is peculiar of the clitoris and the bulbs and allows for engorgement with blood and volume expansion during sexual arousal. The labia minora and glans clitoris are composed of nonerectile vascular tissue, which also is found surrounding the urethral orifice and within the walls of the vagina. A region of the anterior wall of the vagina overlying the mid-urethra has been identified as the Grafenberg spot (or G-spot), an area that is particularly sensitive to tactile stimulation in some women.

The female sexual reflex is mediated by five components: (1) the receptors of the clitoral complex and vulva; (2) somatic afferents (terminal divisions of pudendal nerves via its dorsal clitoral and perineal branches); (3) spinal cord segments S2–S4; (4) visceral efferents (pelvic parasympathetic fibers) via nervi erigentes running in pelvic ganglia; and (5) effectors (erectile or spongy tissue of the clitoral complex) and secretory responses from sub-bulbar and urethral glands. Parasympathetic stimulation causes dilation of arterioles (dorsal and deep arteries of the clitoris) supplying erectile tissue, which becomes engorged. Erection of the clitoral complex is accompanied by swelling of the vulva with changes to the distal vagina and urethra accompanied by a secretory response of the latter structures.

The female sexual response cycle consists of a sequence of physical and emotional changes that occur as a person becomes sexually aroused and participates in sexually stimulating activities, including intercourse and masturbation. Erotic stimuli initiate a series of physiologic changes that have collectively been termed the *sexual response cycle* and are divided into four distinct phases: (1) *excitement/arousal phase* with subjective pleasure and excitement; (2) *plateau phase* during which there is intensification of the changes in phase 1; (3) *orgasm*, a variable, transient peak sensation of intense pleasure, creating an altered state of consciousness; and (4) *resolution phase*, when sexual excitement declines back to baseline levels.

Brain centers deemed particularly important to the integration of sexual desire and arousal responses for women include the medial amygdala, the stria terminalis, the ventromedial nucleus of the hypothalamus, and the paraventricular nucleus (PVN). The nitric oxide (NO)/cyclic guanosine monophosphate (cGMP) pathway contributes to clitoral erection and vaginal vasodilation with sexual arousal. NO activates guanylate cyclase, which produces cGMP. cGMP activates numerous downstream effectors, the net effect of which is to sequester calcium and to reduce contraction of smooth muscle in the clitoral and vaginal circulation and within the vaginal wall.

Hormone levels in the body affect female sexual function. Estrogens maintain female genital tissue integrity and thickness. Levels of estradiol influence both central and peripheral nerve transmissions and regulate nitric oxide synthase (NOS) expression. Testosterone is also important, being related with sexual arousal, libido, sexual responsiveness, genital sensation, and orgasm.

See ExpertConsult.com for more information about anatomy and physiology of female sexual organs.

> **KEY POINTS: ANATOMY, PHYSIOLOGY, AND SEXUAL RESPONSE CYCLE**
>
> - The distal vagina is the site of female sexual response, and it shares blood supply and innervation with the clitoris and urethra.
> - The clitoris, distal vagina, and urethra (the clitoral complex) respond as a unit during sexual activity with their overlying highly vascular skin.
> - There are two types of sexually responsive vascular tissue in the clitoral complex: erectile and nonerectile.
> - The Grafenberg spot (G-spot), which is located in the anterior wall of the vagina overlying the mid-urethra, is particularly sensitive to tactile stimulation in some women.
> - The female sexual response cycle refers to the sequence of physical and emotional changes that occur on sexual arousal and engagement in sexually stimulating activities.
> - The linear sexual response cycle models (excitement/arousal, plateau, orgasm, and resolution) may not be applicable to all women.

EVALUATION OF SEXUAL WELLNESS

History Taking

Patients are usually reluctant to discuss sexual health–related issues with their physicians. Health care providers should bring up the topic of sexual health because only approximately 18% of women with sexual issues will seek medical advice about sexual dysfunction (Kaplan, 1979). Certain barriers, such as a lack of adequate training and confidence in the topic, a perception that there are few treatment options, a lack of adequate clinical time to obtain a sexual history, patients' hesitancy to initiate the conversation, and the underestimation of the prevalence of sexual dysfunction, can preclude an interactive dialogue about sexual health between the patient and the physician (Bachmann, 2006; Frank et al., 2008).

Clinical conversations should acknowledge the contributions of sexuality, relationships, and sexual behavior to overall health (Latif and Diamond, 2013). By using a "broader, sex-positive, health-focused framework" with patients, physicians can encourage communication about sexuality. Sexual health promotion has become increasingly less stigmatized, and the focus has shifted toward a more holistic view that promotes sexual health as a right for all women and men (American College of Obstetricians and Gynecologists [ACOG], 2017).

Assessment of female sexual (dys)function is best approached using an integrated approach addressing biologic, psychological,

sociocultural, and interpersonal factors (Table 74.1) (Bitzer et al., 2013; Fugl-Meyer et al., 2013; Latif and Diamond, 2013).

When discussing female sexual response, physicians should emphasize the wide range of complex normal experiences. In 1966, Masters and Johnson described female sexual response as a linear model with four phases of response: excitement, plateau, orgasm, and resolution. Basson (2002b) described a "Sexual Response Circle", which incorporates psychological and social aspects into female sexual function, such as emotional intimacy and emotional satisfaction as well as sexual desire and physical satisfaction. **Therefore, a discussion of sexual responsiveness with a patient should include the importance of not only sexual stimuli, but also factors such as emotional intimacy and relationship satisfaction.**

The PLISSIT Model of Assessment and Treatment

Annon described the PLISSIT model of assessment for female sexual function, which may increase the efficiency of information gathering in the primary health care setting and also incorporates implications for specialized therapeutic approaches to be followed in that particular patient (Annon, 1976). PLISSIT stands for Permission, Limited Information, Specific Suggestions, Intensive Therapy. Permission stands for the discussion with the patient around normalization of sexual behaviors. Limited Information could include information about behaviors that may increase arousal, including foreplay and a discussion of medical conditions or medications that could be contributing to the problem. Specific Suggestions could include use of lubricants, vaginal estrogen, and position changes. Intensive Therapy would be referral to a specialist, such as a sex therapist or couple's counselor, if appropriate (Annon, 1976). Table 74.2 summarizes the steps of the PLISSIT model.

Assuring the patient that it is not uncommon or abnormal to mention questions or concerns about sexual life might be helpful to initiate the discussion about sexual health issues. Afterwards, simple screening questions may be asked to understand the need for further evaluation. Examples could include the following:

- "Sexuality is such an important part of our overall health. I would like to ask you some questions about that now. Is that okay with you?"
- "Are you currently sexually active?"
- "With men, women, or both?"
- "Do you have any concerns about your sexual health?"

Clinicians can screen all patients, regardless of age, with the help of a validated sex questionnaire or during a routine review of systems. A simple, integrated screening tool to use is the Brief Sexual Symptom Checklist for Women (BSSC-W), created by the International Consultation in Sexual Medicine (Hatzichristou et al., 2010). Although recommended by the ACOG (ACOG, 2017), the BSSC-W is not validated. The questionnaire includes four questions that gather personal information regarding an individual's overall sexual function satisfaction, the problem causing dysfunction, how bothersome the symptoms are, and the willingness to discuss it with her provider (Table 74.3) (Hatzichristou et al., 2016).

The use of basic, broad, open-ended, and gender-neutral questions in a routine history gathering can also help the clinician disclose issues that may require further exploration. Furthermore, it will be helpful to discriminate between different types of female sexual dysfunction (FSD). The following are examples of such questions:

- "Are you sexually active?"
- "Are you sexually satisfied?"
- "Do you have questions or concerns about sexual functioning?"
- "Do you think your partner is satisfied?"
- "Do you have orgasms?"
- "Are you satisfied with the frequency of sexual activity?"
- "Does your vagina lubricate enough?"

After the screening questions, further information about the factors (partners, sexual practices, protection from sexually transmitted infections [STIs], past history of STIs, prevention of pregnancy) that

TABLE 74.1 Biopsychosocial Model of Assessing Sexual (Dys)Function

Biologic factors	Medications Hormonal status Neurobiology Physical health Aging
Psychological factors	Depression Anxiety Self-image Substance abuse History of sexual abuse, trauma
Sociocultural factors	Upbringing Cultural norms and expectations Religious influences
Interpersonal factors	Relationship status/quality Partner's sexual function Life stressors

Modified from Bitzer J, Giraldi A, Pfaus J. Sexual desire and hypoactive sexual desire disorder in women. Introduction and overview. Standard operating procedure (SOP Part 1). *J Sex Med* 2013;10(1):36–49; Fugl-Meyer KS, Bohm-Starke N, Damsted Petersen C, et al. Standard operating procedures for female genital sexual pain. *J Sex Med* 2013;10(1):83–93; Latif EZ, Diamond MP. Arriving at the diagnosis of female sexual dysfunction. *Fertil Steril* 2013;100(4):898–904.

TABLE 74.2 PLISSIT Model of Assessment

STEPS	EXAMPLES OF WHAT TO SAY TO PATIENTS
Permission Give the patient permission to speak about her sexual health and to do what she is already doing sexually (or may want to do).	"This is important. Thank you for sharing. Many postmenopausal women report a decrease in sexual desire."
Limited information Provide basic accurate sex education (e.g., female sexual response cycle, impact of aging on sexual function, anatomy).	"Sexual desire changes with age. After menopause, you may experience more responsive desire than spontaneous desire."
Specific suggestions Provide simple suggestions to increase sexual function (e.g., lubricant use, vibrator use, ways to increase emotional intimacy).	"Your responsive sexual desire may benefit from being more planful with sexual activity. Talk with your partner about how to be more intentional sexually."
Intensive therapy Validate the patient's concerns and refer her to a subspecialist.	"Your sexual health is important. I'd like to refer you to someone with expertise in sexual health."

Modified from Faubion SS, Rullo JE. Sexual dysfunction in women: a practical approach. *Am Fam Physician* 2015;92(4):281–288.

TABLE 74.3 Brief Sexual Symptom Checklist for Women

Please answer the following questions about your overall sexual function:

1. Are you satisfied with your sexual function?
___ Yes ___ No
If No, please continue
2. How long have you been dissatisfied with your sexual function?
3. The problem(s) with your sexual function is: *(mark one or more)*
Problem with little or no interest in sex
Problem with decreased genital sensation (feeling)
Problem with decreased vaginal lubrication (dryness)
Problem reaching orgasm
Problem with pain during sex
Other:
4. Which problem is most bothersome (circle)?
5. Would you like to talk about it with your doctor?

---

might have an influence on female sexual (dys)function can be elaborated via comprehensive history taking (Table 74.4). The precise nature of the sexual concern, any associated symptoms, chronology, presumed or defined trigger events, exacerbating or relieving factors, and previously attempted treatments should be elicited (Kingsberg and Althof, 2009). The ACOG has published recommendations about how to question the patient about these details and how to end the history taking in an interactive and constructive manner (ACOG, 2017). If the clinician does not have training for in-depth discussion of sexuality, an appropriate referral to a specialist should be considered (Goldstein and Alexander, 2005).

Questionnaires

Validated questionnaires/surveys/scales can be used to assess female sexual functioning. However, it should be noted that survey instruments cannot replace a detailed history and physical examination. In 2000, the Female Sexual Function Index (FSFI) was developed based on the *Diagnostic and Statistical Manual of Mental Disorders (DSM-IV-TR)* definitions (American Psychiatric Association [APA], 2000) of sexual dysfunction and the Consensus Report of the International Consensus Development Conference on Female Sexual Dysfunction (Basson et al., 2000). It is a brief, 19-item, multidimensional self-report instrument that assesses six domains of sexual function: desire, arousal, lubrication, orgasm, satisfaction, and pain. The target population consists of heterosexual and homosexual women. It is available for premenopausal and postmenopausal women and women with medical and sexual disorders. It refers to the past 4 weeks, and administration time varies between 10 and 15 minutes (Rosen et al., 2000).

Although it is validated for use in research, it is not yet used in clinical practice. However, the questions are quite useful and may be helpful to clinicians in obtaining a more comprehensive sexual history. How to interpret FSFI scores in the clinical setting has yet to be determined, but the individual responses to each question may be very informative when evaluating a sexual complaint. Each domain of FSFI is scored on a scale of 0 to 6 points with the exception of the desire domain (scored from 1.2 to 6) and the satisfaction domain (scored from 0.8 to 6). The instrument thus has a range of 2 to 36, with 36 representing a "perfect" score. The maximum total score is 36, and higher scores indicate better sexual functioning. A total FSFI score of less than 26.55 is considered at risk for sexual dysfunction (Rosen et al., 2000).

An abbreviated version (six items) also has been validated in premenopausal and postmenopausal women and has been proposed as a tool for screening women likely to have FSD (Chedraui et al., 2012; Isidori et al., 2010). The FSFI also has been validated for use in patients with cancer, in whom strong psychometric properties have been reported (Bartula and Sherman, 2015; Baser et al., 2012) in addition to women with chronic pelvic pain (CPP) (Verit and Verit, 2007). A specific cutoff for the diagnosis of hypoactive sexual desire disorder (HSDD) using the two-item desire domain of the FSFI was reported; on a scale of 2 to 10, women with a score of 6 or higher on this domain were unlikely to carry the diagnosis (Gerstenberger et al., 2010).

The Female Sexual Distress Scale (FSDS) is a 12-item scale that assesses subjective distress associated with sexual dysfunction in women (Derogatis et al., 2002). A revised version with an additional 13th question about distress related to low sexual desire was developed to improve discriminative value in women with HSDD (Derogatis et al., 2008). Both versions have been validated and found to be reliable in distinguishing female patients with and without sexual dysfunction (Rosen, 2002). Table 74.5 summarizes selected sexual functioning questionnaires/scales that have been utilized and clinically tested in the context of female sexual (dys)functional assessment (Hatzichristou et al., 2016).

In addition, the history should focus on systemic comorbidities, medications, and surgeries that may potentially influence neurologic, endocrine, vascular, or psychological function can affect sexual function. There are several correlating factors and conditions that may put some women at an increased risk for sexual dysfunction. Although menopause may seem like a direct risk for sexual dysfunction, there has not been a study with statistically significant results documenting a universal decline in sexual function in menopausal and postmenopausal women (Basson, 2008). Chronic medical conditions, such as diabetes, hypertension, overactive bladder (OAB), multiple sclerosis, spinal cord injury (SCI), and major depressive disorder, can contribute to FSD. Table 74.6 provides a list of possible systemic comorbidities that might potentially influence and/or were found to be associated with the domains of FSD (Clayton and Groth, 2013; Shifren et al., 2008).

Medications can interfere with sexual function by alteration of mood and libido, such as antidepressants, antipsychotics, and sedatives; by alteration of blood flow to the genitals decreasing arousal and/or lubrication, such as certain antihypertensives or antiestrogens; or by increasing sex hormone–binding globulins (SHBGs) and therefore decreasing free testosterone levels such as with oral contraceptives. Oral contraceptives are another medication group that have been thought to affect sexual function, but the majority of evidence reveals that only a small minority of women actually experience such a side effect. Illicit drug use and alcoholism also are associated with FSD. Excessive tobacco abuse may lead to vascular insufficiency and decreased genital blood flow (Clayton, 2007).

Urogynecologic and obstetric conditions, such as endometriosis, fibroids, infections, pelvic organ prolapse (POP), and previous hysterectomy, are associated with sexual dysfunction. Difficult vaginal delivery, episiotomy, or vaginal surgery may also impair sexual function via genital denervation and/or dyspareunia. Surgical castration, which can be employed for a variety of benign and malignant gynecologic conditions, may affect female sexual function adversely, particularly in premenopausal women (Clayton, 2007; Kammerer-Doak and Rogers, 2008).

Evaluation of the Partner

Involvement of the sexual partner is of utmost importance in the management of FSD. The partner of a woman who has sexual dysfunction is likely to have sexual issues of his or her own (Chedraui et al., 2009; Fisher and Rosen, 2005). There is robust evidence that treatment of erectile dysfunction in the male partner of heterosexual couples leads to positive changes in the female partner's sexual life (Conaglen et al., 2010). Treatment or referral to a specialist should be considered for a partner with sexual health problems.

Physical Examination

A thorough physical examination, including a focused internal and external pelvic examination, is important to identify cause(s)

TABLE 74.4 ACOG Committee Recommendations for Comprehensive Sexual History Taking

Partners	Are you currently sexually active? (Are you having sex?) • If no, have you ever been sexually active? In recent months, how many sex partners have you had? In the past 12 months, how many sex partners have you had? Are your sex partners men, women, or both? • If a patient answers "both," repeat the first two questions for each specific gender.
Practices	I am going to be more explicit here about the kind of sex you have had over the past 12 months to better understand if you are at risk for sexually transmitted infections (STIs). What kind of sexual contact do you have or have you had? • Genital (penis in the vagina)? • Anal (penis in the anus)? • Oral (mouth on penis, vagina, or anus)?
Protection from STIs	Do you and your partner(s) use any protection against STIs? • If not, could you tell me the reason? • Are you comfortable asking your partner to use condoms? • If so, what kind of protection do you use? • How often do you use this protection? • If "sometimes," in what situations or with whom do you use protection? Do you have any other questions, or are there other forms of protection from STIs that you would like to discuss today?
Past history of STIs	Have you ever been diagnosed with an STI? • When? • How were you treated? • Have you had any recurring symptoms or diagnoses? Have you ever been tested for human immunodeficiency virus (HIV) or other STIs? Would you like to be tested? Has your current partner or have any former partners ever been diagnosed or treated for an STI? • Were you tested for the same STI(s)? • If yes, when were you tested? • What was the diagnosis? • How was it treated?
Prevention of pregnancy	Are you currently trying to become pregnant? Are you concerned about getting pregnant? Are you using contraception or practicing any form of birth control? Is your partner supportive of your using birth control? Do you need any information on birth control?

COMPLETING THE HISTORY

What other things about your sexual health and sexual practices should we discuss to help ensure your good health?
What other concerns or questions regarding your sexual health or sexual practices would you like to discuss?

Modified from Committee on Gynecologic Practice. Committee Opinion No. 706. Sexual Health. *Obstet Gynecol* 2017;130(1):e42–e47.

TABLE 74.5 Summary of Selected Questionnaires/Scales Used to Evaluate Female Sexual (Dys)Function

QUESTIONNAIRE/SCALE	TARGET POPULATION	ITEMS	DOMAINS	COMMENTS
Female Sexual Function Index (FSFI) (Rosen et al., 2000)	Premenopausal and postmenopausal women (heterosexual and homosexual)	19 and 6	Desire, arousal, lubrication, orgasm, satisfaction, and pain	• The most extensively studied, the most widely used • Available in multiple languages • Validated, abbreviated (6 items) version also available, which can be used for screening • Validated version for use in patients with cancer and chronic pelvic pain also available

TABLE 74.5 Summary of Selected Questionnaires/Scales Used to Evaluate Female Sexual (Dys)Function—cont'd

QUESTIONNAIRE/SCALE	TARGET POPULATION	ITEMS	DOMAINS	COMMENTS
Profile of Female Sexual Function and Personal Distress Scale (PFSF) (Derogatis et al., 2004)	Postmenopausal women with low sexual desire	37	Desire, arousal, orgasm, sexual pleasure, sexual concerns, sexual responsiveness, sexual self-image	• Specifically designed to measure sexual desire and related distress in oophorectomized women with low libido • Available in multiple languages, can be useful for assessing therapeutic change in multicentric trials
Sexual Function Questionnaire (SFQ) (Quirk et al., 2002)	Women (heterosexual and sexually active during past 4 weeks)	28	Desire, arousal, orgasm, pain, enjoyment, and partner relationship	• Good internal consistency, test-retest reliability, and known group validity for female sexual arousal disorder and HSDD
Female Sexual Distress Scale-Revised (FSDS-R) (Derogatis et al., 2008)	Women (premenopausal and postmenopausal dissatisfied with their sexual function)	13 and 1	Distress about sexual life (relationship-based)	• Available in multiple languages • Single-item form can be used to screen midlife women for potential sexually related distress
Sexual Interest and Desire Inventory (SIDI) (Sills et al., 2005)	Women (premenopausal with low desire)	13	Hypoactive sexual desire disorder	• Available in multiple languages • Focused on assessing the severity of and treatment response for HSDD
Pelvic Organ Prolapse/Urinary Incontinence Sexual Questionnaire (PISQ) (Rogers et al., 2001)	Women with pelvic organ prolapse, urinary incontinence, or fecal incontinence	31 and 12	Behavioral and emotive, physical, and partner-related	• Has an IUGA-revised, shorter version (PISQ-IR) • Only questionnaire developed and validated to address sexual issues in women with urinary incontinence and pelvic organ prolapse
Female Genital Self-Image Scale (FGSIS) Herbenick et al., 2010)	Female genital self-image on sexual function and behavior	4	Feeling and beliefs about genital region	• Designed to assess a patient's genital self-image of sexual function and behavior • Validation studies have been conducted in a nationally representative sample of US women
Arizona Sexual Experience Scale (ASEX) (McGahuey et al., 2000)	Heterosexual women	5	Desire, arousal, vaginal lubrication, ability to orgasm, satisfaction from orgasm	• Available for both sexes • Can be used as a screening tool
Brief Index of Sexual Functioning for Women (BISF-W) (Taylor et al., 1994)	Heterosexual women	22	Sexual thoughts/desires, arousal, frequency of activity, receptivity/initiation, pleasure/orgasm, relationship satisfaction, sexual problems	• Ease of administration and scoring • Suitable for use in both clinical and nonclinical samples • Moderate test-retest reliability and internal consistency; needs further development
Golombok Rust Inventory of Sexual Satisfaction (GRISS) (Rust and Golombok, 1986)	Heterosexual women	28	Avoidance, nonsensuality, infrequency, vaginismus, anorgasmia, noncommunication, dissatisfaction	• Available for both sexes • Good reliability and validity • Mainly used to compare the efficacy of different treatment methods

Modified from Hatzichristou D, Kirana PS, Banner L, et al. Diagnosing sexual dysfunction in men and women: sexual history taking and the role of symptom scales and questionnaires. *J Sex Med* 2016;13(8):1166–1182.
HSDD, hypoactive sexual desire disorder; IUGA, International Urogynecological Association.

TABLE 74.6 Medical Conditions That Can Affect Female Sexual Function

MEDICAL CONDITION	POSSIBLE IMPACT ON FEMALE SEXUAL FUNCTION
Coronary artery disease	May affect pelvic perfusion, arousal disorder
Dermatologic conditions (e.g., lichen sclerosus, lichen planus, eczema)	Genital pain, problems with lubrication
Diabetes mellitus	Low desire
Hypertension	Low desire
Hypothyroidism	Problems with lubrication and orgasm
Malignancy and its treatment (breast, anal, colorectal, bladder, gynecologic)	Problems with desire, arousal, orgasm, and genital pain
Neuromuscular disorders, spinal cord injury, multiple sclerosis	Problems with desire, arousal, orgasm, and genital pain
Parkinson disease, dementia	Low desire
Urinary incontinence	Desire, arousal and pain domains can be affected.

Modified from Faubion SS, Rullo JE. Sexual dysfunction in women: a practical approach. *Am Fam Physician* 2015;92(4):281–288.

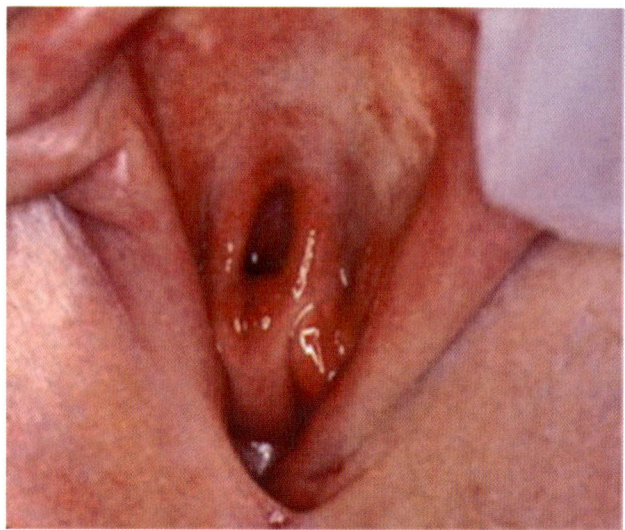

Fig. 74.4. Atrophic vulva. Slightly enlarged clitoris owing to loss of estrogen, with a pale, thin vulvar vestibule. Typical physical examination findings for vaginal atrophy include loss of labial or vulvar fullness, minimal vaginal moisture, pallor of urethra or vagina, narrow introitus, and loss of vaginal rugae. Placing a piece of pH paper on the vaginal wall until it is moistened can test vaginal pH. The pH of an estrogenized vagina ranges from 3.5 to 5.0. A vaginal pH of 4.5 or greater in the absence of infection or recent semen in the vaginal vault can be an indicator of vaginal atrophy caused by estrogen deficiency. (From Apgar BS, Brotzman GL, Spitzer M. Colposcopy: *Principles and practice: An integrated textbook and atlas.* Philadelphia, PA: WB Saunders; 2002.)

of sexual dysfunction. The pelvic examination is especially important for women with dyspareunia or vaginismus. Relatively more common examination findings in female patients with sexual dysfunction include vaginal atrophy (Fig. 74.4), vaginal dryness, genital tract infection, vulvar dermatoses (Figs. 74.5 and 74.6), pelvic floor muscle (PFM) dysfunction, adnexal/genital masses, or deep pelvic pain (Frank

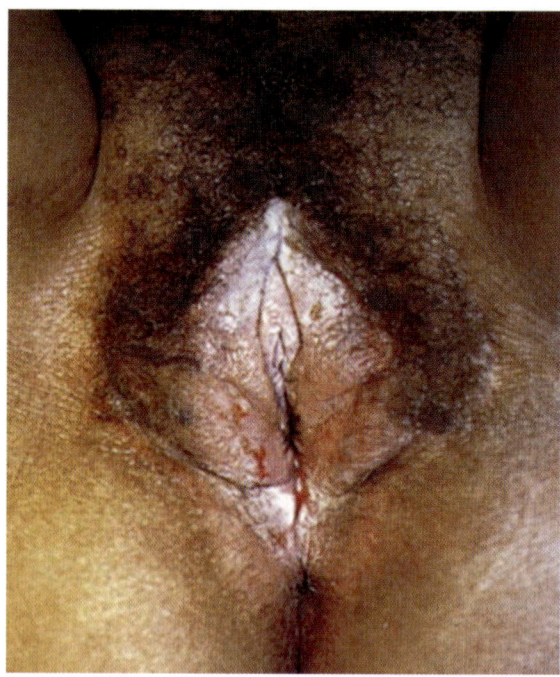

Fig. 74.5. Vulvar lichen sclerosus. Hypertrophic plaques, edema, loss of normal architecture, introital narrowing, and perineal involvement. It is important to evaluate for evidence of vulvar dermatoses when women complain of dyspareunia. Lichen sclerosus is a chronic, progressive inflammatory skin condition of unknown etiology that commonly affects the labia minora and/or labia majora, but can extend to the perineum and around the anus. Dyspareunia is often a late symptom caused by introital stenosis, fissuring, or labial agglutination. (From Moreland A, Kohl P. Genital and dermatologic examination. In: Morse SA, ed. *Atlas of sexually transmitted diseases and AIDS.* 4th ed. Philadelphia, PA: Saunders; 2011:1–23).

et al., 2008). A normal pelvic examination can also be reassuring and informative to a patient.

The external pelvic examination begins with visual inspection of the mons pubis, labia majora, labia minora, clitoris, and vulvar vestibule. Often, this is best accomplished gently with a gloved hand and a cotton swab. This inspection may reveal changes in pubic hair distribution, redundancy of the labia, atrophy of the external genitalia, and vulvar skin lesions (see Figs. 74.4 to 74.6). Inspection may also reveal redness and pain typical of vestibulitis, a flattening and pallor of the labia that suggests estrogen deficiency, or POP.

The internal pelvic examination begins with palpation of the PFMs, urethra, and anus. Bimanual examination of the vagina may reveal ovarian mass(es) and/or palpable abnormalities in the adnexal region. The size and flexion of the uterus or tenderness in the vaginal fornix may be indicative of endometriosis (Goldstein and Alexander, 2005). POP and urethral hypermobility should also be assessed by vaginal inspection (with the help of a speculum) and palpation (during resting and straining). The PFMs should voluntarily contract and relax and are not normally tender to palpation.

Neurologic examination of the pelvis will involve evaluation of sensory and motor function of both lower extremities and include a screening lumbosacral neurologic examination. Lumbosacral examination includes assessment of PFM strength, anal sphincter resting tone, voluntary anal contraction, and perineal sensation. If abnormalities are noted in the screening assessment, a complete comprehensive neurologic examination should be performed. Neuropathy involving the genitals can be evaluated by application of heat/cold stimuli, vibration, and/or application of a toothpick or small pin. Considering the association between lower urinary tract symptoms (LUTS) and sexual health issues, a simple assessment for urinary incontinence (UI) (e.g., clinic stress test, Q-tip test) is also warranted.

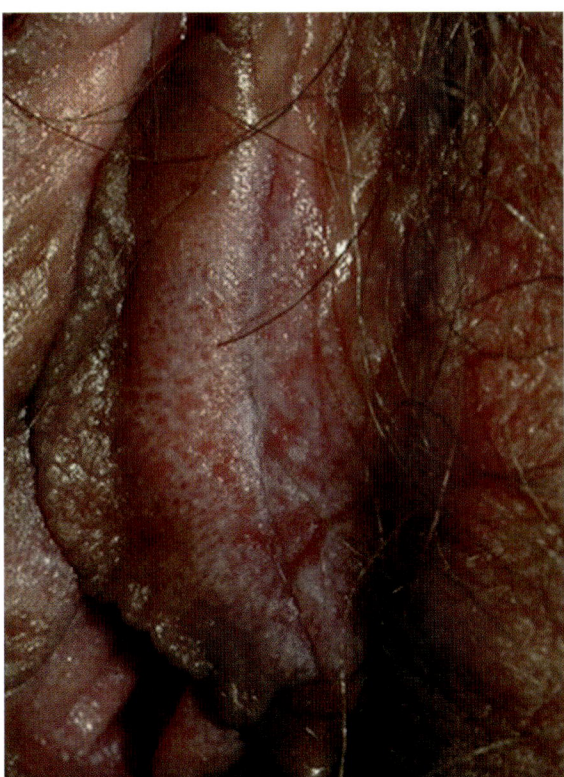

Fig. 74.6. Vulvovaginal lichen planus. Wickham striae is the most classic and only pathognomonic finding of vulvar lichen planus as evident by white, reticulate, lacy papules. This is a chronic, desquamative, erosive dermatitis that can result in severe destruction of the vulvar tissues and stenosis of the vaginal opening. Symptoms most often develop in women 50 to 60 years of age and include severe pruritus or vulvar pain, soreness, or burning. Vulvar lichen planus can involve the labia minor and vestibule. The anus is rarely affected. Lesions can be isolated or diffuse. (From Mirowski GW, Goddard A. Treatment of vulvovaginal lichen planus. *Dermatol Clin* 2010;28[4]:720).

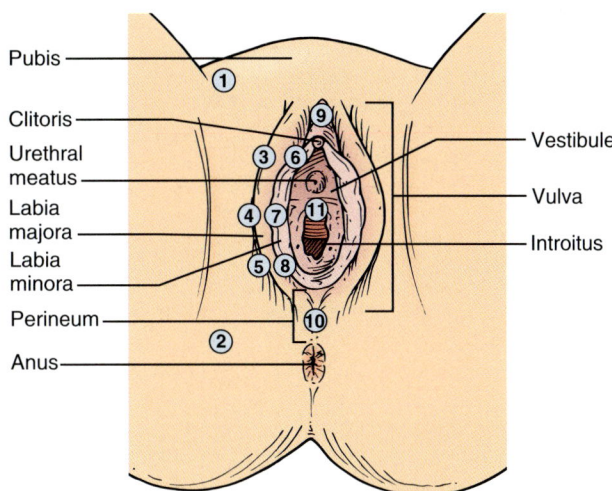

Fig. 74.7. Cotton swab testing for vulvodynia. Check clockwise: *1–2*, inner thigh; *3–5*, labia majora; *6–8*, interlabial sulcus; *9*, clitoris and hood; *10*, perineum; *11*, vestibule. (From Shah M, Hofstetter S. Vulvodynia. *Obstet Gynecol Clin North Am* 2014;41[3]:456.)

Sexual function is associated with normal PFM function (Kegel, 1952; Shafik, 2000). The PFMs, particularly the pubococcygeus and iliococcygeus, are responsible for involuntary contractions during orgasm (Kegel, 1952). Women with strong or moderate PFM contractions were found to have higher orgasm and arousal domain scores of the FSFI compared with women with weak PFM contractions (Lowenstein et al., 2010). Orgasm and arousal functions may be associated with PFM strength, with a positive association between pelvic floor strength and sexual activity and function (Kanter et al., 2015; Wehbe et al., 2010).

PFM activity can be categorized as normal, overactive (high tone), underactive (low tone), and nonfunctioning. Normal PFMs are those that can voluntarily and involuntarily contract and relax (Haylen et al., 2010; Messelink et al., 2005). Overactive PFMs are those that do not relax and possibly contract during times of relaxation for micturition or defecation. This type of dysfunction can lead to voiding dysfunction, defecatory dysfunction, and dyspareunia (Messelink et al., 2005). Underactive PFMs, which cannot contract voluntarily, may lead to incontinence (urinary and/or fecal) and POP. Nonfunctioning muscles are completely inactive (Messelink et al., 2005).

Digital rectal/vaginal palpation is the most commonly employed method to evaluate PFM tone, squeeze pressure during contraction, symmetry, and relaxation. During the examination, the physician should ask the patient to contract as much as she can to evaluate the maximum strength and sustained contraction for endurance. This assessment can be also done invasively via pressure manometry or dynamometry. There are no validated scales to quantify PFM strength (Messelink et al., 2005). However, certain scales can be used to quantify pelvic floor tenderness. Lukban and Whitmore (2002) described a zero to 4 numbered scale that evaluates tenderness in the pelvic floor: (1) comfortable pressure associated with the examination, (2) uncomfortable pressure associated with the examination, (3) moderate pain associated with the examination that intensifies with contraction, and (4) indicating severe pain with the examination and inability to perform the contraction maneuver because of pain.

Localized vulvodynia can be diagnosed using the Q-tip test, in which pain is "provoked" in the vestibule, interlabial sulci, introitus, or around the clitoris with light touch from a moistened cotton swab (Fig. 74.7). Pain may be prevented or reduced with the use of topical 5% EMLA (2.5% lidocaine + 2.5% prilocaine) cream applied to the painful areas 10 minutes before intercourse (Wright and O'Connor, 2015).

Generalized vulvodynia is defined as "unprovoked" stinging, burning, irritation, rawness, or pain anywhere on the vulva that is not explained by another condition. In generalized vulvodynia, physical examination is often normal, or there may be areas of tenderness, hyperesthesia, or hypesthesia (Wright and O'Connor, 2015).

Laboratory Tests

Laboratory evaluation for FSD is rarely indicated unless there is a suspicion for a specific medical condition that might explain the patient's sexual problems. Serum chemistry, lipids, and glycosylated hemoglobin can be assayed, because these are more widely available and might reveal common problems (such as diabetes mellitus) that might potentially influence female sexual function. The normal range of testosterone levels has not been established in women, and testosterone levels do not correlate with libido in females. Therefore, random testosterone measurement is worthless in the evaluation of FSD. Furthermore, there are no data to justify serum testosterone measurement for FSD unless there is a concern about hyperandrogenic/hypoandrogenic state (Meston and Frohlich, 2001; Nappi et al., 2005). If a hormonal abnormality is suspected based on the systemic evaluation of the patient, then a screening blood workup can be done to rule out prolactinoma, thyroid dysfunction, and adrenal disorders. If adrenal insufficiency is suspected, measurement of dehydroepiandrosterone sulfate (DHEA-S) is useful because of isolated adrenal production (Pauls et al., 2005).

There is some suggestion that free testosterone levels less than the lowest quartile may be associated with androgen insufficiency syndrome, which can manifest itself by symptoms of decreased sexual interest and well-being, fatigue, persistent postmenopausal vasomotor symptoms despite estrogen replacement, and lack of motivation (Nappi et al.,

TABLE 74.7 Methods to Assess Vulvovaginal Blood Flow

Method	Description
Oxygen perfusion and heat dissipation in vaginal wall (Levin, 2006)	Heated electrode held by a suction cup onto the vaginal wall; the more blood in the vaginal wall, the greater the amount of oxygen diffusion and heat clearance from the electrode.
Vaginal photoplethysmography (Sintchak and Geer, 1975)	Menstrual tampon-size probe with light source (infrared diode) and photo transistor; diode illuminates vaginal tissue, and photo transistor picks up light that is backscattered from the vaginal wall and the blood circulating within it; the amount of light backscattered is dependent on the volume of blood within the vaginal wall.
Oxygen perfusion in labia minora (Sommer et al., 2001)	Device consisting of heated oxygen electrode attached by a single-sided adhesive ring on minor labia; the more blood present, the greater the amount of perfused oxygen.
Labial photoplethysmography (Prause et al., 2005)	Light source and photo transistor built in a plastic clip that is attached to labia majora.
Thermistor clip (Henson et al., 1978)	Labial temperature is assessed using a thermistor clip attached to labia minora; temperature is assumed to be related to blood flow.
Thermal imaging (Kukkonen et al., 2007)	Human skin emits electrochemical energy, including infrared radiation, which is registered with thermal imaging; genital temperature is assumed to be related to blood flow.
Doppler ultrasonography (Garcia et al., 2005)	Pulse of ultrasound is sent into tissue using ultrasound transducer; sound echoes from parts of the tissue, and the echoes are recorded and displayed as an image.
Laser Doppler imaging (Waxman and Pukall, 2009)	Measures superficial skin blood flow; based on the principle that the frequency of light changes when it interacts with an object in motion (e.g., blood); changes in frequency of light are converted in an electric signal that is processed to an image.
Magnetic resonance imaging (Maravilla and Yang, 2008)	Detects changes in tissue engorgement, which is reflected as increased signal intensity.
Combined clitoral and vaginal photoplethysmography (Gerritsen et al., 2009)	Clitoral photoplethysmograph is built into a silicon shield attached to the lower side of vaginal photoplethysmograph.

Modified from Levin RJ, Both S, Georgiadis J, et al. The physiology of female sexual function and the pathophysiology of female sexual dysfunction (Committee 13A). *J Sex Med* 2016;13(5):733–759.

2005; Pauls et al., 2005). Despite the fact that estrogen deficiency can lead to urogenital atrophy and vascular insufficiency, both of which can contribute to impairment in female sexual function, routine measurement of estrogen levels within the context of FSD workup was not found to be useful. Likewise, progesterone, measured either alone or in combination with estrogen, has very limited diagnostic/prognostic utility in FSD (Davis et al., 2004; Meston and Frohlich, 2001).

Physiologic Measures of Sexual Function

There are many physiologic monitoring parameters of sexual arousal, which could potentially assist in the diagnosis of organic diseases contributing to sexual dysfunctions (Woodard and Diamond, 2009). Recordings at baseline and after sexual stimulation can determine pathologic changes that occur with arousal (Marthol and Hilz, 2004). Estrogen-dependent vaginal hyperperfusion results in increased vaginal secretions that are important for lubrication. Hypoestrogenism is associated with significant decreases in clitoral, vaginal, and urethral blood flow and histologic changes of thin mucosal layers. Thus, any interference with this process can contribute to FSD (Woodard and Diamond, 2009).

Genital blood flow can be measured with vaginal photoplethysmography, which is the most widely studied and most validated physiologic test used in assessment of female sexual function (Woodard and Diamond, 2009). This method uses a vaginal light source on an acrylic tampon to illuminate the vaginal microcirculation and determine the level of vaginal engorgement. Most studies comparing genital responses of women with and without sexual dysfunction have used vaginal photoplethysmography that measures vaginal pulse amplitude (VPA). In most of these studies, women who met the criteria for sexual dysfunction showed no difference in genital response compared with women without sexual problems (Levin et al., 2016). However, women with medical disorders that are likely to impair sexual response as a result of disease-related neurovascular damage had impaired genital response (lower VPA) in response to sexual stimulation (Levin, 2006).

Diagnostic sensitivity of vaginal photoplethysmography has been variable, although it seems to be most sensitive in patients with arousal disorder (Meston and Frohlich, 2001). However, it lacks an absolute scale, and there are no data regarding normal values. Therefore, it is not possible to decide on genital response abnormality based solely on vaginal photoplethysmography results.

Other methods of assessment of genital blood flow have been used in the research setting, including the use of a radioactive tracer (xenon-133), measures of heat dissipation (the oxygen-temperature method), use of vaginal and labial thermistors for temperature assessment, thermographic photography of the genitals during different phases of the sexual response, duplex Doppler sonography and laser Doppler perfusion imaging of genital blood flow, and magnetic resonance imaging (MRI) (Levin et al., 2016). Table 74.7 provides a summary of the methods that have been tested to assess vulvovaginal perfusion in FSD.

Measurement of vaginal lubrication, volume, pressure, and compliance can also be performed. A neurophysiologic examination could evaluate for neurogenic etiologies by measuring the bulbocavernosus reflex and pudendal evoked potentials; genital sympathetic skin response; warm, cold, and vibratory perception thresholds; and pressure and touch sensitivity of the external genitalia (Marthol and Hilz, 2004).

The muscle activity of the pelvic floor can be assessed with electromyography and biofeedback (Woodard and Diamond, 2009). Studies monitoring PFM activity by electromyography have shown some evidence for deviant PFM tone or strength in women with sexual pain disorders. Increased resting electromyography activity and stronger contractile responses to vestibular pressure have been observed (Gentilcore-Saulnier et al., 2010), but some studies have reported lower muscle strength (White et al., 1997).

Many of these methods of physiologic assessment may be beneficial toward our understanding of female sexual physiology and dysfunctions. However, most are invasive, poorly defined, and lack standardization, validity, and reliability. At this time, they are primarily used for research purposes.

> **KEY POINTS: EVALUATION OF SEXUAL WELLNESS**
>
> - Health care providers should bring up the topic of sexual health as female patients are usually reluctant to discuss sexual problems with their physicians.
> - The Brief Sexual Symptom Checklist for Women can be used to screen patients for sexual dysfunction.
> - The Female Sexual Function Index may be helpful to clinicians in obtaining a more comprehensive sexual history.
> - A thorough physical examination is important to identify cause(s) of sexual dysfunction.
> - Laboratory evaluation is rarely indicated unless there is a specific concern for a medical condition that might be contributory for the sexual dysfunction.
> - Physiologic tests that might be used in assessment of female sexual function lack standardization, validity, and reliability.

Definitions of Sexual Dysfunctions in Female Patients

The *International Classification of Diseases, 10th Edition (ICD-10-CM)* by the World Health Organization (WHO, 1992) and the *Diagnostic and Statistical Manual of Mental Disorders (fourth edition with text revision or fifth edition; DSM-IV-TR and DSM-5)* by the APA have been the most widely used systems internationally to define sexual dysfunctions in the female (Table 74.8) (APA 2000, 2013). Currently, the *DSM-5* and *ICD-10-CM* represent two officially sanctioned systems with international influence. The *ICD-10-CM* is focused on the definition of medical conditions, and the *DSM-5* is a document that primarily defines psychiatric conditions. In the *ICD-10-CM*, disorders are coded as either organic or as nonorganic. The organic FSD codes are vaginismus and dyspareunia of organic etiology. On the other hand, the nonorganic FSD codes include lack of sexual desire, sexual aversion or lack of sexual enjoyment, failure of genital response, orgasmic dysfunction, nonorganic vaginismus, nonorganic dyspareunia, excessive sexual drive, and two nonspecific codes (similar to the "not otherwise specified" codes in the *DSM-IV*).

DSM-5 Definitions of Sexual Dysfunctions in Women

Regarding the *DSM-5* definitions and criteria for sexual dysfunctions in women, all disorders except genito-pelvic pain-penetration disorder require that the symptoms meet the *DSM-5* definition of that condition, have been present for 6 months on at least 75% of sexual occasions, cause clinically significant distress, are not a consequence of a nonsexual mental disorder or of a severe relationship distress or other significant stressors, and are not attributable to the effect of a medication or illness.

Female Sexual Interest–Arousal Disorder

Lack of or significantly decreased sexual interest or arousal is manifested by at least three of the following characteristics: (1) absent or decreased interest in sexual activity; (2) absent or decreased sexual or erotic thoughts or fantasies; (3) no or decreased initiation of sexual activity and typically unreceptive to a partner's attempts to initiate; (4) absent or decreased sexual excitement or pleasure during sexual activity in almost all or all (approximately 75% to 100%) sexual encounters (in identified situational contexts or, if generalized, in all contexts); (5) absent or decreased sexual interest or arousal in response to any internal or external sexual or erotic cues (e.g., written, verbal, or visual); or (6) absent or decreased genital or nongenital sensations during sexual activity in almost all or all

TABLE 74.8 Definitions of Female Sexual Dysfunction

DSM-IV-TR	DSM-5
Sexual desire disorders: **Hypoactive sexual desire disorder:** Deficiency or absence of sexual fantasies and desire for sexual activity **Sexual aversion disorder:** Aversion to and active avoidance of genital sexual contact with a sexual partner. **Sexual arousal disorders:** **Female sexual arousal disorder:** Persistent or recurrent inability to attain or to maintain until completion of the sexual activity, an adequate lubrication-swelling response or sexual excitement.	**Female sexual interest or arousal disorder:** Lack of or significantly reduced sexual interest or arousal as manifested by three of the following: 1. Absent or reduced interest in sexual activity 2. Absent or reduced sexual or erotic thoughts or fantasies 3. No or reduced initiation of sexual activity and unreceptive to partner's attempts to initiate 4. Absent or reduced sexual excitement or pleasure during sexual activity in almost all or all (75%–100%) sexual encounters 5. Absent or reduced sexual interest or arousal in response to any internal or external sexual or erotic cues (written, verbal, or visual) 6. Absent or reduced genital or nongenital sensations during sexual activity in almost all or all (75%–100%) sexual encounters
Orgasmic disorder: **Female orgasmic disorder:** Persistent or recurrent delay in, or absence of, orgasm after normal sexual excitement.	**Female orgasmic disorder:** Presence of either of the following on all or almost all (75%–100%) occasions of sexual activity: 1. Marked delay in, marked infrequency of, or absence of orgasm 2. Markedly reduced intensity of orgasmic sensations
Sexual pain disorders: **Dyspareunia:** Genital pain that is associated with sexual intercourse. **Vaginismus:** Recurrent or persistent involuntary contraction of the perineal muscles surrounding the outer third of the vagina when vaginal penetration with a penis, finger, tampon, or speculum is attempted.	**Genitopelvic pain or penetration disorder:** Persistent or recurrent difficulties with one or more of the following: 1. Vaginal penetration during intercourse 2. Marked vulvovaginal or pelvic pain during intercourse or penetration attempts 3. Marked fear or anxiety about vulvovaginal or pelvic pain in anticipation of, during, or because of vaginal penetration 4. Marked tensing or tightening of pelvic floor muscles during attempted vaginal penetration

(approximately 75% to 100%) sexual encounters (in identified situational contexts or, if generalized, in all contexts).

Female Orgasmic Disorder

This disorder is manifested by either of the following symptoms and experiences on almost all or all (approximately 75% to 100%) occasions of sexual activity (in identified situational contexts or, if generalized, in all contexts): (1) marked delay in, marked infrequency of, or absence of orgasm; or (2) markedly decreased intensity of orgasmic sensations.

Genito-Pelvic Pain-Penetration Disorder

This disorder manifests as persistent or recurrent difficulties with at least one of the following: (1) vaginal penetration during intercourse; (2) marked vulvovaginal or pelvic pain during vaginal intercourse or penetration attempts; (3) marked fear or anxiety about vulvovaginal or pelvic pain in anticipation of, during, or as a result of vaginal penetration; or (4) marked tensing or tightening of the PFMs during attempted vaginal penetration.

International Consultation on Sexual Medicine Definitions of Sexual Dysfunctions in Women

The International Consultation on Sexual Medicine (ICSM), which consists of a large number of international experts in the field of sexual dysfunction, has provided insight for the terminology of FSD that could be applied independent of etiology. The last consultation took place in 2015, and the latest ICSM document focusing on the definitions of sexual dysfunctions in women was published in 2016 (McCabe et al., 2016). The definitions provided in this document represented the synthesis of *DSM-5*, *DSM-1V-TR*, and *ICD-10-CM* explanations and some new definitions developed during the consensus meeting. It has been highlighted that some of the new definitions were not mature and subject to future revision. Additionally, many definitions were not based on a sufficient level of evidence and represented merely expert clinical opinion; hence it was not possible to assign a reliable grade of recommendation for each.

Hypoactive Sexual Desire Dysfunction

Hypoactive sexual desire dysfunction manifests as persistent or recurrent deficiency or absence of sexual or erotic thoughts or fantasies and desire for sexual activity.

Female Sexual Arousal Dysfunction

Female sexual arousal dysfunction manifests as persistent or recurrent inability to attain or maintain arousal until completion of the sexual activity.

Female Orgasmic Dysfunction

Female orgasmic dysfunction is characterized by (1) marked delay in, marked frequency of, or absence of orgasm and/or (2) markedly decreased intensity of orgasmic sensation.

Female Genital-Pelvic Pain Dysfunction

This disorder manifests as persistent or recurrent difficulties with at least one of the following: (1) vaginal penetration during intercourse; (2) marked vulvovaginal or pelvic pain during genital contact; (3) marked fear or anxiety about vulvovaginal or pelvic pain in anticipation of, during, or as a result of genital contact; or (4) marked hypertonicity or overactivity of PFMs with or without genital contact.

Persistent Genital Arousal Disorder

Persistent genital arousal disorder manifests as spontaneous, intrusive, and unwanted genital arousal (tingling, throbbing, pulsating) in the absence of sexual interest and desire. Any awareness of subjective arousal is typically, but not invariably, unpleasant. The arousal is unrelieved by at least one orgasm, and the feeling of arousal persists for hours or days.

Postcoital Syndrome (Postorgasmic Illness Syndrome)

This disorder manifests as negative feelings, experiences, and/or physical symptoms such as headache, malaise, fatigue, and other symptoms after sexual activity.

Hypohedonic Orgasm

Hypohedonic orgasm manifests as lifelong or acquired decreased or low level of sexual pleasure with orgasm.

Painful Orgasm

This disorder manifests as the occurrence of genital and/or pelvic pain during or shortly after orgasm.

Epidemiology of Female Sexual Dysfunction

There is limited literature on the prevalence and incidence of FSD. Furthermore, there exists considerable heterogeneity in the methodology of the relevant studies. Available data are difficult to interpret and compare because of differences in the following: (1) the tools used to assess sexual (dys)function (e.g., tick box, diagnostic interviews, nonvalidated assessment measurements, validated assessment measurements); (2) the way information is collected (face-to-face interviews, mail questionnaires, telephone interviews); (3) the definition and classification of sexual dysfunction (3rd, 4th, and 5th edition of *DSM*); (4) the population from which the sample was drawn (e.g., general population, clinical population presenting for treatment of sexual dysfunction, those who have access to the Internet); and (5) terms of the age strata studied, medical history, and socioeconomic and cultural background of the study cohorts.

Burri and Spector found that 5.8% of women reported symptoms consistent with a diagnosis of FSD, and 15.5% of them had lifelong FSD. **Hypoactive sexual desire was the most prevalent sexual complaint (21.4%), followed by problems in arousal (11.4%), satisfaction (10.4%), orgasm (8.8%), and lubrication (8.7%)** (Burri and Spector, 2011). The 5-year incidence study conducted by Kontula and Haavio-Mannila included Finnish women between 18 and 74 years of age. Herein, decreased sexual desire was the most commonly encountered problem, with an incidence of approximately 20% in women younger than 25 years of age and an incidence of 70% to 80% in women 55 to 74 years of age (Kontula et al., 1995). Findings from the Australian Longitudinal Study of Health and Relationships revealed that 36% of women reported at least one new sexual health–related problem during the previous 12 months. Lacking interest in having sex (26%) and taking too long to reach orgasm (11%) were the most common problems. Failure of orgasm (10%), vaginal dryness (9%), not finding sex pleasurable (8%), feeling anxious about the ability to perform sexually (6%), experiencing physical pain during intercourse (5%), and coming to orgasm too quickly (2%) were the other sexual issues having been reported in this patient cohort (Smith et al., 2012).

Interest and Desire

The prevalence of interest and desire-related FSD ranges between 40% and 50% among women older than 65 years of age in most recent studies (McCabe et al., 2016). Laumann et al. investigated the prevalence of sexual dysfunction in the United States. In their cohort of 1749 women between 18 and 59 years of age, the prevalence of lack of interest in sex was in the range of 27% to 32% (Laumann et al., 1999). According to the Global Study of Sexual Attitudes and Behaviors (GSSAB), which included 27,500 individuals, approximately one-half of whom were women 40 to 80 years of age, lack of interest in sex varied from 17% in Northern Europe to 34% in Southeast Asia

(Nicolosi et al., 2004). West et al. (2008) conducted a cross-sectional study of 2207 US women 30 to 70 years of age and found that the overall prevalence of HSDD) was 8.3%. In the Prevalence of Female Sexual Problems Associated with Distress and Determinants of Treatment Seeking [PRESIDE] study, Shifren et al. (2008) reported the overall prevalence of FSD associated with low desire to be 37.7% in a study involving 50.001 US women and 31.531 respondents 18 to 102 years of age who were evaluated by validated questionnaires. In this study, 8.9% of women 18 to 44 years, 12.3% of women 45 to 64 years, and 7.4% of women older than 65 years of age exhibited low desire accompanied by clinically significant distress (HSDD). On the other hand, Hayes et al. (2008) reported a lower overall prevalence, with 16% of Australian women reporting low desire-associated sexual dysfunction in a postal survey that was administered to a random sample of 356 Australian women 20 to 70 years of age. Similarly, the prevalence of low sexual desire was 19% in a large-scale Danish study including women 16 to 67 years of age (Eplov et al., 2007). **In the Women's International Study of Health and Sexuality (WISHeS), Leiblum et al. demonstrated that the prevalence of HSDD ranged from 14% in premenopausal women to 26% in surgically postmenopausal women 20 to 49 years of age.** Furthermore, HSDD was associated with significantly lower sexual and partner satisfaction and significant decrements in general health status, including aspects of mental and physical health (Leiblum et al., 2006).

Arousal

The prevalence of lubrication problems was found to be 12% in the study conducted by Fugl-Meyer et al., who investigated a representative sample of Swedish adults between 18 and 74 years of age (Fugl-Meyer et al., 1999). The rate of female sexual arousal disorder (FSAD) found in the general US population was 5.4% (Shifren et al., 2008). Safarinejad reported a prevalence rate of 30% for arousal disorder among 2626 adult Iranian women 20 to 60 years of age. Furthermore, there was a positive association between the prevalence of arousal disorder and low level of education, low level of physical activity, psychological problems, chronic disease, lower marriage age, and menopausal status (Safarinejad, 2006). In the same study, the significant positive correlation between age and the prevalence of arousal disorder was highlighted (24% in age group 20 to 39 years vs. 35% in age group 50 to 60 years) (Safarinejad, 2006). On the contrary, Laumann et al. (1999) did not detect a relationship between increased age and the prevalence of arousal disorder. Nicolosi et al. (2004) reported the overall prevalence of lubrication difficulties as 16% in the GSSAB. However, in East and Southeast Asia, this ratio increased to 28%. McCool et al. (2016) published a systematic review of the observational studies assessing the prevalence of FSD in premenopausal women and estimated the prevalence of lubrication difficulties as 20.6%.

Orgasm

The prevalence of orgasmic dysfunction varies between 16% and 25% (Fugl-Meyer et al., 1999; Gruszecki et al., 2005; Laumann et al., 1999; Richters et al., 2003). However, 37% of the patients in the Iranian cohort had orgasmic disorder always or often during sexual intercourse (Safarinejad, 2006). Similarly, Kontula et al. (1995) from Finland reported a relatively high prevalence of orgasmic disorder. In the studies from the United States, Australia, and Iran, older women reported a higher prevalence of orgasmic disorder. In the GSSAB, the inability to reach orgasm was the second most frequent FSD, with the highest prevalence in Southeast Asia (34%) and the lowest in Northern Europe (10%) (Nicolosi et al., 2004). In a large-scale epidemiologic survey including a representative sample of 50,002 US women, orgasmic problems were reported in one-fifth of the respondents (Shifren et al., 2008).

Dyspareunia and Vaginismus

Dyspareunia is relatively uncommon in premenopausal women (approximately 5%). However, its prevalence is known to increase among postmenopausal women, ranging between 12% and 45% (Gregersen et al., 2006). Australian and British studies have reported prevalence rates for dyspareunia as low as 1% to 2% (Barlow et al., 1997; Smith et al., 2003). Other studies found that dyspareunia was present in as many as 14% to 27% of women (Gruszecki et al., 2005; Laumann et al., 1999; Richters et al., 2003). The GSSAB reported pain during sexual intercourse to range from 5% in Northern Europe to 22% in Southeast Asia (Nicolosi et al., 2004). In the Ghanaian study conducted by Amidu et al. (2010), 68.1% of the women were found to have vaginismus. Similarly, Ghanbarzadeh et al. (2013) from Iran reported that 54% of the women felt pain during intercourse.

> **KEY POINTS: DEFINITIONS AND EPIDEMIOLOGY**
>
> - The *ICD-10* (WHO), *DSM-1V-TR* (APA), and *DSM-5* (APA) are the most widely used systems to define sexual dysfunctions in the female patient.
> - There are terminological differences between *ICD* and *DSM* definitions of female sexual dysfunction.
> - The ICSM consensus statement about the definitions of female sexual dysfunction represents a synthesis of *ICD* and *DSM* explanations approved by a panel of experts.
> - There is significant heterogeneity in the quality of the literature about the epidemiology of female sexual dysfunction.
> - Hypoactive sexual desire is the most prevalent type of female sexual dysfunction.

SPECIAL POPULATIONS

LGBTQ

Over the past decade, transgender and gender-diverse people have gained greater visibility in society, and consequently health care providers are increasingly co-opting with clinical needs for this population. A person's experienced gender is a fundamental and very important aspect of one's sense of self.

The health care needs in the transgender population vary from gender transition–related hormone therapy to surgeries, fertility, and routine urologic and urogynecologic services (Unger, 2015).

The language used and the attention to the pronouns is critical for this vulnerable population. The impact of gendered language is responsible for health disparities experienced by transgender and nonbinary people (Table 74.9). A simple adjustment in the framing and language use can significantly improve the care provided (Daphna et al., 2018).

Transgender people compose 0.6% of the adult US population, with rising numbers of younger people identifying as transgender, nonbinary, or gender nonconforming over the past decade. Compared with cis-gender individuals, transgender and gender-nonconforming individuals suffer poorer health outcomes that largely stem from societal discrimination and violence. Nearly 20% of transgender people have reported being refused medical care because of their gender identity. Furthermore, 33% reported a negative experience with a health care provider over the past year, and 23% reported avoiding necessary medical care (such as cervical cancer screening) for fear of discrimination (Grant et al., 2011).

The lack of knowledge of how sexual and gender identities intersect with health care needs may lead to a clinician not being able to fully care for an LGBTQ patient. This unfamiliarity can inhibit the clinician's ability to make appropriate risk assessments for diseases or provide information on the latest available gender therapies for patients. Despite the growing social acceptance, one in five transgender patients seeking health care are still turned away by health care providers (Snowdon et al., 2013).

It is essential to collect accurate sexual orientation and gender identity while taking medical history to identify and address potential health disparities among LGBTQ populations. When these data are

TABLE 74.9 Basic Terminology Related With Transgender People

Gender identity: The sense of one's own gender as "male," "female," "genderqueer," and so on. Gender identity is not restricted to physical anatomy or lived social roles and refers to the broader sense of gender one has of himself or herself.
Cis Female: Person assigned female at birth who identifies as a woman
Trans Female: Person assigned male at birth who identifies as a woman
Cis Male: Person assigned male at birth who identifies as a man
Trans Male: Person assigned female at birth who identifies as a man
Nonbinary: Person who does not identify as a man or a woman, whose gender identity may not be accurately described using rigid binary gender definitions
Queer: A more flexible, less prescriptive alternative term for one's sexuality that is used over traditional categories such as "gay" or "lesbian"
Bottom surgery: Genital reassignment surgery
Top surgery: Breast reduction or reconstruction surgery
MSM: Man who has sex with a man
WSW: Woman who has sex with a woman

TABLE 74.10 Most Common Cancer Types Affecting the LGBTQ Population

Anal
Breast
Cervical
Colorectal
Endometrial
Lung
Prostate

not gathered in the everyday clinical practice, there may be missed opportunities to discuss prevention, early detection, and screening for LGBTQ subgroups who may be at an increased risk for certain cancers.

There are some specific conditions more common in the LGBTQ population. For example, gay, lesbian, and bisexual adults and youth are at increased risk for depression, anxiety, suicide, and substance abuse. Lesbian and bisexual women are more likely to be obese than straight women. In addition to these general mental and physical health disparities, the LGBTQ community also has increased risks for some cancers (Table 74.10) (Quinn et al., 2015). Anal cancer disproportionately affects gay and bisexual men as a result of human papillomavirus (HPV) and HIV infection. Breast cancer may affect lesbian and bisexual women at greater rates than heterosexual women. A possible explanation for this higher incidence is the fact that lesbian and bisexual women more commonly experience a variety of breast cancer risk factors such as reduced pregnancy rates, smoking, and obesity. Furthermore, some studies suggest lesbian and bisexual women are less likely to get mammography examinations because of barriers to health care coverage and negative relationships with health care providers (Hart and Bowen, 2009). HPV not only contributes to higher rates of anal cancer among men who have sex with men, but also to higher rates of cervical cancer among lesbian and bisexual women. This health disparity and lack of health education is the reason for an increased risk for cervical cancer in woman who have sex with women and trans men. There is a mistaken belief that they are not at risk for cervical cancer, and therefore they are less prone to undergo Papanicolaou (Pap) testing (Quinn et al., 2015).

The higher incidence of lung cancer in HIV-infected individuals and the higher prevalence of smoking in LGBTQ individuals are the reasons for the increase in lung cancer compared with the general population.

The lower PSA testing among homosexual African-Americans compared with heterosexual African-Americans might be the reason for a higher incidence of prostate cancer in these subjects (Heslin et al., 2008).

It is unclear whether the incidence of prostatic carcinoma is truly lower in the trans female population, possibly caused by estrogen therapy and androgen suppression, or the screening rates are lower in this population, leading to decreased detection. Research in rodent models exploring the effects of combined exogenous estrogen and testosterone on the prostate has revealed a possible estrogenic link to prostate carcinogenesis and progression of prostate cancer. Estrogen and testosterone treatment regimens were shown to transform human prostate epithelium derived from normal human prostate progenitor cells using a tissue recombinant model, and to drive adenocarcinoma in the tissue graft (Sharif et al., 2017).

Gender Dysphoria and Hormonal Treatment

The two major goals of hormonal therapy are to reduce endogenous sex hormone levels and replace them with the sex hormones consistent with the individual's gender identity in the same fashion as in the hormone replacement treatment of hypogonadal patients. This hormonal "inversion" is the baseline treatment to reduce the secondary sex characteristics of the individual's designated gender and help the development of the sexual characteristics of the gender identity.

In trans males, the hormonal treatment basically follows the general principle of hormone replacement treatment of male hypogonadism. Parenteral or transdermal preparations can be used to achieve testosterone values in the normal male range (typically between 320 and 1000 ng/dL). Similar to androgen therapy in hypogonadal men, testosterone treatment in transgender males results in increased muscle mass and decreased fat mass, increased facial hair and acne, male pattern baldness in those genetically predisposed, and increased sexual desire (Hembree et al., 2017)

In **transgender males,** testosterone will result in clitoromegaly, temporary or permanent decreased fertility, deepening of the voice, cessation of menses (usually), and a significant increase in body hair, particularly on the face, chest, and abdomen.

The hormone regimen for **transgender females** is more complex than the transgender male regimen. The estrogen and antiandrogen treatment induces physical changes within the first 3 to 12 months of the treatment. Trans females experience decreased sexual desire, reduction of spontaneous erections, mild reduction of facial and body hair, increased breast tissue growth, and redistribution of body fat.

Because of the possible side effects and complications of the hormonal suppression and replacement therapy (Table 74.11), a thorough pretreatment screening and appropriate regular follow-up monitoring are recommended for both transgender females and males (Tables 74.12 and 74.13).

The clinical monitoring should include weight, blood pressure, and a systemic physical examination, and it should assess routine health questions such as tobacco use and symptoms of depression. Special attention should be given to the side effects of sex steroids such as deep vein thrombosis and pulmonary embolism.

Fertility in Transgender People

Gender-affirming procedures have a devastating and irreversible effect on the reproductive potential of transgender people. Gender-affirming hormones adversely affect fertility, and gender affirmation surgery may involve the removal of gonads (Martinez, 2017). Thus, fertility preservation options should be discussed with all trans people before medical and surgical transition. Based on recent studies, approximately 47% of transgender individuals desire to have a child to whom they

| TABLE 74.11 | Risks Associated With Sex Hormone Treatment |

Estrogen
Thromboembolic disease *(very high risk)*
Cerebrovascular disease, coronary artery disease, breast cancer, hypertriglyceridemia, cholelithiasis *(moderate risk)*
Testosterone
Erythrocytosis (hematocrit >50%) *(very high risk)*
Severe liver dysfunction, coronary artery disease, cerebrovascular disease, hypertension, breast or uterine cancer *(moderate risk)*

| TABLE 74.12 | Recommended Follow-Up for Trans Male Patients |

- Evaluate the patient every 3 months in the first year and then one to two times per year to monitor for appropriate signs of virilization and for development of adverse reactions.
- Measure serum testosterone every 3 months until levels are in the normal physiologic male range.
- Measure hematocrit or hemoglobin at baseline and every 3 months for the first year and then one to two times per year. Monitor weight, blood pressure, and lipids at regular intervals.

| TABLE 74.13 | Recommended Follow-Up for Trans Female Patients |

Measure serum testosterone and estradiol every 3 months.
- Serum testosterone levels should be 50 ng/dL.
- Serum estradiol should not exceed the peak physiologic range: 100–200 pg/mL.
For individuals on spironolactone, serum electrolytes, particularly potassium, should be monitored every 3 months in the first year and annually thereafter.
Routine cancer screening is recommended, as in nontransgender individuals.

are genetically related (Tornello and Bos, 2017). About 37% of trans men wish to have their gametes preserved before gender-affirmation procedures, and 15% to 51% of trans women seek to have children depending on their sexual orientation (De Sutter et al., 2002; Wierckx et al., 2012). Fertility preservation is best addressed before any hormonal treatment and/or genital-related surgery is undertaken.

A prolonged period on gender-affirming hormones will progressively affect semen quality, with increased frequency of oligozoospermia, asthenozoospermia, teratozoospermia, and azoospermia. Restoration of spermatogenesis is possible after stopping hormonal treatment, but the time to restoration is uncertain, and discontinuing hormone therapy may lead to undesirable effects from increased endogenous testosterone production.

Semen cryopreservation using specimens obtained from masturbation is a standard fertility preservation protocol that has been in use for decades. This is an easy and inexpensive method to collect semen in cis males. However, the ejaculation could cause a major distress in trans women (Hamada et al., 2015). The anti-androgen treatment might also play a role in this distress, making the erections and the ejaculation more troublesome. In these cases, the semen can be obtained with electro-ejaculation or surgically with a direct sperm retrieval from the testicles or epididymis. The testicular sperm extraction (TESE) has been well studied in azoospermic patients postchemotherapy, with a 42% to 65% success rate (Meseguer et al., 2003). Unfortunately, the success rate in azoospermic transgender individuals in unknown.

The quality and quantity of cryopreserved sperm determines the pregnancy outcomes. Also, the assisted reproductive method plays a major role in the pregnancy success rate. If there is a good volume and quality of sperm, a direct intrauterine insemination can be used successfully. Conversely, poor quality and volume of sperm has a better chance of a successful pregnancy with in vitro fertilization (IVF) or intracytoplasmic sperm injection (ICSI).

In trans men, the effect of testosterone on ovaries is inconclusive. The common belief that long-term exposure to testosterone could induce polycystic ovary syndrome (PCOS) was not supported by recent studies (Spinder et al., 1989). In terms of reproduction, androgen therapy does not appear to disturb the ovarian follicular pool.

Malignancies in Female Transgender Patients

Recent studies found gender identity to be relevant to **cancer screening**. Trans men were less likely to be up to date on Pap tests than cis women. Trans men and gender-nonconforming individuals were also shown to have significantly lower proportions of regular Pap tests in an Internet-based convenience sample. **Gender-identity disparities** in cancer screenings persist beyond known sociodemographic and health care factors. It is critical that gender-identity questions are included in cancer and other health-related surveillance systems to create knowledge to better inform health care practitioners and policy makers of appropriate screenings for trans and gender-nonconforming individuals. It was found that, of trans men who do receive Pap tests, they were ten times more likely than cis women to have inadequate tests (i.e., the cell sample taken was insufficient for laboratory testing), which may be associated with increased risk for developing high-grade cervical lesions at a later date.

The current literature is inconclusive about the real **incidence of prostate cancer in trans females,** what the screening and diagnostic pathway should be, and what treatment to recommend in this unique population. According to the sparse literature, the incidence of prostate cancer in trans females is quite rare and is still presented as case reports rather than larger series. In one of the largest European studies on 2306 trans female patients, Gooren and Morgant reported only one case of prostate cancer, for an incidence of 0.04%. This low incidence can be a result of the following:
- Marginalization and lack of access to health care
- Inappropriate screening
- Inconsistent follow-up
- Low level of androgenic hormonal milieu

Because of the prolonged anti-androgen treatment, it is possible that any foci of prostate cancer that might develop will be kept in a quiescent phase for a prolonged period. When these foci become clinically relevant, it presents as castration resistant and as a more aggressive disease.

According to other studies, however, if a low-risk disease is present, this might be driven by estrogenic stimulation. The estrogens can affect prostate cell growth potential. **PSA and diagnosis** of prostate cancer in trans females and in the population under hormonal suppression therapy should be interpreted with caution. Gooren suggests the value of 1 ng/mL as a threshold in subjects who are under prolonged hormone-suppression treatment.

Prostate biopsy is not contraindicated after vaginoplasty. The biopsy can be safely performed through the neovaginal cavity, and the images and technique do not differ much from the traditional transrectal approach used in cis males. **Similarly, radical prostatectomy** is not contraindicated after gender-affirming surgery. Particular attention should be paid during the surgical dissection because the traditional anatomic landmarks may be less clear than usual.

Theoretically, **radiation therapy** is also feasible in transgender patients diagnosed with prostate cancer after vaginoplasty. Caution should be exerted to the target radiation field as the traditional anatomic landmarks might be different from that of the cis male. Patients should be aware of the risk for neovaginal stenosis caused by radiation, from any dose being administered to the neovagina. A more intense vaginal dilation program should be recommended in trans females after pelvic irradiation.

Sexuality and Disability

Sexuality and sexual function are important to people with disabilities just as they are to their able-bodied counterparts. Unfortunately, the knowledge about sexual and reproductive health among people with disabilities is frequently inadequate. Society may still perceive people with disabilities negatively and stereotypically. They could be seen either as asexual or as hypersexual and unable to control their sexual urges (Esmail et al., 2010). Additionally, there is increased reporting of dating violence and sexual abuse and assault of the physically disabled (Jemta et al., 2008).

Adolescents and young adults with physical disabilities are less active socially, and they have difficulties in developing intimate relationships. Thus, despite a greater need for sexual and reproductive health education and service delivery than people without disabilities, dedicated services regarding sexuality and physical disabilities are scantly reported.

Historically, society has ignored or minimized the issue of sexuality in people with disabilities. The physically disabled, especially those with more severe impairments, experience poor body image, lower emotional well-being, and lower sexual self-esteem and satisfaction (McCabe et al., 2003).

Special consideration is needed for females with spinal cord injuries. These patients commonly experience impairment of genital sensation, vaginal lubrication, and orgasm. Also, incontinence, pain, and spasticity are common (Ferreiro-Velasco et al., 2005).

Participants in a UK study on female sexuality after SCI reported a range of physical consequences such as reduced libido, arousal, satisfaction, and orgasm. Also, bladder, bowel, and pelvic floor dysfunction; pain; spasticity; and autonomic dysreflexia were common. Altered vaginal sensation (absent, reduced, fluctuating, or position dependent) was frequently reported. After SCI, some participants reported that sensation improved over time. However, complete vaginal sensory loss was devastating and affected participants' view of intercourse (Thrussell et al., 2018).

According to the National Spinal Cord Injury Statistical Center, there are 270,000 Americans with a spinal cord injury. The majority of the spinal trauma occurs in men (80%). Therefore, literature on FSD after SCI is sparse. Sexuality in women with SCI is treated as a minority of minorities and suffers a total lack of attention.

In her study, Fritz et al. (2015) point out that sexual activity and womanhood continues to be important after a SCI. The study demonstrates that despite the physical limitation caused by the injury, most women desire and engage in relationships and see sex as an important part of their lives.

There are some important changes in the sexual activity after the trauma, such as dissatisfaction with current sexual life, that represent major challenges in female sexual life (Consortium for Spinal Cord Medicine, 2010):

- **Physical barriers** related to SCI could produce lack of bladder and bowel control; pain; weakness; pressure ulcers; and sensory loss.
- **Faster aging process:** Female SCI patients believe that they age faster than able-bodied women.
- **Lack of specific sexual education** such as knowledge of possible positions that could be adopted. The treating physician should discuss the sexual function and the different available options for sexual activity in subjects with SCI. The sexual education should go beyond merely discussing the possibility of pregnancy or discussing the appropriate birth control.
- **Pregnancy:** Often the SCI occurs at the peak reproductive age. Knowing the possibilities of childbearing is a relevant factor in the "womanhood" of these patients.
- **Sexual confidence:** There is a need to learn how to develop the confidence to pursue intimate relationships and motherhood after SCI (Kreuter et al., 2011).

> **KEY POINTS: SPECIAL POPULATIONS**
>
> - It is important to question sexual orientation and gender identity during history taking to identify potential health disparities and sexual problems among LGBTQ populations.
> - Transgender females and males should be screened and monitored for the possible side effects of cross-sex hormonal therapy.
> - As gender-affirming procedures and hormonal therapy may have potentially irreversible effects on their fertility capacity, fertility preservation options should be discussed with transgender patients before proceeding with medical and surgical transition.
> - It is not uncommon for females with SCIs to experience problems with genital sensation, vaginal lubrication, and orgasm as well as chronic genital pain and spasticity.
> - Despite all the limitations and disabilities that might have been caused, sexual health/functioning of patients with SCI should not be ignored/overlooked.

FEMALE SEXUAL INTEREST DISORDER

Approximately 40% of women suffer some form of sexual dysfunction in their lifetime (Laumann et al., 1999; Shifren et al., 2008). The most prevalent sexual dysfunction in women across all ages is a lack of sexual desire, which was previously referred to HSDD in the *DSM-IV-TR* (APA, 2000) and female sexual interest and arousal disorder in the *DSM-5* (APA, 2013). The overall prevalence of low sexual desire with distress in premenopausal and postmenopausal women ranged from approximately 8% to 19%. With aging, the intensity of sexual desire generally decreases, whereas the distress associated with low desire decreases. Accordingly, the prevalence of low sexual desire, sexually related personal distress, and HSDD (meeting the diagnostic criteria) were 88%, 15.5%, and 13.6%, respectively, in an Australian cross-sectional study of 1548 women between 65 and 79 years of age (Zeleke et al., 2016).

Associations have also been drawn between distressing low sexual desire and lower health-related quality of life (QoL), as well as psychosocial factors such as dissatisfaction with sex life, partner, or marriage and negative emotional states, including frustration, hopelessness, anger, poor self-esteem, and loss of femininity (Hayes et al., 2007; Leiblum et al., 2006; West et al., 2008). A large-scale survey including more than 2000 US women revealed that those with HSDD had statistically significant decrements in mental aspects of overall health (Leiblum et al., 2006). Biddle et al. showed that postmenopausal women with a lack of sexual desire experienced more health burdens and were more likely to report fatigue, depression, memory problems, back pain, and a lower QoL (Biddle et al., 2009).

Definition

The *ICD-10-CM* defines HSDD as an "absence or marked reduction in desire or motivation to engage in sexual activity as manifested by any of the following: (1) reduced or absent spontaneous desire (sexual thoughts or fantasies); (2) reduced or absent responsive desire to erotic cues and stimulation; or (3) inability to sustain desire or interest during sexual activity. Symptoms are evident over a period of at least several months and are not secondary to a sexual pain disorder. Additionally, sexual symptoms should be associated with clinically significant distress (WHO, 2016).

The International Society for the Study of Women's Sexual Health (ISSWSH) defines HSDD as any of the following for a minimum of 6 months (Parish et al., 2016):

- Lack of motivation for sexual activity as manifested by decreased or absent spontaneous desire (sexual thoughts or fantasies); or decreased or absent responsive desire to erotic cues and stimulation or inability to maintain desire or interest through sexual activity

- Loss of desire to initiate or participate in sexual activity, including behavioral responses such as avoidance of situations that could lead to sexual activity, that is not secondary to sexual pain disorders
- And is combined with clinically significant personal distress that includes frustration, grief, guilt, incompetence, loss, sadness, sorrow, or worry.

HSDD is not secondary to physical and/or emotional abuse, dissatisfaction with the partner, or intrusion of life stressors that can be affected by psychological and/or lifestyle changes. Therefore, relationship issues (e.g., significant relationship conflict) should be ruled out as a primary causative factor before arriving at the diagnosis of HSDD (Goldstein et al., 2017). HSDD may be lifelong or acquired and generalized or situational.

According to the *DSM-IV-TR*, HSDD was defined as "persistently or recurrently deficient (or absent) sexual fantasies and desire for sexual activity that causes marked distress or interpersonal difficulty not related to a medical or psychiatric condition or the use of a substance or medication" (APA, 2000). On the other hand, HSDD and FSAD have been combined into one disorder, now called *female sexual interest/arousal disorder* (FSIAD) in the *DSM-5* (APA, 2013). This revision was based on data suggesting that sexual response is not always a linear process and that the distinction between desire and arousal may be artificial (Basson, 2001; Binik et al., 2010). Diagnosis requires a minimum duration of approximately 6 months, and loss of desire needs to be associated with personal distress rather than partner or relationship issues.

Pathophysiology

The pathophysiology of low sexual desire is complex and should be considered in the context of the biopsychosocial approach. Biologic factors such as common systemic comorbidities (e.g., hypertension, hypothyroidism, and diabetes mellitus) (Basson and Schultz, 2007) and their treatment modalities (including antihypertensives such as calcium channel blockers and angiotensin-converting enzyme inhibitors) (Finger et al., 1997) have been associated with decreased sexual desire. Pregnancy, breastfeeding, or a postmenopausal state can also be associated with decreased libido.

Aging can have a negative influence on sexual desire. It has been shown that middle-aged women had the highest prevalence of decreased desire with distress (Rosen et al., 2012). Neuroendocrine changes of aging (such as declining testosterone, loss of estrogen) can decrease sexual desire. Although lower testosterone levels have been associated with decreased sexual desire, there is no level of testosterone that can accurately predict HSDD (Davis et al., 2005). Likewise, an association can be drawn between low sexual desire and decreased estradiol levels; however, not all patients with HSDD have low estradiol levels (Goldstein et al., 2017). Furthermore, the intensity and duration of the genital stimulation may need to be higher as a result of the diminished genital sensation that commonly occurs in middle-aged and postmenopausal women (Kingsberg et al., 2015). Hypoestrogenism may induce vulvovaginal atrophy and dyspareunia, which eventually leads to decreased sexual desire (Levine et al., 2008).

Psychiatric conditions (e.g., depression and anxiety) and their treatment (e.g., selective serotonin reuptake inhibitors [SSRIs] and anxiolytics) are also associated with decreased sexual desire. Sexual abuse and trauma in childhood and puberty, perceived stress, distraction, self-focused attention or anxiety, personality disorders, and body image or self-consciousness have all been shown to negatively affect desire (Brotto et al., 2010).

Cultural, social, and religious values and beliefs can negatively influence women's sexual desire, especially in women raised in highly conservative cultures or religions (Kingsberg and Rezaee, 2013). Relationship factors such as conflict or a partner's sexual dysfunction (e.g., erectile dysfunction and premature ejaculation in a male partner) (Rubio-Aurioles et al., 2009), stressors such as financial problems, career-related issues, and familial obligations can also contribute to decreased sexual desire (Kingsberg et al., 2015).

The neurophysiologic background of HSDD has not been completely unrevealed. Sexual desire is the result of a delicate

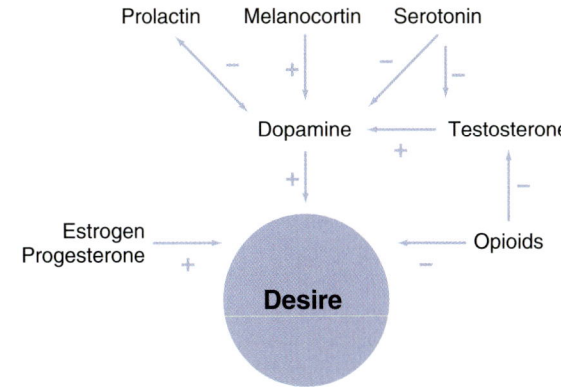

Fig. 74.8. Excitatory and inhibitory effects of neurotransmitters and hormones on sexual desire. (Data from Clayton AH. The pathophysiology of hypoactive sexual desire disorder in women. *Int J Gynaecol Obstet* 2010;110[1]:7–11.)

balance between neuromodulators of excitatory pathways (e.g., dopamine, norepinephrine, melanocortins, oxytocin, vasopressin) and inhibitory pathways (e.g., serotonin, opioids, endocannabinoids, prolactin) (Fig. 74.8). Decreased activity level in the brain regions associated with sexual arousal (e.g., medial orbitofrontal region and periaqueductal gray matter) and a lack of disinhibition of brain regions involved in cognitive processing (e.g., left brain) in women with HSDD can impair vaginal vasocongestion and lubrication and eventually cause orgasmic failure.

Evaluation

Health care providers should initiate the general discussion and assessment of sexual concerns because patients are often reluctant to bring up the topic. **It has been shown that 73% of premenopausal women and 81% of postmenopausal women never mentioned their desire problems to a health care provider** according to survey results including 450 premenopausal and postmenopausal women with self-reported low sexual desire (Kingsberg, 2014).

A variety of screening instruments can be used to help identify women who suffer from low desire. **In particular, the Decreased Sexual Desire Screener is a validated, five-question, self-administered survey that helps identify generalized acquired HSDD in both premenopausal and postmenopausal women** (Table 74.14). This screener is a useful adjunct to the patient history and physical examination in the diagnosis of HSDD (Clayton and Balon, 2009). It was found to be easy to use by clinicians who are not specialized in sexual medicine and had greater accuracy when compared with an expert clinician interview (Goldfischer et al., 2008). Because the *DSM-5* diagnostic category of FSIAD combines the prior *DSM-IV-TR* disorders of HSDD and FSAD, screening and assessment should also include inquiry of difficulties with genital and nongenital excitement and arousal.

Women indicate yes/no responses to the five questions. The purpose of questions 1 to 4 is to determine the presence/absence of HSDD. If the patient responds yes to all the questions, this is consistent with generalized acquired HSDD. The purpose of question 5 is to help determine whether the etiology of HSDD is primary or secondary. If screening suggests the presence of HSDD, the next steps should include gathering more information about patient's experience of low desire, including onset, duration, behavioral adaptation and avoidance, and level of distress.

A complete medical history is essential to identify contributing factors that may reveal the cause of low sexual desire. A variety of systemic comorbidities and urogynecologic problems might interfere with sexual desire (Table 74.15). Psychiatric conditions should be identified, as relatively more prevalent ones such as depression and anxiety disorder have been associated with HSDD. Presence of depression increases the risk for sexual dysfunction in the range of 50% to 70%. On the other hand, problems related to sexual function

TABLE 74.14 Decreased Sexual Desire Screener

1. In the past, was your level of sexual desire or interest good and satisfying to you?	○ Yes	○ No
2. Has there been a decrease in your level of sexual desire or interest?	○ Yes	○ No
3. Are you bothered by your decreased level of sexual desire or interest?	○ Yes	○ No
4. Would you like your level of sexual desire or interest to increase?	○ Yes	○ No
5. Please check all the factors that you feel may be contributing to your current decrease in sexual desire or interest:		
a. An operation, depression, injuries, or other medical conditions	○ Yes	○ No
b. Medications, drugs, or alcohol you are currently taking	○ Yes	○ No
c. Pregnancy, recent childbirth, menopausal symptoms	○ Yes	○ No
d. Other sexual issues you may be having (pain, decreased arousal, or orgasms)	○ Yes	○ No
e. Your partner's sexual problems	○ Yes	○ No
f. Dissatisfaction with your relationship or partner	○ Yes	○ No
g. Stress or fatigue	○ Yes	○ No

- If the patient answers *no* to any of the questions 1–4, then she does not qualify for the diagnosis of generalized acquired hypoactive sexual desire disorder (HSDD).
- If the patient answers *yes* to all of the questions 1–4, and your review confirms *no* answers to all of the factors in question 5, then she does qualify for the diagnosis of generalized acquired HSDD.
- If the patient answers *yes* to all of the questions 1–4 and *yes* to any of the factors in question 5, then decide whether the answers to question 5 indicate a primary diagnosis other than generalized acquired HSDD. Comorbid conditions such as arousal or orgasmic disorder do not rule out a concurrent diagnosis of HSDD.

Reprinted with permission from *J Sex Med*
Data from Clayton AH, Goldfischer ER, Goldstein I, et al. Validation of the decreased sexual desire screener (DSDS): a brief diagnostic instrument for generalized acquired female hypoactive sexual desire disorder (HSDD). *J Sex Med* 2009;6(3):730–738; Goldfischer ER, Clayton AH, Goldstein I, et al. Decreased sexual desire screener (DSDS) for diagnosis of hypoactive sexual desire disorder in women. *Obstet Gynecol* 2008;111:109.

TABLE 74.15 Conditions That Are Associated With Low Sexual Desire

Hypertension
Diabetes mellitus (type 1 and type 2) (Pontiroli et al., 2013)
Metabolic syndrome (Trompeter et al., 2016)
Hypothyroidism, hyperthyroidism (Krysiak et al., 2016; Atis et al., 2011)
Hyperprolactinemia (Kadioglu et al., 2005)
Renal failure
Spinal cord injury (Hajiaghababaei et al., 2014)
Multiple sclerosis (Mohammadi et al., 2013)
Neuromuscular disorders
Parkinson disease
Dementia
Vulvar dermatoses
Postmenopausal status
Polycystic ovary syndrome (Janssen et al., 2008)
Malignancy (breast cancer and its treatment) (Panjari et al., 2011; Fobair and Spiegel, 2009)
Depression

are associated with a 130% to 210% increased risk for depression (Atlantis and Sullivan, 2012). **Given this significant bidirectional relationship, every patient with HSDD should be screened for depressive symptoms.**

Medications should be noted, because certain classes of drugs (e.g., SSRIs, antipsychotics, antihypertensives) may negatively influence desire (Table 74.16). Other examples include medications that lower testosterone production (combined hormonal contraceptives); chemical ovarian suppression by gonadotropin-releasing hormone analogues and exogenous glucocorticoids; drugs with antiandrogenic activity (spironolactone, cyproterone acetate, flutamide, and finasteride); drugs that increase SHBG levels, and hence lowering free testosterone levels (oral estrogens, combined hormonal contraceptive, tamoxifen, and thyroxine); and drugs that increase serum prolactin levels (antipsychotics).

Overlap of female sexual disorders is not uncommon, and concurrent sexual problems might exacerbate low desire, such as HSDD impairing arousal that impairs orgasm or may lead to pain (e.g., attempting penetrative intercourse without adequate lubrication caused by lack of interest and/or orgasmic failure) or hypoestrogenism-related vaginal dryness leading to persistent dyspareunia, which eventually interferes with sexual desire. A temporal relationship between the onset of sexual complaints might provide an idea about the primary versus secondary nature of low sexual desire. Lifelong versus acquired HSDD should be discriminated as well as situational versus generalized (occurs in all settings with all partners) forms of the disorder. Prior sexual function and relationship/interpersonal issues should also be sought. Urogynecologic history should cover information about conditions that might influence a woman's willingness to engage in sexual activity such as menstrual cycles in premenopausal women, menopausal vasomotor symptoms, STIs, LUTS, UI, fecal incontinence, POP, and high-tone pelvic floor dysfunction (Clayton et al., 2018a).

Many women will ask whether their form of contraception, especially combined oral contraceptives (COCs), may be contributing. COCs may decrease libido as a result of antiandrogenic effects and a decrease in lubrication, whereas decreased fear of pregnancy and improvement in certain gynecologic conditions, such as dysmenorrhea, menorrhagia, or endometriosis, might augment sexual desire. The use of oral contraceptives and low sexual desire has been a matter of debate for a long time, with some studies supporting an association (Bitzer et al., 2003; Wallwiener et al., 2010) and others failing to identify any cause-effect relationship (Burrows et al., 2012; Pastor et al., 2013). The presence of menstrual irregularities may give a clue about possible hormonal disorders (e.g., hyperprolactinemia and hypothyroidism) that interfere with sexual desire.

A history of pelvic surgery (such as bilateral salpingo-oophorectomy before natural menopause), pelvic trauma, or radiotherapy involving pelvic organs may point to an anatomic source because these factors may be associated with pelvic pain and altered ovarian function.

Physical examination is not necessary to arrive at the diagnosis of HSDD. However, it can provide valuable information to discover the factors that may be contributing to diminished sexual interest.

TABLE 74.16 Classes and Examples of Medications That Might Be Associated With Low Sexual Desire

Anticonvulsants	Carbamazepine Phenytoin Primidone
Cardiovascular medications	Angiotensin-converting enzyme inhibitors Amiodarone Beta-blockers (atenolol, metoprolol, propranolol) Calcium channel blockers Clonidine Digoxin Diuretics (hydrochlorothiazide, spironolactone) Lipid-lowering agents
Hormones	Antiandrogens (flutamide) Gonadotropin-releasing hormone agonists Oral contraceptives
Analgesics	Nonsteroidal anti-inflammatory drugs Opiates
Psychotropic medications	Antipsychotics Anxiolytics (alprazolam, diazepam) Selective serotonin reuptake inhibitors Serotonin norepinephrine reuptake inhibitors Tricyclic antidepressants
Illicit drugs	Amphetamine Cocaine Heroin Marijuana
Others	Histamine receptor antagonists Alcohol Indomethacin Ketoconazole Chemotherapeutic agents

Modified from Clayton AH, Kingsberg SA, Goldstein I. Evaluation and management of hypoactive sexual desire disorder. *Sex Med* 2018;6(2):59–74.

Signs of hormonal insufficiency, such as vulvovaginal atrophy, may result in dyspareunia and negatively affect sexual desire. Genital sensory changes (sensitivity to pressure with a cotton swab around the vestibule in vulvodynia); macroscopic signs of vulvar dermatoses (e.g., lichen sclerosus, lichen planus); abnormal neurologic examination findings (tenderness at ischial spine suggestive of pudendal nerve disorder or changes in anal sphincter tone/bulbocavernosus reflex latency suggestive of lumbosacral spinal pathology); PFM overactivity/tenderness; urethral hypermobility; positive cough stress test; and POP are some of the important physical examination findings that might shed light to the underlying cause and possible treatment pathway of low sexual desire (Kingsberg et al., 2005).

Laboratory evaluation is rarely helpful in the workup of low sexual desire. There are no biomarkers that can reliably confirm or exclude HSDD. Laboratory tests may only be considered in patients who exhibit signs and symptoms of hormonal dysregulation. Women with physical findings suggestive of hyperprolactinemia or thyroid disease should have prolactin levels and thyroid function tests measured, respectively. Androgen levels have not been shown to correlate with sexual function (Davis et al., 2005; Santoro et al., 2005). Furthermore, currently available testosterone assays are unreliable at the lower levels usually seen in women. As a result, measuring serum testosterone levels in women presenting with low sexual desire will not provide meaningful clinical guidance.

Treatment

The treatment of HSDD involves psychosocial and biologic approaches. It is recommended to sequence treatment that gives priority to the most distressing aspect of the problem (Brotto et al., 2016). An office-based incremental counseling may be helpful using the PLISSIT model, which is basically a stepped approach specifically designed for health care providers in the primary setting (Annon, 1976). According to this incremental model, women are given permission (P) to discuss their problems and emotions. Then, the practitioner provides limited information (LI), which includes basic sexual function education and/or resources, and specific suggestions (SS) for addressing the problem in the form of directives and advice. If the individual needs more intensive treatment (IT) for HSDD, then the practitioner can refer her for individual or couple's therapy.

Initially, modifiable factors that are thought to be playing a role in HSDD should be addressed. Taking control over these conditions (e.g., disease states, medications) will have a positive influence regarding the amelioration of sexual dysfunction. If HSDD persists despite correction of modifiable factors, further treatment can be applied in the form of psychological therapy and medications that exert their effect through central nervous system (CNS) or hormonal pathways (Fig. 74.9).

Psychological Treatment

The most commonly employed psychological interventions that are used to treat HSDD are behavioral therapy, cognitive behavioral therapy (CBT), and mindfulness therapy. Modifying thoughts, beliefs, behaviors, and emotions that interfere with desire represent the common target of each psychological modality. Behavior therapy utilizes education, communication skills training, and sensate focus exercises to tackle sexual complaints (Sarwer and Durlak, 1997). Questions during the assessment address cognitive function, sexual behavior, and skills of the couple (Brotto et al., 2016). Sensate focus therapy involves sensual touching exercises and aims to reduce anxiety and avoidance of sexual activity, improve sexual communication between partners, and improve intimacy by reintroducing sexual activity in an incremental way. It is more effective when HSDD is associated with penetration-related anxiety and associated behavioral avoidance (Masters and Johnson, 1970).

CBT aims to modify thoughts and behaviors that inhibit sexual thoughts in a sexual situation (Meston and Bradford, 2007). Through this process, patients learn to identify and challenge the unrealistic beliefs that keep them away from sexual activity. McCabe (2001) reported that CBT was effective in 44.4% of women with sexual health concerns. Likewise, Trudel et al. (2001) found that 74% of women with HSDD were improved with CBT, and this benefit was durable in 64% at 1-year follow-up.

The goal of mindfulness therapy is to encourage participants to connect and engage with their sexuality by learning and practicing a variety of mindfulness exercises (Brotto et al., 2014). It has been shown to help decrease cognitive distraction during sexual activity and increase awareness of pleasurable sensations when used in the setting of HSDD (Brotto et al., 2008b).

Medical Treatment

Flibanserin is currently the only U.S. Food and Drug Administration (FDA)-approved medication that can be used for the management of premenopausal women with low sexual desire. All of the other medical treatment options that can be applied in patients diagnosed with HSDD are used off-label. Several other drugs are currently under clinical development and may enter the HSDD armamentarium in the future.

Hormones

The increase in FSD during menopause is partly a result of decreasing levels of estrogens, which have been associated with vulvovaginal atrophy. Replacing estrogens via exogenous sources is the most

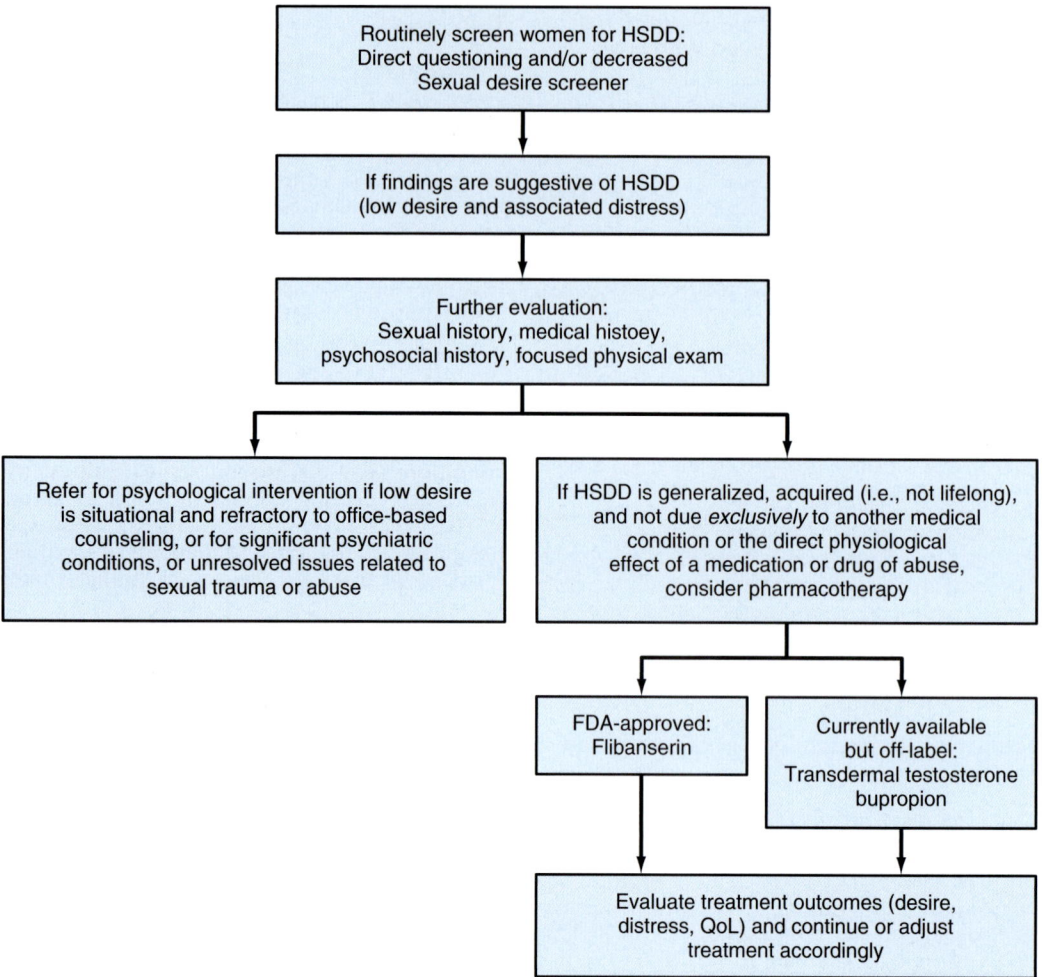

Fig. 74.9. Treatment algorithm for hypoactive sexual desire disorder. (Data from Clayton AH, Kingsberg SA, Goldstein I. Evaluation and management of hypoactive sexual desire disorder. *Sex Med* 2018b;6[2]:59–74.)

straightforward approach to ameliorate hypoestrogenism-related sexual issues (Clayton and Hamilton, 2010). A meta-analysis covering 192 randomized controlled trials, related with estrogen replacement therapy (ERT) in postmenopausal women, showed that estrogens, alone or in a combination form, remain an effective therapy for relieving the symptoms associated with sexual dysfunction (Nelson et al., 2007), especially pain with sexual activity. Vestergaard et al. demonstrated that long-term (5 years) ERT significantly improved libido and dyspareunia (Vestergaard et al., 2003). Ospemifene is a novel selective estrogen receptor modulator with indication for the treatment of vulvovaginal atrophy and dyspareunia in postmenopausal women. A daily dose of 60 mg has been shown to be safe and effective in the treatment of women who have low sexual desire secondary to vaginal atrophy and dyspareunia (Cui et al., 2014; Goldstein et al., 2014). However, the International Society of Sexual Medicine Consensus concluded that, although topical vaginal estrogen is currently the first-line therapy for vulvovaginal atrophy, available evidence does not support the use of systemic estrogen therapy for FSD (e.g., HSDD) (Santoro et al., 2016).

Substantial evidence suggests that testosterone therapy positively influences overall sexual wellness in postmenopausal women with low desire with improvement in the number of sexual events reported as satisfactory, sexual desire, pleasure, arousal, and frequency of orgasm as well as a reduction in personal distress (Braunstein, 2007b; Davis et al., 2008; Somboonporn et al., 2005). In their randomized placebo-controlled study, Braunstein et al. (2005) showed that statistically significant increases in sexual desire and frequency of satisfying sexual encounters were achieved among the group of women who received the 300-μg/day dose. Similarly, positive results were reported by Buster et al., who assessed the efficacy and safety of the 300-μg/day testosterone patch during 24 weeks of administration in surgically menopausal women with HSDD who were already on estrogen therapy. In this study, testosterone treatment significantly increased the number of satisfying sexual events and sexual desire, and decreased sexually related personal distress (Buster et al., 2005). A recent systematic review and meta-analysis of seven randomized placebo-controlled studies enrolling over 3000 postmenopausal women with HSDD revealed that transdermal testosterone (with or without concomitant estrogen therapy) treatment led to significant increases in sexual desire, sexual activity, satisfying sexual events, and orgasms and a significant decrease in personal distress (Achilli et al., 2017).

While being approved for use in postmenopausal women in the European Union, concerns about long-term safety have precluded FDA approval of testosterone treatment in postmenopausal women with low sexual desire (Snabes and Simes, 2009). Peripheral conversion of exogenously administered testosterone by endogenous aromatases to estrogen and the resultant causal possibility of cardiovascular adverse events and development/progression of breast cancer represented the main issues that are being questioned with regard to the safety of long-term testosterone use in women (Brand et al., 2009; Laughlin et al., 2010). The Nurses' Health Study suggested that methyltestosterone users may be at increased risk for breast cancer (Ness et al., 2009), whereas other studies denied such an association (Davis, 2011). A phase III long-term study showed that testosterone transdermal gel did not increase cardiovascular events or breast cancer, even in high-risk women (White et al., 2012).

Oral formulations are not recommended as they are subject to significant intraindividual/interindividual variations in absorption, which might lead to supraphysiologic levels and consequently negative effects on lipid metabolism and hepatotoxicity. Transdermal administration avoids first-pass liver effects; hence it does not lead to alterations in lipid metabolism (Davis et al., 2012). The most common formulation used is a transdermal 1% testosterone cream (0.5 g cream, 5 mg testosterone daily) applied to skin of the arms, abdomen, or legs. Testosterone patches and gels that are originally formulated for men should be used with extreme caution in women, because accurate dosing is difficult. Likewise, testosterone injections and implants are also available but may lead to adverse effects as a result of irreversibly high, supraphysiologic serum testosterone levels. Women prescribed off-label testosterone therapy should be cautiously monitored for potential side effects; lipids and liver function should be regularly assessed (Kingsberg et al., 2015) during the course of treatment. It should also be noted that efficacy may not emerge for several weeks, and treatment should not be continued beyond 6 months in the absence of any clinical benefit (Davis et al., 2016).

The potential side effects of exogenous testosterone administration include signs of virilization, such as development of acne, hirsutism, deepening of the voice, and androgenic alopecia (ACOG, 2011). However, these effects are dose-related and can be avoided if hormone levels are kept in the female physiologic range. In the long-term safety study including women with surgically induced menopause, the most common side effects of transdermal testosterone treatment were application site reactions and unwanted hair growth (Nachtigall et al., 2011).

Tibolone is a synthetic steroid sex hormone with estrogenic, androgenic, and progestogenic effects. Wu et al. randomized 48 postmenopausal women to tibolone versus estrogen-progesterone hormone replacement therapy (HRT) for 12 weeks. As a result, tibolone was found to be superior to HRT in improving sexual parameters, including general sexual satisfaction, sexual interest, sexual fantasies, sexual arousal, and orgasm, with decreased frequency of vaginal dryness and dyspareunia (Wu et al., 2001). Another study compared tibolone to transdermal estradiol (E_2)/norethisterone (NETA) in naturally postmenopausal women with FSD. Both treatment modalities increased the frequency of sexual events and reduced sexuality-related personal distress. However, the increase in total FSFI score was more profound in the tibolone group when compared with that achieved in the E_2/NETA group (Nijland et al., 2008).

Regarding oral dehydroepiandrosterone (DHEA), systematic reviews and meta-analyses have found no statistically significant benefit of its systemic administration within the context of FSD (Elraiyah et al., 2014).

Bupropion

Bupropion is a dopamine and norepinephrine reuptake inhibitor and nicotinic acetylcholine receptor antagonist that is used as an antidepressant and smoking-cessation aid. It is also used as an off-label medical treatment for HSDD. **It has been found superior to placebo in improving sexual desire and decreasing distress in nondepressed premenopausal women with HSDD** (Modell et al., 2000; Segraves et al., 2001). In the randomized, double-blind, placebo-controlled study including 232 premenopausal women with depression, significant increase in sexual desire and decrease in distress were achieved with bupropion (150 mg/day) treatment (Safarinejad et al., 2010). **Bupropion has also been shown to be effective in reversing SSRI-induced sexual dysfunction in premenopausal women, as statistical improvements in desire have been achieved with bupropion SR 300 to 400 mg/day** (Clayton et al., 2004). A Cochrane review supports the addition of bupropion in higher dosages (150 mg twice daily) for the treatment of antidepressant-induced sexual dysfunction in women (Taylor et al., 2013).

The most common adverse effects of bupropion in placebo-controlled clinical trials for major depression or smoking cessation were tremor (13.5%), agitation (9.7%), dry mouth (9.2%), constipation (8.7%), excessive sweating (7.7%), dizziness (6.1%), and nausea/vomiting (4%). Treatment discontinuation rate caused by adverse events was approximately 10% (GlaxoSmithKline, 2016).

Buspirone

Buspirone is a 5-HT_{1A} partial agonist that is approved as an anxiolytic for the management of generalized anxiety disorder and for the short-term relief of symptoms of anxiety. It is one of the off-label treatment alternatives for HSDD. **It has been shown that buspirone minimized the negative effect of selective serotonin reuptake inhibition on sexual function when it was coadministered with SSRIs for the treatment of depression.** Fifty-eight percent of individuals treated with buspirone (20 to 60 mg/day) reported an improvement in sexual function compared with 30% treated with placebo (Landén et al., 1999).

Similar to bupropion, specific safety data of buspirone in women with HSDD is lacking. The most common adverse events in placebo-controlled anxiety disorder trials were dizziness (9%), nervousness (4%), nausea (3%), and headache (3%). Approximately 1 in 10 patients discontinued buspirone because of adverse effects.

Flibanserin

Flibanserin (Valeant Pharmaceuticals North America LLC, Bridgewater, NJ), dosed at 100 mg PO once daily at bedtime, is a nonhormonal, centrally acting, postsynaptic 5-HT_{1A} receptor agonist and 5-HT_{2A} receptor antagonist that results in a decrease in serotonin activity and an increase in dopamine and norepinephrine activity. It is believed to enhance sexual desire by stimulating excitatory elements of brain function and diminishing the inhibitory response to sexual cues (Kingsberg and Woodard, 2015). Approximately 50% of women with HSDD respond to flibanserin, and it may take up to 8 weeks for efficacy to emerge. **Flibanserin is currently the only FDA-approved treatment for acquired, generalized HSDD in premenopausal women.** Phase III trials have demonstrated that flibanserin was significantly superior to placebo with regard to the improvement in sexual desire, decrease in sexually related distress, and increase in the number of satisfying sexual events (Katz et al., 2013; Valeant Pharmaceuticals, 2015). **In the pivotal clinical trials of flibanserin in premenopausal women with HSDD, results of which led to FDA approval, the rate of subjective improvement in sexual desire was significantly higher (54% to 58% in the flibanserin group vs. 40% to 48% in the placebo group) in the treatment arm when compared with the placebo arm.** Although similar results have been obtained in postmenopausal women, flibanserin has not yet been approved for the treatment of HSDD in this population (Simon et al., 2014).

Regarding its safety profile, the most common adverse events in premenopausal women were dizziness (9.2%), somnolence (8.3%), nausea (6.5%), and fatigue (3.7%). Most of the side effects were transient or episodic and were mild to moderate in severity. The discontinuation rate caused by adverse effects was 13% and 6% in patients treated with flibanserin and placebo, respectively (Flibanserin Advisory Committee. https://www.fda.gov/media/93087/download. Katz et al., 2013; Simon et al., 2014; Flibanserin Medication Guide, 2015).

Because somnolence and dizziness were the most common adverse events having been reported in flibanserin clinical trials, safety concerns related to alcohol consumption have been raised during the FDA review process, and several additional investigations had to be carried out to clarify the potential hazards of this possible interaction. Incidence of hypotension- and syncope-related adverse events in flibanserin-treated patients was low for self-reported alcohol users (0.7%) and alcohol nonusers (0.3%) in the post hoc analysis of five randomized, placebo-controlled flibanserin trials. Alcohol use did not increase the rate of adverse events in the three pivotal clinical trials. Furthermore, ethanol ingestion did not have a significant effect on somnolence, drowsiness, orthostatic blood pressure changes, vertigo, hypotension, or syncope in an alcohol interaction study that was carried out after FDA approval (Fisher and Pyke, 2017), **Nevertheless, because of ongoing concerns about the risk for hypotension and/or syncope caused by flibanserin-alcohol interaction, the flibanserin package insert indicates that alcohol use is contraindicated in women taking flibanserin** (Valeant Pharmaceuticals, 2016). **Risk Evaluation and Mitigation Strategy**

(REMS) (https://www.addyirems.com/AddyiUI/rems/home.action) was deemed necessary for the prescription of flibanserin. According to REMS, health care providers must review the drug's prescribing information, review a Prescriber and Pharmacy Training Program, complete a Knowledge Assessment Form, and submit the Prescriber Enrollment Form online before prescribing flibanserin. A similar certification and enrollment process is necessary for the pharmacies that are to dispense flibanserin (Valeant Pharmaceuticals, 2016).

The potential interaction between flibanserin and combined oral contraceptive pills has also been studied since flibanserin was FDA-approved in the premenopausal setting. Flibanserin was not found to cause clinically significant alterations in the pharmacokinetic properties of a combination of ethinyl estradiol and levonorgestrel in a study including healthy premenopausal women (Noll et al., 2016).

Others

The combination of sublingual testosterone with a phosphodiesterase type 5 inhibitor (PDE5I) (Emotional Brain BV, Almere, The Netherlands) or a 5HT$_{1A}$ receptor agonist (Emotional Brain BV) have also been tested for the medical treatment of low sexual desire in women. Both are proposed to increase sexual motivation through testosterone; however, the addition of the PDE5I is thought to increase vascular response (Poels et al., 2013), whereas addition of a 5HT$_{1A}$ receptor agonist is thought to act centrally by releasing sexual inhibition (van Rooij et al., 2013).

Bremelanotide (AMAG Pharmaceuticals, Inc, Waltham, MA), a melanocortin receptor agonist formulated as a subcutaneous injection, is another agent that is being investigated for the treatment of low desire and is also postulated to work through CNS mechanisms (Portman et al., 2014). Bremelanotide (1.25 and 1.75 mg) was found to demonstrate significantly superior clinical efficacy when compared with placebo in a randomized study of women with HSDD and/or FSAD in terms of the measures of sexual desire and arousal and in the number of satisfying sexual events. The most common adverse events were nausea (22% to 24%), flushing (14% to 17%), and headache (9% to 14%) (Clayton et al., 2016). Phase III clinical trials in premenopausal women with HSDD have demonstrated significant improvement in desire domain score of FSFI with bremelanotide treatment (1.75 mg, administered subcutaneously through an auto-injector before anticipated sexual activity) (Clayton et al., 2017; Derogatis et al., 2017).

> **KEY POINTS: HYPOACTIVE SEXUAL DESIRE DISORDER**
> - Pathophysiology of low sexual desire involves biologic, psychological, and social elements.
> - The Decreased Sexual Desire Screener can be utilized to identify generalized acquired HSDD.
> - Concurrent sexual problems involving other aspects of sexual function might exacerbate low desire.
> - A variety of systemic comorbidities and urogynecologic problems might interfere with sexual desire.
> - Flibanserin is currently the only FDA-approved treatment for acquired, generalized HSDD in premenopausal women.
> - All of the other medical treatment options for HSDD (including hormones) are used off-label.

Female Orgasmic Disorder

Female orgasmic disorder (FOD) is defined by a marked delay in orgasm, infrequency or absence of orgasm, or less intense orgasm for at least 6 months in 75% to 100% of sexual interactions (APA, 2013). FOD can be lifelong (primary) or acquired (secondary), generalized or situational, psychological or combined.

FOD is the second most common sexual dysfunction among women, closely following HSDD. Reported prevalence rates of FOD range from 16% to 28% in the United States, Europe, and Central/South America to 30% to 46% in Asia. **FOD can be diagnosed concurrently with at least one other sexual dysfunction** (Lewis et al., 2010). **It has been estimated that among women with FOD, 31% also report difficulties with sexual arousal, 18% with lubrication, 14% with desire, 12% with pain, and 0.9% with vaginismus** (Nobre et al., 2006).

The *DSM-5* definition of FOD does not contain the *DSM-IV-TR* criterion requiring that difficulty with orgasm occur despite "a normal excitement phase." This revision was based on the fact that FOD can occur despite intact arousal. Another difference between the *DSM-5* and *DSM-IV-TR* with regard to the definition of FOD is that the *DSM-5* considers the intensity of orgasm in addition to the frequency and latency aspects of the problem, which were already included in *DSM-IV-TR* (Basson et al., 2003).

To arrive at the diagnosis of FOD, it is necessary to rule out medical conditions, pharmacologic interventions (SSRIs, other psychotropic medications), and psychosocial issues (e.g., severe interpersonal distress, life stressors) that might cause orgasmic difficulties (APA, 2013; Carey, 2006). Moreover, insufficient stimulation must also be ruled out before assigning the diagnosis of FOD. A woman whose sexual partner suffers from erectile dysfunction and/or premature ejaculation, thus depriving her of sufficient stimulation to reach orgasm, cannot be assigned an FOD diagnosis. About one-half of women who do not consistently reach orgasm during sexual activity do not report distress (Shifren et al., 2008). However, for orgasmic problems to be named as FOD, it must cause significant distress and interpersonal difficulty.

Subjective experiences of orgasm and the type and intensity of tactile stimulation that is required to provoke an orgasm can show significant variation. Orgasm triggered by clitoral stimulation has been accepted as a normal variation in sexual response (Harris et al., 2008). Furthermore, although most women can reach orgasm through masturbation, orgasm during partnered sexual activity is less frequent (Garcia et al., 2014) as many women might need additional manual stimulation to orgasm during coitus. Therefore, FOD should not be diagnosed solely on the basis of a failure to experience orgasm during sexual intercourse in the absence of additional clitoral stimulation FOD (APA, 2013; Laan et al., 2013; Meston et al., 2004).

Assessment

A comprehensive sexual history is essential to diagnose and characterize FOD. The nature and onset of the problem should be carefully assessed as well as the other aspects of female sexual function, because FOD often accompanies problems with interest and arousal. Women with lifelong generalized anorgasmia tend to be younger and have never experienced orgasm in any context. Lifelong anorgasmia may suggest that the patient is unfamiliar or uncomfortable with self-stimulation or sexual interaction with her partner, or lacks adequate sex education (Laan et al., 2013). On the other hand, in women with acquired anorgasmia, who have achieved orgasm in the past but have a distressing current inability to reach orgasm, inadequate stimulation, contextual factors, or physiologic factors are usually the cause of orgasmic dysfunction (Kingsberg et al., 2017). In the generalized subtype, FOD occurs with all stimulations, situations, and partners, whereas in the situational subtype, it only occurs within specific conditions. Psychological subtype denotes specific cognitive, affective, or relational factors that are implicated with orgasmic difficulties, in the absence of medical conditions or substance contributors. For the combined subtype, psychological factors together with medical conditions or substance abuse contribute to the development of orgasmic problems.

It is also crucial to understand the degree of bother and distress associated with FOD. Frequency of orgasm during partnered sexual activity has been accepted as a significant predictor of overall sexual satisfaction (Philippsohn et al., 2009).

During clinical evaluation, certain conditions that might increase the risk for FOD should be kept in mind and sought for. Among the risk factors for anorgasmia are lower socioeconomic status; lower educational level; poorer physical health status (de Lucena and Abdo, 2014); cognitive/affective factors such as anxiety disorder (Bradford and Meston, 2006); depression (Shifren et al., 2008); body image misbeliefs (Sanchez and Kiefer, 2007); negative thinking styles (Nobre et al., 2008); relationship adjustment issues such as conflicts, dissatisfaction, and sexual communication (Kelly et al., 2006) or intimacy problems (Burri and Spector, 2011); being exposed to restrictive and conservative attitudes (because of religious or cultural misbeliefs) about sexuality (Kelly et al., 1990); history of sexual abuse or childhood maltreatment (Rellini and Meston, 2007); feeling guilty about sex; sexual inexperience; and the absence or deficiency of sex education during childhood or adolescence (de Lucena and Abdo, 2014).

Certain medical conditions (Bitzer et al., 2013; Kingsberg et al., 2013) including hypothyroidism, arthritis, hypertension, chronic pain, asthma, diabetes, coronary heart disease, malignancies (breast, colorectal, gynecologic), neuromuscular disorders, SCIs, and multiple sclerosis, might also have a negative impact on orgasmic functioning. Additionally, medications such as amphetamines, digoxin, antiandrogens, narcotics, antipsychotics, barbiturates, lithium, SSRIs (Montejo-Gonzalez et al., 1997), tricyclic antidepressants, chemotherapeutics, and antihypertensives (Clayton et al., 2009), can have a similar negative effect. It is often unclear whether it is the medical condition per se, the treatment, or the psychological side effects of such conditions that impair orgasmic response. Likewise, the factors associated with the indications for medication usage (e.g., nerve damage, anxiety, and depression) also affect orgasmic function. Therefore, it is not always possible to realize the actual impact of drugs on FOD.

Validated questionnaires that contain orgasm domains or orgasm-specific items (FSFI, Changes in Sexual Functioning Questionnaire, Brief Index of Sexual Function for Women), can also be used while evaluating patients who experience orgasmic problems. **Questionnaires alone are not sufficient to diagnose FOD. However, they can be used to track progress of the orgasmic function and monitor treatment response.**

Psychosocial Treatment

Several psychosocial treatment strategies for FOD, mainly in the form of cognitive and behavioral psychotherapies, have been evaluated in clinical trials. The majority of the relevant literature dates back to the 1980s. A recent systematic review has supported the efficacy of psychosocial interventions in the treatment of FOD (Frühauf et al., 2013).

It has been recommended that the partner should be actively involved in the assessment and treatment process in cases in which the orgasm problems are acquired or happen only during partnered sex (Laan et al., 2013). The PLISSIT modeled approach can be used while addressing orgasmic disorder. Primary care providers can apply this approach to provide initial support to uncomplicated cases of sexual dysfunction caused mainly by lack of education or need for permission to overcome fears or myths (Haeberle, 2010).

Education

Education is the hallmark of any treatment modality addressing FOD. Informing the patient and/or the partner about female sexual anatomy, physiology, and response as well as how orgasm can be climaxed via different stimulation techniques constitutes the first step of treatment (Kilmann et al., 1983).

Directed Masturbation and Sensate Focus

Directed masturbation is a behavioral technique involving self-awareness and exploration home exercises that are conducted in a progressive fashion (4 to 16 weekly therapy sessions) and aim to make the patient familiarize herself with her genitals and other erotic areas of her body. It has shown well-established efficacy when administered in a variety of modalities: group, individual, couples therapy, and bibliotherapy. Eventually, patients become more aware of sexually arousing stimuli and utilize self-knowledge to masturbate and reach orgasm (Heiman and LoPiccolo, 1988). It has been evaluated in clinical trials and was found to be effective in relieving the symptoms and distress associated with FOD (Andersen, 1981; Morokoff and LoPiccolo, 1986). The success rates for directed masturbation training in women with primary anorgasmia are usually high and show some variation depending on the type of orgasm-triggering stimulation: 60% to 90% with masturbation, and 33% to 85% with partnered sexual activity (Heiman, 2002). CBT can be combined with directed masturbation training in an effort to increase clinical efficacy. Riley and Riley (1978) demonstrated that the percentage of patients achieving the ability to orgasm was significantly higher in the group of patients who received CBT (sensate focus and supportive psychotherapy) plus directed masturbation when compared with those who were treated with conventional CBT only (90% vs. 53%).

Sensate focus consists of graded exposure from nonsexual to sexual touching to acquaint sexual pleasure with trust and effective communication between the couple. It can also be applied within the context of FOD. Similarly, it involves home exercises and active participation of the patient (Kingsberg et al., 2017). Directed masturbation training plus sensate focus was shown to be more effective than directed masturbation training alone (Heiman and Meston, 1997).

Mindfulness and Yoga

Mindfulness and yoga practice may be considered as possible adjuncts to directed masturbation and sensate focus. Herein, attentional focus is directed to "being in the moment without judgment." In their study that utilized the FSFI as the assessment tool, Dhikav et al. (2010) showed that younger women with sexual health–related issues improved maximally in terms of their quality of orgasm and satisfaction with 12 weeks of yoga.

Coital Alignment Technique

The coital alignment technique focuses on maximizing glans clitoris stimulation and aims to increase the frequency of the woman achieving orgasm simultaneously with her male partner during vaginal intercourse. Herein, the male partner is taught about ways to augment clitoral stimulation during the act of penetrative vaginal sexual intercourse (Eichel et al., 1988). In this coital position, the man positions his pelvis above the pubic bone of his partner. The woman stretches her legs and folds them around his. Penetration of the penis is less deep but the glans clitoris is more strongly stimulated with each thrust than with conventional intercourse. Clinical trials, which have included patients with primary anorgasmia, have shown that this technique was more effective than a waiting list control group and as effective as directed masturbation (Eichel et al., 1988; Hurlbert and Apt, 1995).

Sexual Enhancement Products

Modifying the type and intensity of physical and psychological sexual stimulation via sexual enhancement products can be an effective way of addressing FOD. Vibrators and sexually explicit media represent the most commonly utilized methods under this heading. These tools can also be used during directed masturbation sessions. A common concern about the use of vibrators is that the woman will be dependent on this type of stimulation to reach orgasm, and eventually avoid partnered sexual intercourse (Marcus, 2011). However, vibrator use has been associated with higher scores on sexual function domains. Additionally, a vibrator can be used during partnered penetrative sexual intercourse (Herbenick et al., 2010).

Medical Treatment

Medical treatment of FOD can be divided into two main categories: treatment of orgasmic disorder in the context of desire and arousal disorders and the treatment of orgasmic disorder in women without desire or arousal disorder.

Women With Female Orgasmic Disorder Together With Desire and Arousal Problems

When an improvement has been achieved in desire and arousal, this will translate into an enhancement in orgasmic function. Medications, which can be used in this context, act via increasing the intensity of the sexual stimulus and/or augmenting the sensitivity of the receptive areas to sexual stimuli. Alternatively, cholinergic activation and/or stimulation of the guanosine monophosphate pathway can be targeted to treat FOD in an indirect fashion. Furthermore, sexual enhancement products (vibrators, erotica) can be utilized in this subset of patients. Vibrators have been widely available in many countries through drug stores, websites, and erotica shops. However, there is only one FDA cleared-to-market device available to treat FSD (EROS Therapy device; UroMetrics, Inc, St Paul, MN). The EROS device is a small battery-powered handheld vacuum device applied gently and directly over the clitoris, causing the clitoris and labia to engorge with blood. Whereas vibrators do not require a prescription and come in a variety of prices, the Eros Therapy device does require a prescription. Billups et al. demonstrated that the EROS Therapy device was successful in terms of increasing the ability to reach orgasm in more than 50% of their patient cohort who had problems related with arousal and satisfaction (Billups et al., 2001).

Phosphodiesterase Type 5 Inhibitors

These drugs inhibit the enzyme (PDE5) responsible for the breakdown of cyclic guanosine monophosphate. The end result is increased blood flow to the vulva and vagina through smooth muscle relaxation and vasodilation. Caruso et al. (2003) demonstrated that sildenafil has a positive impact on arousal and orgasmic function in their randomized double-blind placebo-controlled study. Nurnberg et al. assessed the efficacy of sildenafil in treating antidepressant-associated FSD in a randomized controlled setting and reported beneficial effects of sildenafil on adverse side effects of SSRI use on orgasmic function (Nurnberg et al., 2008.)

Hormones

Systemic testosterone treatment (either alone or in combination with systemic/intravaginal estrogens) and tibolone (Nijland et al., 2008), (a synthetic steroid available in Europe that provides a mixture of estrogenic, progestonic, and androgenic actions), have a positive influence on all aspects of female sexual response (desire, arousal, and orgasm) in postmenopausal women with low testosterone/low estrogen levels. They achieve this therapeutic effect via CNS-related mechanisms (testosterone's excitatory effect on the limbic system) and changing the hormonal milieu of the vulvovaginal complex (Wierman et al., 2014). In their systematic review, which was conducted in 2014 and focused on testosterone treatment in HSDD, Reis et al. (2014) concluded that androgenic supplementation with transdermal testosterone (patch, gel) was effective in terms of increasing the level of sexual desire, the ability to experience orgasm, and eventually the degree of satisfaction.

Treatment with local or systemic estrogen also has positive effects for orgasmic dysfunction. Increased cellularity of the vaginal epithelium, augmented genital blood flow, and enhanced lubrication provide improvement in all four domains of FSD. Addressing dyspareunia and arousal problems with intravaginal estrogen might also have an indirect beneficial effect on orgasmic issues (Cappelletti and Wallen, 2016).

However, it should be noted that more research is warranted about the safety and efficacy of hormonal treatment in women with FOD as the primary complaint. The majority of available data originate from studies actually concentrating on other aspects of female sexual response and reporting indirect, secondary outcome about orgasmic function.

Women With Female Orgasmic Disorder Who Report Subjectively Sufficient Arousal

The goal of any medical treatment in this context would be to increase the arousal stimulation in intensity and frequency. Sexual enhancement products (vibrators, erotica) can also be used for this purpose.

Oxytocin

Oxytocin can be used on-demand in patients with intact arousal but orgasmic failure. It is a short-acting drug and exerts its effect via working synergistically with sex hormones to facilitate muscle contractions during orgasm. Oxytocin, which can be considered as a facilitator of arousal and orgasm, is normally secreted into the bloodstream from the paraventricular nucleus of the hypothalamus during arousal and orgasm (Magon et al., 2011).

Medication-Induced Female Orgasmic Disorder

SSRIs, which represent the cornerstone of pharmacotherapy for depression, have the potential to adversely affect various aspects of the female sexual response cycle, including desire, arousal, and/or orgasm, with estimates of 30% to 70% of patients on SSRIs reporting some degree of sexual dysfunction (Serretti and Chiesa, 2009). First, it is important to investigate the onset of a patient's sexual dysfunction. Depression itself may lead to sexual dysfunction, and treatment with an SSRI may actually be helpful, although this may take weeks of therapy. On the other hand, if sexual side effects are detected, it is recommended to wait for tolerance to develop, provided that the SSRI is successfully treating the depressive symptoms (Laan et al., 2013). Tolerance usually occurs within 14 to 120 days. After the development of tolerance, some patients will experience spontaneous resolution or marked improvement in their orgasmic complaints, and others will keep having distressing orgasmic delays or failures (Haberfellner and Rittmannsberger, 2004). Regarding the women who have persistent orgasmic dysfunction beyond 3 to 6 months, additional approaches such as reducing the dose of SSRI or switching to another antidepressant medication can be considered. Switching to medications with positive noradrenergic effects, such as serotonin-norepinephrine reuptake inhibitors, or to medications such as buproprion or mirtazapine may reduce sexual side effects (Serretti et al., 2009).

> **KEY POINTS: FEMALE ORGASMIC DISORDER**
>
> - Medical conditions, pharmacologic interventions, and psychosocial issues, which might cause orgasmic difficulties, should be ruled out before arriving at the diagnosis of FOD.
> - A comprehensive sexual history (involving details about the nature and onset of the problem) is essential to diagnose and characterize FOD.
> - FOD often accompanies problems with interest and arousal.
> - Education (about sexual anatomy, physiology, and wellness) is the hallmark of any treatment modality addressing FOD.
> - Directed masturbation and sensate focus, coital alignment, and mindfulness techniques represent the psychosocial treatment options for FOD.
> - More research is warranted about the safety and efficacy of hormonal treatment in women with FOD.

FEMALE SEXUAL AROUSAL DISORDER

In 2017, the ICSM Committee focused on the distressing complaints of hypoactive sexual desire, impaired arousal, and orgasmic problems (Kingsberg et al., 2017). The Committee chose to use the *DSM-IV-TR* (APA, 2000) classifications of female sexual disorders (FSD) instead of those from the *DSM-5* (APA, 2013). This is consistent with the recommendations of the ICSM Committee on Definitions (McCabe et al., 2016) and a recent article on nomenclature by the ISSWSH (Parish et al., 2016). The Committee suggested that separating desire and arousal allows an easier way to characterize the assessment and treatment of each dysfunction, rather than combining them as seen in the new and controversial diagnosis of FSIAD (APA, 2013). We will follow this approach and acknowledge that there is often significant overlap and comorbidity among all *DSM-IV-TR* diagnoses. However, treatment is typically focused on the primary disorder identified by the woman.

The ICSM definition for FSAD is *a persistent or recurrent inability to attain or maintain arousal until completion of the sexual activity, an adequate subjective assessment of her genital response (clinical principle)* (McCabe et al., 2016). As mentioned earlier, FSAD was merged with HSDD in the *DSM-5* (APA, 2013) and is now known as FSIAD (Sungur et al., 2014). On one hand, neither version of the *DSM* categories and their criteria appears to fully correspond with women's subjective experience; on the other hand, experts in the field have not reached a consensus on FSIAD (Kingsberg et al., 2017).

Female sexual arousal has been described since the 1970s. This is a debated topic given the lack of concordance between subjective sexual arousal and genital arousal. A woman's perception about her genital responses is defined as subjective sexual arousal, whereas genital arousal refers to the physiologic activation such as vaginal lubrication and vasocongestion. Lack of concordance leads to a weak relation between subjective and objective sexual responses (Kingsberg et al., 2017). Recent strategies focused on the external genitalia (and, to a lesser extent, on the central processing of sex stimuli) have suggested that the various components composing female sexual arousal might be processed differently in women's appraisal of sexual arousal.

Interview Assessment of Sexual Arousal

Understanding of a woman's subjective experience is crucial in identifying a problem with sexual arousal. During the initial assessment, a semistructured interview could be helpful to define the patient's concepts of sexual arousal, including erotic mental images, emotions of sexual excitement, pleasurable genital sensations, and noticing physical changes such as vaginal lubrication. Table 74.17 presents examples of helpful questions as suggested by the Female Sexual Dysfunction—Medical and Psychological Treatments Committee (Kingsberg et al., 2017).

Potential Treatments for the Psychosocial Aspects of Female Sexual Arousal Disorder

Following the ICSM Committee (Kingsberg et al., 2017), a careful clinical evaluation is mandatory to create a proper treatment plan for a woman with difficulty getting or staying subjectively aroused during sexual situations. Investigation of the cause should focus on at least one of the following factors:

1. Are cultural or religious factors causing sex guilt and inhibition?
2. Is the problem with arousal specific to the partner and associated with problems in a dyadic relationship?
3. Does the woman have many distracting cognitions during sex, and what kinds of thoughts interfere (insecurity about attractiveness or ability to please the partner sexually, memories of past sexual trauma, or other issues)?
4. Is the woman under high levels of stress, and/or does she have poor stress management skills?
5. Does the woman tend to focus on negative affect that might be related to her genetic disposition or her developmental attachment issues?
6. If the woman is older than 40 years of age, does she lack a sexual partner or have a partner whose ill health or erectile dysfunction limits sexual activity and pleasure?

Women's sexuality could be affected by cultural or religious concerns. However, there is no treatment to lessen women's guilt and negative views of sexuality. Christensen et al. described how using online role-playing games may be helpful in identifying a potential role of a member of the clergy or of a local community leader having a moderate stance on sexual pleasure who might be more effective in decreasing guilt than a mental health professional from outside the community (Christensen et al., 2013).

Incorporating mindfulness training into sex CBT approaches (Brotto and Basson, 2014; Brotto et al., 2008a) may improve attention during sex. Learning to focus on pleasurable sensations while avoiding distractions by negative thoughts and feelings during sex can improve satisfaction. Indeed, asking each partner to focus on his or her own bodily sensations while noticing any negative thoughts and refocusing attention on physical feelings could be viewed as training mindfulness.

Mindfulness meditation can help women in stress management, although data are scarce. Improved nutrition and exercise, if applicable, also may have a positive influence on women's sexual function because of enhanced well-being, increased feelings of attractiveness, and decreased distraction from negative thoughts about body image during sex. Depression or anxiety disorders have often been regarded as poor prognostic factors for sex therapy. Although studies on this topic are scarce, treating attachment and mood disorders may play a role in FSAD.

PHARMACOTHERAPY FOR FEMALE SEXUAL AROUSAL DISORDER

Hormonal Therapy

Testosterone and Selective Tissue Estrogenic Activity Regulator

In 2012, Davis et al. demonstrated that transdermal testosterone patch therapy can improve sexual desire and arousal (level of evidence 1) (Davis et al., 2012; Kingsberg et al., 2017). These results were aligned with the study performed by Tuiten et al. (2000) that demonstrated an enhanced genital arousal in hypogonadotropic hypogonadal women after a treatment with testosterone undecanoate

---

TABLE 74.17 Examples of Helpful Questions as Suggested by the Female Sexual Dysfunction–Medical and Psychological Treatments Committee

How often do you notice yourself feeling sexually excited?
What situations help you feel excited (e.g., seeing an attractive person, engaging in sexual caressing, viewing erotic images, or reading an erotic story)? It might be useful to note that Ogi Ogas and Sari Gadam analyzed Internet usage of men and women. In their book, *A Billion Wicked Thoughts: What the Internet Tells Us About Sexual Relationships* (New York, NY: Dutton, Penguin Group; 2011), they described a gender difference. Women are more easily aroused by narrative stories, whereas men look for visual images.
Do you sometimes have sexual fantasies?
Is there a particular type of scenario in a fantasy or story that arouses you?
How easy is it to get aroused with your current sexual partner? (Partner-specific problems can signal relationship issues rather than a generalized sexual problem.)
What sensations do you notice in your genital area when you feel excited (e.g., warmth, tingling, pleasure, increased wetness)?
Do you ever have erotic dreams?
Do you believe that your sexual excitement is healthy? (Guilt about sex can inhibit arousal. Some women, raised in a culture with a strong double standard restricting female sexuality, might rarely or never have felt sexually aroused [Laan et al., 1994]. Women who had a sexually traumatic experience in childhood also might have difficulty feeling sexual excitement [Wylie et al., 2006]).
If you used to get aroused more easily, what do you think is interfering now?

Modified from Kingsberg SA, Althof S, Simon JA, et al. Female Sexual Dysfunction—Medical And Psychological Treatments, Committee 14. *J Sex Med* 2017;14(12):1463–1491.

40 mg/day orally during an 8-week period. Testosterone seems to act independently from the estrogens (Pessina et al., 2006) and has a direct effect on the vagina and genital structures.

Tibolone is a selective tissue estrogenic activity regulator and acts differently in multiple organs because of the dissimilar steroid properties of its metabolites (Nappi and Cucinella, 2015). It has been used in postmenopausal women and it enhanced mood and libido, but further research is needed (Biglia et al., 2010; Davis, 2002).

Nonhormonal Therapy

Phosphodiesterase Type 5 Inhibitors

The use of vasoactive drugs such as PDE5Is in women is based on the notion that an increase in blood flow to the clitoris and vagina might improve sexual function like that seen in men with erectile dysfunction (Chivers and Rosen, 2010). The data for PDE5Is from clinical randomized controlled trials for FSAD have been reviewed and found to be contradictory and ultimately lacking in efficacy (Nappi and Cucinella, 2015; Chivers and Rosen, 2010).

In 2004, Pfizer (New York, NY) ended its program of testing sildenafil in women, perhaps resulting from the conflicting findings in medically healthy women (Major, 2004). However, data suggest a potential therapeutic role for these vasoactive agents in well-established medical conditions interfering with genital neurovascular substrates such as type 1 diabetes, SCI, multiple sclerosis, and FSAD secondary to SSRI use (level of evidence 2) (Kingsberg et al., 2017).

Prostaglandins

Topical alprostadil (prostaglandin E_1) is a vasodilatory agent that acts on smooth muscle relaxation. Indeed, prostaglandins enhancing the activity of sensory afferent nerves, improve sensation. Kielbasa and Daniel did not identify consistent or reproducible results of beneficial effects (Kielbasa and Daniel, 2006).

L-Arginine

L-arginine is the nitric oxide precursor. Its combination with yohimbine, an adrenergic antagonist, in women with FSAD could significantly increase physiologic measures of sexual arousal (vaginal photoplethysmography) but had no effect on subjective measures of arousal or affect (Meston and Worcel, 2002).

Dopamine Agonists

Dopaminergic drugs have a direct effect on the brain and therefore could have a positive influence on sexual arousal and desire. Apomorphine is a nonselective dopamine agonist that acts on D_1 and D_2 receptors. Caruso et al. (2004) reported significant improvement of sexual function in a group of premenopausal women with FSAD after sublingual apomorphine. Furthermore, Bechara et al. (2004) showed that the use of apomorphine before and after vibrator use significantly improved arousal and lubrication but did not improve orgasm.

Bupropion

Bupropion is an antidepressant with dopamine and norepinephrine reuptake inhibition; it has no serotonergic effect and has been shown to have prosexual effects, with improvement in all domains of sexual dysfunction compared with placebo (Levin, 2014; Segraves et al., 2004).

In a Cochrane Database Systematic Review of management of SSRI-induced sexual dysfunction, five high-quality randomized trials, including 579 participants, found improvement in sexual rating scores with the use of bupropion 150 mg twice daily (level of evidence 2) (Kingsberg et al., 2017; Taylor et al., 2013).

Oxytocin

Oxytocin is a neuropeptide involved in parturition and lactation, but it seems to have a potential role as an agent of arousal and orgasm.

TABLE 74.18 Leiblum and Nathan Criteria for Female Persistent Genital Arousal Disorder in Women

Physiologic sexual arousal (genital and breast vasocongestion and sensitivity) persists for an extended period (from hours to days) and does not remit on its own.
The signs of physiologic sexual arousal do not remit with ordinary orgasmic experience.
The signs of physiologic sexual arousal are experienced in the absence of subjective feelings of sexual desire and arousal.
The symptoms of sexual arousal can be triggered by sexual-related stimulus but also by nonsexual cues or no stimulus at all.
These symptoms are perceived as intrusive and unwanted, leading at least to some degree of distress.

Behavioral studies have demonstrated that it might be responsible for prosocial behaviors in humans such as positive physical contact and communication methods with a partner (Grewen et al., 2005).

Female Persistent Genital Arousal Disorder

The ICSM definition for female persistent genital arousal disorder (FPGAD) is a spontaneous, intrusive, and unwanted genital arousal (i.e., tingling, throbbing, pulsating) in the absence of sexual interest and desire. Any awareness of subjective arousal is typically, but not invariably, unpleasant. The arousal is unrelieved by at least one orgasm, and the feeling of arousal persists for hours or days (McCabe et al., 2016) In 2001, Leiblum and Nathan defined this syndrome according to the following criteria reported in Table 74.18.

PGAD must be distinguished from hypersexuality (Kafka, 2010) (a symptomatic cluster characterized by out-of-control sexual thoughts and behaviors, accompanied by subjective feelings of sexual desire) and clitoral priapism (engorgement of the clitoris that is experienced with significant pain) (Goldmeier et al., 2009).

Psychosocial Characterization and Etiologic Factors

Characterization of women with PGAD is complicated, and evidence is limited (Kingsberg et al., 2017). Psychologically, women with PGAD present a negative appraisal of genital sensations (Leiblum and Seehuus, 2009) and are more likely to be depressed and to have panic attacks, or to present a history of sexual victimization (Leiblum et al., 2007). Furthermore, patients with PGAD seem to be associated with a sexually conservative thinking style accompanied by a maladaptive cognitive and emotional functioning during sexual activity (Carvalho et al., 2013). Scores on the FSFI showed that women with PGAD are not sexually dysfunctional but lack a satisfactory sexual life (Leiblum and Seehuus, 2009).

Data on the etiology of PGAD are poor. Studies on the biologic underpinnings of PGAD underline the role of physical defects such as the presence of a periclitoral mass (Bedell et al. 2014), pelvic varices (Thorne and Stuckey, 2008), or Tarlov cysts (Komisaruk and Lee, 2012). Use of venlafaxine or the discontinuation of an SSRI (Leiblum and Goldmeier, 2008; Mahoney and Zarate, 2007) could be involved in the PGAD etiology.

Biologic versus psychological factors may lead to different subsets of cases and variants. However, the exact proportion in which this happens is unknown.

Treatment Targets

Improvement of PGAD symptoms has been described in case series with duloxetine (Philippsohn et al., 2012), pregabalin, and varenicline. Electroconvulsive therapy also has been successfully applied (Korda et al., 2009) and reported in some small studies. CBT targeting anxiety management, response prevention, and dyadic issues has been shown to improve sexual and emotional symptoms (Hiller and Hekster, 2007).

> **KEY POINTS: FEMALE SEXUAL AROUSAL DISORDER**
>
> - FSAD is a persistent or recurrent inability to attain or maintain arousal until completion of the sexual activity.
> - In the *DSM-5*, FSAD is merged with HSDD and is called *female sexual interest/arousal disorder (FSIAD)*.
> - Defining the patient's concepts of sexual arousal should be the first step while assessing FSAD.
> - Testosterone therapy, which has a direct effect on genital structures, can improve sexual desire and arousal.
> - Treatment with PDE5Is can be considered in patients whose arousal disorder is associated with medical conditions interfering with genital neurovascular supply.
> - Leiblum criteria should be used while defining FPGAD.

GENITOPELVIC PAIN AND PENETRATION DISORDER

Pain and Sex

Sexual pain is common and can have many repercussions for women and their partners. Vaginal and vulvar pain is a commonly neglected health problem in women. These conditions are frequently ignored by health care providers, poorly understood, and often mismanaged. Pain during sexual intercourse might originate from any dysfunction of the vulva, vagina, cervix, uterus, adnexa, PFMs, and the nerves that innervate these structures. The following list provides descriptions of the common genitopelvic pain and penetration disorders.

- **Dyspareunia:** pain during intercourse
- **Vaginismus:** involuntary contraction of the musculature of the vagina that interferes with intercourse
- **Vulvodynia:** vulvar discomfort, described as burning pain, occurring in the absence of relevant visible findings (Moyal-Barracco and Lynch, 2004)
- **Localized vulvodynia:** pain localized in a particular part of the vulva (e.g., vestibule, vaginal entrance)
- **Generalized vulvodynia:** pain affecting the entire vulvar region
- **Provoked vulvodynia:** pain triggered by an external stimulation
- **Unprovoked vulvodynia:** spontaneous pain, unrelated to any specific stimulation

The most common type of vulvodynia is localized to the vestibulum and is related to sexual intercourse. This type of provoked vulvodynia leads to dyspareunia (painful intercourse). According to the International Society for the Study of Vulvovaginal Disease (ISSVD) terminology classification, this common subtype of vulvodynia is called *provoked vestibulodynia (PVD)*. It is estimated that 12% of women in the general population are affected by this condition (Goldstein et al., 2009). PVD is frequently associated with other pain syndromes. Frequently documented comorbidities are irritable bowel syndrome (IBS) and fibromyalgia (Arnold et al., 2006).

Provoked Vestibulodynia

Primary

Primary PVD is pain experienced since the first attempt of any type of vaginal penetration (e.g., tampons or sexual activity). This condition has an early onset, the duration of the pain is longer, and the women are less likely to have had children. These patients also have a positive family history of the same condition. Frequently there is also an association with enuresis and dysmenorrhea (Bornstein et al., 2001). The presence of local signs of inflammation is less common.

Secondary

Secondary PVD is pain experienced after a certain period pertaining to vaginal penetrative activities that previously were pain free. This condition is typically acquired and has a late onset. Larger areas of vestibule are involved in the pain process. The clitoral hood is the area with the most severe pain (Bornstein et al., 2001). Secondary PVD appears to be more frequent than primary PVD (65% vs. 35%) (Nguyen et al., 2015), and primary PVD appears to be more frequent in Hispanic women (Bornstein et al., 2001).

Pathogenesis

The cause of PVD is multifactorial in nature and not completely understood. Vaginal secretions seem to play an important role in at least some of these conditions (Jayaram et al., 2015). According to some studies, it appears that human epididymis protein 4 (HE-4) and secretory leukocyte protease inhibitor (SLPI) are reduced in women with PVD compared with control women (Jayaram et al., 2015). Further, the subgroup of patients who experienced constant vulvar pain had markedly lower levels of HE-4 and SLPI compared with the subgroup who experienced pain only during sexual intercourse. These findings play an important role in our understanding of the protease-activated receptor 2 (PAR-2) pathway's influence on pain sensitization in women with PVD. The same pathway is also known to be activated in pain sensitization in cancer patients. Specifically, unopposed protease activity, which can result in decreased ability to inhibit PAR-2 activation, coupled with nerve fiber density changes at the level of the vulvar vestibule may be explanatory for the pain sensitization occurring in women with PVD.

An important difference between primary and secondary PVD is in the nerve fiber density and the presence of inflammation. Primary PVD patients appeared to have greater nerve fiber density and a thicker vulvar vestibule compared with the secondary group. Thus, this subgroup of patients presents with a greater peripheral and central involvement. One potential explanation for the increased nongenital sensitivity found in women with PVD in general, and in women with primary PVD in particular, could be that women with primary PVD are genetically predisposed to factors that contribute to an increased generalized pain response (Lam and Schmidt, 2010).

Additionally, **hypertonicity of PFMs appears to be highly prevalent in patients with PVD** (Morin et al., 2014; Pukall et al., 2016). Pelvic muscle dysfunction in patients with PVD can present with decreased muscular strength and reduced speed of contraction, coordination, and endurance.

Brain activity is also associated with recurrent and chronic pain. Pain is multidimensional involving physical sensations, thoughts, and emotions. Brain regions thought to influence the motivational aspects of pain include the anterior cingulate gyrus (ACC), an area that provides an interface between emotions and rational cognitions. The anterior insula, an area involved in many conscious behaviors, is also involved in the motivational aspects of pain. Somatosensory areas (SI, SII) and the posterior insula process pain's sensory components. The prefrontal cortex (PFC) and amygdala, both involved in processing affect and negative emotions, process the emotional aspects of pain. Specific areas in the brainstem, the periaqueductal gray (PAG), and the medulla are thought to integrate descending signals from the brain to the dorsal horn cells of the spinal cord (Tracey and Mantyh, 2007).

Patients with PVD might develop changes of **central sensitization** in the CNS (Foster et al., 2005). This phenomenon is characterized by higher excitability of the central nociceptive circuits in a number of chronic pain syndromes and could maintain chronicity or even be the main etiologic factor.

Clitoris and Clitorodynia

One possible presenting sign of vestibulodynia might originate from the clitoris (Lam and Schmidt, 2010). Clitoral pain is greatly underdiagnosed and undertreated (Parada et al., 2015). Many health care providers completely neglect the physical examination of the clitoris. In gynecology training programs, physical examination of the clitoris is uncommon and not routinely taught. Interestingly, urology residency programs routinely teach physical examination of the male genitalia, specifically the penis and foreskin, but the examination of the clitoris is totally neglected. The foreskin and clitoral hood have basically the same function and very similar pathologic changes. Clitoral adhesions can reduce an adequate drainage of keratinaceous desquamation. Smegma and squamous

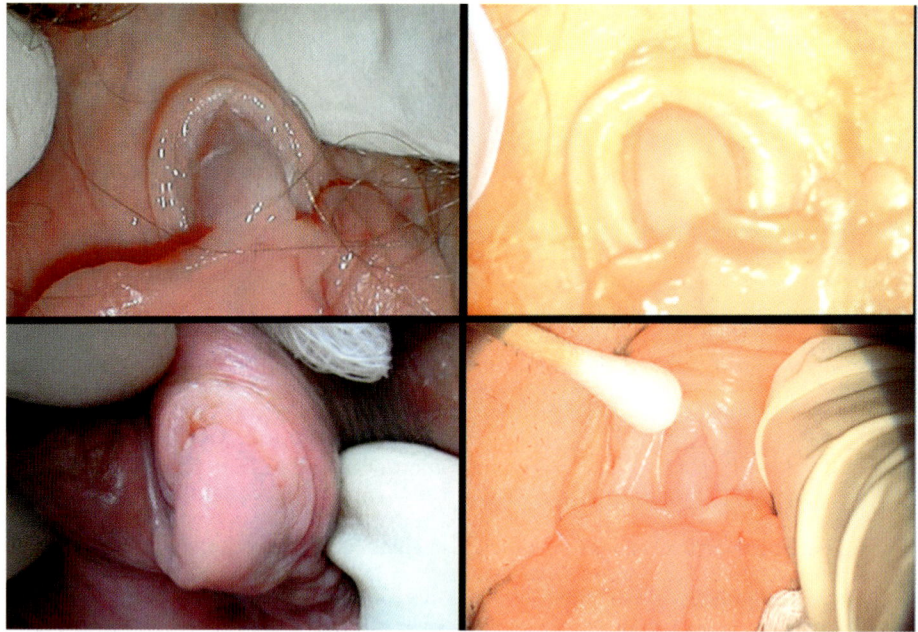

Fig. 74.10. Absent clitoral glans adhesions when the prepuce was retracted to the balanopreputial sulcus and full visualization of the corona. (Aerts L, Rubin RS, Randazzo M, et al. Retrospective study of the prevalence and risk factors of clitoral adhesions: women's health providers should routinely examine the glans clitoris. *Sex Med* 2018;6[2]:115–122.)

cells can accumulate underneath the prepuce, resulting in smegmatic pseudocysts and/or keratin pearls with a subsequent irritation. Erythematous changes and infection of the clitoris is a common cause of pain known as *clitorodynia*. Besides pain, clitoral adhesions could represent a risk factor associated with yeast infection, urinary tract infection, genital trauma, and lichen sclerosus. According to Aerts, of 1265 patients examined in their clinic who underwent a vulvoscopy, 23% presented with some degree of clitoral adhesions (Aerts et al., 2018).

Clinical Presentation (Fig. 74.10)

Menopause and Dyspareunia

Menopause induces changes in vaginal epithelium and is commonly associated with atrophy. Between 10% and 40% of postmenopausal women experience discomfort caused by vulvovaginal atrophy that requires treatment, and approximately 40% of women with vaginal atrophy report dyspareunia (North American Menopause Society [NAMS], 2013).

Sexual activity in menopausal women is not insignificant. A literature review showed that 22% of married women 70 to 79 years of age report that they still have sexual intercourse (Schneidewind-Skibbe et al., 2008).

Vaginal atrophy may present with some or all symptoms of: dryness, burning and sexual symptoms of lack of lubrication, discomfort or pain, and impaired function. Urinary symptoms of urgency, dysuria, and recurrent urinary tract infections can also be observed. According to current terminology, this condition should be referred as genitourinary syndrome of menopause (GSM) (Portman and Gass, 2014).

Murina et al. (2016) stated that many menopausal women with complaints of dyspareunia have vestibular tenderness with more pronounced atrophic changes in this region rather than in the vagina.

Previous Genitourinary Surgery

The use of synthetic mesh in POP surgery is being closely scrutinized because of serious concerns regarding life-changing complications such as erosion, pain, infection, bleeding, dyspareunia, organ perforation, and urinary problems (de Mattos Lourenco et al., 2019). **Mesh complications can occur several years after the procedure** (Arsene et al., 2015). **Most randomized trials evaluating POP surgery using synthetic mesh failed to report on clinically important outcomes and to evaluate medium- and long-term efficacy and safety.**

The sexually active women in the study were relatively satisfied. Interestingly, it was observed that women with a mesh complication, although not statistically significant, appeared to be more satisfied with their sex life. A possible explanation might be that after recovery of a complication, the mere fact of being able to have sexual intercourse again or the absence of pain might be a big relief. Women with a mesh complication were more frequently sexually active. An explanation may be that more sexual activity increases the risk for exposure, as friction is a risk factor for exposure. Further research is needed to investigate whether this observation is a real phenomenon or related to low numbers.

According to a cross-sectional study of 128 women who had vaginal mesh surgery, the sexually active women were relatively more satisfied with their sex life despite mesh-related complications compared with the group of non–sexually active patients (Kowalik et al., 2019). Also, women with a mesh complication were more frequently sexually active. The authors are hypothesizing that more sexual activity increases the risk for exposure, as friction is a risk factor for exposure.

Energy-based devices using radiofrequency and laser technologies have gained popularity as therapies for vaginal atrophy, UI, and vaginal prolapse. The technology is used by both medical and surgical specialties including dermatology, plastic surgery, gynecology, and genitourinary specialties. More recently, **cosmetic or "rejuvenating" nonsurgical procedures** using these same radiofrequency and laser technologies are growing in popularity. Vaginal "rejuvenation" is a descriptive nonscientific term used by the medical device and cosmetic industries for nonsurgical vaginal cosmetic procedures or therapies. It is used to treat symptoms related to menopause or UI, or to improve sexual function (FDA, 2018). Complications such as vaginal burns, scarring, dryness, infection, altered sensation, dyspareunia, adhesions, scarring, recurrent pain, or vaginal stenosis may occur over time. These could cause sexual dysfunction or worsening QoL as a result of radiofrequency and laser vaginal procedures for vaginal rejuvenation (ACOG, 2007).

In July 2018, the FDA issued a public notification regarding significant risks related to devices marketed for use in medical procedures for vaginal rejuvenation. There is a growing number of manufacturers marketing vaginal rejuvenation devices to women and claiming these procedures will treat conditions and symptoms related to menopause, UI, or sexual function. The procedures use lasers and other energy-based devices to destroy or reshape vaginal tissue. These products have serious risks and do not have adequate evidence to support their use for these purposes. Additionally, these procedures are also being marketed for cancer patients who experience an early menopause, eluding the possibility of treating this condition. According to the FDA, this is a dangerous procedure and without a proven benefit in a vulnerable population.

Laser vaginal rejuvenation can produce vaginal burns, scarring, dyspareunia, and CPP. These procedures may be particularly appealing to women who are not candidates for conventional FDA-approved treatments to relieve vaginal dryness and are thus seeking alternative nonhormonal options. Women considering treatment for vaginal symptoms should speak to their doctor about the potential and known benefits and risks of all available treatment options.

Treatment

Education

Discussions with patients related to vulvar hygiene habits, avoidance of irritants, behavior modification, stress-decreasing techniques, and education about sexual function and pain pathophysiology appear to have a relevant role. According to Fowler (2000), an emphasis on the patient's education resulted in a positive response in 21% of patients with PVD and an improvement in pain scores in 56% of the study cohort after 6 to 36 months of treatment.

Biofeedback

PVD has been shown to present heightened PFM tone, which encompasses an active (contractile) component and a passive (viscoelastic) component. The assistance of visual feedback of muscle activity is particularly relevant in women with pain because more than 50% of women without symptoms have difficulty achieving an adequate PFM contraction with only verbal instructions. Glazer et al. were first to develop an electromyographic (EMG) biofeedback protocol for women with vulvar pain and showed that 52% of the sample reported pain-free sexual intercourse after 16 weeks of treatment in a prospective study (Bo et al., 1990).

Dilators and Insertion Techniques

The use of vaginal dilators can help women with dyspareunia to control their fear of pain and promote pelvic floor relaxation during insertion (Idama and Pring, 2000). Little is known about treatment duration and the possible benefit of using dilators in conjunction with other treatments.

Electrical Stimulation

Electrical stimulation is a therapeutic modality widely used in physical therapy and pain management. The stimulation improves muscle proprioception, local blood circulation, and decreases nociceptive signal flows. Additionally, there is an increase in secretion of endorphins. Two prospective studies showed a significant improvement in dyspareunia and sexual function in women with PVD after domiciliary electrical stimulation and in-clinic electrical stimulation combined with home PFM exercises (Nappi et al., 2003; Vallinga et al., 2015).

Manual Therapy

Manual therapy is typically considered the cornerstone of physical therapy. This consists of stretching, massage, and myofascial techniques (Rosenbaum et al, 2008). The aim of this therapy is to facilitate muscle relaxation, release tensions and trigger points, improve blood circulation and mobility in the pelvic-perineal region, adjust postural imbalances, and increase the vaginal opening and desensitize the area.

Multimodal Physical Therapy

Multimodal interventions represent current practice in physical therapy in women with PVD and consist of a combination of manual therapy, stretching, PFM control exercises with or without biofeedback, and education (Hartmann et al., 2007).

Topical Therapy

According to the NAMS, nonhormonal lubricants and moisturizers in combination with regular sexual activity should be considered first-line therapies, but women often find these products inadequate (NAMS, 2013). Estrogen is known to affect inflammatory neuropeptides involved in chronic pain, in which the lack of estrogen is associated with an increased density of sympathetic, parasympathetic, and sensory nerve fibers in the vulva. Acute or chronic estrogen administration may decrease the total and sympathetic fiber numbers. Topical therapy is more effective than systemic therapy in reducing the density of vaginal autonomic and sensory nerve fibers (Griebling et al., 2012). Apparently, estrogen replacement targeted to the vestibule appears to be more effective in reducing the sensitivity compared with vaginal application (Murina et al., 2016).

Surgery

Vestibulectomy is a surgical procedure that can be used to treat PVD and specifically in case of vestibulodynia. According to Goetsch (2007), 79% of participants who underwent vestibulectomy had a significant decrease of pain compared with only 48% for those who received nonsurgical treatments and 12% who did not receive any treatment (eFig. 74.11).

Multidisciplinary and Multimodality Approaches

Because of the multifactorial nature of PVD, multidisciplinary and multimodality approaches have been increasingly proposed to deal with chronic vulvar pain conditions (Goldstein et al., 2016). Thus, a combined approach would better address all factors contributing to the pain and associated psychosexual and relational difficulties and provide greater benefit to patients.

> **KEY POINTS: GENITOPELVIC PAIN AND PENETRATION DISORDER**
>
> - Pain during sexual intercourse can originate from any dysfunction of internal/external genital organs, PFMs, or the nerves that innervate these structures.
> - Approximately 10% of the women are affected by PVD, which is frequently associated with other pain syndromes such as irritable bowel syndrome and fibromyalgia.
> - Postmenopausal atrophic changes in the vagina lead to dyspareunia.
> - Biofeedback can be utilized to treat vulvodynia, especially in patients with hypertonic pelvic floor overactivity.
> - Multimodal physical therapy, which consists of manual therapy, stretching, pelvic floor exercises, biofeedback, and education, represents the mainstay treatment in women with PVD.
> - Optimal treatment of chronic vulvar pain conditions requires the integrated effort of various medical/surgical disciplines.

LOWER URINARY TRACT DYSFUNCTION AND FEMALE SEXUAL DYSFUNCTION

LUTS are the subjective indicator of a disease or change in condition as perceived by the patient, caretaker, or partner and may lead him or her to seek help from health care professionals (Abrams et al., 2002).

In 2017, the International Consultation on Incontinence-Research Society (ICI-RS), a multidisciplinary group of health care professionals, took part in a think tank questioning on how LUTS affect sexual function in men and women (Apostolidis et al., 2017; Rantell et al., 2017). Following this think tank, we will discuss the effect of LUTS on sexual dysfunction in the female population. In 2012, the 5th International Consultation on Incontinence estimated that, of the world's population, 46% of adults (older than 20 years of age) experience LUTS, 11.8% complain of OAB symptoms, 8% suffer from some type of urinary incontinence (UI), and 4% are estimated to have severe stress urinary incontinence (SUI) (Abrams et al., 2013).

Sexual Lifestyle and Communication

Sexual health is a state of physical, emotional, mental, and social well-being in relation to sexuality; it is not merely the absence of disease, dysfunction, or infirmity (WHO, 2006). Over the past 30 years, three National Surveys of Sexual Attitudes and Lifestyles demonstrated that sexual lifestyles and practices have significantly changed (Mercer et al., 2013). In women, age is related to a reduction in sexual frequency and range of practices. Furthermore, certain sexual behaviors and lifestyles have become increasingly more common, such as sexual experience with a same-sex partner and having anal sex (Table 74.19).

Communication about sexual function and LUTS has always been problematic (Rantel et al., 2017). Relief rather than embarrassment is achieved after health care professionals inquire (Penson et al., 2000). An American obstetrician and gynecologist survey reported that 63% of clinicians ask if the patient is sexually active, but only 40% routinely inquire about sexual problems (Sobecki et al., 2012). Indeed, women seem to prefer to discuss sexual problems with a nurse rather than with a physician (Farrell and Belza, 2012). Dyer and das Nair (2013) reported several common themes on why health care professionals do not talk about sex: "opens a can of worms," lack of time/resources/training, concern about knowledge and ability, worry that it will cause offense, personal discomfort, lack of awareness about sexual issues, and opposite gender/race/age concerns.

Epidemiology

Following the 2017 International Urogynecological Association (IUGA) and International Continence Society (ICS) Joint Report, it is reported that more than 40% of women will experience a sexual problem over the course of their lifetime (Rogers et al., 2018). A sexual complaint could lead to personal distress or interpersonal difficulties reaching a level of a diagnosable sexual disorder. Recent epidemiologic surveys place the prevalence of diagnosable sexual disorders at approximately 8% to 12% (Shifren et al., 2008).

The effects of pelvic floor disorders (PFDs) including UI and POP on sexual function remain debatable (Fashokun et al., 2013; Handa et al., 2008; Rogers, 2013). This variability can be attributed partly to the heterogeneity of the populations studied and the methodology and type of questionnaires used, and can also be attributed partly to the complexity of human sexual function, which is subject to a host of influences. Despite conflicting published data, **in general most PFDs are thought to negatively affect sexual health. Handa et al. (2008) showed that dyspareunia, low sexual arousal, and infrequent orgasm are associated with pelvic floor symptoms. Up to 45% of the women with UI and/or LUTS complain of sexual dysfunction, with 34% reporting hypoactive sexual desire, 23% reporting sexual arousal disorder, 11% reporting orgasmic deficiency, and 44% reporting sexual pain disorders (dyspareunia or noncoital genital pain)** (Salonia et al., 2004). Lowenstein et al. reported that sexual function is related to women's self-perceived body image and degree of bother from POP, especially in women with stage 2 or greater POP (Jelovsek and Barber, 2006; Lowenstein et al., 2009a; Zielinski et al., 2012) and particularly in the domains of sexual desire and satisfaction. CPP may cause dyspareunia in 16% to 25% of women, often leading to sexual avoidance (Kingsberg and Knudson, 2011). In women with PFDs, there is a positive association between pelvic floor strength and sexual activity and function (Kanter et al., 2015), highlighting that high PFM tone and sexual dysfunction are related (Bortolami et al., 2015). Resolution of symptoms after successful treatment of PFDs often improves sexual function and/or women's well-being as measured on pelvic floor condition specific measures.

Etiology and Classification

Multiple systemic aspects such as endocrine, neurologic, cardiovascular, dermatologic, and psychiatric disorders; surgical and medical complications; and cancer may lead to central and peripheral changes in cell-to-cell communication, changes in endocrine milieu, disruption in the homeostasis of neurotransmitters and signal molecules, tissue damage, organ damage, vascular changes, and neurologic changes that predispose to FSD (Rantell et al., 2017). The IUGA/ICS 2017 Joint Report disclosed a list of symptoms either volunteered by or elicited from the individual, or described by the individual's caregiver (Haylen et al., 2010). Sexual symptoms may occur in combination with other pelvic floor symptoms such as UI or POP or with pelvic pain. We will discuss the FSD symptoms related with LUTS, POP, and pain.

Lower urinary tract sexual dysfunction symptoms:
1. Coital UI: UI occurring during or after vaginal intercourse
2. Orgasmic UI: UI at orgasm
3. Penetration UI: UI at penetration (penile, manual, or sexual device)
4. Coital urinary urgency: feeling of urgency to void during vaginal intercourse
5. Postcoital LUTS: worsened urinary frequency or urgency, dysuria, suprapubic tenderness
6. Receptive urethral intercourse: having a penis penetrating one's urethra (urethral coitus)

Prolapse-specific symptoms:
1. Abstinence as a result of POP: nonengagement in sexual activity resulting from prolapse or associated symptoms
2. Vaginal wind (flatus): Passage of air from the vagina (usually accompanied by sound)
3. Vaginal laxity: feeling of vaginal looseness
4. Obstructed intercourse: vaginal intercourse is difficult or not possible because of obstruction by genital prolapse or shortened vagina, or pathologic conditions such as lichen planus or lichen sclerosus

Pain symptoms:
1. Dyspareunia: complaint of persistent or recurrent pain or discomfort associated with attempted or complete vaginal penetration (Haylen et al., 2010)

TABLE 74.19 Change in Sexual Practices Over the Past 30 Years

Sexual Behavior	1990	2010
Number of partners over lifetime	3.7	7.7
Number of occasions of SA in the past month	6.1	4.8
Vaginal sex in the past month	76.3%	69.6%
Given or received oral sex in past month	65.6%	75.1%
Anal sex in the past year	6.5%	15.1%
Sexual experience with same sex partner	3.7%	16%
Masturbated in past 4/52	n/a	32.9%

Modified from Rantell A, Apostolidis A, Anding R, et al. How does lower urinary tract dysfunction affect sexual function in men and women? ICI-RS 2015-Part 1. *Neurourol Urodyn* 2017;36(4):949–952.

2. Superficial (introital) dyspareunia: complaint of pain or discomfort on vaginal entry or at the vaginal introitus
3. Deep dyspareunia: complaint of pain or discomfort on deeper penetration (mid- or upper vagina)
4. Vaginismus: recurrent or persistent spasm of vaginal musculature that interferes with vaginal penetration
5. Dyspareunia with penile vaginal movement: pain that is caused by and is dependent on penile movement
6. Vaginal dryness: complaint of reduced vaginal lubrication or lack of adequate moisture in the vagina
7. Hypertonic PFM: A general increase in muscle tone that can be associated with either elevated contractile activity and/or passive stiffness in the muscle (Basson et al., 2004; Raina et al., 2007)
8. Noncoital sexual pain: pain induced by noncoital stimulation
9. Postcoital pain: pain after intercourse such as vaginal burning sensation or pelvic pain
10. Vulvodynia: vulvar pain of at least 3 months duration, without a clear identifiable cause, which may have potentially associated factors (Bornstein et al., 2016; Di Biase et al., 2016).

Clinical Signs and Investigations

The genital examination is often informative and in women with sexual dysfunction could have a therapeutic effect. A focused genital examination is highly recommended in the presence of dyspareunia, vaginismus, neurologic disease, genital arousal disorders, history of pelvic trauma, or acquired or lifelong orgasmic disorder (Haylen et al., 2011). The internal examinations are generally best performed with the woman's bladder empty (Haylen et al., 2010). Examination should be performed and described including vaginal length, caliber, and mobility; presence of scarring and/or pain and estrogenization; and whether or not there is vaginal or labial agglutination. The location of any vaginal pain should be noted. POP should be evaluated as it may affect body image and vaginal symptoms during sexual activity (Toozs-Hobson et al., 2012). If the patient has had an operation in which a synthetic mesh is utilized, then mesh may be felt in the vagina that may or may not be associated with symptoms (Haylen et al., 2011). Bimanual examination may reveal a pelvic mass or unusual tenderness by vaginal examination together with suprapubic palpation. PFM examination may elicit signs pertaining to FSD. If dyspareunia, vaginismus, or history of pelvic trauma are present, completing internal examinations is difficult and may be impossible. Assessing for the presence of vulvar pain via a gentle, introital palpation, or performing a "Q-tip touch test" of the introitus is recommended before any internal examination.

Measurement of sexual activity and function is largely limited to self-reporting and the use of sexual diaries or event logs, clinician-administered interviews, or questionnaires. A daily log of sexual thoughts and activities is helpful to evaluate sexual function (Rogers et al., 2018). Record individual sexual events or activities classifying them as a "sexually satisfying event (SSE)" or not (Rogers et al., 2018).

Physical examinations aim to evaluate different causes of sexual dysfunction and should include vascular, neurologic, musculoskeletal, and hormonal systems investigations.

LOWER URINARY TRACT SYMPTOMS AND FEMALE SEXUAL DYSFUNCTION: LINKS AND TREATMENTS

Urinary Incontinence and Overactive Bladder

Women with UI have a prevalence of FSD estimated to range between 26% and 47% (Geiss et al., 2003; Nusbaum and Gamble, 2001; Ozel et al., 2006; Sacco and Tienforti, 2013). All forms of UI are associated with FSD of all phases of the sexual cycle affecting all the individual domains of sexual function and satisfaction (Aslan et al., 2005; Cohen et al., 2008; Norton and Brubaker, 2006; Sen et al., 2007). **The loss of urine significantly impairs the QoL of women, who are forced to organize exhausting strategies to prevent or mask stains and/or odors causing a generalized apathy, feelings of guilt, and depressive attitude** (Simonelli et al., 2008). Thus, several studies showed a correlation between UI and major depression, which has a three-times higher incidence in incontinent patients than in continent patients (Ko et al., 2005). Specifically, women with UI feel threatened in their femininity, expressing feelings of shame, inadequacy, and reduced self-esteem (Melville et al., 2005) and subsequently a communicative and emotional inability with a strong sense of isolation (Salloum, 2005). **The lack of libido and reduced level of self-esteem because of a fear of uncontrolled leakage are the main factors in women with UI and FSD** (Brubaker et al., 2009). **The presence of severe UI doubled the odds for reduced libido, vaginal dryness, and dyspareunia** (WHO, 1992) **compared with noninconincontinent women.**

As reported by the ICI-RS, large epidemiologic studies, such as the EpiLUTS study, suggest associations between OAB and sexual dysfunctions (Apostolidis et al., 2017; Coyne et al., 2011;). However, the literature is partially contradictory. In a large treatment outcomes study, only 37% of the female participants claimed a negative sexual and relationship impact of OAB in their lives. Moreover, in a multivariate analysis, OAB was not a predictor of loss of interest in sex in female participants as opposed to male participants. Improvement of OAB symptoms was followed by a similar improvement in sex lives only in 19% of the patients, with another 11% reporting a deterioration (Sand et al., 2006). By contrast, in other published studies in which the subjects used tolterodine, there were beneficial effects of both the immediate-release (IR) and extended-release (ER) formulations on sexual health outcomes. Sexual desire, arousal, vaginal lubrication, orgasm, and orgasm satisfaction improved for up to 6 months of treatment (Hajebrahimi et al., 2008; Rogers et al., 2008, 2009).

Nilsson et al. (2011) evaluated women with UI and/or urinary urgency (the key symptom of OAB) and their partners and reported that 22% of men and 43% of women stated that the female urinary symptoms impaired their sexual life. Salonia et al. (2004) found that 47% of patients who reported a hypoactive sexual desire had SUI, and 46% of those who reported orgasm problems also had significant symptoms of OAB with urgency urinary incontinence (UUI). Yip et al. (2003) found that patients with SUI or OAB have a decreased QoL measured with King's Health Questionnaire (KHQ) (Kelleher et al., 1997), less sexual satisfaction, and poorer marital relations than controls (Yip et al., 2003). Sacco et al. (2012) reported that, among women with UI and/or OAB, those with UUI and mixed urinary incontinence (MUI) reported worse FSD as compared with those with SUI or with dry OAB. Women with urodynamically proven detrusor overactivity incontinence appeared in this and other studies to have the worst female sexual function (Barber et al., 2002; Kim et al., 2005; Yip et al., 2003). Mechanisms associated with the impact of OAB on female sexual function can be the fear of leakage during stimulation and intercourse, coital UI during orgasm, the need to interrupt intercourse to void, urgency and frequency after coitus, dyspareunia, and pelvic floor dysfunction.

The 11% to 45% of patients with UI suffered the fear of urine leakage during intercourse (Rogers et al., 2001). **Moran et al. (1999) found that 11% of 2153 women had UI during intercourse.** A questionnaire was helpful in detecting this symptom. **Specifically, 70% reported urine leakage during penetration, 20% only during orgasm, and 11% during both penetration and orgasm. A SUI was present in 80% of women with UI during penetration, in 93% of women with UI during orgasm, and in 92% of women with UI during both phases.** The pathophysiology leading to UI during intercourse is not clear (Sacco and Tienforti, 2013). A hypothesis is that during penetration, the displacement of the anterior wall of the vagina and bladder neck or increase of the intra-abdominal pressure loss can cause SUI. Detrusorial simultaneous contractions and urethral relaxation were demonstrated in urodynamic studies during orgasm (Vierhout and Gianotten, 1993).

Although SUI surgery is thought to improve sexual function (Brubaker et al., 2009; De Souza et al., 2012; Vierhout and Gianotten, 1993), data reporting sexual function after surgical repair are limited and conflicting (Srikrishna et al., 2010). A recent meta-analysis showed that in two studies, women who underwent retropubic and trans-obturator sling intervention and completed the Pelvic Organ Prolapse Urinary Incontinence Sexual Questionnaire (PISQ-12) showed an increase in sexual function of 2.40 points after transobturator compared with retropubic sling intervention (95% CI, −2.48 to −2.32; I2 = 35%, $P < .00001$). However, two other studies composed of 183 women comparing the same techniques, but using the FSFI, did not show a statistically significant difference (95% CI, −1.77 to 3.78; I2 = 0%, $P = .48$). The authors concluded that the impact of UI surgery on sexual function is uncertain because of the imprecision of the effect and inconsistency among studies. Only limited evidence on the impact of the transobturator versus the retropubic sling was found (Bicudo-Fürst et al., 2018).

However, it is important to underline that vaginal sling procedures may have a potential negative effect on FSF as a result of damage to vascular and/or neural genital structures or de novo dyspareunia (Sacco and Tienforti, 2013; Serati et al., 2009). Baessler et al. reported that dyspareunia was a severe indication for removing the posterior intravaginal synthetic sling (Serati et al., 2009). Bekker et al. (2012) described the autonomic and somatic pathways in relationship to sling surgery in 14 adult female dissected hemipelves after tension-free vaginal tape (TVT) or transobturator tape (TOT) procedures were performed. They concluded that the dorsal nerve of the clitoris was not disturbed during placement of the TOT, but the autonomic innervation of the vaginal wall was disrupted by the TVT procedure, which could lead to an altered lubrication-swelling response.

In a meta-analysis performed by Jha et al. (2012), sexual function was unchanged in 55.5% of women, improved in 31.9%, and deteriorated in 13.1% after surgery for SUI. The resolution of coital incontinence is closely correlated to a patient's degree of sexual satisfaction, and preoperative coital incontinence has been suggested as a prognostic factor for improvement of sexual function after surgery (Lonnee-Hoffmann et al., 2013).

As reported by the ICI-RS, improvements in women's sexual function after successful treatment of either OAB/UI or SUI suggest indirect effects of lower urinary tract dysfunction (LUTD) on sexual function (Apostolidis et al., 2017). Improvement of secondary parameters as a result of OAB/UI (leakage during intercourse, intercourse interruption caused by urgency, pain during intercourse) and of factors that have a negative effect on the satisfaction of the sexual relationships and on patients' self-image (embarrassment associated with OAB/UI, fear of leakage during stimulation and intercourse, postcoital worsening of OAB) may also result in improvement of FSD (Coyne et al., 2007; Hajebrahimi et al., 2008). In the case of SUI, surgical or conservative restoration of continence is commonly associated with improvement of sexual function as demonstrated by most prospective studies (Filocamo et al., 2011; Glavind et al., 2014; Kamalak et al., 2014; Narin et al., 2014; Serati et al., 2015), literature reviews (Fatton et al., 2014), and meta-analyses (Jha et al., 2012). **The cure of coital incontinence, achieved in 90% of surgically treated cases, is thought to be a major predictor of sexual improvement** (Fatton et al., 2014; Glavind et al., 2014; Kamalak et al., 2014), **with improvements in coital pain** (Kamalak et al., 2014) **and in partner-related aspects** (Narin et al., 2014; Roos et al., 2014) also reported to be associated with postsurgery sexual function beneficial effects.

The use of neuromodulation to treat refractory LUTD could shed some light in the mechanisms connecting LUTD to FSD. Almost all studies show that sacral neuromodulation (SNM) improves LUTS and sexual function irrespective of the cause of LUTD (Gaziev et al., 2013; Gill et al., 2011; Pauls et al., 2007; Signorello et al., 2011). Their findings suggest that **neural and vascular changes may be common in LUTD and FSD**. In this respect, women with refractory OAB and nonobstructive urinary retention were found to have abnormal pudendal nerve function, which showed a trend toward improvement after SNM (Parnell et al., 2015). Neurally augmented sexual function was achieved by percutaneous epidural spinal cord space stimulation, resulting in reproducible pleasurable genital stimulation, increased frequency of sexual activity and lubrication, and improved orgasmic function (Meloy and Southern, 2006). Active neurostimulation could also increase the vaginal pulse amplitude with both erotic and nonerotic stimuli (van Voskuilen et al., 2012). Whether neurovascular changes proposed in the four-theory complex to explain associations between male LUTS and ED also apply for LUTD and FSD needs be further researched (Kohler and McVary, 2009).

Pelvic Organ Prolapse

POP is associated with different LUTS such as SUI, UI, urgency, and frequency that are present in 40%, 34%, 29%, and 30% of women, respectively (Swift et al., 2005). Women with prolapse may present with a wide range of LUTS such as SUI, UI, urgency, frequency, and urge incontinence have been reported in 40%, 34%, 29%, and 30% of women with POP, respectively (De Boer et al., 2011; Grody, 1998). Understanding the relationship between POP and pelvic floor symptoms is a crucial step in the management of patients. The symptoms are largely subjective in nature (Ghoniem et al., 2008). Contradictory results have been reported regarding the association of POP with LUTS and sexual dysfunction (Broekhuis et al., 2010; Burrows et al., 2004; Ellerkmann et al., 2001; Ghetti et al., 2005; Gutman et al., 2008; Salvatore et al., 2011).

Cetinkaya et al. (2013) demonstrated that there is no significant correlation between POP stages and the PISQ-12. In a recent cross-sectional observational study, Athanasiou et al. (2012) evaluated the effect of POP on FSF in 101 women compared with 70 women without POP, and found that female sexual function was poorer in the POP group than in the control group, but did not correlate with an increasing grade of POP. Handa et al. (2004) found that POP was not associated with any sexual complaint. Weber et al. (1995) reported that women with POP and/or UI have a similar sexual function as women without these PFDs. On the other hand, Novi et al. (2005) **compared sexual function of women with POP to that of women without POP using the PISQ, and reported that mean PISQ scores in sexually active women with POP were significantly lower compared with controls, with significant difference in satisfaction with sexual relationship, actual frequency of intercourse, and ability to achieve orgasm with masturbation, but no difference in the desired frequency of intercourse, initiation of sexual activity, rate of anorgasmia, or subjective assessment of partner satisfaction.** Digesu et al. (2005) observed that FSD was related to uterine displacement, likely leading the cervix to obstruct penile penetration.

Options for prolapse repair include abdominal versus vaginal approaches and native tissue versus grafted repairs. A native tissue repair is one that uses a patient's own structures to repair the vaginal defect. These surgeries most commonly include anterior and posterior repairs (colporrhaphy), uterosacral vault suspensions, and sacrospinous fixations (Thompson and Rogers, 2016). For most women, native tissue repairs result in improved or unchanged sexual function (Azar et al., 2008; Jha et al., 2015; Komesu et al., 2007). A 2014 meta-analysis of the impact of native tissue repair on sexual function using standardized questionnaires included nine studies that showed improvement in sexual function after prolapse repair (Jha et al., 2015). Eight studies evaluating dyspareunia showed that women were 4.8 times more likely to have improvement in pain or unchanged symptoms than increased pain postoperatively (Jha et al., 2015). A systematic review of anterior repair comparing native tissue with biologic graft and polypropylene mesh included 12 randomized trials (Maher et al., 2013). Anterior native tissue repair versus biologic graft showed no difference in dyspareunia rates postoperatively, but the repairs with a graft showed lower recurrent prolapse rates (Thompson and Rogers, 2016). Repair of the posterior compartment of the vagina has been associated with increased concern for postoperative dyspareunia (Thompson and Rogers, 2016). A systematic review comparing posterior native tissue repair with biologic grafting showed no difference in the rate of dyspareunia (Maher et al., 2013)

Grafts can be used for the repair of POP. Graft repairs for anterior, posterior, and apical descent can use vaginal and abdominal approaches. Polypropylene mesh has gained favor in prolapse repair for its durability and low-risk profile. Conversely, biologic grafts have fallen out of favor because of their higher risk for recurrent prolapse. Many surgeons consider sacrocolpopexy the gold standard for surgery addressing apical prolapse (Thompson and Rogers, 2016). Sexual function after sacrocolpopexy can remain unchanged or can be improved after surgery (Geller et al., 2011; Handa et al., 2004;

Price et al., 2011; Sarlos et al., 2008). The Society of Gynecologic Surgeons performed a systematic review on adverse events after vaginal prolapse repair using graft materials from 1950 through 2010. From the 70 articles reporting on dyspareunia after transvaginal mesh placement for prolapse, the incidence was 9.1% (Abed et al., 2011). The incidence was similar regardless of whether synthetic and biologic grafts were used for repairs. This systematic review is limited because most studies did not measure preoperative rates of dyspareunia and did not consistently use validated measurements (Thompson and Rogers, 2016).

Bladder Pain Syndrome/Interstitial Cystitis

Sexual dysfunction issues have been reported among women with BPS/IC and can contribute to reduced QoL in these patients (Sacco and Tienforti, 2013). Pelvic pain caused by inflammation of the bladder wall and neuropathic dysfunction, dyspareunia, and fear of pain during intercourse are particularly frequent among these patients and may cause resistance to penetration and consequent pelvic floor overactivity, vulvodynia, and vaginismus (Peters et al., 2008).

Sacco et al. (2012) showed that women with BPS reported the greatest adverse impact on FSF, mostly as a result of sexual pain, followed by those with urodynamic DO, clinical diagnosis of UUI, MUI and SUI; dry OAB; and voiding-phase LUTS. These results were aligned with those of Peters et al. (2007). CPP is significantly associated with FSD (Ottem et al., 2007; Verit et al., 2006) in terms of HSDD, sexual arousal disorder, orgasmic disorder, and sexual pain disorder.

SELF-IMAGE/BODY IMAGE CONNECTED TO FEMALE SEXUAL DYSFUNCTION AND LOWER URINARY TRACT SYMPTOMS

The ICI-RS reported that body image problems could be associated with sexual problems. Sparse data are available on correlations between self-image and SD in women with LUTS. Sexual function was found to be affected by body image perception in women with POP (Lowenstein et al., 2009a). In neuro-urologic patients, the presence of an indwelling catheter had a negative impact on female sexuality and QoL. Urinary tract reconstruction restored QoL and markedly improved sexual function by improving self-image, self-esteem, and the ability to cope (Watanabe et al., 1996). In women undergoing surgery for SUI, the goals of improving sexuality and body image are predictors of post-treatment sexual function improvement (Lonne-Hoffman et al., 2013), but there is still no available literature on the impact of urgency or MUI on patients' self-image and its possible associations with sexual function. The impact of using pads and diapers on patients' self-image and sexual function also has not been studied.

> ### KEY POINTS: LOWER URINARY TRACT DYSFUNCTION AND FEMALE SEXUAL DYSFUNCTION
>
> - Almost one-half of the women with UI and/or LUTS suffer from various types of sexual dysfunction.
> - Sexual symptoms may occur in combination with other pelvic floor symptoms such as UI, POP, or pelvic pain.
> - UI negatively affects sexual function via interfering with libido and self-esteem.
> - Mid-urethral sling procedures can lead to FSD via neurovascular insult affecting the genital organs or postoperative de novo dyspareunia.
> - Resolution of UI after medical and/or surgical treatment may also have a significant positive effect on various domains of female sexual wellness.
> - Sexually active women with POP can have problems with sexual satisfaction, decreased frequency of intercourse, and inability to achieve orgasm with masturbation.

CONCLUSION

Female sexual function and dysfunction are important aspects of urologic practice. Urologists should be aware of the urologic ramifications of sexual issues and vice versa. Appropriate treatment (or referral) of women with sexual concerns will improve patient satisfaction and treatment compliance.

REFERENCES

The complete reference list is available online at ExpertConsult.com.

PART VII
Male Genitalia

75 Surgical, Radiographic, and Endoscopic Anatomy of the Retroperitoneum

Drew A. Palmer, MD, and Alireza Moinzadeh, MD

Anatomic knowledge of the retroperitoneum is critical for urologists in the clinic and the operating room. This chapter provides a thorough description of retroperitoneal anatomy, including the genitourinary organs, musculature, bony structures, fasciae, vessels, lymphatics, neural structures, and gastrointestinal viscera. See Table 75.1 for a review of the anatomic and surgical history of the retroperitoneum.

The retroperitoneum can be described as the entirety of the structures contained anteriorly by the posterior reflection of the peritoneum, posteriorly by the abdominal wall, cranially by the diaphragm, and caudally by the extraperitoneal pelvic structures (Fig. 75.1). The last term must be distinguished from *extraperitoneal space*, which includes the retroperitoneum and the space that circumferentially surrounds the abdominal cavity (Miralis and Skandalakis, 2009, 2010a-d).

The contents of the retroperitoneum include the **kidneys, ureters, adrenals, pancreas, portions of the duodenum, ascending colon, descending colon, mesentery, arterial structures including the aorta and its branches, venous structures including the inferior vena cava (IVC) and its tributaries, lymphatics, lymph nodes, sympathetic trunk, and lumbosacral plexus** (Fig. 75.2 and Box 75.1; also see Fig. 75.1).

BODY SURFACE LANDMARKS

The ability to identify abdominal organs using physical examination is useful for clinical diagnosis and operative planning. The location of the kidneys can be estimated based on their relationship to the bony structures of the posterior abdominal wall (Fig. 75.3). The upper pole of the left kidney is typically located at the level of the 11th rib. The right kidney lies lower than the left, with its upper pole at the level of the 12th rib. The lower poles of the kidneys are between the L3 and L4 vertebrae, and **the renal hila are approximately at the level of L1.**

POSTERIOR ABDOMINAL WALL
Flank Muscles (Figs. 75.4 to 75.7 and Table 75.2)

The most superficial of the flank muscles is the **external oblique**, which lies beneath the subcutaneous fascia. It originates from ribs 5 through 12, and its muscle fibers travel inferomedially inserting at the iliac crest and ending in the midline at the linea alba. **The inferior border of the aponeurosis of the external oblique forms the inguinal ligament.** Deep to the external oblique lies the **internal oblique**, which originates from the lumbodorsal fascia and the iliac crest. It travels superomedially, inserting at the lower ribs and linea alba. Each of these muscle layers is invested in a layer of fascia. The **transversus abdominis** muscle, named because of the *transverse* direction of its muscle fibers, lies deep to the internal oblique. Deep to the transversus abdominis muscle lies the **transversalis fascia**, which crosses the midline anteriorly and fuses with the lumbodorsal fascia posteriorly. These flank muscles function to flex, extend, and rotate the trunk and provide compression of the abdominal contents.

Psoas, Iliacus, Quadratus Lumborum, and Erector Spinae (Fig. 75.8; also see Figs. 75.4 to 75.7 and Table 75.2)

The **psoas major** muscle arises from the 12th thoracic vertebra to the 5th lumbar vertebra to attach to the lesser trochanter of the femur after traveling along the pelvic brim posterior to the inguinal ligament. The psoas minor muscle, which may be absent in some individuals, originates at T12 and L1 and inserts at the pelvic brim and iliopubic eminence. The psoas major functions in flexion of the thigh at the hip joint and is innervated by the anterior rami of L1, L2, and L3. The **iliacus** muscle originates at the caudal aspect of the iliac fossa and the lateral sacrum to insert at the lesser trochanter of the femur. It functions in flexion of the thigh at the hip joint along with the psoas major. The **quadratus lumborum** lies posterior and medial to the psoas muscle and assists with lateral bending of the trunk and stabilization of the 12th rib. Its origin is at L5 and the iliac fossa, and it attaches to the inferior border of the 12th rib and the transverse processes of L1-L4. The **erector spinae (sacrospinalis)** is a large group of back muscles that function to extend the spine.

Spine

The spine consists of 7 cervical vertebrae, 12 thoracic vertebrae, 5 lumbar vertebrae, the sacrum, and the coccyx. Each vertebra has a large weight-bearing area called the **vertebral body** and a posterior and lateral arch that forms the vertebral foramen (eFig. 75.9 on ExpertConsult.com). The **spinous process** projects posteroinferiorly, and the **transverse processes** project posterolaterally. The lumbar vertebrae are the most clinically significant in regard to the retroperitoneum. They are larger than the other vertebrae with generally long, thin transverse processes.

The vertebral column levels have different relationships with the spinal cord segmental levels at different locations within the spinal column. For example, the sacral spinal cord segmental levels typically begin between vertebral column level T12 and L1 in adults. Discussions of spinal cord injury must specify vertebral column level versus spinal segmental level.

10th, 11th, and 12th Ribs

The lower ribs protect the retroperitoneal structures from traumatic injury. **Fracture of these lower ribs should lead to a high clinical suspicion for injury to the retroperitoneal structures** (eFig. 75.10 on ExpertConsult.com). The lower ribs differ from the upper ribs given their shorter length with less pronounced angulation. The 10th rib articulates with the body of the vertebra at its head and the

Text continued on p. 1665

TABLE 75.1 Anatomic and Surgical History of the Retroperitoneum

Morgagni	1761	Described retroperitoneal lipoma found at autopsy
Cloquet	1817	Studied perirenal fascia
Bogros	1823	Studied surgical anatomy of iliac area
Lobstein	1829	First use of term *retroperitoneal tumor*
Broca	1850	Discovered retroperitoneal tumors at autopsy
Moynier	1850	Discovered retroperitoneal tumors at autopsy
Treitz	1853	Stated theory of "absorption"; described retroduodenopancreatic fascia
Dickinson	1871	Described teratomatous tumor similar to dermoid teratomas commonly found in the ovary
Toldt	1879, 1893	Theory of conjoined visceral fasciae
Zuckerkandl	1883	Described posterior renal fascia
Bassini	1889	Described retroperitoneal cystadenoma that resembled pseudomucinous cystadenoma of ovary
Rogie	1894	Described retroperitoneal anatomy
Gerota	1895	Described anterior renal fascia
Poirer et al.	1923	Studied lobulation of adipose tissue in pararenal and perirenal areas
Drouet	1941	Studied subperitoneal area
Baumann	1945	Described embryology of renal area
Altmeir and Alexander	1961	Described extraperitoneal compartments above pelvic brim
Stevenson and Ozeran	1969	Subdivided anatomy of extraperitoneal pelvis into posterior, anterior, inferior, and superior spaces
Meyers et al.	1972	Descriptions of anterior and posterior pararenal and perirenal spaces
Wickham	1979	Operated in a pneumoretroperitoneum for endoscopic removal of ureteric stone
Hureau et al.	1990, 1991	CT study of extraperitoneal spaces
Korobkin et al.	1992	Used CT to study anatomy and fluid collections in retroperitoneal space
Gaur	1992	Performed retroperitoneal videoscopic renal surgery
McDougall et al.	1994	Performed retroperitoneal videoscopic renal surgery

CT, Computed tomography.
Data from Skandalakis JE, Colborn GL: *Skandalakis' surgical anatomy: the embryological and anatomic basis of modern surgery*, Athens, Greece, 2004, Paschalides Medical Publications.

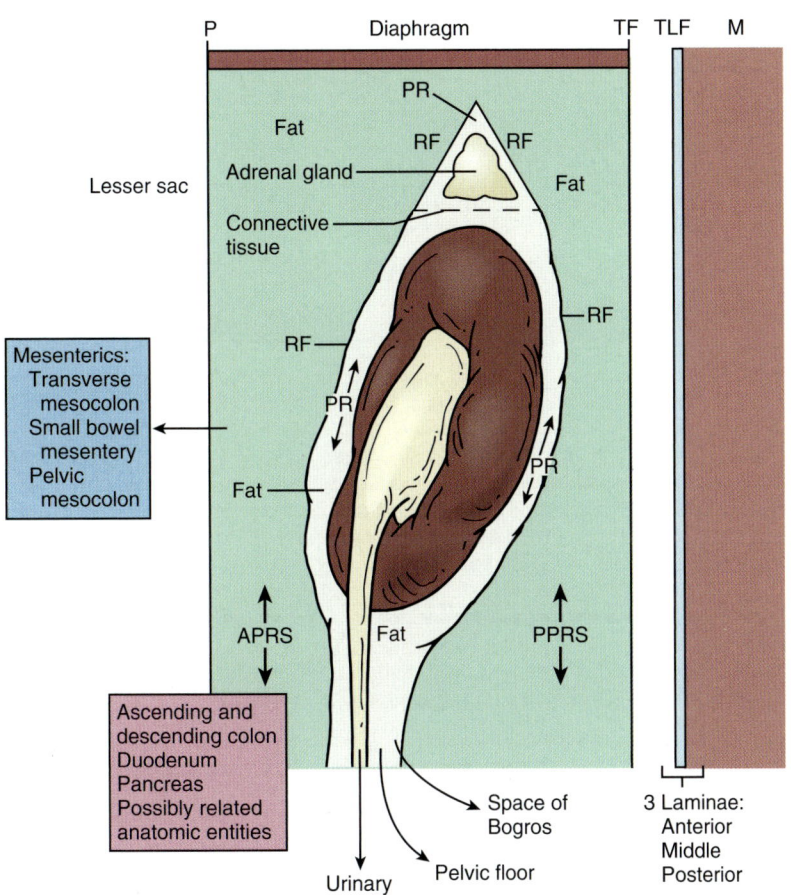

Fig. 75.1. Diagram of retroperitoneal spaces. *APRS*, Anterior pararenal space; *M*, muscles; *P*, peritoneum; *PPRS*, posterior pararenal space; *PR*, perirenal space; *RF*, renal fascia (Gerota fascia); *TF*, transversalis fascia; *TLF*, thoracolumbar fascia. (Modified from Skandalakis JE, Colborn GL: *Skandalakis' surgical anatomy: the embryological and anatomic basis of modern surgery*, Athens, Greece, 2004, Paschalides Medical Publications, p 155.)

1660 PART VII Male Genitalia

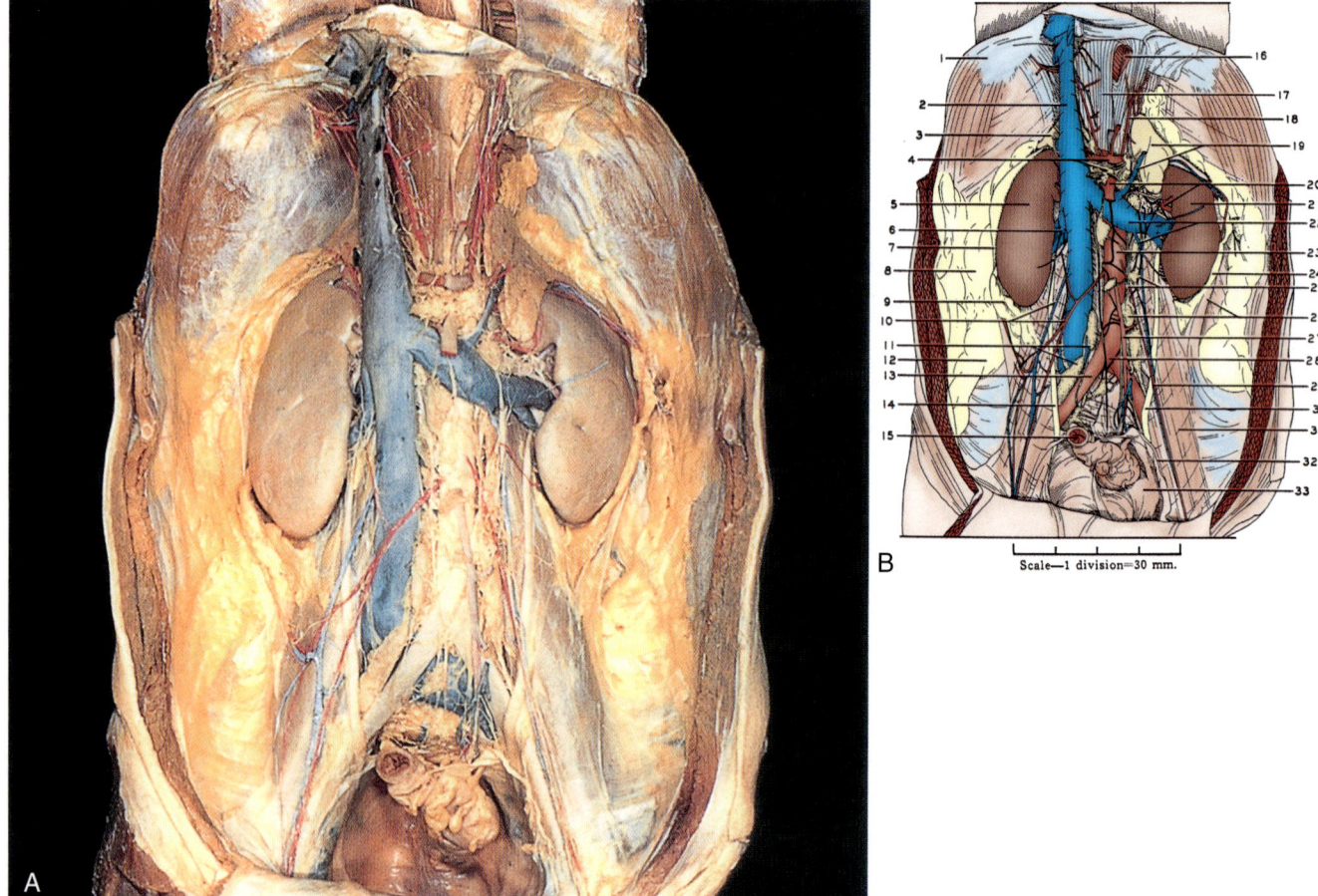

Fig. 75.2. (A) Dissected retroperitoneum. The anterior perirenal (Gerota) fascia has been removed. (B) *1,* Diaphragm. *2,* Inferior vena cava. *3,* Right adrenal gland. *4,* Upper pointer, celiac artery; lower pointer, celiac autonomic nervous plexus. *5,* Right kidney. *6,* Right renal vein. *7,* Gerota fascia. *8,* Pararenal retroperitoneal fat. *9,* Perinephric fat. *10,* Upper pointer, right gonadal vein; lower pointer, right gonadal artery. *11,* Lumbar lymph nodes. *12,* Retroperitoneal fat. *13,* Right common iliac artery. *14,* Right ureter. *15,* Sigmoid colon (cut). *16,* Esophagus (cut). *17,* Right crus of diaphragm. *18,* Left inferior phrenic artery. *19,* Upper pointer, left adrenal gland; lower pointer, left adrenal vein. *20,* Upper pointer, superior mesenteric artery; lower pointer, left renal artery. *21,* Left kidney. *22,* Upper pointer, left renal vein; lower pointer, left gonadal vein. *23,* Aorta. *24,* Perinephric fat. *25,* Aortic autonomic nervous plexus. *26,* Upper pointer, Gerota fascia; lower pointer, inferior mesenteric ganglion. *27,* Inferior mesenteric artery. *28,* Aortic bifurcation into common iliac arteries. *29,* Left gonadal artery and vein. *30,* Left ureter. *31,* Psoas major muscle covered by psoas sheath. *32,* Cut edge of peritoneum. *33,* Pelvic cavity. (Reproduced from the Bassett anatomic collection, with permission from Dr. Robert A. Chase.)

Chapter 75 Surgical, Radiographic, and Endoscopic Anatomy of the Retroperitoneum

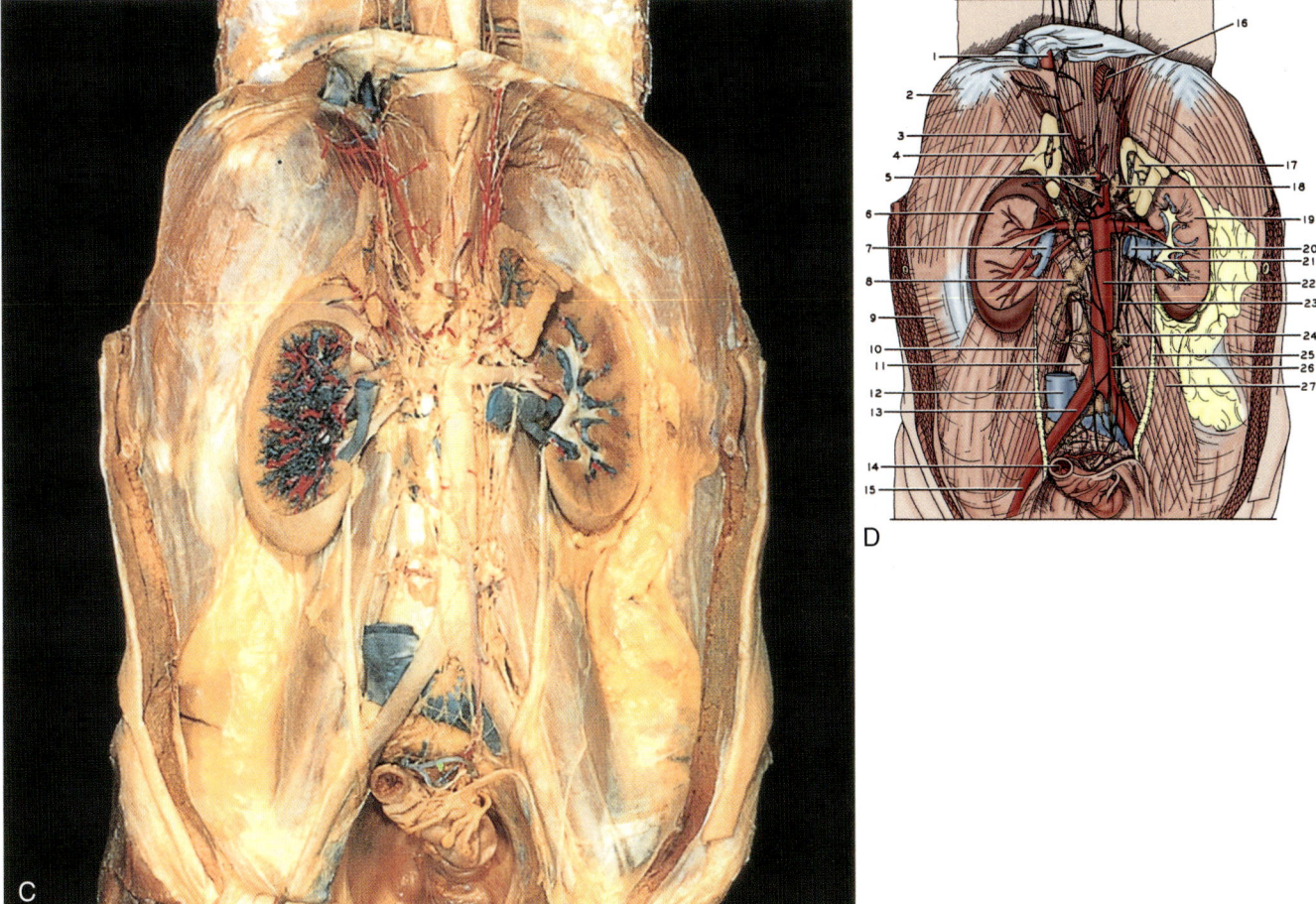

Fig. 75.2., cont'd (C) Dissected retroperitoneum. The kidneys and adrenal glands have been sectioned, and the inferior vena cava has been excised over most of its intra-abdominal course. (D) *1*, Inferior vena cava (cut). *2*, Diaphragm. *3*, Right inferior phrenic artery. *4*, Right adrenal gland. *5*, Upper pointer, celiac artery; lower pointer, superior mesenteric artery. *6*, Right kidney. *7*, Upper pointer, right renal artery; lower pointer, right renal vein (cut). *8*, Lumbar lymph node. *9*, Transversus abdominis muscle covered with transversalis fascia. *10*, Right ureter. *11*, Anterior spinous ligament. *12*, Inferior vena cava (cut). *13*, Right common iliac artery. *14*, Sigmoid colon (cut). *15*, Right external iliac artery. *16*, Esophagus (cut). *17*, Left adrenal gland. *18*, Celiac ganglion. *19*, Left kidney. *20*, Upper pointer, left renal artery; lower pointer, left renal vein (cut). *21*, Left renal pelvis. *22*, Aorta. *23*, Aortic autonomic nervous plexus. *24*, Inferior mesenteric ganglion. *25*, Left ureter. *26*, Inferior mesenteric artery. *27*, Psoas major muscle covered by psoas sheath. (Reproduced from the Bassett anatomic collection, with permission from Dr. Robert A. Chase.)

BOX 75.1 Organs and Structures of the Retroperitoneum

ORGANS
Kidneys (PR)
Ureters (PR)
Adrenal glands (PR)
Portions of the duodenum (SR)
Ascending colon (SR)
Descending colon (SR)
Pancreas (SR)

VESSELS AND LYMPHATICS
Abdominal aorta (and its branches)
Inferior vena cava (and its tributaries)
Ascending lumbar veins
Portal vein
Lumbar lymph nodes
Lumbar lymphatic trunks
Cisterna chyli

NERVES
Branches of the lumbosacral plexus
Sympathetic trunk
Autonomic plexuses
Autonomic ganglia

PR, Primarily retroperitoneal; *SR*, secondarily retroperitoneal.
Data from Miralis P, Skandalakis JE: Surgical anatomy of the retroperitoneal spaces—part I: embryogenesis and anatomy. *Am Surg* 75(11):1091–1097, 2009.

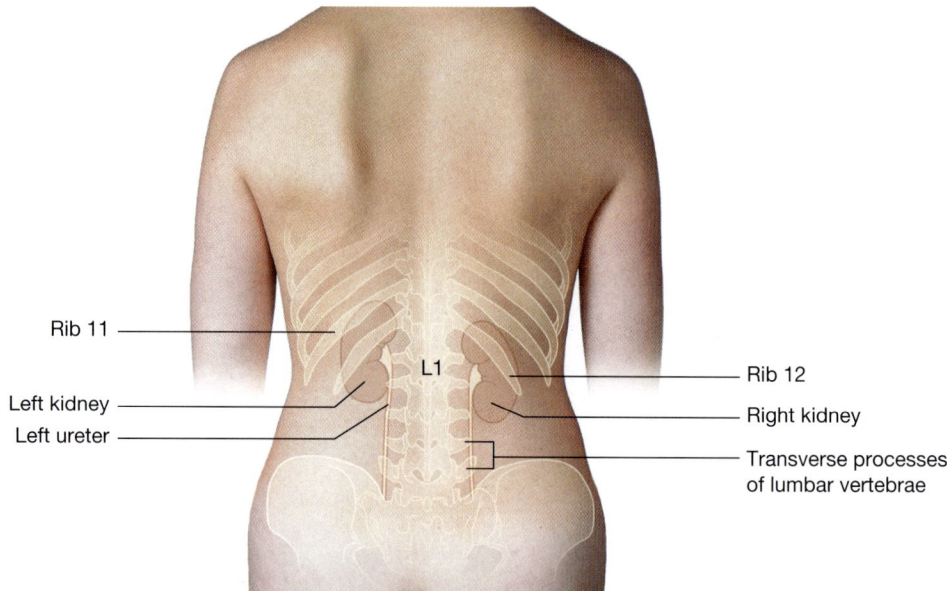

Fig. 75.3. Posterior view of the abdominal region of a woman with projections of the kidneys and ureters. (From Drake RL, Vogl AW, Mitchell AWM: *Gray's anatomy for students,* ed 2, Philadelphia, 2010. Churchill Livingstone.)

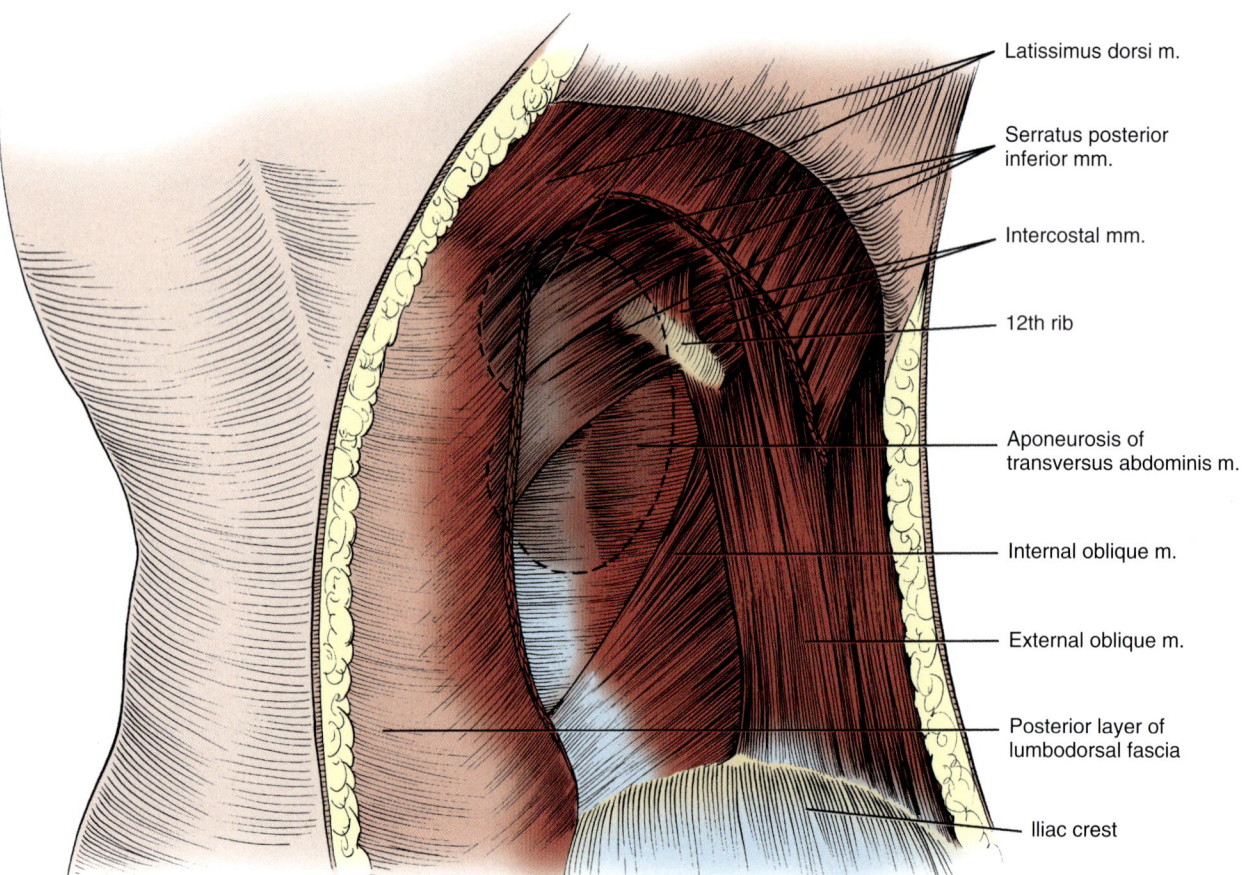

Fig. 75.4. Posterior abdominal wall musculature, superficial dissection. A section of the latissimus dorsi muscle has been removed. The location of the right kidney within the retroperitoneum is shown by the *dashed outline.*

Chapter 75 Surgical, Radiographic, and Endoscopic Anatomy of the Retroperitoneum   1663

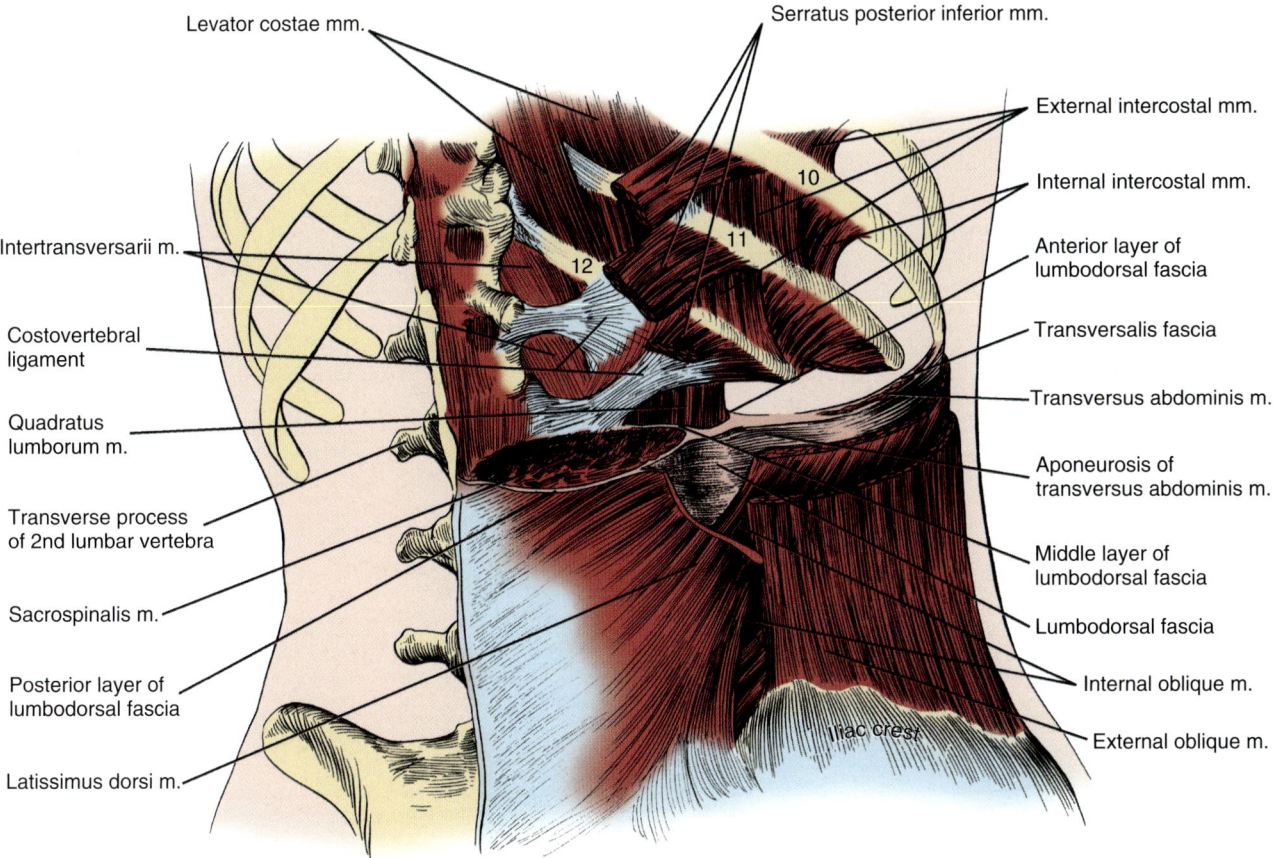

Fig. 75.5. Posterior abdominal wall musculature, intermediate dissection. The sacrospinalis muscle and three anterolateral flank muscle layers are seen in cut section, and the three layers of the lumbodorsal fascia posteriorly can be appreciated.

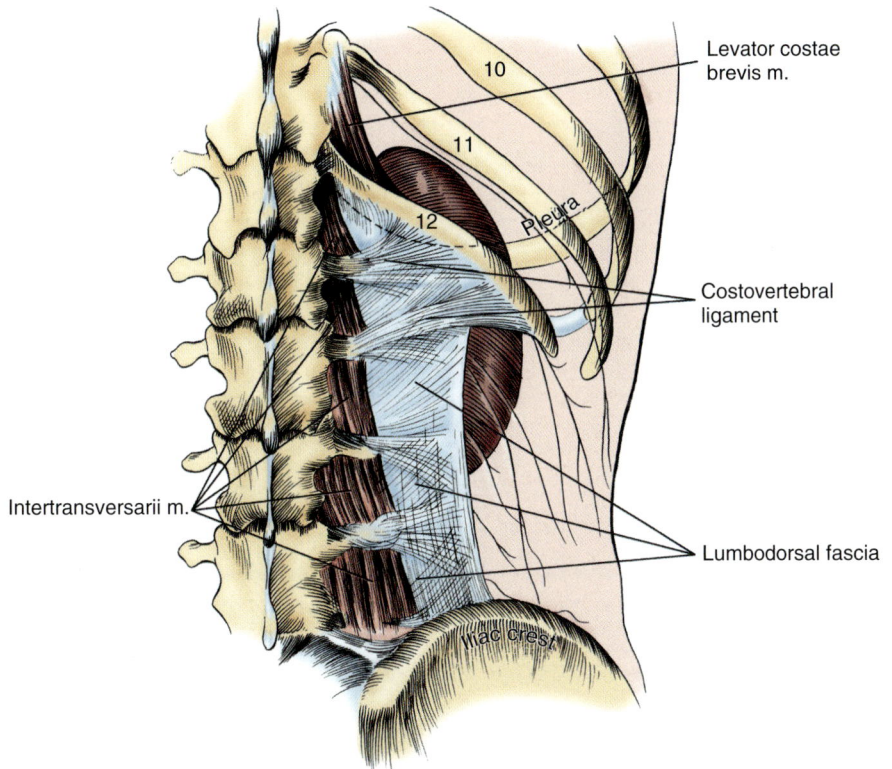

Fig. 75.6. Posterior abdominal wall musculature, deep dissection. The lumbodorsal fascia and costovertebral ligament are visualized arising from the transverse processes of the lumbar vertebrae. The relationship of the kidney and pleura is also shown.

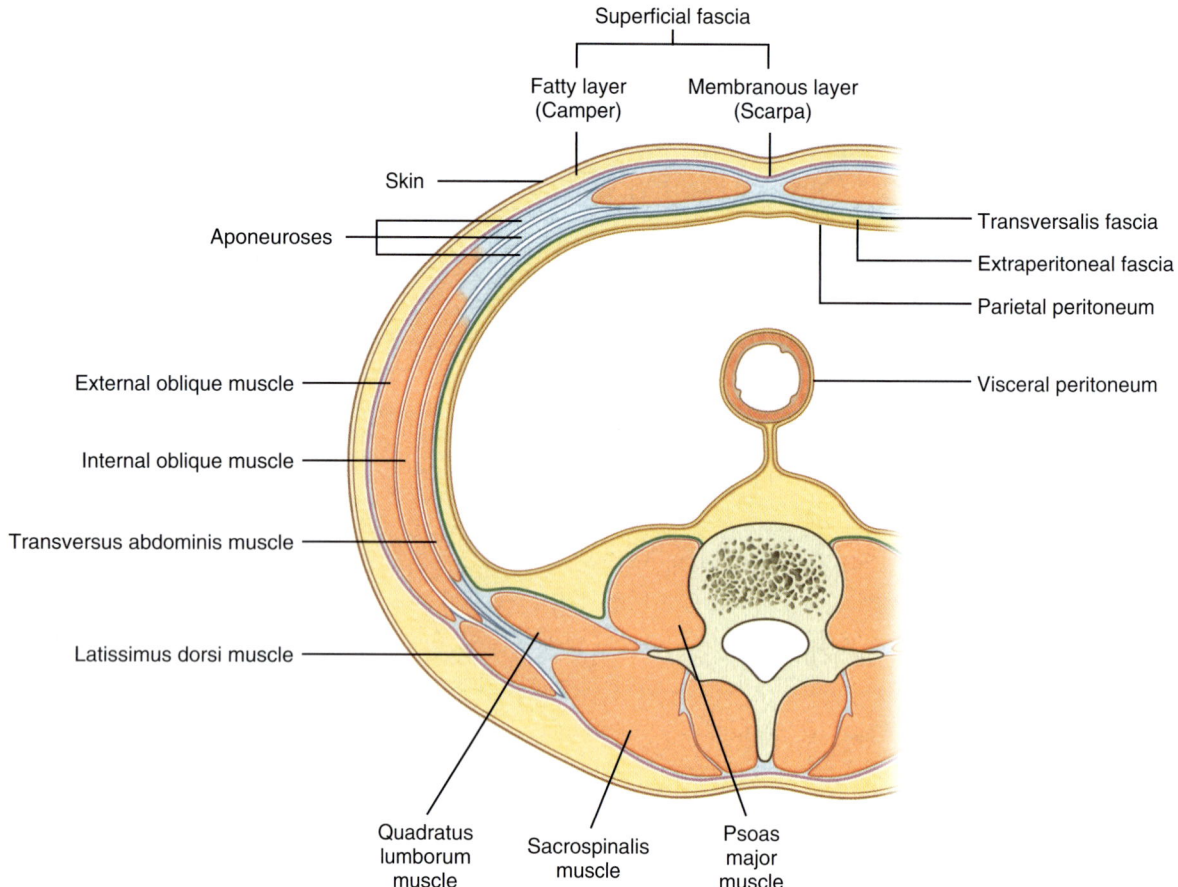

Fig. 75.7. Transverse section showing layers of the lateral flank musculature. (From Drake RL, Vogl AW, Mitchell AWM: *Gray's anatomy for students,* ed 2, Philadelphia, 2010, Churchill Livingstone.)

TABLE 75.2 Musculature of the Posterior and Lateral Abdominal Wall

MUSCLE	ORIGIN	INSERTION	FUNCTION
Erector spinae	Sacrum and vertebrae	Lower ribs and vertebrae	Extension of spine
External oblique	Ribs 5–12	Lateral lip of iliac crest, aponeurosis ending in linea alba	Compress abdominal contents, flexion of trunk
Internal oblique	Lumbodorsal fascia, iliac crest, inguinal ligament	Lower four ribs, aponeurosis ending in linea alba, pubic crest	Compress abdominal contents, flexion of trunk
Transversus abdominis	Lumbodorsal fascia, medial lip of iliac crest, ribs 7–12	Aponeurosis ending in linea alba, pubic crest	Compress abdominal contents
Psoas major	T12-L5 vertebrae	Lesser trochanter of femur	Flexion of hip
Psoas minor	T12 and L1 vertebrae	Pelvic brim, iliopubic eminence	Weak flexion of lumbar vertebral column
Iliacus	Iliac fossa, sacrum	Lesser trochanter of femur	Flexion of the hip
Quadratus lumborum	5th lumbar vertebra, iliac crest	L1-L4 vertebrae, 12th rib	Depress and stabilize 12th rib, lateral bending of trunk

Modified from Drake RL, Vogl AW, Mitchell AWM: *Gray's anatomy for students,* Philadelphia, 2005, Churchill Livingstone.

Chapter 75 Surgical, Radiographic, and Endoscopic Anatomy of the Retroperitoneum **1665**

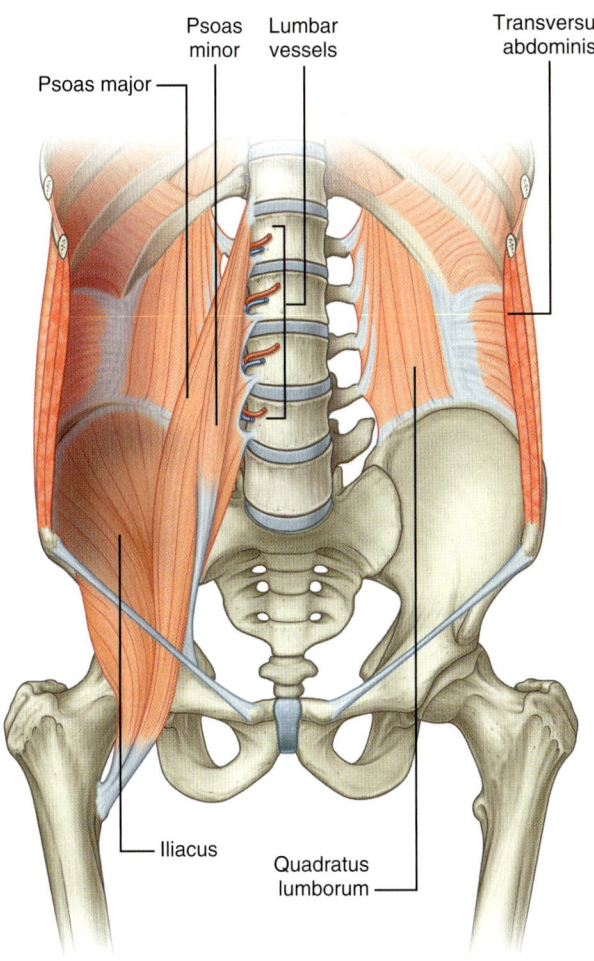

Fig. 75.8. Muscles of the posterior abdominal wall. (From Drake RL, Vogl AW, Mitchell AWM: *Gray's anatomy for students,* ed 2, Philadelphia, 2010, Churchill Livingstone.)

transverse process at its neck. The 11th rib lacks a neck and does not articulate with the transverse process. The angle of the 11th rib is less pronounced than that of the upper ribs. The 12th rib has no angle and is shorter than the other ribs. **Its inferior border is attached to the transverse processes of L1 and L2 by the costovertebral (lumbocostal) ligament, which can be incised to allow for increased mobility for greater exposure of the upper retroperitoneum during posterior approaches.** Similar increased mobility may be achieved by dividing a thick, fibrous band known as the intercostal ligament found between other ribs.

The 11th and 12th ribs must be distinguished from the other ribs because they have no anterior connection with the sternum and are often referred to as *floating ribs*. These ribs are of clinical significance during palpation for the marking of a surgical incision.

The intercostal vessels and nerves travel between the internal intercostal and innermost intercostal muscles within the costal groove on the caudal margin of the superior rib (Fig. 75.11). The vein is the most superior structure with the artery running inferior to it. The intercostal nerve is the most inferior of the three structures and is often not protected by the costal groove.

LUMBODORSAL FASCIA

The **lumbodorsal (thoracolumbar) fascia** is composed of three distinct layers that invest the posterior abdominal wall musculature (Fig. 75.12). **These three layers merge into one as they travel laterally. A common access point to the retroperitoneum is near the tip of the 12th rib, where all layers have merged into one.** This single layer of lumbodorsal fascia merges with the aponeurosis of the transversus abdominis muscle anterolaterally. The **posterior lamella** originates medially from the spinous process of the lumbar vertebrae and covers the erector spinae muscles. The **middle lamella** separates these erector spinae muscles from quadratus lumborum. The anterior lamella covers the ventral surface of quadratus lumborum. Extending medially, the **anterior lamella** attaches to the vertebral transverse process and is continuous with the fascia that invests the psoas muscle.

The retroperitoneum can be entered without incising muscle using a dorsal lumbotomy incision (Fig. 75.13). This approach

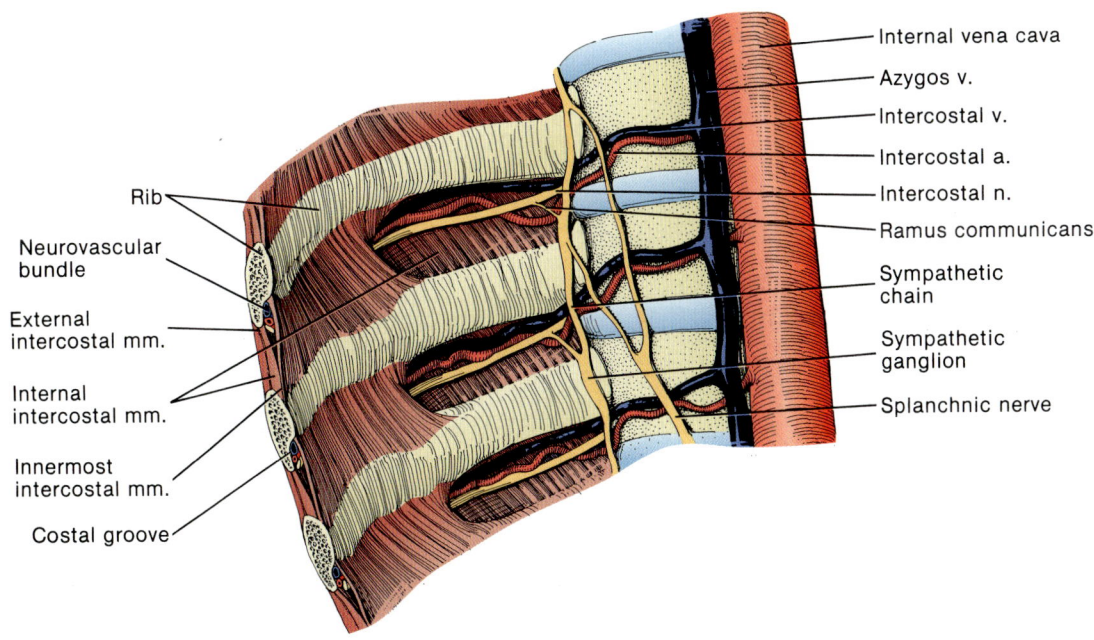

Fig. 75.11. Intercostal neurovascular bundle. (From MacLennan GT: *Hinman's atlas of urosurgical anatomy,* ed 2, Philadelphia, 2012, Saunders.)

uses a vertical incision through the lumbodorsal fascia lateral to the erector spinae and quadratus lumborum muscles (eFig. 75.14 on ExpertConsult.com).

RETROPERITONEAL FASCIAE AND SPACES

Derived from the mesoderm, the primitive mesenchyme differentiates to form a subcutaneous layer, a body layer, and a retroperitoneal layer. The retroperitoneal layer forms three strata in late fetal development: the outer stratum, intermediate stratum, and inner stratum (eFig. 75.15 on ExpertConsult.com). Historically, the retroperitoneum

> **KEY POINTS: ORGANS AND BOUNDARIES OF THE RETROPERITONEUM**
>
> - Retroperitoneal contents include the kidneys, ureters, adrenals, pancreas, portions of the duodenum, ascending colon, descending colon, mesentery, vasculature, lymphatics, and nervous structures.
> - The retroperitoneum is contained anteriorly by the posterior reflection of the peritoneum and posteriorly by the abdominal wall.
> - It is contained cranially and caudally by the diaphragm and the extraperitoneal pelvic structures, respectively.
> - The intercostal vessels and nerves travel between the internal intercostal and innermost intercostal muscles within the costal groove on the caudal margin of the superior rib.
> - The lumbodorsal fascia merges anterolaterally with the transversus abdominis muscle and is composed of three layers that cover the posterior abdominal wall musculature.

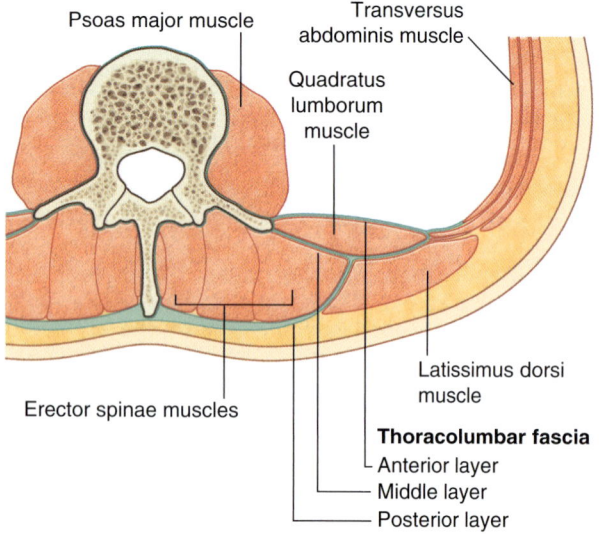

Fig. 75.12. Lumbodorsal fascia and the deep back muscle. (From Drake RL, Vogl AW, Mitchell AWM: *Gray's anatomy for students,* ed 2, Philadelphia, 2010, Churchill Livingstone.)

has been divided embryologically based on these three strata (Tobin, 1944). The **outer stratum** covers the epimysium of the abdominal wall muscles and becomes the transversalis fascia. The **intermediate stratum** is associated with the genitourinary organs, and the **inner stratum** is associated with the gastrointestinal organs (MacLennan, 2012). The aim is not to have the reader memorize what each embryologic stratum becomes during development. **Rather, these embryologic strata categorize the retroperitoneal fasciae, which compartmentalize various spaces within the retroperitoneum.**

Transversalis Fascia and Posterior Pararenal Space

The outer stratum forms the **transversalis fascia**, which lies deep to the transversus abdominis muscle and superficial to the preperitoneal fat and peritoneum. Posterior to the kidney, the transversalis fascia remains anterior to the fascia surrounding the quadratus

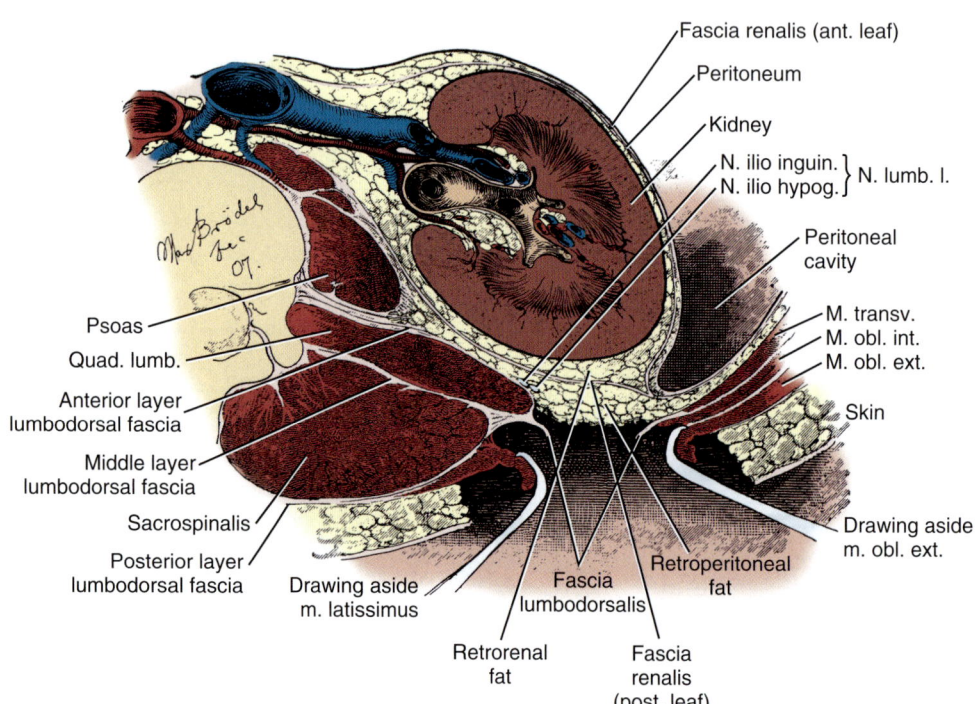

Fig. 75.13. Transverse section through the kidney and posterior abdominal wall showing the lumbodorsal fascia incised. Through such a lumbodorsal incision, the kidney can be reached without incising muscle. (From McVay C: *Anson & McVay surgical anatomy,* ed 6, Philadelphia, 1994, Saunders.)

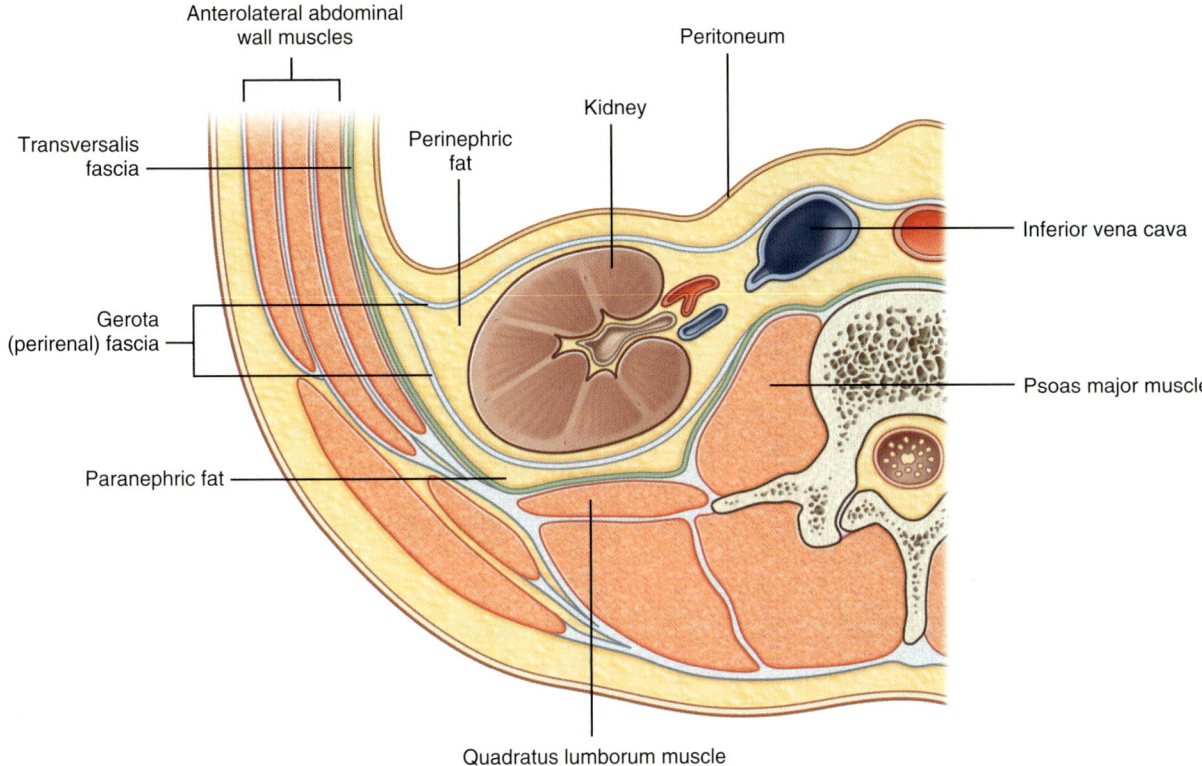

Fig. 75.16. Organization of the fasciae and fat surrounding the kidney. (From Drake RL, Vogl AW, Mitchell AWM: *Gray's anatomy for students,* ed 2, Philadelphia, 2010, Churchill Livingstone.)

lumborum and psoas muscle (Fig. 75.16). **It may fuse medially with the posterior lamina of Gerota fascia, which is of clinical significance during retroperitoneal dissection because this fascia must be incised to allow access to the renal hilum.** This fusion creates the medial boundary of the **posterior pararenal space.** The anterior boundary is formed by the posterior lamina of Gerota fascia, and the posterior and lateral boundaries are formed by the transversalis fascia (Tobin, 1944).

Gerota Fascia (Renal Fascia) and Perirenal Space

The **anterior lamina** (fascia of Toldt or prerenal fascia) and the **posterior lamina** (fascia of Zuckerkandl or retrorenal fascia) of the renal fascia are derived from the intermediate stratum, which embeds the genitourinary organs. **They help to form the boundaries of the retroperitoneal spaces: the posterior pararenal space, perirenal space, and anterior pararenal space** (Figs. 75.17 and 75.18; also see 75.16). The two laminae together form the **renal fascia,** eponymously named *Gerota fascia,* after the Romanian anatomist Dimitrie D. Gerota (1867–1939). The **perirenal space** contains the adrenal, kidney, ureter, perirenal fat, renal vascular pedicle, and gonadal vessels. The perirenal fat is finer and lighter yellow than the coarser yellow-orange pararenal fat. This color distinction can be helpful during colon mobilization for retroperitoneal surgery. The anatomy of the adrenal, kidney, and ureter is discussed in detail in their respective chapters.

The posterior lamina of Gerota fascia is thicker and more frequently visualized radiographically than the anterior lamina. These two layers merge laterally to form the **lateroconal fascia,** which separates the anterior and posterior pararenal spaces and continues anterolaterally deep to the transversalis fascia. There is some controversy regarding the medial and inferior extents of the perirenal space. Historically, it was assumed that there was no communication between the right and left perirenal spaces. However, based on in vivo cases and cadaveric injection studies, **there may be some communication across the midline below the level of the renal hilum** (Lim et al., 1998).

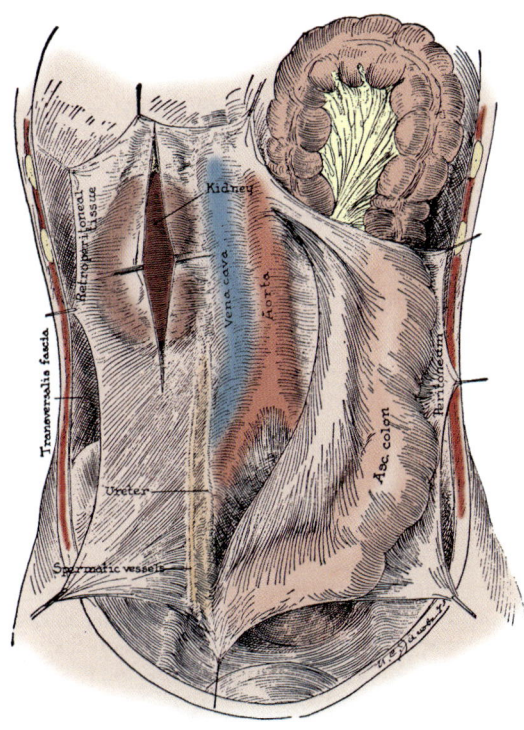

Fig. 75.17. Anterior view of Gerota fascia on the right side, split over the right kidney (which it contains) and showing inferior extension enveloping the ureter and gonadal vessels. The ascending colon and overlying peritoneum have been reflected medially. (From Tobin CE: The renal fascia and its relation to the transversalis fascia. *Anat Rec* 89:295–311, 1944.)

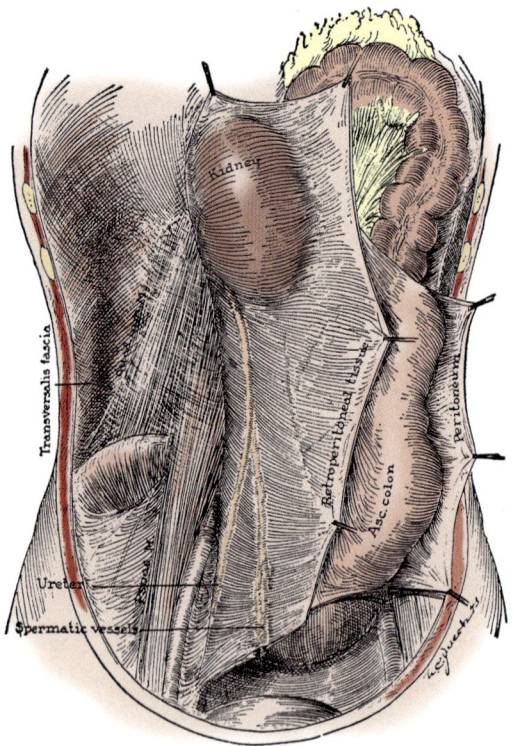

Fig. 75.18. Posterior view of Gerota fascia on the right side, rotated medially with the contained kidney, ureter, and gonadal vessels, exposing the muscular posterior body wall covered by the transversalis fascia. (From Tobin CE: The renal fascia and its relation to the transversalis fascia. *Anat Rec* 89:295–311, 1944.)

In addition, there has been no consensus on the patency and caudal extent of the perirenal space. Previously, it was suggested that the perirenal space is closed inferiorly by the fusion of Gerota fascia. However, in vivo cases and cadaveric injection studies demonstrated that the **perirenal space has a conelike shape that is open at its inferior extent in the extraperitoneal pelvis** (Lim et al., 1998). These boundaries are of clinical significance in the pathology of urologic disease because they function to contain perinephric fluid collections, which include urine (traumatic or iatrogenic urinary extravasation, obstructive uropathy with calyceal rupture), blood (traumatic or iatrogenic perinephric hematoma, ruptured aneurysm), or purulence (perinephric abscess or infected urinoma).

Anterior Pararenal Space and Inner Stratum

The **anterior pararenal space** is formed by the anterior lamina of the renal fascia posteriorly and the posterior layer of parietal peritoneum anteriorly (eFig. 75.19 on ExpertConsult.com). Clinically, this space is significant because it can be developed to gain access to the kidney anteriorly when followed medially from the **white line of Toldt**. This classic landmark is created during embryogenesis when the inner stratum forms a multilayer fusion fascia with the primary dorsal peritoneum during the rotation and posterior attachment of the gastrointestinal viscera (eFig. 75.20 on ExpertConsult.com). **During this event, the white line of Toldt is formed at the lateral border of the fusion of the colonic mesentery with the posterior peritoneum.**

The anterior pararenal space contains the secondarily retroperitoneal organs: the ascending and descending colon, pancreas, and second and third portions of the duodenum. These organs are intraperitoneal at one point during embryogenesis; however, they become retroperitoneal secondarily as they attach to the posterior abdominal wall when the inner stratum fuses with the primary dorsal peritoneum.

> **KEY POINTS: RETROPERITONEAL FASCIAE AND SPACES**
>
> - The boundaries of the posterior pararenal space are the posterior lamina of Gerota fascia anteriorly and the transversalis fascia posteriorly and laterally.
> - The anterior and posterior laminae of Gerota fascia form the boundaries of the perirenal space, which has a conelike shape that is open caudally in the extraperitoneal pelvis.
> - Perinephric fluid collections can expand caudally because of the opening in the perirenal space.
> - The white line of Toldt represents the lateral border of the fusion of the colonic mesentery with the posterior peritoneum.

GASTROINTESTINAL VISCERA AND MESENTERY

The nonurologic structures within the retroperitoneum include the pancreas and parts of the duodenum and the colon (Figs. 75.21 and 75.22). The **pancreas** consists of four parts and has endocrine and exocrine functions. The head lies anterior to the IVC and is surrounded by the second portion of the duodenum. This portion is of concern for potential injury during right kidney procedures. The neck connects the head to the body, which crosses the abdomen anterior to the aorta and the origin of the superior mesenteric artery (SMA). **The tail of the pancreas is closely associated with the spleen and must be accounted for during left retroperitoneal surgery because of its proximity to the upper pole of the left kidney and left adrenal.** In addition, the stomach is anterior to the upper pole of the left kidney and must be accounted for during transperitoneal left renal surgery (eFig. 75.23 on ExpertConsult.com).

The **duodenum** is 20 cm to 25 cm in length and can be divided into four distinct parts. The first (superior) portion is intraperitoneal and extends from the pylorus to the neck of the gallbladder. The second (descending) and third (horizontal or inferior) portions of the duodenum are contained within the retroperitoneum. **The second, descending portion of the duodenum is critical to the urologist because of its proximity to the right renal hilum. The duodenum may be mobilized medially using a *Kocher maneuver* to expose these right-sided retroperitoneal structures.** During left-sided retroperitoneal surgery, as the colon is reflected medially the mesentery thins and the duodenum can be encountered. The common bile duct and the main pancreatic duct combine to enter the second portion of the duodenum at the ampulla of Vater (hepatopancreatic ampulla). The third portion of the duodenum crosses the body from right to left and lies posterior to the SMA and anterior to the aorta. The fourth and final portion ascends and becomes intraperitoneal as it transitions into the jejunum.

As with the duodenum, portions of the colon are secondarily retroperitoneal because they developed intraperitoneally but fused with the posterior abdominal wall during embryogenesis. The **ascending colon** and hepatic flexure overlie the right-sided retroperitoneal structures, and the splenic flexure and **descending colon** cover the left-sided retroperitoneal structures. To gain access to the kidneys transperitoneally, the ipsilateral colon must be reflected medially in most instances. This can be performed by mobilizing the colon at the white line of Toldt, which visually represents the transition from the colonic visceral peritoneum to the posterior parietal peritoneum. **Care must be taken to divide the hepatocolic and splenocolic ligaments sharply when necessary to avoid iatrogenic injury to the liver and spleen, which is often due to excessive retraction during attempts to obtain adequate exposure.**

Recent investigations have begun to classify the mesentery as a distinct organ that has intestinal, vascular, immunologic, and endocrine function. Initial early depictions of the mesentery by Leonardo Da Vinci showed a continuous structure from the small bowel to the colon. However, in the late 1800s, a fragmented mesenteric model was adopted with no mesentery associated with the ascending or descending colon (Coffey and O'Leary, 2016). **Continuity of the mesentery from the ileocecal level to the rectosigmoid level was**

Chapter 75 Surgical, Radiographic, and Endoscopic Anatomy of the Retroperitoneum **1669**

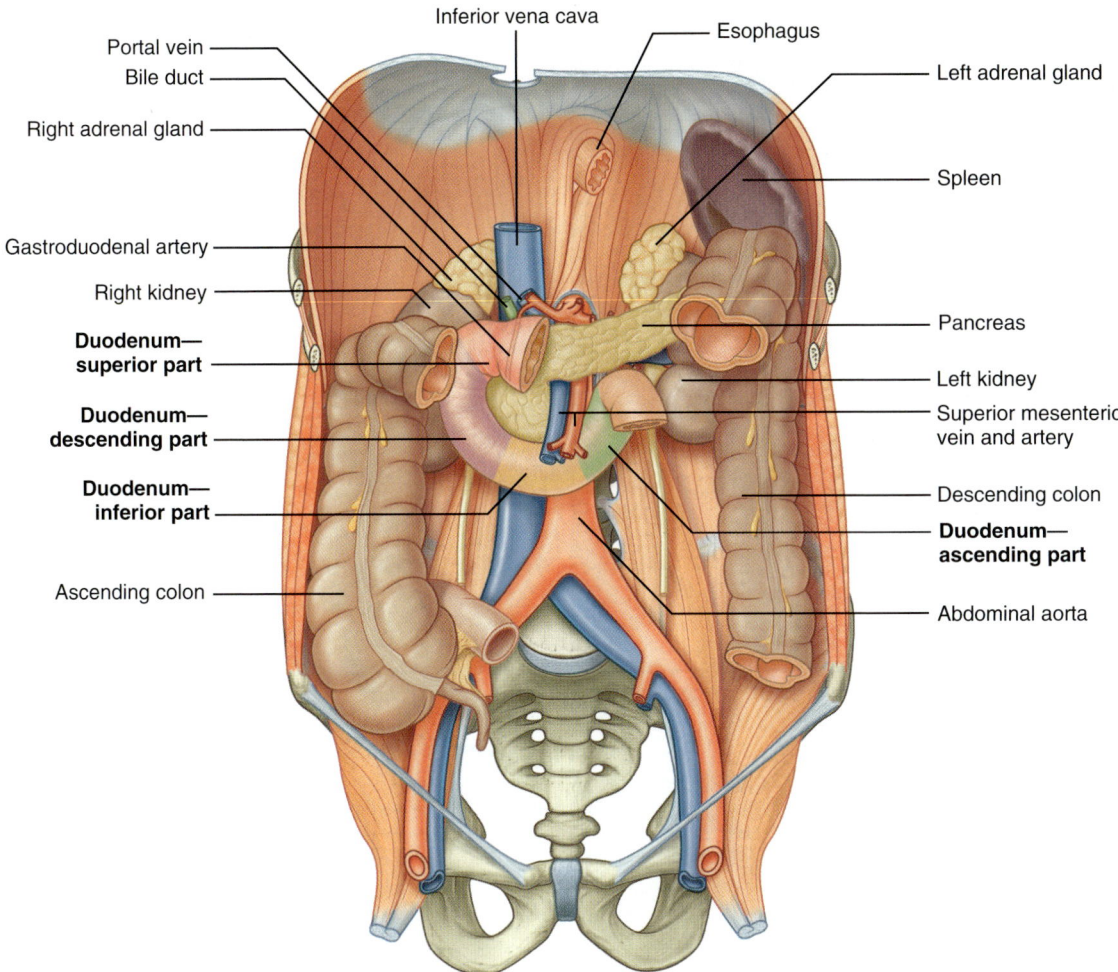

Fig. 75.21. Colon, duodenum, and pancreas within the retroperitoneum. (From Drake RL, Vogl AW, Mitchell AWM: *Gray's anatomy for students,* ed 2, Philadelphia, 2010, Churchill Livingstone.)

established in an observational cohort study of patients undergoing total abdominal colectomy for colon cancer (Culligan et al., 2012).

The function of the mesentery is linked with its physiology and anatomy. It acts as a scaffolding for the small and large intestines, suspending these structures from the posterior abdominal wall. As the mesentery is the first barrier between the intestines and the body, it also acts as a sampling reservoir for systemic immune responses. **Mesenteric nodes regulate the cell-mediated immune response with the adjacent intestinal mucosa.** Although the mesenteric component of the enteric nervous system is poorly understood at this time, it houses the postganglionic nerves from the main abdominal ganglia (Coffey and O'Leary, 2016).

Several mesenteric disease processes are of important clinical significance to the practicing urologist. **Internal herniation resulting from surgically created mesenteric defects can cause a potentially life-threatening postoperative complication.** After bowel segment isolation, it is imperative that small defects in the mesentery are closed primarily because the risk of herniation is higher in these cases. Vascular mesenteropathies are also of clinical significance as vascular compromise of the mesenteric arteries can result in loss of an intestinal segment used for urinary diversion, ureteral interposition, or bladder augmentation (Coffey and O'Leary, 2016).

VASCULATURE
Arterial System

Arterial structures have three layers: the tunica intima (intima), tunica media (media), and tunica externa (tunica adventitia or adventitia)

as shown in eFig. 75.24 on ExpertConsult.com. The **intima** consists of a layer of endothelial cells surrounded by subendothelial connective tissue. The **media** layer contains vascular smooth muscle cells and elastic connective tissue that control the caliber of the vessel. This layer is surrounded by the internal and external elastic laminae. The **adventitia** is the connective tissue sheath surrounding the vessel. It contains the nerves that control vasomotor tone and the *vasa vasorum* (Latin, "vessels of the vessels"), which are smaller vessels that supply the walls of larger vessels.

The major arterial structures of the retroperitoneum include the abdominal aorta (eFig. 75.25 on ExpertConsult.com and Fig. 75.26) and its branches (Fig. 75.27 and Table 75.3). Entering the abdomen through the aortic hiatus of the diaphragm at the level of T12, the **abdominal aorta** courses centrally and to the left of the IVC. The first branches are the paired **inferior phrenic arteries,** which supply the inferior surface of the diaphragm (eFig. 75.28 on ExpertConsult.com). The **superior adrenal artery** branches from the inferior phrenic artery and supplies the ipsilateral adrenal gland. **The superior arterial blood supply to the adrenal is constant; however, the middle and inferior arteries to the adrenal are variable. These arteries vary in number and location with the most common variant being the middle adrenal artery arising from the aorta and the inferior adrenal arising from the renal artery.**

The next branch of the abdominal aorta is the **celiac artery** (celiac trunk or truncus coeliacus), which is a short, unpaired artery that arises anteriorly at the midline at the level of T12. It gives origin to the left gastric, splenic, and common hepatic arteries, which supply the abdominal esophagus, stomach, duodenum, spleen, liver, and pancreas. Of surgical anatomic significance, the splenic vessels course

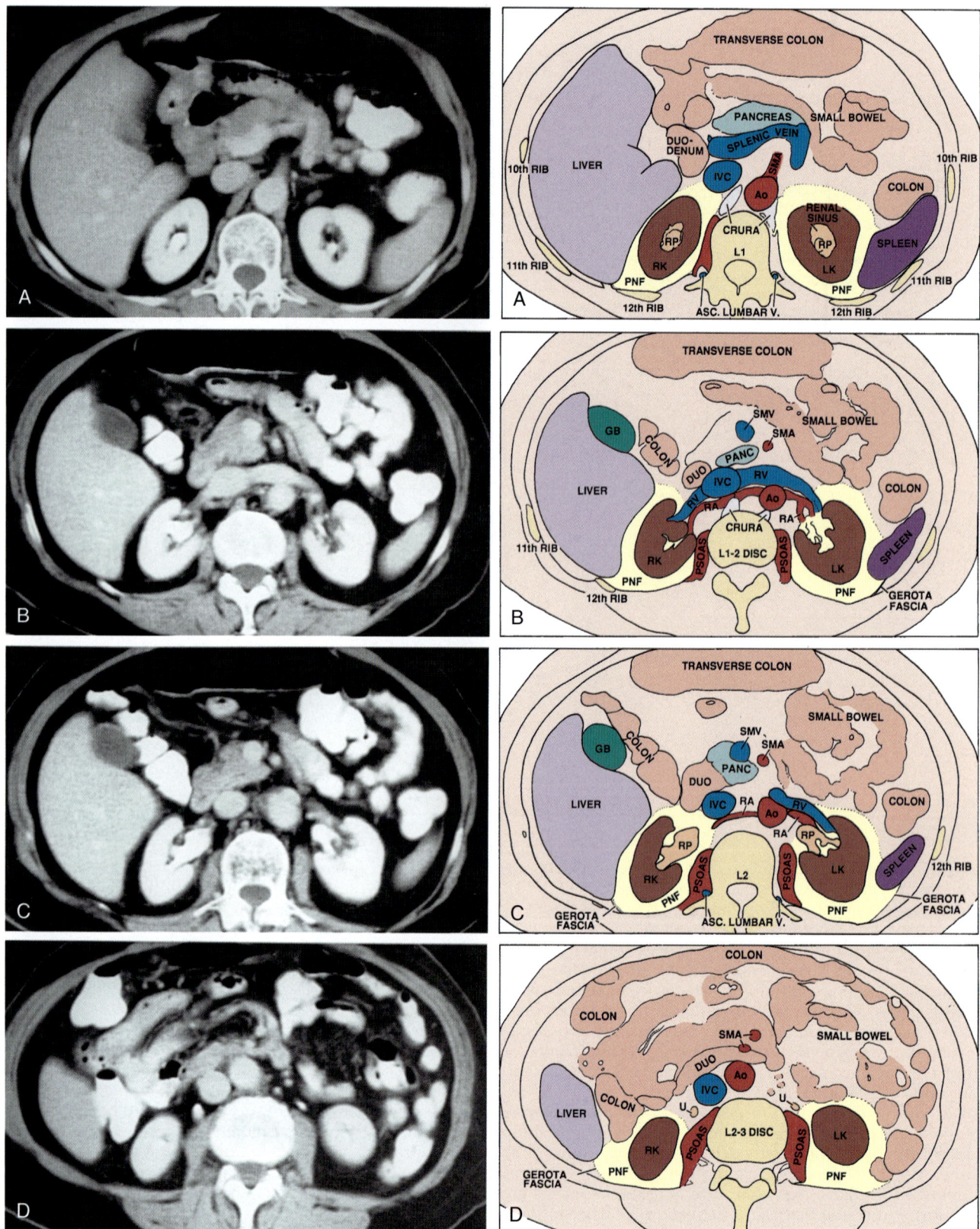

Fig. 75.22. Cross-sectional anatomy of the upper abdomen at the level of the kidneys demonstrated with transverse sections obtained by computed tomography. Sections are arranged from most cephalic to caudal. (A) Section through the upper poles of the kidneys, superior to the renal vascular pedicles. (B) Section through the level of the renal arteries and veins. (C) Slightly more inferior section showing the renal pelves and relationship of the duodenum to the right renal hilum. (D) Section through the lower poles of the kidneys showing the upper ureters. *Ao,* Aorta; *DUO,* duodenum; *GB,* gallbladder; *IVC,* inferior vena cava; *LK,* left kidney; *PANC,* pancreas; *PNF,* perinephric fat; *RA,* renal artery; *RK,* right kidney; *RP,* renal pelvis; *RV,* renal vein; *SMA,* superior mesenteric artery; *SMV,* superior mesenteric vein; *U,* ureter.

Chapter 75 Surgical, Radiographic, and Endoscopic Anatomy of the Retroperitoneum **1671**

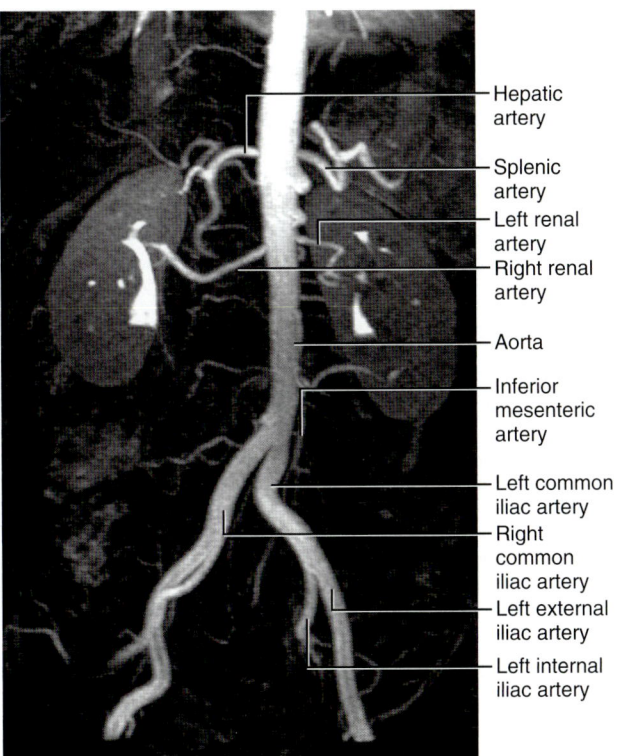

Fig. 75.26. Computed tomography angiogram of the abdominal aorta and its branches. (From MacLennan GT: *Hinman's atlas of urosurgical anatomy*, ed 2, Philadelphia, 2012, Saunders.)

on the cephalad aspect of the body and tail of the pancreas. When the inferior pancreatic edge is mobilized off the anterior renal fascia during adrenal or renal transperitoneal surgery, knowledge of the anatomic relationship between the splenic vessels and the pancreas is important to prevent vascular injury. The next branches are the paired middle adrenal arteries, which supply the ipsilateral adrenal gland as noted earlier.

The **superior mesenteric artery (SMA)** branches next off the aorta, arising anteriorly in the midline at approximately the level of the middle adrenal arteries at L1-L2. It supplies the pancreas (inferior pancreaticoduodenal artery), small intestine, and most of the large intestine (ileocolic, right colic, and middle colic arteries). **The middle colic artery anastomoses with the left colic artery off the inferior mesenteric artery (IMA) via the marginal artery of Drummond. This anastomosis forms an important SMA-to-IMA collateral circulation that allows for the IMA to be sacrificed without colonic ischemia** (Walker, 2009). However, despite the presence of this collateral circulation, injury to the SMA during left-sided retroperitoneal surgery may lead to severe bowel ischemia.

The paired **renal arteries** are the next branch of the aorta (eFig. 75.29 on ExpertConsult.com). These classically arise at the L1-L2 vertebral levels. The inferior adrenal arteries branch off the renal arteries to supply the ipsilateral adrenal gland. There is considerable variation in the location, size, and number of renal arteries, with at least one quarter of cases manifesting with supernumerary renal arteries. There is no clear consensus on whether supernumerary arteries are more common on the right or the left. In a study out of India examining 37 cadavers, 23 (62.2%) were found to have supernumerary renal arteries on the right with 21 (56.8%) on the left (Budhiraja et al., 2013). There are variations between genders as well, with renal arteries in female patients being approximately 5 mm smaller on average than male patients based on CT angiographic

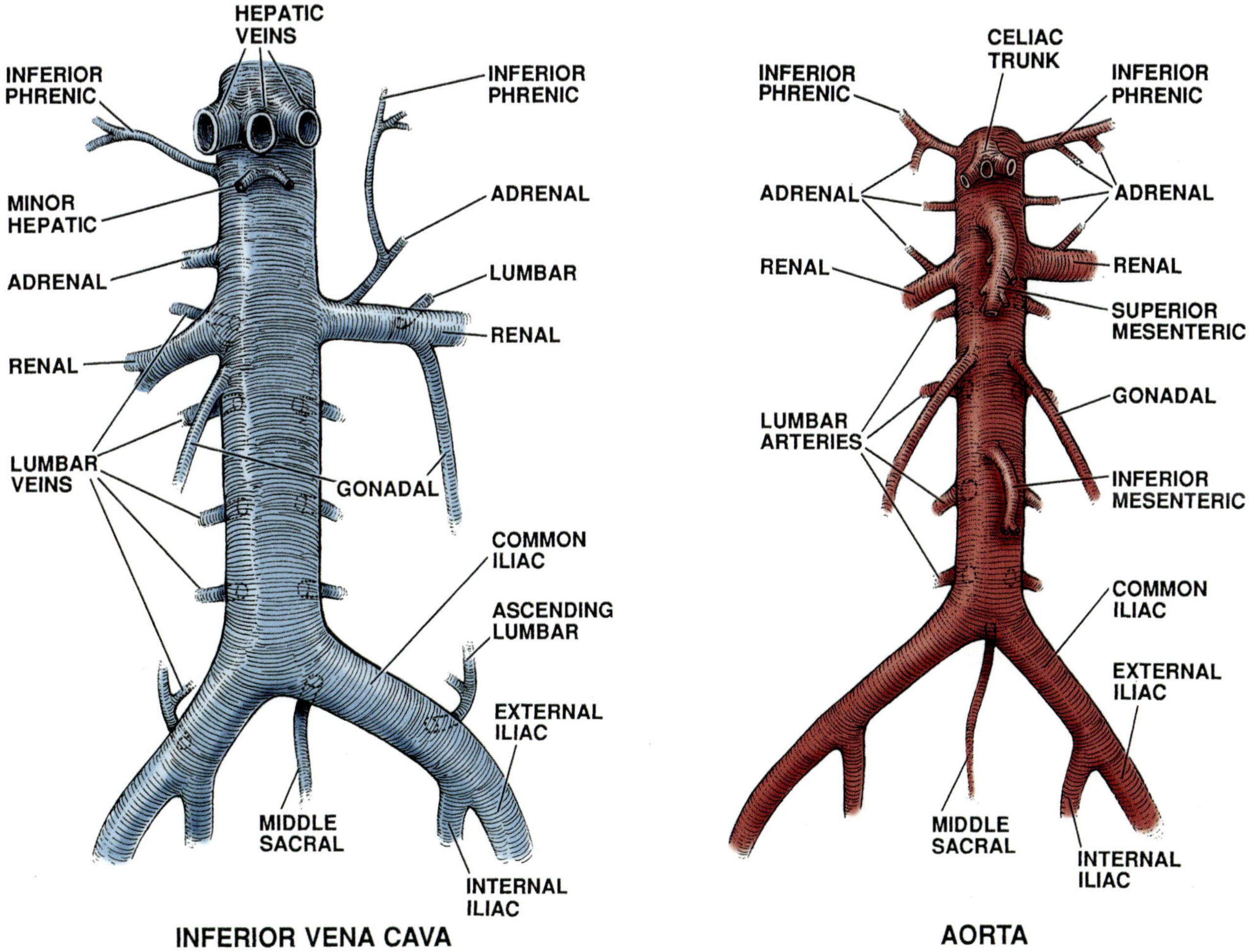

Fig. 75.27. Inferior vena cava and its tributaries and abdominal aorta and its branches.

TABLE 75.3 Branches of the Abdominal Aorta

ARTERY	BRANCH	ORIGIN	SUPPLIES
Celiac trunk	Anterior	Immediately inferior to aortic hiatus of diaphragm	Abdominal foregut
Superior mesenteric artery	Anterior	Immediately inferior to celiac trunk	Abdominal midgut
Inferior mesenteric artery	Anterior	Inferior to renal arteries	Abdominal hindgut
Middle adrenal arteries	Lateral	Immediately superior to renal arteries	Adrenal glands
Renal arteries	Lateral	Immediately inferior to superior mesenteric artery	Kidneys
Testicular or ovarian arteries	Paired anterior	Inferior to renal arteries	Testes in male and ovaries in female
Inferior phrenic arteries	Paired lateral	Immediately inferior to aortic hiatus	Diaphragm
Lumbar arteries	Posterior	Usually four pairs	Posterior abdominal wall and spinal cord
Median sacral arteries	Posterior	Just superior to aortic bifurcation, pass inferiorly across lumbar vertebrae, sacrum, and coccyx	
Common iliac arteries	Terminal	Bifurcation usually occurs at level of L4 vertebra	

Modified from Drake RL, Vogl AW, Mitchell AWM: *Gray's anatomy for students*, Philadelphia, 2005, Churchill Livingstone, p 331.

studies (Turba et al., 2009). The specific anatomic variations are discussed in depth in Chapter 84.

The **gonadal arteries** are the next paired branch of the aorta, typically arising anterolaterally from the aorta below the renal arteries. They may emerge from the renal artery in some variations, in which case they course with the gonadal vein. In males, the gonadal arteries are called the **testicular arteries,** and in females, they are called the **ovarian arteries.** The testicular arteries typically run anterior to the psoas, IVC, genitofemoral nerve, and ipsilateral ureter as they travel toward the internal inguinal ring.

The ovarian arteries arise from the anterolateral aspect of the aorta below the renal arteries. They travel anterior to the ureter and course medially as they pass through the infundibulopelvic ligament (suspensory ligament of the ovary) to the ovary. **There are extensive collaterals to the gonads in both sexes, allowing for ligation of the testicular and ovarian arteries without gonadal ischemia.**

The paired **lumbar arteries** arise posteriorly, adjacent to the bodies of the upper four lumbar vertebrae. They supply the posterior body wall and spine. In some instances, a fifth pair of lumbar arteries is present, arising from the middle sacral artery.

The **inferior mesenteric artery (IMA)** arises from the anterior aorta in the midline at the level of L3-L4 and supplies the colon from the splenic flexure to the upper rectum. The branches of the IMA are the left colic, sigmoid, and superior hemorrhoidal (rectal) arteries. The **sigmoid artery** branches into two to three inferior left colic arteries. As previously mentioned, the colonic branches of the IMA anastomose with the SMA via the marginal artery of Drummond and preclude colonic ischemia with IMA ligation. **The superior hemorrhoidal artery has collateral circulation with the inferior and middle hemorrhoidal arteries, which branch off the internal iliac arteries. These collaterals provide blood supply to the rectum and prevent ischemia during IMA ligation.**

Before bifurcation, the **median sacral** (middle sacral) artery arises from the posterior aspect of the aorta and courses over the fifth lumbar vertebra and sacrum. This vessel may be sacrificed if necessary without end-organ ischemia. At the fourth lumbar vertebra, the aorta bifurcates to form the **common iliac arteries.** No named branches are given off as these arteries enter the pelvis and divide to form the internal and external iliac arteries.

The ureter has a variable arterial supply that changes proximally and distally. **Most often, the renal artery supplies the proximal ureter, and the internal iliac artery, including its branches, the superior and inferior vesical arteries, supply the distal ureter. The middle ureter is typically supplied by the aorta; however, it may also be supplied by the common iliac, gonadal, uterine, middle rectal, and vaginal arteries. In general, the abdominal (proximal) ureter receives its blood supply medially, and the pelvic (distal) ureter receives its blood supply from a lateral direction.**

Venous System

Although not as well defined, the layers of the venous system are similar to that of the arterial system. The layers from innermost to outermost are the intima, internal elastic lamina, media, external elastic lamina, and adventitia. As in the arterial system, the intima is composed of a layer of endothelial cells with subendothelial connective tissue. In the venous system, the internal and external elastic laminae are often poorly defined even in larger caliber vessels. The media layer of veins is significantly smaller than that of arteries and contains less vascular smooth muscle. Conversely, the venous adventitia is larger than the venous media and functions similar to the adventitia of the arterial system.

The venous system also differs from the arterial system with the presence of valves that prevent retrograde flow. These valves are typically bicuspid, and they function to maintain the full venous blood flow toward the heart.

The major retroperitoneal venous structure is the **inferior vena cava (IVC),** formed from the confluence of the **common iliac veins,** inferior and to the right of the aortic bifurcation (see Fig. 75.27). The IVC ascends anterior to the vertebral bodies and to the right of the aorta through the retroperitoneum (eFigs. 75.30 and 75.31 on ExpertConsult.com). The infrarenal portion runs parallel and inferior to the aorta. On its ascent, the IVC becomes more anterior, and at the level of the diaphragm the great vessels are separated by the right crus of the diaphragm. **The IVC then enters the thorax through the central tendon of the diaphragm at the level of T8 and drains into the inferior aspect of the right atrium.**

The venous system is more variable than the arterial system; however, many venous structures run parallel with their arterial equivalent. The **median (middle) sacral vein** runs with its respective artery and typically drains into the left common iliac vein; however, it may enter into the angle created by convergence of the two common iliac veins. Avoiding these veins during fixation of the proximal limb of mesh during sacral colpopexy procedures is critical.

The **ascending lumbar veins** drain the posterior abdominal wall and run posterior to the psoas muscle and lateral to the spinal column (eFig. 75.32 on ExpertConsult.com). They connect with the ipsilateral **lumbar veins,** which are variable in number and location compared with their arterial equivalents. These veins may assume a plexiform arrangement anterior to the vertebral bodies. **As the ascending lumbar veins enter the thorax, they become the hemiazygos vein on the left and the azygos vein on the right.**

In males, the **gonadal veins (testicular veins)** receive drainage from the pampiniform plexus, which is the venous complex that emerges from the testes. The testicular veins ascend through the retroperitoneum medially, running lateral to the respective artery and anterior to the ipsilateral ureter. The left testicular vein typically enters the inferior aspect of the left renal vein at a right angle; however, it may enter the IVC directly. The right testicular vein typically enters into the right anterolateral aspect of the IVC; however, it may enter into the right renal vein in up to 10% of cases. **These anatomic differences have clinical significance because the increased length and perpendicular entry of the left testicular vein into the left renal vein may account for the increased incidence of left-sided varicoceles.** This anatomic configuration may result in some element of increased back pressure in the left testicular vein compared with the right side. With the relative rarity of unilateral right-sided varicocele, a sudden-onset right varicocele should increase suspicion for a renal or retroperitoneal malignancy causing obstruction and poor venous outflow (e.g., right side renal cell cancer with venous thrombus). This clinical scenario should warrant retroperitoneal imaging to rule out malignancy. Further clinical significance exists with this anatomic distinction after mobilization of the colon in transperitoneal retroperitoneal surgery. During the identification of the ureter on the right, the plane is developed lateral to the gonadal, which leaves the gonadal vein in a medial position. If the plane medial to the gonadal vein is developed, there is a risk of injury to the IVC and with elevation of the kidney avulsion of the gonadal may occur.

The **ovarian veins** receive drainage from the pampiniform plexus adjacent to the ovarian hilum and travel through the infundibulopelvic ligament. As with the gonadal veins in males, the left ovarian vein enters the left renal vein, and the right ovarian vein empties into the anterolateral wall of the vena cava.

The **renal veins** course anteriorly to the renal arteries and empty into the lateral aspects of the vena cava at the level of L1. The right and left renal veins differ in length and tributaries with the right being shorter and typically having no tributaries. In rare cases, the right gonadal vein or a lumbar vein may empty into the right renal vein. In one-sixth of cases, the renal vein is duplicated on the right side. The left renal vein is longer and typically receives the left gonadal vein at its caudal margin. At least one lumbar vein enters the left renal vein at or near the ostia of the gonadal vein. **The left adrenal vein is situated at the superior margin of the renal vein and, in most patients, inserts into the renal vein just medial to the gonadal vein.** The left adrenal vein occasionally is joined by the left inferior phrenic vein. The **right adrenal vein** is short, is single, has no tributaries, and drains directly into the posterolateral aspect of the vena cava. Although variable, the right inferior phrenic vein also typically drains into the superior portion of the IVC.

The gastrointestinal venous drainage does not mirror the arterial system as directly as the aforementioned venous structures. **The portal venous system receives venous blood from the bowel, spleen, pancreas, and gallbladder to be emptied into the liver** (Fig. 75.33). The **superior mesenteric vein (SMV)** receives venous drainage from the small intestine and the large intestine proximal to the splenic flexure. Tributaries of the SMV include the right gastroepiploic, anterior and posterior inferior pancreaticoduodenal, jejunal, ileal, ileocolic, right colic, and middle colic veins. The SMV is joined by the splenic vein to form the **portal vein**. The tributaries of the **splenic vein** are

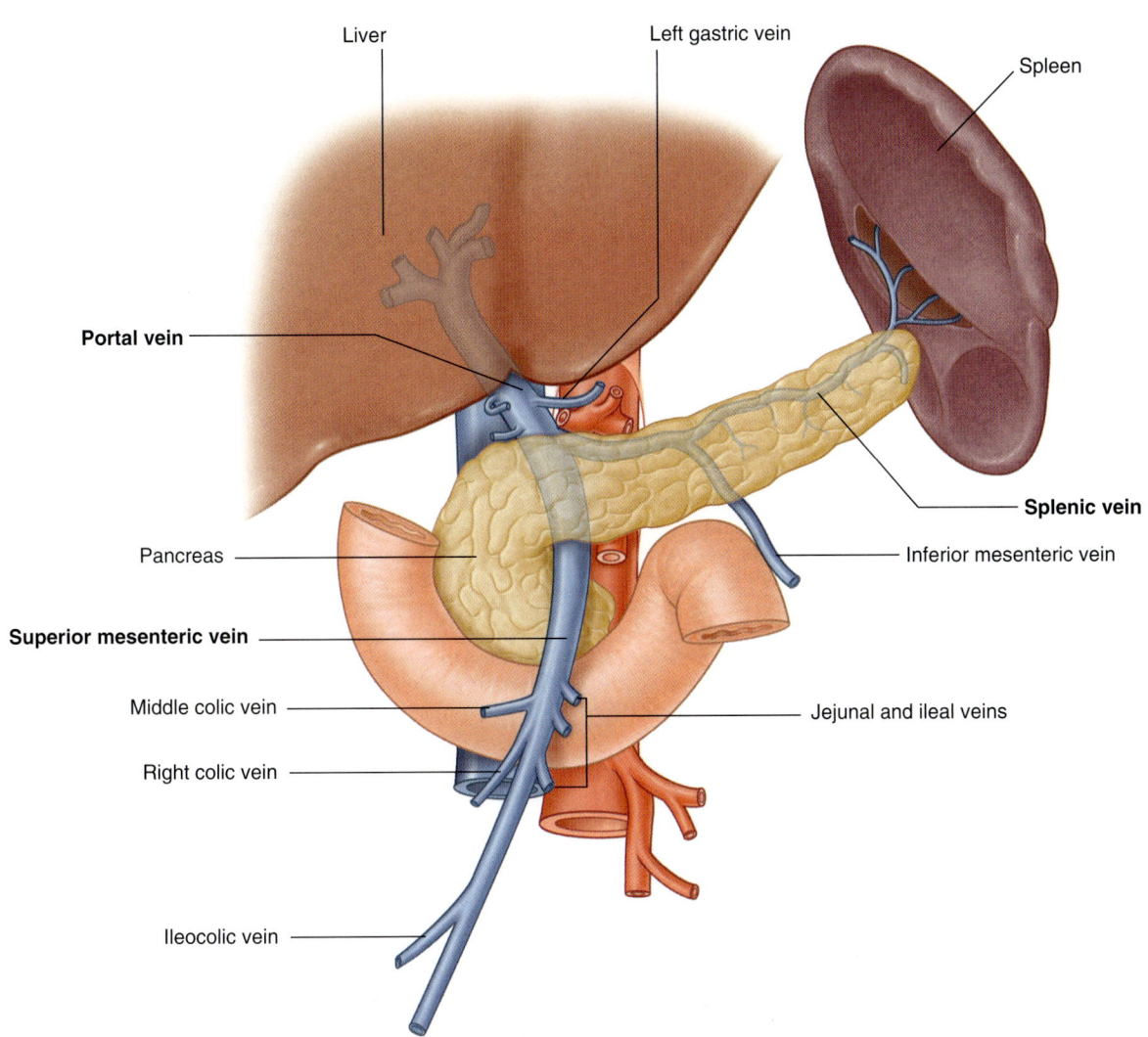

Fig. 75.33. Portal vein and its tributaries. (From Drake RL, Vogl AW, Mitchell AWM: *Gray's anatomy for students*, ed 2, Philadelphia, 2010, Churchill Livingstone.)

the inferior mesenteric, short gastric, left gastroepiploic, and pancreatic veins. The **inferior mesenteric vein** (IMV) drains into the SMV instead of the splenic vein in 40% of cases (Feller and Woodburne, 1961). The IMV receives the venous drainage from the colon distal to the splenic flexure. When the colon is reflected medially for left-sided retroperitoneal surgery, the IMV can often be identified within the mesocolon. Also during re-operative retroperitoneal procedures, the IMV can potentially be mistaken for the gonadal vein during colon mobilization as the mesentery may be adherent to the Gerota fascia.

The portal vein splits into right and left branches, and the venous blood enters the endothelial lined hepatic sinusoids. After passing through these sinusoids, the venous blood leaves the liver through the hepatic veins, which enter the anterior aspect of the IVC before it crosses the diaphragm into the thorax. There are two groups of hepatic veins: the upper group, typically larger in caliber, and the lower group, which are typically smaller. **Occlusion of these hepatic veins can lead to Budd-Chiari syndrome, which is a form of progressive liver failure that often manifests rapidly with jaundice, ascites, abdominal pain, and hepatomegaly.**

> ### KEY POINTS: RETROPERITONEAL VASCULATURE
> - The blood supply to the adrenal artery arises from the inferior phrenic artery, the aorta, and the renal artery.
> - The renal hila are at the level of L1, and the renal veins are anterior to the renal arteries.
> - The paired gonadal arteries typically arising anterolaterally from the aorta below the renal arteries.
> - The SMA to IMA collateral circulation occurs via the marginal artery of Drummond, which allows the IMA to be sacrificed without colonic ischemia.
> - In general, the proximal ureter receives its blood supply medially, and the distal ureter receives its blood supply from a lateral direction.
> - The left gonadal vein enters left renal vein at a right angle and the right gonadal vein enters into the IVC directly; this anatomic distinction results in higher rates of varicoceles on the left.

LYMPHATIC SYSTEM

The lymphatic channels line tissue spaces and transport lymph to specialized areas of lymphoid tissue called lymph nodes. **The nodes typically have multiple afferent lymphatics and a single efferent lymphatic that drains into larger lymphatic vessels. Lymph generally flows cephalad from right to left until it returns to the venous circulation at the left innominate (brachiocephalic) vein.** Lymphatic fluid from the head, neck, right thorax, right arm, and right heart drains into the right innominate vein.

The lymphatic fluid from the pelvis and lower extremities drains into the internal iliac, external iliac, common iliac, obturator, and sacral nodes. These nodal regions then drain cephalad toward the lumbar nodes, whose efferent lymphatics form the lumbar trunks (Parker, 1935). The lumbar nodes are of considerable interest to the urologist because they provide the primary lymphatic drainage for structures supplied by lateral aortic arterial branches: the kidneys, adrenals, ureters, and gonads (Fig. 75.34). **For anatomic classification, three groups of lumbar nodes can be defined: left lumbar (aortic), interaortocaval (interaorticovenous), and right lumbar (caval) nodal groups.**

The left lumbar group includes the preaortic, left para-aortic (periaortic), and retroaortic nodes. The preaortic nodes are located anterior to the abdominal aorta, around the major anterior arterial branches that supply the gastrointestinal tract. The celiac, superior mesenteric, and inferior mesenteric nodes receive lymphatic drainage based on the anatomy of the similarly named arteries that supply the corresponding abdominal viscera. The efferents of these lymphatics coalesce to form the intestinal trunk. The left para-aortic region includes the nodes lateral to the midline of the aorta and medial to the left ureter. The retroaortic nodes are variably present and located between the aorta and vertebrae. The interaortocaval nodal group extends from the midline of the IVC to the midline of the aorta.

The right lumbar group includes the precaval, right paracaval, and retrocaval nodes. The precaval nodes are located on the anterior wall of the IVC. The right paracaval region includes the area lateral to the midline of the IVC, extending to the right ureter. The retrocaval nodes are present between the vena cava and the psoas muscle.

The testes are significant because they are embryologically retroperitoneal and have retroperitoneal blood supply and primary lymphatic drainage. In a practical discussion of testis malignancy, the three significant nodal regions are the left para-aortic, interaortocaval, and right paracaval. Elegant studies of early metastasis demonstrated the drainage pattern of the testes. **The left testis drains to the left para-aortic nodes with some drainage to the interaortocaval nodes.** There is no significant drainage to the right paracaval nodes, which is consistent with the general direction of lymphatic flow from right to left. **The right testis drains primarily to the interaortocaval nodes with some drainage to the right paracaval nodes.** The left para-aortic region receives a small but appreciable amount of lymphatic drainage from the right testis, consistent with the aforementioned right-to-left flow.

The efferent lymphatics of the lateral lumbar nodes coalesce to form the right and left lumbar trunks. Posterior to the right side of the abdominal aorta and anterior to the L1 and L2 vertebrae, these trunks come together at a saccular dilated structure known as the **cisterna chyli**. This marks the beginning of the **thoracic duct**, which runs cephalad posterior to the aorta and empties into the left innominate vein.

> ### KEY POINTS: RETROPERITONEAL LYMPHATIC SYSTEM
> - Testes are embryologically retroperitoneal and have retroperitoneal blood supply and primary lymphatic drainage.
> - The lymph of the left testis drains to the left para-aortic nodes with some drainage to the interaortocaval nodes.
> - The right testis drains primarily to the interaortocaval nodes with some to the right paracaval nodes and a small amount to the left para-aortic region.
> - The lymphatic drainage of the testicles is consistent with global lymphatic flow from right to left.

NERVOUS STRUCTURES

The nervous structures of the retroperitoneum can be divided into the autonomic nervous system and the somatic nervous system. The autonomic system supplies efferent and afferent innervation to the abdominal viscera, blood vessels, and smooth muscle. The somatic system supplies efferent and afferent innervation to skeletal muscle, skin, and peritoneum.

Autonomic Nervous System

The general structure of the **autonomic nervous system** consists of two nerves with two cell bodies. The **preganglionic neuron** has a cell body within the central nervous system and an axon that extends into the peripheral nervous system, synapsing with another neuron within a ganglion. The second neuron is referred to as a **postganglionic neuron,** and its axon enters the structure in which it provides innervation. One caveat to this general structure is the neural anatomy of the adrenal gland. **The preganglionic fibers synapse directly with the cells of the adrenal medulla, resulting in release of catecholamines. The adrenal can be considered a specialized ganglion of the autonomic nervous system.**

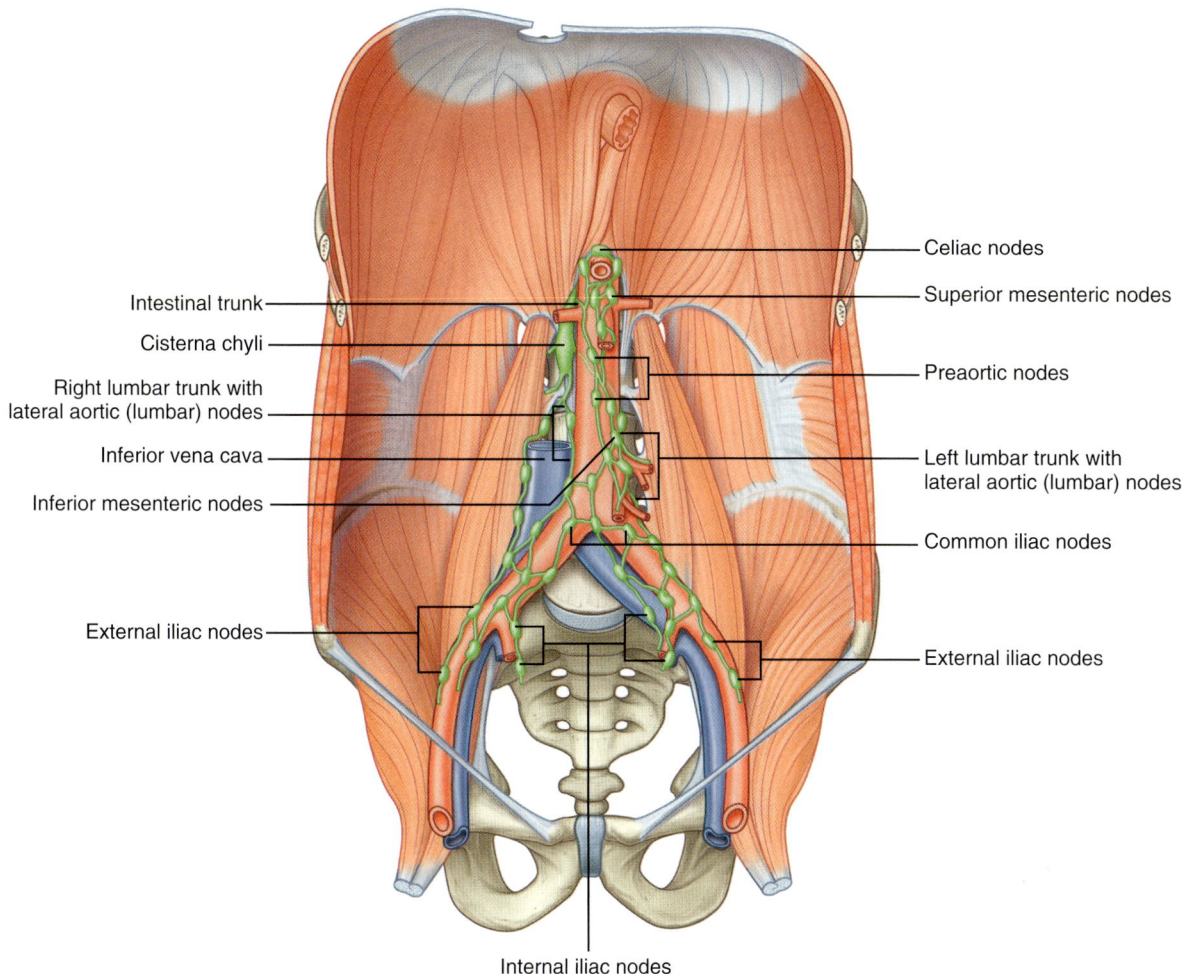

Fig. 75.34. Retroperitoneal lymphatics. (From Drake RL, Vogl AW, Mitchell AWM: *Gray's anatomy for students*, ed 2, Philadelphia, 2010, Churchill Livingstone.)

The autonomic system can be divided further into the parasympathetic and sympathetic nervous systems. The **parasympathetic nervous system** has craniosacral outflow because the preganglionic fibers originate from cranial nerves III, VII, IX, and X and from the ventral rami of the second, third, and fourth sacral nerves. The preganglionic fibers from S2-S4 form the pelvic splanchnic nerves, which provide parasympathetic innervation to the pelvic and abdominal viscera, which often contain the postganglionic parasympathetic fibers within their walls. The vagus nerve (cranial nerve X) also provides preganglionic parasympathetic fibers to the thoracic, abdominal, and pelvic viscera.

In contrast to the parasympathetic system, the preganglionic fibers of the **sympathetic nervous system** originate between the first thoracic and the second lumbar vertebral levels. These fibers exit the spinal cord from T1 to L2 through the ventral root and course through the corresponding spinal nerve and anterior rami into the ipsilateral sympathetic trunk (Fig. 75.35). The fibers then run medial to the psoas muscle along the anterolateral aspect of the spine. **The paired sympathetic trunks are in close proximity to the lumbar arteries and veins, which cross them perpendicularly.** The preganglionic fibers can synapse within the ganglia of the sympathetic trunk and send forth postganglionic fibers to the body wall and lower extremities. The preganglionic fibers also may leave the trunk as splanchnic nerves to synapse with the ganglia of the autonomic plexuses of the aorta (Fig. 75.36).

The first and largest of these plexuses is the celiac plexus, which contains paired ganglia that lie lateral to the celiac artery. Much of the autonomic innervation to the kidney, adrenal, renal pelvis, and ureter runs through this plexus. Some of the autonomic innervation for the testes passes through this plexus and travels caudally with the testicular artery. The renal autonomic plexus is continuous with the celiac plexus and forms adjacent to the renal arteries. It contains the aorticorenal ganglion, which is an inferior extension of the celiac ganglion.

Much of the sympathetic innervation to the pelvic viscera travels through the superior and inferior hypogastric plexuses, which are contiguous. The superior hypogastric plexus originates at the caudal extent of the abdominal aorta and extends to the anterior surface of the fifth lumbar vertebra. **Extensive retroperitoneal dissection that causes disruption of these plexuses may result in loss of seminal vesicle emission or failure of bladder neck closure, resulting in retrograde ejaculation.**

Confusion may arise with the term *splanchnic* used for nerves of the parasympathetic and the sympathetic systems (see Fig. 75.35). For clarification, the thoracic splanchnics (greater, lesser, and least), lumbar splanchnics, and sacral splanchnics carry sympathetic fibers from the paired sympathetic trunks to the autonomic plexuses, whereas the pelvic splanchnics carry parasympathetic fibers from the sacral outflow.

Somatic Nervous System

The somatic sensory and motor nerves of the lower abdomen and lower extremities originate in the retroperitoneum. They form the lumbosacral plexus from the anterior rami of the lumbar and sacral nerves along with T12 (eFig. 75.37 on ExpertConsult.com).

1676 PART VII Male Genitalia

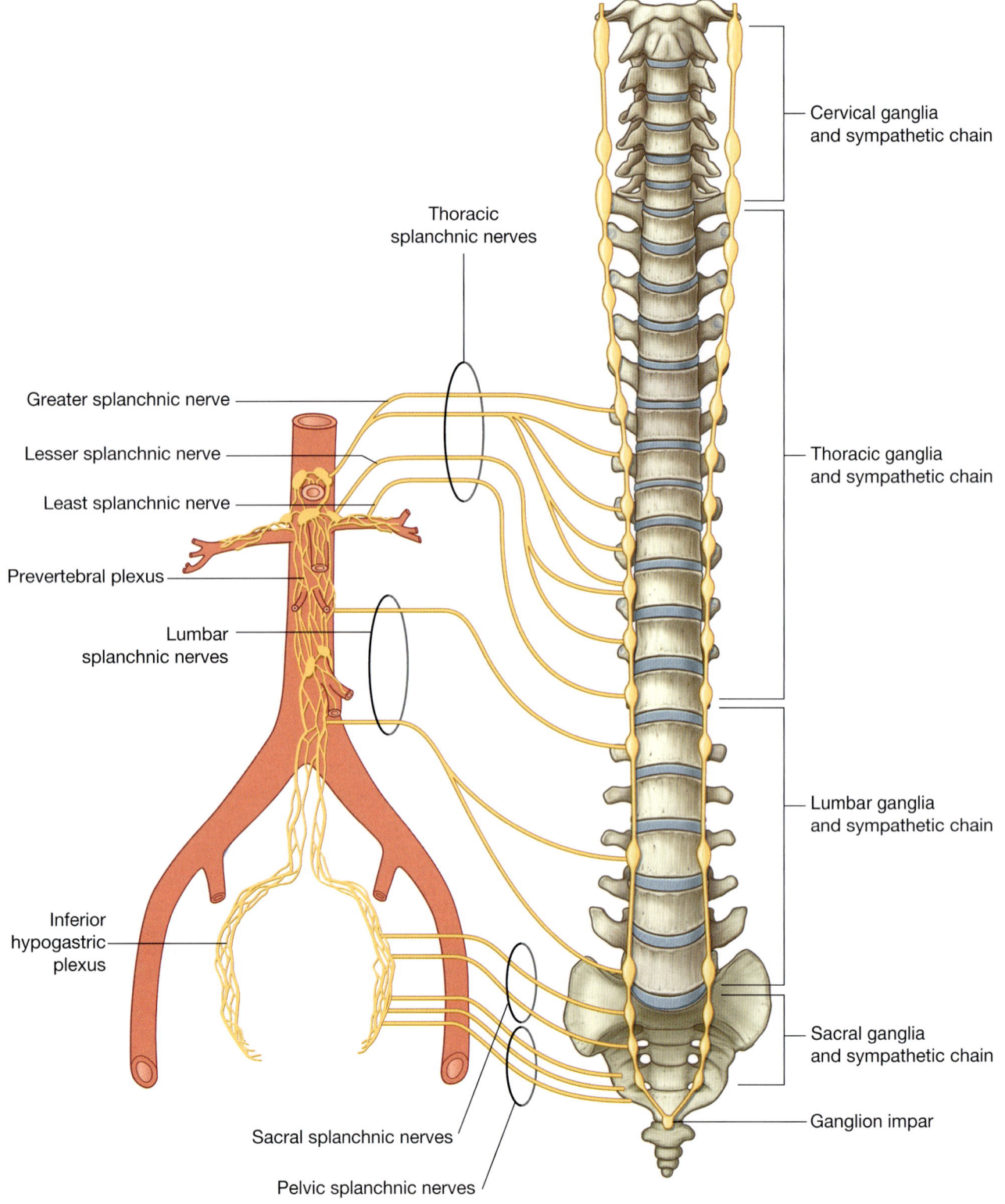

Fig. 75.35. Sympathetic chain and splanchnic nerves. (From Drake RL, Vogl AW, Mitchell AWM: *Gray's anatomy for students,* ed 2, Philadelphia, 2010, Churchill Livingstone.)

The nerves arising from this plexus are close to the psoas muscle, with the superior nerves piercing the muscle, whereas the inferior nerves travel medial to the muscle body (Fig. 75.38). This plexus provides the cutaneous sensory innervation to the lower extremities (Fig. 75.39 and Table 75.4).

The **subcostal nerve** is an extension of the 12th thoracic nerve and runs inferior to the 12th rib. The **ilioinguinal and iliohypogastric nerves** arise from the anterior ramus of L1. These three nerves run laterally over the anterior aspect of the quadratus lumborum and travel through the transversus abdominis to run deep to the internal

Chapter 75 Surgical, Radiographic, and Endoscopic Anatomy of the Retroperitoneum 1677

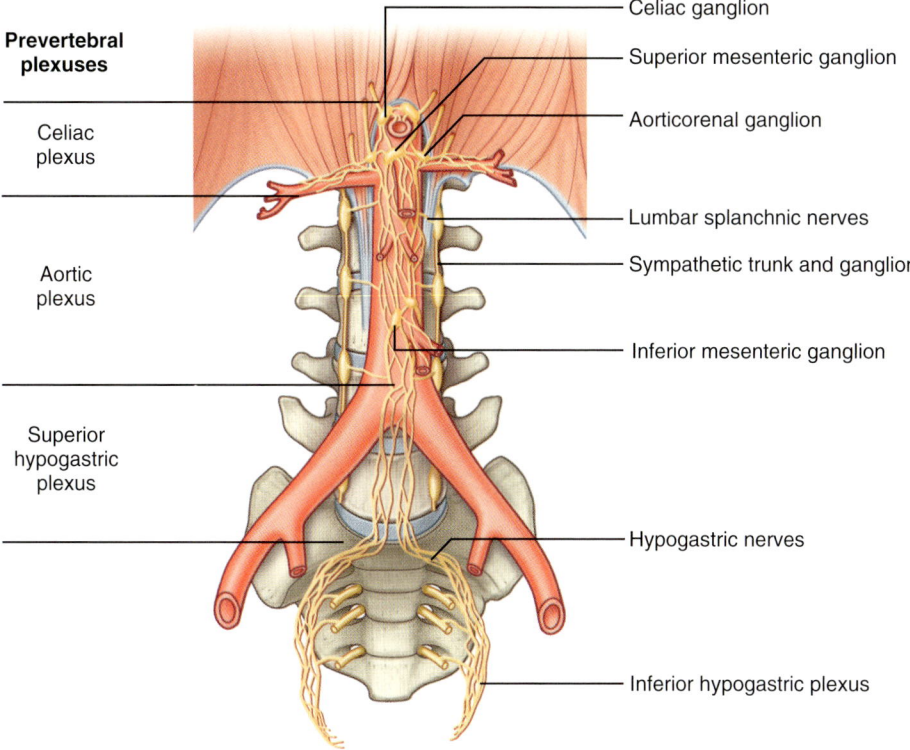

Fig. 75.36. Autonomic plexuses associated with branches of the aorta. (From Drake RL, Vogl AW, Mitchell AWM: *Gray's anatomy for students,* ed 2, Philadelphia, 2010, Churchill Livingstone.)

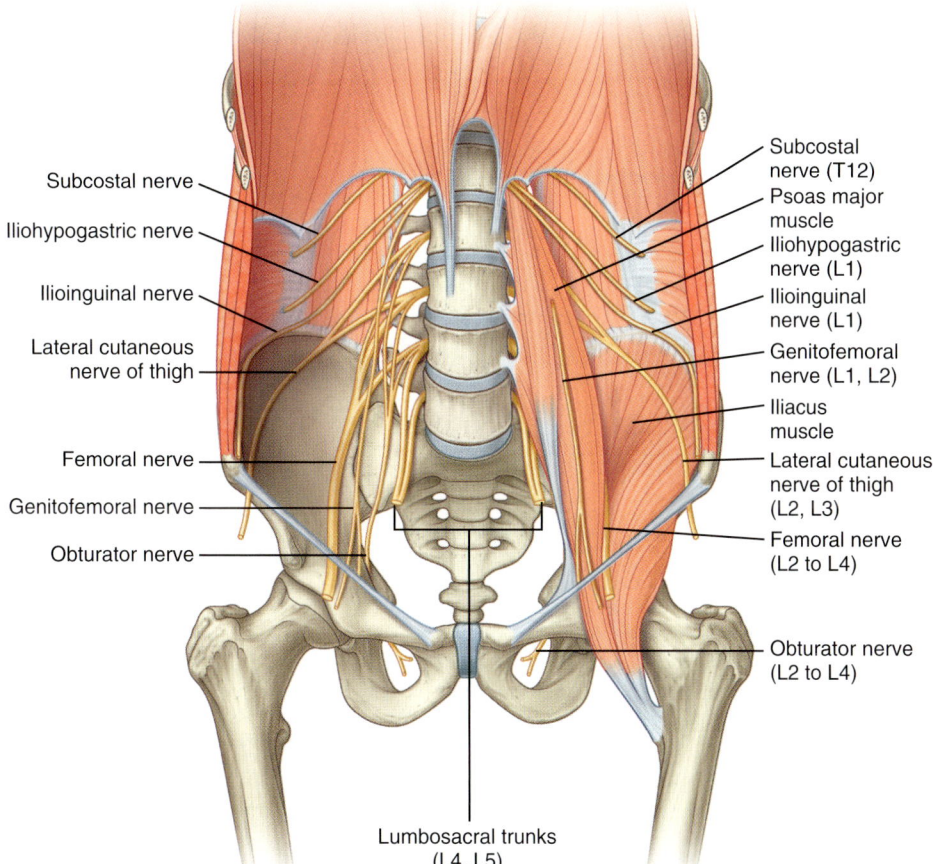

Fig. 75.38. Lumbar plexus in the posterior abdominal region. (From Drake RL, Vogl AW, Mitchell AWM: *Gray's anatomy for students,* ed 2, Philadelphia, 2010, Churchill Livingstone.)

1678 PART VII Male Genitalia

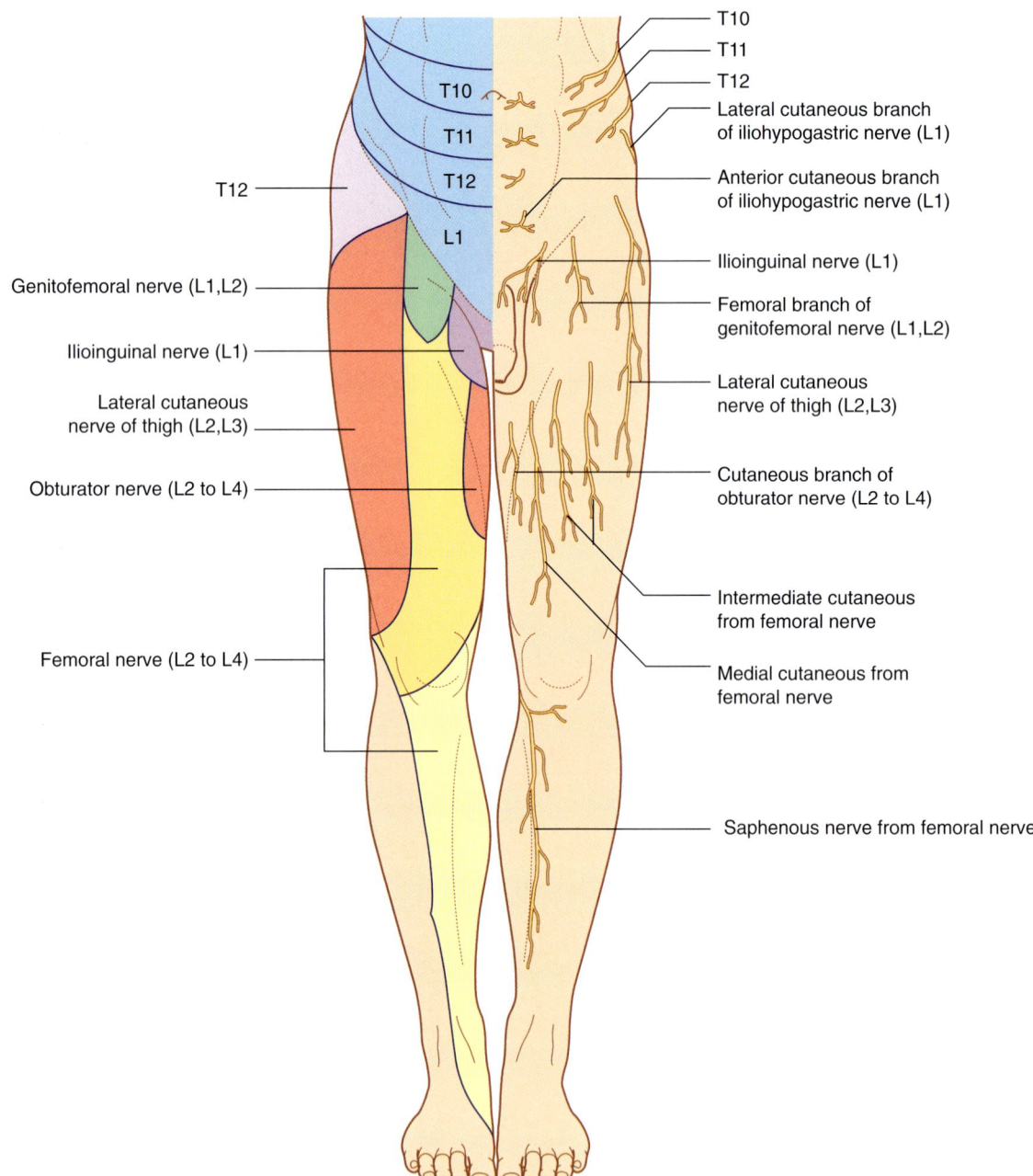

Fig. 75.39. Cutaneous distribution of the nerves from the lumbar plexus. (From Drake RL, Vogl AW, Mitchell AWM: *Gray's anatomy for students,* ed 2, Philadelphia, 2010, Churchill Livingstone.)

TABLE 75.4 Branches of the Lumbosacral Plexus

BRANCH	ORIGIN	SPINAL SEGMENTS	MOTOR FUNCTION	SENSORY FUNCTION
Subcostal	Anterior ramus T12	T12	Muscles of abdominal wall	Skin over hip
Iliohypogastric	Anterior ramus L1	L1	Internal oblique and transversus abdominis	Posterolateral gluteal skin and skin in pubic region
Ilioinguinal	Anterior ramus L1	L1	Internal oblique and transversus abdominis	Skin in upper medial thigh and the skin over either the root of the penis and anterior scrotum or the mons pubis and labium majus
Genitofemoral	Anterior rami L1 and L2	L1, L2	Genital branch: male cremasteric muscle	Genital branch: skin of anterior scrotum or skin of mons pubis and labium majus Femoral branch: skin of upper anterior thigh
Lateral cutaneous nerve of the thigh	Anterior rami L2 and L3	L2, L3	None	Skin on anterior and lateral thigh to the knee
Obturator	Anterior rami L2-L4	L2-L4	Obturator externus, pectineus, and muscles in medial compartment of thigh	Skin on medial aspect of thigh
Femoral	Anterior rami L2-L4	L2-L4	Iliacus, pectineus, and muscles in anterior compartment of thigh	Skin on anterior thigh and medial surface of leg

Modified from Drake RL, Vogl AW, Mitchell AWM: *Gray's anatomy for students*, Philadelphia, 2005, Churchill Livingstone.

oblique muscle. They provide innervation to the muscles of the abdominal wall and sensory innervation to the posterolateral gluteal skin, upper medial thigh, and genitalia.

The **genitofemoral nerve** originates from L1 and L2 and courses anterior and parallel to the psoas muscle. The nerve typically divides near the level of the inguinal ligament. The **femoral branch** passes under the inguinal ligament and enters the femoral sheath to supply sensation to the upper anterior thigh. The **genital branch** enters the inguinal canal at the deep internal ring to provide motor innervation to the cremaster muscle. This motor component allows for contraction of the muscle during the cremasteric reflex. In addition to the motor component, the genital branch supplies sensation to the anterior scrotum in males and the mons pubis and labium majus in females. The genitofemoral nerve may be injured during a psoas hitch procedure (suture placement) and laparoscopic varicocelectomy (ligation). The **lateral cutaneous nerve of the thigh** (lateral femoral cutaneous nerve) arises from L2 and L3 and provides sensory innervation to the anterior and lateral thigh.

The **obturator nerve** originates from the anterior rami of L2-L4 posterior to the psoas muscle and courses inferiorly to the obturator canal. **The function of the obturator nerve includes hip adduction via motor innervation to the medial thigh compartment, which is of clinical significance during lateral transurethral resection and pelvic lymph node dissection.** Electrocautery employed during a transurethral resection of bladder tumor (TURBT) procedure may result in obturator nerve stimulation with subsequent rapid, forceful hip adduction. If this potential event is not anticipated and accounted for, severe bladder perforation may occur.

With its origin from the anterior rami of L2-L4, the **femoral nerve** provides efferent motor input to the muscles of the anterior thigh as well as the iliacus and pectineus, which are responsible for knee extension and hip flexion, respectively. The femoral nerve also gives sensory innervation to the skin over the anterior medial lower extremity. Compression of the femoral nerve may occur intraoperatively with placement of retractor blades inferolaterally against the inguinal ligament. Compression injury may result in a motor palsy to the quadriceps muscle, impairing extension at the knee. In addition, a stretch injury to the femoral nerve may occur with prolonged hip flexion in low lithotomy position used during minimally invasive pelvic surgery.

The **sciatic nerve** receives input from L4-S3 and provides the bulk of motor and sensory input to the lower extremities, including motor innervation to the posterior thigh compartment and all muscles in the leg and foot. Injury to this nerve may occur secondary to prolonged hip hyperflexion used during a high lithotomy position for vaginal and urethral procedures.

See ExpertConsult.com for Videos 75.1, 75.2, 75.3, and 75.4, which show procedures related to this chapter.

> ### KEY POINTS: NERVOUS STRUCTURES
> - The parasympathetic autonomic nervous system has craniosacral outflow, and the postganglionic fibers are often contained within the walls of the innervated viscera.
> - The preganglionic sympathetic nervous system fibers exit from the spinal cord from T1 to L2 and may synapse within the sympathetic trunk or within the autonomic plexuses.
> - The somatic nervous system provides sensory and motor innervation to the pelvis and lower extremities through the lumbosacral plexus.

SUGGESTED READINGS

Drake RL, Vogl AW, Mitchell AWM: *Gray's anatomy for students*, 2nd ed, Philadelphia, 2010, Churchill Livingstone.
MacLennan GT: *Hinman's atlas of urosurgical anatomy*, 2nd ed, Philadelphia, 2012, Saunders.
Smith JA, Howards SS, Preminger GM: *Hinman's atlas of urologic surgery*, 3rd ed, Philadelphia, 2012, Saunders.

REFERENCES

The complete reference list is available online at ExpertConsult.com.

76
Neoplasms of the Testis

Andrew J. Stephenson, MD, MBA, FRCSC, FACS, and Timothy D. Gilligan, MD, MS, FASCO

Neoplasms of the testis comprise a morphologically and clinically diverse group of tumors, more than 95% of which are germ cell tumors (GCTs). GCTs are broadly categorized as seminoma and nonseminoma (NSGCT) because of differences in natural history and treatment. GCT is a relatively rare malignancy, accounting for 1% to 2% of cancers among adult males in the United States. Approximately 95% of GCTs arise in the testis, and 5% are extragonadal in origin. With the development of cisplatin-based chemotherapy and the integration of surgery, GCTs have become a model of a curable neoplasm and serve as a paradigm for the multidisciplinary treatment of cancer (Einhorn, 1981). In the era before cisplatin, the cure rate for patients with advanced GCT was 5% to 10%. Currently, the long-term survival for men with metastatic GCT is 80% to 90%. With the successful cure of patients, an important treatment objective is minimizing treatment-related toxicity without compromising curability. Mortality from GCT is due to inherent resistance to platin chemotherapy and the failure to fully eradicate residual disease elements in the early course of therapy.

Non-GCT tumors of the testis are rare and include sex cord-stromal tumors, lymphoid and hematopoietic tumors, tumors of the collecting duct and rete testis, and tumors of the testicular adnexa. A classification of testis neoplasms is outlined in Table 76.1.

GERM CELL TUMORS

Epidemiology

In 2018 an estimated 9310 men were diagnosed with testis cancer in the United States, and 400 will die from this disease (Siegel et al., 2018). **In the United States, testis cancer is the most common malignancy among men aged 20 to 40 years and the second most common cancer after leukemia among males aged 15 to 19 years** (Howlader et al., 2017). Testis tumors are most common between the ages of 15 and 55. The incidence rate rises rapidly after puberty, peaking at ages 25 to 35, and then slowly declines such that men aged 50 to 54 years have the same incidence as males aged 15 to 19. **The incidence of bilateral GCT is approximately 2%** (Fossa et al., 2005). The majority of bilateral GCTs are metachronous and occur over an average interval of 5 years. Discordant histology between primary tumors occurs in 30% to 50% of patients (Kopp et al., 2017).

The incidence of testis cancer varies significantly according to geographic region; **rates are highest in Scandinavia, Western Europe, and Australia-New Zealand, intermediate in the United States and United Kingdom, and lowest in Africa and Asia** (Trabert et al., 2015). **The incidence of testis cancer in the United States in non-Hispanic whites is 3.6 times higher than the incidence in blacks, 2.5 times higher than the incidence in Asians and similar to but slightly higher than in Hispanics** (Howlader et al., 2017).

The incidence of GCT appears to be increasing worldwide (Huyghe et al., 2003; Rosen et al., 2011; Shanmugalingam et al., 2013; Znaor et al., 2014). In the United States, the age-adjusted incidence rate has increased from 3.73 per 100,000 in 1975 to 6.35 per 100,000 in 2014 (Howlader et al., 2017). Incidence has increased for seminomas and nonseminomas (Bray et al., 2006a; Trabert et al., 2015). **A stage migration of GCT has been observed in several countries partially because of an increased awareness and earlier diagnosis.** Between 1973 and 2014, the percentage of tumors diagnosed at a localized stage increased from 55% to 68% in the United States. **Only about 13% of men are seen initially with distant metastatic disease.**

Risk Factors

There are five well-established risk factors for testis cancer: white race, cryptorchidism, family history of testis cancer, a personal history of testis cancer, and germ cell neoplasia in situ (GCNIS), also referred to as intratubular germ cell neoplasia (ITGCN) (Stevenson and Lowrance, 2015). Infertile and subfertile men also have a higher incidence of testis cancer (Doria-Rose et al., 2005; Hanson et al., 2016). **Numerous studies have reported that recent increases in testis cancer incidence can be largely attributed to birth-cohort effects, which implies that diet and/or other environmental factors play a major role in GCT carcinogenesis** (Bray et al., 2006a,b; Huyghe et al., 2003; Liu et al., 1999; McGlynn et al., 2003; McKiernan et al., 1999; Richiardi et al., 2004; Verhoeven et al., 1970). **Specific environmental factors have not been definitively identified but there is evidence of an association between early exposure to endocrine-disrupting chemicals and an increased risk of testicular germ cell tumors** (Bonde et al., 2016; Giannandrea and Fargnoli, 2017).

Men with cryptorchidism are 4 to 6 times more likely to be diagnosed with testis cancer in the affected gonad, but the relative risk falls to 2 to 3 if orchidopexy is performed before puberty (Dieckmann and Pichlmeier, 2004; Wood and Elder, 2009). **A meta-analysis of cryptorchidism studies reported that the contralateral descended testis is also at slightly increased risk (RR 1.74 [95% CI, 1.01–2.98])** (Akre et al., 2008). Men with a first-degree relative with testis cancer have a substantially increased risk of testis cancer, and the median age at diagnosis in these men is 2 to 3 years younger than in the general population (Mai et al., 2009). An individual's relative risk for testis cancer is 8 to 12 with an affected brother compared with 2 to 4 in those with an affected father (Hemminki and Chen, 2006; Sonneveld et al., 1999; Westergaard et al., 1996). Men with a history of testis cancer are at a 12-fold increased risk of developing GCT in the contralateral testis, but the 15-year cumulative incidence is only 2% (Fossa et al., 2005).

Most GCTs arise from a precursor lesion called GCNIS (Williamson et al., 2017). Exceptions to this are prepubertal germ cell tumors (which can rarely occur after puberty), ovarian cystic teratomas, dermoid cysts, and spermatocytic tumors (previously referred to as spermatocytic seminomas) (Cheng et al., 2017; Williamson et al., 2017). GCNIS is present in adjacent testicular parenchyma in 80% to 90% cases of invasive GCT and is associated with a 50% risk of GCT within 5 years and 70% within 7 years (Dieckmann and Skakkebaek, 1999; Montironi, 2002; Skakkebaek et al., 1982). **Between 5% and 9% of patients with GCT have GCNIS within the unaffected contralateral testis, although the incidence of contralateral GCNIS increases to about 36% in men with testicular atrophy or cryptorchidism** (Dieckmann and Loy, 1996; Dieckmann and Skakkebaek, 1999). Gene expression profile analysis indicates that GCNIS develops before birth from an arrested gonocyte (Hussain et al., 2008; Sonne et al., 2009). In men with a history of GCT, the finding of testicular microlithiasis on ultrasound of the contralateral testis is associated with an increased risk of

TABLE 76.1 2016 World Health Organization Classification of Testis Neoplasms

GERM CELL TUMORS OF THE TESTIS

Germ cell tumors derived from germ cell neoplasia in situ
    Noninvasive germ cell neoplasia
    Germ cell neoplasia in situ
    Specific forms of intratubular germ cell neoplasia
    Seminomatous tumors of a single histologic type (pure seminoma)
    Seminoma
    Seminoma with syncytiotrophoblast cells
    Nonseminomatous germ cell tumors of a single histologic type
    Embryonal carcinoma
    Yolk sac tumor, postpubertal type
    Trophoblastic tumors
    Choriocarcinoma
    Nonchoriocinomatous trophoblastic tumors
    Placental site trophoblastic tumor
    Epithelioid trophoblastic tumor
    Cystic trophoblastic tumor
    Teratoma, postpubertal type
    Teratoma with somatic-type malignancy
    Nonseminomatous germ cell tumors of more than one histologic type
    Mixed germ cell tumors
    Germ cell tumors of unknown type
    Regressed germ cell tumors
Germ cell tumors unrelated to germ cell neoplasia in situ
    Spermatocytic tumor
    Teratoma, prepubertal type
    Dermoid cyst
    Epidermoid cyst
    Well-differentiated neuroendocrine tumor (monodermal teratoma)
    Mixed teratoma and yolk sac tumor, prepubertal type
    Yolk sac tumor, prepubertal type

SEX CORD-STROMAL TUMORS OF THE TESTIS

Pure tumors
Leydig cell tumor
Malignant Leydig cell tumor
Sertoli cell tumor
Malignant Sertoli cell tumor
Large cell calcifying Sertoli cell tumor
Intratubular hyalinizing Sertoli cell neoplasia
Granulosa cell tumor
Adult granulosa cell tumor
Juvenile granulosa cell tumor
Tumors in the fibroma-thecoma group
Mixed and unclassified sex cord-stromal tumors
Mixed sex cord-stromal tumor
Unclassified sex cord-stromal tumor

Data from Williamson SR, Delahunt B, Magi-Galluzzi C, et al.: The World Health Organization 2016 classification of testicular germ cell tumours: a review and update from the International Society of Urological Pathology Testis Consultation Panel. *Histopathology* 70:335–346, 2017.

GCNIS (Karellas et al., 2007). **However, the significance of microlithiasis in the general population is unclear;** a study of 1500 army volunteers found a 5.6% prevalence of microlithiasis, yet fewer than 2% of those with microlithiasis developed GCT within 5 years (DeCastro et al., 2008).

Pathogenesis and Biology

The carcinogenesis of GCTs is poorly understood (Looijenga et al., 2011; Sheikine et al., 2012; Turnbull and Rahman, 2011). As noted earlier, testicular GCTs develop from a precursor lesion, GCNIS, which in turn appears to develop from arrested primordial germ cells or gonocytes that failed to differentiate into prespermatogonia (Hussain et al., 2008; Looijenga et al., 2011; Rajpert-de Meyts and Hoei-Hansen, 2007). These transformed primordial germ cells are thought to then lay dormant until after puberty when they are stimulated by increased testosterone levels.

The increased incidence of testis cancer that started in the first half of the 20th century has been accompanied by an increased incidence of other male reproductive disorders such as hypospadias, cryptorchidism, and subfertility (Rajpert-de Meyts and Hoei-Hansen, 2007; Sonne et al., 2008). These findings led to the hypothesis that testis cancer and these other disorders resulted from a testicular dysgenesis syndrome, which in turn resulted from environmental and/or lifestyle factors and genetic susceptibility (Akre and Richiardi, 2009; Xing and Bai, 2018). Although this hypothesis remains controversial, the increasing incidence of testis cancer supports the presence of environmental and/or lifestyle risk factors. The strongest epidemiologic evidence supports a role for prenatal exposure but there is no strong evidence identifying specific chemicals (Bonde et al., 2016). Increased prenatal estrogen exposure has been hypothesized as a risk factor but this is controversial (Martin et al., 2008). Similarly, mothers of testis cancer patients have been reported to have higher blood levels of polychlorinated biphenyls and other persistent organic pollutants (Hardell et al., 2003, 2006). Epidemiologic studies have also reported associations between testis cancer and prior exposure to organochloride pesticides as well as to firefighting and aircraft maintenance occupations (McGlynn and Trabert, 2012; McGlynn et al., 2008; Purdue et al., 2009). There is stronger evidence that reduction in androgen activity can result in features of testicular dysgenesis syndrome, including cryptorchidism, hypospadias, and impaired spermatogenesis, but a direct link between reduced androgen signaling and GCNIS remains hypothetical (Hu et al., 2009; Sonne et al., 2008).

Evidence of environmental and lifestyle factors contributing to testis cancer includes the rapid rise in its incidence as well as findings that second-generation immigrants' risk is similar to their country of birth. In addition, mothers of children with testis cancer (but not the testis cancer patients themselves) have been found to have higher blood levels of certain organic pollutants compared with other mothers (Sonne et al., 2008). Evidence for genetic factors includes the clustering of testis cancer in some families, the extreme difference in the rate of testis cancer in black and white Americans, and the finding of susceptibility loci on chromosomes 5, 6, and 12 in case-control studies (Mai et al., 2009). In addition, specific polymorphisms of certain genes, including the gene encoding c-KIT ligand, have been associated with an increased risk of testis cancer (Blomberg Jensen et al., 2008; Kanetsky et al., 2009; Sheikine et al., 2012; Turnbull and Rahman, 2011). Gonocytes depend on KIT ligand for survival and the gene for this protein is located on the short arm of chromosome 12. **An increased number of copies of genetic material from the short arm of chromosome 12 is a universal finding in postpubertal testicular and extragonadal germ cell tumors except for spermatocytic tumors** (Cheng et al., 2017). Between 70% and 80% of GCTs have an extra copy of chromosome 12 in the form of an isochromosome 12p (i[12p]), whereas the remainder show gain of 12p sequences detectable with fluorescence in situ hybridization (Mayer et al., 2003). Thus a connection between mutations or polymorphisms in c-KIT ligand and GCT has biologic plausibility.

One of the most striking features of GCTs is their sensitivity to cisplatin-based chemotherapy, which enables cure in the vast majority of patients with widely metastatic disease. The specific biologic basis of this acute vulnerability to chemotherapy remains incompletely understood but is thought to derive from the close relationship between GCTs and embryonal stem cells and gonocytes, which have a low threshold for undergoing apoptosis in response to DNA damage (Mayer et al., 2003; Schmelz et al., 2010). Gene expression analysis has found an upregulation of numerous genes that facilitate apoptosis, including *FasL*, *TRAIL*, and *Bax* while *BCL-2* is downregulated (Schmelz et al., 2010). Expression patterns of genes controlling the G1/S-phase checkpoint in GCTs appear to promote induction of apoptosis (Schmelz et al., 2010). In addition, GCTs lack transporters to export cisplatin from the cell and have a reduced ability to repair cisplatin-induced DNA damage (Mayer et al., 2003). GCTs have high intrinsic levels of wild-type p53 protein (which plays a role in mediating cell cycle arrest and apoptosis), and p53 mutations in GCTs are rare, yet differences have not been consistently found in p53 status when comparing chemo-sensitive and chemo-resistant germ cell tumors (Burger et al., 1998; Houldsworth et al., 1998). Similarly, expression of the anti-apoptotic protein BCL-2 is low in germ cell tumors but BCL-2 levels do not distinguish chemo-sensitive and chemo-resistant cell lines (Mayer et al., 2003). A small fraction of GCTs are resistant to chemotherapy, and the basis of that resistance remains obscure (Veenstra and Vaughn, 2011). Impaired DNA mismatch repair and activating *BRAF* mutations have been associated with treatment failure (Honecker et al., 2009; Looijenga et al., 2011; Sheikine et al., 2012; Veenstra and Vaughn, 2011).

Approximately 5% of postpubertal GCTs are extragonadal in origin, and most develop in midline anatomic locations (retroperitoneum and mediastinum are most common). There are two main competing theories regarding the pathogenesis of extragonadal GCTs. The first hypothesizes that they originate from germ cells that mis-migrated along the genital ridge and were able to survive in an extragonadal environment. The second theory proposes a reverse migration from the testis to extragonadal locations (Chaganti and Houldsworth, 2000).

Primary mediastinal NSGCTs differ in several ways from those originating in the testis or retroperitoneum (Moran and Suster, 1997a,b, 1998; Moran et al., 1997a). First, they are less sensitive to chemotherapy and have a poor prognosis with a 5-year overall survival of about 45% (Bokemeyer et al., 2002). Mediastinal NSGCTs are more likely to have yolk-sac-tumor components and thus to be associated with elevations in serum α-fetoprotein (AFP) (Bokemeyer et al., 2002; Kesler et al., 2008; Moran et al., 1997a). They are also associated with Klinefelter syndrome and with hematologic malignancies that carry extra copies of the short arm of chromosome 12, as seen in adult GCT (Bokemeyer et al., 2002; McKenney et al., 2007). **In contrast, mediastinal seminomas carry a similar prognosis to testicular seminomas, and mature teratomas of the mediastinum have low metastatic potential and can generally be cured surgically** (Allen, 2002; Horner et al., 2009; International Germ Cell Cancer Collaborative Group, 1997). **Primary retroperitoneal GCTs are indistinguishable biologically from testicular GCTs and carry the same prognosis.**

Histologic Classification

The histologic classification of postpubertal GCT is outlined in Table 76.1 (Williamson et al., 2017). **GCTs are broadly classified as GCNIS-derived and non-GCNIS–derived. The majority of postpubertal GCTs are GCNIS derived. For clinical purposes, GCNIS-derived GCTs are divided into seminoma and NSGCT, and the relative distribution of each is 52% to 56% and 44% to 48%, respectively** (McGlynn et al., 2005; Powles et al., 2005). **NSGCTs include embryonal carcinoma (EC), yolk sac tumor, teratoma, and choriocarcinoma subtypes, either alone as pure forms or in combination as mixed GCT with or without seminoma.** Most NSGCTs are mixed tumors composed of two or more GCT subtypes. GCTs that contain both NSGCT subtypes and seminoma are classified as NSGCT even if the NSGCT component represents a tiny proportion of the tumor.

Germ Cell Tumor Neoplasia in Situ

With the exception of spermatocytic tumor, postpubertal invasive GCTs arise from GCNIS. GCNIS consists of undifferentiated germ cells that have the appearance of seminoma that are located basally within the seminiferous tubules. The tubule usually shows decreased or absent spermatogenesis and normal constituents are replaced by GCNIS. The presence of GCNIS in an orchiectomy specimen in men with testis cancer does not carry any prognostic implications with regard to the risk of relapse (von Eyben et al., 2004). GCNIS is much less frequent in pediatric GCTs (Cheville, 1999).

Seminoma

Seminoma is the most common type of GCT. On average, seminomas occur at an older average age than NSGCT, with most cases diagnosed in the fourth or fifth decade of life (Cheville, 1999). Grossly, seminoma is a soft tan to white diffuse or multinodular mass (Fig. 76.1A). Necrosis may be present but is usually focal and not as prominent as other GCTs. Seminomas consist of a sheet-like arrangement of cells with polygonal nuclei and clear cytoplasm, with the cells divided into nests by fibrovascular septae that contain lymphocytes (Fig. 76.1B) (Ulbright, 2005). Syncytiotrophoblasts, which stain positive for human chorionic gonadotropin (HCG), can be identified in about 15% of cases but are of no clear prognostic significance (Cheville, 1999). Lymphocytic infiltrates and granulomatous reactions are often seen, and seminomas appear to be associated with an increased incidence of sarcoidosis (Rayson et al., 1998; Tjan-Heijnen et al., 1998). Seminomas may be confused with solid-pattern EC, yolk sac tumor, or Sertoli cell tumors (Ulbright and Young, 2008). Although immunohistochemical staining plays a limited role in diagnosing GCTs, seminomas are typically negative for CD30, positive for CD117, and strongly positive for placental alkaline phosphatase (PLAP). Anaplastic seminoma was a previously recognized subtype of seminoma, but this distinction is of no clear biologic or clinical significance and is no longer recognized. Seminoma arises from GCNIS and is considered to be the common precursor for the other NSGCT subtypes (Ulbright, 2004). This ability of seminoma to transform into NSGCT elements has important therapeutic implications for the management of seminoma (discussed later) (Ulbright, 2004).

Spermatocytic Tumor

Spermatocytic tumor (previously referred to as spermatocytic seminoma) used to be classified as a subtype of seminoma but is now considered a distinct entity from seminoma and other GCTs. It is rare and accounts for less than 1% of GCTs. Unlike other GCTs, spermatocytic tumor does not arise from GCNIS, is not associated with a history of cryptorchidism or bilaterality, does not demonstrate i(12p), and does not occur as part of mixed GCTs (Ulbright, 2005). The lack of association of spermatocytic tumors with GSNIS is similar to juvenile YST and teratoma. Histopathologically, they differ from seminoma in that they do not stain for OCT 3/4, PLAP, or glycogen (PAS stain), nuclei are round, minimal lymphocytic infiltration is present, and three distinct cell types are present, including small lymphocyte-like cells, medium-size cells with dense eosinophilic cytoplasm and a round nucleus, and large mono- or multi-nucleated cells (Aggarwal and Parwani, 2009). The peak incidence is the sixth decade of life (Chung et al., 2004; Eble, 1994). It is a benign tumor (only three documented cases of metastases) and is almost always cured with orchiectomy (Chung et al., 2004; Horn et al., 2011). An exception to this rule are the rare cases of "spermatocytic tumor with sarcoma," which exhibit elements of sarcomatous differentiation, and an anaplastic variant, both of which are associated with widely metastatic chemotherapy-resistant disease and poor prognosis (Dundr et al., 2007; Narang et al., 2012; Wetherell et al., 2013).

Embryonal Carcinoma

EC consists of undifferentiated malignant cells resembling primitive epithelial cells from early stage embryos with crowded pleomorphic nuclei (Ulbright, 2005). Grossly, EC is a tan to yellow neoplasm that often exhibits large areas of hemorrhage and necrosis. The microscopic appearance of these tumors varies considerably, and they may grow in solid sheets or in papillary, glandular-alveolar, or tubular patterns (Fig. 76.1C). In some cases, syncytiotrophoblasts are identified. EC is an aggressive tumor associated with a high rate

Chapter 76 Neoplasms of the Testis 1683

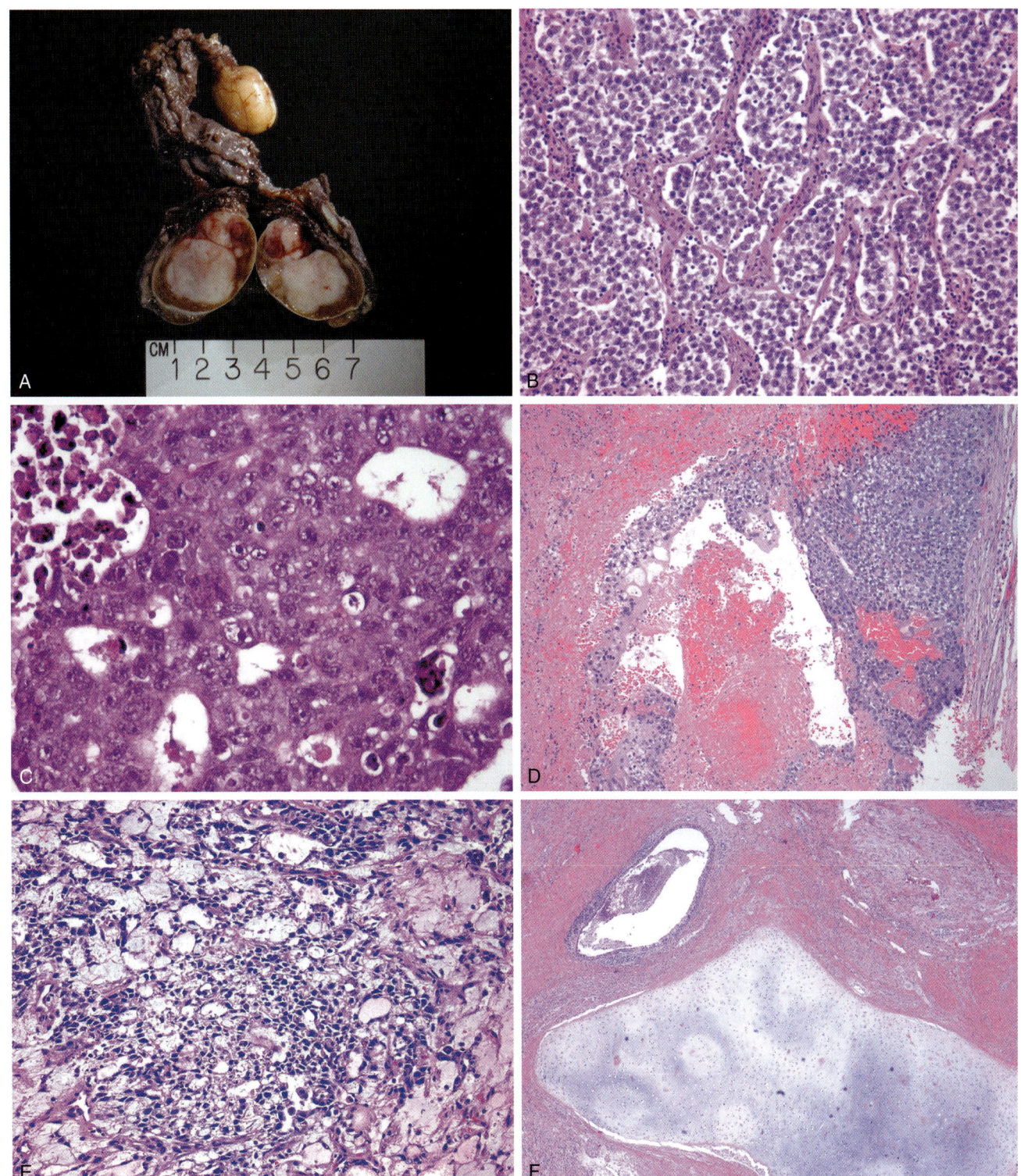

Fig. 76.1. (A) Gross section of testis containing seminoma. (B) Seminoma (H&E stain). (C) Embryonal carcinoma (H&E stain). (D) Choriocarcinoma (H&E stain). (E) Yolk sac tumor (H&E stain). (F) Teratoma (H&E stain).

of metastasis, often in the context of normal serum tumor markers. **EC is the most undifferentiated cell type of NSGCT, with totipotential capacity to differentiate to other NSGCT cell types (including teratoma) within the primary tumor or at metastatic sites.** As discussed later, the presence and proportion of EC has been associated an increased risk of occult metastases in clinical stage (CS) I NSGCT. EC typically stains for AE1/AE3, PLAP, and OCT3/4 and do not stain for c-Kit.

Choriocarcinoma

Choriocarcinoma is a rare and aggressive tumor that typically is seen with extremely highly elevated serum HCG levels and disseminated disease. They are typically poor-risk (stage IIIC) at diagnosis because of the serum HCG level and/or nonpulmonary organ metastases (Alvarado-Cabrero et al., 2014). **Choriocarcinoma commonly spreads by hematogenous routes,** and common sites of metastases include lungs, liver, and brain (Allen, 2002; Alvarado-Cabrero et al., 2014; Osada et al., 2004; Tinkle et al., 2001; Yokoi et al., 2008). Microscopically, the tumor is composed of syncytiotrophoblasts and cytotrophoblasts, and the former stain positively for HCG (Fig. 76.1D; Cheville, 1999). Seminoma and EC may also contain syncytiotrophoblasts. Areas of hemorrhage and necrosis are prominent. As in gestational trophoblastic disease, testicular choriocarcinoma is prone to hemorrhage, sometimes spontaneously and immediately after chemotherapy is initiated; such bleeding can be catastrophic, particularly when it occurs in the lungs or brain (Kandori et al., 2010; Motzer et al., 1987; Yokoi et al., 2008). In addition, choriocarcinomas are associated with hormonal disturbances, most likely because of highly elevated serum HCG. Stimulation of receptors for thyroid stimulating hormone and luteinizing hormone (LH) by HCG (which shares an identical alpha-subunit) can result in hyperthyroidism and elevated androgen production (Ulbright, 2005). Hyperprolactinemia has also been reported.

Yolk Sac Tumor

Pure yolk sac tumors (sometimes called endodermal sinus tumors) represent a very small fraction of adult gonadal and retroperitoneal GCTs but are more common in mediastinal and pediatric GCTs (Cao and Humphrey, 2011; Moran and Suster, 1997b; Moran et al., 1997a; Rossen et al., 2009; Ulbright, 2005). Mixed GCTs often include elements of yolk sac tumor, which consists of a reticular network of medium-sized cuboidal cells with cytoplasmic and extra-cytoplasmic eosinophilic, hyaline-like globules (Epstein, 2010). Yolk sac tumors may grow in a glandular, papillary, or micro-cystic pattern. A characteristic feature is the Schiller-Duval body, which resembles endodermal sinuses, and is seen in roughly half of cases (Fig. 76.1E). Cytoplasmic and extracellular eosinophilic hyaline globules are another characteristic histologic feature and are present in up to 84% of cases. **Yolk sac tumors almost always produce AFP but not HCG.**

Teratoma

Teratomas are tumors that contain well or incompletely differentiated elements of at least two of the three germ cell layers: endoderm, mesoderm, and ectoderm. Characteristically, all components are intermixed. Well-differentiated tumors are labeled mature teratomas, whereas those that are incompletely differentiated (i.e., similar to fetal or embryonal tissue) are called immature teratomas. **In adolescent and adult males, there is no clinical significance to the distinction between mature and immature teratomas, and histopathologists do not typically distinguish between the two entities** (Williamson et al., 2017). Mature teratomas may include elements of mature bone, cartilage, teeth, hair, and squamous epithelium, a fact that most likely explains the name *teratoma*, which roughly means "monster tumor," in Greek (Fig. 76.1F). The gross appearance of teratoma depends largely on the elements within it; most tumors have solid and cystic areas. **Teratomas are generally associated with normal serum tumor markers, but they may cause mildly elevated serum AFP levels.** Approximately 47% of adult mixed GCTs contain teratoma, but pure teratomas are uncommon (Geldart et al., 2002; Leibovitch et al., 1995).

In men, teratomas have a histologically benign appearance but are frequently found at metastatic sites in patients with advanced NSGCT. **Teratoma is resistant to chemotherapy.** Thus, given its frequent presence at metastatic sites in advanced NSGCT, patients with residual masses after chemotherapy require consolidative surgical resection. The inherent chemo-resistance of teratoma is a limitation to treatment strategies for NSGCT that use chemotherapy alone.

Despite their benign histologic appearance, teratomas contain many genetic abnormalities frequently found in malignant GCT elements, including aneuploidy, isochrome 12p (i[12p]), and widely variable proliferative capacity (Castedo et al., 1989; Sella et al., 1991). Studies have also shown that cystic fluid from teratoma frequently contains HCG and AFP, confirming its malignant potential (Beck et al., 2004; Sella et al., 1991). The genetic instability of teratoma has important clinical implications. **Teratomas may grow uncontrollably, invade surrounding structures, and become unresectable** (Logothetis et al., 1982). **On rare occasions, teratoma may transform into a somatic malignancy such as rhabdomyosarcoma, adenocarcinoma, or primitive neuroectodermal tumor** (Comiter et al., 1998; Little et al., 1994; Motzer et al., 1998). These tumors are called "teratoma with somatic-type malignancy" or "teratoma with malignant transformation." These tumors frequently have abnormalities of chromosome 12 or i(12p), indicating their origin from GCT. Malignant transformation is highly aggressive, resistant to conventional chemotherapy, and associated with a poor prognosis (Comiter et al., 1998; El Mesbahi et al., 2007). Only 4% of teratoma with somatic-type malignancy arise within the testis. The majority arise at metastatic sites, usually within 3 to 4 years after completion of chemotherapy as a consequence of unresected teratoma (Magers et al., 2014; Rice et al., 2014). Last, unresected teratoma in patients with advanced NSGCT may result in late relapse (Sheinfeld, 2003). All of these events may have lethal consequences.

Accurate characterization of GCTs is essential for successful treatment and consideration for expert pathology review may be considered. A study of orchiectomy specimens reviewed at Indiana University from outside institutions revealed a 31% discrepancy in histologic subtype and a change in lymphovascular invasion (LVI) status in 22% of cases (Harari et al., 2017). These differences in pathological assessment between expert and community pathologists may have important treatment implications.

KEY POINTS: GERM CELL TUMORS

- GCT is the most common solid malignancy among males age 20 to 40 years.
- Bilateral GCT occurs in 2% of men. Metachronous lesion is the most common presentation.
- Incidence of GCT is highest in Caucasians and lowest in African-Americans.
- Cryptorchidism, personal or family history of GCT, and GCNIS are the known risk factors for GCT.
- Orchidopexy for cryptorchidism performed before puberty is associated with a decreased risk of GCT.
- Postpubertal GCTs other than spermatocytic tumors universally contain extra copies of genetic material from the small arm of chromosome 12. In 70% to 80% of cases, this consists of an extra copy of the short arm of 12 appearing as an isochromosome (i[12p]), whereas in the remaining cases, this genetic material can be demonstrated with fluorescent in situ hybridization. This genetic marker may be used in the diagnosis of GCT (e.g., for carcinomas of unknown primary) and non-GCT somatic malignancy arising from malignant transformation of teratoma.
- Approximately 5% of GCT originate at extragonadal sites, most commonly mediastinum and retroperitoneum. Primary mediastinal NSGCTs are associated with poor prognosis.
- Teratoma is histologically benign. Teratoma at metastatic sites is believed to arise from differentiation of metastatic non-teratoma GCT elements.
- Teratoma is resistant to chemotherapy.
- Teratoma is histologically benign but genetically unstable. Thus it has unpredictable biology. Although uncommon, teratoma has the capacity to grow rapidly or undergo malignant transformation of its ectodermal, mesodermal, and/or endodermal elements to form a non-GCT somatic malignancy.

Initial Presentation

Signs and Symptoms

The most common presentation of testis cancer is a painless testis mass. Acute testicular pain is less common and is caused by rapid expansion of the testis resulting from intra-tumor hemorrhage or infarction caused by rapid tumor growth. Pain is more commonly associated with NSGCT; these tumors tend to be more vascular and exhibit more rapid growth compared with seminomas. Patients frequently report a history of testicular trauma, although incidental trauma is likely responsible for bringing the testis mass to the patient's attention for the first time. Patients may also complain of vague scrotal discomfort or heaviness. **Regional or distant metastasis at diagnosis is present in approximately two-thirds of NSGCTs and 15% of pure seminomas, and symptoms related to metastatic disease are the presenting complaint in 10% to 20% of patients.** Bulky retroperitoneal metastasis may cause a palpable mass, abdominal pain, flank pain resulting from ureteral obstruction, back pain because of involvement of the psoas muscle or nerve roots, lower extremity swelling resulting from compression of the inferior vena cava, or gastrointestinal (GI) symptoms. Pulmonary metastasis may present with dyspnea, chest pain, cough, or hemoptysis. Metastasis to supraclavicular lymph nodes may be seen as a neck mass. **Approximately 2% of men have gynecomastia,** resulting from either elevated serum HCG levels, decreased androgen production, or increased estrogen levels (most commonly seen in men with Leydig cell tumors). **Although approximately two-thirds of men with GCT have diminished fertility, it is an uncommon initial presentation.**

Physical Examination

The physician should carefully examine the affected and the normal contralateral testis, noting their relative size and consistency and palpating for any testicular or extra-testicular masses. Atrophy of the affected or contralateral testis is common, particularly in patients with a history of cryptorchidism. Any firm area within the testis should be considered suspicious for malignancy and should prompt further investigations. A hydrocele may accompany a testis cancer and impair the examiner's ability to evaluate the testis. In this case, a scrotal ultrasound to evaluate the testis is warranted. The patient should also be examined for any evidence of palpable abdominal mass or pain, inguinal lymphadenopathy (particularly if he has had prior inguinal or scrotal surgery), gynecomastia, and supraclavicular lymphadenopathy, and auscultation of the chest for intrathoracic disease.

Differential Diagnosis

The differential diagnosis of a testis mass includes epididymo-orchitis, torsion, hematoma, or para-testicular neoplasm (benign or malignant). Other diagnostic possibilities include hernia, varicocele, or spermatocele, although these usually can be distinguished from a testis mass by physical examination. **A firm intratesticular mass should be considered cancer until proven otherwise and should be evaluated further with a scrotal ultrasound. In patients with a presumptive diagnosis of epididymo-orchitis, patients should be re-evaluated within 2 to 4 weeks of completion of an appropriate course of oral antibiotics.** A persistent mass or pain should be evaluated further with a scrotal ultrasound.

Diagnostic Delay

Diagnostic delay is a well-recognized phenomenon of this disease, with patients and physicians contributing to this delay. Testis cancer patients are typically young and may be less inclined to seek medical evaluation for symptoms because of denial, ignorance, or limited access. **Prior studies show that up to one-third of testis tumors are initially misdiagnosed as epididymitis or hydrocele** (Bosl et al., 1981). For patients with signs or symptoms from metastatic GCT, these may become the focus of the treating physician, resulting in the failure to diagnose GCT. These patients may be subjected to inappropriate treatment, diagnostic tests, and unnecessary surgery with subsequent delays in definitive therapy. Case reports describe patients undergoing exploratory laparotomy, neck dissection, or mastectomy for unsuspected metastatic GCT. The interval of delay is associated with advanced clinical stage, suboptimal response to chemotherapy, and diminished survival. Moul et al. (1990) reported a decrease in survival in GCT patients treated from 1970 to 1987 with a diagnostic delay greater than 16 weeks, though a significant survival difference was not observed among patients treated in the cisplatin era. Stephenson et al. (2004) reported a higher proportion of men requiring intensive chemotherapy (multiple regimens, high-dose, and salvage chemotherapy) among those with a treatment delay greater than 30 days resulting from unnecessary exploratory laparotomy.

Diagnostic delay can be avoided by efforts to improve patient and physician education. Physicians must consider the diagnosis of GCT in any male age 15 to 50 years with a firm testis mass, midline retroperitoneal mass, or mass in the left supraclavicular fossa.

Diagnostic Testing and Initial Management
Scrotal Ultrasound

In men with a testis mass, hydrocele, or unexplained scrotal symptoms or signs, **scrotal ultrasonography should be considered an extension of the physical examination because it widely available, inexpensive, and noninvasive.** With high-frequency transducers (5–10 MHz), intratesticular lesions as small as a few millimeters can be identified and readily distinguished from extra-testicular pathology. On ultrasound, the typical GCT is hypoechoic and two or more discrete lesions may be identified (Fig. 76.2). Heterogeneous echotexture within a lesion is more commonly associated with NSGCT, because seminomas usually have a homogenous echotexture. The presence of increased flow within the lesion on color Doppler sonography is suggestive of malignancy, although its absence does not exclude GCT. The association between testicular microlithiasis and GCT is not clearly defined, and this finding alone should not prompt further evaluation (DeCastro et al., 2008). **Given the 2% incidence of bilateral GCT, both testes should be evaluated sonographically, although bilateral tumors at diagnosis is a rare (0.5% of all GCT) and metachronous presentation is more common** (Fossa et al., 2005).

In men with advanced GCT and a normal testicular examination, scrotal ultrasonography should be performed to rule out the presence of a small, impalpable scar or calcification, indicating a "burned-out" primary testis tumor. GCTs are one of the most common neoplasms to undergo spontaneous regression; seminoma is the most frequent subtype (Balzer and Ulbright, 2006). Radical orchiectomy should be performed in those patients with sonographic evidence of intratesticular lesions (discrete nodule, stellate scar, coarse calcification) because GCNIS and residual teratoma are frequently encountered. Men with advanced GCT with normal testes on physical examination and sonographic evaluation are considered to have primary extragondal GCT.

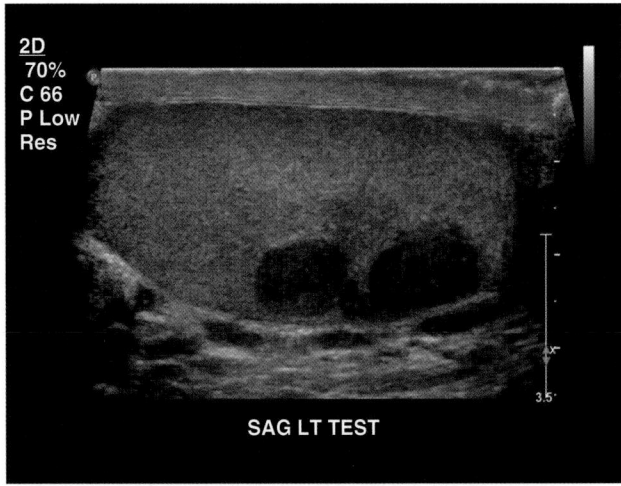

Fig. 76.2. Sagittal view of left testis showing multinodular hypoechoic intratesticular lesion confirmed to be pure seminoma at orchiectomy.

The presence of small (<10 mm), impalpable intratesticular lesions in the absence of disseminated GCT or elevated serum tumor markers represents a diagnostic dilemma. The majority of these lesions are benign (testicular cysts, small infarcts, Leydig cell nodules, or small Leydig cell or Sertoli cell tumors), although up to 20% to 50% may represent small GCT (usually seminoma) (Connolly et al., 2006; Hindley et al., 2003; Muller et al., 2006; Shilo et al., 2012). The risk of malignancy increases with the size of the lesion, from 50% for lesions smaller than 1 cm to 80% or more for lesions 1 to 2 cm (Carmignani et al., 2005). Management options include inguinal orchiectomy, testis-sparing surgery involving inguinal exploration and excision (with frozen section analysis to rule out GCT), and close observation with serial sonographic evaluation (with exploration of growing lesions). Intraoperative ultrasonography is useful during surgical exploration of the testis to locate the lesion.

Magnetic Resonance Imaging

In cases in which the sonographic findings are equivocal or suboptimal, magnetic resonance imaging (MRI) with enhancement is a helpful tool to distinguish between testicular versus extratesticular lesions and neoplastic versus non-neoplastic entities (Park et al., 2011).

Serum Tumor Markers

Testis cancer is one of the few malignancies associated with serum tumor markers (lactate dehydrogenase [LDH], AFP, and HCG) that are essential in its diagnosis and management. Serum tumor marker levels should be obtained at diagnosis, after orchiectomy, to monitor for response to chemotherapy, and to monitor for relapse in patients on surveillance and after completion of therapy.

At diagnosis, AFP levels are elevated in 50% to 70% of low-stage (CS I, IIA, IIB) NSGCTs and 60% to 80% of advanced (CS IIC, III) NSGCTs. EC and yolk sac tumors secrete AFP. Choriocarcinomas and seminomas do not produce AFP. Patients with pure seminoma in the primary tumor with an elevated serum AFP are considered to have NSGCT. The half-life of AFP is 5 to 7 days. AFP levels may also be raised in patients with hepatocellular carcinoma, cancers of the stomach, pancreas, biliary tract and lung, non-malignant liver disease (infectious, drug-induced, alcohol-induced, autoimmune), ataxic telangiectasia, and hereditary tyrosinemia.

HCG levels are elevated in 20% to 40% of low-stage NSGCTs and 40% to 60% of advanced NSGCTs. Approximately 15% of seminomas secrete HCG. HCG is also secreted by choriocarcinoma and EC. Levels above 5000 IU/L are usually associated with NSGCT. The half-life of HCG is 24 to 36 hours. HCG levels may be elevated in cancers of the liver, biliary tract, pancreas, stomach, lung, breast, kidney, and bladder. The alpha-subunit of HCG is common to several pituitary tumors, thus **immunoassays for HCG are directed at the beta-subunit. Cross-reactivity of the HCG assay with LH may cause false-positive HCG elevations in patients with primary hypogonadism.** Elevated serum HCG results caused by hypogonadism will normalize within 48 to 72 hours after the administration of testosterone, and this can be done to distinguish between true- and false-positive HCG results. Marijuana use may also cause false-positive HCG results.

LDH levels are elevated in approximately 20% of low-stage GCT and 20% to 60% of advanced GCT. LDH is expressed in smooth, cardiac, and skeletal muscle. Lymphoma may also cause elevated LDH levels. Of the five isoenzymes of LDH, LDH-1 is the most frequently elevated isoenzyme in GCT. LDH-1 levels are correlated with the chromosome arm 12p copy number, which is frequently amplified in GCT. The magnitude of LDH elevation correlates with the bulk of disease. As a nonspecific marker for GCT, its main use is in the prognostic assessment of GCT at diagnosis. The serum half-life of LDH is 24 hours.

Patients suspected of having a GCT should have blood drawn for serum AFP, HCG, and LDH before orchiectomy to aid in the diagnosis and to help interpret post-orchiectomy tumor marker levels. For staging purposes, it is relevant to know whether pre-orchiectomy serum tumor marker levels are declining after orchiectomy and, if so, how quickly. The results of serum tumor marker assays should not be used to guide decision-making about whether to perform a radical orchiectomy, because AFP or HCG levels in the normal range do not rule out GCT. A significantly elevated serum AFP can establish the diagnosis of NSGCT in a patient whose histopathological diagnosis is pure seminoma because seminomas do not produce AFP. However, borderline-elevated values should be interpreted cautiously. **In rare patients who are seen initially with a testis, retroperitoneal, or mediastinal primary tumor and whose disease burden has resulted in a need to start treatment very urgently, substantially elevated serum AFP and/or HCG may be considered sufficient for diagnosis of GCT.** For such rare, medically unstable patients, treatment need not be delayed until histology results permit a tissue diagnosis. However, these patients should undergo radical orchiectomy after the completion of chemotherapy because the testis is a sanctuary site for malignant GCT because of the blood-testis barrier, and the testis frequently contains residual invasive GCT, teratoma, and/or GCNIS (Geldart et al., 2002).

Radical Inguinal Orchiectomy

Patients suspected of having a testicular neoplasm should undergo a radical inguinal orchiectomy with removal of the tumor-bearing testicle and spermatic cord to the level of the internal inguinal ring. **A transscrotal orchiectomy or biopsy is contraindicated because it leaves the inguinal portion of the spermatic cord intact and may alter the lymphatic drainage of the testis, increasing the risk of local recurrence and pelvic or inguinal lymph node metastasis.** Because of the rapid growth of GCT, orchiectomy should be performed in a timely manner, and delays greater than 1 to 2 weeks should be avoided.

Radical orchiectomy establishes the histologic diagnosis and primary T stage, provides important prognostic information from the tumor histology, and is curative in 80% to 85% and 70% to 80% of CS I seminoma and CS I NSGCT, respectively.

Histopathological examination of the testis should identify the histologic type of the tumor (see Table 76.1; Williamson et al., 2017), tumor size, multifocality, local tumor invasion (rete testis, tunica albuginea, tunica vaginalis, epididymis, spermatic cord, scrotum), primary T stage (Table 76.2; Amin et al., 2017), presence of GCNIS, invasion of blood or lymphatic vessels (termed lymphovascular invasion [LVI]), and the surgical margin status. For patients with mixed GCT, each individual tumor subtype should be identified, including its relative proportion. Because of the relative rarity of GCT and the importance of primary tumor histology for treatment decision making, review of primary tumor specimens by experienced pathologists is recommended (Krege et al., 2008a). One high-volume GCT center reported that among 221 consecutive second-opinion reviews of orchiectomy cases, the pathological stage was changed in 23%, mostly because of changes in whether lymphovascular and/or spermatic cord invasion were present (Harari et al., 2017). Most significantly, 23% of stage T2 and 35% of T3 tumors were downstaged. In addition, 31% had changes in histologic subtype.

Testis-Sparing Surgery

Testis-sparing surgery (or partial orchiectomy) is highly controversial and has no role in the patient suspected of having a testicular neoplasm with a normal contralateral testis. However, it may be considered for organ-confined tumors smaller than 2 to 3 cm (up to 30% of testicular volume) in patients with synchronous bilateral tumors or tumor in a solitary testis with sufficient testicular androgen production. It may also be considered for suspected benign tumor or indeterminate lesion. Benign histology may be encountered in up to 80% of testicular lesions smaller than 3 cm with a long duration of symptoms (>6 months) (Giannarini et al., 2010). Testis-sparing surgery is seldom feasible for larger tumors (>3 cm) because a complete excision frequently leaves insufficient residual testicular parenchyma for preservation. **When testis-sparing surgery is performed, intraoperative frozen section analysis can distinguish between benign and malignant histology in the vast**

TABLE 76.2 TNM Staging of Testicular Tumor: American Joint Committee on Cancer and Union Internationale Contre le Cancer

PRIMARY TUMOR (T)[a]
The extent of primary tumor is usually classified after radical orchiectomy and, for this reason, a *pathological* stage is assigned.

pTx	Primary tumor cannot be assessed
pT0	No evidence of primary tumor (e.g., histologic scar in testis)
pTis	Intratubular germ cell neoplasia (carcinoma in situ)
pT1	Tumor limited to testis and epididymis without vascular/lymphatic invasion; tumor may invade into tunica albuginea but not tunica vaginalis
pT2	Tumor limited to testis and epididymis with vascular/lymphatic invasion or tumor extending through tunica albuginea with involvement of tunica vaginalis
pT3	Tumor invades spermatic cord with or without vascular/lymphatic invasion
pT4	Tumor invades scrotum with or without vascular/lymphatic invasion

REGIONAL LYMPH NODES (N)
Clinical (as Determined by Noninvasive Staging)

NX	Regional lymph nodes cannot be assessed
N0	No regional lymph node metastasis
N1	Metastasis with lymph node mass ≤2 cm in greatest dimension; or multiple lymph nodes, none more than 2 cm in greatest dimension
N2	Metastasis with lymph node mass, >2 cm, but not more than 5 cm in greatest dimension; or multiple lymph nodes, any one mass >2 cm but not more than 5 cm in greatest dimension
N3	Metastasis with lymph node mass >5 cm in greatest dimension

Pathologic (pN) (as Determined by Pathologic Findings of RPLND Without Prior Chemotherapy or Radiotherapy)

pNX	Regional lymph nodes cannot be assessed
pN0	No regional lymph node metastasis
pN1	Metastasis with lymph node mass ≤2 cm in greatest dimension and ≤5 nodes positive, none more than 2 cm in greatest dimension
pN2	Metastasis with lymph node mass >2 cm but not more than 5 cm in greatest dimension; or >5 nodes positive, none more than 5 cm; or evidence of extranodal extension of tumor
pN3	Metastasis with lymph node mass >5 cm in greatest dimension

DISTANT METASTASIS (M)

MX	Distant metastasis cannot be assessed
M0	No distant metastasis
M1	Distant metastasis
M1a	Nonregional nodal or pulmonary metastasis
M1b	Distant metastasis at site other than nonregional lymph nodes or lung

SERUM TUMOR MARKERS (S)

SX	Marker studies unavailable or not performed
S0	Marker study levels within normal limits
S1	LDH <1.5 × N[b] *and* HCG (MIU/mL) <5000 *and* AFP (ng/mL) <1000
S2	LDH 1.5-10 × N *or* HCG (MIU/mL) 5000–50,000 *or* AFP (ng/mL) 1000–10,000
S3	LDH >10 × N *or* HCG (MIU/mL) >50,000 *or* AFP (ng/mL) >10,000

STAGE GROUPING

GROUP	T	N	M	S (SERUM TUMOR MARKERS)
Stage 0	pTis	N0	M0	S0
Stage I	pT1-4	N0	M0	SX
Stage IA	pT1	N0	M0	S0
Stage IB	pT2	N0	M0	S0
	pT3	N0	M0	S0
	pT4	N0	M0	S0

Continued

TABLE 76.2 TNM Staging of Testicular Tumor: American Joint Committee on Cancer and Union Internationale Contre le Cancer—cont'd

GROUP	T	N	M	S (SERUM TUMOR MARKERS)
Stage IS	Any pT/Tx	N0	M0	S1-3
Stage II	Any pT/Tx	N1-3	M0	SX
Stage IIA	Any pT/Tx	N1	M0	S0
	Any pT/Tx	N1	M0	S1
Stage IIB	Any pT/Tx	N2	M0	S0
	Any pT/Tx	N2	M0	S1
Stage IIC	Any pT/Tx	N3	M0	S0
	Any pT/Tx	N3	M0	S1
Stage III	Any pT/Tx	Any N	M1	SX
Stage IIIA	Any pT/Tx	Any N	M1a	S0
	Any pT/Tx	Any N	M1a	S1
Stage IIIB	Any pT/Tx	N1-3	M0	S2
	Any pT/Tx	Any N	M1a	S2
Stage IIIC	Any pT/Tx	N1-3	M0	S3
	Any pT/Tx	Any N	M1a	S3
	Any pT/Tx	Any N	M1b	Any S

[a]Except for pTis and pT4, extent of primary tumor is classified by radical orchiectomy. Tx may be used for other categories in the absence of radical orchiectomy.
[b]N indicates the upper limit of normal for the LDH assay.
AFP, α-Fetoprotein; *HCG*, human chorionic gonadotropin; *LDH*, lactate dehydrogenase; *RPLND*, retroperitoneal lymph node dissection.
Data from AJCC: Testis. In Edge SE, Byrd DR, Compton CC, editors: *AJCC Cancer Staging Manual*, ed 7, New York, 2010, Springer, pp 469–473.

majority of cases (Elert et al., 2002; Tokuc et al., 1992). **Biopsies of the adjacent testicular parenchyma should be performed to rule out the presence of GCNIS. For patients with GCNIS, adjuvant radiotherapy to the residual testis using doses of at least 20 Gy is usually sufficient to prevent the development of a GCT while preserving Leydig cell function (and thereby testicular androgen production).** Radiation at these doses causes permanent sterility of the treated testis. Leydig cell function may decline over time, and up to 40% will require supplemental testosterone (Petersen et al., 2002). The German Testicular Cancer Study Group reported no cases of local recurrence over a median follow-up of 91 months in 46 patients with small, organ-confined tumors who underwent testis-sparing surgery and received adjuvant radiotherapy for GCNIS (Heidenreich et al., 2001). In contrast, recurrent testis cancer developed in 4 of 5 men who did not receive adjuvant radiotherapy. Adjuvant radiotherapy may be delayed after testis-sparing surgery if fathering a child is desired, although close follow-up is mandatory (Giannarini et al., 2010).

Contralateral Testis Biopsy

Between 5% and 9% of patients with GCT have GCNIS in the normal contralateral testis (Dieckmann and Skakkebaek, 1999). In patients with an atrophic testis, history of cryptorchidism, or age less than 40 years, the risk of GCNIS in the contralateral testis has been reported in up to 36% (Dieckmann and Loy, 1996). Thus an open inguinal biopsy of the contralateral testis may be considered in patients with risk factors for GCNIS or those with suspicious lesions on preoperative ultrasound (Motzer et al., 2006).

Suspected Extragonadal Germ Cell Tumor

Approximately 5% of GCTs are extragonadal (Bokemeyer et al., 2002). Thus GCT should be considered in any male with a midline mass and a normal testicular examination. Of the patients with metastatic GCT without a testis mass, only one-third definitively have a primary extragonadal GCT. The majority of these cases represent a "burned-out" primary testicular tumor that has undergone spontaneous regression as 30% to 50% have evidence of GCNIS in the testis and one-third have sonographic evidence of a "burned-out" tumor on the basis of a scar or coarse calcification (Scholz et al., 2002; Ulbright and Young, 2014). GCT should be considered in any young male with a midline mass. The presence of elevated serum AFP and/or HCG with a normal testicular evaluation is sufficient for the diagnosis of GCT, and histologic confirmation by biopsy is not necessary before starting treatment. In cases of normal serum tumor markers, biopsy of the mass should be performed to confirm the diagnosis of GCT before commencing treatment. A biopsy showing poorly differentiated carcinoma represents a diagnostic dilemma if a primary tumor site cannot be confirmed. In this scenario, the diagnosis of extragonadal GCT with malignant transformation may be considered and supported by the expression of i(12p) in biopsy specimens.

Patients with suspected extragonadal GCT should undergo inguinal orchiectomy at some point during their treatment course if the pattern of metastasis is consistent with a right- or left-sided testicular primary or if there is sonographic evidence of a "burned-out" primary tumor.

> **KEY POINTS: DIAGNOSIS AND WORK-UP**
>
> - A solid intratesticular mass in a postpubertal male should be considered a GCT until proven otherwise.
> - With rare exceptions, inguinal orchiectomy with high ligation of the spermatic cord should be performed in men suspected of having GCT. Trans-scrotal orchiectomy or biopsy are to be condemned.
> - Testis-sparing surgery for GCT is a consideration in highly select patients who have a small tumor in either a solitary testis or synchronous bilateral testis masses, where preservation of the affected testis will provide the patient with sufficient testicular androgen production.
> - Diagnostic delay is common in GCT, and approximately one-third of cases are initially misdiagnosed.
> - If elevated before orchiectomy, serum tumor marker levels should be measured after orchiectomy to determine if levels are declining, stable, or rising. Preorchiectomy serum tumor marker levels should not be used in management decisions.

Clinical Staging

The prognosis of GCT and initial management decisions are dictated by the clinical stage of the disease, which is based on the histopathological findings and pathological stage of the primary tumor, post-orchiectomy serum tumor marker levels, and the presence and extent of metastatic disease as determined by physical examination and staging imaging studies. In 1997 an international consensus classification for GCT was developed by the American Joint Committee on Cancer (AJCC) and Union Internationale Contre le Cancer (UICC) (see Table 76.2). The AJCC and UICC staging systems for GCT are unique because, for the first time, a serum tumor marker category (S) based on post-orchiectomy AFP, HCG, and LDH levels is used to supplement the prognostic stages as defined by anatomic extent of disease. **The AJCC and UICC staging systems were updated in 2002, and the new systems consider the presence of LVI in the primary as pT2 in an otherwise organ-confined tumor. CS I** is defined as disease clinically confined to the testis, **CS II** indicates the presence of regional (retroperitoneal) lymph node metastasis, and **CS III** represents non-regional lymph node and/or visceral metastasis.

Staging Imaging Studies

GCT follows a predictable pattern of metastatic spread that has contributed to its successful management. **With the exception of choriocarcinoma, the most common route of disease dissemination is via lymphatic channels from the primary tumor to the retroperitoneal lymph nodes and subsequently to distant sites. Choriocarcinoma has a propensity for hematogenous dissemination. The retroperitoneum is the initial site of metastatic spread in 70% to 80% of patients with GCT.** Detailed mapping studies from retroperitoneal lymph node dissection (RPLND) series have increased our understanding of the testicular lymphatic drainage and identified the most likely sites of metastatic spread (Sheinfeld, 1994). **For right testis tumors, the primary drainage site is the inter-aortocaval lymph nodes inferior to the renal vessels, followed by the paracaval and para-aortic (PA) nodes. The primary "landing zone" for left testis tumors is the PA lymph nodes, followed by the interaortocaval nodes** (Donohue et al., 1982). **The pattern of lymph drainage in the retroperitoneum is from right to left.** Thus contralateral spread from the primary "landing zone" is common with right-sided tumors but is rarely seen with left-sided tumors and usually is associated with bulky disease. **More caudal deposits of metastatic disease usually reflect retrograde spread to distal iliac and inguinal lymph nodes secondary to large volume disease and, more rarely, aberrant testicular lymphatic drainage. Retroperitoneal lymphatics drain into the cisterna chyli behind the right renal artery and right crus of the diaphragm.** Thus retrocrural lymph node metastasis may be visible in patients with retroperitoneal disease. From there, lymphatic spread occurs via the thoracic duct to the posterior mediastinum and left supraclavicular fossa.

Clinical Staging of the Abdomen and Pelvis

All patients with GCT should undergo staging imaging studies of the abdomen and pelvis. Computed tomography (CT) imaging with oral and intravenous contrast is the most effective, noninvasive means of staging the retroperitoneum and pelvis. CT imaging also provides a detailed anatomic assessment of the retroperitoneum to identify anatomic anomalies that may complicate subsequent RPLND, such as a circum-aortic or retro-aortic left renal vein, lower pole renal artery, or retrocaval right ureter. MRI is an alternative to CT, although it is associated with longer examination times, higher cost, and less availability.

Enlarged retroperitoneal lymph nodes are found on CT in approximately 10% to 20% of seminomas and 60% to 70% of NSGCT. The retroperitoneum continues to be the most difficult area to accurately stage clinically. **A consistent 25% to 35% rate of pathologically involved retroperitoneal lymph nodes has been a "normal" CT scan.** A size cutoff of 10 mm is frequently used to identify enlarged lymph reported for CS I NSGCT in the presence of a "normal" CT scan despite the improvements in CT imaging over the last 4 decades (Fernandez et al., 1994). There is no consensus regarding size criteria for retroperitoneal lymph nodes that constitutes nodes, but false-negative rates up to 63% have been reported when this size criterion is used. Among patients with CS IIA and IIB disease, clinical overstaging by CT (i.e., pathologically negative lymph nodes at RPLND despite enlarged lymph nodes on CT) is reported in 12% to 40% of patients.

An understanding of the primary drainage sites for left- and right-sided tumors has led to efforts to increase the sensitivity of abdominal-pelvic CT imaging by decreasing the size criteria for clinically positive lymph nodes in the primary landing zone. Leibovitch et al. (1995) showed that using a size cutoff of 4 mm in the primary landing zone and 10 mm outside this region was associated with a sensitivity and specificity for pathologic stage II disease of 91% and 50%, respectively. In a similar study, Hilton et al. (1997) reported a sensitivity and specificity of 93% and 58%, respectively using a cutoff of 4 mm for lymph nodes in the primary landing zone that were anterior to a horizontal line bisecting the aorta. **Based on this evidence, retroperitoneal lymph nodes 5 to 9 mm in size in the primary landing zone should be viewed with suspicion for regional lymph node metastasis, particularly if they are anterior to the great vessels on transaxial images (Fig. 76.3).** Because of the rapid growth of GCT, it is advisable to base management decision on CT imaging studies performed within 4 weeks of the initiation of treatment.

Malignant GCT accumulate fluorodeoxyglucose (FDG) and several studies have investigated positron emission tomography (FDG-PET) in the staging of GCT at diagnosis and assessing response after chemotherapy. Several small pilot studies suggested that FDG-PET can identify retroperitoneal metastasis in low-stage seminoma and NSGCT more precisely than CT (Albers et al., 1999). In a prospective trial of centrally reviewed FDG-PET studies in 111 contemporary patients with CS I NSGCT on surveillance, relapse was observed in 33 of 87 patients who were PET-negative with an estimated relapse-free rate of 63% (Huddart et al., 2007). The investigators concluded the FDG-PET is not sufficiently sensitive to accurately stage CS I NSGCT. De Wit et al. (2008) also reported that FDG-PET yielded only slightly better results than CT as a primary staging tool for low-stage NSGCT. **Thus there is currently no role for FDG-PET in the routine evaluation of NSGCT and seminoma at the time of diagnosis.**

CS II disease is subclassified based on the size of regional lymph node(s) as determined by abdominal-pelvic imaging into IIA (enlarged retroperitoneal lymph nodes ≤ 2 cm), IIB (enlarged retroperitoneal lymph nodes > 2 cm but ≤ 5 cm), and IIC (enlarged lymph nodes > 5 cm).

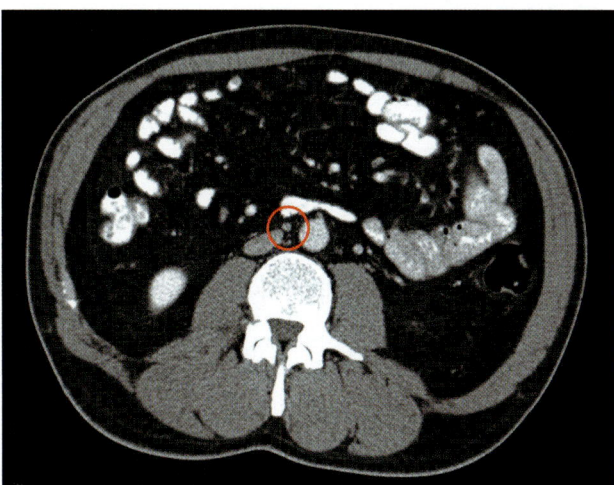

Fig. 76.3. Postorchiectomy computed tomography image of abdomen-pelvis in a patient with right testicular nonseminoma germ cell tumor showing 7-mm lymph node in primary landing zone. The lymph node was involved with teratoma at retroperitoneal lymph node dissection.

Pathological Staging of the Abdomen and Pelvis

In select European centers performing open RPLND and most laparoscopic RPLND series, RPLND is performed in patients with CS I or IIA NSGCT, largely as a staging procedure without curative intent, to identify the presence of regional lymph nodes and determine the need for subsequent chemotherapy (Albers et al., 2003, 2008; Bhayani et al., 2003; Janetschek et al., 2000; Nelson et al., 1999, 2007; Nielsen et al., 2007). Pathological N stage differs from clinical N stage in that the former considers the number of lymph nodes involved:

pN0: no regional lymph node metastasis
pN1: ≤5 lymph nodes involved, none > 2 cm
pN2: >5 lymph nodes involved and/or any lymph node 2–5 cm
pN3: any lymph node > 5 cm

In patients with pathological stage II disease (pTany, pN1-3, M0), the risk of occult metastases (and relapse after RPLND) is closely related to the burden of regional lymph node metastasis (10%–30% of pN1 vs. 50%–80% for pN2-3). The pathological N stage cannot be applied to RPLND specimens from patients who have received prior chemotherapy.

Chest Imaging

All patients with GCT should undergo chest imaging before management decisions. Thoracic metastasis in the absence of retroperitoneal disease and/or elevated serum tumor markers is uncommon, particularly for seminoma. Thus routine chest CT imaging may be associated with a high rate of false-positive findings, which may complicate subsequent therapy (Horan et al., 2007). Thus it is reasonable to obtain chest radiographs at the time of diagnosis as an initial staging study and CT should be performed in patients with elevated post-orchiectomy serum tumor markers, evidence of metastatic disease by physical examination or abdominal-pelvic CT imaging, or abnormal or equivocal findings on chest x-ray (CXR). It may be reasonable to perform chest CT imaging in patients with CS I NSGCT with evidence of LVI or EC predominance because some studies have reported a high rate of hematogenous metastasis to the lung in the setting of a negative CT for retroperitoneal metastasis (Hermans et al., 2000; Sweeney et al., 2000). Mediastinal or hilar lymphadenopathy in the absence of retroperitoneal disease should raise the index of suspicion of non-GCT cause such as lymphoma or sarcoidosis, and histologic confirmation of GCT by mediastinoscopy and biopsy should be performed before initiating systemic therapy (Hunt et al., 2009).

Visceral metastasis to bone and brain is uncommon in GCT in the absence of symptoms or other clinical indicators of disease. As such, there is no role for routine bone scintigraphy or brain CT imaging at the time of diagnosis. A notable exception to this is brain CT imaging for patients with a highly elevated HCG (>10,000 mU/mL) because these levels are often associated with metastatic choriocarcinoma, which has a propensity for brain metastases.

Serum Tumor Markers

Post-orchiectomy AFP, HCG, and LDH levels are important for staging, prognosis, and treatment selection. **Thus all patients should have serum tumor markers drawn after orchiectomy to assess for appropriate decline according to half-life in those with elevated levels before orchiectomy. The presence of newly elevated and/or rising serum tumor marker levels after orchiectomy indicates the presence of metastatic disease, and these patients should receive induction chemotherapy.** In setting of a negative metastatic evaluation and slowly declining markers (i.e., not according to half-life), patients should be monitored closely and have levels checked periodically until levels normalize or begin to rise. Stable AFP or HCG levels slightly above the normal range should be interpreted cautiously, and other causes for serum tumor marker elevation should be ruled out before management decisions are made. As with staging imaging studies, management decisions should be based on serum tumor marker levels measured within 4 weeks of the initiation of treatment.

Prognostic Classification of Advanced Germ Cell Tumor

An international, retrospective pooled analysis of 5202 patients with advanced NSGCT treated between 1975 and 1990 with platin-containing chemotherapy regimens (cisplatin or carboplatin) identified AFP, HCG, and LDH levels at the initiation of chemotherapy, the presence of nonpulmonary visceral metastasis, and primary mediastinal NSGCT as significant and independent prognostic factors for progression and survival (International Germ Cell Cancer Collaborative Group, 1997). In 660 patients with advanced seminoma, only the presence of nonpulmonary visceral metastasis was an important predictor of progression and survival (International Germ Cell Cancer Collaborative Group, 1997).

Based on these analyses, the International Germ Cell Cancer Collaborative Group (IGCCCG) risk classification for advanced GCT was developed (Table 76.3) (International Germ Cell Cancer Collaborative Group, 1997). **The IGCCCG risk group should be determined for each patient with metastatic GCT, and this should be used to guide treatment decision making on the choice of chemotherapy (discussed later).** It should be emphasized that this classification applies only to advanced GCT patients at the time of diagnosis and is not applicable to patients with relapsed GCT. It is also based on the post-orchiectomy serum tumor marker levels at the start of chemotherapy, not pre-orchiectomy levels.

Approximately 56%, 28%, and 16% of advanced NSGCT patients are classified as good-, intermediate-, and poor-risk by IGCCCG criteria, and the 5-year progression-free and overall survival rates for these patients are 89% and 92%, 75% and 80%, and 41% and 48%, respectively. There is no poor-risk category for seminoma. Approximately 90% and 10% of advanced seminoma patients are classified as good- and intermediate-risk by IGCCCG criteria, and the 5-year progression-free and overall survival rates for these patients is 82% and 86%, and 67% and 72%, respectively. Van Dijk et al. (2006) recently published a meta-analysis of 10 studies of 1775 NSGCT patients treated after 1989 and reported pooled 5-year survival estimates of 94%, 83% and 71% for good-, intermediate-, and poor-risk patients by IGCCCG criteria. These results represent a significantly improved survival compared with the original study (particularly for those classified as poor-risk) and are attributed to more effective therapy and more experience in treating NSGCT patients.

The TNM system does incorporate marker levels (S0-3) and nonpulmonary visceral metastasis in the staging of testis cancer. However, this system does not consider the differences in prognosis between seminomas and NSGCT with nonpulmonary visceral metastasis. In the TNM, these would be classified as stage IIIC but IGCCCG would classify the former as intermediate risk and the latter as poor risk. As such, the IGCCCG system is preferentially used for prognostic assessment and the selection of chemotherapy.

Sperm Cryopreservation

Although infertility is an uncommon presentation for GCT, up to 52% of men have oligospermia at diagnosis and 10% are azoospermic (Williams et al., 2009). The germinal epithelium is exquisitely sensitive to platin-based chemotherapy and radiation therapy. Almost all patients will become azoospermic after chemotherapy, and 50% and 80% of patients with normal semen parameters at diagnosis will return to these levels within 2 and 5 years, respectively (Bokemeyer et al., 1996; Feldman et al., 2008). Recovery of spermatogenesis after radiation therapy for seminoma may take to 2 to 3 years or more (Fossa et al., 1999). Retroperitoneal lymph node dissection may result in ejaculatory dysfunction in 80% or more of patients undergoing a full, bilateral template dissection without nerve sparing. **Given the impact of treatments for testis cancer on fertility, men who are undecided or are planning future paternity are recommended to undergo sperm cryopreservation before treatment is initiated.** Sperm banking can be done before or after radical orchiectomy.

TABLE 76.3 International Germ Cell Cancer Collaborative Group Risk Classification for Advanced Germ Cell Tumor

NONSEMINOMA	SEMINOMA
GOOD PROGNOSIS	
Testicular/retroperitoneal primary	Any primary site
and	and
No nonpulmonary visceral metastases	No nonpulmonary visceral metastases
and	and
Good markers—all of:	Normal AFP, any HCG, any LDH
AFP <1000 ng/mL and	
HCG <5000 IU/L (1000 ng/mL) and	
LDH <1.5 × upper limit of normal (N)	
56% of nonseminomas	90% of seminomas
5-year PFS 89%	5-year PFS 82%
5-year survival 92%	5-year survival 86%
INTERMEDIATE PROGNOSIS	
Testicular/retroperitoneal primary	Any primary site
and	and
No nonpulmonary visceral metastases	Nonpulmonary visceral metastases
and	and
Intermediate markers—any of:	Normal AFP, any HCG, any LDH
AFP ≥1000–10,000 ng/mL and ≤10,000 ng/mL or	
HCG ≥5000–50,000 IU/L and ≤50,000 IU/L or	
LDH ≥1.5 × N and ≤10 × N	
28% of nonseminomas	10% of seminomas
5-year PFS 75%	5-year PFS 67%
5-year survival 80%	5-year survival 72%
POOR PROGNOSIS	
Mediastinal primary	No patients classified as poor prognosis
or	
Nonpulmonary visceral metastases	
or	
Poor serum markers—any of:	
AFP >10,000 ng/mL or	
HCG >50,000 IU/L (10,000 ng/mL) or	
LDH >10 × upper limit of normal	
16% of nonseminomas	
5-year PFS 41%	
5-year survival 48%	

AFP, α-Fetoprotein; HCG, human chorionic gonadotropin; LDH, lactate dehydrogenase; PFS, progression-free survival.
Data from International Germ Cell Consensus Classification: a prognostic factor-based staging system for metastatic germ cell cancers. International Germ Cell Cancer Collaborative Group. *J Clin Oncol* 15:594–603, 1997.

KEY POINTS: STAGING

- Testicular GCT follows a predictable pattern of spread from the primary tumor to retroperitoneal lymph nodes and then to distant metastatic sites.
- The primary landing zone for left-sided tumors is the para-aortic and left renal hilar lymph nodes and for right-sided tumors is the inter-aortocaval and paracaval lymph nodes.
- CT imaging is the optimal modality for staging the retroperitoneum, although false-negatives occur in 25% to 35% and 14% to 20% of patients with CS I NSGCT and seminoma, respectively, when a 1-cm cutoff is used.
- Chest x-ray and CT chest are acceptable staging modalities in the absence of retroperitoneal lymphadenopathy or elevated serum tumor marker levels. If serum tumor markers are persistently elevated or CT abdomen and pelvis shows evidence of metastatic disease, then a chest CT should be performed.
- Rising post-orchiectomy serum tumor marker levels indicate the presence of metastatic GCT and these patients should receive chemotherapy.
- The IGCCCG risk classification is used to evaluate the prognosis of patients with metastatic GCT and dictates the selection of chemotherapy. For NSGCT, IGCCCG risk is assigned based on the post-orchiectomy serum tumor marker levels, mediastinal primary tumor, and the presence of nonpulmonary visceral metastases. For seminoma, IGCCCG risk is assigned based on the presence of nonpulmonary visceral metastases only.
- Sperm cryopreservation should be offered to all patients before RPLND, chemotherapy, or radiation therapy because of the potential effects of these treatments on fertility.

required with earlier diagnosis and proper management. After orchiectomy, staging imaging studies, serum tumor marker status, and treatment plans should be performed/developed as rapidly as can be reasonably accomplished.

The probability of cure even in the presence of metastatic disease has also led to an aggressive approach with regard to the administration of chemotherapy and the performance of post-chemotherapy surgery to resect residual masses. Chemotherapy is generally administered regardless of low white blood cell counts or thrombocytopenia, and nephrotoxic chemotherapy (cisplatin) is often administered even in the presence of moderate-to-severe renal insufficiency (Bajorin et al., 1993; Bokemeyer et al., 1996; de Wit et al., 2001; Einhorn et al., 1989; Loehrer et al., 1995; Nichols et al., 1998; Williams et al., 1987). Similarly, an aggressive surgical approach is taken to resect all sites of residual disease after chemotherapy for NSGCT, even if this involves multiple anatomic sites. The young age and generally good health of GCT patients permits an aggressive treatment approach if needed.

Serum tumor markers strongly influence the management of GCTs, particularly NSGCT. As discussed, **elevated serum AFP or HCG after orchiectomy indicates the presence of metastatic disease and these patients are preferentially given chemotherapy.** For patients receiving chemotherapy, rising serum tumor markers levels during or after therapy generally indicates refractory or relapsed disease, respectively. As discussed, serum AFP, HCG, and LDH levels at the initiation of chemotherapy are important prognostic factors and influence the selection and duration of chemotherapy regimens (International Germ Cell Cancer Collaborative Group, 1997).

Testis cancer is a relatively rare disease and general urologists and general oncologists do not typically treat a large volume of GCT patients. In addition, the treatment algorithms are relatively complex and nuanced and the data supporting certain treatments, such as RPLND, are based on data from a relatively small number of surgeons who have performed a large number of these operations (Donohue et al., 1993, 1995; Heidenreich et al., 2003; Stephenson et al., 2005b;

Treatment

Therapeutic Principles

The management of GCTs is governed by the potential for rapid growth and for cure in almost all patients. **This translates into a need for rapid diagnosis and staging and expeditious application of appropriate treatment so as not to have patients die unnecessarily or suffer side effects from treatment that would not have been**

Williams et al., 2009). The majority of urology residents in the United States complete their training having performed 2 or fewer RPLND procedures (Lowrance et al., 2007). Several studies have reported improved survival when the treatment was provided at high-volume institutions (Aass et al., 1991; Collette et al., 1999; Harding et al., 1993; Feuer et al., 1994; Joudi and Konety, 2005; Suzumura et al., 2008). Therefore, whenever possible, GCT patients should be treated at a high-volume centers and RPLND should be performed by surgeons who are experienced with this operation.

Contrasting Seminoma and Nonseminoma Germ Cell Tumor

For treatment purposes, the distinction between seminoma and NSGCT holds great importance. Compared with NSGCT, seminoma has a relatively favorable natural history. In general, seminoma tends to be less aggressive, to be diagnosed at an earlier stage, and to spread predictably along lymphatic channels to the retroperitoneum before spreading hematogenously to the lungs or other organs. **At diagnosis, the proportion of patients with CS I, II, and III disease is 85%, 10%, and 5%, respectively, for seminoma and approximately 33%, 33%, and 33% for NSGCT** (Powles et al., 2005). **Seminoma is also associated with a lower incidence of occult metastasis among patients with CS I (10%–15% vs. 25%–35% for NSGCT) and a lower risk of systemic relapse after treatment of the retroperitoneum (1%–4% after radiotherapy for seminoma vs. 10% after RPLND for NSGCT)**, which has important implications for the use of chemotherapy. Seminoma is less likely to have elevated serum tumor markers and does not range as high as in NSGCT. Serum tumor markers are also not used in the IGCCCG risk classification of seminoma.

Compared with NSGCT, **seminoma is exquisitely sensitive to radiation therapy and platin-based chemotherapy**. Regarding the former aspect, substantially lower radiation doses are required to eradicate seminoma compared to other solid tumors. As such, **radiation therapy is a standard treatment option for CS I and IIA-B seminoma but has no role in NSGCT**, with the exception of treatment for brain metastases. Seminoma only accounts for 10% of advanced GCT cases despite the fact it accounts for 52% to 56% of all GCTs. A poor prognosis IGCCCG risk category does not exist for advanced seminoma and more than 90% of metastatic cases are classified as good risk (compared with 56% for NSGCT) (International Germ Cell Cancer Collaborative Group, 1997). **The risk of teratoma at metastatic sites is generally not a consideration for advanced seminoma, which has important implications for the management of residual masses after chemotherapy. However, the potential for seminoma to transform into NSGCT elements is an important consideration in the management of patients who fail to respond to chemotherapy or who relapse after radiation therapy. Of patients with metastatic seminoma who relapse after treatment, approximately 10% to 15% have NSGCT elements at the site(s) of relapse. An autopsy study has shown that 30% of patients who die from seminoma have NSGCT elements at metastatic sites** (Bredael et al., 1982).

The risk of teratoma at metastatic sites has a substantial effect on treatment algorithms for NSGCT and necessitates the frequent use of post-chemotherapy surgery (PCS) in patients with advanced disease. The risk of teratoma in the retroperitoneum in low-stage NSGCT has also influenced many clinicians to favor RPLND over chemotherapy in situations in which the risk of occult distant metastases is low. As discussed, teratoma is not sensitive to chemotherapy and the outcome of patients with metastatic teratoma is related to the completeness of surgical resection.

Because GCTs are almost always cured, numerous clinical trials have been conducted in an attempt to minimize treatment and avoid any unnecessary therapies in an effort to reduce short- and particularly long-term side effects and toxicity. One such approach has been to limit the number of patients who receive two interventions ("double-therapy"): either surgery or chemotherapy and not both. **However, because NSGCTs are usually mixed tumors and teratoma often exists at metastatic sites with other GCT elements, "cure" often requires chemotherapy to kill the chemosensitive components and surgery to remove teratomatous components**. It is widely accepted that the successful integration of systemic therapy and post-chemotherapy surgery is a major contributing factor to the improved cure rates for metastatic GCT seen over the past several decades. Although minimizing unnecessary treatment is an important goal, chemotherapy, radiation therapy, and CT imaging are associated with an increased lifetime risk of secondary malignant neoplasms (SMN) and/or cardiovascular disease (Brenner and Hall, 2007; Meinardi et al., 2000; Tarin et al., 2009; van den Belt-Dusebout et al., 2007; Zagars et al., 2004). In contrast, RPLND is associated with a substantially more favorable long-term toxicity profile when performed by experienced surgeons.

> **KEY POINTS: SEMINOMA VS. NONSEMINOMA**
>
> - Compared with NSGCT, seminoma is associated with an indolent natural history with a lower incidence of metastatic disease and lower rates of occult retroperitoneal and distant metastases in patients with CS I and IIA-B, respectively.
> - No poor-risk prognostic category exists for metastatic seminoma, and substantially more patients are classified as good-risk by IGCCCG criteria compared with NSGCT.
> - Seminoma is associated with increased sensitivity to radiation therapy and platin-based chemotherapy compared with NSGCT.
> - Serum HCG is elevated in only 15% of patients with metastatic seminoma, and serum tumor marker levels are not used to guide treatment decisions.
> - Teratoma at metastatic sites is less of a concern for seminoma compared with NSGCT but should be considered in patients who fail to respond to conventional therapy.

Germ Cell Neoplasia in Situ

GCNIS is diagnosed by testicular biopsy performed for the investigation of infertility, contralateral testis biopsy in patient with GCT, or within the affected testis in a patient undergoing testis-sparing surgery. The rationale for treatment of GCNIS is based on the high risk of developing invasive GCT (Dieckmann and Skakkebaek, 1999; Skakkebaek et al., 1982). Treatment options include orchiectomy, low-dose radiotherapy, and close observation. The choice of therapy should be individualized based on the patient's desire for future paternity, the presence or absence of a normal contralateral testis, and the patient's desire to avoid testosterone replacement therapy. **Radical orchiectomy is the most definitive, although low-dose radiotherapy (≥ 20 Gy) is associated with similar rates of local control with the prospect of preserving testicular endocrine because of the relative radio-resistance of Leydig cells compared with germinal epithelium** (Dieckmann et al., 2003; Heidenreich et al., 2001; Montironi, 2002). **However, testosterone replacement therapy is ultimately required in up to 40% of patients, and patients should be monitored after radiotherapy for adequate testicular androgen production** (Heidenreich et al., 2001; Petersen et al., 2002). To preserve testicular endocrine function, dose reductions less than 20 Gy have been investigated, but cases of recurrent GCNIS have been observed (Classen et al., 2003; Dieckmann et al., 2003). For patients with a normal contralateral testis who desire future paternity, radical orchiectomy is preferred as scatter to the contralateral testis from radiotherapy may impair spermatogenesis. For patients with abnormal semen parameters but sufficient for assisted reproductive techniques, close surveillance with periodic sonographic evaluation of the testis is a reasonable strategy with deferred therapy until successful pregnancy and/or GCT. Another option for these patients is testis exploration, sperm harvesting, and cryopreservation for assisted reproductive techniques, and radical orchiectomy followed by testosterone replacement therapy.

Patients with GCNIS scheduled to receive cisplatin-based chemotherapy represent a unique circumstance because chemotherapy may reduce (but not eliminate) the risk of GCT. A recent study estimated the risk of testicular GCT after chemotherapy in a patient with GCNIS to be 21% and 45% and 5 and 10 years, respectively (Christensen et al., 1998). These patients may be treated by low-dose radiotherapy after completion of chemotherapy or they may undergo testis biopsy 2 years or more after chemotherapy with therapy reserved for patients with evidence of GCNIS (Krege et al., 2008a).

> **KEY POINTS: GERM CELL NEOPLASIA IN SITU**
>
> - GCNIS is a precursor lesion for GCT and is associated with a 50% risk of developing an invasive GCT within 5 years.
> - Radical orchiectomy or low-dose (≥ 20 Gy) radiation therapy is an effective treatment option for GCNIS.

Nonseminoma Germ Cell Tumor

Clinical Stage I Nonseminoma Germ Cell Tumor

Approximately one-third of NSGCT patients have CS I with normal post-orchiectomy serum tumor markers. **The optimal management of these patients continues to generate controversy as the long-term survival associated with surveillance, RPLND, and primary chemotherapy approaches 100%.** Contributing to the controversy is the fact that occult metastases in the retroperitoneum or at distant sites are present in only 20% to 30% of patients overall. Thus any intervention after orchiectomy, with the potential for short- and long-term morbidity, represents overtreatment for the 70% to 80% of patients with disease limited to the testis. Most centers employ a risk-adapted approach based on the probability of occult metastatic, although surveillance is the preferred approach at select centers, regardless of a man's risk.

Risk Assessment. Numerous studies have attempted to identify histopathological factors within the primary tumor that predict for the presence of occult metastasis. **The most commonly identified risk factors for occult metastasis are LVI and a predominant component of EC.** The definition of EC predominance in the literature varies from 45% to 90%. **The reported rate of occult metastasis (based on observed relapses on surveillance or lymph node metastasis at RPLND) with LVI and EC predominance varies from 45% to 90% and 30% to 80%, respectively** (Albers et al., 2003; Alexandre et al., 2001; Heidenreich et al., 1998; Hermans et al., 2000; Nicolai et al., 2004; Roeleveld et al., 2001; Sogani et al., 1998; Stephenson et al., 2005a; Sweeney et al., 2000; Vergouwe et al., 2003). **In the absence of these two risk factors, the risk of occult metastasis is less than 20%.** Other identified risk factors include advanced pT stage, absence of mature teratoma, absence of yolk sac tumor, presence of EC (regardless of the percent composition), percentage of MIB-1 staining, tumor size, and patient age. In a pooled analysis of 23 studies assessing predictors of occult metastasis in CS I NSGCT, Vergouwe et al. identified LVI (odds ratio [OR] 5.2), MIB-1 staining > 70% (OR 4.7), and EC predominance (OR 2.8) as the strongest predictors, and these factors were present in 36%, 55%, and 51% of patients, respectively (Vergouwe et al., 2003).

As discussed previously, the results of abdominal-pelvic CT imaging should be considered when formulating treatment recommendations because a size cutoff of 1 cm is associated with a high false-negative rate. Retroperitoneal lymph nodes greater than 5 to 9 mm in the primary landing zone should be viewed with suspicion for regional lymph node metastasis.

Numerous risk groups and prognostic indices have been proposed based on the presence/absence of several of these risk factors, most commonly on the basis of LVI and EC predominance (Albers et al., 2003; Alexandre et al., 2001; Freedman et al., 1987; Heidenreich et al., 1998; Hermans et al., 2000; Nicolai et al., 2004; Read et al., 1992; Sogani et al., 1998; Stephenson et al., 2005a). **Patients classified as low- vs. high-risk based on LVI and EC predominance applies to the risk of occult metastatic disease in patients with CS I and should not be confused with the IGCCCG risk classification for metastatic NSGCT** (discussed previously). Only one of these prognostic models has been prospectively validated, and none have considered the results of staging CT imaging (Freedman et al., 1987; Read et al., 1992). Four recent prospective studies suggest that LVI and EC predominance is associated with risks of occult metastasis between 35% and 55%, which are substantially lower than the risks reported in older series (Kollmannsberger et al., 2015). A contemporary surveillance series from Princess Margaret Hospital reported a relapse rate of 52% among patients with LVI and/or pure EC (Sturgeon et al., 2011). Similarly, a series from British Columbia and Portland, Oregon, reported that LVI was associated with a relapse rate of 50%, whereas the relapse rate associated with EC predominance was 33% (Kollmannsberger et al., 2010). Likewise, a population-based surveillance study from Scandinavia reported a 42% relapse rate in patients with LVI (Tandstad et al., 2009). Last, only 18% of CS I NSGCT patients treated by RPLND in a randomized trial had retroperitoneal lymph node metastasis despite the fact that 42% had evidence of LVI in the primary tumor (Albers et al., 2008). This lower-than-expected rate of occult metastasis may be due to greater scrutiny of staging CT imaging for abnormal lymph nodes and/or stage migration.

Surveillance. The rationale for surveillance is based on the fact that 70% to 80% of patients with CS I NSGCT are cured by orchiectomy alone and the ability to salvage virtually all relapsing patients with chemotherapy based on the long-term cure rates achieved for chemotherapy for good-risk metastatic NSGCT (International Germ Cell Cancer Collaborative Group, 1997). Surveillance offers the potential of reducing treatment-related toxicity by restricting treatment to those with a proven need for it. Surveillance series have reported overall and disease-specific survival rates indistinguishable from those seen with RPLND and primary chemotherapy. As a result, initial surveillance is regarded as a standard treatment option for CS I NSGCT. The disadvantages of surveillance are that it is associated with the highest risk of relapse, the need for long-term (>5 years) surveillance, the potential for SMN because of intensive surveillance CT imaging (Brenner and Hall, 2007; Tarin et al., 2009), and the more intensive therapy required to treat patients at the time of relapse than if they had received treatment at diagnosis. In the National Cancer Database between 2004 and 2013, surveillance was the most frequently employed treatment approach for NSGCT patients with CS IA (75%) and CS IB (48%) (Weiner et al., 2017).

Published surveillance series have reported results on more than 3000 men, with a mean relapse risk of 28% and 1.2% cancer-specific mortality. The 11 largest series are summarized in Table 76.4 (Colls et al., 1999; Daugaard et al., 2003; Francis et al., 2000; Freedman et al., 1987; Gels et al., 1995; Hao et al., 1998; Kollmannsberger et al., 2010; Read et al., 1992; Sogani et al., 1998; Sharir et al., 1999; Sturgeon et al., 2011; Tandstad et al., 2009, 2010). More than 90% of relapses occur within the first 2 years, but late relapses (>5 years) are seen in up to 1% of patients (as many as 5% in some reports) (Daugaard et al., 2003; Sturgeon et al., 2011). In more contemporary series, 65% to 75% of relapses are contained in the retroperitoneum, with or without elevated serum tumor markers (Sturgeon et al., 2011; Tandstad et al., 2009). Induction chemotherapy is the most common treatment used for relapsing patients because most will have bulky (>3 cm) retroperitoneal lymphadenopathy, elevated serum tumor markers, or distant metastasis. However, patients with normal serum tumor markers and relapses limited to non-bulky (< 3 cm) retroperitoneal lymphadenopathy may be managed initially with RPLND (Stephenson et al., 2007).

The surveillance schedule employed in published series is highly variable, and no schedule has been demonstrated superior to another in terms of survival. Given that the vast majority of relapses will occur within the first 2 years, surveillance imaging and testing is intense in years 0 to 2, with less frequent testing in years 3 to 5. The risk of late relapse mandates surveillance beyond 5 years, but whether such surveillance should include CT scans is controversial. The frequency of abdominal-pelvic CT imaging varies across multiple series from 2 to 13 or more scans within the first 5 years of follow-up. A randomized trial of 2 vs. 5 CT scans in years 1 to 2 reported no significant differences in survival, IGCCCG risk category at relapse, or clinical stage at relapse (Rustin et al., 2007). Noncompliance with the prescribed surveillance schedule has been reported in

TABLE 76.4 Surveillance Series for Clinical Stage I Nonseminoma Germ Cell Tumor

STUDY	PATIENTS	RELAPSES (%)	MEDIAN FOLLOW-UP (MONTHS)	MEDIAN TIME TO RELAPSE (MONTHS)	% SYSTEMIC RELAPSE[a]	GCT DEATHS (%)
Freedman et al., 1987	259	70 (32)	30	NR	61%	3 (1.2)
Read et al., 1992	373	100 (27)	60	3 (1.5–20)	39%	5 (1.3)
Gels et al., 1995	154	42 (27)	72	4 (2–24)	71%	2 (1)
Sogani et al., 1998	105	27 (26)	136	5 (2–24)	37%	3 (3)
Sharir et al., 1999	170	48 (28)	76	7 (2–21)	79%	1 (0.5)
Colls et al., 1999	248	70 (28)	53	NR	73%	4 (1.6)
Francis et al., 2000	183	52 (28)	70	6 (1–12)	54%	2 (1)
Daugaard et al., 2003	301	86 (29)	60	5 (1–171)	66%	0
Ernst et al., 2005; Hao et al., 1998	197	58 (29)	54	6 (2–135)	22%	0
Kollmannsberger et al., 2010b	223	59 (26)	52	NR	NR	0
Sturgeon et al., 2011	371	104	76	7	33	3 (0.8)
Tandstad et al., 2009 (97% were LVI negative and thus low risk)	350	44 (13)	56	8	27%	1 (0.3)
Tandstad et al., 2010 (96% were LVI negative and thus low risk)	129	19 (15)	123	8	37%	0

[a]Systemic relapse defined as relapse with elevated serum tumor markers and/or relapse in tissue other than retroperitoneal lymph nodes.
LVI, Lymphovascular invasion.

35% to 80% of patients in published series (Hao et al., 1998; Howard et al., 1995).

The majority of relapses will be detected by CT imaging or by elevated STM. CXR and physical examination rarely detect relapses and may be of limited clinical utility. Patients with lymphovascular invasion are more likely to have elevated STM at relapse compared with those without lymphovascular invasion (61% vs. 38%), whereas the latter are more likely to have relapses detected by surveillance CT imaging (48% vs. 41%) (Kollmannsberger et al., 2015). Although late relapses occur in a small proportion of patients, the treatment of these relapses with chemotherapy, surgery, or a combination of the two appears to be as successful as those with early relapses (Rice et al., 2014).

Retroperitoneal Lymph Node Dissection. The rationale for RPLND for CS I NSGCT is based on several factors: (1) the retroperitoneum is the most common site of occult metastatic disease and the risk of associated systemic disease is low, (2) 15% to 25% incidence of retroperitoneal teratoma (which is resistant to chemotherapy) in those with occult metastasis, (3) low risk of abdominal-pelvic recurrence after full, bilateral template RPLND, thereby obviating the need for routine surveillance CT imaging, (4) high cure rates after RPLND alone for patients with low-volume (pN1) retroperitoneal malignancy and teratoma (pN1-3), (5) avoidance of chemotherapy in more than 75% of more of patients if adjuvant chemotherapy is restricted to those with extensive retroperitoneal malignancy (pN2-3), (6) high salvage rate of relapses with good-risk, induction chemotherapy, (7) low short- and long-term morbidity when a nerve-sparing RPLND is performed by experienced surgeons. **In low-stage NSGCT, the therapeutic focus is the retroperitoneum, for which RPLND provides most the effective control with the lowest rates of serious long-term morbidity.** The disadvantages of RPLND are that all patients undergo major abdominal surgery, it requires the availability of experienced surgeons and thus may not be deliverable to all patients, and it is associated with the highest rate of double therapy. In recent years, rates of RPLND have decreased nationally for CS IA (14%) and CS IB (16%) (Weiner et al., 2017).

A summary of the 7 largest RPLND series for CS I NSGCT are listed in Table 76.5 (Albers et al., 2008; Donohue et al., 1993; Hermans et al., 2000; Nicolai et al., 2004; Richie, 1990; Stephenson et al., 2005b; Williams et al., 2009). The rate of pathological stage II in these series ranges from 19% to 28% and an estimated 66% to 81% of these patients were cured after RPLND alone (Al-Ahmadie et al., 2013; Donohue et al., 1993; Hermans et al., 2000; Nicolai et al., 2004; Rabbani et al., 2001; Stephenson et al., 2005a; Sweeney et al., 2000). **The long-term cancer-specific survival with RPLND (+/- adjuvant chemotherapy) approaches 100%, and the risk of late relapse is negligible. Most RPLND series have reported retroperitoneal recurrences in less than 2% of patients, demonstrating its efficacy for control of the retroperitoneum** (Donohue et al., 1993; Hermans et al., 2000; Stephenson et al., 2005b). Rates of relapse after RPLND for retroperitoneal teratoma are low regardless of pathological stage, and adjuvant chemotherapy is not recommended (Liu et al., 2015).

A full, bilateral template dissection is associated with the lowest risk of abdominal-pelvic recurrence (<2%) and the highest rate of antegrade ejaculation (>90%) when nerve-sparing techniques are employed (Donohue and Foster, 1998; Eggener et al., 2007; Jewett, 1990; Stephenson et al., 2005b; Subramanian et al., 2010). For this reason, it is now considered by many to be the standard of care for primary RPLND (Stephenson et al., 2011). A recent randomized trial of primary RPLND (+ adjuvant BEPx2 for pathological stage II) vs. BEPx1 chemotherapy for CS I NSGCT showed a significant improvement in 2-year progression-free survival with chemotherapy (99% vs. 92%), although no GCT deaths were observed in either arm (Albers et al., 2008). The local recurrence rate was 11% in patients with histologically negative retroperitoneal lymph nodes at RPLND, which was substantially higher than the local recurrence rate among all patients from experienced centers. The 191 patients undergoing RPLND in this trial were treated in 1 of 61 centers in Germany. Thus the relative inexperience of surgeons and unilateral templates likely contributed to these poor results. **Thus patients who opt for RPLND should have this procedure performed by experienced surgeon with a full, bilateral template dissection. Otherwise, patients should go on surveillance or receive primary chemotherapy.**

RPLND is a curative procedure in 60% to 90% of patients with pN1 disease and up to 100% of patients with teratoma only (regardless of the extent of lymph node involvement) (Pizzocaro and Monfardini, 1984; Rabbani et al., 2001; Richie and Kantoff, 1991; Sheinfeld et al., 2003; Stephenson et al., 2005; Williams et al., 1987). The risk of relapse in patients with pN2-3 disease is greater than 50% (Socinski et al., 1988; Stephenson et al., 2005b; Vogelzang et al., 1983; Williams et al., 1987). With 2 cycles of adjuvant chemotherapy (most commonly BEPx2 or EPx2), relapses are reduced to 1% or less (Albers et al., 2003; Behnia et al., 2000; Kondagunta et al., 2004). **A randomized trial of adjuvant chemotherapy vs. observation after RPLND for**

TABLE 76.5 Summary of Published Series of Retroperitoneal Lymph Node Dissection for Clinical Stage I Nonseminoma Germ Cell Tumor

	PATIENTS	PS II (%)	% TERATOMA IN RETROPERITONEUM	% RELAPSE, PS I	% RELAPSE, PS II	% ADJUVANT CHEMOTHERAPY	GCT DEATHS (%)
Donohue et al. (Donohue et al., 1993).	378	113 (30)	15%	12%	34%	13%	3 (0.8)
Hermans et al. (Hermans et al., 2000).	292	67 (23)	NR	10%	22%	12%	1 (0.3)
Nicolai et al. (Nicolai et al., 2004).	322	61 (19)	NR	NR	27%	NR	4 (1.2)
Stephenson et al. (Stephenson et al., 2005b).	297	83 (28)	15%	6%	19%	15%	0
Williams et al. (Williams et al., 2009).	76	37 (49)	NR	5%	11%	NR	0
Albers et al. (Albers et al., 2008).	173	31 (19)	NR	9%	***	19%	0
Richie et al. (Richie, 1990).	99	35 (35)	NR	6%	15%	15%	0

GCT, Germ cell tumor; NR, not reported; PS, pathologic stage.

pathological stage II showed a significant reduction in the risk of relapse (6% vs. 49%), but no difference in overall survival (Williams et al., 1987). Adjuvant chemotherapy and observation are acceptable treatment options for patients with pathological stage II disease, and patients should be informed of the risk of relapse after RPLND and the potential benefits and risks of these approaches.

Primary Chemotherapy. In contradistinction to adjuvant chemotherapy given for pathological stage II disease after RPLND, primary chemotherapy refers to treatment administered to men with CS I NSGCT after orchiectomy. The goal of primary chemotherapy is to minimize the risk of relapse and to allow men to avoid RPLND and induction chemotherapy (for those who relapse on surveillance). The rationale for primary chemotherapy is based on the efficacy of 2 cycles of chemotherapy to eradicate micrometastatic disease when given as adjuvant therapy after RPLND and the 20% to 25% need for chemotherapy despite RPLND (either as adjuvant or for treatment of relapse) (Behnia et al., 2000; Hermans et al., 2000; Kondagunta and Motzer, 2007; Nicolai et al., 2004; Stephenson et al., 2005). Primary chemotherapy offers patients the greatest chance of being relapse free with any single treatment modality, and it can be delivered at community-based institutions (Tandstad et al., 2009, 2010). The disadvantages of primary chemotherapy are (1) it does not treat retroperitoneal teratoma and thus exposes patients to the potential for chemo-resistant and/or late relapse (discussed later), (2) long-term surveillance CT imaging of the retroperitoneum is required, and (3) all patients are exposed to chemotherapy and the potential risk of late toxicity (cardiovascular disease and secondary malignancies among others). The risk of late toxicity from 1 or 2 cycles of chemotherapy is poorly defined, although there appears to be no safe lower limit. Rates of primary chemotherapy in the United States for CS IA (13%) and CS IB (37%) NSGCT are substantially lower than in Europe (Weiner et al., 2017).

Primary chemotherapy has been investigated in more than a dozen published series, including five that used BEPx1 (Table 76.6; Abratt et al., 1994; Albers et al., 2008; Amato et al., 2004; Bohlen et al., 1999; Chevreau et al., 2004; Cullen et al., 1996; Dearnaley et al., 2005; Gilbert et al., 2006; Huddart and Reid, 2018; Huddart et al., 2017; Oliver et al., 2004; Ondrus et al., 1998; Pont et al., 1996; Tandstad et al., 2009, 2010). In men with LVI and/or EC predominance, it is possible to reduce the recurrence rate from 30% to 60% down to about 2% to 3%. A total of 1551 subjects were included in the 14 series summarized in Table 76.6, and a total of 38 relapses and 7 deaths were reported. The overall relapse rate was thus 2.4% and the overall mortality rate was 0.45%, but 18% of relapsing patients died. **Primary chemotherapy is thus associated with the lowest risk of relapse, but these relapses are less amenable to salvage therapy** because they are chemo-resistant, particularly if they have received a regimen other than standard dose BEP. In contrast, patients who relapse after RPLND or on surveillance are chemotherapy naïve and are cured with chemotherapy in virtually all cases. However, the overall cure rate (>99%) is similar with both approaches. Although relapses are uncommon with primary chemotherapy, almost all occur in the retroperitoneum. This mandates the use of surveillance CT abdominal-pelvis imaging in the follow-up of these patients. Many European institutions prefer primary chemotherapy with BEP to RPLND, as the latter is primarily used as a staging procedure performed without curative intent (Honecker et al., 2018; Krege et al., 2008a).

For men undergoing primary chemotherapy, major guidelines now recommend BEPx1 (Gilligan et al., 2018; Honecker et al., 2018). Series investing BEPx1 have accrued over 1000 patients and have reported a relapse rate of 2.3% and a mortality rate of 0.2% (n = 2), which is not appreciably different from the rate seen with BEPx2 (Huddart and Reid, 2018).

Treatment Selection for Clinical Stage I Nonseminoma Germ Cell Tumor. There are no randomized trials that compare the standard treatment approaches for CS I NSGCT. A recent phase III, randomized trial compared BEPx1 with unilateral, modified-template RPLND (with BEPx2 for patients with pathological stage II disease) (Albers et al., 2008). Although a statistically significantly reduced risk of relapse was reported with BEPx1 (HR 0.13; 95% CI 0.02–0.55), no cancer-specific deaths were reported in either arm. This trial has been criticized as it compared two non-standard treatment approaches for CS I NSGCT (Sheinfeld and Motzer, 2008).

Given the excellent long-term survival with surveillance, RPLND, and primary chemotherapy, it is inappropriate to recommend any specific treatment option because there are relative advantages and disadvantages of each approach in terms of treatment-related toxicity, the need for subsequent treatment, and intensity of surveillance testing and imaging. Likewise, patient preferences may vary and should be considered. **Several clinical practice guidelines for CS I NSGCT have been published, and surveillance is generally recommended to low-risk patients and either surveillance, RPLND, or primary chemotherapy to those at high-risk** (Albers et al., 2005; Honecker et al., 2018; Hotte et al., 2008; Krege et al., 2008a; Motzer et al., 2006; Stephenson et al., 2011). Recently, Nguyen et al. (2010) developed a decision-analysis model that considered cancer outcomes, treatment-related toxicity, and patient preferences for important post-treatment outcomes to define the optimal treatment for CS I NSGCT. Surveillance is associated with the highest quality-adjusted survival when the estimated risk of relapse is less than 33% to 37%,

TABLE 76.6 Published Series of Primary Chemotherapy for Clinical Stage I Nonseminoma Germ Cell Tumor

	PATIENTS	REGIMEN	MEDIAN FOLLOW-UP (MONTHS)	RELAPSES (%)	TIME TO RELAPSE (MONTHS)	GCT DEATHS (%)
Abratt et al., 1994	20	BEPx2 (E 360)	31	0	-	0
Cullen et al., 1996	114	BEPx2 (E 360)	48	2 (1.8)	7, 18	2 (1.8)
Pont et al., 1996	29	BEPx2 (E 500)	79	2 (2.7)	8, 27	1 (3.5)
Ondrus et al., 1998	18	BEPx2 (E 360)	36	0	-	0
Amato et al., 2004	68	CEBx2 (E 360)	38	1 (1.5)	21	0
Bohlen et al., 1999	58	BEPx2 (E 360) PVBx2 (20 pts)	93	2 (3.4)	22, 90	0
Chevreau et al., 2004	40	BEPx2 (E 360)	113	0	-	0
Oliver et al., 2004	148	BEPx1 (n=28); BEPx2 (n=46), BOPx2 (n=74).(E: 360)	33	6 (4.1)	Not reported	2 (1.4)
Dearnaley et al., 2005	115	BOPx2	70	3 (1.7)	3, 6, 26	1 (0.9)
Gilbert et al., 2006	22	BEPx1	120	1	-	0
Albers et al., 2008	191	BEPx1 (E 500)	56	2 (1.0)	15, 60	0
Tandstad et al., 2009	382	BEPx1 (n=312), BEPx2 (n=70) (E 500)	56	7 (1.8)	Range: 8–36	0
Tandstad et al., 2010	100	PVBx1 (n=40) or PVBx2 (n=60)	116	5	1, 9, 10, 27, 126	0
Huddart et al., 2017	246	BEPx1	39	7 (2.8)	5, 7, 8, 10, 12, 13, 27	1

E 360 refers to an etoposide dose of 360 mg/m (Siegel et al., 2018)/cycle, E 500 refers to an etoposide dose of 500 mg/m (Siegel et al., 2018)/cycle.

and active treatment (RPLND or primary chemotherapy) is favored when the risk of relapse is greater than 46% to 54% (Nguyen et al., 2010).

Clinical Stage IS Nonseminoma Germ Cell Tumor

CS IS defined as the presence of elevated post-orchiectomy serum tumor markers without clinical or radiographic evidence of metastatic disease. Studies of primary RPLND for CS IS NSGCT have reported that 37% to 100% of patients subsequently required chemotherapy for retroperitoneal metastasis, persistently elevated serum tumor markers, or relapse (Davis et al., 1994; Saxman et al., 1996). There is consensus that these patients should be treated similar to those with CS IIC-III and receive induction chemotherapy. The cancer-specific survival after chemotherapy for CS IS is greater than 90% (Culine et al., 1996; International Germ Cell Cancer Collaborative Group, 1997). Slightly elevated and stable serum tumor marker levels after orchiectomy in patients without clinical evidence of disease should be interpreted cautiously as they may represent false positives for disseminated NSGCT.

Clinical Stage IIA and IIB Nonseminoma Germ Cell Tumor

The optimal management of CS IIA-B NSGCT is controversial. RPLND (+/- adjuvant chemotherapy) and induction chemotherapy (+/- post-chemotherapy RPLND) are accepted treatment options with survival rates exceeding 95%. There are no randomized trials comparing these treatment approaches. In a prospective, multi-center, non-randomized trial of RPLND and 2 cycles of adjuvant chemotherapy versus induction chemotherapy, no significant differences in recurrence (7% for RPLND vs. 11% for chemotherapy) or overall survival were observed (Weissbach et al., 2000). A single-institution, non-randomized, retrospective comparison of RPLND (and 2 cycles of adjuvant chemotherapy for pathological stage II) and induction chemotherapy reported a significant reduction in the risk of recurrence with induction chemotherapy (98% vs. 79%), but cancer-specific approached 100% with both modalities (100% vs. 98%), RPLND patients received fewer cycles of chemotherapy (mean 4.2 vs. 1.4), and 51% of RPLND patients avoided chemotherapy (Stephenson et al., 2007).

The arguments in favor of RPLND for CS IIA-B are (1) 13% to 35% of patients have pathologically negative lymph nodes and thus avoid chemotherapy (Donohue et al., 1995; Pizzocaro, 1987; Stephenson et al., 2007; Weissbach et al., 2000), (2) approximately 30% have retroperitoneal teratoma that is resistant to chemotherapy (Foster et al., 1996; Stephenson et al., 2007), (3) long-term cancer-specific survival is 98% to 100% with RPLND +/- adjuvant chemotherapy (Donohue et al., 1995; Pizzocaro, 1987; Stephenson et al., 2007; Weissbach et al., 2000), (4) 10% to 52% avoid any chemotherapy (Donohue et al., 1995; Pizzocaro, 1987; Stephenson et al., 2007; Weissbach et al., 2000), and (5) ejaculatory function is preserved in 70% to 90% of patients (Donohue et al., 1995; Richie and Kantoff, 1991; Weissbach et al., 2000). The disadvantages of RPLND are (1) additional therapy is required in 48% or more of patients, (2) 13% to 15% have persistence of disease after RPLND and require a full induction chemotherapy regimen, and (3) high-quality RPLND may not be deliverable at all institutions (Stephenson et al., 2007; Weissbach et al., 2000).

The arguments in favor of induction chemotherapy are (1) 60% to 78% of patients achieve a complete response and avoid post-chemotherapy surgery, (2) treatment can be delivered at community-based institutions, and (3) cancer-specific survival is 96% to 100% (Culine et al., 1997; Debono et al., 1997; Horwich et al., 1994; Lerner et al., 1995; Logothetis et al., 1987; Ondrus et al., 1992; Peckham and Hendry, 1985; Socinski et al., 1988; Stephenson et al., 2007; Weissbach et al., 2000). The disadvantages of chemotherapy are (1) all patients are exposed to the risk of long-term toxicity of chemotherapy and (2) those who do not undergo post-chemotherapy RPNLD are at risk of relapse with chemorefractory GCT.

Given that 13% to 35% of patients with CS IIA NSGCT have pathologically negative lymph nodes (thus a false-positive CT result), patients with indeterminate lesions on staging abdominal-pelvic CT imaging who are at otherwise low-risk for metastatic disease may be observed closely initially to clarify subsequent treatment decisions.

Treatment considerations for CS IIA-B NSGCT include the risk of occult systemic disease, risk of retroperitoneal teratoma, short- and long-term treatment-related morbidity, and the need for double-therapy. The latter consideration is of least importance but has strongly influenced opinion regarding the optimal treatment of these patients. As discussed earlier, because metastatic NSGCT frequently exists as chemo-sensitive malignant GCT and chemoresistant teratoma, "cure" often requires the combination of chemotherapy and surgery.

Experience with primary RPLND in low-stage NSGCT for over the last 2 decades has identified parameters associated with systemic relapse. As with CS IS NSGCT, the presence of elevated post-orchiectomy AFP and HCG is associated with an increased risk of systemic relapse after RPLND. Rabbani et al. (2001) reported relapses after RPLND in 4 of 5 patients (80%) with elevated post-orchiectomy AFP or HCG compared with 7 of 45 (16%) with normal serum tumor markers. Stephenson et al. identified the presence of elevated serum tumor markers (HR 5.6, $P < 0.001$) and retroperitoneal lymphadenopathy >3 cm (HR 12.3, $P < 0.001$) as significant predictors of systemic relapse after RPLND (Stephenson et al., 2005b). **Thus there is consensus that CS IIA-B NSGCT patients with elevated AFP or HCG or bulky lymph nodes (>3 cm) should receive induction chemotherapy.**

The presence of retroperitoneal teratoma is a limitation to any strategy for metastatic NSGCT that uses chemotherapy alone as it is resistant to chemotherapy. Overall, approximately 20% of CS IIA-B patients have retroperitoneal teratoma, and this increases to 30% to 35% in those with teratoma in the primary tumor (Donohue et al., 1995; Foster et al., 1996; Stephenson et al., 2005b). Residual microscopic teratoma may remain dormant and clinically silent throughout a patient's lifetime. It may also exhibit slow growth, which can be detected on surveillance CT imaging and be amenable to cure by surgical resection. However, growing teratoma syndrome, malignant transformation, and late relapse are the most serious (although rare) sequelae of unresected teratoma. **Thus RPLND is preferred as initial therapy in those patients at risk for retroperitoneal teratoma who are at otherwise low risk for systemic disease (normal serum tumor markers, lymphadenopathy <3 cm).**

Clinical Stage IIC and III Nonseminoma Germ Cell Tumor

Induction chemotherapy with cisplatin-based regimens is the initial approach used for the treatment of CS IIC and III NSGCT. As discussed previously, induction chemotherapy is also the preferred approach for CS IS and CS IIA-B with elevated post-orchiectomy AFP and HCG. The specific regimen and number of cycles is based on the IGCCCG risk stratification (see Table 76.3) (International Germ Cell Cancer Collaborative Group, 1997).

The development of cisplatin-based chemotherapy represents the most important advancement in the treatment of GCT. Before the identification of cisplatin, complete responses to chemotherapy were achieved in 10% to 20% of patients, and the cure rate was only 5% to 10% (Einhorn, 1990). Long-term cure is now anticipated in 80% to 90% of patients with metastatic GCT. Randomized trials have evaluated the efficacy and safety of various drug combinations to determine the optimal regimen based on the IGCCCG risk (Debono et al., 1997).

The initial landmark study was conducted at Indiana University using cisplatin-vinblastine-bleomycin (PVBx4) in the 1970s and reported complete responses in 74% of patients and more than 70% of long-term survivors (Beck et al., 2005). When it was demonstrated that etoposide could cure some patients with relapse after PVB chemotherapy, PVBx4 was compared with bleomycin-etoposide-cisplatin (BEPx4) in a multi-center randomized trial. No significant difference in overall survival was seen between the two regimens (2-year survival 80%, $P = 0.11$), but BEPx4 was associated with less neuromuscular toxicity and was subsequently adopted as the standard regimen (Williams et al., 1987).

Chemotherapy for Good-Risk Nonseminoma Germ Cell Tumor.
After BEPx4 became the standard regimen for advanced GCT, subsequent trials focused on reducing toxicity for patients with good-risk features and improving outcomes for those with intermediate- and poor-risk disease. **For good-risk patients, two randomized trials have shown that BEPx3 is not inferior to BEPx4** (de Wit et al., 2001; Einhorn et al., 1989; Saxman et al., 1998). With 184 patients enrolled in the US study, 92% of patients were continuously disease free in each arm with a minimum follow-up of 1 year, and 4 deaths in each arm at 10 years were reported in a later analysis (Einhorn et al., 1989; Saxman et al., 1998). Similarly, an international European trial comparing BEPx3 with BEPx4 in more than 800 IGCCG good-risk patients reported similar outcomes with respect to 2-year progression-free (90% vs. 89%) and overall survival (97% in each arm) (de Wit et al., 2001). With these studies, BEPx3 became the standard regimen for good-risk GCT.

To reduce toxicity, investigators have studied the effect of omitting bleomycin and substituting carboplatin for cisplatin. **All of the randomized trials in which a cisplatin regimen has been compared with a carboplatin regimen have reported superior outcomes with cisplatin** (Bajorin et al., 1993; Bokemeyer et al., 1996, 2004; Horwich et al., 1997, 2000). **The issue of whether bleomycin can be safely omitted from cisplatin-based regimens in good-risk patients is much less clear and is one of the few remaining controversies in the management of advanced GCT.** The rationale for omitting bleomycin is based on the risk of pulmonary complications (including pulmonary fibrosis) and Raynaud phenomenon. All of these studies have shown a trend toward superiority for the bleomycin-containing regimen, although no significant survival advantage has been shown in any of the trials (Bosl et al., 1988; Levi et al., 1993). EPx3 is inferior to BEPx3 (Loehrer et al., 1995). A European randomized trial comparing BEPx4 with EPx4 (with reduced doses of etoposide) reported a significantly higher complete response rate (95% vs. 87%, $P = 0.008$) with BEPx3, but no difference in overall survival (de Wit et al., 1997). Most recently, a French randomized trial comparing BEPx3 with EPx4 (using conventional doses of etoposide) failed to show a statistically significant difference in the risk of relapse or survival between the two regimens (Culine et al., 2007). **Thus BEPx3 and EPx4 are accepted regimens for advanced GCT patients with good-risk features by IGCCCG criteria, and the 5-year overall survival is 91% to 94%** (International Germ Cell Cancer Collaborative Group, 1997; van Dijk et al., 2006).

Chemotherapy for Intermediate- and Poor-Risk Nonseminoma Germ Cell Tumor.
BEPx4 has been the standard regimen for advanced GCT with intermediate- and poor-risk features since 1987 and the corresponding 5-year survival rate was 79% and 48%, respectively, at the time these risk categories were defined in the 1990s (International Germ Cell Cancer Collaborative Group, 1997). More recent data from an analysis of 10 trials enrolling 1775 patients with disseminated NSGCT suggest that survival in these groups has increased to 83% and 71%, respectively (van Dijk et al., 2006). Ifosfamide-based regimens using either etoposide-ifosfamide-cisplatin (VIPx4) and vinblastine-ifosfamide-cisplatin (VeIPx4) have been investigated in randomized trials compared with BEPx4 (de Wit et al., 1998; Hinton et al., 2003; Nichols et al., 1998). The multi-center US trial reported results on nearly 300 men with advanced GCT, with 13%, 23%, and 64% classified as good-, intermediate-, and poor-risk by IGCCCG criteria, respectively (Hinton et al., 2003; Nichols et al., 1998). Comparing BEPx4 with VIPx4, the 2-year survival was 71% vs. 74% and the 5-year survival was 57% vs. 62%, neither of which was significantly different statistically (Nichols et al., 1998). The European study closed prematurely because the results of the US study became available. Nevertheless, with 84 patients enrolled and over 7 years median follow-up, progression-free survival was similar (85% with VIP and 83% with BEP), and overall survival at 5 years exceeded 80 percent (de Wit et al., 1998). **Because VIPx4 resulted in more high-grade hematologic and urologic toxicity, BEPx4 has remained the standard regimen for intermediate- and poor-risk GCT. However, these trials** showed that comparable cancer outcomes could be achieved when ifosfamide is substituted for bleomycin. **Thus VIPx4 may be substituted for BEPx4 in patients with compromised pulmonary function and to patients in whom extensive chest surgery will likely be performed to remove residual disease after chemotherapy** (Kesler et al., 2008).

High-dose chemotherapy (HDCT) using carboplatin-etoposide–based regimens with autologous stem cell support (also termed stem-cell rescue) has been investigated as an alternative to BEPx4 in patients with poor prognosis GCT. The rationale for HDCT is hypothesis that increasing dosage may overcome chemotherapy resistance. The most widely studied regimens have included carboplatin-etoposide alone or in combination with cyclophosphamide, ifosfamide, paclitaxel, or thiotepa (Beyer et al., 1996; Bokemeyer et al., 2002; Einhorn et al., 2007; Kondagunta et al., 2007; Kollmannsberger et al., 2009; Lorch et al., 2007). Carboplatin is used in HDCT regimens because of dose-limiting nephrotoxicity and neuropathy with cisplatin. A randomized trial in 219 patients with intermediate- (21%) and poor-risk (79%) GCT randomized to BEPx4 vs. BEPx2 followed by 2 cycles of high-dose carboplatin-etoposide-cyclophosphamide and autologous stem cell support showed no significant difference in the 1-year durable complete responses rate (48% vs. 52%, $P = 0.5$) or overall survival (Motzer et al., 2007). The 2-year and 5-year survival for patients in both arms was 83% and 71%, respectively. However, toxicity was more severe for patients receiving HDCT. A smaller randomized trial also failed to demonstrate an improved survival with HDCT compared with standard-dose regimens as first-line therapy for patients with poor-prognosis metastatic GCT (Droz et al., 2007).

More recently, investigators have studied whether outcomes can be improved through intensification of chemotherapy in patients with a prolonged time-to-normalization of serum AFP and/or BHCG during the first 6 weeks of chemotherapy (Fizazi et al., 2014). Longer time to normalization and longer half-life of AFP and BHCG have been shown to be adverse prognostic markers in studies (Fizazi et al., 2004; Massard et al., 2013). A randomized controlled trial enrolled 263 patients and 254 had tumor marker assessment. Of these, 203 (80%) prolonged time-to-normalization of at least one of the markers after one cycle of BEP and were randomly assigned to either standard care with three more cycles of BEP or a dose-dense regimen using two cycles of paclitaxel, bleomycin, etoposide, cisplatin, and oxaliplatin followed by two cycles of cisplatin, ifosfamide, and bleomycin. Three-year progression-free survival was longer in the dose-dense arm (59% vs. 48%, HR = 0.66, 95% CI = 0.44–1.00, $P = 0.05$), but there was no significant difference in overall survival ($P = 0.34$). **As a result, BEPx4 remains the standard first-line regimen in patients with intermediate- and poor-risk disease.**

Management of Post-Chemotherapy Residual Masses in Nonseminoma Germ Cell Tumor. To assess the response to first-line, cisplatin-based chemotherapy, patients are re-staged with serum tumor markers and imaging studies of the chest-abdomen-pelvis (including other sites of disease if present before chemotherapy). **Patients are classified into the following categories based on their response to chemotherapy:** (1) complete response (CR), defined by normalization of serum tumor markers and resolution of radiographic disease (usually defined as residual masses ≤1 cm); (2) normalization of serum tumor markers with persistent radiographic tumor (partial remission–marker negative); (3) partial remission–marker positive; and (4) disease progression. **Approximately 5% to 15% of patients fall into categories 3 and 4 and are typically managed with second-line (also termed salvage) chemotherapy** (de Wit et al., 1997; Debono et al., 1997; Einhorn et al., 1989; Mead et al., 1992). **Between 38% and 68% of patients have residual masses larger than 1 cm after first-line chemotherapy, and there is clear consensus that they should undergo post-chemotherapy surgery (PCS)** (Albers et al., 2005; Honecker et al., 2018; Krege et al., 2008b; Motzer et al., 2006). The management of patients with complete serologic and radiographic response is controversial, with some guidelines advocating close observation and others recommending PCS if pre-chemotherapy mass size is greater than 3 cm (Albers et al., 2005; Honecker et al., 2018; Krege et al., 2008b).

The role of PCS for residual masses in metastatic NSGCT is well established, and its rationale is based on several factors. **Multiple large series of patients undergoing PCS for residual masses after first-line chemotherapy have consistently reported evidence of persistent GCT elements in the resected specimens in 50% or more. On average, histology of resected specimens will demonstrate necrosis, teratoma, and viable malignancy (with or without teratoma) in 40%, 45%, and 15% of cases respectively (Table 76.7)** (Albers et al., 2004; Carver et al., 2007; Debono et al., 1997; de Wit et al., 1997; Gerl et al., 1995; Hartmann et al., 1997; Hendry et al., 2002; Sonneveld et al., 1998; Spiess et al., 2006; Stenning et al., 1998; Steyerberg et al., 1995, 1998; Toner et al., 1990). For primary mediastinal NSGCT, residual masses after first-line chemotherapy contain viable malignancy in up to 53% of cases (Sarkaria et al., 2011). The 5-year overall survival of patients with complete resection of viable malignancy (with or without further chemotherapy) ranges from 45% to 77% (Carver et al., 2007; Donohue et al., 1998; Fizazi et al., 2001, 2008; Fox et al., 1993; Gerl et al., 1995; Hartmann et al., 1997; Spiess et al., 2006; Stenning et al., 1998; Toner et al., 1990). In contrast, if left unresected, residual viable malignancy is destined to relapse and only 25% to 35% of patients will achieve durable remissions to second-line chemotherapy.

As discussed earlier, teratoma is resistant to chemotherapy and is present at metastatic sites in 15% of more of patients with disseminated NSGCT. The presence of metastatic teratoma is a limitation to any strategy for NSGCT that uses chemotherapy alone and necessitates the integration of chemotherapy and PCS in the majority of patients with metastatic GCT. Unresected teratoma has the potential to exhibit rapid growth (growing teratoma syndrome), undergo malignant transformation, or cause late relapse, all of which may have lethal consequences. **The outcome of metastatic teratoma is related to the completeness of surgical resection, and long-term survival is reported in 75% to 90% of patients who undergo PCS for residual teratoma** (Carver et al., 2007; Hartmann et al., 1997; Sonneveld et al., 1998; Stenning et al., 1998; Toner et al., 1990). Last, infield retroperitoneal relapse occurs in fewer than 2% of patients

TABLE 76.7 Histology of Post-chemotherapy Residual Masses

STUDY	PATIENTS	NECROSIS	VIABLE MALIGNANCY +/− TERATOMA	TERATOMA ONLY
Steyerberg et al., 1995	556	45%	13%	42%
Carver et al., 2007	504	49%	11%	39%
Hendry et al., 2002	330	25%	9%	66%
Debono et al., 1997	295	25%	7%	67%
Spiess et al., 2006	236	41%	17%	42%
Albers et al., 2004	232	35%	31%	34%
Toner et al., 1990	185	47%	16%	37%
Steyerberg et al., 1998	172	45%	13%	42%
Stenning et al., 1998	153	29%	15%	55%
deWit et al., 1997	127	35%	9%	56%
Oechsle et al., 2008	121	45%	21%	34%
Sonneveld et al., 1998	113	46%	9%	45%
Gerl et al., 1995	111	47%	12%	41%
Hartmann et al., 1997	109	52%	21%	27%

after a full, bilateral template RPLND, largely eliminating the need for radiographic surveillance of the abdomen and pelvis (Carver et al., 2007).

Approximately 6% to 8% of PCS specimens contain evidence of non–germ cell tumor malignancy, arising from malignant transformation of teratoma (Carver et al., 2007; Little et al., 1994; Toner et al., 1990). The most common histology is rhabdomyosarcoma, and the presence of i(12p) or abnormalities of chromosome 12 in most specimens confirms its origin from GCT (Motzer et al., 1998). **As with teratoma, the outcome of patients with malignant transformation is related to the completeness of surgical resection because they are generally resistant to GCT-specific chemotherapy regimens.** With complete resection, approximately 50% to 66% of patients will survive, whereas the vast majority of patients with incomplete resection will experience rapid progression and death from GCT (Carver et al., 2007; Comiter et al., 1998; Little et al., 1994; Lutke Holzik et al., 2003; Motzer et al., 1998). Chemotherapy specific to the transformed histology (e.g., sarcoma-specific regimen) has been investigated in two small series in select patients with measurable disease limited to one histology. Partial responses are observed in a total of 11 of 24 patients, 6 of whom are alive (Donadio et al., 2003; El Mesbahi et al., 2007).

Patients with necrosis only in the PCS specimens have a favorable prognosis, with relapse rates of 10% or less reported in most series (Carver et al., 2007; Hartmann et al., 1997; Mano et al., 2017; Stenning et al., 1998; Toner et al., 1990). Investigators have sought to identify factors that reliably predict for a high probability of necrosis to obviate the need for PCS in all patients with residual masses. In an early study, Donohue et al. (1987) reported that 0 of 15 patients without teratoma in the primary tumor and who achieved a 90% or greater reduction in the size of the residual mass with chemotherapy had no evidence of viable malignancy or teratoma at PCS. In contrast, 7 of 9 patients (78%) with teratoma in the primary tumor experiencing a similar reduction in the size of the metastasis with chemotherapy had evidence of viable malignancy and/or teratoma (Donohue et al., 1987). **The absence of teratoma in the primary tumor, the percentage reduction in the retroperitoneal mass with chemotherapy, and the size of the residual mass have consistently been identified as predictors of necrosis in PCS specimens** (Albers et al., 2004; Fossa et al., 1992; Stomper et al., 1991; Steyerberg et al., 1995, 1998; Toner et al., 1990). However, despite statistical modeling using these and other factors, a consistent false-negative rate for necrosis of 20% has been reported (Steyerberg et al., 1995, 1998; Vergouwe et al., 2001). **Thus the presence of necrosis only in the retroperitoneum cannot be predicted with sufficient accuracy to safely obviate the need for PCS in patients with residual masses. An important concept is that the absence of teratoma in the primary tumor does not reliably exclude its presence in the retroperitoneum** (Beck et al., 2002; Toner et al., 1990). Investigators have also investigated the utility of FDG-PET in the prediction of the histology of residual masses after first-line chemotherapy. The utility of FDG-PET in the prediction of retroperitoneal histology for NSGCT is limited by the fact that teratoma is not FDG-avid. In a prospective study of 121 patients with residual masses after induction chemotherapy, the predictive accuracy of FDG-PET (56%) for viable malignancy or teratoma was no better than CT (55%) or post-chemotherapy serum tumor markers (56%) (Oechsle et al., 2008). **Thus FDG-PET has no role in the assessment of NSGCT patients with residual masses after chemotherapy.**

Approximately 26% to 62% of patients will experience a serologic and radiographic complete response to first-line chemotherapy (Dearnaley et al., 1991; Debono et al., 1997; Ehrlich et al., 2010; Einhorn et al., 1989; Kollmannsberger et al., 2010a; Mead et al., 1992; Stenning et al., 1998). **The optimal management of these patients is controversial.** Advocates of PCS for these patients argue that residual mass size (or percentage reduction with chemotherapy) cannot be used to reliably exclude the presence of residual disease within the retroperitoneum. **Numerous studies have demonstrated that, on average, patients with residual masses 20 mm or smaller have a 30% and 6% incidence of teratoma and viable malignancy, respectively (Table 76.8;** Beck et al., 2002; Fossa et al., 1989, 1992; Oldenburg et al., 2003; Toner et al., 1990; Stephenson et al., 2007; Steyerberg et al., 1995; Stomper et al., 1991). In an analysis of 295 patients with GCT managed at Indiana University after induction chemotherapy, 77 (26%) experienced a complete serologic and radiographic response to chemotherapy and 92% were alive at 5 to 10 years with an observational strategy (Debono et al., 1997). This result highlights the therapeutic benefit of PCS for patients with residual masses. **However, it should be emphasized that patients with complete serologic and radiographic response after induction chemotherapy represent a small minority of the overall population, indicating that observation is a reasonable option for only a select group of patients.** Recently, two studies have confirmed the low risk of relapse (4% to 10%) and 97% to 100% cancer-specific survival in patients with residual masses smaller than 1 cm who were observed without PCS (Ehrlich et al., 2010; Kollmannsberger et al., 2010). However, the majority of these patients were good risk by IGCCCG criteria and did not have teratoma in the primary tumor, highlighting their select nature.

Approximately one-third of patients have residual masses at multiple anatomic sites (the retroperitoneum, chest, and left supraclavicular fossa are the most common), and these patients should undergo resection of all sites of measurable residual disease (Gerl et al., 1994; Hartmann et al., 1997; McGuire et al., 2003; Toner et al., 1990). Although some centers have described performing simultaneous RPLND, thoracotomy, and/or neck dissection, our practice is to perform infradiaphragmatic and supradiaphragmatic resections as separate procedures. **Discordant histology between anatomic sites is reported in 22% to 46% of cases** (Masterson et al., 2012; Toner et al., 1990). In general, the histology of PCS specimens from non-retroperitoneal sites is more likely to show necrosis (60%) and less likely to show viable malignancy (10%) and teratoma (30%) (Gerl et al., 1994; Hartmann et al., 1997; Steyerberg et al., 1997; Toner et al., 1990). In addition to the size of residual masses and the number of anatomic sites, the presence of necrosis in post-chemotherapy RPLND specimens is highly predictive of necrosis at other sites (Steyerberg et al., 1997). Of patients undergoing PCS for residual masses at different sites, only 33 of 245 (13%) who

TABLE 76.8 Histology of Post-Chemotherapy Residual Masses Less Than 20 mm

STUDY	PATIENTS	SIZE	NECROSIS	VIABLE MALIGNANCY +/− TERATOMA	TERATOMA ONLY
Steyerberg et al., 1995	275	≤20 mm	65%	5%	30%
Steyerberg et al., 1995	162	≤10 mm	72%	4%	24%
Oldenburg et al., 2003	87	≤20 mm	67%	7%	26%
Fossa et al., 1992	78	<20 mm	68%	4%	29%
Fossa et al., 1989	37	≤10 mm	67%	3%	30%
Stephenson et al., 2007	36	≤5 mm	69%	6%	25%
Toner et al., 1990	21	≤15 mm	81%	7%	12%
Stomper et al., 1991	14	≤20 mm	36%	14%	50%

had necrosis in the RPLND specimen had either viable malignancy or teratoma at other sites (Brenner et al., 1996; Gerl et al., 1994; Masterson et al., 2012; McGuire et al., 2003; Steyerberg et al., 1997; Tiffany et al., 1986; Tognoni et al., 1998). **Thus RPLND should be performed before PCS at other sites because the probability of residual disease in the retroperitoneum is highest and RPLND histology is a strong predictor of histology at other sites.** Observation of small residual masses at other sites is a reasonable option if the histology of the RPLND specimen is necrosis.

As mentioned, the 5-year survival for patients with viable malignancy in PCS specimens is 45% to 77%. The role of postoperative chemotherapy in this setting is controversial. Fox et al. (1993) reported that 14 of 27 patients (70%) undergoing PCS for viable malignancy were free of recurrence with adjuvant chemotherapy versus 0 of 7 patients who were observed. In an international pooled analysis of 238 patients with viable malignancy in PCS specimens, Fizazi et al. (2001) identified pre chemotherapy IGCCCG intermediate- and poor-risk disease, incomplete resection, and greater than 10% viable malignancy in PCS specimens as important prognostic factors. Patients with 0, 1, and 2 to 3 risk factors had a 5-year overall survival of 100%, 83%, and 51%, respectively. Overall, a significant improvement in 5-year relapse-free survival was observed with postoperative chemotherapy (73% vs. 64%, $P < 0.001$), but no difference in 5-year overall survival (74% vs. 70%, $P = 0.7$). In a subset analysis, patients with 1 risk factor had an improved 5-year survival with postoperative chemotherapy (88% vs. 56%, $P = 0.02$), but those with 0 (100% survival, with or without chemotherapy) and 2 to 3 risk factors (55% vs. 60%) did not. In a confirmatory study, this prognostic index was validated for relapse-free and overall survival, and no significant difference in these endpoints was observed among the patients who did and did not receive postoperative chemotherapy (Fizazi et al., 2008). **A complete resection of residual masses is the most critical determinant of outcome for patients with viable malignancy in PCS specimens after first-line chemotherapy. Immediate postoperative chemotherapy or surveillance may be reasonable options depending on the completeness of resection, IGCCCG risk group, and percent of viable cells.** There is no consensus on the appropriate chemotherapy regimen and the number of cycles that should be used in this setting.

The importance of PCS was highlighted in a randomized trial of BEPx3 vs. EPx4 in 257 men with good-risk metastatic NSGCT (Culine et al., 2007). As part of this trial, PCS was not dictated by protocol and only 52% underwent PCS, which frequently involved resection of residual mass only. Overall, 14 of 20 (70%) relapsing patients and 7 of 14 (50%) of those who died from GCT either did not undergo PCS or relapsed in the retroperitoneum after an inadequate RPLND. **These results suggest a substantial proportion of deaths from GCT may be prevented by the appropriate integration of chemotherapy and surgery.**

Relapsed Nonseminoma Germ Cell Tumor

The treatment of relapsing NSGCTs depends upon what treatment the patient has previously received and, in certain cases, the location of the relapse. Patients who have never received chemotherapy have a much more favorable prognosis than patients who have already been treated with chemotherapy for disseminated disease.

Chemotherapy-Naïve Nonseminoma Germ Cell Tumor Relapse. Chemotherapy-naïve relapses occur in men with CS I NSGCT managed with either surveillance or RPLND and in the men with CS IIA-B NSGCT treated with RPLND alone. Serum tumor markers are elevated 60% to 75% of the time in CS I patients who relapse on surveillance (Alexandre et al., 2001; Gels et al., 1995; Read et al., 1992; Sharir et al., 1999). **In general, these patients are treated with induction chemotherapy, with the specific regimen and duration of therapy determined by IGCCCG risk, and cure rates exceed 95%. Select CS I patients on surveillance who relapse in the retroperitoneum with non-bulky (<3 cm) and normal serum tumor markers may be treated by induction chemotherapy or RPLND (particularly if teratoma were present in the primary tumor)** (Stephenson et al., 2007). The rationale for RPLND is to avoid or minimize the toxicity of chemotherapy, and long-term cure rates approach 100% with RPLND with or without adjuvant chemotherapy (Stephenson et al., 2007). CS I, IIA, and IIB patients who relapse after RPLND will usually do so in the lungs or mediastinum. Almost all of these patients are cured with first-line chemotherapy. The majority of relapses during surveillance or after RPLND occur within the first 2 years (Albers et al., 1995, 2008; Colls et al., 1999; Daugaard et al., 2003; Francis et al., 2000; Freedman et al., 1987; Gels et al., 1995; Kollmannsberger et al., 2010a; McLeod et al., 1991; Read et al., 1992; Sharir et al., 1999; Sogani et al., 1998; Stephenson et al., 2005b; Williams et al., 2009; Zuniga et al., 2009). For the rare patient relapsing more than 2 years after orchiectomy or RPLND with normal tumor markers, biopsy or surgical resection should be strongly considered because of the likelihood of teratoma (Michael et al., 2000; Oldenburg et al., 2006). **Although the time-to-relapse is an important determinant of outcome in relapsing patients who have received prior chemotherapy, chemotherapy-naïve patients who relapse more than 2 years after initial treatment have a similar prognosis to those who relapse earlier.**

Post-Chemotherapy Nonseminoma Germ Cell Tumor Relapse—Early. Men who relapse after previously receiving first-line chemotherapy are treated with second-line (also termed salvage) chemotherapy. **The majority of relapses occur within 2 years of completing initial treatment, and these are classified as early relapse** (Culine et al., 2007; de Wit et al., 1998; Michael et al., 2000; Motzer et al., 2007; Nichols et al., 1998). **Relapses occurring more than 2 years after the completion of initial therapy are classified as late relapse and differ substantially in terms of prognosis and therapy (discussed later).** A subset of early relapsing patients who appear to have a particularly unfavorable prognosis are those who fail to achieve a complete response to first-line therapy or who relapse within 6 months of achieving a complete response; these patients are frequently termed incomplete responders (Fossa et al., 1999). **In an international pooled analysis of 1984 patients from 38 centers with relapse after first-line chemotherapy who received second-line chemotherapy, median progression-free and overall survival were 10 months and 41 months, respectively** (Lorch et al., 2010). **Incomplete response to induction chemotherapy (HR 1.4–1.9), primary mediastinal NSGCT (HR 3.0), nonpulmonary visceral metastasis (HR 1.3), and elevated AFP (HR 1.3–2.0) and HCG (HR 1.5) were associated with increased risk of progression with second-line chemotherapy.**

As discussed earlier, etoposide and ifosfamide were demonstrated to have substantial activity in patients with relapse after first-line chemotherapy, and this led to the investigation of VIPx4 as a second-line regimen for relapse GCT after PVBx4 (Einhorn, 1990; Loehrer et al., 1986). VeIPx4 was also studied as a second-line regimen in men who had received prior etoposide from BEP regimens (Loehrer et al., 1998). Studies of VIPx4 and VeIPx4 reported long-term remission rates of 23% to 35% and overall survival rates of 32% to 53% (Loehrer et al., 1998; McCaffrey et al., 1997; Pico et al., 2005). Studies of paclitaxel in the early 1990s showed activity in relapsed GCT. This led to the development of the TIP regimen (paclitaxel, ifosfamide, and cisplatin), and relapse-free survival has been reported in 36% to 47% of patients (Kondagunta et al., 2005; Mardiak et al., 2005; Mead et al., 2005). **TIPx4, VIPx4, and VeIPx4 have never been compared in a randomized trial, and all are considered standard second-line regimens.**

HDCT has also been investigated as a second-line (and third-line) regimen in patients with GCT relapse, although its role as second-line therapy is controversial. Indiana University has amassed the largest, single-institution series involving 184 consecutive patients with metastatic GCT that progressed after first- (73%) or second-line chemotherapy (27%), 94% of whom received 2 or more courses of HDCT (Einhorn et al., 2007). Over a median follow-up of 4 years, 63% of patients were continuously disease free, including 70% and 45% of patients who received HDCT as second- and third-line therapy, respectively. An international matched-pair analysis comparing 74 patients treated at a single institution who received 2 to 3 cycles of VIP followed by 1 cycle of HDCT using carboplatin-etoposide-ifosfamide to 119 patients treated at multiple centers throughout

Europe who received standard-dose, second-line chemotherapy using a variety of regimens, reported a 10% improvement in event-free and overall survival with HDCT (Beyer et al., 2002). HDCT was compared with standard-dose, second-line chemotherapy in a randomized controlled trial enrolling 280 patients from 43 institutions. Patients in the standard-dose arm received VIPx4 or VeIPx4, depending on whether they received prior etoposide during first-line therapy. Patients in the HDCT arm received VIP/VeIPx3 followed by 1 cycle of high-dose carboplatin-etoposide-cyclophosphamide (Pico et al., 2005). Over a median follow-up of 45 months, there were no significant differences in complete and partial response rates (56% in both arms) or the 3-year event-free (35% vs. 42%, P = 0.16) and overall survival (53% in both arms).

There are several potential explanations for the lack of benefit of HDCT in the randomized trial despite the favorable results reported in the two non-randomized studies. First, the results from single-arm trials may be subject to selection bias from differences in case-mix. In addition, the results achieved at high-volume institutions with unique experience with HDCT may not be reproducible at other institutions. Alternatively, the treatment strategy employed in the randomized trial may have been suboptimal in that 3 cycles of standard-dose chemotherapy and only 1 cycle of HDCT were given. The treatment philosophy at Indiana University is to take patients to HDCT as quickly as possible, limit the number of cycles of standard-dose chemotherapy so that patients are able to better tolerate HDCT, and to give 2 cycles of HDCT. In the randomized trial, only 73% of patients assigned HDCT were able to receive it, and toxic deaths on the HDCT arm were twice as common as the standard-dose arm (7% vs. 3%). In the Indiana University series, 94% of patients were able to receive 2 cycles of HDCT, and the treatment-related death rate was 2.7%. **Although HDCT as second-line therapy can cure a significant number of patients, the failure to demonstrate an improvement in survival compared with standard-dose regimens in 3 randomized trials (2 as first-line therapy and 1 as second-line therapy) suggests it should not be considered a standard approach.** Currently, HDCT should only be offered at specialized centers with extensive experience.

Treatment options for high-risk patients with relapse (e.g., incomplete responders) include standard-dose, second-line chemotherapy or HDCT (if administered at a specialized, high-volume institution). Standard-dose, second-line chemotherapy is the preferred approach for patients who relapse more than 6 months after first-line chemotherapy. **Special mention is made of patients with declining or normalized serum tumor markers during first-line chemotherapy with enlarging (usually cystic) masses. These patients are considered to have growing teratoma syndrome. In these rare cases, chemotherapy is temporarily interrupted and patients are taken for surgical resection. With complete surgical resection, the long-term prognosis for these patients is favorable** (Andre et al., 2000; Logothetis et al., 1982; Spiess et al., 2007).

For patients relapsing after second-line chemotherapy, subsequent options include HDCT (if not given previously) and regimens including various combinations of the following agents: gemcitabine, paclitaxel, oxaliplatin, and irinotecan (Bokemeyer et al., 2008; De Giorgi et al., 2006; Nicolai et al., 2009; Oechsle et al., 2011; Pectasides et al., 2004; Veenstra and Vaughn, 2011).

Management of Post-Salvage Chemotherapy Residual Masses.
Patients with serologic complete response to second-line chemotherapy with residual masses should undergo post-salvage chemotherapy surgical resection (PSCS). Patients undergoing PSCS differ from those undergoing PCS of residual masses after first-line chemotherapy in several ways. A complete resection of residual masses is feasible in only 56% to 72% of patients (compared with 85% or more after first-line therapy) (Cary et al., 2015; Debono et al., 1997; Eggener et al., 2007; Fox et al., 1993; Hartmann et al., 1997; Stenning et al., 1998). The histology of PSCS specimens is characterized by higher rates of viable malignancy (38%–53%) and lower rates of necrosis (26%) and teratoma (21%–34%) compared with those after first-line chemotherapy. The long-term survival of patients is also substantially poorer with 5-year survival rates of 44% to 61% in most series (Donohue et al., 1998; Fox et al., 1993; Hartmann et al., 1997; Stenning et al., 1998). **Patients with viable malignancy in PCSC specimens have a particularly poor prognosis, and their survival is not improved with the use of postoperative chemotherapy.**

Desperation Surgery.
The majority of patients with progressive disease despite first- and second-line chemotherapy have a dismal prognosis. **However, a highly select group of patients with rising serum tumor markers who are deemed to have resectable disease limited to a single site (usually the retroperitoneum) may be candidates for salvage surgery, commonly referred to as "desperation surgery."** Although published studies are limited to small, single-institution case series, 47% to 60% will have normalization of serum tumor markers postoperatively, and long-term survival is reported in 33% to 57% of patients after desperation surgery with or without postoperative chemotherapy (Albers et al., 2000; Beck et al., 2005; Eastham et al., 1994; Murphy et al., 1993; Wood et al., 1992). Up to 50% of patients undergoing "desperation surgery" have necrosis or teratoma on final pathology.

Post-Chemotherapy Nonseminoma Germ Cell Tumor Relapse—Late.
Late relapse after chemotherapy is defined as that occurring more than 2 years after treatment. Roughly 3% of NSGCT patients experience a late relapse (Oldenburg et al., 2006; Ronnen et al., 2005). Because late relapse is rare, a biopsy should be performed to confirm the diagnosis, particularly when serum AFP and HCG are normal. **Late relapses can be divided into three histopathological categories: viable malignancy (54%–88%; yolk sac tumor most common), teratoma (12%–28%), and malignant transformation (10%–20%; adenocarcinoma most common)** (Baniel et al., 1995; George et al., 2003; Gerl et al., 1997; Michael et al., 2000; Sharp et al., 2008).

Risk factors for late relapse have not been definitively identified, but a history of prior relapse and presence teratoma in PCS specimens (potentially for incomplete resection) are associated with an increased risk (Gerl et al., 1997; Shahidi et al., 2002). Most men with a late relapse have only one site of disease. The majority of late relapses occur in the retroperitoneum (50%–72%), 17% occur in the lungs, 9% in the mediastinum, 7% in the neck, and 4% in the pelvis (Baniel et al., 1995; Dieckmann et al., 2005; George et al., 2003; Gerl et al., 1997; Oldenburg et al., 2006; Sharp et al., 2008). **Thus failure to control the retroperitoneum in the initial treatment phase is a major risk factor for late relapse.** Serum AFP and HCG are elevated in about 50% and 25% of late relapses (Oldenburg et al., 2006). Patients with elevated serum tumor markers as the only manifestation of late relapse should be monitored closely until there is measurable disease (George et al., 2003).

Until recently, late relapse has been associated with a worse prognosis than early relapses, although contemporary data suggest these patients may have a similar probability of cure. **In general, late relapse is resistant to chemotherapy and the outcome is related to the ability to render patients disease free by complete surgical resection** (Dieckmann et al., 2005; George et al., 2003; Gerl et al., 1997; Oldenburg et al., 2006; Shahidi et al., 2002; Sharp et al., 2008).

The importance of surgery is related to the fact that teratoma and malignant transformation are inherently chemo-insensitive, and viable malignancy is usually present in the setting of prior chemotherapy (thereby, platin resistant). Of 32 patients with late relapse at Indiana University who received chemotherapy, only 6 (19%) achieved a complete response. Of the 49 patients treated initially with surgery, 45 (92%) were rendered free of disease (22 [45%] by surgery alone) and 29 (59%) are in complete remission. Overall, 69 (85%) patients achieved a disease-free state, and 58% are disease-free over a median follow-up of 25 months (George et al., 2003). In the Memorial Sloan-Kettering experience, the 5-year cancer-specific survival was 60% and patients who had a complete surgical resection at the time of late relapse (60%) and a significantly improved survival compared with those without complete resection (40%) (79% vs. 36%, P < 0.001) (Sharp et al., 2008). The presence of symptoms and multifocal disease at late relapse were associated with inferior survival. In a German study of 72 patients with NSGCT and late relapse, 35 (49%) were in complete remission at last follow-up, most of whom were treated with a combination of chemotherapy and surgery (Dieckmann et al., 2005). The most favorable chemotherapy results for late relapse are with the TIP regimen (Kondagunta et al., 2005). **An aggressive surgical approach to resect all disease is appropriate either as the primary treatment or, in the setting of unresectable disease, after chemotherapy.**

> **KEY POINTS**
> - The optimal management of CS I NSGCT is controversial. Surveillance, primary RPLND, and primary chemotherapy with BEPx2 are accepted treatment options with long-term survival rates approaching 100% for each.
> - A risk-adapted approach based on the presence of LVI and EC predominance is recommended. Surveillance is recommended to patients without these risk factors and active treatment (RPLND or BEPx2) is recommended to those with LVI and/or EC predominance. A non–risk-adapted approach is employed at some centers, whereby surveillance is the recommended approach for all patients.
> - Surveillance is not recommended to patients who are anticipated to be poorly compliant with follow-up imaging and clinical evaluation. The standard treatment approach to patients who relapse on surveillance is induction chemotherapy based on the IGCCCG risk. However, select patients with normal serum tumor marker levels and non-bulky (<3 cm) retroperitoneal adenopathy may also be managed by RPLND.
> - BEPx1 is the standard regimen used for patients with CS I NSGCT who choose to receive chemotherapy.
> - A full, bilateral template with nerve sparing is the recommended approach for primary RPLND. Attempts at preserving ejaculatory function should not compromise oncologic efficacy. RPLND should be performed only by surgeons experienced with the procedure.
> - Adjuvant chemotherapy after primary RPLND for pathological stage II disease is associated with a substantial reduction in the risk of relapse but no difference in long-term survival compared with an observational strategy with induction chemotherapy at the time of relapse. Adjuvant chemotherapy is usually recommended to patients with extensive retroperitoneal metastasis (pN2-3) and those anticipated to be noncompliant with postoperative cancer surveillance imaging and testing.
> - Induction chemotherapy and primary RPLND are accepted treatment options for patients with CS IIA-B NSGCT, with long-term cure in 95% or more. Induction chemotherapy is favored in patients with a high risk of occult metastasis disease on the basis of elevated post-orchiectomy serum tumor markers and/or bulky (>3 cm) retroperitoneal lymphadenopathy.
> - The management of patients with CS IS, IIC, and III NSGCT is induction cisplatin-based chemotherapy. The specific regimen and number of cycles is dictated by IGCCCG risk criteria. Patients with good-risk disease should receive BEPx3 or EPx4, and those with intermediate- and poor-risk disease should receive BEPx4. With risk-appropriate chemotherapy and post-chemotherapy surgery, the survival of patients with good-, intermediate- and poor-risk disease is 89%–94%, 75%–83%, and 41%–71%, respectively.
> - Post-chemotherapy resection of all residual masses is based on the incidence of residual cancer (either viable malignancy or teratoma) in 50% or more of patients.
> - The use of adjuvant chemotherapy is controversial in patients with viable malignancy in residual masses after first-line chemotherapy.

Seminoma

Clinical Stage I Seminoma

Approximately 80% of patients with seminoma are CS I, and this is the most common presentation of testis cancer. **The management of these patients has undergone substantial changes over the past 2 decades, and surveillance, primary radiotherapy, and primary chemotherapy with single-agent carboplatin are now accepted treatment options.** Recent efforts have focused on reducing the therapeutic burden. **Platin-based chemotherapy and infradiaphragmatic radiotherapy are associated with an increased risk of late cardiovascular toxicity and secondary malignant neoplasms (SMN)** (Travis et al., 2005; van den Belt-Dusebout et al., 2007; Zagars et al., 2004). Minimizing target volume and dose have been investigated to reduce the toxicity of radiotherapy. Carboplatin is associated with less neurotoxicity, ototoxicity, and nephrotoxicity compared with cisplatin, but the risks of cardiovascular disease and SMN are largely unknown. In many instances, the short-term efficacy and safety of these approaches has been validated by randomized trials. **The long-term cancer control with each of these modalities approaches 100%.**

Primary Radiotherapy. Until the turn of the century, the mainstay of treatment for CS I seminoma had been primary radiotherapy to the retroperitoneum and ipsilateral pelvis, termed dog-leg (DL) configuration. Published series of radiotherapy for CS I are listed in Table 76.9 (Classen et al., 2004; Fossa et al., 1989, 1999; Jones et al., 2005; Oliver et al., 2005; Tandstad et al., 2011; Warde et al., 1995, 2005). **The optimal radiation dose has not been defined and most centers use 25 to 35 Gy in 15 to 20 daily fractions** (Fossa et al., 1989, 1999; Warde et al., 1995). Long-term cancer-specific survival approaches 100%, and progression-free probability between 95% and 97% is reported (Fossa et al., 1989, 1999; Kollmannsberger et al., 2010; Tandstad et al., 2011; Warde et al., 1995, 2005). **In-field recurrence after DL radiotherapy is less than 1%,** obviating the need for routine surveillance abdominal-pelvic CT imaging. Inguinal metastases are uncommon in those without prior inguinal or scrotal surgery. **The most common sites of recurrence are the thorax and left supraclavicular fossa. Virtually all recurrences are cured with first-line chemotherapy.** Select patients with isolated inguinal relapse may be salvaged with radiotherapy or surgical resection. **The surveillance of patients after DL radiotherapy consists of regular clinical assessment, chest x-ray, and serum tumor markers.**

Most patients experience some acute side effects with adjuvant radiotherapy, which typically include transient nausea, vomiting, and diarrhea, which are usually mild and self-limited. Acute grade II to IV hematologic toxicity occurs in 5% to 15% (Fossa et al., 1999). Moderate and severe late gastrointestinal (GI) toxicity (usually chronic dyspepsia or peptic ulcer disease) is reported in 5% and less than 2% of patients, respectively. The testicular germinal epithelium is exquisitely sensitive to ionizing radiation, and scatter dose to the contralateral testis may be significant despite protective shielding. After DL radiotherapy, persistent oligospermia is reported in 8% (Fossa et al., 1999). The issue of late cardiac toxicity and SMN is particularly germane for these patients given the long anticipated life expectancy. **The actuarial risk of developing SMN is estimated to be 18% at 25 years after radiotherapy for seminoma** (Travis et al., 2005). Secondary leukemia is linked with radiotherapy and chemotherapy, whereas an excess of the upper GI tract, bladder, and possibly pancreas cancers is associated with radiotherapy.

To reduce the toxicity of radiotherapy, efforts to minimize the target volume and dose have been evaluated in randomized trials. The Medical Research Council (MRC; United Kingdom) conducted a randomized trial of DL vs. para-aortic (PA) radiotherapy for CS I seminoma (Fossa et al., 1999). The rationale for omitting radiotherapy to the ipsilateral pelvis is based on the low rate (1%–3%) of pelvic lymph node involvement in patients without prior inguinal or scrotal surgery. Restricting radiotherapy to the PA strip may reduce the risk of SMN and improve the recovery of spermatogenesis. The 3-year relapse-free survival (96% vs. 97%) and overall survival (99% vs. 100%) in the PA vs. DL arms were similar, but patients receiving PA radiotherapy had an improved short-term recovery of spermatogenesis

TABLE 76.9 Summary of Radiation Therapy Series for Clinical Stage I Seminoma

	PATIENTS	MEDIAN FOLLOW-UP	TARGET VOLUME	MEDIAN DOSE (GY)	GCT DEATHS (%)	RELAPSE (%)	IN-FIELD RELAPSE (%)	PELVIC RELAPSE (%)
Fossa et al., 1989	365	109 months	Dogleg	40	4 (1)	13 (4)	1 (0.3)	0
Warde et al., 1995	194	97 months	Dogleg	25	0	11 (6)	0	0
Warde et al., 2005	282	106 months	Dogleg	25	0	14 (5)	—	—
Fossa et al., 1999	242	54 months	Dogleg	30	0	9 (4)	0	0
Fossa et al., 1999	236	54 months	Para-Aortic	30	1	9 (4)	2 (0.8)	4 (1.7)
Classen et al., 2004	721	61 months	Para-Aortic	26	2 (0.3)	26 (4)	8 (1.1)	13 (1.8)
Jones et al., 2005	313	61 months	Para-Aortic	30	1 (0.3)	10 (4)	3 (1)	6 (2)
Jones et al., 2005	312	61 months	Para-Aortic	20	0	11 (4)	2 (0.6)	3 (1)
Oliver et al., 2005, 2011	904	78 months	Para-Aortic	20-30	1 (0.1)	32 (4)	3 (0.3)	10 (1.6)
Tandstad et al., 2011	481	73 months	Dogleg	25	0	4 (1)	2 (0.6)	—
Kollmannsberger et al., 2010	159	65 months	Para-Aortic	25	0	4 (2)	—	2 (1)

TABLE 76.10 Summary of Surveillance Series for Clinical Stage I Seminoma

STUDY	PATIENTS	MEDIAN FOLLOW-UP	GCT DEATHS (%)	RELAPSE (%)	RPN RELAPSE (%)	CS IIC-III RELAPSE (%)	SYSTEMIC RELAPSE (%)
Daugaard et al., 2003	394	—	0	69 (17)	—	—	—
Warde et al., 2005	348	106 months	1 (0.3)	55 (16)	—	—	—
Warde et al., 1995	172	50 months	1 (0.6)	27 (16)	24 (89)	5 (19)	1 (4)
von der Maase et al., 1993	261	48 months	1 (0.4)	49 (19)	46 (94)	12 (24)	1 (2)
Aparicio et al., 2003	143[a]	52 months	0	23 (16)	19 (84)	—	3 (13)
Horwich et al., 1992	103	62 months	0	17 (17)	17 (100)	3 (18)	1 (6)
Choo et al., 2005	88	145 months	0	17 (19)	15 (88)	3 (18)	2 (12)
Aparicio et al., 2005	100[b]	34 months	0	6 (7)	6 (100)	—	0
Tandstad et al., 2011	512	60 months	0	65 (14)	65 (100)	—	—
Kollmannsberger et al., 2010	313	34 months	0	47 (19)	—	—	—

[a]Patients with lymphovascular invasion or clinical stage ≥ T2 excluded
[b]Patients with tumor size > 4 cm or rete testis invasion excluded
CS, Clinical stage; *GCT*, germ cell tumor; *RPN*, retroperitoneal.

(although no difference was seen at 3 years). However, the PA arm experienced a significant increase in the rate of pelvic recurrence (2% vs. 0, $P = 0.04$). The small but significant risk of pelvic recurrence necessitates the use of routine surveillance pelvic CT imaging with the associated increased cost and radiation exposure (Brenner and Hall, 2007).

The MRC and the European Organisation for the Research and Treatment of Cancer (EORTC) also conducted a randomized trial of 20 vs. 30 Gy PA radiotherapy for CS I seminoma (Jones et al., 2005). The 5-year relapse-free survival (96% vs. 97%) and overall survival (99.6% vs. 100%) were similar, but patients receiving 20 Gy experienced less acute GI toxicity, leukopenia, and lethargy (though results were similar at 12 weeks). Further follow-up is necessary to assess the durability of these results.

Surveillance. Given the potential for late toxicity with DL radiotherapy, the 80% to 85% cure rate after orchiectomy, and the more than 90% cure rates achieved with platin-based chemotherapy for advanced seminoma, surveillance has been evaluated at several centers. Compared with NSGCT, surveillance for CS I seminoma is complicated by the limited utility of serum tumor markers to detect relapse and the need for long-term surveillance CT imaging because 10% to 20% of relapses occur 4 years or more after diagnosis (Chung et al., 2002). In the National Cancer Database, the majority of contemporary CS I seminoma patients (60%) are placed on surveillance (Matulewicz et al., 2016).

The largest surveillance series for CS I seminoma are listed in Table 76.10 (Aparicio et al., 2003, 2005; Choo et al., 2005; Daugaard et al., 2003; Horwich et al., 1992; Kollmannsberger et al., 2010c; Tandstad et al., 2011; von der Maase et al., 1993; Warde et al., 1995, 2005). **The 5-year relapse-free survival ranges from 80% to 86%, and cancer-specific survival approaches 100%. Eighty-four to 100% of patients relapse in the retroperitoneum, and 18% to 24% of patients have bulky retroperitoneal disease and/or distant metastases at the time of recurrence** (Aparicio et al., 2003; Choo et al., 2005; Horwich et al., 1992; von der Maase et al., 1993; Warde et al., 1995). DL radiotherapy is employed for treatment of relapse in 73% to 88% of patients, and cure rates of 70% to 90% are reported. Almost all patients who relapse outside the retroperitoneum are cured with first-line chemotherapy. Compared with NSGCT, the median time to relapse is longer for CS I seminoma (14 months vs. 4–8 months.), and a greater proportion of patients will relapse 5 years or more after diagnosis (Kollmannsberger et al., 2015).

To detect and treat recurrences at an early stage, patients on surveillance should be followed with clinical assessment, chest x-ray, serum tumor markers, and CT abdominal-pelvic imaging. Surveillance schedules employ assessments every 2 to 4 months in years 1 to 3, every 6 months in years 4 to 7, then annually thereafter. The necessary frequency of CT imaging is poorly defined, and centers obtain this every 4 to 6 months in years 1 to 3, every 6 months in years 4 to 7, then annually thereafter. A recent MRC trial suggested that the frequency of surveillance CT imaging in low-risk CS I NSGCT in years 0 to 2 may be safely reduced from 5 to 2 without affecting survival or burden of therapy (Rustin et al., 2007). It is unclear whether these findings can be safely applied to surveillance for seminoma. Long-term follow-up is mandatory given the higher incidence of relapse after 5 years compared with NSGCT (Chung et al., 2002). Surveillance CT imaging detects the majority of relapses among CS I seminoma patients (>85%), less than 5% of relapses are detected by elevated HCG levels, and almost no relapses are detected by chest x-ray or physical assessment (Kollmannsberger et al., 2015).

To better select patients for active treatment, investigators have endeavored to identify prognostic factors for occult metastasis. In a pooled analysis of 3 large surveillance series from the 1980s, tumor size larger than 4 cm and rete testis invasion were significant predictors of relapse in multivariable analysis (Warde et al., 2002). Unlike NSGCT, LVI has not been identified as a significant predictor of relapse for CS I seminoma. The 5-year relapse rate for patients with 0, 1, and 2 risk factors was 12%, 16%, and 32%, respectively. Twenty-one percent of patients in this cohort had rete testis invasion and tumor size greater than 4 cm. Primary radiotherapy or carboplatin for all "high-risk" patients would still expose two-thirds of CS I seminoma patients (who are cured by orchiectomy) to unnecessary therapy. However, prospective validation of these risk factors is currently lacking.

Primary Chemotherapy With Single-Agent Carboplatin. Primary chemotherapy with 1 to 2 cycles of single-agent carboplatin has also been investigated as an alternative to primary radiotherapy with the potential for reduced late toxicity. The rationale for single-agent carboplatin is based on the 65% to 90% reported complete response rates observed among patients with advanced seminoma (Horwich et al., 2000), and its reduced toxicity compared with cisplatin. Oliver et al. (1994) first described the use of 1 to 2 cycles of carboplatin in 78 patients and reported only 2 relapses and no deaths (Oliver et al., 1994). The published studies of carboplatin in CS I seminoma are listed in Table 76.11 (Aparicio et al., 2003, 2005, 2011; Dieckmann et al., 2000; Kollmannsberger et al., 2010c; Reiter et al., 2001; Steiner et al., 2002; Tandstad et al., 2011). No deaths from seminoma have been observed, and 3- to 5-year relapse-free rates are 91% to 100%.

The MRC and EORTC conducted a randomized, phase III clinical trial of 1 cycle of carboplatin vs. 20 to 30 Gy PA radiotherapy in 1477 patients with CS I seminoma (Oliver et al., 2005, 2011). Over a median follow-up of 6½ years, the 5-year relapse-free survival was similar (94.7% vs. 96%), and only 1 death was observed in the PA radiotherapy arm. In this trial, patients receiving carboplatin experienced less lethargy and time away from work than those receiving radiotherapy, and acute grade III to IV hematologic toxicity was observed in 4% of patients. Since this study was completed, a pooled analysis of 185 patients who relapsed after adjuvant carboplatin reported 5-year disease-free survival of 82% and 5-year overall survival of 98%, indicating that these patients are salvageable and do not have an unexpected rate of chemotherapy-resistant disease at relapse (Fischer et al., 2017). Fifteen percent of relapses occurred after 3 years, so a minimum of 5 years of surveillance is recommended.

A concern with one cycle of carboplatin is the potential for inadequate dosing, leading to an increased risk of relapse. A higher relapse rate with 1 vs. 2 cycles has been seen when comparing different studies, and a higher risk of relapse was reported among patients receiving an inadequate dose of carboplatin in the MRC/EORTC trial (Dieckmann et al., 2000; Oliver et al., 2008). More recently, a SWENOTECA study of 1118 men reported that a single dose of carboplatin reduced the risk of relapse in men with risk factors by only about 50% (Tandstad et al., 2016). In men with tumors larger than 4 cm, the risk of relapse was 19% with surveillance and 9.7% with a single dose of carboplatin, whereas the figures were 13.6% and 9.1% for men with rete testis invasion. A German study similarly reported only a 50% reduction in risk of relapse for men with large tumors when one cycle of carboplatin was administered (Dieckmann et al., 2016). Overall, the risk of relapse in this study was 5% with one cycle of carboplatin and 1.5% with two cycles. As a result of these and other studies, guidelines are divided on whether one or two cycles of carboplatin should be administered to men receiving primary chemotherapy for CS I seminomas (Dieckmann and Anheuser, 2016; Gilligan et al., 2018; Honecker et al., 2018). Moreover, the relatively small benefit seen with a single dose of carboplatin has led some to question this agent's use altogether for stage I disease (van de Wetering et al., 2018). Regardless of the number of cycles, the optimal dosing of carboplatin is calculated by the formula

$$7 \times (\text{Glomerular filtration rate [GFR, mL/min]} + 25) \text{ mg}$$

(Calvert and Egorin, 2002). Carboplatin dosing should not be based on estimated GFR. Thus it is recommended to base 1 cycle of carboplatin dosing on the results of radioisotope renal scans or administer 2 cycles of therapy.

Given the low overall risk of relapse with CS I seminoma, the lack of prospectively validated markers to identify a high-risk population, and the potential for late toxicity with radiotherapy and carboplatin, many clinical practice guidelines now recommend surveillance as the preferred approach (Gilligan et al., 2018; Honecker et al., 2018; Krege et al., 2008a). Surveillance enables 80% to 85% of patients to avoid treatment-related toxicity, and relapses are effectively salvaged with DL radiotherapy in most cases. However, surveillance must be continued more than 5 years, and frequent CT imaging is required. For noncompliant patients or those unwilling to accept surveillance, primary radiotherapy or primary chemotherapy with 2 cycles of carboplatin are recommended.

Clinical Stage IIA and IIB Seminoma

Approximately 15% to 20% of seminoma patients have CS II disease, 70% of whom have CS IIA-B. DL radiotherapy using 25 to 30 Gy (including a 5 to 10 Gy boost to involved areas) is

TABLE 76.11 Summary of Adjuvant Chemotherapy Series for Clinical Stage I Seminoma

	PATIENTS	MEDIAN FOLLOW-UP	NO. CYCLES	GCT DEATHS (%)	RELAPSE (%)
Oliver et al., 2011	573	78 months	1	0	27 (5)
Steiner et al., 2002	108	60 months	2	0	2 (2)
Reiter et al., 2001	107	74 months	2	0	0
Dieckmann et al., 2000	93	48 months	1	0	8 (9)
Dieckmann et al., 2000	32	48 months	2	0	0
Oliver et al., 1994	78	51 months	2[a]	0	2 (2)
Aparicio et al., 2003	60	52 months	2	0	2 (3.3)
Aparicio et al., 2005	214	34 months	2	0	7 (4)
Tandstad et al., 2011	188	62 months	1	0	7 (4)
Kollmannsberger et al., 2010	73	33 months	1-2	0	1 (2)

[a]33% of patients received 1 cycle of carboplatin.
GCT, Germ cell tumor.

employed at most centers. The higher radiation doses administered to CS IIA-B patients is generally well tolerated with acute grade III to IV GI toxicity reported in 8% to 10% (Classen et al., 2003). Prophylactic radiation to the left supraclavicular fossa is no longer practiced because less than 3% of patients are likely to benefit (Chung et al., 2003; Zagars and Pollack, 2001). Long-term disease-free survival rates of 92% to 100% for CS IIA and 87% to 90% for CS IIB have been reported, with in-field recurrences reported in 0 to 2% and 0 to 7% of cases, respectively (Chung et al., 2004; Classen et al., 2003; Zagars and Pollack, 2001). Adding single-agent carboplatin to 30 Gy DL radiotherapy reduced the relapse rate from 30% to 6% in one series, although further data are required to assess the utility of this approach (Patterson et al., 2001). **Relapses are cured in almost all cases with first-line chemotherapy, and disease-specific survival approaches 100%. Routine surveillance CT imaging is not necessary after complete resolution of disease.**

Induction chemotherapy using first-line regimens (BEPx3 or EPx4) is an accepted alternative to DL radiotherapy. The Spanish Germ Cell Cancer Study Group recently reported on the use of BEPx3 or EPx4 in 72 patients with CS IIA-B seminoma (Garcia-del-Muro et al., 2008). Overall, 83% of patients achieved a serologic and radiographic complete response, and only 1 (1.3%) had residual mass larger than 3 cm, and the 2 patients who underwent PCS for residual masses had necrosis only in the resected specimens. Overall, the 5-year relapse-free and overall survival was 90% and 95%, respectively. The SWENOTECA group similarly reported that there were no relapses among 73 CSIIA/B patients treated with cisplatin-based chemotherapy, whereas there were 3 relapses (10%) among 29 patients treated with radiotherapy. **Induction chemotherapy is preferentially given to patients with bulky (>3 cm) and/or multiple retroperitoneal masses as the risk of relapse is lower than DL radiotherapy** (Chung et al., 2004; Garcia-del-Muro et al., 2008; Patterson et al., 2001).

Primary RPLND is an accepted intervention for NSGCT patients with CS IIA and IIB disease who have negative serum tumor markers. RPLND has not been accepted as a standard treatment for CS IIA and IIB seminoma for largely historical reasons. With recognition of the late toxicity of primary chemotherapy and radiotherapy, there is renewed interest in defining the role of primary RPLND for these patients. The rationale for RPLND is further supported by the recognition that metastatic disease is usually limited to the retroperitoneum in the majority of patients with CS IIA (>90%) and IIB (>85%) seminoma, suggesting RPLND alone may cure these patient without the need for systemic therapy. Two prospective trials in the United States and Germany are investigating the role of primary RPLND as treatment for CS IIA with or without IIB seminoma or as treatment for isolated retroperitoneal relapses for CS I seminoma patients on surveillance or after carboplatin primary chemotherapy.

Clinical Stage IIC and III Seminoma

As with NSGCT, patients with CS IIC and III seminoma are treated with induction chemotherapy, with the regimen and number of cycles determined by the IGCCCG risk. Ninety percent of patients with advanced seminoma are classified as good-risk and should receive either BEPx3 or EPx4 chemotherapy. Complete radiographic responses are reported in 70% to 90% of patients, and the 5-year overall is 91% (Gholam et al., 2003; International Germ Cell Cancer Collaborative Group, 1997; Loehrer et al., 1987; Mencel et al., 1994). Only 10% of advanced seminomas have nonpulmonary visceral metastasis (classified as intermediate-risk by IGCCCG criteria). With BEPx4 chemotherapy, the 5-year overall and progression-free survival is 79% and 75%, respectively (International Germ Cell Cancer Collaborative Group, 1997). Single-agent carboplatin in advanced seminoma is associated with inferior survival compared to cisplatin-based regimens (Bokemeyer et al., 2004).

Management of Post-Chemotherapy Residual Masses. After first-line chemotherapy, **58% to 80% of patients have radiologically detectable residual masses** (De Santis et al., 2004; Duchesne et al., 1997; Flechon et al., 2002; Fossa et al., 1997; Herr et al., 1997; Motzer et al., 1987; Puc et al., 1996). **Spontaneous resolution of these masses is reported in 50% to 66% of cases (30%–50% for masses >3 cm), and the median time to resolution is 12 to 18 months** (De Santis et al., 2004; Flechon et al., 2002). **The histology of residual masses is necrosis and viable malignancy in 90% and 10% of cases, respectively** (De Santis et al., 2004; Flechon et al., 2002; Herr et al., 1997; Puc et al., 1996; Ravi et al., 1999). **PCS for seminoma is technically difficult (and frequently not feasible) because of the desmoplastic reaction that occurs after chemotherapy with resultant increased perioperative morbidity** (Mosharafa et al., 2003). Surgical complete resections in post-chemotherapy seminoma are reported in only 58% to 74% of patients (compared with 85% or more after first-line chemotherapy for NSGCT) (De Santis et al., 2004; Flechon et al., 2002; Herr et al., 1997; Puc et al., 1996; Ravi et al., 1999). Adjunctive procedures such as nephrectomy are required in 38% to 51% of patients. **Teratoma and malignant transformation are much less of a concern with advanced seminoma.** As such, the management of post-chemotherapy residual masses differences substantially for seminoma compared with NSGCT.

Investigators have endeavored to identify factors associated with a high risk of viable malignancy to justify PCS. **Post-chemotherapy radiotherapy has no role in the management of residual masses** (Duchesne et al., 1997). **The size of residual masses is an important predictor of viable malignancy; 13% to 55% of discrete residual masses larger than 3 cm contain viable malignancy compared with 0 to 4% for masses less than 3 cm** (De Santis et al., 2004; Flechon et al., 2002; Herr et al., 1997; Puc et al., 1996). **Recently, FDG-PET has been found to be a useful adjunct to CT imaging to select patients for PCS** (De Santis et al., 2004). In a prospective study, the specificity and sensitivity of a positive FDG-PET for masses greater than 3 cm was 100% and 80%, respectively. Recently, rates of false-positive FDG-PET results have been reported in 22% to 78% of patients; the accuracy of a negative FDG-PET result remains high. The risk of a false-positive FDG-PET result is higher if the study is completed within 4 to 6 weeks after completion of chemotherapy because of inflammation or residual nonviable malignancy. Thus FDG-PET should be delayed until at least 6 weeks after completion of chemotherapy. **There is consensus that patients with discrete residual masses greater than 3 cm should be evaluated further with FDG-PET at least 6 weeks after completion of chemotherapy, and those who are PET-negative and those with masses smaller than 3 cm should be observed.**

There is controversy regarding the appropriate management of patients with FDG-positive residual masses larger than 3 cm given the reported rates of false-positive FDG-PET imaging. Close observation with repeat FDG-PET imaging in 6 to 8 weeks has been advocated by some, although its role is unproven. Close observation with delayed intervention for growing masses has also been advocated because only 14% to 20% of these patients will relapse with most identified within 4 to 6 months of completion of chemotherapy. In the Indiana University experience, this approach of observation with delayed intervention was associated with durable disease control in only 9 of 36 patients with a 72% relapse rate after PC-RPLND (Rice et al., 2014). Although a survival advantage associated with PCS for metastatic seminoma has yet to be definitely proven, there is a therapeutic benefit to upfront PC-RPLND: it enables an immediate assessment of tumor response and further chemotherapy can be administered in a timely fashion. PCS is also therapeutic for the rare advanced seminoma patient with metastatic teratoma, which is reported to be present in up to one-third of residual masses larger than 3 cm after chemotherapy. In the study by Herr et al. (1997), all 6 patients who had complete resection of viable malignancy were disease free over a median follow-up of 45 months. In contrast, 4 of 6 patients with unresected viable malignancy died of seminoma despite additional chemotherapy and/or radiotherapy (Herr et al., 1997). **For patients with FDG-PET positive residual masses larger than 3 cm, strong consideration should be given for PC-RPLND, particularly those with residual masses after second-line chemotherapy.**

Historically, resection of the residual mass only was advocated rather than completion of a full, bilateral RPLND. In the Indiana University experience, this approach was associated with a 33% local relapse rate (Rice et al., 2014). As such, consideration should be given to performing a full, bilateral, or accepted modified template dissection (as is used at PC-RPLND NSGCT) if it is technically feasible to do so.

Relapsed Seminoma

Chemotherapy-Naïve Seminoma Relapse. Chemotherapy-naïve relapse occurs in men with CS I seminoma on surveillance and in those with CS I-IIB seminoma treated with primary radiotherapy. **For the former patients, DL radiotherapy is employed for treatment of relapse in 73% to 88% of patients and cure rates of 70% to 90% are reported. Patients with bulky (>3 cm) retroperitoneal masses and systemic relapse should receive first-line chemotherapy and salvage rates approach 100%. First-line chemotherapy cures virtually all patients who relapse outside the retroperitoneum after primary radiotherapy.** Patients who relapse after single-agent carboplatin are considered to have chemotherapy-naïve relapse and should receive first-line cisplatin-base chemotherapy.

Post-Chemotherapy Seminoma Relapse—Early. An estimated 15% to 20% of advanced seminoma patients relapse after induction chemotherapy, including 10% who achieve an initial complete response (International Germ Cell Cancer Collaborative Group, 1997; Loehrer et al., 1987; Mencel et al., 1994). In general, patients with incomplete response to first-line chemotherapy or relapse after an initial major clinical response have a poor prognosis with long-term survival rates of 20% to 50% (Gholam et al., 2003; Miller et al., 1997; Vuky et al., 2002). The small number of patients with seminoma who require second-line chemotherapy has limited the evaluation of unique treatment strategies and relapsing patients are treated on regimens that were largely developed for NSGCT relapse. In two small studies, the efficacy of VeIPx4 as second-line chemotherapy was evaluated in 36 patients with relapsed seminoma. Overall, 30 patients (83%) achieved a complete response to chemotherapy (with or without PCS) and 21 (53%) were continuously free of recurrence over a median follow-up of 72 to 84 months (Miller et al., 1997; Vuky et al., 2002). Vuky et al. (2002) also evaluated HDCT in 12 advanced seminoma patients with an incomplete response to first-line chemotherapy and 6 patients (50%) achieving a complete response have remained free of recurrence. **An important consideration for advanced seminoma patients who relapse after first-line chemotherapy is the potential for teratoma at the site of relapse. Thus patients with normal serum tumor markers should undergo biopsy before starting second-line chemotherapy.**

Post-Chemotherapy Seminoma Relapse—Late. In most published series, pure seminoma accounts for fewer than 8% of late relapse events (Baniel et al., 1995; George et al., 2003; Ronnen et al., 2005; Sharp et al., 2008). However, Dieckmann et al. recently (2005) reported a series of 122 patients with late relapse, of whom 50 (41%) had pure seminoma at diagnosis. Only 6 (12%) of these patients had received prior first-line chemotherapy and the majority had received single-agent carboplatin or radiation therapy at diagnosis. Long-term cancer control was achieved in 88% of patients. **Thus late relapse of seminoma may have a favorable prognosis, particularly among patients without prior exposure to cisplatin.**

Brain Metastases

About 1% of men with disseminated GCT have brain metastases detected before initiating chemotherapy and between 0.4% and 3% will develop brain metastases after first-line chemotherapy (Fossa SD et al., 1999; International Germ Cell Cancer Collaborative Group, 1997; Raina et al., 1993). **Brain metastases are associated with choriocarcinoma and should be suspected in any patient with a very high serum HCG level** (Fossa et al., 1999; Gremmer et al., 2008; Kollmannsberger et al., 2000; Nonomura et al., 2009; Salvati et al., 2006). **Choriocarcinomas are highly vascular and tend to hemorrhage during chemotherapy and death rates of 4% to 10% resulting from intracranial hemorrhage have been reported** (Kollmannsberger et al., 2000; Nonomura et al., 2009). Management of these patients must consider this risk and neurologic changes must be evaluated expeditiously.

KEY POINTS

- The optimal management of CS I seminoma is controversial. Surveillance, primary radiotherapy (20–30 Gy to the para-aortic region +/− ipsilateral pelvis), and primary chemotherapy with carboplatin (1–2 cycles) are accepted treatment options with long-term survival rates approaching 100% for each.
- Prognostic factors for occult metastases in CS I seminoma are not as well developed as for NSGCT. Given the overall low-risk of occult metastases (15%–20%), the inability to identify a high-risk population on the basis of histopathological factors in the primary tumor, and the potential for late toxicity with primary radiotherapy, surveillance has become the recommended treatment approach for CS I seminoma.
- Surveillance is not recommended to patients who are anticipated to be poorly compliant with follow-up imaging and clinical evaluation. The standard treatment approach to patients who relapse on surveillance is DL radiotherapy (25–35 Gy), although patients with bulky retroperitoneal lymphadenopathy or distant metastases should receive IGCCCG risk-appropriate first-line chemotherapy.
- Primary radiotherapy and primary chemotherapy with single-agent carboplatin are associated with similar rates of cure and survival. PA radiotherapy and carboplatin require periodic CT imaging in the surveillance of recurrent disease after treatment; this is not required for DL radiotherapy.
- DL radiotherapy (25–35 Gy) and first-line chemotherapy (BEPx3 or EPx4) are accepted treatment options for CS IIA-B seminoma patients with non-bulky (<3 cm) retroperitoneal lymph node metastasis. First-line chemotherapy (BEPx3 or EPx4) is recommended for bulky (>3 cm) and/or multifocal retroperitoneal metastases.
- The treatment of patients with CS IIC and III seminoma is first-line cisplatin-based chemotherapy and the specific regimen and number of cycles is dictated by IGCCCG risk criteria. Patients with good-risk disease should receive BEPx3 or EPx4, and those with intermediate-risk disease should receive BEPx4.
- Patients with discrete, residual masses larger than 3 cm after first-line chemotherapy should undergo further evaluation with FDG-PET imaging. Patients with PET-positive residual masses should undergo post-chemotherapy surgical resection. Residual masses that are PET-negative or less than 3 cm can be safely observed after chemotherapy.

The 5-year overall survival in patients with brain metastases is 33% and 57% for those with disseminated NSGCT and seminoma, respectively (International Germ Cell Cancer Collaborative Group, 1997). **Men who relapse in the brain after achieving a complete response to chemotherapy appear to have a worse prognosis than those with brain involvement at diagnosis**, with overall survival rates of 39% to 44% for isolated brain metastases and 2% to 26% for those with brain metastases in association with other sites of disease (Fossa et al., 1999; Gremmer et al., 2008; Hartmann et al., 1607; Kollmannsberger et al., 2000; Nonomura et al., 2009; Salvati et al., 2006). Case studies and pooled analyses of GCT patients with brain metastases have reported outcomes with various treatment strategies, but there are no randomized trials to clearly define optimal management (Fossa et al., 1999; Gremmer et al., 2008; Hartmann et al., 1607; Kollmannsberger et al., 2000; Nonomura et al., 2009; Salvati et al., 2006; Spears et al., 1992). Treatment strategies have included chemotherapy, surgical resection, whole-brain radiation therapy, and stereotactic radiosurgery, with most patients receiving multi-modal therapy. **Patients with brain metastases at diagnosis should receive BEPx4 chemotherapy followed by resection of residual masses.** The benefit of radiation therapy in this setting is unclear (Fossa et al., 1999; Hartmann et al., 1607; Kollmannsberger et al., 2000). At our institution, radiation therapy is only considered for patients with unresectable residual lesions not amenable to stereotactic radiosurgery because of the concerns of radiation-induced neurotoxicity (Doyle and Einhorn, 2008). **Patients who relapse in the brain after first-line chemotherapy should be treated with second-line chemotherapy followed by resection and/or radiation therapy** (Fossa et al., 1999; Hartmann et al., 1607).

> **KEY POINT: BRAIN METASTASES**
>
> - Brain metastases are associated with choriocarcinoma and should be suspected in any patient with a very high serum HCG level. Choriocarcinomas are highly vascular, and there is a risk of hemorrhage during chemotherapy. Patients with metastatic choriocarcinoma to the brain are at risk of intracranial hemorrhage and should be monitored for such when chemotherapy is started.

Treatment Sequelae

Testis cancer treatment sequelae can be divided into late and early complications. Complications from orchiectomy and retroperitoneal lymph node dissection will not be reviewed here except to note that the main issues after RPLND are midline scar, ejaculatory dysfunction, small bowel obstruction, and perioperative complications. There also is an increased incidence of hypogonadism after orchiectomy for GCT.

Early Toxicity

Cisplatin-based chemotherapy is associated with numerous early complications and side effects, including fatigue, myelosuppression, infection, peripheral neuropathy, hearing loss, diminished renal function, and death. The toxic death rate has ranged from 0 to 2.4% during chemotherapy for good-risk disease and from 3% to 4.4% during standard first-line chemotherapy for intermediate- and poor-risk disease (Culine et al., 2007, 2008; de Wit et al., 1998, 2001; Nichols et al., 1998; Toner et al., 2001). The impact of chemotherapy and radiation therapy on spermatogenesis has been discussed previously. Most men are able to father children after treatment for GCT, but paternity rates are lower for men treated with radiation therapy and/or chemotherapy (Brydoy et al., 2005; Huyghe et al., 2004). Early complications of radiation therapy include fatigue, nausea and vomiting, leukopenia, and dyspepsia (Fossa et al., 1999; Jones et al., 2005; Oliver et al., 2005).

Late Toxicity

Numerous long-term sequelae have been reported in GCT survivors, including peripheral neuropathy, Raynaud phenomenon, hearing loss, hypogonadism, infertility, secondary malignant neoplasms, and cardiovascular disease (Brydoy et al., 2009; Fossa et al., 2009; Rossen et al., 2009). Symptoms of Raynaud phenomenon and peripheral neuropathy have been reported in 20% to 45% and 14% to 43% (Brydoy et al., 2009; Rossen et al., 2009). Significant hearing loss and/or tinnitus after cisplatin-based chemotherapy is reported in 20% to 40% of patients and can be documented via audiometry in 30% to 75%. Hypogonadism has been documented in about 10% to 20% of patients treated with orchiectomy alone, 15% to 40% of patients treated with radiation therapy, and 20% to 25% of men treated with first-line chemotherapy regimens (Lackner et al., 2009; Nord et al., 2003).

Large population-based studies of GCT survivors have reported an increased risk of death from GI and cardiovascular diseases after radiation therapy and an increased risk of death from infections, cardiovascular, and pulmonary diseases after chemotherapy (Fossa et al., 2007). Patients treated with both radiation and chemotherapy have the highest risk of death from nonmalignant causes. The increased cardiovascular disease incidence and mortality in GCT survivors is particularly well documented (Fossa et al., 2007; 2009; Huddart et al., 2003; Meinardi et al., 2000; van den Belt-Dusebout et al., 2007). The causes of these cardiovascular complications are not well understood, but putative contributing factors are radiation- or chemotherapy-induced vascular injury, chemotherapy-induced cardiac injury, and metabolic syndrome (Altena et al., 2009; Nuver et al., 2005).

The risk of second malignant neoplasms is a particular concern. The incidence of non–germ cell malignancies is 60% to 100% higher in GCT survivors treated with cisplatin-based chemotherapy or radiation therapy compared with the general population and 200% higher in patients who received both radiation and chemotherapy (Richiardi et al., 2007; Travis et al., 2005). The risk of death from non–germ cell malignancies in GCT survivors treated with radiation or chemotherapy is less well defined but appears to be doubled compared with the general population (Fossa et al., 2004). The frequent use of body CT imaging in the surveillance of patients after therapy is another source of radiation that may increase the risk of secondary malignant neoplasms (Brenner and Hall, 2007; Chamie et al., 2008; Tarin et al., 2009).

> **KEY POINT: LATE EFFECTS**
>
> - All treatments for GCT (surgery, radiotherapy, and chemotherapy) are associated with risks of early and late toxicity. The most concerning late complications are cardiovascular disease and SMNs. With the successful cure of patients (even those with advanced disease), an important treatment objective is minimizing treatment-related toxicity without compromising curability.

NON–GERM CELL TUMORS

Sex Cord-Stromal Tumors

Sex cord-stromal tumors are rare, making up approximately 0.4% to 4% of testis neoplasms, and the term refers to neoplasms containing Leydig cells, Sertoli cells, granulosa cells, or thecal cells (Banerji et al., 2016). **Approximately 90% of these tumors are benign and 10% are malignant.** Histologic criteria have been developed to help distinguish between benign and malignant histology and include tumor size larger than 5 cm, necrosis, vascular invasion, nuclear atypia, high mitotic index, increased MIB-1 expression, infiltrative margins, extension beyond the testicular parenchyma, and DNA ploidy (Cheville et al., 1998; Kim et al., 1985). Most malignant cases are associated with at least 2 of these features. **However, the presence of metastatic disease is the only reliable criteria for making this distinction.**

Leydig Cell Tumors

Leydig cell tumors account for 75% to 80% of sex cord-stromal tumors. There is no association with cryptorchidism. Most of these tumors occur in adult males between 30 and 60 years, although approximately one-fourth occur in children. Adults may initially be seen with painless testis mass, testicular pain, gynecomastia (as a result of androgen excess and peripheral estrogen conversion), impotence, decreased libido, and infertility. Children usually have a testis mass and isosexual precocious puberty (prominent external genitalia, pubic hair growth, and masculine voice).

Diagnostic workup should include serum tumor markers and testicular ultrasound. The sonographic appearance of these tumors is variable and is indistinguishable from GCT. In the presence of gynecomastia, infertility, depressed libido, or precocious puberty, LH, FSH, testosterone, estrogen, and estradiol should also be drawn (these should be measured after orchiectomy if the diagnosis is not suspected preoperatively). Once the diagnosis is confirmed, patients should undergo CT chest-abdomen-pelvis for staging purposes.

In the past, radical inguinal orchiectomy was the initial treatment of choice. If the diagnosis is suspected preoperatively, testis-sparing surgery may be considered for lesions smaller than

3 cm with intraoperative frozen section histologic confirmation given the 90% incidence of benign histology (Carmignani et al., 2006, 2007). **Completion orchiectomy should be performed if GCT histology is seen (either on intraoperative frozen section or final pathology) or if malignant features (listed earlier) are present on final pathological examination of the resected tumor.** Testis-sparing surgery for small tumors without malignant histologic risk factors is associated with similar survival and a low risk of local recurrence that may be successfully treated with completion orchiectomy (Laclergerie et al., 2018; Nicolai et al., 2015; Paffenholz et al., 2018). Given the rarity of these tumors, they are often not suspected preoperatively, and most patients undergo radical orchiectomy. Benign lesions are usually small, yellow to brown, well circumscribed, without areas of necrosis of hemorrhage. Histologically, the tumors consist of uniform, polygonal cells with round nuclei. Reinke crystals are present in 25% to 40% of cases and appear as densely eosinophilic needle-like or rhomboid structures within the cytoplasm. These tumors must be distinguished from Leydig cell hyperplasia that occur in atrophic testes and adjacent to GCTs, in which Leydig cells infiltrate between seminiferous tubules without displacing or obliterating them. Malignant behavior has not been reported in a prepubertal patient. Older patients are more likely to have malignant tumors.

The most frequent metastatic sites are the retroperitoneum and the lung. Patients with CS I disease with at least 1 malignant histologic feature may be safely observed. Those with 2 or more malignant features or retroperitoneal metastases should undergo RPLND, although high rates of progression are observed in those with pathologically involved nodes (Mosharafa et al., 2003; Nicolai et al., 2015; Silberstein et al., 2014). **Metastatic Leydig cell tumors are resistant to chemotherapy and radiation therapy, and survival is poor** (Mosharafa et al., 2003). Ortho-para-DDD, a potent inhibitor of steroidogenesis, may produce partial responses in metastatic patients with excess androgen production, but cure is not possible (Schwarzman et al., 1989). Surveillance is recommended for those without clinical or pathological features suggestive of malignancy. There are no widely accepted criteria for follow-up, but patients should be monitored at regular intervals with clinical assessment, hormonal profile (including LH, follicle-stimulating hormone [FSH], testosterone, estrogen, estradiol), and CT imaging of the chest-abdomen-pelvis for 2 years. Persistent Leydig cell dysfunction and hypogonadism may occur after excision of the primary tumor, and up to 40% of men may require testosterone supplementation postoperatively (Conkey et al., 2005).

Sertoli Cell Tumor

These tumors constitute less than 1% of testis neoplasms. The median age at diagnosis is 45 years, but rare cases in children have been reported. In rare cases, these tumors are associated with Peutz-Jeghers syndrome and androgen insensitivity syndrome and are frequently bilateral (either synchronous or metachronous). There is no association with cryptorchidism. Gynecomastia is evident in up to one-third of patients. **As for Leydig cell tumors, testis-sparing surgery can be considered for tumors smaller than 3 cm given the high incidence of benign histology (90%). For tumors larger than 3 cm or if intraoperative frozen section or final pathological analysis reveals germ cell tumor or malignant features, radical inguinal orchiectomy should be performed.** The tumors are well circumscribed, yellow-white or tan, with uniform consistency. Microscopically, the tumors contain epithelial elements resembling Sertoli cells with varying amounts of stroma organized into tubules. These tumors may be misinterpreted as seminomas leading to errors in the selection of treatment. **Diagnostic workup, staging studies and criteria for treatment, surveillance, and follow-up are similar to that for Leydig cell tumors with similar outcomes** (Nicolai et al., 2015; Silberstein et al., 2014).

Granulosa Cell Tumors

Granulosa cell tumors of the testis are exceedingly rare. The juvenile type is benign and is the most frequent congenital testis tumor (most frequently occurring in infants younger than 6 months of age), accounting for 7% of all prepubertal testicular neoplasms. The adult-type resembles granulosa cell tumors of the ovary. Gynecomastia and increased estrogen secretion are common. Testis-sparing surgery may be considered for tumors smaller than 3 cm if the diagnosis is suspected preoperatively. Otherwise, radical inguinal orchiectomy is recommended. Treatment of the primary tumor is curative as these tumors appear to have limited metastatic potential.

Gonadoblastoma

Gonadoblastoma is a mixed germ cell-sex cord-stromal tumor composed of seminoma-like germ cells and sex cord cells showing Sertoli differentiation. They occur almost exclusively in patients with dysgenic gonads and intersex syndromes. Eighty percent of affected individuals are phenotypic females, usually with primary amenorrhea. The remainder of patients are phenotypic males, almost always with cryptorchidism (with the dysgenic gonad in the inguinal or abdominal location), hypospadias, and some form of female internal genitalia. **These tumors should be considered an in situ form of malignant GCT; approximately 50% will develop an invasive GCT (usually seminoma, although yolk sac tumor and EC can occur)** (Ulbright, 2004). Gonadoblastomas do not metastasize but the malignant GCT elements may. **Bilateral orchiectomy is required because of the risk of bilateral tumors (40%)** (Scully, 1970). For patients with malignant GCT, subsequent workup for metastatic disease and appropriate treatment should be initiated.

Miscellaneous Testis Neoplasms

Dermoid and Epidermoid Cyst

These rare benign neoplasms that are thought to arise from benign germ cells with retrained embryonic properties or from displaced metaplastic mesothelial cells (Ye and Ulbright, 2012). Grossly, they are well-circumscribed, unilocular cystic masses filled with keratinized debris that may have a laminated appearance that gives them the characteristic "onion peel" or target appearance on ultrasound. They are typically smaller than 3 cm and do not exhibit flow or enhancement on Doppler US and MRI, respectively. Dermoid cysts are differentiated from epidermoid cysts by the presence of adnexal structures such as glandular elements, adipose tissue, and cartilage. Dermoid and epidermoid cysts are distinguished from teratoma by the absence of GCNIS in the adjacent testis. **Enucleation or partial orchiectomy may be performed, although the lesion should be thoroughly sampled by a pathologist to rule out GCT or GCNIS.**

Adenocarcinoma of the Rete Testis

Adenocarcinoma of the rete testis is a rare but highly malignant neoplasm arising from the collecting system of the testis. The usual presentation is a painless testis mass with hydrocele. More than 50% of patients have metastatic disease, and the overall median survival is 1 year. RPLND may be curative in patients with limited retroperitoneal lymph node metastasis. Chemotherapy and radiation therapy are ineffective.

Testicular "Tumor" of the Adrenogenital Syndrome. This non-neoplastic entity is derived from hyperplasia of remnant adrenal steroid cells that migrate to the scrotum during descent of the testis in utero or from pluripotent stem cells within the testis. The hyperplasia occurs as a consequences of ACTH stimulation in response to deficiency of cortisol or aldosterone in patients with C-21- hydroxylase (90%) or C-11-hydroxylase deficiency. Increased LH production at puberty can also stimulate the growth of these cells. The median age at presentation is 22 years; one-third are children. It may be the initial presentation in up to 18% of patients. Bilateral testicular masses are present in 83% of cases and typically develop near the testicular hilum. Corticosteroid therapy typically induces regression or stabilization of these masses. Surgical intervention may be necessary for persistent symptoms and/or evidence of testicular damage because of chronic obstruction (Ozisik et al., 2017; Ulbright and Young, 2014).

Secondary Tumors of the Testis

Lymphoma

Primary testicular non-Hodgkin lymphoma (NHL) is a rare tumor and represents only 1% to 2% of all cases of lymphoma. Most commonly, lymphoma involves the testis through dissemination from extratesticular sites (Ulbright, 2004). Eighty-five percent of cases occur in men over age 60. **NHL is the most common testicular neoplasm in men over age 50. Bilateral testicular involvement occurs in 35% of cases.** It usually is seen as a painless testicular mass in an older male. Approximately 25% of men have systemic symptoms (fever, night sweats, weight loss). Central nervous system involvement at diagnosis is reported in 10% of men. The initial treatment is radical inguinal orchiectomy. Men with testicular NHL should be referred to hematology-oncology for staging investigations and subsequent therapy. Most cases are associated with systemic disease and the overall prognosis is poor.

Leukemic Infiltration

The testis is a frequent site of relapse in boys with acute lymphocytic leukemia. The majority of boys are in complete remission at the time of testicular enlargement. **The diagnosis can usually be made by biopsy, and orchiectomy is unnecessary. Local control can be achieved with low-dose radiotherapy (20 Gy), and treatment should include the contralateral testis because of the frequent risk of bilateral involvement.** Overall, the prognosis is poor because most have associated systemic disease.

Metastases

Metastases to the testis are rare. Bilateral involvement occurs in 15% of patients. The most common primary tumors are prostate, lung, melanoma, colon, and kidney cancer. Although treatment is largely dictated by the primary tumor, orchiectomy may be considered for palliative reasons.

TUMORS OF THE TESTICULAR ADNEXA

Paratesticular tumors are rare and account for approximately 5% of intrascrotal neoplasms, roughly 75% of which arise from the spermatic cord.

Adenomatoid Tumor

Adenomatoid tumor is of mesothelial origin and is the most common paratesticular tumor, 75% of which involve the epididymis (although these tumors may also arise within the testicular tunics or the spermatic cord). The most common presentation is a small (0.5–5 cm), painless paratesticular mass detected on routine examination in a male in their third or fourth decade. **These tumors are benign and managed by inguinal exploration and surgical excision.** On microscopic examination, these tumors are composed of epithelial-like cells, which contain vacuoles and fibrous stroma.

Cystadenoma

Cystadenoma of the epididymis corresponds to benign epithelial hyperplasia. The lesions are usually multicystic, the walls of which are studded with nodules of epithelial cells arranged in a glandular or papillary configuration. **Approximately one-third of cases, which are usually bilateral, occur in patients with von Hippel-Lindau syndrome.** The lesions are usually small and painless and are detected on routine examination in a young adult.

Mesothelioma

Paratesticular mesothelioma arises from the tunica vaginalis and usually is seen as a painless paratesticular mass or tunical vegetations in association with a hydrocele. These tumors most commonly occur in older adults but may be encountered in any age group. **Benign and malignant mesothelioma have been described, with the distinction based on atypia, mitotic activity, and invasion** (Ulbright, 2004). Well-differentiated papillary mesotheliomas are usually solitary exophytic nodules distinguished from malignant cases by a focal exophytic papillary growth without evidence of invasion. Malignant cases may be associated with asbestos exposure and represent less than 5% of all malignant mesothelioma cases. Metastatic spread is typically lymphatic to inguinal, pelvic, and retroperitoneal lymph nodes. **Treatment is radical inguinal orchiectomy and hemiscrotectomy.** Retroperitoneal, pelvic, and inguinal lymph node dissection may be considered in patients with malignant tumors without widespread metastatic disease. The role of chemotherapy for these tumors is poorly defined. Overall, prognosis of malignant cases is poor with a median survival less than 2 years (Recabal et al., 2017).

Sarcoma

Sarcomas of the spermatic cord, epididymis, and testis are the most common genitourinary sarcomas in adults. **Liposarcoma is the most common histologic subtype in adults**, followed by leiomyosarcoma, malignant fibrous histiocytoma, rhabdomyosarcoma, and fibrosarcoma (Coleman et al., 2003; Dotan et al., 2006; Rodriguez et al., 2014; Ulbright, 2004). **Embryonal rhabdomyosarcoma is the most common histologic subtype in men under age 30.** Sarcomas most commonly arise from the spermatic cord and are located in the intrascrotal region; primary mesenchymal tumors of the testis are exceedingly rare. These tumors usually present as a painless, palpable mass and most are large (>5 cm) (Dotan et al., 2006). Ultrasonography will demonstrate a solid mass, although it cannot distinguish between benign and malignant pathology. **As such, any solid mass in the scrotum external to the tunica albuginea should be explored through an inguinal approach and biopsy performed.** Liposarcomas of the spermatic cord in the inguinal canal may be mistaken for inguinal hernia or lipoma, and CT or MRI is helpful to distinguish between these entities.

The majority of patients have localized disease at diagnosis. **Sarcomas should be managed initially through an inguinal approach with wide excision of the spermatic cord and testis with high ligation. Patients with an initial incomplete resection should under repeat wide excision** (Coleman et al., 2003). **The primary pattern of failure is local, particularly for liposarcoma** (Ballo et al., 2001; Khandekar et al., 2013; Montgomery and Fisher, 2003). As such, some have advocated for postoperative radiation therapy for all paratesticular sarcomas, particularly for liposarcomas and for those tumors where the adequacy of local control is in doubt (Ballo et al., 2001; Hazariwala et al., 2013). **However, the efficacy of this approach is debated** (Coleman et al., 2003; Fagundes et al., 1996; Khandekar et al., 2013). Systemic chemotherapy should be given to patients with evidence of retroperitoneal or distant metastases. **In the presence of a normal metastatic evaluation, patients with sarcomas other than liposarcoma should undergo RPLND and postoperative chemotherapy should be given to patients with retroperitoneal lymph node metastasis** (Dang et al., 2013). Given that the lymphatic drainage of the spermatic cord includes the ipsilateral pelvis, inguinal, and retroperitoneal lymph nodes, consideration should be given to treat these areas with lymphadenectomy or radiation therapy. The long-term survival of men with paratesticular sarcoma is approximately 50%, with liposarcoma having the most favorable prognosis and malignant fibrous histiocytoma and leiomyosarcoma having the least favorable prognosis (Coleman et al., 2003; Rodriguez et al., 2014).

SUGGESTED READINGS

Albers P, Siener R, Krege S, et al: Randomized phase III trial comparing retroperitoneal lymph node dissection with one course of bleomycin and etoposide plus cisplatin chemotherapy in the adjuvant treatment of clinical stage I Nonseminomatous testicular germ cell tumors: AUO trial AH 01/94 by the German Testicular Cancer Study Group, *J Clin Oncol* 26:2966–2972, 2008.

Albers P, Weissbach L, Krege S, et al: Prediction of necrosis after chemotherapy of advanced germ cell tumors: results of a prospective multicenter trial of the German Testicular Cancer Study Group, *J Urol* 171:1835–1838, 2004.

Beck SD, Foster RS, Bihrle R, et al: Long-term outcome for patients with high volume retroperitoneal teratoma undergoing post-chemotherapy surgery, *J Urol* 181:2526–2532, 2009.

Calaway AC, Einhorn LH, Masterson TA, et al: Adverse surgical outcomes associated with robotic retroperitoneal lymph node dissection among patients with testicular cancer, *Eur Urol* 2019.

Carver BS, Shayegan B, Serio A, et al: Long-term clinical outcome after postchemotherapy retroperitoneal lymph node dissection in men with residual teratoma, *J Clin Oncol* 25:1033–1037, 2007.

Fizazi K, Oldenburg J, Dunant A, et al: Assessing prognosis and optimizing treatment in patients with postchemotherapy viable nonseminomatous germ-cell tumors (NSGCT): results of the sCR2 international study, *Ann Oncol* 19:259–264, 2008.

Fossa SD, Gilbert E, Dores GM, et al: Noncancer causes of death in survivors of testicular cancer, *J Natl Cancer Inst* 99:533–544, 2007.

Gilligan T, Beard C, Carneiro B, et al: *NCCN Guidelines Version 2.2018 Testicular Cancer*. In. nccn.org: National Comprehensive Cancer Network, 2018.

Gilligan TD, Seidenfeld J, Basch EM, et al; American Society of Clinical Oncology: American Society of Clinical Oncology Clinical Practice Guideline on uses of serum tumor markers in adult males with germ cell tumors, *J Clin Oncol* 28:3388–3404, 2010.

Hanna NH, Einhorn LH: Testicular cancer—discoveries and updates, *N Engl J Med* 371:2005–2016, 2014.

Harari SE, Sassoon DJ, Priemer DS, et al: Testicular cancer: the usage of central review for pathology diagnosis of orchiectomy specimens, *Urol Oncol* 35:605.e9–605.e16, 2017.

Honecker F, Aparicio J, Berney D, et al: ESMO Consensus Conference on testicular germ cell cancer: diagnosis, treatment and follow-up, *Ann Oncol* 29:1658–1686, 2018.

Huddart RA, Reid AM: Adjuvant therapy for stage IB germ cell tumors: one versus two cycles of BEP, *Adv Urol* 2018:8781698, 2018.

International Germ Cell Consensus Classification: a prognostic factor-based staging system for metastatic germ cell cancers. International Germ Cell Cancer Collaborative Group, *J Clin Oncol* 15:594–603, 1997.

Kvammen O, Myklebust TA, Solberg A, et al: Long-term relative survival after diagnosis of testicular germ cell tumor, *Cancer Epidemiol Biomarkers Prev* 25:773–779, 2016.

Motzer RJ, Amsterdam A, Prieto V, et al: Teratoma with malignant transformation: diverse malignant histologies arising in men with germ cell tumors, *J Urol* 159:133–138, 1998.

Oldenburg J, Aparicio J, Beyer J, et al; On behalf of SWENOTECA (Swedish Norwegian Testicular Cancer group), the Italian Germ Cell Cancer Group (IGG), Spanish Germ Cell Cancer Group (SGCCG): Personalizing, not patronizing: the case for patient autonomy by unbiased presentation of management options in stage I testicular cancer, *Ann Oncol* 26:833–838, 2015.

Oliver RT, Mead GM, Rustin GJ, et al: Randomized trial of carboplatin versus radiotherapy for stage I seminoma: mature results on relapse and contralateral testis cancer rates in MRC TE19/EORTC 30982 study (ISRCTN27163214), *J Clin Oncol* 29:957–962, 2011.

Rabbani F, Farivar-Mohseni H, Leon A, et al: Clinical outcome after retroperitoneal lymphadenectomy of patients with pure testicular teratoma, *Urology* 62:1092–1096, 2003.

Spiess PE, Kassouf W, Brown GA, et al: Surgical management of growing teratoma syndrome: the M. D. Anderson cancer center experience, *J Urol* 177:1330–1334, discussion 34, 2007.

Stephenson A, Eggener SE, Bass EB, et al: Diagnosis and treatment of early stage testicular cancer: AUA guideline, *J Urol* 202:272–281, 2019.

Stephenson AJ, Bosl GJ, Motzer RJ, et al: Retroperitoneal lymph node dissection for nonseminomatous germ cell testicular cancer: impact of patient selection factors on outcome, *J Clin Oncol* 23:2781–2788, 2005.

Trabert B, Chen J, Devesa SS, et al: International patterns and trends in testicular cancer incidence, overall and by histologic subtype, 1973-2007, *Andrology* 3:4–12, 2015.

Travis LB, Fossa SD, Schonfeld SJ, et al: Second cancers among 40,576 testicular cancer patients: focus on long-term survivors, *J Natl Cancer Inst* 97:1354–1365, 2005.

Treglia G, Sadeghi R, Annunziata S, et al: Diagnostic performance of fluorine-18-fluorodeoxyglucose positron emission tomography in the postchemotherapy management of patients with seminoma: systematic review and meta-analysis, *Biomed Res Int* 2014:852681, 2014.

Verrill C, Yilmaz A, Srigley JR, et al; Members of the International Society of Urological Pathology Testicular Tumor Panel: Reporting and staging of testicular germ cell tumors: the International Society of Urological Pathology (ISUP) testicular cancer consultation conference recommendations, *Am J Surg Pathol* 41:e22–e32, 2017.

Williamson SR, Delahunt B, Magi-Galluzzi C, et al; Members of the ISUP Testicular Tumour Panel: The World Health Organization 2016 classification of testicular germ cell tumours: a review and update from the International Society of Urological Pathology Testis Consultation Panel, *Histopathology* 70:335–346, 2017.

REFERENCES

The complete reference list is available online at ExpertConsult.com.

77
Surgery of Testicular Tumors
Stephen Riggs, MD, Kris Gaston, MD, and Peter E. Clark, MD

Testicular cancer is a model of success in the treatment of solid tumor malignancies. It is highly chemosensitive in addition to being one of the most surgically curable malignancies. In the modern era, surveillance after orchiectomy for clinical stage I non-seminomatous germ cell tumor (NSGCT) results in cure rates of up to 88% (Daugaar et al., 2014). Patients with low volume pathologic stage II NSCGCT enjoy a 60% to 80% disease-free survival with primary retroperitoneal lymph node dissection (RPLND) alone (Donohue et al., 1993; Stephenson et al., 2007). Even those patients deemed to have refractory disease after primary chemotherapy can achieve durable long-term cure rates of around 45% with various salvage chemotherapy regimens (Petrelli et al., 2017). What is paramount in the treatment of this disease is an active collaboration and multimodal approach that includes surgeons, medical personnel, and radiation oncologists. In this chapter, we describe the management and decision-making process, operative techniques, and outcomes for testicular cancer surgery. This chapter should provide the urologist with a foundation regarding the role of surgery in primary and advanced testicular cancer from orchiectomy, to primary or post-chemotherapy RPLND (PC-RPLND).

MANAGEMENT OF TESTIS MASS

History and Physical Examination, Ultrasonography, and Preorchiectomy Evaluation

Any man with a testicular mass should undergo a prompt and complete evaluation, particularly younger men in the age group most susceptible to testicular cancer. The critical components to that evaluation include a detailed history focused particularly on the growth rate of the lesion and any associated symptoms, a careful physical examination, ultrasound of the scrotal contents, and appropriate serologic studies (Bosl et al., 1981; Honig et al., 1994; Jacobsen et al., 2000; Petersen et al., 1999; Richie, 1993; Robson et al., 1965; Sandeman, 1979; Simon et al., 2001; Thornhill et al., 1987). Because testis cancer is often rapidly progressive, timely diagnosis and management is critical to minimizing the intensity and morbidity of therapy necessary to effect a cure (Chapple et al., 2004; Gascoigne et al., 1999; Oliver, 1985; Moul, 2007; Post and Belis, 1980). The physical examination should include examination of the supraclavicular lymph nodes, the breasts, abdomen, and, in particular, focus on the scrotal contents and characterization of the mass. Although an ultrasound of the testicles is not mandatory, it can more fully characterize the mass and radiographically document its laterality (Goddi et al., 2012; Horstman et al., 1992; Shah et al., 2010). Perhaps the most important role for ultrasound, however, is to document the characteristics of the contralateral testicle, because the incidence of bilateral synchronous testicular masses is approximately 1% of patients (Bokemeyer et al., 1993; Che et al., 2002: Coogan et al., 1998; Fossa et al., 2005; Hentrich et al., 2005; Holzbeierlein et al., 2003; Pamenter et al., 2003). Serum tumor markers should be obtained because these can further bolster the diagnosis of a germ cell tumor, provide important staging information, and will serve as a baseline for follow-up after orchiectomy. Placement of a testicular prosthesis can be considered and should be discussed in advance of surgery (Clifford et al., 2018; Dieckmann et al., 2015; Yossepowitch et al., 2011).

Radical Orchiectomy

In patients in whom a testicular malignancy is suspected, radical orchiectomy is the diagnostic and therapeutic treatment of choice. The approach is via an inguinal incision, allowing for early control of the spermatic cord and complete removal of the ipsilateral testis, epididymis, and spermatic cord to the level of the internal inguinal ring.

Technique

After adequate anesthesia, the patient is positioned supine on the operating room table. Skin preparation should include at a minimum the abdomen to a level cranial to the umbilicus, inferiorly to the mid-thigh bilaterally, and the genitalia posteriorly to the level of the perineum. The patient should be sterilely draped so that the scrotum, ipsilateral anterior superior iliac spine, and pubic tubercle are all adequately exposed. Examination under anesthesia can typically locate the external inguinal ring, which facilitates identification of the medial-most aspect of the inguinal canal.

A 3- to 5-cm incision is made in a transverse orientation over the inguinal canal following Langer lines. This size incision is typically adequate for delivery of the mass; however, if this is inadequate, the incision can be extended over the scrotum. This can be done in a hockey-stick fashion, or the original incision can be rotated in a more caudally directed orientation aiming toward the scrotum from the outset. The subcutaneous tissues are now separated, exposing the external oblique fascia and external inguinal ring. The external oblique fascia is now incised along the course of the inguinal canal for approximately 4 cm. If needed, self-retaining instruments such as a Weitlaner or Gelpi forceps can be used to aid with exposure. Once the fascia is incised, the ilioinguinal nerve should be prospectively identified and preserved as it courses over the anterior aspect of the spermatic cord within the inguinal canal. Once the nerve is displaced, the spermatic cord can be mobilized at approximately the level of the pubic tubercle and encircled with a Penrose drain. The external spermatic fascia and cremasteric fibers that surround the spermatic cord should be divided and traction applied to deliver the testicle/testicular mass superiorly into the incision. This can be facilitated by upward pressure on the ipsilateral hemiscrotum. With the testicle/testicular mass delivered into the operative field the gubernaculum is divided and the spermatic cord dissected superiorly to the level of the peritoneal reflection at the internal inguinal ring. The vas deferens should be separated from the remainder of the gonadal vessels at this level, and both structures should be ligated and divided separately. Nonabsorbable sutures are preferred for ligation with a 1- to 2-cm suture tail to facilitate later identification and excision of the gonadal vessel stump during RPLND. Some surgeons make a specific effort to drop the ligated stump of the spermatic cord into the preperitoneal space deep to the internal inguinal ring to facilitate subsequent dissection at the time of RPLND. Separating the vas deferens from the remaining gonadal vessels is also helpful in this regard because the vas deferens does not have to be removed at the time of RPLND.

After the spermatic cord has been divided, the wound is irrigated and carefully inspected for hemostasis. The ilioinguinal nerve should be positioned safely in the bed of the inguinal canal and external oblique aponeurosis then reapproximated. The subcutaneous tissues should be closed in one to two layers followed by skin closure. Sterile dressings are then applied and often a scrotal support with fluff dressings is added, which aids in reducing scrotal swelling and hematoma formation for the first 2 to 3 days postoperatively.

Partial Orchiectomy

With the success of therapy for testis cancer and the high probability of long-term survival there has been increasing focus on minimizing long-term treatment related side effects while not compromising treatment efficacy (Carmignani et al., 2004; Haas et al., 1986; Jacobsen et al., 1981; Klein et al., 1985; Kressel et al., 1988; Robertson, 1995; Skakkebaek, 1975). **In highly select patients, partial orchiectomy can be considered in cases in which the tumor is polar, measures 2 cm or less, and in which the contralateral testicle is compromised or absent.** If the malignant nature of a testicular mass is not clear, an inguinal exploration with early control of the spermatic cord and excisional biopsy with or without frozen section analysis can be performed. However, this should only be considered in patients for whom the risks of being anorchic outweigh the risks of increased local tumor recurrence. In general, for patients with a normal contralateral testicle attempts at elective testis-sparing surgery should not be made.

Technique

The initial approach to a partial orchiectomy is identical to a radical operation. Once the testicle/testicular mass is delivered into the operative field, the testicle should be isolated from the wound with sterile towels. Intraoperative ultrasonography can be used if necessary to localize the mass. The potential need for hypothermia has been raised by some investigators but can likely be omitted as long as resection times are minimized to less than 30 minutes (Giannarini et al., 2010). After the mass is localized, the tunica albuginea is sharply incised with a scalpel. The approach will vary depending on the mass's location. A vertical incision along the long axis of the testicle is generally preferred for an approach from the ventral midline, whereas incisions medial or lateral to the ventral midline ideally should be oriented horizontally, minimizing injury to the segmental arteries that course just deep to the tunica albuginea.

The mass should then be excised, ideally including a small rim of normal seminiferous tubules to facilitate a negative surgical margin. There is some debate on how to manage the remnant testicle if a germ cell tumor (GCT) is confirmed and the surrounding parenchyma demonstrates intratubular germ cell neoplasia. Many advocate proceeding to radical orchiectomy with these findings, whereas others would recommend only routine adjuvant radiation therapy to the remnant testicle to reduce the risk of local recurrence. The individual surgeon's assessment of this risk will in part dictate whether a frozen section analysis is done to direct whether to preserve the testicle. If the testicle is preserved, then the tunica albuginea is closed with absorbable sutures and the testicle fixed in the dependent aspect of the scrotum at three points, typically including the gubernaculum and scrotal septum.

Traditionally patients who underwent partial orchiectomy for a histologically confirmed GCT underwent 18 to 20 Gy of adjuvant radiotherapy to reduce the risk of local tumor recurrence (Giannarini et al., 2010; Heidenreich et al., 2001; Krege et al., 2008). Thus in patients with a solitary testicle, the main benefit of organ sparing was the preservation of Leydig cell function because spermatogenesis will be permanently compromised. More recently, however, a small series of 27 men who underwent partial orchiectomy, 17 (63%) of which were shown to have GCT, suggested that select patients can be observed with a low risk of recurrence, even in the face of carcinoma in situ (Lawrentschuk et al., 2011). Thus it may be that, in the future, more patients with partial orchiectomy for GCT may be observed. This is an area that requires more investigation. **What is not debated is that any patient who develops ipsilateral local recurrence of GCT should undergo completion radical orchiectomy regardless of prior adjuvant therapy or residual testicular function.**

Delayed Orchiectomy

The majority of cases of testicular cancer are diagnosed via radical orchiectomy. **However, a minority of cases may present with diffuse metastatic and/or symptomatic GCT that requires early initiation of systemic chemotherapy** (Ondrus et al., 2001). In these circumstances, diagnosis may be pursued via biopsy of a metastatic site or even made presumptively based on the clinical features with or without serologic studies. For such cases, a delayed radical orchiectomy is recommended for all patients regardless of response to therapy in the retroperitoneum or elsewhere resulting from the discordant response rates to chemotherapy between the testis and other sites (Leibovitch et al., 1996; Miller et al., 2013; Ondrus et al., 2001; Simmonds et al. 1995; Snow et al., 1983).

The role of delayed orchiectomy for patients with an apparent retroperitoneal/extragonadal primary GCT is more controversial. Studies have biopsied the testicle in such patients and demonstrated intratubular germ cell neoplasia in up to 42% (Daugaard et al., 1992). If such patients are observed after chemotherapy, there is approximately a 5% rate of metachronous testicular cancer during follow-up (Hartmann et al., 2001). **For patients in whom the retroperitoneal disease lateralizes with a distribution strongly suggestive of a testicular primary, a radical orchiectomy on that side has been advocated.** This is based at least in part on a small cohort series of patients with presumed extragonadal GCT who underwent delayed orchiectomy after completing chemotherapy (Brown et al., 2008); 71% of the specimens demonstrated histologic evidence of teratoma or necrotic tissue suggestive of a "burned-out primary" or a complete response to therapy. Should observation be chosen for patients with an apparent extragonadal GCT, follow-up should include careful, regular monthly testicular self-examination and regular practitioner physical examination.

Postorchiectomy Evaluation

After orchiectomy, the clinical stage is determined based on the pathologic findings combined with radiographic and serologic studies. Typically contrast-enhanced computed tomography (CT) with intravenous and oral contrast is used to image the retroperitoneum, although in some cases magnetic resonance imaging (MRI) can be an alternative approach. In general, neither fluorodeoxyglucose-labeled positron emission tomography (PET) nor lymphoangiography play an important role in the initial diagnosis and staging of GCTs. Assessment of serum tumor markers (α-fetoprotein, beta human chorionic gonadotropin, and lactate dehydrogenase) should be repeated after surgery, and the trend in values also aids in guiding subsequent management.

KEY POINTS: MANAGEMENT OF THE TESTIS MASS

- Radical orchiectomy, including early control of the spermatic cord and complete removal of the ipsilateral testis, epididymis, and spermatic cord to the level of the internal inguinal ring, is the diagnostic and therapeutic treatment of choice in patients in whom a testicular malignancy is suspected.
- In highly select patients, partial orchiectomy can be considered in cases in which the tumor is polar, measures 2 cm or less, and in which the contralateral testicle is compromised or absent.
- For the rare patient with diffuse metastatic and/or symptomatic GCT requiring early initiation of systemic chemotherapy, diagnosis may be pursued via biopsy of a metastatic site or even made presumptively based on the clinical features and/or serologic studies. For such cases, a delayed radical orchiectomy is recommended for all patients regardless of response to therapy in the retroperitoneum.

RETROPERITONEAL LYMPH NODE DISSECTION

Testicular cancer has a predilection for spread to the retroperitoneal lymph nodes in a predictable fashion. The landing sites for right- or left-sided primary tumors are illustrated in Fig. 77.1 (Beveridge et al., 2016; Donohue et al., 1982; Ray et al., 1974; Weissbach and Boedefeld, 1987). RPLND is an important part of the management of testicular tumors in several clinical settings, which are discussed across this chapter. However, the technical aspects of the surgery are very similar no matter what the disease state. The following is a list of terms used to describe RPLND based on the timing and whether primary systemic therapy has been used.

- Primary RPLND: After orchiectomy for high-risk clinical stage (CS) 1 or low-volume CS II (N1) NSGCT with normal STMs
- PC-RPLND: Refers to an RPLND performed after induction chemotherapy. Although there remains some debate (see later discussion), this is often performed when there is a residual mass > 1 cm in the retroperitoneum and the STMs post-chemotherapy are normal.
- Salvage PC-RPLND: RPLND performed after both induction and salvage chemotherapy
- Desperation PC-RPLND: RPLND performed after chemotherapy where there is elevated STMs
- Reoperative RPLND: RPLND performed after a prior RPLND
- Resection of late relapse: RPLND performed for relapse of disease > 24 months after a complete response (CR) from primary chemotherapy

Preoperative Planning

The urologic surgeon must review the patient's abdominal CT scan for the location of any retroperitoneal (RP) masses as well as delineating the patient's RP anatomy (e.g., duplicated renal vessels). Careful review of the films helps avoid unplanned intraoperative consultation

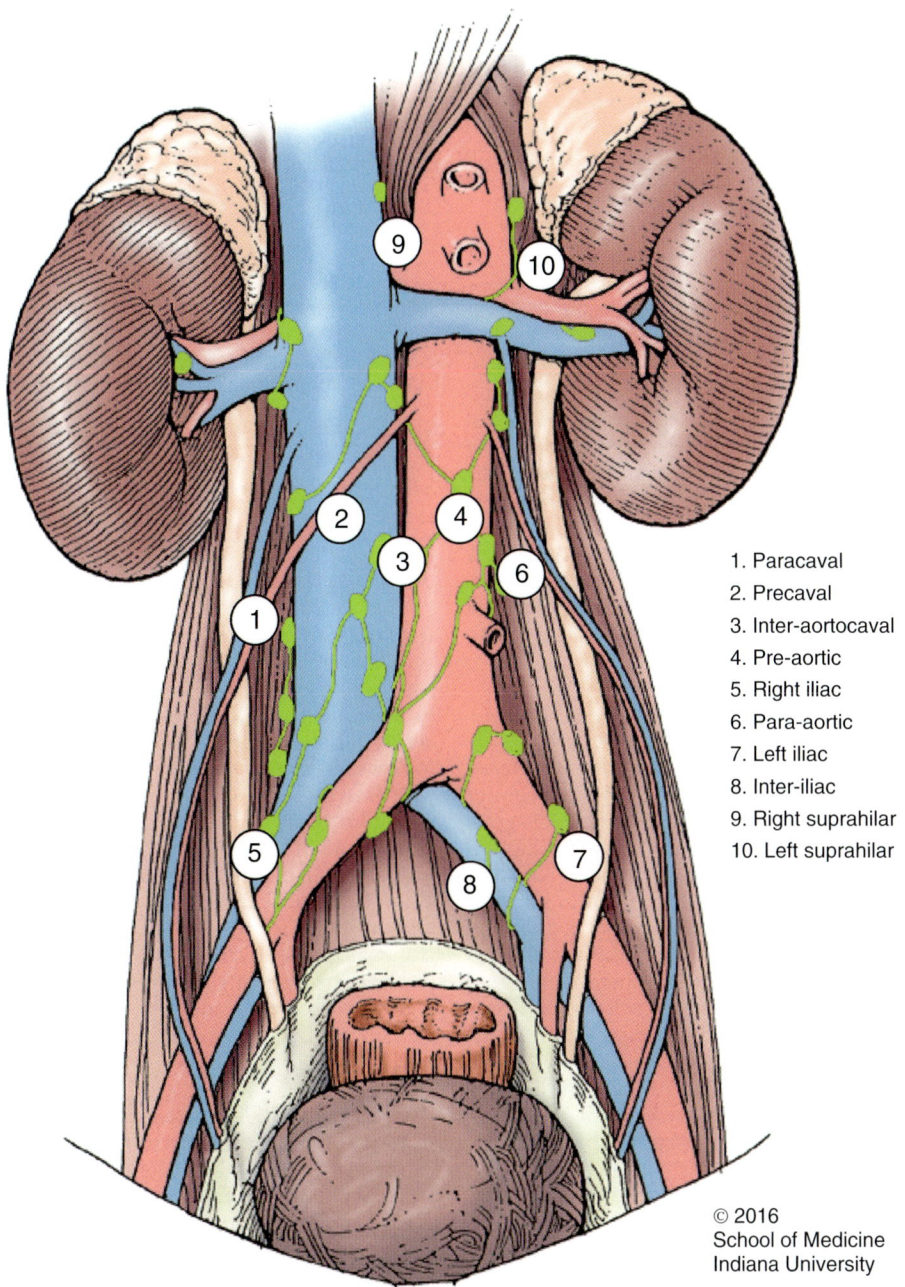

1. Paracaval
2. Precaval
3. Inter-aortocaval
4. Pre-aortic
5. Right iliac
6. Para-aortic
7. Left iliac
8. Inter-iliac
9. Right suprahilar
10. Left suprahilar

© 2016
School of Medicine
Indiana University

Fig. 77.1. Retroperitoneal lymph node regions. (Copyright 2016 Section of Medical Illustration in the Office of Visual Media at the Indiana University School of Medicine. Published by Elsevier Inc. All rights reserved.)

of other surgical services. We prefer a scan within 6 weeks of surgery and STMs within 7 to 10 days. No preoperative bowel preparation is required. Preoperative sperm banking should be offered and recommended to all patients who desire future paternity. Pulmonary toxicity occurs in approximately 11% of patients who received first-line chemotherapy with bleomycin as compared with 1.7% in those receiving non–bleomycin-based regimens. In addition, the probability of grade 3 or grade 4 toxicity is fivefold higher for those receiving bleomycin (Necchi et al., 2017). **Therefore special attention should be given to these patients. Pulmonary function tests should be obtained preoperatively, and if any deficits are noted, these patients should be referred to a pulmonologist for evaluation before proceeding to surgery. Equally as important, the anesthesia team should be alerted, and this should clearly be communicated to all personnel for pre-, intra-, and postoperative management.** Specific recommendations for intraoperative management include (1) low fraction of inspired oxygen (FiO_2) and (2) conservative fluid replacement. We have found that there is no substitute for direct communication at the time of the surgical time-out to ensure the surgical plan and nuances are understood by all who are involved in the operative team.

Preoperative chest CT should be performed in all patients with prior lung lesions as well as those planning to undergo simultaneous lung resection. In addition, identification of inferior vena cava (IVC) thrombus is important because total occlusion can be managed with resection of the IVC (Beck and Lalka, 1998) and incomplete occlusion with allograft reconstruction as needed.

Surgical Technique

For an open RPLND the patient is placed in the supine position with the arms in a T position slightly below a 90-degree angle. An orogastric tube is almost always adequate for gastric decompression. A midline incision is carried from the level of the xyphoid to a couple of centimeters below the umbilicus. For the more traditional intraperitoneal approach, the peritoneal cavity is entered sharply and the round ligament is divided, and the falciform toward the superior IVC is released to avoid hepatic injury from retraction. More recently an extraperitoneal approach for select patients has been advocated (Kim et al., 2012; Syan-Bhanvadia et al., 2017). For this approach, a similar incision is used with care taken to release the peritoneum from the fascia starting at the infraumbilical portion of the incision. Proponents of the latter approach suggest it offers length of stay (LOS) and earlier return of bowel function.

Exposure of the Retroperitoneum

Once the peritoneum is entered, a self-retaining retractor is placed to aid exposure. An incision is started from the tip of the cecum to the medial aspect of the inferior mesenteric vein (Fig. 77.2, *green dotted line*). If full mobilization of the bowels is desired, followed by placement of the bowels on the chest, then the peritoneal reflection (white line of Toldt) is incised up the ascending colon to the level of the foramen of Winslow (see Fig. 77.2, *right purple dotted line*). In cases with large left-sided tumors, the inferior mesenteric vein can be divided to aid in exposure of the left retroperitoneum (see Fig. 77.2, *left purple dotted line*). If a modified left sided approach is being performed, then the peritoneal reflection (white line of Toldt) of the descending colon is incised.

The plane between the mesentery and retroperitoneal fat is developed. Identification of the plane may be facilitated by identification of the gonadal vein and ureter and staying anterior to these structures. The duodenum and inferior surface of the pancreas are freed from the anterior surface of the renal vessels, IVC, and aorta. Liberal use of clips in this area helps reduce the chance of a postoperative chylous leak.

Split and Roll Technique (Video 77.1)

We prefer to start over the left renal vein or vena cava at this level in a top-down approach. The cephalad end of the lymphatics at the

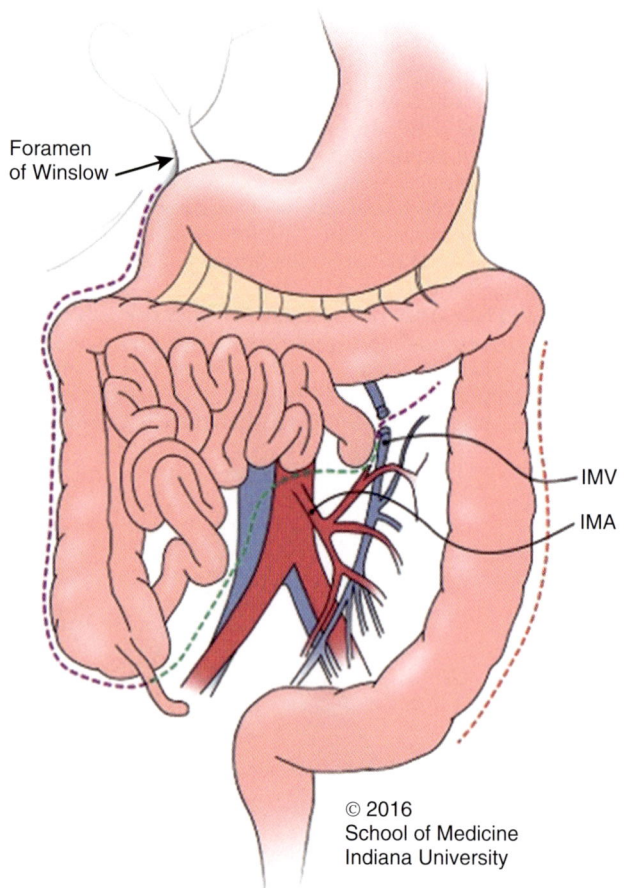

Fig. 77.2. Exposure of the retroperitoneum. *IMA*, Inferior mesenteric artery; *IMV*, inferior mesenteric vein. (Copyright 2016 Section of Medical Illustration in the Office of Visual Media at the Indiana University School of Medicine. Published by Elsevier Inc. All rights reserved.)

level of the renal veins should be ligated. Understanding retroperitoneal anatomy and landmarks is crucial, and although we tend to start on the aorta, the size of the mass and ease of dissection often dictates the flow of the case. If the surgeon does come down the aorta, the postganglionic sympathetic nerves should be accounted for on the anterior surface of the aorta in addition to the superior hypogastric plexus. One advantage of starting on the aorta may be the ability to use the postganglionic sympathetic nerves emanating from the right side to identify the superior hypogastric plexus. The goal is to identify this plexus and avoid injury. The split is started at the 12 o'clock position on the aorta just below the left renal vein, and this plane is continued caudally to identify the IMA (Fig. 77.3). In nerve-sparing techniques it is vitally important to identify and preserve the postganglionic nerves at the level of IMA (or sooner) before proceeding caudally.

Left Para-Aortic Packet

Dissection of the left para-aortic lymphatic packet in a template dissection is facilitated by rolling the descending colon medially (through division of the white line of Toldt). In a bilateral dissection with the small bowels pushed cephalad or placed on the chest, the dissection moves through the mesenteric root. The left gonadal vein is divided, where it crosses the ureter or it is moved medially. A small retractor can be used to pull the ureter laterally to help avoid injury. The anterior split along the aorta and iliac vessels proceeds caudally to the crossing of the ureter, which will include about one-half of the left common iliac artery. The tissue is then rolled laterally, and the lumbar arteries up to the renal hilum are doubly

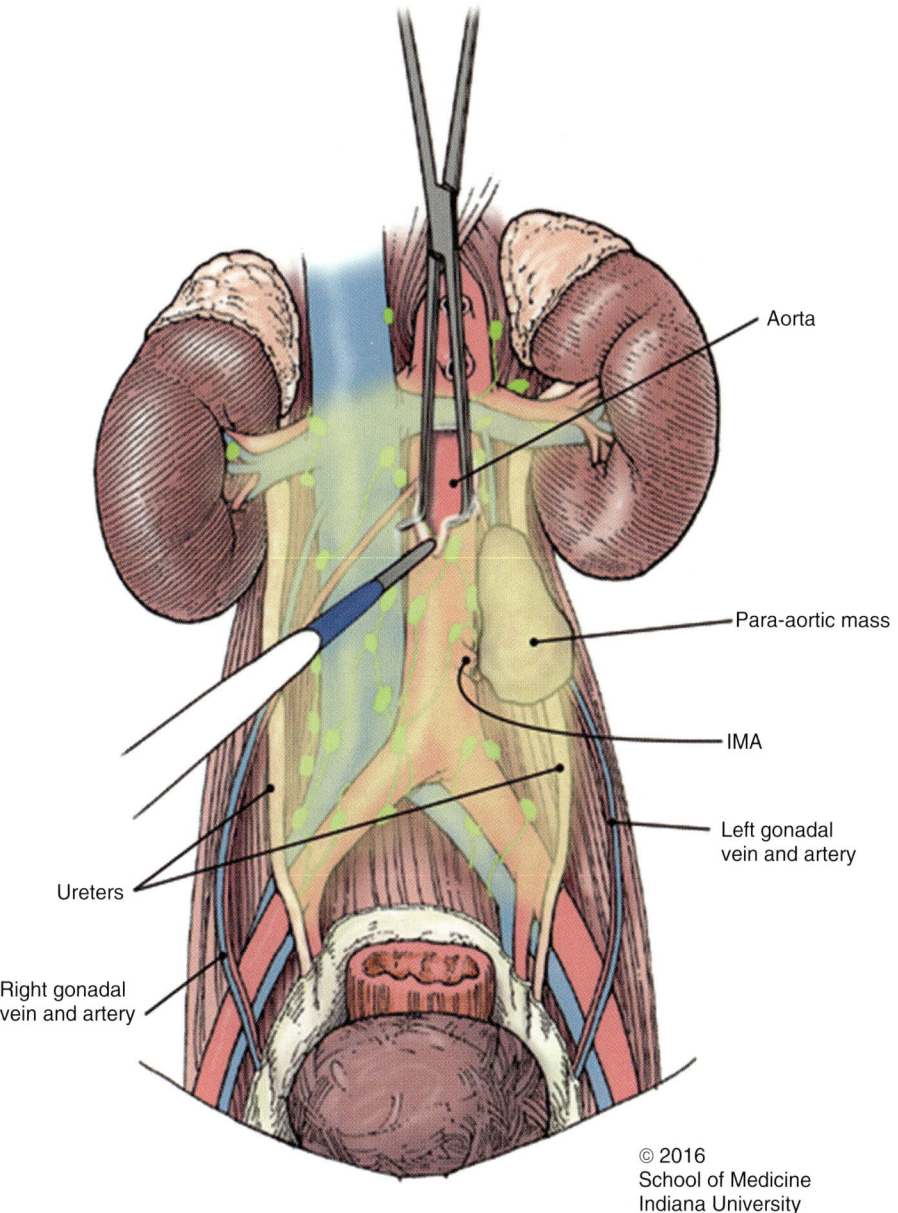

Fig. 77.3. The split-and-roll technique. *IMA*, Inferior mesenteric artery. (Copyright 2016 Section of Medical Illustration in the Office of Visual Media at the Indiana University School of Medicine. Published by Elsevier Inc. All rights reserved.)

ligated. There are usually three pairs of lumbar arteries in equal distance from the hilum to the common iliac vessels. Importantly, the second pair usually comes off at the level of the IMA, thus acting as a landmark to facilitate localization (Beveridge et al., 2016).

Interaortocaval Packet

In a right-sided nerve-sparing procedure, the next step is a split-and-roll on the anterior surface of the IVC including ligation of the gonadal vein. If a non–nerve-sparing procedure is performed and if one starts on the aorta first, then the medial side of the aorta can be controlled before proceeding to the IVC side of the dissection. Dissection should proceed caudally along the IVC until the bifurcation of the iliac vessels and then the right common iliac artery is followed up until the crossing of the right ureter is reached. As with the left side, the gonadal vein on the right can be ligated at the level of its crossing of the ureter and the ureter placed gently in a retractor and held laterally to reduce risk of injury. Dissection should now be performed with the goal of controlling the medial and lateral lumbar veins, which are variable in number and location. A clear knowledge of the anatomy during this portion is critical to safety and efficiency as well as to the ability to spare the nerves. Usually there are two or three lumbar veins. A superior right lumbar vein should be looked for just below or posterior to the renal veins. A common lumbar vein is usually centrally located (between superior and inferior lumbar veins) and is the largest tributary. It can often cross under the aorta to the contralateral side, so it may require additional para-aortic ligation. Equally important is the spatial relationship of the IMA, common lumbar vein, and postganglionic sympathetic nerves. The common lumbar vein can usually be found adjacent to the level of the IMA, and the postganglionic parasympathetic nerve (second-infrarenal lumbar splanchnic nerve) usually crosses to the anterior surface of the aorta at this level. It is important therefore that this is prospectively identified and carefully dissected away in a nerve-sparing procedure (Beveridge et al., 2016).

After control of the medial aspect of the IVC, the medial aspect of the aorta is controlled and the tissue is rotated medially in the interaortocaval space. This requires identification and ligation of the

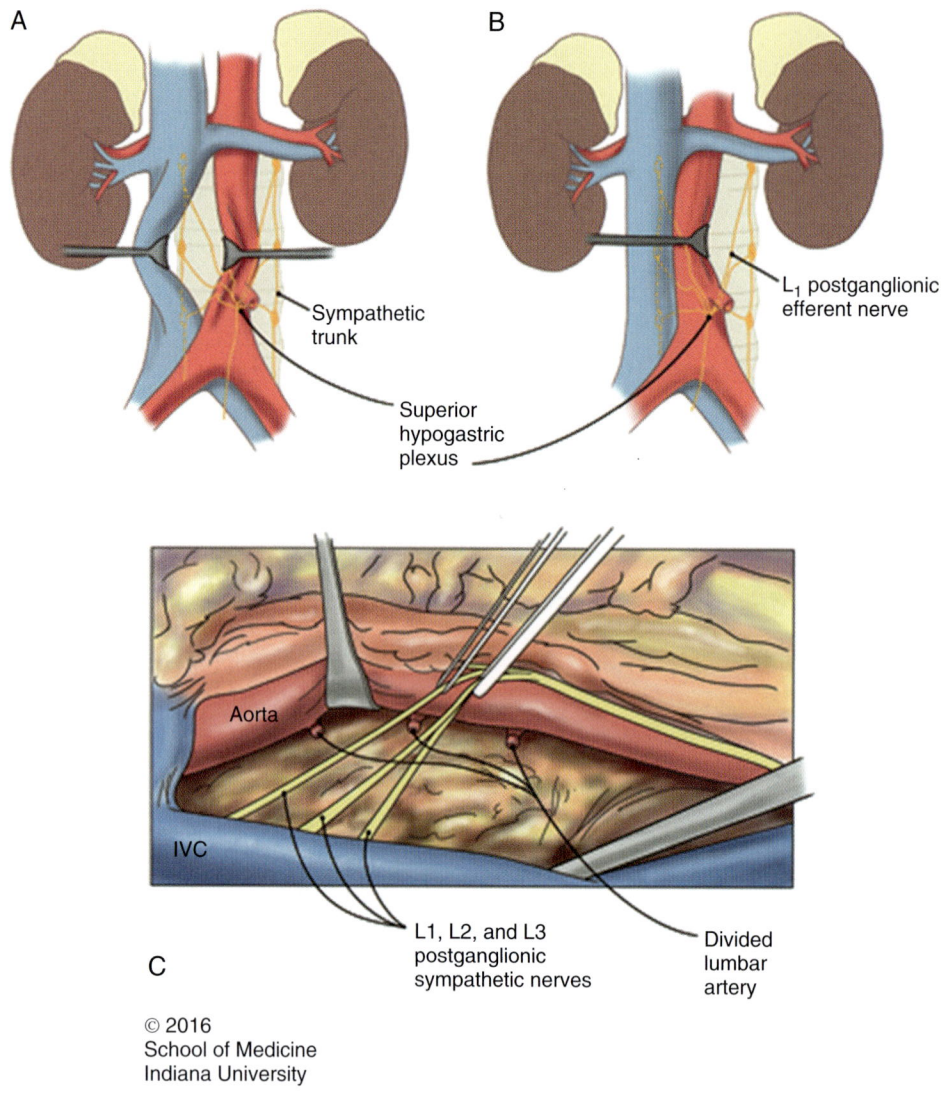

Fig. 77.4. Nerve-sparing technique. (A) Location of right-sided postganglionic sympathetic nerves. (B) Location of left-sided postganglionic sympathetic nerves. (C) Right-sided nerve-sparing technique with ligated lumbar arteries. *IVC,* Inferior vena cava. (Copyright 2016 Section of Medical Illustration in the Office of Visual Media at the Indiana University School of Medicine. Published by Elsevier Inc. All rights reserved.)

three medial lumbar arteries (Fig. 77.4). At this point the anterior and lateral attachments of the desired lymph node packet are fully released. The tissue is now ready to be pulled caudal by release of the lymphatics toward the crus of the diaphragm and anterior spinous ligament in the interaortocaval space at the level of the right renal artery and vein. Care should be taken to ligate the cephalad level of the lymphatics at this point to prevent a postoperative chylous leak. The surgery continues to proceed caudally, exposing the anterior spinous ligament to the level of the left common iliac vein. The surgeon must pay attention to entry and re-entry of lumbar vessels into the body wall as well as clear identification of the right renal artery and any accessory renal arteries.

Right Paracaval Packet

The right paracaval packet is often the smallest and easiest to remove. If a bilateral dissection is performed in a split and roll maneuver, it is often fruitful to release the packet at the level of the right renal artery to allow it to begin passing medially underneath the vena cava en-bloc with the interaortocaval packet. The packet often tapers down to essentially nothing at the level of the right renal vessels. The packet is then released from the psoas muscle, avoiding injury to the genitofemoral nerve to the level of the right common iliac vessel and ureteral crossing. The urologist must take care to identify the right parasympathetic trunk that usually sits posterior and lateral to the IVC. It is often mistaken for lymphatic tissue or vessels but should be preserved, particularly in a nerve-sparing RPLND.

Gonadal Vein

To remove the residual gonadal vein to the previously removed testicle, the peritoneum overlying it should be incised. In addition, the ureter (which is often previously freed) should be swept off from its posterior location. A left gonadal vein that is identified through the mesentery must be passed under the sigmoid before moving toward the inguinal canal. After mobilization of either vein, gentle traction facilitates resection down to the internal ring, where the suture from the previous orchiectomy should be encountered.

Nerve Sparing

The anatomy of the four postganglionic efferent sympathetic fibers (L1 through L4) involved in antegrade ejaculation are variable. From a surgical perspective some of the nerve fibers are often fused, creating

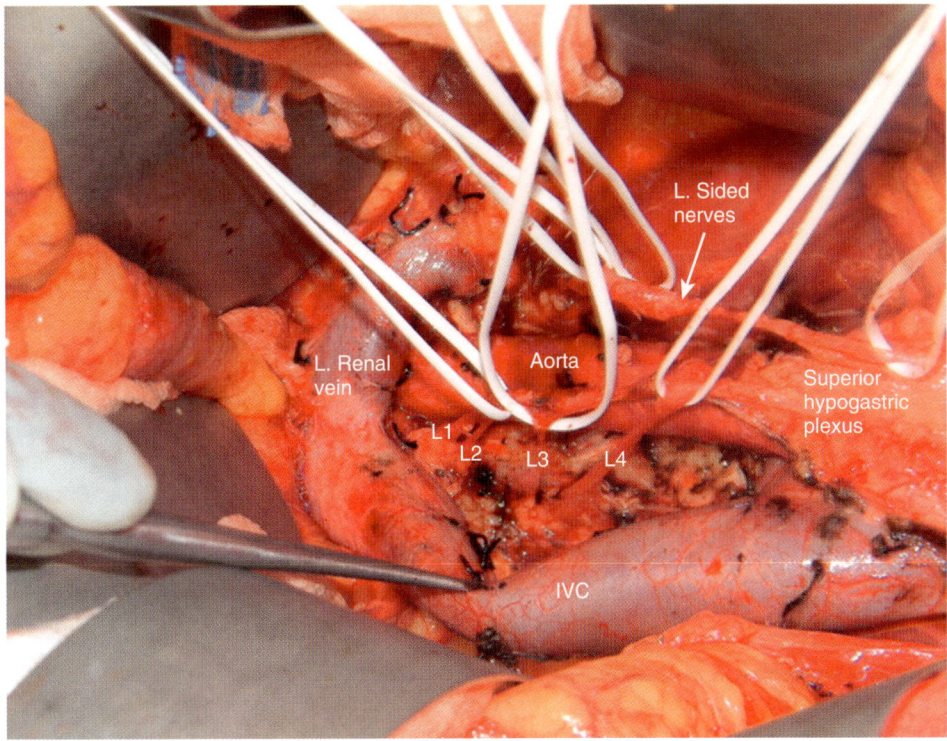

Fig. 77.5. Bilateral nerve-sparing technique. *IVC*, Inferior vena cava; *L.*, left; *L1 through L4*, right-sided postganglionic sympathetic nerves.

essentially three efferent fibers exiting the right sympathetic chain underneath the IVC as well as three para-aortic fibers exiting the left parasympathetic chain. Both course toward and along the anterior surface of the aorta (Fig. 77.5).

The left-sided postganglionic nerves can be identified at the lateral border of the aorta, emanating from underneath the left renal vein, and around the left common iliac artery. The relationship of the nerves posterior to the left renal vein and first lumbar artery are important. In addition, the more inferior nerves usually are located around the left gonadal artery and move toward the IMA (Beveridge et al., 2016). Sharp or blunt dissection helps to sweep the tissue away from these nerves as they course anteriorly on the aorta toward the hypogastric plexus. Fibers can be tagged with vessel loops to facilitate dissection if desired.

Right-sided postganglionic nerve fibers are best identified during dissection of the precaval tissue and medial isolation of the lumbar veins. The postganglionic fibers course from beneath the IVC obliquely toward the superior hypogastric plexus (see Figs. 77.4A and 77.5). Sharp and blunt dissection can facilitate separation from the lymph node packet. Attention should be given to the right superior lumbar vein because the nerve often courses beside this as well as the common lumbar trunk. Care must be taken when ligating these vessels to avoid concomitant injury to the right-sided nerves (Beveridge et al., 2016).

Once all fibers have been isolated the lymph node packet must be sequentially passed around the web of postganglionic fibers as it is released from the body wall. Care must be taken during this portion of the procedure to avoid inadvertent injury.

Closure and Postoperative Care

After completion of the RPLND, the resection bed should be inspected for any residual lymphatic tissue, lymph leak, and hemostasis. Any lymph leaks that are encountered can be clipped or suture ligated with fine suture. Irrigation of the wound with warm irrigation is performed to facilitate identification of any bleeding vessels in spasm. Some advocate reapproximation of the posterior parietal peritoneum to prevent bowel adhesion to the great vessels and retroperitoneum. Consideration can also be given to reapproximation of the root of the mesentery that some feel may decrease the risk of volvulus. No matter how the urologist deals with the peritoneum and root of the mesentery, the bowel should be inspected for inadvertent injury in addition to inspection of the liver, stomach, and pancreas.

We do not routinely leave a surgical drain, but it should be considered in large-volume retroperitoneal, retrocrural, or bowel resection. In these cases, because of the propensity for large-volume third-spacing, a nonsuction drain is left in place and removed when the output has remained serous and less than 100 mL/24 hours on a regular diet.

In the absence of complicating factors, the patients are left without a nasogastric tube and given clear liquids beginning the evening of surgery. The patients are advanced as tolerated to regular low-fat diet through postoperative days 1 and 2. Transition to oral narcotics and use of non-narcotic analgesia (Toradol, Tylenol, gabapentin) is aggressively pursued to reduce narcotic use and ileus. Ambulation is mandatory day 1 along with significant time spent out of bed in a chair. Patients are typically discharged 3 to 5 days after surgery with a target discharge of day 3 depending on their ability to tolerate oral intake and manage their pain. Of course, with any surgery, patients with larger, more complex surgery tend to have a protracted course, and individualization of the postoperative care plan should always trump enhanced any standardized postoperative recovery algorithm.

AUXILIARY PROCEDURES

Auxiliary procedures typically occur in the post-chemotherapy setting and should rarely be required during primary RPLND. The incidence of auxiliary procedures at the time of PC-RPLND ranges from 23% to 45% in the literature (Beck et al., 2009; Heidenreich et al., 2009; Winter et al., 2012). **The most common auxiliary procedure is nephrectomy followed by vascular interventions. The larger the volume of the residual retroperitoneal mass, the greater the need for possible auxiliary procedures.**

TABLE 77.1 Risk Factors and Indications for Nephrectomy at Postchemotherapy Retroperitoneal Lymph Node Dissection[a]

STUDY	PATIENTS UNDERGOING NX, N (INCIDENCE %)	TIME PERIOD	INDICATIONS/RISK FACTORS
Macleod et al., 2016	20 (10)	2007–2012	Older age Year of surgery Comorbidities
Cary et al., 2013	265 (14.8)	1980–1997	RP mass size Year of surgery Primary tumor site Salvage chemotherapy Elevated markers
Djaladat et al., 2012	12 (14.1)	2004–2010	Left-sided hilar mass
Heidenreich et al., 2009	7 (4.6)	1999–2007	Encasement of renal vessels/ureter
Stephenson, 2006	32 (5)	1989–2002	Salvage RPLND Desperation RPLND Redo RPLND Late relapse
Nash et al., 1998	162 (19)	1974–1994	Involvement of renal structures Venous thrombus Poor renal function Combination of above

[a]Not all studies performed formal statistical analyses for predictive risk factors because of small sample size.
Nx, Nephrectomy; *RP*, retroperitoneal; *RPLND*, retroperitoneal lymph node dissection.

Nephrectomy

Nephrectomy is the most common auxiliary procedure, ranging from 5% to 31% (Table 77.1). Renal salvage can be an important issue in advanced RPLND cases because of the primary lymphatic drainage of the testes being in the location of the great vessels near the renal hilum. **Left-sided metastatic testes cancer cases particularly put the left kidney at risk because of its primary lymphatic drainage being at the para-aortic/left renal hilum.** Nephrectomy may have a particularly higher risk in settings such as salvage RPLND, desperation RPLND, and reoperative RPLND. The incidence of concomitant nephrectomy in the setting of retroperitoneal node dissection has been decreasing over the last 3 decades. According to a database review at Indiana University from 1980 to 2007, the overall incidence of nephrectomy was 14.8% (Cary et al., 2013). In this review the authors stratified their data finding the incidence from 1980 to 1988 was 17%, 1989 to 1997 was 19%, 1998 to 2002 was 14%, and 2002 to 2007 was 8%. Histologic stratification of the results of RPLND requiring nephrectomy found it was needed in 10% of cases with fibrosis, 15% with teratoma, and 20% for cases with residual viable cancer. Overall the authors found the strongest predictor of nephrectomy was a residual post-chemotherapy retroperitoneal mass greater than 10 cm (OR 9.30, 95% CI 3.8–22.7). These findings were consistent when compared with a privately insured national US cohort of patients who underwent RPLND between 2007 and 2012, in whom the adjunctive nephrectomy rate was 10% (Macleod et al., 2016). Daneshmand et al. reported the University of Southern California experience with RPLND between 2004 and 2010 and found a 14% adjunctive nephrectomy rate (83% of which were on the left vs. 17% right) (Djaladat et al., 2012). Major risk factors for nephrectomy include bulky disease, especially in cases of a left-sided, greater-than-10-cm residual mass post-chemotherapy, salvage RPLND, desperation RPLND, and repeat RPLND. A major concern with nephrectomy is the possible need for adjuvant/salvage platinum–based salvage chemotherapy in the setting of residual/recurrent disease. With patients in this setting potentially receiving 4 to 8 cycles of cisplatin (primary/salvage chemotherapy), nephrectomy can lead to late-stage chronic kidney disease, which may limit options for future systemic therapy. However, because of the typically young age of this patient population, the renal reserve is typically more than adequate to avoid renal replacement therapy.

Major Vascular Reconstruction

When performing PC-RPLND, surgical planning must always include the need for vascular reconstruction because there can be extensive post-chemotherapy fibrosis involving the great vessels. **Unintentional subadventitial aortic injury can lead to life-threatening hemorrhage and possible intraoperative death. Therefore surgical planning for the need for vascular control and possible intervention with vascular replacement is imperative.** According to data from the University of Southern California, 15% of patients needed vascular procedures, of which 40% required aortic resection, 30% requiring cavotomy/caval resection, 20% requiring iliac resection, and 10% required renovascular resection with repair (Djaladat et al., 2012). Retrospective data out of a high-volume German Center found that out of 185 patients who underwent PC-RPLND, 16 (8.6%) underwent vascular surgery, including aortic resection and replacement, complete or partial resection of the IVC with thrombectomy, and resection and replacement of the iliac vessels (Heidenreich et al., 2017). With adequate expertise, small vessel wall injuries may be repaired with bovine/porcine pericardial patches/grafts, mitigating the need for bypass or replacement of the vessel. However, if complete vessel resection is required, a polytetrafluoroethylene (PTFE) or Dacron graft can be used (Fig. 77.6).

Testes cancer, in addition to displaying post-chemotherapy fibrosis requiring venal caval resection/replacement, can directly invade the wall of the vessel with venous and arterial thrombus formation. According to a database review from Indiana University from 1990 to 2010, about 6% of patients at the time of PC-RPLND have intraluminal thrombus (Johnston et al., 2013). Of these patients, nearly all were involving the vena cava and/or renal vein. However, there was one aortic thrombus that required resection and grafting.

Inferior Vena Cava Resection

Vena caval repair after planned and unplanned venotomy can be performed by interposition bypass replacement, patch venoplasty, or lateral venorrhaphy and primary repair. **When possible, primary repair of the vena cava is preferred because of the low-pressure nature of the IVC with an increased risk of thrombosis compared with the arterial high-pressure system** (see Fig. 77.6). Primary repair can be performed in selected cases in which this does not experience with post-chemotherapy RPLND identified 30 patients that underwent IVC reconstruction, 23 of which were complete IVC resections with only 4 patients undergoing IVC reconstruction using a PTFE graft. On multivariable analysis, retroperitoneal size and International Germ Cell Consensus Classification Group (IGCCCG) intermediate/poor risk group were associated with the need for an IVC intervention. According to their study, masses greater than 5 cm had a 20% IVC intervention rate compared with only 2.7% for those masses less than 5 cm (Winter et al., 2012). At Indiana University for many years the standard protocol with IVC resection was ligation. Data in 65 patients with IVC resection and ligation found that at long-term follow-up only 1 patient had chronic venous sequelae (Beck and Lalka, 1998). Retrospective data from the University of Southern California identified 47 patients who underwent IVC reconstruction in which 27 underwent PTFE grafting and the remainder underwent primary repair or patch venoplasty (Quinones-Baldrich et al., 2012). At a mean follow-up of 3½ years only one IVC went on to develop thrombosis. Vena caval repair/reconstruction is safe and effective at reducing lower extremity edema compared with acute ligation; however, there generally also appears to be no significant long-term effects from ligation in this young population. If possible, because of lack of complications and less operative time required, a primary repair or lateral venorrhaphy is preferred if less than 25% narrowing is expected. If more than 25% narrowing is expected, patch venoplasty or interposition graft should be considered (see Fig. 77.6). Patch venoplasty is particularly useful if the circumferential wall does not have to be completely resected to remove tumor. Most commonly commercially available substances for patch venoplasty consist of bovine and porcine pericardium. Also, if xenografts are not desired, cadaveric donor vein can be used.

Aortic Reconstruction

Aorta dissection in PC-RPLND, especially with seminomatous disease, can be life-threatening if vascular principles are not followed. Small injuries to the aorta can be repaired with primary repair. Unlike venous reconstructive options that can include ligation and resection without reconstruction, significant aortic injury almost always requires grafting. **It is imperative to have a multidisciplinary surgical team immediately available for possible intervention. The most common injuries occur with subadventitial dissection of densely adherent masses, which required aortic replacement with a polytetrafluoroethylene (PTFE) or Dacron graft** (see Fig. 77.6). Any long duodenal serosal injury with aortic injury should be considered for grafting to reduce the risk of delayed aortoduodenal fistula (Donohue and Foster, 1994).

Beck et al. reported their experience at Indiana University over a 30-year span involving 1200 patients and found that approximately 1% required aortic replacement (Beck et al., 2001). Nearly two-thirds of these patients had salvage chemotherapy or were undergoing desperation RPLND with elevated tumor markers at the time of surgery. In this high-risk setting, 33% were disease free at a mean follow-up of 34 months, and there were no graft-related complications. Therefore, especially in the high-risk setting for relapse with little systemic chemotherapeutic options available, aortic resection can be used to obtain complete resection if needed and maximize the patient's opportunity to be cured of their disease.

Hepatic Resections

According to the 1997 IGCCCG nonpulmonary visceral metastases are considered poor risk with a 48% 5-year survival. It is estimated that about 6% of advanced metastatic testes cancer patients have liver metastases (International Germ Cell Consensus Classification, 1997). RPLND of poor risk nonpulmonary liver disease is usually considered after primary, salvage, or third-line chemotherapy. Therefore RPLND requires all disease resection, including residual liver disease identified by cross-sectional imaging.

Unfortunately, liver histology at the time of liver resection can be discordant with retroperitoneal histology. A database review at Indiana University found 59 cases of hepatic resection, and of these cases, the overall rate of histologic discordance between

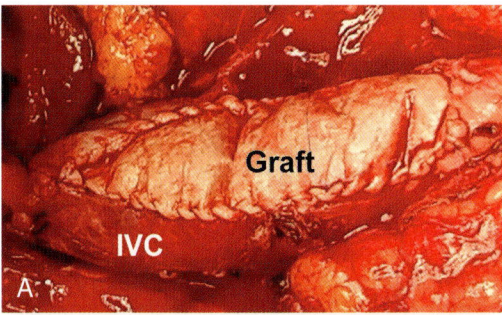
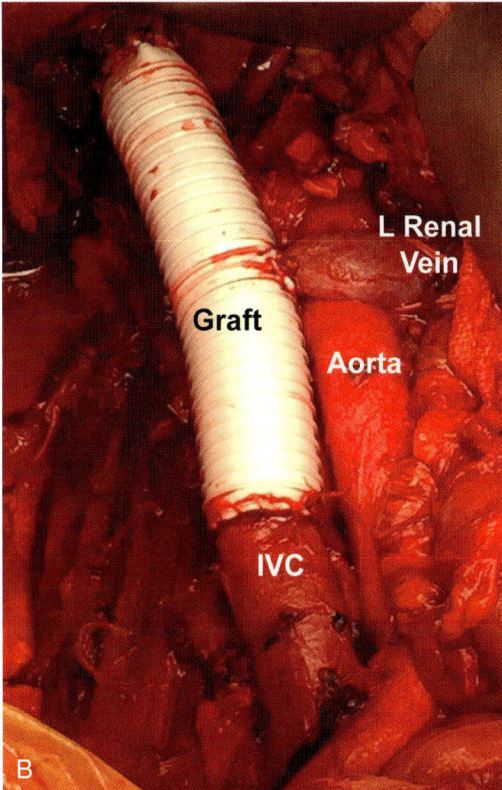
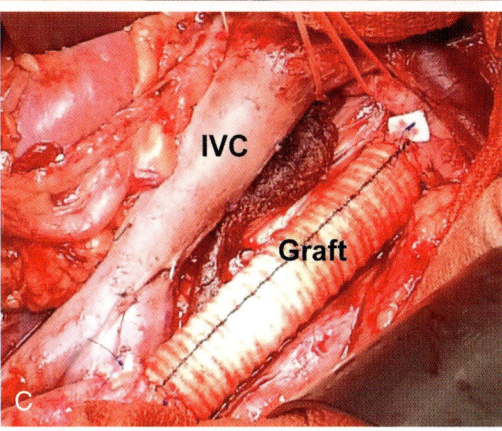

Fig. 77.6. Examples of vascular reconstruction at the time of PC-RPLND. (A) Autologous patch graft of the inferior vena cava (IVC). (B) Synthetic graft replacing a segment of the IVC with anastomosis of the left renal vein. (C) Synthetic graft replacing a portion of the aorta.

cause significant venous obstruction from intraluminal narrowing (Mansukhani et al., 2017). Obviously in the unstable patient with life-threatening bleeding, caval ligation or lateral venorrhaphy should be considered. Historically 5% to 10% of PC-RPLND cases require resection of the vena caval wall or entire abdominal vena cava resulting from fibrosis, direct invasion, and/or tumor thrombus. A German retroperitoneal and liver histology was 51%, with 73% of all liver specimens containing necrosis only. Retroperitoneal necrosis is highly predictive of hepatic necrosis (94%) (Jacobsen et al., 2010). This discordance was also characterized from another high-volume center, who reviewed their database from 1990 to 2015 and concluded that residual liver masses in the absence of marker positive disease should undergo resection or ablation (Pietzak et al., 2018). Data from the Memorial Sloan Kettering Cancer Center (MSKCC) identified 36 patients, of which 29 (81%) presented with a liver mass at initial diagnosis and 17 (47%) received salvage chemotherapy before surgery. Teratoma and viable GCT was found in 8 (22%) and 5 (14%) of PC-RPLND specimens, respectively. For the liver resection specimens, this was 5 (14%) and 4 (11%), respectively. Among patients who had either teratoma or viable GCT on PC-RPLND, 29% (95% CI 0.10–0.56) had teratoma or viable GCT on liver resection as well. The rate of benign versus malignant histologic discordance was 21% (95% CI 0.06–0.46), with 4 of 19 patients having either teratoma or viable GCT on liver resection when only fibrosis/necrosis was found in their PC-RPLND. At some hepatobiliary centers of excellence, liver biopsy with intraoperative open microwave ablation may be performed if liver masses are present, in which resection would lead to undue morbidity. Multi-institutional data from four high-volume centers comparing liver resection to ablation found more morbidity with resection but no difference with respect to recurrence, except for a higher recurrence rate in percutaneous liver-ablated patients (Groeschl et al., 2014). Therefore if the residual liver lesion is less than 3 cm and not amenable to safe resection, open microwave ablation at the time of RPLND may be a safe alternative. However, there are no studies with a large cohort of GCT patients to recommend this as an alternative to extirpation except in cases of undue morbidity with liver resection. Of course, management in the post-chemotherapy and salvage setting must be individualized because some smaller lesions in difficult locations may have to be biopsied and observed.

Pelvic Resections

Pelvic disease in metastatic testes cancer is rarely observed outside of prior groin surgery, repeat RPLND, or late relapsed disease. Data from Indiana University from 1990 to 2009 identified 2722 patients who underwent RPLND, of which 134 had pelvic disease: 14% had prior groin surgery, 98% had prior chemotherapy, 19.4% underwent prior RPLND, and 24% had late-stage relapse (Jacob et al., 2017). Surgical intervention included pelvic excision alone in 27.6%, pelvic excision with primary RPLND in 1.5%, or pelvic excision with PC-RPLND in 70.9%. Median pelvic mass size was 6.5 cm. Histology was 55% teratoma, residual germ cell in 21%, sarcomatous transformation in 6%, and necrosis in 16.5%. The fibrosis rate at pelvic excision is less than 50% compared with PC-RPLND specimens alone; therefore complete resection should be undertaken whenever feasible.

Similar data from MSKCC were found when they reviewed 2186 patients who underwent RPLND between 1989 and 2011, 44 (2%) of whom underwent pelvic excision at the time of RPLND (Alanee et al., 2016). Median size on imaging was 4 cm. Histology revealed teratoma in 15/44 (34%) and viable tumor in 5/44 (11%) patients. At a median follow-up of 46 months, 40/44 (91%) patients were living without disease recurrence. Thus, although patients in both of these series tended to present with higher-volume disease, surgery was curative in the majority of patients after chemotherapy.

Management of Supradiaphragmatic Disease

Approximately 10% to 20% of patients with a diagnosis of testes cancer have evidence of supradiaphragmatic disease at presentation or go on to intrathoracic spread at some point during their illness. Thoracic disease can be the result of hematogenous spread leading to pulmonary metastases or by lymphangitic spread to the mediastinal and cervical lymph nodes. Approximately 80% of mediastinal metastases are in the lower to middle mediastinum (Kesler et al., 2011). Anterior mediastinal disease is worrisome for a primary GCT of the mediastinum. **Multiple studies have looked at the concordance in histology between retroperitoneal and thoracic disease and, as is the case with liver disease, there is substantial discordance ranging from 25% to 50%** (Besse et al., 2009; Gels et al., 1997; Gerl et al., 1994; Steyerberg et al., 1997). Retrospective data from Indiana University regarding metastatic testes patients with thoracic spread of testes cancer from 1980 to 2006 identified 431 patients who underwent 640 post-chemotherapy surgical procedures to remove lung (n = 159), mediastinal (n = 136), and lung and mediastinal (n = 136) disease within 2 years of chemotherapy (Kesler et al., 2011). The overall median survival was 23.4 years, with 295 (68%) patients alive and well after an average follow-up of 5.6 years. There was no survival difference in patients who underwent removal of lung or mediastinal metastases. Pathologic categories of resected residual disease were necrosis (21.5%), teratoma (52.7%), persistent NSGCT (15.0%), and degenerative non–germ cell cancer (10.1%). Multivariable analysis identified older age at time of diagnosis ($P = 0.001$), non–germ cell cancer in testes specimen ($P = 0.004$), and pathology of residual disease ($P < 0.001$) as significant predictors of survival. **Extrapolating from this data it is generally recommended to resect any residual disease greater than 1 cm.**

Steyerberg et al. in a multi-institutional study identified 215 patients undergoing thoracotomy for residual thoracic masses after platinum-based chemotherapy for testes cancer (Steyerberg et al., 1997). Necrosis was found in 116 patients (54%), mature teratoma in 70 (33%), and residual viable GCT in 29 (13%). Necrosis was found at thoracotomy in 89% of those patients with necrosis found in the RPLND specimen. **Therefore, in general, thoracic management should be deferred until after RPLND because, if fibrosis is found in the retroperitoneum, observation of the mediastinal masses may be warranted as a result of the high rate of concordant fibrosis with the lungs in that circumstance. For these reasons, a multidisciplinary team of specialists should be involved in the care of these complex patients.**

Resection of Retrocrural Disease

Resection of retrocrural disease can be extremely challenging from a traditional midline incision. For this reason, other options include a thoracoabdominal approach, left thoracotomy approach, and thorascopic dissection with or without the assistance of robotics. Depending on level of expertise, any of these options can be used to resect retrocrural disease. Without advanced laparoscopy/robotics, a thoracotomy can be used to resect residual retrocrural disease. However, thoracotomy has substantial morbidity and convalescence; therefore efforts to have a combined thoracoabdominal approach avoiding thoracotomy have been employed.

Fadel et al. (2000) reported on 18 patients who had simultaneous resection of retroperitoneal and posterior mediastinal masses using this approach between 1993 and 1999. After standard retroperitoneal lymph node dissection through a midline laparotomy, an incision parallel to the right crus of the diaphragm was made and extended anteriorly through the muscular portion. Excellent exposure of the lower posterior mediastinum was obtained. Masses located higher than vertebra T8 were resected by extending this incision anteriorly and performing a partial sternal division. A complete median sternotomy can be done to allow subcarinal dissection, as well as pulmonary or anterior mediastinal mass resection. There were no perioperative deaths; 3 patients had minor postoperative complications. After a median follow-up of 3.2 years, the overall 5-year survival rate was 92%, and the 5-year disease-free survival rate was 87% (Fadel et al., 2000). Kessler et al. at Indiana have used a transdiaphragmatic approach on 60 patients with a low complication rate (Fig. 77.7). **Deciding to do a retrocrural dissection at the same time as RPLND may be less morbid to the patient; however, if more extensive thoracic resection is required (i.e., pulmonary metastectomy, mediastinal resection), the consideration should be made for a staged procedure because of prolonged anesthesia and potential increased risk of complications with a single-stage approach.**

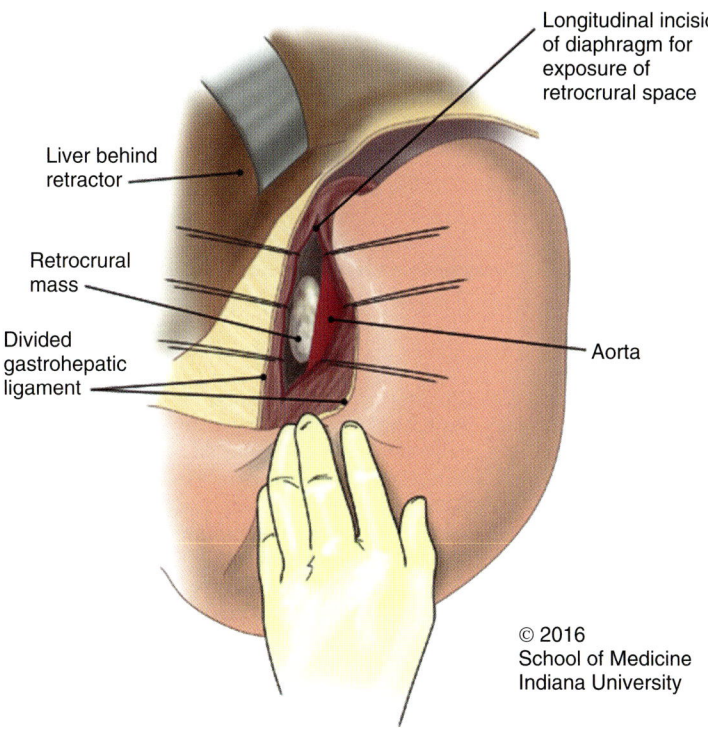

Fig. 77.7. Transabdominal, transdiaphragmatic approach to retrocrural mass. (Copyright 2016 Section of Medical Illustration in the Office of Visual Media at the Indiana University School of Medicine. Published by Elsevier Inc. All rights reserved.)

KEY POINTS: AUXILIARY PROCEDURES

- The most common auxiliary procedure during RPLND is nephrectomy, particularly for left-sided or larger masses in the post-chemotherapy or other higher risk settings.
- Surgical planning is critical to success or RPLND in high-risk settings such as after systemic chemotherapy. This is particularly critical for those who may require an en-bloc aortic replacement.
- When possible, primary reconstruction of the IVC is preferred to grafting when a venotomy or partial excision is required.
- Histologic discordance between the liver and retroperitoneum is common, and the decision to perform hepatic resection should be individualized using a multidisciplinary care team.
- There is frequent histologic discordance between disease in the thoracic cavity and retroperitoneum. In general, thoracic masses should be managed after RPLND is completed, and masses greater than 1 cm should be considered for resection unless the retroperitoneum harbored only fibrosis.
- Retrocrural dissection may be a consideration at the time of RPLND; however, if more extensive thoracic resection is required, a stage approach may be preferable.

SURGICAL DECISION MAKING

This section focuses on the controversies and decision-making process for RPLND in the primary and post-chemotherapy setting and the role for adjuvant chemotherapy after RPLND. The indications for primary RPLND, including its advantages and disadvantages compared with other management strategies, are addressed in another chapter and are not discussed here.

Management of Clinical Complete Remission to Induction Chemotherapy

Roughly 70% of patients who are treated with cisplatin-based chemotherapy for clinical stage II or higher GCT achieve a complete radiographic (defined as no residual mass > 1 cm) and serologic remission. The management for these patients remains controversial, but the fundamental options are observation or performing PC-RPLND.

Those who favor observation for a patient with a complete response to chemotherapy point out the excellent long-term overall and recurrence-free survival for patients who are managed by surveillance (Ravi et al., 2014). For example, a study of 141 men, most of whom were IGCCCG good risk, with a clinically complete response to chemotherapy managed with observation found a 15-year recurrence-free survival (RFS) rate of 90% and cancer-specific survival (CSS) of 97% (Ehrlich et al., 2010). Another similar study of 161 patients with a shorter, median 4½-year follow-up also reported excellent oncologic outcomes with surveillance alone after chemotherapy with RFS of 93.8% and CSS of 100% (Kollmannsberger et al., 2010). Because of these excellent results, investigators at Indiana University and many other major centers observe men who achieve a radiologic (residual mass <1 cm) and serologically complete response after cisplatin-based chemotherapy for stage II or higher disease.

Those who favor performing PC-RPLND in all patients with a history of retroperitoneal metastases regardless of response to chemotherapy point to a risk of harboring residual viable disease even with small residual masses. For example, in a report of 532 patients undergoing PC-RPLND at MSKCC, 154 had a residual mass 1 cm or less on cross-sectional imaging after chemotherapy (Carver et al., 2006). In this group of men with a clinically complete response to chemotherapy, 22%, 1%, and 5% had teratoma, teratoma/GCT, and GCT, respectively, in their final pathologic specimen at the time of surgery.

The debate continues in large part because the natural history of microscopic residual teratoma after cisplatin chemotherapy remains

TABLE 77.2 Management of Patients Experiencing a Clinical Complete Remission to Induction Chemotherapy

	EHRLICH ET AL., 2010	KOLLMANNSBERGER ET AL., 2010	KARELLAS ET AL., 2007
Management	Observation	Observation	PC-RPLND
No. patients	141	161	147
Follow-up (yr)	15.5	4.3	3
Good risk (%)	77	94	98
DFS (%)	91	94	97
CSS (%)	97	100	NR

CSS, Cancer-specific survival; DFS, disease-free survival; NR, not reported; PC-RPLND, post-chemotherapy retroperitoneal lymph node dissection.

unknown. Proponents of PC-RPLND despite a clinical CR argue microscopic teratoma residing in the retroperitoneum may eventually lead to growing teratoma syndrome, late disease relapse, or malignant transformation that is typically chemotherapy resistant and difficult to salvage. Conversely, those who favor observation would argue that microscopic teratoma behaves in an indolent fashion in the majority of cases. The debate is further complicated by the observation that retrospective studies examining either approach (Table 77.2) appear to have similar excellent results, suggesting both can be successful provided patients are appropriately selected (Carver et al., 2006, Ehrlich et al., 2010, Kollmannsberger et al., 2010). The debate will therefore likely continue until it can be demonstrated **(1) whether performing PC-RPLND can prevent cancer-related deaths for patients after a clinically complete response to chemotherapy and (2) if the number needed to treat to prevent one death is sufficiently low to justify the potential morbidity of PC-RPLND.**

Use of Modified Templates in Primary Retroperitoneal Lymph Node Dissection

Historically RPLND included the removal of all the lymphatic tissue included within the bounds of contemporary bilateral infrahilar templates plus resection of the tissue in the interiliac region inferiorly to the level of the bifurcation of the common iliac arteries (Ray et al., 1974), often with the addition of the suprahilar tissue bilaterally (Donohue et al., 1982). The dissection often was done through a thoracoabdominal incision and was associated with significant perioperative morbidity, and the majority of patients were rendered anejaculatory (Donohue and Rowland, 1981). Despite the morbidity, the scale of the dissection was thought necessary to offer the optimal opportunity to cure the patient in an era in which curative chemotherapy for GCT was not yet available.

Beginning in the 1970s and continuing through the 1980s, the advent of curative cisplatin-based chemotherapy (Einhorn and Donohue, 1977)**, the recognition of the distinct patterns of lymphatic spread of right-sided versus left-sided disease** (Donohue et al., 1982; Ray et al., 1974; Weissbach and Boedefeld, 1987)**, and the development of surgical techniques to spare the postganglionic sympathetic nerve fibers responsible for ejaculatory function** (Colleselli et al., 1990; Donohue et al., 1990; Jewett et al., 1988) **revolutionized the management of GCT and the approach to RPLND.** Increasingly the surgical approach to RPLND focused on decreasing the morbidity associated with the operation while maintaining its oncologic efficacy. An important advance in this regard was the development of modifications to the historically wide dissections before these interventions.

The first such attempts at detailing alternative templated modifications to traditional RPLND were pioneered by Ray et al. (1974). This report of 283 patients who underwent RPLND at MSKCC over three decades detailed a transition from full bilateral dissections to modifications that included a focus on the primary landing zones for right- versus left-sided tumors. **This seminal work set the stage for subsequent work and refinement of the modified templates still in use today.**

In 1982 an important pathologic mapping study by Donohue et al. (1982) on 104 patients with pathologically positive lymph nodes at the time of primary RPLND was able to identify a relatively predictable pattern to lymphatic spread of GCT in the retroperitoneum. These included the observation that left-sided tumors typically metastasize to the left para-aortic region, whereas the primary "landing zone" for right-sided tumors was the interaortocaval and precaval spaces. Although spread to the contralateral area and the suprahilar regions was rare, the incidence increased as the bulk of retroperitoneal disease increased. Spread to the interiliac region was very rare. This study provided further confirmation of the modified template concept proposed earlier by Ray et al. (1974) on patients who did not have bulky disease in the retroperitoneum. These findings were further reinforced by a study from Weissbach and Boedefeld in 1987 on 214 patients with nonbulky pathologic stage II disease in which a reduced template of the para-aortic and preaortic regions in left-sided tumors was proposed, with intraoperative frozen section used to identify those patients who should go on to a more formal full template dissection.

The sum of these and other template-based studies was the adoption of a less morbid and more efficient approach to RPLND using modified templates. Examples of the boundaries of full bilateral compared with a modified template dissection are shown in Fig. 77.8. **Most authors now agree that the interiliac region and the suprahilar regions can generally be omitted in the absence of bulky retroperitoneal disease.** Omission of the suprahilar dissection reduces the risk of chylous ascites, renal injury, and pancreatic and/or duodenal injuries. The omission of the interiliac region, when combined with the omission of the contralateral retroperitoneal space, can help preserve antegrade ejaculatory function in the majority of men. **However, the omission of the contralateral retroperitoneal space remains controversial.**

Data that argue against the use of modified unilateral templates include a report by Eggener et al. (2007) from MSKCC, who presented data from a series of 500 patients who underwent primary RPLND for clinical stage I or IIA GCT. Suprahilar dissection was generally omitted in this series, but a full template was otherwise applied across all patients. There were 191 patients (38%) who had pathologic stage II disease. The authors analyzed the anatomic location of the positive nodes in these patients relative to varying modified templates that have been published and noted that 3% to 23% of patients would have had a positive node that would not have been resected, depending on which modified template was analyzed. This extra-template node positivity was more prevalent for right-sided than left-sided tumors. On the basis of this and similar data, the authors recommended that a full bilateral infrahilar nerve-sparing RPLND be the standard for all patients with clinical stage I or IIA GCT.

The most ideal method to resolve the debate between modified/unilateral template versus full bilateral templated dissections for primary RPLND for clinical stage I or IIA disease would be a prospective randomized trial, but no such trial has been completed. Published results of both approaches have shown excellent results with overall and cause specific survival rates approaching 100% (Table 77.3; Donohue et al., 1993; Hermans et al., 2000; Nicolai et al., 2004; Stephenson et al., 2005). Therefore proving a substantive difference between approaches would be difficult. Attempts to compare across series is complicated not only by the usual caveats of such an approach but also varying approaches to the use of adjuvant chemotherapy

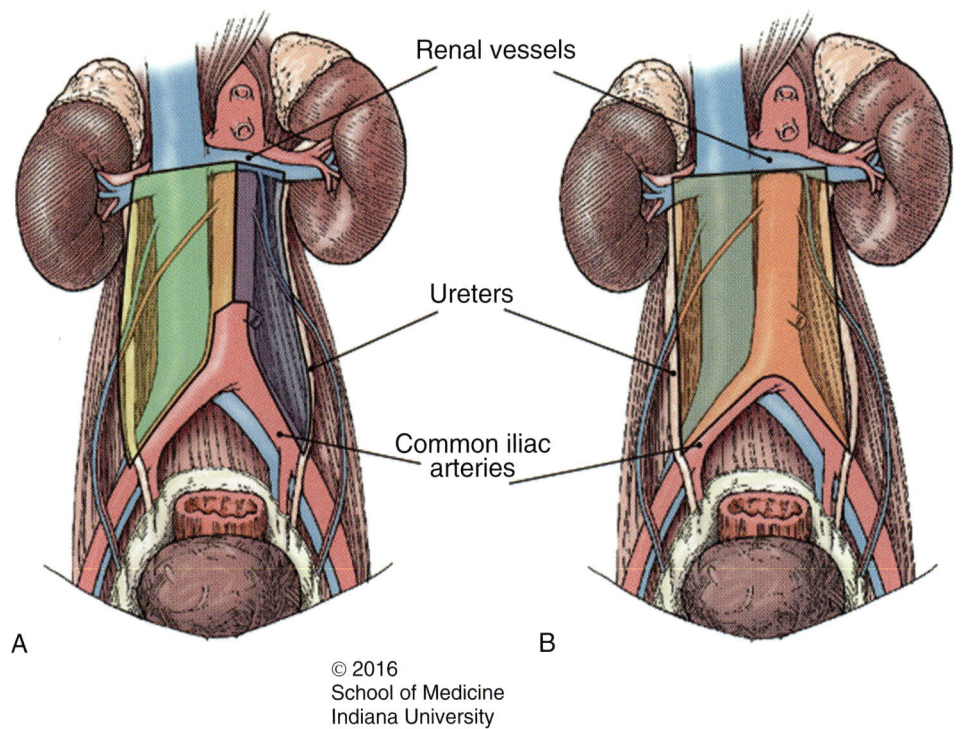

Fig. 77.8. Retroperitoneal lymph node dissection templates. (A) Modified unilateral templates—right-sided shaded in yellow, left-sided shaded in purple. (B) Modified bilateral template—shaded area. (Copyright 2016 Section of Medical Illustration in the Office of Visual Media at the Indiana University School of Medicine. Published by Elsevier Inc. All rights reserved.)

TABLE 77.3 Selected Primary RPLND Series

STUDY	NO. PATIENTS	NO. pN+ (%)	RECURRENCE RATE FOR pN0 (%)	RECURRENCE RATE FOR pN+ MANAGED WITH RPLND ALONE (%)	FOLLOW-UP (YR)	CSS (%)
Donohue et al., 1993a	378	112 (29.6)	31 (12)	22 (34)	6.2	99.2
Stephenson et al., 2005	308	91 (29.5)	NR (7)	NR (34)	4.9	99.7
Hermans et al., 2000	292	66 (22.4)	23 (10.2)	7 (22.6)	3.8	100.0
Nicolai et al., 2004	322	60 (20)	NR	NR	7.2	98.8

CSS, Cancer-specific survival; *NR*, not reported; *pN+*, histologically positive lymph nodes; *pN0*, histologically negative lymph nodes; *RPLND*, retroperitoneal lymph node dissection.

for those patients who ultimately are found to have pathologically positive nodes. For example, in a series by MSKCC that showed a high proportion of patients being cured by surgery (Stephenson et al., 2005), a high proportion of patients with pN2 disease were treated with adjuvant chemotherapy. In one of the studies from Indiana University (Donohue et al., 1993), most of the patients with node-positive disease were randomized on study to observation or adjuvant chemotherapy. However, in a different study from the same institution (Hermans et al., 2000), all pN1 and most patients pN2 patients were observed, while chemotherapy was confined to those patients at relapse or who harbored pN3 disease at the time of surgery. These challenges therefore preclude a definitive "one-size-fits-all" approach to template selection in primary RPLND. From the work summarized here it is clear that with appropriate patient selection, excellent surgical technique, and the judicious use of adjuvant chemotherapy excellent results can be expected for the majority of patients. **Whether it should be mandatory to use either a full bilateral template or a modified/unilateral template to achieve such results remains unclear.**

Use of Modified Templates in Retroperitoneal Lymph Node Dissection After Chemotherapy

Unlike primary RPLND, for patients undergoing PC-RPLND the standard of care in most instances is a resection of the residual mass and a full bilateral infrahilar RPLND. This has been the standard since the first reported experience with PC-RPLND by Donohue et al. in 1982. Although the majority of the viable GCT and/or teratoma was located in the appropriate primary landing zone, given the frequent contralateral crossover in the setting of bulky initial disease and the difficulty of detecting viable residual neoplasm intraoperatively, the authors emphasized the importance of a complete resection (Donohue et al., 1982). **This has remained the standard of care because it provided excellent control of the retroperitoneum, albeit at the cost of significant potential morbidity and frequent ejaculatory dysfunction in patients for whom a nerve-sparing approach was not feasible.**

Because of the potential morbidity of PC-RPLND, a number of groups have explored the potential to apply modified unilateral templates to PC-RPLND in a manner analogous to the primary setting (Beck et al., 2007; Carver et al., 2007; Ehrlich et al., 2006; Heidenreich et al., 2009; Herr, 1997; Rabbani et al., 1998; Steiner et al., 2008; Wood et al., 1992). A summary of the results is shown in Table 77.4 demonstrating that this approach, if appropriately applied, can be done safely with encouraging oncologic results. Despite a high degree of variability in the reported rates of positive nodes outside of a standard full bilateral template the in-field and out-of-field retroperitoneal recurrences rates remained low and, in all but one report, the CSS was 98% to 100% (when reported). Nevertheless, the application of modified unilateral templates in the setting of PC-RPLND is critically reliant on proper patient selection. Although no universal consensus exists, based on the reports to date patients who are potential candidates for modified template PC-RPLND should probably meet the following criteria:

1. Well-defined lesion measuring 5 cm or less confined to the primary landing zone of the primary tumor on imaging before and after chemotherapy (Fig. 77.9 shows representative CT examples)
2. Normal post-chemotherapy STMs
3. IGCCCG good/intermediate risk

After selection criteria, such as those outlined, have been reported in PC-RPLND with excellent local control, including in-field retroperitoneal recurrence rates of 0 to 1% and CSS rates of 98% to 100% at a follow-up of 2.6 to 10.4 years antegrade ejaculation was maintained in more than 85% of men (Beck et al., 2007; Cho et al., 2017; Heidenreich et al., 2009; Steiner et al., 2008). Such excellent results are encouraging and warrant further study. However, as is the case with primary RPLND, there have been no prospective, randomized comparative studies of full bilateral versus modified unilateral template approaches to PC-RPLND. Strict adherence to the criteria described is critical for patient selection and, in general, full, bilateral infrahilar dissection with resection of the residual mass remains the standard of care for the majority of PC-RPLNDs.

Adjuvant Chemotherapy for Pathologic Stage II Disease at Primary Retroperitoneal Lymph Node Dissection

Patients who have no lymph node metastases at the time of primary RPLND can be safely observed without additional therapy. However, there is less consensus on the role for adjuvant chemotherapy for

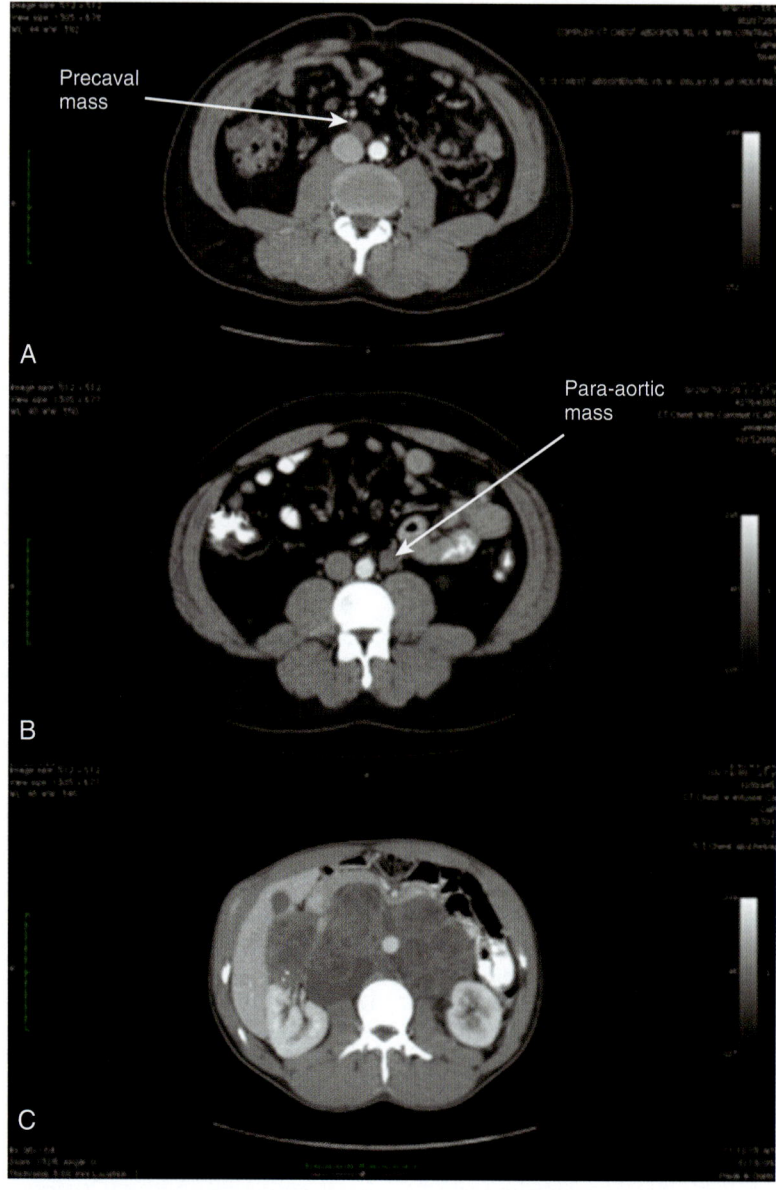

Fig. 77.9. Computed tomography images of post-chemotherapy residual retroperitoneal masses. (A) This patient could be considered a candidate for modified right template post-chemotherapy retroperitoneal lymph node dissection (PC-RPLND). (B) This patient could be considered a candidate for modified left template PC-RPLND. (C) This patient would require an extensive bilateral PC-RPLND.

TABLE 77.4 Studies Evaluating the Use of Modified Unilateral Templates in Post-Chemotherapy Retroperitoneal Lymph Node Dissection

STUDY	NO. PATIENTS	N+ OUTSIDE TEMPLATE (%)	N+ OUTSIDE TEMPLATE & MACROSCOPIC DISEASE	IN-FIELD RP RECURRENCE AFTER B/L RPLND (%)	IN-FIELD RP RECURRENCE AFTER U/L RPLND (%)	PRESERVATION OF EJACULATION IN TEMPLATES	FOLLOW-UP (YR)	CSS
Wood et al., 1992	113	14 (21.4)	9 (8)	NA	NA	NA	NA	NA
Herr, 1997	62	NR	NR	1 (4)	1 (2.7)	NR	6	89%
Rabbani et al., 1998	50	12 (24)	1 (2.6)	1 (2.6)	1* (9.1)	50%	4-5	96%-100%
Ehrlich et al., 2006	50	9 (18)	1 (2)	0	0	NA	4.4	NR
Beck et al., 2007	100	NA	NA	NA	0	NR	2.6	100%
Steiner et al., 2008	102	NA	NA	NA	1(1)	94%	7.8	99%
Carver et al., 2007a	269	20-86 (7-32)	50 (18.6)	NR	NR	NR	3.75	NR
Heidenreich et al., 2009	152	NA	NA	1 (1.9)	0	85%	3.25	98%
Cho et al., 2017	100	7	7	0	0	NR	10.4	99%

*Occurred in patient who underwent tumorectomy only.
B/L, Bilateral; CSS, cancer-specific survival; NA, not applicable; N+, histologically positive lymph nodes; NR, not reported; RP, retroperitoneal; RPLND, retroperitoneal lymph node dissection; U/L, unilateral.

those patients with pathologically positive lymph nodes at the time of surgery. On the one hand, it has been demonstrated that roughly 70% of patients with pN1 or pN2 disease can be cured with surgery alone and, even for those patients who recur, the majority can be successfully salvaged with chemotherapy if they relapse (Donohue et al., 1993, 1995; Nicolai et al., 2004; Stephenson et al., 2005). However, for those patients who do relapse, the salvage chemotherapy required is more intensive, typically at least one more cycle of bleomycin, etoposide, and cisplatin or two more cycles of etoposide and cisplatin, than if the therapy were given in an adjuvant setting. Conversely, adjuvant chemotherapy has been shown to virtually eliminate the risk of disease relapse for patients with pN1 or pN2 disease after primary RPLND (Behnia et al., 2000, Kondagunta et al., 2004; Williams et al., 1987). However, its universal application across all such men would subject 70% of them "unnecessarily" to the potential toxicity of chemotherapy. The ideal, then, would be if clinicians could accurately predict which patients were at the highest risk for subsequent relapse and confine adjuvant chemotherapy to that high-risk group.

Attempts to accurately define a high-risk group for disease relapse in the setting of positive nodal metastases after primary RPLND have met with mixed results. The most obvious potential predictor of relapse would be the bulk of nodal involvement. There have been some early studies suggesting that microscopic lymph node disease involvement had a lower recurrence rate than macroscopic disease (Fraley et al., 1985; Vugrin et al., 1981). In a prospective, randomized trial of adjuvant chemotherapy, analysis of the observation arm demonstrated patients with microscopic nodal disease had a recurrence rate of 40%, those with macroscopic nodal disease less than 2 cm recurred at a 53% rate, whereas those with disease greater than 2 cm recurred at a rate of 60% (Williams et al., 1987). Although these results were not significant (likely because of relatively small sample size), they remain intriguing. At least two retrospective reports on patients with clinical stage II NSGCT managed with RPLND alone reported that larger lymph node metastatic burden was associated with higher recurrence rates (Donohue et al., 1995; Weissbach et al., 2000). Conversely, several other studies that have compared outcomes between pathologic stages IIA and IIB disease for patients managed with observation have not found a difference in recurrence rates (Al-Ahmadie et al., 2013; Donohue et al., 1993; Nicolai et al., 2010; Pizzocaro and Monfardini, 1984). These conflicting results may be, at least in part, due to differences in patient selection for adjuvant therapy and other potential unmeasured confounders inherent in retrospective studies.

There have been a variety of other histologic variables tested for their prognostic ability to predict disease recurrence. These include such parameters as the number of positive nodes as a proportion of the number removed (Al-Ahmadie et al., 2013; Beck et al., 2005), the histologic type of GCT in the metastases (Al-Ahmadie et al., 2013; Beck et al., 2005), and the presence or absence of extranodal extension (Al-Ahmadie et al., 2013; Beck et al., 2007). **None of these have proven reliable enough that they can accurately predict those who are at high risk for recurrence and warrant up-front adjuvant therapy. The one exception is that the finding of only teratoma in the retroperitoneum is associated with very low relapse rates, and therefore additional therapy other than observation is not warranted** (Liu et al., 2015).

Given the absence of a reproducible and reliable predictor for disease recurrence, most centers rely on the nodal staging to determine the approach to adjuvant chemotherapy. **There is relatively broad consensus that many patients with pN1 disease at primary RPLND who are reliable can be safely managed with observation. The management of pN2 disease is more controversial with some centers advocating two cycles of adjuvant chemotherapy** (Kondagunta and Motzer, 2007), **whereas others would manage many of these patients with observation** (Beck and Foster, 2006; Jacobsen et al., 2007).

HISTOLOGIC FINDINGS AT POST-CHEMOTHERAPY RETROPERITONEAL LYMPH NODE DISSECTION AND SURVIVAL OUTCOMES

The three major histologic findings (fibrosis/necrosis, teratoma, and viable GCT) and their frequencies at the time of RPNLD have been reported in multiple series. Although there has been some evolution over time because of refinement in chemotherapy regimens resulting in a decreasing frequency of viable GCT at PC-RPLND, **the current relative frequencies of fibrosis, teratoma, and viable GCT are generally around 40%, 45%, and 15%, respectively** (Albers et al., 2004; Carver et al., 2006; Donohue et al., 1998; Hendry et al., 2002; Spiess et al., 2007; Steyerberg et al., 1995).

Outcomes by Histology

The outcomes after PC-RPLND vary depending on the type of histology encountered. The CSS outcomes after the finding of teratoma or fibrosis in the modern era are excellent, with the group of biggest concern being those with a finding of viable GCT (Table 77.5). There has been some debate on the distribution of histology after BEP × 3 or EP × 4 for good risk disease, but, in general, the long-term survival after PC-RPLND has been similar (Cary et al., 2015; Kundu et al., 2015). The variability in reported histology and outcomes likely is a product of era of treatment, pretreatment risk stratification, and length of follow-up.

Fibrosis/Necrosis

The finding of necrosis/fibrosis only at PC-RPLND portends an excellent prognosis with CSS and RFS approaching 95% (Carver et al., 2007; Donohue and Foster, 1994; Maroni et al., 2008). It can be inferred from this finding that systemic chemotherapy has rendered all malignant cells nonviable and that most likely all other subclinical metastatic deposits have been likely cleared with a low likelihood of subsequent disease recurrence.

Teratoma

Contemporary studies also suggest excellent outcomes after a histologic finding of teratoma after PC-RPLND with expected RFS rates of 80% to 90% and CSS of 85% to 95% (Carver et al., 2006; Donohue and Foster, 1994; Jansen et al., 1991; Liu et al., 2015). In this setting somatic type malignancy and mediastinal primaries are associated with an increased risk of recurrence (Carver et al., 2007; Jansen et al., 1991; Loehrer et al., 1986).

Viable Malignancy

Persistent disease at the time of PC-RPLND suggests primary resistance to systemic treatment. This finding is associated with 50% to 70% long-term survival rate, which is reduced as compared

---

> **KEY POINTS: SURGICAL DECISION MAKING**
>
> - Although there remains some debate in the literature, in general, patients who have a complete response to chemotherapy should be observed.
> - Modified templates can be used for primary RPLND in select patients who have low-stage, low-volume retroperitoneal disease.
> - In general, the standard of care for PC-RPLND is a full, bilateral infrahilar retroperitoneal dissection with nerve sparing where technically feasible.
> - The use of modified templates in the post-chemotherapy setting should be confined to the fraction of patients who meet highly strict selection criteria.
> - Patients who are found to have only teratoma at the time of RPLND have a very low risk for subsequent relapse and likely do not require adjuvant chemotherapy.
> - The use of adjuvant chemotherapy for patients found to have pN+ at RPLND is controversial, but in general pN1 disease can often be observed, while the use of adjuvant chemotherapy for those with pN2 should be individualized.

TABLE 77.5 Survival Outcomes by Histologic Findings at Post-Chemotherapy Retroperitoneal Lymph Node Dissection

STUDY	NO. PATIENTS	FOLLOW-UP (YR)	RFS	CSS
FIBROSIS				
Donohue and Foster, 1994	150	>2	NR	93
Eggener et al., 2007a[a]	36	4.3	NR	85
Carver et al., 2007c	113	NR	95	NR
Maroni et al., 2008	184	4	92.1	NR
TERATOMA				
Loehrer et al., 1986	51	NR	61	82.3
Jansen et al., 1991	26	7.7	88.5	88.5
Donohue and Foster, 1994	273	>2	NR	93.4
Eggener et al., 2007[a]	15	4.3	NR	77
Carver et al., 2006	210	3	85.4	94
Beck et al., 2009	99	3.5	76.8	98
VIABLE MALIGNANCY				
Jansen et al., 1991	23	7.9	54.5	64
Fox et al., 1993	133	3	30.8	42.8
Donohue et al., 1998	122	9	39	51.5
Fizazi et al., 2001	238	7.2	64	73
Eggener et al., 2007a[a]	10	4.3	NR	56
Spiess et al., 2007	41	3.9	50	71
Kundu et al., 2010	90	NR	62	71

[a]All patients received salvage chemotherapy before post-chemotherapy retroperitoneal lymph node dissection.
CSS, Cancer-specific survival; *NR*, not reported; *RFS*, recurrence-free survival.

with the finding of fibrosis or teratoma (Donohue et al., 1998; Fizazi et al., 2001, 2008; Jansen et al., 1991; Kundu et al., 2010; Spiess et al., 2007).

In a multi-institutional review of 238 patients with viable malignancy at PC-RPLND, Fizazi et al. (2001, 2008) determined three factors associated with worse prognosis: (1) incomplete resection, (2) 10% or greater viable malignancy, and (3) IGCCCG intermediate/poor risk group stratification at initial diagnosis. Patients in the favorable risk group (i.e., none of the factors mentioned earlier) demonstrated a 90% 5-year progression-free survival (PFS) and 100% 5-year OS. Those patients with one risk factor were deemed "intermediate risk" (5-year PFS 76%, 5-year OS 83%), and those with two or three risk factors were deemed "poor risk" (5-year PFS 38%, 5-year OS 51%). Unfortunately, these factors and risk group stratification on follow-up analysis (Fizazi et al., 2008) did not predict response to chemotherapy and thus remain only prognostic.

Adjuvant Chemotherapy

The use of adjuvant chemotherapy after the finding of viable malignancy at PC-RPLND remains an area of debate. Historically the use of adjuvant chemotherapy has been recommended; however, the exact regimen has been variable with a duration that usually consists of two cycles. Fizazi et al. (2001, 2008) found that adjuvant chemotherapy was associated with a statistically superior PFS but not OS. As noted above, the indices of complete resection, less than 10% viable tumor, and IGCCCG risk group status are associated with PFS and OS but do not predict response to chemotherapy. Recommendations for the use of adjuvant chemotherapy should remain individualized considering original IGCCCG risk group stratification, pathology, and extent of surgical resection. Adjuvant chemotherapy in the NCCN guidelines is currently recommended for incomplete resection as well as intermediate and poor risk disease (Motzer et al., 2015). Similarly, the European Association of Urology guidelines advocate adjuvant chemotherapy after incomplete resection but not in IGCCCG good risk disease where there is less than 10% viable tumor (Albers et al., 2015). However, because of the lack of randomization, firm data to support the use of adjuvant chemotherapy after single-line chemotherapy are lacking. Finally, use of two cycles of adjuvant chemotherapy after second-line or salvage chemotherapy is not recommended because it does not appear to improve outcomes (Fox et al., 1993; Kundu et al., 2010).

> **KEY POINTS: HISTOLOGIC FINDINGS AT POST-CHEMOTHERAPY RETROPERITONEAL LYMPH NODE DISSECTION AND OUTCOMES**
>
> - Approximately 90% long-term survival can be expected among patients with fibrosis and/or teratoma only at PC-RPLND. This number is reduced to 50% to 70% for patients demonstrating viable GCT at PC-RPLND.
> - Recommendations for adjuvant chemotherapy in patients with residual viable GCT should be individualized, considering original IGCCCG risk group stratification, completeness of resection. and percentage of viable tumor remaining at PC-RPLND.
> - Adjuvant chemotherapy is not needed for patients with either fibrosis/necrosis or teratoma on final pathology after PC-RPLND.

POST-CHEMOTHERAPY RETROPERITONEAL LYMPH NODE DISSECTION IN HIGH-RISK POPULATIONS

Salvage Retroperitoneal Node Dissection

Salvage node dissection occurs in a subset of particularly high-risk metastatic testes cancer patients who have demonstrated some degree of platinum resistance and have typically undergone at least 7 to 8 cycles of chemotherapy with first- and second-line chemotherapy to achieve testes serum tumor marker resolution. Classically, histology after RPLND after first-line chemotherapy demonstrates viable

TABLE 77.6 Post-Chemotherapy Retroperitoneal Lymph Node Dissection in High-Risk Populations

STUDY	NO. PATIENTS	TERATOMA (%)	FIBROSIS (%)	VIABLE MALIGNANCY (%)	FOLLOW-UP (YR)	CSS OR OS
SALVAGE						
Fox et al., 1993	163	NR	NR	55	5	36.7[a]
Donohue et al., 1998	166	NR	NR	NR	9.7	61.4
Eggener et al., 2007a	71	21	51	28	5	74
HDCT						
Rick et al., 2004	57	16	38	46	7.3	65
Cary et al., 2011	77	33.8	27.3	39	4.2	71
DESPERATION						
Donohue et al., 1998	150	NR	NR	NR	9.7	66
Ravi et al., 1998	30	26.7	27.6	46.7	4.8	57
Albers et al., 2000	30	11	25	64	11	57
Beck et al., 2005c	114	34.2	12.3	53.5	6	53.9
Ong et al., 2008	45	25	17	58	4.3	69
REDO						
McKiernan et al., 2003	56	37.5	28.6	33.9	4.1[b] 2.4[c]	56
Sexton et al., 2003	21	67	24	24	4.7	63
Heidenreich et al., 2003	18	33.3	44.4	22.2	1.9	89
Willis et al., 2007	54	35	9	56	5	94.2
Pedrosa et al., 2014	203	34	14.8	51.2	5	61.2
LATE RELAPSE						
Baniel et al., 1995a	81	19	0	81	4.8	56.8
George et al., 2003	83	71	0	78	2.4	74.7
Dieckmann et al., 2005	72	NR	NR	NR	NR	58.3
Sharp et al., 2008	75	19	3	78	4.5	61

[a]Includes only patients with viable malignancy in the survival analysis.
[b]Follow-up for post-chemotherapy retroperitoneal lymph node dissection.
[c]Follow-up for primary retroperitoneal lymph node dissection.
CSS, Cancer-specific survival; *HDCT*, high-dose chemotherapy; *NR*, not reported; *OS*, overall survival.

malignancy in about 20% of cases. **In the salvage setting the rate of viable GCT can be at least double the rate seen after primary chemotherapy with worse overall survival** (Table 77.6). In a study of 16 patients who underwent salvage RPLND, histopathology from the retroperitoneum demonstrated necrosis in 25% of cases, 31% of cases had teratoma, and 44% of cases harbored residual viable tumor (Alqasem et al., 2016). The OS after salvage RPLND ranges from 60% to 75% (Donohue et al., 1998; Eggener et al., 2007; Fox et al., 1993).

RPLND after third-line chemotherapy is extremely rare. Indiana University has the greatest experience in this setting reporting on 92 patients that underwent PC-RPLND after high-dose chemotherapy and stem cell transplantation (Cary et al., 2015). Histology at the time of PC-RPLND was necrosis in 26%, teratoma in 34%, and residual viable cancer in 38%. At a mean follow-up of 80 months, the 5-year OS was 70%. Obviously, such results require great care in patient selection and emphasize the need for treatment decision making in a multidisciplinary fashion because RPLND can still have a significant role for such high-risk patients (Albany et al., 2018).

Desperation Retroperitoneal Node Dissection

In general, one of the main indications for RPLND after first-, second-, or third-line chemotherapy is the normalization of serum tumor markers. **Desperation RPLND occurs in a special limited setting of persistently elevated STMs despite chemotherapy and should never be undertaken outside of a multidisciplinary setting because this subset of patients are at a particularly high risk of relapse and progression** (Albany et al., 2018). Histology in the studies of patients who underwent desperation RPLND are listed in Table 77.6. Beck et al. reported the outcomes of 116 patients who underwent desperation RPLND with a median follow-up of 6 years, and the 5-year OS was 53.9% (Beck et al., 2005). In this report, on multivariate analysis poor OS was independently associated with patients who underwent desperation RPLND after salvage chemotherapy, patients with an elevated beta hCG before surgery, and patients undergoing repeat RPLND. On the contrary, patients with initially declining STMs after first-line chemotherapy but subsequently plateaus at a detectable level had a greater than 75% chance of having fibrosis or teratoma in the specimen. In this setting, however, fibrosis in the RPLND specimen may portend a worse prognosis because this could indicate the patient has elevated tumor markers resulting from disease outside the retroperitoneum (Ong et al., 2008). Normalization of tumor markers after RPLND was the only variable linked to increased OS in this setting. Who should undergo desperation RPLND? It should generally never be done in the setting of rising tumor markers with rapid doubling times or progressive metastatic disease in multiple sites because this is clearly an indication for salvage chemotherapy or third-line high-dose chemotherapy.

Multi-institutional outcomes of desperation RPLND are in Table 77.6. **Desperation RPLND should be done in patients with limited metastatic disease sites (optimally only retroperitoneal but may include thoracic or liver sites) that are completely resectable at the time of RPLND (non-staged), declining/plateauing serum tumor markers, and patients with elevated tumor markers who have exhausted all chemotherapeutic options with resectable disease.**

Reoperative Retroperitoneal Node Dissection

Reoperative or "redo" RPLND is usually performed because of technical failure of the first operation leaving behind residual disease at primary staging RPLND or PC-RPLND. This is the main reason RPLND should be performed by experienced high-volume surgeons and, if done minimally invasively by a laparoscopic or robotic approach, the rules of complete dissection must be the same as in the open setting. Despite the preponderance of data demonstrating superior outcomes by high-volume surgeons, data from the American Board of Urology recertification process shows that most RPLNDs are performed by urologists who have performed only one RPLND (Flum et al., 2014). Urologists who performed more than two RPLNDs per year were in the top 25% and 3 RPLNDs per year were in the top 10%. This lack of volume and experience may be one of the factors that contribute to inadequate RPLND.

The largest contemporary series identified 203 patients at a single institution undergoing reoperative RPLND for recurrent retroperitoneal GCT after initial retroperitoneal lymph node dissection with local relapse (Pedrosa et al., 2014). On multivariate analysis, two factors highly associated with local recurrence were incomplete lumbar vessel division at initial resection ($P < 0.01$) and teratoma histology in the reoperative specimen ($P = 0.01$). Only active cancer at reoperation ($P < 0.01$), M1b stage ($P = 0.01$) and salvage chemotherapy before reoperation ($P = 0.02$) were associated worse oncologic outcomes. Several other studies have supported that incomplete surgical control of the retroperitoneum is the main cause of relapse as most recurrences are within the primary landing zone (Heidenreich et al., 2005; McKiernan et al., 2003). Willis et al. (2007), in a series of reoperative RPLND, found 46% of recurrences were retroaortic or retrocaval and omitted at the time of RPLND. Reoperative RPLND can be technically challenging with higher complications and worse overall cancer specific outcomes (see Table 77.6). There is a higher incidence of residual viable GCT with somatic-type malignancies in 15% to 20% of the specimens. **Reoperative RPLND can lead to poor oncologic outcomes and greater surgical complications; therefore thorough dissection of the retroperitoneum and complete mobilization of the great vessels at the time of RPLND is mandatory and cannot be overemphasized.**

Late Relapse

Late relapse is defined as a recurrence outside the setting of observation occurring 24 months or more after primary management of GCT with initial complete response. Such recurrence after CR is rare and only occurs in 2% to 4% of patients (Baniel et al., 1995; Gerl et al., 1997). The retroperitoneum is the most common site of late relapse (Baniel et al., 1995). Greater than 80% of late relapses have GCT with yolk sac as the dominant histology and additionally a higher incidence of somatic-type malignancy (Baniel et al., 1995; George et al., 2003; Michael et al., 2000; Sharp et al., 2008). **For these reasons, if the recurrent disease is deemed resectable, RPLND should be undertaken as first choice because the dominant histology is usually resistant to chemotherapy. Chemotherapy should be reserved for patients with widespread metastatic or unresectable disease in an attempt to decrease tumor burden and make the disease resectable.** Reported OS is nearly 60% and should be performed in highly select cases. Based upon reported series, factors negatively affecting OS after late relapse PC-RPLND include viable GCT, somatic-type mutation, having received prior salvage chemotherapy, and undergoing incomplete resection of the specimen (Baniel et al., 1995; Michael et al., 2000; Sharp et al., 2008).

SURGICAL OUTCOMES, FUNCTIONAL CONSIDERATIONS, AND COMPLICATIONS OF RETROPERITONEAL LYMPH NODE DISSECTION

Lymph Node Counts

Lymph node counts have been proposed as a measure of surgical quality and shown to be associated with oncologic outcomes in a number of malignancies (Herr et al., 2002; Le Voyer et al., 2003; Schwarz and Smith, 2006, 2007; Stein et al., 2003). A similar concept has been proposed for RPLND but has met with mixed results. One study out of MSKCC has suggested that increased lymph node counts are associated with increased node positivity for primary RPLND (Thompson et al., 2010). However, in other reports there was no significant association between lymph node counts and node positivity (Liberman et al., 2010; Nayan et al., 2015; Risk et al., 2010). In many such reports there is a wide variability in the reported number of nodes removed. In a number of disease states it is well recognized that multiple factors can influence the nodal count at surgery, including how the tissue is submitted, processed, and analyzed by pathology that have little to do with surgical quality.

Retroperitoneal Lymph Node Dissection and Fertility

Fertility in Patients Undergoing Retroperitoneal Lymph Node Dissection

Because testicular cancer predominantly affects young men, the issue of fertility after therapy can be particularly important. Although RPLND does not affect testicular function or spermatogenesis, subfertility is a common finding in men with testicular cancer. When taking into consideration all stages, abnormal semen parameters have been reported in as high as 40% to 60% of newly diagnosed men (Fossa et al., 1985; Foster et al., 1994; Hansen et al., 1991; Lange et al., 1987). This is important to keep in mind when attempting to report paternity rates for men after therapy for GCT. With these caveats in mind, the rates of live birth in a small cohort of men after therapy for GCT managed with orchiectomy and primary RPLND was reported as 36% (Ping et al., 2014).

Ejaculatory Dysfunction and Retroperitoneal Lymph Node Dissection

Antegrade ejaculation of semen is a complex physiologic process that requires coordinated neurologic input. In particular, **the smooth muscle contraction of the vas deferentia, seminal vesicles, and prostate that results in seminal emission and prostate glandular secretion as well as the subsequent closure of the bladder neck preventing retrograde ejaculation is critically reliant on input from the postganglionic sympathetic fibers that emanate from L1 to L4.** These fibers then coalesce at or below the IMA in the

---

> **KEY POINTS: POST-CHEMOTHERAPY RETROPERITONEAL LYMPH NODE DISSECTION IN HIGH-RISK POPULATIONS**
>
> - In the salvage setting the rate of viable GCT at PC-RPLND can be at least double of what is seen after primary chemotherapy with worse overall survival. Although PC-RPLND can still play a role in this setting, it should be done after multidisciplinary decision making.
> - Desperation RPLND should never be undertaken outside of a multidisciplinary setting because this subset of patients are at a particularly high risk of relapse and progression.
> - Desperation RPLND should be done in patients with limited metastatic disease sites that are completely resectable at the time of RPLND, declining/plateauing serum tumor markers, and patients with elevated tumor markers that have exhausted all chemotherapeutic options with resectable disease.
> - Reoperative RPLND is associated with poor oncologic outcomes and greater surgical complications; thorough dissection of the retroperitoneum and complete mobilization of the great vessels at RPLND is mandatory and cannot be overemphasized.

hypogastric plexus before traveling caudally in the interiliac space at the sacral promontory (Donohue et al., 1990).

Because the L1-L4 postganglionic sympathetic fibers course through the retroperitoneum, they were frequently surgically removed, thereby rendering the man anejaculatory at the time of RPLND before the advent of template modification and prospective nerve preservation (Donohue et al., 1991). With a goal of improving ejaculatory function several key modifications to RPLND were made. **The first was a recognition that in carefully selected patients, as discussed previously, a modified unilateral template dissection could be performed that preserved the sympathetic fibers in the majority of men without significantly compromising oncologic outcomes** (Pizzocaro et al., 1985; Weissbach et al., 1985). Early studies in which modified unilateral template RPLND was performed without prospective nerve-sparing demonstrated between 75% and 87% preservation of antegrade ejaculation (Fossa et al., 1985; Pizzocaro et al., 1985; Weissbach et al., 1985). A more recent study shows that with further surgical refinement a 97% rate of antegrade ejaculation in patients after modified, unilateral RPLND without nerve sparing can be achieved (Beck et al., 2010).

The second modification to RPLND that significantly improved postoperative ejaculatory function was a series of studies that demonstrated the postganglionic fibers could be prospectively identified and preserved during RPLND (Jewett and Torbey, 1988). Since the early studies these nerve sparing techniques have been further refined such that current series report preservation of antegrade ejaculation with meticulous prospective sympathetic nerve sparing at 90% to 100% (Beck et al., 2010; Donohue et al., 1990; Heidenreich et al., 2003; Jewett and Torbey, 1988). The initial studies by Jewett and Torbey (1988) reported an anejaculatory period in the immediate postoperative period that subsequently resolved. Later studies have shown that with further refinement the period of transient postoperative anejaculation is no longer apparent (Donohue, 1993), possibly by avoiding undue traction on the nerves and subsequent neuropraxia.

With the development of modified unilateral templates and prospective nerve preservation, ejaculatory function can now be preserved in more than 90% of men undergoing RPLND, particularly in the primary setting. **Indeed paternity rates for men who underwent a nerve-sparing, primary RPLND have been reported as high as 75%** (Beck et al., 2010). Because of the significant and prolonged effect of chemotherapy on spermatogenesis and fertility, the rates of paternity in the PC-RPLND setting have not been well established (Lampe et al., 1997). **Importantly, these approaches to preserving ejaculatory function have not lead to any appreciable decrement in oncologic control.** With follow-up between 10 months and 5 years, only one retroperitoneal recurrence has been reported in the series highlighted here (Beck et al., 2010; Donohue et al., 1990, 1993; Fossa et al., 1985; Heidenreich et al., 2003; Jewett and Torbey, 1988; Pizzocaro et al., 1985; Weissbach et al., 1985).

Complications of Retroperitoneal Lymph Node Dissection

The overall complication rate for primary RPLND has been reported to range from 10.6% to 24% (Baniel et al., 1994; Heidenreich et al., 2003; Subramanian et al., 2010). Historically, complication rates after PC-RPLND appear to occur more frequently in the range of 20% to 30% (Baniel et al., 199; Subramanian et al. 2010; Wells et al., 2017) but may be less common at more experienced centers (Cary et al., 2015). Variability in reported data and expected outcomes is highlighted by the finding that the mean number of RPLNDs performed annually by board-certified urologists is 1 (Flum et al., 2014). Table 77.7 summarizes reported complications for primary and PC-RPLND.

Pulmonary Complications

Major pulmonary complications after primary RPLND are rare. However, in PC-RPLND pulmonary complications have been reported to occur in 3% to 5% but may be decreasing with time as surgical teams become aware of the use of bleomycin and its associated risk of pulmonary toxicity (Baniel et al., 1994, 1995; Cary et al., 2015; Heidenreich et al., 2003; Subramanian et al., 2010). **It cannot be overstated that patients treated with bleomycin-containing regimens for induction chemotherapy are at increased risk for acute respiratory distress syndrome and prolonged postoperative ventilation. The incidence of bleomycin-related perioperative pulmonary complications can be minimized by avoiding aggressive intraoperative and postoperative intravenous fluid resuscitation and keeping the FiO$_2$ as low as safely possible.** As stated previously, the anesthesia team must be notified and skilled in managing patients receiving prior bleomycin. In addition, the postoperative team, including the nursing staff in the PACU and surgical ward must be notified that tachycardia is common after RPLND and that it should not be used as an isolated indicator for fluid management. Finally, nasal cannula O$_2$ should be used judiciously with tolerance for lower FiO$_2$ levels (i.e., S02 88-90).

TABLE 77.7 Complications of Retroperitoneal Lymph Node Dissection

	PRIMARY RPLND			PC-RPLND	
	BANIEL ET AL., 1994	HEIDENREICH ET AL., 2003	SUBRAMANIAN ET AL., 2010	BANIEL ET AL., 1995B	SUBRAMANIAN ET AL., 2010
No. patients	478	239	112	603	96
Overall complications (%)	10.6	19.7	24	20.7	32
Major complications (%)	8.2	5.4	3	NS	8
Mortality (%)	0	0	0	0.8	1
Major pulmonary (%)	1.9	0.8	0.9	5.1	3.1
Minor pulmonary (%)	0.2	0.4	3.6	5.1	3.1
Chylous ascites (%)	0.2	2.1	2	2	2
Symptomatic lymphocele (%)	0.2	1.7	0	1.7	1
Ileus (%)	NR	2.1	17.9	2.2	20.8
Wound infection (%)	4.8	5.4	0.9	4.8	4
Pulmonary embolism (%)	0	0.8	0.9	0.1	3.1
Ureteral injury (%)	0.2	0.4	0.9	0.9	0
Small bowel obstruction (%)	2.3	0.4	2.7	2.3	1.8
Postoperative hemorrhage (%)	0	0.8	0	0.3	1

NR, Not reported; *NS*, not studied; *PC-RPLND*, post-chemotherapy retroperitoneal lymph node dissection; *RPLND*, retroperitoneal lymph node dissection.

Ileus

The reported rates of postoperative paralytic ileus vary widely but can occur up to 21% of the time in primary or PC-RPLND. Use of an extraperitoneal approach may significantly decrease this possibility (Syan-Bhanvadia et al., 2017). We do not advocate routine use of a nasogastric tube and, unless there are extenuating circumstances, always provide some enteric feeding on postoperative day 1.

Lymphocele

The exact rates of lymphoceles after RPLND is unknown because most are subclinical. Symptomatic lymphoceles are very rare and have been reported to occur in up to 1.7% of cases (Baniel et al., 1994, 1995; Heidenreich et al. 2003; Subramanian et al., 2010). Presenting symptoms are usually characterized by a sense of abdominal fullness or flank pain secondary to ureteral compression. Cross-sectional imaging demonstrates a thin-walled cystic lesion located within the resection bed. Air within the lymphocele and/or a rim of enhancement should raise concern for an infection. Treatment for symptomatic or infected lymphoceles is carried out by percutaneous drainage. Antibiotics should be reserved for those who are perceived to be infected, and in this case consideration should also be given to leaving a drain. **Prevention of lymphocele occurs through meticulous surgery with care to clip or ligate lymphatic channels as noted previously.**

Chylous Ascites

Chylous ascites is the accumulation of lipid-rich lymph fluid within the peritoneal cavity. It has been reported to occur in 0.2% to 2.1% of patients undergoing primary RPLND and 2% to 7% of patients undergoing PC-RPLND with lower rates in more recent series (Baniel et al., 1994, 1995; Cary et al., 2015; Evans et al., 2006; Heidenreich et al., 2003; Subramanian et al., 2010). The most common presenting symptoms are an increase in abdominal girth, fullness, anorexia, and weight gain. If the ascites is large, the patients may complain of dyspnea secondary to diaphragmatic restriction. **Diagnosis is usually made through clinical suspicion and cross-sectional imaging such as a CT scan. The fluid is classically a milky color when paracentesis is performed. In addition, it usually has a high protein content (>3 g/dL) as well as a triglyceride level that is two-eight times that of serum.**

Suprahilar resections are thought to carry a higher risk for chylous ascites because of disruption of the cisterna chyli and its contributing lymphatics. The location of the cisterna chyli is variable but generally lies at the level of the L1-L2 vertebral bodies at or just above the level of the renal vessels. Most consistently it has been reported to be located posterior to the aorta behind the left crus of the diaphragm, but a distinct cisterna chyli is believed to be present only about half of the time (Leibovitch et al., 2002).

Patients presenting with symptomatic chylous ascites should first undergo paracentesis without leaving a drain. If rapid accumulation occurs, we leave a drain and cap it off for interval release. In addition, the patient should be given a very low-fat, high-protein diet with replacement of medium chain triglycerides and use of intramuscular octreotide. Octreotide has not been shown in the urologic literature to reduce lymph fluid, but it has demonstrated efficacy-reducing chylous leaks after hepaticopancreaticobiliary surgery (Kuboki et al., 2013; Shapiro et al., 1996). Persistent high-volume leak is rare. If initial dietary modifications fail to adequately address the leak, then the next step is to make the patient NPO and institute parenteral nutrition. If after this the chylous drainage remains significant, then options for management include continued observation or attempted invasive intervention. The latter includes lymphangiogram/lymphoscintigraphy with consideration to percutaneous embolization, peritoneovenous shunt, and surgical exploration. The consideration of invasive options should be reserved as a last resort in high-volume leaks that have not improved over several days to weeks or when electrolyte abnormalities and protein loss are unmanageable with conservative efforts. After resolution of chylous ascites, a low-fat diet should be continued for at least 4 weeks after resolution with gradual reinstitution of a regular diet.

Venous Thromboembolism

The incidence of venous thromboembolism (VTE) after RPLND, although not known with great precision, is thought to be low. Most likely this is secondary to the young, otherwise healthy population who usually undergo RPLND. After primary RPLND, VTE complications have been reported to occur in less than 1% of cases (Baniel et al., 1994; Heidenreich et al., 2003; Subramanian et al., 2010). After PC-RPLND the rates range from 0.1% to 3.1% (Baniel et al., 1995, Cary et al., 2015; Subramanian et al., 2010).

Patients undergoing RPLND should receive sequential compression devices in the preoperative holding area. Early ambulation on postoperative day 0 should be encouraged along with significant periods of time out of bed to chair. The specific use of prophylactic subcutaneous low-dose unfractionated heparin or low-molecular-weight heparin has not been studied after RPLND. However, it has been well documented to reduce VTE rates in patients undergoing surgery in general (Collins et al., 1988; Kakkar et al., 1993). In addition, contemporary reports on patients receiving first-line bleomycin chemotherapy have a deep venous thrombosis (DVT) rate of 12.7%, suggesting that post-chemotherapy patients may have an increased risk (Gizzi et al., 2016). We advocate for pharmacologic thromboprophylaxis in patients undergoing RPLND, especially those with a history of VTE, hypercoagulable conditions, obesity, and prior chemotherapy (particularly those who have received bleomycin).

Neurologic Complications

Peripheral nerve injury has been reported, albeit rarely (Baniel et al., 1995, Cary et al., 2015). All cases are presumed to be secondary to patient positioning or potentially secondary to retractor position (femoral neuropraxia). Careful positioning and discussion with the operative team is important to minimize the possibility of this complication. Post-chemotherapy patients with bulky mediastinal or RP disease may have an increased risk of paraplegia (Kesler et al., 2003).

Mortality

Morality after primary RPLND is excessively rare (Baniel et al., 1994; Capitanio et al., 2009; Heidenreich et al., 2003, Subramanian et al., 2010). In addition, mortality after PC-RPLND is also rare, reported to be less than 1% and, when reported, most often secondary to pulmonary embolism, duodenal fistula, myocardial infarction, and chylous ascites (Baniel et al., 1995; Capitanio et al., 2009; Cary et al., 2015; Subramanian et al., 2010).

RETROPERITONEAL LYMPH NODE DISSECTION IN UNIQUE SITUATIONS

Post-Chemotherapy Retroperitoneal Node Dissection for Seminoma

Pure seminoma is an exquisitely chemosensitive cancer that has been shown to have complete response rates from 70% to 90% with platinum-based chemotherapy even in widely metastatic disease (Loehrer, Birch et al. 1987, 1997, Gholam, Fizazi et al. 2003). **Therefore, it is rare to have residual retroperitoneal masses after chemotherapy. Retroperitoneal node dissection in this setting can be extremely difficult due to dense desmoplastic fibrosis with viable tumor found in only 10% of cases (Herr, Sheinfeld et al., 1997; Ravi, Ong et al., 1999; Flechon, Bompas et al., 2002).** The desmoplastic fibrosis in post-chemotherapy RPLND for seminoma has been well demonstrated to cause more operative complications compared with RPLND for nonseminomatous disease (Fossa et al., 1987; Friedman et al., 1985; Mosharafa et al., 2003). **RPLND in the pure seminoma post-chemotherapy patient must be carefully**

> **KEY POINTS: SURGICAL OUTCOMES, FUNCTIONAL CONSIDERATIONS, AND COMPLICATIONS OF RETROPERITONEAL LYMPH NODE DISSECTION**
>
> - Through the use of modified templates and bilateral nerve-sparing techniques, preservation of antegrade ejaculation should be expected in most patients undergoing primary RPLND. These techniques can be used during PC-RPLND with similar outcomes, although this is not always possible in cases of large retroperitoneal masses.
> - Although major complications are rare following primary RPLND, bleomycin related pulmonary toxicity should always be considered in those undergoing PC-RPLND. Perioperative attention to FiO_2, judicious fluid management, and communication with anesthesia is critical to minimize the potential for respiratory distress syndrome
> - Although rare, chylous ascites can be a challenging complication to manage. Careful attention to retroperitoneal lymphatic anatomy with ligation of lymphatic channels is thought to minimize the risk of this complication

selected because of the low incidence of viable cancer, absence of teratoma that can be seen in nonseminomatous disease, and high fibrosis rate resulting in difficult and potentially morbid surgery.

In a study from MSKCC, 55 patients who had pure seminoma underwent post-chemotherapy RPLND or biopsy obtaining tissue for correlation and found that for masses larger than 3 cm only 30% had viable cancer or teratoma (Herr et al., 1997). On the contrary, all patients had fibrosis on tissue obtained from masses smaller than 3 cm. From this data, the standard of care is now to observe all masses less than 3 cm in patients treated with platinum-based chemotherapy for pure seminoma. It was also recommended that all patients with masses greater than 3 cm undergo PC-RPLND. Unfortunately, 70% of patients with residual masses larger than 3 cm have fibrosis in the PC-RPLND setting and still undergo a potentially morbid procedure. Data from Indiana University regarding observation of residual masses in 21 patients post-chemotherapy for pure seminoma found that there was no correlation with residual masses size and disease relapse/progression. The authors recommended observing all masses unless they demonstrated serologic or radiographic progression. Given the controversy, alternatives have been sought that could better identify which patients may be harboring residual viable GCT. **It is in this setting in which FDG-PET scans have been shown to play a role in testes cancer decision making, specifically on whether RPLND is indicated on post-chemotherapy retroperitoneal masses greater than 3 cm in the setting of pure seminoma after chemotherapy.** DeSantis et al. (2004) studied the role of PET in such residual masses and correlated the findings by histology or radiographic/serologic progression. Out of 51 patients with residual masses, all 19 masses larger than 3 cm and 35 (95%) of 37 with residual lesions of 3 cm or smaller were correctly predicted by FDG-PET. For masses larger than 3 cm, the specificity was 100%, sensitivity 80%, positive predictive value 100%, and negative predictive value was 96%. For masses smaller than 3 cm, the specificity was 74%, sensitivity 70%, positive predictive value 37%, and negative predictive value were 92%. **Residual masses less than 3 cm have a fibrosis rate that is nearly 100% historically and with a low negative predictive value on PET scan, there is little to no role for PET imaging of masses smaller than 3 cm. However, for masses greater than 3 cm, PET is a useful adjunct in the clinical decision to obverse versus surgically treat.** Some oncology guidelines have added PET scan for pure seminoma post-chemotherapy masses greater than 3 cm and observation for masses less than 3 cm (Motzer et al., 2015) or as a general tool for suspicious retroperitoneal masses after chemotherapy (Albers et al., 2015). **Masses greater than 3 cm that are PET avid should be treated by PC-RPLND, salvage chemotherapy, or high-dose chemotherapy (HDCT) with stem cell transplantation.** There is some controversy as to whether patients with a residual PET-avid retroperitoneal mass after chemotherapy for pure seminoma should undergo RPLND versus salvage chemotherapy because residual seminoma in the PC-RPLND specimen is an ominous prognosis. Rice et al. reported the Indiana University experience with 36 patients who underwent PC-RPLND after primary or salvage chemotherapy for pure seminoma and found there was a 54% 5-year cancer specific survival with a mean time from PC-RPLND to death of 6.9 months (Rice et al., 2014). Only 9 of 36 patients remained continuously free of disease. HDCT has demonstrated a 92% overall survival in the second line setting and 64% in the third- or fourth-line setting with pure seminoma and in this subset should be considered as an alternative to consolidative surgery (Agarwala et al., 2011). In general, PC-RPLND in the pure seminoma setting should only be performed for PET-avid masses that are easily resectable in very limited select cases that could spare the morbidity of HDCT or in patients who are chemotherapy ineligible.

Post-Chemotherapy Retroperitoneal Node Dissection for Sex Cord Stromal Tumors

Sex cord stromal tumors (SCSTs) are exceedingly rare, accounting for less than 5% of testes neoplasm. SCST consists of Leydig cell, Sertoli cell, and granulosa cell tumors in pure or mixed histology. Because these are rare tumors, challenges in management exist because there are few large case series to extrapolate data. Adult granulosa cell tumors are the rarest tumor of the testes with less than 50 cases reported in the literature. From a clinicopathologic standpoint, outside of metastatic disease it can be challenging to appropriately diagnose a malignant sex cord stromal tumor. Generally, malignant behavior is correlated with older age of diagnosis, tumor size greater than 4 cm, necrosis, mitotic rate greater than 3–5/10 high-powered fields, moderate to severe nuclear atypia, infiltrative tumor margins/invasion of adjacent structures, and lymphovascular invasion (Dilworth et al., 1991; Kim et al., 1985; Kratzer et al., 1997; Rove et al., 2015; Young et al., 1998). Multiple factors may be present or one or two (Kim et al., 1985; Rove et al., 2015; Young et al., 1998). Some authors suggest, if two or more pathologic variables are present, to categorize such tumors as malignant (Kratzer et al., 1997; Silberstein et al., 2014). **However, in general, prospectively classifying a given tumor as benign or malignant histologically remains challenging.**

Behavior of Sertoli cell and Leydig cell tumors can be difficult to categorize because few centers have any high-volume experience in this subset of patients. For example, Banerji et al. (2016) reviewed a national cancer registry from 1998 to 2011 and out of 79,120 cases of testicular cancer, found a total of 315 (0.39%) Sertoli cell and Leydig cell tumors (Banerji et al., 2016), demonstrating how exceedingly rare these tumors are found. Osbun et al. (2017) used SEER data between 2004 and 2012 to better characterize Sertoli cell and Leydig cell tumors. According to this SEER data only 0.6% of testes tumors had Sertoli cell (n = 31) or Leydig cell (n = 76) histology. Only 3% of germ cell neoplasm patients were African-American, whereas 23% of Sertoli cell and 24% of Leydig cell tumor patients were African-American. Sertoli cell and Leydig cell tumor patients were typically older compared with GCT. Leydig cell tumors most commonly presented with stage I disease (98.5%), whereas patients with Sertoli cell tumors presented at higher stages (35% with stage II/III). Cancer-specific mortality was the highest in the Sertoli cell tumors (32%) compared with the Leydig cell (2%) and GCT in general (7%). This data and others consistently show that Sertoli cell tumors can have aggressive behavior.

Because of low incidence of SCST, the role of RPLND in this subgroup is not well established. As discussed previously, according to SEER data, Leydig cell tumors are predominantly early stage compared with 35% of Sertoli cell tumors presenting at a more advanced stage and generally portending a worse prognosis (Osbun et al., 2017). **It has been difficult to determine if RPLND can treat limited metastatic spread for SCSTs.** Mosharafa et al. (2003) reported data from Indiana University on RPLND for SCSTs in 17 patients. Eight patients had stage II to III disease, of whom 6 (75%) died from metastatic disease despite additional therapies (Mosharafa et al., 2003). Yuh et al. (2017) presented data from the California cancer registry that identified 67 patients with SCST. Nine patients underwent RPLND. Data on outcomes demonstrated that, in patients with stage II disease, the cancer-specific and overall survival was only 30%. Presence of metastatic disease was the only predictor of survival. **In summary, there is no conclusive evidence in the literature that RPLND affects survival in the metastatic setting regarding malignant SCSTs, and therefore it likely plays only a limited role in this subset of germ cell neoplasms.**

KEY POINTS: RETROPERITONEAL LYMPH NODE DISSECTION IN UNIQUE SITUATIONS

- Patients with a residual retroperitoneal mass less than 3 cm in size after chemotherapy for pure seminoma should be observed as the probability of viable GCT is very low.
- An FDG-PET scan is indicated to assess for viable GCT in post-chemotherapy residual retroperitoneal masses more than 3 cm in patients with pure seminoma.
- An FDG-PET–avid retroperitoneal mass greater that 3 cm after chemotherapy for seminoma should be treated by PC-RPLND, salvage chemotherapy, or HDCT with stem cell transplantation.
- The role for RPLND for malignant SCSTs remains unknown because it does not appear to improve survival for these neoplasms.

CONCLUSION

The management of testicular cancer has evolved and now represents one of the great success stories in oncology. With modern therapeutic approaches, cure can now be expected in more than 90% of men diagnosed with testis cancer. Although much of this success is due to the advent of cisplatin based multiagent chemotherapy, surgery retains a central and critical role in the management of this disease. The urologist is typically the physician who first diagnoses testis cancer and often is the one who helps shepherd patients through their cancer journey. It is vital that the urologic surgeon understand the nuances of testis cancer management and work within the framework of a multidisciplinary team to ensure the best care for the patient. Indeed, success is now measured not only by the survival of the patient, but also by accomplishment of this with the least morbidity and treatment burden necessary. Thus refinements in surgery have sought to improve the quality of life and to avoid long-term sequelae while maintaining oncologic efficacy. The urologist therefore remains a key element in the management of testicular malignancies, and surgery (including RPLND) retains a central role in the successful management of this disease.

REFERENCES

The complete reference list is available online at ExpertConsult.com.

78 Laparoscopic and Robotic-Assisted Retroperitoneal Lymphadenectomy for Testicular Tumors

Mohamad E. Allaf, MD, and Louis R. Kavoussi, MD, MBA

Germ cell tumors (GCTs) are the most common malignancy in men between the ages of 15 and 35 years old (Carver and Sheinfeld, 2005). Testicular cancer is also one of the most curable solid-organ neoplasms, primarily because of an excellent multimodal treatment paradigm that includes effective platinum-based chemotherapy and surgery (Einhorn, 1981). **Although contemporary survival rates for GCTs are more than 90%, cure rates and patient morbidity depend on selection of the management options.** Retroperitoneal lymph node dissection (RPLND) plays a major role in the management of patients with GCTs. The role of surgery continues to evolve because of advances in chemotherapy regimens, clinical staging modalities, and continued surgical innovation (Albers et al., 2008; Allaf et al., 2005; Sheinfeld and Herr, 1998).

Primary chemotherapy is favored in Europe, whereas RPLND traditionally has been the management strategy of choice in the United States for high-risk patients with clinical stage I nonseminomatous germ cell tumor (NSGCT). RPLND can accurately stage the retroperitoneum and positively identify patients harboring metastases. In addition, patients with pathologic stage I disease are spared the toxicity and morbidity of any additional therapy because 90% or more experience long-term disease-free survival with surgery alone. Patients with pathologic stage II disease can learn more about the extent of their disease and make informed decisions regarding further therapy after RPLND. For patients in this group who harbor small-volume retroperitoneal disease (pN1), a properly performed RPLND can be curative in approximately 70% of men, so chemotherapy also can be avoided in this setting (Donohue et al., 1993; Rabbani et al., 2001; Richie and Kantoff, 1991). Because the retroperitoneum is the most frequent site of chemoresistant malignant GCT and teratoma, both of these processes are minimized with RPLND (Baniel et al., 1995). Some groups advocate RPLND as the treatment of choice for all men with clinical stage I NSGCT with teratoma in the orchiectomy specimen given the increased propensity of harboring teratoma in the retroperitoneum (Sheinfeld et al., 2003). RPLND eliminates these chemoresistant elements and maximizes therapeutic efficacy.

Traditionally, RPLND for GCTs has been performed via an open transabdominal or thoracoabdominal approach. Over the past two decades, minimally invasive approaches for the treatment of various malignancies have emerged and become popular. Since the early 1990s, retroperitoneal laparoscopic surgery has been used with proven benefits related to reducing perioperative morbidity, improving cosmesis, and shortening convalescence without compromising oncologic efficacy (Allaf et al., 2004; Cadeddu et al., 1998; Permpongkosol et al., 2005). Laparoscopic RPLND (L-RPLND) and more recently robotic-assisted RPLND (RA-RPLND) are technically demanding procedures that are increasingly being performed by experienced surgeons aiming to minimize morbidity while duplicating the open technique. **Given that untreated retroperitoneal disease and late relapses in the retroperitoneum are fatal and can be chemorefractory, it is paramount that, as in open RPLND, a complete "cleanout" of lymph nodes is performed** (Baniel et al., 1995; Borge et al., 1988; Carver et al., 2005; Whitmore, 1979).

In this chapter, the evolution of L-RPLND and RA-RPLND is summarized. Controversies surrounding their use, surgical techniques, outcomes, and associated complications are discussed. The focus is on the management of low-stage NSGCTs and the role of these minimally invasive approaches after chemotherapy.

RATIONALE AND EVOLUTION

In an effort to decrease the morbidity associated with open RPLND, shortly after the introduction of laparoscopic renal surgery in 1991, several reports emerged documenting the feasibility of L-RPLND in the management of clinical stage I NSGCT (Klotz, 1994; Rukstalis and Chodak, 1992; Stone et al., 1993). Larger retrospective series followed, suggesting decreased blood loss, shorter hospital stays, and faster return to normal activity compared with open RPLND, with preservation of antegrade ejaculation in more than 95% of patients (Gerber et al., 1994; Janetschek et al., 1994, 1996). An early multi-institutional retrospective analysis demonstrated preservation of antegrade ejaculation in all patients, short hospital stays (<3 days), and return to normal activity at 2 to 3 weeks postoperatively (Gerber et al., 1994). **The abbreviated convalescence allows patients who are candidates to receive chemotherapy with minimal delay.** These attractive early results encouraged others to investigate L-RPLND as a viable treatment option for low-stage NSGCT.

STAGING LAPAROSCOPIC RETROPERITONEAL LYMPH NODE DISSECTION AND CONTROVERSY

Of all laparoscopic applications to surgical urology, L-RPLND has caused the most controversy. This controversy is due to the technical difficulty of RPLND in general, the limited number of cases, and lack of interest at traditional centers of excellence. Laparoscopy is an access technique with the internal procedure being performed the same as with an open incision. Experience drives an equivalent dissection. In all early series and some contemporary studies, L-RPLND was used as a staging procedure (Bianchi et al., 1998; Janetschek et al., 2000). Patients not harboring occult metastases were identified and spared exposure to chemotherapy without undergoing open RPLND. In this form, L-RPLND was performed without retrocaval or retroaortic dissection, and chemotherapy was given to all patients harboring metastatic disease (including patients with pN1 disease). The decision to omit dissection behind the great vessels was based on the belief of a lack of isolated positive lymph nodes in this area (Holtl et al., 2002). Within this paradigm, the procedure was routinely aborted if positive lymph nodes were encountered, and chemotherapy was instituted in these cases (Bianchi et al., 1998; Nelson et al., 1999). **In contemporary series, this approach has been abandoned, and L-RPLND has evolved into a therapeutic procedure duplicating the open approach in its intent** (Allaf et al., 2005; Hyams et al., 2012; Steiner et al., 2008).

The use of restrictive template boundaries coupled with the universal use of chemotherapy in men harboring pathologic stage II disease generated criticism of published L-RPLND series. The controversy regarding the use of "staging" L-RPLND hinges on mapping studies demonstrating increased multifocality and contralateral disease in the presence of positive retroperitoneal nodes (Donohue et al., 1982;

Eggener et al., 2007; Ray et al., 1974; Weissbach and Boedefeld, 1987). Critics argue that the liberal use of chemotherapy would not prevent relapses and compensate for incomplete resection.

DUPLICATION OF OPEN RETROPERITONEAL LYMPH NODE DISSECTION

At centers with experienced staff, an exact replication of the open template is performed on all patients with NSGCT undergoing L-RPLND with wide templates and complete excision of retroaortic and retrocaval tissue, rendering the procedure a staging and a therapeutic operation. Some groups perform a bilateral dissection on all patients, whereas others reserve bilateral dissection for patients with lymph node involvement (Allaf et al., 2005; Steiner et al., 2008).

DEVELOPMENT OF ROBOTIC-ASSISTED RETROPERITONEAL LYMPH NODE DISSECTION

Robotic technology has become ubiquitous within the urologic oncology community, and it is believed to have facilitated a minimally invasive approach to complex urologic operations such as radical prostatectomy and partial nephrectomy. Robotic technology has been shown to increase use of partial nephrectomy, likely because of perceived ease in facility of this complex laparoscopic procedure (Patel et al., 2013). Given the wide range of robotic procedures performed by urologists and given that L-RPLND requires a complex laparoscopic skill set, small case series of RA-RPLND have emerged demonstrating safety and feasibility (Davol et al., 2006; Pearce et al., 2017; Williams et al., 2011).

SURGICAL TECHNIQUE

L-RPLND and RA-RPLND are technically challenging procedures associated with a steep learning curve and should be undertaken by experienced surgeons who are comfortable and adept with advanced vascular techniques and open surgery in case of conversion. The indications for primary L-RPLND and RA-RPLND are identical to the indications for open RPLND and include clinical stage I or IIA disease, negative serum tumor markers, and the absence of comorbidities that would preclude safe surgery. In the postchemotherapeutic setting, these procedures have been limited mainly to small-volume residual disease; however, experienced surgeons have excised bulky tumors. **The surgical template for the procedure is dictated by laterality and intraoperative findings. Surgical margins should not be compromised to minimize morbidity or to preserve ejaculation or because of technical constraints. The extent of the node dissection can be expanded based on intraoperative findings.**

Preoperative Patient Preparation and Technical Considerations

All patients considered candidates for L-RPLND and RA-RPLND must be fully informed of all treatment options, including open RPLND, chemotherapy, and surveillance. All potential complications should be discussed, including bleeding requiring blood transfusion; injury to adjacent organs (liver, bowel, gallbladder, kidney, ureter, pancreas, major vascular structures); and orthopedic, neurologic, or pulmonary complications as well as conversion to open surgery because of complications or incomplete resection (Allaf et al., 2005; Winfield, 1998). Patients interested in future fertility are educated regarding preoperative sperm banking. Some surgeons advocate a low-fat diet 1 to 2 weeks before surgery to reduce the risk of chylous ascites, but data regarding this practice are not definitive. Patients undergo a mechanical bowel preparation the afternoon before surgery and take only clear liquids until midnight to decompress the bowels. Preoperative antibiotics are given before surgery, and antiembolism devices are placed on the lower extremities to minimize deep vein thrombosis.

Laparoscopic Approach

Standard laparoscopic instruments are used throughout this procedure (e.g., atraumatic graspers, scissors, clip appliers, irrigation/suction device, and laparoscopic paddle retractor). Radiolucent polypropylene clips (Hem-o-lok, Weck Closure Systems, Triangle Park, NC) may minimize artifact on postoperative imaging of the retroperitoneum. In addition, a needle driver loaded with suture and adjunct hemostatic agents such as gelatin matrix (FloSeal Matrix Hemostatic Sealant, Fusion Medical Technologies, Fremont, CA) or oxidized cellulose (Surgicel, Ethicon, Piscataway, NJ) should be readily available in case of vascular injury. Sealing devices such as ultrasonic shears and bipolar devices should be used with caution and can be unreliable in sealing large lymphatic channels. A laparoscopic retractor is particularly useful for medial retraction of the bowel and alleviates the need to position the patient in a modified flank position. A gauze sponge placed in the abdomen can be helpful in tamponading bleeding.

Although some surgeons use an extraperitoneal approach (Hara et al., 2004; Hsu et al., 2003), most prefer a transperitoneal approach because of the larger and more familiar working space. **In addition, a transperitoneal approach facilitates bilateral dissection when warranted by allowing access to all four quadrants.**

Patient Positioning and Port Placement for Laparoscopic Retroperitoneal Lymph Node Dissection

After general anesthesia is induced, an orogastric tube and Foley catheter are inserted. The patient may be placed in the modified flank position (45 degrees) with the side of dissection elevated, but we prefer the supine position because it makes transitioning to a bilateral dissection less cumbersome and does not require patient repositioning (Fig. 78.1 and Video 78.1). Great care is taken to pad all pressure points to minimize the risk of nerve injury or rhabdomyolysis because these surgeries may require a longer time than their open counterpart. The patient must be secured to the operating table because tilt is needed to use gravity to help shift the bowel out of the operative field.

After intraperitoneal access is achieved (via a Veress needle or Hasson technique), four equally spaced, 12 mm trocar (10 mm inner working diameter) laparoscopic ports are placed in the midline beginning 1 cm below the xiphoid process (Fig. 78.2). The umbilicus may not be incorporated as a port site. The large port size is essential to allow for the convenient introduction of larger (10/12-mm) instruments from varying angles. An additional 5-mm port may be placed

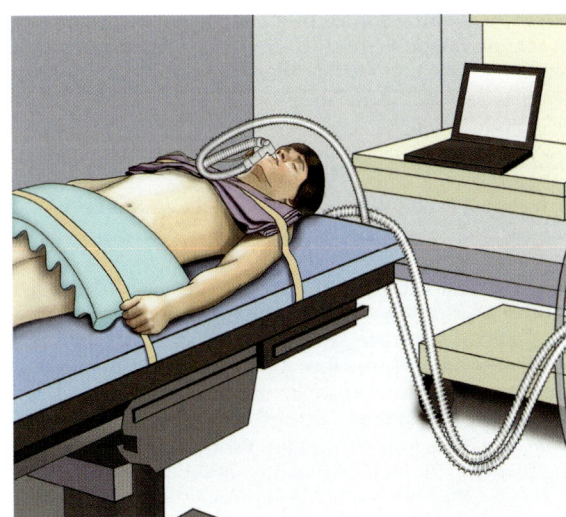

Fig. 78.1. Patient positioning during laparoscopic retroperitoneal lymph node dissection. The arms are tucked, and the patient is padded and secured in a relatively supine position.

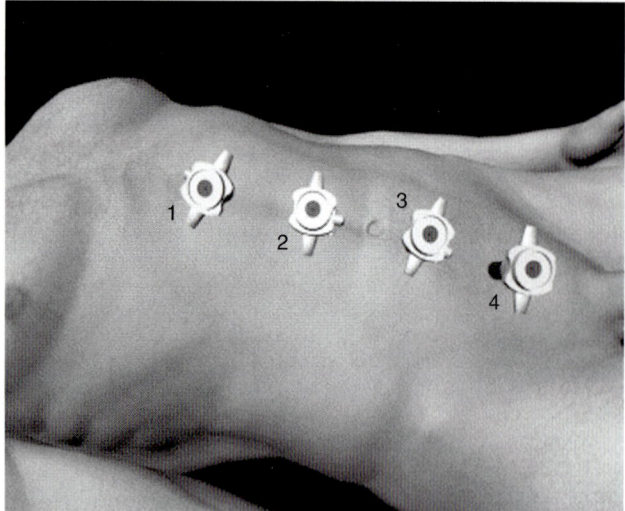

Fig. 78.2. Port placement for laparoscopic retroperitoneal lymph node dissection. Four 10/12-mm, equally spaced trocars are placed in the midline.

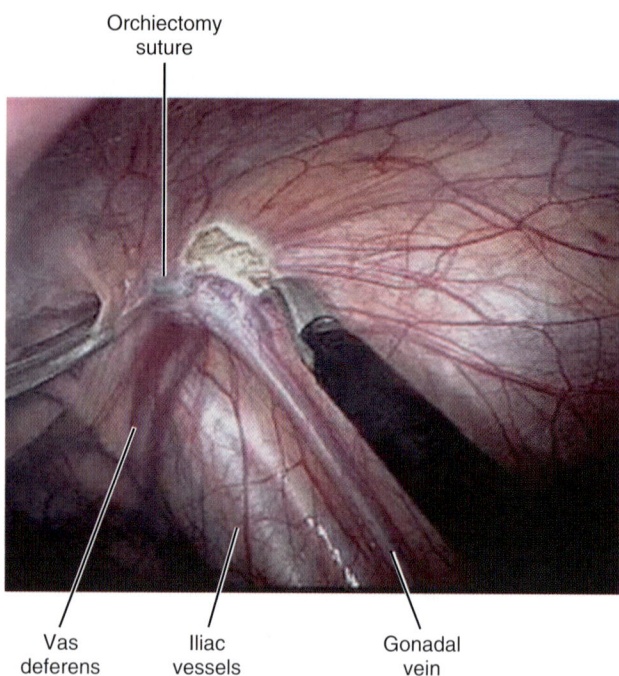

Fig. 78.3. Incision of posterior peritoneum circumferentially around the inguinal ring.

in the midaxillary line midway between the iliac crest and ribs for additional retraction if needed. The bed is rotated maximally to allow optimal medialization of the bowel away from the operative field.

Right-Sided Dissection

The ascending colon is mobilized by incising the white line of Toldt from the pelvis and around the hepatic flexure. The second portion of the duodenum is identified and kocherized, providing exposure of the retroperitoneum including the medial para-aortic space on the left.

Spermatic Cord Dissection

The camera is moved to the second-from-the-bottom trocar (trocar 3 in Fig. 78.2) to facilitate visualization during dissection of the spermatic cord stump. The peritoneum medial to the spermatic cord is incised, and the vas deferens is transected. The peritoneum is incised circumferentially around the inguinal ring (Fig. 78.3). With gentle traction on the cord, fibrous attachments and scar are incised until the suture on the spermatic cord is identified. The attachments are cut, and the cord is followed proximally along with surrounding nodal and fibroadipose tissue to the inferior vena cava (IVC). The ureter must be identified at all times to prevent inadvertent thermal injury. The spermatic vein and artery are ligated proximally and transected. The specimen is placed in an endobag and dropped on the contralateral side of the abdomen.

Lymphadenectomy

Although templates should be individualized to each case, we advocate removal of the right common iliac, paracaval, interaortocaval, preaortic, and medial para-aortic nodes (Fig. 78.4). Occasionally in obese patients (or during a full bilateral dissection), the leftmost border of the dissection must be performed after rotating the table contralaterally to optimize exposure. The camera should be moved to the port second from the top. A paddle retractor is placed in the lowest trocar to protect and sweep the bowel medially.

The testicular vein stump is identified and minimally manipulated to prevent pseudoaneurysm formation with subsequent rupture. The tissues overlying the IVC are gently lifted and carefully incised longitudinally (Fig. 78.5). It is swept off the IVC in a "split-and-roll" fashion. Blunt dissection aids in further separating these lymphatic tissues toward and overlying the common iliac vessels inferiorly and renal hilum superiorly. Care must be taken to avoid injury of lower pole renal arteries, which are present in approximately 20% of cases, and accessory vessels crossing anterior to the IVC. The renal hilum is dissected to separate all fibroadipose tissue from the renal vein and artery as far under the IVC as possible. Next, the ureter is traced to its crossing over the common iliac vessels, and the lymphatic packet is separated from both of these structures. The "split" tissue along the IVC is "rolled" medially to expose the retrocaval space. Lumbar vessels are identified, clipped, and divided to allow splitting of the posterior lymphatic tissues (Fig. 78.6). After this splitting is accomplished, the tissues are released from their attachment to the spine and delivered laterally. Great care is taken to separate the lymph nodes from the sympathetic chain and postganglionic nerve fibers. The aorta is identified next, and the tissues overlying it are similarly split to the level of the inferior mesenteric artery and rolled medially to enter the retroaortic space. The lumbar arteries may be controlled if additional mobility is needed to mobilize the interaortocaval packet posteriorly. The aorta can be medially retracted, facilitating para-aortic node excision with careful preservation of the sympathetic chain laterally. The interaortocaval nodes finally are removed to complete the dissection.

An important technical point is to leave a long stump on the aorta/vena cava side when ligating lumbar vessels so that they can be grasped and controlled in the event a clip dislodges. Lumbar vessels that retract into the iliopsoas uncontrolled usually can be managed with pressure or a figure-of-eight suture placed deep into the muscle. Lacerations of the IVC and aorta may occur during this operation but in most cases do not mandate open conversion. Direct pressure usually prevents excessive hemorrhage and can achieve hemostasis without the need for additional maneuvers. Adjunct hemostatic agents also can be used successfully in this circumstance. If the bleeding persists or in the case of arterial bleeding, direct pressure can be used temporarily before definitive repair is undertaken with intracorporeal suturing.

Left-Sided Dissection

The peritoneum is incised lateral to the descending colon and along the splenic flexure. The colorenal ligaments are severed, and the bowel is bluntly dissected medially. The lateral attachments of the spleen are incised, and the tail of the pancreas is swept medially to ensure wide exposure of the retroperitoneum, including the medial paracaval space.

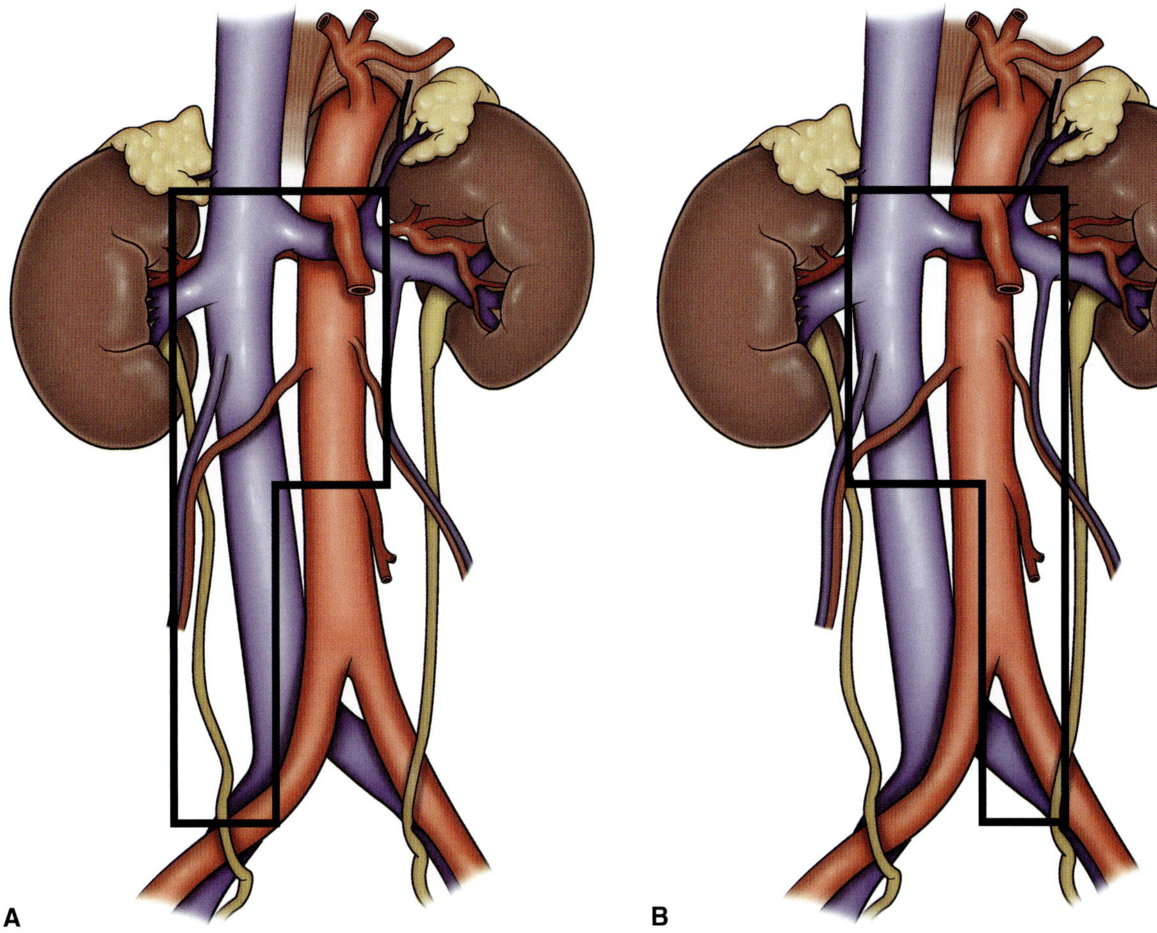

Chapter 78   Laparoscopic and Robotic-Assisted Retroperitoneal Lymphadenectomy for Testicular Tumors   1737

Fig. 78.4. Suggested templates for right (A) and left (B) therapeutic laparoscopic retroperitoneal lymph node dissection. These templates can be expanded or contracted based on each patient's tumor.

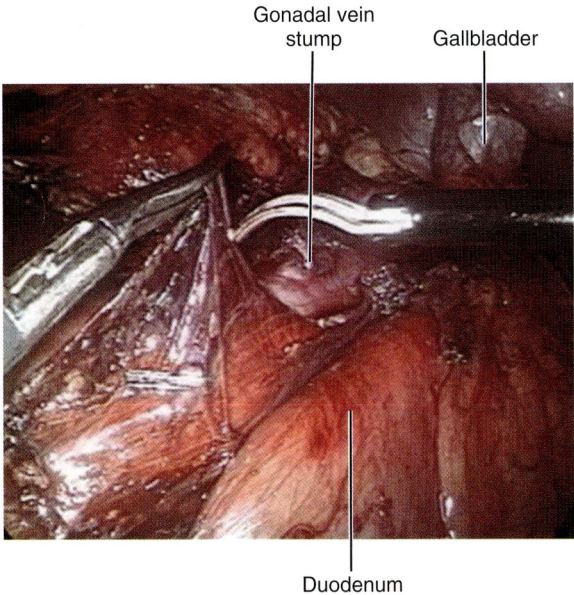

Fig. 78.5. Fibrofatty tissue overlying the inferior vena cava being incised to initiate the "split-and-roll" technique. The duodenum has been reflected medially, and the spermatic vein stump has been clipped and divided.

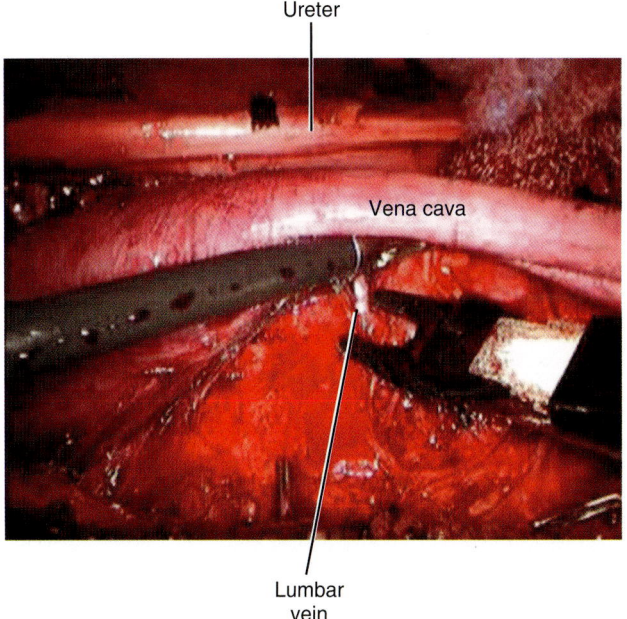

Fig. 78.6. The inferior vena cava is retracted to allow for lumbar vein ligation. Paracaval and precaval lymph nodes have been cleared.

Spermatic Cord Dissection

Analogous to what is done on the right side, the spermatic cord stump suture is identified after circumscribing the peritoneum at the inguinal ring. The spermatic vein along with adjacent lymph nodes is traced proximally to the renal vein and the artery to the aorta, where they are ligated and cut. The cord is placed in an endobag for removal at the conclusion of the procedure.

Lymphadenectomy

We advocate removal of the left common iliac, para-aortic, preaortic, interaortocaval, and medial paracaval lymph nodes (see Fig. 78.4). The dissection can be expanded as needed. Lumbar veins draining into the renal vein are clipped and divided to allow full dissection of the renal hilum. The vein is cleaned off medially to the junction of the vena cava. A paddle retractor in the lowest trocar aids in dissection. The renal artery is completely freed of all lymphatic tissues. Clips are generously used to avoid postoperative leakage of lymph. The tissues overlying the aorta are split from the renal hilum to the level of the inferior mesenteric artery. Care should be taken to identify the right spermatic artery to avoid avulsion. In contrast to the tissues overlying the vena cava, the preaortic space may include postganglionic sympathetic nerves; care must be taken to separate the nodal tissue while preserving these nerves (Fig. 78.7). The ureter and common iliac vessels are separated from all fibroadipose tissue. The preaortic tissues are rolled medially down to the lumbar arteries. The lumbar vessels are controlled and cut, allowing excision of the retroaortic lymph nodes. The vena cava is identified, and with use of a "split-and-roll" approach, the paracaval, precaval, and interaortocaval lymph nodes are removed in the same manner as for a right-sided dissection. Care should be taken to identify any right-sided renal arteries to avoid inadvertent ligation. In patients who have had chemotherapy, it may be necessary to ligate and transect the inferior mesenteric artery. If suspect nodes are detected, the node dissection can be expanded to perform a complete bilateral dissection; this can be performed from the same side using retraction.

At the conclusion of the operation, the lymph nodes are placed in an endobag and extracted. Each packet should be placed in a separate sac during dissection to help increase yield of nodal evaluation and count. The retroperitoneum is irrigated with warm water, and lymphostasis and hemostasis are ensured. The bowel and adjacent organs (liver, gallbladder, kidneys, ureters, pancreas, and spleen) are inspected carefully for injury. The trocar sites are closed with fascial sutures. A drain is not routinely used.

Bilateral Laparoscopic Retroperitoneal Lymph Node Dissection

Bilateral dissections may be performed when necessary and usually can be undertaken without a change in patient positioning. When the side of primary tumor is completed with the templates described, a small amount of tissue is left just medial to the contralateral ureter and inferiorly toward the common iliac vessels. These tissues are dissected free, and a bilateral dissection is completed. It is easier to approach a bilateral dissection from the right side.

Robotic-Assisted Retroperitoneal Lymph Node Dissection Port Placement and Technique

For RA-RPLND, we place the patient in a modified flank position, and the port locations are similar to the locations used in robotic renal surgery, with the ports shifted slightly caudally to assist in the iliac nodal dissection (Fig. 78.8). Use of the robotic fourth arm is preferred for improved retraction, leaving the surgeon two working instruments. The newer-generation robotic systems allow for improved multiquadrant access, facilitating wider dissection templates. One or two 12-mm assistant ports may be used, depending on surgeon preference. The general steps of the operation mirror the open and laparoscopic techniques. The robotic clip applier allows the surgeon to articulate the instrument while placing clips and can be particularly helpful in securing select lumbar vessels. Depending on body habitus, dissection of the spermatic cord to the orchiectomy suture may require re-docking of the robotic arms and triangulating them toward the inguinal ring for a more direct approach to this area, although this rarely is required.

An alternative technique has been described and entails placement of the patient supine and in a steep Trendelenburg supine position with the robot docking from the patient's head (de Cobelli et al., 2013). The ports are placed in positions similar to robotic-assisted radical prostatectomy, but the field of dissection is reversed (toward the head). This allows access to the entire retroperitoneum without changing patient position or challenging the limitations of the working envelope of the robotic arms (Stepanian et al., 2017).

POSTOPERATIVE CARE

Patients are extubated and transferred to the recovery area without nasogastric tube drainage. The patient may ambulate and resume

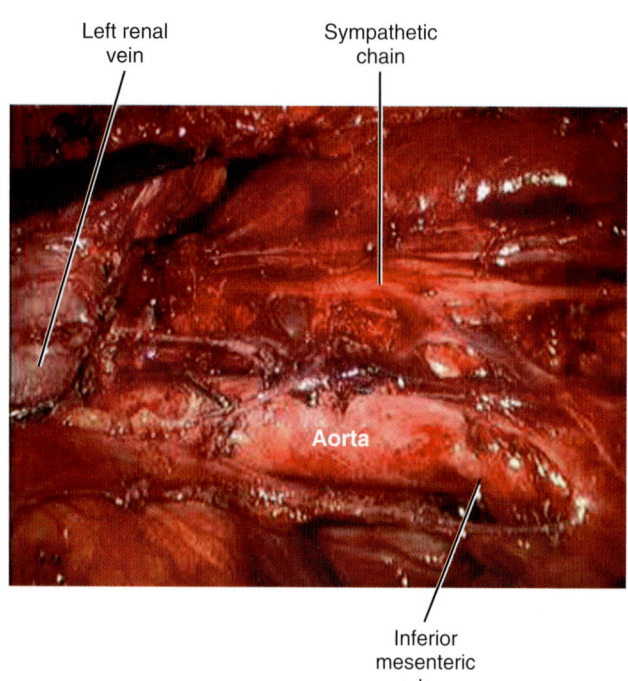

Fig. 78.7. The sympathetic chain and efferent nerves are seen spared, whereas para-aortic and preaortic lymph nodes have been removed.

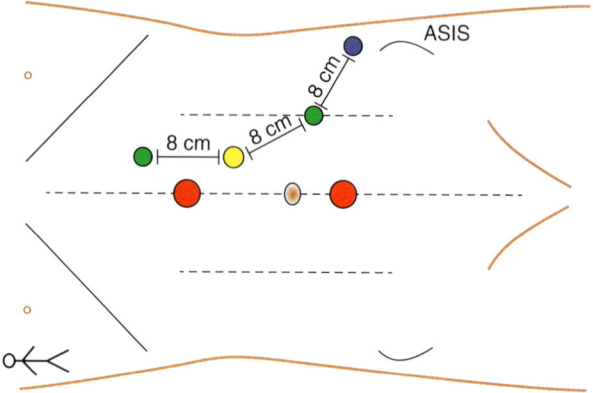

Fig. 78.8. Port placement for robotic-assisted retroperitoneal lymph node dissection. *Yellow* indicates camera port, *green* indicates 8-mm robotic ports, and *red* indicates 12-mm assistant ports. *ASIS*, Anterior superior iliac spine.

a liquid diet the night of surgery. **Postoperative tachycardia may occur secondary to sympathetic stimulation** (Bahnson et al., 1989). Most patients can be discharged on postoperative day 1. Some surgeons advocate consumption of a low-fat diet for 1 to 2 weeks postoperatively.

PROSPECTIVE NERVE-SPARING TECHNIQUES

As in open RPLND, nerve-sparing techniques involve prospectively identifying, dissecting, and preserving the sympathetic chains, hypogastric plexus, and postganglionic fibers. With experience, these tissues can be readily identified as more fibrous compared with lymphatic tissue. On the right side, the postganglionic sympathetic fibers are most easily identified behind the IVC as they cross anterior to the aorta to insert in the hypogastric plexus. Their takeoff from the sympathetic chains is always near lumbar veins, so great care should be taken when clipping lumbar vessels. On the left side, it is easiest to identify the postganglionic sympathetic nerves at the ganglia as they leave the sympathetic chain and dissect them prospectively as they course anterior to the aorta before joining the hypogastric plexus. Care should be taken to avoid energy sources such as electrocautery when dissecting nerve fibers (Abdel-Aziz et al., 2006; Bhayani et al., 2003; Peschel et al., 2002; Steiner et al., 2008).

COMPLICATIONS

The most common reason for conversion to an open procedure is uncontrollable bleeding, and vascular injury is cited as the most common intraoperative complication (Abdel-Aziz et al., 2006; Bhayani et al., 2003; Kenney and Tuerk, 2008; Neyer et al., 2007). Although bleeding and open conversion occurred frequently in older series, it is less common in more recent series. **In most contemporary series, the open conversion rate is less than 5%, but it has been reported to be as high as 11.8%** (Cresswell et al., 2008; Neyer et al., 2007; Nielsen et al., 2007; Rassweiler et al., 2000; Skolarus et al., 2008). **Conversion to an open procedure should never be viewed as a failure, and surgeons should be familiar with open RPLND should it be required.** Injury to major abdominal viscera also has been reported but appears to be a rare event (Kenney and Tuerk, 2008; Neyer et al., 2007).

Postoperative complication rates of 9% to 25% have been reported in contemporary series (Albqami and Janetschek, 2005; Cresswell et al., 2008; Neyer et al., 2007; Nielsen et al., 2007; Skolarus et al., 2008). Reported complications include chylous ascites, ileus, lymphocele, nerve injury, pulmonary embolus, *Clostridium difficile* colitis, retroperitoneal hematoma, and ureteral injury (Kenney and Tuerk, 2008). Retrograde ejaculation is a potential long-term source of morbidity for patients undergoing open RPLND and L-RPLND. **The rates of retrograde ejaculation have been consistently low with the laparoscopic approach and range from 0 to 14%** (Albqami and Janetschek, 2005; Cresswell et al., 2008; Neyer et al., 2007; Nielsen et al., 2007; Skolarus et al., 2008; Steiner et al., 2008). **With meticulous ligation of lymphatic channels, the incidence of chylous ascites should be less than 2%.** A summary of the morbidity of L-RPLND in the management of clinical stage I NSGCT is provided in Table 78.1. Although it is difficult to compare these data retrospectively with published open RPLND series, they appear to compare favorably. In one study of open primary RPLND, a 6% transfusion rate with a mean length of stay of 6 days was reported (Subramanian et al., 2010). Similar to L-RPLND, vascular injury was the most common intraoperative complication (4.5% of cases); 2 patients developed chylous ascites (1.8%) and 14 (12.5%) had an ileus. Antegrade ejaculation in this group of patients was 80%, and 7 patients (6.3%) required reoperation (for small bowel obstruction [2 patients], incisional hernia repair [4 patients], and ureteral reconstruction [1 patient]); 2 patients required nephrectomy, 1 for a dysplastic kidney and the other for oncologic reasons.

The morbidity and open conversion rate of L-RPLND after chemotherapy is higher and seems to depend on surgeon experience

TABLE 78.1 Perioperative and Morbidity Outcomes of L-RPLND for Clinical Stage I NSGCT

STUDY	NO. PATIENTS	OR TIME (MEAN, MIN)	OPEN CONVERSION	EBL (ML)	LENGTH OF STAY (DAYS)	MAJOR INTRAOPERATIVE COMPLICATIONS	MAJOR POSTOPERATIVE COMPLICATIONS	ANTEGRADE EJACULATION
Hyams et al., 2012	91	NA	4	200	2.1	7	2	87 (95.7%)
Steiner et al., 2008	42[a]	323	0	125	4.8	0	2 (lymphoceles)	36 (85.7%)
Skolarus et al., 2008	19	250	0	145	1.5	0	4 (lymphoceles)	23/26[b] (88.5%)
Cresswell et al., 2008	79	177	1	NR	6	1 (bleeding with open conversion)	7 (1 lymphocele, 5 ureteral stenosis/injury, 1 pulmonary embolus)	78 (98.7%)
Albqami and Janetschek, 2005	103	217	3	144	3.6	3 (bleeding with open conversion)	0	217 (100%)
Bhayani et al., 2003	29	258	2	389	2.6	2 (bleeding with open conversion)	2 (1 lymphocele, 1 compartment syndrome)	28 (96.6%)
LeBlanc et al., 2001	20	230	0	<50	1.2	0	0	20 (100%)

[a]Data include 21 patients with clinical stage II disease.
[b]Ejaculation data given only as percentage of all patients (included are 7 patients with nonclinical stage I disease).
EBL, Estimated blood loss; *L-RPLND*, laparoscopic retroperitoneal lymph node dissection; *NA*, not available; *NR*, not reported; *NSGCT*, nonseminomatous germ cell tumor; *OR*, operating room.

level as well. Early series cited major complication rates of more than 50% (Palese et al., 2002) and high conversion rates (Rassweiler et al., 1996). However, similar to primary L-RPLND, more recent series from experienced centers show improvement in these parameters (Permpongkosol et al., 2007; Steiner et al., 2004). Steiner et al. (2004) reported on 68 L-RPLND procedures performed after chemotherapy and reported no open conversions. In another more limited report including 17 patients who underwent L-RPLND after chemotherapy, the authors reported no complications, transfusions, or open conversions (Maldonado-Valadez et al., 2007). Studies report preservation of antegrade ejaculation with experience (Albqami and Janetschek, 2005; Corvin et al., 2005; LeBlanc et al., 2001).

RESULTS AND CURRENT STATUS

There are no randomized trials comparing open RPLND and L-RPLND. Retrospective assessments suggest that patients undergoing L-RPLND have a significantly shorter hospital stay, decreased blood loss, greater quality-of-life scores, and faster return to normal activities (Abdel-Aziz et al., 2006; Janetschek et al., 1996; Poulakis et al., 2006). Results of RA-RPLND are limited to early reports demonstrating feasibility. Early comparative data comparing RA-RPLND and L-RPLND suggest parity between these approaches in terms of safety, perioperative complications, and nodal yields (Harris et al., 2015; Tselos, 2018).

Laparoscopic Retroperitoneal Lymph Node Dissection for Clinical Stage I Disease

Published reports of L-RPLND with long-term follow-up suggest that it is an effective treatment option for patients with low-stage NSGCTs (Table 78.2). The staging accuracy of L-RPLND has been documented and consistent with open series in that 25% to 30% of men with clinical stage I NSGCT are found to harbor occult nodal disease. **A study with a mean follow-up of 7 years included 87 patients with clinical stage I disease and revealed a 9% and 0 relapse rate for patients with pN0 and pN+ disease, respectively, with all patients alive and free of disease at last follow-up** (Cresswell et al., 2008). The two retroperitoneal recurrences (2.5%) in this series occurred outside the dissection template, and all patients with pN+ disease were administered adjuvant chemotherapy. Examination of other large L-RPLND series confirms these findings, and recurrence rates and their patterns in this patient population are comparable with those of open RPLND series. The recurrence rate of patients found to have negative lymph nodes at L-RPLND is reported between 0 and 10%, which compares favorably with open RPLND series (Donohue et al., 1993; Hermans et al., 2000).

Despite the favorable long-term outcomes, the practice of universal chemotherapy in the adjuvant setting in patients with clinical stage I disease who are also harboring metastatic disease at L-RPLND has been the focus of critics who question the therapeutic efficacy of the technique. Approximately 70% of men found to have pN1 disease and who undergo a properly performed RPLND are cured and can avoid chemotherapy (Donohue et al., 1993; Rabbani et al., 2001; Richie and Kantoff, 1991). However, patients found to have pN1 disease can opt to receive two cycles of chemotherapy in the adjuvant setting with excellent long-term results rather than risk receiving three or four cycles of chemotherapy should they experience relapse. The decision to administer chemotherapy to patients with pN1 disease is a matter of preference and factors in the philosophy of the urologist and medical oncologist as well as the patient.

A report of 120 patients undergoing L-RPLND at one of four institutions in the United States included 10 patients with pathologic stage II disease who underwent surveillance (Nielsen et al., 2007). At a mean follow-up of 34.8 months, none of the patients had experienced a retroperitoneal recurrence. **Additional reports omitting chemotherapy for patients with pN1 disease who underwent L-RPLND support its therapeutic efficacy, but further studies and follow-up are required** (Nicolai et al., 2018; Skolarus et al., 2008; Steiner et al., 2008).

The adequacy of L-RPLND also can be evaluated by examining patients found to have pathologic stage I disease. If L-RPLND were inadequate, certain patients with pathologic stage II disease would be mislabeled as having pathologic stage I disease, and a retroperitoneal

TABLE 78.2 Oncologic Outcomes of Published L-RPLND Series for Patients With Clinical Stage I NSGCT

STUDY	NO. PATIENTS	FOLLOW-UP (MEAN, MONTHS)	NODE YIELD	N0/N+	NO. PN+ RECEIVING ADJUVANT CHEMOTHERAPY	NO. RECURRENCES[a]	DISEASE-FREE SURVIVAL
Hyams et al, 2012	91	38	26.1	N0: 63 N1: 21 N2: 7	21 (75%)	N0: (2 PU, 1 BC, 2 distant) N+: 0	100%
Steiner et al, 2008	21	17	22	N0: 16 N+: 5	0 (0%)	N0: 1 (PU) N+: 0	100%
Skolarus et al, 2008	19	23.7	23.8	N0: 13 N1: 6	5 (83.3%)	N0: 0 N+: 0	100%
Cresswell et al, 2008	79	84	14	N0: 60 N+: 19	19 (100%)	N0: 8 (3 PU, 2 RP, 1 PS, 1 BC) N+: 0	100%
Albqami and Janetschek, 2005	103	62	NR	N0: 77 N+: 26	26 (100%)	N0: 5 (3 PU, 1 RP, 1 BC) N+: 0	100%
Bhayani et al, 2003	29	72	20	N0: 17 N+: 12	10 (83.3%)	N0: 2 (PU, BC) N+: 1 (M)	100%
LeBlanc et al, 2001	20	15	9.8 (Rt) 17.7 (Lt)	N0: 14 N+: 6	6 (100%)	N0: 0 N+: 0	100%

[a]Recurrences: *BC*, isolated biochemical; *PS*, port site; *PU*, pulmonary; *RP*, retroperitoneal, outside of template.
L-RPLND, Laparoscopic retroperitoneal lymph node dissection; *Lt*, left; *NSGCT*, nonseminomatous germ cell tumor; *pN+*, histologically positive lymph nodes; *Rt*, right.

recurrence would result. This supposition has not occurred because no retroperitoneal recurrence has resulted in a series of therapeutic L-RPLND where a full dissection has been performed (Bhayani et al., 2003; Nielsen et al., 2007; Porter and Lange, 2003; Skolarus et al., 2008; Steiner et al., 2008). The therapeutic efficacy of L-RPLND will continue to be tested as more patients found to have pathologic stage II disease are choosing observation after this technique with good results (Nicolai et al., 2017).

Laparoscopic Retroperitoneal Lymph Node Dissection for Clinical Stage II

Fewer reports exist examining the role of L-RPLND for patients with clinical stage II NSGCTs as a primary modality or in the postchemotherapeutic setting. Data regarding the use of primary L-RPLND in patients with clinical stage IIA disease are limited. Several authors have reported on the use of L-RPLND in the postchemotherapeutic setting (see Table 78.2). Albqami and Janetschek (2005) reported their experience with 59 patients with stage IIB or IIC disease who underwent L-RPLND after chemotherapy: of the 43 patients with preoperative stage IIB disease with a mean follow-up of 53 months, one experienced a recurrence 24 months postoperatively along the external iliac nodes, outside the original template. Another group (Maldonado-Valadez et al., 2007) reported on 17 patients and demonstrated the feasibility of L-RPLND after chemotherapy: viable tumor was found in 3 patients, 2 of whom experienced retroperitoneal recurrences. Full bilateral RPLND, which is typically recommended in this setting, was not performed in these series (Stephenson and Sheinfeld, 2004).

Keeping in line with the goals of open RPLND performed after chemotherapy, Steiner et al. (2008) performed bilateral nerve-sparing L-RPLND on 19 postchemotherapy patients with stage IIB disease. The authors found teratoma in 4 patients, necrosis/fibrosis in 14 patients, and active tumor in 1 patient. This study included 2 patients with clinical stage IIA disease who underwent L-RPLND without adjuvant chemotherapy. No retroperitoneal recurrences were noted in either group at 17 months of follow-up.

SUMMARY

L-RPLND and RA-RPLND have been demonstrated to be feasible, safe, and effective treatment options for men with clinical stage I NSGCT when performed at large-volume institutions by experienced surgeons. These approaches have evolved into therapeutic operations duplicating the open procedure, with reports demonstrating efficacy and minimal morbidity. Data regarding these procedures for clinical stage II disease and for patients who have received chemotherapy are limited and associated with a longer learning curve.

KEY POINTS

- L-RPLND and RA-RPLND aim to decrease operative morbidity while duplicating the open approach.
- The most common reason for conversion to an open procedure is bleeding, although this is a rare complication (<5%).
- L-RPLND and RA-RPLND are effective treatment options for patients with low-stage NSGCTs.
- Reports omitting chemotherapy for patients with N1 disease who underwent L-RPLND and RA-RPLND support its therapeutic efficacy.
- Traditional centers of excellence should consider offering minimally invasive node dissection to provide patient-focused modern care.

SUGGESTED READINGS

Allaf ME, Bhayani SB, Link RE, et al: Laparoscopic retroperitoneal lymph node dissection: duplication of open technique, *Urology* 65:575–577, 2005.

Nicolai N, Tarabelloni N[2], Gasperoni F, et al: Laparoscopic retroperitoneal lymph node dissection for clinical stage I nonseminomatous germ cell tumors of the testis: safety and efficacy analyses at a high volume center, *J Urol* 199:741–747, 2018.

Nielsen ME, Lima G, Schaeffer EM, et al: Oncologic efficacy of laparoscopic RPLND in treatment of clinical stage I nonseminomatous germ cell testicular cancer, *Urology* 70:1168–1172, 2007.

Steiner H, Zangerl F, Stohr B, et al: Results of bilateral nerve sparing laparoscopic retroperitoneal lymph node dissection for testicular cancer, *J Urol* 180:1348–1352, discussion 1352–1353, 2008.

Stepanian S, Patel M, Porter J: Robot-assisted laparoscopic retroperitoneal lymph node dissection for testicular cancer: evolution of the technique, *Eur Urol* 70(4):661–667, 2017.

REFERENCES

The complete reference list is available online at ExpertConsult.com.

79 Tumors of the Penis

Curtis A. Pettaway, Sr., MD, Juanita M. Crook, MD, FRCPC, and Lance C. Pagliaro, MD

Cancers of the penis are uncommon tumors that are often devastating for the patient and frequently diagnostically and therapeutically challenging for the urologist. Although rare in North America and Europe, penile malignant neoplasms constitute a substantial health concern in many African, South American, and Asian countries.

Any discussion of penile cancers must begin by addressing premalignant and malignant tumors of the penis. A description of these lesions establishes their anatomic, etiologic, and histologic relationship to squamous cell carcinoma, which is the most common malignant tumor of the penis, as well as to other malignant neoplasms that involve the penis. Developments in the causes of various premalignant and malignant penile tumors are reviewed in this chapter.

In this chapter, we review the epidemiology, cause, and natural history of squamous carcinoma and its contemporary management. **Reports have confirmed the importance of pathologic stage and histologic features of the primary tumor as well as the presence and extent of lymph node metastasis in determining prognosis and treatment planning for penile squamous carcinoma** (McDougal, 1995; Pizzocaro et al., 1997; Ravi, 1993a; Slaton et al., 2001; Theodorescu et al., 1996). In addition, developments in staging of the disease, including novel imaging modalities and the use of dynamic sentinel node biopsy (DSNB), and modified surgical approaches to improve staging accuracy and reduce potential morbidities are presented. The selection of patients for organ-preserving surgical strategies is discussed.

The role of radiation therapy as a primary treatment and a palliative measure is reviewed. Contemporary developments in chemotherapy as well as in combination therapy with multiple therapeutic modalities are also discussed. A contemporary scheme for the management of the inguinal region, based on histologic and clinical features, is presented.

Finally, the various nonsquamous malignant neoplasms that may involve the penis are reviewed and discussed.

PREMALIGNANT CUTANEOUS LESIONS

Please see ExpertConsult.com for a discussion of premalignant cutaneous lesions (including eFig. 79.1) and virus-related dermatologic lesions.

Carcinoma in situ (Penile Intraepithelial Neoplasia)

Carcinoma in situ of the penis (penile intraepithelial neoplasia, also known as PEIN or PIN) has been well recognized since its first description by Queyrat in 1911. **Carcinoma in situ (CIS) of the penis is called *erythroplasia of Queyrat* (EQ) by urologists and dermatologists if it involves the glans penis and prepuce or Bowen disease (BD) if it involves the penile shaft or the remainder of the genitalia or perineal region.** Kopf and Bart described a third entity, bowenoid papulosis (BP), a condition having a histologic appearance similar to that of carcinoma in situ but a benign course, in 1977. These three lesions fall under the category of penile intraepithelial neoplasia (i.e., PeIN or PIN) but have distinct clinical presentations and characteristics (Porter et al., 2002). The incidence of HPV infection in two small series of penile dysplasia or carcinoma in situ was approximately 90% (Krusrup et al., 2009; Rubin et al., 2001).

More information about this topic is available online at ExpertConsult.com.

EQ originally described by Queyrat in 1911 consists of a red, velvety, well-marginated lesion of the glans penis or, less frequently, the prepuce of the uncircumcised man (Aragona et al., 1985). It may ulcerate and may be associated with discharge and pain. On histologic examination the normal mucosa is replaced by atypical hyperplastic cells characterized by disorientation, vacuolation, multiple hyperchromatic nuclei, and mitotic figures at all levels. The epithelial rete extends into the submucosa and appears elongated, broadened, and bulbous. The submucosa shows capillary proliferation and ectasia with a surrounding inflammatory infiltrate that is usually rich in plasma cells. These microscopic features distinguish EQ from chronic localized balanitis. Progression to invasive carcinoma can occur in 10% to 33% of patients (Bleeker et al., 2009; Buechner, 2002).

In 1912 Bowen described an intraepithelial neoplasm of the skin associated with a high occurrence of subsequent internal malignant disease as a distinct entity. BD, BP, and EQ are histologically similar (Graham and Helwig, 1973) (see eFig. 79.1C on ExpertConsult.com). All three lesions are characterized by the noninvasive changes of CIS. **Visceral malignant disease is not associated with EQ, and subsequent case-control studies have shown no association of BD with internal malignant tumors** (Anderson et al., 1973). Thus penile CIS does not warrant a specific search for internal malignant tumors.

BD is characterized by sharply defined plaques of scaly erythema on the penile shaft. Crusted or ulcerated variants can occur. The appearance can be confused with BP, nummular eczema, psoriasis, and superficial basal cell carcinoma. If it is not treated, then invasive carcinoma may arise in about 5% of patients (Buechner, 2002). **When all cases of CIS are considered, metastasis is extremely rare but has been reported** (Eng et al., 1995).

Treatment is based on proper histopathologic confirmation of malignancy with multiple biopsies of adequate depth to rule out invasion. When lesions are located on the foreskin, circumcision or excision with a 5-mm margin is adequate for local control (Bissada, 1992). In this regard, lesions on the glans penis are more difficult to treat by excisional strategies while maintaining normal penile anatomy. Recently several groups have described the technique of glans resurfacing for penile squamous carcinoma of the glans penis. In this technique the epithelium and subepithelial tissue of the glans penis are completely dissected off the underlying spongiosal tissue. The resulting defect is then closed with a skin graft. Early follow-up reveals very low rates of local recurrence (Hadway et al., 2006; Shabbir et al., 2011b). Alternative strategies include topical 5-fluorouracil cream (Goette, 1974; Graham and Helwig, 1973; Lewis and Bendl, 1971), 5% imiquimod cream (Danielson et al., 2003), and ablation with Nd:YAG (Frimberger et al., 2002a; Landthaler et al., 1986), potassium titanyl phosphate (KTP) 532-nm, or carbon dioxide lasers (Rosemberg and Fuller, 1980; Tietjen and Malek, 1998; van Bezooijen et al., 2001). Such strategies have been shown to produce excellent cosmetic and functional results. Historically radiation therapy has be used to treat tumors that were resistant to topical treatment, especially among patients who are not surgical candidates (Grabstald and Kelley, 1980; Kelley et al., 1974; Mazeron et al., 1984; McLean et al., 1993).

Information about kaposi sarcoma is available online at ExpertConsult.com.

> **KEY POINTS: VIRUS-RELATED DERMATOLOGIC LESIONS**
>
> - HPV infection among men is associated with penile carcinoma as well as with cervical dysplasia and carcinoma among female partners.
> - Imiquimod cream is now the standard topical treatment of choice for condyloma.
> - Giant condyloma of Buschke Lowenstein are locally progressive HPV-related tumors that are nonmetastatic but require complete excision and follow-up. The potential for co-existing or malignant degeneration to squamous carcinoma has been shown.
> - Penile carcinoma in situ (CIS) is an intraepithelial malignant process manifesting as three differing clinical entities, including bowenoid papulosis, Bowen disease, and erythroplasia of Queryrat.
>   - Bowenoid papulosis occurs on the shaft of young men in most cases and does not progress to invasive disease.
>   - Progression to invasive carcinoma in men with BD and EQ may occur in 5% to 33% of patients, respectively, if it is not treated.
>   - Metastasis has rarely occurred.
>   - Cancer eradication with organ-preserving strategies is the goal of therapy.
> - A diagnosis of penile Kaposi sarcoma is often associated with human herpesvirus 8 and should prompt an investigation into whether the patient is also infected with HIV or otherwise immunosuppressed.

SQUAMOUS CELL CARCINOMA

Invasive Carcinoma

Penile carcinoma accounts for 0.4% to 0.6% of all malignant neoplasms among men in the United States and Europe; it may represent up to 10% of malignant neoplasms in men in some Asian, African, and South American countries (Gloeckler-Ries et al., 1990). **Trends in penile cancer incidence have suggested differing patterns with decreasing rates in many countries, including Finland, the United States, India, and other Asian countries** (Frisch et al., 1995; Maiche, 1992; Yeole and Jussawalla, 1997). However more recently in Denmark, the Netherlands, and the United Kingdom rates have actually increased. In the latter countries increasing exposure to human papillomavirus and decreasing rates of childhood circumcision were suggested as potential factors (Arya et al., 2013; Baldur-Felskov et al., 2012; Graafland et al., 2011a).

Penile cancer is a disease of older men, with an abrupt increase in incidence in the sixth decade of life (Persky, 1977). In two studies the mean ages were 58 years (Gursel et al., 1973) and 55 years (Derrick et al., 1973). The tumor is not unusual in younger men; in one large series, 22% of patients were younger than 40 years and 7% were younger than 30 years (Dean, 1935); the disease has also been reported in children (Kini, 1944; Narasimharao et al., 1985). The Surveillance, Epidemiology, and End Results (SEER) database reveals the age standardized incidence rate of penile cancer between the years of 2000 and 2004 among US white, black, and Hispanic men to be 0.8, 0.9, and 1.1 per 100,000, respectively. However, this same rate was substantially higher among Puerto Rican Hispanic men at 2.8 per 100,000 (Colon-Lopez et al., 2012).

Two studies suggest that mortality in penile cancer may differ in part in relation to race and ethnicity. Rippentrop et al. (2004) found factors independently predictive of worsened survival in penile cancer to be higher stage at diagnosis, age older than 65 years, African-American ethnicity, and disease within lymph nodes. These researchers demonstrated a statistically significant disease-specific risk of death that was 2.2-fold higher in African-American patients than in white patients. Another more recent study using data from the Puerto Rico Cancer Registry and SEER data showed that when compared with US whites, US Hispanics, and African Americans, Puerto Rican men exhibited 1.8 to 3 times higher penile cancer mortality (Colon-Lopez et al., 2012). The reasons for these disparities are unknown but could include differences in cancer biology, health care access, or treatment. Such differences deserve further study.

Etiology

The incidence of carcinoma of the penis varies according to circumcision practice, hygienic standards, phimosis, number of sexual partners, HPV infection, exposure to tobacco products, and other factors (Barrasso et al., 1987; Maden et al., 1993; Maiche, 1992; Misra et al., 2004).

Neonatal circumcision has been well established as a prophylactic measure that virtually eliminates the occurrence of penile carcinoma because it eliminates the closed preputial environment where penile carcinoma develops. The chronic irritative effects of smegma, a byproduct of bacterial action on desquamated cells that are within the preputial sac, have been proposed as a causative agent. Although definitive evidence that human smegma itself is a carcinogen has not been established (Reddy and Baruah, 1963), its relationship to the development of penile carcinoma has been widely observed. Improper hygiene can lead to buildup of smegma beneath the preputial foreskin, with resulting inflammation. Healing by fibrosis leads to phimosis of the preputial skin, which tends to perpetuate the cycle. Phimosis is found in 25% to 75% of patients described in most large series. Reddy et al. (1984) studied the foreskins of 26 men undergoing circumcision because of phimosis and found epithelial atypia in one-third of the specimens.

Carcinoma of the penis is rare among the Jewish population, for whom neonatal circumcision is a universal practice (Licklider, 1961). Similarly, in the United States, where neonatal circumcision is widely practiced, penile cancer represents less than 1% of male malignant neoplasms. Among noncircumcising tribes of Africa and within Asian cultures in which circumcision is not practiced, penile cancer may amount to 10% to 20% of all male malignant neoplasms (Dodge, 1965; Narayana et al., 1982). Data from most large series show that penile cancer is rare among neonatally circumcised individuals but more frequent when circumcision is delayed until puberty (Frew et al., 1967; Gursel et al., 1973; Johnson et al., 1973). Adult circumcision appears to offer little or no protection from subsequent development of the disease (Maden et al., 1993). **These data suggest that the critical period of exposure to certain causative agents may have already occurred at puberty and certainly by adulthood, rendering later circumcision relatively ineffective as a prophylactic tool for penile cancer.**

Population-based data reveal that although neonatal circumcision is highly protective for invasive penile cancer, it does not afford the same level of protection for CIS. Schoen et al. (2000) evaluated the incidence of invasive penile cancer or CIS during a 10-year period and found only 2 cases of 89 (2.3%) occurring among neonatally circumcised men, whereas of 118 men with CIS, 16 cases were noted among 102 men who were circumcised at birth for an incidence of 15.7%. In consideration that the protective effects of circumcision on invasive penile cancer are likely to be mediated by avoidance of phimosis, it is noteworthy that another study associated phimosis with the development of invasive penile cancer but not CIS (Hung-fu et al., 2001).

Male circumcision has also been shown to be effective against HIV type 1 (HIV-1) infection. This effect was shown to be specific by Reynolds et al. (2004). There was no protective effect of circumcision for other sexually transmitted diseases, such as herpes simplex virus type 2 infection, syphilis, or gonorrhea.

HPV infection and exposure to tobacco products are associated with development of penile cancer. Epidemiologic data provided the first clues to a relationship between a sexually transmitted agent and cancer by demonstrating that the wives or ex-wives of men with penile cancer had a threefold higher risk of cervical carcinoma (Graham et al., 1979). Further investigation revealed that the male partners of women with cervical intraepithelial neoplasia had a significantly higher incidence of penile intraepithelial neoplasia

(Barrasso et al., 1987). These same male patients were also found to have a greater incidence of HPV infection.

Polymerase chain reaction and in situ hybridization have provided increased evidence for a causative role of HPV by identifying specific DNA sequences from different HPV types in primary penile lesions (malignant and benign) but not in normal foreskins (Iwasawa et al., 1993; Varma et al., 1991). More than 40 types of HPV infect genital sites. HPV types 6 and 11 are most commonly associated with nondysplastic lesions such as genital warts, but these are also noted in nonmetastatic verrucous carcinomas. In contrast, HPV types 16, 18, 31, 33, 45, 52, 58 are the more common types associated with in situ and invasive carcinomas (Petrosky et al., 2015). **HPV-16 appears to be the most frequently detected type in primary carcinomas and has also been detected in metastatic lesions** (Iwasawa et al., 1993; Varma et al., 1991; Wiener and Walther, 1995). As noted previously, the HPV genome encodes oncoprotein E6, which complexes with the tumor suppressor protein TP53, and oncoprotein E7, which binds the retinoblastoma (RB) protein, thus affecting cell cycle regulation (Griffiths and Mellon, 1999; Levi et al., 1998; Munger et al., 1989; zur Hausen, 1996) via the p14ARF/MDM2/p53 and p15INK4a/cyclin D/Rb pathways (Bleeker et al, 2009). Maden et al. (1993) **found that the incidence of HPV infection directly correlated with the number of lifetime sexual partners, which was also related to risk of penile cancer.** Another recent study found that HIV infection was a risk factor for HPV infection (Olesen et al., 2017).

Poblet et al. (1999) reported on two patients with coexisting HIV-1 and HPV infection and postulated that HIV-1 could synergize with HPV to increase the progression of HPV penile lesions into penile carcinoma. Although there is evidence supporting this effect in cervical and anal neoplasia, definitive proof for penile cancer awaits further study (Northfelt, 1994).

Although HPV infection is probably an important factor in the development of penile cancer, its presence is not invariable (31% to 63% of patients with penile carcinoma test positive) (Backes et al., 2009; Wiener and Walther, 1995), **indicating that additional factors may be involved in the development of the disease or its subtypes.** Additional evidence includes a study by Rubin et al. (2001) who noted that overall, 42% of penile carcinomas were HPV positive and varied by pathologic subtype. Only 34.9% and 33.3% of keratinizing and verrucous carcinomas, respectively, were positive, whereas 80% and 100% of basaloid and warty tumor subtypes, respectively, exhibited HPV DNA. Other non–HPV-dependent molecular events leading to penile carcinogenesis have been described, including silencing of the CDK2NA locus via promoter hypermethylation, the expression of genes that target the INK4a/ARF locus, other gene mutations affecting TP53, and p14ARF, and MDM2 overexpression (reviewed in Bleeker et al, 2009; Ferreux et al., 2003).

Four studies have shown a significant association between exposure to cigarette smoke and development of penile cancer (Daling et al., 1992; Harish and Ravi, 1995; Hellberg et al., 1987; Maden et al., 1993). Hellberg et al. (1987) studied the smoking history of 244 men with penile cancer and matched controls. They found a significantly increased odds ratio for penile cancer based on whether an individual had smoked, and the risk increased with the number of cigarettes smoked. This observation held even when the presence of phimosis was controlled. **Harish and Ravi (1995) extended these observations by showing that all forms of tobacco products, including cigarettes, chewing tobacco, and snuff, were significantly and independently related to the incidence of penile cancer subsequent to multivariate regression analysis.** It has been hypothesized that tobacco products can act in the presence of HPV infection or bacteria associated with chronic inflammation to promote malignant transformation. These same risk factors are also common to other anogenital carcinomas (Daling et al., 1992; Maden et al., 1993).

Penile trauma may be another risk factor for penile cancer. The development of carcinoma in the scarred penile shaft after mutilating circumcision has been reported as a distinct entity (Bissada et al., 1986). Furthermore, Maden et al. (1993) found a greater than threefold risk of penile cancer in men with penile tears and rashes. A case-control study also revealed an odds ratio of 18:1 for the development of penile cancer for those men reporting a penile injury 2 years before the onset of the disease (Hung-fu et al., 2001).

Lichen sclerosus (also known as balanitis xerotica obliterans) is a risk factor for the development of penile cancer. **Studies have shown the incidence of subsequent cancer with long-term follow-up to be between 2.3% and 9% of men with LS** (Depasquale et al., 2000; Micali et al., 2001). Velazquez and Cubilla (2003) studied LS occurring in association with penile cancer and noted its presence distinctly among the subset of penile carcinomas that were not associated with HPV.

Larger studies performed in areas where the disease is endemic, incorporating the many risk factors for penile cancer into a multivariate analysis, are clearly needed to define which factors independently confer risk. Thus far, no convincing evidence has been found linking penile cancer to other factors such as occupation, other venereal diseases (gonorrhea, syphilis, and herpes), marijuana use, or alcohol intake (Maden et al., 1993).

Prevention

The role of routine neonatal circumcision as a preventive strategy for penile cancer has been, to say the least, a controversial topic. The position of the American Academy of Pediatrics has changed over time with accumulating evidence from one of denial of any medical benefits (Schoen et al., 1989) to the more moderate position stating, **"There are potential medical benefits of newborn circumcision"** (Shapiro, 1999), to the most recent statement published in August 2012, which states, "Evaluation of current evidence indicates that the health benefits of newborn male circumcision outweigh the risks and that the procedure's benefits justify access to this procedure for families who choose it." Specific benefits in their data review included prevention of urinary tract infections, penile cancer, and transmission of sexually transmitted infections, including HIV (American Academy of Pediatrics Task Force on Circumcision, 2012).

Any argument against circumcision must consider that penile carcinoma represents the only neoplasm for which there exists a predictable and simple means of prophylaxis to spare the organ at risk (Dagher et al., 1973). Although circumcision can obviate the disease, especially where facilities for daily hygiene may be lacking, it may not be as important in countries where good hygiene is practiced. Frisch et al. (1995) reported a falling incidence of penile cancer (from 1.15 per 100,000 men to 0.82 per 100,000 men) in the Danish population, which has a circumcision rate of only 1.6%. They attributed this trend to improved hygiene because the incidence of dwellings having a bath facility increased from 35% in the 1940s to 90% in the 1990s. Thus considering the benefits of circumcision (including the prevention of infections, HIV infection and its transmission, and penile and cervical cancer), enhanced education about the potential benefits of circumcision, especially in developing countries, seems rational (Kinkade et al., 2005; Reynolds et al., 2004; Schoen et al., 1989).

Although neonatal circumcision and good hygiene to prevent the occurrence of phimosis represent important penile cancer prevention strategies, additional efforts to prevent malignant transformation include avoidance of HPV infection, and avoidance of tobacco products. Thus modifiable behaviors can potentially prevent penile cancer (Bleeker et al., 2009; Griffiths and Mellon, 1999; Harish and Ravi, 1995; Levi et al., 1998; Maden et al., 1993; Munger et al., 1989).

As mentioned previously, HPV vaccination should play an emerging role in the future with respect to preventing transmission of HPV between males and females and, potentially, penile cancer. Three prophylactic HPV vaccines are available (HPV 16/18 vaccine Cervarix [GlaxoSmithKline], the quadrivalent HPV 16/18/6/11 vaccine Gardasil, and Gardasil 9 HPV 16/18/6/11/31/33/45/52/58 [Merck Sharp & Dohme]), and the efficacy of preventing HPV infection among HPV-negative young women and men has been demonstrated (Bleeker et al., 2009; Block et al., 2006; Giuliano et al., 2011, Harper et al., 2004; Petrosky et al., 2015; Villa et al., 2005). Future efforts should focus on gaining more widespread use of such vaccines to prevent HPV-related disease.

> **KEY POINTS: EPIDEMIOLOGY, ETIOLOGY, AND PREVENTION**
>
> - Penile cancer is rare in developed countries and varies worldwide with age, circumcision, HPV exposure, and lifestyle/hygiene practices.
> - Recent epidemiologic data from the United States suggest a disparity in incidence and outcome of penile cancer for Puerto Rican Hispanic men.
> - Risk factors for development of penile cancer include lack of neonatal circumcision, phimosis, HPV infection, exposure to tobacco products, penile LS, and, potentially, penile trauma.
> - Penile cancer represents a preventable disease in most cases via neonatal circumcision, HPV vaccination, and/or behavior modification.

Natural History

Carcinoma of the penis usually begins with a small lesion that gradually extends to involve the entire glans, shaft, and corpora. The lesion may be papillary and exophytic or flat and ulcerative; if it is untreated, penile autoamputation may occur as a late result. The rates of growth of the papillary and ulcerative lesions are similar, but the flat, ulcerative tumor has a tendency toward earlier nodal metastasis and is associated with poorer 5-year survival rates (Dean, 1935; Marcial et al., 1962; Ornellas et al., 1994). Lesions larger than 5 cm (Beggs and Spratt, 1964) and those extending over 75% of the shaft (Staubitz et al., 1955) are also associated with an increased incidence of metastases and a decreased survival rate. However, others have not found a consistent relationship among lesion sizes, presence of metastases, and decreased survival (Ekstrom and Edsmyr, 1958; Puras et al., 1978).

Buck fascia acts as a temporary natural barrier to local extension of the tumor, protecting the corporeal bodies from invasion. Penetration of Buck fascia and the tunica albuginea permits invasion of the vascular corpora and establishes the potential for vascular dissemination.

The earliest route of dissemination from penile carcinoma is metastasis to the regional femoral and iliac nodes. A detailed description of lymphatic drainage of the penis is found elsewhere in this text and is well documented in the literature (Dewire and Lepor, 1992). Briefly, the lymphatics of the prepuce form a connecting network that joins with the lymphatics from the skin of the shaft. These tributaries drain into the superficial inguinal nodes (the nodes external to the fascia lata). The lymphatics of the glans join the lymphatics draining the corporeal bodies, and they form a collar of connecting channels at the base of the penis that drain by way of the superficial nodes. The superficial nodes drain to the deep inguinal nodes (those deep to the fascia lata). From there, drainage is to the pelvic nodes (external iliac, internal iliac, and obturator). Penile lymphangiographic studies demonstrate a consistent pattern of drainage that proceeds from superficial inguinal to deep inguinal to pelvic node sites without evidence of ipsilateral drainage (Cabanas, 1977, 1992). Multiple cross-connections exist at all levels of drainage so that penile lymphatic drainage is bilateral to both inguinal areas.

Metastatic enlargement of the regional nodes eventually leads to skin necrosis, chronic infection, and death from inanition, sepsis, or hemorrhage secondary to erosion into the femoral vessels. Clinically detectable distant metastatic lesions to the lung, liver, bone, or brain are uncommon and are reported to occur in 1% to 10% of patients in most large series (Beggs and Spratt, 1964; Derrick et al., 1973; Johnson et al., 1973; Kossow et al., 1973; Puras et al., 1978, reviewed in Pettaway et al., 2010; Staubitz et al., 1955). Such metastases usually occur late in the course of the disease after the local lesion has been treated. Distant metastases in the absence of regional node metastases are unusual.

Carcinoma of the penis is characterized by a relentless progressive course, causing death for the majority of untreated patients within 2 years (Beggs and Spratt, 1964; Derrick et al., 1973; Skinner et al., 1972). Rarely, long-term survival occurs, even with advanced local disease and regional node metastases (Beggs and Spratt, 1964; Furlong and Uhle, 1953). No report of spontaneous remission of carcinoma of the penis is known; 5% to 15% of patients have been reported to develop a second primary neoplasm (Beggs and Spratt, 1964; Buddington et al., 1963; Gursel et al., 1973), and one series reported secondary carcinoma in 17% of patients (Hubbell et al., 1988).

Modes of Presentation

Signs

It is the penile lesion itself that usually alerts the patient to the presence of penile cancer. The presentation ranges from a relatively subtle induration or small excrescence to a small papule, pustule, warty growth, or more luxuriant exophytic lesion. It may appear as a shallow erosion or as a deeply excavated ulcer with elevated or rolled-in edges. Phimosis may obscure a lesion and allow a tumor to progress silently. Eventually, erosion through the prepuce, foul preputial odor, and discharge with or without bleeding call attention to the disease.

Penile tumors may arise anywhere on the penis but occur most commonly on the glans (48%) and prepuce (21%). Other tumors involve the glans and prepuce (9%), the coronal sulcus (6%), or the shaft (<2%) (Sufrin and Huben, 1991). This distribution of lesions may be the result of constant exposure of the glans, coronal sulcus, and interior prepuce to irritants (e.g., smegma, HPV infection) within the preputial sac, whereas the shaft is relatively spared.

Rarely, a mass, ulceration, suppuration, or hemorrhage in the inguinal area may be caused by nodal metastases from a lesion concealed within a phimotic foreskin. Urinary retention or urethral fistula from local corporeal involvement is a rare presenting sign.

Symptoms

Pain does not develop in proportion to the extent of the local destructive process and usually is not a presenting complaint. Weakness, weight loss, fatigue, and systemic malaise occur secondary to chronic suppuration. On occasion, significant blood loss from the penile lesion, the nodal lesion, or both may occur. Because local disease and regional disease are usually far advanced by the time distant metastases occur, presenting symptoms referable to such metastases are rare.

Diagnosis

Delay

Patients with cancer of the penis, more than patients with other types of cancer, seem to delay seeking medical attention (Lynch and Krush, 1969). In large series, 15% to 50% of patients delayed medical care for more than a year (Buddington et al., 1963; Dean, 1935; Gursel et al., 1973; Hardner et al., 1972). Explanations include embarrassment, guilt, fear, ignorance, and personal neglect. This level of denial is substantial, given that the penis is observed and handled on a daily basis.

Delay on the part of the physician in initiating diagnosis and treatment may also be considerable. In some instances patients have been given prolonged courses of antibiotics or topical antifungal preparations before being referred for biopsy. Although some studies show that the difference in survival rates between patients with early presentation and those with later presentation is negligible (Ekstrom and Edsmyr, 1958; Johnson et al., 1973), other series show decreased survival with longer delay (Hardner et al., 1972). It appears logical that earlier diagnosis and treatment should improve outcome.

Examination

At presentation most lesions are confined to the penis (Derrick et al., 1973; Johnson et al., 1973; Skinner et al., 1972). The penile lesion is assessed with regard to size, location, fixation, and involvement of the corporeal bodies. Inspection of the base of the penis and scrotum is necessary to rule out extension into these areas. Rectal and bimanual examination provides information about perineal body involvement and presence of a pelvic mass. Careful bilateral palpation of the inguinal area for adenopathy is extremely important.

> **KEY POINTS: NATURAL HISTORY AND PRESENTATION**
>
> - Penile cancer often begins on the surface of the glans penis or in the preputial area, where it progressively enlarges.
> - Delay in seeking medical attention and then in subsequent definitive biopsy is common.
> - Examination of the penile primary tumor and the inguinal region is critical to treatment planning.
> - Metastasis occurs by embolization of tumor deposits from the penile tumor through penile lymphatics to the inguinal lymph nodes.
> - Distant metastases occur late in the history of the disease.

Biopsy

Confirmation of the diagnosis of carcinoma of the penis and assessment of the depth of invasion, the presence of vascular invasion, and the histologic grade of the lesion by microscopic examination of a biopsy specimen are mandatory before the initiation of any therapy. This provides insight into the therapeutic options for treatment of the primary lesion as well as the likelihood of nodal metastases in patients with no palpable adenopathy (Lopes et al., 1996; McDougal, 1995; Theodorescu et al., 1996).

Biopsy may be a separate procedure from definitive surgical treatment. A dorsal slit is frequently necessary to gain adequate exposure of the lesion for satisfactory biopsy. An alternative approach to treatment is biopsy with frozen-section confirmation followed by definitive resection or ablation. Velazquez et al. (2004) demonstrated the shortcomings of superficial diagnostic biopsies in a study evaluating specimens from 57 patients. There was difficulty in delineating the extent of depth in 91% of patients, discordance with the histologic grade in 30% of patients (specifically with verrucous and mixed histologic patterns), and failure to detect any cancer in 3.5% of patients with well-differentiated cancers. The importance of obtaining an adequate biopsy specimen cannot be overemphasized.

Histologic Features

Most tumors of the penis are squamous cell carcinomas demonstrating keratinization, epithelial pearl formation, and various degrees of mitotic activity. The normal rete pegs are disrupted. Invasive lesions penetrate the basement membrane and the surrounding structures. Subsequent to review of 61 cases from Memorial Sloan Kettering Cancer Center, Cubilla et al. (2001) classified the histologic types as follows: usual type, 59% of cases; papillary, 15%; basaloid, 10%; warty (condylomatous), 10%; verrucous, 3%; and sarcomatoid, 3%. Both of the basaloid and sarcomatous types were associated with aggressive behavior; 5 of 7 patients with these histologic patterns exhibited metastasis, and 5 of 8 (63%) died. In contrast, the verruciform histologic patterns were more favorable (1 patient with metastasis and no deaths). The typical squamous histologic type was intermediate in biologic potential; 14 of 26 patients exhibited metastases, and 13 of 36 (36%) died.

The basaloid variant, in addition to its aggressive behavior as noted previously, is associated with HPV expression in approximately 80% of cases (Cubilla et al., 1998, 2001; Gregoire et al., 1995; Rubin et al., 2001).

More recently HPV expression has been used to classify penile cancers into morphologically and molecularly distinct subtypes that include HPV-related (basaloid, warty, warty-basaloid, papillary basaloid, clear cell, lymphoepithelioma-like) and non–HPV-related (usual, verrucous, papillary [not otherwise specified], cuniculatum, pseudoglandular, pseudoglandularhyperplastic, adenosquamous, sarcomatoid). This new classification system has subsequently been adopted by the World Health Organization. The classification allows HPV-associated penile cancer to be recognized not only by the demonstration of p16, but also by its associated histologic features (Moch et al., 2016; Sanchez et al., 2015).

Squamous cell carcinomas have classically been graded using the Broders classification to define the level of differentiation on the basis of keratinization, nuclear pleomorphism, number of mitoses, and several other features (Broders, 1921; Lucia and Miller, 1992). This grading system was originally designed for squamous carcinoma of the skin and has been adapted by pathologists for penile squamous carcinoma. Four grades were originally described, but it is common for authors to modify this to a three-grade system by combining grades (Maiche et al., 1991). Low-grade lesions (grade 1 and grade 2) constitute 70% to 80% of the reported cases at diagnosis, whether a three- or four-grade system is used (Maiche et al., 1991). These well-differentiated lesions show cords of atypical squamous cells projecting downward from a hyperkeratotic epidermis. The lower-grade carcinomas typically demonstrate keratin, prominent intercellular bridges, and keratin pearls, characteristics that are absent in high-grade tumors. Almost half the tumors originating in the shaft are poorly differentiated (grade 3 and grade 4, depending on scale), whereas only 10% of tumors located in the prepuce are high-grade tumors (Maiche et al., 1991). Thus grade and stage are often correlated.

Several studies have emphasized the association of high-grade disease with regional nodal metastases (Fraley et al., 1989; Heyns et al., 1997; McDougal, 1995; Ravi, 1993a; Theodorescu et al., 1996). Overall, there is a significant body of agreement as to the histologic features that characterize high tumor grade (grade 3 and grade 4) and its correlation with nodal metastasis. However, as noted previously, most tumors are of lower grades. Histologic features that would better stratify the prognosis for patients with invasive, low- to intermediate-grade penile cancers would be of value for management of patients.

Slaton et al. (2001) found that describing the percentage of poorly differentiated cancer in the primary penile tumor specimen correlated with lymph node metastasis. In this study, a semiquantitative system that estimated the amount of high-grade cancer (i.e., ≤50% vs. >50%) was significantly associated with nodal metastases and was more predictive than the Broders three-grade system in stratifying those with or without nodal metastasis.

However, Chaux et al. (2009) questioned these findings as they examined 117 specimens among patients undergoing primary tumor therapy and lymph node dissection. More than 50% of the tumors were actually heterogeneous with respect to grade, and among these tumors any proportion of grade 3 cancer was associated with lymph node metastasis. These disparate findings point to at least three problems with respect to grading and prognosis, including (1) lack of a uniform system, (2) reproducibility of interpretation, and (3) intratumoral heterogeneity of tumor components.

Vascular invasion by tumor cells has significant prognostic importance but may not be specifically mentioned in pathology reports. When vascular invasion is present, it provides valuable information. Four studies have assessed its presence or absence, and it was an important predictor of nodal metastasis in all the reports (Fraley et al., 1989; Heyns et al., 1997; Lopes et al., 1996; Slaton et al., 2001). **Thus the pathologist should specifically comment on the presence or absence of vascular invasion in the surgical specimen.**

Perineural invasion was recently found to be present in 36% of cases analyzed in a multi-institutional data set of 134 patients and was a strong predictor of lymph node metastasis (Velazquez et al., 2008).

Laboratory Studies

The results of laboratory tests in patients with penile cancer are often normal. Anemia, leukocytosis, and hypoalbuminemia may be present in patients with chronic illness, malnutrition, and extensive

> **KEY POINTS: BIOPSY AND HISTOLOGIC FEATURES**
>
> - Adequate tumor biopsy is essential to diagnosis and treatment planning.
> - Squamous carcinoma histologic subtypes has recently been classified into two major groups by their relationship to HPV and show distinct morphologic features and clinical behavior.
> - Pathologic description of anatomic structures invaded (i.e., stage), the grade, and the status of vascular and perineural invasion provide important information to assess the risk of metastasis.

suppuration at the area of the primary and inguinal metastatic sites. Azotemia may develop secondary to urethral or ureteral obstruction.

Hypercalcemia without detectable osseous metastases has been associated with penile cancer (Anderson and Glenn, 1965; Rudd et al., 1972). In a review from Memorial Sloan Kettering Cancer Center (Sklaroff and Yagoda, 1982), 17 of 81 patients (20.9%) were hypercalcemic. Hypercalcemia seems to be largely a function of the bulk of the disease. It is often associated with inguinal metastases and may resolve after excision of involved inguinal nodes (Block et al., 1973). **Parathyroid hormone and related substances may be produced by tumor and metastases that activate osteoclastic bone resorption** (Malakoff and Schmidt, 1975). Medical treatment of hypercalcemia includes aggressive saline hydration to restore the extracellular fluid volume and to promote sodium and calcium excretion. The administration of diuretics is performed if volume overload is suspected. Bisphosphonates (e.g., pamidronate, etidronate, and zoledronic acid) have become first-line therapy because they possess demonstrated efficacy as antiresorptive agents and are relatively safer than mithramycin, an older agent (Morton and Lipton, 2000; Videtic et al., 1997). For severe hypercalcemia associated with neurologic manifestations, the antiresorptive bisphosphonates can be combined with an agent that produces calciuria, such as calcitonin, to rapidly lower serum calcium levels.

Radiologic Studies

Primary Penile Tumor. In patients with penile cancer the primary tumor and the inguinal lymph nodes are readily assessed by palpation. However, Horenblas et al. (1991) found that physical examination incorrectly established the actual pathologic stage in 26% of cases, with understaging in 10% and overstaging in 16%. It is clear that more accurate means of staging for penile tumors is needed.

Penile ultrasonography was performed on 16 patients referred for primary therapy by Horenblas et al. (1994). With use of a 7.5-MHz linear array small parts transducer they found that the ultrasound appearance of cancer was invariably hypoechoic. However, ultrasound examination often underestimated the thickness of tumors and could not delineate invasion into the subepithelial connective tissue of the glans penis from corpus spongiosum involvement (i.e., glanular stage T1 vs. glanular stage T2). However, the tunica albuginea separating the corpus cavernosum from the glans was easily identified in all patients, and the sensitivity for detecting corpus cavernosum invasion was 100%. This study confirmed the value of ultrasonography in assessing the primary tumor, as reported by others (Dorak et al., 1992; Yamashita and Ogawa, 1989).

Several studies have assessed the role of magnetic resonance imaging (MRI) in evaluating the normal penis and its involvement by cancer. Vapnek et al. (1992) described the MRI appearance of the normal corpus cavernosum, corpus spongiosum, tunica albuginea, and Buck fascia. Of six patients with urethral cancer, the disease was accurately staged in five (83%). De Kerviler et al. (1995) used gadolinium contrast-enhanced MRI to compare clinical and MRI findings with tumor pathologic stage. Clinical examination correctly staged six of nine tumors; MRI was correct in seven of nine cases but was not useful for clinical T1 lesions. Compared with MRI and ultrasonography, computed tomography (CT) has poor soft-tissue resolution and has not been useful for imaging the extent of the primary tumor (Vapnek et al., 1992).

Lont et al. (2003) directly compared physical examination with ultrasonography and MRI to assess their ability to determine the tumor stage. They evaluated 33 patients with penile squamous cell carcinoma, all of whom underwent ultrasound examination, MRI, and physical examination of the primary tumor. Findings were correlated with histologic evaluation of the specimens obtained at surgery with a focus on determining the invasion of the corpus cavernosum. The respective positive predictive value, sensitivity, and specificity for the study were as follows—physical examination: 100%, 86%, 100%; ultrasound examination: 67%, 57%, 91%; and MRI: 75%, 100%, 91%. This comparative study concluded that physical examination is reliable in determining corporeal invasion and that additional tests are mainly of value when physical examination cannot be properly performed.

The technique of artificial erection (by intracorporeal injection of prostaglandin E_1) may augment the use of contrast-enhanced MRI in staging of the primary tumor. A study by the European Institute of Oncology evaluated nine patients to compare clinical, pathologic, and MRI staging (Scardino et al., 2004). MRI aided by artificial erection and contrast enhancement was shown to be of value because it correlated with pathologic stage in eight of nine cases, whereas physical examination correlated with only five of nine cases. Another recent study from the UK supports these findings among a cohort of 100 men with penile cancer where the sensitivity and specificity of detecting tumor invasion of the tunica albuginea was 82% and 79%, respectively (Hanchanale et al., 2016). These data suggest that this novel MRI approach could be beneficial in staging of glanular tumors, specifically when physical examination findings are equivocal. **Thus, for small-volume glanular lesions, imaging studies add virtually no additional information to palpation in most patients. However, for lesions thought to invade the corpus cavernosum, contrast-enhanced MRI (perhaps augmented with artificial erection) may provide unique information, especially when physical examination findings are equivocal and organ-sparing techniques are being considered.**

Inguinal and Pelvic Region

Current Imaging Strategies Among Clinical Node-Negative Patients. The ability to noninvasively determine the presence or absence of inguinal and pelvic metastases in patients with penile cancer remains problematic because physical examination exhibits varying reliability based on the grade and stage of the primary tumor as well as body habitus of the patient. CT and MRI techniques have depended on lymph node enlargement for detection of metastases but are unable to define the internal architecture of normal-sized nodes. Because CT and MRI have similar accuracy in determining lymphadenopathy in other cancers, CT has often been the imaging modality chosen in penile cancer to examine the inguinal and pelvic areas as well as to rule out more distant metastases.

Horenblas et al. (1991) compared the ability of physical examination, CT, and lymphangiography to assess the inguinal region in patients who were surgically staged or had prolonged follow-up. In 102 patients with a 39% prevalence of positive nodes, the sensitivity and specificity of physical examination were 82% and 79%, respectively. CT and lymphangiography were performed in patients who were thought to have metastases. The sensitivity of lymphangiography was only 31%, but there were no false-positive results. Similarly, the sensitivity and specificity of CT were 36% and 100%, respectively. The combination of CT and lymphangiography performed simultaneously demonstrated equally poor sensitivity. Only one-fifth of patients had positive nodes detected with either test. **On the basis of these data the authors concluded that CT and lymphangiography offer no useful additional information over physical examination, especially in patients with no palpable adenopathy.** An important caveat is that CT may have a role in examination of the inguinal region in obese patients or in those who have had prior inguinal surgery, in whom the physical examination may be unreliable.

Insights in the field of nanoparticle technology have been applied to imaging of genitourinary malignant neoplasms to enhance detection of microscopic metastases. Ferumoxtran-10 particles (size, 35 nm), administered at a dose of 2.6 mg of iron per kilogram of body weight intravenously combined with MRI, were capable of imaging microscopic metastasis in lymph nodes that were less than or equal to 1 cm. Tabatabaei et al. (2005) evaluated lymphotropic nanoparticle-enhanced MRI (LNMRI) in seven patients with penile cancer who subsequently underwent groin dissection. Five of seven patients had no palpable adenopathy. LNMRI was highly sensitive and detected positive nodes in all five of these patients. The size range of the metastases was less than 1 cm in four patients. Unfortunately, no confirmatory studies were performed using this agent, and the compound is not currently available for routine use.

Squamous carcinoma was shown to take up the radiopharmaceutical fluorodeoxyglucose (FDG) and to be amenable to detection using combination positron emission tomography (PET) and CT. Scher et al. (2005) evaluated PET/CT among 13 patients with penile cancer who received injections of FDG. Five of the 13 patients had metastatic disease, and FDG-PET/CT detected it in 4 of them (80% sensitivity). However, in a follow-up study from the Netherlands, PET/CT was used in patients who were clinically node negative to determine the sensitivity among patients scheduled to undergo inguinal staging procedures. Among 5 patients with proven nodal metastasis, PET/CT was positive in only 1 (i.e., sensitivity of 20%) (Leijte et al., 2009a).

Among a similar cohort reported from this same group, ultrasound-guided needle aspiration was also shown to have limited sensitivity as well, detecting only 9 of 23 patients with proven metastases (sensitivity of 39%; Kroon et al., 2005a). Thus, among clinically node-negative patients, no current imaging modality has been shown to be sufficiently sensitive to detect microscopic metastases.

Current Imaging Strategies Among Clinical Node-Positive Patients. Recent data among patients with proven inguinal metastases suggest that additional imaging may be of value in determining those patients with advanced disease who may do poorly when treated with surgery alone or could in fact exhibit occult distant metastases.

Graafland et al. (2011) evaluated the CT scan findings among a cohort of biopsy-proven patients with metastatic inguinal adenopathy to define if scan parameters could determine those with poor prognostic features subsequent to lymphadenectomy. They found that central necrosis or an irregular nodal border was highly sensitive and specific for any of the poor prognostic features including three or more positive nodes, extranodal extension (ENE) of cancer, or positive pelvic nodes.

In contrast to the clinically node-negative disease setting, one study has shown the potential value of PET/CT among patients with proven inguinal metastases. Graafland et al. (2009) studied PET/CT among 18 patients with biopsy-proven inguinal metastases and found PET/CT to have a sensitivity and specificity of 91% and 100%, respectively, for detecting pelvic lymph node metastases. In that study, PET/CT also identified several patients with distant metastases that were unsuspected. Thus, if confirmed, PET/CT may become an important study for detecting pelvic and distant metastasis.

In general, distant metastases occur late in the course of the disease, usually in patients with recognized significant inguinal and pelvic adenopathy. The most common metastatic sites are the lung, bone, and liver. Currently, in addition to chest, abdominal, and pelvic CT, radionuclide bone scintigraphy may be indicated to stage the extent of disease in patients thought to have widespread metastases (Vapnek et al., 1992).

KEY POINTS: RADIOLOGIC STUDIES

- Soft-tissue detail of penile tumors is best imaged by MRI.
- Physical examination provides the most reliable staging information for small distal lesions.
- Penile MRI especially performed in combination with artificial erection may provide unique staging information when physical examination findings are equivocal.
- Physical examination of the inguinal region remains the clinical gold standard for evaluating the presence of metastasis in the nonobese patient.
- CT or MRI can be useful in evaluating the inguinal region of obese patients and in those who have had prior inguinal surgery.
- Among patients with proven inguinal metastases, CT scan of the abdomen and pelvis may help to determine those patients with poor prognostic features for cure with surgery alone.
- PET/CT may be useful among patients with clinically detected inguinal metastases to define the presence of pelvic or distant metastasis.

Penile Cancer Staging

Eighth Edition TNM Penile Staging System. The seventh edition of the American Joint Committee on Cancer (AJCC) and Union for International Cancer Control (UICC) TNM staging system was published in 2010 and was the consensus method for staging penile cancer (Edge et al., 2010) until the recent publication of the eighth edition TNM staging system (Table 79.1 and Fig. 79.2) (Pettaway et al., 2017). The eighth edition retains clinical and pathologic components

TABLE 79.1 Definition of Primary Tumor

T CATEGORY	T CRITERIA
TX	Primary tumor cannot be assessed
T0	No evidence of primary tumor
Tis	Carcinoma in situ (penile intraepithelial neoplasia)
Ta	Noninvasive localized squamous cell carcinoma
T1	Glans: Tumor invades lamina propria Foreskin: Tumor invades dermis, lamina propria, or dartos fascia Shaft: Tumor invades connective tissue between epidermis and corpora regardless of location All sites with or without lymphovascular invasion or perineural invasion and is or is not high grade
T1a	Tumor is without lymphovascular invasion or perineural invasion and is not high grade (i.e., grade 3 or sarcomatoid)
T1b	Tumor exhibits lymphovascular invasion and/or perineural invasion or is high grade (i.e., grade 3 or sarcomatoid)

TABLE 79.1 Definition of Primary Tumor—cont'd

T CATEGORY	T CRITERIA
T2	Tumor invades into corpus spongiosum (either glans or ventral shaft) with or without urethra invasion
T3	Tumor invades into corpora cavernosum (including tunica albuginea) with or without urethral invasion
T4	Tumor invades into adjacent structures (i.e., scrotum, prostate, pubic bone)

CLINICAL N (CN)

cN CATERGORY	cN CRITERIA
cNX	Regional lymph nodes cannot be assessed
cN0	No palpable or visibly enlarged inguinal lymph nodes
cN1	Palpable mobile or unilateral inguinal lymph node
cN2	Palpable mobile or bilateral inguinal lymph nodes
cN3	Palpable fixed inguinal nodal mass or pelvic lymphadenopathy unilateral or bilateral

PATHOLOGIC N (PN)

pN CATEGORY	pN CRITERIA
pNX	Lymph node metastasis cannot be established
pN0	No lymph node metastasis
pN1	≤2 unilateral inguinal metastases, no extranodal extension
pN2	≥3 unilateral inguinal metastases or bilateral metastases
pN3	Extranodal extension of lymph node metastases or pelvic lymph node metastases

DEFINITON OF DISTANCE MESTATSIS (M)

M CATEGORY	M CRITERIA
M0	No distant metastasis
M1	Distant metastasis present

AJCC PROGNOSTIC STATE GROUPS

WHEN T IS ...	AND N IS ...	AND M IS ...	THEN THE STAGE GROUP IS ...
Tis	N0	M0	0is
Ta	N0	M0	0a
T1a	N0	M0	I
T1b	N0	M0	IIA
T2	N0	M0	IIA
T3	N0	M0	IIB
T1-3	N1	M0	IIIA
T1-3	N2	M0	IIIB
T4	Any N	M0	IV
Any T	N3	M0	IV
Any T	Any N	M1	IV

Modified from Pettaway CA, Srigley JR, Brookland RK et al: Penis. In Amin MB, Edge SB, Greene FL, et al, editors: *AJCC cancer staging manual*, 8th ed, New York, 2017, Springer, pp 699–712.

for staging but further refines categories defined in the seventh edition. Table 79.2 provides changes incorporated into the eighth edition TNM staging based upon recent evidence (Pettaway et al., 2017).

Tumor Grading. Incorporation of the WHO/International Society of Urologic Pathology Grading System. Tumor grade has traditionally been based on modifications of the Broder's grading system and consists of either a 3- or 4-grade system, in which grade 1 means well differentiated, grade 2 means moderately differentiated, grade 3 means poorly differentiated, and grade 4 means undifferentiated (Cubilla et al., 2016; Edge et al., 2010). The World Health Organization (WHO) has recently adopted the 3-tiered WHO/International Society of Urological Pathology (ISUP) grading system. Using this classification any proportion of anaplastic cells is sufficient to categorize a tumor as grade 3 (Cubilla et al., 2016).

Definition of the Primary Tumor

Stage Ta Definition. In the seventh edition TNM category Ta referred to "non-invasive verrucous carcinoma." This term was misleading to some pathologists who thought this would apply to all cases of verrucous carcinoma. The great majority of verrucous carcinomas are destructive, but the invading front is smooth and pushing with the depth of invasion often difficult to assess. In the current classification, the Ta category is expanded and applies to (1) pure (well or completely sampled) verrucous carcinomas with no overt destructive invasion and (2) noninvasive papillary, warty, basaloid, or mixed carcinomas. These rare, noninvasive surface-based tumors are somewhat analogous to noninvasive (pTa) papillary urothelial neoplasms.

Stage T1 Definition: Anatomic Detail. In the seventh edition structures between the epidermis and the tunica albuginea were designated by the term "subepithelial connective tissue. In the eighth edition the specific layers are designated according to where the tumor is located (i.e., glans penis, foreskin, or shaft).

Stage T1 Definition: Inclusion of Perineural Invasion. Recent data have validated the seventh edition TNM primary tumor pathologic designations stage T1a and T1b as having different capacities for metastasis to inguinal nodes. In a series reported by Sun et al. (2015) including two cohorts, the incidence of inguinal metastases was 10.5% to 18.1% for pT1a tumors versus 33.3% to 50% for pT1b tumors. In addition to lymphovascular space involvement and high tumor grade, the presence of perineural invasion has also been shown to be significantly associated with inguinal lymph node metastasis and is now included as a criterion to define pT1b (Velazquez et al., 2008).

Stage T2-T4 Definition Changes. In the seventh edition TNM corpora spongiosum and cavernosum were grouped as T2 tumors. However, recent studies provide a justification for the separation of tumors invading the corpus spongiosum (CS) from those invading the corpora cavernosa (CC) as pT2 and pT3 tumors, respectively. In two cohorts invasion into the CS versus CC was associated with improved disease-specific survival (77.7% vs. 52.6%, respectively)

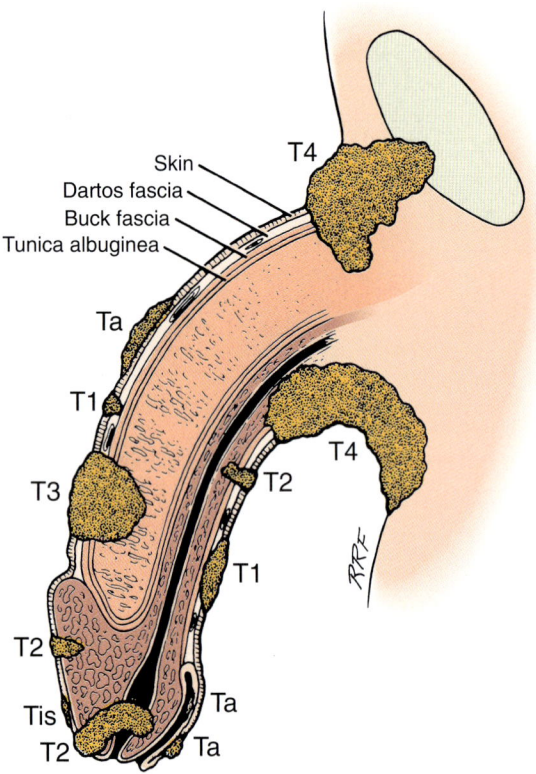

Fig. 79.2. Because treatment decisions for inguinal node dissections are based in part on the pathologic characteristics of the primary lesion (see section on treatment of inguinal nodes), determining the anatomic structure invaded is required. This diagram illustrates primary tumor (T) staging using the eighth edition TNM system.

TABLE 79.2 Eighth Edition American Joint Committee on Cancer: Summary of Penile Cancer Staging Revisions to the Seventh Edition

CHANGE	DETAILS OF CHANGE	LEVEL OF EVIDENCE
Histologic Grade (G)	The three-tiered World Health Organization (WHO)/International Society of Urological Pathology (ISUP) grading system has been adopted. Any proportion of anaplastic cells is sufficient to categorize a tumor as grade 3.	III
Definition of Primary Tumor (T)	Ta definition is now broadened to include noninvasive localized squamous carcinoma.	II
Definition of Primary Tumor (T)	T1a and T1b have been separated by an additional prognostic indicator (the presence or absence or perineural invasion).	III
Definition of Primary Tumor (T)	T1a or T1b are described by the site where they occur on the penis and are designated glans, foreskin, or shaft. Anatomic layers invaded are described for the three locations.	I
Definition of Primary Tumor (T)	T2 definition includes corpus spongiosum invasion.	II
Definition of Primary Tumor (T)	T3 definition now involves corpora cavernosum invasion.	II
Definition of Regional Lymph Nodes (N)	pN1 is defined as ≤2 unilateral inguinal metastases, no extranodal extension.	II
Definition of Regional Lymph Nodes (N)	pN2 is defined as ≥3 unilateral inguinal metastases or bilateral metastases.	II

Modified from Pettaway CA, Srigley JR, Brookland RK et al: Penis. In Amin MB, Edge SB, Greene FL, et al, editors: *AJCC cancer staging manual*, 8th ed, New York, 2017, Springer, pp 699–712.

and a lower incidence of inguinal lymph node metastasis (33%–35% vs. 48.6%–52.5%, respectively) (Leijte et al., 2008a; Sun et al, 2015). Urethral invasion previously designated as stage T3 does not appear to have prognostic significance independent of CS or CC involvement (Leijte et al., 2008) and had been removed from the eighth edition primary tumor staging.

Extensive tumors invading adjacent structures such as the scrotum, prostate, or pubic bone are designated as stage T4 and are less common but may require major amputative procedures, neoadjuvant chemotherapy before surgery, or palliative radiotherapy if unresectable.

Pathologic Stage N1-N2 Definitions. Recent series have suggested refinements to the seventh edition AJCC TNM lymph node definitions to better stratify the prognosis of patients with inguinal lymph node metastasis (Li et al., 2015; Sun et al., 2015). Data from Li et al. revealed that the 3-year disease-specific survival of patients with 1 to 2 unilateral inguinal metastases with no ENE as similar to patients with a single node of the same characteristics (89% to 90%). By migrating patients with 1 to 2 nodes into the pN1 category, this places more patients into a low-risk category and avoids the need for adjuvant chemotherapy recommended for pN2 patients according to the EAU guidelines (Hakenberg et al., 2015).

Alternatively, patients with more than 3 positive unilateral inguinal nodes or bilateral metastasis (pN2) have distinctly worse 3-year disease-specific survival compared with those with 2 or fewer unilateral inguinal nodes (60% pN2 vs. approximately 90% pN1) (Li et al., 2015).

Based upon two series the pN3 category remains defined as the presence of ENE or positive pelvic nodes. This group has an ominous 3-year cancer-specific or relapse-free survival ranging from 32% to 33% (Li et al., 2015; Zhu et al., 2011). In this scenario adjuvant chemotherapy is a strong consideration according to the EAU guidelines (Hakenberg et al., 2015).

Considering that the pathologic status of inguinal nodes is the driving factor determining survival, stage groupings (i.e., stage 0 to stage IV; see Table 79.1) in the eighth edition TNM use the extent of nodal involvement as the major consideration. Thus the strength of the unified AJCC-UICC eighth edition TNM system (2017) is that it provides not only an accurate assessment of the primary tumor based on clinical staging (examination, biopsy) but also clinical and improved pathologic descriptors of lymph node status to predict outcome.

In the TNM staging system the primary tumor stage is assigned by biopsy (or even more reliably by complete resection) and additional prognostic factors within the primary tumor now included in the TNM system (i.e., tumor grade, the presence of vascular or perineural invasion, corpora cavernosum involvement). In most cases, the presence of palpable adenopathy, along with the histologic features of the primary tumor, determines the need for additional imaging studies. Positive fine-needle aspiration of palpably enlarged inguinal nodes or fine-needle biopsy of pelvic adenopathy identified by CT can assist in assigning nodal stage before therapy. In patients requiring surgical staging (palpable lymph nodes or those with adverse primary tumor histologic features), pathologic nodal status assigned according to eighth edition TNM stage provides valuable prognostic information. The suggested diagnostic criteria for current TNM staging are listed in Table 79.3.

> **KEY POINTS: STAGING**
>
> - Clinical and pathologic factors related to the presence and extent of lymph node involvement determine survival and should be recorded.
> - The current, eighth edition unified TNM staging system represents a consensus document that includes clinical and pathologic descriptors that provide important prognostic information.

Differential Diagnosis

A number of penile lesions must be considered in the differential diagnosis of penile carcinoma. They include condyloma acuminatum, Buschke-Löwenstein tumor, and balanitis xerotica obliterans, as well as a number of infectious lesions (e.g., chancre, chancroid, herpes, lymphopathia venereum, granuloma inguinale, tuberculosis). These diseases can be identified by appropriate skin tests, tissue studies, serologic examinations, cultures, or specialized staining techniques.

SURGICAL MANAGEMENT OF THE PRIMARY TUMOR

Organ Preservation

Surgical amputation of the primary tumor remains the oncologic gold standard for rapid definitive treatment of the penile primary tumor; local recurrence rates range from 0 to 8% (de Kernion et al., 1973; Horenblas et al., 1992; McDougal et al., 1986). Whereas amputation is often necessary for bulky stage T2 to T4 tumors, it has been shown to decrease sexual quality of life (Opjordsmoen and Fossa, 1994). This is relevant because approximately 55% of penile cancer patients are 60 years of age or younger and 30% are 55 years of age or younger (Narayana et al., 1982).

It is generally accepted that patients with penile primary tumors exhibiting favorable histologic features (stages Tis, Ta, T1; grade 1 and grade 2 tumors) are at a lower risk for metastases. These patients are also best suited for organ-sparing or glans-sparing procedures (Solsona et al., 2004). The goal of treatment is to preserve glans sensation where possible or at least to maximize penile shaft length. Such approaches include topical treatments (5-fluorouracil or imiquimod cream for Tis only), radiation therapy, Mohs surgery, limited excision strategies, and laser ablation (Alnajjar et al., 2012; Crook et al., 2009; Minhas et al., 2005; Sanchez-Ortiz and Pettaway, 2003; Solsona et al., 2004). This section focuses on novel insights into surgical strategies to achieve organ preservation. Radiation-based strategies are discussed later in the section on radiation therapy for the primary lesion.

TABLE 79.3 Carcinoma of Penis: Suggested Diagnostic Procedures to Assign TNM Stage

PRIMARY TUMOR (T)
Clinical examination
Incisional-excisional biopsy of lesion (or complete resection) and histologic examination for grade, anatomic structure invaded, and presence of vascular or perineural invasion

REGIONAL AND JUXTAREGIONAL LYMPH NODES (N)
Clinical examination
CT, if inguinal adenopathy is palpable[a]
CT/PET may be considered for bulky inguinal adenopathy[b]
Superficial inguinal node dissection or dynamic sentinel node biopsy (as indicated for high grade, vascular or perineural invasion, or invasive histologic pattern)
Aspiration cytology (as indicated)

DISTANT METASTASES (M)
Clinical examination
Biochemical determinations (liver functions, calcium)
CT scan of the chest, abdomen, pelvis; bone scintigraphy; or CT/PET scan (as indicated)

CT, Computed tomography; *PET*, positron emission tomography.
[a]CT should also be performed in obese patients and those who have had prior inguinal surgery, whose physical examination findings may be unreliable.
[b]CT/PET scans coregistered to correlate uptake with anatomic location.

Circumcision and Limited Excision Strategies

Circumcision, limited excisions of the glans, and glans removal with sparing of the penile shaft represent surgical strategies to maintain function and penile length. Historically, data on circumcision and limited excision of glanular lesions have been associated with recurrence rates from 11% to 50% (McDougal et al., 1986; Skinner et al., 1972). However, the grade, size, and exact location of the lesion and the status of surgical margins were often unavailable in such reports.

Recent reports have suggested that conservative surgery may be performed safely in well-selected patients with discrete tumors by intraoperative frozen-section analysis (Bissada et al., 2003; Davis et al., 1999; Minhas et al., 2005; Pietrzak et al., 2004). In addition, several studies have challenged the dictum establishing that a 2-cm surgical margin is required for all patients undergoing partial penectomy (Agrawal et al., 2000; Hoffman et al., 1999). After performing a prospective histologic analysis of 64 penectomy specimens, Agrawal et al. (2000) concluded that tumor grade highly correlated with microscopic tumor spread. The maximum proximal histologic extent was 5 mm for grade 1 and grade 2 tumors and 10 mm for grade 3 tumors. Furthermore, "skip" lesions were not encountered. After performing a retrospective pathologic review of 12 penectomy specimens, Hoffman et al. (1999) also found 7 patients with disease of pathologic stage T1 or greater with microscopic margins measuring less than 10 mm. None of these patients had disease recurrence at a mean follow-up of 32.4 months. Pietrzak et al. (2004) documented the use of various techniques in a series of 39 patients to excise the tumor and to reconstruct or graft the glans and distal penis. With a mean follow-up of 16 months, only 1 patient (2.5%) who underwent a partial glans resection had a local recurrence. There were two early complications with grafts and two late complications with graft overgrowth intruding on the urethral meatus. Minhas et al. (2005) similarly performed either wide local excision or glans penis removal in 51 patients with margins of 0 to 10 mm in 48% and less than 2 cm in 98% of patients. With a median follow-up of 26 months, a local recurrence rate of 4% to 6% was noted. Limitations of this approach include proximal and distal deeply invasive tumors, high-grade tumors, and patients with poor health status who would not be candidates for salvage procedures if they experienced recurrence. A follow-up series from this same group that included 179 patients having undergone a variety of organ-sparing procedures including glansectomy, excisions, and distal corporectomy was recently reported (Philippou et al., 2012). With a mean follow-up of 43 months, the incidence of recurrence was 8.9% (16 patients). Local relapse did not affect disease-specific survival. These results seem to suggest that a 2-cm margin may not be necessary for small tumors of lower grade in the presence of a negative frozen section. However, patients managed with limited excision techniques should be considered to be at a higher risk for local recurrence until longer-term follow-up and additional surgical series are available.

Another recent technique used in the surgical management of carcinoma in situ of the glans penis is *glans resurfacing*, also known as *glans stripping*. In this technique, subdermal dissection of the skin and subepithelial connective tissue off the underlying corpora spongiosa is performed. Shabbir et al. (2011a) described this procedure in 25 patients with clinical carcinoma in situ of the glans; they performed either a total or partial removal of all the glans surface tissue. Positive surgical margins were noted in 48% of patients overall but in only 20% of those having total removal. At a mean of 29 months, 5 patients underwent re-excision for unexpected invasive disease at the margin. One of 25 patients exhibited a clinical recurrence. Topical therapy was used for isolated positive margins with CIS. Important considerations for this procedure are to document the absence of invasive cancer, to use topical therapy as an adjunct in the case of residual CIS at a margin, and to perform careful follow-up.

Mohs Micrographic Surgery

Mohs microsurgery has historically had a positive impact on the management of penile CIS and small, superficially invasive tumors. As originally described by Mohs et al. (1985), it involves layer-by-layer complete excision of the penile lesion in multiple sessions (fixed tissue technique), with microscopic examination of the undersurface of each layer. Its sequential microscopic guidance offers improved precision and control of the negative margin while maximizing organ preservation. In a series of 29 consecutive cases of penile squamous cell carcinoma, the primary tumor was eradicated in 23 (92%) of 25 patients available for follow-up. Local recurrences were highly associated with tumor size (3 cm), advanced stage, and failure of previous definitive therapy (Mohs et al., 1992). These excellent results using a fixed tissue technique have not been reproduced with the currently used frozen-section methodology. Shindel et al. (2007) treated 33 patients with stage Tis (26 patients), T1 (4 patients), T2 (7 patients), and T3 (4 patients) penile cancer. Five procedures were terminated with positive margins. Of 25 patients with mean follow-up of 58 months, 8 (32%) developed recurrence. However, 7 of 8 were retreated successfully with Mohs surgery. One patient who had progression of his disease died from it. **Thus Mohs microsurgery, as currently performed, may offer no additional benefit over surgical excision with intraoperative frozen-section assessment of margin status.**

Laser Ablation

The four most widely used laser energy sources are the CO_2, argon, Nd:YAG, and KTP lasers (Carpiniello et al., 1987; Malloy et al., 1988; von Eschenbach et al., 1991). Although the CO_2 laser has been widely used previously, the superficial depth of penetration (limited to 0.1 mm) makes it less than optimal for the treatment of penile CIS or small T1 tumors. When the CO_2 laser is used, local recurrence rates have been shown to be as high as 50% (Bandieramonte et al., 1988; van Bezooijen et al., 2001). Conversely, the Nd:YAG laser results in protein denaturation at a depth of up to 6 mm by emitting at a wavelength of 1060 nm. Overall recurrence rates after laser ablation have been reported to be 7.7% for penile CIS and have ranged from 10% to 25% for T1 lesions (Malloy et al., 1988; Tietjen and Malek, 1998; Windahl and Hellsten, 1995), but results from more contemporary series using the Nd:YAG laser exclusively have been more encouraging. **Frimberger et al. (2002a) treated 29 men with CIS and stage T1 tumors, combining Nd:YAG laser ablation with tumor base biopsies to ensure negative surgical margins. Only two recurrences (6.9%) were reported at a mean follow-up of 46.7 months, which is comparable to recurrence rates after partial penectomy.** In an effort to reduce the incidence of positive surgical margins, Frimberger et al. (2002b) have proposed the use of autofluorescence and 5-aminolevulinic acid–induced fluorescence for targeting of frozen-section biopsy specimens.

Laser ablation is feasible and may achieve results equivalent to those of extirpative surgery, especially when it is performed in well-selected patients in conjunction with frozen-section biopsies. In addition, laser ablation has been associated with high rates of resumption of sexual activity (75%) and overall satisfaction (78%) (Windahl et al., 2004). However, until additional long-term studies become available, laser ablation should be performed with the understanding that local recurrences may develop and that close surveillance and patient self-examination are necessary for early detection. Although well-selected patients who develop small recurrent lesions may be candidates for repeated laser ablation, recurrences are best treated with wide local excision or partial amputation.

Contemporary Penile Amputation

Penile amputation remains the standard therapy for patients with deeply invasive or high-grade cancers. **Partial (Video 79.1) or total penectomy should be considered in patients exhibiting adverse features for cure by organ-preservation strategies. These are consistently associated with tumors of size 4 cm or more, grade 3 lesions, and those invading deeply into the glans urethra or corpora cavernosa** (Gotsadze et al., 2000; Kiltie et al., 2000; Mohs et al., 1992). Because recurrence rates are higher with organ-preserving strategies, compliance with follow-up is also a consideration in

TABLE 79.4 Treatment of the Primary Penile Tumor

STAGE	TREATMENT
Tis (glans)	Laser therapy, glans resurfacing; alternative: topical therapy
Ta, Tis (foreskin, shaft skin)	Surgical excision to achieve negative margin; alternatives: laser therapy, topical therapy (Tis only)
Ta, T1 grade 1-3 (glans)	Therapy based on size and position of lesion as well as potential side effects, excision, glans resurfacing procedures, glansectomy, radiotherapy (not indicated for Ta)
Ta, Tl grade 1-3 (foreskin, shaft)	Complete surgical excision to achieve negative margin
T2 (glans) without gross cavernosum involvement	Total glansectomy with or without corpora cavernosa transection to achieve negative surgical margins, partial penectomy, radiotherapy
T2 (corporeal invasion), T3	Partial or total penectomy
T4 (adjacent structures)	Consider neoadjuvant chemotherapy with surgical consolidation for responding patients if baseline resectability is a concern
Local disease recurrence after conservative therapy	Complete surgical excision to achieve negative surgical margins; may require partial or total penectomy; select patients with superficial low-grade recurrences may be candidates for repeat penile-conserving procedure
Radiotherapy	Select patients with T1-T2 tumors involving glans, coronal sulcus <4 cm

recommending organ preservation versus amputation. Fortunately, the survival of most patients with recurrences that are detected and treated early is not adversely affected (Lont et al., 2006).

On the basis of contemporary results, organ preservation strategies should be discussed with patients exhibiting optimal tumor characteristics (stages Tis, Ta, T1; grade 1 and grade 2 tumors) to assist them in making informed decisions about therapy. (See Table 79.4 for treatment modalities for the primary penile tumor.)

> **KEY POINTS: SURGICAL TREATMENT OF THE PRIMARY TUMOR**
>
> - Patients with small lesions of low grade and stage (Tis, Ta, T1; grade 1 and grade 2) are the optimal candidates for organ preservation to maintain sexual quality of life.
> - The goals of organ preservation are to maintain glanular tissue for sensory purposes when possible and/or to maintain penile length when glans penis preservation is not possible.
> - Surgical modalities include limited excision strategies, Mohs surgery, and laser ablation.
> - Local recurrence rates overall after organ preservation are higher than with traditional amputation; however, when local recurrences are detected and treated, early survival does not appear to be adversely affected.
> - Amputation remains the standard for large or deeply invasive lesions, to gain rapid tumor control.

TREATMENT OF THE INGUINAL NODES

The presence and the extent of metastasis to the inguinal region are the most important prognostic factors for survival in patients with squamous penile cancer. These findings affect the prognosis of the disease more than do tumor grade, gross appearance, and morphologic or microscopic patterns of the primary tumor.

Unlike with many other genitourinary tumors, which mandate systemic therapeutic strategies once metastasis has occurred, lymphadenectomy alone can be curative and should be performed. The biology of squamous penile cancer is such that it exhibits a prolonged locoregional phase before distant dissemination, providing a rationale for the therapeutic value of lymphadenectomy.

However, because of the morbidity of traditional lymphadenectomy, especially among patients with clinically negative groins, contemporary controversial issues include (1) the selection of patients for lymphadenectomy versus careful observation; (2) the types of procedures to correctly stage the inguinal region with low morbidity; and (3) multimodal strategies to improve survival among patients with bulky inguinal metastases.

In this rare disease, prospective randomized trials have not been performed to answer many of these questions. However, with the use of retrospective and prospective clinicopathologic data from several centers, treatment strategies are presented using the available data.

Contemporary Indications for Inguinal Lymphadenectomy
Prognostic Significance of the Presence and Extent of Metastatic Disease

Table 79.5 reveals data collected from 24 surgical series during a 37-year period. Patients proved to have no evidence of inguinal metastases on the basis of histologic examination of the inguinal nodes or repeated normal examination findings over time; the average 5-year survival rate was 73% (46% to 100%). In patients with resected inguinal metastases the 5-year survival averaged 60% (0 to 86%), but this varied widely and was directly attributable to the extent of nodal metastasis (see Table 79.5). This point is illustrated in several series shown in Tables 79.5 and 79.6. Patients with minimal nodal metastases (usually two or less) exhibited 5-year survivals that ranged from 72% to 88% compared with 0 to 50% when a greater degree of nodal involvement was present (see Table 79.6).

The extent of cancer in a lymph node was also of prognostic significance. Ravi (1993a) noted ENE of cancer in lymph nodes 4 cm in size, and only 1 of 17 patients (6%) undergoing lymphadenectomy survived 5 years. Finally, pelvic lymph node involvement has been a particularly ominous finding with respect to long-term survival; the combined results of several small series reveal an average 5-year survival of 14% when pelvic nodal metastases are present (Table 79.7). Taken together, these data suggest that the pathologic criteria associated with long-term survival after attempted curative surgical resection of inguinal metastases (i.e., 80% 5-year survival) include minimal nodal disease (up to two involved nodes in most series), unilateral involvement, no evidence of ENE of cancer, and absence of pelvic nodal metastases.

Presence of Palpable Adenopathy as a Selection Factor for Inguinal Dissection

One can conclude from these data that it is advantageous to find and to treat nodal metastasis at the earliest possible opportunity. Data in Table 79.5 suggest that the presence of palpable adenopathy is associated with proven nodal metastasis in about 43% of cases on average (range 8% to 64%). In the remainder, lymph node enlargement is secondary to inflammation. Persistent adenopathy after treatment of the primary lesion and 4 to 6 weeks of antibiotic therapy is most often the consequence of metastatic disease. Similarly, the development of new adenopathy during follow-up is much more likely to be caused by tumor than inflammatory response. Thus historically a course of antibiotics was recommended for patients

TABLE 79.5 Carcinoma of the Penis: Prognostic Indicators for Survival

		CLINICAL AND PATHOLOGIC CHARACTERISTICS OF INGUINAL ADENOPATHY			5-YEAR SURVIVAL RATES (%)	
SERIES	NO. OF PATIENTS	PERCENTAGE WITH PALPABLE NODES	PERCENTAGE CLINICALLY FALSE POSITIVE (NODES PALPABLE, HISTOLOGIC FINDINGS NORMAL)	PERCENTAGE CLINICALLY FALSE NEGATIVE (NODES NONPALPABLE, HISTOLOGIC FINDINGS ABNORMAL)	INGUINAL NODES NEGATIVE[a]	INGUINAL NODES RESECTED AND POSITIVE[b]
Ekstrom and Edsmyer, 1958	229	33	48	—	80[c]	42
Beggs and Spratt, 1964	88	35	36	20	72.5	45
Thomas and Small, 1968	190	—	64	20	—	26
Edwards and Sawyers, 1968	77	—	—	0	68	25
Hanash et al., 1970	169	—	58[d]	2[d]	77[e]	—
Kuruvilla et al., 1971	153	39	63	10	69	33
Hardner et al., 1972	100	42	41[d]	16[d]	—	—
Gursel et al., 1973	64	53	60[d]	—	58	—
Skinner et al., 1972	34	29	40	—	75 / 87[f]	20 / 50[f]
de Kernion et al., 1973	48	54	38[d]	—	84[g]	55[g]
Derrick et al., 1973	87	29	52	—	53 / 76[f]	22 / 55[f]
Johnson et al., 1973	153	—	—	—	64.4	21.8
Kossow et al., 1973	100	51	49	25	—	—[h]
Puras et al., 1978	576	82	47	38[b]	89	67[i] / 29[j]
Cabanas, 1977	80	96	65	100	90	70[k] / 50[l] / 20[m]
Fossa et al., 1987	79	—	—	13	90	80[n] / 20[o]
Srinivas et al., 1987	199	63	14[p]	18	74	82[q] / 54[r] / 40[s] / 12[t]
McDougal et al., 1986	65	—	—	66	100	83[u] / 66[v] / 38[w]
Young et al., 1991	34	24	27	42	77	0

TABLE 79.5 Carcinoma of the Penis: Prognostic Indicators for Survival—cont'd

SERIES	NO. OF PATIENTS	CLINICAL AND PATHOLOGIC CHARACTERISTICS OF INGUINAL ADENOPATHY			5-YEAR SURVIVAL RATES (%)	
		PERCENTAGE WITH PALPABLE NODES	PERCENTAGE CLINICALLY FALSE POSITIVE (NODES PALPABLE, HISTOLOGIC FINDINGS NORMAL)	PERCENTAGE CLINICALLY FALSE NEGATIVE (NODES NONPALPABLE, HISTOLOGIC FINDINGS ABNORMAL)	INGUINAL NODES NEGATIVE[a]	INGUINAL NODES RESECTED AND POSITIVE[b]
Horenblas et al., 1993	110	36	26	40	100	38
Ravi, 1993a	201	53	8	16	95	81[x] 50[y] 86[z] 60[aa]
Ornellas et al., 1994	414	50	51[aa]	39	87	29
Theodorescu et al., 1996	40	70	35	—	46	45
Puras-Baez et al., 1995	272	—	—	—	89	38

[a]On histologic or repeated physical examination.
[b]On histologic examination of adenectomy specimen.
[c]Majority of patients received prophylactic or preoperative radiation therapy to inguinal area.
[d]Histologic classification based on node biopsy, not node dissection.
[e]Corrected 5-year survival (i.e., patients dying before 5 years without evidence of disease are excluded).
[f]Patients dying free of cancer before 5 years are considered surgical cures.
[g]Three-year survival.
[h]Omitted.
[i]Positive findings in inguinofemoral nodes.
[j]Positive findings in inguinofemoral and pelvic nodes.
[k]Single inguinal node with positive findings.
[l]More than one inguinal node with positive findings.
[m]Three-year survival with positive findings in inguinal and pelvic nodes.
[n]N1-2.
[o]N3.
[p]After antibiotic therapy.
[q]One node positive.
[r]One to six nodes positive.
[s]More than six nodes positive.
[t]Bilateral nodes positive.
[u]Adjunctive adenectomy.
[v]Immediate therapeutic adenectomy.
[w]Delayed therapeutic adenectomy.
[x]One to three positive nodes.
[y]More than three positive nodes.
[z]Unilateral.
[aa]Some lymph node dissection done without antibiotic pretreatment.

TABLE 79.6 Five-Year Survival (%) Related to Extent of Nodal Metastasis

SERIES	NO. OF PATIENTS	NO. OF POSITIVE NODES	
		≤2	>2
Fraley et al., 1989	31	88%	7%
Johnson and Lo, 1984a	22	85%[a]	13%
Srinivas et al., 1987	119	82%	20% 54%[b]
Graafland et al., 2010	152	73%	27%
Ravi, 1993b	21	81%[c]	50%[d]
Pandey et al., 2006	102	76%[c]	8%[e] 0%[f]

[a]Approximate.
[b]A subset with one to six positive nodes.
[c]One to three positive nodes.
[d]More than three positive nodes.
[e]Four to five positive lymph nodes.
[f]More than five positive lymph nodes.

TABLE 79.7 Five-Year Survival Related to Pelvic Node Metastases

AUTHOR	NO. OF PATIENTS WITH POSITIVE NODES	5-YEAR SURVIVAL NO. (%)
de Kernion et al., 1973	2	1 (50)
Horenblas et al., 1993	2	0 (0)
Srinivas et al., 1987	11	0 (0)
Pow-Sang et al., 1990	3	2 (66)
Kamat et al., 1993	6	2 (33)
Ravi, 1993a	30	0 (0)
Lopes et al., 2000	13	5 (38)
Lont et al., 2007	25	4 (16)
Zhu et al., 2008	16	1 (6)
TOTAL	108	15 (14)

with suspicious nodes to potentially discern metastasis from cancer (Srinivas et al., 1987).

However, several authors have raised the issue that this causes a significant delay and could affect survival, especially among patients who are likely to be truly positive because of the stage or grade of the primary tumor (Kroon et al., 2005b; Pettaway et al., 2007). An alternative approach for such patients is to perform fine-needle aspiration cytology of palpable nodes either at the time of or immediately after treatment of the primary tumor. In the case of a positive result, definite therapy can be planned without a 4- to 6-week delay. Saisorn et al. (2006) reported a 93% sensitivity and a 91% specificity in 16 patients with palpable adenopathy (mean size 1.47 cm) undergoing fine-needle aspiration before lymphadenectomy. The recommendation for this procedure among patients with palpable nodes was also incorporated in the European Association of Urology (EAU) Penile Cancer Guidelines. **Thus, although treatment of the primary tumor and a period of antibiotics are useful to help sterilize the inguinal region, this practice is no longer advocated as a tool to select patients who either should or should not undergo lymphadenectomy.** Should the fine-needle aspiration result be negative, depending on clinical suspicion, close observation, repeat aspiration, or excisional biopsy is performed because the false-negative rate of fine-needle aspiration cytology was 20% to 30% in two other, older series (Horenblas et al., 1991; Scappini et al., 1986).

Evolving Indications for Lymphadenectomy in Patients Without Palpable Adenopathy

Immediate Versus Delayed Surgery

Considering the value of early detection and treatment of metastasis, **should inguinal lymphadenectomy (ILND) be routinely performed in patients with clinically normal groin examination findings at the time of presentation of the primary lesion?** This was the most controversial issue in the management of patients with squamous penile cancer previously; however, the pendulum has moved toward earlier lymphadenectomy in selected patients with penile cancer. As noted, the cure rate with ILND when nodes are positive for malignancy may be as high as 80%. A cure rate of this magnitude with surgery in the face of regional nodal metastases parallels the urologist's experience with testicular cancer, in which retroperitoneal lymphadenectomy provides cure in many patients with minimal nodal metastasis. In contrast, for other common genitourinary malignant neoplasms—bladder, prostate, and kidney—surgical cure in the presence of regional nodal metastases is rare. Given that node dissection can cure metastatic penile cancer, why is there debate about whether the procedure should be performed, especially given that regional node dissections are often advocated in other malignant neoplasms when evidence of their efficacy is marginal at best?

Morbidity Versus Benefit

The reluctance to advocate automatic ilioinguinal lymphadenectomy (IILND) in all patients with penile cancer stems from the substantial morbidity the procedure can produce, as opposed to the relatively limited postoperative morbidity of pelvic or retroperitoneal lymphadenectomies. Early complications of phlebitis, pulmonary embolism, wound infection, flap necrosis, and permanent and disabling lymphedema of the scrotum and lower limbs were frequent after inguinal and ilioinguinal node dissections (Fraley et al., 1989; Johnson and Lo, 1984a; McDougal et al., 1986; Skinner et al., 1972). **Postoperative complications have been reduced by improved preoperative and postoperative care; advances in surgical technique; plastic surgical consultation for myocutaneous flap coverage; and preservation of the dermis, Scarpa fascia, and saphenous vein, as well as modification of the extent of the dissection** (Bevan-Thomas et al., 2002; Catalona, 1988; Coblentz and Theodorescu, 2002; Colberg et al., 1997; Nelson et al., 2004). In the University of Texas MD Anderson Cancer Center experience, the incidence and severity of lymphedema and skin edge necrosis were significantly decreased (Table 79.8; Fig. 79.3; Bevan-Thomas et al., 2002).

Furthermore, experience has suggested that lymphadenectomy in the setting of microscopic disease may be less likely to produce complications than node dissection in the presence of bulky nodal metastases (Coblentz and Theodorescu, 2002; Fraley et al., 1989; Ornellas et al., 1994). This is presumably because of the reduced amount of lymphatic tissue removed, preservation of venous drainage, and less blood supply compromised. Together these factors affect the viability of skin flaps and lymphatic flow.

Mortality after ILND has been reported in association with surgery performed concomitantly with penectomy and after palliative inguinal dissection. In both scenarios it was related to sepsis (Bevan-Thomas et al., 2002). An operative mortality of 3.3% was reported in earlier series (Beggs and Spratt, 1964). However, Johnson and Lo (1984a) and others (Coblentz and Theodorescu, 2002; Nelson et al., 2004; Ornellas et al., 1994; Ravi, 1993b) have reported no mortality in more recent series. Appropriate selection of patients along with routine preoperative antibiotic therapy and wound care to avoid septic complications has minimized this event.

Clearly, lymphadenectomy is not a trivial concern, even though morbidity appears to be decreasing. If a policy of routine lymphadenectomy were adopted in all patients with clinically negative lymph nodes, the average risk of false-negative examination findings (metastasis is actually present) would be approximately 29%, with wide-ranging variation (see Table 79.5). Stated another way, an average of 70% of patients could be subjected to the morbidity of ILND with no benefit. Potential reasons for false-negative examination findings include obesity, preexisting edema, and changes from prior therapy (radiation, inguinal surgery).

TABLE 79.8 Lymphadenectomy Complications in Four Surgical Series

	JOHNSON AND LO (1984b)	RAVI (1993b)	ORNELLAS ET AL. (1994)	BEVAN-THOMAS ET AL. (2002)
No. of dissections	101	405	200	106
Period	1948–1983	1962–1990	1972–1987	1989–1998
COMPLICATIONS (%)				
Skin edge necrosis	50	62	45	8[a]
Lymphedema	50	27	23	23[b]
Wound infection	14	17	15[c]	10
Seroma formation	16	7	6	10
Death	0	1.3	Not stated	1.8

[a]Significantly lower than in the three other reported series (all $P = 0.0001$).
[b]Significantly lower than in the series of Johnson and Lo ($P = 0.0001$).
[c]Incidence among 85 lymphadenectomies performed by Gibson-type incision.
Modified from Bevan-Thomas R, Slaton JW, Pettaway CA: Contemporary morbidity from lymphadenectomy for penile squamous cell carcinoma: the MD Anderson Cancer Center experience. *J Urol* 167:1638–1642, 2002.

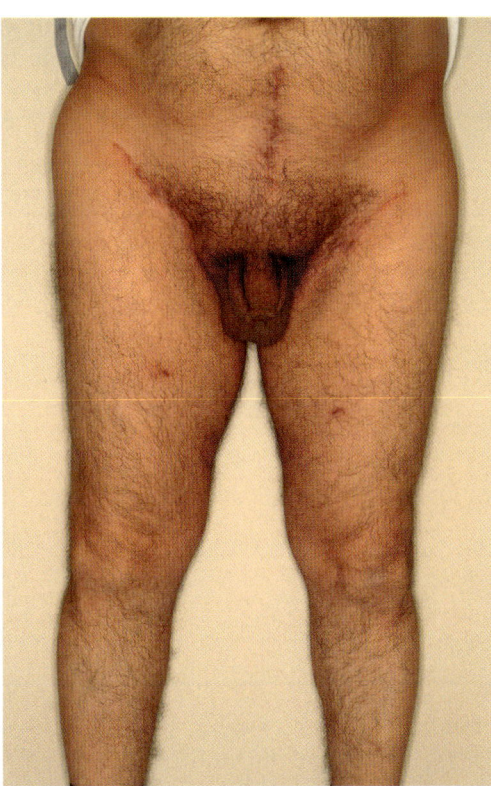

Fig. 79.3. Postoperative appearance after contemporary lymphadenectomy. The patient's status is after right ilioinguinal lymphadenectomy and left superficial inguinal dissection for stage T2N1M0 squamous penile cancer. Mild edema is visible on the left 10 months after surgery. Patient remains without disease at 9 years.

One alternative to immediate lymphadenectomy for all patients has been to observe patients with normal findings on inguinal examination. Lymphadenectomy is subsequently reserved for those patients who develop palpable lymph nodes. **The relevant question then becomes this: Can a delayed therapeutic dissection effectively salvage patients who have inguinal recurrence?**

Several studies have analyzed the survival of men undergoing early versus delayed lymphadenectomy according to pathologic evaluation of nodal status. McDougal et al. (1986) reported a series of 23 patients with invasive primary lesions and nonpalpable nodes; 9 patients were treated with immediate adjunctive lymph node dissection (6 had positive findings), and 14 were treated with surveillance and delayed lymph node dissection. The 5-year survival in the node-positive immediate adjunctive lymphadenectomy group was 83% (5 of 6 patients), whereas in the surveillance group the 5-year survival was 36% (5 of 14 patients). However, only 1 patient in the surveillance group had a node dissection. Presumably, the other 9 patients had progressed to inoperable local tumor or distant disease before presentation, emphasizing the role of careful, frequent follow-up and the difficulty of enforcing it. A third subset in this series had palpable nodes at presentation and had immediate therapeutic lymph node dissection, with 10 of 15 patients (66%) surviving 5 years (McDougal et al., 1986). The best results were from immediate adjunctive lymph node dissection (83%), with the next best from immediate therapeutic lymphadenectomy (66%). The worst results were from the surveillance and delayed lymphadenectomy group (36%), in whom dissection was delayed until palpable nodes developed. The interval of opportunity for cure in this third group appears to have been lost.

Similarly, Fraley et al. (1989) reported that immediate adjunctive lymphadenectomy resulted in a 5-year disease-free survival in 6 of 8 node-positive patients (75%) compared with 1 of 12 patients (8%) who had been observed and then treated with delayed lymphadenectomy when nodal enlargement occurred. Six other patients in that series also had unresectable adenopathy after initial surveillance, and all died of their disease. Although only 2 of 6 patients who had immediate lymphadenectomy had more than 2 positive nodes, all the patients treated by delayed lymph node dissection had 3 or more positive nodes.

Three other series suggest that early lymphadenectomy for varying degrees of "suspicious" or clinically positive nodes improves survival compared with the "surveillance" or delayed intervention approach in patients with clinically negative nodes (Johnson and Lo, 1984b; Kroon et al., 2005b; Ornellas et al., 1994). A series from the University of Texas MD Anderson Cancer Center compared 5-year disease-free survival of 14 patients undergoing early lymphadenectomy for clinically suspicious and histologically node-positive disease with that of 8 patients who were observed and later underwent lymphadenectomy when clinical nodal enlargement was undisputed (Johnson and Lo, 1984b). The primary tumors were of similar stage. The 5-year disease-free survival was 57% for early lymphadenectomy compared with 13% for delayed node dissection. The number of involved nodes in the immediate lymphadenectomy group (median, 2) was half that of the delayed lymphadenectomy group (median, 4), and no patient with more than 2 positive nodes survived more than 5 years.

Kroon et al. (2005b) from the Netherlands Cancer Institute compared survival of 20 patients found to have positive lymph nodes subsequent to prophylactic DSNB with that of 20 patients who underwent delayed inguinal dissection after proven nodal metastasis. The 3-year survival for patients detected during close surveillance was only 35% compared with 84% ($P = 0.0017$) for those undergoing early dissection. Pathologic evaluation of involved lymph nodes revealed ENE of cancer among 19 of 20 patients in the delayed group versus only 4 of 20 patients ($P = 0.001$) in the early group. Thus, despite careful follow-up, survival was adversely affected by the extent of cancer in involved lymph nodes.

A single large study from India disputes the magnitude of the value of early prophylactic dissection. Ravi (1993b) performed early prophylactic dissection in 113 patients with invasive penile cancer and compared the 5-year survival with that of 258 similarly staged patients who were initially observed. In the "early" group, 20 patients (18%) were found to have metastases, and all patients survived 5 years. The recurrence rate in the observed group was only 8% (21 patients). However, the 5-year survival in the patients who experienced recurrence was only 76% (compared with 100% in the early lymphadenectomy group). The enhanced survival of patients undergoing surveillance in India compared with other countries is probably attributable to patient selection factors, strict adherence to follow-up schedules, and aggressive treatment approach for recurrent disease (a combination of radiation and surgical resection) (Ravi, 1993a).

Thus six series reveal an improvement in survival for patients undergoing early therapeutic versus delayed therapeutic dissection. Furthermore, five of the six series show that delayed therapeutic dissection can rarely salvage patients who experience recurrence. Taken together, these data suggest that a policy of immediate adjunctive or early lymphadenectomy gives greater assurance that surgical intervention will occur when tumor volume is small (see Table 79.4) (Fossa et al., 1987; Fraley et al., 1989; Johnson and Lo, 1984a; Kroon et al., 2005b; Ravi, 1993b; Srinivas et al., 1987).

Impact of Primary Tumor Histologic Features on Predicting Occult Nodal Metastasis

Although early lymphadenectomy improves survival in patients with inguinal metastases, the challenge remains to identify those patients who are truly lymph node negative to avoid the morbidity of traditional lymphadenectomy. **Data gained from analysis of a variety of histopathologic variables within the primary penile tumor allow the classification of patients into higher and lower risk groups for lymph node metastasis** (Ficarra et al., 2006; Lopes et al., 1996; McDougal, 1995; Solsona et al., 2001; Theodorescu et al., 1996).

Patients with primary tumors exhibiting CIS or verrucous carcinoma have little or no risk for metastasis. Only 2 cases of metastasis in association with CIS have been reported, and none of 47 cases

TABLE 79.9 Penile Carcinoma: Corporeal Invasion and Incidence of Lymph Node Metastasis

STUDY	NO. OF PATIENTS	NO. OF POSITIVE NODES (%)	CLINICAL N STAGE
McDougal et al., 1986	23	11 (48)	N0
Fraley et al., 1989	29	26 (90)	N0
Theodorescu et al., 1996	18	12 (67)	N0
Villavicencio et al., 1997	37	14 (38)	N0
Lopes et al., 1996	44	28 (64)	NS
Heyns et al., 1997	32	15 (47)	NS
Solsona et al., 1992	42	27 (64)	NS

N, Node; NS, not specified.

TABLE 79.10 Penile Carcinoma: Incidence of Nodal Metastasis for Stage T1, Grade 1, and Grade 2 Primary Tumors

AUTHOR	STAGE AND GRADE	NO. OF PATIENTS	NO. OF PATIENTS WITH METASTASIS (%)
Theodorescu et al., 1996	T1, G1	8	2 (25)
Solsona et al., 1992	T1, G1	19	0 (0)
McDougal, 1995	T1, G1-G2	24	1 (4)
Heyns et al., 1997	T1, G1-G2	9	1 (11)
Hungerhuber et al., 2006	T1, G1-G2	13	1 (8)
TOTAL		73	5 (7)
Solsona et al., 1992	T1, G2	4	1 (25)
Solsona et al., 2001	T1, G2	4	1 (25)
Naumann et al., 2008[a]	T1, G2	16	7 (44)
Hughes et al., 2010	T1, G2	105	9 (9)
TOTAL		129	18 (14)

[a]Five tumors in node-positive group had lymphatic or venous invasion.

of penile verrucous carcinoma have been shown to metastasize (Avrach and Christensen, 1976; Eng et al., 1995; Johnson et al., 1985; Seixas et al., 1994). Thus patients with both Tis and Ta penile cancer are included in the low-risk group for inguinal metastases (Solsona et al., 2001, 2004).

In contrast, patients with corporeal invasion (stage pT2) in the penile tumor exhibit a high risk for metastasis. The average risk for inguinal metastasis among 225 patients in 7 different series was 59% (Table 79.9). **The risk for metastasis among patients exhibiting corporeal invasion was similar regardless of whether palpable adenopathy was present.**

Stage T1 penile cancers exhibit involvement of the subepithelial connective tissue only and lack involvement of the corpus spongiosum, corpora cavernosa, or urethra (Edge et al., 2010). Similarly staged tumors historically have been associated with a 4% to 14% incidence of nodal metastasis (Hall et al, 1998; Solsona et al., 1992; Villavicencio et al., 1997). Theodorescu et al. (1996) noted one exception to this relatively low rate of metastatic disease; 58% of patients (14 of 24) with pT1 primary tumors and initially negative nodes on clinical assessment subsequently developed inguinal nodal metastases. These data suggest that other variables present within the penile cancers of the cohort of patients studied (i.e., tumor grade and presence of vascular invasion) may have modified the effect of tumor stage on metastasis.

Several authors have evaluated the risk of nodal metastasis for stage T1 lesions according to tumor grade (Table 79.10). Among 73 patients with T1 grade 1 or grade 2 primary tumors, metastasis occurred in only 5 patients (7%). Recent data from Naumann et al. (2008), however, suggested that among T1 grade 2 tumors specifically, the risk of metastases could be higher than previously described. Among four series reporting specifically on the T1 grade 2 subset, in 129 initially node-negative patients, metastases occurred in 18 (14%) (see Table 79.8). However, 5 patients in this subset also exhibited either lymphatic or venous invasion (an adverse prognostic feature, see later). Ficarra et al. (2006) developed the first penile cancer nomogram using data from 175 patients. Based on tumor thickness and growth pattern, patients with T1 grade 2 tumors exhibited metastatic rates of 5% to 20%. Thus grade 2 tumors represent a heterogeneous group in which the histologic criteria used to describe grade 2 and the presence or absence of other poor prognostic features ultimately determine prognosis (Cubilla, 2009). In this regard the EAU guidelines assigned patients with T1 grade 2 tumors to the intermediate-risk category in which the risk of lymph node metastasis is greater than 16% (low risk) and less than 68% (high risk) (Pizzocaro et al., 2010; Solsona et al., 2004).

The presence of vascular invasion as a prognostic indicator of inguinal lymph node metastasis in squamous penile cancer is now evident (Ficarra et al., 2005; Fraley et al., 1989; Heyns et al., 1997; Lopes et al., 1996; Slaton et al., 2001). Lopes et al. (1996) studied the prognostic value of lymphatic invasion in 146 patients with penile cancer. In a univariate analysis, clinical nodal stage, tumor thickness, lymphatic and venous embolization, and urethral infiltration were associated with lymph node metastasis. However, subsequent to multivariate analysis, only venous and lymphatic invasion remained significant predictors for positive lymph nodes. Data from the University of Texas MD Anderson Cancer Center revealed that vascular invasion was absent in all patients with T1 tumors (Slaton et al., 2001). These patients were also lymph node negative at surgery. In contrast, patients with stage pT2 primary tumors exhibited nodal metastasis in 75% of cases (15 of 20) when vascular invasion was present but in only 25% of cases (3 of 12) when it was absent.

Ficarra et al. (2005, 2006) developed a nomogram predicting inguinal lymph node involvement including the variables of tumor thickness, growth pattern, grade, venous or lymphatic invasion, corpus spongiosum or cavernosum involvement, urethral involvement, and palpable lymph nodes. The most important variables were venous or lymphatic invasion and the presence of palpable nodes in multivariate analysis. The concordance index of the nomogram was very good at 0.876. Zhu et al. (2010) also developed a nomogram to predict inguinal lymph node metastasis among 110 patients with clinically negative lymph nodes from 1990 to 2008. The variables included in their model were T stage, grade, lymphovascular invasion (LVI), and tumor p53 expression. Similar to Ficarra et al. LVI was the only variable that showed independent prognostic value. This nomogram exhibited a concordance index of 0.79 and actually provided superior ability to stratify patients when compared with the European Association of Urology risk classification system. However, neither of these nomograms has been externally validated, and they are not in routine use. This is likely due to the complexity of the nomogram variables included.

The presence of perineural invasion (Velazquez et al., 2008) and the microscopic front pattern of invasion (Guimares et al., 2006) have also been shown in recent studies to provide independent information with which to stratify a patient's risk of lymph node metastasis. In

TABLE 79.11 Prognostic Molecular Markers of Lymph Node Status and Survival in Penile Cancer: Current Status

MARKER	ROLE	LYMPH NODE STATUS	SURVIVAL
Human papillomavirus (HPV) p16^{INK4a}	High-risk (HR) types affect TP53 and RB function. Increased expression with HR-HPV	Contradictory studies	Increased survival[a]. Increased survival, decreased recurrence[b]
TP53	Altered or mutated expression, increased proliferation, altered apoptosis, dedifferentiation	Preliminary data correlated with increased metastasis	Correlated with decreased survival[c]
CDKN2A	Inhibits RB function, enhancing proliferation	Not established	Not established
Squamous cell carcinoma antigen (TA-4)	Serum marker function unknown	Correlates with grossly evident metastases	No role
Ki-67	Nuclear protein associated with cycling cells	Predicts increased risk	No role
E-cadherin	Epithelial cell adhesion molecule lost in progression	Low expression associated with nodal metastasis	Low expression predicts worse survival
MMP-9	Matrix metalloproteinase family facilitates invasion	No role	High expression predicts recurrence

RB, Retinoblastoma.
Modified from Muneer A, Kayes O, Ahmed HU, et al.: Molecular prognostic factors in penile cancer. *World J Urol* 27:161–167, 2009. With additional references below:
[a]Djajadiningrat RS, Jordanova ES, Kroon BK, et al.: Human papillomavirus prevalence in invasive penile cancer and association with clinical outcome. *J Urol* 193:526–531, 2015.
[b]Gunia S, Erbersdobler A, Hakenberg OW, et al.: p16(INK4a) is a marker of good prognosis for primary invasive penile squamous cell carcinoma: a multi-institutional study. *J Urol* 187(3):899–907, 2012.
[c]Ferrandiz-Pulido C, Masferrer E, Toll A, et al.: mTOR signaling pathway in penile squamous cell carcinoma: pmTOR and peIF4E over expression correlate with aggressive tumor behavior. *J Urol* 190 (6):2288–2295, 2013.

fact the variable perineural invasion is has now been added to the eighth edition TNM staging system (Pettaway et al., 2017).

Molecular Prognostic Markers

Analysis of gene expression in penile cancer will likely have future practical implications with respect to the prediction of lymph node metastasis or survival. A review by Muneer et al. (2009) described the status of several genes evaluated in tissue or serum that could have future prognostic implications with respect to predicting lymph node status or survival (Table 79.11).

Several genetic pathways have been associated with the development of SCC of the penis, including p16 and p53 (Poetsch et al., 2011, Yanagawa et al., 2008).

The p16 gene encodes the protein p16INK4A, and increased expression of this protein has been seen as a late event after HPV infection and causes inactivation of the cell cycle cascade. In cervical carcinoma, increased expression of p16INK4A has been associated with malignant transformation in HPV-positive cancers (Doorbar, 2006).

The tumor suppressor gene p53 encodes a transcription factor that normally blocks cell cycle progression. When altered by deletion or mutation, it results in a loss of inhibition and malignant growth. Further characterizations of the mechanisms involved are needed.

Recently other pathways involved in penile cancer progression and correlated with adverse outcomes include epithelial-mesenchymal transition (with molecular markers such as increased expression of vimentin, matrix metalloproteinases, and loss of E-cadherin), increased expression of CD44, and the mammalian target of rapamycin (MTOR) (da Cunha et al., 2011; Ferrandiz-Pulido et al., 2013; Minardi et al., 2012; Muneer et al., 2009). Although routine evaluation of many of these molecular markers is currently not indicated because of lack of validation, there is a growing evidence that determining the HPV/p16 status of tumors may be useful for prognostic purposes. In recent studies the expression of high-risk HPV and p16 have been correlated with enhanced disease-specific survival (Djajadiningrat et al., 2015; Gunia et al., 2012). This is especially the case for assessing p16 status in tumors via immunohistochemistry, which is routinely available and is highly correlated with high-risk HPV positive tumors (Stankiewicz et al., 2011). In addition, counseling for female partners of males with HPV-associated penile cancers may be indicated.

Standardization of methodologies for assessment of gene expression and the lack of large tissue banks with well-annotated clinical data for validation studies hamper efforts to rigorously evaluate the potential usefulness of such biomarkers. Prospective multi-institutional studies analyzing pathologic and molecular features are needed to further validate which pathologic and molecular variables best stratify a patient's risk for metastasis and survival.

Evolving Indications for Expectant Management of the Inguinal Region

Data reviewed in the preceding paragraphs along with consensus guidelines demonstrate that **patients with primary tumors exhibiting CIS, verrucous carcinoma (Ta), and stage T1, grade 1 tumors exhibit a relatively low incidence of positive lymph nodes overall (0 to 16%) and are optimal candidates for watchful waiting strategies** (Pizzocaro et al., 2010; Pompeo et al., 2009).

Recommendations for the management of T1 grade 2 tumors varied based on quoted rates of subsequent metastases (see Table 79.10). The former EAU guideline (Solsona et al., 2004), although classifying such cases in the intermediate-risk group, recommended observation for T1 grade 2 tumors that lacked vascular invasion and exhibited a superficial growth pattern (i.e., absence of any other adverse features). This guideline was recently modified to recommend an inguinal staging procedure for this group of patients (Hakenberg et al., 2015; Pizzocaro et al., 2010). Given the low rate of metastases of 9% overall in a recent study among 105 patients, we agree with the Société Internationale d'Urologie/International Consultation on Urological Diseases (ICUD) recommendation that these patients may also be considered for observation (Hughes et al., 2010; Pompeo et al., 2009;

TABLE 79.12 Penile Carcinoma: Suggested Follow-Up for Patients With No Evidence of Inguinal Adenopathy Who Do Not Undergo Initial Lymphadenectomy

YEAR	INTERVAL	
	LOW-RISK GROUP[a]	HIGH-RISK GROUP[b]
1–2	3 months	2 months
3	6 months	4 months
4	6 months	6 months
5+	Annually	Annually

[a]Primary tumor stage Tis, Ta, and T1a.
[b]Primary tumor stage T1b or greater.

see Table 79.10). The T1 grade 2 grouping should correspond to the AJCC TNM seventh edition stage T1a classification (Edge et al., 2010, Hakenberg et al., 2015). These tumors lacked LVI and were not poorly differentiated. In two series consisting of 183 total patients the rates of metastases were 10.5% and 18% (Sun et al., 2015). Given that the eighth edition TNM T1a tumor staging definition excludes any tumors with perineural invasion or any proportion of anaplastic cells we anticipate that the eighth edition T1a classification (Pettaway et al., 2017) would represent an even lower-risk group of patient harboring micrometastatic disease.

The incidence of metastases among patients with AJCC stage T1b or greater tumors (see Table 79.1) as a group ranged from 33% to more than 50% in two recent collected series (Sun et al., 2014), so an inguinal staging procedure appears warranted. In addition, noncompliant patients with invasive primary tumors should be offered an inguinal staging procedure versus observation. Table 79.12 provides a guideline for more intensive follow-up of high-risk patients, especially within the first 2 years. **It is imperative for the patient and the physician to adhere to such follow-up agreements and to be willing to intervene immediately if initial inguinal parameters change.** Leijte et al. (2008) have documented that only one-third of patients who were initially node negative but who subsequently develop an inguinal recurrence survive 5 years.

Indications for Modified and Traditional Inguinal Procedures

Modified Procedures

In patients with no evidence of palpable adenopathy who are selected to undergo inguinal procedures by virtue of adverse prognostic factors within the primary tumor, the goal is to define whether metastases exist with minimal morbidity for the patient. A variety of treatment options for this purpose have been reported and include fine-needle aspiration cytology, node biopsy, sentinel lymph node biopsy, extended sentinel lymph node dissection, dynamic sentinel lymph node biopsy, superficial dissection, and modified complete dissection. The technical aspects of many of these procedures are beyond the scope of this chapter but may be found in the references by Horenblas et al. (2000) and Spiess et al. (2009).

Fine-Needle Aspiration Cytology. The experience with aspiration of clinically negative inguinal nodes guided by either lymphangiography or ultrasonography is limited. Scappini et al. (1986) performed fine-needle aspiration cytology under pedal or penile lymphangiography for nodal localization in 29 patients. Of 20 patients who had lymphadenectomy for histologic confirmation, there was complete agreement between aspiration cytology and histologic results. However, 2 of 9 patients whose cytologic analysis was negative subsequently died of metastatic disease, a presumptive 20% false-negative result. A series from Horenblas et al. (1991) also found that the sensitivity of fine-needle aspiration cytology was approximately 71% in 18 patients with clinically negative lymph nodes. This finding and the technical difficulty with lymphangiography make aspiration less practical as a staging technique for patients with no palpable lymph nodes. Kroon et al. (2005a) described fine-needle aspiration cytology guided by ultrasonography as a preliminary study to surgical staging with DSNB. Thirty-four groins in 27 patients with clinically negative groins were found to have suspicious nodes by ultrasound examination and were aspirated. However, the sensitivity of the technique was only 39% subsequent to surgical staging. **Thus, at present, fine-needle aspiration cytology of clinically negative groins does not exhibit high enough sensitivity to be relied on as a staging modality.** However, direct aspiration of palpable inguinal nodes is easily performed, exhibited a sensitivity of 93%, and, if positive, provides immediate information with which to advise patients about further treatment (Saisorn et al., 2006).

Sentinel Lymph Node Biopsy, Extended Sentinel Lymph Node Dissection, and Node Biopsy. The concept of sentinel lymph node biopsy as described by Cabanas (1977) is predicated on detailed penile lymphangiographic studies that have demonstrated consistent drainage of the penile lymphatics into a sentinel node or group of nodes located superomedial to the junction of the saphenous and femoral veins in the area of the superficial epigastric vein. In this series, when this sentinel node was negative for tumor, metastases to other ilioinguinal lymph nodes did not occur. Metastases to this node indicated the need for a complete superficial and deep inguinal dissection.

The accuracy of the sentinel node histology to identify inguinal node metastases was, however, questioned by a number of reports (Fowler, 1984; Perinetti et al., 1980; Wespes et al., 1986). Because nodal metastases became palpable within 1 year of sentinel node biopsy with normal findings in some patients in these series, a false-negative biopsy result must be presumed. In one large series, 5 of 41 patients (12%) with normal findings on sentinel node biopsy subsequently developed inguinal node metastases (Fossa et al., 1987). In Cabanas's series (1992), 3 of 31 patients with negative sentinel nodes died of disease, suggesting a false-negative rate for identifying metastases of 10%. McDougal et al. (1986) reported a 50% false-negative rate with inguinal node biopsy. A report by Pettaway et al. (1995), in which additional nodes around the sentinel node area were also removed, revealed that even this extended dissection was associated with a false-negative rate of 25%. The authors hypothesized that false-negative inguinal node biopsies were the result of anatomic variation in the position of the sentinel node within the inguinal field. **Thus biopsies directed to a specific anatomic area can be unreliable in identifying microscopic metastasis and are no longer recommended.**

Dynamic Sentinel Node Biopsy. DSNB offers the potential for precise localization of the sentinel node with the lowest morbidity of any surgical staging technique (Kroon et al., 2005c). The goal of DSNB is to define where in the inguinal lymph node field the sentinel lymph node resides through use of a combination of visual (vital blue dyes) or gamma emission (hand-held gamma probe) techniques at the time of surgery.

The technique has been studied in patients with malignant melanoma and breast and vulvar carcinomas who required evaluation of the regional lymph nodes (Albertini et al., 1996; Gershenwald et al., 1999; Levenback et al., 1994; Morton et al., 1992). The technique involves intradermal injection of a vital blue dye (isosulfan blue or patent blue dyes) or technetium-labeled colloid adjacent to the lesion. The dye (or radioactive tracer) is transported by the afferent lymphatics to a specific node in the regional nodal basin. This node is designated the sentinel lymph node.

Several studies evaluating the results of DSNB as a staging tool in penile cancer are now available. Kroon et al. (2004) updated the Netherlands Cancer Institute experience, describing their experience using the combination of preoperative lymphoscintigraphy and intraoperative intradermally injected blue dye in 123 patients with penile cancer. They identified a sentinel node in 98% of patients, for a sensitivity rate of 82% and a false-negative rate of 18% (6 patients). Four of the 6 patients subsequently died of disease progression. Spiess et al. (2007) also noted a false-negative rate of 25% among 31 patients undergoing DSNB. The Netherlands Cancer Institute group subsequently instituted several changes, including (1) routine serial sectioning of the involved lymph nodes along with cytokeratin immunohistochemistry, (2) routine exploration of groins with low or no signal subsequent to preoperative or intraoperative studies, and (3) inguinal ultrasonography with fine-needle aspiration to detect subtle architectural changes (nonpalpable) in positive lymph nodes that could result in the redistribution of lymphatic flow (Kroon et al., 2005a).

In a multicenter update that included patients assessed with the modified DSNB protocol from two high-volume centers (the Netherlands Cancer Institute and St. George's Hospital in London) the false-negative rate was 7% (6 patients) among 323 patients (Leijte et al., 2009b). Three of 6 patients with recurrence (50%) either died or developed distant metastases. **Thus DSNB, when performed at high-volume centers using a standardized protocol, has an acceptable sensitivity, but deaths from penile cancer among initially node-negative patients still occurred.** This limits the applicability of this strategy to larger centers with experienced surgeons and nuclear medicine specialists.

Superficial and Modified Complete Inguinal Dissection. Superficial inguinal and modified complete dissections have been proposed as staging tools for the patient without palpable inguinal lymphadenopathy. Superficial node dissection involves removal of those nodes superficial to the fascia lata. A complete IILND (removal of those nodes deep to the fascia lata contained within the femoral triangle as well as the pelvic nodes) is then performed if the superficial nodes are positive at surgery by frozen-section analysis. The rationale for superficial dissection is that two series have shown no positive nodes deep to the fascia lata unless superficial nodes were also positive (Pompeo et al., 1995; Puras-Baez et al., 1995). Furthermore, Spiess et al. (2007) showed that among the lymph node–negative cohort of patients undergoing DSNB followed by completion superficial dissection, no patient with a negative superficial dissection experienced recurrence, with more than 3 years of follow-up. A complete modified inguinal dissection was originally proposed by Catalona (1988) and involves smaller skin incision, limited field of inguinal dissection, preservation of the saphenous vein, and thicker skin flaps. This technique also avoids having to transpose the sartorius muscle to cover exposed femoral vessels. Unlike in superficial dissection, deep nodes within the fossa ovalis are also removed. Two reports involving 21 patients have confirmed the value of this technique, when it is properly performed, for identifying microscopic metastases with minimal morbidity (Colberg et al., 1997; Parra, 1996).

Thus either superficial or complete modified inguinal dissection should adequately identify microscopic metastases in patients with clinically normal inguinal examination findings, without the need for a pelvic dissection if the inguinal nodes are negative. The disadvantage of the modified dissections is the higher overall complication rate (12% to 35%) when compared with DSNB (5% to 7%) (Kroon et al., 2005c; Spiess et al., 2009).

Limited dissections have the following advantages: more information is provided than by biopsy of a single node or group of nodes; the possibility of not identifying the sentinel node is limited by removal of all potential first-echelon nodes; and the dissection is readily performed by any surgeon experienced in inguinal surgery without the need for specialized equipment.

Minimally Invasive Inguinal Lymphadenectomy Using Laparoscopy or Robotic Techniques. The laparoscopic and robotic approaches to the inguinal region offer the potential for removing all of the inguinal lymph nodes at risk for disease while minimizing complications. The technical details of the contemporary procedure and early results have been described (Matin et al., 2013; Sotelo et al., 2007; Tobias-Machado et al., 2007). The results of laparoscopic and robotic ILND have been comparable with those of open inguinal lymph dissection with comparable node counts achieved in both. A single case of inguinal recurrence reported at 12 to 33 months of follow-up and minor complications in about 20% of patients have been reported (Sotelo et al., 2009). However, in one study using a laparoscopic approach with more than 600 days of follow-up, Master et al. (2012) noted minor complications in 27% of patients, with major complications noted in 14.6%. These were mainly infectious in nature and were managed with intravenous antibiotics or incision and drainage. Among 41 dissections there was only a single case of skin edge necrosis. Matin et al. (2013), using a robotic-assisted approach, noted in a phase 1 pilot study that inguinal dissection appeared equivalent to an open approach in 18 of 19 (94.7%) patients when verified by a second surgeon using an open incision to inspect the same groin. Another recent study compared the complication rates and outcomes among 35 patients undergoing open inguinal lymph node dissection versus the robotic approach (n = 33 patients [Kumar and Sethia, 2017]). They also found that lymph node yields were similar for both approaches; however, the wound complication rate was much higher in the open group when compared with the robotic group (68% versus 6%, respectively). There were no local recurrences in either group; however, the open group follow-up was 71 months versus only 16 for the robotic group. Minimally invasive approaches are promising as inguinal staging procedures and appear reasonable in experienced hands for staging clinically negative groins. However, further validation with larger patient numbers and longer follow-up to better determine efficacy among node positive patients are required to determine whether this is an acceptable oncologic procedure. Among those patients who are clinically node negative, data on complication rates compared with traditional approaches or DSNB will help to better determine its place as a staging tool.

Traditional Inguinal and Ilioinguinal Lymphadenectomy

In patients with resectable metastatic adenopathy, the potential therapeutic value of lymphadenectomy justifies the morbidity of treatment. The goals are to eradicate all obvious cancer, to provide coverage for exposed vasculature, and to provide rapid wound healing (primary closure or myocutaneous flap coverage). Several issues remain with respect to surgical decision making.

Should ILND be bilateral rather than unilateral for patients with unilateral adenopathy at initial presentation of the primary tumor? The answer to this question is yes. The anatomic crossover of penile lymphatics is well established, and bilateral drainage is the rule. In 43 of 54 patients (79%) undergoing intraoperative lymph node mapping at the Netherlands Cancer Institute, lymphatic drainage from the penis was bilateral (Horenblas et al., 2000). The contralateral node dissection may be limited to the area superficial to the fascia lata if no histologic evidence of positive superficial nodes is found at surgery by frozen-section analysis. Clinical support for a bilateral procedure is based on the finding of contralateral metastases in more than 50% of patients so treated, even if the contralateral nodal region was normal on palpation (Ekstrom and Edsmyr, 1958).

Should bilateral ILND be performed in patients with unilateral lymphadenopathy some time after the initial presentation and treatment of the primary tumor? It is generally believed that bilateral node dissection in this setting is not necessary. The recommendation of unilateral rather than bilateral node dissection with delayed presentation of unilateral lymphadenopathy is supported by the elapsed disease-free interval of observation on the normal side. If one assumes that nodal metastases will enlarge at the same rate, the clinical palpation of nodal metastases, if present in both groins, should appear at approximately the same time. The absence of clinical adenopathy on one side despite prolonged observation suggests freedom from disease on that side (Ekstrom and Edsmyr, 1958). However, this concept may not apply to all patients with delayed recurrence. Horenblas et al. (2000) noted that in patients with two or more unilateral metastases, contralateral occult metastases were noted in 30% of cases. Thus, in patients with a bulky unilateral recurrence, a contralateral inguinal staging procedure should be considered. With the current treatment recommendations for bilateral inguinal staging procedures in men at high risk for metastasis and the definition of low-risk groups for metastasis by use of available prognostic markers, this scenario should rarely occur.

Should pelvic lymphadenectomy (PLND) be performed in all patients with inguinal metastases, considering its potential for added morbidity and relatively low therapeutic value? This issue remains controversial, but recent data suggest that PLND may be omitted in select patients with limited inguinal metastases (Lont et al., 2007; Pizzocaro et al., 2010; Zhu et al., 2008). Patients with inguinal nodal metastases are at increased risk for spread to the pelvic nodes. Ravi (1993b) found no pelvic nodal metastases when inguinal nodes were negative but found positive pelvic nodes in 17 of 75 patients (22%) with one to three positive inguinal nodes and in 13 of 23 patients (57%) with more than three positive inguinal nodes. Srinivas et al. (1987) also found a similar correlation. Horenblas et al. (1993) showed that among patients with a single inguinal lymph node involved without extracapsular extension, the incidence of pelvic metastases was rare; they recommended avoiding pelvic dissection in such patients. Zhu et al. (2008) found that the sensitivity of CT for pelvic lymph node metastasis was only 37.5%. Use of the Cloquet node in predicting a positive pelvic node was only about 30% sensitive as well. Important predictors were the number of positive nodes and lymph node size. Two contemporary studies addressing this issue have found a 0 to 12% incidence of pelvic lymph node metastasis when patients exhibited only one or two positive inguinal nodes, especially when extracapsular extension was absent and/or size was less than 3.5 cm (Lont et al., 2007; Zhu et al., 2008). Additional factors noted in these studies included the grade of the nodal metastasis and its TP53 status. Thus patients with only a single small lymph node metastasis discovered at the time of inguinal dissection (i.e., no extracapsular extension, not high grade) may be at very low risk for pelvic metastasis and are potentially the optimal candidates in whom PLND can be avoided.

With respect to efficacy, the 5-year survival for patients with positive pelvic nodes averages around 14% (see Table 79.6). However, data from some of the smaller series suggest that in selected instances 5-year survival can occur in patients treated with surgery alone. In the series reported by Ravi (1993b), however, patients with even a single positive pelvic node did not survive 5 years (0 of 8 patients). The difficulty in determining the potential independent value of PLND as a therapeutic procedure is related to the small numbers of patients reported, the coexisting extensive inguinal adenopathy in patients with resectable pelvic nodes, and the failure to specify sites of relapse in patients undergoing IILND (i.e., inguinal versus pelvic versus distant site).

Thus, for patients undergoing ILND for curative intent (i.e., in whom preoperative studies reveal no pelvic adenopathy), PLND should routinely be considered in patients with two or more positive inguinal lymph nodes or when extracapsular nodal extension is present. PLND in this setting serves as an effective staging tool for identifying those patients at increased risk for pelvic metastases in whom adjunctive therapy should be considered (Lont et al., 2007; Pizzocaro et al., 2010). Given the aforementioned indications, PLND can be performed simultaneously with ILND in the setting of higher-volume inguinal metastases or as a secondary procedure after inguinal pathology is available. Alternatively, if pelvic nodal metastases are proven before lymphadenectomy (based on clinical findings), consideration should be given to neoadjuvant chemotherapeutic strategies followed by surgery or clinical trial enrollment (Leijte et al., 2007; National Comprehensive Cancer Network [NCCN], 2018; Pagliaro et al., 2010).

Risk-Based Management of the Inguinal Region

A contemporary schema for management of the inguinal region is presented in Fig. 79.4. Assumptions for these guidelines are that the primary tumor has been adequately controlled, the pathologic stage of the primary tumor is available, and an inguinal examination has been performed. CT of the abdomen and pelvis as well as chest radiography or other imaging studies should also be performed as clinically indicated.

Very Low-Risk Patients

Because the incidence of inguinal metastasis is anecdotal at best for patients with stage Tis or Ta primary tumors, observation is reasonable for those patients with normal inguinal examination findings (see Fig. 79.4A, *left*). For patients with palpable adenopathy, a course of antibiotics should reveal those whose adenopathy is related to infection versus metastasis. A persistently palpable node should undergo fine-needle aspiration cytology; if the result is negative, an excisional

> **KEY POINTS: TREATMENT OF THE INGUINAL NODES**
>
> - The presence and extent of inguinal metastases determine survival in penile cancer.
> - Patients with persistent palpable inguinal adenopathy should undergo an ultrasound or CT-guided inguinal biopsy followed by management appropriate for the clinical scenario.
> - On the basis of the histologic features of the primary tumor, the risk of lymph node metastases can be assessed in patients with no palpable adenopathy based upon the TNM staging system. DSNB, superficial ILND, or close follow-up can be recommended based on TNM stage and other histologic features.
> - Factors associated with a high cure rate in surgically treated patients include no more than two inguinal metastases, unilateral involvement, no ENE of cancer, and the absence of pelvic metastases. Patients with higher volumes of disease should be considered for adjuvant or neoadjuvant therapy.
> - Morbidity of lymphadenectomy is decreasing in contemporary series.
> - Superficial ILND reliably determines the presence of microscopic inguinal metastases without the need for specialized facilities but can have significant morbidity.
> - Modified DSNB techniques to determine microscopic inguinal disease exhibit low morbidity, have been validated externally in higher-volume centers, and are now a recommended procedure in such centers.
> - Laparoscopic and robotic ILND obtains lymph node yields that are comparable with those of open techniques when used in selected patients and are an appropriate staging procedure in clinically lymph node negative patients. Additional studies with larger patient numbers and longer follow-up are required before routine adoption into clinical practice among patients with clinically positive inguinal lymph nodes.
> - PLND is now recommended when more than one inguinal lymph node exhibits metastasis or when ENE of cancer is present.

biopsy is recommended. If the biopsy finding is abnormal, ipsilateral inguinal dissection with contralateral superficial or modified complete dissection is performed. DSNB is an option in experienced centers.

Low- to Intermediate-Risk Patients (American Joint Committee on Cancer Stage T1a)

Several earlier series have combined patients with stage T1 grade 1 and grade 2 tumors and have found them to exhibit less than a 10% incidence of inguinal metastasis (see Fig. 79.4A, *right*; see also Table 79.10). However, the incidence of metastasis among strictly T1 grade 2 tumors (25% to 44%) may be higher, and variable recommendations have been made. The recent EAU guidelines recommend inguinal staging for T1 grade 2 tumors (also stage T1a) among patients with clinically negative lymph nodes (Hakenberg et al., 2015). However, observation is also an option for compliant patients in this setting (ICUD penile cancer guidelines found in Pompeo et al., 2009; NCCN penile cancer guidelines, 2018). Similar patients with palpable nodes on initial presentation should undergo fine-needle aspiration cytology. If the nodes are positive, the patients then undergo lymphadenectomy, as in Fig. 79.4A. If they are negative, then either excisional biopsy and/or planned lymphadenectomy are reasonable options.

High-Risk Patients (American Joint Committee on Cancer Stage T1b or Higher)

For the high-risk cohort, the incidence of inguinal metastasis ranges from 30% to approximately 70% (see Fig. 79.4B). According to the recent guidelines, there is consensus that patients with poorly differentiated tumors, lymphovascular or perineural invasion, or pT2 or greater tumors should undergo an inguinal staging procedure (Hakenberg et al., 2015; NCCN penile cancer guidelines, 2018). The surgical approach depicted in Fig. 79.4B is designed to maximize detection and treatment for those with proven nodal metastasis while limiting the morbidity of those with negative lymph nodes at surgery. Thus surgical staging is indicated even in those patients with clinically normal inguinal examination findings. **In this setting, antibiotic use minimizes the risk of inguinal wound infections or septic complications after control of an infected primary tumor, rather than influencing the decision for surgical staging.**

Patients with normal inguinal examination findings are offered bilateral superficial dissection, complete modified dissection, or DSNB (with the last offered in experienced centers). If frozen-section results reveal no metastasis, the procedure is concluded. For DSNB the results are based on permanent sections; thus further therapy is planned at a second setting if needed. If either side is positive, an ipsilateral inguinal dissection is performed. Pelvic dissection in the setting of a patient with no palpable adenopathy who is discovered to have positive inguinal metastasis at frozen section is optional and based on pathologic findings (Lont et al., 2007; Zhu et al., 2008). Patients with unilateral resectable adenopathy that is strongly suggestive of metastasis should undergo an ipsilateral ilioinguinal dissection and a contralateral superficial or complete modified dissection. Frozen-section analysis then determines if deep inguinal or pelvic nodes should be excised. DSNB is another option in managing the contralateral node-negative side. Palpable adenopathy of less than 4 cm was arbitrarily selected as a cutoff point for surgery as monotherapy because nodal metastases larger than 4 cm are associated with ENE of cancer (Ravi, 1993a).

For patients with bilateral palpable nodes that are strongly suggestive of metastasis, preoperative fine-needle aspiration cytology can be helpful for counseling of the patient as to the likelihood of the extent of surgery. For patients with negative results of fine-needle aspiration cytology, a staged surgical approach starting with superficial dissection is performed. Subsequent procedures in this setting depend on the results of frozen-section analysis. For patients requiring IILND

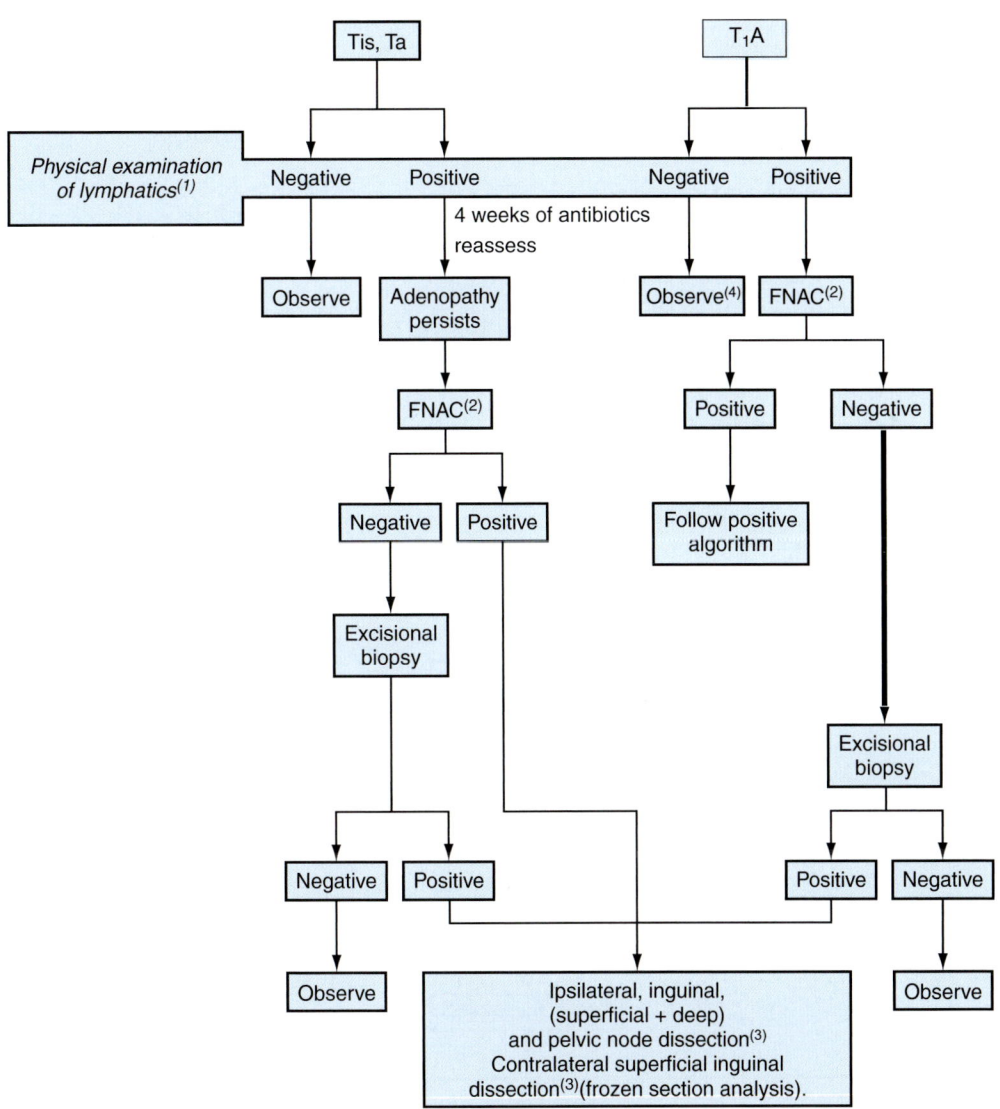

1) Includes physical examination and/or imaging studies.
2) Fine-needle aspiration cytology.
3) If 2 or more positive ipsilateral inguinal nodes or extranodal extension found.
4) Alternative DSNB at experienced centers, superficial dissection if noncompliant patient.

Fig. 79.4. Management of regional disease. (A) Very low risk (left side) and low-intermediate risk (right side).

Continued

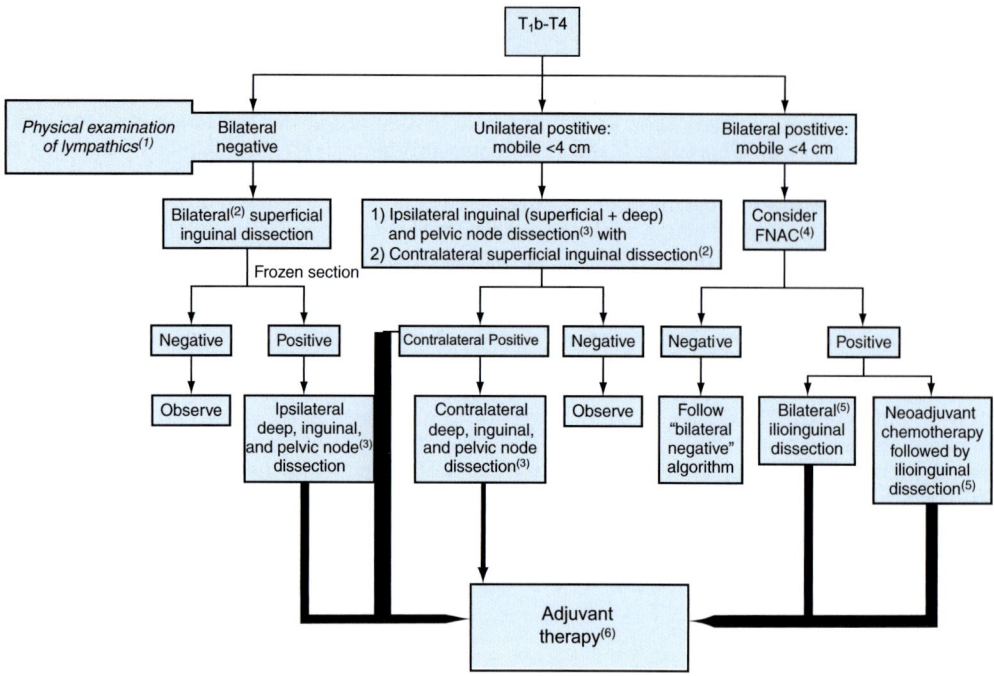

1) Includes physical examination and/or imaging studies.
2) Complete modified dissection and dynamic sentinel node biopsy (DSNB, experienced centers) acceptable.
3) If >2 positive inguinal nodes or extranodal extension of cancer.
4) Fine-needle aspiration cytology.
5) Either approach is acceptable.
6) Consider if >2 positive lymph nodes, or bilateral metastases, extranodal extension of cancer or positive pelvic lymph nodes.

B

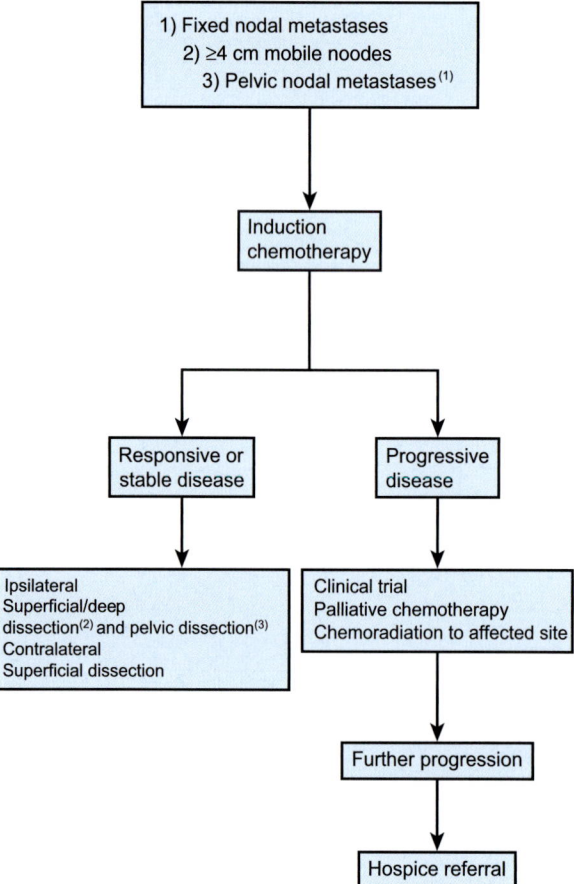

(1) Subsequent to preoperative imaging studies.
(2) May require resection skin, fascia, or muscle.
C (3) Postoperative adjuvant chemoradiation ≥ positive inguinal nodes, bilateral positive comma nodes or pelvic nodes.

Fig. 79.4., cont'd (B) High-risk and lower-volume metastatic patients. (C) Bulky metastatic and distant disease.

because of metastases, adjuvant chemotherapy should be considered for those exhibiting more than two positive lymph nodes, ENE of cancer, or pelvic nodal metastasis (Hakenberg et al., 2015). An alternative approach to consider among patients with bilateral metastases is neoadjuvant chemotherapy followed by surgical resection as described by Pagliaro et al. (2010) and recently incorporated into the NCCN Penile Cancer Guidelines 2018.

Bulky Adenopathy and Fixed Nodal Metastasis

Survival in patients with bulky adenopathy and fixed nodal metastasis is related to complete eradication of extensive disease (see Fig. 79.4C). **This task is difficult to achieve with surgery, chemotherapy, or radiation therapy alone. The combination of surgery and chemotherapy has shown some benefit in advanced penile carcinoma** (Bermejo et al., 2007; Corral et al., 1998; Dickstein et al., 2016; Leijte et al., 2007; Pagliaro et al., 2010; Pizzocaro et al., 1997). The optimal integration and timing of such therapy are unknown. A reasonable approach in this cohort of patients is to use neoadjuvant chemotherapy followed by an aggressive surgical resection for patients demonstrating either response to therapy or stable disease. The neoadjuvant approach could improve surgical resectability and avoid obstacles in the administration of chemotherapy resulting from delays in postoperative healing. The prognosis is poor in patients exhibiting progression while they are receiving chemotherapy. Palliative groin dissection is a consideration but rarely provides significant palliation (Leijte et al., 2007, Wang et al., 2015). Hemipelvectomy in patients without distant metastases was reported before the development of effective chemotherapy (Block et al., 1973) and is no longer used. Endoluminal vascular stents have also been reported to have transient success in preventing vascular erosion by tumor (Link et al., 2004). Clinical trials of novel systemic strategies and radiation therapy to affected areas provide the next level of care. With further progression, supportive care provided by hospice services can provide valuable support to patients with end-stage disease.

RADIATION THERAPY

Radiation Therapy for the Primary Lesion

Primary radiation therapy has curative potential and may permit preservation of penile form and function. If local control is not achieved, salvage surgery may still be curative, and therefore in a subset of men with penile cancer, initial radiation represents a reasonable treatment strategy. External-beam radiotherapy and interstitial brachytherapy can be used to treat the primary penile tumor. Before radiation therapy, circumcision is necessary to expose the lesion, to allow resolution of any surface infection, and to prevent preputial edema and subsequent phimosis. In many cases, circumcision may also significantly debulk the primary tumor.

External-Beam Radiotherapy

External-beam radiotherapy has several advantages. It is widely available, delivers a homogeneous dose, and does not require the same interventional technical skills required for delivery of effective brachytherapy. In a review, Crook et al. described contemporary dose- fractionation ranging from 60 Gy in 25 fractions over 5 weeks to 74 Gy in 37 fractions over 7.5 weeks (Crook et al., 2009). This contrasts with the lower doses of 50 to 55 Gy cited in older series (McLean et al., 1993; Neave et al., 1993). One of the challenges of external-beam radiotherapy is to position the penis consistently for treatment so that it is accessible by the radiation beam while not implicating adjacent normal tissues and structures. This can be achieved by positioning the patient supine on the treatment couch and encasing the penis in a vertical position in a block of wax or Perspex with a central cylindric chamber. The block is bivalved for ease of application and air gaps should be minimal. If penile edema develops during treatment, a larger chamber size may have to be selected. The second consideration involves the physical nature of megavoltage radiation beams, which relatively spare the skin surface and deliver the prescribed radiation dose at a depth in tissue. Penile cancer is of cutaneous origin and requires full treatment of the skin surface. Wax and Perspex are tissue-equivalent materials, so the choice of these in fabricating an immobilization device effectively boluses the penis and brings the full dose to the skin surface.

Table 79.13 is adapted from Crook et al. (2009) and describes the efficacy of external-beam radiotherapy and interstitial brachytherapy with respect to local control, cause-specific survival, complications, and penile preservation. The data represent retrospective reviews of single institution series collected over many years, during which time staging systems and treatment techniques evolved. The data often represent a range of doses and fractionation schemes, which permits only limited conclusions regarding optimal dose and fractionation. **Five-year local control rates among patients treated using a variety of techniques ranged from 55% to 70% with penile preservation rates of 39% to 66%. Thus primary external-beam radiotherapy affords at least a 50% chance to control the primary tumor and avoid penile amputation.** Furthermore, surgical salvage, when necessary, can be achieved in most cases by partial or total amputation. Cause-specific survival ranged from 58% to 96% depending on primary tumor stage and lymph node status.

Prognostic factors for improved local control among patients treated with external-beam radiotherapy include dose above 60 Gy, treatment time not exceeding 45 days, and daily fraction size of 2 Gy. Lower control rates are seen with stage T3 tumors, those more than 4 cm in diameter, and high-grade lesions (Crook et al., 2009; Gotsadze et al., 2000; Sarin et al., 1997). This suggests that the minimum tumor dose should be at least 66 Gy in 2-Gy fractions over a period of 6.5 weeks (45 days). Hypofractionated courses (fraction size >2 Gy) may be associated with increased toxicity.

External beam radiotherapy is most frequently considered in patients who are not surgical candidates by virtue of age or comorbidities, or those presenting with locoregionally advanced disease in which the primary region would be treated in contiguity with the nodal regions, including both groins and the pelvis.

Brachytherapy

Interstitial brachytherapy using the isotope iridium-192 is as an alternative to external-beam radiotherapy. Penile brachytherapy involves a temporary implantation of interstitial needles in a parallel array through and around the tumor (Video 79.2). These can then be either manually loaded with iridium-192 wire or seeds to deliver a classic low-dose rate (LDR; 50–60 cGy/h) treatment or connected to an automated afterloader with a high-activity iridium-192 source for pulse dose rate (PDR) brachytherapy. This delivers an hourly pulse equivalent to the hourly dose rate of LDR brachytherapy. High-dose rate (HDR) brachytherapy is evolving as an option because of the wider availability of HDR equipment and increased convenience.

Low-Dose Rate Brachytherapy. Gerbaulet and Lambin reported successful local control in 82% of 109 patients, with long-term survival rates of 75% to 80% in those with tumor-free regional lymph nodes (Gerbaulet and Lambin, 1992). Rozan et al. (1995) reviewed 184 patients from multiple centers, with 5- and 10-year disease-free survival rates of 78% and 67%, respectively. Although 22% of patients required a prior circumcision or local excision, only 4% underwent total penectomy. The most frequent late side effects were soft tissue ulceration (22%) or meatal stenosis (30%). Factors predicting for late side effects were dose greater than 60 Gy, volume greater than 30 cc, and an implant with more than 2 planes of needles.

Crook et al. reported on 67 patients treated between 1989 and 2007 with iridium-192 delivered by 17- to 19.5-gauge steel needles held in a three-dimensional parallel array by predrilled acrylic plastic templates (Crook et al., 2009). In the early years of the experience, manually afterloaded iridium-192 wires were used but in later years PDR brachytherapy has been preferred because of advantages in radiation safety and protection with radiobiological equivalence to the traditional iridium-192 wires. A median of six needles (range 2–9) were arranged in 2 parallel planes and delivered a prescribed dose of 60 Gy over 4 to 5 days. With a median follow-up of 4 years

TABLE 79.13 Selected Series of Studies Reporting Local Control (LC) of Disease, Cancer-Specific Survival (CSS), Complications, and Penile Preservation for Men Treated With External-Beam Radiation Therapy (Xrt) or Brachytherapy (BT) as Primary Treatment for Penile Cancer

STUDY	#	TYPE	DOSE Gy/fr	F/U (mo)	LC 5y	CSS 5y	COMPLICATION	PENILE PRESERVATION 5-year
EXTERNAL BEAM								
McLean et al., 1993	26	XRT	35/10–60/25	116 (84–168)	62%	69%	7/26 unspecified	66% crude
Neave et al., 1993	20	XRT	50–55	36 mo min	70%	58%	10% stenosis	60%
Sarin et al., 1997	59	XRT	60/30	62 (2–264)	55%	66%	3% necrosis 15% stenosis	50% crude
Gotsadze et al., 2000	155	XRT	40–60	40	65%	86%	1 necrosis 5 stenoses	65%
Zouhair et al., 2001	23	XRT	45–74 @ 1.8–2 Gy	70	57%	—	10% stenosis	39%
Ozsahin et al., 2006	33	XRT/BT	52	62 (2–454)	44%	—	10% stenosis	52%
Azrif et al., 2006	41	XRT	50–52 /16	54	62%	96%	8% necrosis 29% stenosis	52%
Mistry et al., 2007	18	XRT	55/16–50/20	62	63%	75%	2 necroses 1 stenosis	66% crude
BRACHYTHERAPY								
Mazeron et al., 1984	50	BT: LDR	60–70	(36–96)	78% crude		3 necroses 19% stenosis	74%
Delannes et al., 1992	51	BT: LDR	50–65	65 (12–144)	86% crude	85%	23% necrosis 45% stenosis	75%
Rozan et al., 1995	184	BT: LDR	63	139	85%	88%	21% necrosis 30% stenosis	78%
Soria et al., 1997	102	BT: LDR	61–70	111	77%	72%		72% (6 years)
Chaudhary et al., 1999	23	BT: LDR	50	21 (4–117)	70% (8 years)		0 necrosis 9% stenosis	70% (8 years)
Kiltie et al., 2000	31	BT: LDR	63.5	61.5	81%	85%	8 necroses 44% stenosis	75%
Crook et al., 2009	67	BT: LDR	60	48 (4–194)	88%	84%	12% necrosis 9% stenosis	88% 5 years 67% 10 years
de Crevoisier et al., 2009	144	BT: LDR	65	68(6–348)	80% 10-yr	92% 10-yr	26% necroses 29% stenoses	72% 10 years
Pimenta et al., 2015	25	BT: LDR	60–65	110 (0–228)	1@ 4 mo	91%	8% necroses 43% stenoses	86%
Kamsu-Kom et al., 2015	27	BT: PDR	60–70	33(6–64)	88% 3-yr	NS	9% necroses 22% stenoses	85%
Seibold et al., 2016	13	BT:PDR		54(13–155)	88%	78%	30% necroses 15% stenoses	100%
Petera et al., 2011	10	BT: HDR	3 Gy bid 42–45	20	100%	100%	0 necrosis 0 stenosis	100%
Sharma et al., 2014	14	BT: HDR	3 Gy bid 51	22 (6–40)	12/14	83% 3-yr	0 necrosis 0 stenosis	93%
Rouscoff et al., 2014	12	BT: HDR	4–4.3 bid 36–39	27(5–83)	11/12	100%	1 necrosis 1 stenosis	11/12
Kellas-Sleczka, et al., 2015	55	BT: HDR	3–3.5 bid 30–54	55(8–154)	73%	NS	0 necrosis 0 stenosis	80%

bid, Twice daily; *F/U,* follow-up; *HDR,* high-dose rate; *LDR,* low-dose rate; PDR, pulse-dose rate; *RT,* radiation therapy.

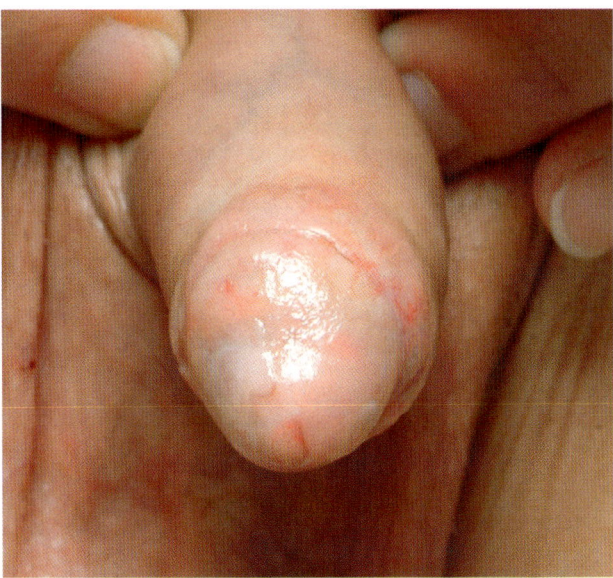

Fig. 79.5. Penile appearance 8 years after low-dose rate brachytherapy for T2N1 squamous cell carcinoma penis. Brachytherapy performed concurrently with inguinal node dissection. 60 Gy delivered over 5 days. Hypopigmented scar at site of original tumor. Minor telangiectasia on glans.

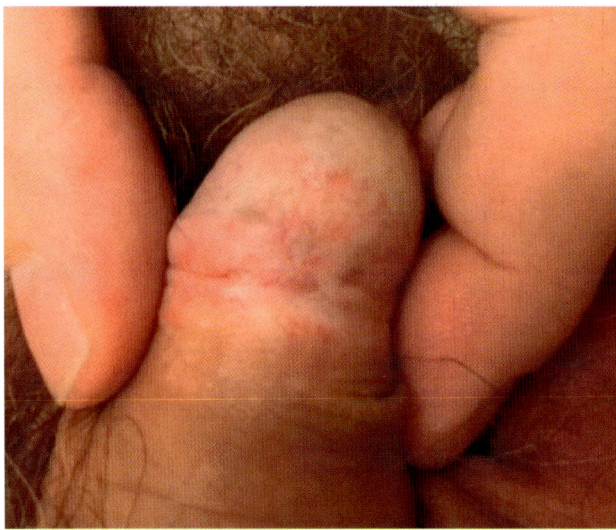

Fig. 79.6. Penile appearnce 5 years after high-dose rate penile brachytherapy, 38.4 Gy in twice daily fractions of 3.2 Gy for 6 days after circumcision and local excision of primary with positive margins (T1 well to moderately differentiated, 8-mm invasion).

(range 0.2 to 16.2), the 10-year actuarial cause-specific survival was 84%. Five- and 10-year penile preservation rates were 88% and 67% (Fig. 79.5). Of 8 local failures, 5 occurred before 2 years and 3 were late, observed at 42, 64, and 90 months. Penectomy was performed for these 8 recurrences as well as 2 necroses; partial penectomy was adequate for 8 patients, whereas 2 required a total penectomy because of insufficient penile length.

Inguinal lymph node status remains an important prognostic factor, even when nonsurgical management of the primary tumor is being considered. Before 2002, prophylactic lymph node dissections were not part of the management algorithm (Crook et al., 2002). Crook et al. reported that 50% of moderately or poorly differentiated tumors treated with brachytherapy recurred regionally or distantly. Subsequently, inguinal lymph nodes have been managed with the same indications as for patients undergoing primary surgery (Hakenberg et al., 2015; NCCN Penile Cancer Guidelines, 2018). Biopsy information provides the required evidence on tumor grade and the presence of lymphovascular invasion.

Overall, in reviewing the literature, **local control** (see Table 79.13) **provided by interstitial brachytherapy appears superior to that provided by external-beam radiotherapy, with 5-year local control rates of 77% to 88%, and 70 to 80% at 10 years. Penile preservation rates are 74% to 88% at 5 years, and 67% to 70% at 8 to 10 years.** Crook et al. (2009) found that a predictor of local failure was needle spacing, with an increase in spacing (range 12 to 18 mm) resulting in decreased local recurrence because of the wider lateral margin achieved. With this consideration, larger tumor size did not predict for local recurrence, although others have reported an increase in local failure in tumors larger than 4 cm and with invasion of the corpora (Kiltie et al., 2000; Mazeron et al., 1984; Soria et al., 1997).

Brachytherapy: High-Dose Rate Interstitial. Manually afterloaded sources such as iridium-192 wires are no longer widely available because of concerns around staff exposure and radiation safety. However, HDR brachytherapy is increasingly common for malignancies such as breast and prostate and is an essential component of curative treatment of cervical cancer. The technique of HDR brachytherapy for penile cancer is similar to that for LDR brachytherapy. Recent publications indicate that 3 Gy given twice daily, a minimum of 6 hours apart, appears safe and effective for total doses of 45 to 51 Gy delivered over $7\frac{1}{2}$ to $8\frac{1}{2}$ days (Petera et al., 2011; Sharma et al., 2014). Although long-term follow-up is still lacking, penile preservation rates are reported between 80% and 100%. The largest report with the most mature follow-up is from Kellas-Slezka et al. (2015), who describe 55 patients with a median follow-up of $4\frac{1}{2}$ years. Treatments were 3.0 to 3.5 Gy twice daily to a median total dose of 49 Gy after biopsy or 36 Gy after previous total gross excision. At 5 years (8–152 months), 22% had local failure, 22% regional, and 5% distant. Penile preservation was achieved in 80%. Although promising, HDR brachytherapy for penile cancer must still be considered to be in evolution; optimal fractionation and homogeneity parameters are yet to be established (Crook et al., 2016; Rouscoff et al., 2014; Fig. 79.6).

Brachytherapy: Surface Mold

For noninvasive or very superficial tumors, a surface mold containing iridium-192 wires can be constructed. Originally reported in the LDR era, the plastic mold is worn in close apposition to the penile shaft for several hours per day for a period of 7 to 10 days for an adequate surface dose of 60 Gy with rapid fall-off at a depth (Akimoto et al., 1997; el-Demiry et al., 1984). Because the depth of tumor invasion can be difficult to ascertain by clinical examination or imaging, and because a dose margin (comparable with the required surgical margin) is advisable beyond visible disease, patients must be carefully selected.

The availability of HDR afterloading has renewed interest in surface mold plesiotherapy. Custom molds can be produced with 3D printing (Helou et al., 2015; Matys et al., 2011). The typical dose is 40 Gy over 5 days with two fractions of 4 Gy per day. The sources are embedded in the mold or applicator to maintain a distance from the skin surface and thus limit the skin dose to tolerable levels while still achieving an appropriate treatment depth. This may be especially suitable for recurrence after laser surgery or topical therapy. The reaction tends to peak at about 3 weeks and takes 6 to 10 weeks to heal (Fig. 79.7). There are no long-term results reported yet.

Adverse Effects Associated With Radiotherapy

Acutely, after radiotherapy or brachytherapy moist desquamation can be expected at the treated site. This will be more extensive after external-beam radiotherapy because of the larger treatment volume. Re-epithelialization occurs in 4 to 8 weeks. Saline soaks and hygiene are important. Intercourse can be resumed when the patient is comfortable, but the use of additional water-based lubrication is recommended.

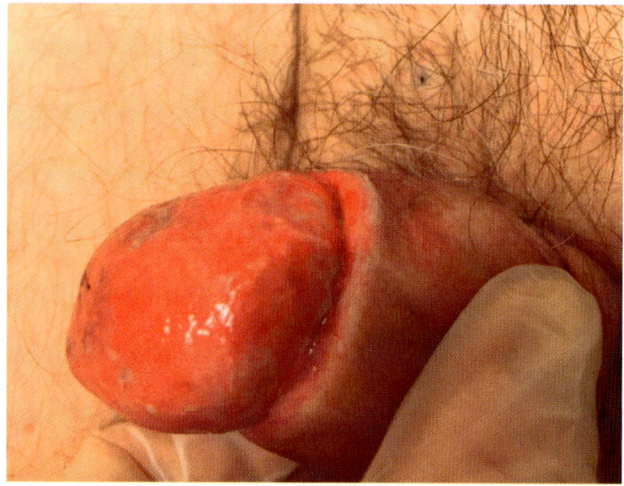

Fig. 79.7. Acute moist desquamation 3 weeks after high-dose rate surface mold brachytherapy for squamous cell carcinoma in situ. 40 Gy over 5 days in twice daily fractions of 4 Gy.

The two most common late side effects associated with radiotherapy are meatal stenosis and soft-tissue ulceration. Soft-tissue ulceration overall is reported in 0 to 8% after external beam radiotherapy and 0 to 26% of after interstitial radiotherapy (see Table 79.13). Persistent ulceration may raise concerns about recurrent cancer. A biopsy may be indicated, but in general, ulceration is flat and superficial, with no raised or exophytic component. The majority will heal over several weeks with conservative management, but healing is slower in patients with diabetes and in those cases that were originally more deeply invasive. Close follow-up and treatment with antibiotics, vitamin E, and steroid creams are recommended. For cases resistant to these measures, hyperbaric oxygen is often effective (Crook et al., 2009; Gomez-Iturriaga et al., 2011).

Meatal stenosis is reported in 10% to 45% of patients and may be related to increased dose per fraction in those treated with external-beam radiotherapy or closer needle spacing and proximity to the meatus after brachytherapy. Meatal stenosis occurs later in follow-up (18 to 24 months) and may be preceded by reports of a weak, deviated, or divided urinary stream. Self-dilatation with a meatal dilator will improve the urinary stream and help to prevent subsequent unyielding fibrotic stenosis. Otherwise, urethral stricture may develop and require a more formal dilation or, in very rare cases, urethroplasty.

The benefits of avoiding a mutilating surgical procedure are clear; penile-sparing options are encouraged whenever appropriate. The side effects of radiation on sexual quality of life would appear modest. Delaunay et al. (2013) approached 21 French patients treated with penile brachytherapy between 1992 and 2009. The response rate to a validated questionnaire was more than 90%. At a median follow-up of 80 months, sexual function was maintained in 59% of those sexually active before brachytherapy. The age of the patient and his partner determined frequency of intercourse. Erections were maintained in 17 of 18 men potent before brachytherapy, although 52% noticed some change in glans sensitivity. A report from Gustave Roussy Institute assessed 39 men with a minimum of 3-year follow-up after brachytherapy (Gambachidze et al., 2017). The response rate to the survey was 60%, median age 63, and median follow-up 5.9 years. Seventy percent maintained sexual activity and erectile dysfunction was mild.

Because brachytherapy irradiates much less of the penile shaft, erectile function is more likely to be preserved than after external-beam radiotherapy. However, for the elderly in whom sexual function is not an issue, partial penectomy may be acceptable, offering a prompt treatment with more rapid healing, conducive to less limitation of activity in the postoperative period.

The organ-sparing benefits of radiation can be compared with surgical choices such as laser therapy, Mohs micrographic surgery, and reconstructive surgery, all of which can provide organ-sparing while minimizing functional loss. This emphasizes the need for multidisciplinary assessment and referral to tertiary-care centers where all options are available. Radiation may be the only solution for a patient with significant comorbidities who is not a surgical candidate.

Finally, as with any organ-sparing approach, extended follow-up is essential and should be emphasized at the time of the original treatment decision. Teaching self-examination and prompt reporting of concerns is also important. Local recurrence can be salvaged surgically without jeopardizing survival. Long-term follow-up is essential because recurrences may be delayed, with up to 1 in 5 local recurrences occurring after 5 years (Crook et al., 2009; Mazeron et al., 1984). Because brachytherapy is a more focal treatment than external beam radiotherapy, salvage options are more likely to result in a partial rather than a total penectomy.

In summary, T1 and T2 tumors smaller than 4 cm with no or minimal extension beyond the coronal sulcus are appropriate for radiotherapy, and with careful planning, complications can be minimized (de Crevoisier et al., 2009). Brachytherapy can provide better local control and penile preservation with faster dose delivery (4 to 5 days rather than 6 to 7 weeks) compared with external beam radiotherapy. For the patient who is an appropriate candidate for a radiation-based approach, the selection of external beam versus brachytherapy may depend on the skill and experience of the radiation oncology team.

The treatment of locally advanced disease is clearly associated with a higher metastatic rate, and the treatment approach must encompass regional nodes. For a locally advanced penile tumor, brachytherapy is not an option. Combined chemoradiotherapy with weekly cisplatin as a radiation sensitizer is standard management in vulvar and cervical squamous carcinoma and is associated with excellent response rates. Chemoradiation may convert a patient with inoperable disease into a surgical candidate or, alternatively, may be used as definitive management, as in cervical cancer (Rose, 2002). Neoadjuvant chemoradiotherapy is being studied in a cooperative international trial, InPACT (International Penile Advanced Cancer Trial) run through ECOG-ACRIN (EA8134; NCT02305654), for patients with clinically positive groin nodes.

Radiation Therapy for the Inguinal Areas

The presence and extent of lymph node involvement is such a key prognostic factor in the management of penile cancer that surgical evaluation of the inguinal regions is recommended for patients selected as per the EAU and NCCN penile cancer guidelines (Hakenberg et al., 2015; NCCN, 2018). Surgical evaluation of high-risk, clinically node-negative patients is recommended so that additional treatment can be tailored to the actual pathology, rather than offering "prophylactic" radiation to the inguinal nodes. A surgical approach to resectable adenopathy is also preferable to obtain the prognostic information of number of involved nodes and presence of extranodal disease. For high-risk groin pathology, consideration should be given to a prophylactic pelvic nodal dissection. InPACT (EA 8134; NCT02305654) will randomize such patients between pelvic node dissection and pelvic chemoradiotherapy.

Preoperative radiation for lymph node metastases from penile cancer has been reported to reduce the incidence of ENE compared with surgery alone (8% vs. 33%; $P < 0.01$) and is associated with a decrease in subsequent groin recurrence (3% vs. 19% $P < 0.03$) in a small series of 33 patients (Ravi, 1993; Ravi et al., 1994). This is consistent with the benefit of radiotherapy used together with surgery or chemotherapy in other squamous malignancies such as vulvar, cervical, or anal carcinomas (Bartelink et al., 1997; Montana et al., 2000; Stehman et al., 2007). Furthermore, there are case reports of remarkable efficacy of chemoradiation for inoperable nodal disease in advanced penile cancer cases (Chhabra et al., 2014; Lapierre et al., 2017; Fig. 79.8A-C). The sequencing of surgery, neoadjuvant chemotherapy and chemoradiation, and the benefits of neoadjuvant treatment, are being investigated for node-positive penile cancer in InPACT (EA 8134; NCT02305654). Four hundred patients with node-positive penile squamous cell cancer will be randomized in the United Kingdom and North America over the next 5 years (http://ecog-acrin.org/clinical-trials/ea8134-educational-materials).

The use of adjuvant radiotherapy improved overall survival (HR 0.58, 95% CI 0.39–0.86). Similarly, data were collected from 4 tertiary referral centers on patients undergoing lymph node dissection from 1980 to 2013 (Tang et al., 2017). Adjuvant pelvic radiation was received by 43% of patients after a positive pelvic node dissection. On multivariate analysis, those without adjuvant pelvic radiotherapy had worse overall survival (HR 1.7; 95% CI 1.01–2.9, $P = 0.04$) and disease-specific survival (HR 1.9; 95% CI 1.09–3.236; $P = 0.02$). Extrapolating from the published literature on vulvar cancer, adjuvant radiotherapy 4500 cGy in 25 fractions over 5 weeks to the ipsilateral groin should be considered for patients with two or more positive nodes and for those with ENE (Hyde et al., 2007). If the pelvic nodes are known to be clear, then the pelvis does not have to be included, but if pelvic node dissection has not been performed, then the radiation volume should extend to include the pelvis. As is the case in vulvar cancer (Lee et al., 2016), HPV-positive patients may derive greater benefit from radiotherapy or chemoradiation for locoregional control.

In summary, inguinal radiotherapy is not recommended as prophylaxis for patients at high risk for inguinal node metastases unless the patient is not a surgical candidate. It should, however, be considered as adjuvant treatment for those with multiple positive nodes or ENE. Chemoradiotherapy may render inoperable disease resectable or can be used definitively. Radiation as a part of a multimodal approach with chemotherapy and surgery among patients with advanced penile cancer is being evaluated in an international prospective randomized trial (InPACT: EA 8134; NCT02305654).

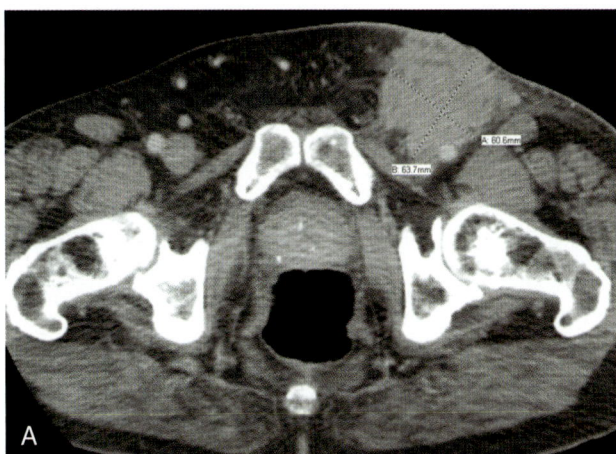
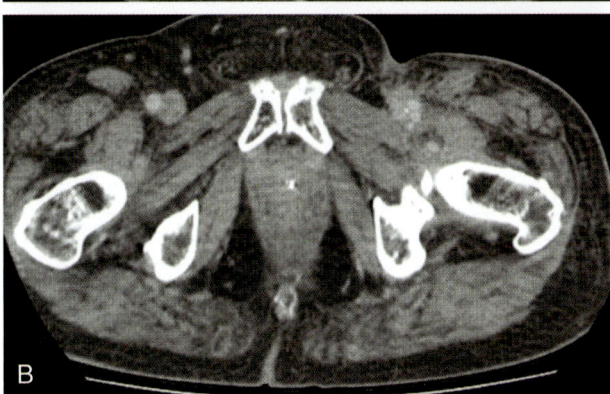
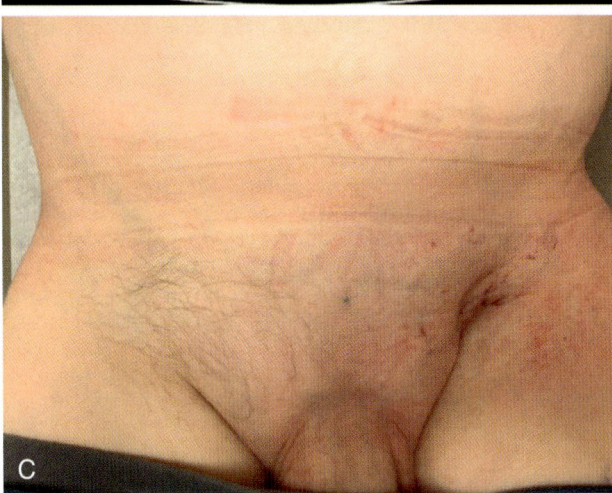

Fig. 79.8. (A) A 70-year-old patient presented with inoperable left inguinal adenopathy from squamous cell carcinoma penis. Treated with concurrent weekly cisplatin chemotherapy (40 mg/m²) and volumetric modulated arc therapy radiotherapy 45 Gy/25 fractions to pelvic nodes and 63 Gy/35 fractions to left groin. PET-CT clear 4 months post-treatment. (B) CT scan 2 years after treatment. (C) Appearance of groin 2 years post-treatment. No leg edema.

> ### KEY POINTS: RADIATION THERAPY
> - Radiation provides an effective penile-preserving approach for T1-T2 squamous cell carcinomas smaller than 4 cm using either external-beam radiotherapy or brachytherapy.
> - Because 20% of recurrences occur after 5 years, continued follow-up is required as salvage penectomy for persistent or recurrent disease may be curative.
> - The criteria for surgical staging of inguinal lymph nodes are the same whether patients undergo primary radiation or primary surgical management.
> - Unresectable lymph nodes may be rendered operable by neoadjuvant chemotherapy or chemoradiation.
> - Integration of radiation, surgery, and chemotherapy in advanced disease is being investigated in a prospective international randomized trial (InPACT: EA 8134).
> - Palliative radiotherapy may be beneficial for metastatic disease.

Palliative radiation ameliorates symptoms in a significant proportion of patients with painful bony metastases, or spinal cord compression, but a standard short course of 5 to 10 fractions is not highly effective for bulky or fixed groin nodes. Although these patients may be elderly and frail, consideration should be given to combined platinum and radiotherapy provided kidney function is adequate with a GFR exceeding 50 mL/min.

Adjuvant radiation has an important role to play for surgically treated pN+ patients. In a review of the National Cancer Data Base from 1998 to 2012, Winters et al. (2017) found 589 patients who underwent inguinal lymph node dissection for stage III penile cancer.

CHEMOTHERAPY

Active Single Agents, Combination Strategies, and Post-Chemotherapy Surgery

Advanced penile cancer presenting as either bulky or unresectable regional disease or visceral metastases at initial presentation or disease recurrence is highly lethal; it is incurable in most cases with either surgery or radiotherapy alone (Hegarty et al., 2006; Ornellas et al., 1994; Ravi et al., 1994). Experience with single-agent or multiagent chemotherapy in this setting is limited: there are few phase II clinical trials and no randomized clinical trials. Several regimens have produced clinically meaningful responses that have occasionally resulted in clearance of disease or facilitated surgical resection.

Single-Agent Chemotherapy

Gagliano et al. (1989) from the Southwest Oncology Group treated 26 patients with low-dose (50 mg/m²) cisplatin and observed responses in 15% and a median overall survival of 4.7 months. In a study from Memorial Sloan-Kettering Cancer Center, 13 patients with extensive disease and either prior radiotherapy or chemotherapy were treated with cisplatin 70 to 120 mg/m^2 every 21 days. Three of 12 evaluable patients (25%) demonstrated responses (one complete and two partial; duration = 2–8 months) (Ahmed et al., 1984).

Initial favorable reports from Japan suggested that bleomycin appeared to be effective in the treatment of penile and scrotal cancer. Ichikawa et al. (1969; 1977) reported a 50% response in 24 previously untreated patients with squamous carcinoma of the penis. A similar report from Uganda documented partial or complete tumor regression in 45% of treated patients (Kyalwazi et al., 1974). A review of 90 patients from the world literature demonstrated similar responses (Eisenberger, 1992). In the study by Ahmed et al. (1984) 14 patients were evaluable for response to single-agent bleomycin. There was one complete response (CR), but the patient died from bleomycin pulmonary toxicity. There were also two partial responses (PRs), for an overall response rate (ORR) of 21%. The median response duration was only 3 months (range 2–4).

Methotrexate produced responses in 8 of 13 patients (61%) treated at Memorial Sloan-Kettering Cancer Center (Ahmed et al., 1984) with one CR. However, median response duration even with the high response rate was 3 months (2–31 months), and one patient died from treatment-related sepsis. Methotrexate had been shown to be active in other reports (Garnick et al., 1979; Mills, 1972). Based on the Ahmed study in which cisplatin, bleomycin, and methotrexate were given sequentially, there did not appear to be any obvious cross-resistance to the three agents. Subsequently a three-drug trial using combination bleomycin, methotrexate, and cisplatin (BMP) was developed.

Combination Chemotherapy

The Southwest Oncology Group reported a phase II study using a modified regimen that reduced the total dose of BMP. Haas et al. (1999) enrolled 45 patients with locally advanced or metastatic penile cancer, including distant metastases. There were five complete and eight PRs among 40 evaluable patients (32.5% response rate). The median duration of response was 16 weeks with an overall survival of 28 weeks (Haas et al., 1999). Although the response rate appeared encouraging, it was still within the 95% confidence intervals previously reported for single agent cisplatin; moreover, there were 5 treatment-related deaths on the study (one from infection and four from pulmonary complications) (Ahmed et al., 1984; Gagliano et al., 1989; Haas et al., 1999). Thus this study failed to confirm the initial high response rate of single agent methotrexate, did not establish superiority of BMP to single agent cisplatin, and found that bleomycin pulmonary toxicity was significant (Haas et al., 1999).

Three additional trials, all employing cisplatin, reveal significant activity while omitting the bleomycin and methotrexate (Table 79.14). Theodore et al. (2008) reported the results of an EORTC phase II study (30992) in which 28 patients with locally advanced or metastatic disease (T3, T4, N1-N3, or M1) received combination cisplatin and irinotecan. Patients were treated in either the neoadjuvant setting for 4 cycles before surgery (T3, N1-N2) or up to 8 cycles (T4, N3, M1 disease). Toxicity was acceptable with no treatment-related deaths. Eight responses were noted (2 complete, 6 partial) for an objective response rate of 30.8% (80% CI 0.188–0.45). Three patients taken to surgery in the neoadjuvant setting were found to have no evidence of residual disease. The authors reported the trial as negative, however, as it was powered to show an ORR not less than 30% by confidence interval.

A phase II clinical trial of neoadjuvant paclitaxel, ifosfamide, and cisplatin (TIP) was conducted at the University of Texas MD Anderson Cancer Center (Pagliaro et al., 2010). Eligible patients exhibited clinical N2-N3 lymph node metastases, no evidence of distant metastases (M0), and no prior chemotherapy. Treatment consisted of 4 courses of TIP followed by bilateral inguinal lymph node dissections, unilateral or bilateral pelvic lymph node dissections, and surgical control of the primary tumor when appropriate. The ORR was 50% and the pathologic CR rate was 10%; 23 of 30 eligible patients completed 4 courses of TIP and 22 of those underwent surgery; 9 patients (30% for the trial, 40.9% of those completing treatment) were alive and disease free at a median follow-up of 34 months; 19 deaths occurred as a result of progressive disease and 2 from unrelated causes. Toxicity was acceptable and no treatment-related deaths occurred (Pagliaro et al., 2010). These data suggest that the TIP regimen has a response rate significantly higher than single-agent cisplatin and is better tolerated than older regimens containing bleomycin or methotrexate. Table 79.13 provides safety and efficacy of cisplatin-containing chemotherapy regimens reported.

A third prospective trial evaluated the combination of docetaxel, cisplatin, and 5-fluorouracil (TPF) in patients with locally advanced or metastatic penile cancer (Nicholson et al., 2013). The response rate was 38.5% (10 of 26 evaluable patients), and 65.5% of patients experienced at least a grade 3 or grade 4 event. The predetermined target response rate of 60% was not reached, and the authors concluded that similar results could be achieved with 5-FU/cisplatin and that the addition of docetaxel resulted in toxicity. By comparison, the objective response rate to 5-FU/cisplatin in one retrospective series was 32% (8 of 25 patients) (Di Lorenzo et al., 2012).

Data from the earlier-mentioned three prospective trials and one retrospective series suggest that patients with advanced, unresectable primary tumors or metastatic disease can benefit from cisplatin-based

TABLE 79.14 Safety and Efficacy of Multidrug Penile Cancer Regimens Without Bleomycin

	CHEMOTHERAPY	RESPONSE RATE	TREATMENT-RELATED DEATH	MEDIAN OVERALL SURVIVAL (mo)
Di Lorenzo et al., 2012[a]	Fluorouracil, 800–1000 mg/m^2/day, days 1–4 continuous infusion Cisplatin, 70–80 mg/m^2, day 1; cycle q3wk	32%	0/25	8
Pagliaro et al., 2010	Paclitaxel, 175 mg/m^2, day 1 Ifosfamide, 1200 mg/m^2, days 1–3 Cisplatin, 25 mg/m^2, days 1–3; cycle q3wk	50%	0/30	17.1[b]
Theodore et al., 2008	Irinotecan, 60 mg/m^2, days 1, 8, 15 Cisplatin, 80 mg/m^2, day 1; cycle q4wk	30.8%	0/28	4.7
Nicholson et al., 2013	Docetaxel, 75 mg/m^2, day 1 Cisplatin, 60 mg/m^2, day 1 Fluorouracil, 750 mg/m^2/day, days 1–5; cycle q3wk	38.5%	0/28	13.9

[a]Retrospective study.
[b]Neoadjuvant setting (N2-3, M0).

chemotherapy, and selected patients with bulky regional lymph node metastases appeared to benefit from post-chemotherapy lymphadenectomy. Negative pathology in lymph nodes was seen after neoadjuvant treatment with TIP (3/30 patients) and irinotecan/cisplatin (3/7 patients). For patients with initially unresectable primary tumors or bulky regional lymph node metastases, neoadjuvant treatment with a cisplatin-containing regimen may be effective and allow curative resection.

Adjuvant Chemotherapy

Historically, combination vincristine, bleomycin, and methotrexate therapy was administered in 12 weekly courses to 17 patients in the postoperative setting (12) or neoadjuvant setting (5) at the Milan National Tumor Institute. The patients treated were at high risk for recurrence with surgery alone; 9 showed extranodal tumor growth, 5 had pelvic nodal involvement, and 5 had bilateral metastases. At follow-up ranging between 18 and 102 months, only 1 relapse had occurred (Pizzocaro and Piva, 1988). Later, reports from this center further confirmed the value of adjuvant chemotherapy. Of 56 node-positive patients, 82% of the 25 patients receiving adjuvant vincristine, bleomycin, and methotrexate (VBM) therapy survived 5 years, compared with 37% of 31 patients treated with surgery alone (Pizzocaro et al., 1995, 1997). In the neoadjuvant treatment group, PRs were noted in 3 of 5 patients with extremely large (6 to 11 cm) nodal metastases. These 3 patients subsequently were completely resected and were free of tumor at intervals ranging from 20 to 72 months. These data have yet to be confirmed and will probably not be further studied given the potential toxicities of bleomycin and methotrexate. A recent contemporary study suggested a potential benefit for the use of adjuvant chemotherapy among penile cancer patients with proven pelvic nodal metastases postsurgery. Sharma et al. (2015) retrospectively studied a multi-institutional cohort of 84 patients (collected from 1978–2013) with pelvic nodal metastases who either did or did not receive adjuvant chemotherapy with published regimens including TIP, TPF (used in later years), and BMP or VBM (used in earlier years). A subset of patients also received adjuvant pelvic radiotherapy. A total of 36 patients received adjuvant chemotherapy (ACT). When compared with the 48 that did not, the ACT cohort was younger, had a lower likelihood of receiving groin or pelvic radiotherapy, were more likely to exhibit inguinal extranodal extension of cancer but had a lower incidence of bilateral metastases. ACT was significantly associated with an 11.6-month survival advantage (21.7 vs. 10.1 months, $P = 0.048$) and was independently associated with reduced all-cause mortality subsequent to multivariate analysis. Thus there is a positive signal that adjuvant chemotherapy may be beneficial at least in the subset of patients with pelvic nodal metastases postsurgery. However, this remains to be confirmed prospectively.

Post-Chemotherapy Surgical Consolidation

Corral et al. (1998) reported on the long-term follow-up of a prospective group of patients treated with BMP. Among the cohort, 21 patients had penile carcinoma with 10/21 (48%) having either N3 or M1 disease. The remainder had either N1 or N2 nodal metastases. Objective responses were noted in 12 patients (57%), and 6 patients in the group (28.5%) eventually achieved disease-free status after chemotherapy alone (2) or followed by surgery (3) or radiotherapy (1). The median survival for patients who were free of disease was 27.8 months and was significantly longer than that of those not achieving disease-free status (6.7 months, $P = 0.004$), suggesting that a multidisciplinary approach to achieve disease-free status could prolong survival. Subsequently Leijte et al. (2007) from the Netherlands Cancer Institute reviewed their experience with neoadjuvant chemotherapy in patients with initially "unresectable" penile cancer. The series included 20 patients treated with 5 different regimens, including (1) single-agent bleomycin, (2) bleomycin, vincristine, methotrexate, (3) cisplatin and 5-fluorouracil, (4) BMP, and (5) cisplatin and irinotecan. The objective responses were evaluable in 19 (one patient died as a result of bleomycin toxicity after 2 weeks) with 12 responses (63%, 2 complete, 10 partial). Surgical procedures included treatment of the primary tumor as well as inguinal and pelvic dissections. Additional soft-tissue resection including bone was sometimes required. Vascularized tissue flaps were used for inguinal reconstruction. Among 12 responders only 9 went to surgery; 2 died of bleomycin-related complications, and the third was deemed unfit for surgery. Eight of 9 responding patients taken to surgery (two were pT0) were free of disease with a median follow-up of 20.4 months. This is in contrast to 3 nonresponders who went to surgery for palliative intent. All 3 died within 4 to 8 months because of locoregional recurrence. The implications from this study were that a response to chemotherapy together with an aggressive surgical procedure provides the optimal scenario for significant palliation or potentially cure.

In a separate study, Bermejo et al. (2007) described the surgical considerations and complications among 10 patients who had either a response or stable disease after combination chemotherapy. The regimens used included (1) BMP, (2) TIP, or paclitaxel and carboplatin. This cohort of patients exhibited bulky inguinal or pelvic metastases before chemotherapy, with the only exclusions being patients with fixed pelvic masses or complete encasement of the femoral vessels. In addition to ilioinguinal lymphadenectomy, resection of the inguinal ligament, the inferior aspect of the rectus abdominis or external and internal oblique muscles, the spermatic cord and ipsilateral testicle, and segments of the femoral artery and vein (with subsequent patch or bypass grafting) were performed to achieve negative margins. Plastic surgery consultation was obtained for wound coverage, including the insertion of monofilament polypropylene mesh for abdominal wall defects and myocutaneous flaps of the sartorius, rectus abdominus, serratus anterior, and latissimus dorsi muscles. Among 5 patients with an objective response to preoperative chemotherapy, 3 were alive and disease free at 48, 50, and 73 months postoperative. Among the 5 patients with stable disease as their best response to chemotherapy, 4 were dead within 7 to 8 months. A single patient treated with paclitaxel and carboplatin achieving only stable disease was alive and disease free at 84 months. These data appear to reinforce the concept that response to preoperative chemotherapy enhances the chance for long-term survival among those undergoing surgical resection. All three pT0 responses at surgery were among patients treated with TIP. Finally, in the prospective phase II study of neoadjuvant TIP for patients with clinical N2-N3 nodal disease (Pagliaro et al., 2010), the patients with an objective response (CR or PR) to neoadjuvant TIP had significantly better overall survival ($P = 0.001$) and time to progression ($P < 0.001$) compared with those who did not. This experience was updated to include a total of 61 patients with 90% of patients receiving the TIP regimen (Dickstein et al., 2016). In all, 39 patients (65%) had either a partial or complete response to chemotherapy. The 5-year survival varied significantly ($P = 0.045–0.001$) among patients achieving a CR/PR (50%), stable disease (25%), and progression (7.7%). In all, 10 patients (16.4%) were rendered pN0 with combined therapy, and 20 patients (33%) were alive and disease free at a median follow-up of 67 months, whereas 32 (52%) died from disease. Long-term survival was associated with response to chemotherapy and favorable pathologic findings after resection.

Taken together these data provide evidence that response to chemotherapy improves resectability and survival. Surgery among patients who do not respond to chemotherapy may occasionally be associated with long-term survival but is more often associated with death resulting from either rapidly occurring locoregional recurrence or distant metastases (Bermejo et al., 2007; Dickstein et al., 2016; Leijte et al., 2007; Pagliaro et al., 2010).

NONSQUAMOUS PENILE MALIGNANT NEOPLASMS

Nonsquamous penile malignant neoplasms are extremely rare. Pathologic descriptions and local and regional treatment options are available; however, outcomes and comparisons are limited to case reports and small retrospective series. Most reports establish the following features: (1) incidence of disease, (2) distinguishing

> **KEY POINTS: CHEMOTHERAPY**
>
> - Neoadjuvant chemotherapy with a cisplatin-containing regimen should be considered for patients with lymph node metastases, as responses in this setting may facilitate curative resection. In the absence of level 1 evidence, the optimal or standard multimodal strategy remains undefined.
> - The use of bleomycin in the treatment of men with metastatic penile cancer was associated with an unacceptable level of toxicity and is discouraged.
> - Surgical consolidation to achieve disease-free status or palliation should be considered in fit patients with a proven objective response to systemic chemotherapy.
> - Among patients who progress through chemotherapy, surgery is not recommended.

pathologic features, (3) treatment recommendations, and (4) parallels (or lack thereof) to the same carcinoma in nongenital locations.

Basal Cell Carcinoma

Although basal cell carcinoma is frequently encountered on other sun-exposed cutaneous surfaces, it is rare on the penis (Fig. 79.9A). Fewer than 30 cases have been well documented (Goldminz et al., 1989; Ladocsi et al., 1998; Nguyen et al., 2006). The lesion can be seen anywhere on the penis but is commonly on the penile shaft. It is slow growing, and delay in diagnosis in one series ranged from 2 months to 50 years (Kim et al., 1994). **Treatment is by local excision, which is virtually always curative** (Goldminz et al., 1989; Hall et al., 1968). Only one case report describes what the authors believe to be the only reported case of metastatic penile basal cell carcinoma (Jones et al., 2000). Nguyen et al. (2006) reported two cases of basal cell carcinoma treated by Mohs surgery.

A benign variant of basal cell carcinoma, the premalignant fibroepithelioma of Pinkus, has been reported to occur on the penile shaft (Heymann et al., 1983). Diagnosis is made at excisional biopsy. Excision has been uniformly curative.

Melanoma and basal cell carcinoma rarely occur on the penis, presumably because the organ's skin is protected from exposure to the sun. Malignant neoplasms arising from the supporting structures of the penis are also rare and include any combination of tumors of smooth or striated muscle or of fibrous, fatty, or vascular tissue. Information about appropriate treatment of these malignant neoplasms is derived from the review of single case reports and small series (Belville and Cohen, 1992).

Melanoma

More than 150 cases of melanoma of the penis have been reported (Fig. 79.9B). Of 1200 melanomas treated at Memorial Sloan Kettering Cancer Center, only 2 were of penile origin (Das Gupta and Grabstald, 1965). At the University of Texas MD Anderson Cancer Center, less than 1% of all primary penile cancers were malignant melanomas (de Bree et al., 1997; Johnson and Ayala, 1973).

Melanoma manifests as a blue-black or reddish brown pigmented papule, plaque, or ulceration on the glans penis. It occurs on the prepuce less frequently. Diagnosis is made by histologic examination of biopsy specimens, which demonstrate atypical junctional cell activity with displacement of pigmented cells into the dermis.

Prognostic characteristics that have been found significant for melanoma in other sites, such as depth of invasion (Clark staging) and thickness of the tumor (Breslow classification), have not been prospectively applied to penile lesions because experience with these lesions is limited. Sanchez-Ortiz et al. (2005) used the AJCC system for classifying cutaneous melanomas in the largest report on melanoma of the penis. This system incorporates elements of the Clark and Breslow staging systems. When this information is favorable, local excision is feasible. Distant metastatic spread has been found in 60% of patients studied (Abeshouse, 1958; de Bree et al., 1997; Johnson et al., 1973) in older series. However, Sanchez-Ortiz found that patients with early stage melanomas had excellent outcomes if primary tumors were of low stage and regional lymph nodes were negative. Hematogenous metastases occur by means of the vascular structures of the corporeal bodies; lymphatic spread to the regional inguinal and pelvic nodes occurs by lymphatic permeation.

Surgery is the primary mode of treatment; radiation therapy and chemotherapy are of only adjunctive or palliative benefit. For stage I melanoma (localized lesion without metastases) and stage II melanoma (metastases confined to one regional area), adequate excision of the primary tumor by partial or total penile amputation together with en bloc bilateral ilioinguinal node dissection has historically been advocated (Bracken and Diokno, 1974; Johnson et al., 1973; Manivel and Fraley, 1988). In reviewing the University of Texas MD Anderson Cancer Center experience plus the literature to date, Sanchez-Ortiz et al. (2005) proposed a treatment algorithm for management of the primary tumor and inguinal lymph nodes. For tumors of the foreskin, circumcision may be adequate. For glans tumors, a partial penectomy was recommended; and for glans-shaft tumors, a partial or total penectomy can be performed. The authors recommend bilateral modified inguinal lymph node dissections in all patients with lesions that are Breslow depth 1 mm or greater, with ulceration, or with Clark level IV or V involvement. Although dynamic sentinel lymph node biopsy techniques are increasingly used in more common sites of melanoma, their use in penile melanoma is unproven as yet. This is likely because of the rarity of the disease (Sanchez-Ortiz et al., 2006).

The prognosis for patients with penile melanoma clearly depends on stage of the primary tumor and the presence or absence of inguinal metastases. Contemporary staging and prognostic factors were reviewed by Sanchez-Ortiz et al. (2005). A report from the Netherlands (van Geel et al., 2007) focused on the concept of mucosal site penile melanomas—glans, meatus, fossa navicularis, and distal urethral. These lesions may appear more aggressive than cutaneous lesions, but greater delay in diagnosis may be a factor. In a pooled, retrospective analysis of 66 cases, the recurrence outcomes were similar for cutaneous melanomas of comparable tumor thickness. Among patients with recurrent or metastatic melanoma, effective immunotherapy based upon immune checkpoint blockade has revolutionized management. A recent study documented a 12-month recurrence-free survival of 70% among patients with resected advanced stage melanoma (stage IIIb-IV) when treated with adjuvant nivolumab (Weber et al., 2017).

Sarcomas

Primary mesenchymal tumors of the penis are rare. A thorough review of 46 such tumors from the Armed Forces Institute of Pathology revealed an equal number of benign and malignant lesions (Dehner and Smith, 1970). The patients ranged in age from newborn to the eighth decade of life. The presenting signs and symptoms of subcutaneous mass, penile pain and enlargement, priapism, and urinary obstruction were the same for benign and malignant lesions. A sarcoma has been reported to masquerade as a Peyronie plaque (Moore et al., 1975).

Malignant lesions were found more frequently on the proximal shaft (Fig. 79.9C); **benign lesions were more often located distally. The most common malignant lesions were those of vascular origin (hemangioepithelioma), followed in frequency by those of neural, myogenic, and fibrous origin** (Ashley and Edwards, 1957). Single case reports of sarcomatous lesions have been published—for example, malignant fibrous histiocytoma (Parsons and Fox, 1988), angiosarcoma (Rasbridge and Parry, 1989), leiomyosarcoma (Planz et al., 1998), epithelioid sarcoma (Leviav et al., 1988), hemangioendothelioma (Kamat et al., 2004), and osteosarcoma (Sacker et al., 1994).

Sarcomas have been classified as superficial when they arise from the integumentary supporting structures and as deep when they develop from the corporeal body supporting structures (Pratt and Ross, 1969). Wide, local surface excision and partial penile amputation for the superficial tumors have been suggested and used successfully

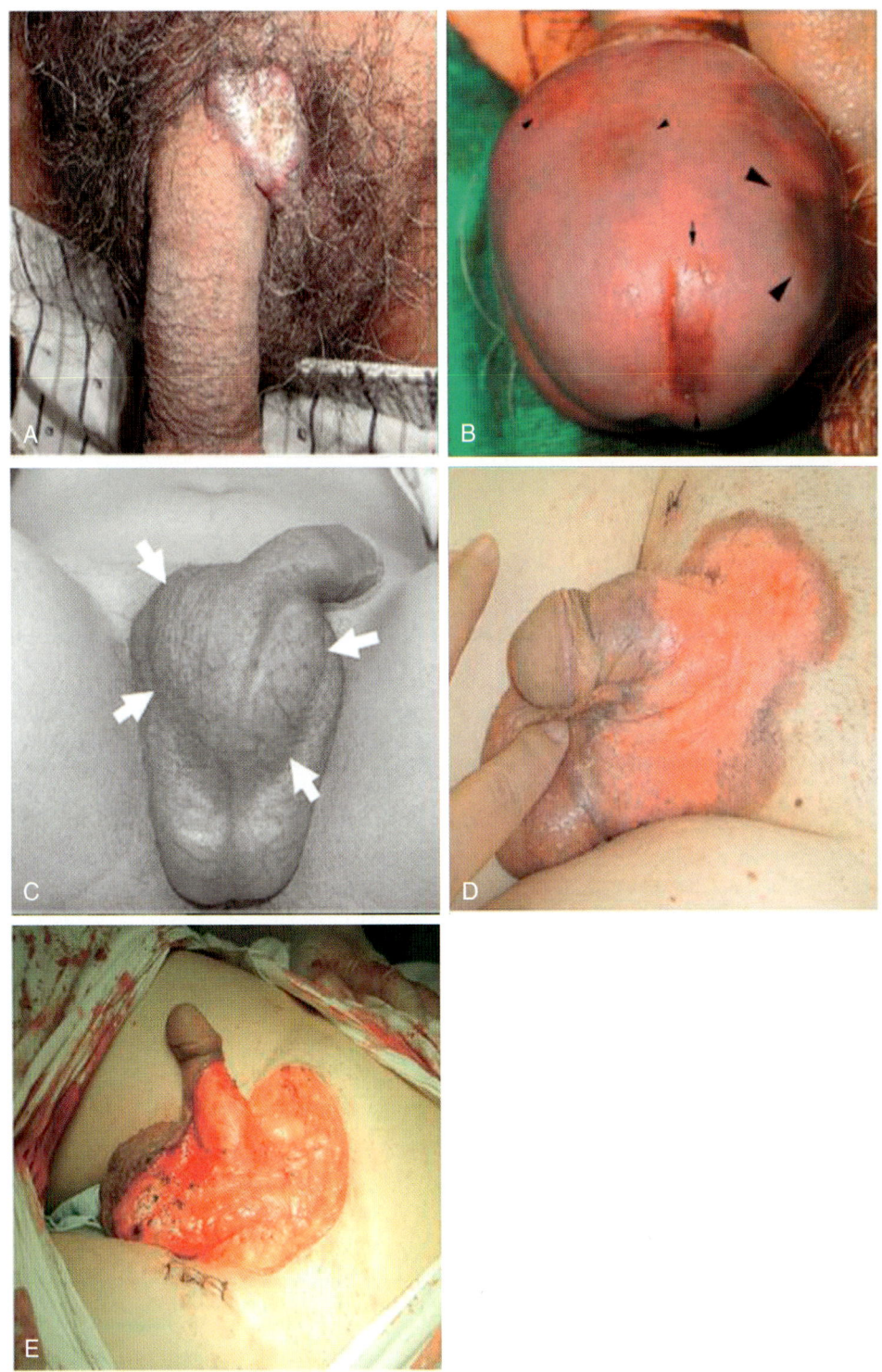

Fig. 79.9. Clinical examination findings from nonsquamous involving the penis. (A) Basal cell carcinoma. (B) Melanoma–superficial spreading type *(large arrowheads)*, melanoma in situ *(arrow)*, and two areas of possible melanosis *(small arrowheads)*. (C) Leiomyosarcoma involving base of penis *(arrows)*. (D) Paget disease involving penile, suprapubic, and left scrotal skin. (E) Surgical defect after Paget disease resection.

in isolated case reports (Dalkin and Zaontz, 1989; Pak et al., 1986). Total penile amputation has been reserved for tumors of deep corporeal origin. **However, local recurrences are characteristic of sarcomas** (Dehner and Smith, 1970). Fetsch et al. (2004), from the Armed Forces Institute of Pathology, have updated their series of 14 cases of leiomyosarcoma with review of the literature. They concluded that small lesions (smaller than 2 cm) were best managed with local resection, whereas deeper-seated tumor often necessitates partial or total amputation. Deep lesions at the base of the penis have the worst prognosis.

Regional metastases are rare. Unless adenopathy is palpable, node dissections are not recommended (Hutcheson et al., 1969). Distant metastases have also been unusual (Dehner and Smith, 1970). This supports aggressive local treatment in anticipation of cure. Radiation therapy and chemotherapy have not been used extensively enough for comment on their efficacy (Fetsch et al., 2004).

Extramammary Paget Disease

Extramammary Paget disease (EMPD) of the penis is rare; however, more recently several large series have been reported from China and Korea (Wang et al., 2008; Yang et al., 2005). EMPD appears grossly as an erythematous, eczematoid, well-demarcated area that cannot be clinically distinguished from EQ, BD, or CIS of the penis. Clinical presentation includes local discomfort, pruritus, and occasionally a serosanguineous discharge involving the penis, the scrotum, the perianal area and the axilla (Figs. 79.9D and E). EMPD in these sites is directly related to the presence of apocrine sweat glands. On microscopic examination, identification is clearly made by the presence of large, round or oval, clear-staining hydropic cells with hypochromatic nuclei (i.e., Paget cells). The cells often stain positively for cytokeratin 7 in addition to carcinoembryonic antigen and show gross cystic fluid protein but are S-100 protein negative (O'Connor et al., 2003). The tumor behaves as a slow-growing intraepithelial adenocarcinoma with cells derived from apocrine glands. With time the cells may become invasive with dermal tumor deposits metastasizing to regional lymph nodes via dermal lymphatics (Hegarty et al., 2011; Park et al., 2001). Penoscrotal EMPD may be associated with other malignancies of the genitourinary tract, such as prostate, bladder, and renal malignancies (Allan et al., 1998; Chanda, 1985; Koh, 1995; Ojeda et al., 1987) and should be evaluated for their presence. In a recent series from MD Anderson Cancer Center among 20 reported patients, 9 (45%) had at least one other malignancy including prostate, bladder, renal, skin, esophageal, and rectal sites. Notably, 8 of the 9 patients were diagnosed with the other cancer before their diagnosis of EMPD.

Two reports from the Far East have added to the case series in the literature: 130 cases of penoscrotal Paget disease from China (Wang et al., 2008) and 36 from South Korea (Yang et al., 2005). In most cases only the skin and dermis must be resected with a gross margin of up to 3 cm. Positive margins may still occur, and frozen sections are recommended to guide the extent of resection (Park et al., 2017; Pettaway, 2017b). However, false-negative frozen-section reports are not uncommon especially in a settings where specialized expertise (i.e., dermatopathologists) is not available to review the cases. Outpatient mapping biopsies may be helpful in determining the approximate tumor-free margin before major resection and can be helpful to the pathologist by providing formalin-fixed paraffin-embedded tissue with which to examine margins before actual resection. In this setting peripheral biopsies away from the obvious tumor are performed sequentially in the outpatient setting until all the margins are negative. In this setting Park et al. (2017) compared EMPD surgical outcomes among cohorts of patients that underwent resection alone versus prior mapping biopsies subsequent to surgical resection. They found that the mapping biopsy cohort exhibited lower rates of positive margins at frozen and permanent section, and this translated into lower 5-year tumor-free rates. Mapping biopsies were independently associated with lower local recurrence rates. Patients with a positive surgical margin are at a higher risk for recurrence, and additional resection is advised. In the series from Hegarty et al. (2011), no recurrences were noted among patients with intraepidermal EMPD with negative surgical margins. Local skin or scrotal flaps (Wang et al., 2008) can be used to cover the defects.

In a minority of cases the tumor may invade deeper structures, necessitating more extensive resection and reconstruction, as reported in case series (Fujisawa et al., 2008; Hatoko et al., 2002). If inguinal adenopathy is present, radical node dissection is advised (Hagan et al., 1975), but prognosis is poor (Yang et al., 2005). Hegarty et al. (2011) described the use of neoadjuvant docetaxel and carboplatin chemotherapy and surgical resection in two patients. One patient was alive with disease at 40 months, and the other had no evidence of disease at 13 months.

Adenosquamous Carcinoma

Adenosquamous carcinoma is a rare tumor characterized by glandular and squamous histologic elements that are independent of the urethral glands. It manifests as a large (5 to 9 cm), firm, and grayish white granular exophytic mass involving the distal shaft or glans. On microscopic examination the glands contain mucin and are positive for carcinoembryonic antigen. In one reported case, the tumor was metastatic to a single inguinal node. This patient was managed with local excision of the primary tumor and a limited inguinal node dissection and lived 9 years after treatment. Other tumors were managed with local excision and surveillance (Cubilla et al., 1996). In only the seventh reported case (Romero et al., 2006), a patient with a bulky primary mass and inguinal lymph nodes underwent total penectomy and delayed ILND and PLND with a final pathologic stage of pT2N3M0 and was free of disease at 5-year follow-up.

Lymphoreticular Malignant Neoplasm

Primary lymphoreticular malignant neoplasms rarely occurs on the penis (Dehner and Smith, 1970). This term is likely a misnomer and when it occurs the penile findings almost always represent an early manifestation of a more systemic process (Chu et al., 2013). **Leukemia may infiltrate the corpora, resulting in priapism** (Pochedly et al., 1974). Given the absence of lymphoid tissue in the penis, **a thorough search for systemic disease is necessary when lymphomatous infiltration of the penis is diagnosed. In a recent report 48 case reports of lymphomatous involvement of the penis were analyzed** (Chu et al., 2013). **The most common type of lymphoma was the diffuse large B cell type with the most common symptoms being a lump on the penis or priapism. Involved additional sites have included lymph nodes, lung, liver, and occasionally the brain thus a search for systemic disease is mandatory.** If the penile lesion is indeed the only identified site, systemic directed toward the disease entity should still be administered. In the case of lymphomatous involvement this included rituxumab-cyclophosphamide, doxorubicin, vincristine, and prednisone as the most common regimen used. A systemic approach is effective therapy for local disease, for potential occult deposits that may exist elsewhere, and for preservation of form and function (Chu et al., 2013; Marks et al., 1988).

Metastases

Metastatic lesions to the penis are relatively rare. Up to the year 2011 approximately 437 cases had been reported (Chaux et al., 2011). Their infrequency is somewhat puzzling when one considers the rich blood and lymphatic supply to the organ and its proximity to the bladder, prostate, and rectal areas frequently involved with neoplasm. It is from these three organs that the majority of metastatic penile lesions originate (Abeshouse and Abeshouse, 1961). The most likely routes of spread are by direct extension, retrograde venous and lymphatic transport, and arterial embolism. Other sources of penile metastases emanate from the gastrointestinal tract, testis, and kidney (Belville and Cohen, 1992).

The most frequent sign of penile metastasis is priapism; penile swelling, nodularity, and ulceration have also been reported (Abeshouse and Abeshouse, 1961; McCrea and Tobias, 1958; Weitzner, 1971). Urinary obstruction and hematuria may occur. The most common histologic feature of penile invasion by metastatic lesions is the replacement of one or both corpora cavernosa, which explains the frequent occurrence of priapism. Solitary cutaneous, preputial, and glandular deposits are less common.

The differential diagnosis includes idiopathic priapism; venereal or other infectious ulcerations; tuberculosis; Peyronie plaque; and primary, benign, or malignant tumors.

Penile metastases represent an advanced form of virulent disease and usually appear rather rapidly after recognition and during treatment of the primary tumor site (Abeshouse and Abeshouse, 1961; Chaux et al., 2011; Hayes and Young, 1967; Mukamel et al., 1987). On rare occasions a long period may elapse between the treatment of the primary lesion and the appearance of penile metastases (Abeshouse and Abeshouse, 1961), or the penile lesion may occur as the initial and only site of metastasis. In one report of 17 patients with penile metastases, 14 patients died of disseminated disease, with a median survival of 5 months after the diagnosis of penile metastases (Chaux et al., 2011).

Because of the association of a penile metastatic lesion with advanced disease, survival after its presentation is limited, and the majority of patients die within 1 year (Chaux et al., 2011; Mukamel et al., 1987; Robey and Schellhammer, 1984). Successful palliative treatment may occasionally be possible in the case of solitary nodules or localized distal penile involvement if complete excision by partial or total amputation succeeds in removing the entire area of malignant infiltration (Spaulding and Whitmore, 1978). The prospect for surgical cure is minimal if proximal corporeal invasion is present. Penectomy is occasionally indicated after failure of other modalities to palliate intractable pain (Mukamel et al., 1987). In such cases obtaining an MRI of the penis to determine the proximal extent of the tumor and the presence of discontinuous tumor satellites can assist in determining the feasibility of surgery and the extent of resection (Gupta and Rajesh, 2014). Pain can also be managed by dorsal nerve section (Hill and Khalid, 1988) along with suprapubic cystostomy diversion used to optimize bladder emptying. In general, radiation therapy has been unsuccessful. Salvage systemic therapy strategies, clinical trials directed toward the primary histology or hospice care represent options to consider in this patient cohort with an overall poor prognosis.

> **KEY POINTS: NONSQUAMOUS MALIGNANT NEOPLASMS**
>
> - Basal cell carcinoma represents a highly curable variant with a relatively low metastatic potential.
> - Sarcomas are prone to local recurrence; regional and distant metastases are rare. Superficial lesions can be treated with less radical procedures.
> - Melanoma is an aggressive form of cancer but can be cured if diagnosed and treated with the appropriate surgical procedure at an early stage. Novel immunotherapy strategies may improve survival in recurrent or advanced disease.
> - EMPD disseminates by intraepidermal spread initially. Wide local excision to achieve negative margins is the therapy of choice. Invasive EMPD can be lethal.
> - Penile metastases most often represent spread from a clinically obvious existing primary tumor. Prognosis is poor, and therapy should be directed toward the primary tumor site histology and local palliation.

REFERENCES

The complete reference list is available online at ExpertConsult.com.

80 Tumors of the Urethra

Christopher B. Anderson, MD, MPH, and James M. McKiernan, MD

BENIGN URETHRAL TUMORS

Benign tumors of the urethra are rare and generally only described in small case reports. Leiomyoma, hemangioma, and fibroepithelial polyp are most frequently reported. Female urethral prolapse and urethral caruncles are benign lesions that can mimic tumors, which will be discussed elsewhere (Fletcher and Lemack, 2008).

Leiomyoma

Leiomyomas are mesenchymal tumors that arise from urethral or paraurethral smooth muscle and are most commonly seen in reproductive-aged women (Pahwa et al., 2012). These tumors often are accompanied by obstructive voiding symptoms, dyspareunia or hematuria, and occasionally are diagnosed incidentally (Cornella et al., 1997). On physical examination they are generally firm, smooth, nontender masses in the anterior vaginal wall or that protrude from the urethral meatus. Cystoscopically they appear as suburothelial lesions without ulceration that often displace or obstruct the urethral lumen. These tumors can grow during pregnancy and regress postpartum, suggesting they are hormonally sensitive (Fry et al., 1988; Kato et al., 2004). They can occur anywhere along the urethra but most commonly arise within the posterior wall (Cicilet et al., 2016). Urethral leiomyomas are hypoechoic with internal vascularity on ultrasound. On magnetic resonance imaging (MRI) they are well-circumscribed tumors that can displace the urethra and vaginal wall. They enhance with contrast and are isointense to muscle on T1 and hypointense on T2, similar to uterine leiomyomas (Del Gaizo et al., 2013; Verma et al., 2014). Surgical excision is curative in nearly all cases and can be accomplished transvaginally or transurethrally depending on size and location. Pathologically, these tumors demonstrate fascicles of smooth muscle cells with uniform, spindle-shaped nuclei that lack atypia or mitotic figures (Goldman et al., 2007).

Hemangioma

Urethral hemangiomas are benign vascular tumors that are thought to arise from angioblastic cells within the urethra. They tend to be more common in men, although there are several reports of female urethral hemangiomas (Manuel et al., 1977; Ongun et al., 2014). There is no obvious age predilection, they can occur as solitary or multiple lesions, and they can grow anywhere along the length of the urethra (Roberts and Devine, 1983). Urinary tract hemangiomas may be associated with the presence of cutaneous hemangiomas or congenital disorders such as Klippel-Trenaunay-Weber syndrome (Terada et al., 2007). The most common symptoms of a urethral hemangioma are intermittent hematuria and bloody urethral discharge (Parshad et al., 2001). They are normally painless, although they can cause pain if they become thrombosed (Tabibian and Ginsberg, 2003). Posterior urethral hemangiomas in males are typically located between the verumontanum and external sphincter and can cause hematospermia and postejaculatory hematuria (Han et al., 2015; Saito, 2008).

The diagnosis of a urethral hemangioma is made by cystoscopy and biopsy. The most common appearance is that of a bluish sessile lesion with associated varicosities, with pathology demonstrating cavernous hemangioma in most cases (Jahn and Nissen, 1991). Because they can sometimes be more extensive than they appear, MRI scans can be used to delineate the extent of the lesion and demonstrates a high signal on T2 similar to hepatic hemangiomas (Hayashi et al., 1997; Jahn and Nissen, 1991). Smaller hemangiomas are treated with transurethral fulguration or laser ablation (Saito, 2008). However, an incompletely ablated or resected hemangioma can recur (Manuel et al., 1977; Uchida et al., 2001). When a hemangioma is more extensive, open excision with urethral reconstruction may be required (Parshad et al., 2001; Roberts and Devine, 1983). Selective embolization has also been used (Murray et al., 1986).

Fibroepithelial Polyp

Urethral fibroepithelial polyps (FEPs) are rare benign tumors of mesodermal origin most commonly found in males (Kumar et al., 2008). Urethral FEPs are usually found in children but can also occur in adults (Kumar et al., 2008; Tsuzuki and Epstein, 2005). Most male FEPs arise within the bulbar and posterior urethra, and the most common clinical presentation in adults is obstructive urinary symptoms, hematuria, dysuria, and rarely urinary retention (Kumar et al., 2008; Tsuzuki and Epstein, 2005). They may protrude from the urethral meatus in women (Aita et al., 2005; Yamashita et al., 2004). Retrograde urethrography and voiding cystourethrography demonstrate a smooth, cylindrical urethral filling defect. On cystoscopy, they usually appear as smooth pink or tan tumors that are connected to the urethra on a stalk.

Transurethral resection of urethral FEPs is usually curative (Kumar et al., 2008). Pathologic examination is required to confirm the diagnosis and rule out a urothelial papilloma. Microscopically they have a fibrovascular core that is surrounded by normal urothelium (Tsuzuki and Epstein, 2005).

MALE URETHRAL CANCER

Epidemiology, Etiology, and Clinical Presentation

Male primary urethral cancer (PUC) is a rare disease that usually manifests after the sixth decade of life and is more common in African Americans than Caucasians (Dalbagni et al., 1999; Rabbani, 2011; Sui et al., 2017; Swartz et al., 2006; Thyavihally et al., 2006; Visser et al., 2012). Based on national cancer registry data, it is estimated that there are 1.3 to 4.3 cases of urethral cancer for every million men (Swartz et al., 2006; Visser et al., 2012). **Most patients with anterior PUC have a history of chronic urethral inflammation with urethral stricture disease being the most common risk factor.** Preexisting stricture disease is present in at least 50% of patients with PUC (Dalbagni et al., 1999; Kaplan et al., 1967). Other risk factors for anterior PUC include sexually transmitted diseases, lichen sclerosis, urethritis, pelvic radiation, trauma, and instrumentation (Agrawal et al., 2017; Anderson and McAninch, 1984; Dalbagni et al., 1999; Gakis et al., 2013; Smith et al., 2007; Thyavihally et al., 2006). Human papillomavirus 16 has been detected in some urethral cancers and may play a role in pathogenesis (Cupp et al., 1996). Arsenic exposure has also been reported to increase the risk of urethral cancer (Tsai et al., 2005).

Presenting symptoms for PUC most commonly include obstructive voiding symptoms, hematuria or bloody urethral discharge, and penile or perineal mass (Dalbagni et al., 1999; Dinney et al., 1994; Kent et al., 2015; Thyavihally et al., 2006). Nearly all patients are

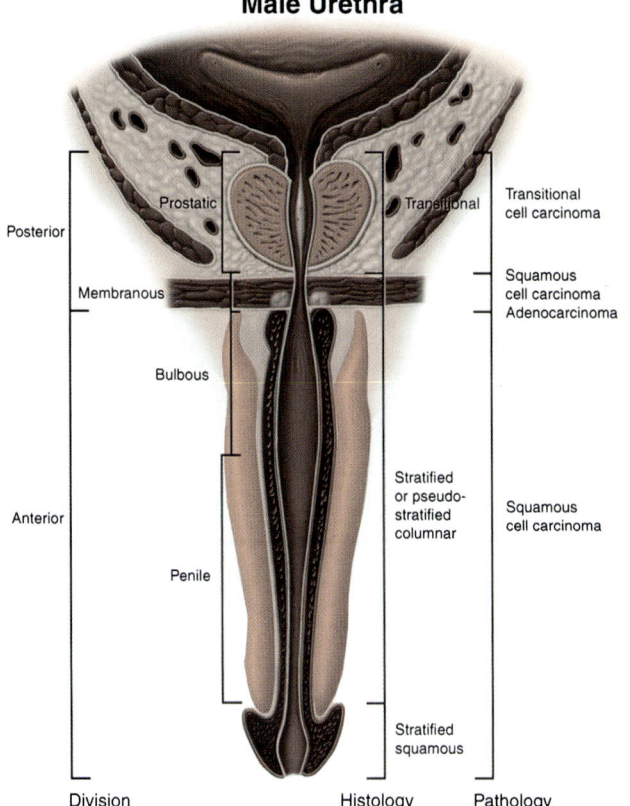

Fig. 80.1. Anatomy of the male urethra with corresponding histology and pathology.

TABLE 80.1 Grading System for Primary Urethral Carcinoma

G	DEFINITION
UROTHELIAL CARCINOMA	
LG	Low grade
HG	High grade
SQUAMOUS CELL CARCINOMA, ADENOCARCINOMA	
Gx	Grade cannot be assessed
G1	Well differentiated
G2	Moderately differentiated
G3	Poorly differentiated

Data from Hansel D, Reuter VE, Bochner B, et al.: Urethra. In Amin MB, editor: *AJCC Cancer Staging Manual*, ed 8, New York, 2017, Springer.

symptomatic at the time of presentation (Dalbagni et al., 1999). The onset of malignant change in a patient with chronic urethral stricture disease may be insidious, and a high index of clinical suspicion is required to diagnose these tumors.

Pathology

The male urethra is approximately 20 cm long and consists of the anterior and posterior urethra. **The anterior urethra includes the bulbar urethra, pendulous urethra, and fossa navicularis, whereas the posterior urethra consists of the prostatic and membranous urethra. The anterior urethra is lined by stratified and pseudostratified columnar epithelium, which transitions to stratified squamous epithelium in the very distal urethra** (Fig. 80.1; Reuter, 2014). **The posterior urethra is lined by urothelium.** Paired bulbourethral glands, or Cowper glands, drain into the bulbar urethra, and several periurethral glands, or glands of Littre, reside along the length of the anterior urethra.

Carcinoma of the male urethra is categorized according to location and histology. Because there is a change in cell type along the length of the urethra, male PUCs vary by site of origin. **Among urethral cancers described in population-level studies, 50% to 80% are urothelial carcinomas, 10% to 30% are squamous cell carcinomas, and 5% to 10% are adenocarcinomas** (Gakis et al., 2016; Rabbani, 2011; Sui et al., 2017; Visser et al., 2012). These large datasets may overestimate the true proportion of urothelial PUCs due to misclassification or miscoding because this histologic class comprises the minority of PUCs in institutional data sets (Dalbagni et al., 1999; Dinney et al., 1994). Other rare cancer types include melanoma and sarcoma (Gakis et al., 2016).

Urothelial carcinomas are graded as either low or high, whereas squamous cell carcinoma and adenocarcinoma are graded as well, moderately, and poorly differentiated (Table 80.1; Hansel et al., 2017). The majority of posterior urethral cancers are urothelial carcinomas, whereas more than 80% of anterior urethral cancers are squamous cell carcinomas (Dalbagni et al., 1999; Dinney et al., 1994; Kaplan et al., 1967; Thyavihally et al., 2006). Adenocarcinoma tends to be more common in the bulbar urethra (Kaplan et al., 1967; Tsai et al., 2005). **Among anterior urethral tumors, 60% are located in the bulbar urethra and 30% are in the pendulous urethra** (Dalbagni et al., 1999; Kaplan et al., 1967; Thyavihally et al., 2006).

Male PUC can spread by direct extension to adjacent structures, including the corpus spongiosum and the periurethral tissues, or it can metastasize through lymphatic spread to regional lymph nodes. **The lymphatics from the anterior urethra drain into the inguinal lymph nodes, although the bulbar urethral can occasionally drain into the external iliac lymph nodes. The posterior urethra drains into the pelvic lymph nodes.** Palpable inguinal lymph nodes occur in approximately 20% to 30% of cases and almost always represents metastatic disease in contrast to penile cancer, in which palpable inguinal nodes can be inflammatory (Dalbagni et al., 1999; Dayyani et al., 2014; Gakis et al., 2016; Rabbani, 2011).

Evaluation and Staging

The tumor, node, metastases (TNM) staging classification is based on depth of invasion of the primary tumor, and presence or absence of regional lymph node involvement and distant metastasis (Table 80.2). Examination under anesthesia with cystoscopy and bimanual palpation of the external genitalia, urethra, rectum, perineum, and inguinal lymph nodes is required to evaluate the extent of local tumor involvement and establish clinical staging. Transurethral or percutaneous needle biopsy of the primary lesion is necessary for a tissue diagnosis. Urine cytology has little utility in diagnosing PUC given its poor sensitivity (Touijer and Dalbagni, 2004). If rectal involvement is suspected, an evaluation of the lower colon with flexible sigmoidoscopy is recommended. **MRI provides superior soft-tissue resolution and is the optimal imaging modality to characterize the local extent of disease** (Fig. 80.2; Stewart et al., 2010). The presence of metastatic disease is best evaluated by a computed tomography (CT) scan or MRI of the abdomen and pelvis. Chest imaging with CT may also be required.

Male Anterior Urethral Cancer

Prognosis

The prognosis of male anterior PUC is variable and is strongly tied to tumor aggressiveness. The 5-year cancer-specific and overall survival for all men with PUC is between 50% and 70%, and 40% and 50%, respectively (Dalbagni et al., 1999; Kent et al., 2015; Rabbani, 2011; Sui et al., 2017; Thyavihally et al., 2006; Visser et al., 2012). Several tumor characteristics are associated with survival, including grade, stage, location, and histology (Gakis et al., 2016; Sui et al., 2017). **Whereas distal urethral tumors are often curable, bulbar tumors have survival rates as low as 20% to 30%** (Dalbagni et al., 1999;

TABLE 80.2	The American Joint Committee on Cancer (AJCC) Urethral Cancer Tumor, Node, Metastases (TNM) Staging System

PRIMARY TUMOR (T) (MALE AND FEMALE)

TX	Primary tumor cannot be assessed
T0	No evidence of primary tumor
Ta	Noninvasive papillary carcinoma
Tis	Carcinoma in situ
T1	Tumor invades subepithelial connective tissue
T2	Tumor invades any of the following: corpus spongiosum, periurethral muscle
T3	Tumor invades any of the following: corpus cavernosum, anterior vagina
T4	Tumor invades other adjacent organs (e.g., bladder)

TRANSITIONAL CELL CARCINOMA OF THE PROSTATE

Tis	Carcinoma in situ, involvement of the prostatic urethra or periurethral prostatic ducts without stromal invasion
T1	Tumor invades urethral subepithelial connective tissue immediately underlying the urothelium
T2	Tumor invades the prostatic stroma surrounding ducts either by direct extension from the urothelial surface or by invasion from prostatic ducts
T3	Tumor invades the periprostatic fat
T4	Tumor invades other adjacent organs (e.g., bladder, rectum)

REGIONAL LYMPH NODES (N)

NX	Regional lymph nodes cannot be assessed
N0	No regional lymph node metastasis
N1	Single regional lymph node metastasis in the inguinal region or true pelvis (perivesical, obturator, internal [hypogastric] and external iliac), or presacral lymph node
N2	Multiple regional lymph node metastasis in the inguinal region or true pelvis (perivesical, obturator, internal [hypogastric] and external iliac), or presacral lymph node

DISTANT METASTASIS (M)

M0	No distant metastasis
M1	Distant metastasis

Data from Hansel D, Reuter VE, Bochner B, et al.: Urethra. In Amin MB, editor: *AJCC Cancer Staging Manual*, ed 8, New York, 2017, Springer.

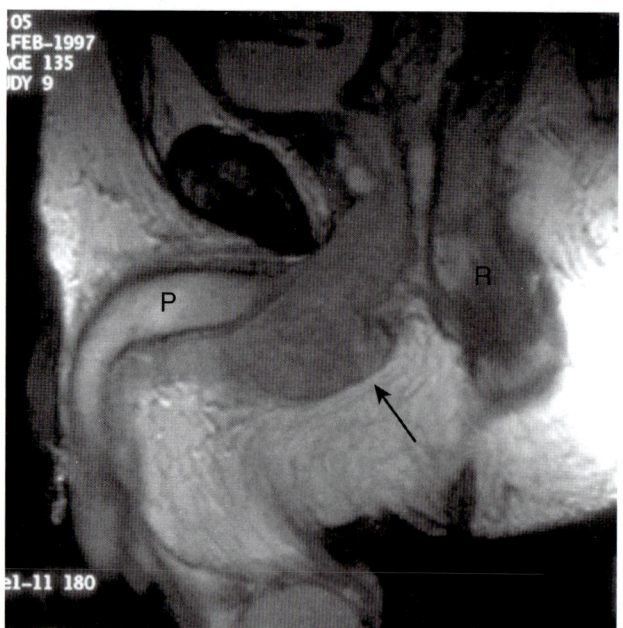

Fig. 80.2. Magnetic resonance image demonstrating a large proximal anterior urethral cancer *(arrow)*. *P*, Penis; *R*, rectum.

Dinney et al., 1994; Thyavihally et al., 2006). One large series reported overall survival rates of 83% for low-stage tumors, 36% for high-stage tumors, 69% for pendulous tumors, and 26% for bulbar tumors (Dalbagni et al., 1999). Similarly, among 29 patients with PUC the 5-year overall survival rates were 67% for low-stage disease, 33% for high-stage, 72% for distal tumors, and 36% for proximal tumors (Thyavihally et al., 2006). **Tumors arising from the proximal urethra tend to be found at more advanced stages** (Gheiler et al., 1998), **although tumor stage is independently associated with survival after controlling for location** (Thyavihally et al., 2006). Tumor grade and location are strongly correlated with stage, which ultimately dictates prognosis. Finally, men with adenocarcinoma may have a more favorable prognosis than other histologic subtypes (Rabbani, 2011; Sui et al., 2017).

Treatment

Aggressive local control is paramount in the management of localized PUC. The optimal method varies according to tumor location; however, there is growing interest in multimodal treatment for patients with advanced-stage disease (Table 80.3).

Carcinoma of the Pendulous Urethra

Tumors of the pendulous urethra and fossa navicularis are usually amenable to surgical resection. Transurethral resection, distal urethrectomy with or without partial penectomy, and total urethrectomy with perineal urethrostomy with or without total penectomy are acceptable treatment options in patients with distal urethral tumors depending on tumor size, location, and stage (Bladder cancer, 2018; Gakis et al., 2013).

Based on a limited number of small case series, surgical monotherapy for patients with distal tumors can successfully achieve local control (Anderson and McAninch, 1984; Gheiler et al., 1998; Kaplan et al., 1967). One series described successful treatment of three patients with low-stage fossa navicularis tumors with distal urethrectomy (Dinney et al., 1994). The same report described 10 patients with pendulous urethral tumors, among whom partial or radical penectomy provided local control in nearly all patients, although the risk of systemic relapse was higher than with tumors originating in the fossa navicularis.

The treatment for distal urethral tumors historically included urethral resection with radical or partial penectomy. **More recently, tumor excision with penile preservation has emerged as an option for select patients** (Gakis et al., 2013). The largest series on penile preservation for patients with distal PUC includes 18 men, most of whom had invasive squamous cell carcinoma and 6 had positive lymph nodes (Smith et al., 2007). Depending on the location and stage of the tumor, treatments included creation of a distal hypospadias with topical 5-fluorouracil (5-FU), distal urethrectomy with two-staged urethroplasty, glansectomy with skin graft reconstruction, and anterior urethrectomy with perineal urethrostomy. Patients with positive margins were treated with additional surgery or adjuvant radiation and no patient experienced a local recurrence. Squamous cell carcinoma in situ (CIS) of the perimeatal glans can extend into the distal urethra (Fig. 80.3) and has been successfully treated with partial glansectomy and distal urethrectomy with urethral reconstruction or penile urethrectomy (Fig. 80.4; Nash et al., 1996).

Partial penectomy with a 1-cm negative margin has been the traditional recommendation for invasive tumors localized to the distal urethra, but excision with a 5-mm negative margin has shown to produce excellent local control (Karnes et al., 2010; Smith

TABLE 80.3 Summary of 2018 National Comprehensive Cancer Network (NCCN) Clinical Practice Guidelines on Primary Urethral Cancer of the Male Anterior and Female Urethra

STAGE		FIRST-LINE TREATMENT OPTIONS	ADJUVANT THERAPY
Tis, Ta, T1		Repeat TUR ± intraurethral BCG or chemotherapy	
Male T2	Pendulous urethra	Partial urethrectomy ± penectomy[a]	If positive margin: Chemoradiotherapy OR Additional surgery OR Chemotherapy
	Bulbar urethra	Urethrectomy ± radical cystectomy[a]	If ≥ pT3 or N+: Chemotherapy OR Chemoradiotherapy
Female T2		Radical cystectomy[a] OR Chemoradiotherapy	
≥ T3	N0	Chemoradiotherapy ± consolidative surgery OR Neoadjuvant chemotherapy with consolidative surgery or radiation OR Radiotherapy	
	N+	Chemoradiotherapy ± consolidative surgery OR Systemic therapy	

[a]Consider neoadjuvant chemotherapy.
BCG, Bacille Calmette-Guérin; TUR, transurethral resection.
Data from Bladder Cancer, NCCN Clinical Practice Guidelines in Oncology, 2018 (website): https://www.nccn.org/professionals/physician_gls/default.aspx.

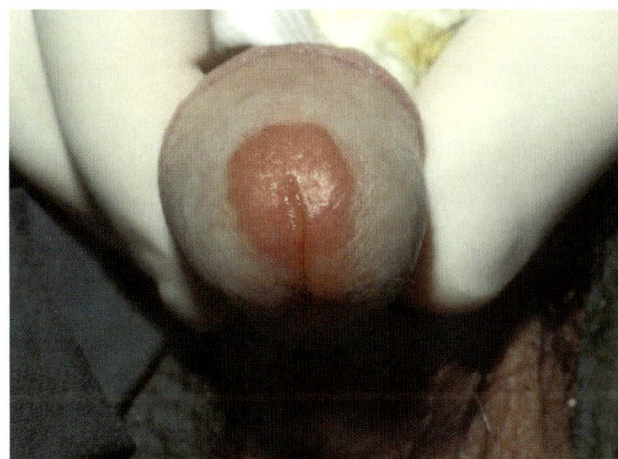

Fig. 80.3. Squamous cell carcinoma in situ of the perimeatal glans extending into the distal urethra.

et al., 2007). If invasive disease extends to or involves the proximal penile urethra, total urethrectomy, with or without penectomy, may be required to obtain a negative margin (Fig. 80.5). The proximal extent of disease must be carefully evaluated if partial urethrectomy is being considered. The risk of local recurrence after resection of a distal urethral tumor is low, but ongoing surveillance is necessary (Kaplan et al., 1967).

As opposed to patients with penile cancer, it is unclear if there is a survival benefit to prophylactic inguinal lymph node dissection in patients with anterior PUC without palpable inguinal lymph nodes. Some institutions have used inguinal sentinel lymph node

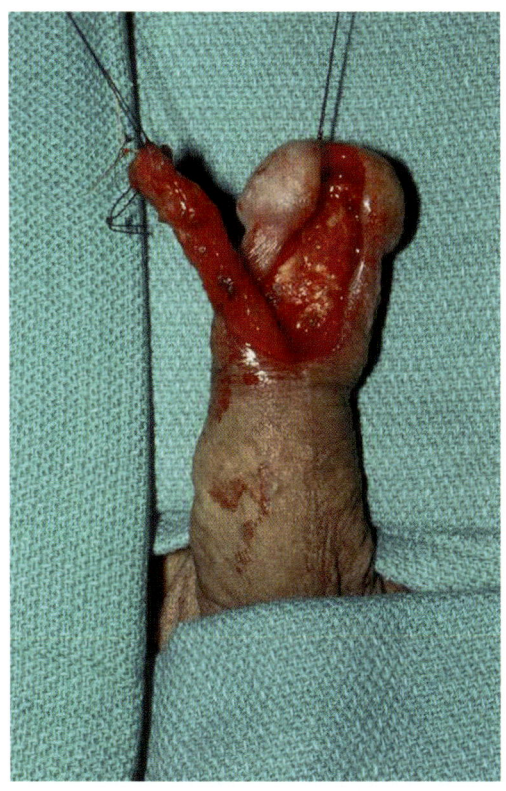

Fig. 80.4. Partial glansectomy and distal urethrectomy (same patient as Fig. 80.3). After a negative margin was obtained, a penile urethrostomy was performed.

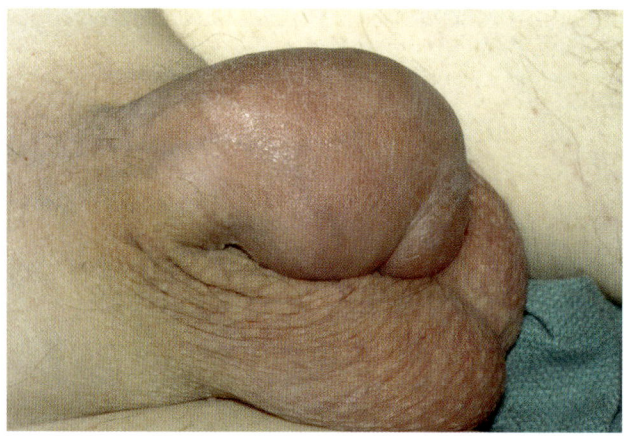

Fig. 80.5. A large penile mass in a patient with urothelial carcinoma of the pendulous urethra.

biopsy to identify patients with low-volume inguinal metastasis, and performed an inguinal lymphadenectomy, if the biopsy is positive (Bracken et al., 1980; Dinney et al., 1994; Smith et al., 2007). Patients with low-volume inguinal lymph node metastasis can be rendered disease free with inguinal lymphadenectomy, providing rationale for aggressive management of inguinal node metastases (Bracken et al., 1980). Certain groups have advocated for prophylactic inguinal lymphadenectomy for advanced stage pendulous PUC with clinically negative inguinal lymph nodes; however, this remains controversial (Karnes et al., 2010; Traboulsi et al., 2016). Prophylactic radiation to the reginal nodal basins should be strongly considered for patients with clinically negative lymph nodes whose primary lesions are being managed with radiotherapy (Bladder cancer, 2018).

Chemoradiation with or without surgical consolidation has emerged as an alternative to surgical resection of advanced urethral tumors (Baskin and Turzan, 1992). The largest series on chemoradiation for male PUC included 29 patients treated with 45 to 55 Gy of external beam radiotherapy combined with systemic 5-FU and mitomycin C (MMC), 12 of whom had squamous cell carcinoma of the pendulous urethra (Kent et al., 2015). Most patients were clinical stage T3 or lymph node positive (N+) and 79% (N = 19) demonstrated a complete response to treatment, including some who were clinically node positive. The 5-year disease-specific survival was 68%, and 6 of 19 complete responders experienced a local recurrence, some of whom could not be salvaged with surgery. **The role of surgical consolidation after a complete response to chemoradiation is unclear at this time, although all patients who responded to primary chemoradiation developed a urethral stricture, often requiring complex urethral reconstruction.** Patients who did not respond to chemoradiation died of disease. The authors recommended surgery for low-stage distal PUC.

Primary radiation therapy has been reserved for patients with early stage lesions of the anterior urethra who refuse surgery. A commonly used technique consists of parallel opposed fields with the penis suspended vertically by a urethral catheter (Heysek et al., 1985). Radiation therapy has the advantage of potentially preserving the penis, but it may result in skin ulceration and necrosis, urethral stricture, and chronic edema. The long-term results of radiotherapy are difficult to evaluate because few reports are available of male patients treated with this modality (Forman and Lichter, 1992; Koontz and Lee, 2010; Raghavaiah, 1978).

Because some patients with distal PUCs will have locally advanced or clinically node-positive disease, surgery with or without systemic therapy has been used with variable success (Dinney et al., 1994; Kaplan et al., 1967). Cases of cure with limited nodal disease have been reported; therefore systemic therapy followed by inguinal lymphadenectomy should be considered in the presence of palpable inguinal lymph nodes. Chemoradiation is also an option for clinically positive inguinal lymph nodes. Control of inguinal nodal disease may also help prevent complications from local invasion such as skin breakdown, wound drainage, and vascular erosion.

Carcinoma of the Bulbar Urethra

Some low-stage lesions of the proximal anterior urethra may be treated by transurethral resection or segmental excision with an end-to-end anastomosis. Patients treated with transurethral resection should be considered for repeat transurethral resection to ensure accurate staging and a complete resection (Bladder cancer, 2018). Unfortunately, there are relatively few patients eligible for limited resection because PUC of the bulbar urethra tends to present at an advanced stage and local control can be difficult (Dinney et al., 1994). **The standard and most aggressive surgical management for advanced-stage bulbar urethral cancer is radical cystoprostatectomy, pelvic lymphadenectomy, and total penectomy.** Depending on the extent of disease, this may require resection of the pubic rami and the adjacent urogenital diaphragm (Dinney et al., 1994). Bladder preservation with urethrectomy and perineal urethrostomy or bladder neck closure and creation of a continent catheterizable stoma may also be an option in select cases (Christopher et al., 2002; Hakenberg et al., 2001). Patients with positive margins or local recurrences should be managed with radiation, with or without chemotherapy. The benefit of more conservative surgical approaches must be weighed against the probability of local relapse or dissemination of disease.

In a cohort of 46 men with PUC treated primarily with surgery alone, the 5-year overall survival for patients with posterior tumors was 26%, and only 4 of 28 patients were free of disease (Dalbagni et al., 1999). This observation led the authors to conclude that surgery alone is inadequate for advanced PUC. Patients with bulbar tumors treated with more aggressive surgical resection may have a more favorable prognosis (Dayyani et al., 2014). Those with involvement of the pelvic lymph nodes have a high risk of recurrence and death (Dinney et al., 1994).

Radical cystectomy with total penectomy is performed with the patient in the dorsal lithotomy position to allow perineal access. Standard transabdominal mobilization of the bladder is completed, except for preservation of the endopelvic fascia and the anterior pubic attachments. A modified λ or inverted U-shaped perineal incision is performed with the apex in the midperineum. The inferior skin flap is mobilized by sharply dividing the intervening subcutaneous tissue and rectourethral muscle. The superior flap is mobilized by sharply incising the subcutaneous tissue to the superficial Colles fascia and then continuing bilaterally to the adductor musculature at the inferior pubic rami. The ischiorectal fossa are developed as in perineal prostatectomy, and a tunnel is bluntly dissected anterior to the rectum, extending from one fossa to the other. Circumferential incision of the skin and dartos fascia at the penoscrotal junction is performed, and the corporeal bodies are mobilized for a short distance proximally from the superior aspect of the symphysis pubis to allow subsequent inferior pubectomy if needed. Care must be taken not to carry this dissection too far proximally to avoid breaching the anterior aspect of a locally advanced tumor. The penis is passed downward through the perineal incision. Wider exposure may be gained by dividing the scrotum in the midline, although the testicles can usually be preserved. The specimen should be delivered en bloc (Fig. 80.6).

Advanced proximal male PUCs, although rare, may require an extensive operation to achieve complete resection with a negative margin. This may include resection of the testicles, inferior pubic rami, and pelvic floor musculature (Fig. 80.7). Reconstruction of the pelvic floor soft tissue defects may require myocutaneous vascularized pedicle flaps. Such resections requires collaboration with orthopedic and plastic surgeons.

Because of the poor outcomes after surgery alone for advanced tumors of the urethra, surgical monotherapy has been deemed inadequate for advanced-stage PUC, particularly of the bulbar urethra, leading to increased interest in multimodal therapy (Bladder cancer, 2018; Dalbagni et al., 1999; Gakis et al., 2013). One option is the use of perioperative chemotherapy. Approximately 30% of patients with PUC in contemporary cohorts are treated with

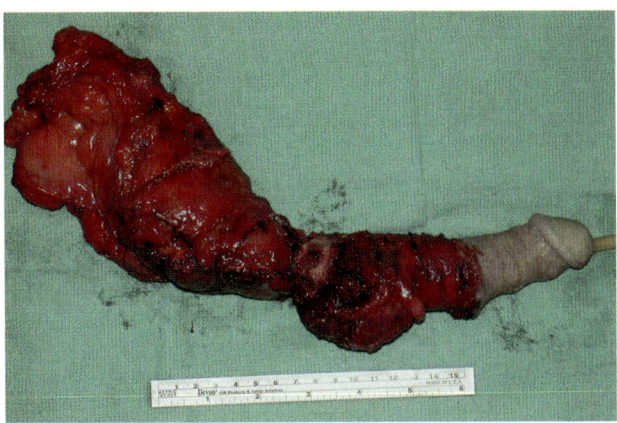

Fig. 80.6. Surgical specimen after radical cystoprostatectomy, urethrectomy, penectomy, and inferior pubectomy for a large bulbomembranous squamous cell carcinoma.

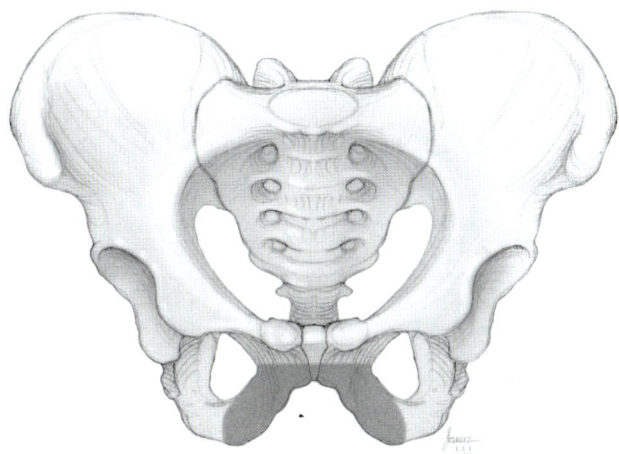

Fig. 80.7. Shaded area outlines the portions of the ischiopubic rami excised at the time of inferior pubectomy during radical excision of bulbomembranous urethral cancer. (Reprinted with permission, Cleveland Clinic Center for Medical Art and Photography. Copyright 2003–2010. All rights reserved.)

perioperative chemotherapy (Gakis et al., 2016). One retrospective study observed that 25% to 33% of patients treated with primarily cisplatin-based neoadjuvant chemotherapy or chemoradiation before surgery had a complete or partial response, and prognosis was highly correlated with response to chemotherapy (Gakis et al., 2015). Chemotherapy before surgery or radiation was associated with better survival for patients with advanced disease compared with surgery alone or surgery plus adjuvant chemotherapy. All patients with locally advanced or clinically node-positive disease treated with neoadjuvant chemotherapy or chemoradiation in this series were alive at 5 years.

A retrospective review of 44 patients with advanced PUC referred for medical oncology evaluation examined the role of cisplatin-based chemotherapy (Dayyani et al., 2013). The study included 28 (64%) females, and squamous cell carcinoma and adenocarcinoma were the most common histologies. All patients but one had at least T3 disease, 43% were N+ and 16% had metastatic disease (M1). Thirty-six patients received one of four platinum-based chemotherapy regimens depending on histologic subtype. Five (14%) were complete responders and 72% of patients achieved a complete or partial response. Surgical consolidation with either urethrectomy or radical cystectomy (RC) was performed in 21 patients. The median overall survival of the entire cohort was 31.7 months, which was higher for the surgical group (46.9 months) compared with the group that did not have surgery (21.7 months). Nine patients initially presented with lymph node–positive disease, four of whom were free of disease after neoadjuvant chemotherapy followed by surgery, although the postchemotherapy pathologic nodal stage was not reported. The authors concluded that neoadjuvant cisplatin-based chemotherapy is a reasonable option for patients with high-risk and locally advanced PUC, which is supported by professional guidelines (Bladder cancer, 2018; Gakis et al., 2013). Adjuvant systemic therapy is an option for patients with locally advanced disease after surgery (Bladder cancer, 2018).

As previously mentioned, chemoradiation therapy with external beam radiation to the external genitalia, perineum, and inguinal lymph nodes with 5-FU plus MMC is an effective treatment option for patients with advanced PUC (Cohen et al., 2008). Patients treated with chemoradiation therapy have similar rates of complete response in the proximal and distal urethra. One group commonly performed consolidative surgery after chemoradiation and found that 7 of 8 patients were ypT0 at surgery (Gheiler et al., 1998). **Given the morbidity of surgery for patients with advanced stage bulbar PUC, chemoradiation is a reasonable alternative for some patients** (Bladder cancer, 2018; Gakis et al., 2013). Surgical consolidation after chemoradiation is recommended by some (Dalbagni et al., 1999). Radiation monotherapy is considered ineffective for bulbar PUC (Bracken et al., 1980; Kaplan et al., 1967).

Professional guidelines recommend radical surgery with or without perioperative chemotherapy, chemoradiation, or radiation monotherapy as treatment options for nonmetastatic bulbar PUC (Bladder cancer, 2018). **Patients with clinically positive lymph should have chemoradiation or chemotherapy followed by surgical consolidation.** There is no high-quality comparative effectiveness research on treatment options for male PUC.

The condition of at least half of patients with advanced disease treated with perioperative chemotherapy will recur (Gakis et al., 2015). After resection of an invasive urethral cancer, there remains a risk of local and/or systemic recurrence at high as 50%, necessitating regular urethral, inguinal, and systemic surveillance (Gakis et al., 2016).

Approximately 10% to 20% of men with PUC have clinically positive lymph nodes, and 5% to 20% have distant metastasis, most commonly to nonregional lymph nodes, liver, lungs, and bone (Dayyani et al., 2014; Gakis et al., 2016; Rabbani, 2011; Sui et al., 2017; Thyavihally et al., 2006). One retrospective cohort observed long-term survival in four of eight patients who presented with metastatic urethral carcinoma that were treated with cisplatin-based chemotherapy and surgical excision of the primary tumor (Dinney et al., 1994).

Male Posterior Urethral Cancer

Prostatic urethral carcinoma is commonly found in patients with a history of bladder cancer. Approximately 20% to 40% of patients with aggressive bladder cancer have synchronous involvement of the prostate at the time of RC, and up to 39% of patients with high-risk non–muscle-invasive bladder cancer (NMIBC) can have recurring problems in the prostate after intravesical therapy (Bruins et al., 2013; Herr and Donat, 1999; Patel et al., 2009). Prostatic urethral biopsies are not consistently performed at the time of transurethral resection of bladder tumor (TURBT), thus the reported range of synchronous prostatic involvement for patients with NMIBC varies widely between 3% and 30% (Bretton et al., 1989; Canda et al., 2004; Gofrit et al., 2009; Orihuela et al., 1989; Palou et al., 1996; Rikken et al., 1987; Schellhammer et al., 1995). However, primary prostatic urethral carcinoma without a history of bladder cancer is rare (Rikken et al., 1987) and comprises fewer than 4% of all prostate cancers (Ende et al., 1963; Tannenbaum, 1975). **Given the rarity of primary prostatic urethral carcinoma, any patients found to have urothelial carcinoma in the prostate should be thoroughly evaluated for coexisting urothelial carcinoma of the bladder and upper tracts.**

Urothelial carcinoma of the prostate can involve the prostatic urothelium, ducts, acini, or stroma and is diagnosed through transurethral resection of the prostate (TURP). Primary posterior male PUC is staged according to the TNM system outlined in Table 80.2. Prostatic urothelial carcinoma commonly presents in the form of carcinoma in situ (CIS) (Schellhammer et al., 1995). Cross-sectional imaging with computed tomography (CT) or MRI is required to evaluate the local extent of disease and to rule out metastasis. Whereas

TABLE 80.4 Summary of 2018 National Comprehensive Cancer Network (NCCN) Clinical Practice Guidelines on Localized Prostatic Urethral Cancer

TYPE	FIRST-LINE TREATMENT OPTIONS
Mucosal	TURP and BCG
Ductal or acinar	TURP and BCG OR Radical cystectomy ± urethrectomy
Stromal invasion	Radical cystectomy ± urethrectomy[a]

[a]Consider neoadjuvant chemotherapy.
Data from Bladder Cancer, NCCN Clinical Practice Guidelines in Oncology, 2018 (website): https://www.nccn.org/professionals/physician_gls/default.aspx.

KEY POINTS: MALE URETHRAL CANCER

- This prognosis of distal anterior male PUC is better than that of proximal anterior PUC, which is often associated with local invasion and distant metastasis.
- Multimodal therapy should be considered for advanced urethral tumors given the poor outcomes after surgery and radiation alone.
- The benefit from prophylactic inguinal lymph node dissection has not been demonstrated in anterior urethral cancer.
- Primary posterior urethral carcinoma is rare, and noninvasive tumors can be effectively managed with TURP and BCG.

patients with superficial or ductal involvement have a 5-year survival rate between 67% and 74%, the 5-year survival rate for bladder cancer patients with stromal involvement drops to 36% (Cheville et al., 1998; Esrig et al., 1996). The prognosis of patients with stromal invasion is related to the primary bladder tumor stage, such that patients with T1 bladder tumors had a 61% 5-year survival rate, and those with muscle invasive or locally advanced bladder tumors had a less than 30% 5-year survival rate (Esrig et al., 1996).

The management of male primary posterior urethral cancer is largely based on the treatment of patients with bladder cancer who have synchronous or metachronous prostatic involvement (Table 80.4). Patients with prostatic urethral involvement were previously classified as stage T4 and historically managed with radical cystectomy (Palou et al., 2013). It was eventually understood that not all patients with prostatic involvement had a poor prognosis, and many could be managed with less aggressive measures (Esrig et al., 1996; Orihuela et al., 1989). **Those with high-grade superficial disease treated with bacille Calmette-Guérin (BCG) can have prostatic response rates of at least 70%** (Bladder cancer, 2018; Canda et al., 2004; Gakis et al., 2013; Gofrit et al., 2009; Orihuela et al., 1989; Palou et al., 2013; Schellhammer et al., 1995). **An extensive TURP before treatment with BCG removes the majority of cancerous urothelium and likely improves exposure of prostatic tissue to BCG and increases response rates** (Gofrit et al., 2009; Orihuela et al., 1989). Although BCG without TURP is an option (Palou et al., 1996). In one study of 23 patients with prostatic urethral involvement who were treated with extensive endoscopic resection and intravesical BCG, there was a 56% complete response rate but a 44% rate of progression, with 7 patients requiring a radical cystectomy (Bretton et al., 1989). However, no progression events occurred within the prostate.

Prostatic ductal involvement has been an indication for cystectomy for some and remains an option in professional guidelines (Bladder cancer, 2018; Orihuela et al., 1989; Taylor et al., 2007). **However, these patients can also be effectively managed with transurethral resection of the prostate (TURP) and BCG, and their prognosis is similar to those with superficial prostatic involvement** (Bladder cancer, 2018; Esrig et al., 1996; Schellhammer et al., 1995). One retrospective series of 11 men with NMIBC and prostatic ductal involvement who were treated with BCG demonstrated a complete response in the prostate of 82% at a median follow-up of 40 months (Palou Redorta et al., 2006). However, there is a risk of progression and understaging mandating close follow-up with repeat prostatic biopsies. **Patients with prostatic urothelial carcinoma invasive into the stroma should be managed with radical cystectomy and pelvic lymphadenectomy with or without perioperative chemotherapy** (Bladder cancer, 2018). Previous studies have evaluated the role of neoadjuvant chemotherapy in patients with advanced-stage disease. A regimen including methotrexate, vinblastine, doxorubicin, and cisplatin (MVAC) has had activity against urothelial carcinoma but not against other histologic types (Scher et al., 1988).

FEMALE URETHRAL CANCER

Epidemiology, Etiology, and Clinical Presentation

Female PUC is a rare malignancy with fewer than 100 cases diagnosed in the United States every year and an estimated annual incidence of 1.5 cases per million women (Champ et al., 2012; Sui et al., 2017; Swartz et al., 2006). One study identified 869 women in the National Cancer Database who were diagnosed with PUC from 2004 to 2013 (Sui et al., 2017). Approximately two-thirds of these patients were older than 60, one-third were black, and PUC was less commonly diagnosed in women than in men. Studies using the Surveillance, Epidemiology, and End Results (SEER) registry found that female PUC is more common in African-American women, and the incidence may be decreasing over time (Swartz et al., 2006). Data from European cancer registries confirm the rare nature of female PUC, its presentation at an advanced age, and a higher incidence of PUC in men (Derksen et al., 2013; Visser et al., 2012).

Given the rarity of the disease, there is relatively little known about the underlying causes of female PUC. Proposed risk factors include leukoplakia, glandular metaplasia, chronic irritation, stricture disease, recurrent urinary infections, caruncles, and human papillomavirus infection (Dalbagni et al., 1998; Fletcher and Lemack, 2008; Milosevic et al., 2000; Murphy et al., 1999; Thyavihally et al., 2005; Wiener et al., 1994). **Female urethral diverticula also may predispose a patient to PUC, with 6% of urethral diverticula harboring a malignancy** (Thomas et al., 2008).

Nearly all women with a PUC present symptomatically (Dalbagni et al., 1998; Dimarco et al., 2004; Johnson and O'Connell 1983; Moinuddin Ali et al., 1988). Common symptoms include hematuria or vaginal spotting, lower urinary tract symptoms, and a vaginal or urethral mass.

Anatomy and Pathology

Knowledge of female urethral anatomy is essential for disease management. The female urethra is approximately 4 cm long (Reuter, 2014). **The proximal third is lined by urothelium and the distal two-thirds are lined by nonkeratinizing stratified squamous epithelium** (Fig. 80.8). Paraurethral (Skene) glands, which are the female homologue of the prostate, surround the urethra and drain via ducts located near the meatus. **The female urethra is divided into an anterior segment (distal one-third) and a posterior segment (proximal two-thirds). This distinction is critical as the distal third can be excised without compromising urinary continence.** The lymphatic drainage differs along the course of the female urethra. **Lymphatics from the posterior urethra generally drain to the pelvic lymph nodes, whereas the anterior urethra drains to the inguinal lymph nodes** (Bracken et al., 1976).

The histology of PUC depends primarily on the site of origin within the urethra. **From population-based studies, there are similar numbers of women with urothelial carcinoma (28%–45%), squamous cell carcinoma (19%–29%), and adenocarcinoma (28%–38%)** (Champ et al., 2012; Derksen et al., 2013; Sui et al., 2017). Adenocarcinoma

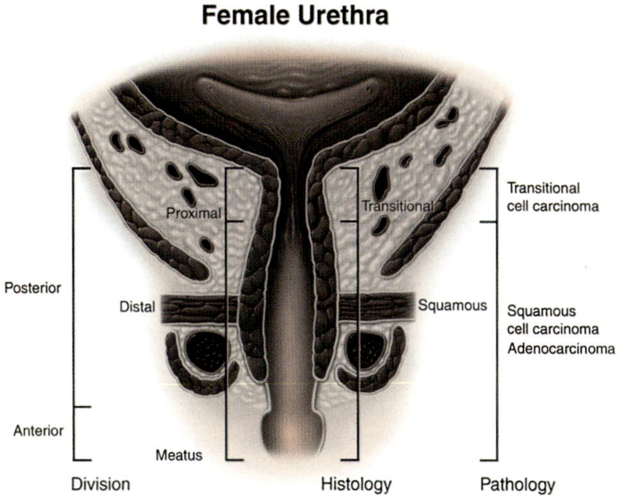

Fig. 80.8. Anatomy of the female urethra with corresponding histology and pathology.

is more likely to occur in women than in men, may be particularly prevalent in African American women, and is the predominant form of cancer found in urethral diverticula (Garden et al., 1993; Sui et al., 2017; Thomas et al., 2008). There are two predominant forms of female urethral adenocarcinoma: mucinous and clear cell (Murphy et al., 1999; Reis et al., 2011). Mucinous adenocarcinoma is more common, can appear microscopically similar to colonic or cervical adenocarcinoma, and may produce carcinoembryonic antigen (Dell'Atti et al., 2018; Kato et al., 1998; Murphy et al., 1999). Clear cell adenocarcinoma is microscopically similar to clear cell carcinomas of the female genital tract, can secrete prostate-specific antigen, and is more commonly found in urethral diverticula (Dodson et al., 1994; Murphy et al., 1999). Some female urethral adenocarcinomas are microscopically similar to prostate adenocarcinoma (Pongtippan et al., 2004). **Female urethral adenocarcinoma likely originates from the Skene gland,** perhaps with the mucinous subtype arising from the proximal gland and the clear cell subtype from the distal gland (Dell'Atti and Galosi, 2018). Others have proposed that female urethral adenocarcinoma can arise from more than one type of urethral tissue, including glandular metaplasia, urothelium, nephrogenic adenoma, and residual müllerian tissue (Alexiev and Tavora, 2013; Murphy et al., 1999). Rare histologic types of female PUC include melanoma, sarcoma, lymphoma, and small cell carcinoma (DiMarco et al., 2004; Grabstald et al., 1966; Grigsby and Corn, 1992).

Evaluation and Staging

The evaluation of women with suspected urethral carcinoma includes a thorough bimanual and pelvic examination to evaluate the clinical extent of disease, with careful attention to potential involvement of the vaginal wall and vulva. The groin should be assessed for adenopathy. Patients should have cystourethroscopy and examination under anesthesia with tumor biopsy, although percutaneous or transvaginal biopsies are alternatives. Cross-sectional imaging is critical to assess the local extent of disease. MRI has superior soft-tissue contrast and gives the best anatomic detail of the pelvis and urethra (Del Gaizo et al., 2013; Surabhi et al., 2013). In addition, MRI can assess local extension and lymph node involvement. Determining the location of the tumor through clinical examination and imaging is critical for treatment decision making. **Approximately one-third of patients have a distal tumor, and the remainder have proximal or pan-urethral tumors** (Dalbagni et al., 1998; Foens et al., 1991; Grabstald et al., 1966; Grigsby, 1998; Johnson and O'Connell, 1983; Kang et al., 2015). Chest radiograph or CT is appropriate to rule out distant metastases. Bone scan may be performed if there is clinical suspicion for bony involvement. Elevated serum prostate-specific antigen has been found in a small number of females with adenocarcinoma and may normalize after successful treatment (Dodson et al., 1994; Pongtippan et al., 2004).

The staging for female urethral cancer is similar to that for male urethral cancer (see Table 80.2). **Approximately 30% to 50% of females with PUC present with locally advanced disease** (Champ et al., 2012; Foens et al., 1991; Grigsby, 1998; Kang et al., 2015; Sui et al., 2017). As compared with men, women tend to present with higher stage and higher grade tumors (Sui et al., 2017). Roughly 20% of women with PUC have clinically enlarged inguinal lymph nodes, which are usually cancerous, and 10% to 20% have metastases to pelvic lymph nodes or distant sites (Bracken et al., 1976; Champ et al., 2012; Derksen et al., 2013; Garden et al., 1993; Milosevic et al., 2000; Sui et al., 2017). Patients with squamous cell carcinoma may be particularly at risk for synchronous or metachronous nodal involvement (Garden et al., 1993). Distant metastatic disease at presentation is rare (Grigsby, 1998).

Prognosis

Female PUC is an aggressive disease with 5-year survival rates of 40% to 60% (Champ et al., 2012; Dalbagni et al., 1998; Dimarco et al., 2004; Grigsby, 1998; Kang et al., 2015; Sui et al., 2017). However, females with PUC do not appear to have an independently increased risk of death compared with males with PUC (Sui et al., 2017). There are several disease characteristics that affect prognosis. In one of the earliest reports of female PUC it was observed that "survival is determined chiefly by the extent of neoplasm," (Grabstald et al., 1966) and **tumor stage has since been strongly associated with survival in numerous studies** (Bracken et al., 1976; Dalbagni et al., 1998; Dimarco et al., 2004; Foens et al., 1991; Kang et al., 2015; Thyavihally et al., 2005). Data from the National Cancer Registry of the Netherlands evaluated 91 females with PUC and reported 5-year overall survival rates of 67%, 53%, and 17% for stage II or less, III, and IV, respectively (Derksen et al., 2013). A retrospective cohort study observed that 5-year overall survival for low- versus high-stage tumors was 78% and 22%, respectively, and high-stage, positive nodal status and pan-urethral location were all negatively associated with survival (Dalbagni et al., 1998). Among the 869 women in a large retrospective cohort from the United States, higher tumor stage and the presence of positive lymph nodes were independently associated with worse survival on multivariate analysis (Sui et al., 2017). Finally, a retrospective cohort study using the SEER dataset identified 722 women with PUC between 1983 and 2008, of whom 359 who could be assessed for cancer survival outcomes (Champ et al., 2012). The observed 5-year overall and disease-specific survival rates were 43% and 53%, respectively, and multivariate analysis revealed that black race, increased age, stage, nodal status, and nonsquamous histology were associated with worse cancer-specific survival. Importantly, when interpreting prognostic factors from the existing literature on female PUC, many case series included patients treated before cross-sectional imaging, in which case they were incompletely staged (Foens et al., 1991).

Tumor location has been shown to affect prognosis, as proximal and pan-urethral cancers have lower survival than distal cancers. Five-year disease-specific survival is 71% for distal, 48% for proximal, and 24% for pan-urethral lesions (Dalbagni et al., 1998), and proximal and pan-urethral involvement are independently associated with worse survival (Dalbagni et al., 1998; Dimarco et al., 2004). **However, it has been noted that proximal and pan-urethral tumors are more likely to be higher stage** (Bracken et al., 1976; Thyavihally et al., 2005).

Several reports have also noted that tumor size is strongly associated with survival. A retrospective study of 44 females with PUC observed 5-year overall survival of 89%, 36%, and 19% for tumors smaller than 2 cm, 2 to 4 cm, and more than 4 cm, respectively (Grigsby, 1998). This study found that size was independently associated with survival, although tumor stage was not included in the model. Similar to tumor location, tumor size is also associated with stage so that lager tumors are more often in a proximal location and have a higher stage (Milosevic et al., 2000). Tumor stage is strongly correlated with grade, size, location, and nodal status;

however, given the small study sizes, multivariate analyses have not always been possible and the independent effects of stage have not been consistently proven.

There is conflicting evidence about the impact of histologic subtype. Several studies have failed to detect any differences in survival based on histologic subtype, recommending similar treatment regardless of histology (Dimarco et al., 2004; Foens et al., 1991). However, two large population-based studies observed that females with squamous cell carcinoma have a lower risk of death compared with nonsquamous histologies (Champ et al., 2012; Sui et al., 2017). Another retrospective cohort study reported 5-year overall survival rates of 64%, 61%, and 31% for squamous cell carcinoma, urothelial carcinoma, and adenocarcinoma, respectively (Derksen et al., 2013). Urethral melanoma, however, does have a poor prognosis (DiMarco et al., 2004).

Treatment

Given the rarity of female PUC, the majority of information on treatment comes from small institutional cohorts or case reports, and there are limited data on the preferred method of treatment or standardized treatment algorithms. Treatment options include surgery, radiation therapy, and chemotherapy, alone or in combination (see Table 80.3). **As with male PUC, there is increasing interest in multimodal therapy for female PUC** (Dayyani et al., 2013; Derksen et al., 2013; Sui et al., 2017), **and the types of operations used vary according to the location and stage of the primary tumor.** Roughly 40% of women with PUC are treated with radiation in some form (Champ et al., 2012). Local excision may be sufficient for the small, low-stage, anterior urethral tumors, whereas proximal and advanced urethral tumors require a more aggressive approach.

Tumors in the **anterior urethra** tend to be low stage, and at least 70% can be cured with local excision alone (Grabstald et al., 1966). Small, noninvasive tumors of the urethra can be managed with endoscopic resection or laser fulguration, with or without adjuvant BCG (Bladder cancer, 2018; Staehler et al., 1985). Anterior urethral tumors not amenable to endoscopic treatment can be treated with surgical resection or radiation (Gakis et al., 2013). **Small, exophytic tumors of the anterior urethra can be surgically excised along with a portion of the anterior vaginal wall via a transvaginal approach.** Frozen section of the proximal urethra should be obtained to ensure a negative margin. In a report from the Mayo Clinic, 26 women with PUC were managed with local resection, the majority of whom had T2 lesions or less in the anterior urethra, and some were also given radiation (Dimarco et al., 2004). The 5-year disease-specific survival for patients who had a partial urethrectomy or endoscopic resection was 81%, but 21% experienced a local recurrence and many could not be salvaged. Small case-series have also observed that many patients selected for partial urethrectomy can be cured with surgery alone (Grabstald et al., 1966; Moinuddin Ali et al., 1988).

Partial urethrectomy is not without the risk of complications, most notably urinary incontinence. Although a portion of the female urethra can be safely excised without sacrificing continence, one series reported that 42% of patients had new or worsening stress incontinence after partial urethrectomy (Dimarco et al., 2004). The risk of meatal stenosis can be minimized by performing a wide spatulation of the urethra.

In select patients with advanced staged anterior tumors, bladder-sparing strategies have been employed. Radical urethrectomy with bladder neck closure and creation of a catheterizable stoma or ileovesicostomy may be an option if a negative margin can be achieved (Dimarco et al., 2004). Radical urethrectomy includes wide resection of all periurethral tissue laterally to the bulbocavernosal muscles, anteriorly to the pubic symphysis, and superiorly to the bladder neck, including the anterior vaginal wall.

Radiation monotherapy is also an effective option for low-stage anterior tumors and is an alternative when urethral preservation is desired and surgical resection would negatively affect functional outcomes (Koontz and Lee, 2010). Radiation can be delivered as external beam, brachytherapy, or combined therapy, using doses between 55 and 70 Gy (Weghaupt et al., 1984). One series of 97 women with PUC treated with radiation therapy included 34 women with invasive tumors of the distal urethra and 13 who had their tumors completely resected before radiation (Garden et al., 1993). Most patients with distal tumors were treated with brachytherapy alone at a median of 60 Gy, and the 5-year survival was 74% if only part of the urethra was involved. The extent of urethral involvement by the primary tumor was the only variable that predicted local control. In another retrospective series of 62 patients treated with combined external and brachytherapy, 68% of patients had an anterior tumor and their 5-year overall survival was 71% (Weghaupt et al., 1984). Finally, in a cohort of 34 women with PUC who were treated with radiation, 9 of whom first had a local tumor resection, the 7-year cancer-specific survival and relapse-free rate were 71% and 85%, respectively, for the 14 patients with distal tumors (Milosevic et al., 2000).

Complication rates after radiation have ranged from 20% to 50%, including urethral stricture, necrosis, fistula, and cystitis (Forman and Lichter, 1992; Garden et al., 1993; Milosevic et al., 2000). Although a higher cumulative dose of radiation increases the risk of complications, the complication rate is less with contemporary radiation techniques (Forman and Lichter, 1992; Garden et al., 1993).

Given the lymphatic drainage of the urethra, patients with anterior PUC are at risk for synchronous or metachronous **inguinal lymph node metastasis.** Up to one-third of patients have or develop inguinal adenopathy at some point during the course of disease (Grabstald et al., 1966; Weghaupt et al., 1984). **Similar to male PUC, there is no clear role for prophylactic inguinal lymphadenectomy for patients with high-risk anterior tumors that have clinically negative inguinal lymph nodes.** However, given the frequent use of prophylactic inguinal lymphadenectomy for vulvar squamous cell carcinoma (Dellinger et al., 2017), there is precedent for such treatment of female urogenital cancers and further study of prophylactic inguinal lymphadenectomy has been advocated (Karnes et al., 2010). **Unlike penile and vulvar cancer, there are no known prognostic factors for the development of inguinal lymph node metastases for PUC.** Prophylactic groin radiation should be considered for patients being treated with primary radiation (Garden et al., 1993). One study suggested prophylactic groin radiation decreased inguinal recurrences; however, recurrences can still occur despite the use of prophylactic radiation (Foens et al., 1991; Milosevic et al., 2000).

Up to 20% of patients experience a recurrence in the inguinal lymph nodes, usually within 2 years of diagnosis (Grabstald et al., 1966; Milosevic et al., 2000). **Patients with clinically palpable inguinal lymph nodes require aggressive treatment because these usually represent metastatic disease, and some of these patients can be cured** (Milosevic et al., 2000; Weghaupt et al., 1984). Treatment options for inguinal lymph node metastases endorsed by professional guidelines include chemoradiation, chemotherapy alone, inguinal lymphadenectomy, and chemoradiation followed by consolidative surgery (Bladder cancer, 2018; Gakis et al., 2013). The technique for inguinal lymphadenectomy is identical to that used for men with penile cancer. Patients with pelvic adenopathy have a poor prognosis and usually die from disease (Grabstald et al., 1966). It is unclear if there is any benefit to pelvic lymphadenectomy for patients with clinically positive pelvic lymph nodes.

Posterior female PUC is more likely to be high stage, involve the entire urethra, and may invade surrounding structures, including the bladder, vagina, and external genitalia (Milosevic et al., 2000). **Despite aggressive treatment with surgery or radiation, the 5-year metastasis-free survival for posterior female PUC is only 24% to 48%** (Dalbagni et al., 1998). **Surgical management usually requires anterior pelvic exenteration.** Anterior exenteration when used alone is associated with low cure rates and a significant risk of local recurrence. In one cohort, 15 of 21 women with posterior or pan-urethral PUC treated with radical surgery died of disease (Grabstald et al., 1966), and a separate group of 26 females with PUC treated with radical cystectomy had a median survival of only 36 months (Dalbagni et al., 1998). Another cohort of 27 women with advanced-stage PUC who were treated with radical surgery alone had a 5-year disease-specific and recurrence-free survival of 52% and 43%, respectively, and a third experienced a pelvic recurrence (Dimarco et al., 2004).

Patients that recur in the pelvis have a poor prognosis and usually die of disease (Dimarco et al., 2004).

Anterior exenteration includes radical cystectomy and urethrectomy along with hysterectomy, oophorectomy, extended pelvic lymph node dissection, and wide or complete vaginal excision, which may be required to obtain negative margins. If the lesion extends into the external genitalia, partial vulvectomy or labial excision may be necessary. Anterior exenteration is performed in a similar fashion to that performed for bladder cancer, with a more extensive perineal portion of the procedure to provide wide urethral margins. The perineal portion is performed by making an inverted U-shaped incision to widely encircle the urethral meatus. This incision can be extended onto the posterior vaginal wall, the labia minora, and continued anteriorly to include the clitoris. En bloc resection of the pubic symphysis and inferior pubic rami may be necessary if obtaining a negative margin at the pubis is not possible (Klein et al., 1983), although intraoperative irradiation may be an alternative to pubic bone resection (Dalbagni et al., 2001).

Radiation monotherapy for proximal urethral carcinoma has yielded similarly poor local control, with 5-year survival rates of 0 to 57% and a median survival of less than 3 years (Dalbagni et al., 1998; Garden et al., 1993; Grabstald et al., 1966; Grigsby, 1998; Narayan and Konety, 1992). In one series, patients with proximal urethral tumors treated with radiation monotherapy experienced a 7-year relapse-free rate of 37% and cancer-specific survival of 20% (Milosevic et al., 2000). Several studies have observed that combined external beam radiation and brachytherapy are more effective at achieving local control for posterior tumors than external beam therapy alone (Foens et al., 1991; Milosevic et al., 2000). This may, in part, be due to dose escalation. After treatment with radiation monotherapy for proximal PUC, up to 50% of women experience a local failure and the length of urethra involved significantly affects local control (Foens et al., 1991; Garden et al., 1993; Milosevic et al., 2000). Almost all failures occur within 2 years of treatment and salvage may not be possible (Bracken et al., 1976; Garden et al., 1993).

Because surgery and radiation have similarly low rates of local control and poor survival outcomes when used alone, there is growing interest in use of multimodal therapy for advanced-stage female PUC (Dalbagni et al., 1998, 2001; Foens et al., 1991; Garden et al., 1993). At least 20% of women with PUC receive a combination of surgery and radiation, which has been increasing over time (Derksen et al., 2013). Neoadjuvant radiation followed by surgery may provide better local control than surgery or radiation alone (Dalbagni et al., 1998; Narayan and Konety, 1992). One small case series of 6 women with advanced-stage PUC were treated with pelvic exenteration with intraoperative radiation therapy as well as postoperative external beam radiation and perioperative chemotherapy (Dalbagni et al., 2001). Two of 6 patients were cured, but 2 experienced a local recurrence, and 4 ultimately died of disease. There are several case reports of excellent cancer control with use of multimodal therapy for female PUC (Awakura et al., 2003; Hara et al., 2004; Licht et al., 1995; Nicholson et al., 2008).

Professional guidelines and several expert groups recommend that women with advanced-stage PUC should be treated with multimodal therapy, including systemic chemotherapy with consolidative radiation, surgery, or radiation followed by surgery (Bladder cancer, 2018; Dalbagni et al., 1998; Garden et al., 1993; Grabstald et al., 1966). The type of chemotherapy should be dictated by the tumor histology. The ideal perioperative systemic therapy for squamous cell carcinoma should be cisplatin based, with regimens including CGI and TIP (Dayyani et al., 2013). Adenocarcinoma has been treated with Gem-FLP, and either M-VAC or GC can be used for urothelial carcinoma. Patients treated with chemoradiation can be given systemic cisplatin, 5-FU, and MMC, alone or in combination, as radiosensitizers. Systemic chemotherapy should be used for metastatic disease. The most common sites of distant metastases are lung, bone, and brain (Grabstald et al., 1966).

Given the poor quality of evidence to support treatment recommendations for female PUC and the inherent confounding by treatment indication present in the literature, treatment should be individualized. However, multimodal treatment should be strongly considered given the aggressive nature of advanced female PUC.

> **KEY POINTS: FEMALE URETHRAL CANCER**
>
> - The three most common histologies for female urethral cancer are urothelial carcinoma, squamous cell carcinoma, and adenocarcinoma.
> - Compared with anterior urethral cancers, posterior cancers are found at a more advanced stage and are associated with worse survival.
> - Radiation and surgical excision are options for low-stage anterior tumors, each with high cure rates.
> - Surgery and radiation therapy for proximal female urethral tumors have poor outcomes when used alone; therefore multimodal therapy is recommended.

URETHRAL RECURRENCE AFTER RADICAL CYSTECTOMY

Male Urethra

After radical cystectomy (RC) there is a risk of recurrence in the remnant urothelium of the urethra and upper urinary tracts. Urothelial recurrence is due to either growth of cancer along the urothelium as an extension of the primary tumor or metachronous tumor development resulting from a field defect (Clark and Hall, 2005; Hardeman and Soloway, 1990). During the early experience with RC, patients often had a prophylactic urethrectomy to eliminate the possibility of a urethral recurrence (UR) (Schellhammer and Whitmore, 1976). However, 64% to 100% of prophylactically removed urethras had no evidence of disease (Lopez-Almansa et al., 1988; Raz et al., 1978; Schellhammer and Whitmore 1976; Spiess et al., 2006; Stockle et al., 1990; Tobisu et al., 1991, 1997; Tongaonkar et al., 1993; Zabbo and Montie, 1984), and when disease was present it was most commonly in the form of CIS (Spiess et al., 2006; Stockle et al., 1990). Over time, surgeons came to understand that the patients with synchronous urethral involvement usually had specific risk factors (Tobisu et al., 1991). Still, the majority of at-risk patients had negative pathology at the time of prophylactic urethrectomy (Tobisu et al., 1991). **Given the low prevalence of synchronous unrecognized urethral involvement, the added morbidity of a urethrectomy to RC, and the growing use of orthotopic urinary diversions, there has been a shift toward urethral preservation** (Beahrs et al., 1984; Tomic and Sjodin, 1992; Zabbo et al., 1984).

The risk of UR after RC ranges from 1% to 15%, with larger series reporting rates near 5% (Table 80.5). Most URs occur within 2 years of RC, although 11% occur after 5 years, and they can rarely present as late as 15 years postoperatively (Clark et al., 2004; Huguet et al., 2008; Sakai et al., 1999). There are several risk factors for UR, including bladder tumor multifocality, presence of CIS, a history of NMIBC, involvement of the prostate with urothelial carcinoma, a positive urethral margin, and a cutaneous diversion (Balci et al 2015; Baron et al., 1989; Donat et al., 2001; Hardeman and Soloway, 1990; Huguet et al., 2003, 2008; Tobisu et al., 1991; Varol et al., 2004). Patients with more risk factors tend to have an increased risk of UR (Tobisu et al., 1991; Tongaonkar et al., 1993). However, using these multiple criteria to select patients for urethrectomy would eliminate as many as 70% of RC patients from orthotopic neobladder (ONB) eligibility (Freeman et al., 1996). Because UR is a rare event, only the highest risk patients should be subjected to a prophylactic urethrectomy.

Prostatic involvement is a strong risk factor for UR. The prostate is involved by urothelial carcinoma in 17% to 40% of RC specimens, most commonly in the prostatic urethra or ducts, but disease can also invade into the prostatic stroma (Donat et al., 2001; Freeman et al., 1996; Hardeman and Soloway, 1990; Huguet et al., 2008; Mazzucchelli et al., 2009; von Rundstedt et al., 2015). Patients with recurrent tumors, tumors located at the trigone or bladder neck, and multifocal tumors are more likely to have prostatic involvement (Mazzucchelli et al., 2009). Stein reported a 5% UR rate among patients with no prostatic involvement but a 15% rate among patients

TABLE 80.5 Male Urethral Recurrences After Radical Cystectomy

STUDY	YEARS	NUMBER	URETHRAL RECURRENCES	TIME TO RECURRENCE	COMMENTS
Beahrs et al., 1984	1965–1974	349	8%		
Zabbo and Montie, 1984	1960–1979	119	6.4%	1–5 yr	
Lopez-Almansa et al., 1988	1975–1984	110	3.8%		
Baron et al., 1989	1977–1987	140	9.1%	Mean 26 mo	
Hardeman and Soloway, 1990	1975–1987	86	15%	Mean 12 mo	
Stockle et al., 1990	1967–1987	273	9.2%		
Tobisu et al., 1991	1963–1987	169	10.6%		
Tongaonkar et al., 1993	1981–1996	177	9%	Mean 13 mo	
Erckert et al., 1996	1969–1994	910	7.4%	Median 17.9 mo	
Nieder et al., 2004	1992–2003	226	3.7%	Mean 12.8 mo	
Donat et al., 2001	1989–1997	246	6.4%	15.2 mo	
Boorjian et al., 2011	1980–2000	1,506	5.6%	Median 13.3 mo	
Hassan et al., 2004	1995–2001	290	1.7%	66 mo	ONB only
Yoshida et al., 2006	1993–2004	77	5%	6–45 mo	ONB only
Huguet et al., 2008	1978–2003	729	4.7%	Median 13.9 mo	
Cho et al., 2009	1986–2004	294	4.4%	Median 17 mo	
Taylor et al., 2010	1980–2004	259	2.3%	Mean 2.3 yrs	ONB only
Mitra et al., 2014	1971–2005	2,029	2.7%	Median 25.3 mo	
Giannarini et al., 2010	1985–2009	479	5%		ONB only
Gaya et al., 2014	1990–2010	234	1.1%		
Balci et al., 2015	1991–2013	287	3.8%	28 mo	
Pichler et al., 2017	2006–2015	177	6.8%		
Perlis et al., 2013	1992–2008	503	3.6%	Median 18 mo	

ONB, Orthotopic neobladder.

with prostatic involvement (Stein et al., 2005). In this cohort, neither multifocality nor CIS were predictive of UR on multivariate analysis. Another group similarly found that prostatic urethral involvement was significantly associated with risk of UR and recommend against ONB for patients with prostatic involvement (Cho et al., 2009).

Preoperative prostatic biopsy has been studied to identify prostatic involvement before RC and select patients for prophylactic urethrectomy. In a cohort of 234 RC patients, a preoperative transurethral prostatic biopsy had a sensitivity of 80.6% and a negative predictive value of 93% for prostatic involvement on final pathology (Gaya et al., 2014). These findings suggested that patients with a negative preoperative biopsy can safely proceed to ONB without additional intraoperative frozen section. Although preoperative prostatic urethral biopsies are reasonably good at diagnosing prostatic involvement, they correlate poorly with the final urethral margin (Kassouf et al., 2008; Lebret et al., 1998; von Rundstedt et al., 2015). **Preoperative prostatic biopsies to determine ONB eligibility have largely been abandoned in favor of intraoperative frozen section** (Donat et al., 2001; Kassouf et al., 2008).

A positive urethral margin is seen in fewer than 7% of RC specimens but is also a strong risk factor for UR (Boorjian et al., 2011; Cho et al., 2009; Donat et al., 2001; Kassouf et al., 2008; Mitra et al., 2014). Among 294 RC patients who experienced 13 URs (4.4%), a positive urethral margin (HR 18.3, 95% confidence interval (CI) 4.6–71.7, $P < 0.001$) was the strongest risk factor for UR after controlling for prostatic involvement and tumor stage (Cho et al., 2009). Still, many URs occur in the absence of a positive apical margin, suggesting additional factors contribute (Donat et al., 2001; Taylor et al., 2010).

Given the low incidence of urethral recurrence, most surgeons feel comfortable proceeding with ONB as long as the frozen-section biopsy of the distal prostatic urethral margin is normal at the time of RC (Freeman et al., 1996; Hassan et al., 2004; Kassouf et al., 2008; Nieder et al., 2004; Stein et al., 2005). Intraoperative frozen section can accurately evaluate the final urethral margin, and up to half of positive margins on frozen section can be converted to negative margins with additional sections (Gaya et al., 2014; Kassouf et al., 2008; Kates et al., 2016). However, if there is concern about the ability of obtaining a negative margin, an ONB should not be performed.

Patients with ONBs have a lower risk of UR than patients with cutaneous diversions. Although this may reflect differences in selection criteria for urinary diversion, some theorize that ONBs are protective against UR because of changes in the local immune response, the antineoplastic effects of ileum, or the continued exposure of the urethra to urine (Freeman et al., 1996; Gakis et al., 2017). When comparing 397 ONB patients with 371 patients with cutaneous diversions, the estimated 5-year risk of UR was 5% and 9%, respectively, equating to a 50% decreased relative risk ($P = 0.035$) (Stein et al., 2005). Diversion type and prostatic involvement were the only two prognostic factors for UR on multivariate analysis. A large retrospective cohort study of 1506 RC patients found that ONB (0.34, 95% CI 0.13–0.86; $P = 0.02$), prostatic involvement (HR 4.89, 95% CI 3.0–7.9; $P < 0.0001$), and bladder tumor multifocality (HR 2.34, 95% CI 1.4–3.9; $P = 0.001$) were significantly associated with UR after adjusting for stage and presence of CIS (Boorjian et al., 2011). Two percent of patients with ONB had a UR, whereas 6% of patients with an ileal conduit had a UR.

Although prior groups have advocated prophylactic urethrectomy in the presence of several risk factors for UR, including multifocal bladder tumors, upper urinary tract tumors, diffuse CIS, involvement of the prostatic urethra, and involvement of the bladder neck, **the strongest indications for prophylactic urethrectomy are a positive urethral margin or gross urethral involvement** (Gaya et al., 2014; Lopez-Almansa et al., 1988; Stockle et al., 1990; Van Poppel and Sorgeloose, 2003; Zabbo and Montie, 1984). A urologist may determine that a patient is at sufficiently high risk to recommend a prophylactic urethrectomy. A staged urethrectomy after RC has similar outcomes compared with a planned urethrectomy at the time of RC (Nelles et al., 2008; Spiess et al., 2006). Still, total urethrectomy after RC with cutaneous diversion can be challenging, particularly with regard to completely excising the proximal urethra from the pelvic floor. The proximal urethra is at risk for positive margins, and incomplete resection can lead to retropubic relapses that are difficult to manage.

Patients who experience a urethral recurrence often have urethral bloody discharge or a palpable mass (Beahrs et al., 1984). Recurrences tend to be proximal but can occur anywhere along the length of the urethra (Stockle et al., 1990; Tongaonkar et al., 1993). Several groups have investigated whether screening for asymptomatic recurrences with urethral cytology improves outcomes for patients with a UR. Cytology is either obtained from a voided sample with an ONB or a catheterized urethral barbotage from patients with a cutaneous diversion. Among 1054 RC patients who had regular urethral cytology assessments, one study found no difference in survival between the 24 patients who presented symptomatically compared with the 13 detected asymptomatically with urine cytology (Clark et al., 2004). Another study similarly found no survival difference between 17 URs detected on cytology compared with 7 who presented symptomatically (Lin et al., 2003). However, a third study found that although patients who presented asymptomatically had a similar time to diagnosis to those with symptoms, an asymptomatic UR tended to be a lower stage and had improved 5-year cancer specific survival compared with a symptomatic recurrence (80% vs. 41%) (Boorjian et al., 2011).

Patients who have a positive cytology or symptoms of urethral bleeding, discharge, or palpable mass require evaluation with urethroscopy and biopsy. There is a risk of false-positive cytology emphasizing the importance confirming a UR with a biopsy before initiating treatment (Lin et al., 2003). Pelvic CT or MRI is necessary to assess the local extent of disease and search for metastasis. The most definitive treatment of a UR is total urethrectomy (Video 80.1). The entire urethra should be removed because incomplete removal of the distal urethra leaves patients at risk for a distal recurrence (Baron et al., 1989; Schellhammer and Whitmore, 1976).

Urethrectomy in patients with a cutaneous diversion can be difficult, with a risk of positive margins proximally given the difficulty of removing the urethral stump from the scarred pelvic floor (Stockle et al., 1990). After an orthotopic diversion radical urethrectomy generally requires conversion to a cutaneous diversion, although subtotal urethrectomy with perineal urethrostomy has been described (Clark et al., 2004).

Patients with noninvasive URs can be managed successfully with endoscopic resection and topical therapy (Erckert et al., 1996; Huguet et al., 2003; Miller and Benson, 1996; Yossepowitch et al., 2003). Intraurethral BCG, although cumbersome to administer, has had high response rates when used for patients with urethral CIS, but not for those with papillary or invasive disease (Giannarini et al., 2010; Huguet et al., 2003; Varol et al., 2004). There is a significant risk of a second UR after endoscopic management necessitating continued surveillance (Yoshida et al., 2006). Radiation therapy has also been used for treatment of UR (Chakrabarti et al., 2013).

Patients who experience an isolated noninvasive UR generally have a favorable prognosis and can usually be salvaged (Beahrs et al., 1984; Clark et al., 2004; Taylor et al., 2010; Tongaonkar et al., 1993; Varol et al., 2004). Patients with invasive URs often have an aggressive disease course with a median survival of 17 months (Baron et al., 1989; Clark et al., 2004). At least one-third of patients with URs have concomitant pelvic or distant recurrences in which case the prognosis is poor (Gakis et al., 2017).

Total Urethrectomy After Cutaneous Diversion

The high lithotomy position provides optimal exposure for total urethrectomy, with the hips and knees gently flexed and the lower limbs abducted in stirrups. A urethral catheter can be placed to assist with urethral dissection. Through a modified λ or midline perineal incision (Fig. 80.9), the subcutaneous tissue and bulbospongiosus muscle are divided in the midline and retracted to expose the corpus spongiosum. The corpus spongiosum is mobilized circumferentially at the level of the bulbar urethra, and traction is applied to facilitate sharp dissection of the urethra distally, thus separating the corpus spongiosum from the adjacent corpora cavernosa. As dissection proceeds distally, the penis becomes inverted, the corpora cavernosa become bowed, and the glans recedes into the phallus. The penis is essentially turned inside out onto the perineum, and the dissection is completed to the base of the glans. To excise the meatus and glandular urethra, the penis is replaced in its anatomic position, and an incision is made around the meatus and extended on each side down the ventral aspect of the glans. The distal urethra is then freed from its investments within the glans, and the isolated pendulous urethra is delivered onto the perineum. The deep spongiosum of the glans penis is reapproximated with 4-0 polydioxanone sutures, and the surface layer is closed with interrupted 4-0 chromic sutures.

Proximal sharp dissection of the urethral bulb is carried out posteriorly and laterally, staying close to the bulb but avoiding entry. Care must be taken with posteriolateral dissection because this is where the bulbar arteries are located. Bothersome bleeding will result if these vessels are not controlled, generally with electrocautery or suture ligature. The urethra is detached from the corporeal bodies anteriorly to the level of the departure of the urethra from the bulb, leaving the specimen attached only by the membranous urethra. Care must be exercised in completing the proximal dissection given the possibility of bowel adhesions to the superior surface of the urogenital diaphragm in patients with cutaneous diversions. This should be done under direct vision, and exposure can be aided by separating the crura of the corporeal bodies in the midline to open the intracrural space. All that remains of the membranous urethra proximally is an ill-defined fibrotic band, which should be completely excised. Frozen-section analysis of this region adds some assurance that a negative proximal margin has been attained. A small suction drain is placed in the urethral bed and brought out through the perineum. The bulbospongiosus muscle, subcutaneous tissue, and skin are closed with interrupted absorbable sutures, and a light pressure dressing is applied. Superficial hematoma, edema along the penile shaft, and infection are uncommon complications.

Total Urethrectomy After Orthotopic Diversion

Total urethrectomy after orthotopic urinary diversion and conversion to a cutaneous diversion is performed through an abdominoperineal approach. The patient is placed in lithotomy position with stirrups that can be adjusted during the procedure. A catheter is placed into the neobladder. Urethrectomy is carried out in a similar fashion to the level of the membranous urethra. Abdominal exploration with lysis of adhesions and mobilization of the orthotopic neobladder is done to the level of the urethral anastomosis. Working from above and below, the urethroneovesical anastomosis is dissected free. A circular area of the pouch adjacent to the anastomosis is excised with the urethra to ensure an adequate margin, and the specimen is delivered through the perineum. Bleeding from the musculature within the tunnel developed during excision of the membranous urethra can be bothersome and is best controlled with suture ligatures or electrocautery.

In most situations, urinary diversion is accomplished with an ileal conduit. This often can be carried out with use of bowel from the ONB, which may be reconfigured when necessary, with care taken to incise the bowel along visible lines of previous closure with preservation of the mesenteric blood supply. The remaining portions of the pouch are excised. If the existing orthotopic diversion has an afferent limb, this segment can be used to construct the conduit without the need for reimplantation of the ureters (Bissada et al., 2004). Conversion to a continent cutaneous diversion may also be possible, depending on intra-abdominal anatomy and the motivation of the patient (Bartoletti et al., 1999; Taylor et al., 2010).

Female Urethra

Urethrectomy at the time of a female RC is relatively easy to perform and has traditionally been a standard part of surgery. However, with the improved understanding of the female continence mechanism and the low rate of urethral involvement at RC, preservation of the urethra and construction of ONBs in women have gained popularity. **Synchronous urethral involvement at the time of radical cystectomy in females is seen in 8% to 13% of patients** (Chen et al., 1997;

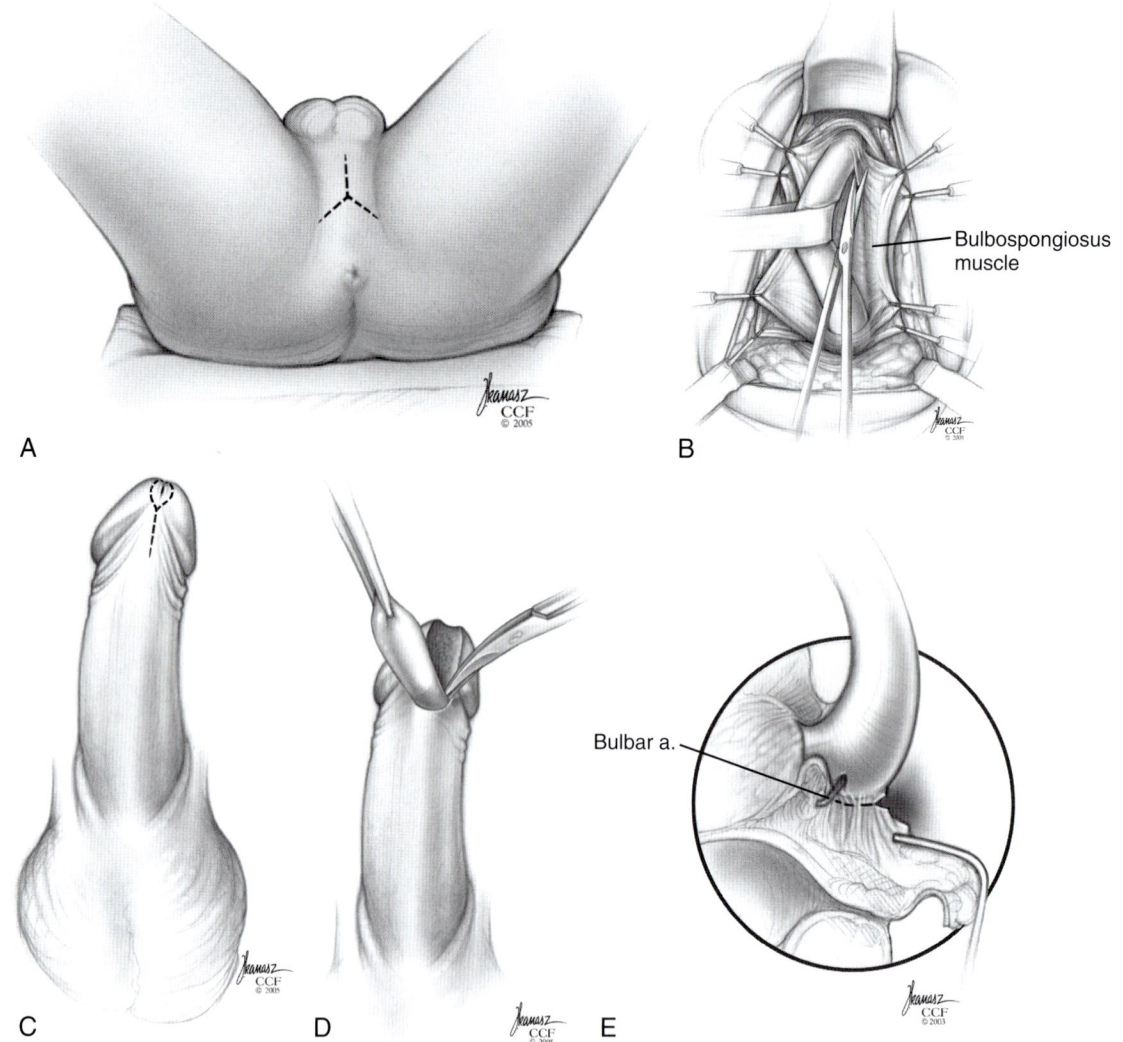

Fig. 80.9. Total urethrectomy after previous cystoprostatectomy. (A) Perineal incision. (B) Division of bulbospongiosus muscle to expose the bulb of the corpus spongiosum and initial dissection of the urethra off of the corporeal bodies. (C) Distal incision circumscribing the urethral meatus. (D) Distal urethral dissection, which then connects to the proximal dissection at the level of the distal shaft. (E) Sagittal view demonstrating posterior bulb dissection and location of the bulbar artery. (Reprinted with permission, Cleveland Clinic Center for Medical Art and Photography. Copyright 2003–2010. All rights reserved.)

Stein et al., 1995). **The main risk factor for female urethral involvement is bladder neck involvement, which is seen in up to 25% of female cystectomy specimens** (Stein et al., 1995). Although nearly all urethral tumors have bladder neck involvement, only 30% to 50% of patients with bladder neck involvement have urethral tumors, suggesting that bladder neck involvement is not an absolute contraindication to urethral preservation (Chen et al., 1997; Stein et al., 1995). Anterior vaginal wall involvement may also increase the risk of urethral involvement, although many patients with vaginal wall invasion also have bladder neck involvement (Maralani et al., 1997; Stein et al., 1995). Direct extension of bladder tumors into the urethra is the most likely cause of urethral involvement, but skip lesions are possible (Chen et al., 1997; Maralani et al., 1997).

There have been several criteria proposed to select women for ONB, including absence of bladder neck, urethral, and anterior vaginal wall involvement, and a negative intraoperative frozen section (Stein et al., 1995, 2007). Intraoperative frozen-section analysis of the urethral stump is an accurate method for determining the presence of cancer, and a positive frozen section can often be converted to negative with additional resection (Jentzmik et al., 2012; Stein et al., 1998). **Most surgeons would consider a negative intraoperative frozen section essential to ONB eligibility** (Stein et al., 2007). Patients with trigonal involvement and positive lymph nodes may still be candidates for ONB as long as the urethral frozen section is negative (Gakis et al., 2015).

A urethral recurrence after ONB in females is a rare event, seen in fewer than 5% of patients (Ali-El-Dein, 2009; Gakis et al., 2015; Pichler et al., 2013; Stein et al., 2008; Stenzl and Holtl, 2003). This is likely due to less at-risk urothelium given shorter female urethral length and the cephalad extension of squamous epithelium after menopause (Stenzl and Holtl, 2003). Urethral recurrences can present with symptoms of obstruction, hematuria, and pain and most commonly occur in the proximal urethra (Gakis et al., 2015; Hrbacek et al., 2015). **Most studies find that URs occur 2 to 4 years postoperatively, although a recent report observed 12 URs that occurred at a median 8 months after RC** (Ali-El-Dein et al., 2004; Gakis et al., 2015; Hrbacek et al., 2015; Pichler et al., 2013; Stein et al., 2008).

One large retrospective cohort study of 180 women who had RC and ONB, approximately 60% of whom had squamous cell carcinoma, demonstrated two URs (1.4%) (Ali-El-Dein, 2009). This highly select group excluded patients having an ONB with trigonal, bladder neck, or vaginal wall involvement and those with a positive intraoperative frozen section. Another large retrospective multi-institutional cohort of 297 highly selected women who had RC and ONB observed seven URs (2.4%) at a median 30 months postoperatively (Gakis et al., 2015). Interestingly, only one UR had a positive final margin at RC, suggesting most recurrences were from skip lesions. Five of the seven URs also had distant or local recurrences, and the 3-year overall survival for all patients with a UR was 25%.

Treatment for local URs most commonly involves urethrectomy and conversion to a cutaneous diversion, although there have been reports on use of BCG (Hrbacek et al., 2015; Jones et al., 2000; Pichler et al., 2013; Stein et al., 2008). Patients with an isolated UR have a good prognosis with curative treatment (Stein et al., 2008). However, many patients with URs also have synchronous pelvic recurrences, distant metastasis, or locally advanced disease, in which case the prognosis is dismal (Hrbacek et al., 2015; Jones et al., 2000).

KEY POINTS: URETHRAL RECURRENCE AFTER RADICAL CYSTECTOMY

- Male urethral recurrence after radical cystectomy is rare, but more common with prostatic involvement, a positive urethral margin, and cutaneous diversions.
- The primary risk factors for female urethral recurrences are bladder neck involvement and a positive urethral margin.
- Most surgeons will proceed with ONB if an intraoperative frozen section of the urethral margin is negative.
- After urethrectomy in patients with ONBs, bowel from the neobladder can often be reconfigured and used for a cutaneous diversion.

ACKNOWLEDGMENTS

Thanks to Dr. Kenneth W. Angermeier and Dr. David S. Sharp, who authored this chapter previously.

REFERENCES

The complete reference list is available online at ExpertConsult.com.

81 Inguinal Node Dissection

Rene Sotelo, MD, Luis G. Medina, MD, and Marcos Tobias Machado, MD, PhD

INTRODUCTION

Inguinal lymph nodes (ILNs) are the primary site for metastasis of invasive penile squamous cell carcinoma (SCC). Despite growing experience in managing penile cancer over the years, surgery remains a cornerstone of treatment. The most important prognostic factor is the involvement of the lymphatics located at the inguinal region (Ornellas et al., 1994; Pettaway et al., 1995; Pizzocaro et al., 2010).

The National Comprehensive Cancer Network (NCCN) recommends bilateral inguinal lymph node dissection (ILND) for all patients, after management of the primary lesions, who are staged as intermediate (T1b) and high-risk (T2 and T3) tumors. Nonpalpable lymph nodes with low-risk primary disease can undergo observation (NCCN, 2018). Additionally, any patient with a positive lymph node on dynamic sentinel node biopsy (DSNB), discussed later in this chapter, should undergo ILND. This recommendation, based on a study by Slaton et al., concluded that patients with T2 disease carry an increased risk for metastasis (42% to 80%) when lymphovascular invasion is present or greater than 50% poorly differentiated cancer is identified in the pathology examination of the primary lesion. However, despite evidence that survival of patients undergoing ILND had a survival benefit (HR 0.79; CI 0.74–0.84, P <0.001), partial adherence to the guidelines has been described, possibly caused by concerns of overtreatment (Slaton et al., 2001; Correa et al., 2018; Pizzocaro et al., 2010).

For patients with a nonpalpable ILN, careful evaluation of prognostic factors for higher risk for inguinal metastasis is crucial. When these factors are present, performing surgical resection of the ILN has been shown to increase survival (Kroon et al., 2005b). On the other hand, for patients with a palpable and resectable ILN, complete cure is possible with or without adjuvant chemotherapy (McDougal et al., 1986; Pizzocaro et al., 2010).

When nodal ulceration or local skin invasion is noted, surgery can be performed for symptom palliation or to avoid death caused by femoral bleeding (Puras-Baez et al., 1995; Ornellas et al., 2008).

In this chapter, we review and discuss the most significant and compelling data regarding anatomy, evaluation, and management of ILNs for penile cancer.

ANATOMIC BACKGROUND
Penile Lymphatics

As a rule, penile carcinoma spreads initially to the ILNs before development of distant metastatic disease (Wood and Angermeier, 2010). Lymphatic spread of disease follows the normal route for penile lymphatic drainage.

Penile lymphatics drain to the superficial and then deep ILNs, and subsequently to the iliac nodes (Pompeo, 2005; Riveros et al., 1967). It is worth mentioning that only anecdotal observations suggested that penile lymphatics may drain directly to the external iliac nodes (Lopes et al., 2000).

The prepuce and skin of the penile shaft drain to the superficial lymphatic system. This consists of a network of vessels that converge dorsally and then divide at the base of the penis to drain into the right and left superficial ILNs, respectively. The glans and frenulum drain into the deep lymphatic system, which consists of large trunks that circle the corona to merge with those from the other side on the dorsum of the penile shaft. They traverse the penis toward the base within Buck fascia, draining through presymphyseal lymphatics into the nodes of the femoral triangle. It is possible for penile cancer to metastasize to the contralateral ILNs because of crossover in the symphyseal region. This fact is critical and guides the surgical approach when considering bilateral inguinal dissection. However, it is accepted that although micrometastases can be found in the contralateral inguinal area, the drainage does not skip levels and usually follows the path from superficial to deep ILNs and from deep ILNs to pelvic lymphatic systems.

Although penile carcinoma metastases to the ILNs confers a poorer prognosis overall, aggressive lymphadenectomy is associated with improved long-term survival and potential cure when lymphatic metastases are present (Horenblas and van Tinteren, 1994; McDougal et al., 1986). Additionally, immediate resection of clinically occult lymph node metastases is associated with improved 5-year survival rates (85% vs. 35%) when compared with delayed resection of involved nodes at the time of clinical detection (Kroon et al., 2005a). Nonetheless, if the tumor has spread to the pelvic nodes, long-term survival is less than 10% (Lapierre et al., 2017).

Urethral Lymphatics

Urethral lymphatic drainage runs parallel to the urethra and is located within the mucosal layer and submucosa (Spirin, 1963). This network is most dense in the area of the fossa navicularis, and these branches join the lymphatics of the glans at the prepuce. The lymphatics of the penile urethra course laterally around the corpora cavernosa to join the vessels proceeding from the glans penis. Bulbar urethral drainage is more variable and may occur along the bulbar artery toward the medial retrofemoral node or may course under the pubis toward the anterior bladder wall, terminating in the retrofemoral and medial external iliac nodes (Wood and Angermeier, 2010).

INGUINAL ANATOMY

The femoral triangle is bounded by the inguinal ligament superiorly, the sartorius muscle laterally, and the adductor longus muscle medially. The floor of the triangle is composed of the pectineus muscle medially and the iliopsoas laterally. The location of the saphenofemoral junction is estimated to be two fingerbreadths lateral and two inferiors from the pubic tubercle.

The ILNs are divided into superficial and deep groups, which are anatomically separated by the fascia lata. The superficial group is composed of 4 to 25 lymph nodes that are settled in the deep membranous layer. The superficial ILNs have been divided into five anatomic groups (Daseler et al., 1948): (1) central nodes around the saphenofemoral junction, (2) superolateral nodes around the superficial circumflex vein, (3) inferolateral nodes around the lateral femoral cutaneous and superficial circumflex veins, (4) superomedial nodes around the superficial external pudendal and superficial epigastric veins, and (5) inferomedial nodes around the greater saphenous vein (Fig. 81.1). Superficial nodes are the first to be affected and therefore play a factor in the selection of the template for the dissection.

The deep ILNs are fewer in number than in the superficial package (1 to 3) and are located medial to the femoral vein in the femoral

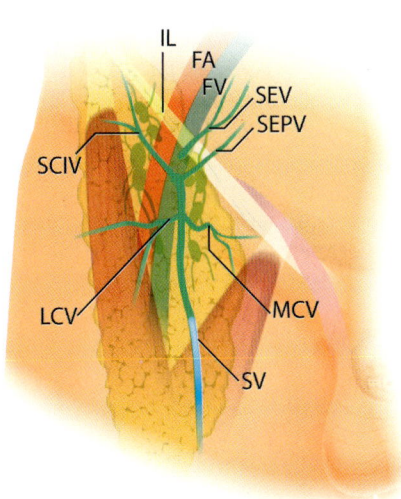
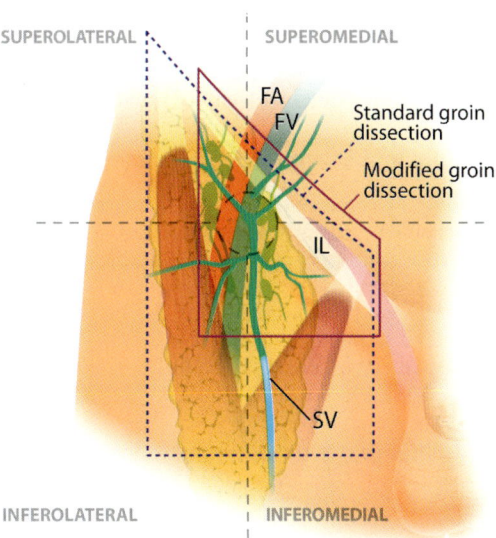

Fig. 81.1. Topographic anatomy plus limits of the standard and modified inguinal lymph node dissections. *IL*, inguinal ligament; *FA*, femoral artery; *FV*, femoral vein; *SEV*, superficial epigastric vein; *SEPV*, superficial external pudendal vein; *MCV*, medial cutaneous vein; *LCV*, lateral cutaneous vein; *SCIV*, superficial circumflex iliac vein.

canal. The node of Cloquet is the most cephalad of this deep group and is situated between the femoral vein and the lacunar ligament. The external iliac lymph nodes receive drainage from the deep inguinal, obturator, and hypogastric groups. The drainage then proceeds on to the common iliac and para-aortic nodes.

The blood supply to the skin of the inguinal region derives from branches of the common femoral artery—the superficial external pudendal, superficial circumflex iliac, and superficial epigastric arteries. Conventional open INLD sacrificed these branches. **Viability of the skin flaps raised during the dissection depends on anastomotic vessels in the superficial fatty layer of Camper fascia that course from lateral to medial along the natural skin lines.** Because lymphatic drainage of the penis to the groin runs beneath Camper fascia, this layer can be preserved and left attached to the overlying skin when the superior and inferior skin flaps are created. Based on this anatomy, a transverse skin incision would compromise this blood supply the least, and serious skin sloughing is prevented in a majority of patients. The femoral nerve lies deep to the iliacus fascia and supplies motor function to the pectineus, quadriceps femoris, and sartorius muscles. In addition, this nerve provides cutaneous sensation to the anterior thigh and should be preserved. Some of the sensory branches of inguinal skin, however, are commonly sacrificed in the regional node dissection.

ENDOSCOPIC ANATOMY OF INGUINAL AREA

Video-endoscopic inguinal surgery has been described as a viable option in patients with low-volume inguinal disease. The most routinely utilized technique is retrograde dissection, initiating at the vertex of the femoral triangle distally and progressing toward the inguinal ligament proximally (Sotelo et al., 2007; Tobias-Machado et al., 2006). To perform this surgery with good results, it is essential to know and understand aspects of endoscopic anatomy.

The first significant anatomic landmarks to identify are the limits of skin, Camper, and Scarpa fascia using a small incision. After that, digital maneuvers are performed to place the trocars.

Insufflation with CO_2 gas and blunt optic dissection allows proper separation of the skin from the lymphatic and vascular elements located beneath it.

The lateral limit of superficial femoral triangle is the fascia of the sartorius muscle, and the medial border is the adductor longus fascia.

Both fascias are externally palpable and easily identified endoscopically. Crossing the medial limit, the Saphena Magna, the great saphenous vein, is identified. In most patients with nonpalpable lymph nodes, it is possible to spare the saphenous vein. Progressive proximal dissection will lead to the fossa ovalis, also referred to as the *saphenous hiatus*, and identification of the accessory saphenous vein and other tributaries of the saphena.

Most nodes are located above the fascia lata, specifically medial to the saphenous-femoral junction, and can be identified by their brown or green coloration. One must be careful to include all areolar tissue between the skin, inguinal cord, and saphenous vein. Preoperative ultrasonographic (US) guidance may be useful to mark the skin above the most prominent nodes. If fluorescence is available, minimally invasive resection can aid to remove suspicious nodes.

Sectioning the fascia lata over the pulse of femoral artery is needed to access the deep node compartment where the deep ILNs lie. This includes all nodal and areolar tissue medial to the femoral vein and lateral to the adductor longus muscle. This resection is continued until Cloquet node (more proximal node located inside the femoral channel) is identified. After this resection has been completed, the most critical structures of femoral triangle are identified.

IMAGING EVALUATION OF INGUINAL AREA

Ultrasonography With Fine-Needle Aspiration Cytology

US of the ILNs can be used to identify neoplastic nodes. Lymph nodes that appear hypoechoic or heterogeneous on US are suspicious of harboring metastases. Some experts can discern better when the normal node architecture is replaced by neoplastic tissue (Goldberg et al., 2005; Clément and Luciani, 2004; Bude, 2004).

Some studies have suggested that in men with penile cancer, fine-needle aspiration cytology (FNAC) of suspicious nodes should be the first investigation in clinically node-negative patients at high risk for occult metastasis. FNAC could also be used in patients with clinically palpable nodes. FNAC is currently performed under US or computed tomography (CT) control. Contemporary studies report a false-negative rate of 20% to 30% (Horenblas et al., 1991).

Although the sensitivity of US-guided FNAC has varied from 50% to 100%, the specificity varies from 90% to 100%. If a tumor is confirmed, therapeutic ILND can be performed instead of DSNB (Saisorn et al., 2006; Kroon et al., 2005b; Van Rijk et al., 2006; Serpa

Neto et al., 2011). If the FNAC is positive, ILND should be performed, and overlying skin and tissues containing the needle tract should be removed with the nodal tissue. If FNAC is negative, it can be repeated if suspicion of lymph node involvement remains.

Computed Tomography and Magnetic Resonance Imaging

Computed tomography (CT) and conventional magnetic resonance imaging (MRI) are unreliable in staging nonpalpable regional lymph nodes as microscopic involvement of lymph node cannot be identified on these studies.

Appropriate staging imaging, including CT of chest, abdomen, and pelvis is recommended in patients with ILN involvement or in patients with clinically suspected pelvic lymph nodes (Horenblas, 2001a, 2001b).

Magnetic Resonance Imaging With Nanotechnology

Preliminary evidence using MRI with iron nanoparticles demonstrated that this imaging modality could detect inguinal metastasis in more than 90% of patients with positive ILN disease. Iron nanoparticles are phagocyted by tumor-associated macrophages, promoting a negative signal in T1 MRI sequences inside the positive nodes (Tabatabaei et al., 2005).

Other studies have suggested that lymphotropic nanoparticle–enhanced MRI (LNMRI) cannot reliably detect micrometastases (Hughes et al., 2009). Furthermore, nanoparticle contrast is rarely available in clinical practice nowadays because of safety concerns such as skin thickening, joint stiffness, and swelling after administration of the contrast (Hughes et al., 2009).

Positron Emission Tomography

Experienced centers have shown that positron emission tomography (PET) has better accuracy over other image methods routinely used such as CT or MRI (Ottenhof and Vegt, 2017; Zhang et al., 2016).

The accuracy of PET/CT for lymph node staging seems to be higher when compared with CT. In groins with normal physical examination, the sensitivity is only 57%. In groins with palpable or enlarged lymph nodes, the sensitivity of PET/CT reaches 96% (Ottenhof and Vegt, 2017). For pelvic lymph nodes and distant metastases, PET/CT is more accurate if inguinal metastases are present. However, these results are based on a very limited number of studies (Ottenhof and Vegt, 2017; Zhang et al., 2016).

In clinical practice today, PET scan is not currently recommended routinely for penile cancer staging.

PENILE CANCER: SURGICAL MANAGEMENT OF REGIONAL LYMPH NODES

In the following sections of this chapter, we will describe the minimally invasive and open techniques for ILND in clinically negative and positive lymph nodes, respectively. It is important to highlight that either technique can be used in each of these clinical scenarios.

PENILE CANCER: NONPALPABLE INGUINAL ADENOPATHY

Approximately 25% of patients with nonpalpable lymph nodes will have lymphatic metastases (Slaton et al., 2001). For nonpalpable lymph nodes, ILND is indicated for intermediate (T1b), and high-risk tumors (T2 and T3) (NCCN, 2018) (Box 81.1). Moreover, there is evidence that **delays in the treatment of the ILNs of more than 12 weeks will negatively impact a patient's chances of survival significantly** (5-year disease specific survival of 64.1% vs. 39.5%) (Chipollini et al., 2017). Lymph node metastases are the most important single predictor for survival in patients with penile cancer; the overall 5-year survival rate for patients with one to three positive

---

BOX 81.1 Indications for Inguinal Lymph Node Dissection in Penile Cancer

- Nonpalpable lymph nodes: intermediate (T1b) and high-risk tumors (T2 and T3)
- Palpable lymph nodes: Lymph nodes less than 4 cm in size with low-risk primary lesions that are positive after fine-needle aspiration or high-risk primary lesions (T1 with high-grade and/or lymphovascular invasion and/or greater than 50% poorly undifferentiated/T2/T3)

ILNs after inguinal lymphadenectomy is about 75.6%, whereas with four to five positive nodes it is 8.4% (Pandey et al., 2006).

Therefore, the standard for both staging and treatment with penile cancer has been ILND, even in patients with no clinical suspicion of lymph node involvement. This procedure, however, has been linked to high rates of morbidity, with complication rates of approximately 55.4% (Gopman et al., 2015). On the other hand, treating all patients with nonpalpable ILNs will result in considerable overtreatment in more than 70% of these cases (Slaton et al., 2001).

Several approaches are being proposed to enhance the patient selection process for ILND, selectively limiting the number of patients to undergo this surgery to those with a higher likelihood of lymph node metastases. (Cabanas, 1977; Pettaway et al., 1995; Leijte et al., 2007; Kumar and Ananthakrishnan, 1998).

Studies assessing predictor factors of lymph node metastasis in patients with penile cancer identified tumor stage, tumor grading, p53 mutation expression, and lymphovascular invasion (Zhu et al., 2010). Other reports in the literature have included molecular factors such as Ki-67, epithelial cadherin, and matrix metalloproteinase, as playing a role in predicting lymph nodes metastasis (Zhu et al., 2007).

Several nomograms have been developed based on these factors to predict lymph node metastasis in an effort to recognize lymph node involvement without performing ILND (Ficarra et al., 2006; Zhu et al., 2007).

Sentinel Lymph Node Biopsy

Physical examination is not reliable when trying to identify ILN metastasis. Using previous experiences reported for melanoma or breast cancer, Cabanas was first to introduce **sentinel lymph node biopsy**, suggesting that lymph node involvement is a stepwise process (Cabanas, 1977). In this technique, he sampled a single node superomedial to the saphenofemoral junction located two fingerbreadths lateral and inferior to the pubic tubercle. He reported that 4% of patients with no clinical suspicion for micrometastasis, were positive for metastasis on SNB. However, even when initial results were encouraging, this approach lost favor after the publication of false-negatives in other experiences throughout the literature (Cabanas, 1977; Catalona, 1980; Perinetti et al., 1980; Srinivas et al., 1991; Wespes et al., 1986).

One of the reasons SNB did not achieve the expected results is the fact that the lymphatic anatomy for penile cancer is not static, and it varies among patients. There is also the possibility that improper pathologic sectioning could be the reason other studies were not able to reproduce Cabanas' results. Subsequently, a **standard extended SN dissection** was suggested (Pettaway et al., 1995). In this modification of the initial SNB technique, all tissue to be resected is located in the area enclosed by the inguinal ligament superiorly, the superior external pudendal vein inferiorly, and the saphenous vein laterally. However, discouraging results for this approach include a false-negative rate of 25% in 20 patients who underwent extended SN dissection, hampering its widespread use (Pettaway et al., 1995).

Furthermore, Kumar and Ananthakrishnan developed another modification of Cabanas' lymph node resection called the **medial inguinal node dissection** in which they resected the most medial node to the groin, but lateral to the pubic tubercle false-negative reported was 8.7%. Yet, the sensitivity was not significantly different when compared with DSNB (Kumar and Ananthakrishnan, 1998).

Dynamic Sentinel Lymph Node Biopsy

Based on our experience with sentinel node biopsies, acknowledging the limitation of the sensitivity of preoperative imaging is important when deciding whether or not ILND surgery should be performed. Advances and improvements in lymphoscintigraphy driven by the work of Morton et al. in melanoma, DSNB was proposed as an alternative method to identify patients who are potentially harboring micrometastasis without clinically palpable nodes (Morton et al., 2006; Leijte et al., 2007).

The pioneers on this area were the Netherlands Group in 1994. The study used radiotracers, such as Technetium-99m nanocolloid, and blue dye injection around the tumor/resection site, and further imaging guidance with lymphoscintigraphy to identify the sentinel lymph node. This technique addresses the previously discussed sentinel node resection criticism that the inguinal lymphatic anatomy is not static. This procedure individualizes the location of the sentinel lymph node, providing an enhanced option for identification and assessment for metastases. Still, misidentification of nodes can still happen when DSNB is performed (4.8% to 19.2%) (Leijte et al., 2007).

The technique has undergone several modifications from its start to the present day. One of these modifications is inclusion of the use of US before the procedure together with fine-needle aspiration of suspicious nodes. Characteristics of suspicious nodes include the presence of necrosis, increased size, abnormal vascularity on Doppler US, a longitudinal/transverse diameter ratio less than 2, and a lack of echogenicity of the hilum of the lymph, with the latter two having relatively high specificity for metastatic nodes (Lam et al., 2008). The introduction of US has overcome the limitation identified by Riveros et al., that some lymph channels can appear deformed as a result of a shift of lymphatic fluid as a consequence of an obstructed node by tumor or necrosis. As a result, the lymph nodes are not visible with other imaging techniques because there is no uptake of contrast material. Ultrasound evaluation of the groin is included in the EAU guidelines for the diagnosis, evaluation, and staging of penile cancer (Leijte et al., 2007; Pizzocaro et al., 2010; Riveros et al., 1967).

There have also been modifications to the sectioning of the pathology slides. In the present day, serial slices (150 micrometers) are done of the entire lymph node to support a more accurate pathologic analysis of the resected node. Since this technique was started, the centers of expertise have been able to develop and finesse their learning curves. This is a critical point of discussion because some centers have not been able to replicate these results. Neto et al. reported that the false-negative rate started to decrease after the first 50 patients, mirroring the findings of other studies like the ALMANAC study for sentinel node biopsy in breast cancer. In that study, they found that 40 patients were required to evidence the value of the sentinel node in for that malignancy. Therefore, achieving proficiency for DSNB in penile cancer can be limited because of the low incidence of this disease, even more in developed countries. As a result, the widespread use of this procedure has been limited to specific centers of expertise. **NCCN guidelines for penile cancer included a recommendation for DSNB only in expert hands** (Leijte et al., 2007; NCCN, 2018; Serpa Neto et al., 2011).

A systematic review and cumulative analysis demonstrated encouraging results regarding this technique for the detection of micrometastasis, as well with a pooled cumulative sensitivity of 84.4% and specificity of 99.4% (Serpa Neto et al., 2011). In expert centers, the false-negative and complication rates have been reported to be 4.8% and 5.7%, respectively (Leijte et al., 2007). These results highlight the importance of expertise in performing this procedure, as other studies have a false-negative rate as high as 22% (Tanis et al., 2002).

Technique

The technique consists of first performing a groin ultrasound. If suspicious nodes are found, FNAC should be performed. If this cytology is positive for malignancy, a bilateral ILND should be performed.

If the cytology is negative or the patient had no suspicious nodes, lymphoscintigraphy is performed. The day before or 4 hours before the start of the procedure, 0.3 to 0.4 mL of technetium nanocolloid (Tc-99m) is injected around the tumor or the base of the penis, and then lymphoscintigraphy is performed. Immediate, dynamic, and static images are obtained with a gamma camera to obtain anterior and lateral views of the sentinel lymph node, which is subsequently marked on the skin surface.

Then, 1 mL of blue dye is injected at the time of the biopsy, intradermally and in a circumferential fashion around the proximal area of the penile shaft. After this, small inguinal incisions are made, and the sentinel lymph node is found using the gamma probe as a guide. The node is resected, and analyzed by the pathologist after paraffin embedding of the entire node. If the results of the pathologic analysis is positive for malignancy, the patient should undergo ILND. Finally, intraoperative palpation of the groin is done to identify nodes that did not have contrast uptake.

Follow-Up

Normally, the follow-up after a DSNB is one follow-up appointment every 2 months for the first 2 years, every 3 months for the third year, and every 6 months up to the fifth year of follow-up. **Ordinarily, most recurrences occur within the first 2 years** (local recurrences: 66.2%, regional recurrences: 86.1%, and distant recurrences: 100%) (Leijte et al., 2008).

In 2007, the Netherlands Cancer Institute reported that after an initial false-negative rate of 19.2%, they were able to decrease it to 4.8% after addition of intraoperative exploration of the groin, fine-needle biopsy, a more extensive pathologic review, and US exploration. However, they were not able to discern what percentage of this was caused by the learning curve of the institution because the study compared one cohort to a historical series (Leijte et al., 2009).

The false-negative rate was associated with lymph vessels rerouting to another ganglion or low uptake of the tracer by the nodes. A meta-analysis by Sadeghi et al. showed that the use of both blue dye and radiotracer improves the detection rate from 88.3% to 90.1% (Sadeghi et al., 2012).

Although the use of the DSNB technique has not been standardized, the EAU guidelines include it in the diagnosis algorithm for evaluation of patients with penile cancer with clinically negative nodes (Pizzocaro et al., 2010). This technique can provide critical information in patient management and surgical decision making. If the DSNB yields positive for malignancy, ILND should be performed.

Superficial Inguinal Lymph Node Dissection (SILND)

For a more accurate assessment of the ILNs, while avoiding high rates of morbidity, a superficial ILN dissection can be considered. This technique consists of removal of the ILNs that are located above the fascia lata with the same template of dissection as the modified ILND (see Modified Inguinal Node Dissection later in the chapter). These nodes are evaluated intraoperatively with frozen section, and if positive for malignancy, a deep ILN dissection is performed.

The rationale is that if the lymph nodes in the superficial compartment are negative, there should be no involvement of the deep package. Pompeo et al. in a prospective study of 50 patients found no cases of deep compartment invasion without positive lymph nodes in the superficial package (Pompeo, 2005). Spiess et al. reported a series of 31 patients with invasive penile cancer who underwent SILND; from those, no recurrences at 3-year follow-up was found in patients without involvement of the superficial compartment (Spiess et al., 2007).

There is debate on the extent of the ILND template (see Modified Inguinal Lymph Node Dissection later in the chapter) and the accuracy of the frozen section to detect malignancy in the nodes. Chipollini et al. in 2018 was the first to evaluate the use of frozen section in penile cancer. In an analysis of 84 patients, they found that frozen section has high specificity (100%), however, the sensitivity is lower (74%). Most false-negative results occurred as a consequence of sampling errors by the pathologist/surgeon, surgeon-related technique, and time limitations. Of note, the rate of accuracy of frozen section is similar when compared with its use in other clinical settings, such as in breast cancer or melanoma (Alperovich et al., 2016; Ariyan et al., 2004). This study also found that a higher body mass index (BMI) is associated with frozen-section false-negatives. Even though it is the only evidence available, this study has some limitations to sample size, the retrospective nature of the study, and the heterogeneity among operators (Chipollini et al., 2018).

Modified Inguinal Lymph Node Dissection

In 1988, Catalona proposed a modified inguinal lymphadenectomy to provide proper diagnostic and therapeutic benefit while decreasing morbidity. In this technique, using a smaller incision, he proposed preservation of the saphenous vein, suggesting that this would decrease lymphatic complications. This modified ILND also excludes the areas lateral to the femoral artery and caudal to the fossa ovalis from the dissection template. It also eliminates the sartorius interposition. **The limits of the modified inguinal lymphadenectomy are the abductor longus muscle medially, the femoral artery laterally, and the inguinal ligament with the fossa ovalis as superior, and inferior limits, respectively** (Catalona, 1988) (see Fig. 81.1).

Since Catalona's implementation of this modified technique, he reported only one case of lymphocele formation and mild lymphedema in all six patients (Catalona, 1988). Several subsequent studies have reported morbidity results using this technique, which include infection (0% to 9.1%), skin necrosis (0% to 8.3%), lymphedema (0% to 100%), seroma (0% to 26.3%), and lymphocele (0% to 22.7%) (Bevan-Thomas et al., 2002; Catalona, 1988; Coblentz and Theodorescu, 2002; d'Ancona et al., 2004; Parra, 1996).

In terms of oncologic outcomes, Lopes et al. reported a 15% recurrence rate when using modified ILND in a 13-patient cohort with 13.2 months of follow-up. This may be in part caused by the lymph nodes with metastatic involvement located in the left lateral quadrant, which should not be eliminated from the template (Lopes et al., 1996). Other studies have shown a false-negative rate between 0% and 5.5% (Bouchot et al., 2004; Coblentz and Theodorescu, 2002; d'Ancona et al., 2004; Parra, 1996).

Endoscopic and Robotic Inguinal Lymphadenectomy

Background

Endoscopic inguinal lymphadenectomy is a more recent technique with the potential for thorough excision of ILNs with decreased morbidity. Bishoff et al. were the first to report the use of endoscopic ILN dissection (Bishoff et al., 2003). In 2006, Tobias-Machado et al. reported 10 patients who underwent bilateral lymphadenectomy for nonpalpable ILNs. Standard open lymphadenectomy was performed on one side, and endoscopic lymphadenectomy on the other. Nodal counts were similar ($P = 0.4$), with a 20% complication rate on the endoscopic side compared with a 70% rate on the open surgery side ($P = 0.01$) (Tobias-Machado et al., 2008). Sotelo et al. reported the outcomes after 14 inguinal endoscopic lymphadenectomies in eight patients with clinical stage T2 SCC of the penis with a median operative time of 91 minutes and an average node yield of 9. Ultrasonic energy is used for the lymph vessel sealing, and postoperatively three lymphoceles were reported but no wound-related complications occurred (Sotelo et al., 2007). In 2011, Tobias-Machado et al. described the single-site video-endoscopic ILND. This consists of a three-port technique for trocar placement (with minimal skin separation between trocars), with the aim to decrease cutaneous complications associated with ILND (Tobias-Machado et al., 2011). This technique raised some concern regarding excessive crowding and clashing of the instruments. In 2011, a detailed analysis of immediate and long-term complications using the Clavien classification system in 29 patients who underwent 41 endoscopic inguinal lymphadenectomy procedures revealed minor complications in 27% (superficial wound infections, seroma, lymphocele, skin edge necrosis, mild-moderate lymphedema), and major complications in 14.6% (death, sepsis, flap necrosis, severe lymphedema, secondary procedure, venous thromboembolism, readmission) (Master et al., 2012). There were no perioperative deaths. Similar experiences have been reported in other series, demonstrating an operative time between 87.86 to 150 minutes, a lymph node yield of 3 to 16 lymph nodes per groin, and a 20% to 73% overall complication rate (Chaudhari et al., 2016; Cui et al., 2016; Pahwa et al., 2013; Pompeo et al., 2013; Yuan et al., 2015; Zhou et al., 2013).

In 2009, the first staged bilateral endoscopic operation performed robotically was reported with the Si DaVinci platform (Josephson et al., 2009). Pathologic examination revealed no metastatic involvement in six superficial and four deep lymph nodes. The contralateral dissection occurred 3 weeks later, and pathologic examination revealed five superficial and four deep negative nodes. There was no wound complication or lower-extremity edema. Sotelo et al. reported performing a concurrent bilateral procedure without repositioning of the robot, which had been identified as a limitation in previous experiences. Metastatic nodes were present bilaterally, with a yield of 19 lymph nodes on the right and 14 on the left (Sotelo et al., 2013). Matin et al. performed a thorough evaluation of the adequacy of a robotic ILN dissection by subsequently opening the incision and having a second surgical oncologist look for residual nodal tissue in 10 patients. The verifying surgeon's role was to inspect the surgical field to ensure that no additional superficial ILNs (above the fascia lata of the thigh) remained within the operative field. If additional tissue was identified at that time, it was removed and sent for pathologic analysis to determine if it was nodal in origin and if it contained metastasis. In one of these groins, two residual lymph nodes were recovered from below Scarpa fascia along the superficial aspect of the inguinal field near the spermatic cord. No metastases were detected in these additional nodes. Among all patients undergoing robotic dissection, 18 of 19 fields (94.7%) were adequately dissected (Matin et al., 2013).

In summary, there is evidence to suggest that the morbidity of an endoscopic ILN dissection is lower than what has been previously reported for the open contemporary series with a similar number of lymph nodes being removed. The applicability of the robot is a more recent development and will need continued prospective evaluation in comparison with standard laparoscopic endoscopic procedures.

Surgical Technique

The patient is positioned on low lithotomy position to allow bilateral groin dissection without repositioning the robot. The assistant stands lateral to the right leg for a right-sided dissection and between the legs for the left side. A Foley catheter is inserted in a sterile fashion, after the inguinal and groin areas have been prepared and draped. Bony and soft tissue landmarks are marked on the skin surface, creating an inverted triangle in which the base is a line connecting the anterior superior iliac spine to the pubic tubercle, along the course of the inguinal ligament. The lateral boundary is the sartorius muscle angling toward the apex. The medial boundary is the adductor longus muscle, again extending toward the apex. These marks aid in correct trocar placement and in delineating the extent of dissection.

A 2-cm incision is made 3 cm below the inferior aspect of the femoral triangle, approximately 25 cm below the inguinal ligament. A white subcutaneous layer is identified, which corresponds to Scarpa fascia. Sweeping finger dissection is used to dissect the potential space beneath the Scarpa fascia to develop the skin flaps at the apex of the triangle in both directions and allow for two additional 8-mm ports to be placed. These two primary robotic 8-mm ports are placed with finger-guided techniques laterally and medially (Fig. 81.2A). A subcutaneous workspace is extended with the endoscope by sweeping with the lens itself (see Fig. 81.2B). The aim of this step is to create a superficial subcutaneous flap under the Scarpa fascia. Alternatively, after the initial finger dissection, a 12-mm Origin balloon port trocar may be used (Origin Medsystems,

Chapter 81 Inguinal Node Dissection 1795

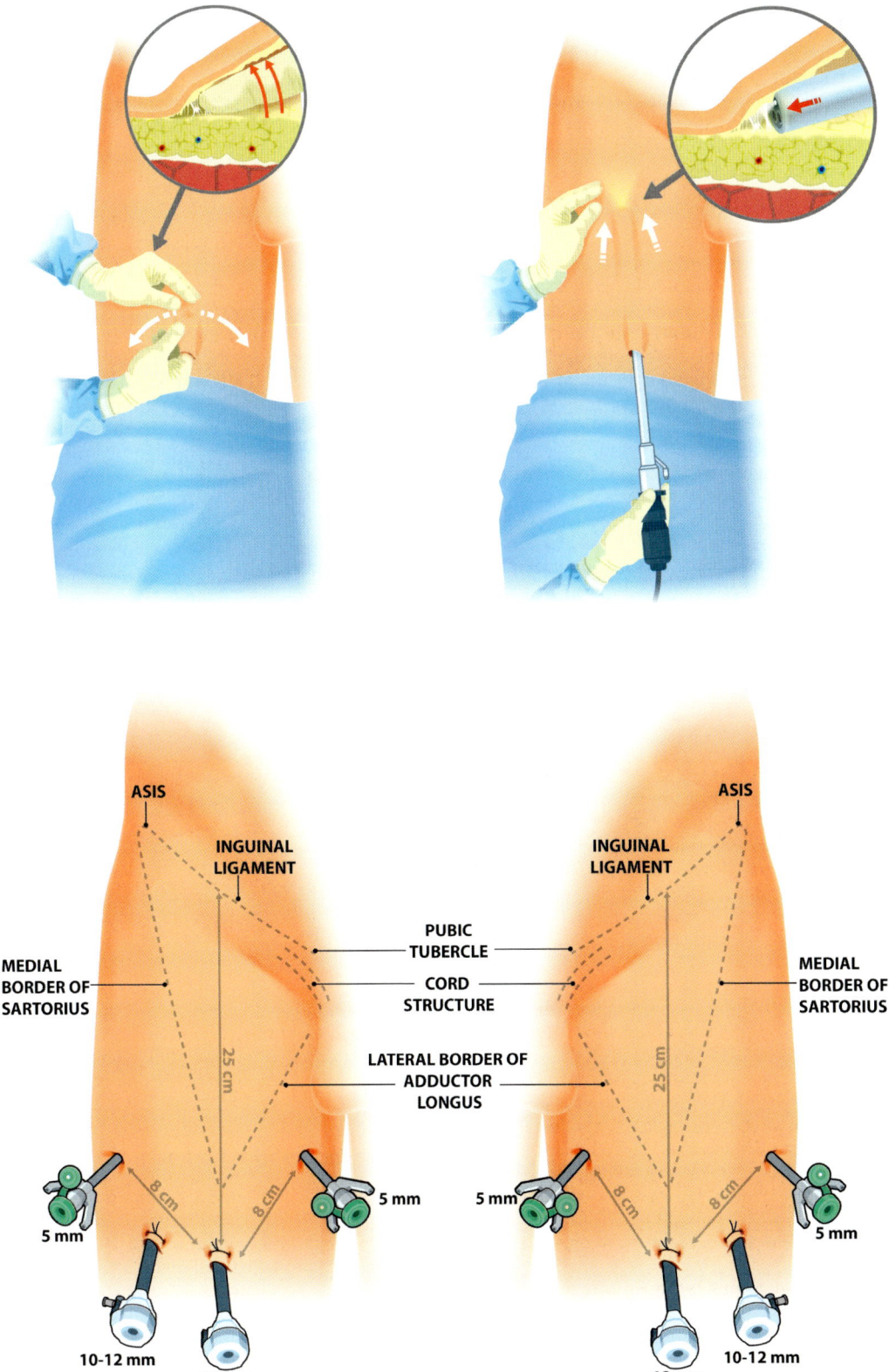

Fig. 81.2. Creation of the working space and trocar placement: *Top left*, Dissection is created by sweeping the finger to find the space below the scarpa at the apex of the dissection. *Top right*, Further extension of the space is done using sweeping movements with the scope. *Bottom left*, Trocar placement for the right side. *Bottom right*, Trocar placement for the left side.

Menlo Park, CA). Insufflation is set at 25 mm Hg for 10 minutes to create the working space (Master et al., 2012); after that, CO₂ insufflation pressure is lowered to 15 mm Hg. A 0-degree 10-mm lens is inserted, and one additional 10-mm assistant port is placed between the camera and primary 8-mm working port on the assistant side. The robot is positioned at 45 degrees contralateral to the first procedure (right side) and ipsilateral to the patient in the second procedure (left side) (see Fig. 81.2C,D).

Instruments that can be used include a bipolar Maryland, or PK forceps (Olympus, Hamburg, Germany) in the left robotic arm, and monopolar scissors or robotic ultrasonic instruments in the right arm to dissect the membranous and lymphatic tissue beneath Camper fascia. Every effort is made to completely develop the anterior working space to the inguinal ligament, which is usually identified at the end of this dissection as being a transverse structure with white fibers, marking the superior limit of the dissection. The boundaries of the dissection extend from the inguinal ligament superiorly, sartorius muscle laterally, and adductor longus muscle medially (Fig. 81.3A). One will be able to spare the saphenous vein in most patients, while the smaller branches of the femoral artery and vein may be clipped and divided. Identification of the adductor longus and sartorius muscles is facilitated by identifying the fascia of the respective muscles and correlating this to the previously made skin markings. The spermatic cord is seen medially. Inadvertent dissection deep to the fascia lata is apparent when reddish muscular fibers are seen.

With blunt dissection, the nodal tissue can be rolled inward on both sides. This maneuver is continued inferiorly as much as possible from both sides to define the inferior apex of the nodal packet. The saphenous vein will be identified as it crosses the internal border of the dissection near the apex of the femoral triangle, and following the vein leads the surgeon to the saphenous arch until its junction with the superficial femoral vein at the fossa ovalis. The dissection continues superiorly, where the packet is dissected off the fascia lata with a combination of sharp and blunt dissection. Typically, the nondominant hand lifts the packet, and the monopolar scissors in the dominant hand advance the dissection. After the fossa ovalis is encountered, the packet is dissected away at its superolateral and superomedial limits, thereby narrowing the packet and pulling it away from the inguinal ligament. At this point, the superficial and deep plane of dissection join and separate the package from the inguinal ligament (see Fig. 81.3B–D).

With the nodal packet circumferentially dissected except for its attachments to the saphenous arch, venous tributaries are clipped. Characteristic pulsations of the femoral artery serve as a nearby landmark. If possible, the packet will be released from the saphenous vein. If not, the vein can be ligated in the saphenous arch with Weck clips (Teleflex, Wayne, Pennsylvania). One must always attempt to preserve the saphenous vein whenever possible, to reduce the risk for postoperative lymphedema (Zhang et al., 2007).

The specimen is removed in a specimen-retrieval bag after extension of the camera trocar incision. Frozen-section results determine whether a deep ipsilateral dissection will be required. While waiting for pathology results, you can begin to create the working space in the contralateral leg.

For the deep ILN dissection, the pneumoperitoneum is reestablished. The fascia lata medial to the saphenous arch is opened to expose the saphenofemoral junction. Inferomedial dissection around the femoral vein enables resection of the deep ILNs (Master et al., 2012) (see Fig. 81.3E). This should be continued to the level of the femoral canal until the pectineus muscle is seen to ensure complete nodal retrieval.

Insufflation pressure is then decreased to 5 mm Hg to confirm hemostasis. It is of great importance that meticulous control of lymphatics and excellent hemostasis be established to reduce the risk for lymphocele and hematoma formation, which could potentially become infected. A closed suction drain is positioned in the most dependent (caudal) portion of the lymphadenectomy field, as the fluid will drain dependently toward the drain when the patient is upright. Trocar incisions are closed in the standard fashion (see Fig. 81.3F). The patient is allowed to ambulate the day of surgery and is given a regular diet. Discharge is planned for the first postoperative day. A compressive elastic girdle, as used for liposuction patients, is used to provide bilateral compression of the groins. In addition, elastic compression stockings are worn simultaneously and are used for 3 months after surgery. Broad-spectrum antibiotics are continued until after the drains have been removed. Drains typically stay in place until the output is less than 50 mL per 24-hour period. All patients receive venous thromboembolism prophylaxis using fractionated or low-molecular-weight heparin.

There are no studies comparing robotic versus laparoscopic techniques to date. There has been no advantage demonstrated of one technique over the other. Theoretically, the ergonomics and the tridimensional view can be an advantage. Additionally, the ability to use indocyanine green (ICG) during groin dissection on the robotic platform, can enhance the surgeon's ability to identify lymphatics and potentially avoid complications (Bjurlin et al., 2017).

For the robotic ILND, the creation of the working space is performed in the same fashion as the one described in the endoscopic technique, however, the size of the ports is different because robotic and assistant ports are 8 and 5 mm in size, respectively. Another shared technical aspect of both techniques is that the ultrasonic instruments available for the laparoscopic and robotic systems do not articulate. Hence, both work in a linear fashion, and this can be cumbersome when different angulations are needed during lymph vessel sealing.

The Xi robotic platform offers several advantages over the Si system, specifically in the capacity of repositioning without modifications of the operative room setting (Fig. 81.4). In addition, the Xi system allows for intraoperative rotation of the camera up and down from the surgeon's console, and the ability to use the camera from any port, which can be beneficial if instrument collisions occur during the dissection. The new Single Port robotic platform can also offer some advantages for this surgery that should be assessed once experience on this system is developed, such as an additional reduction of skin complications without increasing the difficulty of the procedure.

PENILE CANCER: PALPABLE INGUINAL ADENOPATHY OR POSITIVE INGUINAL LYMPH NODES

Primary ILND for patients with palpable nodes is indicated for lymph nodes less than 4 cm, with a low-risk primary lesion, that are positive after FNA/excisional biopsy, or that are high-risk primary lesions. It is also indicated for lymph nodes greater than 4 cm that are mobile and positive for malignancy after percutaneous biopsy (neoadjuvant chemotherapy is an option for this group as well) (NCCN, 2018) (see Box 81.1).

Surgery for Curative Purposes

Radical ILND is indicated for patients with palpable positive nodes and may be curative if disease is limited to ILNs. However, a "therapeutic curative window" exists, and it is mainly associated with the volume of inguinal metastases. Patients who have unilateral limited metastases without extranodal extension of cancer or pelvic metastases are potentially curable (Johnson and Lo, 1984a, 1984b; Spratt, 2000; Srinivas et al., 1987).

Radical Inguinal Lymph Node Dissection

The patient is positioned with the thigh abducted and externally rotated with support under the flexed knee.

The dissection is limited superiorly by a line drawn from margin of the external ring to the anterior superior iliac spine, laterally, by a line drawn from the anterior superior iliac spine extending 20 cm inferiorly, and medially by a line drawn from the pubic tubercle 15 cm down the medial thigh.

The most utilized incision is an oblique 2-cm section below and parallel to the inguinal ligament extending from the lateral to the medial limit of the dissection. If an area of the overlying skin is

Chapter 81 Inguinal Node Dissection 1797

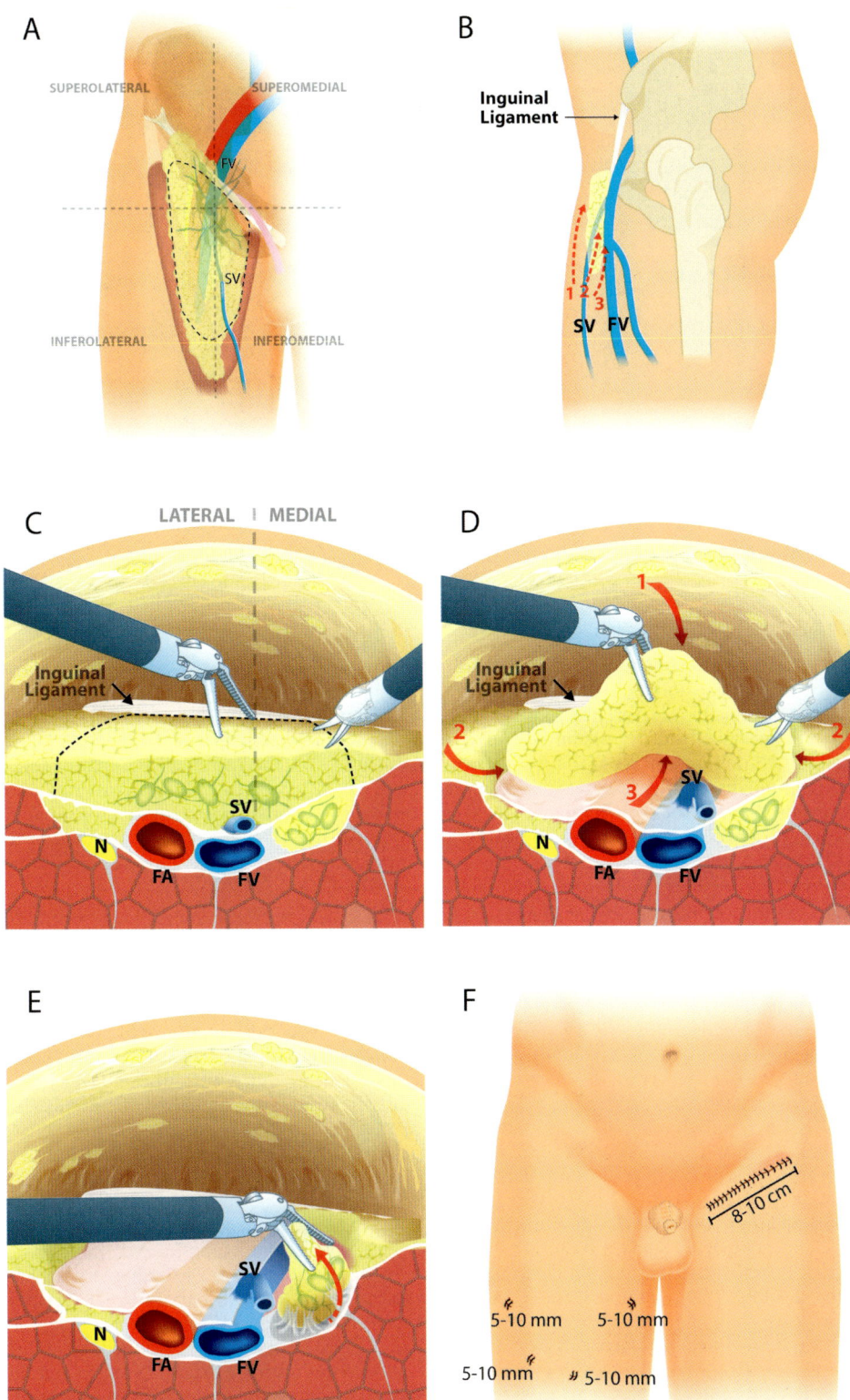

Fig. 81.3. (A) Limits of the endoscopic inguinal lymph node dissection. (B) Lateral view of the steps to perform a nodal inguinal node dissection. (C) Superficial lymph node dissection. (D) Superficial package being removed along with saphenous vein preservation. (E) Deep lymph node dissection resection. (F) Graphic representation of the surgical wounds after open inguinal lymph node dissection *(right)* and inguinal lymph node dissection *(left)*. *1*, Superficial package. *2*, Management/dissection around the saphenous vein. *3*, Deep inguinal package resection. *FA*, femoral artery; *FV*, femoral vein; *N*, femoral nerve; *SV*, saphenous vein.

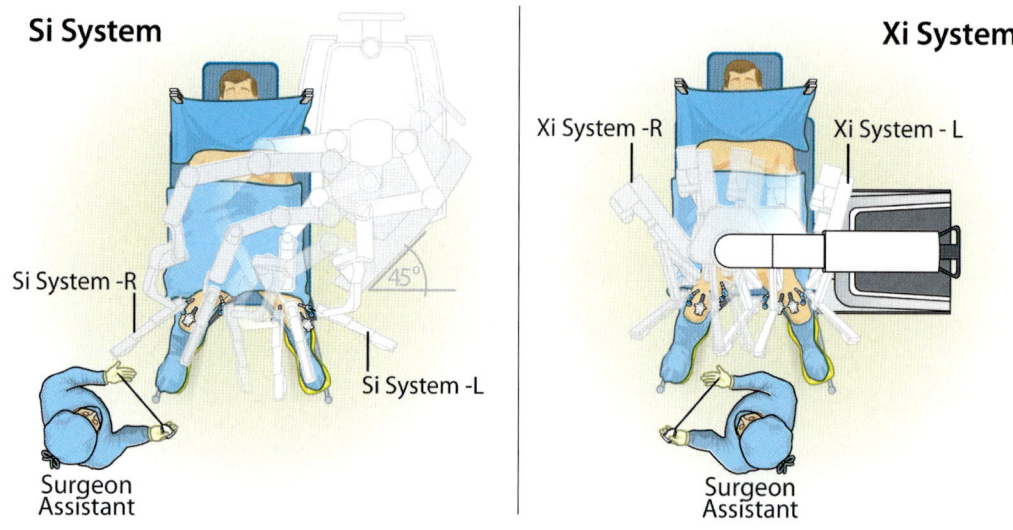

Fig. 81.4. Assistant and robotic dock positioning for robotic inguinal lymph node dissection for the robotic SI system *(left)* and Xi system *(right)*.

involved by the disease or adherent to a palpable node, an elliptical incision is made around the involved skin and then extended medially and laterally (Fig. 81.5). Alternatively, in this case, the incision may be extended superiorly from the lateral border of the ellipse and inferiorly from the medial border to make a single S-shaped incision for concomitant iliac and inguinal dissections. Superior and inferior skin flaps are developed in the plane just below Scarpa fascia. The superior flap is elevated 3 cm cephalad above the inguinal ligament and the inferior flap to the limit of the dissection.

Another option, described by Ornellas et al. in 1991, is to make a large Gibson incision and dissect inferiorly (Ornellas et al., 1991). The advantages reported are minimized skin devascularization, because the superior border of incision remains intact, and this permits easy access to concomitant iliac dissection if necessary.

The fat and areolar tissues are dissected from the external oblique aponeurosis and the spermatic cord to the inferior border of the inguinal ligament, forming the superior boundary of the lymph node packet. The inferior angle is the apex of the femoral triangle, where the long saphenous vein is identified and divided. In patients with minimal metastatic disease, it may be feasible and beneficial to spare the saphenous vein. Dissection is deepened through the fascia lata overlying the sartorius muscle laterally and the fascia covering the adductor longus muscle medially. At the apex of the femoral triangle, the femoral artery and vein are identified, and the dissection is continued superiorly along the femoral vessels. Cutaneous perforating arteries are ligated as they are encountered on the surface of the femoral artery. The saphenous vein is divided at the saphenofemoral junction, and the dissection is continued superiorly to include the deep ILNs medial and lateral to the femoral vein until the femoral canal (see Fig. 81.5). The anterior aspects of the femoral vessels are dissected, but lateral surface of the femoral artery is not exposed. This avoids injury to the femoral nerve and the deep femoral artery.

After the femoral triangle is dissected, the sartorius muscle is mobilized from its origin at the anterior superior iliac spine and either transposed or rolled 180 degrees medially to cover the femoral vessels (Barofsky maneuver). The muscle is sutured to the inguinal ligament superiorly, and its margins are sutured to the muscles of the thigh immediately adjacent to the femoral vessels. The femoral canal can be closed by suturing the shelving edge of the inguinal ligament to Cooper ligament, being careful not to compromise the lumen of the external iliac vein or to injure the inferior epigastric vessels in the process. Primary closure of the dissection is usually possible with minimal or no further mobilization of the excision margins. When circumstances demand a large area of skin resection, a primary closure may be performed using scrotal skin rotation flaps (Skinner, 1974), an abdominal wall advancement flap (Tabatabaei and McDougal, 2003), or a myocutaneous flap based on the rectus abdominis or tensor fascia lata (Airhart et al., 1982) (Fig. 81.6). Closed-suction drains are placed under the subcutaneous tissue. During closure, the skin flaps are sutured to the surface of the exposed musculature to decrease dead space. The skin is closed with absorbable subcutaneous sutures or staples (see Fig. 81.3F).

In contemporary series, early minor complications have been reported in about 50% of radical dissections (Bevan-Thomas et al., 2002; Bouchot et al., 2004; Nelson et al., 2004; Spiess et al., 2009). These consist primarily of lymphocele, wound infection or necrosis, and lymphedema. Major complications, such as debilitating lymphedema, flap necrosis, and lymphocele requiring intervention, occur in 5% to 20% of patients (Bevan-Thomas et al., 2002; Nelson et al., 2004). Deep venous thrombosis (DVT) or pulmonary embolism (PE) has been reported in 5% of patients (Johnson and Lo, 1984a, 1984b; Ravi, 1993; Spiess et al., 2009). Efforts to minimize lower-extremity lymphedema include early use of compression stockings and saphenous vein preservation when feasible.

Adjuvant Chemotherapy

A study of more than 200 patients with penile cancer reported a relapse rate of 45% in patients treated with surgery versus 16% in those who received adjuvant chemotherapy after surgery (Pizzocaro et al., 1996). The authors concluded that adjuvant chemotherapy can improve the results of radical surgery significantly. However, most of the patients in need of adjuvant treatment, such as patients with bilateral metastases or pelvic involvement, had poorer outcomes.

In a study of 13 patients with radically resected node metastases treated with adjuvant chemotherapy, 3 of 8 patients were cured, 4 progressed, and 1 died from chemotherapy-related pulmonary toxicity. The authors concluded that **adjuvant chemotherapy can increase survival compared with surgery alone but that the risk for toxicity is high** (Hakenberg et al., 2006).

A literature review demonstrated that, after ILND, the 5-year survival rate for men is 90% to 100% with negative ILNs, 80% for those with one positive node or unilaterally positive nodes, 50% for two or more unilaterally positive nodes, and 10% for bilaterally positive nodes, extranodal extension, or positive pelvic nodes (Pow-Sang et al., 1979; Srinivas et al., 1987).

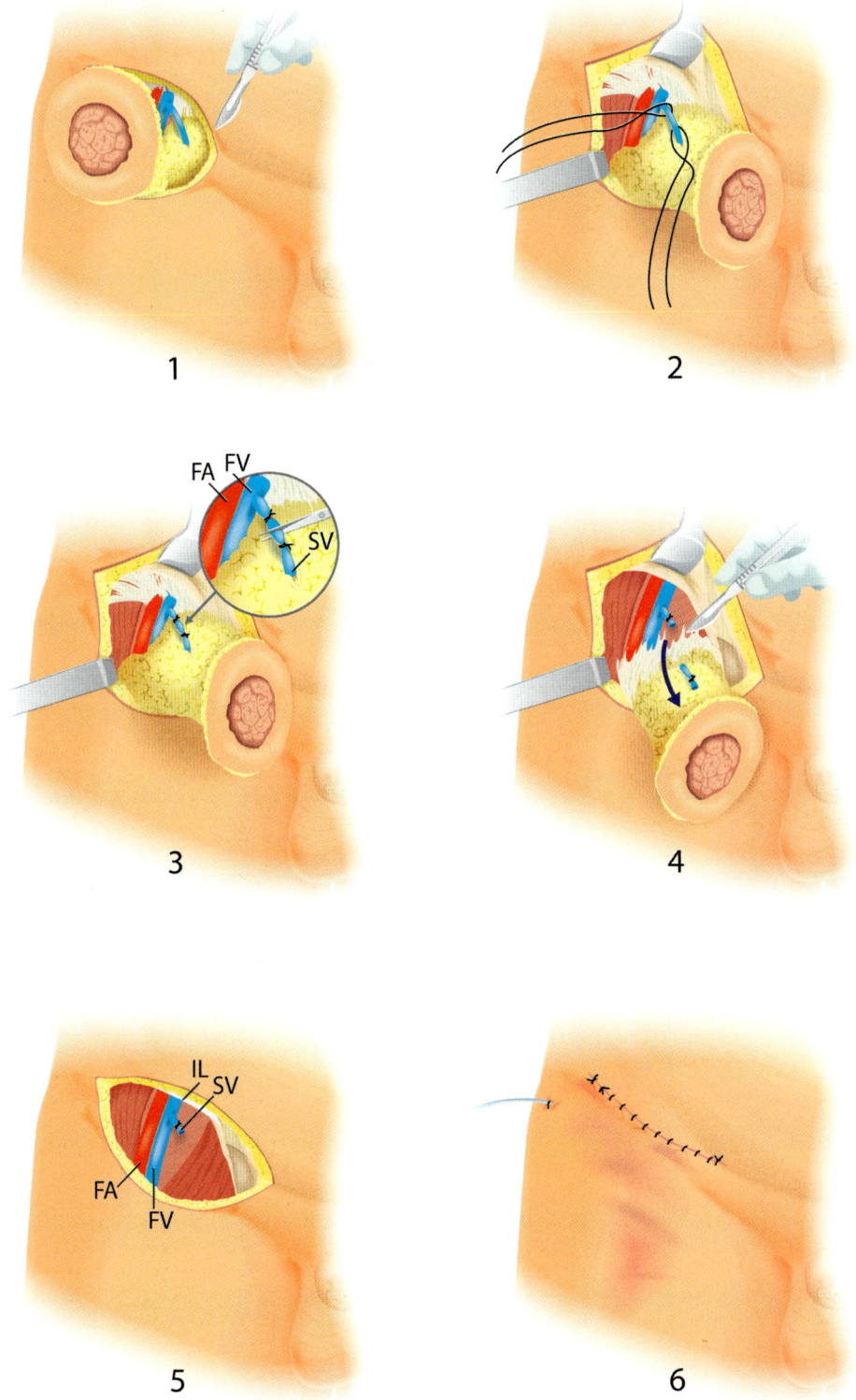

Fig. 81.5. Graphic representation of an inguinal lymph node dissection plus resection of an inguinal metastasis. *1,* Incision is made marking the borders of the metastatic lesion. *2,* Saphenous vein is detected. *3,* Saphenous vein is ligated. *4,* Skin along with the metastatic lesion and the lymph nodes is removed en bloc. *5,* Final setup of the anatomy after resection. *6,* Wound is closed in a traditional aseptic fashion.

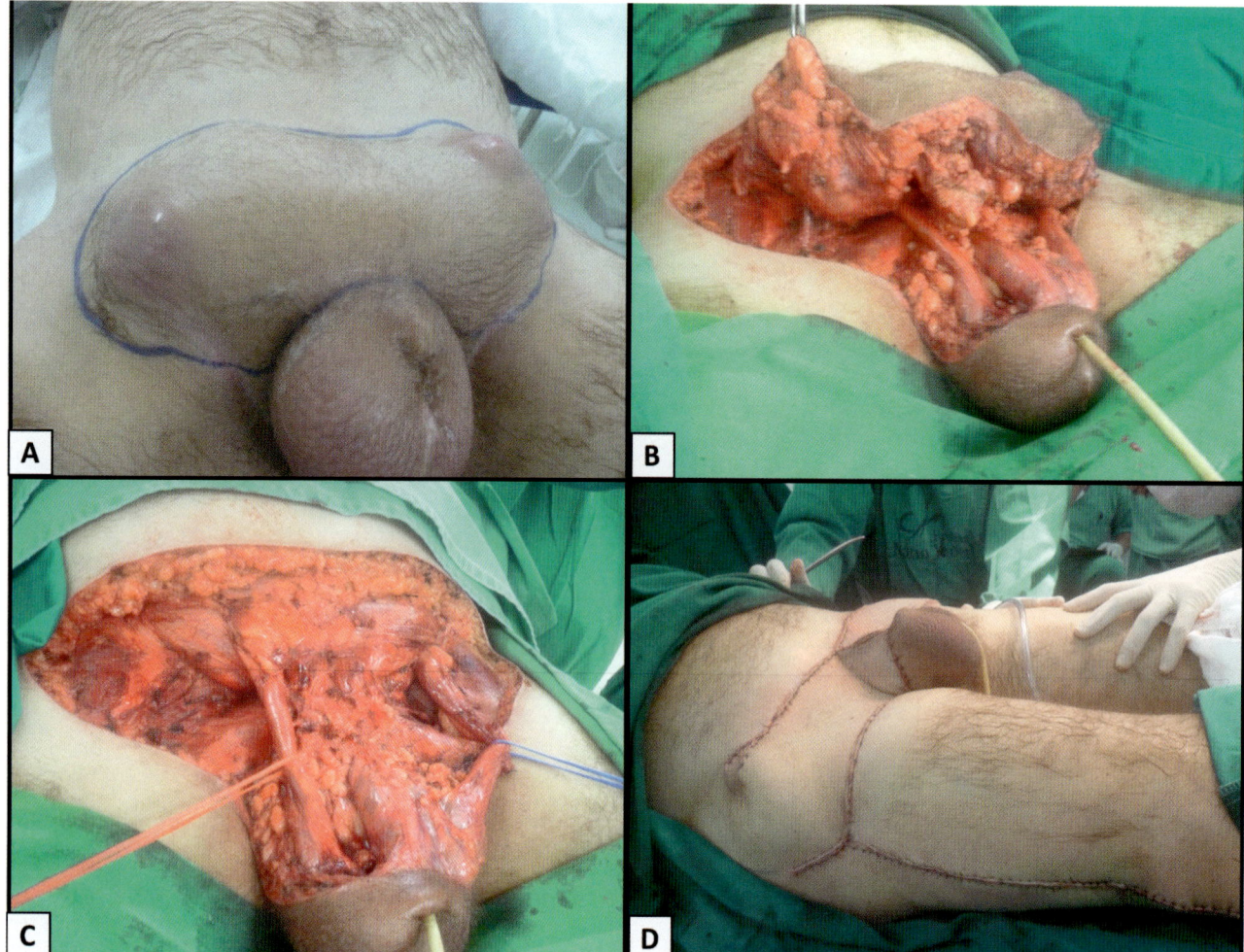

Fig. 81.6. (A) Area to be resected is delineated. (B) Incision including skin and ulcerated nodes plus dissection of the area with inguinal cord and femoral vessels skeletonized. (C) Further incision and removal en bloc of the piece is made. (D) Further vertical incision in lateral position of legs bilaterally to skin muscular fascia lata flap to cover the defect. Final aspect.

It has been suggested that adjuvant therapy is advisable when there are two or more positive nodes, extranodal extension of cancer, or pelvic node metastasis (Solsona et al., 2004).

Surgery for Palliative Purposes

Infiltrative or coalescent inguinal disease left untreated can result in significant local complications such as infection, abscess, foul-smelling drainage, and life-threatening vascular hemorrhage (Koifman et al., 2013).

Palliative surgery can offer a better short-term quality of life by removing infected and painful disease, however, cure is rarely achieved. One study included 24 patients who underwent a palliative dissection, of whom 21%, 8%, and 4% survived 1, 2, and 3 years, respectively (Srinivas et al., 1987).

In very select cases, an extra-anatomical arterial bypass can be performed to prevent femoral hemorrhage or death (Ferreira et al., 2008).

Considering surgery as monotherapy for this disease stage is inadequate because it only addresses the genital and inguinal area, thereby, distant metastases are not being treated. Several series have described multimodal approaches utilizing systemic chemotherapy and surgery in patients with bulky inguinal metastases. The available data are limited to retrospective reviews, and in most of these cases, patients had either initial or recurrent bulky metastases treated with systemic chemotherapy and then subsequently underwent a surgical procedure (Ornellas et al., 2008; Pizzocaro and Piva, 1988).

The feasibility of performing aggressive surgical resection and reconstruction in the postchemotherapy setting has been described and with no perioperative deaths (Chen et al., 2004). In a series from MD Anderson Cancer Center, the incidence of complications was greater among those undergoing a palliative dissection (67%) when compared with prophylactic (35%) or therapeutic (36%) dissections (Bevan-Thomas et al., 2002).

The available literature suggests that the optimal candidates for postchemotherapy surgical consolidation in advanced penile cancer are those with a significant response to therapy, who are fit for surgery, and whose inguinal disease is free from infection (Ornellas et al., 2008).

PREPARATION OF THE PATIENT BEFORE SURGERY

Antibiotics

Antibiotic therapy for at least 4 weeks after treatment of the primary lesion of the penis has been advised to allow complete resolution of septic lymphadenitis (Catalona, 1980; Crawford and Daneshgari, 1992).

Some authors recommend prophylactic antibiotics considering this surgery as a contaminated procedure and the inflammatory reaction in the lymph nodes (Horenblas, 2001a, 2001b).

It has been said that, for palpable disease, **30% to 50% of these nodes are secondary to associated inflammatory conditions and not to metastases.** Traditionally, it was stated that the timing to differentiate between infection and metastasis was 6 weeks of antibiotic treatment. However, recent evidence from Chipollini et al. revealed that **late ILND and positive node disease are significant factors for recurrence and decreased survival** (Chipollini et al., 2017). Precaution must be taken in this regard; percutaneous biopsy may be an option for these cases or antibiotic therapy if an overlying infection is confirmed.

The most frequent microorganisms isolated in inguinal wounds include gram-negative, *Staphylococcus*, diphtheroids, and *Peptostreptococcus*. It has been suggested that proper sterilization of the surgical field before the procedure would decrease wound colonization and therefore decrease the risk for postoperative wound infection. The most utilized broad-spectrum antibiotics have been ampicillin with an aminoglycoside or ciprofloxacin. In patients with preoperative cellulitis or infection of the inguinal region, bacterial cultures should be obtained, and culture-specific–guided oral antibiotics should be given before surgical management (Spiess et al., 2009).

Anticoagulation

Heparin may increase the risk for wound hematoma and serous wound drainage because of continued extravasation of lymph (Tomic et al., 1994). In one study on patients who underwent ILND for melanoma, heparin did not reduce the DVT incidence. However, the total volume and duration of wound drainage was significantly greater in the group treated with low-dose heparin (Arbeit et al., 1981).

However, some authors still advocate using routine low-molecular-weight heparin, starting the evening before surgery and continuing while the patient is on bed rest. Early ambulation is highly recommended as well (Spiess et al., 2009).

In patients with a recent history of DVT or pulmonary embolism (PE), a therapeutic dose of low-molecular-weight heparin followed by oral anticoagulants should be restarted (Spiess et al., 2009).

The use of intermittent compression devices or compression stockings immediately before anesthetic induction to prevent venous stasis has also been recommended (Crawford and Daneshgari, 1992).

Bowel Cleansing

It has been suggested that a low-residue diet and a cleansing enema the day before surgery can minimize the risk for wound contamination. However, there is no evidence for the benefit for bowel preparation, and it is not routinely recommended (Spratt, 2000).

POSTOPERATIVE CARE OF PATIENTS AFTER INGUINAL LYMPHADENECTOMY

Bed Rest

Past literature suggested that after ILND, the patient should be maintained on bed rest for 7 days, with both legs elevated (Crawford, 1984; Ekstrom and Edsmyr, 1958). Lymph flow increases with motion in the lower limb, whereas immobilization permits the regeneration of lymphatics or the opening of anastomotic lymphatics (Dewire and Lepor, 1992). More recent papers recommend early or immediate ambulation after ILND (Milathianakis et al., 2005; Spiess et al., 2009; Tobias-Machado et al., 2007). If a myocutaneous flap has been used, mobilization should be restricted in the early postoperative period (48 to 72 hours) to avoid compromising the blood supply to the flap (Thomas et al., 1995).

Dietary Considerations

There are no dietary restrictions for patients. Patients who present with high drainage of lymph fluid should be recommended restricted fluid intake and decreased saturated fat consumption (Lv et al., 2017).

Antibiotics

Prophylactic antibiotics should be continued for 1 week after surgery, or until all wound drains have been removed (Loughlin, 2006).

Anticoagulation (see Preparation of the Patient Before Surgery)

Compressive Dressings and Stockings

It has been suggested that the wound should be made as airtight as possible, suction drains can be used routinely, and the application of pressure by heavy dressings on the thin flaps is to be avoided (Master et al., 2012; Tobias-Machado et al., 2008). Efforts to minimize lower-extremity lymphedema include early ambulation, and the use of elastic stockings and sequential compression devices. It is advised that individually fitted elastic stockings be worn for at least 6 months after surgery (Leone et al., 2017; Rabe et al., 2018).

Drainage

It has been suggested that lymphorrhea and seroma can be prevented by postoperative suction drainage and that the drains should be removed when the 24-hour output becomes less than 50 mL, usually between 3 to 15 days postoperatively (Loughlin, 2006; Tobias-Machado et al., 2006). Colonization and spread of bacteria along these drains may increase the risk for infection if the drains stay in place for an extended period (Chintamani et al., 2005).

There is a theoretical risk that the presence of a suction drain may prolong and intensify the inflammatory phase and may also prevent leaking lymphatics from closing, thus facilitating seroma formation (Jain et al., 2004).

COMPLICATIONS OF INGUINAL LYMPHADENECTOMY

ILND carries an overall high complication rate when compared with other surgical procedures, however, most of these complications are not severe or life-threatening. Regardless, the burden of mental distress, cost, and morbidity is considerably high, and some may argue unnecessary. This is why patient selection is critical, and extensive evaluation of the patient for micrometastasis assessment is recommended for all patients with penile cancer.

The complication reports of this procedure vary as there is no standard method for reporting these in the literature. This leads to different nomenclatures for the same complications, limiting accurate analysis and development of preventative and management strategies. Overall, the complication rate is 55.4%, of which 65.7% of complications are classified as minor using the Clavien-Dindo classification system. Number of lymph nodes removed has been shown to be a predictive factor for overall and major complication rate (Gopman et al., 2015).

The wound complications reported are largely wound infections, cellulitis, necrosis of the graft, or wound breakdown. Wound-related issues compose 0.6% to 43% of complications in some series (Gopman et al., 2015; Koifman et al., 2013; Stuvier, 2013). Antibiotics that target gram-negative rods, *Staphylococcus* group, *Diphteroids*, or *Peptostreptococcus* are recommended (ampicillin/gentamycin or ampicillin/ciprofloxacin). As previously mentioned, the type of incision, reservation of the fatty tissue within the Camper fascia, and proper preoperative care is important to prevent wound complications. The use of anticoagulants has been discussed previously (see Postoperative Care of Patients After Inguinal Lymphadenectomy).

An attempt to reduce wound complications with the introduction of endoscopic techniques has also been performed. The last prospective comparison study published by Kumar and Sethia showed that with endoscopic procedures there are a higher mean number of nodes retrieved (9.36 vs. 7.1), increased mean number of nodes involved (1.24 vs. 0.57), and fewer major complications (5% vs. 68%). However, concern was raised because of the heterogeneity between the groups compared (Heyns, 2009; Kumar and Sethia, 2017).

It has been suggested that the main advantage of minimally invasive techniques is a decreased rate of wound complications as a result of a smaller surgical incision size. Care must be taken on accomplishing the central surgical principle of preserving Camper fascia as well avoiding ischemic complications of the skin. Gopman

TABLE 81.1 Survival of Men With Squamous Cell Carcinoma of the Penis After Inguinal Lymph Node Dissection

	MONTHLY INTERVAL			
	YEARS 1–2	YEAR 3	YEAR 4	YEAR 5
Low-risk primary lesion: G1–2, Tis, Ta, T1, no vascular invasion	3	4	6	12
High-risk primary lesion: G3, T2–3, vascular invasion	2	3	6	12
Penile preserving treatment	3	6		
Partial penectomy	6	12		
Pathologically N0 (at SNB)	4	6	12	12
Pathologically N1 (at SNB)	3[a]	4[a]	6[a]	12[a]

[a]Includes ultrasonography with fine-needle aspiration cytology, computed tomography, and chest radiograph.
SNB, sentinel node biopsy.

et al. lead a multicenter study including more than 300 patients undergoing ILND and found, after a multivariate logistic regression analysis, that the sartorius flap transposition was a predictor of wound complications. Age was also reported to increase the likelihood of major infection complications (Gopman et al., 2015).

Lymphatic complications and seromas contribute significantly to the morbidity associated with the procedure. They are reported throughout the literature as lymphorrhea, lymphedema, or lymphoceles (2.4% to 26.5%) (Gopman et al., 2015; Koifman et al., 2013). The question has been raised whether drainage with or without suctioning systems should be used, although no difference as been found on this matter. However, there is a theoretical rationale to believe that suctioning systems may prolong and intensify the inflammatory phase postoperatively and prevent lymphatics from closing, resulting in more lymphatic complications. Saphenous preservation has been proposed as one mechanism by which lymphatic complications can be reduced, as preserving the saphenous vein can improve the circulation of the region. A study of vulvar carcinoma reported that this sparing technique could avoid 30% of the overall complication rate (Zhang et al., 2000). Cui et al. in 2016 published a randomized comparison of patients undergoing saphenous vein sparing and ligation. In this study, the authors report that short- and long-term lymphedema were reduced significantly by more than 25% (Cui et al., 2016; Heyns, 2009).

In addition, the type of mechanism used for management of lymph vessels intraoperatively has been extensively evaluated. Some studies advocate the use of electrocautery, and others argue that ultrasonic energy may be superior. In an experiment carried out by Gallo et al., they found that ultrasonic energy was strong enough to obliterate the thoracic duct in cases of chylous ascites, and this is the reason it has been used in other series (Gallo et al., 2002; Sotelo et al., 2009).

A clinical trial presented by Adwani and Ebbs (2006) showed no benefit between ultrasonic energy and regular coagulation. Fibrin sealant was also proposed with the intention of sealing leaking capillaries and obliterating dead space where accumulation of fluids can occur and develop into a lymphocele and seroma. A meta-analysis based on clinical trials on this subject for breast cancer found no difference in the formation of collections, drainage volume, or length of stay (Carless and Henry, 2006)

Mobilization and the use of compressive techniques have been previously discussed in this chapter. Other complications such as DVT, thrombophlebitis, myocardial infarction, and neuropraxias have also been reported in the literature (Adwani and Ebbs, 2006; Heyns, 2009).

ONCOLOGIC RESULTS AND FOLLOW-UP AFTER SURGERY

Oncologic Control

In SCC of the penis with no ILN metastases, the reported 5-year survival rate varies from 40% to 100%, with an average survival rate

TABLE 81.2 Follow-Up Protocol for Men With Penile Squamous Cell Carcinoma

AUTHOR	YEAR	5-YEAR OVERALL SURVIVAL (%) NODE-NEGATIVE	5-YEAR OVERALL SURVIVAL (%) NODE-POSITIVE
Beggs and Spratt	1964	72.5%	19.3%
Johnson and Lo	1984	74%	–
Srinivas et al.	1987	85%	32%
Pow-Sang et al.	1979	80%	62.5%
Ornellas et al.	1991	87%	29%
Ravi	1993	95%	53%
Lopes et al.	1996	–	40.3%
Pandey et al.	2006	95.7%	51.1%

of approximately 75% (Djajadiningrat et al., 2014). In patients with lymph node metastases that were removed surgically, the reported 5-year survival rate varies from 0% to 80%, with an average rate of 60% (Djajadiningrat et al., 2014). This wide variation depends on the extent of nodal metastases. In men with minimal node metastases (one to two nodes) the reported 5-year survival rate varies from 75% to 90%, compared with an average of approximately 25% (7% to 50%) in those with more than two involved nodes, and 5% to 10% in those with extranodal extension of cancer, lymph nodes larger than 4 cm in diameter, or pelvic node metastases (Johnson and Lo, 1984a, 1984b; Spratt, 2000) (Table 81.1).

The data demonstrates that in node-positive patients, ILND may be curative in approximately 20% to 60% of cases. However, it is also clear that even in node-negative men, ILND does not guarantee 5-year survival, with treatment failure varying from 5% to 20% (Johnson and Lo, 1984a, 1984b).

Follow-Up

Previous studies noted that recurrences mainly occur within the first 2 years after treatment of the primary penile lesion (66.2% to 100%) (Leijte et al., 2008).

Based on other proposed follow-up protocols in the literature, the following protocol is suggested (Table 81.2):

Despite all the evidence presented, some physicians are reluctant to proceed with immediate ILND because of concerns over the high complication rate of this surgical procedure. In a recent report on 454 patients registered between 2000 and 2003 in the National Penile Cancer Register in Sweden, ILND was performed in only 50%

KEY POINTS

- The most important independent prognostic factor related to cancer-specific survival in SCC of the penis is lymph node metastasis.
- Immediate ILND is associated with improved survival compared with salvage surgery for clinically detectable disease.
- For centers of excellence with expertise in penile cancer and ILND, DSNB can be performed with a false-negative rate of less than 5%.
- Superficial and modified ILNDs are options in the initial management of the inguinal region in patients with nonpalpable disease. These techniques have less morbidity than radical ILND.
- Endoscopic inguinal lymphadenectomy has been demonstrated to have less morbidity than open ILND and remove a comparable number of lymph nodes.
- Radical ILND is indicated for palpable disease, with potential for cure in inguinal-only disease, and for palliation of pain, infection, or hemorrhage in selected patients.
- Adjuvant chemotherapy can aid in more favorable outcomes in patients with positive inguinal disease.
- Pelvic metastasis do not occur in patients with negative ILNs.

of those considered at high risk for inguinal metastases according to EAU guidelines (G2–3 pT1 primary tumor) (Persson et al., 2007).

Selecting patients for ILND according to risk groups may be useful in guiding decision making, but it has its limitations. Leijte et al. reported that in the low-risk group (G1T1), the incidence of node metastases was only 6%. However, in the intermediate-risk group (G2T1) the incidence was 54%, and in the high-risk groups (G3T1, G1–3T2–3) it was only 37%, suggesting that 46% to 63% of these patients do not have ILN metastases (Leijte et al., 2007). Other recent studies have shown that the current EAU risk stratification guidelines have a low accuracy for predicting lymph node involvement, with the result that up to 82% of patients may undergo unnecessary prophylactic lymphadenectomy (Hegarty et al., 2006; Novara et al., 2008).

REFERENCES

The complete reference list is available online at ExpertConsult.com.

82
Surgery for Benign Disorders of the Penis and Urethra

Ramón Virasoro, MD, Gerald H. Jordan, MD, FACS, FAAP (Hon), FRCS (Hon), and Kurt A. McCammon, MD, FACS

Improvements in microsurgery, tissue transfer techniques, and tissue handling have expanded the repertoire of the urologic surgeon and, in particular, the genitourinary reconstructive surgeon. Urologists are now able to reconstruct congenital and acquired genitourinary abnormalities with greater facility. Microvascular and microneurosurgical techniques have made it possible to construct a phallus that allows a patient to void while standing and to enjoy erotic sensibility. Because the phallus has erotic sensibility and protective sensation, the patient can eventually have a prosthetic implantation that allows an acceptable sexual life. This chapter discusses the general principles of male genital reconstructive surgery; specifics include male urethral surgery, surgery for congenital and traumatic penile lesions, and complex fistula and obliterative issues associated with the posterior urethra.

GENERALITIES OF RECONSTRUCTIVE SURGICAL TECHNIQUES

With any surgical procedure, including reconstructive procedures of the external genitalia, there are basic rules and surgeons' biases regarding the best way to perform a certain operation. In this section, the differences are highlighted.

Reconstructive surgery is performed with all efforts aimed at minimizing tissue injury and promoting healing. Adequate visualization is essential. Surgical loupes are used by almost all surgeons performing adult and pediatric reconstructive genital reconstructive surgery. A headlight or suction with attached light often adds to visualization, especially in deep perineal surgery. **In penile cases, such as reconstruction of the fossa navicularis or correction of penile curvature, bipolar cautery is commonly used.** With cautery, the electrical charge is grounded either to a pad (monopolar) or to the opposite tong of the forceps (bipolar). In most instances, the field effects of the electricity are more confined with bipolar cautery. Because electricity is dissipated by conductors (in the case of human tissue, vessels, and nerves), there is a possibility of damage to these delicate structures. In other cases, monopolar cautery can be used in the superficial structures, but bipolar cautery is better during dissection around the corpus spongiosum, elevation of penile and scrotal flaps, division of the perineal intracorporal space, and dissection of the dorsal neurovascular structures. The same principles apply when harvesting oral mucosal grafts for the purpose of genitourinary reconstruction.

Appropriate instruments for genitourinary reconstructive surgery can commonly be found in a plastic surgery tray or on the peripheral vascular tray in the typical operating room. Some examples are fine tenotomy scissors, fine forceps, various skin hooks, and delicate needle holders. Sharp scissors that cut with minimal collateral trauma are essential. These instruments minimize tissue injury from manipulation and permit more precise dissection. For urethral surgery, a set of bougie à boule sizers is essential to check the caliber of the urethral lumen. McCrea urethral sounds are a good addition to the typical van Buren sounds available in the usual operating room. For calibration, sounds do not replace the need for bougie à boule calibrators. For posterior urethral reconstruction, a sound to pass through the cystostomy tract and prostate to find the proximal end for the reconstruction is often helpful; we currently use a Haygrove sound. Some centers use the cystoscope for this purpose, and often it suffices. Some centers use a hollow Haygrove (Gelman Urethral Sound, CS Surgical, Slidell, LA), which allows the passage of the flexible cystoscope to better visualize the bladder neck (Gelman and Wisenbaugh, 2015).

The choice of suture material evolves on the basis of the surgeon's experience and bias. However, there are some common principles with which most surgeons would agree. **First, in urethral surgery, absorbable suture is the rule.** Typical choices for most surgeons are braided absorbable sutures or the family of monofilament absorbable sutures. Chromic suture is rarely used because the choices of other absorbable sutures seem superior. The caliber of suture should be the smallest possible to align the tissue tension free. There is no reason to use suture that is stronger than the tissue. For a flap or graft repair, 4-0 to 6-0 suture is usually adequate. For primary anastomosis of the corpus spongiosum and urethra or for a posterior urethral reconstruction, 3-0 and 4-0 suture may be appropriate. The needle should be tapered if possible except when, as in urethroplasty, for example, severe spongiofibrosis or scarring is present. Some typical choices are taper needles, such as RB-1, TF, and SH-1, and cutting needles, such as P-3 and PC-3. The UR-6 half-circle taper needle that is often used in radical prostatectomy can be helpful for deep perineal anastomosis of the urethra.

Surgical position and retraction are critical to attaining good results. If possible, procedures are done with the patient supine or prone. Many procedures previously done with the patient in the lithotomy position can be done with the patient in the frog-leg or split-leg position. For penile surgery, a Scott retractor with stay hooks (Lone Star Medical Products, Houston, TX), the Jordan-Bookwalter perineal retractor set (CS Surgical, Slidell, LA; J. Hugh Knight Instrument Company, New Orleans, LA), or the Omni-Tract perineal retractor (Omni-Tract Surgical, Division of Minnesota Scientific, St. Paul, MN) is helpful. Lithotomy or exaggerated lithotomy position is used only for the minimal time necessary. With appropriate padding for the foot and positioning without pressure on the back of the leg, complications in the low-lithotomy position are minimal. When the patient is in the supine, split-leg, and low-lithotomy positions, venous compression stockings can be used. The controversy in positioning revolves around the use of the exaggerated lithotomy position. We prefer to use this position for all bulbar and posterior urethral reconstructions. Other surgeons use a lower lithotomy position. We find the more exaggerated position to be safe and believe it provides unequaled access to the deep perineal structures (Angermeier and Jordan, 1994). Details of positioning, as we do it, are described later. To minimize the patient's time in the exaggerated position, all graft harvesting or flap elevation is done with the patient in the flat supine position.

In addition to proper diagnosis and planning, the surgical technique is important for the overall success of reconstructive surgery. In contrast to the results of extirpative surgery, the results of reconstructive surgery depend on methods that minimize tissue damage and maximize wound healing. The key ingredients are adequate visualization, appropriate choice of suture, delicate tissue handling, appropriate positioning, and adequate retraction.

PRINCIPLES OF RECONSTRUCTIVE SURGERY

Many techniques in reconstructive surgery require the transfer of tissue. Skin is one of those tissues, and **its properties vary from**

> **KEY POINTS: RECONSTRUCTIVE SURGICAL TECHNIQUES**
>
> - Reconstructive surgery is performed with all efforts aimed at minimizing tissue injury and promoting healing. Loupe magnification is used by almost all surgeons performing adult and pediatric reconstructive surgery. For deep exposure, a headlight or lighted suction is advantageous. Instruments must be delicate because reconstructive surgery employs small sutures and small needles.
> - The choice of suture material evolves on the basis of the surgeon's experience. However, absorbable materials are the rule, and the caliber of sutures should be the smallest possible to align the tissue tension free.
> - The choice of surgical positioning is the surgeon's preference.
> - Proper diagnosis and planning of the surgical technique are important for the success of reconstructive surgery.

individual to individual and from place to place on the same individual. Variable characteristics such as color, texture, thickness, extensibility, innate skin tension, and blood supply can be useful in various situations. Mucosa from different sources have been used in genitourinary reconstructive surgery with excellent results. Different anatomic sites have inherent characteristics.

The term *tissue transfer* implies the movement of tissue for purposes of reconstruction. In contrast to extirpative surgery, **the transfer of tissue for reconstruction requires an intimate knowledge of the anatomy of the donor and the recipient sites as well as of the principles that allow the tissue to survive after it is transferred.**

The skin can be used as a model. The superficial layer of the skin is termed the *epidermis* (thickness 0.8 to 1 mm). The deep layer of the skin is termed the *dermis*. The dermis has two layers: a superficial layer, the adventitial dermis (also called the papillary or periadnexal dermis, depending on the anatomy), and a deep layer, the reticular dermis. For genitourinary reconstruction, skin without adnexal structures is often used. Other tissues commonly transferred for genitourinary reconstruction include bladder and oral mucosa as well as rectal. The bladder epithelium is the superficial layer of the bladder; the deep layer of the bladder is termed the *lamina propria*, with superficial and deep layers. The oral mucosa is the superficial layer of much of the oral cavity, which also has a deeper layer termed the *lamina propria*, again with superficial and deep layers.

All tissue has physical characteristics: extensibility, inherent tension, and the viscoelastic properties of stress relaxation and creep. The physical characteristics of a transferred unit are primarily a function of the helical arrangement of collagen along with the elastin cross-linkages. The collagen-elastin structure is suspended in a mucopolysaccharide matrix that influences the viscoelastic properties.

The epidermal (or epithelial) layer is a covering—the barrier to the "outside"—and is adjacent to the superficial dermis, or superficial lamina. At approximately this interface is the superficial plexus. In the case of skin, the plexus is the intradermal plexus. There are some lymphatics in the superficial dermal or tunica layer. On the undersurface of the deep dermal layer or deep lamina is the deep plexus. In the case of skin, this is the subdermal plexus. The deep dermis contains most of the lymphatics and greater collagen content than found in the superficial dermal layer. The deep, or reticular, dermis is generally thought to account for the physical characteristics of the tissue.

Grafts

Tissue can be transferred as a graft (Fig. 82.1). **The term *graft* implies that tissue has been excised and transferred to a graft host bed, where a new blood supply develops by a process termed *take*. Take requires approximately 96 hours and occurs in two phases.**

The initial phase, imbibition, requires about 48 hours. During that phase, the graft survives by "drinking" nutrients from the adjacent graft host bed, and the temperature of the graft is less than the core body temperature. **The second phase, inosculation, also requires about 48 hours and is the phase in which true microcirculation is reestablished in the graft.** During that phase, the temperature of the graft increases to core body temperature. The process of take is influenced by the nature of the grafted tissue and the conditions of the graft host bed. Processes that interfere with the vascularity of the graft host bed interfere with graft take.

Split-Thickness Skin Graft

If a graft is a split-thickness skin graft (STSG) unit, it carries the epidermis or the covering. The graft also exposes the superficial dermal (intradermal or intralaminar) plexus. In most grafts, the superficial plexus comprises small but numerous vessels, which **convey favorable vascular characteristics to a split-thickness unit.** The unit has few lymphatics, and **the physical characteristics are not carried, which accounts for the tendency of split-thickness units to be brittle and less durable.** The reticular dermis is not carried with the split-thickness unit (Jordan, 1993).

A mesh graft is usually an application of the split-thickness graft. After the harvest of a sheet graft, the sheet is placed on a carrier that cuts systematically placed slits in the graft. These slits can expand the graft by various ratios (i.e., 1.5:1, 2:1, 3:1). For most genital reconstructive surgery, the slits are not for expansion but rather to allow subgraft collections to escape; in some cases, the slits allow the graft to conform better to irregular graft host beds (e.g., the testes in STSG scrotal construction). It has also been proposed that mesh grafts take readily because of increased levels of growth factors, possibly as a function of the slits. In general, full-thickness skin grafts (FTSGs) are not meshed (Jordan, 1993; Schreiter and Koncz, 1983).

Full-Thickness Skin Graft

If a graft is a FTSG unit, it carries the covering and the superficial dermis or lamina with all the characteristics attributable to that layer. However, it also carries the deep dermis or deep lamina. In skin, the subdermal plexus is exposed. In most cases, **the plexus is composed of larger vessels that are more sparsely distributed. The graft is fastidious in its vascular characteristics.** A full-thickness unit carries most of the lymphatics, and the physical characteristics are likewise carried with the transferred tissue (Devine et al., 1976; Jordan, 1993; Wessels and McAninch, 1996). Comparing the grafts that are most commonly used in genitourinary reconstructive surgery, **the STSG has favorable vascular characteristics but tends to contract and be brittle when mature. The FTSG tends to have more fastidious vascular characteristics, but it does not contract as much and is more durable when mature** (see Fig. 82.1A).

There is a difference between genital full-thickness skin (penile and preputial skin grafts) and extragenital full-thickness skin. This is probably a reflection of the increased mass of the graft in extragenital skin grafts. This increased mass makes the graft more fastidious, and the poor results reported with urethral reconstruction with extragenital FTSGs are probably due to poor or ischemic take (Jordan, 1993; Webster, 1987; Webster et al., 1984). The posterior auricular graft (Wolfe graft) is an exception to the rule concerning extragenital skin. The postauricular skin is thin and overlies the temporalis fascia and is thought to be carried on numerous perforators. The subdermal plexus of this graft mimics the characteristics of the intradermal plexus, and the total mass of the graft is more like that of the split-thickness unit.

Dermal Graft

The dermal graft has been used for years to augment the tunica albuginea of the corpora cavernosa. When it is harvested, the graft exposes the intradermal plexus and the deep dermal plexus. The dermal graft takes readily (is not fastidious) and has the physical

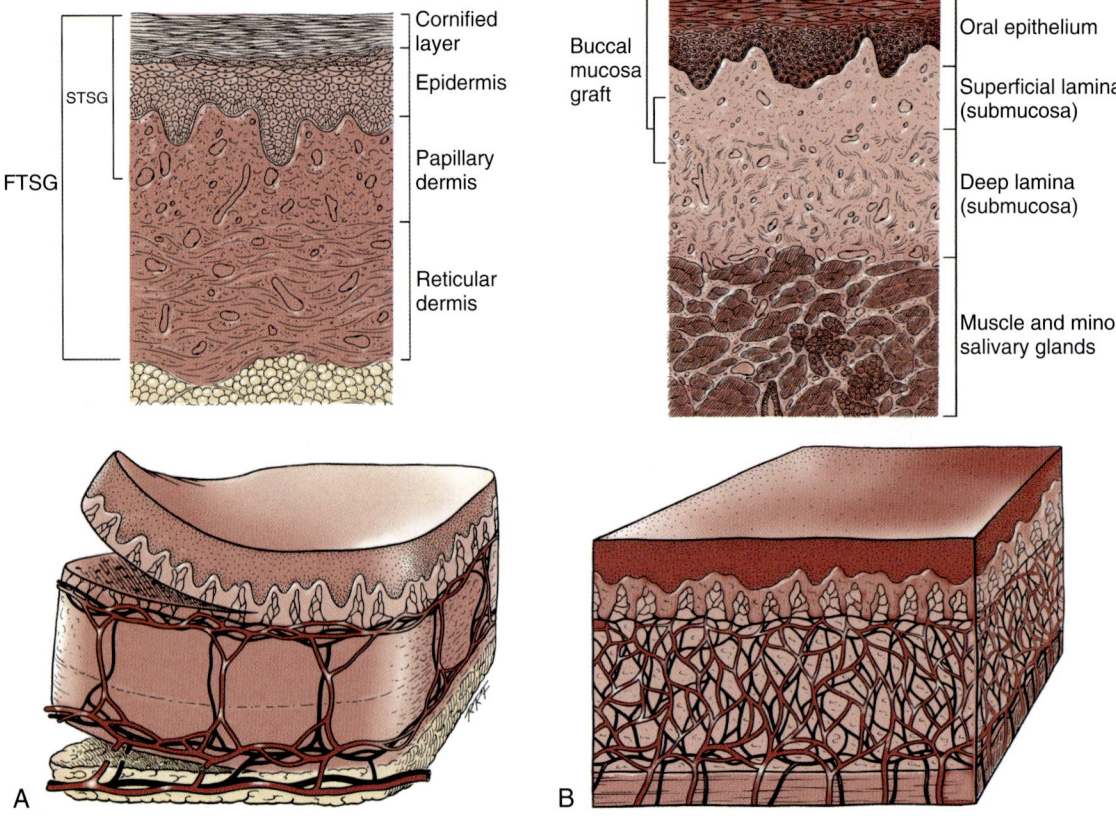

Fig. 82.1. Cross-sectional diagrams (histologic appearance above, microvasculature below) of the skin. (A) Cross-sectional diagrams of skin. (B) Cross-sectional diagrams of oral mucosa. *FTSG*, Full-thickness skin graft; *STSG*, split-thickness skin graft. (From Jordan GH, Schlossberg SM: Using tissue transfer for urethral reconstruction. *Contemp Urol* 13:23, 1993.)

characteristics of normal skin. When it is properly prepared, the tunica vaginalis graft is essentially peritoneum. The tendency of peritoneum to take readily is well documented in the literature that examines adhesion formation and in the urology literature concerning the application of peritoneal grafts for reconstruction of the urinary tract. The literature fails to define accurately what the surgeon can expect regarding physical characteristics (Jordan, 1993).

Oral Mucosa Grafts

Oral mucosal grafts (OMGs) consist of nonkeratinized mucosa and are thought to have optimal vascular characteristics (Humby, 1941; Memmelaar, 1947). **OMGs have a panlaminar plexus. The OMG can be thinned, provided that a sufficient amount of deep lamina is carried to preserve the physical characteristics and not affect the vascular characteristics** (see Fig. 82.1B).

According to dental terminology, there are three types of OMG: buccal mucosal graft (BMG), overlying the buccinator muscle in the cheeks; the labial mucosa graft, overlying the mandible; and the lingual mucosa graft, overlying the caudal aspect of the tongue. The lingual, labial, and buccal grafts vary in thickness and in substance.

The enthusiasm for the BMG seems well founded: it is easy to harvest and handle, is resilient to infections, and is accustomed to a wet environment. The fact that the graft has a "wet epithelial" surface is likewise thought to be a favorable characteristic for many cases of urethral reconstructive surgery. Over the last decade, OMGs have become the new recommended source for urethral reconstruction (Bhargava and Chapple, 2004).

A systematic review of the literature regarding the use of oral mucosa in the reconstruction of urethral defects associated with stricture and hypospadias/epispadias by Markiewicz et al. (2007) revealed a total of 22 studies using OMG only for the reconstruction of urethral defects attributed to stricture, with an overall success rate of 76.4%. A total of 17 studies have assessed OMG in a strictly hypospadias/epispadias population, with an average success rate of 66.5%.

A series by Fichtner et al. (2004) reporting the use of "buccal mucosal" onlay grafts with midterm and long-term results seems to suggest durability for these grafts. In that series, 67 patients were described, all with follow-up exceeding 5 years and some with 10 years of follow-up. All failures occurred within 12 months of the original procedure. More recent studies showed equal results with buccal and lingular grafts (Sharma et al., 2013).

Because the labial mucosal grafts are thin, some surgeons prefer that donor site for reconstruction of the fossa navicularis (Jordan, 1993).

Vein Grafts

As described in the urologic literature, vein grafts are perhaps not true grafts according to the terminology used in this chapter. Vein patches are widely used in vascular surgery. The premise is that the vein survives by endothelial direct perfusion and re-establishment of vein wall blood flow by perfusion of the vasa vasorum. At the present time, vein "grafts" are being widely used for replacement of defects of the tunica albuginea of the corpora cavernosa. The pertinent points with regard to the transfer of vein patches to the corpora cavernosa and their long-term behavior have been inferred from the current vascular literature. Dermal grafts have been tried for urethral reconstruction, also with generally poor results.

Other Grafts

In the bladder epithelial graft, there is a superficial and a deep plexus; however, the plexuses are connected by many more perforators. **Bladder epithelial grafts tend to have more favorable vascular characteristics.**

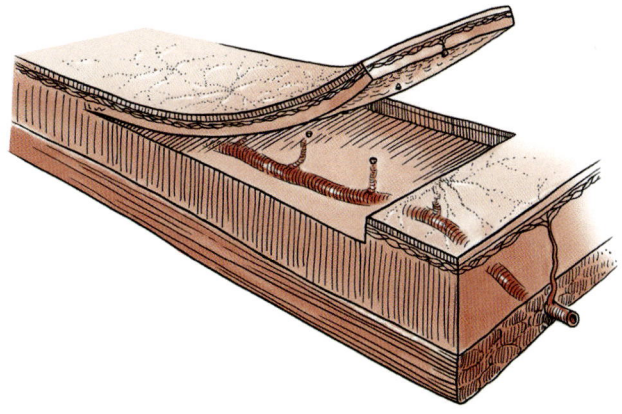

Fig. 82.2. Random flap. The arterial perforators have been interrupted, and flap survival depends on the intradermal and subdermal plexuses.

Rectal mucosal grafts also have been proposed for urethral reconstruction, but little is known about their graft take. In general, the vascularity of the bowel mucosa is based on the vascularity of the underlying muscle, with the mucosa carried on perforators. Little is found in the literature regarding the process of take of these grafts.

Tunica vaginalis grafts have proven useful for small defects of the tunica albuginea of the corpora cavernosa, but aneurysmal dilation tends to develop when they are used for larger defects. Tunica vaginalis grafts have been tried for urethral reconstruction with uniformly poor results.

Flaps

Tissue can be transferred as a flap. **The term *flap* implies that the tissue is excised and transferred with the blood supply either preserved or surgically reestablished at the recipient site. Flaps can be classified by numerous criteria. Flaps can be classified on the basis of their vascularity and characterized as either random flaps** (Fig. 82.2) **or axial flaps** (Fig. 82.3).

Random Flaps

A *random flap* is a flap without a defined cuticular vascular territory. The flap is carried on the dermal or laminar plexuses; the dimensions of random flaps can vary widely from individual to individual and from body site to body site.

Axial Flaps

The term *axial flap* means that there is a defined vessel in the base of the flap. There are three types of axial flaps. The direct cuticular axial flap is a flap based on a vessel superficial to the superficial layer of the deep body wall fascia (see Fig. 82.3A). The classic example of a direct cuticular flap is the groin flap. A musculocutaneous flap (Fig. 82.4A) is based on the vascularity to the muscle. **The overlying skin paddle is carried on perforators.** If the muscle alone is carried as a flap, the overlying skin survives as a random unit. **The fasciocutaneous system of vascularity (Fig. 82.4B) is similar to the musculocutaneous system.** However, the deep blood supply is carried on the fascia (deep and superficial layers), and the overlying skin paddle is based again on perforators. One can transfer a fascial flap based on the deep blood supply associated with the flap; the overlying skin, if it is not carried with the flap, remains as a random unit (Cormack and Lamberty, 1984; Ponten, 1981; Tolhurst and Haeseker, 1982). It has been argued that fascia is relatively avascular and cannot serve as the "blood supply" to the fasciocutaneous unit. Actually, the fascial layer acts as a trellis: the vessels are carried much like the limbs of a vine (Jordan, 1993).

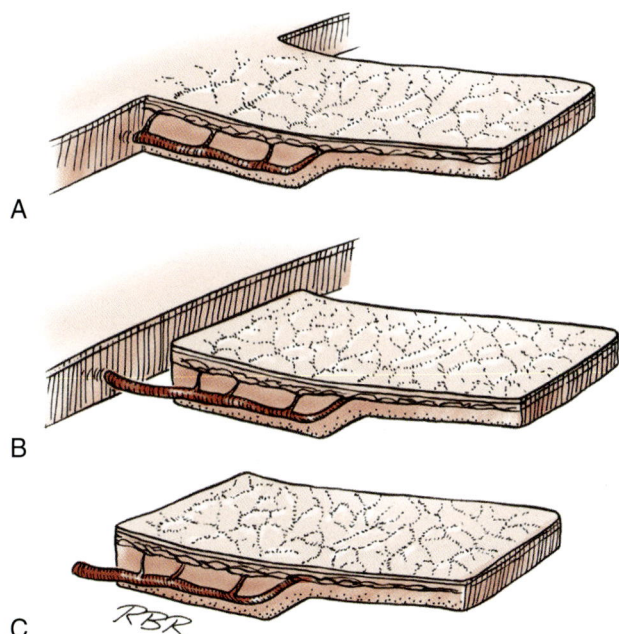

Fig. 82.3. Axial flaps. Large vessels enter the base of the flaps. Survival depends on these vessels and on the random distal vascularity. (A) Peninsula flap. The vascular continuity and the cuticular continuity in the flap base are intact. (B) Island flap. The vascular pedicle is intact; the cuticular continuity has been divided. These axial vessels are unsupported (dangling). (C) Microvascular free-transfer flap. The free-flap cuticular and vascular connections are interrupted at the base of the flap. Vascular continuity is reconstituted in the recipient area by a microsurgical anastomosis. (From Jordan GH, McCraw JB: Tissue transfer techniques for genitourinary reconstructive surgery. *AUA Update Series* 7:lesson 10, 1988.)

Peninsular Flap

A flap also can be classified by the elevation technique. A peninsular flap is a flap in which the vascular continuity and the cuticular continuity of the flap base are left intact (see Figs. 82.2 and 82.3A).

Island Flap

An island flap (see Fig. 82.3B) **is a flap in which the vascular continuity is maintained; however, the cuticular continuity is divided. A true island flap is elevated on dangling vessels. The microvascular free-transfer flap (free flap)** (see Fig. 82.3C) **has the vascular continuity and the cuticular continuity interrupted. The vascular continuity is then reestablished at the recipient site.**

The terminology is confusing. In genitourinary reconstructive surgical procedures, we tend to use the term *island flap*. As already mentioned, a true island flap is elevated on dangling vessels. However, the usual case is that a skin island or paddle is elevated either on the muscle, as in the gracilis musculocutaneous flap, or on the fascia, as in local genital skin flaps. The term *island flap* is not synonymous with the terms *skin island* and *skin paddle*. The usefulness of these flaps and grafts is illustrated in the discussion of surgical techniques later in this chapter. There is continued interest in the use of tissue-cultured grafts or "manufactured" grafts. The likelihood of someday being able to use off-the-shelf grafts or sheets of cultured material successfully is not far in the future (Atala, 2002; Bhargava et al., 2004; Chen et al., 1999; El-Kassaby et al., 2003; Rotariu et al., 2002).

SURGICAL ANATOMY OF THE PENIS AND MALE PERINEUM

More details about this topic are available online at ExpertConsult.com, including eFigs. 82.5 to 82.13.

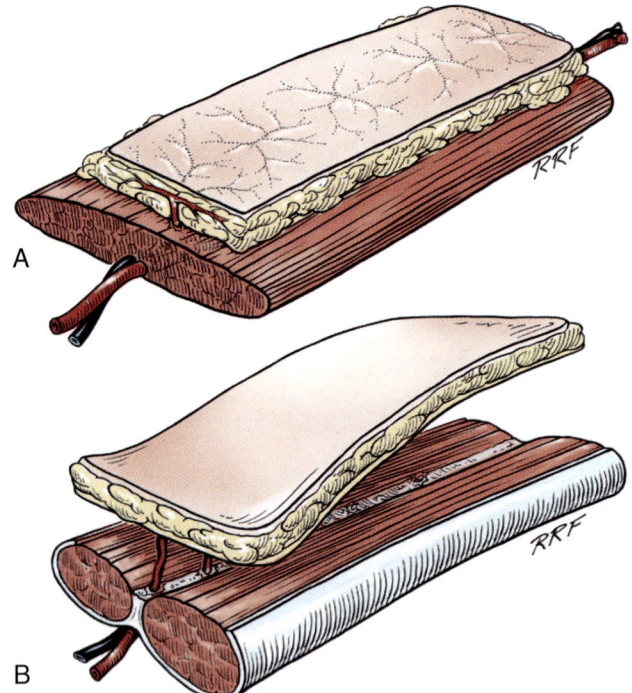

Fig. 82.4. (A) Musculocutaneous flap. Musculocutaneous perforators from the artery to a muscle vascularize the skin and overlying subcutaneous fat. They may be transferred as free flaps but are usually transferred locally, left attached to the vascular pedicle. (B) Fasciocutaneous flap. Perforating blood vessels from rich plexuses on the superficial and deep aspects of the fascia connect to perforator vessels that communicate with the microvasculature of the overlying paddle. In genital reconstruction, these flaps are based on the dartos fascia of the penis or are free flaps from the forearm. (From Jordan GH, McCraw JB: Tissue transfer techniques for genitourinary reconstructive surgery. *AUA Update Series* 7:lesson 10, 1988.)

SELECTED PROCESSES

Urethral Hemangioma

Although **urethral hemangioma is a rare condition, it is usually persistent** and offers a challenge to the surgeon when excision is deemed necessary. Patients typically present with hematuria or a bloody urethral discharge and occasionally with obstructive symptoms. The lesions may be single or multiple, and the urethral meatus is a common location. Although the diagnosis is often made with cystoscopy, which readily visualizes the dilated blood vessels, the lesion often extends beyond the point at which it is seen with cystoscopy.

Because all reported cases of urethral hemangioma have been benign, management depends on the size and location of the lesion. Asymptomatic lesions do not require treatment and should be observed because hemangiomas can regress spontaneously. Symptomatic lesions that require treatment must be completely excised to prevent recurrence.

Although electrofulguration has been reported as a possible treatment of urethral hemangioma, it should be used only to control an acute episode. For smaller lesions, laser treatment has been successful and produces less scarring. Lasers that are used for this purpose include argon, potassium titanyl phosphate (KTP) (532 nm), and neodymium:yttrium-aluminum garnet (Nd:YAG). The preferred treatment of larger lesions is open excision and urethral reconstruction; in some cases, this means circumferential reconstruction. Tubed graft reconstruction should be avoided; tubed flap reconstruction or tubed construction with mixed tissue transfer could be considered, although staged reconstruction is probably preferable. In addition, good initial success has been reported with polidocanol as a sclerosing agent for extensive urethral hemangiomas.

> ### KEY POINTS: PRINCIPLES OF RECONSTRUCTIVE SURGERY
>
> - Many of the techniques in reconstructive surgery require the transfer of tissue. Tissue transfer implies the movement of tissue for purposes of reconstruction. All tissue has extensibility, inherent tension, and the viscoelastic properties of stress relaxation and creep. These physical characteristics are important in predicting the behavior of transferred tissue.
> - A graft is tissue that has been excised and transferred to a graft host bed, where a new blood supply develops by a process termed *take*. A flap is tissue that has been excised and transferred with the blood supply preserved or surgically re-established at the recipient site. Grafts that have been successfully used for primary urethral reconstruction are the FTSG, the OMG, the bladder epithelial graft, and the rectal mucosal graft. The OMG has numerous vascular properties that make it desirable for urethral reconstruction. The issue of desiccation and hypertrophic growth, in the case of the bladder epithelial graft, has limited its use in the distal urethra.
> - FTSGs and STSGs have been used for penile reconstruction. The results with STSGs are so good that FTSGs are rarely used for coverage of the penis. In complex cases, microvascular free-transfer technology has become a mainstay. For urethral reconstruction, skin islands based on the dartos fascia or tunica dartos have been effectively used. The dermal graft has been used for years to augment the tunica albuginea of the corpora cavernosa.
> - The behavior of almost all forms of transfer can be predicted by examining histologic features and recognizing which layers provide which characteristics to the tissue.

Reactive Arthritis/Reiter Syndrome

Reactive arthritis is characterized by a classic triad of arthritis, conjunctivitis, and urethritis. In addition, **some patients have had an episode of diarrhea that preceded the development of arthritis.** However, the classic triad is not present in most cases, and patients present with only arthritis affecting the knees, ankles, and feet in an asymmetrical distribution. The history of urethritis is obtained on detailed questioning.

Urethral involvement is usually mild and self-limited and constitutes a minor portion of the disease. In approximately 10% to 20% of patients, a glanular lesion is present. Referred to as **circinate balanitis**, this lesion **is diagnostic of reactive arthritis** and typically appears as a shallow, painless ulcer with gray borders. Occasionally, the lesion appears as small, red macules, 1 to 2 mm in diameter. When the urethritis is mild and self-limited, no treatment is necessary.

In rare cases, urethritis causes severe inflammation with necrosis of the mucosa, producing uncompromising stricture disease. We have been unsuccessful in excision and replacement of the urethra in these cases. Alternatively, we perform a perineal urethrostomy (PU) and excise the entire distal urethra. This approach may decrease the rheumatic manifestations associated with reactive arthritis.

Lichen Sclerosus

Lichen sclerosus (LS), previously known as balanitis xerotica obliterans (BXO), is a chronic inflammatory, hypomelanotic, lymphocyte-mediated skin disorder, which, in men, involves the prepuce and glans and frequently leads to phimosis, meatal stenosis, and urethral strictures (Stewart et al., 2014).

The reported incidence of LS in the western population is 1 per 300 persons; however, the worldwide prevalence may be substantially different (Datta et al., 1993; Dogliotti et al., 1974; Jacyk and Isaac, 1979; Wallace, 1971). A recent publication showed the incidences in black and Hispanic male populations to be double the incidence among white males (Kizer et al., 2003). In men, LS seems to peak between ages 30 and 50; however, LS has been described in people of all ages, from infants to elderly adults (Kizer et al., 2003; Tasker and Wojnarowska, 2003). LS is commonly found at the time of circumcision when performed after the neonatal period (Garat et al., 1986; Ledwig and Weigland, 1989; McKay et al., 1975; Meuli et al., 1994; Rickwood et al., 1980). **LS is the most common cause of meatal stenosis and appears as a whitish plaque that may involve the prepuce, glans penis, urethral meatus, and fossa navicularis. If only the foreskin is involved, circumcision may be curative** (Akporiaye et al., 1997). In our experience, LS usually begins as a meatal or perimeatal process in a circumcised patient, but it may involve other areas of the preputial space in uncircumcised patients. In uncircumcised men, the prepuce becomes edematous and thickened and often may be adherent to the glans (Bainbridge et al., 1971). Diagnosis of LS remains primarily clinical and histologic, although an assay for circulating autoantibodies to extracellular matrix protein 1 (ECM-1) was recently shown to be a possible indicator of disease severity (Oyama et al., 2004). Several reports have suggested an association with chronic infection by a spirochete, *Borrelia burgdorferi* (Dillon and Ghassan, 1995; Shelley et al., 1999; Tuffanelli, 1987).

The first report of what was probably LS was published by Weir in 1875. He described a case of vulvar and oral "ichthyosis" (Weir, 1875). The term *balanitis xerotica obliterans* was first applied by Stühmer in 1928. Freeman and Laymon showed that BXO and LS were probably the same process (Freeman and Laymon, 1941; Laymon and Freeman, 1944). In 1976 the International Society for the Study of Vulvar Disease devised a new classification system unifying the nomenclature and proposed the term *lichen sclerosus* (Friedrich, 1976).

The SIU/ICUD Consultation on Urethral Stricture convened in Morocco in 2010 recommended that the accepted term for this condition is LS and the term *balanitis xerotica obliterans* should no longer be used (Level A) (Stewart et al., 2014).

The cause of LS has not been defined. Many mechanisms have been proposed. Koebner phenomenon relates the development of LS to trauma to an affected area (Lee and Phillips, 1994). A proposed mechanism is an autoimmune event. Autoantibodies to ECM-1 were detected in the serum of 67% of patients with LS and only 7% of control subjects, which would imply an autoimmune process (Oyama et al., 2003). Reports of LS associated with vitiligo, alopecia areata, thyroid disease, and diabetes mellitus also suggest a possible autoimmune basis. Reported oxidative damage of lipids, DNA, and protein in patients with LS may explain the mechanism of sclerosus, autoimmunity, and carcinogenesis of LS (Sander et al., 2004).

An infectious cause was previously implicated (Ross et al., 1990; Tuffanelli, 1987), but a more recent case-control series found no association (Edmonds and Bunker, 2010). It has also been proposed that LS has a genetic origin, based on the observation of a familial distribution of cases (Marren et al., 1995). There have been reports of concomitant existence of the disease in identical twins (Fallic et al., 1997; Thomas and Kennedy, 1986) and nonidentical twins (Cox et al., 1986), with coexistence of dermatosis. The disease also has been seen in mothers and daughters (Shirer and Ray, 1987). Studies on the human leukocyte antigen (HLA) have suggested a genetic component in patients with LS (Marren et al., 1995).

The combination of topical steroids and antibiotics may help stabilize the inflammatory process. Conservative therapy may be warranted in patients whose meatus can easily be maintained at 14 to 16 Fr (Staff, 1970). In these cases, intermittent catheterization with lubrication of the catheter and meatal dilator with 0.05% clobetasol (Temovate) may be adequate treatment. Long-term antibiotic therapy may also be helpful to improve inflammation because secondary infection of the inflamed tissue may occur. We have typically used tetracycline, but a trial of long-term penicillin or advanced-generation erythromycin therapy may be warranted (Shelley et al., 1999). This nonsurgical approach to treatment is used in patients who are not good surgical candidates for other medical reasons or in older patients and in younger patients who demonstrate stable disease. Secrest et al. (2008) proposed a link between hypogonadism and LS in male patients. These authors consistently showed diminished testosterone levels in patients with LS and analyzed whether replacement androgen therapy would be helpful.

Surgery is indicated in young patients with severe meatal stenosis. Because patients with long-standing meatal stenosis often have severe proximal urethral stricture disease, retrograde urethrography should be performed before therapy is initiated. A simple meatotomy is generally ineffective in patients with LS. Morey et al. (2007) showed that an extended meatotomy in patients with refractory stenosis was successful in 14 of 16 patients (87%). Malone (2004) described a ventral/dorsal meatotomy with an inverted V-shaped relaxing incision with the apex of the V close to the proximal limit of the dorsal meatotomy.

The cause of stricture disease associated with LS is unclear. Possible causes include iatrogenic stricture resulting from repeated instrumentation and pressure voiding associated with meatal stenosis, causing secondary intravasation of urine into the glands of Littre (Fig. 82.14). In cases of early LS with only meatal involvement resulting in stenosis of the fossa navicularis, prompt reconstruction seems to be successful in the long term and seems to avoid the sequelae of panurethral

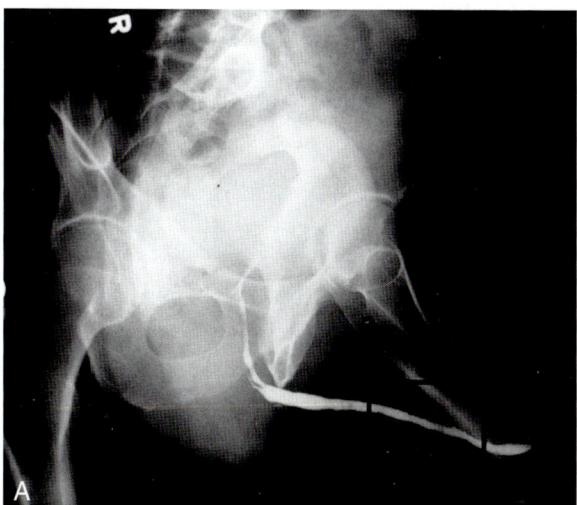
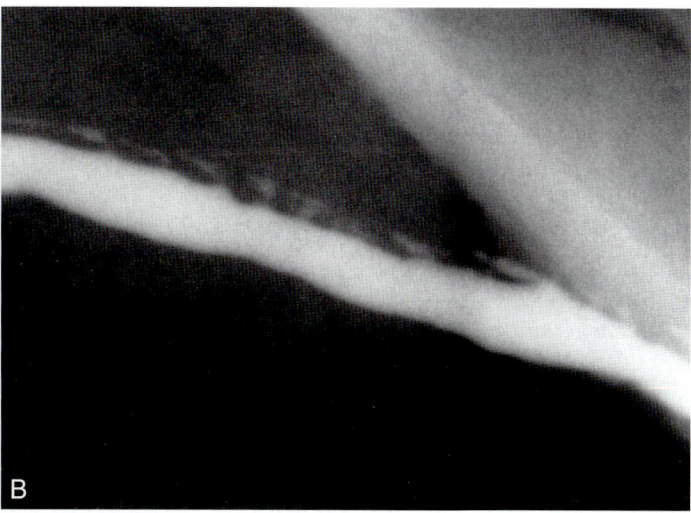

Fig. 82.14. (A and B) Urethrography in a patient with urethral stricture disease associated with lichen sclerosus. The intravasation of contrast material into the dilated glands of Littre during voiding is illustrated. (From Jordan GH: Management of membranous urethral strictures via the perineal approach. In McAninch J, Carroll P, Jordan GH, editors: *Traumatic and reconstructive urology*, Philadelphia, 1996, Saunders.)

stricture disease. Most surgeons believe that because LS is a disease of genital skin, better tissue for reconstruction is the oral mucosa; techniques are discussed later (Bracka, 1999; Mundy, 1994). Long-standing cases with a long length of urethral stricture are amenable to techniques of reconstruction but are challenging. Except in the case of urethral stricture disease confined only to the meatus and fossa navicularis, staged oral graft reconstruction, at least in the short term to midterm, seems to provide superior durable results. This may also be true in cases confined to the meatus and fossa navicularis, because an analysis of patients reconstructed with the ventral transverse skin island technique showed a 50% recurrence rate even in those patients. The weakness of this analysis is that the data did not include biopsy proof that all patients had LS (Virasoro et al., 2007).

We also see patients with a buried penis. This phenomenon occurs when the skin of the penile shaft has been lost because of severe inflammation, and the penis is trapped in the penopubic and scrotal area. These patients are often profoundly overweight, and many are diabetic; they have often had prior surgical procedures. Management of these patients is complex and ultimately determined by their desire and need for functional reconstruction. In some patients with severe urethral stricture disease, we have completely reconstructed the urethra; in others, we have simply performed a perineal urethrostomy. Perineal urethrostomy is usually technically straightforward because the rule in most patients with LS is to spare the proximal anterior urethra. We have proposed that, in many cases, the sparing of the proximal anterior urethra demonstrates the distribution of the glands of Littre for a given patient. Younger patients have requested mobilization and release of the penis with placement of an STSG. However, because the inflammation involves the glans penis (which is not removed), the secondary inflammation may also involve the skin graft. Lifelong monitoring of these patients for the secondary effects of inflammation is necessary.

Finally, **several reports have suggested the development of squamous cell carcinoma in patients with a long history of LS** (Doré et al., 1990; Pride et al., 1993).

Amyloidosis

Amyloidosis of the urethra, although a rare disease, should be considered in the evaluation of any patient with a urethral mass. Patients may present with hematuria, dysuria, or urethral obstruction. Because the differential diagnosis includes urethral neoplasm, cystoscopy with transurethral biopsy is indicated. When the diagnosis is made, treatment should be based only on symptoms. Most patients can be observed expectantly and do not require aggressive treatment. Some patients require treatment for urethral stricture. Progression and recurrence are rare (Crook et al., 2002; Dounis et al., 1985; Walzer et al., 1983).

Urethrocutaneous Fistula

A urethrocutaneous fistula is a tract lined with epithelium that leads from the urethra to the skin. The size of a fistula can vary from pinpoint to large. **Urethral fistula may be a complication of urethral surgery or develop secondary to periurethral infection associated with inflammatory strictures or treatment of a urethral growth** (condyloma or papillary tumor). **Treatment of a urethral fistula must be directed not only to the defect but also to the underlying process that led to its development.** Treatment varies according to the cause of the fistula. In cases of urethral reconstruction, especially reconstruction for hypospadias, fistula often occurs or recurs because of distal obstruction and high-pressure voiding. In addition, in some cases in which multiple attempts at fistula closure have been attempted and failed, the tissues adjacent to the fistula are so scarred that staged reconstruction is needed to import "better tissue."

After urethral surgery, fistulae can develop immediately or as delayed complications. An early fistula is the result of poor local healing, possibly secondary to hematoma, infection, or tension with closure. In addition, breakdown of the urethra or overlying skin closure, or both, could occur. Occasionally, with aggressive local care and continued urinary diversion, the fistula closes spontaneously.

Several techniques are used for fistula closure. Endoscopic and radiographic evaluation of the urethra must be performed before the repair in all cases. If the fistula is small and closure of the hole does not decrease the lumen of the urethra, a button of skin is removed from around the fistula, and its edges are cut flush with the urethral wall. The urethra is closed with small (6-0 or 7-0) absorbable sutures, inverting the epithelial edge, and the repair is tested to ensure that it is watertight. We prefer either polyglycolic acid (Vicryl) or polydioxanone suture. Subsequent layers are designed and closed to avoid superimposed suture lines. Without question, the safest diversion is a suprapubic catheter. However, in many cases, a silicone stent that reduces pressure during voiding for 7 to 14 days suffices. The operating microscope can be useful for the closure of small fistulae, allowing the use of 8-0 polyglycolic acid suture and limiting the size of the associated skin incision.

If the fistula is so large that simple closure would compromise the lumen of the urethra, local flaps often are required. However, if the adjacent tissues are thin and poorly visualized, closure of the fistula may become a staged urethral reconstruction as mentioned earlier. For larger fistulae, a suprapubic tube for diversion is probably prudent. Mobilization of flaps, such as the tunica dartos flap, may be necessary to secure adequate tissue interposition and avoidance of superimposed suture lines.

Fistulae associated with inflammatory strictures occur as periurethral tracts and develop secondary to high-pressure voiding of infected urine. As multiple tracts develop, this problem becomes what is known as a "watering pot perineum." Repair requires suprapubic drainage, and treatment of the infection requires incision and drainage of any abscesses present. We widely excise the fistula tracts and associated inflammatory tissue and wait 4 to 6 months before repairing the underlying stricture. Flap reconstruction, if donor tissues are available, may be used. However, a staged graft procedure (discussed later) is also an excellent choice. Caution is warranted in a patient with urethral fistulae but without a history of chronic obstructive voiding symptoms. In many cases, fistula or periurethral abscess may be the hallmark symptom of urethral carcinoma.

Urethral Diverticulum: Male

A congenital diverticulum is a transitional cell epithelium–lined pouch that is the result of either a distention of a segment of the urethra or the attachment of a structure to the urethra by a narrow neck (i.e., a müllerian remnant). **In male patients, a congenital anterior urethral diverticulum may result from incomplete development of the urethra,** with a defect in only the ventral wall and subsequent distention of this segment by the hydraulic force of the voiding stream (Bedos and Cibert, 1989; Ozgok et al., 1994; Valdivia et al., 1986). The downstream lip of the defect may serve as a valvular obstruction, increasing the pressure in the lumen, and subsequently the diverticulum enlarges. **Another possible cause is injury of the urethra, which may cause an intraspongiosal hematoma.** This hematoma could create a paraurethral space and subsequent diverticulum or fistula. These defects can also be associated with urethral strictures (Bryden and Gough, 1999). It has also been suggested that congenital diverticula may represent giant cystic dilation of Cowper ducts (Gil-Vernet, 1977; Jiminez Cruz and Rioja Sanz, 1993). We do not favor this proposed cause because the diverticula seem to be slightly more distal than the expected location of Cowper ducts, and in our experience with reconstruction of a considerable number of these diverticula, no proximal limb of the ducts seems to exist in them. In many cases, endoscopic unroofing of the diverticulum remedies the voiding symptoms; although after unroofing, the patient commonly may note postvoid dribbling. Open repair essentially excises the redundancy of the urethra associated with the diverticulum. If the lumen is compromised, dorsal onlay by either graft or flap can be useful.

A congenital diverticulum in the prostatic urethra may be a large remnant of the müllerian duct associated with defects of diminished virilization. However, it often occurs in proximal hypospadias and represents an enlarged utricle (Devine et al., 1980). **These diverticula may not be demonstrated with voiding urethrography but are demonstrated with cystoscopy or retrograde urethrography. The tip of a urethral catheter tends to catch in this opening, necessitating the use of something to direct the catheter tip toward the true lumen. Other than necessitating caution during evaluation, these diverticula do not usually cause problems or require treatment unless they are very large.

Large utricles can accumulate urine with voiding and then decompress after voiding. If they are large enough, the stasis of urine can be associated with recurrent urinary tract infection or difficult-to-manage "incontinence." A surgical approach to small lesions can be through a suprapubic incision, possibly opening the bladder to go through the center of the trigone. However, large diverticula can be approached trans-sacrally (Peña and Devries, 1982). Although this is a complex procedure, it is associated with much less morbidity than an abdominal or a perineal approach and provides superior exposure. We excise the diverticulum after exposing and dissecting its communication with the urethra. After ensuring that there is no distal obstruction to interfere with healing, we close the urethra.

Diverticula of the female urethra are covered in Chapter 90.

Paraphimosis, Balanitis, and Phimosis

Paraphimosis, or painful swelling of the foreskin distal to a phimotic ring, occurs if the foreskin remains retracted for a prolonged time. Swelling is sufficient to make reduction of the foreskin over the glans difficult. **In a very young child, paraphimosis is often seen after the foreskin has been traumatically reduced during an examination or sometimes by overzealous parental attempts at hygiene.** Traumatic, sudden reduction of a tight foreskin should be avoided in all ages and circumstances. To reduce a paraphimosis, gentle steady pressure must be applied to the foreskin to decrease the swelling; with a child, this is best accomplished in a quiet room by a parent squeezing it in the hand. Elastic wrap may be helpful in some cases. Putting an ice pack on the area for a short time before gentle compression is helpful as an analgesic. When the swelling has been reduced, the surgeon can push against the glans with the thumbs, pulling on the foreskin with the fingers. Because paraphimosis tends to recur, a dorsal slit at a minimum or a circumcision should be carried out as an elective procedure at a later date. Occasionally a patient has acute paraphimosis that has been present for many hours to days; this is typically seen in an adolescent who is reluctant to reveal the problem to his parents. In these cases, reduction may be impossible, and paraphimosis should be dealt with by emergency dorsal slit or circumcision. Considerable postoperative edema is the rule in these cases.

Balanitis, or inflammation of the glans, can occur as a result of poor hygiene from failure to retract and clean under the foreskin. The subsequent swelling makes cleaning more difficult, but the inflammation usually responds to local care and antibiotic ointment. Oral antibiotic therapy occasionally may be necessary. Balanoposthitis is a severe form of balanitis and occurs when the phimotic band is tight enough to retain inflammatory secretions, creating a preputial cavity abscess. Occasionally, an emergent dorsal slit is required.

Phimosis, or the inability to retract the foreskin, can result from repeated episodes of balanitis. In older patients, balanitis may be a presenting sign of diabetes. In these cases, circumcision may be warranted.

Urethral Meatal Stenosis

A small urethral meatus in a newborn probably would not be called to a urologist's attention unless the stenosis is associated with other congenital deformities (e.g., hypospadias) or causes voiding difficulties or urinary tract infection (Allen and Summers, 1974). If the urethral meatus of a boy appears exceptionally narrow and there are associated symptoms, a meatotomy should be considered. For this decision to be made, voiding should be observed to note that the meatus opens as a full, forceful stream is passed. If the stream is narrow and excessively forceful, stenosis is probably present. The occluding skin is generally a thin layer that sometimes can be seen to pouch out, with the meatus opening at the dorsal lip as the child voids. **Meatal stenosis in a boy appears to be a consequence of circumcision that then allows subsequent ammoniacal meatitis.** If the child is seen with ammoniacal meatitis, we usually start meatal dilation with 0.05% clobetasol cream. Within a week, the process seems to abate. Anecdotally, the fusion of the ventral-meatal skin that causes meatal stenosis can be avoided. Parents must be counseled about the cause—that is, a wet diaper pressing for prolonged periods against the tip of the glans.

A ventral urethral meatotomy sometimes can be accomplished with the use of local anesthesia. In a young child, general anesthesia is the preferred approach, avoiding trauma to the child, the parents, and the urologist. It is important to insert the anesthetic needle into the skin fold from the underside so that the tip of the needle can be observed and controlled. If insertion is from the outside, the needle passes through both layers of the fold, and a wheal cannot be raised because of leakage of the anesthetic solution. After the meatotomy, the edges of the cut seal together unless they are kept open. The tip of a meatal dilator is the best instrument for this purpose. The child's parents are instructed to separate the edges gently with the tip of the dilator three times a day for 7 to 10 days. The surgeon should observe the parents carry out this procedure. Pediatric meatal dilators (see later product reference) are available; however, the tip of an ophthalmic antibiotic tube also works well, and the antibiotic ointment can be used as the lubricant.

Meatal stenosis occurs in adults after inflammation, specific or nonspecific urethral infection, and trauma (especially in association with indwelling catheters, urethral instrumentation, or radical prostatectomy in some cases). It also may be the result of the failure of a previous hypospadias repair. To perform a ventral meatotomy in a normally developed penis in adolescents and adults, it is often necessary to place sutures to approximate the urethral mucosal edge to control bleeding. This step usually requires three sutures: one at the apex and one on either side. We have found a dilator made by Cook Urological (Spencer, IN; Catalog No. 073406, adult 6 to 34 Fr; No. 073403, pediatric 6 to 10 Fr) to be helpful in keeping the meatus open. In some cases, it may be necessary to perform a dorsal rather than a ventral meatotomy. This procedure can be accomplished as a Y-V-plasty after the excision of any scarred ridge of neourethra. Dorsal meatotomy, although effective in opening the meatus, often creates a cosmetically suboptimal shape of the meatus. In an adult, it is unusual for the meatal stenosis to be an isolated finding. The stricture process usually involves the fossa navicularis to some extent as well.

Circumcision

Controversy continues regarding whether neonatal circumcision should or should not be performed (Poland, 1990; Schoen, 1990). Much attention has been focused on this issue, but despite this, many boys in the United States are circumcised. Ritual circumcision will continue; however, in ritual circumcision, it is not necessary to remove the skin but only to draw blood. **It is important not to circumcise any boy with a penile abnormality (e.g., hypospadias, chordee) that may require the foreskin during repair. Circumcision is indicated in a young boy who has had recurrent urinary tract infections thought to be associated with the redundant preputial skin.**

Most circumcisions performed just after birth are done with the Gomco clamp or one of the plastic disposable devices made for this purpose. Care should be taken to free the foreskin from the glans completely and to apply appropriate tension when the foreskin is pulled into the clamp. To prevent either a too generous or an inadequate circumcision, we find it useful to mark the foreskin carefully so that the correct level is ascertained. At our center, we perform neonatal circumcision with a penile block for anesthesia.

The most common complication is bleeding as a result of inadequate control with vascular compression. Application of an epinephrine-soaked sponge may help in controlling minimal venous bleeding. Infection can also occur and responds to local care. Any resulting skin separation should be repaired after the inflammation resolves. Minimal separation may be amenable to healing by secondary intention. Sometimes too much skin is removed, or the urethra is included in the clamp, resulting in a fistula. In many, if not most, cases in which excess skin is removed, closure can still be accomplished with aggressive frenuloplasty along with remaining skin closure by transposition of the remaining skin. If the entire penis is "scalped," it may be best managed with an STSG or with reapplication of the excised foreskin after it is prepared properly as a graft. In complicated cases, burying the penis in the scrotum and repairing it at a later date may be prudent. **Monopolar electrocautery should be avoided in a neonatal circumcision because penile loss from the field distribution of the current can occur. The use of monopolar cautery with a Gomco or similar clamping device must be avoided because devastating loss of tissue can occur.**

A newborn who lost his penis because of a circumcision mishap should not be gender reassigned. Our experience with phallic construction includes many children and youths who had been converted to a female after a circumcision accident. As they passed through puberty, they realized that this sexual assignment was wrong. Most of these boys could undergo reconstruction in such a manner as to preserve reproductive function.

In adults, circumcision can be done with local anesthesia, by blocking the dorsal nerves at the base of the penis and circumferentially infiltrating the superficial layers of the penile base. In men and older boys, we favor a sleeve circumcision. With the foreskin in its retracted position, a marking pen outlines an incision, leaving a small preputial cuff. This mark should go straight across the base of the frenulum. This incision is made and carried through the dartos fascia to the superficial lamina of the Buck fascia. The foreskin is reduced, and a second incision is marked, following the outlines of the coronal margin and the V of the frenulum on the ventral side. The frenulum usually retracts into a V. In some cases, the frenulum can be lengthened by closing the edges of the V in a longitudinal orientation for a short length (frenuloplasty). If frenuloplasty is done, the proximal incision does not have to follow the V of the retracted frenulum because the ventral skin is straight. We make the skin incision and fulgurate bleeding vessels with bipolar cautery as the incision is deepened and the skin edge is mobilized. In older boys and men, the vessels are more substantial and not easily sealed by compression, no matter how vigorous. Circumcision clamps can be ineffective and are not recommended even though larger sizes are available. After the sleeve of preputial skin has been removed, hemostasis is obtained, and the skin edges are reapproximated.

In younger boys, some surgeons may consider this sleeve procedure to be tedious and difficult. If this is the case, after the skin is marked, a dorsal slit is made through both layers of the prepuce back to the level of the corona. After the marks, the two layers of the preputial skin are incised. Bleeders are controlled, and the skin edges are reapproximated.

Complications are uncommon. Most patients develop some hyperesthesia of the glans, which resolves. A hematoma is probably the most common immediate complication. Some patients notice minor cosmetic imperfections that are functionally insignificant. One of the most distressing problems we see is a patient who complains that the surgeon has removed too much skin. To avoid this occurrence, a circumcision should be done precisely, and, whatever the procedure to be carried out, the incisions should first be marked with the skin lying undistorted on the shaft. Adults requesting circumcision must be carefully evaluated from a psychosexual standpoint because many of these patients who are the most persistent in requesting circumcision become the most dissatisfied after the surgery.

Circumcision has been shown in numerous studies to provide protection for men in areas where human immunodeficiency virus (HIV) is very prevalent (Auvert et al., 2005; Bailey et al., 2007; Gray et al., 2007). Circumcision has consistently been shown in well-conducted, randomized controlled trials to reduce the risk of HIV acquisition in heterosexual African men by 50% to 60%. Similar prospective trials have not been performed in developed countries; however, retrospective data among heterosexual men in the United States showed a similar approximately 50% reduction in HIV prevalence among men with known exposure, suggesting the data may be extrapolated to this population. In addition, male circumcision has been shown to reduce the risk for acquisition of herpes simplex virus type 2, human papillomavirus, genital ulcer disease, and some sexually transmitted bacterial infections (Tobian et al., 2014).

There is a biologic rationale for reduction in the spread of sexually transmitted infections, particularly HIV, with circumcision. Superficial Langerhans cells, CD4+ T cells, and CD8+ T cells are rich and less well protected by keratin on the inner aspect of the male foreskin and frenulum. When the foreskin is retracted during intercourse, this large and susceptible surface area is exposed allowing contact with HIV-infected secretions and subsequent risk for infection. Uncircumcised men have also been shown to have an increased frequency of genital ulcers and increased frequency of microtears during intercourse, both of which increase HIV transmission.

Despite the well-demonstrated benefit of circumcision in heterosexual men, the same benefit has not been shown for men who have sex with men (MSM). A large meta-analysis of more than 53,000 MSM did not demonstrate a statistically significant protection against HIV (Millett et al., 2008). Subgroup analysis demonstrated a trend toward reduced prevalence of HIV among MSM performing predominantly insertive rather than receptive anal intercourse, and others have corroborated these findings.

Transitional Urologic Care for the Patient With Failed Hypospadias and Epispadias Repair

Failed Hypospadias Repair

In treatment of a patient in whom hypospadias repair has failed, it is important to obtain all available records to help determine what may have contributed to his complications. **A hypospadias repair may fail because of an inadequate correction of chordee or an inadequate urethra, with a stricture, fistula, or diverticulum** (Winslow et al., 1986). **It is often readily apparent from the records that not all aspects of the hypospadias deformity** (i.e., ventrally displaced meatus, ventral chordee, and some expression of inadequacy of ventral tissue fusion) **were addressed in the previous repairs.** Adults with urethral strictures who have had hypospadias surgery as children are often seen. Depending on the age of the patient and the preference of the treating urologist, a variety of different techniques may have been used to repair the original hypospadias. Many of these patients have persistent chordee and a subcoronal meatus. Adults also have been seen who have had long-standing evidence of urethral fistula. In addition, some patients may have clinical findings not related to hypospadias that should have been recognized previously, especially when hypospadias is part of an overlying intersex problem. In the past, problems associated with previous failures were caused by errors in design, technique, or postoperative care (Devine et al., 1978). **With more modern techniques available and with most hypospadias treated by surgeons with considerable experience, failures often are associated with perioperative infections or other factors that adversely affect wound healing.** At the present time, complex hypospadias repair failures are encountered with much less frequency, and most that are encountered are in patients who had previous procedures more than 15 to 20 years ago. Complications in these patients resulted not from poorly designed surgery at the time but rather from the "state of the art" at the time.

Evaluation of a failed hypospadias repair includes retrograde urethrography, voiding cystourethrography, and cystoscopy. In an older patient, a reliable preoperative assessment of residual chordee can be made on the basis of the history and photographs taken at home. In younger patients, complete evaluation of more complex situations with use of anesthesia may be necessary.

In an adult patient, a detailed discussion must occur regarding the positive and negative aspects of the various approaches. Patients who were initially operated on before the late 1970s probably underwent either a graft or some form of repair using almost exclusively ventral tissue. Some of these patients still have the remnants of a dorsal hood or enough dorsal skin for a dorsal transverse penile skin island type of reconstruction to be performed.

We believe that surgical correction of complex cases requires an aggressive approach by the surgeon (Secrest et al., 1993). However, with the advent and very common use of the tubed incised plate repair, initially described by Snodgrass (1999), the nature of failures is different, and the approaches also are remarkably different. Based on our observations, the number of failed surgeries is less, the nature of graft salvage techniques is remarkably different, and the method of addressing residual curvature is different. It is possible to reincise the "urethral plate" and tubularize it if the plate is not scarred and possible to graft the plate dorsally if it is; if the tissues are badly scarred, many surgeons revert to staged reconstruction (Snodgrass et al., 2009). The use of flaps has a place in corrective procedures, and the excision of scarred tissues causing residual curvature likewise has its place. However, plication or corporoplasty techniques for correction of residual curvature have, for the most part, become the standard of care. Graft techniques for correction of curvature are used but with far less frequency than in years past.

Failed Epispadias Repair

Residual genital defects in men who have had exstrophy/epispadias repaired as children can cause functional, aesthetic, and psychologic problems. The effects of these problems are compounded in men who have undergone urinary diversion and who must wear stomal appliances, although with the improvement of continent diversions, this is less of a factor. Successful reconstruction is possible except in the most severe forms of bladder exstrophy or cloacal exstrophy—when the penis or the halves of the bifid penis are truly inadequate. Even then, if normal testes are present, the success of newer techniques of phallic construction (see subsequent discussion) should lend support to considering the option of raising such a child as a boy, possibly preserving his reproductive potential through puberty. In these very difficult cases, we think that the parents must be presented with both options, gender reassignment versus eventual phalloplasty. Remarkable progress has been made in the treatment of difficult cases (Gearhart et al., 1994; Hendren, 1979; Jeffs, 1979; Johnston, 1975; Mitchell and Bagli, 1996; Perovic et al., 1992; Snyder, 1990) and in techniques of primary closure. However, many patients need further genital surgery because they experience the hypertrophic growth spurt of the penis associated with puberty.

The goals of reconstructive surgery in male patients with exstrophy or epispadias are to produce a dangling penis with erectile bodies of satisfactory length and shape to allow sexual function and to construct a urethra that serves as a conduit for the passage of urine and ejaculate. However, experience has shown that in a patient with a diverted exstrophy and only a bladder remnant, construction of a urethra that is essentially defunctionalized is difficult. These urethras eventually seem to fibrose and stenose. The bladder neck remnant becomes a cyst that is often colonized. Bouts of virulent epididymitis or the formation of what is really a bladder neck remnant abscess begin to occur. We have seen two patients who developed carcinoma of the prostate in a bladder neck remnant. The diagnosis in these patients was difficult, and the resultant surgery was even more difficult. Neither patient did well from the standpoint of treatment of the carcinoma. Both were seen before the aggressive use and better understanding of prostate-specific antigen.

Many patients who have undergone surgery as children do not present for correction of inadequacies of the external genitalia until after they have completed puberty and realize that their situation has not improved and is not likely to improve. Some have been in sexual situations and have encountered problems. We employ a systematic approach to accomplish the reconstruction necessary to correct the anatomic defects in these patients (Devine et al., 1980; Winslow et al., 1988). Sequential surgery is undertaken beginning with the simplest procedure that would achieve the desired functional result.

Lower abdominal wall scarring can be corrected or defects can be closed by fashioning peripenile flaps that are shaped like a W. In many patients, there may be wide diastasis recti that is really a ventral hernia. Anchoring of meshes or Gore-Tex can be difficult, and we have resorted to a fibular bone microvascular free transfer in several cases to reconstruct the continuity of the pubis, allowing effective closure of the abdominal hernia.

With more effective contemporary primary closure techniques, the adult reconstructive surgeon's place is primarily in the correction of hernia or in the patient who has an inadequate penis because of deformity, scarring, or improper gender reassignment.

KEY POINTS: SELECTED PROCESSES

- Urethral hemangioma is a rare condition that is usually persistent. It can present a significant challenge to the surgeon. All reported cases of urethral hemangioma have been benign, and management depends on the size and location of the lesion.
- Reactive arthritis is characterized by a classic triad of arthritis, conjunctivitis, and urethritis. Urethral involvement is usually mild, self-limited, and a minor portion of the disease.
- LS previously was referred to as balanitis xerotica obliterans. Diagnosis is made through biopsy. LS is thought to be possibly premalignant for the development of squamous cell carcinoma of the glans. It is the most common cause of meatal stenosis. Management of patients with LS-related stricture is complex, and results are suboptimal. The management is determined by the desire of the patient and the need for functional reconstruction.
- Amyloidosis is a rare disease of the urethra and should be considered in the evaluation of any patient with a urethral mass. Patients present with hematuria, dysuria, or urethral obstruction.
- A urethrocutaneous fistula is a tract lined with epithelium that leads from the urethra to the skin. It may be a complication of urethral surgery or develop secondary to periurethral infection associated with inflammatory strictures or treatment of a urethral growth. Treatment of the urethral fistula must be directed not only to the defect but also to the underlying process that led to its development.
- A congenital urethral diverticulum is a transitional cell epithelium–lined pouch that is the result of either a distention of a segment of the urethra or the attachment of a structure to the urethra by a narrow neck. In male patients, "congenital" anterior urethral diverticulum may result from incomplete development of the urethra or possibly may be the result of straddle trauma that led to an intracorporeal spongiosal hematoma. Congenital diverticulum in the prostatic urethra is a remnant of the müllerian duct.
- Paraphimosis is a painful swelling of the foreskin distal to a phimotic ring. It occurs when the foreskin has been retracted and not reduced. Edema forms in the distal skin.
- Urethral meatal stenosis in a young boy appears to be a consequence of circumcision. The circumcision allows the development of ammoniacal meatitis, which can heal with a membrane across the ventral portion of the meatus. Controversy continues regarding whether neonatal circumcision should or should not be performed. If it is going to be performed, the circumcision must be adequate. The most common complication of neonatal circumcision, in our opinion, is when it is inadequately done.
- A patient with failed hypospadias repair can be complex. Many are victims of the technology of the time when they had their initial reconstruction. All patients with urethral involvement should be evaluated as if they have urethral stricture disease.
- Advanced techniques for the reconstruction of the exstrophy-epispadias complex have led to much better functional results and less need for secondary exstrophy reconstruction. Secondary exstrophy reconstruction is aimed at the area of the escutcheon, the dorsal base of the penis, the penile shaft, the urethra, and the penoscrotal junction.

URETHRAL STRICTURE DISEASE

The term *urethral stricture* refers to fixed anatomic narrowing of the urethra so that the lumen will not accommodate instrumentation without disruption of the urethral mucosal lining. A stricture involving the urethra that is surrounded by the corpus spongiosum is considered an anterior urethral stricture, and the associated scarring may be associated with a scarring process involving the spongy erectile tissue of the corpus spongiosum (spongiofibrosis) (Fig. 82.15). The spongy erectile tissue of the corpus spongiosum underlies the urethral epithelium, and the scarring process extends through the tissues of the corpus spongiosum in some cases and into adjacent tissues. **Contraction of this scar reduces the urethral lumen.** For example, if a normal urethra measures 30 Fr, its diameter is 10 mm, and the area of the lumen is approximately 78 mm^2. If scarring has resulted in a urethra that measures 15 Fr, the lumen is only 55 mm^2, or 29% reduced. It is evident that scar contraction caused by urethral stricture disease can be asymptomatic for a while, but because the lumen is further reduced, it can be associated with marked voiding symptoms.

In contrast, posterior urethral "strictures" are not included in the common definition of urethral stricture. *Posterior urethral injury* (PUI) and *posterior urethral stenosis* are more appropriate terms, according to the last International Consultation of Urologic Diseases in Urethral Stricture, held in Marrakesh in 2010 (Gómez et al., 2014; Latini et al., 2014). Posterior urethral stenosis is an obliterative process in the posterior urethra that has resulted in fibrosis and is generally the effect of distraction in that area caused by either trauma or radical prostatectomy. Although the distraction defect can be lengthy in some cases, the actual process involving the tissues of the urethra is usually confined. By consensus of the World Health Organization (WHO) conference in 2004 and later by International Consultation on Urological Diseases (ICUD) in 2010, the term *stricture* is limited to the anterior urethra. Distraction defects are processes of the membranous urethra associated with pelvic fracture. Other narrowings of the posterior urethra are termed *urethral contractures* or *stenosis* (Bhargava et al., 2004; Herschorn et al., 2014).

Urethral Anatomy

Although urethral anatomy is described in the earlier section on anatomy, it is useful to re-emphasize key anatomic points. **The bulbous urethra is eccentrically placed in relation to the corpus spongiosum and is much closer to the dorsum of the penile structures** (see eFig. 82.6). As one moves distally, the pendulous or penile urethra becomes more centrally placed within the corpus spongiosum.

The genital skin has a dual (proximal and distal) and bilateral blood supply, forming a fasciocutaneous system (see eFig. 82.10). The corpus spongiosum receives blood from the common penile artery, the terminal branch of the internal pudendal artery (see eFig. 82.12). The corpus spongiosum also has a dual blood supply: a proximal blood supply and a retrograde blood supply through the dorsal arteries as they arborize in the glans penis.

Etiology

Any process that injures the urethral epithelium or the underlying corpus spongiosum to the point that healing results in a scar can cause a urethral stricture.

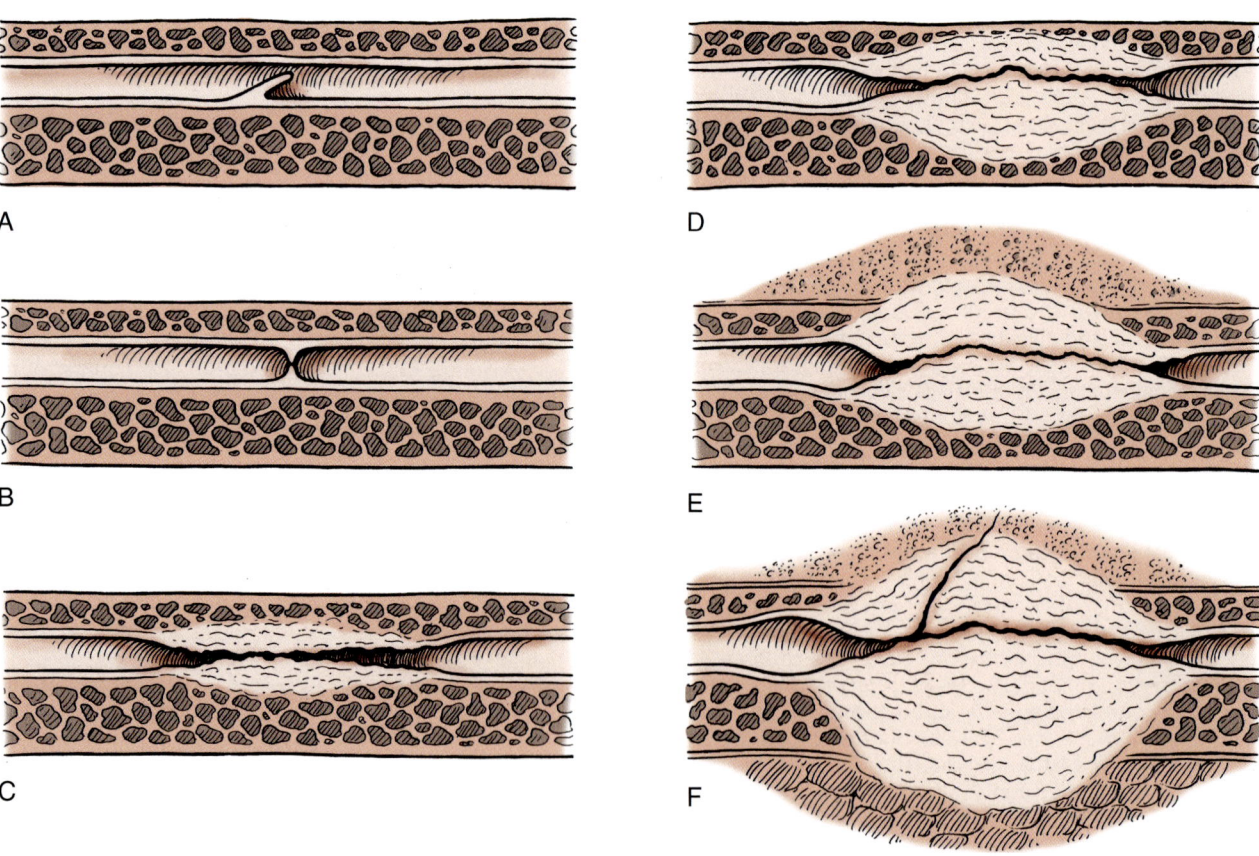

Fig. 82.15. The anatomy of anterior urethral strictures includes, in most cases, underlying spongiofibrosis. (A) Mucosal fold. (B) Iris constriction. (C) Full-thickness involvement with minimal fibrosis in the spongy tissue. (D) Full-thickness spongiofibrosis. (E) Inflammation and fibrosis involving tissues outside the corpus spongiosum. (F) Complex stricture complicated by a fistula. This can proceed to the formation of an abscess, or the fistula may open to the skin or the rectum. (From Jordan GH: Management of anterior urethral stricture disease. *Probl Urol* 1:199–225, 1987.)

Latini et al. (2014) proposed a broad categorization of urethral stricture disease into iatrogenic, traumatic, inflammatory, and idiopathic causes. A recent meta-analysis of etiology found that most common causes are idiopathic (33%) and iatrogenic (33%), followed by post-traumatic (19%) and inflammatory (15%) (Fenton et al., 2005).

Iatrogenic

Iatrogenic urethral strictures can be the result of urethral instrumentation, either diagnostic or therapeutic. Diagnostic cystoscopy and urethral dilation are common causes of urethral stricture. Transurethral procedures such as transurethral resection of bladder tumors (TURBTs) and transurethral resection of the prostate (TURP) also cause strictures of the urethra either by direct insult of the frail mucosa or from inflammation and subsequent ischemia related to the technique, the caliber of the instruments, and the time of the procedure. In addition, the perioperative catheter may play a role in the cause of potential strictures in those settings (Jørgensen et al., 1986). The material, insertion technique, and time of indwelling catheters are closely associated with urethral stricture development. Again, the mechanism of injury may be due to injury, pressure necrosis, or inflammation/infection. In our experience, catheter-related urethral stricture disease is very prevalent in low- and middle-income countries (LMIC) (McCammon and Virasoro, personal communication). The use of silicone catheters and hydrophilic coating for intermittent catheterization may help in reducing this empirical cause.

Traumatic

Urethral strictures can be the result of blunt or penetrating trauma. With straddle and deceleration trauma, the corpus spongiosum is crushed against the inferior rami of the pubis. This trauma to the urethra often goes unrecognized until the patient experiences voiding symptoms resulting from the obstruction of the stricture or scar. In most cases of straddle trauma, reconstruction of the bulbar urethral injury is possible (Park and McAninch, 2004). Finally, posterior urethral injuries, traumatic by definition, result in obliterative or near-obliterative defects that are associated with extensive fibrosis interposed between the distracted ends of the urethra. Another cause of posterior urethral stenosis is prostate cancer treatment.

Inflammatory

Inflammatory strictures associated with gonorrhea were the most commonly seen in the past and are less common now. With the advent of prompt and effective antibiotic treatment, gonococcal urethritis progresses less often to gonococcal urethral strictures. The place of *Chlamydia* and *Ureaplasma urealyticum* (i.e., nonspecific urethritis) in the development of anterior urethral strictures is unclear. No clear association between nonspecific urethritis and the development of anterior urethral stricture has been established.

As mentioned earlier, there is a definite association between the development of an inflammatory stricture and LS. LS usually begins with inflammation of the glans and inevitably causes meatal stenosis, if not a true stricture of the fossa navicularis. The cause of this distal penile skin and urethral inflammation is unknown. Some evidence suggests that the progression of the stricture eventually to involve the anterior urethra extensively may be due to high-pressure voiding that causes intravasation of urine into the glands of Littre, inflammation of these glands, and, perhaps, microabscesses and deep spongiofibrosis. Whether the urethral changes and eventual fibrosis are also related to bacterial injury has not been well defined. Although the use of antibiotics seems to limit obstructive voiding symptoms in these patients, to our knowledge the literature does not show resolution of the stricture process with the use of antibiotics.

Idiopathic

Iatrogenic trauma to the urethra still exists, but with the development of small endoscopes and the limitation of indications for cystoscopy in boys, we see fewer iatrogenic strictures today than in the past. The place of idiopathic urethrorrhagia with regard to strictures in children is unclear; some question whether it may be a cause of strictures in young boys regardless of whether the child underwent an endoscopic procedure (Rourke et al., 2003). No specific inciting factor has been identified as causing idiopathic urethrorrhagia. Histologic results from a patient of ours with resolving urethrorrhagia showed portions of tissues covered in part by squamous epithelium; other parts were covered by transitional epithelium; there were several areas of denuded epithelium with acute hemorrhage and neutrophilic infiltration; a few foci of microcalcification were shown; several mucus glands were found within the submucosal connective tissue as well as a few collections of amorphous material, likely mucin. These areas stained negatively with a special stain for amyloid. There was no evidence of viral cytopathic effect or malignancy. We did not see evidence of bacterial infection or viral inclusions. However, we have seen an increase in strictures associated with LS, and those strictures clearly behave much more like inflammatory strictures than traumatically induced isolated scars.

Congenital

The entity known as a congenital stricture is difficult to understand. In embryologic development, if a stricture is found at a natural place where a fusion of structures occurs (i.e., the posterior and anterior urethra), a congenital stricture may be a reasonable assumption. However, the term *congenital stricture* is used by some authors to define a stricture for which there is no identifiable cause. We propose that it is reasonable to define a stricture as congenital only if it is not an inflammatory stricture, it is a short-length stricture, and it is not associated with a history of or potential for urethral trauma. These criteria limit the term *congenital stricture* to strictures of the anterior urethra found in infants before they attempt erect ambulation. So defined, congenital strictures are the rarest encountered.

Diagnosis and Evaluation

Patients who have urethral strictures most often have obstructive voiding symptoms or urinary tract infections such as prostatitis and epididymitis. Some patients also experience urinary retention. However, on close inquiry, most of these patients are found to have tolerated notable voiding obstructive symptoms for a long time before progressing to complete obstruction.

When a patient cannot void, an attempt commonly is made to pass a urethral catheter. If the catheter does not pass, the nature of the obstruction is determined by dynamic retrograde urethrography. Most cases are managed with acute dilation, but there are many instances in which this is not the best course for the patient. When there is doubt, we determine the nature of the stricture, when possible, and selectively place a suprapubic cystostomy catheter to treat the acute situation and allow time for a more appropriate treatment plan to be devised. The practice of blind passage of filiforms and blind dilation without knowledge of the anatomy of the urethral stricture is condemned. Although detailed imaging is not always available, flexible endoscopy is almost universally available in the United States. The stricture can be visualized, and guidewire placement under direct vision can be attempted.

For an appropriate treatment plan to be devised, it is important to determine the location, length, depth, and density of the stricture (spongiofibrosis). The length and location of the stricture can be determined with radiography, urethroscopy, and ultrasonography. The depth and density of the scar in the spongy tissue can be deduced from the physical examination, the appearance of the urethra in contrast-enhanced studies, and the amount of elasticity noted on urethroscopy. The depth and density of fibrosis are difficult to determine objectively. The absolute length of spongiofibrosis may not be evident on ultrasound evaluation. Ultrasound examination can augment contrast-enhanced studies and is accurate in determining the length of narrow-caliber annularity (Morey and McAninch, 1996b). Contrast studies of the urethra are best carried out by or under the direct supervision of the surgeon responsible for treatment of the patient.

McCallum and Colapinto (1979a, 1979b) described the use of dynamic radiographic studies and emphasized the need for these studies to be dynamic as opposed to static (Fig. 82.16). At our center, imaging includes dynamic studies that are performed during retrograde injection of contrast material and while the patient is voiding. Even with gentle technique, extravasation during retrograde urethrography is possible in patients in whom the urethra is markedly inflamed. For this reason, contrast studies should be carried out with contrast material that is suitable for intravenous injection and used either directly from the bottle or diluted according to the manufacturer's guidelines. Contrast materials that have been thickened with lubricating jelly or anesthetic gels can be a source of problems and offer little with regard to enhancement of radiographic studies, and they do not make the studies more comfortable. Real-time ultrasound evaluation of the urethra after it has been filled with a lubricating jelly or saline has been described by Morey and McAninch (1996a, 1996b). However, it is a misconception that ultrasonography always directly visualizes the spongiofibrosis. Morey and McAninch (1996a, 1996b) believed that ultrasonography of the bulbous urethra possibly more accurately determines the length of the stricture, which could be important in considering an anastomotic repair. If the patient is not in steep lateral oblique position for retrograde urethrography, the length of the stricture will be underestimated. Finally, during contrast-enhanced urethrography, more than one projection may be necessary to visualize the stricture. Magnetic resonance imaging (MRI) is also being explored as an adjunct to the evaluation of urethral stricture and pelvic fracture urethral injuries (PFUIs). In our experience, the use of MRI for routine strictures or pelvic fracture urethral distraction defects is not beneficial. In the case of urethral tumors, we have found MRI to be invaluable. The experience of others is commensurate with ours (Pavlica et al., 2003). In a pelvic fracture urethral distraction defect, the alignment of the two urethral ends can be defined clearly.

Endoscopic examination may be necessary after contrast studies. The flexible cystoscope has simplified this evaluation, and when local anesthesia is used, there is little discomfort associated with it. The scope can be passed to the stricture, and it often is unnecessary to pass it beyond that level. In addition, it is not always necessary, and usually not beneficial, to dilate the stricture at the time of the initial endoscopic evaluation. Pediatric endoscopic equipment has proven to be extremely valuable for examination of the urethra proximal to a narrow-caliber area without the need to dilate the narrowest area. In a patient who cannot void and has a suprapubic tube, combined contrast studies with endoscopy are helpful in defining the stricture anatomy (Fig. 82.17).

It is imperative to evaluate the urethra completely proximal and distal to the stricture with endoscopy and bougienage during surgery to ensure that all the involved urethra is included in the reconstruction. Although hydraulic pressure generated by voiding may keep segments proximal to the stricture patent, unless these segments are included in the repair, they are at risk for contraction after obstruction of the narrow-caliber segment is relieved with reconstruction. For this reason, any abnormal areas of the urethra that are proximal to a narrow-caliber segment of the stricture must be treated with suspicion. If the lumen does not appear to demonstrate evidence of diminished compliance, we presume that area to be uninvolved in active stricture disease. However, coning down of the urethra suggests its involvement in the scar.

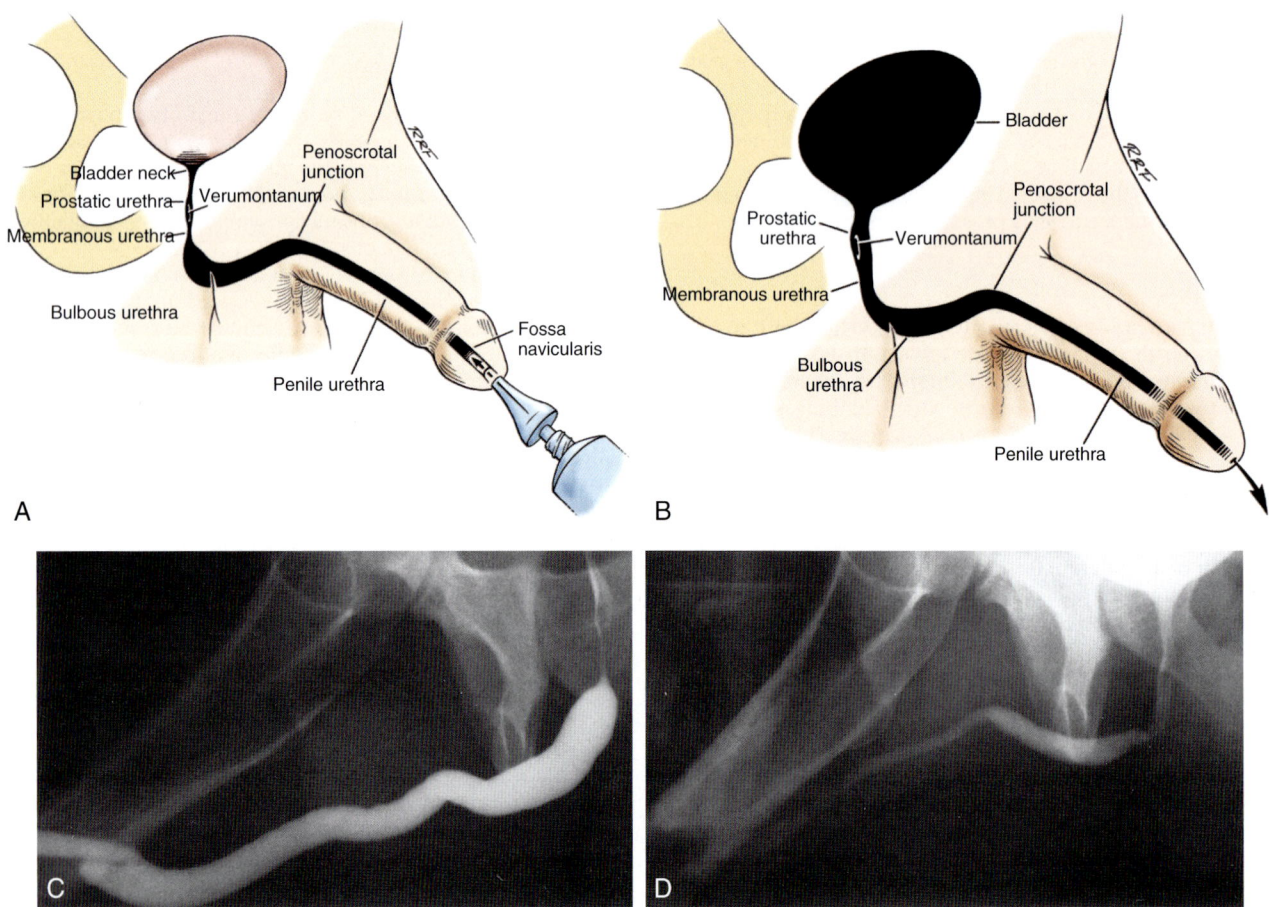

Fig. 82.16. (A) Representation of a dynamic retrograde urethrogram with the criteria of McCallum illustrated. (B) Representation of a dynamic voiding urethrogram with the criteria of McCallum illustrated. (C) Normal retrograde urethrogram. (D) Normal voiding urethrogram. (A and B, Modified from McCallum RW: The adult male urethra. *Radiol Clin North Am* 17:227–244, 1979.)

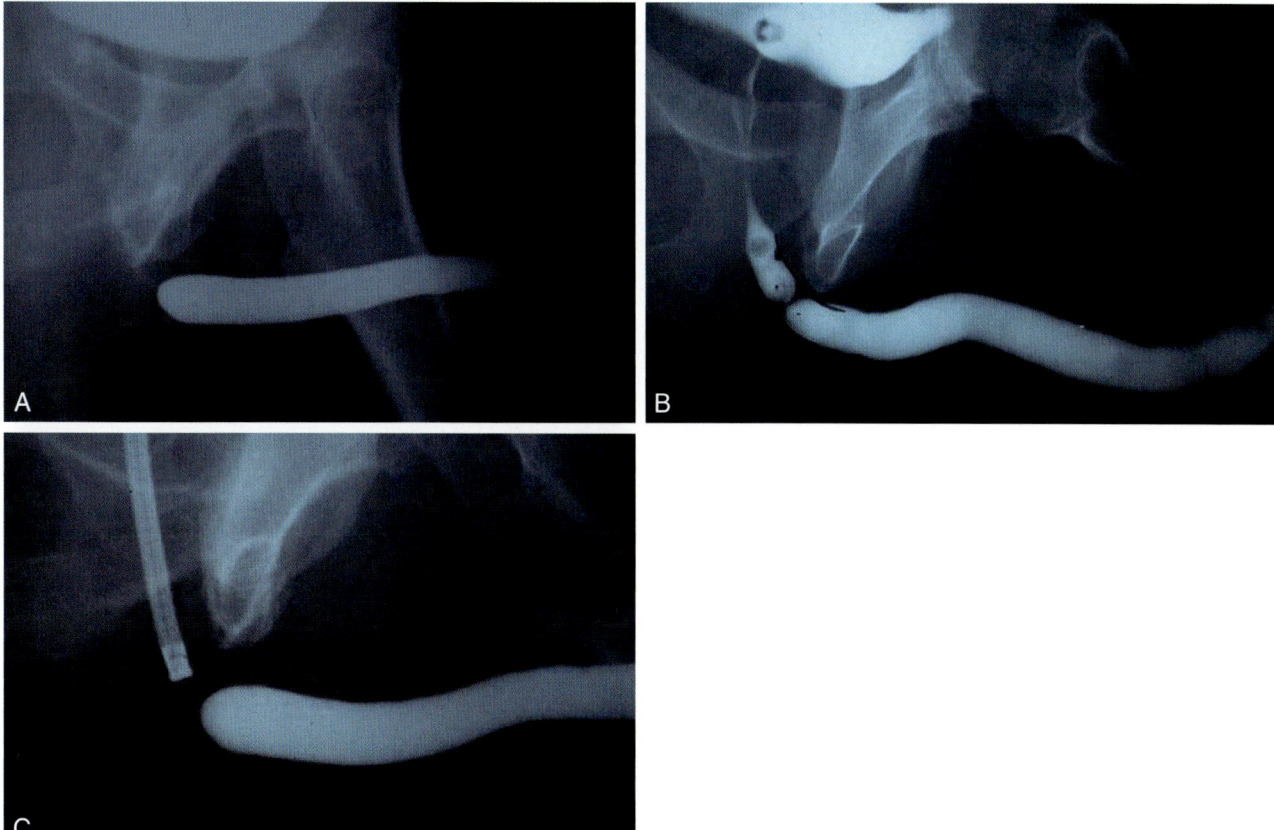

Fig. 82.17. Series of radiographs demonstrating the usefulness of the combination of contrast enhancement with endoscopy. (A) A retrograde urethrogram shows a totally obliterative process involving the proximal bulbous urethra. (B) The patient was successful in relaxing to void; however, there is suggestion of a wide-caliber annular area proximal to the obliterative process of the bulbous urethra. (C) Endoscopy through the suprapubic cystostomy tube clarifies the anatomy of the proximal urethra and demonstrates the length of the obliterative process.

In some patients, the urethra proximal to a narrow area may remain confusing with regard to its potential for continued constriction after reconstruction. In select patients, we have found it useful to place a suprapubic tube to defunctionalize the urethra. After 6 to 8 weeks, if there is to be constriction of an area that was hydrodilated with voiding, the tendency for that constriction to occur should become apparent.

Decision Making

Once the stricture and patient specifics have been evaluated, the next step in the decision-making algorithm is determining if treatment is to be palliative or curative. The assessment and decision-making algorithm in urethral stricture surgery is predicated upon several main factors. First, the surgeon should have a good understanding of the role of radiologic and endoscopic evaluations to fully characterize the anatomy of the stricture. Second, he or she should be familiar with the available techniques and their uses and limitations. Last, patient and surgeon should agree upon a desired outcome of any intervention and understand the long-term goals and expectations. Curative procedures should be attempted when possible and desired. Palliative procedures are acceptable if that is the recognized goal of treatment.

Treatment

Although the treatment of urethral stricture disease dates to the foundations of urology, significant progress made during the last 50 years allows many of the most complex strictures to be reliably reconstructed in one stage. In the past, a concept known as the reconstructive ladder was used as a treatment guideline for urethral strictures. That concept was based on the principle that the simplest procedure should always be attempted first, and sometimes repeated after failure, before moving on to more complex approaches. This approach is considered archaic in modern urethral reconstruction.

The patient and the physician must have a good understanding of the goal of treatment before the treatment choice is made. Treatment options should be discussed with the patient, with care taken to emphasize the anticipated outcome with regard to potential cure. Some patients may prefer stricture management and choose to have periodic dilations in the office, at home, or in the hospital rather than undergo technically detailed open surgery. Others may have cure as a goal and choose surgical management. Many surgical procedures today have short-term and midterm results approaching long-term success rates of more than 90% to 95% for many strictures.

Dilation

Urethral dilation is the oldest and simplest treatment of urethral stricture disease, and for a patient with an epithelial stricture without spongiofibrosis, it may be curative. **The goal of this treatment, a concept that is frequently forgotten, is to stretch the scar without producing more scarring.** If bleeding occurs during dilation, the stricture has been torn rather than stretched, possibly further injuring the involved area.

The least traumatic method to stretch the urethra is to use soft techniques over multiple treatment sessions. We believe that the safest method of urethral dilation currently available involves the use of urethral balloon-dilating catheters. These catheters may be attached to a filiform tip or passed over a guidewire or may come with an integral coudé tip. For initial dilation, we favor the use of balloons placed over wires that have been passed through the stricture under endoscopic control.

Dilation can be curative and, in the literature, in correctly selected patients, has short-term and midterm efficacy rates equal to internal urethrotomy. Selection criteria are discussed in the following section on internal urethrotomy. The literature does not compare internal urethrotomy and dilation in randomized selection, and we do not have a true comparison but rather comparison by retrospective analysis (Steenkamp et al., 1997).

Internal Urethrotomy

Internal urethrotomy refers to any procedure that opens the stricture by incising it transurethrally. The urethrotomy procedure involves incision through the scar to healthy tissue to allow the scar to expand (release of scar contracture) and the lumen to heal enlarged. The goal is for the resultant larger luminal caliber to be maintained after healing.

With epithelial apposition, wound healing occurs by primary intention. Internal urethrotomy does not provide an epithelial approximation but rather aims to separate the scarred epithelium so that healing occurs by secondary intention. In healing by secondary intention, epithelialization progresses from the wound edges. As it progresses from the wound edge, epithelialization slows. In an effort to aid epithelialization, nature invokes the forces of wound contraction, not to be confused with scar contraction. Wound contraction closes the wound defect and limits the size of the area that requires epithelialization, hastening the healing of the surface defect. However, in the case of internal urethrotomy, wound contraction merely tries to reapproximate the edges of the scar, putting a race into effect. If epithelialization progresses completely before wound contraction significantly narrows the lumen, the internal urethrotomy may be a success. If wound contraction significantly narrows the lumen before completion of epithelialization, the stricture has recurred. Dubey et al. (2005) showed the extent of luminal narrowing to be a predictor of success with internal urethrotomy: the narrower the percent of narrowing, the worse the outcome, with a cutoff of 74% narrowing.

Many surgeons have learned to perform internal urethrotomy by making a single incision at the 12 o'clock position. However, this location may be questioned on the basis of the location of the urethra within the corpus spongiosum. Examination of a cross section of the corpus spongiosum demonstrates that the thinnest portion of the anterior aspect is from 10 o'clock to 2 o'clock. The distance between the anterior wall of the urethra and the corpora cavernosa is likewise short in the bulbous urethra, and a single incision at 12 o'clock could rapidly penetrate the corpus spongiosum and extend into the triangular ligament. Although it may not enter the corpora cavernosa, a deep cut could enter the intracrural space. Distally, although the anterior aspect of the corpus spongiosum is thicker, a deep incision in the more distal aspects of the anterior urethra would enter the corpora cavernosa, and these incisions have been associated with erectile dysfunction (ED) thought to be due to local cavernosal veno-occlusive dysfunction. Vigorous incisions at 10 o'clock and 2 o'clock in the bulbous urethra risk the same problem. If deep spongiofibrosis is present, stricture cure is impossible by internal urethrotomy, and these deep incisions are unnecessary.

The most common complication of internal urethrotomy is recurrence of stricture. Less commonly noted complications of internal urethrotomy include bleeding (almost always associated with erections immediately after the procedure) and extravasation of irrigation fluid into the perispongiosal tissues. These complications are rare today because of the less frequent use of aggressive internal urethrotomy as a treatment modality for urethral strictures. Normal saline should be used as the irrigant when direct visual internal urethrotomy is performed. In addition, with the use of deep urethrotomy incisions, another complication can be creation of a fistula between the corpus spongiosum and the corpora cavernosa and cavernosal veno-occlusive dysfunction.

A major problem with assessing the success rates of internal urethrotomy is that the nature of the strictures that have been treated with internal urethrotomy has been poorly reported. In addition, the literature is unclear regarding the goal of internal urethrotomy. For many, an internal urethrotomy is successful if it offers temporary relief. In many cases, internal urethrotomy has been reported as successful despite the fact that it has been associated with eventual stricture recurrence. Rosen et al. (1994) and later Santucci et al. (2001) showed that actuarial curative success rate of internal urethrotomy is approximately 20%. Evaluations by Pansadoro and Emiliozzi (1996) et al. showed the curative success rate of direct visual internal urethrotomy to be approximately 30% to 35%. Their analysis also showed that there is virtually no increase in success rate with a second internal urethrotomy. **The data show that strictures at the bulbous urethra that are less than 1.5 cm in length and not associated with dense, deep spongiofibrosis (i.e., straddle injuries) can be managed with internal urethrotomy, with a 74% moderately long-term success rate.** The study by Pansadoro and Emiliozzi (1996) did not have any long-term successes for treated strictures outside the bulbous urethra. The variables associated with success of internal urethrotomy have been verified by other studies (Heyns et al., 1998). Many studies have shown that the success of reconstruction is diminished by multiple prior urethral dilations and internal urethrotomy (Albers et al., 1996; Boccon-Gibod, personal communication, 2005; Heyns et al., 1998 Stone et al., 1983). Success rates with internal urethrotomy are not equal to success rates of open urethral reconstruction (Mandhani et al., 2005). Numerous analyses have sought to compare the cost effectiveness of the practice of internal urethrotomy initially before consideration of open reconstruction. The analyses differ in method and in findings (Rourke and Jordan, 2005; Wessells, 2009; Wright et al., 2006).

Several techniques have been employed to oppose the process of wound contraction and to prevent stricture recurrence. One method is to leave an indwelling Foley catheter for 6 weeks after urethrotomy in the hope that the urethra will mold around the catheter as it heals. However, studies have shown that the failure rate of long-term catheterization after internal urethrotomy is similar to that seen with 3 to 7 days of catheterization, and even 6 weeks is insufficient time to oppose the forces of wound contraction.

Another technique used to oppose the forces of wound contraction after internal urethrotomy is home self-catheterization or home urethral obturation. After internal urethrotomy, patients generally have an indwelling catheter placed for 3 to 5 days. When the catheter is removed, the patient is started on a urethral obturation regimen. Most regimens require more frequent catheterizations early in the recovery period, with a tapering schedule during the next 3 to 6 months. Anecdotally, many surgeons have reported an improved cure rate with self-catheterization combined with internal urethrotomy. However, it has been our experience that the stricture inevitably recurs when the patient stops self-obturation, regardless of how long it has been used. That being understood, this approach can effectively manage the problems when it is combined with a urethral dilating regimen in a properly motivated patient. Colchicine, because it binds tubulin, has been used along with internal urethrotomy (Carney et al., 2007). Initial findings in a nonrandomized study also suggest that, perhaps by pharmacologically blocking tubulin and possibly wound contracture, the results of internal urethrotomy may be better. Mitomycin C with its antifibroblast and anticollagen activity when injected submucosally has been shown to decrease the risk of recurrence after a urethrotomy (Mazdak et al., 2007).

Lasers

More details on this topic are available online at ExpertConsult.com.
The results of laser urethrotomy are mixed. However, with the advent of new lasers and experience with them, future data may show better results.

Stents

Urethral stents (removable or permanently implantable) are another modality used in opposing the forces of wound contraction

after internal urethrotomy or dilation. Removable urethral stents are designed to prevent the process of epithelialization from incorporating the stent into the urethral wall and are left in place for 6 months to 1 year before they are removed. The greatest experience with these removable stents comes from Israel (Yachia and Beyar, 1991), where success in small series is reported. The Memokath stent is not currently available in the United States. It is a removable stent made of nitinol with varying success rates.

Most experience with permanently implantable stents comes from Europe and the United Kingdom. Milroy (1993) reported a success rate of 84% at 4½ years with use of the permanently implantable UroLume (Ashken et al., 1991; Badlani et al., 1995; Brandes and McAninch, 1998; Jordan, 1997; Krah et al., 1992; Milroy and Allen, 1996; Milroy et al., 1988, 1989; Rousseau et al., 1987; Sarramon et al., 1990; Shah et al., 2003; Sigwart et al., 1987; Sneller and Bosch, 1992; Tillem et al., 1997; Verhamme et al., 1993). The UroLume, made of an alloy, is designed to be incorporated into the wall of the urethra and corpus spongiosum. Available data show that the stent is best employed for relatively short strictures of the bulbous urethra associated with minimal spongiofibrosis. However, these are the strictures that are most successfully reconstructed with open techniques that offer better long-term success rates. The North American Study Group 11-year data showed that of 179 patients originally enrolled in the North American Study, 24 patients completed 11 years of follow-up. The overall success rate for all patients enrolled at 11 years is less than 30% (Shah et al., 2003). A 10-year follow-up study from the Netherlands (De Vocht et al., 2003) reported results thought to "weaken the optimistic early results"; of 15 patients implanted, only 2 were satisfied with their stent at 10 years.

Permanently implantable stents are associated with unique complications. The stents must be **placed only in the bulbous urethra,** and when placed beyond the area of the scrotal urethra, placement has been associated with pain on sitting and intercourse. Some patients (particularly young patients) **complain of perineal pain,** often with vigorous activity, even after implantation of the stent in the deep bulbous urethra. In addition, **longer bulbous strictures require two stents that are overlapped.** These **stents can migrate** away from each other, leaving a gap between them where recurrence of stricture is inevitable. When this occurs, the stricture recurrence is excised, and a third stent is placed to span the gap.

The UroLume stent has been taken off the market and is currently not available for implantation. However, many patients still have UroLume stents, and many of these will need treatment.

Open Reconstruction

If curative techniques are to be employed, then consideration must be given to anastomotic urethroplasty and substitution urethroplasty techniques. There is currently no clear evidence as to which procedure is best for all strictures; however, if stratified by stricture length, cause and site of stricture several recommendation are clear.

Excision and Reanastomosis. The most dependable technique of anterior urethral reconstruction is the complete excision of the area of fibrosis, with a primary reanastomosis of the normal ends of the anterior urethra (Fig. 82.18; Russell, 1914). The best results are achieved when **the following technical points are observed: the area of fibrosis is totally excised; the urethral anastomosis is widely spatulated, creating a large ovoid anastomosis; and the anastomosis is tension free.**

The success of this procedure relies on vigorous mobilization of the corpus spongiosum. With vigorous mobilization, dissection of Buck fascia to improve compliance, development of the intracrural space, and detachment of the bulbospongiosus from the perineal body, significant lengths of stricture can be excised and reanastomosed. Strictures of 1 to 2 cm are generally easily excised with reanastomosis. In some cases, strictures 3 to 5 cm can be totally excised, and a primary reanastomosis of the anterior urethra can be performed. For very proximal short-length bulbous strictures, tension-free anastomosis can be facilitated by the dissection of the membranous urethra (Fig. 82.19). As a rule, the closer the stricture is to the membranous urethra, the longer it can be and still be reconstructed

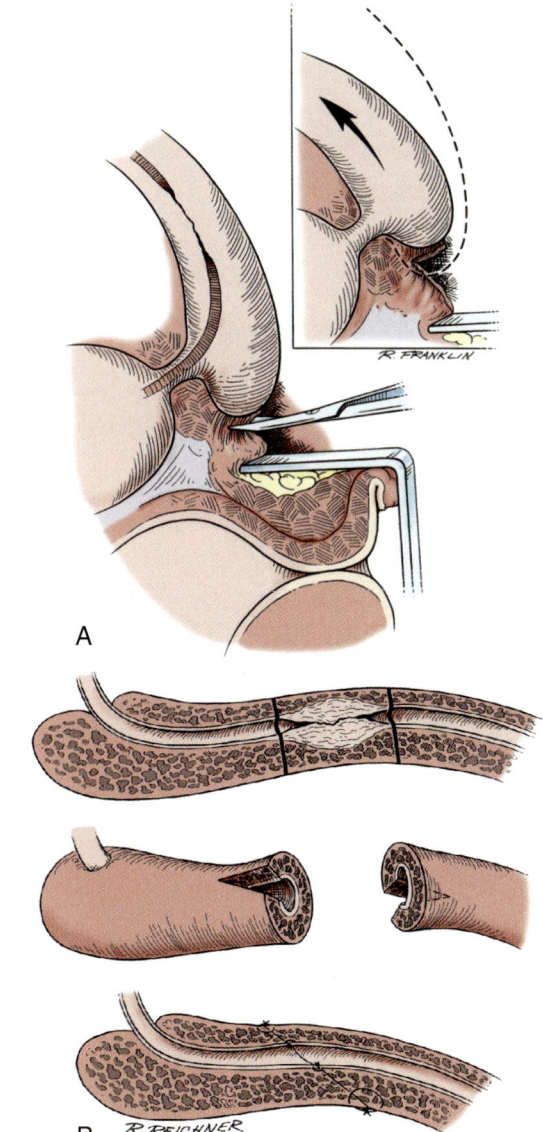

Fig. 82.18. Techniques for excision and primary reanastomosis of anterior urethral stricture. (A) The bulbospongiosus is released from its attachment to the perineal body. The arteries to the bulb are not divided. This technique allows the urethra to be mobilized distally. This technique combined with development of the intracrural space can shorten the path of the urethra by approximately 1 to 1.5 cm. (B) Technique of a primary spatulated anastomosis after excision of an anterior urethral stricture. (From Jordan GH: Principles of plastic surgery. In Droller MJ, editor: *Surgical management of urologic disease: an anatomic approach*, Philadelphia, 1992, Mosby, pp 1218–1237.)

with anastomotic techniques. For many proximal strictures, a single-layer anastomosis is preferable. When the length of stricture precludes total excision of fibrosis with primary anastomosis, tissue transfer is required. Morey and Kizer (2006) studied a series of patients who had stricture excision with anastomosis for strictures up to 5 cm and pointed out that younger patients have more compliant tissue, allowing the limits to be stretched.

DeCastro et al. (2002) reported an interesting variant of excision with anastomosis for anterior stricture. In that case report, a patient had two independent areas of stricture apparently separated by totally normal urethra and corpus spongiosum. The authors excised both areas of stricture independently with respective anastomosis of each site. Although this case was successful, we think that the authors' considerable experience allowed them to achieve a successful result,

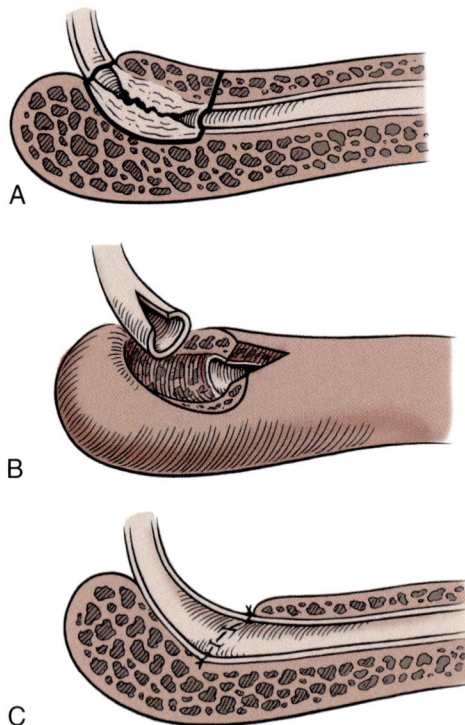

Fig. 82.19. Technique of excision of very proximal bulbous urethral stricture with reanastomosis. This technique is facilitated by dissection of the membranous urethra. (A) The area of the stricture is defined for excision. (B) The stricture is excised, and both ends of the urethra are spatulated on the dorsal aspect. (C) The anastomosis is complete.

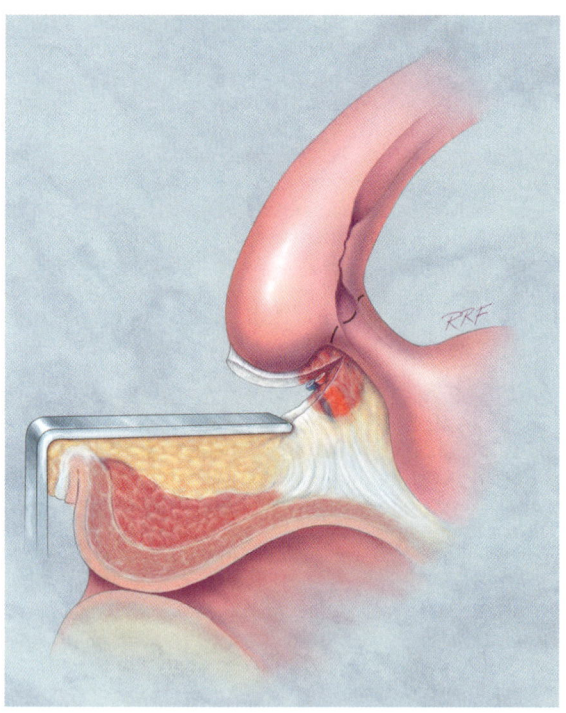

Fig. 82.20. Diagrammatic representation of the dissection of the proximal corpus spongiosum, bulbospongiosum, and membranous urethra. The customary technique for dividing the urethra through the juncture of the membranous urethra with the proximal bulbous urethra—to perform an excision of stricture with a primary anastomosis. In this illustration, the proximal vasculature has been ligated and divided. The urethra can then be divided at the distal-most limits of the membranous urethra.

and a safer reconstruction with use of onlay or augmented onlay may have been better.

Vessel-Sparing Technique. Jordan et al. (2007) first reported the use of a vessel-sparing excision and reanastomosis of the bulbar urethra. The dissection is similar to the standard excision and reanastomosis (Fig. 82.20): the triangular ligament is divided, and the intracrural space is developed, the space between the membranous urethra and the proximal vasculature is developed, and these vessels are preserved (Fig. 82.21). The urethra is divided with the stenotic segment excised, the ends are spatulated, and the reanastomosis is performed. Andrich and Mundy (2012) described an alternative vessel-sparing technique for proximal strictures in which a longitudinal dorsal stricturotomy is performed and the stricture is excised from within the urethra without disrupting the spongiosum. After stricture excision, the ventral urethra is reapproximated primarily, and the longitudinal dorsal stricturotomy is closed horizontally, preserving the vasculature. Preserving the proximal blood supply to the bulbar urethra is advantageous in patients whose distal blood supply is compromised by trauma, previous surgery, or hypospadias. Another theoretical advantage would be a decrease in the risk of ED and potential decreased risk for erosion if subsequent artificial sphincter implantation were probable.

Further studies must be done to confirm the initial excellent results with the vessel-sparing technique and prove the theoretical advantages (Andrich and Mundy, 2012; Gur and Jordan, 2008; Jordan et al., 2007; Virasoro et al., 2015).

Graft Onlay. Four grafts that have been successfully used for primary urethral reconstruction are the FTSG, bladder epithelial graft, OMG, and rectal mucosal graft. OMGs, as mentioned earlier, can be taken from the cheek (buccal), the lip (labial), and the undersurface of the tongue (lingual). STSGs have been used for staged anterior urethral reconstruction (Burger et al., 1992; Devine et al., 1976; El-Kassaby et al., 1996; Hendren and Crooks, 1980; Hendren and Reda, 1986; Humby, 1941; Jordan, 1993; Memmelaar, 1947; Pressman and Greenfield, 1953; Ransley et al., 1987; Schreiter and Koncz, 1983; Webster et al., 1984; Wessels and McAninch, 1996). The characteristics and microvascularity of some of the grafts were discussed earlier in Principles of Reconstructive Surgery.

Graft reconstruction of the urethra was almost abandoned in favor of flap reconstruction techniques. However, since the late 1990s, there has been a resurgence of interest in the use of grafts (Wessells and McAninch, 1996) and, specifically, the use of BMGs (Barbagli et al., 2003; Bhargava and Chapple, 2004; Bhargava et al., 2004; Dubey et al., 2005; Elliott et al., 2003; Hellstrom et al., 1996; Kellner et al., 2004; Weinberg et al., 2002; Xu et al., 2004). **Grafts have been employed most successfully in the area of the bulbous urethra, where the urethra is invested by the bulk of the ischiocavernosus muscles. However, the use of grafts other than in the area of the bulbous urethra and, in some cases, the use of tubed reconstruction are reported in increasing numbers.** The grafts can be applied to the ventrum of the urethra; however, a ventral urethrotomy seems to be advantageous only if use of the spongioplasty maneuver is contemplated (Fig. 82.22). The spongioplasty procedure requires that the corpus spongiosum adjacent to the area of the stricture be relatively normal and free of fibrosis. Data support the superiority of results with the dorsal onlay technique and other reports showing no difference in success. In the past, we preferred to use lateral graft onlay (see Fig. 82.22B) or dorsal graft onlay (see Fig. 82.22C). Placement of the urethrostomy laterally allows exposure of the urethra while cutting through the corpus spongiosum, where it is relatively thinner, limiting bleeding and maximizing exposure. In addition, in the bulbous urethra, the graft can be sutured to the underlying muscle bed in the hope of improving graft–host bed immobilization and approximation.

The Monseur urethral reconstruction was applied in only a few select centers (Monseur, 1980). In this technique, the urethrostomy was made through the stricture on the dorsal wall. The edges of the stricture were sutured open to the underlying triangular ligament or corpora cavernosa, or both. Barbagli et al. (1995) subsequently modified the Monseur technique (Fig. 82.23). In their modification,

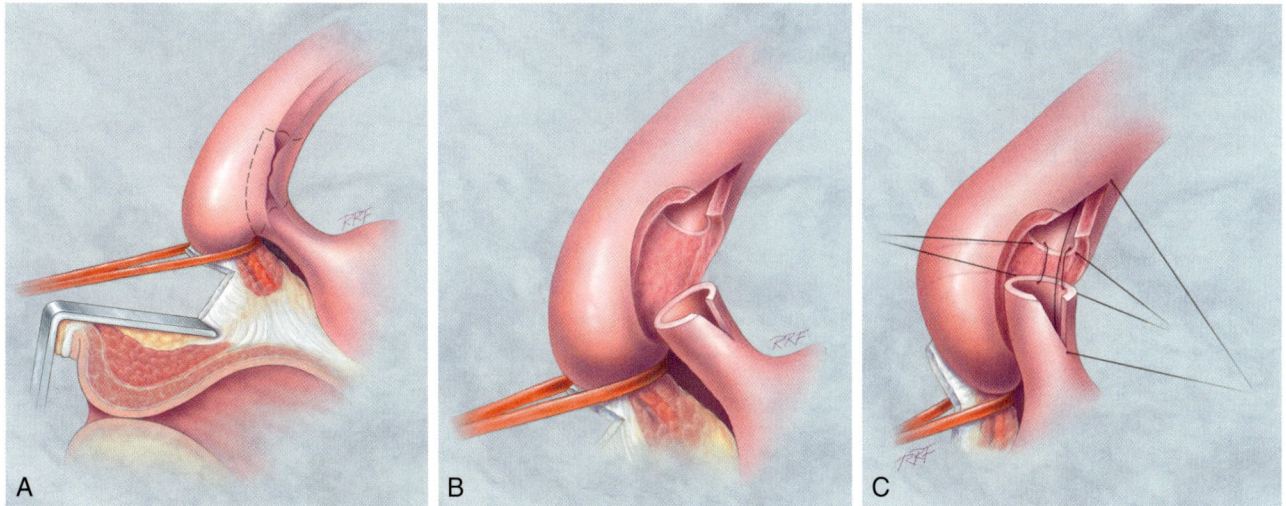

Fig. 82.21. Technique of vessel-sparing excision with primary anastomosis. The proximal corpus spongiosum, bulbospongiosum, and area of the proximal vessels and membranous urethra have been dissected. (A) Dissection of the space between the proximal vasculature and the membranous urethra is illustrated. In this technique, the arteries to the bulb can be preserved, and the membranous urethra can be divided at its juncture with the bulbous urethra. The area of proximal stricture can be excised. (B) The stricture has been excised before placement of the anastomotic sutures. (C) Anastomotic sutures are placed to effect the spatulated anastomosis. At this center, customarily we alternate polydioxanone sutures with Monocryl; however, any acceptable absorbable suture can be used. The membranous urethra is spatulated on the dorsum as is the proximal bulbous urethra.

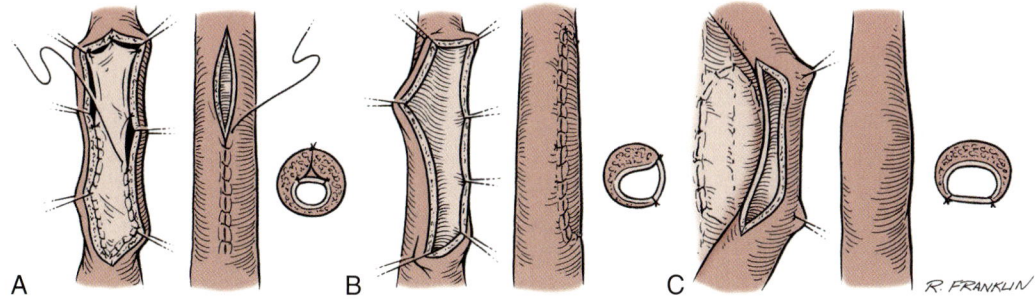

Fig. 82.22. Various techniques of graft onlay. (A) Ventral onlay with spongioplasty. (B) Lateral onlay with quilting to the ischiocavernosus muscle. (C) Dorsal onlay with spread fixation of the graft.

the urethrostomy is performed through the stricture on the dorsal wall. In the area of the urethrostomy, a graft is applied and spread fixed to the triangular ligament or corpora cavernosa, or to both. The edges of the stricturotomy are sutured to the edges of the graft and to the adjacent structures. The results of this technique are excellent. The ventral and dorsal graft onlay techniques can be used with stricture excision and strip anastomosis (augmented anastomotic procedure) (Fig. 82.24). For proximal strictures, the vessel-sparing technique of augmented anastomosis depends on the surgeon's ability to excise the scarred epithelium and underlying corpus spongiosum tissue without the need to divide the corpus spongiosum completely.

Another option is the two-staged application of a mesh STSG, BMG, or posterior auricular FTSG. In the first stage of the staged graft procedure, a medium-thickness STSG, a BMG, or a Wolfe graft is placed over the dartos fascia. If the graft is placed immediately onto the tunica albuginea or corpora cavernosa, the inability to mobilize the graft makes second-stage tubularization difficult. However, there is an advantage to having at least a midline strip of the graft adherent to the corpora cavernosa. At a later date, second-stage surgery is performed to tubularize the graft. Although Schreiter and Noll (1989), who first described the procedure of mesh STSG, often proceeded to the second stage within 3 to 4 months, we wait 12 months between the first-stage and second-stage surgeries if an STSG is used. According to studies in the United States and Europe, this procedure has been determined useful for select cases. In the United States, its use has mostly been confined to the most difficult cases, with single-stage reconstruction still applied to most cases. As already mentioned, staged graft techniques have been used effectively in complicated patients with hypospadias. Staged buccal graft operations have been successful in patients with LS with midterm follow-up. In addition, in complicated patients with hypospadias, staged buccal grafts and posterior auricular skin grafts have been successfully employed (Fig. 82.25).

Flap Onlay. Numerous applications of genital skin islands, mobilized on either the dartos fascia of the penis or the tunica dartos of the scrotum, have been proposed for the repair of urethral stricture disease. In the past, these "flap operations" were considered separate procedures. We suggest that all these procedures are different applications of a single concept, as proposed by the microinjection studies of Quartey (1983). Skin islands can be viewed as passengers on fascial flaps, and the design of flaps for urethral reconstruction can be paralleled to the design of flaps for reconstruction in general.

There are **three important considerations for the use of flaps in urethral reconstruction: the nature of the flap tissue, the**

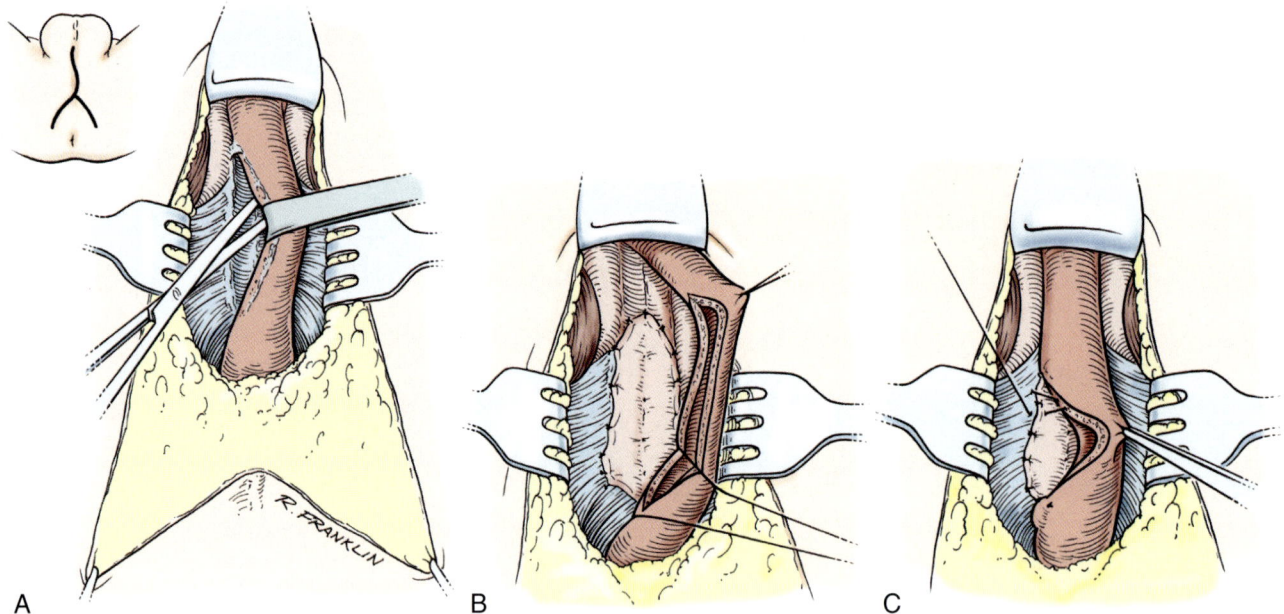

Fig. 82.23. Technique of dorsal graft onlay popularized by Barbagli. (A) The corpus spongiosum is detached from the triangular ligament and corpora cavernosa. (B) A dorsal urethrostomy is performed. The graft is spread fixed to the corpora cavernosa. Note the pie-crusting incision. (C) The edges of the stricturotomy are sutured to the graft and to the corpora cavernosa.

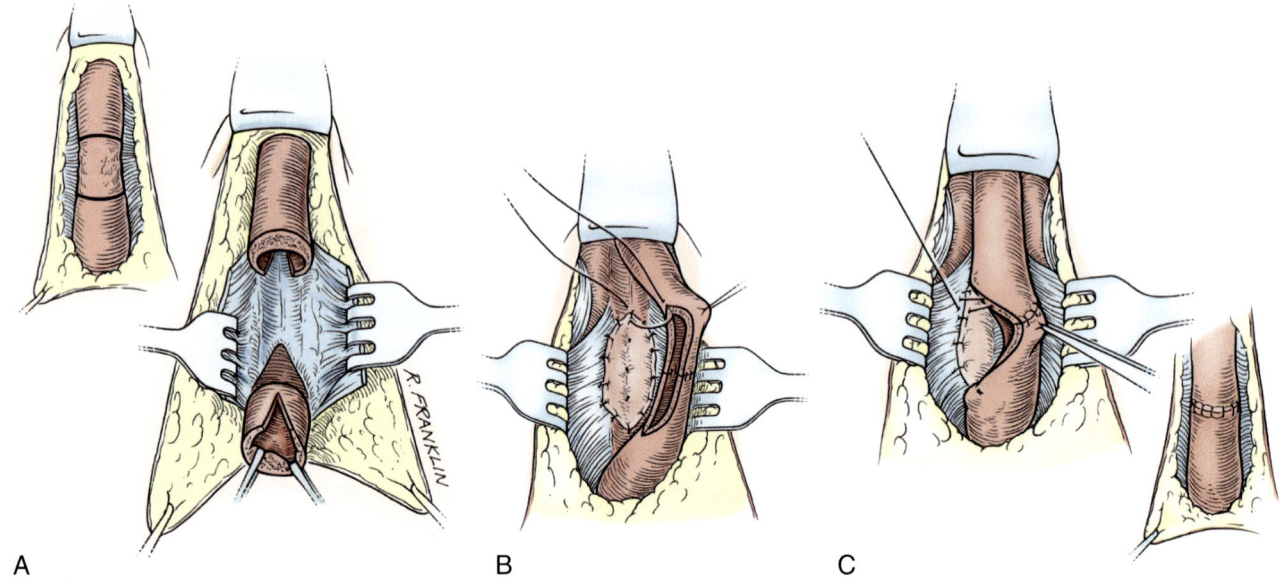

Fig. 82.24. Technique of augmented anastomosis with graft onlay. (A) The corpus spongiosum is detached from the triangular ligament and the corpora cavernosa. The area of spongiofibrosis is identified and marked, and the area of the narrowest caliber stricture is excised. The urethral ends are spatulated on the dorsum. (B) A two-layer floor strip anastomosis is performed, and the graft is spread fixed to the corpora cavernosa. Note the pie-crusting incisions and the mattress sutures. (C) The edges of the stricturotomy are sutured to the graft and to the corpora cavernosa.

vasculature of the flap, and the mechanics of flap transfer. The skin must be nonhirsute for urethral reconstruction. **In addition, for donor site consideration, it is most convenient to use the areas of redundant nonhirsute genital skin.**

If the redundancy is dorsal, the skin island can be oriented transversely and mobilized on the dorsal dartos fascia after the techniques described by Duckett and Standoli in 1984 (Fig. 82.26) (Duckett, 1984, 1992; Duckett et al., 1993; El-Kassaby et al., 1986). If there is redundancy of the ventral skin, the skin island can be mobilized as a ventral longitudinal island. These islands can be either vigorously mobilized on a ventrolaterally oriented dartos fascial flap for transposition to the perineum or less vigorously mobilized and transposed and inverted into a pendulous urethral stricture defect (Fig. 82.27; Orandi, 1972). Ventral islands can be oriented transversely (Fig. 82.28) and longitudinally. Longer skin islands can be mobilized by orienting the island ventrally and transversely at the distal extent. This "hockey stick" orientation allows islands 7 to 9 cm (Fig. 82.29). For distal strictures of the anterior urethra, including

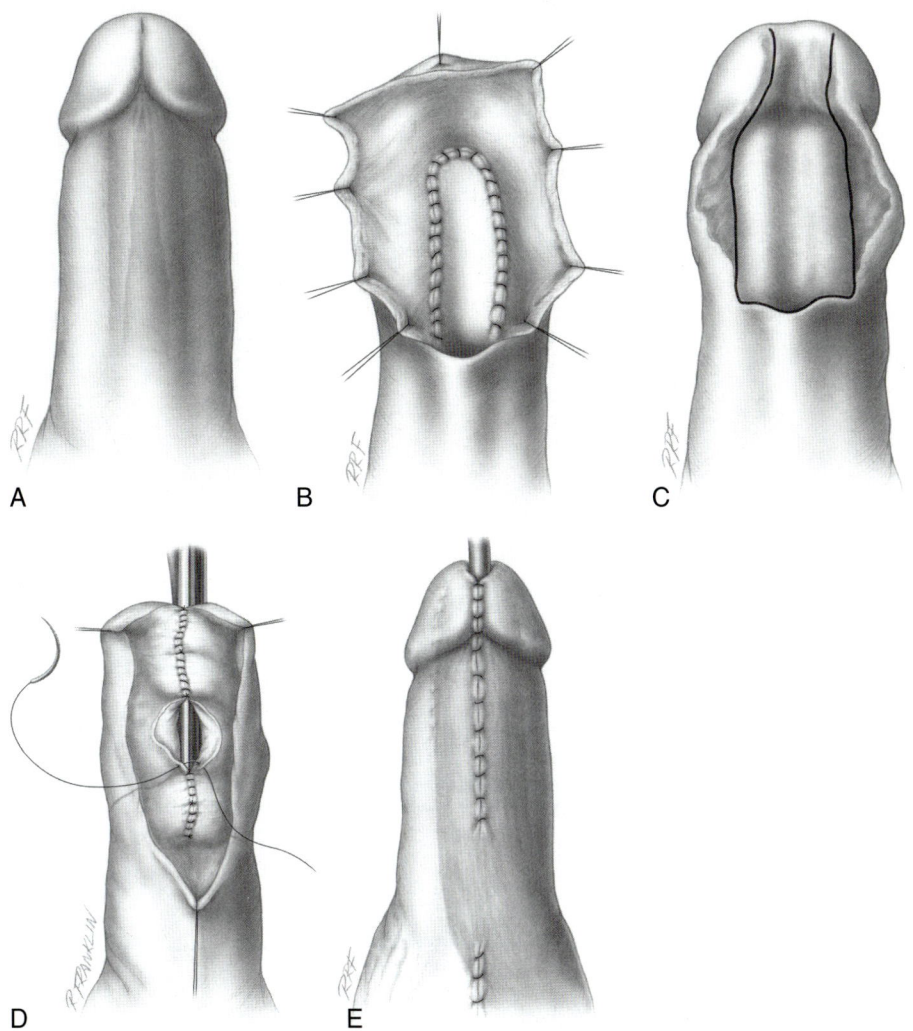

Fig. 82.25. Staged reconstruction of a distal anterior urethral stricture. (A) The appearance of the penis with the urethra (shaded area shows the location of a tight stenosis of the fossa navicularis that extends into the distal pendulous urethra). (B) The distal narrow stricture of the fossa navicularis has been excised, and stricturotomy into the normal urethra proximal to the excised tissue has been performed. A buccal graft has been applied to the defect, but the bolster dressing has not yet been applied. (C) After 6 months, the graft is mature. The illustration shows a Tiersch tube ready for closure. (D) The Tiersch tube is closed with a watertight suture line. The distal urethra is usually calibrated to create a urethral lumen of approximately 28 Fr. (E) Glans reconstruction and closure of the distal shaft has been performed (shaded area shows the tunica dartos flap that carries a parietal tunica vaginalis island). The flap is mobilized in this case from left hemiscrotum and transposed to cover the entire area of the urethral reconstruction.

the fossa and meatus and the pendulous urethra, the islands can be advanced to reconstruct to the level of the meatus by either developing glans wings or elevating the ventral glans.

Where there is general redundancy to the penile skin, the islands can be oriented circumferentially. These "circular skin islands" are mobilized on the entire penile dartos fascia, and the mechanics of transposition suggest that they are most efficient when they are ventrally based, with the pedicle split dorsally. In some cases, circular skin islands 15 cm can be obtained (El-Kassaby et al., 1986; McAninch, 1993; Miller and McAninch, 1993). The so-called Q flap circular island design can provide even longer islands, sometimes necessary for complex long-length anterior urethral reconstruction (Morey et al., 2000).

Augmented Anastomosis. **It is often beneficial to combine the excision of the stricture with a skin island onlay** (Fig. 82.30) **or a graft onlay in an augmented anastomosis** (see Fig. 82.24). We have found that **segments of very narrow caliber (nearly or totally obliterating) are difficult.** These segments can often be completely excised; a roof or floor strip anastomosis of the urethra is performed, and the remaining urethrotomy defect is filled with either a graft or a skin island onlay. In some patients, there are relatively large nonhirsute areas of the scrotal skin that can be elevated on the tunica dartos of the scrotum. This flap has been maligned in the literature in the past. However, we and others have extensive experience with these flaps and, in select cases, have had very good results. The fascial flap must be based laterally, and so oriented, these flaps have been shown to be extremely reliable. Because the tunica dartos has a significant muscle component, the skin island must be carefully tailored. If these skin islands are correctly tailored at the outset, they are not attended with diverticular development as was sometimes believed in the past. Scrotal skin islands are not our first choice; however, for difficult cases, they remain a reasonable option.

These procedures using skin islands oriented on the penile dartos fascia have also been useful for reconstruction of the fossa navicularis (Armenakas et al., 1998; Blandy and Tresidder, 1967; Brannen, 1976; Cohney, 1963; De Sy, 1984; Jordan, 1987). In the past, meatal

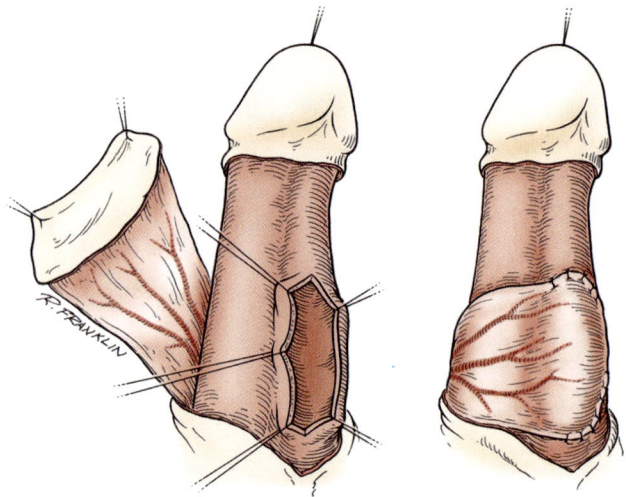

Fig. 82.26. A dorsal transverse island of penile skin applied to a stricture of the urethra. The flap has been elevated on the dartos fascia, and a lateral incision into the urethra has been made. The flap is secured in place *(right)*. (From Jordan GH: Management of anterior urethral stricture disease. In Webster GD, editor: *Problems in urology*, Philadelphia, 1987, Lippincott, p 217.)

strictures and strictures of the fossa navicularis were managed with repeated dilations or sequential meatotomies. Because these meatotomies were seldom successful in the long term, techniques were developed that allowed the spatulation of random penile skin flaps into the meatotomy defects. These procedures functionally improved the results; however, the cosmetic appearance of the penis was suboptimal. With the use of skin islands elevated on the dartos fascia, excellent functional and cosmetic results became the norm. The design of these islands must take into consideration the location of hair on the shaft of the penis and the mechanics of flap transfer (i.e., transposition vs. advancement) (Figs. 82.31 and 82.32). In addition, full-thickness skin has been used to reconstruct the fossa navicularis; however, when they can be avoided, skin grafts are not considered appropriate for reconstruction in cases of LS. As already mentioned, there is question about the use of skin islands in general in patients with LS.

The literature is clear that onlay procedures (graft or flap) are associated with a higher success rate than tubularized grafts or tubularized skin islands (Hendren and Crooks, 1980). **Tubularized grafts and skin islands should be avoided, if possible. When tubularized segments cannot be avoided, the length of these segments can be limited by combining aggressive mobilization and excision. Without question, tubularized flaps provide better results than tubularized grafts.** Where extremely long segments of the anterior urethra require reconstruction, a flap can be used distally and augmented by graft onlay proximally (Wessells et al., 1997). Where tubed reconstruction is required, in a small series with only short follow-up, the combination of a graft spread fixed to reestablish the "urethral plate" with flap onlay seems perhaps to be better than tubed flap reconstruction, even when it is employed in the onlay-tube-onlay configuration (Morey, 2001).

More recently, Kulkarni et al. (2012) published their approach to a single-stage panurethral reconstruction. Through a perineal incision and invaginating the penis, they described using a dorsal graft from the proximal bulbar urethra to the meatus. The mean stricture length was 14 cm, and mean follow-up was 59 months. The overall success rate was 83.7%; for primary repairs, the success rate was 86.5% compared with 61.5% in patients who failed a previous urethroplasty. Most of the recurrences the authors described were proximal.

A flap procedure that can be used as an alternative to STSGs when nonhirsute skin is unavailable is the epilated midline genital skin island. Similar to a STSG, this procedure must be viewed as a staged procedure, with the epilations being the initial stage or stages.

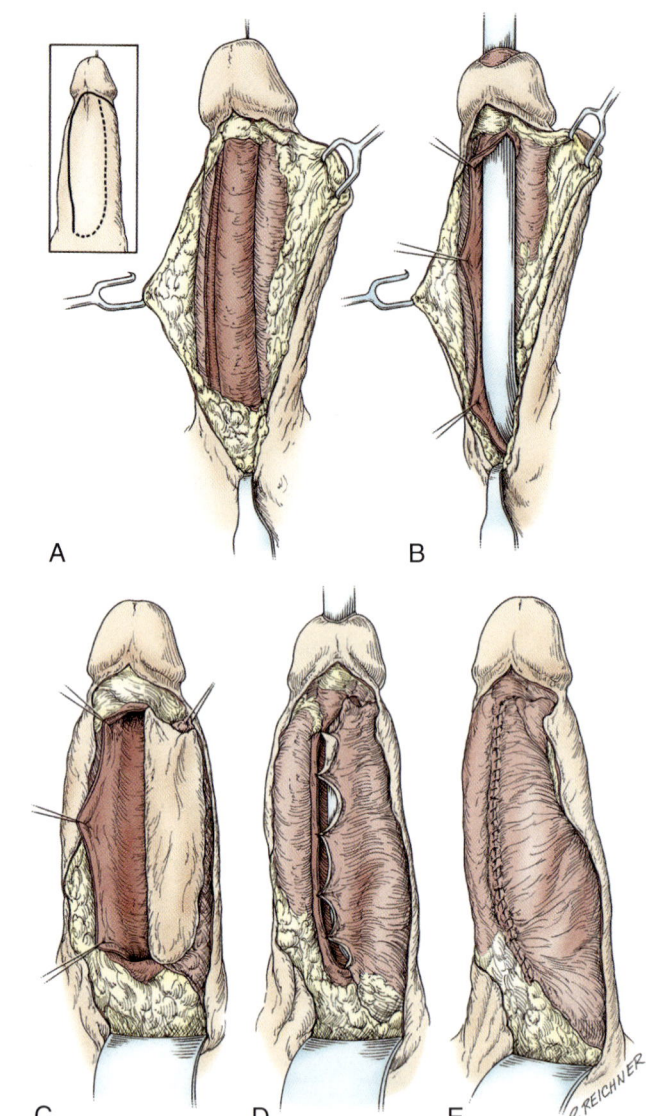

Fig. 82.27. Penile longitudinal skin island. The incisions to be made to mobilize the flap are demonstrated in the *inset*. The heavy line is the primary incision made full thickness through the dartos fascia and superficial Buck fascia lateral to the corpus spongiosum. (A) Dissection elevates the dartos fascial flap well past the corpus spongiosum in the midline. (B) A lateral urethrostomy placed to face the flap has opened the entire length of the stricture. (C) The skin paddle of the flap has been developed by making the incision outlined by the dotted line *(inset)* and undermining the skin lateral to it. The medial edge of the flap has been fixed to the edge of the stricturotomy. (D) The flap is inverted into the defect. (E) A watertight subepithelial suture line has been completed with a running absorbable monofilament suture. The skin will be closed with subcutaneous sutures and interrupted cutaneous sutures. (From Jordan GH: Management of anterior urethral stricture disease. In Webster GD, editor: *Problems in urology*, Philadelphia, 1987, Lippincott, p 214.)

Epilation can be accomplished with either a narrow-gauge needle and monopolar cautery or epilation needles and machines. The interval between the epilations must be 6 to 8 weeks, and urethral reconstruction cannot be accomplished until 10 to 12 weeks after the last epilation. The actual stricture repair involves elevation of the midline skin island, based on the dartos fascia of the penis and the tunica dartos of the scrotum. As with nonhirsute scrotal skin islands in general, the importance of meticulous tailoring of the scrotal portion of the island cannot be overemphasized.

Mundy (1994) analyzed a large series of urethral reconstructions. His data showed that when follow-up is limited to 1 year, the

Fig. 82.28. A ventral transverse skin island is elevated on the penile dartos fascia, inverted to the area of the perineum where flap onlay is accomplished. (A) The skin island is elevated on the dartos fascia. (B) The appearance of the flap transposed to the area of the perineum for onlay in a proximal bulbous urethral stricture.

Fig. 82.29. Ventral skin island for long bulbous stricture. The skin paddle of the flap is developed on the ventral midline of the penis and can be extended around the penile shaft at its distal end. (A) The paddle of the flap has been incised, and its pedicle has been elevated. This pedicle includes Buck fascia and dartos fascia, denuding the tunica of the corpus spongiosum and the corpora cavernosa. The pedicle (the dartos fascia bilaterally) is based on the superficial external pudendal vessels and the internal pudendal vessels in the scrotum. Development of this pedicle allows the flap to be moved to any area of the urethra. (B) The flap has been passed through a tunnel beneath the scrotum developed by dissection along the corpus spongiosum. A laterally placed urethrostomy has opened the urethral stricture. (C) The deep edge of the flap is secured by the suture techniques previously described. (D) Anastomosis of the flap has been completed. The pedicle can be seen extending beneath the scrotum. (From Jordan GH, McCraw JB: Tissue transfer techniques for genitourinary surgery, part III. *AUA Update Series* 7:lesson 11, 1988.)

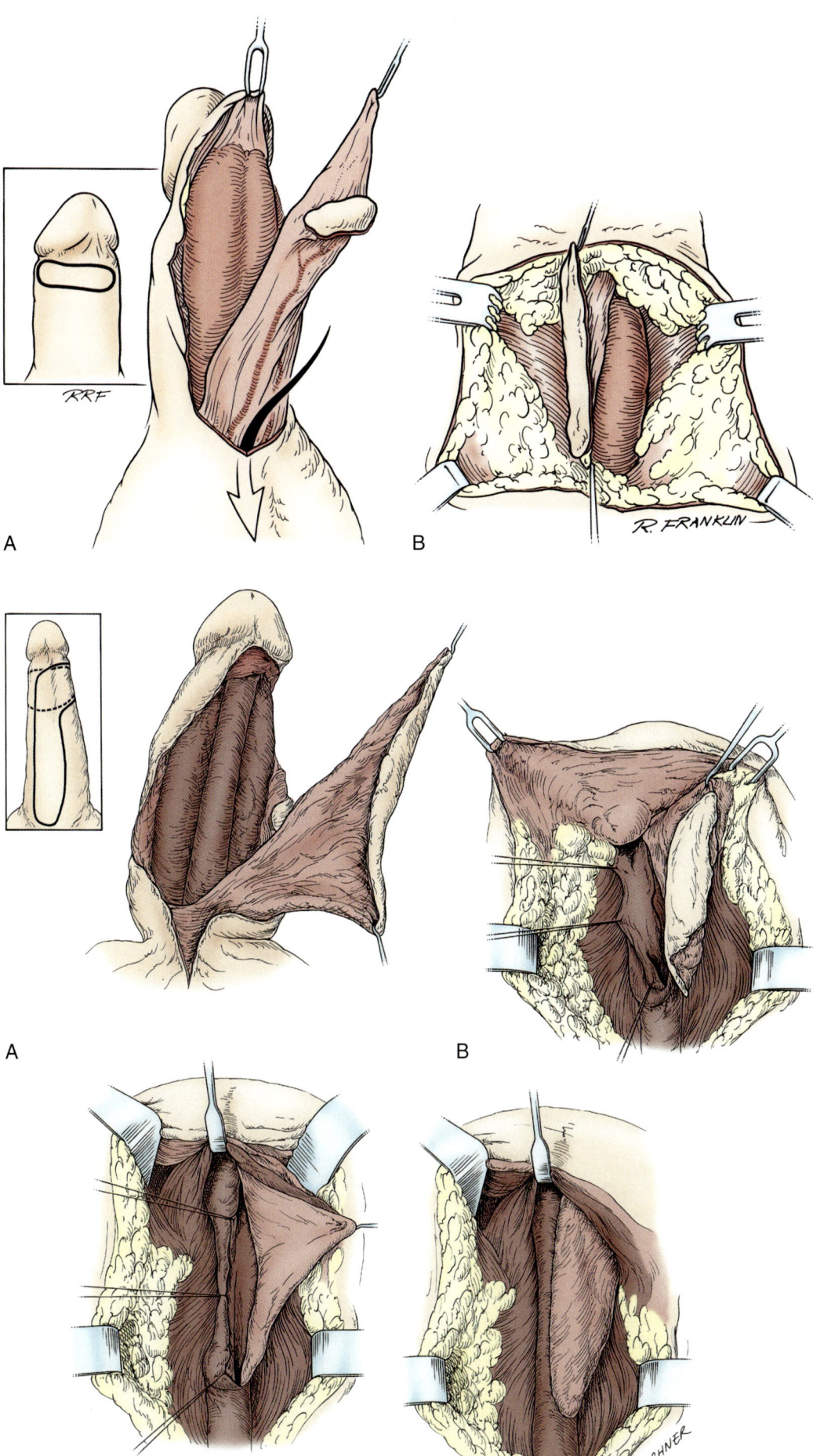

1826 PART VII Male Genitalia

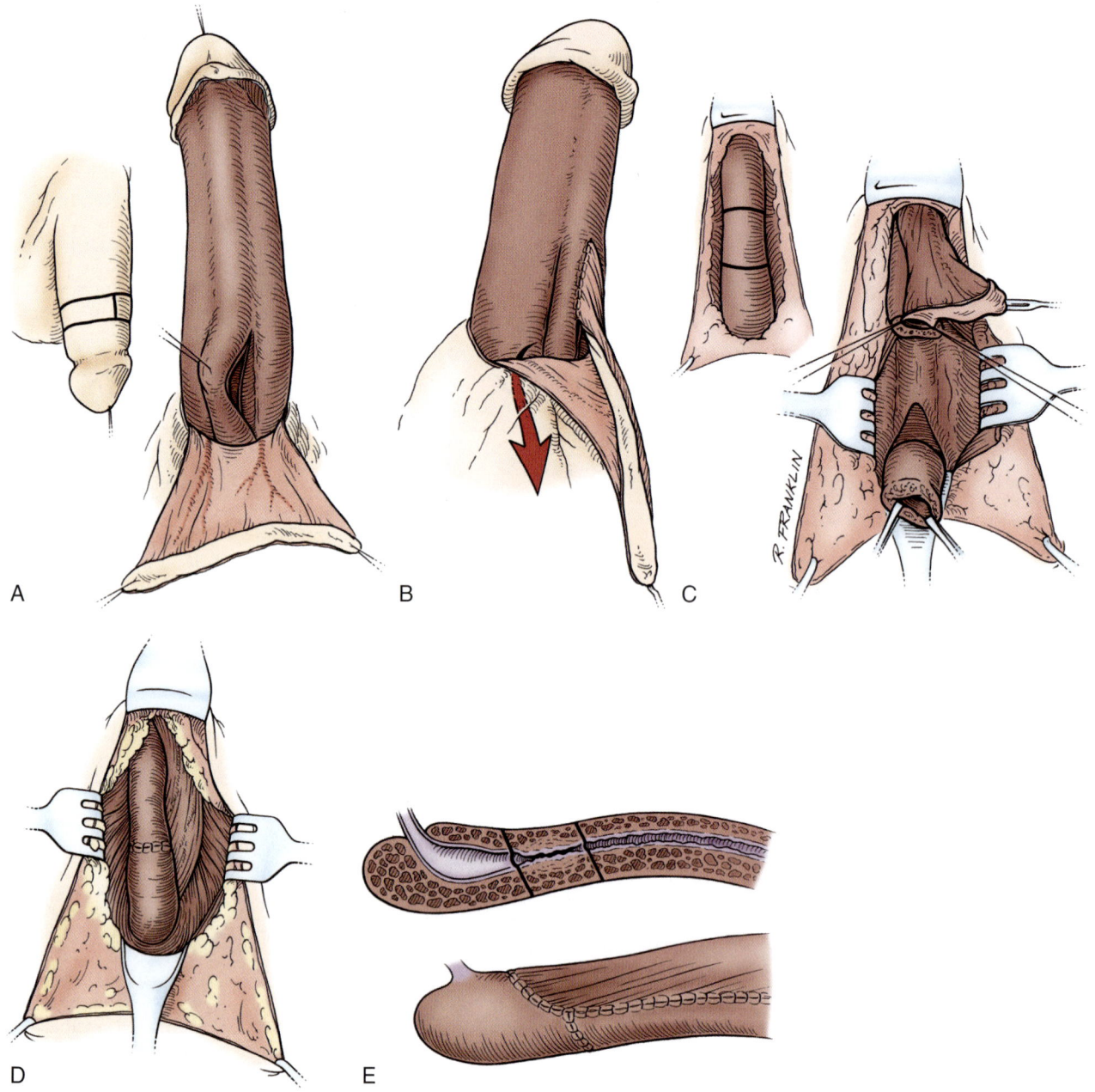

Fig. 82.30. Reconstruction in a patient with a long anterior urethral stricture with a relatively short narrow-caliber section (technique of augmented anastomosis with circular skin island). (A) A circular skin island is elevated on the dartos fascia. The patient is positioned flat on the table. (B) The skin island onlay is begun, the rest of the flap is placed into the perineal dissection, and the penis is closed; the patient is then repositioned in the lithotomy position. (C) The flap is retrieved through the perineal dissection. The narrow-caliber section is excised, and the urethra is spatulated on the dorsum. (D) The onlay is completed, and the floor strip anastomosis is closed. (E) Schematic of the surgery. (From Stack RS, Schlossberg SM, Jordan GH: Reconstruction of anterior urethral strictures by the technique of excision and primary anastomosis. *Atlas Urol Clin North Am* 5:11–21, 1997.)

success rate with tissue transfer clusters is about 95%. However, with longer follow-up, there is deterioration over time. **With excision and primary anastomosis, the success seen at 1 year seems to be more durable and does not appear to deteriorate at the same rate with time.** We have reported our long-term data for excision and primary anastomosis with anterior urethral stenosis in 220 patients with a mean follow-up of 44 months; three recurrences were noted, two within the first 6 months and a third at 4 years. The rate of postoperative ED is 2%, with patients with severe straddle injuries being at increased risk. **In a meta-analysis of graft onlay procedures compared with flap procedures, Wessells and McAninch (1998) showed equivalent results for graft operations and flap procedures,** and graft onlay procedures are technically far easier to perform. There are some cases in which flap reconstruction would be expected to provide superior results (i.e., radiation strictures, patients with multiple operations, pendulous strictures). However, with the increased knowledge gained by the enthusiastic application of graft reconstruction, a paradigm for anterior reconstruction has been redefined. Although grafts have been used successfully for all segments of the anterior urethra, many authors think that, all other

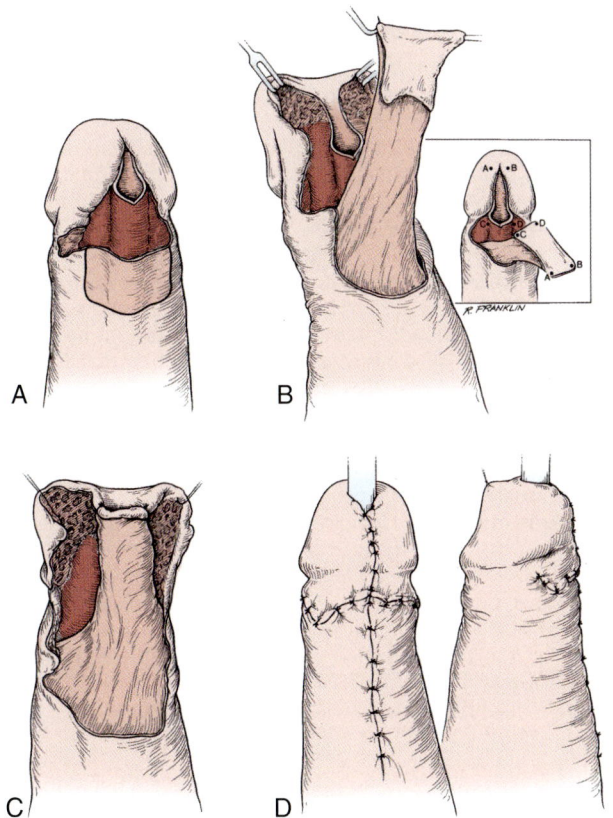

Fig. 82.31. Technique of reconstruction of the fossa navicularis after Jordan. (A) The ventral corpus spongiosum is exposed, and the urethra is opened ventrally through the area of stenosis. A transverse ventral skin island is outlined on the distal penile skin. (B) The skin island is elevated on the ventral dartos fascia. (C) The skin island is transposed and inverted into the meatotomy defect *(inset, B)*. (D) Appearance of the penis closed after the procedure. (A to C, From Jordan GH: Reconstruction of the fossa navicularis. *J Urol* 138:1210, 2987. D, From Jordan GH: Reconstruction of the meatus–fossa navicularis using flap techniques. In Schreiter F, editor: *Plastic-reconstructive surgery in urology*, Stuttgart, 1999, Georg Thieme pp 338–344.)

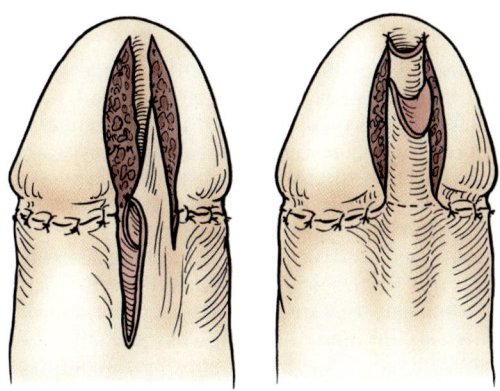

Fig. 82.32. Technique after De Sy, in which a ventral longitudinal skin island is advanced into the meatotomy defect. The skin island is developed by de-epithelialization of a portion of the longitudinal flap. (From Jordan GH: Management of anterior urethral stricture disease. *Probl Urol* 1:199–225, 1987.)

variables being equivalent, flaps are best suited for distal reconstruction, and grafts are best for proximal reconstruction (Greenwell et al., 1999).

Postoperative ED is an important issue. Our rates for anterior urethral anastomotic reconstruction were quoted earlier. **In an analysis by Coursey et al. (2001), 200 patients who underwent urethroplasty were studied. Overall, the rate of ED after urethroplasty was approximately equal to the rate after circumcision. Longer-segment reconstructions were associated with a higher risk of postoperative ED, although the patient's erectile function improved over time in many cases.**

Special mention is needed regarding reconstruction for strictures associated with LS. With the advent of flap techniques, many centers embraced these techniques for these strictures. However, analysis of results from patients with LS treated at several large centers showed a very high recurrence rate. Consequently, these centers adjusted the techniques by applying staged graft techniques (see Fig. 82.25). Staged graft techniques using skin grafts also had a very high recurrence rate in many analyses. **Theoretically, because LS is a skin condition, the use of skin as a flap, single-stage graft, or staged graft does not preclude involvement of the skin with the inflammatory process** (Akporiaye et al., 1997; Lee and Phillips, 1994). **Surgeons at numerous centers believe that staged oral graft techniques should be employed for reconstruction of strictures associated with LS.** Short-term follow-up results suggest better success with this approach. Long-term follow-up results are unavailable. In a review of our experience in patients with a fossa navicularis stricture and LS, we noted a 50% recurrence in the stricture with a ventral transverse skin island (Virasoro et al., 2007).

Perineal Urethrostomy. Complex urethral strictures resulting from LS, previous failed reconstructions, or failed hypospadias repairs are among the most challenging problems, requiring surgical expertise and good clinical judgment to select the appropriate intervention (Myers et al., 2011). These patients usually have a long history of multiple urethral instrumentations, urethral reconstructions or both. Particularly those patients with multiple failed hypospadias repairs or LS can be emotionally devastated; sexual function is diminished and quality of life is negatively affected (Barbagli et al., 2010; Kulkarni et al., 2009). Referral to reconstructive centers often occurs after many options have been exhausted, and appropriate procedure selection is paramount. Pananterior urethral reconstruction with multiple grafts, in one or more stages, is technically feasible and has fair success rates but may not be the optimal solution for these patients (Dubey et al., 2005). In addition, in elderly patients with significant comorbidities and high surgical risk, a complex and prolonged reconstructive surgery may not be indicated. Even for healthy and/or young patients, staged reconstruction may not represent the best option, because success rates are decreased in this group with multiple failed urethroplasties (Myers et al., 2011). For those patients a simpler and more effective urethral procedure such as perineal urethrostomy (PU) may be appropriate. The creation of a perineal urinary diversion is simple and effective (Myers and McAninch, 2011). Challenging cases are those patients who have stricture disease that continues into the proximal bulbar and/or the membranous urethra. In these instances, traditional PU cannot be successfully performed. In addition, patients with prior pelvic radiation and history of LS have a higher rate of restricture at the PU (Levine et al., 2007; Myers et al., 2011). PU creation using BMG is an alternative for these patients. This technique allows the surgeon to bring the urethrostomy to the surface of the perineum instead of burying the skin to the urethral opening. In addition, by inserting tissue into the neomeatus, it decreases the probability of circumferential scarring of the urethrostomy (Kamat, 2008). Our group, in abstract form, previously described this method (Davies et al., 2008), and more recently a combined series was published (DeLong et al., 2017).

The patient is repositioned into high lithotomy. The lower abdomen, genitalia, and perineum are prepped with betadine solution and draped in the usual fashion. An inverted U incision is created and deepened, and the bulbospongiosus muscle is identified and divided in the midline. Corpus spongiosum is freed from the triangular ligament proximally and from the corpora cavernosa distally. Once the necessary mobilization is achieved, the corpus spongiosum is transected transversely and a dorsal urethrotomy is made until healthy mucosa is encountered.

Adequate mobilization allows a healthy ventral urethra to be brought out to perineal skin rather than creating a channel comprising inwardly mobilized skin. Normal urethral mucosa is visualized, and proximal calibration of the lumen is determined with bougie à boule to 30 Fr. The distal urethra is closed and allowed to retract.

At our most recent series (Delong et al., 2017) a total of 44 patients met inclusion criteria. Mean patient age was 60 (range 44–81) years. All strictures were panurethral. Causes were unknown in 16 patients (36%), failed hypospadias repair in 6 (14%), LS in 10 (23%), iatrogenic in 7 (16%), Fournier in 3 (7%), urethral cancer in 1 (2%), and penile cancer in 1 (2%). Mean follow-up was 45 (range 6–136) months. Overall success was 80%; 9 patients recurred, of which 4 had a successful revision, 2 are awaiting potential revision, and 3 are being managed with periodic dilations.

Complex anterior urethral strictures involving the proximal bulbous urethra represent a challenging problem. BMG perineal urethrostomy is a reproducible, viable alternative in appropriately selected patients with encouraging midterm results.

KEY POINTS: URETHRAL STRICTURE

- The term *urethral stricture* refers to anterior urethral disease and is a scarring process that involves the epithelium and the spongy erectile tissue of the corpus spongiosum. Contraction of the scar reduces the urethral lumen. Posterior urethral strictures are more correctly referred to as PFUIs; strictures of the prostatic urethra or bladder neck are properly referred to as contractures or stenoses.
- The anterior urethra is invested by the corpus spongiosum, and, as it proceeds proximally, it is eccentrically placed in relation to the corpus spongiosum. The genital skin has a dual and bilateral blood supply, forming a fasciocutaneous vascular system. The vascularity of the corpus spongiosum is based on the common penile artery.
- In general, most anterior urethral strictures are the result of trauma. Inflammatory strictures associated with gonorrhea are rarely seen; however, strictures associated with LS have behavior similar to inflammatory strictures.
- Patients who have urethral strictures most often have obstructive voiding symptoms or urinary tract infections such as prostatitis and epididymitis. Patients with urinary retention, on close inquiry, have tolerated notable voiding obstructive symptoms for a long time.
- To devise an appropriate treatment plan, it is important to determine the length, location, depth, and density of the spongiofibrosis. This determination can be done with a combination of contrast-enhanced studies, endoscopy, and selective ultrasonography. It is imperative to evaluate the urethra completely proximal and distal to the stricture with endoscopy. A pediatric cystoscope is useful.

KEY POINTS: TREATMENT OF URETHRAL STRICTURE

- In the treatment of urethral stricture disease, the patient and the physician must have a good understanding of the goals of treatment before the treatment choice is made.
- Urethral dilation is the oldest and simplest treatment of urethral stricture disease. However, the goal of dilation is to stretch the scar atraumatically. Dilation is seldom used curatively.
- Internal urethrotomy refers to any procedure that opens the stricture by incising it transurethrally. The factors that contribute to success of internal urethrotomy have been defined as follows: internal urethrotomy should be reserved for strictures of the bulbous urethra; the stricture should be less than 1.5 cm in length; and the stricture should not be associated with dense deep spongiofibrosis. Many studies have shown that repeated dilation and internal urethrotomies diminish the success rate of eventual open urethral reconstruction.
- Numerous lasers have been used for anterior urethral strictures. The results of laser urethrotomy are mixed.
- Excision with primary anastomosis has proven to be the gold standard for repair of anterior urethral strictures. Previously, excision with primary anastomosis was thought to be a relatively limited procedure and applicable only for strictures smaller than 1.5 to 2 cm. However, with better understanding of the anatomy, longer strictures have been successfully addressed with excision and primary anastomosis.
- Some strictures require tissue transfer, and grafts and flaps have been successfully employed. A meta-analysis by Wessells and McAninch (1998) showed that the results of graft reconstruction and flap reconstruction are equivalent. The complexity of flap procedures is greater than that of graft procedures. The concept of augmented anastomosis can be used with graft and flap onlay and is thought to provide better results than just pure onlay in many cases. When flaps are employed for urethral reconstruction, conceptually all become one operation with multidimensional application.
- Perineal urethrostomy is a viable option in selected patients, and the addition of BMG may be useful in those with very proximal bulbar strictures.

PELVIC FRACTURE URETHRAL INJURIES

PFUIs are the result of blunt pelvic trauma and accompany about 10% of pelvic fracture injuries. Although total disruption of the urethra is possible with a straddle injury, these injuries most commonly involve only the bulbous urethra. However, the ensuing spongiofibrosis can be associated with complete obliteration of the urethra. **Distraction injuries are unique to the membranous urethra.** Pelvic fracture distraction injuries of the membranous urethra have been compared with plucking an apple (prostate) off its stem (the membranous urethra). This analogy implies that the injury most frequently occurs at the apex of the prostate. However, experience shows that this is not the case, and the most frequent point of distraction is at the departure of the bulbous urethra from the membranous urethra (Andrich and Mundy, 2001; Mouraviev and Santucci, 2005). The distraction can involve all or any portion of the membranous urethra between the departure of the bulbous urethra and the apex of the prostate. In postpubescent male patients, the injury seldom involves the prostatic urethra. In prepubescent male patients in whom the prostatic urethra is more fragile, the injury can extend into that area.

Total distraction of the entire circumference of the urethra appears not to occur with many injuries. Instead, a strip of epithelium is left intact. In these patients, the placement of an aligning catheter may allow the urethra to heal virtually unscarred or with an easily managed stenosis. Because of flexible endoscopy equipment, the placement of an aligning catheter is straightforward. If distraction is complete, the catheter aligns the obliterated urethral ends, and reconstruction is facilitated. Because of the ready availability of flexible cystoscopes, some centers acutely evaluate these injuries only with endoscopy. Clinicians who are enthusiastic for this approach believe that not only can the injury be completely evaluated but also the entire process, including the placement of an aligning catheter, is expedited (Kielb et al., 2001). **Aligning catheters are just what the name implies—a guide, not a mechanism for placing traction on the bladder and prostate.** Aligning catheters also seem to act as a drain as the pelvic hematoma liquefies, and perhaps the presence of the catheter may allow more rapid and complete resolution of the process (Cohen et al., 1991; Herschorn et al., 1992; Mouraviev et al., 2005; Rehman et al., 1998). Close follow-up after a voiding trial is essential because many of these patients experience stricture formation after removal of the aligning catheter and require definitive repair (Leddy et al., 2012). Some patients who have undergone primary endoscopic realignment have delayed surgical repair and increased unsuccessful endoscopic treatments, which has led some to recommend against its routine use (Tausch et al., 2014).

Evaluation

As with the repair of any stricture or stenosis, it is important to define the precise anatomy of the pelvic fracture injury before treatment is undertaken (McCallum and Colapinto, 1979a, 1979b); this includes the depth, density, length, and location. In pelvic fracture urethral distraction defects, the depth and density of fibrosis are predictable. Although the location of the distraction injury has been shown to be an important factor in continence after reconstruction, this information should be a factor only in counseling of patients before the reconstruction and not in the treatment approach. The length of the defect is an important consideration and must be determined as precisely as possible.

Contrast studies are a first-line tool for the evaluation of PFUI. A cystogram outlines the bladder and provides information about rostral displacement of the proximal urethra. A lack of contrast material in the posterior urethra gives some information, albeit inconclusive, about the integrity of the bladder neck.

When the patient is successful in relaxing to void and the cystogram outlines the posterior urethra, a simultaneous retrograde urethrogram outlines the length of the injury defect. However, this situation is the exception rather than the rule, and retrograde urethrography is most useful for determining whether the anterior urethra is normal. If the anterior urethra is normal, **a successful anastomotic repair is ensured, from our experience and that of others.** A primary anastomosis has been demonstrated possible even with some involvement of the anterior urethra. Even in cases of prior failed posterior urethral reconstruction, primary anastomotic repair is often feasible, although the failure rate is slightly higher in these cases (Chapple and Pang, 1999; Flynn et al., 2003; Koraitim, 2003; Shenfeld et al., 2004). **Primary anastomosis is unquestionably the goal in all patients until it is proven impossible to perform.**

When the proximal urethra is not visualized on a simultaneous cystogram with urethrogram, endoscopy through the suprapubic tract in combination with retrograde urethrography can be used to outline the defect. After the endoscopic appearance of the bladder neck is assessed, the flexible endoscope can be advanced through the bladder neck and into the posterior urethra to the level of the obstruction. **The appearance of the bladder neck on contrast studies or on antegrade endoscopy does not accurately predict the ultimate function of the bladder neck after urethral reconstruction** (Iselin and Webster, 1999). A simultaneous retrograde urethrogram outlines the anterior urethra, with the space not visualized representing the injury defect.

Some authors have advocated MRI for the evaluation of patients with PFUIs. We have had little experience with MRI for that purpose; however, we have found the information obtained on the few studies that we have done to be useful. In these cases, there was the question of bone interposition into the injury defect, and MRI outlined this. We evaluated a case in which the prostatic urethra appeared obliterated. On MRI, one could easily see that the prostate was not only distracted from the membranous urethra but also distracted from the bladder. This information was essential to planning of subsequent reconstruction in this case. It would seem intuitively obvious that knowing the length of distraction would be helpful in determining the precise approach and steps necessary for reconstruction. However, the literature is unclear on this matter (Andrich et al., 2003; Koraitim, 2004), and the surgeon must be prepared to exercise all options of reconstruction in almost all such cases (McCallum and Colapinto, 1979a, 1979b).

Repair

The timetable for the reconstruction of PFUIs is determined by the type and extent of associated injuries. If possible, it is desirable to proceed within 3 to 6 months after trauma. However, orthopedic injuries of the lower extremities often necessitate a delay in proceeding with urethral reconstruction (Brandes and Borrelli, 2001; Follis et al., 1992; Mundy, 1991).

In most cases, PFUIs are not long, and the resultant obliteration is amenable to a technically straightforward mobilization of the corpus spongiosum with a primary anastomotic technique. The classic reconstruction consists of a spatulated anastomosis of the proximal anterior urethra to the apical prostatic urethra. However, experience has demonstrated that anastomosis of the proximal anterior urethra to any segment of the posterior urethra (apical, prostatic, or below) can be successfully accomplished by a widely spatulated anastomosis in which optimal epithelial apposition is achieved. About 10% of PFUIs are associated with more complex injuries and can be associated with fistulae (most commonly urethral rectal fistulae). Reconstruction of these injuries is technically more demanding.

Several series support the concept that the bulk of PFUIs, even the most difficult cases, can be managed by the perineal approach (Flynn et al, 2003; Koraitim, 1985, 1997; Morey et al., 1996; Webster and Sihelnik, 1985; Webster et al., 1983, 1990). A transpubic or an abdominal-perineal approach, as pioneered by Waterhouse et al. (1973), in our experience, is unnecessary for the reconstruction of distraction injuries. In addition, pubectomy can be associated with long-term sequelae, including shortening of the penis, destabilization of erection, and destabilization of the pelvis, resulting in a chronic pain syndrome with exercise. However, some surgeons continue to rely heavily on the transpubic approach (Das et al., 2004; Koraitim, 1997).

Alternatively, the above-and-below approach has merit when concomitant surgery is planned in the region of the bladder neck. We have found, and Iselin and Webster (1999) reported, that the competence of the bladder neck is difficult to assess accurately before the reestablishment of urethral continuity. In the past, great reliance was placed on whether the bladder neck was closed or open on cystography. However, contrast material may opacify the prostatic urethra when the bladder neck is more than adequately competent for continence. Similarly, confidence has been placed in the appearance of the bladder neck on endoscopic examination through the suprapubic tube. Again, even when an obvious scar is noted to involve the bladder neck, follow-up of these patients after urethral reconstruction establishes continuity of the urethra and finds many patients with more than adequate continence. Other patients are believed to have incontinence secondary to scar incarceration of the bladder neck, caused by the extensive fibrosis left behind by resolution of the hematoma. However, in our experience, this is an infrequent occurrence, and the appearance of the bladder neck by any modality available is not predictive of continence. It is currently our practice to reestablish the continuity of the urethra and, when there are concerns about continence, to forewarn the patient before the urethral reconstruction. If these patients find that they experience inadequate continence postoperatively, the problem is addressed in a subsequent procedure (Bhargava et al., 2004).

At the time of reconstruction, before the patient is placed in the lithotomy position, endoscopy is performed through the meatus and again through the suprapubic tube sinus. Endoscopy on the table is designed to ensure that there is no concomitant vesicolithiasis. The endoscopy is performed with a rigid endoscope, which is manipulated through the suprapubic tube sinus and the bladder neck and positioned against the area of total obliteration. On gentle manipulation of the endoscope, if the impulse of the endoscope tip is felt on the patient's perineum, the impulse is palpable when the perineum is opened, and an instrument is manipulated through the bladder neck during reconstruction. If the impulse is not palpable perineally at this time, it may not be palpable during dissection. If unable to pass the sound easily, the creation of a temporary vesicostomy allows the surgeon to position an instrument reliably through the bladder neck, because it allows the surgeon to identify the bladder neck palpably before instrumentation of the posterior urethra. This maneuver has eliminated the occurrence of false passages with use of a sound such as the Haygrove staff through the suprapubic site and has eliminated the occurrence of anastomosis to false passage.

As we mentioned previously, some centers use the cystoscope for this purpose, and often it suffices well, and even some centers use a hollow Haygrove (Gelman Urethral Sound, CS Surgical) that allows the passage of the flexible cystoscope through to better visualize the bladder neck (Gelman and Wisenbaugh, 2015).

We prefer the use of the exaggerated lithotomy position for the perineal approach (Fig. 82.33). This position is safe and provides

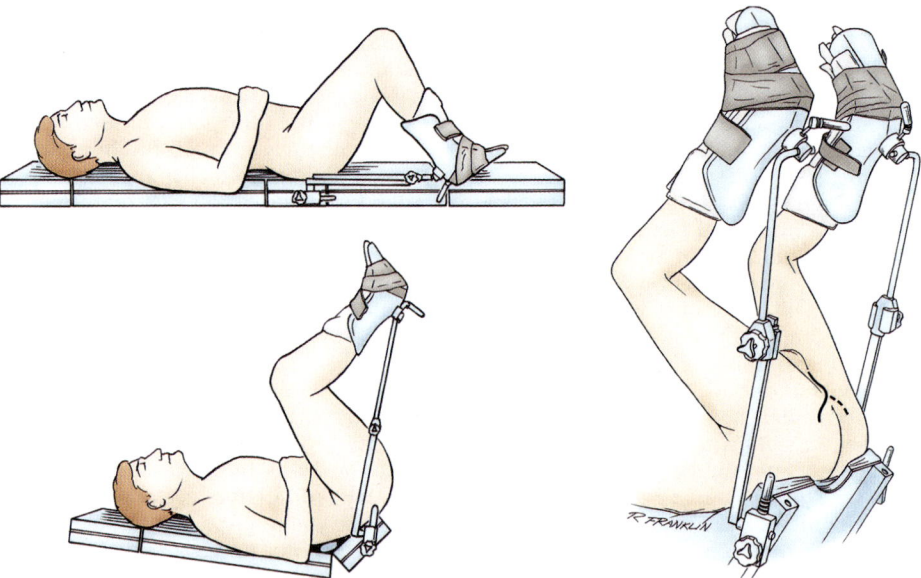

Fig. 82.33. Patient placed in an exaggerated lithotomy position. The hips have been rotated into position by elevation of the buttocks portion of a specially modified table. The legs are suspended from boot-style stirrups with as little flexion of the hips and knees as allowed by the design of the stirrups. (From Angermeier KW, Jordan GH: Complications of the exaggerated lithotomy position: a review of 177 cases. *J Urol* 151:866–868, 1994.)

optimal exposure to the area of the membranous and apical prostatic urethra (Angermeier and Jordan, 1994). The legs are carefully positioned in Allen-style or Guardian-style stirrups. Care is taken to avoid pressure on the lateral aspects of the lower extremities and calf muscles. The patient's hips are elevated into position by raising the buttocks portion of the operating table. The boots are positioned to avoid stretch injuries of the common peroneal nerves (see Fig. 82.33).

After the patient is correctly positioned, the perineal approach to reconstruction begins with an incision and dissection anterior to the transverse perineal musculature (anterior perineal triangle). This is in contrast to the approach posterior to the transverse perineal musculature (posterior anal triangle), which is useful for perineal prostatectomy. We use a λ-shaped incision (Fig. 82.34) that is carried sharply down to the midline fusion of the ischiocavernosus musculature (see Fig. 82.34A), then beneath the scrotum, to expose the uninvested portion of the corpus spongiosum. We then place a self-retaining ring retractor.

The fusion of the ischiocavernosus musculature is divided, and the musculature is cleanly dissected from the corpus spongiosum and bulbospongiosum (see Fig. 82.34B to D). The corpus spongiosum is detached from the triangular ligament and corpora cavernosa (see Fig. 82.34E), the bulbospongiosum is detached from the perineal body, and the dissection is carried farther down to the infrapubic space. Posterior detachment of the bulbospongiosum is carried anteriorly, and the dissection is eventually carried through the area of fibrosis (see Fig. 82.34F).

In some cases, the proximal blood supply is encountered and must be controlled. We have found that these arteries are easily controlled with a sharp-tipped hemostat and monopolar cautery. Suture ligature should be avoided in the arteries to the bulbospongiosum because of their proximity to the nerves as they are coursing into the corpora cavernosa. Recently, vessel sparing repair of a PFUI has been described with good result (Gomez et al., 2016).

We divide the triangular ligament and vigorously develop the intracrural space down to the pubis (Fig. 82.35). If the dorsal vein is encountered, it is ligated and divided. It is important to ensure that the arteries were not rolled into the intracrural space if the tissues were dislocated during trauma. The penetration of the cavernosal arteries or the dorsal arteries, or both, into this space is commonly seen. If there is doubt about the nature of the vessels encountered, Doppler sonography should be performed. When the pubis is exposed, the periosteal elevator can be gently introduced onto the retropubic surface, releasing and allowing the descent of the tissues from beneath the pubis.

We introduce a Haygrove staff into the suprapubic sinus and through the bladder neck to the distal limits of the posterior urethra (see Figs. 82.34G and H). The impulse is palpated, and the fibrosis is resected until normal tissue planes are encountered. The tissue is submitted for histologic examination. The tip of the Haygrove staff is eventually concealed only by the normal urethral epithelium, at which point we open the epithelium and control it with either a skin hook or a stitch. We perform endoscopy to ensure that the urethrotomy is at the distal limits of the posterior urethra. If a tension-free anastomosis is determined impossible, we mobilize the corpus spongiosum beneath the scrotum from its attachment to the corpora cavernosa. Aggressive mobilization of the corpus spongiosum is the last maneuver undertaken because it is thought to have possible ill effects on the retrograde blood supply, which, in a patient with pelvic fracture, may be tenuous. Meticulous detachment of the investment of Buck fascia from the corpus spongiosum increases the compliance of the corpus and limits the need for aggressive mobilization.

The surgeon should try to avoid the creation of chordee during the repair of a distraction injury. To prevent chordee, the attachment cannot be carried beyond the area of the penoscrotal attachment. However, it is warranted in some cases to counsel patients preoperatively that they may have some chordee after aggressive mobilization that results in a primary anastomotic repair. Primary anastomotic repairs have success rates in the high 90% range. If a technique of tissue transfer is needed, the long-term cure rates may eventually be only in the mid-80% range. Most of these patients are young. Successful, durable reconstruction is paramount. If chordee results, it is most often mild and not disabling sexually; it is probably a fair trade for optimizing the urethral reconstruction. Development of the intracrural space—mobilization of the corpus spongiosum, infrapubectomy, and, if needed, rerouting of the corpus spongiosum—shortens the course that the corpus spongiosum must traverse and allows reconstruction without attendant chordee.

The proximal urethrotomy is spatulated so that it accepts at least a 32-Fr bougie à boule, and 10 to 12 anastomotic sutures are placed

Chapter 82 Surgery for Benign Disorders of the Penis and Urethra   1831

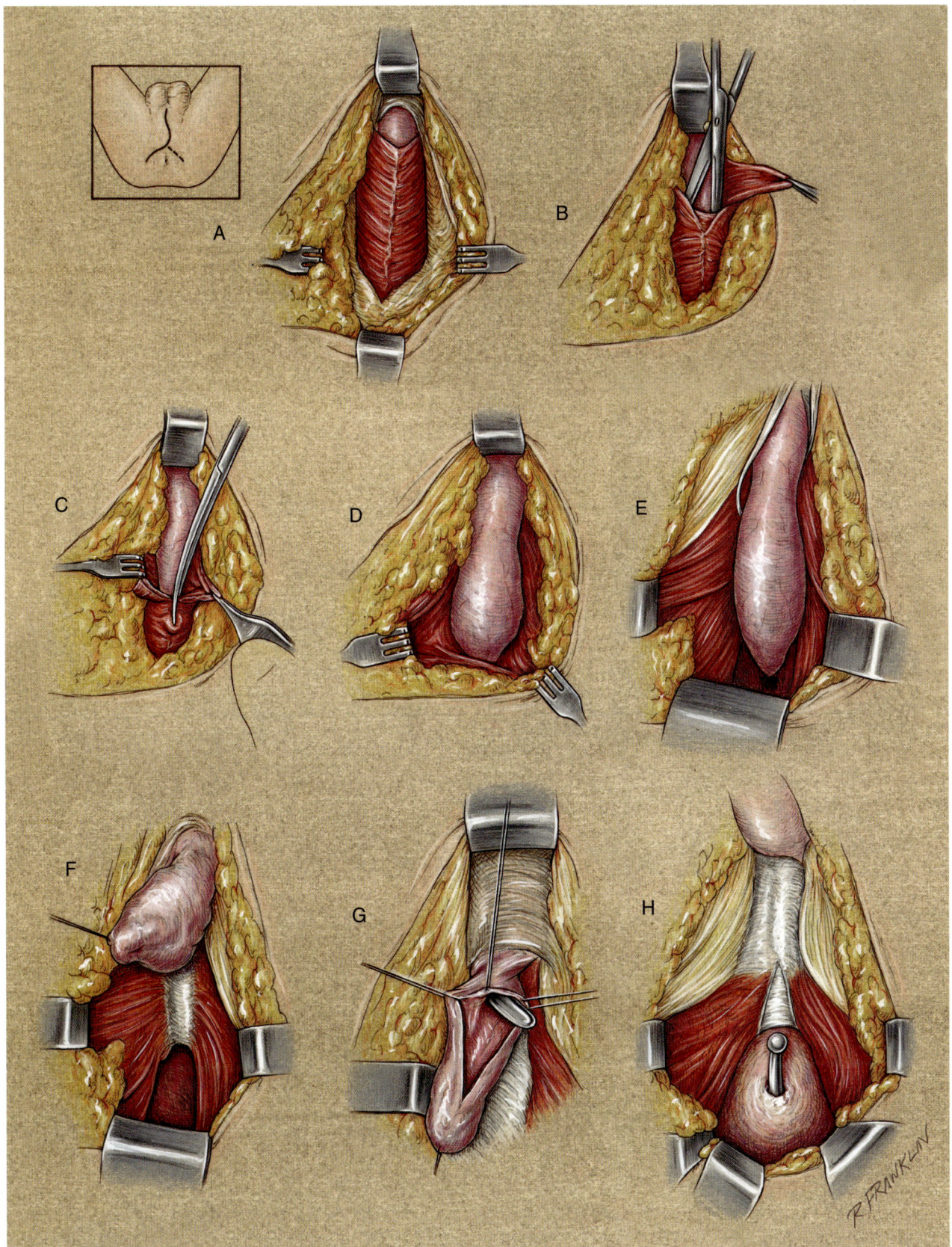

Fig. 82.34. Perineal repair of a membranous urethral stricture. A λ-shaped incision extends from the midline of the scrotum to the ischial tuberosities. (A) Colles fascia has been opened to expose the midline fusion of the ischiocavernosus muscles and the tunica of the corpus spongiosum distal to the edge of the muscles. (B) The scissors are introduced to develop the space between the muscle and the bulb of the urethra. (C) An incision is made in the midline with the scissors, exposing the length of the bulb. (D) The ischiocavernosus muscle is retracted to expose the full length of the bulb. (E) The self-retaining retractor is placed to expose the inferior fascia of the genitourinary diaphragm. The bulb of the corpus spongiosum (bulbospongiosum) can be mobilized to gain access to the fibrosed area of the urethra. (F) The fibrosed urethra is incised, freeing the bulb. (G) The anterior urethra is opened to make an adequate lumen. (H) The Haygrove staff has been passed through the suprapubic cystostomy. Resection of the fibrotic distraction defect has allowed it to pass into the perineum.

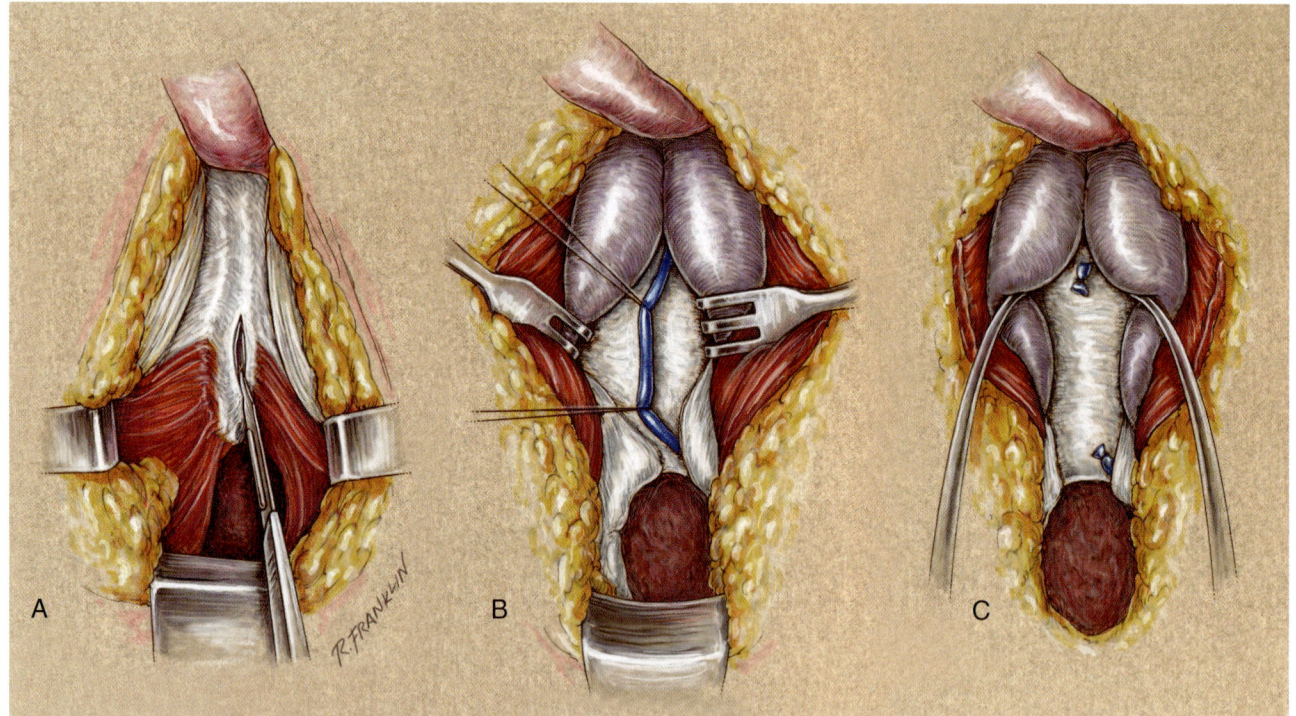

Fig. 82.35. Division of the triangular ligament and development of the intracrural space. (A) When the prostatic urethra is displaced and the arc that the urethra must traverse must be shortened, that length can be shortened by incision of the triangular ligament. (B) Incision and mobilization of the perichondrium and periosteum of the symphysis pubis to allow placement of retractors without trauma to the erectile bodies. Lateral displacement of the crura exposes the dorsal vein of the penis; after careful identification, the vein can be ligated and divided. (C) Completion of the dissection affords additional exposure for resection of the fibrosis that surrounds the apex of the prostate and the proximal end of the disrupted urethra. (From Jordan GH: Reconstruction of the meatus–fossa navicularis using flap techniques. In Schreiter F, editor: *Plastic-reconstructive surgery in urology*, Stuttgart, 1999, Georg Thieme, pp 338–344.)

and tagged to allow identification of their position in the proximal anastomosis. We have used a combination of 3-0 Monocryl and 3-0 polydioxanone sutures for this purpose. No special needles are required for the placement of these sutures. However, a Heaney needle driver and a Ravitch needle driver can be useful in difficult cases. After spatulation of the proximal urethrotomy and placement of the sutures, we spatulate the proximal portion of the anterior urethra. The spatulation is continued until the urethrotomy accepts a 30-Fr to 32-Fr bougie à boule and the anastomotic sutures are placed in their respective locations. Before seating the anastomosis, we introduce a soft silicone (Silastic) ribbed urethral stenting catheter through the anastomosis under direct vision. The wound is copiously irrigated to reduce the clot around the area of the anastomosis, and the anastomosis is seated.

Next, we reattach the corpus spongiosum to the corpora cavernosa and the bulbospongiosum to the perineal body. We place a small suction drain deep to the closure of the ischiocavernosus musculature and Colles fascia and a second one superficial to that closure and beneath the subcutaneous closure.

In cases in which the proximal urethra is significantly distracted in a rostral direction, the surgeon must be prepared to perform infrapubectomy (Fig. 82.36) or corporal rerouting, or both (Fig. 82.37). Performance of the infrapubectomy, along with the development of the intercrural space, allows exposure of the apical prostatic urethra. When the prostatic urethra remains rostrally displaced, the impulse of the sound or instrument placed through the cystostomy tract into the bladder neck is often not readily apparent. In these situations, it is reassuring to be able to palpate the bladder neck and the properly placed sound before embarking on a dissection beneath the pubis. In addition, if the rostral distraction is significant, the path of the anterior urethra over the hilum of the penis into the infrapubectomy often does not allow a tension-free anastomosis, and the infrapubectomy can be continued beneath one side of the corpora cavernosa, allowing rerouting of the corpus spongiosum (see Fig. 82.37).

Postoperative Management

We use a small soft silicone (Silastic) stenting catheter. Urine is diverted via the suprapubic cystostomy, and the urethral catheter is plugged and serves as a stent only. After the reconstruction, patients are initially kept in the hospital for 24 to 48 hours and then ambulated and discharged. Patients are discharged on a regimen of oxybutynin and a suppressive antibiotic only if the preoperative urine culture was positive.

A voiding trial with contrast material is performed between 21 and 28 days postoperatively. Patients are directed to stop taking oxybutynin 24 hours before the voiding trial. In anastomoses that are technically straightforward, the trial is performed at 21 days, and in cases with more rostral distraction of the proximal urethra, the trial is delayed for 3 to 5 days longer. The trial involves removing the urethral catheter, filling the patient's bladder with contrast material, and instructing him to void. We do not use pericatheter retrograde urethrography to evaluate patients who have undergone urethral reconstruction. The voiding film is examined to ensure that there is no extravasation and that the reanastomosis appears widely patent. A urine culture specimen is also obtained. Approximately 6 months postoperatively the patients are evaluated with flexible endoscopy. At that time, we consider the reconstruction to be mature, and it should be widely patent.

We have almost completely replaced postoperative retrograde studies with flexible endoscopy.

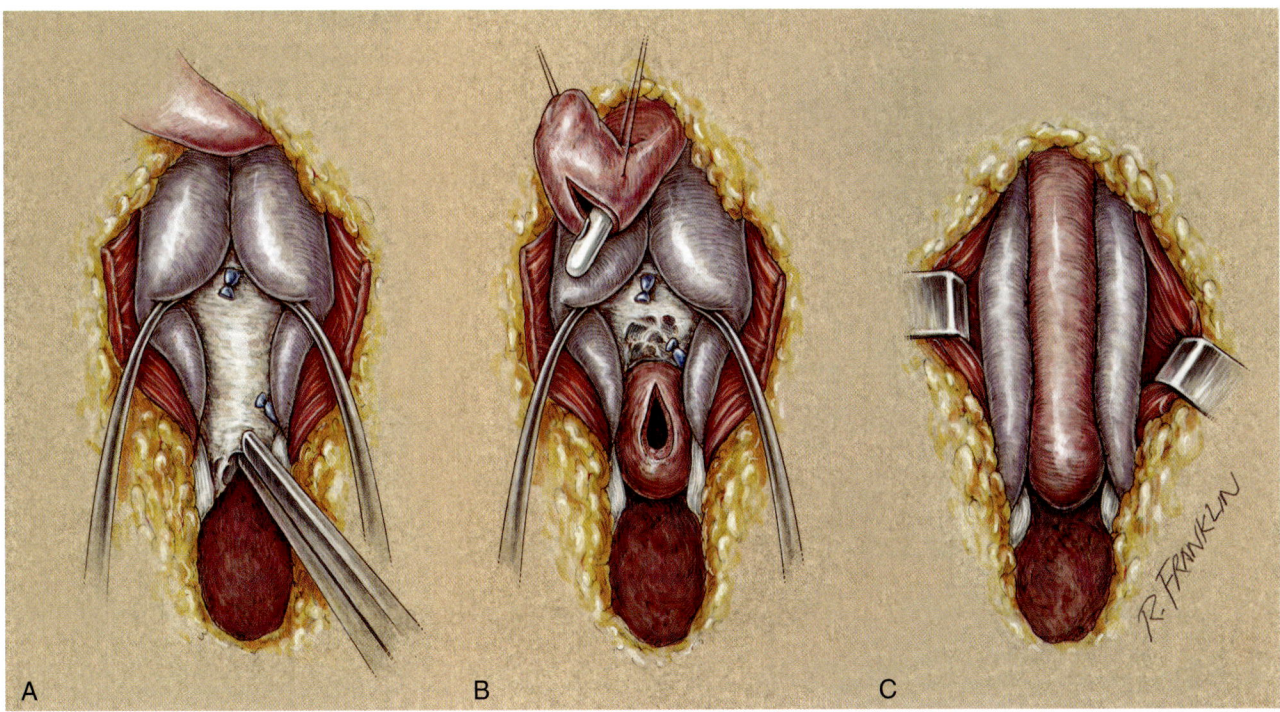

Fig. 82.36. Infrapubectomy. If the prostate is elevated behind the symphysis pubis (A), the inferior aspect of the symphysis is resected with a Kerrison rongeur. As much of the bone can be removed as necessary (B) to afford a simple approximation of the ends of the urethra (C).

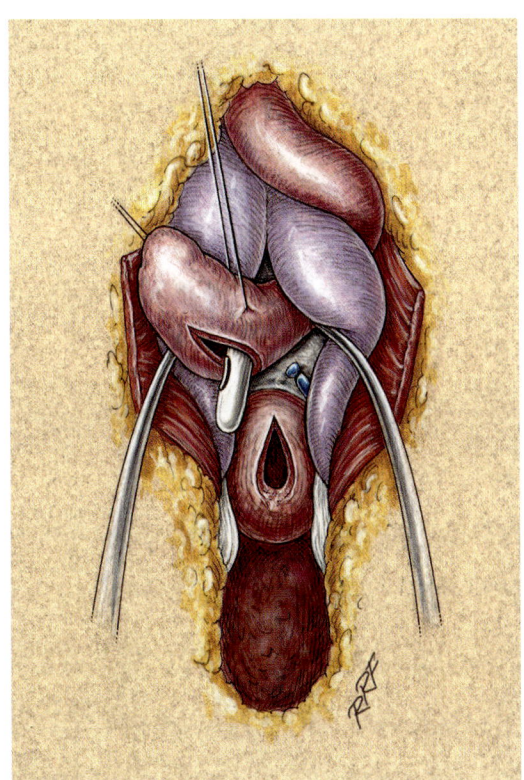

Fig. 82.37. Resection of the pubis and rerouting of the urethra around the crus. When the prostate is markedly displaced, it may be necessary to expand the infrapubectomy. Sometimes, despite separation of the crura to the full extent possible, the two ends of the urethra do not meet when they are brought directly through the crus. It is necessary to bring the urethra lateral to one of the crura to make up this length.

With the use of the techniques discussed or similar techniques, curative rates for reconstruction of posterior PFUIs are in the high 90% range. In large centers, failures are not due to technical problems (i.e., anastomotic restenosis). In general, **failures are indicative of ischemia of the proximal corpus spongiosum with ensuing stenosis of the mobilized corpus spongiosum.** This occurs because, with mobilization, the corpus spongiosum, in essence, becomes a flap with the vascular pedicle being the retrograde vascularity from the arborization of the dorsal arteries through the glans (Fig. 82.38).

We have studied this phenomenon in trauma patients and have arrived at conclusions that we believe allow us to predict the patients at risk for this ischemic atrophy phenomenon. Initially, we used pudendal angiography to study all trauma patients who seemed to be at risk for bilateral deep internal pudendal artery injury at the time of trauma. These were patients who had evidence of injury to the dorsal penile nerves, patients in whom reconstruction had failed at other centers, patients with lateral impact pelvic fractures, and patients whose pelvic fractures were of the "windswept" variety (Brandes and Borrelli, 2001). We found that many patients had evidence of either unilateral or bilateral pudendal artery lesions, but that most had evidence of vascular reconstitution. **Patients with an intact pudendal artery on one side often were potent and were reliably cured with reconstruction. Patients with only reconstituted vessels, either unilateral or bilateral, never were potent but were reliably reconstructed.** We found that these patients were optimal candidates for penile arterial revascularization to improve potency. Because we noted this relationship to potency, we began evaluating patients with duplex ultrasonography. We found that patients with normal unilateral or bilateral pudendal arteries demonstrated normal arterial parameters on duplex evaluation. Patients with only reconstituted bilateral or unilateral arteries never had normal arterial parameters on duplex ultrasonography.

This information allows us to proceed to pudendal angiography only in patients with abnormal arterial parameters on duplex ultrasonography; patients with normal findings on ultrasonography

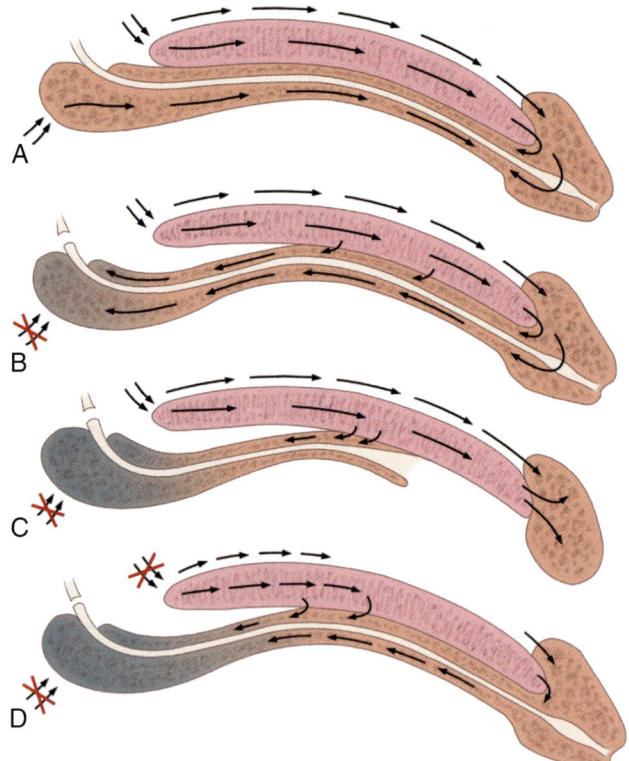

Fig. 82.38. Diagrammatic representation of the deep vasculature of the penis. (A) In the normal situation, through the common penile artery, flow is directed to the tip of the penis with arborization into the spongy erectile tissue of the glans penis. This provides retrograde flow into the corpus spongiosum. If the arteries of the bulb are intact, there is also antegrade arterial flow to the corpus spongiosum. (B) With interruption of the arteries to the bulb and mobilization of the corpus spongiosum, all flow to the corpus spongiosum is retrograde through the common penile arterial system. (C) In hypospadias, the distal corpus spongiosum may have been interrupted, with proximal mobilization of the corpus spongiosum and division of the arteries to the bulb. Even if the common penile circulation is intact to the tip of the penis, it may not adequately provide retrograde vascularity to the corpus spongiosum; ischemic stenosis can ensue. (D) In the case of injury to the common penile artery, with elevation of the proximal corpus spongiosum and division of the arteries to the bulb, blood flow to the proximal corpus spongiosum may be inadequate, leading to ischemic necrosis or ischemic stenosis.

an anastomotic technique. Although the above-and-below approach is used when concomitant bladder neck surgery is performed, the inability to identify these patients accurately has led us to perform bladder neck surgery at a second setting. We have abandoned a transpubic approach as applied to posterior urethral distraction injuries.

Although we favor primary reconstruction of posterior urethral distraction injuries, other authors choose to manage these injuries endoscopically (Barry, 1989). We have found that the endoscopic management of PFUIs is not a simple procedure and must be undertaken only by a skilled and experienced surgeon. Many of these procedures can be categorized as a "cut-for-light" procedure. Although some surgeons report success, most cut-for-light procedures are not done with sufficient precision to allow adequate realignment of the urethra. We have seen many disasters that have resulted from these procedures and in most cases condemn the use of these modalities. In addition, no cut-for-light series compares favorably, with regard to long-term success rates, with series from large centers that use primary anastomotic techniques (Levine and Wessells, 2001).

In 1989 Marshall described his method of using stereotactic techniques for endoscopic alignment of the ends of the urethra. He emphasized the length of time it takes to obtain precise alignment before undertaking the endoscopic portion of the procedure. In his procedure, he passed a wire through the aligned ends of the urethra, minimally dilating the channel and widening it with transurethral resection. The scar is stabilized by a period of self-catheterization. Although technically feasible, this approach has limited applicability for most patients. Patients whose medical condition, age, or concomitant orthopedic injury prevents them from being placed in the exaggerated lithotomy position or reconstructed using a transpubic approach may be managed with this technique.

In children, the goals of surgery are the same as in adults. In our experience, most children can undergo reconstruction by the same perineal exposure as used in adults. Exposure is more difficult, but nonetheless perineal anastomosis can be done (Hafez et al., 2005). However, the posterior, sagittal transsphincteric approach has been proposed as a better approach in children (Mathews et al., 1998; Peña and Hong, 2004). We agree that the posterior approach is an elegant method of exposure; however, with this approach, we have observed that surgeons tend to resort to techniques of substitution reconstruction where primary anastomosis could be done and, in our opinion, is superior. With our growing experience using the vessel-sparing approach to anterior urethral reconstruction—primary anastomosis and augmented anastomosis—we have extended the technique to select patients with pelvic fracture urethral reconstruction and have found the approach feasible with good results in a small number of patients. However, the advantage has not been proven.

predictably do well with reconstruction. Our data also show that patients do well with reconstruction if they have at least one side that is reconstituted, and the only patients at risk for ischemic stenosis are patients with bilateral complete obstruction of the internal pudendal vessels. In such patients, we perform penile arterial revascularization to augment the vascularity and, with that accomplished, proceed to urethral reconstruction (Davies et al., 2009; Jordan, 2005; Zuckerman et al., 2012). In many cases of pelvic fracture urethral distraction defects, ED is a consequence of the injury, although ED clearly results from the reconstructive surgery in some patients. We think that the incidence of injury to the pudendal arteries is drastically under-reported and under-recognized. We and others believe that in many of these cases, the cause of ED is vascular (Brandes and Borrelli, 2001). However, there are at least a portion of patients with neurogenic ED after PFUI; some men experiencing ED after PFUI have normal arterial inflow (Metze et al., 2007; Shenfeld et al., 2003).

Summary

Using the maneuvers outlined, we have found that almost all distraction injuries can be reconstructed through a perineal approach with

> **KEY POINTS: DISTRACTION INJURIES OF THE URETHRA**
>
> - Urethral distraction injuries are the result of blunt pelvic trauma and accompany about 10% of pelvic fracture injuries. In many injuries, there does not appear to be total distraction of the entire circumference of the urethra; instead, a strip of epithelium may be left behind.
> - The use of aligning catheters acutely is controversial, but most clinicians would agree that the aligning catheter, at the very worst, facilitates subsequent reconstruction and, at best, often leaves the patient with an endoscopically manageable stenosis.
> - As with any stricture, it is important to define the precise anatomy. The combination of contrast-enhanced studies with endoscopy and selective MRI is useful. The appearance of the bladder neck on contrast-enhanced studies or on antegrade endoscopy is not predictive of ultimate function of the bladder neck. Simultaneous reconstruction of the bladder neck and the posterior urethra is usually not undertaken at the present time.

VESICOURETHRAL DISTRACTION DEFECTS (VESICOURETHRAL STENOSIS)

Enthusiastic use of radical prostatectomy has led to increasing experience with patients who have had total obliteration of vesicourethral anastomosis. In some patients, there is distraction of the vesicourethral anastomosis with either a totally obliterating distraction defect or severe anastomotic stenosis. With increased use of robotic-assisted laparoscopic techniques we have seen a decrease in the number of significant anastomotic stenoses, and other authors have shown this as well (Breyer et al., 2010). This improvement may be secondary to reduction in anastomotic urine leaks, better mucosal apposition, and the running anastomosis allowed with the magnification and dexterity using the robotic approach.

As with other defects, it is important to determine the length of the defect accurately. This can be accomplished by simultaneous cystography with retrograde urethrography, simultaneous retrograde urethrography, and antegrade endoscopy through the suprapubic tube, or both.

Numerous options are available for the management of these complex patients. Many of these patients have other medical problems, and it has been our observation that many have thick and small bladders, possibly contributing to the difficulty with the initial surgery. The ever-present issue of body habitus also must be considered and, in our opinion, contributes to problems with the initial anastomosis. An indwelling suprapubic tube must always be considered an option. In a patient who is significantly overweight, the results of aggressive reconstruction have not been good. The place for endoscopic techniques is covered later in this section; however, in the case of short-length distractions, we have had success with aggressive incisions at the 3 o'clock and 9 o'clock positions followed in approximately 3 weeks with repeated incisions. Whether the holmium laser is better than the cold knife can be debated; the hot knife is unnecessary. If the urologist must "core through" to establish continuity, endoscopic procedures are not appropriate, in our opinion, except as discussed later. Vanni et al. (2011) published their experience with radial urethrotomy and intralesional injection of mitomycin C. They had an initial success rate of 72% in patients with recalcitrant strictures.

In some cases, a continent catheterizable bladder augmentation may be a better operation than aggressive functional reconstruction; in an obese patient, construction of a functional catheter channel can be difficult. Diversion must also be entertained, and in patients in whom functional reconstruction is not an obvious choice, it becomes a primary option.

If functional reconstruction is deemed possible, we think it is a reasonable choice, and our technique is as follows. We place the patient in a low-lithotomy position and use an abdominal-perineal combined approach. We make a lower midline incision, exposing the bladder and dissecting it from the lateral sidewall and further mobilizing the anterior bladder from beneath the pubis as aggressively as can be safely undertaken from above. We then open the peritoneum and develop the retrovesical space, again taking care to complete the dissection as safely as can be accomplished from above.

A second surgeon begins the perineal dissection by a curvilinear perineal incision similar to that used for a radical perineal prostatectomy. The dissection is posterior to the transverse perineal musculature (posterior anal triangle) and carried along the anterior rectal wall to the area where fibrosis is encountered from the prior radical prostatectomy dissection. The impulse of the perineal surgeon's finger can usually be felt adjacent and lateral to the area of fibrosis and distraction at this point. In addition, the abdominal surgeon places a finger at the limits of the retrovesical dissection from above to provide another palpable landmark and to ensure a safe dissection anterior to the rectal wall and posterior to the bladder and trigone. The perineal dissection is joined to the abdominal dissection, and the rectal wall is completely peeled off the area of fibrosis associated with the distraction defect. We place drains between the rectum and the distraction defect, encircling the area of fibrosis.

The dissection beneath the pubis is made easier by the excision of an ellipse of the rim of the superior pubic ramus. Total pubectomy is not required. Partial pubectomy can be performed with the reciprocating attachment of the Aesculap surgical drilling device (Aesculap, Tuttlingen, Germany); this makes placement of the sutures technically straightforward and improves the exposure for the dissection and resection of the distraction fibrosis.

At this point, the bladder is opened, and the area of the bladder neck is determined. A sound is placed and advanced to the area of obliteration; this allows us to resect the well-defined area of fibrosis completely. The urethral stump is exposed and opened, and the site of the neobladder neck, having been identified, is opened. We marsupialize the bladder epithelium as described by Eggleston and Walsh (1985), place anastomotic sutures in the urethral stump, and pass a stenting catheter.

Before the vesicourethral anastomosis is seated, the omentum is mobilized and placed between the posterior wall of the anastomosis and the anterior rectal wall. We seat the anastomosis and wrap the omentum around the area of anastomosis, tagging it into place. The lateral vesical spaces are drained with closed suction drains, and a suprapubic tube is left in place when the vesicostomy is closed. More recently we have been doing this procedure purely perineally with similar outcomes.

Postoperative care is the same as for a radical prostatectomy. Patients are discharged when their drainage and ambulation allow and their diet has been resumed. We evaluate patients 4 to 6 weeks postoperatively, with the stenting urethral catheter removed and the bladder filled by way of the suprapubic tube.

Our series continues to grow, and we continue to have excellent success in reconstruction. We have some patients who deem their continence adequate for their lifestyle; in the others, we have been successful with the placement of an artificial sphincter.

COMPLEX FISTULA OF THE POSTERIOR URETHRA

The increase in the performance of radical prostatectomy has also led to an increased incidence of vesicorectal or vesicourethrorectal fistulae. In most cases, these are small and managed by a transperineal, transanal-transsphincteric, or posterior approach. However, some cases are complex, with the fistulae associated with large granulated cavities. The problem is magnified when radiation (brachytherapy, external beam therapy, or both) is part of the equation. With radiation fistulae, surgeons at many centers use diversion with ileal conduit or bowel pouch instead of functional reconstruction. These cases have also been managed with the approach described earlier for vesicourethral distraction problems. However, the omentum serves an even more important purpose in these cases. In addition, with the increasing application of "minimally invasive" modalities for carcinoma of the prostate (i.e., brachytherapy, combined brachytherapy with external beam irradiation, higher dose external beam irradiation, and cryotherapy), the magnitude of complexity of these problems of prostatic urethral fistulae, granulated cavities, and severe rectal injury continues to increase. We have tried to approach these problems aggressively, with preservation of function where possible.

In many of these cases, salvage prostatectomy can be combined with rectosigmoid resection. In some cases, we have successfully reanastomosed the bladder to the membranous urethra. Preservation of continence has been mixed. In cases in which vesicourethral anastomosis is impossible, a urachal-peritoneal flap combined with a rectus abdominis muscle flap is used to bolster the closed bladder neck and to keep the closed bladder neck from sticking to the back of the pubis. The bladder is augmented, and a continent catheterizable channel is developed. In some cases, the continuity of the colon cannot be reestablished, and a colostomy is performed as distally on the descending portion of the colon as possible. Whenever continuity of the colon can be reestablished, a J-pouch coloanal anastomosis is done. Omentum is used to envelop the rectal closure or to separate the rectal closure from the vesicourethral anastomosis. The combined abdominal-perineal approach that was previously described provides excellent safe exposure for management of these complex situations. The morbidity associated with this approach has been acceptable.

Zinman reported a 10-year experience with the management of rectourethral fistulae (Vanni et al., 2009). The series comprised 33 patients who had fistulae and who had not undergone irradiation and 33 patients who had undergone irradiation. Mean follow-up for the entire series was about 20 months. The review was a retrospective review taken from office records and hospital records. All fistulae were repaired by an anterior transperineal approach using gracilis muscle interposition flaps and in some cases with a buccal graft. In this series, 100% of the nonirradiated fistulae were successfully closed with a mean follow-up of 20 months, 85% of the irradiated fistulae were closed in a single stage, and 12% required an additional procedure, with an ultimate closure rate of about 97%. In the nonirradiated group, there were no urethral strictures noted with long-term follow-up; five recurrent strictures were noted in the irradiated group. In the nonirradiated group, 91% of the patients had their bowel undiverted. In the irradiated group, 39% had long-term bowel diversion. Zinman believes that the use of muscle interposition flaps are integral to achieving good results, and the use of buccal mucosal grafts, where needed to augment the closure of the urinary tract, was also believed to be invaluable (Vanni et al., 2009). An estimation of ultimate urinary and bowel function is integral to the determination of the plan for reconstruction or diversion, or both. Also, the surgical approach chosen facilitates and limits options (i.e., of the bowel, the urethra, or tissue interposition) (Lane et al., 2006).

> **KEY POINTS: VESICOURETHRAL DISTRACTION DEFECTS AND COMPLEX FISTULAE OF THE POSTERIOR URETHRA**
>
> - Vesicourethral distraction defects are a complication of radical prostatectomy.
> - There are many options for management of these complex patients. An indwelling suprapubic tube must always be considered a long-term option. Likewise, in some cases, a continent catheterizable bladder augmentation may be a better operation than aggressive functional reconstruction. If functional reconstruction is deemed reasonable, we have employed an above-and-below technique, in which laparotomy is combined with a posterior perineal triangle dissection.
> - The interposition of omentum has been used for distraction defects and for complex fistulae. This approach allows safe mobilization of the rectum from the area of the distraction scar or from the fistula site.
> - When radiation is added, the complexity of reconstruction is magnified. The effects of radiation must be allowed to settle; tissue interposition is the rule, and functional reconstruction is impossible in many cases. Some think that diversion, in the case of patients who have received radiation, is the safest and best option.
> - Careful consideration of ultimate urinary and bowel function is integral to proper planning of surgery.

CURVATURES OF THE PENIS

Normal elasticity and compliance of all tissue layers of the penis are critical for erectile function, tumescence, and rigidity. Tissues must expand in all dimensions as the penis engorges with blood; eventually, the tissues of the tunica albuginea and the septal fibers of the corpora cavernosa are stretched to the limits of their compliance, and tumescence is converted to rigidity. In the normal penis, the tissues are symmetrically elastic, and the erection is straight. In curvature of the penis, there is relative asymmetry of one aspect of the erect penis. In some cases, this condition arises from diminished compliance of one aspect of the tunica albuginea or outright foreshortening of one aspect of the erectile bodies.

The term *chordee* means curvature, but it is commonly used as if it refers to the tissues causing the curvature. This misuse of the term is seen in the statement "the chordee was resected"; properly phrased, the statement should be "the chordee can be corrected by resecting the inelastic tissues that are causing the chordee."

Curvatures of the penis can be congenital or acquired. Some confusion also exists in common usage of the term *congenital curvature of the penis*. The terms *congenital curvature of the penis* and *chordee without hypospadias* have often been used interchangeably. We prefer to reserve the term *chordee without hypospadias* for patients in whom the meatus is properly located on the tip of the glans penis; a ventral curvature is associated with abnormalities of the ventral fascial tissues or corpus spongiosum, or both. It has long been recognized that hypospadias is a condition that is associated in some patients with either a diminutive penis or a micropenis. Although a small penis is not diagnostic of hypospadias, it is highly unusual for a patient with hypospadias to have an exceptionally large erect penis. In contrast, other congenital curvatures of the penis (ventral, lateral, or dorsal) are inevitably associated with the finding of a large erect penis. Because **the trauma that results in acquired curvature is virtually always associated with intercourse, the occurrence of acquired curvature is nil before the onset of puberty.** We have seen some patients in whom there was a history of trauma during vigorous masturbation, but these patients are the exception. Similar to congenital curvatures of the penis, acquired curvatures may be dorsal, lateral, ventral, or complex.

Types of Congenital Curvature of the Penis

More information about this topic is available online at Expert Consult.com.

Chordee Without Hypospadias in Young Men

More information on this topic is available online at Expert Consult.com.

Congenital Curvatures of the Penis

Patients with congenital curvature of the penis can have ventral, lateral (which is most often to the left), or, unusually, dorsal curvature. Photographs of the erect penis demonstrate a smooth curvature that generally involves the entire pendulous portion of the penile shaft.

Patients are usually otherwise healthy young men between the ages of 18 and 30 years. Many of these patients have noticed curvature before passing through puberty but have presumed it to be normal. However, with puberty, they discover that the curvature is not normal; or they become sexually active and discover that the curvature impedes their efforts; or they notice increasing curvature as they pass through puberty, and this, in their minds, clearly would preclude sexual intercourse. Occasionally, a patient waits until he is older than 30 years to deal with the anomaly; even less often, a younger adolescent may discuss his genitalia with his parents.

In circumcised patients, we make an incision through the circumcision scar, which in many cases is displaced well down on the penile shaft. However, even with relatively significant displacement of the circumcision scar on the shaft of the penis, the reincision should be through the circumcision scar. The penis is degloved by dissection of the layer immediately superficial to the superficial lamina of Buck fascia.

An artificial erection is obtained with normal saline infusion or pharmacologic agents. We do not routinely recommend a tourniquet device because constricting devices can conceal the proximal limits of the curvature; this is of most significance in cases of ventral curvatures, which frequently extend proximally. Occasionally, some element of perineal pressure is initially required, but these are patients with normal erectile function, and venous occlusive function is normal. The artificial erection demonstrates the character of the curvature and the location of maximal curvature. In patients with ventral curvature, there may be some illusion of thickening of the dartos and Buck fascia, and in these patients, the fibrous tissue is mobilized and completely excised. The corpus spongiosum is detached from the corpora cavernosa and mobilized from the glans to the penoscrotal junction.

After these tissues are excised, the artificial erection is repeated, and occasionally a patient has complete straightening. However, most patients experience a differential elasticity between the dorsal and the ventral aspects of the corporeal bodies, and although the curvature may have been lessened, it persists unless further procedures are done to straighten the penis.

In an adult patient with persistent curvature, there are two options for surgical correction: (1) to lengthen the ventral aspect of the penis by making transverse incisions in the ventral tunica and placing an autologous tissue graft (we currently use the small intestinal submucosal graft at our institution), and (2) to shorten the dorsal aspect of the penis by elevating the neurovascular bundle, excising an ellipse or ellipses from the dorsum of the tunica albuginea, and closing the defects in watertight fashion (Nesbit procedure [Nesbit, 1965]). **Because the size of the erect penis is usually not a problem in these cases of congenital curvature, we have chosen the second option and strenuously discourage ventral grafting in these patients.** The recovery period after this procedure is much shorter, and the variabilities of graft take do not have to be considered. In addition, when a graft is used, there is always the possibility, although uncommon, of the development of graft-induced veno-occlusive dysfunction. **In a 2000 consensus conference sanctioned by the WHO, the committee on Peyronie disease and congenital curvature of the penis agreed that most, if not all, cases in men with the classic finding of congenital curvature of the penis were best managed with plication or corporoplasty techniques but not grafting techniques** (Jardin et al., 1999; Lue, 2004). This consensus was reiterated at the next WHO conference. It is preferable to shorten the longer aspect of the penis in patients with congenital curvature. However, **if the patient falls into the category of chordee without hypospadias and shortness of the penis is an issue, we selectively use incisions with grafts to correct the curvature** (Devine and Horton, 1975).

After the decision has been made to proceed with excisions of ellipses of dorsal tunica, Buck fascia can be elevated in concert with the dorsal neurovascular structures by beginning just lateral to the corpus spongiosum and carrying the dissection dorsally across the midline. Alternatively, the tunica can be exposed by excising the deep dorsal vein of the penis and opening the inner lamina of Buck fascia. Elevation of the neurovascular structures is done by dissecting from the dorsal midline laterally around to the corpus spongiosum and from the coronal margin to the penopubic junction, limiting the effects of stretching the dorsal structures with exposure of the dorsum of the penis.

An artificial erection is obtained to plan the proposed ellipse excisions. We prefer to use several small ellipses rather than try to correct the curvature with one large ellipse. The first ellipse is usually positioned at the point of maximal concavity. The edges of the planned ellipse are apposed with a Prolene suture. The artificial erection is repeated to assess the effects of that excision. If there is good straightening in that area of the shaft, the incisions are again well marked, the plicating sutures are removed, and the ellipses of tunica are made with a sharp scalpel blade. By dissection in the space of Smith and removal of only an ellipse of tunica, the ellipses are carefully excised to avoid damage to the underlying erectile tissue or can be merely closed under the reapproximated edge of the defect in the tunica albuginea. The edge of the ellipse is reapproximated with a combination of interrupted 4-0 polydioxanone sutures and a watertight running 4-0 polydioxanone suture.

After closure, we repeat the artificial erection to assess the results of the first ellipse with the others. A final artificial erection should demonstrate the penis to be perfectly straight. In cases of ventral curvature or when complex curvatures are associated with an element of ventral curvature, a minimal degree of dorsal curvature after correction is acceptable. In most cases, as the sutures dissolve, the penis either remains minimally dorsiflexed or becomes perfectly straight.

The Buck fascia is closed. Two small suction drains are placed superficial to the Buck fascia but deep to the dartos fascia. We replace the skin sleeve, with its edges apposed with interrupted small Vicryl or Monocryl sutures. In all patients, we place a small Foley catheter and a small suction drain, and both are removed on the first postoperative day. Depending on the amount of edema and drainage, patients are discharged from the hospital on the evening of the first postoperative day or early the second postoperative day.

A congenital lateral curvature of the penis is often associated with some complexity of curvature; patients frequently notice lateral curvature in association with a ventral or, less commonly, a dorsal curvature. However, some patients present with only lateral curvature, with the right side larger than the left, and curvature to the left.

In some cases, a repair of the lateral curvature can be approached through a small incision at the point of maximal curvature. Laterally placed incisions on the penile shaft are not cosmetically optimal. We prefer a degloving incision after exposure of the deep penile structures; the point of maximal concavity is then marked. Prolene sutures are placed, and an artificial erection is performed again. The size of the ellipse is assessed, and the ellipse is excised and closed as discussed earlier.

As mentioned, most cases of lateral curvature are associated with complex curvatures. In these patients, the correction of the curvature is similar to that described for patients with ventral curvature, with incision through the circumcision scar with the skin reflected. In contrast to a ventral curvature, with a lateral curvature, the entire dorsal neurovascular bundle does not have to be reflected; it is seldom required and it is not considered beneficial to excise the deep dorsal vein in approaching the dorsum of the penis. The postoperative care is the same as described for a ventral curvature. Uncommonly a patient has a congenital dorsal curvature of the penis; for this, the repair is best accomplished by mobilizing the lateral aspect of the corpus spongiosum to allow small ellipses lateral to the midline to be positioned on the ventrum of the penis, by the technique described before.

Although described as a method for plication for curvature associated with Peyronie disease, corporoplasty, a procedure described by Yachia (1993), is also useful for the correction of congenital curvatures. The procedure consists of longitudinal incisions in the tunica albuginea with transverse closure. The "long side" is plicated without the need for excision; however, the plication is durable in that the tunica is opened and closed with a resulting scar, rather than reliance only on the strength of sutures as originally described by Nesbit (1965). With this technique, closure is done with absorbable monofilament suture.

Acquired Curvatures of the Penis

Acquired curvatures of the penis inevitably follow trauma to the penis. Many of these cases are associated with Peyronie disease, also believed to be associated with trauma to the penis during intercourse (Bella et al., 2007). Patients occasionally have had vigorous internal urethrotomy, with the incision extended outside the urethra and corpus spongiosum and involving the tunica of the corporal bodies, causing scarring that is significant enough to be associated with curvature.

Acquired Curvatures of the Penis From Causes Other Than Peyronie Disease

When a young man presents with an acquired curvature of the penis, one must always consider Peyronie disease. However, many men do not have true Peyronie disease. These patients, on close questioning, reveal a history of minimal lateral curvature of the penis and a clear memory of a lateral buckling injury that occurred during intercourse. In some cases, the patient remembers hearing a "snap" and notices immediate detumescence and significant ecchymosis of the penis. These patients are often referred with a diagnosis of Peyronie disease, but a diagnosis of curvature secondary to penile fracture is more accurate. Because of the noticeable events associated with fracture of the penis, many patients are seen with an acute injury, and reconstruction can be accomplished at that time.

Occasionally, a patient or his primary care physician ignores the stigmata of the trauma (often described as "minimal" by patients), and the patient has a noticeable lateral scar that causes indentation of the lateral aspect of the penis and, in some cases, curvature. Patients who had preexisting lateral curvature may notice that their penis has been straightened by the trauma, but they are disturbed by the concavity caused by the scar. In others, the small linear scar causes a significant lateral curvature.

Another group of patients seek medical attention after a similar buckling trauma to the penis but without associated detumescence or ecchymosis. These patients report noticing that their erections were painful for a period after the trauma, and then a nodule developed in the lateral aspect of the penis. Eventually, they develop a lateral linear scar that has led to curvature and indentation at the site. We refer to this injury as a subclinical fracture of the penis.

The lesion of a subclinical fracture of the penis is believed to be due to the disruption of the outer longitudinal layer of the tunica albuginea during the buckling trauma. The inner, circular layer is not disrupted and maintains the blood-tight continuity of the corpus spongiosum. Another possible scenario is that both layers of the tunica albuginea are disrupted, but the overlying Buck fascia maintains its integrity. Some patients notice a pop with intercourse and a period of pain with erections, followed by curvature of the penis—usually dorsal. These patients probably tear the septal insertion completely. These patients have a similar presentation to patients with Peyronie disease.

Patients usually have normal erectile function after subclinical or clinical fracture of the penis; there does not appear to be an association with concomitant global cavernosal veno-occlusive dysfunction. However, the association of cavernosal veno-occlusive dysfunction and trauma of the penis continues to be seen, and some patients have significant problems with erectile dysfunction after fracture-type injuries of the penis. These injuries are not associated with shortening of the penis. In most cases, the lack of erectile dysfunction and penile shortening help distinguish these patients from patients with Peyronie disease. If a detailed history leads one to suspect blighted erectile function, erectile function should be evaluated before proceeding with surgery. We evaluate these patients with duplex ultrasonography and selectively with dynamic infusion cavernosometry and cavernosography.

Although foreshortening of the penis is a characteristic of neither the injury nor the resulting scar in either of these injuries, these patients are not ideal candidates for contralateral plication procedures. This treatment would result in bilateral scars, which would cause bilateral indentations of the penis. Although the penis would have been straightened by the correction, most patients are upset by the cosmetic and functional result of a near-circumferential indentation of the penis. Instead, we excise the scar and place a graft to replace the corporotomy defect caused by the scar excision. Because these scars are on the lateral aspect of the penis, minimal mobilization of Buck fascia, associated dorsal neurovascular structures, and corpus spongiosum is required at the site.

The results of the surgical correction described have been extremely effective. Successful correction with a single operation has been achieved in all patients treated at our institution.

PENILE TRANSPLANTATION

General

The principal techniques of penile reconstruction were originally developed for treatment of trauma patients, and these patients were often victims of war injuries. In 1936 Bogaraz described a technique for phallic construction in a series of war-injured patients, and in 1944 Frumkin followed with a series from the Soviet Union. Aware of the work in the Soviet Union, Gillies and Harrison (1948) reported on a series of patients in whom they had accomplished penile reconstruction while stationed at a major hospital in the outskirts of London during World War II. In this series, numerous patients had a complete absence of the penis.

> **KEY POINTS: CURVATURES OF THE PENIS**
>
> - Curvatures of the penis can be acquired or congenital. Congenital curvatures of the penis can be categorized as chordee without hypospadias or congenital curvature of the penis.
> - In general, chordee without hypospadias is a forme fruste of hypospadias. Although the meatus may not be abnormally placed, these patients usually have findings suggestive of hypospadias (i.e., malformation of the ventral structures of the penis). These patients are not characterized by large erect penises. In contrast, patients with congenital curvature of the penis seem to have exceptionally large erect penises.
> - The entity of congenital curvature of the penis seems to be related to nonsymmetrical expansion of the erectile bodies, which must expand significantly during tumescence. Reconstruction in these patients generally is best accomplished by excision with plicating closure or pure plication techniques. The use of grafts is not recommended because of the unusual but real occurrence of graft-induced veno-occlusive dysfunction in certain patients.

Initially, all procedures for phallic construction involved delayed formation and transfer of tubed abdominal flaps. These tubes were produced from random flaps of skin and because of their size were based on a tenuous blood supply. To allow new vascular patterns to become established in the transferred tissue, they were formed in stages, with a "delay" between the stages. In the "tube-within-a-tube" design, the inner tube allowed the placement of a baculum during intercourse, and the outer tube provided skin coverage. Patients voided through a proximal urethrostomy. This approach continued to be the "state-of-the-art" phallic construction and penile reconstruction until 1972, when Orticochea described total reconstruction of the penis using the gracilis musculocutaneous flap. In 1978 Puckett and Montie reported a series in which they constructed the penis with a tubed groin flap. In the early cases in this series, the flap was transferred in delayed fashion to the area of the penile stump. Later in the series, a microvascular free-transfer technique was employed.

In 1984 Chang and Hwang popularized the forearm flap, based on the radial artery, for phallic construction. Biemer (1988) reported a modification of the forearm flap, which was also based on the radial artery; in 1990, Farrow et al. reported their "cricket bat" modification of the radial forearm flap. At the present time, forearm flaps are the most commonly employed method for total phallic construction and penile reconstruction.

The forearm flap is usually harvested from the nondominant forearm. Preoperatively, the Allen test is used to screen patients carefully for arterial insufficiency. This test involves palpation of the radial and ulnar arteries in the wrist, with the patient making a tight fist to express blood from his hand. As he opens his hand, the fingers are pale, but if palmar circulation is normal and both arteries are patent, the fingers turn pink when one of the arteries is released. On the basis of either the Allen test or the patient's history, if there is any doubt about the integrity of the radial and ulnar arteries or the palmar arch, upper extremity angiography is performed.

As described, the forearm flap is a fasciocutaneous flap vascularized by the radial artery; however, the ulnar artery also vascularizes the forearm fascia and most of the forearm skin. The radial artery arises as a continuation of the brachial artery and proximally lies beneath the belly of the brachioradialis muscle, becoming more superficial at the wrist. The ulnar artery is also a continuation of the brachial artery and vascularizes a similar area of skin and underlying adipose tissue. The vascularity of the overlying skin is achieved by way of the underlying (antebrachial) fascia, which is the superficial fascia investing the musculature of the forearm.

The forearm flap can be elevated and transferred on the superficial fascia. The lateral and medial antebrachial cutaneous nerves appear proximally beneath the fascia. The cephalic, basilic, and medial antebrachial veins are also included in the flap and constitute a portion of the venous drainage. In some patients, the vena comitans is the dominant venous drainage system. At the time of flap transfer, it is imperative to assess the vena comitans and the superficial veins to determine which is the dominant system in the individual patient.

The various modifications of the forearm flap do not represent changes in the technique of flap elevation; rather, they are modifications in the design of the skin island and the relative position of the urethral paddle in relation to the skin that eventually becomes shaft coverage. Each of these modifications has advantages in different situations.

In the forearm flap as described by Chang and Hwang (1984), the shaft is covered with the radial aspect of the skin paddle. A de-epithelialized strip is made, and a second skin island, on the ulnar aspect of the skin paddle, is tubed to form the urethra. The urethral tube is rolled within the tube of skin to form a tube-within-a-tube design. In the white population, this flap has demonstrated a tendency to lead to ischemic stenosis of the lateral paddle, where the urethra is constructed.

In the cricket bat modification, the urethral tube extends distally, closely overlying either the radial or the ulnar artery. We have experience with elevation of the cricket bat modification on both arteries. Proximal to the urethral strip, a broader portion of the skin paddle provides coverage of the shaft. The urethral portion is tubed and transposed by inverting it into the center of the shaft portion of the skin paddle. The advantage of this modification lies in centering the urethral portion over the respective artery, in contrast to the Chinese design, in which the ulnar aspect is far distal from the radial artery, with the potential for ischemic stenosis or loss of that portion. The cricket bat modification has been useful in trauma patients, particularly in patients who have a significant stump of erectile bodies and urethra left after the injury.

The modification by Biemer (1988) also centers the urethral portion of the flap over the artery. As described by Biemer, the flap is elevated on the radial artery and includes a vascularized piece of the radial bone intended to provide rigidity to the new penis. However, the inclusion of cartilage and bone has not been universally successful, and rigidity in these flaps is obtainable by the use of either an externally applied or an internally implanted prosthesis. If the bone is not elevated, the Biemer flap design can be elevated on either the radial or the ulnar artery. At our center, we most often elevate the flap on the ulnar artery, in a modification of the Biemer design.

Modifications of the Biemer design also include the glans construction technique that was originally described by Puckett and Montie (1978). In the original Biemer design, a central strip becomes the urethra, and lateral to that strip, two de-epithelialized portions and two lateral islands (lateral aspects of that skin paddle) are fused dorsally and ventrally to cover the shaft. With the modification of Puckett et al. (1982), a large island is left distally and flared back over the tip of the tubed flaps, creating the illusion of a glans penis. The Biemer design, especially when it is combined with Puckett's design for glanular construction, offers the best cosmetic results (Fig. 82.39).

There are several disadvantages to the use of a forearm flap for phallic construction. The major disadvantage of forearm flaps is the obvious donor site deformity. We have reconstructed the donor site with FTSGs taken from the area of the inguinal crease or buttock, and the cosmetic result is far superior to that obtained when the donor site is reconstructed with STSG (even thick split-thickness skin). In addition, morbidity can be reduced with mobilization of the intact forearm skin to reduce the grafting requirement and attempts to minimize the step between the skin and muscle bed. A second disadvantage lies in the **possibility of the development of cold intolerance in the hand of the donor side.** Early in our experience with the forearm flap, we reconstructed the radial artery with an interposition vein graft. We have since abandoned this procedure in most of our series and have not seen cold intolerance in our patients. Another disadvantage occurs in male and virilized transgender patients **when the forearm skin is hirsute, because the hair can be problematic** if it is included in the portion of the flap used for urethral construction. In such patients, we try to identify the potential for the problem and refer them for epilation before surgery.

McRoberts and Sadove (2002) proposed the use of the fibular osteocutaneous flap for phallic construction. The fibula is elevated on the periosteal vessel along with the overlying skin paddle. As they described, urethral reconstruction is by tubed graft techniques, and their procedure had a 100% urethral complication rate. Kim et al. (2009) used a radial forearm osteocutaneous flap in 40 patients with reasonable results, although for many patients the incorporation of bone did not provide sufficient rigidity for sexual function over time. For patients who need vascularized tissue only to cover the shaft of the penis, we have used the upper lateral arm flap. This is a fasciocutaneous flap, and its cutaneous vascular territory is centered on the radial collateral artery. The skin of the lateral upper arm is thin, with little subcutaneous adiposity. To mark the location of the lateral intramuscular septum and the course of the superior radial collateral artery, we draw a line joining the insertion of the deltoid with the lateral epicondyle. We begin the dissection posteriorly, elevating the superficial fascia until the posterior lateral portion of the intramuscular septum has been identified. A potential disadvantage of this flap lies in the fact that the entire venous drainage depends on the vena comitans, and although superficial veins do traverse the flap, none of them seems to provide significant venous drainage. We have found the flap to be completely reliable so far, with no losses secondary to venous insufficiency.

This flap has also been used for total phallic construction. For this purpose, the flap is expanded by tissue expander and elevated across the elbow, and the distal flap is elevated on the recurrent radial artery. As with the forearm flap, the donor site of an upper lateral arm flap can be disfiguring. However, because the scar is on the upper arm, it is more easily concealed beneath a shirtsleeve than a scar in the forearm. All the flaps described allow microneurosurgical coaptation of the flap cutaneous nerves with recipient nerves. With total phallic construction, the cutaneous nerves can be attached either to the dorsal nerves of the penis or to the dorsal nerves of the clitoris in a transsexual patient. When these nerves are unavailable, the nerves can be coapted to the pudendal nerve, which in most patients requires an interposition graft. These nerves are thought to provide the best restoration of erogenous cutaneous sensibility. We have also coapted the flap's cutaneous nerves to the ilioinguinal nerves, which provides sensation to the inner aspect of the thigh and the lateral aspect of the scrotum, and have achieved a reasonable degree of erogenous sensibility. The ilioinguinal nerve is also thought to provide a better degree of protective sensation (albeit less erogenous sensation) compared with the dorsal nerves (Monstrey et al., 2009).

In most patients, the deep inferior epigastric vessels are the recipient vasculature for flap transfer. These vessels are medial branches of the iliac system and lie on the dorsal (deep) aspect of the rectus abdominis muscle. The artery usually remains deep to the muscle, although an early penetration of the artery into the muscle can be observed in some patients. The artery classically bifurcates at the level of the umbilicus and is generally accompanied by two or more venae comitantes. These vessels have been elevated by several methods, and Lund et al. (1995) described their elevation for penile revascularization with laparoscopic techniques. When the deep inferior epigastric vessels are used, it is often necessary to include a saphenous vein for further venous runoff.

In some patients, these vessels are unavailable, and we have used a saphenous interposition graft to the superficial femoral artery. With use of this technique, we mobilize the saphenous vein well down the upper aspect of the thigh and then attach the vein to the femoral artery, making a temporary arteriovenous fistula. The fistula is divided, with the saphenous vein becoming the venous runoff and the interposition graft providing the arterial inflow. This system of recipient vessels is greatly inferior to a direct arterial anastomosis; because of this, in a few patients we have divided the profunda femoris vessel and vigorously dissected it from its other branches. We have then performed an end-to-end (artery-to-artery) anastomosis of the ulnar artery to the profunda femoris. However, the long-term consequences to the patient of dividing the profunda femoris are

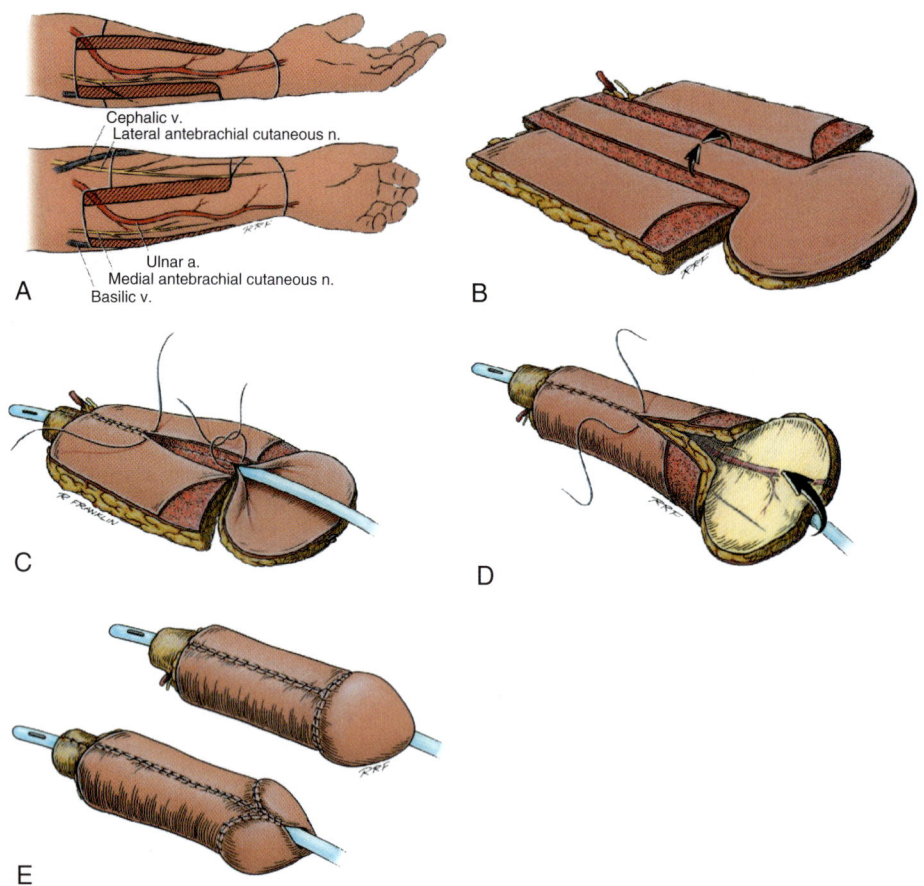

Fig. 82.39. (A) Schematic diagram of an ulnar forearm flap, modified Biemer design, on the patient's left (usually nondominant) forearm. (B) Schematic of the elevated flap. The flap has been divided into skin islands by de-epithelializing the strips. Laterally are the shaft skin islands, medially is the urethral skin island, and distally is the integral glans after the design of Puckett. (C) Schematic of the configuration of the flap. Notice the urethral skin island has been tubularized to the level of the neomeatus. The lateral shaft skin islands are now in the process of being tubularized over the tubularized urethra. (D) Schematic of the phallic flap as it is further configured. This view is of the dorsum. The ventral skin island has been closed over the urethra, and the dorsal skin islands are being collected. The integral glans will then be reflected over the dorsum of the flap. (E) The appearance of the phallus after it is totally configured and transposed to the area of the "penis." *a.*, Artery; *n.*, nerve; *v.*, vein.

unclear. Immediate reconstruction of the profunda does not appear to be advantageous because the dissection required to mobilize the profunda femoris to become a recipient vessel requires the division of numerous proximal branches, and these would not be reconstructed with an immediate reconstruction of the profunda femoris. Mention of this as a potential means of "creating" recipient vessels is not to recommend the procedure because the procedure may yet have unacceptable long-term consequences. Another option in extreme cases is to use the superficial femoral vein, which could be reconstructed with a vein interposition. When the "classic" recipient vessels are unavailable, these other methods may be acceptable. However, we strenuously caution concerning their use because the long-term consequences are unknown. We believe that division of the superficial femoral artery with immediate reconstruction is the preferable choice.

In the latter part of our series, we included the routine transfer of gracilis muscle to cover the area of the urethral anastomosis, increasing the vascularity to that area and significantly altering the incidence of anastomotic fistula and stricture formation. We also elevated a bipedicled flap from the area of the penile shaft base, which is transposed beneath the phallic flap. This flap provides increased bulk and some modicum of scrotal construction, and when it is combined with the gracilis muscle, its thickness provides excellent coverage for the juncture of the flap with the base of the neoscrotum.

Mobilization of a tunica dartos flap with tunica vaginalis pedicle, or a Martius flap in a transgender patient, may obviate the necessity to elevate and transpose a gracilis muscle flap.

During the phallic construction procedure, urine is diverted by means of a suprapubic cystostomy tube, and the urethra is stented with a No. 14 soft silicone (Silastic) catheter. A voiding study is usually performed between the third and fourth postoperative week.

Outcomes after forearm free-flap phalloplasty have now been reported from several centers. Even in centers of excellence for phallic construction, complications and reoperations seem to be the rule rather than the exception. Monstrey et al. (2009) reported the largest single-stage radial forearm phalloplasty series with 289 patients over 15 years. Urologic complications were seen in 41% of patients, the most common being fistula in 25%, stricture in 8.7%, and both in 9% of patients. Stricture treatment in this series required a multitude of procedures to achieve a patent urethra; however, fistulae healed spontaneously in most cases. Tactile sensation was achieved in all patients, and many were sexually active.

Similarly, Garaffa et al. (2010) published a series from the United Kingdom on 112 patients undergoing total phallic construction with a radial forearm free flap. Reconstructions at this center are performed in stages rather than a single stage. The urethral anastomosis is deferred until several months after the flap has demonstrated stability.

At a median 26 months of follow-up, 99% of patients who had achieved urethral continuity were voiding anatomically through the phallus. Despite staging the procedure, strictures still developed in 10% and fistulae in 24% of patients. Most patients (71.5%) developed phallus sensation.

Vascular complications and graft loss are the most feared morbidities associated with free-flap phalloplasty. These are rare events with rates of total flap loss ranging from 0.6% to 5% and higher rate of partial loss or limited skin necrosis (Garaffa et al., 2010; Leriche et al., 2008; Monstrey et al., 2009). Occasionally, minimal loss of the phallus is amenable to local wound care, but more often these cases require debridement and split-thickness skin grafting for coverage.

Rigidity for intercourse in a patient with phallic construction is usually achieved by either an externally applied or a permanently implanted prosthesis. Prosthetic implantation is never undertaken until 1 year after phallic construction because protective sensibility must be demonstrated in the flap. When the flap is transferred, it is, by definition, rendered insensate. At about 3 to 4 months after reconstruction, as nerve regeneration occurs, sensation becomes noticeable. In addition, the urethra must be patent and proved to be durable before prosthetic implantation is undertaken.

At our center, we have a large series of patients with internally implanted devices. We have implanted hydraulic and articulated prostheses encased in Gore-Tex neocorpora. These devices are anchored to the ischial tuberosity and the pubis by anchoring the neocorpora to these bone structures. In most patients, we implant two cylinders or rods. Early in our series, we had problems with hematoma and seroma formation and subsequent infection. However, since modifying our antibiotic regimen and including the routine use of suction drains with the implant procedure, we have had excellent success with implantation. At the present time, we place the antibiotic-coated (Inhibizone) AMS 700CXR (American Medical Systems, Minnetonka, MN). The Titan prosthesis (Coloplast, Humlebaek, Denmark) with hydrophilic coating and narrow base has also been used.

The largest published series describing the use of a mechanical prosthesis in a neophallus is from Belgium, where a variety of prostheses have been put in 129 patients from 1996 through 2007 (Hoebeke et al., 2010). The proximal prosthesis was fixed to the pubic rami using either a Dacron sheath or permanent stitches through a rear tip extender. At a mean 30 months of follow-up, 41.1% of patients needed revision or explant for infection (11.9%), malfunction (13%), erosion/malposition (22.7%), or leak (9.2%). Complications are higher than seen for implants into normal corpora, which would be expected given that the neophallus has had extensive prior surgery, is not as well vascularized, and the device may be used more frequently in this traditionally young patient population.

We also have implanted testicular prostheses in many patients. In patients in whom we have used a hydraulic device, we have implanted the pump in one neohemiscrotum and a testicular prosthesis in the opposite one.

Other options for phallic construction include the use of latissimus dorsi flap. This flap's characteristics allow for adequate size of the phallus as well as allows for good urethral reconstruction and ease of penile implant. A free sensate osteocutaneous fibula flap was initially described in 1993 and has been well accepted and has been shown to have good cosmetic as well as functional outcomes.

With the increase in vascularized composite allotransplantation (VCA) penile transplantation has become a concept that must be explored. There have been a number of reported successful transplants and certainly more will follow. Obviously, there are many issues to consider with regard to penile transplantation. Not only the medical concerns associated with VCAs but religious, personal, emotional, and cultural issues will have to be researched and considered as penile transplantation becomes more of a mainstay.

Reconstruction After Trauma

In many ways, the problems of trauma patients are more challenging to solve than the problems of patients who require total phallic construction. We have treated a large number of patients who have had devastating injuries to the penis after complicated prosthetic surgery or surgery to correct penile curvatures of Peyronie disease. The goal in these patients is to preserve the penile structures and function as much as possible and correct the deficiencies that are imposed on the patient by the trauma.

Acutely, urine must be diverted, necrotic tissue must be carefully debrided, and any foreign bodies that may have been implanted must be removed. Vigorous acute wound management stabilizes the wounds and allows active granulation to progress. In all trauma patients, an attempt should be made to save as many of the penile structures as possible.

Approximately 3 to 6 weeks after trauma, primary reconstruction can be undertaken, although we have elected to wait 4 to 6 months in some patients, depending on the situation. When significant adjacent tissue loss has occurred, the adjacent areas must be well reconstructed before proceeding with either phallic construction or penile reconstruction.

In a trauma patient, well-vascularized tissues must be eventually transposed to the adjacent area, and reconstruction of these areas can be accomplished with numerous flaps. For groin reconstruction, the tensor fascia lata flap has been useful. The rectus femoris flap, characteristically long and large, can be transposed to the area of the lower abdomen and has been an extremely useful flap for inguinal and lower abdominal reconstruction. The gracilis muscle is an excellent flap for reconstruction of the perineum and the groin. Alternatively, the posterior thigh flap can be used for reconstruction of the groin and perineum and, in some cases, transposed to the lowermost portion of the lower abdomen. The rectus abdominis flap is a useful flap and can be elevated with a vertical or transverse skin paddle. In addition, the flap can be transposed to either the ipsilateral or the contralateral side. Care must be taken in a patient who has had lower abdominal external beam irradiation.

Variations of the flap designs described for complete phallic construction have been successfully applied in select patients for penile reconstruction. An example is one patient who sustained an injury to his penis from a shotgun blast. The blast injured a large portion of the patient's right corpus cavernosum, and most of the penile skin was either destroyed or used for urethral reconstruction. In this patient, a flap based on the Chinese design was elevated. However, because the urethral reconstruction was accomplished with a penile skin island, the ulnar portion of the flap was not needed for that purpose. The ulnar portion was de-epithelialized and tubularized to form bulk and a new right corporeal body. This patient is now sexually active, and the bulk of the tube's dermal section gives adequate support to his penis for intercourse.

Another patient required only distal urethral construction and glans reconstruction. For this patient, we based a flap on the Biemer design to construct a glans. The proximal portions of the flap were de-epithelialized, allowing fixation of the neoglans on the tips of the corporeal bodies, and an excellent functional and cosmetic result was achieved for this patient. The versatility of free-flap technology allows the solution of complex issues with reasonably acceptable functional and cosmetic results.

Female-to-Male Transgender

Female-to-male transgender patients present a unique challenge, and no patient should be considered for definitive reassignment surgery without having undergone complex screening and evaluation by a team consisting of mental health professionals as well as surgeons who are skilled in undertaking transgender surgery. It is imperative that an ongoing, stable, therapeutic relationship be established between the patient and a mental health professional at the time of definitive gender reassignment surgery. At our institution, the Harry Benjamin criteria (Ramsey, 1996) are strictly adhered to, and surgery is accomplished by a team of urologists, plastic surgeons, and gynecologists.

In most patients, the first stage of female-to-male transgender surgery consists of bilateral salpingo-oophorectomy, hysterectomy, vaginectomy, and urethral lengthening with colpocleisis. Even in virginal patients, our surgeons have become skilled at accomplishing a hysterectomy and bilateral salpingo-oophorectomy by way of transvaginal surgery. We perform a vaginectomy at the same operation, leaving the anterior vaginal wall to be transposed as a random flap to lengthen the female urethra and allow colpocleisis. Lengthening of the female urethra brings the base of the native urethra up to what will be the base of the phallic flap; along with the transfer of gracilis muscle, it has significantly altered our surgical results with regard to urethral anastomotic fistula and stricture. Urine is diverted with a suprapubic tube, and a voiding trial is performed in approximately 21 days. Patients are generally in the hospital for 2 to 3 days and return 3 to 4 months later for phallic construction.

For phallic construction in a transgender patient, we elevate a bipedicled flap of skin, as already described, from the area where the phallic structure will be implanted and transpose it to the undersurface of the neopenis. The patient is generally in the hospital for 10 to 14 days after total phallic construction, and a voiding trial with contrast material is done at about 28 days postoperatively. After 1 year, when erogenous sensibility is demonstrated and the urethra is proved to be durable, prosthetic implantation is considered.

KEY POINTS: TOTAL PENILE RECONSTRUCTION AND FEMALE-TO-MALE TRANSGENDER

- The principal techniques of penile reconstruction originally were developed for treatment of victims of war injuries. Initially, all of the procedures involved delayed tissue transfer. In 1978 Puckett and Montie reported a series of phallic reconstructions in which a groin flap was transferred by microvascular free-transfer techniques to the area of the penis. The phallus was insensible, but this represented the first free-flap reconstruction for phallic construction. In 1984 Chang and Hwang popularized use of the forearm flap. This flap has been modified by numerous individuals.
- We prefer to use an ulnar forearm flap with a combined Puckett modification of the flap and Biemer modification of the glans. These flaps allow sensible phallic construction that lets the patient stand to void and permits eventual prosthetic implantation because the phallus has protective and erogenous sensibility.
- The techniques employed in transgender patients are not different from techniques employed in trauma patients. The shapes of the skin paddles often must be tailored to the individual patient.

SUGGESTED READINGS

Aboseif SR, Breza J, Lue TF, et al: Penile venous drainage in erectile dysfunction: anatomical, radiological and functional considerations, *Br J Urol* 64:183–190, 1989.

Akporiaye LE, Jordan GH, Devine CJ Jr: Balanitis xerotica obliterans (BXO), *AUA Update Series* 16:166–167, 1997.

Chapple C, Barbagli G, Jordan G, et al: Consensus statement on urethral trauma, *BJU Int* 93:1195–1202, 2004.

Chapple CR, Pang D: Contemporary management of urethral trauma and the post-traumatic stricture, *Curr Opin Urol* 9:253–260, 1999.

Coursey JW, Morey AF, McAninch JW, et al: Erectile function after anterior urethroplasty, *J Urol* 166:2273–2276, 2001.

Devine CJ Jr, Blackley SK, Horton CE, et al: The surgical treatment of chordee without hypospadias in men, *J Urol* 146:325–329, 1991.

Fichtner J, Filipas D, Fisch M, et al: Long-term outcome of ventral buccal mucosa onlay graft urethroplasty for urethral stricture repair, *Urology* 64:648–650, 2004.

Heyns CF, Steenkamp JW, de Kock ML, et al: Treatment of male urethral strictures: is repeated dilation or internal urethrotomy useful?, *J Urol* 160:356–358, 1998.

Iselin CE, Webster GD: The significance of the open bladder neck associated with pelvic fracture urethral distraction defects, *J Urol* 162:34–51, 1999.

Jordan GH: The application of tissue transfer techniques in urologic surgery. In Webster G, Kirby R, King L, et al, editors: *Reconstructive urology*, Oxford, UK, 1993, Blackwell Scientific, pp 143–169.

Levine J, Wessells H: Comparison of open and endoscopic treatment of posttraumatic posterior urethral strictures, *World J Surg* 25:1597–1601, 2001.

McCallum RW, Colapinto V: The role of urethrography in urethral disease. Part I. Accurate radiological localization of the membranous urethra and distal sphincters in normal male subjects, *J Urol* 122:607–611, 1979a.

McCallum RW, Colapinto V: The role of urethrography in urethral disease. Part II. Indications for transsphincter urethroplasty in patients with primary bulbous strictures, *J Urol* 122:612–618, 1979b.

McRoberts JW, Chapman WH, Answell JS: Primary anastomosis of the traumatically amputated penis: case report and summary of literature, *J Urol* 100:751–754, 1968.

Morey AF, Metro MJ, Carney KJ, et al: Consensus on genitourinary trauma: external genitalia, *BJU Int* 94:507–515, 2004.

Pansadoro V, Emiliozzi P: Internal urethrotomy in the management of anterior urethral strictures: long-term followup, *J Urol* 156:73–75, 1996.

Quartey JK: One stage penile/preputial cutaneous island flap urethroplasty for urethral stricture: a preliminary report, *J Urol* 129:284–287, 1983.

Rourke KF, McCammon KA, Sumfest JM, et al: Open reconstruction of pediatric and adolescent urethral strictures: long-term follow-up, *J Urol* 169:1818–1821, discussion 1821, 2003.

Webster GD, Mathes GL, Selli C: Prostatomembranous urethral injuries: a review of the literature and a rational approach to their management, *J Urol* 130:898–902, 1983.

REFERENCES

The complete reference list is available online at ExpertConsult.com.

83 Surgery of the Scrotum and Seminal Vesicles

Dorota J. Hawksworth, MD, MBA, Mohit Khera, MD, MBA, MPH, and Amin S. Herati, MD

SURGICAL ANATOMY OF THE SCROTUM

Scrotal Wall

A detailed understanding of the scrotal anatomy is critical in the operative planning of scrotal and pelvic surgeries. Knowledge of scrotal wall anatomy enables safer access into the scrotum for common scrotal procedures, facilitates identification of surgical planes during surgical debridement, and allows for multilayer closures.

The scrotal skin is rugated because of its underlying attachment to the dartos muscle, deeply pigmented, and hair-bearing. In contrast with other parts of the body, the scrotum is elastic and highly-temperature regulated to enable spermatogenesis.

Scrotal Contents

Scrotal contents are maintained in their position within the scrotal cavity by the spermatic cord and gubernacular attachments. The testicle is intimately encased by the tunica albuginea, and protected by the layers of tunica vaginalis, internal and external spermatic fascia (separated by a layer of cremasteric muscle), and ultimately covered by the dartos layer and scrotal skin. **The dartos fascial layer acts as a barrier to the spread of necrotizing fasciitis to deeper structures in the scrotum (Figs. 83.1 and 83.2).** The epididymis originates from the efferent ducts of the rete testis in mediastinum testis. It is located along the posterolateral aspect of the testis, with its head (caput) located superiorly, the body (corpus) along the longitudinal axis of the testis, and the tail (cauda) at the inferior testicular pole. The vas deferens begins as continuation of the cauda epididymis, travels along the spermatic cord into the pelvis, where it becomes ampulla of the vas, joins with seminal vesicles (SVs), and forms the proximal ejaculatory duct. Two nonfunctional, vestigial structures may be encountered in the scrotum: the appendix testis over the upper pole of the testis and the appendix epididymis attached to the head of the epididymis.

Vasculature

The scrotum is highly vascularized, with blood supply provided anteriorly from the superficial external pudendal artery and deep external pudendal artery, and posteriorly from the posterior scrotal artery. Venous drainage follows the arterial supply draining into the external pudendal vein and posterior scrotal vein, which empty into the great saphenous vein and to the internal iliac veins, respectively.

In addition to temperature regulation, **the thin, highly vascular nature of the scrotal skin allows increased transdermal medication absorption, up to 40 times the absorption of other parts of the body** (Nieschlag and Behre, 2010). This absorptive quality of the scrotal skin was utilized in testosterone supplementation; however, the necessity of frequent scrotal hair clipping made continued application of scrotal testosterone patches cumbersome for patients, and this formulation of testosterone is no longer available. Additionally, the scrotal skin is high in 5α-reductase enzyme, and as result, high dihydrotestosterone levels were seen with scrotal transdermal testosterone therapy (Ahmed et al., 1988).

The blood supply to the testis arises from the aorta as the testicular artery, from the internal iliac artery as the artery to the ductus deferens, and from the external iliac artery as the cremasteric artery. The epididymis is nurtured by the superior epididymal artery from the testicular artery and from the inferior epididymal artery, arising as branches off the deferential artery and distal branches of the testicular artery. Although the majority of the blood supply (~84%) to the epididymis comes from the superior epididymal artery, **the superior epididymal artery can be sacrificed to gain additional testicular mobilization during vasectomy reversal because of the vascular anastomoses between the superior and inferior epididymal artery** (Strittmatter and Konrad, 1989). Understanding the blood supply to the epididymides is important in the surgical treatment of epididymal disease.

Important anastomoses are also present cranial and caudal to the testis. Cranially, thin-caliber anastomoses are often present in the spermatic cord between the testicular artery and the deferential artery approximately 10 cm above the testis (Strittmatter and Konrad, 1989). At the level of the cauda of the epididymis, anastomoses form between the testicular artery, deferential artery, and cremasteric artery. **This redundancy of blood supply to the testis allows viability of the testis if one or two of the arteries are injured or ligated.**

Innervation

The scrotum is innervated by autonomic and somatic nerve fibers. Three groups of converging autonomic nerve fibers contribute to the autonomic innervation of the testes: (1) superior spermatic nerves, from the renal and mesenteric plexi, which follow the testicular artery, (2) middle spermatic nerves, from the superior hypogastric plexus, which travel adjacent to the vas as it enters the internal spermatic ring, and (3) inferior spermatic nerves, which originate from the inferior hypogastric plexus (Patel, 2017). The inferior spermatic nerve fibers fuse with the middle spermatic nerve fibers at the prostate-vesical junction, run within the spermatic cord along the vas deferens, and ultimately penetrate the epididymis and testis (Sosa et al., 2009; Patel, 2017). In addition to the sensory fibers contained in the autonomic spermatic nerves, afferent fibers of these nerves are also important in the endocrine control of the testis. Sosa et al. demonstrated the endocrine control over testis function by modulating androgen release in adult male rats via exposure of autonomic ganglia to adrenoreceptor agonists and antagonists (Sosa et al., 2009). Exposure of the inferior mesenteric plexus ganglia to noradrenaline resulted in significantly higher serum testosterone levels compared with untreated ganglia in the control male rats; however, noradrenaline exposure to the superior mesenteric ganglia did not influence testosterone concentrations.

The scrotum is also innervated by somatic nerves, including ilioinguinal and genitofemoral nerves. The genital branch of the genital femoral nerve is positioned on the inferolateral aspect of the spermatic cord and innervates the anterolateral scrotal skin, the tunica vaginalis, and the cremaster muscles (Ducic and Dellon, 2004; Zorn et al., 1994). In contrast, the ilioinguinal nerve sits on the anterior of the cremasteric muscles and innervates the anterior scrotal skin (Wijsmuller et al., 2007). An understanding of the course of these nerves is important in scrotal denervation procedures, which are discussed later in this chapter.

PREOPERATIVE CONSIDERATIONS

Hair removal from the surgical field facilitates exposure, reduces surgical site infection, enables suturing, and eases the application

1844 PART VII Male Genitalia

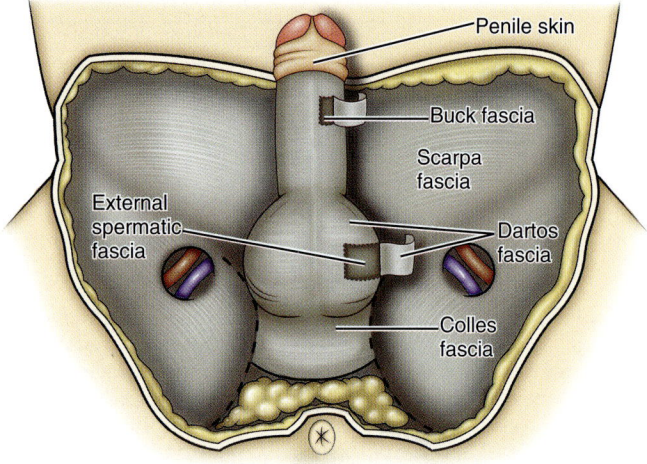

Fig. 83.1. Anatomic barriers to the spread of infection. (Modified from Kavoussi PK, Costabile RA. Disorders of scrotal contents: orchitis, epididymitis, testicular torsion, torsion of the appendages, and Fournier gangrene. In: Chapple CR, Steers WD, eds. *Practical urology: essential principles and practice.* London: Springer-Verlag; 2011.)

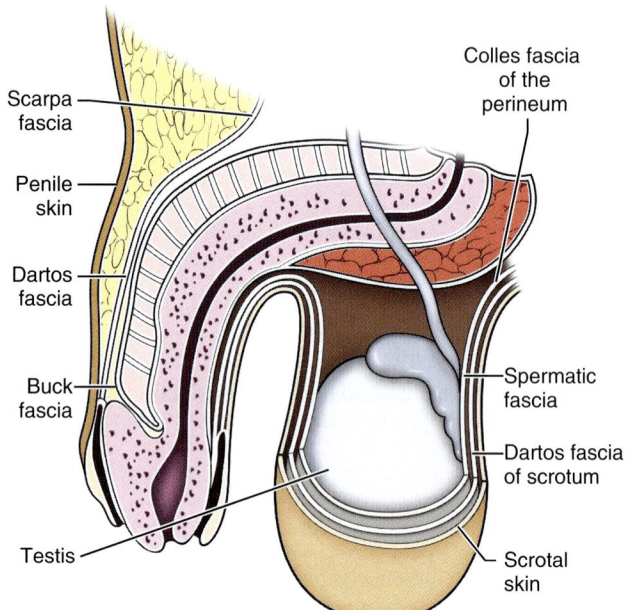

Fig. 83.2. Sagittal view of anatomic barriers to the spread of infection. (Modified from Kavoussi PK, Costabile RA. Disorders of scrotal contents: orchitis, epididymitis, testicular torsion, torsion of the appendages, and Fournier gangrene. In: Chapple CR, Steers WD, eds. Practical urology: essential principles and practice. London: Springer-Verlag; 2011.)

of wound dressing (Alexander et al., 1983; World Health Organization, 2016). The methods of epilation include clippers and razors. Although most hospitals encourage the use of clippers, Grober et al. (2013) showed a lower rate of skin trauma and improved shave quality of razors over clippers ($P < 0.05$). **Scrotal hair should be removed using a disposable razor on the day of surgery.**

The scrotal skin is cleansed of bacteria using an antiseptic such as iodine solutions and chlorhexidine gluconate. Although a 2015 Cochrane review showed lower infection rates with a chlorhexidine scrub compared with alcohol-based povidone iodine paint, the studies analyzed were of small sample sizes and of poor methodologic quality (Dumville et al., 2015). The choice of antiseptic product should be based on cost and patient allergy profile.

According to the American Urological Association (AUA) Best Practice Statement on Urologic Surgery Antimicrobial Prophylaxis, genital surgical procedures should be prophylaxed with a single dose of intravenous cephalosporin or clindamycin for patients who possess risk factors for infection, such as advanced age, anatomic abnormalities of the urinary tract, poor nutritional status, smoking, chronic corticosteroid use, immunodeficiency, externalized catheters, colonized endogenous/exogenous material, distant coexistent infection, and prolonged hospitalization (Wolf et al., 2008).

The choice of anesthetics can include local, regional, spinal, and/or general anesthetics. The combination of spermatic cord block and local infiltration of anesthetic allows for the successful in-office completion of a number of scrotal procedures (Alom et al., 2017; Fuchs, 1982; Magoha, 1998). Regardless of whether the scrotal surgery is performed in the operating theater or in an office setting, preincisional injection of a local anesthetic with 0.5% lidocaine without epinephrine is recommended to control postprocedural pain (Leach, 1996).

Surgical Approaches to Scrotal Contents
Access Into the Scrotum

The approach to scrotal surgery depends on the etiology. Benign diseases of the scrotum are approached through a scrotal incision, whereas possible malignant conditions are approached through an inguinal incision. To prevent tumor seeding during the inguinal approach, the spermatic cord is isolated and clamped with noncrushing clamps until frozen-section biopsies confirm the presence of neoplasia. Scrotal hypothermia can be utilized once the spermatic cord is clamped; however, animal models show impaired testicular function and greater testicular histopathologic change associated with cold ischemia compared with warm ischemia over a 5-week period (Goldstein and Waterhouse, 1983; McNamara et al., 2014). If no malignancy is detected on frozen section, then the testis and spermatic cord can be spared and the remainder of the surgery can be performed.

Access into the scrotum can be obtained with either a transverse or a median raphe scrotal incision. Common to all techniques, dissection must be performed with attention to obtain hemostasis when the tunica vaginalis is bluntly taken off of the scrotal wall and to not injure the testis, epididymis, or other cord structures when making the incision into the tunica vaginalis to access intrascrotal contents. Obstructive azoospermia can result from injuries to the epididymis and/or vas deferens during hydrocelectomy, thus great care should be taken to avoid these structures opening and excising the hydrocele sac (Ross and Flom, 1991).

SURGERIES OF THE SCROTUM
Scrotal Wall
Cyst/Tumor Excision

Scrotal sebaceous cysts and epidermal inclusion cysts, like any other skin cystic lesions, are either managed conservatively or with surgical resection, if not infected. The standard ellipsoid resection yields excellent outcomes and with good cosmetic results (Noel et al., 2006). If the scrotal lesion has any signs of infection, it is either managed solely with a course of antibiotics or with incision and drainage (I&D) in addition to systemic therapy. This can be easily performed in a clinic or emergency room setting with minimal analgesia and morbidity. Once the infection resolves, patients often require surgical excision, as recurrence is quite high.

Partial/Total Scrotectomy

Partial scrotectomy is performed uncommonly and is mostly required in an infectious process caused by Fournier gangrene (FG). Urgent surgical debridement is of essence as tissue gangrene can spread as quickly as 2 to 3 cm/hour, and delay can result in significant increase in patient mortality (Paty and Smith, 1992). Repeat debridement should be performed every 24 to 48 hours as all visibly necrotic tissue must be removed (Fig. 83.3A). On average, patients require up to 4 repeat debridement procedures (Norton et al., 2002). Treatment of patients with FG requires a multidisciplinary approach, to include trauma, general, and colorectal surgeons, and intensive care and infectious disease specialists. Extension of gangrene to the anorectal region may necessitate fecal diversion with a colostomy and is an important consideration in the preoperative planning of FG patients.

Partial scrotectomy is also required in patients who had an inadvertent scrotal violation during an evaluation and/or treatment of a nonseminomatous germ cell tumor of the testis. To prevent tumor contamination and local recurrence, partial scrotectomy is required following a trans-scrotal tumor aspiration, biopsy, exploration, and/or orchiectomy.

Other scrotal nonmalignant conditions (such as hidradenitis suppurativa, postradiation lymphedema, penoscrotal Paget disease, and primary lymphangitis) may also require extensive surgical excision. Finally, partial scrotectomy can also be performed for cosmesis to reduce the level of scrotal descent.

Total scrotectomy is less commonly performed than partial scrotectomy. It is often required when there is extensive involvement of scrotal skin with FD, in malignant processes, and in extensive trauma-related damage. If an extensive amount of scrotal skin is removed and an immediate reconstruction is not performed, the testes are placed into medial thigh pockets with loose wound approximation until the scrotum can be reconstructed.

Scrotal Reconstruction

Reconstruction of the scrotum depends on the extent of the defect and on the availability of suitable local tissue. Following surgical debridement, patients can be left with significant scrotal defects. Small scrotal defects can be successfully treated with wet-to-dry dressing changes. Larger scrotal defects are managed with negative-pressure wound therapy with a vacuum-assisted closure (VAC) device (VAC KCI, San Antonio, TX). Negative-pressure therapy hastens recovery by evacuating bacteria and edema, improving angiogenesis, and promoting granulation of the wound bed. These changes hasten recovery time, reduce the surface area of the wound, and improve the likelihood of skin graft take (Scherer et al., 2002; Silberstein et al., 2008).

Scrotal wound closure for FG depends on the wound size and spread of gangrene beyond the scrotum (Fig. 83.3B–E). Small defects, involving less than one-half of the scrotum, can heal by secondary intention. This process can be potentially further facilitated by loose approximation of skin edges with nonabsorbable monofilament suture and VAC therapy. Larger defects, involving more than one-half of the scrotum, can be closed with local advancement flaps with either use of remaining scrotum or thigh tissues. The remaining scrotal skin and dartos can be undermined and stretched to cover much larger defects (Por et al., 2003). It has been reported that defects up to 96 cm^2 can be replaced with the remaining scrotal skin (Silberstein et al., 2008). If scrotal flaps are impossible to perform because of lack of local tissue, fasciocutaneous flaps obtained either from the superomedial or anterolateral thigh have been described and can be used with good cosmetic results (Lin et al., 2016; Mello and Helene Júnior, 2018; Oufkir et al., 2013). Meshed split-thickness skin grafts can also be used for coverage of scrotal defects, although they are inferior to thigh flaps, as more significant contracture-related effects occur with their application (Karian et al., 2015) (Fig. 83.4).

Testis

Hydrocelectomy

Hydroceles arise from the accumulation of fluid between the parietal and visceral layers of the tunica vaginalis. Congenital hydroceles arise from persistent drainage of peritoneal fluid through a patent processus vaginalis (communicating hydrocele), with a higher prevalence of congenital hydrocele among preterm neonates. The processus vaginalis, which arises embryologically from the peritoneum, normally closes by the second year of life, with 80% of congenital hydroceles spontaneously resolving by 18 months of age (Osifo and Osaigbovo, 2008). In contrast, acquired hydroceles form as a result of an imbalance between the production and reabsorption of fluid within the tunica vaginalis. Acquired hydroceles are among the most common benign scrotal conditions affecting adult men older than 40 years of age. In an ultrasound study of 40 asymptomatic men, 86% of the hemiscrotums evaluated had at least a minimal amount of peritesticular fluid (Leung et al., 1984). This fluid can consist of peritoneal fluid, lymph fluid, abscess, blood, bile, cerebrospinal fluid, or urine (Dagur et al., 2017).

Hydroceles generally present as a painless bulge in the groin and may extend along the spermatic cord and into the inguinal canal. They do not require treatment unless there is associated discomfort, cosmetic concerns, or an underlying malignancy. Urgent treatment may be necessary in the setting of a pyocele with associated clinical symptoms of infection. High-resolution B-mode ultrasonography and color Doppler ultrasonography play important roles in distinguishing among the various causes of fluid accumulation and often guide the surgical approach.

Various approaches are available for performing the hydrocelectomy including excisional and plication techniques. **In general, excisional techniques are associated with the lowest rates of recurrence and should be reserved for chronic, large, multiloculated and thick-walled hydroceles** (Rodriguez et al., 1981). Excisional techniques include the Jaboulay technique, the bottleneck procedure, the window operation, and the simple excision technique.

Lord Plication. Thin-walled and smaller volume hydroceles are often amenable to a plication procedure. The Lord plication technique involves opening the hydrocele sac along its anterior surface, extruding the testis through the aperture, and plicating the sac using interrupted, radially placed chromic sutures in a circumferential fashion (Fig. 83.5) (Lord, 1964). As no excision is performed, this technique carries the lowest risk for hematoma postoperatively and does not benefit from drain placement.

Jaboulay (Winkelman) Technique. The Jaboulay technique involves resecting a portion of the parietal tunica albuginea, everting the parietal layer of the tunica behind the testis, and approximating the opposing parietal tunical edges to each other without compressing the spermatic cord. Alternatively, once the excess tunica vaginalis is excised and the bleeding edges have been cauterized, the cut edges can be oversewn with a 3-0 chromic suture (Fig. 83.6).

Bottleneck Technique. The bottleneck procedure entails trimming all but a 2-cm circumferential segment of tunica around the testis and cord structures and tacking the tunical edges to each other, leaving the sac open (Fig. 83.7).

Window Technique. A less commonly used approach involves a 4-cm anterior scrotal wall incision to reach the parietal layer of the tunica vaginalis. Blunt dissection is performed to separate the tissue overlying the parietal layer away from the tunica vaginalis. Following a stab incision into the tunica to drain the hydrocele fluid, a 2.5 × 2.5-cm cruciate incision, or a "window," is made into the parietal layer of the tunica vaginalis (Nigam, 1984). The flaps of the cruciate incision are everted and stitched with a 2-0 chromic suture.

Aspiration and Sclerotherapy

William of Saliceto first described the instillation of sclerosing agents into the scrotum using sugar and ginger in the thirteenth century (Bullock and Thurston, 1987). Sclerosing agents re-emerged in 1975 as a cost-effective, office-based alternative to hydrocelectomy and spermatocelectomy, and aspiration and sclerotherapy (AS) of hydroceles and spermatoceles remains a viable option for nonsurgical patients (Moloney, 1975). **Because of the high recurrence rate (78% to 86%) associated with aspiration alone, a sclerosing agent should be used to reduce the risk for hydrocele recurrence** (Lund et al., 2014; Roosen et al., 1991). Various sclerotherapy agents have been reported in the literature including doxycycline, tetracycline, alcohol, polidocanol, ethanolamine oleate, and sodium tetradecylsulfate (STDS)

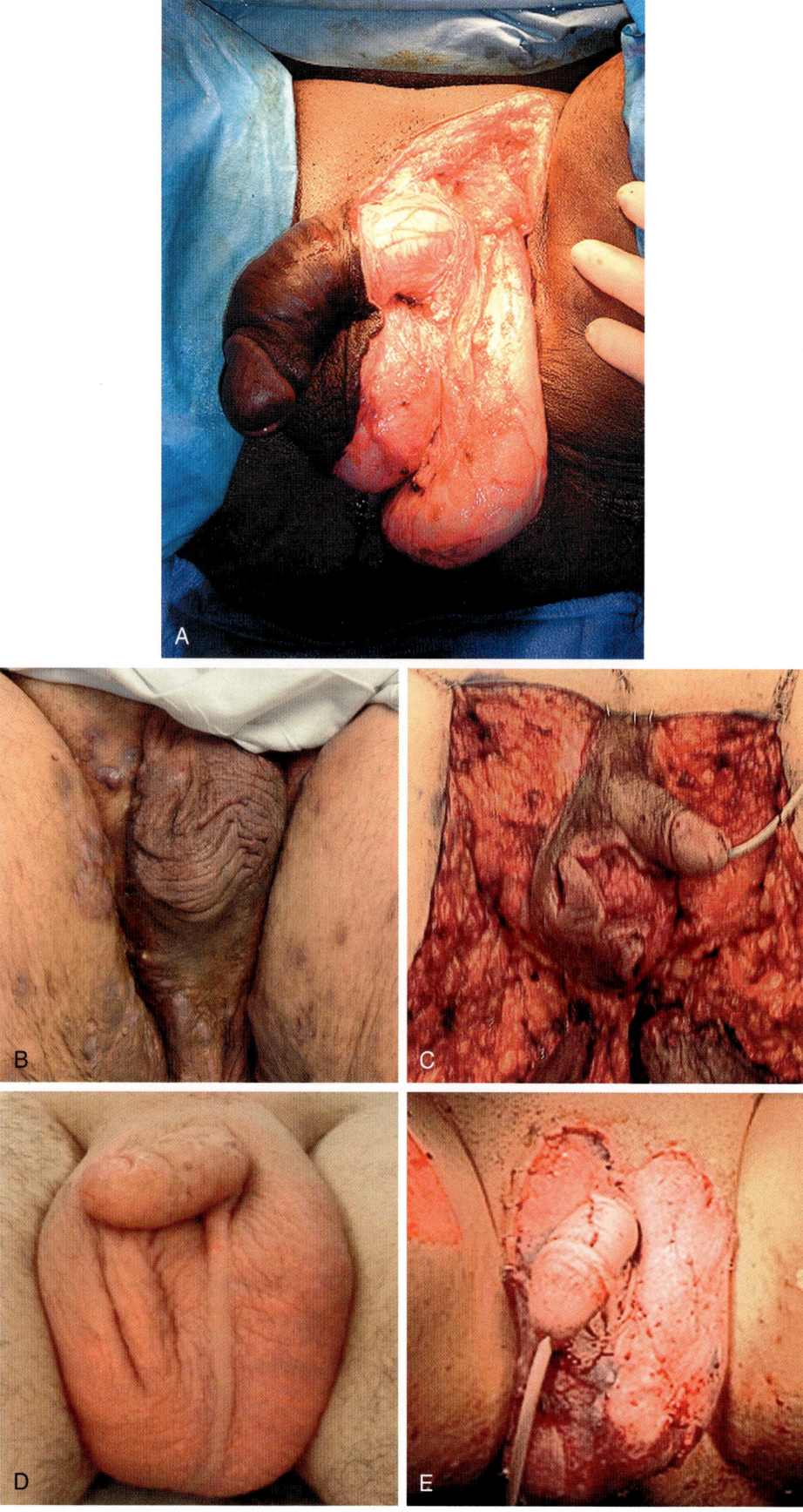

Fig. 83.3. (A) Aggressive debridement of Fournier gangrene. (B to E) Wide excision of hidradenitis suppurativa of the perineum. (B) Before. (C) After. Use of excision and split-thickness skin graft for lymphedema of the penis and scrotum. (D) Before. (E) After. (A, From Kavoussi PK, Costabile RA. Disorders of scrotal contents: orchitis, epididymitis, testicular torsion, torsion of the appendages, and Fournier gangrene. In: Chapple CR, Steers WD, eds. *Practical urology: essential principles and practice*. London: Springer-Verlag; 2011.)

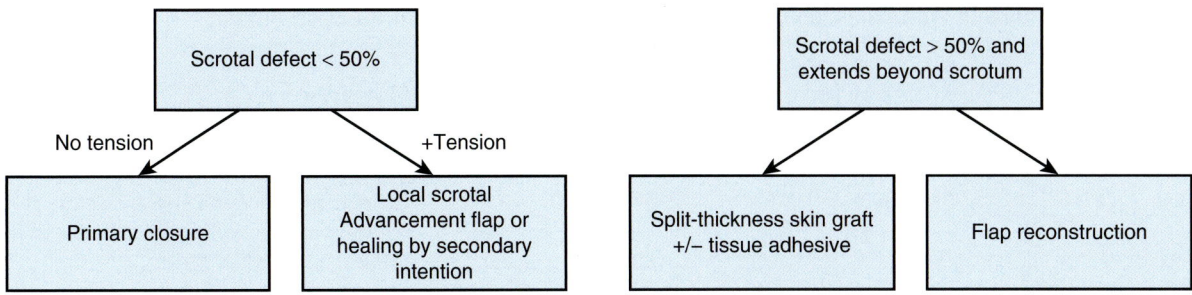

Fig. 83.4. Algorithm for the management of scrotal reconstruction following scrotal debridement. (Modified from Karian LS, Chung SY, Lee ES. Reconstruction of defects after Fournier gangrene: a systematic review. *Eplasty.* 2015;15:e18. eCollection 2015.)

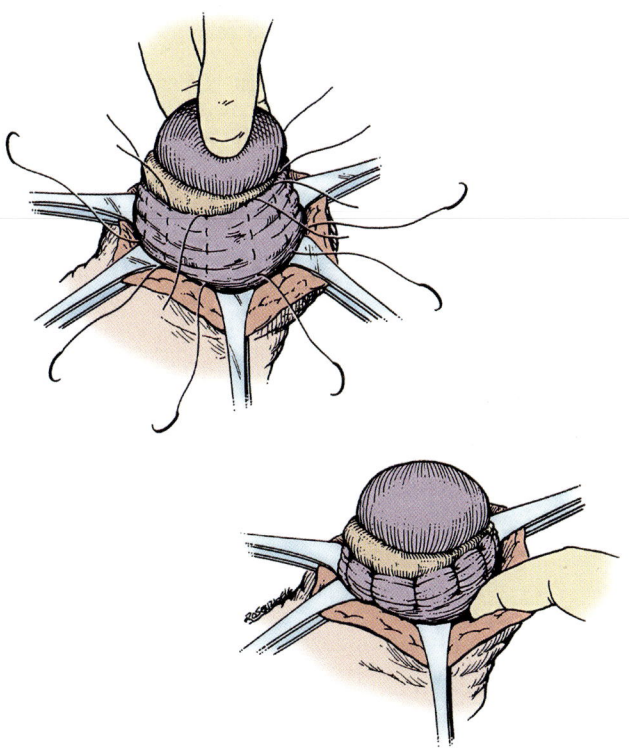

Fig. 83.5. Lord plication technique.

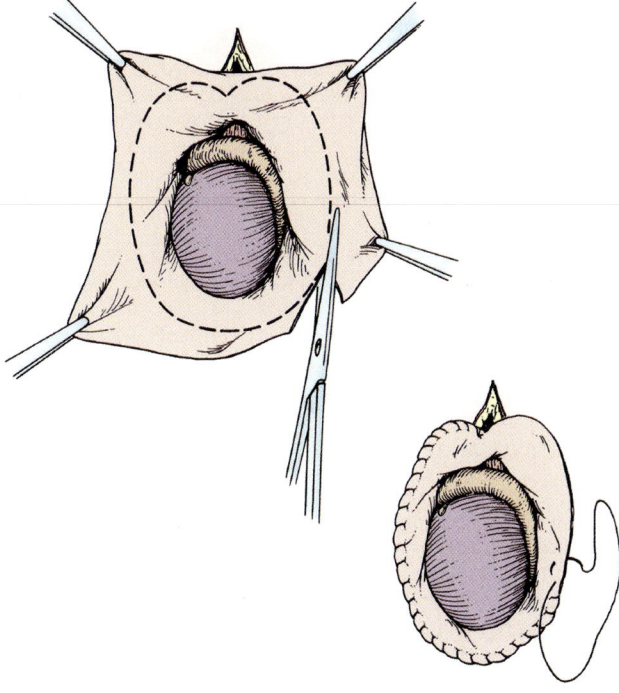

Fig. 83.7. Simple excision of the thick-walled hydrocele sac and oversewn edges.

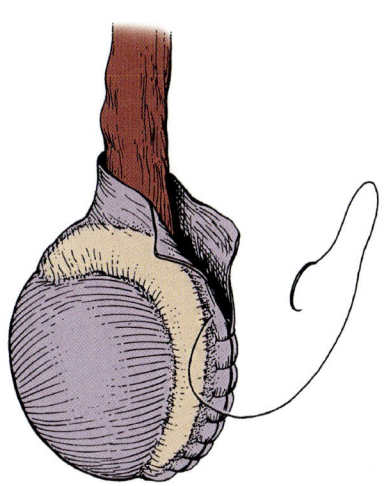

Fig. 83.6. Jaboulay technique for excision of thin, floppy sacs.

(Beiko et al., 2003; Braslis and Moss, 1996; Daehlin et al., 1997; Francis and Levine, 2013; Jahnson et al., 2011; Lund et al., 2014; Shan et al., 2011; Shokeir et al., 1994; Tammela et al., 1992). **Single-procedure success rates vary with the various sclerosing agents and can range from 33% to 85%; however, the best success rates are associated with the use of tetracycline and polidocanol** (see Table 83.1 for comparisons of success rates using various sclerosing agents).

Technique

To perform AS, the affected hemiscrotum is cleansed and prepped with chlorhexidine. Local anesthetic is injected to the site of aspiration and the spermatic cord blocked before aspiration with a mix of 1% lidocaine and 0.25% bupivacaine. Once the skin and spermatic cord are adequately anesthetized, a 16- to 19-gauge angiocatheter is inserted into the sac in either the lateral or anterior and superior aspects of the scrotum. Plastic cannulas are less likely to slip out of the sac and are preferred. The angiocatheter is preconnected to a 60-cc Luer-Lock syringe with connector tubing to maintain a closed system. The fluid is analyzed microscopically to determine if sperm are present. Fluid should also be sent for culture or cytology if clinical

TABLE 83.1 Sclerosants With Associated Single-Procedure and Retreatment Success Rates

SCLEROSANT	SINGLE-PROCEDURE SUCCESS RATE	RETREATMENT SUCCESS RATE	REFERENCE
Polidocanol	54%–67%	83%–89%	(Jahnson et al., 2011; Lund et al., 2014; Sigurdsson et al., 1994)
Tetracycline	57%–85%	57%–90%	(Bullock and Thurston, 1987; Daehlin et al., 1997; Levine and DeWolf, 1988; Shokeir et al., 1994)
Doxycyline	84%	88%	(Francis and Levine, 2013)
Sodium tetradecylsulfate	62%–76%	94%–96%	(Beiko et al., 2003; Braslis and Moss, 1996; Khaniya et al., 2009; Rencken et al., 1990)
99.5% Alcohol	76%	98%	(Shan et al., 2011)
5% Ethanolamine oleate	68%	98%	(Tammela et al., 1992)

suspicion is present for infection or malignancy. Once all the fluid is drained and the volume recorded, sclerotherapy can be performed by injecting the sclerosing agent into the collapsed sac and massaging it. If recurrence occurs in the weeks following AS, the procedure can be repeated or the patient can proceed to hydrocelectomy.

Limitations of AS include pain, multiple treatments necessary for cure, and diminished efficacy for multiloculated hydrocele sacs and large hydrocele sacs (>750 cc) (Francis and Levine, 2013). Comparisons of AS with hydrocelectomy correction confirm the lower success rates (76% vs. 84%, respectively) and lower satisfaction rates (75% vs. 87.5%, respectively) for AS, a first-line option (Beiko et al., 2003). However, complications and costs are less with AS compared with open repair, and repeat treatments may improve the success rate up to 94% (Beiko et al., 2003; Braslis and Moss, 1996; Khaniya et al., 2009).

Simple Orchiectomy

Bilateral simple orchiectomy continues to be a treatment option for patients with hormonally-responsive metastatic prostate cancer who would like to avoid medical androgen deprivation therapy (ADT). From 1991 to 1998, orchiectomy procedures for ADT decreased by 10.2%, and use of gonadotropin-releasing hormone (GnRH) agonist increased 29.6% over the same period (Shahinian et al., 2005). However, with a threefold increase in overall economic burden of cancer treatment over the last two decades, which has partly been driven by the rising cost of medical castration, decreasing reimbursement, and survival advantage conferred with orchiectomy over medical castration, surgical castration is regaining its foothold as a viable treatment option in the setting of advanced prostate cancer (Elkin and Bach, 2010; Elliott et al., 2010; Krahn et al., 2014; Lin et al., 2011; Weight et al., 2008). In a retrospective review of patients with locally advanced and metastatic prostate cancer who were treated with either a luteinizing hormone–releasing hormone (LHRH) agonist or simple orchiectomy, surgical castration was associated with a lower rate of PSA rebound ($P = 0.02$), tumor progression-free survival ($P < 0.001$), and overall survival rate ($P < 0.001$) (Lin et al., 2011). In addition to the cost savings of surgical over medical castration, Potosky et al. showed a lower rate of gynecomastia (LHRH agonist, 24.9% vs. orchiectomy, 9.7%; $P < 0.01$) and higher quality of life because of less physical discomfort and anxiety regarding their prostate cancer in surgically castrated men than in men treated with an LHRH agonist (Potosky et al., 2001). Nevertheless, patients must be counseled on the potential negative impact on self-image associated with orchiectomy procedures (Anderson et al., 2008; Saylor and Smith, 2009).

Several options are available to maintain the esthetics of patients undergoing bilateral orchiectomy for androgen deprivation, including the placement of testicular prostheses and an epididymal-sparing orchiectomy (both of which are described later in this chapter). Epididymal-sparing orchiectomy with epididymoplasty in one study compared patient satisfaction scores between conventional orchiectomy and subepididymal orchiectomy, with significantly higher satisfaction associated with the subepididymal approach (Bapat et al., 2011).

Unilateral simple orchiectomy can also be performed in patients with severe testis trauma or prolonged ischemia caused by testicular torsion, when testis salvage is impossible. Much less commonly, orchiectomy can also be performed in patients with chronic orchalgia. This indication however, lacks level-one evidence and should be utilized only in patients who have failed all other available conservative treatments.

Technique

The simple orchiectomy procedure can be performed through a scrotal incision or through an inguinal incision for patients with orchalgia. **An inguinal approach is associated with better pain-related outcomes in patients with orchalgia.** The improved pain-control arises from resection of more proximal segments of the ilioinguinal, iliohypogastric, and genitofemoral nerves along with the other cord structures to maximize the likelihood of pain relief (Fig. 83.8). In a small retrospective review of 24 patients with orchalgia, Davis et al. showed better pain control with a higher rate of cure associated with an inguinal approach (Davis et al., 1990). The authors showed a 73% cure rate of orchalgia and a 27% rate of improved pain when orchiectomy is performed via an inguinal incision compared with a 55% cure and a 33% improved rate associated with scrotal orchiectomy. Yamamoto et al. demonstrated a similar cure rate of 75% albeit in a smaller cohort of four patients (Yamamoto et al., 1995).

If a scrotal approach is used, a single vertical midline incision in the median raphe or bilateral transverse incisions can be used to access the scrotum. Once all the fascial and tunical layers have been opened, the spermatic cord is divided into two bundles that are double-clamped proximally and distally. The spermatic cord is divided between the two clamps, and the proximal stump is suture-ligated with 2-0 vicryl ties.

If the patient elects epididymis-sparing orchiectomy, rather than dividing the spermatic cord, the testis is sharply dissected off the epididymis using an operating microscope. Attention must be paid to locate and suture-ligate the superior, middle, and inferior epididymal arteries that perforate the testis. To obtain additional hemostasis, the longitudinal epididymal edges are approximated with a 4-0 chromic suture; however, the ends of the suture should be left untied. The caput and cauda of the epididymis are then adjoined by tying the free ends of the 4-0 chromic suture together (Issa et al., 2005).

Testicular Prosthesis Placement

Because of the psychological effects of an empty scrotum following an orchiectomy or as a consequence of testicular atrophy secondary to a maldescended testis, consideration should be given to the insertion of a testicular prosthesis. Although early testicular prostheses were composed of the alloy Vitalium (Girsdansky and Newman, 1941),

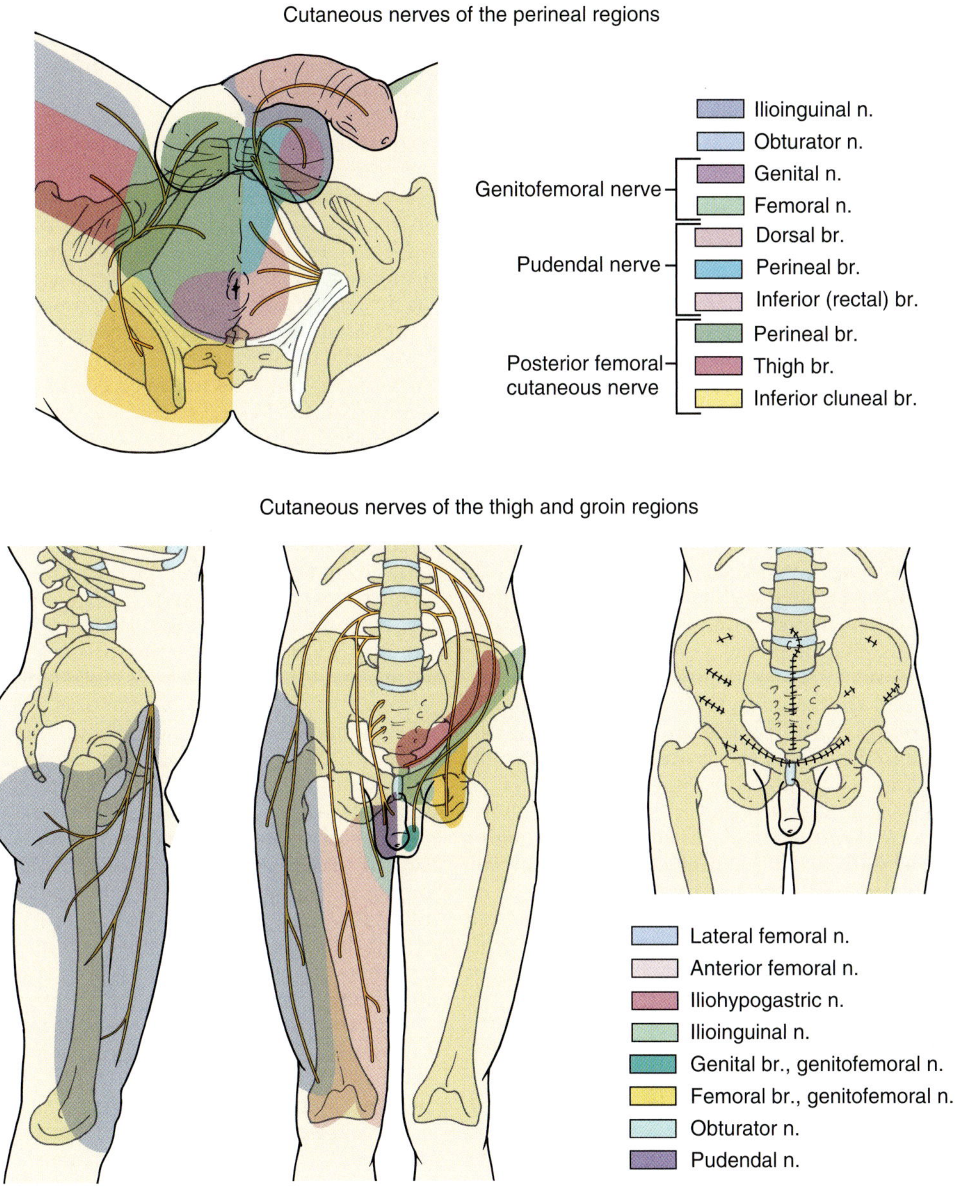

Cutaneous nerves of the perineal regions

- Ilioinguinal n.
- Obturator n.
- Genitofemoral nerve
  - Genital n.
  - Femoral n.
- Pudendal nerve
  - Dorsal br.
  - Perineal br.
  - Inferior (rectal) br.
- Posterior femoral cutaneous nerve
  - Perineal br.
  - Thigh br.
  - Inferior cluneal br.

Cutaneous nerves of the thigh and groin regions

- Lateral femoral n.
- Anterior femoral n.
- Iliohypogastric n.
- Ilioinguinal n.
- Genital br., genitofemoral n.
- Femoral br., genitofemoral n.
- Obturator n.
- Pudendal n.

Fig. 83.8. Distribution of cutaneous nerves of the scrotum, perineum, thigh, and groin regions. (Courtesy A. Lee Dellon, MD, PhD, from Dellon.com.)

lucite (Rea, 1943), and glass (Hazzard, 1953), the only FDA-approved testicular prosthesis is a silicone implant called the Coloplast Torosa (Coloplast, Minneapolis, MN). The Torosa (Fig. 83.9) comes in sizes ranging from extra-small to large and are inflatable with sodium chloride U.S.P. solution, which can be injected into the prosthetic via an injection port. However, the injection port should not be pierced more than five times intraoperatively and should be accessed postoperatively.

Similar to other prosthetic implantation surgeries, strict antiseptic technique is critical during testicular prosthesis insertion. The prosthetics can be inserted via an inguinal, high-scrotal or trans-scrotal incision. The choice of approach often depends on the indication of the orchiectomy, with an inguinal insertion most commonly performed simultaneous to radical orchiectomy and for pediatric patients who have thin scrotal walls (Kogan, 2014; Zaontz et al., 1990). In the absence of malignancy or compromised scrotum, the decision to perform a high-scrotal or scrotal incision depends on surgeon preference; however, the high-scrotal incision into a subdartos pouch carries a lower risk for infection, erosion, and pain secondary to reduced contact between the prosthetic and the suture

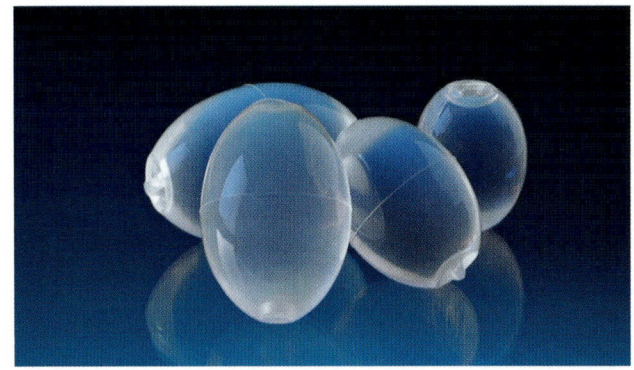

Fig. 83.9. Testicular prostheses. (Image obtained from https://www.coloplastmd.com/products/torosa-testicular-implants/).

line (Libman et al., 2006). The prosthesis can also be placed via a trans-scrotal incision into a suba dartos pouch or into the tunica vaginalis if performed concurrently with a simple orchiectomy for nonsalvageable testicular torsion or during simple orchiectomy for ADT (Bush and Bagrodia, 2012; Lucas et al., 2017).

EPIDIDYMIS

Excision of Epididymal Cysts and Spermatoceles

Epididymal cysts and spermatoceles arise from the cystic accumulations of semen in the epididymal tubules, rete testes, or efferent ductuli. Although most spermatoceles form idiopathically, some can arise from infectious or traumatic processes resulting in inflammation. Similar to the indications for hydrocele repair, spermatoceles and epididymal cysts should only be surgically treated if there is discomfort, infection, disability caused by size, or infertility (Kauffman et al., 2011; Rioja et al., 2011). Epididymal cysts and spermatoceles are common benign findings on scrotal sonography. Leung et al. identified epididymal cystic lesions in approximately 31% of 20- to 39-year-old men and up to 43% of asymptomatic 40- to 59-year-old men (Leung et al., 1984). **Men of reproductive age should be counseled on the risk for obstructive azoospermia associated with epididymal cyst surgery, particularly if the epididymal cyst is located in the corpora or cauda of the epididymis** (Sheynkin et al., 1998).

The preoperative considerations and surgical approach to epididymal cyst excision and spermatocelectomy are similar to that of hydrocelectomy. The most common approach is via a trans-scrotal incision and dissection to the level of the tunica vaginalis. **Once the tunica vaginalis is sharply opened and the epididymal cyst or spermatocele is exposed, an attempt should be made to dissect the cyst or spermatocele down to its stalk and to ligate it with a 5-0 or 6-0 absorbable suture** (Kauffman et al., 2011). If the epididymal cyst or spermatocele cannot be completely dissected off the testis, a portion of the cyst wall can be unroofed and the tunic of the epididymis should be reapproximated with a 4-0 absorbable suture to cover the defect (Rioja et al., 2011). Hemostasis should be obtained with bipolar cautery.

Epididymal Tumor Excision

In contrast with epididymal cystic diseases, tumors of the epididymis with malignant potential should be approached via an inguinal incision to avoid disruption of the natural lymphatic drainage patterns. The spermatic cord is isolated and clamped with noncrushing clamps until frozen-section biopsies confirm the presence of neoplasia (Ting et al., 2018). If preoperative percutaneous biopsy confirms that an epididymal mass is benign, the epididymal tumor can be removed via a trans-scrotal approach. A microsurgical approach with 10× to 25× magnification is recommended to avoid injury to the testicular blood supply (Kauffman et al., 2011; Ting et al., 2018).

> **KEY POINTS: SURGERY OF THE SCROTAL CONTENTS**
>
> - High-resolution ultrasonography is used to evaluate scrotal fluid collection as it may identify intratesticular malignancy and thus guide surgical approach.
> - Excisional hydrocelectomy techniques are associated with the lowest recurrence rates.

VAS DEFERENS

Vasectomy

Vasectomy is a safe, effective, and permanent method of male contraception. In 2015, approximately 520,000 men in the United States underwent a vasectomy (Ostrowski et al., 2018). Worldwide, usage of vasectomy varies by country and can exceed 10% of men in countries such as Australia, Bhutan, Canada, the Netherlands, New Zealand, the Republic of Korea, Great Britain, and the United States (Pile and Barone, 2009). **Contemporary analysis of vasectomy trends demonstrates that >80% of vasectomies are performed on 25- to 44-year-old men, in an office setting, and by a urologist** (Ostrowski et al., 2018).

Despite the simplicity and efficacy of vasectomy, significant gender gaps remain between the prevalence of male vasectomy and female tubal ligation. Anderson et al. analyzed the 2006–2008 National Survey of Family Growth data and found a 13.1% (95% confidence interval [CI] 0.104–0.163) reported rate of vasectomy compared with a 21.1% (95% CI 0.178–0.249) reported rate of tubal ligation (Anderson et al., 2012). This disparity in contraceptive methods likely reflects differing family-planning priorities, insurance with lower Medicaid coverage of vasectomies, and marital status, with more unmarried women undergoing tubal ligation than unmarried men undergoing vasectomy (Eeckhaut, 2015; Pile and Barone, 2009; White et al., 2014).

Although the majority of vasectomies are performed in an outpatient clinic setting, the same approach to preoperative planning should be undertaken as for any other surgical procedure performed in an operating theater. **Before the vasectomy, initial in-person or telephonic preoperative consultation should be conducted and should include a review of medical and surgical history, physical examination, and genitourinary examination.** Patients should also be counseled on the potential need for repeat vasectomy if the postvasectomy semen analysis (PVSA) demonstrates persistent live sperm, the potential for recanalization of the two vasal ends resulting in pregnancy, and the 1% to 2% risk for chronic scrotal pain that can ensue. Following the discussion of procedure risks, benefits, and vasectomy alternatives, an informed consent form should be signed preoperatively.

Vasectomy is performed with local anesthesia with or without oral sedation. If the patient declines local anesthesia or if the surgeon believes that local anesthesia will not be adequate for a particular patient, then vasectomy may be performed with intravenous sedation or general anesthesia (Sharlip et al., 2012). The choice of local anesthesia is based on surgeon preference and formulation availability and may include 1% or 2% lidocaine without epinephrine, or a mixture of either with bupivacaine as a 50-50 mix. More recent availability of long-acting anesthetics such as EXPAREL (Pacira Pharmaceuticals Inc, Parsippany, NJ) have also been used, providing significant short- and long-term pain relief, although they may be cost-prohibitive (Alom et al., 2017). The smallest available needle should be used for injection of the local anesthetic, and the AUA Panel recommends that smaller gauge needles (25- to 32-gauge) cause less injection site–related pain and that topical anesthetic cream should not be used as a sole source of anesthesia (Sharlip et al., 2012).

Vasectomy consists of two key surgical steps, and these include vas isolation and its occlusion. With many approaches to both, it is important to emphasize that the surgeon should perform a vasectomy according to his or her established and trained technique, which should be readjusted when and if a significantly higher than expected failure rate is encountered.

Methods of Vas Isolation

Methods of vas isolation consist of conventional vasectomy (CV) and minimally invasive vasectomy (MIV), which includes a no-scalpel vasectomy (NSV), and are related to procedure-associated risk for infection, bleeding, and pain. It is recommended that vas isolation is performed using one of the MIV techniques, as data indicate less procedure-associated discomfort and fewer complications (Sokal et al., 1999).

CV may be still used in patients with a history of prior scrotal surgery or trauma or with a challenging anatomy such as thick, tight scrotal skin, associated varicocele, hydrocele, or spermatocele or under any other conditions when vas isolation with use of MIV cannot be safely performed.

Conventional Vasectomy

This technique implies that the area of scrotal dissection is much larger than with any of the MIV techniques. Depending on surgeon preference, a 1.5- to 3-cm single vertical, median raphe incision or bilateral paramedian scrotal incisions are made. Although there are no studies demonstrating the advantage over a single incision versus bilateral incisions, the single incision seems to carry fewer side effects and is associated with decreased procedure time. Despite this, many surgeons advocate bilateral incisions, as this helps them avoid potential for grasping and transecting the same vas deferens twice. When performing a vasectomy through a single incision, a gentle tug on the vas during its isolation will move the ipsilateral testis, and this will ensure that one vas is not occluded twice. When using a single midline scrotal incision, the skin opening should be performed at the level of penoscrotal junction or between the penoscrotal junction and the top of the testis. When performing bilateral scrotal incisions, they should be placed at the level of the penoscrotal junction or higher, to access the straight aspect of the vas deferens. Making skin openings in lower locations provides access to smaller-diameter convoluted vas, which is overall much more difficult to manipulate during the vasectomy and in the future, during a potential vasectomy reversal.

After infiltration of adequate anesthesia, the vas is firmly grasped and trapped between the surgeon's thumb, index, and middle fingers using a three-finger grasp. The same hand is used to isolate the bilateral vasa. To ease the initial identification of the vas, a few drops of fluid over the scrotal skin may be used for lubrication. Additional anesthetic can be administered after identification of the vas, assuring proper analgesia over the precise location of the planned skin incision. Anesthetic usually takes effect within a few seconds, but testing appropriate analgesia can be easily performed by grasping the skin with an Adson pickup. The patient should be informed that the sensation of tugging and touch is expected, but sharp pain should not be experienced. Additional anesthetic medication should be injected subcutaneously if the patient reports sharp pain and/or appears in significant discomfort.

The skin incision is made over the vasal sheath, longitudinally, down to the vas. During CV, there are no special instruments used, and the vas is usually grasped with a towel clamp or an Allis forceps. While pulling the vas out of the wound, use of a few overlapping clamps may be helpful to avoid its falling back into the scrotum. Adjacent structures should be avoided, and only vas deferens should be occluded. A small segment of vas is removed, and the remaining free vasal ends are occluded. After inspection and assurance that there is no bleeding, the vas ends are dropped back into the scrotum. The methods of vasal occlusion, with or without tissue interposition, are discussed later in this section.

The same procedure is performed on the contralateral side. The skin incisions are closed with an absorbable suture, especially with larger skin openings, as skin edges commonly bleed and cause undue concern to patients.

Minimally Invasive Vasectomy

The term *MIV* describes any vasectomy technique that utilizes a small (≤10 mm) skin opening and minimal vasal dissection. Minimally invasive vasectomy is performed with the use of special vas dissecting instruments (Fig. 83.10) and/or ring-tipped vas clamps (Fig. 83.11). The initial approach is the same as described earlier for CV (however, the size of the incision is limited to <10 mm). The vas is isolated by elevating it to the level of the anterior scrotal skin with manual pressure using the three-finger grasping method.

The MIV technique can be performed using an open- or closed-access approach. In the open approach, just like in the CV, a small skin incision is made with a scalpel, the perivasal tissues are minimally dissected, and then vas is grasped with a clamp. In the closed approach, the vas is grasped with a vas clamp before making an incision. Once this is done, the surgeon can release the vas and use his or her nondominant hand to manipulate the clamp. The incision is made afterward, and the remainder of the procedure is the same as for all approaches. The MIV incisions may be left open, as they are much smaller and carry less bleeding risk.

No-Scalpel Vasectomy

The NSV is the initial MIV technique, developed in China in 1974 and described by Dr. Shunqiang Li (Li et al., 1991). **It is important**

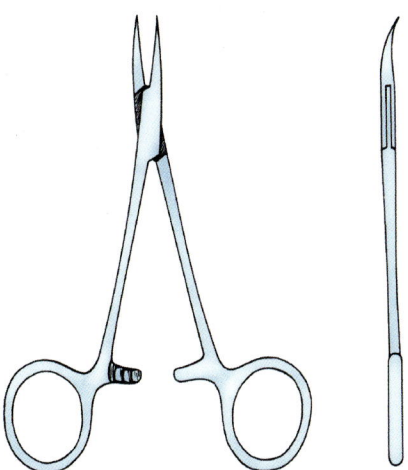

Fig. 83.10. Sharp, curved mosquito hemostat. (From Li S, Goldstein M, Zhu J, et al. The no-scalpel vasectomy. *J Urol* 1991;145:341–344.)

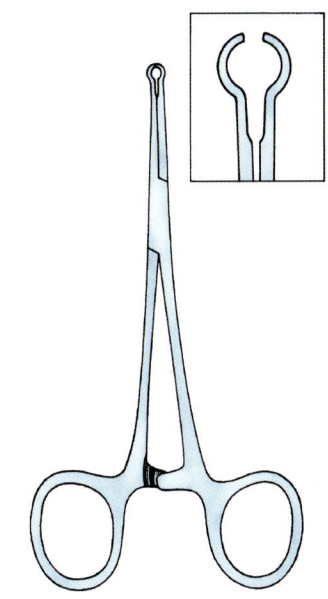

Fig. 83.11. Ring-tipped vas deferens fixation clamp. The cantilevered design prevents injury. (From Li S, Goldstein M, Zhu J, et al. The no-scalpel vasectomy. *J Urol* 1991;145:341–344.)

to emphasize that NSV represents strictly a vas isolation technique and does not specify the vas occlusion method. The vas is grasped with the ring-tipped vas clamp and after a proper anesthesia, the skin overlying the vas is punctured and spread with a sharp, curved mosquito hemostat (Figs. 83.12 and 83.13). This spreading maneuver is continued until the vas is encountered, at which point the anterior vasal wall is pierced with the hemostat and lifted through the skin opening (Figs. 83.14 and 83.15). The partially transected vas is regrasped with the ring clamp, and its posterior wall is dissected and divided to strip the vas of its sheath (see Figs. 83.13 and 83.14). After vas occlusion, the ends are dropped back into the scrotum. The skin perforation(s) can be closed with an absorbable suture or may be left open as the puncture openings are <10 mm.

There are many methods of vas occlusion, and vasectomy success and ultimately failure rates are directly related to the choice of occlusion technique.

In the United States, complete division of the vas with or without excision of its segment is used. Following the vas division, its free ends may be separated by one of many techniques used alone or in combination, including fascial interposition (FI), suture ligation, vas clipping or folding, and mucosal cauterization (MC). **Fascial interposition uses a layer of the internal spermatic fascia to cover**

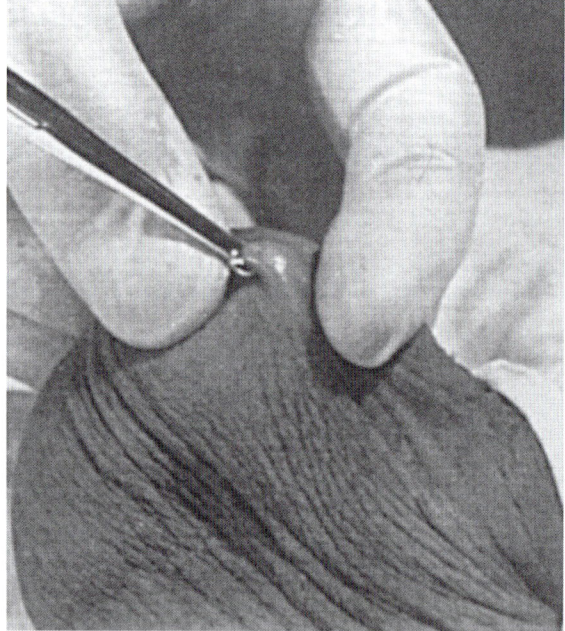

Fig. 83.12. Vas fixed in the ring clamp. The scrotal skin is tightly stretched over the most prominent portion of the vas. (From Li S, Goldstein M, Zhu J, et al. The no-scalpel vasectomy. *J Urol* 1991;145:341–344.)

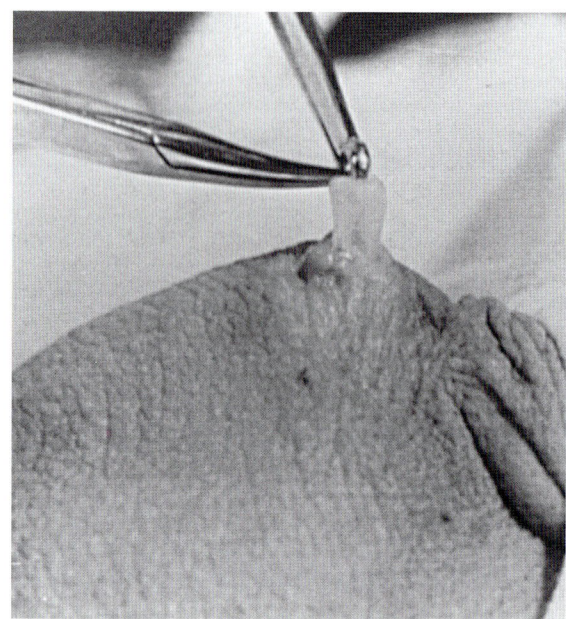

Fig. 83.14. Delivery of the clean vas. (From Li S, Goldstein M, Zhu J, et al. The no-scalpel vasectomy. *J Urol* 1991;145:341–344.)

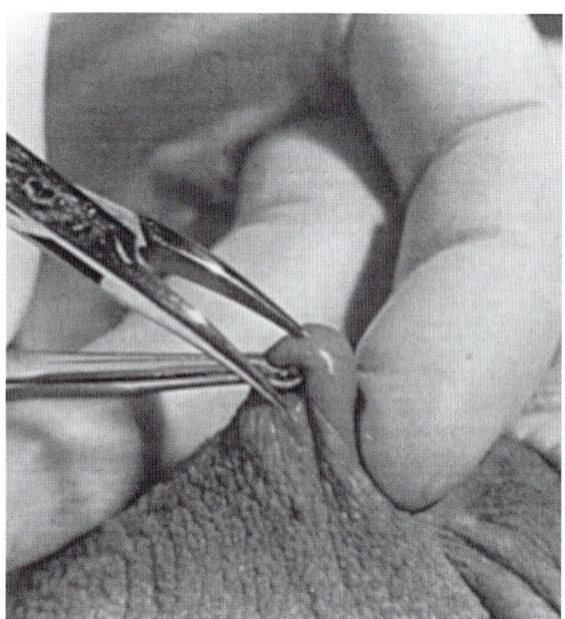

Fig. 83.13. Puncture of the skin, vas sheath, and wall into the lumen. (From Li S, Goldstein M, Zhu J, et al. The no-scalpel vasectomy. *J Urol* 1991;145:341–344.)

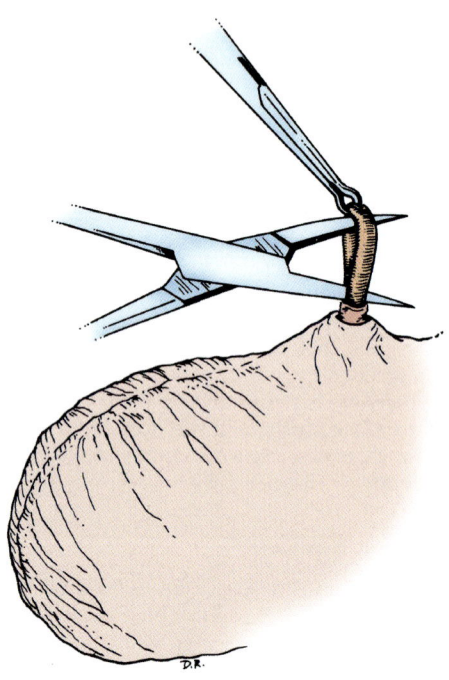

Fig. 83.15. Dissection of the testicular artery away from the vas deferens.

one of the vas ends and is usually used in combination with one of the other occlusion techniques.

Suture ligation is usually applied to both vasal ends. One to three ligating sutures about 1 cm away from the cut edge are usually placed. Clips may be used instead of the suture material to ligate the free vas edges. The vas folding-back technique is utilized at times to prevent the free edges from facing each other and thus possibly recanalizing. MC involves direct application of thermal or electrical cautery to the vas lumen and edge for about a few millimeters to 1.5 cm.

A partial ligation (open-ended) technique may also be used when the abdominal vas is ligated by one of the techniques described earlier, while the testicular vas is left open, and both are separated by FI. This technique is believed to limit the postvasectomy pain likely resulting from epididymal back pressure. This approach may also improve the chances of potential future vasectomy reversal, as presence of sperm granuloma forming at the open vasal end has been associated with improved reversal outcomes (Errey and Edwards, 1986).

The only nondivisional extended cautery technique of vas occlusion (Marie Stopes International technique) does not use vas division and is not commonly used in the United States. This technique involves a 2.5- to 3-cm electrocoagulation of the anterior vas full-thickness and posterior vas partial-thickness. This technique was developed in the United Kingdom as a vasectomy technique that could be easily utilized in Third World conditions (Black et al., 1989).

The current AUA guidelines recommend one of the four methods of vas occlusion that, in large numbers of patients and performed by different surgeons, consistently produce occlusive failure rates (OFR) ≤1%. The following three vas division methods, in addition to the nondivisional approach with extended cautery (OFR = 0.64%), are recommended: (1) MC with FI and without clips or ligatures (OFR = 0.0% to 0.55%); (2) MC without FI and without ligatures/clips (OFR = 0.0% to 0.60%); and (3) open-end vasectomy with the unoccluded testicular end while the abdominal end is occluded with MC and FI (OFR = 0.0% to 0.50%) (Sharlip et al., 2012).

Routine excision of the vasal segment is performed by the majority of surgeons, but, depending on personal preference, training, and outcomes, its excision is not absolutely necessary. It is recommended, that, if excision is performed, a segment of 1.0 cm in length should be adequate.

It is recommended that fresh semen specimen should be tested 8 to 16 weeks postoperatively, with the ultimate choice of proper timing of the initial test left to the surgeon. Before this testing, patients should perform at least 10 to 20 ejaculations, keeping in mind that older men have been found to have lower and slower rates of sperm clearance (Griffin et al., 2005). **If the initial PVSA has persistent motile sperm, a repeat testing is recommended in 6 months. If this trend continues at the 6 month PVSA, the procedure is considered a failure, and arrangements for a repeat procedure should be made** (Sharlip et al., 2012).

Need for use of an alternative contraceptive method until confirmation of procedure success should be emphasized at time of prevasectomy counseling and later, during the discussion of postprocedure instructions. Couples may stop using other contraceptive methods once the PVSA demonstrates azoospermia or only rare nonmotile sperm (RNMS or ≤100,000 nonmotile sperm/mL). **Despite an initial negative PVSA, recanalization can occur and pregnancy rates following a successful vasectomy are at a rate of 0.05%** (Philp et al., 1984a).

Vasectomy Reversal

Vasectomy reversal, performed microscopically is currently a standard of practice and is offered to patients who had a vasectomy in the past and wish to proceed with a natural conception again. A detailed discussion of this topic is provided in a separate chapter.

> **KEY POINTS: VASECTOMY**
> - There is no one vasectomy technique that is 100% effective.
> - Before the vasectomy, initial in-person or telephonic preoperative consultation should be conducted and include review of medical and surgical history, physical examination, and genitourinary examination.
> - Vasectomy success is directly related to the choice of occlusion technique.
> - Complete division of the vas with or without excision of its segment should be utilized.
> - It is recommended that if excision of the vasal end is performed, a segment of 1.0 cm in length should be adequate.
> - Partial ligation (open-ended) technique may improve the chances of potential future vasectomy reversal.
> - Couples may stop using other contraceptive methods once the PVSA demonstrates azoospermia or only rare nonmotile sperm (RNMS or ≤100,000 nonmotile sperm/mL).

SURGICAL MANAGEMENT OF CHRONIC SCROTAL PAIN

Pain is a subjective sensation that originates from noxious stimuli activating nociceptors that transmit ascending signals from the peripheral nervous system toward the central nervous system. Scrotal pain is multifactorial, and its cause often cannot be determined. Chronic scrotal pain is defined as constant or intermittent pain that lasts longer than 3 months and interferes with activities of daily living, and it accounts for up to 4.8% of urologic clinic visits (Ciftci et al., 2010; Sigalos and Pastuszak, 2017). An understanding of the diseases that cause pain in the scrotum, knowledge of the nerve locations in the scrotum, and a systematic approach to the patient with chronic scrotal pain can identify patients who will respond favorably to a surgical approach.

Chronic scrotal pain can originate from the testis, epididymis, pampiniform plexus, sperm extravasation following vasectomy, hematoma following a surgical procedure, or proximal injuries to the ilioinguinal, iliohypogastric, genitofemoral, pudendal, and/or sympathetic nerves (Masarani and Cox, 2003). Scrotal pain can also be referred from the pelvic floor, prostate, or other visceral organs that share nerve pathways with the ilioinguinal, genitofemoral, pudendal, and sympathetic nerves (Tan and Levine, 2017). A comprehensive review of the common causes and treatment of all etiologies of chronic scrotal pain is beyond the scope of this chapter. Rather, the surgical management of intrascrotal abnormalities is discussed. Multiple algorithms are available for patients with chronic scrotal pain (Fig. 83.16).

Surgical Management of Intrascrotal Pain

Acute and Chronic Epididymitis

Most cases of acute epididymitis resolve with conservative measures (rest, scrotal support, elevation, and ice packs), antibiotics, and/or nonsteroidal anti-inflammatory drugs (NSAIDs). Rarely, acute bacterial infections of the epididymis may present as local softening (malacia) of the epididymis suggesting an abscess (Banyra and Shulyak, 2012). Epididymal abscesses that do not respond to antimicrobial therapy should be drained or surgically debrided.

Some patients develop chronic epididymitis despite adequate therapy. Chronic epididymitis is defined as epididymitis that lasts longer than 6 weeks. **Although surgical resection is a treatment option, epididymitis patients treated with epididymectomy often have poor outcomes with persistence of pain, thus surgical management should be considered as a last resort option** (Padmore et al., 1996; Sweeney et al., 1998).

Following a failed trial of medical therapy, the indications for surgical treatment of epididymal disease with partial or total epididymectomy include postvasectomy epididymal engorgement, intractable epididymal pain, severe acute or chronic epididymitis, and symptomatic epididymal cysts. The likelihood of pain control is significantly improved if a palpable abnormality, such as a mass, cyst, or granuloma, is present in the epididymis (Tan and Levine, 2017). **If epididymectomy is performed for epididymitis, patients should be counseled preoperatively on the low likelihood of complete cure of their pain and the potential need for orchiectomy.**

Epididymectomy for Palpable Abnormalities of the Epididymis

In contrast with the poor surgical outcomes of epididymectomy for epididymitis, outcomes are more favorable for patients who have palpable abnormalities of the epididymis, such as epididymal cyst, and undergo partial or complete epididymectomy (Calleary et al., 2009). Epididymectomy performed for cystic dilation, granulomatous, or tender swollen epididymides can be performed by ligating the efferent tubules draining into the caput of the epididymis. The corpora and cauda of the epididymis are sharply dissected from the testis. If a partial epididymectomy is performed, then the remaining proximal and distal stumps of the epididymis are suture-ligated to reduce extravasation of sperm.

Microsurgical Spermatic Cord Denervation

For nonspecific chronic scrotal pain that localizes to the testis and/or epididymis or pain that originates after a vasectomy, a spermatic cord block can identify patients who will respond favorably to microsurgical denervation of the spermatic cord (MDSC) (Benson et al., 2013). **Moreover, the degree of pain relief following a spermatic cord block correlates with the degree of pain relief from MDSC.** Microsurgical denervation of the spermatic cord can be performed via a 4-cm incision over the external inguinal ring.

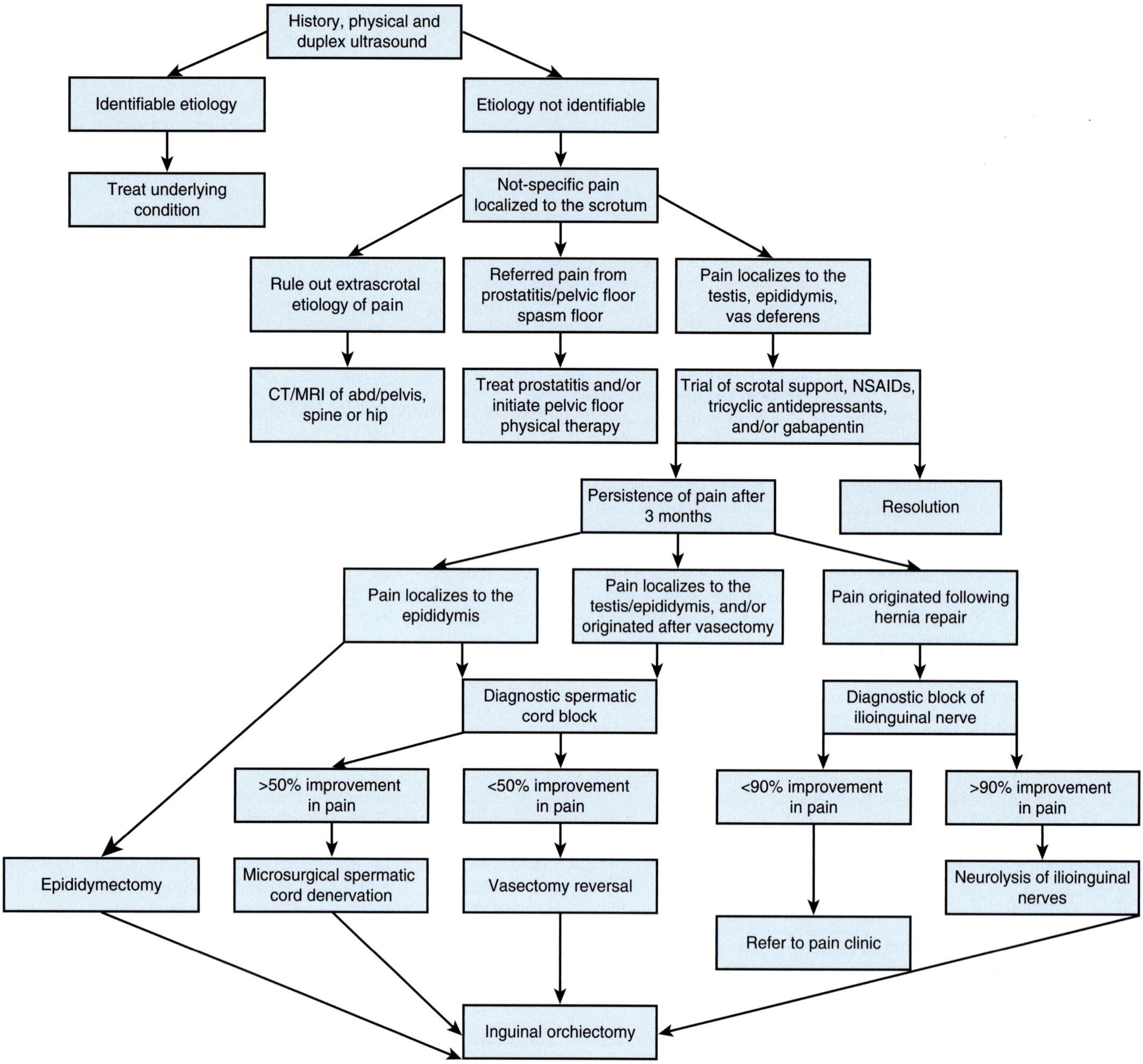

Fig. 83.16. Algorithm of chronic orchalgia evaluation and management. (Modified from Tan WP, Levine LA. What can we do for chronic scrotal content pain? *World J Mens Health* 2017;35(3):146–155).

Once the spermatic cord is isolated at the level of the external inguinal ring, the ilioinguinal nerve is isolated and suture ligated with a 4-0 silk suture (Tan et al., 2018). The genital branch of the genitofemoral nerve can also be identified and ligated at this level. Using an operative microscope with 4× to 20× magnification and a micro-Doppler to distinguish arterial pulsations, arteries of the cremaster muscle and spermatic cord are isolated. Lymphatic vessels are also spared to avoid hydrocele formation. All remaining spermatic cord structures, including pampiniform vessels, vas deferens, and cremaster muscle fibers are subsequently divided with electrocautery.

Denervation can also be performed via a vertical paramedian scrotal incision to isolate the spermatic cord. Similar to the subinguinal approach, lymphatic vessels and arteries of the cremaster and spermatic cord are spared. Parekattil et al. demonstrated a reproducible pattern of scrotal nerve distribution in 56 patients (Parekattil et al., 2013). In decreasing order of nerve density, nerves were located in the cremasteric muscle fibers (mean 19.1 nerves per patient), perivasal tissue and vasal sheath (mean 9.4 nerves per patient), and posterior periarterial/lipoma (mean 3.3 nerves per patient) (Fig. 83.17). In

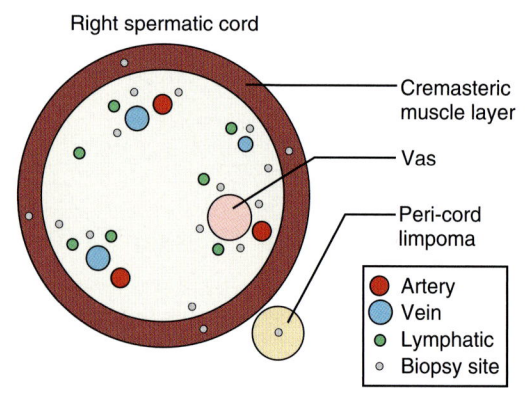

Fig. 83.17. Spermatic cord neural anatomy. (From Parekattil SJ, Gudeloglu A, Brahmbhatt JV, et al. Trifecta nerve complex: potential anatomical basis for microsurgical denervation of the spermatic cord for chronic orchialgia. *J Urol* 2013;190:265–270).

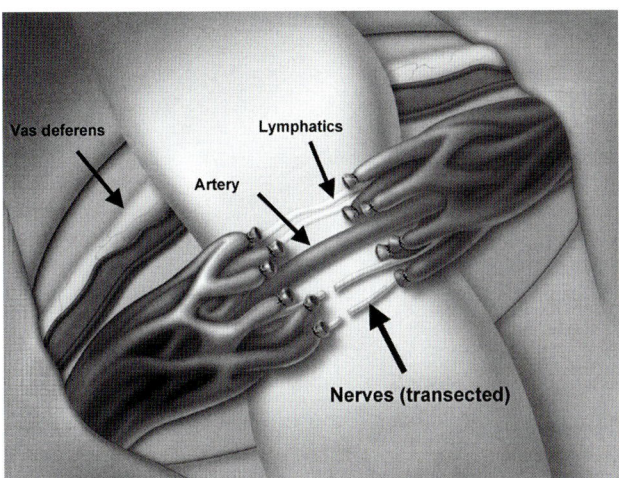

Fig. 83.18. Microsurgical denervation. The goal is to transect all branches of the genitofemoral nerve while preserving the vas deferens, vasal vessels, testicular artery, and lymphatics.

another nerve distribution study by Oka et al., immunohistochemical staining for nerve markers isolated sensory and sympathetic nerves to the perivasal sheath and spermatic fascia (Oka et al., 2016). **Therefore, if a scrotal approach to spermatic cord denervation is utilized, the posterior periarterial/cord lipoma should also be transected to improve the likelihood of pain control (Fig. 83.18).**

Varicocelectomy

Clinical and subclinical varicocele veins are a common physical examination and sonographic finding and are present in 15% of the general male population (Meacham et al., 1994). Despite their ubiquity in the general male population, varicocele veins should remain high in the differential for orchalgia (Peterson et al., 1998). In a review of varicocelectomy procedures performed for orchalgia, Shridharani et al. showed complete resolution of pain in 85% of men and partial resolution of pain in 6% of men who underwent microsurgical repair (Shridharani et al., 2012). In contrast, nonmicrosurgical repair of varicocele veins was associated with a 76.5% rate of complete resolution of pain and a 13% partial resolution of pain.

Retractile Testis and Intermittent Testicular Torsion

Ascent of one or both testes is a rare phenomenon beyond puberty, but it can occur and can be associated with pain and male infertility (Caucci et al., 1997). Equally rare, but a consideration in the differential for testicular pain is the presence of intermittent testicular torsion (ITT). **ITT is characterized by acute, short-duration (<2 hours) scrotal pain with rapid, spontaneous resolution of pain** (Creagh et al., 1988; Eaton et al., 2005). **Nausea and vomiting may be present in one-fourth of patients with ITT.**

Orchiopexy is recommended for retractile testes and ITT given the low morbidity of surgical treatment, excellent outcomes in pain relief, and reduction in risk for testicular infarction (Eaton et al., 2005; Hayn et al., 2008; Pogorelic et al., 2013). Several approaches to orchiopexy are available, including suture fixation of the tunica albuginea of the testis to the tunica vaginalis, and placement of the testis in an extravaginal dartos pouch (Benson and Lotfi, 1967; Frank and O'Brien, 2002; Ritchey and Bloom, 1995).

Technique

Testicular Fixation With Suture. Testicular fixation is performed by accessing the testis and spermatic cord via a midline or transverse incision and dissecting down to the tunica vaginalis. Once the parietal layer of the tunica vaginalis pouch is opened to expose the testis and spermatic cord, the testis is fixed by suturing the tunica albuginea to the dartos muscle with an absorbable 3-0 suture.

Dartos Pouch Procedure. The dartos pouch procedure is carried out by accessing the cranial aspect of the hemiscrotum through a transverse incision. Dissection is carried down to the tunica vaginalis. The parietal layer is opened to externalize the spermatic cord and testis. A subdartos tunnel is developed between the dartos and external spermatic fascia with blunt dissection caudally toward the dependent portion of the scrotum. The testis is then positioned in the pouch and secured in place via a purse-string suture around the spermatic cord as it exits the cremaster window (Redman and Barthold, 1995).

Testicular fixation with suture is not without risk. Recurrent torsion may occur after a successful testicular fixation with suture, despite the use of nonabsorbable suture. **In a retrospective review by Mor et al. (2006), ipsilateral intravaginal torsion occurred at a rate of 2.2% following prior fixation with suture** (Mor et al., 2006). Repeat torsion occurred in the orchiopexied testis 4 to 17 years subsequent to repair. **Segmental or complete infarction of the testis can occur by entrapping the intratesticular arteries at the lower pole of the testis** (Jarow, 1991). Furthermore, animal studies examining the impact of transparenchymal suture fixation have shown an inflammatory reaction and impaired spermatogenesis in rat and hamster testes fixed with chromic and nylon suture (Bellinger et al., 1989; Dixon et al., 1993; Lotan et al., 2005). Bellinger et al. identified intratesticular abscess formation in 76% of rat testes orchiopexed with catgut suture; 88% had tubular necrosis, and 82% had no spermatogonia (Bellinger et al., 1989). In contrast, 94% of testes fixed with a dartos pouch had normal spermatogenesis. The negative impact on spermatogenesis may be diminished by placement of the testis in a dartos pouch or fixation with polytetrafluoroethylene (PTFE) suture (Steinbecker et al., 1999). There is currently no consensus on the ideal fixation method; however, based on animal data, we recommend dartos pouch placement for patients who wish to preserve fertility.

> **KEY POINTS: SURGERY OF THE SCROTAL CONTENTS**
>
> - Patients with chronic orchalgia have better pain-related outcomes when their simple orchiectomy is performed via an inguinal approach.
> - Men of reproductive age should be counseled on the infertility risks before undergoing an epididymal surgery.
> - Epididymectomy performed for chronic epididymitis should be performed as a last resort option, as it has poor outcomes and is associated with persistence of pain.

COMPLICATIONS OF SCROTAL SURGERY

Bleeding and Postoperative Hematoma

Postoperative bleeding is the main complication of scrotal surgery. This complication is most commonly self-limiting, and the accumulated hematoma should be drained only if it is very large, is infected, or continues to enlarge. The continued bleeding is most commonly caused by incomplete ligation of the spermatic artery and can be controlled via a small subinguinal incision. Through this few-centimeter subinguinal incision, the cord can be pulled up and re-ligated. Retroperitoneal hemorrhage in this setting is very rare but potentially lethal and should be promptly recognized and addressed, especially if significant decrease in patient's hematocrit is noted in a setting of an expanding hematoma. If the spermatic cord is retracted into the retroperitoneum, the subinguinal incision may not suffice and should be extended into the retroperitoneum.

Chronic Scrotal Pain

Risk for chronic scrotal pain following vasectomy and affecting a patient's quality of life is reported to be about 2% (Choe and Kirkemo, 1996; Leslie et al., 2007). The reports however, are of poor quality and variable definitions, and only few men ultimately require surgical treatment of their chronic scrotal pain.

Early/Late Vasectomy Failure

Vasectomy failure is defined as either occurrence of pregnancy or failure to achieve azoospermia or RNMS following vasectomy. Early vasectomy failure is usually caused by technical failure, where only one vas has been occluded properly.

If the initial PVSA met success criteria and the patient subsequently is noted to have motile sperm and/or reported conception, this failure usually occurs later and oftentimes is associated with recanalization, and it may occur in approximately 1 in 2000 vasectomies (Davies et al., 1990; Philp et al., 1984a, 1984b).

Epididymal/Vasal Injury or Ligation With Resulting Infertility

Although injury to the epididymis and vasa differentia are known complications of hydrocele and spermatocele correction, few studies have examined the short- and long-term sequelae of hydrocelectomy and aspiration and sclerotherapy (AS). Shan et al. evaluated the impact of AS on the change in semen parameters at 6 and 12 months postinterventionally. The authors found deterioration of sperm concentration, motility, and morphology at 6 months, but return to baseline levels at 12 months (Shan et al. 2011).

Hydrocele Recurrence

Hydrocele recurrence after successful repair ranges from 0% to 2%, regardless of a choice of operative technique (Ku et al., 2001; Rodriguez et al., 1981). Resolution of hydrocele following AS is reported to be 85% to 96%, although repeat procedures may be required to achieve higher success rates.

Infection

Infection commonly results from the pre-existing hematoma. This may be either treated conservatively with antibiotics or with more aggressive wound exploration, irrigation, and hematoma evacuation. If the initial incision is reopened, it should be left open to allow maximal drainage and healing via secondary intention.

Sperm Granuloma

The inflammatory nodule at site of vasectomy is common and not considered a complication of surgery. Initially, for up to 3 months, the nodule may be symptomatic, and treatment with anti-inflammatory analgesics on an as-needed basis in addition to patient reassurance should suffice. The incidence rate of the persisting symptomatic nodule has been reported at rates <5% (Sharlip et al., 2012). In cases of prolonged postprocedural pain localized to the terminal ends of the transected vasa, repeat vasectomy or excision of the vasal edges may be offered with successful outcomes.

ANATOMY AND EMBRYOLOGY OF SEMINAL VESICLES

SV anatomy was first described by Gabriele Fallopius in 1561 with a further, more detailed study and description continued in the late 19th century (Brewster, 1985).

The SVs are paired male reproductive organs that produce about 60% of the seminal fluid (Ndovi et al., 2007). The organs are located posteriorly to the prostate and fuse with the ampulla of the vas deferens to form the ejaculatory ducts that empty into the prostatic urethra via the verumontanum (Fig. 83.19). The arterial supply to the SVs originates from the vesiculodeferential artery, a branch off the umbilical artery (Braithwaite, 1952; Clegg, 1955).

Developmentally, the SVs begin as bilateral dorsolateral bulbous dilations of the distal mesonephric ducts at about 12 weeks' gestation, and continue to form multiple diverticula by the end of 16 weeks (Fig. 83.20A–C). Subsequently, the vesicles elongate, develop multiple diverticula, and become highly convoluted. The seminal epithelium differentiates into the principal (secretory) and basal cells at birth, with the latter decreasing in numbers until 18 years of age.

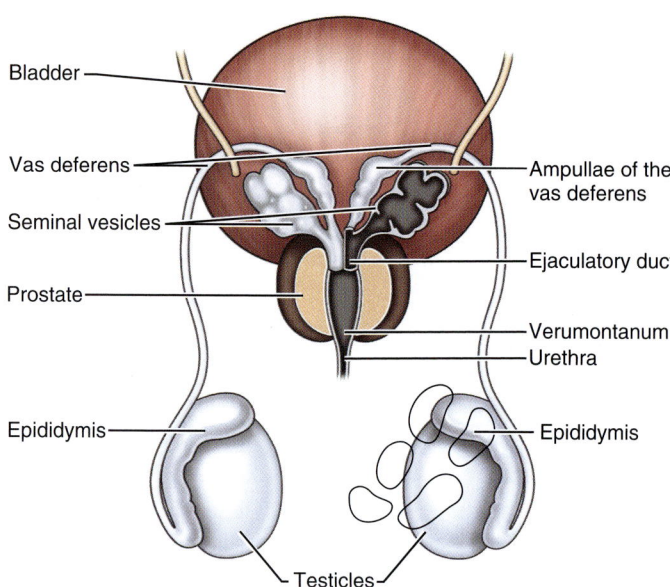

Fig. 83.19. Posterior view of seminal vesicle anatomy in relation to the lower genitourinary tract (bivalved areas in dark gray).

The size of the SVs varies with age and has been assessed historically with autopsy studies, transrectal ultrasonography (TRUS) (Fig. 83.21AB), and more recently cross-sectional imaging (Figs. 83.22 and 83.23AB) and prostatectomy pathology specimens (Mann, 1974). Rosenberg et al. assessed the SV length, width, and volume from pathology specimens of men who underwent transperitoneal robotic-assisted laparoscopic radical prostatectomy (Rosenberg et al., 2009). The authors found the average SV to be 31 ± 10.3 mm long with an average volume 7.1 ± 5.2 mL. Moreover, statistically significant size discrepancy was noted, with the right SV more often larger than the left SV ($P = 0.0003$).

SURGICAL APPROACHES TO SEMINAL VESICLES

The majority of procedures on SVs are performed in conjunction with radical cystectomy or prostatectomy. As a result, traditional approaches to unilateral or bilateral SV surgery have mirrored those for pelvic neoplasms.

Anterior

The transvesical transtrigonal anterior approach has been traditionally utilized when large benign SV masses or cysts are present or when an ectopic ureteral drainage is established into an SV cyst (Politano et al., 1975) (Fig. 83.24AB).

This is the most direct approach to the SVs. Following an infraumbilical midline incision and entry into the space of Retzius, the anterior bladder wall is entered via a vertical/longitudinal incision. Self-retaining retractor is placed to expose the posterior bladder wall. **Ureteral catheters or feeding tubes should be placed bilaterally to easily identify and avoid potential ureteral injury.** A longitudinal incision in the trigone, avoiding the bladder neck is made. Stay sutures may be placed into the cut edges of the posterior bladder wall to aid with further exposure. Once the muscular bladder wall is transected, the ampullae of the vas deferens will be visible below the level of the bladder neck. The SV may be removed where it joins with the vas deferens, or it may be removed together with the ampulla of the vas (Hinman, 1998). Pulling the vas medially helps identify the ipsilateral SV. Once resection is completed, the posterior bladder wall should be closed with a two-layer closure, with a 2-0 or 3-0 vicryl suture to the muscularis and a smaller, 4-0 vicryl to the bladder

Chapter 83　Surgery of the Scrotum and Seminal Vesicles　**1857**

The perivesical anterior approach is useful in pediatric patients with a large SV cyst, and especially when a nephroureterectomy is planned at time of seminal vesiculectomy. A midline or Pfannenstiel incision is utilized for exposure. The bladder is dissected off of the lateral sidewall on the side ipsilateral to the SV cyst. When an SV cyst is identified, the SV needs to be completely dissected all the way down to the junction with the prostate. It can be ligated with a 2-0 absorbable suture and a ligating clip, carefully avoiding the ureter superiorly and the vas deferens, which runs superior and medial to the SV. Once the SV is removed, a standard abdominal closure can be completed. A closed suction pelvic drain and a Foley catheter can be maintained for the next 24 hours postoperatively and safely removed afterwards, provided there was no bladder injury at time of surgery and/or no excessive drain output has been observed.

Transperitoneal anterior approach can be performed either via an open or laparoscopic/robotic approach. This approach is useful for bilateral SV cysts or benign masses. Following a standard entry into the pelvis, a transverse incision is made through the retroperitoneum, where the retroperitoneum joins the bladder wall in the cul-de-sac. The space between the bladder and the rectum is gently developed (Fig. 83.25AC). The SVs and the ampullae of the vas deferens are identified over the posterior bladder wall. The SVs are then dissected off of the bladder, ligated and resected.

The transperitoneal/laparoscopic approach was initially described by Kavoussi in conjunction with the perineal prostatectomy at time of the laparoscopic pelvic lymph node dissection (Kavoussi et al., 1993). Although awaiting the results of frozen section on the lymph nodes, the SVs and ampullae of the vasa deferentia are dissected free. If the frozen pathology section shows no evidence of nodal involvement, the patient is repositioned and perineal prostatectomy is performed. This procedure was further modified for use during the transperitoneal/robotic approach (Fig. 83.26AC), which has increased in utilization with the advent of robotic surgery. Nowadays, the majority of pelvic urologic surgeries are performed via this approach.

Perineal

This approach is most commonly utilized at the time of the perineal radical prostatectomy. The perineal approach is limited in the incision size, possibly making the dissection of the ampulla of the vasa deferentia and SVs difficult. The limited visibility may result in injury to the neurovascular bundles or in incomplete removal of the SVs. The risk for injury to the neurovascular bundle can be minimized by maintaining the plane of dissection as close to the midline as possible. In an effort to facilitate the approach to the SVs, the laparoscopic seminal vesical dissection has been described.

Posterior

The transcoccygeal approach (Fig. 83.27A–D) is the least used approach and the least familiar to urologists, however it may be useful in patients who have had previous suprapubic or perineal surgeries or for those who may not tolerate supine or lithotomy positioning.

In preparation for this approach, the patient is positioned in the prone jackknife position (Kreager and Jordan, 1965). The skin incision is made in an L-shape fashion, proceeding vertically from mid-sacrum and turning down at the tip of the coccyx toward the gluteal cleft, 3 cm away from the rectum. The deeper tissues are dissected down to the lateral side of the coccyx, and once the gluteus maximus muscle fibers are identified and moved over to the side, the rectosigmoid is encountered and carefully dissected off of the sacrum. The lateral rectal wall ipsilateral to the side of the SV lesion is dissected free and moved over medially until prostate is encountered. Next, superiomedial dissection should reveal the ampulla of the vas in midline and the SV lateral to it.

At completion of surgery, a Penrose drain is placed into the resection area and brought out through a separate skin incision. If no significant drainage is observed over the next 2 to 3 days, it

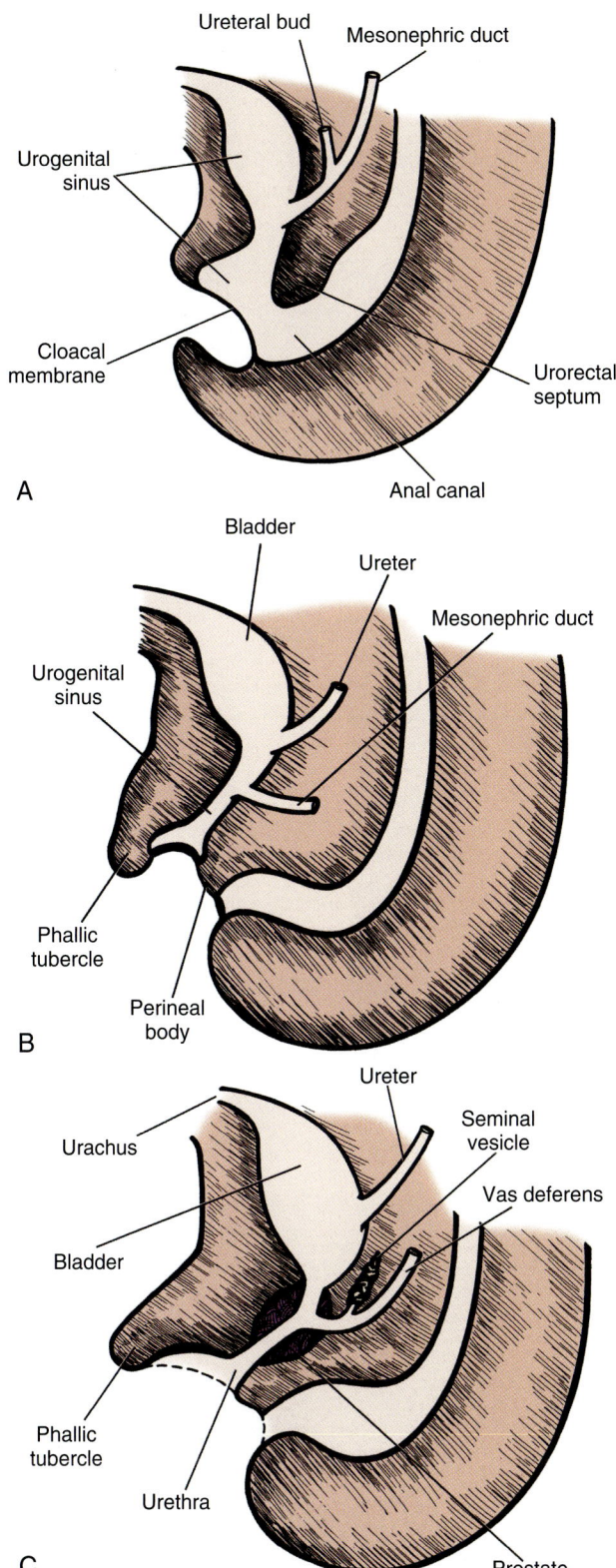

Fig. 83.20. Intrauterine (fetal) development of the seminal vesicles. (A) Week 5. (B) Week 8. (C) Week 13. (Redrawn from Langman J. *Medical embryology*. 4th ed. Baltimore, MD: Williams & Wilkins; 1981:242–243.)

mucosa. The anterior bladder wall should be closed in a similar fashion. A closed suction pelvic drain should be placed and Foley catheter should be maintained postoperatively. Ureteral stent(s) may be placed if there is suspicion of ureteral injury; however, stent placement is not the standard of practice on uncomplicated cases.

Text continued on p. 1862

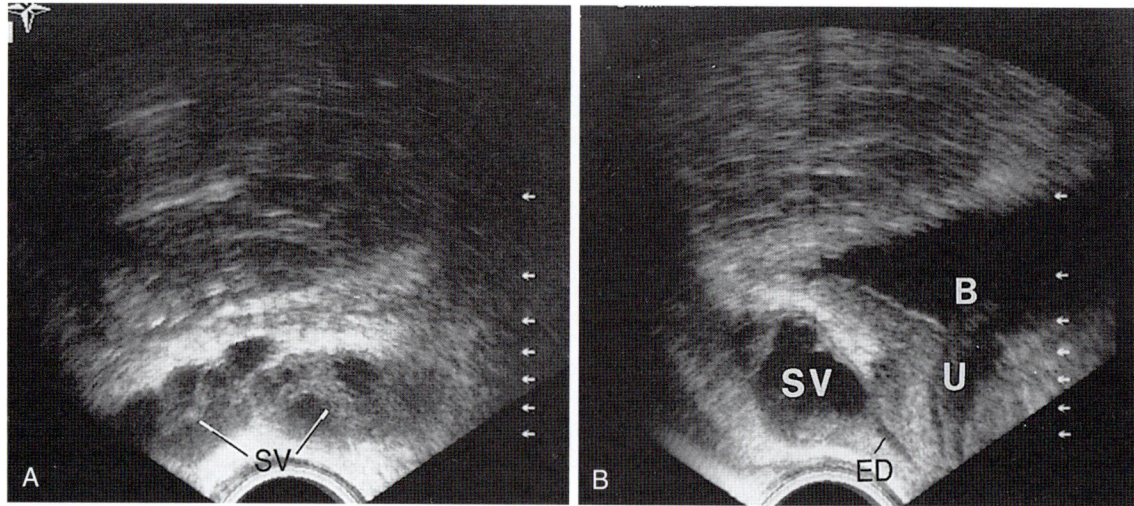

Fig. 83.21. Transrectal ultrasound examination of normal seminal vesicles. (A) Transverse view. (B) Sagittal view. *B*, bladder; *ED*, ejaculatory duct; *SV*, seminal vesicle; *U*, urethra.

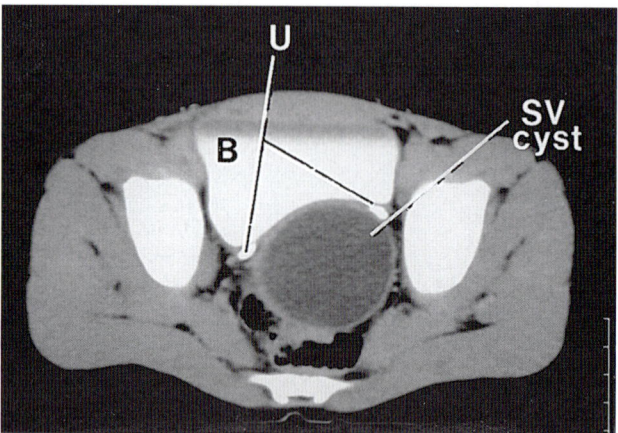

Fig. 83.22. Computed tomography scan of seminal vesicle *(SV)* cyst. *B*, bladder; *U*, ureters.

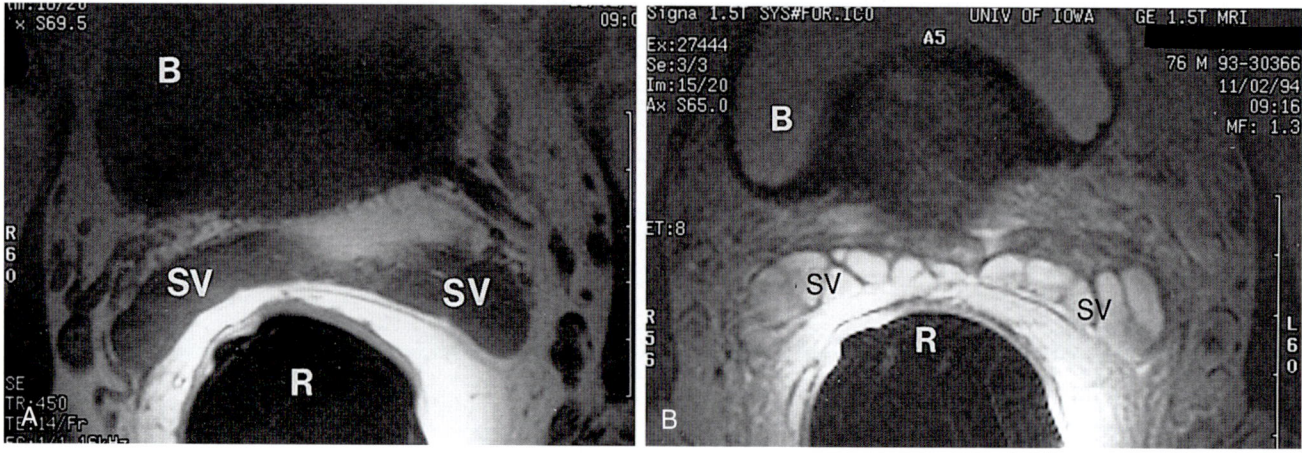

Fig. 83.23. Transaxial magnetic resonance imaging of normal seminal vesicles (SV) with endorectal coil. (A) T1-weighted image. (B) T2-weighted image. *B*, Bladder; *R*, rectum.

Chapter 83 Surgery of the Scrotum and Seminal Vesicles **1859**

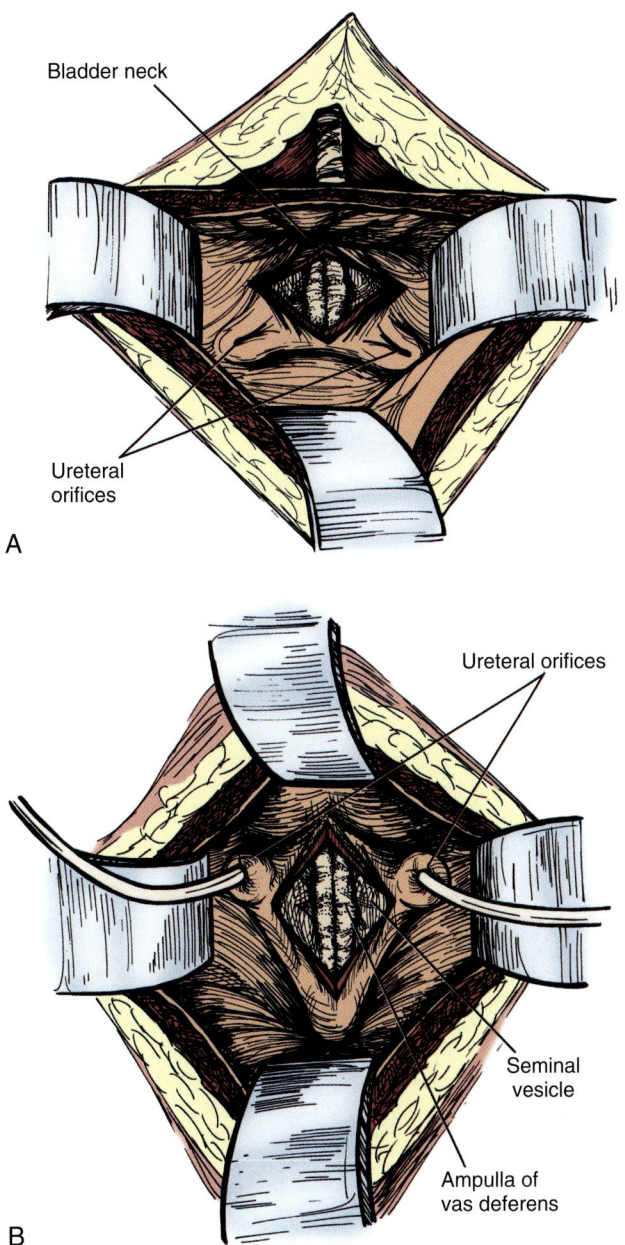

Fig. 83.24. Transvesical approach to seminal vesiculectomy. (A) Vertical incision between the ureteral orifices. (B) Transverse incision 2 cm superior to the bladder neck below the ureteral orifices. (Redrawn from Hinman F Jr. *Atlas of urologic surgery.* Philadelphia, PA: Saunders; 1989.)

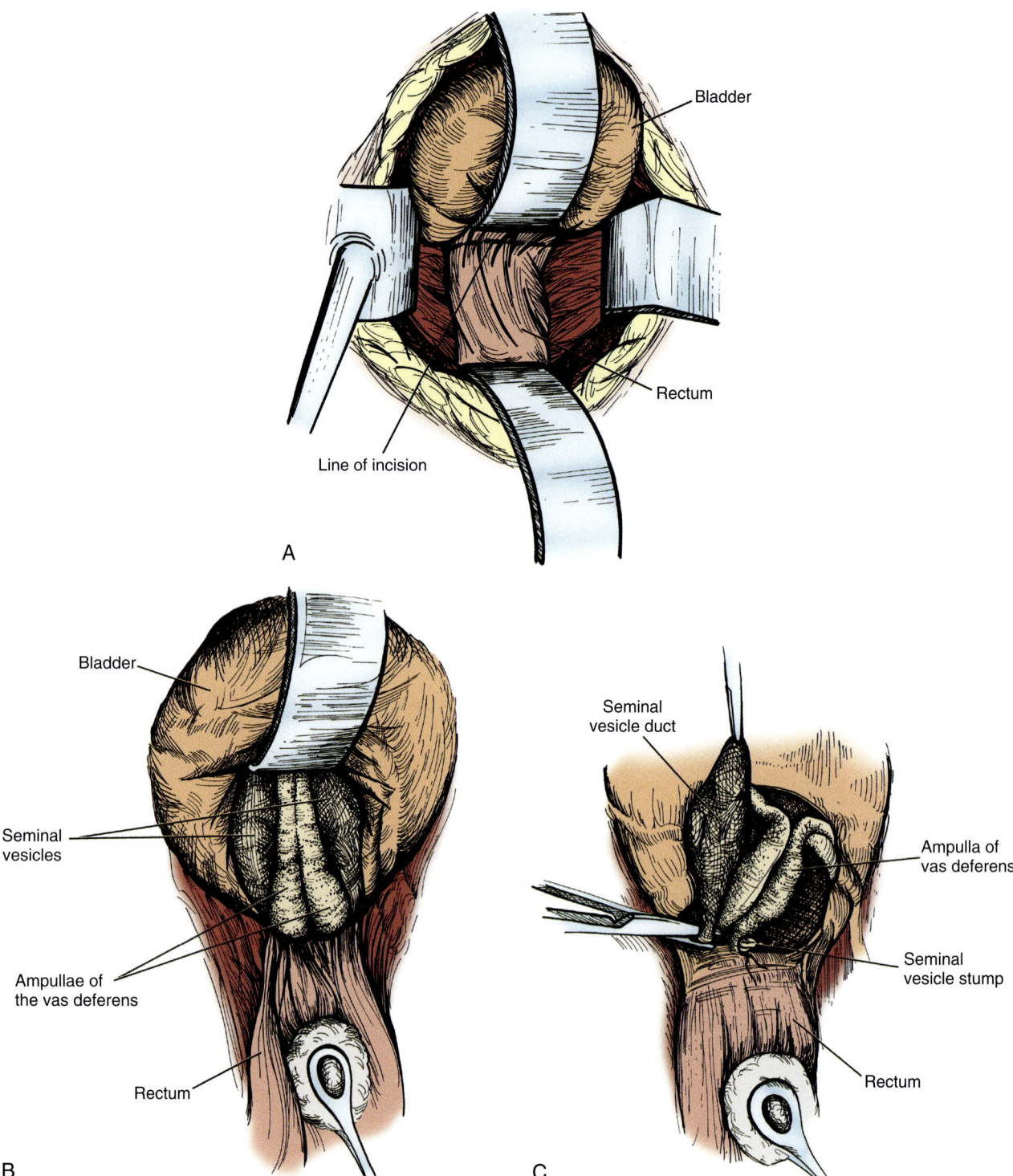

Fig. 83.25. Retrovesical approach to seminal vesiculectomy. (A) Incision line between base of bladder and peritoneal reflection over the rectum. (B) Caudal dissection reveals the ampullae of the vas deferens on the midline and seminal vesicles immediately lateral to them. (C) The duct of the seminal vesicle is ligated and transected. (Redrawn from Hinman F Jr. *Atlas of urologic surgery.* Philadelphia, PA: Saunders; 1989.)

Chapter 83 Surgery of the Scrotum and Seminal Vesicles 1861

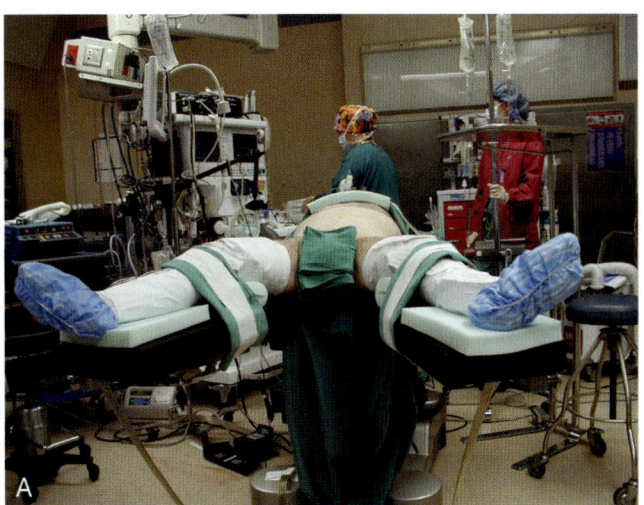

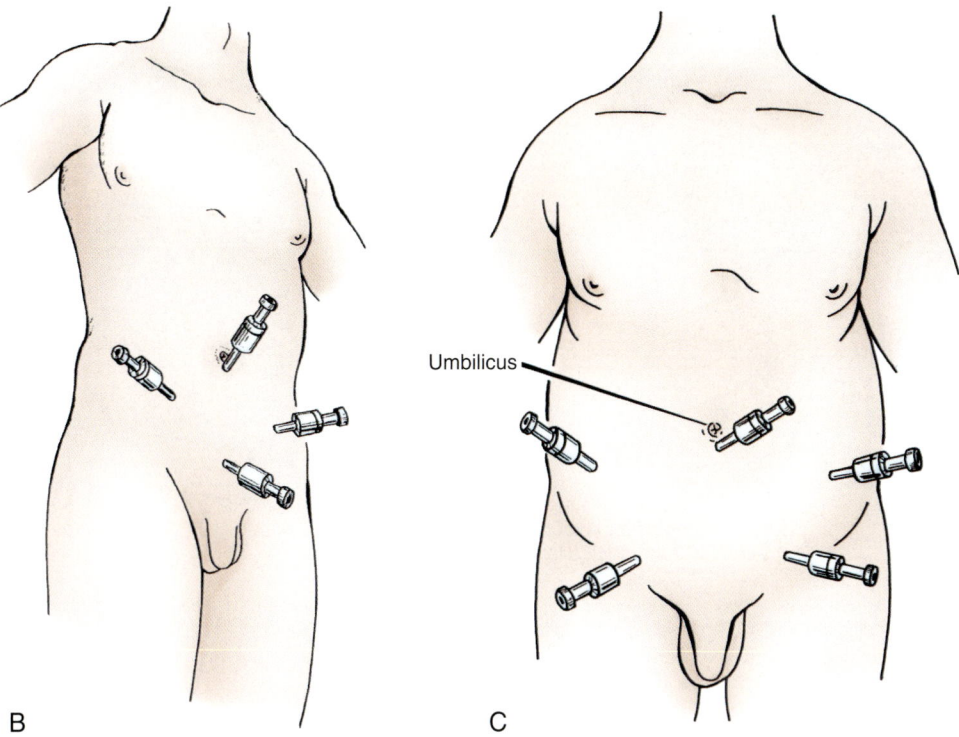

Fig. 83.26. (A) Positioning of the patient for laparoscopic seminal vesicle dissection. (B) Diamond configuration of laparoscopic ports. (C) Inverted U-shaped configuration of laparoscopic ports in obese patients. (From Winifield HN. Laparoscopic pelvic lymph node dissection for urological pelvic malignancies. *Atlas Urol Clin North Am* 1993;1:33–47.)

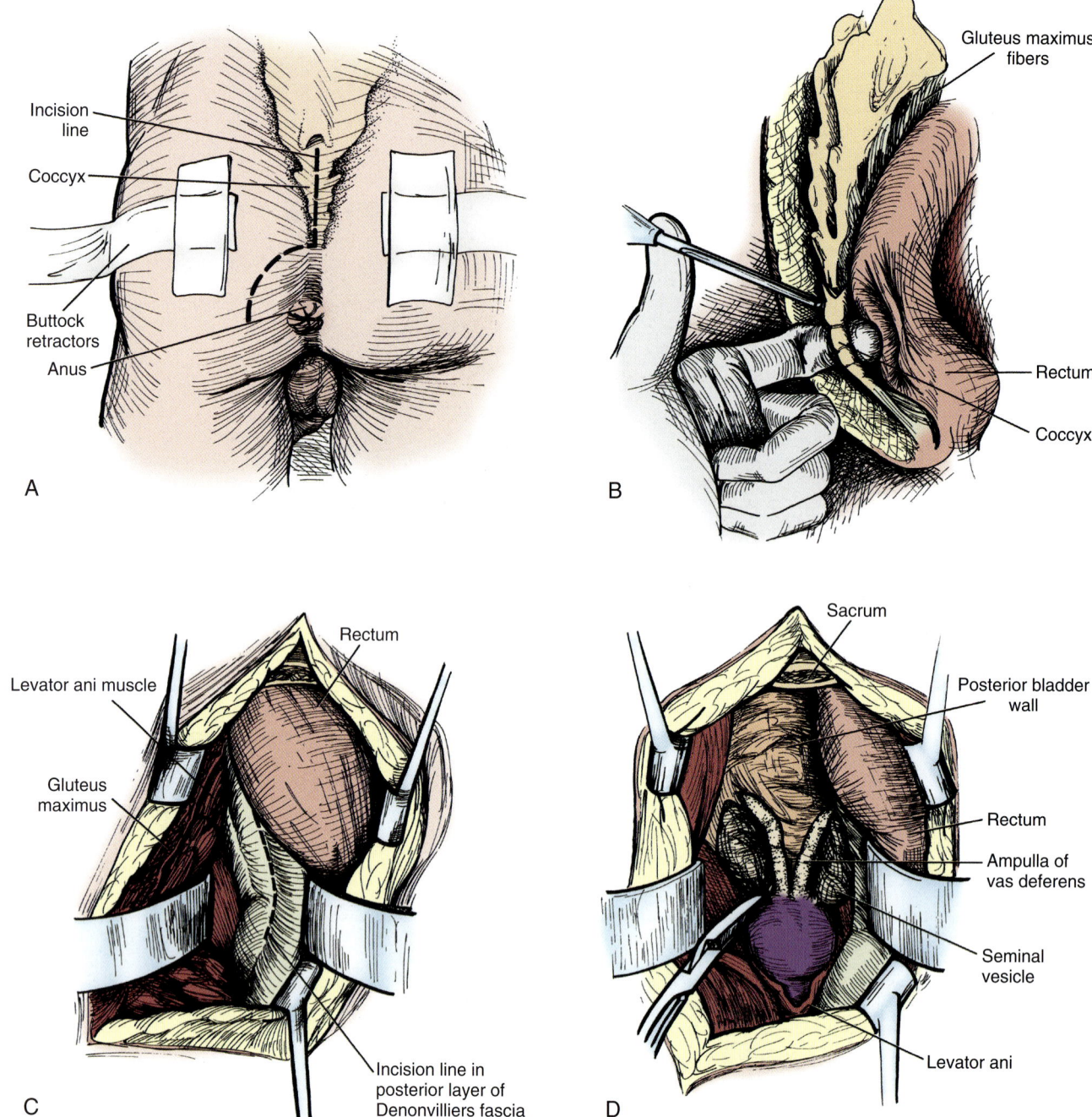

Fig. 83.27. Transcoccygeal seminal vesiculectomy. (A) Incision line over the lower sacrum on coccyx surrounding the anus. (B) Dissection of the coccyx. (C) Incision of Denonvilliers fascia after the rectum has been displaced. (D) Exposure of the prostate and seminal vesicles. (Redrawn from Hinman F Jr. *Atlas of urologic surgery.* Philadelphia, PA: Saunders; 1989.)

should be removed postoperatively. The rectum should be carefully inspected for injury and imbricated in two layers if such injury is encountered. Once the rectum is placed back into its anatomic position, the incision should be closed in layers.

SURGERIES OF THE SEMINAL VESICLES

Seminal Vesicle Cyst Management

Seminal vesicle cysts (SVCs) are rare lesions, with a prevalence of about 0.005% in men, and they can have either a congenital or acquired etiology (Sheih et al., 1990). Congenital SVCs are commonly related to abnormalities of the mesonephric (Wolffian) duct, and the acquired cysts usually result from ejaculatory duct obstruction as further sequelae of infection, urethral inflammation, or ejaculatory duct stones. The vast majority of SVCs are asymptomatic. Symptoms associated with SVCs include hematospermia, terminal hematuria, lower abdominal or lumbosacral pain, and testicular and perineal discomfort. Symptomatic cysts may also result in obstruction-related hydronephrosis and problems with urination or defecation. They are usually associated with ipsilateral renal agenesis and ectopic ureter and require surgical management.

The management of SVCs depends mainly on their size and clinical symptoms. The vast majority of cases involving small cysts and those that are asymptomatic or cause only mild symptoms are usually treated conservatively, with only occasional percutaneous drainage or transrectal or transurethral cyst aspiration.

Surgical excision is generally indicated for the treatment of large SVCs associated with significant clinical symptoms. The first case of symptomatic SVC surgical removal was reported in 1914, when Zinner described their association with other anomalous developments along with their open surgical resection (Zinner, 1914). Currently, SVC excision is either performed laparoscopically or with use of robotic-assisted technology. Both techniques significantly reduce rates of morbidity and hospital stay, and they allow for more accurate dissection of surrounding structures (McDougall et al., 2001; Scarcia et al., 2016).

Transurethral Endoscopic Treatments

Transurethral treatment constitutes the preferred approach to SVCs, persistent hematospermia, or ejaculatory duct obstruction and/or stones, as it is much less invasive, faster, and associated with fewer complications.

Li et al. (1991) demonstrated that transurethral endoscopic unroofing can be safely performed with use of a standard resectoscope. A 1-cm-long, 1-cm-wide, and 1-cm-deep tissue can be resected from the bladder neck to the verumontanum. Once the SVC is unroofed in such fashion, it can be irrigated with saline and cauterized with a loop electrode. This approach was reported to provide easy access to the cyst with very little overall trauma and bleeding. Furthermore, it was associated with few complications and rapid recovery (Wang et al., 2015).

Transurethral seminal vesiculoscopy has been reported for evaluation and treatment of ejaculatory duct and SV disease. The majority of these cases were performed with a semirigid ureteroscope following dilation with a ureteral serial dilator. Holmium laser was shown to be safe and effective in incision of obstructed ejaculatory ducts, coagulation of hemorrhagic mucosa, and fragmentation of the ejaculatory duct or SV stones (Oh and Seo, 2016). When performed during infertility workup and treatment, vesiculoscopy was associated with initial detection of sperm in 66% of patients. This, however, significantly decreased after 6 months, proving that the reobstruction rate was high in this patient population either because of their underlying etiology or secondary to the procedure risks (Li et al., 2013; Tang et al., 2016).

Transrectal Ultrasound–Guided Aspiration

SVs with a width greater than 1.5 cm and an ejaculatory duct diameter greater than 2.3 mm on transrectal ultrasound (TRUS) are suggestive of obstruction (Smith et al., 2008). However, TRUS findings must be interpreted with caution as dilated SV on TRUS does not necessarily demonstrate ejaculatory duct obstruction, and patients with ejaculatory duct obstruction do not always have dilated SVs (Smith et al., 2008). Further investigation is often needed with SV aspiration to confirm obstruction.

Seminal Vesicle Tumor Excision

Primary SV tumors are extremely rare. Both benign and malignant tumors can appear as complex solid cystic retrovesical masses and oftentimes are asymptomatic. If symptoms occur, they are similar to those resulting from other pathologic SV entities (i.e., SVCs, stones, inflammatory disease, metastatic lesions) and are thus difficult to differentiate. Thorough preoperative evaluation with abdominal and pelvic imaging is the initial step in evaluation. Because of its multiplanar technology and excellent tissue contrast, MRI is the most accurate tool currently used (Kim et al., 2009). When imaging is inconclusive or unspecific, TRUS-guided biopsy should be performed to obtain a more precise histopathologic description of the suspicious lesion. Preoperatively, the benign nature of the SV lesion should be distinguished from the malignancy, as the latter can potentially require more radical treatment approaches (Monica et al., 2008).

The benign tumors of SV include cystadenomas, hydatid cysts, papillary adenomas, and amyloid depositions, and malignant primary SV lesions include mixed epithelial-stromal tumors (MESTs), also known as phyllodes tumors, adenocarcinomas, sarcomas, carcinoids, and primary seminomas (Lorber et al., 2011).

All SV tumors are resected either using open or laparoscopic surgery. Over the years, as described earlier in this chapter, open approaches became replaced by laparoscopic and robotic ones, specifically because of the lower risk for complications and shorter hospital stays. The open surgical approach most commonly applied is transvesical, as this enables full exposure to SVs without damaging the pelvic nervous plexus and blood supply to the bladder and rectum (Takayasu et al., 2015). The laparoscopic approach has been previously described in the management of SV cysts, and it is currently applied in the treatment of SV solid tumors (Kavoussi et al., 1993; Zhang et al., 2013; Zhu et al., 2013). Furthermore, with the advent of robotic-assisted technology, nerve-sparing vesiculectomy has been demonstrated to achieve safe and optimal perioperative and oncologic outcomes (Campi et al., 2015).

Primary adenocarcinoma of the SV has been reported in about 60 cases worldwide, and because of its rarity, standard treatment guidelines are not available (Sollini et al., 2014).

A multimodal approach is utilized in the management of this malignant tumor, with radical surgical excision as a mainstay of treatment. The majority of cases present late, with local metastatic disease, mainly to the bladder and prostate. As a result of this late presentation, with metastatic disease, most publications describe radical excision (radical prostatectomy, radical cystoprostatectomy, partial cystectomy, total pelvic exenteration with ileal conduit for urinary diversion, and sigmoid colostomy) with bilateral lymphadenectomy followed by various adjuvant therapies to include hormonal manipulation, radiotherapy, and chemotherapeutic agents (Katafigiotis et al., 2016).

Another extremely rare but highly malignant lesion of the SVs is the yolk sac tumor. Currently, only two case reports of this rare malignant cause of hematospermia have been described. The multimodal approach of chemotherapy, radiotherapy, and radical surgical removal have been described, but because of its rarity, it has not been accepted as a standard of care (Benson et al., 1978; Gill et al., 2015).

> **KEY POINTS: SURGERY OF THE SEMINAL VESICLES**
> - SVs produce about 60% of the ejaculate fluid.
> - Surgical approaches to unilateral or bilateral seminal vesicles mirror those for pelvic neoplasms.
> - Symptomatic SV cysts may be associated with ipsilateral renal agenesis and ectopic ureter.
> - Transrectal ultrasound-guided aspiration of an SV must be performed to confirm ejaculatory duct obstruction, as the SV may be dilated from a nonobstructive cause.
> - Benign and malignant tumors of SVs are very rare.
> - MRI provides the most accurate radiographic evaluation of SV lesions.

COMPLICATIONS OF SEMINAL VESICLE SURGERY

SV surgery mimics surgical approaches to the prostate, and thus carries potential for similar complications.

Bladder Injury

Anterior dissection of the SVs carries a small risk for bladder injury. When recognized, this can be easily closed with absorbable sutures in two layers (mucosal and muscular), and, with prolonged bladder drainage, they heal without significant consequences.

The transvesical approach to the SV places patients at a higher risk for urinary leak, as the bladder sustains two planned transverse incisions, both to the anterior and posterior bladder wall. Prolonged catheterization and consideration of pelvic drain placement is strongly advised in these cases.

Endoscopic Surgery Complications

Potential complications associated with the endoscopic approach to SVs may result in epididymitis and postvoid dribbling caused by urinary reflux and urinary tract infection (Goluboff et al., 1995).

Laparoscopic/Robotic Surgery Complications

Injuries inherent to laparoscopic and robotic surgical approaches, although uncommon these days, can be devastating when they occur and may rapidly result in case termination or conversion to an open one. These include but are not limited to: trocar injury to blood vessel/bowel, abdominal wall bleeding, extraperitoneal insufflation, and gas embolism.

Neurovascular Bundle Injury

Neurovascular bundles (NVBs) run immediately lateral to the tips of SVs, and thus any surgical approach will place them at risk for injury. The NVB may result in transient or permanent erectile dysfunction, thus cautious dissection in this area should be performed.

Rectal Injury

Rectal injury is very rare, but when it happens, the same repair principles as for an injury sustained at time of radical prostatectomy should be applied. In the absence of gross fecal spillage, primary repair is acceptable. Debridement of any devitalized tissue, followed by a double-layer repair (mucosal and muscular) is recommended. For larger injuries, gross fecal spillage, or if the surgeon is concerned about viability of the rectal repair, temporary diverting colostomy in addition to the rectal defect repair is strongly advised. This risk can be minimized by approaching the SVs from an anterior approach.

Ureteral Injury

In general, ureters enter the posterior bladder wall, anterolateral to the tips of the SVs and cross to the midline above the trigone. If ureteral injury is suspected during posterior dissection of the SVs, intravenous indigo carmine or on-the-table retrograde ureterogram may be performed to confirm it. Once the injury is confirmed, the ureteroneocystostomy should be performed in the standard fashion. The cut end of the ureter should be pulled into the bladder, spatulated, and sutured into the bladder mucosa. If tension on the anastomosis is encountered, a Boari flap or a psoas hitch may be further used to ease the tension. Stent placement is advised following reconstruction.

SUGGESTED READINGS

Oesterling JE: Scrotal surgery: a reliable method for the prevention of postoperative hematoma and edema, *J Urol* 143:1201–1202, 1990.

Parekattil SJ, Gudeloglu A, Brahmbhatt JV, et al: Trifecta nerve complex: potential anatomical basis for microsurgical denervation of the spermatic cord for chronic orchialgia, *J Urol* 190:265–270, 2013.

Schlegel PN, Goldstein M: No-scalpel vasectomy, *Semin Urol* 10:252–256, 1992.

Tan WP, Levine LA: What can we do for chronic scrotal content pain?, *World J Mens Health* 35:146–155, 2017.

Weinberg AE, Liu JJ, Sandelien M, et al: Epididymal sparing bilateral simple orchiectomy: cost-effectiveness and aesthetic preservation for men with metastatic prostate cancer, *Urol Pract* 3:112–117, 2016.

REFERENCES

The complete reference list is available online at ExpertConsult.com.

PART VIII

Renal Physiology and Pathophysiology

84

Surgical, Radiologic, and Endoscopic Anatomy of the Kidney and Ureter

Mohamed Aly Elkoushy, MD, MSc, PhD, and Sero Andonian, MD, MSc, FRCS(C), FACS

Anatomy of course does not change, but our understanding of anatomy and its clinical significance does change.
— Frank H. Netter, MD

Anatomy provides a roadmap for surgical procedures. This chapter presents the normal anatomy of the kidney and ureter. To make it more interesting for urologists, we provide clinical, radiologic, surgical, and endoscopic correlations. Of course, the human body never ceases to amaze explorers with its variations from the "normal." With modern imaging technology, it has become possible to create three-dimensional (3D) virtual reality of each patient before surgical procedures. However, the surgeon is advised to be cautious of the minute anomalies not appreciated on perioperative imaging studies.

KIDNEYS

Surface Anatomy and Relationships

The kidneys are paired ovoid, reddish-brown retroperitoneal organs situated in the posterior part of the abdomen on each side of the vertebral column. The kidneys lie on the psoas muscles; thus the **longitudinal axes** of the kidneys are oblique *(arrows,* eFig. 84.1 on the Expert Consult website), with the upper poles more medial and posterior than the inferior poles. Therefore, during percutaneous renal access, the lower pole of the kidney lies laterally and anteriorly relative to the upper pole. In addition, the medial aspect of each kidney is rotated anteriorly at an angle of approximately 30 degrees. The exact **position** of the kidney within the retroperitoneum varies during different phases of respiration, body position, and presence of anatomic anomalies. For example, the kidneys move inferiorly approximately 3 cm (one vertebral body) during inspiration and during changing body position from supine to the erect position. The position of the kidneys in the supine end-expiration is described here. Because of the inferior displacement of the right kidney by the liver, the right kidney sits 1 to 2 cm lower than the left kidney. Therefore the right kidney resides in the space between the top of the 1st lumbar vertebra to the bottom of the 3rd lumbar vertebra, whereas the left kidney occupies a space between the 12th thoracic vertebra and the 3rd lumbar vertebra.

Each kidney measures 10 to 12 cm in length, 5.0 to 7.5 cm in width, and 2.5 to 3.0 cm in thickness. Each adult male kidney weighs approximately 125 to 170 g; the kidney is 10 to 15 g smaller in females. The right kidney is slightly shorter and wider because of downward compression by the liver. The kidneys are relatively larger in children and have more prominent fetal lobulations, which generally disappear by the first year of life. In addition, the adult kidney's lateral contour may have a focal renal parenchymal bulge known as a **dromedary hump,** which is more common on the left side and has no pathologic significance. These dromedary humps are thought to be caused by the downward pressure from the liver or the spleen.

The **posterior relationships** of the kidneys are detailed in eFig. 84.2. Superiorly, the kidneys are related to the inferior edge of the diaphragm and the ribs. The right kidney is related to the 12th rib, and the left kidney is related to the 11th and 12th ribs. When the lower ribs are fractured during trauma, associated renal lacerations could occur. The upper poles of the kidneys come close to the diaphragm and underlying pleural cavity containing the lungs; thus any violations of the diaphragm during excision of large renal masses could lead to pleural tears and pneumothorax. Furthermore, **percutaneous access** to the upper pole of the kidneys above the 11th rib (10th intercostal space) is associated with increased risk for injuring pleura and even lungs. Therefore, when possible, subcostal (below the 12th rib) or 11th intercostal space (between the 11th and 12th ribs) access should be achieved (eFig. 84.3). More inferiorly, the kidneys are related to the psoas major muscle medially and the quadratus lumborum and aponeurosis of the transversus abdominis muscles laterally. The subcostal nerve and vessels and the iliohypogastric and ilioinguinal nerves descend obliquely across the posterior surfaces of the kidneys (Fig. 84.4).

Because the kidneys are retroperitoneal organs, they are related **anteriorly** to other retroperitoneal and intraperitoneal organs (eFig. 84.5). The right kidney is related superiorly to the liver (intraperitoneal and retroperitoneal bare portions) and superomedially to the adrenal gland. Inferiorly, the right kidney is related to the small intestine and hepatic flexure of the colon, and medially it is related to the second stage of the duodenum and head of the pancreas. The parietal peritoneum bridging the upper pole of the right kidney to the liver forms the **hepatorenal ligament.** Therefore excessive downward traction of the right kidney may cause capsular tear of the liver and may lead to excessive intraoperative bleeding. The left kidney is related to the stomach and spleen superiorly, adrenal gland superomedially, jejunum and splenic flexure of the colon inferiorly, and tail of the pancreas with splenic vessels medially. The parietal peritoneum bridging the upper pole of the left kidney to the spleen forms the **splenorenal ligament.** If excessive downward pressure is applied to the left kidney, splenic capsular tears may occur, leading to hemorrhage from the spleen.

The kidneys are surrounded by a smooth, tough fibrous capsule, which is easily removed under normal conditions. Each kidney and its vessels are surrounded by a **perinephric fat** that extends into its hollow vertical cleft, the **renal hilum,** which is the entrance to a space within the kidney called the **renal sinus.** The kidneys and adrenal glands, including the perirenal fat surrounding them, are enclosed by a condensed, membranous layer of **renal (Gerota) fascia,** which continues medially to fuse with the contralateral side (eFig. 84.6). This fascia extends inferomedially along the abdominal ureter as a **periureteral fascia.** The Gerota fascia encasing the kidneys, adrenal glands, and abdominal ureters is closed superiorly and laterally and serves as an anatomic barrier to the spread of malignancy and a means of containing perinephric fluid collections. Because it is open inferiorly, perinephric fluid collections can track inferiorly into the pelvis without violating the Gerota fascia.

The Gerota fascia is further surrounded by a layer of condensed fat called the **paranephric fat,** which is most obvious posteriorly and represents the extraperitoneal fat of the lumbar region. Superiorly,

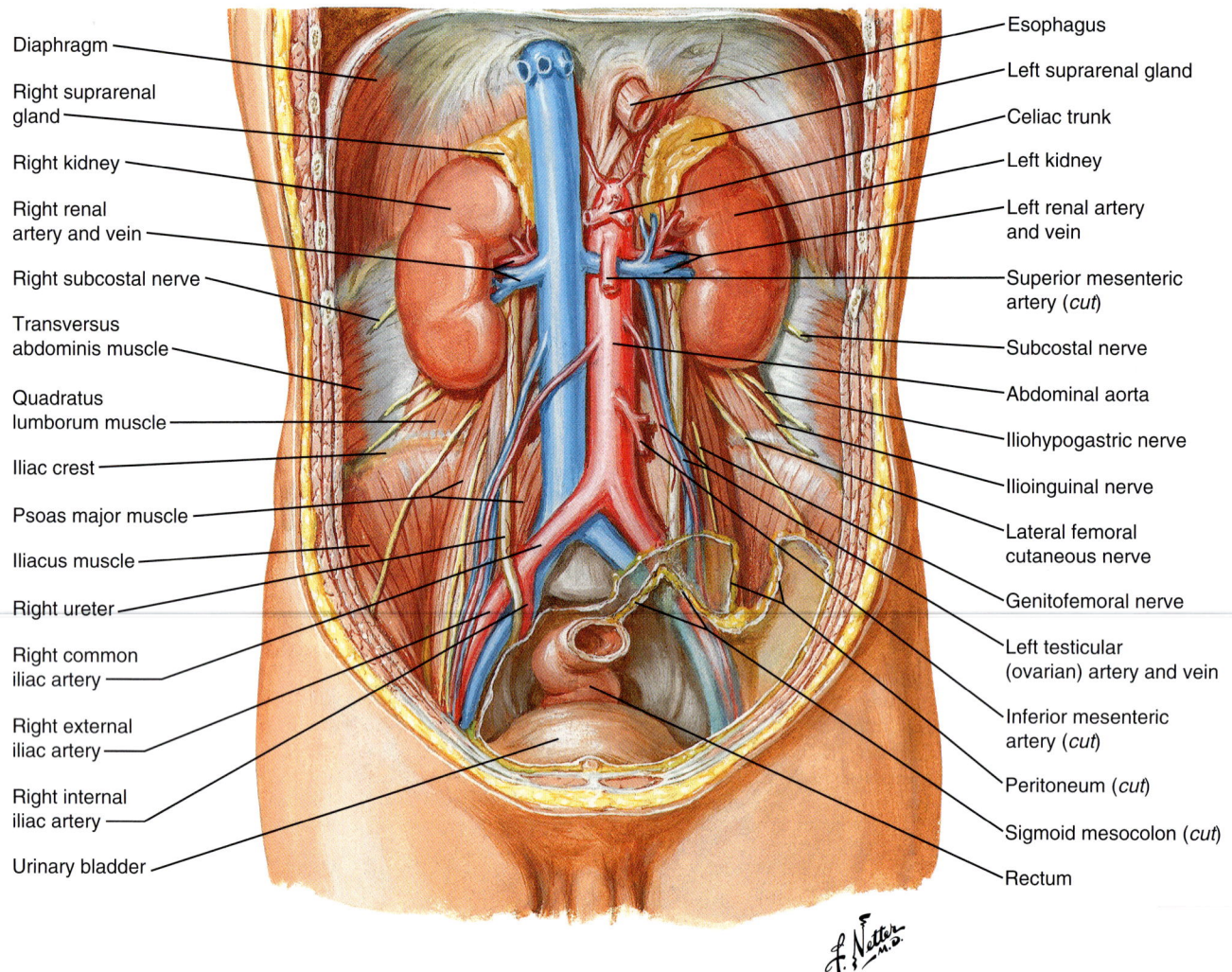

Fig. 84.4. Posterior abdominal wall showing great vessels, kidneys, and adrenal glands. (Copyright 2016 Elsevier Inc. All rights reserved. www.netterimages.com.)

the Gerota fascia is continuous with the diaphragmatic fascia on the inferior surface of the diaphragm, and inferiorly, the anterior and posterior layers of the Gerota fascia are loosely attached. The Gerota fascia is attached with the paranephric fat by collagen bundles. Therefore the kidneys are relatively kept fixed in position by these collagen bundles, the Gerota fascia, and paranephric fat.

The relationships of the kidneys have important **surgical implications**. To access the kidneys, adrenals, or abdominal ureters, the Gerota fascia must be opened. To access the kidneys transperitoneally, the colon must be mobilized from the **white line of Toldt**, which is the lateral reflection of posterior parietal peritoneum over the ascending and descending colon. To access the right renal hilum, the second stage of the duodenum and head of pancreas must be carefully mobilized using the Kocher maneuver. To access the left renal hilum, the tail of the pancreas together with the spleen and splenic vessels must be mobilized medially.

Gross and Microscopic Anatomy

Two distinct regions can be identified on the cut surface of a bisected kidney: the cortex, which is a pale outer region, and the medulla, which is a darker inner region (eFig. 84.7). The renal medulla is divided into 8 to 18 striated, distinct, conically shaped areas that are frequently called renal pyramids. The apex of the pyramids forms the renal papilla, and each papilla is cupped by an individual minor calyx. The base of the pyramids is positioned at the corticomedullary boundary. The cortex and the medulla containing the renal pyramids could be differentiated on renal imaging studies (eFig. 84.8). Furthermore, these renal papillae could be inspected endoscopically (eFig. 84.9).

The renal cortex is approximately 1 cm in thickness and covers the base of each renal pyramid peripherally and extends downward between the individual pyramids to form the **columns of Bertin** (see eFig. 84.7). Interlobar arteries traverse these columns of Bertin from the renal sinus to the peripheral cortex and decrease in diameter as they move peripherally. Therefore percutaneous access to the collecting system is usually performed through a renal pyramid into a calyx to avoid these columns of Bertin containing larger blood vessels. The pyramids and their associated cortex form the lobes of the kidney. The lobes are visible on the external surfaces of the kidneys in fetuses, and evidence of the lobes may persist for some time after birth.

The functional unit of the kidney is the nephron (Fig. 84.10). Approximately 0.4 to 1.2 million nephrons are found in each adult kidney. The nephron consists of a glomerulus, which is composed of a capillary tuft surrounded by epithelial cells and the thin, fibrous Bowman capsule. The glomerulus filters the blood at a rate of 125 mL/min, the glomerular filtration rate, which is considered an index of renal function. The filtrate passes into the Bowman space and then into the proximal convoluted tubule, through the thin and thick limbs of the loop of Henle, to the macula densa adjacent to the glomerulus, and into the distal convoluted tubule. It then enters the collecting tubules and the ducts of Bellini. After absorption of approximately 90% of this filtrate, the remaining part constitutes

Chapter 84 Surgical, Radiologic, and Endoscopic Anatomy of the Kidney and Ureter   1867

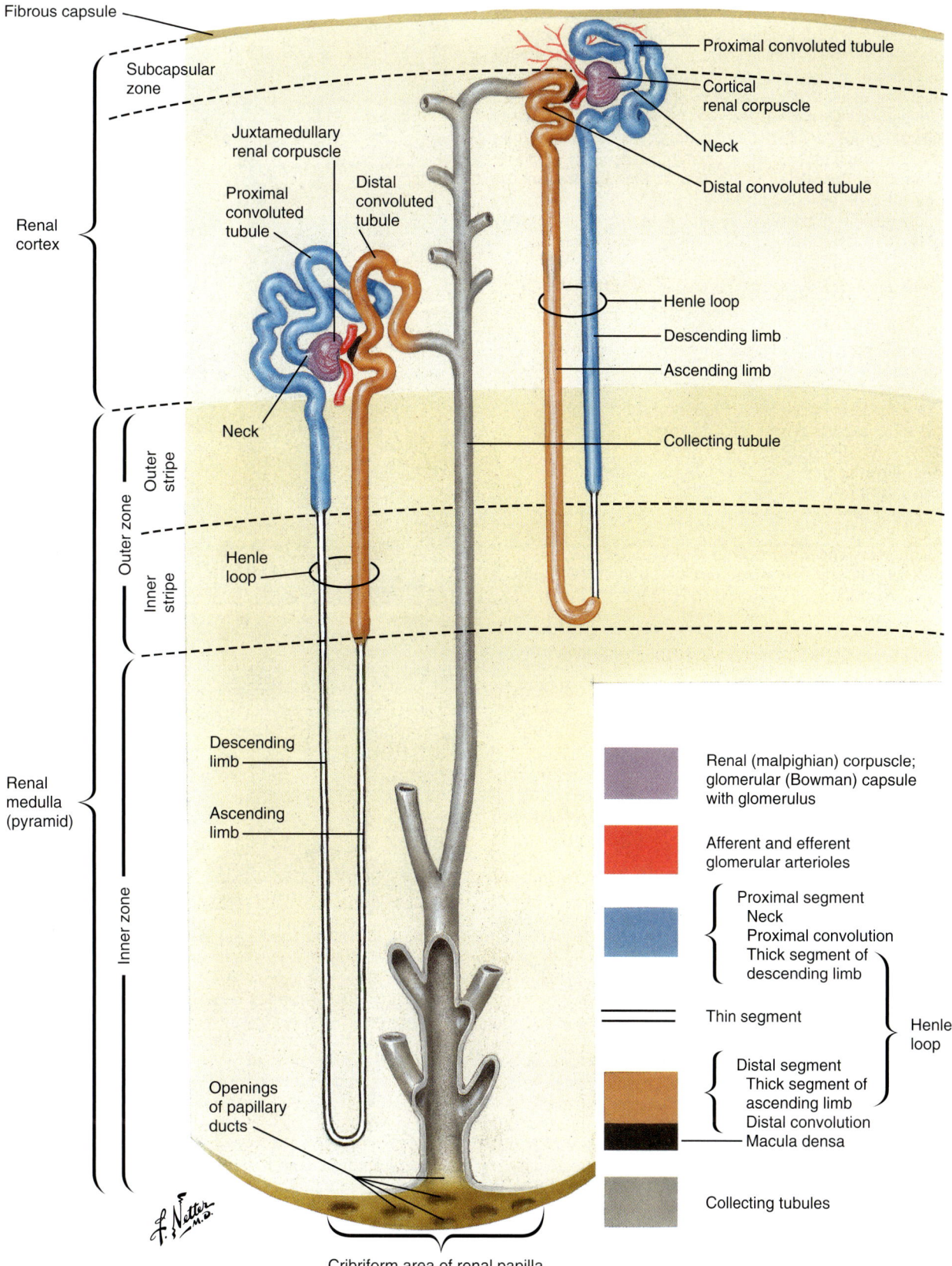

Fig. 84.10. Schematic diagram of the microanatomy of the kidneys. (Copyright 2016 Elsevier Inc. All rights reserved. www.netterimages.com.)

the urine, which drips from the collecting ducts into the calyces, then to the renal pelvis, ureter, and bladder. Three layers separate the filtered blood from the Bowman space: a single layer of endothelial cells, a thin glomerular basement membrane, and a layer of podocytes on the other side of that basement membrane. The proximal and distal convoluted tubules and the loop of Henle are lined by a single layer of cubical epithelial cells. The cells lining the collecting ducts are cubical to columnar and are more resistant to damage than those of the renal tubules. The calyces, pelvis, ureters, bladder, and urethra are lined by transitional epithelium, the urothelium, which may change and give rise to a transitional cell carcinoma of the urinary tract or urothelial carcinoma.

KEY POINTS: THE KIDNEY

- Because the kidneys lie on the psoas muscles, the longitudinal axes of the kidneys are oblique, with the upper poles more medial and posterior than the inferior poles.
- The Gerota fascia envelops the kidney and the adrenal gland on all aspects except inferiorly, where it remains open.
- From anterior to posterior, the renal hilar structures are the renal vein (V), renal artery (A), renal pelvis (U for ureter), and posterior segmental artery (A)—making the mnemonic VAUA.
- The kidney is divided into cortex and medulla. The medullary areas are pyramidal, more centrally located, and separated by segments of cortex, the columns of Bertin.
- Each renal pyramid terminates centrally in a papilla. Each papilla is cupped by a minor calyx. A group of minor calyces join to form a major calyx. The major calyces combine to form the renal pelvis.

Radiologic Anatomy of the Renal Parenchyma

In a well-prepared plain kidney-ureter-bladder (KUB) radiograph, the renal shape, margins, dimensions, and location can be identified. Both kidney shadows are clearly visible and can be assessed with regard to their position and morphology. The psoas muscle line could also be appreciated; it disappears with retroperitoneal effusions. Radiopacities, calcifications, and radiolucencies could be identified (eFig. 84.11). In gray-scale ultrasonography, the renal cortices of newborn kidneys are isoechoic or hyperechoic to the liver and splenic parenchyma, because of the presence of loops of Henle and proportionately greater volume of glomeruli in the cortex than in adults (Hricak et al., 1983; Kasap et al., 2006). In adults, the normal kidneys have smooth margins and are isoechoic to the liver. However, renal cortices and pyramids are usually hypoechoic to the liver, spleen, and renal sinus.

Compared with renal size, cortical thickness, or parenchymal thickness, cortical echogenicity correlates strongly with severity of pathologic changes in renal parenchyma, such as glomerular sclerosis, tubular atrophy, interstitial fibrosis, and inflammation ($r = 0.28$–0.35) (Moghazi et al., 2005). However, this correlation coefficient is still low with subsequent poor predictive value of renal echogenicity.

Compared with renal parenchyma, the renal sinus appears hyperechoic because of the presence of hilar adipose tissue, blood vessels, and lymphatics (eFig. 84.12). On unenhanced computed tomography (CT), the renal parenchyma is homogeneous, with a density ranging from 30 to 60 Hounsfield units (HU) that increases up to 80 to 120 HU after intravenous contrast injection. After 20 to 30 seconds of contrast injection, the arterial CT phase is reached, and the corticomedullary CT phase appears after 30 to 70 seconds, when contrast accumulates in the renal cortex. The nephrographic CT phase, after 80 to 120 seconds, equally enhances renal cortex and medulla and is considered to be the optimal phase for detection of renal neoplasms. Finally, the excretory CT phase, more than 3 minutes after contrast injection, shows the opacified pelvicalyceal system, ureter, and bladder (Fig. 84.13). Magnetic resonance imaging with T1 and T2 relaxation sequences provides information regarding

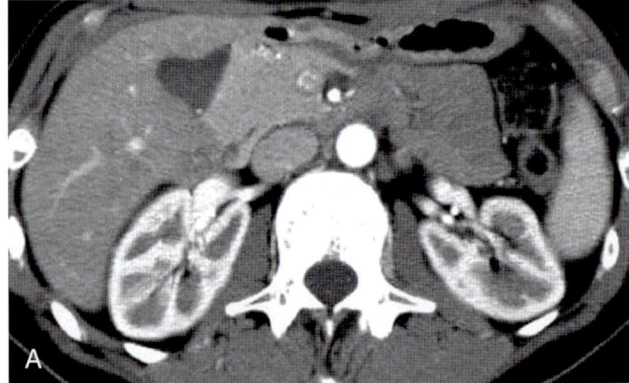
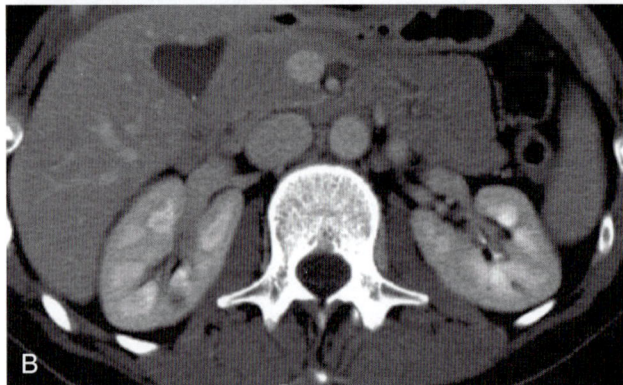
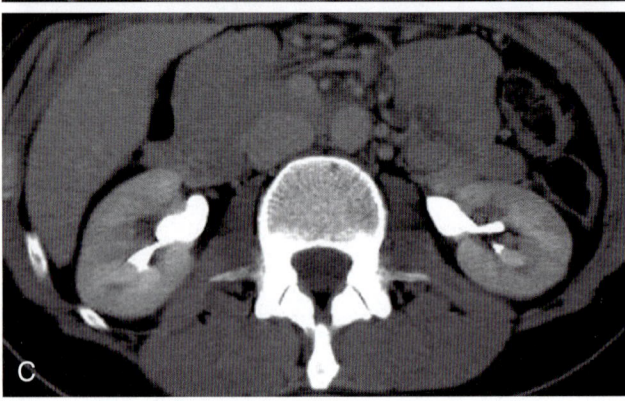

Fig. 84.13. Computed tomography of normal renal parenchyma. (A) The corticomedullary phase shows high contrast in the renal cortex after 30 to 70 seconds of contrast injection. (B) The nephrographic phase shows renal cortex and medulla with equal enhancement after 80 to 120 seconds of contrast injection. (C) The excretory phase shows the opacified urinary tract after more than 180 seconds. (From Quaia E, Martingano P, Cavallaro M, et al.: Normal radiological anatomy and anatomical variants of the kidney. In Quaia E, editor: *Radiological imaging of the kidney (medical radiology/diagnostic imaging)*, New York, 2011, Springer, pp 17–78.)

lipid or fat content and enhancement characteristics of tissues. T1-weighted sequences show the renal cortex much brighter than the renal medulla, whereas the cortex is slightly less intense than the medulla on T2-weighted sequences. The renal pelvis containing fat appears hyperintense on T1- and T2-weighted sequences. After injection of contrast, the nephrographic and excretory phases start after 60 to 90 and 120 seconds of contrast injection, respectively (see eFig. 84.8).

Renal cortex and medulla perform different physiologic functions and are affected by different pathophysiologic processes. Therefore assessment of the degree of separation between these two compartments by imaging studies is important. Normal corticomedullary differentiation (CMD) is visible by ultrasound or T1-weighted and T2-weighted MRI. However, assessment of CMD by CT requires injection of a contrast agent because both compartments have the same density (~30 HU). CMD decreases or disappears in patients with chronic kidney disease and acute kidney injury, without clear correlation with the level of serum creatinine (Semelka et al., 1994). However, upon restoration of renal function, CMD has been shown to reappear by MRI (Chung et al., 2001). Recently, imaging studies such as 3D CT and MRI have been used to calculate renal parenchymal volumes to assess functional parenchymal volume. Studies using customized imaging software have demonstrated a high correlation between measurements of renal and cortical volumes and renal function (Coulam et al., 2002; Vivier et al., 2008). Renal glomerular filtration correlate better with MR measurements of renal volume ($r = 0.86$) than renal bipolar length ($r = 0.78$) (Cheung et al., 2006).

Of all congenital anomalies encountered in newborns, 20% to 30% affect the kidneys and ureters (Schedl, 2007). Anomalies of number, rotation, ascent, and/or fusion may be encountered. Radiologically, renal malrotation is identified because the renal pelvis appears to arise centrally instead of its medial origin from the kidney. Some calyces are located medial to the renal pelvis, a hallmark of rotational anomalies. These renal calyces appear distorted with or without obstruction (eFig. 84.14). Arrest or exaggeration of normal ascent of the kidneys gives rise to renal ectopia and is usually associated with malrotation. Despite the ureteral length being appropriate for the kidney position, the impaired drainage results in urinary stasis and increased chances of infection and stone formation. Moreover, blood supply to the ectopic kidney is also aberrant, originating from adjacent vessels (see eFig. 84.14). A kidney may cross the midline and fuse with the opposite kidney (crossed-fused ectopia). The ureter from the ectopic lower kidney crosses the midline and usually inserts into the bladder in its normal position. The two kidneys may fuse by an isthmus at their lower pole, giving rise to the horseshoe kidney (eFig. 84.15). It is usually positioned low in the abdomen because of its arrest by the origin of the inferior mesenteric artery. The isthmus may contain a fibrotic band or functional renal parenchyma. This kidney is usually subjected to other anomalies, especially ureteropelvic junction obstruction (UPJO), vascular anomalies, duplication anomalies, stone formation, and urinary tract infections.

> **KEY POINTS: RADIOLOGIC ANATOMY OF RENAL PARENCHYMA**
>
> - Although normal kidneys are isoechoic to the liver, renal cortices and pyramids are hypoechoic to the liver, spleen, and renal sinus.
> - Echogenicity correlates to the severity of pathologic changes in renal parenchyma.
> - The renal parenchyma is homogeneous on unenhanced CT.
> - T1-weighted sequences show the renal cortex much brighter than the renal medulla, whereas the cortex is slightly less intense than the medulla on T2-weighted sequences.
> - Blood supply to an ectopic kidney originates from adjacent vessels.

Renal Vasculature

The renal pedicle classically consists of a single artery and a single vein that enter the kidney via the renal hilum (Fig. 84.16). The renal arteries arise from the aorta at the level of the intervertebral disk between the L1 and L2 vertebrae, where the longer right renal artery passes posterior to the inferior vena cava (IVC). Renal arteries give branches to the adrenal glands, renal pelves, and proximal ureters. **After entering the hilum, each artery divides into five segmental end arteries that do not anastomose significantly with other segmental arteries. Therefore occlusion or injury to a segmental branch causes segmental renal infarction. Nevertheless, the area supplied by each segmental artery could be independently surgically resected.** The renal artery usually divides to form anterior and posterior divisions. The anterior division supplies roughly the anterior two-thirds of the kidney, and the posterior division supplies the posterior one-third of the kidney. Typically, the anterior division divides into four anterior segmental branches: apical, upper, middle, and lower. The posterior segmental artery represents the first and most constant branch, which separates from the renal artery before it enters the renal hilum. A small apical segmental branch may originate from this posterior branch, but it arises most commonly from the anterior division. The posterior segmental artery from the posterior division passes posterior to the renal pelvis while the others pass anterior to the renal pelvis. **If the posterior segmental branch passes anterior to the ureter, UPJO may occur.** In 25% to 40% of kidneys, anatomic variations in the renal vasculature have been reported. **Supernumerary renal arteries** are the most common variation, with reports of up to five arteries, especially on the left side. The main renal artery may manifest early branching after originating from the abdominal aorta and before entering the renal hilum. These prehilar arterial branches should be detected in patients undergoing evaluation for donor nephrectomy. An accessory renal artery may arise from the aorta, between T11 and L4, and terminate in the kidney. Rarely, it may also originate from the iliac arteries or superior mesenteric artery. Accessory renal arteries are seen in 25% to 28% of patients and are considered the sole arterial supply to a specific portion of the renal parenchyma, commonly the lower and occasionally the upper pole of the kidney. These accessory renal arteries may contraindicate laparoscopic donor nephrectomy and result in severe bleeding if they are injured during endopyelotomy for UPJO. Multiple renal arteries that arise from the aorta or iliac arteries are frequently seen in horseshoe and pelvic kidneys. In approximately 5% of patients, the main and accessory right renal arteries pass anterior to the IVC.

There is a longitudinal avascular plane (line of Brodel) between the posterior and anterior segmental arteries just posterior to the lateral aspect of the kidney through which incision results in significantly less blood loss. However, this plane may have various locations that necessitate its delineation before incision either by preoperative angiography or intraoperative segmental arterial injection of methylene blue. This has important surgical implications. For example, during percutaneous access into the kidney, posterior calyces along the line of Brodel are preferred. Furthermore, during anatrophic nephrolithotomy **(Boyce procedure)**, an incision is made through this avascular plane.

At the renal sinus, each **segmental artery branches into lobar arteries,** which further subdivide in the renal parenchyma to form **interlobar arteries** (eFig. 84.17). These interlobar arteries progress peripherally within the cortical **columns of Bertin** to give the **arcuate arteries** at the base of the renal pyramids at the corticomedullary junction. Note the close relationship of the interlobar arteries to the infundibuli of minor calyces. **Interlobular arteries** branch off the arcuate arteries and move radially, where they eventually divide to form the **afferent arterioles** to the glomeruli. Each afferent arteriole supplies a glomerulus, one of approximately 2 million glomeruli, where urinary filtrate leaves the arterial system and is collected in the glomerular (Bowman) capsule. Blood returns from the glomerulus via the efferent arteriole and continues as either secondary capillary networks around the urinary tubules in the cortex or descends into the renal medulla as the vasa recta.

The **renal venous** drainage correlates closely with the arterial supply, with the exception that unlike the arterial supply, venous drainage has extensive collateral communication through the venous collars around minor calyceal infundibula (eFig. 84.18 and Figs. 84.19 and 84.20). Furthermore, the interlobular veins that drain the postglomerular capillaries also communicate freely with perinephric veins through the subcapsular venous plexus of stellate veins. The **interlobular veins** progress through the arcuate, interlobar, lobar, and segmental veins paralleling their corresponding arteries. Three to five segmental renal veins eventually unite to form the renal vein. Because the venous drainage communicates freely forming extensive collateral venous drainage of the kidney, occlusion of a segmental venous branch has little effect on venous outflow. The **right and left renal veins** lie anterior to the right and left renal arteries and drain into the IVC. Whereas the right renal vein is 2 to 4 cm long, the left renal vein is 6 to 10 cm. The longer left renal vein receives the left suprarenal (adrenal) vein and the left gonadal (testicular or ovarian) vein. The left renal vein also may receive a **lumbar vein,** which could be easily avulsed during surgical manipulation of the

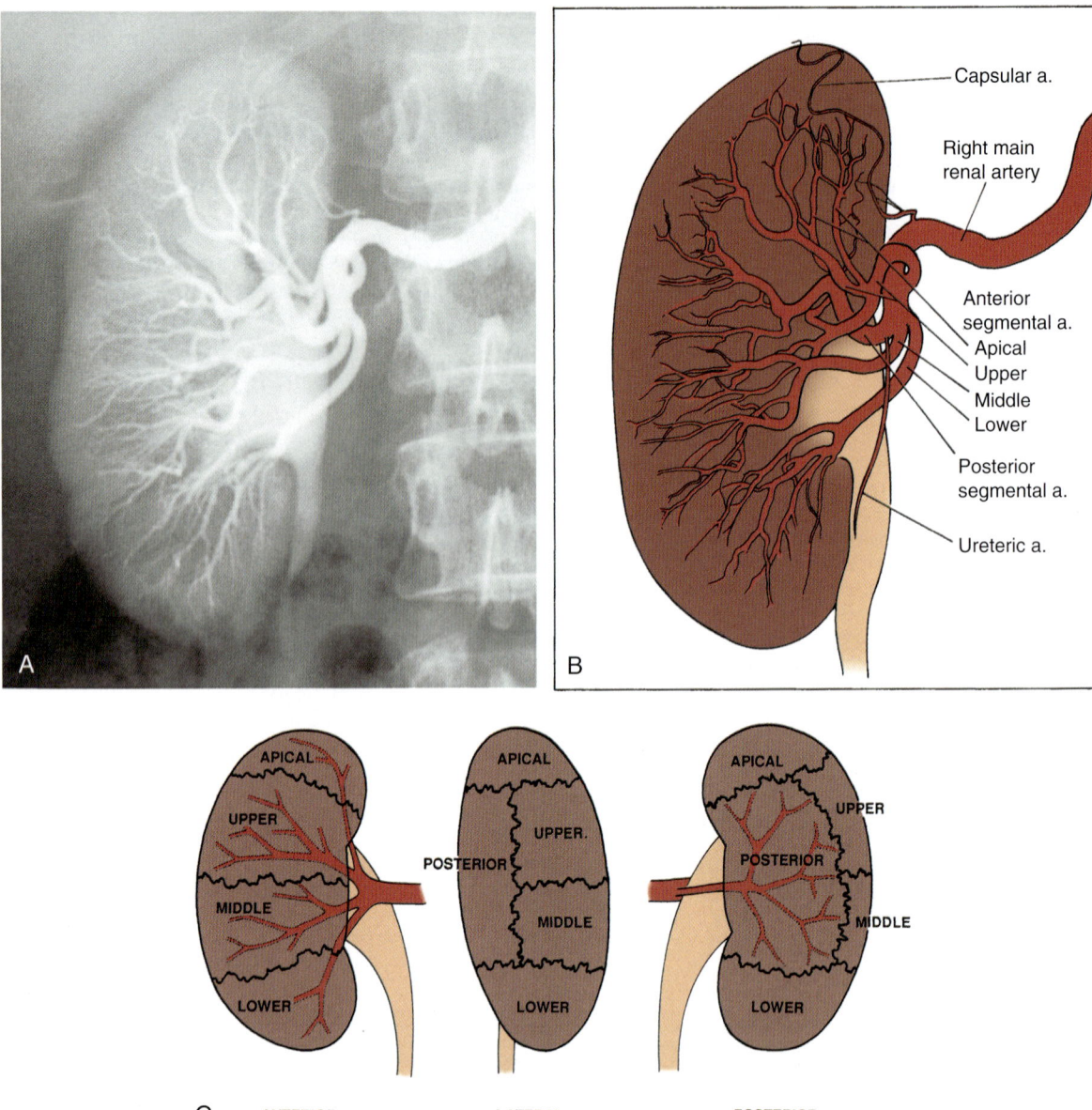

Fig. 84.16. Blood supply of the kidney. (A and B) Segmental branches of the right renal artery demonstrated by renal angiogram. (C) Segmental circulation of the right kidney shown diagrammatically. Note that the posterior segmental artery is usually the first branch of the main renal artery and it extends behind the renal pelvis. *a*, artery.

left renal vein (Beveridge et al., 2016). The left renal vein traverses the acute angle between the **superior mesenteric artery** anteriorly and the aorta posteriorly. In thin adolescents, the left renal vein may get compressed between the superior mesenteric artery and aorta, causing **nutcracker syndrome.** In approximately 15% of the patients, supernumerary renal veins are seen and often are retroaortic when present on the left. Accessory renal veins are more common on the right side, and the most common anomaly of the left renal venous system is the circumaortic renal vein, reported in 2% to 16% of patients. The retroaortic renal vein is less commonly seen than the circumaortic vein, in which the left renal vein bifurcates into ventral and dorsal limbs, which encircle the abdominal aorta. In the retroaortic renal vein, the single left renal vein courses posterior to the aorta and drains into the lower lumbar segment of the IVC.

In terms of imaging studies, Doppler ultrasonography clearly identifies renal arteries at their origin from the abdominal aorta (see eFig. 84.12). However, the main renal artery is often difficult to identify at baseline ultrasonography. Therefore computed tomography angiography (CTA) is currently considered the gold standard to assess renal arteries, with 100% sensitivity for identification of renal arteries and veins. The 3D volume-rendered CTA has emerged as a fast, reliable, and noninvasive modality that can reliably and accurately depict the number, size, course, and relationship of the renal vasculature. Arterial branches down to the segmental branches could be identified, but vessels smaller than 2 mm could be missed (see eFig. 84.15). Magnetic resonance arteriography uses no ionizing radiation, does not require arterial access, and includes different imaging techniques to visualize renal vasculature. Contrast material can give faster, better resolution and more accurate images without artifacts.

Lymphatic Drainage of the Kidney

Interstitial fluid leaves the kidney by either a superficial capsular or a deeper hilar network (eFig. 84.21). Renal lymphatics are embedded in the periarterial loose connective tissue around the renal arteries and are distributed primarily along the interlobular and arcuate arteries in the cortex. The arcuate lymphatic vessels drain into hilar lymphatic

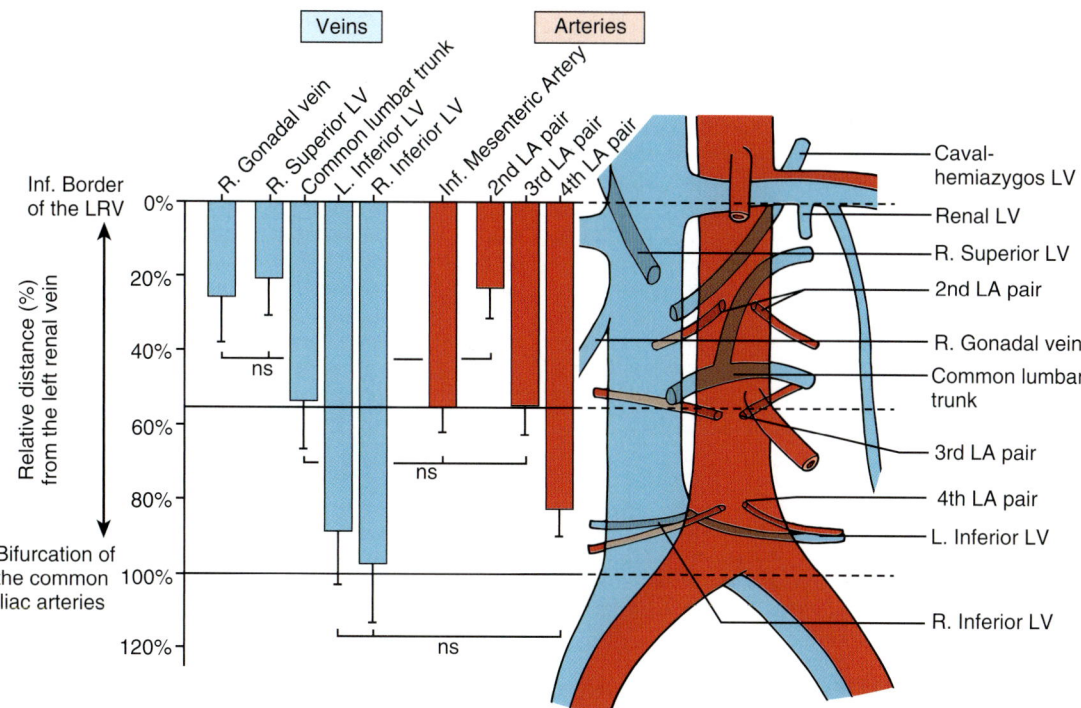

Fig. 84.19. Relative position of infrarenal lumbar arteries (*LA*) and lumbar veins (*LV*), right (*R.*) gonadal vein and inferior (*Inf.*) mesenteric artery. *Dotted lines* demarcate the inferior border of the left renal vein, origin of inferior mesenteric artery (IMA), and bifurcation of common iliac arteries. Superior vessels, including right gonadal vein, right superior lumbar vein (*LV*), the second pair of lumbar arteries, middle vessels, including common lumbar trunk, IMA, and the third pair of lumbar arteries, were significantly different in position from inferior vessels, including left (*L.*) and right inferior lumbar veins, and the fourth pair of lumbar arteries. No significant difference in position was observed in each vessel grouping (superior vessel group of right gonadal vein vs. right superior lumbar vein vs. second pair of lumbar arteries). (Modified with permission from Beveridge TS et al. Retroperitoneal lymph node dissection: anatomical and technical considerations from a cadaveric study. *J Urol* 196: 1764–1771, 2016.)

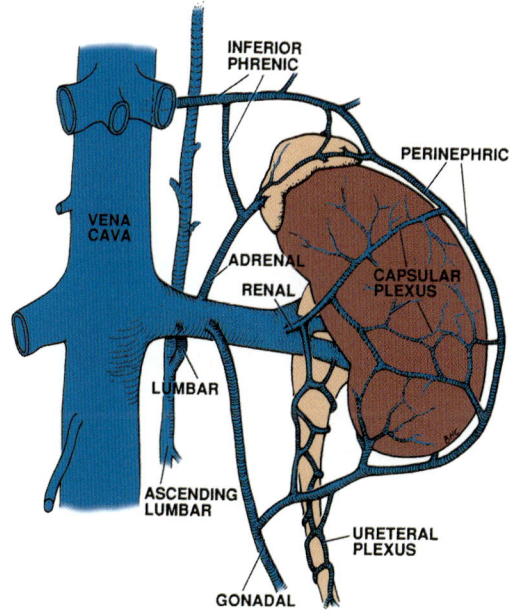

Fig. 84.20. Venous drainage of the left kidney showing potentially extensive collateral circulation.

KEY POINTS: RENAL VASCULATURE

- Each kidney is commonly supplied by a single renal artery, which arises directly from the abdominal aorta, and a single renal vein usually drains directly to the IVC.
- Each renal artery divides into five segmental branches: posterior, apical, upper, middle, and lower segmental arteries.
- The progression of arterial supply to the kidney is as follows: renal artery → segmental artery → interlobar artery → arcuate artery → interlobular artery → afferent arteriole → glomerulus → efferent arteriole.
- The veins anastomose freely throughout the kidney, whereas the arterial supply does not.
- Anatomic variations in the renal vasculature are common in 25% to 40% of kidneys.
- CTA is currently the gold standard to assess renal arteries. Accessory renal arteries are seen in 25% to 28% of patients and are considered the sole arterial supply to a specific portion of the renal parenchyma.
- Anomalies of renal veins are less common than those of the renal arteries.

vessels through interlobar lymphatics. As these lymphatics exit the renal hilum, they join branches from the renal capsule, perinephric tissues, renal pelvis, and upper ureter, where they empty into lymph nodes associated with the renal vein. Afterward, the lymphatic drainage varies considerably between the two kidneys. Left lymphatic drainage primarily goes into the left lateral para-aortic lymph nodes (between the inferior mesenteric artery and diaphragm), with occasional additional drainage into the retrocrural nodes or directly into the thoracic duct above the diaphragm. Right renal lymphatic drainage primarily goes into the right interaortocaval and right paracaval lymph nodes (between the common iliac vessels and diaphragm), with occasional additional drainage from the right kidney into the retrocrural nodes or the left lateral para-aortic lymph nodes.

Innervation of the Kidney

The kidney can function well without neurologic control, as evidenced by the successful function of transplanted kidneys (eFig. 84.22). Sympathetic preganglionic nerves originate from the eighth thoracic through first lumbar spinal segments, with contributions mainly from the celiac plexus and a lesser contribution from the greater splanchnic, intermesenteric, and superior hypogastric plexuses. Postganglionic sympathetic nerve fiber distribution generally follows the arterial vessels throughout the cortex and the outer medulla. These postganglionic fibers travel to the kidney via the autonomic plexus surrounding the renal artery. In addition, parasympathetic fibers from the vagus nerve travel with the sympathetic fibers to the autonomic plexus along the renal artery. The renal sympathetics cause vasoconstriction, and the parasympathetics cause vasodilation.

PELVICALYCEAL SYSTEM

Understanding the collecting system anatomy is of utmost importance for appropriate radiologic interpretation and performance of different endourologic procedures. The upper pole of the kidney usually contains three calyces and less commonly two, whereas three or four calyces could be identified at the interpolar region and two or three calyces at the lower pole (Fig. 84.23). These calyces vary considerably not only in numbers but also in size and shape because of the different numbers of papillae they receive. A calyx may receive a single papilla, two, or even three. Compound papillae are often found in the polar regions of the kidney. The upper pole is usually drained by a single midline calyceal infundibulum, and the lower pole is drained by either a single midline calyceal infundibulum or by paired calyces. The hilar region is drained by anterior and posterior rows of paired calyces. The pelvicalyceal system may have the configuration of either a true pelvis or divided double calyceal pelvis. The true pelvis is the classic type in which the calyces drain directly through elongated necks into an elongated pelvis. This pelvis may be completely imbedded within the renal sinus (intrarenal pelvis) or mostly outside it (extrarenal pelvis). The renal pelvis is roughly pyramidal, with the base facing the parenchyma and the apex funneling down into the ureter. It usually has a capacity of 3 to 10 mL of urine.

In a divided (duplex) pelvis, it is divided at the hilum into upper and lower portions and drains a higher number of calyces than a normal pelvis. Its lower part is usually shorter but larger and often drains the hilar and the lower pole calyces. Therefore there is no direct connection between the upper and lower calyces. This usually becomes apparent during the excretory phase of a CT urogram or on retrograde pyelography. During percutaneous endoscopic evaluation of the kidney, the existence of a duplex pelvis should be considered if upper or lower pole calyces cannot be accessed through a particular calyceal access. Duplex systems are easier to recognize on retrograde nephroureteroscopy. When a duplex system is suspected during ureteroscopy, retrograde pyelography could be performed to illustrate the anomalous pelvicalyceal system.

Radiologic Anatomy of the Collecting System

After an iodinated contrast agent is injected for intravenous urography, nephrotomograms appear after 60 to 90 seconds that represent

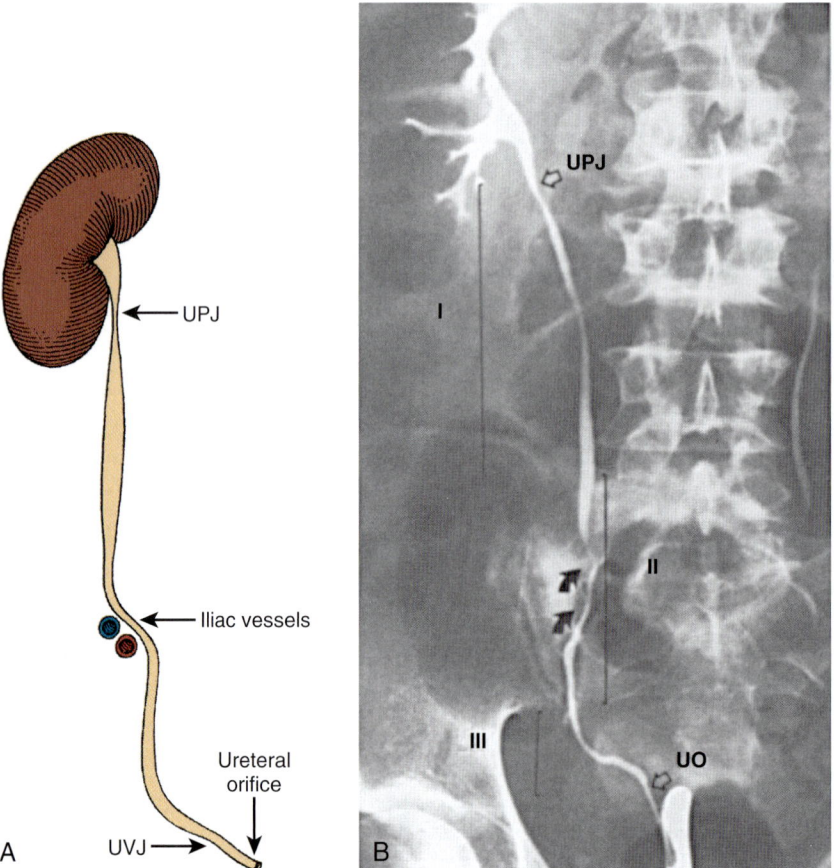

Fig. 84.23. (A) The ureter demonstrating sites of normal functional or anatomic narrowing at the ureteropelvic junction (*UPJ*), the iliac vessels, and the ureterovesical junction (*UVJ*). (B) The right ureter, illustrated by retrograde injection of contrast material. *I*, Upper or proximal ureter, extending to the upper border of the sacrum; *II*, middle ureter, extending to the lower border of the sacrum; *III*, distal or lower ureter, traversing the pelvis to end in the bladder; *UO*, ureteric orifice in the bladder; *UPJ*, ureteropelvic junction. *Arrows* indicate the course of the common iliac artery and vein.

contrast material within the renal tubules. Fifteen minutes after contrast injection, a panoramic radiograph of the whole urinary tract can be obtained; the bladder finally appears 20 to 30 minutes after contrast injection. Absence of contrast excretion 24 hours after intravenous contrast injection indicates a nonfunctioning kidney. **The pelvicaliceal anatomy is variable, and no simple rule defines calyceal organization.** Currently, CT urography has replaced intravenous urography, and multidetector CT provides the ability to obtain thin (<1 mm) collimated data of the entire urinary tract during a short single breath-hold (Van Der Molen et al., 2008). Magnetic resonance urography (MRU) has two consecutive phases: a static-fluid phase and an excretory phase. The static-fluid MRU is ideally indicated for evaluation of the obstructed or dilated collecting system. The practicability of excretory MRU depends on renal function, and its quality could be improved by a low-dose furosemide diuretic. Congenital variants of the pelvicalyceal system are common, representing approximately 4% of the population. The renal pelvis may be completely intrarenal, completely extrarenal, or a combination of both (Friedenberg and Dunbar, 1990). The infundibula insert directly into the extrarenal pelvis, giving the impression of a dilated pelvis. Receiving the tip of renal papilla, the renal calyx is a concave structure with two side projections, the fornices, which surround the papilla of the renal medulla. Multiple single calyces fail to divide completely, forming a larger compound calyx that normally can be observed in the upper and lower poles of the kidneys. Each kidney contains an average of 7 to 9 calyces, although this number may vary considerably from 4 to 19 or even more. Megacalycosis represents a nonobstructive asymptomatic congenital dilation of some or all renal calyces, while the renal pelvis and ureter are normal. It involves all calyces uniformly and usually is associated with a greater number of calyces than normal. Calyceal diverticula represent a focal extrinsic dilation of a renal calyx that is connected to the calyceal fornix and projects into the renal cortex, not into the medulla. The renoureteral unit may show duplication anomalies, including a bifid renal pelvis and complete or incomplete ureteral duplication. Two separate pyelocalyceal collecting systems may be present in one kidney, ranging from a bifid pelvis to a bifid ureter (ureteropelvic duplication).

URETERS

The ureters are bilateral muscular retroperitoneal ducts with narrow lumens that carry urine from the kidneys to the urinary bladder (see Fig. 84.23). Each ureter runs inferiorly as a narrow continuation of its renal pelvis at the UPJ, passing over the pelvic brim at the bifurcation of the common iliac artery. They then run along the lateral wall of the pelvis to enter the urinary bladder. In adults, the ureter is 22 to 30 cm in length with a diameter of 1.5 to 6 mm; in neonates it measures 6.5 to 7.0 cm long. In the retroperitoneum, the ureter is situated just lateral to the tips of the transverse processes of the lumbar vertebrae. The ureters occupy a sagittal plane that intersects the tips of the transverse processes of these lumbar vertebrae. The ureter is arbitrarily divided into proximal (upper), middle (over the sacrum), and distal (lower) segments. However, according to international anatomic terminology the ureter consists of abdominal (from renal pelvis to iliac vessels), pelvic (from iliac vessels to the bladder), and intramural segments.

The abdominal parts of the ureters are adherent to the retroperitoneum throughout their entire course and extend from the renal pelvis to the pelvic brim. From the back, the surface anatomy of the ureter corresponds to a line joining a point 5 cm lateral to the L1 spinous process and the posterior superior iliac spine. Normally, three constrictions could be identified radiologically in each ureter: at its junction with the renal pelvis (UPJ), where it crosses the iliac vessels, and during its passage through the wall of the urinary bladder (intramural ureter) or ureterovesical junction (see Fig. 84.23). These constricted areas are potential sites of obstruction by ureteral calculi.

Posteriorly, both ureters descend anterior to the psoas major muscle and then cross the ventral surface of the transverse processes of the third to fifth lumbar vertebrae and enter the pelvis at the bifurcation of the common iliac vessels (see eFigs. 84.4 and 84.5).

The bifurcation of the common iliac vessels is used intraoperatively as a landmark to look for the ureter. The genitofemoral nerve runs on top of the psoas major muscle behind the ureter. The right ureter begins behind the descending part of the duodenum, where it is crossed by the gonadal vessels (testicular or ovarian), which is called "water under the bridge." The left ureter is covered at its origin by the initial part of the jejunum. The gonadal vessels cross the left ureter after running parallel to it for a small distance. The inferior mesenteric artery and its terminal branch, the superior rectal artery, follow a curved course close to the left ureter. Therefore, as the left ureter approaches the pelvis, it is crossed by the left colic vessels, the sigmoid colon, and its mesocolon. Just above the entry to the pelvis, the ureter is still covered by peritoneum by virtue of the ureteral fold. This location at the pelvic brim represents one of the most common areas of ureteral injury. Furthermore, the close relationship of the ureter with the terminal ileum, appendix, right and left colons, and sigmoid colon makes it susceptible for encroachment of inflammatory and malignant processes, resulting in clinical presentations ranging from microhematuria to ureteral obstruction or even fistulae.

The pelvic segment of the ureter is approximately 15 cm long—half of its total length. At the pelvic inlet, it crosses the common iliac vessels near their bifurcation. This crossover point is usually at the bifurcation of the common iliac artery into the internal and external iliac arteries, making this a useful landmark for pelvic procedures. The ureter then runs downward and laterally toward the ischial spine on the lateral pelvic wall along the anterior border of the greater sciatic notch, dorsally accompanied by the internal iliac artery and its visceral branches and the venous plexuses as well. It is still closely related to the posterior parietal peritoneum. At the ischial spine, the ureter turns medially to descend in the endopelvic fascia with branches of the hypogastric nerves. At the lateral wall of the pelvis, this part of the ureter crosses the obturator artery, vein, and nerve. In males, the vas deferens loops medially over this part while the ureter passes the ampulla of the vas deferens and the seminal vesicles just before it enters the bladder. In females, the descending part of the pelvic segment of the ureter courses posterior to the ovary to form the posterior boundary of the ovarian fossa. The ureter then passes through the base of the broad ligament and swings in a convex curve to cross under the uterine vessels ("water under the bridge") in a sagittal direction approximately 1.5 to 2 cm adjacent to the supravaginal part of the uterine cervix. The terminal ureter runs forward, accompanied by the neurovascular bundle of the bladder and passes the anterior vaginal fornix just before entering the bladder. This close proximity of the ureter to the uterine vessels is the cause of ureteral injuries during gynecologic procedures. In the case of vaginal surgery, there is a high risk for injury, especially for the left ureter that crosses the anterior vaginal fornix closer than the right ureter.

Near the bladder, the terminal ureter is enveloped by a muscular layer, the Waldeyer sheath, and then pierces the bladder wall obliquely as the intramural segment (eFig. 84.24). The length of this intramural part of the ureter in adults is 1.2 to 2.5 cm, and in neonates it is approximately 0.5 to 0.8 cm long. The Waldeyer muscle bundles of the ureter coalesce with those of the detrusor muscle of the bladder wall. Therefore reflux of urine from the bladder to the ureter is prevented during increased intravesical pressure, such as during micturition. Another important feature of the 3D course of the ureter that is critical to appreciate and follow during rigid ureteroscopy is the angulation of the ureter as it courses through the retroperitoneum. When approached from the retrograde direction, the ureter courses anterolaterally as it goes along the lateral pelvic wall. Then, as it crosses the pelvic brim, it angulates posteriorly to continue as the proximal ureter. Following the 3D course of the ureter along a safety guidewire reduces the risk for perforation, especially in patients with large impacted stones.

Radiologic Anatomy of the Ureter

The ureter could be delineated by excretory urography during expiration, because it may be kinked during inspiration as a result of downward movement of the kidney (Friedenberg and Dunbar, 1990).

For radiologic purposes, radiologists describe three segments of the ureter: a proximal portion extending from its origin down to the upper border of the sacroiliac joint, a middle portion lying over the sacroiliac joint, and the remaining segment from the lower border of that joint to its entrance into the bladder, which represents the distal portion of the ureter.

The course of the ureter and its bilateral symmetry are subject to great variability. It may descend laterally away from the margin of the transverse processes or be displaced medial to the renal pedicle. A medially displaced right ureter might normally be seen in young black males (Adam et al., 1985). The right ureter may run medially behind the vein at the level of third lumbar vertebra before it returns to its lateral position. **The entire length of the ureter is rarely seen in a single film of the excretory urography because of its peristaltic activity.** Otherwise, ureteral atony or obstruction should be suspected (Mellins, 1986). Similarly, crossing vessels may compress the ureter and simulate areas of stricture. **Therefore the diagnosis of a ureteral stricture should not be based on a single film of excretory urography with the presence of ureteral dilatation proximal to the site of narrowing.** Ureteral duplication may be complete or incomplete (partial). Complete duplication results from the development of a second ureteric bud, and the two ureters are inserted into the bladder separately. The partial type results from redundant duplication of the single ureteric bud in which the two ureters join together above the bladder to from a single stump draining into the bladder. Complete ureteral duplication with a common or ectopic entry of the upper pole moiety is less common than incomplete duplication. The ureter draining the upper segment of the kidney prevalently inserts in the bladder inferior and medial to the ureter draining the lower segment of the kidney (Weigert-Meyer rule). These ectopic orifices are prone to ureteroceles and/or vesicoureteral reflux. The lower moiety of the completely duplicated system is generally normal. Ureteral duplication also may be bilateral. Triple moiety may be observed. In diagnosis of renal or ureteral displacement, CT scans have replaced lateral views of conventional radiography. In a standard lateral view, the normal renal collecting system should not project anterior to the spine and the ureter stays behind the anterior margin of the vertebral bodies until the level of L4. After this, the ureter lies anterior to the vertebral body by approximately one-fourth the width of the vertebral body (Friedland et al., 1983). In elderly patients with atherosclerotic vessels, ureteral narrowing at the pelvic brim at its crossing to the common iliac vessels may produce a posterior indentation that may appear as an extrinsic filling defect. Dilation proximal to that point may be differentiated from obstruction by the absence of pelvicalyceal dilation without delay in emptying on prone or erect films (Friedenberg and Dunbar, 1990). Medial displacement of both pelvic ureteral segments may result from retroperitoneal fibrosis or pelvic lipomatosis, or it may appear after abdominoperineal surgery. However, medial displacement and concavity of a single pelvic ureter may result from enlarged hypogastric nodes, a bladder diverticulum, or aneurysmal dilation of the hypogastric artery. Nevertheless, this may be a normal finding in adult women if only the right ureter is affected due to the uterine tilt to the left. In older men, benign prostatic hyperplasia may result in elevation of the bladder floor enough to cause the intramural segment of the ureter to curve superiorly, giving a characteristic "fish hook" or "hockey stick" appearance on excretory urography (Olsson, 1986).

> **KEY POINTS: RADIOLOGIC ANATOMY OF THE URETER**
>
> - It is important to have the patient empty the bladder to evaluate the distal ureter appropriately.
> - Radiologically, the ureter is divided into three segments: a proximal portion from UPJ to the sacroiliac joint, a middle portion lying over the sacroiliac joint, and a distal portion from the lower border of that joint to its entrance into the bladder.
> - The entire length of the ureter is rarely seen on a single film of the excretory urography because of its peristaltic activity.

Arteries, Veins, and Lymphatic Drainage of the Ureters

The abdominal portion of the ureter is supplied mainly by arterial branches medially from the main renal arteries (eFig. 84.25). However, this segment may be uncommonly supplied by branches arising from the abdominal aorta or gonadal arteries. These branches approach the ureters medially and divide into ascending and descending branches, forming a longitudinal anastomosis on the ureteral wall. However, despite this anastomotic plexus, ureteral ischemia is not uncommon if these small and delicate ureteral branches are disrupted. Surgeons are trained to handle ureters gently to avoid unnecessary lateral retraction and removing periureteral adventitial tissues containing the blood supply to minimize ureteral ischemia and subsequent stricture. The mid-ureter is supplied by branches arising posteriorly from the common iliac arteries. The blood supply to the distal ureter comes laterally from the superior vesical artery, a branch of the internal iliac artery. Therefore the blood supply of the ureter is medially in the proximal part, posteriorly in the midportion, and laterally in the distal portion. Therefore endoureterotomy should be performed laterally in the proximal ureter, anteriorly in the midportion, and medially in the distal ureter. Another important surgical caveat is to control the obliterated umbilical artery before mobilizing the most distal aspect of the ureter as it enters the bladder.

Veins draining the abdominal part of the ureters drain into the renal and gonadal veins. **Venous drainage of the mid- and distal ureters is into the common and internal iliac veins.** The lymphatics of the ureter form plexuses within its muscular and adventitial layers. The lymphatics from the left abdominal ureter drain into the left para-aortic lymph nodes, and the lymphatics from the right abdominal ureter drain into the right paracaval and interaortocaval lymph nodes. Lymphatic vessels from the middle part usually drain into the common iliac lymph nodes, whereas lymphatics from its intrapelvic part drain into the common, external, and internal iliac lymph nodes.

> **KEY POINTS: URETERS**
>
> - The course of the ureter begins posterior to the renal artery and continues along the anterior edge of the psoas muscle.
> - The gonadal vessels cross anterior to the ureter in this region (water under bridge). The ureter next passes over the bifurcation of the common iliacs into the internal and external iliacs.
> - The blood supply of the proximal ureter is medially, mid-ureter is posteriorly, and distal ureter is laterally.

Nerve Supply of the Ureter

The ureter receives a rich autonomic nerve supply that originates from the celiac, aortorenal, and mesenteric ganglia, together with the superior and inferior hypogastric (pelvic) plexuses. The sympathetic supply to the ureter arises from the preganglionic fibers of the 11th and 12th thoracic and 1st lumbar segments. Parasympathetic vagal fibers supply the upper part of the ureter via the celiac plexus, and the lower portion is supplied by the sacral segments S2 to S4. Therefore afferent nerves from the upper portion of the ureter reach the spinal cord with the sympathetic fibers between T11 and L1 and those from the lower ureter travel via the pelvic plexus between S2 and S4. These fibers conduct afferent sensory stimuli from the ureters and have a minor, if any, role in the control of ureteral motility. This is because excised portions of the ureter continue to contract without nervous control and denervation of the lower portion of the ureter does not result in reflux. As mentioned earlier, the peristalsis of the ureter originates from pacemakers in the minor calyces. Thus the exact role of autonomic input of the ureters is unclear. Distention of the renal capsule and the collecting system causes stimulation of renal pain fibers that carry signals through the sympathetic nerves, thus resulting in visceral-type referred pain in the flank, groin, or scrotal (labial) regions.

Microscopic Anatomy of the Ureter

The ureter consists of three distinct layers. The innermost is the mucosa, the middle muscular layer is the muscularis, and the outer layer is the adventitia. The mucosa consists of transitional epithelium, which has four to six layers of cells when the ureter is contracted. These cells encircle a large number of junctional complexes containing a consistent level of keratin precursors that is responsible for the waterproof property of this layer. The mucosa also contains many longitudinal folds that give the empty ureter a characteristic stellar outline. The epithelium rests on a layer of connective tissue, the lamina propria, which contains the blood vessels and nerve fibers to the ureter (eFig. 84.26).

The muscular wall of the ureter consists of two longitudinal layers separated by a middle circular layer that may not be distinct from each other, especially in the abdominal segment of the ureter. Mostly, these muscle fibers appear to be spirally arranged by the light microscopy. However, in the distal ureter, the inner spirals are steep and the outer spirals are horizontal, thus appearing as inner longitudinal and outer circular layers in cross section. These smooth muscle layers are contiguous with the smooth muscle covering the minor renal calyces, where the pacemaker is located to initiate the rhythmic peristalsis to deliver urine.

The outermost layer, the adventitia, consists of a dense network of collagen and elastic fibers, including many blood vessels and unmyelinated nerve fibers among them. This layer is continuous proximally with the capsule at the renal pelvis while it is thickened distally by a specialized muscle fibers and fibrous tissue to form the Waldeyer sheath.

In a normal kidney, the UPJ does not differ histologically from the renal pelvis. However, in an obstructed kidney, the longitudinal muscle fibers are significantly increased with more collagen deposits around the muscle fibers in addition to attenuation of muscle bundles, leading to the physiologic obstruction known clinically as UPJO.

Endoscopic Anatomy of the Ureter and Pelvicalyceal System

Once the cystoscope is inside the bladder neck, the trigone can be seen as a raised, smooth triangle. The apex of that triangle is situated at the bladder neck, and its base is formed by the interureteral ridge or Mercier bar, extending between the two ureteric orifices. The interureteral ridge is more prominent in males than females, and the ureteric orifices are symmetrically located along it, approximately 1 to 2 cm from the midline. The trigone is the most vascular part of the bladder and is formed by an extension of the longitudinal muscle fibers of the ureters over the detrusor muscle. Therefore it appears cystoscopically to be more deeply colored than the rest of the bladder.

The normal ureteric orifice may appear as a volcano or a horseshoe that is prominent and obvious on endoscopy. However, it may look like a slit that can be identified with only meticulous examination. It is pushed out laterally during bladder filling and may vary in position and appearance. In a normal bladder, the ureteric orifices are usually surrounded by prominent mucosal vessels (Bagley et al., 1985).

The ureteric orifices are classified according to their position or configuration. They are normally located at the medial aspect of the trigone (position A). However, they may be located at the lateral wall of the bladder or at its junction with the trigone (position C) or in between positions A and C (position B) (Lyon et al., 1969). In terms of configuration, grade 0 indicates a normal ureteric orifice that looks like a cone or a volcano. Grades 1, 2, and 3 describe stadium, horseshoe, and golf-hole orifices, respectively. **The higher the grade of the orifice, the higher the tendency to be laterally located and to reflux** (eFig. 84.27).

The intramural ureter represents the narrowest part of the ureter, with an average diameter of 3 to 4 mm. It extends from the ureteric orifice for approximately 1.5 cm, posterolaterally for 0.5 cm, and then obliquely through the detrusor hiatus for approximately 1 cm (Politano, 1972). Being the narrowest ureteral segment, the intramural ureter may have to be dilated before ureteroscopy. The other ureteral narrowing areas at the pelvic brim and UPJ are identified endoscopically by being stenotic and relatively nondistensible. However, they are relatively wider than the intramural segment. They can be easily instrumented with enough pressure from the irrigation fluid. The pulsating iliac vessels could be seen endoscopically as the ureters cross the pelvic brim and angulate posteriorly in the proximal portion.

The proximal ureter goes straight up to the UPJ; the ureter lies on the psoas major muscle, with the appearance of a typical stellate nondistended ureter. The UPJ could be identified easily endoscopically during its frequent opening and closing. The UPJ merges into the wider and more dependent part of the renal pelvis. The respiratory movement of the kidney could be seen by endoscopy after passing the relatively fixed UPJ. The kidneys lie on the diaphragm, and thus they are affected by the respiratory movements. **Therefore, during ureteroscopy, the tidal volume could be decreased to minimize renal excursions during respiration.** Moreover, the physiologic ureteral contractions or peristalsis can be observed endoscopically. It is important to wait for the ureter to relax before pushing the ureteroscope to avoid mucosal trauma (Andonian et al., 2008b, 2010b).

The UPJ represents the apex of the funnel-shaped or conical normal renal pelvis. An extrarenal pelvis is usually larger and has longer major calyceal infundibula than an intrarenal pelvis. In the renal pelvis, the flexible ureteroscope first faces the ostia of the major calyces, which look like circular openings separated by carinae. Then the flexible ureteroscope enters a long tubular infundibulum that branches into the minor calyces. These infundibula usually connect the ostia of major calyces with their apex. For a flexible ureteroscope to pass from the axis of the upper ureteral segment to the axis of the lower infundibulum, it should deflected 140 (104 to 175) degrees at the ureteroinfundibular angle (Bagley and Rittenberg, 1987).

A circular muscle layer extends around the base of the papilla to help expel urine jets from papillary ducts. The renal papillae appear endoscopically as protruding discs surrounded by calyceal fornices, paler in color than the pink friable epithelium covering the papillae. Each papilla represents the apex of a renal pyramid, receiving the papillary ducts of Bellini that drain the pyramids. These ducts are minute openings that become more dilated and obvious with distal obstruction (Andonian et al., 2008a, 2010a).

Segmental and interlobar branches of the renal artery, together with major intrarenal tributaries of the renal vein, run in close relation with the anterior and posterior surfaces of the major caliceal infundibula as well as the necks of minor calices (Sampaio, 2009). Therefore, if infundibulotomy must be performed, it should be performed in either the superior or inferior quadrants, which are free of major vessels. Anatomically, the following sequence is recommended if more

---

> **KEY POINTS: ENDOSCOPIC ANATOMY**
>
> - The trigone is the most vascular part of the bladder and is formed by an extension of the longitudinal muscle fibers of the ureters over the detrusor muscle.
> - Both ureteric orifices are rarely seen in a single endoscopic view.
> - The interureteral ridge is more prominent in males than females, and the ureteric orifices are symmetrically located along it, approximately 1 to 2 cm from the midline.
> - The intramural ureter represents the narrowest part of the ureter, with an average diameter of 3 to 4 mm.
> - The extrarenal pelvis is usually larger and has longer major calyceal infundibula than the intrarenal pelvis.
> - The renal papillae appear endoscopically as protruding discs surrounded by calyceal fornices, paler in color than the pink friable epithelium covering the papillae.
> - If infundibulotomy needs be performed, it should be performed in either the superior or inferior quadrants, which are free of major vessels. Anterior infundibular incision should be avoided to avoid injuring of large intrarenal blood vessels leading to severe bleeding.

than one infundibular incision is necessary: the first two incisions should be done, respectively, in the superior and inferior quadrants, the third incision between the superior and posterior quadrants, and the fourth between the inferior and posterior quadrants. Further incision would be performed in the posterior quadrant, avoiding anterior incisions as much as possible (Sampaio, 2009).

See Videos 84.1, 84.2, 84.3, 84.4, 84.5, and 84.6 for procedures related to this chapter.

SUGGESTED READINGS

Drake RL, Vogl W, Mitchell AWM: *Gray's anatomy for students*, Philadelphia, 2005, Churchill Livingstone.

Frober R: Surgery illustrated: surgical anatomy of the ureter, *BJU Int* 100:949–965, 2007.

Hinman F, Stempen PH: *Atlas of urosurgical anatomy*, Philadelphia, 1993, WB Saunders.

Moore KL, Dalley AF, Agur AM: *Clinically oriented anatomy*, 6th ed, Philadelphia, 2010, Lippincott Williams & Wilkins, pp 292–365.

Netter FH: *Atlas of human anatomy*, 5th ed, Philadelphia, 2010, Saunders.

Quaia E, Martingano P, Cavallaro M, et al: Normal radiological anatomy and anatomical variants of the kidney. In Quaia E, editor: *Radiological imaging of the kidney*, New York, 2011, Springer, pp 17–78.

Sampaio FJB: Renal anatomy: endourologic considerations, *Urol Clin North Am* 27:585–607, 2000.

Silverman SG, Leyendecker JR, Amis SE: What is the current role of CT urography and MR urography in the evaluation of the urinary tract? *Radiology* 250:309–323, 2009.

REFERENCES

The complete reference list is available online at ExpertConsult.com.

85

Physiology and Pharmacology of the Renal Pelvis and Ureter

Dana A. Weiss, MD, and Robert M. Weiss, MD

The function of the ureter is to transport urine from the kidney to the bladder. Under normal conditions, ureteral peristalsis originates with electric activity at pacemaker sites located in the proximal portion of the urinary collecting system (Bozler, 1942; Constantinou, 1974; Gosling and Dixon, 1974; Hurtado et al., 2010; Lammers et al., 1996; Tsuchida and Yamaguchi, 1977; Weiss et al., 1967, 2006; Zhang and Lang, 1994). The electric activity is then propagated distally and gives rise to the mechanical event of peristalsis, ureteral contraction, which propels the bolus of urine distally. Efficient propulsion of the urinary bolus depends on the ureter's ability to completely coapt its walls (Woodburne and Lapides, 1972). Urine passes into the bladder by way of the ureterovesical junction (UVJ), which, under normal conditions, permits urine to pass from the ureter into the bladder, but not from the bladder into the ureter.

CELLULAR ANATOMY

The primary functional anatomic unit of the ureter is the ureteral smooth muscle cell. The cell is extremely small, approximately 250 to 400 μm in length and 5 to 7 μm in diameter. The **nucleus is ellipsoid and contains a darkly staining body, the nucleolus, and the genetic material of the cell. Surrounding the nucleus is the sarcoplasm, which contains the structures involved in cell function. Frequently in close relation to the nucleus, mitochondria** in the cytoplasm **perform many of the nutritive functions of the cell. Endoplasmic or sarcoplasmic reticulum dispersed in the cytoplasm serves as Ca^{++} storage sites.**

Dispersed in the sarcoplasm are the **contractile proteins, actin and myosin**. Depending on the local calcium ion (Ca^{2+}) concentration, they interact to produce contraction or relaxation. **Any process that leads to a significant increase in the Ca^{2+} concentration in the region of the contractile proteins results in contraction; conversely, any process that leads to a significant decrease in the Ca^{2+} concentration in the region of the contractile proteins results in relaxation.** Actin is dispersed throughout the sarcoplasm in hexagonal clumps and is interspersed with the less numerous clumps of more deeply staining myosin. Dark bands along the cell surface are referred to as *attachment plaques* that, along with dense bodies dispersed in the cytoplasm, serve as attachment devices for the actin.

Around the periphery of the cell are numerous cavitary structures, some of which open to the outside of the cell and are referred to as *caveolae*. These **caveolae contain a cytoskeletal protein, caveolin, and a variety of signal transduction molecules and receptors for growth factors and cytokines** (William and Lisanti, 2004). A double-layer cell membrane surrounds the cell. The inner plasma membrane surrounds the entire cell, but the outer basement membrane is absent at areas of close cell-to-cell contact, referred to as intermediate junctions.

DEVELOPMENT OF THE URETER

The ureter, a 25- to 30-cm tube extending from the renal pelvis to the bladder, **arises as an outpouching from the mesonephric duct.** This begins on embryonic day 10.5 (E10.5) in mice and E28 in humans. Signals from the metanephric mesenchyme, stroma, and angioblasts induce the ureteral bud to arise from the mesonephric duct, invade the metanephric mesenchyme, and undergo branching. The nephric (mesonephric or Wolffian) duct cells express a number of surface receptors, including RET, FGFR, AT_2R, and ALK (Fig. 85.1). RET signaling is induced by glial cell line–derived neurotrophic factor (GDNF), **derived from adjacent metanephrogenic mesenchyme** (Pepicelli et al., 1997; Sainio et al., 1997; Shakya et al., 2005), and leads to a rearrangement of the nephric duct cells (Woolf and Davies, 2013). This movement of cells is regulated by the transcription factors ETV4 and ETV5 (Kuure et al., 2010; Yosypiv, 2013; see Fig. 85.1). GDNF-RET signaling is a major pathway in the development of the ureter (Woolf and Davies, 2013) and may be potentiated by neuropeptide Y (NPY) (Choi et al., 2009; Constantini, 2012; Shakya et al., 2005). GDNF signals through the *c-Ret* receptor tyrosine kinase (Vega et al., 1996) and leads to activation of the RAS/ERK MAP kinase, P13K-Akt, and PLC Y-Ca^{++} pathways, which results in increased phosphatidylinositol 3-kinase (P13-kinase) activity and Akt/PKB phosphorylation (Tang et al., 2002). The upregulation of Spry1 by Ret acts as a negative feedback loop (Basson et al., 2006). The expression of GDNF and *c-Ret* is activated by a transcription factor present in the metanephric mesenchyme, paired box 2 *(Pax-2)* (Brophy et al., 2001; Clarke et al., 2006), which is increased by angiotensin II (AT2) (Zhang et al., 2004). A number of other growth factors, including transforming growth factor-β (TGF-β), hepatocyte growth factor (HGF), and fibroblast growth factors (FGF-1, -2, -7, and -10), transcription factors including *Foxd1* and *Wnt11*, and matrix molecules such as heparin sulphate proteoglycans, laminins, integrins, and matrix metalloproteinases (MMP-9) are involved in stimulation or inhibition of growth and branching of the ureteral bud (Basson et al., 2006; Bush et al., 2004; Chen et al., 2004; Davies et al., 1995, 2001; Majumdar et al., 2003; Mendelsohn et al., 1999; Pohl et al., 2000; Qiao et al., 1999, 2001; Sakurai et el., 2003; Takemura et al., 2002).

The nephric ducts also express ALK receptors, which are activated by activins and BMPs (TGF-β family members), **leading to activation of SMADs, which inhibit ureteric bud outgrowth and ureteral development** (Maeshima et al., 2006). Activin A inhibits GDNF-induced ureteral bud formation, and this is accompanied by inhibition of cell proliferation, reduced expression of pax-2, and decreased phosphorylation of PI3-kinase and MAP kinase in the Wolffian duct. The tip of each ureteral bud is capable of inducing adjacent metanephric mesenchyme to undergo mesenchymal-to-epithelial transition (MET) with the formation of the nephron (Ekblom, 1989). Antagonists of the anti-branching factors activin and BMP4 are Gremlin-1 and follistatin, respectively (Woolf and Davies, 2013).

Programmed cell death, or apoptosis, is involved in branching of the ureteric bud and subsequent nephrogenesis. Inhibitors of caspases, which are involved in the apoptotic signaling pathway, **inhibit ureteral bud branching** (Araki et al., 1999). During development, the ureteral lumen is obliterated, and then it recanalizes (Alcaraz et al., 1991; Russo-Gil et al., 1975). **It appears that angiotensin (Ang) acting through the AT2 receptor is involved in the recanalization process** (Yerkes et al., 1998) and in the inhibition of aberrant ureteral budding (Oshima et al., 2001). Knockout mice for the *ATR2* gene have congenital anomalies of the kidney and urinary tract, including duplicated collecting systems with a hydronephrotic upper pole moiety, multicystic dysplastic kidneys, megaureters, and ureteropelvic junction (UPJ) obstructions. Mutant mice lacking AT2 type I receptors fail to develop a renal pelvis and lack

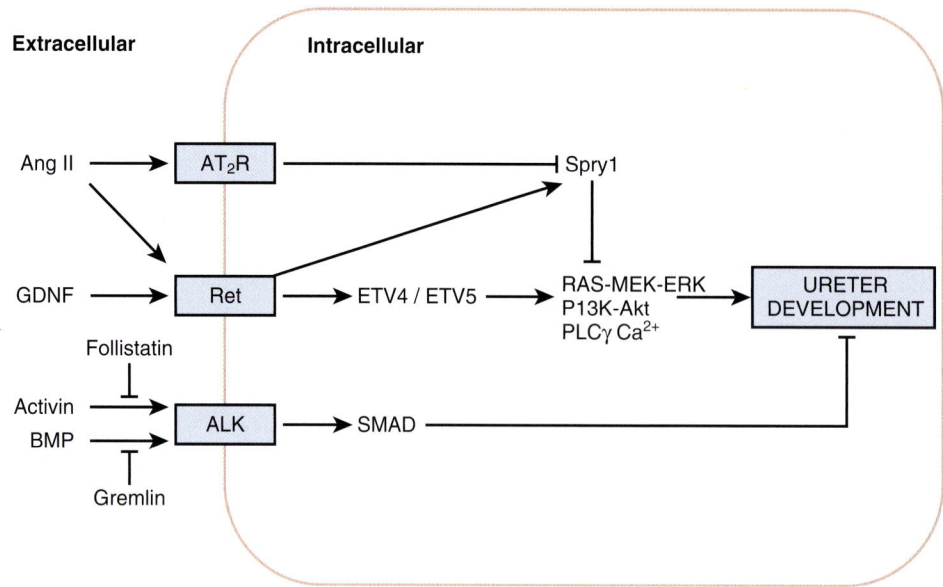

Fig. 85.1. Schematic representation of selected pathways involved in ureter development.

ureteral peristaltic activity (Miyazaki et al., 1998). Angiotensin II acting via AT2 type I receptors also is involved in ureteric bud cell branching, a process that depends on phosphorylation of the EGF receptor (Iosipiv and Schroeder, 2003; Yosypiv et al., 2006) and can stimulate in vitro branching morphogenesis by directly acting on the ureteric bud (Song et al., 2011). In addition, AT2 induces the expression of the GDNF/c-Ret/Wnt11 pathway and represses Spry1 during ureteric bud branching (Song et al., 2010; Yosypiv et al., 2008). Ureteric branching also is promoted by AT2-induced signaling through PI3K/Akt and ERK (Song et al., 2011; Yosypiv, 2013). Some GDNF targets upregulated by AT2 include transcription factors (Etv4, Etv5), signaling molecules (Vsnl1), and receptors (Crlf1) (Song et al., 2011).

Another player in regulating normal ureter development is Brg1 (or SMARCA4). Brg1 is an epigenetic regulator and is part of the switch/sucrose nonfermentable (Swi/Snf) chromatin-remodeling complex. Global loss of Brg1 results in embryonic lethality (Bultman et al., 2000). Brg1 has been shown to be upstream of p63, Pparγ, and sonic hedgehog. Ablation of Brg1 leads to ureter malformation (Weiss et al., 2013).

Calcineurin, a Ca^{++}-dependent serine/threonine phosphatase, also appears to be an essential signaling molecule in urinary tract development. Mutant mice in which calcineurin function is removed are noted to have reduced proliferation of smooth muscle and mesenchymal cells in the developing urinary tract with abnormal development of the renal pelvis and ureter with resultant defective pyeloureteral peristalsis (Chang et al., 2004).

ELECTRIC ACTIVITY

The electric properties of all excitable tissues depend on the distribution of ions on the inside and the outside of the cell membrane and on the relative permeability of the cell membrane to these ions (Hodgkin, 1958). The ionic basis for electric activity in ureteral smooth muscle has not been fully described; however, many of its properties resemble those in other excitable tissues.

Resting Potential

When a ureteral muscle cell is in a nonexcited or resting state, the electric potential difference across the cell membrane, transmembrane potential, is referred to as the resting membrane potential (RMP). The RMP is determined primarily by the distribution of potassium ions (K$^+$) across the cell membrane and by the permeability of the membrane to K$^+$ (Hendrickx et al., 1975). In the resting state, the K$^+$ concentration on the inside of the cell is greater than that on the outside of the cell, that is,

$$[K^+]_i > [K^+]_o,$$

and the membrane is preferentially permeable to K$^+$. Because of the tendency for the positively charged K$^+$ ions to diffuse from the inside of the cell, where they are more concentrated, to the outside of the cell, where they are less concentrated, an electric gradient is created, with the inside of the cell membrane more negative than the outside (Fig. 85.2A). The electric gradient that is formed tends to oppose the further movement of K$^+$ outward across the cell membrane along its concentration gradient, and an equilibrium is reached.

If the membrane in the resting state were exclusively permeable to K$^+$, the measured RMP of the ureteral smooth muscle cell would approximate −90 mV, the K$^+$ equilibrium potential, as predicted by the Nernst equation:

$$E_k = -RT/nF \ln[K^+]_i/[K^+]_o$$

where E_k is the potential difference attributable to the concentration difference of K$^+$ across the cell membrane, R is the molar gas constant, T is the absolute temperature, n is the number of mols of K$^+$, and F is the faraday (Nernst, 1908). However, **in the ureter and in other smooth muscles, the RMP is considerably less than the K$^+$ equilibrium potential, with values of −33 to −70 mV, the inside of the cell being negative with respect to the outside** (Kuriyama et al., 1967). Studies from single isolated ureteral cells show spontaneous transient hyperpolarizations with the RMP transiently becoming more negative (Imaizumi et al., 1989). This phenomenon appears to be due to spontaneous release of Ca^{2+} from the sarcoplasmic reticulum with activation of tetraethylammonium (TEA) and charybdotoxin sensitive Ca^{2+}-dependent K$^+$ channels (I$_{K[Ca]}$). Although the low resting potential of ureteral cells may be explained in part by a relatively small resting K$^+$ conductance (Imaizumi et al., 1989), it also may be due to the contribution of other ions.

One such ion that could account for the relatively low RMP of the ureter and other smooth muscles is the sodium ion (Na$^+$) (Kuriyama, 1963). In the resting state, the Na$^+$ concentration on the outside of the cell membrane is greater than that on the inside, that is, [Na$^+$]$_o$ > [Na$^+$]$_i$. If the resting membrane were somewhat permeable to Na$^+$, the concentration and the electric gradient would support an inward movement of Na$^+$ across the cell membrane, with a resultant decrease in the electronegativity of the inner surface of the cell membrane (see Fig. 85.2B).

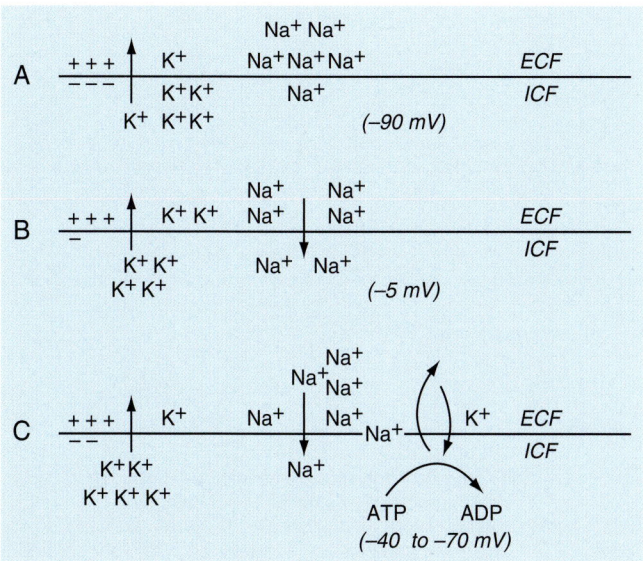

Fig. 85.2. Ionic basis for the resting membrane potential (RMP) in smooth muscle. In the resting state, the K^+ concentration inside the cell is greater than the K^+ concentration outside the cell, and the Na^+ concentration outside the cell is greater than the Na^+ concentration inside the cell. (A) Electrochemical changes that would occur if the membrane were solely permeable to potassium. Potassium would diffuse from the inside of the cell, where it is more concentrated, to the outside of the cell, where it is less concentrated. The outward movement of the positively charged K^+ ions would make the inside of the cell membrane negative with respect to the outside of the cell membrane. (B) Electrochemical changes that would occur if the resting membrane were also permeable to sodium. An inward movement of Na^+ along its concentration gradient would make the inside of the cell membrane less negative with respect to the outside of the cell membrane than is depicted in A. (C) Pump mechanism for extruding Na^+ from within the cell against concentration and electrochemical gradients. Inward movement of K^+ is coupled with outward movement of Na^+. This mechanism helps to maintain a steady state of ion distribution across the cell membrane and a stable RMP. *ADP*, Adenoside disphosphate; *ATP*, adenosine triphosphate; *ECF*, extracellular fluid; *ICF*, intracellular fluid. (A to C, From Weiss RM: Ureteral function. *Urology* 12:114, 1978.)

If such an inward movement of Na^+ went unchecked, the RMP would be expected to decrease to a level lower than that actually observed, and the concentration gradient for Na^+ may become reversed. To maintain a steady-state ion distribution across the cell membrane with $[K^+]_o < [K^+]_i$ and $[Na^+]_o > [Na^+]_i$ and to prevent the transmembrane potential from becoming lower than the measured ureteral RMP, an active mechanism capable of extruding Na^+ from within the cell against a concentration and electrochemical gradient is required (see Fig. 85.2C). Such an outward Na^+ pump that is coupled with an inward movement of K^+ derives its energy requirements from the dephosphorylation of adenosine triphosphate (ATP) (Casteels, 1970). Na^+-Ca^{2+} exchange also may play a role in Na^+ extrusion, especially when the Na^+ pump is inhibited (Aickin, 1987; Aickin et al., 1987; Lamont et al., 1998).

The dynamic processes illustrated in Fig. 85.2 enable the ureter in its resting state to maintain a relatively low RMP. In addition to the mechanisms described, the distribution of chloride ions (Cl^-) across the cell membrane and the relative permeability of the membrane to Cl^- may affect the maintenance of the RMP in the ureter and other smooth muscles (Kuriyama, 1963; Washizu, 1966). Activation of Ca^{2+}-activated Cl^- channels (ClCa) also can decrease the membrane potential and therefore depolarizes the membrane (Verkman and Galietta, 2009).

Action Potential

The transmembrane potential of an inactive or resting ureteral cell remains stable until it is excited by an external stimulus (electric, mechanical, or chemical) or by conduction of electric activity (action potential) from an already excited adjacent cell. **When a ureteral cell is stimulated, depolarization occurs, with the inside of the cell membrane becoming less negative than it was before stimulation. If a sufficient area of the cell membrane is depolarized rapidly enough to reach a critical level of transmembrane potential, referred to as the threshold potential, a regenerative depolarization, or action potential, is initiated.**

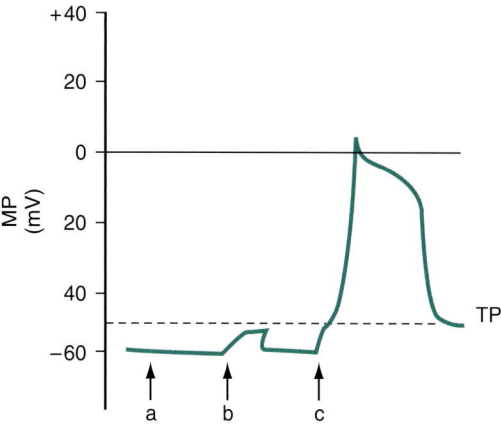

Fig. 85.3. Response of ureteral transmembrane potential to stimuli. At *arrow a*, a weak stimulus is applied that does not alter the resting membrane potential (*MP*). At *arrow b*, a stimulus is applied that decreases the transmembrane potential but not to the level of the threshold potential (*TP*) (subthreshold stimulus). At *arrow c*, a stimulus is applied that decreases the transmembrane potential to TP, and an action potential is initiated (suprathreshold stimulus). (From Weiss RM: Ureteral function. *Urology* 12:114, 1978.)

The changes that occur are diagrammatically depicted in Fig. 85.3. If a stimulus is very weak, as shown by *arrow a*, the transmembrane potential may remain unchanged. A slightly stronger, yet subthreshold, stimulus may result in an abortive displacement of the transmembrane potential, but not to such a degree that an action potential is generated (*arrow b*). If the stimulus is strong enough to decrease the transmembrane potential to the threshold potential, the cell becomes excited and produces an action potential (*arrow c*). The **action potential, which is the primary event in the conduction of the peristaltic impulse**, has the capability to act as the stimulus for excitation of adjacent quiescent cells and, through a complicated chain of events, **gives rise to the ureteral contraction.**

When the ureteral cell is excited, its membrane loses its preferential permeability to K^+ and becomes more permeable to Ca^{2+} ions that move inward across the cell membrane primarily through fast L-type Ca^{2+} channels and gives rise to the upstroke of the action potential (Fig. 85.4A) (Imaizumi et al., 1989; Kobayashi, 1965; Kuriyama and Tomita, 1970; Lang, 1989, 1990; Smith et al., 2002; Sui and Kao, 1997a, 1997b). L-type Ca^{2+} channels are inhibited by the calcium channel blocker nifedipine, and by cadmium (Cd^{2+}), and are potentiated by barium (Ba^{2+}). As the positively charged Ca^{2+} ions move inward across the cell membrane, the inside of the membrane becomes less negative with respect to the outside and may even become positive at the peak of the action potential, a state referred to as overshoot. Na^+ ions also may play a role in the upstroke of the ureteral action potential (Kobayashi, 1964, 1965; Muraki et al., 1991). The rate of rise of the upstroke of the ureteral action potential is relatively slow, 1.2 ± 0.06 V/sec in the cat (Kobayashi, 1969). This compares with a 610-V/sec rate of rise in dog cardiac Purkinje fibers (Draper and Weidmann, 1951) and a 740-V/sec rate of rise in skeletal muscle (Ferroni and Blanchi, 1965). The slow rate of upstroke rise of the ureteral action potential accounts for the slow conduction velocity in the ureter.

After reaching the peak of its action potential, the ureter **maintains its potential for a period of time (plateau of the action potential) before the transmembrane potential returns to its resting level (repolarization)** (Kuriyama et al., 1967). The plateau phase

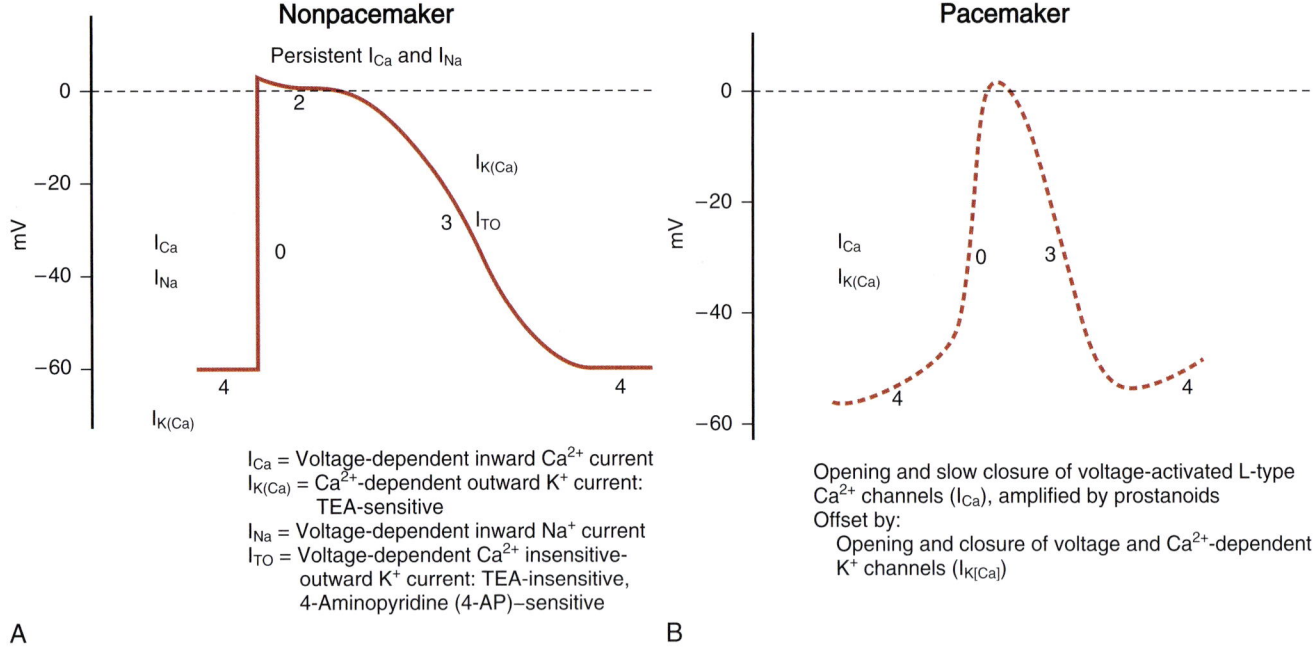

Fig. 85.4. Schematic representation of ionic currents in (A) nonpacemaker *(solid line)* and (B) pacemaker *(dashed line)* action potentials: (0) upstroke or depolarization phase; (2) plateau phase; (3) repolarization phase; and (4) resting potential of the nonpacemaker cell and spontaneous depolarization phase of the pacemaker cell. A spontaneous decrease in the transmembrane potential of pacemaker cells accounts for their spontaneous activity. (*TEA*, Tetraethyl ammonium.)

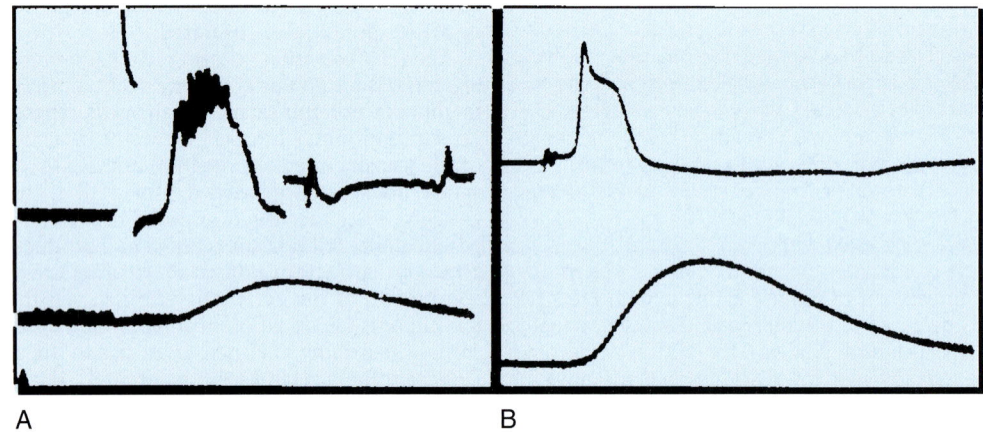

Fig. 85.5. Intracellular recordings of ureteral action potentials (upper tracings) and isometric recordings of contractions (lower tracings) in response to electrical stimuli. Action potentials precede contractions. (A) Guinea pig ureter; oscillations on the plateau of the action potential. (B) Cat ureter; no oscillations on the plateau of the action potential. (A and B, From Weiss RM: Ureteral function. *Urology* 12:114, 1978.)

of the guinea pig action potential is superimposed with multiple oscillations, a phenomenon not observed in the rat, rabbit, or cat (Figs. 85.5A and B; Bozler, 1938). The plateau phase appears to depend on the persistence of an inward Ca^{2+} current and on Na^+ influx through a voltage-dependent Na^+ channel (see Fig. 85.4A; Imaizumi et al., 1989; Kuriyama and Tomita, 1970; Sui and Kao, 1997b). Also involved in the plateau formation is the maintenance of depolarization by an inward calcium-dependent chloride current ($I_{Cl[Ca]}$), which is countered by outward voltage-gated and Ca^{2+}-activated K^+ currents (K_{Ca}) (Smith et al., 2002). There are species differences in the ionic currents involved in the formation of the action potential with the Ca^{2+} activated chloride current present in the rat but not in the guinea pig ureter. The inward Cl^- current can be inhibited by niflumic acid and by Ba^{2+} (Smith et al., 2002). The oscillations on the plateau of the guinea pig action potential appear to depend on the repetitive activation of an inward Ca^{2+} current (Kuriyama and Tomita, 1970) and of a Ca^{2+}-dependent outward K^+ current (Imaizumi et al., 1989). Prolongation of the inward calcium current and the duration of the action potential correlate with an increase force of contraction (Burdyga and Wray, 1999b).

The activation of a Ca^{2+}-dependent K^+ current that is involved in repolarization is mainly due to Ca^{2+} release from the endoplasmic reticulum that is triggered by the influx of extracellular Ca^{2+} through voltage-dependent Ca^{2+} channels. The increase in intracellular Ca^{2+} concentration during the upstroke and plateau of the action potential finally may activate the outward Ca^{2+}-dependent K^+ current ($I_{K[Ca]}$) to such a degree that repolarization occurs with return of the transmembrane potential to its resting level (see Fig. 85.4A; Imaizumi et al., 1989; Sui and Kao, 1997c). The $I_{K(Ca)}$ is sensitive to inhibition by TEA. TEA increases the amplitude and duration of in vitro ureteral contractions (Floyd et al., 2008). A voltage-dependent, Ca^{2+}-insensitive outward K$^+$ current (I$_{TO}$) also appears to be involved in the repolarization (Imaizumi et al., 1990; Lang, 1989). These currents are TEA insensitive and 4-aminopyridine (4-AP) sensitive. In the rat but not the guinea pig ureter there is a late TEA, Cd^{2+}, and Ca^{2+}-insensitive outward K$^+$ current, which also is involved in the repolarization process. The duration of the action potential in the cat ranges from 259 to 405 msec (Kobayashi and Irisawa, 1964).

KEY POINTS

- The RMP of the ureteral cell is approximately −33 to −70 mV and is determined primarily by the distribution of K$^+$ ions across the cell membrane and the relatively selective permeability of the resting cell membrane to K$^+$.
- When excited by a suprathreshold stimulus, the membrane becomes less permeable to K$^+$ and more permeable to Ca^{2+}, which moves inward across the cell membrane and provides the ionic mechanism for the development of the upstroke of the action potential.
- After reaching the peak of its action potential, the membrane maintains a depolarized state—plateau of the action potential—for a period of time before the membrane potential of the activated cell returns to its resting level (repolarization).
- The plateau appears to be related to a persisting inward Ca^{2+} current and to an influx of Na$^+$. Repolarization of the membrane is related to a renewed increase in permeability to K$^+$.

Pacemaker Potentials and Pacemaker Activity

Electric activity arises in a cell either spontaneously or in response to an external stimulus. If the activity arises spontaneously, the cell is referred to as a pacemaker cell. Pacemaker cells differ from nonpacemaker cells in that their transmembrane resting potential is lower (less negative) than that of nonpacemaker cells (Lang and Zhang, 1996) and does not remain constant but rather undergoes a slow spontaneous depolarization (see Fig. 85.4B). If the spontaneously changing membrane potential reaches the threshold potential, the upstroke of an action potential occurs. The **ionic conduction underlying pacemaker activity in the upper urinary tract is due to the opening and slow closure of voltage-activated L-type Ca^{2+} channels** (Santicioli et al., 1995a). This is opposed by the opening and closure of voltage and Ca^{2+}-dependent K$^+$ channels. It has been suggested that prostaglandins and excitatory tachykinins, released from sensory nerves, help maintain autorhythmicity in the upper urinary tract through maintenance of Ca^{++} mobilization (Lang et al., 2002a; Nguyen et al., 2016). **Tetrodotoxin and blockers of the autonomic nervous system, parasympathetic and sympathetic, have little effect on peristalsis, suggesting that autonomic neurotransmitters have little role in maintaining pyeloureteral motility** (Lang et al., 2001; 2002b). Changes in the frequency of action potential development may result from a change in the level of the threshold potential, a change in the rate of slow spontaneous depolarization of the resting potential, or a change in the level of the resting potential.

Bozler (1942), using small extracellular surface electrodes, demonstrated the characteristic slow spontaneous depolarization of pacemaker-type fibers in the proximal portion of the isolated ureter of a unicalyceal upper collecting system. In a multicalyceal kidney, Morita et al. (1981), using extracellular electrodes, recorded low-voltage potentials that appeared to be pacemaker potentials from the border of the pig minor calyces and the major calyx with the contraction rhythm varying between each calyx. Multiple pacemakers fire simultaneously as coupled oscillators or individually as pacemaker activity shifts from one site to another along the renal pelvis of the unicalyceal kidney or the pelvicalyceal border of the multicalyceal pig and sheep kidney (Constantinou and Yamaguchi, 1981; Constantinou et al., 1977; Golenhofen and Hannappel, 1973; Lammers et al., 1996).

Gosling and Dixon (1971, 1974) provided morphologic evidence of specialized pacemaker tissue in the proximal portion of the urinary collecting system and described species differences. **In species with a multicalyceal system, such as the pig, sheep, and human, the "pacemaker cells" are located near the pelvicalyceal border** (Dixon and Gosling, 1973). In species with an unicalyceal system, such as the dog, cat, rat, rabbit, and guinea pig, the "pacemaker cells" extend from the pelvicalyceal border to the UPJ. These **atypical smooth muscle cells that give rise to pacemaker activity**, in contrast to typical smooth muscle cells, have less than 40% of their cellular area occupied by contractile elements and demonstrate sparse immunoreactivity for smooth muscle and actin (Klemm et al., 1999; Lang et al., 2001). These atypical smooth muscle spindle-shaped cells are 90 to 230 µm in length, and their electrical activity consists of simple waveforms of alternating depolarizing and repolarizing phases that occur at a relatively rapid frequency of 8 to 15/min (Fig. 85.6A; Klemm et al., 1999; Tsuchida and Suzuki, 1992). Pacemaker potentials have a lower resting membrane potential (RMP), a slower rate of rise, and a lower amplitude than action potentials recorded from nonpacemaker cells. In the guinea pig these atypical, presumably pacemaker cells make up more than 80% of the cells at the pelvicalyceal junction, about 15% of the cells in the proximal renal pelvis, but are not present in the distal renal pelvis or ureter (Klemm et al., 1999). Electrical recordings correlate with histologic findings in that pacemaker potentials were not observed in the distal renal pelvis or ureter (Klemm et al., 1999).

Driven action potentials that fire at lower frequency (3–5/min) than pacemaker potentials are recorded from longer (150–400 µm) spindle-shaped typical smooth muscle cells (Fig. 85.6B; Klemm et al., 1999). Most muscle cells of the ureter (100%), distal renal pelvis (97.5%), and proximal renal pelvis (83%) are typical nonpacemaker smooth muscle cells with typical action potentials. Lang et al. (1998) described fibroblast-like cells resembling the interstitial cells of Cajal (ICCs), which serve as pacemaker cells in the intestine, in the proximal portion of the guinea pig renal pelvis. These "ICC-like" cells are irregular shaped with oval nuclei and many branching interconnecting processes and contain numerous mitochondria, caveolae, and prominent endoplastic reticulum. The "ICC-like" cells in the guinea pig are not immunoreactive for α-smooth muscle actin, which is present in typical smooth muscle cells, or for C-kit, a tyrosine kinase receptor that is expressed in intestinal ICC pacemaker cells (Klemm et al., 1999). The immunoreactivity to C-kit appears to be species specific as "ICC-like" cells that are immunoreactive to antibodies raised against the C-kit proto-oncogene are present in the upper urinary tract of a number of mammals (Lang and Klemm, 2005; Metzger et al., 2005). Electrical recordings from these cells demonstrate action potentials with properties intermediate to pacemaker and driven action potentials. Intermediate action potentials in the guinea pig have a single spike, a plateau without the superimposed spikes seen in driven action potentials, and a rapid repolarization phase (Fig. 85.6C). Intermediate action potentials are noted in 11% to 17% of cells at the pelvicalyceal junction and the proximal and distal renal pelvis (Lang et al., 2001). These **"ICC-like" cells (telocytes) in the upper urinary tract do not appear to be primary pacemaker cells but rather may provide for preferential conduction of electrical signals from pacemaker cells to typical smooth muscle cells** of the renal pelvis and ureter (Klemm et al., 1999). In the mouse ureteropelvic junction c-KIT–positive "ICC-like" cells have been identified that show high-frequency spontaneous transient inward currents that often occur in bursts and sum to produce long-lasting large inward currents (Lang et al., 2007b). **It is postulated that in the absence of a proximal pacemaker that these "ICC-like" cells could act as pacemaker cells and trigger contractions in adjacent smooth muscle cells in the ureteropelvic junction. Thus atypical smooth muscle cells and "ICC-like" cells may play a pacemaker role in the initiation and propagation of pyeloureteric peristalsis** (Lang et al., 2006, 2007a).

c-KIT is a tyrosine kinase receptor that promotes cell migration and proliferation of melanoblasts, hematopoietic progenitors, and

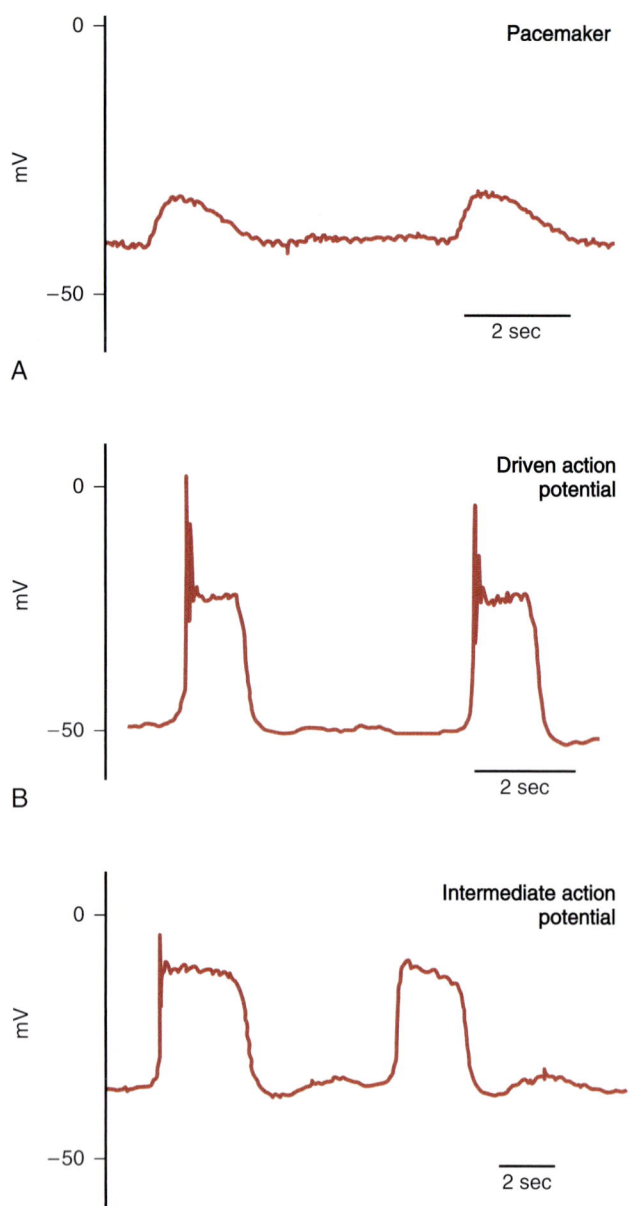

Fig. 85.6. Action potentials in the upper urinary tract of the guinea pig. (A) Pacemaker potentials. (B) Driven action potentials, which fire at a lower frequency than pacemaker potentials, recorded from longer spindle-shaped typical smooth muscle cells. (C) Intermediate action potentials, from "ICC-like cells," have a single spike, a plateau, and a rapid depolarization phase. (Modified with permission from Klemm MF, Exintaris B, Lang RJ: Identification of the cells underlying pacemaker activity in the guinea pig upper urinary tract. *J Physiol (Lond)* 519:867, 1999.)

et al., 2005). Incubation of isolated cultured embryonic murine ureters with antibodies that neutralize c-KIT activity altered ureteral morphology and inhibited unidirectional peristalsis. These data suggest that c-KIT–containing cells, which are most probably "ICC-like" cells, have an important role in pyeloureteric peristalsis. c-KIT–positive cells have been identified in the human ureter (Metzger et al., 2004; van der Aa et al., 2004) and in the human UPJ (Solari et al., 2003). In the presence of obstruction, c-KIT–positive ICC-like cells at the UPJ have been reported decreased (Solari et al., 2003; Yang et al., 2009) or increased (Koleda et al., 2012).

More recently, **hyperpolarization-activated cation-3 channels (HCN3)** were shown to be expressed at the pelvis-kidney junction and to play a role in the development of pacemaker activity. Uncoordinated peristalsis was demonstrated in renal pelvis-ureter explants that were treated with an HCN3 channel blocker (Hurtado et al., 2010). Furthermore, it has been shown that hedgehog signaling controls KIT and HCN3 expression and that the hedgehog signaling pathway is required for the development of pacemaker function and coordinated peristalsis in the mouse ureter (Cain et al., 2011). Inhibition of either c-KIT or HCN3 results in impaired ureteral peristaltic activity, suggesting that both are required for normal ureteral function.

Although the primary pacemaker for ureteral peristalsis is located in the proximal portion of the collecting system, other areas of the ureter may act as **latent pacemakers.** Under normal conditions, the latent pacemaker regions are dominated by activity arising at the primary pacemaker sites. When the latent pacemaker site is freed of its domination by the primary pacemaker, it, in turn, may act as a pacemaker. To demonstrate latent pacemaker sites, Shiratori and Kinoshita (1961) transected the in vivo dog ureter at various levels. Before transection, peristaltic activity arose proximally from the primary pacemaker. When the ureter was transected at the UPJ, antiperistaltic waves of lower frequency than the previous normoperistaltic waves originated from the UVJ. Division of the ureter at the UVJ did not affect the normoperistaltic waves. After division of the midureter, the normoperistaltic waves in the upper segment remained unchanged, and the lower segment demonstrated antiperistaltic waves, which originated at the UVJ at a frequency less than that of the normoperistaltic waves in the upper segment. Thus cells at the UVJ of the dog may act as pacemaker cells when freed of control from the primary proximally located pacemaker. Latent pacemaker cells are present throughout the ureter (Imaizumi et al., 1989; Meini et al., 1995).

Propagation of Electric Activity

Excitable cells possess resistive and capacitative membrane properties similar to those of a cable or core conductor. The transverse resistance of the membrane is higher than the longitudinal resistance of the extracellular or intracellular fluid; this allows current resulting from a stimulus to propagate along the length of the fibers. The spread of current is referred to as *electrotonic spread* (Hoffman and Cranefield, 1960). The space constant (λ) determines the degree to which the electrotonic potential dissipates with increasing distance from an applied voltage. In a cable, this relation is expressed by

$$P = P_o e^{-X/\lambda}$$

where X is the distance from the applied voltage, P is the displacement of the membrane potential at X, P_o is the displacement of the membrane potential at the site of the applied voltage, e is the base of the natural logarithm, and λ is the space constant. Thus the electrotonic potential decreases by 1/e in 1 space constant. The space constant of the guinea pig ureter measured by extracellular stimulation is 2.5 to 3 mm (Kuriyama et al., 1967).

The time constant τ_m is expressed by

$$\tau_m = RC$$

where R is the membrane resistance and C is the membrane capacity. The time constant τ_m signifies that a small displacement of potential

primordial germ cells. Mice expressing mutant inactivating c-KIT alleles lack intestinal ICCs and have abnormal intestinal peristalsis and develop bowel obstruction, showing that **c-KIT is important in the development of pacemaker activity and peristalsis of the gut** (Der-Silaphet et al., 1998). Pezzone et al. (2003) identified c-KIT–positive cells in the mouse ureter. They suggested that the difference from previous studies in the guinea pig upper urinary tract in which c-KIT positivity was not identified in ICC-like cells (Klemm et al., 1999) may be due to species differences, the c-KIT antibody used, and/or the fixation methods. **c-KIT expression** was noted to be **upregulated in the embryonic murine ureter before its development of unidirectional peristaltic contractions** (David is decreased by $1/e$ of its value in 1 τ_m. The time constant of the guinea pig ureter measured by extracellular stimulation is 200 to 300 msec (Kuriyama et al., 1967).

The ureter acts as a **functional syncytium**. Engelmann (1869, 1870) showed that stimulation of the ureter produces a contraction wave that propagates proximally and distally from the site of stimulation. Under normal conditions, **electric activity** arises proximally and is **conducted distally from one muscle cell to another across areas of close cellular apposition referred to as intermediate junctions** (Libertino and Weiss, 1972; Uehara and Burnstock, 1970). The similarity of these close cellular contacts to nexuses, which have been shown to be low-resistance pathways for cell-to-cell conduction in other smooth muscles (Barr et al., 1968), suggests that a similar mechanism for conduction may be present in the ureter. **Gap junctions consisting of groups of channels in the plasma membrane of adjacent smooth muscle cells enable exchange of ions and small molecules and play a role in electrical coupling between adjacent cells and in electromechanical coupling** (Gabella, 1994; Santicioli and Maggi, 2000). 18β-Glycyrrhetinic acid, a gap junction inhibitor, inhibits cell-to-cell electrical coupling in guinea pig renal pelvis and ureter and dissociates electrical and mechanical events (Santicioli and Maggi, 2000). **Conduction velocity in the ureter is 2 to 6 cm/sec** (Kobayashi, 1964; Kuriyama et al., 1967); it has been shown to vary with temperature, the time interval between stimuli (van Mastrigt et al., 1986), and with the pressure within the ureter (Tsuchiya and Takei, 1990). This is in comparison with conduction velocities ranging from 1.5 to 2 m/sec in cardiac Purkinje fibers (Rosen et al., 1981), and myelinated nerves can conduct at speeds up to 150 m/sec. Conduction in the ureter is similar to that in cardiac tissue, even to the extent that the Wenckebach phenomenon (a partial conduction block) has been demonstrated in the ureter as it has been in specialized cardiac fibers (Weiss et al., 1968).

CONTRACTILE ACTIVITY

The contractile event depends on the concentration of free sarcoplasmic Ca^{2+} in the region of the contractile proteins, actin and myosin. Any process that results in a significant increase in Ca^{2+} in the region of the contractile proteins favors the development of a contraction; any process that results in a significant decrease in Ca^{2+} in the region of the contractile proteins favors relaxation (Fig. 85.7).

Contractile Proteins

In skeletal muscle, Ca^{2+} appears to act as a derepressor. It is thought that in the relaxed state, a regulator system, consisting of the proteins troponin and tropomyosin, prevents the interaction of actin and myosin. In the relaxed state, the troponin that is attached to the tropomyosin is inactive, and the tropomyosin prevents the interaction between actin and myosin. With activation, there is an increase in the sarcoplasmic Ca^{2+} concentration. The Ca^{2+} binds to the troponin, producing a conformational change that results in the displacement of tropomyosin, thus allowing interaction of actin and myosin and the development of a contraction.

In smooth muscle, on the other hand, Ca^{2+} appears to act as an activator. The most widely accepted theory suggests that **phosphorylation of myosin is involved in the contractile process** and that a troponin-like system does not constitute the primary regulatory mechanism, as it does in skeletal and cardiac muscle. **With excitation, there is a transient increase in the sarcoplasmic Ca^{2+} concentration** from its steady-state concentration of 10^{-8} to 10^{-7} M to a concentration of 10^{-6} M or higher. At this higher concentration, Ca^{2+} **forms an active complex with the Ca^{2+}-binding protein calmodulin** (Cho et al., 1988; Watterson et al., 1976). Calmodulin without Ca^{2+} is inactive (Fig. 85.8). **The Ca^{2+}-calmodulin complex activates a calmodulin-dependent enzyme, myosin light-chain kinase** (see Fig. 85.8). **The activated myosin light-chain kinase**, in turn, **catalyzes the phosphorylation of the 20,000-dalton light chain of myosin** (Fig. 85.9). **Phosphorylation of the myosin light chain allows actin

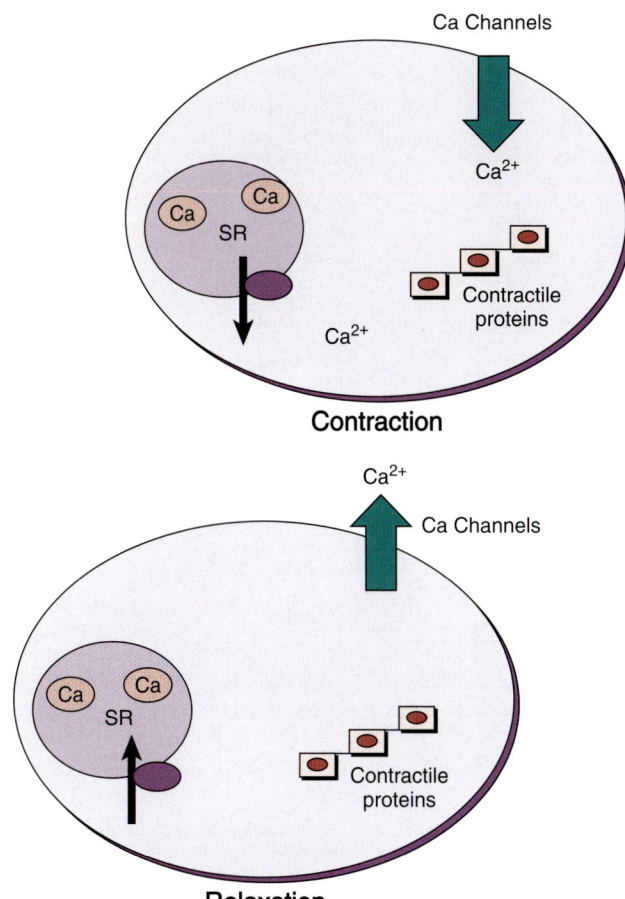

Fig. 85.7. Schematic representation of calcium ion movements during contraction and relaxation. *SR*, Sarcoplasmic reticulum.

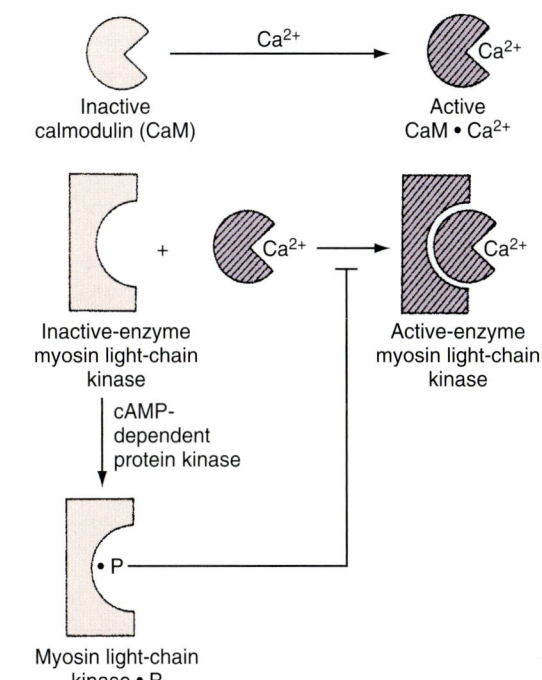

Fig. 85.8. Schematic representation of the contractile process in smooth muscle. Calmodulin is activated by Ca^{2+}. The activated calcium-calmodulin complex activates the enzyme myosin light-chain kinase, which phosphorylates the light chain of myosin. Phosphorylation of myosin light-chain kinase decreases the rate of activation of the enzyme by the Ca^{2+}-calmodulin complex.

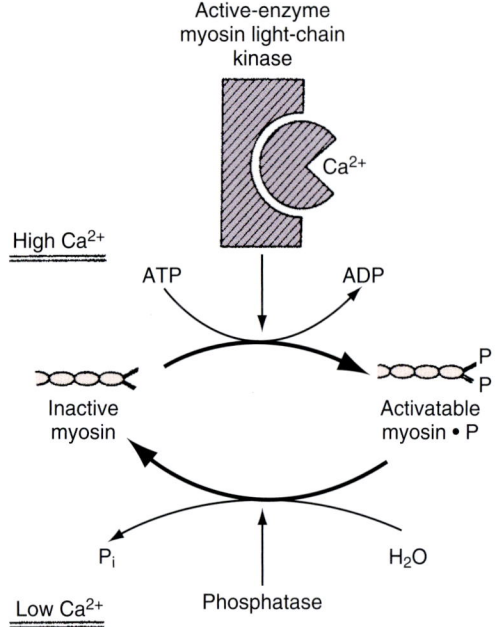

Fig. 85.9. Schematic representation of the contractile process in smooth muscle. The activated enzyme myosin light-chain kinase catalyzes the phosphorylation of myosin. Myosin must be phosphorylated for actin to activate myosin ATPase.

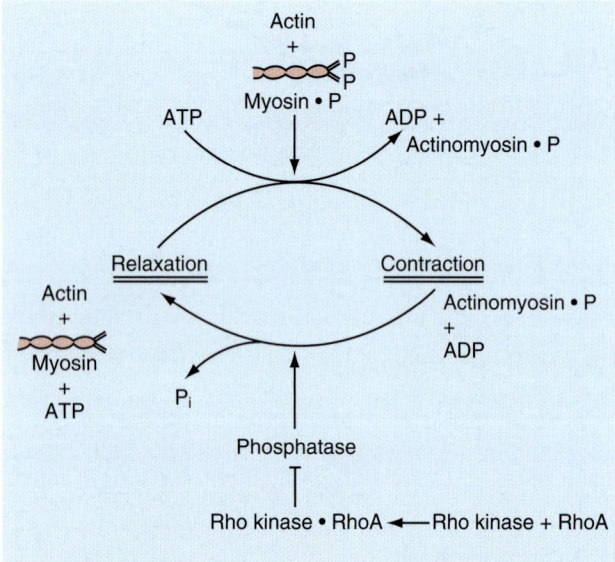

Fig. 85.10. Schematic representation of the contractile process in smooth muscle. Actin activates ATPase activity of phosphorylated myosin. This allows interaction of actin and myosin with the development of a contraction. A phosphatase dephosphorylates phosphorylated myosin to lead to relaxation. Rho kinase combines with RhoA to inhibit the phosphatase, leading to sustained contraction.

to activate myosin Mg^{2+}-ATPase activity, leading to hydrolysis of ATP and the development of smooth muscle tension or shortening (Fig. 85.10). Actin cannot activate the ATPase activity of the dephosphorylated myosin light chain.

When the Ca^{2+} concentration in the region of the contractile proteins is low, the myosin light-chain kinase is not active, because calmodulin requires Ca^{2+} to activate the enzyme. This prevents activation of the contractile apparatus, because the myosin light chain cannot be phosphorylated, a process that must precede tension development. Furthermore, a phosphatase dephosphorylates the myosin light chain, thus preventing actin activation of myosin ATPase activity, and relaxation results.

A Rho/Rho kinase signaling pathway affects contractility by altering the Ca^{2+}-sensitivity of the contractile system (Somlyo and Somlyo, 2003). The Rho-kinase pathway is involved in ureteral contractions in a number of species (Hong et al., 2005; Levent and Buyukafsar, 2004; Shabir et al., 2004). RhoA, a small GTP-binding protein, binds to Rho-kinase and causes its migration to the cell membrane, where it becomes maximally active (Ishizaki et al., 1996; Leung et al., 1995). Rho-kinase inhibits myosin phosphatase by phosphorylation of its regulatory subunit, MYPT1 (myosin targeting subunit of myosin light chain phosphatase), which prevents dephosphorylation of myosin light chain, which in turn leads to Ca^{2+} sensitization of the smooth muscle with subsequent increase in contractility (Borysova et al., 2011) (see Fig. 85.10). Y-27632, an inhibitor of Rho-kinase, decreases spontaneous and EFS-induced contractile responses of in vitro rat and human ureteral segments without causing changes in calcium (Hong et al., 2005; Shabir et al., 2004).

Evidence indicates that phosphorylation of the enzyme myosin light-chain kinase by a cyclic adenosine monophosphate (cAMP)-dependent protein kinase (see Fig. 85.8) decreases myosin light-chain kinase activity by decreasing the affinity of this enzyme for calmodulin (Adelstein et al., 1981).

Although Ca^{2+} is required for most smooth muscle contractile events, there is evidence that Ca^{2+}-independent contractions can occur (Yoshimura and Yamaguchi, 1997). Carbachol, a muscarinic cholinergic agonist, and phorbol ester, which activates protein kinase C (PKC), can induce contraction in Ca^{2+}-depleted bladder strips that can be inhibited by a PKC inhibitor, H7. It is suggested that activation of PKC coupled with agonist stimulation of the muscarinic receptor can induce a Ca^{2+}-independent contraction. Furthermore, activation of Rho-kinase affects smooth muscle contractility without causing changes in calcium.

Calcium and Excitation-Contraction Coupling

The mechanical event of ureteral peristalsis follows an electric event to which it is related. The Ca^{2+} involved in the ureteral contraction is derived from two main sources. Because smooth muscle cells have a very small diameter, the **inward movement of extracellular Ca^{2+} into the cell through L-type voltage-dependent Ca^{2+} channels during the upstroke of the action potential provides a significant source of sarcoplasmic Ca^{2+}** (Brading et al., 1983; Floyd et al., 2008; Hertle and Nawrath, 1989; Maggi and Giuliani, 1995; Maggi et al., 1994a; Yoshida et al., 1992; see Fig. 85.7). This inward movement of Ca^{2+} across the cell membrane is the major source of calcium used for contraction in most smooth muscles. Na^+-Ca^{2+} exchange, with an outward movement of Na^+ and an inward movement of Ca^{2+}, also plays a role in the ureteral contraction (Lamont et al., 1998). Furthermore, in response to an excitatory impulse, Ca^{2+} release from tightly bound storage sites (i.e., the endoplasmic or sarcoplasmic reticulum) also increases the Ca^{2+} concentration in the sarcoplasm (Burdyga and Wray, 1999a; Burdyga et al., 1998; Lang et al., 2002b). Calcium may be released from the sarcoplasmic reticulum (SR) of smooth muscle by an inositol trisphosphate (IP_3)–induced release mechanism or by Ca^{2+}-induced Ca^{2+} release (CICR) (Somlyo and Somlyo, 1994). These processes appear to be species dependent. CICR, which involves ryanodine receptors, appears to be the sole mechanism for calcium release from the SR in the guinea pig ureter, whereas the SR store in the rat ureter appears to be exclusively under the control of IP_3 receptors (Burdyga et al., 1995). IP_3 and ryanodine receptors are expressed in the human ureter (Floyd et al., 2008). The opening of caffeine-sensitive ryanodine receptors produces small local elevations of Ca^{2+} that are termed Ca^{2+} sparks (Nelson et al., 1995). In addition to providing a source of calcium for contraction, Ca^{2+} released from the SR activates Ca^{2+}-sensitive surface membrane channels and modulates membrane excitability (Carl et al., 1996; Imaizumi et al., 1989). Calcium-activated outward potassium currents (K_{Ca}) or STOCs (spontaneous transient outward currents) and calcium-activated inward chloride currents (Cl_{Ca}) or STICs (spontaneous transient inward currents) have been identified in smooth muscles.

These currents affect membrane potential and thus affect calcium entry through L-type Ca^{2+} channels in the membrane. The Ca^{2+}-activated chloride currents are present in rat but not guinea pig ureteral smooth muscle (Burdyga and Wray, 2002). Thus some Ca^{2+} released from SR results in contraction, but caffeine-induced release of SR Ca^{2+} in the form of Ca^{2+} sparks increases outward potassium currents (K_{Ca}) or STOCS with an inhibitory effect on action potentials and contractility (Borysova et al., 2007). At least in the guinea pig ureter this increase in the outward potassium current hyperpolarizes the membrane and determines the refractory period, which is important in determining the frequency of ureteral peristalsis (Burdyga and Wray, 2005).

Support for use of a dual source of Ca^{2+} in the ureter has been provided by Vereecken et al. (1975), who noted that it took approximately 45 minutes for spontaneous contractions of isolated guinea pig ureters to cease when the tissue was placed in a Ca^{2+}-free medium. They interpreted this to indicate that some of the Ca^{2+} involved in the contractile process is derived from tightly bound intracellular stores. They also noted that recovery of the contractile response to electric stimuli was almost immediate when the tissue was returned to a physiologic solution containing a normal concentration of Ca^{2+}. This suggests that free extracellular Ca^{2+} entering the cell during excitation also provides a source of Ca^{2+} for the contractile machinery. A similar conclusion was reached by Hong et al. (1985). There is, however, some evidence that Ca^{2+} release from the sarcoplasmic reticulum may not play a significant role in ureteral contractions, at least in the guinea pig (Maggi et al., 1994a, 1995, 1996), and some perturbations of contractility may be related to movements of ions other than Ca^{2+}. The increase in developed force in the guinea pig ureter with intracellular acidification and decrease with intracellular alkalinization appear to result from modulation of outward K^+ currents rather than effects on inward Ca^{2+} currents (Smith et al., 1998). That is, alkalinization (increasing intracellular pH) enhances outward K^+ currents, and this reduces excitability; acidification has the opposite effect. Relaxation results from a decrease in the concentration of free sarcoplasmic Ca^{2+} in the region of the contractile proteins. The decrease in sarcoplasmic Ca^{2+} can result from the uptake of Ca^{2+} into intracellular storage sites (Maggi et al., 1994a, 1995) or from extrusion of Ca^{2+} from the cell (Burdyga and Magura, 1988).

Urothelial Effects on Contractile Activity

Furchgott (1999) showed in blood vessels that the endothelium produced a factor that had a relaxing action on the smooth muscle layer of the blood vessel. This factor was originally termed endothelium-derived relaxing factor (EDRF) and was subsequently shown to be nitric oxide (NO). Mastrangelo et al. (2003) showed that the urothelium of rat ureter produced NO, which inhibited contractile responses of the rat ureter. It was shown that the urothelium inhibited spontaneous contractions of isolated rat ureteral segments and that removal of the urothelium potentiated the stimulatory effects of neurokinin A, vasopressin, carbachol, bradykinin and angiotensin II (Mastrangelo and Iselin, 2007). In intact ureteral segments cyclooxygenase inhibitors potentiated the stimulatory effects of neurokinin A, vasopressin, carbachol, bradykinin, and angiotensin II. Cyclooxygenase inhibitors had no effect on the responses to these agents in urothelium-free ureters. These data suggest that the inhibitory effects of the urothelium on ureteral contractile events may involve the participation of a urothelial cyclooxygenase product such as prostacyclin.

Second Messengers

The functional response to a number of hormones, neurotransmitters, and other agents is mediated by *second messengers*. The agonist, or first messenger, interacts with a specific membrane-bound receptor (Alquist, 1948; Furchgott, 1964); the agonist-receptor complex then activates or inactivates an enzyme that leads to alteration of an amount of a second messenger within the cell. These **second messengers include cAMP, cyclic guanosine monophosphate (GMP), Ca^{2+}, inositol 1,4,5-trisphosphate (IP_3), and diacylglycerol (DG).** They

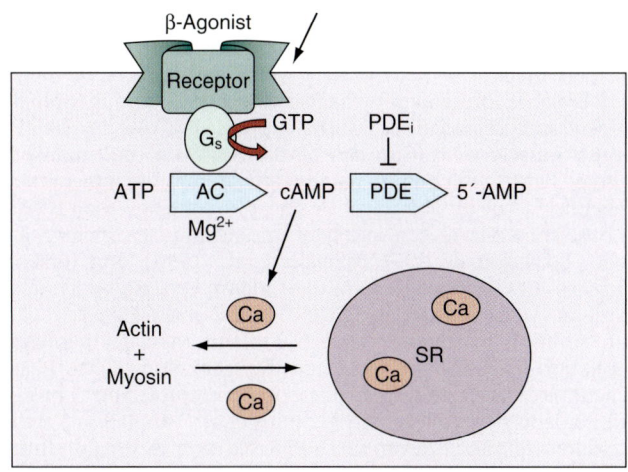

Fig. 85.11. Schematic representation of the role of cAMP in β-adrenergic agonist–induced relaxation of smooth muscle. Agonist combines with receptor on the outer side of the cell membrane. The receptor-agonist complex, in turn, via a stimulatory G-protein, G_s, activates the enzyme adenylyl cyclase (AC) on the inner surface of the cell membrane, which in the presence of Mg^{2+} GTP results in the conversion of ATP to cAMP. cAMP is postulated to cause an increased uptake of Ca^{2+} into intracellular storage sites with a resultant decrease in Ca^{2+} in the region of the contractile proteins that results in relaxation. cAMP may also have other actions (not shown) that inhibit the contractile process. The enzyme phosphodiesterase (PDE) degrades cAMP to 5′AMP and is inhibited by PDE inhibitors such as theophylline and papaverine. SR, Sarcoplasmic reticulum.

mediate the functional response to the agonist (first messenger) through a process that frequently involves protein phosphorylation.

cAMP mediates the relaxing effects of β-adrenergic agonists in a variety of smooth muscles (Andersson, 1972; Triner et al., 1971; Vesin and Harbon, 1974). According to this concept, a β-adrenergic agonist, such as isoproterenol, serves as the first messenger and combines with a receptor on the outer surface of the cell membrane (Fig. 85.11). Isoproterenol itself does not enter the cell. The β-adrenergic agonist-receptor complex activates the enzyme adenylyl cyclase on the inner surface of the cell membrane in close morphologic relation to the receptor. **In the presence of magnesium (Mg^{2+}) and a guanine nucleotide (GTP), adenylyl cyclase catalyzes the conversion of ATP to cAMP within the cell.**

A stimulatory guanine nucleotide–regulatory protein, or G protein (G_s), acts as a functional communication between the agonist-receptor complex and the catalytic or active unit of the enzyme adenylyl cyclase. cAMP acts as a second, or "internal," messenger of the response elicited by the β-adrenergic agonist. It has been suggested that the increase in cAMP through activation of an enzyme, that is, a protein kinase, and phosphorylation of proteins leads to the uptake of Ca^{2+} into intracellular storage sites (i.e., the endoplasmic or sarcoplasmic reticulum) with the resultant decrease of free sarcoplasmic Ca^{2+} in the region of the contractile proteins (Andersson and Nilsson, 1972). The decrease in sarcoplasmic Ca^{2+} in the region of the contractile proteins leads to relaxation of the smooth muscle. β-adrenoceptor induced relaxation of smooth muscle also may be due to the opening of Ca^{2+}-activated K^+ channels (Ferro, 2006; Uchida et al., 2005).

cAMP levels may be increased within the cell in two ways. One is by increasing synthesis, which involves activation of the enzyme adenylyl cyclase; the other is by decreasing degradation. **The degradation of cAMP involves activation of an enzyme, phosphodiesterase, thus agents that either increase adenylyl cyclase activity, such as the β-adrenergic agonist isoproterenol, or decrease phosphodiesterase activity, that is, phosphodiesterase inhibitors such as theophylline and papaverine, increase intracellular cAMP levels and cause smooth muscle relaxation** (see Fig. 85.11).

Weiss et al. (1977) demonstrated the presence of adenylyl cyclase and phosphodiesterase activities in the ureter. They showed in the ureter that isoproterenol stimulates adenylyl cyclase activity and theophylline inhibits phosphodiesterase activity. These two agents that relax ureteral smooth muscle would be expected to increase cAMP levels: isoproterenol by increasing synthesis and theophylline by decreasing degradation. Further support of **a role for cAMP in smooth muscle relaxation** can be derived from the finding that dibutyryl cAMP, which more readily diffuses into the intact cell and is less likely to be broken down by phosphodiesterase than is cAMP, has been shown to relax a variety of smooth muscles, including the ureter (Takago et al., 1971; Wheeler et al., 1990), and forskolin, which activates the catalytic subunit of adenylyl cyclase, which relaxes the ureter (Hernández et al., 2004; Wheeler et al., 1986).

In addition to receptors and G proteins that are involved in stimulation of adenylyl cyclase and the formation of cAMP, as in the actions of β-adrenergic agonists, other receptors and G proteins inhibit adenylyl cyclase activity (Londos et al., 1981). Some actions of α_2-adrenergic and muscarinic cholinergic agonists involve stimulation of these inhibitory G proteins (Gi) with subsequent inhibition of adenylyl cyclase activity.

Another cyclic nucleotide, **cGMP, also causes smooth muscle relaxation. cGMP is synthesized from GTP by the enzyme guanylyl cyclase and is degraded to 5'-GMP by a phosphodiesterase.** Phosphodiesterase activity that can degrade cAMP and cGMP has been demonstrated in the canine ureter, and various inhibitors can preferentially inhibit the breakdown of one or the other cyclic nucleotide (Stief et al., 1995; Weiss et al., 1981). Insulin has been shown to activate cAMP phosphodiesterase activity in the ureter (Weiss and Wheeler, 1988), and 8-bromo-cGMP has been shown to cause relaxation of a number of smooth muscles (Schultz et al., 1979), including the ureter (Cho et al., 1984). BAY 41-2272, a soluble guanylyl cyclase stimulator, has been shown to relax isolated human ureteral segments (Miyaoka et al., 2014).

NO stimulates soluble guanylyl cyclase activity and causes smooth muscle relaxation (Dokita et al., 1991, 1994). **Nitric oxide synthase (NOS) converts L-arginine to NO and L-citrulline in a reaction that requires nicotinamide adenosine dinucleotide phosphate (NADPH). There are three NOS isoforms. Neuronal NOS (nNOS) is present in neuronal tissues and is Ca^{2+} and NADPH dependent** (Bredt and Snyder, 1990). It is thought that with neuronal excitation, there is an increase in Ca^{2+} concentration within nerves that leads to the synthesis of NO from L-arginine. NO released from the nerve **activates the enzyme guanylyl cyclase in the smooth muscle cell with the resultant conversion of GTP to cGMP and thus smooth muscle relaxation** (Fig. 85.12). **Endothelial NOS (eNOS), is Ca^{2+} and NADPH dependent** (Sessa, 1994). Similar to neuronal NOS, eNOS produces small amounts of NO for prolonged periods of time. An **inducible NOS isoform (iNOS), is NADPH dependent but Ca^{2+} independent** and has been identified in ureteral smooth muscle (Smith et al., 1993). iNOS produces large amounts of NO for short periods of time.

NOS-containing nerves have been demonstrated in the human ureter (Goessl et al., 1995; Iselin et al., 1998; Stief et al., 1996), and NOS has been demonstrated in the pig UVJ (Hernández et al., 1995; Phillips et al., 1995) and in the upper ureter and calyces of pigs and humans (Iselin et al., 1998; 1999). NOS colocalizes with vasoactive polypeptide and NPY in nerves supplying the human ureter (Iselin et al., 1997; Smet et al., 1994). NOS localizes to parasympathetic and sensory nerves but not to adrenergic neurons. In primary cultures of rat ureteral cells NO production was detected in urothelial but not in smooth muscle cells (Mastrangelo et al., 2003). These cells contain eNOS and iNOS.

There is evidence that the NO pathway is involved in human ureteral relaxation (Iselin et al., 1997; Stief et al., 1996). The NO donor, SIN-1, relaxes human ureteral segments, an action that is inhibited by the **guanylyl cyclase inhibitor methylene blue.** NO donors also inhibit agonist-induced contractions of isolated pig calyceal and rat, pig, and human intravesical ureteral segments, actions that are associated with an increase in cGMP. Furthermore, NO has been shown to be involved in nonadrenergic, noncholinergic-induced relaxation of the pig UVJ (Hernández et al., 1995).

Some actions of **α_1-adrenergic and muscarinic cholinergic agonists** and a number of other hormones, neurotransmitters, and biologic substances are associated with an increase in intracellular Ca^{2+} and are related to changes in inositol lipid metabolism. These agonists **combine with a receptor on the cell membrane, and the agonist-receptor complex, via a process that involves a G protein, activates an enzyme, phospholipase C, that leads to the hydrolysis of polyphosphatidylinositol 4,5-bisphosphate (PIP$_2$) with the formation of two second messengers, IP$_3$ and DG** (Berridge, 1984; Fig. 85.13). IP$_3$ mobilizes Ca^{2+} from intracellular stores (i.e.,

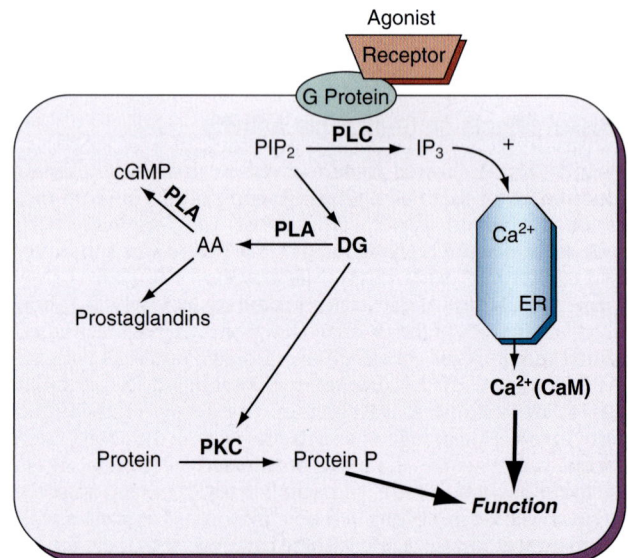

Fig. 85.13. Schematic representation of the role of inositol lipid metabolism in smooth muscle function. The agonist combines with the receptor on the outer side of the cell membrane. The receptor-agonist complex in turn activates the enzyme phospholipase C (*PLC*), which leads to the hydrolysis of polyphosphatidylinositol 4,5-bisphosphate (*PIP$_2$*), with the formation of two second messengers, inositol 1,4,5-trisphosphate (*IP$_3$*) and diacylglycerol (*DG*). The activation of PLC involves a G protein. IP$_3$ mobilizes calcium from intracellular stores (i.e., endoplasmic reticulum), and this leads to a functional response. DG binds to an enzyme, protein kinase C (*PKC*), which results in phosphorylation of proteins and a subsequent functional response. DG also activates PLA, and is a source of AA, the substrate for prostaglandin synthesis. AA then stimulates guanylyl cyclase (*GC*) activity to form cGMP. *AA*, Arachidonic acid; *ER*, endoplasmic reticulum; *PLA*, phospholipase A.

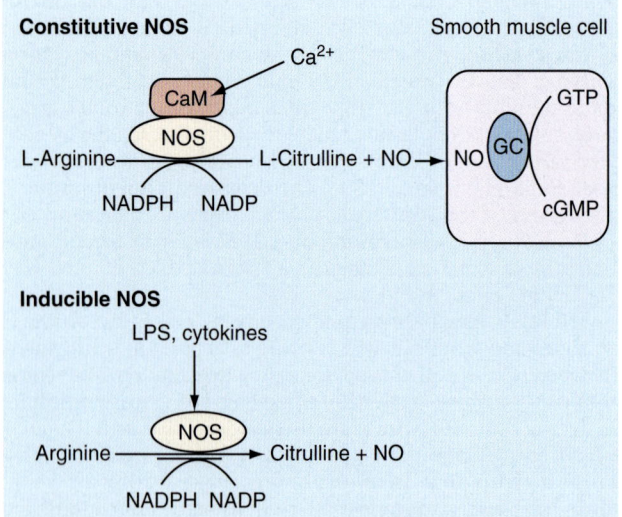

Fig. 85.12. Schematic representation of inducible and constitutive nitric oxide synthase (*NOS*). *CaM*, Calmodulin; *GC*; guanylyl cyclase; *LPS*, lipopolysaccharide.

endoplasmic or sarcoplasmic reticulum) with an initiation of a cascade of events through the calmodulin branch of the Ca^{2+} messenger system. In smooth muscles, **IP$_3$ is thought to be involved in brief contractile responses or in the initial phase of sustained responses** (Park and Rasmussen, 1985).

The other second messenger, **DG, binds to an enzyme, PKC,** translocates to the cell membrane, and, by reducing the concentration of Ca^{2+} required for PKC activation, results in an increase in this enzyme's activity. The **actions of PKC involve the phosphorylation of proteins** (Nishizuka, 1984; see Fig. 85.13). The **PKC branch of the Ca^{2+} messenger system is thought to be responsible for the sustained phase of the contractile response in smooth muscle** (Park and Rasmussen, 1985) and is responsive to hormonally induced changes in intracellular Ca^{2+}. PKC has been implicated in Ca^{2+}-independent smooth muscle contractions (Yoshimura and Yamaguchi, 1997). Numerous PKC isoforms have been identified. The functional activity and specificity of function of these isoforms appear to be determined primarily by the state of phosphorylation of the isoenzyme and its subcellular localization (Dempsey et al., 2000).

DG also activates the enzyme phospholipase A, which serves as a source of arachidonic acid, the substrate for prostaglandin synthesis (Mahadevappa and Holub, 1983). Arachidonic acid, in turn, may stimulate guanylyl cyclase activity with the subsequent formation of cGMP (Berridge, 1984) (see Fig. 85.13), and this would explain the Ca^{2+}-dependent increase in cGMP levels associated with muscarinic cholinergic and α$_1$-adrenergic agonist–induced contractions in smooth muscle. The observed increases in cGMP levels follow, rather than precede, the onset of contractions induced by these agonists.

Thus a group of second messengers are involved in the transduction of the signal that is initiated when an agonist combines with a specific receptor on the cell membrane of the smooth muscle. This process of **signal transduction** ultimately results in the functional response to the agonist.

ROLE OF THE NERVOUS SYSTEM IN URETERAL FUNCTION

Some smooth muscles have a specific innervation of each smooth muscle fiber, whereas other, syncytial-type smooth muscles lack discrete neuromuscular junctions and depend on a diffuse release of transmitter from a bundle of nerves with a subsequent spread of excitation from one muscle cell to another. **The ureter is a syncytial type of smooth muscle without discrete neuromuscular junctions** (Burnstock, 1970).

Because peristalsis may persist after transplantation (O'Conor and Dawson-Edwards, 1959) or denervation (Wharton, 1932), because spontaneous activity may occur in isolated in vitro ureteral segments (Finberg and Peart, 1970), and because normal antegrade peristalsis continues after reversal of a segment of ureter in situ (Melick et al., 1961), it is apparent that **ureteral peristalsis can occur without innervation.** However, analysis of the data in the literature clearly indicates that the **nervous system plays at least a modulating role in ureteral peristalsis, and nerves are present in the muscular layer and adventitia of the ureter, especially the distal ureter** (Vernez et al., 2017). Autonomic innervation does not appear to have a direct effect on peristalsis but may indirectly modulate peristalsis via activation of sensory nerve nicotinic receptors and the release of calcitonin gene-related peptide (CGRP) or via closure of K$_v$7 channels located on interstitial cells within the renal pelvis (Nguyen et al, 2013). Morita et al. (1987) have provided evidence that the autonomic nervous system may affect urine transport through the ureter by affecting peristaltic frequency and bolus volume. Catecholamine fluorescence and acetylcholine (ACh) release studies indicate that the human ureter is supplied by sympathetic (noradrenaline-containing) and parasympathetic (ACh-containing) neurons (Del Tacca, 1978; Duarte-Escalante et al., 1969).

Parasympathetic Nervous System

Although the role of the parasympathetic nervous system in the control of ureteral peristalsis has not been well defined, muscarinic cholinergic receptors have been demonstrated in the ureter of a number of species including the human (Hernández et al., 1993; Latifpour et al., 1989, 1990; Sakamoto et al., 2006). There are five cloned muscarinic subtypes: M$_1$ to M$_5$. The excitatory muscarinic receptors, M$_1$, M$_3$, and M$_5$, work through an excitatory G protein, Gq, and increase intracellular calcium by generating 1-, 4-, 5-trisphosphate (IP$_3$) and 1-, 2-DG. The inhibitory muscarinic receptors, M$_2$ and M$_4$, work through an inhibitory G protein, Gi, with inhibition of adenylyl cyclase (van Koppen and Kaiser, 2003; Wu et al., 2000). Carbachol induced contractile responses are primarily mediated via the M$_3$ receptor subtype (Tomiyama et al., 2003b). It has been suggested that M$_2$ receptor activation may inhibit smooth muscle relaxation that results from activation of adenylyl cyclase (Hegde et al., 1997). There is a higher density of M$_2$ than M$_3$ muscarinic receptors in the human ureter (Sakamoto et al., 2006).

Acetylcholinesterase-positive nerve fibers have been demonstrated in the equine ureter (Prieto et al., 1994). The cholinergic innervation is especially rich in the distal and intravesical ureter (Hernández et al., 1993). Furthermore, ACh has been shown to be released from isolated guinea pig, rabbit, and human ureters in response to electric field stimulation (Del Tacca, 1978), and this release is inhibited by the neural poison tetrodotoxin. These data suggest, but do not prove, that the parasympathetic nervous system has at least a modulatory role in the control of ureteral activity.

The prototypic cholinergic agonist is ACh, which serves as the neurotransmitter at (1) neuromuscular junctions of somatic motor nerves (nicotinic sites); (2) preganglionic parasympathetic and sympathetic neuroeffector junctions (nicotinic sites); and (3) postganglionic parasympathetic neuroeffector sites (muscarinic sites). ACh synthesis involves

$$\text{Acetyl CoA} + \text{Choline} \xrightarrow{\text{choline acetyltransferase}} \text{ACh}$$

where CoA is coenzyme A. The ACh is stored in vesicles within the synaptic terminal; its release depends on the influx of Ca^{2+} into the terminal, which presumably causes vesicle fusion with the presynaptic terminal membrane, thereby expelling ACh into the synaptic cleft. ACh subsequently is hydrolyzed by acetylcholinesterase. The muscarinic effects of cholinergic agonists can be blocked by atropine. The effects of nicotinic agonists can be blocked by nondepolarizing ganglionic blocking agents or by high concentrations of the nicotinic agonist, which may cause ganglionic blockade by desensitization of receptor sites after an initial period of ganglionic stimulation.

Cholinergic agonists, including ACh, methacholine (Provocholine), carbamylcholine (carbachol), and bethanechol (Urecholine), in general have been observed to have an excitatory effect on ureteral and renal pelvic function; that is, they increase the frequency and force of contractions (Hernández et al., 1993; Longrigg, 1974; Maggi and Giuliani, 1992; Morita et al., 1986, 1987b; Prieto et al., 1994; Rose and Gillenwater, 1974; Vereecken, 1973). The excitatory effect of carbachol on isolated canine ureter is mediated by the excitatory M$_3$-receptor subtype and carbachol-induced inhibition of potassium chloride (KCl)–induced contractions of longitudinal canine ureteral preparations is mediated primarily via the inhibitory M$_4$-receptor subtype (Tomiyama et al., 2003b). ACh also has been shown to increase the duration of the guinea pig and rat ureteral action potential (Ichikawa and Ikeda, 1960; Prosser et al., 1955) and the number of oscillations on the plateau of the guinea pig ureteral action potential (Ichikawa and Ikeda, 1960).

Nicotinic agonists, such as nicotine, tetramethylammonium, and dimethylphenylpiperazinium, cause an initial stimulation of nicotinic receptors followed by desensitization of the receptor sites; the receptors then become unresponsive to nicotinic agonists and also to endogenous ACh, with a resultant transmission blockade. Nicotine, as would be expected, has been shown to have excitatory (Boyarsky et al., 1968), biphasic (Labay and Boyarsky, 1967; Satani, 1919), or inhibitory (Prosser et al., 1955; Vereecken, 1973) actions on the ureter.

Anticholinesterases prevent the hydrolysis of ACh by cholinesterases and thus increase the duration and intensity of ACh action at muscarinic and nicotinic receptor sites. With prolonged administration in high doses, they can result in desensitization blockade at nicotinic sites. The effects of **anticholinesterases**, such as **physostigmine and neostigmine**, parallel the excitatory effects of ACh and other parasympathomimetics on the ureter (Satani, 1919; Vereecken, 1973).

Atropine is a competitive antagonist of the muscarinic effects of ACh. The inhibitory effects of atropine may be preceded by a transitory stimulatory effect on muscarinic receptors. Although atropine has been shown to inhibit the excitatory effects of parasympathomimetic agents (Longrigg, 1974; Vereecken, 1973) and physostigmine (Macht, 1916a) on a variety of ureteral and calyceal preparations, the majority of studies have shown that atropine has little direct effect on ureteral activity in a number of species (Butcher et al., 1957; Gibbs, 1929; Gould et al., 1955; Reid et al., 1976; Vereecken, 1973; Washizu, 1967), including humans (Kiil, 1957). Even when atropine has been observed to inhibit ureteral activity, its effects are frequently minimal and inconsistent (Ross et al., 1967), thus providing little rationale for its use in the treatment of ureteral colic. Reports of the direct effects on ureteral activity of two other parasympathetic blocking agents, methantheline and propantheline, also have been inconsistent (Draper and Zorgniotti, 1954; Kiil, 1957; Reid et al., 1976).

Sympathetic Nervous System

The sympathetic nervous system appears to modulate ureteral activity as evidenced by the demonstration of adrenergic receptors in the ureter (Latifpour et al., 1989, 1990; Morita et al., 1994), the identification of catecholaminergic neurons in the ureter as determined by labeling tyrosine hydroxylase as a marker (Edyvane et al., 1994), and the demonstration that catecholamines are released from the ureter (Weiss et al., 1978) and renal calyx (Longrigg, 1975) in response to electric field stimulation.

According to the general consensus, **agents that primarily activate α-adrenergic receptors, such as norepinephrine and phenylephrine, tend to stimulate ureteral and renal pelvic activity** (Danuser et al., 2001; Hannappel and Golenhofen, 1974; Hernández et al., 1992; McLeod et al., 1973; Morita et al., 1987a; Nguyen et al., 2013; Rivera et al., 1992; Rose and Gillenwater, 1974; Santicioli and Maggi, 1998; Vereecken, 1973), and **agents that primarily activate β-adrenergic receptors, such as isoproterenol and orciprenaline, tend to inhibit ureteral and renal pelvic activity** (Ancill et al., 1972; Danuser et al., 2001; Finberg and Peart, 1970; Hannappel and Golenhofen, 1974; Hernández et al., 1992; McLeod et al., 1973; Rivera et al., 1992; Rose and Gillenwater, 1974; Vereecken, 1973; Weiss et al., 1978).

The ureter contains excitatory α-adrenergic and inhibitory β-adrenergic receptors that have been demonstrated with receptor-binding techniques (Latifpour et al., 1989, 1990). In the human ureter, renal pelvis and calyces $α_{1D}$- and $α_{1A}$-adrenoceptor subtypes are more prevalent than the $α_{1B}$-adrenoceptor subtype (Itoh et al., 2007; Karabacak et al., 2013; Sigala et al., 2005). The highest density of $α_1$-adrenoceptors is found in the distal ureter with the relative density being $α_{1D} > α_{1A} > α_{1B}$. This is in accord with the finding that phenylephrine, an α-adrenergic agonist, induces a greater contractile force in isolated human ureteral segments obtained from the distal than the proximal ureter (Sasaki et al., 2011). The expression of $α_1$-adrenoceptors is species dependent with a higher density of $α_{1A}$-adrenoceptors in the mouse ureter and a higher density of $α_{1D}$-adrenoceptors in the dog and hamster ureter (Kobayashi et al., 2009a, b; Tomiyama et al., 2007). The $α_{1A}$-adrenoceptor subtype is the primary receptor subtype that participates in the contraction of the mouse, hamster, and human ureter (Kobayashi et al., 2009c; Sasaki et al., 2008, 2011; Tomiyama et al., 2007). $α_{1A}$-Adrenoceptors appear to be more involved in the maintenance of baseline ureteral tonus than in the potentiation of ureteral peristaltic activity (Morita et al., 1987a; Tomiyama et al., 2002).

Norepinephrine, primarily an α-adrenergic agonist (although it also can stimulate β-adrenergic receptors), increases the force of electrically induced ureteral contractions (Weiss et al., 1978). When administered in the presence of **phentolamine** (Regitine), **an α-adrenergic blocking agent,** norepinephrine, decreases the force of ureteral contractions (Weiss et al., 1978). A similar reversal of action occurs in the in vivo ureter (McLeod et al., 1973) and can be explained by norepinephrine's primary action on inhibitory β-adrenergic receptors when the excitatory α-adrenergic receptors are blocked. Propranolol (Inderal), a β-adrenergic antagonist, potentiates the increase in contractile force induced by norepinephrine (Weiss et al., 1978). This can be explained by norepinephrine's acting more exclusively on excitatory α-adrenergic receptors when the inhibitory β-adrenergic receptors are blocked. Furthermore, **isoproterenol, a β-adrenergic agonist,** depresses contractility (Weiss et al., 1978). These data provide evidence for excitatory α-adrenergic and inhibitory β-adrenergic receptors in the ureter and are in accord with the observations of McLeod et al. (1973) and Rose and Gillenwater (1974) on in vivo ureters.

Further support for the presence of excitatory α-adrenergic and inhibitory β-adrenergic receptors in the ureter includes the demonstration of adenylyl cyclase activity in the ureter (Weiss et al., 1977; Wheeler et al., 1986) and the finding that the ureters of rabbits depleted of catecholamines by the administration of reserpine undergo greater degrees of deformation when a given intraluminal pressure is applied than would result from the application of the same pressure load to the ureters of normal, non–reserpine-treated animals (Weiss et al., 1974). Finally, electric stimulation with high-intensity, high-frequency, short-duration stimuli has been shown to release neurotransmitter, presumably from intrinsic neural tissue within the wall of the ureter (Weiss et al., 1978) and renal calyx (Longrigg, 1975).

Norepinephrine, the chemical mediator responsible for adrenergic transmission, is synthesized in the neuron from tyrosine. After its release from the nerve terminal, some of the norepinephrine combines with receptors in the effector organ, leading to a physiologic response. The greatest percentage of the norepinephrine is actively taken up (reuptake or neuronal uptake) into the neuron. Neuronal reuptake regulates the duration that norepinephrine is in contact with the innervated tissue and thus regulates the magnitude and duration of the catecholamine-induced response. Agents such as cocaine and imipramine (Tofranil), that inhibit neuronal uptake, potentiate the physiologic response to norepinephrine (Boyarsky and Labay, 1969). Tyramine, whose adrenergic agonist effects are due primarily to the release of norepinephrine from adrenergic terminals, also has a stimulatory effect on the upper urinary tract (Boyarsky and Labay, 1969; Finberg and Peart, 1970; Longrigg, 1974). The enzymes monoamine oxidase and catechol-O-methyltransferase provide degradative pathways for norepinephrine.

The α-adrenergic antagonists phentolamine and phenoxybenzamine (Dibenzyline) have been shown to inhibit the stimulatory effects of norepinephrine and other α-adrenergic agonists in a variety of preparations (Finberg and Peart, 1970; Gosling and Waas, 1971; Hannappel and Golenhofen, 1974; Hernández et al., 1992; Longrigg, 1974; McLeod et al., 1973; Rose and Gillenwater, 1974; Vereecken, 1973; Weiss et al., 1978). The α-adrenergic antagonist, doxazosin, has been shown to slightly reduce spontaneous contractility of in vitro pig ureter and to inhibit the contractile effects of epinephrine and phenylephrine (Nakada et al., 2007). Tamsulosin inhibited the contractility of human ureters in vitro (Rajpathy et al., 2008) and in vivo (Davenport et al., 2007). Silodosin, a selective $α_{1A}$-receptor antagonist, was more effective in inhibiting electrical field stimulation (EFS)–induced contractions of human and rat isolated ureters than tamsulosin, a selective $α_{1A/D}$-receptor antagonist, or prazosin, a nonselective α-adrenergic receptor antagonist (Villa et al., 2013).

The β-adrenergic subtypes involved in ureteral relaxation are species specific; $β_1$-adrenoceptors in rats, $β_2$-adrenoceptors in rabbits, mainly $β_3$-adrenoceptors in dogs, and $β_2$- and $β_3$-adrenoceptors in pigs and humans (Park et al., 2000; Tomiyama et al., 1998, 2003a; Wanajo et al, 2004). All three β-adrenergic receptor subtypes are expressed in the human ureter (Matsumoto et al., 2013; Park et al., 2000). Immunohistochemical studies show that the β-adrenergic receptors are expressed in the smooth muscle and the urothelium of the human ureter (Matsumoto et al., 2013) and the expression of $β_1$, $β_2$, and $β_3$ are decreased in the dilated ureter (Shen et al., 2017). A relatively specific $β_3$-adrenoceptor agonist, TRK-380, relaxes in vitro human ureteral segments, and it has been suggested that the $β_3$-agonist mirabegron may do the same (Matsumoto et al., 2013).

A synthesized β_2-/β_3-adrenoceptor agonist, KUL-7211, was a more potent relaxant of isolated dog ureteral segments than the α-adrenergic antagonists, tamsulosin and prazosin; the calcium channel blocker, verapamil; and the phosphodiesterase inhibitor, papaverine (Wanajo et al., 2005). KUL-7211 also is a potent relaxant of the pig ureter (Wanajo et al., 2011). Intraluminal isoproterenol has been shown to lower renal pelvic pressures during ureteroscopy, with the presumption that this would decrease intrarenal backflow that has potential harmful effects (Jakobsen, 2013; Jung et al., 2008). In the rabbit renal pelvis β_2-adrenergic agonists inhibit contractile activity of the distal renal pelvis and β_1-adrenergic agonists potentiate contractile activity of the proximal renal pelvis (Kondo et al., 1989).The β-adrenergic antagonist propranolol has been shown to block or attenuate the inhibitory effects of β-adrenergic agonists, such as isoproterenol, in a variety of preparations (Longrigg, 1974; McLeod et al., 1973; Rose and Gillenwater, 1974; Vereecken, 1973; Weiss et al., 1978).

Sensory Innervation and Peptidergic Agents in the Control of Ureteral Function

Sensory nerves can play a sensory afferent and motor efferent role in a given tissue. Tachykinins and CGRP are neurotransmitters released from peripheral endings of sensory nerves (Maggi, 1995). **Tachykinins stimulate and CGRP inhibit electrical and contractile activity. Capsaicin-sensitive sensory nerves are located in the ureter** (Ammons, 1992; Dray et al., 1989; Maggi and Meli, 1988; Maggi et al., 1986) and contain the tachykinins, substance P, neurokinin A, and neuropeptide K (Hua et al., 1985; Sann et al., 1992), as well as CGRP (Gibbins et al., 1985; Sann et al., 1992; Tamaki et al., 1992). Release of prostaglandins and neuropeptides from sensory nerves plays a role in the maintenance of peristalsis (Nguyen et al., 2016). Immunoreactivity for tachykinins and CGRP is less in the human than in the guinea pig ureter (Edyvane et al., 1992; 1994; Hua et al., 1987; Su et al., 1986). Capsaicin in low doses inhibits ureteral activity, presumably because of the release of CGRP, but in high doses it increases ureteral activity, presumably because of release of the tachykinins neurokinin A, neuropeptide K, and substance P (Hua and Lundberg, 1986). Capsaicin administration to neonatal rats causes degeneration of CGRP-containing sensory nerves in the ureter that is accompanied by an increase in sympathetic innervation (Sann et al., 1995). Because nerve growth factor (NGF) is responsible for increased sensory and noradrenergic innervation, capsaicin-induced degeneration of sensory nerves decreases NGF uptake into sensory neurons with a resultant increase in the amount of NGF available for stimulating sympathetic innervation (Schicho et al., 1998). The excitatory effects of the tachykinins are more prominent in the renal pelvis than in the ureter, and the inhibitory effects of CGRP are more prominent in the ureter than in the renal pelvis (Maggi et al., 1992b). The excitatory effects of tachykinins involve excitation of NK-2 receptors in the human, pig, and guinea pig ureter, pig intravesical ureter, and guinea pig renal pelvis (Bustamante et al., 2001; Jerde et al., 1999; Nakada et al., 2001; Patacchini et al., 1998). The inhibitory actions of the neurotransmitter CGRP appear to involve multiple mechanisms (Maggi and Giuliani, 1991; Maggi et al., 1994b). By opening ATP-sensitive K$^+$ channels, CGRP causes membrane hyperpolarization with a resultant blocking of voltage-sensitive Ca^{2+} channels that are involved in generation of the ureteral action potential and ureteral contraction (Maggi et al., 1994c; Meini et al., 1995; Santicioli and Maggi, 1994). CGRP-induced ureteral relaxation also may result from stimulation of adenylyl cyclase activity with a resultant increase in cAMP (Santicioli et al., 1995b). The action of CGRP on the ureter may be regulated by an endopeptidase that degrades the CGRP released from the sensory nerves (Maggi and Giuliani, 1994). Histochemical studies show that the tachykinins and CGRP colocalize in the same nerves in the ureter (Hua et al., 1987).

Renal pelvic sensory nerves contain substance P (SP) and CGRP. Increases in renal pelvic pressure result in the release of SP and a subsequent increase in afferent renal nerve activity. CGRP potentiates the afferent renal nerve activity responses to SP by retarding the metabolism of SP, thus resulting in increased amounts of SP available for potentiating afferent renal nerve activity (Gontijo et al., 1999). Prostaglandins also contribute to sensory receptor activation (Kopp et al., 2000).

Nonadrenergic, noncholinergic (NANC) excitatory neurotransmission is functional in the pig intravesical ureter (Bustamante et al., 2000; 2001). In the presence of agents that block adrenergic neurotransmission, muscarinic cholinergic receptors, NO synthase activity, prostaglandin synthesis, and A_1/A_2 adenosine receptors, EFS induced (5 H$_z$) contractions that were potentiated by the tachykinins SP and neurokinin A and that were inhibited by a sensory neurotoxin, capsaicin, and by a NK$_2$ receptor antagonist, GR94800. The EFS-induced contractions were abolished by tetrodotoxin, providing evidence that the contractions were neurogenic in origin. It has been suggested that tachykinins, especially neurokinin A, released from capsaicin-sensitive afferent nerves and activating NK$_2$-receptors are involved in NANC excitatory neurotransmission.

Peptidergic neurons containing NPY and vasoactive intestinal polypeptide (VIP) also are present in the ureter (Allen et al., 1990; Edyvane et al., 1992; Prieto et al., 1997). VIP and pituitary adenylate cyclase–activating polypeptide (PACAP) have been shown to relax pig intravesical ureteral segments through a cAMP-dependent mechanism (Hernández et al., 2004). Edyvane et al. (1994) have provided evidence for at least four, and possibly six, different immunohistochemical populations of nerve fibers in the human ureter. The predominant types include noradrenergic nerves containing NPY, neurons containing NPY and vasoactive polypeptide, neurons containing substance P and CGRP, and neurons containing CGRP. NPY potentiates the excitatory effects of norepinephrine on the ureter (Prieto et al., 1997). Rare coexistences also were observed between CGRP and vasoactive polypeptide, CGRP and NPY, and CGRP and tyrosine hydroxylase, a marker of noradrenergic neurons. These investigators demonstrated regional differences in the innervation of the ureter, with a more extensive innervation noted in the lower than in the upper ureter. There also is evidence that adenosine relaxes the pig intravesical ureter through a process independent of NO (Hernández et al., 1999).

Hydrogen sulfide (H$_2$S), which is synthesized from cystathione by the enzyme cystathione γ-lyase (CSE), has been shown to relax the pig intravesical ureter via K$_{ATP}$ channel activation (Fernandes and Hernández, 2016; Fernandes et al., 2014). H$_2$S is an activator of transient receptor potential A1 (TRPA1) expressed in CGRP-positive sensory nerves and interstitial cells in human ureter (Weinhold et al., 2017). TRPA1 agonists and H$_2$S inhibit EFS-induced contractions in the ureter.

Purinergic Nervous System

Burnstock et al. (1972) postulated that ATP could act as an excitatory transmitter in the bladder. It was subsequently shown that ATP is released along with acetylcholine in response to nerve stimulation (Kasakov and Burnstock, 1982) and that the excitatory response in the bladder is mediated through P2X receptors (Theobald, 1995). ATP activation of P2X purinoceptors promotes influx of extracellular Ca^{2+} into the muscle cells with resultant contraction. **Although there is no evidence for ATP mediating contractions in the ureter, there is evidence to suggest that ATP is involved in nociceptive processes.** P2X receptors are present in the ureter (Lee et al., 2000), and P2Y$_4$ receptors are present in ureteral urothelium (Shabir et al., 2013). ATP is released from the urothelium of human and guinea pig ureter in response to ureteral distention (Calvert et al., 2008; Knight et al., 2002) and stimulates sensory nerves that contain purinergic receptors (Calvert et al., 2008; Rong and Burnstock, 2004). Two classes of mechanosensitive afferent fibers have been identified in the guinea pig ureter (Cervero and Sann, 1989). It would appear that one group of fibers are tension receptors that respond to normal ureteral peristalsis, whereas the other is involved in the signaling of noxious events such as kidney stones and increased intraluminal pressures. Both groups are chemosensitive, excited by K$^+$, bradykinin, and capsaicin (Sann, 1998). Because ureteral distention and exogenous ATP increase afferent nerve discharge (Rong and Burnstock, 2004), ATP may be involved in signaling visceral pain with ureteral dilatation, that is, renal colic (Burnstock, 2006, 2009). It has been proposed that ureteral distention causes release of ATP from the urothelium, which in turn activates purinoceptors on suburothelial nociceptive sensory nerves. Consistent with this postulation ATP has been shown to be released with distention of isolated human ureteral segments, and this was accompanied by staining of P2X(3) and capsaicin receptors (Calvert et al., 2008).

MECHANICAL PROPERTIES

Mechanical characteristics of muscle are commonly assessed by defining force-length and force-velocity relations. Isometric force-length measurements depend on the number of linkages between the contractile proteins, actin and myosin, that are brought into action during contraction. Force-velocity relations depend on the rate of formation and breakdown of linkages between the contractile proteins. Interventions may affect force-velocity relations, with or without affecting force-length relations. In addition to these methods of assessing mechanical properties of the ureter, the bidimensional nature of the ureter has lent itself to studies of pressure-length-diameter relations.

Force-Length Relations

Force-length relations express the relation between the force developed by muscle when it is stimulated under isometric conditions and the resting length of the muscle at the time of stimulation. With stretching of the ureter (muscle lengthening), the resting force (i.e., the tension present when the muscle is not excited) increases at a progressive rate (Weiss et al., 1972). The force developed during isometric contraction also increases with elongation until a length is reached at which the maximal contractile force is achieved. With further lengthening, the developed force decreases (Thulesius et al., 1989; Weiss et al., 1972). The ureter at this length is overstretched, or beyond the peak of its force-length curve. Ureteral resting tension is high at the length at which maximal contractile force is developed.

Because the ureter is a viscoelastic structure (Weiss et al., 1972), **the resting or contractile force developed at any given length depends on the direction in which the change in length is occurring and on the rate of length change** (Vereecken et al., 1973; Weiss et al., 1972). **This is referred to as hysteresis;** for the ureter, at any given length, the resting force is less and the contractile force is greater when the ureter is allowed to shorten than when the ureter is being stretched (Fig. 85.14).

When the ureter is stretched, the resting force increases. **If the length is kept constant at its new longer length after a stretch, changes occur that result in a decrease in the resting force, or stress relaxation** (Fig. 85.15; Weiss et al., 1972). Within certain limits, when the ureter is stretched to a length beyond the peak of the force-length curve—that is, when the ureter is stretched to a length at which the contractile force declines in the face of increasing muscle length—the degree of stress relaxation may be such that, within a period of time, the developed force no longer declines, even though the increased length is kept constant (Weiss et al., 1972). Stress relaxation can thus be considered a compensatory mechanism of a viscoelastic structure to stretch.

Force-Velocity Relations

Force-velocity curves depict the relation between the load and the velocity of shortening. A typical force-velocity curve, as predicted by Hill's equation (Hill, 1938) for muscle shortening, has a hyperbolic configuration (Fig. 85.16; Biancani et al., 1984). From the force-velocity curve, one can extrapolate the **maximal velocity of shortening (V_{max}), which represents the velocity of shortening at zero load (i.e., at isotonic conditions).** V_{max} is determined by the level at which the force-velocity curve crosses the ordinate. V_{max} values in the ureter are in the range of 0.5 to 0.7 lengths per second (Biancani et al., 1984). The force-velocity curve intersects the abscissa at zero shortening, that is, at isometric conditions at which the load is great.

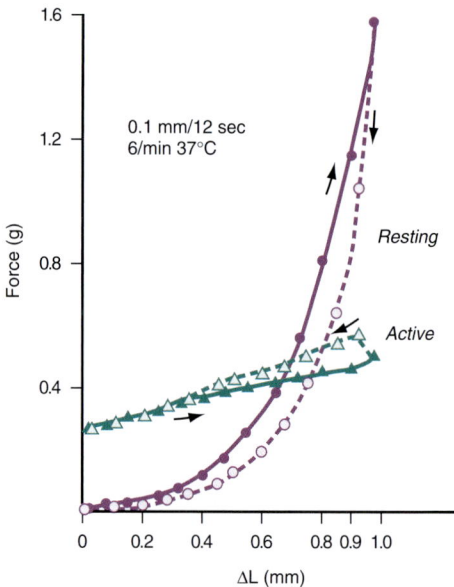

Fig. 85.14. Hysteresis. Resting and contractile (active) force of cat ureter during muscle lengthening and shortening. Force is on the ordinate; change in length (ΔL) is on the abscissa. *Solid symbols* and *solid lines* show data obtained during muscle lengthening. *Open symbols* and *dashed lines* show data obtained during muscle shortening. *Circles* show resting force, and *triangles* show active or contractile force. The length and the direction of length change influence resting and contractile force. (From Weiss RM, Bassett AL, Hoffman BF: Dynamic length-tension curves of cat ureter. *Am J Physiol* 222:388, 1972.)

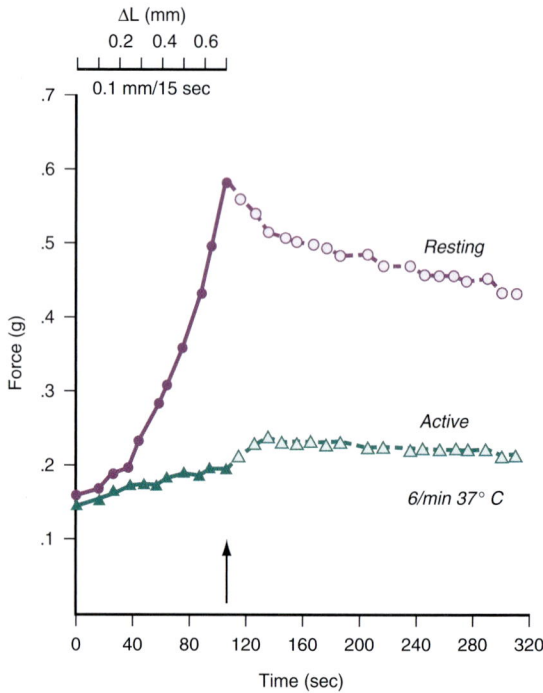

Fig. 85.15. Stress relaxation. The resting and contractile (active) force of cat ureter is on the ordinate, the time from the onset of stretching is on the lower abscissa, and the change in length (ΔL) is on the left upper corner abscissa. Muscle is stretched by a given amount and then held at a fixed length. *Solid symbols* and *solid lines* show data obtained during muscle lengthening; *open symbols* and *dashed lines* show data obtained after stretching has ceased *(arrow)* and muscle is maintained at a constant length. Resting force decreases when muscle is held at a constant length after a stretch (stress relaxation). Contractile (active) force increases during this period of time. (From Weiss RM, Bassett AL, Hoffman BF: Dynamic length-tension curves of cat ureter. *Am J Physiol* 222:388, 1972.)

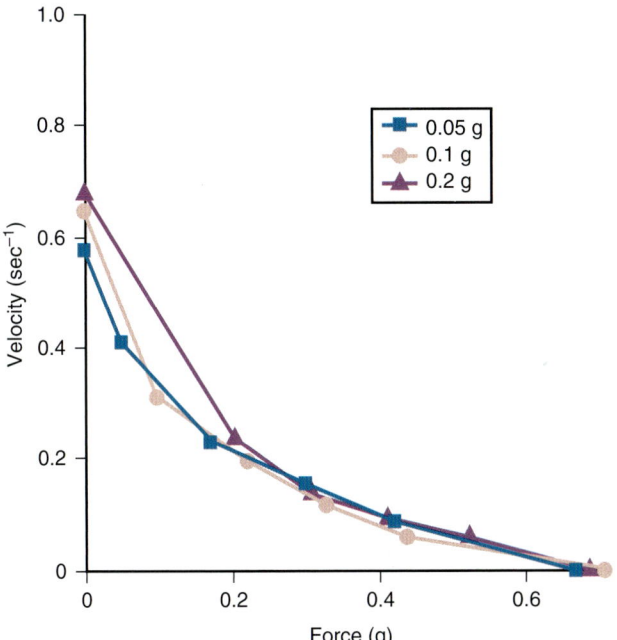

Fig. 85.16. Force-velocity relation of guinea pig ureter. Specimens were stretched by three different preloads (0.05, 0.1, and 0.2 g). The velocity of shortening on the ordinate is plotted as a function of the total load lifted on the abscissa. V_{max} is obtained by extrapolating the experimental curves to intersect the ordinate. Isometric force is given by data points where velocity equals zero. (From Biancani P, Onyski JH, Zabinski MP, et al.: Force-velocity relationships of the pig ureter. *J Urol* 131:988, 1984.)

Shortening depends on the total load lifted, with the ureter shortening to a lesser extent with heavier loads. At conditions near those of zero load, that is, conditions of free shortening (isotonic conditions), the in vitro guinea pig ureter shortens by 25% to 30% of its initial length (Biancani et al., 1984).

Pressure-Length-Diameter Relations

Ureteral muscle fibers are arranged in a longitudinal, circumferential, and spiral configuration (Tanagho, 1971), although there is evidence that it is primarily longitudinal in the rat (Spronk et al., 2014). Because longitudinal and diametral deformation of the ureter are interrelated, simultaneous studies of length and diameter changes in response to an intraluminal pressure load are another means of assessing the mechanical properties of a tubular structure. After application of an intraluminal pressure, the ureter increases in length and diameter, a process known as *creep* (Biancani et al., 1973). Deformation in response to a given intraluminal pressure load is greater in vitro than in vivo; this difference is partially negated if the in vivo preparation is pretreated with reserpine to suppress adrenergic influences (Weiss et al., 1974). Such data provide support for a role of the adrenergic nervous system in the control of ureteral function.

URINE TRANSPORT

Physiology of the Ureteropelvic Junction

At normal urine flows, the frequency of calyceal and renal pelvic contractions is greater than that in the upper ureter, and there is a relative block of electric activity at the UPJ (Morita et al., 1981). At these flows, the renal pelvis fills; as renal pelvic pressure rises, urine is extruded into the upper ureter, which is initially in a collapsed state (Griffiths and Notschaele, 1983). **Ureteral contractile pressures that move the bolus of urine are higher than renal pelvic pressures, and a closed UPJ may be protective of the kidney in dissipating backpressure from the ureter. As the flow rate increases, the block at the UPJ ceases and a 1:1 correspondence between pacemaker and ureteral contractions develops** (Constantinou and Hrynczuk, 1976; Constantinou and Yamaguchi, 1981).

UPJ obstruction can be due to multiple causes. There may be areas of narrowing or valvelike processes (Maizels and Stephens, 1980) or mucosal folds (Takeyama and Sakai, 2007). Alternatively, there may be no gross narrowing at the UPJ, and abnormal propagation of the peristaltic impulse creates the obstruction. In these instances, there appears to be a functional obstruction at the UPJ, because a large-caliber catheter can be passed readily through the UPJ, even though urine transport is inadequate. Murnaghan (1958) related the functional abnormality to an alteration in the configuration of the muscle bundles at the UPJ, and Foote et al. (1970) observed a decrease in musculature at the UPJ. Hanna (1978), in an electron microscopic study of severe UPJ obstructions, noted abnormalities in the musculature of the renal pelvis and disruption of intercellular relations at the UPJ. Increased accumulation of collagen has been described in the region of the UPJ with obstruction (Murakumo et al., 1997), and it has been suggested that differences in types I and III collagen in the region of the obstructed UPJ may be age dependent (Yoon et al., 1998). Increases in smooth muscle myosin heavy-chain isoforms also have been described in congenital UPJ obstruction (Hosgor et al., 2005). Studies also have shown a decrease in nerves and in nerve growth factor mRNA expression in UPJ obstruction specimens compared with controls (Murakumo et al., 1997; Wang et al., 1995). An increase in apoptosis of smooth muscle cells in the region of congenital UPJ obstruction has been reported to accompany a decrease in smooth muscle and nerve terminals and an increase in collagen and elastin (Cutroneo et al., 2011; Kajbafzadeh et al., 2006). In addition, changes in the differentiation of the urothelial cells at the level of the UPJ have been suspected as a contributor to pathogenic obstruction. Overexpression of annexin A7 and A11, EGFR, and keratin 5 and a decrease in uroplakin III have been described with UPJ obstruction (Hou et al., 2014). A murine knockout of Cld-4, a claudin involved in tight junctions of the urothelium, was found to develop hydronephrosis in utero as a result of hyperplasia and thickening of the urothelium (Fujita et al., 2012), whereas deficiency in the miR-143/145 cluster of miRNA led to hydronephrosis resulting from abnormal ureteral peristalsis (Medrano et al., 2014). Furthermore, persistent TGF-β in the UVJ region may be associated with primary megaureter (Ozturk et al., 2016). c-KIT–positive ICC-like cells, which appear to aid in the propagation of electrical impulses from pacemaker cells to typical ureteral smooth muscle cells, have been reported to be decreased (Senol et al., 2016; Solari et al., 2003; Yang et al., 2009), increased (Koleda et al., 2012), or unchanged (Apoznanski et al., 2013) at the obstructed UPJ. Defective contractility of UPJ segments obtained at the time of pyeloplasty has been described (Pontincasa et al., 2006). As a corollary to the finding that the signaling pathway is involved in the development of the ureteropelvic junction, it was found that two downstream transcription factors of Shh, Gli3 and Teashirt3, are significantly decreased in the setting of UPJ obstruction (UPJO) (Chen et al., 2016) and that deletion of the Shh receptor *Patched 1* (*Ptch1*) causes obstructive hydronephrosis in mice (Sheybani-Deloui et al., 2017). A vessel or adhesive band crossing the UPJ may potentiate the degree of dilatation in any of the forms of UPJO.

The differences in the reported findings suggest a histopathologic spectrum in the group of cases referred to as UPJOs. **It appears possible that, at least in some instances, disruption of cell-to-cell propagation of peristaltic activity results in impairment of urine transport across the UPJ.**

The effects of diuresis and obstruction appear to be complementary and additive with respect to the development of renal pelvic and calyceal dilatation, and input and output must be considered when predicting whether or not dilatation will occur. Some UPJs can handle urine flow regardless of the magnitude of diuresis, others cause dilatation at even the lowest flows, and still others can handle low flows but cause massive dilatation at high flows, thus leading to the clinical presentation known as Dietl's crisis (Fig. 85.17).

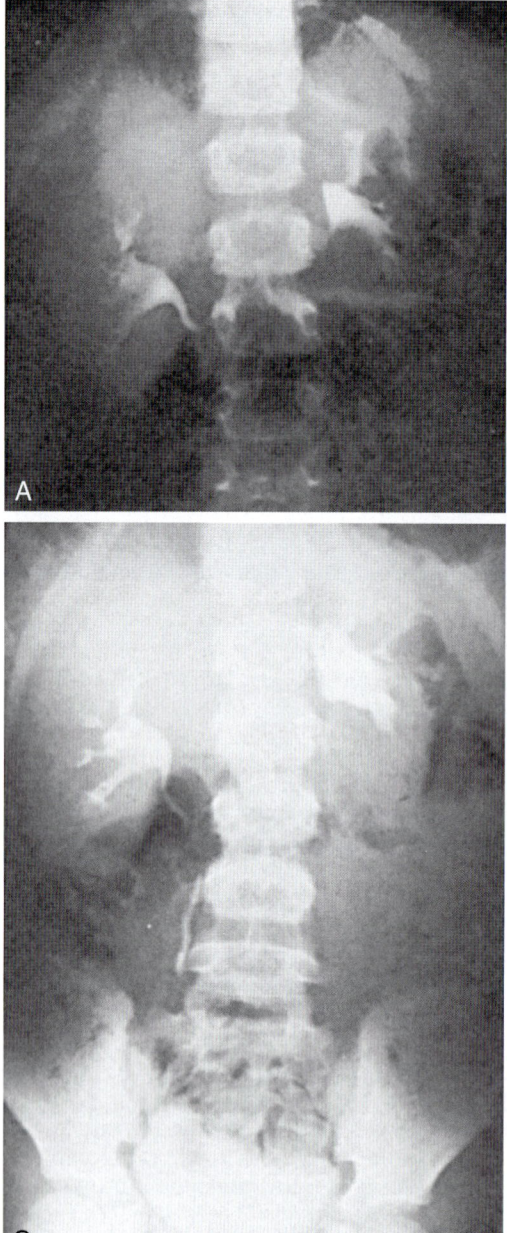
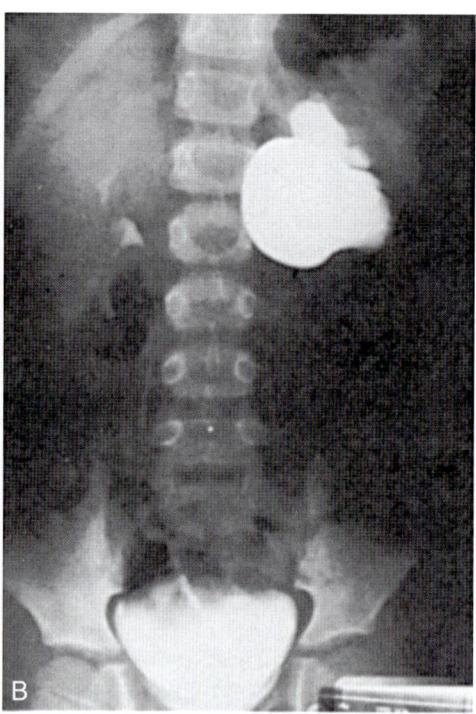

Fig. 85.17. Although no longer commonly used, intravenous pyelograms (IVPs) could demonstrate obstruction induced by a large diuresis. (A) IVP shows essentially normal upper urinary tracts. (B) Film from the same child taken immediately after a cardiac angiogram, which produces a massive diuresis. (C) IVP 6 weeks after the angiogram. (A to C, From Weiss RM: Clinical implications of ureter physiology. *J Urol* 121:401, 1979.)

Propulsion of Urinary Bolus

The theoretical aspects of the mechanics of urine transport within the ureter have been described in detail by Griffiths and Notschaele (1983); these are depicted in Fig. 85.18.

At normal flow rates, as the renal pelvis fills, a rise in renal pelvic pressure occurs, and urine is extruded into the upper ureter, which initially is in a collapsed state. The contraction wave originates in the most proximal portion of the ureter and moves the urine in front of it in a distal direction. The urine that had previously entered the ureter is formed into a bolus. To propel the bolus of urine efficiently, the contraction wave must completely coapt the ureteral walls (Griffiths and Notschaele, 1983; Woodburne and Lapides, 1972), and the pressure generated by this contraction wave provides the primary component of what is recorded by intraluminal pressure measurements. **The bolus that is pushed in front of the contraction wave lies almost entirely in a passive, noncontracting part of the ureter** (Fung, 1971; Weinberg, 1974).

Baseline, or resting, ureteral pressure is approximately 0 to 5 cm H_2O, and superimposed ureteral contractions ranging from 20 to 80 cm H_2O occur two to six times per minute (Kiil, 1957; Ross et al., 1972). The urine traverses the UVJ to enter the bladder; when functioning properly, the UVJ ensures one-way transport of urine. The bolus is forced into the bladder by the advancing contraction wave that then dissipates at the UVJ.

As with any tubular structure, the ureter can transport a set maximal amount of fluid per unit time. Under normal flows, in which bolus formation occurs, the amount of urine transported per unit time is significantly less than the maximal transport capacity of the ureter. At extremely high flows, as are employed in perfusion studies (Whitaker, 1973), the ureteral walls do not coapt, and a continuous column of fluid, rather than a series of boluses, is transported.

When transport becomes inadequate, stasis of urine occurs with resultant ureteral dilatation. **Inadequate transport can result either from too much fluid entering the ureter per unit time or from too little fluid exiting the ureter per unit time.** Input and output must be considered in predicting whether ureteral dilation will occur. For example, a minor degree of obstruction to outflow causes more dilation at high flow rates than at low flow rates. Even a normal, nonobstructed ureter impedes urine transport if the rate of flow is great enough.

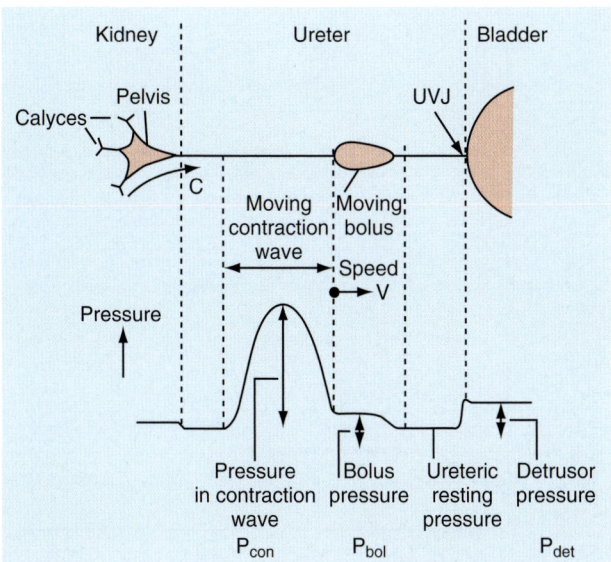

Fig. 85.18. Schematic representation of a single bolus in the ureter moving away from the renal pelvis and toward the bladder. *Arrow C* indicates the direction of bolus transport. The corresponding distribution of pressure within the urinary tract is shown in the lower tracing. UVJ, Ureterovesical junction. (From Griffiths DJ, Notschaele C: The mechanics of urine transport in the upper urinary tract. *Neurourol Urodyn* 2:155, 1983.)

Changes in ureteral dimensions that occur in pathologic states may result in inefficient urine transport, even if the contractile force of the individual fibers is unchanged. The Laplace equation expresses the relation between the variables that affect intraluminal pressure:

$$T = PR$$

and

$$P = T/R$$

where T = wall tension, P = internal pressure, R = radius of a cylinder.

An increase in ureteral diameter can decrease intraluminal pressure and result in inefficient urine transport. Such dimensional changes may, at least theoretically, be deleterious (Griffiths, 1983). Another factor may be the histologic composition of the dilated ureter, as evidenced by the description of different amounts of type I and type III collagen in primary obstructed and refluxing megaureters (Lee et al., 1998).

Effect of Diuresis on Ureteral Function

With increasing urine flow rates, the initial response of the ureter is to increase peristaltic frequency. After the maximal frequency is achieved, further increases in urine transport occur by means of increases in bolus volume (Constantinou et al., 1974; Morales et al., 1952). At relatively low flow rates, small increases in flow result in large increases in peristaltic frequency. At higher flow rates, relatively large increases in flow result in only small increases in peristaltic frequency. As the flow rate continues to increase, several of the boluses coalesce, and finally the ureter becomes filled with a column of fluid and dilates. At these high flow rates, urine transport is through an open tube.

Effects of Bladder Filling and Neurogenic Vesical Dysfunction on Ureteral Function

Ureteral dilatation can result either from an increase in fluid input or from a decrease in fluid output from the ureter. The relation between ureteral intraluminal pressure and intravesical pressure is important in determining the efficacy of urine passage across the UVJ into the bladder. In the case of the normal ureter under normal physiologic rates of flow, ureteral contractile pressure exceeds intravesical pressure, resulting in passage of urine into the bladder. In the dilated, poorly contracting ureter or in the normal ureter at extreme flow rates, the ureter does not coapt its walls to form boluses, and the baseline pressure in the column of urine within the ureter must exceed intravesical pressure for urine to pass into the bladder.

The pressure within the bladder during the storage phase is paramount in determining the efficacy of urine transport across the UVJ. This is the pressure that the ureter must work against for the longest period of time. During filling of the normal bladder, sympathetic impulses and the viscoelastic properties of the bladder wall inhibit the magnitude of the intravesical pressure rise, that is, the tonus limb. With filling, the normal bladder maintains a relatively low intravesical pressure (McGuire, 1983) that facilitates the transport of urine across the UVJ and prevents ureteral dilatation. In the noncompliant fibrotic bladder and in some forms of neurogenic vesical dysfunction, the bladder is autonomous, and relatively small increases in bladder volume result in large increases in intravesical pressure with resultant impairment of ureteral emptying. The ureter initially responds to its decreased ability to empty by increasing its peristaltic frequency (Fredericks et al., 1972; Rosen et al., 1971; Zimskind et al., 1969). Ultimately, stasis occurs with the development of ureteral dilatation. **The ureter has been shown to decompensate when sustained intravesical pressure approaches 40 cm H_2O** (McGuire et al., 1981).

Physiology of the Ureterovesical Junction

Griffiths (1983) has analyzed the factors involved in urine transport across the UVJ. Under normal conditions and at normal flow rates, the contraction wave, which occludes the ureteral lumen, propagates distally with the urine bolus in front of it. When the bolus reaches the UVJ, the pressure within the bolus must exceed intravesical pressure for the bolus of urine to pass across the UVJ into the bladder. Under these conditions, in which the contraction wave is able to coapt the ureteral wall and move the urinary bolus distally, the pressure generated by the contraction wave exceeds the pressure within the urinary bolus. The contracted ureteral ring just proximal to the ureteral orifice at the UVJ is relevant in the antireflux mechanism (Roshani et al., 1996). As the bolus is ejected into the bladder, the distal ureter retracts within its sheaths; this telescoping of the ureter within its sheaths aids in decreasing UVJ resistance to flow and thus facilitates urine passage into the bladder (Blok et al., 1985). The UVJ does not relax (Weiss and Biancani, 1983). **Impediment of efficient bolus transfer across the UVJ into the bladder can occur when there is an obstruction at the UVJ, when intravesical pressure is excessive, or when flow rates are so high as to exceed the transport capacity of the normal UVJ.** Under such conditions, in which the bolus of urine cannot pass freely into the bladder, the pressure within the bolus increases and may exceed the pressure in the contraction wave proximal to it. This results in an inability of the contraction wave to completely occlude the ureter; there is retrograde flow of urine from the bolus, and only a fraction of the urinary bolus passes across the UVJ into the bladder. Griffiths (1983) has presented theoretical evidence to show that a similar situation of impaired bolus transport across the UVJ would be expected if the ureter were wide or weakly contracting, even if the UVJ were perfectly normal. The wider and more weakly contracting the ureter, the lower the UVJ resistance must be not to interfere with bolus transport. The resistance to flow at the UVJ has been variously attributed to forces in the trigone (Tanagho et al., 1968) and to detrusor pressure (Coolsaet et al., 1982).

The theoretical considerations outlined by Griffiths (1983) have direct clinical implications. **If the UVJ is obstructed (i.e., has an abnormally high resistance to flow) or if the detrusor pressure is excessive, large boluses occurring at high-flow conditions would not be completely discharged into the bladder, because the contraction wave pushing the bolus would be forced open and intraureteral reflux would occur.** Such obstruction at the UVJ would be detected by perfusion studies as popularized by Whitaker (1973) (i.e., the Whitaker test). On the other hand, Griffiths' (1983) theory suggests that a similar breakdown of bolus discharge into the bladder can occur in the wide or weakly contracting ureter at high flow rates even if the UVJ is normal, and that such a condition would go undetected by a Whitaker perfusion test.

There is evidence that gravity may assist urine transport and that the erect position may aid urine transport across the UVJ, especially in individuals with dilated upper tracts (Schick and Tanagho, 1973). From a practical standpoint, George et al. (1984) suggested that bed rest may be deleterious to renal function in individuals with urinary retention and wide upper urinary tracts.

PATHOLOGIC PROCESSES AFFECTING URETERAL FUNCTION

Effect of Obstruction on Ureteral Function

General

The effect of obstruction on ureteral function depends on the degree and duration of the obstruction, on the rate of urine flow, and on the presence or absence of infection. After the onset of obstruction, a backup of urine occurs within the urinary collecting system, along with an associated increase in baseline (resting) ureteral intraluminal pressure and an increase in ureteral dimensions, that is, an increase in both length and diameter (Fig. 85.19; Biancani et al., 1976; Rose and Gillenwater, 1973). The increase in intraluminal pressure depends on the kidney's continued production of urine that cannot pass beyond the site of obstruction; the increase in ureteral dimensions results from the increased ureteral intraluminal pressure and the increased volume of urine retained within the ureter. A transient increase in the amplitude and frequency of the peristaltic contraction waves accompanies these initial dimensional and ureteral baseline (resting) pressure changes (Hammad et al., 2011; Rose and Gillenwater, 1978). There also is a decrease in the velocity of electrical impulses that correlates with decreased peristaltic activity (Hammad et al., 2011). With time, as the ureter fills with urine, the peristaltic contraction waves become smaller and are unable to coapt the ureteral wall. Urine transport then becomes dependent on hydrostatic forces generated by the kidney (Rose and Gillenwater, 1973). Superimposed infection may result in a complete absence of contractions in the obstructed ureter and contributes to impairment of urine transport (Rose and Gillenwater, 1973).

Within a few hours after the onset of obstruction, the intraluminal baseline ureteral pressure reaches a peak and then declines to a level only slightly higher than the normal baseline pressure. This occurs at a time in which dimensional changes remain stable (Biancani et al., 1976). The decrease in ureteral pressure can be attributed to changes in intrarenal hemodynamics, such as a reduction in renal blood flow (Vaughan et al., 1971), with resultant decreases in the glomerular filtration rate and intratubular hydrostatic pressure (Gottschalk and Mylle, 1956). Fluid reabsorption into the venous and lymphatic systems and a decrease in wall tension also may play a role in the reduction in baseline ureteral pressure (Rose and Gillenwater, 1978). The persistence of dimensional changes in the face of a decrease in intraluminal pressure depends on the hysteretic properties of the viscoelastic ureteral structure (Fig. 85.20; Biancani et al., 1973, 1976; Vereecken et al., 1973; Weiss et al., 1972).

As the obstruction persists, there is a gradual increase in ureteral length and diameter, which reaches considerable dimensions. This occurs even though ureteral pressure remains at a relatively low and constant level. This process, observed in viscoelastic structures, is referred to as creep (Biancani et al., 1973). A continued, albeit small, urine production is required for the continuing increase in intraureteral volume. Such changes account for the relatively low intrapelvic pressures clinically observed in the massively dilated, chronically obstructed upper urinary tract (Backlund et al., 1965; Djurhuus and Stage, 1976; Struthers, 1969; Vela-Navarrete, 1971); and in experimentally produced obstruction (Koff and Thrall, 1981a;

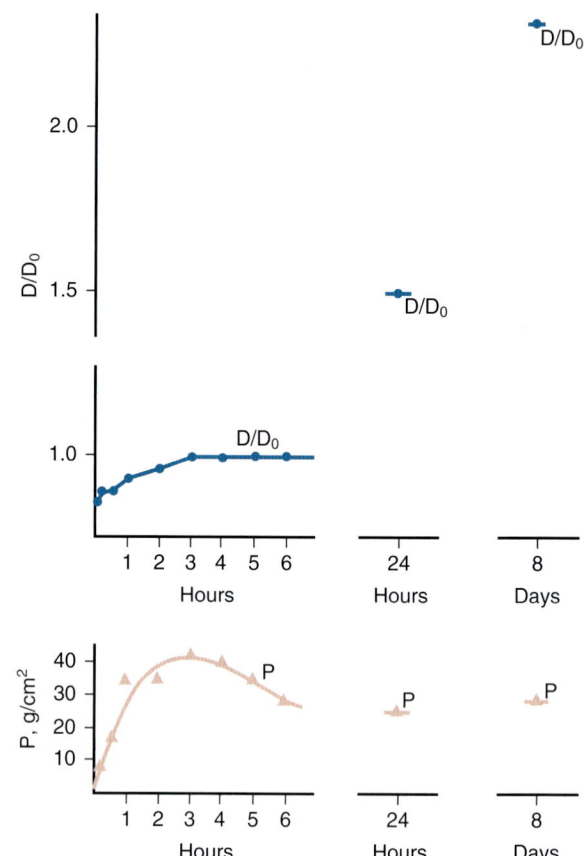

Fig. 85.19. Intraluminal pressure and diameter changes after obstruction of rabbit ureter. The time from the onset of obstruction is on the abscissa. The change in diameter (D/D_0) is on the upper ordinate, and the intraluminal pressure is on the lower ordinate. During the initial 3 hours of obstruction, intraluminal pressure increased to reach a maximum and was associated with an increase in diameter. Between 3 and 6 hours after the onset of obstruction, pressure declined, although diametral deformation persisted. After 6 hours, pressure remained essentially unchanged, although the diameter continued to increase. Each data point represents the mean ± standard error of mean (SEM). D, Diameter during deformation; D_0, initial diameter; P, intraluminal pressure. (Modified from Biancani P, Zabinski MP, Weiss RM: Time course of ureteral changes with acute and chronic obstruction. *Am J Physiol* 231:393, 1976.)

Schweitzer, 1973). One could postulate that with prolonged complete obstruction, the total cessation of urine output ultimately occurs. A subsequent decrease in ureteral dimensions would depend on whether urine is reabsorbed and on the mechanical properties of the ureter at that time.

To determine the effect of obstruction on the contractile properties of the ureter, a rabbit model in which the ureter is totally obstructed for 2 weeks has been employed (Biancani et al., 1982; Hausman et al., 1979). After 2 weeks of obstruction, the cross-sectional muscle area increases by 250%, ureteral length by 24%, and ureteral outer diameter by 100%. In addition to undergoing **muscle hypertrophy**, in vitro segments from obstructed ureters develop greater contractile forces, in longitudinal and circumferential directions, than segments from control ureters (Fig. 85.21). With experimental obstruction at the UPJ there also is an increase in the frequency and amplitude of spontaneous mechanical contractions of the renal pelvis and an increase in the amplitude of phenylephrine and 5-HT–induced contractions (Ekinci et al., 2004). Determination of stress (force per unit area of muscle) provides a means of determining whether the observed increases in developed force result from an increase in contractility or from an increase in muscle mass alone. The increases in force were associated with an increase in maximal active

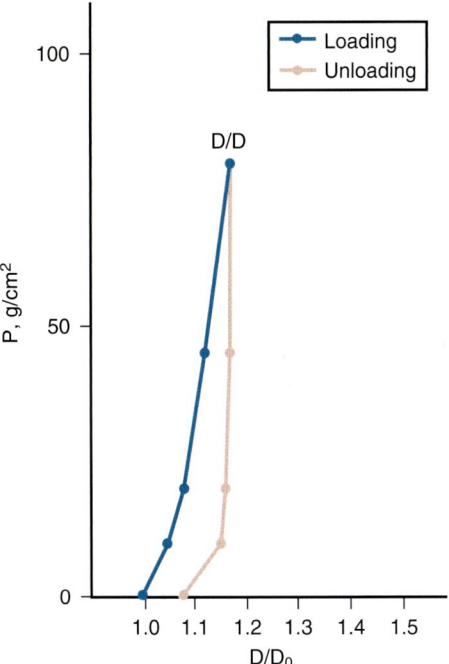

Fig. 85.20. Demonstration of hysteretic properties of ureter show that dimensional changes depend on intraluminal pressure and on the direction of change of that pressure. At comparable pressures, deformations are greater during ureteral emptying than during ureteral filling. The *blue line* shows data obtained during loading; the *pink line*, data obtained during unloading. *D*, Diameter during deformation; D_0, initial diameter; *P*, intraluminal pressure in grams per square centimeter. (Modified from Biancani P, Zabinski MP, Weiss RM: Time course of ureteral changes with acute and chronic obstruction. *Am J Physiol* 231:393, 1976.)

circumferential stress but no change in maximal active longitudinal stress (Fig. 85.22). Because there is an increase in circumferential stress and no change in longitudinal stress, the sum of the stresses (total stress) or overall contractility increases after 2 weeks of obstruction. For these differences in longitudinal and circumferential stresses to occur after obstruction, rotation of muscle bundles must occur; otherwise, longitudinal and circumferential stresses would increase equally. The rotation could result from the greater increase in diameter than in length after obstruction, from remodeling of the muscle fibers, or from both. In addition to an increase in EFS-induced ureteral contractions with obstruction, carbachol, phenylephrine, and KCl also caused a greater increase in contractions in obstructed ureters, and the Rho-kinase inhibitor, Y-27632, has a more pronounced effect in inhibiting these contractile events in the obstructed ureter (Turna et al., 2007; Yalcin et al., 2013). The expression of the two Rho kinase isoforms, ROCK-1 and ROCK-2, is increased in the obstructed ureter (Turna et al., 2007).

Thus the ureter dilated after 2 weeks of obstruction is not mechanically decompensated but rather undergoes changes that result in an increase in contractility. **Despite the muscle hypertrophy and the increase in contractility, it is clinically and experimentally evident that the obstructed, dilated ureter is less able than the normal ureter to generate the contractile pressures required for urine transport** (Rose and Gillenwater, 1973). The decrease in the ability to generate an intraluminal pressure despite an increase in contractility results from the increase in ureteral diameter that occurs after obstruction and can be explained by the **Laplace relation**:

$$\text{Pressure} = \frac{\text{stress} \times \text{wall thickness}}{\text{radius}}$$

Although contractility (stress) increases after 2 weeks of obstruction, the decrease in the wall's thickness-to-radius ratio, resulting from the marked increase in intraluminal diameter and thinning of the muscle layer, accounts for the decrease in pressure. A longer

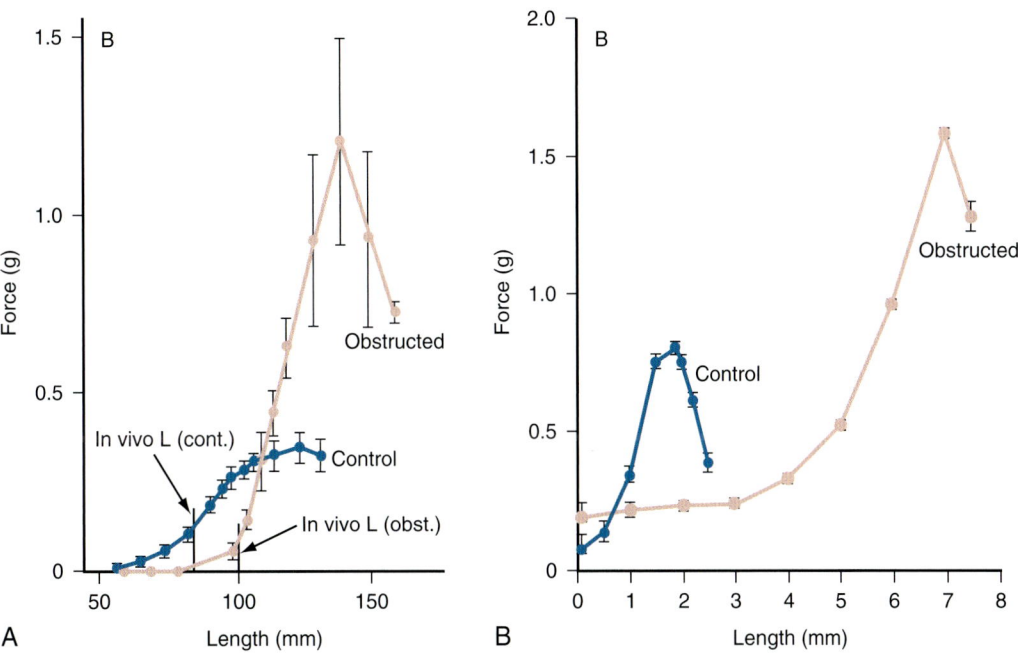

Fig. 85.21. (A) Active (contractile) longitudinal force-length relations of control *(blue circles)* and obstructed *(pink circles)* rabbit ureters. Each data point represents mean ± SEM. (B) Active (contractile) circumferential force-length relations of obstructed *(pink circles)* and control *(blue circles)* ureteral rings. Vertical bars correspond to in vivo lengths of control and obstructed segments. (A, From Hausman M, Biancani P, Weiss RM: Obstruction induced changes in longitudinal force-length relations of rabbit ureter. *Invest Urol* 17:223, 1979. Copyright by Williams & Wilkins, 1979. B, From Biancani P, Hausman, M, Weiss RM: Effect of obstruction on ureteral circumferential force-length relation. *Am J Physiol* 243:F204, 1982.)

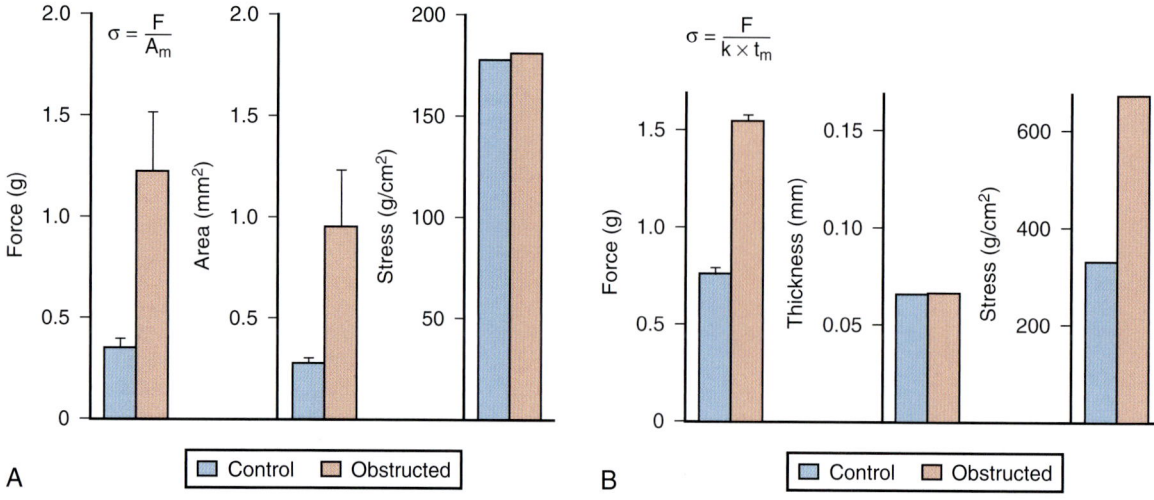

Fig. 85.22. (A) Longitudinal force, cross-sectional muscle area, and longitudinal stress at the length of maximal active force development. (B) Circumferential force, average muscle thickness, and circumferential stress at the length of maximal active force development. A_m, Cross-sectional muscle area; σ, stress; F, force; t_m, average thickness of muscle layer, a constant. (From Weiss RM, Biancani P: A rationale for ureteral tapering. *Urology* 20:482, 1982.)

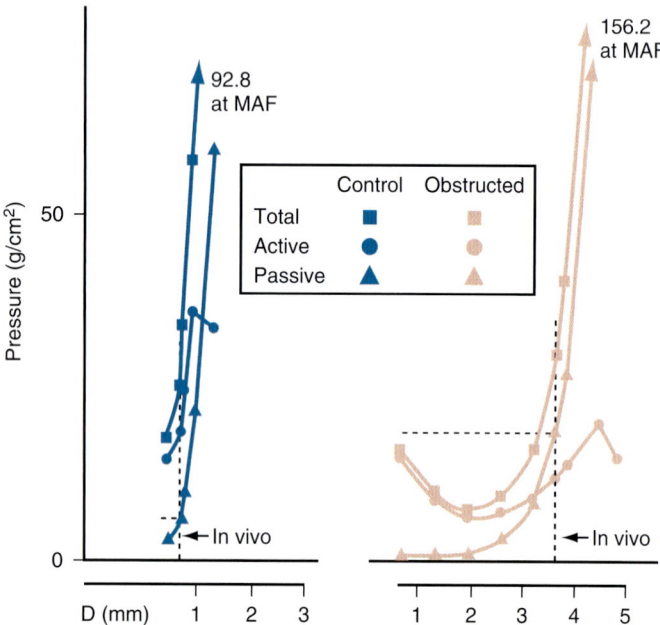

Fig. 85.23. Pressure-diameter relationships of control and obstructed ureters. Calculated total, active, and passive pressures are shown as a function of intraluminal diameter (*D*). In vivo passive pressures are indicated by *horizontal dashed lines* and in vivo dimensions by *vertical dashed lines*. (Modified from Biancani P, Hausman M, Weiss RM: Effect of obstruction on ureteral force-length relations. *Am J Physiol* 243:F204, 1982.)

duration of obstruction or the presence of infection may alter these relations.

Estimates of intraluminal pressures as a function of diameter (pressure-diameter curves) can be calculated from in vitro circumferential force-length data (Fig. 85.23; Biancani et al., 1982; Weiss and Biancani, 1982) and provide insight as to how obstruction interferes with urine transport. The validity of such calculations is supported by their correspondence to actual in vivo measurements (Biancani et al., 1976; Rose and Gillenwater, 1973). The obstructed ureter at in vivo dimensions has a higher resting (baseline) pressure and a lower contractile (active) pressure than does a control ureter. In the control ureter, the total (active plus passive or resting) pressure developed at all diameters exceeds the passive pressure marked by the horizontal dotted line, and thus the generated active or contractile pressures are able to fully coapt the ureteral lumen and propel the urine bolus. In the obstructed ureter at diameters less than 3.3 mm, the passive pressure, as marked by the horizontal dotted line, exceeds the total pressure. The contraction ring therefore is incapable of contracting below this diameter, and the pressure in the whole ureter remains approximately uniform and equal to the passive pressure. The principal effect of the contraction wave in the obstructed dilated ureter is to slightly reduce the ureteral volume and thereby slightly raise the overall resting pressure. Thus, although the obstructed ureter is able to develop greater circumferential contractile forces than the control ureter, the expected intraluminal pressure generated by the obstructed ureter would differ little from baseline (resting) pressure, and the contraction wave occurring during propagation of peristalsis would be incapable of coapting the ureteral lumen and propelling the urine bolus in an effective manner.

The calculated active pressure in the obstructed ureter estimates the pressure that would develop if the whole ureter contracted simultaneously and uniformly throughout its whole length, rather than the pressure measured in a peristaltic contraction wave, which involves contraction of only a small segment of ureter at a given time. The fact that the calculated pressures in the obstructed ureter are, if anything, a slight overestimate of expected pressures only further supports the conclusion that **the obstructed ureter is incapable of coapting its lumen and efficiently propelling the urine bolus. If, however, the urine were removed from the lumen of the ureter (e.g., by relieving the obstruction), the ureter obstructed for 2 weeks would be able to immediately coapt its lumen and produce pressures comparable with those of control ureters.** This can be appreciated from Fig. 85.24, in which the total pressure in the obstructed ureter near zero diameter can be seen to be comparable with the total pressure in the control ureter at a similar diameter. Thus **2 weeks of obstruction results in an increase in ureteral contractility but a decrease in contractile intraluminal pressures.** This decrease in the ability to generate an active intraluminal pressure and to coapt the ureteral lumen impairs urine transport in the obstructed ureter. In a mouse model it has been shown that erythropoietin accelerates return of ureteral peristaltic activity after release of obstruction. In addition, erythropoietin levels increased in the obstructed ureter, suggesting a compensatory mechanism (Jansson et al., 2015).

Obstruction of the fetal ureter also is accompanied by an increase in ureteral weight, smooth muscle mass, extracellular matrix, and the frequency and amplitude of spontaneous ureteral contractile

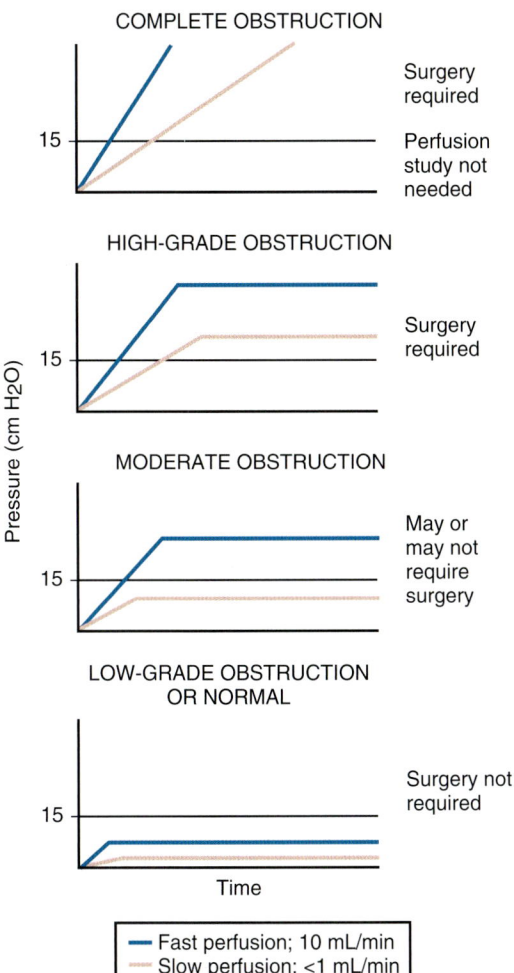

Fig. 85.24. Schematic representation of data that can be obtained with perfusion studies. A fast perfusion rate, 10 mL/min, would be used in a standard Whitaker test. A slow perfusion rate, less than 1 mL/min, would be closer to more physiologic rates of flow. (From Weiss RM: Clinical implications of ureteral physiology. *J Urol* 1979;121:401.)

activity (Santis et al., 2000). Obstructed and refluxing dilated ureters have an increase in type I and type III collagen and an increased ratio of collagen to smooth muscle (Gearhart et al., 1995; Lee et al., 1998). Obstruction also has been shown to alter the hierarchic organization of the multiple coupled pacemakers that normally coordinate peristaltic activity (Constantinou and Djurhuus, 1981; Djurhuus and Constantinou, 1982). Such disruption causes discoordination of pelvic contractility with resultant incomplete emptying of the renal pelvis that contributes to upper urinary tract dilatation. Retrograde propagation of electrical activity or absence of electrical activity has been observed distal to an experimental obstruction (Hammad et al., 2011).

Physiologic Methodologies for Assessing Clinical Obstruction

A variety of radiographic methodologies, the rationale for whose use is based on physiologic principles, are employed in the evaluation of upper urinary tract dilatation and obstruction. Description of these examinations, which include diuretic urograms, diuretic MR urography, diuretic ultrasonography, diuretic radionuclide renograms, pulsed Doppler sonographic assessment of renal vascular resistance, and ultrasonographic evaluation of ureteral peristalsis, is beyond the scope of this chapter. The best methods now available for differentiating obstructive from nonobstructive dilatation depend on assessing the efficacy of urine transport. When transport becomes inadequate, urine stagnates and dilatation occurs. **Dilation depends** on the compliance of the system and can result either from too much fluid entering the system per unit time or from too little fluid exiting the system per unit time. The properly functioning upper urinary tract should transport urine over the entire range of physiologically possible flow rates without undergoing marked deformational changes or increases in intraluminal pressure of a magnitude that would be deleterious to the function of the ureter, renal pelvis, or kidney.

Measurement of basal or resting intraluminal pressures does not help in differentiating obstructive from nonobstructive dilation because the pressures may be low even when obstruction is present (Backlund et al., 1965; Struthers, 1969; Vela-Navarrete, 1971). The values obtained vary with the state of hydration, the degree of renal function, the severity and duration of obstruction, and the compliance of the system. **Perfusion studies are used in an attempt to differentiate dilated systems that are obstructed from dilated systems that are not obstructed** (Backlund and Reuterskiöld, 1969a, 1969b; Reuterskiöld, 1969, 1970; Whitaker, 1973, 1978). The technique involves cannulating the dilated upper urinary tract and perfusing the system at a rate of 10 mL/min. Pressures are measured after the achievement of steady-state conditions, which occur when an equilibrium is reached between the flow into and out of the system. Fluoroscopic monitoring aids in the interpretation of the data. **The basic hypothesis in perfusion studies is that if the dilated upper urinary tract can transport 10 mL/min (a fluid load greater than it would ever be expected to handle during usual physiologic states) without an inordinate increase in pressure, any degree of obstruction that is present is not clinically significant.** Whitaker concluded from a large clinical experience that under these flow conditions, a pressure less than 15 cm H_2O correlates with a nonobstructive state, whereas pressures greater than 22 cm H_2O invariably correlate with clinically significant obstruction (Whitaker, 1978; Witherow and Whitaker, 1981). With this definition, minor degrees of obstruction could go undetected; however, **the presumption is that if at high flows the hydrostatic pressure in the system is not at a level that would produce renal deterioration, then lower, more physiologic flows surely will be tolerated.** The high flows are used to stress the system and thus to detect the slightest propensity to obstruction. The interpretation of data obtained by perfusion studies is schematically shown in Fig. 85.25.

To obtain relevant information, strict adherence to detail is required in the performance of perfusion studies. Care must be taken to ensure that an equilibrium state has been reached before making pressure measurements. Extrinsic factors that affect the resistance to flow, such as the needle size, length and compliance of extrinsic tubing, viscosity of the perfusion fluid, temperature, and flow rate, must be considered when quantitative data are obtained (Toguri and Fournier, 1982). Furthermore, the bladder should be continuously drained to eliminate the bladder's effect on urine transport.

When performed and interpreted properly, perfusion studies may provide clinically relevant information in select cases. The basic problem in the interpretation of data with this and other diagnostic methods is the definition of "clinically relevant obstruction"—that is, just how much resistance to flow or increase in pressure is required to produce renal functional or anatomic deterioration as a function of time, taking into account the compliance of the system (Koff and Thrall, 1981b). Also, it is theoretically possible that the wide or weakly contracting ureter at high flow rates may interfere with bolus transport even if the UVJ is normal (Griffiths, 1983). Such an obstructive process would not be detected by perfusion studies.

These theoretical considerations provide a rationale for **ureteral tapering** (Hendren, 1970). The Laplace relation provides a possible explanation for anticipated improvement in function resulting from tapering. With ureteral tapering, muscle thickness and the ability of the ureteral fibers to contract (stress) are unchanged. The decrease in radius resulting from tapering itself, according to the Laplace relation, could account for higher intraluminal pressures, which could improve urine transport. Thus the tapered ureter may coapt its walls more readily and generate higher intraluminal pressures, even though the material has not changed (Weiss and Biancani, 1982). Although the possibility of deleterious effects of the wide "nonobstructed" ureter

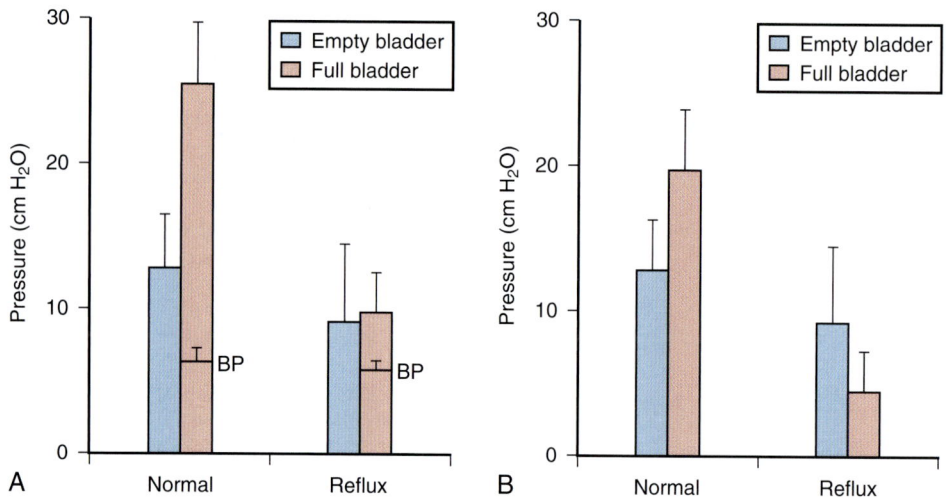

Fig. 85.25. (A) Ureterovesical junction pressures. Bladder pressure is approximately 0 cm H₂O with the bladder empty and is labeled BP with the bladder full. (B) Pressure gradient across the ureterovesical junction, obtained by subtracting the bladder pressure from the ureterovesical junction pressure. (From Weiss RM, Biancani P: Characteristics of normal and refluxing ureterovesical junctions. *J Urol* 129:858, 1983.)

remains controversial, urologists should consider such effects when interpreting data obtained with the present modalities for diagnosing obstruction and when determining management.

Relation Between Vesicoureteral Reflux and Ureteral Function

Factors that have been implicated in the development of vesicoureteral reflux (VUR) include (1) anatomic and functional abnormalities at the UVJ, (2) inordinately high intravesical pressures, and (3) impaired ureteral function. The normal intravesical ureter is approximately 1.5 cm in length and takes an oblique course through the bladder wall. It is composed of an intramural segment surrounded by detrusor muscle and a submucosal segment that lies directly under the bladder urothelium (Tanagho et al., 1968). The relation between the length and the diameter of this intravesical segment of ureter appears to be a factor in the prevention of VUR. Paquin (1959) noted that the normal ratio of intravesical tunnel length to ureteral diameter was 5:1, and Tanagho et al. (1969) noted that the ratio was 1.4:1 in children with VUR. The 5:1 ratio may be an overestimation, and a more recent study reported the proportion of intravesical ureteral length to intravesical ureteral diameter to be 2.23:1 (Oswald et al., 2003b). The ratio of intravesical ureteral length to ureteral diameter is smaller in the fetus: 0.69:1 and 1.23:1 in 11- and 20-week old fetuses, respectively (Oswald et al., 2003a). Reflux may occur when the intravesical tunnel is destroyed. Trigonal function also may be a factor in the prevention of VUR. Tanagho et al. (1965) created VUR in the cat by disruption of the trigone and by sympathectomy. The development of VUR in individuals with bladder outlet obstruction and neurogenic vesical dysfunction provides evidence that increased intravesical pressures also may be a factor in certain instances of reflux.

A significant percentage of units with VUR improve spontaneously with age. In a study by Jorgensen et al. (1984), 35% of young pigs had VUR that disappeared with age. In the pig, significant growth and organization of smooth muscle and increase in innervation occurs during the postnatal period, and this may be the anatomic correlate of maturation of the UVJ during infancy and the spontaneous functional disappearance of reflux (Pirker et al., 2007).

Although an abnormality of the UVJ is the primary etiologic factor in most cases of reflux, evidence suggests that decreased ureteral peristaltic activity can be a contributory factor. This may explain why a normal ureter may not reflux even when reimplanted into a bladder without a submucosal tunnel (Debruyne et al., 1978) or why a defunctionalized refluxing ureter may cease to reflux when a proximal diversion is taken down (Teele et al., 1976; Weiss, 1979).

The observation that VUR may temporarily cease after ureteral electric stimulation (Melick et al., 1966) further supports this possibility.

Even the mildest forms of VUR are associated with a decreased frequency of ureteral peristalsis (Kirkland et al., 1971; Weiss and Biancani, 1983). Although this may offer further evidence that decreased peristaltic activity is a possible etiologic factor in the development of reflux, an alternative interpretation is that the decreased peristaltic activity reflects changes in ureteral or renal function resulting from the reflux. Finally, **the success rate of antireflux procedures is lower with poorly functioning dilated ureters, and, although this may be related to technical factors, decreased peristaltic activity may be another reason for failure.**

Studies in normal and mildly refluxing systems have shown that there is a high-pressure zone in the distal ureter, with a resultant pressure gradient across the UVJ (Weiss and Biancani, 1983). Although the cause of the UVJ gradient is not known, the weight of the fluid within the bladder compressing the intravesical ureter may be a factor. Another causative factor may be bladder or trigonal tension involving myogenic or neurohumoral mechanisms. With bladder filling, there is an increase in the amplitude of the high-pressure zone that is greater in nonrefluxing than in refluxing systems. With bladder filling, the resultant UVJ-bladder pressure gradient increases in nonrefluxing systems, whereas it decreases and may disappear in refluxing systems (Fig. 85.26; Weiss and Biancani, 1983). This decrease in pressure gradient may correspond to the time when reflux occurs and may be related to lateralization of the ureteral orifice and shortening of the intravesical tunnel. More recent studies have shown a decrease in basal and maximum pressures at the UVJ of refluxing ureters that correlated with histologic changes (Arena et al., 2007). The histologic changes included a degree of smooth muscle deterioration and atrophy, an increase in collagen deposition, and fewer c-KIT–positive ICC-like cells at the UVJ in patients with VUR (Arena et al., 2007; Oswald et al., 2004; Schwentner et al., 2005). Matrix metalloproteinase-1 (MMP-1) production and the number of CD68+ macrophages are increased, whereas S-100–positive myelinated nerves are decreased in the distal portion of refluxing ureters (Oswald et al., 2004; Radmayr et al., 2010). MMP-1 cleaves collagen and is frequently seen in collagen-rich regions. Some MMPs can damage nerves. CD68+ macrophages presumably phagocytize cells undergoing apoptosis. TGF-β1 levels were found to be higher and VEGF levels lower in refluxing ureters (Izol et al., 2014). Furthermore, deletion of fibroblast growth factor receptor 2 was associated with a high incidence of VUR in newborn mice (Narla et al., 2017). A heterozygous null mutation in odd-skipped related 1 (*Osr1*), a transcriptional repressor involved in maintaining the mesenchymal stem cell population, is

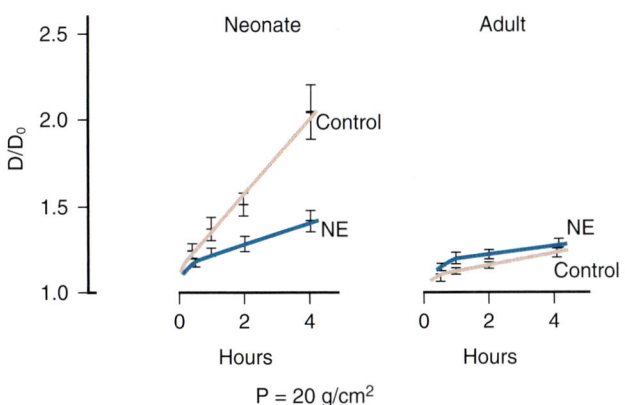

Fig. 85.26. Changes in diameter of neonatal and adult rabbit ureteral segments as a function of time after the application of a constant intraluminal pressure (P) of 20 g/cm². Diametral deformation (D/D₀) of control neonatal ureters was significantly greater than that of control adult ureters. Norepinephrine (10^{-5} M) decreased the diametral deformation of the neonatal ureters but had no significant effect on the deformation of the adult ureteral segments. D, Diameter during deformation; D₀, initial diameter. (From Akimoto M, Biancani P, Weiss RM: Comparative pressure = length − diameter relationships of neonatal and adult rabbit ureters. *Invest Urol* 14:297, 1977.)

associated with a 21% incidence of VUR and a shortened intravesical tunnel in newborn mice and has been considered a candidate gene in the development of VUR in humans (Fillion et al., 2017). *Pax2*, a nuclear transcription factor involved in the development of the urinary tract, was increased in refluxing human ureters (Zheng et al., 2015). Contraction of the longitudinal muscles at the UVJ also may function as an active antireflux mechanism (Schwentner et al., 2005).

Effect of Infection on Ureteral Function

Infection within the upper urinary tract may impair urine transport. Pyelonephritis in the monkey has been associated with decreased peristaltic activity (Roberts, 1975). Furthermore, Rose and Gillenwater (1973) have shown that infection can potentiate the deleterious effects of obstruction on ureteral function. In 1913 Primbs showed that *Escherichia coli* and staphylococcal toxins inhibited contractions of in vitro guinea pig ureteral segments. **A number of studies have confirmed that bacteria and *E. coli* endotoxin can inhibit ureteral activity** (Grana et al., 1965; King and Cox, 1972), although these findings have not been universal (Struthers, 1976; Thulesius and Araj, 1987). Uropathogenic *E. coli* (UPEC) decreased phasic and potassium induced contractions of isolated human and rat ureteral segments (Floyd et al., 2010). These inhibitory changes were due to activation of K⁺ channels with resultant inhibition of calcium entry through voltage dependent L-type calcium channels. UPEC also caused impairment of urothelial barrier function. Urothelial cells show an increased expression of iNOS in response to bacterial invasion. Activation of iNOS leads to the formation of NO a known smooth muscle relaxant, and this may contribute to inhibitory effects of infection on ureteral contractility (Poljakovic and Persson, 2003).

In humans, irregular peristaltic contractions with an often-decreased amplitude have been recorded with infection, and an absence of activity has been noted in the more severe cases (Ross et al., 1972). Furthermore, ureteral dilation has been reported to result from retroperitoneal inflammatory processes secondary to appendicitis, regional enteritis, ulcerative colitis, or peritonitis (Makker et al., 1972). Infection also may reduce the compliance of the intravesical ureter and permit reflux to occur in situations in which the UVJ is intrinsically of marginal competence (Cook and King, 1979).

Effect of Calculi and Stents on Ureteral Function

Factors that affect the spontaneous passage of calculi are (1) the size and shape of the stone (Ueno et al., 1977); (2) intrinsic areas of narrowing within the ureter; (3) ureteral peristalsis; (4) hydrostatic pressure of the column of urine proximal to the calculus (Sivula and Lehtonen, 1967); **and (5) edema, inflammation, and spasm of the ureter at the site at which the stone is lodged** (Holmlund and Hassler, 1965).

In an attempt to understand the physiologic processes that contribute to or hinder the passage of stones through the ureter, Crowley et al. (1990) created acute ureteral obstruction in the dog with an intraluminal balloon catheter and measured intraluminal ureteral pressures and peristaltic activity above and below the acutely obstructed site. The peristaltic rate and baseline, peak, and delta (peak minus baseline) pressures increased proximal to the site of obstruction. In contrast, the peristaltic rate remained unchanged distal to the obstruction, despite decreases in the baseline, peak, and delta pressures. It has been suggested that failure of transmission of effective peristalsis across the site of obstruction may hinder stone passage. Implantation of an artificial calculus in a rat ureter resulted in an increase in the amplitude of contractions, a decrease in the rate of contractions, and a decrease in baseline pressure (Laird et al., 1997). These changes persisted for a period after spontaneous passage of the calculus. It was suggested that the increased motility caused by a stone contributes to the visceral pain associated with ureteral stone passage.

Two factors that appear to be most useful in facilitating stone passage are an increase in hydrostatic pressure proximal to a calculus and relaxation of the ureter in the region of the stone. In support of the theory that hydrostatic pressure facilitates stone passage, artificial concretions with holes were shown to move more slowly in the rabbit and dog ureter than those without holes (Sivula and Lehtonen, 1967). Furthermore, ureteral ligation proximal to a concretion, which decreases hydrostatic pressure by decreasing urine output and decreases peristaltic activity proximal to a stone, hampers stone passage (Sivula and Lehtonen, 1967).

With respect to the potential facilitative effect of ureteral relaxation on stone passage, spasmolytic agents phentolamine, an α-adrenergic antagonist, and orciprenaline and isoproterenol β-adrenergic agonists have been shown to dilate the ureteral lumen or decrease ureteral wall tension at the level of an artificial concretion and thus permit increased fluid flow beyond the concretion (Miyatake et al., 2001; Peters and Eckstein, 1975). **Pharmacologic data can be interpreted to imply that ureteral relaxation in the region of a concretion could aid in stone passage.** Agents such as theophylline (Green et al., 1987; Weiss et al., 1977), with strong relaxant effects on the ureter, have potential value in facilitating stone passage. It also has been reported that local aminophylline facilitates ureteroscopy and transureteral lithotripsy (Barzegarnezhad et al., 2012) and that endoluminal administration of isoproterenol reduces renal pelvic pressures during flexible ureterorenoscopy (Jakobsen, 2013) and facilitates passage of ureteral access sheaths during ureterorenoscopy in a pig model (Lildal et al., 2016). In a rabbit in vivo model rolipram, a cAMP-specific PDE inhibitor (PDE4 inhibitor), caused a more marked ureteral relaxation than did the nonspecific PDE inhibitors, papaverine and theophylline, and without the circulatory side effects seen with the nonspecific PDE inhibitors (Becker et al., 1998). Because the relaxant effect of rolipram was similar in human and rabbit in vitro ureteral segments, it was suggested that rolipram could potentially be beneficial in the treatment of renal colic and in the facilitation of stone passage (Becker et al., 1998). Rolipram also has been shown to relax pig intravesical ureteral segments (Hernández et al., 2004). In addition to the PDE4 inhibitor rolipram, PDE5 inhibitors (cGMP-specific PDE inhibitors) relax in vitro pig, sheep, and human ureteral segments (Al-Aown et al., 2011; Kuhn et al., 2000; Kyriazis et al., 2015; Liatsikos et al., 2013). The relaxant effects of PDE4 and PDE5 inhibitors were paralleled by an increase in cAMP and cGMP, respectively. Gratzke et al. (2007) showed that PDE5 inhibitors reversed KCl-induced increases in tension of isolated human ureteral segments, with a rank order of efficacy (most efficient to least) of vardenafil (Levitra), sildenafil (Viagra), then tadalafil (Cialis). Species differences in PDE subtypes may exist. Although the nonspecific PDE inhibitor papaverine decreased the frequency of ureteral peristalsis in the pig, the PDE4 inhibitor, rolipram, had no effect (Danuser et al., 2001).

A combination of the calcium channel blocker nifedipine, which causes ureteral relaxation and the corticosteroid deflazacort, which reduces edema, was shown to facilitate spontaneous passage of 1-cm or smaller distal ureteral stones (Borghi et al., 1994; Porpiglia et al., 2000). Spontaneous expulsion of 79% of stones (average size 5.8±1.8 mm) occurred in an average of 7 days in patients treated with nifedipine and deflazacort compared with spontaneous passage of 35% of stones (average size 5.5±1.4 mm) within an average of 20 days in untreated patients (Porpiglia et al., 2000). In a subsequent study, this same group showed that nifedipine and the α-adrenergic antagonist tamsulosin, when combined with deflazacort, increased the rate of spontaneous passage of lower ureteral calculi, and that, in addition, tamsulosin, a selective $α_{1A/1D}$-adrenergic receptor antagonist, reduced the time to spontaneous expulsion (Porpiglia et al., 2004, 2006). They showed that tamsulosin alone was effective in facilitating expulsion of distal ureteral stones, and that this effect was potentiated by steroids. Steroids alone were ineffective. $α_1$-Adrenergic receptors are present throughout the human ureter with the greatest quantity of $α_1$-adrenergic receptors being in the distal ureter (Sigala et al., 2004, 2005). $α_{1D}$ mRNA was expressed throughout the human ureter, with significantly greater amounts than the $α_{1A}$- and $α_{1B}$-receptor subtypes in the proximal and distal ureter. $α1_{A/1D}$-Adrenergic receptors are present in the distal ureter. **A number of other studies have noted an increased spontaneous stone expulsion rate and expulsion rate after ESWL, a decrease in renal colic, and an improved tolerance of ureteral stents with the administration of tamsulosin and other α-adrenergic antagonists** (Al-Ansari et al., 2010; Autorino et al., 2005; Cervenakov et al., 2002; Dellabella et al., 2003; De Sio et al., 2006; El Said et al., 2015; Gravas et al., 2007; Gravina et al., 2005; Kupeli et al., 2004; Liatsikos et al., 2007; Liu et al., 2015; Losek and Mauro, 2008; Lu et al., 2012a; Resim et al., 2005; Sur et al., 2015; Yencilek et al., 2010; Yilmaz et al., 2005). Yilmaz et al. (2005) reported that doxazosin and terazosin were equally effective in facilitating stone passage, and Dellabella et al. (2005) reported that tamsulosin was more effective than the calcium channel blocker nifedipine in facilitating stone expulsion. Naftopidil, an $α_{1D}$-adrenergic receptor antagonist, also has been reported to be effective in facilitating the expulsion of intramural ureteral stones (Lu et al., 2012b), although others have failed to show effectiveness of naftopidil in medical expulsive therapy (MET) (Cho et al., 2017). Furthermore, a large multicenter analysis failed to show effectiveness of either nifedipine or tamsulosin in aiding stone passage (Pickard et al., 2015).

Indwelling ureteral stents are frequently used to bypass an obstructing ureteral calculus and/or to dilate the ureter to facilitate subsequent ureterorenoscopy. A variety of α-adrenergic antagonists have been used to ameliorate stent-induced discomfort (Beddingfield et al., 2009; Damiano et al., 2008; Dellis et al., 2014). In addition to ureteral dilation, stents decrease ureteral activity, increase tissue inflammation and decrease expression of GLi1, a downstream target of Shh signaling (Janssen et al., 2017).

Effect of Diabetes on Ureteral Function

In cases of diabetes, changes in bladder function affect the ureter. In addition, there is some evidence of a direct effect of diabetes on the ureter. The length and velocity of movement of the urinary bolus is decreased in the streptozotocin (STZ) diabetic rat (Watanabe and Miyagawa, 2002). Although the frequency of contractions of in vitro segments of the renal pelvis and ureter of STZ-induced diabetic rats are unchanged, the amplitude of contractions is increased in comparison with renal pelvic and ureteral segments from control sucrose-induced diuretic rats (Davidson and Lang, 2007). Capsaicin is known to release tachykinins from sensory nerves and it is postulated that a supersensitivity of the upper urinary tract of STZ-induced diabetic rats to the sensory neurotoxin capsaicin, and to the sensory excitatory neuropeptides substance P and neurokinin A, results from a sensory neuropathy (Davidson and Lang, 2007).

Effect of Age on Ureteral Function

Clinically, the response of the ureter to pathologic conditions varies with age. **More marked degrees of ureteral dilatation are observed in the neonate and young child than in the adult.** Experimental data corroborating this clinical impression can be derived from observed age-dependent differences in the response of in vitro ureteral segments to an intraluminal pressure load. The neonatal rabbit ureter undergoes a greater degree of deformation in response to an applied intraluminal pressure than does the adult rabbit ureter (Akimoto et al., 1977). Furthermore, norepinephrine decreases the diametral deformation of the neonatal rabbit ureter in response to an applied intraluminal pressure but has little effect on the deformation of the adult rabbit ureter (Fig. 85.27). Thus the in vitro neonatal rabbit ureter appears to be more compliant and more sensitive to norepinephrine than the adult rabbit ureter.

Age also affects the response of the ureter to β-adrenergic agonists; with aging there is a decrease in the relaxant response to the β-adrenergic agonist isoproterenol (Wheeler et al., 1990). The relaxant response to β-adrenergic agonists is related, in part, to cAMP levels. It has been shown that with aging there is a decrease in the enzymatic activities involved in the synthesis of cAMP (Wheeler et al., 1986) but no change in the enzymatic activities involved in cAMP degradation (Cho et al., 1988). These data suggest that the decrease in the ability of isoproterenol to relax the ureter with aging is due to a decrease in the ability of isoproterenol to activate adenylyl cyclase, the enzyme involved in cAMP synthesis. Developmental differences in the response of the ureter to metabolic inhibitors are evident, with cyanide causing a larger decrease in force in the adult than in the neonatal guinea pig ureter (Bullock and Wray, 1998a, 1998b). Furthermore, the response to 5-HT$_2$ is greater in a young than an old pig ureter (Lim et al., 2018).

A progressive increase in ureteral cross-sectional muscle area is observed in the guinea pig between 3 weeks and 3 years of age. This is in accord with the findings of Cussen (1967), who noted in a human autopsy study of subjects ranging in age from 12 weeks' gestation to 12 years, a progressive increase in the population and a small increase in the overall size of the individual smooth muscle cells with age. In addition, an irregular increase in the number of elastic fibers was observed with increasing age.

The contractility of the ureter also is affected by age. The maximal active force of isolated guinea pig ureteral segments increases between 3 weeks and 3 years of age (see Fig. 85.27) (Hong et al., 1980). The increase in force developed between 3 weeks and 3 months of age seems to be attributable to an increase in contractility, because there is an associated increase in active stress (force per unit area of muscle). The increase in force developed between 3 months and 3 years of age can be explained by an increase in muscle mass alone because there is no change in active stress between these two age groups (see Fig. 85.27).

Although changes in the force-length relations of guinea pig ureter occur with age, the force-velocity relations do not change with age (Biancani et al., 1984). Thus, although ureteral contractility increases during early development, as shown by an increase in force per unit area of muscle, or stress, no significant change is apparent in the rate of the driving reactions that control the contractile process, that is, no change in shortening, velocity, work, or power.

EFFECT OF PREGNANCY ON URETERAL FUNCTION

Hydroureteronephrosis of pregnancy begins in the second trimester of gestation and subsides within the first month after parturition. It is more severe on the right side, and the ureteral dilatation does not occur below the pelvic brim. Roberts (1976) **has presented a strong case in favor of obstruction as the etiologic factor in the development of hydroureteronephrosis of pregnancy, whereas other investigators have suggested a hormonal mechanism for the ureteral dilatation of pregnancy** (van Wagenen and Jenkins, 1939).

Roberts (1976) emphasized the following: (1) Elevated baseline (resting) ureteral pressures consistent with obstructive changes have been recorded above the pelvic brim in pregnant women, and these pressures decrease when positional changes permit the uterus to fall away from the ureters (Sala and Rubi, 1967). (2) Normal ureteral contractile pressures recorded during pregnancy suggest that

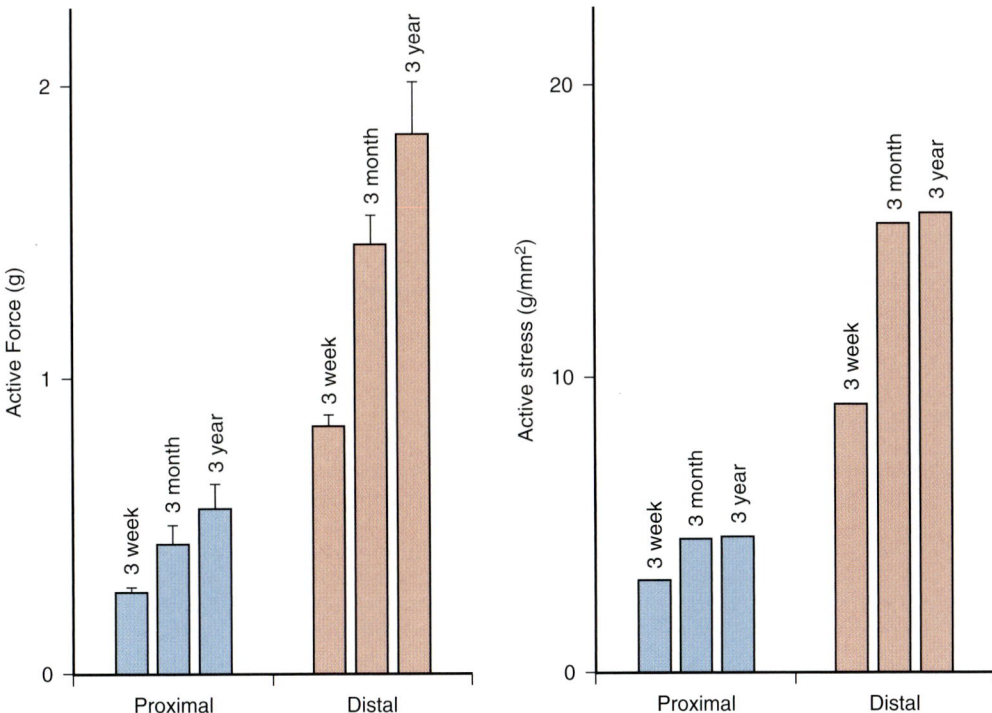

Fig. 85.27. Maximal active (contractile) force and maximal active stress of proximal and distal guinea pig ureteral segments as a function of age.

hormonally induced ureteral atony is not the prime factor in ureteral dilatation of pregnancy. (3) Women whose ureters do not cross the pelvic brim (i.e., those with pelvic kidneys or ileal conduits) do not develop hydronephrosis of pregnancy. (4) Hydronephrosis of pregnancy usually does not occur in quadrupeds, whose uterus hangs away from the ureters (Traut and Kuder, 1938). (5) Elevated ureteral pressures in the pregnant monkey return to normal when the uterus is elevated from the ureters at laparotomy or when the fetus and placenta are removed from the uterus.

Observed hormonal effects on ureteral function have been used to implicate a hormonal mechanism in the ureteral dilatation of pregnancy, although difficulties in interpretation arise from inconsistencies in the data. Several studies have shown an inhibitory effect of **progesterone** on ureteral function (Kumar, 1962). Progesterone has been noted to increase the degree of ureteral dilatation during pregnancy and to retard the rate of disappearance of hydroureter in postpartum women (Lubin et al., 1941). Other studies, however, have failed to demonstrate an effect of progesterone on ureteral activity in animals (McNellis and Sherline, 1967) or in humans (Lapides, 1948), and still others have failed to induce changes in ureteral activity in women through the administration of estrogens, progesterone, or a mixture of these drugs (Clayton and Roberts, 1973; Marchant, 1972). Although some have noted that estrogens increase ureteral activity (Hundley et al., 1942), the majority of investigators have failed to observe an effect of estrogens in animal models (Abramson et al., 1953) or in humans (Kumar, 1962). Thus **obstruction appears to be the primary factor in the development of hydronephrosis of pregnancy,** although some evidence suggests that a combination of hormonal and obstructive factors is involved (Fainstat, 1963).

EFFECT OF DRUGS ON THE URETER

This section provides an assessment of the effects of the major classes of drugs on ureteral function. Many of the studies referred to were performed in animal models, and extrapolation of the data to the intact human ureter is often difficult. In the clinical situation, the relatively sparse blood supply to the ureter limits the distribution of drugs to the ureter, and the pharmacokinetics are different in the laboratory than in the clinic. In addition, many drugs with potential usefulness in the management of ureteral abnormalities have potential untoward side effects when used in concentrations required to affect the ureter.

To assess the effect of drugs on the ureter, it is necessary to understand the anatomic, physiologic, and biochemical properties of the ureter, in addition to understanding the principles of drug action. For a drug to elicit a given response, it is necessary to achieve and maintain an appropriate concentration of that drug at its site of action. Factors that can influence the achievement of an effective concentration of drug at a site of action are (1) the route of administration and cellular distribution of the drug; (2) the dosage of the drug administered; (3) the biotransformation, including metabolism and excretion, of the drug; (4) the binding of the drug to plasma and tissue proteins; and (5) the effects of age and disease on the absorption, distribution, metabolism, and elimination of the drug.

The literature contains considerable confusing and conflicting information concerning the effects of drugs on the ureter. To some extent, the discrepancies in the available data are due to poorly controlled experimental procedures or to attempts to compare dissimilar functional responses of the ureter with a given drug. To simplify the present section, no attempt is made to analyze the validity of each pharmacologic study or to rationalize discrepancies in the literature; rather, an overview is presented with an attempt to provide a consensus that, at times, may be prejudiced by personal bias. Furthermore, discussion of drugs related to the nervous system, pregnancy, and a variety of pathologic states is included in earlier sections of this chapter, and will not be duplicated in this section.

Histamine and Its Antagonists

Histamine has a dual action on smooth muscle; it may (1) release catecholamines from sympathetic nerve endings or (2) act directly on receptors within the smooth muscle. In addition, **histamine may have excitatory or inhibitory effects on ureteral function.** The majority of studies have shown an excitatory effect of histamine on ureteral function (Benedito et al., 1991; Borgstedt et al., 1962; Sharkey et al., 1965; Smita et al., 2006; Vereecken, 1973), a finding that may be species dependent (Tindall, 1972). **Histamine's excitatory effect on the ureter and UVJ appears to be mediated by H$_1$ receptors** as they are inhibited by the H$_1$-receptor antagonists mepyramine, pheniramine, and dimethindene but not by the H$_2$-receptor antagonists cimetidine and ranitidine (Benedito et al., 1991; Dodel et al., 1996; Smita et al., 2006). An H$_1$ agonist, 2-(2-pyridyl)ethylamine, increases ureteral contractility (Dodel et al., 1996). The H$_1$ inhibitor, pheniramine, has no effect on spontaneous activity of isolated goat ureter (Smita et al., 2006). The excitatory effect of histamine on the sheep UVJ is partially blocked by scopolamine, suggesting an indirect stimulatory action of histamine on intramural parasympathetic nerves. H$_1$ histamine receptors are expressed in the smooth muscle and urothelium of the human ureter (Floyd et al., 2008). The antihistamines diphenhydramine (Benadryl) and tripelennamine have been shown to inhibit the effects of histamine on the ureter (Borgstedt et al., 1962; Sharkey et al., 1965). **The H$_2$ receptor mediates inhibitory effects of histamine.** Histamine and the H$_2$-receptor agonist impromidine relax precontracted ureteral segments, actions that are inhibited by the H$_2$-receptor antagonist cimetidine (Dodel et al., 1996).

Serotonin

Serotonin (5-hydroxytryptamine, 5-HT) usually has been reported to stimulate the ureter (Dodel et al., 1996; Hauser et al., 2002; Hernández et al., 2003; Lim et al., 2018; Vereecken, 1973), although serotonin has been reported to inhibit ureteral contractility (Mazzella and Schroeder, 1960), or to have no effect (Finberg and Peart, 1970) on a variety of ureteral preparations. In the pig ureter the contractile effects appear to be mediated by 5-HT$_2$ receptors (Hauser et al., 2002; Hernández et al., 2003), specifically the 5-HT$_{2A}$ subtype (Lim et al., 2018). Gidener et al. (1999) showed that 5-hydroxytryptamine induces concentration-dependent contractions of isolated human ureteral segments. Tetrodotoxin, guanethidine, and phentolamine had an inhibitory effect on 5-HT–induced contractions of pig isolated intravesical ureteral segments, suggesting that part of the contractile effects of 5-HT are indirectly mediated through release of norepinephrine from sympathetic nerves (Hernández et al., 2003).

Kinins

The kinins—kallidin, eledoisin, and bradykinin—increase the frequency of contraction and baseline intraluminal pressure of the dog ureter (Boyarsky et al., 1966a, b; Labay and Boyarsky, 1966). Although bradykinin has been reported to increase the contractility of pig intravesical ureter via excitation of bradykinin B2 receptors (Ribeiro et al., 2016), it has been reported to decrease the contractile force of the sheep ureter (Kaygisiz et al., 1995).

Angiotensin

Angiotensin has a stimulatory effect on the ureter. Angiotensin II (AT2) and mRNA for angiotensinogen, a principal precursor of AT2, renin, angiotensin-converting enzyme (ACE), and the type I angiotensin receptor are expressed in the human ureter (Santis et al., 2003). The AT2 type I receptor also is expressed in the rat ureter (Paxton et al., 1993). Losartin, an AT2-receptor antagonist, decreases the amplitude and frequency of spontaneous contractions of human ureteral segments (Jankovik et al., 2016). AT2 induces phasic contractions of rat ureteral segments, an effect that is inhibited by losartan (Fujinaka et al., 2000).

Narcotic Analgesics

Morphine has been reported to increase ureteral tone or the frequency and amplitude of ureteral contractions or both in a variety of experimental preparations and in humans (Macht, 1916b; Gruber, 1928; Ockerblad et al., 1935; Vereecken, 1973). Others, however, have failed to observe an effect of morphine on ureteral function (Gould et al., 1955; Kiil, 1957; Ross et al., 1967; Weinberg and Maletta, 1961).

Meperidine (Demerol) appears to have a similar excitatory effect on the activity of the intact dog ureter (Sharkey et al., 1968). Kiil (1957), however, failed to observe an effect of meperidine on ureteral peristalsis in humans. **If one considers only the effects on ureteral activity, there is no basis to preferentially favor morphine or meperidine in the treatment of renal colic. Both agents may have ureteral spasmogenic effects that theoretically would detract from their value in the management of ureteral colic. They certainly do not have potentially valuable spasmolytic actions. Their efficacy in treating colic depends on their central nervous system (CNS) actions, which decrease the perception of pain.**

Prostaglandins

Prostaglandins are derived from fatty acids and have a variety of biologic actions in various systems of the body. Their effects vary with the species, type of prostaglandin, endocrine status of the tissue, experimental conditions, and origin of the smooth muscle. **The "primary" prostaglandins (PGs), PGE$_1$, PGE$_2$, and PGF$_{2\alpha}$, are synthesized from the fatty acid arachidonic acid by enzymatic reactions involving two cyclooxygenase (COX) isoforms, COX-1 and COX-2** (Vane, 1998). In most tissues COX-1 is constitutively expressed and is involved in the regulation of normal physiologic processes, whereas COX-2 is induced in response to processes such as inflammation and mitogenesis (Mitchell and Warner, 1999). **These enzymatic reactions can be inhibited by indomethacin and aspirin, and by a number of COX-1 and COX-2 inhibitors.** COX-1 and COX-2 receptors have been identified in the human ureter (Chaignat et al., 2008).

Prostaglandin E$_2$ acts via four G-protein–coupled receptors, PTGER$_{1-4}$, and prostaglandin F$_{2\alpha}$ acts via PTGFR. PTGER$_1$ and PTGER$_3$ induce smooth muscle contractions, PTGER$_1$ via activation of phosphatidylinositol hydrolysis and PTGER$_3$ via cAMP inhibition. Prostaglandin receptors PTGER$_1$ and PTGFR$_3$ are highly expressed in human ureter urothelium and muscle (Oll et al., 2012). PTGER2 and PTGER4 induce smooth muscle relaxation via cAMP stimulation.

PGE$_1$ inhibits the activity of the dog (Abrams and Feneley, 1976; Boyarsky et al., 1966b; Wooster, 1971) and guinea pig ureter (Vermue and Den Hertog, 1987). PGE$_1$ inhibition of ureteral activity in the guinea pig is associated with an increase in cAMP levels (Vermue and Den Hertog, 1987). In the ureter, PGE$_1$ activates adenylyl cyclase, and this may account for the increase in cAMP (Wheeler et al., 1986). Johns and Wooster (1975) suggested that the inhibitory effects of PGE$_1$ on ureteral activity depended on the sequestration of Ca^{2+} at the inner surface of the cell membrane, with a resultant increase in outward K$^+$ conductance and hyperpolarization of the membrane.

Although reports have indicated that PGE$_2$ relaxes the ureter (Vermue and Den Hertog, 1987), other reports describe an excitatory action of PGE$_2$ on sheep (Thulesius and Angelo-Khattar, 1985), dog (Boyarsky and Labay, 1969), and human (Angelo-Khattar et al., 1985; Cole et al., 1988) ureters and on renal pelvic smooth muscle (Lundstam et al., 1985). Although PGE$_2$ relaxes normal porcine ureter, it increases the contractility of acutely obstructed porcine ureters (Ankem et al., 2005; Lowry et al., 2005) and chronically obstructed human ureters. In human ureteral preparations PGE$_1$ and PGE$_2$ have been shown to decrease spontaneous contractions, whereas **PGF$_{2\alpha}$** increased ureteral contractility (Abrams and Feneley, 1976). In human renal pelvis and ureter there is a higher concentration of PGF$_{2\alpha}$ than PGE$_2$ (Zwergel et al., 1991). **PGF$_{2\alpha}$** increased contractility of porcine ureteral segments (Ankem et al., 2005). The prostanoid PGI$_2$ is synthesized in the urothelium of the ureter (Ali et al., 1998). COX inhibitors such as indomethacin have been shown to inhibit the activity of rat (Davidson and Lang, 2000), guinea pig (Davidson and Lang, 2000), sheep (Thulesius and Angelo-Khattar, 1985), and human ureters (Angelo-Khattar et al., 1985; Cole et al., 1988) and renal pelvic smooth muscle (Davidson and Lang, 2000; Lundstam et al., 1985; Santicioli et al., 1995a; Zhang and Lang, 1994).

Indomethacin has been employed in the management of ureteral colic (Flannigan et al., 1983; Holmlund and Sjöden, 1978; Jönsson et al., 1987). The beneficial effects probably are due to indomethacin's inhibition of the prostaglandin-mediated vasodilatation that occurs subsequent to obstruction (Allen et al., 1978; Sjöden et al., 1982). The vasodilatation theoretically would result in an increase in glomerular capillary pressure and a subsequent increase in pelviureteral pressure. Indomethacin, by reducing pelviureteral pressure and thus pelviureteral wall tension, may eliminate some of the pain of renal colic that is dependent on distention of the upper urinary tract. An upregulation of COX-2 mRNA and protein with obstruction supports the potential use of selective COX-2 inhibitors in the treatment of obstructive ureteral disease (Nakada et al., 2002). **A potential problem with the use of indomethacin for the treatment of renal colic is that prostaglandin-mediated vasodilatation aids in preserving renal function; thus indomethacin may provide pain relief, but it may be potentially deleterious to renal function** (Kristova et al., 2000; Perlmutter et al., 1993).

The nonspecific COX inhibitor, diclofenac, and the selective COX-2 inhibitors, NS-398 and celecoxib, have been shown to be equipotent in inhibiting agonist-induced contractions of isolated pig and human ureter (Mastrangelo et al., 2000; Nakada et al., 2000). Diclofenac also has been shown to relax human ureteral segments that were precontracted with KCl (Sivrikava et al., 2003). NS-398 inhibition of ureteral contractility also may involve blockade of voltage-dependent calcium channels (Lee et al., 2010). The COX-2 selective inhibitor celecoxib, and indomethacin-inhibited porcine ureteral contractility and TNF-α induced prostanoid release (Jerde et al., 2005). Diclofenac, but not the COX-2 selective inhibitor valdecoxib, decreased the contractile amplitude of electrically stimulated in vitro human ureteral segments and valdecoxib decreased the contractility of normal, but not obstructed, ureters of the pig in vivo (Chaignat et al., 2008). Species differences may exist with COX-2 as the primary enzyme involved in synthesizing PGs in the guinea pig upper urinary tract, and COX-1 the primary enzyme involved in PG synthesis in the rat upper urinary tract (Davidson and Lang, 2000).

Chronic obstruction upregulates COX-2 activity in the human ureter (Nakada et al., 2002). With stretch of the porcine ureter there is COX-2 induction in the urothelial and smooth muscle layers, with a more significant induction in the urothelium (Jerde et al., 2006). The stretch-induced upregulation on COX-2 expression in the urothelium of the obstructed mouse ureter is mediated via phosphatidylinositol 3-kinase (PI3K) (Owusu-Ofori et al., 2013). PI3K also mediates stretch-induced activation of protein kinase C (Owusu-Ofori et al., 2013). In the normal rat ureter COX-1, but not COX-2, mRNA was detected, and after obstruction there was an increase in COX-2 mRNA and protein expression, but no change in COX-1 expression (Norregaard et al., 2006). In addition to an increased synthesis of prostanoids with obstruction, there is a decrease in prostanoid degradation contributing to the increase in prostanoids with obstruction. 15-Hydroxyprostaglandin dehydrogenase (PGDH), the enzyme responsible for prostaglandin degradation, is suppressed in the human ureter with obstruction (Jerde et al., 2004). The dilated ureter after obstruction has an increase expression of COX-2, PGE$_2$, TGF-β$_1$, α-smooth muscle actin (α-SMA), fibrosis, apoptotic cells, and proliferation cell nuclear antigen (PCNA) (Chuang et al., 2007). The administration of the COX-2 selective inhibitor celecoxib abolished the expression of COX-2 and PGE$_2$, decreased the expression of TGF-β$_1$ and α-SMA, decreased apoptotic cells and fibrosis, but increased the expression of PCNA in the smooth muscle of the dilated obstructed ureter (Chuang et al., 2007). These investigators concluded that the COX-2 inhibitor may ameliorate, in part by inhibition of COX-2 and TGF-β$_1$ expression, ureteral damage resulting from obstruction.

CARDIAC GLYCOSIDES

Ouabain, a cardiac glycoside, has an effect on ureteral activity that appears to be species dependent. In the isolated cat ureter, ouabain produces a marked increase in contractility, which usually is followed by a late decrease in excitability (Weiss et al., 1970). In the guinea pig ureter, ouabain inhibits activity without a preliminary potentiation of contractility (Hendrickx et al., 1975; Washizu, 1968). The inhibitory effects of ouabain are accompanied by a shortening of the action potential duration, a decrease of the number of oscillations on the plateau of the guinea pig action potential, and a decrease in the RMP.

Calcium Antagonists

Because Ca^{2+} is necessary for the development of the action potential and contraction of the ureter, agents that block the movement of Ca^{2+} into the cell would be expected to depress ureteral function. Voltage-dependent Ca^{2+} channel antagonist–binding sites (receptors) have been demonstrated in the ureter, and their density decreases with age (Yoshida et al., 1992). These dihydropyridine-sensitive, **L-type, voltage-dependent Ca^{2+} channels appear to provide the main inward current for generation of the ureteral action potential and the phasic contractile response** (Aickin et al., 1984; Brading et al., 1983; Imaizumi et al., 1989; Lang, 1989; Shuba, 1977). Potassium-induced ureteral contractions depend on the inward movement of Ca^{2+} through L-type voltage-dependent Ca^{2+} channels (Maggi and Giuliani, 1995). The dihydropyridine Ca^{2+} channel agonist Bay K 8644 has an excitatory effect on ureteral activity (Floyd et al., 2008; Maggi et al., 1994a) and potentiates K^+-induced contractions. The Ca^{2+} channel blockers (CCB) verapamil, D-600 (a methoxy derivative of verapamil), diltiazem, and nifedipine have been shown to inhibit ureteral activity (Davenport et al., 2006; Golenhofen and Lammel, 1972; Hertle and Nawrath, 1984; Hong et al., 1985; Maggi et al., 1994a; Sakanashi et al., 1985, 1986; Vereecken et al., 1975). More recently, the new CCB benidipine was shown to inhibit the contractility of the distal ureter (at lower concentration than in the proximal ureter) in goats, and inhibited the amplitude rather than the frequency of contractions (Mathew et al., 2017). These inhibitory effects are accompanied by decreases in the duration of the action potential, the number of oscillations on the plateau of the guinea pig action potential, excitability, and the rate of rise and amplitude of the action potential. High concentrations of verapamil and D-600 cause a complete cessation of electric and mechanical activity.

Potassium Channel Openers

Potassium channel openers such as cromakalim, nicorandil, BRL 38227, and PFK217-744b hyperpolarize smooth muscle membranes and **inhibit renal pelvic and ureteral activity** (Floyd et al., 2008; Kontani et al., 1993; Maggi et al., 1994c; Smita et al., 2006; Weiss et al., 2002). Glibenclamide, a blocker of K^+/ATP channels, on its own, had no effect on contractility (De Moura and De Lemos Neto, 1996). The inhibitory effects of cromakalim and nicorandil are prevented by glibenclamide, providing evidence that ATP-sensitive K^+ channels are involved in these processes (Maggi et al., 1994c; Smita et al., 2006). Activation of these K+ channels may reduce the probability of the opening of voltage-sensitive Ca^{2+} channels, inhibit agonist induced increases in inositol-1, 4,5-trisphosphate, or reduce Ca^{2+} sensitivity of contractile elements processes that are important in the generation of the ureteral action potential and the contractile response (Cook and Quast, 1990; Quayle et al., 1997).

The tricyclic antidepressant amitriptyline (Elavil) has been shown to relax isolated pig and human ureteral strips by opening potassium channels (Achar et al., 2003). This relaxation response is inhibited by 4-aminopyridine (4-AP), a voltage-dependent K^+ channel blocker. Nicorandil, a K^+ channel opener and NO donor, stimulates guanylyl cyclase activity with formation of cGMP and hyperpolarizes the smooth muscle with resultant relaxation of rabbit, guinea pig, and human ureter (Klaus et al., 1989; 1990; Weiss et al., 2002). The relaxant effects of nicorandil can be inhibited by the K_{ATP} antagonist glibenclamide and the guanylyl cyclase inhibitor methylene blue (Weiss et al., 2002).

Endothelins

Endothelins are potent vasoconstrictor peptides that exist in three isoforms: ET-1, ET-2, and ET-3. These peptides interact with their specific receptors: ET_A, ET_B, and ET_C. Endothelin binding sites (receptors) have been identified in the ureter and renal pelvis (Eguchi et al., 1991; Latifpour et al., 1995; Wada et al., 2001), where they are primarily of the ET_A subtype (Latifpour et al., 1995; Wada et al., 2001). Endothelins have been shown to initiate contractions in isolated guinea pig and porcine ureters (Eguchi et al., 1991; Maggi et al., 1992a) and increase the contractile force of renal pelvis smooth muscle (Wada et al., 2001). ET-1 acting on the ETA receptor increased contractile force of rat, mouse, and human renal pelvis smooth muscle (Grisk et al., 2010; Steinbach et al., 2016). COX-1 and rho kinase (ROCK) activity are required for ET-1 effects on renal pelvic contractility. ET-1, ET-2, and ET-3 increased tonic contractions and intraluminal pressures in isolated human ureteral segments. These actions were inhibited by BQ123, an ET_A-receptor antagonist, and BQ788, an ET_B-receptor antagonist. ET-1 and ET-3 inhibited spontaneous phasic activity of the isolated human ureteral segments, an action that was not blocked by either ET_A- or ET_B-receptor antagonists (Jankovic et al., 2011). Diabetes upregulates the expression of ureteral endothelin receptors (Nakamura et al., 1997).

Antibiotics

Ampicillin causes relaxation of the ureter and antagonizes the stimulatory effects of barium chloride ($BaCl_2$), histamine, serotonin, and carbachol on the ureter, thus suggesting that its action is directly on the smooth muscle (Benzi et al., 1970b). Chloramphenicol, the isoxazolyl penicillins, and gentamicin also have spasmolytic effects on the ureter (Benzi et al., 1970a, 1971, 1973). The tetracyclines, on the other hand, potentiate the contractile effects of $BaCl_2$ on the ureter (Benzi et al., 1973).

SUGGESTED READINGS

Biancani P, Hausman M, Weiss RM: Effect of obstruction on ureteral circumferential force-length relations, *Am J Physiol* 243:F204, 1982.

Biancani P, Zabinski MP, Weiss RM: Time course of ureteral changes with acute and chronic obstruction, *Am J Physiol* 231:393, 1976.

David SG, Cebrian C, Vaughan ED Jr, et al: C-kit and ureteral peristalsis, *J Urol* 173:292, 2005.

Floyd RV, Borisova L, Bakran A, et al: Morphology, calcium signaling and mechanical activity in human ureter, *J Urol* 180:398, 2008.

Griffiths DJ, Notschaele C: The mechanics of urine transport in the upper urinary tract. I. The dynamics of the isolated bolus, *Neurourol Urodyn* 2:155, 1983.

Griffiths DJ: The mechanics of urine transport in the upper urinary tract. 2. The discharge of the bolus into the bladder and dynamics at high rates of flow, *Neurourol Urodyn* 2:167, 1983.

Klemm MF, Exintaris B, Lang RJ: Identification of the cells underlying pacemaker activity in the guinea pig upper urinary tract, *J Physiol* 519:867, 1999.

Koff SA, Thrall JH: The diagnosis of obstruction in experimental hydroureteronephrosis: mechanism for progressive urinary tract dilation, *Invest Urol* 19:85, 1981b.

Lang RJ, Davidson ME, Exintaris B: Pyeloureteral motility and ureteral peristalsis: essential role of sensory nerves and endogenous prostaglandins, *Exp Physiol* 87:129, 2002.

Lang RJ, Hashitani H, Tonta MA, et al: Spontaneous electrical and Ca2+ signals in typical and atypical smooth muscle cells and interstitial cell of Cajal-like cells of mouse renal pelvis, *J Physiol* 583:1049, 2007a.

Lang RJ, Tonta MA, Zoltkowski BZ, et al: Pyeloureteric peristalsis: role of atypical smooth muscle cells and interstitial cells of Cajal-like cells as pacemakers, *J Physiol* 576:695, 2006.

McGuire EJ, Woodside JR, Borden TA, et al: Prognostic value of urodynamic testing in myelodysplastic patients, *J Urol* 126:205, 1981.

Weiss RM, Tamarkin FJ, Wheeler MA: Pacemaker activity in the upper urinary tract, *J Smooth Muscle Res* 42:103, 2006.

Weiss RM: Clinical implications of ureteral physiology, *J Urol* 121:401, 1979.

Weiss RM: Ureteral function, *Urology* 12:114, 1978.

Woolf AS, Davies JA: Cell biology of ureter development, *J Am Soc Nephrol* 24:19, 2013.

REFERENCES

The complete reference list is available online at ExpertConsult.com.

86 Renal Physiology and Pathophysiology Including Renovascular Hypertension

Thomas Chi, MD, and Meyeon Park, MD, MAS

Urologic disease states often result in intrinsic renal dysfunction. To provide comprehensive care to the patient, urologists must have a thorough understanding of renal physiology and pathophysiology. The aim of this chapter is to highlight the most clinically relevant aspects of these topics as they relate to urologic practice. We organize this broad topic in a clinically relevant fashion by separating renal function into three main categories: filtration and filtrate transport, hormonal regulation, and blood flow. Physiology and pathophysiology are presented together to encourage their understanding as multiple facets of one system, rather than as separate knowledge silos. Principles of physiology and pathophysiology in the kidney can direct therapeutic intervention on many levels for the practicing urologist.

GLOMERULAR FILTRATION

The fundamental function of the kidney is to filter blood. **Renal blood flow (RBF) makes up 20% of cardiac output with the body at rest, and the average adult circulates nearly 5 L of blood per minute for cardiac output.** From that perspective, the kidney's capacity for continuous filtration is remarkable. In addition, the complex handling of solutes by the kidney is a critical component of maintaining homeostasis.

After blood passes from the main renal artery, it travels through smaller and smaller branching interlobar, arcuate, and interlobular arteries until it reaches the afferent arteriole. At that point, blood enters the glomerular capillary at the glomerular apparatus. Here, passive filtration occurs across the glomerular membrane, after which blood exits the glomerular apparatus via the efferent arteriole. **The glomerular filtration rate (GFR) is a reflection of the movement of the filtrate across the membrane and an estimate of hydraulic and oncotic pressure differences between the glomerular capillary and the Bowman space.** It can also be affected by membrane permeability and is represented as

$$GFR = LpS \times (\Delta Hydraulic\ pressure - \Delta Oncotic\ pressure)$$

where Lp = glomerular permeability and S = glomerular surface area. Although renal plasma flow, glomerular permeability, and oncotic pressure influence GFR, the greatest determinant is the hydraulic pressure. Thus, in the setting of acute urinary obstruction, GFR can quickly deteriorate.

Because GFR cannot be directly measured, it is estimated based on renal clearance. The ideal substrate to accurately reflect GFR would be one that has a stable plasma concentration, is freely filtered across the glomerulus, and is not secreted, reabsorbed, metabolized, and synthesized once in the renal tubule. Under these circumstances, the amount of this substrate excreted would be a direct reflection of its filtration and thus a measurement of the GFR. Although inulin and radiolabeled dyes have been used to measure GFR based on these characteristics, their required intravenous administration makes them impractical for use (Perrone et al., 1990). Plasma cystatin C is an endogenous protein that has also been shown to measure renal function (Filler et al., 2005). Clearance of cystatin C is not affected by tubular secretion or excretion and is less affected by muscle mass than serum creatinine, but this test is not yet universally available for clinical use. Endogenous creatinine measurement therefore remains the most clinically relevant marker used as an estimate of GFR. Compared with inulin, some creatinine is secreted from the proximal tubule. Therefore creatinine may overestimate true GFR, and this inaccuracy is magnified as GFR declines, given that tubular secretion will increase under these circumstances (Shemesh et al., 1985; Fig. 86.1). Under some circumstances, a 24-hour collection of urine for creatinine clearance can be a useful measure of kidney function, but this relies on a patient being in steady state. Pragmatically speaking, however, measurement of serum creatinine is the most common approach to estimating GFR.

With use of plasma creatinine to estimate GFR, two mathematical formulas have been widely accepted: the Cockcroft-Gault and the Modification of Diet in Renal Disease (MDRD) formulas (Cockcroft and Gault, 1976). The Cockcroft-Gault formula is as follows:

$$CrCl = \frac{(140 - age) \times (IBW\ in\ kg)}{[PCr\ (mg/dL) \times 72]} \times 0.85\ (women)$$

The Cockcroft-Gault equation generally overestimates creatinine clearance and is no longer widely used clinically for purposes other than drug dosing estimates. The MDRD formula seen below is more accurate comparatively and accounts for severe renal impairment:

$$GFR(mL/min/1.73\ m^2) = 186 \times (PCr\ [mg/dL])^{-1.154} \times (age)^{-0.203} \times (0.742\ if\ female) \times (1.210\ if\ African\text{-}American)$$

Cockgroft-Gault and MDRD equations are less accurate in individuals with normal or only mildly reduced GFR (Levey, 1990). A more recent equation called CKD-EPI may be preferable for use in the general population and in older individuals and may improve risk prediction for chronic kidney disease (CKD) and adverse events associated with CKD (Rose, 1987). Many laboratories that automatically report eGFR have converted to use of CKD-EPI equation to do so (Manjunath et al., 2001).

$$GFR = 141 \times min(SCr/\kappa, 1)^\alpha \times max(SCr/\kappa, 1)^{-1.209} \times 0.993^{Age} \times 1.018[if\ female] \times 1.159[if\ black]$$

$$\kappa = 0.7\ if\ female$$
$$\kappa = 0.9\ if\ male$$

$$\alpha = -0.329\ if\ female$$
$$\alpha = -0.411\ if\ male$$

min = The mininum of SCr/κ or 1
max = The maximum of SCr/κ or 1

SCr = serum creatinine (mg/dL)

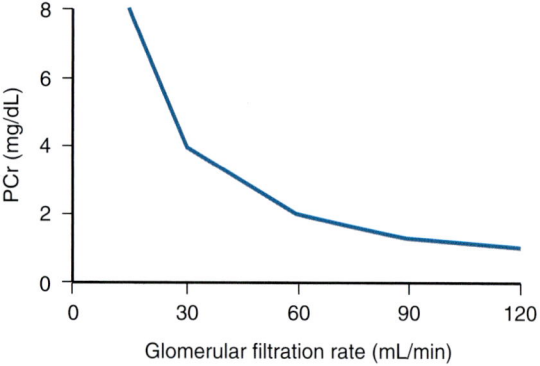

Fig. 86.1. Relationship between serum creatinine and glomerular filtration rate. *PCr*, Plasma creatinine.

> **KEY POINTS**
> - GFR reflects total renal function.
> - GFR can be approximated by creatinine clearance.
> - Formulas based on patient's age, weight, and serum creatinine can best estimate GFR.

Nephron Anatomy

After the filtrate passes the glomerular apparatus into the renal tubule, solutes pass in and out of the tubule. Reabsorption describes movement from tubular lumen back to the blood, and secretion indicates movement from the blood into the tubular lumen. Transport mechanisms occur in a transcellular and paracellular fashion. The renal tubule is divided into anatomic segments, in which different overall functions take place (Fig. 86.2). **Starting at the proximal convoluted tubule (PCT), approximately 60% of the glomerular filtrate is reabsorbed. Under normal circumstances the PCT reabsorbs 65% of the filtered sodium, potassium, and calcium; 80% of filtered phosphate, water, and bicarbonate; and 100% of the filtered glucose and amino acids.** The PCT is also responsible for the generation of ammonia from glutamine, which is necessary for urinary acidification (Michoudet et al., 1994; Nagami, 2004).

After the proximal convoluted tubule comes the loop of Henle (Fig. 86.3), which comprises the thin descending limb, the thin ascending limb, the medullary thick ascending limb, and the cortical thick ascending limb. Although each segment differs in specific activity, the overall function of the loop of Henle is reabsorption of 25% to 30% of the filtered sodium (Na^+) and creation of a highly concentrated medullary interstitium, the basis of counter-current exchange (Figs. 86.4 and 86.5). The thin descending limb is highly water permeable, whereas the thin and thick ascending limbs are water impermeable.

The distal tubule comprises first the distal convoluted tubule and the connecting tubule. In these segments significant sodium and calcium reabsorption occur. After this, the collecting tubule is encountered, in which the cortical and medullary collecting tubules demonstrate slightly different functions. Both handle transport of Na^+ via principal cells and acid loads via intercalated cells as well as potassium (K^+) via both cell types. In the medullary collecting tubule, however, tight regulated control of water and urea permeability exists, allowing for this area of the collecting tubule to concentrate urine to a much greater level than plasma.

Filtrate Transport

Sodium

Most of the kidney's total Na^+ reabsorption occurs in the proximal convoluted tubule (Fig. 86.6). Secondary active and passive

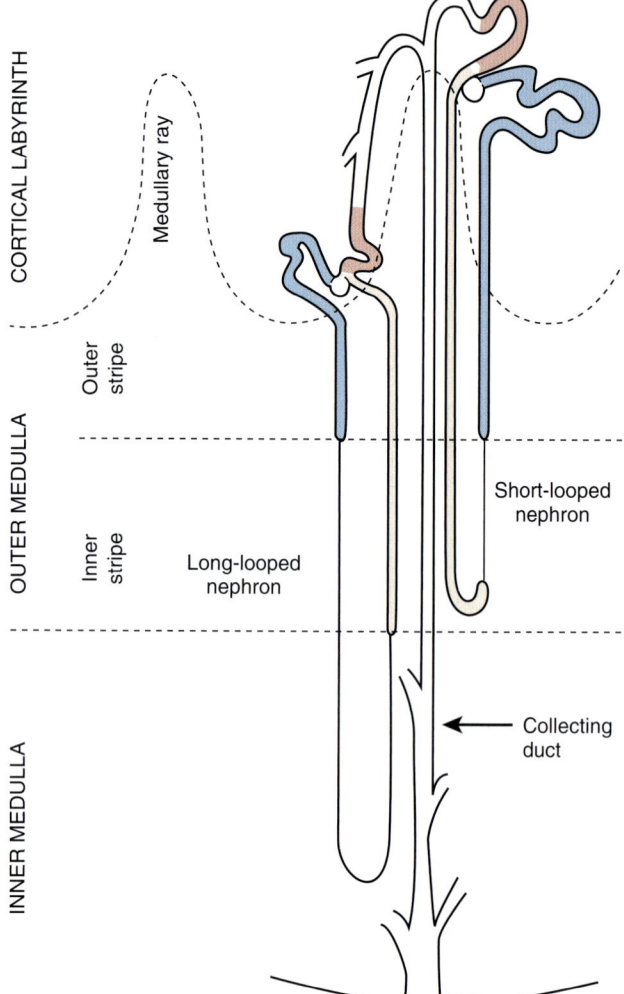

Fig. 86.2. Organization of the renal tubule. (From Knepper MA, Gamba F: Urine concentration and dilution. In Brenner BM, editor: *Brenner and Rector's the kidney*, ed 7, Philadelphia, 2004, WB Saunders, p 601.)

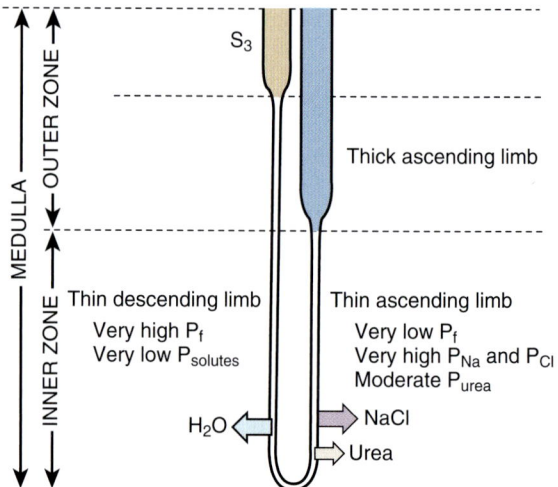

Fig. 86.3. Anatomy of the loop of Henle. (From Moe OW, Baum M, Berry CA, Rector FC Jr.: Renal transport of glucose, amino acids, sodium, chloride, and water. In Brenner BM, editor: *Brenner and Rector's the kidney*, ed 7, Philadelphia, 2004, WB Saunders, p 431.)

Chapter 86 Renal Physiology and Pathophysiology Including Renovascular Hypertension

KEY POINTS

- The nephron has different functional segments that control homeostasis.
- Most resorption of bicarbonate and ions occurs in the proximal tubule.
- The architecture of the loop of Henle allows a highly hypertonic interstitium to develop, which is crucial to maximal urinary concentration.

mechanisms account for this movement (Adrogue and Madias, 2000). In secondary active reabsorption, an Na-K ATPase at the basolateral cell membrane exchanges three intracellular Na^+ for two extracellular K^+ ions, lowering the intracellular sodium levels. Na^+ then enters the tubule cell via coupled transport or an Na^+/H^+ antiporter. In passive reabsorption, Na^+ moves paracellularly into the intercellular space mediated through active chloride (Cl^-) transport that creates an electrochemical gradient, driving Na^+ out of the tubular lumen into the intercellular space.

An additional 25% to 35% of Na^+ reabsorption occurs in the thick ascending limb of the loop of Henle. Similar to the proximal convoluted tubule, a basolateral Na-K ATPase pump keeps intracellular Na^+ levels low. Na^+ is also transported by the NKCC2 transporter on the apical membrane. This functions by Cl^- being pumped across the basolateral membrane via a Cl^-/K^+ cotransporter. K^+ is then recycled back into the tubular lumen through an apical membrane K^+ channel (ROMK), where it can then be used by the NKCC2 transporter. Thus Na^+ reabsorption is linked to K^+ transport. In the

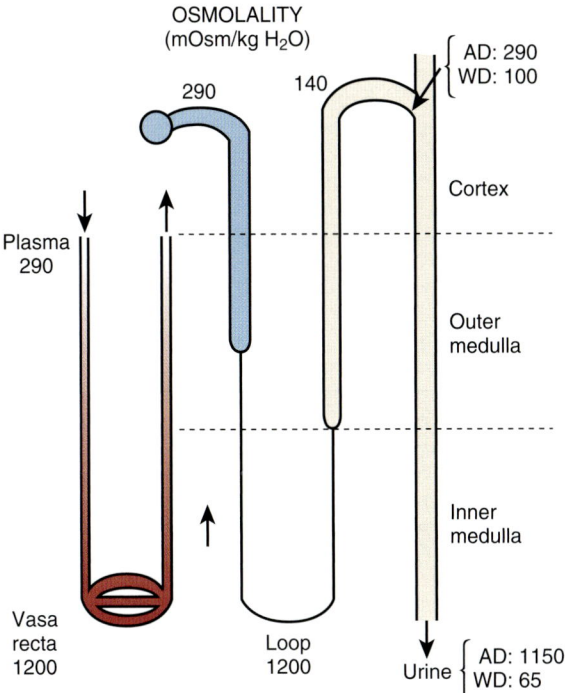

Fig. 86.4. Countercurrent mechanism in the renal tubule. *AD,* Antidiuresis; *WD,* water diuresis. (From Knepper MA, Gamba F: Urine concentration and dilution. In Brenner BM, editor: *Brenner and Rector's the kidney,* ed 7, Philadelphia, 2004, WB Saunders, p 604.)

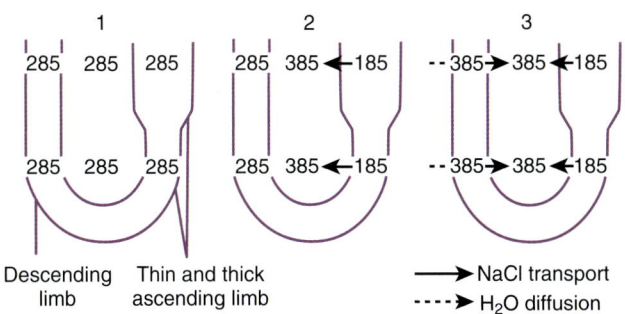

Fig. 86.5. Role of active NaCl transport in initiating countercurrent multiplication. In step 1, at time zero, the fluid in the descending and ascending limbs and the interstitium is isosmotic to plasma. In step 2, NaCl is transported out of the ascending limb into the interstitium to a gradient of 200 mOsm/kg. In step 3, the fluid in the descending limb equilibrates osmotically with the hyperosmotic interstitium, primarily by water movement out of the tubule. Dilution of the interstitium by this water movement is prevented by continued NaCl transport out of the ascending limb. The result is the creation of an osmotic gradient between the ascending limb and the relatively hyperosmotic descending limb and interstitium.

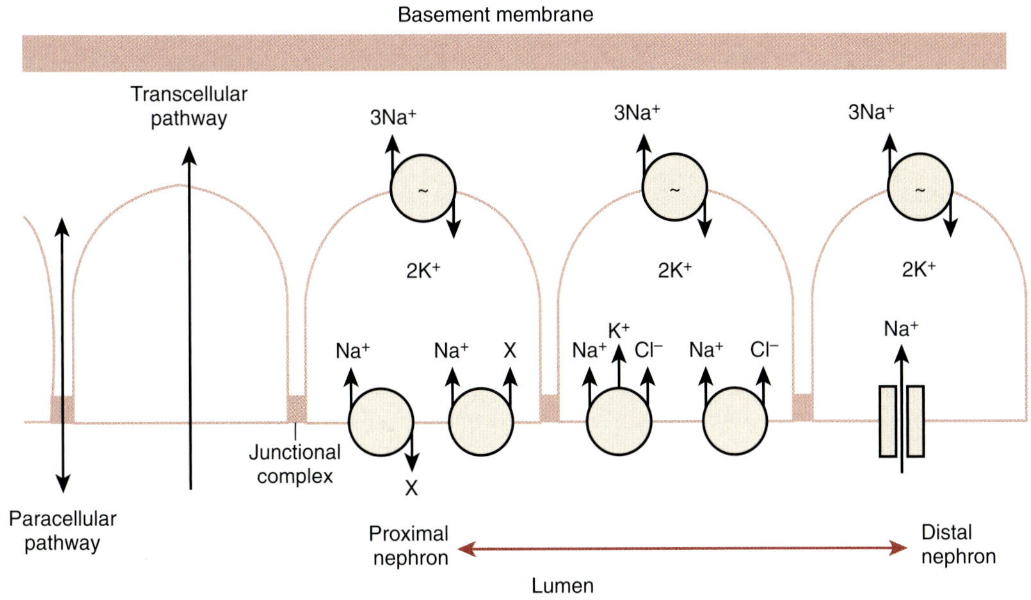

Fig. 86.6. Mechanisms of sodium reabsorption in the proximal tubule. (From Moe OW, Baum M, Berry CA, Rector FC Jr.: Renal transport of glucose, amino acids, sodium, chloride, and water. In: Brenner BM, editor: *Brenner and Rector's the kidney,* ed 7, Philadelphia, 2004, WB Saunders, p 414.)

thick ascending limb, this Na+ reabsorption facilitates creation of a high interstitial concentration gradient that allows for urinary concentration in the collecting duct. Therapeutically, NKCC2 transporters are the active target of loop diuretics that bind the Cl− receptor, thereby decreasing NaCl reabsorption, leading to diuresis.

The distal convoluted tubule then reabsorbs an additional 5% to 10% of sodium filtered through the glomerulus (Loffing and Kaissling, 2003). A basolateral Na-K ATPase pump and Na+/Cl− (NCC) cotransporter in addition to an Na+/H+ exchange transporter in the membrane of the lumen are found here. The NCC transporter is directly inhibited by thiazide diuretics. One consideration is that this therapeutic mechanism of action works in a complementary fashion to loop diuretics. Loop diuretics increase Na+ delivery to the distal convoluted tubule by inhibiting NKCC2 activity in the thick ascending limb. This leads to increased Na+ reabsorption and thus a blunted response over time to loop diuretics. This can be mitigated with simultaneous administration of thiazide diuretics.

Sodium transport also occurs in the principal cells of the collecting tubule. Passive reabsorption takes place through ENaC1, a luminal sodium channel. Active Na+ transport via basolateral Na-K ATPase pumps (as described earlier) also exists in these cells. In the principal cells, aldosterone can increase the number of open ENaC1 channels, and amiloride can block its activity. Prostaglandin E_2 (PGE_2) inhibits Na reabsorption, and thus agents that decrease PGE_2 production, including nonsteroidal antiinflammatory drugs, can cause clinical signs of sodium retention.

The pathological state of sodium imbalances in the body are driven by free water excess relative to sodium content. Sodium largely resides in the extracellular space, and therefore water balance across the intra- and extracellular space of the body (regulated by antidiuretic hormone, or ADH) is a major determinant of hyponatremia and hypernatremia as opposed to total body sodium content. Hyponatremia can lead to seizures, altered mental status, coma, and even death but is rarely symptomatic until serum sodium is below 120 mEq/L. Hyponatremia occurs when the kidney fails to excrete appropriate solute-free urine. This can occur because of states of reduced GFR, diuretic use that impairs NaCl reabsorption, or in syndrome of inappropriate ADH. Excessive free water intake above the level of the kidney's ability to clear free water can sometimes cause hyponatremia, although this is relatively uncommon except in states of reduced eGFR or psychiatric conditions (Goh, 2004).

Hypernatremia can often seem similar to hyponatremia, with tremors, lethargy, coma, and death being late symptoms after restlessness, nausea, and vomiting. Most patients with an intact thirst mechanism and access to water will consume adequate free water to prevent hypernatremia. Therefore it often is seen in the very young and old or in hospitalized patients. Other causes of hypernatremia include excess extrarenal water loss or sodium intake, Cushing syndrome, primary hyperaldosteronism, and diabetes insipidus.

Evaluation of the patient with sodium imbalances should always start with a determination of fluid status. Clinical assessment should include evaluation of skin turgor, blood pressure including orthostatics, jugular venous distention, and looking for an abdominal fluid wave or respiratory crackles. Urinary sodium greater or less than 20 can be used as a measure of urinary osmolality in the evaluation. For example, in hyponatremia, with hypovolemic patients a low urinary sodium would be expected. If high, then a renal source including diuretic overdose, renal tubular acidosis, or mineralocorticoid deficiency may be suspected (Figs. 86.7 and 86.8).

Treatment of hyponatremia and hypernatremia should be aimed at identifying and correcting the underlying cause, with correction by appropriate fluids as needed. Patients with acute severe hyponatremia symptomatic with confusion, convulsions, or coma, may require an initial bolus of hypertonic (3%) saline (about 1 cc/kg/h). Use of fluid restriction with or without administration of fluids (hypertonic versus isotonic) should be determined by the electrolyte-free water

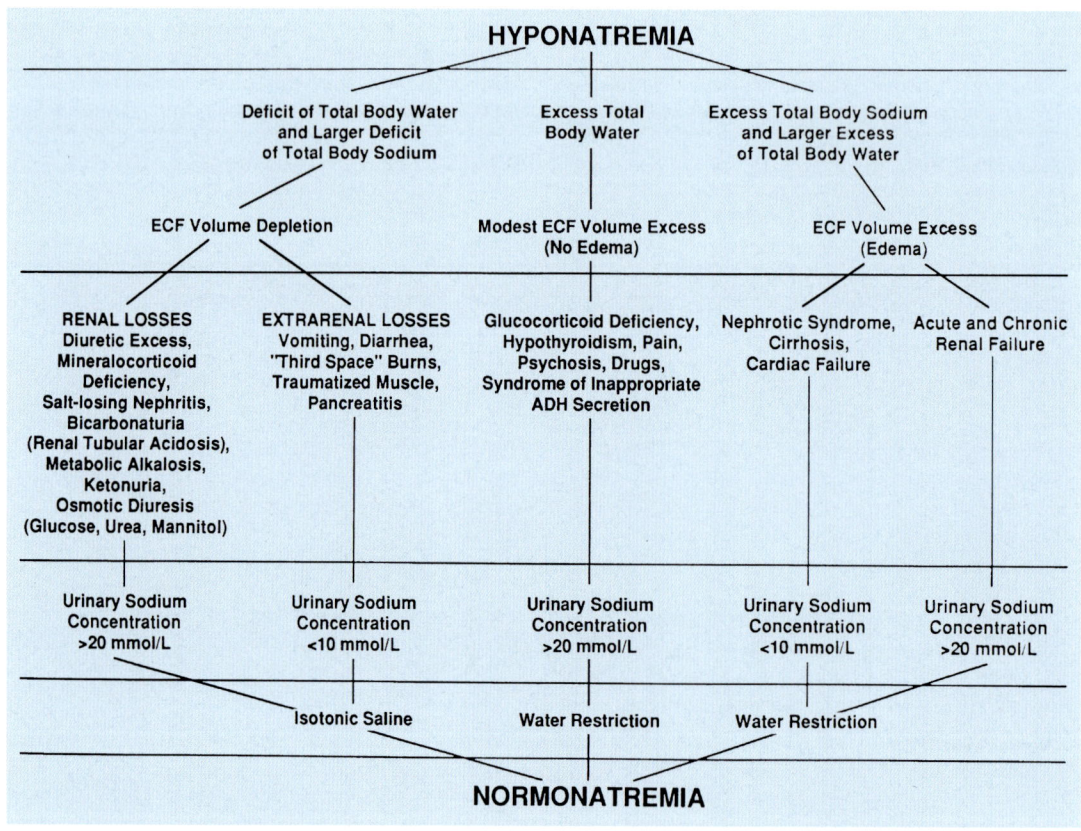

Fig. 86.7. Clinical approach to patient with hyponatremia. *ADH*, Antidiuretic hormone; *ECF*, extracellular fluid. (From Berl T, Anderson RJ, McDonald KM, Schrier RW: Clinical disorders of water metabolism. *Kidney Int* 10:117–132, 1976.)

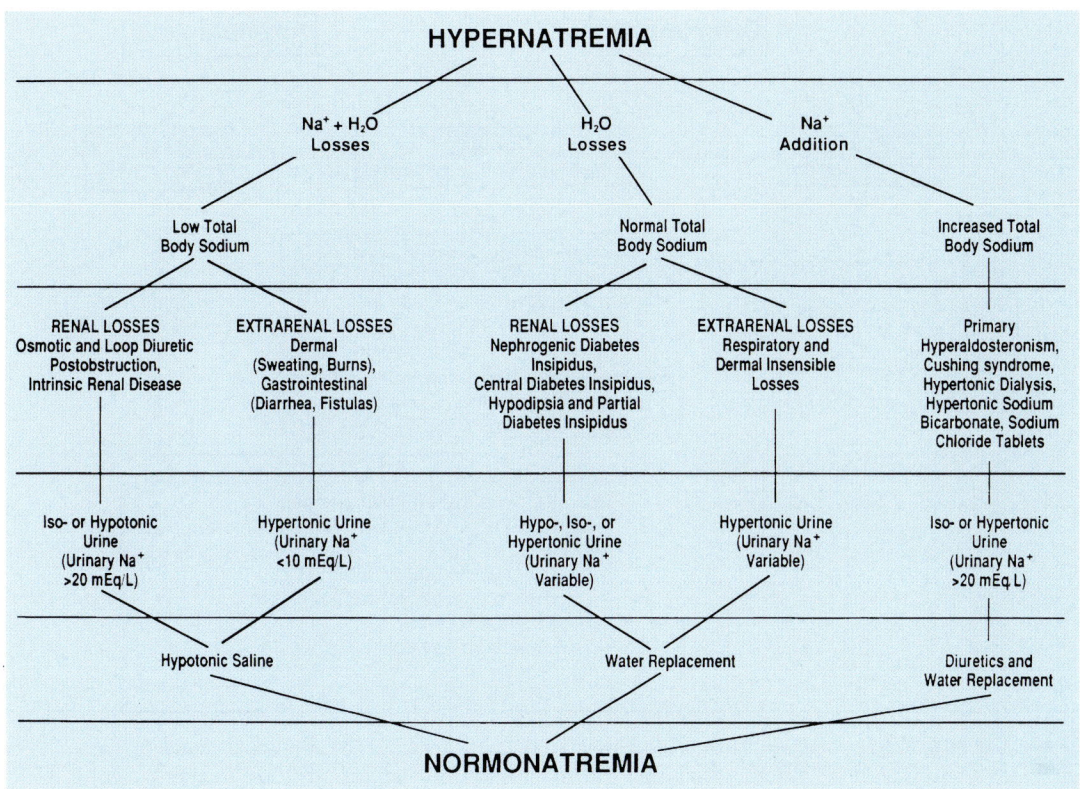

Fig. 86.8. Clinical approach to patient with hypernatremia. (From Berl T, Anderson RJ, McDonald KM, Schrier RW: Clinical disorders of water metabolism. *Kidney Int* 10:117–132, 1976.)

clearance, measured by the rate of urine sodium and potassium excretion (Fig. 86.9).

$$EFWC = Vol_{urine} \times (1 - (Na^+ + K^+)_{urine} / Na^+_{serum})$$

where Vol_{urine} stands for the urine volume, $(Na^+ + K^+)_{urine}$ for sodium and potassium in urine, and Na^+_{serum} for serum sodium concentration.

Fluid overload in correction of hyponatremia is unlikely to occur in the absence of heart failure or cirrhosis but may be further reduced by simultaneous administration of a loop diuretic such as furosemide, which causes excretion of hypotonic fluid. The serum sodium concentration should be raised to no more than 6 to 8 mEq/L in the first 24 hours, at a rate of no more than 0.5 to 1 mEq/L per hour, and the target goal should be 120 to 125 mEq/L. To avoid overcorrection, subcutaneous or intranasal administration of DDAVP may be required to mitigate the brisk excretion of free water that can occur in some causes of hyponatremia as soon as fluid replacement begins. Total sodium deficit to reach this point can be calculated as

$$(\text{Volume of distribution}) \times \text{Body weight (kg)} \times (125 - \text{Plasma [Na]})$$

where volume of distribution is 0.5 for men and 0.6 for women. If the hyponatremia is severe but chronic, the rate of correction should not exceed 8 to 12 mmol/L/day; otherwise a cerebral demyelination syndrome may occur (Martin, 2004). During acute intervention for severe hyponatremia, frequent electrolyte measurements and patient reassessment are required, usually in an intensive care unit setting. Aggressive therapy should be discontinued when the serum sodium concentration is raised 10% or symptoms subside. At that point, water restriction and reversal of underlying causes should suffice. This is also the best approach for therapy of asymptomatic hyponatremia. Patients with associated hypovolemia should have this corrected with the appropriate volume of normal saline. In hypernatremia, hypovolemia should be initially corrected with half-normal saline. If the patient is awake and not symptomatic, oral hydration with water is sufficient. Otherwise, intravenous (IV) therapy should be started with the goal of slowly lowering plasma osmolality to no more than 2 mOsm/L/h to avoid cerebral edema. The water deficit can be calculated as

$$(\text{Volume of distribution}) \times \text{Body weight (kg)} \times (\text{Plasma [Na]}/140 - 1)$$

where, again, volume of distribution is 0.5 for men and 0.6 for women. For patients with central diabetes insipidus, desmopressin (a synthetic exogenous vasopressin) can be given intranasally. For nephrogenic diabetes insipidus, the underlying cause (lithium, hypercalcemia) should be treated. If polyuria persists while the kidney recovers, therapy includes modest sodium restriction, thiazide diuretics, and nonsteroidal anti-inflammatory drugs (Pattaragarn and Alon, 2003; Sasaki, 2004).

> **KEY POINTS**
> - Sodium imbalances should be evaluated in the context of fluid status.
> - The best tools to determine the cause of a sodium disorder are the history, volume status, and urinary sodium.
> - Severe sodium deficit or excess must be corrected slowly.

Potassium

Potassium transport intersects closely with sodium. In the proximal convoluted tubule, its reabsorption is passive, occurring by the paracellular route in a parallel direction as sodium and water movement. At the level of the collecting tubule, potassium transport is handled by the same basolateral Na-K ATPase pump that manages

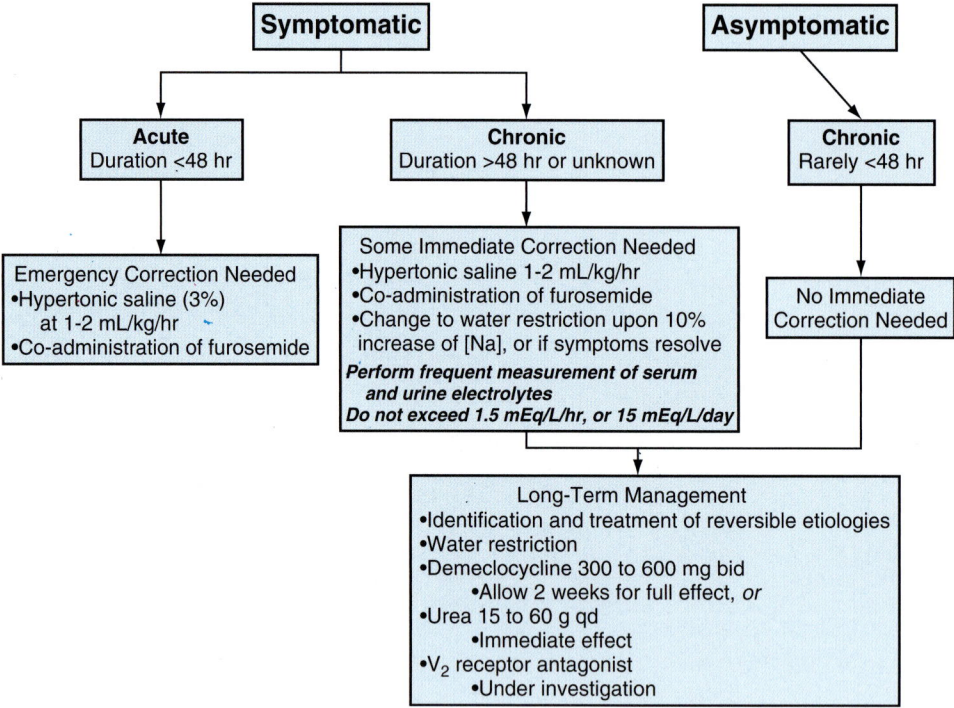

Fig. 86.9. Therapy of hyponatremia. (From Halterman R, Berl T: Therapy of dysnatremic disorders. In Brady H, Wilcox C, editors: *Therapy in nephrology and hypertension,* Philadelphia, 1999, WB Saunders, p 261.)

sodium transport (Wang, 1995). Changes in sodium availability and movement thus alter potassium secretion, such as can be induced with aldosterone. In addition, K+ channels exist whose density in the luminal membrane is altered by antidiuretic hormone (ADH). In the cortical collecting tubule, a net secretion of K+ is the usual state, although H-K ATPase pumps become activated during periods of potassium depletion resulting in reabsorption of potassium in the tubule along with H+ secretion and an accompanying metabolic alkalosis (Khanna and Kurtzman, 2001).

Hypo- and hyperkalemia can cause neuromuscular dysfunction leading to cardiac arrhythmias and death. The majority of potassium resides intracellularly, and regulating urinary K+ excretion and moving K+ between the intra- and extracellular space are primary strategies for treating potassium imbalances. **Urinary excretion can be increased in the kidney through increased aldosterone, a high sodium load in the distal tubule, and by acidosis.**

Hypokalemia is most commonly caused by gastrointestinal and renal loss as well as system alkalosis leading to intracellular shift of K+. Other causes include medications (e.g., diuretics, laxatives, amphotericin, theophylline), postobstructive diuresis, and states associated with elevated aldosterone levels (e.g., adrenal adenoma, Cushing syndrome, adrenal cancer). Potassium supplementation in an oral or parenteral form of up to 40 mEq/h is the most common treatment while any underlying cause is addressed.

Hyperkalemia is most commonly caused by impaired potassium renal excretion and systemic acidosis driving extracellular movement of potassium. Evaluation includes a careful history as well as assessment for cardiac symptoms and electrocardiogram (ECG). Hemolysis should be ruled out as a spurious cause of hyperkalemia. Once confirmed, treatment should be dictated by severity and acuity of elevation as well as clinical signs and symptoms. Mildly elevated K+ levels with no accompanying ECG changes can be managed with dietary restriction of potassium and reversal of underlying causes. The presence of ECG changes (classically short QT interval, peaked T waves, and ventricular arrhythmias) warrants urgent intervention. This includes sodium bicarbonate, insulin with glucose, and nebulized albuterol to drive potassium into the intracellular space. Kayexalate as a potassium-binding exchange resin can be used to reduce potassium stores and hemodialysis can be used for emergent and complete potassium removal. Calcium gluconate can be given to stabilize cardiac myocytes while hyperkalemia-induced ECG changes are addressed.

> **KEY POINTS**
> - Potassium is primarily intracellular.
> - Serum potassium levels reflect total body potassium, as well as the equilibrium between intra- and extracellular potassium.
> - Symptomatic hyperkalemia requires urgent intervention to prevent cardiac dysfunction.

Water

Water reabsorption in the PCT is a passive process, driven by the reabsorption of other solutes and the subsequent osmotic gradient that develops between the lumen and intercellular space (Fig. 86.10). Water transport is not a direct source of pathology, but its movement dictates solute concentrations (sodium in particular) and gradients. Therefore water movement can indirectly cause pathological solute imbalances, whereas insufficient solute intake can be a cause of hyponatremia if relatively excess water is consumed (Mallie et al., 1997). The majority of water reabsorption occurs in the late PCT. As with Na+ movement, water can also move either transcellularly or paracellularly. Transcellular movement accounts for 80% of water reabsorption and occurs through the specialized water channel aquaporin-1 (AQP-1) (Kwon et al., 2001). Paracellular movement accounts for only 20% of water reabsorption and occurs across the tight junctions between cells.

The water permeability of the cortical collecting tubule is low in the basal state. However, it can be greatly increased in the presence of ADH. This is due to the insertion of preformed AQP-2 water channels into the luminal membrane, which allows water to be passively reabsorbed and equilibrate with the cortical interstitium through basolateral AQP-3 and AQP-4 channels (Agre et al., 2002). This is important for the development of highly concentrated final urine, because it decreases the volume of ultrafiltrate delivered to the medullary collecting tubule (MCT), where most of the final concentration of urine occurs.

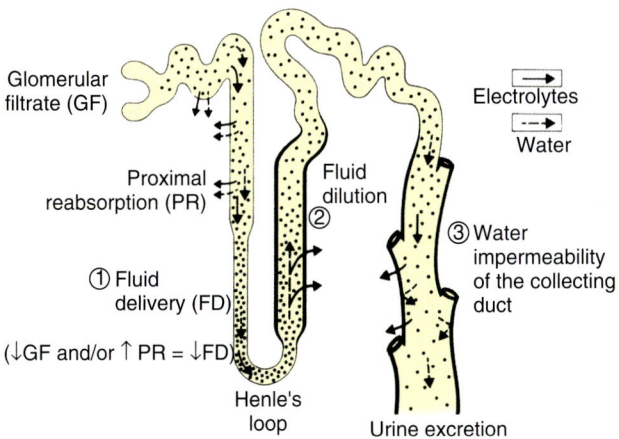

Fig. 86.10. The components of the normal urine dilution mechanisms. (Redrawn from Berl T, Schrier RW: Water metabolism and the hypo-osmolar syndrome. In Brenner BM, Stein JH, editors: *Sodium and water homeostasis*, New York, 1978, Churchill Livingstone, pp 1–23.)

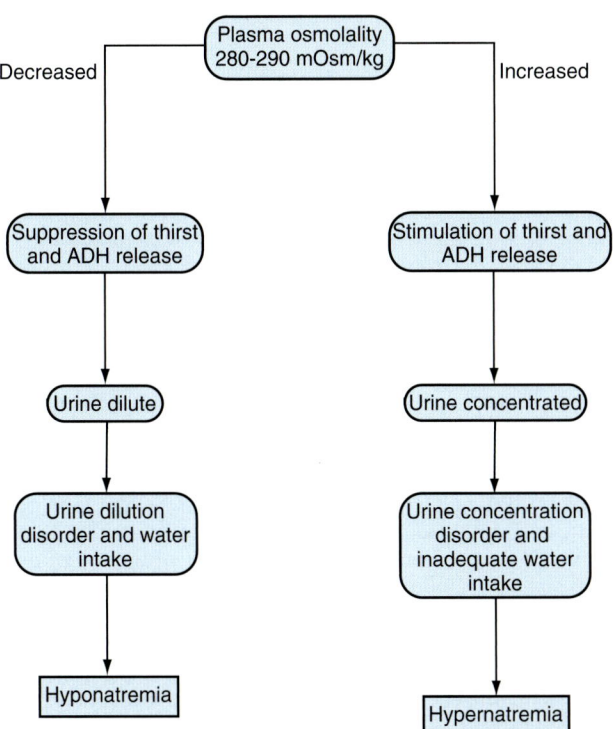

Fig. 86.11. Flowchart illustrating the development of disorders of water metabolism. *ADH*, Antidiuretic hormone.

The MCT is relatively impermeable to water in the basal state, but under the influence of ADH, permeability increases in the inner MCT and outer MCT by the insertion of AQP-2 water channels. This allows water to move out of the tubule into the hyperosmolar interstitium, and urine concentration occurs. Thirst is the primary mechanism that regulates body water intake. ADH, or vasopressin, can dysregulate this water sensitivity (Fig. 86.11). Produced in the posterior pituitary gland, it regulates free water excretion by increasing passive water reabsorption in the collecting duct. It does so by interacting with the V2 receptor, which then leads to insertion of aquaporin-2 (AQP-2) into the principal cell luminal membrane. AQP-2 allows entry of water back into the cell and from there passively into whole body circulation (Leung et al., 2005). ADH also increases urea reabsorption, sodium reabsorption, potassium excretion, prostaglandin synthesis, ACTH secretion, systemic vascular resistance, and release of factor VIII and von Willebrand factor from vascular endothelium (which has the net effect of increasing sodium). ADH release is caused by hyperosmolality (mostly a reflection of increased serum sodium concentration) and decreased effective circulating volume (as in heart failure or cirrhosis) (Miller, 1994; Robertson, 1987). Desmopressin is an analogue of vasopressin used to treat adult nocturia by taking advantage of water reabsorption to reduce urine production at night. Serum sodium must be closely monitored during its use.

> **KEY POINTS**
>
> - Water movement dictates solute concentrations, **especially** important for sodium balance.
> - Regulation of water movement is highly dependent on antidiuretic hormone.
> - Insertion of aquaporin channels facilitates water reabsorption.

Calcium

Calcium reabsorption occurs mostly in the proximal convoluted tubule (approximately 75%) followed by the thick ascending loop of Henle (15%) and the distal convoluted tubule (10%–15%) (Fig. 86.12) (Friedman and Gesek, 1993). In the proximal convoluted tubule and the loop of Henle, transport is primarily passive across the paracellular route via the claudin-2 calcium tight junction channel and the claudin-16 channel, respectively (Amasheh et al., 2002). This movement is driven by the voltage difference between the luminal and extraluminal spaces and tied tightly to sodium concentrations. In contrast, in the distal convoluted tubule calbindin D_{28} is an intracellular binding protein that binds calcium after it is transported into the cell via the $ECaC_1$ channel. This binding process keeps intracellular levels of calcium low and allows for continued inward calcium movement. On the basolateral side, calcium leaves the cell via either a Ca^{2+}/H^+ (PMCA) or Na^+/Ca^{2+} (NCX) exchanger. Parathyroid hormone and calcitriol/vitamin D act in the distal tubule to increase calcium reabsorption. **Hypercalciuria in the context of renal stones most often represents a renal leak of calcium, although it can also be associated with a renal phosphate leak, a sign of hyperparathyroidism, or a dietary-dependent absorptive issue.** For stone prevention, hypercalciuria is treated with thiazide diuretics to decrease urinary calcium excretion.

Acid-Base Balance

Renal physiology is critical to maintaining homeostatic acid-base balance (Corey, 2005). **Although the body's primary three mechanisms to maintain acid load balance are buffers in the blood, CO_2 excretion by the lungs, and H^+ excretion by HCO_3^-, the kidney acts mostly by regulating transport of H^+ and HCO_3^-. Bicarbonate is the main buffer regulated by the kidney, and approximately 80% of filtered bicarbonate is resorbed in the proximal convoluted tubule** (Fig. 86.13; Kildeberg, 1983). Of the remaining 20%, approximately half is resorbed in the thick ascending loop of Henle and half in the collecting duct. In all locations, its movement is closely tied to H^+ movement. In the proximal convoluted tubule and loop of Henle, as H^+ is secreted via the Na^+/H^+ antiporter, carbonic anhydrase catalyzes the combining of HCO_3^- with H^+ within the lumen, forming H_2O and CO_2. Water and carbon dioxide then diffuse into the intracellular space, where carbonic anhydrase again catalyzes the conversion back to H^+ and HCO_3^-. Bicarbonate is then secreted back into vascular circulation across the basolateral membrane through a Na^+-coupled transporter. Thus carbonic anhydrase inhibitors such as acetazolamide can be used to reduce HCO_3^- reabsorption and increase Na^+ and water excretion (Kaunisto et al., 2002; Puscas et al., 1999).

Acid-base movement also occurs in the collecting duct in types A and B intercalated cells. In these areas, H^+ ATPase and H^+-K^+ ATPase pumps as well as HCO_3^-/Cl^- move hydrogen and bicarbonate in and out of the intracellular space. In type A cells, the proton pumps exist on the luminal membrane and the bicarbonate transports on the basolateral membrane. This results in a net movement of protons

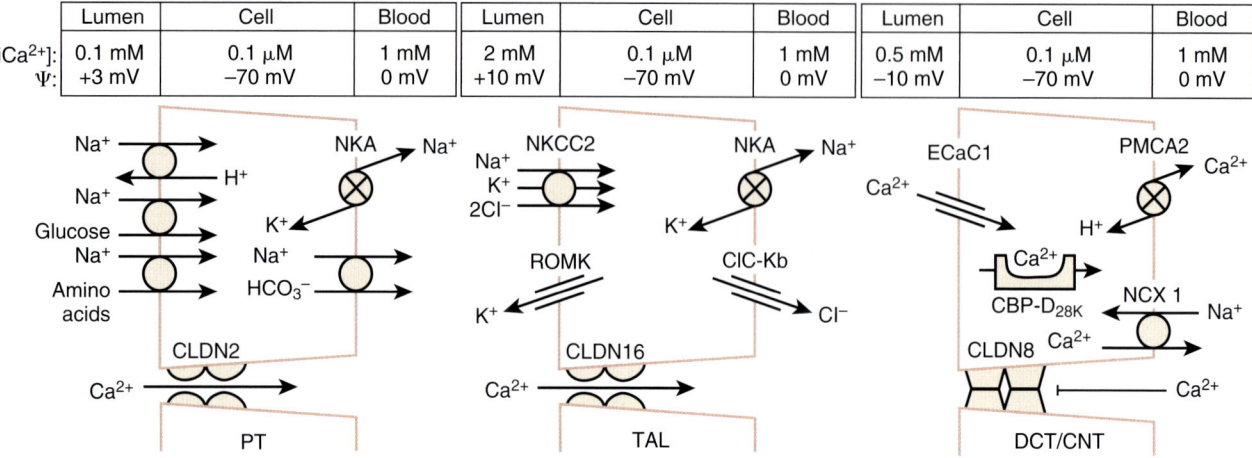

Fig. 86.12. Absorption of calcium by the renal tubule. *CNT,* Connecting tubule; *DCT,* distal convoluted tubule; *PT,* proximal tubule; *TAL,* thick ascending limb. (From Yu SLY: Renal transport of calcium, magnesium, and phosphate. In Brenner BM, editor: *Brenner and Rector's the kidney,* ed 7, Philadelphia, 2004, WB Saunders, p 538.)

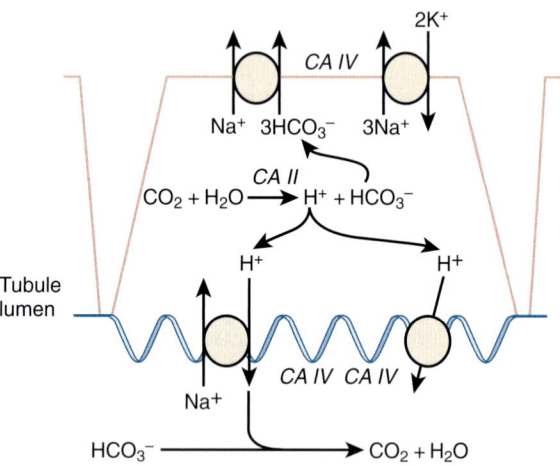

Fig. 86.13. Reabsorption of bicarbonate in the renal tubule. *CA,* Carbonic anhydrase. (From Hamm LL. Renal acidification mechanisms. In Brenner BM, editor: *Brenner and Rector's the kidney,* ed 7, Philadelphia, 2004, WB Saunders, p 500.)

into the lumen, causing acidification of the urine. In type B cells, the pumps and transports exist in opposite locations (i.e., proton pumps are basolateral and bicarbonate transporters are luminal), driving net loss of bicarbonate and systemic acidification. Predominance of type A versus type B activity depends on systemic states of metabolic acidosis and alkalosis, where their activity occurs in response to balance these potentially pathological states.

Regulation of H+ secretion occurs through multiple biochemical and hormonal actions upon the earlier-mentioned system. **Volume depletion** leads to Na retention and enhanced HCO_3^- absorption, with a net loss of H+. **Elevated PCO_2,** as seen in chronic respiratory acidosis (see later), will lead to a renal response of increased H+ secretion (Epstein and Singh, 2001). **Reduced GFR** will reduce the amount of filtered HCO_3^-, leading to increased H+ excretion. **High aldosterone levels** indirectly increase H+ excretion by increasing Na+ absorption. **Low potassium and low chloride** increase HCO_3^- reabsorption and can maintain chronic metabolic alkalosis.

The kidney as a source of acid-base imbalances is usually derived from excess bicarbonate loss (metabolic acidosis) or impaired bicarbonate excretion (metabolic alkalosis). Renally derived metabolic acidosis caused by excess bicarbonate loss results in systemic acidemia, marked by an acidic arterial pH, low serum HCO_3^-, and low PCO_2. The low CO_2 is caused by compensatory respiratory alkalosis (Foster et al., 2001; Levraut and Grimaud, 2003; Madias and Adrogue, 2003). Renal defects in tubular H+ secretion can also cause a family of acid-base imbalance disorders collectively called renal tubular acidosis (RTA) (Roth and Chan, 2001). These are associated with urinary acidification and classified as types I, II, and IV based on causative mechanism. In type II RTA, bicarbonate is unable to be resorbed in the proximal tubule leading to HCO_3 loss into the urine in the distal tubule and therefore a systemic acidosis (de Mello-Aires and Malnic, 2002; Igarashi et al., 2002). Type IV RTA is caused by dysfunctional cation exchange in the distal tubule that leads to decreased H+ and K+ secretion (Uribarri et al., 1994). **The RTA most relevant to urologic practice is type I RTA, or distal RTA. In type I RTA, H+ is unable to be secreted in the distal nephron, resulting in a hyperchloremic metabolic acidosis marked by a high urinary pH of more than 5.5 and low serum HCO_3 and low urinary citrate.** Type I RTA is associated with recurrent calcium phosphate stone formation, likely driven by the low urinary citrate, high urinary pH, and hypercalciuria. Potassium citrate supplementation and urinary alkalinization are the primary forms of treatment to prevent urinary stone formation (Domrongkitchaiporn et al., 2002).

> **KEY POINTS**
>
> - Physiologic chemical reactions require a narrow range of serum pH.
> - Acid is excreted through the lungs and the kidney.
> - Type I RTA (distal) is the only type associated with renal stones.
> - In acid-base disorders, first determine whether the kidney (HCO_3) or lungs (PCO_2) are responsible for the primary disorder; then determine whether the compensatory response is appropriate.

Additional Solutes

Several additional solutes are handled in the kidney but are less clinically relevant to urologic practice than sodium, potassium, calcium, water, and bicarbonate (Moe et al., 2004). **Glucose** in the filtrate is normally completely reabsorbed. This occurs via a combination of passive Na+ reabsorption and a low-capacity, high-affinity 2Na+/glucose transporter called SGLT-1. When plasma levels of glucose are excessive, however, the reabsorptive capacity of the kidney for glucose is overloaded, and it will be found in the urine. Filtered **phosphate** is mostly reabsorbed in the proximal convoluted tubule through an Na+-phosphate cotransporter. When a renal phosphate leak exists, a secondary increase in renal calcitriol synthesis occurs, leading to increased intestinal calcium absorption and hypercalciuria. This phosphate leak is treated with phosphate supplementation to prevent a relatively uncommon but clinically significant source of recurrent calcium-based urinary stones. **Magnesium** is also filtered in the kidney, where it is reabsorbed partially in the proximal and distal tubule and mostly (60%–70%) in the thick ascending loop of Henle (Konrad et al., 2004; Voets et al., 2004). **Urea** exists in a high concentration in the interstitium. This facilitates an osmotic gradient that is responsible for water reabsorption and urinary concentration. The outer medullary collecting tubule is relatively impermeable to urea, in the basal state and under ADH stimulation. In contrast, the inner medullary collecting tubule has a high basal permeability for urea, largely because of the urea transporters UT-A1 and UT-A3 located mostly on the basolateral cell membrane. Short-term regulation is under the influence of ADH, which can increase urea permeability as much as fourfold through an increased number of urea transporters. Longer-term regulation can be affected by protein intake (Yang and Bankir, 2005).

Renal Hormone Effects

The kidney is involved in regulating systemic vascular tone, red blood cell production, and bone mineralization through its interaction with various hormones.

Vasoconstriction

Multiple hormones are involved in regulating vasoconstriction. **One important factor is the renin-angiotensin system where, in response to decreased renal blood flow, the kidney converts prorenin into renin and releases renin into circulation** (Dworkin and Brenner, 2004; Vaughan and Laragh, 1975). Renin in turn converts angiotensin I to angiotensin II via angiotensin-converting enzyme (ACE) **primarily in the lungs** (Romero et al., 1973). **Angiotensin II** interacts with the AT1 and AT2 receptors in the kidney, leading to vasoconstriction of the efferent arteriole, aldosterone release, and retention of sodium (Carey, 2005; Kaschina and Unger, 2003; Pimentel et al., 1995). The net effect of angiotensin II is to increase systemic vascular resistance and maintain GFR when renal blood flow is reduced (Arima, 2003; Bumpus et al., 1976; Romero et al., 1974).

Outside of the renin-angiotensin system other agents play important roles as well. **Norepinephrine** acts through the α_1 receptor to vasoconstrict all major renal blood vessels (Albanese et al., 2004). Its use as a blood pressure support agent is thus associated with preservation of renal function. **Endothelin** release, stimulated by angiotensin II, antidiuretic hormone, thrombin, cytokines, reactive oxygen species, and shearing forces acting on the vascular endothelium, causes vascular smooth muscle cell vasoconstriction (Bhangdia et al., 2003; Perez del Villar et al., 2005). In addition, it increases aldosterone secretion, stimulates atrial natriuretic peptide, decreases renal blood flow and GFR, and increases sodium excretion (Evans et al., 2004; Fellner and Arendshorst, 2004). It is the most potent vasoconstrictor currently known. **Vasopressin** directly stimulates vasoconstriction via the V1 receptor on blood vessel walls (Knepper et al., 1994; Segarra et al., 2002). At low doses, it preserves renal blood flow, whereas at high doses, it can lead to renal ischemia. It is therefore used as a blood pressure support medication at low doses in the setting of septic shock to increase systemic vascular resistance while preserving renal function (Baylis, 1987; Holmes et al., 2001; Malay et al., 2004). **Atrial natriuretic peptide** is released by the atria in response to stretching of the atrial wall in states of volume expansion (Fig. 86.14). It increases GFR and natriuresis by afferent arteriolar vasodilation and efferent arteriolar vasoconstriction as well as sodium reabsorption inhibition in the medullary collecting duct, respectively (Kim et al., 2002; Koda et al., 2005; Laragh, 1985; Sward et al., 2004, 2005; Zeidel et al., 1988).

Vasodilation

Two gases act as hormones at the level of the kidney to stimulate vasodilation. **Nitric oxide (NO)** is synthesized by the actions of the enzyme nitric oxide synthase (NOS) (Albrecht et al., 2002; Arnal et al., 1999; Cai et al., 2001; Chander et al., 2005; Harris et al., 2003). Vascular shear stress leads to NOS expression, which in turn upregulates NO production (Davis et al., 2004). NO diffuses to vascular smooth muscle cells, where it activates soluble guanylyl cyclase (sGC), producing 3',5'-cyclic guanosine monophosphate (cGMP). Subsequently, cGMP activates cGMP- and 3',5'-cyclic adenosine monophosphate (cAMP)-dependent protein kinases (PKG and PKA, respectively), leading to smooth muscle relaxation (Kawashima et al., 2001; Rudic et al., 1998; Schnermann and Levine, 2003). NOS inhibition increases renal vascular resistance and decreases the glomerular filtration rate (Schnermann et al., 1998; Takeda et al., 2004; Wang et al., 2003). **Carbon monoxide (CO)** is produced by heme oxygenase, an essential enzyme that catalyzes heme degradation, resulting in the formation of CO as well as iron and biliverdin (Gabbai, 2001; Hill-Kapturczak et al., 2002; Miyazono et al., 2002; Mustafa and Johns, 2001; Nakao et al., 2005; Ohta et al., 2000; Rodriguez et al., 2003; Sikorski et al., 2004; Wang et al., 2003; Zou et al., 2000). Increased CO production produces vasodilation in the kidney and can counteract catecholamine-induced vasoconstriction. In addition, CO has documented antiinflammatory, antioxidant, and cytoprotective actions.

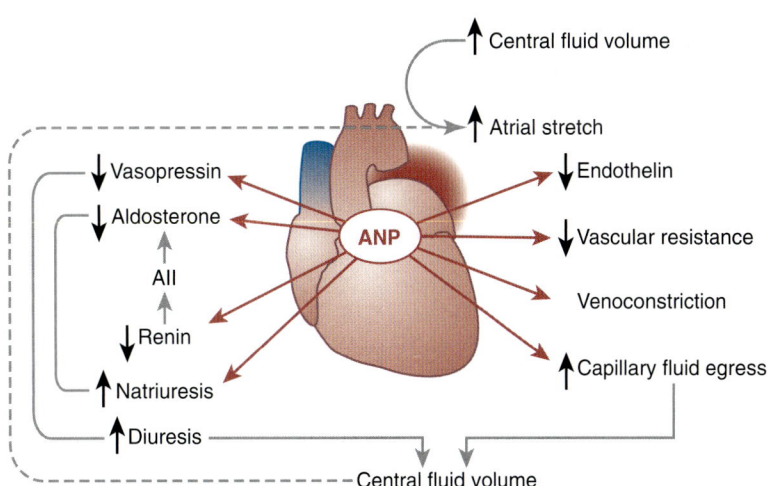

Fig. 86.14. Schematic representation of the fundamental biologic processes of atrial natriuretic peptide (ANP). *AII*, Angiotensin II.

> **KEY POINTS**
> - The renin-angiotensin system is one of multiple chemical mediators that act on renal vascular tone to control renal blood flow.
> - Endothelin is the most potent vasoconstrictor.
> - NO and CO are potent vasodilators.

Red Blood Cell Production

The kidney is the major organ involved in monitoring and regulating red blood cell (RBC) levels. It does so via erythropoietin (EPO). **Basal RBC production is roughly 10 RBCs/h, but this rate can be greatly increased during times of anemia or hypoxia** (Arany et al., 1996). **The kidney is responsible for the majority of EPO production (90%), whereas the liver may contribute a smaller amount (10%).** Kidney-derived EPO is produced by a subpopulation of interstitial fibroblasts, and possibly proximal tubular cells, in response to decreased O_2 tension (Suda et al., 1984). Under hypoxic conditions, the alpha subunit of the regulatory protein hypoxia-inducible factor-1 (HIF-1) is exposed. Binding of HIF-1α with HIF-1β, hepatic nuclear factor-4 (HNF-4), and p300 turns on erythropoietin transcription (Juul et al., 1998; Mikami et al., 2005; Munugalavadla and Kapur, 2005; Wang et al., 1995). In certain malignancies, such as renal cell carcinoma, erythropoiesis is enhanced because of a mutation in the von Hippel-Lindau (VHL) gene (Wiesener et al., 2002). As a result, there are constitutively increased levels of HIF-1 and polycythemia. In states of chronic inflammation and renal insufficiency, erythropoiesis is decreased (Suehiro et al., 2005). Thus anemia is common in the later stages of renal failure. This is due to decreased EPO levels as a result of a reduction in the number of functional EPO-producing cells within the kidney (Muta and Krantz, 1993). Recombinant human erythropoietin (rHuEPO) has been shown to be an effective treatment for this type of anemia (Bennett et al., 2008; Patel et al., 2004).

Bone Mineralization

The kidney plays an important role in the regulation of **vitamin D** activity. The major source of vitamin D is through dermal synthesis of the precursor compound cholecalciferol (vitamin D_3), or through dietary intake of vitamin D_3–fortified foods. Vitamin D_3 has minimal biologic activity. In the liver it is hydroxylated through the action of 25-hydroxylase to form 25-hydroxycholecalciferol (calcidiol). The calcidiol molecule is bound to vitamin D binding protein and transported to the kidney, where it is filtered and reabsorbed by renal tubular cells. In the tubular cell, vitamin D_3 is also hydroxylated by 1α-hydroxylase and 24α-hydroxylase to produce either inactive 24,25-dihydroxycholecalciferol or 1,25-dihydroxycholecalciferol (calcitriol), the biologically active form that is 100 times more potent than calcidiol (Portale et al., 1989; Young et al., 2004). Calcitriol production is regulated by calcidiol levels as well as the 1α-hydroxylase levels (Tuohimaa et al., 2005). These are, in turn, determined by parathyroid hormone (PTH) and plasma phosphate levels (increased enzyme activity) and serum calcitriol levels (decreased enzyme activity). However, unregulated calcitriol synthesis can occur in macrophages in granulomatous conditions such as sarcoidosis and tuberculosis, and in prostate epithelial and cancer cells. **Calcitriol functions through a single intracellular vitamin D receptor (VDR) to regulate gene transcription. Its primary function is the maintenance of serum calcium and phosphorus levels.** The four main target organs are the intestine (increases intestinal absorption of calcium, and to a lesser extent, phosphorus), the bones (regulates osteoblast activity, and in combination with PTH, allows for osteoclast activation and bone resorption), the kidney (increases reabsorption of calcium), and the parathyroid gland (suppresses PTH release) (Lowe et al., 1992). In total, vitamin D contributes to normal bone mineralization by maintaining normal serum calcium and phosphorus levels through increased intestinal absorption of calcium and phosphorus and increased renal reabsorption of calcium.

PTH production is directly influenced by serum calcium levels (Fig. 86.15). Its synthesis, secretion, and degradation is regulated through calcium-sensing receptors located on parathyroid cells. During periods of hypocalcemia, PTH synthesis and secretion are increased while degradation is decreased. The opposite occurs during hypercalcemia. In addition, calcitriol has a suppressive effect on PTH synthesis and parathyroid cell proliferation, mediated through vitamin D receptors located on the surface of parathyroid cells (Broadus et al., 1980). Hyperphosphatemia also directly stimulates PTH release, primarily in advanced renal insufficiency. PTH exerts its activity through PTH/PTHrP receptors, which are localized primarily in the kidneys and bone (Pfister et al., 1997). In the bone it stimulates bone resorption and increases serum calcium and phosphorus levels when administered continuously, whereas it leads to increased bone formation and mineral density when given intermittently.

In the kidney, the effects of PTH are threefold. First, it increases active calcium reabsorption at the level of the distal tubule. Second, it decreases phosphate reabsorption in the proximal convoluted tubule (and the distal tubule, to a lesser degree) through its action on the sodium phosphorus cotransporter. Third, it stimulates calcitriol production by increasing 1α-hydroxylase levels while decreasing 24α-hydroxylase levels. **Overall, PTH maintains normal serum calcium and phosphorus levels by increasing bone resorption, increasing renal reabsorption of calcium and excretion of phosphorus, and stimulating production of calcitriol.**

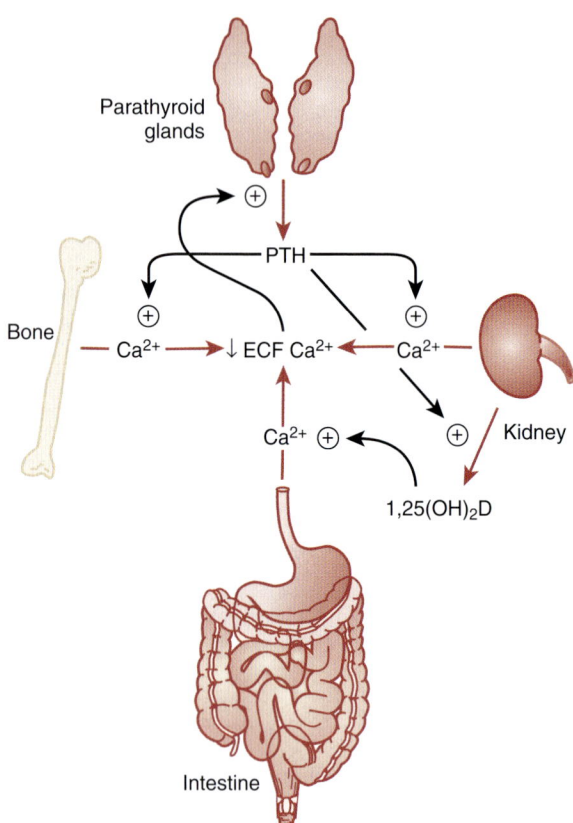

Fig. 86.15. Effects of vitamin D and parathyroid hormone (PTH) on calcium homeostasis. *ECF*, Extracellular fluid. (From Yu SLY: Renal transport of calcium, magnesium, and phosphate. In Brenner BM, editor: *Brenner and Rector's the kidney*, ed 7, Philadelphia, 2004, WB Saunders, p 536.)

> **KEY POINTS**
> - Renal physiology influences bone metabolism through several hormonal actions.
> - In the kidney, vitamin D is hydroxylated into calcitriol, which helps maintain systemic calcium and phosphate levels.
> - PTH influences the kidney to increase calcium reabsorption.

PATHOPHYSIOLOGY AND MANAGEMENT OF RENOVASCULAR HYPERTENSION

Pathophysiology

Renovascular disease refers to states in which reduced perfusion of the kidney exist. This may occur in the absence of hypertension. For example, in ischemic nephropathy, reduced GFR is associated with reduced renal blood flow beyond levels of renal autoregulatory compensation (Chonchol and Linas, 2006; Garcia-Donaire and Alcazar, 2005; Jacobson, 1988; Meyrier et al., 1998; Novick and Fergany, 2002; Novick et al., 1996). In contrast, renovascular hypertension is a clinical syndrome marked by a rise in arterial pressure with or without associated ischemic and hypertensive renal injury (Ploth, 1995; Pohl, 1993, 1999). Its most common cause is renal artery stenosis (RAS), defined as narrowing of the renal artery by more than 50% of its natural luminal diameter (Derkx and Schalekamp, 1994; Dworkin and Cooper, 2009). RAS can be unilateral or bilateral and is separated into two major subtypes. Atherosclerotic RAS accounts for 60% to 80% of cases and fibromuscular dysplasia the remainder. Other rare causes of renovascular hypertension include arterial aneurysm, arteriovenous malformation, extrinsic renal artery compression, neurofibromatosis type 1, and Williams syndrome. **Although affecting only 5% of hypertensives, renovascular disease has been estimated to be the cause of renal failure in 5% to 15% of those older than 50 years of age and may account for as much as 10% to 20% of the end-stage renal disease population** (Mailloux et al., 1994; Svetkey et al., 1991; van Ampting et al., 2003).

Atherosclerotic renal artery disease predominantly affects men and women aged 40 to 70 years (Caps et al., 1998a; Greco and Breyer, 1997; Pohl and Novick, 1985). The proximal third of the renal artery is usually involved, and in 70% to 80% of the patients there is an aortic plaque impinging on the renal ostium, whereas the remaining 30% exhibit non-ostial narrowing usually 1 to 3 cm distal to the renal artery ostium (Caps et al., 1998b; Crutchley et al., 2009).

In contrast to atherosclerotic renal artery disease, **there are four types of fibromuscular dysplasia: medial fibroplasia, perimedial fibroplasia, intimal fibroplasia, and medial hyperplasia** (Table 86.1). Medial, perimedial, and intimal fibroplastic lesions may affect the renal artery with an incidence of 30%, 5%, and 5%, respectively, and they represent 70% to 85%, 10% to 25%, and 10%, respectively, of all fibrous renal artery diseases. Medial hyperplasia, the fourth type of fibrous dysplasia, constitutes only 2% to 3% of all fibrous dysplastic lesions (Eddy, 2000; Olin, 2007; Olin and Sealove, 2011; Olin et al., 2012; Slovut and Olin, 2004).

Medial fibroplasia occurs almost exclusively in women between 25 and 50 years of age. This lesion has the characteristic **"string of beads"** appearance on angiography and usually involves both renal arteries (Fig. 86.16). **The lesions involve the distal half of the main renal artery and may extend into the branches.** Histologically, the lesions are characterized by the growth of fibroblasts in the media covered by fibrous connective tissue in the stenotic areas and thinned-out medial tissue in the aneurysmal areas, thus creating the string-of-beads appearance on angiography. **These patients are not likely to progress to complete occlusion, nor are they likely to experience a decrease in their overall renal function.**

Perimedial fibroplasia also occurs almost exclusively in women, but they are younger (between 5 and 15 years of age). The stenosis **occurs classically in the midrenal artery**, although it may extend into the distal renal artery and its branches. Similar to medial fibroplasia, angiography may demonstrate a string of beads. However, unlike

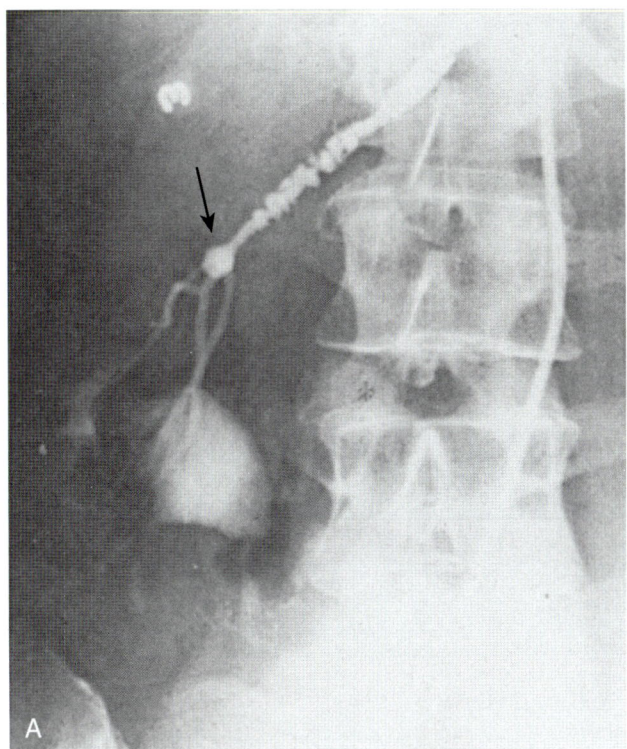

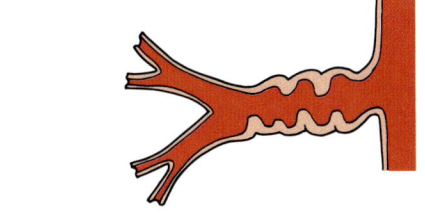

Fig. 86.16. Arteriogram and schematic diagrams of medial fibroplasia. (A) Right renal arteriogram demonstrating weblike stenosis with interposed segments of dilatation (large beads) typical of medial fibroplasia ("string-of-beads" lesion) *(arrow)*. (B) Schematic diagram of perimedial fibroplasia. (A, From Novick AC: Renal vascular hypertension in children. In Kelalis PP, King LR, Belman AB, editors: *Clinical pediatric urology*, Philadelphia, 1984, Saunders. B, From Pohl M: Renovascular hypertension and ischemic nephropathy. In Schrier RW, editor: *Atlas of diseases of the kidney: hypertension and the kidney*, vol 3, Hoboken, NJ, 1999, Wiley-Blackwell [chapter 3, figure 3-5].)

TABLE 86.1 Frequency and Natural History of Fibrous Renal Artery Diseases

LESION	FREQUENCY, %[a]	RISK OF PROGRESSION	THREAT TO RENAL FUNCTION
Intimal fibroplasia and medial hyperplasia	10	++++	++++
Perimedial fibroplasia	10–25	++++	++++
Medial fibroplasia	70–85	++	—

[a]Frequency relates to frequency of only the fibrous renal artery diseases.
From Pohl M. Renovascular hypertension and ischemic nephropathy. In Schrier RW, editor: *Atlas of diseases of the kidney: hypertension and the kidney*, vol 3, Hoboken, NJ, 1999, Wiley-Blackwell (chapter 3, figure 3-4).

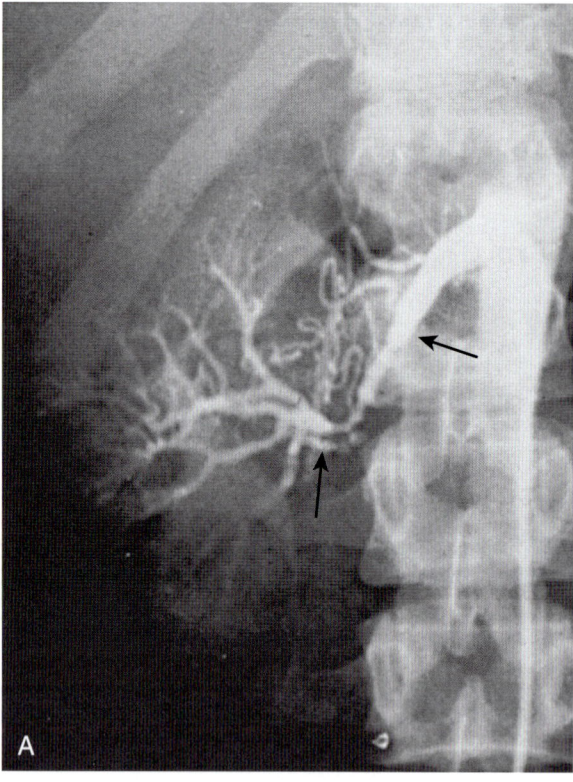

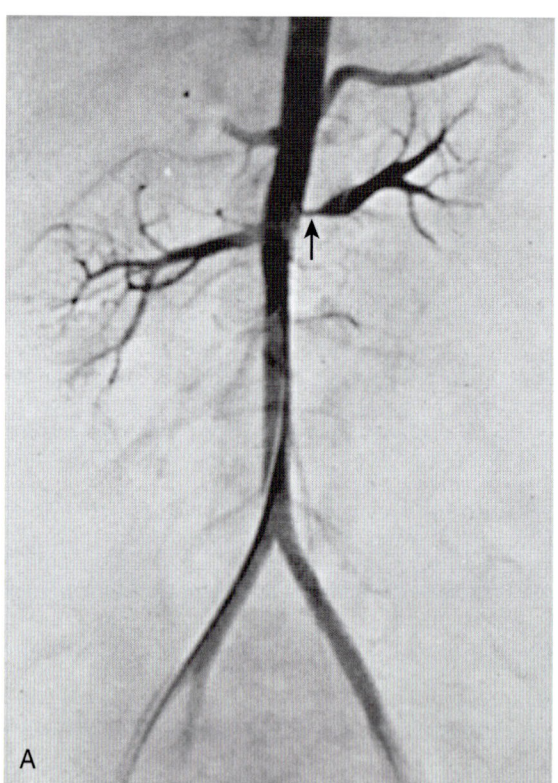

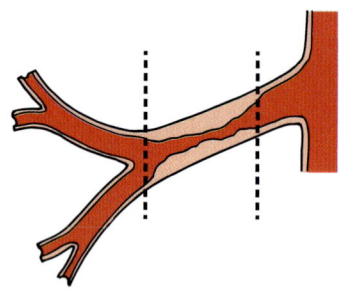

Fig. 86.17. Arteriogram and schematic diagram of perimedial fibroplasia. (A) Selective right renal arteriogram shows a tight stenosis in the midportion of the renal artery *(arrows)* with a small string-of-beads appearance, typical of perimedial fibroplasia. (B) Schematic diagram of perimedial fibroplasia. (A, From Novick AC: Renal vascular hypertension in children. In Kelalis PP, King LR, Belman AB, editors: Clinical pediatric urology, Philadelphia, 1984, Saunders. B, From Pohl M: Renovascular hypertension and ischemic nephropathy. In Schrier RW, editor: *Atlas of diseases of the kidney: hypertension and the kidney*, vol 3, Hoboken, NJ, 1999, Wiley-Blackwell [chapter 3, figure 3-6].)

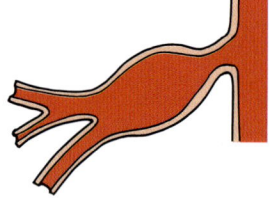

Fig. 86.18. Arteriogram and schematic diagram of intimal fibroplasia. (A) Selective right renal arteriogram demonstrates a localized, highly stenotic, smooth lesion involving the distal renal artery, from intimal fibroplasia. (B) Schematic diagram of intimal fibroplasia. Aortogram of a 6-year-old boy in (A) demonstrates proximal left renal artery stenosis *(arrow)* from intimal fibroplasia. (A, From Novick AC: Renal vascular hypertension in children. In Kelalis PP, King LR, Belman AB, editors: *Clinical pediatric urology*, Philadelphia, 1984, Saunders. B, From Pohl M: Renovascular hypertension and ischemic nephropathy. In Schrier RW, editor: *Atlas of diseases of the kidney: hypertension and the kidney*, vol 3, Hoboken, NJ, 1999, Wiley-Blackwell [chapter 3, figure 3-7].)

> **KEY POINTS**
> - RAS is the most common cause of renovascular hypertension.
> - Atherosclerotic vascular disease accounts for two-thirds of cases of RAS.
> - Four types of fibromuscular dysplasia can also cause RAS. Of these types, medial fibroplasia is the most common and least likely to progress over time.

medial fibroplasia, the aneurysmal "beads" in perimedial fibroplasia that never exceed the diameter of the main renal artery (Fig. 86.17). Histologically, there is widespread collagen deposition in the outer half of the media. **If left untreated, perimedial fibroplasia often progresses to renal occlusion and loss of renal function.**

Intimal fibroplasia accounts for 10% of the cases of fibromuscular dysplasia and occurs predominantly in children and younger adults. Histologically, there is collagen deposition within the intimal arterial layer. This form of fibroplasia may be complicated by disruptions of the internal elastic lamina and hence **may result in dissection, arterial wall hematoma, and renal infarction** (Fig. 86.18). The lesions are usually in the proximal renal artery; however, they may also occur in the mid- or distal renal artery and **without intervention are likely to progress and result in loss of renal function.**

Medial hyperplasia is a rare disease, often angiographically indistinguishable from intimal fibroplasia. Histologically, there is smooth muscle cell hyperplasia with no associated fibrosis.

Diagnosis

Renovascular hypertension should be suspected in the presence of the following signs and symptoms (Working Group on Renovascular Hypertension, 1987):
1. Severe or refractory hypertension with evidence of grade III or IV hypertensive retinopathy (Davis et al., 1979)
2. Abrupt onset of moderate to severe hypertension, particularly in a normotensive or previously well-controlled hypertensive (Ram et al., 1995)

3. Onset of hypertension before age 20 (early onset) or after age 50 (late onset), particularly in those without a family history of hypertension (Spitalewitz and Reiser, 2000)
4. Unexplained worsening of renal function with or without hypertension or in association with the use of ACE inhibitors or angiotensin II receptor blockers (ARBs) or with a reduction of blood pressure (BP) to the current accepted norm with the use of other antihypertensive agents (Hricik and Dunn, 1990)
5. Paradoxic worsening of hypertension with the use of diuretics
6. Unexplained recurrent episodes of heart failure—"flash" pulmonary edema
7. The presence of a systolic-diastolic abdominal bruit that radiates to both flanks
8. The presence of diffuse vascular disease and/or evidence of cholesterol embolization

Because effective BP control may be achieved in most patients with renovascular hypertension, and **it remains uncertain whether the correction of an underlying vascular lesion results in long-term BP control or preservation of renal function,** testing for renovascular hypertension should be pursued only if revascularization is being seriously considered. Some screening techniques pose risks to those with compromised renal function and may be associated with significant morbidity.

The now-classic dog experiments performed by Goldblatt et al. in 1934 led to our current understanding of the pathogenesis of renovascular hypertension. Use of a clamp allowed control of the degree of RAS in each kidney separately in the dog model. Blood pressure was monitored in the dogs after clamping the renal artery to one or both kidneys and to one kidney after the removal of the contralateral kidney. Subsequently, **two animal models of renal hypertension have become the hallmark for all studies on experimental renovascular hypertension.** They are the two-kidney, one-clip hypertension model (Fig. 86.19), in which one renal artery is clipped and the other renal artery is left unaltered (2K1C), and the one-kidney, one-clip hypertension model (Fig. 86.20), in which one renal artery is clipped and the contralateral kidney is removed. In the two-kidney model, hypertension is mediated by angiotensin II driving aldosterone secretion and in turn sodium retention (Caravaggi et al., 1976; Imamura et al., 1995). Renin secretion in the normal contralateral kidney is suppressed and under a higher perfusion pressure is able to excrete most of the excess salt and water. Because there is limited sodium retention, there is no significant feedback inhibition of renin secretion in the stenotic kidney. Thus it continues to secrete AII and the vasoconstriction and hypertension is maintained. **This form of hypertension may be managed with reversal of the RAS, with ACE inhibition, or with angiotensin receptor blockade** (Michel et al., 1986). In contrast to the two-kidney model, the absence of a normal contralateral kidney prevents natriuresis and diuresis in response to RAS. Thus there is volume expansion, and renin secretion is suppressed in the clipped kidney because of feedback inhibition. Volume expansion remains, and there is sustained hypertension in spite of the decreased vasoconstriction associated with the now-suppressed RAS (Vasuvattakul et al., 1992). The one-kidney model is driven by volume expansion and sodium retention with normal circulating levels of AII.

Multiple screening tests for renovascular hypertension exist (Canzanello and Textor, 1994; Mann and Pickering, 1992; White et al., 2006). Intravenous pyelography (IVP), measurement of plasma renin activity, and renal scintigraphy were used in the past (Pedersen, 1994; Rene et al., 1995; Setaro et al., 1991; van Jaarsveld et al., 1997), but they have been replaced by more sensitive and specific techniques. Currently, the noninvasive screening tests that provide the highest sensitivity and specificity are magnetic resonance angiography (MRA) (de Haan et al., 1996; Klatzburg et al., 1994; Postma et al., 1997; Sommer et al., 1992), spiral (helical) computed tomography (CT) (Kim et al., 1998; Olbricht et al., 1995), and duplex Doppler ultrasonography (Hoffman et al., 1991; Kaplan-Pavlovcic and Nadja, 1998; Kliewer et al., 1994; Stavros and Harshfield, 1994). Concerns regarding the possibility of gadolinium-induced nephrogenic systemic fibrosis raise the need for caution for MRA use in patients with unstable or reduced renal function (GFR <30 mL/min), although it has the greatest sensitivity and specificity (100% and 71%–96%, respectively) of the three tests (Rieumont et al., 1997; Schoenberg et al., 1998; Tan et al., 2002). CT angiography has a sensitivity of 98% and a specificity of 94% for detecting renovascular lesions, but the sensitivity and specificity of CT angiography decline (93% and

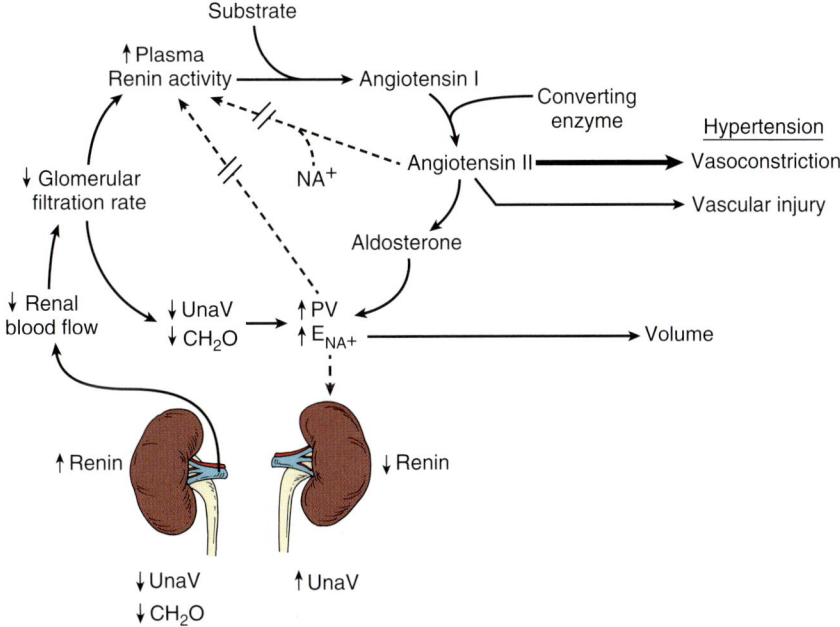

Fig. 86.19. The renin system in the setting of unilateral renal artery stenosis with a normal contralateral kidney characterized by (1) high peripheral plasma renin activity, (2) contralateral suppression of renin release, and (3) a decrease in ipsilateral renal blood flow (RBF). The resultant hypertension is mediated by angiotensin II-induced vasoconstriction. (From Vaughan E, Laragh J: New concepts of the renin system and vasoconstriction-volume mechanisms: diagnosis and treatment of renovascular and renal hypertensions. *Urol Clin North Am* 2:240–241, 1975, figure 2.)

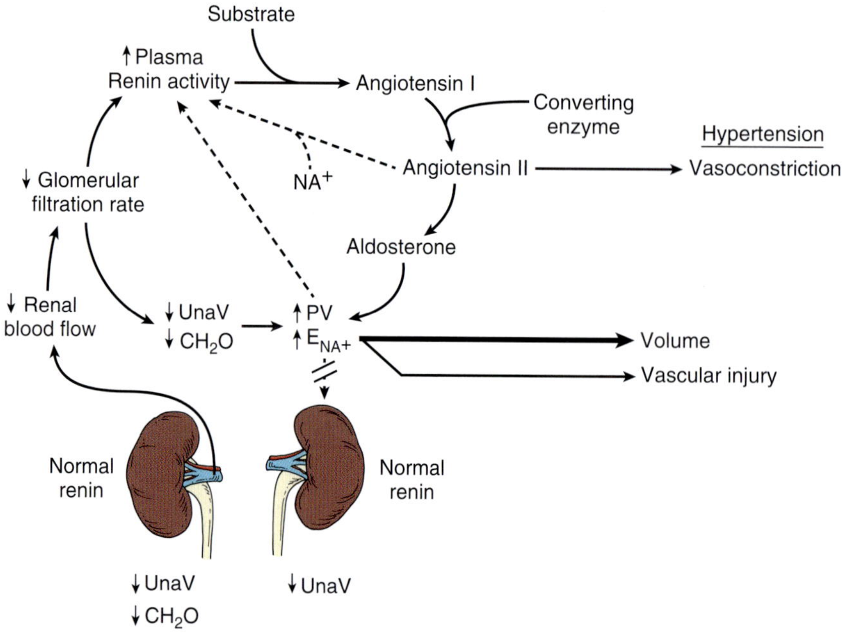

Fig. 86.20. The renin system in the setting of unilateral renal artery stenosis (or parenchymal disease) with an abnormal contralateral kidney. Disease in the opposite kidney limits sodium excretion, thereby allowing volume (sodium) retention, which feeds back to lower the peripheral renin to normal or subnormal values. In addition, contralateral renin secretion continues so that contralateral renin suppression does not occur. The hypertension is maintained by an inappropriate interaction of vasoconstriction and volume with the volume factor predominating. (From Vaughan E, Laragh J: New concepts of the renin system and vasoconstriction-volume mechanisms: diagnosis and treatment of renovascular and renal hypertensions. *Urol Clin North Am* 2:240–1, 1975, figure 2.)

81%, respectively) in the presence of renal insufficiency (serum creatinine >1.7 mg/dL), and the risk of dye-induced nephrotoxicity increases. Comparatively, duplex Doppler ultrasonography provides many advantages. It can demonstrate bilateral disease, does not require the discontinuation of antihypertensive therapy or the exposure to potentially nephrotoxic contrast, and is accurate for those with renal failure (Radermacher et al., 2001; Williams et al., 2007). Despite these advantages, the use of duplex Doppler ultrasonography is limited by the fact that it is time consuming, is highly operator dependent, and is a technically difficult test to perform (Olin et al., 1995). If suspicion for a renovascular lesion remains high despite a negative noninvasive screening test, conventional renal angiography and intraarterial digital subtraction angiography (DSA) remain the gold standard for diagnosing renovascular disease and are indicated particularly if intervention is contemplated (Dunnick et al., 1989; Hawkins et al., 1994).

> **KEY POINTS**
> - Suspect renovascular hypertension in patients with severe or abrupt-onset hypertension who otherwise have no risk factors for high blood pressure.
> - Two models of renovascular hypertension were established with classic dog model experiments: the two-kidney, one-clip and one-kidney, one-clip models.
> - Noninvasive diagnostic imaging, including MR angiography, CT angiography, and duplex ultrasonography, should be first-line screening to diagnose RAS.

Management

Medical Therapy

Control of BP in those with renovascular hypertension may be achieved in more than 90% of patients with medical therapy alone (Aurell and Jensen, 1997; Hirsch et al., 2006). Because of the severity of the hypertension, however, therapy generally requires multiple antihypertensive medications. Although all classes of antihypertensives may be used (Franklin and Smith, 1985), drugs that inhibit AII production **(ACE inhibitors)** or block its receptor site **(ARBs) have been shown to be particularly efficacious** because the hypertension is often the result of activation of the renin-angiotensin system (Hollenberg, 1987; Ishidoya et al., 1995; van de Ven et al., 1999). When used as monotherapy, ACE inhibitors may control BP in 80% of patients, and when combined with a diuretic, control may be increased to almost 90%. **Medical therapy may reduce BP below a critical level and induce ongoing renal ischemia** distal to the arterial lesion, resulting in tubular atrophy, interstitial fibrosis, glomerulosclerosis, and progressive loss of function in the affected kidney(s). **Although these changes are more likely to be observed with antihypertensives that inhibit angiotensin or block its receptors than with others,** this is not uniformly seen in clinical practice (Tullis et al., 1999). In addition, with the exception of medial fibromuscular dysplasia, all forms of RAS can progress in severity despite medical therapy (Safian and Textor, 2001; Schreiber et al., 1984; Strandness, 1994; Wollenweber et al., 1968). Therefore **renal function should be closely monitored whenever antihypertensive agents are used in patients with renovascular hypertension** (Baboolal et al., 1998), particularly when they are combined with a diuretic. In addition to monitoring the serum creatinine concentration and estimated GFR or creatinine clearance, renal sizes and cortical blood flow velocity by duplex scanning should be assessed, because they may more quickly provide evidence of irreversible nephron loss (Rimmer and Gennari, 1993). ACE inhibitors and ARBs, particularly in the setting of volume contraction, may also result in acute (usually reversible) renal failure in 10% to 20% of those with either bilateral RAS or RAS affecting a solitary kidney.

Percutaneous Intervention

Percutaneous transluminal renal artery angioplasty (PTRA) is an angiographic technique by which stenotic renal arteries are dilated

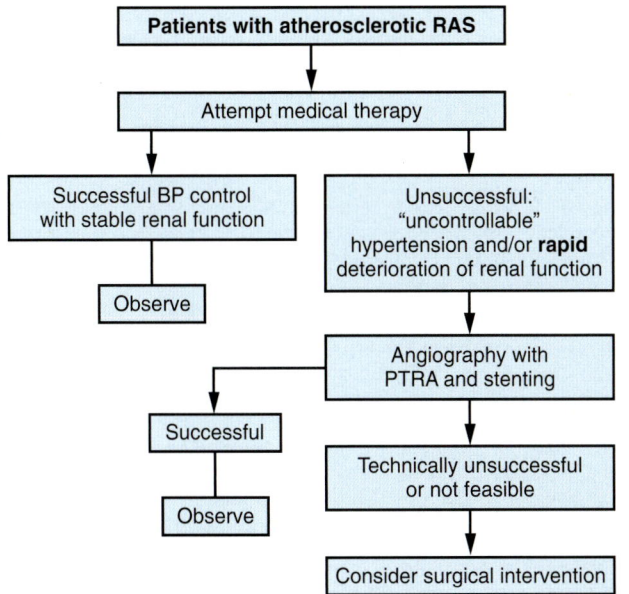

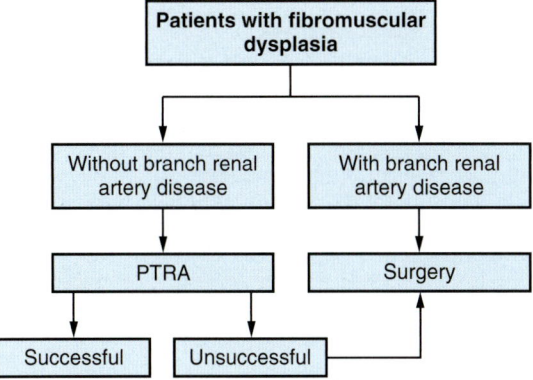

Fig. 86.22. Algorithm for the management of patients with fibromuscular dysplasia. *PTRA*, Percutaneous transluminal renal angioplasty.

Fig. 86.21. Algorithm for the management of patients with arteriosclerotic renal artery stenosis (RAS). *BP*, Blood pressure; *PTRA*, percutaneous transluminal renal angioplasty.

with a balloon-tipped catheter (Kidney and Deutsch, 1996; Libertino and Beckmann, 1994; Sos, 1991). Lesions that are most amenable to PTRA include those that are less than 10 mm in length, are partially occluded, and do not involve the ostium (Fig. 86.21; Geyskes, 1988; Tuttle et al., 1998; van de Ven et al., 1995). After successful PTRA, an improvement in BP may be seen as quickly as 4 to 6 hours after the procedure but is more commonly seen after 48 hours, although the maximal antihypertensive effect may not be observed for several weeks (Bonelli et al., 1995; Canzanello et al., 1989; O'Donovan et al., 1992; Ramsay and Waller, 1990; van Jaarsveld et al., 2000). In general, the absence of an early antihypertensive response suggests that a long-term improvement of hypertension is unlikely (Webster et al., 1998). PTRA without stenting has proved successful for patients with underlying fibromuscular dysplasia (Fig. 86.22; Dorros et al., 1995,1998a,b; Mousa et al., 2012; Plouin et al., 1998). In contrast, successful PTRA in patients with unilateral atherosclerotic RAS is technically more difficult to achieve (technical success rates may be as low as 70%), and rates of cure or long-term improvement of hypertension have not been consistent. Although the placement of an intraluminal stent may increase success rates (Harden et al., 1997; Iannone et al., 1996; Marana et al., 1998; Marshall et al., 1990; Rees, 1999; Rees et al., 1991; Rundback et al., 1998), **the restenosis rate remains at about 15% to 25%** (Blum et al., 1997; Boisclair et al., 1997; Isles et al., 1999; Rocha-Singh et al., 2005). **The effects on BP after PTRA in patients with bilateral RAS have been disappointing as well**, in part, because of the frequent presence of ostial or completely occluded lesions. **Even when technically successful, the restenosis rate after PTRA is significant** (30% for nonostial and 50% for ostial lesions) and may occur shortly after the procedure (15% to 30% within 2 years) with recurrence of uncontrolled or accelerated hypertension.

Although the results of many earlier studies suggest that PTRA with stenting may cure or improve control of hypertension, three more recent randomized studies raise questions about the effectiveness of revascularization with stenting for BP control. The Stent Placement and Blood Pressure and Lipid-lowering for Prevention of Progression of Renal Dysfunction Caused by Atherosclerotic Ostial Stenosis of the Renal Artery **(STAR)** trial enrolled 140 patients with BP controlled to less than 140/90 mm Hg, and with a renal ostial lesion greater than 50%, and prospectively randomized the patients to either renal artery stenting and medical therapy or medical therapy alone. At the end of follow-up, **there was no difference in the degree of BP control** (Bax et al., 2009; Corriere et al., 2008). In the Angioplasty and Stenting for Renal Artery Lesions **(ASTRAL)** trial, 806 patients with atherosclerotic RAS were randomized to undergo revascularization and medical therapy or to undergo medical therapy alone. After a median follow-up of **34 months, there was no difference in BP control between the two groups**, although the number of antihypertensive medications required was slightly higher in the medically managed group (ASTRAL Investigators et al., 2009). The Cardiovascular Outcomes and Renal Atherosclerotic Lesions (CORAL) study was a multicentered, open-label, randomized controlled trial that compared medical therapy alone with medical therapy plus renal artery stenting in patients with atherosclerotic RAS and elevated BP, chronic kidney disease, or both. **Medical therapy consisted of an ARB, a calcium channel blocker, a statin, a diuretic, and other medications as necessary.** Overall, a reduction of systolic BP of a mean of 15 to 16 mm Hg was achieved in both groups with **an average of 3.4 medications, not different in either group.** In addition, for all three studies, no long-term preservation of renal function was shown with vascular stenting. These studies raise the question of whether the risk of stenting for RAS is worth the potential benefit regarding BP control or prevention of renal failure, although many believe that a subset of patients may benefit from endovascular intervention (Cooper et al., 2014; Ives et al., 2003; Korsakas et al., 2004; Krijnen et al., 2004; Nordmann et al., 2003).

Surgical Treatment

With the advent of ACE inhibitors, angiotensin receptor blockade, statins, and PTRA, **the need for surgical revascularization and reconstruction of the renal artery has diminished.** However, an indication for surgical intervention in a select group of patients remains (Bhatt et al., 2014). Patients with RAS with concomitant aneurysmal or occlusive aortic disease in which surgery is indicated may benefit from surgical intervention to correct both lesions if the aortic disease cannot be repaired without correcting the renal occlusive disease as well. Surgery is also indicated in patients with macroaneurysms of the renal artery associated with the stenosis because rupture of these lesions may occur if they are larger than 4 cm. Patients who exhibit malignant/accelerated or uncontrollable hypertension, who do not tolerate medical therapy, or who show rapid deterioration of renal function (1 to 6 months before presentation) with serum creatinine remaining between 1.5 and 3.0 mg/dL may also benefit from surgical intervention (Textor, 1998). Although PTRA can still be performed under most circumstances in these latter groups, for an ostial lesion greater than 10 mm in length, there may still be a role for surgical revascularization. Therefore there remains a group of patients who will require surgical intervention (Middleton, 1998; Novick et al., 1987).

KEY POINTS

- Medical management for renovascular hypertension is the mainstay of therapy.
- Percutaneous intervention to treat RAS may be effective, but growing evidence calls into question its efficacy to control blood pressure or prevent renal failure long term.
- Although surgical treatment is no longer first-line therapy for RAS, its role still exists for the appropriately selected patient.

SUGGESTED READINGS

HORMONAL
Delles C, Klingbeil AU, Schneider MP, et al: The role of nitric oxide in the regulation of glomerular haemodynamics in humans, *Nephrol Dial Transplant* 19:1392–1397, 2004.

Lariviere R, Lebel M: Endothelin-1 in chronic renal failure and hypertension, *Can J Physiol Pharmacol* 81:607–621, 2003.

Robertson GL: Physiology of ADH secretion, *Kidney Int Suppl* 21:S20–S26, 1987.

RENAL TUBULAR FUNCTION
Cockcroft DW, Gault MH: Prediction of creatinine clearance from serum creatinine, *Nephron* 16:31–41, 1976.

Shemesh O, Golbetz H, Kriss JP, et al: Limitations of creatinine as a filtration marker in glomerulopathic patients, *Kidney Int* 28:830–838, 1985.

Wang T: Role of iNOS and eNOS in modulating proximal tubule transport and acid-base balance, *Am J Physiol Renal Physiol* 283:F658–F662, 2002.

SODIUM, WATER, AND POTASSIUM IMBALANCES
Kaschina E, Unger T: Angiotensin AT1/AT2 receptors: regulation, signaling and function, *Blood Press* 12:70–88, 2003.

Miller M: Inappropriate antidiuretic hormone secretion, *Curr Ther Endocrinol Metab* 5:186–189, 1994.

Yeates KE, Singer M, Morton AR: Salt and water: a simple approach to hyponatremia, *CMAJ* 170:365–369, 2004.

ACID-BASE
Corey HE: Bench-to-bedside review: fundamental principles of acid-base physiology, *Crit Care* 9:184–192, 2005.

Levraut J, Grimaud D: Treatment of metabolic acidosis, *Curr Opin Crit Care* 9:260–265, 2003.

Roth KS, Chan JC: Renal tubular acidosis: a new look at an old problem, *Clin Pediatr (Phila)* 40:533–543, 2001.

RENOVASCULAR HYPERTENSION
ASTRAL Investigators, Wheatley K, Ives N, et al: Revascularization versus medical therapy for renal-artery stenosis, *N Engl J Med* 361:1953–1962, 2009.

Bax L, Woittiez AJ, Kouwenberg HJ, et al: Stent placement in patients with atherosclerotic renal artery stenosis and impaired renal function: a randomized trial, *Ann Intern Med* 150:840–848, 2009.

Cooper CJ, Murphy TP, Cutlip DE, et al: Stenting and medical therapy for atherosclerosis renal-artery stenosis, *N Engl J Med* 370:13–22, 2014.

Dworkin LD, Cooper CJ: Renal-artery stenosis, *N Engl J Med* 361:1972–1978, 2009.

Slovut DP, Olin JW: Fibromuscular dysplasia, *N Engl J Med* 350:1862–1871, 2004.

REFERENCES

The complete reference list is available online at ExpertConsult.com.

87 Renal Insufficiency and Ischemic Nephropathy

Joshua Augustine, MD, Alvin C. Wee, MD, Venkatesh Krishnamurthi, MD, and David A. Goldfarb, MD

ACUTE KIDNEY INJURY

Acute kidney injury (AKI) in is defined by an acute rise in serum creatinine (SCr) and/or an acute decline in urine output. This abrupt decline in kidney function occurs over hours to days and results in the accumulation of byproducts of metabolism and the dysregulation of electrolyte homeostasis, acid/base, and volume status. Changes in blood urea nitrogen (BUN) and SCr have been used as surrogate markers for changes in kidney function. BUN can be altered by other factors and may be disproportionately elevated in states of volume depletion, in hypercatabolic states, or in marked increased in protein loads seen with gastrointestinal bleeding or total parenteral nutrition. Creatinine is a metabolite of muscle and is used to calculate the estimated glomerular filtration rate (GFR), using GFR equations that also account for age, gender, and black race. The two equations most commonly used and often reported with routine lab values include the Modification of Diet in Renal Disease (MDRD) and the Chronic Kidney Disease Epidemiology Collaboration (CKD-EPI) equations (Levey et al., 1999, 2009). The CKD-EPI equation is a modification of the MDRD formula and is less likely to underestimate true GFR in patients with early stages of chronic kidney disease (CKD) (Levey et al., 2009). It is more predictive of mortality associated with CKD than the MDRD equation (Matsushita et al., 2012).

Because of its dependence on muscle mass, SCr may overestimate kidney function in cases of muscle wasting, such as in patients with cirrhosis or prolonged intensive care unit (ICU) stays (Schetz et al., 2014; Skluzacek et al., 2003). Alternatively, at extremes of high muscle mass, SCr may underestimate kidney function. Another marker of kidney function that has been compared with SCr is the measurement of cystatin C, a low-molecular-weight protein that is a member of the cystatin superfamily of cysteine protease inhibitors (Newman et al., 1995). Unlike creatinine, cystatin is not secreted by renal tubules, although it does undergo renal tubular metabolism. Cystatin C does not appear to be as strongly correlated with muscle mass and thus may improve the accuracy of estimating kidney function in patients with extremes of muscle mass and nutrition, such as patients with cirrhosis (Pöge et al., 2006). However, cystatin C levels appear to be altered in states of inflammation, thyroid disease, and smoking, making it an imperfect replacement for SCr (Knight et al., 2004; Manetti et al., 2005). Combining formulas that estimate GFR using both SCr and cystatin C leads to improved precision and accuracy compared with using either variable alone (Inker et al., 2012). Online calculators that allow for combining of such formulas are available. See The National Kidney Foundation website at https://www.kidney.org/professionals/KDOQI/gfr_calculator.

It is also important to recognize that changes in SCr may lag in appearance after an episode of AKI. For example, contrast nephropathy, which may induce kidney injury immediately after contrast exposure, is often associated in a change in SCr evident only after 24 to 48 hours (Rich et al., 1990). **For this reason, it is inappropriate to estimate GFR using a single SCr value in a hospitalized patient whose SCr is fluctuating.** For example, a patient whose SCr doubles from 1 to 2 mg/dL in 24 hours may have advanced kidney failure with lower clearance than a patient with a stable SCr of 2 mg/dL. Conversely, a patient recovering from AKI or after kidney transplantation with an SCr falling from 6 mg/dL to 3 mg/dL in 24 hours has a better GFR than would be reflected by a stable SCr of 3 mg/dL. Such fluctuation in kidney function can create challenges in drug dosing in the hospital setting (Lewis et al., 2016). In addition, drug dosing has historically relied on outdated methods of measurement of kidney function, such as SCr alone or the calculation of creatinine clearance using formulas such as Cockcroft-Gault. The Cockcroft-Gault formula uses patient weight but does not account for morbid obesity, which may positively skew the estimation of creatinine clearance well above the true GFR (Bouquegneau et al., 2016).

Another method occasionally used to estimate kidney function in the hospital setting is a 24-hour urine collection for creatinine clearance. Twenty-four–hour urine is often imprecise and may result in errors related to over- or undercollection. It may be used to assess kidney function in a patient who is suspected of having impaired kidney function beyond that reflected by the SCr alone, or to screen for renal recovery in a patient with nonoliguric AKI. However, in addition to errors in collection, the percentage of creatinine excreted in the tubules can vary and tends to be a higher percentage of total creatinine excretion at lower levels of GFR. Tubular secretion of creatinine may account for more than a third of creatinine measured in the urine and thus may artificially inflate creatinine clearance relative to true GFR (Doolan et al., 1962).

The gold standard for evaluating kidney function is a measurement of GFR using a marker of pure glomerular filtration (Stevens et al., 2009). Inulin has been used historically but is no longer available in the United States. GFR is more often measured by nuclear medicine testing using iothalamate or other isotopes. Few hospitals routinely use nuclear measurement of GFR, but it has been a valuable tool particularly in research designed to derive estimation formulas. It has also been used in some kidney transplant centers to evaluate kidney function in living kidney donor candidates.

One set of criteria used to define AKI is known as the Risk, Injury Failure, Loss of kidney function, and End-stage kidney disease (RIFLE) criteria (Bellomo et al., 2004; Table 87.1), which divides AKI and chronic kidney failure into stages based on severity and duration. The Kidney Disease: Improving Global Outcomes (KDIGO) definition of AKI is also widely used and is described in Table 87.2. Contrasting from the RIFLE criteria, KDIGO includes an acute rise in SCr more than 0.3 mg/dL within 48 hours as a definition of AKI, along with a rise in SCr of at least 1.5 times baseline within 7 days, or urine volume below 0.5 mL/kg/h for 6 consecutive hours (KDIGO, 2012). Unlike RIFLE, the KDIGO criteria do not include scoring related to prolonged kidney failure or end-stage renal disease (ESRD).

Use of these AKI definitions does not account for the cause of AKI, which may be rapidly correctable in cases of volume depletion, or more severe and sustained in cases of intrinsic ischemic kidney injury. Therefore staging alone has some prognostic capability but should optimally be subdivided into cause of AKI. In addition, it is not always clear whether a patient had a normal baseline SCr before AKI, or developed "acute on chronic" kidney injury with underlying CKD. Patients with CKD have a greater risk for AKI (Chawla et al., 2012). AKI may develop before a hospital admission, with an elevation in SCr on presentation, thus affecting definitions that use the change in SCr from admission to a later hospital date. Regardless, it is recommended that the practitioner identify AKI early in its course because even small changes in SCr may indicate a significant change in kidney function. Early consultation with nephrology may also improve outcomes in hospitalized patients with AKI (Balasubramanian et al., 2011).

TABLE 87.1 The Risk, Injury Failure, Loss of Kidney Function, and End-Stage Kidney Disease (RIFLE) Criteria for Acute Kidney Injury

RIFLE CRITERIA: STAGES	
Stage 1	Increase in serum creatinine 50%–99% OR Urine output < 0.5 mL/kg/h for 6–12 h
Stage 2	Increase in serum creatinine of 100%–200% OR Urine output < 0.5 mL/kg/h for 12–24 h
Failure	Increase in serum creatinine ≥ 200% OR Increase in serum creatinine > 0.5 mg/dL to > 4 mg/dL OR Urine output < 0.3 mL/kg/h for >24 h or anuria for >12 h OR Initiation of renal replacement therapy
Loss	Need for renal replacement therapy for >4 weeks
End stage	Need for renal replacement therapy for >3 months

TABLE 87.2 The Kidney Disease: Improving Global Outcomes (KDIGO) Definition of Acute Kidney Injury

KDIGO CRITERIA: STAGES	
Stage 1	Increase in serum creatinine ≥ 0.3 mg/dL or 50%–99% OR Urine output < 0.5 mL/kg/h for 6–12 h
Stage 2	Increase in serum creatinine of 100%–200% OR Urine output < 0.5 mL/kg/h for 12–24 h
Stage 3	Increase in serum creatinine ≥ 200% OR Increase in serum creatinine ≥ 0.3 mg/dL to ≥ 4 mg/dL OR Urine output < 0.3 mL/kg/h for > 24 h or anuria for ≥ 12 h OR Initiation of renal replacement therapy In patients < 18 y/o: a decline in estimated glomerular filtration rate < 35 mL/min/1.73 m^2

TABLE 87.3 Cause of Hospital-Acquired Acute Kidney Injury in 748 Patients in Thirteen Tertiary Care Centers in Madrid, Spain

CAUSE	PERCENTAGE
Acute tubular necrosis	45
Prerenal disease	21
Acute on chronic kidney disease (primarily resulting from acute tubular necrosis or prerenal)	13
Obstructive disease	10
Glomerulonephritis or vasculitis	4
Acute interstitial nephritis	2
Atheroembolic disease	1

A classic way to divide AKI is by "prerenal," "intrinsic," and "postrenal" or obstructive causes. However, prolonged prerenal physiology may lead to intrinsic kidney ischemia and injury, such as is seen with prolonged hepatorenal syndrome (HRS). Prolonged obstruction can also lead to intrinsic kidney damage. **The greatest proportion of hospital acquired AKI is secondary to acute tubular necrosis (ATN).** A Spanish analysis of 748 cases of AKI in 13 tertiary care hospital centers revealed that ATN accounted for 45% of all AKI (Liaño et al., 1996). Alternatively, immune-mediated AKI from glomerulonephritis or acute interstitial nephritis accounted for less than 10% of cases (Table 87.3).

Prerenal Kidney Injury

Prerenal AKI is caused by new renal hypoperfusion that leads to a fall in GFR typically with urinary sodium avidity, as noted by a reduction in urinary sodium or the fractional excretion of sodium (FeNa) in the urine. **The hallmark of prerenal disease is its reversibility after treatment of the underlying cause, with absence of structural damage to the kidney if treatment promptly.** Recovery of renal function within 24 to 72 hours of volume resuscitation or correction of renal hemodynamics helps to define prerenal AKI in isolation.

The kidney can maintain normal renal blood flow and GFR with systemic perfusion pressures as low as 55 to 60 mm Hg under normal conditions (Walsh et al., 2013), although such autoregulation of kidney blood flow may be compromised in CKD, making patients with chronic disease more susceptible to AKI. In the setting of low systemic blood pressure, renal angiotensin II, which has selective vasoconstriction on the efferent (postglomerular) arteriole, and vasodilatory prostaglandins, which dilate the afferent (preglomerular) arteriole, play an important role in maintaining glomerular hydrostatic pressure and GFR. **Drugs that inhibit angiotensin, such as angiotensin-converting enzyme (ACE) inhibitors and angiotensin receptor blockers (ARBs), exert a vasodilatory effect on the efferent arteriole and thus reduce glomerular pressure and filtration fraction.** Such agents are of great value in treatment of diabetic nephropathy and congestive heart failure and help to reduce proteinuria and convey renal protection in proteinuric kidney disease. However, they may increase the risk of prerenal AKI as well as hyperkalemia during periods of hypotension and hypoperfusion and are thus often held in the hospital setting after identification of AKI. In addition, drugs that inhibit prostaglandins such as nonsteroidal anti-inflammatory drugs (NSAIDs) can contribute to the risk of prerenal and intrinsic AKI (Whelton, 1999).

Although prerenal AKI may often occur as a result of volume depletion such as after hemorrhage or GI losses, it can also occur in instances of total body overload. For example, **congestive heart failure and cirrhosis often occur with total body overload, edema and/or ascites and yet are defined by prerenal AKI typically with a low urine sodium concentration and low FeNa.** Other causes of prerenal AKI related to volume overload include third spacing related to low albumin states, sepsis, and burn injury. These conditions can create a reduction in "effective" circulating volume. Such prerenal states are difficult to manage because administration of crystalloid only worsens total body volume overload and third spacing. **Treatment is directed toward treating the underlying disease states in an effort to optimize systemic hemodynamics and renal perfusion.** In heart failure, paradoxically, prerenal AKI may improve with diuresis using agents such as loop diuretics. Improvement in right heart function (Testani et al., 2010) and reduction in venous back pressure on the kidneys (Bock and Gottlieb, 2010) may explain improved kidney function with diuresis in heart failure.

The sympathetic nervous system and the renin-angiotensin cascade are activated in prerenal AKI in the face of reduced blood flow. In addition, hypotension is a powerful stimulus for the release of antidiuretic hormone (ADH) from the posterior pituitary gland. ADH release is triggered by baroceptor activation in response to low systemic blood pressure, and it causes free water retention even in the face of normal or low serum sodium concentrations (Bankir et al., 2017). ADH binds to V2 receptors in the distal collecting tubule of the kidney, leading to increased transcription and insertion of aquaporin-2 water channels and free water absorption, often leading to hyponatremia. **The most common cause of hyponatremia in the hospital setting is related to such "hypovolemic" hyponatremia, as** opposed to other conditions such as the syndrome of inappropriate ADH secretion (SIADH). It is important to assess volume status through measurements of urine sodium, FeNa in the urine, and other measures such as orthostatic blood pressure monitoring. **In hyponatremia related to volume depletion, urinary sodium, and FeNa tend to be low (UNa < 20 mEq/L, FeNa < 1%).** Serum sodium levels correct quickly with volume repletion, typically with the use of normal saline or other isotonic crystalloid therapy. Hyponatremia in patients with volume overload but ineffective circulating volume is also typically associated with low urine sodium. It is more difficult to manage and often requires diuresis and free water restriction. Tolvaptan, an arginine vasopressin receptor antagonist, blocks the V2 receptor and leads to a rapid water diuresis in patients with a high ADH response. It has been used in patients with SIADH and in patients with congestive heart failure (Konstam et al., 2007). The use of tolvaptan has been curtailed somewhat by the rapid correction of serum sodium that can be seen, high cost of the agent, and a "black box" warning against its use in patients with liver impairment, leading to avoidance in cirrhotic patients.

HRS represents a unique and severe form of prerenal AKI in patients with cirrhosis, acute hepatitis, or any acute form of hepatic decompensation. HRS can be seen in the hospital setting, and the risk increases with additional known risk factors, including bacterial peritonitis and gastrointestinal bleeding (Wu et al., 2006). Dilation of the splanchnic vasculature mediated by nitric oxide appears to drive HRS pathophysiology (Iwakiri, 2007). Temporary improvement in AKI associated with HRS has been associated with the use of albumin, along with midodrine, an α_1 agonist, which mediates vasoconstriction, and octreotide, a somatostatin analogue that decreases splanchnic blood flow (Angeli et al., 1999). Terlipressin, a vasopressin analogue, has been shown to improve renal function in HRS relative to midodrine and octreotide (Cavallin et al., 2015), but it can cause intestinal ischemia and is currently not available in the United States. The gold standard therapy for HRS is liver transplantation, which can result in reversal of HRS pathophysiology and recovery of kidney function (Gonwa et al., 1991). Prolonged HRS, however, may result in permanent kidney injury, and the decision to allocate a kidney allograft with a liver (simultaneous liver kidney transplantation) is in part related to the duration of AKI related to HRS. Recent guidelines for combined liver kidney allocation define advanced AKI with an eGFR of 25 mL/min or less and/or dialysis dependence for 6 consecutive weeks as an appropriate duration of AKI to warrant a combined liver and kidney transplant rather than liver transplant alone (Formica et al., 2016).

Postrenal Kidney Injury

Obstruction of the urinary tract can be a cause of AKI and can be acute or chronic, complete or partial, and involve any area of the lower urinary tract. Obstructive uropathy often occurs in the outpatient setting, and patients often are seen in the clinic or hospital with functional impairment (Gottlieb et al., 1997). Unilateral obstruction may initially go unnoticed in terms of kidney function and changes in SCr, although patients may gradually lose function in a single kidney, rendering them with reduced kidney mass and GFR. Chronic obstruction, whether partial or complete, may lead to tubule-interstitial atrophy and fibrosis, with irreversible loss of kidney function (Klahr, 1991). Patients may develop a distal renal tubular acidosis, with hyperkalemia, mild sodium wasting, and reduced serum bicarbonate levels (Batlle and Arruda, 2018). The duration of obstruction predicts recovery of kidney function, and ideally obstruction should be relieved as soon as possible and within a week of onset at most (Better et al., 1973).

Bilateral obstruction presents dramatically, often with oligoanuria, advanced kidney failure, and electrolyte perturbations. **Common causes of bilateral obstruction include congenital posterior urethral valves in a younger population, bladder dysfunction including neurogenic bladder, and prostatic disease in men. Oligoanuria is a diagnostic sign that suggests complete obstruction and is an uncommon feature of AKI overall.** Other causes of anuric AKI include shock, which is readily apparent upon presentation, severe ATN, bilateral vascular occlusion, hemolytic-uremic syndrome, or severe cases of crescentic glomerulonephritis such as anti–glomerular basement membrane (GBM) disease.

A kidney ultrasound is a sensitive test for identifying hydronephrosis related to obstruction. However, there is a high false-positive rate, which can vary depending upon the index of suspicion (Kamholtz et al., 1989). The negative predictive value is high, although false-negative tests may also be seen with early obstruction. In addition, **metastatic malignancies involving the ureters or retroperitoneal fibrosis may mask hydronephrosis by restricting the ability of the ureters to expand** (Somerville et al., 1992). Further imaging may be indicated, such as computed tomography (CT) scanning, with noncontrast imaging if there is suspicion or concern for kidney stones. A simple bladder scan may reveal a distended bladder resulting from bladder outlet obstruction. Foley catheter placement relieves obstruction related to bladder outlet obstruction and allows for sampling of the urine for urinalysis (UA) and culture. Dilation at the level of the ureteropelvic junction with minimal bladder filling is more typically a result of a kidney stone or ureteropelvic malignancy.

One challenge that urologists commonly face after the relief of obstructive uropathy is "postobstructive diuresis." This usually represents an appropriate response to prolonged obstruction with elimination of excess fluid and sodium. However, there may be dysregulation with inappropriate water loss resulting from tubular injury or an osmotic effect created by excretion of elevated blood urea nitrogen (Schlossberg and Vaughan, 1984). This is a condition that typically lasts 24 to 72 hours and can result in dehydration and hypernatremia, as well as electrolyte wasting. Generally it is recommended to replace one-half of the urine output using hypotonic solutions, such as one-half normal saline and to monitor electrolytes closely during this interval. Intravenous (IV) replacement with free water in dextrose may be appropriate in hypernatremic patients.

Intrinsic Kidney Injury

Acute Tubular Necrosis Resulting From Ischemic Injury

Overall, AKI may occur in 2% to 7% of hospitalized patients in tertiary care centers, and the incidence in surgical or medical ICUs may exceed 25% to 35%. **The type of AKI in hospitalized patients is ATN in the majority of cases** (Myers and Moran, 1986; Uchino et al., 2005). Hypoperfusion and ischemic injury most commonly cause ATN in the hospitalized setting related to operative bleeding and intraoperative hypotension, sepsis, and shock.

Contrast Nephropathy

Contrast-induced tubular injury (contrast nephropathy) is common in the hospital setting. It is a type of ATN that is generally reversible but can contribute to patient morbidity, mortality, and long-term kidney impairment. Patients who develop contrast nephropathy are more likely to be older with more comorbidities, including diabetes. Despite general reversibility of AKI, one analysis found a higher 30-day mortality rate in patients with contrast nephropathy than those without after controlling for other factors (Giacoppo et al., 2015). Iodinated contrast, particularly with higher osmolarity, has been shown to induce renal vasoconstriction and medullary ischemia and also cause direct toxic effects at the proximal renal tubules (Persson et al., 2005). Contrast nephropathy may occur with a low FeNa (<1%) because of constrictive or renal tubular obstructive effects (Schwab et al., 1989). An increase in SCr is generally observed at 24 to 48 hours after contrast exposure, and the AKI is typically nonoliguric. Muddy brown casts may be seen on urinary sediment.

Risk factors for contrast nephropathy include older age, preexisting CKD, diabetic nephropathy, congestive heart failure, hemodynamic instability, high osmolar contrast (Lautin et al., 1991), **NSAID usage, higher volume of contrast, and volume depletion before contrast exposure.** Preventive measures should be used in patients with CKD. NSAIDs, which can induce vasoconstriction, should be avoided for 24 hours before contrast exposure. Generally, diuretics are held before the procedure as well to avoid volume depletion. **The use of isotonic IV fluids before and after contrast is a staple in the prevention of contrast nephropathy despite only limited data on protection** (Jurado-Román et al., 2015; Luo et al., 2014). There are various strategies related to IV hydration, but in general normal saline is given either in bolus form at 3 mL/kg for an hour or 1 mL/kg for 6 to 12 hours before contrast exposure, followed by 1 to 1.5 mL/kg for 4 to 12 hours after contrast exposure. Sodium bicarbonate solutions may be used, although studies have been mixed in terms of any additional benefit over normal saline. Outcomes with the use of N-acetylcysteine have also been mixed. One large randomized trial with a 2×2 design was unable to demonstrate benefit with either sodium bicarbonate or N-acetylcysteine compared to standard normal saline administration (Weisbord et al., 2018). Iso-osmolar contrast agents (e.g., iodixanol) are preferred in patients with preexisting kidney disease, with slight benefit seen in one recent meta-analysis (Eng et al., 2016). Limiting contrast volume to the lowest amount possible is recommended in high risk patients, and diagnostic angiography may often be performed with minimal contrast (10–20 mL).

One important differential diagnosis in patients with AKI after arterial instrumentation is atheroembolic kidney injury. Atheroembolic disease should be suspected in patients who have other evidence of embolic injury such as lesions in fingers or toes (e.g., "blue toe syndrome") or symptoms of gut ischemia such as pain, nausea, and vomiting. Patients may develop transient eosinophilia (Scolari et al., 2007) and hypocomplementemia (Lye et al., 1993). The natural history is different from contrast nephropathy, in that kidney injury may be gradual and unremitting, exhibiting a stuttering pattern and progressing to advanced kidney failure. On biopsy, needle-shaped clefts from cholesterol emboli that dissolve during fixation may be seen. These clefts are often surrounded by inflammatory cells, including eosinophils.

Pigment-Related Kidney Injury

Pigment injury related to hemoglobin or myoglobin may be suspected in the appropriate clinical situation, such as severe hemolysis or muscle breakdown related to trauma, toxicity, or surgical injury, causing rhabdomyolysis. Muscle breakdown is associated with elevation in creatine phosphokinase (CPK) in the bloodstream along with high levels of phosphorus, potassium, and uric acid related to cellular breakdown. Metabolic acidosis is common and hypocalcemia can be severe related to cellular entry, and phosphorus binding is often seen. Myoglobin may cause positive testing for blood by urine dipstick testing in the absence of true hematuria. Myoglobinuria may also be seen early in the course and can contribute to the production of red-brown–tinged urine. The risk of AKI is related to the severity of muscle injury as well as volume status. Early aggressive fluid resuscitation may prevent or limit the extent of kidney injury after muscle injury. Forced alkaline diuresis with bicarbonate based therapy is controversial and requires close monitoring of arterial pH and serum calcium levels every 2 hours ideally in an ICU setting. Bicarbonate therapy may worsen hypocalcemia and promote calcium-phosphorus precipitation.

In urology, two specific clinical circumstances have been identified in association with rhabdomyolysis. The first relates to protracted exaggerated lithotomy positioning, as used in urethral stricture surgery (Anema et al., 2000; Vijay et al., 2011) and robotic-assisted radical prostatectomy (Keene et al., 2010). Gluteal muscles are often affected, and long exposure to lithotomy positioning greater than 5 hours appears to convey greater risk for muscle injury. Attention to padding, positioning, and any maneuver that can reduce the duration of exaggerated positioning help prevent this complication. A second type of surgery that has been associated with rhabdomyolysis is laparoscopic nephrectomy, including after living kidney donor surgery (Deane et al., 2008; Glassman et al., 2007; Kuang et al., 2002). Prolonged lateral decubitus positioning appears to be a risk factor for downside iliopsoas muscle injury, and risk factors also include high body mass index. Unusually severe muscle pain early after surgery along with darkened red-brown urine should prompt an early evaluation with blood CPK levels and measurement of kidney function. As stated earlier, aggressive volume resuscitation may prevent or curtail kidney injury.

Tumor Lysis Syndrome

Tumor lysis syndrome (TLS) is a condition seen in the presence of high tumor burden that may cause AKI in part because of precipitation of uric acid crystals in renal tubules causing urate nephropathy. TLS is most commonly seen after treatment for high-grade lymphomas and leukemias but has also been reported in cases of solid tumors, including renal cell and transitional cell carcinomas (Lin et al., 2007; Norberg et al., 2014). Prophylactic use of agents such as rasburicase, a urate-oxidase enzyme that converts uric acid to allantoin, has greatly reduced the incidence of urate nephropathy associated with TLS. Hyperphosphatemia with subsequent hypocalcemia and calcium-phosphate deposition remain features of TLS and may contribute to AKI by causing nephrocalcinosis. Renal replacement therapy may be required if the calcium-phosphorus product (Ca × Phos) exceeds 70 mg^2/dL^2 (Coiffier et al., 2008; Howard et al., 2011). Potassium levels may also become critically high. Cardiac monitoring and frequent assessment of electrolytes are essential in the management of TLS.

Drug Toxicity as a Cause of Acute Kidney Injury

Nephrotoxic pharmacologic agents are a common source of kidney injury through direct toxic effects or by causing inflammation (interstitial nephritis). Drugs and agents known to cause direct tubular toxicity are shown in Table 87.4. Some, like aminoglycosides, amphotericin B, cisplatin, and ifosfamide, cause renal proximal tubular toxicity, which is cumulative with repeated dosing. Patients with proximal tubular toxicity may initially have a "Fanconi syndrome," with evidence of proximal tubular wasting, including acidosis with an alkaline urine (proximal renal tubular acidosis), phosphorus wasting, and renal glycosuria.

TABLE 87.4 Drugs/Agents Known to Cause Direct Renal Tubular and Interstitial Toxicity

Antibacterial/antifungal/antiviral
- Aminoglycosides
- Amphotericin B
- Polymyxin, colistin
- Vancomycin
- Acyclovir
- Foscarnet
- Cidofovir
- Indinavir
- Ritonavir
- Tenofovir
- Pentamidine

Iodinated contrast

Nonsteroidal anti-inflammatory drugs

Chemotherapeutic agents
- Cisplatin
- Carboplatin
- Ifosfamide
- Gemcitabine
- Methotrexate

Immunosuppressive/immunomodulating therapy
- Cyclosporine
- Tacrolimus
- Intravenous immunoglobulin

Psychotropics
- Lithium

Mannitol

Zoledronic acid

Some examples of agents recently identified as causing nephrotoxicity include a number of chemotherapeutic agents that have shown great promise in treating and stabilizing various metastatic malignancies. For example, tyrosine kinase inhibitors, including sorafenib and sunitinib, inhibit vascular endothelial growth factor (VEGF), and are known to cause hypertension, proteinuria (typically subnephrotic), and AKI in certain patients. Inhibition of VEGF has been shown to predispose animal models to thrombotic microangiopathy (TMA) (Eremina et al., 2008), and TMA has been a finding on kidney biopsy in patients with tyrosine kinase inhibitor–related kidney injury (Bollée et al., 2009). **Tyrosine kinase inhibitors are approved for the treatment of metastatic renal cell carcinoma, and urologists involved with treatment should be aware of the potential nephrotoxicity associated with such agents.**

Another newer group of chemotherapeutic agents that may induce AKI are the so-called checkpoint inhibitors, which are immunomodulatory agents designed to enhance the immune response against various malignancies. One class, known as programmed cell death receptor-1 (PD-1) inhibitors, includes medications such as nivolumab and pembrolizumab. These agents are used in metastatic renal cell and urothelial carcinomas, along with other malignancies. PD-1 inhibitors may cause immune mediated side effects including skin rash, colitis, hepatotoxicity, and pneumonitis. They are also known to cause AKI with acute interstitial nephritis (AIN) and occasionally immune complex glomerular disease manifesting with heavy proteinuria (Cortazar et al., 2016; Izzedine et al., 2017). **AKI associated with these agents may require cessation of drug therapy and/or corticosteroid treatment.**

Recent epidemiologic data have also linked proton pump inhibitors (PPIs) to acute and chronic kidney disease. PPIs have long been known to cause AIN in a small percentage of patients (Geevasinga et al., 2006). More recently, studies of large patient populations have linked PPIs to CKD and ESRD (Lazarus et al., 2016; Xie et al., 2016). Duration of PPI usage appeared to correlate with risk. It is not entirely clear whether such studies are flawed by residual confounding, but there may be incidences of subacute AIN that go undetected in some patients. It appears prudent to limit PPI usage in patients who can otherwise be managed with dietary changes and/or the use of histamine-2 receptor antagonists. Alternatively, patients with a history of peptic ulcer or esophageal ulceration would likely retain benefit that exceeds risk with maintenance PPI therapy.

In general, interstitial nephritis is common in the hospital setting and can occur acutely (AIN), often related to antibiotic therapy, or chronically, often related to the long-term use of NSAIDs. Table 87.5 lists common drugs associated with AIN. The acute presentation is classically described as including a rash, fever, and eosinophilia. However, a report on AIN in 128 patients described a rash in only 15%, fever in 27%, and eosinophilia in only 23%, and these findings were less common in AIN related to NSAIDs or PPIs (Baker and Pusey, 2004). Urinary eosinophils are commonly measured but are neither sensitive nor specific for AIN (Muriithi et al., 2013). The most common urinary findings are pyuria and hematuria, although a bland urine sediment does not exclude AIN. Thus the diagnosis of AIN requires a high index of suspicion. Sterile pyuria and white cell casts on urine sediment support the diagnosis, and confirmation is made by kidney biopsy. A Spanish registry analysis found AIN in 12.9% of those biopsied for AKI, and the prevalence of AIN appeared to be increasing in the more recent era, particularly in elderly patients (Goicoechea et al., 2013).

Non–drug-related AIN may be seen in various infections and rheumatologic diseases, including systemic lupus, sarcoidosis, and Sjögren syndrome. **Another emerging disease entity that may cause AIN is so-called IgG-4 related disease, characterized by an inflammatory infiltration predominantly containing IgG-4–positive plasma cells.** Manifestations may include pancreatitis, lymphadenopathy, salivary or orbital involvement, cholangitis, and involvement of other organ systems. **Patients may have AKI related to retroperitoneal fibrosis, which can mimic the appearance of a tumor and cause obstructive uropathy.** IgG-4–related disease may also cause intrinsic kidney injury with a dense AIN displaying a nodular pattern of inflammation on biopsy that can mimic tumor infiltration (Saeki et al., 2010). Patients with kidney involvement often have extrarenal manifestations. Serum IgG-4 levels are elevated in the majority of patients, and serum complement levels are often low, suggesting complement activation. Treatment with corticosteroid therapy and other immunosuppressive agents has been proven effective (Khosroshahi et al., 2015).

Renal Vein Thrombosis

Renal vein thrombosis is a condition occasionally seen in nephrotic patients and patients with malignancy. Renal vein thrombosis is most commonly associated with membranous glomerulonephritis and is more common with glomerular disease associated with malignancy. Loss of anticoagulation factors such as anti-thrombin III and an increase in procoagulant factors predispose nephrotic patients to venous clotting (Loscalzo, 2013). **The classic clinical findings include flank pain (usually unilateral), microscopic or gross hematuria, elevated lactate dehydrogenase (LDH), and an enlarged, swollen kidney on imaging.** Severe AKI is seen in cases of bilateral acute renal vein thrombosis.

Urologists may see renal vein thrombosis associated with renal cell carcinoma with renal vein involvement or external compression or postoperative thrombosis related to manipulation of the renal circulation (partial nephrectomy or renal transplantation). Catheter-directed local thrombolytic therapy has been used with success in cases of AKI (Kim et al., 2006) and in renal transplantation (Fulton et al., 2011). In cases of renal malignancy, nephrectomy with removal of the tumor thrombus is usually the therapy of choice.

Clinical Approach to the Differential Diagnosis of Acute Kidney Injury

Distinguishing among prerenal, intrinsic, and postrenal causes of AKI should be feasible with appropriate attention to the history, physical, laboratory, and imaging results. A thorough history and physical examination to assess volume status, cardiovascular hemodynamics, potential nephrotoxic insults, and evidence of systemic disease should be undertaken in patients with AKI. All interventions and drug therapies surrounding an AKI event should be outlined against the timeline of changes in kidney function. Risk factors associated with AKI such as advanced age, heart failure, liver failure, baseline CKD, diabetes, and recent surgery should be identified. Exposures including radiocontrast and potential inciting pharmacologic agents may offer clues as to the cause. In perioperative AKI,

TABLE 87.5 Drugs Known to Cause Acute Interstitial Nephritis

Antibiotics
  Penicillins
  Cephalosporins
  Sulfonamides
  Ciprofloxacin
  Rifampin
Nonsteroidal anti-inflammatory drugs
  Including cyclooxygenase-2 inhibitors
Proton pump inhibitors
Checkpoint inhibitor chemotherapeutic agents
Allopurinol
Loop and thiazide diuretics
Anticonvulsants
  Phenytoin
  Carbamazepine
  Phenobarbital
Indinavir
Cimetidine
Mesalamine

the duration of the procedure, blood loss, hemodynamic instability, integrity of the urinary tract, and intraoperative drug treatment are critical to review.

Vital signs and hemodynamic parameters should be assessed, including the measurement of orthostatic hypotension, correctly performed, which may identify volume depletion and prerenal AKI. Hypertension and third spacing of volume identify patients who would benefit from diuresis or possible renal replacement therapy. Daily weights and accurate intake and output are essential in the management of AKI in hospitalized patients. Central venous pressure monitoring may also be beneficial, particularly after major surgery and in an ICU setting.

Examination of the UA and urinary studies is fundamental to the evaluation of the patient with AKI (Perazella and Parikh, 2009). A basic UA may distinguish between various causes of AKI. A urine sediment should also be examined. The nephrologist may assist in identifying cells and casts after urine cytospin because relying on automated laboratory reporting of urinary casts from UA samples is unreliable (Cavanaugh and Perazella, 2018). Heavy proteinuria, hematuria, and red cell casts on urinary sediment are classic findings of acute glomerulonephritis, which may require a prompt biopsy and institution of immunosuppressive therapy. Proteinuria can further be quantified by a spot urinary protein to creatinine or albumin to creatinine ratio or by 24-hour urine collection. Nephrotic range proteinuria (>3.5 g protein/24 h) is highly suggestive of glomerular disease and typically prompts a biopsy, unless there is a high suspicion for diabetic nephropathy or a contraindication to biopsy. Alternatively and more commonly in the hospital setting, a bland urine is noted on UA, and "muddy brown" casts may be seen on urine microscopy, helping to confirm the diagnosis of ATN. Sterile pyuria and hematuria in association with white blood cell casts on urine microscopy is suggestive of AIN and should prompt a careful review of medication exposure and consideration for kidney biopsy and/or treatment. Tuberculosis, chlamydia, ureaplasma, and mycoplasma are infectious agents that may also cause sterile pyuria.

The urine sodium and FeNa are helpful in delineating prerenal physiology in AKI. Typically, a urine sodium under 20 mEq/L and a FeNa under 1% are markers of a prerenal state and are usually associated with a bland UA (Table 87.6). The FeNa is superior to measurement of urinary sodium alone because it does not vary by urinary volume. Low sodium and FeNa may also be seen in shock, heart failure, HRS, contrast nephropathy, rhabdomyolysis, or acute GN. One caveat to urinary sodium analysis is that patients on diuretic therapy may have higher values despite volume depletion. An alternative measurement that may be undertaken is the fractional excretion of urea (FeUrea) (see Table 87.6). FeUrea is typically less than 35% in prerenal disease and 50% to 65% in ATN (Carvounis et al., 2002; Pépin et al., 2007). Renal reabsorption of urea relies on intact proximal tubular function and may not be accurate in the face of hyperglycemia or other causes of osmotic diuresis.

Imaging is typically incorporated in the evaluation of AKI. As mentioned earlier, renal ultrasound is instrumental in identifying most cases of obstructive uropathy and can also identify chronic changes that may be seen after prolonged kidney injury and CKD. Total kidney size reduction and loss of cortical echogenicity correlate with tubular atrophy and interstitial fibrosis and may guide intervention. For example, a chronically obstructed kidney that is small and atrophied may not recover significant function after ureteral stenting or surgical intervention. CT imaging with low radiation dose is a highly sensitive test to identify or confirm stone disease and can be used in the absence of IV contrast in patients with AKI. **CT has improved sensitivity in identifying kidney stones relative to plain abdominal radiography and avoids the contrast required for IV urography** (Pfister et al., 2003).

Management of Acute Kidney Injury

The management of AKI focuses on reversing any prerenal condition, restoring and maintaining euvolemia, and eliminating nephrotoxic drugs when clinically appropriate. Early consultation with a nephrologist improves the outcome of AKI in some studies of critically ill patients (Mehta et al., 2002; Ponce et al., 2011). During the initial evaluation, it is imperative to search for reversible causes such as volume depletion, obstruction, and vascular occlusion. A trial of parenteral hydration with isotonic fluids may correct AKI secondary to prerenal causes (Prowle et al., 2014). Thereafter fluid status should be monitored vigilantly to maintain euvolemia. In patients with oliguria, special attention must be provided to avoid excessive hydration and volume overload, which could precipitate the need for renal replacement therapy.

Diuretic therapy is commonly used in patients with AKI and volume overload. **Response to diuretic therapy may depend on the severity of kidney injury, but diuretic therapy used appropriately neither hinders nor hastens recovery from AKI.** Response to diuretic therapy is a favorable prognostic sign in AKI (Cosentino, 1995). When dosing loop diuretics such as furosemide, a response to an IV bolus can be assessed within 60 minutes of administration. If there is no significant augmentation in urine output, the dose should be increased to find the threshold dose for a given patient. If a dose response is established, IV furosemide may be dosed every 6 to 8 hours at the amount required to elicit a diuretic response. Alternatively, a continuous infusion may be administered. For example, if a patient responds to 60 mg of IV furosemide bolus, he or she may be converted to a 10 mg/h continuous infusion. Continuous infusions increase the area under the curve of therapeutic efficacy, allowing for more consistent dosing. In one comparison study of heart failure patients there was a trend for increased dosage requirement with bolus dosing compared with continuous therapy, and there was a trend for fewer complications with continuous infusion as well (Felker et al., 2011).

Bumetanide and torsemide are alternative loop diuretic agents and have the advantage of increased potency and improved oral bioavailability compared with furosemide. Torsemide also exhibits a longer duration of action compared with furosemide. Comparison of dosing of loop diuretics is shown in Table 87.7. Ethacrynic acid is occasionally used when patients have exhibited drug allergies to the sulfonamide component of loop diuretics. However, ethacrynic acid may be more ototoxic than the sulfonamide diuretics at high doses, and it is difficult to administer intravenously because of the relative insolubility. **Patients who fail to respond to high doses of loop diuretics may respond to the addition of a low dose of thiazide diuretic, such as metolazone 2.5 to 5 mg/d.** Distal sodium absorption may be augmented, particularly in patients on chronic loop diuretic therapy, and an impressive increase in diuresis may be observed by combining loop and thiazide diuretic therapy. Close monitoring of electrolytes is essential with such dual diuretic therapy because hypokalemia and metabolic alkalosis are common side effects. If there is minimal response to high-dose loop diuretic therapy combined with a thiazide in an oliguric patient, then dialysis or ultrafiltration therapy should be considered.

Other agents such as low-dose dopamine and fenoldopam have not been shown to improve outcomes in AKI. One randomized trial assigned 328 critically ill patients to low-dose dopamine (2 µg/kg/min) versus placebo. There were no differences in renal recovery, need for dialysis, hospital stay, or mortality between groups (Bellomo et al., 2000). Even "renal" dose dopamine may precipitate cardiac arrhythmias and should be used with caution. A large randomized trial using fenoldopam, a selective dopamine receptor-1 agonist, similarly did not show any improvement in AKI compared with placebo (Bove et al., 2014). The study included 667 cardiac surgical patients with early AKI who were randomized to fenoldopam versus placebo. There were no differences in rates of dialysis or mortality, and patients on fenoldopam had a higher rate of hypotension.

TABLE 87.6 Formulas for the Fractional Excretion of Sodium and Urea

FeNa, % = UNa × SCr / SNa × UCr × 100
FeUrea, % = Urea × SCr / SBUN × UCr × 100

B, Blood; *BUN*, blood urea nitrogen; *Cr*, creatinine; *Fe*, fractional excretion; *Na*, sodium; *U*, urine.

TABLE 87.7 Comparison of Dosing, Bioavailability, and Half-Life of Various Loop Diuretics

DRUG	BIOAVAILABILITY	EQUIVALENT DOSING	DURATION OF ACTIVITY	DOSING INTERVAL
Furosemide oral	50% with variability	40 mg	6 h	Daily to q6h
Furosemide IV	100%	20 mg	6 h	Daily to q6h
Bumetanide oral	80%–90%	1 mg	6 h	Daily to q12h
Bumetanide IV	100%	1 mg	6 h	Daily to q12h
Torsemide oral	80%–90%	20 mg	8–12 h	Daily to q12h
Torsemide IV	100%	20 mg	8–12 h	Daily to q12h
Ethacrynic acid oral	100%	50 mg	6 h	Daily to q8h
Ethacrynic acid IV	100%	50 mg	6 h	Daily to q8h

IV, Intravenous.

Electrolyte abnormalities are common after AKI, and hyperkalemia is the most common and dangerous electrolyte abnormality in the AKI setting (Fordjour et al., 2014; Hoorn et al., 2013). If serum potassium levels exceed 6 mEq/L, an electrocardiogram (ECG) should be obtained and evaluated. Peaked T waves may be observed with broadening of the PR interval, which may lead to QRS broadening and the potential for maturation into a sine waveform. The goals for treatment of hyperkalemia in the face of ECG changes include stabilization of the cardiac conduction system, shifting potassium intracellularly, and eventual elimination of excess potassium from the body. Stabilizing the cardiac membrane may be achieved by immediate administration of calcium salts. Shifting potassium into cells may be accomplished by insulin therapy (usually with glucose to prevent hypoglycemia), sodium bicarbonate, or β_2-adrenergic agonist therapy. A cationic binding resin such as sodium polystyrene sulfonate (SPS) may be used to augment potassium excretion in the gut. SPS appears to have modest efficacy (Hagan et al., 2016). There are reported cases of intestinal necrosis with SPS, with or without the concomitant use of sorbitol (Goutorbe et al., 2011). Its use should be avoided in patients with postoperative ileus, intestinal obstruction, or active colitis.

Two newer agents have been approved that augment the excretion of potassium and are the first agents available since SPS was approved for use in 1958. Patiromer is a nonabsorbed polymer that exchanges potassium for calcium in the gastrointestinal tract. It has efficacy in dropping potassium levels over days by approximately 0.75 mEq/L in patients with CKD, with minimal adverse effects including constipation and hypomagnesemia (Bushinsky et al., 2015; Weir et al., 2015). It is taken in powder form mixed with water and must be separated from other oral medications. However, because of its delayed onset of action, patiromer is not indicated for the treatment of severe acute hyperkalemia. A second agent, sodium zirconium cyclosilicate (ZSC), was approved for use in the United States in 2018. It is also a nonabsorbed inorganic cation exchange agent that works in the gastrointestinal tract by exchanging potassium for hydrogen and sodium. It also can lower potassium over 48 hours and is not approved for emergent treatment of severe hyperkalemia but holds promise as an agent with minimal adverse effects (Hoy, 2018).

Despite medical intervention, dialysis therapy may be required for patients with severe, persistent AKI. The indications for initiation of dialysis therapy include volume overload, severe hyperkalemia, severe metabolic acidosis, pericarditis, selected poisonings and drug overdoses, and uremic symptomatology. There are disparate outcomes from studies examining the utility of starting dialysis earlier in the course of AKI in the ICU setting. One study in patients with septic shock and advanced failure by RIFLE criteria (see Table 87.1) were randomized to early renal replacement therapy within 12 hours versus delaying more than 48 hours if there was no urgent indication for dialysis. Mortality rates were similar at 90 days between groups, and dialysis was avoided altogether in 38% of the delayed group (Barbar et al., 2018). A theoretical concern exists that the dialysis treatment may have a detrimental impact on recovery of AKI. A drop in urine output is often seen during and after intermittent dialysis therapy, and hypotension often occurs during therapy. There may be a greater risk for ischemic injury during dialysis treatment, and efforts should be made to avoid exacerbating hypotension and hemodynamic instability. Slower, continuous dialysis modalities are often used in the ICU setting, particularly in hypotensive patients or in patients dependent on pharmacologic vasopressor support.

> **KEY POINTS: ACUTE KIDNEY INJURY**
>
> - AKI is defined by an acute rise in SCr and/or an acute decline in urine output. This abrupt decline in kidney function occurs over hours to days and results in the accumulation of byproducts of metabolism and the dysregulation of electrolyte homeostasis, acid/base, and volume status.
> - A classic way to divide AKI is by "prerenal," "intrinsic," and "postrenal" or obstructive causes. The hallmark of prerenal disease is its reversibility after treatment of the underlying cause, with absence of structural damage to the kidney if treatment promptly.
> - Prolonged prerenal physiology may lead to intrinsic kidney ischemia and injury. The greatest proportion of hospital-acquired AKI is secondary to ATN.
> - Nephrotoxic pharmacologic agents are a common source of kidney injury through direct toxic effects or by causing inflammation (interstitial nephritis).
> - Examination of the UA and urinary studies, including measurement of electrolytes and protein concentration, are fundamental to the evaluation of the patient with AKI.

CHRONIC KIDNEY DISEASE

CKD is defined as kidney impairment sustained beyond 3 months with a reduction in GFR, structural abnormalities in the kidneys, and/or proteinuria (often defined specifically by albuminuria). As described earlier, estimations in GFR may be derived from the MDRD and CKD-EPI equations and should be used when kidney function and SCr are at steady state. The 2012 KDIGO guidelines included albuminuria in the definition of CKD to emphasize the prognostic implications related to abnormal urinary protein excretion. For example, a patient with diabetic nephropathy who has a GFR of 60 mL/min/1.73 m^2 and is excreting 3 g/day of albuminuria is more likely to progress to ESRD than a patient with a GFR of 45 mL/min/1.73 m^2 related to prior kidney injury and no albuminuria. The interplay between albuminuria and GFR as outlined by the 2012 KDIGO guidelines is shown in Fig. 87.1.

The presence of CKD has implications in terms of greater risk for AKI, and recognizing that CKD is a risk factor for AKI should lead to measures taken to prevent AKI in the hospital or office setting. Precautions should be taken in CKD patients to avoid nephrotoxic drugs, avoid or limit iodinated contrast exposure, and to dose medications appropriately with adjustment for level of kidney function. Conversely, it is important to recognize that AKI often leads

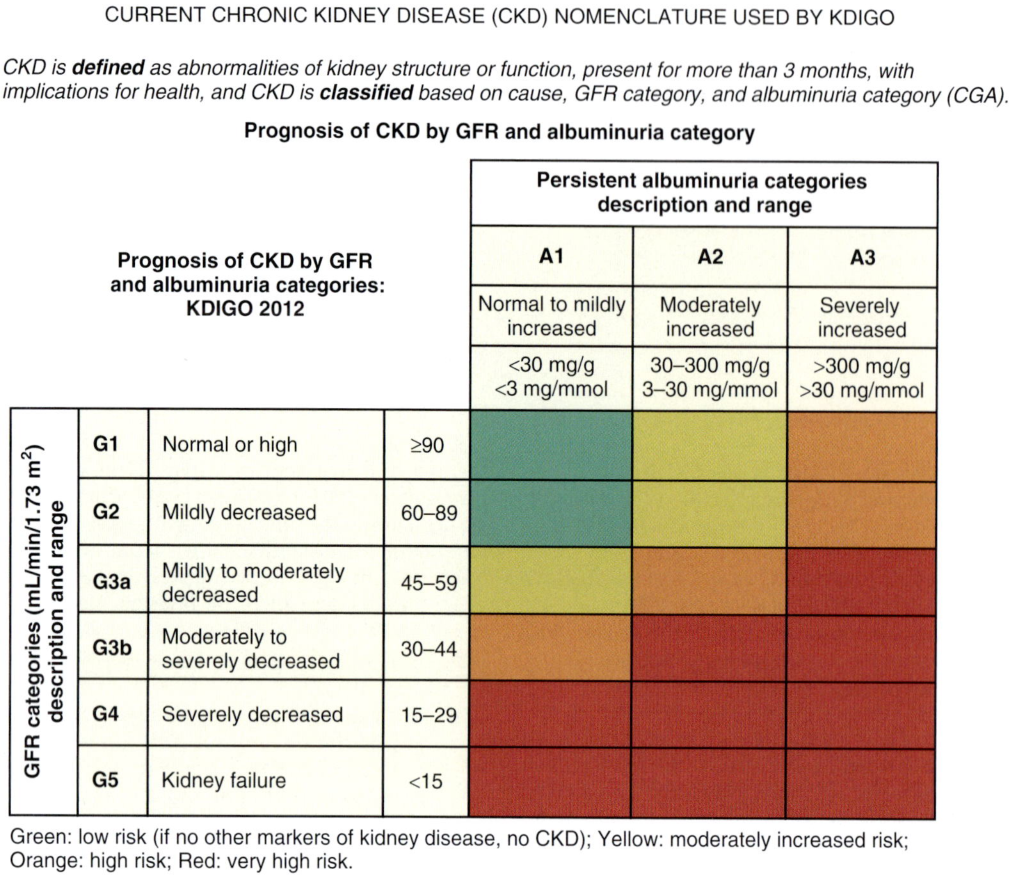

CURRENT CHRONIC KIDNEY DISEASE (CKD) NOMENCLATURE USED BY KDIGO

*CKD is **defined** as abnormalities of kidney structure or function, present for more than 3 months, with implications for health, and CKD is **classified** based on cause, GFR category, and albuminuria category (CGA).*

Prognosis of CKD by GFR and albuminuria category

Prognosis of CKD by GFR and albuminuria categories: KDIGO 2012			A1: Normal to mildly increased (<30 mg/g, <3 mg/mmol)	A2: Moderately increased (30–300 mg/g, 3–30 mg/mmol)	A3: Severely increased (>300 mg/g, >30 mg/mmol)
GFR categories (mL/min/1.73 m²)	G1	Normal or high	≥90		
	G2	Mildly decreased	60–89		
	G3a	Mildly to moderately decreased	45–59		
	G3b	Moderately to severely decreased	30–44		
	G4	Severely decreased	15–29		
	G5	Kidney failure	<15		

Green: low risk (if no other markers of kidney disease, no CKD); Yellow: moderately increased risk; Orange: high risk; Red: very high risk.

Fig. 87.1. Chronic kidney disease (CKD) risk for progression based on Kidney Disease: Improving Global Outcomes (KDIGO) 2013 classification of glomerular filtration rate (GFR) and albuminuria. (From KDIGO Committee: KDIGO 2012 Clinical Practice Guideline for the Evaluation and Management of Chronic Kidney Disease. *Kidney Int Suppl* 3[1]:2012.)

to CKD that will require monitoring after renal recovery (Lewington et al., 2013; Pannu, 2013).

Deficits in nephron number may predispose to progressive kidney disease and hypertension. Nephron number averages approximately 600,000 ± 200,000 per normal kidney. Loss of kidney mass through ablation or partial nephrectomy may trigger progressive glomerular injury in the remnant kidney. The injury is associated with hyperfiltration, glomerular hypertrophy, and systemic hypertension (Brenner and Mackenzie, 1997). Proteinuria appears to correlate with degree of nephron loss and time from the loss (Novick et al., 1991). Reduced birth weight or solitary kidney from birth may similarly lead to kidney injury over time because of low nephron number (Bhathena et al., 1985; Hughson et al., 2003; Lopes and Port, 1995). In general, monitoring of kidney function, albuminuria, and blood pressure should be undertaken after loss of kidney mass. This includes living kidney donors, although the typical natural history in kidney donors is an improvement in GFR and lack of proteinuria in the years after donation (Fehrman-Ekholm et al., 2011). The development of albuminuria should lead to targeted therapy in patients with reduced renal mass. The use of ACE inhibitors or ARBs appears to be protective and can reduce proteinuria in a "remnant kidney" model (NDT 9: 131, 1994), (Novick and Schreiber, 1995).

The causes of progressive CKD parallel the most common causes of ESRD. Table 87.8 lists the incident causes of ESRD from the US Renal Data System (USRDS, 2013). Diabetes mellitus and hypertension account for the largest percentage of cases (63%) followed by glomerular diseases (14%). A caveat to such reporting is that many patients go without kidney biopsy and lack a definitive cause of ESRD. **Genetic disease or other occult kidney diseases may commonly go undiagnosed or unrecognized, resulting in the labeling of "hypertensive" kidney disease in the absence of a definitive**

TABLE 87.8 Incidence of Reported Causes of End-Stage Renal Disease

DIAGNOSIS	PERCENTAGE
Diabetes mellitus	38
Hypertension	25
Glomerulonephritis	14
Cystic kidney disease	5
Urologic disease	2
Other/missing/unknown	15

diagnosis. This is particularly common in the black community, in which the diagnosis of hypertensive kidney failure is increasingly being recognized to correlate with genetic risk of CKD.

Accordingly, special mention should be made to the identification of genetic risk for CKD in a subset of black patients, which relates to variants in apolipoprotein genetics. Polymorphisms in the genes that encode apolipoprotein L1 (APOL1) are found in patients of sub-Saharan African ancestry, and two separate variants have been identified: G1 and G2. These gene variants appear to convey protection against African sleeping sickness caused by *Trypanosoma* parasitic infection, whether inherited as a single or dual variant (Vanhamme et al., 2003). Inheritance of two *APOL1* gene variants of any combination (G1/G1, G1/G2, or G2/G2) appears to greatly increase the risk of CKD related to hypertensive kidney disease, focal sclerosis, diabetic nephropathy, lupus nephritis, and human immunodeficiency virus associated nephropathy (HIVAN) in patients of African descent (Cohen et al., 2017; Larsen et al., 2013;

Parsa et al., 2013). Two gene variants are found in approximately 13% of the black population (Friedman et al., 2011) and explain to a large extent the increased risk of CKD and ESRD seen in blacks in the United States (Freedman et al., 2018). Although APOL1 is a circulating protein, it has also been localized to the podocyte, proximal tubule, and vasculature of the kidney (Madhavan et al., 2011). The idea that the integrity of the kidney may be affected by APOL1 gene variation is suggested by studies in kidney transplantation, which demonstrate reduced allograft survival when kidneys came from deceased donors with high-risk gene variants (Freedman et al., 2016). The long-recognized risk of inferior transplant outcomes with kidneys from black deceased donors also appears to be entirely explained by the disproportionate risk related to the smaller percentage of donors with two APOL1 gene variants (Julian et al., 2017).

Glomerulonephritis

Glomerulonephritis is evolving in terms of accuracy of diagnosis and identification of cause. The diagnosis of focal segmental glomerulosclerosis (FSGS) may represent a primary immune process or a secondary pattern of injury. Secondary forms of FSGS may develop for many reasons, including loss of renal mass such as after partial or total nephrectomy, genetic risk such as *APOL1* gene variants in blacks, a consequence of morbid obesity (Goumenos et al., 2009), or as a consequence of other prior drug or immune-mediated injury. In addition, primary FSGS may be familial rather than immune mediated. Familial FSGS is suggested by a positive family history of disease and an onset of nephrotic syndrome at a very young age (Sadowski et al., 2015). Identifying such secondary or genetic forms of FSGS is critical because these patients would not be expected to benefit from immunotherapy with medications such as corticosteroids or calcineurin inhibitors. Diffuse podocyte effacement on electron microscopic biopsy in the absence of genetic association may alternatively point to a primary FSGS for which immunotherapy would potentially convey benefit (De Vriese et al., 2018). Such primary FSGS patients are more likely to be young adults, Caucasian, and have heavy proteinuria in the nephrotic range.

Nephrotic syndrome is a clinical presentation that may be caused by FSGS or other primary or secondary glomerular diseases. It is characterized clinically by a urinary protein excretion of greater than 3.5 g/day, hypoalbuminemia, and peripheral edema. Primary diseases that may cause nephrotic syndrome include FSGS; minimal change disease, which is especially common in children; membranous nephropathy; and certain types of membranoproliferative diseases. Secondary nephrotic syndrome may be seen in secondary FSGS related to infection such as HIV infection, lupus-associated membranous nephropathy, hereditary diseases, and amyloid or light chain deposition caused by monoclonal proteins.

Abnormal monoclonal proteins in the absence of defined myeloma or amyloidosis may be seen with variable nephrotic and nephritic presentations in the kidneys and has been termed *monoclonal gammopathy of renal significance (MGRS)* (Leung et al., 2012). Accordingly, testing for monoclonal proteins as a potential cause of glomerular disease is essential, with risk for MGRS increasing with age. Serum and urine electrophoresis along with measurements of free light chains kappa and lambda may detect low level monoclonal proteins that may be involved in renal glomerular or tubular pathology. Treatment with agents used to treat myeloma may be indicated even in the absence of other organ disease if renal pathology is present (Sethi and Rajkumar, 2013).

Membranous nephropathy is one of the most common causes of nephrotic syndrome in adults. The diagnosis and treatment of membranous nephropathy have improved because of the discovery of a target antibody against a podocyte protein that is positive in 70% to 80% of idiopathic membranous disease cases. The antibody targets the M-type phospholipase A2 receptor (PLA2R), a transmembrane receptor that is highly expressed in glomerular podocytes (Beck et al., 2009). This antibody may be identified in the glomerulus on kidney biopsy by immunofluorescence or immunohistochemistry staining and may be detected in the circulation by ELISA or other methods. Monitoring of PLA2R Ab titers is useful to guide treatment of membranous nephropathy because clearance of the antibody often precedes a reduction in proteinuria and is predictive of remission (Beck et al., 2011). Reemergence of antibodies may also predict disease recurrence (Ruggenenti et al., 2015). Other antibodies have been identified that are present in a minority of membranous cases, including one targeting thrombospondin type-1 domain-containing 7A (THSD7A), another podocyte transmembrane protein. THSD7A antibodies have been detected in 10% of patients with membranous who lack antibodies to PLA2R (Ren et al., 2018). Some cases of membranous nephropathy with antibodies against THSD7A have been associated with malignancy, and clearance of the antibody leading to remission of glomerular disease has been described with the use of chemotherapy targeting the malignancy directly (Hoxha et al., 2016).

End-Stage Renal Disease Demographics and Treatment Options

There continues to be a steady growth of ESRD patients on renal replacement therapies (RRTs) throughout the world. In the United States the incidence rate for ESRD in 2016 was 373 new cases per million people (US Renal Data System, 2018). The prevalence of ESRD patients has continued to increase since 2006, and the number of patients with ESRD in the United States in 2016 was approximately 726,000. The number of kidney transplants performed annually in the United States has increased slightly and in 2016 was just more than 20,000, with approximately one-third of transplants coming from living kidney donors. Rates of living donation have declined slightly since 2004 and remained relatively level in more recent years. In 2016, 87% of patients with incident ESRD in the United States started hemodialysis, 10% started on peritoneal dialysis, and 3% received a preemptive kidney transplant (before any dialysis therapy). By the end of 2016, 63% of prevalent ESRD patients were on hemodialysis, 7% were on peritoneal dialysis, and 30% had a functioning kidney transplant. **Although home hemodialysis is a modality that has demonstrated improved survival** (Mailloux et al., 1996) **and cost effectiveness** (McGregor et al., 2000), **only 2% of hemodialysis patients received home treatments in 2016.**

Poor long-term survival of ESRD patients is illustrated by comparing the expected remaining lifetime on dialysis or transplant with the general US population. The expected survival for dialysis patients was less than one-third of those age-matched in the general population, whereas the expected survival in transplant patients was 69% to 85% of that in the general population. The adjusted mortality rate in patients on dialysis was 164 per 1000 patient-years, whereas the rate in transplant recipients was 29 per 1000 patient-years. Importantly, however, survival is improving for patients on dialysis and with transplantation. Between 2001 and 2016, adjusted mortality rates decreased in dialysis patients by 29%. Such improved survival is contributing to the growing prevalence of ESRD patients. This improvement in survival was similar to that seen in non-dialysis patients on Medicare with diabetes and cancer. In transplant patients, the adjusted mortality rates between 2001 and 2016 decreased by 40%. The transplant population is aging. In 2001, 8% of transplant recipients were over the age of 65, and in 2016 the rate increased to 24% (USRDS, 2018).

Outcome comparisons suggest that kidney transplantation is still the best overall treatment for ESRD patients, despite advances in dialysis care and modalities. The time on dialysis (vintage) has an impact on transplant outcomes, with inferior outcomes seen with longer dialysis vintage (Meier-Kriesche et al., 2000). This finding likely relates in part to progressive vascular disease on dialysis therapy but also reflects socioeconomic status and timeliness of listing (Schold et al., 2010). Patients who progress to stage IV CKD with an estimated or measured GFR of 20 mL/min/1.73 m^2 or less are eligible for active transplant listing in the United States and should be counseled and referred for transplant evaluation. Patients at advanced age or with severe medical comorbidities or problems with medical adherence may be excluded from transplant listing. **For those approved, preemptive transplantation, before initiation of dialysis therapy, should be the goal. Because of long waiting times for deceased donor**

Atherosclerotic Renal Artery Stenosis

Atherosclerotic renal artery stenosis, a recognized cause of severe, secondary hypertension and impaired renal function, is present in approximately 7% of individuals older than 65 years (Hansen et al., 2002) and in 40% to 50% of patients with atherosclerotic disease in other vascular beds (Miralles et al., 1998). Clinically relevant complications, specifically resistant hypertension and/or renal atrophy with progressive decline in renal function, develop in 15% to 20% of cases of atherosclerotic renal artery stenosis (Caps et al., 1998; Chabova et al., 2000). In addition, atherosclerotic renal artery stenosis appears to be an independent risk factor for adverse cardiovascular events and increased cardiovascular mortality. In 3 recent studies, patients with atherosclerotic renal artery stenosis had between a two- and fivefold increases in mortality compared with healthy age-matched normotensive control patients (Conlon et al., 2001; Edwards et al., 2005; Johansson et al., 1999). Moreover, the increased risk profile appears to remain despite anatomic correction of atherosclerotic renal artery stenosis.

Atherosclerotic renal artery stenosis accounts for 90% of the lesions that impede blood flow within the renal artery. Fibromuscular dysplasias, vasculitides, congenital bands, and intrinsic and extrinsic causes make up the remaining 10% of causes. Atherosclerosis typically involves the ostium and proximal one-third of the renal artery and can also involve the adjacent aorta. Involvement of segmental renal arteries and higher-order branches is uncommon. Because atherosclerosis is a systemic condition, atherosclerotic renal artery stenosis most often occurs in patients with risk factors for atherosclerosis, such as hypertension, hyperlipidemia, diabetes mellitus, and tobacco use.

Early studies determined the prevalence of renal artery disease in autopsy series. In patients older than 60 years and with a history of hypertension, moderate to severe renal artery stenosis was found in approximately 50% of patients (Holley et al., 1964; Schwartz et al., 1964). Because atherosclerosis-related complications are a leading cause of death, autopsy studies may overestimate the prevalence of atherosclerotic renal artery disease but nonetheless suggest a direct relationship to increasing patient age and severity of hypertension.

The clinical prevalence of atherosclerotic renal artery stenosis, which is frequently identified in patients with cerebrovascular, coronary, and peripheral arterial disease depends on the radiographic definition (percent of renal artery luminal narrowing), imaging technique, and the patient population being studied. In a general population of patients older than 65 years of age the prevalence was noted to be 6.8%, when assessed with duplex Doppler ultrasonography (Hansen et al., 2002). In a systematic review of studies using more sensitive imaging techniques and defining atherosclerotic renal artery stenosis as at least 50% luminal narrowing, the prevalence ranged between 10.5% in consecutive patients undergoing coronary angiography to 54.1% in patients with congestive heart failure (de Mast et al., 2009). In patients with underlying atherosclerotic conditions, atherosclerotic renal artery stenosis can be anticipated in approximately 10% to 20% of cases. With these sensitive imaging techniques the prevalence of bilateral atherosclerotic renal artery stenosis is 4.2%, in contrast to 0.8% when identified by duplex ultrasonography (de Mast et al., 2009; Hansen et al., 2002).

Pathophysiology of Hypertension in Atherosclerotic Renal Artery Stenosis

Basic Concepts in Arterial Physiology. Blood flows throughout the circulatory system primarily because of differences in total fluid energy but from a functional standpoint, blood flow can be attributed to differences in pressure gradients. A pressure gradient is maintained by cardiac contractions and elasticity of the arterial system. The basic concept that describes the relationship between blood pressure (and/ or flow) and blood vessel diameter follows Pouiseuille's law, which states that the **pressure difference** between two points along a tube is directly proportional to the flow velocity (Q), length of tube (L),

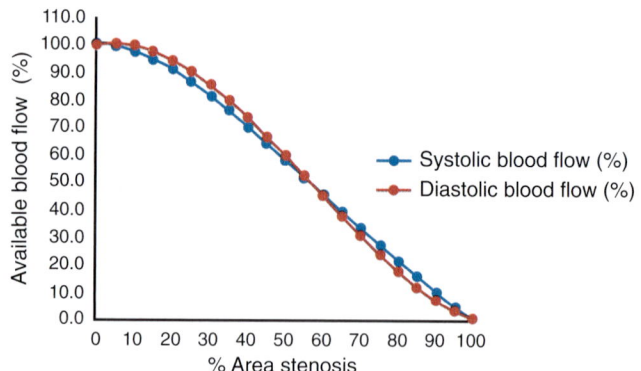

Fig. 87.2. Relationship of blood flow to increasing arterial stenosis.

and fluid viscosity (η) and is inversely proportional to the second power of the radius of the tube.

$$\text{Pouiseuille's law} = \Delta P = Q8L\eta/r^2$$

Viewed simplistically, this relationship shows that as the radius (or diameter) of a tube decreases, the difference in pressure increases exponentially. Therefore, as the diameter of a blood vessel decreases, the decline in pressure, ΔP, increases.

The second important concept relates to the relationship between luminal diameter and cross-sectional area. The cross-sectional area of a tube, which is equal to that of a circle, is expressed as $A=\pi r^2$. This can be further expanded to consider diameter or $A=\pi (d/2)^2$ or $\pi d^2/4$. Again showing that as the diameter of a vessel decreases, the luminal area decreases by the square of the diameter reduction. Early experiments have conclusively shown that clinically significant vascular stenosis, specifically those that cause a pressure drop, occur when the luminal area is reduced by more than 70%, also expressed as "70% stenosis" (May et al., 1963; Fig. 87.2). This corresponds to a diameter reduction of approximately 50% because such a diameter reduction will result in a reduction in cross-sectional area to 25% of the original area.

Given that a constant amount of fluid (blood) circulates through the vascular system, another basic assumption is that blood flow (volume of blood per time) is maintained in all parts of the circulatory system. Extending from the Bernoulli equation, as the diameter of tube decreases, the velocity of the moving fluid increases to maintain the conservation of energy principle of flowing fluids. Importantly, these concepts are based on laminar flow of frictionless fluids through rigid tubes, markedly different from the human circulatory system. Flow is maintained in human arteries by increasing velocity until a critical level of stenosis or approximately a 70% decrease in area. Beyond 70%, flow begins to decrease rapidly, and beyond a 90% stenosis flow and velocity are reduced, compatible with "trickle-flow" (Fig. 87.3).

Based upon this relationship, flow decreases markedly at critical levels of stenosis (>70%). Under normal systolic blood pressures (120 mm Hg) there is an approximately 40- to 60-mm Hg pressure drop to the level of the afferent arterioles within the kidney (Fig. 87.4).

De Bruyne et al. (2006) have shown that as the degree of stenosis increases to approximately 50%, the pressure in the renal artery distal to stenosis is 60 to 70 mm Hg. It is likely therefore that at this lower perfusion pressure, the pressure and flow, at the afferent arteriole reaches precipitously low levels, thus initiating the pathophysiologic processes.

The pathophysiologic basis for hypertension resulting from impaired renal blood flow was first elegantly described more than 75 years ago (Goldblatt et al., 1941). These initial studies stimulated numerous experiments that outlined the hormonal basis for the kidney's role in blood pressure control. Adding to these initial studies, it is now well outlined that a reduction in renal perfusion leads to a decrease in glomerular filtration. Consequently, the reduction in distal tubular sodium chloride (NaCl) delivery to the macula densa

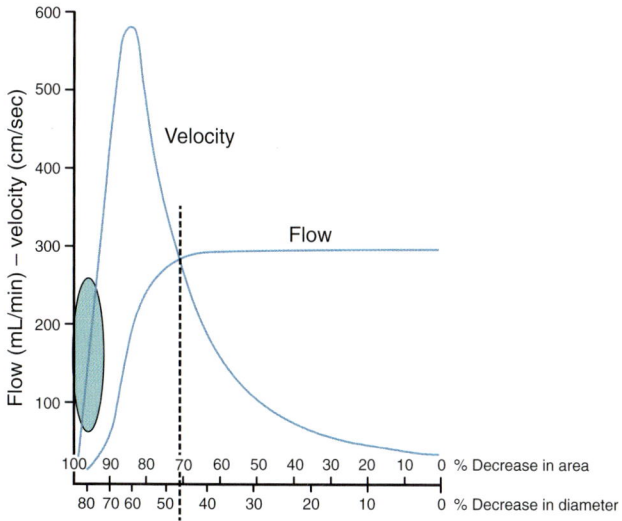

Fig. 87.3. Correlation of percent diameter reduction with increases in blood flow velocity (cm/sec) and reduction in volume flow (mL/min) in arteries. Note that a high-grade (>95%) diameter-reducing stenosis causes volume flow to decrease toward zero, whereas the velocity within the stenosis may be minimally elevated.

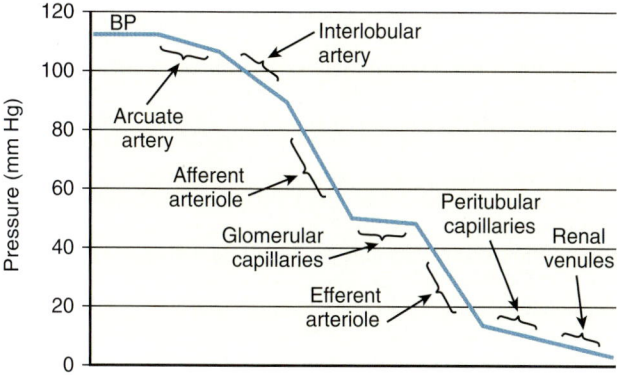

Fig. 87.4. Hydraulic pressure profile in the renal vasculature based on a variety of micropuncture studies in superficial nephrons of the rat and squirrel monkey as well as values obtained by micropuncture of juxtamedullary nephrons in the rat. For these latter studies, the arcuate artery was perfused with whole blood at normal arterial pressures, and hydraulic pressures were measured at downstream sites, including the interlobular artery, the proximal and distal portions of the afferent arteriole, the glomerular capillaries, the proximal and late segments of the efferent arteriole, the peritubular capillaries, and the renal vein.

cells of the juxtaglomerular apparatus initiates an epithelial response that consists of activation of multiple mitogen-activated protein kinases and stimulation of cyclooxygenase-2 activity and induction of cyclooxygenase-2 expression. This is subsequently followed by the appearance in the juxtaglomerular interstitium of prostaglandin E2 and the suppression of adenosine. Prostaglandin E2 activates receptors on granular cells which then results in adenylate cyclase activation and phosphokinase A-mediated renin secretory and transcriptional activation (Schnermann et al., 2003).

Renin, in turn, cleaves hepatically-produced angiotensinogen to produce angiotensin I, which is then converted by the angiotensin converting enzyme in the pulmonary vasculature to angiotensin II. In addition to causing hypertension via its potent vasoconstrictive effects, angiotensin II stimulates adrenal synthesis of aldosterone, which further results in sodium and fluid retention.

In the classic 2-kidney, 1-clip model, increased renin release from the affected kidney leads to hypertension and sodium retention. However, the contralateral (unaffected) kidney senses increased perfusion pressure, which, in turn, promotes a natriuresis and volume loss. **Therefore maintenance of hypertension in unilateral renal artery stenosis and normal contralateral kidney is driven primarily by renin and angiotensin. In contrast, in the setting of bilateral renal artery stenosis or renal artery stenosis affecting a solitary kidney, sodium and volume retention are not modified to the extent of having a normal contralateral kidney. Renin and angiotensin levels do not remain elevated, and hypertension remains sodium and volume dependent.**

Given the transient elevation in renin and angiotensin, several other pressor pathways participate in the development of hypertension. These pathways include sympatho-adrenergic activation, oxidative stress pathways, and impaired vasodilatory responses within the kidney and systemic microcirculation (Lerman et al., 2001).

Pathophysiology of Ischemic Nephropathy in Atherosclerotic Renal Artery Stenosis

A reduction in renal perfusion resulting from atherosclerotic renal artery disease, which in turn leads to renal parenchymal loss and declining renal function, describes a condition known as ischemic nephropathy. Several interrelated pathophysiologic mechanisms are likely responsible for the renal structural and functional changes that occur in atherosclerotic renal artery disease. The impairment in microvascular blood flow, in combination with conditions that contribute to the atherosclerotic milieu, such as hypercholesterolemia, diabetes mellitus, and hypertension, lead to vascular dysfunction, which is mediated by endothelial injury, reduced bioavailability of nitric oxide, and increased vascular tone resulting from the predominance of vasoconstrictors, primarily angiotensin II. Concomitant cellular activation leads to migration of mononuclear cells and release inflammatory mediators including nuclear factor kappa-B (NF-κB). Upregulated tubular and glomerular expression of profibrotic factors, including transforming growth factor β (TGF-β), tissue inhibitor of metalloproteinase-1, and plasminogen activator inhibitor-1 leads to structural changes of tubulointerstitial fibrosis, vascular changes and/or glomerulosclerosis (Chade et al., 2003; Lerman et al., 2009).

Changes in intrarenal blood flow have been identified using blood oxygen level–dependent (BOLD) magnetic resonance imaging (MRI) analysis. Gloviczki et al. (2013) found that in cases of severe renal artery stenosis in which tissue hypoxia may occur, there is preferential redistribution of blood flow away from the renal cortex and toward the medulla. At the same time, there are changes in metabolic processes to preserve oxygen (Eirin et al., 2013).

Studies sampling renal vein blood from patients with atherosclerotic renal artery stenosis compared with those with essential hypertension found multiple markers reflecting active inflammation, suggesting kidney injury and reduced function. Endothelial progenitor cells expressing the markers CD34 and KDR were sequestered in kidneys with atherosclerotic renal artery stenosis, whereas levels of E-selectin, vascular cell adhesion molecule-1, and several inflammatory molecules were increased (Eirin et al., 2013).

In summary, atherosclerotic renal artery stenosis, in combination with other atherosclerotic risk factors, results in progressive loss of renal function through a complex interplay between inflammatory and immune responses, angiotensin II, oxidative stress, vascular rarefaction, and fibrosis. These molecular and cellular level processes ultimately lead to renal atrophy and diminished renal function.

Diagnostic Evaluation of Atherosclerotic Renal Artery Stenosis

Clinical Features. The primary goal when undertaking diagnostic evaluation for suspected atherosclerotic renal artery stenosis is to identify patients who, if found to have a lesion, are most likely to benefit from treatment. Given that most patients with atherosclerotic renal artery stenosis are asymptomatic, the decision to pursue diagnostic assessment, particularly with invasive studies, should be driven by the probability that renovascular disease is a significant contributor to the patient's condition and will result in potential clinical consequences. If blood pressure and renal function are satisfactorily controlled with medical therapy, further diagnostic evaluation may not lead to treatment gains.

In general, the clinical criteria that should prompt evaluation are (1) early onset of hypertension (age < 30 years), (2) accelerated hypertension, (3) severe hypertension, or (4) hypertension resistant to optimal medical therapy, (5) asymmetric kidney size with more than 1.5 cm difference in craniocaudal length, (6) unexplained loss of kidney function, (7) rapid or recurrent decline in GFR in association with systemic blood pressure reduction, and (8) decline in GFR (SCr at least 30% from pretreatment level) after initiation of ACE inhibitors or ARBs. In addition, although most likely unrelated to atherosclerosis, all children with unexplained hypertension should be screened for renal artery stenosis.

Other clinical features that are often present in patients with atherosclerotic renal artery stenosis are typical for patients with systemic atherosclerotic disease. These include advanced age; atherosclerotic risk factors, including hypertension, CKD, hyperlipidemia, diabetes mellitus, tobacco exposure; and history of atherosclerotic disease in the coronary, cerebral, and/or the peripheral arterial circulation. On physical examination these patients often have severe hypertension and may also have fewer common signs, such as diminished lower extremity pulses, peripheral edema, and abdominal bruits.

To generate uniformity, the American Heart Association proposed the following classification scheme in patients with renal artery disease (Rocha-Singh et al., 2008):

Grade I: Renal artery stenosis present, but no clinical manifestations (normotensive and normal renal function)
Grade II: Renal artery stenosis present, but patients have medically controlled hypertension and normal renal function
Grade III: Renal artery stenosis present and patients have evidence of abnormal renal function, medically refractory hypertension, or evidence of volume overload

Laboratory Features

Apart from decreased GFR, patients with atherosclerotic renal artery stenosis typically do not have notable laboratory abnormalities. The urine analysis is likely to be unremarkable. On routine chemistry panels, patients may have low or low normal serum potassium because of aldosterone secretion.

Ritchie et al. (2014) retrospectively reviewed 467 patients with at least 50% atherosclerotic renal artery stenosis and noted that nearly half of their patient group was asymptomatic. One or more "high-risk presentations," defined as flash pulmonary edema, refractory hypertension (>140 mm Hg systolic and/or >90 mm Hg diastolic) despite use of 3 or more different classes of antihypertensive agents, or rapidly declining kidney function (SCr level more than 1.2-fold or 1.14 mg/dL greater than baseline within the previous 6 months) was present in 51% of the patients, and 30% to 40% had a history of angina, previous myocardial infarction, cerebrovascular accident/transient ischemic attack, peripheral arterial disease, or diabetes (Ritchie et al., 2014)

These data underscore a guiding principle for diagnostic evaluation in atherosclerotic renal artery stenosis. Patients who are asymptomatic, have normal renal function, and have satisfactory blood pressure control likely do not need evaluation. Alternatively, patients who fail to improve or who decline while on medical therapy may benefit from additional diagnostic testing.

Radiographic Assessment of Atherosclerotic Renal Artery Stenosis

Radiographic evaluation of suspected atherosclerotic renal artery stenosis should begin with noninvasive imaging studies. Given the wide availability, low cost, ease to the patient, and diagnostic accuracy, **duplex ultrasonography should be considered the screening test of choice.** Duplex ultrasonography combines anatomic information (B- or brightness-mode and color Doppler imaging) with acquisition of blood flow.

The primary diagnostic advantage of duplex ultrasonography is the ability to accurately determine blood flow velocity. A duplex ultrasonographic examination for renal artery stenosis should be done by an experienced technologist, and patients should undergo an overnight fast to minimize bowel gas. Imaging is performed from anterior and flank (lateral decubitus) approaches, with attention directed to the perirenal aorta, looking for aneurysmal change, stenosis, or occlusion. The lateral decubitus position may aid in the obese patients and/or in the setting of excessive bowel gas. Peak systolic velocity in the aorta is recorded. Subsequently each renal artery is imaged, and velocities and waveforms are recorded from the proximal, mid, and distal segments of the renal arteries. Duplex ultrasonography with color-flow and Doppler imaging is used to determine the patency and phasicity of the renal veins. Velocity measurements within the superior, mid, and lower poles of the kidneys are used to calculate resistive indices and acceleration times. Last, the duplex ultrasonographic study determines renal parenchymal anatomic details including kidney size, parenchymal thickness and echogenicity, and potentially unanticipated findings such as masses, calculi, and/or hydronephrosis.

The most commonly measured duplex ultrasonographic parameters include peak systolic velocity (PSV), end diastolic velocity (EDV), and adjacent aortic peak systolic velocity. The ratio of velocity in the main renal artery to the aorta (renal aortic ratio, RAR) and resistive index within the renal parenchyma (RI = [(PSV−EDV)/PSV]) can be derived from these measurements. In addition, arterial blood flow characteristics such as tardus/parvus, acceleration time, and acceleration index can be determined within the main, accessory, and intraparenchymal renal arteries.

The accuracy of duplex ultrasonography for the diagnosis of renal artery stenosis varies according to predetermined velocity thresholds, which in turn, depend on individual vascular laboratory experience. AbuRahma et al. (2012) reviewed their institution's large experience and found that a PSV of 285 cm/s or a RAR of 3.7 alone had the best overall accuracy in diagnosing at least 60% stenosis when compared with angiography. Using these thresholds, these investigators were able to achieve more than 80% accuracy. Lower velocity thresholds, although more sensitive, were less accurate. These findings reinforce the notion that clinicians should recognize the expertise in their individual vascular laboratories and use the data to screen patients who require more invasive examination.

Computed tomography (CT) and magnetic resonance imaging (MRI) have sensitivity of more than 90% in detecting atherosclerotic renal artery stenosis, and MRI has a specificity of 91% (Eklof et al., 2006). CT and MRI provide excellent anatomic detail; however, the blood flow changes that result from the stenosis cannot be determined. The functional consequences of these lesions may be indirectly determined by the findings of parenchymal atrophy. Another drawback of CT is the cost and need for intravenously administered radiographic contrast agents. Because many patients with suspected atherosclerotic renal artery disease may have co-existent renal insufficiency, administration of iodinated contrast agents raises concerns of contrast nephropathy. Patients with estimated glomerular filtration rate (GFR) below 50 mL/min should receive IV hydration before contrast administration and those with GFR below 30 mL/min should not receive iodinated contrast as part of a diagnostic procedure (contrast should be reserved for use during a therapeutic procedure). Administration of IV gadolinium for magnetic resonance angiography (MRA) in patients with GFR below 30 mL/min should be avoided because it is associated with the development of nephrogenic systemic fibrosis.

Renal arteriography, the "gold standard" for the diagnosis of atherosclerotic renal artery stenosis, can also provide detailed imaging of the aorta, segmental renal arteries, and intrarenal vasculature. Digital subtraction improves resolution and allows a reduction in the amount of contrast material. Angiography is an invasive study with risks of bleeding from arterial puncture, arterial dissection, arterial spasm, and thromboembolism. Additionally iodinated contrast material cannot be administered in patients with contrast allergy or significant renal dysfunction, and use of carbon dioxide may reduce the amount of contrast.

Two additional diagnostic studies that warrant discussion are radionuclide renography and plasma renin determination. With radionuclide or nuclear renography, a radiopharmaceutical agent, either diethylenetriaminepentaacetic acid (DTPA) or mercaptoacetyltriglycine (MAG 3), is administered intravenously, and images are reviewed to determine a renal functional difference, delay in time to peak uptake of the radioisotope, or delayed excretion of the isotope. Additional imaging after administration of captopril, an ACE inhibitor, may show decreased function (GFR), suggesting the influence of angiotensin II maintaining glomerular filtration. Radionuclide renography has largely fallen out of favor because of its unreliability. In addition to diagnostic limitations in patients with diminished renal function (SCr > 2.0 mg/dL) or bilateral arterial disease, these imaging studies have poor sensitivity and specificity (Vasbinder et al., 2001). Currently the primary role of renography in evaluating patients with hypertension may be to determine differential function before recommending nephrectomy.

Plasma renin activity or determination of renin level from the renal vein has been suggested to be highly diagnostic for the presence of renal artery stenosis, but these studies are limited by their invasiveness and stringent testing conditions. The patient's volume status must be optimized, concurrent medications must be addressed, and blood pressure must be tightly controlled. Last, and as mentioned previously, renin may be elevated early in the course of atherosclerotic renal artery stenosis and likely declines over time as other pathophysiologic processes maintain the hypertensive state.

Therapeutic Options for Atherosclerotic Renal Artery Stenosis

Medical Management. Medical management makes up the foundation of atherosclerotic renal artery stenosis treatment. The general objectives of therapy are control of blood pressure, preservation of renal function, and prevention of atherosclerosis-related complications. Antihypertensive treatment with ACE inhibitors or ARBs are the first-line approach for blood pressure control and for their beneficial effect on cardiovascular risk reduction (Heart Outcomes Prevention Evaluation Study Investigators, 2000). Use of these agents may initiate concerns of renal insufficiency from loss of glomerular filtration as a result of blockade of the AII-induced efferent arteriolar constriction. However, significant renal function decline is uncommon in most series and, when it occurs, is almost diagnostic of renal artery stenosis. If additional antihypertensive agents are needed, beta-blockers, diuretics, and calcium-channel blockers can be added.

Given the presence of systemic atherosclerosis, many patients with atherosclerotic renal artery stenosis also have pre-existing cardiovascular risk factors, including essential hypertension, diabetes mellitus, dyslipidemia, and smoking. Established additional related therapies include glycemic control, statins, antiplatelet agents, and lifestyle modifications, including tobacco cessation.

Procedural Management. Whether all patients with atherosclerotic renal artery stenosis should undergo renal revascularization in addition to medical therapy remains a controversial practice, although recent trials do not support this procedure. Renal revascularization, with open surgical renal artery bypass and percutaneous transluminal angioplasty with or without stent placement, has been the subject of several randomized prospective trials. Numerous single-center retrospective studies have reported on various techniques of open surgical revascularization and have shown durable long-term patency rates (Cambria et al., 1996; Cherr et al., 2002; Darling et al., 1999; Fergany et al., 1995; Hansen et al., 2000; Marone et al., 2004; Paty et al., 2001). Notwithstanding these results, open surgical renal artery repair is associated with considerable perioperative mortality (5%) and morbidity (20%) rates and therefore is generally reserved for young patients and those with hemodynamically significant atherosclerotic renal artery stenosis and significant juxtarenal or suprarenal aortic disease (Edwards et al., 2009).

Renal revascularization with percutaneous transluminal renal artery angioplasty (PTRA) has been compared with medical therapy in three randomized controlled trials, none of which showed improved renal function, hypertension management, or survival with PTRA (Plouin et al., 1998; van Jaarsveld et al., 2000; Webster et al., 1998). These trials enrolled small numbers of patients, excluded patients with severe renal functional impairment, had extensive crossover between treatment groups, and did not use current medical therapy, thus making the results difficult to apply to current practice.

When compared with PTRA alone, percutaneous transluminal renal artery angioplasty with stenting (PTRS) was found to have superior technical success rates, increased patency rates, and decreased restenosis rates, leading to widespread adoption of PTRS as the standard endovascular management for atherosclerotic renal artery stenosis during the 1990s and early 2000s (Liang et al., 2013; van de Ven et al., 1999). A comparison of PTRS and medical management for atherosclerotic renal artery stenosis has been the subject of several randomized controlled trials. In three of these trials, which were presented or published in 2009, nearly 1000 patients with atherosclerotic renal artery stenosis were enrolled and followed for 2 to 4 years (Bax et al., 2009; Kumbhani et al., 2011; Wheatley et al., 2009). Aside from a slight reduction in number of antihypertensive medications, no significant improvement in systolic or diastolic blood pressure, renal function decline, or adverse cardiovascular events was seen with PTRS and medical management in comparison with medical management alone. Despite the randomized prospective design, these trials have faced several criticisms, including discrepancies in atherosclerotic renal artery stenosis diagnosis, flaws in the intention-to-treat analysis, and inclusion of patients with wide-ranging degrees of stenosis.

The NIH sponsored Cardiovascular Outcomes in Renal Atherosclerotic Lesions, or CORAL, trial attempted to correct these limitations and definitively answer whether revascularization of hemodynamically significant atherosclerotic renal artery stenosis in hypertensive patients prevents adverse cardiovascular and renal events when added to optimal medical therapy (Cooper et al., 2014). **The CORAL study enrolled 947 patients with atherosclerotic renal artery stenosis and hypertension between 2005 and 2010 and randomly assigned these patients to medical therapy plus renal artery stenting or medical therapy alone. After a median follow-up period of 43 months, the rate of the primary composite end point, made up of cardiovascular and renal sequelae, was not significantly different between participants who underwent stent placement in addition to medical therapy versus those who received medical therapy alone (Cooper et al., 2014). Although the limitations of these studies continue to be debated, the conclusions reached by the CORAL study reliably show the lack of benefit of renal artery stenting in most patients with atherosclerotic renal artery stenosis.**

Complications of PTRS, although generally less frequent than those seen with open surgical revascularization, can still account for significant morbidity. Periprocedural mortality rate is approximately 0.7%, and renal artery complications range from 1% to 10% (Kumbhani et al., 2011).

In contrast to asymptomatic patients who are found to have high-grade atherosclerotic renal artery stenosis, a subgroup of patients who appear to benefit from renal artery revascularization are those with flash pulmonary edema. As stated earlier, randomized prospective trials included mostly asymptomatic patients. Ritchie et al. (2014) evaluated outcomes between medical management alone compared with medical management plus percutaneous renal artery revascularization with stent placement in patients with high-risk clinical presentation, defined as flash pulmonary edema, rapidly declining renal function, or refractory hypertension. In this large analysis, flash pulmonary edema appeared to be an adverse prognostic marker with increased risk of death and cardiovascular events in medically treated patients, whereas the combination with renal artery revascularization reduced the risk of death (Ritchie et al., 2014).

Nonatherosclerotic Renal Artery Diseases

Fibromuscular Dysplasia

Fibromuscular dysplasia (FMD) is a nonatherosclerotic, noninflammatory vascular disease that most often affects small to medium arteries. Unlike atherosclerosis, FMD mostly involves the **mid- to distal renal artery** and can affect segmental renal artery branches. FMD has a female predominance and typically occurs in patients between 20 and 60 years of age but can occur in older and pediatric patient populations. Asymptomatic patients are most often diagnosed on imaging studies. Symptomatic patients can experience sequelae of arterial disease such as stenosis, occlusion, arterial dissection, or aneurysm. Although FMD can occur in any arterial bed in the body, involvement of the renal artery is most common.

Epidemiology of Renal Artery Fibromuscular Dysplasia. Because many patients with FMD remain asymptomatic, the true prevalence of FMD is difficult to assess. The overall prevalence can be estimated from the evaluation of renal donors, a suitable representation of healthy adult population. The prevalence of FMD in renal donors ranges between 2.6% to 6.6% with the variance most likely resulting from differences in imaging technique and patient populations (Cragg et al., 1989; McKenzie et al., 2013; Neymark et al., 2000). Bilateral renal artery involvement is seen in approximately one-third of FMD cases (McKenzie et al., 2013; Olin et al., 2011). FMD has a marked female preponderance: nearly **90% of cases occur in women.** Several causative factors, including hormonal and environmental causes, have been proposed for the development of FMD; however, the prevailing thought is that FMD is idiopathic.

Histopathology of Fibromuscular Dysplasia. FMD is classified according to the affected layer of arterial wall; specifically, the intima, media, and adventitia. FMD involving the media occurs most commonly and can be further subdivided into medial fibroplasia, perimedial fibroplasia, and medial hyperplasia. The latter two conditions are very uncommon, whereas **medial fibroplasia accounts for 90% of all types of FMD.** Medial fibroplasia is characterized by multiple diaphragm-like thickened areas of media that result in segments of arterial stenosis and poststenotic dilatation, typically seen as a "string of beads" appearance on CT angiography (Fig. 87.5).

Accounting for the remaining 10% of cases of FMD, intimal fibroplasia is due to collagen deposition within the intima with resultant fragmentation of the intimal layer. On angiography, intimal fibroplasia often appears as a concentric stenosis and, occasionally, as a long, diffuse narrowing.

Clinical Presentation. As mentioned previously, the diagnosis of renal artery FMD is often made in asymptomatic patients undergoing abdominal imaging for other reasons. The most common symptomatic presentation is **a middle-age woman with new-onset or difficult-to-control hypertension.** Other clinical presentations of renal artery FMD include flank pain and/or hematuria, both of which can result from dissection or occlusion of the renal artery and aneurysmal changes involving the artery. Interestingly, unless dissection occurs, medial fibroplasia rarely results in renal dysfunction. Intimal and perimedial fibroplasia may be associated with renal dysfunction, arterial dissection, and progression to occlusion (Stokes et al., 1996).

Diagnostic Evaluation. As with atherosclerotic renal artery stenosis, angiography remains the gold standard to diagnose and evaluate renal artery FMD. Catheter-based angiography provides excellent resolution of the main and segmental renal arteries and can identify luminal changes such as aneurysm formation and dissection that may affect the smaller vessels. More recently intravascular ultrasound has been used as an adjunct to angiography and can depict pressure gradients and even provide virtual histology of the arterial lumen (Prasad et al., 2009). CT and MRA are able to suggest the diagnosis of FMD in main renal vessels but are limited by poor visualization along branch renal vessels.

Management of Fibromuscular Dysplasia. The primary treatment goals in patients with renal artery FMD are control of hypertension and prevention of secondary complications of hypertension. Because ischemic nephropathy is not a sequela of FMD, preservation of renal function is not a consideration in the treatment of FMD. The primary factors in considering which patients with FMD merit treatment are patient age, temporal relationship between onset of hypertension and diagnosis of FMD, adequacy of blood pressure control with anti-hypertensive agents, and duration of hypertension.

Asymptomatic, normotensive patients with renal artery FMD should be followed for the development of hypertension. Young, otherwise healthy patients in whom FMD is diagnosed proximate to the onset of hypertension should be referred for PTRA, which provides immediate and long-term blood pressure control in nearly 75% of patients (Davies et al., 2008; Trinquart et al., 2010). Patients in whom hypertension has been present for many years should be continued on antihypertensive medications as long as blood pressure control is satisfactory. Dopper ultrasound–based surveillance of kidney length and cortical thickness should be done once or twice per year.

If blood pressure control becomes difficult, medication side effects become intolerable, or renal size or function decrease, PTRA should be performed (Olin, 2011). Balloon angioplasty alone is a very effective treatment for renal artery FMD, thereby making stent placement unnecessary. Surgical revascularization is reserved for cases not amenable to percutaneous approaches such as those with aneurysms or FMD involving distal extrarenal branches. Indications for stent placement in FMD are inability to eliminate a pressure gradient with angioplasty alone and intimal dissection.

Treatment success is fairly similar between PTRA and surgery. Approximately 50% of patients have cure of hypertension, but the complications are markedly fewer after PTRA. Major complication rates after PTRA are approximately 12%, in contrast to 17% after surgery (Trinquart, 2010).

Restenosis can occur after PTRA, particularly if the angioplasty was inadequate. Most instances of restenosis can be successfully treated with repeat angioplasty. Use of intravascular ultrasound (IVUS) in this setting can document resolution of a pressure gradient. Similar to patients on antihypertensive medications, patients are advised to continue with routine surveillance for recurrence of hypertension and for Doppler ultrasound of renal length and cortical thickness. Routine use of aspirin (81 mg) is advised for all patients with renal artery FMD (Olin, 2011).

> **KEY POINTS: CHRONIC KIDNEY DIEASE**
>
> - CKD is defined as kidney impairment sustained beyond 3 months with a reduction in GFR, structural abnormalities in the kidneys, and/or proteinuria.
> - There continues to be a steady increase in the number of patients with ESRD on RRTs throughout the world. Outcome comparisons suggest that kidney transplantation is still the best overall treatment for ESRD patients, despite advances in dialysis care and modalities.
> - Hemodynamically significant narrowing in the renal artery, or renal artery stenosis, can result in secondary hypertension and/or diminishing renal function.
> - Atherosclerotic vascular disease accounts for 90% of causes of renal artery stenosis, and fibromuscular dysplasias account for the remaining 10%.
> - Renal artery stenosis can lead to renal parenchymal loss and diminished renal function, a condition known as *ischemic nephropathy.*
> - Although the limitations of these studies continue to be debated, the conclusions reached by the CORAL study reliably show the lack of benefit of renal artery stenting in most patients with atherosclerotic renal artery stenosis.

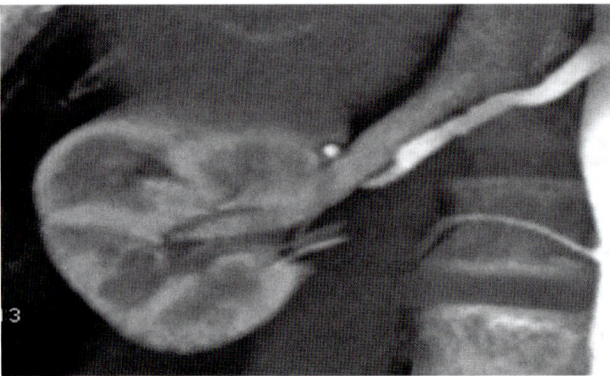

Fig. 87.5. "String of beads" appearance of the right renal artery typical of fibromuscular dysplasias.

SUGGESTED READINGS

Bax L, Woittiez AJ, Kouwenberg HJ, et al: Stent placement in patients with atherosclerotic renal artery stenosis and impaired renal function: a randomized trial, *Ann Intern Med* 150(12):840–848, W150–841, 2009.

Beck LH, Bonegio RG, Lambeau G, et al: M-type phospholipase A2 receptor as target antigen in idiopathic membranous nephropathy, *N Engl J Med* 361(1):11–21, 2009.

Cavanaugh C, Perazella MA: Urine sediment examination in the diagnosis and management of kidney disease: core curriculum 2019, *Am J Kidney Dis* 2018.

Chawla LS, Kimmel PL: Acute kidney injury and chronic kidney disease: an integrated clinical syndrome, *Kidney Int* 82(5):516–524, 2012.

Cooper CJ, Murphy TP, Cutlip DE, et al: Stenting and medical therapy for atherosclerotic renal-artery stenosis, *N Engl J Med* 370(1):13–22, 2014.

Freedman BI, Limou S, Ma L, et al: APOL1-Associated Nephropathy: a key contributor to racial disparities in CKD, *Am J Kidney Dis* 72(5S1):S8–S16, 2018.

Goicoechea M, Rivera F, López-Gómez JM: Increased prevalence of acute tubulointerstitial nephritis, *Nephrol Dial Transplant* 28(1):112–115, 2013.

Khosroshahi A, Wallace ZS, Crowe JL, et al: International consensus guidance statement on the management and treatment of IgG4-related disease, *Arthritis Rheumatol* 67(7):1688–1699, 2015.

Liaño F, Pascual J: Epidemiology of acute renal failure: a prospective, multicenter, community-based study. Madrid Acute Renal Failure Study Group, *Kidney Int* 50(3):811–818, 1996.

May AG, De Weese JA, Rob CG: Hemodynamic effects of arterial stenosis, *Surgery* 53:513–524, 1963.

REFERENCES

The complete reference list is available online at ExpertConsult.com.

88. Urologic Complications of Renal Transplantation

Mohammed Shahait, MBBS, Stephen V. Jackman, MD, and Timothy D. Averch, MD

Renal transplantation is the most cost-effective treatment for patients with end-stage renal disease and improves their chances of survival and their quality of life. Nevertheless, kidney transplantation is associated with a distinct array of urologic complications that must be managed promptly to prevent deterioration of graft function and improve graft survival. Urologic complications after renal transplantation are the most common surgical adverse event; overall rates range between 8% and 9.5%. These complications have been associated with high morbidity and increased care cost. The majority of the urologic complications are related to the transplanted ureter and ureterovesical anastomosis. The goal of this chapter is to review the major urologic complications encountered after kidney transplant and help the urologist to manage these complications.

HEMATURIA

Hematuria during the immediate postoperative period is typically related to the ureterovesical anastomosis. **In the majority of the cases, hematuria resolves over several days and rarely requires bladder irrigation.** Hematuria is observed more commonly after Leadbetter anastomosis compared with other types of anastomosis (Alberts et al., 2014).

Conversely, persistent hematuria after allograft biopsy is caused by an arteriovenous collecting system fistula. Duplex ultrasound (US) establishes the diagnosis and can be confirmed by magnetic resonance angiography. **Fortunately, in 70% of the cases, fistulas tend to resolve spontaneously; when they do not, highly selective embolization is indicated** (Branchereau et al., 2016).

The evaluation of asymptomatic microscopic hematuria (AMH) in transplant recipients follows the American Urology Association guidelines for AMH; the biggest difference is adding BK virus as part of the differential diagnosis. This may be suspected by viral cytopathic changes seen on cytology and confirmed by urine BK virus titers (Davis et al., 2012).

URETERAL STENT MANAGEMENT

Timing of Stent Removal

Several randomized clinical trials confirmed the utility of the routine use of a ureteral stent across the ureteovesical anastomosis during renal transplantation to decrease the incidence of urine leak and stricture of the ureter (Bassiri et al., 1995; Benoit et al., 1996; Dominguez et al., 2000; Kumar et al., 1998; Osman et al., 2005; Pleass et al., 1995). On the other hand, ureteral stent insertion is associated with an intrinsic risk of bacterial colonization. This risk can be substantial because 27% of the ureteral stents are colonized regardless of the indwelling time, and subsequent urinary tract infection (UTI) may pose a significant risk for graft infection and graft failure (Bonkat et al., 2012).

Several measures can be taken to improve outcome and decrease transplant stent-related complications such as infection and idiosyncratic stent-related complications. In a recent meta-analysis, early stent removal, defined by removal of the stent before the third postoperative week (before day 15), has been shown to reduce the incidence of UTI (RR 0.45, 95% CI 0.29–0.70; I^2 = 13%) without discernible effect on the incidence of urine leak and stenosis (Thompson et al., 2018).

Nevertheless, a case-by-case approach to the timing of stent removal for every patient must take into consideration surgeon satisfaction with the anastomosis and the patient's related risk factors such as diabetes, transplant revision, and presence of UTI.

Retained Stent

A retained stent can be due to a technical error during the ureteroneocystostomy closure in which the anastomosis suture inadvertently has caught the stent or because of stent encrustation. If the suture holds the stent, then leaving the stent until the suture dissolves is an option versus endoscopic stitch transection.

Stent encrustation is a significant problem for stents left for extended periods, with an incidence ranging from 0 to 5.7% (Guleria et al., 1998; Lynch et al., 2007). **Because of renal allograft denervation, kidney transplant recipients rarely manifest the classical symptoms of ureteral obstruction.** A transplant recipient with an encrusted stent usually presents with a progressive decline in renal function, a decrease in urine output and recurrent UTIs. In a rare instance, patients may experience a poorly characterized ache over the allograft because of irritation of peritoneum.

Prevention

Stent encrustation is a prime example of Reasons' Swiss Cheese Model of system failure and can be attributed to a chain of errors such as lack of documentation regarding stent insertion and poor team communication, as well as inadequate patient counseling about the temporary function of the stent, expected complications, and the importance of timely follow-up for stent removal. Different methods have been proposed to ensure timely removal; log books, stent cards, computerized tracking registry, web-based stent registry, and Smartphone application have been proposed and studied, yet none have yet been shown to be completely reliable (Ather et al., 2000; Lynch et al., 2007; McCahy et al., 1996; Molina et al., 2017; Sabharwal et al., 2014; Tang et al., 2008).

Diagnosis and Treatment

Computed tomography (CT) scan should be obtained in all patients with stent encrustation to assess encrustation burden and distribution, which will help guide the surgical approach (Fig. 88.1). **The first step of management is typically a urinary diversion by a nephrostomy tube, which will allow for decompression of the renal collecting system, improvement in renal function as well as antegrade access.** Different combinations of percutaneous nephrolithotomy, retrograde intrarenal renal surgery, and extracorporeal wave shock lithotripsy have been described to treat the encrusted transplant stent (Veltman et al., 2010; Wu et al., 2014).

KEY POINTS: HEMATURIA AND URETERAL STENT MANAGEMENT

- Majority of post-op hematuria is self-limiting.
- Consider duplex US for severe or persistent hematuria after renal biopsy to rule out AV fistula.
- Ureteral stent decreases ureteral stricture and urinary leak.
- Individualized stent removal after 3 weeks post-transplantation.

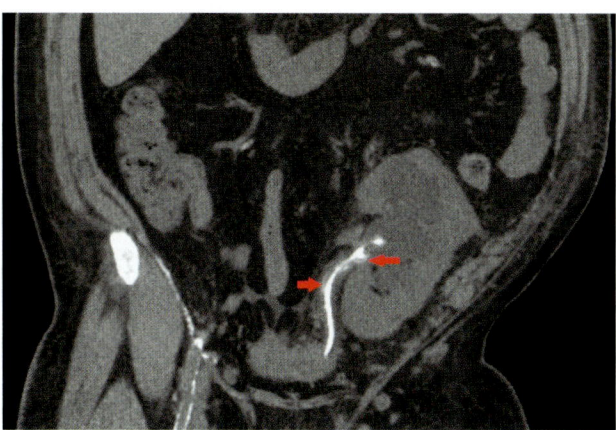

Fig. 88.1. Encrusted ureteral stent. Computed tomography scan demonstrates deposition of stone-like material *(arrows)* in the upper ureter. It is no longer functional (i.e., side holes and lumen are occluded).

BOX 88.1 Additional Causes of Urinary Leak

- An excessively long ureter
- Premature removal of bladder and/or ureteric drainage
- Technical problem such as suture dehiscence, ureteric twisting, or kinking
- Acute urine retention/bladder catheter obstruction
- Necrosis of renal parenchyma
- Parenchymal perforation during double-J stent placement

TABLE 88.1 Common Causes of Ureteral Obstruction

EARLY URETERAL OBSTRUCTION (<3 MONTHS)
Technical error during ureteroneocystostomy anastomosis
Forgoing ureteral stent
Anastomosis edema
Redundant ureter
Extrinsic compression (lymphocele, hematoma, abscess)

LATE URETERAL OBSTRUCTION (>3 MONTHS)
Stones
Ureteral strictures
Lymphocele
Fibrosis related to immunosuppressant medications

URINARY LEAK

Urine leak is the most common early urologic complication after renal transplantation, with an incidence ranging from 1.2% to 8.9% (Dinckan et al., 2007; Lempinen et al., 2015; Streeter et al., 2002). **Compromising the blood supply to the distal ureter during organ procurement is the main risk factor for ureteral necrosis and urine leak.** This has been observed more frequently in advanced donor age, extended criteria donors, allograft with multiple arteries, and failure to re-implant the lower polar artery (Branchereau et al., 2016; Rahnemai-Azar et al., 2015).

Additional causes for urine leak can be related to bladder dysfunction and other technical issues, which are outlined in Box 88.1.

Diagnosis

Early urine leak can be manifested as high fluid output from the drain with a concomitant decrease in urine output and an elevated serum creatinine. Alternatively, if the drain has been removed or omitted by the surgeon at the time of surgery, urine leak can be evident as a fluid leak from the wound, wound dehiscence, scrotal swelling, and/or pelvic or abdominal pain. US or non-enhanced CT scan can establish the diagnosis of fluid collection. The diagnosis can be confirmed by analysis of the content of collection sampled by CT/US-guided aspiration or fluid from the drain or the wound discharge. If the fluid is urine, the creatinine in the fluid will be significantly higher than the serum creatinine.

Treatment

The initial goal of treatment of a urine leak after transplantation is to divert urine away from the region of extravasation, improve graft function, and ameliorate the patient's general status. This can be achieved by a Foley catheter and a percutaneous nephrostomy tube. A nephrostomy tube can be used to perform an antegrade nephrostogram and characterize the leak further. In addition, it provides access for antegrade stent placement. Retrograde stent placement has also been proposed when a double-J stent was not placed at the time of surgery. However, retrograde insertion can be challenging because of the angulation required to access the neoureteral orifice, edema of the orifice, and the potential to further disrupt the anastomosis. If a substantial urinoma forms or causes ureteral obstruction or there is evidence of infection, then percutaneous drainage is recommended. In the instance of a small anastomotic leak, periodic contrast studies are performed to asses for healing every 1 to 2 weeks. A Foley catheter can be used to help facilitate healing in instances of a urine leak. The Foley catheter and nephrostomy tube can be removed when the leak is resolved. Patients should follow up diligently because they have the potential to develop ureteral stenosis in the future. The success rate of the endourologic management of the urine leak after kidney transplant ranges between 36% and 87% at a mean follow-up of 35 months (Alcaraz et al., 2005; Berli et al., 2015; Bhagat et al., 1998; Campbell et al., 1993; Matalon et al., 1990; Nie et al., 2009; Swierzewski et al., 1993; Tillou et al., 2009).

Early exploration and reconstructive surgery should be offered to patients with a proximal large leak, or persistent leak despite maximal drainage. The rationale for early surgical intervention is the low success rate of conservative management, the lack of intraabdominal adhesion, the minimal degree of postoperative fibrosis, and the decreased risk of subsequent ureteric stenosis. If the ureter remnant has an adequate blood supply, a tension-free ureteroneocystostomy should be attempted. Otherwise, other options should be entertained such as ureteroureteral anastomosis using the patient's native ipsilateral ureter, a bladder flap, or a pyelovesicostomy (Branchereau et al., 2016).

URETERAL STRICTURE

Strictures are the predominant cause of ureteral obstruction in patients greater than 3 months posttransplantation. They affect 1% to 9% of patients; early ureteral obstruction can be due to technical faults during the construction of the ureteroneocystostomy, such as not using a ureteral stent, anastomotic edema, redundant ureter length or extrinsic compression by lymphocele, hematoma, or abscess (Table 88.1; Faenza et al., 1999; Pereira et al., 2011).

The primary cause of ureteral stricture development is ischemia. Other causes for stricture development are related to urine leak, a component of graft rejection phenomena, or chronic infection. Also, BK and cytomegalovirus have been linked to ureteral stricture formation. Ureteral stricture development rates do not show a difference across the variety of types of the urinary anastomosis (Karam et al., 2004).

Diagnosis

The diagnosis of ureteral stricture should be considered when any deterioration of renal function is observed, especially when it is associated with hydronephrosis of the renal transplant. Hydronephrosis may be less than expected because of the inability of the system to expand secondary to surrounding fibrosis. Antegrade nephrostogram or a Whitaker test may be needed to establish the diagnosis.

Treatment

The priority in the management of ureteral obstruction is to decompress the collecting system and allow the allograft to recover. Nephrostomy, nephroureteral stent, antegrade stent, or retrograde stent placement can be used. Retrograde stent insertion can be cumbersome because of the location of the neoureteral orifice, location of stricture, and ureteral tortuosity. Antegrade nephrostomy helps to obtain a detailed antegrade nephrostogram of the pathology and provides versatile access for various endoscopic tools (Fig. 88.2; Duty et al., 2015; Orvieto et al., 2006). Once a stent is in place, retrograde exchange is usually straightforward, making long-term nephrostomy unnecessary in conservatively managed strictures.

The decision to proceed with endoscopic or surgical management depends on several factors: patient performance status, the presence of comorbidities, and length and location of the stricture.

Endoscopic options include double-J stent insertion, ureteral balloon dilation, and different variations of endoureterotomy (i.e., cold knife, holmium laser). In a small case series, the intermediate-term success rate of antegrade double-J stent insertion was 33% (Bhagat et al., 1998). Balloon dilation is associated with a 3-year success rate of 51% (range 44% to 62%) (Bachar et al., 2004; Bromwich et al., 2006; Juaneda et al., 2005).

Several series have reported on the efficacy of different techniques of endoureterotomy in treating allograft ureteral stricture, with success rate of 79%, 78%, and 55% for holmium laser endoureterotomy, Acucise balloon cutting device, and electrocautery with the T loop of a resectoscope, respectively (Duty et al., 2015).

With respect to these results, definitive open surgical repair remains the most effective treatment modality with superior long-term results when compared with endoscopic management. Open surgical reconstructive options vary, depending on the size and location of the stricture and consist of allograft ureter reimplantation, ureter-ureteral anastomosis using ipsilateral native ureter, Boari flap, appendix or ilium interposition or pyelovesicostomy (Adani et al., 2015). Recently, different series reported on the translation of different open ureteral reconstructive options to robotic-assisted laparoscopic surgery with a comparable short-term outcome (Benamran et al., 2017; Hauser et al., 2011).

> **KEY POINTS: URETERAL STRICTURE**
>
> - Strictures are the predominant cause of ureteral obstruction in patients greater than 3 months posttransplantion.
> - The primary cause of ureteral stricture development is ischemia.
> - Stricture should be suspected in patients with hydronephrosis and decreased graft function.
> - A variety of endourologic treatment options have been described to treat ureteral strictures; however, open reconstructive surgery offers superior long-term results.

VESICOURETERAL REFLUX

Several modifications of the ureterovesical anastomosis have been described to replicate an antireflux mechanism. Nevertheless, on voiding cystography, the incidence of vesicoureteral reflux (VUR) can be evident in 50% to 86% of the cases, whereas the incidence of symptomatic or clinically significant VUR is less than 1% and independent of the ureterovesical anastomosis technique (Masahiko et al., 2000; Ostrowski et al.,1999). The clinical sequelae of VUR are unclear; in one study it was found that, at 5 years, patients with VUR had a higher incidence of hypertension and trended toward an increased susceptibility for urosepsis (Mastrosimone et al., 1993).

VUR can be related to a technical error during the ureteroneocystostomy anastomosis, bladder outlet obstruction, or high-pressure urine storage secondary to either detrusor overactivity or reduced bladder compliance.

Diagnosis

Patients with recurrent urinary tract infections should be evaluated for VUR by voiding cystography. Once the diagnosis of VUR is established, a comprehensive workup to rule out bladder outlet obstruction and high-pressure urine storage is recommended.

Treatment

Therapy should be focused on the underlying cause for the symptomatic reflux. Patients with high-pressure urine storage or bladder outlet obstruction can be treated in the usual fashion. In rare cases, the reflux itself can be addressed.

Traditionally, the standard treatment for VUR involved revision of the anastomosis or ureter-reimplantation to the ipsilateral native ureter. However, endoscopic submucosal injection of various composites, either Teflon or Macroplastique, is a less invasive alternative. The success rate of submucosal injection depends on the grade of reflux; it reaches 90% in grades I and II disease, whereas it is only 30% in high-grade disease. Thus an endoscopic submucosal injection should be attempted only in patients with clinically significant low-grade VUR. **On the other hand, patients with high-grade reflux or failed previous endoscopic treatment with persistent symptoms are best managed by reconstructive surgery** (Elder et al., 2006; Pichler et al., 2011; Seifert et al., 2007; Stenberg et al., 1995; Yucel et al., 2010).

LYMPHOCELE

A lymphocele is a pseudocyst with lymph content covered by a hard fibrous capsule around the graft. Lymphocele is radiographically evident in 0.6% to 33.9% of recipients. However, the incidence of symptomatic lymphocele ranges from 0.03% to 26%. A lymphocele most frequently develops within the first 6 months after transplantation with a peak incidence at 6 weeks (Dubeaux et al., 2004; Ebadzadeh et al., 2008).

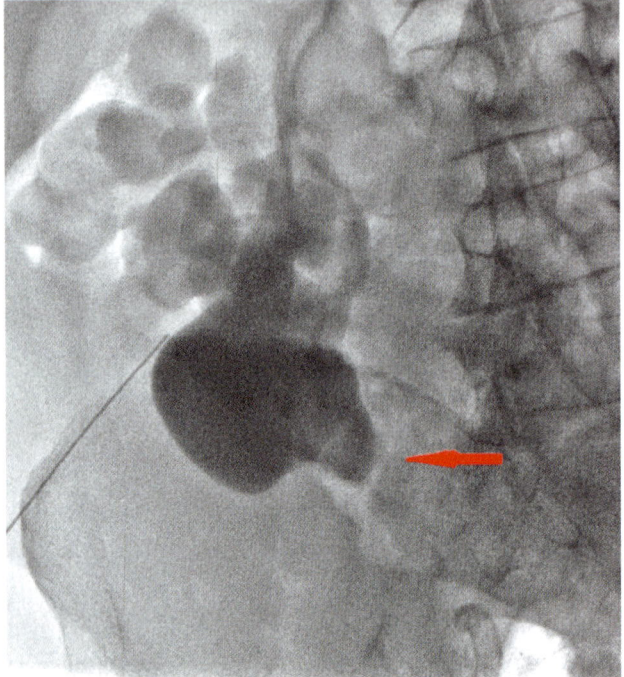

Fig. 88.2. Proximal ureteral stricture. Antegrade nephrostogram reveals hydronephrosis in the allograft without visualization of the ureter.

Lymphoceles occur mainly because of extensive dissection of the lymphatics around the iliac vessels of the recipient or renal vessels of the donor occuring during the time of organ procurement surgery or back table preparation. Other factors found to be associated with lymphocele formation include obesity, recipient age, duration of dialysis treatment, warm ischemia time, use of prophylaxis low-molecular-weight heparin, delayed graft function, acute rejection, redo-transplant, and the use of mTOR inhibitors (Cash et al., 2012; Dean et al., 2004; Goel et al., 2004; Huber et al., 2007; Khauli et al., 1993; Martinez-Ocana et al., 1995; Mokos et al., 2010; Pengel et al., 2011; Stephanian et al., 1992; Tiong et al., 2009).

The majority of patients with lymphocele are asymptomatic. However, large lymphoceles may present as unilateral lower limb edema, deterioration of graft function, symptoms related to bladder compression, fever, and deep vein thrombosis as a consequence of compression of the external iliac vein.

Diagnosis

Confirmation of the presence of a fluid collection around the graft can be determined on US examination or CT scan. Biochemical and microbiological analysis of the fluid from the lymphocele can be obtained directly from the drain or the aspirate using a US-guided/CT-guided fine-needle percutaneous aspiration. This should be performed to differentiate lymphocele from urinoma, seroma, or abscess.

Treatment

As mentioned earlier, the majority of lymphoceles are asymptomatic, and no treatment is required because they tend to resolve spontaneously. Treatment for lymphoceles is necessary in less than 15% of the cases. Primary treatment modalities include aspiration with or without sclerotherapy, drain placement, and laparoscopic or open decortication surgery with possible peritoneal window. The success rate for aspiration alone, sclerotherapy using different composite, drain placement, laparoscopic, and open surgery is 41%, 69%, 50%, 92%, and 84%, respectively. **Open drainage should be considered in patients with wound complications and those with a small lymphocele adjacent to vital renal structures** (Lucewicz et al., 2011; Ulrich et al., 2010; Zagdoun et al., 2010; Zietek et al., 2007).

NEPHROLITHIASIS

The estimated incidence of kidney stones in kidney transplant recipients is 1.0%. The mean time to stone onset is 28 ± 22 months. The most common stone composition is calcium-based stones (67%), followed by struvite stones (20%) and uric acid stones (13%) (Branchereau et al., 2018; Cheungpasitporn et al., 2016).

Several factors favor stone formation in kidney transplant patients, such as secondary hyperparathyroidism, recurrent urinary tract infections, and metabolic abnormalities such as hypercalciuria, hyperuricosuria, hypocitraturia, or hyperoxaluria. In addition, the deleterious effect of certain immunosuppressive medications on the urine environment has been noted; for example, cyclosporine induces chronic hyperuricemia, and calcineurin inhibitors cause hyperoxaluria and hypocitraturia (Stapenhorst et al., 2005).

Treatment

The treatment of kidney stones in transplant patients follows the algorithm of stone management in native kidneys. In asymptomatic patients with a nonobstructing stone less than 4 mm, observation with serial US and creatinine level has been shown to be a feasible option. When growing or symptomatic, extracorporeal wave shock lithotripsy, retrograde intrarenal surgery, percutaneous nephrolithotomy and various combinations of these approaches have been described in treating urolithiasis in transplant allograft (Challacombe et al., 2005; Gupta et al., 2007; Klingler et al., 2002).

After management of the stone, patients should be followed for development of silent hydronephrosis after ureteral instrumentation. Patients should undergo comprehensive metabolic screening to identify and treat underlying metabolic abnormalities.

LOWER URINARY TRACT COMPLICATIONS

Voiding Dysfunction

Voiding dysfunction is common after renal transplantation. Because the majority of patients are oliguric before transplant, low urine volume may conceal bladder outlet obstruction or incontinence symptoms pretransplant. An intricate interaction between a small bladder capacity (<300 mL), preexisting anatomic abnormalities, and the direct effect of the immunosuppression on bladder function by decreasing bladder mass play a significant role in voiding dysfunction in kidney transplant recipients (Karam et al., 2011; Shenasky, 1976).

Evaluation of patients with voiding dysfunction should include a detailed history of urologic and neurologic disorders and previous urologic surgeries and be supported by a complete urologic and gynecologic physical exam. Assessing the symptoms using standardized questionnaires from the International Continence Society and the International Prostate Symptom score, and using a voiding diary is desirable. The indication for further testing such as uroflowmetry, urodynamic testing, and cystoscopy depends on individual risk factors and symptoms.

Small Bladder After Transplant

The bladder capacity in anuric recipients tends to grow gradually to reach normal capacity after kidney transplantation. **As a result, efforts to increase the bladder capacity before transplantation by bladder rehabilitation or surgical augmentation are unnecessary.**

If the bladder symptoms affecting the quality of life of the recipients, patients may benefit from the standard spectrum of treatments from anticholinergics and botox to bladder capacity is insufficient, or there is evidence of high storage pressure, or lower urinary tract augmentation or urinary diversion using an ileal conduit.

Benign Prostatic Hyperplasia

Benign prostatic hypertrophy (BPH) is a disease of aging men and as such is more common in the renal transplant population compared with the general population. It can be challenging to detect in anuric patients. The estimated 3-year incidence of BPH among renal transplant patients is 9.7% and has been shown to be associated with an increased risk of urinary tract infection and graft loss (Hurst et al., 2009; Tsaur et al., 2009).

If the preoperative evaluation or intraoperative findings are suggestive of the presence of significant BPH, precautionary measures should be considered, such as starting patients on an alpha-blocker and aggressive treatment of constipation before removing the Foley catheter. In selected cases, insertion of a suprapubic tube at the time of transplant can be performed.

Surgical resection of the prostate before transplantation while the patient is still anuric or oliguric may increase the risk of developing a bladder neck contracture or a urethral stricture secondary to the lack of urine during healing. Transurethral resection of prostate (TURP) or holmium enucleation of the prostate has been reported to be safe and effective in this subset of patients if performed at least 3 weeks posttransplant. **It is crucial to avoid TURP in the first 2 weeks and in the presence of a ureteral stent after the transplant because it has been associated with devastating complications such as sepsis and death** (Pedraza et al., 2004; Reinberg et al., 1992; Volpe et al., 2013).

Urine Incontinence

The estimated prevalence of urinary incontinence among female recipients is 28% (Heit et al., 2004). The diagnosis and treatment of stress incontinence in transplant patients are similar to nontransplant patients. Several reports have described the feasibility and safety of tension-free vaginal tape (TVT), transobturator tape (TOT), sacral neuromodulation, and laparoscopic sacrocolpopexy in female recipients (Rouffilange et al., 2017).

Limited reporting in the literature supports the feasibility of insertion of an artificial urinary sphincter prosthesis in kidney transplant patients after radical prostatectomy (O'Malley et al., 1999).

GENITOURINARY MALIGNANCIES

Renal Cell Carcinoma

The incidence of renal cell carcinoma (RCC) is higher in transplant recipients than in the general population. RCC represents 4.6% of posttransplant cancers compared with 3% of tumors in the general population. However, only 10% occurred in kidney grafts (Fig. 88.3). The mean time to develop a de novo tumor in the graft is 131 months (Chapman et al., 2013; Hickman et al., 2018; Penn, 1995).

Tillou et al. (2012) analyzed the histology subtype of de novo RCC in kidney grafts and found that papillary carcinomas are reported in 56% of kidney graft tumors, and low-grade tumors (Fuhrman grades 1 and 2) accounted for 65% of nonpapillary kidney graft tumors.

The treatment of RCC in kidney transplant patients is similar to RCC in the general population (Fig. 88.4).

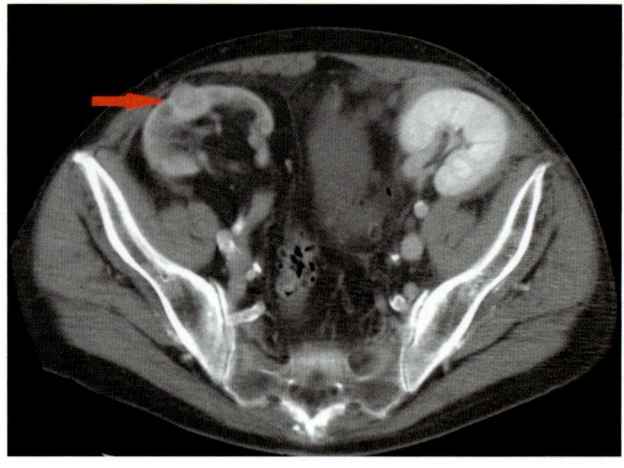

Fig. 88.3. Renal mass in transplanted kidney. Computed tomography scan reveals exophytic renal mass in nonfunctioning allograft in an 80-year-old patient. Biopsy was performed and low-grade papillary renal cell carcinoma, type 1 was found. Cryotherapy was used to ablate this mass.

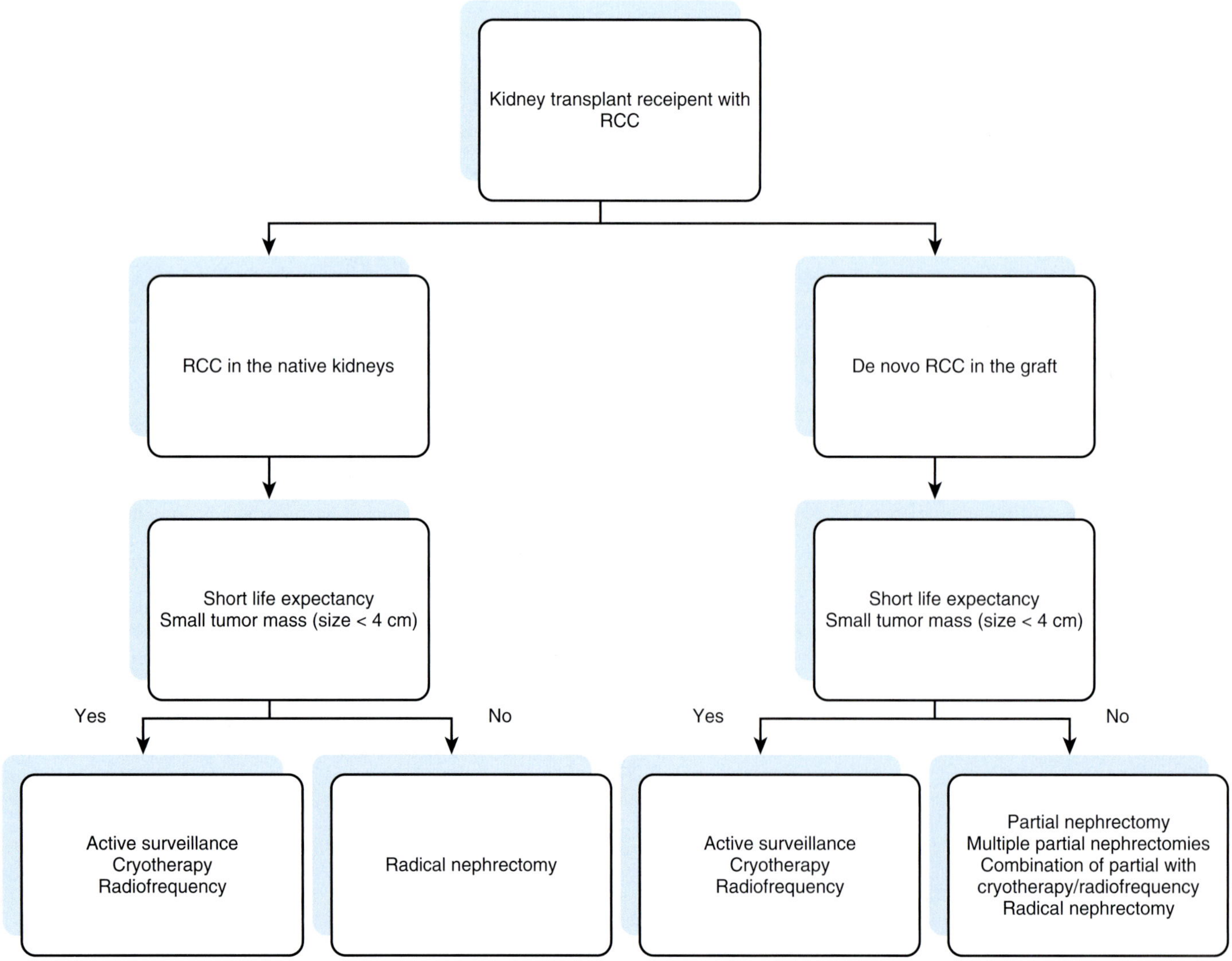

Fig. 88.4. Renal cell carcinoma management in kidney transplant patients.

No specific recommendations exist regarding modifications to the immunosuppressive regimen after diagnosing malignancy in recipients. However, in the case of metastatic RCC originating from the graft, some authors have proposed stopping immunosuppression medications after the allograft nephrectomy to help the recipient immune system recover and reject the donor-associated cancer cells.

Despite the high incidence of RCC, the Kidney Disease: Improving Global Outcomes (KDIGO) guidelines do not endorse screening of the native kidneys posttransplantation because no evidence exists that the benefits of screening outweigh any potential harm. **However, consider screening high-risk recipients with a previous history of RCC, analgesic nephropathy, tuberous sclerosis, or known acquired cystic disease** (Kasiske et al., 2010).

Prostate Cancer

The incidence of prostate cancer in kidney transplant recipients is similar to that in the general population. However, the performance of PSA testing in transplant patients is not similar to the general population. The preoperative workup for the older male recipient generally includes a PSA. Nevertheless, no definite national recommendation exists for or against prostate cancer screening in recipients, except following the current guidelines for prostate cancer screening in the general populace (Hickman et al., 2018; Kasiske et al., 2010).

Management of prostate cancer in kidney transplant recipients poses a challenge for the treating physician because of the risk of direct or indirect injury to the transplanted kidney that may occur as a result of its anatomic proximity to the surgical or radiation field. In addition, recipients are maintained on immunosuppressive medications that put them at increased risk of infection, lymphocele, impaired wound healing, and wound complications.

In a recent meta-analysis, the majority of kidney transplant patients with prostate cancer who underwent treatment had organ-confined disease, and Gleason score of 6 or less. **The most common modality of treatment is surgical extirpation by any approach, followed by radiation therapy and then active surveillance, which was underused** (Marra et al., 2018). The variety of prostate cancer treatment modalities in kidney transplant recipients provide comparable oncologic outcomes to those observed in the nontransplant patients (Sierra et al., 2016).

Bladder Cancer

Kidney transplant patients are at a significantly increased risk of developing bladder cancer compared with the general population (SIR = 3.18; 95% CI: 1.34–7.53; *P* = 0.008). Bladder cancer in kidney transplant patients is aggressive and tends to be associated with higher recurrence rates, progression, and metastasis. Therefore an aggressive surveillance regimen is necessary. The mean time between transplantation and bladder cancer diagnosis ranges between 2.8 and 4 years (Buzzeo et al., 1997; Wallerand et al., 2010; Yan et al., 2011).

Bladder cancer management in kidney transplant recipients is challenging because of immunosuppression and high overall comorbidity. **Intravesical bacillus Calmette-Guerin can be used in selected patients with high-risk non-muscle-invasive bladder cancer.** Muscle invasive bladder cancer can be treated with chemoradiotherapy or radical cystoprostatectomy and urinary diversion. During cystectomy with lymph node dissection, care must be taken to avoid injury to the graft vessels or blood supply to the ureter or the ureter itself (Demirdag et al., 2017; Hickman et al., 2018; Moses et al., 2013; Prabharasuth et al., 2013; Tomaszewski et al., 2011).

KEY POINTS: GENITOURINARY MALIGNANCIES

- Most of the kidney tumors develop in the native kidneys and are low-grade tumors.
- Active surveillance, radiation, and surgery (open and minimally invasive) are reasonable options to treat prostate cancer in kidney transplant patients.
- Kidney transplant recipients have a three-fold risk of urothelial carcinoma (UC) compared with the general population, and it is biologically more aggressive.

CONCLUSION

In conclusion, renal transplant patients are at risk for multiple urologic complications as described. The management, in most instances, mirrors the management of these issues in the general population with some special considerations as discussed. Diligence in recognition and treatment of these issues by the urologist is important to ensure the optimal survival of graft and host.

See Videos 88.1 and 88.2 for procedures related to this chapter.

SUGGESTED READINGS

Arpali E, Al-Qaoud T, Martinez E, et al: Impact of ureteral stricture and treatment choice on long-term graft survival in kidney transplantation, *Am J Transplant* 18(8):1977–1985, 2018.

Boissier R, Hevia V, Bruins HM, et al: The risk of tumour recurrence in patients undergoing renal transplantation for end-stage renal disease after previous treatment for a urological cancer: a systematic review, *Eur Urol* 73(1):94–108, 2018.

Branchereau J, Timsit MO, Neuzillet Y, et al: Management of renal transplant urolithiasis: a multicentre study by the French Urology Association Transplantation Committee, *World J Urol* 36(1):105–109, 2018.

EAU guidelines on renal transplantation: 2017. (website): http://www.uroweb.org/guideline/renal-transplantation/.

Hevia V, Zakri RH, Taylor CF, et al: Effectiveness and harms of using kidneys with small renal tumors from deceased or living donors as a source of renal transplantation: a systematic review. *Eur Urol Focus* 5(3):508–517, 2019.

Thompson ER, Hosgood SA, Nicholson ML, et al: Early versus late ureteric stent removal after kidney transplantation. *Cochrane Libr* 2018 Jan 1.

REFERENCES

The complete reference list is available online at ExpertConsult.com.

PART IX: Upper Urinary Tract Obstruction and Trauma

89. Management of Upper Urinary Tract Obstruction

Stephen Y. Nakada, MD, FACS, FRCS(Glasg.), and Sara L. Best, MD

Technologic advances evolve the diagnostic and therapeutic alternatives available in the contemporary management of upper urinary tract obstruction. The obstructive processes may be intrinsic, extrinsic, congenital, or iatrogenic, and in many patients the cause of obstruction may not be immediately evident. Making an accurate diagnosis of obstruction is paramount for therapeutic treatment.

The treatments for upper tract obstruction range from ureteral stent placement to ileal interposition. Myriad skills are required for total surgical management of upper urinary tract obstruction. Not surprisingly, endourology, laparoscopy, and robotics continue to be more prominent in the surgical management of upper urinary tract obstruction. As a result of the wide array of available treatments, the urologist must have an understanding of the indications and risks of all the alternatives.

This chapter provides a state-of-the-art presentation of the diagnostic and therapeutic management strategies for patients with upper urinary tract obstruction. The chapter is organized by the anatomic location of obstruction. The cause, diagnosis, indications for intervention, risks, and therapeutic options (including endoscopic, laparoscopic, robotic, and open approaches) are thoroughly reviewed.

EVALUATION OF UPPER TRACT OBSTRUCTION

The use of computed tomography (CT) scanning and renal ultrasound in emergency departments and for various screening purposes has led to frequent suspicion of upper tract obstruction (Davis et al., 2012; Smith-Bindman et al., 2014). Moreover, the widespread use of noncontrast, low-dose CT scans may necessitate follow-up imaging (Zagoria and Dixon, 2009). After low-dose CT, the urologist can use ultrasound, diuretic renography, CT urography, retrograde pyelography, Whitaker tests, and ureteroscopy to delineate the precise cause and subsequent treatment strategy of upper tract obstruction. For each disorder we will discuss the recommended approach to the upper tract evaluation.

URETEROPELVIC JUNCTION OBSTRUCTION

The diagnosis of ureteropelvic junction (UPJ) obstruction (UPJO) describes a functionally significant impairment of urinary transport from the renal pelvis to the ureter. Although most cases are congenital, the problem may not become clinically apparent until much later in life (Jacobs et al., 1979). Acquired conditions such as stone disease, postoperative or inflammatory stricture, or urothelial neoplasm may also manifest clinically with symptoms and signs of obstruction at the level of the UPJ. Similarly, extrinsic obstruction can occur at this level. This section focuses primarily on the diagnosis and treatment of "congenital" UPJO, although these techniques may be applied to the management of certain acquired conditions, such as urinary stones.

Pathogenesis

Congenital UPJO usually results from intrinsic disease. A frequently found defect is the presence of an aperistaltic segment of the ureter, perhaps similar to that found in primary obstructive megaureter. In these cases, histopathologic studies reveal that the spiral musculature normally present has been replaced by abnormal longitudinal muscle bundles or fibrous tissue (Allen, 1970; Foote et al., 1970; Gosling and Dixon, 1978; Hanna et al., 1976; Fig. 89.1). This results in failure to develop a normal peristaltic wave for propagation of urine from the renal pelvis to the ureter. Recognition that this type of segmental defect is often responsible for UPJO is of utmost importance clinically because such ureters may appear grossly normal at the time of surgery and, in fact, may often be calibrated to 14 Fr or greater. Further studies in the cause of UPJO have shown decreased density of interstitial cells of Cajal at the UPJ in children, but less so in cases involving solely intrinsic UPJO (Koleda et al., 2012; Solari et al., 2003). In addition, cytokine production in the urothelium has also been proposed to exacerbate UPJO (Chiou et al., 2005). Other experimental studies have implicated transforming growth factor-β, epidermal growth factor expression, nitric oxide, and neuropeptide Y in UPJ stenosis (Knerr et al., 2001; Yang et al., 2003). A less frequent intrinsic cause of congenital UPJO is true ureteral stricture. Such congenital ureteral strictures are most frequently found at the UPJ, although they may be located at sites anywhere along the lumbar ureter. Abnormalities of ureteral musculature have been implicated as electron microscopy has demonstrated excessive collagen deposition at the site of the stricture (Hanna et al., 1976).

Intrinsic obstruction at the UPJ may also result from kinks or valves produced by infoldings of the ureteral mucosa and musculature (Maizels and Stephens, 1980). In these patients the obstruction may actually be at the level of the proximal ureter. This phenomenon appears to result from retention or exaggeration of congenital folds normally found in the ureter of developing fetuses. In some of these patients the defects are bridged by ureteral adventitia. Grossly, this can manifest as external bands or adhesions that appear to be causing the obstruction. In fact, Johnston et al. (1977) reported that lysis of external adhesions can at times reestablish flow without pyeloplasty. In the majority of patients, these bands or adhesions are likely to be a secondary phenomenon associated with intrinsic obstruction, thus operative pyeloplasty would usually be most effective. The presence of these kinks, valves, bands, or adhesions may also produce angulation of the ureter at the lower margin of the renal pelvis in such a manner that as the pelvis dilates anteriorly and inferiorly, the ureteral insertion is carried further proximally. In these patients the most dependent portion of the pelvis is inadequately drained, and the apparent high insertion of the ureteral ostium is actually a secondary phenomenon (Kelalis, 1976). In at least some patients, however, the high insertion is likely the primary obstructing lesion because this phenomenon is found more frequently in the presence of renal ectopia or fusion anomalies (Das and Amar, 1984; Zincke et al., 1974). Thus a high insertion can have implications in the

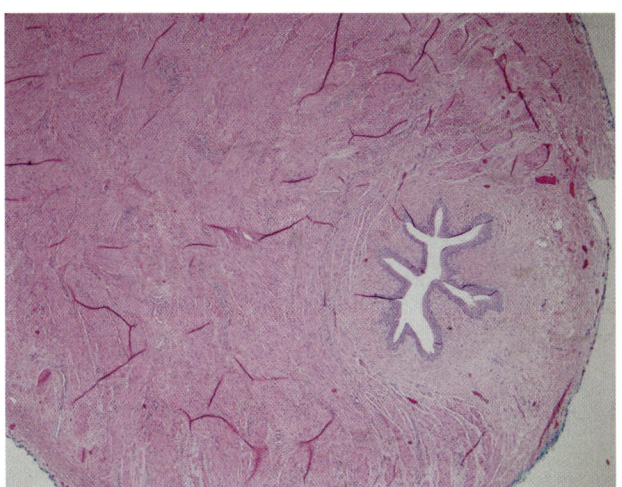

Fig. 89.1. The microphotograph is taken through the ureteropelvic junction. There is marked attenuation of smooth muscles and smooth muscle in disarray and hypertrophy surrounding the urothelial lining.

subsequent surgical management, particularly endourologic approaches.

Controversy persists regarding the potential role of "aberrant" vessels in the cause of UPJO. Significant crossing vessels have been noted in up to 63% of patients with UPJO but in as little as 20% of individuals with normal kidneys (Quillin et al., 1996; Richstone et al., 2009; Zeltser et al., 2004). Although these lower pole vessels have often been referred to as aberrant, these segmental vessels, which may be branches from the main renal artery or arise directly from the aorta, are usually normal variants (Stephens, 1982). In some patients, these lower pole vessels cross the ureter posteriorly and truly have an aberrant course. Historically, it has been believed that the associated vessel alone does not cause the primary obstruction (Hanna, 1978). In fact, the true cause is an intrinsic lesion at the UPJ or proximal ureter that causes dilation and ballooning of the renal pelvis over the polar or aberrant vessel. Recent studies using three-dimensional (3D) multidetector row CT demonstrated that the precise location of crossing vessels did not correspond to the obstructive transition point in patients with UPJO (Lawler et al., 2005). In contrast, one group found improvement in patients undergoing only ligation of crossing vessels (Keeley et al., 1996). Richstone et al. (2009) reviewed histopathology from 95 patients with UPJO and found that 43% of 65 patients with a crossing vessel had no intrinsic abnormality. Another histopathologic study identified only increased inflammation at the point of crossing vessels (Cancian et al., 2017). Regardless, the presence of crossing vessels most certainly has been shown to have a detrimental effect on the success rates of endopyelotomy (Nakada et al., 1998; Van Cangh et al., 1994). UPJO with concomitant anatomic anomalies such as horseshoe kidney and pelvic kidney also present surgical challenges. **Notably, the increased use of laparoscopic and robotic pyeloplasty has decreased the need for preoperative assessment of crossing vessels; this can be addressed at the time of pyeloplasty.**

UPJO may also result from acquired lesions. In children, vesicoureteral reflux can lead to upper tract dilation with subsequent elongation, tortuosity, and kinking of the ureter. In some patients these changes may only mimic the radiographic findings of true UPJO. However, true UPJO can definitely coexist with vesicoureteral reflux, although it may be difficult to determine whether the anomalies are merely coincident or whether the upper tract ureteral obstruction has resulted from the reflux (Lebowitz and Johan, 1982). Diuretic renography remains the first-line modality for differentiating between UPJO and reflux. Other acquired causes of obstruction at the UPJ include benign lesions such as fibroepithelial polyps (Berger et al., 1982; Macksood et al., 1985), urothelial malignancy, stone disease, and postinflammatory or postoperative scarring or ischemia. For these acquired diseases, the surgical techniques discussed in this section may be useful adjuncts for management of the obstruction as long as the primary problem is also addressed where appropriate. For instance, fibroepithelial polyps can be managed using retrograde ureteroscopy and holmium laser excision (Lam et al., 2003a).

Patient Presentation and Diagnostic Studies

UPJO, although most often a congenital problem, can manifest clinically at any time of life. Historically, the most common presentation in neonates and infants was the finding of a palpable flank mass. However, **the use of maternal prenatal ultrasonography has led to a dramatic increase in the number of asymptomatic newborns being diagnosed with hydronephrosis, many of whom are subsequently found to have UPJO** (Bernstein et al., 1988; Wolpert et al., 1989). A fraction of cases may also be found during evaluation of azotemia, which may result from bilateral obstruction in a functionally or anatomically solitary kidney. UPJO may also be incidentally found during studies performed to evaluate unrelated anomalies such as congenital heart disease (Roth and Gonzales, 1983). In older children or adults, intermittent abdominal or flank pain, at times associated with nausea or vomiting, is a frequent presenting symptom. Hematuria, either spontaneous or associated with otherwise relatively minor trauma, may also be an initial symptom. Laboratory findings of microhematuria, pyuria, or frank urinary tract infection may also bring an otherwise asymptomatic patient to the urologist. Rarely, hypertension may be a presenting finding (Riehle and Vaughan, 1981).

Radiographic studies should be performed with a goal of determining the anatomic location and the functional significance of an apparent obstruction. Historically, excretory urographic findings include delay in function associated with a dilated pelvicalyceal system. If the ureter is visualized, it should be of normal caliber. In some patients, symptoms may be intermittent, and urography findings between painful episodes may be normal. In such cases, the study should be repeated during an acute episode when the patient is symptomatic (Nesbit, 1956). Today, provocative testing with diuretic renography may allow accurate diagnosis in most patients. The patient should be well hydrated and the study then performed after injection of furosemide, 0.3 to 0.5 mg/kg (Malek, 1983; Fig. 89.2). Studies have recently shown using P40, or the percentage of maximal tracer at 40 minutes, that the sensitivity of renal scan can be increased from 49% to 73% (Liu et al., 2017).

Noncontrast CT scan is commonly obtained for patients with acute flank pain (Dalrymple et al., 1998; Fielding et al., 1997; Vieweg et al., 1998; Fig. 89.3). **Moreover, contrast-enhanced CT scans provide detailed anatomic and functional information to aid in diagnosis of UPJO** (Fig. 89.4). In fact one study showed contrast-enhanced CT can be a surrogate test for renography when assessing patients for UPJO repair (Ark et al., 2016). Ultrasonography and CT scanning also have a role in differentiating acquired causes of obstruction such as radiolucent calculi or urothelial tumors. **In neonates and infants, the diagnosis of UPJO has usually been suggested either by routine performance of maternal ultrasonography or by the finding of a flank mass. In either setting, renal ultrasonography is usually the first radiographic study performed. Ideally, ultrasonography should be able to visualize dilation of the collecting system to help differentiate UPJO from multicystic kidney and determine the level of obstruction.** UPJO and multicystic kidneys are distinguishable in the majority of patients by ultrasound alone. With UPJO, the pelvis is visualized as a large, medial sonolucent area surrounded by smaller, rounded sonolucent structures representing dilated calyces. At times, dilated calyces will be seen connecting to the pelvis via dilated infundibula (Fig. 89.5). More recently, Dias et al. (2013) have shown that prenatal renal pelvis dilation can predict the need for surgical repair of the UPJ.

Occasionally, a solid-appearing renal cortex can be seen surrounding the sonolucent areas or separating the dilated calyces. In contrast, the cysts of multicystic kidneys are visualized as various-sized sonolucent areas in random distribution. Although the cysts may be connected, this is rarely visualized sonographically. Furthermore, little solid tissue is seen, and what is present has a random distribution

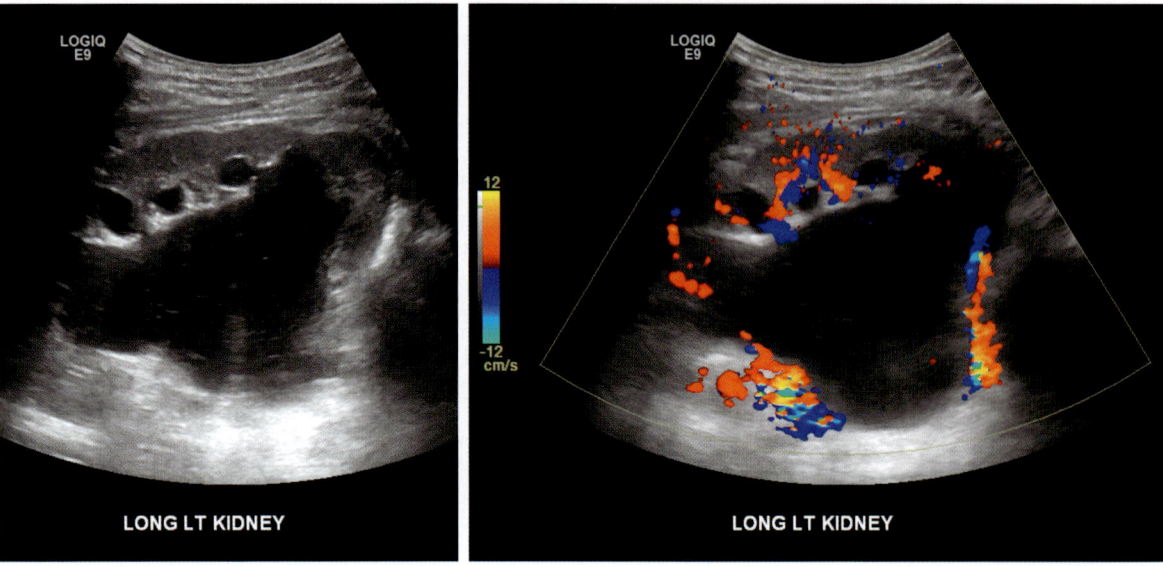

Fig. 89.2. Typical ultrasound image of ureteropelvic junction obstruction, with dilated renal pelvis and infundibula and calyces, including color Doppler images. Note, the ureter is not visualized in this image.

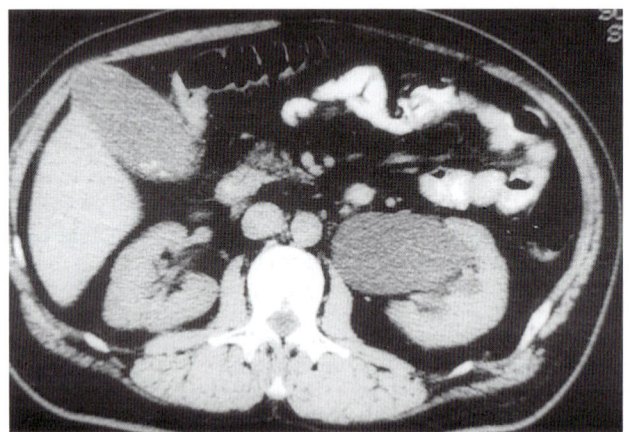

Fig. 89.3. Noncontrast computed tomography scan performed as the initial radiographic study in a patient with left flank pain revealed hydronephrosis to the level of the ureteropelvic junction (UPJ). No calculus was visualized, and a presumed diagnosis of UPJ obstruction was considered. This proved correct on subsequent radiographic studies.

among the cysts. Rarely a large, centrally located cyst may cause confusion in the diagnosis (King et al., 1984a). In this setting, a renal scan should be performed. Specifically, a technetium^{99m}-diethylenetriamenepentaacetic acid (^{99m}Tc-DTPA) scan allows differentiation of these two entities. Multicystic kidneys rarely reveal concentration of this isotope. When uptake is seen, the areas of functioning tissue are initially discrete and are usually medial to the bulk of the mass, which remains a "cold" area. In contrast, neonatal kidneys with UPJO usually exhibit good concentration of the isotope. Furthermore, even with severe obstruction in which only a cortical rim remains, uptake of the isotope will be seen peripherally in the cortex, again helping to differentiate this from multicystic kidney (King et al., 1984a).

Diuretic renography is effective in predicting recovery of function in cases in which intravenous urography has revealed nonvisualization. Diuretic renography allows quantification of the degree of obstruction and can help differentiate the level of obstruction. Today, ^{99m}Tc-mercaptoacetyltriglycine (^{99m}Tc-MAG3, or MAG3) is the preferred isotope over ^{99m}Tc-DTPA or radioiodinated Hippuran because of favorable imaging and dosimetry considerations (Roarke and Sandler, 1998). **Diuretic renography remains a reliable study for diagnosing UPJ and ureteral obstruction because it provides quantitative data regarding differential renal function and obstruction, even in hydronephrotic renal units.** Diuretic renography is noninvasive and readily available in most medical centers. Ideally, diuretic renography can be used to follow patients for functional loss, most effectively when a standard protocol is used. The diuretic is given 20 minutes into the study to allow time for filling of the collecting system. One study found diuretic renography to be useful in children to rule out concomitant UPJO with associated high-grade reflux (Stauss et al., 2003). There is evidence that diuretic renography using MAG3 is a most accurate study for patients with UPJO after therapeutic intervention (Niemczyk et al., 1999; Fig. 89.6).

The diagnosis of UPJO can generally be made with a high degree of certainty on the basis of the clinical presentation and the results of any one or more of the imaging studies already cited. It is preferable to have a combination of anatomic and functional studies, such as retrograde pyelogram and diuretic renography, to best plan therapy. Retrograde pyelography thus retains a role for confirmation of the diagnosis and for demonstration of the exact site and nature of obstruction before repair. In most cases, this study is performed at the time of the planned operative intervention to avoid the risk of introducing infection in the face of obstruction. However, retrograde pyelography is used emergently whenever the UPJO requires acute decompression, such as in the setting of infection or compromised renal function. **If cystoscopic retrograde manipulation has been unsuccessful or may be hazardous, particularly in neonates or infants, placement of a percutaneous nephrostomy is an alternative. This also facilitates antegrade studies that will help define the nature and exact anatomic site of obstruction.** It also allows decompression of the system in patients with associated infection or compromised renal function and allows assessment of recoverability of renal function after decompression. **When there remains some doubt as to the clinical significance of a dilated collecting system, placement of a percutaneous nephrostomy tube also facilitates dynamic pressure perfusion studies.** First described by Whitaker in 1973, the renal pelvis is continuously perfused at 10 mL/min with normal saline solution or dilute radiographic contrast solution under fluoroscopic control through a nephrostomy tube. Renal pelvic pressure is monitored during the infusion, and the pressure gradient across the UPJ is determined. The bladder is continuously drained with an indwelling catheter to prevent transmission of intravesical

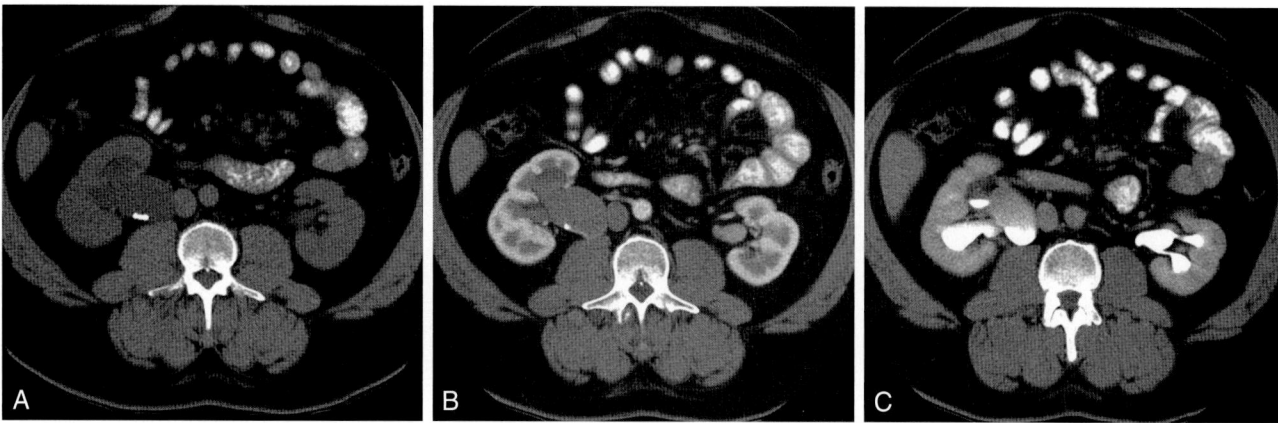

Fig. 89.4. (A) Contrast-enhanced computed tomography scan identifies a classic ureteropelvic junction (UPJ) appearance in early phase imaging. (B) Early images reveal normal nephrogram and delayed filling of the obstructed, dilated UPJ. (C) Delayed images demonstrate holdup of contrast drainage on the right compared with the normal left side.

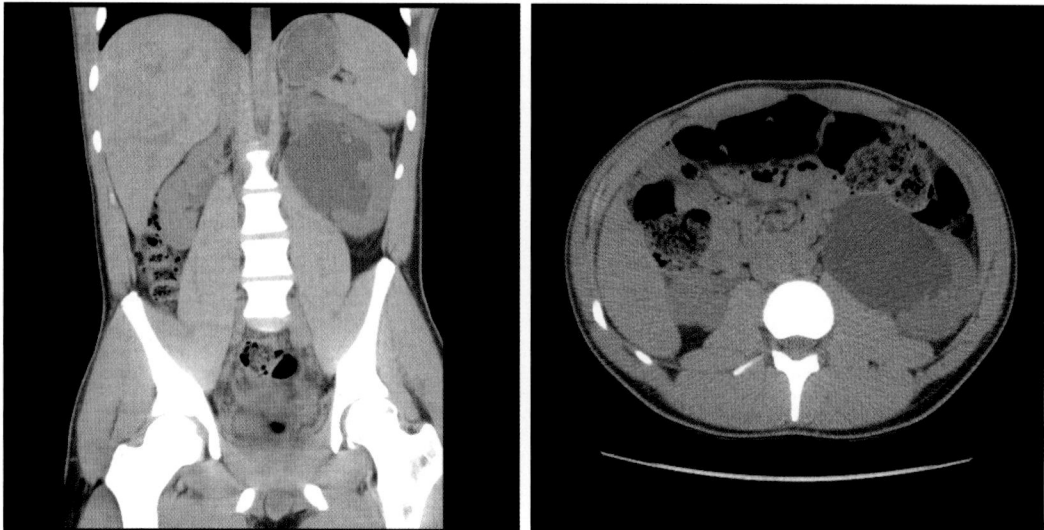

Fig. 89.5. Noncontrast computed tomography of left ureteropelvic junction obstruction, typical coronal and axial image.

pressures. Renal pelvic pressure ranging up to 12 to 15 cm H_2O during this infusion suggests a nonobstructed system. In contrast, pressures in excess of 15 to 20 cm H_2O are suggestive of a functional obstruction. Although equivocal studies were a concern, a recent study identified equivocal pressures in less than 5% of cases (Lupton and George, 2010; O'Reilly, 1986).

Although pressure perfusion studies can often provide valuable information regarding the functional significance of an apparent obstruction, these studies can at times be inaccurate. This inaccuracy may be a result of variations in renal pelvic anatomy and compliance (Koff et al., 1986) or positional variations (Ellis et al., 1995). Moreover, the procedure is invasive and should be reserved for cases that are nondiagnostic using less invasive methods (Lupton BJUI 2014). The urologist must collate the clinical presentation and results of all diagnostic studies performed to identify the best clinical intervention.

Indications and Options for Intervention

Contemporary indications for intervention for UPJO include the presence of symptoms associated with the obstruction, impairment of overall renal function or progressive impairment of ipsilateral function, development of stones or infection, or, rarely, causal hypertension. The primary goals of intervention are relief of symptoms and preservation of renal function. Traditionally, such intervention should be a reconstructive procedure aimed at restoring nonobstructed urinary flow. This is especially true for neonates, infants, or children in whom early repair is desirable because these patients will have the best chance for improvement in renal function after relief of obstruction (Bejjani and Belman, 1982; Roth and Gonzales, 1983; Wolpert et al., 1989). However, timing of the repair in neonates remains controversial (DiSandro and Kogan, 1998; Hanna, 2000; Koff, 1998, 2000; Shokeir and Nijman, 2000), mostly because of difficulty in defining those kidneys truly at risk for functional obstruction. In a prospective study of 104 neonates with primary unilateral hydronephrosis suspected of being caused by UPJO, after a mean follow-up of 21 months, only 7 (7%) required pyeloplasty for functional obstruction, defined as a progression of hydronephrosis or a 10% reduction in differential glomerular filtration rate on serial ultrasonography and diuretic renography (Koff and Campbell, 1994). All treated patients had a return of renal function to predetermination levels, supporting selective nonoperative management of neonatal hydronephrosis.

UPJO may not become apparent until middle age or later (Jacobs et al., 1979). Occasionally, if the patient is asymptomatic and the physiologic significance of the obstruction seems indeterminate, careful observation with serial follow-up renal scans

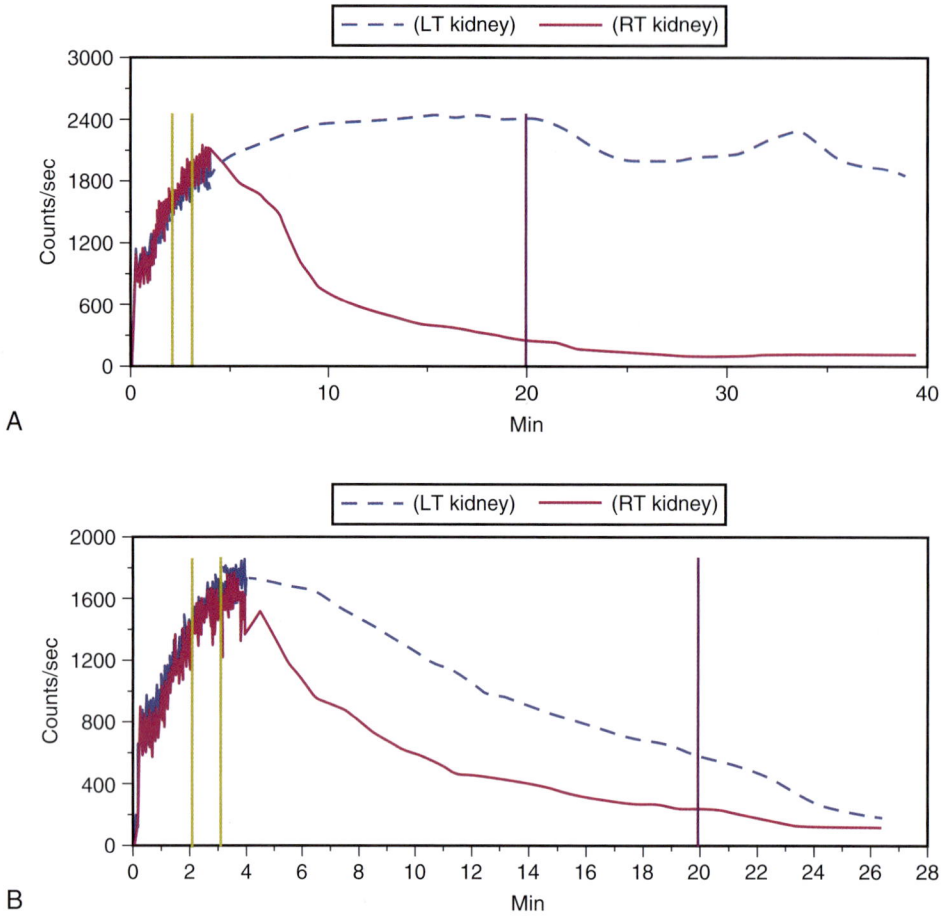

Fig. 89.6. (A) ^{99m}Tc-mercaptoacetyltriglycine (MAG3) diuretic renography revealing functional ureteropelvic junction obstruction of the left kidney, with a T$_{½}$ greater than 40 minutes. Furosemide was administered 20 minutes into the study *(vertical purple line)*. (B) Follow-up study reveals normal renal drainage after robotic pyeloplasty with spontaneous drainage before furosemide administration.

is appropriate. Gurbuz et al. (2011) observed minimally symptomatic UPJO and found 29% required surgery over a 4-year period. Gulur et al. (2009) noted that 3 of 14 patients with UPJO lost less than 10% renal function over a mean of 44 months of observation. However, the majority of affected patients ultimately benefit from reconstructive intervention (Clark and Malek, 1987; Jacobs et al., 1979; O'Reilly, 1989). **When intervention is indicated, the procedure of choice has historically been open dismembered pyeloplasty; however, less invasive endourologic incisional procedures have emerged as an alternative, particularly in secondary UPJO** (Brannen et al., 1988; Cohen et al., 1996; Conlin, 2002; Gerber and Kim, 2000; Kletscher et al., 1995; Lechevallier et al., 1999; Motola et al., 1993a; Nadler et al., 1996; Nakada, 2000; Tawfiek et al., 1998; Thomas et al., 1996). **More recently, laparoscopic and robotic pyeloplasty has gained acceptance as primary therapy in most major centers** (DiMarco et al., 2006; Jacobs et al., 2013; Rassweiler et al., 2007).

Although success rates with most endourologic techniques have not proven comparable with those of pyeloplasty, it has been suggested that the success rates may be improved with careful patient selection. In an important prospective study, Van Cangh et al. (1994) achieved an overall success rate for endopyelotomy of 73%. However, these investigators found the presence of crossing vessels to be a major determinant of outcome (42% success rate in the setting of a crossing vessel vs. 86% success without a crossing vessel). Furthermore, when endopyelotomy was applied to patients with "a high degree of obstruction," the success rate was only 60% compared with an 81% success rate for those patients with "low-grade" obstruction. When patients with a crossing vessel and a high degree of obstruction were excluded from analysis, the success rate improved to 95%, which is comparable with that of open pyeloplasty. However, other studies have suggested a less important role for these factors with regard to their impact on a successful outcome (Danuser et al., 1998; Gupta et al., 1997; Nakada et al., 1998). Also, the incisional approach may be favored in patients who are poor surgical candidates or in patients poorly suited to an abdominal approach (ElAbd et al., 2009). In most primary UPJO, minimally invasive pyeloplasty has become a common procedure in adults and in many centers for children as well (Jacobs et al., 2013). A more recent study showed a 10-fold increase in the rate of minimally invasive pyeloplasties, whereas open pyeloplasties decreased 40% and endopyelotomies remained stable over a 9-year period (Jacobs et al., 2017a). A recent comparative effectiveness study showed a higher treatment failure rate for endopyelotomy compared with open or minimally invasive pyeloplasty, which were equivalent (Jacobs et al., 2018).

Although the indications for intervention for UPJO are similar regardless of technique, it is critical to discuss the risks and benefits of each available option with patients. As a result of studies linking crossing vessels to hindered endourologic successes, there is increased interest in intraoperative management of primary UPJO by either an open, laparoscopic, or robotic approach (Conlin, 2002). **Notably, for secondary UPJO, it remains reasonable to recommend an open or laparoscopic approach to any patient in whom primary endourologic management has failed and an endourologic approach to those in whom open or laparoscopic repair has failed.** The results of endourologic management after failed pyeloplasty remain excellent (Canes et al., 2008; Jabbour et al., 1998; Patel et al., 2011).

Rarely, nephrectomy may be the procedure of choice. Indications for nephrectomy as primary therapy include diminished function or nonfunction of the involved renal moiety and a normal contralateral kidney on the basis of radiographic and nuclear studies. These patients may be symptomatic with urinary tract infections or pain. In such cases, ultrasonography or CT scanning is typically performed and will reveal only a thin shell of parenchyma remaining. **Renography can provide quantitative measures of renal function, and, in general, kidneys with less than 15% to 20% differential function are considered nonsalvageable in adults.** If the potential for salvageability of function is still unclear, an internal stent or percutaneous nephrostomy may be placed for temporary relief of obstruction and renal function studies subsequently repeated. Nephrectomy may also be considered for patients in whom the obstruction has led to extensive stone disease with chronic infection and significant loss of function in the face of a normal contralateral kidney. Removal of the kidney may also be chosen over reconstruction for patients in whom repeated attempts at repair have already failed and in whom further intervention would therefore be extremely complicated. This option should be considered only when the contralateral kidney is essentially normal.

Options for Intervention

Endourologic Management. Endourologic management of UPJO was introduced by Ramsay et al. in 1984 as a "percutaneous pyelolysis" and then popularized in the United States by Badlani et al. (1986), who coined the term *endopyelotomy*. **Although various nuances in the technique have been described** (Korth et al., 1988; Ono et al., 1992; Van Cangh et al., 1989), **the basic concept of the endopyelotomy is a full-thickness lateral incision through the obstructing proximal ureter, from the ureteral lumen out to the peripelvic and periureteral fat.** A stent is placed across the incision and is left to heal, in keeping with the original work of Davis in 1943, who performed an "intubated ureterotomy" to repair UPJO. Subsequently, alternative techniques using a retrograde approach to the UPJ were developed. The retrograde approach most used today is the ureteroscopic approach, typically using the holmium laser to incise the UPJ under direct visual control. Alternatively, a cautery wire balloon endopyelotomy, which incises the UPJ under fluoroscopic control, or percutaneous endopyeloplasty may be used (ElAbd et al., 2009; Gill et al., 2002). Recently, Vaarala et al. (2008) reported a small series of 64 patients who underwent either antegrade or retrograde cold knife or cautery wire balloon endopyelotomy. In this study, success rates ranged from 79% to 83%, without statistically significant differences among the three treatments. Transplantation complications are particularly suited to endoscopic management, either antegrade or retrograde (Gdor et al., 2008b; Schumacher et al., 2006). **As far as efficacy is concerned, there continues to be little evidence for significant differences among endopyelotomy techniques. The differences lie in technical considerations and complications.**

Operative intervention for UPJO has historically provided a widely patent, dependently positioned, well-funneled UPJ. In addition, the option to reduce the size of the renal pelvis is readily available with this approach. Although formal pyeloplasty has stood the test of time with a published success rate of nearly 95%, endourologic alternatives to standard operative reconstruction are still used (Clark et al., 1987; ElAbd et al., 2009). **The advantages of endourologic approaches include reduced hospital stays and postoperative recovery. However, the success rate does not approach that of open, laparoscopic, or robotic pyeloplasty. Furthermore, whereas open, laparoscopic, or robotic pyeloplasty can be applied to almost any anatomic variation of UPJO, consideration of any of the less invasive alternatives requires that the surgeon take into account the degree of hydronephrosis, ipsilateral renal function, concomitant calculi, and possibly the presence of crossing vessels.**

Percutaneous Antegrade Endopyelotomy

Indications and Contraindications. The indications to intervene for any patient with UPJO include the presence of symptoms, progressive or overall impairment of renal function, development of upper tract stones or infection, or, rarely, causal hypertension. Historically, a percutaneous approach for definitive management of UPJO was offered only to those patients undergoing percutaneous removal of associated stones or to those in whom open pyeloplasty had previously failed. However, encouraging results ultimately led many centers to offer percutaneous endopyelotomy as primary therapy for almost any patient with UPJO. **Even with the acceptance of laparoscopic and robotic pyeloplasty, percutaneous endopyelotomy remains appropriate for patients with UPJO and concomitant pyelocalyceal stones requiring percutaneous access, which can then be managed simultaneously. Contraindications to a percutaneous endopyelotomy are similar to the contraindications to any endourologic approach and include a long segment (>2 cm) of obstruction, active infection, and untreated coagulopathy.** Often these cases can also be managed robotically (Pedro and Buchholz, 2018). Whereas the impact of crossing vessels is controversial, the mere presence of crossing vessels is not a contraindication to an endopyelotomy (Lam et al., 2003b; Motola et al., 1993b; Nakada et al., 1998). However, significant entanglement of the UPJ by crossing vessels can occasionally be identified, and this may render any endourologic approach unsuccessful. Vessel entanglement can be reliably identified with 3D helical CT (Kumon et al., 1997; Fig. 89.7).

Patient Preparation. Patients undergoing a percutaneous endopyelotomy undergo preoperative evaluation and preparation as if they were undergoing any percutaneous, laparoscopic, or open renal intervention. The evaluation includes an assessment for any comorbidity that may increase the risk of anesthesia. Sterile urine should be ensured at the time of definitive intervention. If upper tract infection cannot be cleared because of obstruction, temporization should be accomplished through use of internal stenting or percutaneous nephrostomy drainage alone. **The patient should be counseled as to the risks and benefits of the procedure, and in particular the fact that the success rate of any endourologic approach, including percutaneous endopyelotomy, may be less than that of formal reconstruction.** Patients should also be counseled of the risk of bleeding requiring transfusion, urinary leak, drainage-related complications, and hydropneumothorax, particularly if upper pole access is used.

Technique. **An endopyelotomy cannot be performed safely by any route until access across the UPJ is established.** This can be accomplished in a retrograde fashion cystoscopically or in an antegrade manner percutaneously. For retrograde access, the UPJ can almost always be traversed using a hydrophilic wire passed through an open-end catheter. Once the hydrophilic wire is successfully positioned

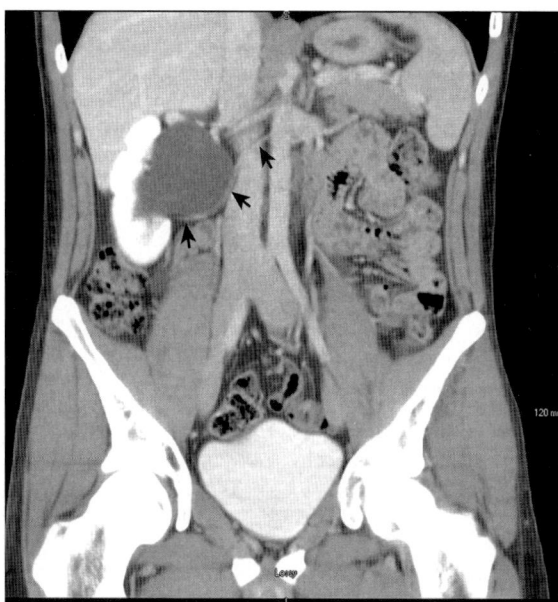

Fig. 89.7. Contrast-enhanced computed tomography scan reveals apparent right ureteropelvic junction obstruction in this patient with right flank pain. A crossing lower pole artery is visible on this coronal section.

in the pyelocalyceal system, the open-end catheter is advanced over it into the renal pelvis. The wire can then be withdrawn so that contrast material can be injected through the open-end catheter to guide subsequent percutaneous access.

With the patient in the prone position, the site for percutaneous access is chosen to allow straightforward access to the UPJ. In general, a midposterior or superolateral calyx is chosen. Typically, the UPJ can be intubated in an antegrade fashion when the tract is initially established with fluoroscopic control. Alternatively, once the tract has been dilated and nephroscopy has been performed, a wire can again be passed in a retrograde fashion through the open-end catheter and grasped from above so that through-and-through access is reestablished. In either case, as soon as access is obtained with one wire, an introducing catheter is used to pass a second wire as a safety wire, so a working and a safety wire are now both in place. At this point, percutaneous access is complete and the endopyelotomy may be performed.

In the original descriptions of the technique from the Institute of Urology in London (Ramsay et al., 1984) and from Long Island Jewish Hospital in New York (Badlani et al., 1986), the endopyelotomy was performed using a cold knife technique under direct vision. With one or two wires in place across the UPJ, a direct vision "endopyelotome" is used. This hook-shaped cold knife may be used to completely incise the UPJ in a full-thickness manner, from the ureteral lumen to periureteral and peripelvic fat. **Rigorous anatomic studies have shown the incision should usually be made laterally because this is the location devoid of crossing vessels** (Sampaio, 1998; Sampaio and Favorito, 1993). However, in cases of high insertion, the incision should instead "marsupialize" the proximal ureter into the renal pelvis, such that an anterior or posterior incision may be required. When such incisions are done under direct vision, any crossing vessel can be directly visualized and avoided. In addition to the endopyelotome, the holmium laser at tissue settings may be used to perform an antegrade endopyelotomy.

Once the incision is complete, stenting is accomplished. There remains no consensus as to the optimal stent size or duration for endopyelotomy. A No. 14/7-Fr endopyelotomy stent may be used, passed in an antegrade fashion with the larger-diameter end of the stent positioned across the UPJ. In some cases, especially when the patient has not been prestented, passage of this large-caliber stent may be difficult. In those instances, a No. 10/7-Fr endopyelotomy stent or even a standard No. 8-Fr internal stent may be used without compromising the ultimate outcome. Once proper positioning of the stent has been determined fluoroscopically, any remaining safety wires are withdrawn. One group showed no difference between larger and standard stents in a porcine study of endopyelotomies (Moon et al., 1995). Alternatively, Danuser et al. (2001) demonstrated improved success rates using a modified 27-Fr stent after percutaneous endopyelotomy at nearly 2 years of follow-up.

In the setting of a high insertion, the incision can often be extended to the dependent portion of the renal pelvis under direct vision, bridging the gap between the lateral wall of the ureter and the medial wall of the pelvis, across the periureteral and peripelvic fat (Fig. 89.8).Once the incision is complete, the stent is already in place and nephrostomy drainage is instituted for 24 to 48 hours.

Postoperative Care. Avoidance of strenuous activity for 8 to 10 days after the procedure is recommended. The ideal stent size, duration of stent placement, and radiographic follow-up after endopyelotomy remain unclear (Canes et al., 2008). One study did report a benefit to larger stents in patients undergoing antegrade endopyelotomy (71% vs. 93%); however, a large-bore (27-Fr) catheter was used for the initial 3 weeks postoperatively (Danuser et al., 2001). On the other hand, Kletscher et al. (1995) reported no benefit to larger stents, as did Hwang et al. (1996). Wolf et al. (1997) reported improved success using larger stents (12 Fr) in endoureterotomy patients in a retrospective review. Regarding stent duration, less is known. The original report and recommendation of 6 weeks by Davis (1943) is still often used, although Mandhani et al. (2003) identified no difference in results when comparing 57 patients stented for 2 weeks versus 4 weeks. Although the need for prophylactic antibiotics while the stent is indwelling is not literature based, many use a daily suppressive dose.

Once the stent is removed, the patient returns 1 month later for clinical follow-up and radiographic evaluation. In general, this includes a history, physical examination, urinalysis, and diuretic renography. If the patient remains asymptomatic and the diuretic renography reveals normal drainage (normal $T_{1/2}$), reevaluation is performed at 6 months and then at 12-month intervals. Most literature indicates that the majority of endopyelotomy failures occur within the first year of the procedure; however, longer-term studies demonstrate failures well beyond that timeframe (Albani et al., 2004; DiMarco et al., 2006; Doo et al., 2007; Nadler et al., 1996). For most adults, 2- to 3-year follow-up is justified because studies indicate that even at 36 months some late failures are identified, but relatively few are identified at 60 months (Doo et al., 2007).

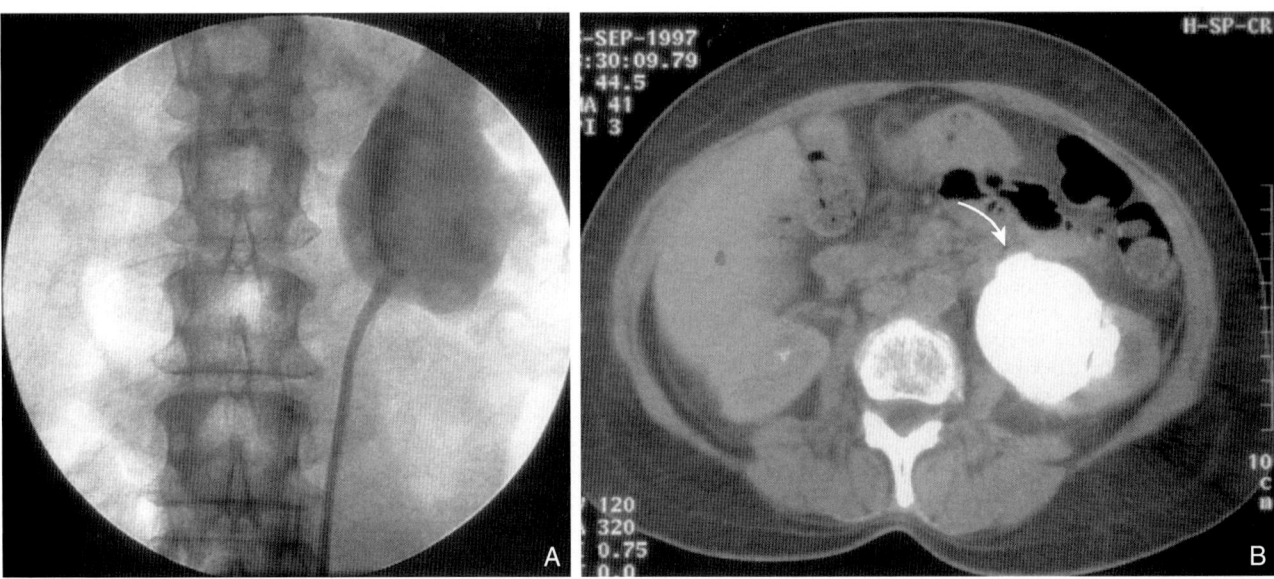

Fig. 89.8. (A) Retrograde study in this patient with left ureteropelvic junction obstruction reveals a "high insertion" of the left ureter. (B) Computed tomography scan in the same patient reveals the ureter inserting on the anatomically anterior aspect of the renal pelvis. A marsupializing incision must be made in a true posterior direction from the ureter into the renal pelvis.

Results. The immediate and long-term results of percutaneous endopyelotomy are well established. Although percutaneous endopyelotomy compares favorably with open operative pyeloplasty in terms of postoperative pain, length of hospital stay, and return to prehospitalization activities (Brooks et al., 1995; Karlin et al., 1988), retrograde endopyelotomy and laparoscopic and robotic pyeloplasty also offer favorable convalescence.

Gerber and Lyon in 1994 reviewed the outcome of percutaneous endopyelotomy in 672 patients reported from 12 centers and found a success rate ranging from 57% to 100% (mean, 73.5%) at follow-up ranging from 2 to 96 months. Currently, success rates approaching 85% to 90% are being reported at experienced centers, with little difference in outcome noted in those patients undergoing the procedure for primary versus secondary UPJO (Kletscher et al., 1995; Motola et al., 1993a; Shalhav et al., 1998). Knudsen et al. (2004) reported long-term results in 80 patients after use of the cold knife and holmium laser for antegrade endopyelotomy, with 55-month follow-up. This series had a success rate of 67%, slightly lower than otherwise reported. DiMarco et al. (2006) reported on 182 antegrade endopyelotomies with a recurrence-free survival over 10 years at a single center as low as 41%. Schumacher et al. (2006) reported on three successful antegrade endopyelotomies in transplanted kidneys in 2006.

When percutaneous endopyelotomy does fail, several options exist, including a retrograde endopyelotomy; repeat percutaneous endopyelotomy; and laparoscopic, robotic, or open operative intervention. There remains a role for CT angiography in failed endopyelotomy, to rule out a crossing vessel. If a significant vessel is found, repeat endopyelotomy is usually not recommended (Nakada, 2000; Nakada et al., 1998; Sampaio, 1998). **Alternatively, operative intervention is typically offered to any patient in whom an endourologic approach has failed.** Studies suggest that the results of laparoscopic pyeloplasty will not be compromised, although Sundaram et al. (2003) reported longer operative times in these circumstances (Conlin, 2002; Gupta et al., 1997; Motola et al., 1993b). Albani et al. (2004) reported contemporary long-term results with various endopyelotomy approaches to have a success rate of 67%, with the majority of failures in the first 32 months. DiMarco et al. (2006) reported long-term follow-up of more than 400 patients undergoing either percutaneous antegrade endopyelotomy or pyeloplasty. The 3-, 5-, and 10-year success rates were superior for pyeloplasty, 85% versus 63%, 80% versus 55%, and 75% versus 41%. Moreover, Rassweiler et al. (2007) compared retrograde laser endopyelotomy with laparoscopic retroperitoneal pyeloplasty in 256 patients in a 10-year single-surgeon experience and found success rates were 73% for laser endopyelotomy compared with 94% for pyeloplasty. One recent literature review for laser endopyelotomy found success rates ranging from 44% to 89% with follow-up ranging from 10 to 63 months (Elmussareh et al., 2017). Kim et al. (2012) reported a 65% success rate in 37 pediatric patients after primary endopyelotomy at 34 months, but a 94% success rate in children at 61 months using secondary endopyelotomy.

Complications. The complications associated with percutaneous endopyelotomy are analogous to those associated with percutaneous nephrolithotomy (Badlani et al., 1988; Bellman, 1996; Cassis et al., 1991; Malden et al., 1992; Weiss et al., 1988), **and hemorrhage is a risk of any percutaneous upper tract procedure, including endopyelotomy.** However, because in patients with UPJO the renal parenchyma is often atrophied and usually thinner than that of a normal kidney, the risk of bleeding may be higher than that of stone patients undergoing percutaneous manipulation. Acute management in this setting is usually conservative to start: bed rest, hydration, and transfusion if necessary. The nephrostomy tube should not be irrigated acutely. Rather, it is preferable to allow the pyelocalyceal system to tamponade the bleeding. When continued bleeding does not respond to these conservative measures, the next step is selective angiographic embolization. **In general, the urologist should have a low threshold to proceeding to angiography, to minimize the need for transfusion and potential exploration. Successful angiographic embolization usually obviates the need for operative intervention.**

Infection is a risk of any urinary tract manipulation including percutaneous endopyelotomy, and all attempts should be made to sterilize the urinary tract before the procedure. Whereas the role of prophylactic antibiotics at the outset of the procedure in the setting of a sterile urine is unproven, most urologists give a second-generation cephalosporin "on call" to the procedure. Consideration should be given to the use of prophylactic antibiotics while the endopyelotomy stent is indwelling for the month after the procedure, especially in women who are more prone to bacteriuria.

Persistent obstruction is rare in the early postoperative period because of the internal stent. Occasionally the stent can be obstructed from blood clots, and continued nephrostomy drainage for a few days typically allows the problem to resolve spontaneously.

Special Considerations. Percutaneous endopyelotomy and **nephrolithotomy remain appropriate when the UPJO is associated with upper tract stone disease because the stones can be managed concomitantly.** In such cases, percutaneous access is established with a wire across the UPJ. The stone should be removed before the endopyelotomy so that stone fragments do not migrate into the peripyeloureteral tissue, as can happen if the endopyelotomy is performed first. Otherwise, localized obstruction may result from fibrosis or granuloma formation (Giddens et al., 2000; Streem, 2000). The urologist must ensure that the UPJO is not a result of edema from the concomitant stone disease, in particular with stone disease in the renal pelvis. In this circumstance, initial management of the stone percutaneously and subsequent radiographic assessment of the UPJ once the stone has been removed are most prudent. In addition, if a nephrostomy tube is retained, a Whitaker test is straightforward and definitive to assess for persistent obstruction. Conversely, UPJO and solitary lower pole calculi do not represent a dilemma regarding UPJ edema, and combined percutaneous management remains most efficient. Alternatively, laparoscopic or robotic pyeloplasty with concomitant stone removal is also effective for these patients. Often the deciding factor between percutaneous and laparoscopic approaches relates to the stone burden present and the experience of the surgeon (Sutherland and Jarrett, 2009). Percutaneous endopyeloplasty is an uncommon hybrid technique described as an endoscopic Heineke-Mikulicz repair performed through a percutaneous tract. Stein et al. (2007) reported 55 patients with short-term follow-up with more than 90% success. Endopyeloplasty may not be effective for secondary UPJO because tissue scarring may inhibit the endoscopic reconstruction. More recently a technique modification was reported requiring no specialized equipment (laparoscopic needle holders and a nephroscope) in 10 patients (Lezrek et al., 2012).

Retrograde Ureteroscopic Endopyelotomy. A ureteroscopic approach to endopyelotomy was first reported in 1985 when Bagley et al. reported a combined percutaneous and flexible ureteroscopic procedure approach for management of an "obliterated" UPJ. Subsequently, Inglis and Tolley (1986) reported a ureteroscopic "pyelolysis" for UPJO. Shortly thereafter, Clayman et al. (1990) reported an initial experience in a small number of patients with ureteroscopic endopyelotomy with a 3-Fr or 5-Fr cutting electrode passed under direct vision using large, rigid or flexible ureteroscopes. In that series, however, an 8-Fr nephrostomy tube was placed at the outset of the procedure and left indwelling for at least 48 hours. Therefore that series still represented a "combined" endourologic approach to endopyelotomy. Stents were routinely left in place for 6 to 8 weeks, after which diagnostic studies were performed. With a mean follow-up approaching 1 year, a success rate of 81% was achieved in 16 patients. However, two patients developed distal ureteral strictures, probably resulting from the larger-diameter rigid instrumentation. Cold-knife ureteroscopic endopyelotomies are still reported. Butani and Eshghi (2008) identified 96% success rates in primary procedures with an average 5-year follow-up, although rigid ureteroscopy and preprocedure stents were necessary.

Advances in instrumentation and technique now allow a ureteroscopic approach to be performed reliably at a single setting (Conlin and Bagley, 1998), and this is now considered the standard. **The main advantage of a ureteroscopic approach is that it allows direct visualization of the UPJ and assurance of a properly situated,** full-thickness endopyelotomy incision without the need for percutaneous access. Another advantage of the ureteroscopic approach is a decrease in cost compared with the use of the cautery wire balloon, assuming ureteroscopic equipment and electroincision or holmium laser are already available. Moreover, the risks and morbidity of percutaneous access are avoided with the ureteroscopic procedure. Gettman et al. (2003) found that the retrograde ureteroscopic endopyelotomy was more cost effective than hot-wire cutting balloon endopyelotomy, antegrade endopyelotomy, and pyeloplasty for treating UPJO when taking into account treatment failures. Another study showed endopyeltomies to be less expensive than minimally invase or open pyeloplasty. Open and minimally invasive pyeloplasty approaches were cost neutral, making minimally invasive pyeloplasty the best option when available (Jacobs et al., 2017b).

Indications and Contraindications. The indications for a ureteroscopic endopyelotomy include functionally significant obstruction, as defined earlier. Contraindications include long areas of obstruction and upper tract stones, which are best managed simultaneously with alternative approaches, usually percutaneously or laparoscopically. Another consideration is that in patients with significant hydronephrosis, the evidence indicates an antegrade endopyelotomy may be more efficacious (Lam et al., 2003b).

Technique. In women, the UPJ can be reached with a 6.9-Fr semirigid ureteroscope, although typically a flexible ureteroscope is used. In men, flexible ureteroscopes are used with ureteral access sheaths and flexible ureteroscopes for most retrograde endopyelotomies.

General anesthesia is used to minimize patient movement during ureteroscopy and the subsequent incision of the UPJ. In preparation for the endopyelotomy, a retrograde pyelogram is performed under fluoroscopic control at the outset of the procedure. A hydrophilic guidewire is passed cystoscopically under fluoroscopic control and coiled in the pyelocalyceal system. The cystoscope is then withdrawn and an access sheath is placed. A flexible ureteroscope is passed alongside the guidewire to the level of the UPJ. If the distal ureter is too narrow to allow easy passage of the ureteroscope, the intramural ureter can be dilated using a 5-mm balloon or a 9- or 10-Fr "introducing" catheter. If the ureter is still too narrow at any point to easily accommodate the ureteroscope, then an internal stent is placed and the procedure postponed for 5 to 10 days to allow passive ureteral dilation. Alternatively, an actively deflecting flexible ureteroscope may be used, and in most cases a ureteral access sheath is useful. The sheath allows for rapid transfer of the ureteroscope for assessment of the UPJ. Once the flexible ureteroscope is passed to the UPJ, a 200-µm holmium fiber is placed through the working channel and the UPJ is incised in the appropriate location, as suggested by the radiographic studies (Figs. 89.9 and 89.10).

Once the UPJ is reached with the ureteroscope, the renal pelvis is drained to assist movement across the UPJ during the incision. When a semirigid ureteroscope is used, the 200- or 365-µm holmium laser fiber is inserted through the working channel as the ureteroscope is positioned at the proximal extent of the UPJ or in the renal pelvis. At a setting of 0.8 to 1.2 J and a frequency of 10 to 15 Hz, the UPJ is incised, usually in a lateral direction, while the ureteroscope is withdrawn back down across the UPJ. This procedure is repeated, and the incision gradually deepened to extend into the peripelvic and periureteral retroperitoneal space. Because this is done gradually and under direct vision, any visualized vessels, and thus potentially significant bleeding, is usually avoided.

The incision is carried caudally into normal ureteral tissue, until the UPJ is widely patent. Injection of contrast material through the ureteroscope can demonstrate extravasation and confirm an adequate depth of incision, although this is usually not necessary because the entire procedure has been performed under direct vision. Balloon dilation up to 24 Fr can also be performed to complete the incision. If any small bleeding points are visualized ureteroscopically, they can be treated by defocusing the holmium laser. Similarly, the balloon can be reinflated to allow tamponade for 10 minutes to see if the bleeding will subside. The ureteroscope is then withdrawn from the ureter while the safety wire is left in place in the renal pelvis for subsequent passage of a stent. Experimental studies have shown that 36-Fr balloon dilation alone can create linear incisions in the UPJ (Pearle et al., 1994). **Although retrograde balloon dilation alone has been reported for treatment of UPJO, long-term follow-up studies have shown a diminishing success rate over time, as low as 42%** (McClinton et al., 1993; Webber et al., 1997).

Once the ureteroscope has been removed, a stent is advanced over the remaining wire using fluoroscopic guidance. A Foley catheter is left indwelling, again to obviate the risk of reflux and extravasation at the site of the endopyelotomy incision and to rapidly identify any significant bleeding. Diuretic renography is performed 4 weeks after stent removal to assess results. Clinical and radiographic follow-up is then continued at 6- to 12-month intervals for 24 to 32 months.

Results. Biyani et al. (1997) described their initial experience with a ureteroscopic approach using holmium laser energy. With a mean follow-up of slightly more than 12 months, they achieved a success rate of 87.5% in a small group of patients. One patient developed a urinoma, which was managed conservatively. In 1998 Renner et al. reported a larger series of patients undergoing ureteroscopic laser endopyelotomy. With a semirigid ureteroscope, the UPJ was incised at a posterolateral location unless vessels were visualized in that area, in which case a contralateral incision was made. Tawfiek et al. (1998) reported the Jefferson Medical College experience with ureteroscopic endopyelotomy. These investigators combined endoluminal ultrasound with their ureteroscopic approach to definitively identify crossing vessels or a ureteropelvic septum, which is present in patients with high-inserting ureters. The authors believed this helped them definitively site their endopyelotomy incision. Different modalities were used for the endopyelotomy, including electrocautery and holmium laser. An 87.5% success rate was achieved in 32 patients. There were no significant bleeding complications, and all patients were discharged within 24 hours of the procedure.

Several investigators have reported success rates of 70% to 80% with follow-up out to 5 years using ureteroscopic holmium laser endopyelotomy (ElAbd et al., 2009; Gerber and Kim, 2000; Matin et al., 2003). Yanke et al. (2008) reported on 128 retrograde ureteroscopic endopyelotomies with a 60% success rate at 20 months; Rassweiler et al. (2007) reported 73% success in 113 patients at 63 months. Improved results (91% success rates) were reported by Conlin (2002) with retrograde endopyelotomy in patients when culling patients with crossing vessels greater than 4 mm using preoperative ultrasonography. Giddens et al. (2000) also published excellent results after culling patients with anterior and posterior crossing vessels from retrograde endopyelotomy using endoluminal ultrasound. However, endoluminal ultrasound is rarely used to identify crossing vessels because similar data can be obtained using less invasive studies (Mitterberger et al., 2008). **Regardless, the best retrograde endopyelotomy success rates still lag behind those of open or laparoscopic pyeloplasty.**

Complications. Complications of this approach have diminished in frequency and severity with the refinement of ureteroscopic instrumentation and the introduction of small-caliber holmium laser fibers. Postprocedural ureteral strictures are rare in contemporary series, and angiographic embolization and nephrectomy are rare when the retrograde approach is used. Most complications are minor and relate primarily to urinary leak, stent migration, and infection (Gerber and Kim, 2000; Tawfiek et al., 1998). Castle et al. (2009) reported on ureteroarterial fistula 2 weeks after retrograde laser endopyelotomy, which could be fulgurated ureteroscopically.

Other Retrograde Techniques. Use of fluoroscopically guided cautery wire balloon for management of UPJO was first reported in a clinical series by Chandhoke et al. in 1993. Ponsky and Streem (2006) reported on 64 patients undergoing either ureteroscopic endopyelotomy or fluoroscopically guided cautery balloon endopyelotomy and found equivalent success rates with both procedures yet higher major complication rates in the cautery wire balloon endopyelotomy, specifically transfusion and selective embolization. ElAbd et al. (2009) reported a higher rate of hemorrhage using this technique compared with direct vision laser incisional approach. **Improved ureteroscopic instrumentation, laser technology, and better outcomes make ureteroscopic endopyelotomy the current retrograde approach of choice.**

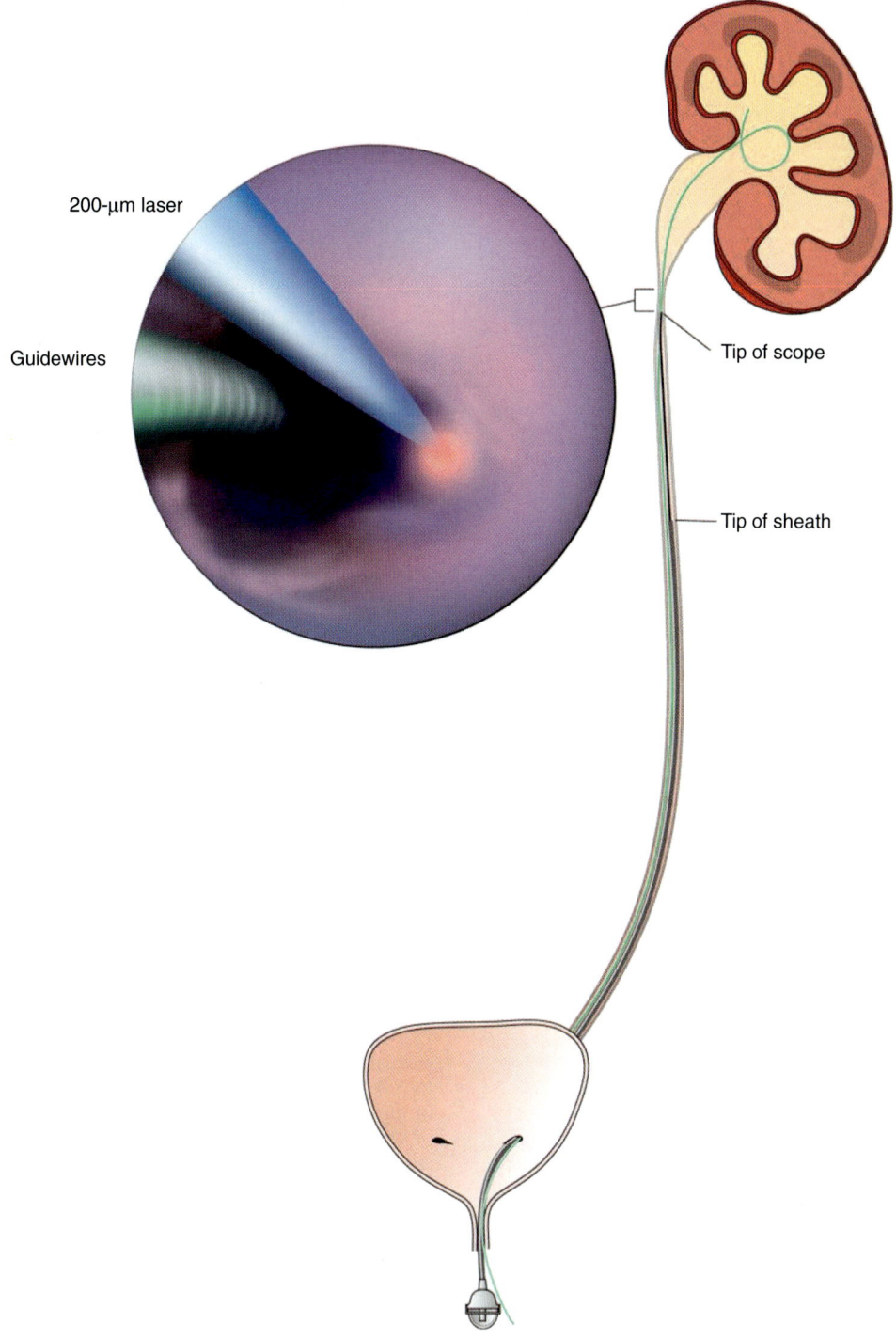

Fig. 89.9. Flexible ureteroscopic endopyelotomy using holmium laser, demonstrating endoscopic view of the ureteropelvic junction *(inset)*. A safety wire is in place, and the ureteroscope is passed through a ureteral access sheath as a lateral incision is being made under endoscopic view, using holmium laser fiber. A properly sited, complete incision is straightforward with this direct visualization technique.

Operative Interventions

Historical Notes. The historical aspects of UPJ repair were previously examined by Kay in 1989 and by Schaeffer and Grayhack in 1986. The first reconstructive procedure was performed by Trendelenburg in 1886; however, the patient died of postoperative complications. In 1891 Kuster divided the ureter and reanastomosed it to the renal pelvis, thus apparently performing the first successful dismembered pyeloplasty. Kuster's technique, however, was prone to recurrent stricture. In 1892 Fenzer applied the Heineke-Mikulicz principle to UPJ repair. This surgical technique involves transverse closure of a longitudinal incision. However, this technique can cause shortening of the suture line on one side, thus resulting in buckling or kinking of the UPJ with recurrent obstruction. In 1916 Schwyzer introduced the Y-V-pyeloplasty, which was subsequently modified by Foley in 1937. However, this technique was best applied to high ureteral insertions and was essentially unsuitable when the UPJ was already in a dependent position. Later on, flap techniques were developed that were more universally applicable including the spiral flap of Culp and DeWeerd (1951) and the vertical flap of Scardino and

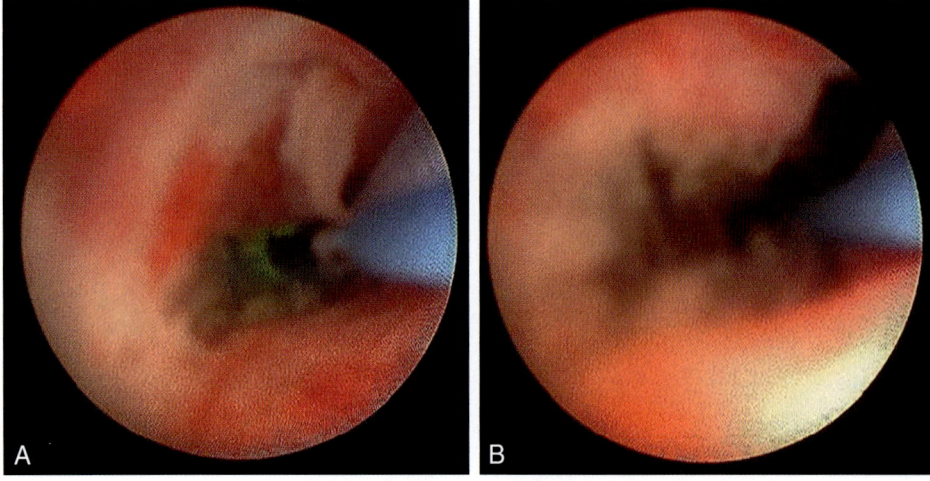

Fig. 89.10. (A) Endoscopic view of ureteropelvic junction (UPJ) stenosis with safety wire and laser fiber during incision. (B) After incision, note full-thickness incision and minimal bleeding with capacious UPJ.

> **KEY POINTS: ENDOUROLOGIC MANAGEMENT OF URETEROPELVIC JUNCTION OBSTRUCTION**
>
> - Contemporary indications for intervention for UPJO include the presence of symptoms associated with the obstruction, impairment of overall renal function or progressive impairment of ipsilateral function, development of stones or infection, or, rarely, causal hypertension.
> - The advantage of endoscopic management is the avoidance of the intra-abdominal approach; however, the success rates do not approach that of laparoscopic or robotic pyeloplasty.
> - Endourologic approaches to UPJO should be carried out under direct visualization.
> - In general, the urologist should have a low threshold to proceeding to angiography in patients with bleeding after endopyelotomy to minimize the need for transfusion and potential exploration. Successful angiographic embolization can obviate the need for operative exploration, which can lead to nephrectomy.

Prince (1953). Thompson et al. (1969) reported the use of a renal capsular flap for complex cases in which an adequate amount of renal pelvis is not available for repair.

In 1949 Nesbit followed the principle of Kuster's dismembered procedure and further modified it by creating an elliptical anastomosis to decrease the likelihood of stricture formation at the site of repair. Also in 1949, Anderson and Hynes described their modifications of this dismembered technique that involved anastomosis of the spatulated ureter to a projection of the lower aspect of the pelvis after a redundant portion was excised. Use of healing by secondary intention was also investigated in the similar time period. The techniques of intubated ureterotomy were popularized by Davis in 1943, but they had been previously described by Fiori in 1905, Albarran in 1909, and Keyes in 1915.

Developments in minimally invasive surgery have led to a dramatic rise in the use of laparoscopic and robotic techniques in the reconstruction of the UPJ (Jacobs et al., 2013). Despite the increased used of minimally invasive techniques, open approaches remain common in many centers, even in adults, with open surgery representing 41% of pyeloplasties performed between 2002 and 2010 in a review of MarketScan surgeries by Jacobs et al. (2017a). Irrespective of surgical approach, several basic principles must always be applied to maximize the success of surgical repair. For any procedure, the resultant anastomosis should be widely patent and completed in a watertight fashion without tension. In addition, the reconstructed UPJ should allow a funnel-shaped transition between the pelvis and the ureter that is in a position of dependent drainage. Because the goal of minimally invasive surgery is to mimic open surgery, the operative principles will be reviewed together with specific technical nuances for each approach.

Before the definitive surgical management, drainage of a kidney with UPJ obstruction is recommended only in select circumstances, including infection associated with the obstruction or azotemia resulting from obstruction in a solitary kidney or bilateral disease. Procedural drainage may be of value in the uncommon scenario of severe, unrelenting pain requiring emergent relief of obstruction. For any of these situations, such drainage can be achieved by placement of an internal ureteral stent or a percutaneous nephrostomy tube. Although most patients do not require preoperative drainage, most urologists place an indwelling ureteral stent at the time of pyeloplasty in adults. Our preference is for routine placement of a soft, inert, self-retaining internal ureteral stent, which is removed 4 to 6 weeks postoperatively. Stents in adults can be easily removed in an outpatient office setting under local anesthesia. Routine use of internal ureteral stents offers several advantages, especially in the early postoperative period. Such practice appears to decrease the amount and length of time of urinary extravasation at the surgical repair site, thereby decreasing the risk of secondary fibrosis. Decreased urinary extravasation also allows earlier removal of external drains. For the uncomplicated pyeloplasty in adult patients, there appears to be no advantage to using a nephrostomy tube and a stent because this may result in a prolonged hospital stay and an increased incidence of infection (Wollin et al., 1989). Instead, nephrostomy tubes may be reserved for complicated procedures such as those required for secondary UPJ obstruction or those associated with active inflammation. However, if a percutaneous nephrostomy tube had been placed preoperatively, it is generally left in place to allow proximal diversion and access for antegrade radiographic studies during the postoperative period.

At the completion of the pyeloplasty procedure, surgeons typically provide external drainage of the surgical bed. Such external drainage may be achieved with a closed suction drain placed near, but not on, the suture line and brought out through a separate stab incision. This practice helps to minimize the risk of urinoma formation leading to possible disruption of the suture line, scarring, or sepsis.

Dismembered Pyeloplasty

Indications. At present, a dismembered pyeloplasty is preferred by most urologists in the surgical repair of UPJ obstruction because this procedure is almost universally applicable to the different clinical scenarios. This approach can be used regardless of whether

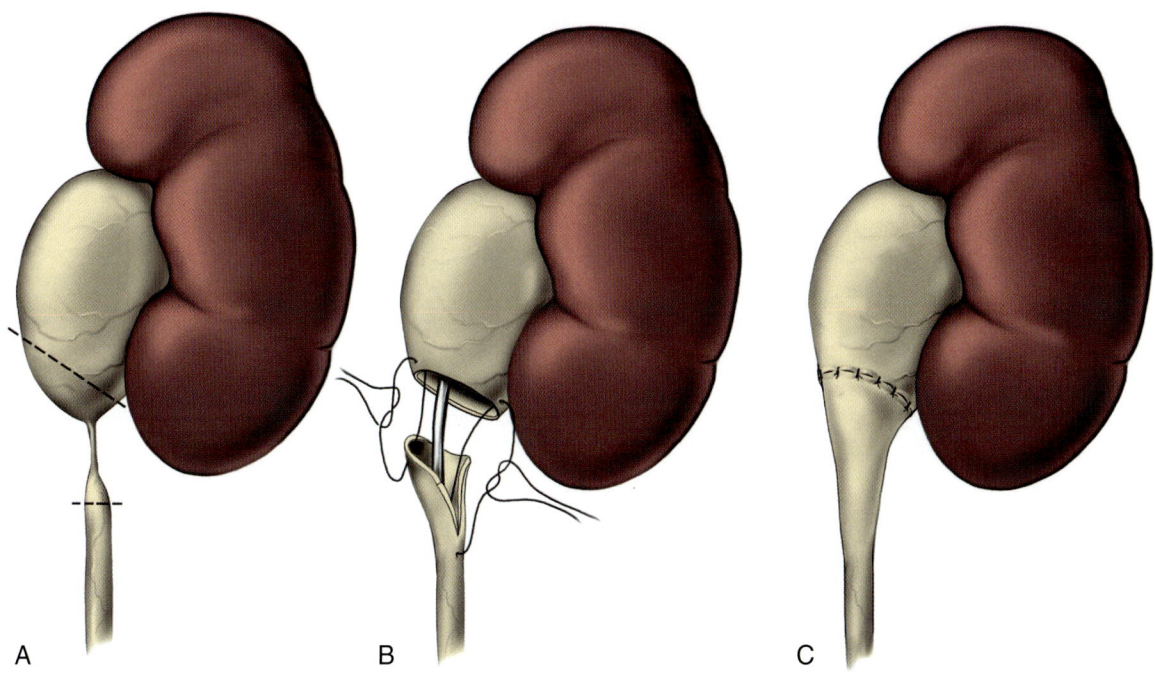

Fig. 89.11. (A) Traction sutures are placed on the medial and lateral aspects of the dependent portion of the renal pelvis in preparation for dismembered pyeloplasty. A traction suture is also placed on the lateral aspect of the proximal ureter, below the level of obstruction. This will help maintain proper orientation for the subsequent repair. (B) Ureteropelvic junction is excised. The proximal ureter is spatulated on its lateral aspect. The apex of this lateral, spatulated aspect of the ureter is then brought to the inferior border of the pelvis while the medial side of the ureter is brought to the superior edge of the pelvis. (C) Anastomosis is then performed with fine interrupted or running absorbable sutures placed full thickness through the ureteral and renal pelvis walls in a watertight fashion. In general, we prefer to leave an indwelling internal stent for adult patients. The stent is removed 4 to 6 weeks later.

the ureteral insertion is high on the pelvis or already dependent. It also permits reduction of a redundant pelvis or straightening of a tortuous proximal ureter. Furthermore, **anterior or posterior transposition of the UPJ can be achieved when the obstruction is due to accessory or aberrant lower pole vessels.** In addition, unlike the flap techniques, **only a dismembered pyeloplasty allows complete excision of the anatomically or functionally abnormal UPJ. A dismembered pyeloplasty is not well suited to UPJ obstruction associated with lengthy or multiple proximal ureteral strictures or to patients in whom the UPJ obstruction is associated with a small, relatively inaccessible intrarenal pelvis.** This surgical repair can be accomplished by either open or minimally invasive techniques; the reconstruction of the UPJ is essentially the same.

Technique. Surgical exposure to the UPJ is achieved by first identifying the proximal ureter in the retroperitoneum. The proximal ureter is then dissected cephalad to the renal pelvis, leaving a large amount of periureteral tissue to preserve the ureteral blood supply. A marking stitch of fine suture can be placed on the lateral aspect of the proximal ureter, below the level of the obstruction, to assist proper orientation for the subsequent repair (Fig. 89.11A). The UPJ tissue is typically excised, and the proximal ureter is then spatulated on its lateral aspect. The apex of this lateral, spatulated aspect of the proximal ureter is brought to the inferior border of the renal pelvis, while the medial side of the ureter is brought to the superior aspect (Fig. 89.11B). The anastomosis is then performed with fine interrupted or running absorbable sutures, placed full thickness through the ureteral and renal pelvic walls, in a watertight manner (Fig. 89.11C). As discussed earlier, our preference for adult patients is to routinely perform the anastomosis over an internal ureteral stent, which is left indwelling.

If the renal pelvis is exceptionally redundant, a "reduction" pyeloplasty can be performed by excising the redundant portion of the pelvis, but this is often unnecessary (Morsi et al., 2013; Stein et al., 1996; Fig. 89.12A). The cephalad aspect of the pelvis is then closed with running absorbable sutures down to the dependent portion, which will subsequently be anastomosed to the ureter. In the event that aberrant or accessory lower pole vessels are found in association with the UPJ obstruction, a dismembered pyeloplasty allows transposition of the UPJ in relation to these vessels (Fig. 89.13).

Surgical Approaches for Pyeloplasty

Open Surgery. Several types of open surgical incisions have been used for a pyeloplasty in the management of UPJO. The preference of many surgeons for the open surgical repair of UPJO is an extraperitoneal flank approach, similar to that used for other open renal operations such as partial nephrectomy. This incision may be subcostal but is usually performed through the bed of the 12th rib or carried anteriorly off its tip. The extraperitoneal flank approach is advantageous in that it is familiar to all urologists and provides excellent exposure without regard to body habitus. An anterior extraperitoneal approach is chosen by some because it allows surgical repair with minimal mobilization of the pelvis and proximal ureter. Alternatively, a posterior lumbotomy provides direct exposure to the UPJ and again allows repair with minimal mobilization of the surrounding structures. Like the anterior extraperitoneal approach, posterior lumbotomy is best suited to relatively thin patients without previous ipsilateral surgery. In the presence of other renal anomalies associated with the UPJ, such as horseshoe or pelvic kidney, anterior extraperitoneal approaches are often preferable, although laparoscopic management may be considered in this setting.

Laparoscopic and Robotic Intervention. Laparoscopic approach to pyeloplasty (Video 90.1) was first introduced in 1993 by Schuessler et al. (1993) and has been developed worldwide as a viable minimally invasive alternative to open pyeloplasty and endopyelotomy. Relative to open pyeloplasty and endopyelotomy, laparoscopic pyeloplasty is associated with greater technical complexity and a steeper learning

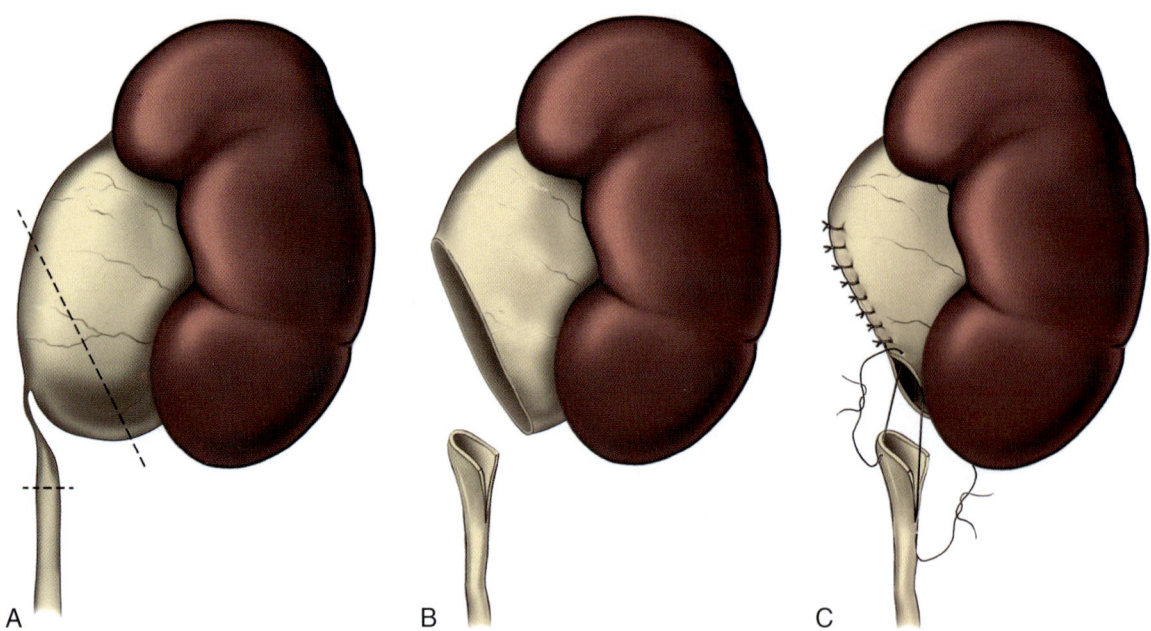

Fig. 89.12. (A) For large or redundant renal pelves, a reduction pyeloplasty is performed by excising the redundant portion between traction sutures. (B) The cephalad aspect of the pelvis is then closed with running absorbable suture down to the dependent portion. (C) The dependent aspect of the pelvis is then anastomosed to the proximal ureter.

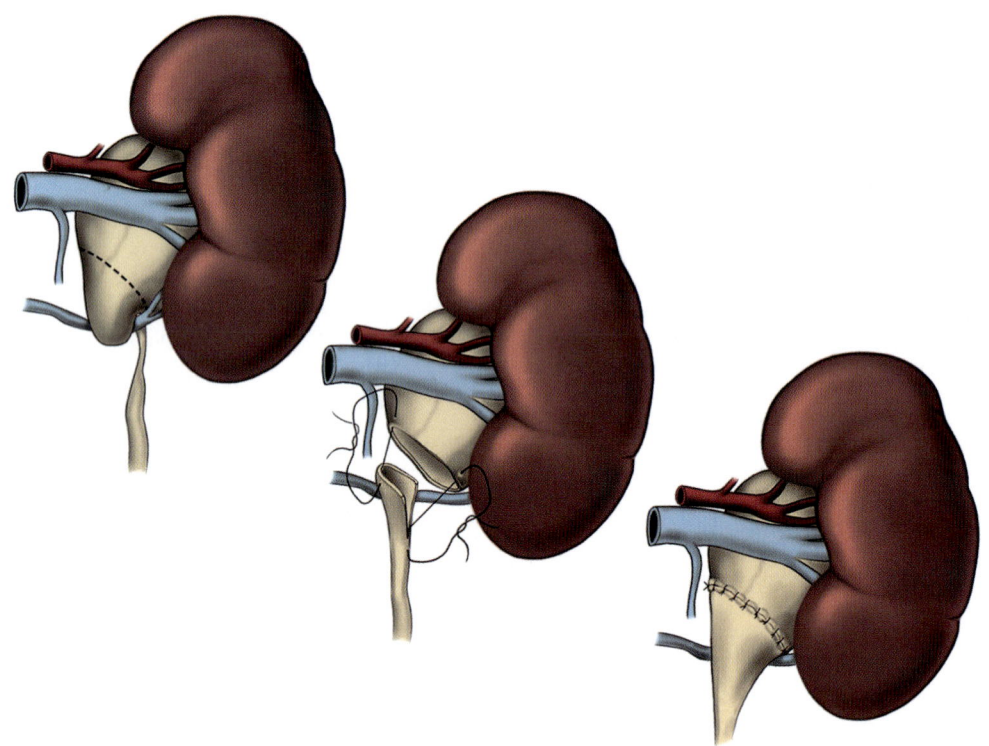

Fig. 89.13. When aberrant or accessory lower pole vessels are found in association with the ureteropelvic junction (UPJ) obstruction, a dismembered pyeloplasty allows transposition of the UPJ in relation to the vessels.

curve. **In the hands of the experienced laparoscopic surgeons, it has been shown to provide lower patient morbidity, shorter hospitalization, and faster convalescence, with the reported success rates matching those of open pyeloplasty (≥90%).** Autorino et al. (2014) conducted a meta-analysis of studies comparing open and minimally invasive pyeloplasty techniques and found they have similar success and complication rates with a weighted mean difference in hospital stay of 2.68 days favoring minimally invasive surgery. Following the similar surgical principles of anatomic dissection and repair used in open pyeloplasty, laparoscopic pyeloplasty has been shown to provide success rates surpassing those of endopyelotomy by approximately 10% to 30%. In the same meta-analysis the authors found that in case series containing more than 100 patients, laparoscopic pyeloplasty was associated with success rates ranging from

94% to 100%, although follow-up intervals tended to be short (Autorino et al., 2014).

The introduction of the surgical robotic platform (Video 90.2), with its shorter learning curve and wristed instrumentation that facilitates the ergonomics of intracorporeal suturing, has led to widespread use of minimally invasive pyeloplasty. Gettman et al. (2002) reported the first patient experience with robotic-assisted laparoscopic pyeloplasty in 2002. Jacobs et al. (2013) reported a 360% increase in the use of minimally invasive pyeloplasty between 2001 and 2009; this is thought to be related, at least in part, to adoption of robotic pyeloplasty at many centers. Similarly, Sukumar et al. (2012) found that the use of minimally invasive pyeloplasty in the United States increased from 2.4% to 55.3% from 1998 to 2009, driven by robotics, which accounted for 45.1% of pyeloplasties performed in 2009. Preoperative, intraoperative, and postoperative techniques are analogous in these approaches; thus the next section refers to laparoscopic and robotic pyeloplasty.

Indications and Contraindications. The indications and contraindications for a laparoscopic repair are similar to those for either an endourologic or an open operative procedure. Indications to intervene include the presence of clinical symptoms of UPJO, the progressive impairment of renal function, and the development of ipsilateral upper tract calculi or infection. Cases requiring the transposition of crossing vessels obstructing the ureteropelvic junction or the size reduction for massively dilated renal pelvis are suitable for the laparoscopic approach. Absolute contraindications to intervene include the presence of uncorrected coagulopathy, the absence of adequate treatment of active urinary tract infection, and the presence of cardiopulmonary compromise unsuitable for surgery. The objective of the laparoscopic surgery is to provide a tension-free, water-tight repair with a funnel-shaped drainage product to relieve clinical symptoms and to preserve renal function.

Techniques. Several laparoscopic techniques for pyeloplasty have been described in the literature including the standard transperitoneal approach (including transmesenteric), retroperitoneal approach, anterior extraperitoneal approach, laparoendoscopic single-site (LESS) approach, and robotic-assisted approach. For each approach, a dismembered Andersen-Hynes pyeloplasty, which is preferred by most surgeons, or one of the nondismembered methods such as Y-V plasty and flap pyeloplasty (Culp) analogous to those described for the open pyeloplasty can be used.

Transperitoneal Laparoscopic Approach. The initial transperitoneal approach to laparoscopic pyeloplasty was first described by Schuessler et al. (1993) and Kavoussi et al. (1993). **This approach has been the most widely used laparoscopic method because of its associated large working space and familiar anatomy.** Before the laparoscopic portion of the procedure, cystoscopy with retrograde pyelography may be first performed to define the anatomy and confirm the diagnosis, followed by placement of a ureteral stent and a urethral Foley catheter. Alternatively, the surgeon may place a stent laparoscopically in an antegrade fashion after incising the UPJ. The patient is placed in a 45-degree lateral decubitus position, and access to the peritoneal cavity is obtained via either the Veress needle or the Hassan access technique. Three to five laparoscopic ports are placed after the creation of CO_2 pneumoperitoneum. Typically the umbilical port is for the laparoscope use. Colonic mobilization to expose the retroperitoneal structures is the initial step of the laparoscopic procedure, although transmesenteric approach without bowel mobilization has been reported if renal pelvis or ureter can be readily recognized through the descending colonic mesentery (Romero et al., 2006). In a nontransmesenteric approach, after medial mobilization of the colon, the ureter is identified and dissected in the cephalad direction to achieve mobilization of the ipsilateral proximal ureter, ureteropelvic junction, and renal pelvis (Fig. 89.14A). Extensive dissection of the ureter and excessive electrocautery use in close proximity to the ureter should be avoided to minimize injury to its vascular supply. At this time, the anatomy of the proximal ureter, renal pelvis, and nearby vasculature are carefully examined to

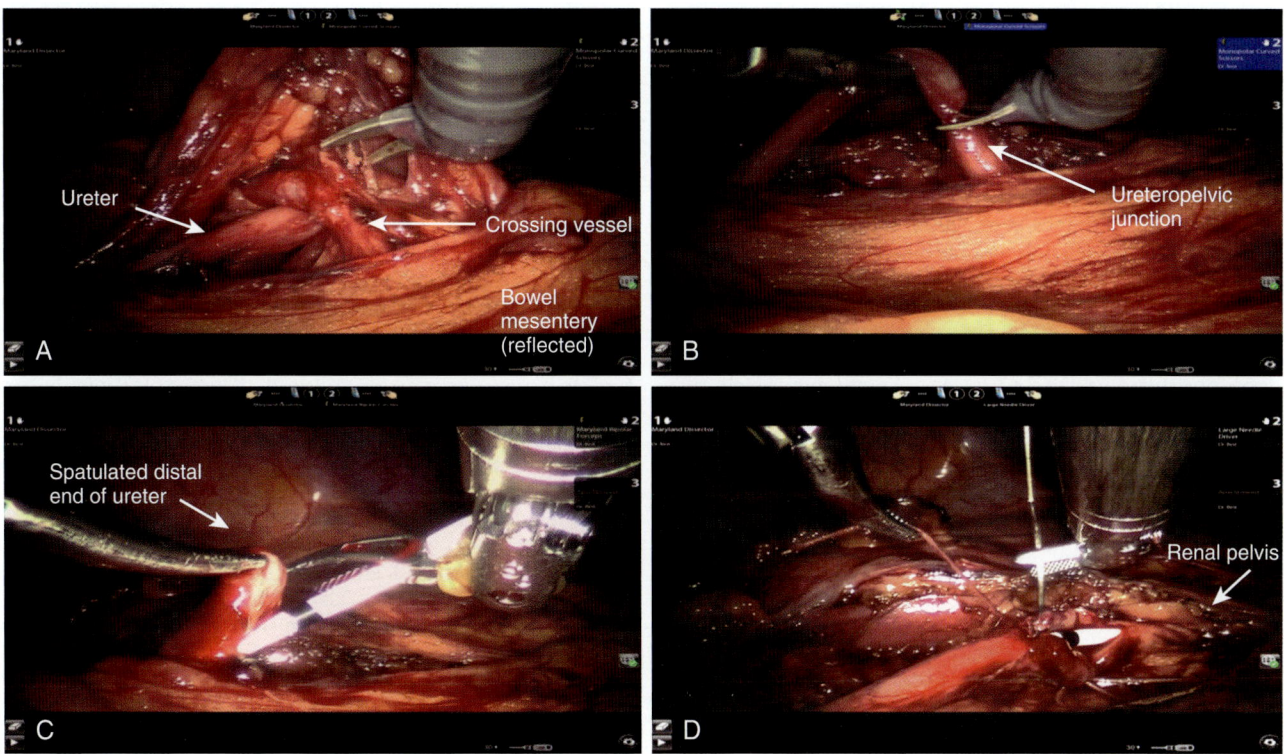

Fig. 89.14. Transperitoneoscopic view of a patient undergoing a right robotic laparoendoscopic single-site pyeloplasty. Patient's head is to the right of the images. (A) A lower pole crossing vessel is being mobilized off the anterior surface of the ureteropelvic junction (UPJ). (B) The right proximal ureter being transected sharply after complete mobilization of the proximal ureter and UPJ. (C) Percutaneous antegrade placement of a double-J ureteral stent through a small puncture in the subcostal region (not shown). (D) Completion of the anterior portion of the ureteropelvic anastomosis.

determine the cause of the UPJO and the appropriate type of surgical repair. The general methods and principles of various types of surgical repair for laparoscopic pyeloplasty are identical to those described for open pyeloplasty.

If dismembered pyeloplasty is to be performed, the renal pelvis is first transected circumferentially above the ureteropelvic junction and the lateral aspect of the proximal ureter is spatulated (Fig. 89.14B). The renal pelvis and proximal ureter are then transposed to the opposite side of the crossing vessel, if such vessel is present, and the ureteropelvic anastomosis is then completed with intracorporeal suturing techniques (Figs. 89.14C and D). If the surgeon opted for antegrade laparoscopic stent placement, this can be accomplished by passing a wire down the ureter though either the upper quadrant port or alternatively, percutaneously after advancing a wire with the help of a 14-gauge angiocatheter passed through the subcostal region. Clamping the Foley catheter and allowing the bladder to fill before wire passage can facilitate this process. After the wire has been placed, a stent can be inserted over the wire using the pusher. Watching for drainage of urine through the stent perforations can be a helpful sign that the distal end of the stent is well positioned in the bladder and is another reason to consider clamping the catheter until the stent is in place. In the presence of redundant renal pelvis, reduction pelvioplasty may be performed by excising redundant renal pelvic tissue and closing the pyelotomy. The actual laparoscopic suturing maneuver can be accomplished either freehand or with a semiautomated device (EndoStitch, US Surgical, Newark, CT). Either continuous running or simple interrupted suturing method may be used in the dismembered laparoscopic pyeloplasty, typically with a 4-0 absorbable suture. A surgical drain is placed after the completion of the anastomosis, and one of the trocar sites is typically used as the drain exit site.

Transmesenteric Modification of the Transperitoneal Approach. In select cases, it may be possible to forgo the initial step of colonic mobilization to reveal the UPJ by instead carefully opening the mesocolonic mesentery directly over the UPJ, being careful to not damage any mesenteric or crossing vessels. After incision of the mesentery, the UPJ is mobilized and reconstructed in the same fashion as the standard retrocolic approach described above. To use the transmesenteric approach approach, the dilated renal pelvis must be well visualized, and this is more often possible in thinner, younger patients with less adipose in their mesenteries. Also, preoperative stent placement typically deflates the renal pelvis and may obscure its visualization in this approach. Because the colon is not reflected, operative times using the transmesenteric approach may be shorter (Castillo et al., 2007; Romero et al., 2006; Shadpour et al., 2012). Some authors have reported a shorter hospital stay in transmesenteric approach patients, theorizing an earlier return of bowel function as a result of minimal bowel manipulation during surgery (Porpiglia et al., 2008; Romero et al., 2006; Shadpour et al., 2012).

Vascular Transposition. An alternative approach has been described to treat an obstruction related to lower pole crossing vessels, also known as the "vascular hitch," in which the lower pole vessels are mobilized and moved to a more cranial position overlying the renal pelvis rather than the UPJ without dismembering the UPJ itself (Sakoda et al., 2011). The majority of the reports on this approach describe its use in the pediatric population, although a series of 42 patients ranging in age from 7 to 69 years reported a 90% success rate (Nouralizadeh et al., 2010). Gundeti et al. (2008) performed vascular transposition procedures in 20 children with a 95% success rate at a mean of 22 months' follow-up. However, Nerli et al. (2009) noted the uncertainty regarding whether the crossing vessels are the sole cause of obstruction as a possible reason for the failure they noted in a 9-year-old on whom they performed a vascular hitch.

Retroperitoneal Laparoscopic Approach. The initial retroperitoneoscopic approach to pyeloplasty was first reported by Janetschek et al. (1996). Cystoscopy with retrograde pyelography and ureteral stent placement are first performed as described earlier. For the retroperitoneal approach, the patient is usually positioned in the flank position with the use of flexion and elevation of the kidney rest. Following Hassan access technique to enter the retroperitoneum, a retroperitoneal working space can be created with balloon dilation. Following CO_2 pneumoretroperitoneum, three to four laparoscopic ports are used to perform the laparoscopic pyeloplasty. The ureter is usually identified early in the procedure, and the dissection, mobilization, and UPJ repair steps are identical to those described for the transperitoneal approach.

Anterior Extraperitoneal Laparoscopic Approach. The anterior extraperitoneal laparoscopic approach to pyeloplasty was first described by Hsu et al. (2003). Cystoscopy with retrograde pyelography and ureteral stent placement are first performed as described earlier. For the anterior extraperitoneal approach, the medial mobilization of the peritoneal sac containing the bowel contents en bloc. Subsequently, full exposure of the anterior aspects of the retroperitoneal structures including the ipsilateral ureter and kidney comes into view. The proximal ureter, UPJ, and renal pelvis are identified, dissected, mobilized, and repaired as in the transperitoneal laparoscopic pyeloplasty. The entire procedure is completed in an extraperitoneal manner. A surgical drain is similarly placed at the end of the procedure.

Robotic-Assisted Laparoscopic Approach. The robotic-assisted laparoscopic pyeloplasty in the experimental setting was first reported by Sung et al. (1999). Its feasibility was subsequently confirmed with worldwide clinical application in recent years (Gettman et al., 2002; Mufarrij et al., 2007; Palese et al., 2005; Schwentner et al., 2007; Yanke et al., 2008). The most widely used robotic system in the clinical setting today is the da Vinci Robot (Intuitive Surgical, Sunnyvale, CA), and the reported benefits of the robot include enhanced 3D vision, motion scaling, tremor reduction, improved dexterity, and increased range of motion. Typically the procedure is performed in a transperitoneal manner providing a larger working space for the robotic arms, although the feasibility of retroperitoneal approach has been demonstrated (Cestari et al., 2010; Kaouk et al., 2008). A ureteral stent may be placed via a cystoscopic retrograde or laparoscopic antegrade manner. In transperitoneal and retroperitoneal approaches, four trocars are typically used in a robotic-assisted procedure including three for the robotic arms (including one for the camera) and one for the surgical assistant to perform suction, irrigation, retraction, and suture introduction. After the initial laparoscopic access and trocar placement, the robotic system is placed in close proximity to the operating table, and the robotic arms are attached to the laparoscope and specifically designed laparoscopic instruments. The surgeon at the console operates via the control of the robotic arms, while the assistant remains at the bedside and performs suction, retraction, exchange of laparoscopic instruments, suture needle introduction, and removal. The general surgical steps are identical to those described for non–robotic-assisted laparoscopic pyeloplasty.

Laparoendoscopic Single-Site Surgery Approach. Since the adoption of laparoscopic and robotic techniques, LESS has been developed in an effort to further decrease surgical invasiveness and improve morbidity (Kaouk et al., 2011). Proponents of the LESS approach suggest it may offer patients improved cosmetic outcomes by decreasing the number of ports from 3 to 5 to a single intra- or periumbilical incision that is often inconspicuous (Fig. 89.15). In LESS, all of the instruments are inserted through a single location. This approach abandons the common laparoscopic principle of triangulation of the ports and results in ergonomic challenges and the clashing of instruments as they compete for space in a limited working envelope. Although this approach increases the level of complexity in performing the procedure, in experienced hands, complication rates of LESS pyeloplasty are similar to those with other minimally invasive approaches (Rais-Bahrami et al., 2013; Tugcu et al., 2013). Pyeloplasty is particularly appealing for LESS, because there is no sizable specimen to be extracted and the incisions can be kept small. However, laparoscopic suturing can be challenging in LESS. Some authors report using an accessory subcostal needlescopic instrument/port to facilitate anastomotic suturing.

Typically, a 2.5- to 3-cm intra- or periumbilical incision is made using the Hassan technique. A variety of purpose-built LESS port devices are commercially available. Alternatively, 3 separate 5-mm ports can be placed in individual incisions inside the umbilicus. A 5-mm laparoscope is commonly used in LESS to reduce instrument

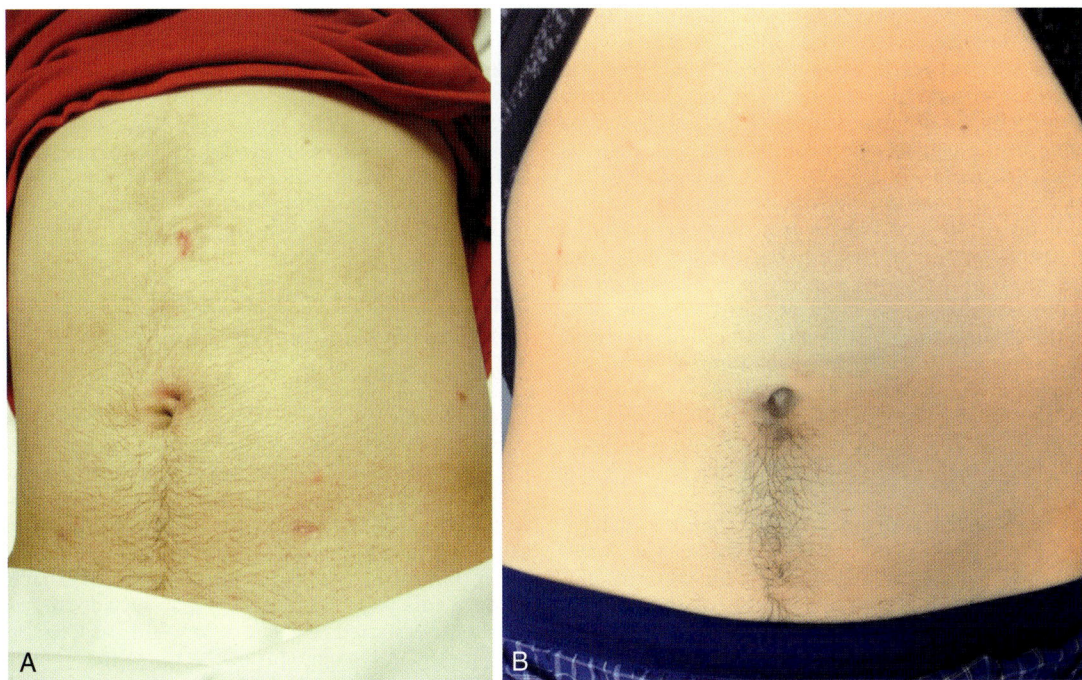

Fig. 89.15. (A) Postoperative photograph of the abdomen of a patient with left-sided laparoscopic dismembered pyeloplasty. Note the four small scars from the laparoscopic procedure. (B) Postoperative appearance of the scar from a right-sided robotic laparoendoscopic single-site pyeloplasty, performed through a single incision at the umbilicus.

conflict and a right-angle adapter for the light cord can also be helpful to reduce external conflicts with other operating instruments. A variety of bent and articulating instruments are available to help reduce instrument conflicts ("swordfighting") inside the abdomen. Some surgeons have found a deflecting laparoscope to be helpful as well.

The technical challenges of LESS suturing have led some urologists to apply the robotic platform to LESS pyeloplasty. Just as the articulating instrumentation can shorten the learning curve and facilitate anastomotic reconstruction in standard robotic pyeloplasties, robotic LESS has been reported by several authors as having ergonomic advantages over standard LESS (Cestari et al., 2012; Desai et al., 2009; Olweny et al., 2012; Stein et al., 2010; Tobis et al., 2013). Purpose-designed equipment for robotic LESS remains limited at this time, but future technologic advances may further adoption of these advanced techniques. Renal functional outcomes of LESS and robotic LESS pyeloplasty have been reportedly excellent, with symptomatic and radiographic success seen in 93% of patients in a recent study by Harrow et al. (2013).

Postoperative Care and Complications. Typically, a clear liquid diet is initiated on postoperative day 1 and advanced rapidly after minimally invasive pyeloplasty. Perioperative prophylactic antibiotic coverage is maintained. The Foley catheter is usually removed 24 to 36 hours postoperatively, and the surgical drain is removed before hospital discharge if the drain output remains negligible. If the drain output increases after the Foley catheter removal, the Foley catheter should be replaced for 7 days to eliminate urinary reflux along the stent in the treated ureter and decrease urinary extravasation at the ureteropelvic anastomosis. The ureteral stent is typically removed 4 to 6 weeks later in an outpatient setting, and follow-up, including the use of imaging studies such as diuretic renography, is performed as for an open pyeloplasty. Most of the complications of laparoscopic pyeloplasty are similar to those of general laparoscopic procedures, including colonic injury, hemorrhage, ileus, pneumonia, congestive heart failure, thrombophlebitis, and urinoma formation. In the first 100 cases of laparoscopic pyeloplasty performed at Johns Hopkins (Jarrett et al., 2002), such complications occurred in 12% of the patients. Another large-scale review involving 189 cases of laparoscopic pyeloplasty identified approximately 2% to 2.3% intraoperative complication rate and 12.9% to 15.8% postoperative complication rate (Rassweiler et al., 2008).

Results

Open Approach. The overall success of open dismembered pyeloplasty has been favorable in the literature. In a retrospective review, Persky et al. (1977) noted that none of their 109 dismembered pyeloplasties for UPJO required subsequent nephrectomy. In another retrospective review involving 111 patients with UPJO undergoing open surgical repair over a 15-year period, Clark and Malek (1987) found 95% success in resolution of clinical symptoms and 91% success in decompression of pelviocaliceal system on urography after one surgical repair. Of the 111 patients with open pyeloplasty, 95 (86%) patients underwent dismembered pyeloplasty. Examining the functional outcomes on the basis of split-function analysis from preoperative and postoperative renal scans, O'Reilly (1989) found that open Anderson-Hynes dismembered pyeloplasty arrests functional deterioration in almost every case and improves function significantly in the majority in 26 consecutive patients with UPJO.

Minimally Invasive Approaches. Most of the published laparoscopic pyeloplasty reports have used the classic Andersen-Hynes dismembered technique because most laparoscopic surgeons attempt to duplicate the well-established principles of open surgery (Bachmann et al., 2006; Eden et al., 2001; Inagaki et al., 2005; Janetschek et al., 2000; Jarrett et al., 2002; Rassweiler et al., 2008; Soulie et al., 2001; Turk et al., 2002). The overwhelming majority of patients in these recent series had primary laparoscopic pyeloplasties, and the mean operative times are in the range of 119 to 252 minutes. In experienced hands, the entire procedure can be consistently performed in less than 3.5 hours (Jarrett et al., 2002), reflecting greater confidence in intracorporeal suturing and knot tying. Perioperative complication rates are low, ranging from 2% to 15.8%, demonstrating the safety of the laparoscopic procedure. Open conversion rates are also low, in the range of 0% to 5.5%. Furthermore, blood transfusion risks are low, limited to anecdotal reports. Postoperative analgesic use is generally minimal. Mean length of hospital stay is about 2.7 days with minimally invasive pyeloplasty, compared with 4.2 days for open (Jacobs et al., 2018). With mean follow-up times of 14 to 26 months, the rates of surgical success (defined as durable clinical and/or radiographic success) reach the range of 87% to 99%; the majority of contemporary series report success rates of greater than 95%. The safety and efficacy of laparoscopic pyeloplasty have also been demonstrated in the pediatric population including patients younger than 1 year (Metzelder et al., 2006).

Most failures from laparoscopic pyeloplasty occur in the first 2 years, although up to 30% of failed cases may occur after 2 years postoperatively (Madi et al., 2008). **For the patients who fail laparoscopic pyeloplasty, open surgery has been used as a salvage procedure, with success rates of approximately 86%** (Thomas et al., 2005). **However, most cases can be well managed with endoscopic intervention such as endopyelotomy, with success rates of approximately 70%** (Varkarakis et al., 2004). Although success rates of pediatric pyeloplasty are typically high in the literature, a recent review of the MarketScan database found that 1 in 9 pediatric patients underwent a secondary procedure, suggesting failure is not rare (Dy et al., 2016).

More data on robotic-assisted laparoscopic pyeloplasty have emerged recently (Table 89.1; Mufarrij et al., 2007; Palese et al., 2005; Schwentner et al., 2007; Yanke et al., 2008). Like the conventional laparoscopic studies, the overwhelming majority of the patients in these recent series had primary robotic-assisted laparoscopic pyeloplasties. The mean operative times are in the range of 100 to 299 minutes. Perioperative complication rates are low (3% to 24%). Open conversion rates are also relatively low (0% to 6.8%). Postoperative analgesic use is generally minimal. Mean length of hospital stay is in the range of 2.2 to 2.8 days. With mean follow-up times of 11 to 39 months, the rates of surgical success (defined as durable clinical and/or radiographic success) are 94.7% to 100%. These results were similar to those from the historic laparoscopic series in the literature. The feasibility of the robotic approach has also been demonstrated in the pediatric patients (Atug et al., 2005b; Lee et al., 2006). The additional reported benefits provided by the robot include better 3D magnification, increased range of motion, and ease of dissection and suturing. However, the value of the robot in the setting of clinical pyeloplasty remains controversial and has been addressed by one recent study (Link et al., 2006). In this study comparing robotic and laparoscopic pyeloplasty in a prospective manner, the mean operative time and total room time for robotic cases were found to be significantly longer than laparoscopic cases by 19.5 and 39 minutes, respectively. Robotic cases were also found to be more costly than laparoscopic cases (2.7 times) because of longer operative time, increased cosumables costs, and depreciation of the robot system. In the hands of experienced laparoscopic surgeons, the use of the robot does not seem to confer significant clinical or cost advantage compared with conventional laparoscopic approach. Beyond cost, additional concerns for the robotic-assisted laparoscopic pyeloplasty include limited instrumentation and need for experienced bedside laparoscopic assistance (Peschel et al., 2004).

Although success rates of pyeloplasty are generally high, late failures can occur and long-term follow-up may be helpful in identifying these patients. DiMarco et al. (2006) reported that success rates of pyeloplasty in their series of 175 patients, defined as absence of radiographic obstruction and flank pain, dropped from 85% at 3 years to 75% at 10 years, lower than they anticipated. A more recent series of robotic pyeloplasties had limited radiographic follow-up (mean 12.2 months) but found an 8-year pyeloplasty failure-free survival of 91.55% at a mean telephone follow-up of 64.8 months (Hopf et al., 2016).

Primary UPJO associated with renal anomalies such as horseshoe kidneys and pelvic kidneys have also been managed with laparoscopic pyeloplasty safely and successfully (Bovie et al., 2004; Hsu et al., 2003; Janetschek et al., 1996). Furthermore, secondary UPJO has similarly been managed with success. In a retrospective review, Sundaram et al. (2003) identified 36 cases of laparoscopic transperitoneal pyeloplasty for secondary UPJO, mostly after failed retrograde or antegrade endopyelotomies. Mean operative time was 6.2 hours, longer than the reported times associated with primary UPJO. Open conversion was necessary in 1 patient, and postoperative complication occurred in 8 patients. With a mean follow-up of 21.8 months, the overall success rate of a greater than 50% decrease in pain, a patent UPJ, and stable or improved function of the affected renal unit was 83% (30 of 36 patients). Shapiro et al. (2009) identified 9 cases of laparoscopic transperitoneal pyeloplasty for secondary UPJO after a failed open procedure. Mean operative time was 204 minutes. At a median follow-up of 66 months, 89% (eight of nine) patients had clinical and radiologic resolution of UPJO, with stable renal function, pain-free status, and patent UPJ.

Special Situations of Laparoscopic and Robotic-Assisted Laparoscopic Management of Ureteropelvic Junction Obstruction

Laparoscopic and Robotic-Assisted Laparoscopic Ureterocalicostomy. Ureterocalicostomy has been completed successfully via laparoscopic and robotic-assisted laparoscopic approaches. Gill et al. (2004) performed laparoscopic ureterocalicostomy in two patients with UPJO associated with small renal pelvis and dilated lower pole calix. In both patients a double-J ureteral stent was first placed into the ipsilateral ureter cystoscopically. With the patient in a 45- to 60-degree flank position, a transperitoneal approach using three or four ports was used to gain access to the ipsilateral renal unit laparoscopically. A circular rim of the tip of the thin lower pole renal parenchyma was identified and excised. The UPJ was transected, followed by ligation of the renal pelvic opening. The ureter was spatulated laterally, and end-to-end ureterocaliceal anastomosis with mucosa-to-mucosa apposition over the preplaced double-J stent was performed with free-hand intracorporeal suturing and knot-tying techniques. The general reconstructive principles are identical to those of open ureterocalicostomy described previously, including the need to achieve tension-free, water-tight, dependent drainage.

The largest series of ureterocalicostomies reports outcomes in 72 procedures, 38 of which were laparoscopic, while the rest were open procedures (Srivastava, 2017). Mean follow-up was 60 months, and 82% of patients had had previous ipsilateral renal surgery. The authors reported a 69.5% success rate, **identifying poor ipsilateral renal function and thin renal parenchyma as risk factors for failure.** This success rate is fairly similar to other "redo" pyeloplasty series, although it contrasts with some smaller ureterocalicostomy series, suggesting the importance of technical and patient factors in the decision to perform this operation. In a series of laparoscopic ureterocalicostomies by Arap et al. (2014), all six procedures remained successful radiographically at a mean of 30 months' follow-up, and there were no major complications.

Casale et al. (2008) reported successful robotic-assisted laparoscopic ureterocalicostomy in 9 pediatric patients, following the identical reconstructive principles described earlier. Mean operative time was 168 minutes, and feasibility of the use of a robot was well demonstrated. All patients were found to have no evidence of obstruction on diuretic radionuclide imaging at 12 months postoperatively.

Laparoscopic and Robotic-Assisted Pyeloplasty With Concomitant Pyelolithotomy. Presence of calculi in the setting of UPJO can be managed laparoscopically with success. In a retrospective review, Ramakumar et al. (2002) reported 20 cases of laparoscopic pyeloplasty with concomitant extraction of renal stones through the pyelotomy site under laparoscopic guidance. In the series, extraction of the caliceal stones was assisted by the use of a flexible cystoscope introduced through a 10- to 12-mm port site. At a mean follow-up of 3 months, 90% of patients were stone free, and 90% patients had patent UPJ radiographically. In another retrospective review, Stein et al. (2008) reported 15 cases of laparoscopic pyeloplasty with concomitant pyelolithotomy, involving the use of laparoscopic graspers, flexible cystoscopes, and/or laparoscopic irrigation. The overall stone-free rate was 80%. Robotic-assisted laparoscopic pyeloplasty with concomitant pyelolithotomy has also been demonstrated in eight patients, using the similar instruments including laparoscopic graspers (Atug et al., 2005a). To complete the pyelolithotomy, one of the robotic arms was temporarily undocked to

TABLE 89.1 Comparative Series of Robotic Versus Laparoscopic Pyeloplasty

AUTHOR, YEAR		n	MEAN AGE (yr)	EBL (mL)	OR TIME (min)	DURATION OF FOLLOW-UP (months)	HOSPITAL STAY (days)	COMPLICATIONS	SUCCESS RATES
Link et al., 2006	LP	10	38.0	NSD	80.7 ± 21.9[a]	5.6		None	100% (authors note short follow-up limits meaning of success)
	RAP	10	46.5	NSD	100.2 ± 9.1[a]	5.6		10% (1 delayed urine leak)	100%
Weise and Winfield, 2006	LP	14	24.5		271	10	2	0	100% (64% "strict" success; no pain and no obstruction on nuclear scan)
	RAP	31	26		299	6	2	0	97% (66% "strict" success)
Kim et al., 2008	LP	58	Peds		196 ± 38		0.9 ± 0.23	3.4%	97%
	RAP	84	Peds		188 ± 45.8		1.5 ± 0.55	0	99%
Hemal et al., 2010	LP	30	28.1	100	145 ± 44	18	5.5 ± 3.8	10%	97%
	RAP	30	24.9	40	99 ± 29	18	2.5 ± 0.8	3.3%	93%
Garcia-Galisteo et al., 2011	LP	33	NR	NR	152.1 ± 23.3	42.5	4.5 ± 1.5	51.5%	93.9%
	RAP	17	NR	NR	121.6 ± 13.3	20.6	2.4 ± 0.5	23.5%	94.1%
Olweny et al., 2012[b]	LP (LESS)	10	35.8	42	188	10	2.6	20	88%
	RAP (LESS)	10	40.3	56	226	3	2.6	10	100%
Kumar and Nayak, 2013	LP	11	25	46	150 (11–200)	NR	2.9	None	100%
	RAP	19	21	54	129 (70–180)	NR	2.8	None	100%

[a]Significant difference, $P = 0.018$.
[b]LESS LP versus LESS RAP.
EBL, Estimated blood loss; LESS, laparoendoscopic single-site surgery; LP, laparoscopic pyeloplasty; NR, not reported; NSD, no significant difference; OR, operating room; Peds, pediatric cases only; RAP, robotic-assisted pyeloplasty.

allow passage of a flexible nephroscope into the renal pelvis to gain visualization of the stones in the collecting system. In this small series, all patients were rendered stone free.

Laparoscopic Dismembered Tubularized Flap Pyeloplasty. Presence of a significant upper ureteral defect after the excision of ureteropelvic junction stricture may also be managed laparoscopically with success. Kaouk et al. (2002) described a case of laparoscopic pyeloplasty for secondary ureteropelvic junction obstruction, in which a 3-cm upper ureteral defect was found following excision of the long stricture. Using a four-port transperitoneal approach, a wide-base renal pelvic flap was created and tubularized to bridge the defect, using intracorporeal freehand suturing techniques. At a 2-month follow-up, excretory urography and diuretic renal scan confirmed a widely patent upper ureter.

Laparoscopic Calicovesicostomy. Presence of a large-capacity bladder in the setting of UPJO associated with a low-lying obstructed renal unit can be managed successfully using an unconventional laparoscopic reconstructive strategy. Hsu et al. (2006) described a case of laparoscopic management of UPJO involving a horseshoe kidney with a unilateral hydronephrotic yet functioning lower pole moiety, ipsilateral ureteral duplication with high bifurcation, and complex anomalous renal vasculature. Rather than performing tedious anatomic dissection and complex ureteral reconstruction in such a scenario as required in conventional laparoscopic pyeloplasty, a nephrotomy was created at the most dependent portion of the hydronephrotic lower pole moiety and then laparoscopically anastomosed to the bladder dome vesicostomy using intracorporeal freehand suturing and knot-tying techniques. At the 4-month follow-up, patent calicovesicostomy was confirmed endoscopically and clinically.

> **KEY POINTS: LAPAROSCOPIC AND ROBOTIC INTERVENTION**
>
> - Transperitoneal laparoscopic approach is the most widely used method because of its associated large working space and familiar anatomy. Retroperitoneal laparoscopic approach and anterior extraperitoneal approach rely on creation of a working space using manual or balloon dilation.
> - Laparoscopic management of UPJO has been shown to provide low perioperative complication rate, short hospital stay, and success rates greater than 95% in the experienced hands.

Other Reconstructive Procedures Involving the Ureteropelvic Junction (Non–Anderson-Hynes)

Although the Anderson-Hynes dismembered pyeloplasty is the most commonly performed technique for reconstruction of the UPJ, other techniques or modifications may be useful in particular situations as dictated by patient anatomy. These variations in many cases may be performed through either open or minimally invasive approaches, depending on the skill level of the surgeon.

Flap Procedures
Foley Y-V-Plasty
Indications. The Foley Y-V-plasty was originally designed for repair of a UPJO secondary to a high ureteral insertion. Like other flap techniques, however, its use has generally been replaced by the more versatile dismembered pyeloplasty. As in other flap techniques, the Foley Y-V-plasty is specifically contraindicated when transposition of lower pole vessels is necessary. In situations requiring concomitant reduction of redundant renal pelvis, this technique is also of little value.

Technique. In Foley Y-V-plasty, the renal pelvis and proximal ureter are first exposed, and a widely based triangular or V-shaped flap is outlined with methylene blue or fine stay sutures. The base of the V is positioned on the dependent, medial aspect of the ipsilateral renal pelvis and the apex at the UPJ. The incision from the apex of the flap (the stem of the Y) is then performed along the lateral aspect of the proximal ureter. The surgical incision in the ureter should be long enough to completely traverse the area of stenosis and extend for several millimeters into the normal-caliber ureter (Fig. 89.16A). The renal pelvic flap and ureterotomy are then created. A fine scalpel blade is used for the initial pelvic incision, after which a Potts or a fine Metzenbaum scissors is used to complete the flap and ureterotomy (Fig. 89.16B). An internal ureteral stent is placed and the repair performed over it. First, the apex of the pelvic flap is approximated to the apex (inferior aspect) of the ureterotomy incision using fine, absorbable suture. The posterior walls are then approximated using fine interrupted or running suture (Fig. 89.16C). Interrupted technique is likely to minimize pursing or buckling of the suture line, as well as local tissue ischemia. Anastomosis of the anterior walls is then performed, thereby completing the surgical repair (Fig. 89.16D).

Culp-DeWeerd Spiral Flap
Indications. The Culp-DeWeerd spiral flap is generally best suited for large, readily accessible extrarenal pelves, in which the ureteral insertion is already in a dependent, oblique position. Although most of these patients are also good candidates for a standard or reduction

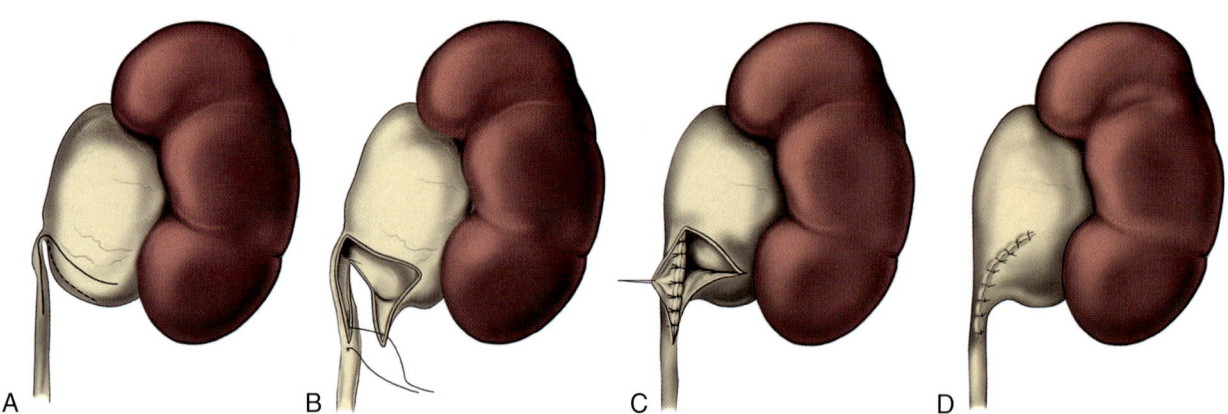

Fig. 89.16. (A) Foley Y-V plasty is best applied to a ureteropelvic junction (UPJ) obstruction associated with a high insertion of the ureter. The flap is outlined with tissue marker or stay sutures. The base of the V is positioned on the dependent, medial aspect of the renal pelvis and the apex at the UPJ. The incision from the apex of the flap, which represents the stem of the Y, is then carried along the lateral aspect of the proximal ureter well into an area of normal caliber. (B) The flap is developed with fine scissors. The apex of the pelvic flap is then brought to the most inferior aspect of the ureterotomy incision. (C) The posterior walls are then approximated using interrupted or running fine absorbable suture. (D) The anastomosis is completed with approximation of the anterior walls of the pelvic flap and ureterotomy.

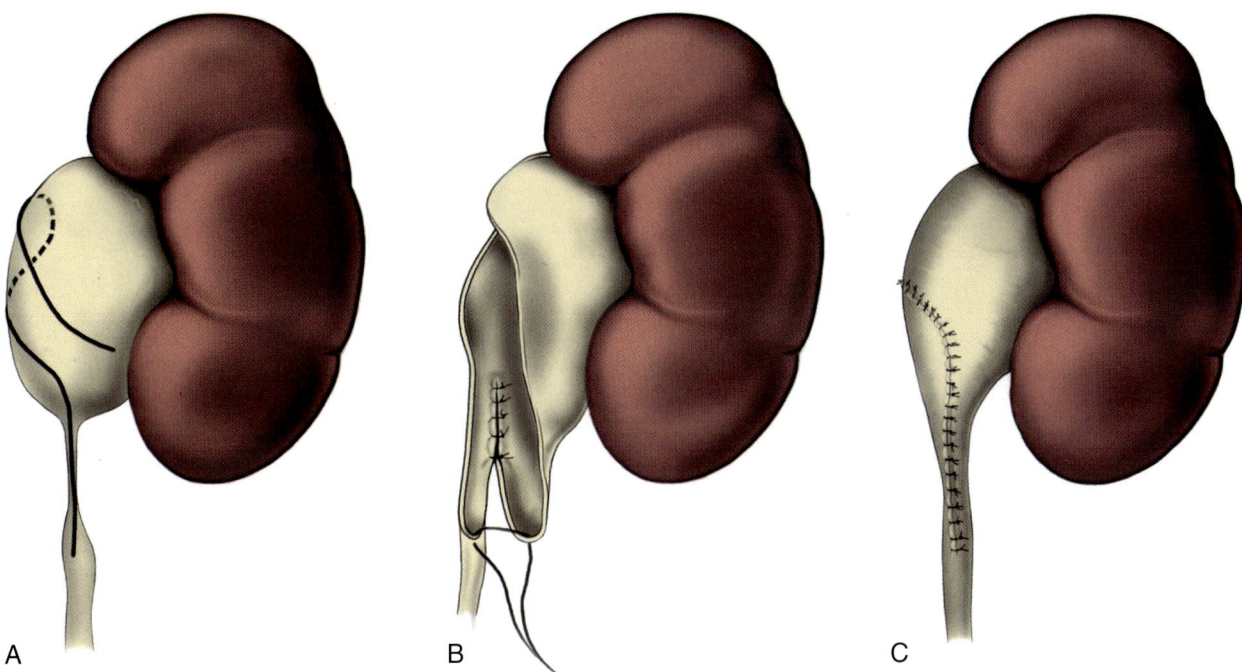

Fig. 89.17. (A) A spiral flap may be indicated for relatively long areas of proximal ureteral obstruction when the ureteropelvic junction (UPJ) is already in a dependent position. The spiral flap is outlined with the base situated obliquely on the dependent aspect of the renal pelvis. The base of the flap is positioned anatomically lateral to the UPJ, between the ureteral insertion and the renal parenchyma. The flap is spiraled posteriorly to anteriorly or vice versa. The anatomically medial line of incision is carried down completely through the obstructed proximal ureteral segment into normal-caliber ureter. The site of the apex for the flap is determined by the length of flap required to bridge the obstruction. The longer the segment of proximal ureteral obstruction, the farther away is the apex because this will make the flap longer. However, to preserve vascular integrity of the flap, the ratio of flap length to width should not exceed 3:1. (B) Once the flap is developed, the apex is rotated down to the most inferior aspect of the ureterotomy. (C) The anastomosis is then completed, usually over an internal stent, again using fine absorbable sutures.

dismembered pyeloplasty, the spiral flap may be of significant value when UPJO and a relatively long segment of proximal ureteral narrowing or stricture occur in the same setting.

Technique. The spiral flap is first outlined with a broad base positioned obliquely on the dependent aspect of the renal pelvis. To maximize preservation of the flap's blood supply, the base is placed in a position anatomically lateral to the UPJ, that is, between the ureteral insertion and the renal parenchyma. The pelvic flap may be spiraled posteriorly to anteriorly or vice versa. In either case, the anatomically medial line of incision (farthest from the parenchyma) is carried down the proximal ureter, completely traversing through the obstructed segment (Fig. 89.17A). Appropriate placement of the apex of the flap is determined by the length of flap needed. This, in turn, depends on the length of proximal ureter to be bridged. The longer the flap required, the farther away the apex will be from the base. However, to preserve vascular integrity of the flap, the ratio of flap length to width should not be greater than 3:1. In general, the outline of the flap should be made longer than what may initially be perceived as necessary because the flap will shrink once the pelvis is incised. If the flap is found to be too long, excess length can be reduced by trimming back the apex, thereby preserving its blood supply. Once the flap is created, the apex is rotated down to the most inferior aspect of the ureterotomy (Fig. 89.17B). The anastomosis with fine absorbable sutures is subsequently performed over an internal stent (Fig. 89.17C).

Scardino-Prince Vertical Flap

Indications. The Scardino-Prince vertical flap technique generally has limited clinical application. It may be appropriately used only when a dependent UPJ is situated at the medial margin of a large, square ("box-shaped") extrarenal pelvis (Fig. 89.18A). Its use in most instances has been replaced by a standard dismembered pyeloplasty, although the vertical flap may be preferable for relatively long areas of proximal ureteral narrowing. The vertical flap technique generally cannot produce as long a flap as the spiral flap.

Technique. The Scardino-Prince vertical flap is similar to the spiral flap technique except that the base of the flap is positioned more horizontally on the dependent aspect of the renal pelvis, between the UPJ and the renal parenchyma. The flap is created by straight incisions converging from the base vertically to the apex on either the anterior or the posterior aspects of the renal pelvis. The site of the apex and the length of the flap are determined by the length of proximal ureter to be bridged. The medial incision is carried down the proximal ureter, completely traversing through the stenotic area and into normal-caliber ureter, using fine scissors (Fig. 89.18B). The apex of the flap is then rotated down and approximated to the most inferior aspect of the ureterotomy. Finally, the flap is closed with interrupted or running fine absorbable sutures (Fig. 89.18C).

Intubated Ureterotomy

Indications. The Davis intubated ureterotomy, which is rarely used today, was developed for surgical repair of lengthy or multiple ureteral strictures. If these strictures are found in association with UPJO, the intubated ureterotomy may be combined with any of the standard pyeloplasty procedures. However, in such a situation, the intubated ureterotomy would be best combined with a spiral flap procedure. Compared with the vertical flap, the spiral flap can be made longer, which allows more of the strictured area to be bridged by a pelvic flap, thereby leaving a shorter area to rely on healing by "secondary intention." In fact, in this specific clinical setting, any flap technique

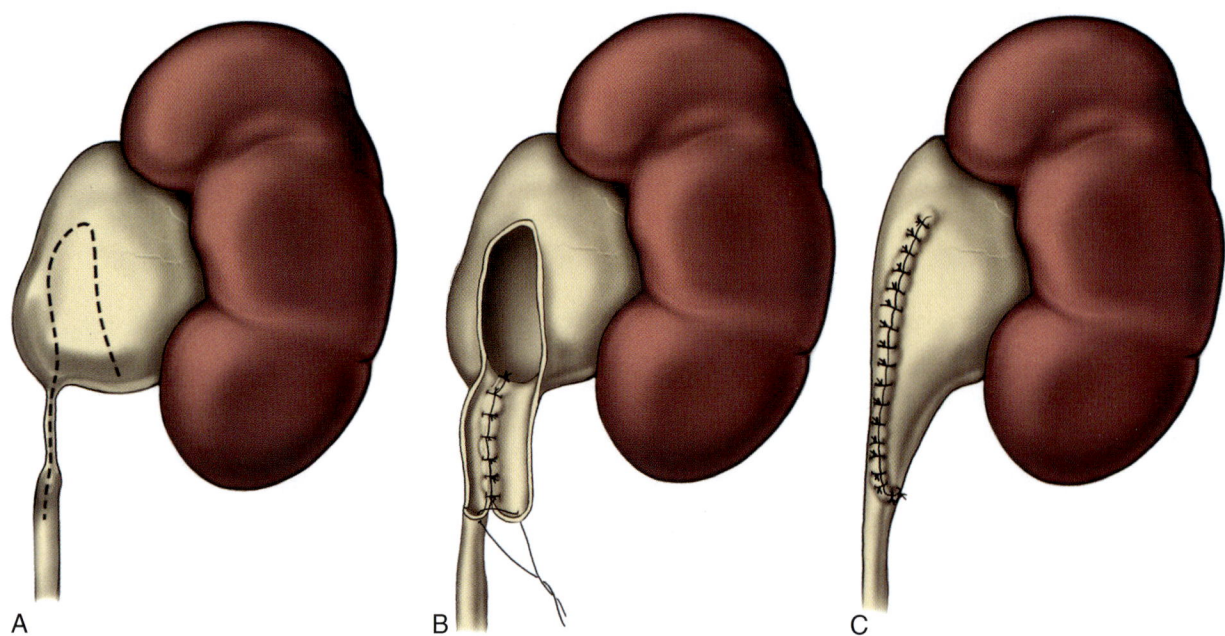

Fig. 89.18. (A) A vertical flap technique may be used when a dependent ureteropelvic junction (UPJ) is situated at the medial margin of a large, box-shaped extrarenal pelvis. In contrast to the spiral flap, the base of the vertical flap is situated more horizontally on the dependent aspect of the renal pelvis, between the UPJ and the renal parenchyma. The flap itself is formed by two straight incisions converging from the base vertically up to the apex on either the anterior or the posterior aspect of the renal pelvis. As for the spiral flap, the position of the apex determines the length of the flap, which should be a function of the length of proximal ureter to be bridged. The medial incision of the flap is carried down the proximal ureter completely through the strictured area into normal-caliber ureter. (B) The apex of the flap is rotated down to the most inferior aspect of the ureterotomy. (C) The flap is then closed by approximating the edges with interrupted or running fine absorbable sutures.

would be preferable to a dismembered repair, at least in regard to blood supply preservation of and subsequent healing.

Technique. A flap is outlined as described previously, with the ureterotomy to be made completely through the long, strictured area (Fig. 89.19A). The flap is then created, with minimal dissection of the ureter to preserve its blood supply. Unlike the uncomplicated pyeloplasties, these cases require routine nephrostomy tube drainage to prevent postoperative urinoma formation. Nephrostomy drainage in these cases also allows access for subsequent antegrade radiographic studies during the postoperative period.

On the basis of the original description, the ureteral intubation is achieved with a stenting catheter that is placed across the stenotic area to the distal ureter or bladder. Proximally, it is brought out through the renal cortex alongside a nephrostomy tube. Currently, most urologists use a self-retaining, soft, inert, internal ureteral stent instead. The apex of the flap is brought over the stent as far down as possible on the ureterotomy, and the flap is closed with either interrupted or running absorbable suture (Fig. 89.19B). The distal aspect of the ureterotomy is then left open for secondary healing via ureteral regeneration (Fig. 89.19C).

An antegrade nephrostogram is usually obtained 6 weeks after the surgery. If there is no extravasation, the ureteral stent is removed cystoscopically and an antegrade radiographic study is repeated. When ureteral patency without extravasation is ensured with such study, the nephrostomy tube is clamped and subsequently removed.

Ureterocalicostomy

Indications. Ureterocalicostomy may be used as a primary reconstructive procedure whenever a UPJO or proximal ureteral stricture is associated with a relatively small intrarenal pelvis (Fig. 89.20A). When the UPJ is associated with rotational anomalies such as horseshoe kidney (Levitt et al., 1981), ureterocalicostomy may be useful to provide completely dependent drainage. Furthermore, ureterocalicostomy is a well-accepted salvage technique for the failed pyeloplasty (Ross et al., 1990).

Technique. The ureter is first identified in the retroperitoneum and dissected proximally with a generous amount of periureteral tissue. For secondary procedures, however, extensive scarring may preclude adequate identification and dissection of the renal pelvis (Fig. 89.20B). The kidney is then mobilized to gain access to the lower pole. An important technical point in ureterocalicostomy is that the parenchyma overlying the lower pole calyx must be resected rather than simply incised because a simple nephrotomy may lead to a secondary stricture (Couvelaire et al., 1964).

The proximal ureter is first spatulated laterally, and the ureterocalyceal anastomosis is completed over an internal stent. Leaving an indwelling nephrostomy tube should also be considered in these cases. The first suture is placed at the apex of the ureteral spatulation and lateral wall of the calyx, and the second suture is placed 180 degrees apart. The remainder of the anastomosis is then performed using an interrupted "open" suture technique. That is, each suture placed is left untied until the final one is in place (Fig. 89.20C). This method seems to provide a more accurate anastomosis under direct vision. When the full set of circumferential sutures has been placed, the sutures are secured down together (Fig. 89.20D). The renal capsule is closed over the cut surface of the parenchyma if possible. However, such closure should not be close enough to the anastomosis to cause extrinsic compression on the anastomosis. Instead, the anastomosis should be covered with perinephric fat or a peritoneal or omental flap (Fig. 89.20E). A follow-up urogram is generally obtained at 1 month after the ureteral stent extraction (Fig. 89.20F).

Reports exist of laparoscopic and robotic ureterocalicostomy (Casale et al., 2008; Gill et al., 2004; Korets et al., 2007). Arap et al. (2014) report 100% success at a mean of 30 months after laparoscopic ureterocalicostomy in 6 patients.

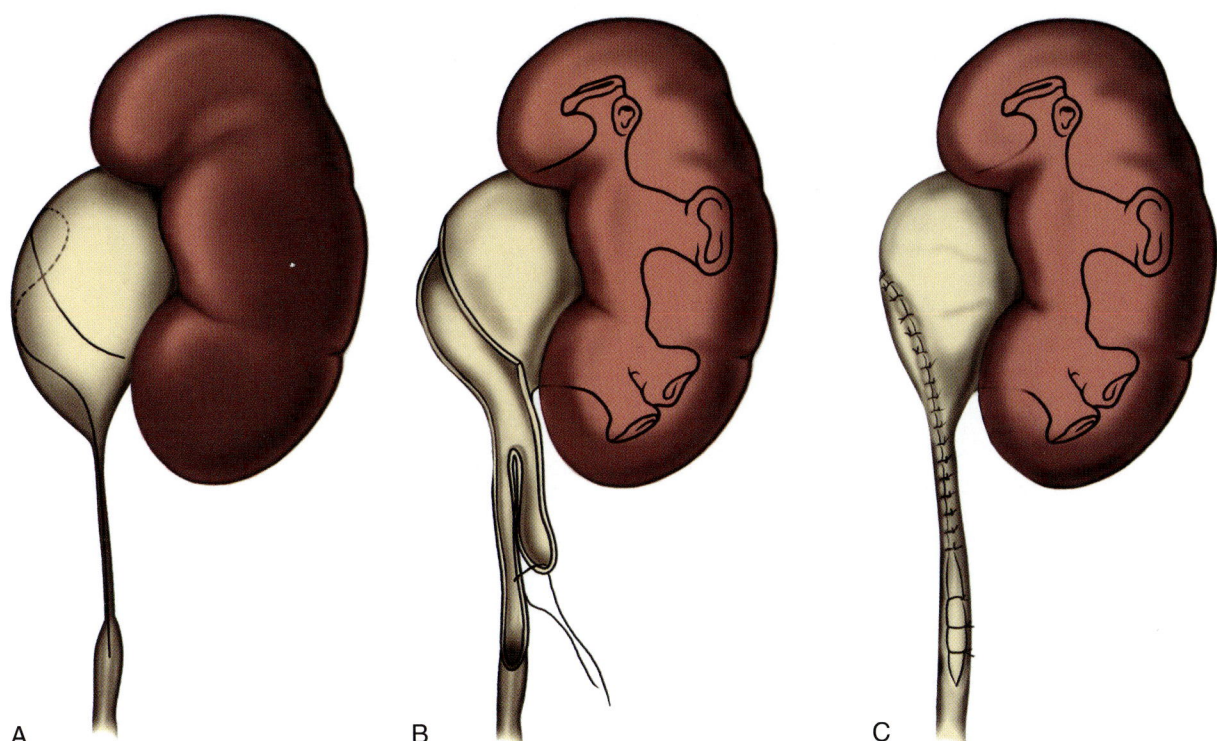

Fig. 89.19. (A) Intubated ureterotomy may be of value when a ureteropelvic junction obstruction is associated with extremely long or multiple ureteral strictures. A spiral flap is outlined and developed as described in Fig. 89.20. The ureterotomy incision will be carried completely through the long strictured areas or through each of the multiple areas of stricture. (B) The flap is developed, taking care to use minimal dissection of the ureter to preserve its blood supply. In contrast to uncomplicated repairs, nephrostomy tube drainage is used routinely. A self-retaining, soft, inert internal ureteral stent is then placed and positioned proximally in the renal pelvis or lower infundibulum and distally in the bladder. The apex of the flap is then brought as far down as possible over the stent on the ureterotomy, and the flap is closed with interrupted or running absorbable suture. (C) The distal aspect of the ureterotomy is left open to heal secondarily by ureteral regeneration. A few fine absorbable sutures may be loosely placed to keep the sides of the ureter in apposition to the stent.

Salvage Procedures. Failed open pyeloplasty is a challenging problem that is usually best managed initially using an endourologic approach. In some cases, such approach may not be applicable. In these cases, successful reconstruction can at times be achieved using one of the flap or dismembered techniques already described. The secondary open operative reconstruction may be significantly aided by the placement of a ureteral catheter to aid intraoperative identification and dissection of the ureter and renal pelvis. In these situations, there is often a relatively long length of proximal ureteral stenosis to repair, and wide mobilization of the kidney and ureter is generally a necessity. This helps to bridge the area of stenosis and allows a tension-free secondary pyeloplasty.

Several other options are available for these secondary and often complex repairs. These surgical alternatives include those generally available for any extensive ureteral problem such as ileoureteral replacement and autotransplantation with a Boari flap pyelovesicostomy. For cases in which function of the involved kidney is already significantly compromised and the contralateral kidney is normal, nephrectomy is considered.

Postoperative Care and Management of Complications. In general, external drains are removed 24 to 48 hours after cessation of urinary drainage, and internal ureteral stents, if placed, are removed on an outpatient basis approximately 4 to 6 weeks after the surgery. If a nephrostomy tube is used, a nephrostogram is obtained no sooner than 7 to 10 days postoperatively, or even later for particularly complicated repairs. If nephrostogram demonstrates a patent anastomosis without obstruction or extravasation, the tube is clamped for 12 to 24 hours and removed if there is no flank pain, fever, or leakage around the tube.

RETROCAVAL URETER

Etiology and Diagnosis

Retrocaval ureter is a rare congenital urologic anomaly. It occurs as a consequence of the persistence of the posterior cardinal veins during embryologic development (Considine, 1966). Its presence should be suspected with the finding of a characteristic S-shaped deformity on intravenous or retrograde pyelography (Fig. 89.21A). Today, a definitive diagnosis can be made noninvasively using 3D CT imaging (Fig. 89.21B; Pienkny et al., 1999). Procedural intervention is indicated in the presence of functionally significant obstruction leading to pain or renal function deterioration.

Operative Intervention

The standard repair of retrocaval ureter is surgical pyelopyelostomy. **In this procedure, the ureter, dilated renal pelvis, and inferior vena cava are identified and dissected using the standard open surgical techniques. The dilated renal pelvis is then transected, after which the ureter is transposed to its normal anatomic position anterior to the vena cava** (Fig. 89.22). Pyelopyelostomy is then performed circumferentially with absorbable sutures in a tension-free, water-tight manner. Surgical drain and internal ureteral stent are typically used.

Laparoscopic Surgical Management

Retrocaval ureter has been managed successfully with the laparoscopic approach in the clinical setting as shown by a series of sporadic case

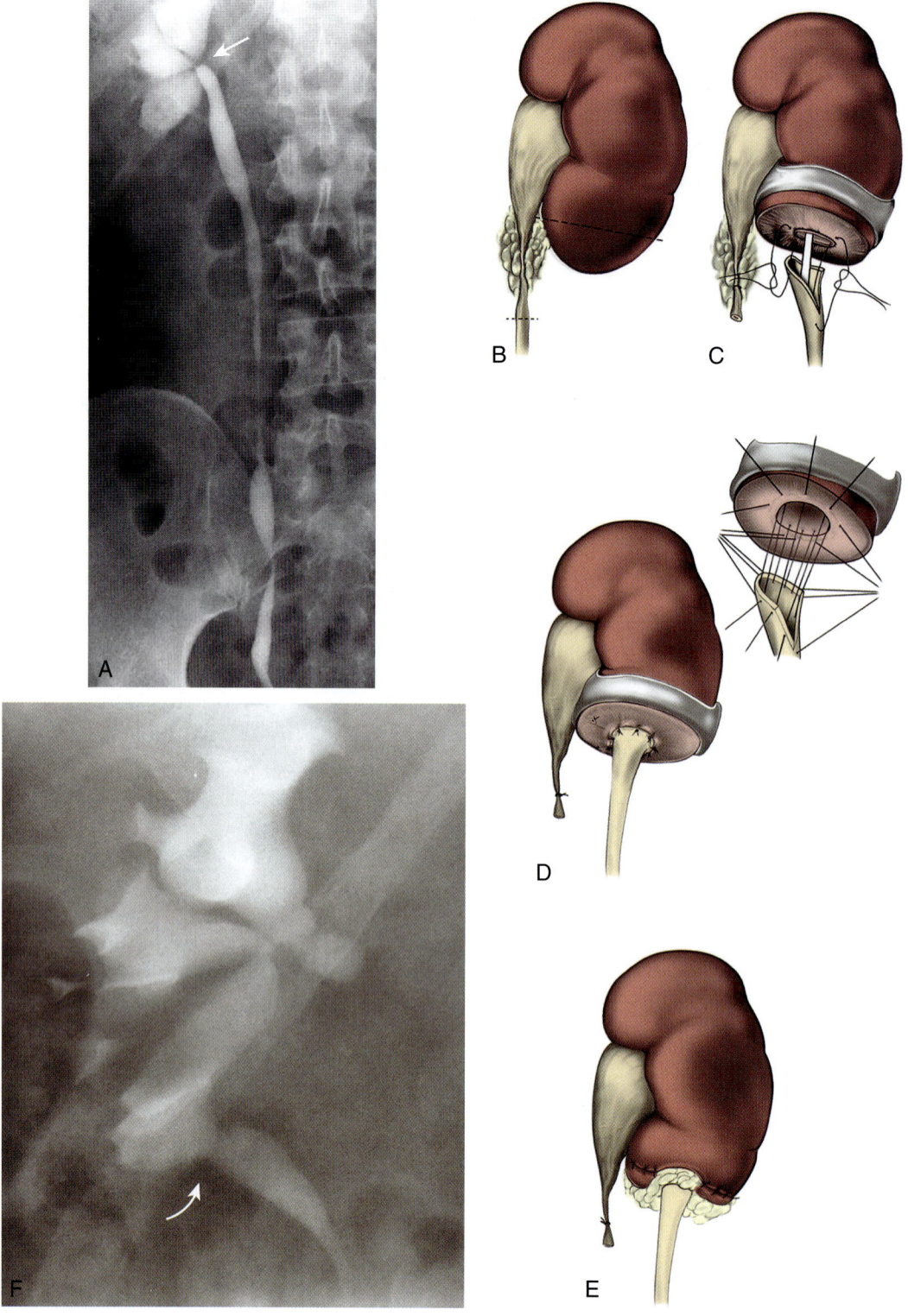

Fig. 89.20. (A) This patient reported progressive right flank pain and was found on this retrograde study to have a ureteropelvic junction obstruction *(arrow)* associated with a small intrarenal pelvis. This situation may be best managed with a ureterocalicostomy. (B) The ureter is identified in the retroperitoneum and dissected proximally as far as possible. The kidney is mobilized as much as necessary to gain access to the lower pole and to subsequently perform the anastomosis without tension. A lower pole nephrectomy is performed, removing as much parenchyma as necessary to widely expose a dilated lower pole calyx. (C) The proximal ureter is spatulated laterally. The anastomosis should subsequently be performed over an internal stent, and consideration should also be given to leaving a nephrostomy tube. The initial sutures are placed at the apex of the ureteral spatulation, and the lateral wall of the calyx with a second suture is placed 180 degrees from that. (D) Anastomosis is then completed in an open fashion, placing each suture circumferentially *(inset)* but not securing them until the anastomosis has been completed. (E) Renal capsule is closed over the cut surface of the parenchyma whenever possible. However, the capsule should not be closed near the anastomosis because that may compromise the lumen by extrinsic compression. Instead, the anastomosis should be protected with a graft of perinephric fat or a peritoneal or omental flap. (F) Intravenous urogram 2 months after right ureterocalicostomy reveals a widely patent ureterocalyceal anastomosis at the lower pole *(arrow)*.

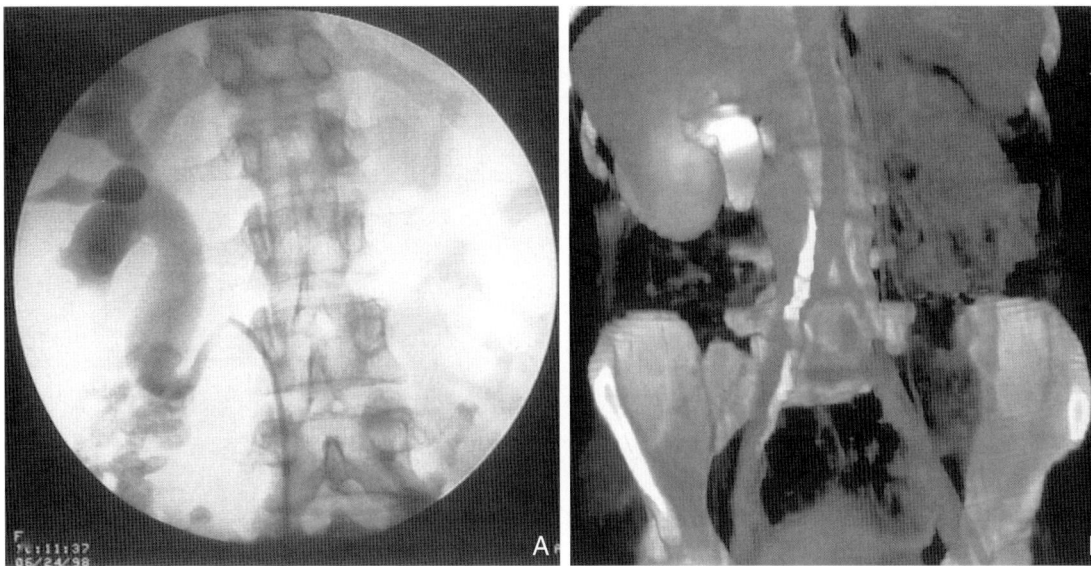

Fig. 89.21. (A) Retrograde pyelography in a patient with right-sided hydronephrosis. This study reveals a typical S-shaped deformity secondary to the ureter coursing laterally to medially posterior to the inferior vena cava. (B) Three-dimensional spiral computed tomography demonstrates the presence of a retrocaval ureter.

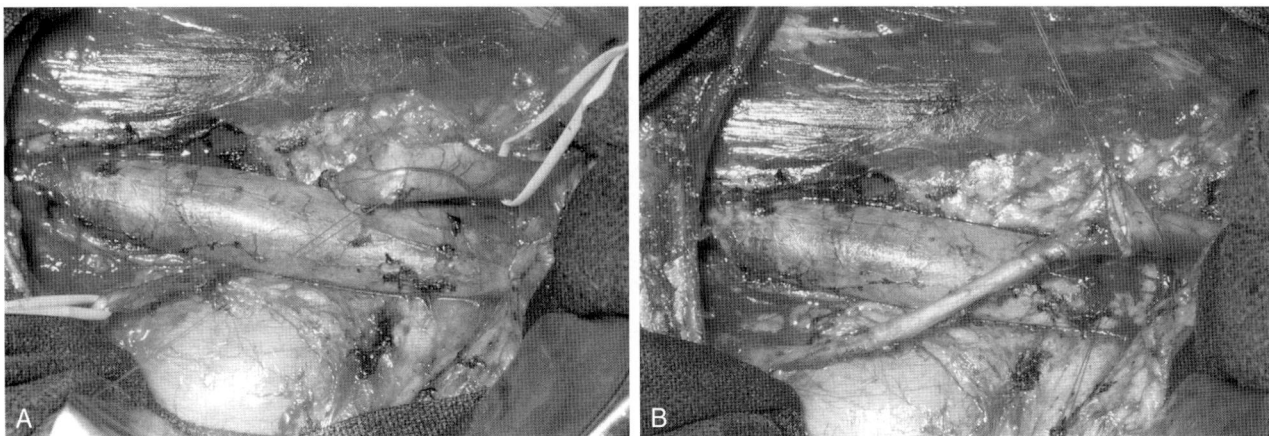

Fig. 89.22. (A) Intraoperative photograph of a patient with retrocaval ureter undergoing surgical repair via a retroperitoneal flank approach. Right side of the photo represents the cephalad direction. Note the dilated proximal right ureter passing behind the inferior vena cava. (B) Right ureteropelvic anastomosis has been completed after transection of the right renal pelvis and transposition of the ureter anterior to the inferior vena cava.

reports (Baba et al., 1994; Gupta et al., 2001; Matsuda et al., 1996; Polascik et al., 1998; Ramalingam et al., 2003; Salomon et al., 1999). Either a transperitoneal or a retroperitoneal approach may be used laparoscopically. A double-J ureteral stent is first placed into the ipsilateral ureter cystoscopically. After transperitoneal or retroperitoneal laparoscopic access, the ipsilateral ureter is identified and mobilized off the inferior vena cava. The ureter is then divided at the most distal segment of the dilated ureter. Redundant segment of dilated proximal ureter and stenotic segment of ureter are excised if present. The ureteral ends are positioned anterolateral to the vena cava, spatulated for 1.5 to 2 cm on opposite ends, and then anastomosed with absorbable sutures using intracorporeal suturing techniques over the stent. Tension-free, water-tight anastomosis is the objective. A surgical drain is then left in place and typically removed within a few days postoperatively, and the ureteral stent is typically removed 4 to 6 weeks postoperatively.

Today retrocaval ureter has been managed successfully with the robotic-assisted laparoscopic approach (Hemal et al., 2008; Mufarrij et al., 2007; Smith et al., 2009). A transperitoneal approach providing a large working space is typically used. The general principles of laparscopic ureteral dissection, division, transposition, and anastomosis are identical to those described in conventional laparoscopic approach. At least four different ports are involved, including three for the robot and one for the surgical assistant providing suction, irrigation, suture introduction, and retraction.

Clinical results with laparoscopic/robotic repair have been favorable, indicating minimal postoperative patient morbidity, short convalescence, and anastomotic patency on short-term radiographic follow-up.

URETERAL STRICTURE DISEASE

Etiology

Common causes of ureteral stricture formation include ischemia, surgical and nonsurgical trauma, periureteral fibrosis, malignancy, and congenital factors (Box 89.1). **Proper evaluation and treatment of a ureteral stricture are essential to preserve renal function and**

> **BOX 89.1 Cause of Ureteral Stricture**
>
> Malignancy (e.g., transitional cell carcinoma, cervical cancer)
> Ureteral calculus
> Radiation
> Ischemia or trauma caused by surgical dissection
> Periureteral fibrosis caused by abdominal aortic aneurysm or endometriosis
> Endoscopic instrumentation
> Renal ablation injury
> Infection (tuberculosis)
> Idiopathic condition

> **KEY POINTS: RETROCAVAL URETER**
>
> - Retrocaval ureter results from the persistence of the posterior cardinal veins.
> - Retrocaval ureter can be diagnosed using retrograde pyelography or CT.
> - Procedural intervention is indicated in the presence of functionally significant obstruction, and open and laparoscopic approaches can be successfully applied.

rule out the presence of malignancy. Although the classic radiographic presentation of a transitional cell carcinoma of the ureter is a radiolucent filling defect within the lumen with the characteristic goblet sign, it may have the same appearance as a benign stricture. In addition, metastatic tumors such as cervical, prostate, ovarian, breast, and colon cancer may appear as a ureteral stricture (Lau et al., 1998). Although the incidence of ureteral strictures in the general population is unknown, it is clear that the **presence of ureteral calculi and associated treatment of stones are risk factors.** Roberts et al. (1998) evaluated 21 patients with impacted ureteral stones and found that impaction for more than 2 months' duration was associated with a 24% incidence of stricture formation. Any ureteral instrumentation can lead to the development of a ureteral stricture. As advances in ureteroscopic technology have provided smaller, more actively deflecting instruments with digital optics, ureteroscopic procedures have become less traumatic and are now associated with a long-term complication rate of less than 5% (Ambani et al., 2013; Delvecchio et al., 2003; Harmon et al., 1997). Alternately, the more prevalent use of access sheaths for upper tract ureteroscopy led to one study documenting ureteral injury in up to 13% of cases involving the smooth muscle layers (Traxer and Thomas, 2013). No other clinical studies have been reported to verify this report. Other causes of benign ureteral strictures include radiation; abdominal aortic aneurysm; infections such as tuberculosis and schistosomiasis; endometriosis; and trauma including iatrogenic injury from previous abdominal or pelvic surgery or post–renal ablation injury (ElAbd et al., 1996; Johnson et al., 2004; Lacquet et al., 1997; Oh et al., 2000; Ramanathan et al., 1998). Patients with presumed idiopathic ureteral strictures should be evaluated with CT scan to rule out the presence of an intrinsic ureteral malignancy or a lesion causing extrinsic compression.

Diagnostic Studies and Indications for Intervention

The presence of obstruction on standard CT can identify ureteral stricture disease, but antegrade or retrograde pyelogram, CT urography, or diagnostic ureteroscopy is typically necessary to define the location and length of the ureteral stricture. Subsequent ureteroscopy with biopsy or barbotage should be performed in any patient in whom the cause of the stricture is not certain. Diuretic renography will provide differential renal function and evaluate the renal unit for functional obstruction. **It is important to assess the renal unit for function before starting treatment because endourologic therapies, in general, require 25% function of the ipsilateral moiety to have reasonable success rates** (Wolf et al., 1997). Once a ureteral stricture is diagnosed, indications for intervention include the need to rule out malignancy, ongoing renal obstruction, recurrent pyelonephritis, and pain associated with functional obstruction.

Endourologic Options for Intervention

Ureteral Stent Placement

Ureteral stent placement is effective acutely in treating most ureteral strictures, in particular intrinsic ureteral strictures. Wenzler et al. (2008) reported good success rates in treating intrinsic ureteral obstruction, with 88% success rates at 26 months. Although intrinsic ureteral strictures can be managed or temporized with ureteral stents, patients with extrinsic ureteral compression eventually require percutaneous drainage or surgical management (Chung et al., 2004; Docimo and Dewolf, 1989).

If the patient is not a candidate for definitive repair or has a poor prognosis, chronic stent placement with periodic stent changes can be considered. In addition, patients undergoing systemic treatments for malignancies can be managed with periodic stent changes. **The use of chronic stent placement must be guarded, particularly when treating ureteral obstruction from extrinsic compression because adequate drainage may be short-lived** (Chung et al., 2004; Docimo and Dewolf, 1989). Careful monitoring of the upper tracts and patient symptoms is warranted in this subgroup of patients. Rosevear et al. (2007) reported an 84% success rate at 16 months in their series using ureteral stents, with 68% of the patients having malignancy. The remainder included patients with retroperitoneal fibrosis (RPF) and other benign extrinsic diseases. **The use of tandem ureteral stent placement (two parallel stents) has been shown to be effective in benign and malignant extrinsic ureteral obstruction** (Elsamra et al., 2013; Yohannes and Smith, 2001). Elsamra et al. (2013) reported on 66 patients managed with tandem ureteral stent placement, with stent failure in 12% of patients with malignant obstruction and none with benign ureteral obstruction. Alternatively, tandem ureteral stent placement may be an excellent option in patients in whom single-stent drainage fails.

After initial reports in 2006, the use of metallic stents in patients with malignant ureteral obstruction has gained popularity (Borin et al., 2006). Liatsikos et al. (2010) reported on 50 patients treated with the full metallic stent, and although concerns arose regarding stent exchange and encrustation, overall the study supported use of the stent at 12-month intervals. Kadlec et al. (2013) reported 5-year data showing good results for use of full-length metal stents with up to a 3-year duration of stent drainage of long-term benign and malignant obstruction in select patients. Expandable metallic mesh stents that allow tissue ingrowth have proven to have problems with encrustation, hyperplastic reactions, and tumor ingrowth (Liatsikos et al., 2009).

Alternatively, Papatsoris et al. (2010) reported using nonmesh thermoexpandable metallic stents with both drainage and therapeutic benefits, although urinary tract infections, stent migration, encrustation, and obstruction were similarly identified. Goldsmith et al. (2012) found a 35% failure rate of metallic stents in 25 patients undergoing stent placement for malignant obstruction. Persistent obstruction, distal stent migration, and subcapsular hematoma were noted, and at the present time there is no clear consensus regarding the benefits of metallic stents. More recently, a systematic review of the literature confers that metallic stents are a viable alternative because of a low migration rate (1%); however, high-quality studies are needed in this area (Khoo et al., 2018).

Balloon Dilation

Retrograde Balloon Dilation. Retrograde dilation of ureteral strictures has historically been part of the urologic armamentarium. The technique was rarely definitive and usually required repeated dilations on a

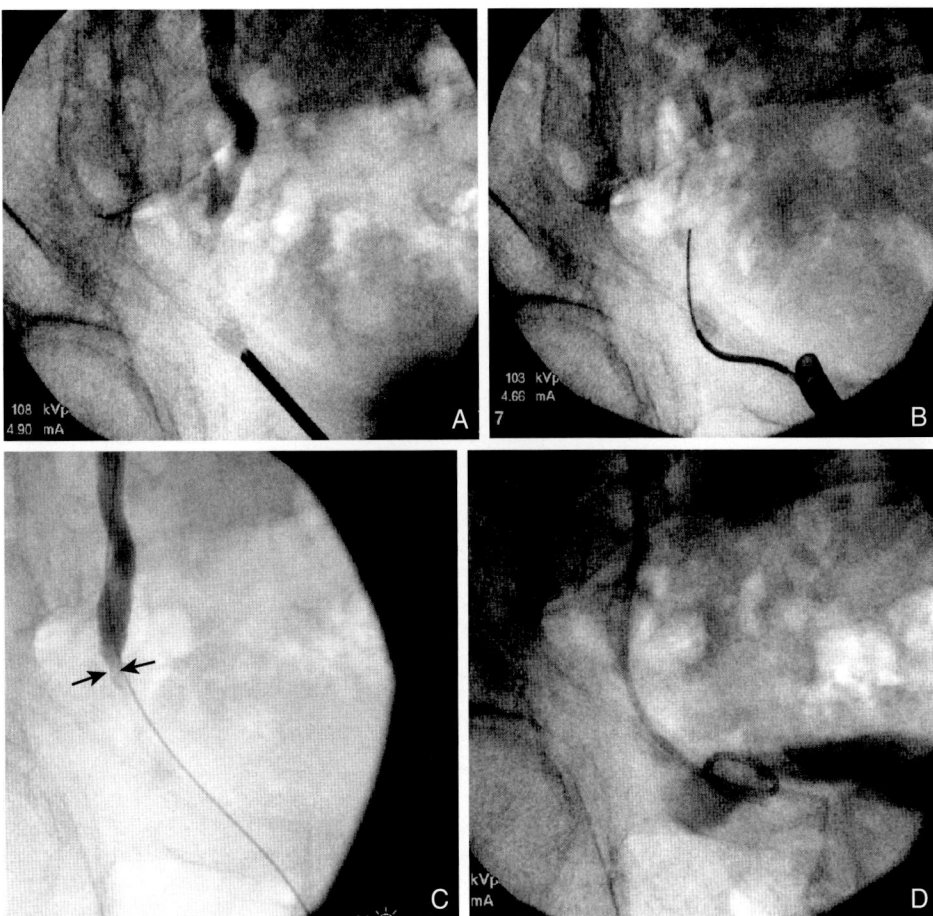

Fig. 89.23. (A) Antegrade and retrograde contrast demonstrating a distal ureteral stricture after prior traumatic ureteroscopic stone procedure. (B) Image demonstrating complex guidewire access across this long and narrow stricture with retained proximal stones. (C) The stricture is greater than 2 cm, and minimal contrast would pass through antegrade. (D) Image after ureteral stent placement. This patient required ureteral reimplantation and stone removal.

regular basis. In the early 1980s angiographic and vascular balloons were introduced into urologic practice, and the technique of balloon dilation with temporary internal stenting became an accepted mode of treatment (Banner et al., 1983; Finnerty et al., 1984).

As for any patient with a ureteral stricture, the indications to intervene include functionally significant obstruction. Contraindications to this approach include active infection or a stricture longer than 2 cm because dilation alone will rarely be successful in this setting. Moreover, any endoscopic technique is likely to fail with strictures greater than 2 cm (Fig. 89.23).

A retrograde approach is indicated whenever access across the strictured area is easily accomplished using transurethral techniques. In general, the procedure begins with a retrograde pyelogram performed under fluoroscopic control to precisely delineate the site and length of stricture. A floppy-tipped guidewire is passed in a retrograde fashion across the strictured area and coiled proximally in the pyelocalyceal system. This is most easily accomplished by passing an open-ended catheter up to the level of the stricture to use as a guide for the hydrophilic or floppy-tipped wire. Passage of the open-ended catheter through the strictured area over the wire will then aid subsequent passage of a balloon catheter. Techniques for bypassing difficult areas of obstruction have been described in detail (Mata et al., 1994).

At this point, the open-ended catheter is withdrawn and replaced with a high-pressure, 4-cm–long, 5- to 8-mm balloon. Under fluoroscopic control, the balloon catheter is positioned across the strictured area, with proper position ensured by visualization of radiopaque markers at the tips of the balloon. Balloon inflation is then begun, and a waist will be visualized at the strictured area, which will disappear with progressive balloon inflation (Fig. 89.24). After 10 minutes of tamponade, the balloon is deflated and withdrawn. A guidewire is still in place, and this is used to pass an internal stent, which is left indwelling for 2 to 4 weeks. Follow-up diuretic renography is usually performed approximately 1 month after stent extraction and at 6- to 12-month intervals thereafter.

Occasionally, access across the involved area cannot be obtained using fluoroscopic control alone. In such cases direct ureteroscopic visualization can aid initial passage of the guidewire, and the procedure can be continued as described. Alternatively, a low-profile balloon can be passed through the ureteroscope and the stricture dilated under direct vision.

Antegrade Balloon Dilation. At times, retrograde access across a strictured area is impossible. In such cases, access can be obtained using an antegrade approach and fluoroscopic control (Banner and Pollack, 1984; Mitty et al., 1983), with or without direct antegrade ureteroscopic visualization (de Jonge et al., 1986). **Percutaneous nephrostomy drainage is established; in cases associated with infection or compromised renal function, percutaneous drainage alone is instituted to allow resolution of infection and return to baseline renal function.** Once that is accomplished, the percutaneous tract is used for access for a fluoroscopically or ureteroscopically guided approach. The procedure is then analogous to a retrograde approach. Under fluoroscopic guidance, an antegrade contrast agent study is used to definitively define the site and length of the stricture. A floppy-tipped guidewire or glidewire is passed antegrade across the level of obstruction; then a balloon catheter is passed, and the

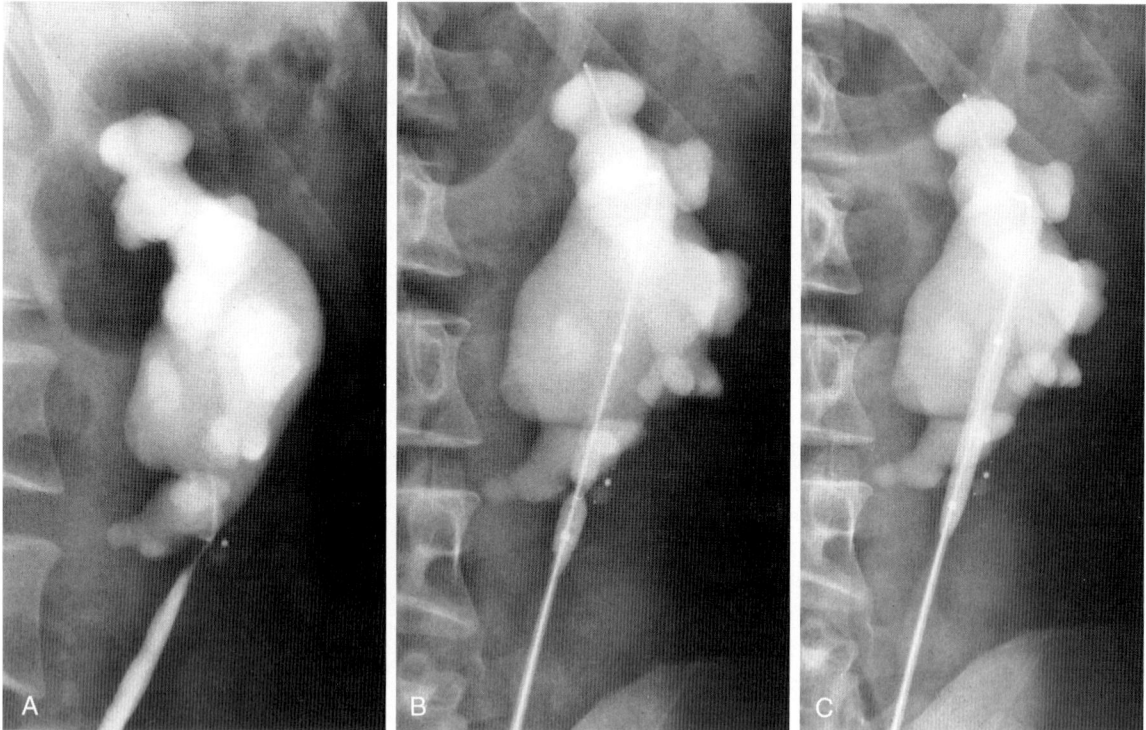

Fig. 89.24. (A) Retrograde study confirms a short stricture at the level of the ureteropelvic junction in this patient with a horseshoe kidney referred after failed ureteroscopic management of a ureteral calculus impacted at that level. (B) The stricture has been traversed with a guidewire, over which a high-pressure balloon has been passed. A waist is evident at the level of the stricture during initial balloon inflation. (C) Balloon inflation and stricture dilation are complete with disappearance of the waist.

balloon is progressively inflated until the waist disappears. The balloon catheter is withdrawn over a wire and replaced with an internal stent, and a nephrostomy tube is also left indwelling. A follow-up nephrostogram is obtained within 24 to 48 hours to ensure proper positioning of a functional internal stent, and at that time the nephrostomy tube can be removed. Alternatively, access can be maintained by the use of an internal-external stent, which can be capped to allow internal drainage.

Results. Initial reports of retrograde and antegrade balloon dilation of ureteral strictures suggested that results were better when the stricture was anastomotic and of relatively short duration and length (Chang et al., 1987; King et al., 1984b; Netto et al., 1990). Goldfischer and Gerber (1997) **reviewed the literature regarding results of balloon dilation of ureteral strictures and found reported success rates ranging from 50% to 76%. In that review, the best results were obtained in patients with iatrogenic, nonanastomotic strictures such as those who had undergone ureteroscopic instrumentation. In that setting, a success rate of 85% was achieved compared with a rate of 50% for anastomotic strictures.** Alternatively, Ravery et al. (1998) found a 40% success rate using retrograde balloon dilation in treating inflammatory ureteral strictures at 16 months' follow-up. Richter et al. (2000) reviewed their results with balloon dilation in 114 patients with a minimum 2-year follow-up. As in other series, balloon dilation was more successful for patients with relatively short strictures. In addition, these authors noted the significance of an intact vascular supply on the success of this procedure. Koukouras et al. (2010) reported antegrade percutaneous balloon treatment of iatrogenic ureteral strictures with 72% success at 1-year follow-up. One series of transplant ureteral strictures in which percutaneous balloon dilation was used in 14 transplant patients demonstrated 79% success at 29 months. Notably, these were short, anastomotic strictures in patients on immunosuppression (Voegeli et al., 1988). Others report endoureterotomy as the primary treatment option in such cases (Duty et al., 2013). In experimental models, balloon dilation created longitudinal incisions similar to endoureterotomy, explaining some of the success seen with use of balloon dilation in ureteral strictures (Nakada et al., 1996).

Endoureterotomy

Endoluminal ureteral incision is a logical extension of balloon dilation for "minimally invasive" management of ureteral strictures. As for balloon dilation, access to and across the strictured area can be obtained in a retrograde or antegrade fashion, although a retrograde approach is preferred because it is less invasive. The antegrade approach is indicated when percutaneous access is already present. The procedure is performed under direct vision using ureteroscopic control or it can be guided fluoroscopically using the hot-wire cutting balloon catheter. In general, radiographic follow-up using diuretic renography is recommended for up to 2 years to detect most late failures (Wolf et al., 1997).

Retrograde Ureteroscopic Approach. A retrograde study is performed under fluoroscopic control at the outset of the procedure. Whenever possible, a floppy-tipped guidewire or hydrophilic glidewire is passed across the level of obstruction as outlined earlier. If a wire cannot be passed across the strictured area using fluoroscopic control alone, the flexible ureteroscope is passed to the level of obstruction, and the guidewire is advanced through the ureteroscope across the involved area under direct vision. The ureteroscope is then withdrawn, but a safety wire is always left in place across the stricture. The ureteroscope is then reintroduced and passed alongside the guidewire to the level of obstruction.

The position for the endoureterotomy incision is chosen as a function of the level of the ureter involved. **In general, lower ureteral strictures are incised in an anteromedial direction, taking care to stay away from the iliac vessels. In contrast, upper ureteral strictures are incised laterally or posterolaterally, again away from the great vessels** (Meretyk et al., 1992; Fig. 89.25).

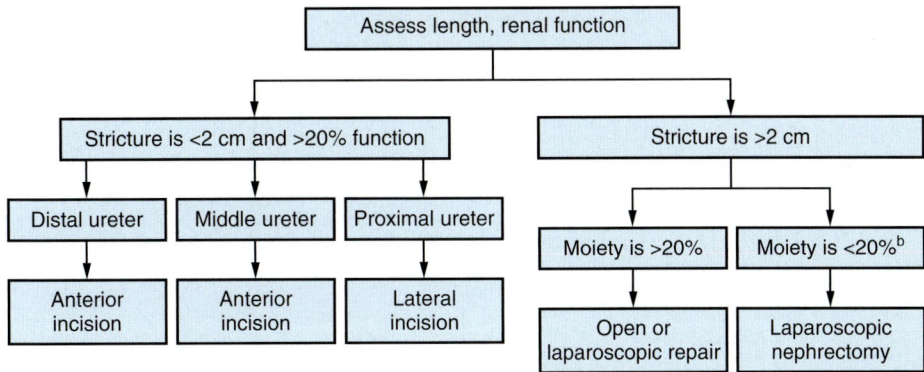

Fig. 89.25. Algorithm for management of benign ureteral stricture disease.

The ureterotomy incision can be performed using a cold knife (Schneider et al., 1991; Yamada et al., 1995), a cutting electrode (Conlin et al., 1996), or a holmium laser. Today, the holmium laser represents the dominant approach to endoscopic incisions. In all cases the incision is made from the ureteral lumen out to periureteral fat in a full-thickness fashion. Proximally and distally, the endoureterotomy should encompass 2 to 3 mm of normal ureteral tissue. In certain instances the stricture must be balloon dilated to gain access across the stricture (Fig. 89.26). Similarly, the strictures may be balloon dilated after endoincision, to enlarge the incision. Once the endoureterotomy incision is complete, the remaining guidewire is used to pass an internal stent. In general, the larger-diameter stents should be considered because larger stents (8 to 12 Fr) have been associated with improved results (Hwang et al., 1996; Wolf et al., 1997). Similarly, Wolf et al. (1997) found benefit in the injection of triamcinolone ureteroscopically after endoureterotomy. Steroids and other biologic response modifiers may eventually have a role in the future in managing select strictures.

Results. The success of holmium laser endoureterotomy ranges from 66% to 83% in series of more than 10 patients with longer than 12 months' follow-up (Gdor et al., 2008b; Hibi et al., 2007; Lane et al., 2006). There is early evidence that strictures related to stone impaction and prior stone treatment may have lower success rates (56% in one series) than typical benign strictures (Gdor et al., 2008a). As ureteroscopy and laser lithotripsy continue to grow, more strictures involving impacted stones may be encountered, and this may become a growing clinical problem. Gdor et al. (2008b) reported 67% success in treating transplant ureteral strictures using the holmium laser at 58 months' follow-up, and more recently Mano et al. (2012) reported an 83% success rate in 26 transplant patients at 44 months' follow-up, with 67% of the patients having undergone initial percutaneous balloon dilation. **The familiarity of ureteroscopy, coupled with relative availability of the holmium laser, makes retrograde laser endoureterotomy an attractive initial management strategy for ureteral strictures less than 2 cm in length.** Meretyk et al. (1992) and Razdan et al. (2005) reported poor results using the retrograde approach in patients with strictures longer than 2 cm.

Antegrade Approach. When direct visual ureteroscopic access to the strictured area cannot be accomplished in a retrograde fashion, an antegrade approach may be used. Nephrostomy tube drainage is instituted, and any associated infection or compromised renal function is allowed to resolve before definitive incision. The percutaneous tract is dilated to a size large enough to allow a working sheath through which a flexible ureteroscope is passed. The procedure is then performed in a fashion analogous to a retrograde approach. A safety wire should be in place at all times alongside the ureteroscope, across the obstructed area and coiled distally in the bladder.

Combined Retrograde and Antegrade Approach. Rarely, a ureteral stricture is associated with an area of complete ureteral obliteration across which a wire cannot be passed to allow subsequent balloon dilation or ureteroscopic endoureterotomy. Typically open or robotic reconstruction is best when possible. In cases where surgery is high risk, a combined retrograde and antegrade approach has been described (Beaghler et al., 1997; Cardella et al., 1985; Conlin et al., 1996; Knowles et al., 2001). This approach should be taken on with caution. The obstructed area is defined radiographically with a simultaneous antegrade and retrograde pyelogram. Endoscopes are passed simultaneously in a retrograde and an antegrade manner, and the two opposing ureteral ends are localized under fluoroscopic guidance. A working guidewire is then passed from one end of the ureter, through and through to the other lumen, using a combination of fluoroscopic and direct visual control. For completely obliterated ureteral segments, this is most easily accomplished using the stiff end of a guidewire passed through a semirigid ureteroscope via the retrograde approach, although when a semirigid ureteroscope cannot be placed, a flexible ureteroscope or even an open-ended ureteral catheter can be used to stabilize the wire from above or below. The ureteral segments are aligned as closely as possible under endoscopic and fluoroscopic guidance, and the light source to one of the ureteroscopes is turned off. The light from the opposite ureteroscope is then used to aid incisional restoration of urinary continuity. The strictured area is then recannulated using the stiff end of a guidewire, a small electrocautery electrode, or holmium laser. Once through-and-through control is obtained with a guidewire, a stent is passed and left in place for 8 to 10 weeks. As with other endourologic approaches to ureteral strictures, success rates are inversely related to the length of the strictured area. **Although success rates may be uncertain, internalization of urinary flow, even when dependent on long-term stent placement, can be a quality-of-life advantage for certain high-risk patients.** Knowles et al. (2001) reported a 90% patency rate at 36 months' follow-up for use of cautery wire balloon incision to treat 10 patients with obliterated distal ureteral segments, 3 of whom required the combined. Bach et al. (2008) reported a retrograde blind (fluoroscopically guided) endoureterotomy with a 61% success rate in patients with subtotal ureteral strictures.

Surgical Repair

Before any surgical repair, it is essential to conduct careful evaluation of the nature, location, and length of the ureteral stricture. Preoperative assessment typically includes an intravenous pyelogram (or antegrade nephrostogram) and a retrograde pyelogram if indicated as the location and length of the stricture heavily influence the options for repair. Other studies such as a nuclear medicine diuretic renogram to assess renal function and ureteroscopy, ureteral barbotage, and/

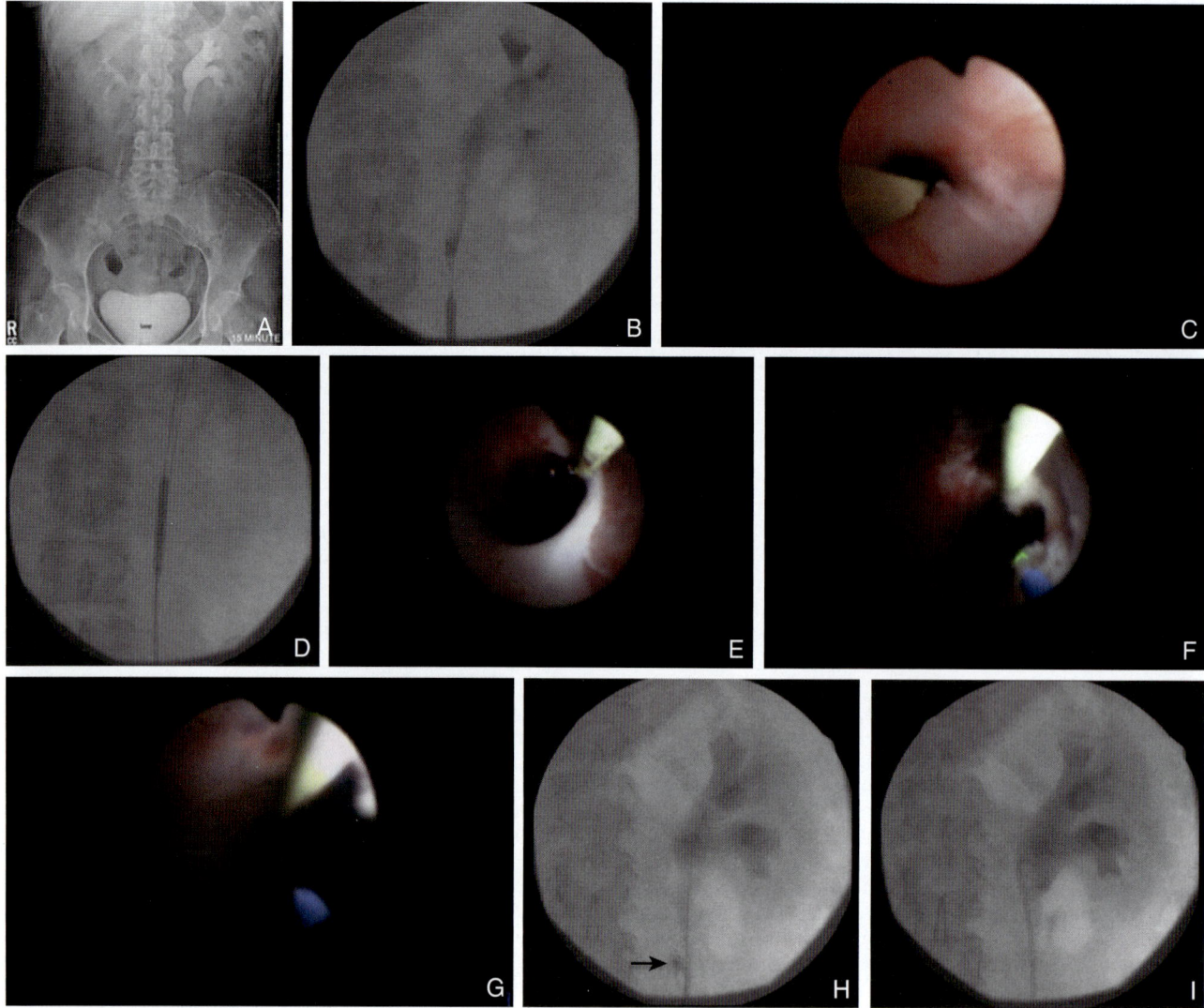

Fig. 89.26. (A) Preoperative excretory urogram showing proximal ureteral stricture after ureteral injury. (B) Fluoroscopic image of flexible ureteroscope at stricture. (C) Corresponding endoscopic image of stricture. (D) Fluoroscopic image of balloon dilation to enable incision of ureteral stricture. (E) Endoscopic image of strictured area after balloon dilation (note resultant full-thickness, lateral incision). (F) Endoscopic view completing laser incision of stricture. (G) Endoscopic view of full-thickness incision. (H) Fluoroscopic image demonstrating extravasation *(arrow)*. (I) Fluoroscopic image after stent placement.

or brushing to rule out carcinoma should be individualized. On the basis of such information, the appropriate surgical procedure can then be planned for the patient (Table 89.2).

Ureteroureterostomy

A short defect involving the upper ureter or midureter, either in the form of stricture or as a consequence of recent injury, is most appropriate for ureteroureterostomy. On the other hand, a lower ureteral stricture is usually best managed by ureteroneocystostomy with or without a psoas hitch or Boari flap. In the transplant setting, a donor ureteral stricture may be managed by a ureteroureterostomy to a healthy, native ureter. Because tension on the anastomosis almost always leads to stricture formation, only short defects should be managed by end-to-end ureteroureterostomy. Determination of whether enough ureteral mobility can be achieved to allow tension-free ureteroureterostomy usually cannot be made until the time of surgery, and thus the urologist must be prepared to pursue other options.

Open Approach. The choice of surgical incision depends on the level of the ureteral stricture. A flank incision is appropriate for the upper ureter. A Gibson or a lower midline incision is suitable for

TABLE 89.2 Bridging Various Ureteral Defect Lengths With Different Reconstructive Surgical Techniques

TECHNIQUE	URETERAL DEFECT LENGTH (cm)
Ureteroureterostomy	2–3
Ureteroneocystostomy	4–5
Psoas hitch	6–10
Boari flap	12–15
Renal descensus	5–8

the middle and lower ureter. If the patient has sustained an iatrogenic ureteral injury from a previous surgery performed through a Pfannenstiel incision, the same incision may be used for the ureteral reconstruction. In such situations, proximal ureteral dissection may be difficult through the Pfannenstiel incision, requiring cephalad extension of the lateral portion of the incision in a "hockey-stick"

KEY POINTS: ENDOUROLOGIC MANAGEMENT OF URETERAL STRICTURES

- Proper evaluation and treatment of a ureteral stricture are essential to preserve renal function and rule out the presence of malignancy. It is critical to assess the renal unit for function before starting treatment because endourologic therapies typically require 25% function of the ipsilateral moiety.
- The use of chronic stent placement for extrinsic ureteral obstruction must be guarded because the drainage is often limited. Innovations in stents and stent techniques have led to long-term success in select patients with malignant ureteral obstruction.
- The indications to intervene for ureteral stricture disease include clinical symptoms and functionally significant obstruction. Contraindications to this approach include active infection or a stricture longer than 2 cm.
- Current available reports and the familiarity of ureteroscopy, coupled with relative availability of the holmium laser, make retrograde laser endoureterotomy an attractive initial management strategy for short ureteral strictures.
- The position for the endoureterotomy incision is chosen as a function of the level of the ureter involved. In general, lower ureteral strictures are incised in an anteromedial direction, taking care to stay away from the iliac vessels. In contrast, upper ureteral strictures are incised laterally or posterolaterally, away from the great vessels.

fashion. Extraperitoneal dissection is usually performed except in cases of transperitoneal surgical ureteral injury.

After surgical incision, the retroperitoneal space is developed as the peritoneum is mobilized and retracted medially. Frequently, the ureter can be easily identified as it crosses the iliac vessels. A Penrose drain or vessel loop may be placed around the ureter to assist its atraumatic handling. Direct handling of the ureter with forceps should be minimized. Care should be taken to preserve its adventitia, which loosely attaches the blood supply to the ureter.

During ureteral dissection and mobilization, enough mobility must be achieved to avoid tension after the excision of the diseased ureter. With a gunshot injury, devitalized tissue and an adjacent segment of normal-appearing ureter should be excised to eliminate late ischemia and stricture formation from the blast effect. Once both ends of the ureter have been adequately trimmed to healthy areas, mobilized, and correctly oriented, they are spatulated for approximately 5 to 6 mm. Spatulation is performed for both ureteral segments at 180 degrees apart. If a grossly dilated ureter is involved, it may be transected obliquely and not spatulated to match the circumference of the nondilated segment. A fine, absorbable suture is placed in the corner of one ureteral segment and the apex of the other, and the two ends of the suture are tied outside the ureteral lumen. The opposite corner and apex are similarly sutured and approximated. The anastomosis may then be completed by running these two sutures continuously and tying them to each other or in an interrupted fashion (Fig. 89.27). A double-J ureteral stent should be placed before completion of the anastomotic closure. Stent placement can be facilitated by passing the wire through one of the side holes in the middle of the stent to straighten and stiffen the stent enough to permit it to pass. Observation of reflux of methylene blue

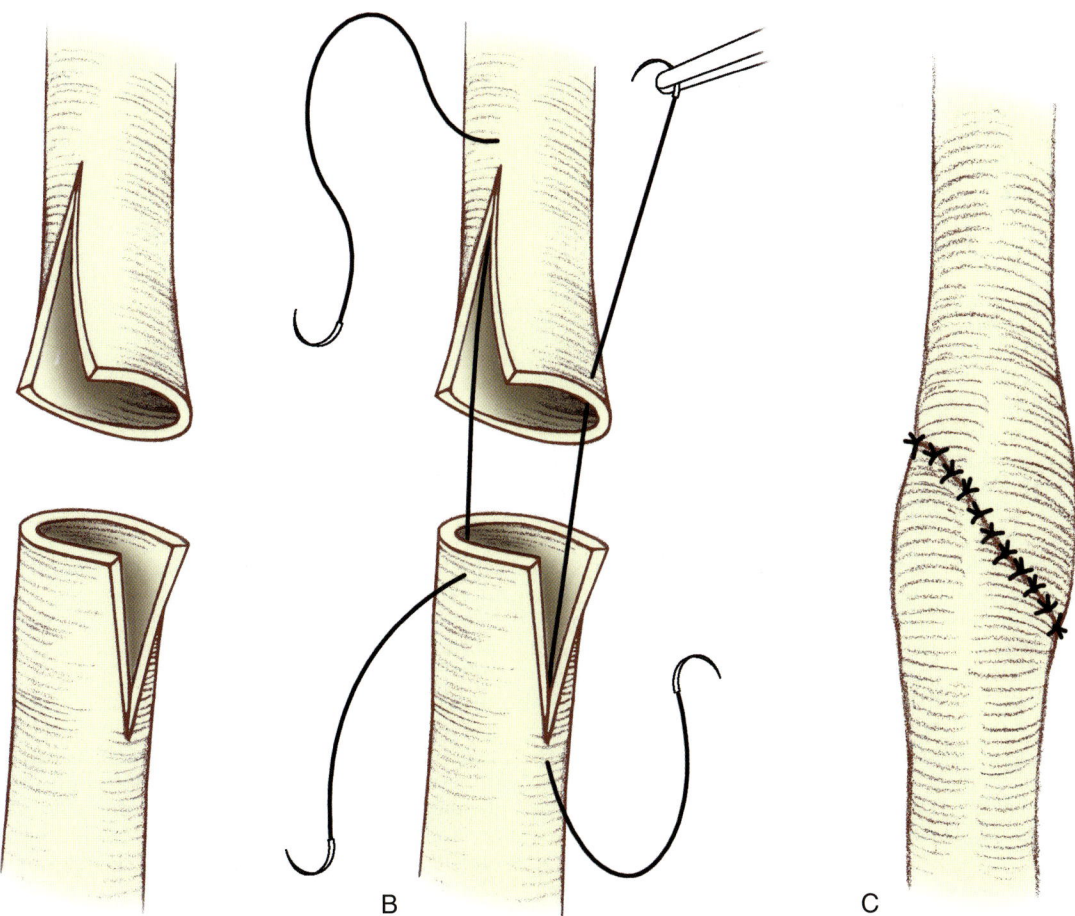

Fig. 89.27. (A) Spatulated ureteral ends. (B) Placement of sutures. (C) End-to-end ureteroureterostomy.

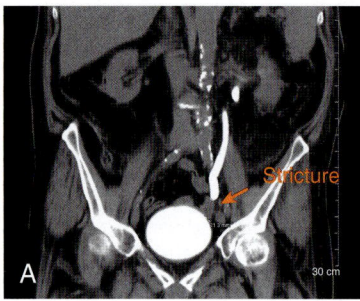 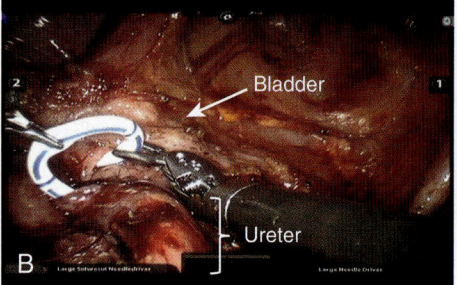 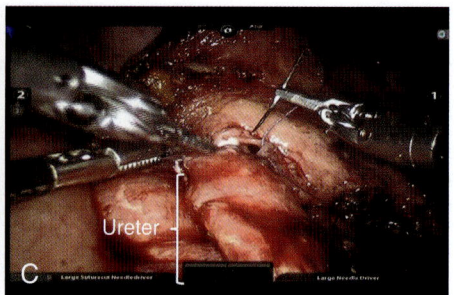

Fig. 89.28. Intraoperative photograph of a patient undergoing a robotic right ureteral neocystostomy for distal ureteral stricture seen in computed tomography urography (A). (B) The distal coil of the ureteral stent being placed through the opening in the bladder after completion of half the ureteral anastomosis. (C) Completing the ureteral anastomosis.

irrigant from the bladder to the ureterotomy can be used to verify the appropriate placement of the distal stent in the bladder. Retroperitoneal fat or omentum may be used to cover the anastomosis.
Laparoscopic or Robotic Approach. A laparoscopic or robotic approach may be offered to patients with ureteral stricture disease. Nezhat et al. (1992) first reported laparoscopic management of an obstructed ureter resulting from endometriosis. In this case, ureteroureterostomy was performed laparoscopically over a ureteral stent after resection of the obstructed ureteral site. Most of the studies since that time consist of single case reports or small series. Several reports of laparoscopic ureteroureterostomy to unobstruct a duplicated system in the pediatric population have appeared (Piaggio et al., 2007; Smith et al., 2009). More recently, the robotic-assisted approach has been applied to laparoscopic ureteroureterostomy in a small number of patients (Lee et al., 2010; Mufarrij et al., 2007; Passerotti et al., 2008). Lee et al. (2010) reported a series of three robotic ureteroureterostomies, all successful by symptom and nuclear renal scan criteria at an average of 24 months. The overall clinical experience in minimally invasive ureteroureterostomy is limited worldwide. However, in the hands of the experienced surgeons, it appears to be a viable minimally invasive approach applicable to almost any patient with a relatively short area of obstruction.
Postoperative Care. The postoperative care of ureteroureterostomy patients is similar, regardless of surgical approach. A surgical drain is placed, and a Foley catheter is generally left indwelling for 1 to 2 days. The surgical drain may be removed if there is minimal output for 24 to 48 hours. If the surgical procedure is not performed entirely in a retroperitoneal manner, it is important to determine the nature of the fluid from the surgical drain, which can be achieved by checking the creatinine level of the fluid. If there is no urinary extravasation, the drain can then be removed. The double-J ureteral stent is removed endoscopically, usually 4 to 6 weeks postoperatively.

The success rate for a tension-free, watertight ureteroureterostomy is high—more than 90% (Carlton et al., 1969; Guiter et al., 1985). If a urinary fistula is suspected, a plain abdominal radiograph should first be obtained to verify the position of the double-J stent. The proximity of a drain to the anastomosis should also be checked because it may exacerbate a leak. If this occurs, suction should be stopped if a suction drain device is used because straight drainage may assist closure of the ureteral leakage site. Reflux from voiding or bladder spasms may also contribute to prolonged urinary extravasation, a problem that can be managed by Foley catheter drainage and anticholinergics. Prolonged urinary leakage from the anastomosis may require the placement of a nephrostomy tube for proximal urinary diversion.

Ureteroneocystostomy

Ureteroneocystostomy in an adult is appropriate for injury or obstruction affecting the distal 3 to 4 cm of the ureter. As is the case in all ureteral repairs, a tension-free anastomosis is critical and thus modifications such as a psoas hitch or Boari flap may be necessary.

Repair of the distal ureter can be accomplished by either open or minimally invasive techniques. Successful laparoscopic application to ureteroneocystostomy has been reported by a variety of investigators (Ehrlich et al., 1993; Gözen et al., 2010; Reddy et al., 1994; Yohannes and Smith, 2001). In the management of distal ureteral stricture, laparoscopic ureteroneocystostomy is usually performed transperitoneally incorporating intracorporeal suturing techniques because it provides a large working space. Ureteral stenting is typically used postoperatively as in open surgery. Although this procedure requires intracorporeal laparoscopic suturing, the overall clinical experience for laparoscopic management of distal ureteral strictures has been increasing over time. Abraham et al. (2011) reported their experience performing laparoscopic ureteral reimplantation in 36 patients and reported success in all patients at a mean of 16 months' follow-up. Overall, the clinical outcomes have been reported favorable to and comparable with those of open surgical data while providing minimal postoperative morbidity, as in many other laparoscopic urologic procedures. LESS neocystostomy has been reported as well (Khanna et al., 2012).

As is the case for many reconstructive urologic procedures, urologists have reported finding the robotic platform useful in neocystostomy (Fig. 89.28; Laungani et al., 2008; Mufarrij et al., 2007; Williams et al., 2009). This procedure can typically be performed using a 4-arm robotic approach with port placement similar to that of a robotic prostatectomy or with ports shifted slightly cephalad. Isac et al. (2013) reported similar success rates for robotic and open neocystostomy with the robotic approach being associated with a significantly shorter hospital stay (3 vs. 5 days, $P = 0.0004$) and less narcotic use (morphine equivalent, mg 104.6 vs. 290, $P = 0.0001$). Musch et al. (2013) reported a robotic approach to be effective even in cases requiring a psoas hitch or Boari flap.

Psoas Hitch

The psoas hitch is an effective method to bridge a defect of the lower third of the ureter, providing an additional up to 5 cm of length compared with simple ureteroneocystostomy. However, a ureteral defect extending proximal to the pelvic brim usually requires more than a psoas hitch alone. Indications include distal ureteral stricture, injury, and failed ureteroneocystostomy (Ehrlich et al., 1978; Prout and Koontz, 1970; Rodo Salas et al., 1991). A psoas hitch may also be used in conjunction with other maneuvers such as a transureteroureterostomy (TUU) in more complicated urinary tract reconstruction. **Generally, a small, contracted bladder with limited mobility is considered a contraindication.** In addition to the preoperative radiographic and endoscopic evaluation described previously, urodynamic studies may provide information regarding bladder capacity and compliance before the surgery. Bladder outlet obstruction or neurogenic dysfunction, if present, must be treated preoperatively.

Relative to Boari flap, the advantages of psoas hitch include increased technical simplicity and decreased risk for vascular compromise and voiding difficulties. The success rate of ureteroneocystostomy with a psoas hitch is greater than 85% in adults and children (Ahn and Loughlin, 2001; Mathews and Marshall, 1997). Complications occur uncommonly but have included urinary fistula, ureteral obstruction, nerve injury, bowel injury, iliac vein injury, and urosepsis.

Boari Flap

When the diseased ureteral segment is too long or when ureteral mobility is too limited to perform a tension-free ureteroureterostomy, a Boari flap may be a useful alternative. Boari first described the use of this technique in the canine model in 1894. **A Boari flap can be constructed to bridge a 10- to 15-cm ureteral defect, and a spiraled bladder flap can reach the renal pelvis in some circumstances, especially on the right side.** As in a psoas hitch, evaluation of bladder function and capacity should be performed preoperatively in addition to the ureteral evaluation. Bladder outlet obstruction and neurogenic dysfunction, if present, should be addressed preoperatively. **A small bladder capacity is likely to be associated with difficult or inadequate Boari flap creation, warranting consideration of alternative methods in the preoperative surgical planning.**

The number of reported patients treated with a Boari flap is small, yet the results are good if a well-vascularized flap is used (Middleton, 1980; Motiwala et al., 1990; Ockerblad, 1947; Scott and Greenberg, 1972; Thompson and Ross, 1974). The most common complication is clearly recurrent stricture formation, resulting from either ischemia or excessive tension on the anastomosis. Rare pseudodiverticulum has also been reported (Berzeg et al., 2003). Mauck et al. (2011) reported success in 9 out of 10 patients with proximal ureteral strictures treated with a Boari flap (+/- simultaneous downward nephropexy) at 12.8 months' mean follow-up.

A series of 98 patients undergoing ureteral reimplantation by Wenske et al. (2013), 76 of whom had a psoas hitch with or without Boari flap, particularly studied postoperative changes in renal function. They found that in 44% of the cases, postoperative eGFR declined in the first 2 years after surgery, despite hydronephrosis resolving in most patients. Interestingly, men and those patients with abnormal preoperative renal function were more likely to experience a loss of function during follow-up. These findings may help counsel patients about their chances of experiencing a renal functional improvement with surgical repair.

Fugita, Dinlenc, and Kavoussi reported three successful cases of laparoscopic Boari flap for distal ureteral obstruction, in which a transperitoneal approach was used (Fugita et al., 2001). Following the same principles in open surgery, the bladder flap was created and anastomosed to the ureteral end over a stent in a tension-free, water-tight manner. Operative time ranged from 120 to 330 minutes, and blood loss ranged from 400 to 600 mL. Two patients were discharged home within 3 days postoperatively, whereas 1 patient was hospitalized for 13 days for *Clostridium difficile* colitis. With a follow-up of more than 6 months, there was radiographically demonstrated patency of the anastomosis. In this report, the information of the length of distal ureteral stricture was not available. More recently, laparoscopic Boari flap assisted by the robot has been successfully performed (Allaparthi et al., 2010; Kozinn et al., 2012; Musch et al., 2013; Schimpf and Wagner, 2009; Yang et al., 2011). Transperitoneal approach was used in all cases reported thus far.

The issue of refluxing versus antirefluxing anastomosis in ureteroneocystostomy in adults has been examined previously. In a retrospective review of adult patients with ureteroneocystostomy, no significant difference in the preservation of renal function or risk of stenosis was identified in the refluxing versus antirefluxing procedures (Stefanovic et al., 1991). However, it is unclear if a nonrefluxing anastomosis decreases the risk of pyelonephritis in an adult patient.

Renal Descensus

Renal mobilization, which was originally described by Popescu in 1964, can provide additional length to bridge a defect in the upper ureter or decrease tension on a ureteral repair (Harada et al., 1964; Passerini-Glazel et al., 1994). A transperitoneal, subcostal, midline, or paramedian incision may be used to gain access to the kidney and the appropriate level of the ureter. Following entry to the Gerota fascia, the kidney is completely mobilized and rotated inferiorly and medially on its vascular pedicle. The lower pole of the kidney is then secured to the retroperitoneal muscle using several absorbable sutures. Up to 8 cm of additional length may be gained using this technique. In such cases the renal vessels—especially the renal vein—limit the extent to which the kidney can be mobilized. As a solution, the technique for division of the renal vein with reanastomosis more inferiorly to the inferior vena cava may be performed but rarely applied clinically. Renal decensus may also be combined with other reconstructive techniques such as a Boari flap to repair panureteral strictures. In addition, laparoscopic techniques have been reported (Sutherland et al., 2011).

Transureteroureterostomy

The initial clinical application of TUU was described by Higgins in 1934. In the management of ureteral stricture, a TUU may be used when ureteral length is insufficient for anastomosis to the bladder (Brannan, 1975). **The only absolute contraindication is insufficient length of the donor ureter to reach the contralateral recipient ureter in a tension-free manner. However, any disease process that may affect both ureters represents a relative contraindication. Absolute contraindications include the presence of a diseased recipient ureter or a donor ureter of inadequate length. Relative contraindications include history of nephrolithiasis, retroperitoneal fibrosis, urothelial malignancy, chronic pyelonephritis, and abdominopelvic radiation. Reflux to the recipient ureter, if present, must be identified and corrected simultaneously.** Therefore a voiding cystogram should be performed preoperatively, in addition to the other imaging and endoscopic studies previously described for thorough evaluation of both ureters.

In performing a TUU, a midline, transperitoneal approach is used to gain access to both ureters. After medial colonic mobilization, the affected ureter is mobilized, preserving the adventitia with the ureteral blood supply, and divided just proximal to the level of obstruction. The contralateral colon is medially mobilized. Only the portion of recipient ureter needed for the anastomosis is exposed, which is generally 5 cm proximal to the level of division of the affected ureter. A tunnel under the sigmoid colon mesentery is created proximal to the inferior mesenteric artery to avoid ureteral tethering by this vessel, after which the donor ureter is then brought through the tunnel to the recipient side. Mobilization of the recipient ureter should be minimized to help preserve the integrity of its vascular supply. An anteromedial ureterotomy is made in the recipient ureter, which is then anastomosed to the spatulated donor ureteral end in a tension-free, watertight manner using either interrupted or running absorbable sutures. A double-J ureteral stent is usually passed from the donor renal pelvis, through the anastomosis and into the bladder. A second ureteral stent may also be placed throughout the length of the recipient ureter if the ureter is found to be adequately large in diameter.

The clinical success of TUU has been demonstrated by multiple investigators. Hendren and Hensle (1980) reported 75 cases of pediatric TUU without compromising a single recipient kidney. Hodges et al. (1980) reported a similar success in a large group of children and adults. However, two patients required revision because of ureteral kinking by the inferior mesenteric artery. The successful application of TUU was further confirmed more recently by Pesce et al. (2001). In two other recent studies, nephrectomy for ureteral stenosis was found to be rarely necessary (Mure et al., 2000; Sugarbaker et al., 2003).

A few reports of successful laparoscopic TUU exist. This may be a viable option in skilled hands, although long-term clinical data to support this technique do not yet exist (Kaiho et al., 2011; Piaggio et al., 2007).

Ileal Ureteral Substitution

Surgical management of long length of ureteral defect or loss, especially the proximal ureter, is particularly challenging (Benson et al., 1990). Reconstruction of the ureter with tissue lined with urothelium is most preferable because urothelium is not absorptive and is resistant to the inflammatory and potentially carcinogenic effects of urine (Harzmann et al., 1986). Incorporation of other tissue in ureteral repair is therefore reserved for situations in which a defect cannot be bridged by other methods or the bladder is unsuitable for reconstruction. In this scenario, ileal interposition has been demonstrated to be a satisfactory option for complicated ureteral reconstruction. On the other hand, the appendix and fallopian tube have been found to be unreliable ureteral substitutes.

Shoemaker reported the first ileal ureter in a woman with tuberculous involvement of the urinary tract in 1909. Later, the metabolic and physiologic effects of the ileal ureter have been investigated in the canine model (Hinman and Oppenheimer, 1958; Martinez et al., 1965). When an isoperistaltic segment of ileum is directly anastomosed to the bladder, reflux and renal pelvic pressure increase are generally seen only during voiding. The retrograde transmission of intravesical pressure is dependent on the length of ileum segment used in interposition and the voiding pressure. In patients with ileal segments longer than 15 cm, Waldner et al. (1999) found no reflux into the renal pelvis in a report involving 19 cases of ileal ureter with refluxing ileovesical anastomosis. Comparing dogs with tapered versus nontapered ileal segments, Waters et al. (1981) found no difference in renal perfusion pressure or metabolic derangements. A large clinical experience in ileal ureter involving 89 patients was reported by Boxer et al. (1979). Only 12% of patients with normal preoperative renal function developed significant metabolic problems postoperatively, and preoperative renal function was identified to be an important prognostic factor.

In a separate study, nearly half of those with a serum creatinine of greater than 2 mg/dL developed hyperchloremic metabolic acidosis, requiring conversion to a conduit (Koch and McDougal, 1985). Patients with bladder dysfunction also experienced more complications. No sufficient clinical data exist to establish the superiority of a tapered segment, a nonrefluxing anastomosis, or a shorter, segmental replacement over a standard ileal substitution (Waters et al., 1981). **Therefore the contraindications to an ileal ureteral substitution are baseline renal insufficiency with a serum creatinine of greater than 2 mg/dL, bladder dysfunction or outlet obstruction, inflammatory bowel disease, or radiation enteritis.**

Before the surgical procedure, a full mechanical and antibiotic bowel preparation is often used. A long midline incision is made. The ipsilateral colon is mobilized medially, and the affected ureter is dissected proximally to the level of healthy tissue. The proximal anastomosis may be performed at the level of the renal pelvis if the entire upper ureter is unhealthy. The length of the ureteral defect is measured, and an appropriate segment of distal ileum is chosen. The segment should be at least 15 cm away from the ileocecal valve, and adequate blood supply should be confirmed before harvesting. The mesentery is usually divided more extensively than with a standard ileal conduit to provide greater mobility. Occasionally, a segment of colon may be more accessible than ileum and is harvested using the similar surgical principles. **In the presence of a scarred or intrarenal pelvis, ileocalycostomy may be performed** (McQuitty et al., 1995). In this circumstance, excision of a piece of lower pole renal parenchymal tissue is helpful in preventing stenosis at the anastomosis, as in a typical ureterocalicostomy. After bowel division, the distal end of the ileal segment is marked for orientation and bowel-to-bowel continuity is reestablished. A small window is made in the colonic mesentery, through which the segment of ileum is delivered laterally. Alternatively, the cecum and ascending colon can be reflected superiorly to avoid mesenteric window creation in performing right ureteral reconstruction. The orientation of the ileal segment is checked to ensure isoperistalsis, and the anastomoses are performed at the level of the renal pelvis or lower pole calyx and at the bladder (Fig. 89.29). Bilateral ileal ureteral substitution

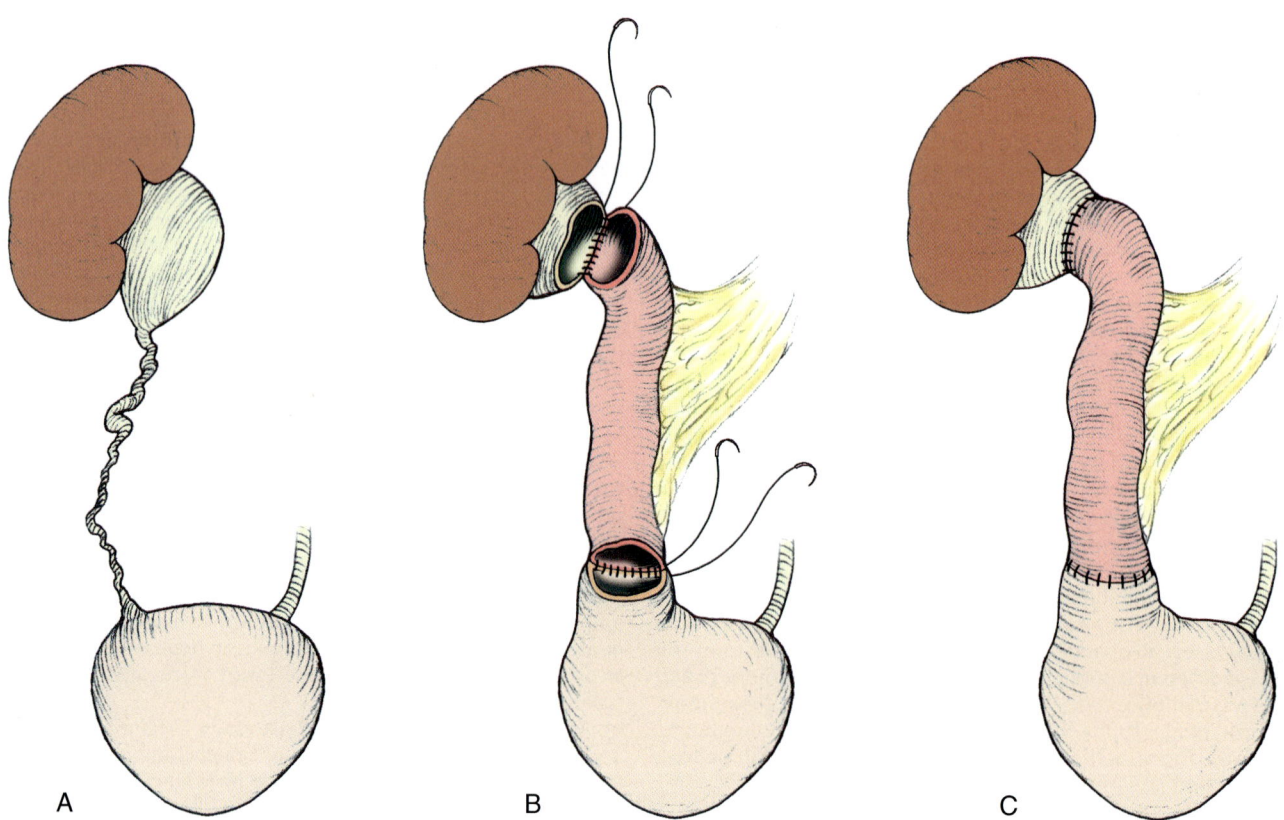

Fig. 89.29. (A) In ileal ureteral substitution, the affected ureter is first identified and dissected; this is followed by removal of the diseased portion. (B) A piece of ileum is brought through the colonic mesentery to bridge the renal pelvis and the bladder. (C) Proximal and distal anastomoses are completed in a full-thickness, watertight, tension-free manner.

may be achieved by using a longer segment that travels intraperitoneally from one kidney to the other and then to the bladder. An alternative to such is to use two separate bowel segments.

Perioperative complications associated with ileal ureter include early urinary extravasation or urinoma formation and obstruction from edema, a mucous plug, or a kink in the segment. Ischemic necrosis of the ileal segment may occur and should be considered if signs of an acute abdomen are present. Significant electrolyte abnormalities and renal insufficiency are unusual if preoperative renal function is normal. **Patients with worsening metabolic abnormalities associated with a progressively dilating ileal ureter should be evaluated for bladder outlet obstruction. Furthermore, malignancy arising from ileal ureter segment has been reported in four cases in the literature** (Austen et al., 2004), **and it is recommended that regular endoscopic examination should be performed starting at postoperative year 3 for early detection of such malignancy.** However, Bonfig et al. (2004) confirmed the safety and reliability of ileal ureter creation for complex ureteral stricture/loss in 43 patients with a mean follow-up of 40.8 months. A more recent study from Wolff et al. (2011) reported long-term follow-up on 17 patients undergoing ileal ureteral substitution (median 174 months) and found that 15 patients still had ileal ureters at the end of the study interval, although 3 patients were later on dialysis. The mean creatinine value at last follow-up was 1.8±0.6 mg/dL.

Larger series with longer follow-up are now appearing in the literature. Kocot et al. (2017) reported outcomes over a mean 54 months in their series of 157 patients. Although functional drainage was not reported, 85% of kidneys displayed a decrease in hydronephrosis, and serum creatinine remained stable or improved in 94%. Hyperchloremic metabolic acidosis requiring pharmacologic treatment was noted in 19.5% of patients. Their conclusion from their 25-year experience with ileal ureteral substitution was that a refluxing anastomosis was typically safe when the ileal segment was anastomosed to a functional bladder but that nonrefluxing reconstruction may be useful in cases in which the urine reservoir is expected to be colonized with bacteria, such as continent cutaneous diversions, to reduce the risk of pyelonephritis. No cases of malignancy in the reconstructed system have been identified.

Minimally Invasive Ileal Ureteral Substitution

The clinical experience in laparoscopic ileal ureteral substitution is limited worldwide, yet this procedure appears to hold significant promise. Gill et al. (2000a) reported successful laparoscopic ileal ureter replacement using a transperitoneal, three-port approach. The feasibility of the laparoscopic approach is affirmed in a more recent publication from Stein et al. (2009), which compared 7 laparoscopic ileal ureters created during the same time period as 7 open procedures. This retrospective comparison found analgesic use and time to convalescence to favor the laparoscopic approach (median morphine equivalents 38.9 vs. 322.2 mg, $P = 0.035$, and 4 vs. 5.5 weeks, $P = 0.03$, respectively). Although median follow-up was short, particularly in the laparoscopic cohort (13 months, range 2–79), the authors report that all procedures were successful by imaging and symptomatic measurements. Since then, several other small case series have been reported favoring the approach.

In addition, several series of robotic-assisted laparoscopic ileal ureter have been published (Brandao et al., 2014; Chopra et al., 2016; Ubrig et al., 2018; Wagner et al., 2008). Of three patients undergoing completely intracorporeal robotic ileal substitution, Chopra et al. (2016) reported one patient had recurrence of urothelial cancer affecting the ipsilateral kidney necessitating later nephroureterectomy; another patient experienced volvulus causing ischemia of the ileal segment postoperative day 4, and this required emergent resection. Although other authors with similarly small series had favorable outcomes, longer follow-up will be needed to assess the outcomes of this approach.

Buccal Mucosa Grafting

The repair of complex, long, or reoperative stricture disease at any position in the ureter remains a challenging prospect, as evidenced by the variety of approaches described to tackle them. The success experienced by surgeons repairing complex urethral strictures using buccal mucosa harvested from the patient's oral cavity has led some surgeons to investigate this tissue as a tool for repairing complex ureteral strictures. This was first reported in humans by Naude in 1999 after working in an animal model, since that time a number of small case series have appeared using this technique in open and minimally invasive approaches, most commonly as an "onlay" similar to urethral repair. A recent multi-institutional series of 19 patients who underwent robotic buccal grafting illustrates the early findings of this technique. Median stricture length was 4 cm, and half of patients had had a prior repair. An omental flap was sewn to the graft to provide blood supply. At a median follow-up of 26 months, 17 of 19 patients remained stricture free (Zhao et al., 2017).

Autotransplantation

In 1963 Hardy performed the first autotransplantation for a patient with proximal ureteral injury. Since then, clinical autotransplantation has been performed for a variety of problems including extensive ureteral loss or stricture (Chuang et al., 1999; Hardy, 1963; Novick and Stewart, 1981; Wotkowicz et al., 2004). Generally, autotransplant is considered when the contralateral kidney is absent or poorly functioning or when other methods for ureteral substitution or repair are not feasible. The kidney is harvested with maximal vessel length as in a typical live donor nephrectomy for allotransplantation, and the renal vessels are anastomosed to the iliac vessels to reestablish renal perfusion. A healthy segment of the proximal ureter is anastomosed to the bladder (Bodie et al., 1986). Alternatively, the ipsilateral renal pelvis may be anastomosed directly to the bladder (Kennelly et al., 1993). Not surprisingly, laparoscopy has been successfully incorporated in autotransplantation for severe ureteral loss. Nephrectomy can be performed laparoscopically as in any typical laparoscopic donor nephrectomy, followed by renal graft retrieval, bench preparation, and autotransplantation in the ipsilateral iliac fossa via a Gibson incision using the standard open surgical techniques (Blueblond-Langner et al., 2004; Fabrizio et al., 2000; Meng et al., 2003). The use of laparoscopy in autotransplantation has been shown to provide reduced postoperative analgesic need and faster recovery because a large open upper abdominal or flank incision for renal harvest is avoided. Laparoscopic nephrectomy in autotransplantation is most commonly performed transperitoneally. However, retroperitoneal approach for such purpose has been applied successfully by Gill et al. (2000b).

URETEROENTERIC ANASTOMOTIC STRICTURE

Incidence and Etiology

Several factors determine the incidence of stricture formation at the anastomosis of the ureter and intestine at the time of urinary diversion. The longest follow-up data available are for urinary conduits, in which the stricture rate is 4% to 9%, and strictures are more common on the left (Anderson et al., 2013; Mattei et al., 2008; Schmidt et al., 1973; Skinner et al., 1980; Westerman et al., 2016). Factors potentially influencing outcome in this population include the technique used for ureteral dissection, the segment of bowel used for the diversion, and the type of anastomosis performed. Because ureteral ischemia is central to the cause of ureteroenteric strictures, careful attention to dissection is necessary to prevent complications. Anderson et al. (2013) found no difference in risk of ureteroenteric anastomotic stricture comparing open versus robotic/lap-assisted radical cystectomy. Another study found most of these strictures were benign (85%) and risk factors included CIS in the ureteral margin (Westerman et al., 2016).

The ureteral blood supply runs parallel to the ureter in the adventitia, and although ureteral mobilization is necessary to approximate the ureter and bowel and prevent tension on the anastomosis, stripping the ureter of its surrounding adventitia can lead to ureteral ischemia and stricture formation. The ileotomy

> **KEY POINTS: SURGICAL REPAIR OF URETERAL STRICTURE**
>
> - Only short ureteral defects may be managed by end-to-end ureteroureterostomy.
> - Distal ureteral stricture may be managed with ureteroneocystostomy with a psoas hitch or Boari flap.
> - Boari flap may be used to bridge a 10- to 15-cm ureteral defect. Small bladder capacity is a contraindication to such flap creation. Care should be taken to ensure adequate vascular supply to the flap.
> - Transureteroureterostomy is contraindicated in the presence of any disease process that may affect both ureters. It is also contraindicated if there is insufficient length of the donor ureter to reach the contralateral recipient ureter in a tension-free manner.
> - Ileal ureter is useful in the presence of extensive ureteral loss. It is contraindicated in cases of baseline renal insufficiency with a serum creatinine of greater than 2 mg/dL, bladder dysfunction or outlet obstruction, inflammatory bowel disease, or radiation cystitis.
> - Autotransplantation is considered when the contralateral kidney is absent or poorly functioning or when other methods for ureteral substitution or repair are not feasible.
> - Laparoscopic or robotic reconstructive techniques in the hands of urologists skilled in these approaches may provide quicker recovery for patients.

technique is also a consideration. Cheng et al. (2011) reported using a shield-shaped ileotomy rather than a slit-shaped incision and found a 4.3% stricture rate compared with 8.3% in a retrospective assessment. Barbieri et al. (2010) reported ureteroileal anastomosis with intraluminal visualization in 118 patients with a 4.2% stricture rate at 15 months, all on the left side. With this approach the conduit is opened on the antimesenteric border to allow for direct visualization of the anastomosis. Moreover, Mattei et al. (2008) reported numerous advantages to routine stenting of ureteroileal anastomosis. **When an ileal conduit is performed, the left ureter is brought underneath the sigmoid mesentery just overlying the aorta. The additional length and dissection needed on the left and the possibility of angulation around the inferior mesenteric artery may lead to a higher incidence of stricture formation on the left** (Barbieri et al., 2010; Mansson et al., 1989).

Controversy exists over the choice of bowel segment used for conduit diversion. One theoretic advantage to the use of colon is the feasibility of performing a nonrefluxing anastomosis. However, the reported incidence of renal deterioration with a nonrefluxing versus a refluxing ureterocolonic anastomosis has been mixed, and there does not appear to be a clear advantage with respect to renal function and colonization with a nonrefluxing anastomosis. The issues influencing stricture formation in continent urinary diversions become even more complex because of the variety of bowel segments, reservoir configurations, and types of anastomoses available for reconstruction. **The reported rate of ureteroenteric anastomotic stricture after continent diversion is 3% to 25%, with the majority occurring within the first 2 years** (Kouba et al., 2007; Lugagne et al., 1997; Weijerman et al., 1998). Despite the paucity of randomized studies, there remains evidence in the literature that the risk of obstruction with a nonrefluxing anastomosis is significantly higher than that of a refluxing anastomosis. Pantuck et al. (2000) compared 60 nonrefluxing ureteroenteric anastomoses with 56 direct, refluxing anastomoses and found the long-term stricture rates to be 13% and 1.7%, respectively. With a mean follow-up of 41 months, there was no significant difference in the two groups with respect to hydronephrosis, pyelonephritis, nephrolithiasis, or renal insufficiency. Similarly, Roth et al. (1996) found a greater than fivefold increase in ureteral strictures in the group undergoing a nonrefluxing anastomosis.

Their data also indicated that the risk of obstruction was unrelated to surgical expertise.

Studer et al. (1995) have reported a randomized study evaluating a nonrefluxing versus a refluxing anastomosis into an isoperistaltic afferent ileal limb. Thirteen percent of nonrefluxing anastomoses resulted in stricture formation, as compared with 3% of refluxing anastomoses. Although there is no clear evidence that reflux into an adult kidney is detrimental, it is clear that obstruction is harmful to renal function. These studies and others support the use of a refluxing anastomosis in low-pressure continent reservoirs.

Kouba et al. (2007) compared the Wallace and Bricker techniques of ureteroileal anastomosis for continent and incontinent diversions and found low rates of stricture (0% to 3%) using both techniques in 186 patients with 34-month follow-up. Notably, with use of the Wallace technique (joined ureters) no strictures were identified, compared with 3.7% in patients undergoing the Bricker technique (separate ureters). The group undergoing the Bricker anastomosis had a higher body mass index than the Wallace group.

Evaluation

Screening of the upper tracts in patients who have undergone any type of urinary diversion may include renal ultrasound, CT, or magnetic resonance imaging (MRI). If a stone or recurrent tumor is suggested, a CT scan or MRI is necessary for a more detailed assessment. In addition, patients with renal colic, recurrent urinary tract infection, or loss of renal function will require evaluation. In patients with hydronephrosis, CT urography, excretory urography, loopogram, or antegrade nephrostogram can provide information on the length and location of a stricture. Diuretic renography is indicated in patients with hydronephrosis to assess differential renal function and confirm the presence of functional obstruction. If hydronephrosis is present but renal function is insufficient for intravenous urogram or renography, placement of a nephrostomy tube and performance of an antegrade nephrostogram are diagnostic and therapeutic. This approach is also useful before endoscopic intervention because it clarifies stricture length, which aids in surgical planning.

Initial Management and Intervention

Not all patients with urinary diversion and hydronephrosis require intervention. **Most patients with a long-term urinary conduit will have an element of chronic hydronephrosis that is not secondary to obstruction. In this population, a decrease in renal function or loss of reflux on a routine loopogram should prompt diuretic renography to quantitatively assess for functional obstruction.** Indications for intervention in patients with diversions and hydronephrosis include pain, infection, and renal insufficiency associated with functional obstruction. Although recurrence of transitional cell carcinoma at the level of the anastomosis is uncommon, the radiographic picture of an irregular mass at the level of the stricture and the rapid progression of obstruction and loss of renal function should prompt further evaluation and intervention (Tsuji et al., 1996).

A particularly challenging subset of patients is those undergoing urinary diversion as part of a pelvic exenteration for gynecologic malignancy. Penalver et al. (1998) reported on 66 patients, 95% of whom had undergone previous pelvic irradiation. Early and late complications at the ureteroenteric anastomosis were 22% and 10%, respectively. Eighty-five percent of the postoperative complications were managed successfully by conservative measures such as percutaneous nephrostomy.

Open or robotic repair has been reported to be highly successful in 1 series of 50 patients (Gin et al., 2017). Open repair was associated with a 33% complication rate and 6-day hospitalization compared with 3-day hospitalization with robotic repair (Gin et al., 2017).

Endourologic Management

Endourologic management of ureteroenteric strictures has evolved in a manner analogous to that for ureteral stricture disease. Although the initial procedures involved simple balloon dilation and stent placement, unsatisfactory results led to incisional techniques using electrocautery; more recently, the laser was applied using fluoroscopic and direct endoscopic control. The current state-of-the-art incisional technique for endoureterotomy includes small-caliber flexible ureteroscopic instrumentation along with holmium laser incision (Cornud et al., 1992; Delvecchio et al., 2000; Laven et al., 2001, 2003; Muench et al., 1987; Schöndorf et al., 2013; Siegel et al., 1982).

Endourologic management of ureteroenteric or ureterocolic strictures, unlike the management of ureteral strictures, still favors antegrade management (Gomez et al., 2017). Accordingly, endourologic procedures typically begin with antegrade percutaneous access. Simple percutaneous drainage is continued to allow relief of any associated infection or obstruction-related renal dysfunction. Once the patient's condition is clinically stable, fluoroscopic control is used to pass a guidewire in an antegrade fashion across the anastomotic stricture, over which a balloon catheter can be positioned and inflated until the waist disappears. Stents are a routine part of endourologic management, and these are typically inserted in this same antegrade fashion. However, because of difficulty with mucous plugging of stents in this setting, many centers routinely use an internal-external stent, which can be easily flushed or changed over a wire. In addition, retrograde looposcopic access can be combined with percutaneous access and antegrade passage of a wire. With through-and-through control, the anastomosis can be visualized fluoroscopically or, preferably, with direct ureteroscopic, looposcopic, or trans-stomascopic visualization. Any number of procedures can then be used for the dilation, including balloon dilation alone, electroincision with an electrode or hot-wire cutting balloon, or holmium laser incision. In all cases, a stent is placed, usually for 4 to 8 weeks.

Balloon dilation of ureteroenteric strictures was one of the first endourologic forms of management used, and fortunately long-term results are available. Notably, short-term reports of use of high-pressure balloon dilation have demonstrated success rates as high as 61% (Ravery et al., 1998). Alternatively, Shapiro et al. (1988) reported balloon dilation for 37 benign ureteroenteric strictures in 29 patients. Only 6 dilations (16%) were considered to have a successful result at least 1 year after interventional treatment, and repeat dilations were often required to maintain ureteral patency. Similarly, Kwak et al. (1995) achieved an overall success rate of less than 30% at 9 months for patients undergoing antegrade balloon dilation of ureteroenteric strictures. More recently, DiMarco et al. (2001) reported a 5% 3-year success rate in 52 balloon dilations of ureteroenteric anastomotic strictures. Recently Schöndorf et al. (2013) reported on 74 patients with ureteroenteric anastomotic strictures with a 26% success rate with endourologic intervention compared with a 91% success rate with open intervention at 29 months. For strictures greater than 1 cm, the endourologic success rate was 6%, compared with a 50% success rate in strictures less than 1 cm. **Endourologic intervention was successful 19% on the left compared with 41% on the right, whereas no difference was noted in sidedness with open repair** (Schöndorf et al., 2013). More recently, one series reported 100% success rate in 7 patients with strictures smaller than 1 cm and overall 71% success rate using antegrade or retrograde balloon or sheath dilation with or without laser incision with 25-month median follow-up (Gomez et al., 2017). These authors eventually advocated for antegrade approach based on their experience.

Metallic stents have also been used for ureteroenteric anastomotic strictures, with acceptable short-term results. Overall, of 30 patients in the published literature, the reported patency rate is greater than 80% with 6- to 22-month follow-up (Kurzer and Leveillee, 2005). **There is a higher incidence of encrustation and stone formation with use of metallic stents for ureteroenteric anastomotic strictures, in addition to the risks of tissue ingrowth, recurrent obstruction, and stent migration** (Gorin et al., 2011; Kurzer and Leveillee, 2005; Ng et al., 2013). This may explain the limited published data regarding use of this approach.

Cautery wire balloon incision has also been reported in patients treated for ureteroenteric strictures (Lin et al., 1999; Schöndorf et al., 2013). For benign strictures, stent-free long-term patency was achieved in only 30% of patients. Meretyk et al. (1991) reviewed the long-term results of endourologic management of ureteroenteric anastomotic strictures at Washington University. In that study, 15 patients with 19 ureteroenteric strictures were followed for an average of 2½ years. An antegrade approach was used most frequently and was usually combined with electroincision. A 57% long-term stent-free patency rate was achieved, even with follow-up longer than 2 years. **Historically long-term patency of most endoscopic procedures approaches has been lower than operative revision, thus these approaches may be used preferentially as the initial intervention in select patients. Definitive operative management is reserved for patients in whom endourologic intervention fails and for patients with strictures longer than 1 cm** (Gin et al., 2017; Kramolowsky et al., 1987, 1988; Schöndorf et al., 2013).

Cornud et al. (1996) reported their long-term results with percutaneous electroincision of ureterointestinal anastomotic strictures and specifically compared the results of fluoroscopic and endoscopic guidance. Twenty-seven patients were followed for longer than 1 year after stent removal, and an overall patency rate of 71% was reported. These investigators found better results when direct endoscopic control was combined with fluoroscopic guidance, compared with fluoroscopic guidance alone. In that report, right common iliac artery damage was reported during electroincision in 1 patient who had the procedure performed under fluoroscopic guidance alone. As a result, direct visual approaches have been favored for the management of ureteroenteric or ureterocolic anastomotic strictures, and the holmium laser has proven to be an excellent incisional tool. Endoureterotomy is typically performed in an antegrade manner, and success rates ranging from 50% to 80% have been reported (Laven et al., 2001; Singal et al., 1997; Watterson et al., 2002). These reports suggest the left side is more resistant to management because the majority of the failures occurred on the left side (Laven et al., 2003; Schöndorf et al., 2013). **When endoscopic incision of a left ureteroenteric stricture is considered, the risk of hemorrhage is a concern because the sigmoid mesentery can be in close proximity. This, taken with the lower success rates of all endoscopic approaches on the left side, supports serious consideration for primary repair when treating left ureteroenteric anastomotic strictures** (Fig. 89.30). In spite of this, Lovaco et al. (2005) reported success treating 25 ureteroenteric strictures with endoureterotomy by an intraluminal invagination technique, with 80% success at more than 50 months' follow-up. This approach increases the distance between the incision site and surrounding vessels and viscera and does not favor left or right strictures.

> **KEY POINTS: URETEROENTERIC STRICTURES**
>
> - Although long-term patency of minimally invasive procedures for ureteroenteric strictures is in the range of 50%, such approaches are still used as the initial intervention, reserving operative management for those patients in whom endourologic intervention fails.
> - When considering endoscopic incision of a left ureteroenteric anastomotic stricture in an ileal conduit, hemorrhage is a concern because the sigmoid mesentery can be in close proximity. With the low success rates of endoscopic approaches in this scenario, these patients may be best treated with definitive repair.
> - Acceptable long-term success rates have been reported with open or robotic repair of ureteroenteric anastomotic strictures. As expected, strictures longer than 1 cm were more likely to recur, and procedures on the left side had lower success rates.

RETROPERITONEAL FIBROSIS
Presentation and Etiology

RPF is typically characterized by the presence of an inflammatory, fibrotic process in the retroperitoneum causing compression of

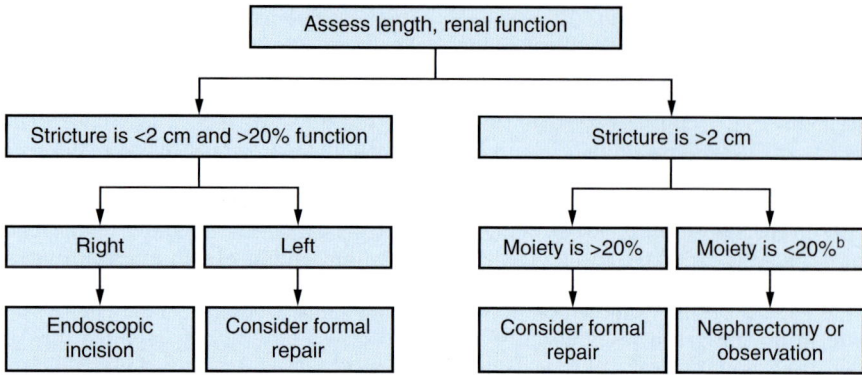

Fig. 89.30. Algorithm for management of ureteroenteric anastomotic stricture disease.

the retroperitoneal structures including the ureters. RPF most commonly affects patients who are 40 to 60 years of age. However, more than 30 cases of RPF have been reported in patients younger than 18 years of age (van Bommel, 2002). RPF cases are rare, have a male predominance, with a male-to-female ratio of 2:1 to 3:1, although one recent outcomes series showed no gender predominance (Jadhav et al., 2017). The true incidence is unknown but has been estimated to be 1 per 200,000 to 500,000 per year.

In general, the retroperitoneal fibrotic mass centers around the distal aorta at L4 to L5 and wraps around the ureters, leading to hydronephrosis via extrinsic compression on the ureters or interference with ureteral peristalsis (Koep and Zuidema, 1987; Lepor and Walsh, 1979). In most patients, the presenting symptom is pain in the lower back and/or flank. The pain, which is typically dull, noncolicky, and unchanged with posture, may radiate to the lower abdomen or groin. Furthermore, the pain is often relieved by aspirin rather than narcotics. Other symptoms include weight loss, anorexia, nausea, generalized malaise, fever, hypertension, and oliguria or anuria. The mass may compress the inferior vena cava, resulting in deep venous thrombosis and lower extremity edema (Rhee et al., 1994). The mass may extend proximally to the renal hilum and encase the renal vein, resulting in renal vein hypertension and subsequent gross hematuria (Powell et al., 2000). Aortic obstruction and involvement of the mediastinum, the biliary system, the mesentery, and the kidney are rare (Azuma et al., 1999; Dejaco et al., 1999; Klisnick et al., 1999; Tripodi et al., 1998). Distal extension to the bifurcation of the iliac vessels may occur, and extension to the spermatic cord with scrotal involvement has been reported (Palmer and Rosenthal, 1999; Schulte-Baukloh et al., 1999). Duration of symptoms before diagnosis is usually 4 to 6 months, and approximately half of the patients have fibrosis that has caused significant ureteral obstruction and symptoms secondary to uremia.

In approximately 70% of patients, the disease is idiopathic. Currently, idiopathic RPF is considered part of the spectrum of chronic periaortitis, a large vessel vasculitis (Pipitone et al., 2012). Ceroid, a complex polymer of oxidized lipids and protein found in atherosclerotic plaques, has been suggested as the antigen initiating the inflammatory response (Parums et al., 1991). Indeed, a higher incidence of aortic aneurysms has been identified in patients with RPF (Breems et al., 2000). RPF usually occurs as an isolated disease entity, but it may occur as part of multifocal fibrosclerosis, a rare syndrome characterized by fibrosis involving multiple organ systems. In such a scenario, the clinical presentation may include RPF, sclerosing mediastinitis, sclerosing cholangitis, orbital pseudotumor, and Riedel thyroiditis (Dehner and Coffin, 1998; Özgen and Cila, 2000). The pathogenesis of these disorders is unknown but appears to be autoimmune.

Among the 30% of RPF patients who have an identifiable cause, drugs such as methysergide (Sansert) and other ergot alkyloids are most commonly associated with RPF. Beta-blockers and phenacetin have also been implicated. The exact pathophysiology of drug-induced RPF remains unknown. Other causes of RPF include malignancies such as lymphoma, the most common malignancy in RPF cases, and multiple myeloma, carcinoid, pancreatic cancer, prostate cancer, and sarcoma (Usher et al., 1977; Webb and Dawson-Edwards, 1967). Radiotherapy for retroperitoneal malignancy is also known to produce a residual fibrotic mass leading to secondary ureteral obstruction. Asbestos exposure has also been associated with RPF in exposed workers in Finland, via gastrointestinal and pulmonary lymphatic drainage (Scheel and Feeley, 2013). In addition, infectious causes such as tuberculosis, *Actinomyces*, gonorrhea, and schistosomiasis have been suggested in the pathogenesis of RPF.

Association of RPF with membranous glomerulonephritis has also been documented in the literature (Mercadal et al., 2000; Shirota et al., 2002). The exact cause remains unclear, although the association has been speculated to be secondary to an unknown antigen triggering systemic immune response that leads to RPF. Association of RPF with ankylosing spondylitis and Wegener granulomatosis has also been reported, further suggesting an underlying immune cause in some patients (Izzedine et al., 2002; LeBlanc et al., 2002).

Pathologically, the typical gross appearance of RPF is that of a smooth, flat, tan, dense mass enveloping the surrounding retroperitoneal structures. It is also known to invade the ureter or psoas muscle. Histologically, the appearance of RPF is that of a nonspecific inflammatory process that varies with the stage of the disease. Early in the disease, affected tissue consists mainly of collagen bundles with capillary proliferation and inflammatory cells including lymphocytes, plasma cells, and fibroblasts. In the later stage, the mass becomes relatively acellular and avascular, consisting of sheets of hypocellular collagen. RPF secondary to malignancy is often histologically indistinguishable from idiopathic RPF, and it can be identified only on the basis of the demonstration of small islands of tumor cells within the fibrotic mass.

Evaluation

In most RPF patients, the clinical symptoms are generally nonspecific, and physical examination is usually unrevealing. Laboratory evaluation may reveal an elevated erythrocyte sedimentation rate (ESR), elevated C-reactive protein (CRP), moderate leukocytosis, anemia, and variable renal insufficiency with associated electrolyte abnormalities. The ESR and CRP are elevated in one-half to two-thirds of patients with idiopathic RPF (Pipitone et al., 2012). If the overall renal function is normal CT urography may be performed. Typical findings include hydronephrosis with medial deviation of the proximal ureter and midureter and a smoothly tapered ureter at the level of obstruction. Urinary obstruction is usually bilateral, but unilateral cases have been described. Uncommonly, there are patients with symptoms of urinary obstruction but little hydronephrosis on imaging.

CT scan typically reveals hydronephrosis associated with a well-delineated retroperitoneal soft tissue mass enveloping the great vessels and the ureters (Fig. 89.31). If the patient has significant renal impairment, a retrograde pyelogram may be performed. **In the radiographic evaluation of RPF, MRI is useful as the fibrotic mass has characteristic T1- and T2-weighted characteristics. RPF is characterized as a diffusely low signal intensity on T1-weighted imaging, although the T2 signal may vary considerably, with high signal intensity consistent with active disease** (Fig. 89.32). With treatment, T2 signal often diminishes and thus provides a measure of therapeutic efficacy. Moreover, gadolinium enhancement may also prove valuable in assessing the response to treatment because associated decreases in gadolinium contrast enhancement should also be expected after appropriate therapy (Cronin et al., 2008). Similarly, contrast enhancement on CT can also be used to monitor therapy, as can positron emission tomography (PET). In fact, PET appears to be the most sensitive imaging study for disease activity and may obviate the need for biopsy (Fernando et al., 2017; Pipitone et al., 2012). In addition, single-stop PET and contrast-enhanced CT has been used for ongoing assessment of patients with RPF (Guignard et al., 2012).

If a kidney is suspected to be nonfunctioning, differential renography should be considered to determine renal function because it may affect surgical planning. Representative biopsy samples of the mass may be obtained percutaneously or at the time of surgery to rule out malignancy if the diagnosis remains uncertain after imaging.

Management

Initial Management

The initial management of RPF depends on the patient's clinical status. Patients with hydronephrosis and uremia should be emergently decompressed by either percutaneous nephrostomy or indwelling ureteral stents. The advantages to placing ureteral stents include the opportunity to perform retrograde pyelograms to evaluate the anatomy as well as the convenience of internal drainage. Ureteral stent placement is usually not difficult to perform in the setting of ureteral obstruction caused by RPF. In a critically ill patient with electrolyte abnormalities and little or no urine output, nephrostomy tube placement is favored. **After renal decompression, the patient should be monitored closely for postobstructive diuresis, renal function status, and appropriate replacement of fluids and electrolytes.**

After the initial management, an attempt to identify the cause of RPF should be made. Methysergide or any other potentially inciting drug, if identified, should be discontinued. Although most patients with malignant RPF have a prior history of malignancy, a thorough evaluation for occult malignancy with careful application of imaging studies is necessary. Biopsy to rule out malignancy, performed percutaneously or at the time of ureterolysis to provide long-term relief of obstruction, should be considered. **However, some believe that in patients with no history of prior malignancy, no classic radiographic features on MRI or CT, and no lymphadenopathy, a biopsy is not essential before medical therapy. This concept has been further strengthened with the use of PET scans** (Fernando et al., 2017).

Medical Management

Once the diagnosis of idiopathic RPF is made, the common primary medical management has been steroid therapy. In the medical literature there are approximately 170 cases of idiopathic RPF treated with steroids that resulted in about an 80% clinical response, including a decrease in size of the mass and improvement in ureteral obstruction or inferior vena cava compression (Adam et al., 1998; Baker et al., 1987; Fry et al., 2008; Higgins et al., 1998; Kearney et al., 1976; van Bommel, 2002). The characteristic clinical response to steroid therapy includes resolution of pain and constitutional symptoms within days after treatment, a rapid fall of ESR, and diuresis. Dose and duration of steroid therapy vary considerably in the literature, but most regimens start with initial doses of 60 mg daily tapered to 5 mg daily. Chronic steroid therapy up to 2 years has been shown to provide significant improvement in clinical symptoms and

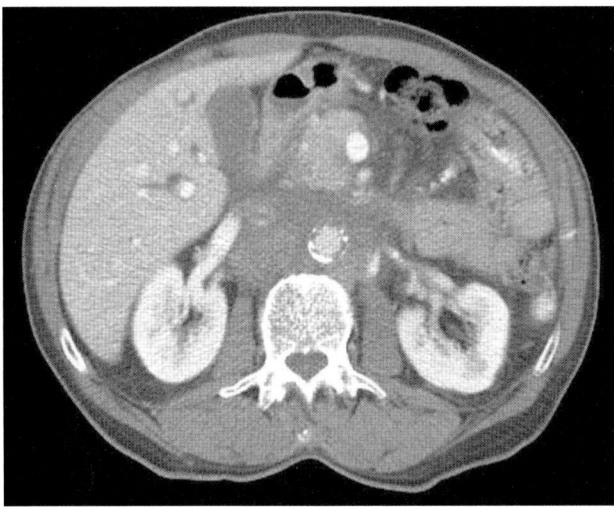

Fig. 89.31. Typical computed tomographic findings of retroperitoneal fibrosis. The study demonstrates the presence of a homogeneous mass obliterating the outline of the great vessels at the lumbar area.

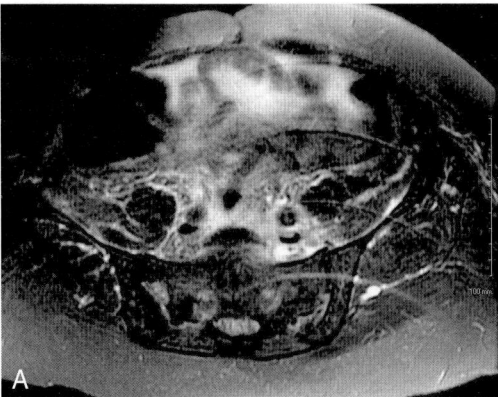 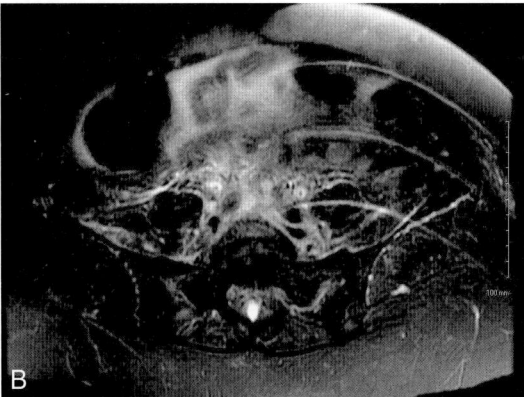

Fig. 89.32. (A) T2-weighted magnetic resonance image of a symptomatic patient demonstrating retroperitoneal fibrosis with enhancement and thus active disease. (B) Same patient after 1 month of medical therapy; note the decrease in enhancement on this corroborative T2-weighted image.

regression of retroperitoneal mass (Kardar et al., 2002), although relapse during tapering occurs in 25% to 50% of patients (Pipitone et al., 2012). Patients who have evidence of active inflammation—manifested by increased ESR, CRP, leukocytosis, or active inflammation on a biopsy—are more likely to respond to steroid therapy.

In addition to steroids, immunosuppressive agents including azathioprine, cyclophosphamide, cyclosporine, colchicine, and mycophenolate mofetil have been described to provide benefit in idiopathic RPF in isolated reports (Grotz et al., 1998; Marzano et al., 2001; McDougal et al., 1991; Vega et al., 2009; Wagenknecht et al., 1981). Medroxyprogesterone acetate, progesterone, and particularly tamoxifen have also been found to be beneficial in idiopathic RPF (Al-Musawi et al., 1998; Benson and Baum, 1993; Clark et al., 1991; Dedeoglu et al., 2000; Pipitone et al., 2012; Puce et al., 2000). The exact mechanisms of action of these medications are unclear, but they are believed to inhibit fibroblastic proliferation leading to clinical response. **Use of immunosuppressive agents is reserved for patients in whom steroid therapy fails, because relapses are as high as 50% during steroid tapering** (Pipitone et al., 2012).

Surgical Management

Ureterolysis may be performed open surgically or laparoscopically, although open surgery has been considered the standard (Elashry et al., 1996; Lindell and Lehtonen, 1988). **When an open surgery is performed, a midline, transperitoneal abdominal incision is made to allow access to both ureters. For laparoscopic or robotic bilateral ureterolysis, the patient is typically placed in the modified flank position and repositioned to the other flank after the first side is complete.** The surgical principles are the same regardless of approach. Placement of ureteral catheters or stents at the beginning of the procedure is advisable to assist identification and dissection of the ureters. **Although hydronephrosis may be unilateral on preoperative assessment, the process is generally bilateral requiring bilateral ureterolysis.** After medial mobilization of the ascending and descending colon, deep biopsies of the mass should be obtained for frozen and permanent section to rule out malignancy and confirm the diagnosis. Dissection should begin at the distal, nondilated ureteral segment to avoid injury to the thin, dilated proximal segment. A right-angle clamp can be placed between the ureter and the retroperitoneal mass along the course of the ureter, and the fibrotic tissue is then incised above the clamp, the so-called "split and roll technique." This is repeated throughout the length of the entrapped ureter, using blunt and sharp dissection techniques to free the affected ureter from its fibrous bed. The ureteral wall may become thin at times after the dissection. An inadvertent ureterotomy should be closed with absorbable suture. Ureteral excision with ureteroureterostomy is usually unnecessary.

After bilateral ureterolysis, the surgeon must physically separate the newly freed ureters from the fibrotic tissue that encased them, lest the obstructive process recur. Several surgical options may be considered to accomplish this goal, but the key principles favor an approach that provides a new healthy tissue layer that is not affected by the fibrotic process, ideally one with good blood supply such as the omentum, as well as a reconstruction that does not kink the ureters. One option is to retract the ureters laterally after they have been released and then close the parietal peritoneum over the fibrotic "bed" that contained them, creating a physical separation that should prevent the ureters from re-entering the retroperitoneum and becoming entrapped again. Some surgeons will accomplish a similar intraperitonealization of the ureter by moving the previously reflected colon behind the mobilized ureter and securing the peritoneal edge of the bowel to the abdominal side wall. It is important not to obstruct or kink the ureter in the closure of the peritoneum at the ureteral hiatus. In a report on a group of patients with idiopathic RPF undergoing intraperitoneal placement of the ureters or lateral retroperitoneal placement of the ureters, no difference in the radiologic or clinical outcome was found (Barbalias and Liatsikos, 1999). In the setting of extensive RPF, a more definitive approach is to surround the ureters with omentum after repositioning them within the peritoneal cavity (Carini et al., 1982; Tresidder et al., 1972). To perform the omental wrap, the omentum is first mobilized from its attachment to the transverse colon, followed by its division along its midline with ligation of the small omental vessels up to the gastric attachment. The short gastric vessels are then divided and ligated at the level of the stomach wall, after which the two halves of the omentum can be retracted laterally on the basis of the right and left gastroepiploic arteries. The entire length of the ureter can be surrounded by omental tissue, which is tacked in place with absorbable sutures (Fig. 89.33A and B). The omentum provides protection of the ureter against recurrent extrinsic compression and vascularity to a potentially ischemic ureter. Steroid therapy may be used postoperatively in an attempt to prevent recurrent upper tract compression. If no ureterotomy occurs during ureterolysis, the previously placed stents may be removed shortly after surgery.

If ureterolysis is impossible to perform because of extensive periureteral fibrosis, renal autotransplantation may be performed if the ipsilateral renal unit demonstrates satisfactory function (Penalver et al., 2001). If no significant renal function can be recovered after an adequate time period of decompression in the presence of the satisfactory contralateral renal function, nephrectomy may be considered.

Outcomes of Ureterolysis

A recent report demonstrated 94% of patients were stent free at 12 months after open ureterolysis (O'Brien and Fernando, 2017). Another report showed good results employing ureterolysis, ureteral reconstruction, or ileal ureter (Jadhav et al., 2017). The first laparoscopic ureterolysis was reported by Kavoussi and Clayman in 1992. Subsequent success with this technique was confirmed by others (Puppo et al., 1994). Another report described an experience with laparoscopic ureterolysis in 13 patients, including bilateral procedure in 7 and unilateral procedure in 6 (Fugita et al., 2001). Preoperative stent placement was performed in all cases before laparoscopy. For each ureter, the laparoscopic procedure was performed using a transperitoneal four-port approach. After incision of the posterior peritoneum and mobilization of the colon, the affected ureter was dissected free from the retroperitoneal fibrotic tissue. Multiple frozen-section biopsies of the periureteral tissue were obtained to rule out malignancy. The edge of the posterior peritoneum was reapproximated to the sidewall underneath the ureter to intraperitonealize the ureter. Laparoscopic ureterolysis was completed successfully in 85% (11) of the cases, with 2 (15%) open conversions resulting from iliac vein injury (in 1 patient) and marked fibrosis (in 1 patient). Mean operative time was 381 minutes for bilateral procedures and 192 minutes for unilateral procedures. Mean use of parenteral analgesics was 59 mg of morphine sulfate equivalent. Mean hospital stay was 4 days. Postoperative complications occurred in 30% (4) of the patients, including epididymitis, umbilical port erythema, prolonged ileus, and urinary retention. Pathology showed fibrous tissue with lymphocytes, plasma cells, macrophages, and fibroblast proliferation in all cases. At a mean follow-up of 30 months, upper tract imaging such as intravenous urography or renal scan showed lack of obstruction in 92% (12) of the patients. A multi-institutional survey that included 17 academic centers identified that centers with a fellowship-trained laparoscopist performed laparoscopic ureterolysis, and in 59% of centers urologists performed the medical management. Notably in this survey the reported laparoscopic success rates were 83% (Duchene et al., 2007).

A more recent retrospective comparison of laparoscopic and open ureterolysis (16 ureters in each group) concluded that the minimally invasive approach was associated with a shorter hospital stay (mean 2.1 vs. 5.9 days, $P = 0.004$) but that success and complication rates were similar with both approaches (Styn et al., 2011).

Robotic ureterolysis for retroperitoneal fibrosis has also been reported. Keehn et al. (2011) treated a total of 21 renal units in 17 patients with robotic ureterolysis and omental wrapping. Fourteen percent recurred and required a secondary surgical intervention, whereas 86% remained patent at a mean follow-up of 20.5 months. They reported one perioperative complication, an enterocutaneous fistula from an unrecognized thermal bowel injury that required bowel resection.

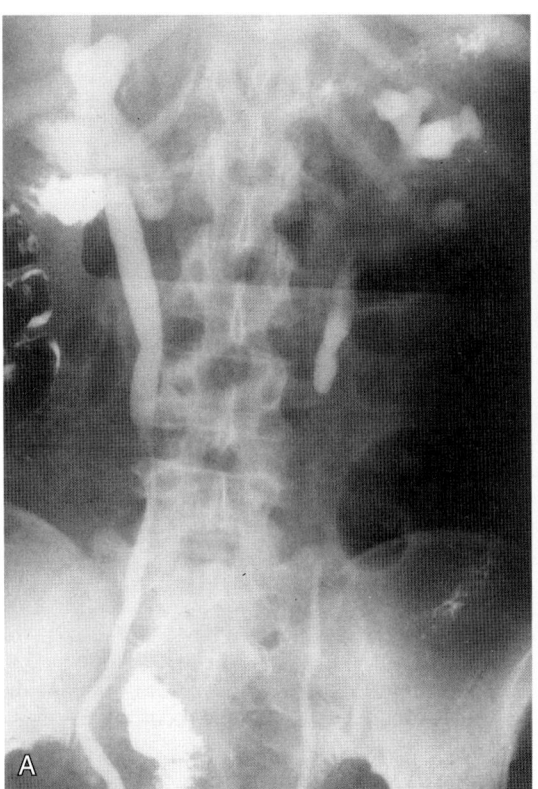
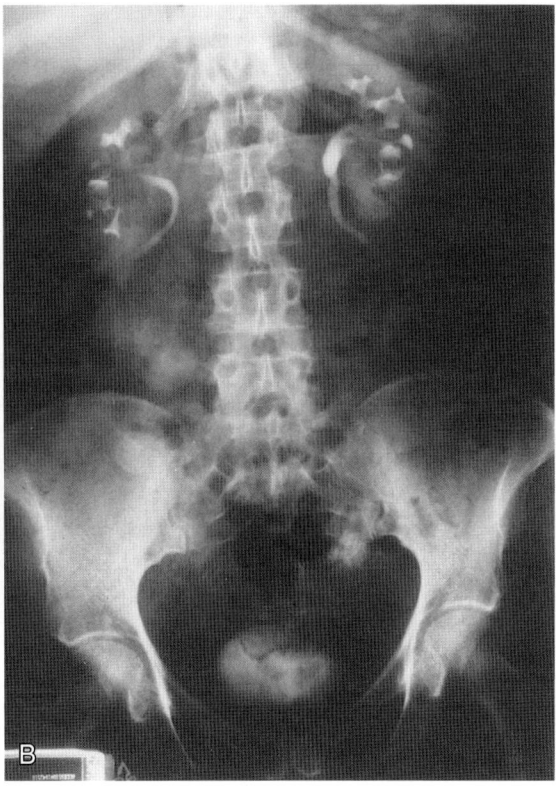

Fig. 89.33. (A) Preoperative intravenous contrast-enhanced radiograph of a patient with idiopathic retroperitoneal fibrosis, showing bilateral hydronephrosis with medial deviation of the ureters. (B) Postoperative radiograph of the same patient after surgical ureterolysis with intraperitoneal omental wrapping.

KEY POINTS: RETROPERITONEAL FIBROSIS

- The retroperitoneal fibrotic mass generally centers around the distal aorta at L4-L5 and wraps around the ureters, leading to hydronephrosis via extrinsic compression on the ureters or interference with ureteral peristalsis. In most cases the disease is idiopathic, associated with chronic aortitis.
- RPF symptoms and signs are usually nonspecific. Laboratory evaluation may show an elevated erythrocyte sedimentation rate, C-reactive protein, moderate leukocytosis, anemia, and variable renal insufficiency associated with electrolyte abnormalities.
- Initial management of RPF in the presence of hydronephrosis and uremia includes emergent decompression by percutaneous nephrostomy or indwelling ureteral stents. After decompression, the patient should be monitored closely for postobstructive diuresis.
- The most common primary medical management of idiopathic RPF has been steroid therapy, with immunosuppressive agents as second line.
- In surgical bilateral ureterolysis, the ureters need to be protected by intraperitonealization or omental wrapping. Both open and laparoscopic techniques may be applied successfully. If ureterolysis is impossible to perform, renal autotransplantation may be performed.

SUGGESTED READINGS

Jarrett TW, Chan DY, Charambura TC, et al: Laparoscopic pyeloplasty: the first 100 cases, *J Urol* 167:1253, 2002.
Khanna R, Isac W, Laydner H, et al: Laparoendoscopic single site reconstructive procedures in urology: medium term results, *J Urol* 187:1702, 2012.
Link RE, Bhayani SB, Kavoussi LR: A prospective comparison of robotic and laparoscopic pyeloplasty, *Ann Surg* 243:486, 2006.
Mufarrij PW, Woods M, Shah OD, et al: Robotic dismembered pyeloplasty: a 6-year, multi-institutional experience, *J Urol* 180:1391, 2008.
Ockerblad NF: Reimplantation of the ureter into the bladder by a flap method, *J Urol* 57:845, 1947.
Pipitone N, Vaglio A, Salvarani C: Retroperitoneal fibrosis, *Best Pract Res Clin Rheumatol* 26:439, 2012.
Razdan S, Silberstein IK, Bagley DH: Ureteroscopic endoureterotomy, *BJU Int* 95(Suppl 2):94, 2005.
Richstone L, Seideman CA, Reggio E, et al: Pathologic findings in patients with ureteropelvic junction obstruction and crossing vessels, *Urology* 73:716, 2009.
Schöndorf D, Meierhans-Ruf S, Kiss B, et al: Ureteroileal strictures after urinary diversion with an ileal segment—is there a place for endourological treatment at all?, *J Urol* 190:585, 2013.
Turner-Warwick RT, Worth PH: The psoas bladder-hitch procedure for the replacement of the lower third of the ureter, *Br J Urol* 41:701, 1969.

REFERENCES

The complete reference list is available online at ExpertConsult.com.

90
Upper Urinary Tract Trauma
Steven B. Brandes, MD, and Jairam R. Eswara, MD

RENAL INJURIES

The kidney is the most commonly injured urologic organ from external trauma. Advances in radiographic staging, improvements in hemodynamic monitoring, and wider use of angioembolization have improved the rates of renal preservation and decreased unnecessary surgery. **The majority of blunt and select penetrating injuries to the kidneys can be safely managed non-operatively. Complications that arise from expectant management can often be successfully managed percutaneously, endoscopically or by selective angioembolization. Absolute indications for immediate renal intervention is hemodynamic instability with no or transient response to resuscitation or a pulsatile or expanding retroperitoneal hematoma.**

Presentation and History

Motor vehicle accidents, falls from heights, and assaults cause the majority of blunt renal trauma. Direct transmission of kinetic energy and rapid deceleration forces place the kidneys at risk. In the United States, blunt trauma accounts for 80% to 90% of all renal injuries, whereas penetrating trauma accounts for 10% to 20%. The kidney is injured in 1% to 5% of all trauma and accounts for 24% of all solid organ injury (Hardee et al., 2013; Hotaling et al., 2012; Meng et al., 1999; Smith et al., 2005). The majority of renal injuries are minor and heal spontaneously. Most renal injuries, 78% to 82%, are low grade (AAST grades I–II) and are managed conservatively with little or no long-term consequence (Keihani et al., 2018; Zinman and Vanni, 2016).

Perhaps the most important information to obtain in the history of blunt renal injury is the mechanism of injury. This should include the speed of the car or the height of the fall, to better determine if significant deceleration injury was a component of the injury pattern. The kidney is particularly vulnerable to deceleration injury. Significant deceleration can cause the kidney to tear at retroperitoneal points of fixation, such as the renal hilum or ureteropelvic junction, resulting in renal artery thrombosis, renal vein disruption, renal pedicle avulsion, or ureteropelvic junction disruption. A more specific history of injury mechanism can be helpful. For example, the majority of the renal injuries after automobile accidents occur in unrestrained drivers upon direct impact on the steering wheel or side impact with the lateral door, often with 30 cm or more of door incursion (Kuan et al., 2007). Eliciting details of the accident from first responders at the scene can increase the level of suspicion for renal injury.

Penetrating renal injuries most often come from gunshot and stab wounds, and the kidneys are injured in approximately 10% of all abdominal penetrating injuries. More than 77% of patients with penetrating renal injuries have associated abdominal injuries. Gunshot wounds make up the majority of the penetrating trauma, with stab wounds a distant second (86% vs. 14%). Penetrating renal injuries have higher rates of significant and persistent renal bleeding, need for renorrhaphy/nephrectomy, and complications when managed nonoperatively. Of all patients sustaining renal trauma, civilian renal gunshot wounds are typically low velocity and occur in approximately 4% (McAninch et al., 1993). Low velocity gunshot wounds cause less damage and are not as devastating as high velocity, unless they penetrate the renal hilum or collecting system. High velocity bullet wounds cause blast effect and often cause delayed tissue necrosis.

Stab wound entry sites that include the upper abdomen, flank, and lower chest, should raise suspicion for possible renal involvement. **Trauma to the anterior axillary line is more prone to damage important renal structures such as the renal hilum and pedicle compared with the posterior axillary line, which more commonly results in parenchymal injury.** Should the weapon be recovered, the size of the blade should be noted, to better understand the depth of the injury and the chance for organ damage.

Physical examination of all body systems must be detailed and complete. In a conscious patient, a thorough history can be taken during the examination. Rapid resuscitation according to American Association for the Surgery of Trauma (AAST) guidelines should be followed for polytrauma. With a blunt mechanism, cervical spine immobilization is mandated until confirmed intact by radiography. Examination of the abdomen, chest, and back must be performed. Indicators of possible renal injury on physical exam include flank ecchymoses, abdominal or flank tenderness, rib fractures, a significant blow to the flank, and penetrating injuries to the low thorax or flank. **It is important to consider concurrent intraabdominal injuries especially to the liver, intestine, and spleen in such trauma. Ipsilateral rib fracture can increase the incidence of significant renal trauma threefold.**

Gunshot injuries can be misleading in that small entrance wounds may underestimate larger tissue destruction within the body. Exit wounds are frequently, but not necessarily, much larger. Soft tissue and bone can alter the bullet's trajectory; thus the projectile may not take a direct path from entrance to exit. Bullet fragments can create secondary missiles, resulting in multiple injury tracts. When radiographs of the chest and abdomen are taken, a small metallic object should be placed at each entrance and exit site, to help define these locations on the films, and thus the path of the bullet.

Hematuria

The best indicators of significant urinary system injury include **gross and microscopic hematuria (>5 red blood cells/high-power field [RBCs/HPF] or positive dipstick finding), especially when associated with acceleration/deceleration injury, penetrating trauma, or hypotension in the field or emergency room (systolic blood pressure <90 mm Hg).**

The degree of hematuria and the severity of the renal injury do not consistently correlate. Gross hematuria has been observed in minor renal contusions, and microscopic hematuria has been seen in some with severe renal injuries. Hematuria was absent in 7% of 420 grade IV renal injuries in a recent analysis (Shariat et al., 2008a), 11% of patients with renal gunshot wounds (Voelzke and McAninch, 2009), and 36% of renal vascular injuries from blunt trauma (Cass, 1983). Also, approximately 50% of injuries to the ureteropelvic junction have no microscopic or gross hematuria. In patients with blunt trauma, microscopic hematuria associated with shock significantly increases the incidence of severe renal injuries (Mee and McAninch, 1989; Mee et al., 1989; Miller and McAninch, 1995; Nicolaisen et al., 1985). In addition, recreational injuries (primarily blunt) have a far lower rate of gross hematuria or microscopic hematuria with hypotension than urban renal trauma, and using hematuria as a criterion for imaging would have missed 23% of grades II to IV injuries (Lloyd et al., 2012).

The first aliquot of urine obtained by catheterization or voiding is used to determine the presence of hematuria. Later urine samples may be diluted by diuresis from resuscitation fluids, resulting in an underestimation or absence of hematuria. Any degree of visible blood in the urine is regarded as gross hematuria. Microscopic hematuria can be detected by dipstick analysis or microanalysis. The dipstick method is rapid and has a sensitivity and specificity for detection of microhematuria of more than 97%, even though a poor correlation with actual urinalysis was noted in a single study (Chandhoke and McAninch, 1988). **Although critical to the initial evaluation of traumatic urinary tract injury, the presence or absence of hematuria should not be the sole determinant in the assessment of a patient with suspected renal trauma.** Mechanism of injury and concurrent injuries should also play a role. Because the significance of hematuria varies with blunt and penetrating mechanisms, the importance of proper detection and staging of renal injuries, usually by computed tomography (CT), must be emphasized.

Classification

The AAST Organ Injury Scaling Committee (Moore et al., 1989) is the most widely used and accepted classification of renal injury (Table 90.1, Fig. 90.1). Based on accurate grading by contrast-enhanced CT, the kidney AAST injury severity scale has been validated in multiple series, as a predictive tool for clinical outcomes, such as the need for surgical or angiographic intervention or the rate of nephrectomy (Phan et al., 2018; Shariat et al., 2007). The organ injury scale for renal trauma was recently updated (Kozar et al., 2018). The

TABLE 90.1 American Association for the Surgery of Trauma Organ Injury Severity Scale for the Kidney

GRADE[a]	TYPE	DESCRIPTION
I	Contusion	Microscopic or gross hematuria, urologic studies normal
	Hematoma	Subcapsular, nonexpanding without parenchymal laceration
II	Hematoma	Nonexpanding perirenal hematoma confined to renal retroperitoneum
	Laceration	<1 cm parenchymal depth of renal cortex without urinary extravasation
III	Laceration	>1 cm parenchymal depth of renal cortex without collecting system rupture or urinary extravasation
IV	Laceration	Parenchymal laceration extending through renal cortex, medulla, and collecting system
	Vascular	Main renal artery or vein injury with contained hemorrhage
V	Laceration	Completely shattered kidney
	Vascular	Avulsion of renal hilum, devascularizing the kidney

[a]Advance one grade for bilateral injuries up to grade III.
Data from Moore EE, Shackford SR, Pachter HL, et al.: Organ injury scaling: spleen, liver, and kidney. *J Trauma* 29:1664–1666, 1989.

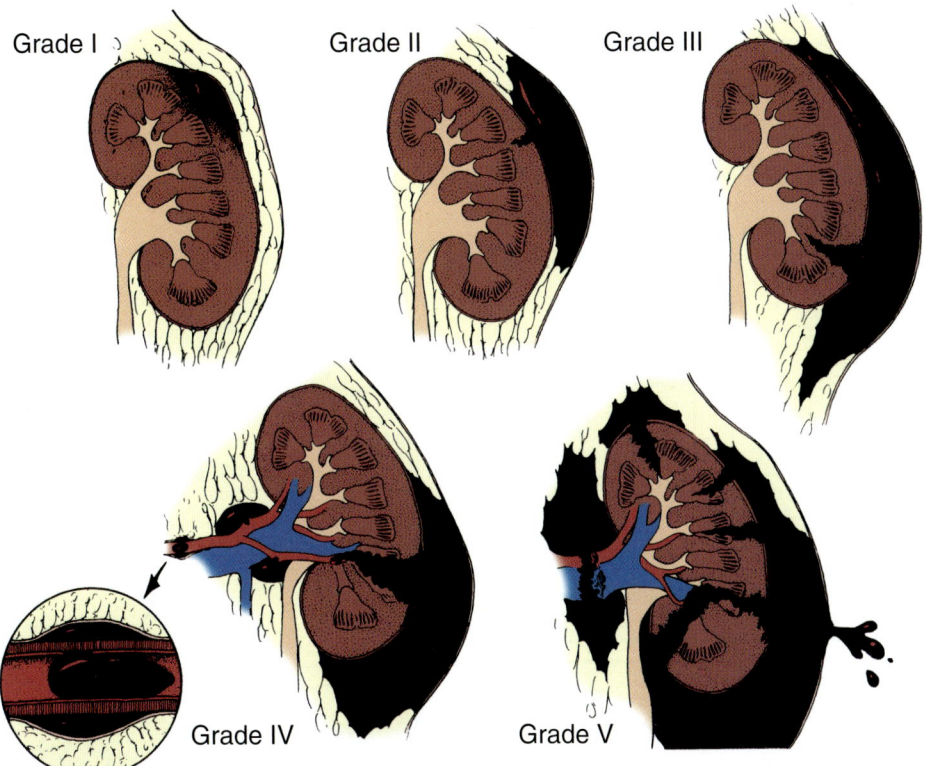

Fig. 90.1. Classification of renal injuries by grade. (Modified from the organ injury scale of the American Association for the Surgery of Trauma. Based on Moore EE, Shackford SR, Pachter HL, et al.: Organ injury scaling: spleen, liver, and kidney. *J Trauma* 29:1661–1664, 1989.)

grading scale remains largely unchanged. However, Grade IV now includes vascular injuries such as arterio-venous malformation or pseudo-aneurysm, and Grade V now includes a devascularized kidney with active bleeding and a shattered kidney with loss of identifiable parenchymal renal anatomy.

Indications for Renal Imaging

Based on the AUA Urotrauma guidelines and EAU Upper Urinary Tract Trauma guidelines published in 2014, the criteria for radiographic imaging include the following (Morey et al., 2014; Serafetinides et al., 2015):

1. **All patients with a penetrating trauma with a likelihood of renal injury (abdomen, flank, ipsilateral rib fracture, significant flank ecchymosis, or low chest entry/exit wound) who are hemodynamically stable enough to have a CT (instead of going directly to the operating room or angiography suite)**
2. **All patients with blunt trauma with significant acceleration/deceleration mechanism of injury, specifically rapid deceleration as would occur in a high-speed motor vehicle accident or a fall from heights**
3. **All patients with blunt trauma and gross hematuria**
4. **All patients with blunt trauma with microhematuria and hypotension (defined as a systolic pressure of less than 90 mm Hg at any time during evaluation and resuscitation)**
5. **All pediatric patients with greater than 5 RBCs/HPF**

The preferred imaging test is an abdominal/pelvic CT using IV contrast with immediate and delayed images.

An extensive prospective study based at San Francisco General Hospital evaluating indications for radiographic imaging continued for more than 25 years. The findings have been updated in three reports (Mee and McAninch, 1989; Miller and McAninch, 1995; Nicolaisen et al., 1985; Fig. 90.2). Based on information from this study, all patients with blunt trauma with gross hematuria and patients with microscopic hematuria and shock (systolic blood pressure <90 mm Hg any time during evaluation and resuscitation) should undergo renal imaging, usually with CT using intravenous (IV) contrast and with delayed films to evaluate urinary extravasation.

Patients with microscopic hematuria without hypotension or acceleration/deceleration injury can be observed clinically without imaging. First noted by Miller and McAninch (1995) but confirmed by several subsequent findings, these patients rarely have a significant injury (<0.0016%) (Cimbanassi et al., 2018). **However, if renal injury is suspected on the basis of history, mechanism of injury, examination, or the patient's subsequent clinical course, imaging should be performed.** It is important to remember that blunt rapid deceleration injuries, such as high-speed motor vehicle accidents or falls from great heights, pose a higher risk for vascular pedicle or ureteral pelvic junction injury.

Penetrating injuries with any degree of hematuria should be imaged. In a report by Carroll and McAninch (1985), 27 of 50 patients with penetrating renal trauma had only microscopic hematuria. Three of these had practically undetectable amounts of microhematuria—0 to 3 RBCs/HPF. Despite this, one of the three had a renal pedicle injury. A more recent study from South Africa showed a stronger correlation between degree of hematuria and severity of injury (Moolman et al., 2012). Microscopic hematuria was associated with grade III or lesser injury in 85% of patients while gross hematuria was noted in 94% of patients with grade III injury or worse.

Pediatric patients (younger than 18 years) sustaining blunt renal trauma generally can be evaluated like adults (Santucci et al., 2004), with a few caveats:

1. Children have an up to 50% higher risk for renal trauma than adults after blunt abdominal injury, such as motor vehicle accidents (Kurtz et al., 2017) and 33% higher risk for high grade injury. Possible explanations are the larger comparative kidney size, less perirenal fat, non-ossified bones, and less relative rib coverage over the kidneys in children (Buckley and McAninch, 2004).
2. Importantly, children often do not become hypotensive with major blood loss, and in the absence of this sign can still have an exsanguinating renal injury. Liberal use of renal imaging is probably warranted. Children have a high catecholamine output after trauma, which maintains blood pressure until approximately 50% of blood volume has been lost.
3. Children have a higher proportion of congenital renal abnormalities such as severe hydronephrosis or uretero-pelvic junction obstruction, which may result in significant renal injury from seemingly minor trauma.

Imaging Studies

Contrast-enhanced CT with immediate and delayed images, is the best method for genitourinary imaging in renal trauma (Bretan et al., 1986; Morey et al., 2014). Quick, highly sensitive, and specific, CT provides the most definitive staging information—parenchymal lacerations are clearly defined; extravasation of contrast-enhanced urine can easily be detected (Fig. 90.3); associated injuries to the bowel, pancreas, liver, spleen, and other organs can be identified; and the degree of retroperitoneal bleeding can be assessed by the size of the retroperitoneal hematoma. Lack of uptake of contrast material in the parenchyma suggests arterial thrombosis (Fig. 90.4) or transection. Detection of fine anatomic detail of the most serious injuries (urinary extravasation, active arterial bleeding, and severe

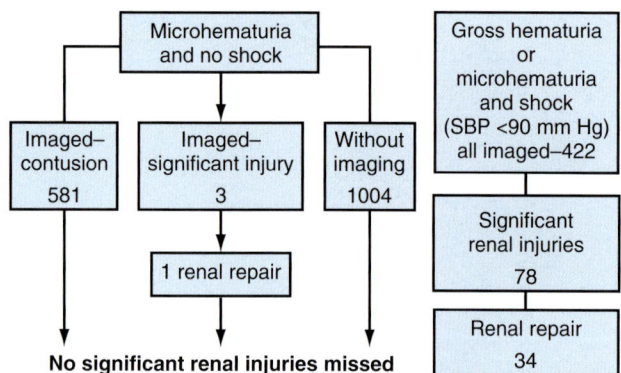

Fig. 90.2. Algorithm demonstrating the results of the authors' study on radiographic assessment of renal injuries. In adults with blunt trauma, imaging studies may be performed selectively. *SBP,* Systolic blood pressure. (From Miller KS, McAninch JW: Radiographic assessment of renal trauma: our 15-year experience. *J Urol* 154:352–355, 1995.)

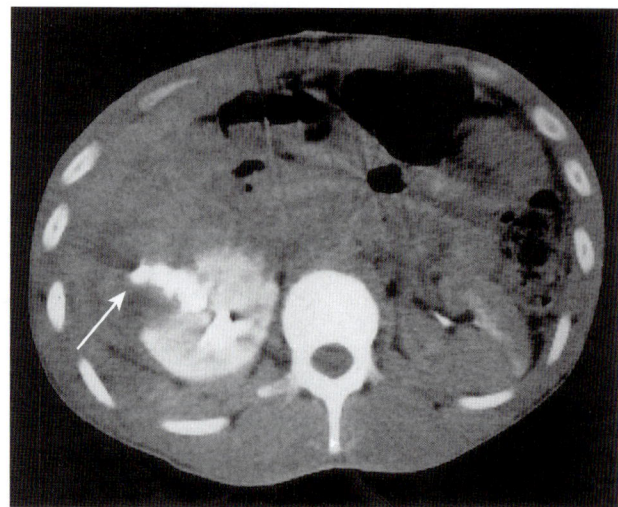

Fig. 90.3. Computed tomography scan of a right renal stab wound (grade IV) *(arrow),* demonstrating extensive urinary extravasation and large retroperitoneal hematoma.

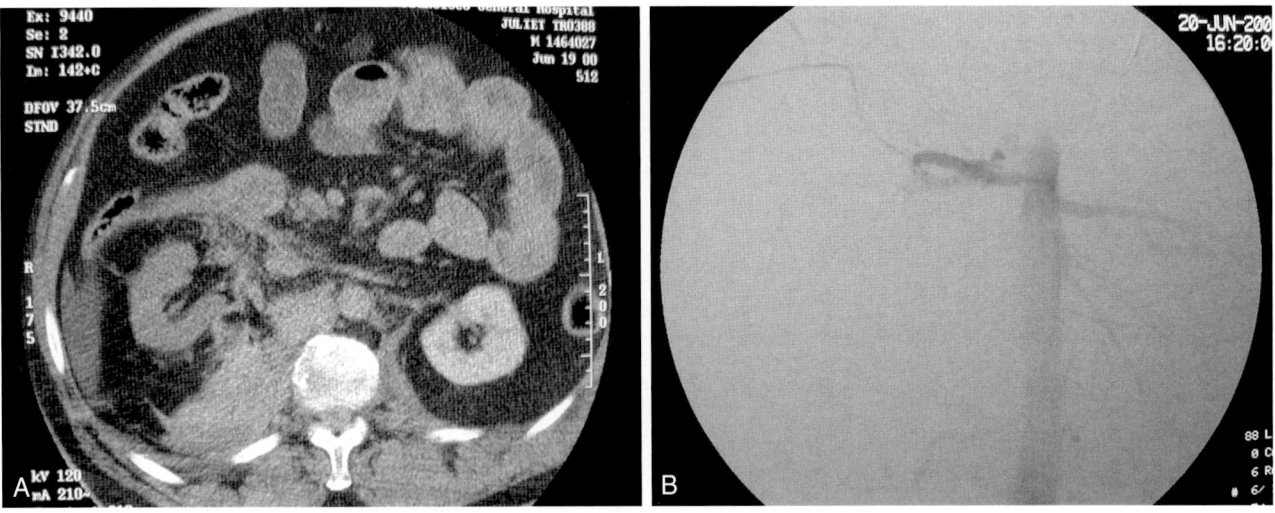

Fig. 90.4. (A) Computed tomography showing right renal artery thrombosis after crush injury. Note poor contrast uptake in right kidney compared with left and diffuse soft tissue injury medial to right kidney in the area of the renal artery. (B) Angiogram showing right renal artery thrombosis after crush injury.

parenchymal/vascular injuries) has improved confidence in our ability to understand which injuries can be managed nonoperatively.

Arteriovenous CT scanning (typically 80 seconds after contrast administration) provides visualization of the kidneys in the nephrogenic phase of contrast excretion and is necessary to detect arterial extravasation. Injury to the renal collecting system may be missed if contrast material has not had time to be excreted into the parenchyma and collecting system adequately. Delayed scanning of the kidneys 10 to 15 minutes after injection of contrast identifies parenchymal lacerations and urinary extravasation accurately and reliably. Expert opinion holds that delayed films may be omitted when the kidneys are deemed normal, and no perinephric, retroperitoneal, pelvic, or perivesical fluid is present (Morey et al., 2014). **Findings on CT that raise suspicion for major injury are (1) medial hematoma, suggesting vascular injury; (2) medial urinary extravasation, suggesting renal pelvis or ureteropelvic junction avulsion injury; (3) global lack of contrast enhancement of the parenchyma, suggesting renal artery occlusion; and (4) the combination of two or more of the following: large hematoma greater than 3.5 cm, medial renal laceration, and vascular contrast extravasation (suggesting brisk active bleeding), which constitute an AAST grade IVb injury** (Dugi et al., 2010).

Patients with grade IVb injuries require open surgery or angioembolization nine times more frequently than those with none or one of these features (Dugi et al., 2010). Also, active extravasation of intravascular contrast seen on CT (i.e., the patients are bleeding so briskly as to be detectable on the vascular phase CT scan) is highly associated with the need for subsequent angioembolization (Nuss et al., 2009; Fig. 90.5). The widespread use and anatomic detail provided by CT imaging has now supplanted the much less sensitive, less specific, and rarely used excretory urography (IV pyelography [IVP]) for grading purposes. The need for delayed-phase contrast-enhanced CT for pediatric trauma patients has been questioned, however (Fuchs et al., 2018).

One major limitation of CT is the inability to define a renal venous injury adequately. With normal arterial perfusion, the parenchyma appears normal and the collecting system may contain contrast material. A medial hematoma accompanying the preceding findings suggests a venous injury. Most venous injuries result in either hemorrhage requiring surgery or angioembolization or tamponade and stop bleeding and thus require no further treatment. The true clinical significance of the insensitivity of CT to renal vein injury is currently unknown.

In contemporary practice, there is a limited role for intraoperative "one-shot" IVP. The indications are uncommon, such as when the

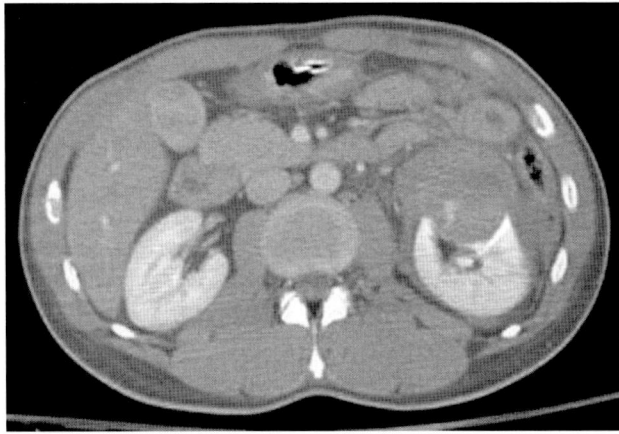

Fig. 90.5. Computed tomography showing left renal fossa hematoma after blunt renal trauma, with bright jet of active extravasation of intravascular contrast indicating brisk active bleeding.

surgeon encounters an unexpected retroperitoneal hematoma surrounding a kidney during abdominal exploration in an unstable trauma patient without a previous CT scan, and are contemplating renal exploration or nephrectomy. **The main purpose of the one-shot IVP is to assess the presence of a functioning contralateral kidney.** It is vital to know if a patient has only one kidney, because urgent surgical exploration of renal injuries often leads to nephrectomy for the injured kidney. **The IVP technique is key to gaining important information and minimizing the time involved. Only a single film is taken 10 minutes after IV injection (IV push) of 2 mL/kg of contrast material.** The study can also be helpful in assessing for urinary contrast extravasation. If the study is normal, exploration of the injured side may be avoided. If findings are not near normal, further imaging is recommended or the kidney explored to complete the staging of the injury.

Morey et al. (1999) reported their experience with one-shot intraoperative IVP for the immediate management of renal injuries. In 50 patients, the film quality was adequate and properly done to avoid renal exploration in 32%. However, it is often difficult to obtain a well performed or timed one-shot IVP because unstable trauma patients are typically hypoperfused. Moreover, most trauma surgeons today use retroperitoneal palpation to assess for the presence of a normal caliber contralateral kidney, and rarely utilize one-shot IVP (Yeung and Brandes, 2012).

Sonography is typically used in the immediate evaluation of abdominal injuries (focused assessment with sonography for trauma [FAST] examination), but has poor specificity in the adult renal patient for renal injuries. FAST is limited by obesity, subcutaneous air and prior abdominal operations. If necessary, sonography can confirm the presence of two kidneys and can detect a retroperitoneal collection. It cannot differentiate between a hematoma and a urine leak.

Angioembolization

Renal arteriography and embolization is a commonly used modality in renal trauma and is increasingly being used for higher-grade injuries (Otsuka et al., 2018). In the correct setting, it can be used to stop significant renal bleeding without the need for laparotomy, and its indications are increasing. It is vital that if angioembolization is used and the local angiography team is experienced, the procedure can be done without delay, and the patient can be monitored and even resuscitated during transport to and in the angiography suite. Superselective embolization therapy for renal trauma may provide an effective and less invasive technique to avoid unnecessary exploration that could otherwise result in nephrectomy. Initial failure is common, between 13% and 88% (Breyer et al., 2008; Sugihara et al., 2012), but subsequent embolization is highly successful in at least one series (Hotaling et al., 2011). A recent survey of urologists and interventional radiologists showed that urologists are more willing to use angioembolization for grade IV and V injuries (Glass et al., 2014). Another study found increasing use of angioembolization for grade IV and highly select V injuries, with hemodynamic instability and grade being independent predictors of surgical treatment (Lanchon et al., 2016).

Traumatic pseudoaneurysms and arteriovenous fistulas are often treated by angiographic embolization with a high expected success rate (Fig. 90.6). A recent study found a pseudoaneurysm rate of 2.5% among all grades of renal trauma with successful angioembolization in 84.6% of patients (Guyot et al., 2017). Endovascular stents have been used with success during angiography in patients with acute renal artery thrombosis occurring from intimal flaps (Goodman et al., 1998). Longer term follow-up and more cases are needed to determine whether this will be a successful management approach, especially considering kidney warm ischemia time, and that most stents require anticoagulation after placement, which may not be possible in a trauma patient.

Nonoperative Management

Significant renal injuries (grades II to V) are found in only 5% of renal trauma cases (Keihani et al., 2018). **Nonoperative management is the standard of care in hemodynamically stable, well-staged patients with AAST grades I to IVa renal injuries, regardless of mechanism** (Dugi et al., 2010; Morey et al., 2014). **Most experts agree that patients with grades IV and V injuries more often require surgical exploration, but even these high-grade injuries can be managed without renal operation if carefully staged and selected** (Fig. 90.7) (Buckley and McAninch, 2006; Santucci and McAninch, 2000; Umbreit et al., 2009; van der Wilden et al., 2013). Interestingly, conservative management of high-grade renal injuries has not been associated with increased length of stay (Hampson et al., 2018) and may even be associated with a shorter length of stay and likely higher renal preservation rate (Sujenthiran et al., 2019).

A trial of expectant management has been advocated for most adult blunt renal parenchymal injuries, many isolated (kidney only) renal stab wounds, and select and isolated renal gunshot wounds.

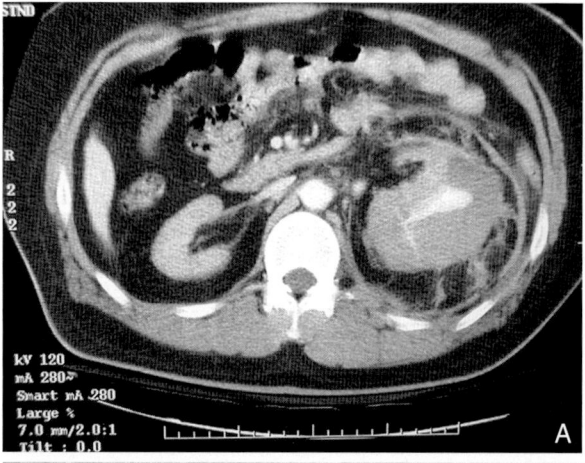
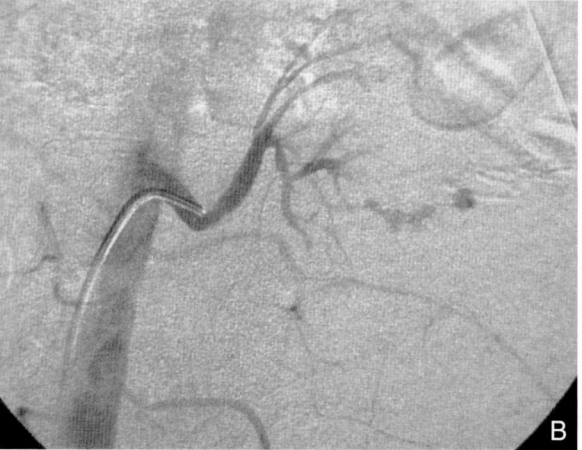
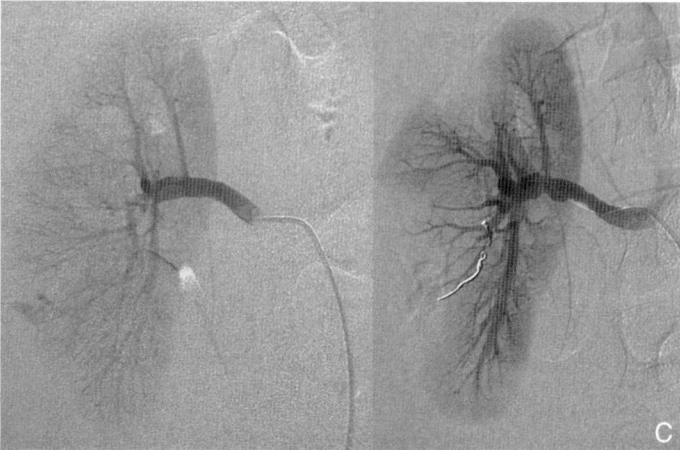

Fig. 90.6. (A) Computed tomography showing left post-traumatic arteriovenous fistula. (B) Angiogram showing left post-traumatic arteriovenous fistula. (C) Angioembolization of right renal laceration: arteriography demonstrating active arterial bleeding. Coil embolization was used to control bleeding. Note the presence of the coil and large, triangular area of infarct.

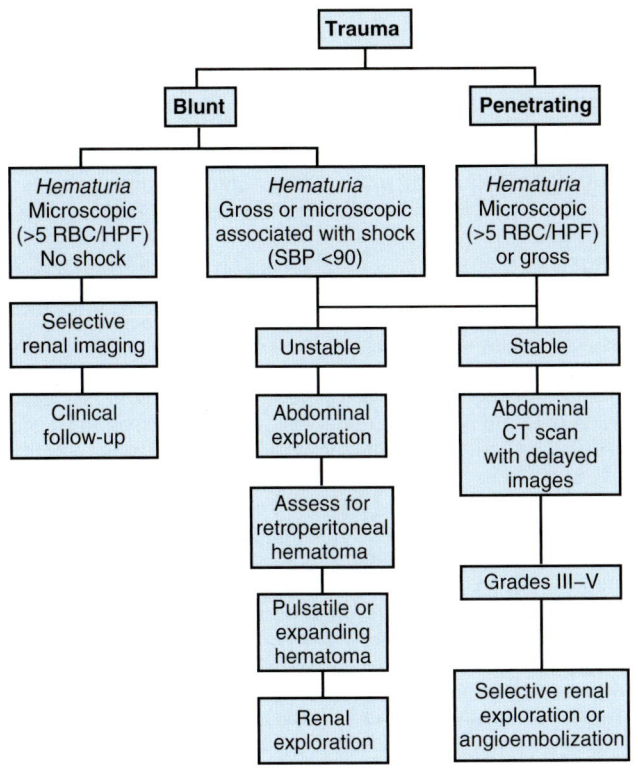

Fig. 90.7. Flow chart for adult renal injuries to serve as a guide for decision making. *CT*, Computed tomography; *IVP*, intravenous pyelography; *RBC/HPF*, red blood cells per high-power field; *SBP*, systolic blood pressure.

Bluntly injured kidneys often heal well when managed conservatively, even in the setting of urinary extravasation and nonviable tissue. Overall, over 90% can be successfully managed without exploration. Even select high-grade injuries can successfully be treated nonoperatively. In a series of six hemodynamically stable, grade V blunt "shattered" kidney injuries, all were treated successfully without surgery (Altman et al., 2000). Patients who are exsanguinating (hemodynamically unstable) from the kidney, however demand exploration and subsequent nephrectomy/renorrhaphy. Those who are hemodynamically stable can in select circumstances be successfully treated without surgery (Moolman et al., 2012). Significant delayed renal bleeding is usually amenable to angioembolization, occurs in 9%. Another series showed a 93% renal salvage rate among patients with grades IV and V injury (May et al., 2016).

Select gunshot or stab wounds isolated to the kidney can be managed nonoperatively in stable patients. In one large series, 55% of renal stab wounds and 24% of gunshot wounds were successfully managed nonoperatively in carefully selected patients with well-staged injuries (McAninch et al., 1991). The AAST GU Trauma Study recently reported managing 57 patients (13%) with isolated, low-velocity gunshot wounds conservatively with few complications (Keihani et al., 2018). High grade penetrating injuries (AAST grade III or IV) are typically managed surgically because of the high rate of delayed bleed (24%) and the necessity to explore for associated intra-abdominal injuries. Stab wounds posterior to the posterior axillary line are less likely to have visceral injuries, and thus more likely to be successfully managed conservatively. The penetrating wound can often disrupt Gerota's fascia significantly, and thus can uncontain the perirenal hematoma. If the injury is isolated to the kidney, however, and no major intra-abdominal structure has been injured, it is safe to manage expectantly. Such patients must undergo frequent serial abdominal exams, particularly in the first 24 hours. Any new tenderness or abdominal guarding warrant abdominal exploration.

Stab injuries have even more evidence to support conservative management. Nonoperative management was successful and resulted in no delayed nephrectomies in a cohort of 108 hemodynamically stable patients with stab wounds (Armenakas et al., 1999). Some blunt and penetrating abdominal trauma may require laparotomy because of associated nonurologic injury, but even in these cases it is not necessary to explore the kidney additionally, especially if Grade 1–3 (Shariat et al., 2008b). The only absolute intraoperative indication for kidney exploration is a pulsatile and expanding retroperitoneal hematoma, that suggests a life-threatening renal artery laceration.

All patients with high-grade injuries selected for nonoperative management should be closely observed with serial hematocrit readings and vital signs. Classic teaching is to prescribe bed rest until gross hematuria resolves. However, this practice is empiric and there is little to no support in the literature for such.

Routine follow up CT imaging for Grade IV–V renal injuries is prudent at 48 to 72 hours post injury, to evaluate for a troublesome urinoma, collection or hematoma. **Recently, there is mounting evidence that significant complications almost always present with symptoms (fever, flank pain, dropping hematocrit, increasing hematuria, etc.)** (Davis et al., 2010). Thus, routine follow-up CT may be unnecessary in the asymptomatic patient. Routine follow-up CT imaging is not needed for uncomplicated Grade I–III injuries because it is unlikely to change management and not cost effective. Although most grade II to IV injuries resolve uneventfully, delayed renal bleeding sometimes can occur (Wessells et al., 1997). Should bleeding persist or delayed bleeding occur, angiography with selective embolization of bleeding vessels can obviate surgical intervention. The patient should be periodically undergo blood pressure monitoring for up to a year post injury, for the rare instance of acute or delayed renovascular hypertension. Delayed bleeding after discharge to home is rare and usually occurs within 2 weeks post injury.

Conservative management rarely fails within the first 24 hours (2.7% of patients). Risk factors for failure include renal injury grade, nonrenal abdominal injuries, and penetrating injuries (Bjurlin et al., 2017). Most patients for whom conservative management fails require only a ureteral stent or angioembolization. The complication rate of nonoperative treatment is much lower than that of aggressive surgical exploration and results in shorter intensive care unit (ICU) stays, shorter hospital stays, lower mortality, and fewer transfusions (Bjurlin et al., 2011). **However, patients who are hemodynamically unstable with no or transient response to resuscitation from the kidney injury require rapid open surgical exploration or in some cases quick expert angioembolization to avoid death.** Although nonoperative management for renal trauma has been increasing, recent study shows that the rate of surgical intervention for renal trauma varies significantly among high-, medium-, and low-volume trauma centers, with high-volume centers intervening in only 12.6% of patients (Dagenais et al., 2016).

Initial observation is warranted for patients with renal injury and urinary extravasation (Morey et al., 2014). **Such injuries often resolve spontaneously in over 90%, unless a renal pelvis avulsion or proximal ureteral avulsion injury is present. Medial extravasation of contrast from the kidney, with lack of contrast in the distal ureteral on delayed CT imaging, suggests UPJ avulsion.** For such patients, prompt intervention is required, either endoscopically or open, depending on the clinical situation. When continued urinary drainage leads to enlarging urinoma, fistula, infection, or signs of chemical peritonitis such as pain, fever, ileus, urinary drainage via ureteral stent and/or urinoma drain are required. In severe renal injuries with continued urinary extravasation, placement of an internal ureteral stent alone for drainage usually prevents prolonged urinary extravasation and decreases the chance of perirenal urinoma formation. On occasion, retrograde placement of ureteral stents is not possible. Examples include concomitant pelvic fracture urethral distraction defects, severe genital trauma prohibiting urethral access, complete ureteral transection, and fractures prohibiting the dorsal lithotomy position. Percutaneous nephrostomy drainage with consideration for antegrade ureteral stent placement is a viable option in these situations.

Fluid collections seen on serial imaging for renal trauma are either hematomas, urinomas, or abscesses. Urinomas can be distinguished from hematomas by their radiographic characteristics: urinomas range from 0 to 20 Hounsfield units (HU), whereas hematomas typically are greater than 30 HU (Federle and Jeffrey, 1983). Also, urinomas enhance with contrast pooling dependently during delayed phase imaging (5 to 20 minutes after IV injection of contrast). Abscesses have rim enhancement and high attenuation fluid (HU >20) on contrasted films (Allen et al., 2012). When the perinephric fluid collection persists despite ureteral stenting or percutaneous nephrostomy drainage, placement of a percutaneous drain can facilitate healing and prevent or treat abscesses.

Operative Management

Indications for renal exploration or speedy angioembolization after trauma can be separated into absolute and relative (Morey et al., 2014). **Absolute indications include (1) hemodynamic instability with no or transient response to resuscitation, (2) expanding/pulsatile renal hematoma (usually indicating renal artery laceration), (3) suspected renal vascular pedicle avulsion, and (4) ureteropelvic junction avulsion.** Relative indications are (1) urinary extravasation with significant renal parenchymal devascularization (older data suggested a higher complication rate than average if watched, but these also can be closely observed), (2) renal injury together with colon/pancreatic injury (these patients have a higher complication rate if their renal injury is not repaired at the time of colon/pancreatic injury, but the renal injury may be closely observed after repair of the enteric injury), (3) arterial thrombosis, and (4) urinary extravasation from parenchymal injury. More recent data suggest that patients with renal devascularization and urine leak actually have excellent outcomes, with only 1 of 18 (6%) patients requiring subsequent intervention during conservative management of segmental renal artery injuries (Elliott et al., 2007). Also, more recent data suggest that concurrent renal and colonic injuries do not have to be managed operatively (Oosthuizen et al., 2018).

Urinary extravasation alone from a grade IV parenchymal laceration can be safely managed nonoperatively with an expectation of spontaneous resolution of more than 90%. Should nonviable tissue constitute more than 25% in association with a parenchymal laceration, urinary extravasation, or both, the potential for complications (i.e., abscess) increases, and thus a threshold for renal exploration should be lower (Alsikafi et al., 2006).

Renal Exploration

Surgical exploration of the acutely injured kidney is best by a transabdominal approach, which allows complete inspection of intra-abdominal organs and bowel. In some reported series of penetrating injuries, nonrenal organ injury has been noted to be as high as 94% (McAninch et al., 1993). Injuries to the great vessels, liver, spleen, pancreas, and bowel can be identified and stabilized, if necessary, before renal exploration.

The surgical approach to renal exploration is shown in Fig. 90.8 (McAninch and Carroll, 1989). The renal vessels are isolated before exploration to provide the immediate capability to occlude them if massive bleeding should ensue when Gerota fascia is opened (Scott and Selzman, 1966). The small bowel is eviscerated and lifted out of the surgical field. This exposes the mid-retroperitoneum. An incision is made over the aorta in the retroperitoneum just superior to the inferior mesenteric artery. The incision is extended superiorly to the ligament of Treitz. Exposure of the anterior surface of the aorta is accomplished and followed superiorly to the left renal vein, which crosses the aorta anteriorly. A vessel loop is placed on the right or left renal vein as necessary. The vein usually must be retracted cephalad, with a vein or-Gil Vernet retractor, to expose the left and right renal arteries beneath. The artery is secured with vessel loops. The right renal vein also can be secured through this incision; but if this proves difficult, reflecting the second portion of the duodenum provides excellent exposure to the vein.

Large hematomas may extend over the aorta and obscure the landmarks for the planned initial retroperitoneal incision. In such instances, the inferior mesenteric vein can be used as an anatomic guide for an appropriate incision. By making the retroperitoneal incision just medial to the inferior mesenteric vein and dissecting through the hematoma, the anterior surface of the aorta can be identified and followed superiorly to the crossing left renal vein.

The kidney is then exposed by incising the peritoneum lateral to the colon, followed by mobilization off Gerota fascia. This maneuver often requires release of the splenic (left) or hepatic (right) attachments of the colon. Gerota fascia is then opened, and the kidney with injury is completely dissected from the surrounding hematoma. Should troublesome bleeding develop, the previously isolated vessels can be temporarily occluded with a vascular clamp or a vessel loop tourniquet.

Is Early Vessel Isolation Necessary? Debate surrounds the method of renal vascular control. Some manadate that control of the renal

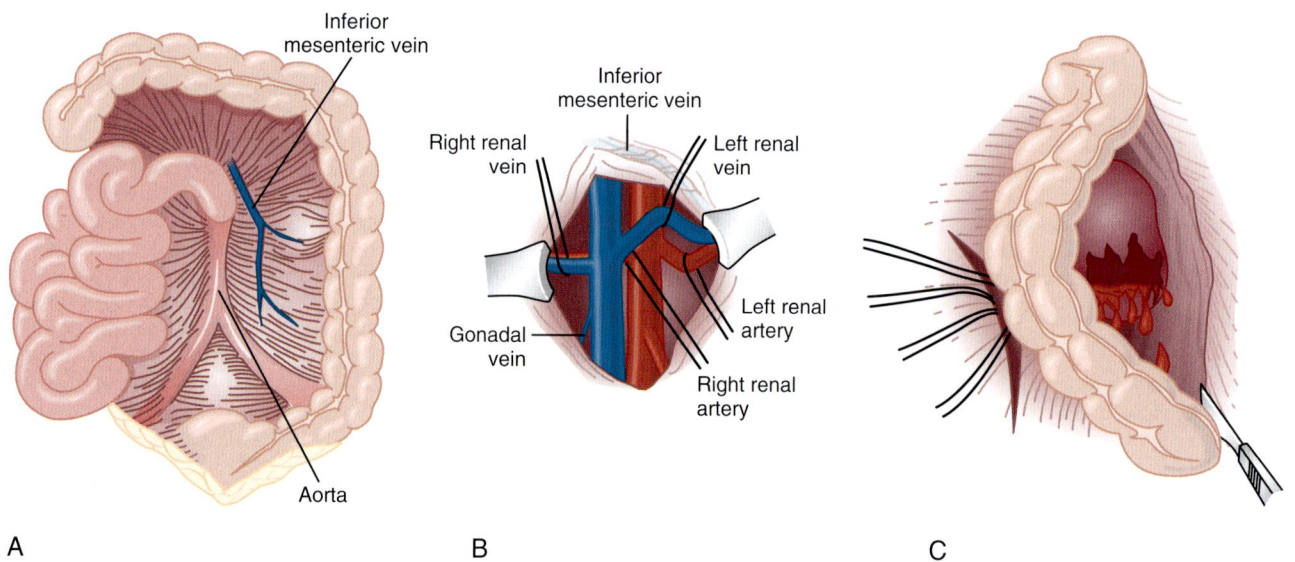

Fig. 90.8. The surgical approach to the renal vessels and kidney. (A) Retroperitoneal incision over the aorta medial to the inferior mesenteric vein. (B) Anatomic relationships of the renal vessels. (C) Retroperitoneal incision lateral to the colon, exposing the kidney.

artery and vein need to be done proximal to the injury site, prior to opening Gerota's fascia. The argument being, that proximal vascular control avoids a potential massive bleed, from release of the tamponade effect. Thus, obtaining early vascular control before opening Gerota fascia can decrease renal loss, depending on the injury site. In a comparative series, the total nephrectomy rate was reduced from 56% to 18% when vascular control was obtained (McAninch and Carroll, 1982). Carroll et al. (1989) reported that the looped vessels only had to be temporarily clamped in approximately 2% of renal explorations. In a series of 133 renal units in which early vessel isolation and control were achieved before opening Gerota fascia, McAninch et al. (1991) found that a renal salvage rate of 89% was possible.

Corriere et al. (1991) reported a series of renal units in which vascular control was obtained only if needed after opening Gerota fascia. In this group, the total nephrectomy rate was 37%. Atala et al. (1991) reported a similar group of patients with a total nephrectomy rate of 36%. Others argue that mobilizing the kidney from Gerota's fascia laterally before proximal control yields equivalent blood loss and renal salvage (Gonzalez, 1999), and that most parenchymal kidney bleeding can be controlled by manual compression and, if need be, a Satinsky clamp across the hilum.

Overall, the goal of kidney exploration is to control the bleeding first, repair the kidney (when possible) and retroperitoneal drainage.

The AUA urotrauma guideline states that the benefit of "primary vascular control in modern series are inconclusive, although older studies suggest that it is beneficial" (Morey et al., 2014). **Regardless of the method of vascular control, when unstable, high grade kidney trauma patients undergo open retroperitoneal exploration, nephrectomy is often the result.**

Renal Reconstruction

The principles of renal reconstruction after trauma include complete renal exposure, measures for temporary vascular control, limited debridement of nonviable tissue, hemostasis by individual suture ligation of bleeding vessels, watertight closure of the collecting system if necessary/possible, re-approximation of the parenchymal defect, coverage with nearby fascio-adipose flaps (Gerota fascia or omentum) if feasible, and liberal use of drains (Fig. 90.9).

Renorrhaphy is illustrated in Fig. 90.10. Note the approximation of the margins of the laceration (3-0 Vicryl or similar suture) with the use of renal capsule over an absorbable hemostatic agent bolster such as Surgicel or Nu-Knit (oxidized rgenerated cellulose; Ethicon, NJ), or Gelfoam (Pfizer, New York, NY).

When polar injuries cannot be reconstructed, a partial nephrectomy can be performed. The open parenchyma should be covered when

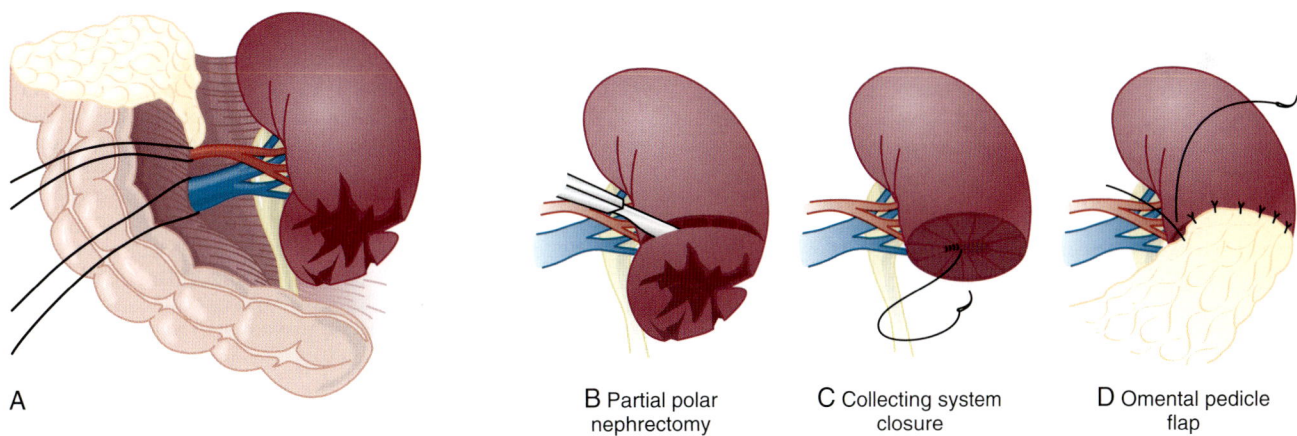

Fig. 90.9. Technique for partial nephrectomy. (A) Total renal exposure. (B) Sharp removal of nonviable tissue. (C) Hemostasis obtained and collecting system closed. (D) Defect covered.

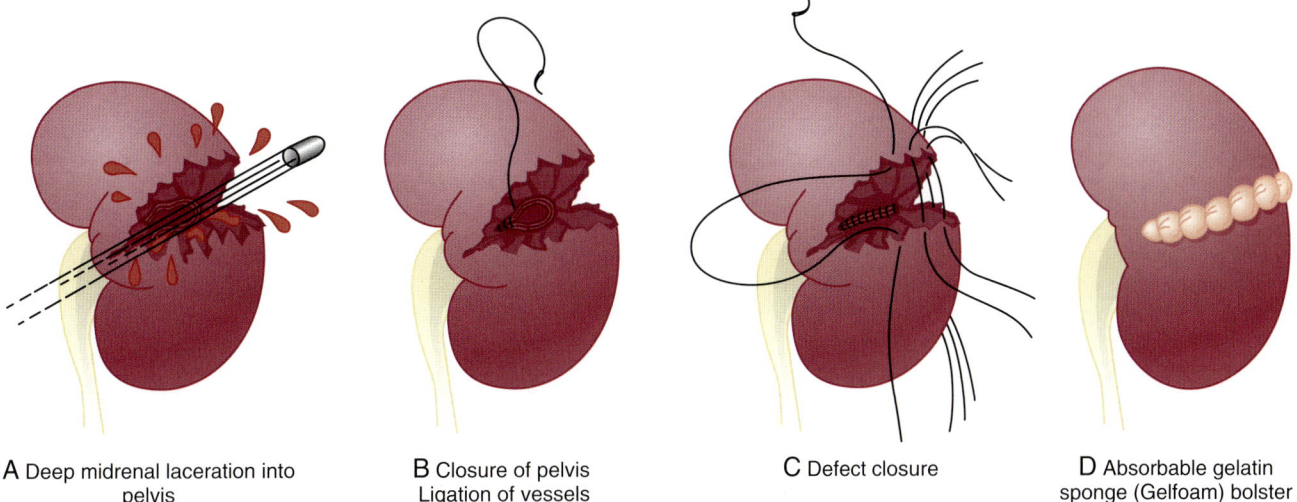

Fig. 90.10. Technique for renorrhaphy. (A) Typical injury in midportion of kidney. (B) Debridement, hemostasis, and collecting system closure. (C) Approximation of parenchymal margins. (D) Sutures tied over gelatin sponge bolster.

possible by a pedicle flap of omentum (see Fig. 90.9). With its rich vascular and lymphatic supply, omentum promotes wound healing and decreases the risk for delayed bleeding and urinary extravasation. Should it not be available, the use of absorbable mesh, peritoneal graft, or retroperitoneal fat also has been successful.

Hemostatic agents such as Floseal, thrombin plus gelatin (Baxter, Deerfield, IL) are potent and have an increasing role in the management of genitourinary trauma (Fig. 90.11). Based on experience from nephron-sparing surgery, gelatin matrix was applied to a porcine model of complex renal trauma and demonstrated less mean blood loss than conventional suture treatment (Hick et al., 2005).

In a high percentage of major renal injuries, intra-abdominal structures are also injured, with the liver and spleen being the most common. Injuries to the colon, pancreas, and stomach also occur frequently. In previous years total nephrectomy was suggested because of the high complication rate with attempted renal salvage. However, renal repair concomitantly with these associated injuries can be successful with few complications (Master and McAninch, 2006; Oosthuizen et al., 2018; Rosen and McAninch, 1994; Wessells and McAninch, 1996). Drains should be used liberally after these repairs.

Renovascular Injuries. Renovascular penetrating or avulsion injuries after trauma are uncommon and often have associated injuries requiring operative intervention. For major renovascular injuries in patients with two kidneys, prompt nephrectomy is advocated. In rare instances in which vascular repair is technically feasible, renal salvage rates are disappointingly low, exemplified by a 33% renal salvage rate for main renal artery reconstruction even in the most expert of hands (Elliott et al., 2007). Vascular repair requires occlusion of the involved vessel with vascular clamps. The lacerated main renal vessels can be repaired with 5-0 nonabsorbable vascular suture (Fig. 90.12).

Main renal artery thrombosis from blunt trauma occurs most often secondary to deceleration injuries. The mobility of the kidney results in stretch on the renal artery, which in turn causes the arterial intima, low in elastic fibers, to disrupt. The consequent thrombus occludes the vessel, rendering the kidney ischemic (Fig. 90.13). **For unilateral arterial thrombosis, revascularization rarely results in a successful salvage or a viable kidney.** As long as the contra-lateral kidney is normal, observation is often the best management. In contrast, for bilateral renal hilar injuries, revascularization should be attempted, as up to 56% of patients can potentially avoid dialysis by prompt intervention (Knudson et al., 2000; Haas and Sprinak, 1998).

Case reports of successful renal revascularization through the use of endovascular stents during angiography offers a promising approach to the problem of blunt trauma renal artery thrombosis caused by the intimal flap (Inoue et al., 2004; Memon and Cheung, 2005). The great disadvantage of this approach has been the inability to safely institute post-stent anticoagulation in the patient with polytrauma.

Surgical revascularization is seldom successful in renal artery thrombosis, and at least 43% of patients with repairs develop hypertension (Haas et al., 1998). Periodic blood pressure monitoring for hypertension for up to a year after injury is thus warranted. Many patients with renal vascular injury are critically injured, with numerous associated organ injuries; time constraints thus limit any attempt at vascular repair.

Penetrating injuries to the renal hilar vessels are uncommon and very challenging. A penetrating injury to the right renal hilum often has associated injuries to the pancreatoduodenal complex, the right renal artery artery, the right renal vein and/or the IVC. Thus, such hilar injuries typically result in nephrectomy. If the patient is stable, surgical repair with fine vascular suture (5-0) can be attempted (see Fig. 90.12). Partial occlusion of the vein is ideal during repair, but in some instances total temporary occlusion with vascular clamps is necessary. On the left, if the injury is proximal to the

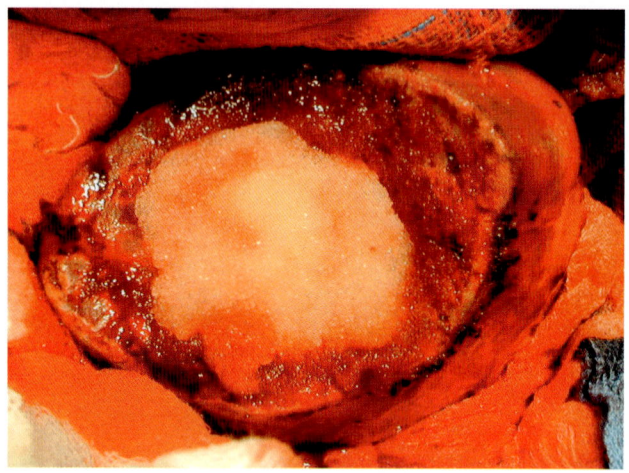

Fig. 90.11. Partial nephrectomy showing excellent hemostasis with use of Floseal (hemostatic agent).

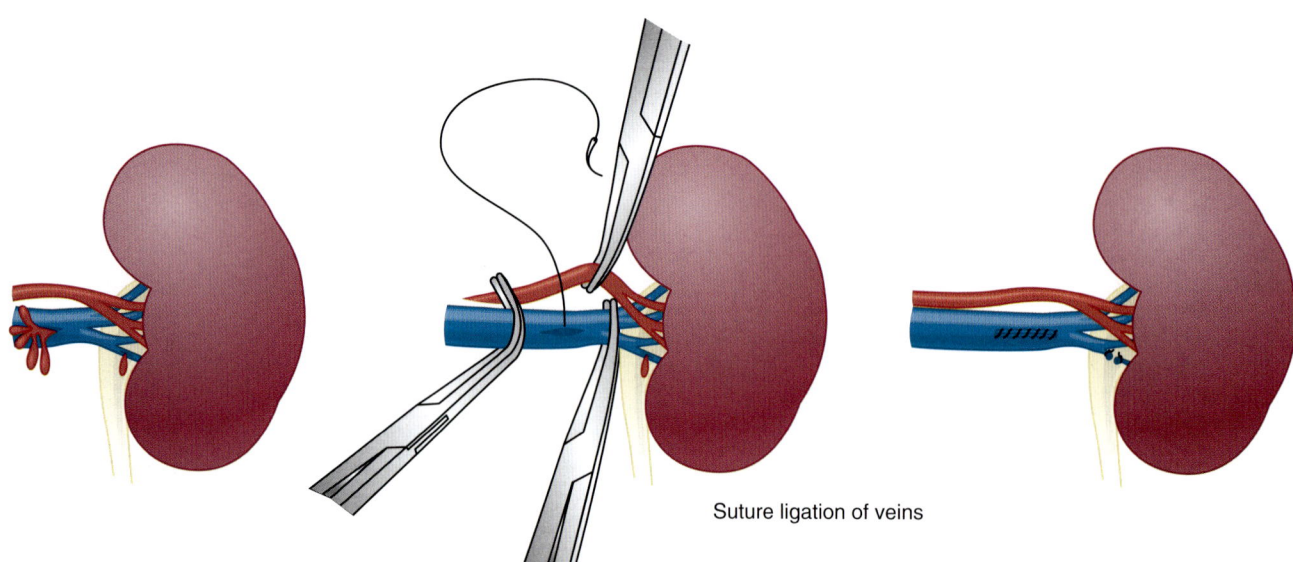

Fig. 90.12. Vascular injuries. *Left,* Venous injuries may occur in the main renal vein or the segmental branches. *Middle,* Repair of main renal vein. *Right,* Ligation of segmental branch can be done safely.

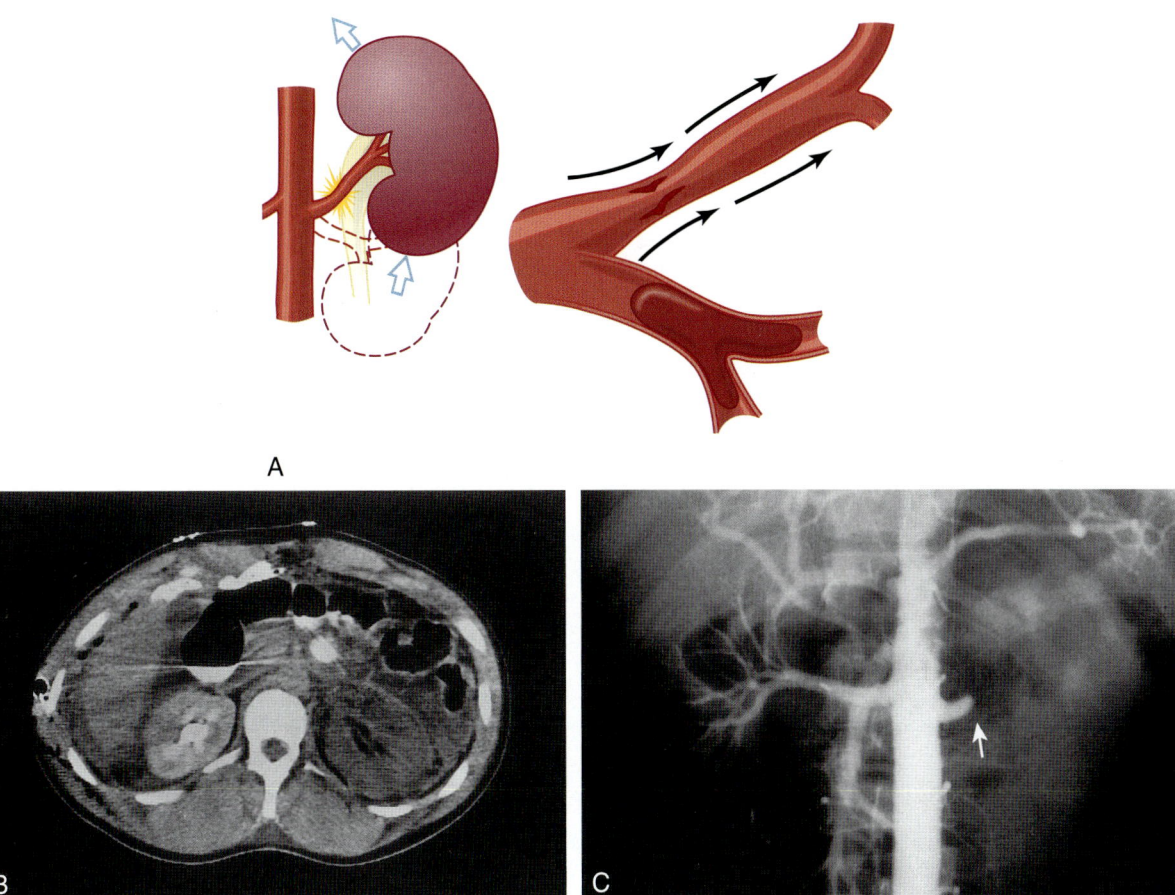

Fig. 90.13. (A) Movement of the kidney from blunt trauma (deceleration injury) causes stretch on the renal artery, resulting in rupture of the arterial intima and formation of a thrombus. (B) Computed tomography of a left kidney with renal artery thrombosis, demonstrating lack of contrast material perfusion to the kidney. (C) Arteriography demonstrating complete occlusion of the left renal artery *(arrow)* secondary to thrombus formation.

gonadal and adrenal branches, the renal vein can be ligated, unlike the right renal vein, which is uncolateralized. For the injured renal artery, the simplest repair possible is warranted, in order to limit ischemic time.

Damage Control

Once exanguinating hemorrhage is controlled and bowel contamination limited, Coburn (1997) and Pursifull et al. (2006) noted the benefit of damage control to improve renal salvage after polytrauma and further benefit was noted by Yeung and Brandes (2011). If there is active oozing from Gerota's fascia, the area around the injured kidney can be packed with laparotomy pads to control bleeding, with a planned return in 24 to 48 hours to explore and evaluate the extent of injury. Furthermore, managing a nonpulsatile, contained, and nonexpanding retroperitoneal hematoma by observation is another method of damage control of the injured kidney. This allows the cold, acidotic, and coagulopathic patient to be stabilized in the ICU before any attempt at potentially lengthy renal reconstruction is attempted. At times, the bleeding kidney can be controlled by angioembolization, after the patient has been being resuscitated. Damage control may allow patients with complex renal injuries to avoid unneeded nephrectomy. However, if the kidney is massively injured, and the patient persistently unstable, a quick damage control nephrectomy can be life saving. Survival predictors in patients undergoing damage control surgery include Glasgow Coma Scale below 8, base excess below −13.9, and low preoperative diastolic pressure (Wang et al., 2014).

Indications for Nephrectomy

The ability to reconstruct an injured kidney depends on numerous factors. In an unstable patient, if damage control is not an option, total nephrectomy would be indicated immediately when the patient's life would be threatened by attempting a renal repair. When Nash et al. (1995) examined the reasons for nephrectomy in patients with renal injuries, 77% required removal because of the extent of parenchymal, vascular, or combined injury. The remaining 23% required nephrectomy in otherwise reconstructable kidneys because of hemodynamic instability. Factors predictive for nephrectomy are high injury severity score, high grade of renal injury, and hemodynamic instability (Davis et al., 2006).

Complications

Persistent urinary extravasation can result in urinoma, perinephric infection, and, rarely, renal loss. These patients are initially administered systemic antibiotics, although data supporting their use do not exist. In a high percentage, the extravasation resolves spontaneously (Matthews et al., 1997). Should it persist, placement of an internal ureteral stent often corrects the problem. The addition of a percutaneous nephrostomy or transcutaneously placed urinoma drain may be required in patients not cured by ureteral stent placement.

Delayed renal bleeding can occur up to several weeks after injury but usually occurs within 21 days. The initial management is bed rest and hydration. Should the bleeding persist, angiography frequently can localize and control the bleeding vessel by embolization.

Perinephric abscess rarely occurs after renal injury; persistent urinary extravasation and urinoma are the typical precursors. Urinary drainage with a ureteral stent with or without percutaneous nephrostomy followed by percutaneous abscess drainage offers a good initial method of management, followed by surgical drainage (rarely) if necessary.

Hypertension is seldom noted in the early postinjury period but can occur later (Monstrey et al., 1989). The basic mechanisms for arterial hypertension as a complication of trauma are (1) renal vascular injury, leading to stenosis or occlusion of the main renal artery or one of its branches (Goldblatt kidney); (2) compression of the renal parenchyma with extravasated blood or urine (Page kidney); and (3) post-trauma arteriovenous fistula. In these instances, the renin-angiotensin axis is stimulated by partial renal ischemia, resulting in hypertension (Cosgrove et al., 1973; Goldblatt et al., 1934).

In addition, patients should be followed for decline in renal function. A retrospective study of renal trauma patients managed nonoperatively showed a postinjury decline in renal function that correlated with severity of injury (Tasian et al., 2010).

> **KEY POINTS: RENAL TRAUMA**
>
> - Expectant management strategies of renal trauma allow for maximal renal preservation.
> - The degree of hematuria and the severity of renal injury do not consistently correlate.
> - Contrast-enhanced CT is the best imaging method to assess and grade for renal trauma.
> - Patients with microscopic hematuria without shock can be observed clinically without imaging studies.
> - Hemodynamically stable, well-staged renal injuries can be conservatively managed (even with high-grade injuries).
> - Selective embolization provides an effective and minimally invasive means to stop active bleeding from parenchymal lacerations and segmental arterial injury.
> - CT findings suspicious for significant renal injury include (1) medial hematoma (vascular pedicle injury), (2) medial urinary extravasation (renal pelvis or ureteropelvic junction injury), (3) lack of contrast enhancement of the parenchyma (main renal arterial injury), and (4) active intravascular contrast extravasation (arterial injury with brisk bleeding).
> - Kidney injuries with hemodynamic instability, despite resuscitation, suggests uncontrolled and ongoing bleeding and warrants immediate intervention (surgery or in selected situations, angioembolization).
> - Kidney injuries with urinary extravasation can often be managed conservatively and resolve spontaneously. Renal pelvis or proximal ureteral avulsion demand prompt intervention.

URETERAL INJURIES

Cause

Acute ureteral injury results from external trauma, open surgery, laparoscopy, and endoscopic procedures. Intraoperative suture ligation, sharp incision and transection, avulsion, devascularization, and heat (e.g., microwave, electrocautery, or vibratory energy) or freezing (e.g., cryoablation) energies can produce ureteral damage. In addition, penetrating stab and gunshot wounds and external injury from high-speed blunt mechanisms contribute to the overall incidence; 95% are penetrating and 5% are blunt injuries. Of all urologic trauma, roughly 1% to 2.5% are ureteral (Presti et al., 1989; Siram et al., 2010). An unrecognized or mismanaged ureteral injury can lead to significant complications, including urinoma, abscess, ureteral stricture, urinary fistula, and potential loss of an ipsilateral renal unit. Increased nephrectomy rates and a prolonged hospital stay are associated with a delayed or missed diagnosis from penetrating ureteral trauma (Kunkle et al., 2006). **Ureteral injuries are often subtle, and clinicians must maintain a high index of suspicion to prevent a delay in diagnosis and comorbidity.**

External Trauma

Damage to the ureter after external violence is rare, occurring in less than 4% of all penetrating and less than 1% of all cases of blunt trauma (Table 90.2). During wartime in the past century, 3% to 15% of urologic injuries involved the ureter, with an average of 5% from World War II up to modern conflicts (Busch et al., 1967; Elliott and McAninch, 2006; Marekovic et al., 1997; Selikowitz, 1977; Serkin et al., 2010). In the nonmilitary setting, a similar 2% to 3% of ureteral injuries are caused by civilian gunshot wounds. **These patients often have significant concurrent injuries and a high degree of mortality that approaches one-third** (Medina et al., 1998). **More than 90% of patients with ureteral injuries have a concurrent abdominal or retroperitoneal organ injury** (Pereira et al., 2010). Associated visceral injury is common—predominantly small (39% to 65%) and large (28% to 33%) bowel perforation (Cinman et al., 2013; Presti et al., 1989). A significant percentage (10% to 28%) of patients with ureteral injuries also have associated renal injuries (Medina et al., 1998; Presti et al., 1989). A smaller percentage (5%) have associated bladder injuries (Medina et al., 1998).

The mechanism by which bullets injure the ureter is thought to be similar to the mechanism by which they injure analogous structures such as blood vessels—that is, not only by direct transection but by disruption of the delicate intramural blood supply. In experimental models, such microvascular damage has been found as far away as 2 cm from the point of transection, although ureters seldom need extensive debridement and can generally be minimally debrided back to a bleeding edge (Amato et al., 1970).

Whereas penetrating trauma imparts a large degree of energy over a small area (as in the course of a bullet), patients with blunt trauma with ureteral injuries are subject to extreme force applied over the entire body, such as during a fall from heights, pedestrian vs. motor vehicle, or high-speed motor vehicle accident. The great degree of energy imparted to the victim is associated with such uncommon injuries as fractured lumbar processes (Evans and Smith, 1976) and thoracolumbar spinal dislocation (Campbell et al., 1992). The presence of massive force injuries in the patient with blunt trauma should always increase the level of suspicion for ureteral injury.

Patients with penetrating trauma with any degree of hematuria or a wound pattern that suggests the possibility of genitourinary injury should be imaged. Patients with blunt trauma with gross hematuria or microhematuria plus hypotension, a history of significant deceleration, or significant associated injuries also should be imaged (Morey et al., 2014; Serafetinides et al., 2015).

TABLE 90.2 American Association for the Surgery of Trauma Organ Injury Severity Scale for the Ureter

GRADE[a]	TYPE	DESCRIPTION
I	Hematoma	Contusion or hematoma without devascularization
II	Laceration	<50% transection
III	Laceration	≥50% transection
IV	Laceration	Complete transection with <2 cm devascularization
V	Laceration	Avulsion with >2 cm devascularization

[a]Advance one grade for bilateral up to grade III.
Data from Moore EE, Cogbill TH, Jurkovich GJ, et al.: Organ injury scaling. III. Chest wall, abdominal vascular, ureter, bladder, and urethra. *J Trauma* 33:337–339, 1992.

Absence of hematuria, however, cannot be relied upon to exclude ureteral injury. Mechanism of injury and physical examination findings must be taken into account. For example, a history of rapid deceleration was found in 100% of patients with ureteropelvic junction (UPJ) injury in one small series (Boone et al., 1993).

Surgical Injury

Any abdominopelvic surgical procedure, whether gynecologic, obstetric, general surgical, or urologic, can potentially injure the ureter. The overall incidence of ureteral injury varies between 0.5% and 10% (Al-Awadi et al., 2005), although more recent studies suggest a lower rate closer to 0.3% for gynecologic surgeries (Wong et al., 2018). A similar study of colorectal surgeries found an overall rate of 0.18% (Eswara et al., 2015b), whereas another found the rate to be 0.6% for open surgeries and 1.0% for laparoscopic surgeries (Marcelissen et al., 2016). Ureteral injury is more commonly associated with thermal injury, whereas bladder injuries are associated with lysis of adhesions. Analysis of 13 published studies concluded that the following procedures contribute to iatrogenic ureteral injuries: hysterectomy (54%), colorectal surgery (14%), pelvic procedures such as ovarian tumor removal (8%), transabdominal urethropexy (8%), and abdominal vascular surgery (6%) (St Lezin and Stoller, 1991). One series reported that repeat cesarean section also can result in a large proportion of ureteral injuries, in this case up to 23% of the reported ureteral injuries at one hospital (Ghali et al., 1999). Historically, open urologic procedures, because they often occur in proximity to the ureters, were also responsible for a significant number (21%) of reported ureteral injuries (Selzman and Spirnak, 1996). However, they are now extremely rare because of improved ureteroscopic techniques and equipment, although a study from Wake Forest questioned whether familiarity with ureteroscopy is leading to increasingly aggressive technique and a rise in ureteral injuries (Romero et al., 2011).

Vascular Surgery. Intraoperative ureteral manipulation resulting in subsequent hydronephrosis is common after aortoiliac and aortofemoral bypass surgery (12% to 20%), but the course is benign in most (St Lezin and Stoller, 1991). Surgical devascularization or inflammation can result in symptomatic ureteral stenosis, often delayed in manifestation by months, occurring in only 1% to 2% of these patients (Adams et al., 1992; Brandes and McAninch, 1999; St Lezin and Stoller, 1991).

In patients undergoing intra-abdominal vascular surgery, risk factors for surgical injury of the ureter include reoperation; placement of a vascular graft anterior to the ureter (Adams et al., 1992); and large, dilated arterial aneurysms that cause retroperitoneal inflammation that can involve the ureter. The majority (up to 85%) of surgical injuries to the ureter after vascular procedures are not recognized immediately (Adams et al., 1992). Postoperative symptoms of missed ureteral injury include flank pain (36% to 90%), fever, ileus, abdominal distention, and urinary fistula (Adams et al., 1992; St Lezin and Stoller, 1991).

Arterioureteral fistulas are a rare and potentially catastrophic condition that should be diagnosed and treated immediately because it can cause life-threatening hematuria. The initial presentation usually consists of either microscopic or gross hematuria. The fistula is typically located between the ureter and ipsilateral iliac artery, although the aorta can be involved. This process is associated with previous pelvic surgery, radiation therapy, long-term indwelling ureteral stents, infection, primary vascular disease, and pregnancy. Placement of an endovascular stent graft bridging the fistula site has been shown to be a safe and effective treatment in multiple series (Araki et al., 2008; Kerns et al., 1996; van den Bergh et al., 2009). Many will have to be repaired primarily, but up to 13% of patients will die of an arterioureteral fistula-related cause.

Robotic and Laparoscopic Surgery. Since the inception of laparoscopic surgery in the 1960s and robotic surgery in the 1990s, ureteral injuries have occurred (Grainger et al., 1990). The explosion of laparoscopic and robotic surgery into other surgical specialties has meant that the incidence of ureteral injury during and after minimally invasive surgery has increased. At one center, the incidence of ureteral injuries from laparoscopy went from 0% of all reported ureteral injuries in the early 1980s to 25% of all the reported ureteral injuries only 5 years later (Assimos et al., 1994). As laparoscopic experience has grown, however, the initially high incidence of injury fell to a baseline of 0.8% on a subsequent review of 1300 laparoscopic urologic procedures (Vallancien et al., 2002). Currently, the reported rate of ureteral injury varies between 0.5% (experienced surgeons) and 14% (inexperienced surgeons) after laparoscopic hysterectomy (Härkki-Siren et al., 1999; Léonard et al., 2007). In a modern series, the rate of ureteral injury after robot-assisted hysterectomy is reported to be the same as it was for laparoscopic and open hysterectomies (0.92% vs. 0.90% vs. 0.96%, respectively) (Petersen et al., 2018). Similarly, no difference was noted between robotic and open sacrocolpopexies (Anand et al., 2014). Interestingly, a recent series comparing laparoscopic and open colectomy found a *lower* rate of ureteral injury with the minimally invasive technique (Zafar et al., 2014).

A large percentage of ureteral injuries after gynecologic laparoscopy occur during electrosurgical or laser-assisted lysis of endometriosis (Grainger et al., 1990). There are three reasons for this: (1) endometrioma can involve the ureter either extrinsically or intrinsically; (2) long-standing endometriosis can cause intraperitoneal adhesion, making ureteral visualization difficult (Ribeiro et al., 1999); and (3) the disease can deviate the ureters medially away from their normal anatomic position (Nackley and Yeko, 2000). A significant number of ureteral injuries also occur during tubal ligation, even when bipolar cautery is used (Grainger et al., 1990).

Technologic advances have allowed for thermoablative treatment of renal tumors that can result in ureteral damage. With experience, the real clinical risks have decreased. A multi-institutional review of 271 thermoablative procedures for small renal tumors reported only one ureteral injury (Johnson and Pearle, 2004). There may be a potentially higher risk for ureteral stricturing associated with ablation of medial or lower pole masses. A study from Massachusetts General Hospital showed a stricture rate of 4% when retrograde irrigation for ureteral cooling was used to protect the ureter during high-risk cases adjacent to the ureter (Eswara et al., 2015a).

In distinction to open surgery, in which at least one-third of ureteral injuries are recognized immediately, fewer injuries to the ureter are immediately identified after laparoscopy (Grainger et al., 1990; Parpala-Spårman et al., 2008). **Therefore, during laparoscopy and robotic surgery, a high index of suspicion for ureteral injury is required.** The symptoms may develop acutely or insidiously, depending on the mechanism. Postoperatively, patients must be monitored for fever, abdominal pain, port site pain, and leukocytosis, which herald the potential for missed ureteral injury (Grainger et al., 1990; Parpala-Spårman et al., 2008). A smaller number of patients with missed ureteral injury present with hematuria or a pelvic mass representing urinoma (Grainger et al., 1990). A low threshold for postoperative imaging is required, especially in those with these symptoms.

Avoiding and Detecting Ureteral Injury. **Avoidance of ureteral injury is predicated on intimate knowledge of its location, especially its relation to the uterine and ovarian arteries, if those structures are going to be ligated, as in a hysterectomy** (Fig. 90.14). Visualization of the ureter in the area of the uterosacral ligaments can be especially difficult, and special care must be taken in this area. It is an axiom that ureteral injury is more likely in cases of uncontrolled bleeding, and adequate intraoperative hemostasis and surgical exposure should further decrease these injuries, even in high-risk cases (Liapis et al., 2001). Intraoperative hydration or diuretic administration has been suggested to enhance ureteral visualization and potentially decrease the risk for injury, although data to support this claim do not exist. Preoperative ureteral stenting can be used to ease identification of the ureter in high-risk cases; however, published data in the gynecologic and colectomy literature are unclear about whether they actually decrease ureteral injuries (Bothwell et al., 1994; Chou et al., 2009; Leff et al., 1982). Although older studies showed no benefit, a more recent review of the National Surgical Quality Improvement Program (NSQIP) showed that stents were associated with a lower rate of ureteral injury after colectomy (Coakley et al., 2018). Ureteral

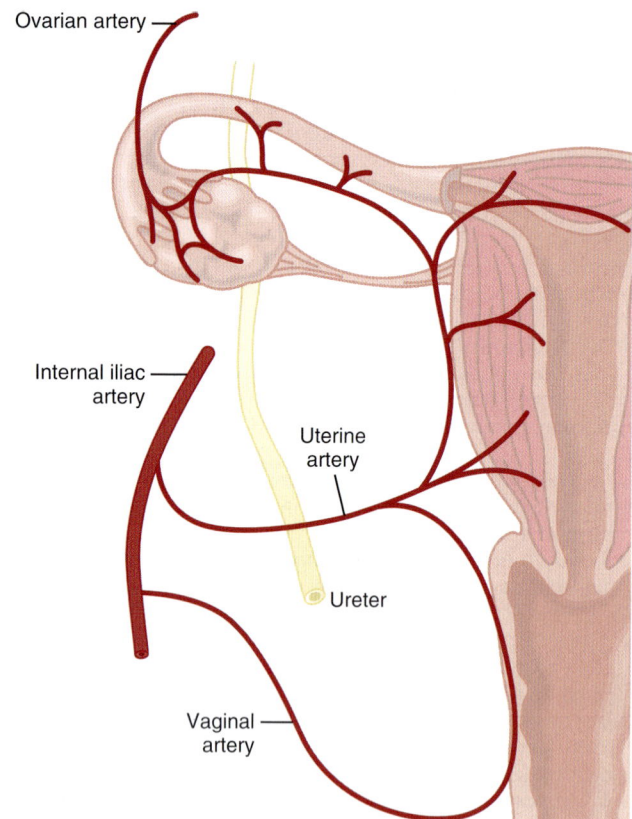

Fig. 90.14. Ureteral anatomy showing relationship to fallopian tube and uterine artery.

stents are not without complications; the rate of anuria after bilateral prophylactic ureteral stent placement has been reported between 1% and 5% (Kyzer and Gordon, 1994; Leff et al., 1982; Sheikh and Khubchandani, 1990), and the rate of iatrogenic ureteral injury during stent placement is 1% (Bothwell et al., 1994). Ureteral stent placement is not always successful; stents cannot be placed on one side in 13% of cases, and total failure to place either catheter can occur in 2% (Bothwell et al., 1994). Lighted fiberoptic ureteral catheters have been used with good effect (Ben-Hur and Phipps, 2000), and smaller 5-Fr models may avoid the complications of ureteral edema and obstruction, which have been reported after the use of larger, older-model lighted stents (Chahin et al., 2002). A 5-year review of the use of lighted stents for laparoscopic colorectal surgery showed no ureteral injuries and no infections (Boyan et al., 2017).

Some authors have advocated maneuvers to check the patency of the ureter after all surgeries in which ureter injury is commonly reported (e.g., hysterectomy). Cystoscopy alone, used to look for the absence of hematuria and the presence of bilateral ureteral jets, is typically a poor predictor of injury. In one decade-long study, cystoscopy missed more injuries than it detected (Dandolu et al., 2003). In another, it increased the detection rate from 30% to 96% (Vakili et al., 2005). Purposefully opening the retroperitoneum before or after hysterectomy has been advocated to avoid ureteral injury or at least allow intraoperative detection. A majority of authors advocate this approach (Cruikshank, 1986; Liapis et al., 2001), yet this may contribute to ureteral devascularization by inadvertent disruption of the delicate distal ureteral blood supply (Nezhat et al., 1995). Digital palpation of the ureter, through the unopened retroperitoneum, is also ineffective (Symmonds, 1976). Some have advocated that grasping the ureter with forceps to evoke ureteral peristalsis can be a measure of an uninjured ureter, but this is highly ineffective and unreliable. Finally, some authors recommend routine injection of 5 to 10 mL of IV indigo carmine methylene blue, or fluorescein dye, or oral phenazopyridine (started pre-surgery) followed by cystoscopy to ensure patency of the ureters after hysterectomy. In 118 patients undergoing laparoscopic hysterectomy, 4 of 4 cases of ureteral occlusion were identified immediately by the lack dye from the ureteral orifice (mostly caused by suture ligation) and repaired immediately without complications (Ribeiro et al., 1999).

IV methylene blue should be avoided in pregnant women and in patients who are taking selective serotonin reuptake inhibitors (SSRIs; e.g., paroxetine, sertraline, fluoxetine, fluvoxamine, citalopram) or serotonin and norepinepherine reuptake inhibitors (SNRIs; e.g., duloxetine, venlafaxine) or monoamine oxidase inhibitors (MAOIs; e.g., isocarboxid, phenelzine). Methylene blue is a potent monoamine oxidase inhibitor and can cause serious serotonin toxicity (and in rare circumstances, serotonin syndrome and death) in patients taking medications that increase serotonin levels. IV methylene blue also should be avoided in patients with glucose-6-phosphate dehydrogenase deficiency because it can cause methemoglobinemia and hemolysis. IV methylene blue can also result in underestimation of blood oxygen saturation by pulse oximetry. IV indigo carmine is safe but has been implicated in case reports of bronchospasm, bradycardia, hypertension, hypotension (most common), and anaphylactoid reactions (Jeon et al., 2012). Indigo carmine is rapidly renal excreted, has a half life of 4 to 5 minutes and appears blue in the urine within 5 to 10 minutes (depending on patient hydration).

Tenuous Ureteral Blood Supply. The distal ureteral blood supply is variable (Daniel and Shackman, 1952). It is estimated by cadaver studies that 10% of females carry a disproportionate amount of their distal ureteral blood supply via uterine artery branches. These branches are necessarily severed when the uterine artery is ligated during the course of a normal hysterectomy. In cadaveric experiments, it was noted that 40% of females have decreased ureteral perfusion after ligating the uterine artery. The resultant hypothesis is that distal ureteral devascularization may be an unavoidable consequence in a small percentage of women after hysterectomy (Michaels, 1948). Ureteral devascularization tends to manifest differently from other ureteral injuries. Patients tend to present late (more than a week after surgery, but as late as 1 to 2 months), usually with ureteral stenosis, urinoma, or even ureterovaginal fistula that was not seemingly present at the time of surgery or the early days after surgery.

Ureteroscopic Injury

Since the first reported ureteral injury after rigid ureteroscopy in 1984, countless ureteral misadventures have resulted (Kaufman, 1984). In fact, ureteroscopic injury was the most common cause of iatrogenic ureteral trauma in some modern series (Johnson and Pearle, 2004). In the late 1980s, an explosion of ureteral injuries coincided with the widespread use of ureteroscopy (Huffman, 1989). Improvements in equipment and operator experience subsequently decreased the rate of ureteral perforation, to a stable average of 7% in the 1990s (range 0% to 28%) (Huffman, 1989), whereas contemporary series report the stricture rate after ureteroscopy as 0.6% (El-Abd et al., 2014).

One factor associated with ureteral injury during ureteroscopy was continued stone basket attempts after recognition of a ureteral tear. Current recommendations are to stop the procedure and place a ureteral stent when ureteral perforations are identified (Chang and Marshall, 1987). The wide use of the holmium:yttrium-aluminum-garnet (Ho:YAG) laser to fragment larger stones before basket manipulation is attempted should further decrease the potential for this complication (Bagley et al., 2004). Extraureteric extrusion of calculi during laser fragmentation or basket retrieval has shown to be a minor complication and only rarely leads to stricture formation (Kriegmair and Schmeller, 1995).

It is also recommended to perform ureteroscopy alongside or over a wire placed up into the renal pelvis (Chang and Marshall, 1987; Flam et al., 1988), although some experts no longer use a safety wire during routine flexible ureteroscopy (Bratslavsky and Moran, 2004). This wire facilitates not only safe ureteroscopy but also placement of a ureteral stent later in the case if necessary. **Factors associated with higher complication rates during ureteroscopy** are longer surgery times, treatment of renal calculi, surgeon inexperience, and previous irradiation (Huffman, 1989), whereas other series have identified stone size, number, and the presence of congenital renal abnormalities (Baş et al., 2017). During stone fragmentation attempts, electrohydraulic lithotripsy (now hardly used) is associated with the highest risk for ureteral injury, followed by the neodymium:yttrium-aluminum-garnet (Nd:YAG) laser and finally by the Ho:YAG laser (Johnson and Pearle, 2004). Factors that are thought to protect against ureteral injury are smaller and flexible ureteroscopes (Flam et al., 1988; Huffman, 1989). Ureteral access sheaths also protect the ureter, but the sheaths can cause ureteral wall injury, especially if the patient did not receive a ureteral stent preoperatively (Traxer and Thomas, 2013). Smaller diameter (≤14-Fr) sheaths are preferred for nonstented ureters.

Diagnosis

Gunshot and Stab Wounds

Hematuria. Hematuria is a nonspecific indicator of urologic injury. Significant ureteral injury can occur in the absence of hematuria (Brandes et al., 2004; Elliott and McAninch, 2006). Because many (25% to 45%) cases of ureteral injury do not demonstrate even microscopic hematuria, a high index of suspicion is required in cases of potential ureteral injury after penetrating trauma (Brandes et al., 1994; Campbell et al., 1992; Palmer et al., 1999; Presti et al., 1989).

Intraoperative Recognition. In an analysis of previously published reports of ureteral injury secondary to violent injury, Armenakas et al. (1999) noted that 93% of injuries were recognized promptly, including 57% that were identified intraoperatively. Every attempt should be made to diagnose these injuries during surgical exploration (Armenakas et al., 1999; Brandes et al., 1994; Medina et al., 1998). Intraoperative detection requires a high degree of suspicion, and there is evidence that vigilance for ureteral injuries may decrease the incidence of missed injuries (McGinty and Mendez, 1977). The trajectory of the knife or missile must be carefully examined during laparotomy and ureteral exploration undertaken in all cases of potential injury. Direct ureteral inspection is necessary in patients suspected to have ureteral injury who undergo laparotomy without adequate pre-surgical imaging. **Direct exploration is typically the most accurate method for diagnosis, but can be difficult because of overlying hematoma.** Care must be taken not to devascularize the ureter during exploration. Intravenous indigo carmine is helpful in identifying ureteral injury by searching for extravasation of blue dye from the injury site. Ureteral integrity can also be tested by retrograde injection of indigo and/or saline though a ureteral stent or pediatric feeding tube, placed by cystoscopy or cystotomy (depending on the clinical situation) (Elliott and McAninch, 2003).

Inadequate exploration or a low index of suspicion in the presence of multiple injuries is often responsible for missed ureteral injury. In a large meta-analysis, analyzing 16 busy trauma centers with 429 ureteral injuries with laparotomy, a collective 11% miss rate of ureteral injury was noted (Kunkle et al., 2006). Another study found that 62% of ureteral injuries were missed after hysterectomy (Blackwell et al., 2018). Delayed diagnosis in these series was associated with a prolonged hospital stay, increased rates of nephrectomy, and death. An unrecognized or undertreated ureteral injury can lead to other significant complications, including urinoma, abscess, ureteral stricture, and urinary fistula.

Vigilance for delayed presentation of ureteral injuries allows detection of initially missed injuries. Fever, leukocytosis, and local peritoneal irritation are the most common signs and symptoms of missed ureteral injury and always should prompt CT examination. Retrograde ureterography is most often used for diagnosing such "missed" ureteral injury, in a stable patient, and has the added benefit of allowing immediate attempt at ureteral stent passage to aid urinary drainage, and avoid or treat urinoma.

Imaging Studies

Computed Tomography. CT urography with delayed images is the best study for detecting ureteral injuries (Kawashima et al., 2001). Ureteral injuries often manifest with absence of contrast in the ureter

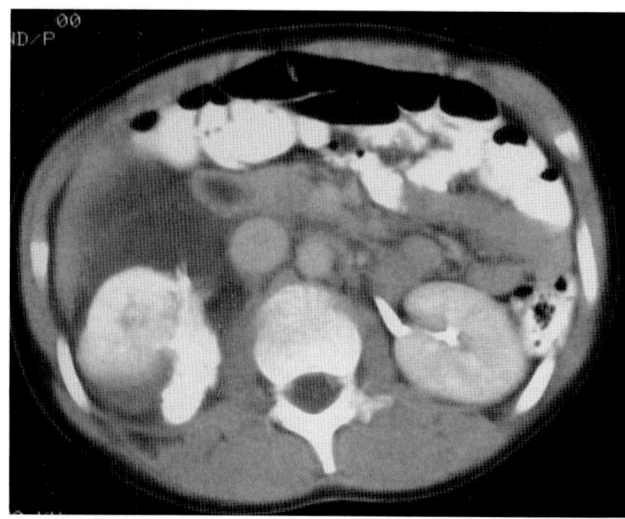

Fig. 90.15. Computed tomography showing right medial extravasation of contrast material in a patient with a renal pelvis laceration.

on delayed images. This underscores the necessity of tracing both ureters throughout their entire course on CT scans obtained to evaluate urogenital injuries (Townsend and DeFalco, 1995). **Because modern CT scanners can obtain images rapidly, before IV contrast dye is excreted in the urine, delayed images must be obtained (10 minutes after contrast injection) to allow contrast material to extravasate from the injured collecting system, renal pelvis, or ureter** (Brown et al., 1998; Kawashima et al., 2001; Mulligan et al., 1998). CT findings suggestive of ureteral injury are contrast extravasation, delayed ipsilateral nephrogram, ipsilateral hydronephrosis, and lack of contrast in the distal ureter, and a periureteral urinoma (Gayer et al., 2002; Siegel, 2002).

In reported series, all patients with significant ureteropelvic laceration, for instance, had either medial extravasation of contrast material or nonopacification of the ipsilateral ureter on CT (Kawashima et al., 2001; Fig. 90.15) or a "circumrenal" contrast extravasation. Delayed images that demonstrate medial or circumrenal extravasation but do not opacify the distal ureter suggest an avulsion injury (Kawashima et al., 1997).

Retrograde Ureterography. Retrograde ureterogram is the most sensitive radiographic test for ureteral injury (Campbell et al., 1992). Although accurate in demonstrating site, presence, and location of extravasation, retrograde ureterography is often time consuming and cumbersome. Thus, it often has a limited role in the acute trauma setting, especially if the patient is unstable. Retrograde ureterography is most commonly used to diagnose initially missed ureteral injuries, because it allows the simultaneous placement of a ureteral stent if possible.

Antegrade Ureterography. In cases in which ureteral injury is discovered, and retrograde stent placement is not possible (usually secondary to a large gap in the two ends of the transected ureter), anterograde ureterography and stent placement at the time of percutaneous nephrostomy placement, should be performed, when possible (Toporoff et al., 1992).

Intravenous Pyelography. Although rarely used today, IVPs still play a role in resource poor countries where CT scans are not readily available (Fig. 90.16). One-shot IVP is often unhelpful, proving nondiagnostic 33% to 100% of the time for ureteral injury, and thus should not be solely used for this purpose (Azimuddin et al., 1998; Brandes et al., 1994; Campbell et al., 1992; Elliott and McAninch, 2003; Palmer et al., 1983; Presti et al., 1989). Findings on IVP that are suggestive of ureteral injury are incomplete visualization of the entire ureter, ureteral deviation or dilation, urinary extravasation, and hydronephrosis. Insensitivity of these usual diagnostic tools and high false-negative rates are some of the reasons why delay of

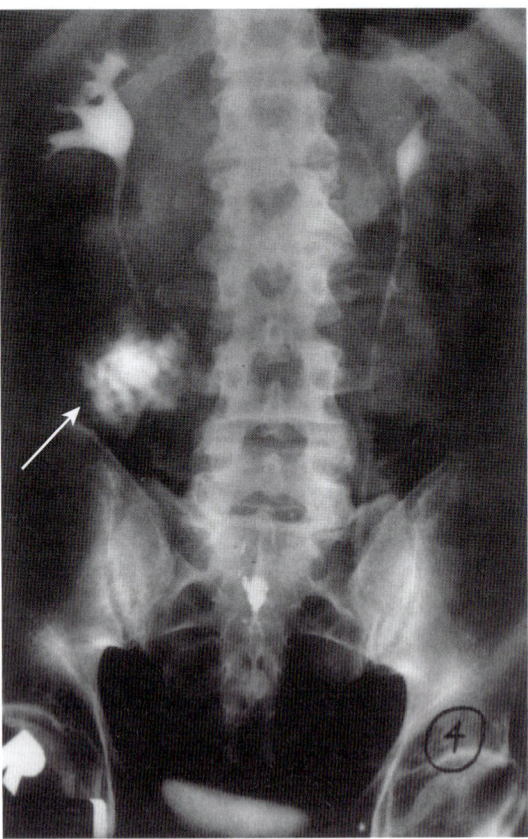

Fig. 90.16. Excretory urography demonstrating extravasation in the upper right ureter consequent to stab wound. Note lack of contrast (arrow) in the ureter below the site of injury, indicating complete ureteral transection.

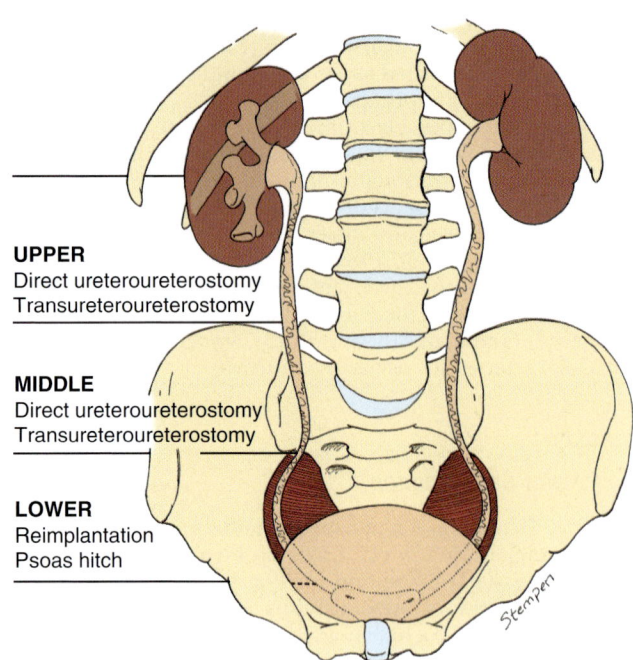

Fig. 90.17. Suggested management options for ureteral injuries at different levels.

detection occurs in 8% to 20% of cases (Brandes et al., 1994; Palmer et al., 1999; Presti et al., 1989).

Management

See Fig. 90.17.

General Principles

When possible, repair of the injured ureter should be performed at the same time as the initial laparotomy, in a stable patient. Immediate repair of the ureter is often not appropriate in the unstable, complex polytrauma patient. Ureteral blood supply is tenuous, and a sequela of imperfect repair can be urine leakage that can result in patient debility, nephrectomy, and, in rare cases, even death. Principles of management of the injured ureter are as follows (Fig. 90.18):

1. Mobilize the injured ureter carefully, sparing the adventitia widely, so as not to devascularize the ureter further.
2. Debride the ureter minimally but judiciously until edges bleed, especially in high-velocity gunshot wounds.
3. Repair ureters with spatulated, tension-free, stented (Palmer et al., 1983) watertight anastomosis, using fine absorbable sutures and retroperitoneal drainage afterward.
4. Retroperitonealize the ureteral repair by closing peritoneum over it if possible.
5. Do not tunnel ureteroneocystostomies but rather create a widely spatulated nontunneled anastomosis.
6. With severely injured ureters, blast effect, concomitant vascular surgery, and other complex cases, consider omental interposition to isolate the repair when possible.
7. If immediate repair is not possible, or the patient hemodynamically unstable, one management option is to ligate the ureter with long silk or polypropylene suture, and plan to repair it later, or place a nephrostomy tube after ICU resuscitation (damage control). The other option is a temporary cutaneous ureterostomy over a single-J stent or pediatric feeding tube with a suture tied around the ureter proximal to the injury site, in order to secure the stent in place, and to prevent urinary leakage.

External Trauma

Contusion. Ureteral contusions, although the most minor of ureteral injuries, can heal with stricture or breakdown later if microvascular injury results in ureteral necrosis. Contusion is not uncommon with proximity gunshot wounds with blast injury. **Severe or large areas of contusion that appear to lack viability should be treated with excision of the damaged area and ureteroureterostomy/ ureteroneocystostomy. In general, intact contused ureters, when identified at laparotomy, are primarily managed by ureteral stenting** (placed by cystoscopy or cystotomy, depending on the clinical setting).

When a missed ureteral contusion later presents as a leak, retrograde imaging with ureteral stent placement should be initially performed. When antegrade stenting is not possible a percutaneous nephrosotmy tube and subsequent antegrade ureteral stent should be placed for 6 weeks, which provides surprisingly good success rates (83% [Toporoff et al., 1992] to 88% [Lang, 1984]).

Upper Ureteral Injuries

Ureteroureterostomy. Ureteral avulsion from the renal pelvis, or even very proximal ureter, can be managed by reimplantation of the ureter directly into the renal pelvis (Fig. 90.19). These can be done open, or in a delayed fashion, laparoscopically, or robotically (Marien et al., 2015; Mufarrij et al., 2007). Ureteroureterostomy, or so-called end-to-end repair, is used in acute injuries to the upper two-thirds of the ureter. It is required commonly—up to 32% of the time in large series (Elliott and McAninch, 2003; Presti et al., 1989) and has a reported success rate as high as 90% (Carlton et al., 1971). For long ureteral strictures that develop in a delayed fashion, some authors now advocate for the use of buccal graft ureteroplasty with 90% success (Zhao et al., 2017). Complications after ureteroureterostomy, usually urine leakage, occur 10% to 24% of the time (Bright and Peters, 1977; Campbell et al., 1992; Medina et al., 1998; Pitts and Peterson, 1981; Presti et al., 1989; Velmahos et al., 1996). Other acute complications include abscess and fistula, which can occur in up to 12% of patients (Lee et al., 2012). Chronic complications,

Chapter 90 Upper Urinary Tract Trauma 1997

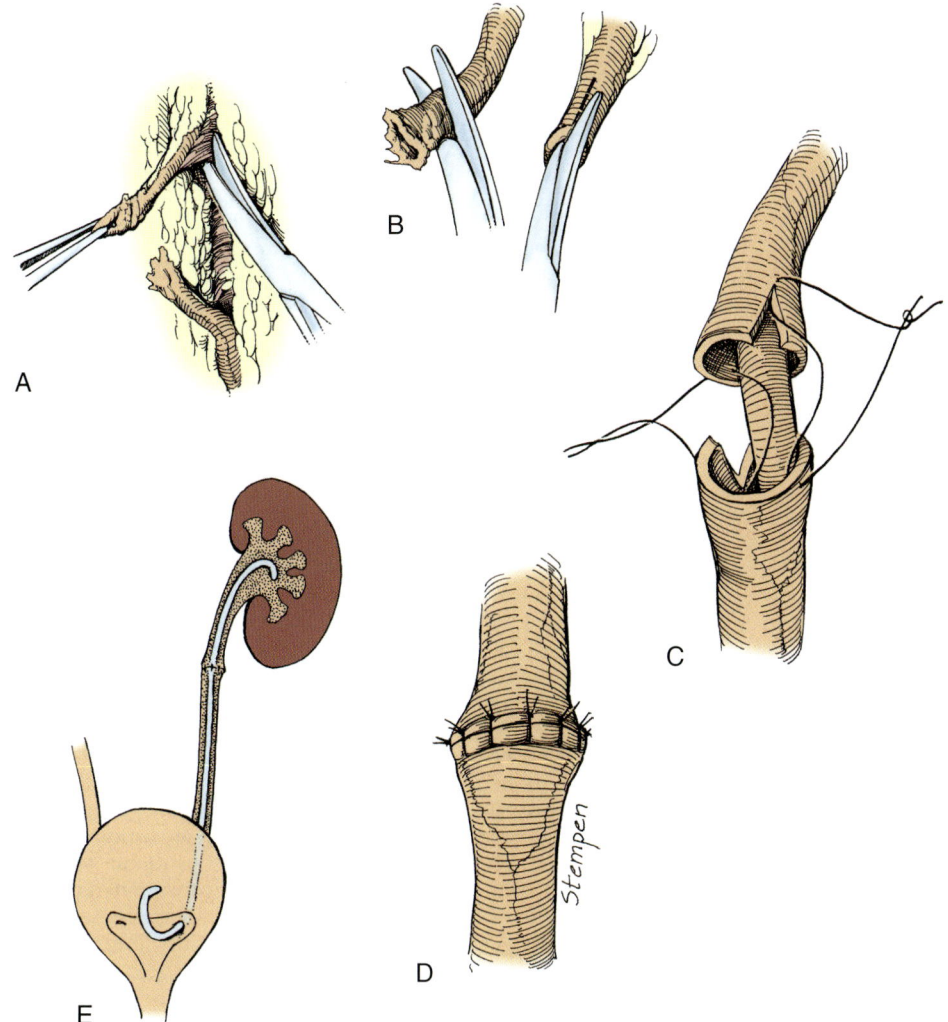

Fig. 90.18. Technique of ureteroureterostomy after traumatic disruption. (A) Injury site definition by ureteral mobilization. (B) Debridement of margins and spatulation. (C) Stent placement. (D) Approximation with 5-0 absorbable suture. (E) Final result.

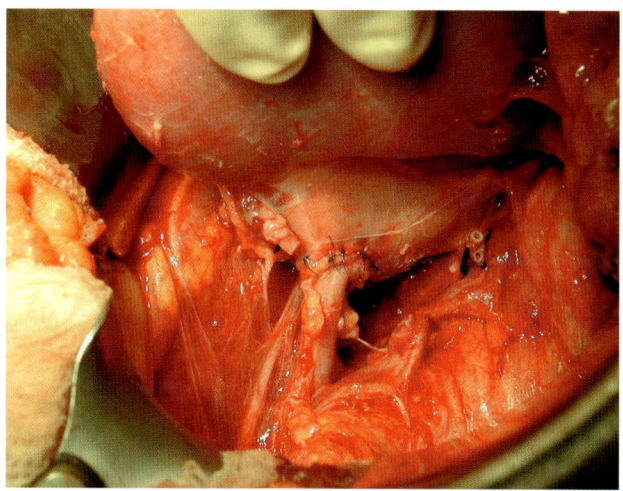

Fig. 90.19. Proximal ureter is spatulated and sutured to the renal pelvis.

usually ureteral stenosis, are less common, involving approximately 5% (Palmer et al., 1999) to 12% (Velmahos et al., 1996) of patients. Interestingly, some authors report prolonged leakage of urine from the drain after UPJ avulsion repair but otherwise did well. Steers et al. (1985) reported that most of their patients had persistent drainage (averaging 12 days) from the retroperitoneal Penrose drain after repair. Routine retroperitonealization of the repair may decrease the time or severity of postoperative urine leakage.

Rarely, ureterocalycostomy, in which the ureteral stump is sewn end-to-side into an exposed renal calyx, also can be used where there is profound damage to the renal pelvis and UPJ (Matlaga et al., 2005). This is a technically challenging case. It can be difficult to find an inferior calyx. Moreover, this technique requires renal surgery equivalent to a partial nephrectomy. Often, the technical complexity of sewing the small, medially located ureter to a large laterally located renal calyx can be difficult or even impossible. Recently, robotics for the non-acute and stable trauma patient can be successfully and safely used for a wide variety of delayed upper urinary tract reconstructions, including dismembered pyeloplasty, ureteroureterostomy, and ureterocalicostomy.

Autotransplantation. Autotransplantation of the kidney has been used after profound ureteral loss or after multiple attempts at ureteral repair have failed. Such surgery is reserved only for a delayed repair in select patients and has no role in the acute trauma patient (Cowan et al., 2015). This maneuver remains the final option before nephrectomy. Despite great efforts, renal units are sometimes lost after autotransplantation, occurring between 5% and 10% (Bodie et al., 1986; Cowan et al., 2015; Eisenberg et al., 2008), although centers with significant transplant experience have reported good results. Early high-grade complications (Clavien III or higher) including bleeding and infection occurred in 15% of patients.

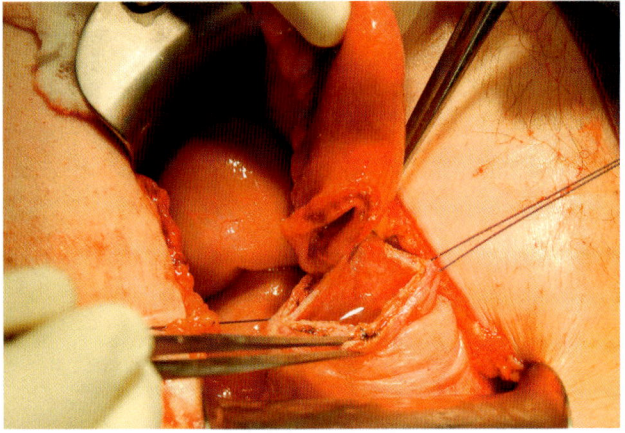

Fig. 90.20. Nontapered distal ileal segment is anastomosed to the bladder in a wide-open, and refluxing fashion.

Bowel Interposition. Delayed ureteral repairs, especially when a very long segment of ureter is destroyed, also can be performed by creation of an ileal "chimney" in much the same way that an ileal conduit is constructed to drain the urine after cystectomy. Success rates for ileal replacement of the ureter have been reported to be 81% (Boxer et al., 1979; Verduyckt et al., 2002) to 100% (Bonfig et al., 2004; Kocot et al., 2017; Matlaga et al., 2003). A review of long-term complications of 99 renal units reported a 3% anastomotic stricture and 6% fistula rate (Armatys et al., 2009). A recent series, and the largest to date, involving 157 patients found that complications were not uncommon (Kocot et al., 2017). Hyperchloremic metabolic acidosis occurred in 20% of patients, pyelonephritis in 9%, and surgical intervention in 4%. Some have successfully used the Monti procedure, in which short segments of small or large bowel are sewn together to make a long, thin tube in ureteral reconstruction (Ali-el-Dein and Ghoneim, 2003; Bao et al., 2017; Ubrig et al., 2001). Laparoscopic and robotic ileal interposition have been described (Brandao et al., 2014; Castillo et al., 2008; Chopra et al., 2016; Gill et al., 2000). The use of appendix in open (Jang et al., 2002) and laparoscopic (Reggio et al., 2009) ureteral substitution has also been reported. Most practitioners create a wide-open, refluxing, ileal replacement of the ureter (Fig. 90.20), because significant clinical reflux is not a problem (Waldner et al., 1999). We often prefer to combine the ileal chimney with an ipsilateral Psoas bladder hitch, in order to shorten the length of the conduit and hypothetically decrease the risk of metabolic and mucus complications. Ileal interposition has *no* role in the acute repair of ureteral injury and should be reserved only for delayed or staged repairs.

Monitoring After Ureteral Repair. There is little consensus in the literature when and how to image for silent hydronephrosis/ureteral obstruction after traumatic ureteral reconstruction. Typically a diuretic renogram or renal ultrasound with doppler imaging for ureteral jets is performed at 4 to 12 weeks and at 1 year post injury. If the patient had severe polytrauma and requires CT imaging for the associated non-renal injuries, then a CT with IV contrast with delayed cuts should be done. Because ureteral injury repairs often happen in the setting of ureteral devascularization, late stenosis can occur and is often clinically silent.

Nephrectomy. Rarely, acute nephrectomy is required to treat ureteral injury after external trauma. Reasons for nephrectomy include hemodynamic instability and associated severe visceral injuries (although damage control without nephrectomy is nearly always preferable) or severe associated injury to the ipsilateral kidney when renal repair is not possible (McGinty and Mendez, 1977). Delayed nephrectomy may be required because of poor renal function (which can sometimes be seen after delayed recognition of an obstructing ureteral injury), severe panureteral injury when ileal ureter or other reconstruction is impossible, or persistent ureteral fistula (especially vascular fistula) despite previous intervention (Ghali et al., 1999).

In general, nephrectomy must be avoided if at all possible no matter the severity of the ureteral injury, and instead a damage control and delayed reconstruction approach be followed.

Midureteral Injuries. The majority of midureteral complete transections (above the iliac vessels), regardless of the mechanism, can be repaired by primary ureteroureterostomy over a stent. When the midureteral injury/defect is very long, however, and the ends of the ureters cannot be brought together without tension, then a transureteroureterostomy (TUU) can be considered.

Transureteroureterostomy. TUU is a rarely used (Presti et al., 1989) but often (90% to 97%) successful (Kawamura et al., 2017; Rainwater et al., 1991; Sugarbaker et al., 2003) technique in adults is transureteroureterostomy (TUU). Pediatric series show a lower success rate of 70% (Mure et al., 2000). This form of repair involves bringing the injured ureter across the midline and anastomosing it end-to-side into the contra-lateral, uninjured ureter (a 2 cm or more ureterotomy in the recipient ureter is advised). TUU has little role in the acute trauma setting and is typically performed as a secondary or delayed procedure. As an alternative, in the acute setting, the injured ureter can be treated in a damage control approach by ligation or diversion to the skin over a stent. It also may be mandated in some cases of middle or distal ureteral injury in which ureteroureterostomy or bladder flap/hitch repair is impossible (usually because of severe bladder scarring, a congenitally small bladder, or very long segment of missing ureter, or pelvic phlegmon) or when there are associated rectal, major pelvic vascular or extensive bladder injuries. Laparoscopic transureteroureterostomy has been performed successfully in the pediatric population (Piaggio and González, 2007).

Relative contraindications to performing a TUU is in patients with a history of urothelial cancer or calculi, genitourinary tuberculosis, pelvic radiation, retroperitoneal fibrosis, or chronic pyelonephritis. At the time of ureteral injury, however, this information is seldom available to the operating trauma surgeon. Caution is required while performing this procedure because it involves surgery on the uninjured, contralateral ureter with the theoretical risk for converting unilateral ureteral injury into (iatrogenic) bilateral ureteral injury.

Lower Ureteral Injuries

Ureteroneocystostomy. Ureteroneocystostomy is used to repair distal ureteral injuries that occur so close to the bladder that the bladder does not need to be brought up to the ureteral stump with a psoas hitch or Boari procedure. For the non-acute trauma patient, and in an elective fashion, robotic ureteroneocystostomy is increasingly common with a success rate of around 95% (Fifer et al., 2014; Gellhaus et al., 2015). Standard principles of ureteroneocystostomy include a long, nontunneled, spatulated, stented anastomosis. Refluxing ureteroneobladder (Minervini et al., 2005) and ureteroileal loop (Wiesner and Thüroff, 2004) anastomoses show no increase in complications related to urine reflux, although these populations of patients are different from the average trauma population and reports do not address whether ureteral implantation into the native bladder is equally safe. A comparison of nonrefluxing and refluxing anastomoses in neobladders found a higher rate of stricture leading to renal deterioration in the nonrefluxing group (Shaaban et al., 2006). As such, we favor nontunneled anastomoses for the trauma patient, because we prefer the very low risk of clinically significant reflux to the higher risk of ureteral obstruction using a tunneled approach.

Psoas Bladder Hitch. The psoas hitch procedure (Fig. 90.21) is a mainstay in the treatment of injuries to the lower third of the ureter and has a high success rate, from 95% to 100% (Ahn and Loughlin, 2001; Middleton, 1980; Riedmiller et al., 1984). We prefer it over ureteroureterostomy in lower ureteral injuries because the tenuous ureteral blood supply may not survive transection. Some authors prefer end-to-end repair in lower ureteral injuries when the distal stump is preserved (Paick et al., 2006). For lower ureteral injuries, the ureteral gap can be bridged by "hitching" (suturing) the apex of the bladder to the ipsilateral psoas muscle and psoas minor tendon. The contralateral superior vesical pedicle is often divided to improve mobilization. When hitching the bladder, it is important not to injure or entrap the genitofemoral nerve in the sutures. The psoas hitch is relatively quick to perform, but is only appropriate in the stable

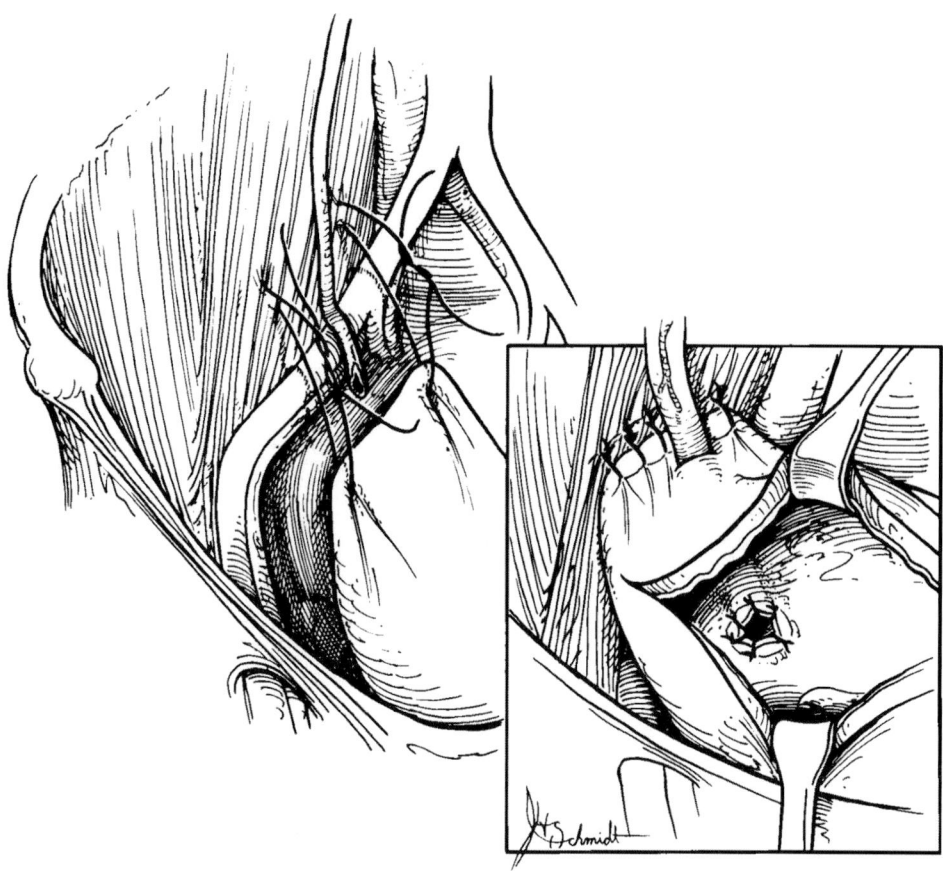

Fig. 90.21. Psoas hitch. Bladder is opened and secured to the psoas muscle to facilitate ureteral anastomosis. (From Hohenfellner M, Santucci RA: *Emergencies in urology*, Heidelberg, Germany, 2007, Springer. Copyright 2007, Dr. Markus Hohenfellner, with permission.)

trauma patient. If the patient is unstable, the procedure should be delayed until a planned and staged repair.

Boari Flap. Injuries to the lower two-thirds of the ureter with long ureteral defects (too long to be bridged by bringing the bladder up in the psoas hitch procedure) can be managed with a Boari flap or a transureteroureterostomy (Fig. 90.22). If the bladder is normal in size and thickness, a long pedicle of bladder can be incised and rotated cephalad and tubularized to bridge the gap to the injured ureter. The procedure is time-consuming, however, and is not appropriate for most acute injuries. It is not commonly performed, but authors report a high success rate with the open or robotic technique (Benson et al., 1990; Stolzenburg et al., 2016).

Partial Transection. Primary repair of a partial transection is used in the majority of ureteral injuries, up to 58% of the time in one large series (Presti et al., 1989). Principles of primary repair involve spatulated, watertight closure, with interrupted or running absorbable suture such as Maxon (polyglyconate), Vicryl (polyglactin 910), or Dexon (polyglycolic acid). The ureteral injury is closed by converting a longitudinal laceration into a transverse one so as not to narrow the ureteral lumen (Heineke-Mikulicz procedure) and retroperitonealize if possible. A ureteral stent and retroperitoneal drain are always placed.

Damage Control. **In cases of ureteral injury after trauma, it is sometimes necessary to treat the injured ureter by deferring definitive treatment until later. This is usually because the patient is too unstable to tolerate the operative time required to complete the repair** (Cass, 1983). Some have suggested that in cases of severe hemorrhagic shock, uncontrollable intraoperative bleeding, or severe colon injury (especially those requiring colectomy), ureteral reconstruction should be delayed until the patient is fully resuscitated and performed as a staged repair (Velmahos et al., 1996).

The four options for damage control in ureteral injuries are (1) do nothing, but plan a reoperation when the patient is more stable, usually within 24 hours; (2) place a ureteral stent into the proximal end of the transected ureter and exteriorize the stent to the skin; (3) mobilize and exteriorize the ureter, as in a cutaneous ureterostomy; or (4) ligate the ureter and plan a staged percutaneous nephrostomy (Hirshberg et al., 1994). In most cases of planned staged repair, we prefer to ligate the proximal end of the damaged ureter, using long silk or polypropylene ties to aid the dissection of the ureteral stump during the second-stage repair. The kidney is then drained percutaneously. We advocate percutaneous (not intraoperative or intra-abdominal) placement of a nephrostomy tube, only once the patient has been fully stabilized and in a delayed fashion. Open nephrostomy placement is too time-consuming and has no role in these unstable patients. Alternatively, a single-J stent or 5-Fr pediatric feeding tube can be placed into the proximal end of the injured ureter, with minimal to no mobilization of the proximal ureter, a nonabsorbale tie placed around the proximal ureter to secure the stent in place, the stent, and the stent end externalized through the abdominal wall into a urostomy pouch (Ball et al., 2005). If possible, appropriate planned ureteric reconstruction should be performed after functional and anatomic imaging.

Surgical Injury

Timing of Repair. Ureteral repair of traumatic injuries should be performed at the time of initial laparotomy, when possible. Immediate repair, however, may not be appropriate in unstable, complex polytrauma patients. Even with immediate recognition, success is not ensured. In small series, patients with immediately repaired ureteral injuries still suffered urine leak, fistula, and even nephrectomy (Grainger

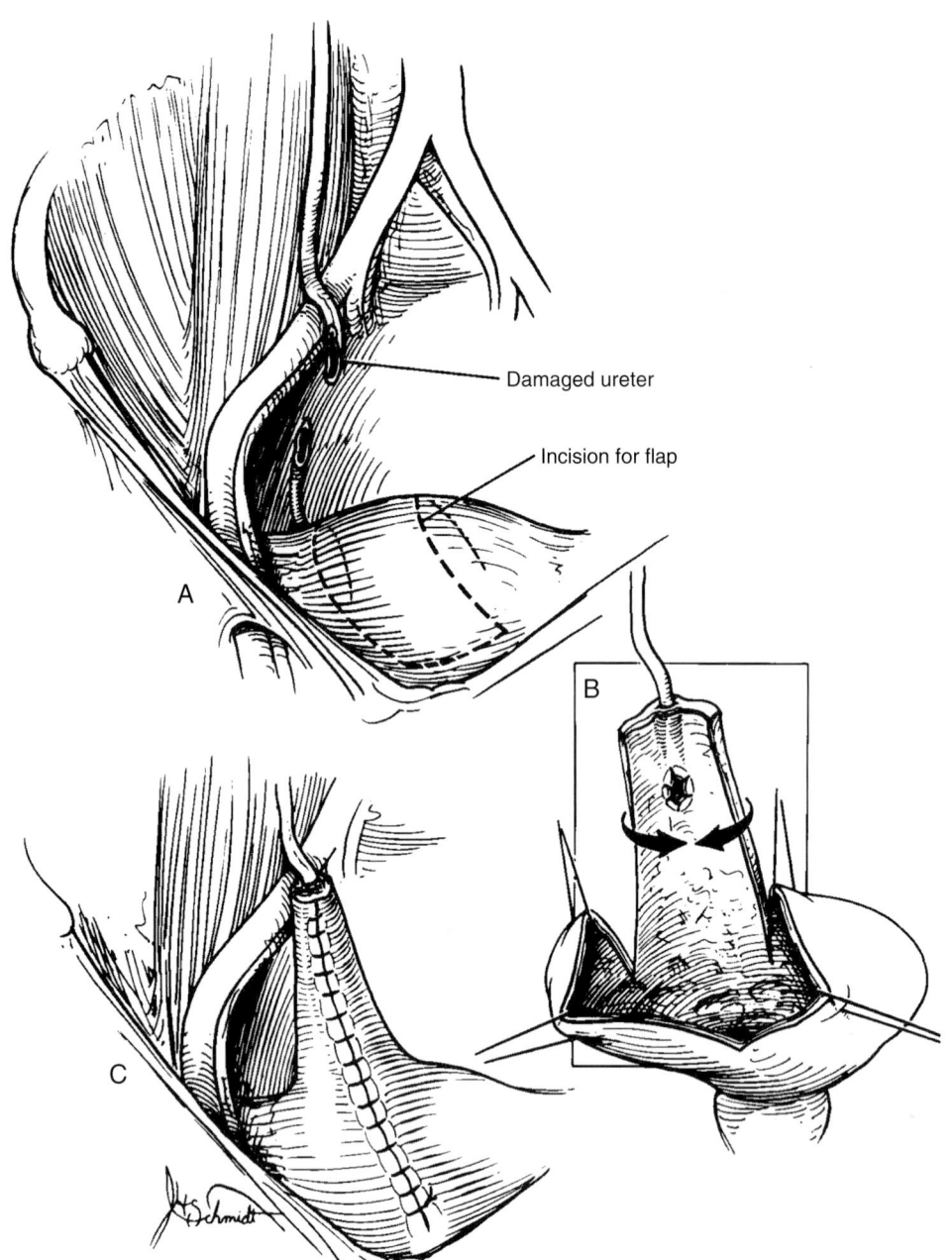

Fig. 90.22. Boari flap. Bladder flap is marked (A), mobilized free (B), tubularized (C). (From Hohenfellner M, Santucci RA: *Emergencies in urology*, Heidelberg, Germany, 2007, Springer. Copyright 2007, Dr. Markus Hohenfellner, with permission.)

et al., 1990; Mandal et al., 1990). The AUA urotrauma guidelines state that injuries diagnosed postoperatively or in a delayed fashion can be considered for immediate repair if the injury is recognized with 1 week (Morey, 2014). Injuries discovered after this 1-week period, should be managed by retrograde ureteral imaging with ureteral stent placement, percutaneous nephrostomy, or both, and definitive repair delayed until a minimum of 6 weeks after injury. This putatively avoids an inflammatory phase, when ureteral repairs are thought to be less reliable. Others recommend immediate repair even when discovered weeks to months, and cite low complication rates, similar to injuries that are recognized immediately (Ghali et al., 1999; Witters et al., 1986). However, delayed diagnosis of ureteral injury increase the complication rate of the repair significantly (Selzman and Spirnak, 1996), from 10% to 40% in one series (Campbell et al., 1992). Some have suggested that delaying the repair (6 or more weeks) avoids this risk by allowing for maximal resolution of perioperative inflammation.

A recent report suggests that even delayed repairs have a slightly higher rate of failure than immediate repair (Eswara et al., 2015b).

Most delayed diagnosed ureteral injuries, are discovered within 6 weeks of surgery (Hatch et al., 1984; Oh et al., 2000), and in one series almost half were discovered more than 6 weeks after the initial surgery (Badenoch et al., 1987). Cure rates appear equal in the early (within 1 week) and late discovery groups (Brandt et al., 2001; Liapis et al., 2001). Another study found no difference between repairs performed immediately, within 1 month, or at 3 months (Li et al., 2012). Overall, it is most prudent to repair the ureteral injury immediately if identified within 1 week or wait at least 6 weeks for inflammation to subside.

Ligation. **Ligation of the ureter discovered intraoperatively should be treated by removal of the ligature and observation of the ureter for viability. If viability is in question, ureteroureterostomy or ureteral reimplantation should be performed** (Assimos et al., 1994;

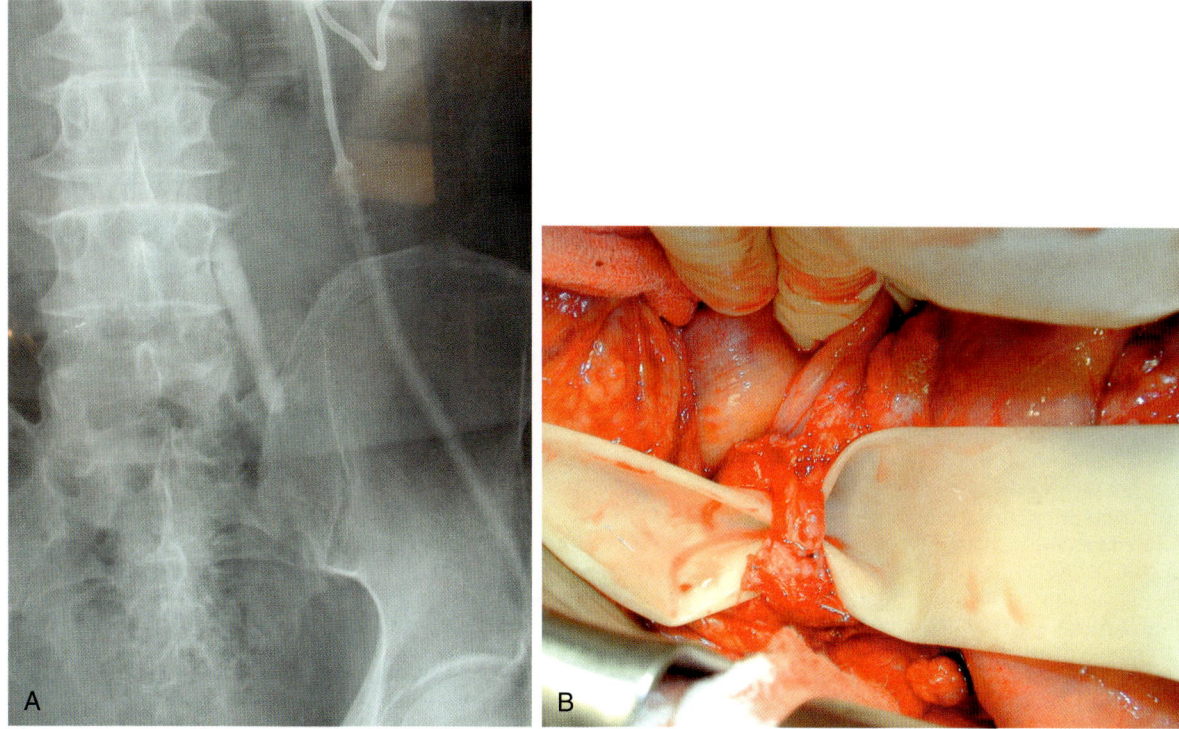

Fig. 90.23. (A) Left nephrostogram showing abrupt midureteral cutoff consistent with (inadvertent) suture ligation of the ureter. (B) Intraoperative view of left midureteral suture ligation.

Brandes et al., 2004; Fig. 90.23). Even if the ureter looks healthy, a ureteral stent should be placed at minimum, either by opening the bladder or by immediate cystoscopic placement.

Transection

Immediate Recognition. Injuries discovered immediately after nonaortic surgery are largely treated in the same way as ureteral injury after external trauma. Most lacerations can be treated with ureteroureterostomy, although additional maneuvers such as omental wrapping of the repair or placement of an ipsilateral nephrostomy tube have been advocated to decrease the potential for urine leakage or breakdown of the repair (Adams et al., 1992). With increasing laparoscopic and robotic popularity, many iatrogenic injuries are now being treated without the need for open conversion (Andrade et al., 2016; Dinlenc et al., 2004; Menderes et al., 2015; Ou et al., 2005). Ureteroscopic ureteroureterostomies for operative ureteral injuries have even been described (Tsai et al., 2000).

Ureteral injuries that occur during vascular graft surgery are a special case. Intraoperative management of these should be primary ureteroureterostomy with isolation of the repair with omentum (Adams et al., 1992). Nephrectomy in cases of ureteral injury should be avoided. Although nephrectomy avoids the potential for postoperative urine leakage around an aortic or iliac vascular graft (Schapira et al., 1981), it is associated with increased mortality. In patients with a ruptured aneurysm, it can increase the mortality rate fourfold, from 3% to 12% (Schapira et al., 1981). We recommend careful repair of the ureteral injury, reserving nephrectomy for patients who develop urine leakage postoperatively.

Delayed Recognition. Intraoperative recognition of ureteral injuries occurs in as few as 34% of patients undergoing open operation (Ghali et al., 1999) and even more rarely during laparoscopic surgery (Grainger et al., 1990). Delayed diagnosis of ureteral injury is most often (66% to 76%) determined by CT urography, or retrograde ureterography (Ghali et al., 1999; Grainger et al., 1990). In a series of 35 ureteral injuries, patients had a variety of signs and symptoms: anuria (14%, most with bilateral injury), urogenital fistula (11%), persistent pain or fever (9%), urinary leakage from the wound (9%), hydronephrosis (3%), and hematuria (3%) (Ghali et al., 1999). Some authors cite a triad of fever, leukocytosis, and generalized peritoneal signs as being most diagnostic for missed ureteral injury (Medina et al., 1998). Repair of these delayed-recognition injuries is controversial. When an incomplete ureteral injury presents in a delayed fashion, the AUA urotrauma guideline recommends retrograde ureteral imaging with ureteral stent placement (Morey, 2014). Reported success of retrograde stent placement varies widely: 5% to 10% (Dowling et al., 1986; Hoch et al., 1975), 20% (Ghali et al., 1999; Oh et al., 2000), and 50% (Cormio et al., 1993). When stent placement is possible, ultimate success rate without the need for eventual open surgery is variable, from as low as 0% to as high as 73% (Dowling et al., 1986; Oh et al., 2000). Usually, failure to place a stent is due to complete obstruction of the ureter or complete ureteral transection with a long defect/gap (Cormio et al., 1993). Some authors have suggested that stenting alone has the highest failure rate in those with multiple previous pelvic operations, radiation therapy, or significant previous ureteral surgery (Chang and Marshall, 1987). The ideal length of time to leave the stent has never been studied in a randomized, prospective, double-blind fashion, but most authors recommend at least 6 weeks (Selzman and Spirnak, 1996). The literature and our experience seem to indicate that a majority of patients will eventually require definitive repair of significant ureteral injuries, whether or not stent placement is possible. If stents cannot be placed, or the patient is so unstable as to preclude a retrograde stent attempt, then a percutaneous nephrostomy should be placed (Morey et. al., 2014). If the nephrostomy alone does not adequately control the urine leak, then further treatment is usually percutaneous urinoma drain placement or open ureteral repair.

Percutaneous nephrostomy tube placement is the single procedure most likely to be successful at draining the collecting system and diverting urine away from the ureteral injury site. In addition, when compared with ureteral stenting, a percutaneous nephrostomy tube allows for decreased periureteral inflammation at the time of the repair and thus more favorable anatomy. Ureteral balloon catheters, which are designed to stop urine from traveling down the ureter, have been advocated if simple stenting does not eliminate associated urine leakage or urinoma, although we often have found them to be ineffective. We think the safest approach is to wait at least 6 weeks for complete healing of the wounds, then attempt open or robotic repair. Some have recommended even longer ureteral drainage and delay until definitive repair, in certain special cases, such as in the presence of ureteroenteric fistula (Bright and Peters, 1977).

Some authors have advocated treating postinjury ureteral stenosis endoscopically with either balloon dilation (Richter et al., 2000) or laser incision (Patel and Newman, 2004; Singal et al., 1997). Others have used endoluminal stents for ureteral obstruction after injury with good results in limited numbers of patients (Wenzler et al., 2008). In general, endoscopic dilation and incision techniques in the long, devascularized, postinjury or postoperative ureteral strictures typically have poor results.

Ureteroscopy Injury

Avulsion. Ureteral avulsion during ureteroscopy is treated in the same manner as ureteral injuries after open or laparoscopic surgery, as detailed in the section on ureteral transection.

Perforation. Ureteral perforation during ureteroscopy can be treated by ureteral stenting, usually with no subsequent complications (Flam et al., 1988; Huffman, 1989). The safest approach is to avoid injury by always performing ureteroscopy over a ureteral guidewire and by placing a second ureteral safety wire that is always in place during ureteroscopy and facilitates ureteral stent placement in the presence of problems. We recognize that some expert centers do not use a ureteral guidewire during ureteroscopy and that some no longer use a safety wire, but we believe that at least a safety wire is most prudent for the majority of practitioners.

KEY POINTS: URETERAL TRAUMA

- Ureteral injury diagnosis requires a low index of suspicion. Absence of hematuria does not reliably rule out ureteral injury.
- Stable patients with suspected ureteral injury should undergo CT urogram with delayed images.
- After penetrating injury, determine the course of the knife or bullet tract to ensure that the ureter is not at risk.
- If delayed recognition is suspected, image with CT urogram or retrograde ureterogram.
- Ureteral repair should be performed in stable patients at the time of laparotomy, when possible.
- Consider damage control, followed by delayed definite repair for unstable patients with ureteral injuries.
- Manage ureteral contusions with stenting or, if severe, resection and primary repair.
- Place a nephrostomy tube for delayed diagnosed injuries that cannot be stented retrograde.
- Retroperitoneal surgery should be undertaken only with constant attention to the location of the ureter. Intraoperatively, the ureter should be exposed and inspected when ureteral injury is suspected.
- See Fig. 90.24.

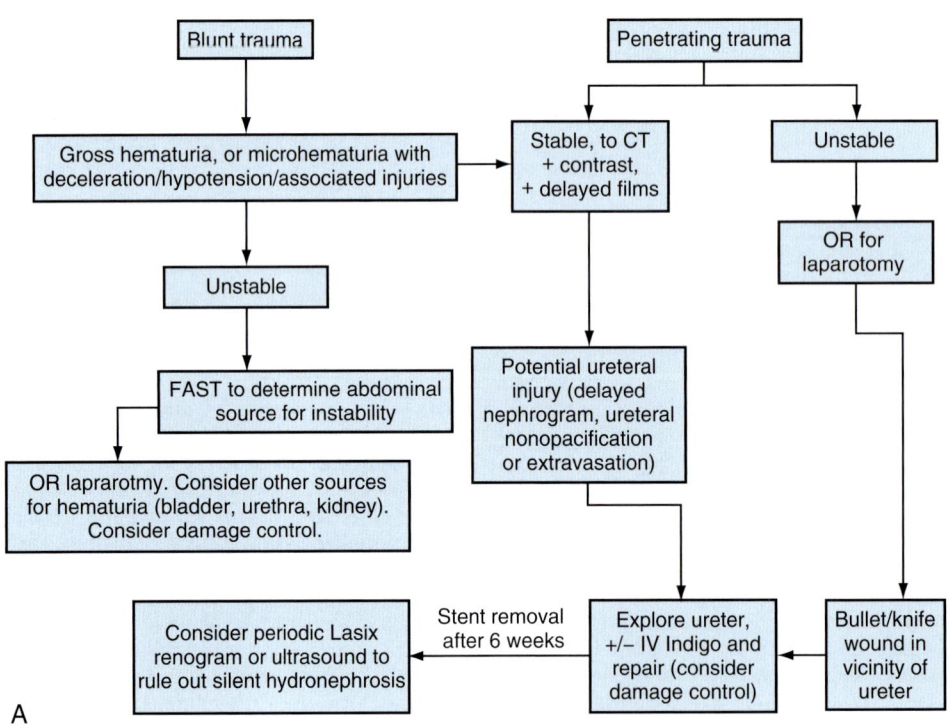

Fig. 90.24. Algorithms for the diagnosis and treatment of ureteral injuries. (A) From external violence.

Chapter 90 Upper Urinary Tract Trauma 2003

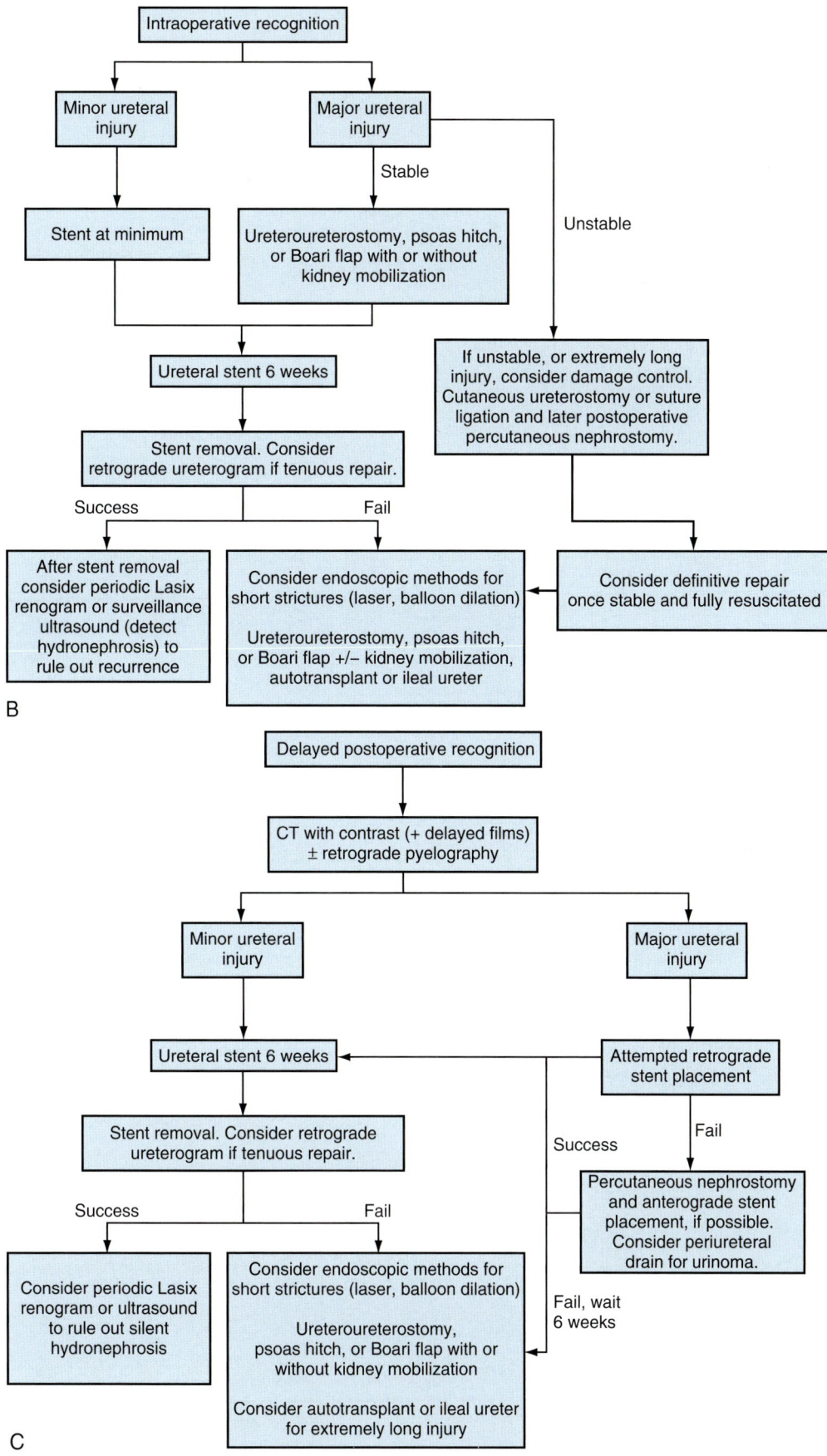

Fig. 90.24, cont'd. (B) Discovered intraoperatively. (C) Discovered postoperatively. *CT,* Computed tomography; *IVP,* intravenous pyelography; *OR,* operating room.

SUGGESTED READINGS

Brandes S, Coburn M, Armenakas N, et al: Diagnosis and management of ureteric injury: an evidence-based analysis, *BJU Int* 94:277–289, 2004.

Bretan PN Jr, McAninch JW, Federle MP, et al: Computerized tomographic staging of renal trauma: 85 consecutive cases, *J Urol* 136:561–565, 1986.

Broghammer JA, Fisher MB, Santucci RA: Conservative management of renal trauma: a review, *Urology* 70:623–629, 2007.

Buckley JC, McAninch JW: Pediatric renal injuries: management guidelines from a 25-year experience, *J Urol* 172:687–690, discussion 690, 2004.

Carroll PR, Klosterman P, McAninch JW: Early vascular control for renal trauma: a critical review, *J Urol* 141:826–829, 1989.

Chandhoke PS, McAninch JW: Detection and significance of microscopic hematuria in patients with blunt renal trauma, *J Urol* 140:16–18, 1988.

Miller KS, McAninch JW: Radiographic assessment of renal trauma: our 15-year experience, *J Urol* 154:352–355, 1995.

Moore EE, Shackford SR, Pachter HL, et al: Organ injury scaling: spleen, liver, and kidney, *J Trauma* 29:1664–1666, 1989.

Morey AF, Brandes SB, Dugi DD, et al: Urotrauma: AUA guideline, *J Urol* 192:327–335, 2014.

Presti JC Jr, Carroll PR, McAninch JW: Ureteral and renal pelvic injuries from external trauma: diagnosis and management, *J Trauma* 29:370–374, 1989.

Santucci RA, Wessells H, Bartsch G, et al: Evaluation and management of renal injuries: consensus statement of the renal trauma subcommittee, *BJU Int* 93:937–954, 2004.

Selzman AA, Spirnak JP: Iatrogenic ureteral injuries: a 20-year experience in treating 165 injuries, *J Urol* 155:878–881, 1996.

Voelzke BB, McAninch JW: The current management of renal injuries, *Am Surg* 74:667–678, 2008.

REFERENCES

The complete reference list is available online at ExpertConsult.com.

PART X
Urinary Lithiasis and Endourology

91 Urinary Lithiasis: Etiology, Epidemiology, and Pathogenesis

Margaret S. Pearle, MD, PhD, Jodi A. Antonelli, MD, and Yair Lotan, MD

Although stone disease is one of the most common afflictions of modern society, it has been described since antiquity. With Westernization of global culture, however, the site of stone formation has migrated from the lower to the upper urinary tract, and the disease once limited to men is increasingly gender blind. Revolutionary advances in the minimally invasive and noninvasive management of stone disease over the past few decades have greatly facilitated stone removal. However, surgical treatments, although they remove the offending stone, do little to alter the course of the disease. Indeed, the overall estimated annual expenditure for individuals with insurance claims corresponding to a diagnosis of nephrolithiasis exceeded $10 billion in 2012, reflecting a nearly fivefold increase since 2000 (Litwin et al., 2005). Given the frequency with which stones recur, the development of a medical prophylactic program to prevent stone recurrences is desirable. To this end, a thorough understanding of the cause, epidemiology, and pathogenesis of urinary tract stone disease is necessary.

EPIDEMIOLOGY OF RENAL CALCULI

The lifetime prevalence of kidney stone disease is estimated at 1% to 15%, varying according to age, gender, race, and geographic location. Around the world prevalence rates vary ranging from 7% to 13% in North America, 5% to 9% in Europe, and 1% to 5% in Asia (Sorokin et al., 2017). **Data from the National Health and Nutrition Examination Survey (NHANES) data sets have demonstrated a linear increase in the prevalence of kidney stones for US adults over the last several decades** (Stamatelou et al., 2003), **with the most recent prevalence estimate of 8.8% for the period 2007 to 2010** (Scales et al., 2012). Tasian et al. (2016) examined temporal trends in nephrolithiasis incidence among a subset of the US population and found a 16% rise in annual stone incidence (from 206 to 239 per 100,000 persons) between 1997 and 2012.

The rise in kidney stone prevalence is a global phenomenon. Data from five European countries, Japan, and the United States showed that the incidence and prevalence of stone disease has been increasing over time around the world (Romero et al., 2010). In a unique data set derived from a series of nationwide surveys conducted by the Japanese Society on Urolithiasis Research, Yasui et al. (2008) found an increase in the age-adjusted annual incidence of first-time stone events from 54.2 per 100,000 in 1965 to 114.3 per 100,000 in 2005. Although the incidence increased in all age groups and in men and women, the age of peak incidence shifted in men from 20 to 49 years in 1965 to 30 to 69 years in 2005 and in women from 20 to 29 years in 1965 to 50 to 79 years in 2005. A population-based analysis from Taiwan using the Longitudinal Health Insurance Database 2005 contains data on all medical benefit claims from 1997 to 2010 for 1 million beneficiaries randomly chosen from the 2005 enrollment file. This analysis showed that the prevalence of stone disease overall was 7.4% (5.8% in women and 9.0% in men), with an overall peak prevalence of 19.4% in 60- to 69-year-old adults (Huang et al., 2013). A similar population-based study in Korea showed that the lifetime prevalence of kidney stones was 3.5% (1.8% in women and 6% in men) (Bae et al., 2014).

It has been suggested that the rise in stone incidence and prevalence seen in the United States and worldwide can be attributed in part to a rise in the detection of asymptomatic calculi through increased use of radiographic imaging, particularly computed tomography (CT) (Boyce et al., 2010; Edvardsson et al., 2013). Edvardsson et al. (2013) identified 5945 incident stone formers in the Icelandic population from 1985 to 2008 and found that the annual incidence of stones increased significantly from 108 per 100,000 in the first 5 years of the study to 138 per 100,000 through the remainder of the study interval ($P < 0.001$). However, they found that the annual incidence of symptomatic stones did not increase significantly, despite significant increases in the incidence of asymptomatic stones in both genders (from 7 to 24 per 100,000 in men, $P < 0.001$, and from 7 to 21 per 100,000 in women, $P < 0.001$).

Gender

Historically, stone disease affected adult men more commonly than adult women. By a variety of indicators, including inpatient admissions, outpatient office visits, and emergency department visits, men were affected two to three times more often than women (Pearle et al., 2005; Soucie et al., 1994). However, recent evidence suggests that the difference in incidence between men and women is narrowing. Using the National Inpatient Sample data set representing hospital discharges, Scales et al. (2007) found that, although overall population-adjusted discharges for a diagnosis of renal or ureteral calculus increased by only 1.6% from 1997 to 2002, discharges for women increased by 17%, while discharges for men decreased by 8.1%. This trend reflects a change in the ratio of male-to-female discharges from 1.7 in 1997 to 1.3 in 2002. Lieske et al. (2006) used the Rochester Epidemiology Project data (including office, emergency department, and nursing home visits and inpatient and outpatient admissions) to compare the age-adjusted incidence of new symptomatic stone disease from 1970 to 2000 and found similar trends with regard to gender. Although the total rate of symptomatic stone disease for each decade in this time period remained relatively flat ($P = 0.33$), the rate of symptomatic stones in men declined by 1.7% per year (age-adjusted $P = 0.019$) but increased in women by 1.9% per year (age-adjusted $P = 0.064$), resulting in an overall decrease in the male-to-female ratio of symptomatic stones from 3.2 to 1.3 ($P = 0.006$) during this time period. Another, more contemporary geographic epidemiologic database, the Marshfield Epidemiologic Study Area Database, showed a decline in the male-to-female ratio for urolithiasis from 1.4 in 1992 to 1.0 in 2008 (Penniston et al., 2011).

Using NHANES data, Stamatelou et al. (2003) reported a slight decrease in the male-to-female ratio of stone disease, from 1.75 (between 1976 and 1980) to 1.54 (between 1988 and 1994), with the most recent NHANES data (2007–2010) revealing a stone prevalence of 10.6% in men and 7.1% in women for a ratio of 1.49, which is only slightly lower than that reported for 1988 to 1994 (Scales et al., 2012). Tasian et al. (2016) used US census and South Carolina Medical Encounter data from 1997 to 2012 to capture temporal trends in nephrolithiasis incidence among South Carolina residents. After adjusting for age and race, they found that the incidence of nephrolithiasis in women increased by an estimated 15% per 5 years (incidence rate ratio [IRR] 1.15, 95% CI 1.14–1.16) but was stable in men (IRR 0.99, 95% CI 0.98–1.00) during this time period. Furthermore, they found a gender differential in age-specific incidence rates: women showed a 10% to 28% increase per 5 years with the highest increase in 10- to 19-year-olds, while men older than 25 years demonstrated less than 5% change in incidence per 5 years.

Walker et al. (2013) retrospectively analyzed their database of 2799 eligible patients (1983 men and 816 women) at a tertiary care stone clinic in the UK and found a male:female ratio of 2.43:1. Furthermore, they noted that the prevalence of risk factors for stone formation differed between men and women in this cohort, with family history, recurrent urinary tract infections, and anatomic abnormalities occurring more commonly in women and gout and bladder outlet obstruction occurring more commonly in men. Likewise, 24-hour urine parameters showed gender disparity, with men excreting greater amounts and having higher urinary concentrations of calcium, oxalate, and uric acid, whereas women had higher citrate levels.

Race and Ethnicity

Racial and ethnic differences in the incidence of stone disease have been observed. **Among US men, Soucie et al. (1994) found the highest prevalence of stone disease in whites, followed by Hispanics, Asians, and African-Americans, who had prevalences of 70%, 63%, and 44% of whites, respectively.** Among US women, the prevalence was highest among whites but lowest among Asian women (about half that of whites). According to the most recent NHANES data set, Hispanics (odds ratio [OR] 0.60, 95% CI 0.49–0.73, P < 0.001) and black non-Hispanics (OR 0.37, 95% CI 0.28–0.49, P < 0.001) were significantly less likely to report a history of stone disease compared with white non-Hispanics (Scales et al., 2012). However, a population-based study of adults and children in South Carolina demonstrated that independent of age and gender the incidence of kidney stones increased an estimated 3% per 5 years in whites (IRR 1.03, 95% CI, 1.02–1.03) compared with 15% for African-Americans (IRR 1.15, 95% CI 1.14–1.17) (Tasian et al., 2016).

Mente et al. (2007) attempted to identify genetic influences on stone disease by comparing stone prevalence among different ethnic groups residing in the same geographic region. Using Europeans (Caucasians) as the reference group, the relative risk of calcium stones was higher in individuals of Arabic (OR 3.8, 95% CI 2.7–5.2), West Indian (OR 2.5, 95% CI 1.8–3.4), West Asian (OR 2.4, 95% CI 1.7–3.4), and Latin American (OR 1.7, 95% CI 1.2–2.4) origin and significantly lower in those of East Asian (OR 0.4, 95% CI 0.3–0.5) and African (OR 0.7, 95% CI 0.5–0.9) descent. Interestingly, despite differences in prevalence of stone disease according to ethnicity, Maloney et al. (2005) observed a remarkably similar incidence of metabolic abnormalities between white and nonwhite stone formers from the same geographic region, although the distribution of abnormalities differed, suggesting that dietary and other environmental factors may outweigh the contribution of ethnicity in determining stone risk.

The gender distribution of stone disease varies according to race. Sarmina et al. (1987) **noted a male-to-female ratio among whites of 2.3 and among African-Americans of 0.65.** Michaels et al. (1994) also noted a reversal of the male predisposition of stone disease in Hispanics and African-Americans, reporting a male-to-female ratio of 1.8 among Asians, 1.6 among whites, 0.7 among Hispanics, and 0.5 among African-Americans, among a group of patients undergoing shockwave lithotripsy. Tasian et al. (2016) corroborated these findings by observing that the estimated changes in incidence of kidney stone disease over time were greater in African-American women than in African-American men. Dall'era et al. (2005) reviewed emergency department records to identify patients with symptomatic renal or ureteral calculi and found a male-to-female ratio of 1.17 among Hispanic patients compared with 2.05 for white patients.

Age

Historically it was relatively uncommon for stones to occur in individuals under age 20. However, over the last few decades stone disease has been increasing at a rate of 5% to 10% annually in the pediatric population (Bonzo and Tasian, 2017). Routh et al. (2010) queried the Pediatric Health Information System Database, which includes inpatient admissions and emergency and outpatient surgery visits for 42 freestanding US pediatric hospitals, for patients treated for stones between 1999 and 2008. After adjusting for increases in total patient volume over this time period, they found that the portion of pediatric patients with urolithiasis increased from 18.4 per 100,000 in 1999 to 57.0 per 100,000 in 2008, representing a mean annual increase of 10.6% (P < 0.0001). Dwyer et al. (2012) analyzed data from the Rochester Epidemiologic Project and identified 207 patients under 18 years of age diagnosed with a symptomatic stone in Olmsted County, Minnesota, between 1984 and 2008. During this 25-year time period the overall incidence of stone disease increased by 4% per year. However, among adolescents 12 to 17 years of age the annual increase was 6%. Although an increase in stone disease among children has been consistently observed, the factors accounting for this trend have not been completely elucidated. It has been suggested that epidemiologic changes, by which risk factors such as obesity and metabolic syndrome that predispose to kidney stones are more often affecting younger generations, may play a role (Alfandary et al., 2018; Kuroczycka-Saniutzcz et al., 2015; Tiwari et al., 2012).

In adults, the incidence of kidney stones peaks in the fourth to sixth decades of life (Johnson et al., 1979; Marshall et al., 1975). Lieske et al. (2006) found a peak incidence in the age group 60 to 69 years in men but observed relatively little change in incidence between 20 and 70 years of age in women, with just a slightly higher incidence in women in the age groups 30 to 39 and 60 to 69.

It has been observed that women show a bimodal distribution of stone disease, demonstrating a second peak in incidence in the sixth decade of life corresponding to the onset of menopause and a fall in estrogen levels (Johnson et al., 1979; Marshall et al., 1975). This finding and the lower incidence of stone disease in women compared with men have been attributed to the protective effect of estrogen against stone formation in premenopausal women because of enhanced renal calcium absorption and reduced bone resorption (McKane et al., 1995; Nordin et al., 1999). Indeed, Heller et al. (2002) identified lower urinary saturation of calcium oxalate and brushite in women compared with men. Moreover, urinary calcium was lower in women than in men until beyond age 50, when it reached equivalence in the two groups. Estrogen-treated postmenopausal women had lower urinary calcium and saturation of calcium oxalate than untreated women.

Fan et al. (1999) found that androgens increased and estrogens decreased urinary and serum oxalate in an experimental rat model, perhaps accounting for the reduced risk of stone formation in women. However, van Aswegen et al. (1989) found lower levels of urinary testosterone in stone formers compared with non–stone-forming control subjects, further confounding the issue.

Geography

The geographic distribution of stone disease tends to roughly follow environmental risk factors; **a higher prevalence of stone disease is found in hot, arid, or dry climates such as the mountains, desert, or tropical areas.** However, genetic factors and dietary influences may outweigh the effects of geography. Finlayson (1974) reviewed several worldwide geographic surveys and found that areas of high stone prevalence included the United States, the British Isles, Scandinavian and Mediterranean countries, northern India and Pakistan, northern Australia, central Europe, portions of the Malay peninsula, and China. Within the United States, Mandel and Mandel (1989a, 1989b) **identified the highest rates of hospital discharges for patients with calcium oxalate stones in the Southeast and for uric acid**

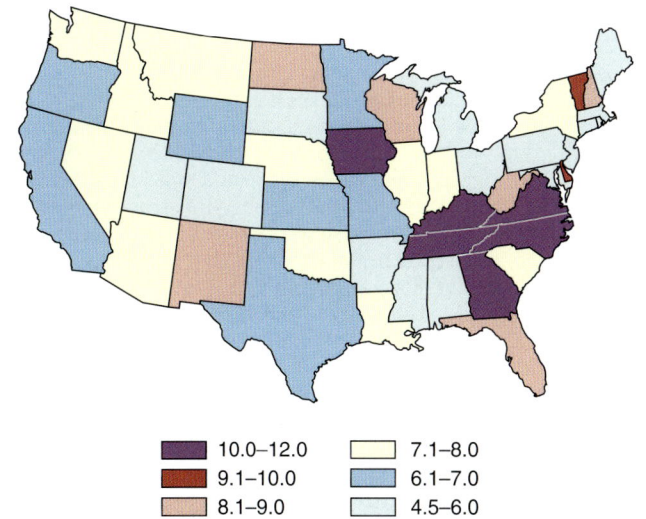

Fig. 91.1. Geographic distribution of urinary tract stone disease in the US veteran population from 1983 to 1986. Data are expressed as urinary tract stone patients per 1000 hospital discharges. (From Mandel NS, Mandel GS: Urinary tract stone disease in the United States veteran population: II. Geographical analysis of variations in composition. *J Urol* 142:1516, 1989.)

stones in the East, among the veteran patient population (Fig. 91.1). Soucie et al. (1994) found increasing age-adjusted prevalence rates in men and women going from north to south and west to east, with the highest prevalence observed in the Southeast. After controlling for other risk factors, the authors determined that ambient temperature and sunlight were independently associated with stone prevalence (Soucie et al., 1996). Unfortunately, the multitude of factors that affect stone formation and the considerable variability in documentation and availability of data in some parts of the world limit our ability to accurately capture true variation in incidence and prevalence of stone disease worldwide (Sorokin et al., 2017).

Climate

Seasonal variation in stone disease is likely related to temperature by way of fluid losses from perspiration and perhaps by sunlight-induced increases in vitamin D. Prince and Scardino (1960) noted the highest incidence of stone disease in the summer months, July through September, with the peak occurring within 1 to 2 months of maximal mean temperatures (Prince et al., 1956). Using data obtained from the Taiwan National Health Insurance Research Database (1999–2003), Chen et al. (2008) analyzed monthly inpatient and outpatient medical benefit claims for a primary diagnosis of renal or ureteral calculi or renal colic and found that the peak incidence of stone-related claims occurred in July through September, with a sharp decline in claims in October. Ambient temperature, atmospheric pressure, and hours of sunshine correlated with monthly stone-related claims, but after adjusting for seasonality, month, and trend, ambient temperature was found to be the most important determinant of stone-related events. The link between seasonal high ambient temperatures and increased risk of kidney stones worldwide has been validated in a systematic review of the literature over a 26-year period (Geraghty et al., 2017).

Tasian et al. (2014) used the MarketScan Commercial Claims data set to perform time-series, nonlinear modeling to estimate the relative risk of kidney stone presentation associated with mean daily temperature in five large metropolitan areas geographically distributed throughout the United States. They noted that as mean daily temperature increased to greater than 10°C, kidney stone presentation in most cities correspondingly increased in the ensuing 10 days. Furthermore, the association between kidney stone presentation and mean daily temperature was greatest at 30°C compared with 10°C and occurred within 3 days of that temperature, with a second peak at 4 to 6 days, indicating that the time interval between hot days and kidney stone presentation is actually short.

The study of military personnel translocated to desert locations has provided a unique opportunity to study the effect of climate on a defined population. Pierce and Bloom (1945) reported that American soldiers in an undisclosed desert location had an increase in symptomatic episodes of renal colic during the summer season. Another study of military personnel who developed symptomatic stones after arrival in Kuwait and Iraq revealed a mean time interval to stone formation of 93 days (Evans and Costabile, 2005). Finally, Parry and Lister (1975) measured urinary calcium and magnesium levels in soldiers before and 10 days after transfer to the Persian Gulf. They noted increased urinary calcium levels from baseline in those soldiers transferred during the summer months but not among those transferred during the "cold season," which was attributed to sunlight-induced increased production of 1,25-dihydroxyvitamin D_3 (1,25$[OH]_2D_3$). Thus it is likely that climate and geography influence the prevalence of stone disease indirectly, through effects on temperature and possibly sunlight.

Ordon et al. (2016), using a population-based, time-series analysis of linked health care databases in Ontario, Canada, showed that the increase in presentation to the emergency department during times of warmer ambient temperature was more pronounced in men than women (RR = 1.64 vs. 1.22, respectively, $P = 0.006$) and in those patients aged 40 to 69 compared with other adult age groups. The pathophysiology responsible for these gender and age differences in response to temperature has not been elucidated but is likely affected by confounders such as differential sunlight exposure, occupation, and hydration status.

Brikowski et al. (2008) constructed two alternate models describing the temperature dependence of stone disease on the basis of reported regional stone prevalence rates and corresponding mean annual temperatures to predict the anticipated change in stone prevalence resulting from global warming. Prevalence rates obtained from the Second Cancer Prevention Survey of 1982 (Soucie et al., 1996) were consistent with a nonlinear, or peaked, relationship between temperature and stone prevalence, whereas a data set from the Veterans Administration that was analyzed by the Urologic Diseases in America project (Pearle et al., 2005) more closely approximated a linear fit. Using a moderate-severity warming model to predict temperature change resulting from global warming in the United States, the authors estimated an increase of 1 to 1.5 million lifetime cases of climate-related nephrolithiasis by 2050. According to the linear model of temperature dependence, the net effect of warming will be a northward expansion of the current-day "stone belt" (which occupies primarily the Southeast region of the United States) into the Midwest, such that by 2050 it will occupy the entire Southeast portion of the country and all of California. The nonlinear model predicts that the zone of elevated stone risk currently located in the Southeast will expand northward to include a band of states from Kansas to Virginia and Northern California, but with the increase in prevalence primarily concentrated south of the temperature threshold.

Fakheri and Goldfarb (2009) later revisited the analysis correlating mean annual temperature and stone prevalence and confirmed that temperature positively correlated with rate of stone prevalence. However, they further established that the temperature dependence of stone disease could be attributed primarily to an effect on men. For every unit degree Fahrenheit increase in temperature, the percentage prevalence rate increased by 0.15 ($R^2 = 0.37$) in men and 0.04 ($R^2 = 0.51$) in women. A hypothesis for the increased incidence of stones related to temperature is that more people are exposed to urban heat islands as a result of progressive urbanization. The effects of urban architecture and infrastructure coupled with reduced vegetation result in cities that are warmer than more rural areas (Goldfarb et al., 2015). A study examining this association that takes into account relevant variables such as fluid intake, diet, and socioeconomic status is lacking.

Occupation

Heat exposure and dehydration constitute occupational risk factors for stone disease as well. Cooks and engineering room personnel, who are exposed to high temperatures, were found to have the highest rates of stone formation among personnel of the Royal Navy (Blacklock, 1969). Likewise, Atan et al. (2005) found a significantly higher incidence of stones among steelworkers exposed to high temperatures (8%) compared with those working in normal temperatures (0.9%). Metabolic evaluation of these two groups of workers showed a higher incidence of low urine volume and hypocitraturia among the workers in the hot area. Borghi et al. (1993) also noted differences in the incidence of stone disease and urinary stone risk factors between workers at a glass plant who were or were not chronically exposed to high temperatures causing massive perspiration. Those exposed to high temperatures exhibited lower urine volumes and pH, higher uric acid levels, and higher urine specific gravity, leading to higher urinary saturation of uric acid. Accordingly, those workers who formed stones had a remarkably high incidence of uric acid stones (38%).

Individuals with sedentary occupations such as those in managerial or professional positions have been found to carry an increased risk of stone formation for unclear reasons (Blacklock, 1969). This finding is consistent with the work of Robertson et al. (1980), who reported an increased risk of stone disease in affluent individuals, countries, and societies, which may be reflective of a more indulgent diet and lifestyle. In addition, those with occupations that limit bathroom access, such as taxi drivers and operating room personnel, have been shown to have an increased risk of stones (Linder et al., 2013; Mass et al., 2014).

Obesity, Diabetes, and Metabolic Syndrome

The association of body size and incidence of stone disease has been extensively investigated. In two large prospective cohort studies of men and women, **the prevalence and incident risk of stone disease directly correlated with weight and body mass index (BMI) in both sexes, although the magnitude of the association was greater in women than in men** (Curhan et al., 1998; Taylor et al., 2005b). Furthermore, they found that obesity and weight gain were independent risk factors for incident stone formation that could not be accounted for by diet alone (Taylor et al., 2005b). Nowfar et al. (2011) used a large all-payer inpatient care data set and found an increased risk of stones with obesity that was more pronounced in women than men. Yoshimura et al. (2016) followed more than 4000 Japanese male gas company workers without stones at baseline for a period of 19 years and found that BMI was independently associated with risk of incident kidney stones. Finally, Semins et al. (2010) using claims data found an increasing risk of kidney stones with increasing BMI, up to a BMI of 30 kg/m^2, at which point the risk stabilized.

Sorensen et al. (2013) investigated the independent effects of caloric intake, physical activity, and BMI on stone risk in 84,225 postmenopausal women with no prior stone history in the Women's Health Initiative Observational Study. They found that in addition to BMI, less physical activity and increased dietary energy intake (more than 2200 kcal/day) were each associated with an increased incident risk of kidney stones, which supports dietary and physical activity components of weight loss counseling as part of an overall kidney stone prevention program.

The constellation of visceral obesity along with hyperlipidemia, hypertriglyceridemia, hyperglycemia, and/or hypertension, known as metabolic syndrome, has been linked to an increased risk for kidney stones. Using the NHANES III (1988–1994) data set, West et al. (2008) found that those with a diagnosis of metabolic syndrome were significantly more likely to report a history of kidney stones compared with healthy subjects (8.8% vs. 4.3%, respectively, $P < 0.001$). Furthermore, they found that the prevalence of a self-reported history of kidney stones increased with the number of metabolic syndrome traits, with the prevalence of kidney stones estimated at 3% for no traits, 7.5% for three traits, and 9.8% for five traits. Multivariate analysis revealed that the presence of four or five metabolic syndrome traits was associated with a more than twofold increase in the odds of a self-reported stone history (OR 2.42, 95% CI 1.57–3.73). Wong et al. (2016) corroborated these findings in a systematic review of six studies comprising 219,255 patients.

Metabolic syndrome has been implicated as a potential precursor of type 2 diabetes mellitus. Taylor et al. (2005a) prospectively studied the association between diabetes and incident kidney stones in three large cohorts (Nurses' Health Study I [NHS I] composed of older women; Nurses' Health Study II [NHS II] composed of younger women; and the Health Professionals Follow-Up Study [HPFS] composed of men) and found that, after adjusting for BMI, diet, and thiazide use, a history of diabetes was associated with an increase in incident kidney stones in women but not men. Conversely, a history of kidney stones was associated with an increase in the incidence of self-reported diabetes for women and men (OR 1.33, 95% CI 1.18–1.50 for older women; OR 1.48, 95% CI 1.14–1.91 for younger women; and OR 1.49, 95% CI 1.29–1.72 for men). In addition, Chung et al. (2011) observed a 1.3-fold higher likelihood of being diagnosed with diabetes among individuals within 5 years of a diagnosis of kidney stones than in a comparison cohort of individuals who did not form stones (95% CI 1.26–1.39, $P < 0.001$). Stone formers with type 2 diabetes have been shown to have higher urinary oxalate and lower urine pH than nondiabetic stone formers (Eisner et al., 2010a).

Although the association between obesity, diabetes, and metabolic syndrome has been explored in the epidemiologic literature, the exact pathophysiologic mechanism responsible for this association has yet to be completely defined; however, a central theme of these comorbidities is a metabolic state of insulin resistance. Evidence linking obesity and insulin resistance with low urine pH and uric acid stones (Maalouf et al., 2004a, 2004b), as well as an association between hyperinsulinemia and hypercalciuria (Kerstetter et al., 1991; Nowicki et al., 1998; Shimamoto et al., 1995), could account for an increased risk of uric acid and/or calcium stones in obese patients. Overweight (BMI 25–30 kg/m^2) has also been shown to be associated with lower urine pH and higher urinary sodium, uric acid, and calcium compared with normal weight (Shavit et al., 2015). Furthermore, evidence suggests that urinary abnormalities may be harder to correct in overweight and obese compared with normal individuals. Astrova et al. (2016) found a significant inverse relationship between BMI and response to potassium citrate in patients with low urine pH and hypocitraturia, with more frequent dose adjustments required to correct these abnormalities in patients with higher BMI.

A study of stone-forming and non–stone-forming participants in the HPFS (599 stone-forming and 404 non–stone-forming men), NHS I (888 stone-forming and 398 non–stone-forming older women), and NHS II (689 stone-forming and 295 non–stone-forming younger women) for whom 24-hour urine studies were collected correlated urinary stone risk profiles with BMI (Taylor and Curhan, 2006). **Subjects with higher BMI excreted more urinary oxalate, uric acid, sodium, and phosphorus than those with lower BMI. Furthermore, similar to other studies, urinary supersaturation of uric acid increased with BMI.**

It has been suggested that the association of obesity with calcium oxalate stone formation is primarily due to increased excretion of promoters of stone formation (Negri et al., 2007; Siener et al., 2004). **In contrast, the association of obesity and uric acid stone formation is primarily influenced by urinary pH.**

Cardiovascular Disease

A number of investigators have explored the association between hypertension and kidney stones. In a recent meta-analysis, Shang et al. (2017) found that patients with nephrolithiasis had a significantly increased risk of hypertension (OR 1.43; 95% CI 1.30–1.56) compared with those without a history of stones, an association that was more pronounced in women (OR 1.43; 95% CI 1.21–1.69) than men (OR 1.31; 95% CI 1.25–1.37). Increased dietary intake of substances associated with hypertension and stone disease, including calcium, sodium, and potassium, has been proposed as a possible explanation for this finding. Indeed, Borghi et al. (1999) observed higher urinary calcium, uric acid, oxalate and supersaturation of calcium oxalate in men and women with hypertension compared with normotensive individuals, and Eisner et al. (2010b) found that hypertensive stone formers excrete about 25 mg/day more calcium than normotensive stone formers.

Stone disease has also been linked to heart disease. One longitudinal study found a 31% higher incidence of myocardial infarction (MI) among those with a history of kidney stones compared with those without stones, even after adjusting for comorbidities, including chronic kidney disease (Rule et al., 2010). In addition, Reiner et al. (2011) documented an association between history of kidney stones and subclinical carotid atherosclerosis in young men and women. Ferraro et al. (2013b) explored the association between kidney stones and risk of heart disease in three large cohort studies, NHS I, NHS II, and HPFS, and found that a history of kidney stones was associated with a modest but significant increase in heart disease in both female cohorts but not in the male cohort. Alexander et al. (2013), in a cohort study of more than 3 million people in Alberta, Canada, found that after adjusting for cardiovascular and other potential confounding variables, those with a history of at least one kidney stone had a higher risk of subsequent cardiovascular events such as acute MI (HR 1.4, 95% CI 1.30–1.51) and stroke (HR 1.26, 95% CI 1.12–1.42) than those without stones, a risk that was greater in younger individuals (age <50 versus ≥50 years, $P < 0.001$) and women ($P < 0.01$). Although the factors responsible for the association between nephrolithiasis and cardiovascular disease have yet to be elucidated, dyslipidemia (high total cholesterol, high triglycerides, and low high-density lipoprotein [HDL]) has been associated with alterations in urine chemistry that can predispose to kidney stone formation (Torricelli et al., 2014).

Chronic Kidney Disease

Epidemiologic studies have demonstrated a link between nephrolithiasis and development of chronic kidney disease (CKD). In a case control study, Vupputuri et al. (2004) demonstrated that patients with a history of kidney stones had a higher risk of CKD (OR 1.9; 95% CI 1.1–3.3) even after controlling for confounding factors. Furthermore, Gillen et al. (2005) demonstrated that stone formers, particularly those with a BMI of at least 27 kg/m^2, had a mean estimated glomerular filtration rate (eGFR) 3.4 mL/min/1.73 m^2 lower (95% CI −5.8–1.1, $P = 0.005$) and were nearly twice as likely to have stage 3 CKD (RR 1.87, 95% CI 1.06–3.30) compared with a group of non–stone-forming controls.

Two prospective cohort studies involving insured, predominantly white individuals demonstrated a higher risk of incident CKD in patients with a history of kidney stones (Alexander et al., 2012; Rule et al., 2009). Likewise, in a multivariate analysis adjusting for other comorbid conditions, Shoag et al. (2014) found that a history of kidney stones was associated with CKD (OR 1.50, 95% CI 1.10–2.04, $P = 0.013$) and end-stage renal disease (ESRD) requiring dialysis (OR 2.37, 95% CI 1.13–4.96, $P = 0.025$), a finding largely accounted for by women as there was no association between kidney stones and CKD or ESRD in men. In a population-based cohort study, El-Zoghby et al. (2012) also found that symptomatic stone formers were at an increased risk of developing ESRD (HR 2.09, 95% CI 1.45–3.01). Further studies are needed to elucidate the relationship between CKD and nephrolithiasis.

Water

The beneficial effect of a high fluid intake on stone prevention has long been recognized. In two large observational studies, fluid intake was found to be inversely related to the risk of incident kidney stone formation (Curhan et al., 1993, 1997). Furthermore, in a prospective, randomized trial assessing the effect of fluid intake on stone recurrence among first-time idiopathic calcium stone formers, urine volume was significantly higher in the group assigned to a high fluid intake compared with the control group receiving no recommendations, and, accordingly, stone recurrence rates were significantly lower (12% vs. 27%, respectively) (Borghi et al., 1996).

Geographic differences in the incidence of stone disease have been ascribed in some cases to differences in the mineral and electrolyte content of water in different areas. Although several investigators reported a lower incidence of stone disease in geographic regions with a "hard" water supply compared with a "soft" water supply, where water "hardness" is determined by content of calcium carbonate (Churchill et al., 1978; Sierakowski et al., 1979), others found no difference. Schwartz et al. (2002) found no association between water hardness and incidence of stone episodes, although they did observe a correlation between water hardness and urinary magnesium, calcium, and citrate levels.

> **KEY POINTS: EPIDEMIOLOGY**
>
> - Upper urinary tract stones occur more commonly in men than women, but there is evidence that the gender gap is narrowing.
> - Whites have the highest incidence of upper tract stones compared with Asians, Hispanics, and African-Americans.
> - Prevalence of stone disease shows geographic variability, with the highest prevalence of stone disease in the Southeast.
> - The risk of stone disease correlates with weight and BMI.
> - Stone disease has been correlated with a number of systemic disorders, including diabetes, metabolic syndrome, cardiovascular disease, and CKD.

PHYSICOCHEMISTRY AND PATHOGENESIS

The physical process of stone formation comprises a complex cascade of events that occurs as the glomerular filtrate traverses the nephron. It begins with urine that becomes supersaturated with respect to stone-forming salts, such that dissolved ions or molecules precipitate out of solution and form crystals or nuclei. Once formed, crystals may flow out with the urine or become retained in the kidney at anchoring sites that promote growth and aggregation, ultimately leading to stone formation. The discussion that follows describes the process of stone formation from a physicochemical standpoint.

State of Saturation

A solution containing ions or molecules of a sparingly soluble salt is described by the *concentration product*, which is a mathematical expression of the product of the concentrations of the pure chemical components (ions or molecules) of the salt. For example, the concentration product (CP) expression for sodium chloride is

$$CP = [Na^+][Cl^-].$$

A pure aqueous solution of a salt is considered *saturated* when it reaches the point at which no further added salt crystals will dissolve. The concentration product at the point of saturation is called the *thermodynamic solubility product* (K_{sp}), which is the point at which the dissolved and crystalline components are in equilibrium for a specific set of conditions. At this point, addition of further crystals to the saturated solution will cause the crystals to precipitate unless the conditions of the solution, such as pH or temperature, are changed.

In urine, despite concentration products of stone-forming salt components such as calcium oxalate that exceed the solubility product, crystallization does not necessarily occur because of the presence of inhibitors and other molecules that allow higher concentrations of calcium oxalate to be held in solution before precipitation or crystallization occurs. In this state of saturation, urine is considered to be *metastable* with respect to the salt. As concentrations of the salt increase further, the point at which it can no longer be held in solution is reached and crystals form. The concentration product at this point is called the *formation product* (K_f).

The solubility product and the formation product differentiate the three major states of saturation in urine: undersaturated, metastable, and unstable (Fig. 91.2). Below the solubility product, crystals will not form under any circumstances, and dissolution of crystals is theoretically possible. At concentrations above the formation product, the solution is unstable and crystals will form. In the metastable range between the solubility product and the formation product, in which the concentration products of most common

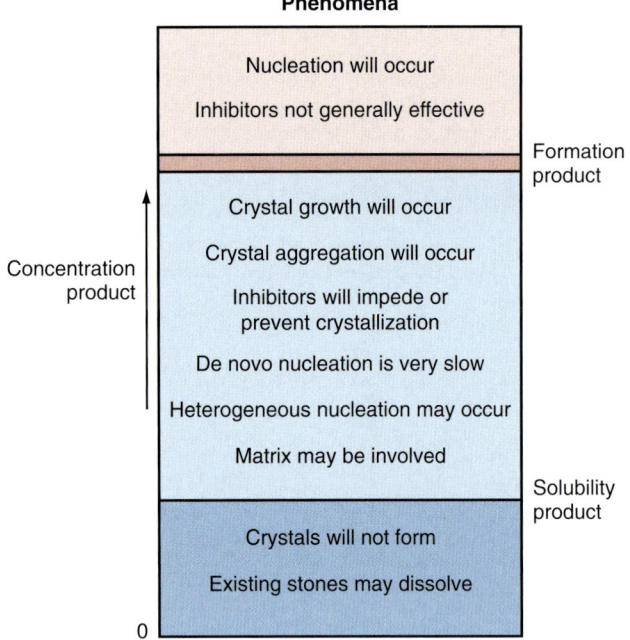

Fig. 91.2. States of saturation. Listed are solid-solution phenomena that are likely to occur at a given range of concentration products. Three general situations are considered: (1) concentrations less than the solubility product (undersaturation), (2) concentrations that are metastable with respect to de novo precipitation (between the solubility product and the formation product), and (3) concentrations that are greater than the formation product (unstable). (From Meyer JL: Physicochemistry of stone formation. In Resnick MI, Pak CYC, editors: *Urolithiasis: a medical and surgical reference*, Philadelphia, 1990, Saunders, pp 11–34.)

stone components reside, spontaneous nucleation or precipitation does not occur despite urine that is supersaturated. In this area modulation of factors controlling stone formation can take place and therapeutic intervention is directed.

In the metastable range of concentration products, although crystal growth can occur on existing crystals, de novo formation of crystals cannot occur in the length of time it normally takes for the filtered urine to reach the bladder. However, crystal formation can occur in this range under certain circumstances. First, in parts of the nephron local concentration products may exceed the formation product for long enough time periods to allow nucleation to occur. Second, local areas of obstruction or stasis in the upper urinary tract may prolong urinary transit time and allow crystal formation to occur in metastable urine. Finally, microscopic impurities or other constituents in the urine can facilitate the nucleation process by adsorption of the crystal components in a geometric way that resembles the native crystal. The energy required for this "heterogeneous nucleation" process is much less than that required for "homogeneous nucleation."

To estimate the state of saturation for any given crystal system such as calcium oxalate or calcium phosphate, Pak and Chu (1973) developed a mathematical formula, the *activity product ratio*, that takes into account urine pH and the ionic activities of all major ion species directly involved in the stone-forming process or those that affect the overall ionic strength of the urine. Finlayson subsequently developed a computer program, EQUIL 2, to measure the state of saturation, which is commonly used today (Werness et al., 1985). The *relative saturation ratio* (RSR) or *concentration product ratio* (CPR) is defined as the ratio of the concentration product of the urine to the solubility product of the specified stone-forming salt. A reduction in the numerator will lead to undersaturation of the urine with respect to the stone-forming salt and consequently reduce the likelihood of precipitation. Thus at RSR values less than 1, crystals will dissolve; at RSR values greater than 1, crystals will form and grow.

Reducing the RSR can be accomplished by reducing the urinary concentrations of the stone components (e.g., calcium or oxalate), by reducing the filtered load, or by increasing urinary reabsorption. In addition, complexation with substances such as citrate reduce available free ionic calcium and decrease the RSR. On the other hand, manipulation of factors such as pH can significantly affect the concentration of ions such as phosphate, the generation of which is highly pH dependent. Manipulation of pH has little effect on oxalate concentration, however, because oxalic acid is a strong acid (pK = 4), and pH changes within the physiologic range will have little effect on oxalate concentration.

Rodgers et al. (2006) introduced another computer program, JESS (Joint Expert Speciation System), to calculate urinary saturation of stone-forming salts as an estimate of the propensity for stone formation, thereby challenging the accuracy of the widely accepted EQUIL 2 computer program. The JESS program recognizes several soluble complexes not taken into account by EQUIL 2, including dicalcium-dihydrogen phosphate and calcium phosphocitrate, whose formation depends on pH and citrate. Consequently, the fraction of ionized calcium, phosphate, and oxalate estimated by JESS will be lower than that estimated by EQUIL 2. To resolve the discrepancy between the two programs, the supersaturation index (SI) according to JESS and the RSR according to EQUIL 2 were compared with experimentally determined urinary saturation of brushite (Pak et al., 2009b) and calcium oxalate (Pak et al., 2009a). The experimentally determined method measures the CPR without using computer-derived ionic activities. By determining the concentration product before and after incubation with a synthetic stone-forming salt, this method directly estimates saturation by measuring the extent of stone growth (in a supersaturated solution) or dissolution (in an undersaturated solution). No significant difference was found between experimentally determined CPR and JESS-derived SI, for either brushite or calcium oxalate. However, EQUIL 2–derived RSR was consistently and significantly higher than CPR and SI, overestimating CPR by about 80% for brushite and 50% for calcium oxalate. **Because CPR is too labor intensive for routine use, SI according to JESS probably provides a more reliable estimation of urinary saturation than RSR derived from EQUIL 2.**

Historically, urinary oxalate has been considered a more important contributor to calcium oxalate stone formation than urinary calcium, because a rise in urinary calcium concentration affected urinary saturation of calcium oxalate less than a rise in oxalate concentration (Nordin et al., 1972; Robertson and Peacock, 1980). Furthermore, at high urinary calcium concentrations the saturation of calcium oxalate reached a plateau that did not exceed the theoretic formation product of calcium oxalate, whereas high oxalate concentrations did, thereby increasing the risk of calcium oxalate crystal formation. Pak et al. (2004), however, challenged the notion that urinary oxalate exerts a greater pathogenetic effect than calcium in calcium oxalate stone formation. They demonstrated that the choice of stability constant used for calculating the RSR determines the relative effects of urinary calcium and oxalate concentration. Using the commonly accepted stability constant of 2.746×10^3 (used in the EQUIL 2 program), the effect of urinary calcium and oxalate proved to be equivalent. Thus they concluded that **urinary calcium and oxalate are important and equal contributors to calcium oxalate stone formation** (Fig. 91.3). As such, reduction in calcium and oxalate will be effective in reducing the RSR, and intervention to prevent stone formation can be directed at either. When these studies were repeated using JESS, the same finding of an equivalent effect of calcium and oxalate on urinary SI of calcium oxalate was found, although the dependence of SI on calcium and oxalate was less marked than was demonstrated for RSR (Pak et al., 2009a).

Nucleation and Crystal Growth, Aggregation, and Retention

In normal human urine, the concentration of calcium oxalate is four times higher than its solubility in water. Urinary factors favoring stone formation include low volume and citrate, whereas increased calcium, oxalate, phosphate, and uric acid increase calcium oxalate supersaturation. Once the concentration product of calcium oxalate

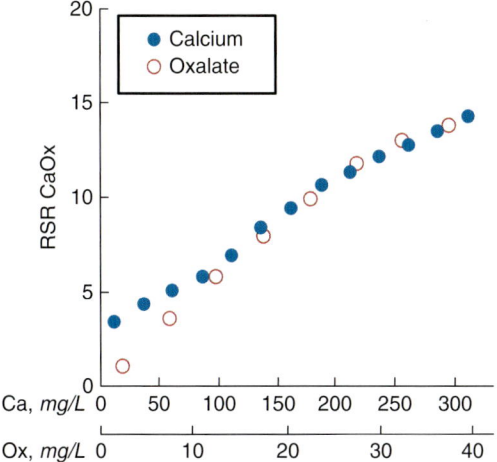

Fig. 91.3. Approximation of the actual relationship between relative saturation ratio (RSR) of calcium oxalate and calcium concentration by the actual relationship between RSR and oxalate concentration. Group mean RSRs of calcium oxalate for each 25 mg/L interval of calcium concentration from 667 patients are shown (●), and group mean RSRs for each 5 mg/L interval of oxalate are depicted (○). (From Pak CY, Adams-Huet B, Poindexter JR, et al.: Rapid communication: relative effect of urinary calcium and oxalate on saturation of calcium oxalate. *Kidney Int* 66:2032–2037, 2004.)

exceeds the solubility product, crystallization can potentially occur. However, in the presence of urinary inhibitors and other substances, calcium oxalate precipitation occurs only when supersaturation exceeds solubility by 7 to 11 times.

Homogeneous nucleation is the process by which nuclei form in pure solution. Nuclei are the earliest crystal structures that will not dissolve. Small nuclei are unstable; below a critical size threshold, dissolution of the crystal is favored over crystal growth. If the driving force (supersaturation level) and the stability of the nuclei are favorable and the lag time to nucleation is sufficiently short compared with the transit time of urine through the nephron, the nuclei will persist. Inhibitors, such as citrate, destabilize nuclei, whereas promoters stabilize nuclei by providing a surface with a binding site that accommodates the crystal structure of the nucleus. In urine, crystal nuclei usually form through heterogeneous nucleation by adsorption onto existing surfaces of epithelial cells (Umekawa et al., 2001), cell debris (Fasano and Khan, 2001), or other crystals (Kok, 1997).

Within the timeframe of transit of urine through the nephron, estimated at 5 to 7 minutes, crystals cannot grow to reach a size sufficient to occlude the tubular lumen. However, if enough nuclei form and grow, aggregation of the crystals will form larger particles within minutes that can occlude the tubular lumen. Inhibitors can prevent the process of crystal growth or aggregation. Magnesium and citrate inhibit crystal aggregation. Nephrocalcin, an acidic glycoprotein made in the kidney, inhibits calcium oxalate nucleation, growth, and aggregation (Asplin et al., 1991; Nakagawa et al., 1987). Tamm-Horsfall mucoprotein, the most abundant protein in urine, inhibits aggregation (Hess et al., 1991), and uropontin inhibits crystal growth (Shiraga et al., 1992). Bikunin, the light chain of inter-α-trypsin, has been shown to be an efficient inhibitor of crystal nucleation and aggregation.

Opposing views regarding the formation and growth of crystal particles have led to controversy over the concept of free crystal particle growth versus fixed particle growth. Although it was initially concluded that free particle stone formation, based solely on growth and aggregation of crystals and subsequent retention in the tubules, was impossible within the normal transit time through the nephron (Finlayson and Reid, 1978), later recalculation using current nephron dimensions, supersaturation, and crystal growth rates determined that crystalline particles can be formed that are large enough to be retained during normal transit time through the kidney (Kok and Khan, 1994). This theory is supported by histologic evidence of crystals occluding the intermedullary collecting ducts in select patients (Evan et al., 2003, 2005, 2006b, 2007, 2008).

Fixed particle growth theory presupposes an anchoring site to which crystals bind, thereby prolonging the time the crystals are exposed to supersaturated urine and facilitating crystal growth and aggregation. Randall (1937) first suspected the renal papilla was the anchoring site for stone formation after he observed subepithelial plaque on the renal papillae of 17% of 429 pairs of kidneys examined at autopsy. He implicated the basement membrane as the site of origin of the plaque and postulated subsequent erosion into the papillary luminal surface, thereby providing a nidus for stone formation. Low and Stoller (1997) found that papillary plaques occurred in 74% of stone formers compared with only 43% of control subjects undergoing endoscopy for conditions unrelated to stone disease.

Evan et al. (2003) validated and refined this theory for the pathogenesis of stone formation based on extensive analysis of papillary plaques derived from biopsies obtained during percutaneous nephrolithotomy in idiopathic calcium oxalate stone formers. **They localized the origin of the plaque to the basement membrane of the thin limbs of the loops of Henle and demonstrated that the plaque subsequently extends through the medullary interstitium to a subepithelial location** (Fig. 91.4). Once the plaque erodes through the urothelium, it is thought to constitute a stable, anchored surface on which calcium oxalate crystals can nucleate and grow as attached stones.

Using high-resolution Fourier transform infrared microspectroscopy and electron diffraction, the crystal component of plaque was determined to be calcium apatite (Evan et al., 2003). Daudon et al. (2007) analyzed more than 5000 stones associated with plaque and also found that carbapatite constituted the main component of the plaque in nearly all cases. Further analysis by Evan et al. (2005) revealed that the deposits consisted of individual laminated particles with mineral and organic layers. All crystals were coated with organic material, and osteopontin was identified on the outer surface of the crystal at the junction of the overlying organic molecular layer, potentially implicating osteopontin in plaque biology (Evan et al., 2005). The apatite crystals appear as spherical units, spherulites, that grow, aggregate, and fuse into larger particles. In the basement membrane, they are embedded in amorphous matrix and may be associated with membrane-bound vesicles. As they migrate into the interstitium, they propagate the mineralization front as they come in contact with collagen and cellular degradation products until they reach the subepithium of the renal papilla, comprising Randall plaque (Khan et al., 2012).

Another intriguing but unproven hypothesis for the origin of the calcium phosphate crystal involves calcifying nanoparticles (CNPs), also known as nanobacteria, which have been implicated in other types of pathologic calcifications such as atherosclerotic plaques (Shiekh et al., 2009). Ciftçioğlu et al. (2008) found an association between presence of CNPs and Randall plaques in kidneys removed for neoplasia. Although not necessarily causative, these findings suggest at least a loose association between CNPs and Randall plaque.

Because this process of calcium phosphate deposition in association with collagen has been observed in atherosclerotic lesions, some investigators have proposed a vascular origin for Randall plaque formation. Stoller et al. (2004) hypothesized that the inciting event in the pathogenesis of stone formation may be vascular injury to the vasa recta near the renal papilla. Repair of damaged vessel walls could involve an atherosclerotic-like reaction that results in calcification of the endothelial wall, followed by erosion into the papillary interstitium and then into the collecting ducts, where it could serve as a nidus for stone formation. Analogous to vascular smooth muscle, which has been shown to undergo transformation to an osteogenic phenotype in the presence of high concentrations of calcium and phosphate, renal tubular epithelial cells in rats have demonstrated a similar potential for osteogenic activity when exposed to high levels of oxalate or calcium oxalate and calcium phosphate crystals (Joshi et al., 2015). This process is thought to be mediated by nicotinamide adenine dinucleotide phosphate (NADPH) oxidase activation and the production of reactive oxygen species.

The pathogenesis of stone formation in other calcium stone formers and in noncalcium stone formers may differ from that of

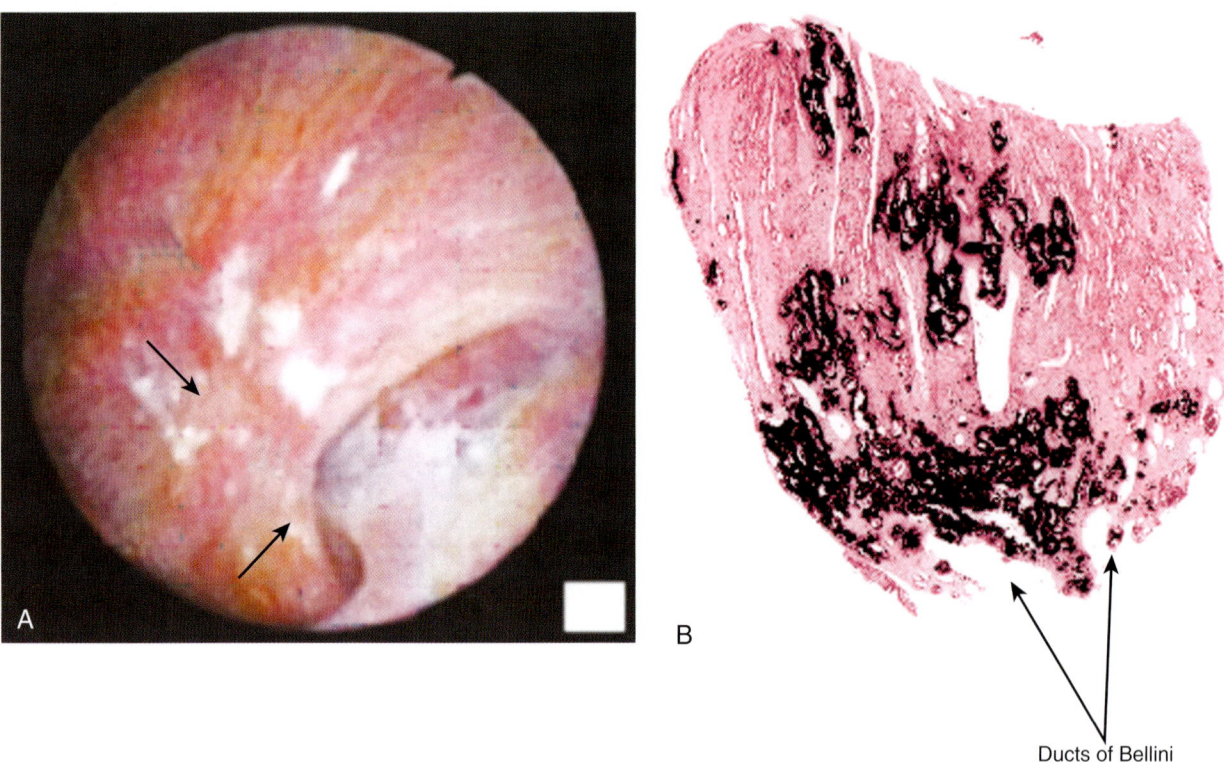

Fig. 91.4. Endoscopic (A) and histologic (B) images of Randall plaques in calcium oxalate patients. (A) Sites of Randall plaques *(arrows)* appear as irregular white areas beneath the urothelium. (B) A low-magnification light-microscopic image of a papillary biopsy specimen. Sites of calcium deposits were stained black by the Yasue metal substitution method for calcium histochemistry. (From Evan AP, Lingeman JE, Coe FL, et al.: Randall's plaque of patients with nephrolithiasis begins in basement membranes of thin loops of Henle. *J Clin Invest* 111:607–616, 2003.)

typical idiopathic calcium oxalate stone formers. Indeed, Randall plaques are not a universal finding in all types of stone formers. **Patients with enteric hyperoxaluria resulting from intestinal bypass for obesity demonstrate no plaque but instead show apatite crystal deposits plugging the inner medullary collecting duct lumens, along with associated epithelial cell damage with interstitial inflammation and fibrosis** (Fig. 91.5; Evan et al., 2003). **Brushite stone formers have been found to have pathology intermediate between idiopathic calcium oxalate stone formers and intestinal bypass patients, demonstrating interstitial apatite plaque *and* apatite plugging of the inner medullary and terminal collecting ducts, along with associated collecting duct injury and interstitial fibrosis** (Fig. 91.6; Evan et al., 2005). The pathogenesis of brushite stones has been postulated by Evan et al. (2005) to occur by way of crystallization of apatite in the collecting ducts, leading to collecting duct injury, cell death, and enlargement of collecting ducts. Interstitial inflammation in response to the injured cells may finally lead to progressive involvement of adjacent renal tissue. Krambeck et al. (2010) hypothesized that some brushite stones may start as calcium oxalate stones until an inciting insult such as infection or shockwave lithotripsy leads to tubular dysfunction, resulting in an alkaline environment, inflammation, and intraductal hyaluronic acid deposition, thereby prompting a transition from calcium oxalate to brushite stones. Ductal plugs have been observed in a number of other metabolic conditions that predispose to renal stone disease, including distal renal tubular acidosis (RTA) (Evan et al., 2007), primary and secondary hyperparathyroidism (Evan et al., 2008), and cystinuria (Evan et al., 2006b).

Historically, the pathogenesis of idiopathic calcium stone formation was thought to originate exclusively in papillary plaques. Evidence in support of this assumption came from the positive correlation between plaque surface area and the number of stones formed (Kim et al., 2005) as well as plaque surface area and 24-hour urine parameters (Kuo et al., 2003a, 2003b). In addition, mapping studies detailing sites of stone attachment on the renal papillae of calcium oxalate stone formers along with micro–computed tomographic analysis of the removed stones suggested that the stones originated on interstitial plaque (Matlaga et al., 2006; Miller et al., 2009, 2010). Thus the prevailing presumption was that the finding of plaques implied an idiopathic cause of calcium stone formation.

More recently, however, the distinction between stone formers with plaques versus those with ductal plugs has been less clear cut. Linnes et al. (2013) demonstrated that 99% of patients from a cohort of 78 patients undergoing consecutive endoscopic stone procedures had Randall plaques, including uric acid stone formers. Furthermore, they observed ductal plugging in 50% of uric acid stone formers. Conversely, ductal plugs were seen in up to 32% (severe in 11%) of the idiopathic calcium oxalate stone formers in the group (Linnes et al., 2013). Not only was tubular plugging more common than previously reported but also it too predictably correlated with urinary stone risk parameters. Furthermore, only 3.6% ± 4.2% of the papillary surface in idiopathic calcium oxalate stone formers, versus 7.4% as previously reported, comprised plaque (Kuo et al., 2003b), and no distinct correlation was found between urinary parameters and plaque coverage (Linnes et al., 2013). The discrepancy between the observations of Linnes et al. (2013) and those of the Indianapolis group may reflect the greater metabolic diversity of the idiopathic calcium oxalate group in Linnes' study, which was not restricted solely to hypercalciuria. In light of these important differences, the role of plaque versus plug in calcium oxalate stone formation may differ according to the underlying metabolic background, such as severe hypercalciuria. Nonetheless, available evidence suggests that the presence of ductal plugs should raise suspicion for a secondary cause of stone disease. Larger studies of demographically and metabolically heterogenous patients are needed to clarify roles of plaques and plugs in idiopathic and other causes of calcium stone formation.

Chapter 91 Urinary Lithiasis: Etiology, Epidemiology, and Pathogenesis **2013**

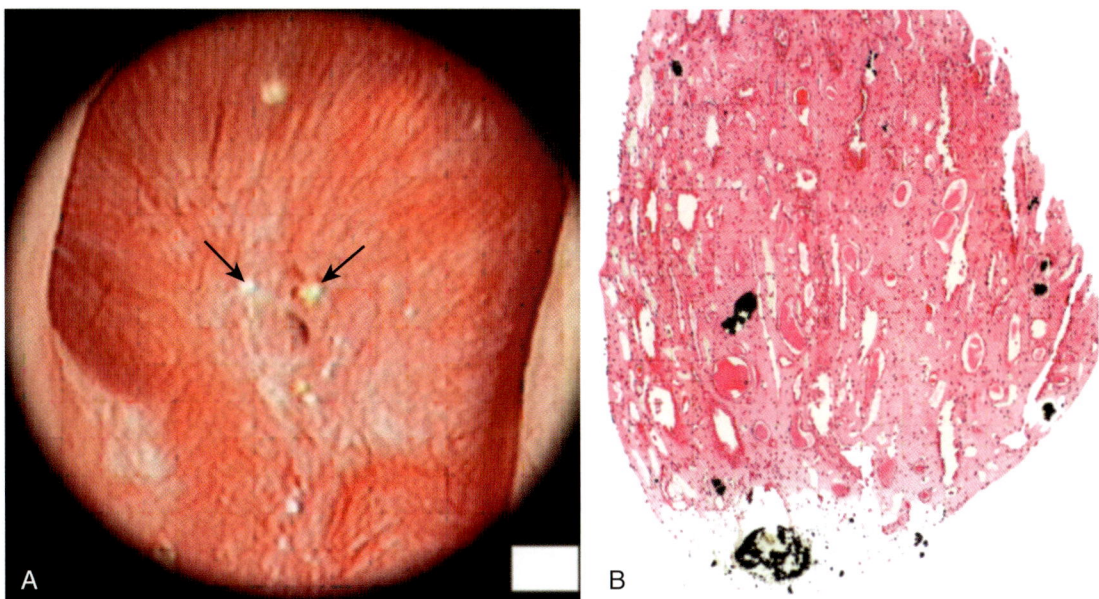

Fig. 91.5. Endoscopic (A) and histologic (B) images of Randall plaques in intestinal bypass patients. (A) Sites of Randall plaques *(arrows)* appear as irregular white areas beneath the urothelium. (B) A low-magnification light-microscopic image of a papillary biopsy specimen. Sites of calcium deposits were stained black by the Yasue metal substitution method for calcium histochemistry. (From Evan AP, Lingeman JE, Coe FL, et al.: Randall's plaque of patients with nephrolithiasis begins in basement membranes of thin loops of Henle. *J Clin Invest* 111:607–616, 2003.)

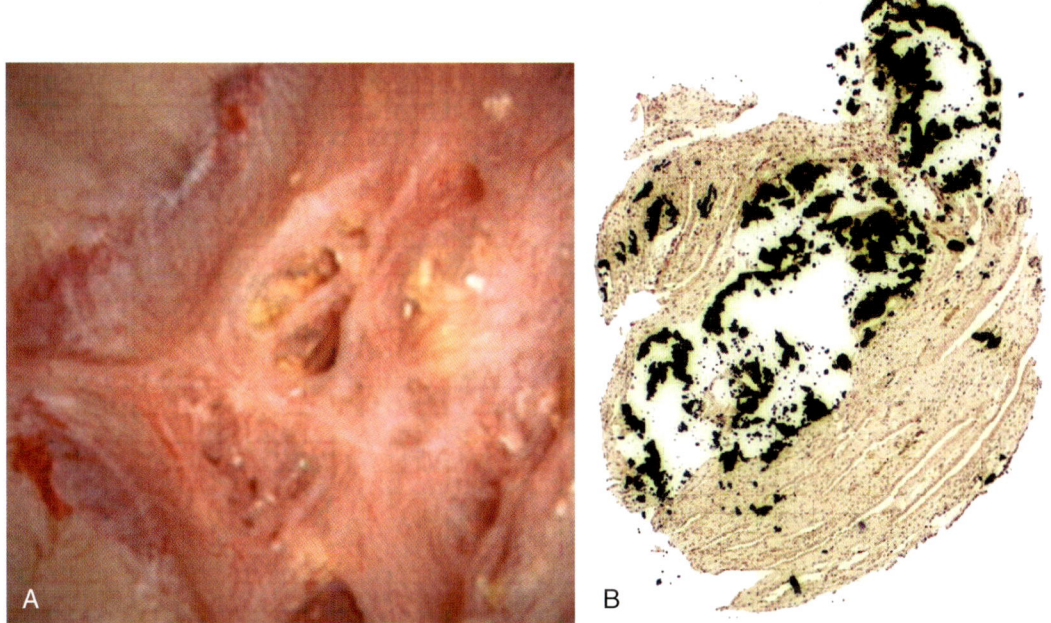

Fig. 91.6. Endoscopic (A) and histologic (B) images of Randall plaques in brushite patients. (A) Sites of Randall plaque appear as irregular white areas of crystalline deposit beneath the urothelium. In addition, a yellowish crystalline deposit is apparent at the opening of the ducts of Bellini. (B) A low-magnification light-microscopic image of a papillary biopsy specimen. Sites of calcium deposits were stained black by the Yasue metal substitution method for calcium histochemistry. A large amount of Yasue-positive material is seen in the ducts of Bellini. (From Evan AP, Lingeman JE, Coe FL, et al.: Crystal-associated nephropathy in patients with brushite nephrolithiasis. *Kidney Int* 67:576–591, 2005.)

Incorporating available clinical and experimental data, Khan et al. (2015) proposed a "unified" theory for the formation of plaques and plugs. They postulated that renal epithelial cells when subjected to oxidative stress induced by excessive urinary excretion of calcium, oxalate, and phosphate and/or decreased production of crystallization inhibitors, de-differentiate into osteoblast-like cells. As a result, calcium phosphate crystals, forming within membrane-bound vesicles, grow and propagate beyond the basement membrane. When the crystals make contact with collagen and membranous degradation products, they form a plaque that extends through the interstitium causing local inflammation and fibrosis further propagating the plaque. Finally, with the assistance of matrix metalloproteinases to breach the papillary surface epithelium, the plaque is exposed to urine in the renal pelvis, which facilitates stone growth. With regard to the formation of plugs in the collecting ducts, Khan et al. (2015) theorized that the plugs formed by supersaturated tubular fluid and pelvic urine slow movement of urine from the ducts to the renal pelvis, thereby promoting crystal formation and aggregation through retention.

Although tissue culture, experimental animal models, and clinical data have provided much insight into the pathophysiology of stone formation, it is likely that our knowledge of these processes will remain incomplete until we have a reliable animal model for stone formation.

Inhibitors and Promoters of Crystal Formation

At the concentrations at which most stone-forming salt components (including calcium, oxalate, and phosphate) are present in urine, urine is supersaturated, thereby favoring crystal formation. However, **the presence of molecules that raise the level of supersaturation needed to initiate crystal nucleation or reduce the rate of crystal growth or aggregation prevents stone formation from occurring on a routine basis.** Although inhibitors have been identified that prevent calcium oxalate and calcium phosphate crystallization, no specific inhibitors are known that affect uric acid crystallization. In addition, interference with the site of adhesion of crystals to the renal epithelium can prevent calculus retention and growth (Kumar et al., 2005).

Whole urine, when added to a solution of calcium phosphate, raises the supersaturation level required to initiate calcium phosphate crystallization (formation product) (Fleisch and Bisaz, 1962). Inorganic pyrophosphate was found to be responsible for 25% to 50% of the inhibitory activity of whole urine against calcium phosphate crystallization. Using different methodology, citrate, magnesium, and pyrophosphate together were noted to account for approximately 20% of the inhibitory activity of whole urine, with citrate as the most important factor (Bisaz et al., 1978).

Citrate acts as an inhibitor of calcium oxalate and calcium phosphate stone formation by a variety of actions. First, it complexes with calcium, thereby reducing the availability of ionic calcium to interact with oxalate or phosphate (Meyer and Smith, 1975; Pak et al., 1982). Second, it directly inhibits the spontaneous precipitation of calcium oxalate (Nicar et al., 1987) and prevents the agglomeration of calcium oxalate crystals (Kok et al., 1986). Although it has limited inhibitory effect on calcium oxalate crystal growth, it has potent activity in reducing calcium phosphate crystal growth (Meyer and Smith, 1975). Third, citrate prevents heterogeneous nucleation of calcium oxalate by monosodium urate (Pak and Peterson, 1986).

The inhibitory activity of magnesium is derived from its complexation with oxalate, which reduces ionic oxalate concentration and calcium oxalate supersaturation (Meyer and Smith, 1975). A recent study showed that magnesium reduced the contact time between calcium and oxalate molecules in vitro, an effect that showed synergism with citrate and was negated by the presence of uric acid (Riley et al., 2013). Grases et al. (2015) performed a turbidimetric assay in synthetic urine to determine the induction time and morphology of calcium oxalate crystal formation in the presence or absence of magnesium, citrate, and phytate. Their results confirmed the inhibitory effects of magnesium, citrate, and phytate and demonstrated the synergistic effects of magnesium and phytate. Pyrophosphate, phosphate, and magnesium have been shown to inhibit crystal growth, but only high concentrations of magnesium and pyrophosphate have been shown to inhibit aggregation (Kok et al., 1988).

Polyanion macromolecules, including glycosaminoglycans, acid mucopolysaccharides, and RNA, have been shown to inhibit crystal nucleation and growth by bonding with surface calcium ions. The most prominent glycosaminoglycan in human urine is chondroitin sulfate (Angell and Resnick, 1989). However, among the glycosaminoglycans, heparin sulfate interacts most strongly with calcium oxalate monohydrate crystals (Yamaguchi et al., 1993). Erturk et al. (2002) used a dye-binding assay to measure urinary glycosaminoglycan concentration and found a significantly lower concentration in stone formers than in controls. Furthermore, recurrent stone formers demonstrated lower levels of glycosaminoglycans than those who had experienced a single stone episode. Although these macromolecular proteins have been shown to inhibit stone aggregation, Reid et al. (2011) demonstrated through nuclear magnetic resonance spectroscopy that glycosaminoglycans and proteins are strongly integrated into the mineral lattice of apatite-predominant phosphate stones. Furthermore, they found that nonphosphate crystals such as calcium oxalate and uric acid did not exhibit composite lattices containing these proteins. These findings are consistent with plaque formation as apatitic foci that develop in a basement membrane environment rich in extracellular matrix proteins and glycosaminoglycans.

Two urinary glycoproteins, nephrocalcin and Tamm-Horsfall, are potent inhibitors of calcium oxalate monohydrate crystal aggregation (Nakagawa et al., 1987). Nephrocalcin is an acidic glycoprotein containing predominantly acidic amino acids that is synthesized in the proximal renal tubules and the thick ascending limb. In simple solution, nephrocalcin strongly inhibits the growth of calcium oxalate monohydrate crystals (Nakagawa et al., 1987), and it has been shown to inhibit nucleation and aggregation of calcium oxalate crystals (Coe et al., 1994). Nephrocalcin has been identified in four isoforms: non–stone formers excrete greater quantities of two isoforms associated with the most inhibitory activity, whereas stone formers excrete urine enriched for the two isoforms lacking inhibitory activity (Nakagawa, 1997). The isoforms with inhibitory activity were found to contain γ-carboxyglutamic acid residues that were lacking in the isoforms isolated from stone formers.

Tamm-Horsfall protein, also known as uromodulin, is expressed by renal epithelial cells in the thick ascending limb and the distal convoluted tubule as a membrane-anchored protein that is released into the urine after cleavage of the anchoring site by phospholipases or proteases. **Tamm-Horsfall is the most abundant protein found in the urine and a potent inhibitor of calcium oxalate monohydrate crystal aggregation, but not growth.** The role of Tamm-Horsfall protein in stone formation is controversial and may depend on the state of the molecule, which determines whether it functions as an inhibitor or a promoter of crystal formation. In alkaline urine it is a strong inhibitor of calcium oxalate monohydrate crystal aggregation, whereas in acidic urine it polymerizes into a configuration that promotes crystal aggregation (Hess, 1992). There are several studies that support the involvement of uromodulin in the regulation of renal tubular calcium reabsorption, including a genome-wide association study (GWAS) that found that a specific uromodulin allele was protective against calcium-containing kidney stones (Gudbjartsson et al., 2010).

A study using a Tamm-Horsfall knockout *(Thp–/–)* mouse model demonstrated spontaneous formation of calcium oxalate crystals in the kidneys of mice fed ethylene glycol and vitamin D, suggesting a protective role of Tamm-Horsfall protein against crystallization of calcium salts (Mo et al., 2004). A subsequent study on more than 250 Tamm-Horsfall protein–null mice demonstrated a consistent phenotype of progressive renal calcification that consisted of hydroxyapatite in the interstitial space of renal papillae resembling the plaques seen in idiopathic calcium oxalate stone formers (Liu et al., 2010). More recent studies have suggested that uromodulin may also regulate TRPV5 and TRPV6, which are channels critical for renal transcellular Ca^{2+} reabsorption (Wolf et al., 2013). Osteopontin, or uropontin, is an acidic phosphorylated glycoprotein expressed in bone matrix and renal epithelial cells of the ascending limb of the loop of Henle and the distal tubule. **Osteopontin has been shown to inhibit nucleation, growth, and aggregation of calcium oxalate crystals, as well as to reduce binding of crystals to renal epithelial cells in vitro** (Asplin et al., 1998; Wesson et al., 1998). In an osteopontin knockout mouse model, intratubular calcium oxalate crystals could be induced in mice exposed to high levels of oxalate by ethylene glycol feeding (Wesson et al., 2003). Interestingly, in a *Thp–/–* mouse model, mice fed ethylene glycol and vitamin D exhibited a dramatic increase in osteopontin levels over baseline but still formed calcium oxalate crystals (Mo et al., 2004). The authors concluded that osteopontin may constitute an inducible inhibitor of calcium oxalate crystallization that works in conjunction with constitutively expressed Tamm-Horsfall protein to prevent crystallization.

Urinary prothrombin fragment 1 (F1) is a crystal matrix protein named for its resemblance to the F1 degradation product of prothrombin. Ryall et al. (1995) purified urinary prothrombin F1 from human urine and used an artificial crystallization system to determine that it was associated with a reduction in crystal aggregation and deposition.

Matrix GLA protein (MGP) is a vitamin K–dependent protein that functions primarily as an inhibitor of vascular calcifications (Khan et al., 2013). MGP gene polymorphism is associated with vascular calcification and myocardial infarction (Herrmann et al., 2000). A single nucleotide polymorphism (SNP) has been shown to be associated with calcium oxalate kidney stone disease in Japanese and Chinese patients (Lu et al., 2012).

Lastly, inter-α-trypsin is a glycoprotein synthesized in the liver that is composed of three polypeptides (two heavy chains and one light chain), of which bikunin makes up the light chain. Bikunin is a strong inhibitor of calcium oxalate crystallization, aggregation, and growth in vitro (Atmani and Khan, 1999; Hochstrasser et al., 1984), and its expression has been shown to be upregulated in a rat model when exposed to oxalate.

Matrix

Renal calculi consist of crystalline and noncrystalline components. The noncrystalline component is termed *matrix*, which typically accounts for about 2.5% of the weight of the stone (Boyce and Garvey, 1956). In some cases, matrix comprises the majority of the stone (up to 65%), usually in association with chronic urinary tract infection (Allen and Spence, 1966; Boyce and Garvey, 1956). The exact composition of matrix is difficult to ascertain because only 25% of it is soluble (Ryall, 1993); however, chemical analysis reveals a heterogeneous mixture consisting of approximately 65% protein, 9% nonamino sugars, 5% glucosamine, 10% bound water, and 12% organic ash (Boyce, 1968). Among the proteins incorporated into the matrix substance are Tamm-Horsfall protein, nephrocalcin, a γ-carboxyglutamic acid–rich protein, renal lithostathine, albumin, glycosaminoglycans, free carbohydrates, and a mucoprotein called matrix substance A (Hess and Kok, 1996). Boyce et al. (1962) found that substance A is immunologically unique and present in the matrix component of all stone formers. Moore and Gowland (1975) determined that substance A is composed of three or four distinct antigens unique to stones that were detected in the urine of 85% of stone formers but in no normal individuals. A study using reverse-phase, high-performance liquid chromatography and tandem mass spectrometry to evaluate calcium oxalate stones identified 68 distinct proteins with 95% confidence, including a significant number of inflammatory proteins (immunoglobulins, defensin-3, clusterin, complement C3a, kininogen, and fibrinogen) (Canales et al., 2008). Comparing the matrix component of 13 calcium oxalate and 12 calcium phosphate stones, these investigators found that inflammatory proteins were the predominant proteins in both stone types, with many proteins in common, suggesting a shared pathogenesis for the two stone types that involves inflammation (Canales et al., 2010).

Okumura et al. (2013) analyzed calcium oxalate stones from 9 patients and found highly heterogeneous electrophoretic mobilities of certain matrix proteins for which they subsequently performed solution protease digestion and proteomic analysis that identified 92 proteins. All stones had some osteopontin, prothrombin F1 fragments, and THP among other proteins, but their amounts were highly variable among individual stones. Furthermore, some stones had leukocyte-derived proteins such as myeloperoxidase and lactotransferrin. Although the exact role of matrix in stone formation, whether as promoter, inhibitor, or passive bystander, has yet to be elucidated, the variability in type and proportion of protein species in this study supports a diverse etiology, likely influenced by heredity, and provides a target for future research.

KEY POINTS: PHYSICOCHEMISTRY AND PATHOGENESIS

- Urine must be supersaturated for stones to form.
- Supersaturation alone is not sufficient for crystallization to occur in urine because of the presence of urinary inhibitors.
- Nephrocalcin, uropontin, and Tamm-Horsfall protein are important inhibitors of crystal nucleation, growth, or aggregation.
- Urinary calcium and oxalate contribute equally to urinary saturation of calcium oxalate.
- Common calcium stones may originate from subepithelial plaques composed of calcium apatite that serve as an anchor on which calcium oxalate stones can grow.
- The noncrystalline component of stones is matrix, which is composed of a combination of mucoproteins, proteins, carbohydrates, and urinary inhibitors.

MINERAL METABOLISM

Calcium

Between 30% and 40% of dietary calcium is absorbed from the intestine, with most being absorbed in the small intestine and only approximately 10% absorbed in the colon (Bronner and Pansu, 1999). By a process of intestinal adaptation, absorption of calcium varies with calcium intake. At times of low calcium intake, fractional calcium absorption is enhanced; during high calcium intake, fractional calcium absorption is reduced. With a calcium-rich diet, a nonsaturable, paracellular pathway for calcium absorption predominates. A saturable, vitamin D–dependent transcellular pathway constitutes the major pathway for intestinal calcium absorption when calcium intake is limited; this pathway is downregulated by a diet replete in calcium (Bronner et al., 1986; Buckley and Bronner, 1980). Because of the saturable component of calcium transport, a larger portion of calcium is absorbed when it is divided into several doses taken hours apart than with a large single dose (Phang et al., 1968). A small amount of calcium is secreted into the lumen of the intestine, thereby reducing net calcium absorption such that, overall, 100 to 300 mg of a total average calcium intake of 600 to 1200 mg daily will be absorbed.

Calcium is absorbed in the ionic state, and incomplete calcium absorption is due in part to formation of soluble calcium complexes in the intestinal lumen. **Therefore substances that complex with calcium, such as phosphate, citrate, oxalate, sulfate, and fatty acids, reduce the availability of ionic calcium for absorption** (Allen, 1982). Calcium readily complexes with phosphate in the intestinal lumen, but because calcium phosphate formation is dependent on pH (pK = 6.1), high luminal pH favors calcium phosphate complexation, thereby reducing calcium availability. On the other hand, calcium oxalate complex formation displays less pH dependence and complex formation is less reversible. Consequently, an oxalate-rich diet reduces calcium absorption. Transcellular calcium absorption is mediated by 1,25(OH)$_2$D$_3$ (calcitriol), which is reported to enhance calcium permeability at the brush border of the intestinal epithelial cells (Fontaine et al., 1981).

The active form of vitamin D, 1,25(OH)$_2$D$_3$, is the most potent stimulator of intestinal calcium absorption. After conversion of 7-dehydrocholesterol in the skin to previtamin D$_3$ promoted by sunlight, previtamin D$_3$ is hydroxylated in the liver to 25-hydroxyvitamin D$_3$, which is further hydroxylated in the proximal renal tubule to 1,25(OH)$_2$D$_3$. The conversion of 25-hydroxyvitamin D$_3$ to 1,25(OH)$_2$D$_3$ is stimulated by parathyroid hormone (PTH) and by hypophosphatemia. **A decrease in serum calcium increases secretion of PTH, which in turn directly stimulates the enzyme 1α-hydroxylase, which is located in the mitochondria of the proximal renal tubule.** After transport via the bloodstream to the intestine, 1,25(OH)$_2$D$_3$ binds to the vitamin D receptor in the brush border membrane epithelial cells to enhance calcium absorption.

Calcitriol acts on the bone and kidney in addition to its action in increasing intestinal calcium absorption. In the bone, 1,25(OH)$_2$D$_3$, along with PTH, promotes the recruitment and differentiation of osteoclasts that subsequently mobilize calcium from the bone. Consequently, the filtered load of calcium and phosphate increases. However, PTH increases renal calcium reabsorption and enhances phosphate excretion, leading to a further net increase in serum calcium, which suppresses further PTH secretion and synthesis of 1,25(OH)$_2$D$_3$. Calcitriol modulates parathyroid function by inhibiting synthesis of PTH through enhanced vitamin D receptor and calcium-sensing receptor (CaSR) expression in the parathyroid glands (Dusso et al., 2005).

PTH is critical in maintaining normal calcium concentration in the extracellular fluid. PTH is an 84–amino acid protein that is the cleavage product of the precursor protein prepro-PTH. **Only mature PTH is secreted from the parathyroid gland, and the most potent stimulus for its secretion is a decrease in serum calcium** (Sherwood et al., 1968). In response to serum calcium levels, the G-protein–coupled extracellular CaSR regulates PTH secretion and renal tubular calcium reabsorption (Devuyst and Pirson, 2007). PTH stimulates mobilization of calcium from bone through the action of osteoclasts, further raising serum calcium and phosphorus. The action of PTH is mediated through changes in cyclic adenosine monophosphate and phospholipase C (Dunlay and Hruska, 1990; Muff et al., 1992). **At the kidney, PTH enhances renal calcium reabsorption and reduces renal tubular reabsorption of phosphate.** It also stimulates synthesis of 1,25(OH)$_2$D$_3$, which leads to enhanced intestinal calcium and phosphate absorption. PTH has no direct effect on intestinal calcium absorption.

Calcium absorption in the kidney is complex, but recent work has begun to elucidate the proteins and mechanisms involved. On average, only 1% to 3% of filtered calcium is excreted in the urine, with most being reabsorbed paracellularly in the renal proximal tubule (60% to 65%) and thick ascending limb of the loop of Henle (25% to 30%). The remaining 8% to 10% of filtered calcium is reabsorbed transcellularly in the distal convoluted tubule (Friedman, 2007).

The paracellular absorption of calcium in the proximal tubule and thick ascending limb of the loop of Henle occurs by several mechanisms. First, calcium travels through paracellular channels found at the tight junctions of epithelial cells in the proximal tubule. The integral membrane proteins of the tight junction include occludin, junctional adhesion molecules, and claudins (Ebnet et al., 2004; Furuse et al., 1993; Hou, 2013). Claudins are a family of proteins with four transmembrane domains (Hou, 2013; Lal-Nag and Morin, 2009), including claudin-2, which has been implicated in paracellular reabsorption of calcium and other cations in the proximal tubule (Muto et al., 2010), and claudin-16 and claudin-19, which form a paracellular channel complex that allows selective cation permeation in the thick ascending limb (Hou et al., 2008, 2009).

Calcium is passively reabsorbed from the lumen of the thick ascending limb of the loop of Henle into the interstitial space through a paracellular pathway driven by a lumen-positive transepithelial voltage gradient (Hou, 2013). The positive luminal voltage occurs as a result of apical potassium secretion and basolateral chloride secretion, as well as by way of a transepithelial NaCl concentration gradient over the cation-selective paracellular channel in the thick ascending limb.

The CaSR plays a role in renal handling of calcium, and its expression predominates in the thick ascending limb. Serum calcium stimulates the CaSR to increase expression of claudin-14, which blocks the calcium channels formed by the claudin-16/19 complex, thereby reducing paracellular calcium reabsorption (Gong et al., 2012; Toka et al., 2012).

Transcellular calcium absorption in the distal convoluted tubule occurs via several mechanisms (Mensenkamp et al., 2006, 2007). Calcium enters the epithelial cells of the distal tubule through a transcellular channel (transient receptor potential vanilloid 5, or TRPV5), which is unique among other channels in the TRP family because of its high calcium selectivity. Calcium flux through TRPV5 into the distal tubule cells is controlled at several levels, including TRPV5 gene expression, feedback inhibition, and trafficking across the plasma membrane. Inactivation of TRPV5 in mice leads to severe hypercalciuria, which is compensated for by increased intestinal calcium absorption resulting from enhanced calcitriol synthesis. Calcium is bound in the cell to a chaperone protein (calbindin-D28k), which facilitates diffusion across the cell from the apical to the basolateral space where calcium can then exit.

Phosphorus

Like calcium, inorganic phosphate absorption is dependent on saturable transcellular and nonsaturable paracellular transport. At low phosphorus concentrations (1 to 3 mmol/L), saturable absorptive transport occurs. At higher phosphorus levels, absorption increases without saturation (Walton and Gray, 1979). Approximately 60% of dietary phosphate is absorbed in the intestine. Active absorption of phosphate from the intestine involves a 1,25(OH)$_2$D$_3$-regulated, sodium-dependent transport process (Danisi and Straub, 1980; Lee et al., 1986). Phosphate absorption is highly pH dependent; low luminal pH reduces while high pH enhances phosphate transport.

Approximately 65% of absorbed phosphate is excreted by the kidney and the remainder by the intestine. In normal healthy adults, 80% to 90% of the filtered load of phosphate is reabsorbed in the renal tubule and 10% to 20% is excreted in the urine. **Regulation of renal phosphate handling is primarily by way of PTH, which inhibits renal tubular reabsorption of filtered phosphate.**

Magnesium

Magnesium is absorbed from the intestine by passive diffusion or active transport, although passive diffusion accounts for most of the net magnesium absorption. Magnesium is absorbed in the large and small intestine, with the majority absorbed from the distal small intestine. Hormonal regulation of magnesium is primarily through vitamin D.

Oxalate

Oxalate metabolism differs markedly from calcium metabolism. Although 30% to 40% of ingested calcium is absorbed from the intestine, only 6% to 14% of ingested oxalate is absorbed (Hesse et al., 1999; Holmes et al., 1995). Oxalate absorption occurs throughout the intestinal tract, with about half or more occurring in the small intestine and half in the colon (Holmes et al., 1995). Although oxalate absorption is difficult to measure directly, it has historically been estimated by urinary oxalate excretion, a relationship that is valid only if there is a linear relationship between ingested and excreted oxalate and if absorbed oxalate is not significantly taken up in the tissues, metabolized, or secreted back into the intestine. Holmes et al. (2001) in fact demonstrated that the relationship between ingested oxalate and absorbed oxalate is curvilinear because of higher absorption of oxalate at low intake than at high intake. Moreover, they showed that oxalate absorption varies widely among individuals, ranging from 10% to 72% of ingested oxalate. A recent study suggested that hyperoxaluric stone formers absorb more oxalate in response to an oral oxalate load than stone formers with normal oxalate excretion (Krishnamurthy et al., 2003). Knight et al. (2007), however, found no difference between normal subjects and stone formers in intestinal absorption or renal handling of oxalate. In patients with small bowel disease or history of intestinal resection and an intact colon, oxalate absorption is markedly increased (Barilla et al., 1978).

Oxalate transport occurs via transcellular and paracellular pathways. Although transport by way of paracellular pathways and some nonmediated transcellular pathways is primarily passive, driven by electrochemical or concentration gradients, transcellular transport is largely actively mediated by membrane carriers. The transport protein responsible for oxalate secretion has been suspected to belong to the SLC26 family of solute-linked carrier (SLC) anion exchangers. A putative anion exchange transporter, SLC26A6, which is expressed in the apical membrane of small intestinal and perhaps colonic epithelial cells, has been implicated in intestinal oxalate transport

(Hatch and Freel, 2005). Evidence suggests that oxalate may be secreted, as well as absorbed, in the intestine (Jiang et al., 2006). In vitro flux studies using intestinal segments of mutant mice lacking SLC26A6 showed enhanced net absorption of oxalate as a result of defective oxalate secretion. Furthermore, in vivo *Slc26a6*-null mice were found to have elevated plasma and urinary oxalate levels, reduced fecal oxalate excretion, and a high incidence of calcium oxalate bladder stones compared with wild-type mice. These findings provide compelling evidence for a possible role of SLC26A6 in oxalate secretion and suggest a potential target for therapeutic agents that modify urinary oxalate absorption.

A number of other factors can influence oxalate absorption, including the presence of oxalate-binding cations such as calcium or magnesium and oxalate-degrading bacteria. Coingestion of calcium- and oxalate-containing foods leads to formation of calcium oxalate complexes, which limits the availability of free oxalate ion for absorption (Hess et al., 1998; Liebman and Chai, 1997; Penniston and Nakada, 2009). Oxalate-degrading bacteria, notably *Oxalobacter formigenes*, use oxalate as an energy source and consequently reduce intestinal oxalate absorption. The mechanism of action of *O. formigenes* in reducing urinary oxalate excretion may not be entirely accounted for by degradation of intestinal oxalate. In vivo and ex vivo studies in *O. formigenes*–colonized rats demonstrated reduced urinary oxalate excretion and net colonic oxalate secretion, suggesting that *O. formigenes* may interact directly with intestinal mucosal cells to stimulate secretion of endogenously derived oxalate (Hatch et al., 2006).

The potential for therapeutic use of probiotics or oxalate-degrading enzyme preparations has been explored in mice models and in several short-term clinical trials. In two knockout mice models, one of which resembles primary hyperoxaluria, administration of an oxalate-degrading enzyme reduced urinary oxalate and prevented nephrocalcinosis (Grujic et al., 2009). Likewise, in a small study of patients with primary hyperoxaluria and normal renal function or varying degrees of renal failure, administration of *O. formigenes* was associated with a reduction in serum and/or urinary oxalate (Hoppe et al., 2006). However, a subsequent randomized trial in 43 patients with primary hyperoxaluria administered oral *O. formigenes* versus placebo failed to show a treatment effect in reducing urinary oxalate (Hoppe et al., 2011). Similarly, although one uncontrolled study (Campieri et al., 2001) of calcium oxalate stone formers with mild hyperoxaluria showed a 24% to 40% reduction in urinary oxalate with the administration of a preparation of mixed lactic acid bacterium species, a randomized, controlled trial (Goldfarb et al., 2007) failed to demonstrate an effect of the same probiotic. At this time, the contribution of *O. formigenes* to the overall risk of stone formation is not fully understood, and although *O. formigenes* is the most potent oxalate-degrading bacterium, other bacterial species have demonstrated oxalate-degrading activity in vitro (Klimesova et al., 2014; Magwira et al., 2012).

Absorbed oxalate is nearly completely excreted in the urine (Hodgkinson and Wilkinson, 1974; Prenan et al., 1982). Urinary oxalate is derived from endogenous production in the liver (from ascorbic acid and glycine) and dietary sources. **Evidence suggests that, on average, half of urinary oxalate is derived from the diet, with the precise amount depending on the relative amount of ingested calcium and oxalate** (Holmes et al., 2001).

It is estimated that between 86% and 98% of oxalate is ultrafilterable. However, renal tubular handling of oxalate has not been clearly defined, although secretion and reabsorption have been suspected. There is evidence from a number of animal models of a secretory pathway for oxalate that likely resides in the renal proximal tubule (Holmes and Assimos, 2004). The SLC26 transport proteins responsible for oxalate secretion include one implicated in intestinal oxalate secretion, SLC26A6. However, no specific transporter has been definitively linked to renal oxalate secretion, and a recent study in a rat model investigating the role of a likely candidate, the basolateral anion exchanger sulfate anion transporter-1 (SAT1, or SLC26A1), found no correlation between changes in renal expression of SAT1 messenger RNA or protein and hyperoxaluria (Freel and Hatch, 2012).

Clinical evidence also supports renal oxalate secretion, although it is not clear if renal handling of oxalate differs between stone formers and non–stone formers (Holmes et al., 2005; Knight et al., 2007; Schwille et al., 1989). Holmes et al. (2005) studied six normal subjects administered increasing oral oxalate loads and found oxalate clearance ratios consistent with renal oxalate secretion, with up to 50% of urinary oxalate accounted for by oxalate secretion at the highest oxalate load. These investigators subsequently compared plasma and urine oxalate levels in idiopathic hypercalciuric stone formers versus normal subjects while fasting and after consuming three low-oxalate meals (Bergsland et al,. 2011). Despite no difference in plasma oxalate between the two groups in either the fasting or fed states, urinary oxalate and fractional excretion was higher in patients than normal subjects. Fractional excretion of oxalate exceeded 1, indicating oxalate secretion, in almost a third of patients and no controls, suggesting that renal oxalate secretion may play a role in regulating plasma oxalate levels.

> **KEY POINTS: MINERAL METABOLISM**
>
> - Calcium absorption occurs primarily in the small intestine at a rate that is dependent on calcium intake.
> - 1,25-Dihydroxyvitamin D_3 is the most potent stimulator of intestinal calcium absorption.
> - PTH stimulates 1α-hydroxylase in the proximal tubule of the kidney to convert 25-hydroxyvitamin D_3 to 1,25$(OH)_2D_3$.
> - PTH enhances proximal tubular reabsorption of calcium and renal phosphate excretion.
> - Intestinal oxalate absorption is influenced by luminal calcium, magnesium, and oxalate-degrading bacteria.

PATHOPHYSIOLOGY OF UPPER URINARY TRACT CALCULI

Classification of Nephrolithiasis

The most common component of urinary calculi is calcium, which is a major constituent of nearly 80% of stones. Calcium oxalate makes up about 60% of all stones, mixed calcium oxalate and hydroxyapatite 20%, and brushite stones 2%. Uric acid and struvite (magnesium ammonium phosphate) each account for approximately 7% of stones, and cystine stones represent only about 1% (Table 91.1; Wilson, 1989). Stones associated with medications and their byproducts, such as triamterene, silica, indinavir, and ephedrine, are uncommon and usually preventable.

TABLE 91.1 Stone Composition and Relative Occurrence

STONE COMPOSITION	OCCURRENCE (%)
CALCIUM-CONTAINING STONES	
Calcium oxalate	60
Hydroxyapatite	20
Brushite	2
NON–CALCIUM-CONTAINING STONES	
Uric acid	7
Struvite	7
Cystine	1–3
Triamterene	<1
Silica	<1
2,8-Dihydroxyadenine	<1

From Pearle MS, Pak YC: Renal calculi: a practical approach to medical evaluation and management. In Andreucci VE, Fine LG, editors: *International yearbook of nephrology*, New York, 1996, Oxford University Press, pp 69–80.

TABLE 91.2 Diagnostic Classification of Nephrolithiasis

CONDITION	METABOLIC/ENVIRONMENTAL DEFECT	PREVALENCE (%)
Absorptive hypercalciuria	Increased gastrointestinal calcium absorption	20–40
Renal phosphate leak	Impaired renal phosphorus absorption	
Renal hypercalciuria	Impaired renal calcium reabsorption	5–8
Resorptive hypercalciuria	Primary hyperparathyroidism	3–5
Hyperuricosuric calcium nephrolithiasis	Dietary purine excess, uric acid overproduction	10–40
Hypocitraturic calcium nephrolithiasis		10–50
Isolated	Idiopathic	
Chronic diarrheal syndrome	Gastrointestinal alkali loss	
Distal renal tubular acidosis	Impaired renal acid excretion	
Thiazide-induced	Hypokalemia	
Hyperoxaluric calcium nephrolithiasis		2–15
Primary hyperoxaluria	Oxalate overproduction	
Dietary hyperoxaluria	Increased dietary oxalate	
Enteric hyperoxaluria	Increased intestinal oxalate absorption	
Hypomagnesiuric calcium nephrolithiasis	Decreased intestinal magnesium absorption	5–10
Idiopathic low urine pH	Low urinary pH	15–30
Cystinuria	Impaired renal cystine reabsorption	<1
Infection stones	Infection with urease-producing bacteria	1–5
Low urine volume	Inadequate fluid intake	10–50
Miscellaneous or no abnormality	NA	<3

Modified from Pearle MS, Pak CY: Renal calculi: a practical approach to medical evaluation and management. In Andreucci VE, Fine LG, editors: *International yearbook of nephrology*, New York, 1996, Oxford University Press, pp 69–80.

Most classification systems for nephrolithiasis differentiate stones on the basis of the underlying metabolic or environmental abnormalities with which they are associated (Table 91.2). A number of pathophysiologic derangements contribute to calcium stone formation, either alone or in combination, including hypercalciuria, hypocitraturia, hyperuricosuria, and hyperoxaluria (Coe et al., 2005). Uric acid, cystine, and struvite stones form in relatively unique settings; uric acid stones form only in an acid urine, cystine stones are the result of impaired renal reabsorption of cystine, and infection stones occur in alkaline urine produced by urease-producing bacteria. For some stones such as cystine, knowledge of the chemical composition of the stone may provide sufficient information to initiate appropriate therapy. However, because of the multiple causes associated with calcium-based stones, an understanding of the underlying metabolic disorders and environmental factors that predispose to stone formation is required to implement a rational treatment plan. Recent investigation into the molecular and genetic causes of stone formation may ultimately translate into newer treatment strategies (Devuyst and Pirson, 2007; Frick and Bushinsky, 2003; Langman, 2004).

Calcium Stones

Hypercalciuria

Hypercalciuria is the most common abnormality identified in calcium stone formers (Bushinsky, 1998; Coe et al., 1992; Pak et al., 1982). However, the role of hypercalciuria in stone formation is controversial because of the overlap in urine calcium levels between stone formers and non–stone formers (Coe et al., 1992; Robertson and Morgan, 1972). Several lines of evidence support a pathogenetic role for hypercalciuria in stone formation. First, hypercalciuria is common in stone-forming patients, occurring in 35% to 65% of patients (Levy et al., 1995). Indeed, treatment strategies aimed at reducing urinary calcium levels are associated with a reduction in stone recurrence rates (Pearle et al., 1999), and medical therapy often fails in patients with persistent hypercalciuria (Strauss et al., 1982). In addition, multivariate analysis of a subset of men and women from three large epidemiologic studies in whom 24-hour urine studies were available revealed that, after adjusting for other factors, the risk of incident stone formation increased with increasing urinary calcium (Curhan et al., 2001). Lastly, recent investigations of Randall plaques as potential precursors to calcium stone formation have shown that plaques occur more commonly in stone formers and their number directly correlates with urine calcium levels and number of stone episodes (Kim et al., 2005; Kuo et al., 2003b).

High urinary calcium concentrations lead to increased urinary saturation of calcium salts (Pak and Holt, 1976) and reduced urinary inhibitory activity by way of complexation with negatively charged inhibitors such as citrate and chondroitin sulfate (Zerwekh et al., 1988). The normal kidney filters approximately 270 mmol of calcium daily and reabsorbs all but 4 mmol (Bushinsky, 1998). However, a variety of conditions lead to elevated urinary calcium levels and increased urinary saturation of calcium salts. Criteria defining hypercalciuria are variable, but **the strictest definition classifies hypercalciuria as greater than 200 mg of urinary calcium/day after adherence to a 400-mg calcium, 100-mg sodium diet for 1 week** (Menon, 1986). **Parks and Coe (1986) defined hypercalciuria as excretion of greater than 4 mg/kg/day or greater than 7 mmol/day in men and 6 mmol/day in women.** However, arguably a threshold level of calcium that separates hypercalciuria from normocalciuria is artificial, as urinary calcium demonstrates a spectrum of effects over its range by which higher or lower calcium levels are associated with a greater or lesser effect.

Historically, the term *idiopathic hypercalciuria* was applied to stone formers for whom classification of their metabolic abnormality was difficult. Calcium transport is regulated at three sites: intestine, bone, and kidney. Dysregulation at any of these sites can lead to hypercalciuria. In 1974 Pak et al. divided hypercalciuria into three distinct subtypes on the basis of unique pathophysiologic abnormalities: absorptive hypercalciuria resulting from increased intestinal absorption of calcium, renal hypercalciuria resulting from primary renal leak of calcium, and resorptive hypercalciuria resulting from increased bone demineralization.

Although historically this classification system was used because of its utility in simplifying the understanding and treatment of specific metabolic derangements, many have argued that hypercalciuria is associated with multiple, interrelated disturbances that cannot be readily separated into a specific organ system (Coe et al., 1992). Furthermore, studies into the molecular mechanisms of stone formation have identified gene mutations that can affect several organ systems, culminating in hypercalciuria (Frick and Bushinsky, 2003; Langman, 2004). Indeed, use of a classification system for hypercalciuria has not been associated with superior therapeutic efficacy and is therefore not routinely implemented in clinical practice. Although improved understanding of the molecular and genetic causes of stone disease may change the categorization and management of stones in the future, for the purposes of this chapter, the standard classification system is used.

Absorptive Hypercalciuria. Absorptive hypercalciuria (AH) is defined as increased urinary calcium excretion (>0.2 mg/mg creatinine) after an oral calcium load. Although fasting urinary calcium is usually normal in AH (<0.11 mg/dL glomerular filtration), severe forms of AH may occasionally be associated with fasting hypercalciuria as well. The underlying pathophysiologic abnormality in AH is increased intestinal absorption of calcium, which occurs in approximately 30% of stone formers. Dietary calcium restriction may normalize urinary calcium in some patients with AH (type II) but not in others (type I). **The added systemic load of calcium caused by intestinal calcium hyperabsorption results in a transient increase in serum calcium, which suppresses serum PTH and results in increased renal filtration of calcium, ultimately leading to hypercalciuria. Because the increase in intestinal absorption of calcium is matched by enhanced renal calcium excretion, serum calcium level remains normal.**

The cause of increased intestinal absorption of calcium has been variously ascribed to vitamin D–independent and dependent processes, as well as to upregulation of the vitamin D receptor (Breslau et al., 1992). However, no proposed mechanism completely accounts for all the findings associated with absorptive hypercalciuria, and there is no clear evidence that upregulation of intestinal calcium absorption is the primary cause. There are several genetic abnormalities that can potentially affect vitamin D activity. The active form of vitamin D, $1,25(OH)_2D_3$, is generated by way of 1-hydroxylation of $25(OH)D_3$ by the gene product of cytochrome P450 (CYP) 27B1 *(CYP27B1)*, which is present in a variety of tissues. The mitochondrial enzyme $1,25(OH)_2D$-24-hydroxylase (CYP24A1), which is present in the intestine and kidney, inactivates both major vitamin D metabolites, $25(OH)D_3$ and $1,25(OH)_2D_3$. Bi-allelic mutations in *CYP24A1* have been shown to reduce activity of the enzyme, resulting in elevated levels of $1,25(OH)_2D_3$, particularly in individuals taking large amounts of vitamin D (Schlingmann et al., 2011). Mutations in this gene are responsible for increased sensitivity to vitamin D supplementation in the autosomal recessive disorder idiopathic infantile hyperkalemia. In adults, recessive mutations in *CYP24A1* have been associated with a syndrome characterized by hypercalcemia, hypercalciuria, nephrocalcinosis, and nephrolithiasis (Dinour et al., 2013; Nesterova et al., 2013). Genome-wide association studies revealed an association between *CYP24A1* variants and serum vitamin D concentrations (Wang et al., 2010). The frequency of $1,25(OH)_2D$-24-hydroxylase deficiency is estimated at 4% to 20% in the general population (Nesterova et al., 2013). However, although these mutations may be common, not all affected individuals demonstrate clinically significant abnormalities.

Hypersensitivity to vitamin D has also been shown to increase intestinal calcium absorption and cause hypercalciuria (Bushinsky and Monk, 1998). Moreover, several studies have linked hypercalciuria and the vitamin D receptor *(VDR)* gene. Jackman et al. (1999) identified a polymorphism in *VDR* in 19 patients with a family history of nephrolithiasis and hypercalciuria, thereby establishing a potential link. Likewise, Scott et al. (1999) identified linkage between a microsatellite marker and the *VDR* locus on chromosome 12q12-q14 in a cohort of 47 French-Canadian pedigrees with idiopathic hypercalciuria and calcium nephrolithiasis.

Other studies, however, failed to confirm the association of *VDR* abnormalities with hypercalciuria (Zerwekh et al., 1995, 1998). Indeed, other genetic loci have been identified in association with AH. Reed et al. (1999, 2002) mapped the locus for an inherited form of AH to chromosome 1q23.3-q24 and found a putative gene (subsequently shown by others to be homologous with the rat soluble adenylate cyclase gene) in this region in 12 unrelated white AH patients.

Another proposed cause of AH is renal phosphate wasting leading to a subsequent increase in active vitamin D. Patients with hereditary hypophosphatemic rickets with hypercalciuria (HHRH) manifest this abnormality, which is characterized by decreased renal reabsorption of phosphate, hypophosphatemia, and a subsequent compensatory increase in vitamin D levels, leading to enhanced absorption of calcium and phosphate from the intestine and hypercalciuria (Tieder et al., 1987). The mutations associated with HHRH are thought to be inherited in an autosomal recessive pattern. Candidate genes for HHRH include *SLC34A1* and *SLC34A3*, which encode sodium-coupled phosphate transporters located in the apical membrane of the renal proximal tubule (NaPi-IIa and NaPi-IIc, respectively) (Devuyst and Pirson, 2007). Renal phosphate leak, however, is a rare cause of nephrolithiasis, affecting at most 2% to 4% of patients (Levy et al., 1995).

Renal Hypercalciuria. The kidney filters approximately 270 mmol of calcium and must reabsorb more than 98% of it to maintain calcium homeostasis (Bushinsky, 1998). Approximately 70% of calcium reabsorption occurs in the proximal tubule, with paracellular pathways predominating (Frick and Bushinsky, 2003; Moor and Bonny, 2016). In renal hypercalciuria, impaired renal tubular reabsorption of calcium results in elevated urinary calcium levels leading to secondary hyperparathyroidism (Coe et al., 1973). Serum calcium levels remain normal because the renal loss of calcium is compensated by enhanced intestinal absorption of calcium and bone resorption as a result of increased secretion of PTH and enhanced synthesis of $1,25(OH)_2D_3$. **High fasting urinary calcium levels (>0.11 mg/dL glomerular filtration) with normal serum calcium values are characteristic of renal hypercalciuria.** The elevated fasting urinary calcium and serum PTH levels can differentiate a primary renal cause from a primary intestinal cause of hypercalciuria.

The actual cause of renal calcium leak is not known. However, alterations in transcellular and paracellular pathways for calcium reabsorption are likely implicated. Studies of several monogenetic disorders associated with hypercalciuria and nephrolithiasis provide insight into the mechanisms involved (Devuyst and Pirson, 2007; Ferraro et al., 2013a; Gambaro et al., 2004; Langman, 2004). In Dent disease (X-linked recessive nephrolithiasis), defects in chloride channel-5 (ClC-5), which is located in the proximal tubule, thick ascending limb, and α-type intercalated cells of the collecting ducts lead to hypercalciuria, proteinuria, nephrolithiasis, nephrocalcinosis, and progressive renal failure. Familial hypomagnesemia with hypercalciuria and nephrocalcinosis (FHHNC) is caused by mutations in claudin-16 (also known as paracellin-1) and claudin-19, members of the claudin gene family of tight junction proteins that are involved in the voltage-driven paracellular reabsorption of magnesium and calcium in the thick ascending limb and distal convoluted tubule (Konrad et al., 2006; Simon et al., 1999). Other claudin abnormalities, including defects in claudin-14, have been associated with nephrolithiasis (Thorleifsson et al., 2009). Finally, Bartter syndrome encompasses a group of autosomal recessive disorders involving dysfunction in the thick ascending limb that is characterized by salt wasting and hypokalemic metabolic acidosis, with variable occurrence of hypercalciuria and nephrolithiasis (Devuyst and Pirson, 2007). This disorder arises from a mutation in any of the genes encoding membrane proteins involved in transepithelial sodium chloride transport across the thick limb of the loop of Henle: *SLC12A1*, which encodes the $Na^+, K^+, 2Cl^-$ cotransporter, NKCC2; *KCNJ*, which encodes the apical renal outer medullary potassium channel, ROMK; *CLCNKB*, which encodes the basolateral chloride channel, ClC-Kb; and *BSND*, which encodes a subunit (Barttin) for the chloride channel proteins ClC-Ka and ClC-Kb.

The CaSR is the main calcium sensor involved in the maintenance of calcium metabolism. Mutations of the genes encoding CaSR *(CASR)*, G protein alpha 11 *(GNA11)*, and adaptor-related protein complex 2 sigma 1 subunit *(AP2S1)* can shift the set point for calcium sensing, leading to hyper- or hypocalcemic disorders (Mayr et al., 2016). Activating mutations in the gene encoding the CaSR have been associated with an autosomal dominant form of hypocalcemia by which a lower set-point for extracellular calcium sensing leads to decreased serum PTH levels, reduced renal calcium reabsorption, and subsequent hypocalcemia and hypercalciuria (Devuyst and Pirson, 2007). A potent activating mutation in the CaSR has been associated with salt-losing nephropathy and secondary hyperaldosteronism (Bartter syndrome type V), which is likely related to dysfunction of ROMK as a result of constitutive activation of the abnormal CaSR (Vargas-Poussou et al., 2002). CaSR regulates calcium reabsorption in the thick ascending limb through changes in paracellular permeability (Loupy et al., 2012).

Loss-of-function polymorphisms in the *CaSR* gene have also been associated with idiopathic nephrolithiasis. Two synonymous single nucleotide polymorphisms (rs6776158 and rs1501899) that significantly reduce renal CaSR messenger RNA levels have been shown to be highly associated with normocitraturic nephrolithiasis (Vezzoli et al., 2010, 2011). Reduced CaSR expression can increase paracellular calcium reabsorption in the thick ascending limb of the loop of Henle, leading to interstitial calcium precipitation and hypocalciuria. Diminished calcium delivery to the collecting duct may affect the cellular mechanism for urinary acidification and concentration, leading to calcium oxalate stone formation. Other mutations in the genes for the Na^+-K^+-$2Cl^-$ cotransporter NKCC2 and the potassium channel ROMK have been associated with autosomal recessive disorders characterized by fasting hypercalciuria and nephrocalcinosis.

Understanding these genetic disorders has the potential to further elucidate the tubular handling of calcium and the pathophysiology of renal hypercalciuria.

Resorptive Hypercalciuria. Resorptive hypercalciuria is an infrequent abnormality most commonly associated with primary hyperparathyroidism. Primary hyperparathyroidism is the cause of nephrolithiasis in about 5% of cases (Broadus, 1989). **Excessive parathyroid hormone (PTH) secretion from a parathyroid adenoma leads to excessive bone resorption and increased renal synthesis of $1,25(OH)_2D_3$, which in turn enhances intestinal absorption of calcium. The net effect is elevated serum and urine calcium levels and reduced serum phosphorus levels.** Although most patients with primary hyperparathyroidism demonstrate hypercalcemia and hypercalciuria, a normal serum calcium level in the presence of an inappropriately high serum PTH value may be seen in some cases, making the diagnosis more difficult. Administration of a thiazide diuretic will enhance renal calcium reabsorption and exacerbate the hypercalcemia, without suppression of PTH production, thereby facilitating the diagnosis ("thiazide challenge") (Eisner et al., 2009).

Primary hyperparathyroidism is associated with nephrolithiasis in less than 5% of affected individuals (Heath et al., 1980; Parks et al., 1980). However, the diagnosis should be suspected in patients with nephrolithiasis and serum calcium levels greater than 10.1 mg/dL (Broadus et al., 1980; Menon, 1986). Serum calcium levels can vary by up to 5%, and patients with mild hyperparathyroidism may exhibit relatively small increases of serum calcium (Yendt and Gagne, 1968). Therefore repeated measurements of serum calcium, along with serum intact PTH, may be necessary to make the diagnosis. Measurement of serum ionized calcium may help in equivocal cases because ionized calcium may be elevated in the setting of normal serum calcium (Yendt and Gagne, 1968). PTH also increases excretion of bicarbonate and phosphorus from the proximal renal tubule, resulting in phosphaturia and mild hyperchloremic acidosis.

Hypercalcemic-Induced Hypercalciuria

Sarcoid and Granulomatous Disease. Additional, rare causes of hypercalciuria include hypercalcemia of malignancy, sarcoidosis, thyrotoxicosis, and vitamin D toxicity. Many granulomatous diseases, including tuberculosis, sarcoidosis, histoplasmosis, leprosy, and silicosis, have been reported to produce hypercalcemia. Among these, sarcoidosis is most commonly associated with urolithiasis. **Macrophages in the sarcoid granuloma, through synthesis of 1α-hydroxylase, increase production of $1,25(OH)_2D_3$, which enhances intestinal absorption of calcium and promotes bone resorption, ultimately leading to hypercalciuria** (Adams et al., 1983, 1985). As such granulomatous diseases manifest absorptive and resorptive hypercalciuria. Pulmonary alveolar cells and lymph node homogenates in patients with sarcoidosis are capable of synthesizing vitamin D, a function usually limited to the kidney. Most patients with sarcoidosis have a suppressed level of PTH secondary to hypercalcemia (Cushard et al., 1972). Sarcoidosis can also be differentiated from other diagnoses by the rapid resolution of hypercalcemia with initiation of corticosteroid therapy (Breslau et al., 1982).

Malignancy-Associated Hypercalcemia. Although primary hyperparathyroidism is the most common cause of hypercalcemia in an outpatient setting, malignancy is the main cause of hypercalcemia in hospitalized patients (Rizzoli and Bonjour, 1992). Measuring intact PTH can help distinguish patients with hyperparathyroidism from those with other causes of hypercalcemia (Burtis et al., 1990). Tumors in patients with humoral hypercalcemia produce a PTH-related protein (PTHrP) whose production is regulated by CaSRs on the cell surface (Chattopadhyay, 2006). Lung and breast cancers account for about 60% of malignancy-associated hypercalcemia, whereas renal cell (10% to 15%), head and neck (10%), and hematologic cancers such as lymphoma and myeloma (10%) account for the rest. Although direct mechanical destruction of bone constitutes one cause of hypercalcemia, many tumors secrete humoral factors, including PTHrP, transforming growth factor-α, and cytokines such as interleukin-1 and tumor necrosis factor, which activate osteoclasts and result in bone lysis and hypercalcemia (Burtis et al., 1990; Edelson and Kleerekoper, 1995; Mundy, 1990). Like PTH, PTHrP increases renal calcium absorption and stimulates osteoblasts to secrete receptor activator of nuclear factor-κB ligand (RANKL), which binds to the RANK receptor on osteoclasts, leading to differentiation of osteoclast precursors into mature osteoclasts and subsequently to enhanced bone resorption and hypercalcemia (Mirrakhimov, 2015). Furthermore, PTHrP stimulates 1-α hydroxylation of $25(OH)_2D_3$, leading to increased production of calcitriol and enhanced intestinal calcium absorption and bone turnover.

Glucocorticoid-Induced Hypercalcemia. Glucocorticoids can significantly alter calcium metabolism through their actions on bone, intestine, and parathyroid glands. Their most potent effect is related to calcium metabolism in bones, where glucocorticoids promote bone resorption and reduce bone formation, ultimately leading to osteopenia with chronic use (Manelli and Giustina, 2000). In addition, they stimulate release of PTH (Fucik et al., 1975). On the other hand, glucocorticoids inhibit intestinal absorption of calcium, which accounts for their effectiveness in preventing hypercalciuria induced by sarcoidosis (Manelli and Giustina, 2000). The net effect probably favors promotion of stone formation because nephrolithiasis is common in patients with Cushing syndrome (Faggiano et al., 2003). In one study, stones were found in 50% of patients with active Cushing syndrome, 27% of cured patients, and 6.5% of controls. Compared with controls, patients with active disease had a significantly higher prevalence of hypercalciuria, hypocitraturia, and hyperuricosuria, but these patients were also at greater risk of obesity and diabetes, which have been linked to stone formation (Faggiano et al., 2003).

Hyperoxaluria

Hyperoxaluria, defined as urinary oxalate greater than 40 mg/day, leads to increased urinary saturation of calcium oxalate and subsequent promotion of calcium oxalate stones. In addition, oxalate has been implicated in crystal growth and retention by means of renal tubular cell injury mediated by lipid peroxidation and the generation of oxygen free radicals (Ravichandran and Selvam, 1990). Membrane injury facilitates the fixation of calcium oxalate crystals and subsequent crystal growth. Antioxidant therapy has been shown to prevent calcium oxalate precipitation in the rat kidney and to reduce oxalate excretion in stone patients (Selvam, 2002). Similarly, calcium oxalate crystal deposition on urothelium in vitro was prevented by free radical scavengers such as phytic acid and mannitol, purportedly by protecting the membrane from free radical–mediated damage (Selvam, 2002; Thamilselvan and Selvam, 1997). Human studies, however, failed to demonstrate increases in markers of oxidative stress or renal injury in normal subjects and stone formers ingesting large doses of oxalate (up to 8 mmol), thus calling into question the importance of oxalate-induced cell membrane damage in calcium oxalate stone formation (Knight et al., 2007).

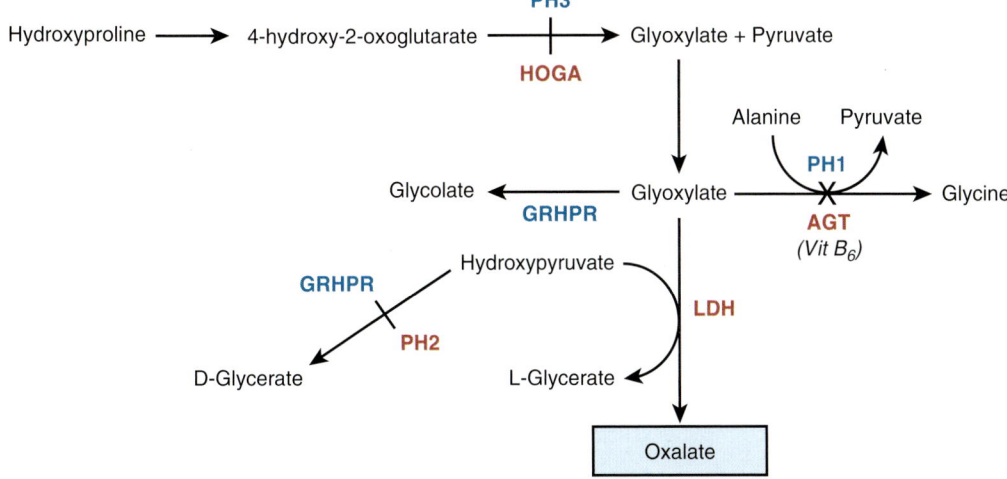

Fig. 91.7. Pathway of oxalate metabolism in the liver. Defects in alanine glyoxylate aminotransferase (AGT) are associated with primary hyperoxaluria type 1 (PH1), defects in glyoxylate reductase/hydroxypyruvate reductase (GRHPR) are associated with primary hyperoxaluria type 2 (PH2), and defects in 4-hydroxy-2-oxoglutarate aldolase (HOGA) are associated with primary hyperoxaluria type 3 (PH3). *LDH,* Lactate dehydrogenase.

Causes of hyperoxaluria include disorders in biosynthetic pathways (primary hyperoxaluria); intestinal malabsorptive states associated with inflammatory bowel disease, celiac sprue, or intestinal resection (enteric hyperoxaluria); and excessive dietary intake or high substrate levels (vitamin C) (dietary hyperoxaluria).
Primary Hyperoxaluria. The primary hyperoxalurias (PHs) are the result of rare autosomal recessive inherited disorders in glyoxylate metabolism by which the normal conversion of glyoxylate to glycine is prevented, leading to preferential oxidative conversion of glyoxylate to oxalate, an end product of metabolism (Fig. 91.7). The markedly high levels of urinary oxalate that ensue (>100 mg/day) lead to increased saturation of calcium oxalate and formation of calcium oxalate complexes and crystals in the renal tubular lumen. Some crystals attach to the surface of renal tubular epithelial cells and further aggregate into stones, whereas others are internalized into tubular cells and then extruded into the renal interstitium, leading to marked nephrocalcinosis (Hoppe et al., 2009). Renal injury may be a consequence of direct cell toxicity from either high oxalate concentration or calcium oxalate crystals, mediated through reactive oxygen species. Renal impairment occurs from recurrent obstructing calcium oxalate stones and as a result of renal parenchymal inflammation and interstitial fibrosis from severe nephrocalcinosis (Mulay et al., 2013). With progressive renal damage, renal elimination of oxalate is impaired, leading to systemic deposition of calcium oxalate crystals, or systemic oxalosis.

Three forms of PH have been identified (types 1, 2, and 3) that differ in the enzyme and intracellular organelle affected. The primary enzyme catalyzing glyoxylate conversion to glycine is the pyridoxal phosphate–dependent alanine-glyoxylate aminotransferase (AGT), which is synthesized in the liver peroxisome. Mutations in this gene (*AGXT*) result in primary hyperoxaluria type 1 (PH1), and patients with this disorder have elevated levels of oxalate and frequently glycolate. ESRD occurs during the second to third decades of life in most patients with PH1, making it the most aggressive form of the disease (Hoppe et al., 2009). Elucidation of the crystal structure of AGT to 2.5 Å has improved the understanding of mutations in the gene for this protein (Zhang et al., 2003). The most common mutation of *AGXT* results in a substitution of glycine by arginine at position 170; in the setting of a proline-to-leucine substitution at position 11 present in a polymorphic minor allele, the enzyme inappropriately targets the liver mitochondria, where it is metabolically inactive, rather than the liver peroxisomes (Fargue et al., 2013a). Patients with this mutation are responsive to pyridoxine therapy because pyridoxine is metabolized to pyridoxal phosphate, an essential cofactor for AGT, which results in an increased enzyme catalytic activity and enhanced peroxisome targeting (Fargue et al., 2013b). At least 178 mutations have been identified in the *AGXT* gene.

Primary hyperoxaluria type 2 (PH2) is associated with a defect in glyoxylate reductase/hydroxypyruvate reductase (GRHPR) in the liver, resulting in hyperoxaluric nephrolithiasis, but with a less aggressive course with regard to renal failure than PH1 (Johnson et al., 2002). Patients with PH2 have elevated urinary levels of L-glyceric acid and oxalate because reduced GRHPR enzyme activity leads to increased hydroxypyruvate and glyoxylate, which are converted by lactate dehydrogenase to L-glyceric acid and oxalate, respectively. A total of 30 mutations have been identified in the *GRHPR* gene (Cochat and Rumsby, 2013).

A third type of primary hyperoxaluria is caused by a defective mitochondrial enzyme, 4-hydroxy-2-oxoglutarate aldolase (HOGA), which is thought to play a role in hydroxyproline metabolism (Belostotsky et al., 2010). Hydroxy-2-oxoglutarate derived from hydroxyproline is converted to pyruvate and glyoxylate in a reaction catalyzed by HOGA. However, the mechanism by which this defect leads to hyperoxaluria has not been established. There are two common pathologic variants, including a 3 bp deletion (c.944_946delAGG, p.Glu315del), which is prevalent in the Ashkenazi Jewish population, and another mutation, c.700+5G > T, which causes missplicing in hepatic RNA (Belostotsky et al., 2010; Williams et al., 2012). Although PH3 is associated with hyperoxaluria and severe hypercalciuria, the recurrent calcium oxalate stone formation seen in early childhood may become clinically silent later in life, and there are no reports of progression to ESRD in these patients (Hoppe, 2012).

If untreated, PH1 inevitably leads to end-stage renal failure, which occurs by age 15 in 50% of affected patients and is associated with an overall death rate of approximately 30% (Cochat et al., 1999). Because the liver is the only organ responsible for detoxification of glyoxylate, combined liver-kidney transplantation is the accepted treatment for most patients with severe PH. Reported 5-year patient survival and liver allograft survival after combined liver-kidney transplantation are 80% and 72%, respectively (Jamieson, 2005). Furthermore, the renal function of survivors reportedly remains stable over time (Cochat et al., 1999; Hoppe and Langman, 2003). Isolated kidney transplantation is the treatment of choice for patients with PH2 and ESRD, because hypoxanthine-guanine phosphoribosyl transferase (HGPRT) is not liver specific. PH3 has not been associated with ESRD, and transplantation in this setting has not been reported.

Genetic testing is available for all three forms of PH, which can provide confirmation of biochemical testing and allows prenatal

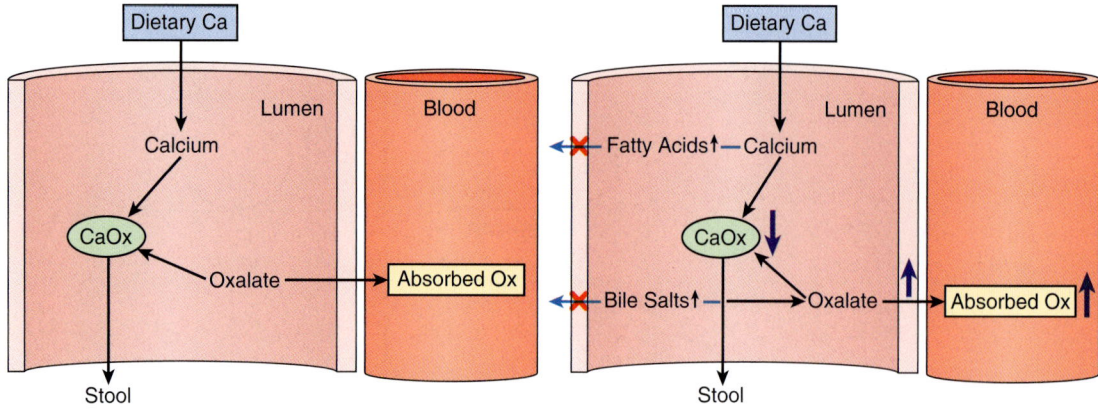

Fig. 91.8. Mechanism of enteric hyperoxaluria. (A) Under normal intestinal and dietary conditions, dietary calcium combines in the intestinal lumen with oxalate, forming a calcium oxalate complex that is excreted in the stool. (B) In malabsorptive conditions, poorly absorbed fatty acids bind cations such as calcium and magnesium in the process of saponification, thereby decreasing calcium-oxalate complex formation and increasing luminal oxalate, which is overabsorbed and excreted in the urine. Poorly absorbed bile salts increase colonic permeability of oxalate, furthering increasing absorbed oxalate.

diagnosis and the confirmation or exclusion of disease in other family members. Because all three forms of PH may remain clinically asymptomatic until adulthood, it is imperative to screen family members. Furthermore, because renal transplantation may constitute a part of the treatment plan for patients with PH1 and PH2, it is imperative to exclude PH in family members before consideration of living-related kidney donation from within the family. One caveat for genetic testing is that not all carriers develop primary hyperoxaluria.

Another inherited cause of calcium oxalate stones associated with hyperoxaluria is mutations in the SAT1 sulphate-oxalate transporter, encoded by *SLC26A1* (Gee et al., 2016). Mutations in this gene may account for suspected inherited hyperoxaluria in patients in whom the three known forms of PH have been excluded.

Enteric Hyperoxaluria. The most common cause of acquired hyperoxaluria is enteric hyperoxaluria. This abnormality is associated with chronic diarrheal states, by which **fat malabsorption results in saponification of fatty acids with divalent cations such as calcium and magnesium, thereby reducing calcium oxalate complexation and increasing the pool of available oxalate for reabsorption** (Earnest et al., 1975; Fig. 91.8). The poorly absorbed fatty acids and bile salts may increase colonic permeability to oxalate, further enhancing intestinal oxalate absorption (Dobbins and Binder, 1976; Hatch and Freel, 2008). A strong relationship between fecal fat and urinary oxalate excretion has been demonstrated in patients with steatorrhea (Fig. 91.9; Worcester, 1996). Dehydration, hypokalemia, hypomagnesiuria, hypocitraturia, and low urine pH also increase the risk of calcium oxalate stone formation in patients with chronic diarrheal syndrome. Malabsorption from any cause can lead to increased intestinal absorption of oxalate. As such, small bowel resection, intrinsic disease, and jejunoileal bypass (Cryer et al., 1975) have been associated with hyperoxaluria.

As the prevalence of obesity in the population has increased, bariatric surgery has become more popular and pervasive. Although jejunoileal bypass for obesity was discontinued in the past in part because of renal failure and nephrolithiasis induced by severe hyperoxaluria, modern bariatric surgery was thought to provide a safer alternative for weight loss. However, a 2005 report from the Mayo Clinic revealed two patients with oxalate nephropathy and renal failure who required dialysis and/or renal transplantation among 23 patients with enteric hyperoxaluria and calcium oxalate stones after Roux-en-Y gastric bypass surgery (Nelson et al., 2005). Since then, a number of retrospective (Asplin and Coe, 2007; Patel et al., 2009), cross-sectional (Maalouf et al., 2010), and prospective (Duffey et al., 2010; Park et al., 2009) studies have shown increased urinary oxalate excretion in non–stone-forming individuals after Roux-en-Y gastric bypass and other malabsorptive bariatric procedures. The rise

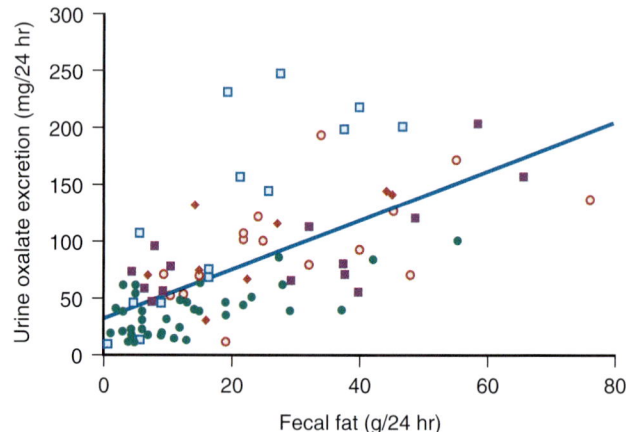

Fig. 91.9. The relationship between fecal fat and urinary oxalate excretion in patients with steatorrhea. Diet oxalate was 300 to 500 mg/day in all but one study, in which it was 55 to 90 mg/day. Diet calcium was 500 to 900 mg/day in all studies when reported. Normal urine citrate was less than 50 mg/day in all studies, except one in which it was less than 34 mg/day. Oxalate = 2.1 × fecal fat + 30.7 (r^2 = 0.4, n = 96, P < 0.001). (From Worcester EM: Stones due to bowel disease. In Coe F, Favus M, Pak C, et al, editors: *Kidney stones: medical and surgical management*, New York, 1996, Lippincott-Raven, pp 883–903.)

in urinary oxalate was shown to develop at least 6 months after bypass surgery (Sinha et al., 2007). To varying degrees, the increase in urinary oxalate was offset by a decline in urinary calcium and uric acid, leading to conflicting effects on urinary saturation of calcium oxalate.

Despite some variation in the observed effect on urinary analytes, an increased rate of stone formation has been reported after gastric bypass surgery. Using a claims database, Matlaga et al. (2009) found that 7.65% of 4639 patients after Roux-en-Y gastric bypass surgery versus 4.63% of 4639 obese controls were diagnosed with kidney stones (P < 0.0001) after a median observation period of 4.6 years and 4.1 years, respectively. In a telephone survey of patients who underwent Roux-en-Y gastric bypass surgery, Haddad et al. (2014) also found a postsurgical rate of symptomatic urolithiasis of 7.3% at a mean follow-up of 7 years, with a 5% rate of de novo symptomatic stones. The median time to presentation of the first symptomatic stone was 3.1 years. The risk appears to be limited to patients undergoing gastric bypass surgery, as another claims study demonstrated a *higher* rate of stone formation in a control group compared with a group of patients undergoing gastric banding (5.97% vs. 1.49%, respectively) (Semins et al., 2009). Indeed, a comparison of 27 patients after Roux-en-Y gastric bypass surgery with 12 patients after gastric banding revealed higher urinary oxalate, lower urinary calcium, and marginally lower urinary citrate in the bypass group compared with the banding group, suggesting that gastric banding is not associated with malabsorption and enteric hyperoxaluria (Penniston et al., 2009).

The cause of the hyperoxaluria observed after gastric bypass surgery has not been fully elucidated. Although loss of *O. formigenes*, an oxalate-degrading bacterium that resides in the intestinal tract, has been suggested as a possible source, the presence of low *O. formigenes* colonization levels in morbidly obese patients before Roux-en-Y gastric bypass surgery argues against this hypothesis (Duffey et al., 2011). Moreover, no significant difference in *O. formigenes* colonization was found between 10 post–bariatric surgery patients and 13 morbidly obese controls (40% vs. 15%, respectively) (Froeder et al., 2012). However, the urinary oxalate response to an oral oxalate load was more pronounced in patients after bariatric surgery than before and greater than the response in morbidly obese controls, suggesting that hyperoxaluria observed after bariatric surgery is due to increased intestinal absorption of dietary oxalate. Indeed, Kumar et al. (2011) prospectively studied 11 morbidly obese subjects before and 6 and 12 months after bariatric surgery (Roux-en-Y gastric bypass or biliopancreatic diversion–duodenal switch) and found significant increases in plasma oxalate, urine calcium oxalate supersaturation, and fecal fat excretion at both time points after surgery. Unlike previous studies, no significant increase in urinary oxalate or decline in urinary calcium was observed, likely as a result of aggressive calcium supplementation postsurgery. However, urinary oxalate was elevated in a 24-hour urine collection obtained after an oral oxalate load at both 6 and 12 months. These findings suggest that the cause of the hyperoxaluria and increased stone risk associated with bariatric surgery is at least in part the result of malabsorption and enteric hyperoxaluria.

Dietary Hyperoxaluria. Overindulgence in oxalate-rich foods such as nuts, chocolate, brewed tea, spinach, potatoes, beets, and rhubarb can result in hyperoxaluria in otherwise normal individuals. The contribution of dietary oxalate to urinary oxalate excretion can range from 24% to 42% (Holmes et al., 2001). In addition, severe calcium restriction may result in reduced intestinal binding of oxalate and increased intestinal oxalate absorption. Ascorbic acid supplementation has been shown to increase urinary oxalate levels by in vivo conversion to oxalate (Traxer et al., 2003), although increased clinical rates of stone formation have not been unequivocally linked to ascorbic acid use (Curhan et al., 1996, 1999).

Recent studies have also implicated *O. formigenes*, an oxalate-degrading intestinal bacterium, as a potential modulator of intestinal oxalate levels (Duncan et al., 2002). Stone formers were found to have reduced levels or absent colonization of *O. formigenes* compared with non–stone-forming control subjects, and individuals lacking the bacteria have been shown to have higher urinary oxalate levels (Mikami et al., 2003; Sidhu et al., 1999; Troxel et al., 2003). In a large case-control study of age- and gender-matched recurrent calcium oxalate stone formers ($n = 274$) and normal subjects ($n = 259$), 17% of stone formers and 38% of normal subjects tested positive for *O. formigenes* (Kaufman et al., 2008). Controlling for confounding factors, the OR for colonization (case vs. control) was 0.3 (95% CI 0.2–0.5). Interestingly, median urinary oxalate levels did not differ between those with or without *O. formigenes* colonization. **Cystic fibrosis patients, many of whom are exposed to prolonged antibiotic use, have also been shown to have absence of *O. formigenes* from the intestinal tract and corresponding elevated urinary oxalate levels** (Sidhu et al., 1998). Likewise, *O. formigenes* colonization was compared between a group of patients with *Helicobacter pylori* treated with antibiotics and a group of patients without *H. pylori*. Among 12 patients positive for *O. formigenes* not treated with antibiotics, 92% of patients remained *O. formigenes*–positive at 1 and 6 months. In contrast, among 19 subjects with *H. pylori* who received antibiotics, only 36.8% remained colonized with *O. formigenes* 1 and 6 months after treatment (Kharlamb et al., 2011). These findings highlight the potential prolonged effect of antibiotic therapy on intestinal colonization of *O. formigenes* and a potential role in modulating stone risk.

Interestingly, a recent case-control study among more than 13 million children and adults using electronic medical record data from the United Kingdom demonstrated that after adjusting for confounding factors, exposure to any of 5 different antibiotic classes 3 to 12 months before the index encounter was associated with an increased likelihood of developing kidney stones (Tasian et al., 2018). Although antibiotic exposure has been postulated by some investigators to account for the decreased *O. formigenes* colonization in some stone formers, the bacterium has been shown to be resistant to some of the antibiotics evaluated in the previous study (Lange et al., 2011), suggesting that the increased stone risk associated with antibiotic exposure may not be mediated solely by *O. formigenes* but may instead be the result of lower diversity of the intestinal microbiome resulting from antibiotic use. Indeed, multivariate logistic regression analysis comparing fecal samples from 52 stone formers and 48 controls subjects revealed that fecal microbial diversity was lower in stone formers than in controls (Chao 1 biodiversity index 1460 vs. 1658 operational taxonomic units, $P = 0.02$) (Ticinesi et al., 2018). Moreover, although 3 taxa were significantly underrepresented in the stone-forming group, *Oxalobacter* abundance did not differ significantly between the two groups. On the other hand, genes involved in oxalate degradation *were* significantly underrepresented among stone formers and correlated inversely with 24-hour urinary oxalate levels ($r = -0.87, P = 0.002$). These finding may account for the lack of benefit of probiotic products containing *O. formigenes* and lactobacilli in reducing urinary oxalate excretion and suggest that gut microbiota, specifically other bacterial species with oxalate-degrading properties, may contribute to risk of stone formation.

Idiopathic Hyperoxaluria. Several studies have suggested that mild hyperoxaluria is as important a factor as hypercalciuria in the pathogenesis of idiopathic calcium oxalate stones (Menon, 1986; Robertson and Hughes, 1993). In some populations, such as those inhabiting the Arabian Peninsula, the prevalence of calcium-containing stones is considerably higher than in the West despite the almost complete absence of hypercalciuria (Robertson and Hughes, 1993). Hyperoxaluria is implicated as the predominant risk factor in this population.

Abnormalities in the metabolism and transport of oxalate may contribute to calcium oxalate nephrolithiasis. Baggio et al. (1986) detected a higher rate of oxalate flux across the red blood cell membrane at steady state in 114 patients with a history of calcium oxalate kidney stones compared with control subjects. Treatment with oral hydrochlorothiazide (50 mg/day), amiloride (5 mg/day), or both restored normal or nearly normal red blood cell oxalate exchange in all of the patients who initially demonstrated increased rates. Up to 50% of the time, however, the abnormality in red blood cell oxalate transport is not associated with hyperoxaluria. Furthermore, Motola et al. (1992) found high rates of oxalate flux in non–calcium oxalate stone formers as well, thus leading some to question the importance of this mechanism in calcium oxalate stone formation.

Hyperuricosuria

Hyperuricosuria is defined as urinary uric acid exceeding 600 mg/day. Up to 10% of calcium stone formers have high urinary uric acid levels as an isolated abnormality, but it is found in combination with other metabolic abnormalities in up to 40% of calcium stone formers (Preminger, 1992). The mechanism by which hyperuricosuria induces calcium oxalate stones is not completely elucidated. Hyperuricosuria has been postulated to increase urinary levels of monosodium urate, which in turn promotes calcium oxalate crystallization through **heterogeneous nucleation, or epitaxial crystal growth** (Coe et al., 1975; Pak and Arnold, 1975). In addition, **the colloidal form of sodium urate has been shown to adsorb naturally occurring macromolecular inhibitors of crystallization, thereby reducing their effectiveness and promoting nucleation of calcium oxalate** (Pak et al., 1977; Robertson et al., 1976). However, some investigators dispute the effect of monosodium urate and attribute **the effect of**

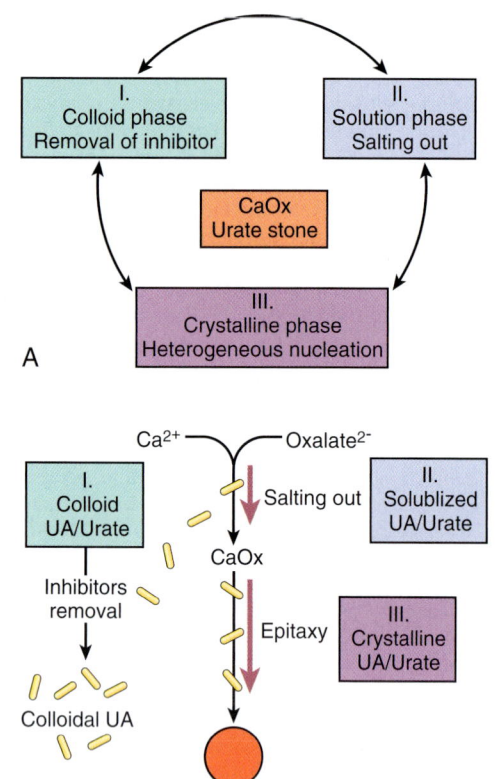

Fig. 91.10. Pathophysiologic mechanisms of hyperuricosuric calcium nephrolithiasis. (A) Mechanisms of sodium urate–induced calcium oxalate crystallization and growth (I) colloidal phase (II) solution phase (III) crystalline phase. (B) (I) Adsorption of inhibitors by colloidal uric acid (II); "Salting-out" of calcium oxalate by soluble urate salts; (III) Heterogenous nucleation (epitaxy) of calcium oxalate crystals by sodium urate nidi. (Data from Moe OW, Xu LHR: Hyperuricosuric calcium urolithiasis. J Nephrol 31:189–196, 2018.)

uric acid on calcium oxalate stone formation to the simple process of "salting out," whereby the solubility of calcium oxalate in solution is decreased by the addition of another salt (Grover and Ryall, 1994; Ryall et al., 1991). Whether any or all of these three pathogenetic mechanisms contributes to uric acid-induced calcium oxalate nephrolithiasis is not clear, but there is compelling evidence in support of each one individually (Fig. 91.10; Moe and Xu, 2018).

The most common cause of hyperuricosuria is increased dietary purine intake. However, acquired and hereditary diseases may also be accompanied by hyperuricosuria, including gout, myeloproliferative and lymphoproliferative disorders, multiple myeloma, secondary polycythemia, pernicious anemia, hemolytic disorders, hemoglobinopathies and thalassemia, complete or partial HGPRT deficiency, overactivity of phosphoribosylpyrophosphate synthetase, and hereditary renal hypouricemia (Halabe and Sperling, 1994). The identification of a urate transporter, the anion exchanger URAT1, in the proximal renal tubule may provide new insight into the causes of hyperuricosuria (Enomoto et al., 2002; Ichida et al., 2004). Mutations in *SLC22A12*, the gene encoding URAT1, have been shown to cause hyperuricosuric hypouricemia (renal uric acid leak) along with exercise-induced acute renal failure and a high risk of kidney stones (Enomoto et al., 2002; Ichida et al., 2004; Iwai et al., 2004; Tanaka et al., 2003).

Not all evidence supports a role for uric acid in calcium oxalate stone formation. Among 3350 male and female participants (2237 stone formers and 1113 non–stone formers) from three large cohort studies who collected 24-hour urine specimens for stone risk analysis, after adjusting for other urinary parameters, urinary uric acid excretion was significantly inversely associated with incident kidney stone formation in men, marginally inversely associated in younger women, and not associated in older women (Curhan and Taylor, 2008). On the other hand, a randomized trial among hyperuricosuric, normocalciuric calcium oxalate stone formers demonstrated a greater than twofold reduction in stone recurrence rates among patients randomized to allopurinol versus those taking placebo (Ettinger et al., 1986). However, the mechanism of action of allopurinol in reducing stone recurrence rates cannot be definitively attributed to its effect in reducing urinary uric acid.

Hypocitraturia

Hypocitraturia is an important and correctable abnormality associated with nephrolithiasis that exists as an isolated abnormality in up to 10% of calcium stone formers and is associated with other abnormalities in 20% to 60% of stone formers (Levy et al., 1995; Pak, 1994). Citrate is an important inhibitor that can reduce calcium stone formation by several mechanisms. First, citrate reduces urinary saturation of calcium salts by complexing with calcium (Pak et al., 1982). Second, citrate directly prevents spontaneous nucleation of calcium oxalate (Sakhaee et al., 1987). Third, citrate inhibits agglomeration and sedimentation of calcium oxalate crystals (Kok et al., 1986; Tiselius et al., 1993a, 1993b), as well as the growth of calcium oxalate and calcium phosphate crystals (Meyer and Smith, 1975). Finally, normal urinary citrate levels can enhance the inhibitory effect of Tamm-Horsfall glycoprotein (Hess et al., 1993).

Hypocitraturia is defined as a urinary citrate level less than 320 mg/day. **Acid-base state is the primary determinant of urinary citrate excretion. Metabolic acidosis reduces urinary citrate levels secondary to enhanced renal tubular reabsorption and decreased synthesis of citrate in peritubular cells** (Hamm, 1990). A study comparing normal subjects and stone formers noted comparable mean serum citrate levels and filtered citrate loads in the two groups; however, 24-hour urinary citrate and the fasting citrate-to-creatinine ratio was significantly reduced and mean tubular reabsorption of citrate was significantly increased in the stone formers compared with control subjects (Minisola et al., 1989).

Indirect evidence for a primarily renal cause of hypocitraturia comes from a study comparing intestinal absorption of citrate in idiopathic hypocitraturic stone formers and normal subjects (Fegan et al., 1992). Oral ingestion of citrate was followed by rapid and efficient absorption in both groups, with 96% to 98% absorbed within 3 hours. As such, hypocitraturia is unlikely to arise from impaired gastrointestinal absorption of citrate in stone formers without overt bowel disease.

Low urinary citrate results from a variety of pathologic states associated with acidosis. Distal RTA is characterized by high urine pH (>6.8), high serum chloride, and low serum bicarbonate and potassium (Preminger et al., 1985). The inability to acidify urine in response to an oral acid (ammonium chloride) load confirms the diagnosis of RTA. Chronic diarrheal states cause intestinal alkali loss in the stool with subsequent systemic acidosis and hypocitraturia (Rudman et al., 1980). Excessive animal protein intake can provide an acid load, reducing citrate levels (Breslau et al., 1988). Indeed, a metabolic study evaluating the effect of a high-protein, low-carbohydrate diet demonstrated a significant reduction in urinary citrate and pH, likely as a result of low citrus and high animal protein intake (Reddy et al., 2002). Diuretics such as thiazides induce hypokalemia and intracellular acidosis (Nicar et al., 1984). Angiotensin-converting enzymes can cause hypocitraturia independently of systemic acidosis or hypokalemia, perhaps as a result of intracellular acidosis (Melnick et al., 1998). Finally, strenuous exercise may induce lactic acidosis (Sakhaee et al., 1987). However, hypocitraturia may also represent an isolated abnormality unrelated to an acidotic state.

Citrate levels in the urine increase in alkalotic states, as well as with elevated levels of PTH, estrogen, magnesium, calcitonin, and vitamin D (Hamm and Hering-Smith, 2002).

Low Urine pH

At low urine pH (<5.5), the undissociated form of uric acid predominates, leading to uric acid and/or calcium stone formation. Calcium oxalate stones form as a result of heterogeneous nucleation with uric acid crystals (Coe and Kavalach, 1974; Pak et al., 1974). Any disorder leading to low urine pH may predispose to stone formation. Chronic metabolic acidosis can lead to low urine pH, hypercalciuria, and hypocitraturia. Acidosis increases bone resorption and produces renal calcium leak (Lemann, 1999; Lemann et al., 2003). Idiopathic low urine pH, previously referred to as "gouty diathesis," refers to stone-forming propensity characterized by low urine pH of unknown cause with or without associated gouty arthritis (Levy et al., 1995).

Renal Tubular Acidosis

RTA is a clinical syndrome characterized by metabolic acidosis resulting from defects in renal tubular hydrogen ion secretion or bicarbonate reabsorption. There are three types of RTA: 1, 2, and 4. **Type 1 (distal) RTA is of particular significance to urologists not only because it is the most common form of RTA but also because it is the form of RTA most frequently associated with stone formation,** which occurs in up to 70% of affected individuals (Van den Berg et al., 1983). Indeed, symptoms associated with nephrolithiasis led to the initial diagnosis of RTA in upward of 50% of cases (Van den Berg et al., 1983).

Acid-base balance is maintained by the kidney through several mechanisms involving the proximal and distal nephron. Because bicarbonate is freely filtered at the glomerulus, the **kidney must reabsorb or regenerate nearly all of the filtered bicarbonate each day** ($\approx$4500 mmol) to maintain its buffering capacity, a process that takes place primarily in the proximal renal tubule (Pohlman et al., 1984). **Furthermore, the kidney must excrete excess acid,** which accumulates from the breakdown of carbohydrates, fats, and proteins and as a result of bicarbonate loss in the stool. Net acid excretion occurs in the distal renal tubule. A defect in either bicarbonate reabsorption or acid excretion will lead to metabolic acidosis.

Filtered bicarbonate (HCO_3^-) is almost completely reabsorbed in the proximal renal tubule through an indirect mechanism involving hydrogen (H^+) secretion (Laing et al., 2005). Carbonic anhydrase in the tubular cells generates H^+ and HCO_3^-, thereby providing H^+ ions that are secreted into the tubular lumen by way of a Na^+,H^+ exchanger in the apical membrane. Sodium (Na^+) pumped out of the proximal tubule cell by the sodium-potassium adenosine triphosphatase (Na^+,K^+-ATPase) exchanger located in the basolateral membrane drives the Na^+,H^+ exchanger in the apical membrane by reducing intracellular sodium. At the same time, HCO_3^- is transferred via a basolateral Na^+,HCO_3^- cotransporter into the plasma. Additional active H^+ secretion into the tubular lumen is accomplished by an apical H^+-ATPase. Luminal H^+ ion combines with filtered HCO_3^- to form H_2CO_3, which is rapidly converted by another form of carbonic anhydrase to H_2O and CO_2, which diffuses back in to the cell. **The net effect is transepithelial HCO_3^- absorption without causing net H^+ secretion or a significant change in urinary pH.**

The distal nephron is the site of net elimination of H^+, although 5% to 10% of filtered bicarbonate is also reabsorbed there in a manner similar to the proximal nephron. **Hydrogen binds with urinary buffers such as titratable acid (mainly phosphate) and ammonia, allowing net elimination of hydrogen in the form of NH_4^+. H^+ excretion occurs through active secretion from α-intercalated cells.** These cells secrete H^+ into the distal tubule using H^+-ATPase and a H^+,K^+-ATPase exchanger (Laing et al., 2005). The intercalated cells also have a Cl^-,HCO_3^- anion exchanger that transports HCO_3^- into the blood. **These active pumps generate a 1000:1 hydrogen ion gradient between the cell and the tubular lumen, allowing reduction of urine pH to as low as 4.5** (Kinkead and Menon, 1995). Another contributing factor is the lack of luminal carbonic anhydrase that prevents the rapid dissociation of carbonic acid catalyzed by the enzyme.

Distal and proximal RTA occurs as a result of impairment of net excretion of acid into the urine (distal or type 1) or of reabsorption of bicarbonate (proximal or type 2). Distinction between these abnormalities provides the basis for classification of RTA into proximal or distal, although both share the characteristic findings of hyperchloremic metabolic acidosis associated with inappropriately high urinary pH.

Type 1 (Distal) Renal Tubular Acidosis. **Type 1 RTA comprises a syndrome of abnormal collecting duct function characterized by inability to acidify the urine in the presence of systemic acidosis.** The classic findings include hypokalemic, hyperchloremic, non–anion gap metabolic acidosis along with nephrolithiasis, nephrocalcinosis, and elevated urine pH (>6.0). Patients with incomplete RTA also demonstrate defective renal acid excretion manifested as failure to lower urine pH below 5.5 after an acid load, but they do not manifest metabolic acidosis and consequently have normal serum electrolytes (Osther et al., 1989).

The most common stone composition associated with distal RTA is calcium phosphate as a result of **hypercalciuria, hypocitraturia, and increased urinary pH** (Pohlman et al., 1984; Van den Berg et al., 1983). The metabolic acidosis promotes bone demineralization, which leads to secondary hyperparathyroidism and hypercalciuria. **Profound hypocitraturia, perhaps the most important factor in stone formation in this setting, is due to impaired citrate excretion as a result of metabolic acidosis** but may also be related to abnormal renal tubular citrate transport or migration of citrate into the mitochondria as a result of intracellular acidosis (Kinkead and Menon, 1995; Osther et al., 1989).

Distal RTA is a heterogeneous disorder that may be hereditary, idiopathic, or acquired, and although most cases are sporadic, autosomal dominant and autosomal recessive patterns of inheritance have been identified (Laing et al., 2005). The inherited forms of distal RTA are associated with growth retardation, nephrocalcinosis, renal calculi, and hypokalemic metabolic acidosis. The autosomal recessive form of the disease is more severe, tends to occur earlier in life, and is associated with mental retardation and sensorineural hearing loss. Children make up one-third of affected individuals and often experience vomiting or diarrhea, failure to thrive, or growth retardation. Secondary distal RTA occurs in association with autoimmune diseases such as Sjögren syndrome and systemic lupus erythematosus, or it may occur with obstructive uropathy, pyelonephritis, acute tubular necrosis, hyperparathyroidism, and idiopathic hypercalciuria.

Distal RTA occurs as a consequence of dysfunction of the α-type intercalated cells, which secrete protons into the urine via an apical H^+-ATPase that is coupled to an anion exchanger (AE1) located at the basolateral membrane (Fig. 91.11; Karet, 2002). Mutations in three genes in the α-type intercalated cells have been implicated in hereditary distal RTA; *SLC4A1* encodes the AE1 Cl^-,HCO_3^- anion exchanger, and *ATP6V1B1* and *ATP6V0A4* encode the B1 and A4 subunits, respectively, of H^+-ATPase. A fourth gene, *CA2*, encodes carbonic anhydrase II, which is found in the proximal tubule, the loop of Henle, and the α-intercalated cells of the collecting duct. Because carbonic anhydrase II affects bicarbonate reabsorption as

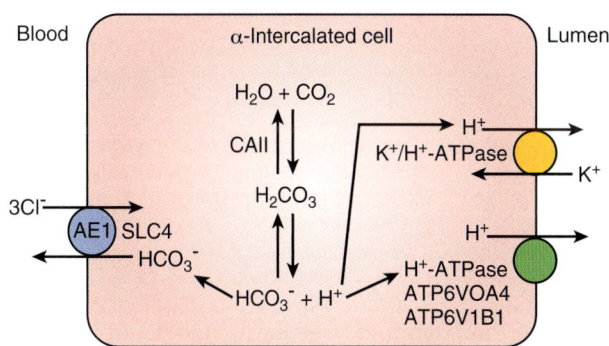

Fig. 91.11. Mechanism of acidification in the collecting duct α-intercalated cell. The α-intercalated cells secrete H^+ into the lumen of the distal tubule and collecting duct by way of an apical H^+-ATPase and possibly an H^+,K^+-ATPase exchanger. Bicarbonate is transported into the blood via a Cl^-,HCO_3^- anion exchanger (AE1) on the basolateral membrane. Defects in the AE1 Cl^-,HCO_3^- anion exchanger or in H^+-ATPase result in failure to acidify the urine in distal RTA. *CAII*, Carbonic anhydrase II.

well as H+ secretion, mutations in *CA2* present a mixed pattern of proximal and distal RTA (Batlle and Haque, 2012).

Mutations in the *SLC4A1* gene are most commonly associated with the autosomal dominant form of distal RTA, which can present in the complete or incomplete form. Hearing loss is not usually a feature of mutations in the *SLC4A1* gene (Batlle and Haque, 2012). Mutations in the *ATP6V1B1* and *ATP6V0A4* genes encoding H+-ATPase have been primarily associated with autosomal recessive distal RTA (Batlle et al., 2006). Recent findings suggest that incomplete distal RTA may be the result of a hypofunctional vacuolar-type H+-ATPAase in heterozygous carriers of a mutation in the B1 subunit (Dhayat et al., 2016; Zhang et al., 2014) of the transporter. Finally, *CA2* mutations are recessive and lead to a mixed proximal-distal RTA picture characterized by bicarbonate wasting, inability to acidify the urine below pH 5.5, and reduced NH_4^+ excretion (Batlle and Haque, 2012).

Type 2 (Proximal) Renal Tubular Acidosis. Proximal RTA is characterized by a defect in HCO_3^- reabsorption associated with initial high urine pH that normalizes as plasma HCO_3^- decreases and the amount of filtered HCO_3^- falls (Laing et al., 2005). With reduced capacity of the proximal tubule to reclaim filtered HCO_3^-, more HCO_3^- is delivered to the distal tubule, which has a limited capacity for bicarbonate reabsorption. Consequently, bicarbonaturia ensues, resulting in reduced net acid excretion and metabolic acidosis. As the filtered HCO_3^- load declines with progressive metabolic acidosis, less bicarbonate reaches the distal tubule until eventually the capacity of the distal tubule is sufficient to handle the load and no further bicarbonate is lost. At steady state, serum HCO_3^- is low (15 to 18 mEq/L) and urine pH is acidic (<5.5).

This syndrome is usually associated with generalized defects in proximal tubule function similar to Fanconi syndrome, with loss of glycogen, protein, uric acid, and phosphate (Rocher and Tannen, 1986). The clinical manifestations of proximal RTA include growth retardation and hypokalemia in children resulting from metabolic acidosis. **Nephrolithiasis is uncommon in this disorder because of relatively normal urinary citrate excretion** (Laing et al., 2005).

Type 4 (Distal) Renal Tubular Acidosis. Type 4 RTA is associated with chronic renal damage, usually seen in patients with interstitial renal disease and diabetic nephropathy. Reduction in glomerular filtration results in hyperkalemic, hyperchloremic metabolic acidosis caused by loss of HCO_3^- in the urine and decreased excretion of ammonium (Pohlman et al., 1984). Aldosterone resistance is commonly associated with type 4 RTA (Davidman and Schmitz, 1988). Because aldosterone contributes to stimulation of distal acidification and H+,K+ exchange, aldosterone resistance results in decreased ammonia generation and further exacerbates hyperkalemia (Davidman and Schmitz, 1988). Patients with type 4 RTA can still generate acidic urine in response to an acid challenge.

Renal stone formation is uncommon in patients with type 4 RTA. **The protection against renal stone formation in these patients may be attributed to reduced renal excretion of stone-forming substances such as calcium and uric acid because of impaired renal function** (Uribarri et al., 1994).

Hypomagnesiuria

Hypomagnesiuria is a rare cause of nephrolithiasis, affecting less than 1% of stone formers as an isolated abnormality, although it can be found in conjunction with other abnormalities in 6% to 11% of cases (Levy et al., 1995; Schwartz et al., 2001). **Magnesium complexes with oxalate and calcium salts, and therefore low magnesium levels result in reduced inhibitory activity. Low urinary magnesium is also associated with decreased urinary citrate levels, which may further contribute to stone formation** (Preminger et al., 1989; Schwartz et al., 2001). Whether low magnesium is the cause or effect of low citrate is not clear. Low magnesium levels occur with poor dietary intake or as a result of reduced intestinal absorption associated with intestinal abnormalities producing chronic diarrheal syndrome.

Although a number of studies in rats have implicated hypomagnesiuria as a factor in stone formation (Rushton and Spector, 1982), others (Borden and Lyon, 1969; Faragalla and Gershoff, 1963; Rattan et al., 1993) have questioned the impact of magnesium (Su et al., 1991). Clinical studies regarding the role of magnesium are contradictory. Schwartz et al. (2001) found that hypomagnesiuric patients had higher stone recurrence rates than patients with normal urinary magnesium. However, other studies found no difference in magnesium excretion between stone patients and controls (Esen et al., 1991; Johansson et al., 1980). The lack of difference in mean magnesium levels may be a result of the small fraction of stone formers with low urinary magnesium levels.

Although magnesium has been shown to increase urinary pH, citrate, and magnesium levels and therefore to decrease urinary saturation of calcium oxalate in vitro (Khan et al., 1993) and in vivo (Curhan et al., 2001), two randomized trials comparing magnesium oxide with placebo or no treatment in stone formers failed to demonstrate clinical benefit (Ettinger et al., 1988; Wilson et al., 1984).

Uric Acid Stones

Most mammals, except humans and Dalmatians, synthesize the hepatic enzyme uricase, which catalyzes the conversion of uric acid to allantoin, the end product of purine metabolism (Bannasch et al., 2004; Yu, 1981). Consequently, humans accumulate significantly higher levels of uric acid in their blood and urine (Watts, 1976; Yu, 1981). Because allantoin is 10 to 100 times more soluble in urine than uric acid, humans are prone to uric acid stone formation. Uric acid makes up 8% to 10% of all kidney stones in the United States and up to 25% in certain regions in Germany (Maalouf et al., 2004a).

Uric acid is a weak acid with a pK_a of 5.35 at 37°C. At that pH, half the uric acid is present as the urate salt and half as free uric acid. Because sodium urate is approximately 20 times more soluble than the free acid, the relative proportion present as free uric acid strongly determines the risk of stone formation. **Urine pH is a critical factor in determining uric acid solubility**; at pH 5, even modest amounts of uric acid exceed uric acid solubility, whereas at pH 6.5, concentrations of uric acid exceeding 1200 mg/L remain soluble (Fig. 91.12; Asplin, 1996). Under normal conditions, the limit of uric acid solubility is approximately 96 mg/L, a level readily exceeded by normal daily uric acid excretion, which averages 500 to 600 mg/L. Consequently, urine may reach supersaturation, particularly at pH less than 6. Low urine pH increases concentrations of sparingly soluble undissociated uric acid, which leads to direct precipitation of uric acid. Uric acid and sodium urate have been implicated as nidi for calcium oxalate stones through heterogeneous nucleation and epitaxial crystal growth, and thus low urine pH is thought to be a risk factor for uric acid, calcium oxalate, and mixed calcium and uric acid stones (Maalouf, 2011).

The process of uric acid stone formation once uric acid crystals precipitate has not been fully elucidated. Although some investigators have suggested that uric acid crystal adhesion to kidney epithelial cells (Koka et al., 2000) and inhibitors such as glycosaminoglycans (Ombra et al., 2003) may play a role in uric acid stone formation, the involvement or importance of these factors in uric acid stone formation is unclear. No urinary inhibitors of uric acid stones formation have been identified (Doizi et al., 2016).

The three main determinants of uric acid stone formation are low pH, low urine volume, and hyperuricosuria (Fig. 91.13). **The most important pathogenetic factor is low urine pH because most patients with uric acid stones have normal uric acid excretion but invariably demonstrate persistent low urine pH** (Pak et al., 2001; Sakhaee et al., 2002). Uric acid stones can develop as a result of congenital, acquired, or idiopathic causes. Congenital disorders associated with uric acid stones involve renal tubular urate transport or uric acid metabolism, leading to hyperuricosuria. Acquired causes of uric acid stones such as chronic diarrhea, volume depletion, myeloproliferative disorders, high animal protein intake, and uricosuric drugs may affect any of the three factors determining uric acid stone formation. Patients with "gouty diathesis" or idiopathic uric acid nephrolithiasis typically demonstrate decreased fractional excretion of urate and do not have gout (Maalouf et al., 2004a). Patients with idiopathic uric acid nephrolithiasis differ from those with hyperuricosuric calcium nephrolithiasis in that the former

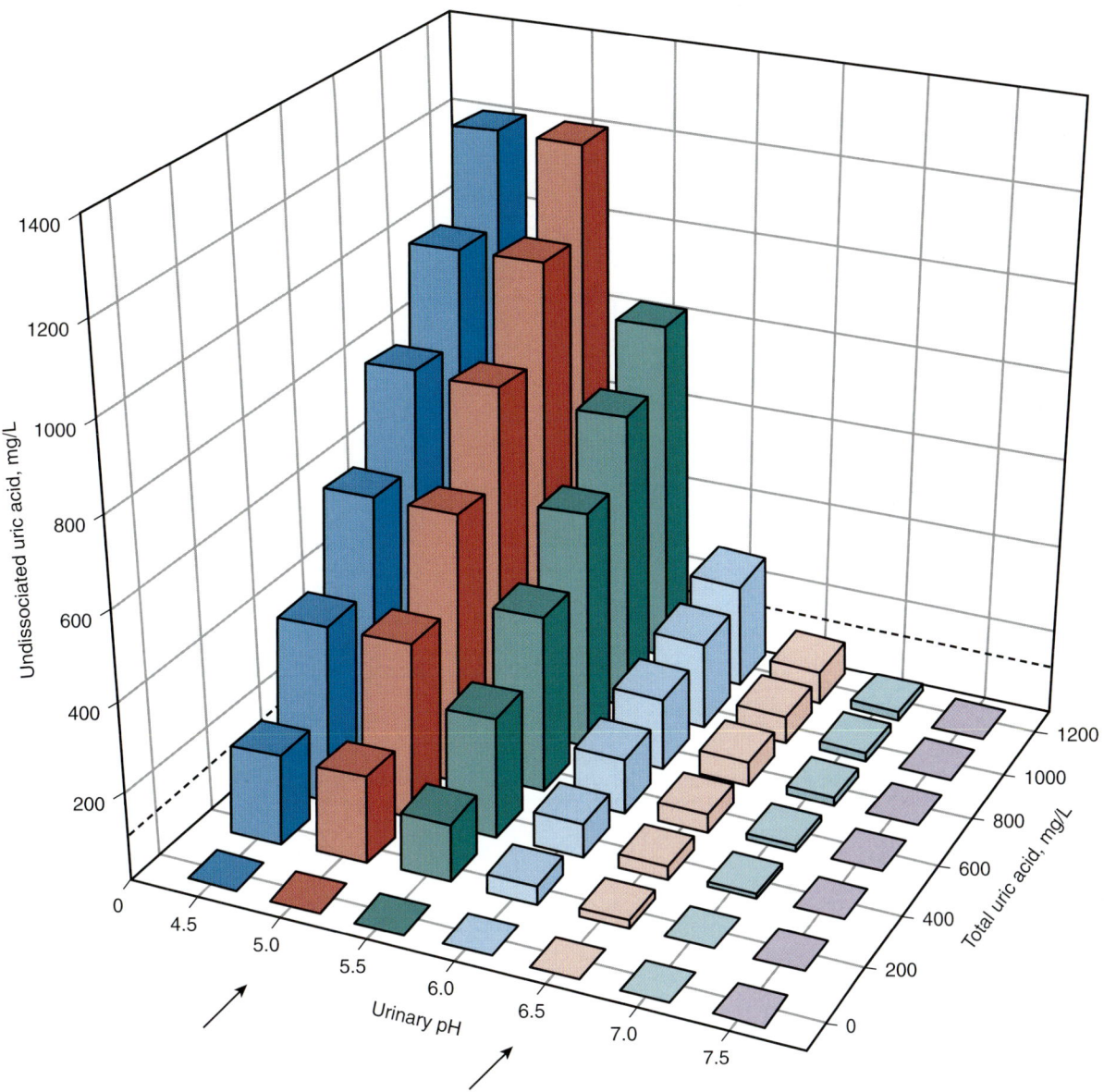

Fig. 91.12. Relationship among undissociated uric acid, total uric acid, and urinary pH. The limit of solubility of undissociated uric acid is depicted by the *dotted line* (≈100 mg/L). Two hypothetical urine pH values are considered *(arrows)*. At low pH (e.g., 5.0), even a modest amount of total urinary uric acid will exceed its solubility. At high pH (e.g., 6.5), even massive hyperuricosuria is well tolerated. (From Maalouf NM, Cameron MA, Moe OW, et al.: Novel insights into the pathogenesis of uric acid nephrolithiasis. *Curr Opin Nephrol Hypertens* 13:181–189, 2004.)

generally have normal urinary uric acid levels and acidic urine, whereas the latter have hyperuricosuria and normal urine pH (Pak et al., 2002). Patients with hyperuricosuria frequently have high urinary sodium and calcium levels leading to increased urinary saturation of sodium urate and calcium oxalate, placing them at risk for calcium oxalate stones (Sorensen and Chandhoke, 2002).

Pathogenesis of Low Urine pH

Although the pathogenesis of low urine pH in idiopathic uric acid stone formers is not known with certainty and may be multifactorial, several potential mechanisms have been proposed. Sakhaee et al. (2002) first observed that normouricosuric individuals with pure uric acid stones were more likely to have diabetes mellitus or to demonstrate glucose intolerance than normal individuals or those with mixed uric acid–calcium oxalate or pure calcium oxalate stones. Furthermore, when a group of normouricosuric uric acid stone formers was placed on a controlled metabolic diet, the urinary pH was lower than that of either normal volunteers or other stone formers (mixed uric acid–calcium oxalate or calcium oxalate). Further investigation revealed that the uric acid stone formers excreted less acid into the urine as ammonium and proportionately more titratable acid and less citrate to maintain normal overall acid-base balance. **This apparent impairment in ammonium excretion in uric acid stone formers has been putatively linked to an insulin-resistant state.**

Supporting this hypothesis, Pak et al. (2003) noted a higher prevalence of uric acid stones and low urinary pH among patients with non–insulin-dependent diabetes mellitus (34%) than among nondiabetic stone formers. Daudon et al. (2006) analyzed 2464 calculi and also found that uric acid stones made up 36% of stones among 272 patients with type 2 diabetes mellitus but only 11% among 2192 patients without type 2 diabetes. Furthermore, uric acid stone formers have been found to share many of the characteristic features of the metabolic syndrome (a condition defined by insulin resistance and high-risk atherosclerotic cardiovascular disease), including hypertriglyceridemia, hyperglycemia, obesity, and

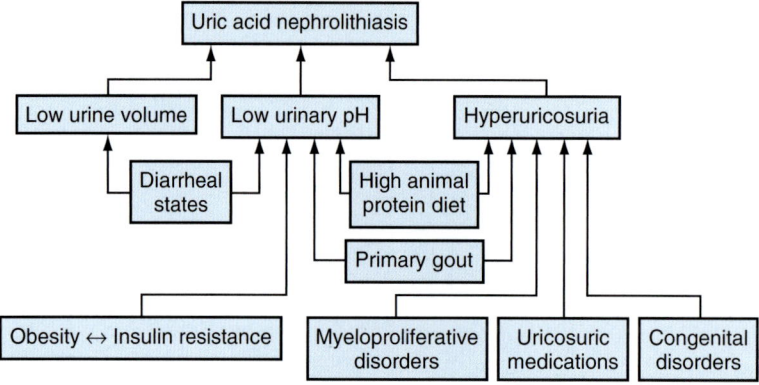

Fig. 91.13. Pathophysiology and etiology of uric acid nephrolithiasis. The three major pathophysiologic mechanisms that contribute to uric acid nephrolithiasis are low urine volume, low urinary pH, and hyperuricosuria. Each of these mechanisms can result from diverse causes. The most important pathogenetic factor is low urinary pH. (From Maalouf NM, Cameron MA, Moe OW, et al.: Novel insights into the pathogenesis of uric acid nephrolithiasis. *Curr Opin Nephrol Hypertens* 13:181–189, 2004.)

hypertension (Pak et al., 2003; Sakhaee et al., 2002). In an elegant series of experiments, Abate et al. (2004) performed hyperinsulinemic euglycemic clamps to measure insulin sensitivity in a diverse group of non–stone-forming normal volunteers and a group of uric acid stone formers and determined that among normal subjects, low urine pH correlated with low rates of glucose disposal (indicating insulin resistance) in both groups, but uric acid stone formers displayed the most severe levels of insulin resistance. This association of insulin resistance with low urinary pH was further corroborated by the finding of a strong inverse association of body weight (known to be associated with peripheral insulin resistance) and urinary pH, even after adjusting for urinary sulfate (a marker of animal protein intake) (Maalouf et al., 2004b).

The mechanism by which insulin resistance leads to low urine pH has not been completely elucidated. However, insulin has been shown in vitro to promote renal ammoniagenesis from the substrate glutamine (Chobanian and Hammerman, 1987; Nissim et al., 1995) and also to stimulate the Na^+, H^+ exchanger (NHE3) in the proximal tubule, which is responsible for either the direct transport or trapping of ammonium in the urine (Klisic et al., 2002). **Impaired ammonium production or excretion as a result of insulin resistance could leave hydrogen ions unbuffered in the urine, thereby leading to reduction in urine pH** (Fig. 91.14).

Acidic urine pH may also be promoted by increased endogenous acid production or by dietary influences. When idiopathic uric acid stone formers and normal subjects were maintained on a fixed, low acid-ash diet, net acid excretion was higher in the former group compared with the latter, implicating higher endogenous acid production (Sakhaee et al., 2002). Furthermore, when controlled for urinary sulfate (a marker of acid intake), net acid excretion was higher in uric acid stone formers and in non–stone formers with type 2 diabetes compared with normal controls (Cameron et al., 2006). These studies suggest that, in the setting of impaired ammonium excretion and increased endogenous acid production resulting from obesity and/or insulin resistance, titratable acids make up the primary urinary buffer, and although acid-base equilibrium can be maintained, it occurs at a lower urine pH than is typically maintained by ammonium, which has a higher pK_a.

Lipotoxicity, a process whereby fat is redistributed into nonadipocyte tissues such as the heart, liver, skeletal muscle, and pancreatic beta cells, resulting in cellular injury, has been implicated in impaired insulin sensitivity, cardiac dysfunction, and hepatic steatohepatitis and has been postulated to play a role in the pathogenesis of chronic renal disease (Bagby, 2004; Wahba and Mak, 2007; Weinberg, 2006). Whether lipotoxicity plays a role in impaired ammonium excretion or increased endogenous acid production leading to low urine pH in uric acid stone formers is unknown (Sakhaee, 2009). However, studies in a rodent model of metabolic syndrome (Zucker diabetic fatty rat) and a proximal tubular cell line demonstrated that renal steatosis may be responsible for the reduced expression and activity of NHE3, the primary mediator of ammonium excretion (Bobulescu et al., 2008, 2009). Interestingly, recent proteomic analysis of the matrix component of uric acid stones identified 242 unique proteins among five stones, with the largest proportion of proteins involved in the inflammation and complement pathways; the most commonly involved metabolic pathways associated with these proteins were the phospholipid and fatty acid pathways (Jou et al., 2012). Finally, in a recent study of 98 stone formers using axial CT imaging to measure visceral fat, multivariable logistic regression analysis revealed that low urine pH (<6) was associated with higher visceral fat area (OR 11.1, 95% CI 2.18–56.3, $P < 0.004$) (Patel et al., 2017). Furthermore, low urine pH (OR 5.87, 95% CI 1.59–58.3, $P = 0.26$) and visceral fat area greater than 48% (OR 5.33, 95% CI 1.05–27.2,

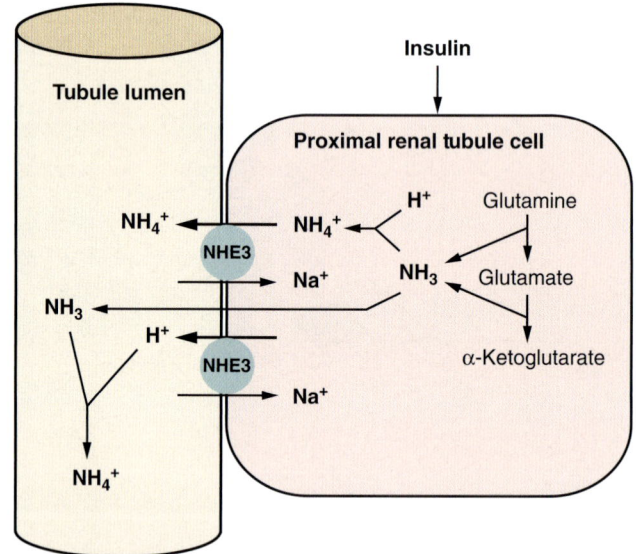

Fig. 91.14. Potential effects of the insulin-resistant state on the generation and secretion of ammonium in the proximal tubule. The deamination of glutamine and glutamate provides ammonia. Insulin stimulates glutamine metabolism, as well as the sodium-hydrogen exchanger NHE3. NHE3 mediates ammonium transport by either directly carrying the ammonium ion or providing the luminal hydrogen ion to trap ammonia. The end product of glutamine metabolism is α-ketoglutarate. (Modified from Maalouf NM, Cameron MA, Moe OW, et al.: Novel insights into the pathogenesis of uric acid nephrolithiasis. *Curr Opin Nephrol Hypertens* 13:181–189, 2004.)

$P = 0.047$) were independently associated with uric acid stone composition.

Dietary content also plays a role in determining urine acidity. Breslau et al. (1988) evaluated 15 normal subjects in a three-way randomized, crossover study involving three 12-day phases of study in which subjects were maintained on a controlled metabolic diet containing vegetable protein, vegetable and egg protein, or animal protein, with increasing sulfate content, respectively, in the three diets. As the fixed acid content of the diets increased, urinary calcium excretion increased from 103 mg/day on the vegetarian diet to 150 mg/day on the animal protein diet ($P < 0.02$). Moreover, the animal protein–rich diet was associated with the highest excretion of undissociated uric acid and lowest excretion of citrate because of the reduction in urinary pH. Urinary crystallization studies revealed that the animal protein diet, when matched for electrolyte composition and quantity of protein with the vegetarian diet, conferred an increased risk of uric acid stones, but because of opposing factors, not of calcium oxalate or calcium phosphate stones.

Hyperuricosuria

Hyperuricosuria is defined as urinary uric acid exceeding 600 mg/day. Hyperuricosuria predisposes to uric acid stone formation by causing supersaturation of the urine with respect to sparingly soluble undissociated uric acid. Patients with gout and urinary uric acid levels less than 600 mg/day had significantly fewer stones than those with uric acid levels greater than 1000 mg/day (Hall et al., 1967; Yu and Gutman, 1967). The causes of hyperuricosuria have been discussed previously but include dietary factors as well as acquired and hereditary diseases and defects in the urate transporter.

Low Urinary Volume

All conditions that contribute to low urinary volume increase the risk of uric acid supersaturation. Borghi et al. (1993) noted high uric acid relative supersaturation in workers exposed to hot temperatures compared with those working in normal temperatures. Likewise, high rates of uric acid stone formation have been found in populations living in warmer climates such as Israel (Shekarriz and Stoller, 2002).

Cystine Stones

Under normal conditions amino acids are freely filtered by the glomerulus and almost completely reabsorbed in the renal proximal tubule. Cystine and the other dibasic amino acids are transported across the apical membrane of the renal proximal tubule and in the jejunum by a sodium-independent heteromeric amino acid transporter (HAT) in exchange for neutral amino acids. The cystine transporter is composed of the rBAT heavy subunit, encoded by *SLC3A1* (Calonge et al., 1994; Pras et al., 1994), which resides on the short arm of chromosome 2, and the bo,+AT light subunit encoded by *SLC7A9* (Feliubadaló et al., 1999) located on the long arm of chromosome 19. The two subunits form a heterodimer that resides in the apical membrane of the proximal tubule cells, and mutations in the genes of either subunit lead to cystinuria. As of 2010, 133 and 95 mutations had been reported in the *SLC3A1* and the *SLC7A9* genes, respectively (Chillaron et al., 2010). Cystinuria is inherited as an autosomal recessive disorder (or rarely autosomal dominant with incomplete penetrance).

Under normal conditions, the fractional excretion of cystine is approximately 0.4% but rises to 100% in cystinuria. Although there is significant loss of other dibasic amino acids, the poor solubility of cystine leads to stone formation. Cystine is a dimer composed of two cysteine molecules linked via a disulfide bond. Cystine is much less soluble than cysteine and is responsible for cystine stone formation. Cystine is reduced intracellularly to cysteine, thereby providing a favorable gradient for continued cystine reabsorption (Broer, 2008). Cystine stones are rare, occurring in the United States and Europe with an incidence of only 1 in 1000 to 1 in 17,000 (Cabello-Tomas et al., 1999; Knoll et al., 2005). In children, cystinuria is the cause of up to 10% of all stones (Erbağci et al., 2003; Faerber, 2001; Knoll et al., 2005).

Several factors determine the solubility of cystine, including cystine concentration, pH, ionic strength, and urinary macromolecules. The main contributor to cystine crystallization is supersaturation because there is no specific inhibitor of cystine crystallization in the urine (Pak and Fuller, 1983). Because of the poor solubility of cystine in urine, precipitation of cystine and subsequent stone formation occur at physiologic urine conditions (Joly et al., 1999). The solubility of cystine is highly pH dependent, with solubilities of 300 mg/L, 400 mg/L, and 1000 mg/L at pH levels of 5, 7, and 9, respectively (Dent and Senior, 1955). Ionic strength also influences solubility, and as much as 70 mg of additional cystine can be dissolved in each liter of solution as ionic strength increases from 0.005 to 0.3 (Pak and Fuller, 1983). Macromolecules such as colloid also increase cystine solubility, although the mechanism is unclear (Pak and Fuller, 1983). Therefore cystine is more soluble in urine than in synthetic solution (Fig. 91.15).

Other factors may contribute to stone formation in cystinuric patients as well. Sakhaee et al. (1989) evaluated 27 patients with documented cystine nephrolithiasis and identified hypercalciuria in 19%, hyperuricosuria in 22%, and hypocitraturia in 44%, which could contribute to formation of not only cystine stones but also calcium or mixed calcium-cystine stones.

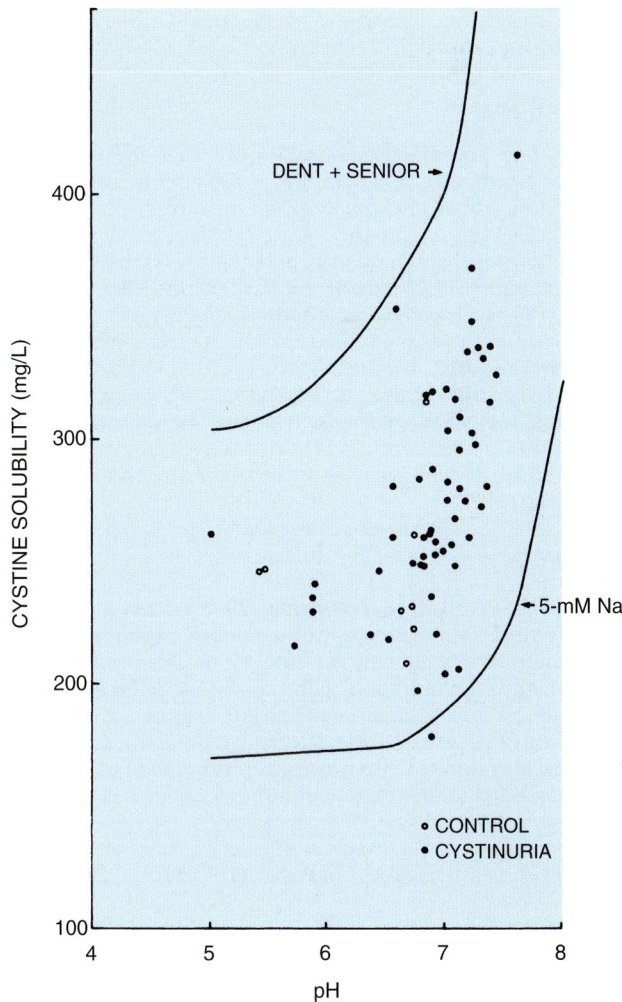

Fig. 91.15. Cystine solubility in urine. Each point represents solubility of cystine determined in a separate urine sample by incubation with an excess of solid cystine. The solubility curve of Dent and Senior (1955) and that obtained in a 5-mM sodium cacodylate solution are plotted for comparison. (From Pak CY, Fuller CJ: Assessment of cystine solubility in urine and of heterogeneous nucleation. *J Urol* 129:1066–1070, 1983.)

Although historically cystinuria was classified on the basis of levels of urinary cystine in obligate heterozygote parents of the proband (Rosenberg et al., 1966), this classification correlated poorly with molecular findings and was subsequently revised by the International Cystinuria Consortium (ICC) to take into account the chromosomal localization of the mutation: type A (chromosome 2), type B (chromosome 19), and type AB (both chromosomes) (Dello Strologo et al., 2002). Homozygotes with the condition exhibit urinary cystine levels as high as 2000 μmol/g of creatinine. Review by the ICC revealed that the average age at first stone diagnosis was 12.2 years, with a mean number of stone episodes of 0.42 and 0.21 per year occurring in men and women, respectively (Dello Strologo et al., 2002). Although mean urinary cystine levels are significantly higher in heterozygotes with type B abnormalities (475 μmol/g creatinine) compared with those with type A abnormalities (70 μmol/g creatinine), there is no difference in stone formation between the two groups, and, in fact, stone formation is uncommon (Dello Strologo et al., 2002).

Although stone formers in general have been found to have a higher likelihood of developing chronic kidney disease (Worcester et al., 2006b), cystine stone formers have been shown to have lower creatinine clearances than other stone formers (Worcester et al., 2006a). A potential explanation for this finding is the observation that cystinuric patients undergo more open surgical procedures, including nephrectomy, than their calcium oxalate stone-forming counterparts (Assimos et al., 2002). Histologically, these patients have been observed to have dilated ducts of Bellini plugged by cystine crystals as well as evidence of cortical glomerulosclerosis and interstitial fibrosis (Evan et al., 2006b).

Infection Stones

Infection stones are composed primarily of magnesium ammonium phosphate hexahydrate ($MgNH_4PO_4 \cdot 6H_2O$) but may in addition contain calcium phosphate in the form of carbonate apatite ($Ca_{10}[PO_4]_6 \cdot CO_3$). A Swedish geologist discovered magnesium ammonium phosphate in guano and named it "struvite" after his mentor, naturalist H.C.G. von Struve (Griffith and Osborne, 1987). Brown (1901) first theorized that bacteria split urea, thereby setting up the condition for stone formation, and he later isolated *Proteus vulgaris* from a stone. Hager and Magath (1925) postulated that a bacterial enzyme hydrolyzed urea, and Sumner (1926) isolated urease from *Canavalia ensiformis*. It is now well established that struvite stones (magnesium ammonium phosphate) occur only in association with urinary infection by urea-splitting bacteria (Griffith and Musher, 1973).

Pathogenesis

The process of urealysis provides an alkaline urinary environment and sufficient concentrations of carbonate and ammonia to induce the formation of infection stones. Because urease is not present in sterile human urine, infection with urease-producing bacteria is a prerequisite for the formation of infection stones. A cascade of chemical reactions generates the conditions conducive to the formation of infection stones. Urinary urea, a constituent of normal urine, is first hydrolyzed to ammonia and carbon dioxide in the presence of bacterial urease:

$$(NH_2)_2CO + H_2O \rightarrow 2NH_3 + CO_2$$

The alkaline urine that results from this reaction (pH 7.2 to 8.0) favors the formation of ammonium:

$$NH_3 + H_2O \rightarrow NH_4^+ + OH^- \ (pK = 9.0)$$

Under physiologic conditions, the alkaline urine would prevent further generation of ammonium. However, in the presence of urease, ammonia continues to be produced, further increasing urinary pH. The alkaline environment also promotes the hydration of carbon dioxide to carbonic acid, which then dissociates into HCO_3^- and

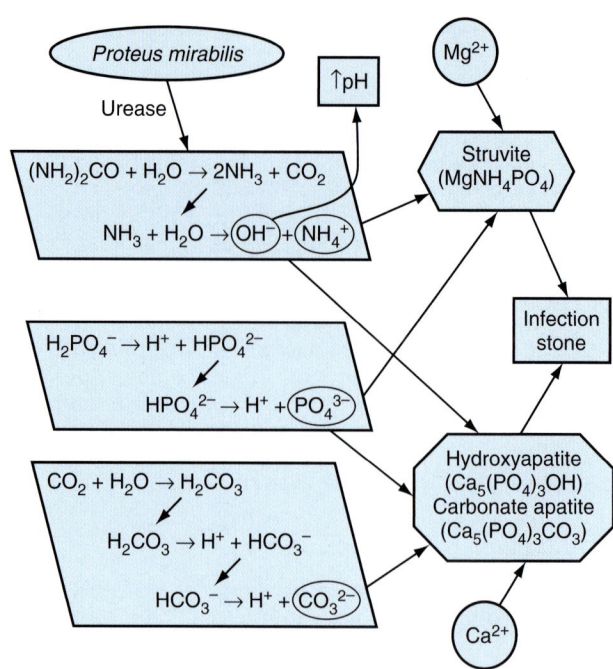

Fig. 91.16. Schematic depicting concurrent events leading to struvite stone formation. (From Johnson DB, Pearle MS: Struvite stones. In Stoller ML, Meng MV, editors: *Urinary stone disease: the practical guide to medical and surgical management*, Totowa, NJ, 2007, Humana Press.)

H^+. Further dissociation of HCO_3^- yields carbonate and another hydrogen ion:

$$CO_2 + H_2O \rightarrow H_2CO_3 \ (pK = 4.5)$$

$$H_2CO_3 \rightarrow H^+ + HCO_3^- \ (pK = 6.3)$$

$$HCO_3^- \rightarrow H^+ + CO_3^{2-} \ (pK = 10.2)$$

The dissociation of hydrogen phosphate under alkaline conditions provides phosphate, thereby completing the generation of constituent ions for infection stone formation:

$$H_2PO_4^- \rightarrow H^+ + HPO_4^{2-} \ (pK = 7.2)$$

$$HPO_4^{2-} \rightarrow H^+ + PO_4^{3-} \ (pK = 12.4)$$

This chemical cascade, along with physiologic concentrations of magnesium, provides the constituents necessary for precipitation of struvite. In addition, the concentrations of calcium, phosphate, and carbonate allow precipitation of carbonate apatite and hydroxyapatite, thereby composing the components of infection stones (Fig. 91.16).

Although infection stones are a direct result of persistent or recurrent infection with urease-producing bacteria, they may also be associated with or exacerbated by urinary obstruction or stasis (Bichler et al., 2002). Therefore growth of infection stones can progress at a rapid rate.

Bacteriology

Although the family Enterobacteriaceae makes up the majority of urease-producing pathogens, a variety of gram-positive and gram-negative bacteria and some yeasts and *Mycoplasma* species have the capacity to synthesize urease (Table 91.3). **The most common urease-producing pathogens are *Proteus*, *Klebsiella*, *Pseudomonas*, and *Staphylococcus* species, with *Proteus mirabilis* the most common organism associated with infection stones.** Although *Escherichia coli* is a common cause of urinary tract infections, only rare species of *E. coli* produce urease (Bichler et al., 2002). A recent multicenter

TABLE 91.3 Organisms That May Produce Urease

ORGANISMS	USUALLY (>90% OF ISOLATES)	OCCASIONALLY (5%–30% OF ISOLATES)
Gram-negative	*Proteus rettgeri* *Proteus vulgaris* *Proteus mirabilis* *Proteus morganii* *Providencia stuartii* *Haemophilus influenzae* *Bordetella pertussis* *Bacteroides corrodens* *Yersinia enterocolitica* *Brucella* species	*Klebsiella pneumoniae* *Klebsiella oxytoca* *Serratia marcescens* *Haemophilus parainfluenzae* *Bordetella bronchiseptica* *Aeromonas hydrophila* *Pseudomonas aeruginosa* *Pasteurella* species
Gram-positive	*Flavobacterium* species *Staphylococcus aureus* *Micrococcus* *Corynebacterium ulcerans* *Corynebacterium renale* *Corynebacterium ovis* *Corynebacterium hofmannii*	*Staphylococcus epidermidis* *Bacillus* species *Corynebacterium murium* *Corynebacterium equi* *Peptococcus asaccharolyticus* *Clostridium tetani* *Mycobacterium rhodochrous* group
Mycoplasma	T-strain *Mycoplasma* *Ureaplasma urealyticum*	
Yeasts	*Cryptococcus* *Rhodotorula* *Sporobolomyces* *Candida humicola* *Trichosporon cutaneum*	

From Gleeson MJ, Griffith DP: Infection stones. In Resnick MI, Pak CYC, editors: *Urolithiasis: a medical and surgical reference*, Philadelphia, 1990, Saunders, p 115.

review of 121 struvite and/or carbonate apatite stones obtained from patients undergoing surgical intervention for stones at four participating centers revealed preoperative urine cultures that grew *Proteus* species in 11.3% and *E. coli* in 15.2% of cases (Flannigan et al., 2018)

Bacteria may be involved in stone formation by damaging the mucosal layer of the urinary tract, resulting in increased bacterial colonization and crystal adherence (Djojodimedjo et al., 2013; Grenabo et al., 1988; Parsons et al., 1984). It has been proposed that ammonium, generated as a result of urealysis, may alter the glycosaminoglycan layer present on the surface of the transitional cell layer and significantly increase bacterial adherence to normal bladder mucosa, further exacerbating infection risk (Parsons et al., 1984). In addition, a study in rats found that injury to the bladder mucosa increased crystal adherence to the bladder wall, a process that was potentiated by the presence of common bacteria such as *Proteus*, *E. coli*, *Enterococcus*, and *Ureaplasma urealyticum* (Grenabo et al., 1988). Another potential mechanism for increased stone formation in the presence of bacteria is the finding that particular bacteria, such as *E. coli* and *Proteus*, may alter the activity of urokinase and sialidase, whereas organisms not typically associated with infection stones do not (du Toit et al., 1992). This altered enzymatic activity may explain the frequent association of *E. coli* with stone formation despite lacking urease activity (Holmgren et al., 1989).

Epidemiology

Although infection stones account for only 5% to 15% of all stones (Levy et al., 1995), they have been thought to be the most common component of staghorn calculi. However, a recent analysis of the composition of 52 staghorn calculi demonstrated that only 44% of stones were infection stones, whereas 56% of stones were metabolic, with calcium phosphate the most common (Viprakasit et al., 2011). Moreover, struvite–carbonate apatite was the most common stone composition among a population of African-American stone formers in Ohio, accounting for one-third of stones in males and nearly half of stones in females in this population (Sarmina et al., 1987). **Because infection stones occur most commonly in those prone to frequent urinary tract infections, struvite stones occur more often in women than men by a ratio of 2 : 1** (Resnick, 1981). Other populations at risk of recurrent infection include the elderly (Kohri et al., 1991), premature infants or infants born with congenital urinary tract malformation, patients with diabetes, and those with urinary stasis as a result of urinary tract obstruction, urinary diversion, or neurologic disorders. Spinal cord–injured patients are at particular risk for infection and metabolic stones because of neurogenic urinary tract dysfunction and hypercalciuria related to immobility. Patients with a functionally complete cord transection are at highest risk of developing a staghorn calculus (DeVivo et al., 1984).

Miscellaneous Stones

Xanthine and Dihydroxyadenine Stones

Autosomal recessive disorders of purine metabolism have been implicated in stone disease. Deficiencies of the enzymes adenine phosphoribosyltransferase (APRT) and xanthine dehydrogenase (XDH) lead to an accumulation of precursors immediately proximal to the site of enzyme action (Rumsby, 2016). XDH deficiency results in accumulation of xanthine and APRT deficiency leads to accumulation of adenine which is metabolized to 2,8-dihydroxyadenine (DHA) by XDH. Xanthine and DHA stones are highly insoluble and completely radiolucent, often resulting in them being mistaken for uric acid stones. Accumulation of DHA leads to stone formation and obstructive nephropathy or crystalline nephritis.

Allopurinol, which inhibits XDH and is consequently used to treat hyperuricemia and hyperuricosuria, can, at high levels, predispose to xanthine stones. This side effect is distinctly uncommon because the drug causes only partial inhibition of the enzyme and rarely reduces serum uric acid to levels lower than 3 mg/dL. Patients with Lesch-Nyhan syndrome who suffer from an inherited deficiency of the purine salvage enzyme HGPRT are occasionally treated with high enough doses of allopurinol to place them at risk for xanthine stones (Cameron et al., 1993).

Children with inherited deficiencies of APRT in infancy can have renal complications and stones (Cameron et al., 1993). The APRT enzyme is encoded by *APRT*, a gene on the long arm of chromosome 16 (16q24) (Fratini et al., 1986). More than 40 mutations have been described, including Met136Thr, which is common in Japanese individuals (Kamatani et al., 1992), whereas a single T insertion in a splice donor site in intron 4 was the most common mutation (40%) in a French cohort (Bollée et al., 2010). Children with APRT deficiency may be difficult to distinguish from those with HGPRT deficiency because the insoluble product excreted, 2,8-dihydroxyadenine, is chemically similar to uric acid. Like xanthine stones, 2,8-dihydroxyadenine stones are extremely insoluble at any pH, but stone formation can be averted by the administration of allopurinol.

Ammonium Acid Urate Stones

Ammonium acid urate stones represent about 1% of all stones (Pichette et al., 1997; Soble et al., 1999). In developing countries, however, endemic ammonium acid urate urolithiasis is still observed because it makes up bladder calculi in children (Vanwaeyenbergh et al., 1995).

Ammonium urate stones are radiolucent and occur in patients with chronic diarrhea, inflammatory bowel disease, ileostomy bowel diversions, laxative abuse, recurrent urinary tract infection, and recurrent uric acid stone formation (Dick et al., 1990; Pichette et al., 1997; Soble et al., 1999). Soble et al. (1999) reviewed their experience with 44 patients identified as having stones composed of ammonium acid urate, although the ammonium acid urate contribution varied from 2% to 60%. Among these patients, 25% had a history of inflammatory bowel disease, 14% had a history of significant laxative abuse, 41% were morbidly obese, 36% had a history of recurrent urinary tract infections, and 21% had a history of recurrent uric acid stones. The subgroup of patients with inflammatory bowel disease and ileostomy as the sole clinical risk factor had the highest mean ammonium acid urate content (39%), and ammonium acid urate constituted the predominant stone type in seven of eight such patients. In a more contemporary series Lomas et al. (2017) identified 111 ammonium acid urate stones in 89 patients and found 22% had a history of prostate surgery with bladder neck contracture. They found no association with laxative use.

Patients with ileostomy after colectomy have markedly reduced urinary volume, pH, and sodium and are not prone to hyperoxaluria as are other individuals with bowel disease because the colon is the main site of dietary oxalate absorption (Kennedy et al., 1982). Therefore these patients are prone to ammonium acid urate and uric acid stones rather than calcium oxalate stones. **The underlying pathophysiologic mechanism of ammonium acid urate stone formation attributable to laxative abuse has been postulated to be dehydration resulting from gastrointestinal fluid loss, causing intracellular acidosis and enhanced ammonia excretion. Because urinary sodium is low in the setting of laxative use, urate complexes with abundant ammonia, thereby leading to urinary supersaturation of ammonium acid urate.**

Bowyer et al. (1979) demonstrated that ammonium acid urate precipitation is favored at pH 6.2 to 6.3. The association of recurrent uric acid stones with ammonium acid urate stones is likely related to the shared risk factors of low urine volume and pH. Soble et al. (1999) identified nine patients with stones of mixed composition, containing uric acid and ammonium acid urate (mean ammonium acid urate content 27%), although 8 of the 9 patients had uric acid as the predominant constituent (range 40% to 95%). They theorized that transient fluctuations in urinary acidity and ammonium and sodium levels may shift the balance between uric acid and sodium- or ammonium-bound urate excretion.

Among the ammonium acid urate stone producers in the study by Soble et al. (1999), obesity (BMI >30) was the most prevalent characteristic in 41% of patients, after excluding patients with inflammatory bowel disease and ileostomy (none of whom was obese). Indeed, a statistically significant correlation was found between BMI and ammonium acid urate content. This is consistent with recent evidence suggesting a correlation between stone risk and obesity (Powell et al., 2000) and between obesity and low urine pH (Maalouf et al., 2004b).

Matrix Stones

The association between urinary proteins and stone formation has long been recognized. Early experiments demonstrated that protein suspensions could promote calcium stone formation (Kimura et al., 1976). Osteopontin and calprotectin have been shown to play a role in forming the matrix structure of urinary calcium stones (Kleinman et al., 2004; Tawada et al., 1999). However, stones composed predominantly of matrix are rare; these "stones" are typically radiolucent and may be mistaken for tumor or uric acid stones depending on the imaging study obtained (Bani-Hani et al., 2005).

The literature regarding matrix stones is sparse, consisting mostly of anecdotal case reports (Allen and Spence, 1966; Bani-Hani et al., 2005; Boyce and King, 1963). The matrix component of calcium-based stones makes up only 2.5% of the dry weight of the stone, whereas pure matrix stones may contain more than 65% protein (Allen and Spence, 1966). Boyce and Garvey (1956) determined that the composition of matrix stones was approximately two-thirds mucoprotein and one-third mucopolysaccharide by weight. Furthermore, they found that the matrix substance in crystalline calculi is closely related to the matrix substance found in matrix calculi. However, it is unclear why some matrix calculi fail to fully calcify. Although some have theorized that reduced urinary calcium levels may account for the preferential formation of matrix stones (Allen and Spence, 1966; Boyce and King, 1959), a recent metabolic evaluation of five patients with matrix stones revealed normal urinary calcium excretion (Bani-Hani et al., 2005). In renal failure patients undergoing dialysis, proteinuria may contribute to an increased risk of matrix stone formation. In these patients, matrix stones have been shown to include microfibrillar protein (Bommer et al., 1979) and β_2-microglobulin (Linke et al., 1986). Recent analysis of the matrix stone from a single patient with *Proteus* urinary tract infection by scanning electron microscopy revealed fibrous netlike laminations containing bacterial, cellular, and crystalline material (Canales et al., 2009). Proteomic analysis identified 33 unique proteins, of which 90% had not been previously reported as components of matrix stones and 70% are considered inflammatory or defensive.

Medication-Related Stones

Drug-induced stones form either directly as a result of precipitation and crystallization of a drug or its metabolite or indirectly by altering the urinary environment, making it favorable for metabolic stone formation (Daudon, 1999). Drugs such as loop diuretics (furosemide, bumetanide) and carbonic anhydrase inhibitors (acetazolamide, topiramate, and zonisamide) contribute to calcium stone formation (Matlaga et al., 2003). Ephedrine (Assimos et al., 1999; Powell et al., 1998), triamterene (Carr et al., 1990; Ettinger et al., 1980), guaifenesin (Assimos et al., 1999), silicate (Farrer and Rajfer, 1984), indinavir (Bruce et al., 1997; Gentle et al., 1997), and ciprofloxacin (Matlaga et al., 2003) have been associated with stones composed of the drug in patients who consumed excessive amounts.

Medications That Directly Promote Stone Formation
Antiretroviral Agents. Indinavir sulfate is a protease inhibitor that has been shown to be effective in increasing CD4+ cell counts and decreasing HIV-RNA titers in patients infected with human immunodeficiency virus (HIV) or who have acquired immunodeficiency syndrome (Wu and Stoller, 2000). However, indinavir poses a risk for indinavir stone formation in treated patients, leading to an estimated incidence of 4% to 13% (Wu and Stoller, 2000). Indinavir is rapidly absorbed from the intestine, achieving peak plasma

concentrations in less than 1 hour. The drug is metabolized in the liver and eliminated primarily in the stool, but about half of the ingested dose of indinavir is excreted essentially unchanged in the urine (Sutherland et al., 1997). In pure form, indinavir is relatively insoluble in aqueous solution, although the solubility is pH dependent. With a pK_a of 5.5, indinavir has a solubility of 0.300 mg/mL at pH 5, 0.035 mg/mL at pH 6.0, and 0.020 mg/mL at pH 7.0 (Daudon et al., 1997; Hermieu et al., 1999). Although indinavir solubility increases significantly at pH levels below 5.5, the standard dose of indinavir in an individual with an average urine volume and pH would produce a urinary concentration of indinavir near the limit of solubility 3 hours after ingestion (Daudon et al., 1997). As such, **individuals taking indinavir on a regular basis are at high risk of producing indinavir stones because of the high urinary excretion and poor solubility of the drug at physiologic urinary pH.** Initiation of indinavir in 54 asymptomatic, indinavir-naive, HIV-positive individuals led to indinavir crystalluria in 67% of subjects (Gagnon et al., 2000). After the first 2 weeks, indinavir crystalluria remained constant at a frequency of approximately 25% of urine sediments examined at each test point.

Indinavir is now an infrequently used antiretroviral agent, replaced with newer generation agents. Kidney stone formation has been associated with a number of newer antiretroviral agents, including lopinavir-ritonavir (Doco-Lecompte et al., 2004), ritonavir-boosted atazanavir (Hamada et al., 2012; Rockwood et al., 2011), nelfinavir (Engeler et al., 2002), and amprenavir (Feicke et al., 2008). Ritonavir-boosted atazanavir, currently one of the more widely used agents, has been shown to have a nearly 7% incidence of stone formation, higher than most of the other new agents (Hamada et al., 2012; Rockwood et al., 2011). Because stone formation associated with these agents is thought to be the result of high urinary excretion and low solubility of the drug in urine, agents with higher excretion rates are associated with higher rates of stone formation; 7% of ritonavir-boosted atazanavir is excreted in the urine unmetabolized versus less than 3% for nelfinavir and amprenavir, which have lower rates of stone formation.

Triamterene. Triamterene is a potassium-sparing diuretic commonly used for the treatment of hypertension. It is an uncommon stone composition, accounting for only 0.4% of 50,000 calculi in one report, with only one-third of the stones composed largely or entirely of triamterene (Ettinger et al., 1980). An evaluation of triamterene stone formers revealed no significant differences between patients and matched control subjects with respect to total recovery of the drug, hourly excretion patterns, and urinary concentrations of triamterene and its sulfate metabolite (Ettinger, 1985). Approximately half of all subjects tested demonstrated urine concentrations of the sulfate metabolite that exceeded the observed solubility limit. One investigation determined that triamterene is more likely to become incorporated into existing stones or stone nidi than to promote stone formation independently (Werness et al., 1982). This may account for the rarity of this stone in nonrecurrent stone formers, as well as the finding that hospitalization rates for urinary stones did not differ between patients prescribed triamterene and hydrochlorothiazide (Jick et al., 1982).

Guaifenesin and Ephedrine. Consumption of large quantities of guaifenesin and ephedrine can lead to stones composed of their metabolites (Assimos et al., 1999; Powell et al., 1998). Most of the patients reported to have these stones are found to have consumed large quantities of over-the-counter preparations of cold medicine for the stimulatory properties of the ephedrine component, and a history of drug abuse is not uncommon (Assimos et al., 1999). Herbal ecstasy and ma huang are also popular ephedrine-containing preparations that are abused for stimulatory properties (Mack, 1997). Unfortunately, chronic ephedrine use leads to tachyphylaxis and prompts the use of increasing doses to achieve a comparable effect. Serious toxicity may result from ephedrine abuse, including death, cardiomyopathy, stroke, hypertension, and seizures.

Silicate Stones. Silica is a common element seen in vegetables, whole grains, seafood, and even drinking water that is easily excreted in the urine (Matlaga et al., 2003). Silicate stones are extremely rare and have been associated with consumption of large amounts of silicate-containing antacids such as magnesium trisilicate (Daudon, 1999; Haddad and Kouyoumdjian, 1986).

Medications That Indirectly Promote Stone Formation. Other medications indirectly promote stone formation by increasing urinary stone risk factors. Corticosteroids, vitamin D, and phosphate-binding antacids can induce hypercalciuria. **Thiazides cause intracellular acidosis and subsequent hypocitraturia** (Nicar et al., 1984). Loop diuretics such as furosemide and bumetanide inhibit sodium and calcium resorption in the thick ascending loop of Henle, which in addition to a diuretic effect results in hypercalciuria (Matlaga et al., 2003). Renal calculi have been identified in up to 64% of low-birth-weight infants receiving furosemide therapy, and stones are consistently composed of calcium oxalate (Hufnagle et al., 1982; Shukla et al., 2001).

Carbonic anhydrase inhibitors such as acetazolamide block resorption of sodium bicarbonate at multiple segments in the nephron, thereby inducing a metabolic acidosis and leading to urinary alkalinization (Parfitt, 1969). **Chronic use results in hypocitraturia, hypercalciuria, and increased risk for calcium phosphate stones** (Matlaga et al., 2003). Topiramate is a widely used drug approved for the treatment of seizures and prophylaxis of migraine headaches but is additionally increasingly used for the treatment of a variety of other disorders, such as obesity, neuropathic pain, alcoholism, type 2 diabetes, cigarette smoking, and cocaine dependence. Topiramate inhibits several isoenzymes of carbonic anhydrase with subsequent stone-potentiating effects (Vega et al., 2007). Although the incidence of calcium stones with topiramate use in adults based on short-term clinical trials was reported as 1.2% to 1.5% in the package insert, this number is thought to be an underestimate. Indeed, a recent retrospective study identified 150 individuals who were treated with topiramate out of 1500 adults in an electronic database from an epilepsy monitoring unit, among whom 75 were successfully contacted and queried regarding their kidney stone history (Maalouf et al., 2011). A total of eight subjects reported a diagnosis of kidney stones since the start of topiramate use, resulting in 10.7% prevalence. Furthermore, 15 patients among the 67 patients without a history of stones from the same study group were evaluated with computed tomographic imaging at an average of 43 months of topiramate use, revealing a 20% prevalence of asymptomatic stones, suggesting the problem is much more prevalent than previously suspected.

The risk of stone formation with topiramate use is related to its action as a carbonic anhydrase inhibitor. A recent cross-sectional study comparing 32 topiramate-treated patients with 50 normal controls revealed systemic metabolic acidosis, increased fractional excretion of bicarbonate, higher urine pH, and lower urinary citrate excretion in the topiramate-treated group (Welch et al., 2006). Likewise, in a short-term longitudinal study of seven patients before and 3 months after initiation of topiramate, significant metabolic acidosis and increased urine pH, bicarbonate excretion, and saturation of calcium phosphate were seen with initiation of the drug (Welch et al., 2006). Furthermore, topiramate-induced hypocitraturia demonstrates a dose-dependent response that additionally correlates inversely with duration of treatment (Kaplon et al., 2011). Zonisamide, a sulfonamide agent that also exerts an antiepileptic effect and has a weak carbonic anhydrase activity, has also been associated with increased risk of kidney stone formation (Zaccara et al., 2011).

Laxative abuse has also been associated with stone formation because persistent diarrhea increases the risk of ammonium acid urate stones. Patients abusing laxatives excrete large amounts of ammonia in the urine to eliminate excess acid, resulting in low urine pH. In the setting of low urine volume resulting from dehydration and low urinary sodium from laxative use, the urine of these patients can be highly supersaturated with respect to ammonium urate (Matlaga et al., 2003; Soble et al., 1999). Last, cytotoxic agents promote a high cell turnover, resulting in urinary excretion of large amounts of uric acid.

Anatomic Predisposition to Stones

Patients with anatomic anomalies associated with urinary obstruction and/or stasis have been noted to have a high incidence of associated stones. It has long been debated whether the predisposition to stone disease is a result of urinary stasis and delayed transit time through the nephron, leading to higher likelihood of crystal formation and retention, or if these patients form stones as a result of the same or unique metabolic abnormalities associated with stone formation.

Ureteropelvic Junction Obstruction

The incidence of renal calculi in patients with ureteropelvic junction obstruction (UPJO) is nearly 20% (Clark and Malek, 1987; David and Lavengood, 1975; Lowe and Marshall, 1984). However, Husmann et al. (1995) **provided several lines of evidence to suggest that patients with UPJO and concurrent renal calculi carry the same metabolic risks as other stone formers in the general population.** First, among 111 adult patients with UPJO and stones for whom long-term follow-up was available, 62% developed recurrent stones after treatment of the UPJO and 43% of the recurrences occurred in the contralateral kidney. These findings suggest that a metabolic predisposition persisted despite correction of the obstruction. Second, 76% of 42 patients with noninfectious stones who underwent a metabolic evaluation demonstrated an underlying metabolic abnormality that could account for the stones, a rate comparable to that of other stone formers (Pak, 1982; Yagisawa et al., 1999). Finally, the type and distribution of metabolic abnormalities identified in these patients were similar to those of the general stone-forming population: hypercalciuria in 46% of patients, hyperuricosuria in 11%, hypocitraturia in 13%, primary hyperparathyroidism in 13%, and RTA in 3% (Pak et al., 1980). Treatment of patients with identifiable abnormalities significantly reduced their rate of recurrence, from 55% in patients managed conservatively to 17% in treated patients.

Matin and Streem (2000) also performed metabolic evaluations before definitive repair in 47 patients with UPJO with or without associated stones. An identifiable abnormality was found in 67% of the stone patients compared with only 33% of the control group; urinary calcium and the incidence of hypercalciuria and hyperuricosuria were significantly higher in the patients with stones compared with the controls, further underscoring the contribution of pathophysiologic background to stone-forming risk in patients with anatomic abnormalities.

Similar findings in two series of children with UPJO and concurrent renal calculi further support a metabolic contribution to stone formation in the presence of renal obstruction. Tekin et al. (2001) prospectively compared children with UPJO with and without stones to a control group of calcium stone formers without UPJO. Both groups of stone formers, those with and without UPJO, exhibited significantly higher urinary levels of citrate and lower levels of oxalate compared with the non–stone-forming children with UPJO. Husmann et al. (1996) reported a 70-fold increased risk of stone formation in the pediatric population with UPJO compared with normal children. Among 22 children who underwent treatment of their stones and UPJO, 68% of patients with nonstruvite stones developed a recurrence after surgical treatment, and a metabolic abnormality was identified in 68%. Among the seven patients with nonstruvite renal calculi who did not experience a recurrence, only 29% had an identifiable metabolic abnormality. Thus correction of the UPJO did not prevent recurrent stones in most patients, further emphasizing the role of underlying metabolic abnormalities in the cause of renal calculi in patients with UPJO.

Horseshoe Kidneys

Horseshoe kidneys occur with a prevalence of 0.25% but have an associated rate of renal calculi of 20% (Cussenot et al., 1992; Janetschek and Kunzel, 1988). Because of the high insertion of the ureter into the renal pelvis, there is a relative impairment of renal drainage, predisposing to UPJO. Therefore the risk of stone formation has been attributed to urinary stasis rather than to metabolic derangements. Raj et al. (2004) reviewed 37 patients with horseshoe kidneys and stones and identified at least one metabolic abnormality in all 11 patients in whom 24-hour urine collections were available. Compared with a group of stone formers with normal renal anatomy, the patients with horseshoe kidneys exhibited a similar distribution of metabolic derangements, with the exception that hypocitraturia was over-represented (55% in the patients with horseshoe kidneys vs. 31% in controls). It seems clear that **although urinary stasis likely contributes to a propensity toward stone formation in patients with horseshoe kidneys, an underlying metabolic abnormality is required for stone formation to occur.**

Caliceal Diverticula

Caliceal diverticula are associated with stones in up to 40% of patients (Middleton and Pfister, 1974). Like stones in horseshoe kidneys, it is unclear whether the stones are caused by local anatomic obstruction and urinary stasis or are due to underlying metabolic factors. Two groups of investigators have addressed this issue. Hsu and Streem (1998) identified metabolic abnormalities, including hypercalciuria, hyperoxaluria, and hyperuricosuria, in 50% of 14 patients with stone-bearing caliceal diverticula. Notably, 64% of patients reported a history of synchronous or metachronous stones at a site distinct from the diverticulum, supporting the idea of underlying metabolic risk as a contributing cause of the stones. In contrast, Liatsikos et al. (2000) compared 49 patients with caliceal diverticula and stones with 44 stone formers without diverticula and found a low rate of metabolic abnormalities in both groups (25% in patients with diverticula and 23% in the control patients). However, the metabolic evaluation in this study involved measurement of only urinary volume, creatinine, calcium, phosphorus, oxalate, and uric acid. Because low urinary pH and hypocitraturia are identified in approximately 10% and 28% of recurrent stone formers, respectively (Levy et al., 1995), the number of metabolic abnormalities reported in this series is likely under-represented. Finally, a study by Matlaga et al. (2007) evaluated 29 patients who underwent percutaneous treatment of stone-bearing calyceal diverticuli and compared their 24-hour urine collections with those of 245 calcium oxalate stone formers and 162 normal controls. The urinary stone risk parameters of the patients with calyceal diverticular stones were similar to those of calcium oxalate stone formers, who demonstrated significantly greater hypercalciuria and higher calcium oxalate supersaturation compared with normal controls. Interestingly, urine aspirated directly from the diverticulum had lower calcium oxalate supersaturation than that of urine obtained from the ipsilateral and contralateral renal pelves. These findings imply that calyceal diverticular calculi arise from a combination of metabolic abnormalities and urinary stasis.

Stones formed in caliceal diverticula are mainly composed of calcium oxalate monohydrate, but they can also contain struvite–carbonate apatite because of an infectious component. Concomitant urinary tract infection is found in up to 40% of cases, with *E. coli*, *Proteus*, and *Pseudomonas* the most frequent pathogens (Daudon et al., 2003; Monreal et al., 1998).

Medullary Sponge Kidney

Medullary sponge kidney (MSK) is a disorder characterized by ectasia of the renal collecting ducts. Nephrocalcinosis and renal calculi are frequent complications of MSK (Ginalski et al., 1990; Lavan et al., 1971; Parks et al., 1982; Sage et al., 1982), but the exact risk factors for stone formation are not clearly understood. Although recurrent infection and urinary stasis within the ectatic tubules pose a risk for stone formation (Ginalski et al., 1990), renal tubular defects, including hypercalciuria, impaired renal concentrating ability, and defective urinary acidification after an ammonium chloride load, have been detected in some MSK patients (Granberg et al., 1971), further potentiating the risk of stone formation. Osther et al. (1988) performed ammonium chloride load tests in 13 patients with MSK and found renal acidification defects in 9 patients: 8 with distal RTA and 1 with proximal RTA. Likewise, Higashihara et al. (1984) reported renal acidification defects in 80% of 11 MSK patients (36% with distal RTA) and impaired concentrating ability in 90% of these 11 patients. The identification of mutations in the hydrogen proton pump genes *ATP6V1B1* and *ATP6V0A4* in two patients with MSK lends further support to an association between MSK and distal RTA (Carboni et al., 2009).

Despite these findings, three studies performed specifically on MSK patients with nephrolithiasis revealed no case of associated RTA (O'Neill et al., 1981; Parks et al., 1982; Yagisawa et al., 2001). O'Neill et al. (1981) identified hypercalciuria as the most common metabolic abnormality in 17 patients with MSK and nephrolithiasis, occurring in 88% of patients and attributed to absorptive hypercalciuria in most cases (59%). The spectrum of abnormalities in these patients was judged to be comparable with that of the general stone-forming population. Other investigators identified hypercalciuria less frequently, in only 9% to 44% of MSK patients with nephrolithiasis. In some cases, the cause of the hypercalciuria was attributed to renal calcium leak by which renal calcium reabsorption was presumed to be impaired by damaged renal tubules (Parks et al., 1982; Yagisawa et al., 2001; Yendt, 1981). Yagisawa et al. (2001) identified hypocitraturia as the most common metabolic abnormality, occurring in 77% of 22 MSK patients. Kinoshita (1990) likewise reported hypocitraturia in 58% of MSK patients. **Thus it appears that although renal acidification defects may be associated with MSK, hypercalciuria and hypocitraturia are likely contributing factors even in the absence of RTA.**

Stones in Pregnancy

Symptomatic stones during pregnancy occur at a rate of 1 in 250 (Lewis et al., 2003) to 1 in 3000 (Butler et al., 2000) pregnant women. Unlike the rest of the population, the incidence of nephrolithiasis in pregnant women did not increase when comparing 1991 to 2000 and 2001 to 2011 (Riley et al., 2014). Similar to stones in nonpregnant women, they occur more commonly in white than African-American women (Lewis et al., 2003). The majority of symptomatic stones occur in the second and third trimesters of pregnancy, heralded by symptoms of flank pain or hematuria (Biyani and Joyce, 2002; Butler et al., 2000; Lewis et al., 2003; Stothers and Lee, 1992). The diagnosis can be difficult in this patient population; up to 28% of women are misdiagnosed with appendicitis, diverticulitis, or placental abruption (Stothers and Lee, 1992).

A number of physiologic changes occur during pregnancy. Physiologic hydronephrosis occurs in up to 90% of pregnant women and persists up to 4 to 6 weeks postpartum (Swanson et al., 1995). Although hydronephrosis may be in part due to the effects of progesterone, compression of the ureters by the gravid uterus is at least a contributory, if not the primary, factor (Gorton and Whitfield, 1997; McAleer and Loughlin, 2004). Dilation is typically greater in the right ureter as a result of the engorged uterine vein and derotation of the enlarged uterus (Biyani and Joyce, 2002). The physiologic dilation may promote crystallization as a result of urinary stasis (Swanson et al., 1995), and the increased renal pelvic pressure has been suggested to increase the likelihood of stone movement and symptoms.

Important physiologic changes in the kidney occur during pregnancy and modulate urinary stone risk factors. Renal blood flow increases, leading to a 30% to 50% rise in glomerular filtration rate, which subsequently increases the filtered loads of calcium, sodium, and uric acid (McAleer and Loughlin, 2004). Hypercalciuria is further enhanced by placental production of $1,25(OH)_2D_3$, which increases intestinal calcium absorption and secondarily suppresses PTH (Biyani and Joyce, 2002; Gertner et al., 1986). Resim et al. (2006) demonstrated that hypercalciuria of pregnancy is a reversible physiologic condition by performing 24-hour urine collections on 25 pregnant women during each trimester and postpartum. Hyperuricosuria has also been reported as a result of increased filtered load of uric acid (Swanson et al., 1995).

Despite increases in a number of stone-inducing analytes, pregnant women have been shown to excrete increased amounts of inhibitors such as citrate, magnesium, and glycoproteins (Maikranz et al., 1987; Smith et al., 2001). Therefore the overall risk of stone formation has been reported to be similar in gravid and nongravid women (Coe et al., 1978; Drago et al., 1982). Although some studies found that the stone composition is similar between gravid and nongravid women, one multi-institutional study found that 74% of stones from pregnant women were composed predominantly of calcium phosphate and 26% were predominantly calcium oxalate (Ross et al., 2008). Meria et al. (2010) compared stone composition in 244 pregnant patients to 5712 age-matched nonpregnant female patients in France and found a significantly higher percentage of calcium phosphate carbapatite stones in pregnant compared with nonpregnant patients (65.6% and 31.4%, respectively, $P < 0.0001$). The higher prevalence of calcium phosphate stones observed in some studies of pregnant women may suggest that changes in pH during pregnancy could contribute to a higher likelihood of calcium phosphate stone formation, although this remains speculative.

> **KEY POINTS: PATHOGENESIS**
>
> - Absorptive hypercalciuria is characterized by normal serum calcium, normal or suppressed PTH, normal fasting urinary calcium, and elevated urinary calcium.
> - Renal hypercalciuria is due to impaired renal calcium reabsorption, which stimulates PTH secretion and leads to fasting hypercalciuria.
> - Resorptive hypercalciuria is primarily due to primary hyperparathyroidism but may be seen with granulomatous diseases that elaborate $1,25(OH)_2D_3$.
> - The most important determinant of uric acid stone formation is low urinary pH.
> - Low urine pH seen in uric acid stone formers is likely due to impaired ammoniagenesis as a result of insulin resistance and excess acid production.
> - In distal RTA, a defective H^+-ATPase accounts for excretion of excess acid into the distal tubule.
> - Formation of infection stones requires alkaline urine that can be achieved only with infection with urease-producing bacteria.

SUGGESTED READINGS

Devuyst O, Pirson Y: Genetics of hypercalciuric stone forming diseases, *Kidney Int* 72:1065–1072, 2007.
Evan A, Lingeman J, Coe FL, et al: Randall's plaque: pathogenesis and role in calcium oxalate nephrolithiasis, *Kidney Int* 69:1313–1318, 2006.
Holmes RP, Assimos DG: The impact of dietary oxalate on kidney stone formation, *Urol Res* 32:311–316, 2004.
Hoppe B: An update on primary hyperoxaluria, *Nat Rev Nephrol* 8:467–475, 2012.
Khan SR: Is oxidative stress, a link between nephrolithiasis and obesity, hypertension, diabetes, chronic kidney disease, metabolic syndrome?, *Urol Res* 40:95–112, 2012.
Maalouf NM, Cameron MA, Moe OW, et al: Novel insights into the pathogenesis of uric acid nephrolithiasis, *Curr Opin Nephrol Hypertens* 13:181–189, 2004.
Matlaga BR, Shah OD, Assimos DG: Drug-induced urinary calculi, *Rev Urol* 5:227–231, 2003.
Miller NL, Evan AP, Lingeman JE: Pathogenesis of renal calculi, *Urol Clin North Am* 34:295–313, 2007.
Pearle MS, Calhoun EA, Curhan GC: Urologic Diseases in America project: urolithiasis, *J Urol* 173:848–857, 2005.
Sakhaee K, Maalouf NM, Sinnott B: Kidney stones 2012: pathogenesis, diagnosis and management, *J Clin Endocrinol Metab* 97:1847–1860, 2012.
Scales CD, Smith AC, Hanley JM, et al: Prevalence of kidney stones in the United States, *Eur Urol* 62:160–165, 2012.
Siva S, Barrack ER, Reddy GP, et al: A critical analysis of the role of gut Oxalobacter formigenes in oxalate stone disease, *BJU Int* 103:18–21, 2009.

REFERENCES

The complete reference list is available online at ExpertConsult.com.

92

Evaluation and Medical Management of Urinary Lithiasis

Nicole L. Miller, MD, and Michael S. Borofsky, MD

EVALUATION OF URINARY LITHIASIS

Urinary stone disease is one of mankind's oldest and longest recognized urologic afflictions. Historic records describing symptoms related to stones and efforts to dissolve them date back to ancient Mesopotamia between 3200 and 1200 BCE (Tefekli and Cezayirli 2013). Some of history's most famous physicians proposed hypotheses for how stones form and diagnostic and treatment recommendations including Hippocrates (460 BCE), Aristotle (384 BCE), and Galen (131 to 200 AD) (Shah, 2002). The understanding of how stones form and the therapies used to treat and prevent them have evolved dramatically in the hundreds of years since these initial descriptions. Nonetheless, despite such efforts, urinary stone disease remains one of the most common urologic conditions. A proper conceptual understanding of the mechanisms by which stones form and the methods by which stone growth may be reduced are necessary for the practicing urologist. Not only are stones likely to recur without identification and modifications of the factors that enabled them to form in the first place, but they may also be indicative of a larger systemic disease. Herein, the basis for a proper stone evaluation and an overview of the available conservative and medical treatments to prevent them are provided.

EPIDEMIOLOGY AND MORBIDITY FROM URINARY LITHIASIS

The prevalence of urinary stone disease is rising at a rapid rate. Recent national estimates from the United States suggest that stones affect 1 in 11 at some point in their lifetime, nearly double the rate it was 15 years earlier (Scales et al., 2012). Historically stone disease tended to affect more men than it did women, but a disproportional increase in stones particularly among younger females has leveled the gender disparity and made it close to equal (Lieske et al. 2006). Several recent estimates of gender distribution of stones between men and women have reported ratios between 1.2 and 1.45 : 1 (Nowfar, 2011; Pearle, 2005; Scales et al., 2007). Although the precise reason for this demographic change is unclear, it does not appear to be a result of a decrease in male stone formation but rather as a significant increase in female stone formation (Pearle, 2005).

The morbidity attributed to stone disease is classically considered in the acute sense where severe colic, emergency medical care, life interruption, missed work, and often surgical treatment are undesired aspects of a single stone episode. However, it is important to consider the long-term impact of stone disease on quality of life, particularly as stone recurrence is quite common. **First-time stone formers often have been estimated to have a 50% risk for recurrence within the subsequent 10 years** (Uribarri, 1989). In two separate studies, Ljunghall and Danielson attempted to measure the incidence of stone recurrence in a Northern European population (Ljunghall, 1984, 1987). A retrospective review estimated the chance of recurrence at nearly 50% at 5 years, whereas a prospective evaluation noted a lower overall rate of 53% within 8 years. Males had both a higher incidence of calculi overall and a higher recurrence rate. Patients had a higher risk for repeat stones in the years immediately after their first episode. It is not completely apparent whether these were preexisting stones that passed later or whether they represent the formation of new calculi.

Recognizing that the risk for stone recurrence can vary greatly from one patient to another, Rule et al. developed the recurrence of kidney stone (ROKS) nomogram to help better predict the risk for a second kidney stone. They found that by taking various demographic and clinical considerations into account, 10-year recurrence risk could be better predicted and ranged from 12% among patients with the lowest risk scores to 56% to those with the highest risk stratification. Significant predictors of stone recurrence included younger age, male sex, family history, prior stone event, nonobstructing renal stones, symptomatic renal pelvis/lower pole stones and uric acid composition. Notably, urinary chemistries were unable to be taken into consideration of the nomogram (Rule et al., 2014).

The effect of stone disease on overall quality of life (QOL) is gaining greater appreciation as patient-reported outcomes measures are increasingly utilized in modern health care systems. This is particularly true among patients with recurrent urinary stones whose health-related QOL has the potential to suffer for a variety of reasons including chronic/episodic pain, frequent clinic visits, recurrent interventions, or side effects from medications or dietary measures being used for prophylaxis. **Application of generic health and well-being questionnaires such as the SF-36 has demonstrated that the health-related QOL for stone formers is lower than the population mean,** with women reporting greater impairment than men (Penniston, 2007a). The National Institutes of Health (NIH)-supported Patient-Reported Outcome Measurement Information System (PROMIS) has also been applied to patients with stone disease. Studies using this tool have shown that stone patients have subjectively worse pain intensity, pain interference, and physical function relative to the general population at various phases of a stone episode (Borofsky et al., 2017; Patel, 2017). A disease-specific health-related QOL measurement system has also been validated for the purpose of studying the effect of stone disease on QOL (Penniston, 2017). To date, this system has proven useful and has led to a number of notable findings including a poorer QOL in cystine versus noncystine stone formers (Streeper et al., 2017) and decreased QOL in patients with asymptomatic stones compared with those with no stones (Penniston, 2016).

> **KEY POINTS**
> - The incidence of nephrolithiasis is increasing.
> - The historic male predominance of stone formers is disappearing.
> - Risk for stone recurrence is variable but has been estimated at 50% between 5 and 10 years.
> - Quality of life for stone formers is poorer than for non–stone formers.

IMAGING FOR URINARY LITHIASIS

Diagnostic imaging is a cornerstone in the evaluation of stone disease. American Urological Association (AUA) guidelines recommend obtaining and/or reviewing imaging studies to quantify stone burden as part of a routine medical evaluation for stone disease (Pearle et al., 2014). An overview of the different imaging modalities used in urology can be found in Chapters 2 to 4, but there are several unique considerations that should be made when looking for stones in particular. Utilization of the most appropriate diagnostic test will depend on the clinical scenario and the resources that are available. Consideration should be made regarding whether or not the patient is symptomatic, if surgery is being planned, and how much detail is needed regarding the potential stones themselves versus the collecting system of the kidneys.

Computed Tomography

Noncontrast computed tomography (CT) imaging is the gold standard in terms of diagnostic accuracy for stones, with a reported sensitivity of 98% and a specificity of 97% (Fulgham et al., 2013). Advantages of CT include the diagnostic certainty, ability to obtain rapid results, and relative ubiquity of CT scanners in medical settings. As a result, CT is the most commonly utilized test for evaluation of flank pain in emergency room settings, with the number of CT scans ordered for kidney stone evaluation having tripled between 1992 and 2009 (Fwu et al., 2013). An additional advantage of CT scanning for stones is the ability to obtain detailed anatomic information about the kidney itself including the presence or absence of hydronephrosis, perinephric stranding, and parenchymal abnormalities.

CT also has the potential to provide insight into stone composition. The classic example of this is for uric acid stones, which are radiolucent on conventional radiography but well visualized on CT. Furthermore, uric acid stones have lower Hounsfield units (HU) relative to other stones, a feature that has been shown to have clinical utility regarding the likelihood of that stone to respond to shock wave lithotripsy (Pareek et al., 2003; Saw et al., 2000). Recently, there is evidence that dual-energy CT may be able to further distinguish stone composition including uric acid, calcium phosphate, cystine, struvite, and calcium oxalate (Ascenti et al., 2010; Boll et al., 2009; Hidas et al., 2010).

CT scans are not without their limitations. They are more expensive than alternative studies and have been estimated to be ten times as expensive as radiographs of the kidneys, ureter, and bladder (KUB) and five times as expensive as a renal ultrasonography (RUS) (Brisbane et al., 2016). They are also not able to visualize 100% of stones with several rare types of calculi that are radiolucent on CT including those made of drugs or bacteria (protease inhibitors and pure matrix). Another significant limitation of CT scans is the associated exposure to ionizing radiation with a mean effective dose of around 10 mSv per scan (Fulgham et al., 2013) (Table 92.1). **Patients with kidney stones are at particular risk for high levels of radiation exposure given the nature of stone recurrence and the potential for additional radiation exposure during surgical treatments and in surveillance.** Ferrandino et al. found that within the first year of an acute stone event, patients underwent an average of four radiographic examinations (mean of 1.2 KUBs, 1.7 CTs, 1 intravenous pyelogram (IVP). Median effective radiation dose per patient was 29.7 mSv with 20% receiving greater than 50 mSv, the recommended yearly dose limit for occupational exposure by the International Commission on Radiological Protection (Valentin and ICRP, 2005).

Low-dose CT scans have been introduced with the intention of preserving the diagnostic accuracy of a regular CT scan with a lower dose of radiation exposure (Fig. 92.1). There is no standard terminology for what a low-dose CT means, but radiation exposure <3 to 4 mSv has been proposed (Fulgham et al., 2013; Gervaise et al.,

TABLE 92.1 Estimated Effective Radiation Dose (mSv) by Type of Examination

IMAGING MODAILTY	EXAMINATION TYPE	EFFECTIVE DOSE (mSv)
Ultrasonography	Abdomen and pelvis	0
MRI	Abdomen and pelvis	0
Conventional radiography		
	KUB	0.7
	KUB with tomograms	3.9
	IVU	3.0
CT		
	Noncontrast abdomen and pelvis	10.0
	Without and with contrast, abdomen and pelvis (2-phase)	15.0
	Without and with contrast, abdomen and pelvis (3-phase)	20.0
	Noncontrast CT, abdomen and pelvis (low-dose protocol)	3.0
	Noncontrast CT, abdomen and pelvis (ultra-low-dose protocol)	<1.0

Modified from Fulgham PF, Assimos DG, Pearle MS, Preminger GM. Clinical effectiveness protocols for imaging in the management of ureteral calculous disease: AUA technology assessment. *J Urol* 189(4):1203-1213, 2013.
CT, Computed tomography; *IVU*, intravenous urogram; *KUB*, kidney, ureter, bladder; *MRI*, magnetic resonance imaging.

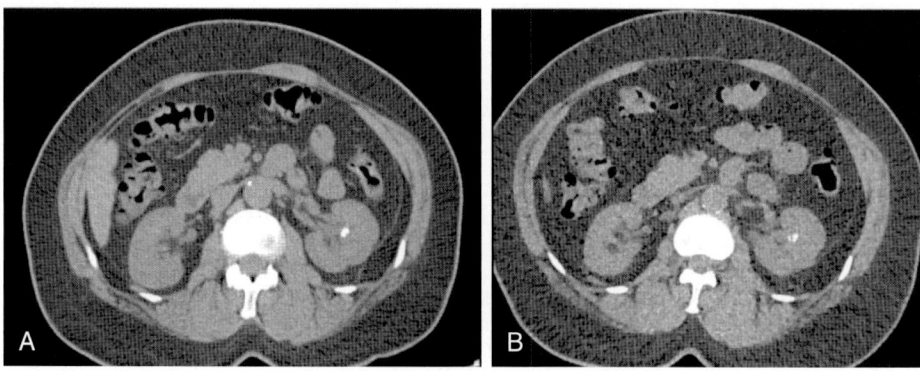

Fig. 92.1. Comparison of standard-dose (A) and low-dose CT (B) for the evaluation of renal stones.

2016). Several studies have demonstrated the ability to maintain a greater than 90% sensitivity and specificity for upper-tract stones using this approach (Liu et al., 2000; Tack et al., 2003). To date, this technique has shown promise but is underutilized for stones. A 2018 report looking specifically at the utilization of CT scans for stones found that despite a near threefold increase in utilization over a four-year period, overall low-dose CT scans only accounted for 7.6% of the CT scans ordered for stone evaluations across the United States (Weisenthal et al., 2018). Body mass index (BMI) is an important factor when considering low-dose CT as accuracy suffers when the BMI is greater than 30 (Fulgham et al., 2013). Ultra-low–dose CT scans (mSV <1) have also been proposed, though to date, studies have found a suboptimal sensitivity and specificity in the 70% range frequently caused by missing small stones 3 mm or less (Glazer et al., 2014; McLaughlin et al., 2014).

Radiography (KUB and IVP)

Plain radiographs of the KUB are the oldest method of identifying stones in the body. Used alone, without contrast, KUB has an estimated sensitivity of 57% and a specificity of 76% (Fulgham et al., 2013). Limitations of this technique include an inability to visualize all stone types, particularly uric acid, and the potential for overlying structures such as bones or bowel gas to interfere with stone identification. IVPs can improve the ability to detect stones through better delineation of the pelvicalyceal and ureteral anatomy, but even so, they have an estimated sensitivity of only 70% despite a better specificity (95%) (Fulgham et al., 2013). Limitations of this approach include the required use of intravenous contrast and a limited degree to obtain information that might offer insight into other causes of symptoms (Dale et al., 2017).

Ultrasound

RUS is one of the most active areas of research in terms of stone imaging. Use of ultrasonography is very appealing as it is widely available, cost effective, and does not expose patients to ionizing radiation. The biggest disadvantage of RUS for stones though remains a poor sensitivity (61%) despite adequate specificity (97%) (Fulgham et al., 2013). RUS may still provide clinical utility, particularly of the kidney itself, where it is an excellent test for hydronephrosis.

Application of Doppler ultrasonography can help find ureteral jets that may not be present in the setting of obstruction. Doppler ultrasonography can also be used to find a twinkling artifact (Fig. 92.2). This finding describes a mosaic of colors that appears over the stone and can help distinguish a stone from other echogenic structures, in turn improving the specificity of stone detection (Cunitz et al., 2014; Simon et al., 2018).

Even when stones are properly identified via ultrasonography, there is potential for misinterpretation of their size (Fowler et al., 2002). Small stones seen on ultrasound were previously found to be misclassified as over 5 mm in nearly one-half of cases because of issues related to interpretation, image acquisition, body habitus, and other patient-specific factors (Ray et al., 2010). One method that may improve the accuracy of stone sizing is measuring the acoustic shadow produced by an echogenic stone rather than the stone itself (Fig. 92.3). Dunmire et al. tested this hypothesis and found that this technique significantly improved the accuracy of measurements, with 78% of measured shadow sizes being accurate within 1 mm of the true stone size when measured in vitro (Dunmire et al., 2016). Several additional methods of RUS optimization have been explored as well including smoothing algorithms, compression of high–signal-intensity regions, and sharpening of contrast at the stone edge to better detect the posterior acoustic shadow. When used together, this has been referred to as S-mode (stone-specific mode) and has been shown to have improved ability to detect stones (78% vs. 61%) and properly size them compared to traditional ultrasonography (Dai et al., 2018).

Other Imaging Modalities

One lesser used but promising technique to find stones is digital tomosynthesis (DT). DT is akin to a conventional abdominal radiograph (KUB) but obtains several low-dose images via a tomographic sweep of the x-ray emitter. Multiple coronal slice images are then reconstructed by digital software. DT has been shown to have improved sensitivity over that of plain KUB for the detection of renal stones and significantly less radiation than a standard noncontrast CT (Mermuys, 2010; Neisius et al., 2014).

The ability of magnetic resonance imaging (MRI) to detect upper urinary tract stones is variable and most commonly is used to infer stones based on a signal void rather than true identification

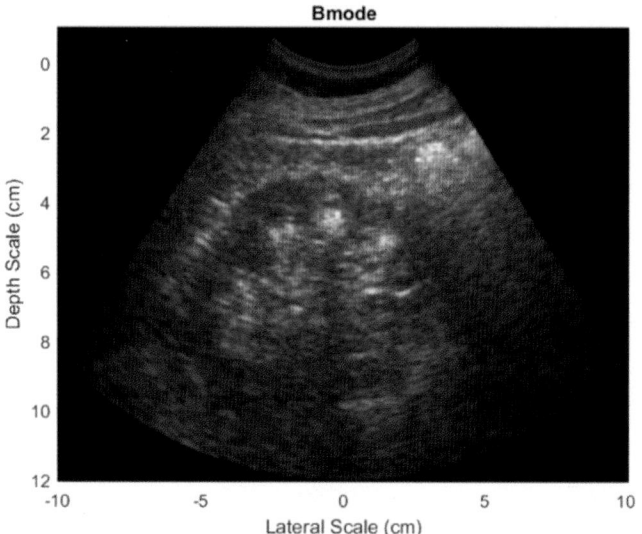
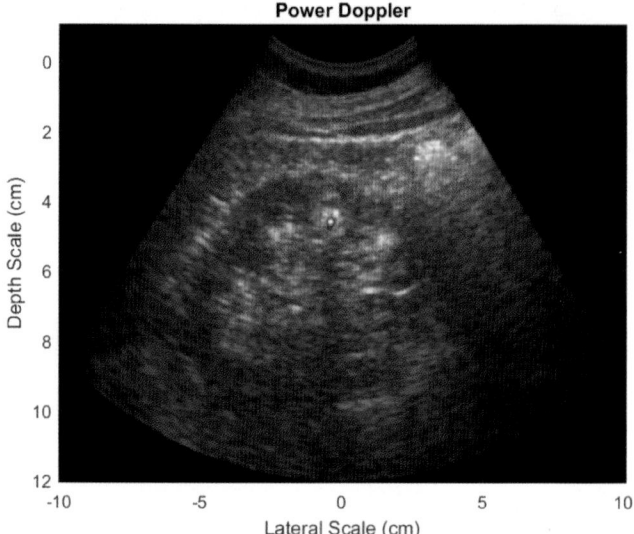

Fig. 92.2. Standard brightness mode *(B-mode)* ultrasound image of a stone in a kidney *(left)* and the same image with the stone identified with the twinkling artifact on power Doppler ultrasound. Twinkling adds color and contrast to the background to make the stone more easily identified in the image. The white brightness of the stone itself is seen in both images, although it is hard to distinguish form other bright objects. With the eye directed to the color on the stone, the shadow behind the stone may also be more obvious. (Courtesy of Bryan Cunitz and Michael Bailey, PhD, University of Washington.)

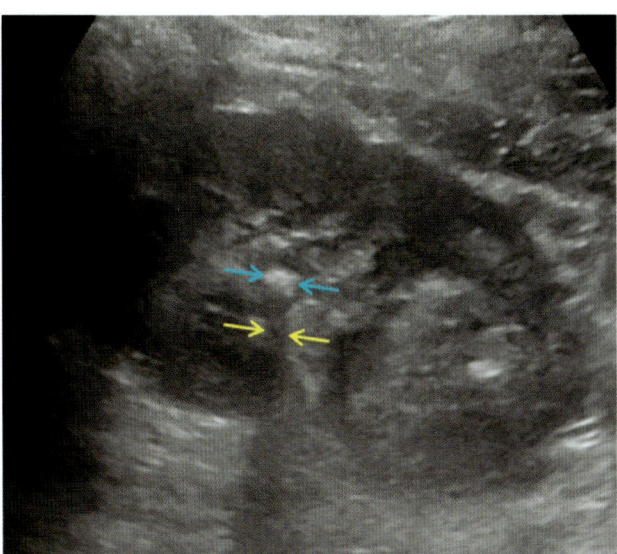

Fig. 92.3. Demonstration of stone shadow seen on ultrasound. Presence of a shadow can not only be used to improve confirmation of stone visualization, it can also improve accuracy of stone measurement. In this example, the hyperechoic area of the stone *(blue arrows)* measures 4.9 mm compared with the shadow, which measures 3.5 mm. Stone size on CT is 3.8 m. (Image courtesy of Barbrina Dunmire and Michael Bailey, PhD. University of Washington.)

of the stone itself (Robson et al., 2003). Nonetheless, sensitivity and specificity of this technique are 82% and 98.3%, respectively (Fulgham et al., 2013). An advantage of MRI is the lack of ionizing radiation, yet the high cost and lengthy time for image acquisition are barriers to widespread adoption of this technique. A common clinical scenario in which MRI may be useful is for evaluation of flank pain during pregnancy, and it is recommended as a second-line imaging test when ultrasonography is nondiagnostic (Coursey et al., 2012, Fulgham et al., 2013).

> **KEY POINTS**
>
> - CT is the gold standard imaging modality for the detection of urolithiasis.
> - Low-dose CT is an attractive option for stone evaluation that can maintain high diagnostic accuracy with less exposure to ionizing radiation.
> - Ultrasound technology continues to evolve with several new modes being developed to improve identification and sizing of stones.

METABOLIC EVALUATION

Through even a rudimentary understanding of the physiologic causes of urinary calculus formation, physicians may offer a straightforward approach to elucidating the metabolic basis of nephrolithiasis for any given patient. This evaluation should be simple to perform, it must be economically viable, and it should provide information that can be applied toward a selective, rational therapy of stone disease (Pak et al., 1980).

Any evaluation should be able to identify associated metabolic disorders responsible for recurrent stone disease. These metabolic problems include distal renal tubular acidosis (RTA), primary hyperparathyroidism, enteric hyperoxaluria, cystinuria, and gouty diathesis. In many of these relatively uncommon conditions, it is generally agreed that selective medical therapy is indicated not only to prevent further stone formation but also to correct underlying physiologic disturbances that may lead to nonrenal complications (Pak et al., 2002, 2003b).

First-Time Stone Formers

Considering that dietary and fluid manipulation alone can reduce rates of stone recurrence, some suggest that first-time stone formers should be provided empirical fluid and dietary recommendations until they suffer a recurrence (Borghi et al., 1996). Indeed, studies of single stone formers placed on a conservative program of high fluid intake alone or combined with avoidance of dietary excess, revealed a low incidence of recurrent stone disease (Hosking et al., 1983). Calling this finding the *stone clinic effect,* Hosking et al. noted metabolic inactivity in nearly 60% of all patients followed for over 5 years.

In comparison, Pak found that single stone formers have an equally high incidence of metabolic abnormalities as recurrent stone formers (Pak, 1982). Furthermore, these derangements are just as severe, leading the authors to conclude that single stone formers should undergo the same evaluation as recurrent stone formers. Similar findings were reported in a series of 182 patients in which one-half of the patients had hypercalciuria or hyperuricosuria and roughly 20% had a systemic disorder that predisposed them to the formation of calculi (Strauss et al., 1982b). The remainder, 29.1%, had no metabolic disorder. Patients with single stones tended to be older when they passed their stones and required a greater rate of intervention to treat the calculus. The recurrence for both groups of patients was very similar (~10% at 3 years). Because the authors did not note substantial differences between solitary and recurrent stone disease, they recommended that first-time stone formers be evaluated similarly to patients with recurrent stone disease. A more recent study comparing the frequencies of metabolic abnormalities between first-time stone formers and recurrent stone formers found no difference between the two groups (Eisner et al., 2012). Approximately 40% of both first-time and recurrent stone formers had hypercalciuria, 45% of both groups had hypocitraturia, and approximately 30% had hyperoxaluria. The authors suggest it is reasonable to perform a full metabolic evaluation in first-time stone formers.

The AUA guideline for the medical management of kidney stones states "clinicians should perform additional metabolic testing in high-risk or interested first-time stone formers" (evidence strength: grade B) (Pearle et al., 2014). **Importantly, the formation of a first stone may be the harbinger of a more severe underlying systemic disorder such as RTA, bone disease, or hypercalcemia resulting from hyperparathyroidism. In such patients, metabolic evaluation is justified solely to make the correct diagnosis to prevent extrarenal complications.** The decision to thoroughly investigate a first-time stone former should ideally be shared by the physician and the patient. Whereas some first-time stone formers will readily accept and follow conservative therapy, others may elect to undergo a thorough evaluation. A "know your numbers approach" has been shown to be quite effective in other chronic diseases such as diabetes mellitus. It is quite reasonable to determine the extent of evaluation according to the estimation of potential/risk for recurrent stone formation (Smith, 1984).

Defining the High-Risk Stone Former

All patients with newly diagnosed kidney or ureteral stones should undergo a screening evaluation that includes a detailed medical and dietary history (Pearle et al., 2014). The purpose of this evaluation is to identify patients at highest risk for stone formation and evaluate for systemic etiologies for kidney stone disease. **Patients identified as high-risk stone formers include those with a family history of stone disease, those with obesity and/or metabolic syndrome, and patients with medical conditions that predispose to stone formation such as gastrointestinal (GI) disease or prior surgical resection resulting in malabsorption, primary hyperparathyroidism, renal tubular acidosis, sarcoidosis, gout, type 2 diabetes mellitus, and urinary tract infection (UTI).** Stone composition when known can also help identify high-risk patients who would benefit from a

> **BOX 92.1 Indications for a Metabolic Stone Evaluation**
>
> Recurrent stone formers
> Strong family history of stones
> Intestinal disease (particularly chronic diarrhea)
> Pathologic skeletal fractures
> Osteoporosis
> History of urinary tract infection with calculi
> Personal history of gout
> Infirm health (unable to tolerate repeat stone episodes)
> Solitary kidney
> Anatomic abnormalities
> Renal insufficiency
> Stones composed of cystine, uric acid, struvite

> **BOX 92.2 Abbreviated Evaluation of Single Stone Formers**
>
> **History**
> - Underlying predisposing conditions (see Box 92.1)
> - Medications (calcium, vitamin C, vitamin D, acetazolamide, steroids)
> - Dietary excesses, inadequate fluid intake, excessive fluid loss
>
> **Multichannel Blood Screen**
> - Basic metabolic panel (sodium, potassium, chloride, carbon dioxide, blood urea nitrogen, creatinine)
> - Calcium
> - Intact parathyroid hormone
> - Uric acid
>
> **Urine**
> - Urinalysis
>   pH >7.5: infection lithiasis
>   pH <5.5: uric acid lithiasis
>   Sediment for crystalluria
> - Urine culture
>   Urea-splitting organisms: suggestive of infection lithiasis
> - Qualitative cystine
>
> **Radiography**
> - Radiopaque stones: calcium oxalate, calcium phosphate, magnesium ammonium phosphate (struvite), cystine.
> - Radiolucent stones: uric acid, xanthine, triamterene
> - Intravenous pyelogram: radiolucent stones, anatomic abnormalities
>
> **Stone Analysis**

metabolic evaluation, such as those with cystine or uric acid stones in whom the likelihood of finding a metabolic abnormality requiring medical therapy is high (Box 92.1).

In addition, the overwhelming consensus is that all children should undergo a full metabolic evaluation because they have been found to have a significant risk for underlying metabolic disturbances (Bartosh, 2004; Coward et al., 2003; Pietrow et al., 2002; Polito et al., 2000; Tekin et al., 2001). Moreover, pediatric patients with metabolic abnormalities have been shown to have recurrence at a higher rate than those without metabolic risk factors (Abhishek et al., 2013). Additionally, these young patients have more at stake, because early, repeated episodes of urinary obstruction, UTI, and repeated radiographic imaging all have associated morbidities.

Race and ethnicity may also play a role in identifying the high-risk stone former. Mente et al. found that compared with Europeans, East Asian and African patients had a decreased relative risk for calcium nephrolithiasis, and Arabic, West Indian, West Asian, and Latin American patients had an increased relative risk (Mente et al., 2007). The authors found differing urinary profiles for a variety of the ethnicities reported when compared with those of Europeans. However, despite the decreased risk for calcium stone formation, patients of African ancestry demonstrated no significant differences in urinary metabolic derangements. A more recent study investigating the prevalence of stones in the United States between 2007 and 2010 found a significantly lower rate of stones in African-Americans, Hispanics, and multiracial persons compared with that in whites (Scales et al., 2012). Although the prevalence of stones in African-Americans remained lower than in whites, the increase in stone prevalence from the previous report (1988 to 1994) to the current report (2007 to 2010) was over 150%. Hsi et al. (2018)investigated race-sex associations with risk among whites and blacks in the southeastern US Southern Community Cohort Study (SCCS) and found that among black men and women, incidence rates were 2.19 and 2.47 per 1000 person-years, respectively. Among white SCCS participants, the corresponding rates were 5.98 and 4.50 per 1000 person-years for men and women, respectively, which are higher than what was previously reported.

Following the assumption that a lower incidence of calculi might imply a significant risk for a metabolic or anatomic abnormality in patients who still manage to make calculi, it seems reasonable to advocate for the performance of a metabolic evaluation for all patients of African-American descent. This suggestion is supported by recent studies that assessed the underlying metabolic abnormalities of nonwhite stone formers. **African-Americans, Asians, and Hispanics appear to have a surprisingly similar incidence of underlying metabolic disturbances when compared with white stone formers. These results suggest that dietary and environmental factors may be as important as ethnicity in the cause of stone disease** (Beukes et al., 1987, Maloney et al., 2005).

Finally, patients with anatomic abnormalities that may increase the risk for stone formation or complicate the treatment of it should be considered for metabolic evaluation. These would include patients with horseshoe kidney, calyceal diverticulum, ureteropelvic junction obstruction, medullary sponge kidney disease, urinary diversion, and solitary kidney.

> **KEY POINTS: SELECTION OF PATIENTS FOR METABOLIC EVALUATION**
>
> - All first-time stone formers should undergo a detailed medical and dietary history.
> - High-risk stone formers include those with GI disease, obesity, metabolic syndrome, diabetes mellitus, primary hyperparathyroidism, renal tubular acidosis, sarcoidosis, gout, and family history of nephrolithiasis.
> - Children should generally be evaluated because of concerns about renal damage and long-term sequelae of stone recurrence.

Screening Evaluation for Newly Diagnosed Stone Formers

In newly diagnosed stone formers, the following screening evaluation should be applied (Box 92.2). A thorough medical history should be obtained for any underlying conditions that may have contributed to the stone disease. Because of the association between bowel disease and calcium oxalate nephrolithiasis (enteric hyperoxaluria), a careful history of bowel habits and bowel disease should be sought (Bohles et al., 1988; Lindsjo et al., 1989; McConnell et al., 2002; Parks, 2003b; Smith et al., 1972; Worcester, 2002). This includes questions regarding chronic diarrhea that could be caused by inflammatory bowel disease (Crohn disease, ulcerative colitis) or irritable bowel syndrome. A history of gout should be elicited because this finding may predispose the patient to hyperuricosuria or gouty diathesis with either uric acid calculi or calcium oxalate stone formation (Grover and Ryall, 1994; Khatchadourian et al., 1995; Kramer and Curhan, 2002). **As described by Pak et al. (2003b), patients with a history of diabetes mellitus may be at an increased risk for developing calcium oxalate and/or uric acid stones, with altered ammonium excretion and acidic urine.**

A thorough surgical history should be obtained focusing particularly on bariatric surgery and surgeries on the intestinal tract. Roux-en-Y gastric bypass surgery has been shown to significantly increase the risk for kidney stones (Matlaga et al., 2009). This study demonstrated a significantly higher rate of stones in obese patients who underwent gastric bypass surgery compared with obese patients who had not (7.65% vs. 4.63%). In contrast with gastric bypass surgery, restrictive bariatric surgeries such as gastric sleeve or gastric band do not seem to increase the risk for kidney stone formation (Chen et al., 2013). Bowel resection, particularly of the small intestines, can lead to malabsorption with an increased risk for kidney stone formation, and patients with prior bowel surgery should be considered for a metabolic evaluation.

In addition, information should be obtained concerning the patient's dietary habits, including fluid consumption and excessive intake of certain foods, and a list of all medications taken. A social history may provide obvious clues regarding a patient's hydration status. Does the patient have access to fluids on a regular basis? Does the patient perform daily tasks that would increase the insensible losses of fluids? Patients on prolonged bed rest demonstrate alterations in urinary chemistry such that urinary calcium and phosphorus excretion increase significantly, leading to significant increases in urinary saturation of calcium phosphate, calcium oxalate, and monosodium urate, particularly during bed rest (Hwang et al., 1988). A family history may reveal a genetic predisposition to urinary calculi if there is a history of close relatives affected by nephrolithiasis. Age of onset of the patient or of affected relatives may give clues regarding genetic disorders such as autosomal recessive cystinuria.

The screening evaluation of newly diagnosed patients with kidney or ureteral stones should also include serum chemistries including electrolytes (sodium, potassium, chloride, bicarbonate), calcium, creatinine, and uric acid (Pearle et al., 2014). **These serum studies are helpful in identifying certain systemic problems** such as primary hyperparathyroidism (high serum calcium and low serum phosphorus), renal phosphate leak (hypophosphatemia), uric acid lithiasis (hyperuricemia), and distal RTA (hypokalemia, decreased serum carbon dioxide). For patients in whom primary hyperparathyroidism is suspected (hypercalcemia), a serum intact parathyroid hormone (PTH) level is also recommended (Pearle et al., 2014). Even mid-range or high-normal PTH in the face of higher serum calcium should lead to the suspicion of primary hyperparathyroidism because under normal circumstances, PTH should be suppressed when serum calcium is elevated.

A voided urine specimen should be obtained for comprehensive urinalysis including dipstick and microscopic analysis to assess urine pH, find indicators of infection, and identify crystals pathognomonic of stone type (Pearle et al., 2014) (Table 92.2). Urinary pH greater than 7.0 is suggestive of infection lithiasis or RTA, whereas a pH less than 5.5 suggests a risk for uric acid stone formation. **The urine sediment should be examined for crystalluria, because particular crystal types may give a clue as to the composition of stones the patient is forming.** Tetrahedral "envelopes" are seen in calcium oxalate lithiasis, and rectangular, "coffin-lid" crystals are often seen in patients with struvite calculi. Hexagonal crystals confirm cystinuria; uric acid crystals may be seen as amorphous fibers or as irregular plates. The microscopic appearances of common calculi are summarized in Fig. 92.4.

When the urinalysis is suggestive of urinary tract infection or the patient is known to have an infection-related stone, a urine culture is useful not only to determine the source of infection but also to identify the presence of urea-splitting bacteria *(Proteus, Pseudomonas, Klebsiella, Staphylococcus aureus,* and *Staphylococcus epidermidis)* **that may predispose to struvite stone formation.** A positive culture also will warrant therapy with appropriate antibiotics before initiation of any surgical procedure to remove the stone. Surgical treatment of a calculus during an active infection will place the patient at great risk for bacteremia or sepsis. **Unfortunately, many infected calculi will harbor bacteria even after treatment with broad-spectrum antibiotics.** Korets et al. evaluated the concordance between preoperative bladder urine cultures with renal pelvic urine cultures and stone cultures in patients undergoing percutaneous nephrolithotomy. They found that despite treatment with culture-specific antibiotics, stone culture was positive in 17 patients (8.6%) who had a positive preoperative bladder urine culture. Another 16 patients had a positive stone culture associated with a negative preoperative bladder culture (Korets et al., 2011). Furthermore, McAleer et al. demonstrated that infection calculi contain large quantities of endotoxin after disintegration (McAleer et al., 2002). In a comparison of infected versus noninfected calculi, infected stones contained 36 times more endotoxin. One-half of the infected calculi grew bacterial cultures that were different from the preoperative urine specimens. The same investigators described how endotoxin can cause a vascular collapse because it induces physiologic changes consistent with those of septic shock.

Finally, the screening evaluation should include review of stone analysis and imaging studies when available (Pearle et al., 2014). As mentioned earlier, stone composition can help identify high-risk patients who would benefit from a metabolic evaluation such as those with cystine or uric acid stones in whom the likelihood of finding a metabolic abnormality requiring medical therapy is high. In addition, calcium phosphate stone composition, particularly brushite, may indicate systemic etiologies of stone formation such as RTA, primary hyperparathyroidism, medullary sponge kidney disease, and the use of carbonic anhydrase inhibitors (Kourambas et al., 2001; Pak and Adams-Huet, 2004). Imaging studies are not only helpful to quantify the existing stone burden, but they also identify patients at greater risk for recurrence or who may have underlying metabolic or anatomic conditions predisposing to stone formation. For example, patients with multiple or bilateral renal calculi at initial presentation may be a greater risk for recurrence. Furthermore, the presence of nephrocalcinosis may be an indicator of RTA, primary hyperparathyroidism, or medullary sponge kidney disease.

TABLE 92.2 Microscopic Appearance of Common Urinary Calculi

CHEMICAL TYPE	APPEARANCE
Calcium oxalate monohydrate	Hourglass
Calcium oxalate dihydrate	Envelope, tetrahedral
Calcium phosphate-apatite	Amorphous
Brushite	Needle shaped
Magnesium ammonium phosphate (struvite)	Rectangular, coffin-lid
Cystine	Hexagonal
Uric acid	Amorphous shards, plates

KEY POINTS: SCREENING EVALUATION FOR NEWLY DIAGNOSED STONE FORMERS

- A complete medical and dietary history should be obtained.
- Patients should be screened for medical diseases that predispose to calculi.
- Serum metabolic panel and urinalysis tests should be performed.
- Urine microscopy for crystals may provide clues to diagnosis.
- Stone analysis may improve the accuracy of further evaluation.
- Basic radiography (plain films) should screen for existing calculi.

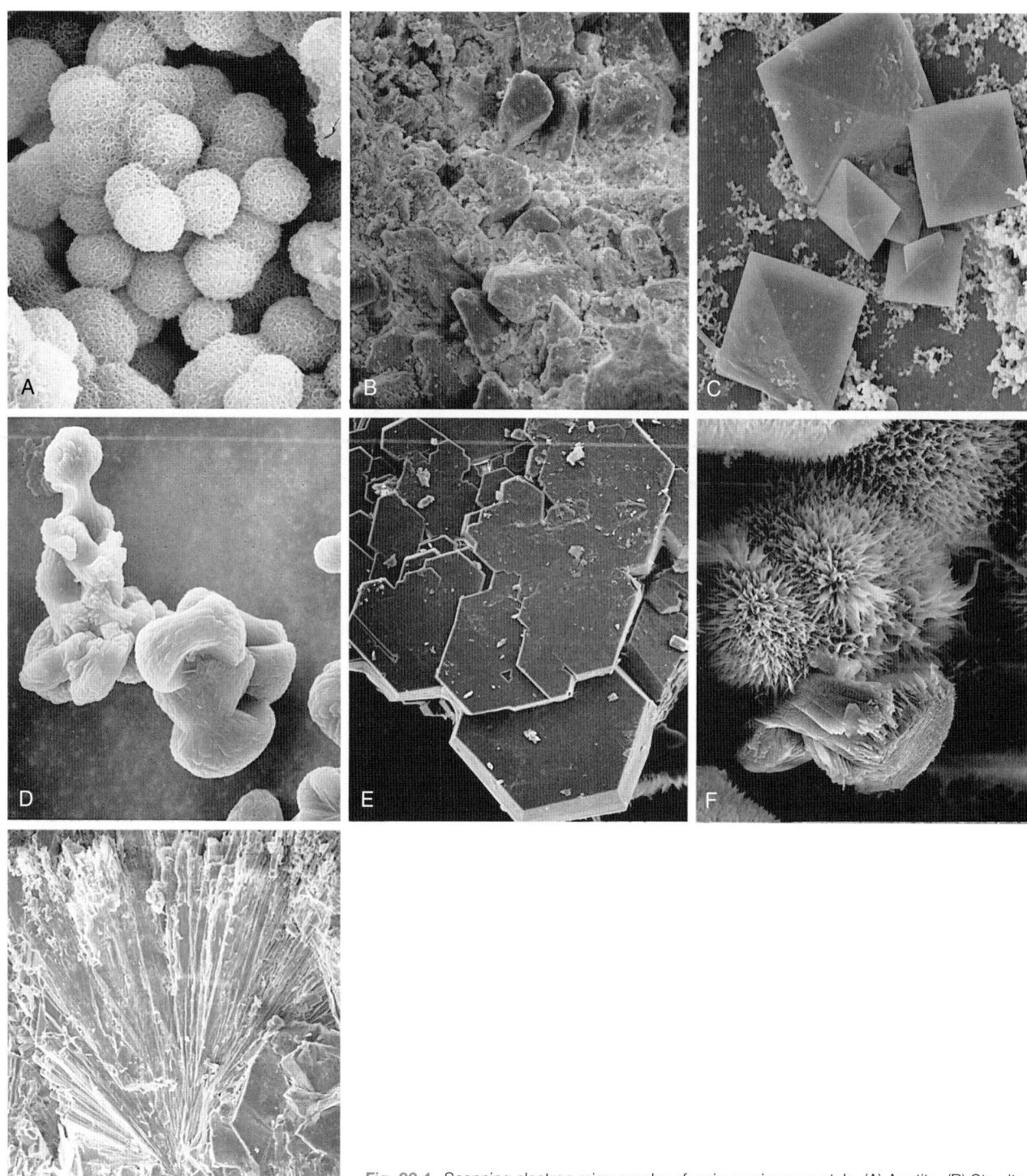

Fig. 92.4. Scanning electron micrographs of various urinary crystals. (A) Apatite. (B) Struvite. (C) Calcium oxalate dehydrate. (D) Calcium oxalate monohydrate. (E) Cystine. (F) Ammonium acid urate. (G) Brushite. (Courtesy of Dr. SR Khan, University of Florida, Gainesville, FL.)

Metabolic Evaluation for High-Risk and Recurrent Stone Formers

The AUA guidelines on the medical management of kidney stones recommends that clinicians perform additional metabolic testing in high-risk or interested first-time stone formers and recurrent stone formers (evidence strength: Grade B) (Pearle et al., 2014). High-risk stone formers were defined in the previous section. The AUA guidelines define recurrent stone formers as patients with recurrent stone episodes and multiple stones at initial presentation. These individuals are thought to benefit from a more extensive diagnostic evaluation as it may provide targeted recommendations for diet and/or medical therapy. Regardless of whether a particular patient requires a full metabolic evaluation, it is prudent to perform at least a screening evaluation combined with a thorough history and physical examination to assess for underlying systemic syndromes that may cause recurrent calculi and extrarenal complications. This assessment also should screen for patients at an increased risk for stone recurrence, as outlined in the previous paragraphs.

In these patients, a more extensive evaluation is recommended. In addition, obese patients with stones, particularly obese women, have a significantly elevated risk for recurrence and should be given consideration for metabolic evaluation (Taylor et al., 2005). Diabetes has been correlated with an increased risk for stone disease, and patients with diabetes and stones, particularly those with poorly controlled diabetes, should be considered for a full metabolic evaluation (Weinberg et al., 2014). Any patients with stones composed of cystine, uric acid, or struvite should undergo a complete metabolic workup.

Pak et al. previously recommended an extensive outpatient ambulatory protocol that included multiple office visits with 24-hour urine collections, laboratory studies, and a fast and calcium load study (Levy et al., 1995; Pak et al., 1980). The purpose of this testing was to delineate between various forms of hypercalciuria such as absorptive versus renal leak hypercalciuria. However, despite its high diagnostic yield and reliability, this testing is no longer recommended as it is cumbersome and has not been shown to change clinical practice (Lein and Keane, 1983; Pak, 1997; Pak et al., 2011; Pearle et al., 2014). Lifshitz et al. advocated for a less complex approach (Lifshitz et al., 1999). All patients undergo a basic metabolic screening, searching for systemic disorders that could pose a long-term health risk. They suggest that all patients should be advised about conservative nonspecific preventive measures. Patients at high risk for forming stones should have a more extensive metabolic evaluation based on two 24-hour urine samples.

Based on expert opinion of the guidelines panel, metabolic testing should consist of one or two 24-hour urine collections obtained on a random diet and analyzed at minimum for total volume, pH, calcium, oxalate, uric acid, citrate, sodium, potassium, and creatinine (Pearle et al., 2014). As indicated by the panel recommendation, there is no clear consensus based on the available literature regarding whether one or two 24-hour urine samples are necessary. A retrospective study by Pak et al. (2001) supports collection of a single 24-hour urine sample. They compared the results of two 24-hour urine samples collected on a random diet and found no significant difference in the excretion of urinary calcium, oxalate, uric acid, citrate, pH, total volume, sodium, potassium, sulfate, or phosphorus. The researchers concluded that the reproducibility of urinary stone risk factors was adequate in repeat samples, and therefore a single 24-hour urine collection was sufficient.

However, other studies have demonstrated a benefit to two separate 24-hour collections citing significant disparities in the results of the two studies. Parks et al. examined more than 1000 patients from both private practice and academic settings noting that within nearly 70% of the comparisons, there were large enough differences that the standard deviation would contain clinically relevant disparities (Parks et al., 2002). The authors therefore conclude that relying on one specimen alone could easily lead to misdiagnosis and, consequently, mismanagement. Healy et al. similarly advocate for two collections based on their study of 813 stone formers who submitted two 24-hour urine collections ≤10 days apart and found that a single 24-hour urine collection may have changed clinical decision making in up to 45% of patients (Healy et al., 2013). Finally, Rivers et al. (2000) recommended collection of two samples while the patient is on differing diets (random and restricted) to discern between absorptive hypercalciuria II and renal leak (hypercalciuria disappears while the patient is on the restricted diet in absorptive hypercalciuria II) (Box 92.3).

> **BOX 92.3 Potential Causes of Erroneous 24-Hour Urine Collection Results**
>
> Error in collection technique (e.g., improper use of preservatives, ice)
> Failure to collect a full 24 hours' worth of urine
> Changes in the patient's diet for the sake of the study
> Intermittent indiscretions in diet
> Failure of specimen to accurately represent typical day
> Bacterial contamination

Despite the guidelines panel recommendations, a recent population-based study found that the prevalence of metabolic testing in high-risk kidney stone formers was only 7.4% (Milose et al., 2014). The benefit of 24-hour urine testing in all recurrent stone formers has also recently been questioned. Hsi et al. cite several limitations of 24-hour urine testing such as complexity of interpretation, need for repeat collections, inability to predict stone recurrence with individual parameters and supersaturation values, unclear rationale of laboratory cutoff values, and difficulty of determining collection adequacy (Hsi et al., 2017). However, there is support for the effectiveness of a targeted approach given that urinary supersaturation values correlate closely with stone type, and a prospective trial has demonstrated that selective dietary recommendations based on 24-hour urine data was more effective than general dietary measures in preventing stone recurrence (Kocvara et al., 1999; Parks et al., 1997).

In an effort to develop alternate strategies to metabolic testing for stone formers, Otto et al. (2017) performed a retrospective study of 392 recurrent calcium oxalate stone formers with 24-hour urine testing and used logistic regression and receiver operating characteristic curve analysis to assess their predictive ability of age, gender, BMI, and comorbidities to detect abnormal 24-hour urine parameters. Essentially they were attempting to define surrogates for metabolic testing that might obviate the cost and burden of 24-hour urine testing while still providing appropriate stone-prevention treatment. They found that age significantly affected urinary calcium, oxalate, citrate, and pH, with older age associated with greater urinary oxalate, lower urinary uric acid, and lower urinary pH. Urinary calcium levels peaked at 40 to 49 years of age, and citrate nadired at 18 to 29 years of age. The study concluded that age, gender, and BMI can be used to predict 24-hour urine abnormalities and may be able to serve as a surrogate for 24-hour urine results.

> **KEY POINTS: METABOLIC EVALUATION FOR HIGH-RISK AND RECURRENT STONE FORMERS**
>
> - High-risk and recurrent stone formers should undergo the screening evaluation.
> - In addition, metabolic testing should consist of one or two 24-hour urine collections obtained on a random diet and analyzed at minimum for total volume, pH, calcium, oxalate, uric acid, citrate, sodium, potassium, and creatinine.
> - Despite guideline recommendations, prevalence of metabolic testing in high-risk stone formers remains low.

24-Hour Urine Collection

The cornerstone of reliable 24-hour urine analysis has been the development of a urine preservation method that allows collection of urine without refrigeration. The patient is then able to submit an aliquot to a central laboratory for an analysis of various stone-forming substances (Nicar et al., 1987). The urinary constituents most commonly assayed include calcium, oxalate, citrate, total volume, sodium, magnesium, potassium, pH, uric acid, and sulfate. Although most of these parameters are self-evident, sulfate is added to the list to assess the volume of protein loading from animal meat. From such determinations, the urinary saturation with respect to stone-forming salts can be calculated.

At present, multiple laboratories offer services focused on simplified, accurate 24-hour urine assessment for stone-forming risk factors. These laboratories provide collection containers with chemical preservatives (obviating iced storage and transport) and extrapolate 24-hour cumulative data from the submission of a small aliquot of the entire collection. After the values of all urinary constituents and saturations have been determined, the physician receives a computer printout that provides a numeric display of the test results (Fig. 92.5). These results should aid the physician in formulating a metabolic/physiologic diagnosis. It may be difficult to make a definitive diagnosis on a single 24-hour urinalysis; therefore repeated evaluation is often

Litholink Laboratory Reporting System™
Patient Results Report

PATIENT	DATE OF BIRTH	PHYSICIAN
Sample, Patient	**06/03/1951**	**Sample, Physician**

Stone Risk Factors / Cystine Screening: Negative (12/03/04)

Values larger, bolder, and more toward red indicate increasing risk for kidney stone formation.

DATE	SAMPLE ID	Vol 24	SS CaOx	Ca 24	Ox 24	Cit 24	SS CaP	pH	SS UA	UA 24
12/04/04	089979	2.35	**12.3**	**375**	**52**	401	.95	6.04	0.6	0.85
12/03/04	089978	2.17	**17.9**	**423**	**61**	471	0.9	5.72	1.6	1.01

ABBR.	ANALYTE	NORMAL RANGE	TREATMENT RECOMMENDATION
Vol 24	Urine Volume	1/d: 0.5 - 4 L	Raise vol at least 2L
SS CaOx	Supersaturation CaOx	6-10	Raise urine vol and cit, lower ox and ca.
Ca 24	Urine Calcium	men <250, women <200	IH, consider Hydrochlorothiazide 25 mg bid or chlorthalidone 25 mg qam, urine Na <100.
Ox 24	Urine Oxalate	20-40	usually dietary; if enteric, consider cholestyramine, oral calcium 1-2 gm with meals; if >80, may be primary hperoxauria.
Cit 24	Urine Citrate	men >450, women >550	consider K citrate 25 bid; if from RTA (urine pH > 6.5) also use K citrate
SS CaP	Supersaturation CaP	0.5-2	Urine usually pH > 6.5, IH common.
pH	24 Hour Urine pH	5.8-6.2	<5.8 consider K or Na citrate 25-30 mEq BID; 6.5, RTA if citrate is low; >8, urea splitting infection.
SS UA	Supersaturation Uric Acid	0-1	urine pH <6, creates UA stones. Treated with alkali
UA 24	Urine Uric Acid	g/day: men <0.800, women <0.750	dietary; if stones are severe and low protein diet fails try allopurinol 200 mg/d

**Cystine Screening: positive result may be seen in patients with homozygous cystinuria and cystine stone disease, some individuals heterozygous for cystinuria without cystine stone disease, or in patients taking medications such as captopril or penicillamine.

Fig. 92.5. Commercial 24-hour urine results are available and simplify the collection and reporting process. (Courtesy of Litholink, Chicago, IL.)

warranted. For example, it is desirable to confirm the presence of hypocitraturia or hyperuricosuria by repeat measurements.

Most patients will require detailed instructions on the proper collection of a complete 24-hour urine specimen. The patient should choose a day when all voids can be completely captured and when the specimen will represent a typical day. The first morning void is discarded, because this represents urine from the previous night and may not have had a predictable starting point. From that point on, all urine must be collected in the appropriate, laboratory-provided container. The canister may need to be kept on ice, and/or preservatives should have been added according to the requirements of the specific laboratory. When the patient awakens the next morning, the first morning void is collected with the rest of the specimen, thereby completing a full 24 hours. Total urinary creatinine should be measured to provide an internal check. Males will be expected to have produced roughly 20 to 25 mg of creatinine for every kilogram of body weight during the 24-hour period. Females generally have less muscle mass and therefore will typically produce 15 to 20 mg of creatinine for every kilogram of body weight in 24 hours. Significant aberrations in total creatinine excretion from these estimated values imply incomplete collection, overcollection, greater-than-expected muscle mass, or less-than-expected muscle mass.

Before and throughout the period of evaluation, the patient is instructed to discontinue any medication known to interfere with the metabolism of calcium, uric acid, or oxalate. These medications include vitamin D, calcium supplements, antacids, diuretics, acetazolamide, and vitamin C. Any current medication for stone treatment (thiazides, phosphate, allopurinol, or magnesium) should be discontinued as well, to better determine the patient's baseline physiology (and pathophysiology). Two random 24-hour urine samples are collected. These 24-hour specimens are obtained with the patient on a random diet, which is reflective of his or her usual dietary intake. It is important to stress to the patient to maintain his or her normal diet and fluid intake during urine collections. An attempt on the patient's part to suddenly eat well or to increase fluid consumption for the sake of the test will only mask the underlying causes of the stone disease.

Economics of Metabolic Evaluation

There is no doubt that the costs associated with the treatment of nephrolithiasis are substantial. Estimations of the annual medical expenditures for stone disease in the United States for 2000 were $2.1 billion, inclusive of $971 million for inpatient services, $607 million for physician office and hospital-based outpatient services, and $490 million for emergency room charges (Pearle, 2005). These calculations are based on a range of nationally available datasets and do not necessarily reflect the additional societal costs of lost productivity and social service support. These costs are clearly not negligible because the peak incidence of urolithiasis occurs in patients between 20 and 60 years of age (the years of highest worker productivity), and an analysis of more than 300,000 beneficiaries from 25 large US employers identified that 30% of patients with urolithiasis missed an average of 19 hours of work and had an additional $3500 in annual medical costs (Saigal et al., 2005).

With the increasing incidence of stone disease, it only can be concluded that the national health care expenditure for urolithiasis will continue to rise. Particularly worrisome is the increasing evidence that obesity confers an increased risk for nephrolithiasis, which is quite sobering considering the epidemic of obesity that is enveloping the United States (Curhan et al., 1998; Ekeruo et al., 2004; Morrill and Chinn, 2004; Rigby et al., 2004; Scales et al., 2012; Strumpf, 2004; Taylor et al., 2005).

With these figures in mind, prudence would dictate that medical prevention could help curb runaway costs and prevent long-term sequelae of recurrent nephrolithiasis. **However, office visits, serum studies, and 24-hour urine studies have their own costs. Is there a break-even point at which the costs of a metabolic evaluation, pharmacologic prophylaxis, and continued office visits are less than the expense of surgical management?**

Chandhoke (2002) compared the cost of medical prophylaxis with the cost of clinically managing recurrent stone episodes. Additionally, he determined the stone recurrence rate without prophylaxis (stone frequency) at which these two treatment approaches became cost-equivalent. This review conducted a cost survey in 10 countries to compare costs of medical prophylaxis and managing recurrent acute stone episodes. Costs of an acute stone episode included an emergency department visit, associated radiographic imaging to confirm diagnosis of a symptomatic stone, and outpatient treatment of upper urinary tract stones that did not pass spontaneously. Costs of medical management included an initial limited metabolic evaluation, drug therapy, a follow-up office visit every 6 months that included a 24-hour urinalysis, and yearly radiographic KUB imaging. Not surprisingly, the costs of medical prophylaxis and managing an acute stone episode varied significantly from country to country. The stone frequency at which costs of these management options became equivalent ranged from 0.3 to 4 stone episodes per year. This study concluded that medical management of a first stone episode is not cost-effective and that individual decisions should be determined by local costs.

Researchers at the University of Texas, Southwestern Medical Center have created a decision tree model to evaluate the cost-effectiveness and stone recurrence rates of common management strategies in stone formers (Lotan et al., 2004). They evaluated four common medical strategies: dietary measures alone (conservative), empirical drug treatment, or directed drug therapy based on simple or comprehensive metabolic evaluation. The model made reasonable assumptions regarding costs for evaluation, medications, emergency treatment, and surgery for stone recurrence. A review of the literature guided estimations of stone recurrence and risk reduction from various medical therapies. They found that first-time stone formers were best treated with a conservative approach because it was the least costly and it yielded a stone formation rate of 0.07 stone per patient yearly. For recurrent stone formers, conservative treatment was less costly than drug treatments but it was associated with a higher stone recurrence rate (0.3 stone per patient yearly). Directed medical therapies were more costly than conservative treatment ($885 to $1187 vs. $258 yearly), but they provided the obvious advantage of decreasing recurrence rates by 60% to 86%.

The authors went on to compare the expense of the simple medical evaluation and associated management as described earlier in this chapter and noted it to be more costly than empirical treatment but also more effective. Importantly, a complete evaluation with attendant treatment offered no advantage in cost or efficacy over empirical treatment or modified simple metabolic evaluation and management. The authors also recommended that first-time stone formers be treated with conservative therapy because it is both cost-effective and efficacious. In contrast, however, **recurrent stone formers should be treated medically after a simplified evaluation, because of the high recurrence rate of stone formation.**

TABLE 92.3 Mineralogic Names of Renal Calculi

RENAL CALCULI	MINERAL NAME
Calcium oxalate monohydrate	Whewellite
Calcium oxalate dihydrate	Weddellite
Calcium hydrogen phosphate dihydrate	Brushite
Tricalcium phosphate	Whitlockite
Carbonite-apatite	Carbonite-apatite
Magnesium ammonium phosphate	Struvite
Cystine	None
Uric acid	None

KEY POINTS: ECONOMICS OF METABOLIC EVALUATION

- Routine performance of a comprehensive metabolic evaluation may not be economically sound if applied to all stone patients.
- Many first-time stone formers may not benefit economically from a metabolic evaluation unless initial screening puts them in a high-risk category.
- Recurrent stone formers are best treated with a metabolic evaluation and directed medical therapy.

STONE ANALYSIS

Stone analysis can provide valuable insight into how and why a patient may have formed a stone. In some instances, a stone analysis may be more practical to obtain than a 24-hour urine collection, and in other cases it can serve as a useful adjunct to serum and urine metabolic evaluation. **The AUA guidelines on medical management of kidney stones recommend obtaining a stone analysis at least once when one is available to help classify patients and guide preventive measures.** They also recommend repeating stone analysis in the event further stones are available, particularly if not responding to treatment as stones are known to vary in composition from event to event.

Because most stones are a mixture of more than one component, the relative ratios or predominance of any particular molecule may have predictive value (Table 92.3). In an analysis of almost 1400 patients who had both stone analysis and a complete metabolic evaluation, Pak et al. noted that calcium phosphate and mixed calcium oxalate–calcium phosphate stones were associated with the diagnoses of RTA and primary hyperparathyroidism (odds ratio [OR], ≥ 2), but not with chronic diarrheal syndromes (Pak et al., 2003b). As the phosphate content of the stone increased from calcium oxalate to mixed calcium oxalate–calcium phosphate, and finally to calcium phosphate, the percentage of patients with RTA increased from 5% to 39%, and those with primary hyperparathyroidism increased from 2% to 10%. Not surprisingly, pure and mixed uric acid stones were strongly associated with a gouty diathesis, and brushite stones were associated with RTA. As expected, a very strong association was found between infection stones and infection and between cystine stones and cystinuria.

Parks et al. also evaluated the clinical significance of calcium phosphate percentage in mixed stones and identified greater numbers of shock wave lithotripsy procedures in patients with high percentages of calcium phosphate. They also identified the potential for calcium oxalate stone formers to convert to calcium phosphate stone formers (Parks et al., 2004). Although the precise mechanism for this change remains unclear, acidification defects from prior shock wave lithotripsy and citrate supplementation have been postulated to be contributing factors (Parks et al., 2004, 2009; Evan et al., 2015a).

There are several different methods of performing a stone analysis. The two most widely recommended and utilized methods are x-ray diffraction or Fourier-transform infrared spectroscopy (Gilad et al., 2017; Mandel et al., 2017; Tiselius et al., 2017). Although highly reliable in optimized settings, real-world data to date has shown heterogeneity in reported findings ranging from 30% to 50% depending on the mineral being evaluated (Krambeck 2010a, 2010b; Siener et al., 2016). Inaccuracies in struvite and calcium phosphate have been identified as particularly challenging (Krambeck, 2010b). One potential reason is the heterogeneity and lack of quality-control standards and best-practice policies for testing. An assessment of stone analysis laboratories across Europe identified only 56% as meeting quality requirements (Siener et al., 2016).

An inherent limitation of these techniques is that they are destructive methods that rely on turning the stone into a powder before analysis. Once the stone is destroyed, the opportunity to evaluate the microstructure and different compositions relative to one another is lost. There is increasing recognition that such information may provide more useful information than previously recognized.

Gross morphologic analysis of stones has been suggested to help elucidate the etiology of stone formation, and a morphologic classification system has been previously described by Daudon et al. (Cloutier et al., 2015; Daudon et al., 1993). This system, which features 6 main types of stones and 22 subtypes, has proved superior to stone composition alone in predicting the likelihood of stone recurrence. Daudon et al. (2018b) also linked stone morphology to metabolic disorders in a published analysis of over 30,000 intact stones. In the study, over one-third harbored Randall's plaque residues. Notably, the rate of such stones increased significantly over three decades and was associated with younger age of onset, higher serum ionized calcium levels, and increased serum osteoclasts providing potential insight into the rising prevalence of stone disease (Letavernier et al., 2015).

Another emerging technique to better appreciate the structure and composition of stones is microCT. MicroCT is a nondestructive imaging technique whereby small structures such as stones can be visualized at 1000 times the resolution of clinical CT scanners (Borofsky et al., 2016a). MicroCT images allow for identification of mineral subtypes with roughly the same accuracy as infrared spectroscopy but preserves the microstructure such that the relationships of the crystals to one another can be analyzed (Fig. 92.6) (Borofsky et al., 2016b). One example of how microCT may improve stone classification is via identification of stones that form on Randall's plaque compared with those that form on ductal plugs (Fig. 92.7) (Williams et al., 2015, 2018).

> **KEY POINTS: STONE ANALYSIS**
> - Stones should be sent for analysis when available.
> - Repeat stone analysis should be performed if stone formation continues, particularly if they are not responding to treatment.
> - Stones commonly have mixed mineral composition.
> - The most common method of stone analysis is x-ray diffraction or Fourier-transform infrared spectroscopy.
> - MicroCT is an emerging method of stone analysis that is nondestructive.

CLASSIFICATION OF NEPHROLITHIASIS

Classification of stone formers is a challenging concept that is under constant evolution as more is learned about the mechanisms by which stones form. Different information can be obtained from the results of stone analysis, evaluation of serum chemistries, and results of 24-hour urine testing. There is also increasing interest and investigation in using endoscopic appearances of the renal papillae as a method to classify patients (Almeras et al., 2016; Borofsky et al.,

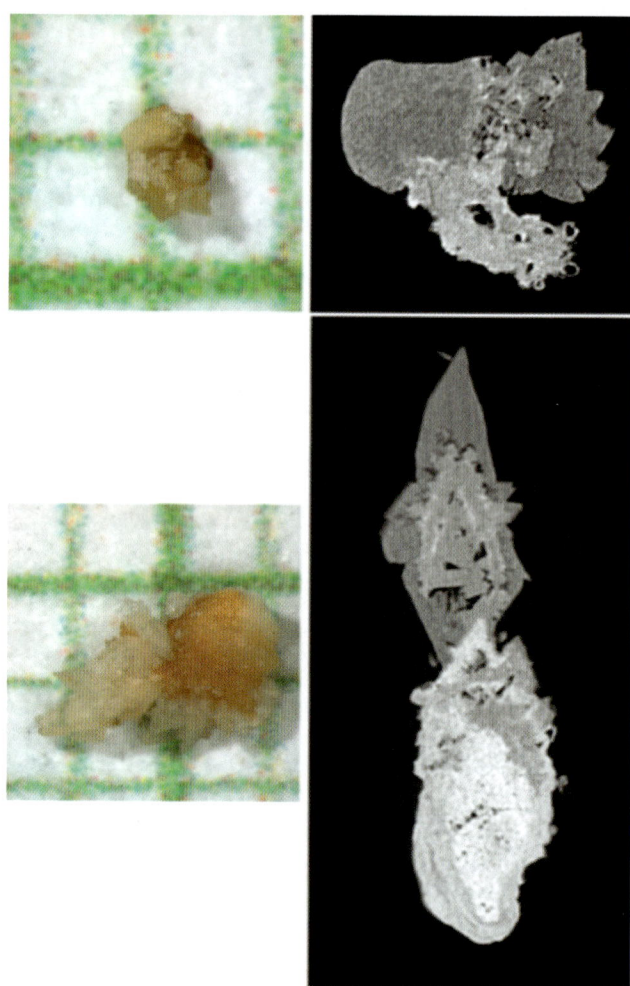

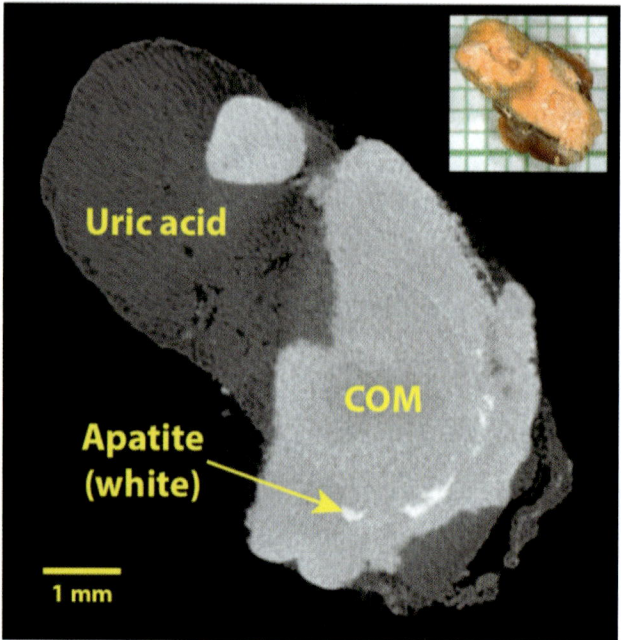

Fig. 92.6. MicroCT appearance of a 7-mm stone removed from the kidney. Note is made of the mixed composition of mineral components with uric acid appearing dark, calcium oxalate monohydrate (COM) slightly brighter, and calcium phosphate (Apatite) white. (Courtesy of Drs. James Williams and James Lingeman, Indiana University School of Medicine.)

Fig. 92.7. MicroCT appearance of stone forming over Randall's plaque *(top)* and ductal plug *(bottom)*. The brighter-appearing regions on the microCT images are calcium phosphate. On the *top right* image, the plaque demonstrates several small cylindrical empty spaces indicative of peritubular calcification within the papillary interstitium over which stones can form. On the *bottom right* figure, a more dense mineral accumulation has formed via accretion and layering forming a ductal plug of calcium phosphate over which a stone may grow. (Courtesy of Drs. James Williams and James Lingeman, Indiana University School of Medicine.)

2016b; Marien and Miller, 2016). Under ideal circumstances, all of these factors are taken into consideration; however, as previously discussed, this can be a taxing process and is not always feasible. Identification of a single metabolic process is not always possible, and at times more than one metabolic abnormality may be identified. The scientific rationale and physiologic processes by which these abnormalities lead to stone formation can be found in Chapter 91.

General Recommendations for Stone Formers

Certain conservative recommendations should be made for all patients regardless of the underlying cause of their stone disease. In a recent study, Ferraro et al. examined dietary and lifestyle risk factors associated with incident kidney stones in men and women (Ferraro et al., 2016b). Using data from the Health Professionals Follow-up Study (HPFS) and the Nurses' Health Study (NHS) I and II, they demonstrated that five modifiable risk factors (fluid intake, BMI, DASH diet, dietary calcium intake, and intake of sugar-sweetened beverages) accounted for greater than 50% of incident kidney stones. The results suggest that preventive measures centered on these factors could substantially decrease the burden of kidney stone disease.

Fluid Recommendations

Low urine volume is perhaps the most important risk factor for kidney stone formation. Increased fluid intake is a powerful tool in preventing stone recurrence for all stone types and likely does so via a decrease in urinary supersaturation of stone components (Pak et al., 1980). In a randomized controlled trial of idiopathic calcium oxalate stone formers, Borghi et al. (1996) demonstrated that increased fluid intake sufficient to maintain a urine volume greater than 2L/day significantly lowered the stone recurrence rate over a 5-year follow-up period compared with a control group (12.1% vs. 27%, $P = 0.008$). High fluid intake has also been found to be protective in relation to stone formation in several large prospective observational studies. In the HPFS, stone incidence was 192 per 100,000 person-years for fluid intake greater than 2.5 L/day compared with 372 per 100,000 person-years for fluid intake less than 1.2 L/day ($P < 0.01$). The NHS I demonstrated similar findings, with stone incidence lower for fluid intake greater than 2.5 L/day (Curhan et al., 1993). Furthermore, researchers at the University of Chicago demonstrated that failure to increase urine output was one of three very strong predictors of relapse for patients followed in a dedicated stone clinic (Strauss et al., 1982a). **Therefore, a mainstay of conservative management for kidney stone prevention is increased fluid intake to achieve a urine output of at least 2.5 L/day.** This recommendation is supported by the American Urological Association and the European Association of Urology (EAU) guidelines for medical management of nephrolithiasis (Pearle et al., 2014; Skolarikos et al., 2015). The economic impact of increasing fluid intake to decrease stones has also been considered. Models based on the French health care system estimated that increased fluid intake could prevent over 11,000 stone events per year and save the health care system almost 50 million euros (Lotan et al., 2012).

Although the concept of increased fluid intake is quite simple, patient compliance with this therapy can be difficult particularly in the long term. Parks et al. (2003) demonstrated in a large series of 2877 university and private practice patients that the average increase in urinary volume was only 0.3 L/day. Khambati et al. (2017) retrospectively investigated factors associated with compliance to increased fluid intake and urine volume following dietary counseling in first-time kidney stone patients. They found the compliance rate of obtaining a urine volume greater than 2.5 L/day was 50.1% at 6 months. Logistic regression found male sex, stone-related surgical procedures, and baseline 24-hour urine volume greater than 1 L/day were associated with greater odds of compliance, and age older than 58 years and presence of lower urinary tract symptoms were associated with lower odds of compliance. There are practical recommendations to help patients achieve increased fluid intake including measuring out the desired fluid intake for the day ahead of time, keeping fluid (preferably water) in one's line of sight while at work or home (at desk, refrigerator, even bathroom while brushing teeth), and keeping a log of fluid intake (Clayman et al., 2018).

Furthermore, smart phone applications and devices have also been developed to improve patient compliance. Mobile health technology including utilization of smart phone applications, fitness trackers, social media engagement, and improved communication methods has been demonstrated to be effective in facilitating health behavior changes across a wide spectrum of diseases (Zhao et al., 2016). This technology has been applied to stone prevention in several ways. The most common stone-related applications are those directed at increasing fluid intake, with over 50 such applications available at the time of this publication. These applications use a variety of behavior change techniques, most commonly control-based theory techniques featuring goal setting, self-monitoring, and behavioral feedback (Conroy et al., 2017). Smart water bottles are another novel technology that has been applied toward promoting fluid intake by tracking the amount of fluid consumed through the bottle over designated periods and communicating data to smart phone–based applications (Borofsky et al., 2018). Other applications related to stone prevention include information-based services, health professional resources, and dietary recording tools. One potential concern related to mobile health applications is accuracy. A review of 42 unique applications directed at kidney stones found that only 36% had clear input from health professionals, and many offered guideline-inconsistent recommendations (Stevens et al., 2015).

The impact of beverages on stone risk has also been studied. A full discussion of citrus and citrate-containing beverages can be found in the hypocitraturia section to follow. However, the effect of beverages other than water can have a considerable influence on overall stone risk. **Epidemiologic data has demonstrated that consumption of sugar-sweetened soda and punch is associated with a higher risk for stone formation, and coffee, tea, beer, and wine are associated with a lower risk for stone formation** (Curhan et al., 1996a, 1998b; Ferraro et al., 2013). The diuretic properties of coffee, tea, and alcohol have been cited as the factor potentially reducing kidney stone risk (Ferraro et al., 2013). Sugar-sweetened beverages contain fructose, and this simple sugar has been shown to increase urinary calcium excretion in both rats and humans and the production and excretion of uric acid in humans (Koh et al., 1989; Milne and Nielsen, 2000; Taylor and Curhan, 2008). Taylor and Curhan's analysis of the HPFS and NHS (I and II) documented that increasing fructose intake correlated with an increasing relative risk for incident stone formation, regardless of BMI, caloric intake, or other risk factors (Taylor and Curhan, 2008). In a randomized controlled trial, Shuster et al. studied 1009 male subjects, who reported consuming at least 160 mL/day of soft drinks (Shuster et al., 1992). One-half of the subjects were randomized to refrain from consuming soft drinks, and the remaining subjects served as controls. The intervention group had an observed 6.4% advantage in actuarial 3-year freedom from recurrence over the control group. One important secondary finding was that those who reported that their most consumed drink was acidified by phosphoric acid but not citric acid had a 15% higher 3-year recurrence-free rate than controls. Meanwhile, those who consumed drinks acidified by citric acid had no increase in stone episodes when compared with controls.

Animal Protein

Nondairy animal protein (meat, fish, poultry, eggs) intake can affect several urinary parameters that may increase kidney stone risk including calcium, uric acid, oxalate, and citrate. Urinary calcium excretion has been shown to increase secondary to animal protein consumption through a mechanism of bone reabsorption and lower tubular calcium reabsorption (Reddy et al., 2002; Frank et al., 2009; Bonny and Edwards, 2013). In addition, high animal protein as a source of purines can deliver an acid load that reduces tubular reabsorption of citrate and hypocitraturia and increases urinary uric acid levels resulting in hyperuricosuria (Breslau et al., 1988; Choi et al., 2004; Kok et al., 1990; Tracy et al., 2014). The effect of high animal protein intake appears to be most harmful when coupled with a diet that is low in calcium (Martini and Heilberg,

2002). The effect of nondairy animal protein on urinary oxalate has yielded conflicting results, with some studies demonstrating no change and others suggesting increased oxalate (Giannini et al., 1999; Holmes et al., 1993; Marangella et al., 1989; Nguyen et al., 2001). In a study evaluating short-term dietary protein restriction in hypercalciuric stone formers, Gianni et al. demonstrated a beneficial effect on urinary parameters including reduced urinary excretion of calcium, phosphate, hydroxyproline, uric acid, and oxalate and increased urinary citrate excretion (Giannini et al., 1999).

Epidemiologic studies have suggested that the incidence of nephrolithiasis is higher in populations in which there is increased animal protein intake. For example, in the northern and western regions of India, animal protein intake is approximately 100% greater than in the southern and eastern regions, and the rate of kidney stones is four times greater. When populations are matched for economic status, the intake of protein and other dietary constituents does not differ in patients with recurrent stones and controls; however, patients with stones secrete greater quantities of calcium in the urine than do controls for a given intake of protein (Wasserstein et al., 1987). The explanation for this finding may be that patients with recurrent nephrolithiasis are more sensitive to the calciuric action of protein than normal subjects (Goldfarb, 1990).

More recent observational studies have reported conflicting results regarding the effect of animal protein intake on kidney stone risk. In the NHS I and II cohorts, no association was demonstrated, and in the HPFS the positive association between animal protein consumption and risk for kidney stone formation was only in men with a BMI less than 25 (Curhan et al., 1997, 2004; Taylor et al., 2004). Ferraro et al. reported that kidney stone risk may vary by protein type (Ferraro et al., 2016). Again using the NHS I and II and the HPFS, they found that subjects in the highest quintile of nondairy animal protein intake had 54 mg/dL lower urinary citrate, 24 mg/dL higher urinary uric acid, lower urinary pH, and higher relative supersaturation for uric acid. Vegetable protein was not associated with risk for stones, and dairy protein was associated with decreased risk in younger women. In addition, a major finding of the study was a strong inverse association between higher dietary potassium intake and risk for stones with a 33% to 56% lower risk for stones for subjects in the highest quintile of potassium intake. **The results of this study suggest that diets high in potassium and lower in animal protein may be effective in preventing kidney stone formation.**

Unfortunately, despite the known alteration in urinary parameters related to the intake of animal protein, few clinical trials have evaluated the effect of animal protein restriction on kidney stone formation. Hiatt et al. conducted a randomized controlled trial of a low–animal protein, high-fiber diet in calcium oxalate stone formers who were followed for over 4 years with food questionnaires and serum and urine chemistry measurements (Hiatt et al., 1996). The control group was instructed only on fluid intake and adequate calcium. They found that the intervention group actually had an increased relative risk for recurrent stone formation compared with the control group and concluded that a low–animal protein, high-fiber diet had no advantage over high fluid intake alone. However, one problem limiting the conclusions of this study is that several participants in the intervention group appeared to have poor compliance with the prescribed diet. Another 4-year randomized trial compared the effect of two diets, a low animal protein–diet and high-fiber diet, to a normal diet in 175 idiopathic calcium stone formers for secondary prevention of calcium nephrolithiasis (Dussol et al., 2008). There was no change in urinary calcium levels or stone recurrence rates for either group compared with the control group. In comparison, Borghi et al. (2002) prospectively randomized hypercalciuric stone formers to either a low-protein, low-salt, moderate-calcium diet or to a low-calcium diet. Although acknowledging that it is difficult to separate the potential effects of the three facets of the first diet, there was a convincing 50% reduction in stone events compared with those patients on the low-calcium diet.

Although increased animal protein induces effects on urinary parameters that should increase kidney stone risk, to date there are no studies demonstrating that restriction of animal protein in isolation reduces stone recurrence. Furthermore, long-term compliance with animal protein restriction may be challenging, particularly in Western populations. **However, more recently the Dietary Approaches to Stop Hypertension (DASH) diet has been evaluated for its effect on kidney stone formation. The DASH diet is rich in fruits and vegetables, moderate in low-fat dairy products, and low in animal protein. In a prospective population-based study, higher DASH scores were associated with a lower risk for kidney stone formation** (Taylor and Curhan, 2009). The inhibitory effect of the DASH diet is likely related to increases in urinary citrate and urine volume (Taylor et al., 2010). Meschi et al. (2004) also showed the benefits of a diet high in fruits and vegetables on urinary parameters. Twelve normal subjects had fruits and vegetables eliminated from their diet, and 26 hypocitraturic calcium-stone formers had their diet supplemented with low-oxalate–containing fruits and vegetables. Compared with normal subjects, the hypocitraturic calcium-stone formers with increased fruit and vegetable intake significantly increased their urinary volume, pH, potassium, magnesium, and citrate. In addition, the supersaturation of calcium oxalate and uric acid fell in the stone formers with increased fruit and vegetable intake. **In summary, patients with calcium oxalate or uric acid stones are most likely to benefit from a diet limiting nondairy animal protein and increasing fruit and vegetable intake** (Pearle et al., 2014, Skolarikos et al., 2015).

KEY POINTS: FLUIDS AND ANIMAL PROTEIN

- Fluid intake over 2.5 L/day is recommended for prevention of recurrent stones.
- Compliance with high fluid recommendations is challenging and can be potentially aided by behavioral changes and mobile health applications.
- Randomized studies have confirmed the advantage of a diet with reduced nondairy animal protein intake.
- A diet high in fruits and vegetables imparts a reduced risk for stone formation over diets high in animal protein.

CALCIUM-BASED CALCULI

Calcium-based calculi are the most common type of stone. A review of nearly 90,000 stone analyses over a 35-year period from Mandel et al. identified primary calcium-based composition in 78% of stones (42% calcium oxalate, monohydrate, 18% calcium oxalate dihydrate, 15% calcium phosphate, 3% brushite) (Mandel et al., 2017). Not surprisingly, this stone type also has the greatest number of potential contributing metabolic factors and therapies.

Not all calcium stones are the same, and the metabolic considerations related to stone composition are considerable. One of the most important distinctions is calcium oxalate versus calcium phosphate (hydroxyapatite) versus brushite stone disease. This is not always a clear distinction as **stones are often composed of more than one mineral subtype.** Traditionally, the stone is classified as a calcium oxalate or calcium phosphate stone based on the dominant mineral subtype in the analysis (Parks et al., 2004). From a clinical and metabolic perspective, this distinction may have relevance. **Calcium phosphate stone disease appears to differ from calcium oxalate stone disease in that it tends to affect women more than men, present at a younger age, and is associated with alkaline urinary pH** (Asplin et al., 1998; Parks et al., 1997, 2004). Furthermore, a high percentage of calcium phosphate in stones has been linked to metabolic abnormalities and nephrocalcinosis (Bhojani et al., 2015; Kacker et al., 2008). Recent epidemiologic studies have demonstrated that young women are the demographic group with the most rapidly rising incidence of stone disease. Calcium phosphate stones are more common in young women, and it has been hypothesized that this is part of the reason stone rates based on gender are becoming more even (Scales et al., 2007; Singh et al., 2015; Kittanamongkolchai et al., 2018).

Brushite is another subtype of calcium stone worth consideration. Brushite is a precursor to hydroxyapatite and is a subtype

BOX 92.4 Medical Conditions Associated With Calcium Nephrolithaisis

Hyperparathyroidism	Primary hyperoxaluria
Hyperthyroidism	Enteric hyperoxaluria
Sarcoidosis	Bowel disease
Vitamin D excess	Chronic pancreatitis
Calcium supplementation	Vitamin C supplements
Prolonged immobilization	Chronic diarrhea
Clinical evidence of bone disease	Lithogenic drugs
	Urinary infection
Malignant neoplasms	Gouty diathesis
Distal renal tubular acidosis	Cystinuria
Medullary sponge kidney	

Modified from Gambaro G, Croppi E, Coe F, et al. Consensus Conference. Metabolic diagnosis and medical prevention of calcium nephrolithiasis and its systemic manifestations: a consensus statement. *J Nephrol* 29(6):715–734, 2016.

of calcium phosphate stones only identified in 2% to 3% of stone analyses (Mandel et al., 2017). Unlike calcium oxalate and calcium phosphate (hydroxyapatite) stones, which are classified using a dominant percentage of mineral, **the unique clinical and metabolic associations with brushite calculi have led some experts to classify a stone former as a brushite stone former if any brushite mineral is identified on stone composition** (Evan et al., 2005). Brushite stones present several unique clinical challenges in that they are among the hardest stones to break and are refractory to shock wave lithotripsy (Klee et al., 1991; Williams et al., 2012b). They are also strongly associated with metabolic abnormalities. A relatively large-scale analysis of 82 brushite stone formers identified metabolic abnormalities in 100% of cases including hypercalciuria in 81% and elevated urinary pH (>6.2) in 62%. Recurrence rates were very high as well, with recurrence demonstrated in 38% of patients at a mean of only 33 months (Krambeck et al., 2010a). The distinct profile of the brushite stone former relative to calcium phosphate (apatite) has been demonstrated both in terms of endoscopy/tissue biopsy and urinary profiles, where brushite stone formers may have higher degrees of hypercalciuria (Evan et al., 2014; Moreira et al., 2013).

In 2016, a consensus statement from 44 international experts in calcium stone disease was published regarding the metabolic diagnosis and prevention of calcium stone disease. Among the numerous issues addressed, one was on proper classification of calcium stone formers. It was recommended that twenty different medical conditions be ruled out before assigning a designation for someone as being an "idiopathic" calcium stone former, a diagnosis of exclusion (Box 92.4) (Gambaro et al., 2016).

Role of Dietary Calcium

The preponderance of evidence now supports the maintenance of moderate calcium intake in the face of calcareous nephrolithiasis (Borghi et al., 2002; Curhan et al., 1993, 1997; Heller et al., 2003; Lewandowski et al., 2001; Martini et al., 2000; Takei et al., 1998; Taylor et al., 2004; Trinchieri et al., 1998). **Older recommendations to significantly restrict calcium intake likely led to an increase in available intestinal oxalate.** As a result, this limitation in dietary calcium may subsequently increase oxalate absorption, thereby raising the supersaturation of calcium oxalate. As noted earlier, a prospective, randomized study has shown that patients on a moderate-calcium diet, combined with salt restriction and moderation of animal protein had one-half as many stone episodes as those who attempted to follow a calcium-restricted diet (Borghi et al., 2002). Review of a large cohort of middle-aged nurses revealed that there was a decreased incidence of nephrolithiasis in subjects who had increased levels of dietary calcium (Curhan et al., 1997). Interestingly, this protection did not remain for those who received increased calcium intake from supplements instead of from dietary sources (i.e., dairy products).

There is further evidence to suggest that calcium supplementation can be safe if attention is paid to preparation and especially to timing. In a review of postmenopausal women, authors demonstrated that initiation of calcium supplementation does not have deleterious effects on urinary calcium, oxalate, or citrate levels. Furthermore, calcium supplement with a meal or combined calcium supplement and estrogen therapy was not associated with a significant increased risk for calcium oxalate stone formation in the majority of postmenopausal osteoporotic patients (Domrongkitchaiporn et al., 2002). Additional work from the same group determined that the timing of calcium supplementation may have positive or negative effects (Domrongkitchaiporn et al., 2004). In a study of healthy male recruits, the authors compared the urinary effects of calcium carbonate supplementation taken with meals versus at bedtime. In both instances, urinary calcium excretion increased equal amounts. However, for those taking the calcium supplement with meals, this increase was offset by an equally significant decrease in urinary oxalate. As a result, there was no increase in urinary supersaturation of calcium oxalate when calcium supplementation was taken with meals, a protection that did not remain for the nighttime bolus ingestion.

Evidence also suggests that the type of calcium supplementation may have an impact on the potential of stone formation. Two long-term studies from researchers in Dallas document that supplementation with calcium citrate does not have a significant impact on stone formation. Calcium citrate is an over-the-counter calcium preparation that provides 950 mg of calcium citrate and 200 mg of elemental calcium in each tablet. As with other available calcium supplements, calcium citrate will significantly increase urinary calcium excretion. Yet, this preparation offers the benefit of also increasing urinary citrate excretion. The concomitant increase in citraturia potentially offsets the lithogenic potential of calcium supplement–induced hypercalciuria and therefore provides a more stone-friendly calcium supplement (Sakhaee et al., 2004).

One clinical trial further studied the effects of long-term calcium citrate supplementation in premenopausal women. This investigation demonstrated that the urinary saturation of calcium oxalate and calcium phosphate (brushite) did not significantly change during calcium citrate therapy. It appears that the lack of calcium supplement–induced hypercalciuria was secondary to the downregulation of intestinal calcium absorption, because of prolonged calcium supplementation and the inhibitory effects of citrate included in the calcium citrate preparation. The results of this long-term calcium citrate trial suggest that calcium supplementation using calcium citrate does not increase the propensity for crystallization of calcium salts within the urine. This protective effect is most likely caused by an attenuated increase in urinary calcium excretion (from a decrease in fractional intestinal calcium absorption), a decrease in urinary phosphorus, and an increased citraturic response (Sakhaee et al., 1994).

KEY POINTS: CALCIUM BASED CALCULI

- Calcium-based calculi are the most common type of urinary stones.
- Calcium oxalate is the most common subtype.
- Calcium phosphate stones are more common in young women and associated with alkaline urinary pH.
- Brushite is a type of calcium phosphate strongly associated with rapid stone growth and recurrence.
- Dietary calcium restriction actually increases stone recurrence risk.
- Calcium supplementation is likely safest when taken with meals.
- Calcium citrate appears to be a more stone-friendly calcium supplement because of the additional inhibitory action of citrate.

HYPERCALCIURIA (>200 mg/day)
Clinical Considerations

Hypercalciuria is the most common metabolic contributor to kidney stone disease (Pearle et al., 2014). The term itself is used to describe an excess of urinary calcium. **There is no exact level at which the amount of calcium in the urine become pathologic; rather, the higher the degree of hypercalciuria, the higher the associated risk for calcium stone formation** (Curhan et al., 2001). A level of >200 mg/day has been recommended based on epidemiologic studies suggesting that over this level, the relative risk for stone formation among both men and women becomes greater than 1 (Curhan et al., 2001). Nonetheless, lowering the levels of urinary calcium even below this may be warranted if stone activity persists at these levels (Coe et al., 2016). The goal of a metabolic evaluation in these cases should be to identify modifiable factors contributing to high urinary calcium.

Resorptive Hypercalciuria (Primary Hyperparathyroidism)

Primary hyperparathyroidism (PHPT) is one of the most common modifiable causes of hypercalciuria in stone formers, with an estimated incidence between 2% and 8% (Rodman and Mahler, 2000). **Patients with PHPT suffer from an overproduction of PTH from either one dominant adenoma or diffuse hyperplasia of all four glands.** Elevated levels of PTH in turn lead to an excess of calcium in the blood and urine from increased bone turnover and intestinal reabsorption (Silverberg et al., 1990). An elevated serum calcium level should trigger suspicion for PHPT as should other factors including a high percentage of calcium phosphate in stone composition, and high urinary calcium level (Pearle et al., 2014). Rarely, patients may develop PHPT as a result of multiple endocrine neoplasia or parathyroid carcinoma (Craven et al., 2008).

Patients with PHPT frequently demonstrate hypercalcemia and elevations of parathyroid hormone (PTH). Several considerations should be made before proceeding with an evaluation for PHPT. First, care should be taken to identify any medications that the patient may be taking that can interfere with calcium and PTH levels. Thiazide diuretics can artificially elevate serum PTH levels and should be held for 2 weeks before measurement (Porpiglia et al., 2015). Lithium is another medication that can raise serum calcium and PTH levels (Albert et al., 2013). Consideration should also be made regarding the timing of the lab draw as recent ingestion of calcium either through supplements or diet has been shown to cause transient elevations in serum calcium levels. For this reason, a fasting serum calcium level is preferred (Siyam and Klachko, 2013).

Unfortunately, some patients may have normocalcemic PHPT. These patients may be hard to distinguish from those with renal leak hypercalciuria, during which serum calcium will be normal but a mild elevation of PTH can occur, creating a secondary hyperparathyroidism. In these instances, the patient can be treated with a 2-week course of a thiazide diuretic, such as chlorthalidone 25 mg daily. If the patient actually has renal leak, the calcium loss should be suppressed and the PTH should return to normal (Aroldi et al., 1979; Barilla and Pak, 1979; Zechner et al., 1981). Those with true primary hyperparathyroidism will continue to circulate elevated levels of PTH and may become mildly hypercalcemic, although this latter feature has been debated in the literature (Farquhar et al., 1990; Klimiuk et al., 1981; Strong et al., 1991).

Parathyroidectomy is the optimum treatment for nephrolithiasis in patients with primary hyperparathyroidism (Fraker 2000). This therapy may include resection of a dominant adenoma or removal of all four hyperplastic glands. After removal of abnormal parathyroid tissue, urinary calcium is expected to return to normal, commensurate with a decline in serum calcium and intestinal calcium absorption. However, these findings are not always dependable, because some patients may suffer from changes in tubular and glomerular functions as a result of long-standing hypercalcemia/hypercalciuria (Farias et al., 1996). Moreover, it is imperative to repeat a 24-hour urinary calcium determination to make sure the hypercalciuria has resolved.

There is no established medical treatment for the nephrolithiasis of primary hyperparathyroidism. Although orthophosphates have been recommended for the disease of mild-to-moderate severity, their safety or efficacy has not yet been proved. These medications should be used only when parathyroid surgery cannot be undertaken. Estrogen has been reported to be useful in reducing serum and urinary calcium in postmenopausal women with primary hyperparathyroidism (Boucher et al., 1989; Coe et al., 1986; Diamond et al., 1996; Herbai and Ljunghall, 1983; Marcus et al., 1984; Orr-Walker et al., 2000; Selby and Peacock, 1986).

> **KEY POINTS: RESORPTIVE HYPERCALCIURIA**
> - An elevated serum calcium level should trigger suspicion for hyperparathyroidism.
> - A high calcium phosphate percentage in stone and elevated urinary calcium may also be indicative of hyperparathyroidism.

Sarcoidosis and Granulomatous Disease

Patients with sarcoidosis and other granulomatous disease are predisposed to hypercalcemia and hypercalciuria. The mechanism by which this occurs is via extrarenal production of calcitriol by 1-alpha hydroxylase, which is produced by macrophages within the granulomas. Low serum PTH despite high serum and urinary calcium may provide clinical suspicion for such a disorder. The mechanism behind this process is further described in Chapter 91. Treatment is typically accomplished using glucocorticoids, which decrease the granulomatous activity and ultimately the hypercalciuria that results from it (Iannuzzi and Fontana, 2011).

Idiopathic Causes of Hypercalciuria

Hypercalciuria used to be distinguished into three broad categories; absorptive, renal, and idiopathic. In absorptive hypercalciuria, urinary calcium levels are elevated as a result of increased calcium absorption by the GI tract. Renal hypercalciuria refers to calcium wasting through the nephron. **Fasting and dietary calcium loading tests used to be recommended as a way to distinguish the various types of absorptive and renal pathophysiologies but have fallen out of favor and are no longer recommended by the AUA guidelines as they are not believed to change clinical practice** (Lein and Keane, 1983; Pak et al., 2011; Pearle et al., 2014). As a result, such patients who have high urinary calcium levels and no identifiable diseases that may be contributing are referred to as having idiopathic hypercalciuria (Coe et al., 2016). Of note, idiopathic hypercalciuria alone is not a disease and can be found in both normal subjects and stone formers (Coe and Favus, 1980; Coe and Bushinsky, 1984).

Calcium Supplementation

The influence of dietary and supplemental calcium and vitamin D remains an incompletely understood process. Administration of exogenous calcium and vitamin D supplements has been found to correlate with higher urinary calcium levels, but the overall effect this may have on stone formation remains unclear (Gallagher et al., 2014; Riggs et al., 1998). In one large randomized controlled trial, 36,000 postmenopausal women were randomized to receive either placebo or 500 mg of calcium carbonate plus 200 units of vitamin D_3 two times a day. At 7 years, the cohort that was prescribed supplementation had a 17% increased rate of stone formation (Wallace et al., 2011). A similar (20%) increased risk was observed as part of the NHS I observational study among women taking supplemental calcium (Curhan et al., 1997). On the contrary, several other large-scale observational studies among younger women and men that have examined the potential association between calcium supplements and stones failed to identify a correlation (Curhan et al., 2004; Taylor et al., 2004). It is suspected that some of the aforementioned discrepancies may have to do with oversupplementation and timing of calcium supplement ingestion at separate times than meals (Pearle et al., 2014). The most recent AUA guidelines on medical management of stones recommends that if a patient with known history of calcium stones is on or is interested in taking calcium supplements, he or she should limit total calcium intake to 1000 to 1200 mg/day and should be advised to perform 24-hour urine testing on and off the supplements. If indeed the urinary supersaturation of the calcium salt in question rises while the patient is taking it, calcium supplementation should be stopped (Pearle et al., 2014).

There is similar controversy over the stone-specific effects of vitamin D supplementation. 1,25 Dihydroxyvitamin D, or calcitriol, is the active form of vitamin D that exerts biologic effects. Correlations between serum calcitriol levels and intestinal calcium absorption have been proven (Wilz et al., 1979) as have correlations between calcitriol and urinary calcium (Halalsheh et al., 2017). One of the reasons it has been difficult to determine the influence of vitamin D administration on stone risk is the fact that most randomized and placebo-controlled studies administer vitamin D with calcium, making the independent risk assessment of the vitamin difficult to quantify. **There are conflicting sentiments about the influence of vitamin D repletion in patients with low vitamin D levels and histories of kidney stones.** Cochrane review meta-analyses have found a 17% increased risk for stone formation among patients taking vitamin D and analogues (Avenell et al., 2014; Bjelakovic et al., 2014). However, few studies have prospectively evaluated the effect of vitamin D supplementation among stone formers with low serum vitamin D levels. Among 29 vitamin D–depleted patients, Leaf et al. (2012) found that supplementation led to an overall increase in serum vitamin D levels without significant change in urinary calcium levels. A subset of patients did have an appreciable rise in urinary calcium, but urinary sodium levels were higher as well, likely reflecting dietary variability over direct effects of vitamin D supplementation (Abt et al., 2017). Johri et al. (2017) found that among 37 vitamin D–deficient stone formers, supplementation resulted in a significant rise in vitamin D levels without a significant rise in urinary calcium levels, though hypercalciuria did occur is several instances. Ferroni et al. randomized patients with a history of calcium stones and low vitamin D to low dose (1000 IU daily) versus high dose (50,000 IU weekly) and found that only the high-dose regimen significantly improved vitamin D levels. Notably, neither regimen led to hypercalciuria. The results of these studies support the notion that vitamin D supplementation can likely be safely administered, though the potential for hypercalcuria to occur in a subset of patients is real, and patients who start therapy should have urine calcium levels monitored after initiation.

Conservative Strategies for Hypercalciuria

Sodium and Hypercalciuria

Dietary sodium increases urinary calcium levels because sodium and calcium share a common transport mechanism in the renal tubule. High sodium intake will result in decreased proximal sodium reabsorption and reduced distal renal tubular calcium reabsorption. The end result is hypernatriuria and hypercalciuria, which are risk factors that contribute to calcium nephrolithiasis. The degree of hypercalciuria has been shown to increase proportionally with the amount of sodium excreted in the urine (Sakhaee et al., 1993). Earlier studies reported that for every 100 mEq increase in dietary sodium, there was a 25- to 40-mg increase in urinary calcium excretion in normal subjects and an 80- to 120-mg increase in hypercalciuric stone formers (Bleich et al., 1979; Burtis et al., 1994; Martini et al., 1998; Muldowney et al., 1982; Phillips and Cooke, 1967; Silver et al., 1983). A more recent study suggests that the effect of sodium on urinary calcium excretion may be slightly overestimated as the investigators found in a short-term randomized controlled trial of hypercalciuric calcium oxalate stone formers a reduction of urinary calcium of approximately 64 mg/day for every 100-mmol reduction in urinary sodium (Nouvenne et al., 2010).

Epidemiologic studies have shown an independent association of dietary sodium consumption with kidney stone formation, particularly in women (Curhan et al., 1993, 1997). A more recent cross-sectional study by Taylor et al. (2009) found that subjects in the highest quartiles of urinary sodium excreted 37 mg/day more urinary calcium than participants in the lowest quartile. **Beyond the risk for stone formation, the adverse effects of high sodium intake and hypercalciuria include decreased bone mineral density and bone loss.** Martini et al. demonstrated that calcium stone formers who ingest large quantities of daily salt are more likely to suffer from decreased bone mineral density (Martini et al., 2000). In this study of 85 patients, all females were premenopausal, underscoring the risks for further osteopenia that they might develop later in life. After adjustment for calcium and protein intakes, age, weight, BMI, urinary calcium, citrate and uric acid excretion, and duration of stone disease, multiple-regression analysis showed that a high sodium chloride intake (≥16 g/day) was the single variable that was predictive of risk for low bone density in calcium stone formers (OR = 3.8).

A 3-month randomized controlled trial by Nouvenne et al. (2010) investigated the effects of a low-sodium diet on idiopathic hypercalciuria in calcium oxalate stone formers. There were 210 patients randomly assigned to a control diet that consisted of recommendations for water intake only or a low-sodium diet that included elimination of kitchen salt and strict limitation of foods containing high quantities of salt in addition to water therapy. They found that the stone formers consuming the low-sodium diet had a reduction in urinary calcium (271 vs. 361 mg/day) and oxalate (28 vs. 32 mg/day) compared with the control group. In addition, a low-sodium diet corrected the idiopathic hypercalciuria in approximately 30% of patients. These findings are supported by an earlier randomized controlled trial performed by Borghi et al. (2002), which found a low-sodium diet, limited to 50 mmol/day of sodium chloride, in conjunction with normal calcium intake and low animal protein reduced urinary calcium excretion in hypercalciuric stone formers. **In addition, when combined with animal protein restriction and moderate calcium ingestion, a reduced-sodium diet decreased stone episodes by roughly 50%. A recommended target for patients with calcium stones is sodium consumption of less than or equal to 100 mEq (2300 mg) per day** (Pearle et al., 2014).

KEY POINTS: IDIOPATHIC HYPERCALCIURIA

- Fasting and calcium-loading tests are no longer routinely recommended to distinguish types of hypercalciuria.
- Calcium and vitamin D supplementation may increase urinary calcium levels, but overall effect on risk for stone-formation risk remains unclear.
- Randomized controlled trials have demonstrated a benefit of dietary sodium restriction in both normal subjects and stone formers.
- The recommended sodium intake for patients with calcium stones is less than or equal to 100 mEq (2300 mg) per day.

Medical Therapy for Hypercalciuria

Thiazides and Thiazide-Like Diuretics

Thiazide diuretics are the preferred medical agent for hypercalciuria. They are among the best-studied medications for stone prevention, with evidence supporting their use both in disease-specific and nonspecific subgroups of stone formers (Borghi et al., 1993; Brocks et al., 1981; Ettinger et al., 1988; Laerum and Larsen, 1984; Mortensen et al., 1986; Ohkawa et al., 1992). As such, they are currently favored by the AUA guidelines and recommended for patients with hypercalciuria and recurrent calcium stones and those suffering from recurrent calcium stones in spite of normal metabolic evaluations (Pearle et al., 2014).

The use of thiazides was first described by Yendt et al. (1966) for the treatment of undifferentiated hypercalciuria. **Thiazides directly stimulate calcium resorption in the distal nephron while promoting excretion of sodium.** A list of available thiazides and other medications used in stone prevention can be found in Table 92.4. This

TABLE 92.4 Dosages of Common Medications Used to Prevent Urinary Calculi

MEDICATION	DOSAGE
Thiazide diuretics	
Hydrochlorothiazide	25 mg PO bid
Chlorthalidone	25–50 mg PO daily
Indapamide	2.5 mg PO daily
Sodium cellulose phosphate	10–15 g/day divided with meals
Orthophosphate	0.5 g PO tid
Potassium citrate	20 mEq PO bid-tid
Allopurinol	300 mg PO daily
Magnesium gluconate	0.5–1 g tid
Pyridoxine (B6)	100 mg PO daily
d-Penicillamine	250 mg PO daily (titrated to effect)
α-Mercaptopropionyl glycine	100 mg PO bid (titrated to effect)
Captopril	25 mg PO tid
Acetohydroxamic acid	250 mg PO bid-tid

TABLE 92.5 Potential Side Effects of Medications Used to Prevent Urinary Lithiasis

MEDICATION	SIDE EFFECT

Thiazide diuretics
  Hydrochlorothiazide
  Chlorthalidone
  Indapamide
	Potassium wasting, muscle cramps, hyperuricosuria, intracellular acidosis, hypocitraturia

Sodium cellulose phosphate (SCP)	GI distress, hypomagnesemia, hyperoxaluria, PTH stimulation
Orthophosphate	Similar to SCP, soft tissue calcification
Potassium citrate	GI upset, hyperkalemia
Allopurinol	Rash, myalgia
Magnesium gluconate pyridoxine (B6)	Diarrhea
d-Penicillamine	Nephrotic syndrome, dermatitis pancytopenia
α-Mercaptopropionyl glycine	Rash, asthenia, rheumatologic complaints, GI distress, mental status changes
Captopril	Rash, cough, hypotension
Acetohydroxamic acid	Thromboembolic phenomena, tremor, headache, palpitations, edema, GI distress, loss of taste, rash, alopecia, anemia, abdominal pain

GI, Gastrointestinal; *PTH*, parathyroid hormone.

table includes indapamide, which is a thiazide-like diuretic that is effective against hypercalciuria (Ceylan et al., 2005). Two double-blind randomized controlled trials have tested the treatment effect of hypercalciuria. Ettinger et al. identified a 90% decrease in predicted rates of stone formation for patients on chlorthalidone (25 or 50 mg daily) relative to placebo or magnesium hydroxide (Ettinger et al., 1988). Laerum and Larsen (1984) found that patients administered hydrochlorathiazide 25 mg two times a day had a 75% likelihood of not forming a stone at a median of 3 years follow-up compared with 45% among patients administered a placebo. A Cochrane review on the topic also identified a protective effect of thiazides. Among 316 patients included from five separate studies, patients on thiazide therapy had a 60% reduction in new stone recurrences relative to those on placebo (Escribano et al., 2009).

Long-term thiazide therapy results in volume depletion, extracellular volume contraction, and proximal tubular resorption of sodium and calcium. Thiazides may increase urinary excretion of magnesium and zinc, but these responses are not consistent. **Potassium losses from thiazide therapy can cause hypocitraturia, as a result of hypokalemia with intracellular acidosis. As a result, potassium supplementation should be considered either in the form of potassium citrate or potassium chloride.** Serum potassium levels should be monitored within 1 to 2 weeks after initiating therapy or adjusting the dose, and particular caution should be exercised for patients who have known potassium deficiencies, are on digitalis therapy, or develop hypocitraturia. Addition of potassium citrate has been documented to prevent occurrence of hypokalemia and hypochloremic metabolic acidosis in patients undergoing long-term thiazide therapy (Odvina et al., 2003).

Amiloride in combination with thiazide (Moduretic) may be more effective than thiazide alone in reducing calcium excretion (Leppla et al., 1983; Maschio et al., 1981). However, this medication does not augment citrate excretion. Because amiloride is a potassium-sparing agent, potassium replacement is not necessary and could, in fact, be problematic. **It is not advisable to provide potassium supplementation to patients receiving a potassium-sparing diuretic.** Although the potassium-sparing effects of amiloride may be beneficial, the use of triamterene, another potassium-sparing agent, should be undertaken with caution because of reports of triamterene stone formation (Watson et al., 1981).

Thiazide therapy has the potential to affect bone mineral density and has been shown to be protective against osteopenia. Pak et al. studied a subset of patients with absorptive hypercalciuria who were treated with a thiazide and potassium citrate and a low-calcium, low-oxalate diet and followed them for a mean of 3.7 years. During the period of treatment, stone formation decreased from 2.94 to 0.05 per year, and bone mineral density increased by 5.7% to 7.1% (Pak et al., 2003b). There is also data showing that patients on thiazide diuretics have a decreased risk for bony fractures. A Cochrane review on this topic identified a 24% reduction in hip fractures among patients taking thiazides (Aung and Htay, 2011).

Side effects of thiazides are typically mild at low doses and often improve with time (Table 92.5). Nonetheless, they can be bothersome and have been estimated to lead to quitting therapy in as many as 1 in 6 patients (ALLHAT, 2002). Side effects that may be experienced include increased thirst, polyuria, cramps, and GI upset. Initiation of a thiazide also has the potential to precipitate gout or diabetes owing to disturbances in serum uric acid and glucose levels (York et al., 2015). Finally, decreased libido or sexual dysfunction can be seen in a small percentage of patients (Derby et al., 2001).

Occasionally, thiazides unmask primary hyperparathyroidism (i.e., "thiazide challenge"). Patients with normal serum calcium may develop elevated serum calcium. Wermers et al. (2007) reported that this occurs an average of 6 years after initiation of thiazide. In this heterogeneous population (3% of whom were known stone formers), hyperparathyroidism was diagnosed in 64% of patients who had persistently elevated serum calcium after the thiazide was stopped (Wermers et al., 2007). Another way a thiazide challenge can be used is to differentiate primary and secondary hyperparathyroidism (Eisner et al., 2009). In patients with nephrolithiasis, hypercalciuria, and elevated serum parathyroid hormone, hydrochlorothiazide 25 mg orally twice daily is administered for 2 weeks. If the parathyroid hormone remains elevated, the diagnosis of primary hyperparathyroidism is confirmed. If it returns to normal, the diagnosis is secondary hyperparathyroidism from renal leak hypercalciuria.

Orthophosphate

Orthophosphate (neutral or alkaline salt of sodium and/or potassium, 0.5 g phosphorus three or four times per day) has been shown to inhibit 1,25-(OH)$_2$D synthesis (Insogna et al., 1989; Van Den Berg et al., 1980). **However, there is as yet no convincing evidence from randomized controlled trials that this treatment restores normal intestinal calcium absorption.** Orthophosphate reduces urinary calcium probably by directly impairing the renal tubular reabsorption of calcium and by binding calcium in the intestinal tract. Urinary phosphorus is markedly increased during therapy, a finding reflecting the absorbability of soluble phosphate. Physicochemically, orthophosphate reduces the urinary saturation of calcium oxalate but increases that of brushite. Moreover, the urinary inhibitor activity is increased, probably owing to the stimulated renal excretion of pyrophosphate and citrate. Although contrary reports have appeared, this treatment program has been reported to cause soft tissue calcification and parathyroid stimulation (Dudley and Blackburn, 1970). Orthophosphate is contraindicated in nephrolithiasis complicated by UTI because of the increased phosphorus load.

Sodium Cellulose Phosphate

Sodium cellulose phosphate, given orally, is a nonabsorbable ion exchange resin that binds calcium and inhibits calcium absorption (Pak, 1973). **Unfortunately, despite early enthusiasm, the use of sodium cellulose phosphate has largely fallen out of favor, and this medication is no longer available in the United States.**

> **KEY POINTS: MEDICATIONS FOR HYPERCALCIURIA**
> - Thiazides and thiazide-like medications are the preferred pharmacotherapy for medical management of hypercalciuria.
> - Potassium levels should be monitored, and potassium supplementation should be coadministered with thiazides.
> - Thiazide therapy may be protective against osteopenia.

HYPOCITRATURIA (<550 mg/day FEMALE, <450 mg/day MALE)

Clinical Considerations

Hypocitraturia is considered one of the more common metabolic diagnoses, probably second only to hypercalciuria. Citrate is an inhibitor of crystal aggregation and can reduce calcium stone risk, particularly of calcium oxalate. The physiology of this process is better elucidated in Chapter 91. When citrate levels are low, stone risks rise. Citrate repletion may reduce stone risk by forming soluble complexes with calcium and reducing supersaturation (Pak et al., 1986b). Defining a normal level of urinary citrate excretion is somewhat controversial, particularly as citrate levels can vary by gender and age. Early studies from Dr. Pak's research group identified hypocitraturia in up to 50% of patients being evaluated for stone disease, and it was often associated with other metabolic abnormalities (Nicar et al., 1983). Despite noting gender differences, Resnick Martin and Pak (1990) define normal urine citrate as greater than 320 mg for both genders. Parks and Coe also noted the importance of urinary citrate for the prevention of calcareous stones and set the limits of normal at higher values, with men greater than 450 mg and women greater than 550 mg daily (Parks, 1986a, 1986b). Hypocitraturia may be a reflection of a systemic disease (distal renal tubular acidosis, chronic diarrhea). It may also occur as a result of medical therapy (thiazides) or urinary tract infection. In many instances, however, hypocitraturia is an idiopathic process.

Conservative Strategies for Hypocitraturia

Citrus Juices

Citrus juices, predominantly lemonade and orange juice, have long been used as an adjunct to water to provide increased urinary volume and increased urinary citrate excretion. Citrate is a weak organic acid, but it can act as a conjugate base when paired with a cation such as sodium or potassium (Kurtz and Eisner, 2011). Oral citrate is absorbed by the intestine and nearly completely metabolized to bicarbonate providing an alkali load that increases urinary pH and citrate excretion. Citrate is an effective inhibitor of calcium oxalate stone formation as it forms soluble complexes with calcium and affects crystal nucleation and growth (Siener, 2016). Using nuclear magnetic resonance spectroscopy, the citrate concentrations of a number of commercially available citrus and citrus-based beverages was assessed (Haleblian et al., 2008). This finding confirmed that natural juices are highest in citrate and potassium content, with grapefruit juice containing the greatest amount of citrate (197.5 mEq/L), followed closely by lemon and orange juice (145.48 and 144.57 mEq/L, respectively). Of the commercially available citrus-based beverages, Crystal Light (Kraft Foods, Northfield, IL) exhibited the highest concentration of citrate (117.2 mEq/L). Citrate in orange and grapefruit juices is complexed mainly by potassium, which results in increased urinary pH, and citrate in lemon juice is in the form of citric acid and therefore does not result in as significant of an alkali load. More recently, malate, another organic anion found in some beverages, has been shown to increase urinary citrate as well (Eisner et al., 2010). Therefore, the amount of alkaline citrate may be more important than the total citrate content of a beverage in terms of raising urinary citrate (Kurtz and Eisner, 2011).

Several studies have investigated the effects of citrus juices on urinary parameters. In a study of 12 hypocitraturic patients, lemonade made from reconstituted lemon juice resulted in a more than twofold rise in urinary citrate levels and corrected the hypocitraturia in seven subjects (Seltzer et al., 1996). Urinary calcium excretion decreased an average of 39 mg daily, whereas oxalate excretion did not change. The lemonade mixture was well tolerated and inexpensive (estimated $2 per week), with only two patients reporting mild indigestion that did not require cessation of therapy. Similar benefits of homemade lemonade therapy were demonstrated in two other studies, with urinary citrate levels increasing at least twofold, and in the study by Kang et al., mean stone burden also decreased by 18% in patients on lemonade therapy (Kang et al., 2007; Aras et al., 2008). Despite these studies suggesting benefit to lemonade therapy, at least three other studies have questioned the benefit (Koff et al., 2007, Odvina, 2006, Penniston, 2007b). Koff et al. (2007) compared reconstituted lemonade (1 oz ReaLemon in ¾ cup of water) to 60 mEq of potassium citrate and found that potassium citrate increased urinary citrate but the lemonade solution did not. Penniston et al. (2007) also examined lemonade therapy alone versus lemonade therapy combined with potassium citrate and found that the combination therapy resulted in increased urinary citrate levels but lemonade therapy alone did not.

Orange juice has been shown to have less citrate content than lemon juice; however, citrate in oranges is complexed with potassium and therefore may have a greater impact on raising urinary citrate. Data from three large cohort studies found that orange juice consumption was associated with a lower risk for stone formation (Ferraro et al., 2013). Wabner and Pak evaluated the effects of orange juice on the urinary parameters of normal subjects and found that compared with potassium citrate, orange juice delivered an equivalent alkali load and caused a similar increase in urinary pH (6.48 vs. 6.75 from 5.71 mg/day) and urinary citrate (952 vs. 944 from 571 mg/day) (Wabner and Pak, 1993). However, orange juice increased urinary oxalate and did not alter calcium excretion, whereas potassium citrate decreased urinary calcium without altering urinary oxalate. Odvina performed a crossover study of 14 patients examining the effects of distilled water, orange juice, and lemonade on urinary citrate levels (Odvina et al., 2006). They found that urinary citrate and pH were significantly increased in response to orange juice (mean increase of 500 mg citrate per day), and no difference was observed for lemonade or water. However, urinary oxalate levels increased in the orange juice arm, which would not be ideal for calcium oxalate stone formers. Although less vigorously studied, other fruit juices (lime, cranberry, black currant, grapefruit, and tomato) have been shown to result in variable increases in urinary citrate (Gettman et al., 2005; Goldfarb and Asplin, 2001; Kessler et al., 2002; McHarg et al., 2003; Tosukhowong et al., 2008; Yilmaz et al., 2010). Perhaps the greatest concern with using fruit juices as a dietary fluid prevention for stone formation is the caloric content. Given that many stone formers are already overweight, obese, or have diabetes mellitus, consumption of large quantities of sweetened fruit juice may actually be detrimental. In this aspect, lemonade is preferable as the sweetener added and caloric content of the beverage can be better controlled.

A number of citrus-flavored low-calorie sodas (orange flavored, lemon/lime flavored) have been shown to have high citrate content, which may aid in stone prevention (Haleblian et al., 2008, Eisner et al., 2010). In addition, the effects on urinary citrate levels of two citrus-based sports drinks, Performance and Gatorade, were compared in 19 non–stone formers. Performance increased mean citrate excretion by 170 mg/day and increased urine pH by 0.31, and Gatorade had no effect on either parameter (Goodman et al., 2009). However, like the fruit juices, the fructose and calorie content of these sports drinks may be too considerable for them to be preferred beverages for stone prevention.

In summary, although several beverages have been shown to increase urinary citrate levels, none has demonstrated superiority. The greatest amount of clinical evidence exists for lemonade therapy, and this is most widely prescribed. **For kidney stone prevention, the absolute amount of fluid consumed per day is more important than the type of fluid. Stone formers should be encouraged to drink at least 3000 mL/day to maintain a urine output greater than 2500 mL/day.**

Medical Therapy for Hypocitraturia

Idiopathic Hypocitraturic Calcium Nephrolithiasis

This entity includes hypocitraturia occurring alone, and in conjunction with other abnormalities (e.g., hypercalciuria or hyperuricosuria). Stones formed in this condition may be composed of calcium oxalate, calcium phosphate, or a combination of the two (Gambaro et al., 2016). Treatment of hypocitraturia is typically accomplished with citrate repletion (Pak et al., 1986b). **Orally ingested citrate salts are metabolized to bicarbonate in the liver. The resulting alkali load in turn inhibits proximal tubular citrate reabsorption, which leads to increased levels of citrate in the urine.** Several commercially available forms of citrate are available. In the United States, potassium citrate is the predominant form that is used. It is available in a wax tablet, as a liquid, and in a crystal/powder form meant to be dissolved (York et al., 2015). The usual therapeutic dose is 30 to 60 mEq/day given in divided doses or as a single evening dose (Berg et al., 1992). Another dosing strategy is ½ mEq/kg/day given in divided doses until the urinary pH is sufficiently alkaline (i.e., pH is 6 to 6.5) (York et al., 2015). Sodium citrate is another formulation that is more commonly used in Europe or reserved for patients with concerns about causing hyperkalemia. Sodium citrate does not lower urinary calcium excretion, perhaps as a result of the increased sodium load associated with this therapy (Preminger et al., 1988; Sakhaee et al., 1983). **Current AUA guidelines recommend that clinicians offer potassium citrate to patients with recurrent calcium stones and low urinary citrate** (Pearle et al., 2014). Additionally, similar to thiazides, potassium citrate is recommended, even in the absence of hypocitraturia or other metabolic abnormalities in recurrent calcium stone formers (Pearle et al., 2014).

Long-term therapy with citrates has been shown to provide a favorable and durable response in alteration of urinary parameters and stone formation rate (Robinson et al., 2009) In a retrospective study published by Robinson et al. of 503 patients on potassium citrate therapy for a mean of 41 months (range 6 to 168), urinary pH and citrate demonstrated significant increases (pH, 5.9 to 6.46; citrate, 470 to 700 mg/day), with substantial improvement in urinary parameters in as short as 6 months of therapy. In addition, potassium citrate decreased the stone formation rate from 1.89 stones per patient per year to 0.46 (Robinson et al., 2009).

Several randomized control trials have evaluated the effect of citrate on new stone formation. Ettinger et al. randomized 64 recurrent calcium oxalate stone formers to either potassium magnesium citrate or placebo and found that the citrate cohort had a 0.16 relative risk for new stone formation relative to the placebo cohort at 3 years (Ettinger et al., 1997). Another randomized control placebo trial from Barcelo et al. found similar results with patients on potassium citrate therapy exhibiting significant reductions in stone formation rate at 3 years (0.1 vs. 1.1 new stones per patient year). **A Cochrane review among predominantly calcium oxalate stone formers found that patients on citrate had a relative risk of 0.26 (95% CI 0.10 to 0.68) for new stone formation compared with patients who were not on citrate** (Phillips et al., 2015).

Citrates are generally well tolerated, though several common side effects exist. The most common side effect is GI upset. The wax matrix tablet has been suggested to reduce this complication, though data supporting this is limited. Taking the medication with water and after meals may reduce GI irritation as well (York et al., 2015). Patients should also be informed that it is common to see the wax component of the potassium citrate tablet in their stool and should be reassured that this does not mean the medication is not being absorbed (Fegan et al., 1992). The aforementioned Cochrane review on citrate therapy did not show a significant difference in GI side effects in patients on citrate, though citrate was associated with an increased number of study dropouts from medication-related adverse events (Phillips et al., 2015). Another potential concern specific to potassium citrate supplementation is hyperkalemia. **Potassium levels should be regularly monitored for patients with renal insufficiency and should be avoided for those on potassium-sparing diuretics.**

One unique side effect that relates directly to stone formation is the effect of citrate therapy on urinary pH. As discussed earlier, citrate therapy raises urinary pH. In some cases, this is a desired effect, particularly among calcium oxalate stone formers, where inhibitors of stone formation may be more effective in alkaline urine. **However, exceedingly alkaline urine also raises the risk for calcium phosphate stone formation, particularly at a pH of 7 or greater** (Coe 2010; Evan et al., 2005, 2015b; Pearle et al., 2014). **Higher utilization of citrate therapy has been postulated as a contributing factor in the rise of calcium phosphate stone disease.** Parks et al. identified a threefold increase in calcium phosphate content of stones over the past three decades and identified an association of this trend with rising urinary pH (Parks 2004) Furthermore, the same group found that patients who transformed their stone content to increased calcium phosphate received more potassium citrate compared with those who did not transform (Parks et al., 2009).

The role of citrate supplementation in patients who form calcium phosphate stones is subsequently controversial. **No randomized controlled trials to date have evaluated the effect of citrate on stone recurrence among patients with calcium phosphate stones, though nonrandomized studies among diseases commonly associated have suggested a benefit** (Gambaro et al., 2016; Preminger et al., 1985). Subsequently, investigation into alternative therapies for such patients has been identified as an opportunity for future research (Gambaro et al., 2016). In the interim, **if citrates are started on a patient with prior calcium phosphate stones, a follow-up 24-hour urine collection is advised, with specific attention directed toward the corresponding urinary citrate levels, pH, and supersaturation. Those whose pH rises in the absence of a significant rise in urinary citrate may not benefit to the same degree as those whose citrate levels rise without production of an exceedingly alkaline urine.**

> **KEY POINTS: HYPOCITRATURIA**
>
> - Citrus juices (particularly lemon and orange) and low-calorie citrus soda with citric acid may decrease stone risk and be an alternative to water.
> - Citrate supplementation is a primary treatment for patients with hypocitraturia and recurrent calcium stones.
> - Common side effects from citrate therapy include GI upset and hyperkalemia.
> - Serum potassium levels should be monitored in patients on citrates.
> - There is controversy as to whether citrates are beneficial in calcium phosphate stone disease as higher urinary pH could increase calcium phosphate stone risk

BOX 92.5 Causes of Acquired Renal Tubular Acidosis	
Obstructive uropathy	Analgesic nephropathy
Recurrent pyelonephritis	Sarcoidosis
Acute tubular necrosis	Idiopathic hypercalciuria
Renal transplantation	Primary hyperparathyroidism

Distal Renal Tubular Acidosis (Type 1)

Patients may have either an acquired or an inheritable version of RTA, with the incomplete version representing a less serious clinical pattern (Box 92.5). Regardless of the actual cause, the laboratory hallmark of this disease is a low urine citrate (hypocitraturia) with an inappropriately high urine pH (Evan et al., 2007). Often, the measured 24-hour urine citrate will be quite diminished, with values less than 100 mg/day. The urine pH will be elevated to 6.5 or above. Hypokalemia is often evident on the serum studies, as is hyperchloremia. A non–anion gap acidosis may be present as well with carbon dioxide values in the mid-teens (Preminger et al., 1985). First-void urine samples can be evaluated to assess urine pH and screen for RTA. Patients with RTA will be unable to acidify urine overnight and should have a urine pH no lower than 5.5.

Distal RTA may manifest as an isolated entity, or it may be the secondary manifestation of a variety of systemic and renal disorders. More than two-thirds of patients with distal RTA are adults, but occasionally children are identified with this disorder. Infants generally present with vomiting or diarrhea, failure to thrive, and growth restriction; children often present with metabolic bone disease and renal stones; and adults frequently present with symptoms attributable to nephrolithiasis and nephrocalcinosis (Fig. 92.8).

Up to 70% of adults with distal RTA have kidney stones (Caruana and Buckalew, 1988). Those patients with onset at an early age or with severe forms of the disorder may develop nephrocalcinosis and eventual renal insufficiency. RTA is more common in women, accounting for nearly 80% of all cases. It is very important to note that secondary RTA can be induced by many common urologic disorders that also may be sought after a diagnosis of acquired RTA. These include obstructive uropathy, pyelonephritis, acute tubular necrosis, renal transplantation, analgesic nephropathy, sarcoidosis, idiopathic hypercalciuria, and primary hyperparathyroidism and can lead to secondary RTA (Buckalew, 1989).

Some patients will have an incomplete variant of the disease with less marked hypocitraturia and a more normal urine pH level. Incomplete variants of distal RTA can be diagnosed with the use of an ammonium chloride loading challenge. In this evaluation, the fasting patient is given ammonium chloride 0.1 g/kg of body weight in crushed granules mixed with a soft drink. Subsequently, hourly measurements of urinary pH and bi-hourly measurements of serum pH or bicarbonate are taken over 4 to 6 hours (Pohlman et al., 1984). If the serum pH falls below 7.32, or the bicarbonate falls below 16 mmol/L but urinary pH remains at or above 5.5, the diagnosis of incomplete distal RTA is confirmed. If at any time the urinary pH falls below 5.5, the diagnosis of incomplete distal RTA is excluded (Preminger et al., 1985, 1987). More recently, a furosemide/fludrocortisone test whereby these two agents are administered simultaneously and urine acidity measured has been tested as an alternative diagnostic test with the potential to be easier to perform and better tolerated by patients (Walsh et al., 2007). Initial experiences have shown promise with excellent sensitivity and negative predictive value relative to the ammonium chloride loading challenge. However, a low specificity means that ammonium chloride testing is still recommended as the gold standard if the diagnosis remains in question (Dhayat et al., 2017; Shavit et al., 2016).

Alkali supplementation (such as potassium citrate), typically in the form of potassium citrate, is a cornerstone of therapy for RTA as it is able to correct the metabolic acidosis and hypokalemia found in the disease (Preminger et al., 1985). In addition, this medication is capable of restoring normal urinary citrate, although large doses (up to 120 mEq/day) may be required in severe acidotic states. With correction of the acidosis, urinary calcium should decline into the normal range. Because urinary pH is generally high to begin with in patients with RTA, the overall rise in urinary pH is small.

Potassium citrate therapy typically produces a sustained decline in the urinary saturation of calcium oxalate (from reduction in urinary calcium and in citrate complexation of calcium). The urinary saturation of calcium phosphate should not increase because the rise in phosphate dissociation is relatively small and is adequately compensated by a decline in ionic calcium concentration. In addition, the inhibitory activity against the crystallization of calcium oxalate and calcium phosphate is augmented because of the direct action of citrate.

Clinical data evaluating the efficacy of potassium citrate in stone management related to RTA is limited. In 1985, Preminger et al. administered 60 to 80 mEq/day of potassium citrate to nine patients with confirmed RTA. At a mean treatment interval of 34 months, none of the patients reported new stones since starting therapy despite reporting a mean of 39.3 stones per patient formed during the 3 years before starting treatment (Preminger et al., 1985).

Chronic Diarrheal States

The full management of enteric stone disease is discussed later in this chapter. Part of the management should involve the use of citrate to correct the acidosis that accompanies the chronic bicarbonate

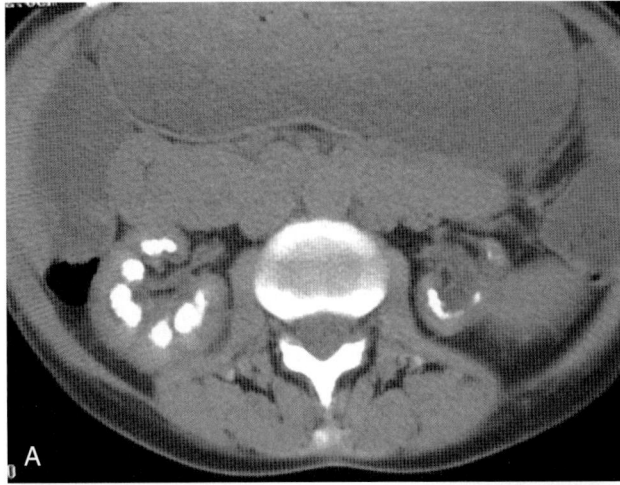
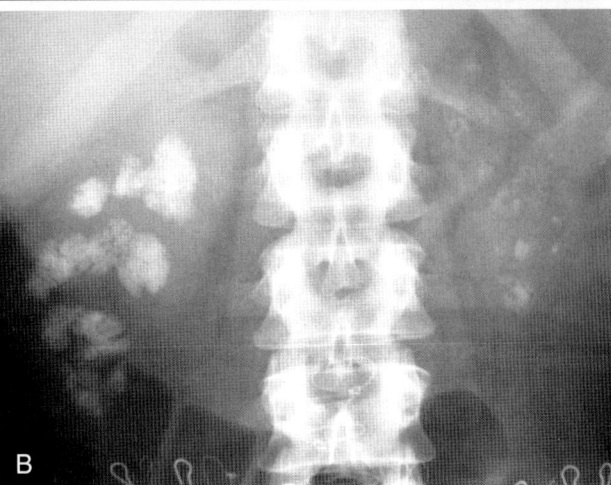

Fig. 92.8. Computed tomography (CT) (A) and plain film (B) of a patient with renal tubular acidosis and renal failure. Both kidneys demonstrate severe calcification of the medullary pyramids consistent with nephrocalcinosis. Note the atrophic left kidney on the CT image (A).

losses with diarrhea. The amount of potassium citrate will depend on the severity of hypocitraturia in these patients, with dosages ranging from 60 to 120 mEq in three or four divided doses.

It is recommended that a liquid preparation of potassium citrate be used rather than the slow-release tablet preparation; the slow-release medication may be poorly absorbed because of rapid intestinal transit time. In addition, frequent dose schedules (3 or 4 times per day) for the liquid preparation is necessary because this form of the medication has a relatively short duration of biologic action.

Thiazide-Induced Hypocitraturia

One of the side effects of thiazide therapy is the development of hypocitraturia. This defect is presumably secondary to the hypokalemia and resultant intracellular acidosis that may develop after prolonged therapy with thiazides (Pak et al., 1985). Therefore it should be a common practice to administer potassium supplementation, preferably in the form of potassium citrate, to patients receiving thiazides for treatment of hypercalciuria. Potassium citrate has been shown to be equally effective as potassium chloride in correcting thiazide-induced hypokalemia. Moreover, the addition of potassium citrate not only prevents a decrease in urinary citrate during thiazide therapy, but may increase citrate excretion (Pak et al., 1985). Because thiazides are still widely used as a diuretic and for the management of hypertension, some patients may present with a stone episode after prolonged therapy with this medication. Stone patients who are treated with thiazides for the control of hypercalciuria should be screened for hypocitraturia (Pak et al., 1985).

HYPEROXALURIA (>40 mg/day)
Clinical Considerations

Hyperoxaluria is one of the more common metabolic abnormalities identified during metabolic evaluations. Like urinary calcium levels, there is no set level above which stone risk suddenly occurs; rather, stone risk rises in line with increases in urinary oxalate levels, even when urinary oxalate levels are in the "normal" range (Curhan et al., 2001). Oxalate is a ubiquitous molecule that originates from both diet and a byproduct of metabolism (Holmes et al., 2001). To date, there is no recognized functional role of oxalate in human metabolism. Elevated urinary oxalate may occur via a variety of mechanisms.

Certain people may be more susceptible to dietary oxalate absorption than others. The importance of dietary oxalate and the possibility of an inheritable sensitivity to oral oxalate loads are debated and are discussed in Chapter 91. It appears increasingly evident that a deficiency of a bacterium found within intestinal flora (*Oxalobacter formigenes*) is a factor in the formation of calcium oxalate calculi (Allison et al., 1986; Barnett et al., 2016; Sidhu et al., 1999; Siener et al., 2013; Troxel et al., 2003). In some patients, the cause of *Oxalobacter* deficiency may be iatrogenic because it is sensitive to a number of commonly prescribed antibiotics (Lange et al., 2012; Tasian et al., 2018). There are ongoing efforts investigating a potential therapeutic role in recolonization of the GI tract with *Oxalobacter*.

Enteric Hyperoxaluria

The term *enteric hyperoxaluria* is used to describe elevations in urinary oxalate levels (>40 mg/day) that occur in the context of and as a result of GI malabsorption and diarrhea. Malabsorption mainly leads to increased oxalate reabsorption as a result of saponification of oral calcium with poorly absorbed fats in the GI tract, although it can also increase stone risk via dehydration, hypokalemia, bicarbonate loss, and hypocitraturia. Further details regarding this pathophysiology can be found in the preceding chapter. Urine oxalate levels can be quite high in this condition well over 60 to 70 mg/day. Furthermore, urinary calcium levels may be quite low (well under 100 mg/day).

Another increasingly common etiology of enteric hyperoxaluria is gastric bypass surgery performed for obesity. **Malabsorptive procedures, such as Roux-en-Y gastric bypass (RYGB) has been shown to increase the risk for stone formation.** Restrictive bariatric surgeries such as lap banding or sleeve gastrectomy may also infer additional stone risk, mainly via dehydration, and the direct risk for stone formation as a result of the procedure is less. Among 277 non–stone formers who underwent pre- and post-RYGB 24-hour urine testing, urinary oxalate levels increased from 28 to 44 mg/day, an increase of 34% (Espino-Grosso and Canales, 2017). As anticipated, urinary citrate levels and volume have also been demonstrated to decrease after RYGB (Park et al., 2009; Valezi et al., 2013). Using claims data, Matlaga et al. identified a 7.65% risk for stone formation within 2 years after RYGB compared with a 4.6% rate in a matched control group of patients with obesity (Matlaga et al., 2009).

Primary Hyperoxaluria

Primary hyperoxaluria (PH) is an extremely rare disorder caused by an inborn error of glyoxalate metabolism. Three genetic types of PH have been described to date. The more common variant, type 1, is caused by a defect of the enzyme alanine glyoxylate aminotransferase (AGXT) via an autosomal recessive inheritance. Type 2 is a less common variant thought secondary to a defect in D-glycerate dehydrogenase (GRHPR). More recently, primary hyperoxaluria type 3 has been described, which occurs as a result of a mutation in the hydroxy-2-oxoglutarate aldolase gene (*HOGA1*) and is inherited in an autosomal recessive manner. Estimates suggest that 70% of patients with PH have PH1, 10% have PH2, 10% have PH3, and 10% have PH from an unidentified genetic cause (Hopp et al., 2015).

The clinical manifestations of the different subtypes of PH have considerable overlap. The disease usually manifests during childhood with early stone formation, tissue deposition of oxalate (oxalosis), and commonly renal failure resulting from nephrocalcinosis. Death can occur before 20 years of age in untreated patients (Williams and Smith, 1968; Leumann and Hoppe, 1999). Metabolic evaluation will reveal high urine oxalate excretion (often over 100 mg/day) and high serum levels of this molecule. PH3 has been suggested to have a milder course and tends to have lower levels of urinary oxalate with decreased risk for developing renal failure and systemic oxalosis. Patients with PH3 are also more likely to have concomitant hypercalciuria (Monico et al., 2011; Williams, 2012a, Hopp et al., 2015).

Conservative Strategies for Hyperoxaluria

A review of a patient's dietary habits may reveal a predisposition for foods that are particularly high in oxalate. Although oxalate cannot be entirely avoided even with the best efforts, recognition and avoidance of high-oxalate foods is a cornerstone in management of urinary hyperoxaluria (Holmes and Assimos, 2004; Holmes et al., 2001, 2016). The contribution of dietary oxalate consumption to urinary oxalate can vary. Some have estimated that only 10% to 20% of urinary oxalate is usually derived from dietary sources (Williams and Wandzilak, 1989). More recently, Holmes et al. found that the contribution of dietary oxalate to urinary oxalate ranged from 24.4% ± 1.5% on a diet of 10 mg/day of oxalate to 41.5% ± 9.1% on a diet of 250 mg/day of oxalate. They also demonstrated that the mean contribution of dietary oxalate increased when calcium consumption decreased (Holmes et al., 2001).

Although dietary oxalate clearly plays a role in increased urinary oxalate, it is difficult to restrict its intake because oxalate is ubiquitous and found in most vegetable matter. However, it is important to avoid large portions of foodstuffs that are rich in oxalate, such as spinach, beets, chocolate, nuts, and tea. **Whereas general advice on a restricted-oxalate intake might be given to patients with recurrent nephrolithiasis, a low-oxalate diet would be most useful in patients with enteric hyperoxaluria, those with underlying bowel abnormalities, or patients who have undergone gastric bypass surgery** (Holmes and Assimos, 2004).

Box 92.6 presents an extensive list of foods containing a high level of oxalate. It is notable that recent work has illustrated similar relationships of dietary intake and urinary excretion of oxalate in a cross-sectional analysis of HPFS and NHS (I and II) for both stone formers and non–stone formers, thereby further adding to the question of the impact that dietary oxalate has on urinary oxalate excretion (Taylor and Curhan, 2004).

BOX 92.6 Foods Containing High Levels of Oxalate	
Black tea	Okra
Cocoa	Berries (some)
Spinach	Chocolate
Mustard greens	Nuts
Pokeweed	Wheat germ
Swiss chard	Soy crackers
Beets	Pepper
Rhubarb	

Repeated concerns have been raised regarding the risk associated with vitamin C (ascorbic acid) ingestion and the possibility of its conversion to oxalate with subsequent urinary excretion. Unfortunately, conflicting evidence has been presented by multiple authors (Curhan 1996b; Curhan et al., 1999; Traxer et al., 2003). In fact, conflicting conclusions have been reported even from the same group of authors, underscoring the need for close scrutiny of presented data. Some of the confusion stems from differences in study end points. Although ingestion of large amounts of vitamin C may demonstrate increases in 24-hour oxalate excretion and therefore calcium oxalate supersaturation, this does not guarantee an eventual increase in the formation of symptomatic calculi. A recent large, prospective cohort of men found that increased ascorbic acid intake was associated with a twofold increased risk for kidney stone formation (Thomas et al., 2013).

In the end, it seems reasonable to avoid heavy dosing of vitamin C. Limiting one's intake to a maximum daily dose of less than 2 g is an easy recommendation to follow (Traxer et al., 2003).

Medical Therapy for Hyperoxaluria

Oxalate avoidance and treatment of any underlying pathophysiologies are the cornerstones for management of idiopathic hyperoxaluria; however, medications may occasionally be useful.

Enteric Hyperoxaluria: Medical Therapy

No randomized controlled trials have been performed regarding treatment of enteric hyperoxaluria to date. Calcium supplementation is one of the primary treatment methods of lowering urinary oxalate levels with several prior studies having shown benefit when supplemental calcium supplements are administered (Hylander et al., 1980; Pang et al., 2012). Typically, over-the-counter calcium supplements have been recommended to provide the patient with up to 1 g/day of calcium in divided doses. Calcium citrate is one formulation commonly used for this purpose that has been shown to not only lower urinary oxalate levels but also raise urinary citrate and pH by providing an alkali load (Harvey et al., 1985). It is important that supplements are administered with meals to maximize oxalate binding potential. It is also important that patients maintain very high fluid intake during calcium treatment to avoid the potential of the calcium supplementation actually increasing overall stone risk.

Another mechanism by which oxalate reabsorption may be reduced in this disease state is via binding of bile salts, which can in turn decrease colonic mucosal irritability and resulting oxalate hyperabsorption. This has been previously attempted with the administration of cholestyramine, a bile acid sequestrant. Although this should be effective in principle and has been demonstrated to be efficacious in animal models of hyperoxaluria, studies testing the efficacy of cholestyramine in human subjects have been less favorable (Nordenvall et al., 1983).

Hypomagnesiuria may also play a role in the elevated levels of urinary oxalate seen in enteric hyperoxaluria. Normally, magnesium has the potential to act as an oxalate binder and can destabilize calcium oxalate crystal formation (Li et al., 1985; Riley et al., 2013). However, the underlying GI issues that can lead to enteric hyperoxaluria may lead to impaired intestinal magnesium absorption as well, leading to hypomagnesiuria and elevated levels of unbound urinary oxalate. Oral magnesium supplements may be administered to correct low urinary magnesium levels; however, caution must be exercised to ensure the supplementation does not provoke further diarrhea. Magnesium supplementation can be administered as magnesium gluconate, oxide, and hydroxide. Optimal dosing has yet to be established. It has also been suggested to have a complementary role when added to potassium citrate therapy for stone prevention (Massey, 2005).

Patients with enteric hyperoxaluria are at risk for stone formation for reasons beyond solely high levels of urinary oxalate as well. It is critical for patients to maintain a high fluid diet at minimum over 2 L/day to combat the additional fluid losses resulting from GI malabsorption. Additionally, potassium citrate supplementation can help correct resulting hypokalemia and metabolic acidosis. As mentioned earlier, preference should be given toward the liquid form of potassium citrate in patients with rapid GI transit times, because the liquid form of this medication may be better absorbed than the slow-release, wax matrix pills.

Medical Therapy for Primary Hyperoxaluria

There are limited treatment options for PH. Pyridoxine (vitamin B_6) is one therapeutic agent that has been studied. It has been shown to be capable of increasing the expression, catalytic activity, and peroxisomal import of AGT (the missing enzyme responsible for PH1) by acting as a cofactor (Fargue et al., 2013). It has also shown some potential benefit in patients with idiopathic hyperoxaluria. In a retrospective study, Ortiz-Alvarado et al. (2011) found that a combination of dietary counseling (low-oxalate diet) and pyridoxine significantly reduced urinary oxalate in patients with idiopathic hyperoxaluria without note of any significant side effects.

Another potential therapy for patients with PH is oral *Oxalobacter formingenes* administration. Conceptually, increased levels of *Oxalobacter* in the gut could help improve intestinal oxalate elimination. A previous study showed promising results after patients with PH were administered enteric-coated capsules containing lyophilized *Oxalobacter* for 4 weeks (Hoppe et al., 2006). However, follow-up studies using modified formulations for longer duration failed to replicate these findings (Hoppe et al., 2017; Milliner et al., 2018).

> **KEY POINTS: HYPEROXALURIA**
> - Urine oxalate reduction may be accomplished by following a low-oxalate diet.
> - GI malabsorption can lead to hyperoxaluria via increased amounts of unbound oxalate and mucosal irritation from excess bile salts.
> - Calcium supplementation with meals can lower urinary oxalate levels in enteric hyperoxaluria.
> - Primary hyperoxaluria is a genetic disease characterized by extremely high urinary oxalate levels.
> - Gut flora *(Oxalobacter formingenes)* likely plays a role in dietary oxalate degradation and can be affected by exposure to antibiotics.

Other Causes of Calcium Stone Formation

Hyperuricosuric Calcium Oxalate Nephrolithiasis

Patients with hyperuricosuria may be prone to the formation of calcium oxalate calculi through the process of heterogeneous nucleation (also referred to as epitaxy) (Coe 1978; Coe and Kavalach, 1974; Pak and Arnold, 1975; Pak et al., 1976). The details of this process are outlined in Chapter 91. These patients give a history of calcium oxalate nephrolithiasis and may have a history of hyperuricemia with symptomatic gout. During metabolic evaluation, these patients will demonstrate hyperuricosuria (>800 mg/day).

There are two pharmacologic approaches to the management of hyperuricosuric calcium nephrolithiasis. The first involves decreasing the production of uric acid. Physicochemical changes ensuing from restoration of normal urinary uric acid include an increase in the urinary limit of metastability of calcium oxalate (Pak et al., 1978). Thus the spontaneous nucleation of calcium oxalate is slowed by allopurinol treatment, probably via inhibition of monosodium urate–induced stimulation of calcium oxalate crystallization (Coe, 1980).

Allopurinol is the most well-studied medication for this purpose and may be used to block the ability of xanthine oxidase to convert xanthine to uric acid (Coe and Raisen, 1973). There are few convincing randomized trials demonstrating the efficacy of allopurinol for the treatment of hyperuricosuria. However, one study by Ettinger et al. does stand out (Ettinger et al., 1986). In this double-blind, prospective, randomized trial, allopurinol was given to 60 patients with hyperuricosuria, normocalciuria, and recurrent calcium oxalate stones. A 6-month grace period was established, during which any new calculus that was passed was not considered to represent failure of therapy. With a follow-up of up to 39 months, new stone events (stone growth or recurrence) occurred in 58% of the patients on placebo and 31% of the patients on allopurinol. The placebo group had 63.4% fewer calculi, whereas the allopurinol group had 81.2% fewer calculi. The mean rate of calculus events was 0.26 per patient per year in the placebo group and 0.12 in the allopurinol group. The allopurinol group had a significantly longer time before the recurrence of stones (Ettinger et al., 1986). This study is the basis for AUA guideline recommendations that clinicians offer allopurinol to patients with recurrent calcium oxalate stones who have hyperuricosuria and normal urinary calcium (Pearle et al., 2014).

Recently, a newer-generation xanthine oxidase inhibitory, febuxostat (80 mg/day), has also been suggested to have similar efficacy in this regard with potentially fewer side effects. In one randomized controlled trial, patients on febuxostat had greater decreases in urinary uric acid from baseline than those on allopurinol or placebo (Goldfarb et al., 2013).

Alternatively, management of hyperuricosuria may be approached by altering the urinary milieu such that uric acid remains in a dissolved state (Pak et al., 1986). Central to this approach would be the obvious advantage of copious amounts of dilute urine to maintain uric acid at a low concentration. Attempts to maintain the urine at a pH above the pKa also may be successful by promoting dissolution of this molecule (Pak et al., 1986). This effect is usually achieved by the use of an alkalinizing agent such as potassium citrate (at a dose of 30 to 60 mEq/day in divided doses). In the study by Pak et al., the treatment produced a sustained rise in urinary pH by 0.55 to 0.85 to the high-normal range. Urinary citrate levels increased by 249 to 402 mg/day. Commensurate with these changes, urinary saturation of calcium oxalate (relative saturation ratio) and the amount of undissociated uric acid decreased significantly. Stone formation decreased from 1.55 per patient-year to 0.38 per patient-year during the mean treatment period of 2.35 years. Stones ceased to form in 16 of 19 patients during treatment.

Hypomagnesuric Calcium Nephrolithiasis (<80 mg)

Hypomagnesuric calcium nephrolithiasis is characterized by low urinary magnesium and is frequently seen in the setting of inflammatory bowel diseases accompanied by other stone-forming factors such as hypocitraturia and low urine volume. Treatment is achieved with magnesium supplementation.

The administration of magnesium salts was first advocated on the theory that it reduced urinary excretion of oxalate. Some magnesium salts increase urinary magnesium excretion and thus produce a more favorable magnesium-to-calcium ratio in the urine, a condition that offers relative protection against stone formation. Magnesium also decreases renal tubular citrate resorption through the chelation of citrate and thus increases urinary citrate excretion. Several treatment studies to date have demonstrated efficacy when using magnesium supplementation for stone prevention (Johansson et al., 1980; Melnick et al., 1971; Prien and Gershoff, 1974). Conversely, at least one randomized trial showed no difference in recurrence rates between treated and untreated patients (Ettinger et al., 1988).

Several magnesium salts have been used for the treatment of stone disease including magnesium oxide, hydroxide, gluconate, and potassium–magnesium citrate. **GI intolerance is the major side effect of magnesium therapy.** At this time, magnesium supplementation is not widely used (Table 92.6).

Uric Acid Stones
Clinical Considerations

The proportion of uric acid stones in increasing. Xu et al. retrospectively analyzed the records of 1516 patients diagnosed with either a calcium or uric acid stone at a university kidney stone clinic from 1980 to 2015 (Xu et al., 2017). **During this time, the proportion of uric acid stones increased from 7% to 14%, and uric acid stone formers were consistently older with higher BMI and lower urinary pH than calcium stone formers.** The strongest clinical discriminant of uric acid versus calcium stones was urinary pH. Perhaps this increase in uric acid stones can be explained by the rise in metabolic syndrome and obesity as major health burdens affecting 30% of the general population in the United States (Cheal et al., 2004; Flegal et al., 2010). The pathophysiology of uric acid nephrolithiasis is explained in detail in Chapter 91 but does deserve some mention to better understand its diagnosis. **There are essentially three main determinants of uric acid stone formation: low urinary pH, hyperuricosuria, and low urine volume.** Disorders known to result in one or more of these urinary abnormalities include chronic diarrheal states, inflammatory bowel disease, ileostomy, myeloproliferative

TABLE 92.6 Physicochemical and Physiologic Effects of Pharmacologic Therapy for Calcium Stone Disease

	SODIUM CELLULOSE PHOSPHATE	ORTHOPHOSPHATE	THIAZIDE	ALLOPURINOL	POTASSIUM CITRATE
Urinary calcium	Marked decrease	Mild decrease	Moderate decrease	No change	Mild decrease
Urinary phosphorus	Mild increase	Marked increase	Mild increase/no change	No change	No change
Urinary uric acid	No change	No change	Mild increase/no change	Marked decrease	No change
Urinary oxalate	Mild increase	Mild increase/no change	Mild increase/mild decrease	No change	No change
Urinary citrate	No change	Mild increase	Mild decrease	No change	Marked increase
Calcium oxalate saturation	Mild decrease/no change	Mild decrease	Mild decrease	No change	Moderate decrease
Brushite saturation	Moderate decrease	Mild increase	Mild decrease	No change	No change

disorders, high animal protein intake, uricosuric medications, primary gout, obesity, metabolic syndrome, type 2 diabetes mellitus, and rare inherited diseases with mutations in the enzymatic pathways for uric acid production such as Lesch-Nyhan syndrome (deficiency of the enzyme hypoxanthine-guanine phosphoribosyltransferase [HGPRT]). Although these congenital and acquired disorders can result in uric acid stone formation, idiopathic uric acid nephrolithiasis is most common. **Idiopathic uric acid nephrolithiasis is characterized by decreased fractional excretion of urate, normal urinary uric acid levels, and acidic urine** (Maalouf et al., 2004).

Low Urine pH

Urine pH is the most important determinant of uric acid solubility. Because there are no known inhibitors of uric acid crystallization, undissociated uric acid will precipitate when the urine becomes supersaturated. The sigmoidal-shaped solubility curve will predict that at a pH of 6.5, more than 90% of all uric acid is ionized and therefore soluble. Fifty percent of uric acid is soluble at a pH of roughly 5.5 (pK$_a$) (Gutman and Yu, 1968). Urine pH <5.5 will increase the urinary content of undissociated uric acid and result in uric acid precipitation. **Low urine pH (<5.5) is the most common cause of uric acid stone formation** (Pak et al., 2002; Sakhaee et al., 2002). **There are essentially two pathogenic mechanisms for low urine pH: increased net acid excretion and reduced renal ammonium excretion** (Cameron et al., 2006; Sakhaee et al., 2002). Patients with uric acid stones and non–stone formers with type 2 diabetes mellitus on controlled diets have been shown to have a net acid excretion 1.5 times the normal and reduced renal ammonium excretion (Cameron et al., 2006; Maalouf et al., 2010) (Fig. 92.9). It has been postulated that the increased net acid excretion may be secondary to differences in gut microflora in diabetics and uric acid stone formers (Larsen et al., 2010). Ammonium is a high-capacity buffer that works to buffer most of the hydrogen secreted by the kidney and maintain acid base hemostasis. Renal proximal tubular cells are the main renal segment for production and secretion of ammonium (Sakhaee, 2014). Animal studies have suggested that renal steatosis may be responsible for the reduced ammonium excretion (Bobulescu et al., 2008). **The impairment in ammonium excretion has been linked to insulin resistance in diabetic uric acid stone formers** (Sakhaee, 2014). **Impaired ammonium production can leave hydrogen ions either unbuffered or buffered by titratable acid, and the result is low urinary pH.**

Diabetes, Obesity, and Metabolic Syndrome

Metabolic syndrome consists of a cluster of disease states—glucose intolerance, elevated blood pressure, dyslipidemia, and central obesity—that increase the risk for developing type 2 diabetes and coronary vascular disease. All of these issues are frequently found in the obese population. Assessment of the overall rise of type 2 diabetes, obesity, metabolic syndrome, and stone disease suggests potential correlation among these states. A number of investigations have shown an increased risk for stone disease in patients with metabolic syndrome (Kadlec et al., 2012; Sakhaee et al., 2012). Cho et al. reported on the stone composition of patients with metabolic syndrome (Cho et al., 2013). Although the most common stone composition was calcium oxalate, these patients had a significantly higher risk for having a uric acid stone compared with patients without metabolic syndrome.

A number of studies have identified an increased risk for stone disease in diabetics (Lieske et al., 2006; Pak et al., 2003; Taylor et al., 2005; Weinberg et al., 2014). Lieske et al. identified an OR of 1.22 for diabetes among stone formers, whereas Taylor et al. found a relative risk of 1.31 to 1.38 of stone formation in patients with diabetes, depending on age and sex (Lieske et al., 2006; Taylor et al., 2005). These studies confirm the earlier work by Pak et al., in which uric acid stones were identified in a statistically significant predominance for patients with diabetes, indicating innate metabolic abnormalities specific to patients with diabetes.

Recent studies suggest that the increased incidence of uric acid stone formation in obese stone formers may be secondary to the production of more acidic urine than in nonobese patients. Combined data from the two largest stone centers in the United States found that urine pH appears to be directly correlated with body size (Maalouf et al., 2004). Furthermore, patients with type 2 diabetes have been found to have lower urinary pH than nondiabetics independent of the formation of uric acid stones (Cameron et al., 2006). When evaluating patients who form uric acid stones, Sakhaee et al. (2002) identified a much higher incidence of diabetes (both types 1 and 2) compared with other groups. Because individuals with diabetes have impaired ammonium excretion, they have been shown to have an increased incidence of uric acid stone formation (Abate 2004; Pak et al., 2003b). Finally, low urine pH has been shown to directly correlate with the number of metabolic syndrome features (Maalouf et al., 2007). From evaluation of 24-hour urinalyses in 148 non–stone-forming patients, a statistically significant linear relationship was identified in which each additional characteristic of metabolic syndrome portended a decrease in urine pH. Additionally, the degree of insulin resistance was also inversely related to urinary pH.

The Curhan group formally studied the association between body size and risk for stone formation (Curhan et al., 1998a). In two large cohorts, the HPFS and the NHS, the prevalence of stone disease history and the incidence of new stone formation were directly associated with weight and BMI. The magnitude of the association was greater in women than in men. Subsequently, Taylor and Curhan performed a subset analysis on the HPFS and NHS cohorts with evaluation of 24-hour urinalyses (Taylor and Curhan, 2006). Higher BMI was found to be associated with increased urinary excretion of oxalate, sodium, uric acid, calcium, and phosphorus, and lower pH. These same cohorts of patients have been continuously followed, and the group from Boston has provided a recent update on the role of obesity and nephrolithiasis. **They demonstrated that increased BMI, larger waist size, and weight gain correlated with an increased risk for stone episodes. This increased stone risk was still more pronounced for women** (Taylor et al., 2005).

In a review of a large national database, Powell et al. examined the serum and 24-hour urine parameters from nearly 6000 patients with a history of nephrolithiasis (Powell et al., 2000). Within this cohort, obese patients had increased urinary excretion of sodium, calcium, magnesium, citrate, sulfate, phosphate, oxalate, uric acid, and cystine combined with a decrease in urinary pH. One study has specifically evaluated the metabolic disturbances of obese patients, defined as a BMI greater than 30 (Ekeruo et al., 2004). It was determined that the most common manifesting metabolic abnormalities among obese patients included gouty diathesis (54%), hypocitraturia (54%), and hyperuricosuria (43%), which manifested at levels that were significantly higher than those found in nonobese stone formers. When present, chemical stone analysis showed a predominance of uric acid calculi, implicating excessively acidic urine in these subjects. Directed medical therapy and dietary recommendations were able to dramatically reduce stone episodes for these patients.

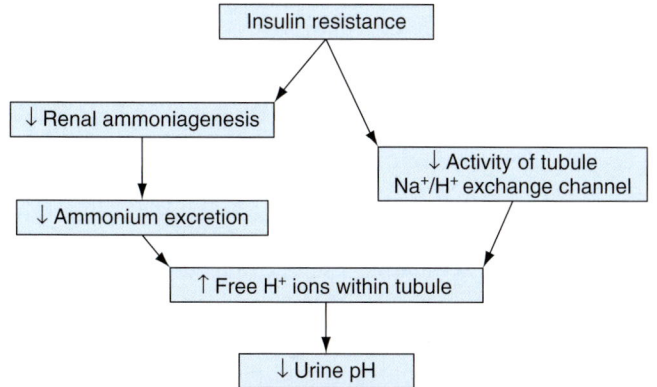

Fig. 92.9. Pathophysiology of low urine pH in patients with insulin resistance. (From Wollin DA, Skolarikos A, Preminger GM: Obesity and metabolic stone disease, *Curr Opin Urol* 27(5):422–427, 2017.)

Diagnosis

The diagnosis of uric acid nephrolithiasis is best made with stone analysis; however, a detailed patient history is important to identify conditions known to increase the risk for uric acid stone formation as described previously (chronic diarrheal states, inflammatory bowel disease, ileostomy, myeloproliferative disorders, high animal protein intake, uricosuric medications, primary gout, obesity, metabolic syndrome, type 2 diabetes mellitus, rare inherited diseases). Uric acid calculi are notoriously radiolucent. Tomography may overcome this difficulty, as can the acquisition of an noncontrast CT scan. Dual-energy CT can be used to distinguish uric acid calculi from calcium stones with a high degree of accuracy (Primak et al., 2007). These stones frequently have an orange/canary yellow appearance, especially when viewed endoscopically. Uric acid stone formers can have a propensity to produce large volumes of very small calculi that may cause obstruction as they pass down the ureter.

Once the diagnosis of uric acid nephrolithiasis is made, a dietary history should be obtained to assess for purine gluttony (high intake of animal protein). 24-hour urine testing is also recommended to evaluate the three main determinants of uric acid stone formation: urine volume, urine pH, and urinary uric acid levels. Often, 24-hour urine collections can underestimate the total amount of uric acid if the specimen pH drops lower than 5.5. In this scenario, the uric acid forms precipitates and settles to the bottom of the collection container. Up to 20% of patients with gout will develop uric acid calculi, prompting examination of serum for hyperuricemia.

Conservative Treatment for Uric Acid Stone Prevention

Low urine volume is a major risk factor for stone formation, and fluid intake is the main determinant of urine volume. Similar to other stone types, uric acid stone formers should maintain fluid intake high enough to achieve a urine volume of at least 2.5 L/day (Pearle et al., 2014). **Uric acid stone formers with hyperuricosuria should be counseled to limit nondairy animal protein as diet-derived purines account for an estimated 30% of urinary uric acid (Pearle et al., 2014).** In addition, these patients should be encouraged to consume foods that confer an alkali load, such as fruits and vegetables, to raise urine pH. In addition, physical activity, weight loss, and glucose control are useful adjuncts for stone prevention in patients with obesity, metabolic syndrome, and/or diabetes mellitus (Torricelli et al., 2014).

Medical Treatment for Uric Acid Stone Prevention

The major goal in the management of uric acid stones is to increase the urinary pH above 5.5, preferably between 6.0 and 6.5 (Khatchadourian et al., 1995). In the past, urine alkalinization has been accomplished with either sodium bicarbonate or various combinations of sodium and potassium alkali therapy. Although sodium alkali may enhance dissociation of uric acid and inhibit uric stone acid formation by raising urinary pH, this medication may be complicated by the development of calcium-containing stones (calcium phosphate and/or calcium oxalate). Potassium citrate is advantageous because it is not only a good alkalinizing agent, but it appears to be devoid of the complication of calcium stones. Potassium citrate should be given at doses sufficient to maintain urinary pH at approximately 6.5 (30 to 60 mEq/day in two or three divided doses). Attempts at alkalinizing the urine to a pH of greater than 7.0 should be avoided because at a higher pH there is a danger of increasing the risk for calcium phosphate stone formation.

Allopurinol should not be routinely offered as first-line therapy in patients with uric acid stones as low urinary pH is by far the predominant risk factor (Maalouf et al., 2004; Pearle et al., 2014). Patients with hyperuricemia and hyperuricosuria, such as may be seen with primary gout, may be an exception. The AUA guidelines also suggest allopurinol may be used as adjunctive therapy in patients in whom alkalinization of the urine is not successful or who continue to form stones despite appropriate alkalinization of the urine. If allopurinol is to be used, the typical dose is 300 mg/day orally. Allopurinol is primarily eliminated by the kidney; therefore, dose reduction is required in patients with impaired renal function. Common side effects include skin rash, muscle pain, nausea, vomiting, and diarrhea. In 2% to 8% of patients, allopurinol can cause adverse reactions ranging from cutaneous hypersensitivity reactions to the potentially life-threatening allopurinol hypersensitivity syndrome (AHS), which causes death in up to 27% of cases. Allopurinol is also reported to be a common cause of Stevens-Johnson syndrome (erythema multiforme exudativum) and complicated renal failure. Adverse reactions were reported in association with higher dosage, renal insufficiency, and diuretic and statin use (Ryu et al., 2013). Finally, hypersensitivity reactions may be increased in patients with decreased renal function who receive thiazides and allopurinol concurrently.

> **KEY POINTS: URIC ACID STONES**
>
> - The proportion of uric acid stones is increasing.
> - The most common cause of uric acid stones is low urinary pH (<5.5).
> - Low urine pH results from increased net acid excretion and reduced renal ammonium excretion.
> - Obesity, metabolic syndrome, and diabetes mellitus increase the risk for uric acid stone formation.
> - Prevention and treatment of uric acid stones centers on reduction of non-dairy animal protein and alkalinization of the urine.

CYSTINURIA

Clinical Considerations

Cystinuria occurs secondary to mutations in the *SLC3A1* gene (located on chromosome 2) and the *SLC7A9* gene (located on chromosome 19), which encode the two subunits of the amino acid transporter, resulting in failure of absorption of dibasic amino acids in the proximal tubule including cystine, ornithine, lysine, and arginine (Pak and Fuller, 1983; Thier et al., 1965). The *SLC3A1* gene encodes the heavy subunit of the renal amino acid transporter (rBAT), which is needed to localize the transporter to the plasma membrane (Eggermann et al., 2012). The *SLC7A9* gene encodes the light subunit of the renal amino acid transporter (b0, +AT), which compromises the catalytic, transporting component. The type of genetic mutation and the mode of inheritance has been used to categorize cystinuria as types A, B, and AB. Cystinuria type A is defined by mutations in the *SLC3A1* gene with autosomal recessive inheritance and high penetrance, meaning increased urinary cystine excretion and kidney stone formation. Cystinuria type B is caused by mutations in the *SLC7A9* gene, which can be inherited as autosomal recessive or autosomal dominant with incomplete penetrance. Type B homozygotes present similar to type A, and carriers (parents, siblings, and children) may have elevated cystine levels but reduced stone formation. In rare cases (1.2% to 4%), patients may have mutations in both genes and be classified as cystinuria type AB. Although no clinical differences have been found between types A and B cystinuria, one benefit of knowing genotype is to estimate recurrence risk in the family.

Cystine has limited solubility in the physiologic range of urine pH, and therefore crystallization occurs when concentrations rise above the saturation point (~250 mg cystine per liter of urine) (Pak and Fuller, 1983). Patients with cystinuria may present with stones at a young age and have affected first-degree relatives. The stones are often yellow and waxy and relatively faint on plain radiography. Staghorn calculi or multiple, filled calyces are common. Historically, a diagnosis of cystinuria was made with the use of a sodium nitroprusside spot test that displays a purple color in the presence of cystine (Smith, 1977). Microscopic analysis of the urine may also demonstrate the pathognomonic hexagonal cystine crystals (see Fig. 92.4). These tests are primarily used to screen for cystinuria as they do not provide a quantitative measurement. Once the diagnosis of cystinuria is made, cystine excretion can be measured by 24-hour urine collection. However, quantitative measurements of cystine can be difficult to perform because of interference from other sulfhydryl-containing compounds (e.g., medications used to treat this disorder) or from significant variances with minor changes in urine pH or creatinine content (Pak and Fuller, 1983). For example, most chromatographic cystine assays cannot distinguish cystine from soluble thiol-cysteine drug complexes. Coe et al. developed a more reliable method of cystine supersaturation measurement known as *cystine capacity* (Coe et al., 2001). The assay involves adding a known amount of solid cystine to the urine of a patient with cystinuria to measure the change in solid phase after incubation. In undersaturated urine, some of the solid-phase cystine will dissolve and thereby reduce the amount that was initially added (positive capacity). In supersaturated urine, the cystine already in the urine precipitates on the added cystine crystals, and the amount of solid phase cystine recovered is greater than what was initially added (negative capacity). In other words, undersaturated urine has positive cystine capacity, and supersaturated urine has negative cystine capacity. Cystine capacity has proved to be equivalent to cystine concentration and supersaturation to predict clinical stone capacity and greatly aids in the diagnosis and management of cystinuria (Nakagawa et al., 2000).

Patients with cystinuria may demonstrate additional metabolic anomalies on 24-hour urine studies (Sakhaee et al., 1989). In a controlled dietary assessment of 27 patients with cystinuria, hypercalciuria was noted in 18.5% of patients and hyperuricosuria in 22.2%. Hypocitraturia was identified in 44.4% and was associated with defective renal acidification in 80% of the patients in whom it was tested. The authors noted that hypercalciuria, hyperuricosuria, and hypocitraturia frequently accompany cystinuria and speculated that these conditions might be renal in origin, rather than a result of dietary or environmental aberrations. They further concluded that these unrelated anomalies may contribute to the formation of calcium and uric acid stones, which sometimes complicate cystine nephrolithiasis. In addition, alkalinizing agents prescribed as treatment for cystinuria may have the effect of raising urine pH and increasing the risk for calcium phosphate stone formation.

Conservative Strategies for Cystine Stone Prevention

The primary goal in the treatment of cystinuria is to decrease the risk for stone formation by lowering cystine concentration (below 250 mg/L) and increasing cystine solubility (Andreassen et al., 2016; Pak and Fuller, 1983). Measures that lower cystine concentration include hydration and dietary measures, and alkalinization of the urine and cystine-binding drugs are used to increase solubility. High fluid intake, although preventive for many different types of stones, is absolutely essential in the prevention of cystine stones. The fluid intake must be high enough for a person to produce at least 3 L/day of urine and evenly distributed throughout the 24-hour period to prevent the physiologic concentration of urine that typically occurs at night. This amount of urine output will dramatically raise the denominator of the concentration fraction and help reduce the supersaturation of urine with respect to cystine. Recommendations for fluid intake vary from 3 to 5 L/day for adults and 3 L/day for children depending on age and weight. In addition, fluid intake must be adjusted during periods of increased insensible losses such as heavy exercise, fever, and high ambient temperature.

In addition to hydration, other dietary measures known to reduce cystine excretion include sodium reduction and protein restriction (Fjellstedt et al., 2001; Lindell et al., 1995; Norman and Manette, 1990; Rodriguez et al., 1995). The AUA guideline on the Medical Management of Kidney Stones recommends that clinicians counsel patients with cystine stones to limit sodium and protein intake (Pearle et al., 2014). Restricting sodium intake to 1 mmol/kg/day has been shown to not only decrease cystine excretion but also increase proximal tubular reabsorption of cystine (Lindell et al., 1995). In fact, Fjellstedt et al. (2001) showed that when sodium citrate was used to alkalinize the urine of patients with cystinuria rather than potassium citrate, the efficacy of other medical interventions, such as the sulfhydryl-containing compound α-mercaptopropionylglycine (Thiola), was diminished. A general recommendation for sodium intake in cystinuric patients is ≤2300 mg/day. Animal protein is rich in amino acids cystine and methionine, which is ultimately metabolized to cystine. Therefore, limiting animal protein such as eggs, fish, chicken, beef, and pork has been suggested as a means of decreasing cystine excretion. Rodman et al. (1984) demonstrated this in a study in which urinary cystine excretion was significantly decreased in homozygous cystinuric patients who were maintained on a low-protein diet of less than 9% of total calories compared with those on a diet in which 27% of total calories were from protein. However, protein restriction should not be recommended in children and adolescents as methionine is an essential amino acid for growth and is limited in plant foods. Furthermore, an effect on cystine stone recurrence of a protein-restricted diet has yet to be demonstrated. Cystinuric patients should be encouraged to consume fruits and vegetables that contain malate and citrate, which may have the effect of raising urine pH.

Medical Therapy for Cystine Stone Prevention

In addition to hydration and the dietary measures discussed earlier, **first-line treatment for cystinuria includes urinary alkalinization, which is best achieved by oral administration of soluble alkali at a dose sufficient to raise the urinary pH to 7.0 to 7.5** (Chow and Streem, 1998; Joly et al., 1999). This treatment strategy attempts to increase the solubility of the filtered cystine to prevent crystal formation. Although sodium bicarbonate, sodium citrate, and potassium citrate all have the ability to alkalinize the urine, **potassium citrate is the preferred alkali in cystine stone formers** as a sodium load may actually increase cystine excretion. The usual dose of potassium citrate is 30 to 60 mEq/day but should be titrated to achieve the goal of a urinary pH of 7.0 to 7.5. Although the pKa of cystine is 8.3, which would achieve greatest solubility for cystine, it is quite difficult to achieve a urine pH this high, and raising the urine pH over 7.5 introduces the risk for calcium phosphate stone formation. Common side effects of potassium citrate include nausea, abdominal pain, vomiting, and diarrhea, which are reduced when patients take the medication with a meal. **Potassium citrate must be used with caution in patients with impaired GI motility as it may lead to gastric ulceration and in patients with impaired renal function or those taking angiotensin-converting enzyme (ACE) inhibitors as hyperkalemia may develop.**

When first-line therapy with hydration, dietary measures, and alkalinization are not enough to prevent cystine stone formation, **second-line therapy consists of agents that increase cystine solubility in urine by formation of a more soluble mixed-disulfide bond (i.e., cystine to drug, rather than cystine to cystine). These agents include α-mercaptopropionylglycine (Tiopronin [Thiola]), D-penicillamine (Cuprimine), and captopril.** Thiols are organosulfur compounds that contain a sulfhydryl group that combines with cystine to form a more soluble drug-cysteine complex.

Introduced in 1963, D-penicillamine was the first thiol drug used in the treatment of cystinuria. Interestingly, very little has been written specifically about this agent and its use in the treatment of cystinuria since the 1960s to 1970s (Combe et al., 1993; Crawhall and Thompson, 1965; Lotz et al., 1966; McDonald and Henneman, 1965). Dahlberg et al. (1977) demonstrated a reduction in stone recurrence, stone passage, and stone growth when D-penicillamine was added to conservative therapy in cystinuric stone formers. Two follow-up studies further demonstrated benefit of thiol drugs. The first study evaluated 27 adult cystine stone formers treated with D-penicillamine or α-mercaptopropionylglycine (Tiopronin) in addition to hydration and alkalinizing agents, and found a significant decrease in stone episodes and urologic procedures (Barbey et al., 2000). The second study conducted in 16 cystinuric patients with long-term follow-up (7 to 141 months) demonstrated that the stone event per patient year decreased from 1.58 to 0.52 (or 65% decrease in yearly stone event rate) when thiol drugs were added to conservative management. Although moderately effective, D-penicillamine has largely been replaced by α-mercaptopropionylglycine (Tiopronin) because of frequent adverse effects including rash, fever, arthralgia, pancytopenia, proteinuria, and nephrotic syndrome. However, there are some long-time cystinuric patients originally started on D-penicillamine who tolerate the drug without significant side effects. One recent study documented 9 in 11 patients without toxicity for an average of 109 months of follow-up after an initial dose escalation (DeBerardinis et al., 2008). Typical doses of D-penicillamine for adults start at 250 mg/day and are titrated to effect.

The second-generation medication to be introduced for the treatment of cystinuria was α-mercaptopropionylglycine (Tiopronin [Thiola]), which was approved by the Food and Drug Administration in 1988 (Hautmann et al., 1977; Johansen et al., 1980; Remien et al., 1975). This agent also contains a sulfhydryl group that forms a disulfide bond with cystine. **α-mercaptopropionylglycine (Tiopronin) is possibly more effective than D-penicillamine and is associated with fewer adverse effects, making it the thiol drug of choice in patients with cystinuria** (Pak et al., 1986a; Pearle et al., 2014). Pak et al. (1986a) showed that among the patients who took both drugs, 30.6% had to stop taking α-mercaptopropionylglycine, whereas 69.4% could not tolerate D-penicillamine. Typical dosages of α-mercaptopropionylglycine (Tiopronin) start at 300 mg, taken orally two times per day, up to as high as 1200 mg/day and titrated to achieve urinary concentrations of cystine less than 250 mg/L urine. Side effects may still occur with α-mercaptopropionylglycine (Tiopronin) including asthenia, GI distress, rash, joint aches, and mental status changes; however, serious adverse reactions requiring cessation of therapy are less common (Pak et al., 1986a).

Finally, the ACE inhibitor captopril has been used to treat cystinuria because it contains a sulfhydryl group and can form a captopril-cysteine disulphide shown to increase cystine solubility in vitro nearly 200 times (Sloand and Izzo, 1987). Although this agent enjoyed early enthusiasm (Streem and Hall, 1989; Cohen et al., 1995), its popularity seems to have waned because of predominantly case-based reports and contradictory results (Michelakakis et al., 1993). Captopril has mainly been used in patients intolerant of other thiols and the recommended dose is 25 mg orally three times daily. Side effects are less severe than the other agents and include fatigue, hypotension, and chronic cough. **Yet, there have been no long-term clinical trials demonstrating the effectiveness of captopril in preventing recurrent cystine stone formation perhaps because its excretion in the urine at maximal doses may not be sufficient to have an effect in binding cystine** (Michelakakis et al., 1993; Pearle et al., 2014).

A novel treatment for the prevention of cystine nephrolithiasis has been studied using the *Slc3a1−/−* mouse model of cystinuria. Zee et al. compared *Slc3a1−/−* mice treated with the nutritional supplement alpha lipoic acid with untreated mice and found alpha lipoic acid was effective in inhibiting cystine stone formation by increasing the solubility of urinary cystine (Zee et al., 2017). The authors postulate that alpha lipoic acid undergoes extensive metabolism resulting in urine metabolites that are ultimately responsible for preventing cystine stone formation. The effect on cystine solubility was also achieved without inducing any change in urinary pH. If the results can be confirmed in human subjects, this could be a promising new therapy for cystinuric patients as the supplement is widely available and has few adverse side effects (Ziegler et al., 2006).

Follow-Up

The goals of care for cystinuric patients include preventing stone formation, preserving renal function, limiting adverse effects of medical therapy, and ensuring patient compliance. The AUA guidelines for the medical management of kidney stones recommends for stone formers an initial 24-hour urine study, a repeat study within 6 months of initiating dietary and/or medical therapy, followed by repeat testing annually or with greater frequency depending on stone activity (Pearle et al., 2014). As mentioned previously, 24-hour measurement of urinary cystine concentration may not be adequate to determine treatment efficacy because most cysteine assays do not distinguish cysteine from soluble thiol-cysteine drug complexes. Therefore, cysteine capacity may be a more effective tool for guiding patient response to therapy. A recent study by Friedlander et al. evaluated urinary cystine parameters including cystine capacity to determine if any could reliably predict clinical stone recurrence (Friedlander et al., 2018). They prospectively followed 48 cystinuric patients using 24-hour urine collections and serial imaging while recording stone activity. Urinary cystine parameters at times of stone activity were compared with those obtained during periods of stone inactivity. Cystine concentration and supersaturation were significantly lower and cystine capacity was significantly higher during stone inactivity than during periods of active stone formation. Cystine capacity proved to be equivalent to cystine concentration and supersaturation to predict clinical stone activity but seemed to be the parameter most reflective of stone-forming potential in any individual urine sample. The authors also suggested that the target value for cystine capacity to prevent stone recurrence should be lowered to 90 mg/L rather than the current recommendation of 150 mg/dL. In addition to maintaining cystine capacity (>90 to 150 mg/dL), treatment goals include 24-hour urine volume (>3 L/day), pH (7.0 to 7.5), and sodium (<100 mmol/day).

Chronic kidney disease has been reported in 5% to 17% of cystinuric patients, with end-stage renal failure occurring in less than 5% (Lindell et al., 1997). Assimos et al. (2002) examined the clinical status of 40 cystinuric patients followed at two medical centers and compared their kidney health to that of 3964 calcium oxalate stone formers enrolled in a database. The mean serum creatinine for stone-forming cystinuric patients was significantly higher than that of the calcium oxalate cohort. Male gender, increasing number of open surgical stone removal procedures, and nephrectomy were significant variables associated with an increased serum creatinine. An alarming number of cystinuric patients had undergone nephrectomy for any reason (14%) versus the patients in the calcium oxalate cohort (3%). These statistics underscore the necessity to regularly monitor renal function in cystine stone formers and actively manage comorbid conditions that may affect renal function such as hypertension and diabetes mellitus.

In addition to preserving renal function, cystinuric patients on thiol drugs must be monitored for adverse effects including neutropenia, thrombocytopenia, anemia, proteinuria, rash, and copper/zinc deficiency. Complete blood count, liver enzymes, and 24-hour urinary protein or urine protein-to-creatinine ratio should be evaluated at least annually in these patients.

Compliance and Quality of Life

The medical management of cystinuria can be quite challenging. Although the array of medication choices is not particularly complicated, it is often difficult to achieve patient compliance (Barbey et al., 2000). Perhaps this is not surprising given the rare hereditary nature of the disease, which results in recurrent stone formation and the risk for chronic stone passage and/or stone treatment (Lindell et al., 1997). A recent study suggests that few patients are able to achieve and maintain targeted goals of medical intervention (Pietrow et al., 2003). Of the 26 patients followed at a dedicated stone center, only 15% achieved and maintained therapeutic success, as defined by urine cystine concentration less than 300 mg/L. An additional 42% achieved therapeutic success but subsequently had failure at an average of 16 months (range 6 to 27). Of these patients, two-thirds were able to regain therapeutic success at an average of 9.4 months (range 4 to 20). However, 19% never achieved therapeutic success, and an additional 23% failed to present to follow-up appointments or provide subsequent 24-hour urine studies, despite having been referred to a tertiary care center. It is very important to note that patient self-assessment of medical compliance was uniformly high regardless of physician perceptions or treatment results.

Given the known challenges of compliance and adherence to prescribed dietary and medical therapy, cystinuric patients may also suffer from decreased health-related quality of life (HRQOL). Streeper et al. used a stone-specific Wisconsin Stone Quality of Life (WISQOL) questionnaire to compare HRQOL in cystine stone formers compared with noncystine stone formers (Streeper et al., 2017). They found that compared with noncystine stone formers, cystine stone formers had significantly lower total WISQOL scores, lower HRQOL scores for subscales (domains) related to social impact, emotional impact, disease impact, and vitality and reported significantly more sleep problems, nocturia, and fatigue.

Efforts to improve compliance and disease management in cystinuric patients include patient education, support groups, and an interdisciplinary approach (urology, nephrology, dietician, pediatrics). The Rare Kidney Stone Consortium (http://www.rarekidneystones.org) facilitates cooperative exchange of information and resources among investigators, clinicians, patients, and researchers to improve care and outcomes for patients with rare stone diseases such as cystinuria. Other patient resources include the International Cystinuria Foundation (http://www.cystinuria.org) and the Cystinuria Support Network (http://cystinuria.net).

KEY POINTS: CYSTINURIA

- Cystinuria is an inherited disease that occurs secondary to mutations in the *SLC3A1* and *SLC7A9* genes resulting in failure of absorption of dibasic amino acids in the proximal tubule including cystine, ornithine, lysine, and arginine.
- Cystinuria manifests when urinary concentrations exceed 250 mg/L.
- Cystinuria may be accompanied by other metabolic abnormalities.
- First-line treatment for cystinuria includes hydration, limitation of dietary sodium/protein, and alkalinization of the urine (potassium citrate).
- Thiol drugs are recommended for cystine stone formers who are unresponsive to dietary modifications and alkalinization.
- α-Mercaptopropionylglycine (Tiopronin) is the thiol drug of choice because it has fewer adverse effects.
- The medical compliance of patients with cystinuria remains a challenge but can be improved with a patient-centered multidisciplinary approach and patient education.

Infection Calculi

The term *infection stone* typically refers to stones that form secondary to infection of the urine with urease-producing bacteria. This can result in stones composed of magnesium ammonium phosphate (struvite) or calcium carbonate apatite. **Infection calculi form in the presence of alkaline urine (pH >7.2) and in an environment rich in ammonia** (Nemoy and Staney, 1971). Urease splits urea into ammonia and carbon dioxide. Ammonia reacts with water to become ammonium and hydroxide ions, which creates an alkaline urine. The ammonium combines with magnesium, phosphate, and water to create magnesium ammonium phosphate (struvite) stones. The carbon dioxide eventually breaks down to carbonate, which combines with calcium and phosphate to form calcium carbonate apatite stones (Fig. 92.10) (Marien and Miller, 2015). Many bacterial organisms are able to produce the urease enzyme (Table 92.7), the most notorious of which is *Proteus mirabilis*. Although most *Escherichia coli* species are not able to split urea, 1.4% of *E. coli* species have been reported as producing urease, and *E. coli* may be associated with struvite calculi, perhaps through a metachronous infection. A recent study by Flannigan et al. retrospectively analyzed data from patients with infection stones over a 4-year period from four different institutions and found that struvite stones were most often heterogeneous in composition (only 13.2% were pure struvite), and urease-producing bacteria were only present in 30% of cases (Flannigan et al., 2018). *Proteus, E. coli,* and *Enterococcus* were the most common bacterial isolates from perioperative urine, and only 40% of patients had a urinalysis that was nitrite-positive, indicating that urinalysis alone is not reliable for diagnosing infection stones, and patients with struvite stones can have urinary tract pathogens other than urease-producing bacteria.

Patients with infection calculi may present with symptoms of acute pyelonephritis, including fevers, chills, flank pain, dysuria, frequency, urgency, and malodorous, cloudy urine. Some patients may exhibit more chronic symptoms of malaise, fatigue, loss of appetite, and generalized weakness. Rarely, infections and obstruction have been long-standing enough to produce xanthogranulomatous

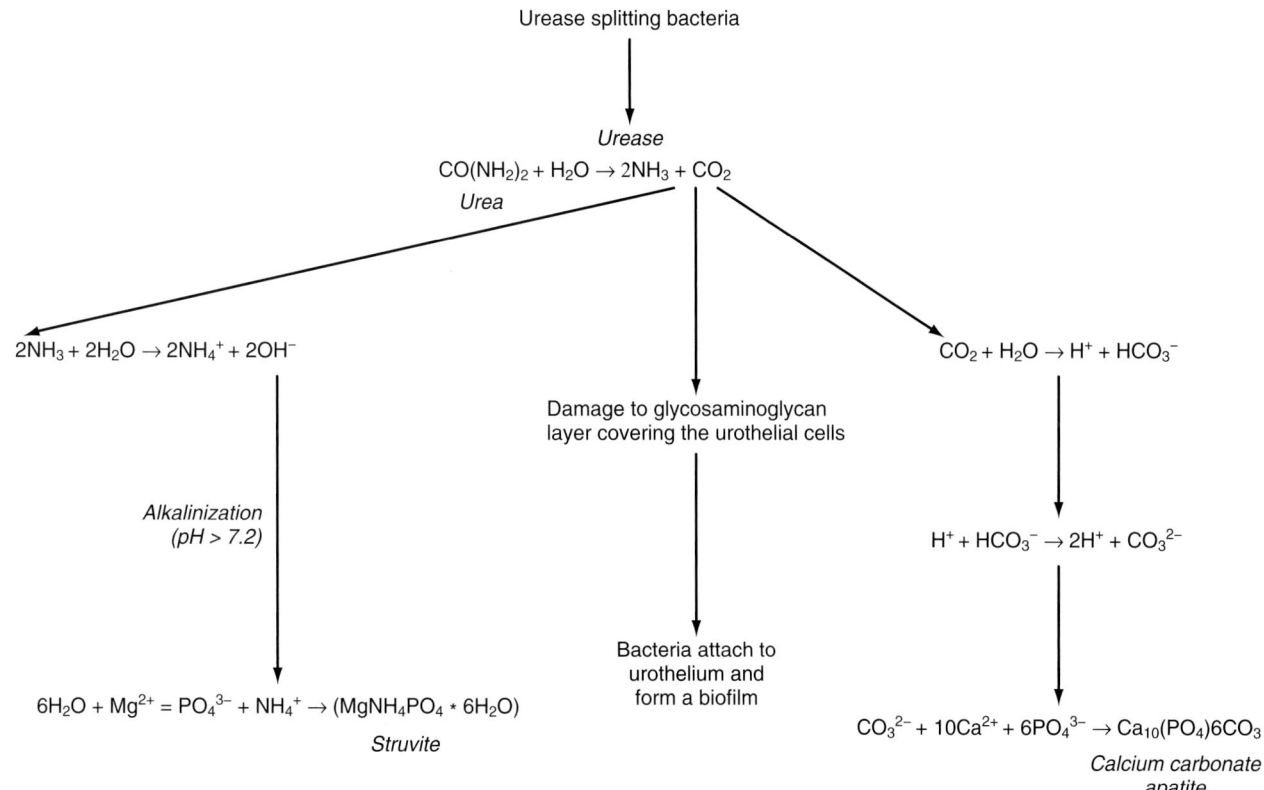

Fig. 92.10. Pathophysiology of infection stone. (Marien T, Miller NL. Treatment of the infected stone. *Urol Clin North Am* 42(4):459–472, 2015.)

TABLE 92.7 Urea-Splitting Organisms

ORGANISMS	USUALLY (>90% OF ISOLATES)	OCCASIONALLY (5%–30% OF ISOLATES)
Gram negative	*Proteus rettgeri* *Proteus vulgaris* *Proteus mirabilis* *Proteus morganii* *Providencia stuartii* *Haemophilus influenzae* *Bordetella pertussis* *Bacteroides corrodens* *Yersinia enterocolitica* *Brucella* spp.	*Klebsiella pneumoniae* *Klebsiella oxytoca* *Serratia marcescens* *Haemophilus parainfluenzae* *Bordetella bronchiseptica* *Aeromonas hydrophila* *Pseudomonas aeruginosa* *Pasteurella* spp.
Gram positive	*Flavobacterium* spp. *Staphylococcus aureus* *Micrococcus* *Corynebacterium ulcerans* *Corynebacterium renale* *Corynebacterium ovis* *Corynebacterium hofmannii*	*Staphylococcus epidermidis* *Bacillus* spp. *Corynebacterium murium* *Corynebacterium equi* *Peptococcus asaccharolyticus* *Clostridium tetani* *Mycobacterium rhodochrous* group
Mycoplasma	T-strain *Mycoplasma* *Ureaplasma urealyticum*	
Yeasts	*Cryptococcus* *Rhodotorula* *Sporobolomyces* *Candida humicola* *Trichosporon cutaneum*	

From Gleeson MJ, Griffith DP. Infection stones. In: Resnick MI, Pak CYC, eds. *Urolithiasis: a medical and surgical reference.* Philadelphia, PA: Saunders; 1990:115.

pyelonephritis, which may cause the failure of an entire kidney or may just affect a portion. Jaeger et al. examined the endoscopic characteristics of renal papillae in struvite stone formers undergoing percutaneous nephrolithotomy and found less Randall's plaque formation than calcium oxalate stone formers and evidence of severe parenchymal and interstitial inflammation compared with other stone formers (Jaeger et al., 2016). The natural history of these stones is associated with progressive morbidity and mortality, with the 10-year mortality rate reported at 28% with nonsurgical management versus 7% with surgical treatment (Koga et al., 1991). Spontaneous fistulae may develop to external surfaces or to peritoneal contents.

The incidence of infection stones has decreased over the past 30 years, likely a result of improved medical care. However, women are more often affected than men (10% to 11% versus 4% in men) as are the elderly, and this is likely a result of increased susceptibility to urinary tract colonization (Daudon et al., 2004; Knoll et al., 2011). Patients with neurogenic bladder, urinary diversion, or history of a foreign body (e.g., forgotten stent, suture material, staple, indwelling stent) are at highest risk for developing infection stones. Struvite calculi can be quite large and take on a typical partial or full staghorn configuration. Urine cultures often will reveal a bacterial pathogen, although, as noted previously, the presence of a sterile urine culture does not preclude the sequestration of bacteria within the calculus itself.

The preferred management of infection (struvite) calculi involves aggressive surgical management with the goal of complete stone clearance. The American Urological Association Nephrolithiasis Guidelines Committee has strongly recommended endoscopic-based procedures (i.e., percutaneous nephrolithotomy) as the first-line therapy for managing complex renal staghorn calculi (Assimos et al., 2016a, 2016b; Preminger, 2005). This report noted that complete elimination of all infected stone material is essential for the prevention of recurrent struvite stone formation.

The medical management of infection calculi centers on the prevention of recurrence, rather than medical dissolution. Thus long-standing effective control of infection with urea-splitting organisms should be achieved if at all possible with improved bladder health, adequate urinary drainage, and monitoring of patients for reinfection with urease-producing organisms (Bichler et al., 2002; Hess, 1990; Pearle et al., 2014). Unfortunately, such control is difficult to obtain in the face of residual calculi because stones often harbor organisms and endotoxin within their interstices (McAleer et al., 2002, 2003; Rocha and Santos, 1969). Antibiotics should be tailored to the predominant organism found on culture and sensitivity screening (Hugosson et al., 1990). Notably, cultures do not always correlate well between a patient's urine and a resuspension of stone material (Fowler, 1984). Therefore strong clinical suspicion is always indicated, and all patients undergoing removal of presumed infection calculi should be covered with broad-spectrum antibiotics that account for local resistance patterns. Although cultures may become negative during treatment, it is important to remember that recurrence of colonization is likely if residual fragments remain within the collecting system.

Acetohydroxamic acid (AHA) is an oral urease inhibitor. It may reduce the urinary saturation of struvite and therefore retard stone formation (Griffith et al., 1978). **When given at a dose of 250 mg three times per day, AHA has been shown to prevent recurrence of new stones and inhibit the growth of stones in patients with chronic urea-splitting infections.** AHA achieves high levels in the urine and can penetrate bacterial cell walls. Randomized and placebo-controlled studies have proven AHA's ability to significantly reduce stone growth (Griffith et al., 1991; Williams 1984). In a randomized, double-blind, placebo-controlled trial of AHA in 210 spinal cord injury patients, Griffith et al. (1988) reported a significant decrease in stone growth for those receiving AHA versus placebo (33% and 60%, respectively). In addition, in a limited number of patients, this agent has caused dissolution of existing struvite calculi (Rodman et al., 1983). According to the AUA guidelines for the medical management of stones, clinicians may offer AHA to patients with residual or recurrent struvite stones only after surgical options have been exhausted (evidence strength Grade B) (Pearle et al., 2014).

The problem with AHA is that a significant percentage of patients, up to 30%, experience side effects including tremor, headache, palpitations, edema, GI distress, loss of taste, rash, alopecia, anemia, and abdominal pain (York et al., 2015). In addition, hemolytic anemia occurs in 3% to 15% of patients, which requires cessation of the medication. **The most severe complication of treatment with AHA is deep venous thrombosis.** Rodman et al. (1987) demonstrated that patients receiving AHA enter into a state of low-grade intravascular coagulation requiring careful follow-up for signs of thrombosis. Furthermore, renal insufficiency increases the risk for toxicity. AHA is contraindicated in patients with creatinine >2.5 and pregnant women and those of childbearing age who are not using birth control (Daudon et al., 2004). In the previously noted randomized studies, 22% to 68% of treated patients had to stop therapy and withdraw from the investigation (Griffith et al., 1988, 1991; Williams et al., 1984). Because of these concerns, AHA is frequently reserved for patients deemed unfit for surgical management.

Controversy exists as to whether patients with infection stones warrant metabolic evaluation with 24-hour urine collections. Resnick (1981) advocated for the performance of a metabolic evaluation for all patients with infection calculi given a high incidence of positive findings. Conversely, Lingeman et al. (1995) studied 22 patients with infection calculi and noted that patients with pure struvite calculi were significantly less likely to have metabolic anomalies on 24-hour urine evaluation than those with mixed compositions of struvite and calcium oxalate. More recently, Iqbal et al. (2016) reviewed their experience with struvite stones. They reported that 60% of pure struvite stone formers and 77% of mixed struvite stone formers had metabolic abnormalities on 24-hour urine collections. The most common abnormalities were hypercalciuria and hypocitraturia. The authors found that with appropriate medical management of both the metabolic abnormalities and the UTI with either AHA and/or suppressive antibiotics, 60% of patients with residual stone demonstrated no stone growth at a median follow-up of 22 months. Therefore, there may be some value for preventing recurrence in performing 24-hour urine collections in patients with struvite stones and appropriately managing their metabolic abnormalities.

> **KEY POINTS: INFECTION CALCULI**
>
> - Women and the elderly are at higher risk for infection calculi.
> - Infection calculi (struvite and calcium carbonate apatite) form as a result of urinary tract infection with urea-splitting microorganisms.
> - Infection calculi form in alkaline urine.
> - Infection calculi commonly produce staghorn stones.
> - Infection calculi are best managed with complete surgical removal.
> - Acetohydroxamic acid (AHA, Lithostat) can effectively inhibit urease, but its widespread use is precluded by significant side effects.
> - Metabolic evaluation should be considered in patients with infection calculi for prevention of recurrence.

Miscellaneous and Drug-Induced Stones

Drug-induced stones represent 1% to 2% of all renal calculi. Several medications have been associated with stone disease and are listed in Box 92.7. There are essentially two mechanisms by which drugs can contribute to stone formation. **The first mechanism involves crystallization of the drug itself in the urine typically secondary to poor solubility and high dosage of the drug. The second mechanism includes drugs that induce stone formation by producing metabolic abnormalities in the urine such as effects on urine pH, citrate, and calcium** (Daudon et al., 2018a).

> **BOX 92.7 Medications Associated With Renal Calculus Formation**
>
> **CALCULI FORMED FROM DRUG**
> Indinavir
> Ephedrine
> Triamterene
> Magnesium trisilicate antacids (silicates)
> Trimethoprim-sulfamethoxazole
>
> **CALCULI PROVOKED BY DRUG**
> Carbonic anhydrase inhibitors
> Topiramate
> Furosemide
> Vitamin C (excess)
> Vitamin D (excess)
> Laxatives

Drug-Containing Calculi

Although many drugs have been reported to crystallize in the urine, the most common are the protease inhibitors used to treat human immunodeficiency virus (HIV), namely indinavir and atazanavir, the antimicrobials sulfadiazine and ceftriaxone, the potassium-sparing diuretic triamterene, and the cough suppressant/stimulant guaifenesin and ephedrine. Bennett et al. reported abuse of ephedrine and guaifenesin taken individually or in combination accounted for nearly 35% of drug-induced stones in the United States (Bennett et al., 2004). Because not all patients who take these drugs develop stones, the formation of drug-induced stones involves not only characteristics specific to the drug but also patient factors. Common patient risk factors include dehydration/low urine volume, acidic urine (low pH), urinary stasis, and altered hepatic function, and drug-specific risk factors include high drug dosage or prolonged drug treatment and poor solubility (Table 92.8).

The classic example of drugs that crystallize in the urine and form calculi include the antiretroviral medications for HIV, namely indinavir and atazanavir (Bach and Godofsky, 1997; Hug et al., 1999; Saltel et al., 2000; Sundaram and Saltzman, 1999). Indinavir is used much less commonly now than atazanavir perhaps largely because of the high incidence of nephrolithiasis seen with indinavir treatment ranging from 7% to 15% of patients in the majority of publications (Daudon et al., 1997; Kopp et al., 1997). One of the greatest difficulties in diagnosing indinavir stones is their radiolucency and inability to visualize on plain film radiography or even stone protocol CT imaging (Gentle et al., 1997; Sundaram and Saltzman, 1999). Lafaurie et al. (2014) examined risk factors for atazanavir-associated stones in a retrospective case-control study comparing 30 HIV-positive patients who formed atazanavir calculi with 90 HIV-positive controls with no history of stone formation but also receiving atazanavir therapy. They identified a previous history of urolithiasis of any type, long duration of atazanavir exposure, and high serum free bilirubin as independent risk factors for atazanavir stone formation. Treatment of these stones centers on aggressive hydration and endoscopic surgical intervention for obstructing stones. Prevention is best accomplished by discontinuing the medication in patients who develop stones, initiating a different antiretroviral agent, and avoiding atazanavir treatment in patients with a history of urolithiasis or with hepatic dysfunction.

As described earlier, triamterene, a potassium-sparing antihypertensive agent, may crystallize in the urinary tract, requiring cessation of this medication (Sorgel et al., 1985; Werness et al., 1982). Two risk factors for triamterene-associated stone formation include high daily drug dosage (150 to 200 mg daily) and low urine pH (<6.0). For this reason, triamterene should be avoided in patients with a history of uric acid nephrolithiasis or those known to have low urine pH such as diabetics. In addition, renal failure has been reported in patients taking a combination of triamterene and thiazide diuretics;

TABLE 92.8 Patient-Dependent and Drug-Specific Risk Factors of Drug-Induced Calculi

Patient-dependent risk factors
Personal or family history of nephrolithiasis
Pre-existing stones
Urinary stasis (malformative uropathy, prostatic hypertrophy)
Underlying lithogenic metabolic abnormalities (e.g., hypercalciuria, hyperoxaluria, hypocitraturia)
Detoxification enzyme pattern
Abnormally low or high urine pH
Urinary tract infection
Environmental factors (e.g., hot temperature)
Low urine output
Drug-specific risk factors of drug-induced calculi or crystal formation and retention
High daily dose of drug
Long-standing treatment
High urinary excretion of the drug and/or its metabolites
Low aqueous solubility of the drug and/or its metabolites
Short half-life of the drug, inducing concentration peaks in urine
Concomitant therapy that causes changes in the pharmacokinetics or metabolism of the drug
Size of drug crystals
Morphology of drug crystals
Interaction between drug crystals and tissue (tubular obstruction, inflammation)

Daudon M, Frochot V, Bazin D, Jungers P. Drug-induced kidney stones and crystalline nephropathy: pathophysiology, prevention and treatment. *Drugs* 78(2):163–201, 2018a.

therefore, triamterene is not recommended as an adjunct to thiazides for treatment of hypercalciuria.

Antibacterial drugs that can crystallize in the urine include the sulfonamides, aminopenicillins, cephalosprins (ceftriaxone), quinolones, and furanes (nitrofurantoin). Sulfadiazine, a first-generation sulfonamide, has largely been used to treat cerebral toxoplasmosis in patients with HIV and chronically immunosuppressed transplant patients (Guitard et al., 2005; Izzedine et al., 2005). Sulfadiazine undergoes fast liver *N*-acetylation with high urinary excretion of both the drug and its metabolites, both of which are poorly soluble. In addition, the *N*-acetylsulfadiazine crystals rapidly aggregate and can form calculi and obstruction of renal tubules (Daudon et al., 2018a). The patient risk factors for sulfadiazine stone formation include low urine volume, low urinary pH, high daily dosing, and urinary stasis. Ceftriaxone stone formation is much more common in children, with incidence varying worldwide from 1% to 8% (Avci et al., 2004; Mohkam et al., 2007; Youssef et al., 2016). Approximately 33% to 67% of ceftriaxone is excreted in the urine as unchanged drug, and it may complex with calcium in the urine to form calcium ceftriaxonate (Chutipongtanate and Thongboonkerd, 2011; Patel, 1984). The best treatment for these types of stones is discontinuation of the medication. If this is not possible, then one should consider aggressive hydration and alkalinization of the urine.

The high incidence of guaifenesin and ephedrine stones in the United States is likely secondary to the abuse of these medications as over-the-counter combination preparations. Ephedrine in particular has been widely abused for its stimulant properties including weight loss, enhanced energy, sexual performance, and euphoria (Daudon et al., 2018a). The dispensing of these over-the-counter medications is not strictly regulated.

Drugs That Induce Metabolic Stone Formation

Carbonic anhydrase inhibitors may be associated with the formation of calcium-based calculi, particularly calcium phosphate (Kondo et al., 1968; Parfitt, 1969). In this scenario, use of the medication creates a chronic intracellular acidosis. This effect, in turn, creates a urinary milieu reminiscent of a distal tubular acidosis with hyperchloremic acidosis, high urine pH, extremely low urinary citrate, and hypercalciuria. Treatment may be accomplished with potassium citrate replacement or, more logically, cessation of the medication.

Topiramate is prescribed for the treatment of refractory epilepsy and recurrent migraine headaches and was recently approved for weight loss. Unfortunately, it may mimic the effect of a carbonic anhydrase inhibitor with resultant metabolic acidosis, hypocitraturia, hypercalciuria, and elevated urine pH (Kossoff et al., 2002; Kuo et al., 2002; Lamb et al., 2004). Potassium citrate has been shown to restore urinary citrate and prevent recurrent stone disease (Kaplon et al., 2011; McNally et al., 2009; Vega et al., 2007; Warner et al., 2008).

Finally, **multiple authors have described calculi that have formed in patients taking over-the-counter supplements containing ephedrine** (Assimos et al., 1999; Bennett et al., 2004; Blau, 1998; Hoffman et al., 2003; Powell et al., 1998; Smith et al., 2004; Whelan and Schwartz, 2004). These calculi are likely radiolucent but have been reported to be "visible" on noncontrast CT. Ephedrine stones have been treated with a variety of methods, including shock wave lithotripsy, endoscopy, and even alkalinization therapy. Because this supplement has a risk for abuse, it may be difficult to effectively interfere with the formation of future stone events.

Ammonium Acid Urate Stones

Ammonium acid urate calculi are infrequently seen in industrialized nations and are often associated with laxative abuse (Dick et al., 1990; Kato et al., 2004). In an earlier series reported in 1999 (Soble et al., 1999), 23 women and 21 men ranging from 20 to 81 years of age (mean 48.7 years) were treated for stones partly composed of ammonium acid urate. Stone composition ranged from 2% to 60% ammonium acid urate (mean 24.1%) of the total stone mass. No patient had a pure ammonium acid urate stone, although 11 (25%) had stones with ammonium acid urate as the predominant crystal. The authors identified one or more potential risk factors for ammonium acid urate for most patients. Of the patients, 25% had a history of inflammatory bowel disease, with 22.7% having undergone ileostomy diversion, 13.6% admitted to a history of significant laxative use or abuse, 40.9% were morbidly obese, 36.4% had a history of recurrent UTIs, and 20.5% had a history of recurrent uric acid stones. Based on these findings, the authors suggested that laxative abuse should not be assumed for all patients with ammonia acid urate calculi, but rather conditions resulting in metabolic acidosis, the prime risk factor for urate stones. A more recent study by Lomas et al. (2017) retrospectively identified 111 stones in 89 patients with at least 10% of the total composition being ammonium acid urate. In addition to the previously described risk factors, they identified patients with prior prostate surgery and bladder neck contracture or a surgically altered bladder to be at increased risk for ammonium acid urate stone formation. Therefore, a full history and metabolic evaluation should be sought for each patient.

Medical treatment for these calculi is determined by the underlying cause of the stone. Those with laxative abuse are strongly encouraged to develop a healthier bowel regimen. Those with chronic infections are treated much like those with struvite calculi. Bowel disease is treated, if possible, while standard recommendations of fluid intake, oral calcium, alkalinization, and oxalate reduction are made. Those with a history of uric acid calculi are also treated in a similar manner with increased fluid intake, protein and salt restriction, alkalinization with potassium citrate, and the possible use of allopurinol.

Medical Management of Bladder Calculi

The pathogenesis of bladder stones has been historically believed to be mainly attributable to urinary stasis, but it is likely that metabolic factors play an underappreciated role in this process as well. Bladder calculi occur in 3% to 8% of men with bladder outlet obstruction secondary to benign prostatic hypertrophy (BPH) (Childs et al.,

2013; Douenias et al., 1991) yet are known to occur in the absence of pathologic BPH. Bladder stones can occasionally occur in women with normal functioning urinary tracts (Rabani, 2016) and young male patients with metabolic stone diseases such as cystinuria and primary hyperparathyroidism (Gurdal et al., 2003; Halalsheh et al., 2017).

In general, the most common mineral composition of a bladder stone is calcium oxalate, calcium phosphate, and uric acid (Childs et al., 2013). Among a series of matched patients undergoing BPH surgery with and without bladder stones, men with stones were more likely to have prior nephrolithiasis and gout. There were also different 24-hour urine profiles between the cohorts, with bladder stone patients having lower urinary pH levels, lower magnesium, and higher uric acid supersaturation. The presence of bladder stones in the setting of urinary obstruction (i.e., bladder outlet obstruction from BPH) is typically an indication for surgical correction of the underlying problem. Nonetheless, it is reasonable to believe that the same preventive therapies that are applied toward renal stone prevention apply to bladder stone prevention in the absence of an identifiable source of mechanical or functional obstruction or stasis.

One particularly challenging etiology that can lead to bladder stone formation is in the case of augmentation cystoplastly and urinary reconstruction using intestine. Patients with intestinally reconstructed bladders have a high potential for stone formation, with estimates ranging from 3% to 52% (Kisku et al., 2015). They are predisposed to bladder stones for a variety of reasons. In addition to urinary stasis, there is potential for stone overgrowth from either built-up mucous or foreign bodies related to catheterization or the surgical procedure itself. Struvite stones may occur in this population as a result of predisposition to urinary tract infection. In such instances, presence of a urea-splitting organism may raise urinary pH and favor stone formation. Urinary pH may also be elevated as a result of the metabolic consequences of incorporating intestinal segments into the urinary tract. In such instances, patients are prone to a hyperchloremic metabolic acidosis with intestinal absorption of ammonium and exchange of bicarbonate into the urine. Finally, urinary oxalates should be measured and can be elevated as a result of intestinal surgery, particularly if the distal ileum has been used, which could lead to enteric hyperoxaluria. Among 83 patients with stones in such instances, a majority (45%) were infectious with 33% mixed and 23% metabolic. Additionally, metabolic abnormalities on 24-hour urine were common, with all patients having alkaline urine and hypocitraturia (Marien et al., 2017). Prevention of stones in these circumstances is challenging. Routine catheterization, irrigation, and monitoring for stone development are critical. High urine outputs are undoubtedly beneficial, whereas other medical treatments remain somewhat controversial, particularly in the case of potassium citrate, when the beneficial effects of citrate must be weighed against the potential for exacerbation of stone formation secondary to exceedingly alkaline urinary pH.

Follow-Up Considerations in the Medical Management of Urinary Lithiasis

An integral part of the medical management of urinary lithiasis is ensuring appropriate follow-up to determine if the goals of therapy have been achieved and maintained (Fig. 92.11). Previously in this

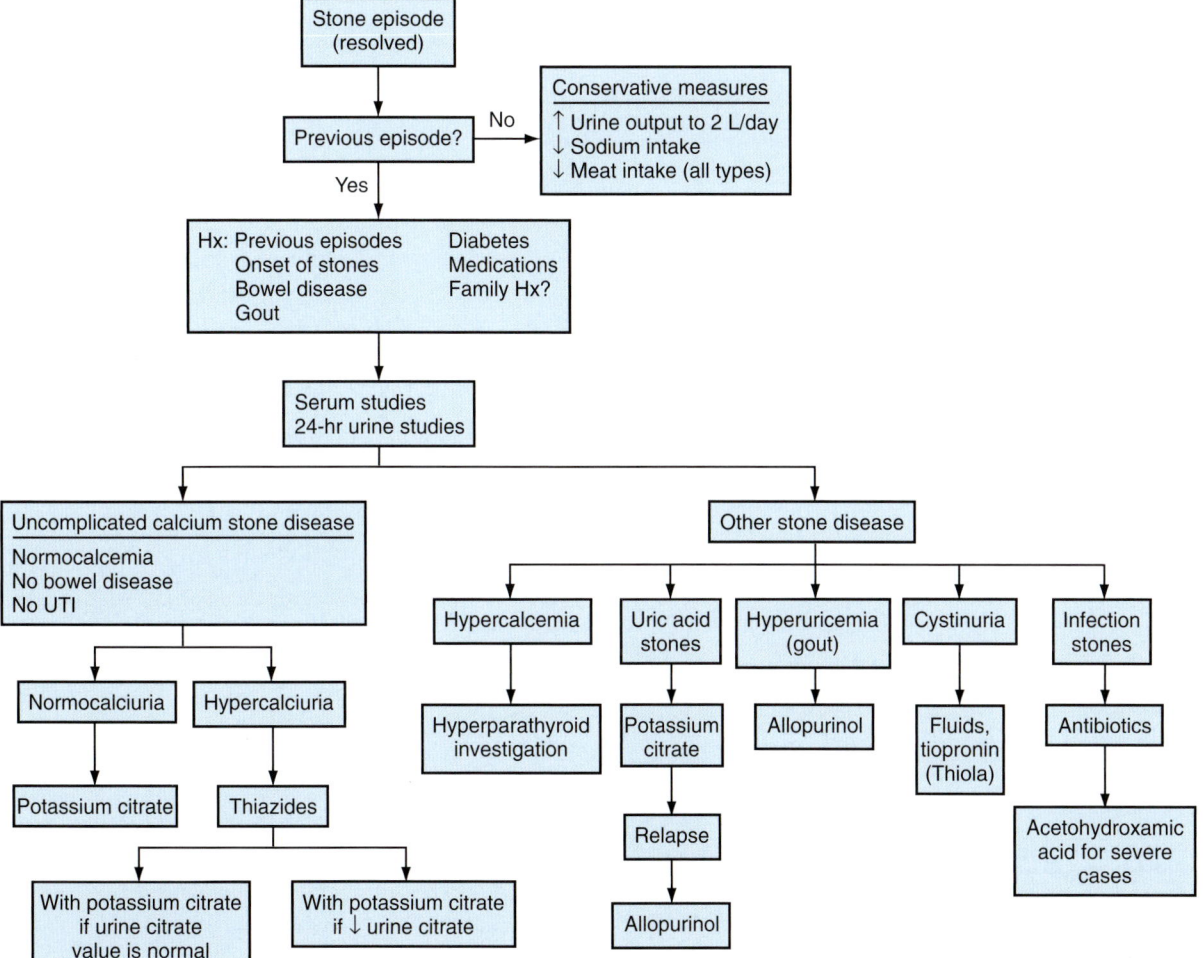

Fig. 92.11. Simplified treatment algorithm for the evaluation and medical management of urinary lithiasis. *Hx*, History; *UTI*, urinary tract infection. (Modified from Pak CY, Britton F, Peterson R, et al: Ambulatory evaluation of nephrolithiasis. Classification, clinical presentation and diagnostic criteria, *Am J Med* 69(1):19–30, 1980.)

chapter, 24-hour urine testing was discussed as part of the metabolic evaluation for high-risk and recurrent stone formers. There is inadequate evidence to define how often these studies should be repeated, however, it is the expert opinion of the AUA Guidelines Panel that a single 24-hour urine sample should be obtained within 6 months of initiation of treatment to assess response to dietary and/or medical therapy. Furthermore, after the initial follow-up, a 24-hour urine collection is recommended annually or with greater frequency, depending on stone activity (Pearle et al., 2014). However, there is significant geographic variation in the quality of secondary prevention. Alruwaily et al. (2015) used Litholink corporation data to identify patients with abnormal urine biochemistries on the initial 24-hour urine collection and then determined if follow-up testing was performed on-treatment. The mean rate on-treatment testing was low at 11.9%, and there was a fourfold variation in the rate across hospital referral regions from 6.6% to 23.4%, with the highest follow-up testing seen in regions with a wealthier, more educated population and those with more primary care physicians.

In addition to ensuring adherence to therapy, it is also critical for the clinician to assess for any adverse effects, particularly as may be seen with pharmacologic therapy. Periodic blood testing is indicated in patients on thiazide therapy, allopurinol tiopronin, and potassium citrate (Pearle et al., 2014). For patients with struvite stones, follow-up should include monitoring for reinfection with urease-producing organisms by obtaining periodic surveillance urine cultures (Pearle et al., 2014). Patients with the highest risk are typically those with urinary diversion or altered lower urinary tract anatomy.

In patients with rapid stone growth or those who are not responding to treatment despite compliance, clinicians should obtain a repeat stone analysis (Pearle et al., 2014). Some patients based on medical history and/or diet may be at risk for more than one stone type, for example, the obese patient who could make both calcium oxalate and uric acid stones. In addition, patients may convert from one stone composition to another as has been reported for calcium oxalate to calcium phosphate stone formation (Mandel et al., 2003).

Recognizing that kidney stones have high potential for recurrence, the AUA and EAU both recommend periodic imaging to assess for new stones. The timing and type of imaging depend both on the presence or absence of existing stones and the stone activity. The AUA recommends annual surveillance for stable patients with plain abdominal radiographs, RUS, or low-dose CT (Pearle et al., 2014). The EAU offers recommendation options for patients with untreated renal stones with initial surveillance imaging at 6 months and then annually, also with plain abdominal radiographs, RUS, or low-dose CT (Turk et al., 2016).

REFERENCES

The complete reference list is available online at ExpertConsult.com.

93
Strategies for Nonmedical Management of Upper Urinary Tract Calculi

David A. Leavitt, MD, Jean J.M.C.H. de la Rosette, MD, PhD, and David M. Hoenig, MD

Further information on kidney and ureteral calculi and the rise of endourology is available online at ExpertConsult.com.

RENAL CALCULI

One of the core tenets of renal stone surgery is to maximize stone removal while minimizing attendant morbidity to the patient. Before the era of endourology, stones were removed via open stone surgery, which provided high stone-free rates but was associated with a high rate of complications. In the early 1980s SWL was developed and proved to have an excellent safety profile while achieving acceptable stone-free rates. During the same time period, PCNL was developed and refined such that it is now considered the gold standard for large and complex kidney stone disease for most patients. Over the last three decades as the technology has improved and the surgical technique diffused, URS has been used with increasing frequency in the treatment of renal stones. More recently, in experienced hands, it has been demonstrated that laparoscopic and robotic-assisted renal stone surgery can be safely used in selected patients with good outcomes. In areas where endourologic technology is widely available, open stone surgery is pursued only 1% of the time or less, and even in developing countries open stone surgery rates have dropped dramatically from 26% to 3.5% (Honeck et al., 2009; Paik and Resnick, 2000).

Thus for most urologists the armamentarium to surgically treat kidney stones consists of four minimally invasive modalities including SWL, URS, PCNL, and laparoscopic or robotic-assisted stone surgery. Staged procedures of a given modality and combinations of different modalities (i.e., "sandwich technique" using SWL and PCNL, and SWL and URS) have been described as well. There appears to be an evolving paradigm shift in the surgical treatment of upper tract stones, with an increasing use of URS, a reciprocal decreasing use of SWL, and a miniaturization in the tract size and instrumentation for PCNL (Lee and Bariol, 2011; Ordon et al., 2014).

Deciding on the optimal treatment for a given patient is not always clear and depends on many variables, which can be broadly lumped into stone-related factors, renal anatomic factors, and clinical factors (Box 93.1). The combination of these factors, availability of technology and equipment, and familiarity of the urologist with the different surgical techniques ultimately determines which treatment is preferred for a given patient. The purpose of this section is to provide a framework to help guide the urologist in matching a given patient's unique clinical situation and renal stone disease characteristics to the most effective and least morbid surgical therapy (Fig. 93.1).

Natural History

The incidence of asymptomatic renal stones has been reported in approximately 10% of screened populations. In one evaluation of just more than 5000 patients undergoing screening computed tomography (CT) colonography, asymptomatic urinary stones were found in 7.8% of patients, with a mean size of 3 mm and an average of two stones per patient (Boyce et al., 2010). In another study evaluating almost 2000 potential kidney donors, asymptomatic renal stones were found in 9.7% of patients (Lorenz et al., 2011). The true natural history of renal calculi, in particular asymptomatic renal calculi, has not been well characterized. Treatment is generally recommended for symptomatic stones, including those associated with pain, infection, obstruction, active stone growth, and significant hematuria. However, the available evidence is less clear on how to approach minimally symptomatic or asymptomatic renal calculi.

Before the era of minimally invasive stone treatments, asymptomatic and minimally symptomatic stones were not actively removed, given the high morbidity associated with treatment. Currently, with the expanding availability of SWL and URS, treatment of small stones can be offered with low surgical morbidity. Although some small, asymptomatic renal stones may never require treatment, a review of the known behavior of such stones suggests that many will grow over time, become symptomatic, and ultimately require treatment.

Nonstaghorn Renal Calculi

A number of studies have reviewed the fate of asymptomatic renal stones while under observation; however, the longest follow-up for any of these series is approximately 10 years, with the majority of them following patients for less than 5 years. Thus the true natural history of asymptomatic renal stones over an extended time period is unknown. Most studies evaluating this type of stone presentation report the rate of spontaneous passage, the rate of intervention, and the rate of stone progression, often defined as stone growth, development of symptoms, or need for intervention.

Hubner and Porpaczy (1990) reviewed the natural history of renal stones in 62 patients managed before the advent of SWL or widespread URS. Of this cohort, spontaneous passage was seen in 16%, whereas 40% required surgical intervention. Stone growth was noted in 45% of patients, urinary tract infection (UTI) occurred in 68%, and pain developed in 51%. Similar results were found by Glowacki et al. (1992), with 32% of initially asymptomatic renal stones becoming symptomatic. Of these patients, half (15%) spontaneously passed their stones, and the calculated 5-year probability of developing symptoms from initially asymptomatic renal stones was 48.5%. Keeley et al. (2001) randomized 228 patients with asymptomatic renal stones to SWL or observation. Spontaneous passage was noted in 17% of the observation group and 28% of the SWL group ($P = 0.06$). There was no difference in the need for additional interventions (analgesics, antibiotics, SWL, stent insertion, URS) between the observation and SWL groups (15% vs. 21%, $P = 0.27$); however, invasive interventions were required only in the observation group. Despite this, there was no appreciable difference in renal function, quality of life, or stone-related symptoms between the two groups, leading the authors to conclude that SWL was not advantageous for small, asymptomatic renal stones.

Burgher et al. (2004) retrospectively reviewed 300 male patients with asymptomatic renal stones with a mean follow-up of 3.26 years. Disease progression, defined as the need for intervention, stone growth, or the development of stone-related pain, was seen in 77% of patients, with 26% of patients requiring surgery. Larger stone size and renal pelvis location were associated with disease progression. All renal pelvis stones and those larger than 15 mm experienced disease progression. The extrapolated risk of intervention

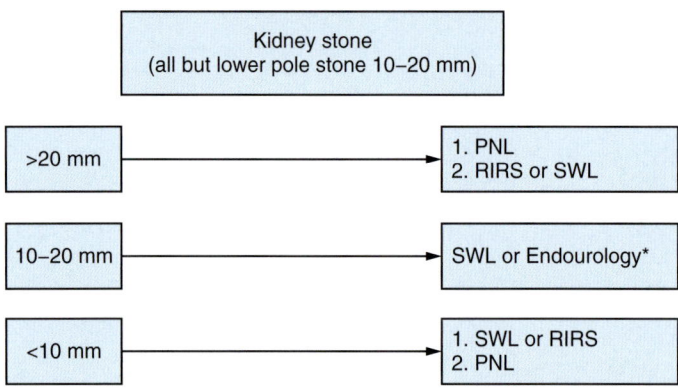

Fig. 93.1. Treatment algorithm: renal stones. *PNL*, Percutaneous nephrolithotomy; *RIRS*, retrograde intrarenal surgery; *SWL*, shock wave lithotripsy; *URS*, ureterorenoscopy. Endourology includes all PNL and URS. RIRS includes retrograde URS. (Modified from Turk et al.: *EAU Guidelines on urolithiasis*, 2017.)

BOX 93.1 Factors Affecting Management of Renal Stones

STONE-RELATED FACTORS
Size
Number
Location
Composition

RENAL ANATOMIC FACTORS
Obstruction or stasis
Hydronephrosis
Ureteropelvic junction obstruction
Calyceal diverticulum
Horseshoe kidney
Renal ectopia or fusion
Lower pole

CLINICAL (PATIENT) FACTORS
Infection
Obesity
Body habitus deformity
Coagulopathy
Juvenile
Elderly
Hypertension
Renal failure or transplant
Solitary kidney
Urinary diversion
Pregnancy
Patient symptoms

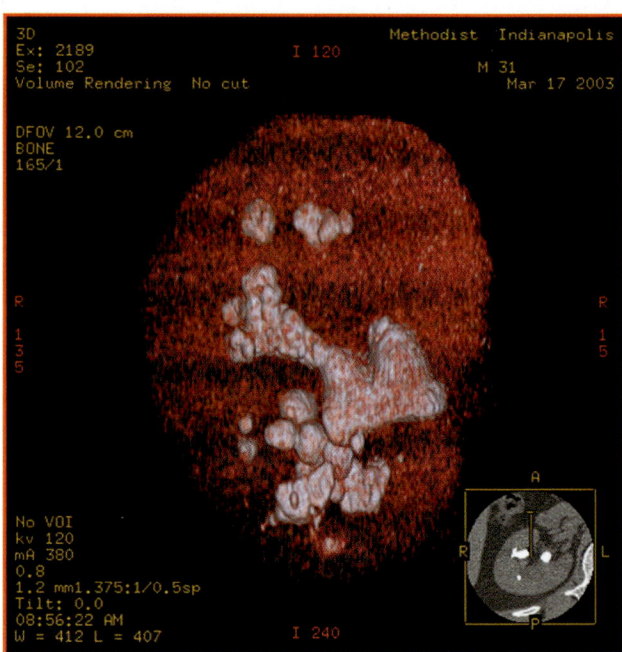

Fig. 93.2. Three-dimensional computed tomography reconstructed image of a staghorn calculus.

at 7 years was 50%. In a similar study by Boyce et al. (2010), 20.5% of initially asymptomatic patients with renal stones became symptomatic over a 10-year period. Koh et al. (2012) found a 20% rate of spontaneous passage, 46% rate of stone progression, and 7.1% rate of intervention.

Inci et al. (2007) showed that approximately one-third of lower pole calculi enlarge, 21% pass spontaneously, and 11% eventually require intervention. Mean stone size was 8.8 mm, and average follow-up was 52 months. No intervention was required in any patient during the first 2 years of observation. In a similar prospective, randomized study, Yuruk et al. (2010) demonstrated an 18.7% intervention rate for asymptomatic lower pole renal stones, with a median time to intervention of 22.5 months. Kang et al. (2013) reported a 29% spontaneous passage rate, 24.5% intervention rate, and 53.6% stone-related-events rate in 347 patients with mean follow-up of 31 months.

Taken together, these studies imply a number of findings about asymptomatic renal stones that can be used to advise patients regarding their ideal care. **First, overall stone disease progression, as defined by the development of stone-related symptoms or stone growth, occurs in as many as 50% to 80% of cases, with a calculated risk of approximately 50% at 5 years. Second, spontaneous stone passage occurs about 15% of the time and is more likely in stones 5 mm in size or smaller. Third, larger stones and those located in the renal pelvis are more likely to become symptomatic.** Finally, the risk of eventual surgical intervention for initially asymptomatic renal stones is approximately 10% to 20% at 3 to 4 years after the stones are initially discovered.

Staghorn Calculi

Staghorn calculi are large renal stones that occupy most or all of the renal collecting system. The name arises from the fact that these branched stones look like the antlers of a deer or stag on imaging (Fig. 93.2). The stones frequently involve the renal pelvis and branch into the surrounding infundibula and calyces. No standardized definitions exist for complete and partial staghorn stones, although most consider complete staghorn stones to occupy the entire renal collecting system, whereas partial staghorn stones occupy less. Struvite composes the majority of staghorn stones, although this configuration of collecting system involvement can include any type of stone (Segura et al., 1994). Before the era of endourology, staghorn stones were not always treated, because the surgical morbidity was high and achieving stone-free status was challenging (Segura, 1997). More recent data have improved our understanding of the natural history of staghorn stones, and the contemporary consensus is that staghorn stones should be treated. **Untreated, staghorn stones are associated with recurrent UTIs, urosepsis events, renal functional deterioration, renal loss, end-stage renal disease, and a higher likelihood of death** (Blandy and Singh, 1976; Koga et al., 1991; Segura et al., 1994; Teichman et al., 1995). **Complete renal function loss in 50% of affected kidneys can occur after 2 years without treatment.** Indeed, the American Urological Association (AUA) guideline on the surgical management of stones (2016) and an older guideline specifically developed for the management of staghorn calculi (2005) advocate for the surgical treatment of staghorn stones in patients healthy enough for treatment, with complete stone removal as the therapeutic goal (Assimos et al., 2016; Preminger et al., 2005).

Pretreatment Assessment

Before the surgical treatment of renal and ureteral stones, a thorough medical history and physical examination, proper imaging studies, and appropriate laboratory tests are necessary in all patients. In some instances, more elaborate laboratory analysis and upper urinary tract anatomic and functional studies may provide important additional information that is useful in surgical decision making.

Medical History

A number of medical and surgical conditions affect urinary calculi formation and have an impact on treatment planning. Medical conditions that predispose to nephrolithiasis formation should be considered in all stone formers (Strauss et al., 1982). Hyperparathyroidism, renal tubular acidosis (type 1), inflammatory bowel disease and chronic diarrhea, prior intestinal resection and gastric bypass surgery, sarcoidosis, cystinuria, metabolic syndrome and diabetes, gout, recurrent UTIs, spinal cord injury, prior urinary tract surgery, anatomic abnormalities, and medullary sponge kidney, among others, are associated with urinary stone formation. In addition to treating symptomatic stones in these patients, medical treatment is often required for the underlying disorder and usually assists in preventing further stone formation.

An understanding of a patient's prior stone surgeries and stone composition is also important. Patients with particularly dense stones (i.e., cystine, calcium oxalate monohydrate, brushite) and obese patients are less well suited for SWL, and complete stone clearance is essential with infectious stones. Failed prior approaches may certainly suggest the need for a more invasive or comprehensive approach for the new presentation, as well as a correction of any anatomic factors that may be associated.

Certainly, all patients, and in particular those with a history of cardiovascular and cerebrovascular disease, need to be risk stratified and medically optimized before any stone therapy. Patients on anticoagulation, those with high cardiovascular risk, and those with recent coronary artery stents may need to remain on anticoagulation or antiplatelet agents perioperatively, which must be considered when selecting the best surgical approach. Consultation with the patient's cardiologist, hematologist, or internist is recommended.

Imaging

Preoperative urinary tract imaging is required in all patients before surgical intervention, to assess stone burden, location, density, obstruction, and anatomic considerations. In the past, plain abdominal radiography and intravenous urography and tomography were routinely used; however, plain abdominal radiography (kidney-ureter-bladder [KUB] study) has limited sensitivity and specificity, and its ability to easily demonstrate a stone is subject to multiple stone and patient anatomic factors. Approximately 10% to 20% of stones are uric acid and hence radiolucent, and roughly a third of ureteral stones occur in the mid-ureter and therefore are screened by the sacroiliac bone structure. In addition, body habitus can influence film quality, as will the presence of bowel contents, which can screen a stone from view (Jackman et al., 2000; Levine et al., 1997).

More recently, noncontrast helical CT has gained widespread acceptance as the imaging modality of choice for urinary stones (Heidenreich et al., 2002). CT visualizes almost all renal stone types and has sensitivities and specificities of greater than 95%, which is considerably better than any other imaging modality, even at low dose protocols and across all body habitus (Chen et al., 1999; Hamm et al., 2001; Pfister et al., 2003; White, 2012; White et al., 2007). In addition, CT has the advantage of providing three-dimensional anatomic information about the kidney and adjacent organs, relevant treatment strategy considerations such as skin-to-stone distance, and stone density characteristics to help guide therapeutic choices (White, 2012).

Routine CT scanning may expose patients to cumulative radiation risks; accordingly, modern low-dose imaging protocols are widely used to adhere to the ALARA ("as low as reasonably achievable") principle and thus reduce the radiation exposure while retaining sufficient anatomic and stone details (Lipkin and Preminger, 2013). Only on occasion are more detailed anatomic and functional studies necessary, such as contrast-enhanced studies or renal scintigraphy.

Renal ultrasound has become a more widely used modality for initial evaluation. Greater experience in its use among urologists and emergency medicine physicians has led to its greater availability as a screening tool to determine whether a CT scan is necessary (Dalziel and Noble, 2013). Ultrasound has a sensitivity of 45% to detect kidney and ureteral stones; furthermore, its use as the primary imaging modality for adults arriving at the emergency department with acute flank pain appears to be safe and may significantly reduce cumulative radiation exposure (Smith-Bindman et al., 2014; Turk et al., 2017). Kocher et al. (2011) reported that use of CT for suspected renal colic had increased from 4% to 42% between 1996 and 2007, although there was no overall increase in stone diagnosis or hospital admissions during the same period of time. Recognition of this overuse of CT scanning has led to the implementation of urinalysis- and renal ultrasound–based algorithms to try to decrease it (Edmonds et al., 2010; Riddell et al., 2014).

Chronic kidney stone formers can also be monitored over time with serial ultrasound examinations as a means to reduce radiation exposure to these patients. The limitations of renal ultrasound include the inability to visualize most ureteral stones and a well-recognized poor correlation between measured and actual stone size and location.

More recently, high-Tesla magnetic resonance imaging (MRI) and magnetic resonance urography are being explored as possible alternatives to CT. Preliminary studies have reported sensitivities, specificities, and diagnostic accuracies of 80% or higher for renal and ureteral stones (Semins et al., 2013).

Laboratory Tests

Preoperative urinalysis and culture are mandatory before any stone surgery, and positive cultures should prompt appropriate treatment before the day of surgery. Administration of preoperative antibiotics for 1 week preceding surgery may reduce associated complications (Bag et al., 2011; Mariappan et al., 2006). Despite appropriate antibiotic therapy, sepsis is still a risk; stone culture and renal pelvis culture are better predictors of postoperative sepsis and infectious complications than bladder urine culture results (Mariappan et al., 2005). Therefore patients with radiographic or clinical histories suspicious for infectious or struvite stones should receive culture-directed or broad-spectrum antibiotics before surgery.

Urinalysis may reveal clues to underlying stone composition based on the presence of crystals, and urinary pH may add useful information about uric acid stones or the presence of urease-producing bacteria.

Assessment of underlying renal function is necessary, and serum creatinine often serves as an adequate evaluation, although it reflects total function only. As stated earlier, prolonged presence of untreated staghorn stones, or a long-term, chronically obstructed kidney can significantly affect function of the affected kidney, and in patients with severe, unrecoverable compromise, nephrectomy rather than stone removal may be the most prudent treatment.

Preoperative serum chemistries are important because they may provide clues to underlying systemic diseases such as renal tubular acidosis or hyperparathyroidism or other metabolic derangements. When PCNL or laparoscopic or open stone removal is contemplated, preoperative complete blood counts should be obtained. Routine assessment of coagulation status using prothrombin time (PT) and activated partial thromboplastin time (APTT) is imperative in patients on anticoagulation therapy, but recent reviews have suggested that routine testing may not be necessary. This has been slow to be adopted in clinical practice because of a lack of prospective, randomized controlled trials (Dzik, 2004).

Stone Factors

When treatment for any patient with a renal stone is being contemplated, the main stone-related factors include stone burden (total number and size of stones), stone location, and stone composition. Unless prior stone composition is known, absolute stone type is difficult to determine preoperatively. Certain predictions regarding stone composition can be made based on CT scan data, with increasing resistance to fragmentation associated with higher Hounsfield unit (HU) measurements. In addition to stone density, patient body habitus, stone burden, and location play important roles in the selection of the optimal surgical approach.

Treatment Decision by Stone Burden

The total kidney stone burden, or total volume of stone(s) requiring treatment, is arguably the most important factor influencing treatment decisions. Problematically, however, there is no standard for reporting kidney stone burden. Accordingly, the following decision analysis is based on the largest single-dimensional stone diameter measured on plain radiography or CT. Based on the available evidence, it is convenient to stratify stone burdens as those up to 1 cm, those between 1 cm and 2 cm, and those greater than 2 cm.

Because staghorn stones reflect additional complexity with respect to treatment because of the volume and the branched nature of the stone, and because there is ample literature specifically regarding staghorn stones, these are discussed separately.

Kidney Stone Burden Up to 1 cm. The majority (50% to 60%) of solitary kidney stones are 1 cm or less in diameter, and many of them are asymptomatic (Cass, 1995; Logarakis et al., 2000; Renner and Rassweiler, 1999). Given enough time, however, many will enlarge or become associated with clinical factors that warrant treatment. Almost all renal stones 1 cm or smaller may be treated with SWL, URS, or PCNL. Laparoscopic or open stone removal is necessary in exceedingly rare cases, most often when there is underlying aberrant anatomy.

SWL has been considered first-line treatment for these smaller kidney stones without complicating clinical or renal anatomic considerations because it is the least invasive modality, achieves reasonably high stone-free rates, and requires the least technical skill. **More recently, flexible URS use, instrumentation, and familiarity are growing within the urologic community. As reflected in the most recent European Association of Urology (EAU) and AUA urolithiasis guidelines, flexible URS is now considered an alternative first-line therapy for kidney stone burden 1 cm or less in size** (Assimos et al., 2016; Turk et al., 2017). Stones with high attenuation on CT (≥900 HU) and those located in lower pole calyces represent special situations for which SWL clearance rates are poor. In these instances, URS or PCNL may be the preferred first-line treatment options or become necessary if SWL fails.

For kidney stones 1 cm or less in diameter, SWL achieves stone-free rates of approximately 50% to 90% and effectiveness quotients of approximately 50% to 70% (Abdel-Khalek et al., 2004; Ackermann et al., 1994; Albala et al., 2005; Galvin and Pearle, 2006; Micali et al., 2009; Tailly et al., 2008). Most of these studies have assessed stone-free outcomes using renal ultrasound or plain radiography. Successful clearance is highest for stones in the renal pelvis and ureteropelvic junction (UPJ; 80% to 88%), favorable for stones in the upper and middle calyces (approximately 70%), and consistently less for lower pole stones (35% to 69%) (Albala et al., 2001; Danuser et al., 2007; Fialkov et al., 2000; Pearle et al., 2005). Stone-free rates with the newer second- and third-generation SWL machines have been somewhat disappointing and have yet to match those seen with Dornier HM3, which is considered the gold standard treatment in SWL. This has been the consequence of downsizing the newer generation lithotripters in an attempt to make them more portable and decrease anesthetic requirements.

Even for kidney stones smaller than 1 cm, myriad circumstances exist for which SWL is contraindicated or is significantly less effective than other modalities. Box 93.2 lists the contraindications for SWL; Box 93.3 describes clinical and renal anatomic factors that make SWL less favorable than URS or PCNL for treating kidney stones.

Over the last decade, technologic advances in flexible endoscope design and instrumentation have facilitated the use of URS, also referred to as *retrograde intrarenal surgery*, for the treatment of kidney stones. Multiple reports have now clearly established URS as a reasonable alternative for the treatment of most kidney stones, especially those smaller than 1 cm. Flexible, rather than semirigid, URS is usually necessary to access most middle and lower calyces. Compared with SWL, URS has the advantage of actively removing stones and thereby expediting stone clearance.

BOX 93.2 Contraindications to Shock Wave Lithotripsy

Pregnancy
Uncorrected coagulopathy or bleeding diathesis
Untreated urinary tract infection
Arterial aneurysm near stone (renal or abdominal aortic aneurysms)
Obstruction of urinary tract distal to stone
Inability to target stone (skeletal malformation)

BOX 93.3 Factors Negatively Affecting Shock Wave Lithotripsy Success

Stone composition (cystine, brushite, calcium oxalate monohydrate, matrix)
Stone attenuation ≥1000 HU
Skin-to-stone distance >10 cm (morbid obesity)
Renal anatomic anomalies (horseshoe kidney, calyceal diverticulum)
Unfavorable lower pole anatomy (narrow infundibulopelvic angle, narrow infundibulum, long lower pole calyx)
Relative or complete patient immobility

Contemporary URS for renal stones 1 cm or smaller offers stone-free rates of approximately 80% to 90%, with recent series reporting even better outcomes. Note that many of these reports are from high-volume stone centers. Thus URS for small renal stones in experienced hands consistently provides stone-free rates superior to those of SWL and requires fewer ancillary procedures to do so.

Sabnis et al. (2013) randomized 70 patients with renal stones smaller than 1.5 cm to either micro-PCNL or URS and found a 94% clearance rate for URS and 97% clearance rate for micro-PCNL. Sener et al. (2014) prospectively randomized patients with lower pole calculi to SWL or flexible URS and found a significantly better stone-free rate with URS (100% vs. 91.5%), whereas the SWL cohort required an average of 2.7 treatment sessions. The Global Ureteroscopy Study, which included an international, multi-institutional cohort of 11,885 patients, reported an 85.6% stone-free rate, although this study included ureteral and renal stones (de la Rosette et al., 2014).

These excellent results contrast sharply to those from the well designed, multicenter, prospective, randomized Lower Pole II study, which reported only a 50% stone-free rate for URS of lower pole stones 1 cm or smaller (Pearle et al., 2005). This difference is believed to be secondary to the use of CT to evaluate stone-free status and the fact that this study accrued patients more than a decade ago, closing in 2003. Since that time, URS has experienced marked technologic advances, which are believed to have made URS safer and better. However, more recent URS series evaluating stone-free status by CT similarly show stone free rates between 50% and 60% (Macejko et al., 2009; Portis et al., 2006; Rippel et al., 2012).

The increased stone clearance of URS compared with SWL comes at the cost of a traditionally higher, albeit low, complication rate. Contemporary ureteroscopic series have shown a noticeably lower rate of complications than in prior years. In the Global Ureteroscopy Study, the overall complication rate was 3.5%, with sepsis (0.3%), ureteral stricture (0.3%), and death (0.02%) occurring rarely (de la Rosette et al., 2014). Similarly low complication rates have been reported by others, with rates of ureteral perforation, avulsion, and stricture rates all below 1%, and often below 0.5% (Butler et al., 2004; Geavlete et al., 2006). **Taken together, the recent literature suggests that URS in experienced hands has an excellent safety profile, with stone-free rates and treatment efficiency superior to SWL for small renal stones.**

PCNL is generally reserved for failures of SWL and URS, or for patients with anatomic considerations that make PCNL vastly superior, such as lower pole stones with acute infundibulopelvic angles or calyceal diverticula. So-called "mini" and "micro" PCNL procedures appear to offer similar stone-free rates as traditional PCNL, but with an overall lower complication rate thought to be secondary to the smaller tract dilation. Such techniques may be ideally suited for stones smaller than 1 cm that require PCNL.

Kidney Stone Burden Between 1 and 2 cm. For renal stones between 1 cm and 2 cm, SWL, URS, and PCNL are the most frequently used treatments, with laparoscopic and open stone removal seldom necessary. Stone location, composition, and density and patient anatomic factors become increasingly relevant as stone burden enlarges and have an important impact on treatment outcomes. Larger stone burdens located in lower pole calyces, increasing skin-to-stone distance, and unfavorable lower renal pole anatomy decrease the success rates of SWL and URS but have limited influence on PCNL outcomes. Thus, for renal calculi between 1 cm and 2 cm, stone-specific and anatomic factors must be carefully considered when weighing the relative outcomes and invasiveness of each procedure (see Fig. 93.1).

As a general principle, the efficacy of SWL decreases while the need for ancillary procedures and re-treatment increases as stone burden enlarges (Drach et al., 1986; El-Assmy et al., 2006; Lingeman et al., 1986; Wiesenthal et al., 2011). The same holds true for URS, although to a lesser degree. Although clearance of residual fragments has been observed up to 2 years after SWL, larger initial stone burdens are associated with larger postoperative residual fragments and higher re-treatment rates (Fig. 93.3).

For stones between 1 cm and 2 cm that are *not* located in the lower pole, SWL had traditionally been recommended as first-line therapy. However, for the reasons discussed in the prior section about expanded use and improved outcomes with URS, the most current AUA and EAU stone guidelines recommend URS and SWL as alternative first-line therapeutic options (Assimos et al., 2016; Turk et al., 2017). In general, SWL outcomes are improved when stones are not located in the lower pole, stone attenuation is less than approximately 900 HU, skin-to-stone distance is less than 10 cm, and the patient has no history of SWL-resistant minerals (cysteine, calcium oxalate monohydrate, brushite). When these factors are present, URS or PCNL should be considered a more desirable initial treatment because SWL is more likely to fail.

SWL treatment success rates exceeding 70% have been reported for stones in the upper (71.8%) and middle (76.5%) calyces (Saw and Lingeman, 1999). Lower pole stone clearance rates range significantly lower, between 37% and 61% (Albala et al., 2001; Riedler et al., 2003; Saw and Lingeman, 1999). Nomograms have been developed to predict SWL treatment success and reflect worse outcomes with increasing stone burden and skin-to-stone distance (Kanao et al., 2006; Tran et al., 2015; Wiesenthal et al., 2011). The nomogram by Kanao et al. (2006) predicts stone-free rates after a single SWL session of 56.8% (11 to 15 mm) and 35.1% (16 to 20 mm) for solitary calyceal stones and 64.4% (11 to 15 mm) and 42.7% (16 to 20 mm) for renal pelvis stones.

URS is a reasonable treatment approach for many kidney stones between 1 cm and 2 cm. In general, URS provides stone-free outcomes that are at least comparable, and often superior, to SWL for such renal stones. Moreover, fewer treatment sessions are usually necessary. The tradeoff, again, is a historically higher rate of complications for URS inherent in its more invasive nature. Grasso (2000) reviewed the outcomes of URS at a single, high-volume stone center and found an overall success rate of 81% after one procedure and 90% after two procedures. Single-procedure treatment success was highest for stones in upper and middle calyces (90%) and lower for stones in the renal pelvis and lower pole calyces (approximately 80%).

URS is also useful as a salvage therapy for failed SWL, rendering 58% of these patients stone free after a single treatment session and up to 76% of patients stone free after two URS sessions (Jung et al., 2006). Unlike SWL, which becomes less effective with increasing skin-to-stone distance, similar URS results have been found in patients with normal, overweight, and obese body mass indexes (BMIs) (Caskurlu et al., 2013).

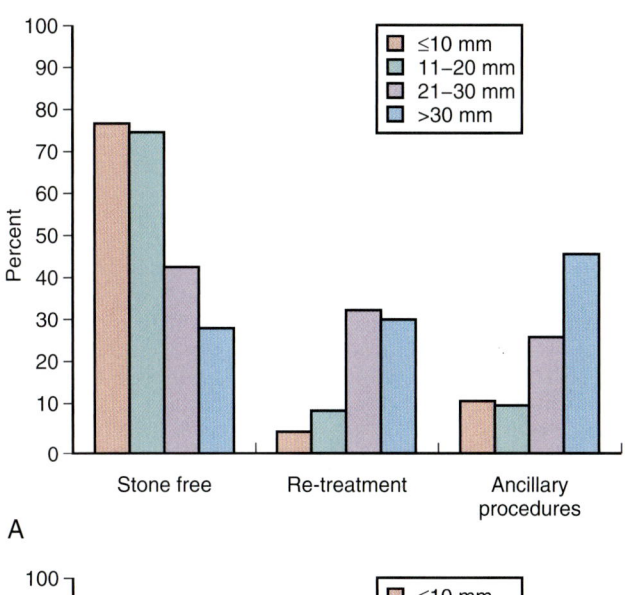

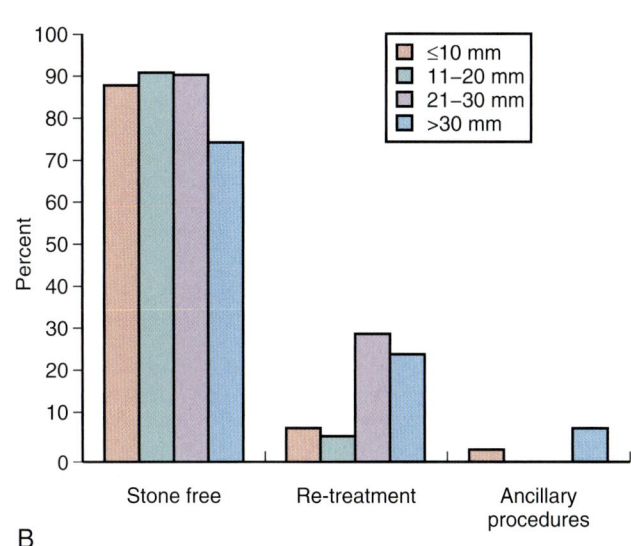

Fig. 93.3. (A) Solitary nonstaghorn calculi treated by shock wave lithotripsy, stratified by size. (B) Solitary nonstaghorn calculi treated by percutaneous nephrolithotomy, stratified by size.

PCNL accomplishes higher stone-free rates and requires fewer auxiliary procedures than SWL or URS for renal stones between 1 cm and 2 cm. The greater invasiveness and higher rate of significant complications of PCNL limit its widespread adoption to the treatment of all renal stones larger than 1 cm. Several series have emerged comparing outcomes among SWL, URS, and PCNL for kidney stones 1 to 2 cm in size (Bas et al., 2014; Resorlu et al., 2013). Success rates were highest for PCNL (91% to 98%), respectable for URS (87% to 91%), and significantly lower for SWL (66% to 86%). As expected, the PCNL groups experienced more overall and serious complications, but they also had the lowest need for additional procedures. The difference in treatment success is even more apparent when comparing SWL (37%) with PCNL (95%) for lower pole stones as demonstrated in the prospective, randomized Lower Pole I study (Albala et al., 2001).

In the last few years, smaller PCNL access sheaths have been used in an attempt to reduce PCNL-related morbidity, and out of this experience have come the terms "mini-perc" and "micro-perc." No precise definitions have been coined, but mini-perc in general refers to PCNL performed through sheaths from 12 Fr to 20 Fr, whereas micro-perc is performed through a 16-gauge needle (Helal et al., 1997; Sabnis et al., 2012).

A few prospective reports with small samples sizes have surfaced evaluating mini-perc and micro-perc (Mishra et al., 2011; Sabnis et al., 2012, 2013). In general, mini-perc has demonstrated equivalent stone clearance to standard PCNL (96% vs. 100%) with a smaller hemoglobin drop, shorter hospital stay, and decreased analgesic requirement. Mini-perc and URS were also found to be essentially the same in terms of stone clearance (100% vs. 97%), whereas URS was associated with a lower hemoglobin drop and less analgesic medication. Similarly, micro-perc and URS showed similar stone clearance (97% vs. 94%) and essentially equivalent blood loss, postoperative pain, and length of stay. Notably, mini-perc and micro-perc techniques are mainly performed in highly specialized, high-volume stone centers. These procedures are of significant interest, although the techniques have not yet been widely adopted by the urologic community at large. Certainly, additional studies with larger sample sizes are necessary to better evaluate these techniques and their learning curves.

Kidney Stone Burden Greater Than 2 cm. PCNL should be considered first-line therapy for kidney stone burdens 2 cm and greater (Assimos et al., 2016; Turk et al., 2017). Unlike URS and SWL, **the success of PCNL is relatively independent of stone location and stone composition.** Stone clearance was once considered independent of stone burden as well, although more recent studies suggest that stone-free rates decrease as stone burdens increase (Desai et al., 2011; Lingeman et al., 1987). Nonetheless, modern-day PCNL is the most efficient means to remove stone burdens 2 cm and greater in a single surgical setting. It is also routinely associated with shorter operative times and a lower likelihood of requiring a staged procedure, which is usually the norm when URS, SWL, or both are used to tackle larger stones. Meanwhile, the complication and re-treatment rates rise noticeably when SWL monotherapy is used to approach these larger stones.

As the most efficient means to remove large stones from the kidney, PCNL has consistently achieved stone clearance rates of at least 75%, and often much higher, when used by many different groups across the world (Albala et al., 2001; de la Rosette et al., 2011; Osman et al., 2005a; Segura et al., 1985). Clearance of lower pole stones is also excellent with PCNL, with a rate that has been reported as high as 95% in the Lower Pole I study (Albala et al., 2001). The superior stone-free rates come as a tradeoff for more frequent and more serious complications after PCNL compared with either URS or SWL. **Overall complication rates between 20% and 30% have been reported, with most contemporary series showing rates of transfusion of 5% to 10%, severe sepsis of 1% or less, delayed bleeding requiring angioembolization of 1% or less, thoracic complications of about 3% or less, organ injury of less than 1% and death of less than 0.3%** (de la Rosette et al., 2011; Michel et al., 2007; Turk et al., 2017). Stone-free rates can be improved and blood loss decreased when flexible nephroscopy is used to augment standard PCNL (Gucuk et al., 2013).

Early after its introduction, SWL was recognized as a suboptimal modality to efficiently clear renal stones 2 cm or greater, as was reported at a National Institutes of Health (NIH) consensus conference (Consensus conference, 1988). Subsequent studies confirmed overall success rates below 30% for stones 3 cm and greater treated with SWL monotherapy (Murray et al., 1995). More recently, stone-free rates of 59% were demonstrated after SWL monotherapy for larger renal stones; however, steinstrasse (23%) and the need for secondary procedures (20%) occurred frequently (El-Assmy et al., 2006). The previously described SWL nomograms predict a stone clearance of 30% or less for renal stones 2 cm or greater (Kanao et al., 2006). When SWL is combined with URS under a single anesthesia, stone clearance rates of nearly 77% can be achieved but require multiple stages (Hafron et al., 2005).

In the late 1990s URS surfaced as a viable, low-morbidity alternative to SWL for large renal stones. One of the first series was reported by Grasso et al. (1998), with a stone-free rate of 76% after a single URS procedure and improving to 91% after a second stage. Unfortunately, at 6 months of follow-up only 60% of patients were completely clear of stones. **Since this report, however, many others have followed, which describe similarly encouraging outcomes, including a mean stone-free rate of 93.7% (77% to 96.7%), an average minor complication rate of 5%, an average major complication rate of 5%, and an average of 1.6 procedures to accomplish such success** (Aboumarzouk et al., 2012a; Bader et al., 2010; Breda et al., 2008, 2009; Mariani, 2008). In many of these studies, stone-free rates were typically evaluated with KUB and/or renal ultrasound. There was no standardization in terms of what size residual fragments were considered insignificant, and patients were therefore categorized as "stone free."

More recently, a few studies have directly compared PCNL with URS for stones 2 cm and larger (Akman et al., 2012a, 2012c; Bryniarski et al., 2012). Overall, stone clearance rates remain consistently higher for PCNL (91% to 96%) than for URS (71% to 93%), and URS cohorts required staged procedures 20% to 30% of the time. **Thus PCNL remains the first-line treatment for kidney stone burdens 2 cm and greater, unless significant comorbidities or contraindications to PCNL are present (frailty, coagulopathy, refusal of transfusion).** In such patients, although less efficient and potentially requiring multiple stages, less invasive alternatives such as URS should be considered.

Staghorn Stones

PCNL is the method of choice for treating partial and complete staghorn kidney stones, with the caveat that poorly functioning or nonfunctioning kidneys and those associated with xanthogranulomatous pyelonephritis may be best managed with nephrectomy. The AUA Nephrolithiasis Guideline Panel and the EAU urolithiasis guidelines recommend PCNL as the first-line therapy for staghorn stones in most patients (Assimos et al., 2016; Preminger et al., 2005; Turk et al., 2017). Stone-free rates are higher with PCNL (78%) than with SWL (22% to 54%) or open surgery (71%). When staghorn stones are discovered, active stone removal should be pursued unless the patient cannot safely tolerate the surgery. **Observation and nonoperative management should be generally discouraged, because the natural history of untreated staghorn stones has shown that they may eventually cause complete loss of function in the affected kidney, can be the cause of recurrent UTIs and sepsis episodes, and are associated with an increased overall mortality** (Blandy and Singh, 1976; Koga et al., 1991; Preminger et al., 2005; Rous and Turner, 1977; Segura et al., 1994; Teichman et al., 1995). However, nonoperative management may not be as harmful as previously suggested, especially for unilateral staghorn stones; and it is a prudent consideration in those of highest surgical and anesthetic risk (Deutsch and Subramonian, 2016). PCNL has proven safe and effective in the adult and pediatric populations (Kumar et al., 2011).

No standardized classification system exists for staghorn kidney stones; however, in general they are defined as branched stones that occupy much of the intrarenal collecting system. Most staghorn stones occupy the renal pelvis and extend into one or more of the surrounding calyces. Historically, staghorn stones have been described as either partial or complete, depending on how fully they occupy the intrarenal collecting system. Multiple other staghorn classification schemes have been developed but have not been widely adopted because they are cumbersome to use and have not yet made a meaningful impact on clinical decision making (Ackermann et al., 1989; Di Silverio et al., 1990; Griffith and Valiquette, 1987; Mishra et al., 2012; Rocco et al., 1984). CT with sagittal and coronal reformatting can provide excellent anatomic and stone dimension details and is valuable in preoperative treatment planning (Nadler et al., 2004; Thiruchelvam et al., 2005).

Infectious stones, those composed of magnesium-ammonium-phosphate (or "struvite"), alone or in combination with calcium carbonate apatite, have long been considered the most frequently occurring composition of staghorn calculi; cystine, uric acid, and calcium oxalate also are able to form staghorn configurations. A more recent report challenged this concept, describing a single-center experience with 52 complete staghorn stones of which 56% were metabolic in nature and 44% were infectious (Gettman and Segura, 1999; Viprakasit et al., 2011). Complete stone clearance is paramount in patients with infectious stones. Incomplete stone removal in these patients can predispose to further UTIs and rapid stone recurrence, because the urease-producing bacteria can persist within the residual stone fragments (Nemoy and Staney, 1971).

Staghorn stones are challenging to treat, frequently require multiple percutaneous access tracts and/or multiple stages, and have high treatment-related morbidity. Surgical strategy should focus on selecting the procedure, or combination of procedures, most likely to render the patient stone free while minimizing morbidity. For most patients, SWL monotherapy should be avoided because it is highly unlikely to be successful and frequently is complicated by steinstrasse. In the only prospective, randomized trial comparing SWL with PCNL for staghorn stones, PCNL provided superior stone-free rates (74% vs. 22%), shorter overall treatment duration, and fewer septic complications (Meretyk et al., 1997).

Combination therapy with multiple endourologic modalities has been used as an alternative to PCNL monotherapy. In one such approach, referred to as sandwich therapy and popularized in the 1990s, staghorn stones were treated first with PCNL, then with SWL for residual or inaccessible stones, and finally with another percutaneous procedure to clear any remaining fragments (Streem et al., 1997). However, outcomes for combination therapy were comparable with those attained with PCNL monotherapy or open nephrolithotomy (Lam et al., 1992b). **Because PCNL allows rapid and effective treatment of large stone burdens, as well as efficient stone clearance rather than requiring spontaneous passage, combined approaches should be based around PCNL as the principal procedure.** The use of flexible nephroscopy during PCNL can improve stone clearance and reduce the number of access tracts necessary by allowing access to calyces unreachable with rigid instruments (Wong and Leveillee, 2002). Flexible nephroscopy is considered a guideline recommendation by the AUA (Assimos et al., 2016). Retrograde flexible URS can be of similar benefit (Marguet et al., 2005).

URS as the sole modality to treat complete staghorn stones is highly unlikely to be successful and has not been reported. URS may be considered an alternative to PCNL for simple partial staghorn stones in patients with favorable anatomy or with contraindications to PCNL, although it often requires multiple stages (Cohen et al., 2013).

Laparoscopic and robotic-assisted techniques have been described in small series for the treatment of complete, or nearly complete, staghorn stones (Giedelman et al., 2012; King et al., 2014). Although these techniques have been shown to be feasible, actual stone-free rates were relatively low (29% to 67%), and the techniques provide no obvious advantage over PCNL for routine staghorn stones in anatomically straightforward situations. In extenuating circumstances, such as ectopic kidneys, laparoscopic or robotic assistance may prove helpful in allowing safe access into the collecting system.

Open nephrolithotomy, once the preferred approach to staghorn stones, is now reserved for rare instances in which complicating factors make PCNL impossible or unlikely to achieve reasonable stone clearance within an acceptable number or combination of procedures. Stone-free rates for open surgery have been reported to be as high as 85%; however, since the rise of endourology and PCNL, superior stone-free rates are routinely achievable with PCNL (Al-Kohlany et al., 2005; Lingeman et al., 1987). In addition, length of hospital stay, the risks for blood transfusions and of renal function loss, and postoperative pain and convalescence favor PCNL over open nephrolithotomy.

Treatment Decision by Stone Localization

Although total stone burden is arguably the most important consideration when deciding how to approach a given patient's stone disease, the location and distribution of stones within the kidney are often the next most important considerations; this is particularly true for stones between 1 cm and 2 cm. The location of stones within the kidney can be simplified to two groups: lower pole stones and non–lower pole stones. Lower pole stones tend to prove the most difficult to treat, especially when the lower pole anatomy is unfavorable (acute infundibulopelvic angle, long infundibular length, narrow infundibular width), because it becomes challenging to reach this location ureteroscopically or to ensure stone clearance with SWL. Because stones within the lower pole are dependently positioned, they are less likely to pass spontaneously after fragmentation by SWL or URS without adjunctive positioning or the use of percussion techniques to assist passage. In addition, the unfavorable anatomic factors may limit passage of fragments even with those adjunctive treatments.

Many studies have evaluated the impact of lower pole stone location on treatment success and complications for a variety of stone treatment modalities. Further discussion of lower pole stones and the influence of lower pole anatomy on treatment outcomes is covered in the section on lower pole calculi. **Stones situated in the lower pole prove more difficult to clear with URS or SWL, and therefore stones 1 cm or larger within the lower pole may be most efficiently treated with PCNL. Stones in a non–lower pole location tend to respond more readily to SWL and URS, making those techniques more competitive with PCNL.**

For non–lower pole renal stones treated with SWL, firm conclusions about treatment outcomes based on differences in non–lower pole renal stone location are difficult to make because the available studies use a variety of different lithotripters and include non-uniform stone burdens and wide variation in the assessment and definition of successful stone clearance. Nevertheless, some patterns emerge when the available data are pooled (Coz et al., 2000; Egilmez et al., 2007; Graff et al., 1988; Khalil, 2012; Kosar et al., 1998; Neisius et al., 2013; Obek et al., 2001; Seitz et al., 2008; Turna et al., 2007). **In general, non–lower pole kidney stone treatment success by SWL tends to be similar for any given stone size regardless of the precise intrarenal location.** That is, stone clearance rates and effectiveness quotients are reported as statistically similar for stones in the renal pelvis, upper pole calyces, and middle calyces within a given study, despite differences in absolute numbers among studies. Thus stone size and composition, rather than stone location, should dictate SWL treatment decisions.

Few recent studies have evaluated URS outcomes based on stone location. With the vast advancements in endourology over the past decade, flexible ureteroscopes can often access all locations within the intrarenal collecting system.

Before the newer-generation flexible ureteroscopes with improved deflection capabilities, lower pole calculi often proved more challenging to access and completely clear. With modern flexible ureteroscopes, however, lower pole stones can be reached in most instances, and small or partially fragmented stones can often be repositioned into more favorable intrarenal locations (e.g., renal pelvis or upper pole). **Excellent stone clearance with URS has been reported for all renal stone locations (>80% to 90%), suggesting that stone size and density, along with patient anatomy, are more important factors than intrarenal stone location when considering URS treatment decisions** (Hussain et al., 2011; Perlmutter et al., 2008; Portis et al., 2006).

Similar to URS, data are sparse with regard to PCNL outcomes based on specific stone location. With the addition of flexible nephroscopy at the time of initial PCNL, much of the kidney and hence stones in many intrarenal locations are accessible through the initial percutaneous tract. However, **some evidence suggests that upper pole calyceal stone location in patients undergoing PCNL is an independent predictor of incomplete stone clearance,** although this study concentrated on single-tract PCNL only (Shahrour et al., 2012). In developing a nomogram to predict stone-free status after PCNL, Smith et al. found that stones within the middle calyx and renal pelvis were more likely to be cleared than stones in an upper or lower calyceal location (Smith et al., 2013). Other than for staghorn stones, upper calyx location was associated with the lowest stone clearance, inferior even to stones within the lower pole.

Results from the PCNL global study demonstrated a higher rate of postoperative complications for large calyceal stones compared with large renal pelvis stones. However, those in the large calyceal stone group had more overall comorbidities and higher American Society of Anesthesiologist scores, which may be significant confounding variables (Xue et al., 2012).

Anterior versus posterior calyceal stone location may also affect PCNL outcomes. When targeting directly into the stone-bearing calyx, anteriorly located calyces require longer tract lengths and traverse more renal parenchyma than posteriorly located calyces. Tepeler et al. (2013) explored this hypothesis in a series in which patients were divided into anterior or posterior calyceal stone location, and found no difference in overall success and complication rates but did note a trend toward increased severe hemorrhagic events in the cohort with anterior calyceal stones.

Treatment by Stone Composition

Stone composition has significant implications with respect to treatment outcomes primarily with SWL, whereas URS, PCNL, and laparoscopic and open stone surgery appear to be only minimally affected. When composition is known, a prior stone analysis can be used to better decide on therapy.

In general, cystine, calcium phosphate (specifically "brushite"), and calcium oxalate monohydrate stones are the most resistant to SWL. The remainder of the common stone types by order of increasing fragility are struvite, calcium oxalate dihydrate, and finally uric acid stones (Pittomvils et al., 1994; Saw and Lingeman, 1999; Zhong and Preminger, 1994).

Zhong and Preminger (1994) showed that brushite and calcium oxalate monohydrate stones' resistance to SWL can be explained by their inherent mechanical properties (higher Young's modulus, greater hardness, and fracture toughness). The resistance of cystine stones to SWL lies in their ductile structure, which conveys a higher resilience to internal crack propagation and a higher deformation capability. **In addition, SWL fragmentation of cystine, brushite, and calcium oxalate monohydrate results in relatively larger stone fragments than other stone compositions, which may negatively affect subsequent stone clearance** (Dretler, 1988; Pittomvils et al., 1994; Rutchik and Resnick, 1998).

In vitro studies have shown that holmium laser lithotripsy fragmentation efficiency is also dependent on stone composition, with the poorest fragmentation seen for calcium oxalate monohydrate stones and moderate fragmentation seen for uric acid and cystine stones (Teichman et al., 1998a). However, this may have little clinical practicality, as a separate study by Teichman et al. (1998b) demonstrated that holmium laser lithotripsy was able to successfully fragment all stone types tested and resulted in no fragments larger than 4 mm. Moreover, when stone basket extraction was added to holmium laser lithotripsy, Wiener et al. (2012) showed that operative time was independent of stone composition.

Stone attenuation values (in Hounsfield units) on CT have been correlated to stone composition, although overlap exists across many stone types. Numerous investigators have shown that **uric acid stones consistently have lower Hounsfield unit values than calcium oxalate monohydrate stones and can be readily discerned from them on helical CT** (Kulkarni et al., 2013; Marchini et al., 2013; Mitcheson et al., 1983; Mostafavi et al., 1998; Nakada et al., 2000). Moreover, uric acid stones tend to display more homogeneous attenuation throughout a given stone than calcium oxalate stones (Marchini et al., 2013). Discriminating between struvite- and calcium-containing stones is usually not possible based on stone attenuation alone, because considerable overlap exists between them.

Even though stone attenuation values are far from perfect in accurately determining stone composition, stone attenuation can be helpful in predicting treatment success with SWL. **Multiple studies now show that attenuation values higher than 900 to 1000 HU are associated with poorer outcomes with SWL** (El-Nahas et al., 2007; Gupta et al., 2005; Joseph et al., 2002; Tran et al., 2015; Wang et al., 2005). Indeed, Gupta et al. (2005) have shown a linear relationship between SWL fragmentation success and stone attenuation, with decreasing fragmentation as stone attenuation increases. Joseph et al. (2002) reported that stone clearance with SWL occurred in just 54.5% of patients with stone attenuation levels above 1000 HU, whereas success was seen in 85.7% of patients when stone attenuation was between 500 and 1000 HU and in all patients with stone attenuation below 500 HU. Ouzaid et al. (2012) showed that a threshold of 970 HU was the most sensitive and specific cutoff value to predict treatment success with SWL. Stones below 970 HU were associated with an SWL treatment success rate of 96%, whereas stones above 970 HU were successfully treated only 38% of the time. Similar to the study by Gupta et al. (2005), this study found a linear association between SWL success and stone attenuation.

Matrix

Matrix renal stones are rare, and unlike most other renal stones in that they are predominantly (approximately 65%, range 42% to 84%) composed of organic proteins, sugars, and glucosamines, whereas other crystalline calculi have only minimal organic material (2.5%) (Boyce and King, 1959). In addition, these stones are soft, gelatinous, and relatively amorphous (Fig. 93.4). Matrix stones can be challenging to diagnose preoperatively because they can mimic upper tract collecting system soft-tissue masses and require a high index of suspicion. Traditionally described as radiolucent, these stones often exhibit either a radiodense calcific center or faint peripheral rim of radiodensity, and both of these signs are frequently visible on preoperative imaging (Fig. 93.5; Bani-Hani et al., 2005; Shah et al., 2009). These stones tend to be large and can assume partial staghorn configurations, and therefore **PCNL is the preferred treatment approach for most matrix renal stones because of its high success rates and low recurrence rates.** Descriptions of successful treatment with URS have been reported (Chan et al., 2010; Rowley et al., 2008; Shah et al., 2009; Stoller et al., 1994b), but SWL is ineffective in these stones, given their soft composition and relative paucity of brittle mineral content.

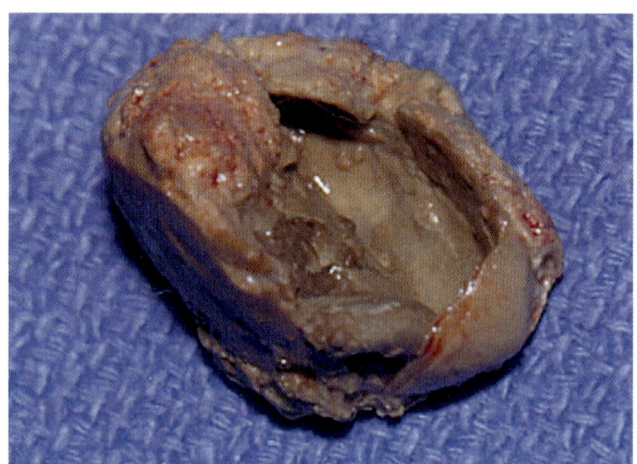

Fig. 93.4. Matrix stone with soft, gelatinous, amorphous consistency and air pocket. (From Bani-Hani AH, Segura JW, Leroy AJ: Urinary matrix calculi: our experience at a single institution. *J Urol* 173:120–123, 2005.)

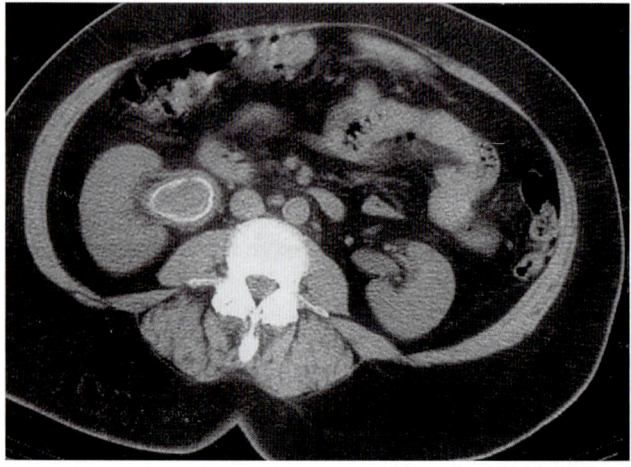

Fig. 93.5. Computed tomography imaging of matrix stone showing radiodense rim and radiolucent center. (From Bani-Hani AH, Segura JW, Leroy AJ: Urinary matrix calculi: our experience at a single institution. *J Urol* 173:120–123, 2005.)

Further details on this topic are available online at Expert Consult.com.

Renal Anatomic Factors

Ureteral Pelvic Junction Obstruction

Ureteropelvic junction obstruction (UPJO) is associated with kidney stones up to 20% to 30% of the time (Berkman et al., 2009; Rutchik and Resnick, 1998). It is vital to, b**efore undertaking any surgical correction, try to distinguish if the UPJO is the underlying disorder with subsequent renal stone formation, or if a renal pelvis or UPJ stone provoked edema at the UPJ, giving the misleading appearance of UPJO when none actually exists.** Although this is not always straightforward, review of CT cross-sectional imaging can provide some insights. For example, when smaller stones are found in calyceal locations with a significantly hydronephrotic renal pelvis and tight UPJ or proximal ureter, UPJO is likely the primary pathology with resulting stone formation. On the contrary, a stone lodged at the UPJ or a renal pelvis stone in close proximity to the UPJ may be the primary pathology causing the obstruction, and no UPJO may actually exist.

If there is any question about primary UPJO or a mimic from a UPJ or renal pelvis stone, then the kidney stones should be treated and no specific therapy should be directed at the UPJ. Rather, 4 to 6 weeks after the stone has been treated, follow-up renal imaging (sonogram, CT, or MRI) can be performed to ascertain if hydronephrosis persists, and if so, further renal functional imaging may be indicated (diuretic renogram). Alternatively, if a nephrostomy tube is in place and the presence of UPJO remains equivocal, then a Whitaker test can be performed. If UPJO is confirmed at that time, only then is UPJ repair recommended.

Similarly, it is important to determine the overall renal function of the affected kidney if it appears atrophic or with thinned parenchyma. If a nonfunctioning or poorly functioning kidney is confirmed, then the simplest option may be nephrectomy rather than simply treating the stone. It is also important to determine if the UPJ has been operated on in the past. Reports have shown that UPJO that recurs after previous endopyelotomy responds favorably to minimally invasive or open pyeloplasty and that UPJO that recurs after previous pyeloplasty responds well to endopyelotomy (Canes et al., 2008; Patel et al., 2011).

A variety of strategies can be used to treat UPJO with concomitant kidney stones, with the ultimate goal of repairing the UPJO and restoring normal renal drainage while simultaneously rendering the patient stone free. PCNL with antegrade endopyelotomy, laparoscopic or robotic pyeloplasty with pyelolithotomy or nephrolithotomy, and retrograde endopyelotomy with URS stone removal have been described. Endopyelotomy should be discouraged when long strictures (>2 cm) are encountered, high UPJ insertions are found, or prior endopyelotomy has been performed and failed.

As a general rule, it is prudent to clear the stone burden before incising the UPJO during endopyelotomy and before completing the UPJ repair with pyeloplasty. This is particularly important for PCNL with antegrade endopyelotomy so that stone fragments do not extrude or settle near the area of the UPJ incision. Stone incorporated in or near the endopyelotomy site can lead to restricturing through granuloma and fibrosis formation (Giddens et al., 2000). Retrograde endopyelotomy with URS stone treatment is also susceptible to this problem because endopyelotomy is necessary as an initial step to allow the ureteroscope access to the kidney, and any subsequent attempts at stone fragmentation or retrieval may result in residual fragments lodging in close proximity to the UPJ.

Over the last decade an increasing number of reports have surfaced describing laparoscopic and robotic pyeloplasty with simultaneous kidney stone removal, and when combined with the available literature on minimally invasive UPJO repair, a number of patterns emerge. There appears to be no difference in operative outcomes, success, or complications of UPJO repair between laparoscopic and robotic pyeloplasty (Braga et al., 2009). Short-term success for laparoscopic and robotic pyeloplasty is excellent at more than 90% and appears superior to that of antegrade endopyelotomy, which is closer to 70% to 80% (Berkman et al., 2009; Knudsen et al., 2004; Rassweiler et al., 2007). Berkman et al. (2009) found PCNL at the time of percutaneous antegrade endopyelotomy to have no effect on success rates of relieving obstruction. Long-term outcomes with endopyelotomy or pyeloplasty are worse than short-term results, with recurrence seen in 25% of pyeloplasties and approximately 60% of endopyelotomies after 10 years (DiMarco et al., 2006).

Laparoscopic, and more recently robotic, pyeloplasty with concurrent renal calculi removal through a pyelolithotomy achieves a stone-free rate of 75% to 100%, and resolution of the UPJO exceeding 90% (Atug et al., 2005; Mufarrij et al., 2008; Ramakumar et al., 2002; Srivastava et al., 2008; Stein et al., 2008; Stravodimos et al., 2014). Laparoscopic graspers, flexible nephroscopes, and wire baskets passed through laparoscopic or robotic trocars, laparoscopic irrigation, and robotic graspers have been used to remove renal stones through the pyelotomy incision. Operative times are approximately 3.5 to 4 hours. In one small series, combined robotic nephrolithotomy and UPJO repair was undertaken and the use of intraoperative ultrasound aided in stone identification within the kidney to direct small nephrolithotomy incisions (Ghani et al., 2014).

In very select cases in which patients have larger, highly complex stone burdens and calyceal anatomy unlikely to permit adequate stone clearance through the standard pyeloplasty incisions, performing standard PCNL first and then performing laparoscopic pyeloplasty under the same anesthetic has been described with encouraging results (Agarwal et al., 2008). However, this approach is associated with longer operative time of almost 4 hours. All patients were stone free by renal sonography at 6 months and demonstrated adequate renal drainage on renogram.

Calyceal Diverticula

Calyceal diverticula are urothelium-lined, nonsecretory, cystic dilations of the intrarenal collecting system that are thought to arise embryonically. They were first described by Rayer in 1841 and were first given the name *calyceal diverticula* in 1941 by Prather. They have a narrow connection to the normal pelvicalyceal system, which is thought to allow for preferential urine filling and poor urine drainage from the diverticulum. Calyceal diverticula are rare, with a reported incidence of 0.2% to 0.6% in patients undergoing intravenous urography (IVU) (Michel et al., 1985; Middleton and Pfister, 1974; Timmons et al., 1975; Wulfsohn, 1980). They may arise from any portion of the pelvicalyceal system, with (approximately) 50% or more originating from the upper pole calyces, 30% from the middle pole calyces or renal pelvis, and 20% stemming from the lower pole calyces (Abeshouse and Abeshouse, 1963; Waingankar et al., 2014).

Stone formation within calyceal diverticula has been reported to occur between 10% and 50% of the time (Middleton and Pfister, 1974; Williams et al., 1969; Yow and Bunts, 1955). A combination of urinary stasis and metabolic derangements is believed to underlie stone development in these structures (Burns et al., 1984; Hsu and Streem, 1998; Liatsikos et al., 2000; Matlaga et al., 2007; Parkhomenko et al., 2017). Hsu and Streem (1998) reported a 50% rate of metabolic abnormalities in 14 patients with stones in calyceal diverticuli. In contrast, Liatsikos et al. (2000) reported that only 25% of patients with calyceal diverticular stones have metabolic abnormalities, compared with 77% of patients without urinary tract anatomic anomalies.

A large percentage of calyceal diverticula are asymptomatic and require no treatment; however, **diverticular stones associated with pain, recurrent infections, hematuria, or a decline in renal function warrant treatment.** Similar to other locations in the kidney, stones within calyceal diverticula have been managed through a variety of approaches, including open surgery, SWL, URS, PCNL, and laparoscopic and robotic modalities. The preferred management approach depends on stone and diverticular anatomic characteristics. Open surgery is primarily of historic interest except in extenuating circumstances, and when undertaken, the diverticulum is marsupialized and cavity lining fulgurated.

SWL has been used to treat calyceal diverticular stones, albeit with modest results, and should not be considered first-line therapy for most symptomatic diverticular stones. Although the underlying pathogenesis is not fully understood, ablation of the calyceal diverticular lining, dilation of the diverticular neck to improve drainage, or both are considered integral to achieving stone clearance and preventing stone recurrence (Cohen and Preminger, 1997). Neither of these is accomplished with SWL. Stone-free rates for SWL are typically poor, ranging from 4% to 58% (Renner and Rassweiler, 1999; Turna et al., 2007). In one of the largest reported series involving SWL of calyceal diverticular stones, Turna et al. (2007) showed a 21% stone-free rate, although 60% of patients did experience symptom relief. Symptom-free status has been achieved in 36% to 86% of patients after SWL across a number of series, with the average closer to 60%; all studies, however, involved relatively few patients. Streem and Yost (1992) reported the highest symptom relief (86%) and stone-free rates (58%) after SWL, and these results appear to be reliant on strict patient selection criteria, including stones smaller than 1.5 cm and large, patent diverticular necks on IVU. With longer follow-up averaging about 24 months (12 to 49 months), the symptom-free rate had declined to 75%, and stone recurrence was witnessed in one patient. In general, with longer follow-up, symptom-free status consistently appears to diminish (Jones et al., 1991a; Streem and Yost, 1992; Turna et al., 2007).

URS is a reasonable first-line treatment approach for patients with small (<2 cm) calyceal diverticular stones arising from an upper or middle calyx, and with a diverticular neck that is short and identifiable (Grasso et al., 1995b; Waingankar et al., 2014). Diverticular stones in these locations are usually accessible via retrograde URS, whereas lower pole diverticular stones present more of a challenge because of angulation. The holmium laser can be used to incise the narrow diverticular neck, fragment stones within, and ablate the diverticular lining. Stone-free rates of 50% to 90% are found in most series, although Auge et al. (2002) found a much lower symptom-free rate of 35% (Auge et al., 2002; Batter and Dretler, 1997; Chong et al., 2000; Fuchs and David, 1989; Grasso et al., 1995b; Legraverend et al., 2013). Adequate diverticular obliteration is lower with the ureteroscopic approach (approximately 20%) than with a percutaneous approach (>70%), hence the need to ensure a patent and well-draining diverticular neck.

In general, most URS failures have occurred in lower pole diverticula, although a small number have occurred in upper pole and interpolar diverticula with unfavorable acute-angle offshoots of the calyceal diverticular neck. Unfortunately, the ostium to calyceal diverticulum cannot be successfully located in up to 25% of cases, and when this occurs the diverticular stones cannot be treated ureteroscopically (Auge et al., 2002; Canales and Monga, 2003). Legraverend et al. reported a 62% stone-free rate, which increased to 84% when residual fragments less than 3 mm were included. Symptom-free rate was 93%. Overall, stone-free rates are superior to those achievable with SWL but inferior to those of PCNL. Furthermore, staged URS procedures are not uncommon in this setting.

PCNL should be considered first-line treatment for most calyceal diverticular stones. Stone-free rates (70% to 100%) and symptom-free rates (77% to 100%) are excellent for PCNL, and the most data supports the efficacy of the percutaneous approach (Al-Basam et al., 2000; Auge et al., 2002; Cohen and Preminger, 1997; Hulbert et al., 1986; Monga et al., 2000; Kim et al., 2005; Krambeck and Lingeman, 2009; Parkhomenko et al., 2017; Shalhav et al., 1998). Diverticular ablation rates are also excellent (>70%) with a percutaneous approach, and the overall success rates appear durable (Monga et al., 2000; Shalhav et al., 1998). Directly puncturing into the calyceal diverticulum is preferable and allows for stone fragmentation and removal, easy fulguration of the diverticular lining, and dilation of the diverticular neck if visible and desired. Ultrasound or CT guidance can be used in selected cases when retrograde contrast instillation does not fill the calyceal diverticulum and when diverticular stones are nonradiopaque (Matlaga et al., 2006a). Posteriorly located diverticuli are particularly well suited for a percutaneous approach because there is usually minimal renal parenchyma between the diverticulum and renal capsule. Anteriorly located calyceal diverticula can also be managed with a percutaneous approach; however, it is often difficult to incise and dilate the diverticular neck secondary to unfavorable angles between the entry vector and the neck.

Laparoscopic and robotic approaches for the treatment of symptomatic stones within calyceal diverticuli have been described and are usually reserved for anteriorly located, symptomatic diverticuli with thin overlying renal parenchyma, which are otherwise not amenable to less invasive endoscopic methods (Akca et al., 2014; Curran et al., 1999; Gluckman et al., 1993; Harewood et al., 1996; Hoznek et al., 1998; Miller et al., 2002; Ruckle and Segura, 1994; Terai et al., 2004; Wyler et al., 2005). Retroperitoneal and transperitoneal approaches have been used; the retroperitoneal method provides easier access to posteriorly located diverticula. Outcomes are superb, with a 100% stone-free rate in those series reporting it as an outcome, approximately a 92% cavity ablation rate, and a 75% to 87% average symptom resolution rate (Basiri et al., 2013; Waingankar et al., 2014; Waxman and Winfield, 2009). The average operative time reported in these studies is approximately 180 minutes, which is longer than for the other surgical approaches. Important common considerations for this approach include the use of intraoperative ultrasound to assist with diverticulum localization, direct cavity lining ablation using electrocautery or argon beam coagulation, and suturing of the diverticular neck when required to manage wide-mouthed diverticulum.

Horseshoe Kidneys and Renal Ectopia

Horseshoe Kidneys. Horseshoe kidneys are the most common renal fusion anomaly, with a reported incidence of 1 in 400 live births (Evans and Resnick, 1981; Pitts and Muecke, 1975). **There is a 15% to 20% incidence of kidney stone disease in horseshoe kidneys.** Most stones are composed of calcium oxalate, and the most common locations are the renal pelvis and posterior lower pole calyces (Evans and Resnick, 1981; Tan et al., 2013). Embryonically, the abnormal medial fusion of the left and right metanephric blastemata creates an isthmus that anchors the fused kidneys at the level of the inferior mesenteric artery, leading to incomplete renal ascent and malrotation (Hohenfellner et al., 1992; Figs. 93.7 through 93.9).

As a result, a number of anatomically important changes are noted. The renal pelvis becomes elongated and anteriorly located, the UPJ has a high insertion into the renal pelvis and is anteriorly situated, and the proximal ureter courses more anteriorly than usual because it must traverse over the isthmus of the horseshoe kidney. **Collectively, these changes are thought to impede normal urinary drainage and to promote urinary stasis and renal stone formation.** These anatomic and functional changes have an impact on the various treatment options for renal stones, and specific horseshoe kidney anatomy, stone location, and stone size must also be considered when choosing the optimal stone treatment. The presence of impaired renal drainage or UPJO should preclude SWL treatment, and other modalities that can address the obstruction, such as PCNL or laparoscopic pyeloplasty, should be pursued. **In general, stones smaller than 15 mm and not situated in the lower pole can be approached with SWL or URS. Stones that fail treatment with SWL or URS and stones larger than 15 mm should be considered for PCNL.** Based on numerous reports, stone clearance and complications in horseshoe kidneys appear to be no different than for PCNL on orthotopic kidneys.

SWL can be considered for stones less than 1.5 cm in diameter located in the renal pelvis or nondependent upper pole and mid-pole calyces. Stone-free rates of 28% to 80% have been reported, with an average closer to 58%. Moreover, multiple treatment sessions are almost always necessary (Elliott et al., 2010; Lampel et al., 1996; Ray et al., 2011; Tan et al., 2013). On average, a higher number of shocks are necessary per treatment session, and a higher re-treatment rate is found versus similar stones in orthotopic, anatomically normal kidneys (Chaussy and Schmiedt, 1984; Drach et al., 1986; Lingeman et al., 1986).

In a series of 11 patients by Vandeursen and Baert (1992), an average of 3.8 treatment sessions per renal unit were required to achieve a 55% stone-free rate, whereas the series by Ray et al. (2011)

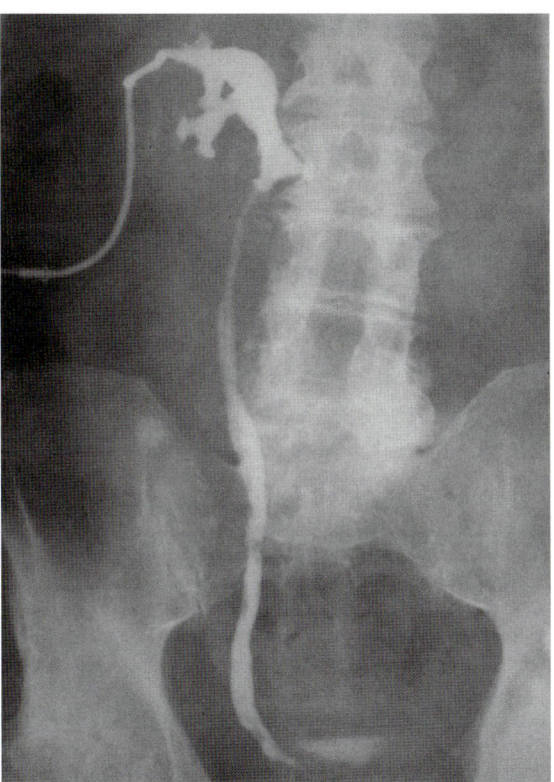

Fig. 93.7. Antegrade nephrostogram obtained after percutaneous nephrolithotomy of a horseshoe kidney via an upper pole access. Note the subcostal nature of the access and the unique calyceal orientation inherent in a horseshoe kidney.

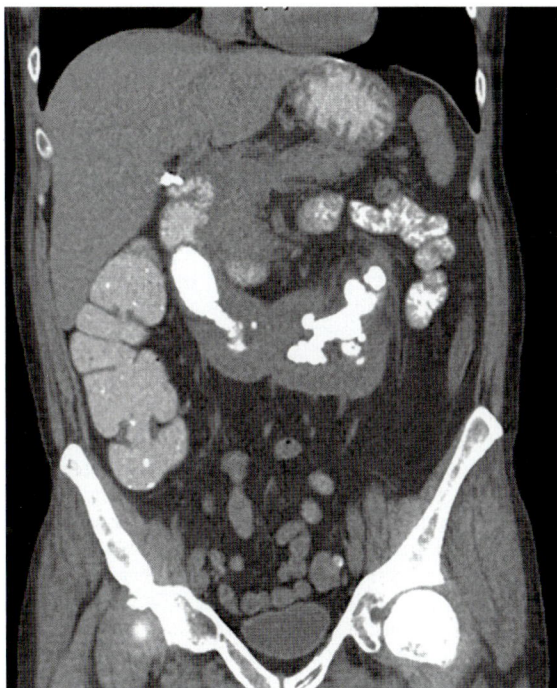

Fig. 93.8. Coronal computed tomographic reconstruction of horseshoe kidney with bilateral staghorn calculi. Note the medial and inferior position of the horseshoe kidney.

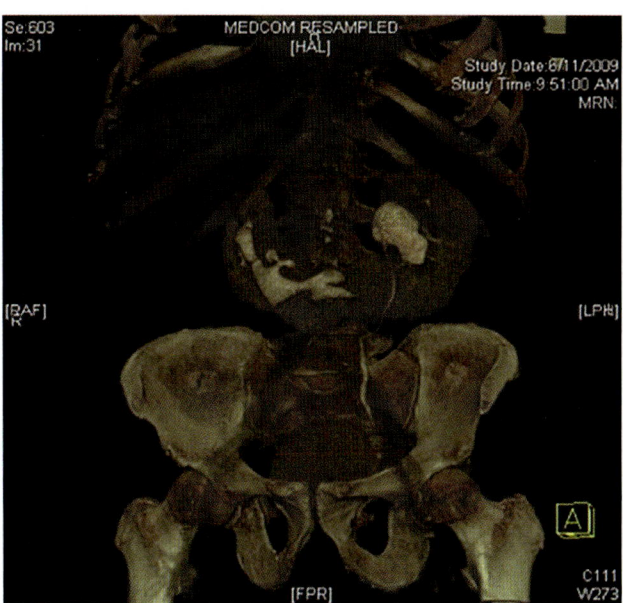

Fig. 93.9. Three-dimensional computed tomographic reconstruction of horseshoe kidney with bilateral staghorn calculi. Note the medial and inferior position of the horseshoe kidney. (From Tan YK, Cha DY, Gupta M: Management of stones in abnormal situations. *Urol Clin North Am* 40:79–97, 2013.)

showed an average of 1.7 SWL sessions for a stone-free rate of 39%. In addition, Ray et al. (2011) reported an abysmal 9.1% stone-free rate and 25% treatment success rate after single-session SWL at 3 months in 41 patients with horseshoe kidneys. In this series, 73% of patients required additional treatments in the form of repeat SWL, PCNL, or URS, and stone-free rate and overall success rate improved to 39.1% and 63.6%, respectively (Ray et al., 2011). The efficiency quotient was disappointing, at 10.5%. Just as SWL efficacy diminishes as stone burden increases in anatomically normal kidneys, so too it diminishes in horseshoe kidneys with increasing stone burden. Sheir et al. (2003) found superior stone-free rates of 79% for stones up to 15 mm, compared with 53% for stones larger than 15 mm. Kirkali et al. (1996) similarly found poor stone-free rates (28%) for stones larger than 10 mm.

Before SWL treatment, UPJO and poor pelvicalyceal drainage must be excluded, because these are not uncommon in horseshoe kidneys and severely curtail SWL success. The more medial and central location of the horseshoe kidney makes it more difficult to properly target calyceal and renal pelvis stones because of the overlying vertebrae, pelvic bones, and bowel gas. Anteromedially located calyceal stones present the greatest difficulty. Positioning patients in the prone position or in the modified supine position can optimize stone targeting and is often necessary for stones situated below the pelvic brim (Gupta and Lee, 2007; Jenkins and Gillenwater, 1988). In addition, long skin-to-stone distances are frequently encountered in horseshoe kidneys, which can also hinder SWL efficacy. When SWL is chosen and skin-to-stone distances are outside of the focal zone of the lithotripter, a "blast path" technique can be used, during which the stone is targeted along the same axis but beyond F2, and relies on shock wave energy transmission past F2 to fragment the stone (Locke et al., 1990).

URS is challenging in horseshoe kidneys because of the high ureteral insertion and tortuous course of the anteriorly displaced ureter. The need for ureteral dilation is not uncommon, and ureteral access sheaths, if able to be placed safely, can significantly expedite repeated entry to and withdrawal from the pelvicalyceal system. Flexible ureteroscopes are almost always necessary to access renal stones in a retrograde fashion, and the use of small-caliber nitinol baskets and holmium laser fibers can minimize loss of URS tip deflection. **Given the aberrant anatomy, ureteroscopy appears to be ideally limited to stone burdens 2 cm or less.** Moreover, staged procedures are common when approaching these stones ureteroscopically, and particularly so among the largest stones. Given the often compromised drainage associated with horseshoe kidneys, fragmented stones should be basket extracted rather than left in situ and left to pass spontaneously.

A number of small retrospective series report favorable surgical outcomes and low morbidity with URS for stone burdens less than

2 cm in horseshoe kidneys (Andreoni et al., 2000; Legemate et al., 2017; Symons et al., 2008; Weizer et al., 2005). No reports focus on larger stone burdens, and none compare URS with SWL or PCNL in a direct fashion. Atis et al. (2013) reviewed outcomes in 20 patients with 25 stones in horseshoe kidneys. Mean stone size was 17.8 mm and stone-free rate after a single procedure was 70%. Weizer et al. (2005) detailed the URS outcomes in 4 patients with horseshoe kidneys and four pelvic kidneys. Mean stone size was 1.4 cm, complete stone clearance was found in 75% of patients, and 88% of patients were symptom free after the procedure. Molimard et al. (2010) reported results in 17 patients with horseshoe kidneys, 4 of whom had undergone failed previous PCNL and 8 of whom had undergone failed prior SWL. In this series, mean stone burden was 16 mm, and an average of 1.5 procedures per patient were required to achieve an 88% stone-free rate, which included residual fragments smaller than 3 mm. In subgroup analysis from the Global Ureteroscopy Study, Legemate et al. (2017) found a 77% and 85% stone-free rate for renal and ureteral stones, respectively, in 43 patients with horseshoe kidneys. Thus URS can render patients stone free more than 70% of the time when stone burdens are less than 2 cm, although a staged approach may be necessary at least half the time.

PCNL is the treatment of choice for stone burdens 2 cm and greater in horseshoe kidneys, with treatment results similar to those obtained in normal kidneys. It is also the preferred method when less invasive methods, such as SWL and URS, fail to adequately treat lesser stone burdens, or when stone density may further decrease expected successful treatment with those methods. Stone-free rates are superior to those achieved with SWL or URS. Overall, an average stone-free rate of 82% to 84% has been reported, with contemporary series describing stone-free rates of 90% or greater with the concomitant use of flexible nephroscopy (Al-Otaibi and Hosking, 1999; Blackburne et al., 2016; Elliott et al., 2010; Esuvaranathan et al., 1991; Gupta et al., 2009b; Janetschek and Kunzel, 1988; Jones et al., 1991b; Ozden et al., 2010; Raj et al., 2003; Shokeir et al., 2004).

Familiarity with the anatomy of the horseshoe kidney is key to safely performing PCNL. Percutaneous access to the horseshoe kidney is often preferentially directed at a posterior upper pole calyx, which results in an access tract situated more medially than those created in orthotopic kidneys. This is because the malrotation of the horseshoe kidney positions the renal pelvis anteriorly and angles the posterior calyces almost directly posteriorly compared with normally positioned kidneys. Percutaneous tracts through the posterior upper pole calyx provide easy access into the renal pelvis and laterally positioned calyces (Elliott et al., 2010).

However, the high insertion of the lower pole, combined with the anteromedially situated calyces, often requires a flexible nephroscope to reach all calyces in the system. In addition, the more anteriorly and centrally positioned horseshoe kidney causes the access tract to be longer, and this may necessitate use of extra-long access sheaths, nephroscopes, and instruments, especially in obese patients. A retrorenal colon may accompany horseshoe kidneys, and given the altered anatomy, preoperative CT is recommended to fully evaluate the safest percutaneous tract. Supracostal access is rarely necessary because the entire horseshoe kidney is often situated below the 12th ribs, and consequently pleural injuries are rare (Raj et al., 2003; Shokeir et al., 2004). The Clinical Research Office of the Endourological Society (CROES) PCNL study group showed that median operative time was longer and percutaneous access more likely to be unsuccessful (5% vs. 1.7%) in horseshoe kidneys than orthotopic kidneys (Osther et al., 2011).

Laparoscopic assistance is only rarely used for stone surgery on horseshoe kidneys, and only a few case reports exist. In general, this adjunctive technique can be useful when particularly large renal pelvis stones exist or when concomitant UPJO exists and pyelolithotomy with or without pyeloplasty is contemplated (Stein and Desai, 2007; Symons et al., 2008; Tan et al., 2013).

Renal Ectopia. Ectopic kidneys are most commonly situated in the pelvis, with the incidence of pelvic kidneys estimated at 1 in 2200 to 1 in 3000 patients. More rarely, ectopic kidneys can be located in the abdomen, in the thoracic cavity, or in a crossed, retroperitoneal location. The approach to kidney stone treatment in these instances should be highly tailored to the specific individual, stone burden, and kidney location, along with any associated kidney drainage impediments. Similarly to horseshoe kidneys, evaluation for impaired renal drainage or UPJO is prudent before embarking down a treatment path, because pelvic kidneys are routinely malrotated and often have a high ureteral insertion or UPJO, which can further hinder stone fragment passage (Gleason et al., 1994). In the appropriate setting, SWL, URS, PCNL, and laparoscopy can be selectively applied to achieve good stone clearance rates.

SWL achieves stone-free rates of 25% to 92%, although multiple treatment sessions are the norm (Gallucci et al., 2001; Semerci et al., 1997; Sheir et al., 2003; Talic, 1996; Theiss et al., 1993; Tunc et al., 2004). With the pelvic kidney shielded posteriorly by the bony pelvis, prone positioning, or rotating the treatment head of the lithotripter anterior to the supine patient, is often necessary to improve shock wave delivery to the pelvic kidney stones when this technique is selected. If treatment with SWL is entertained for stones in ectopic kidneys, renal functional studies evaluating renal drainage (e.g., renography) are recommended, because the presence of impaired kidney drainage is a relative contraindication to proceeding with SWL. Ureteroscopy has also been described for pelvic and ectopic kidneys with stone-free rates of 75% after a single setting, showing that URS and SWL can achieve similar outcomes, but URS is more efficient (Bozkurt et al., 2014; Singh et al., 2017; Weizer et al., 2005). This is likely because of the active fragment removal with URS, whereas SWL requires spontaneous drainage of fragments, which can be problematic in a poorly draining ectopic kidney. Ureteral access sheaths can greatly facilitate re-entry into the ectopic kidney; however, their placement should be undertaken with caution because the associated ureters can be tortuous and perhaps prone to injury with sheath advancement.

Stones within pelvic kidneys present unique challenges to performing PCNL because clear access to the kidney is seldom encountered. Nonetheless, stone clearance rates are better for PCNL than for SWL, at least in part because of active stone extraction and the ability to perform flexible nephroscopy. Traditional posterior access is hampered by the bony pelvis, and even when it can be safely accomplished can result in debilitating femoral neuropathy (Monga et al., 1995). Patients must usually be in the supine position, and safe access into the collecting system is rarely feasible without CT or laparoscopic assistance, although it has been described ultrasonographically. Desai and Jasani (2000) report a technique exploiting transperitoneal ultrasound guidance for supine PCNL in pelvic kidneys in which the ultrasound probe is used to target the kidney and maneuver intervening intra-abdominal contents out of the way of the proposed access tract (Desai, 2009). In this series of 16 patients, 1 experienced a bowel injury. Given its limitations, this method is unlikely to prove successful in overweight or obese patients. Rare case reports of transhepatic, transiliac, and trans-sciatic punctures have been described; however, such approaches should be considered only in the highly selected patient and done in conjunction with CT guidance and the interventional radiologist (Matlaga et al., 2006b).

Laparoscopic assistance has been used during PCNL to ensure a safe percutaneous access tract into the kidney by mobilizing and displacing any overlying intestines and directly observing the needle puncture into the kidney (Fig. 93.10). This was first described by Eshghi et al. (1985), and others have followed suit since then (Elbahnasy et al., 2011; El-Kappany et al., 2007; Gowel et al., 2006; Holman and Toth, 1998; Maheshwari et al., 2004; Matlaga et al., 2006b). Excellent stone-free rates are reported and overall morbidity is low. Most of these techniques use a Trendelenburg position to mobilize the intestines during a transperitoneal procedure. To minimize the risks of urinary leakage to the peritoneal cavity, appropriate postoperative drain placement is recommended. Zafar and Lingeman (1996) have described a simultaneous laparoscopic nephrostomy closure and ureteral catheter placement during pelvic kidney PCNL, thereby avoiding the need for an intra-abdominal drain. An entirely extraperitoneal approach to minimize the risk of intraperitoneal leakage has also been described (Holman and Toth, 1998).

Purely laparoscopic or robotic approaches to pelvic and ectopic kidneys provide high success with low morbidity and are particularly

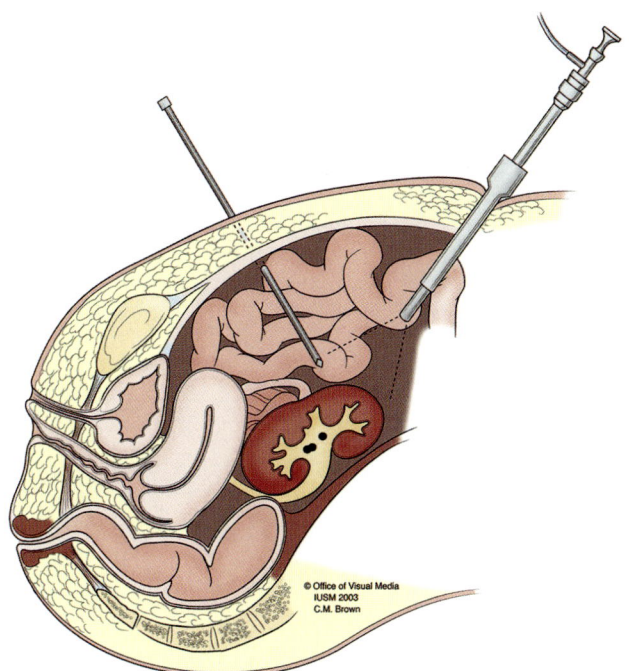

Fig. 93.10. Laparoscopy-assisted percutaneous nephrolithotomy technique in which the bowel is reflected off the ectopic kidney before radiographically and laparoscopically guided percutaneous access. (Copyright 2003, Indiana University Medical Illustration Department.)

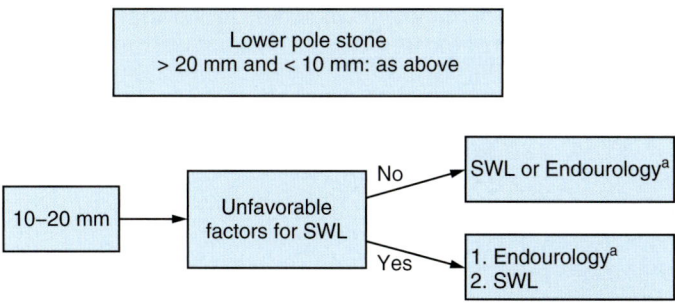

[a]The term 'Endourology' encompasses all PNL and URS interventions.

Fig. 93.11. Treatment algorithm: lower pole stones. *PNL*, Percutaneous nephrolithotomy; *RIRS*, retrograde intrarenal surgery; *SWL*, shock wave lithotripsy; Endourology includes all PNL and URS. RIRS includes retrograde URS. (Modified from Turk et al.: *EAU Guidelines on urolithiasis*, 2017.)

appealing treatment options when simultaneous repair of UPJO is planned (Chang and Dretler, 1996; El-Bahnasy et al., 2011; Hoenig et al., 1997; Kamat and Khandelwal, 2004; Nayyar et al., 2010). The concept is the same as for horseshoe kidneys: a pyelotomy is made to clear renal pelvis stones, and a flexible nephroscope and stone basket are then inserted through one of the laparoscopic trocars to access and clear calyceal stones. Stone-free rates of 80% to 100% have been reported (Atug et al., 2005, Masson and Hoenig, 2008; Ramakumar and Segura, 2000). Most authors use a transperitoneal approach, although Gaur et al. (1994) detail a retroperitoneal approach.

For kidney stones in ectopic and horseshoe kidneys, SWL is a reasonable treatment option when stones are smaller than 1.5 cm and there is no UPJO or demonstration of poor renal drainage. URS may also be reasonable for stone burdens less than 2 cm, although they may require multiple treatment sessions. For stone burdens of 2 cm or more, PCNL or laparoscopy should be the initial treatment; a combination of the two procedures is expected for pelvic kidneys. When UPJO is confirmed, laparoscopy is the treatment of choice because it can address the stones and provides the highest success rate for UPJ repair.

Lower Pole Calculi

The preferred treatment of lower pole renal calculi has generated appreciable controversy over the last few decades (Armagan et al., 2015; Bozzini et al., 2017; Chan et al., 2017; Donaldson et al., 2015; Kandemir et al., 2017; Raman and Pearle, 2008; Sener et al., 2015; Soliman et al., 2016; Tolley and Downey, 1999; Yuruk et al., 2010). Regarding non–lower pole intrarenal calculi, stones within the lower pole tend to have worse surgical stone clearance rates compared with other locations when stratified by size and composition. The management strategy for lower pole stones continues to evolve as ureteroscopic capabilities improve, percutaneous stone removal instrumentation miniaturizes, and the limitations of the newer generations of shock wave lithotripters become more evident (Fig. 93.11; see also Fig. 93.1).

As discussed previously in the section on stone factors, overall stone burden is the main driver of treatment decisions for lower pole stones. Treatment decisions are most conveniently divided into stone burdens less than 1 cm, stone burdens of 1 to 2 cm, and stone burdens greater than 2 cm (see Figs. 93.1 and 93.11). Lower pole kidney stone burdens 2 cm or larger are best approached with PCNL because the collective evidence shows that PCNL offers a considerably higher stone-free rate in a single procedure than URS or SWL. For lower pole stone burdens of 1 cm to 2 cm, PCNL remains the most efficient treatment option, although it is more invasive, and is preferred when prior URS or SWL attempts have been unsuccessful. Ureteroscopy is the treatment modality of choice when PCNL is completely or relatively contraindicated and is a reasonable first-line option in experienced hands. In general, SWL results are disappointing for lower pole stone burdens over 1 cm, and therefore SWL should not be recommended as an initial treatment modality for such stones. For lower pole stones 1 cm or less, stone characteristics and patient factors become relatively more important than for larger stone burdens and should be incorporated into treatment recommendations. Stone burdens 1 cm or less in size may be reasonably approached with any modality including observation if completely asymptomatic, although future stone disease progression is likely. Lower-density stones, in nonobese patients without acute lower pole infundibulopelvic angles are among the few in the lower pole for which SWL provides a reasonable chance of success. Meanwhile, URS, with improved ureteroscopes and accessory instrumentation, has allowed better access into the lower pole and improved outcomes. Finally, PCNL should be used for stones that have failed less invasive treatment modalities or are extremely large or dense.

Historically, shortly after its clinical dissemination, it was realized that SWL provided unsatisfactory results for larger lower pole stones (Consensus conference, 1988). In fact, multiple series over the last 20 years have shown stone-free rates of approximately 50% or less for lower pole stones 1 to 2 cm and less than approximately 30% for lower pole stones larger than 2 cm (Table 93.1). It was hypothesized that the gravity-dependent nature of the lower pole and certain lower pole anatomic characteristics may impede stone clearance (Elbahnasy et al., 1998; Sampaio and Aragao, 1992, 1994). Sampaio and Arago executed a series of elegant anatomic studies to better define the anatomy of the lower pole by creating polyester resin endocasts of the pelvicalyceal collecting system using adult cadaveric kidneys. They hypothesized that a number of different lower pole anatomic features may reduce stone passage, including a narrow lower pole infundibulum (width <4 mm), an acute lower pole infundibulopelvic angle (<90 degrees), and multiple lower pole infundibula rather than a single infundibulum (Fig. 93.12). Similar findings have been demonstrated in subsequent investigations, suggesting that lower pole infundibular length greater than 3 cm, infundibular width less than 5 mm, and infundibulopelvic angle less than 70 degrees inhibit lower pole stone clearance during SWL (Elbahnasy et al., 1998; Madbouly et al., 2001; Manikandan et al., 2007; Sabnis et al., 1997; Sumino et al., 2002). Other studies have shown no effect of lower pole anatomy on stone clearance after SWL (Albala et al., 2001; Sorensen and Chandhoke, 2002).

TABLE 93.1 Treatment Outcomes for Lower Pole Calculi

STUDY	SHOCK WAVE LITHOTRIPSY	URETEROSCOPY	PERCUTANEOUS NEPHROLITHOTOMY
LOWER POLE CALCULI <1 CM			
Lingeman et al., 1994	74		100
Elashry et al., 1996		87	
Elbahnasy et al., 1998	52	62	
Grasso and Ficazzola, 1999		82	
Gupta et al., 2000	72		
Kourambas et al., 2000		85	
Albala et al., 2001	63		100
Hollenbeck et al., 2001		82	
Schuster et al., 2002		79	
Sorensen and Chandhoke, 2002	74		
Pareek et al., 2005	47		
Pearle et al., 2005[a]	35	50	
Kumar et al., 2014	72	88	
Sener et al., 2014	92	100	
LOWER POLE CALCULI 1 TO 2 CM			
Lingeman et al., 1994	56		89
Grasso and Ficazzola, 1999		71	
Saw and Lingeman, 1999	55		
Gupta et al., 2000	51		
Albala et al., 2001	23		93
Hollenbeck et al., 2001		63	
Madbouly et al., 2001	57		
Schuster et al., 2002		64	
Sorensen and Chandhoke, 2002	41		
Sumino et al., 2002	54		
Kuo et al., 2003[a]		31	76
Yuruk et al., 2010	55		97
El-Nahas et al., 2012	68	87	
Singh et al., 2014	54	86	
Burr et al., 2015	25	93	
Soliman et al., 2016	76		96 (mini-PCNL)
Chan et al., 2017	36	67	67
Kandemir et al., 2017		87	83 (micro-PCNL)
Bozzini et al., 2017	62	82	87
LOWER POLE CALCULI >2 CM			
Lingeman et al., 1994	33		94
Grasso et al., 1998		76	
Grasso and Ficazzola, 1999		65	
Albala et al., 2001	14		86
El-Anany et al., 2001		60	

[a]Computed tomography–measured outcome.

In an attempt to improve stone clearance rates after SWL of lower pole calculi, a number of supplemental therapies have been proposed and examined. McCullough (1989) anecdotally reported that postural drainage may assist in the elimination of retained fragments from dependent calyces. Brownlee et al. (1990) subsequently treated patients with residual lower pole fragments with controlled inversion therapy, using intravenous hydration, inversion, and percussion. D'a Honey et al. (2000) reported a pilot study to determine whether mechanical percussion with inversion therapy and furosemide-induced diuresis can move stone fragments out of the lower pole of the kidney. At a mean time of 63 days after SWL, this group reported an 83% stone passage rate. In a subsequent study, Pace et al. (2001) compared the effectiveness of mechanical percussion, inversion, and furosemide-induced diuresis with observation for elimination of lower calyceal fragments after SWL. They reported that 40% of patients with residual lower pole fragments treated with this regimen became stone free compared with 3% in the observation group; the observation group was then treated with this regimen as part of a crossover design, and 43% were rendered stone free.

Chiong et al. (2005) performed a similar study and showed that percussion, diuresis, and inversion therapy improved stone-free rates after SWL for lower pole stones. A recent Cochrane review included the studies by Pace et al. and Chiong et al. and concluded that overall evidence was limited, but that percussion, diuresis, and inversion

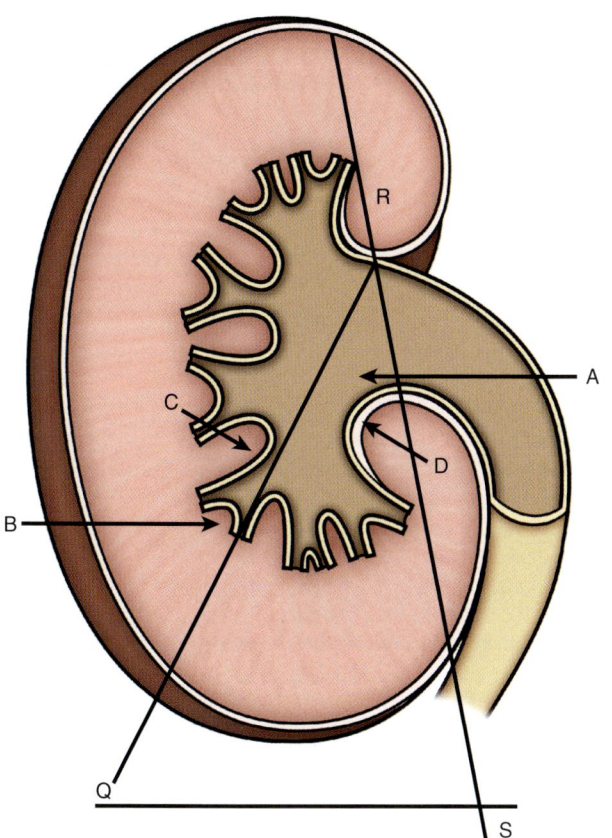

Fig. 93.12. Measurement scheme for lower pole anatomy. Lower pole infundibular length: measure A to B. Lower pole infundibular width: measure C to D. Lower pole infundibulopelvic angle: measure QRS angle. (From Albala DM, Assimos DG, Clayman RV, et al.: Lower pole I: a prospective randomized trial of extracorporeal shock wave lithotripsy and percutaneous nephrostolithotomy for lower pole nephrolithiasis—initial results. *J Urol* 166:2072–2080, 2001.)

were safe, were well tolerated, and appeared to modestly aid in stone passage after SWL (Liu et al., 2013). Other authors have reported lower pole irrigation techniques as adjuncts to SWL (Graham and Nelson, 1994; Nicely et al., 1992). More recently, pharmacotherapy with potassium citrate and thiazide diuretics has been described (Arrabal-Martin et al., 2006; Soygur et al., 2002). However, at this point in time none of these techniques has gained widespread acceptance.

The superiority of PCNL over SWL in clearing lower pole stones first became widely evident in a meta-analysis performed by Lingeman et al. in 1994. **In this report, PCNL achieved an overall 90% stone-free rate compared with 60% for SWL.** Subgroup analysis stratified by stone burden showed that stones 10 mm or smaller had a 74% clearance rate with SWL and 100% clearance rate with PCNL, whereas stones 10 to 20 mm had a 56% clearance rate with SWL and an 89% clearance rate with PCNL (see Table 93.1). An even larger difference was appreciated for lower pole stones larger than 2 cm, for which stone-free rates were 94% for PCNL and only 33% for SWL. On regression analysis, increasing stone size was associated with decreasing stone clearance for SWL but had no demonstrable effect on PCNL.

After these retrospective data, a number of prospective trials ensued confirming the dominance of PCNL over SWL for the vast majority of lower pole stones (Albala et al., 2001; Yuruk et al., 2010). In the multicenter, prospective, randomized Lower Pole I study by Albala et al. (2001), stone-free rates as evaluated by nephrotomograms at 3 months after treatment were 95% for PCNL and only 37% for SWL. Stone-free rates for SWL were particularly low for stones 10 mm and larger: 23% for stones 1 to 2 cm, and 14% for stones larger than 2 cm. Yuruk et al. (2010) randomized 90 patients with lower pole stones 2 cm or smaller to SWL, PCNL, or observation. PCNL achieved a 97% stone-free rate compared with a 55% stone-free rate with SWL when patients were assessed at 3 months after treatment. As an additional component of this study, dimercaptosuccinic acid (DMSA) renal scintigraphy was performed in all patients, and a higher percentage of SWL patients (16%) were found to have developed renal scarring compared with the PCNL cohort (3%). These SWL patients had received three treatment sessions with an average of 1863 shocks per session. Ozturk et al. retrospectively reviewed 221 SWL, 144 PCNL, and 38 URS procedures and showed a 94% success rate with PCNL, a 76% success rate with SWL, and a 73% success rate for URS (Ozturk et al., 2013). Bozzini et al. (2017) completed a prospective, randomized comparison among SWL, URS, and PCNL for lower pole stones less than 2 cm and found overall stone-free rates of 62% (SWL), 82% (URS), and 87% (PCNL) on CT at 3 months after surgery.

In an analogous fashion, SWL has been compared with URS for lower pole stone treatment, and the most contemporary results favor URS, although this was not always the case. In the seminal prospective, multicenter randomized trial by Pearle et al. (2005) comparing URS with SWL for lower pole stones 1 cm or smaller, stone-free status was accomplished in 50% of URS cases and only 35% of SWL cases, although the difference was not found to be statistically significant. Not unexpectedly, the convalescence time was less, and the health care–related quality of life measures were better for the SWL cohort (Pearle et al., 2005). More recently, Sener et al. (2014) performed a single-center randomized trial comparing SWL with URS for lower pole stones 1 cm or less in diameter. Treatment success was defined as stone-free or residual fragments less than 3 mm, and patients with acute infundibulopelvic angles (<30 degrees) were excluded. Stone-free status was achieved in 100% of URS cases and 91.5% of SWL cases, although an average of 2.7 SWL sessions per patient were necessary.

Recent series evaluating outcomes for lower pole stone burdens of 1 to 2 cm further highlight the ascendency of URS over SWL, especially with respect to treating increasing lower pole stone burden. Stone-free rates of 85% and higher have been reported for single-session URS compared with 54% to 83% for multisession SWL (Chan et al., 2017; El-Nahas et al., 2012; Resorlu et al., 2013; Singh et al., 2014). Moreover, re-treatment rates and auxiliary treatment rates are consistently higher for SWL, whereas complication rates are commensurate between the two modalities. These studies echo the results of Pearle et al. (2005), because voiding symptoms and convalescence time are more favorable for SWL than URS.

Since the early reports of URS for lower pole calculi in the mid and late 1990s, endourology has witnessed considerable progress in instrument design and surgical technique. These, in turn, have made URS more effective than SWL in treating lower pole stones (Elashry et al., 1996; Grasso and Ficazzola, 1999). Smaller ureteroscopes with improved tip deflection and better stone manipulation instruments aid in accessing and fragmenting lower pole stones. Nitinol stone baskets have been used to reposition stones from the lower pole to more optimal intrarenal positions for lithotripsy, such as the middle or upper pole calyces (Kourambas et al., 2000). Stone-free rates approaching and exceeding 90% have been reported when stones were repositioned out of the lower pole, compared with stone-free rates closer to 80% when stones were fragmented in situ within the lower pole (Kourambas et al., 2000; Schuster et al., 2002). Furthermore, contemporary URS outcomes appear to depend on lower pole infundibulopelvic angle, as was shown by Resorlu et al. (2012b), who found that URS was successful in 91% of cases when the angle was greater than 45 degrees versus only 65% of the time with more acute angles. In this same study, infundibular length and width did not affect URS outcomes.

Given the advancements in ureteroscopic design and technique, a number of investigators have sought to compare URS and PCNL for lower pole stones (Armagan et al., 2015; Bozkurt et al., 2011; Bozzini et al., 2017; Jung et al., 2015; Kandemir et al., 2017; Kirac et al., 2013, Kuo et al., 2003). The Lower Pole Study Group compared URS and PCNL for lower pole stones of 1 cm to 2.5 cm. PCNL achieved a 71% stone-free rate, whereas URS achieved a 37% stone-free rate as determined by CT. The length of hospitalization was shorter for those undergoing URS; however, overall convalescence was not statistically different and was attributed to ureteral stent–related morbidity in the URS cohort (Kuo et al., 2003). Bozkurt et al. (2011) retrospectively compared outcomes between PCNL and URS for lower pole stones of 1.5 cm to 2 cm. Single-stage stone-free rates of 93% (PCNL) and 89% (URS) were appreciated. The PCNL group required more blood transfusions, but otherwise complications were similar between groups. It is important to recognize that this was not a randomized study, and patients with unfavorable lower pole anatomy (acute infundibulopelvic angles, small infundibular width) were preferentially treated with PCNL.

The same group also retrospectively compared URS with mini-PCNL for stones smaller than 1.5 cm and found equivalent stone-free rates of 89% between the two modalities. Not surprisingly, operative time, mean fluoroscopy time, and length of hospital stay were longer for PCNL (Kirac et al., 2013). Taken collectively, these data suggest that URS performed by clinicians experienced with the technique can produce excellent stone-free rates approaching those of PCNL. **The key to excellent URS outcomes appears to be careful patient selection, which includes those patients with favorable lower pole anatomy (nonacute lower infundibulopelvic angle, wide lower pole infundibulum).**

Not enough data exist to determine the optimal place for mini- and micro-PCNL in the treatment of lower pole stones, although initial results are encouraging in terms of stone clearance and overall morbidity.

KEY POINTS: RENAL CALCULI

- Stones that are symptomatic, obstructing, or associated with infections should be treated, with the goal of complete stone clearance.
- SWL success is highest in stones 1 cm or smaller, 800 to 900 HU or lower, with shorter skin-to-stone distances, and in a non–lower pole location.
- PCNL offers the highest successful stone treatment for stones larger than 2 cm (including staghorn configuration), across all density measurements, and in all intrarenal locations.
- URS offers excellent success for all stone locations, although it may have decreased effectiveness in the lower pole.
- Staghorn stones should be treated if the patient can tolerate surgery.
- The outcomes of PCNL and URS are relatively independent of the patient's BMI, whereas SWL success falls more sharply with increasing obesity.

URETERAL CALCULI

Just as for renal calculi, the **urologists's armamentarium to surgically treat ureteral stones consists of four minimally invasive modalities including SWL, URS, PCNL, and laparoscopic or robotic-assisted stone surgery.** Open ureteral stone surgery is rarely performed when access to minimally invasive modalities exists and is often reserved for instances in which less invasive options have failed. There appears to be an evolving paradigm shift in the surgical treatment of upper tract stones, with an increasing use of URS and a reciprocal decreasing use of SWL for upper urinary tract stone disease (Lee and Bariol, 2011; Ordon et al., 2014). Determining the optimal treatment for a given patient is not always straightforward and depends on stone-related factors, clinical factors, and technical factors (Box 93.4). It is the interplay of these factors and the familiarity of the urologist with each surgical technique that ultimately determine the best treatment modality for a given patient. The purpose of this section is to provide a framework to help guide the urologist in matching a given patient's unique clinical situation and ureteral stone disease characteristics to the most effective and least morbid surgical therapy (Fig. 93.13).

BOX 93.4 Factors Affecting Management of Ureteral Stones

STONE-RELATED FACTORS
Location
Size
Composition
Degree of obstruction

CLINICAL FACTORS
Symptom severity
Patient's expectations
Associated infection
Solitary kidney
Abnormal ureteral anatomy
Coagulopathy
Obesity

TECHNICAL FACTORS
Available equipment
Cost

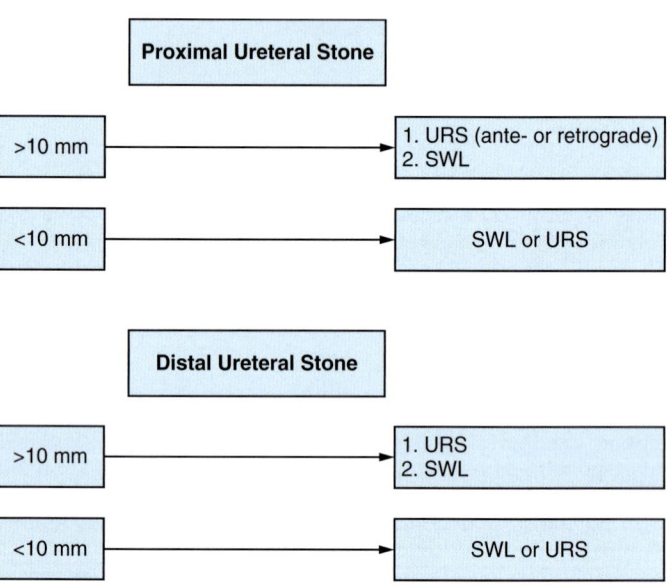

*Upgraded following panel consensus.

Fig. 93.13. Treatment algorithm: ureteral stones. *SWL,* Shock wave lithotripsy; *URS,* ureterorenoscopy. (Modified from Turk et al.: *EAU Guidelines on urolithiasis,* 2017.)

Natural History

When a renal calculus begins to pass, it moves from the kidney into the UPJ and into the ureter proper. At that point, depending on the size of the stone relative to the ureter throughout its course, the stone will begin to obstruct the kidney. The first manifestation of this is an increase in the intra–collecting system pressure, which will stretch the renal pelvis, calyces, and renal capsule. It is during this phase that the traditional colic of a stone episode begins.

This increase in intraluminal pressure will increase the hydrostatic pressure exerted on the walls of the renal pelvis and ureter, which can cause the failure of normal peristalsis. Pressure further increases at that point, with direct transmission to the nephron tubules, with a resulting drop in the glomerular filtration rate (GFR). Pressure will subsequently decrease to the levels present before obstruction developed, usually within 12 to 24 hours. Accordingly, the renal colic episode caused by a stone is often limited to severe pain from the acute renal stretch, followed by gradual resolution of the pain. Further movement of the stone down the ureter can relieve the pressure and reobstruct further distally, explaining the intermittent nature of renal colic as a stone passes.

Long-term obstruction can cause permanent damage to the kidney's function; therefore, regardless of the absence of pain or infection, a stone must either pass spontaneously or be surgically treated. Key to the passage of a stone is ureteral peristalsis, not hydrostatic pressure (Lennon et al., 1997). When the ureter is not otherwise obstructed, **the chief determinant of stone passage is the diameter of the stone in its transverse orientation** (Ueno et al., 1977). Next most important is the location of the stone within the ureter at presentation, with a review of the literature demonstrating **a 71% chance of passage of a distal ureteral stone versus 22% for proximal stones** (Morse and Resnick, 1991). Additional evidence supports the idea that the likelihood of spontaneous passage may be directly related to stone location at the time of presentation (Coll et al., 2002; Hubner et al., 1993).

With respect to size as a predictor of spontaneous passage, meta-analysis of the available literature (as described in the AUA ureteral stone guidelines) demonstrates a 68% chance of passage for stones 5 mm or smaller, and an estimated 47% chance for stones 6 to 10 mm in size (Preminger et al., 2007). More recent, albeit smaller, prospective, randomized studies suggest an approximately 80% spontaneous passage rate for stones 10 mm or less at 4 weeks after stone presentation. These rates may be enhanced with medical expulsive therapy (MET) using either calcium channel blockers (such as nifedipine) or, more commonly, α-receptor blockers (such as tamsulosin); however, the utility of MET remains controversial (Furyk et al., 2016; Hollingsworth et al., 2016; Pickard et al., 2015; Ye et al., 2017). **There appears to be limited, if any, benefit with MET for stones less than 5 mm. For distal ureteral stones 5 mm and greater, there may be up to a 57% increase in spontaneous stone passage with MET, as well as a shorter time to stone passage and a potential reduction in pain medication needed during stone passage** (Table 93.2).

Pretreatment Assessment

The pretreatment assessment, including medical history, imaging, and laboratory testing, for ureteral stones is similar to that for renal stones, and the reader is directed to the previous section on this topic in the renal calculi section of this chapter. Particular attention should be directed toward the duration of symptoms, given the fact that long-term obstruction can result in irreversible nephron loss. Any suggestion of fever in the setting of a ureteral stone strongly suggests the presence of infection proximal to the point of obstruction, and, regardless of how the patient appears at presentation, there should be a low threshold to proceed with urgent or immediate urinary tract drainage.

Specific symptoms may give clues to the course of the episode: New-onset urgency and frequency may herald a stone at the ureterovesical junction (UVJ) irritating the bladder, or the sudden relief of flank pain may indicate either passage or forniceal rupture as the pressure in the collecting system dramatically decreases. Assessment of renal function is paramount because ureteral stones are often obstructing at the time of presentation, and therefore renal function may be impaired by obstruction, dehydration, or a combination of both. The associated physiologic stress of an acutely obstructing stone can lead to white blood cell (WBC) demargination and an elevated serum WBC count. Thus leukocytosis in these patients may or may not represent an actual infection. In addition, urinary tract stones frequently lead to pyuria and leukocyte esterase positivity on urinalysis, and these findings do not always represent an active UTI. However, if there is any concern regarding an associated UTI, then the immediate focus should be on urinary tract decompression rather than definitive stone surgery.

Stone Factors

Treatment Decision by Localization

Proximal and Mid-Ureter. The chief determinant of the optimal treatment for calculi in these locations is size. As previously mentioned, those which are more proximal and greater in size are significantly less likely to pass spontaneously. There is a paucity of data on the effectiveness of MET use in proximal and mid-ureteral stones, although since many of these stones do migrate distally, presumptive use of MET is not contraindicated (Hollingsworth et al., 2006, 2016; Seitz et al., 2009; Ye et al., 2017).

For stones that do not move in a reasonable time frame, or in the setting of recurring severe pain, or if the patient prefers, surgical therapy is indicated. Primary options include SWL and URS, although PCNL and antegrade nephroscopy may be indicated for select cases. Pooled data, as evaluated in the 2007 AUA ureteral stone guidelines, have defined outcomes in proximal and mid-ureteral stones (of all sizes) in patients who underwent SWL, with overall 82% and 73% treatment success rates, respectively (Preminger et al., 2007). In consideration of proximal ureteral stones that are 1 cm or smaller, SWL success rises among these pooled series to 90% (85% to 93%), and 84% (65% to 95%) for mid-ureteral stones. For stones larger than 1 cm, rates of complete stone clearance drop in both groups, to 68% for proximal and 76% for mid-ureter stones. Updated systematically reviewed data from the 2016 AUA Guideline on the Surgical Management of Stones show overall ureteral stone

TABLE 93.2 Likelihood of Spontaneous Stone Passage

STUDY	NO. OF PATIENTS	NO. REQUIRING INTERVENTION (%)	NO. PASSING STONE (%)
STONE SIZE <5 MM			
Miller and Kane, 1999	59	4 (7)	55 (93)
Hussain et al., 2001	9	0 (0)	9 (100)
Coll et al., 2002	114	29 (25)	85 (75)
Kupeli et al., 2004	15	12 (80)	3 (20)
Furyk et al., 2016	114 (placebo)	4 (2.8)	102 (81.9)
	125 (tamsulosin)	1 (0.7)	110 (87)
STONE SIZE ≥5 MM			
Miller and Kane, 1999	16	8 (50)	8 (50)
Hussain et al., 2001	15	6 (40)	9 (60)
Coll et al., 2002	73	42 (58)	31 (42)
Furyk et al., 2016	41 (placebo)	4 (7.6)	25 (61)
	36 (tamsulosin)	4 (8)	30 (83)

TABLE 93.3 Ureteroscopic Treatment Outcomes for Proximal Ureteral Calculi

STUDY	NO. OF PATIENTS	MEAN STONE SIZE (mm)	STONE-FREE RATE (%)
Lam et al., 2002	31	8.2	97
Sofer et al., 2002	194	12.0	97
Aghamir et al., 2003	115	>10	75
Sozen et al., 2003	36	7.4	83
Fong et al., 2004	51	9.0	90
Wu et al., 2005	39	15.1	92
Lee et al., 2006	20	18.5	35
Preminger et al., 2007	2242	<10	80
		>10	79
Perez Castro et al., 2014	2611	81 mm^2	85

TABLE 93.4 Ureteroscopic Treatment Outcomes for Distal Ureteral Calculi

STUDY	NO. OF PATIENTS	MEAN STONE SIZE (mm)	STONE-FREE RATE (%)
Pearle et al., 2001	32	6.4	91
Sofer et al., 2002	348	10.3	99
Zeng et al., 2002	180	6–20	93
Aghamir et al., 2003	247	<10	96
Sozen et al., 2003	464	8.8	95
Preminger et al., 2007	5952	<10	97
		>10	93
Perez Castro et al., 2014	4446	67 mm^2	94

treatment success rate with SWL to be 64% for stones smaller than 10 mm, and 62% for stones larger than 10 mm (Assimos et al., 2016).

Similarly, the guidelines pooled numerous studies to evaluate outcome success for URS for these locations and sizes, demonstrating an overall success of 81% for proximal and 86% for mid-ureteral stones (Preminger et al., 2007). Calculi 1 cm or smaller again demonstrated higher success rates in both groups than did larger stones. In the updated 2016 AUA stone guidelines, success rates of 93% for stones smaller than 10 mm and 83% for stones larger than 10 mm were reported (Assimos et al., 2016). A further breakdown of selected studies assessing stone-free rates after ureteroscopy for proximal ureteral stones is shown in Table 93.3.

The likelihood of postoperative results requiring additional procedures was 1.5 with SWL for these larger stones, and only 1.07 for URS. Of related interest, the cost-efficiency of management of proximal ureteral stones has been shown to be superior for URS when compared with SWL, when used as the initial treatment procedure (Lotan et al., 2002).

For very large proximal ureteral calculi not amenable to either SWL or URS (including large or dense stones, severe inflammatory response at the site of stone impaction that prevents passage of a guidewire from below, or associated ureteral pathology), **a percutaneous and antegrade approach may be ideal** (Maheshwari et al., 1999). Depending on the exact location within the ureter and calyx for percutaneous entry, such stones may be amenable to either rigid or flexible endoscopy. The opportunity to clear stone fragments using the access tract may offer optimal success for these challenging stones.

Last, laparoscopic and robotic ureterolithotomy have been described for proximal and mid-ureteral calculi, with success rates for stone clearance in selected cases of 93% to 100% (Hemal et al., 2010; Yasui et al., 2013). Significant discussion regarding such an approach, in many cases significantly more invasive than SWL, URS, or PCNL with antegrade endoscopy, should be undertaken with the patient when considering this option.

Stones in a mid-ureteral location are typically handled in much the same way as proximal calculi, although some considerations relative to the pelvic anatomy apply. With respect to SWL, the presence of the bony structures lying posterior to the ureter at this level can interfere with fluoroscopic or plain film imaging of the stone, as well as pose challenges to positioning the patient so that shock wave energy does not pass through the bone. Oblique or prone positioning may be required for SWL at this level.

Finally, URS for the mid-ureteral stone can often be accomplished with a semirigid ureteroscope; however, limitations caused by the iliac vessels, particularly in male patients, may be encountered. In addition, proximal migration of these stones can sometimes present a challenge with semirigid instrumentation. **The availability of flexible ureteroscopes and the skills to perform flexible URS will improve the overall success rates and decrease complications** (Perez Castro et al., 2014).

Distal Ureter. As discussed earlier, distal stones are most likely to pass with observation or MET (Assimos et al., 2016; Hollingsworth et al., 2016; Preminger et al., 2007; Turk et al., 2017). The most typical site for impaction in this region of the ureter is at the UVJ; stones reaching this location often cause significant irritative symptoms because of stimulation of the bladder, a clinical sign that helps localize them. When stones fail to pass, once again surgical therapy is indicated.

SWL and URS remain the mainstays of treatment of distal ureteral stones. Once again, the AUA ureteral stone guidelines present a detailed review of pooled studies to identify success rates in both procedures. Among reviewed series using SWL for distal ureteral stones, the overall success rate was 74%. For stones 1 cm or smaller, an overall success rate of 86% was noted, whereas stones larger than 1 cm yielded a success rate of 74% (Preminger et al., 2007). In the updated AUA stone guideline from 2016, success for distal ureteral stones less than and greater than 1 cm was 74% and 71%, respectively (Assimos et al., 2016).

In the same 2007 AUA stone guidelines, URS for distal ureteral calculi was shown to yield a 94% overall success rate, with stones 1 cm or smaller at 97% and more than 1 cm at 93% success rate (Preminger et al., 2007). In the updated 2016 AUA stone guidelines, URS accomplished stone-free rates of 94% and 92%, respectively, for stones less than and greater than 1 cm (Assimos et al., 2016). A further breakdown of selected studies assessing stone-free rates after ureteroscopy for distal ureteral stones is shown in Table 93.4.

When SWL is compared with URS for the distal stone, reviewing the combined data for SWL in this fashion, the variation must be considered in lithotripters used that would affect overall outcomes in the multitude of series. In one randomized controlled trial comparing SWL with URS for distal ureteral calculi up to 15 mm, SWL was equally as effective as URS (100% in both groups), although this series used only the highly effective HM3 lithotripter (Pearle et al., 2001).

All Locations. Additional factors to consider in addition to stone-free success rates in the choice of therapy include the following:
- Complications of therapy such as sepsis, steinstrasse, ureteral stricture, and ureteral injury
- Anesthetic requirements

- Bleeding risk in patients with anticoagulation or antiplatelet therapy
- Recovery expectations
- Potential need for adjunctive procedures
- Previously placed ureteral stent

Treatment Decision by Stone Burden

As described earlier, SWL success for ureteral stones at all locations is significantly affected by the total stone burden, just as it is for renal calculi: the larger the stone(s), the less effective the treatment (Assimos et al., 2016; Preminger et al., 2007). As a specific example, the success rates for SWL at the distal ureter were 86% for stones 1 cm or smaller and 74% for those larger than 1 cm, and such differences held true for all locations. In contrast, URS had a much smaller degree of variation in terms of success based on stone burden: 97% success for stones 1 cm or smaller and 93% for those larger than 1 cm.

In a cost-comparison study of the management of ureteral calculi, Lotan et al. (2002) demonstrated that URS was associated with a lower cost than SWL for proximal stones, even before factoring in the higher adjunctive procedure rate associated with SWL. The prospective comparison of SWL to URS for distal stones by Pearle et al. (2001) showed that the overall complication rate was lower for SWL (9%) compared with URS (25%), although this was shown to mostly be related to urinary retention or significant colic requiring emergency evaluation or admission for pain control (and more likely to be clarified as a "minor" complication in the current literature).

Treatment by Stone Composition

As discussed earlier with respect to renal calculi, stone composition, if known or able to be predicted radiologically, can be useful in selecting the most appropriate therapy. Brushite (calcium phosphate) stones, calcium oxalate monohydrate, and cysteine stones are more resistant to SWL therapy and can be expected to have better rates at all sizes and locations with URS (Ahmed et al., 2008; Rudnick et al., 1999). Similarly to renal calculi, assessment of ureteral stone density based on the Hounsfield units on CT scan can offer valuable predictive ability as to the stone-free rate using SWL (El-Nahas et al., 2007; Gupta et al., 2005; Joseph et al., 2002; Wang et al., 2005). In identical fashion as well, skin-to-stone distance—reflected in body habitus—can be measured on the CT scan, again allowing more informed prediction of SWL success.

Therefore, where possible to obtain prior stone composition data or prediction of composition based on radiologic studies, this should be undertaken to best inform the patient regarding choices of therapy.

It is imperative to tailor therapy choices to the individual patient, after careful discussion of outcomes of treatment: success rates, adjunctive procedures, and treatment-related morbidity. Patient factors (body habitus, coagulation status, medical comorbidities) and stone factors (location, burden, composition) must be considered when selecting the optimal treatment for ureteral calculi.

Ureteral Anatomic Factors

Megaureter

Congenital megaureter most often is seen in children and usually represents an abnormality of the distal ureter or UVJ, in which there is either an aperistaltic segment (causing obstruction) or incompetent UVJ (causing reflux), which yields dilation of the ureter. The first description of this condition in the literature was by Caulk in 1923. Subsequently, a number of attempts to classify megaureter were undertaken, culminating in the consensus of a committee made up of members of the American Academy of Pediatrics, Society of Pediatric Urological Surgeons, and the Society for Pediatric Urology. These criteria have remained the most comprehensive system for classifying the megaureter (Stephens, 1977). Under this system, megaureters can be identified as refluxing, obstructed, and nonrefluxing and nonobstructed.

The majority of megaureters that are obstructed or refluxing are discovered when symptomatic during childhood and may require surgical repair. Reports of nonoperative, conservative management have been published, suggesting that some of these will resolve with the evolution of the UVJ as the child grows (Oliveira et al., 2000; Pitts and Muecke, 1974). The most typical operative repair has been ureteral reimplantation with, or without, tapering, but a recent report suggests that short-segment megaureters may be able to be successfully managed with endoureterotomy (Christman et al., 2012).

Megaureter has been associated with stones in the pediatric population and rarely the adult population (Rosenblatt et al., 2009). Management strategies significantly depend on the patient's surgical history, if any, and on recognition of any intrinsic ureteral obstruction that exists independent of the stone's location. Previously reimplanted ureters may be difficult to access in retrograde fashion, limiting the ability to place stents or approach stones via URS. In addition, an obstructed megaureter must be expected to lead to difficulties passing fragments after URS is performed.

Guidance as to ideal management is limited because only case reports or small series have been reported in adults. In a nonobstructed megaureter, MET, SWL, and URS are viable initial strategies. In the obstructed megaureter, strategies to manage the stone and the underlying pathology have included the following:
- Retropulsion of the stones to the kidney, treatment of the stones via PCNL, and repositioning the patient to perform ureteroneocystostomy (Kumar et al., 2014)
- Ureterolithotomy with ureteroneocystostomy, open (Demirtas et al., 2013; Solinas et al., 2010) or robotic-assisted laparoscopic (Hemal et al., 2009)
- Ureteroscopy with endoureterotomy (in short-segment cases <3 cm), which would make concomitant ureteroscopic treatment of stone possible (Christman et al., 2012)

Clearly, when considering stone treatment in patients with a megaureter, one must choose a strategy that will account for the stone and the underlying ureteral pathology.

Duplicated Collecting System

Duplication anomalies of the collecting system arise from ureteral bud abnormalities during gestation, occurring with an incidence of approximately 0.8% and following the Weigert-Meyer "rule" (Schlussel, 2007). This principle explains that in complete duplications, separate ureters enter the bladder with the more medial and inferior orifice draining the upper pole, whereas the more lateral and superior orifice drains the lower pole. In incomplete duplications, there is only one ureteral orifice on that side within the bladder, with a variable level of bifurcation of the separate ureters, which lead to the upper and lower moieties.

There are limited reports describing URS management of stones in partially or completely duplicated systems, but it is clear that ureteroscopy for these systems is little different from the more common single ureter. In the setting of a complete duplication, retrograde pyelography should be performed for each orifice to confirm which ureter contains the stone to be treated, and then treatment proceeds as usual.

In partial duplications, retrograde pyelography should be performed to locate the level of bifurcation in addition to the stone, with recognition of the fact that an intramural ureter location of the division of the two systems is most common (Rich, 1988). This can potentially inhibit visualization if the retrograde catheter is past the point of bifurcation. In this situation, ureteroscopy, after dilation of the ureteral orifice when necessary, can be used to directly inspect for the other moiety of the second ureter. In such cases, simultaneous stenting of upper and lower pole ureteral segments may be necessary.

Ureteral Stricture or Stenosis

The presence of intrinsic ureteral obstruction certainly affects the selection of ideal stone treatment in a number of ways. First, an untreated stricture or stenosis precludes fragment passage and hence creates an expectation of SWL failure. Second, the mechanism that is chosen to deal with the obstruction may facilitate and/or dictate how the stone will be managed. Finally, the physical properties of the stricture may mandate a particular course of action.

Most important, not every narrow point that is encountered in the ureter reflects a pathologic stricture, particularly when a stone may be impacted there. Inflammatory reaction and ureteral spasm may account for a significant portion of apparent obstructions encountered. In these situations, it is critical to recognize that overdilation of the ureter via endoscopic approach may cause localized ureteral injury (Eshghi, 1988). Despite this concern, balloon dilation of the ureter, when required for ureteroscopy, is safe and effective in the vast majority of patients (Huffman and Bagley, 1988). If the area of obstruction is thought to reflect spasm, placing a stent to allow passive dilation facilitates a second-stage procedure in pediatric and adult patients (Hubert and Palmer, 2005; Rubenstein et al., 2007).

When a definite stricture is present, underlying causes must be considered. Methods of dealing with ureteral strictures are covered elsewhere in this text and may provide the primary guidance for dealing with a ureteral stricture; a post-ureteroscopy stricture is obviously significantly different from a radiation-induced one.

Endoureterotomy can be performed at all levels of the ureter; however, it will have a lower rate of long-term success in longer strictures (Wolf et al., 1997). Few data have been reported on the concomitant use of ureteroscopic laser lithotripsy at the time of an endoureterotomy or endopyelotomy, although there is a recognized potential for stone fragments to come to rest in the periureteral space and cause granulomatous inflammatory reaction and recurrent stricture (Dretler and Young, 1993). It is possible that, if URS is the preferred management strategy, endoureterotomy should be undertaken as a first stage, with placement of a ureteral stent to allow healing, and subsequent URS to manage the stone at a second stage.

Alternatively, consideration may lead one to proceed with open, laparoscopic, or robotic-assisted laparoscopic treatment for the stricture and the stone in the same session. Numerous reports of laparoscopic and robotic-assisted ureterolithotomy have been reported, and the identical techniques and approaches used for management of a ureteral stricture can be used to also treat a ureteral stone in the same session (Dogra et al., 2013; Nasseh et al., 2013; Singh et al., 2013).

Technical Factors

Further information on this topic is available online at Expert Consult.com.

> **KEY POINTS: URETERAL CALCULI**
>
> - Conservative therapy has its greatest success in stones 5 mm or smaller but may still see fair success rates in stones up to 10 mm.
> - Medical expulsive therapy (alpha-blockers) appear to be most effective for distal ureteral stones 5 mm or larger.
> - Fever, or the presence of clinical or laboratory signs of UTI, may herald impending sepsis, a life-threatening condition; emergent drainage and decompression with either stent or nephrostomy should be undertaken.
> - SWL and URS are considered first-line therapies for stones at all locations within the ureter, although a higher rate of ancillary procedures should be expected with stones larger than 10 mm.
> - Positioning challenges may be present for SWL in the mid-ureteral stone, requiring prone or oblique positioning for a clear blast path to the stone.

Clinical Factors for Upper Urinary Tract Calculi

Complete treatment planning for upper tract stones must incorporate the relevant clinical factors for a given patient, in addition to the stone-specific and anatomic factors (see Boxes 93.1 and 93.4). Certain patient conditions, anatomic aberrations, and underlying comorbidities assume significant importance in counseling patients on the relative risks and benefits of the different treatment options, because each can influence surgical outcomes and complications. Therefore a tailored approach to the individual patient is best.

Urinary Tract Infection

UTIs are common in the setting of upper tract calculi and should be adequately treated before any stone treatment. Offending bacteria may reside deep within stones and prove impossible to eradicate without complete stone removal. Because of this, it may be difficult to completely sterilize the urine before stone surgery, in which case at least a short course of preoperative, culture-directed antibiotics is recommended. When infectious stones are suspected, every attempt at complete removal of stones should be undertaken because residual fragments commonly harbor bacteria that can serve as a nidus for recurrent UTIs and promote rapid stone regrowth (Bichler et al., 2002). **Therefore PCNL and URS, when active stone extraction is possible, are preferred over SWL, in which stone clearance relies on physiologic stone passage and may take months to reach completion.**

The rate of sepsis after PCNL or SWL is approximately 1% when preoperative urine cultures are negative. However, when preoperative bacteriuria exists or there is evidence of distal obstruction, the rate of sepsis associated with SWL for staghorn stones increases substantially (2% to 56%), and SWL should not be pursued (Lam et al., 1992a; Meretyk et al., 1992, 1997; Zink et al., 1988).

A UTI associated with an obstructing upper tract stone (ureteral or renal) represents a true urologic emergency and requires emergent urinary tract drainage. This is accomplished by either ureteral stenting or percutaneous nephrostomy. Attempts to definitively treat the obstructing stone should be postponed until the patient is stabilized and the infection is completely treated. Measures to treat the stone before patient stabilization and clearance of the infection risk worsening sepsis and death. In these instances, a urine culture from the obstructed segment is helpful to guide subsequent antibiotic therapy.

Renal Function

Assessment of underlying renal function becomes most important when there is suspicion that nephrectomy rather than stone removal is the treatment of choice. This scenario is encountered most frequently with staghorn stones, a history of recurrent pyelonephritis or renal abscess episodes, or xanthogranulomatous pyelonephritis and with chronic, relatively asymptomatic renal obstruction from ureteral stones. Renal imaging can provide clues to poor underlying renal function, including renal cortical atrophy or thinned renal parenchyma. In these instances, further functional renal studies, such as diuretic renography, can be used to quantify remaining renal function. In equivocal cases, temporary relief of obstruction with ureteral stenting or percutaneous nephrostomy is warranted, after which renal function can be reassessed. **The general consensus is that symptomatic upper tract stones located in renal units with approximately 15% or less split function should be considered for nephrectomy, and stone-specific, nephron-sparing treatments should not be pursued.**

A considerable body of evidence exists evaluating the effects of SWL and PCNL on renal function, whereas there is a relative paucity of data surrounding URS effects on renal function (Kartha et al., 2013; Sninsky et al., 2014; Wood et al., 2011). It is believed that URS induces minimal renal parenchymal damage, and although few studies have evaluated this directly at a histologic or biochemical level, no change in long-term renal function has been reported even after multiple URS treatments (Lee and Bagley, 2001; Sninsky et al., 2014). More robust and in-depth data exist and have consistently shown that SWL and single–access tract PCNL do not appear detrimental to total renal function over the long term (Canes et al., 2009; Chandhoke et al., 1992; El-Tabey et al, 2014; Lee and Bagley 2001; Sninsky et al., 2014). These results have been repeatedly shown in patients with renal insufficiency and with solitary kidneys for SWL

(Chandhoke et al., 1992; Cass, 1994; Eassa et al., 2008; El-Assmy et al, 2008; Krambeck et al., 2008a; Kulb et al., 1986; Zanetti et al., 1992) and PCNL (Agrawal et al., 1999; Alken, 1982; Canes et al., 2009; Kuzgunbay et al., 2010; Marberger et al., 1985; Schiff et al., 1986; Singh et al., 2001; Unsal et al., 2010). Renal scintigraphy and single-photon emission computed tomography (SPECT) evaluation of kidneys after PCNL have also confirmed no changes in total renal function, although new focal cortical defects and reduced renal functional activity were seen in a minority of patients at the site of percutaneous renal access (Akman et al., 2012a; Unsal et al., 2010). The effects of multi–access tract PCNL on renal functional outcomes are mixed; some investigators suggest no effect on renal function (Moskovitz et al., 2006), and others demonstrate renal deterioration (El-Tabey et al., 2014).

Considering the available evidence, as long as adequate renal function exists and nephrectomy is not being entertained, stone treatment decisions should not, in general, be based on renal function. Rather, they should be based on stone-specific characteristics, renal anatomic factors, and other more relevant clinical factors.

Solitary Kidney

The main considerations in treating stones in congenitally, surgically, and functionally solitary kidneys include having a lower threshold to treat asymptomatic renal stones and ensuring sufficient renal drainage after stone treatment. Because only one kidney exists or is functioning, a single, obstructing stone leads to total urinary obstruction and demands urgent attention. **It is for this reason that proactive treatment of asymptomatic stones, which may otherwise be observed when two functioning kidneys exist, is recommended in solitary kidneys.** The perils of complete ureteral obstruction, especially with concomitant UTI, can be life-threatening for patients with solitary kidneys. In the setting of clinical instability, UTI, or electrolyte abnormalities, initial urinary decompression via ureteral stenting or percutaneous nephrostomy drainage should be undertaken. Once the patient is clinically stable, and after treatment of any associated infection, definitive stone treatment may be pursued following the strategies outlined in the ureteral calculi section. Although not mandatory based on any meaningful evidence, it is highly advocated to place a ureteral stent after ureteroscopic manipulation, because temporary ureteral edema and occlusion caused by spasm or fragments can result in acute kidney injury and anuria.

Morbid Obesity

A BMI above 40 kg/m^2 is considered morbid obesity by the World Health Organization. Obesity, and in particular morbid obesity, can pose physiologic and technical challenges that must be accounted for when recommending stone treatment to such patients (Freedman et al., 2002; Giblin et al., 1995). Proper preoperative medical optimization and risk stratification are imperative, because obesity has been linked to a number of medical conditions that increase anesthetic risk, including cardiovascular disease, diabetes mellitus type II, and obstructive sleep apnea (among others). **Ureterorenoscopy and PCNL outcomes appear to be relatively independent of obesity status, whereas those after SWL are drastically worse.**

SWL is frequently suboptimal in morbidly obese patients, and in some cases it is actually impossible because patients may exceed the weight limitations of the lithotripter table or gantry. Many studies have shown increasing BMI to be a negative prognosticator for stone-free status after SWL (Ackermann et al., 1994; Portis et al., 2003). Moreover, the significant adipose tissue found in the morbidly obese can attenuate x-ray through-transmission, making it difficult to localize stones with fluoroscopy. If the stone is visible but located beyond the F2 focus of the lithotripter, a blast path technique may be used in which the stone is targeted along the same axis as the F2 focal point and relies on high pressures, although slightly defocused, generated beyond F2 to fragment the stone (Locke et al., 1990; Whelan et al., 1988). Given this, it is often necessary to use higher energy settings in obese patients, and lithotripters offering the highest peak pressures and longest focal length are preferred.

Skin-to-stone distance, or the distance between the SWL transducer and stone, has emerged as an important factor affecting SWL outcomes and is readily measured on axial CT slices. In general, the larger the skin-to-stone distance, the worse the fragmentation during SWL. Many studies have shown that **SWL outcomes worsen when skin-to-stone distance exceeds 10 cm** (El-Nahas et al., 2007; Foda et al., 2013; Pareek et al., 2005; Wiesenthal et al., 2011). Furthermore, Pareek et al. (2005) found that skin-to-stone distance was a stronger predictor of stone-free status than BMI. Perks et al. (2008) reviewed SWL in 111 patients with solitary stones 5 to 20 mm in size and found the best treatment success (91%) for skin-to-stone distances below 9 cm and stone attenuation below 900 HU, and the least successful treatment (41%) for skin-to-stone distances greater than 9 cm and stone attenuation exceeding 900 HU.

More recently, excessive visceral fat, as measurable on noncontrast CT, has proved to be a useful prognosticator for SWL outcomes. Indeed, increasing abdominal circumference, visceral fat, subcutaneous fat, and perirenal and pararenal fat are associated with decreasing stone-free rates after SWL (Juan et al., 2012). Taking this one step further, Zhou et al. (2013) demonstrated that increasing visceral fat was an independent predictor of uric acid stones. Hence a trial of urinary alkalinization is recommended in obese patients with radiolucent stones, a low urinary pH, and no other indications for urgent decompression.

PCNL in the morbidly obese is feasible and reportedly safe but also requires some technical modifications. Extra-long instruments (fascial dilators, access sheath, nephroscope, stone graspers) may become necessary, and mobility around the collecting system from a given access tract may be hindered by the long tract length. **Most available data confirm that stone-free rates are not affected by obesity, although there is some suggestion that stone-free rates are lower, and major complication rates are higher, in the morbidly obese** (Koo et al., 2004; Pearle et al., 1998). El-Assmy et al. (2007) and Kuntz et al. (2014) found no difference in stone-free rates, complications, auxiliary procedure rates, or length of stay among patients stratified by BMI, and proved that "tubeless" PCNL could be performed safely in these individuals. The CROES PCNL global study found equivalent stone-free rates for normal, overweight, and obese cohorts (approximately 80%), but significantly lower stone-free rates for the morbidly obese group (65.6%) (Fuller et al., 2012). Overall complication rates did not differ either among groups, although a greater percentage of major complications (Clavien-Dindo III to V) were found in the morbidly obese (10.5%) relative to the other groups (3.5% to 3.9%).

Initial reports suggested URS success and safety did not appear to change in the morbidly obese (Dash et al., 2002; Natalin et al., 2009; Preminger et al., 2007). More recent data from a systematic review (Ishii et al., 2016) and from the global ureteroscopy study (Krambeck et al., 2017) point toward a small decrease in stone-free rates and an increase in re-treatment rates and postoperative complications in the morbidly obese. However, total complications remained relatively low (3%–9%), and overall treatment success with URS remained relatively high, between 73% and 83%. **Accordingly, URS may be the preferable treatment modality for obese patients without exceedingly complex or large stone burdens.** Chew et al. (2013) performed a multicenter trial comparing URS in patients with normal BMIs with those considered overweight or obese; no significant difference was found in stone-free rates. Aboumarzouk et al. (2012c) performed a systematic review of URS in obese patients (mean BMI 42.2 kg/mm^2) and found an excellent pooled stone-free rate (87.5%), mean operative time (97.1 minutes), and complication rate (11.4%).

Old Age and Frailty

Recently the concept of frailty has gained considerable attention in the surgical literature, although it has been somewhat slow to permeate into the field of urology. There is mounting evidence to suggest that the degree of frailty a patient exhibits, rather than his or her chronologic age, is a more robust predictor of postoperative complications (Makary et al., 2010; Revenig et al., 2014). At present, there are limited data on the effects of frailty on stone treatment outcomes; however, extrapolating from the available frailty literature in other fields, the frailest of patients may be better served with less invasive stone treatments (URS or SWL). Resorlu et al. (2012a) conducted a multicenter, retrospective review of PCNLs in elderly patients and found that a higher Charlson Comorbidity Index score was associated with a significantly higher rate of severe medical complications and hemorrhage. Similarly, many elderly patients have less physiologic reserve to handle an acute, obstructing stone event well, or to successfully tolerate a drawn-out trial of passage. In these instances, a more direct treatment strategy with early relief of urinary obstruction is prudent.

A number of groups have looked at PCNL outcomes in elderly populations and have found essentially unchanged surgical success, albeit with a higher rate of complications. Doré et al. (2004) reviewed PCNL outcomes in 201 patients age 70 and older and found a stone-free rate of 70.8%. Early work by Stoller et al. (1994a) showed that PCNL was safe in patients older than 65 years but was associated with more frequent blood transfusions (26% vs. 14%). Akman et al. (2012b) compared URS and PCNL outcomes in patients older than 65 years and reported excellent stone-free rates (93% for URS, 96% for PCNL), reasonable operative times (65 minutes for URS, 41 minutes for PCNL), and acceptable complication rates (10.7% for PCNL, 7.1% for URS). In the largest published series on the topic, no difference was appreciated in stone-free rates (79% vs. 82%) or length of hospitalization in elderly (median age 74 years) versus younger (median age 49 years) cohorts, but there was a higher overall complication rate (19.9% vs. 6.6%) in the elderly (Okeke et al., 2012).

SWL in the elderly is feasible as well, but it may be associated with an increased risk of perinephric hematoma. Dhar et al. (2004) found a 1.67-times increased risk of hematoma formation after SWL with every 10-year increase in patient age, although subsequent studies have not consistently borne this out. Reports on treatment success with SWL in the elderly are mixed, showing a trend toward lesser success for renal stones and no effect on ureteral stones (Abe et al., 2005; Delakas et al., 2003; Ng et al., 2007). Furthermore, URS does not appear to confer any known additional surgical risks to the elderly.

Spinal Deformity or Limb Contractures

Patients with spinal deformities and limb contractures present a number of challenges that can be anticipated preoperatively. Despite its minimally invasive nature, SWL is often unsuccessful, and with high re-treatment and auxiliary procedure rates, because it can be difficult or impossible to properly position these patients on the lithotripter table. Moreover, stone targeting may be fraught with difficulties, as scoliosis and abnormal pelvic anatomy can preclude an acceptable shock wave blast path. Fragment passage can also be hindered by aberrant renal location and associated poor upper tract drainage. Few contemporary reports exist, but older studies show only modest stone-free results in this population, along with a frequent need for multiple treatment sessions (Lazare et al., 1988; Neuwirth et al., 1986).

PCNL and URS are good alternatives to SWL, and both have been used with good success, although special considerations are necessary with each (Goumas-Kartalas et al., 2010; Resorlu et al., 2012c; Rubenstein et al., 2004). For URS, patient anatomy may preclude rigid instrument use (cystoscope and ureteroscope). The use of ureteral access sheaths is encouraged, if they can be safely placed, because they can provide rapid re-entry into the otherwise challenging-to-access upper collecting system. PCNL remains the preferred method of stone treatment in many of these patients, particularly with large and complex stone burdens. Stone clearance rates with PCNL are no different than in the general population, although there is a greater need for secondary procedures. Furthermore, PCNL in these circumstances is associated with a higher rate of infectious complications (Culkin et al., 1990; Goumas-Kartalas et al., 2010; Nabbout et al., 2012; Symons et al., 2006). Given the abnormal anatomic relationships in these patients, preoperative CT of the abdomen and pelvis is essential in planning optimal renal access and may reveal the need for ultrasound guidance, CT guidance, or potentially even laparoscopic guidance in selected situations to avoid bowel or solid organ injury (Matlaga et al., 2003a).

Uncorrected Coagulopathy

Uncorrected coagulopathy is a contraindication to SWL and PCNL; however, URS can be successfully undertaken in such circumstances with little to no increase in surgical morbidity. When coagulopathies have been corrected, patients should be considered candidates for SWL and PCNL, assuming no other contraindications exist. Many instances of life-threatening retroperitoneal hemorrhage have been reported after SWL use in patients on continuous anticoagulant and antiplatelet agents (Alsaikhan and Andonian, 2011; Katz et al., 1997; Ruiz and Saltzman, 1990; Sare et al., 2002; Streem and Yost, 1990; Zanetti et al., 2001).

For patients with imperative indications to remain on antiplatelet therapy (e.g., recent coronary artery stenting) or anticoagulant agents (e.g., high-risk atrial fibrillation, venous thromboembolic disease, or mechanical cardiac valves), URS with holmium:yttrium-aluminum-garnet (Ho:YAG) laser lithotripsy is the treatment modality of choice. Since Grasso and Chalik (1998) first reported the safe use of URS and Ho:YAG laser lithotripsy in patients with uncorrected coagulopathies, numerous other reports have followed recapitulating not only the safety but also the high efficacy of URS in these challenging scenarios (Aboumarzouk et al., 2012b; Turna et al., 2008; Watterson et al., 2002). Ho:YAG laser lithotripsy is preferred and is considered safer than other intracorporeal lithotripters (Watterson et al., 2002).

Prior Renal Surgery

Prior renal surgery or trauma can lead to fibrosis, scarring, and deformity of the intrarenal collecting system, which in turn can complicate renal stone surgery. This situation is less frequently encountered today because fewer open stone surgeries are performed worldwide. **Prior renal surgery is not a contraindication to any form of renal stone surgery and presents no new specific concerns. Thus all treatment modalities may be employed as necessary, given appropriate indications (SWL, URS, PCNL).** Certain precautions should be taken, however; the possibility of poor renal drainage should be entertained, because previous surgery can predispose to infundibular stenosis, iatrogenic UPJO, and ureteral stenosis. If obstruction is found or suspected, a treatment modality other than SWL should be chosen. URS and PCNL may be used as previously described. During URS an infundibulotomy may be necessary to adequately access a stone trapped behind an area of infundibular stenosis. Nevertheless, stone-free rates of 79% after a single URS and 92% after a secondary URS have been described (Osman et al., 2012).

PCNL after prior open kidney surgery and after prior SWL has been described by multiple investigators. For the most part, prior renal surgery (open or SWL) has no effect on PCNL complication rates (Gupta et al., 2009a; Resorlu et al., 2010; Tugcu et al., 2008; Yuruk et al., 2009; Zhong et al., 2013). A single recent retrospective study found a higher need for renal angioembolization to control postoperative bleeding in patients with previous open nephrolithotomy; however, this finding has not been corroborated by others (Yesil et al., 2013). The effect of prior open surgery on stone-free rates is less consistent; some studies show rates that are worse (Gupta et al., 2009a), and others show unchanged rates (Resorlu et al., 2010; Tugcu et al., 2008).

Prior SWL therapy can make salvage PCNL more difficult, as evidenced by longer operative times and lower stone-free rates (Yuruk et al., 2009; Zhong et al., 2013). This is the presumed result of stone fragment scattering after SWL and the tendency for some of the stones to embed suburothelially within the renal parenchyma. In fact, the more ineffective the prior SWL attempt (i.e., less fragmentation), the better the expected results from the following PCNL. Bon et al. (1993) found a 92% success rate for nonfragmented stones compared with a 64% success rate in patients with numerous fragments.

Urinary Diversion

Renal and ureteral stones in patients with urinary diversions present unique obstacles. Adequate preoperative imaging is essential to provide details on the anatomy of the urinary diversion and provide clues to possible routes to access the stone. It may also suggest the presence of urinary stasis and obstruction within the diversion, which, if present, should also be addressed to minimize the risk of stone recurrence. In general, SWL, PCNL and antegrade URS, retrograde URS, or a combination thereof can be exploited.

As in other instances, SWL should not be used in the setting of urinary obstruction. However, without urinary obstruction, a single session of SWL can achieve success rates of 60% to 65% (Deliveliotis et al., 2002; El-Assmy et al., 2005). Retrograde URS is usually confined to flexible instruments, and redundant ileal conduits and large-capacity urinary reservoirs with some form of nonrefluxing ureteral anastomosis often require flexible instruments to locate the ureteral "orifices." Successful access to the upper urinary tract has been reported up to 75% of the time in urinary diversions, with a much lower rate seen in Indiana pouches (Hyams et al., 2009). Loopograms or pouchograms can aid in locating ureteral insertions when upper tract reflux exists. Alternatively, intravenous indigo carmine or contrast can be used as well. For patent ureteroenteric anastomoses, the judicious use of ureteral access sheaths can facilitate upper tract re-entry and protect the anastomotic site.

For larger stone burdens and when retrograde access is not possible, PCNL becomes the treatment modality of choice, with a reported stone-free rate of 75% to 88% (El-Nahas et al., 2006; Hertzig et al., 2013; Wolf and Stoller, 1991). In addition, percutaneous access can allow antegrade URS to achieve access to the ureter when retrograde techniques fail. Complication rates of 8% to 30% have been reported for percutaneous approaches to stones in these patients. Percutaneous access may require ultrasound guidance if retrograde or antegrade contrast filling of the pelvicalyceal system is not possible.

Renal Transplants

The general consensus is to remove upper tract stones within renal transplants, because the consequences of an obstructing stone can be devastating. Indeed, because of the lack of innervation in renal transplants, obstructing stones do not manifest with typical renal colic. Rather, vague graft site discomfort, fevers, oliguria, hematuria, or rising creatinine may be the only presenting signs.

SWL has been described for stones in transplant kidneys and is an option for stones smaller than 1.5 cm; however, high re-treatment rates and auxiliary procedure rates should be expected (Challacombe et al., 2005; Klingler et al., 2002). Given that the renal allograft is located near the bony pelvis, prone positioning is often necessary. Antegrade and retrograde URS have been used to successfully treat transplant kidney and ureteral stones. Angled catheters and guidewires are often indispensable in achieving retrograde access, and prior placement of a percutaneous nephrostomy tube can facilitate antegrade URS and obviate the need for percutaneous tract dilation (Hyams et al., 2012). Stone-free rates of 67% to 92% have been reported, although no large series exist (Basiri et al., 2006; Del Pizzo et al., 1998).

PCNL remains the preferred treatment choice for large-burden stones (>1.5 cm) or if less invasive methods have failed. Stone-free rates ranging from 77% to 100%, similar to rates in the general population, have been reported (He et al., 2007; Krambeck et al., 2008b; Rifaioglu et al., 2008). When obtaining percutaneous access to transplant kidneys, CT or ultrasound guidance is advisable because there is a risk for intervening bowel. Furthermore, some reports describe difficulty with percutaneous access secondary to a fibrous capsule that develops around certain transplanted kidneys and may require use of metal fascial dilators to overcome. Percutaneous access with a 16-Fr peel-away sheath has been illustrated; this mini-PCNL technique is thought to carry a lower risk of surgical bleeding and still be of significant usefulness for these stones (He et al., 2007).

Duration of Ureteral Stone Presence

As discussed in the natural history section on ureteral calculi, after the initially reversible physiologic changes seen with acute ureteral obstruction, chronic ureteral obstruction can ultimately lead to permanent renal damage. Patients attempting to spontaneously pass a ureteral stone should be intermittently imaged to evaluate for persistent or worsening hydronephrosis and stone location and passage. The exact duration of renal blockage beyond which irreversible kidney damage begins is unknown in humans. Furthermore, it is possible that a ureteral stone may cause intermittent obstruction rather than permanent obstruction, and how this ultimately influences renal function is also not known. Despite this uncertainty, in general active stone treatment of any form is recommended when obstruction has persisted for approximately 4 to 6 weeks (Assimos et al., 2016; Singal and Denstedt, 1997). Continued renal blockage after this time may lead to irreversible kidney damage (Vaughan and Gillenwater, 1971). Moreover, at least one prior small prospective study showed the vast majority (95%) of stones that spontaneously pass, do so in the first 6 weeks (Miller and Kane, 1999). Holm-Nielsen et al. (1981) reported that of 134 patients with unilateral ureteral stones, one-third of the patients with obstruction lasting more than 4 weeks developed irreversible renal damage. Similarly, Kelleher et al. (1991) found that sequential renal scintigraphy performed on 76 patients with obstructive ureteral calculi demonstrated an 18% incidence of reduced renal function (defined as a decrease in relative function greater than 7%).

KEY POINTS: CLINICAL FACTORS

- Definitive stone treatment should be undertaken only in the setting of sterile urine, although a negative urinalysis may be an applicable surrogate to negative culture.
- Morbid obesity significantly decreases SWL success rate.
- Kidneys with inherent drainage problems, such as those with UPJO, infundibular stenosis, or ectopic or horseshoe configuration, must have the underlying obstruction managed in addition to treatment of the stone.
- In kidneys with poor (<15%) function, nephrectomy may be the optimal treatment.
- Active treatment should be strongly considered for ureteral stones that have not passed after 4 to 6 weeks.

Evaluation of Outcome

Assessment and Fate of Residual Fragments

In the era of open stone surgery, residual fragments of any size suggested a failed procedure. In the modern era with the rise of endourology and the frequent use of SWL, URS, and PCNL, postoperative residual fragments are common. However, the definition and optimal management of residual fragments continue to generate controversy.

With the increasing popularity of SWL in the 1980s and the observation that many patients retained small fragments of questionable clinical relevance after such therapy, the concept of **clinically insignificant residual fragments (CIRF)** was introduced and would become incorporated into the definition of a successful treatment outcome (Newman et al., 1988). These fragments were initially, and arbitrarily, defined as residual fragments 4 mm or less in diameter that were nonobstructive, noninfectious, associated with sterile urine, and in an otherwise asymptomatic patient (Newman et al., 1988). Since then, the term has been applied to fragments of various sizes, with most studies using a cutoff between 2 mm and 4 mm.

Therefore, since the introduction of SWL, treatment outcomes for patients with renal calculi have been reported by two different terms: stone-free rate and success rate. The stone-free rate is self-explanatory, but the success rate includes patients who are stone free as well as those with CIRF. These different methods of reporting treatment results, the lack of a standard definition for CIRF, and the various modalities used for assessing postprocedural stone-free status (KUB studies, nephrotomography, ultrasonography, CT) make the comparison of endourologic stone outcomes difficult. Further complicating matters is the fact that stone fragment passage after SWL is not immediate; as many as 85% of patients have radiologic evidence of residual fragments several days after SWL (Drach et al., 1986). Although most fragments pass spontaneously during the first 3 months after SWL, continued clearance can occur for more than 24 months after treatment (Chaussy and Schmiedt, 1984; Graff et al., 1988; Kohrmann et al., 1993).

In an attempt to better characterize the clinically meaningful success of any given stone treatment, Clayman et al. (1989) introduced the effectiveness quotient:

$$\frac{\% \text{ Stone free}}{100\% + \text{Re-treatment} + \% \text{ Auxiliary procedures}} \times 100$$

The effectiveness quotient accounts for the re-treatment rate, stone-free rate, and number of ancillary procedures and is useful in comparing results among different treatment modalities. For example, the study by Netto et al. (1991) compared PCNL and SWL for the treatment of stones in lower pole calyces. The PCNL group had a 93.6% stone-free rate with no need for re-treatment, whereas the SWL group had a 79.2% success rate with a 41.6% re-treatment rate. The relative success rates for PCNL and SWL were not significantly different; however, a significant difference was appreciated when comparing the effectiveness quotients (93.7% for PCNL vs. 55.9% for SWL).

The term *clinically insignificant residual fragments* may be a misnomer because **many small residual fragments eventually become clinically significant and symptomatic by dislodging and causing obstruction, serving as niduses for further stone growth, or acting as a source for persistent infections** (Candau et al., 2000; Delvecchio and Preminger, 2000; Streem et al., 1996; Zanetti et al., 1997). Streem et al. (1996) reported that 43% of initially deemed CIRF became symptomatic at a mean follow-up of 23 months. Moreover, complete stone removal appears to decrease the risk of stone recurrence (Newman et al., 1988; Patterson et al., 1987; Singh et al., 1975). Stone recurrence rates of 6% to 15% have been reported for patients rendered stone free after SWL, compared with rates of 17% to 80% when residual fragments remained (Beck and Riehle, 1991; Fuchs et al., 1991; Graff et al., 1988; Nakamoto et al., 1993; Newman et al., 1988; Nijman et al., 1989; Zanetti et al., 1991). Residual fragments are most likely to pass when located within the ureter and least likely to pass when located in the lower pole.

In a large review on SWL by Rassweiler et al. (2001), CIRF were found to spontaneously pass in 25%, remain stable in 55%, and become clinically significant in 20% of patients, with anywhere from 4% to 25% of patients requiring a subsequent intervention to address the residual fragment. A similar spontaneous passage rate of 25% to 30% has been reported by others (Candau et al., 2000; Streem et al., 1997). **When the findings from the available prospective data are pooled, the probability that CIRF after SWL later become clinically significant increases with lower pole fragments, increasing fragment burden, increasing fragment number, and longer follow-up** (Khaitan et al., 2002; Osman et al., 2005b; Streem et al., 1996).

Many investigators have noted that, **after SWL, residual fragments are commonly localized to lower pole calyces no matter where the stone was treated in the kidney** (Drach et al., 1986; Graff et al., 1988; Kohrmann et al., 1993; Liedle et al., 1988; Zanetti et al., 1991). The incidence of stone recurrence is greater in the lower pole calyces after SWL than it is after PCNL (Carr et al., 1996; Kohrmann et al., 1993; Zanetti et al., 1991). Furthermore, at 1-year follow-up there is a significantly greater rate of new stone formation in those treated with SWL, and the recurrent stones are more likely to be in the lower calyces. A plausible explanation for these results is that fine debris, undetectable by imaging, persists after SWL and, because of gravity, settles in the most dependent calyces and serves as a nidus for new stone formation. Supporting this hypothesis are the results from Carr et al. (1996) showing that de novo stone formation occurs significantly more often after SWL (22%) than PCNL (4%).

Stone-free rates after PCNL vary widely from 40% to well above 90%. However, as with SWL reporting, the definition of stone free is not consistent across studies (Park et al., 2007; Skolarikos and de la Rosette, 2008). Raman et al. (2009) found an 8% rate of residual fragments by CT scan, with approximately half located in the lower pole. Of the patients with residual fragments, 43% developed a stone-related event at a median of 32 months after initial PCNL. Fragments larger than 2 mm in greatest diameter were more likely to undergo a secondary procedure and independently predicted a postoperative stone-related event. Similarly, fragments located in the renal pelvis and ureter were associated with a stone event on multivariate analysis but also were associated with the highest likelihood of spontaneously passing (Ganpule et al., 2009; Raman et al., 2009). In another retrospective study, Emmott et al. (2018) showed a 45% rate of residual fragments after PCNL, and of these patients almost one-third (31%) had a subsequent stone-related event (21% required re-intervention, 9% required no intervention) at a median time of approximately 20 months after initial PCNL.

Few investigators have evaluated the destiny of residual fragments after URS. The recent meta-analysis by the AUA and EAU revealed that residual fragments occur in 6% of cases for distal ureteral stones, 14% of cases for mid-ureteral stones, and 19% of cases for proximal ureteral stones (Preminger et al., 2007). The limited data in which CT was used to evaluate residual fragment status after URS have shown stone-free rates of only 50% to 54% (Pearle et al., 2005; Portis et al., 2006). Expanding the definition of treatment success to also include fragments 2 mm or smaller improves the success rate to 62% to 84% (Macejko et al., 2009; Portis et al., 2006; Rippel et al., 2012). Schatloff et al. (2010) found that patients with residual fragments after semirigid ureteroscopy were significantly more likely to experience unanticipated medical visits (3% vs. 30%) and exhibited a trend toward more ancillary procedures (0 vs. 7%) and more frequent rehospitalization (0 vs. 10%). Over a 19-month period after URS, Rebuck et al. (2011) reported a 20% rate of unplanned stone events, a 22% rate of spontaneous passage, and a 57% rate of persistent residual fragments (≤4 mm). A retrospective, multicenter study of 232 ureteroscopy patients with residual fragments showed almost half of these patients (44%) experienced a subsequent primary stone event (15% required no intervention, 29% required intervention) (Chew et al., 2016).

In patients with infection-related calculi, the consequence of residual fragments is particularly harmful. Residual fragments may harbor offending bacteria and thus predispose to persistent infection. Furthermore, stone regrowth has been reported in up to 75% of such patients after SWL, compared with 10% of patients who experienced complete stone removal (Beck and Riehle, 1991; Zanetti et al., 1991).

For patients with metabolic stone disease, complete stone removal does not prevent stone recurrence, but it does prolong the intervals between symptomatic events and treatment (Chow and Streem, 1998). Thus residual stones, including small stones, may not have an immediate clinical relevance but are likely to affect the patient's well-being in the long term.

The sensitivity of the method used to detect remaining fragments has important effects on the reported incidence and size of residual fragments. As stated, plain radiography, nephrotomography, ultrasonography, intravenous urography, and CT have all been used to evaluate residual fragments. Plain radiography, ultrasonography, and CT are used most frequently in contemporary practice. In the current era with the recognition that repeated radiation exposure from CT may be harmful, the routine use of CT scan for follow-up studies should be done cautiously and only when necessary. Some of this concern can be tempered with the use of low-dose and ultra-low–dose protocols for CT, although widespread availability of these modalities is limited.

In early studies investigating stone clearance after SWL, plain radiography was commonly used to determine stone-free status for radiopaque calculi and could detect opaque stone fragments as small as 2 mm (Thornbury and Parker, 1982). Plain radiography has a sensitivity of approximately 60% for detecting urinary stones (Assi et al., 2000; Ege et al., 2004; Johnston et al., 2009; Mutgi et al.,

1991). However, Denstedt et al. (1991) reported that for patients with large renal calculi treated by a combination of PCNL and SWL, plain radiography overestimated stone-free rates by 35% and 17%, respectively, compared with flexible nephroscopy. Nephrotomography, although becoming obsolete in many centers, has proved superior to plain radiography in detecting residual fragments (Goldwasser et al., 1989; Hjollund Madsen, 1972; Schwartz et al., 1984).

Traditionally, ultrasonography has been inferior to plain radiography in detecting urinary calculi, with particular deficiency in detecting ureteral stones (Older and Jenkins, 2000; Yilmaz et al., 1998). The sensitivity of ultrasonography to detect urinary calculi over the last decade has ranged from 24% to 57% (Fowler et al., 2002; Ulusan et al., 2007; Viprakasit et al., 2012), although these results were potentially confounded because CT scans and ultrasounds were rarely done on the same day and infrequently performed by a dedicated uro-ultrasonographer. Kanno et al. (2014) recently reported a 70% ultrasound sensitivity in detecting renal stones when the ultrasound was done the same day as the CT, average patient BMI was 23, and all ultrasounds were performed by experienced ultrasonographers. Therefore, even under the most favorable circumstances, ultrasound may still miss up to 30% of renal stones.

Despite its shortcomings, in detecting ureteral stones, ultrasound is highly effective in diagnosing hydronephrosis. In fact, some advocate for ultrasonography after all ureteroscopic procedures because silent obstruction has been reported to occur in certain, albeit rare, instances (Weizer et al., 2002). A prospective study comparing the relative efficacy of abdominal radiography and renal ultrasonography versus excretory urography for the evaluation of asymptomatic patients 1 month after SWL treatment demonstrated that the combination of ultrasonography and abdominal radiography was as good as or better than intravenous urography in identifying residual stone fragments and hydronephrosis, suggesting that **routine radiologic evaluation of asymptomatic patients after SWL could be limited to abdominal radiography and ultrasonography** (Coughlin et al., 1989).

Although flexible nephroscopy may be considered the gold standard for assessment of residual stones after PCNL, its routine use has been challenged by studies showing the high sensitivity of CT in detecting residual stones after PCNL. Pearle et al. (1999) noted that CT had 100% sensitivity for detecting residual stones after PCNL in 36 patients evaluated with both CT and flexible nephroscopy. Selective use of flexible nephroscopy based on positive CT findings would have avoided an unnecessary procedure in 20% of patients. In a retrospective study of 121 patients who underwent CT after PCNL (including 59% stone-free patients and 16% patients with fragments of 1 to 3 mm), Waldmann et al. (1999) reported that routine nephroscopy would not have been required in 75% of cases. Given its wide availability and high sensitivity, CT is becoming more popular for the evaluation of residual stone fragments after PCNL. However, this must be balanced with the need to minimize unnecessary radiation exposure in patients, and when available, strong consideration for low- and ultra-low–dose CT is prudent.

> **KEY POINTS: RESIDUAL FRAGMENTS**
>
> - Many small residual fragments eventually become clinically significant and symptomatic.
> - In the setting of infectious stones, residual stones portend a future of UTIs and stone recurrence; therefore aggressive treatment with removal of fragments is usually indicated.
> - Risks for stone recurrence are higher in the setting of residual stone fragments, because stone growth on an existing crystal matrix is harder to prevent than spontaneous nucleation of new stones.

SUGGESTED READINGS

Albala DM, Assimos DG, Clayman RV, et al: Lower Pole I: a prospective randomized trial of extracorporeal shock wave lithotripsy and percutaneous nephrostolithotomy for lower pole nephrolithiasis-initial results, J Urol 166(6):2072–2080, 2001.

Assimos D, Krambeck A, Miller NL, et al: Surgical management of stones: American Urological Association/Endourological Society guideline, PART I, J Urol 196:1153–1160, 2016.

Assimos D, Krambeck A, Miller NL, et al: Surgical management of stones: American Urological Association/Endourological Society guideline, PART II, J Urol 196:1161–1169, 2016.

de la Rosette J, Assimos D, Desai M, et al: The Clinical Research Office of the Endourological Society percutaneous nephrolithotomy global study: indications, complications, and outcomes in 5803 patients, J Endourol 25(1):11–17, 2011.

de la Rosette J, Denstedt J, Geavlete P, et al: The Clinical Research Office of the Endourological Society ureterorenoscopy global study: indications, complications, and outcomes in 11,885 patients, J Endourol 28(2):131–139, 2014.

Lingeman JE, Siegel YI, Steele B, et al: Management of lower pole nephrolithiasis: a critical analysis, J Urol 151(3):663–667, 1994.

Pearle MS, Lingeman JE, Leveillee R, et al: Prospective, randomized trial comparing shock wave lithotripsy and ureteroscopy for lower pole caliceal calculi 1 cm or less, J Urol 173:2005–2009, 2005.

Pearle MS, Nadler R, Bercowsky E, et al: Prospective randomized trial comparing shock wave lithotripsy and ureteroscopy for management of distal ureteral calculi, J Urol 166:1255–1260, 2001.

Preminger GM, Assimos DG, Lingeman JE, et al: AUA guideline on management of staghorn calculi: diagnosis and treatment recommendations, J Urol 173(6):1991–2000, 2005.

Preminger GM, Tiselius HG, Assimos DG, et al: 2007 Guideline for the management of ureteral calculi, J Urol 178:2418–2434, 2007.

Semins MJ, Trock BJ, Matlaga BR: The safety of ureteroscopy during pregnancy: a systematic review and meta-analysis, J Urol 181:139–143, 2009.

Tan YK, Cha DY, Gupta M: Management of stones in abnormal situations, Urol Clin North Am 40:79–97, 2013.

Turk C, Neisius A, Petrik A, et al; European Association of Urology (EAU) Guidelines Office: European Association of Urology guidelines on urolithiasis, 32nd ed, London, 2017, EAU Annual Congress.

REFERENCES

The complete reference list is available online at ExpertConsult.com.

94

Surgical Management for Upper Urinary Tract Calculi

Brian R. Matlaga, MD, MPH, and Amy E. Krambeck, MD

EXTRACORPOREAL SHOCK WAVE LITHOTRIPSY

Methods and Physical Principles

In extracorporeal shock wave lithotripsy (SWL) a source external to the patient's body generates a shock wave. Specifically, the energy source rapidly deposits pulses of energy into a fluid environment, which results in the generation of a shock wave. **Shock waves are surfaces that divide material ahead, not yet affected by the disturbance from that behind, which has been compressed as a consequence of energy input at the source** (Sturtevant, 1996). These waves move faster than the speed of sound, and the stronger the initial shock, the faster the shock wave moves. **Shock wave behavior is characteristic of the propagation of nonlinear waves.** Although the shock waves in lithotripters generate large pressures, they are relatively weak in that they induce only slight compression and deformation of a material. **The shock wave lithotripter uses weak, nonintrusive waves that are generated externally, transmitted through the body, and focused onto the stone. The shock waves build to sufficient strength only at the target, where they generate enough force to fragment a stone.**

Generator Type

The three primary types of shock wave generators are electrohydraulic (spark gap), electromagnetic, and piezoelectric.
Electrohydraulic (Spark Gap) Generator. In the electrohydraulic shock wave lithotripter, a spherically expanding shock wave is generated by an underwater spark discharge (Cleveland et al., 2000). High voltage is applied to two opposing electrodes; the resulting spark produces a vaporization bubble. The bubble expands and collapses rapidly producing a high-energy pressure wave. **The resulting shock wave occurs at F1 (the electrode) located on an ellipsoid, which focuses the wave on the stone target (F2).** Fig. 94.1 shows a hemiellipsoid reflector and a spark gap typical of those used in the older electrohydraulic machines.

The clear advantage of this generator is its effectiveness in breaking kidney stones (Lingeman, 1997). **Disadvantages are the substantial pressure fluctuations from shock to shock.** As the electrode deteriorates, it wears down. With a 1-mm displacement of the electrode tip off F1, the F2 can shift up to 1 cm off the initial stone target.
Electromagnetic Generator. The electromagnetic generators produce a magnetic field in either a flat plane or around a cylinder. The flat plane waves are focused by an acoustic lens (Fig. 94.2); the cylindric waves are reflected by a parabolic reflector (Fig. 94.3) and transformed into a spherical wave. Fig. 94.2 shows a system that uses a water-filled shock tube containing two conducting cylindric plates separated by a thin insulating sheet. When an electrical current is sent through one or both of the conductors, a strong magnetic field is produced between the conductors, moving the plate against the water and thereby generating a pressure wave. The *magnetic pressure* causes a corresponding pressure (shock wave) in the water. The shock front produced is a plane wave that is of the same diameter as the current-carrying plates. **The energy in the shock wave is concentrated onto the target by focusing it with an acoustic lens.** The electromagnetic system that uses a cylindric source (see Fig. 94.3) also has a cylindric coil surrounded by a cylindric membrane that is pushed away from the coil by the induction of a magnetic field between the two components. In both systems the pressure pulse has only one focal point (F2) that is positioned on the target.

Electromagnetic generators are more controllable and reproducible than electrohydraulic generators because they do not use a spark gap generator. Another advantage of the electromagnetic generators is it will deliver several hundred thousand shock waves before requiring servicing, thereby eliminating the need for frequent electrode replacement. Electromagnetic lithotripters introduce energy into the body over a large skin area, causing less pain; however, they also generate a high-energy density at the stone (F2). This high-energy density at F2 has resulted in an increased rate of subcapsular hematoma formation over the older electrohydraulic models. The rate of subcapsular hematoma formation for the Storz Modulith (Storz Medical, Tägerwilen, Switzerland) has been suggested to be 3.1% to 3.7% (Dhar et al., 2004). Piper et al. (2001) suggested that perinephric hematomas may occur in up to 12% of patients treated with a DoLi S lithotripter (Dornier Medical Systems, Kennesaw, GA), which is higher than what has been reported for the original HM3 electrohydraulic lithotripters (Chaussy and Schmiedt, 1984; Knapp et al., 1987).
Piezoelectric Generator. The piezoelectric lithotripter also produces plane shock waves with directly converging shock fronts. A capacitor is fired through a collection of several hundred to several thousand piezoceramic elements positioned on a reflector, often shaped like a satellite dish (Fig. 94.4). Each element produces a limited power shock front that is focused on the same F2.

The advantages of piezoelectric generators include the focusing accuracy, a long service life, and the possibility of an anesthetic-free treatment because of the relatively low-energy density at the skin entry point of the shock wave (Marberger et al., 1988). The piezoelectric energy sources produce some of the highest peak pressures of any lithotripter currently available. However, **the actual energy delivered to the stone per shock wave is several orders of magnitude lower than that delivered by an electrohydraulic machine because of the extremely tiny volume of F2, making poor stone comminution a disadvantage of this technology.**

Imaging Systems

There are three basic designs used by lithotripter manufacturers for stone localization. They are fluoroscopy alone, ultrasonography alone, and the combination of ultrasonography and fluoroscopy.
Fluoroscopy Alone. The original Dornier HM3 lithotripter used two x-ray converters arranged at oblique angles to the patient and 90 degrees from each other to localize the stone effectively at F2. To reduce the cost of lithotripters, an adjustable C-arm has been subsequently introduced on many devices. Furthermore, in an attempt to develop multifunctional operating rooms and tables, the fluoroscopic systems used by lithotripter manufacturers have become more standardized. The fluoroscopic system typically consists of a high-quality digitized x-ray imaging system mounted on a rotatable C-arm with an isocentrically integrated shock wave source. Because the shock wave head can be rotated out of the field of the fluoroscopic system, the table can be used for other routine urologic fluoroscopic applications.

The primary advantages of fluoroscopy still include its familiarity to most urologists, the ability to visualize radiopaque calculi throughout the urinary tract, the ability to use iodinated contrast

Chapter 94 Surgical Management for Upper Urinary Tract Calculi **2095**

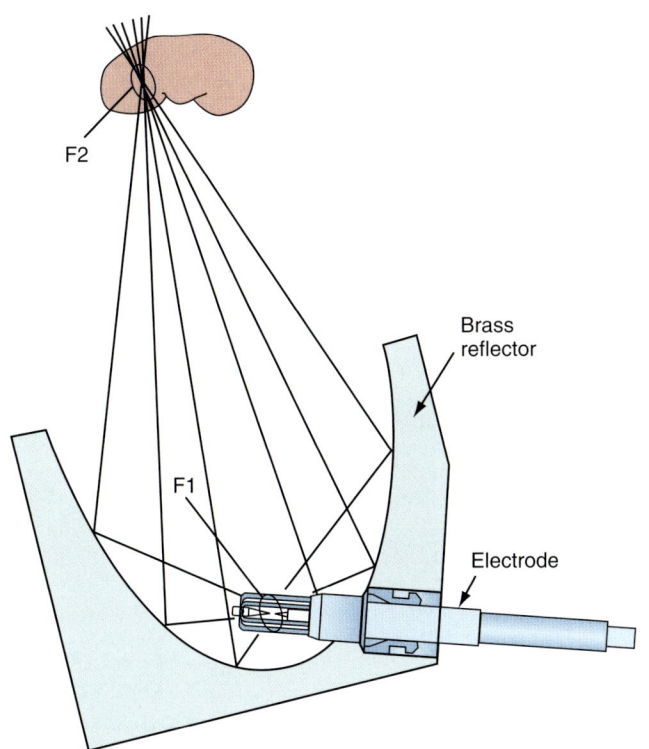

Fig. 94.1. Schematic view of an electrohydraulic shock wave generator. An electrode is used to generate a shock wave. *F1*, Focus 1; *F2*, focus 2.

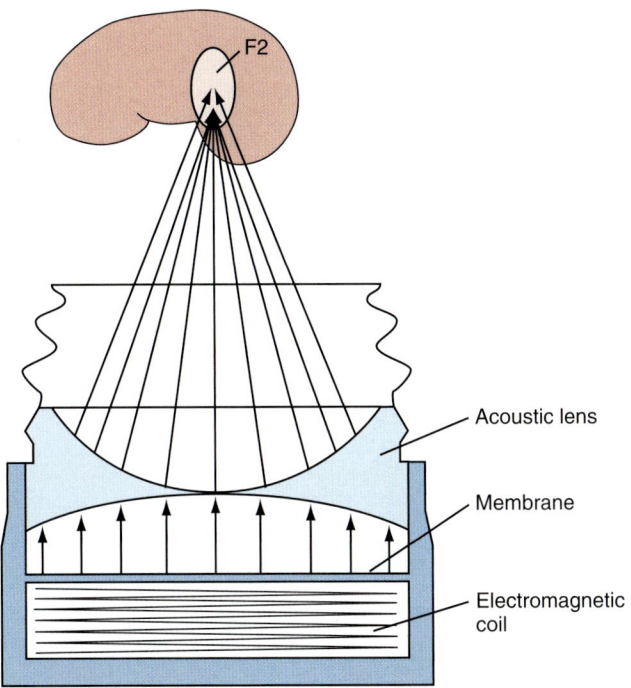

Fig. 94.2. Schematic view of an electromagnetic shock wave generator that uses an acoustic lens to focus the shock wave. An electromagnetic coil is used to generate the shock wave. *F2*, Focus 2.

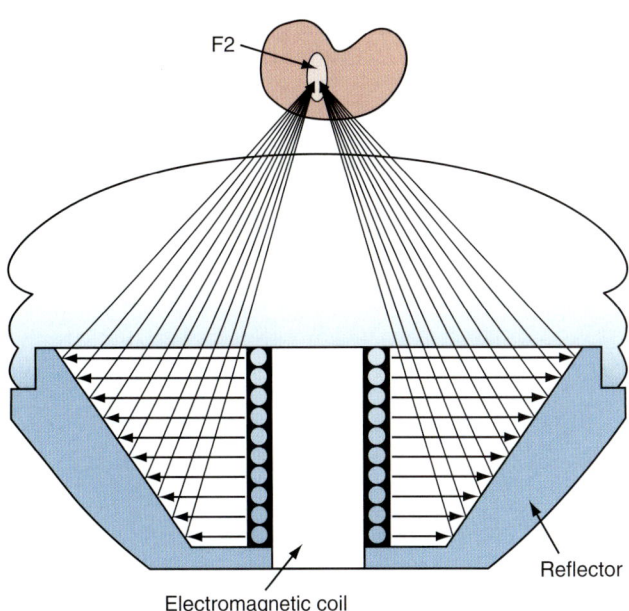

Fig. 94.3. Schematic view of an electromagnetic shock wave generator that uses a parabolic reflector to focus the shock wave. An electromagnetic coil is used to generate the shock wave. *F2*, Focus 2.

agents to aid in stone localization, and the ability to display anatomic detail. The disadvantages include the exposure of the staff and patient to ionizing radiation, the high maintenance demands of the equipment, and the inability to visualize radiolucent calculi without the use of radiographic contrast agents.

Ultrasonography Alone. Ultrasonic localization was initially designed to aid multifunctional lithotripters for treatment of urinary and biliary stones. It is presently used in several low-cost machines because it is inexpensive to manufacture and maintain compared with fluoroscopic systems. Another major advantage of this technology is in the treatment of children and infants when concern exists about the dose of ionizing radiation. In addition, ultrasonography can localize slightly opaque or nonopaque calculi.

Despite its advantages, ultrasound imaging has a number of significant disadvantages. Sonographic localization of a kidney stone requires a highly trained operator, and many urologists are not comfortable or familiar with identifying stones ultrasonically. Complicating the issue of stone detection is the fact that it is almost impossible to view a kidney stone in areas such as the middle third of the ureter or when there is an indwelling ureteral catheter. Furthermore, once a stone is fragmented, it is difficult to identify each individual stone piece. Unfortunately, these disadvantages tend to overshadow the advantages of ultrasound imaging.

Combination of Ultrasonography and Fluoroscopy. As the demand for interdisciplinary lithotripters has increased, the lithotripsy industry has responded, in some cases combining ultrasonography and fluoroscopy for stone localization. There are clearly advantages to these setups, but each system has a drawback that limits one of the functions of the system.

Stone Fragmentation

A typical pressure pulse generated by an electrohydraulic shock wave lithotripter is shown in Fig. 94.5. The pressure wave involves **an initial short and steep compressive front with pressures of approximately 40 megapascals (MPa) that is followed by a longer, lower amplitude negative (tensile) pressure of 10 MPa, with the entire pulse lasting for a duration of 4 microseconds.** The ratio of the positive to negative peak pressures is approximately 5:1. (Cleveland et al., 2000; Müller, 1990). **Stone fragmentation during SWL, also called comminution, occurs as a result of mechanical stressors created by two mechanisms that can occur simultaneously or separately: (1) directly by the incident shock wave or (2) indirectly by the collapse of bubbles.** The different mechanical stresses that result from SWL and contribute to stone fragmentation are as follows: spall fracture, squeezing, shear stress, superfocusing, acoustic cavitation, and dynamic fatigue (Fig. 94.6).

Spall fracture, also known as spallation, is the calescence of microcracks within a stone resulting in comminution. The

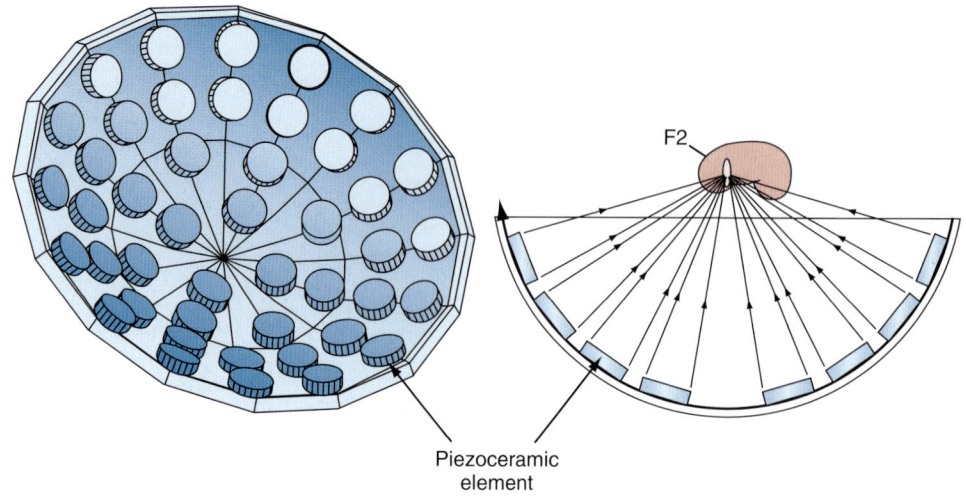

Fig. 94.4. Schematic view of a piezoelectric shock wave generator. Numerous polarized polycrystalline ceramic elements are positioned on the inside of a spherical dish. *F2*, Focus 2. The focal plane at the focus *(circles)*.

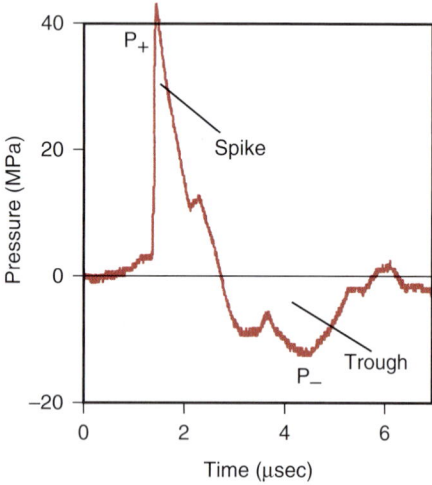

Fig. 94.5. A typical pressure pulse at the lithotripter focus (F2) as measured by a polyvinylidene difluoride membrane hydrophone. First, there is a steep positive pressure front of about 40 MPa, which is followed by a negative pressure of 10 MPa, with the entire pulse lasting for a duration of 4 μsec. (From Coleman AJ, Saunders JE, Preston RC, et al.: Pressure waveforms generated by a Dornier extracorporeal shock wave lithotriptor. *Ultrasound Med Biol* 13:651–657, 1987.)

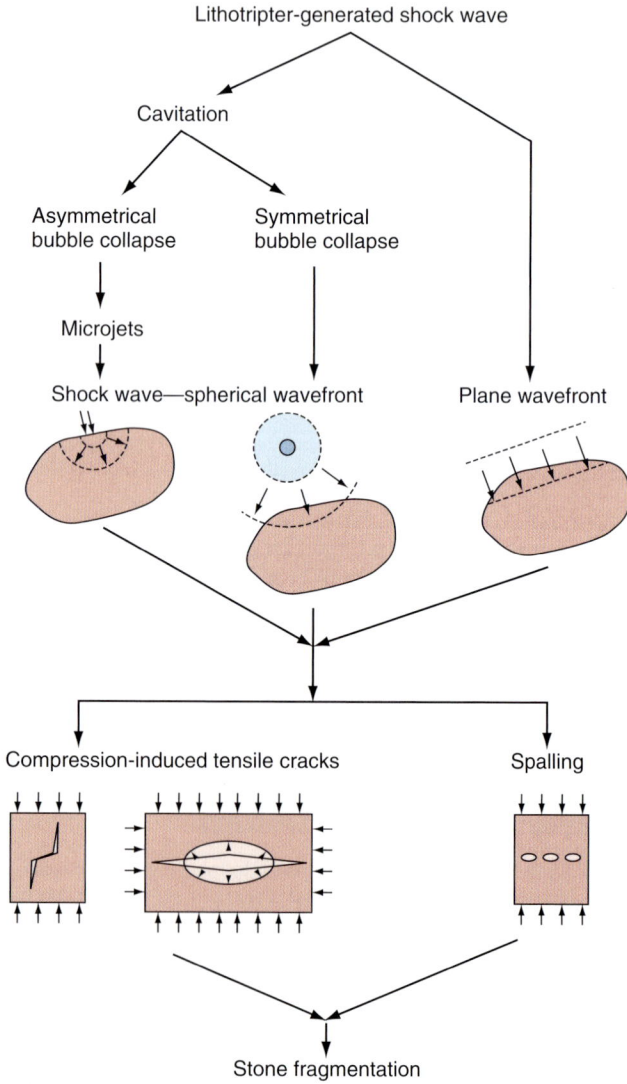

Fig. 94.6. Summary of how the various mechanical forces generated by a lithotripsy shock wave may cause a kidney stone to fracture. (Reproduced with permission from Dr. Bradley Sturtevant.)

fragmentation plan is perpendicular to the applied stress. Once the shock wave enters the stone, it will be reflected at sites of impedance mismatch, such as the distal stone-urine interface. As the shock wave is reflected, it is inverted in phase to a tensile (negative) wave. Fragmentation occurs when the tensile wave exceeds the tensile strength of the stone. Because they are a brittle material, kidney stones are theorized more likely to fail under tension rather than compression (Johrde and Cocks, 1985).

The second mechanism for stone breakage, *squeezing-splitting* or *circumferential compression*, occurs because of the difference in sound speed between the stone and the surrounding fluid (Eisenmenger, 1998). The shock wave inside the stone advances faster through the stone than the shock wave in the fluid outside the stone. The shock wave in the fluid outside the stone produces a circumferential force on the stone, resulting in a tensile stress at the proximal and distal ends of the stone. It has been theorized that squeezing should be enhanced when the entire stone falls within the diameter of the focal zone; thus a wider F2 or focal zone in a lithotripter may be of benefit.

The third mechanism is shear stress. Shear stress will be generated by shear waves (also termed *transverse waves*) that develop as the shock wave passes into the stone. The shear waves propagate through the stone, which results in shifting of molecules perpendicular or transverse to the wave. Mathematical modeling has demonstrated that shear waves are a more power force in stone comminution than the spall effect (Sapozhnikov et al., 2007). However, the intensity of the shear wave is dependent on the width of F2 or focal zone with larger focal zones being more beneficial.

The fourth mechanism for stone breakage, superfocusing, is the amplification of stresses inside the stone because of the geometry of that stone. The shock wave that is reflected at the distal surface of the stone can be focused by either refraction or diffraction from the corners of the stone to create areas of high stress in the interior of the stone (Gracewski et al., 1993; Xi and Zhong, 2001). The regions of high stress (tensile and shear) depend on the geometry of the stone and elastic properties.

The fifth mechanism for SWL stone breakage is cavitation (Coleman et al., 1987; Crum, 1988; Vakil and Everbach, 1993; Zhong and Chuong, 1993; Zhong et al., 1993). *Cavitation* is the formation and subsequent collapse of bubbles. The negative pressure in the trailing part of the shock pulse causes bubble formation. As these bubbles grow, they oscillate in size for about 200 microseconds and then collapse violently, giving rise to high pressures and temperatures. This release of energy is generally in the form of a positive and negative wave that can create all the comminution mechanisms described. However, in the presence of a boundary, a liquid jet, also termed a *cavitation microjet*, forms inside the bubble during the collapse (Crum, 1979, 1988). If the cavitation microjet is near the surface of a stone, it creates a locally compressive stress field in the stone, which propagates into the stone interior.

The final mechanism of stone fragmentation to be considered is the accumulation of damage induced by SWL that eventually destroys the structure of the stone. Essential to this process are nucleation, growth, and coalescence of flaws within the stone caused by a tensile or shear stress. Because renal calculi are not homogeneous but rather have either a lamellar crystalline structure bonded by an organic matrix material or an agglomeration of crystalline and noncrystalline material there are numerous sites of preexisting flaws (microcracks). All of the fracture mechanisms described have the potential to generate progressive damage to the interior of the stone. By use of a mathematical model taking, Lokhandwalla and Sturtevant (2000) were able to calculate the number of shock waves required for comminution to occur in a typical calcium oxalate monohydrate calculus. The values they determined had a range of two orders of magnitude (30 to 3000 shocks), which is well within the clinical dose presently used to treat patients.

Bioeffects: Clinical Studies

Acute Extrarenal Damage

SWL induces acute injury in a variety of extrarenal tissues (Evan et al., 1991, 1998). Although rarely clinically significant, SWL has been associated with trauma to organs such as the liver and skeletal muscle, as evidenced by elevated levels of bilirubin, lactate dehydrogenase, serum aspartate transaminase, and creatinine phosphokinase within 24 hours of treatment (Lingeman et al., 1986; Parr et al., 1988; Ruiz Marcellan and Ibarz Servio, 1986). Such laboratory parameter changes begin to normalize within 3 to 7 days of SWL treatment and are normalized by 3 months. There have also been reports of surrounding visceral injuries after SWL, such as perforation of the colon, hepatic hematoma, splenic rupture, pancreatitis, and abdominal wall abscess. Extrarenal vascular complications have been reported to occur as well, such as rupture of the hepatic artery, rupture of the abdominal aorta, and iliac vein thrombosis. Thoracic events, such as pneumothorax and urinothorax, have even been described. Fortunately, these events are exceedingly rare and have generally been presented as isolated incidents.

Early clinical studies noted that shock waves could induce a cardiac arrhythmia, an observation that led to electrocardiographic synchronization with R-wave triggering on the Dornier HM3 device (Chaussy and Schmiedt, 1984). However, later clinical studies with non–water bath lithotripters have concluded that SWL is safe to the electrophysiology of the heart and gating to the cardiac rhythm is unnecessary.

Although a shock wave lithotripter focuses its waves and peak pressure on the stone (the focal zone, or F2), it is known that high acoustic pressure does extend beyond this zone (Fig. 94.7). Therefore it is reasonable to expect that organs other than the kidney are exposed to stresses sufficient to cause injury. One such organ is the pancreas; a retrospective follow-up study from the Mayo Clinic suggests that patients who underwent SWL for the treatment of kidney stones in 1985 were at increased risk for developing diabetes mellitus compared with controls (Krambeck et al., 2005). The development of diabetes was related to the total number of shock waves and the power level of the lithotripter. Although these data are provocative, there were a number of limitations of the study, including that the stone disease of the SWL cohort was more severe than that of the control cohort; a family history of diabetes was not ascertained for either group; and the data for the SWL group were collected by self-report questionnaire, whereas the control group was examined by chart review. A follow-up study by Rashed et al. in 2017, also a retrospective review, noted an increase in blood serum glucose levels, diagnosis of diabetes, and prescription of antidiabetic therapy after SWL. However, several other groups have subsequently investigated the association of diabetes mellitus and SWL and have not noted an association (Chew et al., 2012, Fankhauser et al., 2015; Makhlouf et al., 2009; Sato et al., 2008). Notably, de Cogain et al. (2012) performed a population-based study of Olmsted County, Minnesota,

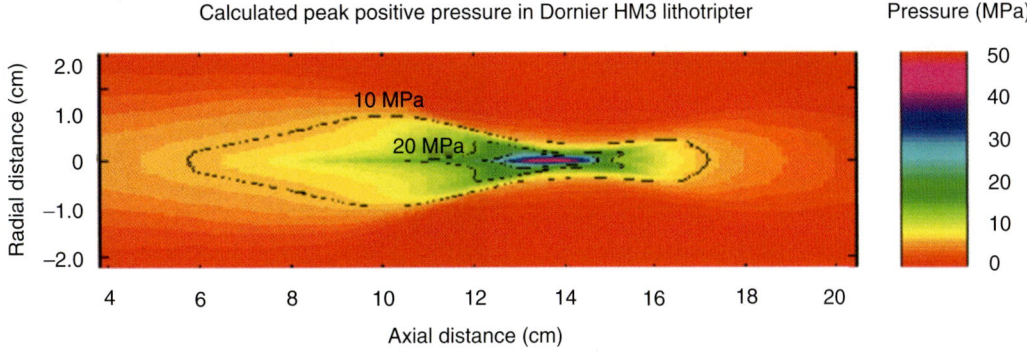

Fig. 94.7. Predicted peak positive pressure in a Dornier HM3 lithotripter. The pressure is not focused to a point but extends over a finite volume.

Acute Renal Injury: Structural and Functional Changes

Almost all patients who undergo SWL for renal stones demonstrate hematuria after approximately 200 shock waves. Hematuria is so common that it may be considered an incidental finding, and its severity is rarely of concern. Although hematuria was initially considered to be a consequence of irritation of the urothelium as stones were fragmented by shock waves, it is now known that damage to the kidney is the most likely source. Morphologic studies in the canine and porcine models have demonstrated that shock waves rupture blood vessels and can damage surrounding renal tubules (Fig. 94.8). In the porcine model SWL-injured vessels ranging in size from the glomerular and cortical capillaries and vasa recta to the larger arcuate and intralobular vessels have been identified after therapeutic levels of shock waves have been received. The resulting hemorrhagic lesion generally extends from cortex to medulla and comprises torn blood vessels with platelet aggregation and red blood cells in the interstitial space (Fig. 94.9). In the setting of a more severe injury induced in the porcine model, complete necrosis of the endothelium and vascular smooth muscle may result. In laboratory studies a typical clinical dose of 2000 shock waves with the Dornier HM3 lithotripter, operated at 24 kV with shock waves delivered at 2 Hz, produces a lesion measuring 5% to 6% of the functional renal volume (Fig. 94.10).

In the clinical setting, there have been reports of moderate-to-severe renal injury occurring after SWL, generally manifesting as a hemorrhagic event. Hematoma rates range from less than 1% to as high as 20%, depending on the type of lithotripter used and the treatment parameters employed, as well as the radiographic modality and timing of imaging follow-up. Some of the third-generation lithotripters have very high peak positive pressures; therefore the rate of reported clinically significant renal hematomas are rising (3% to 12%) (Kohrmann et al., 1995; Piper et al., 2001; Thuroff et al., 1988; Ueda et al., 1993). The appearance of renal hematomas can range in severity from a mild contusion localized within the renal parenchyma to a large hematoma (Fig. 94.11) associated with

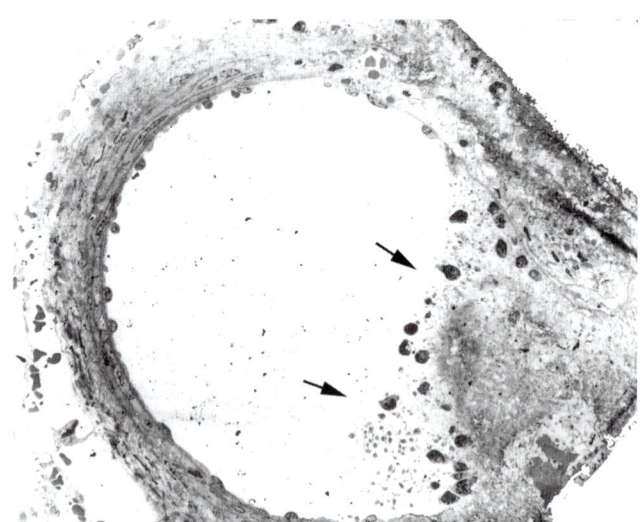

Fig. 94.9. Low-magnification transmission electron micrograph demonstrating injury to a medium-sized artery located within F2 of a pig treated with 2000 shock waves at 24 kV. The shock wave-induced injury to the right side of this vessel resulted in a rupture site that permitted extravasation of blood into the nearby interstitium. The site of injury in the vessel wall is plugged with a clot *(arrows)*.

Fig. 94.8. Macroscopic photomicrograph of a coronal section through the kidney of a juvenile pig (~6 weeks old) treated with 2000 shocks at 24 kV by an unmodified Dornier HM3 lithotripter and examined 4 hours after treatment. The region of intraparenchymal hemorrhage has been colored red by an automated computer color recognition program. Note that the lesion involves multiple papillae and in some regions extends through the cortex to the renal capsule, where a subcapsular hematoma may develop.

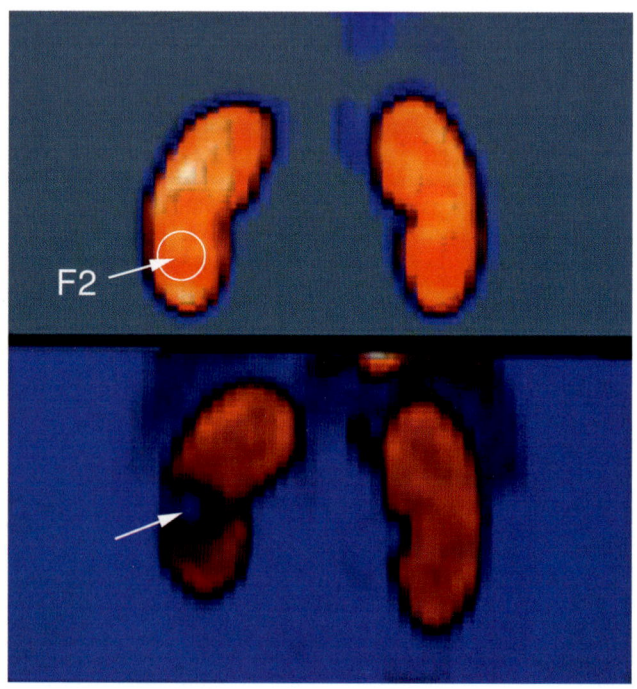

Fig. 94.10. Shock wave lithotripsy-treated and control kidneys imaged by positron emission tomographic scanning before and immediately after treatment with 3500 shock waves to the lower pole, at level six, with a DoLi 50 device. The site of focus 2 (F2) (lower pole) on the shocked kidney shows a 50% reduction of renal blood flow *(arrow)*.

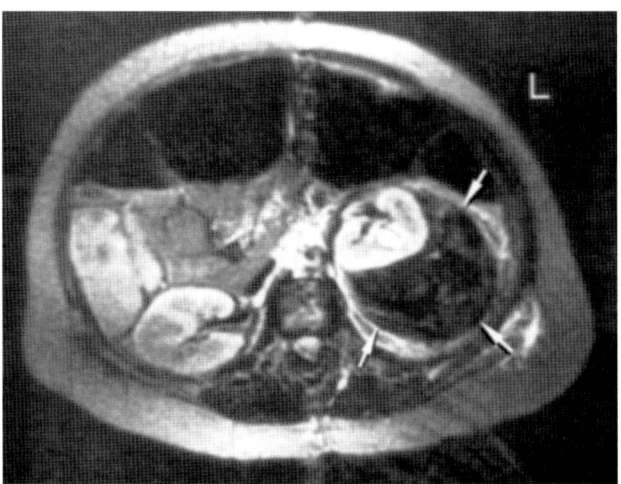

Fig. 94.11. Magnetic resonance image taken 24 hours after shock wave lithotripsy with 1200 shocks at 22 kV (by an unmodified Dornier HM3 lithotripter) shows a large subcapsular hematoma (arrows) in the treated (left) kidney.

TABLE 94.1 Potential Long-Term Concerns Regarding Shock Wave Lithotripsy (SWL)

Condition	Overall Findings/Conclusion
Hypertension	No large-scale evidence to support an association between SWL and the development of hypertension
Chronic kidney disease	No evidence to support an association between SWL and the development of chronic kidney disease
Diabetes mellitus	No large-scale evidence to support an association between SWL and the development of diabetes mellitus
Increased rate of stone recurrence	Likely an association between SWL and subsequent stone events of patient not rendered stone free
Male fertility	Sperm quality decreases immediately post-SWL for distal ureteral stones but normalizes by 3 months postoperatively
Female fertility	Data inconclusive and limited

BOX 94.1 Acute Renal Side Effects: Risk Factors for Shock Wave Lithotripsy

Age	Diabetes mellitus
Obesity	Coronary heart disease
Coagulopathies	Preexisting hypertension
Thrombocytopenia	Body mass index >30 or <21.5

severe bleeding, possibly necessitating blood transfusion or rarely even angiographic embolization. Although some hematomas may persist for many months to years, it has been reported that most resolve within weeks and without long-term sequelae.

Several risk factors for the development of a post-SWL hematoma have been identified (Box 94.1). Dhar et al. (2004) reported that the probability of a subcapsular hematoma increased 2.2 times for every 10-year increase in the patient's age. Knapp et al. (1988) found patients with existing hypertension to be at increased risk for the development of a perinephric hematoma as a consequence of SWL. In particular, those patients having unsatisfactory control of their hypertension at the time of SWL had the highest incidence of hematoma formation. Additional risk factors for renal hemorrhage were diabetes mellitus, coronary artery disease, and obesity, all of which suggest a link to a vascular disorder. More recently, Nussberger et al. (2017) found no difference in the presence of hypertension, diabetes mellitus, or history of anticoagulant/antiplatelet usage between patients with and without renal hematoma on routine ultrasound after SWL with a third-generation lithotripter. However, the authors found that patients with a high body mass index (BMI >30) or a low BMI (<21.5) were at a greater risk of hemorrhage compared with other patients.

Chronic Renal Injury: Structural and Functional Changes

It is well accepted that shock waves damage blood vessels in the human and animal model, and the resulting hemorrhage initiates an inflammatory response that ultimately leads to scar formation in the animal model. In animal studies parenchymal fibrosis, a precursor to renal scarring, is seen as early as 1 month after SWL, and scar formation also has been reported to be a dose-dependent phenomenon. In the clinical, long-term setting there are **four chronic concerns thought to potentially be associated with SWL treatment. These concerns are development of renovascular hypertension, a decrease in overall renal function, an increase in the rate of stone recurrence, and a decrease in fertility** (Table 94.1).

The possibility that SWL may be associated with significant changes in systemic blood pressure was first suggested by Peterson and Finlayson (1986) and has been investigated by others. Multiple initial reports indicated a probable association between SWL and the development of hypertension (Lingeman et al., 1987; Williams et al., 1989) or even more specifically diastolic hypertension (Lingeman et al., 1990). Janetschek et al. (1997) performed a prospective study that demonstrated age was a significant risk factor for post-SWL hypertension, with an increase in intrarenal resistive index observed in patients 60 years of age and older. However, multiple subsequent studies have failed to demonstrate an association between SWL and the development of new-onset hypertension. de Cogain et al. (2012) used a population-based cohort in Olmsted County, Minnesota and found no association between SWL and the development of de novo hypertension. A more recent meta-analysis reviewed 30 studies focusing on SWL and the development of hypertension (Fankhauser et al., 2015). The follow-up period was 12 to 240 months, and the number of patients ranged from 35 to 1758. Only 6 of the 30 studies found an increase in hypertension after SWL, and the remaining 24 found no association. A subcapsular hematoma can induce hypertension; however, such changes are generally transient. **Transient changes in blood pressure control, frequent visits to the physician surrounding the stone event, pain, and broad definitions of hypertension may account for the many varied study results; however, based on the current literature, there is no strong evidence associating SWL with development of hypertension.**

Another potential concern surrounding SWL is its effect on long-term renal function. Williams et al. (1988) found a **significant decrease in the percentage of effective renal plasma flow 17 to 21 months after SWL for patients with two kidneys**. Orestano et al. (1989) noted that patients receiving more than 2500 shocks had a reduction in creatinine clearance and a prolongation of ^{131}I-Hippuran transit time 30 days after SWL in the treated kidney; in some cases, similar findings were noted in the contralateral kidney. Lingeman et al. (1990) reported that patients with a solitary kidney demonstrated elevated serum creatinine levels 5 years after SWL. These observations stand in contrast to the early reports by Chaussy and Fuchs (1986), which suggest a significant increase in renal function 3 months to 1 year after SWL. A longer follow-up study of patients treated in Munich failed to demonstrate any long-term change in renal function after SWL (Liedle et al., 1988). More recent reports have found no association between permanent decrease in renal function and SWL. A meta-analysis included 14 studies from 1992 to 2012 that focused on renal function and SWL, of which 7 were retrospective and 7 prospective (Fankhauser et al., 2015). Follow-up for the studies ranged 15 months to 17 years. None of the studies found evidence for an increase in chronic kidney disease after SWL. Thus, **based on the current literature, there is no evidence to indicate SWL is associated with long-term renal dysfunction.**

Another significant concern is that **stone recurrence rates may be higher after SWL because of residual stone debris** (Pearle et al., 2005). A study by Carr et al. (1996) documented new stone formation in 298 consecutive patients who initially were determined to be stone free after SWL and compared those recurrence rates with those of 62 patients treated by percutaneous nephrolithotomy (PCNL). The Carr study data showed a significant increase in the rate of new stone formation within 1 year of SWL treatment compared with PCNL. The authors suggested that fine sand debris generated from SWL treatment remained in the kidney and gravity acted to position it as a nidus in the calyceal system. Subsequent surgical stone research has demonstrated that residual fragments after endoscopic stone procedures result in a higher recurrence rate (Chew et al., 2016); thus the lower stone-free results after SWL compared with other treatment modalities for certain stone sizes and locations must be taken into consideration (Assimos et al., 2016a). **If SWL has a higher residual fragment rate after treatment, then it is likely to result in higher stone recurrence rates.**

Finally, the effect of SWL on the reproductive system has yet to be fully elucidated. During SWL the female reproductive organs, as well as the female and male reproductive organ vascular supplies, are directly exposed to SWL when ureteral stones are treated. Early in vitro studies have demonstrated that sperm are sensitive to the effects of SWL. Multiple investigators have demonstrated a decrease in sperm vitality and change in morphology when semen samples are exposed to SWL (Andressen et al., 1996), of which two investigators have even noted a dose-dependent change in the quality of the semen sample (Kaller et al. 1988; Ohmori et al. 1993). Clinically, the effects of SWL on sperm quality and function are not so clearly observed. The first study on male fertility and SWL was performed by Puppo et al. (1990), who analyzed 10 men before and after SWL of a distal ureteral stone and noted no change in their semen analyses. A follow-up study by Andressen et al. (1996) of 10 men undergoing SWL of a distal ureteral stone found a decrease in sperm motility and density from preoperatively to postoperatively. A more extensive study of 62 men treated with SWL for distal ureteral calculi and 62 men treated with SWL for proximal ureteral calculi compared semen analyses results from preoperatively, to 1 week postoperatively, to 3 months postoperatively (Sayed, 2006). This study found that sperm density and mobility decreased 1 week postoperative in the men treated with distal ureteral SWL from preoperatively but did not change in the men treated with SWL for a proximal ureteral stone. However, all abnormal findings normalized to baseline by 3 months postprocedure. A more recent meta-analysis of 6 studies focusing on male fertility after SWL confirms that there is a decrease in sperm concentration and motility with an increase in hematospermia after SWL; however, all findings normalized by 3 months postprocedure (Radfar et al., 2017). There are limited data focusing on female fertility after SWL. Two retrospective studies of women after SWL were of minimal benefit in determining effects of SWL on fertility. One study focusing on 67 women after SWL found that only 10 were actually trying to conceive (Vieweg et al., 1992). Another questionnaire study of 39 women found that only 10 reported pregnancy with successful delivery of 11 babies (Erturk et al., 1997). Both studies concluded that SWL did not adversely affect fertility in the female patient. However, based on the low number of women actually trying to conceive who are mentioned in the current available literature, no definitive conclusions can be made regarding the effects of SWL on female fertility.

Mechanism for Tissue Injury

The mechanism for the traumatic effects of SWL is not known, although Delius et al. (1988) have speculated that the violent collapse of cavitation bubbles generated by the shock waves is primarily responsible for the cellular changes. This cavitation concept is based on data showing that cavitation bubbles are present during shock wave application and that lithotripter shock waves can cavitate water and blood in vitro (Coleman, 1987). Zhong et al. (2001) suggested that the expansion of bubbles in a vessel leads to rupture of the wall of that blood vessel, which has been tested and proven in an in vitro setting.

Bailey et al. (2005) used a novel detection system to demonstrate cavitation of tissue in vivo. Their data found pooling of fluid in tissue at sites of cavitation, suggesting that **once blood vessels have been ruptured and blood has collected in pools, there is a greater potential for cavitation to occur. The pooling of blood provides a large fluid-filled space for cavitation bubbles to grow and collapse.**

Techniques to Optimize Shock Wave Lithotripsy Outcome

First and foremost proper patient selection is necessary for a successful SWL procedure. Selecting patients based on stone size, composition, skin-to-stone distance, stone location, Hounsfield units, and Triple D score are paramount. Proper patient selection is covered elsewhere in this volume. For device-specific variables, the urologist has the ability to control a number of lithotripter parameters that may affect the ultimate treatment outcome (Box 94.2). These parameters include the acoustic output and focal volume that are employed, optimal coupling, the number of shock waves administered, the rate at which they are dispensed, and the power or voltage that is used. In addition, other intraoperative factors that may affect stone breakage can be controlled, such as anesthetic technique.

Although all lithotripters generate waveforms that are fundamentally similar, lithotripters may be distinguished from one another by the peak pressure and the size of their focal zone at F2. In vitro studies suggest that the focal width generated by a lithotripter affects stone breakage; a wider focal width increases the likelihood of stone breakage (Sapozhnikov et al., 2007). Because the kidney tends to move, as a consequence of respiratory motion, the stone may move in and out of a narrow focal zone. Furthermore, when the focal zone is narrower than the stone, the stress inside a stone is reduced. For the stone to be subjected to the full force of shear stress, the outer surface of the stone must be subjected to high-pressure shock wave energy, which will not occur with a small focal zone (Sapozhnikov et al., 2007). This assessment is supported by clinical studies comparing large focal zone lithotripters (Dornier HM3) with intermediate zone lithotripters (Siemens Lithostar Plus), and small focal zone lithotripters (Storz Modulith SLX) in which the large focal zone devices had the lowest retreatment rate, whereas the small zone devices had the highest (Dhar et al., 2004).

The present generation of lithotripters has dry treatment heads, which make them smaller and more easily transportable. However,

---

BOX 94.2 Factors That Induce the Degree of Renal Trauma Associated With Shock Wave Lithotripsy

AGGRAVATING FACTORS
Number of shocks
Period of shock wave administration: Shorter period increases damage
Accelerating voltage: Higher voltage increases damage
Type of shock wave generator: First- versus second-/third-generation devices
Kidney size: Juvenile versus adult
Preexisting renal impairment

MITIGATING FACTORS
Pretreatment with 100 to 500 shocks at low energy level to reduce lesion size
Treatment at a slow rate of shock wave delivery (≤60 shocks/min)

they require a coupling medium, such as gel or oil, to join the patient to the device. Optimal coupling permits the efficient transfer of energy from the lithotripter to the patient; poor coupling will reduce stone breakage. Most commonly, energy transfer through a coupling medium is attenuated by air pockets in the coupling interface. Air pockets covering as little as 2% of the coupling area diminish stone comminution by 20% to 40% (Pishchalnikov et al., 2006). Decoupling and recoupling, which may occur during repositioning of a patient during SWL, can generate large-volume air pockets in the coupling medium (Li et al., 2012; Neucks et al., 2008; Pishchalnikov et al., 2006). With current available lithotripters, it is not possible to actively monitor coupling during treatment; however, such technology may be beneficial in future generation lithotripters. A study using video cameras placed in the head of a Dornier Doli SII lithotripter to detect air pockets in the coupling gel demonstrated that air bubbles could be actively monitored and that the presence of air bubbles affected the number of shock waves needed for stone fragmentation (Bohris et al., 2012). One measure to limit coupling defects is by altering how the agent is applied. Coupling has been found to be improved by delivering a large volume of gel as a mound dispensed from the stock jug and allowing the gel to spread on contact between the treatment head and the skin. The type of coupling media is also an important factor to consider. One study of five different coupling agents found that water-soluble lubricating jelly required the least amount of shocks for stone fragmentation, whereas local anesthetic cream (EMLA) and petroleum jelly required the greatest number of shocks (Cartledge et al., 2001).

During an SWL treatment session the urologist can directly control the rate at which shock waves are delivered and the number of shock waves dispensed. In vitro and animal studies have shown that slowing the shock wave delivery rate to less than 120 SW/min improves stone fragmentation (Greenstein and Matzkin, 1999; Paterson et al., 2002). The first clinical randomized trials also demonstrated better stone-free rates when SWL was performed at 60 SW/min as compared with 120 SW/min (Madbouly et al., 2005; Pace et al., 2005). These findings were confirmed in a literature review and meta-analysis of randomized controlled trials evaluating different shock wave delivery rates: a rate of 60 shocks per minute was found to break stones more effectively than 120 shocks per minute (Semins et al., 2008). More recently, a systematic review and network meta-analysis based on 13 randomized clinical trials found that success rates of SWL procedures at low (60–70 shocks/min) (odds ratio [OR] 2.2, 95% confidence interval [CI] 1.5–2.6) and intermediate-frequency (80–90 shocks/min) (OR 2.5, 95% CI 1.3–4.6) are significantly higher than at high (100–120 shocks/min) frequency (Kang et al., 2016). Furthermore, there was no significant difference in outcomes between low- and intermediate-frequency SWL procedures. **Cavitation is thought to play a role in improved results at lower SWL rates, because the dynamic bubbles are given a longer time interval to dissipate with a slower rate. At a higher rate the bubbles build on the surface of the stone forming a barrier to SW energy transmission and thus act as an energy draw from subsequent shocks** (Choi et al., 1993). The disadvantage of a slow rate is, of course, a longer treatment time, particularly if the number of shock waves being delivered is predetermined. Slowing the rate has also been shown to be protective of the kidney vasculature in the animal model (Evan et al., 2007). However, clinical studies in humans have found no difference in complication rates across different SWL frequency ranges (Kang et al., 2016). Despite the conflicting findings between animal studies and human outcomes it is generally recommended that **the lowest number of shock waves needed to fragment the stone be used to reduce the risk of renal injury. To minimize overtreatment physicians are encouraged to not use a preset treatment number but to instead image the stone frequently during the SWL treatment and discontinue shock wave delivery once the stone shows adequate fragmentation.**

Another parameter urologists adjust is the energy setting on the machine. Increasing the power setting on most electromagnetic lithotripters actually narrows the focal zone, which, as discussed earlier, decreases stone breakage and may also increase the risk for renal injury and renal hematoma (Connors et al., 2000). **In vitro**

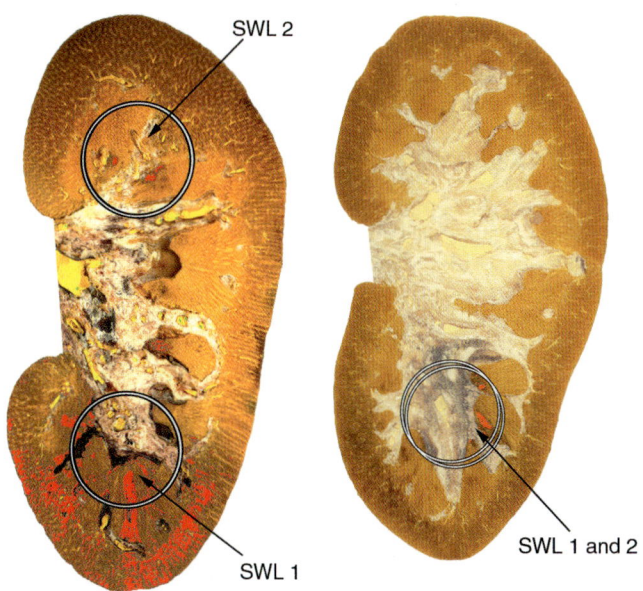

Fig. 94.12. On the left is a coronal section of a kidney from an animal treated with 2000 shocks at 24 kV first to the lower pole (shock wave lithotripsy [SWL] 1) and then an additional 2000 shocks at 24 kV to the upper pole (SWL 2) of the same kidney. The typical lesion *(in red)* is seen at the lower pole; however, a greatly reduced lesion is seen on the upper pole. These data suggest that a pretreatment protocol may reduce the lesion induced by a clinical dose of shock waves. At right, lesion size is shown in an animal first treated at the lower pole with 500 shocks at 12 kV (SWL 1) and then treated again at the lower pole with 2000 shocks at 24 kV (SWL 2). A greatly reduced lesion is also noted for this protocol.

and in vivo studies have demonstrated a benefit of "ramping up" the energy of the lithotripter by not only improving stone fragmentation but also decreasing renal injury effects (Fig. 94.12). In the stone phantom model (Zhou et al., 2004) and the porcine model (Connors et al., 2009; Maloney et al., 2006; Willis et al., 2006) energy-ramping protocols have demonstrated superior stone fragmentation over standard fixed treatments. Furthermore, clinical studies have demonstrated that pretreatment with a lower energy for the first 100 shocks and gradual ramping of the lithotripter energy level as the treatment progresses has resulted in higher stone-free rates (Demirci et al., 2007; Lambert et al., 2010). In the study by Lambert et al. (2010) patients were randomized to receive 500 shocks at 14 kV, 1000 at 16 kV, and 1000 at 18 kV or to a standard 18 kV for 2500 shocks. The ramping group had a significantly higher stone-free rate at 1 month compared with the standard group (81% vs. 48%). In addition, the ramping group demonstrated lower levels of beta2 microglobulin and microalbumin, markers of renal injury, 1 week postoperative compared with the standard group. Such protective effects of ramping protocols have been previously noted in the porcine model. Renal lesion size has been shown to be decreased after pretreatment with low-energy shock waves (100 to 2000 at 12 kV followed by 24 kV) (Willis et al., 2006). Interestingly, Connors et al. (2009) demonstrated in a pig model that the voltage that is initiated is less important than the actual ramping up or halt in treatment, because pretreatment groups with 100 shock waves at 18 or 24 kV had significantly smaller lesions than just treating with 2000 shock waves at 24 kV without pretreatment. The reduction in renal injury is thought to be secondary to vasoconstriction because the same beneficial effect was blocked when dopamine was administered (Willis et al., 2006). A recent study of 418 patients treated with either a fixed or ramping protocol during SWL and followed with ultrasound imaging found that significantly fewer renal hematomas occurred in the ramping group (5.6% vs. 13%) (Skuginna et al., 2016). Handa et al. (2012) reported that a pause in treatment, when switching from low-energy to high-energy settings, is not necessary provided that the delivery of low-energy shock waves lasted at least 4 minutes.

Current generation lithotripters have been specifically developed so that treatment can be delivered without anesthesia. **The discomfort experienced during SWL is related directly to the energy density of the shock wave as it passes through the skin and the size of the focal point.** To minimize treatment discomfort the lithotripters were designed with wider aperture, which will spread the acoustic field across a broader area of the patient's skin, reducing skin surface pain. However, this wider aperture resulted in a narrow focal zone, which had a deleterious effect on stone breakage. Interestingly, the higher pressures used with these newer machines also have the potential to result in higher adverse event rates. Any movement during the SWL procedure, either by the patient because of pain or discomfort or by the kidney or stone through respiratory movement can adversely affect SWL outcomes by decreasing the number of shocks actually delivered to the stone. The kidney may move up to 50 mm during respiration, which is significant considering stone fragmentation can be reduced substantially with just 10 mm of motion in the bench top model (Cleveland et al., 2004). A study by Sorensen et al. (2012) that reviewed ultrasound videos during SWL found that only 60% of shock waves were delivered to the stone and mean stone motion was 15 mm. To reduce stone motion, urologists can perform SWL with general anesthesia, which will control the patient's respiratory rate and volume. Two clinical studies compared the outcome of SWL performed with intravenous sedation and SWL performed with general endotracheal anesthesia. General anesthesia yielded significantly better outcomes: 78% to 87% stone-free rates versus 51% to 55% with intravenous sedation (Eichel et al., 2001; Sorensen et al., 2012). Because general anesthesia is associated with superior outcomes, this may be the anesthesia of choice for SWL, unless contraindicated for medical reasons. High-frequency jet ventilation is an alternative form of ventilation during general anesthesia that may also be beneficial during SWL. One clinical study found that when high-frequency jet ventilation was used, there was minimal respiratory movement, and patients undergoing SWL required fewer shocks with lower total energy to achieve stone fragmentation (Mucksavage et al., 2010).

Adjuncts to Improve Shock Wave Lithotripsy Outcomes

Although successful SWL starts with appropriate patient selection and proper surgical technique, a few adjunctive measures may help to facilitate stone passage and limit patient morbidity in the postoperative period. Currently, the American Urological Association (AUA) guidelines do not recommend the placement of ureteral stents at the time of SWL because stent placement has not been shown to improve stone passage rates and only increases patient morbidity (Assimos et al., 2016b). However, the use of medical expulsive therapy and percussion diuresis and inversion (PDI) therapy have been found to be beneficial (Box 94.3).

Kupeli et al. (2004) evaluated the use of alpha-blockers for 2 weeks after SWL in 48 patients. The authors found a significant improvement in stone-free rates in the patients treated with alpha-blockers compared with SWL alone (70.8% vs. 33.3%). Subsequent studies have demonstrated similar improvements in stone-free rates (Bhagat et al., 2007; Georgiev et al., 2011; Gravina et al., 2005), and recent meta-analysis of multiple different alpha-blockers shows similar benefits regardless of the type of alpha-blocker used (Skolarikos et al., 2015; Yang et al., 2017). Other investigators have found that the use of alpha-blockers in the SWL postoperative setting resulted in decreased time to fragment clearance (Kobayashi et al., 2008), and improvements in overall pain control (Georgiev et al., 2011; Gravas et al., 2007; Resim, 2005), which has been confirmed with a recent meta-analysis. Based on these studies and a limited side effect profile of alpha-blockers, they appear to be a beneficial pharmacologic tool in the immediate post-SWL period.

Another novel mean to facilitate stone fragment passage is PDI therapy. The general concept is some type of diuretic—either drinking copious amounts of fluid or taking a diuretic agent (e.g., furosemide)—is employed and the patient is placed in a prone Trendelenburg position while the flank is percussed for approximately 10 minutes. Percussion of the flank can be manual or using a mechanical device such as a chest physiotherapy vibrator. PDI is generally performed at least weekly for several weeks. Randomized prospective trials comparing PDI after SWL for fragments less than 4 mm in the lower pole versus observation alone found a higher stone-free rate (40% vs. 3%) with PDI (Pace et al., 2001). Another study randomized patients to SWL + PDI vs. SWL alone for stones smaller than 2 cm and found that stone-free rates were higher in the PDI group (62.5% vs. 35.4%) (Chiong et al., 2005).

Future Direction

Improving visual coupling of SWL may improve overall outcomes and stone-free results by increasing the percentage of shock waves impacting the stone at F2. The Visio-Track (VT) locking system has the potential to increase stone fragmentation rates and decrease fluoroscopy time. The VT is a hand-held probe with an infrared stereovision, which allows triangulation of the stone location. The VT is used with ultrasound-guided lithotripters and allows the lithotripter to "lock on" to the stones location during treatment. The preliminary data for the VT system have demonstrated a significantly higher stone-free rate when VT-SWL was used versus standard ultrasound-guided SWL (79.5% vs. 54.5%) (Abid et al., 2015).

Ultrasonic propulsion of renal and ureteral calculi is another measure thought to potentially improve outcomes with SWL. Focused ultrasound has emerged as a technology that can expel small stones or stone fragments from the urinary system (Sorensen et al., 2013). Harper et al. (2013) reported an in vitro study that effectively and rapidly migrated stone material through a urinary system using ultrasound. As a next step a handheld device has been developed that uses a higher amplitude and larger pulses of ultrasound than standard diagnostic ultrasound to physically manipulate stones in vivo (Harper et al., 2014). The stone-pushing technology has been demonstrated to be safe with minimal tissue destruction in the porcine model (Connors et al., 2014). The first human clinical trial occurred in 2016, aimed to reposition stones 10 mm or less in 15 subjects (Harper et al., 2016). Stones were successfully repositioned in 93% of subjects with a mean skin to stone depth of 11 cm. Ultrasonic propulsion also demonstrated a collection of stones rather than a solid stone in 5 subjects, which the subjects then passed after fragment relocation. Potential future uses of this technology would be to assist in expulsion of residual stone fragments after SWL or movement of a stone from an unfavorable (lower pole of the kidney) or painful location (ureter) to a more favorable location (the renal pelvis) before SWL treatment (Fig. 94.13).

Poor stone-free results with later-generation lithotripters has led investigators to explore other forms of ultrasound stone fragmentation. A newly developed mode of lithotripsy has demonstrated promising initial results. Excessive bubble production through cavitation can block the surface of the stone from subsequent shock waves and protect the stone from further comminution. Burst wave lithotripsy uses sinusoidal short bursts of focused ultrasonic pulses to fragment stones. The short bursts of ultrasound eliminate the blocking effect

---

BOX 94.3 Ways to Improve Shock Wave Lithotripsy Outcomes

Appropriate coupling
Water-soluble lubricant applied by hand
Decrease rate to low (60–70 shocks/min) or intermediate (80–90 shocks/min)
Image frequently and stop shocking once fragmented
　Do not use a preset number of shocks
Ramping protocol
　Treat with low power escalating to higher levels
General anesthesia
Do not use a ureteral stent
Consider alpha-blockers for medical expulsive therapy
Consider percussion, diuresis, inversion therapy

of surface cavitation and improve stone fragmentation with lower F2 pressures. In vitro studies of burst wave lithotripsy indicate that the technology can fragment struvite and uric acid stones in seconds and calcium oxalate monohydrate stones in 10 minutes to very small fragment sizes (<2 mm) with low peak pressures of 4 mPa (Maxwell et al., 2015). In the porcine model, bust wave lithotripsy can fragment stones at less than 12 mPa and at a faster rate, less than 200 Hz (May et al., 2017). As a comparison, standard SWL uses pressures of 30 to 100 mPa and less than 2 Hz. Furthermore, because burst wave lithotripsy is ultrasound guided, it is designed to provide real-time feedback so the development of cavitation in the tissue can be identified and treatment subsequently halted, thus preventing tissue damage (Maxwell et al., 2015). Initial porcine studies in which burst wave lithotripsy was used at 21 treatment sites found that renal injury did occur in the form of focal tubular damage, as well as cellular fragmentation and necrosis similar to SWL (May et al., 2017). However, the area was minimal at less than 0.1% of the renal functional volume. When the treatment was allowed to progress at extreme doses, extended pressures, and large areas of cavitation, the damage was still confined to only 1% of the kidney (Fig. 94.14). Based on initial animal and in vitro studies, burst wave lithotripsy is an advancing technology that has the potential to revolutionize the future of SWL.

> **KEY POINTS: SHOCK WAVE LITHOTRIPSY**
>
> - Shock waves fragment stones via multiple different mechanisms, including compressive and tensile forces.
> - SWL is associated with anatomic injury to the kidney; however, extensive studies in humans have not indicated long-term adverse effects.
> - Adverse outcomes with SWL are associated with high peak pressures at F2.
> - The effectiveness of SWL can be enhanced by ensuring optimal coupling of the patient to the lithotripter, treating at a slow to intermediate rates (60 shocks/min), ramping the power settings, and treating with general anesthesia.
> - The adverse effects of SWL may be reduced by initiating treatment at low power settings and slowly ramping up the power to standard treatment energy.

PERCUTANEOUS NEPHROLITHOTOMY

Preparation of the Patient

The initial evaluation of the patient who is being considered for PCNL should be a complete history and physical examination. A complete medical history will **identify patients with an absolute contraindication to PCNL, such as uncorrected coagulopathy, as well as those with an active, untreated urinary tract infection**

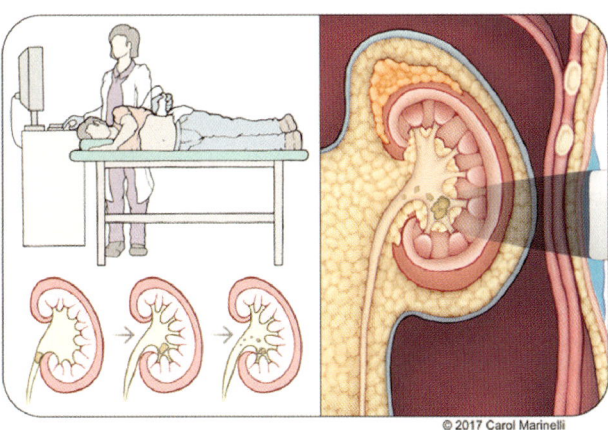

Fig. 94.13. Proposed use of ultrasonic propulsion to reposition a stone to a more favorable location for subsequent shock wave lithotripsy.

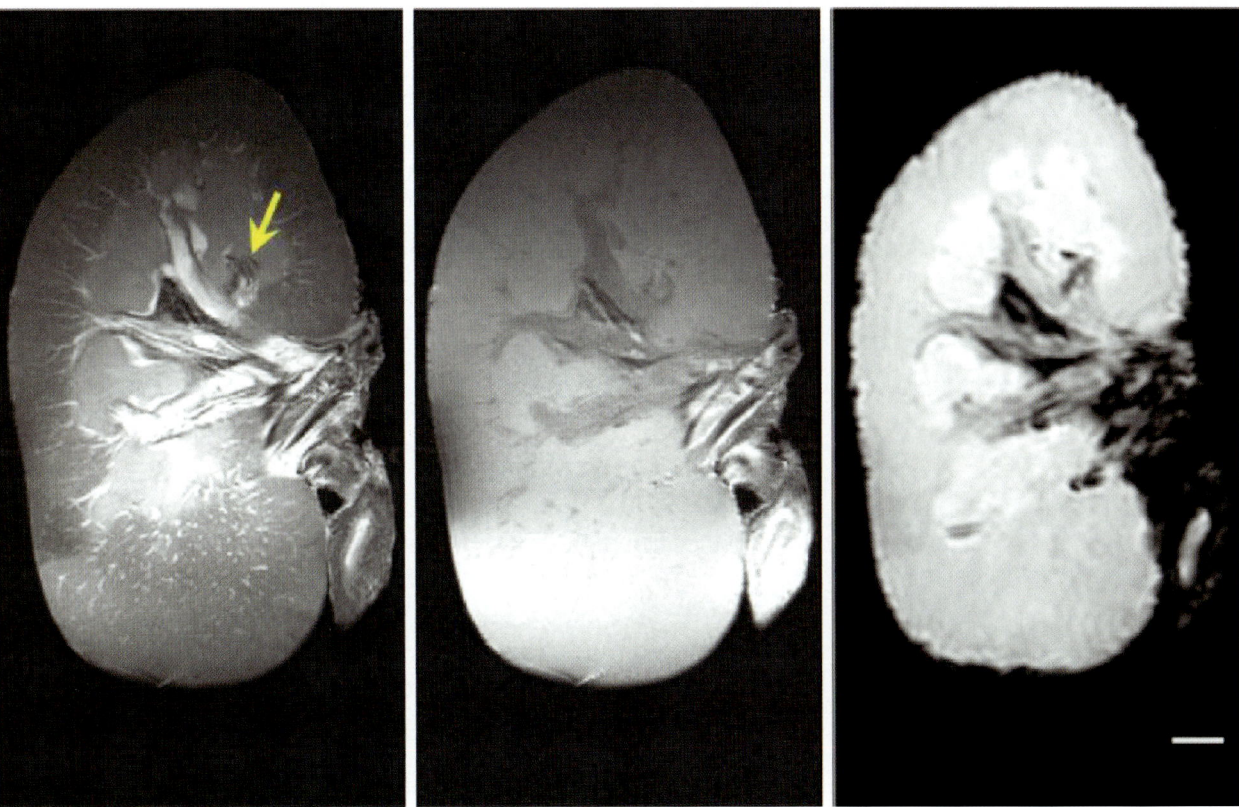

Fig. 94.14. MRI images of a porcine kidney after burst shock wave lithotripsy. *Arrow* indicates small area of renal damage and hemorrhage.

(UTI). The placement of a percutaneous nephrostomy drain, without manipulation of the calculus, may be an appropriate therapy if the stone is associated with obstruction of the renal unit and sepsis. If it is medically feasible, **aspirin and other antiplatelet or anticoagulation medications should be discontinued before surgery.** In patients with a higher risk for thrombotic complications, bridging therapy with short-acting may be necessary.

Preoperative laboratory evaluation of patients scheduled for PCNL should include a complete blood cell count as well as serum electrolyte determinations and renal function tests. A urine culture should be obtained if there is suspicion of infection; perioperative antibiotics can be appropriately tailored to culture-specific organisms. Typing and screening of the patient's blood should be considered, although preoperative crossmatching usually is not necessary.

The standard usage of helical computed tomography (CT) to evaluate the patient with urolithiasis has eliminated the need to perform preoperative intravenous urography or retrograde pyelography. **In most cases, the decision to perform PCNL may be based on the stone burden displayed on the CT images.** The main advantage of CT is the ability to assess the spatial relationship of the kidney relative to the stone and that of the kidney in relation to adjacent peritoneal and retroperitoneal structures. For example, CT permits identification of structures such as a retrorenal colon, or a liver or spleen that may be in the projected access trajectory. Patients with ectopic kidneys, congenital and iatrogenic (e.g., resulting from renal allograft, autotransplantation), as well as patients with dysmorphic body habitus because of congenital malformations such as spinal dysraphism may also benefit from cross-sectional imaging before PCNL; intra-abdominal structures, such as the bowel, may be located between the skin and the renal access point in such cases. Retrograde pyelography can be performed at the time of the surgical procedure, acquiring information about calyceal anatomy that may aid in selecting the targeted puncture site. Radionuclide scanning may be necessary in selected patients, particularly those harboring an extensive stone burden or an atrophic kidney, to evaluate differential renal function.

Antibiotics

Although data to support the need for antibiotic prophylaxis during PCNL are limited because of the lack of randomized controlled clinical trials, it is generally accepted that antibiotic prophylaxis reduces infectious complications. Institutional antibiograms aid in the selection of a most appropriate perioperative antimicrobial regimen. Importantly, it has been reported that urinary calculi may harbor bacteria even though bacteriuria is only intermittently present. In addition, **the fragmentation of stones, despite sterile urine, may release preformed bacterial endotoxins and viable bacteria that place the patient at risk for septic complications.** Therefore patients who have radiographic or clinical features suggestive of struvite, or in whom infection is suspected, should receive broad-spectrum antibiotics before surgery to reduce the risk for sepsis. For patients with indwelling stents, too, a course of antibiotic prophylaxis, particularly for gram-positive organisms, may be beneficial before instrumentation.

Anesthesia

PCNL can be performed after the administration of general, epidural, or local anesthesia. Typically, general anesthesia is preferred; however, local anesthesia may be an option when general anesthesia is contraindicated. A local anesthetic, such as lidocaine, can be delivered into the access tract by use of an 8.3-Fr anesthetic injection catheter with multiple side holes or with a dual-lumen ureteral access catheter or using a 23-gauge spinal needle with injection along the access tract to the renal capsule. Regional anesthesia (e.g., epidural, spinal) can be used for percutaneous procedures, but several problems may be associated with these regional anesthetic techniques. First, a relatively high block is necessary to eliminate all renal pain, and second, distention of the renal pelvis during PCNL may cause a vasovagal reaction that is not always prevented by regional anesthesia. **In cases in which upper pole puncture is contemplated, general anesthesia is preferred because it permits control of respiratory movements,** which is essential to minimize the risk for pulmonary complications. **A close relationship between the surgeon and the anesthesia team is essential to optimize the outcome of a PCNL procedure.** The anesthesiologist should be aware that pulmonary injuries, including hydrothorax and pneumothorax, can occur during PCNL; to that end, the anesthesiologist should monitor airway pressures, end-tidal carbon dioxide levels, and oxygen saturation and should auscultate the lungs frequently. Acute anemia from blood loss or dilution also may occur, emphasizing the need for frequent hemodynamic assessments. Because of the large amounts of fluids administered to the patient during nephroscopy there is a potential risk for hypothermia. Warming of irrigation fluids as well as patient warming devices may attenuate this risk.

Stone Removal

The fundamental techniques of gaining and maintaining percutaneous access, including imaging modalities and patient positioning (prone versus supine), are reviewed in Chapter 12.

After the nephrostomy access has been appropriately dilated and the Amplatz sheath positioned, the urologist can proceed with stone removal by endoscopic techniques. **Physiologic solutions should be used for irrigation during PCNL to minimize the risk for dilutional hyponatremia in the event of large-volume extravasation.** The height of the irrigant during rigid nephroscopy should not be excessively elevated, which will minimize intrapelvic pressure and fluid absorption through pyelovenous backflow. The use of an Amplatz working sheath also prevents elevated intrapelvic pressures. Rigid nephroscopy is performed initially, and small stones may be grasped with rigid graspers or stone baskets and extracted intact through the Amplatz sheath. Larger stones, though, require fragmentation before extraction. Several intracorporeal lithotripsy techniques are available and are reviewed elsewhere in this chapter.

Rigid nephroscopy is the preferred method for stone removal; however, only the simplest intrarenal collecting systems can be completely inspected with a rigid nephroscope through a single access. Therefore **flexible nephroscopy should be used during every PCNL to survey the entire intrarenal collecting system for residual stone fragments.** With an Amplatz sheath in place, pressurization of irrigation fluid during flexible nephroscopy can be used to adequately distend the collecting system and to improve visualization. The entire collecting system should be examined systematically, including the proximal ureter. Injection of contrast material through the flexible nephroscope and occasional fluoroscopy is helpful in maintaining orientation and verifying that each calyx has been inspected. Small stone fragments can be removed with a stone basket passed through the flexible instrument, and larger stones can be fragmented with laser or electrohydraulic lithotripsy (EHL). Alternatively, fragments may be flushed or manipulated into the renal pelvis, where they may be retrieved more easily with rigid instruments. The goal of PCNL is complete or nearly complete clearance of stone material at the time of the primary procedure, which greatly simplifies secondary procedures.

Multiple different sizes and shapes of nephrostomy tubes are currently available for use at the time of PCNL. The role of nephrostomy tube drainage is to aid in healing of the nephrostomy tract, promote hemostasis, prevent urinary extravasation, drain infection, and allow re-entry if necessary. Recently, tubeless (ureteral stent is left instead of nephrostomy tube) and even totally tubeless (no drainage device used) PCNL have been introduced and popularized. Comparison of nephrostomy tube size, shape, and tubeless and totally tubeless procedures is presented in Chapter 12.

Technique Modifications

In an attempt to decrease morbidity association with PCNL, modifications have been made to the size of the renal access tract, resulting in the new designations of "mini-percutaneous nephrolithotomy," "ultra-mini-percutaneous nephrolithotomy," and "micro-percutaneous nephrolithotomy." These smaller diameter access procedures have been reported to be associated with longer operative times because of the need to fragment stones into small pieces. However, blood loss and transfusion rates with mini-PCNL are lower compared with those with standard PCNL. Although all of the recent technique modifications work to decrease overall patient morbidity, because of technical limitations with the mini-, ultramini-, and micro-PCNL their exact role in the treatment of upper tract nephrolithiasis is uncertain and continues to be defined. Selection among these procedures is reviewed in Chapter 93.

> **KEY POINTS: PERCUTANEOUS NEPHROLITHOTOMY**
>
> - Critical preoperative steps include correcting underlying coagulopathy and close attention to preoperative microbiologic studies and perioperative antibiotic therapy.
> - Complete stone removal generally requires both rigid and flexible nephroscopy and a corresponding armamentarium of rigid and flexible lithotrites.
> - There is an increasing role for smaller caliber dilation/instrumentation approaches such as mini-, micro-, and ultramini-PCNL. Their ultimate place in the spectrum of therapies is not yet well defined, but they appear to be associated with less bleeding and pain. However, the efficiency of stone clearance also may be reduced.

Special Situations

Calyceal Diverticula

Treatment of calculi within a calyceal diverticulum can be difficult, and percutaneous removal has the reported highest treatment success rate of all endourologic minimally invasive treatment modalities (Krambeck and Lingeman, 2009). Percutaneous access into stone-bearing diverticula poses several unique problems. Direct puncture is often difficult because of the small size of the cavity and the frequent occurrence of calyceal diverticula in the upper pole of the kidney. After successful puncture is achieved, negotiation of a guidewire into the renal pelvis is often not possible. A similar situation can occur when a stone fills a calyx so completely that a guidewire cannot be passed through the infundibulum into the renal pelvis or in the rare case of infundibular stenosis. To overcome these difficulties, a special access technique is required.

If the calculi are visible on fluoroscopy, it is often preferable to puncture directly onto the stone. **Direct puncture into the diverticulum allows use of rigid instruments that provide superior visualization compared with flexible instruments that are used in an indirect approach** (Fig. 94.15). Once the diverticulum is punctured with an access needle, a guidewire is coiled within the diverticulum. It is important to ensure that not only the floppy tip of the wire but also the solid core is coiled within the diverticulum so that sufficient stabilization is provided for proper placement of coaxial dilators. A safety wire is then passed through a coaxial dilator or dual-lumen catheter. With two guidewires coiled within the diverticular lumen, dilation of the tract can be performed safely. Care should be taken to avoid perforation of the back wall of the diverticulum. If a balloon dilator is used, once the balloon is inflated, the working sheath should be passed over the balloon so that it rests as closely as possible to the diverticulum. In small diverticula, this results in the placement of the sheath outside the diverticulum. An 11-Fr alligator forceps is passed through the rigid nephroscope and used to follow the wire and gently spread renal parenchyma to allow entry into the calyceal diverticulum under direct vision. Stone material is then extracted. Careful inspection of the urothelium with the rigid nephroscope, and in cases of a large diverticulum, a flexible nephroscope as well, is performed in an effort to identify a flattened renal papilla, which suggests an obstructed calyx rather than a diverticulum. The neck of the diverticulum is often difficult to identify because it can be diminutive. Methylene blue injected through the ureteral catheter can facilitate visualization of the ostium. Once a guidewire is passed into the renal pelvis, the neck of the diverticulum can be balloon dilated or incised. Alternatively, if the ostium is not identified, fulguration of the urothelium may be accomplished by a resectoscope equipped with a roller-ball electrode.

Horseshoe Kidney

The horseshoe kidney presents several anatomic issues that should be considered before PCNL. The unique location and orientation of the horseshoe kidney are due to the incomplete cephalad migration and malrotation of the kidney, a consequence of the entrapment of the isthmus under the inferior mesenteric artery. The ureteropelvic junction (UPJ) is commonly deformed because of the high insertion of the ureter into a typically elongated renal pelvis. The course of the proximal ureter is similarly aberrant; it drapes ventrally over the

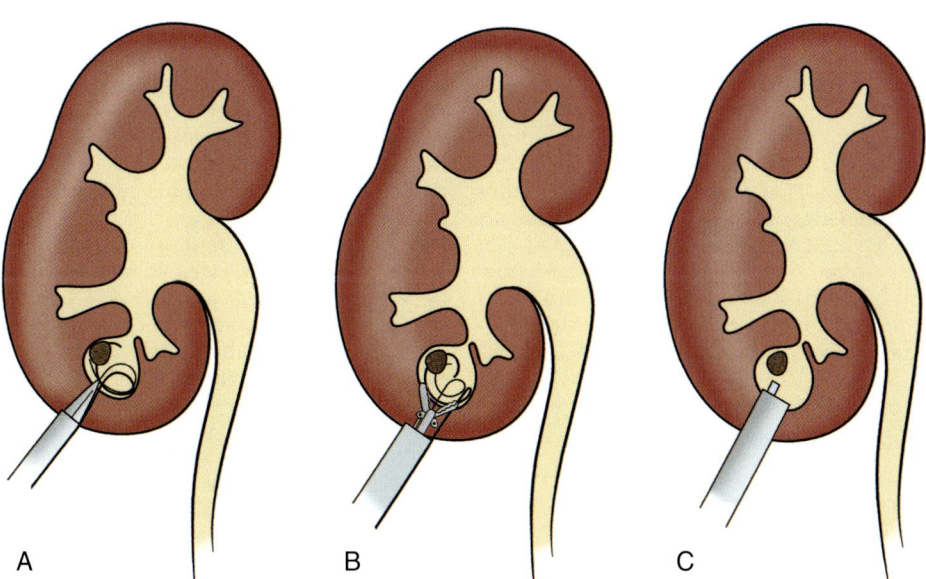

Fig. 94.15. Access into small diverticula. (A) Balloon dilator is advanced as far as possible without perforating the back wall of the diverticulum. The working sheath is placed just outside the diverticulum. (B) Alligator forceps spread the parenchyma and allow advancement of the nephroscope under vision into the diverticulum. The working sheath is then advanced over the nephroscope and into the diverticulum (C).

renal symphysis, where it may be compressed by the vessels that supply the lower pole and isthmus. Ureteral obstruction that may result from these anomalies can give rise to hydronephrosis, urinary stasis, sepsis, and calculi formation.

In considering PCNL in a horseshoe kidney, the characteristic lower and centrally oriented position of the kidney, the orientation of the collecting system, and the abnormal blood supply should be taken into account. Therefore **a puncture of the dorsal or dorsolateral aspect of the kidney will be well away from major renal vessels. The lower pole calyces lie within a coronal plane, angled medially, and are seldom suitable for direct puncture. However, the upper pole calyces are more posterior and lateral and are often subcostal, providing a convenient and relatively safe route for PCNL access.** The standard site for PCNL (inside the posterior axillary line just caudad to the 12th rib) is punctured, but the angle of the puncture is caudad rather than cephalad. Because most of the calyces of horseshoe kidneys point either dorsomedially or dorsolaterally, they are more favorably positioned for puncture than are normal renal units. Because of the malrotation of the kidney, the renal pelvis may be more anteriorly located, and the length of the nephrostomy tract often exceeds the length of the rigid nephroscope, necessitating the use of flexible nephroscopy or multiple accesses. Flexible nephroscopy also may be required to gain access to the lower medial calyces, where stones are often found.

Transplantation and Pelvic Kidneys

Urolithiasis is uncommon in patients who have undergone renal transplantation; factors that may predispose transplant recipients to form calculi include metabolic abnormalities, foreign bodies (nonabsorbable suture material, forgotten stents), recurrent infection, and papillary necrosis. On occasion, calculi may be present in the donor. Renal allografts present a unique anatomic situation for PCNL. The most common surgical anatomy is for the donor left kidney to be placed extraperitoneally into the recipient's right iliac fossa; alternatively, the right kidney is transplanted in the left iliac fossa. In either case, the renal pelvis is located medially, requiring that the kidney be rotated 180 degrees on its axis. Thus the posterior calyces point anteriorly and, consequently, an anterior approach to the kidney is similar to a posterior approach to native kidneys. In the usual percutaneous approach to a transplanted kidney the patient is placed in the lithotomy position, which allows simultaneous cystoscopic access to the bladder. A ureteral catheter is inserted for instillation of contrast material. Access is most safely established (i.e., avoiding intraperitoneal contents) into the lower pole with the skin puncture as caudal as possible. Percutaneous access to transplanted kidneys is actually facilitated by their superficial location. However, scar formation around the graft may make the initial needle puncture and tract dilation more difficult.

Patients with ectopic pelvic kidneys necessitate a different and more complicated approach for PCNL as a result of their unique anatomy. The pelvic kidney is retroperitoneal, posterior to the peritoneum and anterior to the sacrum. Interposing bowel loops between the kidney and the anterior abdominal wall prevent a direct puncture through the anterior abdominal wall. Laparoscopic-assisted PCNL technique for access to the kidney may be required. Alternatively, if laparoscopy will not be used to assist guidance and reflect intervening organs away from the anticipated course of percutaneous access, percutaneous access could be obtained using CT guidance (Fig. 94.16).

Staghorn Calculi or Complex Stones

Patients suffering from staghorn calculi or complex renal calculi remain a challenging problem for the practicing urologist. **Many staghorn stones are composed of struvite. The goal for patients with staghorn calculi should be stone free, because if all of the infected stone debris is not evacuated, urea-splitting bacteriuria may persist, which can ultimately lead to eventual stone regrowth.** PCNL techniques incorporating the use of flexible nephroscopy may provide for complete or nearly complete clearance of stone material at the time of the primary procedure.

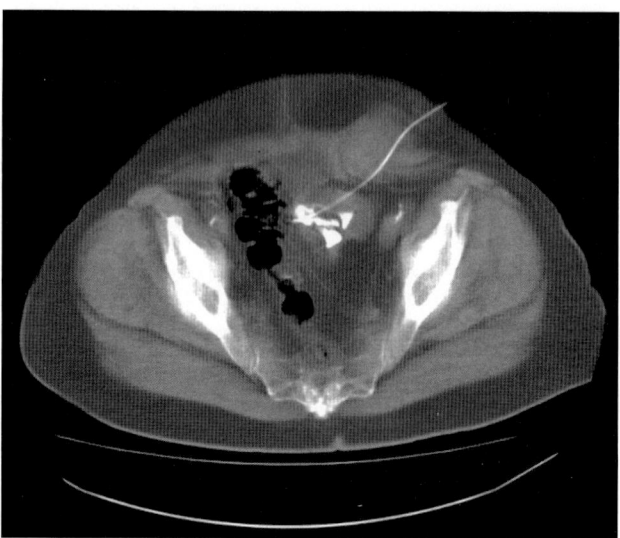

Fig. 94.16. Computed tomography–guided percutaneous access of a renal transplant for subsequent percutaneous nephrolithotomy procedure.

In general, if a single access tract is to be used in treating complex branching stones, the upper pole is preferred. An upper pole access allows for treatment of the upper pole, renal pelvis, and many lower pole stones using the rigid nephroscope. Midcalyceal stones can then be treated using a flexible nephroscope and holmium laser. When pressurized irrigant is used, the debris and fragments created by the holmium laser in most cases wash out the access sheath or into the renal pelvis, where it can be retrieved with the rigid nephroscope and suction.

Morbid Obesity

Patients with morbid obesity present technical as well as anesthetic challenges during any surgical intervention. General anesthesia may be a special concern for obese patients in the prone position because of restricted respiratory capacity that may require higher ventilation pressures intraoperatively. Multiple studies have not demonstrated an increase in overall morbidity in the obese patient undergoing PCNL. Pearle et al. (1998) were the first to examine the issue of PCNL among the obese and found that performing standard prone PCNL was not associated with an increased risk for morbidity; in fact, complication and transfusion rates as well as the length of hospitalization were no different compared with those in nonobese patients. However, a multi-institutional study of 3709 PCNL procedures performed across the globe found that complication rates were not associated with BMI, but patients with a higher BMI were more likely to have comorbid conditions, including chronic anticoagulation, and a lower overall stone-free rate (Fuller et al., 2012).

Positioning the morbidly obese patient for PCNL can be difficult; and in particular for large patients, two surgical tables may have to be secured together. Excessive body size may also be associated with rhabdomyolysis secondary to crush injuries from placement in the lateral approach; if this technique is used, care must be taken to minimize muscle crush injury. An important challenge in performing PCNL in the morbidly obese patient is the long distance from the skin to the collecting system, which may exceed the length of the working sheath or the length of the rigid nephroscope. Extralong Amplatz working sheaths (≥20 cm) and extralong rigid nephroscopes are now available that can overcome this challenge. Alternatively, the Amplatz sheath can be secured by a suture, allowing easy retrieval even when it migrates under the skin. On occasion, when the long Amplatz sheath is not sufficient to reach the kidney, an incision can be made through the subcutaneous tissue to the muscles of the flank and the PCNL tract created from the level of the muscle sheath. Another possibility is to dilate the tract and place a nephrostomy tube for 1 week to let the tract mature. In some cases, maturation of the tract allows the kidney to fall back posteriorly closer to the skin, allowing the use of standard nephroscopic instrumentation. Flexible nephroscopy also can be performed through the mature tract, reducing the necessity of rigid nephroscopy.

After stone removal, if a nephrostomy tube is placed, consideration should be given to the type of nephrostomy tube used. Tube displacement can occur in morbidly obese patients, so balloon-type catheters or re-entry Malecot catheters may be preferable. Alternatively, if a Cope loop catheter is used, placement of a ureteral catheter should be considered to ensure that access to the kidney is not lost should the nephrostomy tube become displaced.

Complications

Even for the most experienced urologist, complications can occur; up to 7% of patients undergoing PCNL suffer a major complication, and minor complications may be encountered in up to 25% of patients (Preminger et al., 2005). **Hemorrhage is a significant complication of PCNL.** Risk for hemorrhage has been associated with stone burden and operative duration. Bleeding from an arteriovenous fistula or pseudoaneurysm that requires angiographic embolization occurs in less than 1% of patients (Keoghane et al., 2013). Other potential complications include sepsis (postoperative temperature > 38.5°C [101.3°F] is found in almost one-fourth of patients undergoing PCNL), adjacent organ injury (bowel, spleen), failed access, and perforation of renal pelvis and ureter. The need for open surgery is rare and mostly reported as part of early experience in various studies. The mortality rate of PCNL is between 0.03% and 0.8% (de la Rosette et al., 2011). When supracostal puncture is performed, the risk for pneumothorax or pleural effusion requiring drainage can vary widely from 1.8% to as high as 8% in historical series (de la Rosette et al., 2011; Picus et al., 1986). Experience of the center performing the PCNL procedure also can contribute to overall complication rates and stone-free results. Opondo et al. (2012) evaluated PCNL performed at 96 centers worldwide. The results of their study found that as their institution case volume increased, so did stone-free rates. Complication rates and duration of stay diminished with increasing case volume after adjusting for stone burden and other cofactors. The highest stone-free results and lowest complication rates were observed in centers with more than 120 cases p1er year.

Because the kidney is an extremely vascular organ, some degree of bleeding occurs during every PCNL. Significant bleeding usually requires cessation of the procedure because of impaired visualization. In most cases the source of hemorrhage is venous, and placement of a nephrostomy tube is usually sufficient to control the bleeding. If bleeding persists despite the placement of a nephrostomy tube, then clamping the tube for a period of time may facilitate the tamponade of any bleeding points. If these measures do not control the hemorrhage, a Kaye nephrostomy tamponade balloon catheter should be placed. The Kaye nephrostomy tube incorporates a low-pressure 12-mm balloon that may be left inflated for prolonged periods to tamponade bleeding from the nephrostomy tract (Kaye and Clayman, 1986). If bleeding persists despite placement of a Kaye catheter, immediate angiography should be performed to identify a possible arteriovenous fistula or false aneurysm. Angiography is diagnostic and therapeutic, because arteriovenous fistulas and false aneurysms are best managed by embolization. In the rare event that bleeding cannot be controlled with angiography, partial nephrectomy may be required.

PCNL can lead to some absorption of irrigation fluid; therefore the use of physiologic irrigating solutions is mandatory. The amount of absorbed fluid depends mostly on the irrigant pressure and the length of the procedure; thus an Amplatz-type open sheath should be used. Larger amounts of fluid absorption may occur in the setting of collecting system perforation. Extravasation usually occurs into the retroperitoneal tissue and may be noted by medial displacement of the kidney during fluoroscopy. Minor perforations are common during PCNL; premature termination of the procedure usually is not necessary when a low-pressure system (e.g., Amplatz sheath) is being used. However, with more significant perforations, termination of the procedure and nephrostomy drainage are advisable. Intraperitoneal extravasation is a less common but potentially more serious complication than retroperitoneal extravasation. Because the patient is prone, abdominal distention may be difficult to recognize, although in such a situation the anesthesiologist generally notes a gradual rise in the patient's diastolic blood pressure with consequent narrowing of the pulse pressure and increase in central venous pressure. In advanced cases of a large-volume extravasation event, ventilation may become difficult because of increased abdominal pressure. Early recognition of major extravasation is crucial. Intraperitoneal extravasation may be treated by vigorous diuresis; alternatively, peritoneal drainage or even laparotomy may be required.

When a supracostal puncture is performed, extravasation of irrigant into the pleural cavity may occur. The use of an Amplatz-type access sheath tends to minimize extravasation into this space because intrarenal pressure remains low. The chest should be examined at the end of PCNL procedures in which a supracostal puncture is used. Fluoroscopy with use of the C-arm is usually sufficient to examine for pneumothorax or hydrothorax, but if the surgeon has a high index of suspicion for a thoracic complication, a chest radiograph may be obtained postoperatively. Should a pneumothorax or hydrothorax occur, aspiration may be sufficient because lung injury is extremely rare. Should the pneumothorax recur, a chest tube should be placed.

Colonic injury is an unusual complication and is often diagnosed on postoperative nephrostogram or CT imaging, although passage of gas or feculent material through the nephrostomy tract, intraoperative diarrhea, and hematochezia or peritonitis are signs of a possible colonic perforation. Typically, the injury is retroperitoneal; thus signs and symptoms of peritonitis are infrequent. If the perforation is extraperitoneal, management may be expectant, with placement of a ureteral catheter or double-J stent to decompress the collecting system and withdrawal of the nephrostomy tube from an intrarenal position to an intracolonic position to serve as a colostomy tube. The colostomy tube is left in place for a minimum of 7 days and removed after a nephrostogram or a retrograde pyelogram shows no communication between the colon and the kidney.

URETEROSCOPIC STONE MANAGEMENT

Basic ureteroscopic techniques and intracorporeal lithotripsy techniques have been reviewed elsewhere. In this section issues of anesthesia and specific points of technique and complications of ureteral stone management are reviewed.

The fundamental initiation of ureteroscopy is the advancement of the ureteroscope into the ureter. When the ureteral orifice is too narrow to accommodate the ureteroscope, dilation may be accomplished with serial dilators, balloons, or even the ureteroscope. The anatomy of male patients may not allow a rigid ureteroscope to be easily passed above the iliac vessels, but a flexible ureteroscope usually can be advanced over a guidewire. The entire ureter can be more easily accessed with a rigid ureteroscope in female patients. Once the stone is visualized, fragmentation with the lithotrite of choice is performed, as described elsewhere in this chapter.

For treatment of ureteral stones, multiple different devices are designed to prevent stone retropulsion from the ureter into the kidney during lithotripsy. These antiretropulsion devices are covered extensively elsewhere in this textbook. Their overall benefit is seen with semirigid ureteroscopy during cases when the surgeon wishes to avoid having to perform flexible nephroscopy of the kidney to retrieve a small fragment that may have traveled proximally at time of treatment of the ureteral stone.

When a retrograde ureteroscopic approach is used to treat patients with intrarenal calculi, two wires are placed initially. The flexible ureteroscope is passed over one working wire in a monorail fashion. Saline is used for irrigation. When an implement is present within the working channel, simple gravity irrigation is inadequate and pressurized irrigation is required. The holmium:YAG laser lithotripter is used in almost all cases. Stones in lower pole calyces can be treated in situ or moved, with flexible graspers or a basket, into a position that allows better visualization. A head-down patient position with the ipsilateral flank elevated may help with stone and fragment visualization because fragments tend to migrate superiorly and are thus more easily localized during treatment. If the stone is large, the collecting system often may become lined with fine dust and debris, which can obscure residual stones. Furthermore, poor visualization may lead to perforation. In such cases, either the irrigant in the intrarenal collecting system may be aspirated through the ureteroscope or a ureteral stent can be placed and the situation approached in a staged fashion.

Fragmentation of stones in situ in the lower pole can be challenging. If the lower pole infundibulum is accommodating, the most straightforward way to treat the stone is to engage it in a nitinol basket and displace it to the renal pelvis or an upper pole calyx. In this way it is generally a straight passage of the scope, with minimal deflection of the tip, which will simplify ureteroscopic laser lithotripsy. Residual fragments also should be more likely to evacuate spontaneously from the kidney.

If ureteral edema or injury is present after stone extraction, a postureteroscopy stent should be placed to prevent colic and obstruction. Multiple meta-analyses have found that for uncomplicated ureteroscopy, a ureteral stent may be safely omitted (Assimos et al., 2016a,b).

The use of a ureteral access sheath as an adjunct to ureteroscopy was initially described as a means to simplify access to the intrarenal collecting system. It was not until more than two decades later that the ureteral access sheath was rediscovered and refined, simplifying the deployment and safety of these devices. The present generation of ureteral access sheaths consists of a hydrophilic outer coating as well as a tapered transition from obturator to sheath, which facilitates their retrograde placement. The walls of the sheaths are designed not only for a slim profile but also for strength and often are reinforced so as to resist kinking. The use of an access sheath can decrease operating room time because it simplifies re-entry of the ureter during repeated ureteroscope insertions. An added benefit of ureteral access sheaths is that the use of a sheath has been reported to maintain low intrapelvic pressures during ureteroscopy (Rehman et al., 2003). In addition, as irrigating fluid drains through the access sheath external to the patient, the need for periodic emptying of the patient's bladder during a prolonged procedure is eliminated. However, potential drawbacks to the ureteral access sheath have been identified. Traxer and Thomas (2013) observed that ureteral injury can occur as a consequence of employing a ureteral access sheath.

Complications

As modern ureteroscopes have become smaller and less traumatic, as safer intracorporeal lithotripters have become widely available, and as a better understanding of the technical principles of ureteroscopy has been developed, the risk of complications arising from the management of ureteral stones has been steadily decreasing.

Fortunately, most of the complications caused by ureteral stones and their management respond favorably to simple drainage of urine with ureteral catheters or stents.

Perforation

As is true with most ureteroscopic complications, the incidence of ureteral perforation has decreased over time, as technology and technique continue to improve. In a series of ureteroscopic procedures reported in 1992, ureteral perforation was reported in approximately 15% of cases. More recent series report a perforation rate of 0 to 4% (Assimos et al., 2016a,b). **A number of actions may result in a ureteral perforation; some of the more commonly encountered scenarios include the splitting of a ureter after balloon dilation, forceful placement of ureteral access sheath, or a traumatic injury from forceful and misdirected manipulation of a stone.** In some cases an intracorporeal device such as a lithotrite or electrocautery can cause full-thickness damage to the ureter. Baskets and grasping devices also may cause injury, because in the process of grasping a stone or lesion it is possible to inadvertently snare part of the ureter, which may result in a perforation. As previously noted, placement of a ureteral access sheath may cause a ureteral perforation. In addition, pressurized irrigation can cause perforation or calyceal rupture. Finally, the risk for a ureteral perforation may be increased in the case of a prolonged ureteroscopic procedure, as visualization may decline because of bleeding and/or debris in the field and surgeon fatigue may develop. Therefore, if the procedure is difficult and not progressing, it is wise for the urologist to stop, place a stent, and plan for a staged procedure.

Adherence to the tenets of safe ureteroscopy will minimize the likelihood of a ureteral perforation. Nonetheless, such a complication may still occur, and it is important for the urologist to be familiar with the treatment of this event. **When a ureteral perforation is recognized, the ureteroscopic procedure should be terminated and a stent placed across the injury.** The risk for perforation underscores the importance of using saline as an irrigant to prevent electrolyte derangements resulting from fluid extravasation. In cases of a severe injury, with significant extravasation of fluid, a percutaneous nephrostomy drain also may be necessary. Urinoma can result from perforation as well and may have to be drained. Antibiotics should be given because of the risk for infected urine and abscess formation. In general, a stent should be left in place for approximately 4 weeks after injury. Subsequent imaging after ureteral stent removal is mandatory to evaluate for a proper healing and adequate drainage.

Stricture

The development of a postoperative ureteral stricture is one of the more serious complications that may occur after ureteroscopy. Approximately two decades ago, the reported incidence of ureteral stricture after ureteroscopy was as high as 10%. More recently, however, the incidence of a postoperative stricture is reported to be 3% to 6% (Assimos et al., 2016a,b). It is likely that the improvements in surgical technology and technique are responsible for this dramatic reduction.

Although the cause of a ureteral stricture is likely multifactorial, there are certain identifiable risk factors. Impacted stones, which are defined by the inability to pass a wire or catheter beyond the stone or stones that have been present and not moved for a prolonged period of time, can induce changes in the ureter, which increases the risk for stricture formation. Ureteral perforation also may increase the risk for stricture formation. It may be that an inflammatory response that results in devascularization and ischemia promotes this process, because such local changes can result in a cicatrization of the ureter. Patients with a history of ureteral surgery, pelvic radiation, and impacted stones are also at greater risk secondary to altered blood flow and poor healing. Devascularization injury can result in ureteral necrosis, which necessitates open or laparoscopic repair. However, some patients develop a ureteral stricture in the presence of no intraoperative misadventures, suggesting that there is much about this process that remains to be elucidated.

To reduce the risk for stricture, care should be taken during all parts of the procedure, because the traumas that may increase the risk for this event are many and varied. **Overly aggressive manipulation of a ureteroscope across a narrow segment of ureter as well as trauma or perforation from injudicious manipulation of intracorporeal devices or lithotrites may increase the risk for stricture. Because of the reported occurrence of a postoperative ureteral stricture even after an uncomplicated ureteroscopy, it is recommended that all patients undergo postoperative imaging after ureteroscopic instrumentation to ensure that such a complication is recognized.** Although most patients with a stricture are symptomatic, some may not be, so postureteroscopy imaging is recommended in all patients to exclude such cases of silent obstruction (Fulgham et al., 2013).

The management of a postureteroscopic ureteral stricture depends primarily on its length and location, although other factors such as the time elapsed since injury, nature of trauma, and patient-specific parameters merit consideration. The treatment of ureteral strictures is discussed elsewhere in this text.

Submucosal Stone and Lost Stone

The submucosal stone and the lost stone represent two points on a continuum of iatrogenic displacement of a ureteral calculus into the wall of the ureter. When the stone migrates only to the submucosa, a problematic complication can develop, because removal of such stones is difficult. If submucosal stones are encountered, laser excision followed by ureteral stent placement is recommended. Submucosal stones are of concern, because they can increase the risk for ureteral stricture formation.

Complete extrusion of a calculus, also known as a lost stone, can occur in the setting of a ureteral perforation. In most cases, if the fragment is completely outside the collecting system, it can be left in place. Attempts to retrieve the stone may exacerbate the injury and increase the risk for significant irrigant extravasation. When an extruded stone is recognized, the procedure should be terminated and a ureteral stent placed. Antibiotics should be administered to prevent the theoretical risk for abscess formation, although such a complication would be rare. One of the most serious sequelae of such an event is the later development of a ureteral stricture; for this reason patients who have calculus extrusion should undergo postoperative imaging, which will confirm the stone location. It is possible that, in the future, the lost stone could be confused for a ureteral stone, and it is important for the patient to be aware that such a situation exists.

Avulsion

Perhaps the most catastrophic complication that can occur during a ureteroscopic procedure is avulsion of the ureter. Fortunately, such a complication is a rare occurrence, reported in less than 0.06% to 0.5% of all cases (Bader et al., 2012). **Ureteral avulsion generally occurs as a consequence of overly forceful manipulation of a large or impacted calculus; however, a scabbard effect also can be created with resulting avulsion at time of scope withdrawal if too large a rigid ureteroscope is forcefully advanced up the ureter.** It has been reported that the proximal third of the ureter may be at greatest risk for avulsion, because it is the portion of the ureter that has the least muscular tissue support. A ureteral avulsion is usually diagnosed when a portion of the ureter is withdrawn from the patient, along with the stone and basket or grasper.

There are a number of maneuvers the urologist can undertake to avoid a ureteral avulsion. **Blind basketing, the removal of a ureteral calculus without the aid of endoscopy, may increase the risk for ureteral avulsion and should never be considered an appropriate method of stone extraction.** In fact, even endoscopically guided basketing should be reserved for small stones only. In general, a safe ureteroscopic procedure relies on the placement of safety and working guidewires. **Before stone in a basket or grasping device is engaged, it should be endoscopically evaluated to determine if it is of a size that would be likely to be extracted out of the ureter. When the stone is engaged in the basket or grasper, the stone and device should both be kept under direct vision as they are extracted so that the size of the stone can be continually compared with the size of the ureteral lumen.** If the stone appears to be too large to be removed intact, it should be fragmented into smaller pieces that may either pass spontaneously or be extracted. If a stone too large to pass through the ureter is inadvertently engaged with a basket or grasping device, it should be released or replaced more proximally. If it is not possible to release the stone, the basket should be disassembled and the ureteroscope passed alongside the basket and the entrapped stone fragmented in situ. The use of a grasping device, rather than a basket, may simplify the release of an entrapped stone. The great benefit of having a safety wire in place is that should a stone become entrapped in the ureter, a ureteral stent may be placed that will passively dilate the upper urinary tract and perhaps permit a more straightforward procedure at a later date.

Should a ureteral avulsion occur, a reasoned and considered approach to the management of the affected patient is advised. Although it may be tempting to perform an immediate primary repair at the time of injury, in general a delayed repair is recommended. The patient should undergo immediate diversion of the renal unit with the placement of a percutaneous nephrostomy drain. In some cases, a urinoma may develop as a consequence of urinary extravasation; these collections are generally amenable to percutaneous drainage. Subsequent ureteral reconstruction techniques depend on the location of the injury and the amount of viable ureter that remains. For extensive injuries the treatment options are generally limited to ileal interposition (ileal ureter) or renal autotransplantation. Although a transureteroureterostomy may be a replacement option for some patients who have a ureteral injury, this repair technique is contraindicated in stone formers. For a more distal ureteral injury, a ureteral reimplantation with either a psoas hitch or Boari flap also may be successful. Nephrectomy has been reported to be an option for these patients as well; however, given the recurrent nature of stone disease and the fact that stone formers may be at increased risk for hypertension and diabetes, this approach is controversial.

INTRACORPOREAL LITHOTRIPSY

Ureteroscopy and PCNL occupy an essential place in the treatment of urinary calculi as increasing technologic advancements allow easier access to stones in all parts of the kidney and ureter. In particular, improvements in ureteroscopic equipment emphasize the need for appropriate and effective miniaturized intracorporeal lithotripsy devices. Although smaller ureteral stones may be extracted intact, larger ureteral stones require lithotripsy to permit the safe extraction of calculus fragments. The fragmentation of renal stones during PCNL requires an approach different from that applied to during ureteroscopy. Although small and flexible endoscopic lithotrites are essential for the occasional difficult-to-approach kidney stone, renal stones can usually be visualized with a rigid nephroscope. In such situations, with a large kidney stone burden, the efficiency of the lithotrite is the most important requirement and size and flexibility are of secondary importance. The urologist who treats patients with urolithiasis thus requires an armamentarium of intracorporeal lithotripsy devices, each maximizing a different quality (e.g., size, flexibility, efficiency).

Four technologies are available for intracorporeal lithotripsy: EHL, laser lithotripsy, ultrasonic lithotripsy, and ballistic lithotripsy. These techniques can be divided into those lithotrites that are flexible (laser lithotripsy and EHL) and those that are rigid (ultrasonic and ballistic lithotripsy). In the following sections, we review the mechanisms, advantages, disadvantages, and surgical techniques of the various flexible and rigid intracorporeal lithotripters.

Flexible Lithotripters

Electrohydraulic Lithotripsy

The EHL probe is essentially an underwater spark plug composed of two concentric electrodes of different voltage polarities separated by insulation. When a current sufficient to overcome the insulative gap is applied, a spark is produced. The spark discharge causes the explosive formation of a plasma channel and vaporization of the water surrounding the electrode. The rapidly expanding plasma causes a hydraulic shock wave followed by formation of a cavitation bubble (Fig. 94.17). Depending on the proximity of the probe to the stone surface, the collapse of the cavitation bubble may be symmetrical (at a distance of ~1 mm from the stone), resulting in a strong secondary shock wave, or asymmetrical (at a distance equivalent to a maximum bubble radius of ~3 mm), leading to the formation of high-speed microjets (Vorreuther et al., 1995; Zhong et al., 1997). **Unlike in SWL the shock wave is not focused, so the stone must be placed where the shock wave is generated.** The first EHL probes developed were of larger diameters (9 Fr) and, because of their size, had a narrow margin of safety. Later improvements in technology allowed the development of smaller probes, from 1.6 to 5 Fr, that were safer and had the ability to be passed through small-diameter,

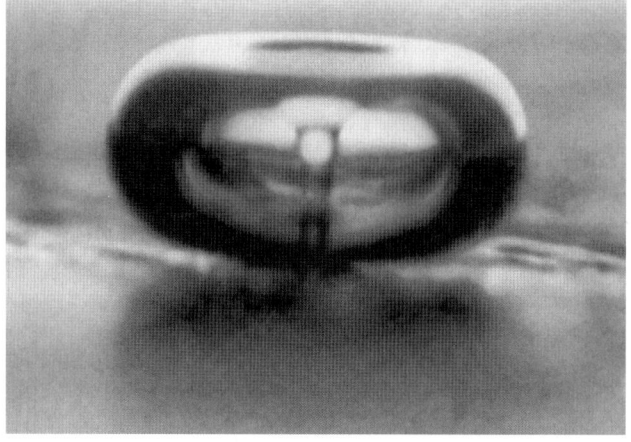

Fig. 94.17. Photograph of liquid microjet produced by an asymmetrically collapsing cavitation bubble. (Courtesy Dr. Larry Crum.)

flexible ureteroscopes without occluding the irrigation or working channel.

Advantages and Disadvantages. EHL was, at one point, a commonly used intracorporeal lithotrite because of its low cost and the flexible nature of its probes. However, the major disadvantage of EHL is its propensity to damage the ureteral mucosa and its association with ureteral perforation. The mechanism of damage caused by EHL is the expansion of the cavitation bubble, and thus injury may occur even when the probe is not in direct contact with the mucosa. The diameter of the cavitation bubble depends on the energy used and can expand to more than 1.5 cm when energies greater than 1300 mJ are employed. Therefore **the risk for perforation is greater with higher energies, such as in treatment of a hard stone.** Primarily because of the propensity for ureteral damage, EHL has become less commonly used as an intracorporeal lithotrite.

Laser Lithotripsy

Laser is an acronym for *light amplification by stimulated emission of radiation*, which is a concise description of how a laser works. Laser energy is produced when an atom is stimulated by an external energy source, which creates a population of electrons in an excited state. These excited or higher energy electrons can release their excess energy in the form of photons or light energy. Laser light differs from natural light in that it is coherent (all photons are in phase with one another), collimated (photons travel parallel to each other), and monochromatic (all photons have the same wavelength). These unique features of laser light allow considerable energy to be transmitted in a highly concentrated manner. Lasers are named after the medium that generates their specific wavelength of light; for example, the laser was developed in 1960 and the first medium used was the ruby. Although the ruby laser could effectively fragment urinary calculi, this continuous-wave laser simply heats the stone until vaporization occurs, which requires the laser to generate heat greater than the melting point of the stone. Consequently, it generated excessive heat and was not appropriate for clinical use. A solution for this problem came with the development of pulsed lasers: the application of pulsed energy results in high-power density at the stone's surface but little heat dissipation. The first widely available laser lithotrite was the pulsed-dye laser, which employed a coumarin green dye as the liquid laser medium. Although the coumarin pulsed-dye laser represented a major advancement in intracorporeal lithotripsy, there were a number of significant drawbacks to this technology: stones of certain composition (calcium oxalate monohydrate, cystine) would not fragment well or even at all; coumarin dye is a toxic agent and required cumbersome disposal procedures; the required eye protection made visualization of the stone and fiber difficult.

Continued technologic advancements eventually led to the development of the holmium:YAG laser. The holmium laser is a solid-state laser system that operates at a wavelength of 2140 nm in the pulsed mode. Pulse duration of the holmium laser ranges from 250 to 350 microseconds and is substantially longer than the pulse duration in pulsed-dye lasers. The holmium laser is highly absorbed by water; because tissues are composed mainly of water, the majority of the holmium laser energy is absorbed superficially, which results in superficial cutting or ablation. **The zone of thermal injury associated with laser ablation ranges from 0.5 to 1.0 mm** (Wollin and Denstedt, 1998). The mechanism of stone fragmentation of the holmium:YAG laser is different from that of the pulsed-dye lasers. **The long holmium:YAG pulse duration produces an elongated cavitation bubble that generates only a weak shock wave,** in contradistinction to the strong shock wave produced by short-pulse lasers. Therefore **holmium laser lithotripsy occurs primarily through a photothermal mechanism that causes stone vaporization** (Wollin and Denstedt, 1998).

Advantages and Disadvantages. The holmium:YAG laser can transmit its energy through a flexible fiber, which facilitates intracorporeal lithotripsy throughout the entire collecting system. However, compared with EHL, the holmium:YAG laser is safer and more efficient. Whereas EHL may cause injury to the ureter even when the probe is activated several millimeters away from the ureteral wall, because of its low depth of penetration the holmium laser may be safely activated at a distance of 0.5 to 1 mm from the ureteral wall. **The ability of the holmium laser to fragment all stones regardless of composition is a clear advantage** over the coumarin pulsed-dye laser. Successful fragmentation of ureteral stones of all compositions has been reported, and perforation and stricture rates are generally low. During PCNL the holmium laser is most helpful in clearing smaller stones (<2 cm) when the use of flexible instruments is required for access to stones in a calyx remote from the nephrostomy site. The **holmium laser is one of the safest, most effective, and most versatile intracorporeal lithotripters.** Further advantages of the holmium laser include its production of significantly smaller fragments compared with other lithotrites. These small fragments are easily irrigated out of the collecting system, which reduces the need for extraction of the fragments with basket or grasping devices. **The holmium laser produces a weak shock wave, which reduces the likelihood of retropulsion of the stone** or stone fragments compared with EHL or pneumatic lithotrites. The degree of retropulsion can be further modulated with both laser fiber size as well as laser settings, such as the pulse duration. Additional advantages of the holmium laser include that the required eye protection for the holmium laser does not compromise the ureteroscopic view of the stone or the fiber. In fact, the holmium laser properties are such that with use of energy levels applied for stone disease (i.e., less than 15 W), the operator's cornea would be damaged only if it were positioned at a distance of 10 cm or less from the fiber (Scarpa et al., 1999).

The major disadvantage of the holmium laser is the initial high cost of the device and the cost of the laser fibers. However, **the holmium laser has multiple soft-tissue applications and can be used to treat patients with benign prostatic hyperplasia, strictures, and urothelial tumors.** In addition, certain models of laser fiber are reusable, so the effective cost of the holmium laser device and reusable fibers may be further controlled.

The thulium fiber laser has emerged as a potential therapeutic alternative to the holmium laser, because it may hold several advantages over the holmium platform. Its laser fibers are smaller, which may permit improved endoscope deflection and irrigation flow. At present, though, its use in lithotripsy remains is not well defined.

Technique. The technique of holmium laser lithotripsy is relatively straightforward and involves placement of the fiber on the stone surface before the laser is activated. Clear vision is essential at all times to ensure the fiber maintains near contact to the stone. After initiation of holmium laser lithotripsy, a short pause is often required because of the "snowstorm effect" created by the scattering of minute stone fragments, which can be cleared by endoscopic irrigation. Caution must be exercised in operating the holmium laser near a guidewire or a basket because **the holmium laser is capable of cutting through metal.** Furthermore, the laser fiber should extend at least 2 mm beyond the tip of the endoscope to avoid destroying the lens system or the working channel of the endoscope. It is preferred that baskets used to stabilize calculi during laser lithotripsy should be composed of nitinol rather than stainless steel because should the holmium laser inadvertently transect the nitinol basket, the material will retain its basket shape and not cause a sharply barbed effect as stainless steel would. Holmium laser fibers are available in a variety of sizes, generally ranging from 200-, 365-, 550-, and 1000-μm diameters as well as end- or side-firing fibers. However, only the 200- and 365-μm fibers are used for flexible intracorporeal lithotripsy, as larger fibers cannot be accommodated in an endoscope's working channel.

Early in the introduction of Holmium laser lithotripsy, it was noted that altering the treatment parameters affected the efficiency of fragmentation and risk of retropulsion. For example, low pulse energy (0.2 J) led to smaller fragments and less retropulsion at the cost of fragmentation efficiency. Some Holmium laser devices can also provide the ability to modulate the pulse duration. A longer laser pulse duration (700 μs or 1500 μs) as compared with a traditional pulse duration (300 μs or 350 μs) has been demonstrated in in vitro studies to provide effective stone comminution while reducing laser fiber tip degradation and stone retropulsion. To maximize efficiency of Holmium laser lithotripsy, shorter pulse durations with higher pulse energy has been recommended because low frequency (5 Hz) and high pulse energy (1.2 J) leads to more efficient stone ablation as manifested by deeper and wider stone fissures.

Laser Lithotripsy Approaches

Fragmentation and Extraction. Initially, ureteroscopic laser lithotripsy relied on an approach whereby stones were broken into fragments and then retrieved from the kidney with basket devices. Often a ureteral access sheath was used to facilitate repeated passages of the ureteroscope as the fragments were extracted. Laser setting requirements for fragmentation with extraction generally rely on combination energy settings such as 0.6 to 1.0 J along with rates of 6 to 10 Hz. In vitro studies as well as clinical practice has demonstrated that these settings create stone fragments that are larger and ideal for removing with extraction devices. A common technique is to begin with a relatively low energy and rate setting (e.g., 0.6 J, 6 Hz) and only increase if necessary. This technique not only maximizes laser tip preservation but also minimizes retropulsion or stone movement during lithotripsy.

A ureteral access sheath may expedite access, fragmentation, and subsequent clearance of the targeted stone. The midportion of the stone is typically targeted first, with the goal of breaking the stone into halves. Beginning in the midportion of the stone additionally maximizes the margin of safety between the laser fiber and the ureteral or renal wall. The generated fragments can then be sequentially further fragmented in the same fashion until they appear to be a retrievable size. A small caliber nitinol grasper or basket is used to effect stone clearance. Active extraction continues until all visible fragments have been cleared.

The process of fragmenting and retrieving kidney stones may hold several advantages. Stone composition may direct metabolic intervention to help prevent future stone episodes; absence of this information may limit the specificity of patient counseling. If residual stone material is left behind at the time of initial stone treatment, patients may also be at increased risk for future stone events. Chew et al. looked at the natural history of asymptomatic stone fragments left behind after URS and found that only 56% of patients required no intervention and remained asymptomatic (Chew et al., 2016).

Dusting. As later-generation holmium consoles were introduced, there developed an ability to increase the pulse rate to much higher levels; pulse rates of 50 Hz became commonplace on 100-watt Holmium lasers. Investigations of the clinical effects of these higher pulse rates found that they yielded smaller stone fragments. Ultimately, an approach developed, termed "dusting," which relied on lower pulse energy and higher pulse frequencies to fragment the stone into fine debris that could be left in situ in the kidney and then spontaneously be expelled by the patient.

A concern with a dusting approach is that there is some uncertainty as to the likelihood of passive fragment clearance. However, a prospective multicenter study of dusting versus fragmentation with stone retrieval for renal stones 15 mm or less in diameter demonstrated that in the short term, there was no difference in readmission rates, reintervention rates, or patients becoming symptomatic from residual fragments. An additional recent study, examining ureteroscopy with lithotripsy for stones 10 to 40 mm noted that active fragment retrieval using a nitinol basket was not associated with improvements in stone-free rates.

Dusting may also confer advantages in patient outcomes. For example, dusting has been associated with shorter operative times because of omission of active fragment retrieval. Another potential advantage for dusting is decrease in use of ureteral access sheaths, which may lead to decreases in ureteral trauma. However, the relationship between such ureteral trauma and subsequent ureteral stricture formation is not yet well defined. Because active retrieval is not performed during dusting, basket-associated complications can be reduced. In addition, because there is less of a need for multiple implements to be passed through the ureteroscope's working channel, there may be greater scope longevity with this approach.

The goal of dusting is to fragment the stone into tiny pieces that resemble "dust" and thus can pass spontaneously. This is accomplished by using the Holmium laser at a very high frequency with very low energy. Typical settings will depend on the laser console being used; for low-power lasers, a rate of 15 or 20 Hz may be upper limit of what can be achieved. However, for higher-power lasers, such as a 100-watt laser, a rate of 50 Hz or even higher may be achieved. The technique of dusting involves moving the laser fiber tangentially from the very edge of the stone and taking care not to break off large fragments from the main stone. As the procedure progresses, the surgeon should continue to treat the edges of the stone circumferentially or from one leading edge to the other.

The other principle involved in dusting is to keep the laser fiber slightly off of the stone, which "defocuses" it and minimizes the mechanical acoustic effect of the laser energy. Accounting for respiratory renal movement is also important. Fine movements of the hand holding the tip of the ureteroscope as it enters into the urethra or a fine movement of the thumb-activated deflecting cables allows the surgeon to "paint" the stone from the edge toward the middle of the stone. At the beginning of the case, the laser energy is typically less than the mass of the stone and the stone does not tend to move very much and stays in place. Once the stone is ablated down to a smaller mass, the laser energy becomes greater than the stone fragment and the stone will start to bounce within the calyx, making it more difficult to shave the stone from the edges. When this happens, one can either extract the remaining pieces or place the laser fiber safely in the middle of the calyx and keep discharging the laser as fragments come into contact with the fiber—a technique known as "popcorning." Fragments may be deemed small enough to pass when they are of 1 to 2 mm. The most commonly used technique to measure stone size is to compare to a structure of known size that is in the surgical field such as a guidewire or laser fiber.

Rigid Lithotripters

Ballistic Lithotripsy

Ballistic lithotripsy relies on energy generated by the movement of a projectile (Fig. 94.18). The initial movement of the projectile can be induced by a variety of stimuli, but once the projectile is in contact with another object, the ballistic energy is transferred to the object. Flexible objects preserve the momentum of the energy, but inflexible objects, such as a stone, fragment on impact (a "jackhammer" effect).

Advantages and Disadvantages. **Ballistic lithotrites provide an effective means for stone fragmentation in the entire urinary tract, with a wide margin of safety.** Successful fragmentation of ureteral stones of all compositions can be accomplished with a ballistic device. Ballistic devices may be especially advantageous when large or hard stones are encountered during PCNL or endoscopic lithotripsy of bladder calculi. In contrast to ureteral stones, kidney stones are easily "pinned down" against the urothelium during ballistic lithotripsy,

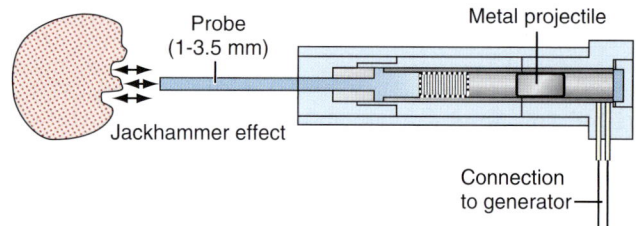

Fig. 94.18. Schematic illustration of the LithoClast (Electromedical Systems, Kaufering, Germany) hand piece mechanism. An oscillating pellet provides ballistic energy to the probe, resulting in a jackhammer-like effect on calculi. (Courtesy Dr. John Denstedt.)

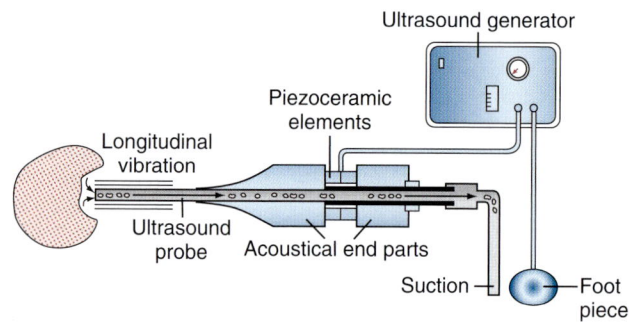

Fig. 94.19. Ultrasound lithotripsy generator and hand piece.

allowing a rapid and more efficient fragmentation method than ultrasonic lithotripsy. Once the bulk of the calculus is fragmented, lithotripsy can be completed with the ultrasonic lithotripter, which can also aspirate minute stone fragments. Compared with EHL, ultrasonic lithotripsy, and laser lithotripsy, ballistic devices have a significantly lower risk for ureteral perforation. Furthermore, because no heat is produced during lithotripsy, the risk for thermal injury to the urothelium is eliminated. An additional advantage of ballistic lithotrites is their relatively low cost and low maintenance because there are may be no disposable costs and the probes have an extremely long life span.

Disadvantages of ballistic devices include the rigid nature of the technology, which requires ureteroscopes or nephroscopes with straight working channels. In addition, **ballistic lithotripsy is associated with a relatively high rate of stone retropulsion** because of their mechanism of action. In some cases, failure to fragment a stone may be related to an inability to trap a ureteral stone in a capacious ureter.

Technique. Like other lithotrites, the ballistic lithotripter should be activated only when there is a clear view of the stone and the probe position can be identified. Fixation of the stone is rarely difficult in the kidney or the bladder but may be a problem in the ureter. Fixation of ureteral stones with a basket or proximal placement of a ureteral occlusion device is sometimes necessary. The goal of ballistic lithotripsy in the ureter is to generate fragments that are small enough to permit spontaneous passage (<2 mm). Larger fragments have to be removed with a basket or grasping device.

Ultrasonic Lithotripsy

Ultrasonic lithotripsy relies on the properties of ultrasound vibrations that fragment brittle renal calculi. The ultrasound probe works by applying electrical energy to excite a piezoceramic plate in the ultrasound transducer (Fig. 94.19). The plate resonates at a specific frequency and generates ultrasonic waves at a frequency of 23,000 to 25,000 Hz. At operating frequencies there is no audible sound, although 98 dB of ultrasonic inaudible noise levels have been measured.

Ultrasound energy is transformed into longitudinal and transverse vibrations of the hollow steel probe, which then transmits the energy to the calculus. The probe tip causes the stone to resonate at high frequency and to break; but when the probe is placed on compliant tissue, such as urothelium, damage is minimal because the tissue does not resonate with the vibrational energy. Although some heat may develop at the end of the probe during lithotripsy, continuous irrigation through the endoscope minimizes any temperature increase at the tip of the probe. Because irrigation may be limited during ureteroscopy, **ultrasonic lithotripsy is more efficient during PCNL because of the greater flow of irrigant through the larger diameter ultrasonic probes that can be used**. The ultrasonic lithotripter system is connected to suction so that debris from the stone is removed continuously with the irrigating fluid during lithotripsy. In addition, the flow of fluid through the hollow probe cools the instrument. Heating of the ultrasound transducer should alert the surgeon to possible occlusion in the probe lumen, an occurrence more commonly encountered with small-diameter probes that are used in the ureter. Ultrasonic probes are available at sizes ranging from 2.5 to 12 Fr. The 2.5-Fr probe is solid and contains no hollow center for suction. Therefore, when it is used in the ureter, heat dissipation is slow.

Stones vary in their susceptibility to destruction with ultrasound. Although the chemical composition of the stone influences the time required for complete disintegration (cystine, calcium oxalate monohydrate, and uric acid being the most resistant to fragmentation), the size, density, and surface structure of the calculus appear to be more important. Smaller stones are more rapidly destroyed, as are rough stones. Smooth-surfaced large stones may be more difficult to fragment.

Advantages and Disadvantages. The major advantage of ultrasonic lithotripsy is the efficient combination of stone fragmentation and simultaneous fragment removal. Fragments smaller than 2 mm are aspirated through the hollow lithotrite along with the irrigation fluid. Larger fragments may be removed with forceps or baskets. The efficiency of this technique coupled with the minimal risk for serious tissue damage has made this technology popular.

However, the rigid nature of ultrasonic probes and their small diameter limit the appeal of this technology in treatment of ureteral stones. A ureteroscope with a straight working channel is required. Furthermore, a relatively large 5-Fr working channel is needed to accommodate the 4.5-Fr hollow probe.

Technique. When ultrasonic lithotripsy is applied during PCNL the stone should first be trapped between the probe and the urothelium. The application of gentle pressure to the stone enhances fragmentation, but the temptation to push too hard should be avoided because calculi can easily be pushed through the urothelium. The risk for perforation increases with smaller or more ruggedly surfaced stones because the force applied to the stone is transferred to a smaller surface area of the urothelium. The risk for perforation is particularly high in the thin-walled renal pelvis or ureter rather than in a calyx that is backed by renal parenchyma.

When ureteral stones are treated, the ureter may have to be dilated to allow passage of the offset rigid ureteroscope. The ultrasonic probe is passed through the working channel and placed directly on the stone. If necessary, the stone can be engaged in a stone basket to prevent proximal migration. As with other intracorporeal lithotripsy devices the goal of treatment is either to fragment the stone completely or to generate fragments that are small enough to be extracted or passed spontaneously.

Combination Ballistic and Ultrasonic Devices

Several manufacturers have introduced combined ultrasonic and pneumatic devices that aim to combine the superior fragmentation ability of the pneumatic component with the ability of the ultrasonic modality to simultaneously evacuate stone fragments. Broadly speaking, the combination devices are used in a similar fashion as the stand-alone units. The target stone is identified, and continuous gentle pressure is applied via the lithotrite, until fragmentation and evacuation occur. These devices have been evaluated in multiple clinical studies. Chu et al. (2013) also investigated whether pneumatic, ultrasonic, or combination devices had an effect on postoperative fever. A study of more than 5000 patients collated through the Clinical Research Office of the Endourological Society found that the lithotrite had no effect (Chu et al., 2013). York et al. performed a prospective randomized controlled trial at nine different centers between 2009 and 2016. The authors compared the Cyberwand, a dual-probe ultrasonic device, the Lithoclast Select, a combination pneumatic and ultrasonic device, and the Stone Breaker, a portable pneumatic device. Ultimately, they found no difference in stone clearance rates, and overall safety and efficacy were comparable. Perhaps the technology of the lithotrite is of secondary importance to the technique of the surgeon.

LAPAROSCOPIC AND ROBOTIC STONE REMOVAL

The surgical technique and outcomes of laparoscopic and robotic stone surgery are discussed in subsequent chapters; the focus of the following section is a brief overview of the role of laparoscopic and robotic procedures in the modern era of stone surgery. The advent of laparoscopic and subsequently robotic renal and ureteral stone removal procedures has provided the urologist with another means to circumvent open stone surgery. However, because of higher morbidity and longer hospitalization, a laparoscopic or robotic approach to stone removal should be considered only if the results with SWL or endoscopic approaches are expected to be poor (Assimos et al., 2016a,b).

In certain cases a laparoscopic or robotic approach may be considered a preferred therapy. Situations that may benefit from a laparoscopic approach include pyeloplasty with pyelolithotomy; patients harboring stones in poorly functioning polar areas or with nonfunctioning kidneys; pelvic kidneys containing a large stone volume, in which laparoscopic techniques can be used to reflect overlying bowel, allowing pyelolithotomy or percutaneous stone removal; and ureterolithotomy for the extremely rare endoscopic failure or large/multiple impacted ureteral calculi. Such procedures can be technically demanding and require a skilled laparoscopic/robotic surgeon to be performed with minimal morbidity. In present practice, the use of laparoscopy and robotics in the treatment of renal calculi continues to be limited; Desai and Assimos (2008) reported that only 1% of patients undergo such an approach, with the most common indication being renal stones with a concomitant UPJ obstruction.

See Videos 94.1, 94.2, 94.3, and 94.4 for procedures related to this chapter.

REFERENCES

The complete reference list is available online at ExpertConsult.com.

Lower Urinary Tract Calculi

Arvind P. Ganpule, MS, DNB, and Mahesh R. Desai, MS, FRCS

HISTORY

The significance of subspecialization in urology was realized centuries ago when Hippocrates said, "I will not cut for stone, even for patients in whom the disease manifest, I will leave this operation to be performed by practitioners" (Herr, 2008). The history of urolithiasis dates back to the Greek, Egyptian, and the Indus Valley civilizations (Ellis, 1979). Shattock (1905) described what may be the earliest known case of lower urinary tract stone disease in a gravesite in Egypt from a 16-year-old boy. This dates back to approximately 4800 BCE (Shattock, 1905). It was well known in those days that the approach to the bladder stone involved a perineal, suprapubic, and transurethral approach (Ellis, 1979). The term *lithotomy* was coined sometime in 276 BCE by the Greek Ammonius; the writings of the same were described by Roman Cornelius Celsius 300 years later (Herr, 2008; Parladidius et al., 2007). Celsius was credited with operating on a patient with the first perineal urethrotomy. It involved restraining the patient in a lithotomy position. He described this as "methodus celsiana." In Italy, Marianas introduced a simple operation that he termed *apparatus minor*. The term *minor* was used because no instruments were used, and the stone was retrieved by a large incision on the anus in the perineum. Subsequently, an *apparatus major* operation was described; the term *major* was used because a large number of instruments were used in the operation (Ellis, 1979).

Jean Civiale is credited for developing the art of lithotrity. He operated on Leopold I for a bladder stone. Sir Henry Thompson was credited with the development of operation of lithotrity. A British excavation revealed a bladder stone in a middle-aged man. It was concluded in the archaeological findings that the stone was most likely formed as a result of bladder outlet obstruction (BOO) (Anderson, 2001).

There has been a paradigm shift in the size and the location of stones seen in the lower urinary tract. In the past 50 years, the incidence of vesical calculus has steadily declined in the Western world. The underdeveloped nations continue to see instances of vesical calculi particularly in children (Schwartz and Stoller, 2000).

ETIOPATHOGENESIS OF BLADDER CALCULI

Bladder stones are the most common manifestation of lower urinary tract lithiasis, **accounting for 5% of all the urinary stone diseases and approximately 1.5% of urologic hospital admissions** in the Western world (Schwartz and Stoller, 2000; Smith and O'Flynn, 1975). Bladder calculi in nonendemic areas are commonly found in adults and are secondary to some other disease process. In endemic areas, the calculi are seen frequently in children and do not exist with other anomalies (Schwartz and Stoller, 2000). The dietary intake and socioeconomic conditions are responsible for its occurrence (Andersen, 1962; Asper, 1984). **Traditionally, the bladder stones are classified as migrant, primary idiopathic, or secondary** (Phillippou et al., 2012). Primary bladder stones usually are described as those that form without any predisposing cause, whereas a secondary cause is found in most patients with certain predisposing causes.

Primary bladder stones are historically associated with nutritional deficiency. These are known to be rampant in undernourished or nutritionally compromised individuals. They are prevalent in North Africa and the Middle East (Ashworth, 1990). The cause for formation of these calculi is believed to be a combination of decreased urine output, alteration in the urine PH, and other metabolic abnormalities. Vitamin deficiency and dietary compromise in the form of deficient animal proteins is responsible for the genesis of these stones. Children in endemic areas consume a cereal-based diet that is poor in animal protein and low in phosphate (Teotia and Teotia, 1990; Thalut et al., 1976; Van Reen, 1980). Low dietary intake of phosphates leads to hypophosphaturia, promoting the precipitation of calcium oxalate and ammonium acid urate. It has been proposed that in endemic areas in addition to the earlier-mentioned factors that a diet rife with oxalates leads to hyperoxaluria, leading to calcium oxalate stones (Teotia and Teotia, 1990). The primary bladder stones are known to form within the first 5 years of life and have a male preponderance (Phillippou et al., 2012). **Primary bladder calculi are most common in children younger than the age of 10 with a peak incidence at 2 to 4 years. The disease is much more common in boys than in girls with ratios ranging from 9:1 to as high as 33:1.** Primary bladder stones are most commonly solitary and rarely recur after removal (Teotia and Teotia, 1990; Van Reen, 1980). The composition of primary bladder stone is commonly ammonium acid urate, calcium oxalate, uric acid, and calcium phosphate (Valyasevi and Van Reen, 1968).

Secondary bladder stones are always associated with an underlying bladder pathology. In the Western world typically they are found in men older than 60 and usually in concert with lower urinary tract obstruction. Bladder calculi are known to occur de novo in the bladder, but sometimes they **may migrate from the upper tract and fail to expel 3% to 17% of bladder calculi** (Douenias et al., 1991; Smith and O'Flynn, 1975). The frequent absence of calcium oxalate in the nucleus of the bladder stones further argues against upper tract origin (Douenias et al., 1991). **The commonly implicated factors are foreign bodies such as migrated intrauterine devices** (Chow, 1997); **intravaginal gynecologic accessories such as pessaries, diaphragms** (Cumming, 1997), **and eroded clips** (Desai and Ganpule, 2017; Tugcu et al., 2009); **and causes leading to significant postvoid residue (BOO resulting from stricture, benign prostatic hyperplasia, neurogenic bladders, urinary diversion, bladders, bladder neck contractions)** (Douenias et al., 1991). A few reported but uncommon causes of intravesical foreign bodies leading to bladder calculi formation are erosion of wire used for cerclage (Ehrenpreis et al., 1986), unrecognized anorectal impalement (Guha et al., 2012), eroded silk sutures used in dorsal vein complex (Miller et al., 1992; Scheidler et al., 1990), migration of brachytherapy seeds (Leapman et al., 2014; Miyazawa et al., 2012), and hair as a nidus after clean intermittent catheterization (Derry and Nuseibeh, 1997).

Long-term urinary catheters are one of the causative factors for bladder stone formation. The incidence is 0.7% to 2.2% in chronic indwelling catheters (Kohler-Ockmore and Feneley, 1996). Retained fragments of burst Foley balloon catheters are responsible for nidus formation (Smith and O'Flynn, 1975). Crystal formation has been implicated in formation of these stones. Homogenous nucleation rarely is to be blamed for crystallization in this entity. Heterogeneous nucleation occurs around the foreign body as a result of infection or because of obstruction with resulting supersaturation (Schwartz and Stoller, 2000).

Among the neurogenic bladder patients, those with spinal cord injury are more prone to form bladder stones (Chen et al., 2001; Ord et al., 2003). In a study by Hall 29% of patients with spinal cord injuries had bladder calculi. The factors implicated included complete neurologic lesion, urinary tract infection caused by *Klebsiella*, and Caucasian race (DeVivo, 1985; Hall, 1989). Thus continuous mucosal injury with resulting chronic inflammation secondary to indwelling Foley or chronic bladder calculi could substantiate the deficiency of glycosaminoglycan layer in these patients (Schwartz and Stoller, 2000).

In a large series, Takasaki et al. (1979) found that 52% of all stones had magnesium ammonium phosphate. In this large series no females had uric acid stones as compared with 7.7% of males.

Drugs have been implicated as a causative factor in a number of locations of urolithiasis. **Triamterene, a diuretic, is associated with urolithiasis** because it inhibits sodium reabsorption in the distal tubule. There have been reports of triamterene-associated urolithiasis in patients with BOO and those keeping high residues (Hollander, 1987). **Indinavir, a protease inhibitor, has been implicated as a causative factor for urolithiasis** (Gentle et al., 1997).

PRESENTATION OF BLADDER STONES

Bladder stones are rarely asymptomatic at the time of presentation. **The most common presentation of bladder calculi is terminal hematuria** (Smith and O'Flynn, 1975). In addition, the patients have a **varied degree of lower urinary tract symptoms,** which include intermittency, frequency, urgency, decreased flow urge incontinence, and abdominal pain (Douenias et al., 1991; Ellis, 1979; Smith and O'Flynn, 1975). Children suffering from bladder stones rarely seek medical attention acutely. There are often preceding symptoms such as passage of cloudy and sandy urine. **Children often experience abdominal discomfort, dysuria, frequency, and hematuria. Pulling the penis, in children, is considered pathognomonic of bladder stone.** In adults, the presentation can be acute urinary retention; however, this is rare in children with primary bladder stone (Ali and Rifat et al., 2005; Teotia and Teotia, 1990).

MANAGEMENT OF BLADDER STONES

The options for treatment of bladder stones are medical management, extracorporeal shock wave lithotripsy, transurethral lithotripsy, suprapubic cystolithotomy, suprapubic cystolithotripsy, and open surgery.

The factors that decide the line of management are size of the stone, stone composition, age of the patient, build of the patient, coexistent location of urolithiasis elsewhere, concomitant BOO, and available expertise or equipment.

Medical Management

Chemo dissolution as a sole treatment for bladder stones is time consuming and not completely efficient. In the current era its role is limited to use in select cases as an adjunct treatment. The treatment of chemodissolution is particularly effective for encrustation over long-term catheters. This can be considered as the treatment modality as well as a prophylactic measure (Phillippou et al., 2012).

Extracorporeal Shock Wave Lithotripsy

Extracorporeal shock wave lithotripsy (ESWL) as a modality of treatment has been considered as an option in patients with bladder calculi with artificial urinary sphincters or a penile prosthesis. Any endoscopic intervention in such a situation is fraught with jeopardizing the integrity of the prosthesis or sphincter device. It has also been considered as a treatment option in stones in neobladders and medically high-risk patients (Bhatia et al., 1994; Delakas et al., 1998; Frabboni, 1998; Hussain, 1994; Kostakopoulos et al., 1996; Millan Rodrigues et al., 2005; Razvi et al., 1996).

The protocol 22 for ESWL includes prone positioning of the patient, which avoids the artifacts from the coccyx and the rectum, and an indwelling catheter in form of a three-way Foley. The bladder is filled up to 150 mL; this enables the localization of the stone. Once the session is over, the bladder is drained. Intermittent irrigation further helps to localize the stone. **The factors that affect the outcome of ESWL in bladder stones include the amount of postvoid residue, the stone composition, and the stone size** (Frabboni, 1998).

Endourologic Approach to Bladder Stone

In the recent years the development of miniaturized endourologic equipment with efficacious energy source has ensured that majority of the bladder stones can be tackled with the endourologic approach.

A few terms that merit mention are the following:
1. Cystolithotomy: intact removal of stone
2. Cystolithotripsy: fragmenting the stone with energy source
3. Cystolitholapaxy: mechanical breakage of the stone (Fig. 95.1)

The transurethral route has been the most popular route for managing bladder stones because of the ease of this approach and robust energy devices that can be deployed. Modern series report the use of the holmium laser, electrohydraulic lithotripter, and lithoclast technology (Isen et al., 2008; Lipke et al., 2004). The lithotrite is slowly falling out of favor because of high incidence of complications such as bladder mucosal injury and perforations (Smith and O'Flynn, 1975).

Recently, laser lithotripsy, particularly with the use of side-firing laser, has become the modality of choice because it offers the possibility of a one-time procedure with minimal complications (Lipke et al., 2004; Teichman et al., 1997). One of the concerns with transurethral access is the possibility of urethral injury because of repeated passage of transurethral instruments. The measures described to decrease the incidence of urethral stricture are use of transurethral Amplatz sheath (Okeke et al., 2004), adequate lubrication, and preoperative meatotomy and use of a suprapubic catheter postoperatively (Sathaye, 2003).

The advantages of the percutaneous approach are safety, efficacy, and potential lesser risk to the urethra (Ikari et al., 1993). Percutaneous nephrolithotomy has been advocated in patients with difficult urethras, such as patients who have undergone previous bladder neck reconstruction or closures. The percutaneous access is created with an Amplatz sheath or a Hassan cannula (Hubscher and Costa, 2011; Ikari et al., 1993). A combination of ultrasonic and pneumatic energy effectively fragments the stones. Placement of an entrapment sac for retrieval of fragments has been described (Tan et al., 2014). **The success rates for this procedure range from 89% to 100% in a single sitting.** The complications include urine leak and persistent hematuria in 1% (Ikari et al., 1993).

Open Surgery for Bladder Stones

Open cystolithotomy is associated with the need for prolonged catherization and hospital stay. Workers have also reported the feasibility of catheterless and drainless cystolithotomy in children with two-layered closure (Rattan et al., 2006). Open approach can also be considered in such situations in which there remains a contraindication for transurethral or percutaneous access to the bladder such as small-capacity bladders and stricture urethra (Miller, 2003).

LOWER TRACT CALCULI IN SPECIAL SITUATIONS

Bladder Outlet Obstruction With Bladder Lithiasis

BOO results in incomplete emptying and nonevacuation of fragments. These two factors are noted in 45% to 79% of all patients diagnosed with vesical calculi. The presence of urolithiasis secondary to BOO forms the absolute indication for treatment of BPH. The theory that secondary bladder calculi are due to outlet obstruction has been challenged. Approximately 1% to 2% of all bladder calculi are associated with BOO, which indicates that infection does play a role in the pathogenesis of bladder stones. All secondary bladder stones do not require treatment for BOO. More than 30% of all bladder stones are associated with infection. The infection is usually by a urea-splitting organism (Douenias et al., 1991).

Millan Rodrigues et al. noted a study that performed a urodynamic examination before and after treatment of bladder calculi found that only half of this subgroup of patients had urodynamic suggestion of BOO.

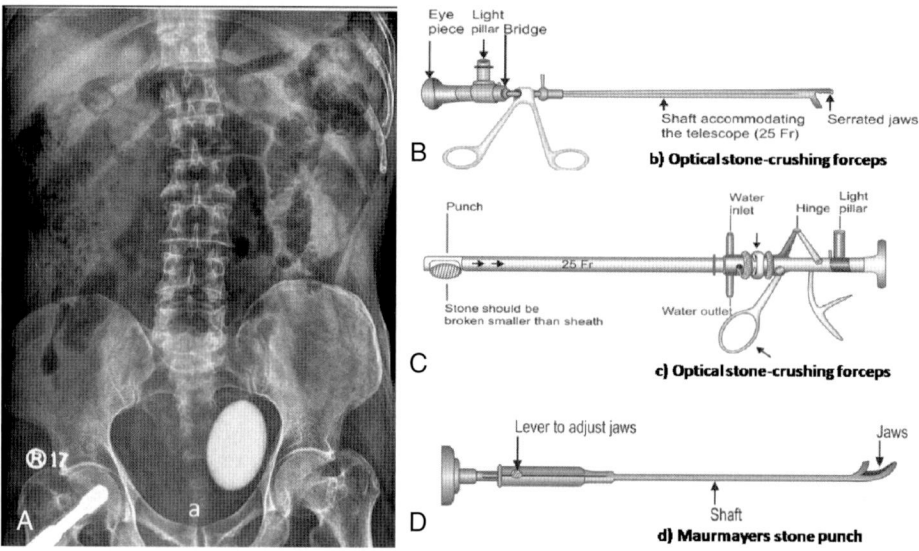

Fig. 95.1. Large bladder stone and cystolitholapaxy equipment used for fragmenting bladder stones. (A) Large bladder stone. (B) Stone-crushing forceps. (C) Optical stone-crushing forceps. (D) Maurmayer stone punch. (Reproduced from Sabnis RB, Patwardhan SK, Ganpule AP, editors: *Urology instrumentation: a comprehensive guide*, New Delhi, India, 2016, Jaypee Publications.)

Douenias, however, found that BOO was the cause of bladder stone in 88% of patients (Douenias et al., 1991; Millan Rodrigues et al., 2005).

Bladder Calculi in Urinary Diversions and Augmented Bladder

Calculi can occur in the upper and lower tracts after augmentation or diversion, and the incidence varies depending upon the type of surgery performed.

The cause of urolithiasis is multifactorial in patients who have urinary diversions. The reasons for stone formation can be divided into persistent bacterial colonization leading to infection, metabolic abnormalities, and anatomic and structural factors (Hensle et al., 2004; Robertson and Woodhouse, 2006). **The common metabolic abnormalities that result in usage of ileum or colon for diversions is hyperchloremic metabolic acidosis, which in turn may cause hypercalciuria because of a decrease in absorption of calcium** (Assimos, 1996). Loss of ileum can lead to enteric hyperoxaluria and diarrhea, which in turn can lead to stone formation (Terai et al., 1995).

Most of the stones in this subset of patients are mainly struvite calculi, which proves that recurrent and persistent urinary tract infections are one of the most important causative factors in these patients (Arif et al., 1999; Beiko and Razvi, 2002; Turk et al., 1999). The organisms responsible for persistence of infections in these patients are urease-producing bacteria such as *Pseudomonas, Proteus,* and *Klebsiella* (Hertzig et al., 2013). The urease leads to alkalinization of urine and promotes crystallization. The mucus in these diversions may also facilitate bacterial growth by aiding in deposition of bacterial biofilm and thereby making the penetration of antibiotics difficult (Blyth et al., 1992; Bruce et al., 1984; Khoury et al., 1997). The use of stomach for diversion helps in reducing the incidence of bladder calculi, but the complications associated with its use, such as hematuria dysuria syndrome and need for long-term proton pump inhibitors, discourages the use of stomach (Kronner et al., 1998). Urinary stasis can occur as the result of stomal stenosis in a case of conduit or poor emptying in a case of continent diversion. This urinary stasis can be a contributory factor for formation of stones. It has been proven that the incidence of calculi has significantly decreased in this subset of patients by shifting from nonabsorbable to absorbable sutures (Arif et al., 1999; Turk et al., 1999).

Surgeries for calculi in patients with urinary diversions require special considerations. Preoperative knowledge of the type of diversion used is important, and it may help in deciding the operative modality. The accurate knowledge of anatomy is important and aids in planning the puncture in percutaneous approach and avoiding bowel injury. In patients in whom the stone in the conduit is due to stomal stenosis, removal of stone alone will lead to recurrence because of persistence of anatomic obstruction. The best treatment modality is concomitant revision of the stoma. In stones in continent diversions, such as those in cutaneous continent pouches, percutaneous approaches is preferable, and any treatment option that may cause injury to the continence mechanism should be avoided. Some authors even advocate ESWL as a treatment modality in these subset of patients, even though the routine use of ESWL in lower tract calculi and in diversions is not commonly practiced (Boyd et al., 1988).

In case of small burden stones in a neobladder, transurethral procedures can be done with minimal injury to the sphincter. However, if the stone burden is large, percutaneous method or open method is preferable (L'Esperance et al., 2004). In percutaneous technique either the Amplatz sheath or laparoscopic trocars can be used (Franzoni et al., 1999; Thomas et al., 1993). Postoperative management of these patients includes adequate drainage of either the stoma or the pouches with a suprapubic catheter or stomal catheter in case of a stoma or per urethral catheter in case of neobladder. The prevention strategies include complete removal of stone, treatment of infection, correction of anatomic abnormalities, and prevention of mucus.

Bladder Calculi in Patients With Spinal Cord Injury

The risk of bladder stone formation increases in patients with neurogenic bladder resulting from spinal cord injury and meningomyelocele. The incidence depends on multiple factors such as level of lesion, the severity of the injury, previous incidence of stones, persistence of infection, and method of urinary drainage (Chen et al., 2001; Sugimura et al., 2008). **For adults with spinal cord injury, the risk of bladder stone formation peaks at 3 months after injury, and within 10 years 15% to 30% of patients have formed at least one stone** (Chen et al., 2001). **Unfortunately this risk quadruples after first stone formation** (Ord et al., 2003). After spinal cord injury two phases are important for calculi formation: the acute phase, in which most patients are immobilized, and the second phase, which is later after recovery. The reason for calculi formation during the acute phase may be immobilization hypercalciuria, which may lead to formation of calcium stones (Naftchi et al., 1980). These stones can occur anywhere in the urinary tract, including the kidney and the bladder. In the recovery phase the main reason for calculi formation is the persistence of infection, which can be caused by either inadequate emptying or the methods deployed in emptying the urine (Burr et al., 1993).

Other causes for stone formation in spinal cord injury patients include the increase in alkalinity of urine coupled with hypocitraturia in spinal cord injury patients. Patients on clean intermittent catheterization were found to have decreased incidence of bladder stones when compared with those on indwelling catheter (Ord et al., 2003). Indwelling Foley catheters should be avoided because they are prone to encrustation and can contribute to the formation of nephrolithiasis. If an indwelling Foley catheter must be used, weekly catheter changes can dramatically reduce catheter encrustation and stone formation. In patients on indwelling catheter the incidence of stones does not vary between those on suprapubic or per urethral catheterization (Ord et al., 2003). The ways to reduce the incidence of bladder calculi in such patients include long-term antibiotic therapy, use of ascorbic acid to acidify the urine, increased fluid intake, routine bladder lavage with antibacterial irrigants, and the use of silicone catheters.

As in the general population, bladder calculi of small to intermediate size (up to 4 cm) may be treated transurethrally by electrohydraulic lithotripsy or Ho:YAG laser lithotripsy, and larger stones can be treated by percutaneous means or by open cystolithotomy (Schwartz and Stoller, 2000). ESWL for bladder stones may be an ideal treatment for spinal cord injury patients who are anesthetic risks or prone to autonomic dysreflexia (Kilciler et al., 2002).

Bladder Calculi After Renal Transplantation

Urolithiasis after renal transplantation is not uncommon and has an incidence of 1% to 1.8% (Kim et al., 2001; Schwartz and Stoller, 2000). Even though renal calculi are more common after transplantation, bladder calculi are common. There are many causative factors for bladder calculi in a post-transplant setting, especially persistent infection with *Proteus* sp. (urease-splitting organism), persistent outflow obstruction, and retained suture material. Immunosuppressive drugs such as calcineurin inhibitors and steroids can also be a contributory factor. The incidence of bladder stones has decreased after the use of absorbable suture (Klein and Goldman, 1997; Lipke et al., 2004).

The first investigation in case of a bladder stone is ultrasonography to rule out the presence of concomitant renal or ureteric calculi. CT scan can be used for confirmation.

The ideal modality of treatment of bladder calculi in a post-transplantation scenario does not differ much from routine situations. The modalities that can be used are cystolitholapaxy, laser, and ESWL (Grasso, 1996; Hahnfeld et al., 1998).

URETHRAL CALCULI

Urethral calculi amount to 0.3% to 1% of all stone disease, and obstructing urethral calculus is a very rare presentation of lower urinary tract urolithiasis (Aegukkatajit, 1999; Larkin and Weber, 1996). In the last few decades, the urethral calculi have become a rarity in the industrialized Western societies, although not so uncommon in and endemic regions of Asia and Middle East (Aegukkatajit, 1999; Amin, 1973; Menon and Martin, 2002; Seltzer et al., 1993). More recent epidemiologic studies have suggested a declining incidence of lower urinary tract bladder and urethral calculi (Trinchieri, 2008).

Urethral calculi have been exceedingly more common in males, with a bimodal age distribution. The first peak occurs in early childhood, and the second peak incidence occurs in the fourth or fifth decades of life (Kamal et al., 2004; Verit et al., 2006). Shorter length of the female urethra and higher peak flow rates in adolescence and younger age groups may have the protective effect for the younger demographic age group (Kamal et al., 2004; Verit et al., 2006).

Pathogenesis and Composition of Urethral Calculi

Urethral stones can be *primary* or *autochthonous*, those that arise de novo in the urethra, or *secondary* or *migratory*, in which the stones from the upper tracts or the bladder migrate into the urethra. The urethral stones are most commonly found proximal to the above-mentioned sites, especially prostatic urethra and less commonly in the pendulous urethra.

The majority of urethral calculi are migratory. Any pathology, either structural or functional, affecting the urethra, such as urethral stricture, meatal stenosis, or benign prostatic hyperplasia, can impede the normal stone passage and result in a migratory calculus, which otherwise would have been cleared (Hegele et al., 2002; Verit et al., 2006).

It was commonly believed that the bladder was the source of migratory calculi (Shanmugam et al., 2000), but recent evidence has suggested that the source of these migratory calculi could as well be the upper urinary tract calculi (Kaplan et al., 2006). The evidence in favor is threefold. First, the composition of these migratory calculi has been predominantly calcium oxalate (85%–90%), which is akin to those found in the upper tracts (Kamal et al., 2004; Verit et al., 2006). Second, patients with urethral calculi had concomitant bladder and upper tract calculi in 2% and 18%, respectively (Kamal et al., 2004). Third, in areas that were endemic for bladder calculi, the incidence of the bladder calculi has decreased considerably because of changes in food and lifestyle, whereas there has been no change in the incidence of urethral calculi, suggesting an origin from the upper tracts (Aegukkatajit, 1999; Kamal et al., 2004; Verit et al., 2006).

Primary Urethral Calculi

Primary urethral calculi are considered primary because they originate at the same site as they are found ultimately. **In reality, they form secondary to obstruction of urethra at any level of urinary stasis in urethral diverticula.** Presence of a foreign body and urinary infection provide a conducive milieu for stone formation (Rivilla et al., 2008; Susco et al., 2008). In the presence of infection stones, the commonly isolated organisms are *Escherichia coli*, *Proteus* spp., and Enterococci (Susco et al., 2008). Most of these stones are small, round, without a core or nucleus, and composed primarily of struvite (magnesium ammonium phosphate), although other types such as calcium phosphate and uric acid have been reported (Verit et al., 2006).

Urethral stricture is the leading cause for the formation of urethral stones as discussed earlier. On the other hand, placement of hair-bearing grafts for the management of urethral stricture or hypospadias has resulted in urethral stones as well. The hair acts as a nidus for precipitation and inspissation of lithogenic salts and results in primary calculi in the urethra (Singh and Hemal, 2001). These stones remain adherent to the hair ball and the urethral mucosa, causing partial obstruction and further stone formation. Attempts at epilation before engraftment have reduced but not eliminated the risk: the follicles persist and lead to hair growth in 3% to 6% of patients (Singh and Hemal, 2001).

The presence of foreign body may also serve as a nidus for stone formation. The advent of brachytherapy as a treatment modality for carcinoma prostate over the last two decades requires the placement of radioactive seeds into the prostate. These seeds can migrate or intrude into the prostatic urethra and may form a nidus for stone formation. Cryoablation causes ischemic necrosis of the gland, and necrosis with persistent inflammation may give rise to stones (Aus et al., 1997; Steinmetz and Barrett, 2006).

Clinical Presentation and Evaluation

The clinical presentation depends on the type and location of the stone. Patients with migratory calculi usually have a history of stone disease, previous surgeries for stone or instrumentation of lower tract, a vague history of flank pain in the preceding 1 or 2 weeks, suggesting origin from the upper tracts, and lower urinary tract symptoms (Verit et al., 2006). **More commonly, urethral calculi patients present with acute painful retention of urine from sudden impaction of the stone. In other patients who are able to void despite the urethral calculus, there occurs weak stream, interrupted stream, or splaying, gross hematuria, and dysuria.** Posterior urethral stones typically have perineal or rectal pain, whereas those in the pendulous urethra have pain at the penile tip. Patients with primary urethral calculi or diverticular calculi have more insidious symptoms of persistent pain during voiding, obstructive lower urinary tract symptoms, chronic pelvic pain, or recurrent urinary tract infections. Women tend to report increased urinary frequency and occasional incontinence (Susco et al., 2008).

Migratory urethral calculi are usually solitary and larger than primary calculi, although urethral steinstrasse has been reported (Atikeler et al., 2005; Verit et al., 2006). Different authors have reported differing location of the stone, with most unanimously reporting the posterior urethral stones to be more common (as high as 88%) than anterior urethral stones (4%–11%) in their series (Amin, 1973; Kamal et al., 2004; Selli et al., 1984; Shanmugam et al., 2000; Sharfi, 1991). Examination may be completely normal in a posterior urethral calculus except for a mild tender prostate, whereas those located in the bulbar or the penile urethra may be palpable as a hard mass along the course of the normal urethra. In females, it is identified as a hard mass in the anterior vaginal wall (Kaplan et al., 2006; Subbarao et al., 1998; Susco et al., 2008). Primary urethral calculi have a more protracted course and insidious symptoms. Examination reveals a urethral diverticulum, if present, and very large diverticula are readily palpable with multiple stones in the perineum (Beatrice et al., 2008; Gallo et al., 2007; Koh et al., 1999; Subbarao et al., 1998; Susco et al., 2008).

Patients with migratory calculi present immediately in view of sudden and drastic onset of the symptoms. Those who are able to void with minimal symptoms and those with urethral diverticula often seek medical attention late with a long history, often up to many years (Gallo et al., 2007; Koh et al., 1999; Susco et al., 2008). Prolonged delays have a more complicated presentation with larger calculi and urethra-cutaneous or urethra-rectal fistulas (Kaplan et al., 2006; Kumar et al., 2012). These fistulous complications are more common in those who cannot report their symptoms because of decreased sensation, especially in infants and those afflicted with spinal cord injuries (Kaplan et al., 2006; Shamsa et al., 2008).

Urine examination reveals gross or microscopic hematuria and presence of infection in cases of primary calculi. Majority of urethral stones are radiopaque and visible on plain radiographs. The density of these stones vary in individual patients, but as against the previous literature, which quotes 40% to be radiopaque, newer studies have suggested an overwhelming majority of 98% of urethral stones to be radiopaque (Kamal et al., 2004; Verit et al., 2006). A retrograde urethrogram can identify the stones as filling defect and has been the mainstay of investigation. A carefully done transrectal ultrasonography can identify the prostatic urethral calculi as a hyperechoic structure with postacoustic shadowing (Aus et al., 1997; Peabody et al., 2012). Similarly, a high-frequency (10-MHz) linear transducer, when placed on the dorsal surface of the penis along its long axis, can screen the entire urethra and identify the calculi (Peabody et al., 2012).

With the advent of ultrasonography, retrograde urethrogram is reserved for cases in which ultrasonography is inconclusive or when a stricture of the urethra is suspected as a cause for the stone. Most authors also agree with the fact that upper tract stones may coexist and therefore advocate ultrasonography of the kidney, ureter, and bladder or a cross-sectional computerized tomography, especially if a strong suspicion exists (Hayashi et al., 2007; Rivilla et al., 2008; Singh and Hemal, 2001; Susco et al., 2008).

Treatment

Treatment of urethral calculi depends on the location within the urethra and the distance from the internal or the external urethral meatus, stone characteristics, the ability of the stone to get pushed into the bladder, and associated structural abnormalities of the urethra, if any. Stones located in the posterior urethra can be pushed back into the bladder for ESWL or intracorporeal fragmentation with mechanical or electrohydraulic lithotripsy. Shockwave lithotripsy after pushback has been reported in the literature and widely followed in the past, albeit with a success rate of only 60% and residual stones (El-Sharif and Prasad, 1995). Intracorporeal laser lithotripsy is least traumatic to the mucosa and has a guaranteed success rate of 85% to 90% (Kamal et al., 2004; Verit et al., 2006). Few authors have innovated with the Microperc armamentarium for fragmenting the urethral calculi (Desai and Ganpule, 2017). It is less traumatic to the urethra, easier to handle because it is less bulky, and has its own learning curve; it still remains to be seen if it can give equivalent success rates. For stones that do not get pushed back into the bladder, in situ fragmentation using laser or pneumatic lithotripsy should be undertaken. Open cystolithotomy remains the last option in the event of failure of endourologic maneuvers (Kamal et al., 2004).

For stones in the anterior urethra, pushback into the bladder is hardly ever possible and is not to be attempted. The distance of the stone from the external meatus and the surface characteristics of the stone are the factors to be considered before contemplating treatment options. Milking the stone out from the meatus is an option, but caution regarding urethral injury should be exercised (Kamal et al., 2004). This should be attempted only for smooth-surfaced stones because the risk of urethral injury with milking is not known (Maheshwari and Shah, 2005). If the stone is large or the surface is rough and irregular, extraction by milking is to be condemned. Few authors have noted success with simple instillation of lidocaine jelly into the urethra for small distal stones (El-Sharif and El-Hafi, 1991; Kamal et al., 2004). In situ lithotripsy is feasible using either electrohydraulic or Swiss lithoclast with a success rate of up to 80% (Kamal et al., 2004). Concerns regarding urethral damage exist and have been offset with the use of Holmium laser lithotripsy (Fig. 95.2; Kamal et al., 2004; Koh et al, 1999; Maheshwari and Shah, 2005; Verit et al., 2006).

For stones located in the fossa navicularis and distal urethral stones, manipulation with a forceps under anesthesia is successful. A ventral meatotomy helps in controlled removal of the stone and actually reduces urethral trauma. For larger and more proximal anterior urethral stones, urethrotomy and stone extraction is advocated. When complicated by urethral stricture or urethra-cutaneous fistula, simultaneous or staged repair should be undertaken (Kamal et al., 2004; Singh and Hemal, 2001). Stones within the diverticula are usually treated with incision of the diverticulum and stone extraction. Diverticulectomy and urethral repair is usually required and can be done either in a same sitting or in a staged fashion (Maheshwari and Shah, 2005; Singh and Neogi, 2006; Subbarao et al., 1998).

Unusual Lower Tract Urolithiasis

Preputial Calculi

These commonly occur in adults (Sharma and Bapna, 1977). The common factors associated are severe phimosis along with poor hygiene and low socioeconomic status (Ellis et al., 1986). The possible causes for preputial stones are inspissation of the smegma, stasis, and resultant precipitation of salts. There can be a combination of factors (Ellis et al., 1986; Winsbury-White, 1954). The accumulated smegma initiates a vicious cycle, which in turn leads to severe phimosis as a result of scarring and inflammation (Mohapatra and Kumar, 1989). A few other unusual mechanisms for causation of preputial calculi are foreign bodies, suture material (Ellis et al., 1986), and extruded bladder calculi (Nagata et al., 1999; Williamson, 1932).

In all the cases, the presentation is lower urinary tract symptoms, most commonly difficulty in passing urine. Other symptoms include dysuria, hematuria, foul-smelling urine, and palpable swelling or calculi (Ellis et al., 1986; Mohapatra and Kumar, 1989; Sharma and Bapna, 1977; Williamson, 1932). Occasional presentation can be urinary retention (Shahi and Ram, 1962). On examination tight phimosis is encountered (Shahi and Ram, 1962; Sharma and Bapna, 1977). If any associated lymphadenopathy is detected, an imaging study may include plain radiography and, if required, CT imaging (Mohapatra and Kumar, 1989; Nagata et al., 1999).

The treatment of preputial calculi involves removal of calculi and the inciting cause. In most cases this requires circumcision and dorsal slit (Shahi and Ram, 1962; Williamson, 1932). The excised skin should be sent for histopathology (Ellis et al., 1986). The calculi

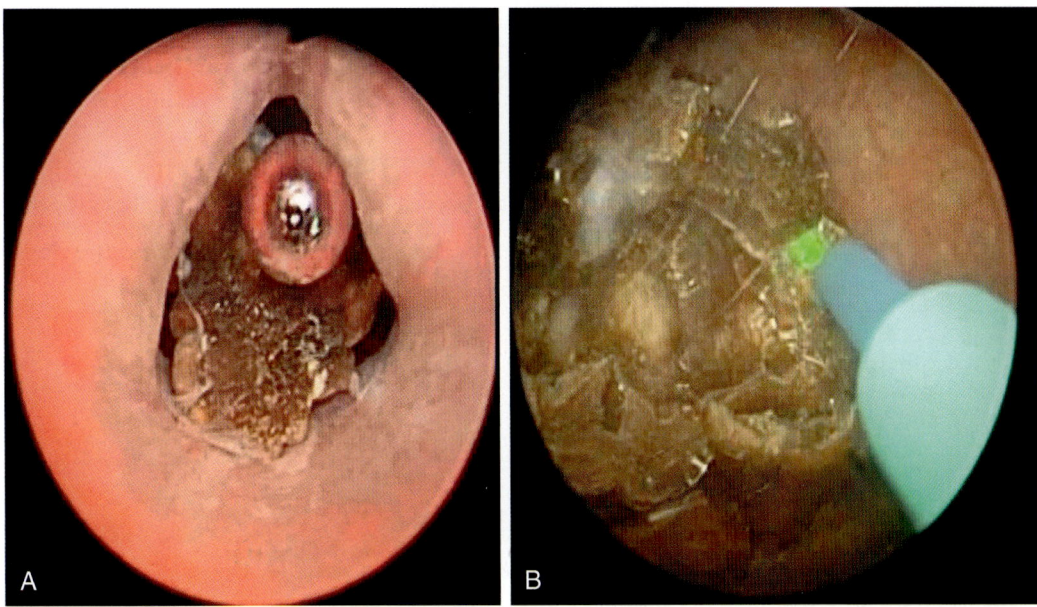

Fig. 95.2. Urethral calculi: diagnosis and management. (A) Cystourethroscopic view of a calculus impacted at the bulbomembranous junction. (B) The stone being fragmented with laser.

are typically multiple, smooth, and rounded, and the commonest stone composition is ammonium magnesium phosphate (Shahi and Ram, 1962; Williamson, 1932).

Prostatic Calculi

In the 19th century, a correlation between the presence of prostatic calculi and pathogenesis of lower urinary tract symptoms was identified (Huggins et al., 1944; Klimas et al., 1985; Moore, 1936; Thomas et al., 1927). With a more widespread use of transrectal ultrasonography for prostatic illnesses, more and more prostatic calculi are identified, 99% of asymptomatic adult men were identified in one study with some degree of prostatic calcification in autopsy studies (Sondergaard et al., 1987).

Etiopathogenesis and Composition. Prostatic calculi can be either prostatic urethral calculus or true prostatic calculi (within the prostate). Prostatic urethral calculus is always migratory and should be managed as any other urethral calculi. True prostatic calculi can be either primary/endogenous (occurring within the acini of the prostate) or secondary/exogenous (reflux of urine into the prostate). The majority of prostatic calculi are composed of calcium phosphate (83%), calcium carbonate phosphate (8.7%), calcium oxalate (4.5%), and mixed calcium stones (4.4%) (Dessombz et al., 2012). Exogenous calculi are caused by reflux of urine and therefore they are fewer in number and larger than primary calculi.

Clinical Presentation. There is a increased prevalence of prostatic calculi in patients with pathologically proven benign prostatic hyperplasia. Different authors report different associations between them, ranging from 40% to 70% (Harada et al., 1979; Kim et al., 2009; Lee et al., 2003; Shoskes et al., 2007). There is no increase in incidence of prostatic carcinoma in patients with prostatic calculi. Indeed, a focused evaluation of areas of calcification/calculi has shown no correlation with the sites of adenocarcinoma (Muezzinoglu and Gurbuz, 2001).

Patients with at least one symptom of prostatitis are 3.2 times more likely to harbor a significant prostatic calculus than the age-matched asymptomatic group, and the size rather than the number of stones that correlated with the symptoms (Geramoutsos et al., 2004). Most studies suggest that prostatic calculi are common in patients with chronic pelvic pain syndrome (CPPS) and are associated with greater inflammation and symptoms (Shoskes et al., 2005, 2007). Moreover, patients with prostatic calculi are more likely to grow *E. coli, Klebsiella,* and other gram-negative pathogens on cultures

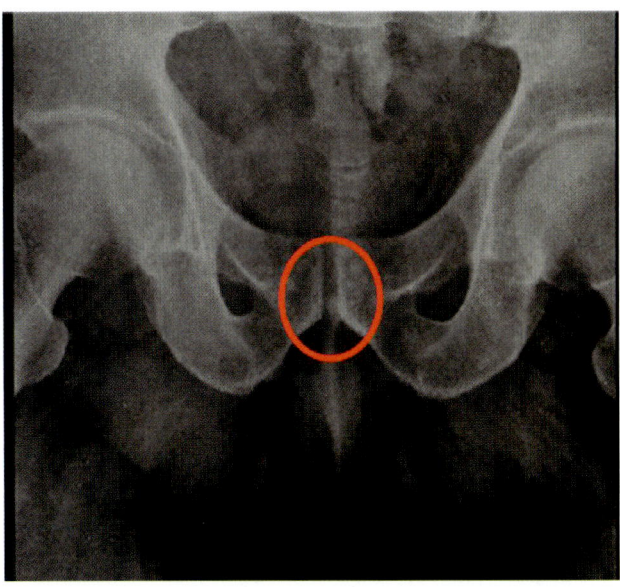

Fig. 95.3. Plain x-ray showing a prostatic urethral calculus. A plain x-ray of the pelvis in a patient with recent onset lower urinary tract symptoms depicts the urethral stone.

and exhibit more white blood cells in expressed prostatic secretions (Shoskes et al., 2007). Other authors have found no conclusive evidence between prostatic infection, inflammation, and prostatic calculi (Sondergaard et al., 1987).

Evaluation and Management. Prostatic calculi are identified primarily with the use of transrectal ultrasonography (TRUS) in the evaluation of lower urinary tract symptoms (LUTS) or prostatomegaly. Ultrasonography-based classification exists for prostatic calculi based on echo pattern in ultrasonography: type A, discrete and multiple small echoes evenly distributed throughout the gland, and type B, coarser and larger, but focal echoes (Harada et al., 1979). **Plain x-ray film shows calculi in 14% of patients** (Fig. 95.3). The role of CT and MRI is not clear. Apart from the use of TRUS, imaging has a limited role in the identification of calculi.

Prostatic calculi identified during transurethral resection of prostate require removal during the procedure using the endoloop; these

KEY POINTS

- Primary bladder calculi are most common in children younger than the age of 10 with a peak incidence at 2 to 4 years. The disease is much more common in boys than in girls.
- The most common presentation of bladder stones is hematuria with lower urinary tract symptoms.
- Children with bladder stones often experience abdominal discomfort, dysuria, frequency, and hematuria.
- Pulling the penis, in children, is considered pathognomonic of bladder stone.
- The options for treatment of bladder stones are medical management, extracorporeal shock wave lithotripsy, transurethral lithotripsy, suprapubic cystolithotomy, suprapubic cystolithotripsy, and open surgery.
- The advantages of percutaneous approach in bladder stones are safety and efficacy and potential lesser risk to the urethra.
- Urethral calculi amount to 0.3% to 1% of all stone disease, and obstructing urethral calculus is a very rare presentation of lower urinary tract urolithiasis.
- More commonly urethral calculi patients present with acute painful retention of urine from sudden impaction of the stone.
- Patients with at least one symptom of prostatitis are 3.2 times more likely to harbor a significant prostatic calculus than the age-matched asymptomatic group.
- The common factors associated with preputial calculi are severe phimosis, poor hygiene, and low socioeconomic status.
- Plain x-ray film shows calculi in 14% preputial calculi in patients.

patients have more symptomatic relief with removal of these calculi compared with those in whom they were not removed (Jeon et al., 2005). They also serve as a surrogate marker for the capsule during the transurethral resection.

SUGGESTED READINGS

Phillippou P, Moraitis K, Massod J, et al: The management of bladder lithiasis in the modern era endourology, *Urology* 79:980–986, 2012.

Schwartz BF, Stoller ML: The vesical calculus, *Urol Clin North Am* 27:333–346, 2000.

REFERENCES

The complete reference list is available online at ExpertConsult.com.

PART XI
Neoplasms of the Upper Urinary Tract

96
Benign Renal Tumors
William P. Parker, MD, and Matthew T. Gettman, MD

Benign renal tumors are an ever-increasing (because of routine axial imaging) and common entity in the urology clinic because of the widespread use of abdominal imaging (Murphy et al., 2009; Patard, 2009). Even among suspected renal cell carcinoma (RCC) cases, 20% of resected masses are benign (Kutikov et al., 2006). As such, benign masses represent a clinically significant and heterogeneous collection of pathologic conditions. These include the simple renal cyst, selected complex renal cysts, oncocytomas, angiomyolipomas (AMLs), cortical and metanephric adenomas, mixed epithelial-stromal tumors, the rarer cystic nephroma, leiomyoma, and other, rarer tumors.

Management of these lesions is based on the perceived risk of RCC, and can vary widely, from no management for the simple renal cyst to selective embolization for larger AMLs and surgical extirpation for solid renal masses. In addition, as the American Urological Association guidelines recognize, renal mass biopsy may have a role in decision making for small renal masses (Campbell et al., 2009), which has been shown to potentially reduce the need for intervention in a significant proportion of patients with benign histology (Richard et al., 2015).

DIAGNOSIS

When symptoms are present, common symptoms are flank pain, a palpable mass, and hematuria; however, most diagnoses result from an incidental renal mass. Although the initial identification of a benign mass is through imaging, such as ultrasonography, computed tomography (CT), or magnetic resonance imaging (MRI), these modalities are imperfect in their identification of benign histology (Canvasser et al., 2017; Gordetsky and Zarzour, 2016; Monn et al., 2015; Pierorazio et al., 2013). Certainly there are clues to a benign entity, such as thin, unenhanced walls in simple cyst disease or macroscopic fat in an AML; however, these are not universal and therefore most diagnoses are made at biopsy or resection. Additional clues to the diagnosis of benign histology include smaller mass size, lack of growth in serial imaging, female sex, and older age; however, none except for lack of growth over time, can reliably rule out malignancy (Ambani et al., 2016; Lane et al., 2007; Pierorazio et al., 2016; Snyder et al., 2006).

In this chapter the most common benign entities are reviewed with specific focus on their cause, diagnosis, and management.

RENAL CYSTS
Epidemiology, Etiology, and Pathophysiology

Renal cysts are by far the most common benign entity encountered in the kidney. **Up to 10% of the population may harbor a renal cyst, with putative risk factors of increasing age, male gender, hypertension, and worsening renal function** (Terada et al., 2004). Renal cysts can be sporadic, acquired, or genetic in their origin. However, beyond their associations with a cause, phenotypically renal cysts are similar. Mechanistically, genetic renal cyst disease is the most well-described cause of renal cyst disease through autosomal dominant polycystic kidney disease (ADPKD) and autosomal recessive polycystic kidney disease (ARPKD).

ADPKD is an inherited renal cystic disease related to alterations in cilia function (ciliopathies); primarily through mutation of *PKD1* and *PKD2*. *PKD1* (polycystin-1) is on the short arm of chromosome 16 and is highly complicated gene that is predisposed to recombination error and thus spontaneous mutation. *PKD2* (polycystin-2) is on the long arm of chromosome 4, and by contrast, is less complicated than *PKD1*. **Together, polycystin-1 and polycystin-2 form a transmembrane complex that is hypothesized to function as a mechanosensor to the flow of urine (through the cilia), regulating intracellular calcium levels based on this flow. Reductions in intracellular calcium levels result in amplification of cyclic adenosine monophosphate levels that upregulate downstream effectors, giving rise to the typical cystic epithelial histology** (Abdul-Majeed and Nauli, 2011; Casuscelli et al., 2009; Rangan et al., 2015). The process by which cysts in ADPKD develop was initially described in microdissection studies, which demonstrated a progression from a diverticulum on the tubular epithelium that ultimately detaches from the tubule to form a true cyst in the interstitium of the kidney (Rangan et al., 2015). Growth of cysts is asynchronous but persistent and radially oriented, with gradual development of large kidneys, renal insufficiency, and mortality based on growth kinetics (Hateboer et al., 1999; Irazabal et al., 2015). **Diagnosis of ADPKD is based on presentation, with the presence of at least 2 unilateral or bilateral renal cysts before age 30, at least 2 cysts in each kidney between ages 30 and 59, or 4 cysts in each kidney in patients 60 years or older.** In addition, patients with ADPKD tend to develop hepatic and pancreatic cysts (Grantham, 2008).

Acquired cystic kidney disease (ACKD) is a special circumstance in which renal cyst development is preceded by the development of chronic and end-stage renal disease (Rahbari-Oskoui and O'Neill, 2017). Development of cysts is largely dependent on the length of time on dialysis, with up to 80% of patients developing cysts after 10 years (Matson and Cohen, 1990). **Unlike the cysts in sporadic and genetic renal cyst disease, ACKD is associated with the development of RCC, with almost 7% developing RCC after 10 years of dialysis** (Ishikawa et al., 2003). Mechanistically, the cysts of ACKD arise from the proximal convoluted tubule (as in clear cell RCC), unlike the cysts of ADPKD and sporadic renal cyst disease, which arise from the distal tubule (Liu et al., 2000).

Natural History

The natural history of renal cyst disease varies with the cause. For example, the kidneys of patients with ADPKD increase in size exponentially over time (~5% in total volume per year). This volume expansion is associated with mass effect and reduction in renal function over time (Grantham et al., 2006). Long-term follow-up of ACKD patients demonstrates that renal volumes can increase to three times their native size by 20 years of dialysis, an increase attributed to the growth of renal cysts (Ishikawa et al., 2003). Meanwhile, sporadic renal cysts increase in size and number over time, with an average growth rate of 1.6 mm/year, although notably growth rates decrease with increasing follow-up (Terada et al., 2008).

Evaluation

Most patients with renal cyst disease are diagnosed incidentally. However, patients can experience pain from local expansion, a palpable mass, hematuria, and, in the case of ADPKD, pulmonary symptoms from mass effect in the kidney. Evaluation is through imaging, which can include ultrasonography, CT, or MRI. The goal of imaging in cystic renal disease is evaluation of malignancy risk as defined by increasing complexity. For example, simple renal cysts are characterized by smooth walls, sharp outlines, and the absence of internal echoes on ultrasonography. Meanwhile, on CT and MRI the hallmark of simple cyst disease is the absence of enhancement (Eknoyan, 2009; Helenon et al., 2018). Although CT and MRI are comparable in most aspects, MRI can help in the evaluation of hyperdense cysts but at the expense of overestimating cyst wall thickness in smaller cysts (Bosniak, 2012).

To aid in the evaluation of renal cyst disease, the Bosniak classification (Table 96.1) is a commonly used method to characterize cysts and their risk of malignancy (Bosniak, 1986). The Bosniak system has been reviewed and validated in multiple studies, and a recent meta-analysis confirmed the utility of this system (Schoots et al., 2017). As outlined in the table, Bosniak I and II lesions require no additional follow-up, whereas Bosniak IIF (Fig. 96.1) lesions should have interval imaging. Notably, Bosniak IIF lesions that are stable on repeat imaging have a less than 1% risk of malignancy, whereas those that increase in complexity have an approximately 85% risk of malignancy (Schoots et al., 2017). Conversely, management of Bosniak III/IV lesions is more involved given the higher risk of malignancy.

TABLE 96.1 Bosniak Classification of Renal Cysts

BOSNIAK CLASSIFICATION	IMAGING CHARACTERISTICS	INCIDENCE OF MALIGNANCY	THERAPY
I	Simple cyst with a hairline thin wall that does not contain septa, calcifications, or solid components. It measures water density in Hounsfield units and does not enhance with intravenous administration of a contrast agent.	1.7%	No therapy or follow-up required
II	Cyst may contain a few hairline thin septa and fine calcifications, or a short segment of slightly thickened calcification may be present in the wall or septa. Uniformly high-attenuation lesions <3 cm (so-called *high-density cysts*) are well marginated and do not enhance with intravenous administration of a contrast agent.	18.5%	No therapy or follow-up required
IIF	Cysts may contain multiple hairline thin septa or minimal smooth thickening of their wall or septa. Their wall or septa may contain calcifications that may be thick and nodular, but no measurable contrast enhancement is present. These lesions are typically well marginated. Totally intrarenal nonenhancing high-attenuation renal lesions ≥3 cm are also included in this category.	18.5%	Repeat imaging to assess stability of size and radiographic characteristics
III	"Indeterminate" cystic masses have thickened irregular or smooth walls or septa in which measurable contrast enhancement is present.	33%	Active surveillance, excision, or ablation
IV	Clearly malignant cystic masses can have all the criteria of category III but also contain enhancing soft-tissue components.	92.5%	Excision or ablation

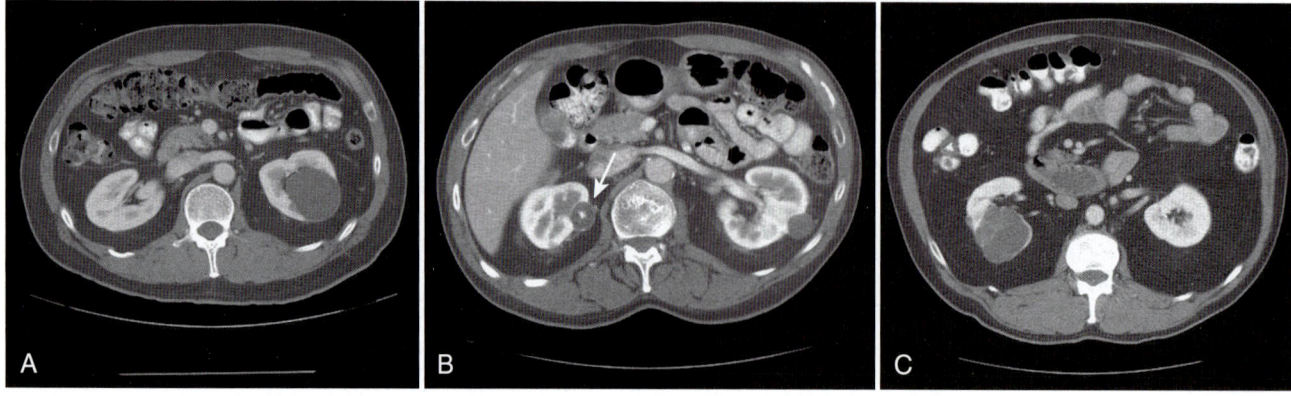

Fig. 96.1. (A) Computed tomography (CT) scan of a Bosniak I renal cyst. (B) CT scan of a Bosniak II renal cyst. Note internal calcification. (C) CT scan of a Bosniak IIF renal cyst. Several thin irregular septations are present within the cyst. (Copyright 2009, C. G. Wood.)

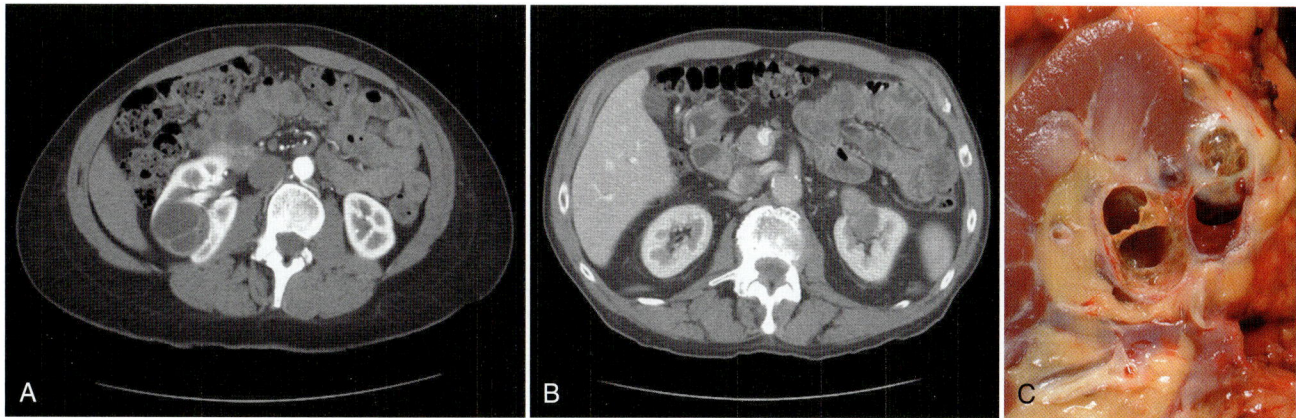

Fig. 96.2. (A) Computed tomography (CT) scan of a Bosniak III renal cyst. Thick, irregular septations are present within the cyst. (B) CT scan of a Bosniak IV renal cyst with a solid enhancing nodule. (C) Bivalved Bosniak IV renal cyst demonstrating a solid component that proved to be conventional renal cell carcinoma. (Copyright 2009, C. G. Wood.)

Management Options

The management of renal cyst disease is based on the risk of malignancy and the associated symptoms. **For most simple renal cysts, no additional follow-up is required, with the maximal intervention of serial imaging recommended for Bosniak IIF lesions.** Patients with ACKD and ADPKD should have serial imaging given the risk of malignancy in ACKD and because of the risk of mass effect, cyst infection, and chronic pain in ADPKD (Grantham, 2008; Ishikawa et al., 2003).

Conversely, surgical resection or ablation is recommended for Bosniak III/IV lesions (Fig. 96.2). Renal mass biopsy has been reported to aid in the evaluation; however, it should be limited to cases in which the risk of intervention is high, because the risk of cyst rupture could alter the radiographic anatomy during follow-up and potential seed the retroperitoneum in the case of true malignancy (Bosniak, 2003; Harisinghani et al., 2003). More recently, however, the concept of active surveillance of cystic renal masses (Bosniak III/IV) has been evaluated. Although most Bosniak III/IV lesions are malignant, they are overwhelmingly low grade and small and associated with excellent cancer-specific survival (Chandrasekar et al., 2018; Kashan et al., 2018; Mousessian et al., 2017). When intervention is selected, and given the low malignant potential of these masses, renal preservation through either partial nephrectomy or ablation should be chosen.

Outside of malignant risk, occasionally renal cysts require treatment because of local symptoms such as pain, infection, hypertension, hemorrhage, or traumatic cyst rupture (Bas et al., 2015; Lai et al., 2017; Mabillard et al., 2017; Yoder and Wolf, 2004; Zerem et al., 2009). **Management can include aspiration, cyst decortication, cyst resection, sclerotherapy, arterial embolization, and even nephrectomy depending on the cause and symptom** (Grodstein et al., 2017; Lai et al., 2017; Mabillard et al., 2017; Yoder and Wolf, 2004; Zerem et al., 2009). A host of therapies have been used in the setting of ADPKD, including nephrectomy for mass effect and renal denervation for chronic pain (Casteleijn et al., 2017; Grodstein et al., 2017). These are challenging cases, particularly in the setting of chronic pain, and recurrence of symptoms is common. Multidisciplinary care with pain management should be employed as a standard.

ONCOCYTOMA

Epidemiology and Etiology

Whereas renal cyst disease is the most common benign renal tumor, oncocytoma is the most common benign enhancing renal mass (Frank et al.. 2003). **Up to 25% of renal masses smaller than 3 cm represent oncocytomas, making them a challenging diagnostic entity in clinical practice** (Shuch et al., 2015). Historically, the benignity of oncocytoma has been questioned; however, genetic studies have confirmed it as a benign renal mass, and reports of metastatic disease (extremely rare) are likely cases of eosinophilic chromophobe RCC (Kuroda et al., 2003; Oxley et al., 2007).

Pathophysiology

Pathologically, oncocytoma represents a diagnostic dilemma resulting from overlapping features with eosinophilic chromophobe RCC, succinate dehydrogenase-deficient RCC, and papillary RCC (Wobker and Williamson, 2017). Grossly, these tumors have a mahogany brown surface, similar to the appearance of normal renal parenchyma, with a variably present central scar (Fig. 96.3A). Histologically, these tumors are classically strongly eosinophilic because of the high mitochondrial density (Renshaw, 2002), with nests and tubular structures common, arising from the distal tubule (see Fig. 96.3B). Nuclei tend to be round and regular with extremely rare mitotic figures (Williamson et al., 2017). **Interestingly, oncocytoma can be associated with perirenal fat invasion and renal vein invasion—findings that carry prognostic significance in RCC but do not in oncocytoma and should not be interpreted as an aggressive pathology** (Hes et al., 2008; Williamson, 2016; Wobker et al., 2016).

When typical features of oncocytoma are present, histology and morphology are sufficient to establish the diagnosis pathologically; however, when morphologic variants are seen, such as the presence of papillary structures or compacted, nested architecture, the International Society of Urologic Pathology (ISUP) recommends use of immunohistochemistry to differentiate oncocytoma from non-benign tumors (such as chromophobe RCC) (Reuter et al., 2014). **In cases in which the diagnostic dilemma is between chromophobe and oncocytoma, cytokeratin-7 (CK7) can be useful. CK7 is rarely positive in oncocytoma, whereas chromophobe RCC tends to be diffusely positive and is recommended by the ISUP to distinguish these entities** (Reuter et al., 2014; Williamson et al., 2017). Other markers used to distinguish include kidney specific cadherin, S100A1,

> ### KEY POINTS: RENAL CYSTS
> - Renal cyst disease is the most common benign renal tumor.
> - ACKD is associated with a significant increase in malignancy risk and should be followed closely.
> - Most cysts require no additional follow-up or therapy.
> - The Bosniak classification is a useful tool to estimate malignancy risk and direct therapy.

and Hale's colloidal iron (Mazal et al., 2005; Rocca et al., 2007; Tickoo et al., 1998). Colloidal iron staining can be variable, making interpretation difficult; however, the hallmark is negative staining for oncocytoma and diffuse reticular staining in chromophobe RCC (Tickoo et al., 1998). Alternatively, when the differentiation is between oncocytoma and non-chromophobe RCC histologies, CD117 and vimentin can be useful, because oncocytoma is positive for CD117 and negative for vimentin, whereas nonchromophobe RCC stains oppositely (Liu et al., 2007; Reuter et al., 2014). The central scar can stain positive for vimentin and CK7, which can cloud the picture if this is not taken into account (Hes et al., 2007). Many other markers have been assessed; however, their clinical utility is still being explored, and only CK7, CD117, and kidney-specific cadherin are supported by the ISUP for the diagnosis of oncocytoma when histology alone is insufficient (Reuter et al., 2014).

Genetically, oncocytoma is typically associated with loss of chromosome 1, X or Y, 14, and 21 along with rearrangement of 11q13 (Cyclin D-1) (Joshi et al., 2015). **In addition, genetic predisposition exists in patients with Birt-Hogg-Dube (BHD) syndrome and renal oncocytosis. BHD syndrome is an autosomal dominant disease characterized by mutations in the folliculin gene on chromosome 17 and is associated with the development of pulmonary cysts (70%–84%) that can be seen as spontaneous pneumothoraces (25%), cutaneous fibrofolliculomas (>90%), and the development of chromophobe RCC and oncocytomas (12%–34%)** (Steinlein et al., 2018). This common developmental pathway of these two tumor types in BHD underscores their histologic similarity. Indeed, there is an intermediary tumor, the "hybrid oncocytoma-chromophobe tumor," which has been described in these and other patients, that argues toward oncocytoma and chromophobe RCC existing on a continuum (Reuter et al., 2014; Steinlein et al., 2018). Oncocytosis is a separate entity from BHD characterized by the presence of numerous, bilateral renal oncocytomas (Fig. 96.4; Giunchi et al., 2016).

Evaluation

Most cases of oncocytoma occur asymptomatically as an unilateral incidental renal mass (5% occur bilaterally) (Amin et al., 1997; Perez-Ordonez et al., 1997). Definitive diagnosis of oncocytoma is typically postoperative; however, there are certain imaging clues to the diagnosis. **Hypervascularity and a central scar on axial imaging can suggest oncocytoma as the diagnosis; however, these alone are insufficient for a definitive diagnosis** (Choudhary et al., 2009). Multiphasic MRI has been studied with some initial promising results; however, larger study is needed to confirm the clinical utility of this approach (Young et al., 2017; Zhong et al., 2017). More recently, research into technetium-99m (^{99m}Tc)-sestamibi single-photon emission computed tomography/x-ray computed tomography (SPECT/CT) has been studied with a sensitivity and specificity of 87.5% and 95.2%, respectively (Gorin et al., 2016). **When suspicion of oncocytoma is high based on imaging, renal mass biopsy has been used with some success** (Schmidbauer et al., 2008). **However, a recent meta-analysis reported a relatively low positive predictive value of 67% for oncocytoma on renal mass biopsy, raising concern about the utility of this approach in the patient with suspected oncocytoma** (Patel et al., 2017).

Management

As most renal oncocytomas are diagnosed after surgical resection (because of perceived risk of RCC), the mainstay of management is

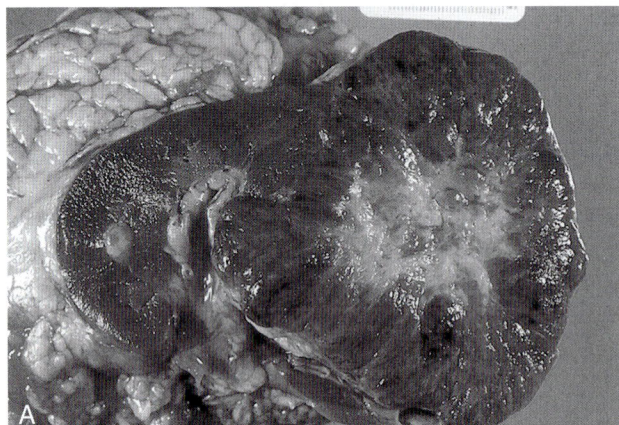
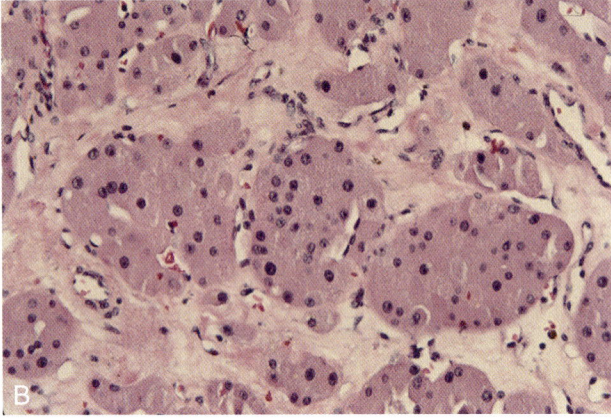

Fig. 96.3. (A) Bivalved renal oncocytoma demonstrating central scar. (B) Oncocytoma with large eosinophilic cells arranged in distinct nests.

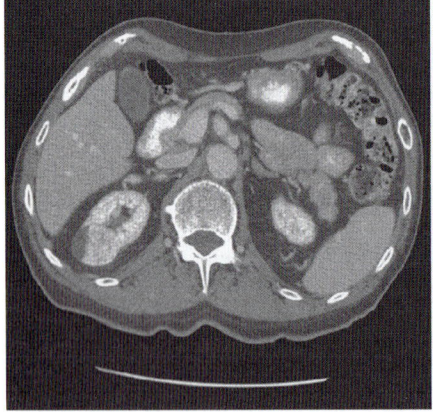 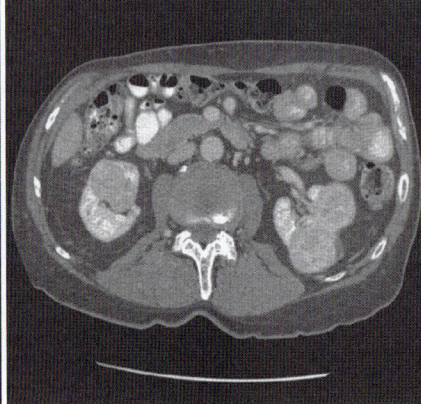 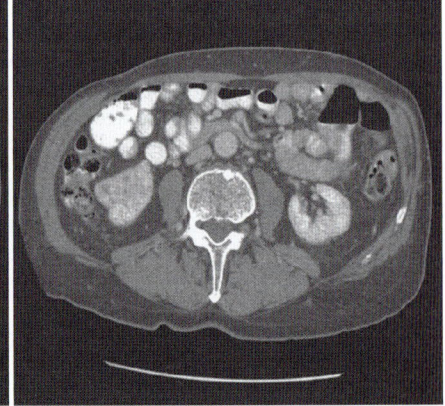

Fig. 96.4. Computed tomography scan of a patient with multiple bilateral oncocytomas. (Copyright 2009, S. F. Matin.)

postsurgical observation. **However, in the setting of diagnosis based on renal mass biopsy, the role of active surveillance has been explored with favorable results** (Liu et al., 2016a and 2016b; Miller et al., 2018; Richard et al., 2016). In evaluation of 90 patients initially managed with active surveillance, only one-third received intervention (either surgery or ablation), mainly because of growth on surveillance, with 100% 5-year cancer-specific survival (Miller et al., 2018). Importantly, in patients with nononcocytic lesions, such as chromophobe RCC, the growth on interval imaging was more rapid, with an average 0.38 cm/year among chromophobe lesions compared with 0.14 mm/year for oncocytomas (Richard et al., 2016). Furthermore, because chromophobe RCC is rarely aggressive, there is little risk in observing a small chromophobe RCC while obtaining these growth kinetics (Leibovich et al., 2018). **Conversely, when oncocytoma is suspected but uncertainty exists or treatment is indicated, nephron-sparing approaches (such as ablation or partial nephrectomy) should be the standard when technically feasible given the benign nature of this disease** (Romis et al., 2004).

KEY POINTS: ONCOCYTOMA

- Renal oncocytoma is the most common benign enhancing renal mass.
- Oncocytomas are histologically similar to chromophobe RCC, and immunohistochemical staining may be required to distinguish the two.
- Oncocytoma is associated with Birt-Hogg-Dube syndrome: characterized by pulmonary cysts, spontaneous pneumothoraces, and fibrofolliculomas.
- When suspected, a percutaneous biopsy may provide a diagnosis when core tissue is available for additional immunohistochemical studies.
- Active surveillance represents a reasonable treatment strategy that minimizes risk and increases certainty based on growth kinetics.

ANGIOMYOLIPOMA

Epidemiology

Initially described in 1900 by Grawitz, AML is a benign renal entity composed of dysmorphic blood vessels, smooth muscle, and adipose tissue (Flum et al., 2016; Grawitz, 1900; Nelson and Sanda, 2002). These tumors can occur sporadically or as part of genetic syndromes: most commonly tuberous sclerosis complex (TSC) and lymphangioleiomyomatosis (LAM). **Epidemiology studies estimate the prevalence at 0.13% in the general population, with a female predisposition and a peak in the fourth and fifth decade** (Eble, 1998; Fujii et al., 1995; Seyam et al., 2008). **Among TSC patients, the prevalence has been reported from 55% to 90%, with an earlier presentation than sporadic cases** (Curatolo et al., 2008; Seyam et al., 2008; Steiner et al., 1993).

Pathophysiology

TSC represents the most well-described heritable cause of AML. **Genetically, TSC arises from mutations in either *TSC1* (encoding hamartin) on chromosome 9q34 or *TSC2* (encoding tuberin) on chromosome 16p13. Inheritance is autosomal dominant; however, penetrance is variable and sporadic mutations are common** (Consortium, 1993; Curatolo et al., 2008; Henske et al., 1995; van Slegtenhorst et al., 1997). Mechanistically, hamartin and tuberin dimerize to inhibit mTOR (Curatolo et al., 2008; Franz, 2011) and therefore inactivating mutations of these proteins result in unregulated mTOR activation. Downstream, this results in protein synthesis, cellular growth, and angiogenesis (Franz, 2011). Beyond the development of AML, these genetic changes result in the variable presence of epilepsy, neurocognitive impairment, autism, cortical tubers, astrocytomas, cardiac rhabdomyomas, retinal hamartomas, hypomelanotic macules, facial/ungual angiofibromas, and shagreen patches (Curatolo et al., 2008; Flum et al., 2016; Franz, 2011). Related to TSC, LAM is a disorder that predominantly affects women and genetically involves mutation of the *TSC1* or *TSC2* (Ferrans et al., 2000; Matsui et al., 2000, McCormack, 2008; Ryu et al., 2006). It can occur in isolation (rarely) or associated with TSC. Common features of LAM include (in addition to TSC features) cystic lung lesions, lymphangioleiomyomas, and chylous effusions (Ferrans et al., 2000; Matsui et al., 2000; McCormack, 2008; Ryu et al., 2006).

Pathologically, AMLs are thought to arise from perivascular epithelioid cells and are often grouped with other perivascular epithelioid cell tumors, or PECOMAs (Bissler and Kingswood, 2004). On gross examination, tumors are well circumscribed with a tan, pink, or yellow surface, depending on the fat content (Flum et al., 2016). As previously noted, tumors are composed of blood vessels, spindle cells, and adipocytes. Vessels are thick-walled and eccentric with spindle cells around the vessels. Adipocytes are mature and without atypia (Flum et al., 2016). The proportion that each of these components contributes to the tumor can, histologically, confuse the diagnosis. **Of special circumstance is epithelioid AML, which is characterized by minimal fat content and an abundance of epithelioid cells** (Park et al., 2007; Sun and Campbell, 2018). **Atypia within the epithelioid cells, the presence of mitotic figures, and necrosis are common and suggest a more aggressive course** (Brimo et al., 2010). **Indeed, metastatic disease has been reported in one-third of reported cases, sporadic and TSC associated** (Bissler and Kingswood, 2004; Cibas et al., 2001; Huang et al., 2007; Kato et al., 2009; L'Hostis et al., 1999; Lee et al., 2018; Limaiem et al., 2008; Martignoni et al., 2000; Matsuyama et al., 2008; Mene et al., 2001; Moudouni et al., 2008; Nelson and Sanda, 2002; Pea et al., 1998; Saito et al., 2002; Tan et al., 2015; Zanelli et al., 2008).

Other diagnoses that can pathologically mimic AML include sarcoma (specifically, fibrosarcoma, leiomyosarcoma, and liposarcoma) and RCC (Wang et al., 2002). Indeed, leiomyosarcomas have been described as arising within an AML, raising concern for potential malignant transformation (Christiano et al., 1999; Ferry et al., 1991). **Importantly, spindle cells have melanocytic features, and therefore melanocyte markers HMB-45 and Melan-A are important immunohistochemical stains to aid in the diagnosis when in doubt** (Eble et al., 1997; Flum et al., 2016). AMLs stain strongly for estrogen receptor β, progesterone receptor, and androgen receptor, which may mechanistically explain the postpubertal female preponderance (Boorjian et al., 2008; Henske et al., 1998; L'Hostis et al., 1999).

Diagnosis

As with most renal masses, patients with AML are often diagnosed incidentally on cross-sectional imaging (Lemaitre et al., 1997; Seyam et al., 2008). However, historically up to 15% of patients have Wunderlich syndrome (spontaneous retroperitoneal hemorrhage) (Eble, 1998; Oesterling et al., 1986, Sooriakumaran et al., 2010; Steiner et al., 1993). Pregnancy has been identified as a risk factor for hemorrhage, likely because of the hormonal receptor positivity of these tumors (Boorjian et al., 2008; Eble, 1998). **Contrary to other benign renal masses, the diagnosis of AML can be made on imaging.** The presence of macroscopic fat on CT or MRI is diagnostic of AML. Ultrasonographically, masses are hyperechoic, similar to some RCCs, making ultrasound less reliable in the diagnosis (Steiner et al., 1993). **On CT the presence of intralesional fat (−15 to −20 Hounsfield units [HU]) on nonenhanced series is diagnostic** (Fig. 96.5A; Bosniak et al., 1988; Jinzaki et al., 1997; Lemaitre et al., 1997; Simpfendorfer et al., 2009). The diagnostic accuracy of CT has been evaluated in different settings. Using a cutoff of −10 HU, Davenport et al. (2011) found a c-index of 0.83 for the diagnosis of AML when the lesion was at least 19 to 24 mm in size. Meanwhile, the finding of 20 pixels with an attenuation of less than −20 HU and at least 6 pixels with an attenuation less than −30 HU was associated with a positive predictive value of 100% (Simpfendorfer et al., 2009). Similar to CT, on MRI the presence of intralesional fat is diagnostic of an AML. **Key findings on MRI include T1 and T2 hyperintensity** (Fig. 96.5B), **enhancement on gadolinium administration** (Fig. 96.5C), **hypointensity on T1 fat-suppressed sequences** (Fig. 96.5D), **and the**

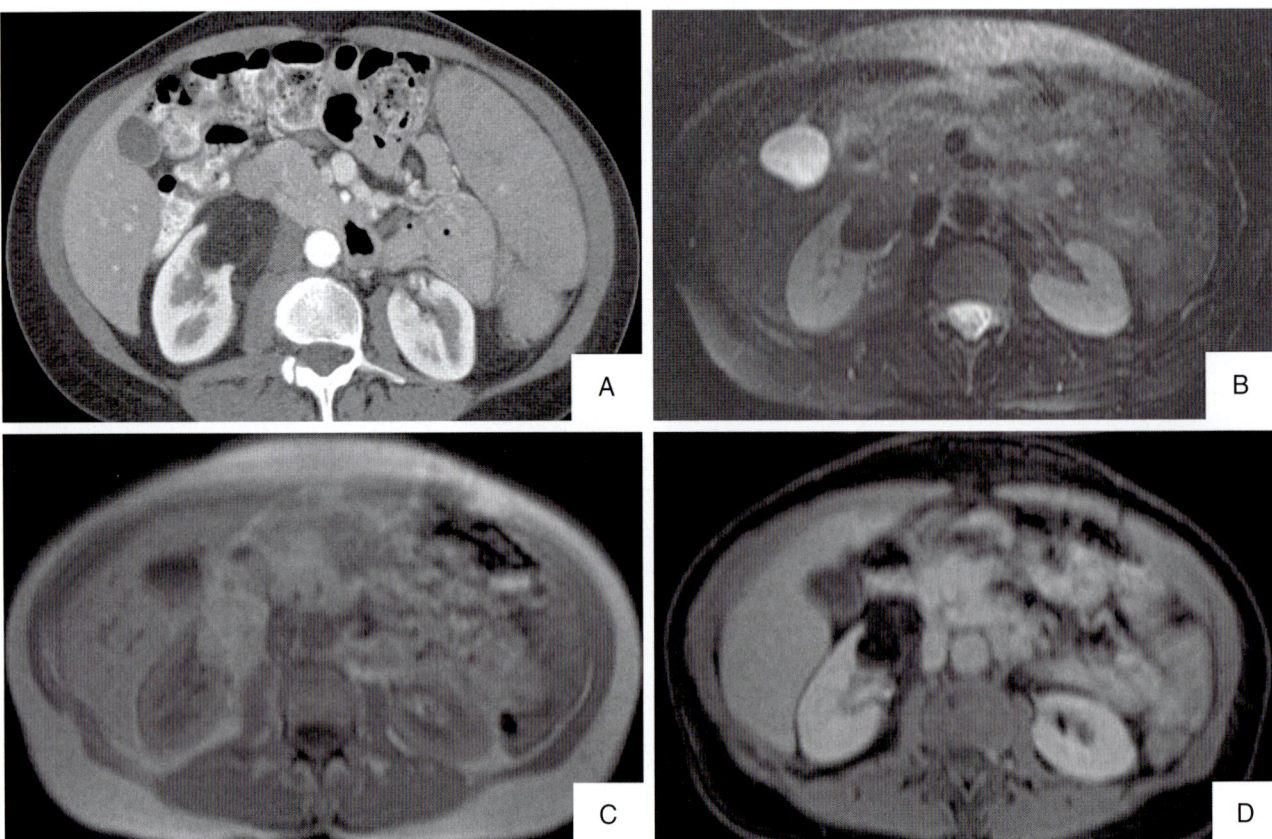

Fig. 96.5. (A) Contrast-enhanced computed tomography demonstrating macroscopic intralesional fat. (B) T2-weighted magnetic resonance imaging (MRI) with hypointensity. (C) Non–contrast-enhanced T1 MRI with hyperintensity of lesion secondary to macroscopic fat. (D) Post-contrast, fat-suppressed T1 image with signal dropout of mainly fat containing lesion, all consistent with classic angiomyolipoma. (From Flum AS, Hamoui N, Said MA, et al.: Update on the diagnosis and management of renal angiomyolipoma. *J Urol* 195[4 Pt 1]:834–846, 2016.)

presence of a dark boundary on in-phase/opposed-phase imaging that is also called an "India ink artifact" (Halpenny et al., 2010; Kim et al., 2006a and 2006b; Silverman et al., 2007).

Although the diagnosis can be confidently made on imaging in most circumstances, fat-poor AML (which resembles RCC), fat-containing RCC, and liposarcoma are unique situations in which the diagnosis can be problematic on imaging. Approximately 4% to 14% of AML do not contain radiographically identifiable fat and appear similar to RCC on standard imaging (hyperdense on noncontrast imaging and enhancing on contrasted series) (Hafron et al., 2005; Jinzaki et al., 1997, 2014; Kim et al., 2004; Lemaitre et al., 1997; Milner et al., 2006; Potretzke et al., 2017; Silverman et al., 2007). **In this setting MRI may be helpful, because lesions appear hyperintense on T1 sequences with subsequent hypointensity on fat-suppression and appear hypointense on T2 because of the preponderance of smooth muscle** (Halpenny et al., 2010; Jinzaki et al., 2014; Kim et al., 2006a and 2006b; Potretzke et al., 2017). When fat-poor AML is considered, percutaneous biopsy has been useful in determining the diagnosis (Lebret et al., 2007; Silverman et al., 2007). Fat-containing RCC is a rare situation; however, when described, intralesional calcification is commonly, although not universally, described, a finding not routinely seen in AML (Hayn et al., 2009; Henderson et al., 1997; Lemaitre et al., 1997; Roy et al., 1998). Finally, very large AMLs may have the appearance of retroperitoneal liposarcomas, with the key difference relating to the impact on the renal parenchyma. As AML arises from the parenchyma, an indentation in the parenchyma can be observed from this site of origination, whereas liposarcomas begin in the retroperitoneum and subsequently envelop and compress the renal parenchyma (Clark and Novick, 2001; Wang et al., 2002).

Management

Once the diagnosis is made, the management of patients with an AML should be individualized on the basis of sporadic versus syndromic AML, the presence of symptoms, and the perceived risk of hemorrhage. Flum et al. (2016) outlined an algorithm for management of AML that summarizes the mainstays of management (Fig. 96.6). Historically, a size of 4 cm or greater and being of childbearing age were used as indications for intervention because of a concern for spontaneous hemorrhage and pain (Blute et al., 1988; De Luca et al., 1999; Dickinson et al., 1998; Lemaitre et al., 1995; Nelson and Sanda, 2002; Oesterling et al., 1986; Preece et al., 2015; Seyam et al., 2008, Steiner et al., 1993). **Based on these series, AML less than 4 cm in size are expected to be asymptomatic and unlikely to bleed, and therefore active surveillance is an option.** Seyam et al. (2008) monitored sporadic and TSC-associated AML and demonstrated an average growth rate of 0.19 cm and 1.25 cm per year, respectively, suggesting relative stability, particularly in the sporadic cases. Furthermore, De Luca et al. (1999) found that, for AMLs less than 5 cm in diameter, 92% remained unchanged in size during follow-up. **Although 4 cm is used as a reasonable cutoff for observation, there are reports of larger AMLs being observed without significant risk** (Bhatt et al., 2016; Danforth et al., 2007; Hadley et al., 2006; Kennelly et al., 1994), **underscoring that 4 cm should not be used as an absolute indication for intervention.** Indeed, Ouzaid et al. (2014) described their experience with 130 AML patients on active surveillance, of whom 29% had masses larger than 4 cm. They found that among lesions larger than 4 cm, 66% remained on surveillance, suggesting overtreatment among patients with lesions larger than 4 cm managed with upfront intervention

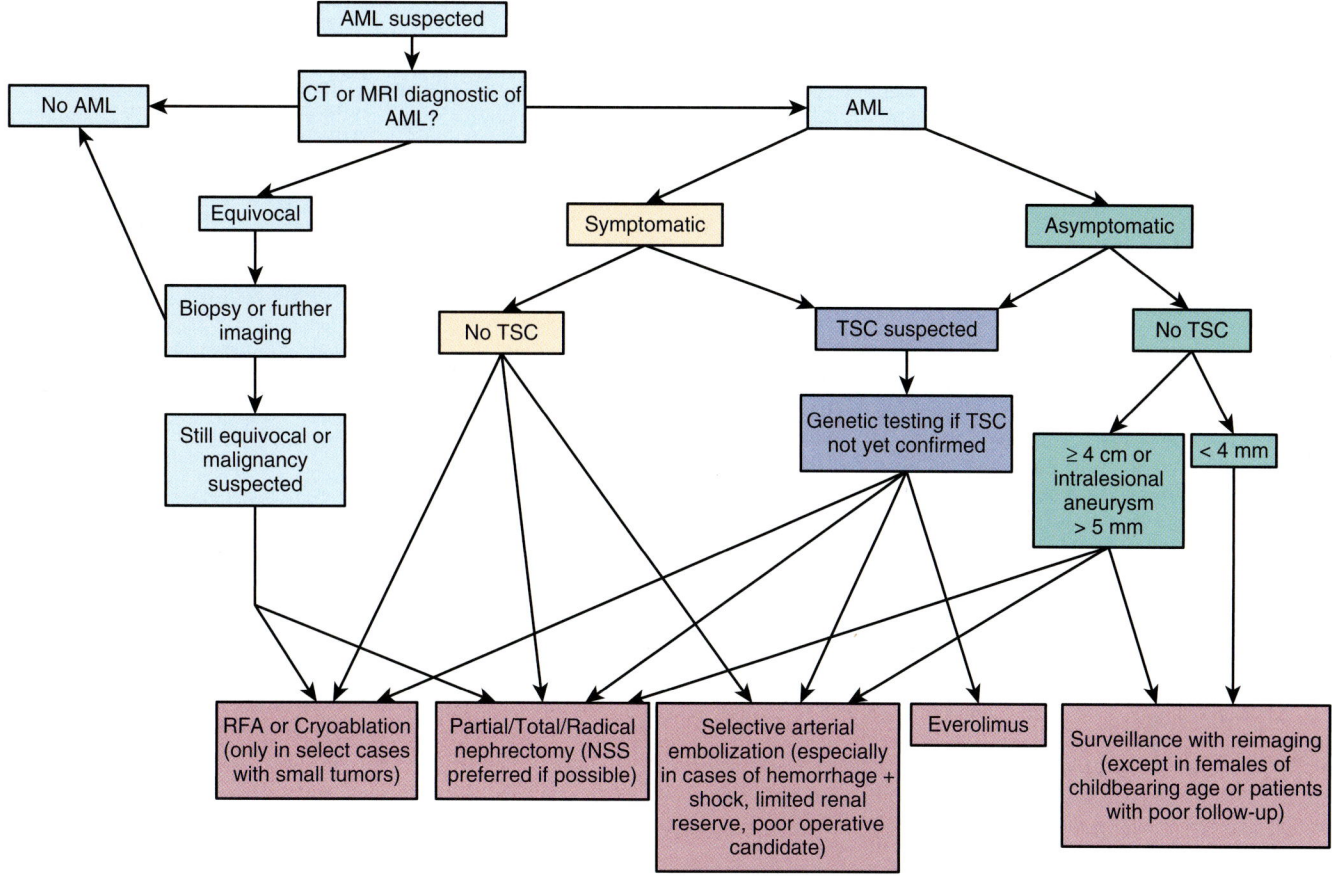

Fig. 96.6. Proposed updated management algorithm for renal angiomyolipoma (AML) by Flum et al. Algorithm represents suggested options. *CT*, Computed tomography; *MRI*, magnetic resonance imaging; *NSS*, nephron sparing surgery; *RFA*, radiofrequency ablation; *TSC*, tuberous sclerosis complex. (From Flum AS, Hamoui N, Said MA, et al.: Update on the diagnosis and management of renal angiomyolipoma. *J Urol* 195[4 Pt 1]:834–846, 2016.)

(Ouzaid et al., 2014). **As retroperitoneal hemorrhage is the overarching concern when observing an AML, Yamakado et al. (2002) identified that the presence of an intralesional aneurysm larger than 5 mm in diameter was predictive of subsequent hemorrhage. As such, when considering observation of a lesion more than 4 cm in size, assessment of intralesional aneurysm size with a thin-slice CT angiogram may improve the risk stratification of these patients. Finally, when considering observation, the reported association of hemorrhage during pregnancy must be considered, and prophylactic intervention in women of child-bearing age is recommended** (Preece et al., 2015). Once surveillance is selected, follow-up should be individualized but generally includes repeat imaging within the first 6 to 12 months with subsequent surveillance intervals determined by interval growth or stability (De Luca et al., 1999; Oesterling et al., 1986; Ouzaid et al., 2014).

When intervention is considered—because of size, concern for RCC, concern for epithelioid AML, or as prophylactic intervention—there are four mainstays of therapy: surgical resection, thermal ablation, embolization, and systemic therapy with mTOR inhibitors. When resection is chosen, nephron-sparing approaches should be performed because of improved renal function and overall mortality (Thompson et al., 2008). **Furthermore, in patients with TSC, where multifocal, bilateral, and recurring lesions are almost universal, nephron sparing is paramount.** Boorjian et al. (2007) evaluated the safety of nephron-sparing approaches in 58 patients with sporadic AML and documented a 3.4% recurrence risk and a 12% complication risk. Reported complications for open and minimally invasive partial nephrectomy in AML are no different than for traditional RCC, suggesting equivalence among well-selected patients (Boorjian et al., 2007; Heidenreich et al., 2002; Liu et al., 2016a and 2016b; Minervini et al., 2007; Msezane et al., 2010; Yip et al., 2000). Ablation is less well studied, with small case series reported using radiofrequency ablation or cryoablation, with acceptable safety (Castle et al., 2012; Makki et al., 2017; Tan et al., 2012) but require more study before routine, noninvestigational use. **Selective arterial embolization has been described as well, although it is more often reserved for the management of acute hemorrhage in AML, in which operative intervention most often results in total nephrectomy** (Chang et al., 2007; Pappas et al., 2006). When used as primary treatment of an AML, a reduction in size noted in most (Bardin et al., 2017; Hocquelet et al., 2014), but interval growth has been reported in up to 40% of patients (Bishay et al., 2010; Chan et al., 2011; Chick et al., 2010; Lee et al., 2009; Ramon et al., 2009, Villalta et al., 2011). Indeed, repeat procedures are not infrequent, often because of pain or bleeding, and can result in total nephrectomy (Hamlin et al., 1997; Han et al., 1997; Kehagias et al., 1998; Lenton et al., 2008; Mourikis et al., 1999). Complications for embolization include potential infection/abscess, postembolization syndrome (characterized by fever, pain, and leukocytosis), and renal infarction (Andersen et al., 2015; Flum et al., 2016; Lee et al., 2009). **When therapeutic embolization to surgery is considered, it is important to note that embolization obligates the patient to continued surveillance (based on recurrence risk), whereas surgery is curative in most sporadic AML cases. Therefore the burden of post-treatment follow-up is different between the two approaches.**

As noted earlier, TSC is associated with mutations that result in activation of the mTOR pathway. Given this molecular understanding of TSC-associated AML, mTOR inhibitors have been explored as systemic therapeutic agents for managing this disease in TSC patients. The first agent explored, sirolimus, has been examined in 4 phase II trials (94 patients) (Bissler et al., 2008; Cabrera-Lopez et al., 2012; Dabora et al., 2011; Davies et al., 2011). Using Response Evaluation

Criteria in Solid Tumors (RECIST) to assess response, the combined 12-month response rate (50% reduction in volume or 30% reduction in longest diameter) was 46.8%. Staehler et al. (2012) assessed the use of sirolimus in 3 patients whose tumors were too large to resect via partial nephrectomy and found that all 3 patients were ultimately able to proceed to partial nephrectomy after therapy. **More recently everolimus has been assessed in a phase III study among TSC- and LAM-associated AML (Bissler et al., 2013). In this study, the authors identified a response rate of 42% (at least 50% reduction in volume), with 80% achieving at least a 30% reduction in size. Furthermore, no patient who had a tumor response suffered progression during follow-up.** The authors recently updated their findings with 4 years of follow-up (Bissler et al., 2017). They found that 92% of patients experienced a response at some point, with only 14.3% experiencing progression and no patient requiring embolization for bleeding or nephrectomy for size increase. **Given these results, everolimus is approved by the US Food and Drug Administration for the treatment of AML in the setting of TSC.** Currently it is unknown how mTOR inhibition may influence sporadic AML cases, and there are ongoing trials assessing the role of everolimus in these patients.

KEY POINTS: ANGIOMYOLIPOMA

- AML is a benign tumor of dysmorphic blood vessels, smooth muscle, and adipose tissue that can be diagnosed definitively on cross-section imaging because of the presence of macroscopic fat.
- Most patients present asymptomatically; however, AML is the most common cause of spontaneous retroperitoneal hemorrhage.
- Tuberous sclerosis is associated with the development of multifocal and bilateral renal AML and is associated with activation of the mTOR pathway.
- Treatment depends on size, presence of symptoms, and pregnancy status and should be tailored to the patient with the goal of renal function preservation.
- The treatment of choice in patients with acute hemorrhage is selective renal angioembolization.
- Everolimus is indicated for the management of larger, multifocal AMLs in patients with TSC and LAM.

PAPILLARY ADENOMA OF THE KIDNEY

Papillary adenoma of the kidney is an entity of some controversy regarding its benignity. **In 2004 the World Health Organization defined papillary adenoma as a low-grade (grade 1–2), well-circumscribed cortical lesion measuring less than 0.5 cm** (Lopez-Beltran et al., 2006). Incidence increases with age, male sex, end-stage renal disease, acquired renal cystic disease, sporadic RCC, and hereditary papillary RCC (Denton et al., 2002; Hughson et al., 1986; Ornstein et al., 2000; Reis et al., 1988; Snyder et al., 2006; Wang et al., 2007; Xipell, 1971).

Histologically, cells are uniform with benign nuclei and are arranged as either tubular, papillary, or tubulopapillary, similar to papillary RCC (Grignon and Eble, 1998; Lopez-Beltran et al., 2006), raising concerns about the potential that papillary adenomas are a premalignant lesion. As shown by Wang et al. in 2007, papillary adenomas are associated with papillary RCC (47%) and are often multifocal when associated with papillary RCC (61%). Furthermore, in analysis of nephrectomy specimens in patients with hereditary papillary RCC, up to 3000 small papillary lesions are predicted per kidney, suggesting a common lineage from papillary adenomas to papillary RCC (Ornstein et al., 2000). **In addition, supporting this concern is the similar immunohistochemical staining (α-methylacyl CoA racemase [AMACR] positivity) and cytogenetic changes (such as trisomy 7 and 17) of papillary adenoma and papillary RCC** (Brunelli et al., 2003; Wang et al., 2007).

Because papillary adenomas are, by definition, less than 1 cm in size, they are often diagnosed pathologically as a concomitant finding with RCC (Wang et al., 2007) **and therefore require no further directed therapy.** Although the diagnosis of papillary adenoma as a benign entity remains controversial, the changing paradigm of active surveillance for small renal masses certainly supports observation of these small lesions when papillary adenoma is considered.

KEY POINTS: PAPILLARY ADENOMA OF THE KIDNEY

- Papillary adenomas are 5 mm or smaller and are therefore not readily diagnosed on imaging.
- Papillary adenomas share common immunohistochemical staining and genetic changes and are found in association with papillary RCC, suggesting a commonality between these disease.

METANEPHRIC ADENOMA

Metanephric adenomas of the kidney is a rare benign epithelial lesion in the kidney that has been described in the literature, mainly through case reports, representing approximately 0.2% of renal masses (Amin et al., 2002; Saremian et al., 2015). **It can present at any age, although peaks in the fifth decade, and is found more often in females (2:1 female:male ratio)** (Bastide et al., 2009; Davis et al., 1995; Jones et al., 1995; Renshaw, 2002; Snyder et al., 2006). As originally described by Davis et al. in 1995, approximately one-half of patients are diagnosed incidentally; the remainder experience symptoms such as flank pain, gross hematuria, a palpable mass, and polycythemia. The cause of polycythemia in metanephric adenoma has been investigated using in vitro cell cultures, which demonstrated the production of erythropoietin, IL-6, IL-8, G-CSF, and GM-CSF (Yoshioka et al., 2007).

Grossly, these appear as well-circumscribed, tan/brown masses that have been reported up to 15 cm (Davis et al., 1995; Jones et al., 1995). On pathologic evaluation, the differential includes Wilms tumor, papillary RCC, and papillary adenomas. Saremian et al. (2015) reviewed 14 reported cases of metanephric adenoma in which histologic findings were described from cytology (either fine-needle aspiration or core-needle biopsy). They found that all cases contained uniform cells with bland nuclei and scant cytoplasm. Where architecture was described, acinar, follicular, tubulopapillary, and glomerular structures were reported. **Importantly, necrosis, atypia, or mitotic figures, features commonly found in Wilms tumors, are not present** (Patel et al., 2009; Saremian et al., 2015). **Although histology may differentiate Wilms tumor from metanephric adenoma, immunohistochemistry may be beneficial in distinguishing papillary RCC from this entity** (Muir et al., 2001; Olgac et al., 2006; Saremian et al. 2015). **Specifically, metanephric adenomas stain positive for Wilms tumor protein WT1 and CD57 and negative for α-methylacyl CoA racemase (AMACR), whereas papillary RCC stains oppositely** (Muir et al., 2001; Olgac et al., 2006). Meanwhile, papillary adenomas are notable for cytokeratin-7 and epithelial membrane antigen positive, whereas metanephric adenomas are negative for these markers (Saremian et al., 2015). Other markers have been explored, including S-100, cytokeratins 8, 18, and 19, and vimentin (Azabdaftari et al., 2008; Skinnider et al., 2005). Together, the description of histologic and immunohistochemical methods to differentiate metanephric adenoma from alternative diagnoses may suggest a role for renal mass biopsy when suspicion is high for such a benign entity (Bosco et al., 2007; Patel et al., 2009).

As previously noted, these tumors are histologically similar to Wilms tumor and have been hypothesized to be the most well-differentiated and mature form of Wilms tumors (Argani, 2005). Supporting this theory is the strong staining for WT1 observed in these tumors (Muir et al., 2001; Olgac et al., 2006). However, the cytogenetics of metanephric adenomas vary widely, and as descriptions are limited to case series, drawing inference from these associations is difficult. Reported mutations include 2p13 (Pesti et al., 2001), gain of chromosome 7 and 17 (Brown et al., 1997), and gain of chromosome 19 (Pan and Epstein, 2010). Because trisomy 7 and

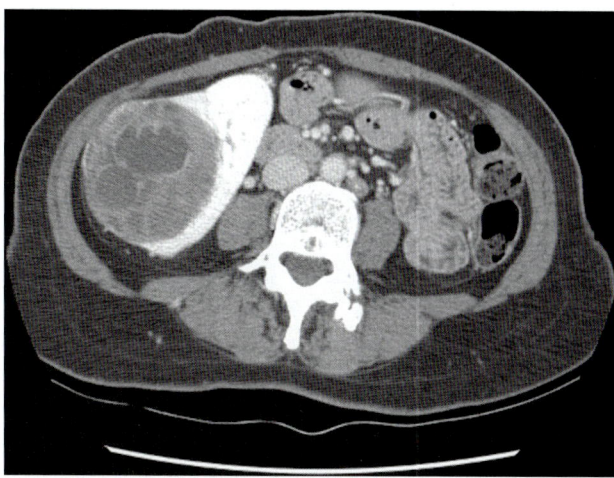

Fig. 96.7. Computed tomography scan showing a metanephric adenoma in a middle-aged woman. (Copyright 2009, S. F. Matin.)

17 are associated with papillary RCC and papillary adenoma and given the histologic similarities of metanephric adenoma to these entities, it has also been suggested that metanephric adenoma may exist on a spectrum with papillary RCC (Blanco et al., 2013; Brown et al., 1997).

On CT, these masses appear may appear hypovascular with minimal enhancement and calcifications (Bastide et al., 2009). Yan et al. (2016) performed a detailed review of radiographic features in nine histologically confirmed metanephric adenomas and found that tumors were isodense on non-contrast phase, with progressive but lower enhancement at each phase of a contrast-enhanced CT. **Notably, enhancement was uniformly less than that of the renal parenchyma; a finding in contrast to RCC, in which rapid hyperenhancement is common** (Fig. 96.7; Yan et al., 2016). Unfortunately, radiographic findings may be insufficient to establish the diagnosis, and as such, these are often diagnosed after surgical resection. When the suspicion is high, renal mass biopsy may be considered, with fine-needle aspiration to perform immunohistochemical staining. Once diagnosed, management is often nephron sparing (such as partial nephrectomy or thermal ablation), because metastatic metanephric adenoma has rarely been described (Drut et al., 2001; Paner et al., 2005; Renshaw et al., 2000).

> **KEY POINTS: METANEPHRIC ADENOMA**
>
> - Metanephric adenoma is a rare, benign enhancing renal mass.
> - Symptoms are present in approximately 50% of patients, with a female predisposition.
> - Metanephric adenoma may exist on a continuum with Wilms tumors and papillary RCC and can be distinguished based on histology and immunohistochemical staining.

MIXED MESENCHYMAL AND EPITHELIAL TUMORS

Cystic nephroma and mixed epithelial and stromal tumors (MESTs) are a group of tumors that are separate but genetically and morphologically related benign lesions in the kidney (Lopez-Beltran et al., 2006; Moch et al., 2016; Montironi et al., 2008; Turbiner et al., 2007; Zhou et al., 2009). Commonalities include a female predilection and frequent expression of estrogen and progesterone receptors (Montironi et al., 2008).

Cystic Nephroma

Cystic nephroma is a rare benign tumor that occurs in youth (boys predominately, 2–3 years of age) and adults (females predominately;

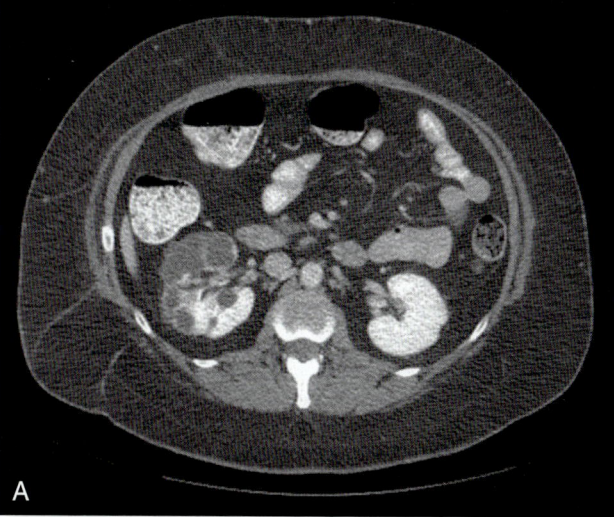

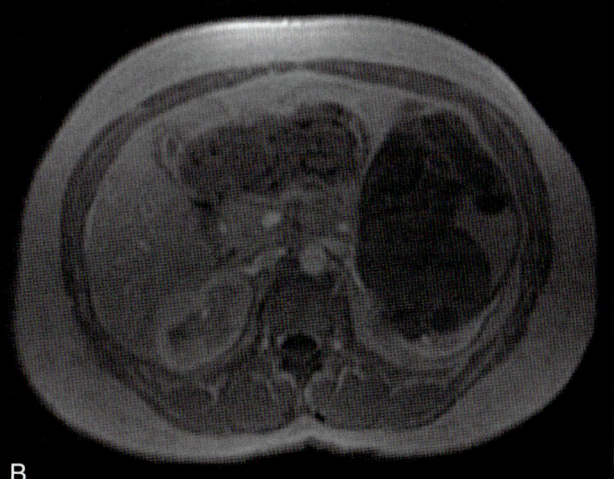

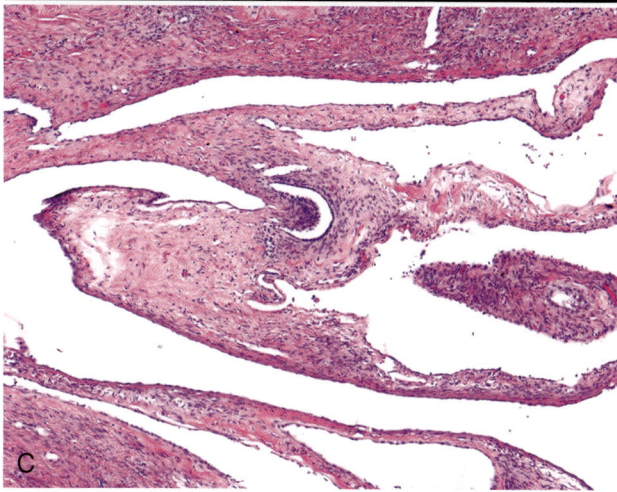

Fig. 96.8. Cystic nephroma. Computed tomography (A) and magnetic resonance imaging (B) scans do not allow reliable distinction from cystic renal cell carcinoma or cystic Wilms tumor. (C) The variably sized cystic spaces are lined by flattened epithelium (low magnification). (Copyright 2009, V. Margulis.)

fourth and fifth decades) (Castillo et al., 1991; Kuzgunbay et al. 2009; Madewell et al., 1983, Montironi et al., 2008, Stamatiou et al., 2008; Tamboli et al., 2000; Upadhyay and Neely, 1989).

Radiographically, tumors are often solitary, central cystic masses with calcifications, extension to the collecting system, and septal enhancement (Figs. 96.8A and B; Madewell et al., 1983; Turbiner et al., 2007). Given this appearance, in children, cystic nephroma is difficult to distinguish from Wilms tumor and is often diagnosed after surgical resection. **Because of the inability to rule out Wilms tumor radiographically, children should be managed as per the Children's Oncology Group Renal Tumor Committee guidelines, with initial radical nephrectomy** (Board, 2002). On histologic evaluation, tumors are encapsulated cystic lesions lined with cuboidal and hobnail epithelium (Fig. 96.8C) in a stroma variably composed of collagen and spindle cell fascicles (Tamboli et al., 2000). Immunohistochemical stains are notable for cytokeratin positivity in the epithelium, which stromal elements stain for CD10, calretinin, inhibin, estrogen, and progesterone (Montironi et al., 2008; Turbiner et al., 2007). **The key finding that differentiates cystic nephroma from Wilms tumor is the lack of blastemal and embryonal elements in the resected tissues** (Joshi and Beckwith, 1989). In adults, management depends on the certainty of the diagnosis; however, the radiographic appearance of an enhancing cystic mass mimics cystic clear cell RCC, and therefore resection is common. In addition, although benign, there have been reports of sarcoma, leiomyosarcoma, rhabdomyosarcoma, pleomorphic sarcoma, and clear cell RCC arising from cystic nephroma, further supporting the role of resection when feasible (Eble and Bonsib, 1998, Montironi et al., 2008; Omar et al., 2006; Sukov et al., 2007).

MIXED EPITHELIAL AND STROMAL TUMORS

MESTs are benign tumors of the kidney that are most often identified in perimenopausal women, often with a history of estrogen replacement, with a peak incidence in the fifth decade (Adsay et al., 2000; Moslemi, 2010). In men this has been reported after long-term hormonal deprivation for prostate cancer (Adsay et al., 2000; Chuang et al., 2018).

On radiologic evaluation, MESTs often appear as a complex cystic mass, such as a Bosniak III-IV lesion, similar to RCC (Fig. 96.9A) (Adsay et al., 2000). As such, the diagnosis can be difficult and is often not made until after resection. Grossly, tumors are identified with a mean size of 6 cm and are encapsulated with solid and cystic components that often extend into the renal pelvis (Fig. 96.9B; Adsay et al., 2000; Michal, 2000; Michal et al., 2004). Because tumors are composed of mesenchymal and epithelial elements, on microscopic evaluation there are cystic components variably lined with cuboidal and columnar epithelium, although urothelium can be seen as well, interspersed in a stroma of spindle cells, smooth muscle fascicles, and collagen bands (Fig. 96.9C; Adsay et al., 2000; Antic et al., 2006; Montironi et al., 2008; Turbiner et al., 2007). Immunohistochemical staining generally reveals estrogen and progesterone positivity in the stromal elements, along with mesenchymal markers such as vimentin, CD 34, and desmin (Adsay et al., 2000). Meanwhile the epithelial components will stain positive for cytokeratin 7 (Montironi et al., 2008).

Importantly, malignant transformation has been observed in primary lesions and as recurrence. These transformations are observed in the stromal elements with sarcomatoid features and poor clinical outcomes are expected (Adsay et al., 2000; Nakagawa et al., 2004; Shen et al., 2007; Yap et al., 2004).

> **KEY POINTS: CYSTIC NEPHROMA AND MIXED EPITHELIAL-STROMAL TUMOR**
>
> - Cystic nephroma and MESTs are biologically related and histologically similar.
> - Frequent expression of estrogen and progesterone receptors in tumor tissue is reported with a female predisposition.
> - Cystic nephroma clinically resembles Wilms tumor, particularly in children.
> - If feasible, a nephron-sparing approach with partial nephrectomy is the preferred management strategy.

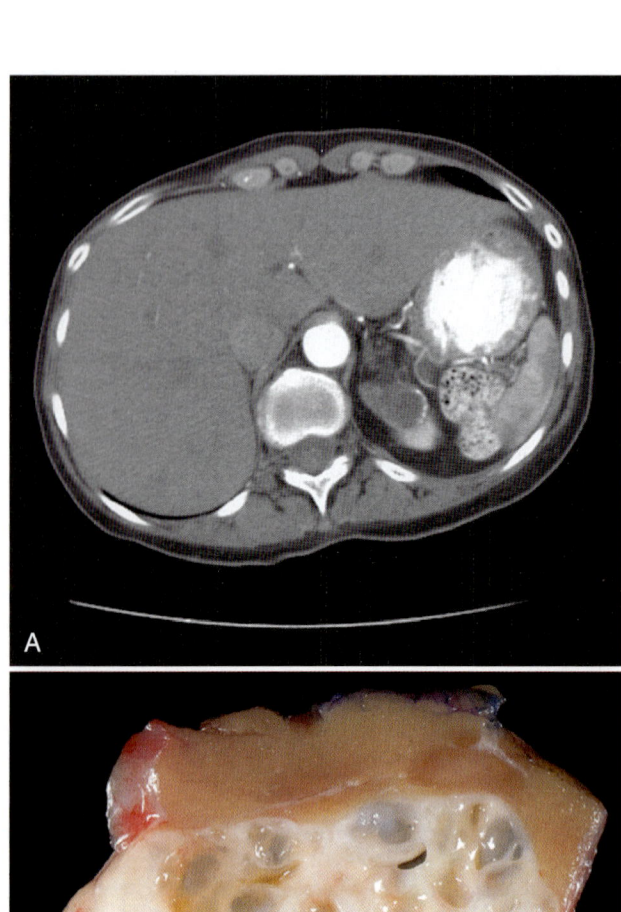
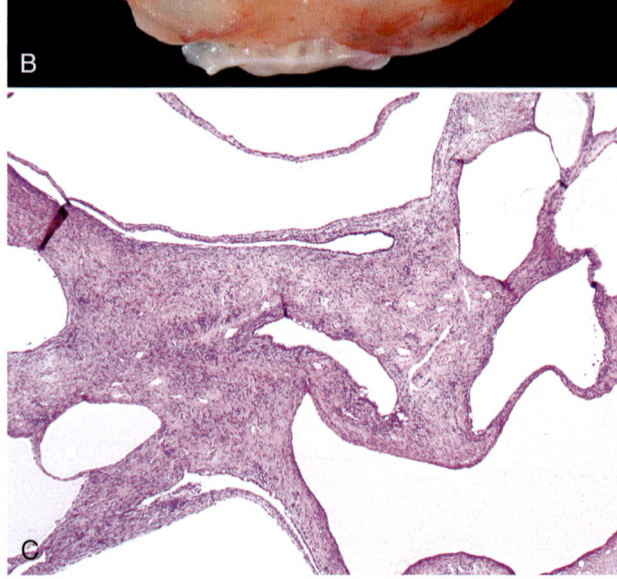

Fig. 96.9. Mixed epithelial and stromal tumor. (A) Computed tomography scan characteristics are not distinguishable from renal cell carcinoma. (B) Gross photograph of a partial nephrectomy specimen demonstrating a well-circumscribed mass composed of variably sized cysts separated by thick white septa. (C) Medium-power magnification shows cysts lined by hobnailed cells and spindle cell stroma. (Copyright 2009, V. Margulis.)

LEIOMYOMA

Leiomyoma is a rare renal tumor of smooth muscle differentiation (Moch et al., 2016). These tumors can arise anywhere in the urinary tract; the bladder is the most common site (Larbcharoensub et al., 2017; Tamboli et al., 2000). **Within the kidney, multiple sites have been described; however, the renal capsule is the most often described location** (Rao et al., 2001; Romano et al., 2017; Steiner et al. 1990; Wells et al., 1981). **They are found more often in women (2:1 predominance), and account for 0.29% of primary renal mass** (Khetrapal et al., 2014).

As leiomyomas arise from the capsule, radiographically they appear as small exophytic masses that are hyperdense on noncontrast CT with hypoenhancement on intravenous contrast administration (Cong et al., 2011). **Although this enhancement is less than that observed with traditional clear cell RCC, chromophobe RCC tends to have hypoenhancement similar to leiomyoma, making the radiologic diagnosis difficult** (Fig. 96.10A; Cong et al., 2011; Steiner et al., 1990).

On gross examination, these tumors appear well circumscribed and firm. Tumors can range in size and may have associated calcifications and focal cystic degeneration. Microscopic examination demonstrates spindle cells that form intersecting fascicles without evidence of hypercellularity, pleomorphism, mitotic figures, or necrosis (Fig. 96.10B; Larbcharoensub et al. 2017; Steiner et al., 1990; Tamboli et al., 2000). Immunohistochemical staining is notable for vimentin and smooth muscle markers desmin and caldesmon (Fig. 96.10C; Larbcharoensub et al., 2017; Romero et al. 2005). Interestingly, leiomyomas can stain for HMB-45 (Bonsib, 1996). Because AML is on the differential for a leiomyoma, the key factors differentiating these entities include the absence of melan-A staining and the absence of adiposity in leiomyomas.

Radiographically, tumors are hyperdense relative to the renal parenchyma on noncontrast imaging, with clear sharp margins (Cong et al., 2011). With contrast administration, homogeneous enhancement is observed, which increases in later phases, except in the setting of large masses, in which hemorrhage or cystic changes may result in heterogeneous patterns. As RCC typically enhances early and heterogeneously, with washout on later phases, these differences may be exploited to differentiate leiomyoma from RCC (Cong et al., 2011). **Management, as with most benign renal masses, depends on the certainty of the diagnosis before intervention, with nephron-sparing approaches preferred when treatment is considered.**

> ### KEY POINTS: LEIOMYOMA
> - Leiomyomas are described along the urinary tract but most often from the renal capsule.
> - Radiologic examination is insufficient to confirm the diagnosis.
> - Nephron-sparing approaches are preferred when technically possible.

OTHER BENIGN RENAL TUMORS

In addition to the commonly identified lesions outlined earlier, a host of other benign lesions have been described, including hemangiomas, lymphangiomas, juxtaglomerular cell tumors, renomedullary interstitial cell tumor, intrarenal schwannoma, and solitary fibrous tumor.

Hemangiomas are vascular lesions that are more often identified in young patients. Although most are sporadic, they can be found in association with syndromes such as Klippel-Trenaunay, Struge-Weber, and systemic angiomatosis. When identified they are often singular, associated with the renal pyramids and pelvis. There is no capsule and on histologic evaluation there are irregular vascular spaces (Tamboli et al., 2000). More recently, a potentially related lesion, renal anastomosing hemangioma (RAH), has been described (Brown et al., 2010; Kryvenko et al., 2011; Kuroda et al., 2016; Omiyale, 2015). Mean age of RAH is older, at 50 years of age with a male predisposition (Omiyale,

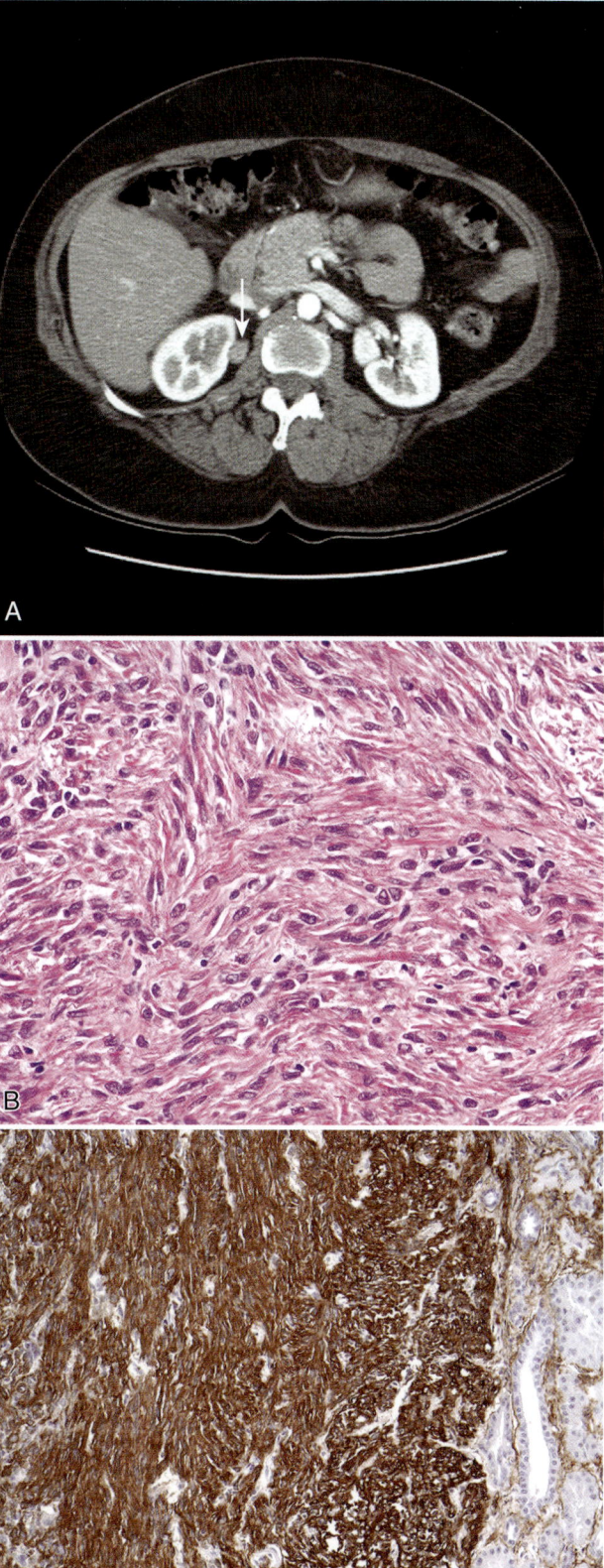

Fig. 96.10. Renal leiomyoma. (A) Computed tomography scan with characteristic appearance of a small renal mass arising from the renal capsule *(arrow)*. (B) Medium-power magnification shows uniform spindle cells with thin cigar-shaped nuclei, without any pleomorphism. (C) Strong positive immunohistochemical staining with smooth muscle actin in the leiomyoma. Note lack of smooth-muscle actin staining in the normal renal tubules on the right. (Copyright 2009, V. Margulis.)

2015). When identified, they have a similar anatomic distribution within the kidney as other hemangiomas, although are more commonly multifocal (Kryvenko et al., 2011; Kuroda et al., 2016; Omiyale, 2015). Because most are diagnosed incidentally at nephrectomy, no specific treatment is required or suggested.

Renal lymphangiomas are rare tumors that arise from a developmental abnormality in which the perirenal lymphatics do not communicate with the rest of the lymphatic system, resulting in dilated, cystic masses around the renal capsule, renal sinus, or peripelvic fat (Mani et al., 2003). Presentation is often incidental; however, compression and involvement of the renal pelvis can cause signs and symptoms of obstructive uropathy, hypertension, hematuria, proteinuria, hemorrhage, and chyluria (Chiu et al., 2004; Kekre et al., 1998, Varela et al., 1998). Treatment depends on presence of symptoms and can include aspiration/sclerosis or surgical excision (Daali et al., 2001; Wildhaber et al., 2006).

Juxtaglomerular cell tumor (also known as *reninoma* or *JGCT*), is a tumor arising from the juxtaglomerular cells of the kidney and was originally described in 1967 by Robertson et al. It is most commonly identified in women in their second and third decades (Kim et al., 2006a and 2006b; Martin et al., 2001; McVicar et al., 1993). **The hallmark of these tumors is overproduction of renin; therefore patients often experience symptoms of hyperaldosteronism, such as polydipsia, polyuria, myalgias, double vision, and headaches** (Haab et al., 1995; Kuroda et al., 2011; McVicar et al., 1993; Rubenstein et al., 2002; Schonfeld et al., 1991). **On examination, hypertension, hypokalemia, and proteinuria are often identified** (Gottardo et al., 2010; Haab et al., 1995; Kuroda et al., 2011; McVicar et al., 1993). Although hypertension is a common finding, Haab et al. (1995) only identified 8 cases of JGCT among 30,000 patients in a hypertension clinic. Imaging typically reveals a small renal mass that is solid and can be hypoechoic on ultrasound and nonenhancing on CT (Gottardo et al., 2010; Mete et al., 2003; Schonfeld et al., 1991; Tanabe et al. 2001). Grossly these tumors are well circumscribed with hemorrhage commonly observed (Martin et al., 2001). On microscopic evaluation, common findings are uniform, packed, polygonal cells with indistinct borders (Kuroda et al., 2011). Staining for intracytoplasmic renin is pathognomonic (Caregaro et al., 1994; Tanaka et al., 1993). **When such small lesions are identified in a young, hypertensive patient, the diagnosis should be considered and confirmed by high plasma renin levels. Once diagnosed, surgical resection results in resolution of symptoms in the majority of patients; however, up to 10% have persistent hypertension because of the development of hypertensive angiopathy** (Kuroda et al., 2011; Squires et al., 1984). A benign post-treatment course is expected, and only one case of metastatic JGCT has been reported (Duan et al., 2004).

Renomedullary interstitial cell tumor is a tumor that arises within the renal medullary tissue. The cells of origin, renomedullary interstitial cells, synthesize prostaglandins; it was therefore thought to be the result of hypertension (Stuart et al., 1976; Zhuo, 2000). These tumors were initially described on autopsy study (Reese and Winstanley, 1958), with a recent report finding an incidence of 44% in unselected adult autopsy specimens (Calio et al., 2016). Importantly, no association between hypertension was identified in this more recent study. Tumors are small (mean 1.7 mm), often multifocal (mean 3 per patient), with spindle/stellate cells in a fibrous background with increasing collagen as age increased (Calio et al., 2016).

Intrarenal schwannomas are exceptionally rare benign renal masses arising from nerve sheath tissue in the renal parenchyma. Patients can present with nonspecific symptoms, such as malaise, weight loss, fever, and abdominal pain (Umphrey et al., 2007). They are well-circumscribed masses that can range in size. Histologically they are composed of spindle cells in a palisading pattern, which stain positive for S-100 (Alvarado-Cabrero et al., 2000; Singer and Anders, 1996).

Solitary fibrous tumor is a rare benign tumor of mesenchymal origin that tends to occur with hematuria, flank pain, and an enlarging mass (Fursevich et al., 2016; Hirano et al., 2009; Kohl et al., 2006; Park et al., 2011). Masses are large with heterogenous enhancement, calcifications, and necrosis on CT that are hard to distinguish from RCC (Cortes et al., 2014; Katabathina et al., 2010). Histologically they are circumscribed and consist of spindle cells and collagen bands and stain positive for CD34, CD99, and BCL-2 (Magro et al., 2002; Wang et al., 2001).

> **KEY POINTS: OTHER BENIGN RENAL TUMORS**
>
> - Multiple rare tumors of the kidney have been described.
> - Radiologic differentiation from renal malignancy is not possible.
> - Reninoma, a benign tumor of the renal juxtaglomerular cell apparatus, is an important but rare cause of secondary hypertension and hypokalemia.

SUGGESTED READINGS

Bissler JJ, Kingswood JC, Radzikowska E, et al: Everolimus long-term use in patients with tuberous sclerosis complex: four-year update of the EXIST-2 study, *PLoS ONE* 12(8):2017. e0180939.
Curatolo P, Bombardieri R, Jozwiak S: Tuberous sclerosis, *Lancet* 372(9639):657–668, 2008.
Eknoyan G: A clinical view of simple and complex renal cysts, *J Am Soc Nephrol* 20(9):1874–1876, 2009.
Flum AS, Hamoui N, Said MA, et al: Update on the diagnosis and management of renal angiomyolipoma, *J Urol* 195(4 Pt 1):834–846, 2016.
Grantham JJ: Clinical practice. Autosomal dominant polycystic kidney disease, *N Engl J Med* 359(14):1477–1485, 2008.
Halpenny D, Snow A, McNeill G, et al: The radiological diagnosis and treatment of renal angiomyolipoma-current status, *Clin Radiol* 65(2):99–108, 2010.
Helenon O, Crosnier A, Verkarre V, et al: Simple and complex renal cysts in adults: classification system for renal cystic masses, *Diagn Interv Imaging* 2018.
Kuroda N, Gotoda H, Ohe C, et al: Review of juxtaglomerular cell tumor with focus on pathobiological aspect, *Diagn Pathol* 6:80, 2011.
Kuroda N, Ohe C, Deepika S, et al: Review of renal anastomosing hemangioma with focus on clinical and pathological aspects, *Pol J Pathol* 67(2):97–101, 2016.
Larbcharoensub N, Limprasert V, Pangpunyakulchai D, et al: Renal leiomyoma: a case report and review of the literature, *Urol Case Rep* 13:3–5, 2017.
Lopez-Beltran A, Scarpelli M, Montironi R, et al: 2004 WHO classification of the renal tumors of the adults, *Eur Urol* 49(5):798–805, 2006.
Moch H, Cubilla AL, Humphrey PA, et al: The 2016 WHO classification of tumours of the urinary system and male genital organs-part a: renal, penile, and testicular tumours, *Eur Urol* 70(1):93–105, 2016.
Montironi R, Mazzucchelli R, Lopez-Beltran A, et al: Cystic nephroma and mixed epithelial and stromal tumour of the kidney: opposite ends of the spectrum of the same entity?, *Eur Urol* 54(6):1237–1246, 2008.
Pappas P, Leonardou P, Papadoukakis S, et al: Urgent superselective segmental renal artery embolization in the treatment of life-threatening renal hemorrhage, *Urol Int* 77(1):34–41, 2006.
Patel HD, Druskin SC, Rowe SP, et al: Surgical histopathology for suspected oncocytoma on renal mass biopsy: a systematic review and meta-analysis, *BJU Int* 119(5):661–666, 2017.
Rahbari-Oskoui F, O'Neill WC: Diagnosis and management of acquired cystic kidney disease and renal tumors in ESRD patients, *Semin Dial* 30(4):373–379, 2017.
Reuter VE, Argani P, Zhou M, et al: Best practices recommendations in the application of immunohistochemistry in the kidney tumors: report from the International Society of Urologic Pathology consensus conference, *Am J Surg Pathol* 38(8):e35–e49, 2014.
Saremian J, Kubik MJ, Masood S: Cytologic features of metanephric adenoma of the kidney: case report and review of the literature, *Lab Med* 46(2):153–158, quiz e130, 2015.
Seyam RM, Bissada NK, Kattan SA, et al: Changing trends in presentation, diagnosis and management of renal angiomyolipoma: comparison of sporadic and tuberous sclerosis complex-associated forms, *Urology* 72(5):1077–1082, 2008.
Steinlein OK, Ertl-Wagner B, Ruzicka T, et al: Birt-Hogg-Dube syndrome: an underdiagnosed genetic tumor syndrome, *J Dtsch Dermatol Ges* 16(3):278–283, 2018.
Sun DZ, Campbell SC: Atypical epithelioid angiomyolipoma: a rare variant with malignant potential, *Urology* 112:20–22, 2018.
Wobker SE, Williamson SR: Modern pathologic diagnosis of renal oncocytoma, *J Kidney Cancer VHL* 4(4):1–12, 2017.
Yan J, Cheng JL, Li CF, et al: The findings of CT and MRI in patients with metanephric adenoma, *Diagn Pathol* 11(1):104, 2016.

REFERENCES

The complete reference list is available online at ExpertConsult.com.

97

Malignant Renal Tumors

Steven C. Campbell, MD, PhD, Brian R. Lane, MD, PhD, and Phillip M. Pierorazio, MD

HISTORICAL CONSIDERATIONS

The introduction of nephrectomy for renal diseases provided the clinical information and histopathologic insight that form the basis of current concepts regarding renal tumors. Wolcott accomplished the first documented nephrectomy in 1861, mistakenly removing a tumor mass he believed was a hepatoma. **Simon performed the first planned nephrectomy in 1869** for persistent ureteral fistula, and this patient survived with cure of the fistula. One year later Gilmore in Mobile, Alabama, successfully accomplished the first planned nephrectomy in the United States for treatment of atrophic chronic pyelonephritis (Herr, 2008). Harris (1882) subsequently reported on 100 renal extirpations, a sufficient number to permit analysis of the clinical and pathologic features of renal disorders that require surgery.

With surgical intervention, tissue became available for histologic interpretation, although there were often serious professional differences of opinion. According to Carson (1928), the first accurate gross description of kidney tumors was from Konig and dates to 1826. In 1855 Robin examined solid tumors apparently arising in the kidney and concluded that renal carcinoma arose from renal tubular epithelium, and Waldeyer supported this interpretation in 1867. Unfortunately, theoretical and practical considerations of renal tumors were confused by Grawitz (1883), who contended that renal tumors arose from adrenal rests within the kidney. He introduced the terminology *struma lipomatodes aberrata renis* as descriptive nomenclature for the tumors of clear cells that he believed were derived from the adrenal glands. He based his conclusions not only on the fatty content of the tumors, analogous to that seen in the adrenal glands, but also on the location of the tumors beneath the renal capsule, approximation to the adrenal glands, and the lack of similarity of the cells to uriniferous tubules.

Subsequent investigators readily embraced the idea that renal tumors truly arose from the adrenal glands. In 1894 Lubarch endorsed the idea of a suprarenal origin of renal tumors, and the term *hypernephroid tumors*, indicating origin above the kidneys, was introduced (Birch-Hirschfeld and Doederlein, 1894). This semantic and conceptual mistake led to the term *hypernephroma*, which predominated in the literature describing parenchymal tumors of primary renal origin. Some clarification of the histopathology of renal tumors was derived from the work of Albarran and Imbert in 1903, and the four-volume contribution of Wolff, written between 1883 and 1928, improved our understanding of renal tumors (Herr, 2008).

The modern era has brought an appreciation that renal cell carcinoma (RCC) includes a number of distinct subtypes derived from the various parts of the nephron, each with a unique genetic basis and tumor biology (Linehan and Ricketts, 2013; Rini et al., 2009a). Other major advances in the past several decades have included the introduction of classic radical nephrectomy (RN) in the 1960s followed by a trend toward less radical approaches, including nephron-sparing surgery and a variety of minimally invasive approaches (Novick, 2007; Robson, 1963; Volpe et al., 2011). A common theme from early understanding to contemporary management of renal tumors **is that RCC remains primarily a surgical disease** and, although immune-based and targeted molecular approaches can occasionally provide durable clinical responses, cure is rarely seen without complete surgical excision (Petrelli et al., 2016; Pindoria et al., 2017). Unfortunately, the incidence of RCC is gradually increasing and, despite a trend toward earlier detection, mortality rates remain high.

CLASSIFICATION

Renal masses can be malignant, benign, or inflammatory (Table 97.1; Srigley et al., 2013), **or they can be classified based on radiographic appearance (simple cystic, complex cystic, solid)** (Table 97.2). These classification schemes have been updated based on current knowledge about the distinct subtypes of RCC and other benign and malignant tumors of the kidney (Srigley et al., 2013). Malignant renal tumors include RCC, urothelial-based malignancies, sarcomas, embryonic or pediatric tumors, lymphomas, and metastases. Benign renal tumors are diverse and present unique diagnostic challenges (see Chapter 96). Inflammatory and vascular entities must also be considered in the differential diagnosis.

Imaging and Clinical Risk Stratification of Renal Masses

Given the wide differential diagnosis of renal masses and current perspectives about tumor biology, clinical evaluation is extremely important in the assessment of the risk of malignancy and metastatic potential of a given renal mass in a specific patient. Clinical evaluation may include patient characteristics and mode of presentation, imaging characteristics, laboratory evaluation, and renal mass biopsy (RMB). A number of composite models and nomograms predict the likelihood of malignancy; however, these models have relatively modest concordance indices for the prediction of malignancy, generally in the range 0.55 to 0.65 (Haggstrom et al., 2013; Karakiewicz et al., 2009; Lane et al., 2007a; Yaycioglu et al., 2013). In these models and a large, systematic review of the data, **the strongest predictors of malignancy are male sex and increasing tumor size** (Pierorazio et al., 2016). In systematic meta-analysis of surgically resected tumors, men have a nearly threefold increased risk of malignancy (effect size 2.71, 95% confidence interval [CI] 2.39–3.02) compared with women. Although benign histology is more common in women, RCC still predominates in both genders.

When considering tumor size, 20% to 30% of renal masses less than 4 cm and 40% of renal masses less than 2 cm are benign (Johnson et al., 2015; Kutikov et al., 2006). The likelihood of malignancy increases per centimeter of tumor diameter (effect size 1.3 per cm increase in diameter, 95% CI 1.22–1.43) (Pierorazio et al., 2016). For example, one study reported that for tumors smaller than 1 cm 46% were benign and only 2% were high-grade RCC, whereas for tumors larger than 7 cm only 6% were benign and 58% were high-grade RCC (Frank et al., 2003). Importantly, many clinical T1a cancers (<4 cm) demonstrate indolent tumor biology. Less than 2% of patients with tumors 4 cm or smaller had or developed metastatic disease in extirpative surgical series (Thompson et al., 2009a; Umbreit et al., 2012). The emerging, prospective active surveillance (AS) literature also supports the indolent nature of small renal masses because 2% or less of patients progress to metastatic disease during short- to intermediate-term follow-up (Jewett et al., 2011; Pierorazio et al., 2015). Given the importance of tumor size in the risk-stratification of tumor biology and the fact that the majority of renal masses are discovered via incidental imaging, the initial discussion of risk stratification focuses on radiographic evaluation.

TABLE 97.1 Renal Masses Classified by Pathologic Features

MALIGNANT		BENIGN

RENAL CELL CARCINOMA (RCC)
• Clear cell RCC
• Multilocular cystic clear cell renal cell neoplasm of low malignant potential
• Papillary RCC
• Chromophobe RCC
• Hybrid oncocytic chromophobe tumor
• Carcinoma of the collecting ducts of Bellini
• Renal medullary carcinoma
• MiT family translocation RCC[a]
  • Xp11 translocation RCC
  • t(6;11) RCC
• Mucinous tubular and spindle cell carcinoma
• Tubulocystic RCC
• Acquired cystic disease–associated RCC
• Clear cell (tubulo) papillary RCC
• Hereditary leiomyomatosis RCC syndrome–associated RCC
• RCC, unclassified
 	
UROTHELIUM-BASED CANCERS
• Urothelial carcinoma
• Squamous cell carcinoma
• Adenocarcinoma
 	
SARCOMAS
• Leiomyosarcoma
• Liposarcoma
• Other sarcomas
	NEPHROBLASTIC TUMORS[a]
	• Nephrogenic rests
	• Nephroblastoma (Wilms tumor)
	• Cystic partially differentiated nephroblastoma
	
	CARCINOMA ASSOCIATED WITH NEUROBLASTOMA
	Neuroendocrine Tumors
	• Carcinoid (low-grade neuroendocrine tumor)
	• Neuroendocrine carcinoma (high-grade neuroendocrine tumor)
	• Primitive neuroectodermal tumor
	• Neuroblastoma
	• Pheochromocytoma
	Hematopoietic and Lymphoid Tumors
	• Lymphoma
	• Leukemia
	• Plasmacytoma
	Germ Cell Tumors
	• Teratoma
	• Choriocarcinoma
	
	METASTASIS
	
	INVASION BY ADJACENT NEOPLASM
		CYSTIC LESIONS
		• Simple cyst
		• Hemorrhagic cyst
		
		SOLID LESIONS
		• Angiomyolipoma
		• Oncocytoma
		• Papillary adenoma (renal adenoma)
		• Metanephric tumors (adenoma, adenofibroma, stromal tumor)
		• Congenital mesoblastic nephroma[a]
		• Cystic nephroma/mixed epithelial stromal tumor
		• Reninoma (juxtaglomerular cell tumor)
		• Renomedullary interstitial tumor
		• Leiomyoma
		• Fibroma
		• Hemangioma
		• Lymphangioma
		• Schwannoma
		• Solitary fibrous tumor
		
		VASCULAR LESIONS
		• Renal artery aneurysm
		• Arteriovenous malformation
		
		PSEUDOTUMOR
		
		INFLAMMATORY
		• Abscess
		• Focal pyelonephritis
		• Xanthogranulomatous pyelonephritis
		• Infected renal cyst
		• Tuberculosis
		• Rheumatic granuloma

[a]More common in childhood or young adults.
Modified from Srigley JR, Delahunt B, Eble et al.: The International Society of Urological Pathology (ISUP) Vancouver Classification of Renal Neoplasia. *Am J Surg Pathol* 37(10):1469–1489, 2013.

Subsequent portions of the chapter cover clinical presentation, renal mass biopsy, and laboratory evaluation.

RADIOGRAPHIC EVALUATION OF RENAL MASSES

Radiographic evaluation of a renal mass remains the strongest predictor of malignancy and metastatic potential (Pierorazio et al., 2016). Several radiographic modalities are currently available for detection and evaluation of renal masses, each with relative strengths and limitations (Kang and Chandarana, 2012). Current guidelines recommend multiphase, cross-sectional imaging to ensure a systematic approach and diligent evaluation of suspected renal masses, given the large differential diagnosis and considerable overlap between benign and malignant renal lesions (Fig. 97.1 and see Table 97.2; Campbell et al., 2017a; Ljungberg et al., 2015; Motzer et al., 2017b).

Intravenous pyelography and renal arteriography are no longer recommended in the routine evaluation of renal masses. Historic features suggestive of malignancy on intravenous pyelography included calcification within the mass, increased tissue density, irregularity of the contours of the kidney, and distortion of the collecting system (Zagoria, 2000); however, the lack of sensitivity and specificity of intravenous pyelography for the detection of parenchymal tumors is well documented (Kang and Chandarana, 2012). Renal arteriography has a limited role in the diagnostic evaluation of renal masses and is primarily reserved for patients with concomitant renal artery disease. In equivocal cases, the presence or absence of neovascularity may help establish the diagnosis of RCC. However, 20% to 25% of RCCs are angiographically indistinct, even though most of these tumors are not truly avascular and demonstrate modest degrees of contrast enhancement on computed tomography (CT).

Multiphasic, cross-sectional imaging provides the most accurate characterization of renal masses while assessing for locally advanced features and intra-abdominal metastases and readily excludes angiomyolipoma by identifying intralesional fat (Davenport et al., 2017). CT and magnetic resonance imaging (MRI) are the most widely used and studied imaging modalities (Berland et al., 2010), whereas ultrasound and contrast-enhanced ultrasound (CEUS) are options for the evaluation of patients with renal masses (Gulati et al., 2015).

A dedicated renal CT remains the most important radiographic test for delineating the nature of a renal mass. CT, with and without the administration of contrast, is necessary to take full advantage of the contrast enhancement characteristics of highly vascular renal

TABLE 97.2 Radiologic and Pathologic Correlates for Renal Masses

SIMPLE CYSTIC	STRONGLY ENHANCING MASS	INFILTRATIVE MASS
Benign cyst	Clear cell RCC	Lymphoma
Parapelvic cyst	Angiomyolipoma	High-grade urothelial carcinoma
Hydronephrosis	Oncocytoma	Sarcomatoid differentiation
Caliceal diverticulum	Papillary RCC (occasionally)	Collecting duct carcinoma
	Chromophobe RCC (occasionally)	Renal medullary carcinoma
		Xanthogranulomatous pyelonephritis
		Metastasis (occasionally)
COMPLEX CYSTIC	**MODERATELY ENHANCING SOLID MASS**	**CALCIFIED MASS**
Cystic RCC	Papillary RCC	RCC
Hemorrhagic cyst	Chromophobe RCC	Urothelial carcinoma
Hyperdense cyst	Clear cell RCC (occasionally)	Benign complex cyst
Benign complex cyst	Oncocytoma	Xanthogranulomatous pyelonephritis
Cystic nephroma	Fat-poor angiomyolipoma	Renal artery aneurysm
Mixed epithelial-stromal tumor	Adenoma/metanephric adenoma	Concomitant nephrolithiasis
Cystic Wilms tumor	Unifocal lymphoma	
Infected cyst/abscess	Sarcoma	
Hydrocalix	Lobar nephronia	
Arteriovenous malformation	Pseudotumor	
Renal artery aneurysm	Infarct	
	Metastasis	
FAT-CONTAINING MASS	**MULTIFOCAL/BILATERAL MASSES**	
Angiomyolipoma	Familial RCC	
Liposarcoma	Metastases	
Lipoma	Sporadic, multifocal RCC (particularly papillary RCC or clear cell RCC)	
	Angiomyolipomas (tuberous sclerosis)	
	Lymphoma	
	Cystic tumors (autosomal dominant polycystic kidney disease)	

RCC, Renal cell carcinoma.
Modified from Simmons MN, Herts BR, Campbell SC: Image based approaches to the diagnosis of renal masses [lesson 39]. *AUA Update Series* 26:382–391, 2007.

parenchymal tumors (Kang and Chandarana, 2012). **Enhancement of greater than 15 to 20 Hounsfield units (HU) is indicative of RCC, although this does not preclude benign histology** (Fig. 97.2; Berland et al., 2010). **Solid masses that also have substantial areas of negative CT attenuation numbers (below −20 HU) indicative of fat are diagnostic for angiomyolipoma (AML)** (Nelson and Sanda, 2002). Patients with an estimated glomerular filtration rate (eGFR) below 45 mL/min/1.73 m^2 undergoing CT with intravenous contrast should be considered for periprocedural hydration. Administration of intravenous contrast should be avoided and alternative imaging pursued if possible in patients with severe chronic kidney disease (CKD) who are nearing dialysis (see Fig. 97.1).

MRI is the alternate standard imaging modality for the characterization of a renal mass (Donat et al., 2013; Kang and Chandarana, 2012). **Enhancement of greater than 20% with intravenous gadolinium-based contrast on MRI is suggestive of RCC** and may be particularly helpful in masses smaller than 2 cm (Fig. 97.3; Rofsky et al., 1991). MRI is also useful for differentiating tissue planes and for defining extent of vascular involvement in many patients with locally advanced RCC. **A significant concern with MRI with gadolinium is the uncommon but potentially serious complication of nephrogenic systemic fibrosis (NSF). NSF is most common in patients on dialysis, with CKD stage 4 and 5, significant acute kidney injury, and/or patients receiving multiple doses of gadolinium-based contrast agents** (Bach and Zhang, 2008). Therefore gadolinium-based contrast should generally be used only in patients with an eGFR greater than 30 mL/min/1.73 m^2 (Agarwal et al., 2009).

Newer macrolytic gadolinium agents appear to have substantially reduced risk of NSF and will probably allow for use of MRI with contrast in patients on dialysis or those with severe CKD in the near future (ACR Committee on Drugs and Contrast Media, 2017).

Ultrasonography is a noninvasive and relatively inexpensive modality that can differentiate cystic versus solid renal masses, and it continues to play an important role for such lesions. **Strict ultrasonographic criteria for simple cysts have been defined and include a smooth cyst wall, a round or oval shape without internal echoes, and through-transmission with strong acoustic shadowing posteriorly. A renal mass that is not clearly a simple cyst by strict ultrasound criteria should be evaluated further with multiphasic, cross-sectional imaging** (Campbell et al., 2017a). CEUS using microbubbles has also shown promise for the characterization and assessment of enhancement of renal masses and may play an important role in patients with CKD in the future (Gulati et al., 2015).

Regardless of imaging modality used, **imaging should comment on renal mass diameter in craniocaudal, transverse, and anteroposterior dimensions; tumor morphology, including involvement of or juxtaposition to the renal hilum, vein, or collecting system; enhancement characteristics; and associated features such as retroperitoneal lymphadenopathy and presence or absence of abdominal metastases.** As discussed earlier, increasing tumor size is the strongest predictor of malignant disease and subsequent metastatic potential (Pierorazio et al., 2016). Solid tumor architecture (versus cystic) is also predictive of malignancy, although many complex cystic masses are RCC (Israel and Bosniak, 2005). Risk-stratification of cystic

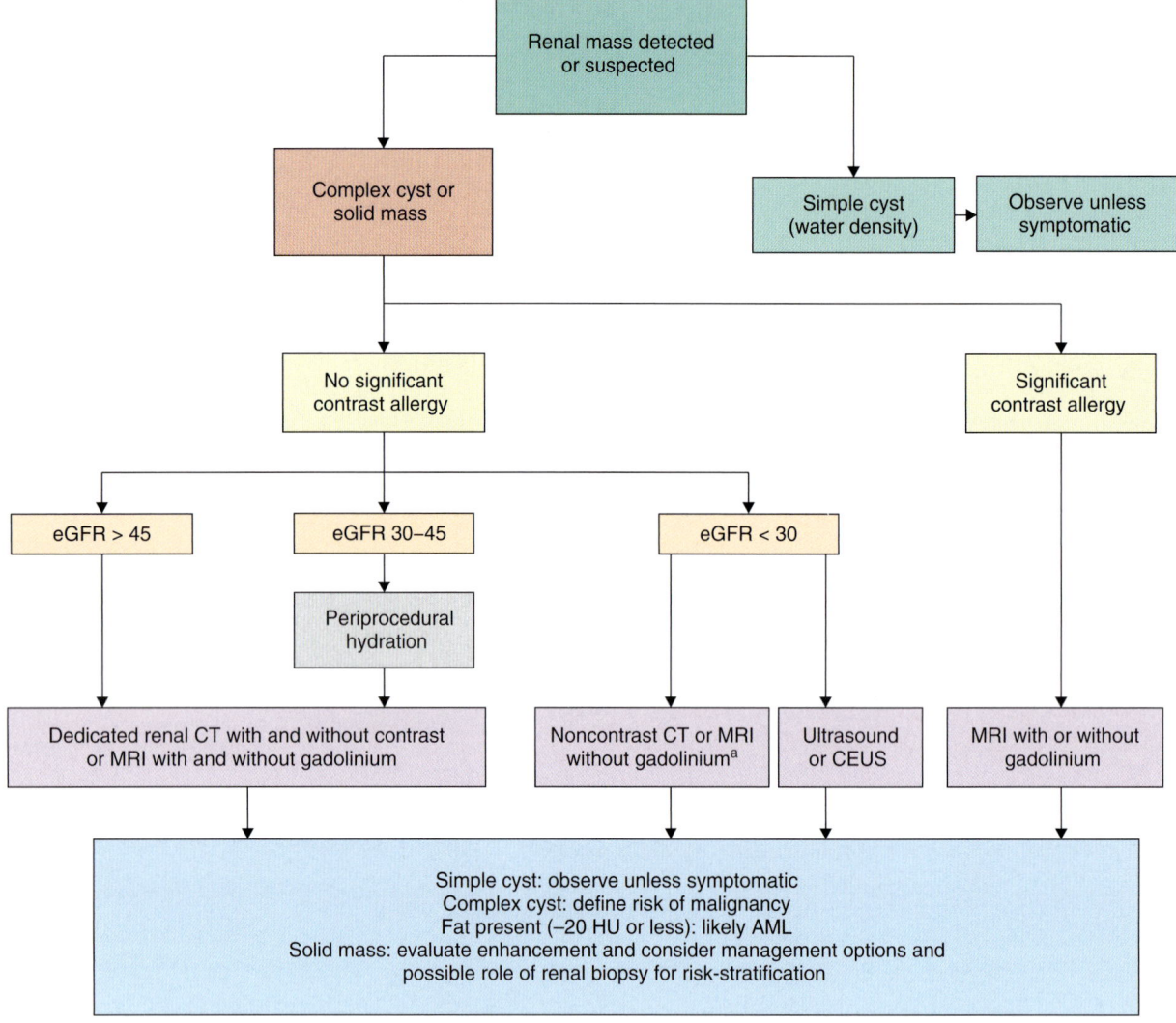

Fig. 97.1. Algorithm for radiographic evaluation of renal masses. *AML,* Angiomyolipoma; *CEUS,* contrast-enhanced ultrasound; *CT,* computed tomography; *eGFR,* estimated glomerular filtration rate in units of mL/min/1.73 m²; *HU,* Hounsfield units; *IV,* intravenous; *MRI,* magnetic resonance imaging. [a]Based on the current literature, non-contrast CT or MRI are preferred over ultrasound or CEUS, although ultrasound-based technologies are reasonable alternatives.

renal masses is discussed below. Tumor location and complexity describe the relationship of the mass with the renal hilum, collecting system, polarity, and endophytic versus exophytic location. Composite complexity profiles include the R.E.N.A.L. (Radius, Endophytic vs. exophytic, Nearness to collecting system, Anterior/posterior, Location relative to polar lines) nephrometry score, the PADUA score, and the C-index (Ficarra et al., 2009b; Kutikov and Uzzo, 2009; Simmons et al., 2010). Tumor complexity may be useful in the selection of nephron-sparing surgery versus RN, surgical approach (open vs. minimally invasive), and assessing for risk of surgical complications (Bruner et al., 2011; Stroup et al., 2012; Tobert et al., 2012). Emerging data indicate that increasing tumor complexity may also correlate with risk of malignancy and aggressive histology (Kutikov et al., 2011; Pierorazio et al., 2016).

Infiltrative growth pattern broadens the differential diagnosis and has prognostic significance; urothelial cancer, lymphoma, infectious processes, and high-grade or sarcomatoid RCC commonly demonstrate infiltrative growth patterns and indistinct borders on imaging. Enhancement patterns can also be suggestive of tumor histology because the papillary subtype of RCC is often hypoenhancing relative to other subtypes of RCC (Pierorazio et al., 2013; Young et al., 2013). However, definitive conclusions cannot be drawn regarding biologic potential based on enhancement pattern alone because significant overlap can exist in imaging characteristics of clear cell RCC, oncocytoma, and subtypes of papillary RCC on cross-sectional imaging (Kopp et al., 2013; Young et al., 2013).

Molecular imaging exploits existing cellular processes and high-affinity radio-labeled molecules to improve diagnostic imaging. Fluorodeoxyglucose positron emission tomography (FDG-PET)-CT is used in a variety of malignancies but has a limited role in RCC because of its high levels of visual conspicuity in the kidney and at the most common sites of metastatic disease (Bagheri et al., 2017). ^{99m}Tc-sestamibi single-photon emission CT (SPECT) has demonstrated promising early results in distinguishing renal oncocytoma and hybrid oncocytic/chromophobe tumors from clear cell RCC and awaits large-scale validation (Gorin et al., 2016). Sestamibi is taken up by mitochondria, which are in abundance in oncocytomas and hybrid oncocytic/chromophobe tumors, and a strong signal is suggestive of these histologies. Additional molecular imaging agents including ^{124}I-girentuximab, which targets carbonic anhydrase IX primarily present on clear cell RCC, and prostate-specific membrane antigen (PSMA, epithelial membrane target) remain in development for RCC (Divgi et al., 2013; Rowe et al., 2015).

Evaluation of Cystic Renal Lesions

The differentiation between benign renal cysts and cystic RCC remains one of the more common and challenging problems in renal imaging (Bosniak, 2012). Simple cysts are thin-walled, fluid-filled structures with a nearly zero risk of malignancy. The risk of malignancy increases with cyst complexity as defined by evaluation of the wall of the lesion; its thickness and contour; the number, contour, and thickness of any septa; the amount, character, and location of any calcifications; the density of fluid in the lesion; the margination of the lesion; and the presence of solid components. **The Bosniak classification scheme was developed based on CT imaging criteria to define renal cystic lesions into categories that are distinct from one another in terms of the likelihood of malignancy** (Table 97.3; Israel and Bosniak, 2005). Bosniak 1 lesions are uncomplicated, simple, benign cysts of the kidney that are straightforward to diagnose on ultrasonography, CT, or MRI. These are by far the most common renal cystic lesions, and **in the absence of associated symptoms, no treatment or surveillance is necessary.**

Bosniak 2 lesions are minimally complex cysts with a low risk of malignancy and include nonenhancing septated cysts, cysts with calcium in the wall or septum, infected cysts, and hyperdense (high-density) cysts (Fig. 97.4; Israel and Bosniak, 2005). Hyperdense cysts are benign lesions, classically less than 3 cm in diameter, with high CT attenuation before contrast administration (>20 HU) because of old, degenerated, or clotted blood. This category is now subdivided to differentiate Bosniak 2 lesions that do not require surveillance from category 2F lesions that mandate surveillance. **Bosniak 2F lesions have a 15% risk of radiographic progression to more complex cysts and a 3% to 10% risk of malignancy** (El-Mokadem

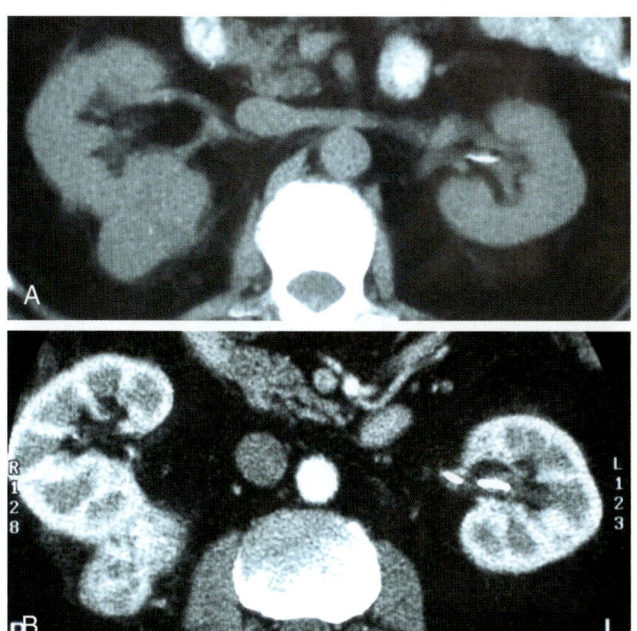

Fig. 97.2. (A) Computed tomography (CT) without administration of contrast shows solid, right posterior renal mass. (B) After administration of the contrast agent, CT shows that the mass enhances more than 20 HU and is thus highly suggestive of renal cell carcinoma (RCC). This mass was excised and confirmed to be clear cell RCC. (Courtesy Dr. Terrence Demos, Maywood, IL.)

TABLE 97.3 Classification of Complex Renal Cysts

BOSNIAK CLASSIFICATION	RADIOGRAPHIC FEATURES	RISK OF MALIGNANCY	MANAGEMENT
I	Water density Homogeneous, hairline thin wall No septa No calcification No enhancement	None	Surveillance not necessary
II	Few hairline septa in which "perceived" enhancement may be present Fine calcification or short segment of slightly thickened calcification in wall or septa No unequivocal enhancement	Minimal	Surveillance not necessary
	Hyperdense lesion: ≤3 cm, well marginated, with no unequivocal enhancement	Minimal	Periodic surveillance
IIF	Multiple hairline thin septa Minimal smooth wall thickening "Perceived" enhancement of wall or septae may be present Calcification may be thick or nodular but must be without enhancement Generally well marginated No unequivocal enhancement	3%–5%	Periodic surveillance
	Hyperdense lesion: >3 cm or totally intrarenal with no enhancement	5%–10%	Periodic surveillance
III	"Indeterminate," thickened irregular or smooth walls or septa in which measurable enhancement is present	50%	Surgical excision[a]
IV	Clearly malignant lesions that can have all the criteria of category III but also contain enhancing soft-tissue components	75%–90%	Surgical excision[a]

[a]Surgical excision should be considered if the patient is in good health. Active surveillance is an option for select patients. Thermal ablation is probably best avoided for cystic lesions because of concern about tumor spillage.

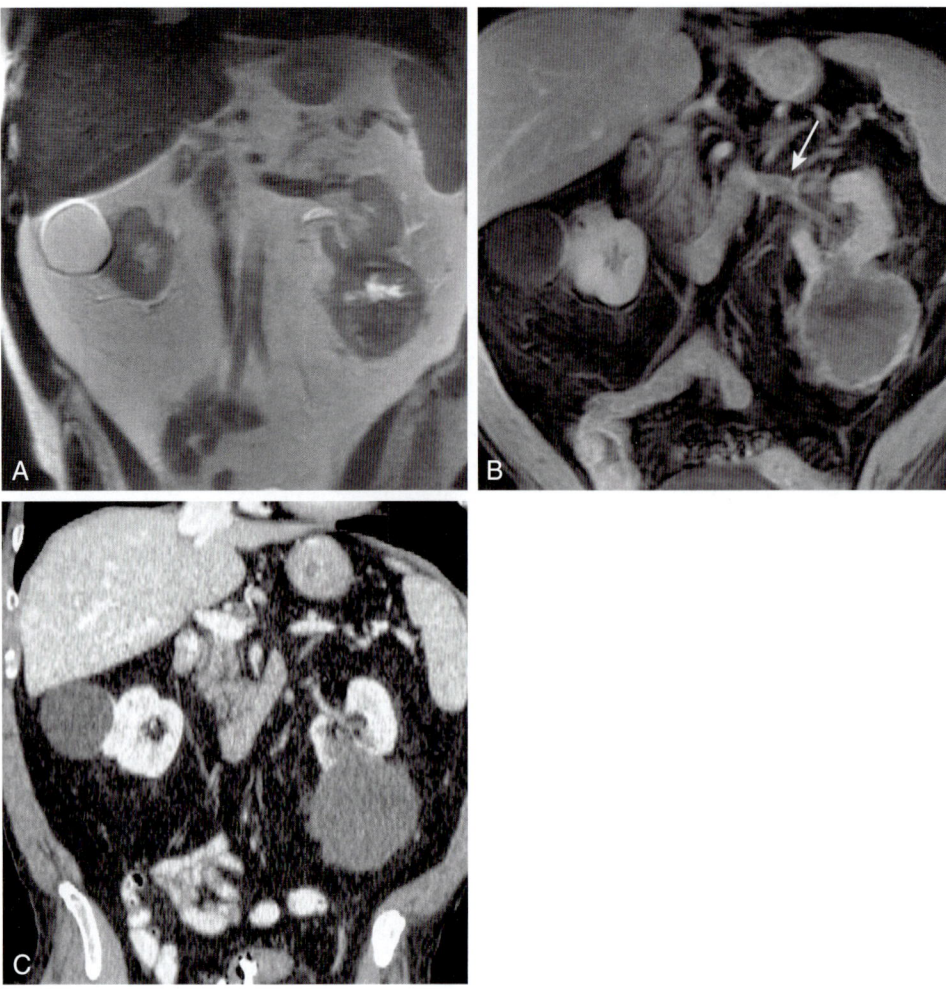

Fig. 97.3. Renal cell carcinoma on pre- and postcontrast magnetic resonance image (MRI) and contrast-enhanced computed tomography (CT). (A) Precontrast, T2-weighted MRI showing a simple cyst in the right kidney and heterogeneous 8.5-cm, lower pole tumor in the left kidney. (B) Postcontrast, fat-saturated, T1-weighted MRI reveals further anatomic details regarding the left renal tumor, including a tumor thrombus *(arrow)* within the renal vein. (C) Contrast-enhanced CT imaging (parenchymal phase) from the same patient also shows the left renal tumor. MRI was performed in this patient because of equivocal findings on the initial CT regarding a renal vein thrombus, which was seen clearly on pre- and postcontrast MRI. (Courtesy Dr. Leena Mammen, Grand Rapids, MI.)

et al., 2014; Graumann et al., 2013; O'Malley et al., 2009; Smith et al., 2012). Diagnostic criteria for Bosniak 2F cysts are detailed in Table 97.3. **A major differentiating factor for complex renal cysts is the presence of unequivocal contrast enhancement, which is not seen in Bosniak 2 and 2F lesions.**

Bosniak 3 lesions are more complex renal cysts that cannot be confidently distinguished from malignant neoplasms (Goenka et al., 2013; Israel and Bosniak, 2005; Smith et al., 2012). The radiographic features include thickened irregular walls or septa, or whenever measurable enhancement can be observed in such structures (Fig. 97.5). **Bosniak 4 lesions have large cystic components; irregular, shaggy margins; and, most important, solid enhancing portions that provide a definitive diagnosis of malignancy** (Fig. 97.6; Israel and Bosniak, 2005). High-quality imaging, preferably CT, and considerable radiologic expertise are required to optimize the characterization of complex renal cystic lesions. In the absence of a mitigating factor such as renal trauma or infection, **surgical exploration is usually indicated in healthy patients with Bosniak 3 or 4 lesions** (Campbell et al., 2017a). Renal mass biopsy or aspiration is rarely performed on cystic lesions because of sampling error, poor diagnostic yield, and risk of tumor spillage (Marconi et al., 2016; Patel et al., 2016b).

RENAL CELL CARCINOMA

Incidence

RCC, which accounts for 2% to 3% of all adult malignant neoplasms, is the most lethal of the common urologic cancers (Siegel et al., 2017). Approximately 64,000 new diagnoses of RCC are made each year in the United States, and 14,400 patients die of disease (Siegel et al., 2017). **Overall, approximately 16 new cases are diagnosed per 100,000 population per year, with a male-to-female predominance of 1.9 to 1** (Siegel et al., 2017). **This is primarily a disease of older adults, with typical presentation between 55 and 75 years of age** (Pantuck et al., 2001b; Siegel et al., 2017; Wallen et al., 2007). However, diagnosis of renal cancer has increased more rapidly in those less than 40 years of age than any other age group (Nepple et al., 2012). Compared with Americans of other races, the incidence and death rates are about 50% lower in Asian-American/Pacific Islanders, and 5% to 10% higher in African-Americans, for unknown reasons (Chow et al., 2013; Lipworth et al., 2006; Siegel et al., 2017; Stafford et al., 2008). **The majority of cases of RCC are sporadic; only 4% to 6% are believed to be familial** (Lipworth et al., 2006; Schmidt and Linehan, 2016).

The incidence of RCC has increased since the 1970s by an average of 3% per year, largely related to more prevalent use of

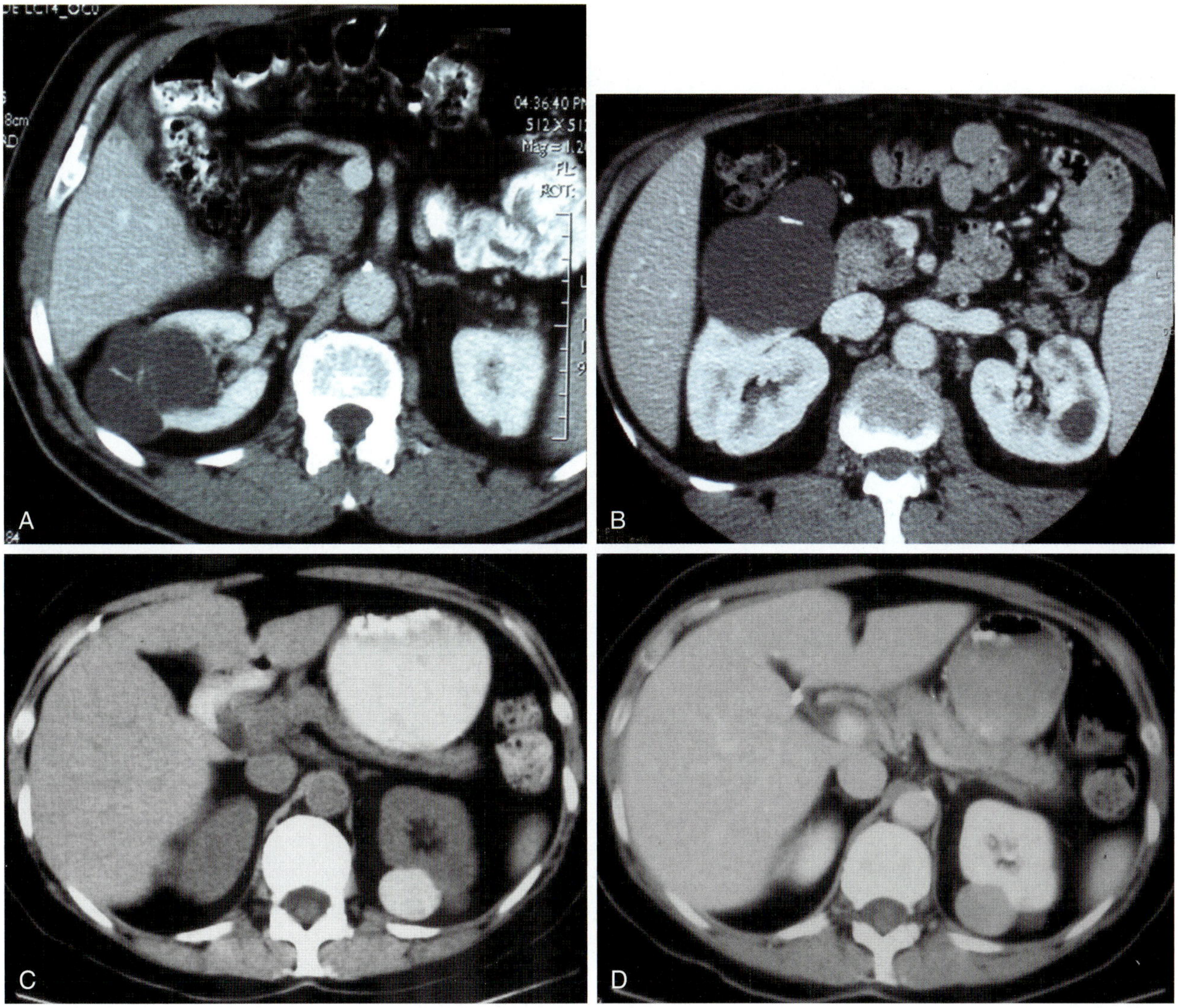

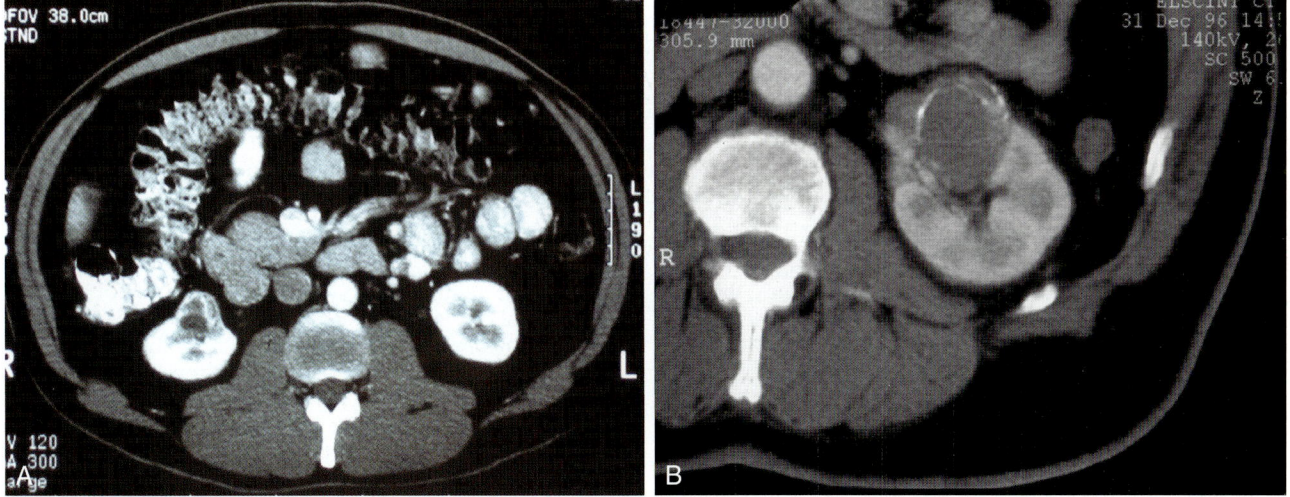

Fig. 97.4. Bosniak category 2 renal cysts. (A) Computed tomography (CT) shows right renal cyst with thin internal septation. (B) CT in another patient shows relatively thin, curvilinear calcification in the septa of the wall of right renal cyst. (C) CT without administration of contrast material shows small, smooth-walled, high-density left renal cyst. (D) CT after administration of contrast material shows no enhancement of the cyst. This is an extreme example of a hyperdense cyst. (Courtesy Dr. Terrence Demos, Maywood, IL.)

Fig. 97.5. Bosniak category 3 cysts. (A) Computed tomography (CT) shows complex right renal cyst with thick, irregular septae and inhomogeneous character. (B) CT shows thick-walled, complex left renal cyst also exhibiting irregular calcification and moderate heterogeneity. (Courtesy Dr. Terrence Demos, Maywood, IL.)

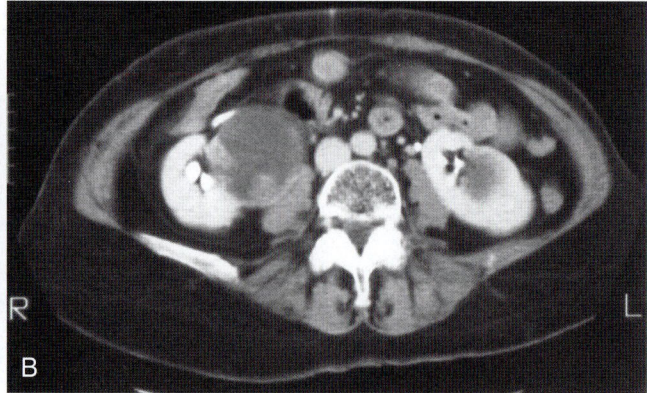

Fig. 97.6. Bosniak category 4 cysts. (A) Computed tomography (CT) shows complex left renal cystic lesion with thick, enhancing walls. (B) CT shows complex right cystic lesion with enhancing nodular areas and inhomogeneity. Both lesions proved to be renal cell carcinoma.

ultrasonography and CT for the evaluation of a variety of nonspecific abdominal complaints (Decastro and McKiernan, 2008; Kummerlin et al., 2008). This trend has correlated with an increased proportion of incidentally discovered and localized tumors and with improved 5-year survival rates for patients with this stage of disease (Kane et al., 2008; Pantuck et al., 2001b; Parsons et al., 2001). However, other factors must also be at play because a steadily increasing mortality rate from RCC per unit population has been observed in all ethnic groups and both genders since the 1980s (Chow et al., 1999; Siegel et al., 2017). This rising mortality rate is particularly troubling because the proportion of advanced tumors has actually decreased (Decastro and McKiernan, 2008; Siegel et al., 2017; Wallen et al., 2007). This suggests that a deleterious change in tumor biology may have occurred during the past several decades, perhaps related to tobacco use, dietary factors and obesity, or exposure to other carcinogens (Hock et al., 2002; Kane et al., 2008; Pantuck et al., 2001b; Parsons et al., 2001).

Although childhood renal tumors represent about 7% of all pediatric cancers, RCC is relatively uncommon in this population. About 90% of renal tumors in children are Wilms tumors or nephroblastomas, with RCC representing only 1% to 6% (Broecker, 2000; Brok et al., 2016). **Although Wilms tumor is much more common in younger children, RCC is as common as Wilms tumor during the second decade of life.** Mean age at presentation for RCC in children is 8 to 9 years, and the incidence is similar in boys and in girls. RCC in children and young adults is more likely to be symptomatic, locally advanced, high grade, and of unfavorable histologic subtypes (Argani et al., 2010; Cook et al., 2006; Estrada et al., 2005; Sanchez-Ortiz et al., 2004b). The most common RCC subtypes are characterized by translocations involving the transcription factor E3 gene *(TFE3)* on chromosome Xp11, which can fuse to other genes leading to increased *TFE3* overexpression. As many as 15% of these tumors occur in children that have received chemotherapy for other malignancies (Brok et al., 2016; Syed et al., 2017). TFE3 protein overexpression leads to a distinct pathologic subtype of RCC that exhibits clear cell and papillary features but may respond to chemotherapeutic or targeted molecular agents (Algaba et al., 2011; Brok et al., 2016). **Most studies suggest that stage for stage, children and young adults with RCC may respond better to surgical therapy,** and a number of long-term survivors have been reported after radical nephrectomy and lymphadenectomy for lymph node–positive disease (Abou El Fettouh et al., 2002; Geller et al., 2008; Sanchez-Ortiz et al., 2004b). **An aggressive surgical approach with formal lymphadenectomy has thus been recommended at the time of radical nephrectomy when RCC is suspected in children or young adults** (Bosquet et al., 2008; Selle et al., 2006).

Etiology

RCCs were traditionally thought to arise primarily from the proximal convoluted tubules, and this is probably true for the clear cell and papillary variants. However, we now know that other histologic subtypes of RCC, such as chromophobe RCC and collecting duct carcinoma, are derived from the more distal components of the nephron (Moch et al., 2016; Pantuck et al., 2001a). **The most generally accepted environmental risk factor for RCC is tobacco exposure, although the associated relative risks have been modest, ranging from 1.4 to 2.5 compared with controls.** All forms of tobacco use have been implicated, and risk increases with cumulative dose or pack-years (Cote et al., 2012; Cumberbatch et al., 2016). Relative risk is directly related to duration of smoking and begins to fall after cessation, further supporting a cause-and-effect relationship (Cumberbatch et al., 2016; Ljungberg et al., 2011). Tobacco use accounts for 20% to 30% of cases of RCC in men and 10% to 20% in women.

Obesity is now accepted as another major risk factor for RCC, with an increased relative risk of 1.07 for each additional unit of body mass index (Bagheri et al., 2016; Bhaskaran et al., 2014; Ito et al., 2017; Renehan et al., 2008). Increased prevalence of obesity has likely contributed to the increased incidence of RCC in Western countries, and it has been estimated that more than 40% of cases of RCC in the United States may be causally linked to obesity (Calle and Kaaks, 2004). Although RCC is more prevalent in patients with higher BMI, increased BMI is also associated with lower stage RCC at presentation, a so-called "obesity paradox" noted in other metabolic disorders and malignancies such as diabetes, CKD, and colon cancer (Bagheri et al., 2016; Choi et al., 2013; Hakimi et al., 2013; Ito et al., 2017). Potential mechanisms linking obesity to RCC include increased insulin-like growth factor-1 expression, increased circulating estrogen levels, and increased arteriolar nephrosclerosis and local inflammation (Calle and Kaaks, 2004; Ljungberg et al., 2011).

Hypertension appears to be the third major causative factor for RCC. Diuretics and other antihypertensive medications have also been implicated, particularly for papillary RCC (Colt et al., 2017). However, the weight of the epidemiologic evidence suggests that it is the underlying disorder, hypertension, rather than the treatment that increases the risk of RCC (Colt et al., 2017; Lipworth et al., 2006; Ljungberg et al., 2011). The proposed mechanisms are hypertension-induced renal injury and inflammation or metabolic or functional changes in the renal tubules that may increase susceptibility to carcinogens (Lipworth et al., 2006; Ljungberg et al., 2011).

Although a number of other potential causative factors have been identified in animal models, including viruses, lead compounds, and more than 100 chemicals such as aromatic hydrocarbons, no specific agent has been definitively established as causative in human RCC (Ishida et al., 2015). The potential role of trichloroethylene exposure has been actively investigated; some studies showed relative risks ranging from twofold to sixfold, but others have argued that inherent biases likely account for these results (Kelsh et al., 2010). Slightly increased relative risks for RCC have been reported for workers in the metal, chemical, rubber, and printing industries and those exposed to asbestos or cadmium, but the data are not particularly convincing (Ljungberg et al., 2011; Mariusdottir et al., 2016).

Case-control studies have shown that RCC is more common among individuals with low socioeconomic status and urban background, although the causative factors have not been defined. The typical modern Western diet, increased intake of dairy products, and increased consumption of coffee or tea have been associated with RCC, but the relative risks have been modest, and conflicting data are available in most instances (Ljungberg et al., 2011). A family history of RCC may also be a factor; one study showed a relative risk of 2.9 for individuals with a first- or second-degree relative with RCC (Gago-Dominguez et al., 2001).

Other potential iatrogenic causes include regular usage of nonsteroidal anti-inflammatory drugs, which was associated with a relative risk of 1.51, whereas aspirin and acetaminophen were not associated with increased risk (Cho et al., 2011). Retroperitoneal radiation therapy, typically administered for Wilms tumor or testicular cancer, appears to be a risk factor for RCC, although the relative risks are low (Romanenko et al., 2000). An increased incidence of RCC is also observed in patients with end-stage renal disease and certain familial syndromes such as tuberous sclerosis, as discussed later (Schmidt and Linehan, 2016).

> **KEY POINTS: INCIDENCE AND ETIOLOGY OF RENAL CELL CARCINOMA**
>
> - RCC accounts for 2% to 3% of adult malignancies, with a male-to-female predominance of 1.9 to 1.
> - RCC typically is diagnosed between 55 and 75 years of age.
> - The incidence of RCC has been rising, largely because of incidental detection.
> - The strongest risk factor for RCC is tobacco exposure, which increases the relative risk by 1.4- to 2.5-fold compared with controls.
> - Hypertension and obesity are also associated with increased prevalence of RCC.
> - Approximately 4% to 6% of RCC is familial in origin.

Familial Renal Cell Carcinoma and Molecular Genetics

Since the early 1990s, several familial syndromes of RCC have been identified, and the tumor suppressor genes and oncogenes contributing to the development of sporadic and familial forms of this malignancy have been characterized (Table 97.4; Nielsen et al., 2016; Schmidt and Linehan, 2016). **The distinct nature of the various subtypes of RCC and advances in molecular genetics have contributed to a major revision in the histologic classification of this malignancy** (see Table 97.1) (Samaratunga et al., 2014; Schmidt and Linehan, 2016; Zhou, 2009). A direct and beneficial impact on patient management has also been achieved, with targeted molecular agents now extending survival for many patients with advanced RCC (Schmidt and Linehan, 2016).

Knudson and Strong recognized that familial forms of cancer may hold the key to the identification of important regulatory elements known as tumor suppressor genes (Knudson, 1971; Knudson and Strong, 1972). **Their observations about the childhood tumor retinoblastoma, in which familial cases tend to be multifocal and early onset, led them to propose a two-hit theory of carcinogenesis. They hypothesized that a gene product that could suppress tumor development must be involved and that both alleles of this "tumor suppressor gene" must be mutated or inactivated for tumorigenesis to occur.** Furthermore, Knudson postulated that patients with familial cancers are born with one mutant allele and that all cells in that organ or tissue are at risk, accounting for the early onset and multifocal nature of the disease. In contrast, sporadic tumors develop only if a mutation occurs in both alleles within the same cell; because each event occurs with low frequency, most tumors develop late in life and in a unifocal manner (Knudson, 1971; Knudson and Strong, 1972). Knudson's hypothesis has proven true for retinoblastoma and a number of other tumor types, including RCC (Schmidt and Linehan, 2016). Identification of familial cases of RCC was particularly important because it allowed linkage analysis between affected family members.

von Hippel-Lindau Disease, VHL Gene, and Genetics of Clear Cell RCC

The familial form of clear cell RCC is von Hippel-Lindau (VHL) disease, an autosomal dominant disorder that occurs with a frequency of 1 per 36,000 people. **Major manifestations include the development of RCC, pheochromocytoma, retinal angiomas, and hemangioblastomas of the brainstem, cerebellum, or spinal cord** (Table 97.5; Schmidt and Linehan, 2016). All of these tumor types are highly vascular and can lead to substantial morbidity. In particular, central nervous system lesions can lead to paralysis or death and retinal lesions to blindness if they are not identified and managed in an expedient manner. Other common or important manifestations of VHL disease include renal and pancreatic cysts, inner ear tumors, neuroendocrine tumors of the pancreas, and papillary cystadenomas of the epididymis (Neumann and Zbar, 1997). Penetrance for all of these traits is far from complete, and some, such as pheochromocytomas, tend to be clustered only in certain families (Table 97.6; Neumann and Zbar, 1997). **RCC develops in about 50% of patients with VHL disease and is distinctive for early age at onset (often in the third to fifth decades of life) and bilateral and multifocal involvement** (Kim et al., 2010; Schmidt and Linehan, 2016). With improved management of the central nervous system manifestations, RCC has now become the most common cause of mortality in patients with VHL disease. Screening for VHL and important considerations for the management of RCC in this syndrome are reviewed later in this chapter.

Early clues to the genetic elements involved in RCC development came from cytogenetics. These studies demonstrated a common loss of chromosome 3 in kidney cancer, particularly the clear cell variant, and led to intensive efforts to find a tumor suppressor gene in this region (Seizinger et al., 1988; Zbar et al., 1987). Reports by Kovacs et al. (1989a) and Cohen et al. (1979) of translocations involving chromosome 3 further implicated this chromosome as an important regulatory element. Sophisticated molecular genetic linkage studies in patients with VHL disease eventually led to the **identification of the *VHL* tumor suppressor gene** (Latif et al., 1993). **The role of this gene as a tumor suppressor for sporadic and familial forms of clear cell RCC has been confirmed** (Schmidt and Linehan, 2016). The *VHL* gene consists of three exons, and it encodes a protein of 213 amino acids. A large number of common mutations or "hot spots" in the gene have been identified, and a direct correlation between genotype and phenotype has been established in some cases (McNeill et al., 2009; Nielsen et al., 2016). For instance, missense mutations (type 2 mutations) that result in a full-length but nonfunctional protein are commonly found in families with VHL disease who develop pheochromocytomas, whereas deletions leading to a truncated protein (type 1 mutations) are typically found in families who do not develop pheochromocytomas (see Table 97.6; McNeill et al., 2009; Nielsen et al., 2016). The identification of this tumor suppressor gene represented a major advance in the field and required close collaboration between urologic oncologists and molecular geneticists (Schmidt and Linehan, 2016).

Subsequent work has focused on the function of the VHL protein and its likely mechanisms of action (Fig. 97.7). The VHL protein is known to bind to elongins B and C and other proteins to form an E3 ubiquitin ligase complex and thereby modulates the degradation of important regulatory proteins (Nielsen et al., 2016; Schmidt and Linehan, 2016; Shen and Kaelin, 2013). **A critically important function of the VHL protein complex is to target the hypoxia-inducible factors-1α and -2α (HIF-1α and HIF-2α) for ubiquitin-mediated degradation, keeping the levels of HIFs low under normal conditions. Inactivation or mutation of the *VHL* gene leads to accumulation of HIFs, most notably HIF-2α** (Shen and Kaelin,

TABLE 97.4 Familial Renal Cell Carcinoma Subtypes

SYNDROME	PREDISPOSING GENE (CHROMOSOME)	RENAL TUMOR HISTOLOGY AND OTHER MAJOR CLINICAL MANIFESTATIONS	RECOMMENDED MANAGEMENT FOR RENAL TUMORS	POTENTIAL THERAPEUTIC TARGETS
von Hippel-Lindau disease (VHL)	*VHL* (3p25)	Clear cell RCC, often multifocal Retinal angiomas Central nervous system hemangioblastomas Pheochromocytoma Other tumors	Active surveillance <3 cm Surgical excision ≥3 cm, preference for nephron-sparing approaches	HIF-VEGF pathway
Hereditary papillary renal carcinoma (HPRC)	*MET* (7q31)	Multiple, bilateral type 1 papillary RCC	Active surveillance <3 cm Surgical excision ≥3 cm, preference for nephron-sparing approaches	MET kinase
Hereditary leiomyomatosis and renal cell carcinoma (HLRCC)	*Fumarate hydratase (FH)* (1q42-43)	Type 2 papillary RCC most common Collecting duct carcinoma Leiomyomas of skin or uterus Uterine leiomyosarcomas Low-grade variants of RCC also seen in children	Surgical excision, preference for PN, but only when wide margins can be achieved	HIF-VEGF pathway; antioxidant response pathway; reductive carboxylation pathway
Succinate dehydrogenase-deficient RCC (SDH-RCC)	*SDHA* *SDHB* (1p36.13), *SDHC* (1q23.3), *SDHD* (11q23.1), *SHDAF2*	SDH-associated RCC (chromophobe, clear cell, type 2 papillary RCC; or oncocytoma), variable aggressiveness Paragangliomas (benign and malignant) Papillary thyroid carcinoma	Surgical excision, preference for PN, but only when wide margins can be achieved	HIF-VEGF pathway; reductive carboxylation pathway
Birt-Hogg-Dube syndrome (BHD)	*Folliculin* (17p11.2)	Multiple chromophobe RCC, hybrid oncocytic tumors, oncocytomas Clear cell RCC (occasionally) Papillary RCC (occasionally) Facial fibrofolliculomas Lung cysts Spontaneous pneumothorax	Active surveillance <3 cm Surgical excision ≥3 cm, preference for nephron-sparing approaches	mTOR pathway
PTEN hamartoma tumor syndrome (Cowden syndrome)	*PTEN* (10q23)	Papillary RCC or other histology Breast tumors (malignant and benign) Epithelial thyroid carcinoma	Active surveillance <3 cm Surgical excision ≥3 cm, preference for nephron-sparing approaches	
Tuberous sclerosis complex (TSC)	*TSC1* (9q34) or *TSC2* (16p13.3)	Multiple renal angiomyolipomas Clear cell RCC (2%-3% incidence) Renal cysts/polycystic kidney disease Cardiac rhabdomyomas Cutaneous angiofibromas Pulmonary lymphangiomyomatosis Neuropsychiatric disorders, including autism spectrum disorder and cognitive disability	AML: surveillance for <3 cm, everolimus for 3–5 cm, consideration for embolization or excision for ≥5 cm, preference for nephron-sparing approaches RCC: surgical excision ≥3 cm, preference for nephron-sparing approaches	mTOR pathway
BAP1 tumor predisposition syndrome	*BAP1* (3p21.2)	Clear cell RCC, can be high grade	Surgical excision, preference for nephron-sparing approaches	To be determined
MiTF-associated cancer syndrome	*MiTF* (3p14.1–p12.3)	Not defined	To be determined	To be determined

AML, Angiomyolipoma; CNS, central nervous system; MiTF, microphthalmia-associated transcription factor; PN, partial nephrectomy; PTEN, pentaerythritol tetranitrate; RCC, renal cell carcinoma.
Modified from Schmidt LS, Linehan WM: Genetic predisposition to kidney cancer. *Sem Oncol* 43:566–574, 2016.

2013). Accumulation of HIF-2α leads to a several-fold upregulation of the expression of vascular endothelial growth factor (VEGF), the primary angiogenic growth factor in RCC, contributing to the pronounced neovascularity associated with clear cell RCC. HIF-2α also upregulates the expression of transforming growth factor-α, platelet-derived growth factor, glucose transporter 1, erythropoietin, and carbonic anhydrase IX, which also promote tumorigenesis (see Fig. 97.7). VHL also upregulates HIF-1α, which also plays a regulatory role, and this remains an important area of investigation (Shen and Kaelin, 2013).

The other three most commonly mutated genes involved in the development of sporadic clear cell RCC are also located on the short arm of chromosome 3, which is affected in more than 90% of clear cell RCC cases (Cancer Genome Atlas Research Network, 2013). Unlike *VHL*, these genes, which include *PBRM1*, *BAP1*, and *SETD2*, are involved in chromatin remodeling and histone methylation (Cancer Genome Atlas Research Network, 2013; Dalgliesh et al., 2010; Farley et al., 2013; Varela et al., 2011). BAP1 mutations occur in up to 14% of sporadic clear cell RCC and are associated with poor prognosis. Germline mutations of BAP1 have been identified in some individuals with early onset, multifocal clear cell RCC and should be considered in such patients who are wild type for VHL (Rai et al., 2016).

Hereditary Papillary Renal Carcinoma Syndrome

Several studies have documented distinct cytogenetic findings in non–clear cell histotypes of RCC; chromosome 3 and *VHL* gene abnormalities are uncommon in these variants (Schmidt and Linehan, 2016). These observations suggested an alternate genetic basis for non–clear cell RCC. Papillary RCC, the second most common histologic subtype of RCC, is characterized by trisomy for chromosomes 7 and 17 as well as abnormalities on chromosomes 1, 12, 16, 20, and Y (Schmidt and Linehan, 2016). In 1995 Zbar et al. reported a second familial syndrome of RCC—hereditary papillary renal carcinoma (HPRC). Median age at diagnosis in the 41 affected members from 10 families was 45 years, and most patients developed multifocal and bilateral papillary RCC. **Type 1 papillary RCC is typically found in this syndrome rather than type 2, which is commonly seen in the hereditary leiomyomatosis and RCC syndrome.** Unlike VHL disease, most patients with HPRC typically do not develop tumors in other organ systems (Schmidt and Linehan, 2016). Mean survival in affected individuals was only 52 years in Zbar's series, although the number of patients dying of RCC was not defined (Zbar et al., 1995). The development of CKD as a result of malignant replacement of the parenchyma and loss of functioning nephrons resulting from various interventions can contribute to morbidity and mortality in this syndrome (Ornstein et al., 2000).

Studies of families with HPRC demonstrate an autosomal dominant mode of transmission, similar to all of the other familial RCC syndromes (Schmidt and Linehan, 2016). Again, molecular linkage analysis in affected families played a key role in the discovery of the involved gene, which was localized to chromosome 7q31. However, in this case, the inciting event is activation of a proto-oncogene, rather than inactivation of a tumor suppressor gene. Missense mutations of the *c-MET* proto-oncogene at 7q31 were found to segregate with the disease, implicating it as the relevant genetic locus (Schmidt et al., 1997). The protein product of this gene is the receptor tyrosine kinase for hepatocyte growth factor, and its activation leads to cellular proliferation and other potential tumorigenic effects (Vira et al., 2007). **Most of the mutations in HPRC have been found in the tyrosine kinase domain of c-MET and apparently lead to constitutive activation** (Schmidt et al., 1997; Sudarshan and Linehan, 2006). Relatively early onset and multifocality in HPRC are due to inheritance of the mutated *c-MET* gene, which places all the cells in the kidney at risk from birth, but the incomplete penetrance and variable clinical course associated with this syndrome suggest

TABLE 97.5 Manifestations of von Hippel-Lindau Disease

TUMOR	AGE OF ONSET, MEAN (RANGE), YEARS	INCIDENCE, %
CENTRAL NERVOUS SYSTEM		
Retinal hemangioblastoma	25 (1–68)	25–60
Endolymphatic sac tumor	22 (12–50)	10–15
Craniospinal hemangioblastoma (overall)	30 (9–70)	60–80
Cerebellum	33 (9–78)	44–72
Brainstem	32 (12–46)	10–25
Spinal cord	33 (11–66)	13–50
VISCERAL		
Renal cell carcinoma	39 (13–70)	25–75
Renal cysts	39 (13–70)	20–60
Pheochromocytoma	27 (5–58)	10–25
Pancreatic neuroendocrine tumors (benign and malignant)	36 (5–70)	11–17
Pancreatic cysts	36 (5–70)	45–75
Epididymal cystadenoma	Unknown	25–60
Broad ligament cystadenoma	Unknown (16–46)	Unknown

Modified from Nielsen SM, Rhodes L, Blanco I, et al.: von Hippel-Lindau disease: genetics and role of genetic counseling in a multiple neoplasia syndrome. *J Clin Oncol* 34(18): 2172–2181, 2016.

TABLE 97.6 Incidence of Major Tumor Types of von Hippel-Lindau Disease by Subtype and Type of Mutation

VHL SUBTYPE	VHL MUTATION TYPE	HIGH RISK	LOW RISK
Type 1	Deletions, insertions, truncations, missense	RCC, CNS/R HB	Pheo
Type 1B	Contiguous gene deletions encompassing *VHL*	CNS/R HB	Pheo, RCC
Type 2A	Missense[a] (e.g., p. Y98H, p. Y112H, p. V116F)	Pheo, CNS/R HB	RCC
Type 2B	Missense (e.g., p.R167Q, p.R167W)	RCC, Pheo, CNS/R HB	–
Type 2C	Missense (e.g., p.V84L, p.L188V)	Pheo	RCC (absent); CNS/R HB

[a]Specific missense mutations arise from a point mutation in a single nucleotide that changes one amino acid in the encoded protein. For example, Y98H indicates that the tyrosine (Y) at position 98 in pVHL has been replaced with a histidine (H).
CNS/R HB, Central nervous system or retinal hemangioblastoma; *Pheo*, pheochromocytoma; *RCC*, renal cell carcinoma; *VHL*, von Hippel-Lindau disease.
Modified from Nielsen SM, Rhodes L, Blanco I, et al.: von Hippel-Lindau disease: genetics and role of genetic counseling in a multiple neoplasia syndrome. *J Clin Oncol* 34(18):2172–2181, 2016.

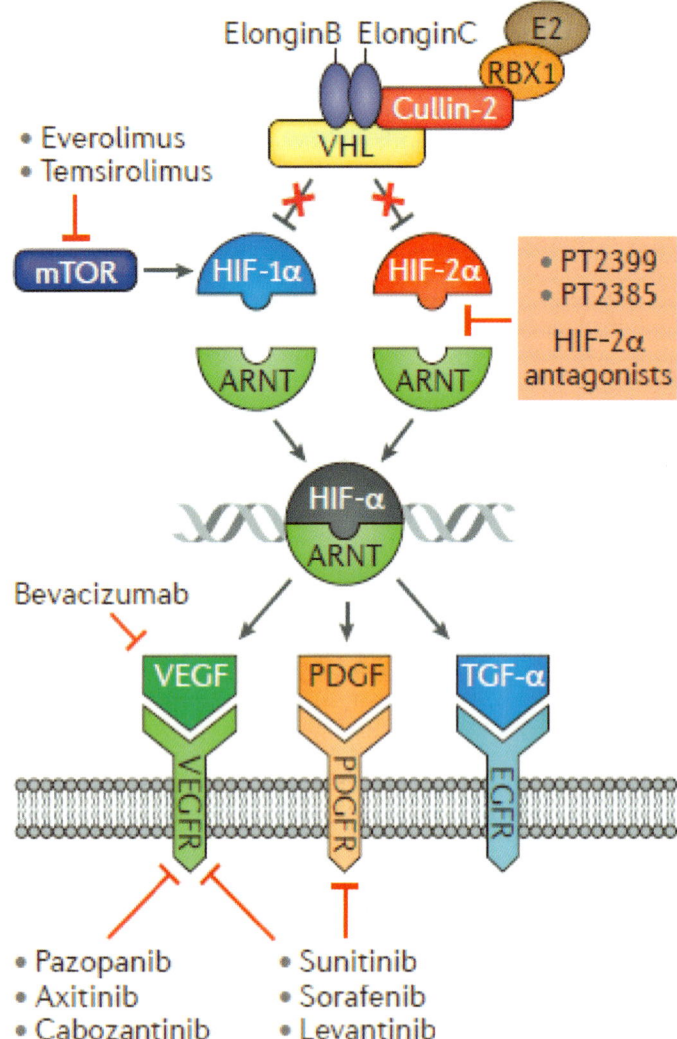

Fig. 97.7. The von Hippel-Lindau (VHL) pathway. The wild-type VHL protein is one component of a complex that targets the hypoxia-inducible factors HIF-1α and HIF-2α for degradation under normoxic conditions. In hypoxia, or with VHL loss (as occurs in clear cell RCC), the HIFs are stabilized, enabling dimerization with aryl hydrocarbon receptor nuclear translocator (ARNT) and increased production of vascular endothelial growth factor (VEGF), platelet-derived growth factor (PDGF), and transforming growth factor-α (TGF-α). These growth factors are involved with angiogenesis, glucose transport, and autocrine and paracrine growth stimulation, respectively. Therapeutic agents for advanced RCC can either sequester VEGF (bevaciumab), block the receptors for VEGF and PDGF (pazopanib, axitinib, cabozantinib, sunitinib, sorafenib, and levantinib), or target the mTOR pathway (temsirolimus and everolimus) to decrease levels of HIF by inhibiting translation of de novo HIF proteins. The novel therapeutic antagonists PT2399 and PT2385 specifically inhibit the dimerization of HIF-2α and ARNT, resulting in reduced HIF-2α downstream gene expression. (Modified from Linehan WM, Ricketts CJ: Kidney cancer in 2016: RCC—advances in targeted therapeutics and genomics. *Nat Rev Urol* 14:76–78, 2017.)

that additional genetic loci or epigenetic phenomena may modulate the phenotype (Schmidt and Linehan, 2016). **Whereas tumors in HPRC tend to be less aggressive than their sporadic counterparts, it is clear that some can metastasize. Schmidt et al. reported *c-MET* mutations in 13% of patients with sporadic papillary RCC, suggesting that this molecular defect also contributes to a subset of this disease population** (Sudarshan and Linehan, 2006; Schmidt and Linehan, 2016). Small molecule inhibitors of the *c-MET* receptor are currently in early clinical trials for the management of HPRC and the subset of patients with sporadic RCC who harbor this mutation (Choueiri et al., 2017b).

Hereditary Leiomyomatosis and Renal Cell Carcinoma

In 2001 Launonen et al. described a familial renal cancer syndrome in which patients commonly develop cutaneous and uterine leiomyomas and type 2 papillary RCC (Launonen et al., 2001; Pithukpakorn et al., 2006; Schmidt and Linehan, 2016). Mean age at diagnosis is in the early 40s. **Renal tumors in this syndrome are unusual for familial RCC in that they are often solitary and unilateral, and they are more likely to be aggressive than other forms of familial RCC.** Collecting duct carcinoma, another highly malignant variant of RCC, has also been observed in this syndrome, which was named **hereditary leiomyomatosis and renal cell carcinoma (HLRCC) syndrome.**

The HLRCC locus was mapped to a region on 1q42-43, and this was later shown to be the site of the fumarate hydratase *(FH)* gene (Pithukpakorn et al., 2006; Schmidt and Linehan, 2016). Again, autosomal dominant inheritance was observed, and *FH* appears to be a tumor suppressor gene rather than an oncogene. *FH* is an essential enzyme in the Krebs cycle of oxidative metabolism. The exact mechanisms by which loss of *FH* expression leads to malignancy are still under investigation, although hypotheses about this date back to the 1920s and the proposed Warburg effect.

Penetrance for RCC in HLRCC is lower than for the cutaneous and uterine manifestations, with only 15% to 20% of patients developing RCC. In contrast, almost all individuals with HLRCC develop cutaneous leiomyomas and uterine fibroids (if female), usually manifesting between the ages of 20 to 35 years. A high proportion of women have had a hysterectomy for fibroids before formal diagnosis of HLRCC, and occasionally leiomyosarcoma has been reported (Pithukpakorn et al., 2006; Schmidt and Linehan, 2016). **Prompt surgical management of the renal tumors is recommended in individuals with HLRCC, given their tendency toward aggressive behavior** (Schmidt and Linehan, 2016). **This is in contrast to most of the other familial syndromes of RCC, for which management tends to be more conservative.** Recent studies have shown the utility of FDG-PET imaging for identification of small foci of metastases in patients with HLRCC, reflecting the increased metabolic activity of these tumors (Carter et al., 2017; Nakatani et al., 2011; Pithukpakorn et al., 2006; Smith et al., 2017). However, not all patients with HLRCC develop aggressive cancers; some younger patients with *FH* mutations have been described with low-grade oncocytic neoplasms that resemble succinate dehydrogenase renal cell carcinoma (SDH-RCC)–associated tumors (Carter et al., 2017; Smith et al., 2017).

Succinate Dehydrogenase Renal Cell Carcinoma

Another syndrome that shares features with HLRCC is SDH-RCC (Ricketts et al., 2012). Affected individuals present with bilateral, multifocal, early onset (<40 years) renal tumors, often along with pheochromocytomas and head and neck paragangliomas. Individuals with germline mutation of one of the multiple genes encoding subunits of the Krebs cycle enzyme succinate dehydrogenase, including *SDHA, SDHB, SDHC, SDHD,* and *SHDAF2,* are at increased risk for RCC (Ricketts et al., 2008, 2012; Vanharanta et al., 2004). Another example of the Warburg effect in cancer, individuals with SDH-RCC can experience early onset and potentially aggressive disease; early studies suggested that about a third of such patients eventually developed metastatic disease (Ricketts et al., 2012). However, more recent reports have demonstrated a good prognosis for a subset of patients with SDH-RCC, particularly when low-grade features predominate. Tumors with high-grade, coagulative necrosis, or sarcomatoid features are more likely to behave aggressively (Gill et al., 2015; Kuroda et al., 2014; Williamson et al., 2015).

Birt-Hogg-Dube Syndrome

Birt-Hogg-Dube (BHD) syndrome, in which patients can develop cutaneous fibrofolliculomas, lung cysts, spontaneous pneumothoraces, and a variety of renal tumors primarily derived from the distal nephron, is named after three Canadian physicians who first described the cutaneous lesions in 1977 (Dal Sasso et al., 2015). **The renal tumors typically include chromophobe RCC, oncocytomas, and hybrid oncocytic tumors that exhibit features of both of these entities** (Boris et al., 2011). However, other forms of RCC, including a substantial proportion of clear cell RCC, have been observed (Dal Sasso et al., 2015). Overall penetrance for renal tumors is 23% to 34%, but when they occur they are often bilateral and multifocal (Dal Sasso et al., 2015; Toro et al., 2008). Average age at renal tumor diagnosis is approximately 50 years. Most renal tumors in BHD syndrome have limited biologic aggressiveness, although metastatic behavior and lethality have been reported.

The *BHD* gene responsible for this syndrome has been mapped to chromosome 17p12q11.2, and the gene product is the tumor suppressor folliculin (Khoo et al., 2001; Toro et al., 2008). Folliculin forms a complex of proteins that interfaces with the mammalian target of rapamycin (mTOR) pathway, and germline mutations in this gene have been found in 88% of kindreds (Toro et al., 2008). When folliculin is lost, mTOR signaling complexes 1 and 2 (mTORC1 and mTORC2) are activated, which leads to increased transcriptional activity and nuclear translocation of *TFE3* (Hasumi et al., 2009; Hong et al., 2010; Liu et al., 2016). An autosomal dominant pattern of inheritance is characteristic and genetic testing is now available (see Table 97.4).

Cowden Syndrome

Cowden syndrome is one of several syndromes that result from germline mutations of the phosphatase and tensin homolog *(PTEN)* tumor suppressor gene, which together are termed PTEN hamartoma tumor syndrome. Individuals with Cowden syndrome carry a 50% lifetime risk of female breast cancer, **34% lifetime risk of RCC,** and 10% lifetime risk of epithelial thyroid carcinoma (Mester et al., 2012; Starink et al., 1986). Patients with clinical features of Cowden syndrome but without *PTEN* mutations were subsequently found to have mutations in *KILLIN*, an adjacent tumor suppressor gene that was also associated with increased incidence of RCC (Bennett et al., 2010). Based on a greater than 31-fold increased risk of RCC, individuals with Cowden or Cowden-like syndrome should be screened with CT or MRI for RCC. **RCC in this syndrome is most often of papillary histology,** although chromophobe and clear cell histology have also been reported (Mester et al., 2012; Shuch et al., 2013).

Tuberous Sclerosis Complex

Tuberous sclerosis complex (TSC) is an autosomal dominant disorder that manifests with characteristic tumors in multiple organ systems (Caban et al., 2017; Schmidt and Linehan, 2016). **Major features include AML, cortical tubers, subependymal nodules or subependymal giant cell astrocytomas (SEGA), pulmonary lymphangioleiomyomatosis (LAM), cardiac rhabdomyomas, and facial angiofibromas.** Renal AML are typically multifocal, bilateral, and often large, occasionally requiring angioembolization or partial nephrectomy (PN) to treat or prevent bleeding from larger (>5 cm) tumors. Germline mutations in either the *TSC1* gene on chromosome 9q34 encoding hamartin or the *TSC2* gene on chromosome 16p13 that encodes tuberin are responsible for the manifestations of TSC (Caban et al., 2017). The TSC1/TSC2 complex normally downregulates the mTOR pathway; mTOR inhibitors (such as everolimus) have shown clinical activity against TSC-associated AMLs (see Chapter 96). RCC, typically clear cell type, can also be seen in a small proportion (2%–3%) of patients with TSC.

Microphthalmia-Associated Transcription Factor–Associated Cancer Syndrome

A germline missense variant (p.E318K) of microphthalmia-associated transcription factor (MiTF) confers a greater than fivefold increased risk (Bertolotto et al., 2011; Yokoyama et al., 2011) of melanoma and RCC in affected individuals. MiTF regulates HIF-1α and is normally suppressed by posttranslational regulatory processes; the mutated version activates HIF-1α, potentially contributing to the development of RCC.

TABLE 97.7 Tumor Biology and Clinical Implications

BIOLOGIC CHARACTERISTIC	CLINICAL IMPLICATIONS
Expression of multidrug resistance	Contributes to chemorefractory nature of RCC
Immunogenic	10%–20% response rate with interferon or IL-2 3%–5% complete response rate with high-dose IL-2 Modulation of PD-1 and other costimulatory molecules can lead to prolonged recurrence-free survival and overall survival
Angiogenic	Vascular invasion can lead to venous tumor thrombus 20%–40% response rates with agents targeting the VEGF pathway (sunitinib, sorafenib, pazopanib, axitinib, bevacizumab, etc.) Prolonged recurrence-free survival and overall survival with some antiangiogenic agents
Dependence on mTOR pathway	Agents targeting mTOR prolong survival in patients with poor-risk RCC (temsirolimus) and demonstrate responses in patients failing prior targeted molecular therapies (everolimus)

IL-2, Interleukin-2; *mTOR,* mammalian target of rapamycin; *PD-1,* programmed death–1; *RCC,* renal cell carcinoma; *VEGF,* vascular endothelial growth factor.

Tumor Biology and Clinical Implications

Resistance to Cytotoxic Therapy

RCC has demonstrated only limited responses to cytotoxic chemotherapeutic agents, contributing to the traditionally poor prognosis for patients with metastatic disease (Motzer and Russo, 2000; Rini et al., 2009b). **Study of the tumor biology of RCC has provided insight into its resistance to chemotherapy and, through elucidation of the VEGF, mTOR, and relevant immunomodulatory pathways, has yielded agents with clinical benefit for advanced disease** (Table 97.7, see Chapter 104) (Rini et al., 2009b). Expression of multidrug-resistance proteins, which act as energy-dependent efflux pumps for a wide variety of hydrophobic cytotoxic compounds, contributes to the chemorefractory nature of advanced RCC. However, the resistance of RCC to cisplatin and other agents that are not extruded by multidrug resistance proteins suggests redundancy in chemotherapy resistance mechanisms.

Immunobiology and Immune Tolerance

Several lines of evidence demonstrate that RCC is immunogenic, and this has stimulated intensive efforts to harness the immune system to improve outcomes for patients with advanced disease (McDermott and Atkins, 2013; Rijnders et al., 2017; Zibelman and Plimack, 2017). Tumor-infiltrating immune cells can be readily isolated from RCC, including cytotoxic T cells, dendritic cells, and helper T cells, which express interleukin (IL)-1 and IL-2 and function as antigen-presenting cells. Study of the molecular mechanisms involved in the interactions of the host immune system with the tumor has yielded insights and effective therapies for RCC (McDermott and Atkins, 2013; Rijnders et al., 2017; Zibelman and Plimack, 2017). Immunotherapy with interferon and high-dose IL-2 was the only effective systemic therapy for RCC in the years before the discovery of the first VEGF-targeted therapies. Newer protocols that activate or maintain the viability of T cells, prime dendritic cells with tumor antigens, or block tumor-induced immunosuppression are now commonly used for metastatic RCC and hold great promise for the future (Brahmer et al., 2012; Rijnders et al., 2017; Zibelman and Plimack, 2017).

Clinical observations such as validated responses to immunotherapy, prolonged disease stabilization, and occasional spontaneous tumor regression support the immunogenicity of RCC. In the past, observed responses of RCC to immunomodulators, such as IL-2 and interferon-α, argued in favor of an important role for the immune system in the biology of RCC (Coppin, 2008; Zibelman and Plimack, 2017). Indeed, high-dose IL-2 remains a treatment with curative potential for patients with metastatic clear cell RCC, with durable and complete regression of disease accomplished in a finite proportion (3% to 5%) of patients (Amin and White, 2013; Coppin, 2008; Zibelman and Plimack, 2017). The estimated incidence of spontaneous regression of RCC is between 0.3% and 1% and is believed to be due to immune surveillance (Oliver, 1989). Most spontaneous regressions have been noted in patients with pulmonary metastases and have occurred after cytoreductive nephrectomy, but regression of primary RCC has also been reported in the absence of any form of treatment (Vogelzang et al., 1992).

Unfortunately, overall response rates with cytokine or other immune-based approaches for RCC were disappointing, typically ranging from 15% to 20%, despite a variety of creative treatment strategies, including the harvesting, ex vivo culturing, and reinfusion of tumor infiltrating lymphocytes. Suboptimal results with these ambitious protocols suggested immune tolerance, likely induced by the tumor (Amin and White, 2013; Zibelman and Plimack, 2017). A number of observations support impaired immune surveillance in RCC and a variety of mechanisms affecting virtually all levels of regulation of the immune system have been implicated, as reviewed previously (Campbell and Lane, 2016). Factors that downregulate effector T cells are particularly important in RCC: cytotoxic T-lymphocyte antigen–4 (CTLA-4) and the programmed death–1 (PD-1) molecule, also known as B7-H1, are glycoprotein receptors expressed on T cells that are central to this process (Fig. 97.8) (Buchbinder and Desai, 2016; Rijnders et al., 2017; Zibelman and Plimack, 2017). Under normal conditions these receptors participate in the regulation of the immune system, essentially serving an inhibitory role to prevent autoimmune diseases from developing. Increased activation of these receptors such as by enhanced programmed death ligand–1 (PD-L1) expression by the tumor leads to downregulation of effector T cells and immune tolerance (Rijnders et al., 2017). Thompson et al. (2006) reported that increased PD-L1 expression by clear cell RCC correlates with aggressive pathologic features and increased risk of disease progression, even after multivariate adjustment.

Recent trials have demonstrated that humanized antibodies that block PD-1 (e.g., nivolumab or pembrolizumab), PD-L1 (e.g., atezolizumab), or CTLA-4 (e.g., ipilimumab) can lead to complete and durable responses for patients with metastatic RCC. Improved overall survival has been documented for nivolumab when compared with everolimus for patients with metastatic RCC who have failed front-line therapy (Motzer et al., 2015). For untreated patients with metastatic RCC with intermediate or high-risk features, combination treatment with nivolumab plus ipilimumab was associated with better survival when compared with sunitinib (Escudier et al., 2017). Another combination approach, pembrolizumab plus axitinib, also appears to be active in untreated patients with metastatic kidney cancer, as it demonstrated better overall survival when compared to sunitinib monotherapy, with benefit observed in all risk groups (Rini et al., 2019). As such, these immune modulators, also known as checkpoint inhibitors, are changing the landscape of metastatic RCC, and we have now moved into a post-TKI era (see Chapters 61 and 104). Side effects of immune modulators can include autoimmune diseases, such as enterocolitis, hepatitis, dermatitis, or pneumonitis, as expected by their mechanism of action (Choueiri et al., 2016; Escudier et al., 2017; Hammers et al., 2017; Motzer et al., 2015; Zibelman and Plimack, 2017).

Angiogenesis and Targeted Pathways

RCC has long been recognized as one of the most vascular of cancers, as reflected by the distinctive neovascular pattern exhibited on renal angiography and robust enhancement observed on dedicated renal CT. The primary angiogenesis inducer in clear cell RCC is VEGF, which is suppressed by the wild-type VHL protein under normal conditions and is dramatically upregulated during tumor development (Gnarra et al., 1996; Iliopoulos et al., 1996). Increased levels of VEGF can be found in the serum and urine of patients with RCC, particularly in patients with hypervascular tumors when compared with hypovascular tumors, suggesting functional relevance (Takahashi et al., 1994).

VEGF is actually a family of ligands consisting of several subtypes, most of which are regulated by HIFs and VHL and bind to one or more of the corresponding VEGF receptor (VEGFR) family members (Lane et al., 2007c). VEGFR-1 (Flt-1) and VEGFR-2 (KDR/Flk-1) are receptor tyrosine kinases that are the target of several multi–tyrosine kinase inhibitors (TKIs) with activity against RCC (Carmeliet, 2005; Hicklin and Ellis, 2005). Upon binding of ligand (VEGF), key tyrosine residues along the intracellular portion of the VEGFR are phosphorylated, which leads to the binding of specific intracellular factors and activation of corresponding signal transduction pathways. Pathways known to be activated by phosphorylation of VEGFRs include the Raf-MEK-Erk and phosphatidylinositol-3-kinase/Akt/mTOR pathways that promote endothelial cell survival and proliferation (Carmeliet, 2005; Hicklin and Ellis, 2005). However, the promiscuity of the interactions between the various ligands, receptors, downstream effectors, and inhibitors can lead to a variety of effects that may be difficult to predict. This promiscuity is likely a major reason that therapeutic agents that appear to have similar modes of action (VEGFR tyrosine kinase inhibitors) are found to have somewhat disparate clinical or off-target effects. In contrast, bevacizumab is a monoclonal antibody that binds to VEGF and sequesters the ligand so that it cannot interact with VEGFR; its clinical activity is therefore almost certainly directly related to this activity.

Given the dependence of RCC on angiogenesis and the absence of generally effective forms of systemic therapies in the previous millennium, it is not surprising that RCC was one of the first malignancies targeted for anti-VEGF approaches when they became available. Promising results were initially reported for bevacizumab for patients with metastatic RCC, as it substantially reduced tumor burden and delayed time to progression when compared to placebo. A clinical niche for bevacizumab when combined with interferon-alpha was defined shortly thereafter (Escudier et al., 2007b; Rini et al., 2008; Yang et al., 2003). A number of multiple kinase inhibitors that target the VEGF pathway were subsequently tested in clinical trials and also approved by the US Food and Drug Administration (FDA) beginning in December 2005 and extending into the current era (see Fig. 97.7 and further details in Chapter 104) (Haddad and Rini, 2012; Motzer et al., 2006, 2013a, 2013b). More recently, cabozantinib, an inhibitor of VEGF as well as MET and AXL, demonstrated significant activity as second-line treatment for metastatic RCC (Choueiri et al., 2015).

Cancer Genome Research

In 2013 the Cancer Genome Atlas Research Network provided a more comprehensive molecular characterization of clear cell RCC that will serve as a solid foundation for future studies in this field. Analyses performed in this landmark study included next-generation sequencing to evaluate the whole genome of 22 tumors and whole-exome sequencing of 417 additional tumors. DNA copy number and genotype, CpG DNA methylation, messenger RNA expression, microRNA expression, and protein expression were also

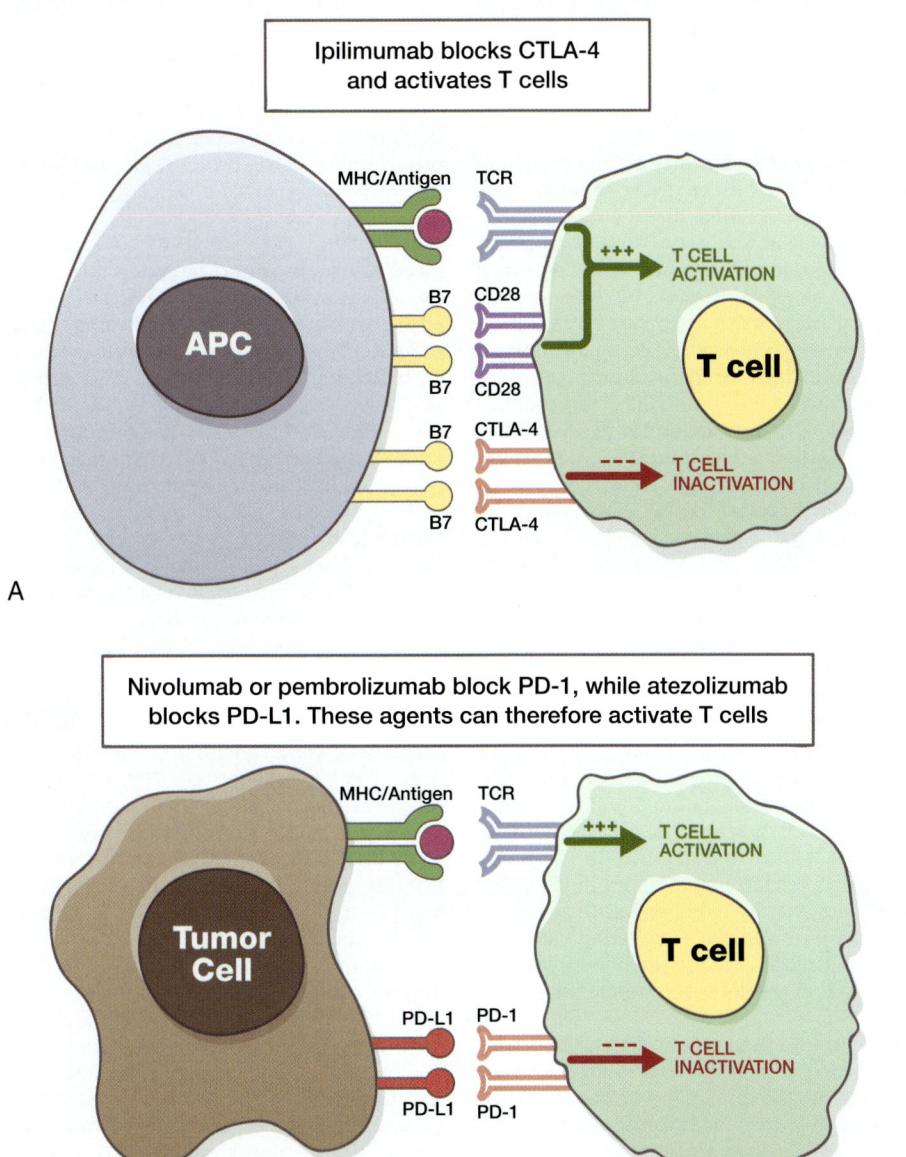

Fig. 97.8. Mechanism of action of checkpoint inhibitors. (A) Interactions between an antigen presenting cell (APC) and the T cell include activating signals and those that inhibit the T cell. Positive signals include interactions between the T cell receptor (TCR) and MHC/antigen complex and those associated with B7 and CD-28. In contrast, interactions between B7 and CTLA-4 inhibit the T cell, and the balance between these positive and negative signals determines whether the T cell becomes activated. The checkpoint inhibitor ipilimumab blocks CTLA-4 and thus tilts the balance in favor of T cell activation. (B) Interactions between the tumor cell and the T cell are also critically important and again comprise positive and negative signals with the former primarily consisting of interactions between the TCR and MHC/antigen complex. Some tumor cells, such as kidney cancer cells, can express PD-L1, the ligand for PD-1, and the resulting interactions between these molecules can suppress the T cell. Nivolumab and pembrolizumab block PD-1, while atezolizumab blocks PD-L1. These checkpoint inhibitors thus can activate the T cells and bolster immune responses to the malignancy.

analyzed in these same tumors, providing a wealth of information about the molecular features of clear cell RCC. The main findings included the identification of alterations in genes controlling cellular oxygen sensing, such as *VHL*, and regulation of chromatin status, such as *PBRM1*, *BAP1*, and *SETD2*.

In total, 19 significantly mutated genes were identified, including the previous genes as well as genes involved in the PI3K/AKT pathway (Dalgliesh et al., 2010). Mutation of the H3K36 methyltransferase *SETD2* was notable in that it is associated with widespread DNA hypomethylation, and complex integrative analyses suggested that mutations involving the switch sucrose nonfermentable (SWI/SNF) chromatin remodeling complex *(PBRM1, ARID1A, SMARCA4)* could have broad effects on other signaling pathways. **Overall, the analyses provide strong evidence for a metabolic shift in aggressive renal cancers,** with downregulation of genes involved in the tricarboxylic acid (TCA) cycle, upregulation of pentose phosphate and glutamine transporter genes, decreased AMPK and PTEN protein levels, and increased acetyl coenzyme A carboxylase protein. **The recurring** theme of metabolic remodeling in clear cell RCC suggests multiple new windows into future targets for disease treatment.

Other Signal Transduction and Cell Cycle Regulation Pathways

Aberrant activation of additional signal transduction pathways in RCC may also contribute to altered cell cycle kinetics, and these pathways represent excellent targets for therapeutic intervention. One such regulatory pathway in RCC is the mTOR pathway, which interfaces with Akt (protein kinase B) and the *PTEN* tumor suppressor gene (Barthelemy et al., 2013; Hudes, 2009). Expression of mTOR is upregulated by various growth factors or by mutation or loss of *PTEN*. Through complex pathways involving a variety of intermediaries, the mTOR pathway leads to increased expression of HIFs and other growth-promoting and potentially tumorigenic sequelae. **Inhibition of mTOR with temsirolimus (Torisel) has yielded prolonged survival in patients with poor-risk, metastatic RCC, and everolimus (Afinitor) has shown efficacy for patients in whom tyrosine kinase inhibitors have failed, confirming the clinical relevance of the mTOR pathway** (see Fig. 97.7) (Hudes et al., 2007; Motzer et al., 2008). Both of these mTOR inhibitors are now also approved by the FDA.

Proliferative index, as defined by proliferating cell nuclear antigen or Ki-67 staining, has correlated with pathologic parameters and clinical outcomes in RCC, suggesting that regulation of the cell cycle plays an important role in the tumor biology of RCC (Bui et al., 2004; Tollefson et al., 2007). Increased expression of transforming growth factor-α and its receptor tyrosine kinase, the epidermal growth factor receptor (EGFR), have been reported in RCC and may contribute to tumorigenesis by promoting cellular proliferation or transformation through an autocrine mechanism. Unfortunately, phase II clinical trials using agents that target EGFR, including erlotinib (Tarceva), gefitinib (Iressa), panitumumab (Vectibix), and lapatinib (Tykerb), demonstrated a lack of substantial activity in patients with advanced RCC (Rini, 2010). Based on these results, agents targeting the EGFR pathway have fallen out of favor for RCC, although selective treatment of patients who overexpress EGFR may still be a consideration within precision medicine trials.

The hepatocyte growth factor and its receptor, the c-*MET* protooncogene, may also contribute to the pathogenesis of RCC (Gibney et al., 2013; Giubellino et al., 2009; Harshman and Choueiri, 2013). The role of activating mutations of the c-*MET* proto-oncogene in the cause of hereditary papillary RCC has already been discussed, but data suggest that upregulated expression of this ligand may also occur in most of the histologic subtypes of RCC (Giubellino et al., 2009; Harshman and Choueiri, 2013). Hepatocyte growth factor is expressed by normal proximal tubular cells, where it is involved in branching tubulogenesis of the developing kidney and regeneration after renal injury. Increased serum levels of hepatocyte growth factor have also been reported in most patients with RCC, independent of histologic subtype, and activation of the receptor by phosphorylation at two sites is associated with cancer progression, making c-Met a potential therapeutic target for papillary and other forms of RCC (Gibney et al., 2013). Cabozantinib, an inhibitor of VEGFR, MET, and AXL, demonstrated a significant clinical benefit versus sunitinib, which primarily targets VEGFR, as first-line treatment for intermediate- to poor-risk RCC, suggesting a potential superiority to dual pathway inhibition (Choueiri et al., 2017a).

Other potential factors involved in RCC pathogenesis include the insulin-like growth factor axis, telomerase, apoptotic factors, and extracellular matrix proteins (Campbell and Lane, 2016).

Pathology

Most RCCs are round to ovoid and circumscribed by a pseudocapsule of compressed parenchyma and fibrous tissue rather than a true histologic capsule. Unlike upper tract urothelial carcinomas, most RCCs are not grossly infiltrative, with the notable exception of collecting duct carcinoma and sarcomatoid variants. Tumor size has averaged between 4 and 8 cm in most series but can vary from a few millimeters to large enough to fill the entire abdomen. Tumors smaller than 3 cm were previously classified as benign adenomas, but small tumors have on rare occasion been associated with metastases (Daugherty et al., 2017; Nguyen and Gill, 2009). Most pathologists agree that, with the exception of oncocytomas and some small (≤5 mm) low-grade papillary adenomas, there are no reliable histologic or ultrastructural criteria to differentiate benign from malignant renal epithelial tumors (see Chapter 96). When they are bivalved, RCCs consist of yellow, tan, or brown tumor interspersed with fibrotic, necrotic, or hemorrhagic areas; few are uniform in gross appearance. Cystic degeneration is prominent in 10% to 25% of RCCs and appears to be associated with a better prognosis compared with purely solid RCC (Bhatt et al., 2016; Jhaveri et al., 2013; Webster et al., 2007). Calcification can be stippled or plaquelike and is found in 10% to 20% of RCCs.

Nuclear features can be highly variable and are an independent prognostic factor for RCC generally and for clear cell and papillary RCC in particular (Delahunt et al., 2014; Fuhrman et al., 1982; Klatte et al., 2010; Sukov et al., 2012). Grading has been based primarily on nuclear size and shape and the presence or absence of prominent nucleoli. Fuhrman's system (Fuhrman et al., 1982) was the most frequently used system for more than three decades but was not reliable for chromophobe RCC and has not been validated for the newer subtypes of renal carcinoma (Cheville et al., 2012; Delahunt et al., 2007; Finley et al., 2011). **A new four-tiered grading system developed by the World Health Organization and International Society of Urological Pathology has been validated for clear cell and papillary RCC** (Delahunt et al., 2014) and is now the recommended grading system for RCC (Table 97.8).

Aggressive local behavior is not uncommon with RCC and can be expressed in a variety of ways. Invasion of the renal capsule, renal sinus, or collecting system is found in approximately 20% of cases, although displacement of these structures is a more common finding. Further spread to involve adjacent organs or the abdominal wall is often precluded by the Gerota fascia, although some high-grade RCCs are able to overcome this natural barrier. **One unique feature of RCC is its predilection for involvement of the venous system, which is found in 10% of cases,** more often than in any other tumor type (Schefft et al., 1978; Skinner et al., 1972). Contiguous

TABLE 97.8 World Health Organization/International Society of Urological Pathology (WHO/ISUP) Grading System for Clear Cell and Papillary Renal Cell Carcinoma

GRADE	DESCRIPTION
1	Nucleoli are absent or inconspicuous and basophilic at 400× magnification
2	Nucleoli are conspicuous and eosinophilic at 400× magnification and visible but not prominent at 100× magnification
3	Nucleoli are conspicuous and eosinophilic at 100× magnification
4	There is extreme nuclear pleomorphism, multinucleated giant cells, and/or rhabdoid and/or sarcomatoid differentiation

Modified from Delahunt B, Srigley JR, Egevad L, et al.: International Society of Urological Pathology grading and other prognostic factors for renal neoplasia. *Eur Urol* 66(5):795–798, 2014.

tumor thrombus can extend into the renal vein and inferior vena cava (IVC) and ascend as high as the right atrium. Many such tumor thrombi are highly vascularized by arterial blood flow (Novick et al., 1990), and some directly invade the wall of the renal vein or vena cava, which correlates with compromised prognosis (Haddad et al., 2014; Schefft et al., 1978; Skinner et al., 1972; Zini et al., 2008).

Most sporadic RCCs are solitary. **Bilateral involvement can be synchronous or asynchronous and is found in 2% to 4% of sporadic RCCs, although it is considerably more common in patients with familial forms of RCC, such as von Hippel-Lindau disease. Multicentricity, which is found in 10% to 20% of cases, is more common in association with papillary RCC and familial RCC** (Cheng et al., 1991; Krambeck et al., 2008; Mukamel et al., 1988; Nguyen et al., 2017). Satellite lesions are often small and difficult to identify by preoperative imaging, intraoperative ultrasonography, or visual inspection; they appear to be the main factor contributing to ipsilateral recurrence after partial nephrectomy (Mukamel et al., 1988). Microsatellite analysis suggests a clonal origin for most multifocal RCC within the same kidney (Junker et al., 2002), but tumor in the contralateral kidney is likely to be an independent growth if it is synchronous or a metastasis if it is asynchronous (Kito et al., 2002; Lane et al., 2009). Comprehensive sequencing of multiple biopsy specimens obtained from primary and metastatic tumors in the same patient has revealed significant intratumor heterogeneity (Gerlinger et al., 2012). These studies suggest that analysis of single biopsy samples may underestimate this inherent heterogeneity and prevent discernment of "driver" mutations from "passenger" mutations, presenting significant challenges to personalized medicine and biomarker development (Beksac et al., 2017; Gerlinger et al., 2012; Hanahan and Weinberg, 2011).

All RCCs are, by definition, adenocarcinomas, derived from renal tubular epithelial cells (Moch et al., 2016; Zhou, 2009; Table 97.9). **Most RCCs share ultrastructural features, such as surface microvilli and complex intracellular junctions, with normal proximal tubular cells and are believed to be derived from this region of the nephron** (Axelson and Johansson, 2013; Kim and

TABLE 97.9 Pathologic Subtypes of Renal Cell Carcinoma

HISTOLOGY[a]	FAMILIAL FORM AND GENETIC FACTORS	GROSS CHARACTERISTICS	MICROSCOPIC PATHOLOGIC CHARACTERISTICS	OTHER CHARACTERISTICS
COMMON SUBTYPES				
Clear cell RCC (70%–80%)	von Hippel-Lindau (VHL) disease VHL gene (3p25) mutation or hypermethylation Chromosome 3p deletions Loss of chromosome 8p, 9p, 14q; gain of chromosome 5q	Typically well-circumscribed, lobulated, golden yellow tumor but can be infiltrative Necrosis, hemorrhage, and cystic degeneration common Venous involvement also common	Hypervascular tumor Nests or sheets of clear cells with delicate vascular network IHC[b]: LMWCKs[c], vimentin, EMA, CA-IX	Originates from proximal tubule Aggressive behavior more common Often responds to targeted molecular therapy and immunotherapy
Papillary RCC Type 1 (5%–10%)	HPRC Altered MET proto-oncogene status present in 81% of sporadic cases Trisomy of chromosome 7 and 17	Fleshy tumor with fibrous pseudocapsule Necrosis and hemorrhage are common	Hypovascular tumor Papillary structures with single layer of cells around fibrovascular cores Basophilic cells with low-grade nuclei IHC[b]: LMWCKs[c], CK7 (type 1 > type 2), AMACR	Originates from proximal tubule Good prognosis Often multicentric Common in ARCD
Papillary RCC Type 2 (5%–10%)	HLRCC Fumarate hydratase (FH) gene (1q42-43) mutation in HLRCC	Fleshy tumor with fibrous pseudocapsule Necrosis and hemorrhage are common	Hypovascular tumor Papillary structures with single layer of cells around fibrovascular cores Eosinophilic cells with high-grade nuclei IHC[b]: LMWCKs[c], AMACR	Originates from proximal tubule Worse prognosis then type 1 papillary RCC; similar or worse prognosis when compared with clear cell RCC
Chromophobe RCC (3%–5%)	Birt-Hogg-Dube (BHD) syndrome Folliculin (FLCN) gene mutation (17p11) Loss of multiple chromosomes (1, 2, 6, 10, 13, 17, 21, Y) TPS3 and PTEN mutations	Well-circumscribed, homogeneous Tan or light brown cut surface	"Plant cells" with pale cytoplasm, perinuclear clearing or "halo," nuclear "raisins," and prominent cell borders (classic subtype) Positive Hale's colloidal iron staining IHC[b]: diffuse CK7 Eosinophilic subtype has dense pink cytoplasm and mitochondrial gene mutations	Originates from intercalated cells of collecting duct Generally good prognosis, although sarcomatoid variant associated with poor prognosis

Continued

TABLE 97.9 Pathologic Subtypes of Renal Cell Carcinoma—cont'd

HISTOLOGY[a]	FAMILIAL FORM AND GENETIC FACTORS	GROSS CHARACTERISTICS	MICROSCOPIC PATHOLOGIC CHARACTERISTICS	OTHER CHARACTERISTICS
Clear cell papillary RCC (~5%)	VHL disease	Well-circumscribed, well-developed capsule	Low-grade clear epithelial cells organized in linear papillae and tubules IHC[b]: diffuse CK7; cuplike CA-IX distribution	Arise in ESRD and VHL Good prognosis, indolent tumor behavior
Unclassified RCC (1%–3%)	Unknown	Varied	Varied	Origin not defined Generally poor prognosis
RARE SUBTYPES (EACH REPRESENTS <1%)				
Carcinoma of the collecting ducts of Bellini (collecting duct carcinoma)	Unknown Multiple chromosomal losses	Firm, centrally located tumor with infiltrative borders Light gray to tan-white	Complex, highly infiltrative cords within inflamed (desmoplastic) stroma High-grade nuclei, mitoses	Originates from collecting duct Poor prognosis May respond to cytotoxic chemotherapy
Renal medullary carcinoma	Associated with sickle cell trait	Infiltrative, gray-white Extensive hemorrhage and necrosis	Poorly differentiated cells with lacelike appearance Inflammatory infiltrate	Originates from collecting duct Dismal prognosis
Hereditary leiomyomatosis and renal cell carcinoma (HLRCC)-associated RCC	HLRCC Fumarate hydratase (FH) gene (1q42-43) mutation	Fleshy tumor with fibrous pseudocapsule Necrosis and hemorrhage are common	Hypovascular tumor Papillary structures with single layer of cells around fibrovascular cores Eosinophilic cells with high-grade nuclei IHC[b]: LMWCKs[c], AMACR	Tendency to metastasize early with extremely poor prognosis Low-grade variant recently described in children
Succinate dehydrogenase-deficient renal carcinoma	SDH-RCC SDHA, SDHB (1p36.13), SDHC (1q23.3), SDHD (11q23.1), SHDAF2	Solitary lesion	Vacuolated eosinophilic or clear cells Shares features with chromophobe RCC, oncocytoma, clear cell RCC, type 2 papillary RCC IHC[b]: Loss of SDHB	Presents in young adults, most often in those with a germline mutation in an SDH gene HIF-VEGF pathway; reductive carboxylation pathway High-grade and low-grade variants have been described
MiT family translocation RCC (includes Xp11 translocation RCC and t(6;11) RCC)	Various mutations involving chromosome Xp11.2 resulting in TFE3 gene fusion	Well-circumscribed, tan-yellow tumor	Variable; often clear cells with papillary architecture IHC[b]: nuclear TFE3	Occurs in children and young adults; accounts for 40% of pediatric RCC t(X;17) presents with advanced stage and often follows indolent course t(X;1) can recur with late lymph node metastases
Acquired cystic disease–associated RCC	VHL gene alterations Chromosome 3p deletion	Cystic degeneration	Cribriform, microcystic or sieve-like architecture Cysts lined with single layer of clear cells IHC[b]: absent CK7	Occurs in patients with ESRD and acquired cystic kidney disease Excellent prognosis

TABLE 97.9 Pathologic Subtypes of Renal Cell Carcinoma—cont'd

HISTOLOGY[a]	FAMILIAL FORM AND GENETIC FACTORS	GROSS CHARACTERISTICS	MICROSCOPIC PATHOLOGIC CHARACTERISTICS	OTHER CHARACTERISTICS
Multilocular cystic clear cell renal neoplasm of low malignant potential	Identical to clear cell RCC	Well-circumscribed mass of small and large cysts	Cysts lined by single layer of low grade clear cells No expansive nodules of tumor cells	Almost uniformly benign clinical behavior
Tubulocystic RCC	Unknown	Multiple small to medium renal cysts with spongy appearance	Enlarged nucleoli (grade 3) Eosinophilic and oncocytoma-like cytoplasm	Favorable prognosis
Mucinous tubular and spindle cell carcinoma	Unknown	Well-circumscribed, tan-white-pink tumors centered in medulla	Mixture of tubules and spindle-shaped epithelial cells; mucin background	Favorable prognosis
Hybrid oncocytic chromophobe tumor	Birt-Hogg-Dube (BHD) syndrome Folliculin (FLCN) gene mutation (17p11)	Well-circumscribed, homogeneous appearance Tan or light brown cut surface	Shares features with chromophobe RCC and oncocytoma; often coexists with these tumors in BHD patients	Generally good prognosis

[a]Sarcomatoid variants of all of these subtypes have been described and are associated with compromised prognosis.
[b]Immunohistochemistry (IHC) using these markers can help to differentiate between RCC subtypes.
[c]Cytokeratin (CK): low-molecular-weight cytokeratins (LMWCKs).
AMACR, Alpha-methylacyl-coenzyme A racemase; *ARCD*, acquired renal cystic disease; *CA-IX*, carbonic anhydrase IX; *CK7*, cytokeratin 7; *EMA*, epithelial membrane antigen; *ESRD*, end-stage renal disease; *HLRCC*, hereditary leiomyomatosis and RCC; *HPRC*, hereditary papillary RCC; *IHC*, immunohistochemistry; *RCC*, renal cell carcinoma; *VHL*, von Hippel-Lindau.
Modified from Eble JN, Sauter G, Epstein JI, et al.: *WHO classification of tumours: pathology and genetics of tumours of the urinary system and male genital organs*, Lyon, France, 2004, IARC Press; Srigley JR, Delahunt B, Eble J N, et al.: The International Society of Urological Pathology (ISUP) Vancouver classification of renal neoplasia. *Am J Surg Pathol* 37(10):1469–1489, 2013; Moch H, Cubilla AL, Humphrey PA, et al.: The 2016 WHO classification of tumours of the urinary system and male genital organs–Part A: renal, penile, and testicular tumours. *Eur Urol* 70(1):93–105, 2016.

Kim, 2002). Chromophobe RCC and two aggressive subtypes of RCC, renal medullary carcinoma and collecting duct carcinoma, appear to be derived from more distal elements of the nephron (Abern et al., 2012; Amin et al., 2017; Davis et al., 2014; Storkel et al., 1997; Zambrano et al., 1999).

Since the early 1990s, the histologic classification of RCC has undergone several major revisions (see Table 97.9) (Algaba et al., 2011; Moch et al., 2016; Srigley et al., 2013; Zambrano et al., 1999; Zhou, 2009). Traditionally, RCC was divided into four histologic subtypes: clear cell, granular cell, tubulopapillary, and sarcomatoid. Based on advances in the molecular genetics of RCC and a more discerning interpretation of histologic and ultrastructural features, a newer classification scheme was proposed (Kovacs, 1993). In this system, granular cell tumors were reclassified into other categories based on distinct histopathologic features, chromophobe RCC was recognized as a new RCC subtype, and sarcomatoid features were categorized as variants of other histologic subtypes rather than a distinct tumor type (Storkel et al., 1997; Weiss et al., 1995; Zambrano et al., 1999). **Current practice is to identify the primary histologic subtype and comment on the presence and extent of sarcomatoid differentiation rather than to separate these tumors into a distinct category, although the prognostic implications have not changed** (Cheville et al., 2004; Moch et al., 2016).

Depending on well-defined histologic and ultrastructural criteria, granular cell tumors were reclassified as papillary RCC, eosinophilic variants of chromophobe RCC, or clear cell RCC. Another important development was the identification of renal medullary carcinoma that is occasionally seen in young African-Americans with sickle cell trait (Abern et al., 2012; Davis et al., 1995). With additional pathologic advances, including electron microscopy, immunohistochemistry, molecular genetics, and cytogenetics, several additional unique subtypes of RCC have been identified since implementation of the 1993 classification system. Based on these findings, an updated classification of malignant epithelial tumors of the kidney was presented by the World Health Organization in 2004 and updated in 2016 (see Tables 97.1 and 97.9; Eble et al., 2004; Moch et al., 2016).

The World Health Organization classification reflects current understanding of RCC not as a single malignant neoplasm, but rather as a group comprising several different tumor subtypes, each with a distinct genetic basis and unique clinical features. Important changes include the addition of several RCC subtypes that were previously grouped within "conventional" or unclassified RCC. One example is MiT family translocation RCC, which has microscopic features of clear cell and papillary RCC and occurs primarily in children and young adults (Argani et al., 2010; Choueiri et al., 2010; Delahunt et al., 2014; Liu et al., 2016). Another is succinate dehydrogenase-deficient RCC, which also occurs in young adults and has favorable prognosis in most instances (Gill et al., 2014; Ricketts et al., 2008). Sophisticated gene expression profiling and proteomic analyses support the individuality of each of these tumor subtypes and hold great promise for differentiating additional subtypes in the future (Jonasch et al., 2012; Moch et al., 2016; Raspollini et al., 2017; Yang et al., 2006). This has clearly been a field in evolution with changes stimulated by basic science advances and astute clinical observation.

Clear Cell Renal Cell Carcinoma

Clear cell RCC accounts for 70% to 80% of all RCCs, representing the garden variety of RCC (Deng and Melamed, 2012; Moch et al., 2016; Storkel et al., 1997). **These tumors are typically yellow and highly vascular,** containing a network of delicate vascular sinusoids interspersed between sheets or acini of tumor cells (Fig. 97.9). **On microscopic examination, clear cell RCC can include clear cells, granular or eosinophilic cells, or mixed types.** Clear cells are typically round or polygonal with abundant cytoplasm containing glycogen, cholesterol, cholesterol esters, and phospholipids, all of which are readily extracted by the solvents used in routine histologic

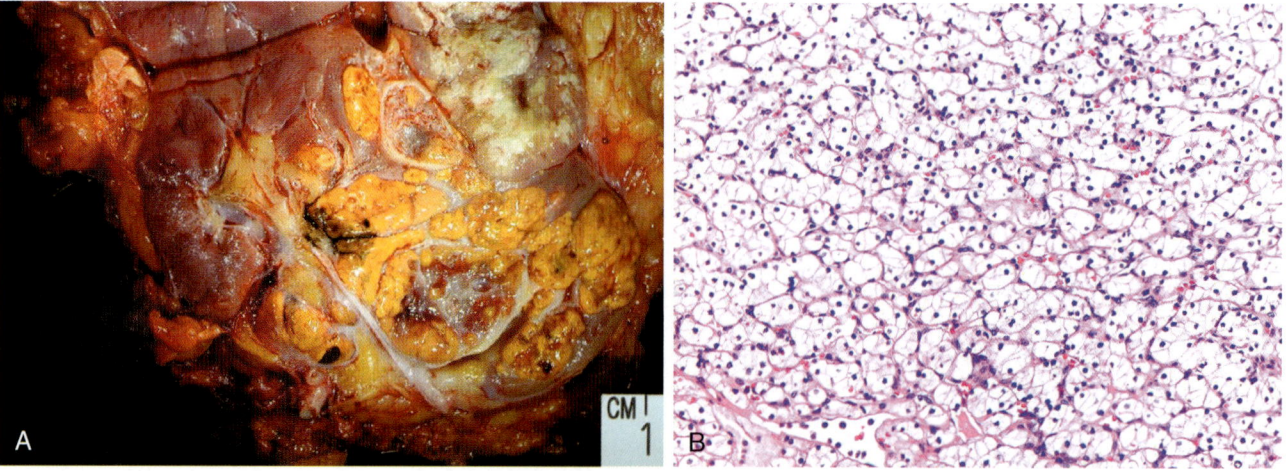

Fig. 97.9. (A) Clear cell renal cell carcinoma (RCC) with typical golden yellow color. (B) Low-power view of typical microscopic appearance of a low-grade clear cell RCC demonstrating a delicate vascular network interspersed within homogeneous nests of cells with clear cytoplasm. (Courtesy Dr. Ming Zhou, Cleveland, OH.)

preparations, contributing to the clear appearance of the tumor cells (Farrow, 1997). Granular cells with eosinophilic cytoplasm and abundant mitochondria can predominate. Three to five percent of clear cell RCCs demonstrate sarcomatoid features, and clear cell RCC is more likely to exhibit venous tumor extension than any other subtype of RCC (Rabbani et al., 2004). **In general, patients with clear cell RCC have a worse prognosis compared with papillary type 1 or chromophobe RCC, even after stratification for stage and grade** (Cheville et al., 2003; Deng and Melamed, 2012). **Paradoxically, clear cell RCC is more likely to respond to VEGF-targeted therapy, checkpoint inhibitors, or high dose IL-2 than other subtypes of RCC, so it typically has a better prognosis when it is metastatic. Chromosome 3 alterations occur in more than 90% of clear cell RCCs, leading to mutation or inactivation of the *VHL*, *PBRM1*, *SETD2*, or *BAP1* genes, which are all present on this portion of the genome** (Cancer Genome Atlas Research Network, 2013; Schmidt and Linehan, 2016). The familial form of clear cell RCC, the VHL syndrome, in which the *VHL* tumor suppressor gene is inactivated, has already been reviewed.

Papillary Renal Cell Carcinoma

Papillary RCC, which was previously designated chromophilic RCC, is the second most common histologic subtype (10%–15%) of all RCCs (Moch et al., 2016). On microscopic examination, most tumors consist of basophilic or eosinophilic cells arranged in papillary or tubular configuration (Fig. 97.10). Gross features of papillary RCC include beige to white color, spherical boundary, and frequent hemorrhage, which may mimic cystic components radiologically. **One unique feature of papillary RCC is its tendency toward multicentricity, which approaches 40% in many series and occurs more commonly in patients with end-stage renal disease and acquired renal cystic disease** (Deng and Melamed, 2012).

Two distinct variants of papillary RCC have been described by characteristic cytogenetics, immunostaining profiles, and gene expression profiling (see Fig. 97.10) (Eble et al., 2004; Pal et al., 2018; Storkel et al., 1997; Yang et al., 2005). **Type 1 papillary RCC, the more common form, consists of basophilic cells with scant cytoplasm; type 2 papillary RCC includes potentially more aggressive variants with eosinophilic cells and abundant granular cytoplasm** (Pal et al., 2018; Pignot et al., 2007).

The Cancer Genome Atlas (TCGA) analysis for papillary RCC demonstrated that many type 1 tumors have activating MET mutations, whereas three subgroups of type 2 were identified that harbor other genetic defects (Cancer Genome Atlas Research Network, 2013). The two subtypes of papillary RCC correspond with two familial RCC syndromes: HPRC syndrome (type 1) and HLRCC syndrome (type 2). **The cytogenetic abnormalities associated with type 1 papillary RCC are characteristic and include trisomy of chromosomes 7 and 17 and loss of the Y chromosome** (Cancer Genome Atlas Research Network, 2013; Kovacs et al., 1989b; Pal et al., 2018). Other common findings include gain of chromosomes 12, 16, and 20 and loss of heterozygosity on chromosome 14 (Deng and Melamed, 2012; Kenck et al., 1996). Papillary RCC is more likely to be hypovascular, perhaps because of the lack of *VHL* mutations that regulate VEGF, the primary proangiogenic molecule in RCC (Blath et al., 1976). As discussed earlier, activating mutations of the c-*MET* protooncogene located on chromosome 7 appears to be common and pathogenic in hereditary papillary RCC (Kenck et al., 1996; Schmidt et al., 1997). Indeed, this genetic defect is now being targeted for novel treatment approaches with the use of cabozatinib (Harshman and Choueiri, 2013; Jonasch et al., 2012).

The prognosis associated with papillary RCC remains controversial. Five-year cancer-specific survival rates for patients with papillary RCC traditionally ranged from 86% to 92%, in part because papillary RCCs often presented with low stage and grade, and most studies in the past were likely enriched in type 1 tumors (Deng and Melamed, 2012; Mancilla-Jimenez et al., 1976). However, more recent studies that have used immunohistochemistry and cytogenetics to define papillary histology contain an increased proportion of high-grade and advanced tumors that, although still in the minority, can prove to be lethal. In part this is due to the ineffectiveness of systemic therapies against metastatic papillary RCC (Amin and White, 2013; Lager et al., 1995; Margulis et al., 2008; Renshaw, 2002). **Current evidence suggests that type 1 papillary RCC carries a better prognosis than clear cell RCC, whereas type 2 papillary RCC is similar or worse than clear cell RCC** (Deng and Melamed, 2012).

Papillary adenomas are small (≤5 mm) tumors that resemble papillary RCC under the microscope, are often well encapsulated and low grade, and are commonly found at autopsy (Algaba et al., 2011). These lesions, which possess many of the same genetic alterations found in larger papillary RCCs, are generally considered benign (see Chapter 96).

Chromophobe Renal Cell Carcinoma

Chromophobe RCC, first described by Thoenes et al. in 1985, is a distinctive histologic subtype of RCC that represents 3% to 5% of all RCCs and appears to be derived from the distal convoluted tubules (Algaba et al., 2011; Davis et al., 2014; Haake and Rathmell,

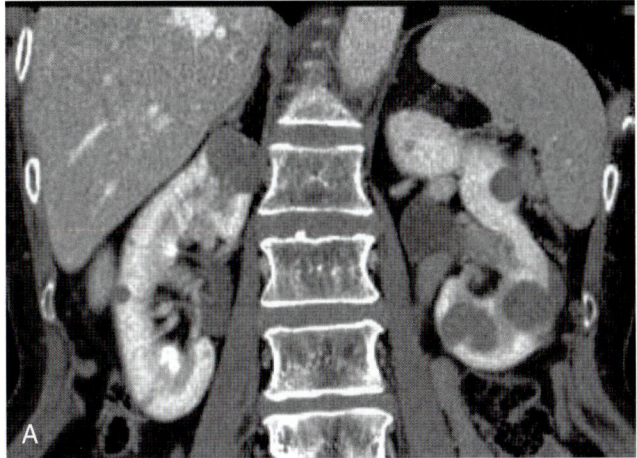
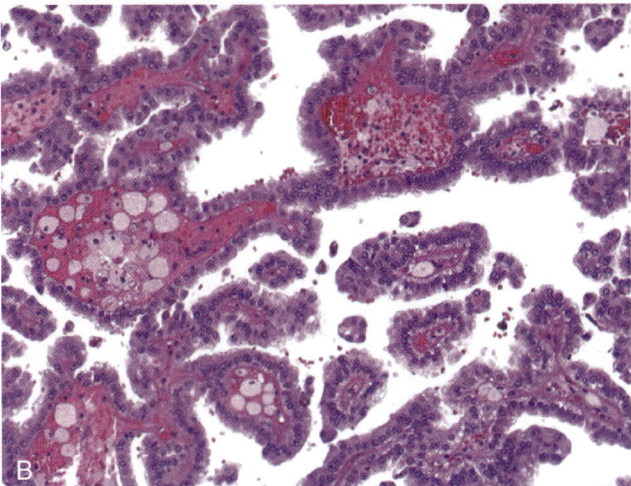
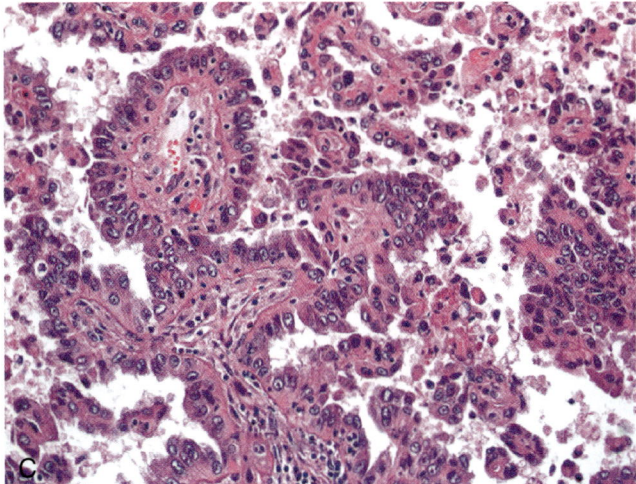

Fig. 97.10. (A) Papillary renal cell carcinoma (RCC) often presents with multiple small, modestly enhancing renal tumors as demonstrated on this computed tomography image. (B) Microscopic appearance of type 1 papillary RCC demonstrating basophilic cells with scant cytoplasm and low-grade nuclei. (C) In contrast, type 2 papillary RCC consists of eosinophilic cells with abundant granular cytoplasm and high-grade nuclei. (Courtesy Dr. Ming Zhou, Cleveland, OH.)

> **KEY POINTS: PATHOLOGY OF RENAL CELL CARCINOMA**
>
> - Clear cell RCC is the most common subtype (70%–80%) of RCC. Origin is the proximal tubule, and hypervascularity and necrosis are frequently present. Typically, these are more aggressive than the other common subtypes of RCC but also more likely to respond to immunotherapy and other targeted molecular therapies.
> - Papillary RCC (10%–15% of RCC) is divided into type 1, an indolent form associated with MET mutations and frequently multifocal, and type 2, which is associated with poorer prognosis.
> - Chromophobe RCC (3%–5% of RCC) is typically an indolent type of RCC that shares some histopathologic features with benign oncocytomas.

2017; Moch et al., 2016; Thoenes et al., 1985). Chromophobe RCC is commonly seen in the BHD syndrome, but most cases are sporadic (Schmidt and Linehan, 2016). The tumor cells typically exhibit a relatively transparent cytoplasm with a fine reticular pattern that has been described as a "plant cell" appearance (Fig. 97.11). Most chromophobe RCCs are resistant to the pigment used during typical hematoxylin and eosin staining, but eosinophilic variants constitute about 30% of cases (Nagashima, 2000; Thoenes et al., 1988). In either case, **a perinuclear clearing or "halo" is typically found and electron microscopic findings consist of numerous 150- to 300-nm microvesicles, which are the single most distinctive and defining feature of chromophobe RCC.** These microvesicles characteristically stain positive for Hale colloidal iron, indicating the presence of a mucopolysaccharide unique to chromophobe RCC (see Fig. 97.11). Immunohistochemistry typically reveals positive staining for pan-cytokeratin, epithelial membrane antigen, and parvalbumin and negative for vimentin and CD10 (Algaba et al., 2011). Multidimensional and comprehensive characterization of 66 primary chromophobe RCC by TCGA confirmed earlier discoveries of hypodiploid DNA content in most cases (Bugert et al., 1997; Davis et al., 2014). **Massive chromosomal losses, including the whole chromosomes 1, 2, 6, 10, 13, and 17 occur in 86% of cases,** and losses of chromosomes 3, 5, 8, 9, 11, 18, and 21 were noted in 12% to 58% of cancers (Davis et al., 2014). Combined mitochondrial DNA and gene expression analysis implicate changes in mitochondrial function as a common feature of chromophobe RCC (Davis et al., 2014).

Most studies suggest a better prognosis for localized chromophobe RCC than for clear cell RCC but a poor outcome in the small subset of patients with sarcomatoid features or metastatic disease (Klatte et al., 2008; Moch et al., 2016; Renshaw et al., 1996). Most early reports suggested a tendency to remain localized despite growth to large size, as well as a predominance of low-grade disease (Thoenes et al., 1988). Subsequent reports have verified that chromophobe RCC generally occurs at an earlier T stage, with more than 90% of patients remaining cancer free for 5 or more years after treatment (Deng and Melamed, 2012; Klatte et al., 2008). Limited data exist regarding treatment of metastatic chromophobe RCC, with most evidence suggesting limited activity of tyrosine kinase inhibitors, mTOR inhibitors, and immune modulators in this population (Kroeger et al., 2013; Tannir et al., 2012). Further clinical evaluation is required to identify effective therapeutic agents for patients with metastatic, non–clear cell RCC.

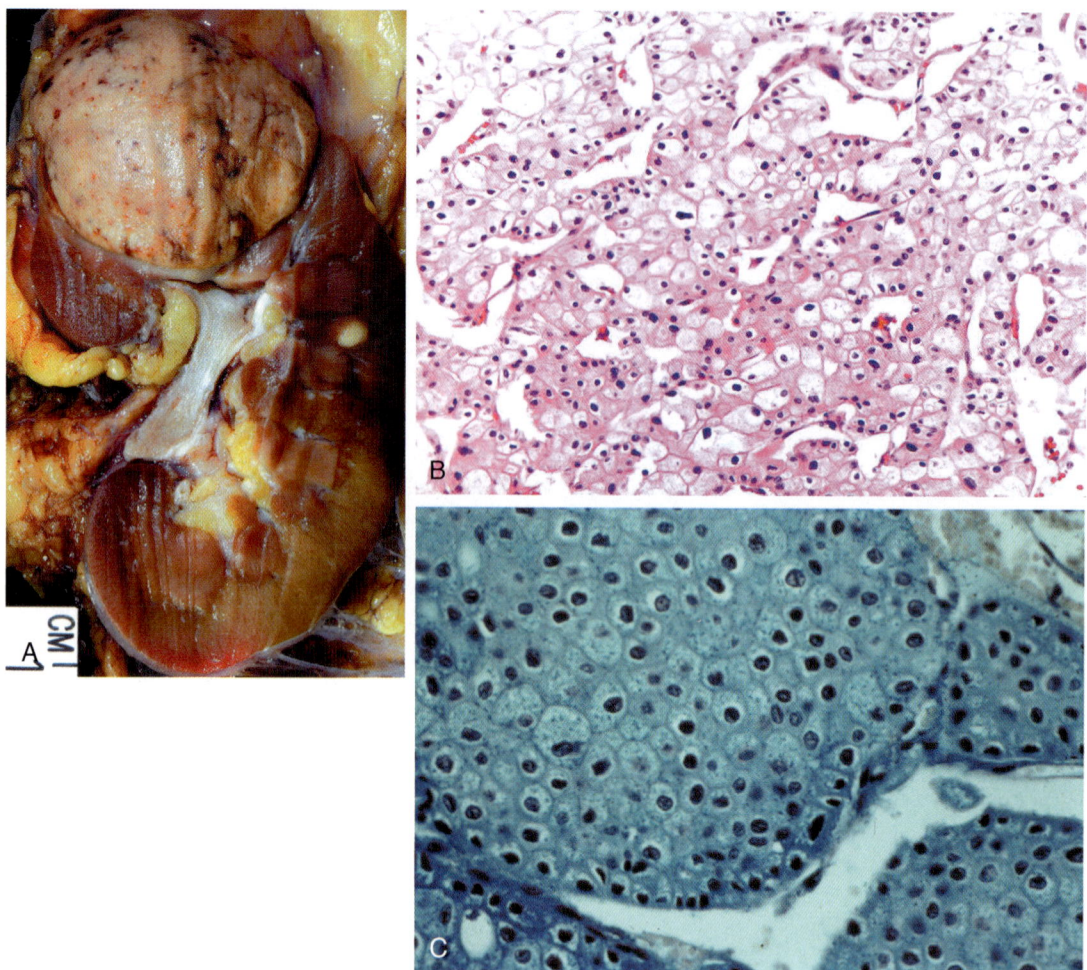

Fig. 97.11. (A) Chromophobe renal cell carcinoma (RCC) typically appears as a well-circumscribed, homogeneous, tan tumor. (B) Chromophobe RCC with admixture of classic (chromophobic) and eosinophilic cells. Characteristic features include distinct cytoplasmic borders, perinuclear "halos," and nuclear "raisins." The classic variant is notable for its "plant cell" appearance. (C) Chromophobe RCC stains positive for Hale colloidal iron and demonstrates multiple microvesicles on electron microscopy. (Courtesy Dr. Ming Zhou, Cleveland, OH.)

Collecting Duct Carcinoma

Carcinoma of the collecting ducts of Bellini is a relatively rare subtype of RCC, with a predictably poor prognosis (Algaba et al., 2011; Moch et al., 2016; Seo et al., 2017; Sui et al., 2017). Small collecting duct carcinomas can arise in a medullary pyramid, but most are large, infiltrative masses, and extension into the cortex is common (Deng and Melamed, 2012; Pickhardt et al., 2001). On microscopic examination, these tumors consist of an admixture of dilated tubules and papillary structures typically lined by a single layer of cuboidal cells, often creating a cobblestone appearance. The characteristic immunophenotype of these tumors is coexpression of low- and high-molecular-weight cytokeratins and *Ulex europaeus* agglutinin-1 reactivity (Rumpelt et al., 1991). Positivity for E-cadherin and c-KIT help to distinguish this entity from aggressive papillary RCC, but this staining profile can also be present in urothelial carcinoma, and differential diagnosis often requires careful examination of multiple sections (Kobayashi et al., 2008). **Most reported cases of collecting duct carcinoma have been high grade, advanced stage, and unresponsive to conventional therapies** (Karakiewicz et al., 2007c; Tokuda et al., 2006; Wright et al., 2009). Reflecting the fact that collecting duct carcinoma may share features in common with urothelial carcinoma, some patients with advanced collecting duct carcinoma have responded to cisplatin- or gemcitabine-based chemotherapy (Dason et al., 2013; Seo et al., 2017). Multimodality therapy, including surgery, systemic therapy, and possibly radiation therapy appear to improve survival compared with nephrectomy alone for metastatic disease (Seo et al., 2017). Early reports of the use of VEGF-targeted agents and checkpoint inhibitors for this aggressive cancer indicate potential clinical benefit (Ansari et al., 2009; Mizutani et al., 2017; Tannir et al., 2012; Yin et al., 2016).

Renal Medullary Carcinoma

Renal medullary carcinoma is an uncommon subtype of RCC that occurs almost exclusively in patients with sickle cell trait. It is typically diagnosed in young African-Americans, often in the third decade of life, and many cases are locally advanced and metastatic at the time of diagnosis (Davis et al., 1995; Moch et al., 2016; Swartz et al., 2002). Most patients do not respond to therapy and succumb to their disease within months, with less than 15% surviving more than 2 years (Shah et al., 2017a). More recent treatment protocols have produced modest improvements compared with a historical report with mean survival of 15 weeks (Davis et al., 1995). Median survival in two relatively large series of patients (159 and 52) reported in 2017 were 8 and 13 months (Ezekian et al., 2017; Shah et al., 2017a). Platinum-based chemotherapy was associated with a 29% objective response rate, with no objective clinical responses seen with targeted therapy in 28 patients (Shah et al., 2017a). This tumor shares many histologic features with collecting duct carcinoma,

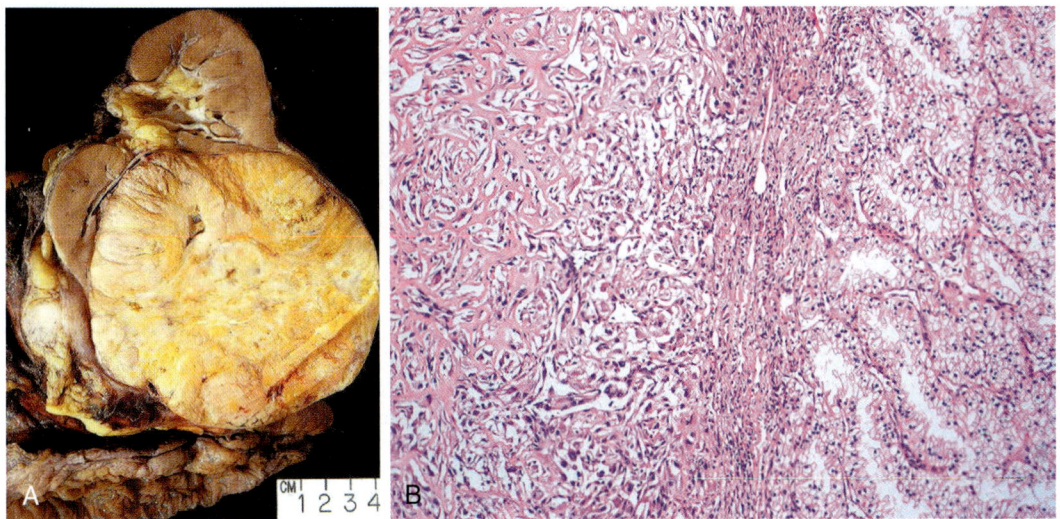

Fig. 97.12. (A) Clear cell renal cell carcinoma (RCC) with sarcomatoid differentiation demonstrating extension into the perinephric fat. (B) High-grade RCC with typical spindle cell appearance on the left indicating a component of sarcomatoid differentiation. (Courtesy Dr. Ming Zhou, Cleveland, OH.)

and many consider it a subtype of collecting duct carcinoma (Algaba et al., 2011; Seo et al., 2017; Swartz et al., 2002). Renal medullary carcinoma is thought to arise from the calyceal epithelium near the renal papillae but is often highly infiltrative. The site of origin (renal papillae) and association with sickle cell trait suggest that a relatively hypoxic environment may contribute to tumorigenesis.

Sarcomatoid and Rhabdoid Differentiation

Sarcomatoid differentiation is found in 1% to 5% of RCCs, most commonly in association with clear cell RCC or chromophobe RCC, but variants of most other subtypes of RCC have been described (Moch et al., 2016; Ro et al., 1987; Shuch et al., 2012; Wei and Al-Saleem, 2017). Most authors now believe that sarcomatoid lesions represent poorly differentiated regions of RCC rather than independently derived tumors (DeLong et al., 1993; Eble et al., 2004) because it is rare to find a truly pure sarcomatoid renal mass. **For this reason, this entity is no longer recognized as a distinct histologic subtype of RCC** (Eble et al., 2004). **Sarcomatoid differentiation is characterized by spindle cell histology, positive staining for vimentin, infiltrative growth pattern, aggressive local and metastatic behavior, and poor prognosis** (Fig. 97.12). Invasion of adjacent organs is common, and median survival has been less than 1 year in most series (Kara et al., 2016; Molina et al., 2011; Ro et al., 1987; Wei and Al-Saleem, 2017). Multimodal approaches should be considered if performance status allows, based on the extremely poor prognosis with surgery alone and selected reports demonstrating modest response rates in patients receiving immunotherapy, chemotherapy, or VEGF-targeted therapy after surgery (Shuch et al., 2012).

Similar to RCC with sarcomatoid differentiation, rhabdoid features can be seen with many of the subtypes of RCC but is not considered a separate subtype. The presence of rhabdoid cells mandates assignment of grade 4 and is generally associated with a poor prognosis (Kara et al., 2016; Przybycin et al., 2014; Zhang et al., 2015). Several studies have implicated a specific molecular mechanism affecting the switch sucrose nonfermentable (SWI/SNF) chromatin remodeling complex in rhabdoid and other de-differentiated subtypes of carcinomas from multiple organs, including the kidney, potentially identifying a target for future therapies for these aggressive cancers (Agaimy et al., 2017).

Unclassified Renal Cell Carcinoma

Unclassified RCC represents a minority of cases (1% to 5%) of presumed RCC with features that remain indeterminate even after careful analysis (Crispen et al., 2010). **Many are poorly differentiated and are associated with a highly aggressive biologic behavior and a particularly poor prognosis** (Amin et al., 2002; Karakiewicz et al., 2007b). Included within this "catch-all" category are occasional cases of RCC with extensive sarcomatoid differentiation and no discernible epithelial component. Advances in molecular diagnostics, such as gene expression profiling, may enable further classification of unusual tumors that previously would have fallen into this category and identify candidate pathways for targeted molecular therapeutics (Jonasch et al., 2012; Yang et al., 2006).

Clinical Presentation

Because of the sequestered location of the kidney within the retroperitoneum, many renal masses remain asymptomatic and nonpalpable until they are locally advanced. With the more pervasive use of noninvasive imaging for the evaluation of a variety of nonspecific symptom complexes, more than 60% of RCCs are now detected incidentally (Beisland, 2017; O'Connor et al., 2011; Silverman et al., 2008). Several studies have shown that such tumors are more likely to be confined to the kidney and a positive impact on survival has been reported, although the contributions of lead and length time biases have not been defined (Beisland, 2017; Decastro and McKiernan, 2008; Kane et al., 2008; Tsui et al., 2000).

Symptoms associated with RCC can be due to local tumor growth, hemorrhage, paraneoplastic syndromes, or metastatic disease (Table 97.10; Hu et al., 2016). Flank pain is usually due to hemorrhage and clot obstruction, although it can also occur with locally advanced or invasive disease. **The classic triad of flank pain, gross hematuria, and palpable abdominal mass is now rarely seen.** This is fortunate because this constellation of findings almost always denotes advanced disease and some refer to it as the "too late triad." Before the advent of ultrasonography and CT, most patients with RCC presented with one or more of these signs or symptoms, and many were incurable. Other indicators of advanced disease include constitutional symptoms such as weight loss, fever, and night sweats, and physical examination findings such as palpable cervical lymphadenopathy, nonreducing varicocele, and bilateral lower extremity edema resulting from venous involvement. A minority of patients present with symptoms directly related to metastatic disease, such as bone pain or persistent cough. **A less common but important presentation of RCC is that of spontaneous perirenal hemorrhage, in which the underlying mass may be obscured.** Zhang et al. have shown that more than 50% of patients with perirenal hematoma of unclear cause have an occult renal tumor, most often AML or

TABLE 97.10 Clinical Presentation of Renal Cell Carcinoma

Incidental presentation
Symptoms of localized or locally advanced disease
    Hematuria
    Flank pain
    Abdominal mass
    Perinephric hematoma
Obstruction of the inferior vena cava
    Bilateral lower extremity edema
    Nonreducing or right-sided varicocele
Symptoms of systemic disease
    Persistent cough
    Bone pain
    Cervical lymphadenopathy
    Constitutional symptoms
    Weight loss/fever/malaise
Paraneoplastic syndromes

KEY POINTS: CLINICAL PRESENTATION OF RENAL CELL CARCINOMA

- Local symptoms of RCC can include flank pain, gross hematuria, and palpable abdominal mass; however, this classic triad of symptoms is now rarely seen.
- The majority of RCC are detected incidentally; early detection is more commonly associated with small primary tumors and localized disease.
- Spontaneous renal hemorrhage can occur with RCC or AML.
- Paraneoplastic syndromes are seen more commonly with metastatic disease; many resolve once the malignant lesion(s) are surgically removed. Hypercalcemia can also be managed with vigorous hydration and diuresis, or with other medical approaches.

RCC (Xie et al., 2017; Zhang et al., 2002). Repeat CT a few months later often provides a definitive diagnosis.

Paraneoplastic syndromes are found in 10% to 20% of patients with RCC and few, if any, nonrenal malignancies are associated with a comparable quantity and diversity of such syndromes. In fact, **RCC was previously referred to as the internist's tumor because of the predominance of systemic rather than local manifestations.** Paraneoplastic syndromes are more common in metastatic disease and less common (almost nonexistent) in patients with small, incidental renal masses (Hu et al., 2016; Moreira et al., 2016). Now, a more appropriate name for RCC would be the radiologist's tumor, given the frequency of incidental detection (Decastro and McKiernan, 2008; Parsons et al., 2001). Nevertheless, it is still important to evaluate for paraneoplastic phenomena because they can be a source of major morbidity and can affect clinical decision making. The most common of these syndromes is elevated erythrocyte sedimentation rate, which accounts for more than 50% of identified paraneoplastic syndromes (Gold et al., 1996). Under normal circumstances, the kidney produces 1,25-dihydroxycholecalciferol, renin, erythropoietin, and various prostaglandins, all of which are tightly regulated to maintain homeostasis. RCC may produce these substances in pathologic amounts, and it may also elaborate a variety of other physiologically important factors, such as parathyroid hormone–like peptides, lupus-type anticoagulant, human chorionic gonadotropin, insulin, and various cytokines and inflammatory mediators. These substances are responsible for the development of paraneoplastic syndromes and often contribute to constitutional symptoms and decline of performance status.

Hypercalcemia has been reported in up to 13% of patients with RCC and can be due to either paraneoplastic phenomena or osteolytic metastatic involvement of the bone (Klatte et al., 2007; Schwarzberg and Michaelson, 2009). The signs and symptoms of hypercalcemia are often nonspecific and include nausea, anorexia, fatigue, and decreased deep tendon reflexes. **Medical management predominates and includes vigorous hydration followed by diuresis with furosemide and the selective use of bisphosphonates, corticosteroids, or calcitonin.** Bisphosphonate therapy is now established as a standard of care for patients with hypercalcemia of malignancy, as long as renal function is adequate (Schwarzberg and Michaelson, 2009). Zoledronic acid, 4 mg intravenously every 4 weeks, appears to be particularly effective in patients with RCC but must be withheld in the presence of renal insufficiency (Lipton et al., 2003; Schwarzberg and Michaelson, 2009). If hypercalcemia proves refractory to bisphosphonates, denosumab therapy can be considered (Hu et al., 2014). More definitive management includes nephrectomy and occasional metastasectomy, depending on the clinical circumstances. Hypercalcemia related to extensive osteolytic metastases is much more difficult to palliate because it is not amenable to surgical approaches, but many such patients may respond to bisphosphonate therapy and focused radiation therapy if limited sites of involvement can be identified (Lipton et al., 2003; Young and Coleman, 2013).

Hypertension and polycythemia are other important paraneoplastic syndromes commonly found in patients with RCC (Moein and Dehghani, 2000; Moreira et al., 2016). Hypertension associated with RCC can be secondary to increased production of renin directly by the tumor; compression or encasement of the renal artery or its branches, effectively leading to renal artery stenosis; or arteriovenous fistula within the tumor. Less common causes include polycythemia, hypercalcemia, ureteral obstruction, and increased intracranial pressure associated with cerebral metastases. Polycythemia associated with RCC can be due to increased production of erythropoietin, either directly by the tumor or by the adjacent parenchyma in response to hypoxia induced by tumor growth (Wiesener et al., 2007).

One of the more fascinating paraneoplastic syndromes associated with RCC is nonmetastatic hepatic dysfunction, or **Stauffer syndrome**, which has been reported in 3% to 20% of cases (Giannakos et al., 2005; Kranidiotis et al., 2009). Almost all patients with Stauffer syndrome have an elevated serum alkaline phosphatase level, 67% have elevated prothrombin time or hypoalbuminemia, and 20% to 30% have elevated serum bilirubin or transaminase levels. Other common findings include thrombocytopenia and neutropenia, and typical symptoms include fever and weight loss. Hepatic metastases must be excluded. Biopsy, when indicated, often demonstrates nonspecific hepatitis and discrete regions of necrosis are also occasionally seen. Elevated serum levels of IL-6 have been found in patients with Stauffer syndrome, and it is believed that this and other cytokines may play a pathogenic role. Hepatic function normalizes after nephrectomy in 60% to 70% of cases. Persistence or recurrence of hepatic dysfunction is almost always indicative of viable tumor and thus represents a poor prognostic finding.

A variety of other less common, but distinct paraneoplastic syndromes associated with RCC include Cushing syndrome, hyperglycemia, galactorrhea, neuromyopathy, clotting disorders, and cerebellar ataxia (Sufrin et al., 1989). **In general, treatment of paraneoplastic syndromes associated with RCC has required surgical excision or systemic antineoplastic therapy to reduce the burden of disease and, except for hypercalcemia, medical therapies have not proved helpful.**

Screening and Clinical Associations

A number of factors make screening for RCC appealing (Carrizosa and Godley, 2009; Diaz de Leon and Pedrosa, 2017). **Most important, RCC remains primarily a surgical disease requiring early diagnosis to optimize the opportunity for cure.** Unfortunately, our ability to salvage patients with advanced disease remains limited. Consistent with these observations, several studies have demonstrated an apparent advantage to early or incidental diagnosis of RCC (Lee et al., 2002; Leslie et al., 2003).

The primary factor that limits the widespread implementation of screening for RCC is the relatively low incidence of RCC in the general population (approximately 16 cases per 100,000 population per year) (Siegel et al., 2017). In this setting a screening test must be almost 100% specific to avoid an unacceptably high false-positive rate, which would lead to unnecessary, expensive, and potentially harmful diagnostic or therapeutic procedures. In addition, even if the test were 100% sensitive and specific, the yield from screening would be so low that it would not be considered cost effective (Carrizosa and Godley, 2009; Rini and Campbell, 2015). Even for populations with established risk factors for RCC, such as male gender, increased age, and heavy tobacco use, generalized screening would be difficult to justify because the increase in relative risk associated with each of these factors is at best twofold to threefold (Carrizosa and Godley, 2009). Another confounding factor is the prevalence of clinically insignificant tumors such as renal adenomas, which are found at autopsy in 10% to 20% of individuals, and other benign or slow-growing tumors (Pantuck et al., 2000; Parsons et al., 2001). There is clearly a risk that such clinically insignificant lesions could be detected, leading to unnecessary evaluation and treatment (Pantuck et al., 2000; Parsons et al., 2001). All these factors recommend against generalized screening efforts for the detection of RCC.

Review of the literature describing the use of dipstick analysis for hematuria and imaging for screening for RCC supports these conclusions (Carrizosa and Godley, 2009; Diaz de Leon and Pedrosa, 2017). Urinalysis is simple and inexpensive, but the yield of RCC in several screening studies has been exceedingly low. In part, this may be because small RCCs are often not associated with hematuria (gross or microscopic) because they are parenchymal rather than urothelial-based malignancies. The incidence of RCC in ultrasound or CT screening studies has ranged from 23 to 300 per 100,000 population, much higher than expected, and an increased proportion of organ-confined tumors has been found in such screened populations compared with historical controls (Carrizosa and Godley, 2009; Turney et al., 2006). However, the incidence of RCC in these studies is still relatively low, and it is unlikely that such efforts would be considered cost effective. Overall, the yield of RCC in such studies is an order of magnitude lower than the yield from prostate-specific antigen–based screening for prostate cancer, and many of the same controversies about lead and length time biases that have plagued the debate about screening for prostate cancer also apply to RCC (Carter et al., 2013). Because of these considerations, it is difficult to justify generalized screening efforts for RCC given the currently available technology.

RCC-related biomarkers in the urine or serum have the potential to distinguish patients with RCC from controls and could play a role for screening in the future (Morrissey and Kharasch, 2013; Rini and Campbell, 2015). Multiple investigations have demonstrated aquaporin-1 levels to be 10-fold higher in patients with RCC (Morrissey and Kharasch, 2013; Sreedharan et al., 2014). Subsequent phase 3 investigation confirmed that aquaporin-1 and perilipin-2 have sensitivity and specificity of at least 95% and at least 91%, respectively, for detection of RCC (Morrissey et al., 2015). Other potential biomarkers include microsatellite alterations in the DNA, *VHL* gene mutations or hypermethylation, upregulation of angiogenic factors (including VEGF), or expression of other RCC-specific proteins such as CA-IX (Jonasch et al., 2012). Further validation of these biomarkers in various clinical settings is needed, and, at least as presently constituted, such approaches would be cost prohibitive for broader populations.

For these reasons, the focus of screening for RCC must be on well-defined target populations, such as patients with end-stage renal disease and acquired renal cystic disease, tuberous sclerosis, and familial RCC (Table 97.11). Eighty percent of patients with end-stage renal disease eventually develop acquired renal cystic disease, and 1% to 2% of this cohort develops RCC (Ishikawa et al., 2010). **Overall, the relative risk of RCC in patients with end-stage renal disease has been estimated to be 5- to 20-fold higher than the general population** (Chen et al., 2015a; Farivar-Mohseni et al., 2006). Fifteen percent of patients with RCC in the setting of end-stage renal disease have metastases at the time of presentation, and many such

TABLE 97.11 Screening for Renal Cell Carcinoma: Target Populations

PATIENTS WITH END-STAGE RENAL DISEASE
Screen only patients with long life expectancy and minimal major comorbidities
Periodic ultrasound examination or CT scan beginning during third year on dialysis

PATIENTS WITH KNOWN VON HIPPEL-LINDAU DISEASE
Obtain biannual abdominal CT or ultrasound beginning at the age of 15–20 years
Periodic clinical and radiographic screening for nonrenal manifestations

RELATIVES OF PATIENTS WITH VON HIPPEL-LINDAU DISEASE
Obtain genetic analysis
 If positive, follow screening recommendations for patients with known von Hippel-Lindau disease
 If negative, less stringent follow-up is required

RELATIVES OF PATIENTS WITH OTHER FAMILIAL FORMS OF RENAL CELL CARCINOMA
Obtain periodic ultrasound or CT and consider genetic analysis

PATIENTS WITH TUBEROUS SCLEROSIS
Periodic screening with ultrasound examination or CT scan

PATIENTS WITH AUTOSOMAL DOMINANT POLYCYSTIC KIDNEY DISEASE
Routine screening not justified

GENERAL POPULATION
Routine screening not justified

CT, Computed tomography.

patients die of malignant progression (Hurst et al., 2011; Ishikawa et al., 2010). Given these considerations, screening for RCC is recommended in this population, which is substantial, representing more than 660,000 patients in the United States alone (National Kidney Foundation, 2016). Concerns about screening this population include short life expectancy, increased incidence of adenomas (20% to 40% vs. 10% to 20% in the general population), complexity of imaging given the altered architecture associated with acquired renal cystic disease, and inevitable cost-related issues. **A reasonable compromise for patients with end-stage renal disease is to target those who are still relatively young and without other major comorbidities, to delay screening until the third year on dialysis, and to take into account gender and type of renal replacement therapy, although data about the last factors are admittedly controversial** (Carrizosa and Godley, 2009). Interestingly, renal transplant recipients remain at increased risk for RCC in the native kidneys, with detection in between 1.4% and 2.3% of patients within 3 years of transplantation, leading to a recommendation for continued periodic radiologic screening even after transplantation (Hurst et al., 2010; Ianhez et al., 2007).

An increased incidence of RCC has also been debated in tuberous sclerosis, an autosomal dominant disorder in which patients can develop adenoma sebaceum (a distinctive skin lesion), epilepsy, mental retardation, and renal cysts and AMLs (see Chapter 96; Henske et al., 2016; Lendvay and Marshall, 2003). Many cases of RCC in this syndrome have been characterized by early onset and multifocality, suggesting a genetic predisposition (Lendvay and Marshall, 2003). In addition, the Eker rat, which is mutant for the rodent homolog of the *TSC2* gene responsible for the development of tuberous sclerosis in humans, develops RCC at high frequency, as do *Tsc2*-deficient knockout mice (Lendvay and Marshall, 2003; McDorman and Wolf, 2002). **Such biologic and clinical observations argue in favor of an increased predisposition for RCC in this syndrome, which is consistent with most, although admittedly not all, relevant demographic data** (Schmidt and Linehan, 2016). **A reasonable conclusion is that periodic renal imaging should be pursued in patients with tuberous sclerosis; such a policy will also facilitate follow-up for the development and progression of AML.**

Screening for RCC in autosomal dominant polycystic kidney disease (ADPKD) has been controversial. Imaging is extremely difficult in this population related to the altered intrarenal architecture, and **more recent studies have found no significantly increased risk of RCC in ADPKD** (Gregoire et al., 1987; Hajj et al., 2009; Jilg et al., 2013; Mosetti et al., 2003). The increased incidence of adenomas and other benign lesions in ADPKD also militates against a potential benefit of screening. **Taken together, these considerations suggest that routine screening for RCC in patients with ADPKD should not be pursued.**

Patients with VHL disease (and other hereditary RCC syndromes) should undergo screening for RCC and other syndrome-associated diseases. VHL should be considered in any patient with early onset or multifocal RCC or RCC in combination with any of the following: a history of visual or neurologic disorders; coexistent pancreatic cysts, epididymal lesions, or inner ear tumors; or a family history of blindness, central nervous system tumors, or renal cancer (Kim et al., 2010; Schmidt and Linehan, 2016). **Patients suspected of having VHL disease, or the appropriate relatives of those with documented disease, should strongly consider genetic evaluation. Patients with germline mutations of the *VHL* gene can be identified and offered clinical and radiographic screening that can identify the major manifestations of VHL disease at a presymptomatic phase, allowing potential amelioration of the considerable morbidity associated with this syndrome** (Nielsen et al., 2016; Schmidt and Linehan, 2016). The VHL alliance has recommended that such patients be evaluated with (1) annual physical examination and ophthalmologic evaluation beginning in infancy; (2) annual estimation of plasma or urinary metanephrines beginning at 5 years of age; (3) MRI of the central nervous system biannually beginning at the age of 16 years; (4) ultrasound examination of the abdomen annually beginning at the age of 8 years, with MRI of the abdomen or functional imaging if biochemical abnormalities are found; (5) the addition of MRI abdomen every other year beginning at age 16; and (6) biannual auditory examinations beginning at age 16 (or earlier if hearing loss, tinnitus, or vertigo) (Nielsen et al., 2016; Schmidt and Linehan, 2016; VHL Alliance, 2016). Less intensive protocols have also been advocated, although all relevant organ systems should be addressed (Fraser et al., 2007). Individuals who are found to be wild type for both alleles of *VHL* also benefit because they can be spared much of the expense and anxiety associated with such intensive surveillance protocols.

Genetic counseling and appropriate testing is also available for patients suspected of having hereditary papillary RCC and other familial forms of RCC and should be discussed with appropriate family members (Schmidt and Linehan, 2016). This should include all patients diagnosed with RCC at 46 years of age or less, based on an increased likelihood of germline mutations in this population (Campbell et al., 2017a; Nguyen et al., 2017; Shuch et al., 2014). Individuals at risk, as defined by the presence of mutations of the *c-MET* proto-oncogene or other relevant genetic alterations, and those with suggestive clinical or family histories should be screened for the development of renal lesions with abdominal ultrasonography or CT at periodic intervals. Further testing may be indicated according to the syndrome involved.

Staging

Until the 1990s, the most commonly used staging system for RCC was Robson's, and this schema is still embedded in the mindset of many older urologists (Robson, 1963; Robson et al., 1969). This classification scheme had several limitations, including the grouping of tumors with lymphatic metastases, a very poor prognostic finding, in stage III along with tumors with venous involvement, many of which can be cured with an aggressive surgical approach (Gershman et al., 2017a; Gettman and Blute, 2002; Leibovich et al., 2003; Nguyen and Campbell, 2006). Further imprecision resulted from the fact that the extent of venous involvement was not delineated in this system, and tumor size, an important prognostic parameter, was not incorporated. The tumor, node, and metastasis (TNM) system proposed by the Union International Contre le Cancer (UICC) and endorsed by the American Joint Committee on Cancer (AJCC) represents a major improvement because it defines the anatomic extent of disease more explicitly (Amin et al., 2017; Decastro and McKiernan, 2008; Leung and Ghavamian, 2002; Nguyen and Campbell, 2006).

The recommended staging system for RCC is the eighth edition of the AJCC TNM classification, which was released in 2016 (Table 97.12; Amin et al., 2017). TNM for RCC has undergone several modifications in the past three decades in an effort to more accurately

TABLE 97.12 International TNM Staging System for Renal Cell Carcinoma

T: PRIMARY TUMOR	
TX	Primary tumor cannot be assessed
T0	No evidence of primary tumor
T1a	Tumor ≤ 4.0 cm and confined to the kidney
T1b	Tumor > 4.0 cm and ≤7.0 cm and confined to the kidney
T2a	Tumor > 7.0 cm and ≤10.0 cm and confined to the kidney
T2b	Tumor > 10.0 cm and confined to the kidney
T3a	Tumor extends into the renal vein or its segmental branches, or invades the pelvicalyceal system, or invades perirenal and/or renal sinus fat but not beyond Gerota fascia
T3b	Tumor grossly extends into the vena cava below the diaphragm
T3c	Tumor grossly extends into the vena cava above the diaphragm or invades the wall of the vena cava
T4	Tumor invades beyond Gerota fascia (including contiguous extension into the ipsilateral adrenal gland)
N: REGIONAL LYMPH NODES	
NX	Regional lymph nodes cannot be assessed
N0	No regional lymph nodes metastasis
N1	Metastasis in regional lymph node(s)
M: DISTANT METASTASES	
MX	Distant metastasis cannot be assessed
M0	No distant metastasis
M1	Distant metastasis present

STAGE GROUPING

Stage I	T1	N0	M0
Stage II	T2	N0	M0
Stage III	T1 or T2	N1	M0
	T3	Any N	M0
Stage IV	T4	Any N	M0
	Any T	Any N	M1

Modified from Edge SB, Byrd DR, Compton CC: *AJCC cancer staging manual*, ed 8, New York, 2016, Springer-Verlag.

TABLE 97.13 Tumor, Node, Metastasis (TNM) Stage and 5-Year Cancer-Specific Survival for Renal Cell Carcinoma

FINDINGS	ROBSON STAGE	TNM (6th ed. 2002)	TNM (7th ed. 2009)	TNM (8th ed. 2016)	5-YEAR SURVIVAL (%)
Organ-confined (overall)	I	T1-2N0M0	T1-2N0M0	T1-2N0M0	70–90
≤4.0 cm	I	T1aN0M0	T1aN0M0	T1aN0M0	90–100
>4.0 cm to 7.0 cm	I	T1bN0M0	T1bN0M0	T1bN0M0	80–90
>7.0 to 10.0 cm	I	T2N0M0	T2aN0M0	T2aN0M0	65–80
>10.0 cm	I	T2N0M0	T2bN0M0	T2bN0M0	50–70
Invasion of pelvicalyceal system	I	T1-2N0M0	T1-2N0M0	T3aN0M0	50–70
Invasion of perinephric or renal sinus fat	II	T3aN0M0	T3aN0M0	T3aN0M0	50–70
Extension into renal vein or branches	IIIA	T3bN0M0	T3aN0M0	T3aN0M0	40–60
Extension into IVC below diaphragm	IIIA	T3cN0M0	T3bN0M0	T3bN0M0	30–50
Extension into IVC above diaphragm or invasion of IVC wall	IIIA	T3cN0M0	T3cN0M0	T3cN0M0	20–40
Direct adrenal involvement	II	T3aN0M0	T4N0M0	T4N0M0	0–30
Locally advanced (invasion beyond Gerota fascia)	IVA	T4N0M0	T4N0M0	T4N0M0	0–20
Lymph node involvement	IIIB	T(Any)N1-2M0	T(Any)N1M0	T(Any)N1M0	0–20
Systemic metastasis	IVB	T(Any)N1-2M1	T(Any)N1M1	T(Any)N1M1	0–10

IVC, Inferior vena cava.
Data from Amin MB, Edge SB, Greene FL, et al.: *AJCC cancer staging manual*, ed 8, New York, 2017, Springer; Bailey GC, Boorjian SA, Ziegelmann MJ, et al.: Urinary collecting system invasion is associated with poor survival in patients with clear-cell renal cell carcinoma. *BJU Int* 119(4):585–590, 2017; Campbell SC, Novick AC, Belldegrun A, et al.: Guideline for management of the clinical T1 renal mass. *J Urol* 182(4):1271–1279, 2009; Haddad H, Rini BI: Current treatment considerations in metastatic renal cell carcinoma. *Curr Treat Options Oncol* 13(2):212–229, 2012; Hafez KS, Fergany AF, Novick AC: Nephron sparing surgery for localized renal cell carcinoma: impact of tumor size on patient survival, tumor recurrence and TNM staging. *J Urol* 162(6):1930–1933, 1999; Kim SP, Alt AL, Weight CJ, et al.: Independent validation of the 2010 American Joint Committee on Cancer TNM classification for renal cell carcinoma: results from a large, single institution cohort. *J Urol* 185(6): 2035–2039, 2011; Lane BR, Kattan MW: Prognostic models and algorithms in renal cell carcinoma. *Urol Clin North Am* 35(4): 613–625, 2008; Leibovich BC, Cheville JC, Lohse CM, et al.: Cancer specific survival for patients with pT3 renal cell carcinoma-can the 2002 primary tumor classification be improved? *J Urol* 173(3):716–719, 2005; Martinez-Salamanca JI, Huang WC, Millan I, et al.: Prognostic impact of the 2009 UICC/AJCC TNM staging system for renal cell carcinoma with venous extension. *Eur Urol* 59(1):120–127, 2011; Thompson RH, Cheville JC, Lohse CM, et al.: Reclassification of patients with pT3 and pT4 renal cell carcinoma improves prognostic accuracy. *Cancer* 104(1):53–60, 2005a.

reflect tumor biology and prognosis. It is important to be cognizant of these changes when comparing studies from different eras (Nguyen and Campbell, 2006). For example, in the sixth edition (2002), stage T1 was subdivided to reflect data demonstrating excellent outcomes for patients with small (≤4 cm), unilateral, confined tumors managed by either PN or RN (Igarashi et al., 2001; Nguyen and Campbell, 2006). In the seventh edition (2009), larger (>7 cm) organ-confined tumors were subdivided into stage T2a (>7 to 10 cm) and T2b (>10 cm) (Table 97.13), supported by a number of studies demonstrating prognostic relevance at the 10-cm breakpoint (Edge et al., 2010; Frank et al., 2005; Klatte et al., 2007).

Other major revisions in 2009 included a reclassification of tumors with adrenal metastasis, venous thrombi, and lymphatic involvement, representing a substantial departure from previous staging paradigms for RCC (Edge et al., 2010). **Contiguous extension of tumor into the ipsilateral adrenal gland is classified as T4 and noncontiguous involvement of either adrenal as M1, reflecting likely patterns of dissemination.** The poor prognosis of adrenal involvement from RCC is well documented and supported this important change (Kirkali et al., 2007; Nguyen and Campbell, 2006; Thompson et al., 2005b; von Knobloch et al., 2009). The favorable prognosis of isolated renal vein thrombi prompted a downgrading from stage T3b to stage T3a in the 2009 version (Leibovich et al., 2005; Margulis et al., 2007b; Moinzadeh and Libertino, 2004; Shvarts et al., 2005). Finally, lymphatic metastases, which previously were subdivided based on the number of involved nodes, were compressed to simplify this aspect of the staging process, because prognostic relevance of the previous version was not observed (Amin et al., 2017). **The only change in the eighth edition (2016) relates to stage pT3a, which now includes invasion of the pelvicalyceal system, based on multiple reports indicating this finding has independent prognostic significance in RCC** (Amin et al., 2017; Bertini et al., 2009; Moch et al., 2009). Continued re-evaluation and validation of the TNM system for RCC has optimized its value to patients and clinicians (Anderson et al., 2011; Bailey et al., 2017; Bhindi et al., 2017; Brookman-May et al., 2011; Chen et al., 2016; Jeon et al., 2009; Kim et al., 2011; May et al., 2017; Verhoest et al., 2009).

TNM staging classically is defined by the most advanced feature demonstrated by the tumor, yet important prognostic information can be lost in the process. Many renal tumors exhibit multiple adverse findings, such as high-level tumor thrombus along with ipsilateral adrenal involvement. Ideally all of the relevant anatomic staging information would be captured, at least parenthetically (e.g., "pT4 [ipsilateral adrenal involvement; also exhibiting IVC thrombus above the diaphragm]"). Future staging systems will need to capture all of this information, because several studies have confirmed a compromised prognosis for patients with multiple adverse factors (Brookman-May et al., 2015; Chen et al., 2016; Ficarra et al., 2007; Leibovich et al., 2005; Shvarts et al., 2005; Terrone et al., 2006).

The clinical staging of renal malignant disease begins with a thorough history, physical examination, and judicious use of laboratory tests (Decastro and McKiernan, 2008; Nguyen and Campbell, 2006). Systemic symptoms such as significant unintended weight loss (>10% of body weight), cachexia, or poor performance status at presentation suggest advanced disease, as do physical examination findings of a palpable mass or lymphadenopathy. A nonreducing varicocele and lower extremity edema suggest venous involvement. Significant anemia, hypercalcemia, abnormal liver function parameters or sedimentation rate, or elevated serum alkaline phosphatase or lactate dehydrogenase level point to the probability of advanced disease (Lane and Kattan, 2008; Nguyen and Campbell, 2006).

The radiographic staging of RCC can be accomplished in most cases with a high-quality abdominal CT scan and a routine chest radiograph, with selective use of MRI and other studies as indicated

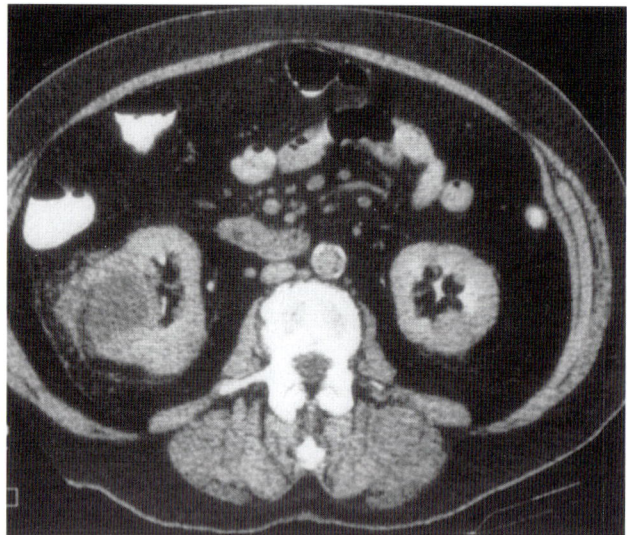

Fig. 97.13. Computed tomography scan after administration of contrast agent shows right renal tumor with perinephric stranding suggesting invasion of the perinephric fat.

(Campbell et al., 2017a; Choyke et al., 2001; Diaz de Leon and Pedrosa, 2017; Herts, 2009; Ng et al., 2008). MRI can be reserved primarily for patients with locally advanced malignant disease, equivocal venous involvement, or allergy to intravenous contrast material (Choyke et al., 2001; Herts, 2009; Zhang et al., 2007). CT findings suggestive of extension into the perinephric fat include perinephric stranding (Fig. 97.13), which is a nonspecific finding, or a distinct, enhancing soft tissue density within the perinephric space, which is a more definitive but uncommon finding (Bechtold and Zagoria, 1997; Herts, 2009). Overall, the accuracy of CT or MRI for detection of involvement of the perinephric fat is low, reflecting the fact that extracapsular spread often occurs microscopically (Choyke et al., 2001; Kamel et al., 2004; Zhang et al., 2007). Ipsilateral adrenal involvement can be assessed with reasonable accuracy through a combination of preoperative CT and intraoperative inspection. Patients with an enlarged or indistinct adrenal gland on CT, extensive malignant replacement of the kidney, or a palpably abnormal adrenal gland are at risk for malignant adrenal involvement and should be managed accordingly (Campbell et al., 2017a; Kobayashi et al., 2008; Lane et al., 2009c; Ng et al., 2008; Paul et al., 2001; Sawai et al., 2002; Weight et al., 2011; Zhang et al., 2007).

Enlarged hilar or retroperitoneal lymph nodes (2 cm or more in diameter) on CT almost always harbor malignant change, but this should be confirmed by surgical exploration or percutaneous biopsy if the patient is not a surgical candidate. Many smaller lymph nodes prove to be inflammatory rather than neoplastic and should not preclude surgical therapy (Campbell et al., 2017a; Choyke et al., 2001; Gershman et al., 2017a; Herts, 2009; Israel and Bosniak, 2003; Ng et al., 2008). MRI can add specificity to the evaluation of retroperitoneal nodes by distinguishing vascular structures, such as lumbar veins, from lymphatic ones (Bassignani, 2006). **MRI is still the premier study for evaluation of invasion of tumor into adjacent structures and for surgical planning in these challenging cases** (Choyke et al., 2001; Diaz de Leon and Pedrosa, 2017; Herts, 2009; Pretorius et al., 2000). Obliteration of the fat plane between the tumor and adjacent organs (e.g., the liver) on CT can be a misleading finding for RCC and should prompt further imaging with MRI. In reality, surgical exploration is often required to make an absolute differentiation.

The sensitivities of CT for detection of renal venous tumor thrombus and IVC involvement are 78% and 96%, respectively (Herts, 2009; Ng et al., 2008). CT findings suggestive of venous involvement include venous enlargement, abrupt change in the caliber of the vein, and filling defects, and the diagnosis is strengthened by demonstration of collateral vessels. Most false-negative findings occur in patients with right-sided tumors in whom the short length of the vein and the mass effect from the tumor combine to make detection of the tumor thrombus difficult (Herts, 2009). Fortunately, most such cases are readily identified and dealt with intraoperatively. **MRI is well established as the premier study for the evaluation and staging of IVC tumor thrombus, although several studies suggest that multiplanar CT is likely equivalent in many patients** (Aslam Sohaib et al., 2002; Diaz de Leon and Pedrosa, 2017; Ng et al., 2008; Pretorius et al., 2000; Zhang et al., 2007). Venacavography is now best reserved for patients with equivocal MRI or CT findings or for patients who cannot tolerate or have other contraindications to cross-sectional imaging. Transesophageal echocardiography also appears to be accurate for establishing the cephalad extent of the tumor thrombus, but it is invasive and provides no distinct advantages over MRI or CT in the preoperative setting (Glazer and Novick, 1997).

Metastatic evaluation in all cases should include a routine chest radiograph, systematic review of the abdominal and pelvic CT or MRI, and liver function tests (Campbell et al., 2017a; Griffin et al., 2007; Herts, 2009; Ng et al., 2008). **Bone scintiscan can be reserved for patients with elevated serum alkaline phosphatase, bone pain, or poor performance status** (Campbell et al., 2017a; Shvarts et al., 2004) **and chest CT scan for patients with pulmonary symptoms or an abnormal chest radiograph** (Campbell et al., 2017a; Choyke et al., 2001). **Patients with locally advanced disease, enlarged retroperitoneal lymph nodes, or significant comorbid disease may mandate more thorough imaging to rule out metastatic disease and to aid in treatment planning** (Campbell et al., 2017a; Choyke et al., 2001; Griffin et al., 2007). Positron emission tomography (PET) has also been investigated for patients with high risk of metastatic RCC, with most studies showing good specificity, but suboptimal sensitivity (Bagheri et al., 2017). At present, its best role is for select patients with equivocal findings on conventional imaging, as an abnormal PET scan may increase the concern about metastatic disease (Bouchelouche and Oehr, 2008; Griffin et al., 2007; Powles et al., 2007). Molecular imaging, using ^{99m}Tc-sestamibi SPECT/CT to distinguish renal oncocytoma and hybrid oncocytic/chromophobe tumors from clear cell RCC or PET imaging with either ^{124}I-girentuximab or prostate-specific membrane antigen (PSMA), is a promising technique that is still under evaluation (Divgi et al., 2013; Gorin et al., 2016; Rowe et al., 2015). **Biopsy of the primary tumor and/or potential metastatic sites is also selectively required as part of the staging process.**

> **KEY POINTS: STAGING AND PROGNOSIS OF RENAL CELL CARCINOMA**
>
> - The TNM staging system has replaced the Robson system (stage I to IV).
> - Tumor (T) stage is based on size and extension of the cancer into renal or extrarenal structures.
> - Pathologic stage is the most important prognostic factor for RCC.
> - Invasion of neighboring organs (T4), involvement of retroperitoneal lymph nodes (N1), and the presence of metastatic disease (M1) confer a poor outcome for patients with RCC.
> - Other important pathologic features include nuclear grade, tumor size, and histologic subtype.
> - Important prognostic factors for cancer-specific survival in patients with RCC include specific clinical signs or symptoms, tumor-related factors, and various laboratory findings.
> - Integrated systems, such as nomograms, often outperform other prediction methods.

Prognosis

Important prognostic factors for cancer-specific survival in patients with nonmetastatic RCC include specific clinical signs or symptoms,

TABLE 97.14 Adverse Prognostic Factors for Renal Cell Carcinoma

CLINICAL	ANATOMIC	HISTOLOGIC
Poor performance status	Larger tumor size	High nuclear grade
Systemic symptoms	Venous involvement	Certain histologic subtypes
Anemia	Extension into contiguous organs, including adrenal gland	Sarcomatoid features
Hypercalcemia		Presence of histologic tumor necrosis
Elevated lactate dehydrogenase	Lymph node metastases	Vascular invasion
Elevated erythrocyte sedimentation rate	Distant metastases and greater metastatic burden	Invasion of perinephric or renal sinus fat
Elevated C-reactive protein		Collecting system invasion
Thrombocytosis		Positive surgical margin
Elevated alkaline phosphatase		

Data from Lane BR, Kattan MW: Prognostic models and algorithms in renal cell carcinoma. *Urol Clin North Am* 35(4):613–625, 2008; Sun M, Vetterlein M, Harshman LC, et al.: Risk assessment in small renal masses: a review article. *Urol Clin North Am* 44(2):189–202, 2017.

tumor-related factors, and various laboratory findings (Table 97.14) (Lane and Kattan, 2008; Meskawi et al., 2012; Sun et al., 2017). Overall, tumor-related factors such as pathologic stage, tumor size, nuclear grade, and histologic subtype have the greatest individual predictive ability. However, an integrative approach, combining a variety of factors that have independent value on multivariate analysis, appears to be most powerful (Campbell and Lane, 2016; Meskawi et al., 2012). Patient-related factors such as age, presence of chronic kidney disease, and comorbidities have a significant impact on overall survival and should be a primary consideration during treatment planning for patients with localized RCC (Campbell et al., 2017a; Hollingsworth et al., 2006; Kutikov et al., 2010).

Clinical findings that suggest a compromised prognosis in patients with presumed localized RCC include symptomatic presentation, unintended weight loss of more than 10% of body weight, and poor performance status (Lane and Kattan, 2008; Sun et al., 2017). Anemia, thrombocytosis, hypercalcemia, albuminuria, elevated serum alkaline phosphatase, C-reactive protein, lactate dehydrogenase, or erythrocyte sedimentation rate, as well as other paraneoplastic signs or symptoms, have also correlated with poor outcomes for patients with RCC (Lane and Kattan, 2008; Magera et al., 2008b; Sun et al., 2017). Although abnormal values are more common in patients with advanced RCC, some of these abnormalities, including hypercalcemia, anemia, and elevated erythrocyte sedimentation rate, were independent predictors of cancer-specific mortality in patients with localized clear cell RCC as well (Magera et al., 2008b).

Pathologic stage has proved to be the single most important prognostic factor for RCC (Kanao et al., 2009; Lane and Kattan, 2008; Leibovich et al., 2005; Sun et al., 2017). The RCC TNM staging system clearly distinguishes between patient groups with different predicted cancer-specific outcomes (see Table 97.13), confirming that the extent of locoregional or systemic disease at diagnosis is the primary determinant of outcomes for this disease. Several studies demonstrate 5-year survival rates of 70% to 90% for organ-confined disease and document a 10% to 15% reduction in survival associated with invasion of the perinephric fat (Lane and Kattan, 2008; Sun et al., 2017). Renal sinus involvement is classified along with perinephric fat invasion as T3a, and several studies suggest that these patients may be at even higher risk for metastasis related to increased access to the venous system (Amin et al., 2017; Bertini et al., 2009; Bonsib et al., 2000; Jeon et al., 2009; Thompson et al., 2005b). Collecting system invasion has also been shown to confer poorer prognosis in otherwise organ-confined RCC and is now incorporated into the T3a category (Amin et al., 2017; Anderson et al., 2011; Chen et al., 2016; Uzzo et al., 2002; Verhoest et al., 2009). Several reports have shown that most patients with contiguous ipsilateral adrenal involvement or noncontiguous adrenal metastasis, which are found in 1% to 2% of cases, eventually succumb to systemic disease progression, suggesting a hematogenous route of dissemination and/or highly invasive phenotype (Sagalowsky et al., 1994; von Knobloch et al., 2009).

Venous involvement was once thought to be a very poor prognostic finding for RCC, but several reports demonstrate that many patients with tumor thrombi can be salvaged with an aggressive surgical approach. These studies document 45% to 69% 5-year survival rates for patients with venous tumor thrombi as long as the cancer is otherwise confined to the kidney (Martinez-Salamanca et al., 2011). Patients with venous tumor thrombi and concomitant lymph node or systemic metastases have markedly decreased survival, and those with tumor extending into the perinephric fat have intermediate survival (Martinez-Salamanca et al., 2011). The most recent versions of the TNM system advocate capturing all such adverse features during the staging process. Some studies suggest that patients with microvascular invasion may have compromised outcomes compared with matched tumors without these features, indicating that even microscopic venous or lymphatic involvement may be a poor prognostic sign (Amin et al., 2017; Feifer et al., 2011; Kroeger et al., 2012).

The prognostic significance of the cephalad extent of tumor thrombus has been controversial, and it is difficult to compare various series because of selection biases and related covariables (Blute et al., 2007; Haddad et al., 2014; Leibovich et al., 2005; Libertino et al., 1987; Wotkowicz et al., 2008). In several series, the incidence of advanced locoregional or systemic disease increased with the cephalad extent of the tumor thrombus, likely contributing to the reduced survival associated with tumor thrombus extending into or above the level of the hepatic veins (Wotkowicz et al., 2008). **Direct invasion of the wall of the vein appears to be a more important prognostic factor than level of tumor thrombus and is now classified as pT3c independent of the level of tumor thrombus** (Hatcher et al., 1991; Zini et al., 2008).

The major drop in prognosis comes in patients whose tumor extends beyond the Gerota fascia to involve contiguous organs (stage T4) and in patients with lymph node or systemic metastases (Amin et al., 2017; Margulis et al., 2007a; Thompson et al., 2005b). **Lymph node involvement is associated with 5- and 10-year survival rates of 5% to 30% and 0 to 5%, respectively** (Crispen et al., 2011; Gershman et al., 2017a; Haddad and Rini, 2012; Lohse et al., 2015; Phillips and Taneja, 2004; Rijnders et al., 2017; Zibelman and Plimack, 2017). **Systemic metastases also portend a particularly poor prognosis for RCC, traditionally with 1-year survival of less than 50%, 5-year survival of 5% to 30%, and 10-year survival of 0% to 5%, although these numbers have improved modestly in the era of VEGF-targeted treatments and checkpoint inhibitors** (Haddad and Rini, 2012; Lohse et al., 2015; Rijnders et al., 2017; Zibelman and Plimack, 2017). Patients presenting with synchronous metastases fare worse, with many patients dying of disease progression within 1 to 2 years (Haddad and Rini, 2012; Heng et al., 2013; Leibovich et al., 2003; Mekhail et al., 2005). **For patients with asynchronous metastases, the metastasis-free interval can be a useful prognosticator because it often reflects the tempo of disease progression** (Maldazys and deKernion, 1986; Mekhail et al., 2005; Motzer et al.,

2004). Other important prognostic factors for patients with systemic metastases include performance status, number and sites of metastases, anemia, hypercalcemia, elevated alkaline phosphatase or lactate dehydrogenase levels, thrombocytosis, and sarcomatoid histology (Heng et al., 2013; Lane and Kattan, 2008). **The presence of bone, brain, and/or liver metastases and multiple metastatic sites have been associated with further compromise in prognosis** (Escudier et al., 2007a; McKay et al., 2014; Mekhail et al., 2005). These factors have been used to effectively categorize patients with metastatic RCC as low, intermediate, and poor risk, with corresponding differences in median survival with systemic therapy (see Chapter 104; Heng et al., 2013; Motzer et al., 2004).

Another significant prognostic factor for RCC is tumor size, which has proved to be an independent prognostic factor for organ-confined and invasive RCC (Amin et al., 2017; Kattan et al., 2001; Kontak and Campbell, 2003; Lane and Kattan, 2008). To a large extent, this is due to a strong correlation between tumor size and pathologic tumor stage, but several studies have demonstrated that tumor size can function as an independent prognostic factor (Crispen et al., 2008; Kattan et al., 2001; Nguyen and Gill, 2009; Sorbellini et al., 2005). Larger tumors are more likely to exhibit clear cell histology and high nuclear grade, and both of these factors correlate with a compromised prognosis (Frank et al., 2003; Lane et al., 2007a; Thompson et al., 2009b). A review of 1771 patients with organ-confined RCC showed 10-year cancer-specific survival rates of 90% to 95%, 80% to 85%, and 75% for patients with pT1a, pT1b, and pT2 tumor, respectively (Patard et al., 2004a). Many other studies have also shown a particularly favorable prognosis for the unilateral pT1a tumors that are now being discovered with increased frequency. In series from the Cleveland Clinic and the Mayo Clinic, such tumors were associated with greater than 95% 5-year cancer-specific survival rates, whether they were managed with nephron-sparing surgery or RN (Butler et al., 1995; Cheville et al., 2001; Lane et al., 2013).

Other important prognostic factors for RCC include nuclear grade and histologic subtype. Almost all the proposed grading systems for RCC have provided prognostic information, and nuclear grade is established as an independent prognostic factor when subjected to multivariable analysis, at least for clear cell and papillary RCC (Ficarra et al., 2009a; Fuhrman et al., 1982; Lane and Kattan, 2008; 2005; Lohse and Cheville, 2005; Lohse et al., 2002; May et al., 2017; True, 2002; Zisman et al., 2001). For a variety of reasons the Fuhrman's classification system has fallen out of favor, and an alternate grading system based on nucleolar morphology is now recommended (see Pathology and Table 97.8; Delahunt et al., 2014).

Histologic subtype of RCC also carries prognostic significance. The presence of sarcomatoid or rhabdoid differentiation or collecting duct, renal medullary, or unclassified histologic subtype denotes a poor prognosis (Deng and Melamed, 2012; Kara et al., 2016; Wei and Al-Saleem, 2017; Zhou, 2009). Several studies suggest that clear cell RCC may have a worse prognosis on average compared with papillary type 1 or chromophobe RCC, although there are clearly poorly differentiated tumors in each of these subcategories that can be lethal (Deng and Melamed, 2012; Leibovich et al., 2010; Lohse et al., 2015; Teloken et al., 2009). Finally, several subtypes of RCC are predictably indolent, including multiloculated cystic clear cell RCC, mucinous tubular and spindle cell carcinoma, and clear cell/papillary RCC.

A variety of molecular factors have correlated with outcomes for RCC in observational studies and may prove to be useful in the future (Jonasch et al., 2012; Keefe et al., 2013). Increased proliferative index as assessed by Ki-67 has correlated with reduced survival in clear cell RCC (Parker et al., 2009). Other factors that may be useful include cell cycle regulators, such as the tumor suppressor gene *p53*, various growth factors and their receptors, including members of the VEGF family, adhesion molecules, and other factors, such as survivin (Campbell and Lane, 2016; Klatte et al., 2009; Parker et al., 2009). Aggressive renal cancers demonstrate downregulation of genes involved in the TCA cycle and upregulation of the pentose phosphate pathway (Cancer Genome Atlas Research Network, 2013). In general, clinical validation has not yet been achieved with any of these factors and they remain primarily investigational (see Tumor Biology and Clinical Implications, and reviewed in Campbell and Lane, 2016).

Several investigators have developed tools that integrate clinical and pathologic factors, improving the predictive capacity for patients with RCC. Incorporation of the strongest predictors into a nomogram is one way to provide an individual assessment of risk that clinicians can use during patient counseling. Kattan et al. (2001) developed the first of these for RCC, and several nomograms have been introduced subsequent to this (Campbell and Lane, 2016; Kattan et al., 2001). One such nomogram incorporating stage, size, grade, and symptoms at presentation has been validated using multi-institutional data sets and appears to outperform several of the other existing prognostic tools for localized RCC (Karakiewicz et al., 2007a; Sun et al., 2017).

Two other integrated staging systems that have been used to risk stratify patients for clinical trials are the UCLA Integrated Staging System (UISS) and the Mayo Clinic Stage, Size, Grade, and Necrosis (SSIGN) score. The UISS was developed based on multivariate analysis revealing three independent prognostic factors for RCC, namely TNM stage, performance status, and tumor grade (Zisman et al., 2001). The UISS was subsequently modified to stratify patients with localized or metastatic disease into cohorts with low, intermediate, or high risk of disease progression and has been validated internally and externally (Cindolo et al., 2008; Parker et al., 2009; Patard et al., 2004b; Tan et al., 2010; Zisman et al., 2002). **The SSIGN score can be used to estimate cancer-specific survival based on TNM stage, tumor size, nuclear grade, and presence of histologic tumor necrosis** (Frank et al., 2002). The SSIGN score has been validated in multiple data sets, but the inclusion of histologic necrosis as a predictor limits its clinical usefulness (Ficarra et al., 2006, 2009a; Fujii et al., 2008; Parker et al., 2017; Zigeuner et al., 2010).

TNM staging systems and prognostic algorithms have different purposes. The TNM staging system is used to provide a universal language for communication between clinicians and patients and is based solely on the anatomic extent of cancer dissemination. **A wealth of literature now supports the notion that algorithms that incorporate multiple predictive elements, such as nomograms and artificial neural networks, outperform risk assessment based on expert opinion or simpler models, such as classic staging systems** (Isbarn and Karakiewicz, 2009; Ross et al., 2002; Shariat et al., 2009; Sun et al., 2017). The development and use of these integrated staging systems can help guide counseling and follow-up of patients with RCC and identify patients more likely to benefit from specific interventions, such as adjuvant treatments.

TREATMENT OF LOCALIZED RENAL CELL CARCINOMA

Localized renal masses have increased in incidence because of widespread use of cross-sectional imaging and now represent a relatively common clinical scenario (Capitanio and Montorsi, 2016; Miller et al., 2010a; Turner et al., 2017). Our perspectives about clinical T1 renal masses have changed substantially in the past two decades. Previously, all were presumed malignant and managed aggressively, mostly with RN. **We now recognize great heterogeneity in the tumor biology of these lesions, and multiple management strategies are available, including RN, PN, thermal ablation (TA), and active surveillance (AS)** (Campbell et al., 2017a; Kunkle et al., 2008; Volpe et al., 2011). Concepts that were once controversial, such as elective PN, are now accepted as standards of care. A greater understanding of the tumor biology and appreciation of the merits and limitations of the various management strategies has facilitated improved management of this patient population (Campbell et al., 2017a; Finelli et al., 2017; Ljungberg et al., 2015; Motzer et al., 2017b).

American Urological Association Guidelines for Renal Mass and Localized Renal Cancer

The 2017 American Urological Association (AUA) Guidelines for Renal Mass and Localized Renal Cancer provide an evidence-based review of this topic, along with comprehensive recommendations

Renal Mass and Localized Renal Cancer[1]

Evaluation/Diagnosis
1. Obtain high quality, multiphase, cross-sectional abdominal imaging to optimally characterize/stage the renal mass.
2. Obtain CMP, CBC, and UA. If malignancy suspected, metastatic evaluation should include chest imaging and careful review of abdominal imaging.
3. Assign CKD stage based on GFR and degree of proteinuria.

Counseling
1. A urologist should lead the counseling process and should consider all management strategies. A multidisciplinary team should be included when necessary.
2. Counseling should include current perspectives about tumor biology and a patient-specific oncologic risk assessment. For cT1a tumors, the low oncologic risk of many small renal masses should be reviewed.
3. Counseling should review the most common and serious urologic and non-urologic morbidities of each treatment pathway and the importance of patient age, comorbidities/frailty, and life expectancy.
4. Physicians should review the importance of renal functional recovery related to renal mass management, including risk of progressive CKD, potential short/long-term need for dialysis, and long-term overall survival considerations.
5. Consider referral to nephrology in patients with a high risk of CKD progression, including those with GFR < 45[2], confirmed proteinuria, diabetics with preexisting CKD, or whenever GFR is expected to be < 30[2] after intervention.
6. Recommend genetic counseling for all patients ≤ 46 years of age and consider genetic counseling for patients with multifocal or bilateral renal masses, or if personal/family history suggests a familial renal neoplastic syndrome.

Renal Mass Biopsy (RMB)
1. RMB should be considered when a mass is suspected to be hematologic, metastatic, inflammatory, or infectious.
2. RMB is not required for: 1) young/healthy patients who are unwilling to accept the uncertainties associated with RMB; or 2) older/frail patients who will be managed conservatively independent of RMB.
3. Counsel regarding rationale, positive/negative predictive values, potential risks and non-diagnostic rates of RMB.
4. Multiple core biopsies are preferred over FNA.

Management

Partial Nephrectomy (PN) and Nephron-Sparing Approaches
1. Prioritize PN for the management of the cT1a renal mass when intervention is indicated.
2. Prioritize nephron-sparing approaches for patients with an anatomic or functionally solitary kidney, bilateral tumors, known familial RCC, preexisting CKD, or proteinuria.
3. Consider nephron-sparing approaches for patients who are young, have multifocal masses, or comorbidities that are likely to impact renal function in the future.

Radical Nephrectomy (RN)
1. Physicians should consider RN for patients where increased oncologic potential is suggested by tumor size, RMB, and/or imaging characteristics. In this setting, RN is preferred if all of the following criteria are met:
1) high tumor complexity and PN would be challenging even in experienced hands;
2) no preexisting CKD/proteinuria; and
3) normal contralateral kidney and new baseline eGFR will likely be > 45[2].

Thermal Ablation (TA)
1. Consider TA an alternate approach for management of cT1a renal masses <3 cm in size. A percutaneous approach is preferred.
2. Both radiofrequency ablation and cryoablation are options.
3. A RMB should be performed prior to TA.
4. Counseling about TA should include information regarding increased likelihood of tumor persistence/recurrence after primary TA, which may be addressed with repeat TA if further intervention is elected.

Active Surveillance (AS)
1. For patients with renal masses suspicious for cancer, especially those <2cm, AS is an option for initial management.
2. Prioritize AS/Expectant Management when the anticipated risk of intervention or competing risks of death outweigh the potential oncologic benefits of active treatment.
3. When the risk/benefit analysis for treatment is equivocal and the patient prefers AS, physicians should repeat imaging in 3-6 months to assess for interval growth and may consider RMB for additional risk stratification.
4. When the oncologic benefits of intervention outweigh the risks of treatment and competing risks of death, physicians should recommend active treatment. In this setting, AS may be pursued only if the patient understands and is willing to accept the associated oncologic risk

Principles Related to PN
1. Prioritize preservation of renal function through efforts to optimize nephron mass preservation and avoidance of prolonged warm ischemia.
2. Negative surgical margins should be a priority. The extent of normal parenchyma removed should be determined by surgeon discretion taking into account the clinical situation; tumor characteristics including growth pattern, and interface with normal tissue. Enucleation should be considered in patients with familial RCC, multifocal disease, or severe CKD to optimize parenchymal mass preservation.

Surgical Principles
1. In the presence of clinically concerning regional lymphadenopathy, lymph node dissection should be performed for staging purposes.
2. Adrenalectomy should be performed if imaging and/or intraoperative findings suggest metastasis or direct invasion.
3. A minimally invasive approach should be considered when it would not compromise oncologic, functional and perioperative outcomes.
4. Pathologic evaluation of the adjacent renal parenchyma should be performed after PN or RN to assess for possible nephrologic disease, particularly for patients with CKD or risk factors for developing CKD.

Factors Favoring AS/Expectant Management

Patient-related	Tumor-related
Elderly	Tumor size <3cm
Life expectancy <5 years	Tumor growth <5mm/year
High comorbidities	Non-infiltrative
Excessive perioperative risk	Low complexity
Frailty (poor functional status)	Favorable histology
Patient preference for AS	
Marginal renal function	

1. Focus is on clinically localized renal masses suspicious for RCC in adults, including solid enhanced tumors and Bosniak 3 and 4 complex cystic lesions. 2. ml/min/1.73m².

Fig. 97.14. Algorithm for evaluation, counseling, and management of patients presenting with a renal mass or localized renal cancer. (From Campbell SC, Uzzo RG, Allaf ME, et al.: Renal mass and localized renal cancer: AUA Guideline, 2017 [website]: https://www.auanet.org/guidelines/renal-mass-and-localized-renal-cancer-new-2017.)

for evaluation, counseling, and management (Fig. 97.14; Campbell et al., 2017a). Novel elements in the guidelines include forsaking the use of index patients based on strong consensus that there are a multitude of factors to take into consideration when evaluating a patient's general health, the oncologic potential of the mass, and important functional issues. Simply put, there are just too many gray zones within each of these vitally important assessments to justify the ongoing use of index patients (Campbell et al., 2017a).

Another major change relates to **increased focus on functional issues, preoperatively and postoperatively, recognizing their importance for cancer survivorship for many patients with localized RCC** (Campbell et al., 2017a; Zabell et al., 2017a). Evaluation should include a serum creatinine-based estimation of glomerular filtration rate (GFR) and assessment for proteinuria, and CKD stage at presentation should be assigned based on these parameters. Presence of proteinuria and reduced baseline GFR have both proven to be strong and independent predictors of functional stability and survival for kidney cancer patients, similar to the general population. Referral to nephrology should be considered in patients at high risk for CKD progression, including those who present with GFR of less than 45 mL/min/1.73 m² or confirmed proteinuria (Tourojman et al., 2016), patients with diabetes and preexisting CKD, or whenever the GFR is expected to be less than 30 mL/min/1.73 m² after intervention.

Other important considerations for the evaluation and counseling of this patient population are summarized in Fig. 97.14. The AUA Guidelines also provide well-defined indications for RN versus PN, updated recommendations for use of TA, and objective criteria related to intelligent use of AS, as outlined in the following sections (Campbell et al., 2017b; Pierorazio et al., 2016a). Many of these perspectives are also supported by other Guidelines from the American Society of Clinical Oncology, European Association of Urology, and National Comprehensive Cancer Network (Finelli et al., 2017; Ljungberg et al., 2015; Motzer et al., 2017b).

Risk Stratification and Renal Mass Biopsy

Overall, about 20% of solid, enhancing, clinical T1 renal masses are benign, most often oncocytomas or atypical AMLs, although the incidence of benign pathology can vary greatly in different populations (Campbell et al., 2017a; Frank et al., 2003; Gill et al., 2010). Young to middle-age women, in particular, are more likely to have benign pathology, as high as 40% in some series (Eggener et al., 2004). One potential explanation is that some benign renal masses, such as cystic nephroma and atypical AML, may be influenced by the hormonal milieu. An even more important determinant of benign pathology is tumor size, with multiple studies confirming this (Campbell et al., 2017b). In the series from Frank et al. (2003), 30% of tumors less than 2 cm were benign, whereas only 9.5% of clinical T1b tumors were benign (reviewed in Johnson et al., 2015). **Tumor size also correlates strongly with biologic aggressiveness for clinical T1 renal masses, as reflected by high tumor grade, locally invasive phenotype, or unfavorable histology.** In Frank's series, such adverse findings were uncommon in tumors less than 4 cm diameter: only 1.7% demonstrated invasion of the perinephric fat, 0.7% had venous involvement, 0.6% had lymph node involvement, and only 15% were high grade. Adverse features such as this were more commonly observed in clinical T1b tumors. Surveillance studies confirm a slow growth rate and low risk of metastasis for many small renal tumors (Bosniak, 1995; Campbell et al., 2017b; Kunkle et al., 2007, 2008).

A recent systematic review indicated that tumor size and male sex were the strongest predictors of malignant pathology. In contrast, the results were inconclusive or not significant for other tumor characteristics, age, body mass index, and incidental presentation (Lane et al., 2007a; Pierorazio et al., 2016). **Current algorithms incorporating clinical and radiographic factors to predict tumor aggressiveness for small renal tumors are very limited in their accuracy, with concordance indices less than 0.65, not much better than a coin flip** (Kutikov et al., 2011; Lane et al., 2007a; Patel et al., 2016a).

Renal mass biopsy (RMB) can substantially improve on this and should be considered for further risk stratification when it may influence management (see Fig. 97.14) (Ginzburg et al., 2014; Haifler and Kutikov, 2017; Jeon et al., 2016; Marconi et al., 2016; Patel et al., 2016b). Recent meta-analyses suggest that RMB is generally safe and accurate (Campbell et al., 2017b; Patel et al., 2016b).

> **KEY POINTS: RENAL MASS BIOPSY**
> - RMB is safe with relatively low rates of hematoma (4.9%), clinically significant pain (1.2%), gross hematuria (1.0%), pneumothorax (0.6%), and hemorrhage requiring transfusion (0.4%).
> - There have been *no* reported cases of RCC tumor seeding in the contemporary literature.
> - A positive biopsy is reliable with high specificity (96%) and positive predictive value (99.8%).
> - The nondiagnostic rate for RMB is approximately 14%, which can be substantially reduced with repeat biopsy.
> - Histologic evaluation of RCC subtype is dependable (>90%), but accuracy for grade is variable (60%–80%).
> - A nonmalignant biopsy result may *not* truly indicate that a benign entity is present.

The downsides of RMB are that it can be nondiagnostic in about 14% of cases, some series have reported occasional false-negative results, and cystic tumors may be at risk for tumor spillage. The AUA Guidelines emphasize the importance of counseling patients about the potential merits and limitations of RMB, and advocates for a utility-based approach (Campbell et al., 2017a; Patel et al., 2016b). **RMB is *not* indicated for young, healthy patients who are unwilling to accept the limitations of RMB, or for older, frail patients who will be managed conservatively even if RMB suggests a potentially aggressive tumor.** Increased use of RMB has been documented over the past decade, and some have advocated for office-based ultrasound-guided RMB, which can be performed by the urologist (Okhunov et al., 2017). **Molecular profiling of RMB samples will also likely play an increasing role in the near future** (Fig. 97.15), analogous to the evaluation of patients with early stage prostate cancer.

Molecular imaging also holds great promise as a noninvasive approach to risk stratification of renal masses (Gorin et al., 2015). PET coupled with administration of radioactively labeled anticarbonic anhydrase-IX monoclonal antibody can provide specificity for the more aggressive subtypes of renal cancer, including clear cell RCC and type 2 papillary RCC (Divgi et al., 2013; Muselaers et al., 2013). Recent studies suggest that sestamibi-based SPECT/CT imaging may allow for identification of benign or less aggressive variants or RCC, such as oncocytomas or hybrid oncocytic/chromophobe tumors (Gorin et al., 2015).

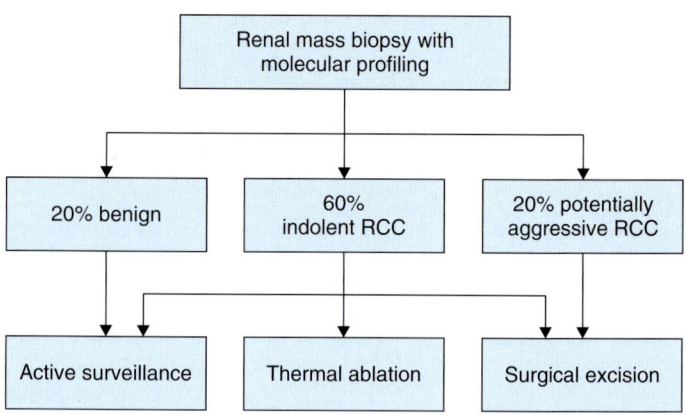

Fig. 97.15. The American Urological Association guideline panel for the management of renal mass and localized renal cancer strongly advocates research priority for renal mass biopsy with molecular profiling to facilitate more rational management. The distribution of benign, indolent, and potentially aggressive RCC can vary based on tumor size, gender, and other patient and tumor characteristics. *RCC,* Renal cell carcinoma.

Renal Function After Partial or Radical Nephrectomy: Survival Implications

Notwithstanding advances in our understanding of the genetics and biology of RCC, **surgery remains the mainstay for curative treatment of this disease.** Simple nephrectomy was practiced for many decades but was supplanted by RN when Robson et al. (1969) established this procedure as the gold standard for the management of localized RCC. RN is still preferred for many patients with localized RCC, such as those with very large tumors, and it should remain a consideration whenever increased oncologic risk is suspected (see Fig. 97.14) (Robson et al., 1969; Tomaszewski et al., 2014). **RN has fallen out of favor for small renal tumors because of concerns about CKD and should only be performed when necessary in this population** (Campbell et al., 2017a; Finelli et al., 2017; Ljungberg et al., 2015; Motzer et al., 2017b).

The main downside of RN is that it predisposes to CKD, which can be associated with morbid cardiovascular events and increased mortality rates. Several studies have shown an increased risk of CKD on longitudinal follow-up after RN, including a landmark study that looked at 662 patients with a solitary tumor, a normal opposite kidney, and a "normal" serum creatinine level—essentially patients who would be considered for elective PN (Huang et al., 2006; Mashni et al., 2015). Huang et al. (2006) found that 26% of such patients had preexisting CKD (GFR <60 mL/min/1.73 m^2), demonstrating that kidney cancer patients are substantially different than the kidney transplant donor population that is often considered analogous. In reality, the donor population is not comparable because it is carefully screened to exclude CKD and related comorbidities. Huang also reported that CKD was much more common after RN than PN: 65% versus 20%, respectively ($P < 0.001$).

Several studies illustrate the potential negative implications of CKD, including a population-based analysis that reported **increased rates of cardiovascular events and death as the degree of CKD worsened,** even after controlling for diabetes and other potential confounding factors (Go et al., 2004). The relative death rates were 1.2, 1.8, 3.2, and 5.9 for subjects with an estimated GFR of 45 to 60, 30 to 45, 15 to 30, and less than 15 mL/min/1.73 m^2, respectively. **These data highlight the potential need to optimize renal function and underscore nephron-sparing as an important** principle in the management of clinical T1 renal masses, particularly small renal masses (Campbell et al., 2017a; Miller et al., 2008).

Multiple retrospective series in the past decade have compared PN and RN for the management of clinical T1 renal masses, almost uniformly concluding in favor of PN (Kim et al., 2012b; Tan et al., 2012; Zabell et al., 2017a). One meta-analysis looked at more than 30 such studies and reported the following statistically significant correlations in favor of PN: (1) 61% lower incidence of severe CKD; (2) 19% reduced overall mortality; and (3) 29% reduced cancer-specific mortality (Kim et al., 2012b). The retrospective nature of these studies naturally raises concern about selection bias, and the third result listed earlier substantiates this. Clearly, PN is not a stronger oncologic intervention than RN, and the only reasonable way to explain an advantage for PN with respect to oncologic outcomes is selection bias. One cannot help but wonder whether selection bias may also be contributing to the improved overall survival associated with PN in these studies (Giordano et al., 2008; Shuch et al., 2013a; Weight et al., 2013). As such, the recent AHRQ systematic review of RCC management concluded that cancer-specific survival was similar among management strategies and attributable to tumor size and stage, whereas overall survival after intervention was related to age and competing comorbidities and was reflected in the selection for specific treatment modalities (Pierorazio et al., 2016a; Zabell et al., 2017b).

A prospective trial of RN versus PN was reported in 2011 that remains controversial. EORTC 30904 randomized more than 500 patients with small (<5.0-cm), unifocal tumors and a normal contralateral kidney to RN versus elective PN. RN showed an advantage in terms of lower perioperative morbidity, whereas PN provided better functional outcomes (Scosyrev et al., 2014; Van Poppel et al., 2011b). Oncologic events were uncommon, as expected for small renal masses, and similar in both groups. Based on prevailing paradigms, we would have expected better overall survival with PN, primarily driven by reduced cardiovascular morbidity. **However, 10-year overall survival was better for RN than PN (81% vs. 76%, respectively, $P < 0.05$), and cardiovascular deaths were less common in the RN group.** This trial had substantial flaws and most thought leaders in the field have preferred to dismiss the primary findings of the study. However, EORTC 30904 has stimulated further research by suggesting that the functional advantage of PN in the setting of a healthy patient and normal contralateral kidney may not be as beneficial as previously believed (Wang et al., 2016; Zabell et al., 2017a).

Subsequent studies have suggested that there may be a difference between CKD resulting from medical causes (CKD-M) and CKD primarily related to surgical removal of nephrons (CKD-S) (Demirjian et al., 2014; Lane et al., 2015; Parker et al., 2015). Patients with CKD caused by hypertension or diabetes will continue to suffer from these comorbidities and will likely experience progressive decline in renal function, eventually affecting survival (Go et al., 2004). However, patients with CKD-S typically do not need further surgery and can stabilize (Weight et al., 2013). This hypothesis was tested in a series of more than 4000 patients with localized RCC managed with PN or RN, including 1182 with preexisting CKD needing surgery (CKD-M/S), 927 who developed CKD only after surgery (CKD-S), and more than 2000 with no CKD even after surgery (Lane et al., 2013a). **The mean annual decline of renal function was 4.7% in patients with CKD-M/S compared with only 0.7% for the CKD-S group, and the survival of patients was CKD-S was significantly improved compared with those with CKD-M/S. Furthermore, the survival of patients with CKD-S was nearly identical to patients with no CKD, particularly if new baseline GFR was more than 45 mL/min/1.73 m²** (Wu et al., 2018).

The functional differences between RN and PN also may not be as great as previously thought. On average, PN saves about 90% of the global renal function and RN about 65% to 70%, but there can be considerable overlap. In a study by Zabor et al. (2016), 49% of patients managed with RN experienced recovery of global renal function to within 5% of their preoperative level within 2 years after surgery (Zabor et al., 2016). Compensatory hypertrophy after RN in adults averages about 20% but may be higher in some cohorts, and RN for kidneys with reduced function will naturally have less functional impact.

Our understanding of functional outcomes after PN and RN and their potential implications on survival has advanced considerably (Kim et al., 2017). However, there is clearly a need for higher quality data in this domain.

> **KEY POINTS: PARTIAL NEPHRECTOMY VERSUS RADICAL NEPHRECTOMY**
>
> - PN is preferred for small renal masses (stage T1a, <4.0 cm) whenever feasible. RN represents gross overtreatment for most such lesions, which often have limited biologic potential.
> - PN is also strongly preferred whenever preservation of renal function is potentially important, such as patients with preexisting CKD or proteinuria, an abnormal contralateral kidney, or multifocal or familial RCC.
> - Larger tumors (clinical stages T1b/T2) have increased oncologic potential and have often already replaced a substantial portion of the parenchyma, leaving less to be saved by PN. In this setting, if a normal contralateral kidney is present, the relative merits of PN vs. RN can be debated.
> - The AUA guidelines provide well-defined oncologic and functional criteria for consideration for RN (see Fig. 97.14). If these criteria are not satisfied, PN should be considered, if feasible.
> - Well-designed randomized, prospective trials will be required to provide higher quality data and allow for more rational management of patients with localized renal tumors.

Radical Nephrectomy

Prototypical RN encompasses the basic principles of early ligation of the renal artery and vein, removal of the kidney with primary dissection external to Gerota fascia, excision of the ipsilateral adrenal gland, and performance of an extended lymph node dissection (LND) (O'Malley et al., 2009b). Controversy has arisen regarding the routine need for many of these practices (Lam et al., 2004). Performance of a perifascial nephrectomy is of undoubted importance during RN for preventing postoperative local tumor recurrence because approximately 25% of clinical T1b/T2 RCCs manifest perinephric fat involvement (Lam et al., 2007; Shah et al., 2017b). Preliminary renal arterial ligation remains an accepted practice; however, in large tumors with abundant collateral vascular supply, it is not always possible to obtain complete preliminary control of the arterial circulation (O'Malley et al., 2009b). **Removal of the ipsilateral adrenal gland is not routinely necessary** in the absence of radiographic adrenal enlargement or local invasion, unless the malignant lesion extensively involves the kidney and/or is locally advanced (Campbell et al., 2017a; Lane et al., 2009c; Weight et al., 2011).

The need for an extensive LND in all patients undergoing RN has also been challenged, and there are several factors that mitigate against a therapeutic benefit of routine LND (Blom et al., 2009; Blute et al., 2017; Crispen et al., 2011; Leibovich and Blute, 2008). RCC metastasizes through the bloodstream independent of the lymphatics in many patients, and the lymphatic drainage of the kidney is highly variable. Therefore even an extensive retroperitoneal LND may not remove all possible sites of metastasis. **Most importantly, a rigorous study by Gershman et al. (2016) was not able to define a cohort of patients that experienced a therapeutic benefit from LND.** Based on these considerations, the AUA Guidelines now recommend that LND should be performed when suspicious lymphadenopathy is identified on imaging or surgical exploration. Beyond this LND can be selectively considered for locally advanced disease, although in all of these settings LND is primarily for staging and prognostic purposes. **There is strong consensus that LND need**

not be performed for most patients with localized kidney cancer and clinically negative nodes (Blom et al., 2009; Campbell et al., 2017a). LND is discussed in greater detail in subsequent sections of this chapter.

Open surgical techniques for RN are described in detail in Chapter 101. **The surgical approach for RN is determined by the size and location of the tumor as well as the body habitus of the patient** (Diblasio et al., 2006). The authors prefer an extended subcostal incision for most patients undergoing open RN, although a midline incision is a reasonable alternative, and the thoracoabdominal approach can be useful for very large and potentially invasive tumors involving the upper portion of the kidney. An extraperitoneal flank incision may be appropriate in elderly patients or patients of poor surgical risk, but exposure can be limiting, particularly for large tumors or those with contentious hilar anatomy (Diblasio et al., 2006; Russo, 2006). In reality, many of these patients are now managed with a minimally invasive approach in this era.

Laparoscopic RN is now established as a less-morbid alternative to open surgery in the management of low- to moderate-volume RCCs with no local invasion, limited or no venous involvement, and manageable lymphadenopathy. Current minimally invasive techniques allow replication of the important tenets of RN, and oncologic and other outcome data reflect this (see Chapter 102) (Berger et al., 2009a; Petros et al., 2015; Wille et al., 2004). Morbidly obese patients, those with a history of previous abdominal surgery, and those with large tumor size may also be considered for minimally invasive renal surgery, although selection of patients must be judicious and surgical expertise and experience should also be taken into account (Campbell et al., 2017b; Feder et al., 2008; Gabr et al., 2008; Tan et al., 2011). **One concern is that minimally invasive RN has become particularly appealing to patients and physicians alike, and this has likely been a major driver in the overuse of RN for small renal masses over the past several years** (Fig. 97.16).

Several studies on outcomes after RN for localized RCC have demonstrated that the risk of postoperative recurrence is stage-dependent, and surveillance protocols should reflect this (Merrill, 2017; Stephenson et al., 2004). In 2013 an AUA Guidelines Panel provided recommendations for the surveillance of patients after renal surgery for localized renal RCC (Donat et al., 2013). Table 97.15 outlines general surveillance considerations that apply to all patients managed for a localized renal mass, including the role of laboratory testing, longitudinal assessment of renal function, and specific indications for central nervous system or bone imaging. Table 97.16 provides stage-specific information for patients managed with surgical excision, particularly the indications for abdominal and thoracic imaging.

Partial Nephrectomy

Nephron-sparing surgery for the treatment of renal tumors was first described by Czerny in 1890, but this approach was infrequently used until the 1980s (reviewed in Herr, 2005). **Interest in PN for RCC has subsequently been stimulated by advances in renal imaging, experience with renal vascular surgery for other conditions, improved methods of preventing ischemic damage, growing numbers of incidentally discovered renal tumors, greater appreciation of the potentially deleterious effects of CKD, and encouraging long-term survival in patients undergoing this form of treatment** (Uzzo and Novick, 2001). Nephron-sparing surgery entails complete local resection of the tumor while optimally preserving normal functioning parenchyma within the involved kidney (Fig. 97.17).

Accepted indications for PN traditionally included situations in which RN would render the patient anephric or at high risk for ultimate need of dialysis (Campbell et al., 2017a; Licht et al., 1994; Russo et al., 2008). This comprised patients with bilateral RCC or RCC involving a solitary functioning kidney. A solitary

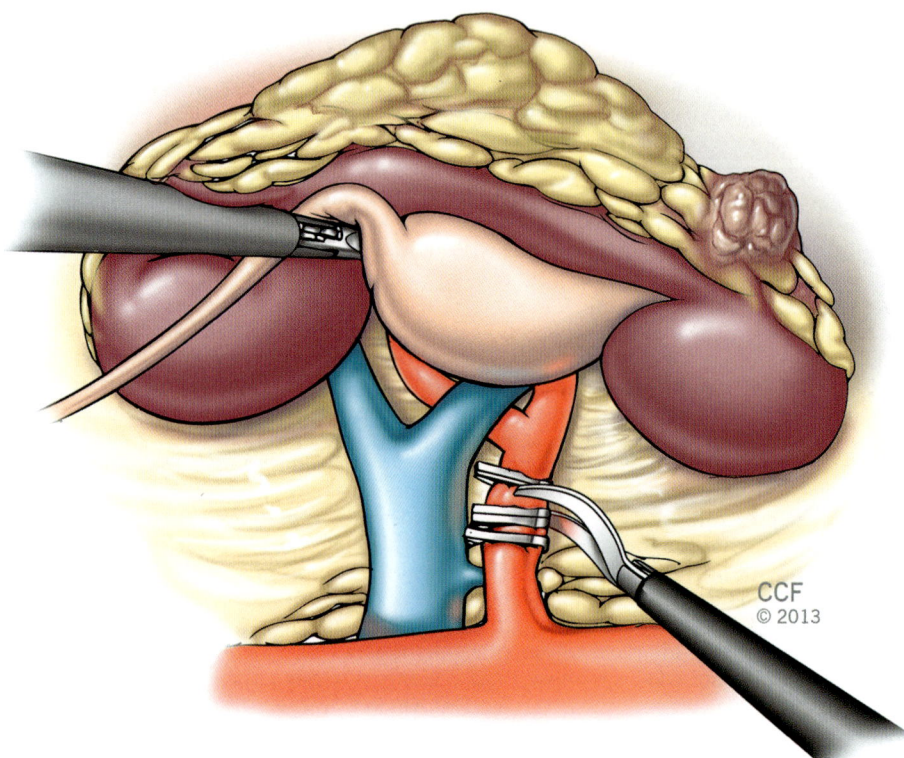

Fig. 97.16. Laparoscopic radical nephrectomy (a retroperitoneal approach is illustrated) provides excellent oncologic outcomes and rapid recovery but predisposes patients to chronic kidney disease. Partial nephrectomy should be prioritized for small renal masses. The 2017 AUA Guidelines provides well-defined criteria for consideration for radical nephrectomy. Patients not meeting these criteria should be considered for partial nephrectomy if feasible.

TABLE 97.15 Surveillance for Clinically Localized Renal Neoplasms: General Considerations

FOLLOW-UP MEASURE	RECOMMENDATION
Physical examination and history	History and physical examination directed at detecting signs and symptoms of metastatic spread or local progression
Laboratory testing	Basic laboratory testing, including BUN/creatinine, urinalysis, and eGFR, for all patients Progressive renal insufficiency or proteinuria should prompt nephrology referral CBC, LDH, LFTs, alkaline phosphatase, and serum calcium per discretion of the physician
Central nervous system imaging	Acute neurologic signs should lead to prompt neurologic cross-sectional imaging of the head or spine based on localized symptoms
Bone scan	Elevated alkaline phosphatase, clinical symptoms such as bone pain, and/or radiographic findings suggestive of a bony neoplasm should prompt a bone scan Bone scan should not be performed in the absence of these signs and symptoms

BUN, Blood urea nitrogen; *CBC*, complete blood count; *eGFR*, estimated glomerular filtration rate; *LDH*, lactate dehydrogenase; *LFTs*, liver function tests.
Modified from Donat SM, Diaz M, Bishoff JT, et al.: Follow-up for clinically localized renal neoplasms: AUA guideline. *J Urol* 190:407–416, 2013.

TABLE 97.16 Surveillance After Radical or Partial Nephrectomy[a]

FOLLOW-UP MEASURE	RECOMMENDATION
LOW-RISK PATIENTS	
Abdominal imaging	**Partial Nephrectomy:** Obtain a baseline abdominal scan (CT or MRI) within 3–12 months after surgery. If the initial postoperative scan is negative, abdominal imaging (US, CT, or MRI) may be performed yearly for 3 years based on individual risk factors. **Radical Nephrectomy:** Patients should undergo abdominal imaging (US, CT, or MRI) within 3–12 months after surgery. If the initial postoperative imaging is negative, abdominal imaging beyond 12 months may be performed at the discretion of the clinician.
Chest imaging	**Partial and Radical Nephrectomy:** Obtain a yearly CXR for 3 years and only as clinically indicated beyond that time period.
MODERATE- TO HIGH-RISK PATIENTS (pT2-4N0Mx or pT[any]N1Mx): PARTIAL OR RADICAL NEPHRECTOMY	
Abdominal imaging	A baseline abdominal scan (CT or MRI) within 3–6 months after surgery with continued imaging (US, CT, or MRI) every 6 months for at least 3 years and annually thereafter to year 5. Imaging beyond 5 years may be performed at the discretion of the clinician. Perform site-specific imaging as symptoms warrant.
Chest imaging	Obtain a baseline chest scan (CT) within 3–6 months after surgery with continued imaging (CXR or CT) every 6 months for at least 3 years and annually thereafter to year 5. Imaging beyond 5 years is optional and should be based on individual patient characteristics and tumor risk factors.

[a]Please also refer to Table 97.15 for general considerations related to surveillance.
CT, Computed tomography; *CXR*, chest x-ray; *MRI*, magnetic resonance imaging; *US*, ultrasound.
Modified from Donat SM, Diaz M, Bishoff JT, et al.: Follow-up for clinically localized renal neoplasms: AUA guideline. *J Urol* 190:407–416, 2013.

---

functioning kidney may be the result of unilateral renal agenesis, prior removal of the contralateral kidney, or irreversible impairment of contralateral renal function by a benign disorder. Another traditional relative indication for PN was represented by patients with unilateral RCC and a functioning opposite kidney affected by a condition that may threaten its future function, such as renal artery stenosis (Campbell et al., 1993), hydronephrosis, calculus disease, or systemic diseases such as diabetes or nephrosclerosis (Campbell et al., 2017a; Finelli et al., 2017; Uzzo and Novick, 2001).

In patients with bilateral synchronous RCC, the general approach has been to perform bilateral PNs whenever feasible, usually as staged procedures, particularly if the tumors are relatively large. When a locally extensive tumor on one side precludes nephron-sparing surgery, an RN is performed on the more involved side along with a contralateral PN (Booth et al., 2008; Nguyen et al., 2008a). Margin width appears to be immaterial as long as the final margins are negative; this is particularly relevant when the tumor is located within the hilum and preservation of renal function is at a premium (Bensalah et al., 2010; Bernhard et al., 2010; Marszalek et al., 2012; Sundaram et al., 2011).

Patients with RCC involving a functionally or anatomically solitary kidney must be advised about the potential need for temporary or permanent dialysis. In the series by Fergany et al. (2006), 3.5% of patients with a solitary kidney managed with PN required temporary dialysis, and 18 of 400 patients (4.5%) eventually progressed to end-stage renal failure. Many of these patients also had preexisting CKD, and in some instances only a small remnant kidney could be preserved because of anatomic considerations. A functioning renal remnant of at least 20% to 30% of one kidney is necessary to avoid end-stage renal failure, although this presumes good functional status of the remaining parenchyma (Uzzo and Novick, 2001). Overall preservation of renal function is thus achieved in the great majority of patients with PN, even in patients with traditional imperative indications (Nguyen et al., 2008a). Local recurrence after PN for imperative indications traditionally ranged from 3% to 5%, because many of these cases were particularly challenging because of hilar tumor location, the need to minimize the amount of excised functional parenchyma, tumor multifocality, or other complexities (Nguyen et al., 2008a; Uzzo and Novick, 2001).

In some patients with absolute indications, PN may not be anatomically feasible and RN followed by dialysis may have to be considered. Renal transplantation may be an option for some of these patients after an appropriate cancer-free interval. An alternative approach is a trial of tyrosine kinase inhibitor (TKI) therapy

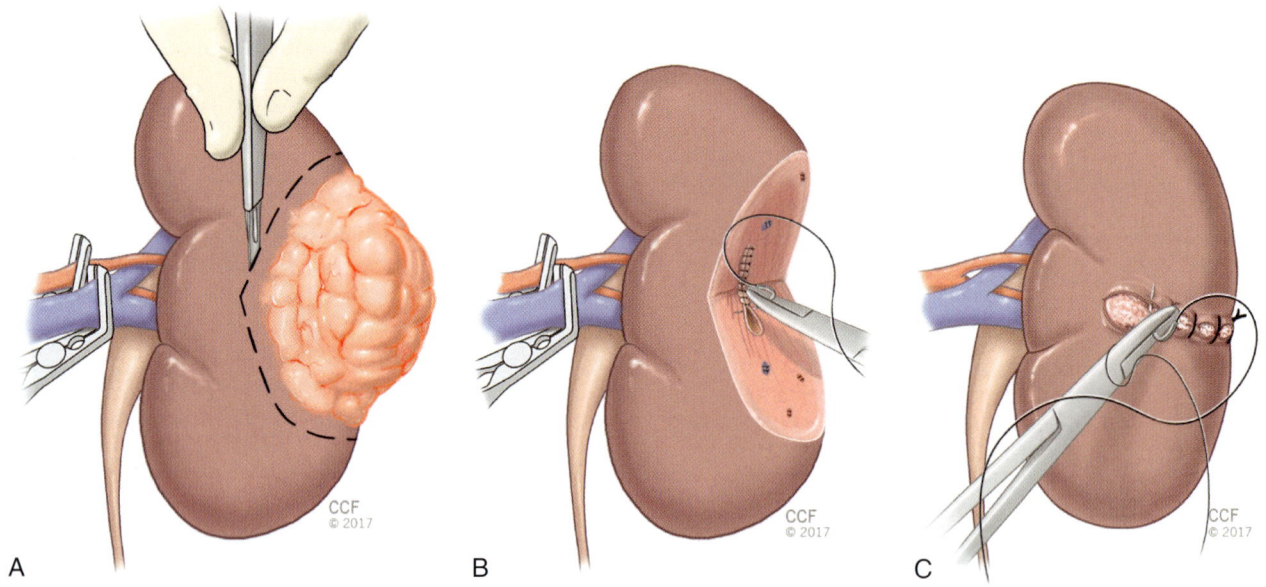

Fig. 97.17. Essential steps in traditional partial nephrectomy as illustrated with open approach. (A) Temporary occlusion of the vascular pedicle and excision of the tumor with a rim of normal parenchyma. (B) Closure of the collecting system and ligation of transected vessels. (C) Capsular reconstruction. (Reprinted with permission, Cleveland Clinic Center for Medical Art and Photography, Copyright 2017. All Rights Reserved.)

in an effort to downsize the tumor and enable PN, which can be successful in appropriately selected patients, particularly those with clear cell histology (Dey et al., 2017; Gorin et al., 2012a; Kroon et al., 2013; Rini et al., 2012; Thomas et al., 2009a; Tobert et al., 2013). Meticulous surgical technique is paramount because TKIs can impair tissue healing, and these agents should be withheld for at least a few half-lives before and after PN (Chapin et al., 2011; Hellenthal et al., 2010; Thomas et al., 2009b). Complications after PN may be more common in this setting, but most are urine leaks that are readily manageable with conservative measures (Rini et al., 2015). Nevertheless, this approach should only be used when truly necessary—upfront surgery should be prioritized whenever feasible (Dey et al., 2017; Rini et al., 2015).

PN is now standard of care for the management of small renal masses (clinical T1a) in the presence of a normal contralateral kidney, presuming that the mass is amenable to this approach (Campbell et al., 2017a; Finelli et al., 2017; Ljungberg et al., 2015; Motzer et al., 2017b). A robust literature demonstrates equivalent oncologic outcomes for PN when compared with RN in appropriately selected patients, and the functional outcomes tilt the balance in favor of PN whenever feasible (Pierorazio et al., 2016a; Russo and Huang, 2008; Thompson et al., 2008; Van Poppel et al., 2011a). Prior experience with "elective" PN for T1a RCC demonstrated local recurrence rates of 1% to 2%, and overall cancer-free survival well over 90% (Campbell et al., 2009). Most local recurrences observed after PN in this setting are a manifestation of undetected microscopic multifocal RCC—most are found distant from the previous tumor bed. Concern about local recurrence after elective PN is counterbalanced by a 1% to 2% incidence of contralateral RCC on longitudinal surveillance, in which case RN would have left the patient with tumor in a solitary kidney (Nguyen et al., 2008a; Russo et al., 2008).

The AUA Guidelines now provide evidence-based recommendations for use of PN (see Fig. 97.14) relative to RN with emphasis on well-defined selection criteria for RN (Campbell et al., 2017b). Tumors that demonstrate features suggesting increased oncologic potential (e.g., large tumor size, aggressive histology on RMB, or concerning imaging characteristics, such as infiltrative appearance) should be considered for RN, and RN is generally preferred in this setting only if *all* of the following criteria are met: (1) high tumor complexity and PN would be challenging even in experienced hands; (2) no preexisting CKD or proteinuria; and (3) normal contralateral kidney and new baseline GFR will likely be >45 mL/min/1.73 m^2. If all of these criteria are not satisfied, PN should be considered, if feasible (Campbell et al., 2017a; Lee et al., 2014; Tomaszewski et al., 2014; Volpe et al., 2013; Wu et al., 2018). Adherence to these Guidelines would greatly reduce overuse of RN.

Evaluation of patients with RCC for PN should include preoperative testing to exclude locally extensive or metastatic disease and additional specific renal imaging to delineate the relationship of the tumor to the intrarenal vascular supply and collecting system. Three-dimensional volume-rendered CT (or MRI) is now established as a noninvasive imaging modality that can accurately depict the renal parenchymal and vascular anatomy in a format familiar to urologic surgeons (Campbell et al., 2017b; Novick, 2009).

Urologic complications, such as urine leak or postoperative bleed, are more common after PN when compared with other management strategies, because the procedure yields a reconstructed organ that is highly vascular (An et al., 2017; Becker et al., 2014; Berg et al., 2017; Jung et al., 2014; Meeks et al., 2008; Pierorazio et al., 2016a). Nevertheless, most such complications are readily manageable with conservative measures (Campbell et al., 2017b; Gonzalez-Aguirre and Durack, 2016). The open and minimally invasive techniques for performing nephron-sparing surgery and paradigms for managing PN-related complications are reviewed in Chapters 101 and 102. R.E.N.A.L. and other nephrometry systems allow for assessment of tumor complexity and risk of complications and have facilitated comparison of evolving surgical techniques for PN in this era (Joshi and Uzzo, 2017; Kutikov and Uzzo, 2009; Simhan et al., 2011; Simmons et al., 2010). In general, margin status and oncologic outcomes associated with laparoscopic or robotic PN appear to be similar to open PN in experienced hands, presuming sensible patient selection (Lane and Gill, 2007; Spana et al., 2011; Tan et al., 2014; Tanagho et al., 2013).

One ongoing controversy in the field relates to the determinants of renal function after PN, which has important implications regarding surgical technique (Mir et al., 2015; Volpe et al., 2015; Zabell et al., 2017a). One of the main objectives of PN is to preserve as much function as possible and the factors that can influence ultimate renal function include the quality of the parenchyma before surgery, the quantity of vascularized parenchyma that can be preserved, and potential deleterious effects of ischemia (Fig. 97.18). **The quality of the parenchyma is for the most part nonmodifiable, essentially setting the ceiling for functional recovery after any intervention.** Most studies that have incorporated the other two factors into multivariable analysis suggest that the number of preserved nephrons is the primary factor determining functional outcomes after PN, while irreversible ischemic injury plays a secondary role (Dong et al., 2017c; Ginzburg et al., 2015; Lane et al., 2011; Mir et al., 2015; Song et al., 2009). Stated another way, as long as prolonged warm ischemia is avoided, most nephrons will recover from the ischemic insult (Kallingal et al., 2016; Mir et al., 2013; Parekh et al., 2013; Shah et al., 2016a; Thompson et al., 2012; Zabell et al., 2017a).

Precise excision of the tumor with a small rim of normal parenchyma along with careful reconstruction of the kidney to minimize devascularization is paramount and can be facilitated by a short ischemic interval to allow for a bloodless field (Bahler et al., 2015; Dong et al., 2017b; Mir et al., 2015; Zabell et al., 2017a). **Hypothermia should be considered for more complex cases or whenever a prolonged ischemic interval (>25–30 minutes) is anticipated, particularly for patients with a solitary kidney or preexisting CKD** (Abdeldaeim et al., 2015; Kaouk et al., 2014; Mir et al., 2015; Zhang et al., 2016). However, other techniques and perspectives, such as the concept of segmental arterial clamping (Desai et al., 2014; Gill et al., 2011, 2012; Shao et al., 2011), have shown promise, and further investigation will be required to address ongoing controversies in this field (see Chapter 102; Campbell et al., 2016; Paulucci et al., 2017; Satkunasivam et al., 2015; Simone et al., 2015).

Increased contact surface area (CSA) between the tumor and normal parenchyma correlates with increased loss of vascularized parenchyma mass because of parenchyma that is excised along with the tumor and devascularization related to reconstruction, both of which are more extensive in this setting (Dong et al., 2017b; Hsieh et al., 2016; Shin et al., 2015). CSA, which can be readily estimated from cross-sectional imaging studies using a simple mathematical formula, thus correlates strongly with functional outcomes after PN (Hsieh et al., 2016).

Surveillance of patients after PN, similar to RN, can be tailored to pathologic tumor stage; the basic recommendations are detailed in Tables 97.15 and 97.16. These protocols should help minimize costs, radiographic exposure, and patient inconvenience while still allowing for detection of most clinically relevant recurrences (Donat et al., 2013).

Patients who undergo nephron-sparing surgery for RCC may be left with a remnant kidney and are at risk for development of long-term functional impairment from hyperfiltration (Grady and Novick, 1996; Novick, 2009). In a study of 14 patients observed for up to 17 years after PN in a solitary kidney, patients with more than 50% reduction in overall renal mass were found to be at increased risk for development of proteinuria, focal segmental glomerulosclerosis (Fig. 97.19), and progressive renal failure (Novick et al., 1990). Development of proteinuria correlated directly with the length of follow-up and inversely with the amount of remaining renal tissue. **If proteinuria or progressive decline in GFR is noted in such patients, nephrology consultation should be obtained. Efforts to ameliorate the damaging effects of renal hyperfiltration have focused on dietary and pharmacologic interventions,** primarily the use of angiotensin-converting enzyme inhibitors along with a low-protein diet (Goldfarb, 1995; Novick and Schreiber, 1995).

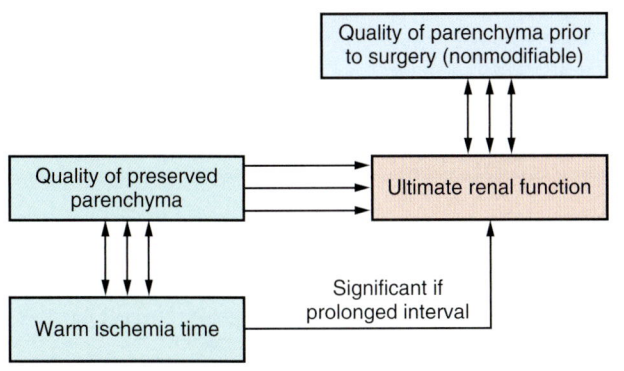

Fig. 97.18. Determinants of renal function after partial nephrectomy. The quality and quantity of preserved parenchyma are the main determinants of renal function after partial nephrectomy, with ischemic injury playing a secondary role as long as limited warm ischemia or hypothermia is used. Prolonged warm ischemia, however, can lead to irreversible loss of nephron function.

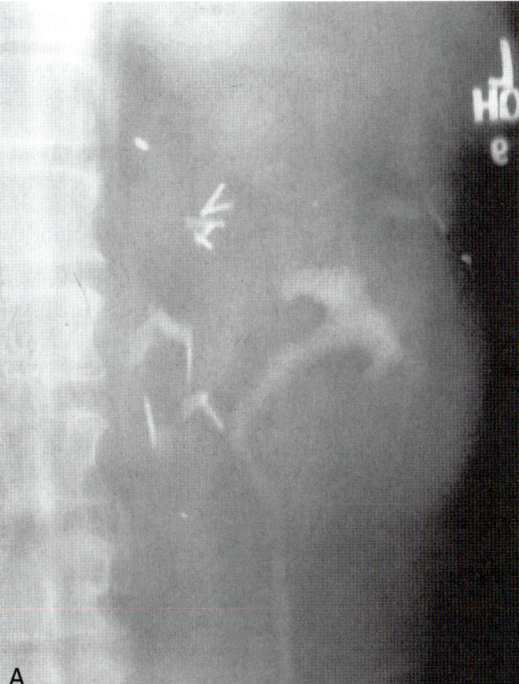

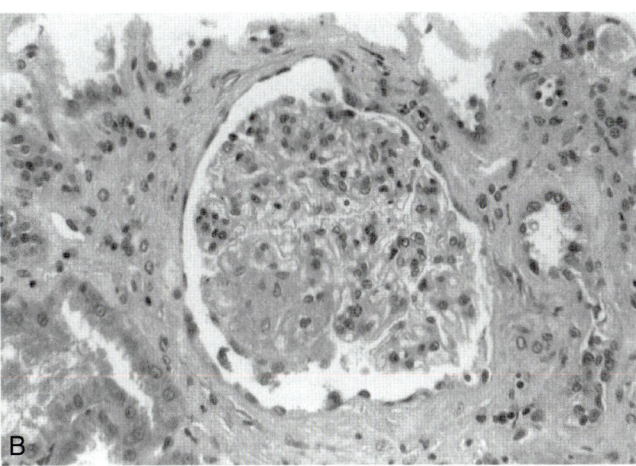

Fig. 97.19. (A) Ten years after partial nephrectomy for a large tumor in a solitary left kidney, imaging shows function of small renal remnant. The patient had developed nephrotic syndrome at this time. (B) Renal biopsy specimen demonstrates focal segmental glomerulosclerosis indicative of hyperfiltration nephropathy.

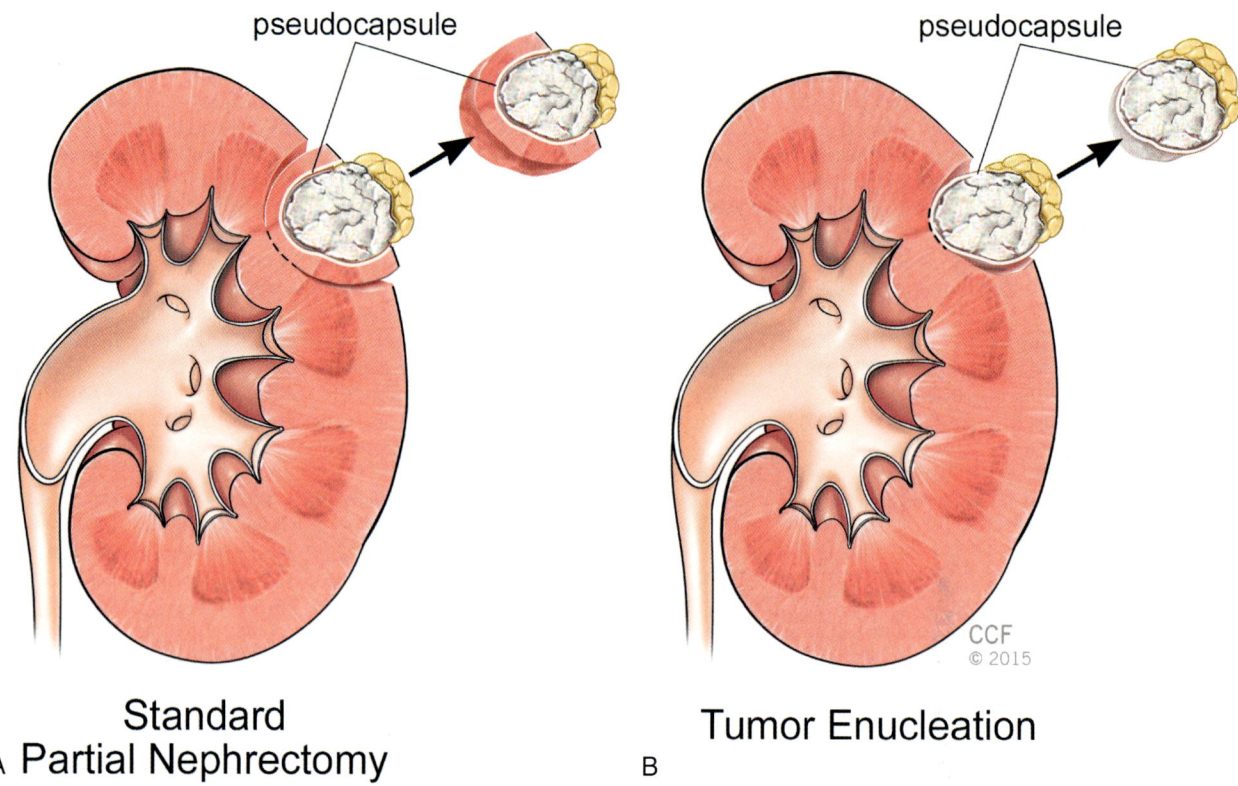

Fig. 97.20. (A) Standard partial nephrectomy is typically performed by strategic sharp dissection through the parenchyma leaving a small rim of normal parenchyma surrounding the mass. (B) Tumor enucleation primarily consists of blunt dissection along the pseudocapsule, yielding a specimen that includes tumor surrounded by pseudocapsule with minimal or no parenchyma in most areas. (Dong W, Gupta GN, Blackwell RH, et al.: Functional comparison of renal tumor enucleation versus standard partial nephrectomy. *Eur Urol Focus* 3[4–5]:437–443, 2017.)

Tumor Enucleation

Tumor enucleation (TE) is well-established for patients with familial kidney cancer, although its role for sporadic RCC remains controversial (Gupta et al., 2015). **TE entails blunt dissection along the pseudocapsule, thereby reducing the amount of normal parenchyma removed with the tumor.** In contrast, standard PN is performed by strategic sharp dissection, intentionally leaving a 2- to 3-mm rim of normal parenchymal adjacent to the tumor (Fig. 97.20). By minimizing dissection into the main substance of the kidney, TE may reduce blood loss, preclude entry into the collecting system, facilitate zero ischemia approaches to PN, and obviate the need for capsular closure. **As such, it may improve functional outcomes, although the bar is set high by standard PN, which typically saves about 90% of the global renal function.** In reality, only patients with severe preexisting CKD would be likely to benefit from the small incremental improvement in functional recovery that TE may provide (Blackwell et al., 2017; Dong et al., 2017a).

The main concern with TE is oncologic, as the basic tenets of surgical oncology would prioritize an approach that avoids the pseudocapsule and reduces the risk of positive surgical margins. Recent studies strongly suggest an increased risk of RCC recurrence after PN when positive margins are present, and 40% to 50% of localized RCC infiltrate into or beyond the pseudocapsule at least to some extent (Azhar et al., 2015; Gupta et al., 2015; Khalifeh et al., 2013; Minervini et al., 2009; Shah et al., 2016b). **However, most reports of TE have described relatively low rates of positive margins and encouraging longitudinal oncologic outcomes** (Carini et al., 2006; Kutikov et al., 2008; Minervini et al., 2011, 2015a; Porpiglia et al., 2016; Serni et al., 2014). Proponents of TE argue that infiltrative tumor within or beyond the pseudocapsule results in an inflammatory reaction that naturally directs dissection away from these danger zones, whereas sharp dissection as per standard PN is essentially blind and may increase the risk of an unrecognized margin in such areas. The basic concept is captured in the latter aspect of the adage, "keep your friends close, and your enemies closer." The other way to explain such findings relates to potential methodological differences in evaluation of margins among various centers and in different settings. **Selection for TE based on favorable imaging characteristics such as homogeneity or encapsulated appearance may also be a contributing factor, and a randomized trial with uniform pathologic assessment will be required to resolve some of these controversies** (Gupta et al., 2015).

In reality, TE is likely performed more often than previously appreciated, even when standard PN is intended. A recent recommendation has been to **standardize recording of the resection technique (enucleation versus standard resection, versus enucleoresection, which is a hybrid of the other two) based on visual inspection of the final gross pathologic specimen.** With enucleation only the pseudocapsule is seen and for standard resection the true tumor contour cannot be appreciated. Such assessments should be taken from the Surface, Intermediate region, and Base of the tumor, and this protocol, which is termed SIB, should facilitate comparison of outcomes for the various approaches to tumor resection (Antonelli et al., 2017; Minervini et al., 2014, 2015b).

In summary, review of the TE literature suggests that this **approach is reasonable for many patients, but selection criteria are not well defined.** Capsular invasion appears to be less common for low-grade tumors and for chromophobe RCC and oncocytomas (Jacob et al., 2015; Volpe et al., 2016b). As expected, high-grade tumors appear to be at risk for recurrence after TE, and RMB can be considered to assess suitability for this approach (Gupta et al., 2015). **The AUA Guidelines emphasize that negative surgical margins should always be a top priority with PN (see Fig. 97.14). Beyond** this overriding principle, the Guidelines state that "the extent of normal parenchyma removed should be determined by surgeon discretion taking into account the clinical situation; tumor characteristics including growth pattern, and interface with normal tissue" (Campbell et al., 2017a).

Thermal Ablative Therapies

TA, including renal cryosurgery and radiofrequency ablation (RFA), are now established as alternate nephron-sparing treatments for patients with localized RCC (Bhagavatula and Shyn, 2017; Kavoussi et al., 2016; Zargar et al., 2016). Both can be administered percutaneously and thus offer the potential for reduced morbidity (Campbell et al., 2017a; Taylor et al., 2017). In the recent meta-analysis associated with the AUA Guidelines, the morbidity profile for TA proved to be favorable, particularly relative to PN, which can be associated with an increased incidence of urologic complications (Campbell et al., 2017b). The effect of TA on renal function is typically limited, and these modalities appear to be reasonable choices for select patients with tumor in a solitary kidney, although PN remains the preferred choice in this setting (Altunrende et al., 2011; Weisbrod et al., 2010).

In general, long-term efficacy of TA is still not as well established as surgical excision, and local recurrence rates with primary TA are somewhat higher than those reported for traditional surgical approaches (Fig. 97.21) (Campbell et al., 2017b; Klatte et al., 2014). Another concern with TA has been risk of inaccurate histologic assessment because tumor heterogeneity may not be captured by RMB (Ball et al., 2015a) and lack of pathologic staging because the tumor is left in situ. **Most local recurrences after TA can be salvaged with repeat ablation, and cancer-specific survival rates for clinical T1a tumors are generally high across all management strategies** (Campbell et al., 2017a). Overall survival is primarily determined by age and general health status, not approach to management.

The traditional candidates for TA have been patients with reasonable life expectancy despite advanced age or significant comorbidities, who prefer a proactive approach but are not optimal candidates for conventional surgery. Although TA is still a reasonable choice for such patients, AS is now more commonly used in this setting. Other candidates for TA include patients with local recurrence after previous nephron-sparing surgery, and those with hereditary renal cancer who present with multifocal lesions for whom multiple PNs may be cumbersome (Johnson et al., 2008; Kavoussi et al., 2016; Liu et al., 2010; Zargar et al., 2016). Patient preference must also be considered, and some patients not fitting these profiles may also select TA, which can be supported as long as balanced counseling about the merits and limitations of these modalities has been provided (Campbell et al., 2017a; Kavoussi et al., 2016).

Tumor size is another important factor in patient selection because success rates appear to be highest for tumors smaller than 2.5 to 3.0 cm, and complication rates are also lower in this setting (Atwell et al., 2013; Campbell et al., 2017a; Tanagho et al., 2012). Some centers report local control rates of 95% to 100% with TA for such small renal masses. In general, success rates with TA appear to be lower for avidly enhancing masses and for clear cell histology, suggesting a potential role for RMB for risk stratification (Lay et al., 2015, 2016). **The 2017 AUA Guidelines advocate for TA as an alternate approach for the management of clinical T1a renal masses smaller than 3.0 cm in diameter,** which can be considered even in healthy patients (see Fig. 97.14; Campbell et al., 2017a).

Experience with renal cryosurgery predates that of RFA and has been more extensive (Nielsen et al., 2016; Zargar et al., 2016). Established prerequisites for successful cryosurgery include rapid freezing, gradual thawing, and a repetition of the freeze-thaw cycle. The mechanism of action consists of immediate membrane and cellular damage followed by microcirculatory failure and ischemia (Zondervan et al., 2016). Intracellular ice irreversibly disrupts cellular organelles and the cell membrane, and delayed microcirculatory occlusion eventually leads to cellular anoxia.

Complete and reliable tissue necrosis with cryoablation is consistently achieved only at temperatures of −19.4°C or lower, which

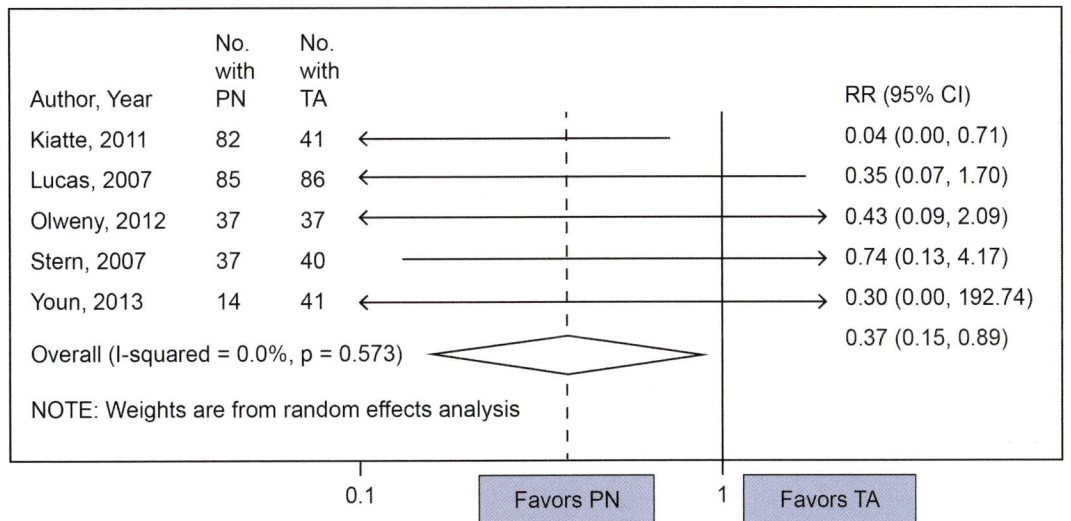

Risk Ratio and 95% Confidence Intervals of Local Recurrence

CI = confidence interval: No = numbers: PN = partial nephrectomy: RR = risk ratio for local recurrence: TA = thermal ablation
Note: The width of the horizontal lines represents the 95 percent confidence intervals for each study. The diamond at the bottom of the graph indicates the 95 percent confidence interval.

Fig. 97.21. Meta-analysis of local recurrence rates after partial nephrectomy (PN) versus primary tumor ablation (TA) incorporating studies with 48 +/− 12 months of follow-up. Risk ratios with 95% confidence intervals are shown for each study and for the overall analysis. Most such recurrences can be salvaged with repeat TA and the observed differences in local recurrence rates were no longer present when secondary ablations were taken into account. (Modified from Campbell SC, Uzzo RG, Allaf ME, et al.: Renal mass and localized renal cancer: AUA Guideline, 2017 [website]: https://www.auanet.org/guidelines/renal-mass-and-localized-renal-cancer-new-(2017).)

occurs about 3 mm inside the leading edge of the iceball as visualized by real-time ultrasonography. **Thus, to ensure complete cell kill, the iceball must extend well beyond the visible margins of the targeted tumor.** In practice, we routinely extend the iceball approximately 1 cm beyond the edge of the tumor, as determined by real-time imaging (Gill et al., 1998). The availability of sophisticated ultrasonography and introduction of finer cryoprobes that allow for more accurate and less traumatic probe placement have contributed to improved efficacy and safety of visceral cryosurgery (Sterrett et al., 2008; Zargar et al., 2016). Further details about techniques required to achieve optimal outcomes with cryoablation are available in Chapter 103.

Clinical experience after primary renal cryoablative therapy suggests successful local control in about 80% to 90% of patients, although many studies provide only limited follow-up (Campbell et al., 2017a; Stein and Kaouk, 2007; Zargar et al., 2016). Diagnosis of local recurrence after TA can be challenging because evolving fibrosis within the tumor bed can be difficult to differentiate from residual cancer. **In general, central or nodular enhancement within the tumor bed on extended follow-up has been considered diagnostic of local recurrence, and the clinical experience with TA has thus far supported this** (Bolte et al., 2006; Weight et al., 2008). However, only a minority of studies have incorporated routine post-therapy biopsies to provide histologic confirmation of oncologic status (Gill et al., 2000; Weight et al., 2008). Other findings that suggest local recurrence include a progressive increase in size of an ablated neoplasm, new nodularity in or around the treated zone, failure of the treated lesion to regress over time, or satellite or port site lesions (Donat et al., 2013). If these features are found, biopsy and possible retreatment should be considered. The **AUA Guidelines for surveillance after TA are outlined in Tables 97.15 and 97.17.**

Other concerns with cryoablation and TA in general, relate to surgical salvage and potential morbidity. Most local recurrences can be salvaged with repeat ablation, although some patients with progressive disease eventually require conventional surgery. **PN and minimally invasive approaches are occasionally precluded in this setting** because of the extensive fibrotic reaction induced by TA (Abarzua-Cabezas et al., 2015; Cross et al., 2017; Jimenez et al., 2016; Karam et al., 2015; Kowalczyk et al., 2009). Complications associated with cryoablation can include renal fracture, hemorrhage, adjacent organ injury, ileus, and wound infection, although major morbidity is decidedly uncommon presuming good patient selection (Sidana et al., 2010; Tsivian et al., 2010; Zargar et al., 2016). As expected, the incidence of treatment failure or complications after TA correlates with tumor size and complexity (Schmit et al., 2013).

The experience with RFA was initially more variable, likely related to variance in surgeon experience, differences in platforms used to perform the procedure, and inability to monitor treatment progress as stringently as cryoablation (Chang et al., 2015; Sterrett et al., 2008). However, as experience with RFA increased, outcomes similar to cryoablation were reported, and the AUA Guidelines Panel concluded that neither modality was notably **superior,** presuming adequate experience and expertise (see Fig. 97.14; Campbell et al., 2017a).

The mechanism of action of RFA is based on high-frequency electrical currents that lead to excitation of ions, frictional forces, and heat, which in turn causes denaturation of intracellular proteins and melting of cellular membranes (Kelly and Leveillee, 2016). These effects are observed at tissue temperatures above 41°C but increase directly with increasing temperature and duration of treatment. Temperatures in excess of 100°C are typically obtained at the tips of the probes, although this rapidly dissipates further away from the tip. Multiple probes or tines are thus typically required to achieve adequate heating of the entire region of interest, and thermosensors can be used to monitor progress, at least in areas of concern (Chang et al., 2015; Kelly and Leveillee, 2016). **Nevertheless, one disadvantage of RFA is that the treatment effect is potentially more difficult to monitor in real time—there is no true "iceball equivalent"** (Chang et al., 2015). Rather, treatment is primarily based on empirical results from previous probe alignments, supplemented by data from strategically placed thermoprobes when necessary (see Chapter 103).

TABLE 97.17 Surveillance After Renal Ablation[a]

FOLLOW-UP MEASURE	RECOMMENDATION
Diagnostic biopsy	Patients should undergo a pretreatment diagnostic biopsy.
Abdominal scan	Cross-sectional scanning (CT or MRI) with and without IV contrast unless otherwise contraindicated at 3 and 6 months after ablative therapy and with continued scanning annually thereafter for 5 years. Imaging beyond 5 years is optional based on individual risk factors.
Chest imaging	Patients who have either biopsy-proven renal cell carcinoma, oncocytoma, a tumor with oncocytic features, nondiagnostic biopsies, or no prior biopsy should undergo annual CXR for 5 years. Imaging (CXR or CT) beyond 5 years is optional based on individual patient risk factors and the determination of treatment success.
Benign biopsy	Radiographic scanning is not recommended with pathologic confirmation of benign disease at or before treatment and post-treatment radiographic confirmation of treatment success and no evidence of treatment-related complications. Oncocytoma is a possible exception for which continued surveillance should be considered.
Repeat biopsy	New enhancement, a progressive increase in size of an ablated neoplasm with or without contrast enhancement, new nodularity in or around the treated zone, failure of the treated lesion to regress over time, or satellite or port site lesions should prompt a repeat lesion biopsy. Observation, repeat treatment, and surgical intervention should be discussed for recurrence.

[a]Please also refer to Table 97.15 for general considerations related to surveillance.
CT, Computed tomography; *CXR,* chest x-ray; *IV,* intravenous; *MRI,* magnetic resonance imaging.
Modified from Donat SM, Diaz M, Bishoff JT, et al.: Follow-up for clinically localized renal neoplasms: AUA guideline. *J Urol* 190:407–416, 2013.

The technology for RFA continues to improve, and most contemporary series report relatively low rates of local recurrence, particularly for small renal masses less than 3 cm in diameter. Again, most local recurrences can be salvaged with repeat ablation, **and cancer-specific survival remains high** (Campbell et al., 2017b). Complications from RFA are uncommon but can include acute renal failure, stricture of the ureteropelvic junction, necrotizing pancreatitis, and lumbar radiculopathy, so careful and judicious selection of patients is essential (Chang et al., 2015; Sterrett et al., 2008).

Other new technologies, including high-intensity focused ultrasound (HIFU), stereotactic body radiation therapy (SBRT), microwave ablation, and laser interstitial thermal therapy, **are also under investigation and may allow for extracorporeal treatment** of small renal tumors in the future (de Senneville et al., 2016; Lin et al., 2014; Nair et al., 2013; Siva et al., 2012; Swaminath and Chu, 2015). However, at present cell kill with these modalities is not sufficiently reliable, and they are best considered developmental (Campbell et al., 2017b).

Active Surveillance

There was once relatively little information about the growth rate of RCC because almost all renal tumors were excised shortly after detection (Jewett et al., 2011; Lane et al., 2012). **The incidental discovery of many small RCCs in asymptomatic elderly patients or those of poor surgical risk provided the opportunity to observe the growth rate of these tumors in patients who were unable or unwilling to undergo surgery** (Chen and Uzzo, 2009; Crispen et al., 2009). Bosniak (1995) reported one of the first series of AS that included 72 small (<3.5 cm) renal tumors in 68 patients who were observed with serial imaging for a mean of 3.3 years. On CT these were solid, enhancing tumors consistent with RCC. During observation these tumors exhibited a median growth rate of 0.36 cm per year. In 32 patients whose tumors grew to larger than 3 cm, surgical excision was performed; all excised tumors were organ confined and most were grade 1. No patients developed metastasis during surveillance.

Subsequent series from several institutions confirmed that many small renal masses will grow slowly (median growth rate 0.09 to 0.34 cm/year) and with a relatively low rate of metastasis (less than 2.0% during 2 to 5 years of follow-up) (Campbell et al., 2017b; Conti et al., 2015; Jewett et al., 2011; Organ et al., 2014; Pierorazio et al., 2015; Smaldone et al., 2012; Uzosike et al., 2017). However, there are potential limitations to this literature (Campbell et al., 2017b). First, most AS series are enriched with small, well-marginated, homogeneous renal masses reflecting selection bias. A substantial proportion (20% or more) of these tumors may have been benign—RMB was often not performed. Finally, in most of these series there is a subpopulation of patients with rapidly growing tumors that appear to have more aggressive characteristics (Uhlman et al., 2013). For instance, in the series from Volpe et al. (2004), 25% of the masses doubled in volume in 12 months and 22% reached a diameter of 4 cm, triggering surgical intervention (Volpe et al., 2004). Salvage of patients with metastatic RCC is unlikely, and in some patients the window of opportunity for PN or TA may be lost.

Nevertheless, these studies suggest that patients with small, solid renal lesions, who are elderly or have increased surgical risk, can safely be managed with observation and serial renal imaging at 6-month or 1-year intervals (Jewett and Zuniga, 2008; Lallas et al., 2015; Ljungberg et al., 2015; Patel et al., 2016c; Volpe, 2016a). In this population, the risk of competing non-cancer causes of death and the risk of intervention often outweigh the risk of RCC progression (Kutikov et al., 2012; Smaldone et al., 2013; Sun et al., 2014). In fact, a number of studies indicate that active treatment of small renal masses in elderly patients may not confer a measurable survival benefit (Campbell et al., 2017b; Lane et al., 2010; Mirza, 2015).

Prospective studies with more prolonged follow-up are now available and provide further support for the use of AS, even in healthy patients when the mass has low malignant potential, such as very small (<2.0 cm), incidentally discovered renal masses (Ahmad et al., 2016; Danzig et al., 2016; Jewett et al., 2011; Ristau et al., 2017). The Delayed Intervention and Surveillance for Small Renal Masses (DISSRM) Registry prospectively enrolls patients with incidentally discovered, solid, small renal masses choosing AS or primary intervention. With a median follow-up of 2 years, and many patients with greater than 5-year follow-up, no patient undergoing AS has died of RCC or developed metastatic disease, while approximately 15% have undergone delayed intervention because of tumor growth or patient preference (Pierorazio et al., 2015). For small renal masses with low oncologic potential a trial of close observation can be considered with deferred RMB or intervention if interval growth is observed (Campbell et al., 2017a). The risk of delayed intervention in this setting appears to be low: most such tumors are readily salvageable, typically with nephron-sparing approaches (Hawken et al., 2016).

TABLE 97.18 Active Surveillance: Imaging Recommendations[a]

FOLLOW-UP MEASURE	RECOMMENDATION
Percutaneous biopsy	Percutaneous biopsy may be considered before active surveillance.
Abdominal imaging	Cross-sectional scanning (CT or MRI) within 3–6 months of active surveillance initiation to establish a growth rate, with continued imaging (US, CT, or MRI) at least annually thereafter.
Chest imaging	Patients with biopsy-proven renal cell carcinoma or a tumor with oncocytic features on active surveillance should undergo annual CXR. Continued surveillance should also be considered by oncocytoma.

[a]Please also refer to Table 97.15 for general considerations related to surveillance.
CT, Computed tomography; *CXR*, chest x-ray; *MRI*, magnetic resonance imaging; *US*, ultrasound.
Modified from Donat SM, Diaz M, Bishoff JT, et al.: Follow-up for clinically localized renal neoplasms: AUA guideline. *J Urol* 190:407–416, 2013.

The AUA Guidelines now provide specific recommendations about AS or expectant management and well-defined criteria for monitoring patients on surveillance (see Fig. 97.14 and Tables 97.15 and 97.18; Campbell et al., 2017a). For small, solid or Bosniak 3-4 complex cystic masses, AS should be considered on option for initial management, and for tumors with reduced malignant potential, such as those smaller than 2.0 cm diameter, this applies to healthy patients too. Shared decision making about AS versus intervention can be complex, and patient and tumor-related factors that favor conservative management are detailed in Fig. 97.14. RMB can also be considered for risk stratification before counseling.

Nephron-Sparing Surgery in von Hippel-Lindau and Other Forms of Familial Renal Cell Carcinoma

RCC in VHL disease differs from its sporadic counterpart in that the diagnosis is typically made at a younger age and there are usually multiple bilateral renal tumors (Bausch et al., 2013; Byler and Bratslavsky, 2014; Linehan and Ricketts, 2013). Although these are generally low-stage tumors, they are capable of progression to metastasis and represent a frequent cause of death in patients with VHL. RCC in VHL is characterized histologically by solid tumors and renal cysts that contain either frank carcinoma or a lining of hyperplastic clear cells representing incipient carcinoma (Fig. 97.22).

The surgical options in patients with bilateral RCC and VHL disease are bilateral nephrectomy and renal replacement therapy or nephron-sparing approaches such as PN or TA to avoid end-stage renal disease. The general philosophy has been to pursue nephron-sparing strategies whenever possible, given the multifocal nature of the disease, even for centrally located tumors (Linehan and Ricketts, 2013; Metwalli and Linehan, 2014). For PN, an enucleative approach is often preferred to optimize preservation of parenchymal mass and function. Although early results of PN were promising, subsequent studies suggested a high incidence of ipsilateral postoperative tumor recurrences (Grubb et al., 2005; Novick and Streem, 1992). It is likely that most of these local recurrences were a manifestation of occult microscopic RCC that was not removed at the time of the original PN.

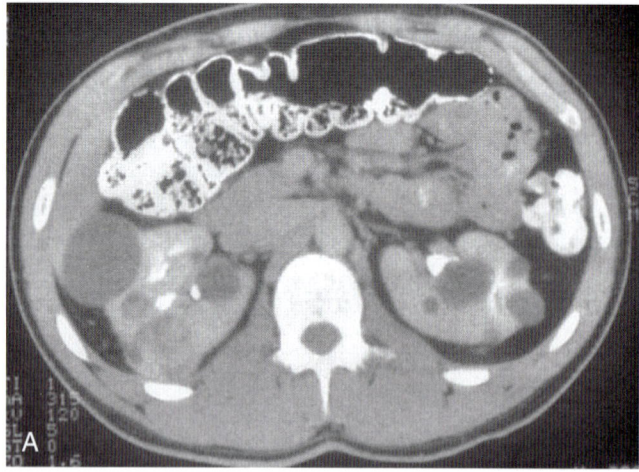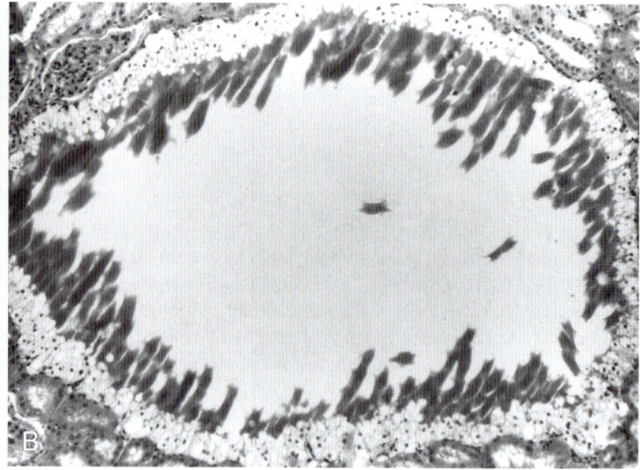

Fig. 97.22. (A) Computed tomography scan after administration of contrast agent shows bilateral solid and cystic renal masses in a patient with von Hippel-Lindau disease. (B) Histopathologic section of one of the renal cysts shows lining of clear cells representing incipient carcinoma.

One multicenter study delineated the long-term outcomes after surgical treatment of localized RCC in 65 patients with VHL (Steinbach et al., 1995). RCC was present bilaterally and unilaterally in 54 and 11 patients, respectively, and RN and PN were performed in 16 and 49 patients, respectively. The 5-year and 10-year cancer-specific survival rates for all patients were 95% and 77%, respectively. The corresponding rates for patients treated with PN were 100% and 81%, respectively. Survival free of local recurrence after PN was 71% at 5 years but only 15% at 10 years, emphasizing the need for long-term surveillance.

Duffey et al. (2004) **at the National Cancer Institute have defined a 3-cm threshold for intervention in patients with VHL.** In their series, 108 patients with VHL and solid renal tumors smaller than 3 cm were observed, and none developed metastatic disease during mean follow-up of 58 months. In contrast, metastases developed in 20 of 73 patients (27%) with tumors larger than 3 cm, and the frequency of metastases increased with increasing tumor size. A 3-cm cut point has thus been proposed to reduce the number of surgical interventions, optimize renal function, and minimize the risk of metastatic disease. **This recommendation also applies to patients with HPRC and BHD syndromes** (Shuch et al., 2012b; Stamatakis et al., 2013). **However, HLRCC is an exception in that tumors in this syndrome are often more aggressive and should be managed accordingly, even when less than 3 cm** (Linehan and Rouault, 2013; Ricketts et al., 2012; Shuch et al., 2012b).

Taken together, these studies suggest that PN can provide effective initial treatment of patients with RCC and VHL but should be withheld until tumor size reaches or eclipses 3.0 cm. After initial management, patients with VHL must be observed closely because most will eventually develop locally recurrent RCC with the concomitant need for repeat renal intervention (Grubb et al., 2005; Ploussard et al., 2007). In this setting, repeat PN can be challenging because of postoperative fibrosis and TA may be considered to reclaim local control (Liu et al., 2010; Metwalli and Linehan, 2014; Shuch et al., 2012b). Targeted agents are now being investigated in an effort to slow disease progression in this syndrome (Shuch et al., 2012b). When removal of all renal tissue is necessary for oncologic reasons, subsequent renal transplantation can provide satisfactory renal replacement therapy and appears to be generally safe despite the tumor diathesis (Goldfarb et al., 1997).

Comprehensive management of patients suspected of having familial RCC should also include genetic counseling and screening for other manifestations of the disease process (as discussed in the earlier section on familial RCC and molecular genetics) (Byler and Bratslavsky, 2014; Ho and Jonasch, 2014; Shuch et al., 2012b). For patients with VHL, identification of pheochromocytoma or central nervous system hemangioblastoma is particularly important before surgical intervention for RCC (Linehan and Ricketts, 2013).

TREATMENT OF LOCALLY ADVANCED RENAL CELL CARCINOMA

Inferior Vena Cava Involvement

One of the unique features of RCC is its frequent pattern of growth intraluminally into the renal venous circulation, also known as venous tumor thrombus. This growth may extend into the IVC with cephalad migration as far as the right atrium or beyond. The absence of metastases in many patients with vena cava extension is an intriguing aspect of this cancer's behavior (Gettman and Blute, 2002; Martinez-Salamanca et al., 2011; Wotkowicz et al., 2008;). **Forty-five to seventy percent of patients with RCC and IVC thrombus can be cured with an aggressive surgical approach, including RN and IVC thrombectomy** (Blute et al., 2004b; Martinez-Salamanca et al., 2011).

> **KEY POINTS: TREATMENT OF LOCALLY ADVANCED RENAL CELL CARCINOMA**
>
> - Forty-five to seventy percent of patients with venous tumor thrombus can be cured with nephrectomy and thrombectomy, including patients with tumor thrombus extending to the cardiac atrium.
> - Thrombus extending into the IVC below the main hepatic veins can be readily managed with isolation of the involved vasculature and removal of the tumor thrombus.
> - Thrombus extending above the main hepatic veins requires more extensive dissection, venovenous bypass, or cardiopulmonary bypass and circulatory arrest.
> - For large tumors with radiographic suspicion of invasion into adjacent structures (cT4), complete excision with en bloc resection of the involved structures provides the only chance of cure.
> - Bulky lymphadenopathy carries a poor prognosis similar to metastatic disease, although surgical resection should be considered if feasible, given careful assessment of disease burden and patient age/comorbidities.
> - High-quality preoperative imaging (CT or MRI) should be obtained in proximity to the anticipated surgery to plan for and achieve intraoperative success.
> - Although locally advanced RCC is still primarily a surgical disease, adjuvant systemic therapy trials should be encouraged and, in select patients, neoadjuvant approaches may be considered.

Overall, involvement of the venous system with RCC occurs in 4% to 10% of patients with RCC. IVC tumor thrombus should be suspected in patients with a renal tumor who also have lower extremity edema, isolated right-sided varicocele or one that does not collapse with recumbency, dilated superficial abdominal veins, proteinuria, pulmonary embolism, right atrial mass, or nonfunction of the involved kidney. **Staging of the level of IVC thrombus is as follows: I, adjacent to the ostium of the renal vein; II, extending up to the lower aspect of the liver and below the hepatic veins; III, involving the intrahepatic portion of the IVC but below the diaphragm; and IV, extending above the diaphragm.** The IVC thrombus level is distinct from the AJCC TNM staging, which distinguishes tumors with thrombi above the diaphragm (stage T3c) from those with IVC thrombi below the diaphragm (stage T3b) and those with thrombi only within the renal vein or its major branches (stage T3a) (Amin et al., 2017). Consequently, the prognostic significance of IVC thrombus level is controversial. However, two large, multicenter retrospective cohort studies confirm tumor thrombus level as an independent predictor of survival and recurrence. The largest cohort of IVC thrombi, composed of 11 international sites and 1215 patients, demonstrates tumor thrombus level as an independent predictor of survival (Martinez-Salamanca et al., 2011). A second cohort of 636 patients from five American centers also confirms tumor thrombus level as a significant predictor of recurrence (Abel et al., 2017).

Microscopic invasion of the wall of the IVC is also a strong predictor of cancer-specific survival (Abel et al., 2017; Rodriguez Faba et al., 2017), with other studies reporting nodal or metastatic involvement, tumor grade, non–clear cell histology, preoperative anemia, and body mass index as predictors of oncologic outcomes (Abel et al., 2014; Blute et al., 2004b; Terakawa et al., 2007). **In all series, a significant proportion of patients with level IV IVC thrombi are cured with surgical resection, typically in the absence of metastases and other adverse features** (Ciancio et al., 2007; Glazer and Novick, 1996; Granberg et al., 2008; Libertino et al., 1987). Along with contemporary systemic therapies, overall survival can reach 40% at 5 years (Dashkevich et al., 2016).

The importance of high-quality preoperative imaging cannot be overemphasized, and imaging should be obtained as close as possible to the date of surgery as progression of the tumor thrombus may mandate important changes in intraoperative management (Blute et al., 2004b; Wotkowicz et al., 2008). MRI, CT, and echocardiography are useful adjuncts in the pre- and perioperative planning settings. **MRI is the preferred diagnostic study at many centers** (Goldfarb et al., 1990; Pouliot et al., 2010); **however, recent literature indicates that an appropriately performed CT can provide essentially equivalent information** (Fig. 97.23; Guzzo et al., 2009; Ng et al., 2008). Administration of contrast during the study often allows tumor thrombus to be differentiated from bland thrombus because the latter does not demonstrate enhancement.

Invasive contrast-enhanced imaging, such as venacavography, is rarely used and reserved for patients in whom MRI and CT findings are equivocal or for whom MRI and CT are contraindicated. Interestingly, vascularization of IVC tumor thrombus is observed in 35% to 40% of cases. Preoperative **renal artery embolization** is not essential nor recommended for the routine management of IVC thrombi because there are little or no measurable objective benefits (e.g., blood loss, complications) in the literature; current data suggest an increased risk of major complications and mortality (Subramanian et al., 2009). In patients with extensive level III or IV thrombi, when adjunctive cardiopulmonary bypass with deep hypothermic circulatory arrest is considered, **preoperative coronary angiography** identifies patients who may benefit from revascularization at the time of bypass (Novick et al., 1990). **Intraoperative echocardiography** can be a valuable adjunct in the operating room to evaluate thrombus extent, monitor embolic phenomenon and cardiac function, and recognize residual tumor during and after resection (Cywinski and O'Hara, 2009; Glazer and Novick, 1997; Kostibas et al., 2017; Shuch et al., 2009; Wotkowicz et al., 2008).

The surgical approach is tailored to the level of IVC thrombus but uniformly begins with early ligation of the arterial blood supply, and in the process the kidney is gently mobilized, leaving it only attached via the renal vein (Blute et al., 2004b; Gorin et al., 2012; Shuch et al., 2009). An alternate strategy whereby the IVC thrombus is addressed before mobilization of the kidney can be considered and may reduce the risk of tumor embolism.

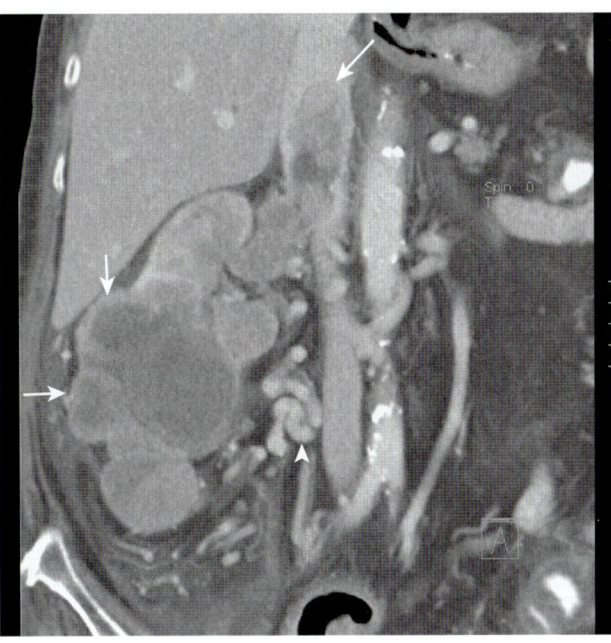

Fig. 97.23. Computed tomography demonstrating right lower pole renal cell carcinoma *(short arrows)* with level III inferior vena cava (IVC) thrombus. The *long arrow* indicates the upper extent of the tumor thrombus within the intrahepatic portion of the IVC. The *arrowhead* indicates extensive retroperitoneal venous collateral vessels associated with restricted flow within the IVC.

In general, level I thrombi are isolated by a Satinsky clamp or vascular stapler (Fig. 97.24A). Care to preserve at least 50% of the lumen of the IVC is essential to prevent downstream vascular complications related to reduced blood flow, and patch grafts should be considered when appropriate (Armstrong et al., 2014; Hyams et al., 2011). Level II thrombi require sequential clamping of the caudal IVC, contralateral renal vasculature, and cephalad IVC along with mobilization of the relevant segment of the IVC and occlusion of lumbar veins. The renal ostium is then opened and the thrombus is removed, all in a bloodless field (Fig. 97.24B). When tumor thrombus invades the wall of the vena cava, aggressive resection of the involved cava and attainment of negative surgical margins are required to minimize the risk of recurrence (Blute et al., 2007; Wotkowicz et al., 2008). IVC grafting or reconstitution is required in some instances, but patients with a completely occluded IVC may not need reconstruction because of established, collateral blood flow (Blute et al., 2007; Hyams et al., 2011; Sarkar et al., 1998). Attempts to remove distal bland thrombus within the IVC or iliac vessels are reasonable, although bland thrombus may be left in situ when resection places the patient at undue risk of complications. When left in situ, ligation of the IVC cephalad to this level or placement of a filter should be considered to prevent pulmonary embolism.

Vascular control for level III and level IV IVC thrombi requires more extensive dissection, venovenous bypass, or cardiopulmonary bypass and hypothermic circulatory arrest. For level III thrombi, mobilization of the liver and exposure of the intrahepatic IVC often allows the thrombus to be mobilized caudad to the hepatic veins, and venous isolation can then proceed as for a level II thrombus (Fig. 97.24C) (Gallucci et al., 2004). Alternatively, the IVC should be clamped above the liver and a Pringle maneuver performed to temporarily occlude the portal triad (Ciancio et al., 2007, 2011). Venovenous bypass is commonly used in these cases but may not be required if adequate collateral flow is present. Level IV IVC thrombi have traditionally been managed with cardiopulmonary bypass and hypothermic circulatory arrest, and this is still the preferred approach

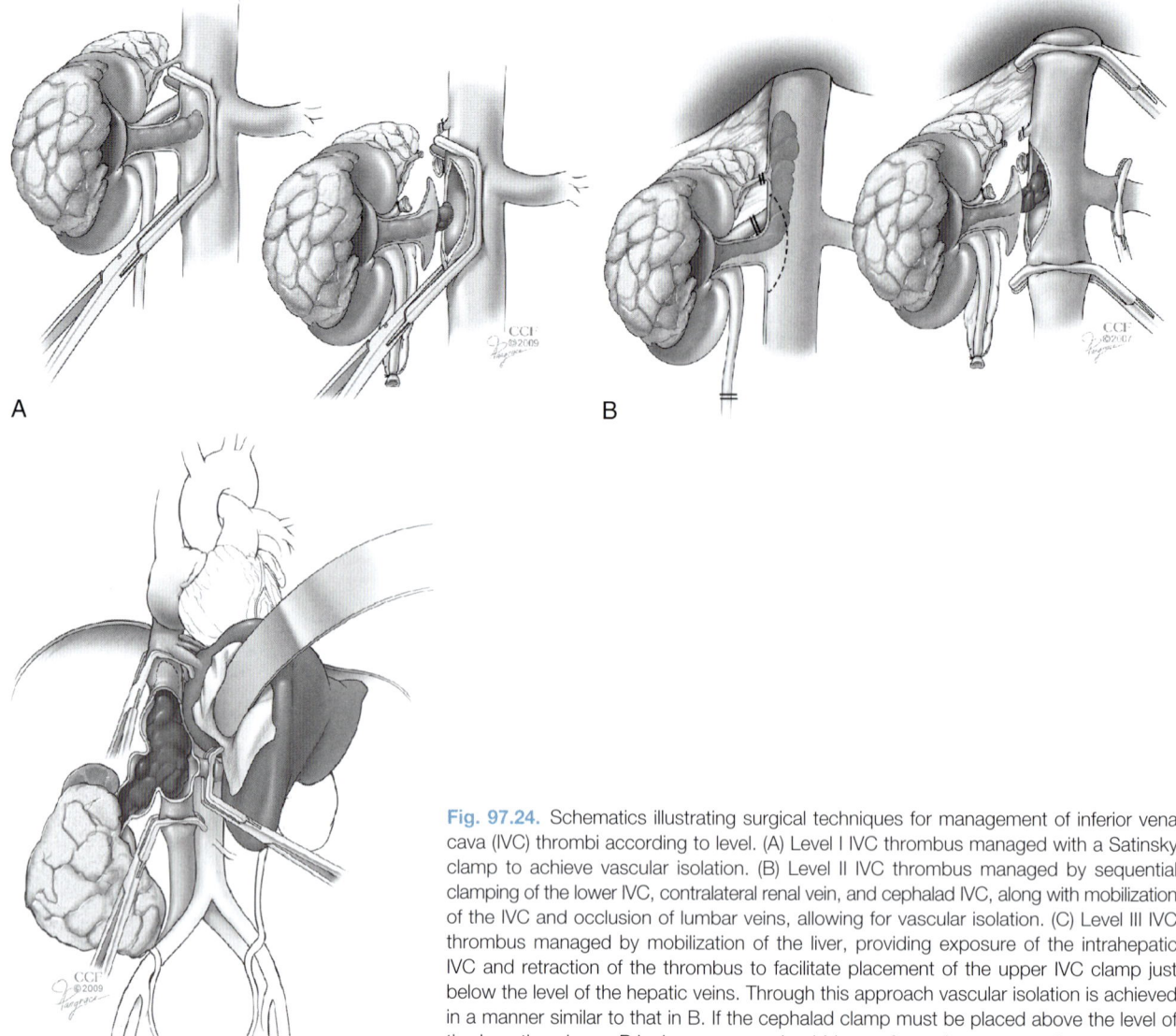

Fig. 97.24. Schematics illustrating surgical techniques for management of inferior vena cava (IVC) thrombi according to level. (A) Level I IVC thrombus managed with a Satinsky clamp to achieve vascular isolation. (B) Level II IVC thrombus managed by sequential clamping of the lower IVC, contralateral renal vein, and cephalad IVC, along with mobilization of the IVC and occlusion of lumbar veins, allowing for vascular isolation. (C) Level III IVC thrombus managed by mobilization of the liver, providing exposure of the intrahepatic IVC and retraction of the thrombus to facilitate placement of the upper IVC clamp just below the level of the hepatic veins. Through this approach vascular isolation is achieved in a manner similar to that in B. If the cephalad clamp must be placed above the level of the hepatic veins, a Pringle maneuver should be performed to temporarily occlude the hepatic blood flow. (Reprinted with permission, Cleveland Clinic Center for Medical Art and Photography, Copyright 2007-2009. All Rights Reserved.)

in complex cases (Blute et al., 2007; Chen et al., 2015b; Gaudino et al., 2016; Wotkowicz et al., 2008). However, many centers are now trying to avoid hypothermic circulatory arrest because of the hypocoagulable state that ensues when coming "off pump," and increased risk of cerebrovascular accident and myocardial infarction associated with this approach (Ciancio et al., 2011; Navia et al., 2012). If the thrombus is mobilized below the atrium, sequential vascular control can often be achieved without opening the heart (Chen et al., 2015b; Ciancio et al., 2010) or advanced veno-veno bypass techniques can be used to access the right atrium and cranial IVC (Gaudino et al., 2016). Further detail about these procedures are provided in Chapter 101.

The risk of morbidity can be substantial for thrombi extending above the diaphragm, and mortality rates associated with RN and IVC thrombectomy as high as 5% to 10% have been reported in some series, depending on patient comorbidities and tumor characteristics (Blute et al., 2004b; Ciancio et al., 2010; Navia et al., 2012). **Patient selection is critical as many patients, especially those with metastatic disease, will have a limited life expectancy** (Ciancio et al., 2010; Culp et al., 2010; Pouliot et al., 2010; Slaton et al., 1997). **However, surgery can impart a significant palliative benefit by preventing pulmonary emboli and minimizing disability from intractable edema, ascites, cardiac dysfunction, or associated local symptoms such as abdominal pain and hematuria.**

Data regarding robot-assisted laparoscopic nephrectomy and IVC thrombectomy are emerging from a few centers around the world. Early data indicate that select patients with level I through III thrombi can undergo safe robotic surgery, although oncologic outcomes remain preliminary and more mature data is needed (Abaza, 2011; Ball et al., 2015b; Chopra et al., 2017).

Locally Invasive Renal Cell Carcinoma

Patients with locally advanced and invasive (stage T4) RCC are uncommon, accounting for less than 2% of surgical series, and usually experience pain, generally from invasion of the posterior abdominal wall, nerve roots, or paraspinous muscles (Karellas et al., 2009; Thompson et al., 2005a). Large tumors are more likely to metastasize than invade adjacent structures (Yezhelyev et al., 2009); only 40% of patients with suspected direct invasion are confirmed pathologically (Margulis et al., 2007a). A familiar scenario is the upper pole renal tumor that appears to be invading the liver, suggesting that partial hepatectomy may be required, yet on exploration the tissue planes are found to be intact. **In evaluation of patients with** large, invasive retroperitoneal masses, a broad differential diagnosis should be considered, including adrenocortical carcinoma, urothelial carcinoma, sarcoma, and lymphoma, in addition to locally invasive RCC.

Because surgical therapy is the only potentially curative management for RCC, extended operations with en bloc resection of adjacent organs are occasionally indicated. Complete excision of the tumor, including resection of the involved bowel, spleen, distal pancreas, or abdominal wall muscles, is the aim of therapy. Consequences of a complete resection of adjacent organs should be considered preoperatively, and careful perioperative management is essential including proper bowel preparation, vaccinations for splenectomized patients, and the need for endocrine replacement for patients with bilateral adrenal involvement.

However, even with an aggressive surgical approach, the prognosis remains poor. In 61 patients with pT4 RCC from MD Anderson Cancer Center, median cancer-specific survival was 37 and 8 months for patients with nonmetastatic and metastatic RCC, respectively (Borregales et al., 2016). Although negative surgical margins were achieved in 63% of patients in another series, 34 of 38 patients (90%) ultimately died of disease at a median of 12 months after surgery (Karellas et al., 2009). For these reasons, neoadjuvant systemic therapy is a valid consideration for patients with potentially unresectable RCC, because it can provide a "litmus test" to identify patients who are destined to progress rapidly (Rini et al., 2012).

Incomplete excision of a large primary tumor, or debulking, is rarely indicated because 1-year survival estimates are only 10% to 20% in this setting (Dekernion et al., 1978; Karellas et al., 2009). Given potential toxicity to adjacent bowel and limited efficacy in small case series (Cox et al., 1970; van der Werf-Messing, 1973), radiation therapy has traditionally played little role in the management of locally extensive RCC. Recent data with contemporary stereotactic radiation techniques are emerging and may alter some of these perspectives (Staehler et al., 2015).

Lymph Node Dissection for Renal Cell Carcinoma

The presence of lymph node metastasis is an important prognostic factor and defines a high-risk subset of patients with advanced RCC (Blute et al., 2004a). **Although lymphadenectomy for RCC provides accurate staging, the therapeutic benefits of routine lymphadenectomy are controversial.** Even in patients with radiographic adenopathy, only 30% to 43% of clinically enlarged lymph nodes contain metastatic disease (Capitanio et al., 2016; Ming et al., 2009; Studer et al., 1990). In a series of patients at high-risk of lymph node metastases, the rates of metastatic nodes were 20%, 29%, and 90% for nodes 7, 10 and 30 mm in size, respectively (Gershman et al., 2016). In addition to the relationship with nodal size, the prevalence of node-positive disease is also stage specific (Blute et al., 2004a; Capitanio et al., 2009; Pantuck et al., 2003; Whitson et al., 2011), and a number of well-recognized pathologic features are associated with lymph node metastases (Table 97.19). These findings were confirmed in a prospective study in which patients with two or more high-risk features were found to be at increased risk (greater than 40%) for nodal involvement (Blute et al., 2004a; Crispen et al., 2011). These features included (1) large primary tumor (>10 cm); (2) clinical stage T3/T4; (3) high tumor grade (grade 3/4); (4) sarcomatoid features; or (5) histologic tumor necrosis. Although these criteria will identify a significant proportion of patients with lymph node metastases, 45% will have positive nodes away from the renal hilum calling into question the extent and templates needed for accurate staging (Fig. 97.25; Crispen et al., 2011).

Most importantly, the EORTC 30881 randomized trial of lymphadenectomy at RN failed to show a survival advantage for most patients undergoing lymphadenectomy (Blom et al., 2009). This study has been criticized for being underpowered to detect a difference in survival because most patients were low risk for nodal metastasis (81% were grade 1 or 2 and 72% were organ confined); and lymph node metastases were present in only 4% of patients undergoing complete lymph node dissection. Contemporary, large retrospective analyses also fail to demonstrate a consistent oncologic benefit to routine lymphadenectomy. For instance, a large series from the Mayo Clinic of nearly 1800 patients failed to show a

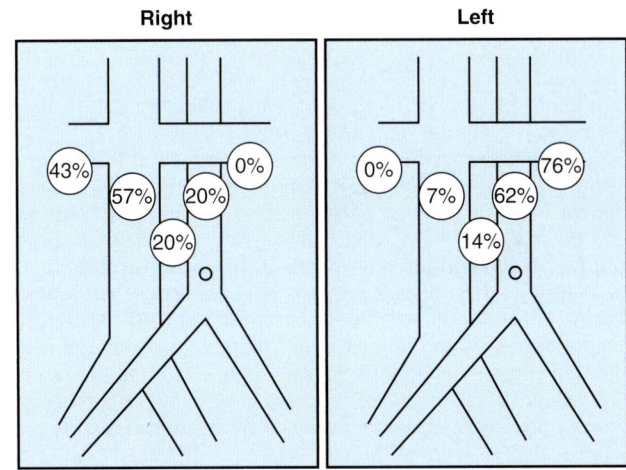

Fig. 97.25. Frequency of lymph node positivity detected at extended lymphadenectomy in patients with lymph node positive renal cancer at nephrectomy. (From Crispen PL, Breau RH, Allmer C, et al.: Lymph node dissection at the time of radical nephrectomy for high-risk clear cell renal cell carcinoma: indications and recommendations for surgical templates. *Eur Urol* 59:18–23, 2011.)

TABLE 97.19 Risk of Regional Lymph Node Metastases in Renal Cell Carcinoma Based on Pathologic Risk Factors

NO. OF RISK FACTORS[a]	PERCENTAGE OF PATIENTS IN THIS RISK GROUP	PERCENTAGE WITH POSITIVE LYMPH NODES IN RETROSPECTIVE SERIES[b]	PERCENTAGE WITH POSITIVE LYMPH NODES IN PROSPECTIVE SERIES[c]
0	44% (729/1652)	0.4% (3/729)	—
1	18% (302/1652)	1.0% (3/302)	—
2	17% (276/1652)	4.4% (12/276)	20% (7/35)
3	13% (209/1652)	12% (26/209)	37% (26/71)
4	7.3% (121/1652)	13% (16/121)	49% (26/53)
5	0.9% (15/1652)	53% (8/15)	50% (5/10)

[a]Risk factors for regional lymph node metastases include: (1) large primary tumor (>10 cm); (2) clinical stage T3/T4; (3) high tumor grade (Fuhrman grade 3 or 4); (4) sarcomatoid features; or (5) histologic tumor necrosis.
[b]Data from (Blute et al., 2004b); lymph node dissection performed in 58% of 1652 patients overall.
[c]Data from (Crispen et al., 2011); lymph node dissection performed in 41% of 415 patients with 2+ risk factors.

therapeutic benefit to lymphadenectomy in patients with nonmetastatic RCC, despite a comprehensive analysis that evaluated several intermediate and high-risk cohorts (Gershman et al., 2017b). However, a large, European study of 1983 patients suggested better cancer-specific survival in patients with large, bulky tumors and sarcomatoid features when a more extensive lymph node dissection was performed (Capitanio et al., 2014). In addition, rare patients with isolated lymph node metastases (analogous to isolated systemic metastases) may experience a durable survival with resection to cancer-free status (Gershman et al., 2017b). Therefore **lymphadenectomy may be performed in patients with clinically suspicious (radiographic or intraoperative) lymphadenopathy for staging purposes and, because of lack of data indicating a reliable therapeutic benefit, need not be performed routinely in patients with localized kidney cancer and clinically negative nodes.**

Local Recurrence After Radical Nephrectomy or Nephron-Sparing Surgery

Local recurrences of RCC can occur after RN and nephron-sparing surgery and present unique challenges. **Local recurrence of RCC after RN, which includes recurrence in the renal fossa, ipsilateral adrenal gland, renal vein stump or adjacent IVC, or ipsilateral retroperitoneal lymph nodes, is an uncommon event, occurring in 2% to 4% of cases** (Margulis et al., 2009). **Risk factors include locally advanced or node-positive disease and adverse histopathologic features** (Esrig et al., 1992; Levy et al., 1998; Sandock et al., 1995). In contrast, local recurrence after RN is rare in patients with organ-confined RCC. **Only about 20% to 40% of local recurrences are isolated; the majority of patients with local recurrence also have systemic disease, and a thorough metastatic evaluation should be pursued** (Eggener et al., 2008; Schrodter et al., 2002).

Surgical resection of isolated local recurrence of RCC after RN should be considered, because it can provide long-term cancer-free status for 30% to 40% of patients (Bandi et al., 2008; Margulis et al., 2009; Master et al., 2005; Yohannan et al., 2010). Complete resection of abdominal recurrence is often a formidable task because the natural tissue barriers are no longer present and invasion of contiguous organs is common. En bloc resection of adjacent organs is often required, and the risk of morbidity can be substantial (Eggener et al., 2008; Gogus et al., 2003; Margulis et al., 2009). Margulis et al. (2009) reported on 54 patients with local recurrence after nephrectomy managed by surgical resection, 69% of whom also received adjunctive systemic therapy. Risk factors associated with cancer-specific death after resection included recurrent tumor size, sarcomatoid features in the recurrence specimen, positive surgical margins, abnormal alkaline phosphatase, and increased lactate dehydrogenase. Patients with 0, 1, and greater than 1 adverse risk features demonstrated cancer-specific survival times of 111, 40, and 8 months, respectively. Intraoperative radiation has not been found to impart an oncologic benefit (Master et al., 2005), but radiation therapy may be of value for palliation of symptomatic local recurrence in patients who are not operative candidates.

Local recurrence in the remnant kidney after PN for RCC has been reported in 1.4% to 10% of patients, and the main risk factors are advanced T stage or high tumor grade (Campbell and Novick, 1994; Krambeck et al., 2008; Lane and Gill, 2007). Historically, positive surgical margins associated with PN were thought to have little impact on recurrence rates and cancer-specific survival (Bansal et al., 2017; Kutikov et al., 2008; Kwon et al., 2007; Yossepowitch et al., 2008;). However, recent data indicate that positive surgical margins, especially in patients with high-grade or high-stage disease may portend worse recurrence-free and metastases-free survival (Khalifeh et al., 2013; Shah et al., 2016b). This phenomenon may reflect expanding indications for PN or evolution of surgical technique to maximize functional renal parenchyma (Kutikov et al., 2008). Most patients with a positive surgical margin are managed with close surveillance rather than reflex completion nephrectomy, although the latter may occasionally be a valid consideration if the margins are grossly involved and the contralateral kidney is cancer-free and functioning well. **Patients with isolated local recurrence after PN can be considered for repeat PN, completion nephrectomy, TA, or AS** (Berger et al., 2009; Bratslavsky et al., 2008; Johnson et al., 2008; Magera et al., 2008a).

As a surgical management strategy, TA carries the highest risk of persistence or local recurrence following a single treatment (Pierorazio et al., 2016a). However, most local recurrences after TA can be salvaged with repeat TA, and there are no differences in metastatic recurrence rates or cancer-specific survival when compared with other treatment pathways, presuming reasonable patient selection. Reported incidences of local recurrence or persistence range between 3% and 10% for cryoablation and between 5% and 20% for RFA (Kunkle and Uzzo, 2008; Levinson et al., 2008; Weight et al., 2008). Management options are similar to those for recurrence after PN, with the caveat that salvage surgery in this setting is often challenging because of the dense inflammatory reaction induced by TA (Kowalczyk et al., 2009; Nguyen et al., 2008).

Neoadjuvant and Adjuvant Therapy for Renal Cell Carcinoma

Unfortunately, recurrence develops in a significant proportion of patients thought to be rendered disease free after surgical resection, primarily because of occult micrometastatic disease. Although postsurgical recurrence is not common in patients with low-stage, organ-confined disease, locally advanced RCC and RCC with other adverse histopathologic features carry a significant risk of recurrence. Various predictive tools can assist in the assessment of the risk in individual patients (Kim et al., 2012), although in general, **distant metastases develop in 20% to 35% and local recurrence in 2% to 5% of patients** (Lane and Kattan, 2008). In view of these findings, a strong rationale for systemic adjuvant therapy exists in high-risk patients.

> **KEY POINTS: TREATMENT OF LOCAL RECURRENCE AND ADJUVANT THERAPY FOR RENAL CELL CARCINOMA**
>
> - Isolated local recurrence after RN occurs in 2% to 4% of patients, and a thorough metastatic evaluation should be pursued. If this evaluation is negative, surgical excision should be considered, although en bloc resection of adjacent organs may be required because of obliteration of tissue planes.
> - Local recurrence after PN is more common at sites distant from the tumor bed and can be managed by repeat PN, completion nephrectomy, TA, or AS.
> - Local recurrence after TA often reflects incomplete tumor eradication; management options include repeat TA, AS, or salvage surgery.
> - Despite a significant likelihood of recurrence of RCC with poor-risk features, there is no established evidence of a benefit for adjuvant therapy in patients who appear to be cancer-free after surgical resection, and observation remains the standard of care.
> - Ongoing adjuvant clinical trials investigating targeted molecular agents, checkpoint inhibitors, and other novel systemic approaches should be supported in an effort to identify an efficacious adjuvant strategy.

Historically, randomized trials of adjuvant therapy failed to demonstrate any survival benefit using a variety of agents including IL-2 (Clark et al., 2003), interferon alpha (Messing et al., 2003; Pizzocaro et al., 2001), medroxyprogesterone acetate (Pizzocaro et al., 1987), and radiation therapy (van der Werf-Messing, 1973). Autologous tumor vaccine–based approaches have also been used to immunize RCC patients in the postoperative setting, again with essentially negative results (Galligioni et al., 1996; Jocham et al., 2004; Wood et al., 2008). The ARISER adjuvant trial investigated girentuximab, a chimeric monoclonal antibody directed against G250, a cell surface antigen expressed by the majority of clear cell RCC; and in 2012, the interim analysis showed no improvement in median disease-free survival and the trial was terminated (Chamie et al., 2017).

The emergence of targeted molecular agents and subsequent responses in metastatic disease led to great enthusiasm for new adjuvant trials in high-risk populations. By 2012 six ongoing adjuvant trials were enrolling worldwide, and, as of early 2019, four had been reported (Table 97.20). The double-blind, phase 3 ASSURE trial reported outcomes for 1934 patients with nonmetastatic, pT1b (high-grade), pT2-4 or N1 RCC randomized to sunitinib, sorafenib, or placebo and failed to demonstrate a recurrence-free survival benefit at 6 years (Haas et al., 2016). Importantly, 45% of patients discontinued therapy because of toxicity. The phase 3 PROTECT trial randomized 1538 patients with pT2 (high grade) or at least pT3, including N1, clear cell RCC to pazopanib versus placebo and demonstrated no benefit in disease-free survival (Motzer et al., 2017a). The phase 3 S-TRAC randomized 615 men with pT2 (high-grade), pT3-4 or

TABLE 97.20 Ongoing or Recently Completed Clinical Trials of Adjuvant Treatment for Renal Cell Carcinoma (RCC)

TRIAL	STUDY GROUPS	TREATMENT DURATION (NO. PATIENTS)	INCLUSION CRITERIA	RESULTS
TARGETED MOLECULAR AGENTS				
Adjuvant Sorafenib or Sunitinib for Unfavorable Renal Cell Carcinoma (ASSURE) (Haas et al., 2016)	Sunitinib vs. sorafenib vs. placebo	1 year (1943 patients)	Clear cell and non–clear cell RCC eligible Stage T2–T4 or stage T1b and G3–G4, or N1 if complete dissection performed	No difference in disease-free or overall survival at 6 years; 45% of patients in treatment arms discontinued therapy because of toxicity leading to early discontinuation of trial
Sorafenib for Patients with Resected Primary Renal Cell Carcinoma (SORCE)	Sorafenib (for 1 or 3 years) vs. placebo	3 years (1711 patients)	Clear cell and non–clear cell RCC eligible Mayo Clinic progression score 3–11	Completed enrollment 2012; awaiting results
Sunitinib vs. Placebo for the Treatment of Patients at High Risk for Recurrent Renal Cell Cancer (S-TRAC) (Ravaud et al., 2016)	Sunitinib vs. placebo	1 year (615 patients)	Predominant clear cell histology eligible High-risk RCC according to UISS[a]	Significantly longer disease-free survival in sunitinib group (6.8 versus 5.6 years; $P = 0.03$) with higher rate of toxic events; no difference in overall survival
Everolimus for Renal Cancer Ensuing Surgical Therapy (EVEREST)	Everolimus vs. placebo	1 year (1545 patients)	Clear cell and non–clear cell RCC eligible Stage T2–T4 or stage T1b and G3–G4, or N1 if complete dissection performed	Estimated study completion, 2021
Adjuvant Axitinib Treatment of Renal Cancer (ATLAS)	Axitinib vs. placebo	3 years (700 patients)	Clear cell predominant (>50%) eligible pT2 and G3–G4, or pT3a and > 4 cm, or pT3b/pT3c/pT4, or N1	No difference in disease-specific or overall survival
Pazopanib as an Adjuvant Treatment for Locally Advanced Renal Cell Carcinoma (PROTECT) (Motzer et al., 2017a)	Pazopanib vs. placebo	1 year (1538 patients)	Clear cell predominant (>50%) eligible pT2 and G3–G4, pT3, pT4, or N1	No benefit in disease-free survival or overall survival
IMMUNOMODULATORY CHECKPOINT INHIBITORS				
A Phase 3 Randomized Study Comparing Perioperative Nivolumab vs. Observation in Patients With Localized Renal Cell Carcinoma Undergoing Nephrectomy (PROSPER RCC)	Neoadjuvant nivolumab for 1 month, followed by nephrectomy, followed by adjuvant nivolumab for 9 months vs. nephrectomy alone; no placebo group	10 months (766 patients)	Up to 15% non–clear cell component; pT2-4, NX, M0; pT any, N1–N2, M0; all grades included	Estimated study completion, 2022

Continued

TABLE 97.20 Ongoing or Recently Completed Clinical Trials of Adjuvant Treatment for Renal Cell Carcinoma (RCC)—cont'd

TRIAL	STUDY GROUPS	TREATMENT DURATION (NO. PATIENTS)	INCLUSION CRITERIA	RESULTS
A Study of Atezolizumab as Adjuvant Therapy in Participants With Renal Cell Carcinoma (RCC) at High Risk of Developing Metastasis Following Nephrectomy (IMmotion010)	Adjuvant atezolizumab vs. placebo	1 year (664 patients)	Clear cell, or non–clear cell with sarcomatoid component; pT2, NX, M0, grade 4; pT3a, NX, M0, grade 3–4; pT3b/c, NX, M0, any grade; pT any, N+, M0, any grade; fully resected M1 disease; selected patients	Estimated study completion, 2024

[a]UISS: UCLA Integrated Staging System (Zisman et al., 2002).
Data from Haas NB, Manola J, Uzzo RG, et al.: Adjuvant sunitinib or sorafenib for high-risk, non-metastatic renal-cell carcinoma (ECOG-ACRIN E2805): a double-blind, placebo-controlled, randomised, phase 3 trial. *Lancet* 387(10032):2008–2016, 2016; Motzer RJ, Haas NB, Donskov F, et al.: Randomized Phase III trial of adjuvant pazopanib versus placebo after nephrectomy in patients with localized or locally advanced renal cell carcinoma. *J Clin Oncol* Jco2017735324, 2017a; Ravaud A, Motzer RJ, Pandha HS, et al.: Adjuvant sunitinib in high-risk renal-cell carcinoma after nephrectomy. *New Engl J Med* 375(23):2246–2254, 2016; Zisman A, Pantuck AJ, Wieder J, et al.: Risk group assessment and clinical outcome algorithm to predict the natural history of patients with surgically resected renal cell carcinoma. *J Clin Oncol* 20(23):4559–4566, 2002.

N1 clear cell RCC to subitinib or placebo (Ravaud et al., 2016). S-TRAC reported a significantly longer disease-free survival in the sunitinib group (6.8 versus 5.6 years) compared with placebo. ATLAS randomized patients to 3 years of axitinib versus placebo and failed to demonstrate an advantage for disease-free survival (Gross-Goupil et al., 2018). Difference in risk profiles of the enrolled patients, average doses of TKI received in the treatment arms, and restriction to clear cell–only patients in some of the trials may account for the observed differences in outcomes. However, in all of these trials patients receiving therapy experienced significantly higher rates of adverse events and there were no differences in overall survival. **Given these results, none of the adjuvant studies in this field is convincingly positive, and the standard of care remains observation if the patient will not consider an adjuvant trial** (Haas and Uzzo, 2018; Ridyard et al., 2019; Sun et al., 2018). More recent trials are testing immunologic modulators, such as check point inhibitors, in the adjuvant setting as the search for an efficacious adjuvant strategy continues (see Table 97.20). Please refer to Chapter 104 for a more detailed discussion of these protocols and their rationale for patients with advanced RCC.

Neoadjuvant therapy, with either VEGF-targeted agents or checkpoint inhibitors, represents a new and promising treatment paradigm with the potential advantages of tumor cytoreduction and eradication of micrometastatic disease. Emerging data from phase 2 studies using pazopanib, sunitinib, sorafenib, or axitinib indicate consistent primary tumor size reduction with average volume reductions of 10% to 31% (Bindayi et al., 2018). In patients with imperative indications for nephron-sparing but in whom surgery is felt to be unsafe, unfeasible, or not optimized, neoadjuvant therapy may facilitate tumor resection (Rini et al., 2015). Further prospective investigation is needed before oncologic outcomes can be evaluated. Six ongoing, early phase neoadjuvant therapy trials are investigating checkpoint inhibitors or other immunomodulatory compounds (Bindayi et al., 2018).

OTHER MALIGNANT RENAL TUMORS

Sarcomas of the Kidney

Sarcomas represent 1% to 2% of all malignant renal tumors in adults, with a peak incidence in the fifth decade of life (Miller et al., 2010a; Vogelzang et al., 1993). Renal sarcoma is less common but more lethal than sarcoma of any other genitourinary site, including the prostate, bladder, and paratesticular region (Russo et al., 1992). **Differentiation of renal sarcoma from sarcomatoid RCC is often difficult based on clinical presentation, radiographic findings, and, in some cases, pathologic analysis.** Identification of any features of the various subtypes of RCC excludes the diagnosis of primary renal sarcoma. The common signs and symptoms associated with renal sarcoma in adults include palpable mass, abdominal or flank pain, and hematuria and are similar to those seen with large, rapidly growing RCC (Economou et al., 1987). Specific findings suggestive of sarcoma rather than RCC include apparent origin from the capsule or perisinuous region, growth to large size in the absence of lymphadenopathy, presence of fat or bone suggestive of liposarcoma or osteosarcoma, and hypovascular pattern, although one notable exception is the hemangiopericytoma, which is highly vascular (Shirkhoda and Lewis, 1987). Renal sarcoma should be suspected in any of these circumstances or in any patient with a very large or rapidly growing renal mass (Table 97.21).

Sarcomas of the kidney, like sarcomas of any other site, are derived from mesenchymal components and are thus free of many of the natural barriers to dissemination that confine other tumor types (Russo et al., 1992). **These tumors are typically surrounded by a pseudocapsule that is often infiltrated with cancer cells,** which can extend for some distance into the surrounding tissues. In many cases this cannot be recognized macroscopically, although it is often manifested in the form of local recurrences, which are common after surgical extirpation, even when wide excision has been performed. **High-grade sarcomas often metastasize, with the lungs being a primary site of spread, and prognosis is poor; some patients die of disease progression in a matter of months. Low-grade sarcomas tend to pursue a more indolent course,** although local recurrences often require repeat resection to prolong survival and minimize morbidity.

In general, **the most important prognostic factors for sarcomas are margin status and tumor grade. The initial resection is the key event because this is the best chance for a long-term cure.** For renal sarcomas this often mandates RN along with en bloc excision of adjacent organs (Brescia et al., 2008; Dotan et al., 2006; Wang et al., 2011). MRI can be useful for preoperative planning by defining tissue planes and proximity to vital structures. This is primarily a surgical disease, and wide excision is the goal with intraoperative monitoring of margin status. Chemotherapeutic agents traditionally used against metastatic sarcomas included doxycycline and ifosfamide, and more recently gemcitabine and docetaxel have been explored. Tyrosine kinase inhibitors and other novel approaches are also being investigated for soft tissue sarcomas, but even in the best

TABLE 97.21 Characteristics of Other Malignant Renal Tumors

TUMOR TYPE	CHARACTERISTICS	MANAGEMENT
Sarcomas	Leiomyosarcoma most common Typically hypovascular Often rapidly growing and occasionally appear to be derived from the renal capsule	Wide local excision with confirmation of negative margins
Renal lymphoma and leukemia	Multiple radiographic patterns described Typically hypovascular Suspect in patients with massive retroperitoneal lymphadenopathy or lymphadenopathy in other regions of the body or atypical locations	Biopsy should be considered Extirpative surgery should be avoided Typically managed with chemotherapy and/or radiation therapy
Metastatic tumors	Most common sources include lung, breast, and gastrointestinal cancers, malignant melanoma, and hematologic malignancies Typically hypovascular and multifocal	Biopsy should be strongly considered Typically managed with systemic therapy or palliative care
Carcinoid	Typically hypovascular May present with carcinoid syndrome Derived from neuroendocrine cells	Surgical excision
Small cell carcinoma of the kidney	Neuroendocrine derivation Typically hypovascular Most locally advanced or metastatic	Multimodal therapy with surgery and platinum-based chemotherapy
Primitive neuroectodermal tumor	Derived from primitive neural crest cells Hypovascular pattern typical Poor prognosis	Multimodal therapy
Wilms tumor	Heterogeneous solid renal mass on computed tomography More common in children, but occasionally seen in adults	Multimodal therapy analogous to treatment protocols for pediatric Wilms tumor

of circumstances response rates are disappointing (Antman et al., 1993; Frezza et al., 2017; Miller et al., 2010b; Ratan and Patel, 2016; Ravi et al., 2015).

The combination of radiation therapy and chemotherapy, which has an established role in the adjuvant setting for the management of sarcomas of the extremity, has not been as effective for renal or retroperitoneal sarcomas (Russo et al., 1992; Shah et al., 2016; Wortman et al., 2016). Recent data indicate that preoperative radiation therapy may reduce the incidence of positive margins (Shah et al., 2016; Wortman et al., 2016), which is particularly important in a disease state where administration of postoperative radiation is anatomically challenging. Intraoperative radiation has demonstrated some benefit for renal and retroperitoneal sarcomas with minimal additional morbidity (Abdelfatah et al., 2017). At present, the role of such adjuvant approaches for the management of renal sarcomas is not well defined, although a multimodal approach is often pursued if performance status allows, given the poor prognosis.

The largest single-institution series of renal sarcomas include only 15 to 41 cases and represent a composite experience extending for a period of several years (Shirkhoda and Lewis, 1987; Wang et al., 2011). In all such series, leiomyosarcoma is the most common histologic subtype, and in many series, liposarcoma is the second most common entity. For retroperitoneal sarcomas, in contrast, the order is reversed with liposarcoma most common (Karakousis et al., 1995). All such series report a poor prognosis; the experience of Srinivas et al. (1984) at Memorial Sloan Kettering Cancer Center is representative. In this series of 16 patients with renal sarcomas, 15 underwent nephrectomy, often with en bloc excision of adjacent organs; 5 received adjuvant radiation therapy and chemotherapy without apparent benefit; and 13 died within 6 months after surgery.

Leiomyosarcoma accounts for 50% to 60% of renal sarcomas, and the cell of origin is the smooth muscle cell of the capsule or other perinephric structures (Fig. 97.26; Deyrup et al., 2004; Moudouni et al., 2001; Wang et al., 2011). Niceta et al. (1974) identified 66 cases of renal leiomyosarcoma in the literature and reported a female predominance with most patients diagnosed in the fourth through sixth decades of life. Renal leiomyosarcoma, like other renal sarcomas, tends to displace rather than invade the parenchyma and is characterized by rapid growth rate, frequent metastasis, and high local and systemic recurrence rates (Deyrup et al., 2004; Kendal, 2007). In the cases reviewed by Niceta et al. (1974), most patients were treated primarily with RN and died within 2 years. In the Mayo Clinic series, 14 of 15 patients with renal leiomyosarcoma died of disease progression within 4 months to 5½ years after surgery (Frank et al., 2000).

Other than leiomyosarcoma, a wide variety of histologic subtypes have been described, and almost every conceivable type of sarcoma has been found in the kidney. **Liposarcoma** is readily distinguished from RCC because of the presence of adipose tissue but is often confused with AMLs or large, benign renal lipomas (Frank et al., 2000). Renal liposarcoma often grows to extremely large size. Response to radiation therapy and cisplatin-based chemotherapy in an adjuvant setting has been reported and should be considered in patients with high-grade disease or positive margins (Belldegrun and DeKernion, 1987).

Osteogenic sarcoma is a rare but distinctive form of renal sarcoma that contains calcium and is often rock hard (Leventis et al., 1997; Micolonghi et al., 1984). Extensive calcification in a large, hypovascular tumor should suggest the diagnosis. The appearance on plain films can mimic a staghorn calculus, but the readily evident mass effect should suggest xanthogranulomatous disease or, more rarely, osteogenic sarcoma. **Less common histologic subtypes include rhabdomyosarcoma, fibrosarcoma, malignant fibrous histiocytoma, and others** (see Table 97.1; Srigley et al., 2013). **Malignant hemangiopericytomas** are notable for their extensive vascularity (Brescia et al., 2008; Chaudhary et al., 2007). Preoperative angioembolization has been described and may simplify surgical excision (Smullens et al., 1982).

Renal Lymphoma and Leukemia

Renal involvement with hematologic malignancies, which include the lymphomas and leukemias, is common, found at autopsy in

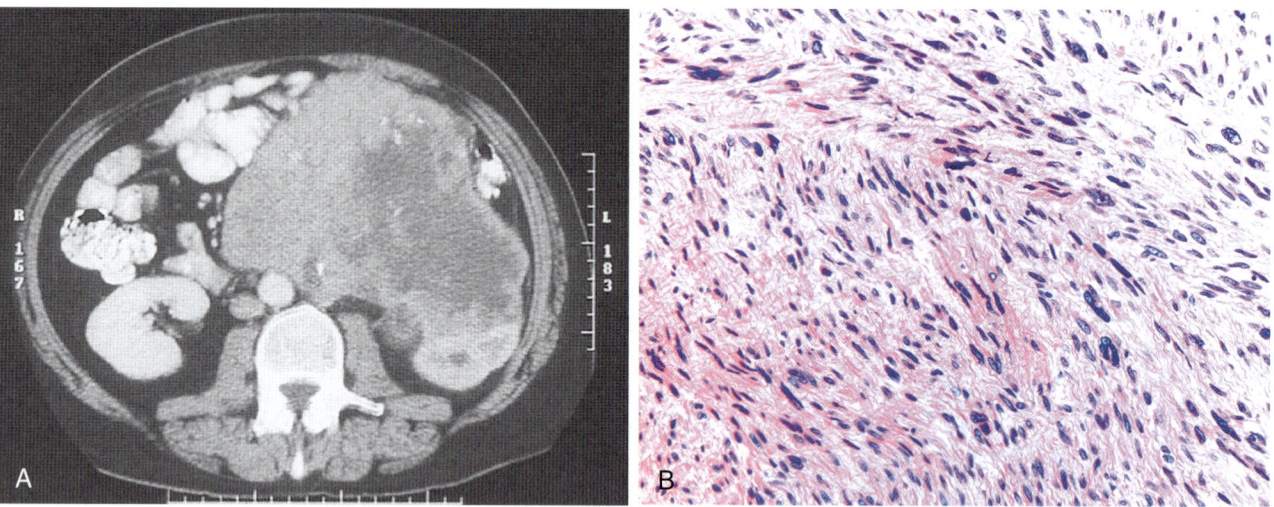

Fig. 97.26. (A) Computed tomography scan demonstrates a large leiomyosarcoma of the left kidney. (B) Microscopic features of leiomyosarcoma include spindle cells, blunt-ended nuclei, and eosinophilic cytoplasm. (Courtesy Dr. Michael McGuire, Evanston, IL and Dr. Ming Zhou, Cleveland, OH.)

approximately 34% of patients dying of progressive lymphoma or leukemia. However, these processes are uncommonly seen in clinical practice because they are often silent and generally occur only as a late manifestation of systemic disease (McVary, 1991; Pollack et al., 1987). The role of the urologist in the evaluation of renal lymphoma or leukemia is critical and can include differentiation from other renal malignant neoplasms, timely provision of a pathologic diagnosis, and preservation of renal function (McVary, 1991).

Renal involvement is more common with non-Hodgkin lymphoma than with Hodgkin disease, and, as with most other forms of extranodal non-Hodgkin lymphoma, histologically diffuse forms predominate over nodular forms (O'Riordan et al., 2001; Pollack et al., 1987). Primary renal lymphoma is rare, with only a few well-documented case reports in the literature (Ahmad et al., 2005; Garcia et al., 2007; Pollack et al., 1987). This is not surprising given the relative paucity of lymphoid tissue in the normal renal parenchyma. Hematogenous dissemination of lymphoma to the kidney is most common and is thought to occur in 90% of cases; direct extension from retroperitoneal lymph nodes accounts for the remainder. Hartman et al. (1982) have shown that the most common pattern of renal involvement consists of multiple small malignant lymphoid nodules interlaced between the individual nephrons. Eventually, these nodules become confluent, forming radiographically detectable masses. At the extreme, they can replace the entire parenchyma, leading to renal failure.

CT scan is the radiographic modality of choice for the diagnosis of renal lymphoma and for monitoring response to therapy, although MRI can be used in patients with renal insufficiency, contrast medium allergy, or in children and young adults in whom lifelong radiation exposure is a consideration (Pollack et al., 1987; Urban and Fishman, 2000). The common radiographic patterns associated with renal lymphoma include multiple distinct renal masses; as a solitary renal mass, which can be difficult to differentiate from RCC; as diffuse renal infiltration; or as direct invasion of the kidney from enlarged retroperitoneal nodes (Ganeshan et al., 2013; Heiken et al., 1983; Sheth et al., 2006; Table 97.22). **Renal lymphoma should be suspected in patients with massive retroperitoneal lymphadenopathy, splenomegaly, or lymphadenopathy in other regions of the body or atypical regions within the retroperitoneum.** Relative to this, the main lymphatic landing zones for RCC should be kept in mind—the interaortocaval region for right RCC and para-aortic region for left RCC—and lymphadenopathy centered outside of these areas should raise suspicion for lymphoma. Any patient with a prior history of lymphoma and a renal mass should

TABLE 97.22 Computed Tomographic Findings Associated With Renal Lymphoma

FINDING	INCIDENCE (%)
Multiple renal masses	45
Solitary renal mass	15
Renal invasion from enlarged retroperitoneal lymph nodes	25
Diffuse renal involvement	10
Predominantly perinephric involvement	5

Data from Heiken JP, Gold RP, Schnur MJ, et al.: Computed tomography of renal lymphoma with ultrasound correlation. *J Comput Assist Tomogr* 7(2):245–250, 1983; Pollack HM, Banner MP, Amendola MA: Other malignant neoplasms of the renal parenchyma. *Semin Roentgenol* 22(4):260–274, 1987.

also be evaluated for renal recurrence rather than for RCC. In general, lymphomas are more common in patients with iatrogenic immune suppression, acquired immunodeficiency syndrome, autoimmune diseases, or graft-versus-host disease, and a history of radiation therapy (McVary, 1991). These clinical associations may also increase the index of suspicion about a diagnosis of systemic lymphoma.

Renal involvement related to leukemia is more common in children, paralleling the demographics of the disease, and is more commonly due to lymphocytic leukemia than the myelogenous forms (Pollack et al., 1987). Leukemia typically involves the kidney in a diffusely infiltrative pattern and most often represents a late manifestation of systemic disease.

If lymphoma or leukemic renal involvement is suspected, consideration should be given to percutaneous biopsy or aspiration to obtain a pathologic diagnosis (Ganeshan et al., 2013; Herts, 2012); if exploratory surgery is necessary, intraoperative biopsy and frozen-section analysis should take priority. **Extirpative surgery should be avoided if renal lymphoma and leukemia are suspected because the primary treatment of these processes is systemic chemotherapy with or without radiation therapy** (McVary, 1991). The classic chemotherapy regimen for non-Hodgkin lymphoma is the CHOP protocol, which includes cyclophosphamide, doxorubicin, vincristine, and prednisolone (Colevas et al., 2000). Recent reports suggest that adding rituximab to the CHOP protocol ("R-CHOP") may improve short-term renal function and long-term survival. Nephrectomy is only indicated in patients with severe symptoms, such as uncontrollable hemorrhage. The other notable exception is the extremely rare patient with primary renal lymphoma in whom a combination of nephrectomy and systemic chemotherapy may represent optimal therapy (Garcia et al., 2007; Hart et al., 2012). Fourteen cases of marginal zone B-cell lymphoma of mucosa-associated lymphoid tissue localized to the kidney have been described, with some apparently cured by surgery alone (Garcia et al., 2007).

Renal lymphoma and leukemia are commonly silent but can be associated with hematuria, flank pain, or progressive renal failure. Fever, weight loss, and fatigue, the so-called B symptoms of lymphoma, are much more common (Zomas et al., 2004). Renal failure can be due to extensive replacement of the functioning parenchyma or bilateral ureteral obstruction associated with enlarged retroperitoneal lymph nodes (McVary, 1991). In reality, renal failure in such patients is more often related to medical causes, such as hypercalcemia or urate nephropathy, which can develop during systemic treatment of advanced disease (Luciano and Brewster, 2014).

Metastatic Tumors

Metastatic tumors are the most common malignant neoplasms in the kidney. Autopsy studies have shown that 12% of patients dying of cancer have renal metastases, making the kidney one of the most common sites for metastatic dissemination (Pollack et al., 1987). **Almost all renal metastases develop through a hematogenous route of spread because of the profuse vascularity of the kidney.** Direct invasion of tumors derived from adjacent organs (such as the pancreas, colon, and adrenal gland) is much less common. **The most frequent sources of renal metastases include lung, breast, and gastrointestinal cancers, malignant melanoma, and the hematologic malignant neoplasms** (Aron et al., 2004; Choyke et al., 1987; Pollack et al., 1987; Tomita et al., 2015; Wu et al., 2014). Of the solid malignant neoplasms, lung cancer is most commonly associated with renal metastases. **Most renal metastases are multifocal, and almost all are associated with widespread nonrenal metastases.** However, renal metastases from lung, breast, and colon carcinomas are notable because they are occasionally large and solitary, making them difficult to differentiate from RCC (Choyke et al., 1987; Pollack et al., 1987; Wu et al., 2014).

The typical pattern of renal metastases consists of multiple small nodules that are often clinically silent, although they can lead to hematuria or flank pain in exceptional circumstances (Pollack et al., 1987). CT typically demonstrates isodense masses that enhance only moderately (5 to 30 HU) after administration of intravenous contrast material (Ahmad et al., 2005). **Renal metastases should be suspected in any patient with multiple renal lesions and widespread systemic metastases or a history of nonrenal primary cancer. If there is uncertainty about the diagnosis, percutaneous renal biopsy usually provides pathologic confirmation** (Sanchez-Ortiz et al., 2004a; Wu et al., 2014). Most patients with renal metastases are managed with systemic therapy or placed on a palliative care pathway, depending on the clinical circumstances. Nephrectomy is almost never required except in extenuating circumstances, such as renal hemorrhage that is refractory to embolization. Patients with a solitary, strongly enhancing renal lesion and a history of organ-confined, nonrenal malignant disease are more likely to have RCC, particularly if the temporal interval between the two diagnoses is substantial (Rybicki et al., 2003; Sanchez-Ortiz et al., 2004a). In one study involving 100 consecutive patients with a renal mass and a history of nonrenal malignancy, none of the 54 patients without other evidence of disease progression had a renal metastasis (Sanchez-Ortiz et al., 2004a).

Other Malignant Tumors of the Kidney

Other malignant tumors of the kidney include adult Wilms tumor and neuroendocrine tumors such as renal carcinoid, small cell carcinoma, and primitive neuroectodermal tumor (PNET). All are relatively uncommon, but each has distinct tumor biology.

Carcinoid is an uncommon renal malignant neoplasm with fewer than 60 cases reported in the English literature (Canacci and MacLennan, 2008; Hansel et al., 2007; Lane et al., 2007b; Romero et al., 2006). Median age at diagnosis is 49 years, and an association with horseshoe kidneys has been reported with increased relative risk of 82-fold compared with normal kidneys (Begin et al., 1998; Romero et al., 2006). Carcinoid tumors are derived from neuroendocrine cells and stain positive for neuron-specific enolase and chromogranin (Lane et al., 2007b). **Measurement of urinary or plasma serotonin or its metabolites can also be diagnostic** (Kulke and Mayer, 1999). **A minority of patients will present with the carcinoid syndrome—episodic flushing, wheezing, and diarrhea** (Lane et al., 2007b; Romero et al., 2006). Unfortunately, CT findings are nonspecific. Many renal carcinoids are small and nonaggressive yet metastases were found in 46% of patients at diagnosis in one review (Romero et al., 2006). Surgical excision is the mainstay of treatment with nephron-sparing surgery preferred if the diagnosis is suspected preoperatively (Kawajiri et al., 2004). Prognosis is generally good, particularly when associated with a horseshoe kidney (Begin et al., 1998). Significant adverse prognostic factors include age older than 40 years, tumor size greater than 4 cm, high mitotic rate, purely solid morphology, metastasis at initial diagnosis, and tumor extending through the renal capsule (Niceta et al., 1974).

Other neuroendocrine tumors, including small cell carcinoma and primary large cell neuroendocrine carcinoma, can occur in the kidney but are even less common than renal carcinoids (Dundr et al., 2010; Lane et al., 2007b; Majhail et al., 2003). Approximately 30 cases of small cell carcinoma of the kidney have been reported for which another primary site could not be identified (Kilicarsalan Akkaya et al., 2003; Kuroda et al., 2014; Mirza and Shahab, 2007). **On pathologic examination, small cell carcinoma has features of neuroendocrine and epithelial neoplasms and must be differentiated from Wilms tumor, PNET, lymphoma, and metastasis from pulmonary small cell carcinoma. Positive staining for neuron-specific enolase, chromogranin, and synaptophysin is characteristic** (Kilicarsalan Akkaya et al., 2003). Preoperative differentiation from RCC is difficult, although a relatively hypovascular pattern may be an indication. Many small cell carcinomas of the kidney are locally advanced or metastatic at presentation, and flank pain or hematuria is common. Multimodal therapy with surgical tumor debulking combined with platinum-based chemotherapy regimens is advocated for extrapulmonary small cell carcinoma in general and may also be useful for the renal manifestation of this malignancy, but the prognosis remains poor (Carranza et al., 2013; Majhail et al., 2003; Mirza and Shahab, 2007).

PNET is related to the Ewing sarcoma family of tumors that are more common in the pediatric population, typically manifesting in the bone or soft tissues of the extremities, trunk, and head and neck and only rarely in the viscera or kidneys (Bartholow and Parwani, 2012; Jimenez et al., 2002; Maly et al., 2004). However, all ages may be affected, and several cases of PNET have been reported in the kidneys of adults (Ellinger et al., 2006; Narayanan et al., 2017; Thyavihally et al., 2008). These tumors are derived from primitive neural crest cells, and positive staining for CD99 in addition to vimentin, cytokeratin, and neuron-specific enolase strongly supports the diagnosis (Ellinger et al., 2006; Gonlusen et al., 2001; Maly et al., 2004). On microscopic examination, renal PNET typically shows small round cells that may form Homer-Wright rosettes (Thyavihally et al., 2008). A characteristic t(11;22)(q24;q12) translocation is highly specific for PNET and can help differentiate it from neuroblastoma or adult Wilms tumor (Jimenez et al., 2002; Parham et al., 2001). Clinical symptoms are nonspecific; CT often demonstrates a heterogeneous ill-defined mass with areas of necrosis, and equivocal enhancement with contrast medium is typical (Doerfler et al., 2001; Narayanan et al., 2017). Renal PNET appears to behave more aggressively than similar tumors at other sites, exhibiting a strong propensity for local recurrence and early metastasis to lymph nodes, lung, liver, and bone (Gonlusen et al., 2001; Parham et al., 2001; Thyavihally et al., 2008). **Multimodal treatment protocols combining tumor debulking, chemotherapy targeted to round cell or Ewing sarcoma family of tumors and radiotherapy to the renal bed are often employed, but prognosis is poor, with 5-year disease-free survival rates of 45% to 55%** (Ellinger et al., 2006; Narayanan et al., 2017; Thyavihally et al., 2008).

Wilms tumor is the most common abdominal malignant neoplasm in children, but 3% of Wilms tumors occur in adults. Of these, 20% are found between the ages of 15 and 20 years, and the remaining 80% are distributed between the third and seventh decades of life (Li et al., 2011; Winter et al., 1996). Adult and pediatric Wilms tumors are histologically similar with a distinctive triphasic pattern consisting of varying amounts of blastema, epithelium, and stroma. **Pathologic staging is the same as for pediatric Wilms tumor.** Adult Wilms tumor typically presents as a heterogeneous intrarenal mass on CT with a relatively hypovascular pattern. Differentiation from RCC can be difficult if not impossible in many cases (Modi et al., 2016; Reinhard et al., 2004; Winter et al., 1996). Clinical presentation of adult Wilms tumor is also similar to that of RCC, and this tends to be an unsuspected pathologic diagnosis in most cases. **Multimodal therapy should be considered, analogous to the treatment protocols for pediatric Wilms tumor** (Li et al., 2011; Modi et al., 2016; Reinhard et al., 2004; Terenziani et al., 2004; Varma et al., 2015). **Prognosis is worse for adults with Wilms tumor than for children** because adults are more likely to present with advanced disease and a sudden drop in performance status (Terenziani et al., 2004; Varma et al., 2015; Winter et al., 1996).

SUGGESTED READINGS

Amin MB, Edge SB, Greene FL, et al, editors: *AJCC cancer staging manual*, ed 8, New York, 2017, Springer.

Bindayi A, Hamilton ZA, McDonald ML, et al: Neoadjuvant therapy for localized and locally advanced renal cell carcinoma, *Urol Oncol* 36(1):31–37, 2017.

Blom JH, van Poppel H, Maréchal JM, et al: Radical nephrectomy with and without lymph-node dissection: final results of European Organization for Research and Treatment of Cancer (EORTC) randomized phase 3 trial 30881, *Eur Urol* 55(1):28–34, 2009.

Blute ML, Boorjian SA, Leibovich BC, et al: Results of inferior vena caval interruption by greenfield filter, ligation or resection during radical nephrectomy and tumor thrombectomy, *J Urol* 178(2):440–445, 2007.

Borregales LD, Kim DY, Staller AL, et al: Prognosticators and outcomes of patients with renal cell carcinoma and adjacent organ invasion treated with radical nephrectomy, *Urol Oncol* 34(237):e219–e226, 2016.

Bosniak MA: The Bosniak renal cyst classification: 25 years later, *Radiology* 262:781–785, 2012.

Campbell S, Uzzo RG, Allaf ME, et al: Renal mass and localized renal cancer: AUA guideline, *J Urol* 198:520–529, 2017.

Cancer Genome Atlas Research Network: Comprehensive molecular characterization of clear cell renal cell carcinoma, *Nature* 499:43–49, 2013.

Capitanio U, Montorsi F: Renal cancer, *Lancet* 387:894–906, 2016.

Ciancio G, Gonzalez J, Shirodkar SP, et al: Liver transplantation techniques for the surgical management of renal cell carcinoma with tumor thrombus in the inferior vena cava: step-by-step description, *Eur Urol* 59:401–406, 2011.

Crispen PL, Breau RH, Allmer C, et al: Lymph node dissection at the time of radical nephrectomy for high-risk clear cell renal cell carcinoma: indications and recommendations for surgical templates, *Eur Urol* 59:18–23, 2011.

Delahunt B, Cheville JC, Martignoni G, et al: International Society of Urological Pathology (ISUP) grading system for renal cell carcinoma and other prognostic parameters, *Am J Surg Pathol* 37(10):1490–1504, 2013.

Diaz de Leon A, Pedrosa I: Imaging and screening of kidney cancer, *Radiol Clin North Am* 55(6):1235–1250, 2017.

Donat SM, Diaz M, Bishoff JT, et al: Follow-up for clinically localized renal neoplasms: AUA guideline, *J Urol* 190:407–416, 2013.

Gershman B, Thompson RH, Moreira DM, et al: Radical nephrectomy with or without lymph node dissection for nonmetastatic renal cell carcinoma: a propensity score-based analysis, *Eur Urol* 71(4):560–567, 2017.

Gupta GN, Boris RS, Campbell SC, et al: Tumor enucleation for sporadic localized kidney cancer: pro and con, *J Urol* 194:623–625, 2015.

Herr HW: Surgical management of renal tumors: a historical perspective, *Urol Clin North Am* 35(4):543–549, 2008.

Joshi SS, Uzzo RG: Renal tumor anatomic complexity: clinical implications for urologists, *Urol Clin North Am* 44:179–187, 2017.

Kang SK, Chandarana H: Contemporary imaging of the renal mass, *Urol Clin North Am* 39:161–170, 2012.

Kelly EF, Leveillee RJ: Image guided radiofrequency ablation for small renal masses, *Int J Surg* 36:525–532, 2016.

Kim SP, Campbell SC, Gill I, et al: Collaborative review of risk benefit trade-offs between partial and radical nephrectomy in the management of anatomically complex renal masses, *Eur Urol* 72:64–75, 2017.

Kutikov A, Uzzo RG: The R.E.N.A.L. nephrometry score: a comprehensive standardized system for quantitating renal tumor size, location and depth, *J Urol* 182(3):844–853, 2009.

Ljungberg B, Bensalah K, Canfield S, et al: EAU guidelines on renal cell carcinoma: 2014 update, *Eur Urol* 67:913–924, 2015.

Marconi L, Dabestani S, Lam TB, et al: Systematic review and meta-analysis of diagnostic accuracy of percutaneous renal tumour biopsy, *Eur Urol* 69:660–673, 2016.

Margulis V, McDonald M, Tamboli P, et al: Predictors of oncological outcome after resection of locally recurrent renal cell carcinoma, *J Urol* 181:2044–2051, 2009.

Massari F, Di Nunno V, Ciccarese C, et al: Adjuvant therapy in renal cell carcinoma, *Cancer Treat Rev* 60:152–157, 2017.

Moch H, Cubilla AL, Humphrey PA, et al: The 2016 WHO classification of tumours of the urinary system and male genital organs – Part A: renal, penile, and testicular tumours, *Eur Urol* 70(1):93–105, 2016.

Pierorazio PM, Patel HD, Johnson MH, et al: Distinguishing malignant and benign renal masses with composite models and nomograms: a systematic review and meta-analysis of clinically localized renal masses suspicious for malignancy, *Cancer* 122(21):3267–3276, 2016.

Pierorazio PM, Johnson MH, Patel HD, et al: Management of renal masses and localized renal cancer: systematic review and meta-analysis, *J Urol* 196:989–999, 2016.

Ravaud A, Motzer RJ, Pandha HS, et al: Adjuvant sunitinib in high-risk renal-cell carcinoma after nephrectomy, *N Engl J Med* 375(23):2246–2254, 2016.

Rijnders M, de Wit R, Boormans JL, et al: Systematic review of immune checkpoint inhibition in urological cancers, *Eur Urol* 72:411–423, 2017.

Ristau BT, Correa AF, Uzzo RG, et al: Active surveillance for the small renal mass: growth kinetics and oncologic outcomes, *Urol Clin North Am* 44:213–222, 2017.

Scosyrev E, Messing EM, Sylvester R, et al: Renal function after nephron-sparing surgery versus radical nephrectomy: results from EORTC randomized trial 30904, *Eur Urol* 65:372–377, 2014.

Srigley JR, Delahunt B, Eble JN, et al: The International Society of Urological Pathology (ISUP) Vancouver classification of renal neoplasia, *Am J Surg Pathol* 37:1469–1489, 2013.

Sun M, Vetterlein M, Harshman LC, et al: Risk assessment in small renal masses: a review article, *Urol Clin North Am* 44:189–202, 2017.

Van Poppel H, Da Pozzo L, Albrecht W, et al: A prospective, randomised EORTC intergroup phase 3 study comparing the oncologic outcome of elective nephron-sparing surgery and radical nephrectomy for low-stage renal cell carcinoma, *Eur Urol* 59:543–552, 2011.

Volpe A, Blute ML, Ficarra V, et al: Renal ischemia and function after partial nephrectomy: a collaborative review of the literature, *Eur Urol* 68:61–74, 2015.

Zabell JR, Wu J, Suk-Ouichai C, et al: Renal ischemia and functional outcomes following kidney cancer surgery, *Urol Clin North Am* 44:243–255, 2017.

Zargar H, Atwell TD, Cadeddu JA, et al: Cryoablation for small renal masses: selection criteria, complications, and functional and oncologic results, *Eur Urol* 69:116–128, 2016.

REFERENCES

The complete reference list is available online at ExpertConsult.com.

98

Urothelial Tumors of the Upper Urinary Tract and Ureter

Panagiotis Kallidonis, MD, MSc, PhD, FEBU, and Evangelos Liatsikos, MD, PhD

EPIDEMIOLOGY

Incidence

Urothelial carcinomas are relatively common: they are the fourth most common tumor. Nevertheless, upper urinary tract carcinomas (UTUCs) make up only 5% to 10% of urothelial tumors (Munoz and Ellison, 2000; Siegel et al., 2013). The annual incidence of the UTUC in Western countries has been estimated at 2 cases per 100,000 inhabitants (Roupret et al., 2011; Soria et al., 2017). The highest incidence is observed in individuals aged 70 to 90, men, and in the Balkan countries, where UTUC represents 40% of all renal neoplasms (Grollman, 2013; Shariat et al., 2011). The incidence of UTUC has risen over the last few decades because of improved diagnostic methods employed in everyday practice (David et al., 2009; McCarron et al., 1983; Munoz and Ellison, 2000; Soria et al., 2017).

The majority of UTUCs are presented in a single renal unit, although up to 5% of patients have bilateral disease (Holmäng and Johansson, 2004). The involvement of the pelvicalyceal system is twice as common as with ureteral tumors. Multifocal presence of UTUC is diagnosed in 10% to 20% of cases. Concomitant carcinoma in situ (CIS) could be diagnosed in 11% to 36% of cases (Soria et al., 2017). Concurrent bladder cancer is diagnosed in 17% of cases (Cosentino et al., 2013). Up to 41% of American men with UTUC have a history of bladder cancer, whereas only 4% of the Chinese men with UTUC have a history of bladder cancer (Singla et al., 2017). Nonetheless, the Asian population seems to be seen initially with a higher-grade disease than other ethnic groups (Soria et al., 2017).

Disease recurrence after treatment involves the bladder in 22% to 47% of cases (Xylinas et al., 2012) and the contralateral upper tract in 2% to 6% (Li et al., 2010). Metachronous UTUC after treated bladder cancer could reach 80% of cases, and most of these occurrences take place in the renal pelvis rather than the ureter (Li et al., 2010; Novara et al., 2009). Approximately 60% of the UTUCs are invasive, and 7% have metastasized at diagnosis (Margulis et al., 2009).

The National Cancer Institute's Surveillance, Epidemiology, and End Results (SEER) database provided interesting data on the epidemiology of UTUC (Raman et al., 2010). The time ranged between 1975 to 2005. The annual incidence rates were 1.88 to 2.06 cases per 100,00 person-years. An increase in the annual incidence of ureteral neoplasms was observed during this period (0.69 to 0.91), while the pelvic lesions showed a slight decrease (1.19 to 1.15). A significantly higher proportion of earlier stage tumors has been observed over the study period. Earlier stage tumors represented only 7.2% of the UTUC cases in 1973 to 1984 and 31% in 1994 to 2005. The National Cancer Data Base (NCDB) for the United States for 1993 to 2005 confirmed the increase in early stage tumors of the ureter and pelvis and further noted an increase in the proportion of high-grade UTUCs (David et al., 2009).

Gender, Race, Age Variations, and Familial Predisposition

UTUCs are twice more frequent in men than in women (Greenlee et al., 2000; Lughezzani et al., 2010). African-Americans develop UTUC twice more often than the Caucasian population (Greenlee et al., 2000). Patients with UTUC are older than patients with urothelial bladder tumors (Melamed and Reuter, 1993) and tend to have worse prognosis (Audenet et al., 2012). Familial/hereditary upper tract tumors should be considered when the patient is younger than 60 years (Audenet et al., 2012).

Mortality Rate

Disease mortality has been related to increasing age, male gender, black non-Hispanic race, and advanced tumor stage (Raman et al., 2011). A SEER-based study evaluated data from 1973 to 1996 and showed 5-year disease-specific survival rates for overall, in situ, localized, regional, and distant disease of 75%, 95%, 88.9%, 62.5%, and 16.5%, respectively (Munoz and Ellison, 2000). Disease-specific annual mortality has been reported to be higher in black men than white men (7.4% vs. 4.9%). The same is true for women over men (6.1% vs. 4.4%) (Munoz and Ellison, 2000). Pathologic features or survival was not correlated to the gender in two multicenter studies (Fernández et al., 2009; Shariat et al., 2011). In addition, disease-specific mortality after radical nephroureterectomy was related to the gender when clinicopathologic features were controlled (hazard ratio (HR) = 1.07, $P = 0.4$). In the same study, advanced stage (pT3) disease was associated with the female gender (odds ratio [OR] = 1.15, $P = 0.03$) (Lughezzani et al., 2010).

> **KEY POINTS: EPIDEMIOLOGY**
>
> - Upper urinary tract carcinomas make up only 5% of the urothelial cancers.
> - The highest incidence is observed in individuals age 70 to 90 years in the Balkan countries, where UTUC represents the 40% of all renal neoplasms.
> - Multifocal presence of UTUC is diagnosed in 10% to 20% of cases.
> - Concurrent bladder cancer is diagnosed in 17% of cases.
> - UTUCs are twice as frequent in men than in women.

RISK FACTORS

Genetic Predisposition

Familial/hereditary UTUCs are linked to hereditary nonpolyposis colorectal carcinoma (HNPCC) syndrome (or Lynch syndrome) (Lynch et al., 1990; Roupret et al., 2008). Patients with HNPCC have mutations in the DNA mismatch repair genes *MLH1* (MutL homolog 1), *MSH2* (MutS protein homolog 2), *MSH6* (MutS protein homolog 6), and *PMS2* (mismatch repair endonuclease PMS2). These patients have a higher likelihood to develop colonic, urothelial, gastric, pancreatic, uterine, sebaceous, and ovarian carcinomas. These urothelial cancers mainly involve the upper urinary tract, whereas the involvement of the bladder remains unclear (Matsuoka et al., 2003; Skeldon et al., 2013; van der Post et al., 2010). Any bladder tumor in this population of patients could have been a result of seeding of the bladder from the upper tract. Patients with HNPCC and UTUC are younger than 60 years (mean age 55 years). Moreover, there is a higher representation of female patients in UTUC patients (Lynch et al., 1990). Suspicion for genetic predisposition should be raised in young patients with UTUC, personal history, or having two first-degree relatives with a cancer related to HNPCC (especially colon or endometrial tumors). A short interview could be helpful in screening these patients according to the European Association of Urology (EAU) guidelines (Fig. 98.1; Audenet et al., 2012). DNA sequencing for the patient and family counseling should be recommended in high-risk patients for HNPCC syndrome (Acher et al., 2010; Roupret et al., 2008).

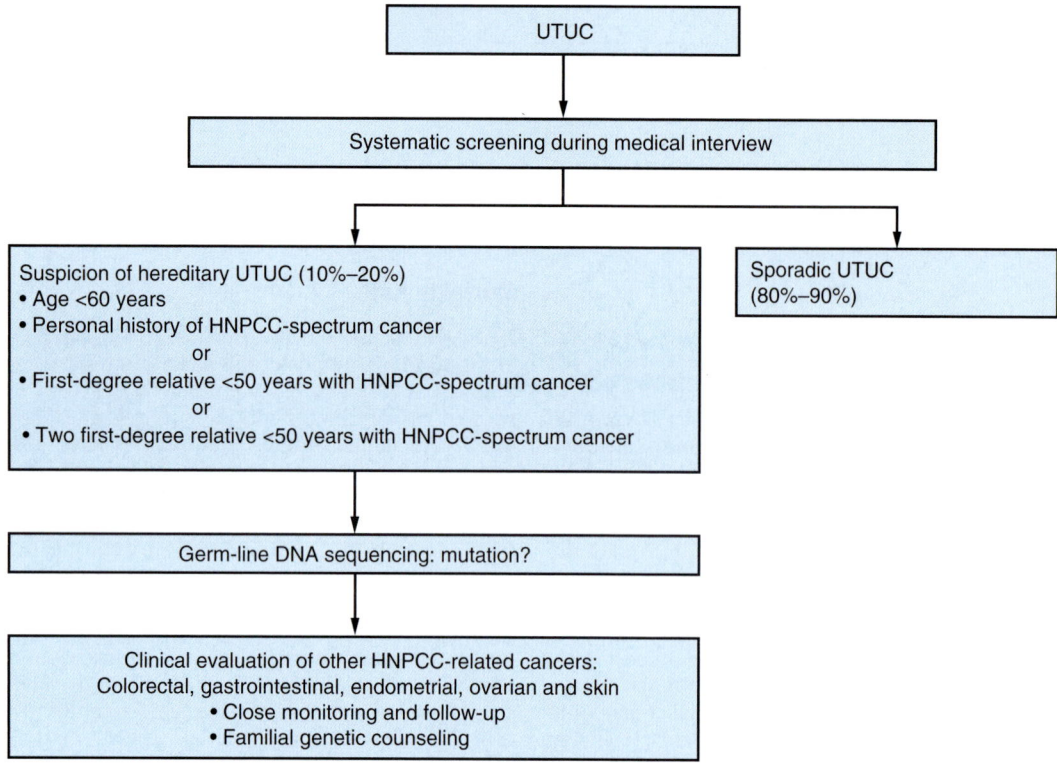

Fig. 98.1. Selection of patients with upper tract urothelial cancer (UTUC) for hereditary screening during the first medical interview. *HNPCC,* Hereditary nonpolyposis colorectal carcinoma. (From Rouprêt M, Babjuk M, Compérat E, et al: European Association of Urology Guidelines on Upper Urinary Tract Urothelial Carcinoma: 2017 Update, *Eur Urol* 73[1]:111–122, 2018.)

Environmental Factors

There are several environmental factors that could contribute to the development of UTUC (Colin et al., 2009).

Tobacco Exposure

The routine use of tobacco increases the relative risk for UTUC from 2.5 to 7 times (Crivelli et al., 2014). Cigarette smoking is a modifiable risk factor and probably the most important one for UTUC. Smoking exposure is complex in terms of mechanism of action for carcinogenesis. A variety of toxic substances are inhaled during smoking and include aromatic amine with arylamine, benzopyrene, and dimethylbenzanthracene. These aromatic amines are metabolized by the body in the carcinogenic N-hydroxylamine. The detoxification of this derivative takes place by several enzyme systems (cytochrome P450s with CYP1A1, glutathione S-transferases, and N-acetyl transferases). Genetic polymorphisms in enzymes that neutralize N-hydroxylamine may reflect susceptibility to the carcinogenic effect of smoking (Hung et al., 2004). The risk for UTUC is modulated by the number of cigarettes consumed daily and the number of years of exposure. An odds ratio (OR) of 2.0 has been calculated for a smoking history of 20 pack-years or less. For heavy smokers such as 60 or more pack-years, the respective OR is 6.2. Smoking cessation results in decreased risk for UTUC with a risk reduction of 60% to 70% with an interruption of smoking for more than 10 years (OR 2.3 for former vs. 4.4 current smokers). The ureter is at higher risk for UTUCs in the smoking population in comparison with the pyelocaliceal system (McLaughlin et al., 1992).

Coffee, Tea, and Yerba Mate

An increased incidence of urothelial cancers has been associated with the consumption of coffee (Ross et al., 1989). Nevertheless, coffee drinkers may also be smokers, so this correlation is probably unsubstantial (Villanueva et al., 2009). A prospective European study into cancer and nutrition included 233,236 subjects with a mean follow-up period of 9.3 years. The investigation showed that the intake of water, coffee, tea, and dairy beverages was not related to urothelial cancer (Ros et al., 2011). In general, there are several studies in the literature evaluating the consumption of coffee or tea as a risk factor for UTUC, and none of them showed any significant correlation (Colin et al., 2009; De Stefani et al., 2007). A traditional beverage in South American countries is yerba mate. The consumption of yerba mate has been considered responsible for urothelial cancer. The beverage could result in providing high levels of polycyclic aromatic hydrocarbons. The risk ratio for urothelial cancer is estimated at 2.2. Nonetheless, currently no study evaluates yerba mate for its potential role in UTUC (De Stefani et al., 2007).

Occupation

UTUC "amino tumors" were related to occupational exposure to carcinogenic aromatic amines. These aromatic substances are still in use in industry in such products as dyes, textiles, rubber, chemicals, petrochemicals, and coal. The aromatic amines benzidine and beta-naphthylane are implicated in carcinogenesis (Colin et al., 2009; Matsuoka et al., 2003; Shinka et al., 1988). Both amines have been banned since the 1960s in most industrialized countries. The average duration of exposure needed to develop UTUC is 7 years, with a latency of up to 20 years after termination of exposure (Colin et al., 2009).

Persons exposed to the chemical, petroleum, and plastic industry have a risk ratio of 4. The same risk has also been identified for those exposed to coal or coke. Persons exposed to asphalt or tar have a risk ratio of 5.5 (Jensen et al., 1988). Polycyclic aromatic hydrocarbons and nitrosamines have been associated with the development of urothelial cancer. An increased risk of 1.3 times for the urothelial cancer with a significant dose effect has been reported (Clavel et al., 1994). Chlorinated solvents (trichloroethylene, tetrachloroethylene) used in metallurgy and printing have been related to urothelial carcinoma genesis with a risk of 1.8.

Aristolochic Acid Nephropathy

Dramatically higher incidence of UTUC has been reported in several studies since the 1950s. These investigations have proposed a 60 to 100 times higher incidence of UTUC in some Balkan rural areas in comparison with the rest of the world. There has been a significant reduction in these rates over the last 3 decades with a reduction in the endemic areas of the incidence of the disease from 57 times to 11 times between 1988 and 1998 (Colin et al., 2009; Stefanovic and Radovanovic, 2008). This endemic nephropathy has been also described as Balkan endemic nephropathy (BEN) and has been related to proximal tubule dysfunction. The latter is responsible for the presence of low-molecular-weight protein and a dense interstitial fibrosis within the glomeruli (Colin et al., 2009; Dragicevic et al., 2007; Grollman et al., 2007; Matsuoka et al., 2003). The special characteristics of the tumors developed in this endemic form of UTUC are the increased occurrence of bilateral disease, the lack of gender predominance, the occurrence in rural areas, and the diagnosis in an earlier age (approximately 10 years earlier) than the UTUC observed in the rest of the world (Colin et al., 2009).

The cause of BEN has been investigated over decades with several hypotheses to explain the association of environmental parameters to the UTUC. Mycotoxin ochratoxin A (OTA) has been investigated as a possible carcinogen related to the development of UTUC for more than 30 years (Colin et al., 2009; Dragicevic et al., 2007; Grollman et al., 2007; Matsuoka et al., 2003). OTA has been confirmed as a carcinogen in animals, but the histologic characteristics of the lesions developed by the toxin are not the same with the BEN UTUC (Colin et al., 2009).

Between 1992 and 1993, 43 patients were hospitalized in Belgium with end-stage renal failure, which was associated with the ingestion of Chinese herbal products (Acher et al., 2010; Audenet et al., 2012; Margulis et al., 2009). A manufacturing error led to the replacement of *Stephania tetracta* by *Aristolochia fangchi* in the mixture of these products. Almost 46% of these patients developed UTUC with similar histologic and genetic characteristics to the UTUC developed in BEN (Cosyns et al., 1999; Nortier et al., 2000). The term "Chinese herb nephropathy" was eventually proposed for this clinical entity. The high prevalence of UTUC in Taiwan and China could be connected to the use of *Aristolochia* in various herbal remedies. The highest incidence in the region is observed on the southwest coast of Taiwan, where 20% to 25% of UTUC cases are reported (Colin et al., 2009).

Specifically, aristolochic acid is found in the plants *Aristolochia fangchi* and *Aristolochia clematitis*. The plants are endemic in these countries and grow as weed in the wheat fields (Grollman et al., 2007). BEN is observed in the Balkan countries as a familial, not inherited, condition related to the dietary exposure to aristocholic acid (Radovanovic et al., 1985; Stefanovic and Radovanovic, 2008). Bladder cancer does not have a higher incidence in the affected families (Petkovic, 1975). The derivative of aristocholic acid, aristolactam, causes a mutation on codon 139 of p53 gene (A:T to T:A). This mutation is predominant in patients with BEN and Chinese herb nephropathy (Colin et al., 2009). Women (HR = 2.2), those with tumor size larger than 3 cm (HR = 2.8), and those with stage T3 or T4 disease (HR = 3.1) have a worse prognosis (Dragicevic et al., 2007).

Analgesics

Phenacetin was suspected for the first time for nephrotoxicity and development of UTUC in 1961 (Holmäng and Johansson, 2004). Phenacetin has been hypothesized to have a direct mutagenic effect and indirectly causes carcinogenesis by inducing nephrotoxicity through papillary necrosis (Colin et al., 2009). The second hypothesis has been confirmed by experimental and epidemiologic evidence (Stewart et al., 1999). The use of phenacetin was abandoned 30 years ago and paracetamol has replaced it. The average latency for the presentation of UTUC was approximately 22 years, and the prevalence of the phenacetin-related UTUC is decreasing (Stewart et al., 1999).

In general, analgesic abuse is an established risk factor for the development of UTUC (Johansson et al., 1974; McCredie et al., 1986; Morrison, 1984). Patients with pelvic and ureteral tumors have been reported to have a history of analgesic abuse in 22% and 11% of the cases, respectively. A latency period of approximately 2 years has been reported (Steffens and Nagel, 1988). Phenacetin is the best-described causative agent in analgesic nephropathy. Nonetheless, most of the patients are usually using combinations of substances, including caffeine, codeine, acetaminophen, and salicylates (De Broe and Elseviers, 1998). The pathognomonic histologic changes observed in analgesic abuse is the thickening of the basement membrane and the scarring of the papilla. When thickening of the basement membrane is observed in UTUC, the physician should be suspicious for analgesic abuse. Up to 15% of the UTUC cases may involve this histologic alteration, and the possibility for contralateral involvement should be considered (Palvio et al., 1987). Tumor grade is correlated to the degree of papillary scarring. On the contrary, the scarring is not associated with the development of squamous metaplasia or cancer (Stewart et al., 1999).

Arsenic

A disproportional incidence of UTUC has been reported in the southwest coast of Taiwan (Tan et al., 2008; Yang et al., 2002). Up to 25% of the UTUCs of the country are diagnosed in this region. The excess of inorganic arsenic in drinking water from artesian wells is a significant risk of UTUC and health problems in several regions worldwide (Tan et al., 2008; Yang et al., 2002). The chronic exposure to arsenic induces a form of peripheral vascular disease known as blackfoot disease. The latter clinical entity causes dry gangrene of the extremities and is related to the increased incidence of UTUC. The UTUC presented in the endemic areas of blackfoot disease has specific characteristics, which include the twice-more-common presentation of UTUC in the female population, the onset of the disease in a younger age (55–60 years), and the twice-more-common presentation of lesions of the ureter in comparison with the renal pelvis. The higher predominance of the disease in women may be related to the exposure of women to arsenic fumes during cooking and probably is related to the inhalation risk along with ingestion risk from the drinking water. The direct relationship of blackfoot disease and UTUC remains unclear (Lamm et al., 2006). Patients with UTUC may never be affected by blackfoot disease. Moreover, there is a high incidence of UTUC (10%–15% of the UTUC incidents) in the northeast regions of Taiwan, where blackfoot disease is not endemic. The association of arsenic and UTUC is not established in the case of UTUC but seems to play a role in bladder urothelial cancer. Nevertheless, arsenic and blackfoot disease are probably not the only relevant risk factors (Lamm et al., 2006).

Chronic Inflammation and Infection

Chronic urinary tract infections facilitate carcinogenesis by weakening the urothelium. The estimated risk for the development of UTUC is 1.5 to 2 greater in these cases (Liaw et al., 1997). The chronic irritation and/or inflammation of the urothelium induced by the stasis and the presence of urine substances may promote carcinogenesis. Thus lithiasis may be implemented in the process. The history of lithiasis is present in 5% to 8% of UTUC cases. Tumor incidence remains low in patients with urinary calculi (Colin et al., 2009). The relative risk of developing UTUC in cases with history of lithiasis ranges between 1.2 and 2.5 (Chow et al., 1997; Liaw et al., 1997). This risk is considered higher in female gender, renal pelvis calcifications, and lithiasis related to hospitalization. Chronic bacterial infection associated with urinary stones and obstruction has been associated with the development of squamous cell cancer (and less frequently adenocarcinoma) (Colin et al., 2009; Spires et al., 1993).

Iatrogenic Factors

Alkylating chemotherapy is known to induce UTUC via the associated metabolites such as acrolein. Chronic exposure to these substances leads to UTUC with epidermoid pathology. The relative risk for the development of urothelial cancer is 3.2 (Brenner and Schellhammer, 1987; McDougal et al., 1981).

Routine use of anthranoid and chemical laxatives has been implicated in the development of UTUC. When these products are used for more than 1 year, a relative risk of 9.62 has been reported. Nevertheless, the mechanism for carcinogenesis remains unclear (Pommer et al., 1999).

Radiotherapy-induced urothelial cancer could develop after the treatment of gynecologic cancers. The relative risk is 1.9, which remains lower than the respective figure for chemotherapy-treated patients. Current literature is lacking on data estimating the risk of UTUC (McDougal et al., 1981).

> **KEY POINTS: RISK FACTORS**
>
> - Familial/hereditary UTUCs are linked to hereditary nonpolyposis colorectal carcinoma syndrome (Lynch syndrome).
> - Tobacco increases the relative risk for UTUC from 2.5 to 7.
> - UTUC "amino tumors" were related to occupational exposure to carcinogenic aromatic amines.
> - Balkan nephropathy is observed as a familial, not inherited, condition related to the dietary exposure to aristocholic acid.
> - Patients with pelvic and ureteral tumors have been reported to have a history of analgesic abuse in 22% and 11% of the cases, respectively.
> - The excess of inorganic arsenic in drinking water from artesian wells is a significant risk factor for UTUC.

HISTOPATHOLOGY

Most the upper urinary tract tumors are urothelial cancer; the pure nonurothelial cancers, such as squamous cell cancers and adenocarcinomas, represent rare conditions (Bennington and Beckwith, 1975; Ouzzane et al., 2011; Sakano et al., 2015; Vincente et al., 1995). Specifically, the urothelial origin of these cancers represents more than 90% of the cases (Rouprent et al., 2018). Variants of urothelial cancer are encountered in approximately 25% of cases (Masson-Lecomte et al., 2014; Rink et al., 2012). These cases correspond to high-grade tumors, and the associated prognosis is worse in comparison with the urothelial cancer (Kim et al., 2017a,b).

Normal Upper Tract Urothelium

The renal pelvis and the ureter derive from the mesoderm and have distinct embryologic origin from the bladder (endodermal origin). The urothelial lining of the upper urinary tract is like the bladder urothelial layer. Nonetheless, the upper tract possesses a significantly thinner muscle layer in comparison with the bladder. On the contrary, the urothelium of the renal pelvis and calyces is relatively abundant. There is a continuity of the epithelial layer from the calyces to the distal ureter. Moreover, the extension of the urothelial layer to the collecting ducts has been proposed (Orsola et al., 2005). The latter possibility could lead to the use of therapeutic measures used for urothelial cancer in the carcinomas originating from the collecting ducts.

Renal Pelvis and Calyces

The pelvic and calyceal walls are lined with transitional epithelium. Two layers of muscle tissue and fibrous connective tissue represent the deeper layers (Dixon and Gosling, 1982). The muscle layers have a spiral, helical arrangement, which originates in the minor calyces.

Ureter

The ureter has two continuous spiraled thin muscle layers. The spiral configuration of the muscle fibers is tighter in the case of the external layer, whereas the internal layer has a looser structure. There is also a third outer longitudinal layer in the lower third of the ureter. These three layers merge with the three muscle layers of the bladder (inner longitudinal, middle circular, and outer longitudinal). The serosa covers the outer muscular layer and is composed of loose connective tissue, blood vessels, and lymphatics (Hanna et al., 1976; Notley, 1978).

Urothelial Neoplasms

Benign Lesions: Papillomas and von Brunn Nests

Papillomas, inverted papillomas, and von Brunn nests are benign lesions. The presentation of synchronous or metachronous UTUCs cannot be excluded. Consequently, close surveillance of these benign lesions is necessary (Chan et al., 1996; Cheville et al., 2000; Matsuoka et al., 2003; Renfer et al., 1988; Stower et al., 1990). Malignancy has been observed in 18% of the inverted papillomas of the ureter (Grainger et al., 1990). Two types of inverted papilloma have been proposed based on the malignant potential of these tumors. The type 1 lesions are benign. The type 2 lesions may be malignant. Current knowledge does not provide an efficient method to distinguish between the two types, and the surveillance of all inverted papillomas is advisable. The follow-up should be extended for at least 2 years from the diagnosis (Asano et al., 2003). Considering this, close follow-up of the inverted papilloma is necessary in all cases.

Metaplastic and Dysplastic Lesions

Current evidence suggests that UTUC develops through a gradual progression of hyperplasia to dysplasia and eventually CIS in a significant proportion of the UTUC cases (Heney et al., 1981; McCarron et al., 1983). The CIS is frequently spread in patches with extension up to the level of the collecting ducts of the kidney (Mahadevia et al., 1983). The severity of urothelial dysplasia could be associated with a worse prognosis because of a greater risk for tumor recurrence in the distal ureter and bladder.

Urothelial Malignant Lesions

Urothelial Carcinoma. Urothelial carcinomas represent more than 90% of the upper urinary tract tumors (Fig. 98.2). Similarly, to the urothelial tumors of the bladder, the morphology of the lesions could be flat (CIS), papillary, or sessile. The distribution in the system could be unifocal or multifocal. Despite the histologic similarity of these lesions to the urothelial bladder cancer, the thinner muscle layers of the renal pelvis and ureter allow for an earlier involvement of the muscle layer in comparison with the bladder. CIS is difficult to diagnose: significant morphologic variations range from whitish plaque to epithelial hyperplasia or a smooth red patch because of increased submucosal vascularity (Fig. 98.3; Melamed and Reuter, 1993). The muscle invasion or invasion to the renal parenchyma or the surrounding adventitia is more likely to take place on the upper tract. Collecting duct carcinoma possesses similar characteristics to UTUC because of the common embryologic origin, but it is considered kidney cancer and not UTUC (Albadine et al., 2010).

Micropapillary Variant of Urothelial Carcinoma. Variants of the urothelial carcinoma could be diagnosed in up to 25% of UTUCs. These variants include squamous cell, glandular, sarcomatoid, micropapillary, neuroendocrine, and lymphoepithelial morphology. All these variants are related to aggressiveness and poor clinical outcome. Nonetheless, there is evidence that the presence of these variants does not predict poor clinical outcome if the remaining clinicopathologic features are considered (Rink et al., 2012). Two studies have proposed that the micropapillary variant is related to inferior progression- and cancer-free survival (Holmäng et al., 2006; Sung et al., 2014). The micropapillary subtype of urothelial carcinoma has a more aggressive progression in the bladder. This histologic variant is rarely diagnosed in the upper urinary tract and is associated usually with advanced disease. Holmäng et al. (2006) reported that 22 out of 26 patients with micropapillary UTUC had T3 stage at presentation. CIS and lymph node (LN) involvement was observed in 64% and 81% of the cases, respectively. Five-year survival was 26.9% and the disease-specific mortality was 77% (Holmäng et al., 2006). Sung et al. (2014) showed in a multivariate analysis that the micropapillary UTUC was an independent predictor of progression-free survival (HR 3.85, $P = 0.003$) and was related to poorer cancer-specific survival than the nonmicropapillary UTUC ($P < 0.001$).

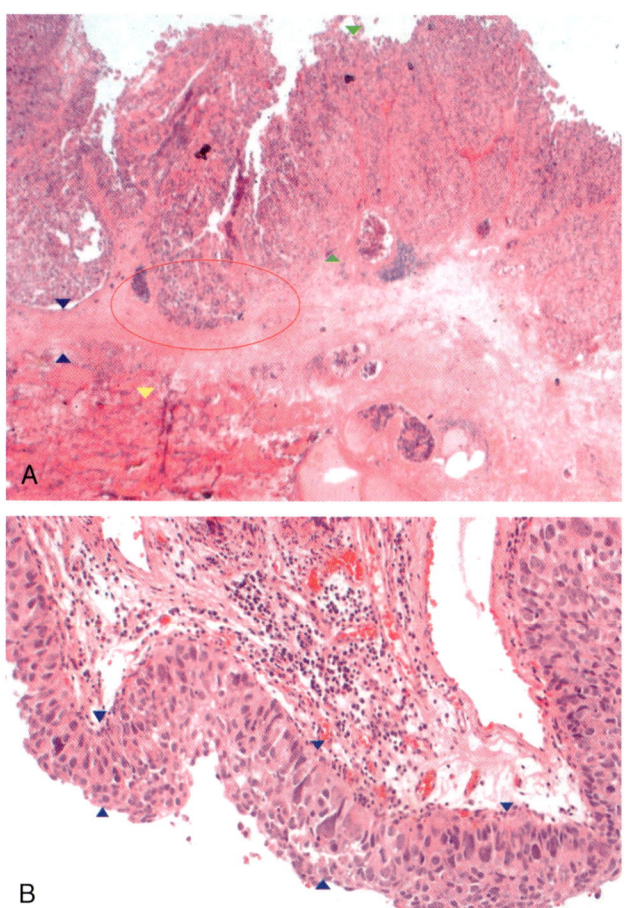

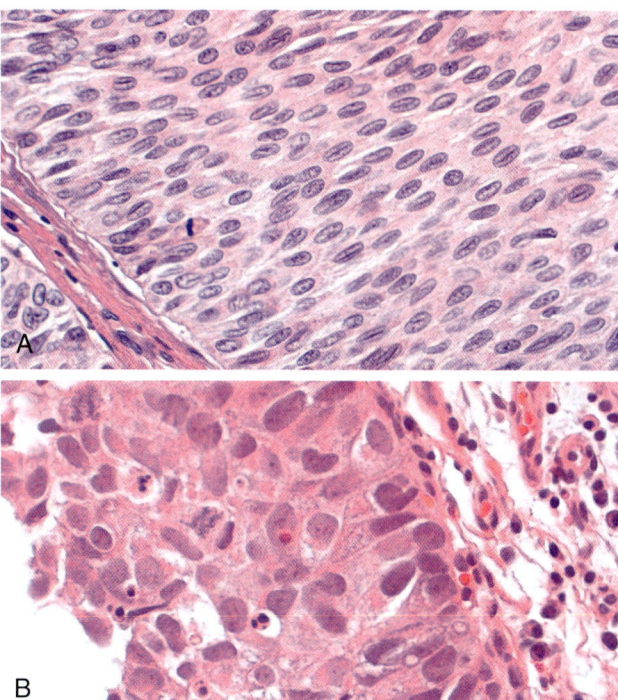

Fig. 98.3. (A) Low-grade urothelial carcinoma. The orientation of the cells is still preserved (hematoxylin-eosin staining, 20×). (B) Carcinoma in situ. The cells are dividing; there is no specific orientation of the cells. Their nuclei are in different phases of mitosis. There are sites of apoptosis (hematoxylin-eosin staining, 20×).

Fig. 98.2. (A) High-grade urothelial carcinoma. Between the *green arrowheads* is the urothelial layer with high-grade carcinoma. Between the *blue arrowheads* is the lamina propria. At the site of the *yellow arrowhead* lies the muscular layer. The *red circle* shows a site of invasion of the carcinoma to the lamina propria (hematoxylin-eosin staining, 2.5×). (B) Carcinoma in situ. Between the *blue arrowheads* is the urothelial layer with carcinoma. The underlying tissue is not infiltrated by carcinoma (hematoxylin-eosin staining, 20×).

Nonurothelial Malignant Lesions

The nonurothelial lesions of the upper urinary tract are rare and characterized by a wide variety of malignancy potential (Ouzzane et al., 2011; Sakano et al., 2015). It is a wide spectrum of lesions ranging from benign to highly malignant tumors. Squamous cell cancers and adenocarcinomas have the higher incidence among all these nonurothelial tumors.

Squamous Cell Carcinoma. Squamous cell carcinomas (SCCs) have an incidence of 0.7% to 7.0% of upper urinary tract cancers (Babaian and Johnson, 1980; Blacker et al., 1985). The abuse of analgesics and the presence of chronic inflammation have been associated with these carcinomas (Stewart et al., 1999). The incidence of SCC is 6 times higher in the renal pelvis than in the ureter. SCCs are usually moderately to poorly differentiated and are already invasive at presentation.

Adenocarcinoma. Adenocarcinomas are observed in less than 1% of renal pelvic tumors. There is a strong association of adenocarcinomas with urinary calculi, long-term obstruction, and inflammation (Spires et al., 1993; Stein et al., 1988). At diagnosis, adenocarcinomas are in an advanced stage and have a poor prognosis.

Other Tumors. Fibroepithelial polyps (Blank et al., 1987; Musselman and Kay, 1986) and neurofibromas (Varela-Duran et al., 1987) are benign rare tumors. Their treatment is simple excision. There are other rare tumors of the upper tract such as neuroendocrine (Ouzzane et al., 2011) and hematopoietic (Igel et al., 1991) tumors as well as sarcomas (Coup, 1988; Madgar et al., 1988). The treatment of these very rare tumors is based on the experience with tumors of similar histology presenting in other organs. Thus these lesions are treated by excision and adjuvant therapy.

> **KEY POINTS: HISTOPATHOLOGY**
>
> - Urothelial carcinomas represent more than 90% of the upper urinary tract tumors. Pure nonurothelial upper urinary tract cancers are rare conditions.
> - Variants of urothelial cancer are encountered in approximately 25% of UTUCs.
> - Papillomas, inverted papillomas, and von Brunn nests are usually benign lesions.
> - UTUC develops through a gradual progression of hyperplasia to dysplasia and eventually carcinoma in situ (CIS) in a significant proportion of UTUC cases.
> - CIS is difficult to diagnose with significant morphologic variations.
> - The muscle invasion or invasion to the renal parenchyma or the surrounding adventitia is more likely to take place on the upper tract.

DIAGNOSIS

Upper urinary tract tumors are associated with several symptoms and signs. The common symptoms include hematuria, dysuria, and flank pain, which are usually related to localized disease. Hematuria is the most common sign of the UTUCs and could be either gross or microscopic. The incidence of hematuria is 56% to 98% of cases (Guinan et al., 1992; Matsuoka et al., 2003; Murphy et al., 1981; Raabe et al., 1992). Flank pain represents the second most frequent symptom and is observed in 20% to 30% of cases. The gradual onset of obstruction and hydronephrosis is associated with the dull nature of the flank pain. A lumbar mass could also be palpated in approximately 10% (Ito et al., 2011; Raman et al., 2011). Acute pain mimicking renal colic could also occur when clots are passing, and the collecting system is acutely obstructed. The incidence of flank pain resulting from malignant obstruction or clot is more prevalent in upper tract tumors than in bladder tumors. This incidence has been reported to be 10% to 40% of cases (Babaian and Johnson, 1980; McCarron et al., 1983; Melamed and Reuter, 1993). Asymptomatic patients represent approximately 15% of cases and are diagnosed as incidental radiologic findings. Advanced disease could be presented with flank or abdominal mass, weight loss, anorexia, and bone pain with similar frequency to the respective signs and symptoms of bladder cancer. These symptoms and signs should prompt rigorous metastatic evaluation and confer a worse prognosis (Ito et al., 2011; Raman et al., 2011). UTUC represents a rare autopsy finding, and the majority of the upper tract lesions are diagnosed before death (Resseguie et al., 1978).

The UTUC has some similarities to the respective bladder tumors. Specifically, ureteral tumors are low grade and low stage in 55% to 75% of cases (Cummings, 1980; Williams, 1991). In addition, most of the tumors are papillary (85%) and the remaining are sessile. Invasion of the lamina propria or muscle (stage T1 or T2) is observed in 50% of papillary and more than 80% of sessile tumors. Invasive tumors are more common in the ureter in comparison with the balder. Renal pelvic tumors involve the lamina propria or muscle in 50% to 60% of cases (Anderstrom et al., 1989; Williams, 1991).

Endoscopy of the Lower Tract

Cystoscopy

Cystoscopy should always be performed because the upper urinary tract tumors are often associated with bladder cancer. During the investigation of a suspicious case, the upper tract should be evaluated when the cytology is positive and the cystoscopy (including the urethra) is negative (Rosenthal et al., 2016; Witjes et al., 2010).

Endoscopy of the Upper Tract

Ureterorenoscopic Evaluation

Flexible ureteroscopy (URS) is the key approach for the visualization of the ureter, renal pelvis, and collecting system. The biopsy of suspicious lesions could also be done with URS. The diagnostic accuracy of excretory or retrograde urography alone can be increased from 75% to 85% to 90% when URS is also performed in conjunction with these studies (Fig. 98.4; Blute et al., 1989; Matsuoka et al., 2003; Streem et al., 1986). Pyelovenous and pyelolymphatic dissemination of the disease with URS has been reported without further confirmation of this phenomenon (Lim et al., 1993). Thus the URS should be performed for diagnosis whenever deemed necessary.

Ureteroscopic biopsies can provide valuable information by determining the tumor grade in 90% of cases. Accurate biopsies

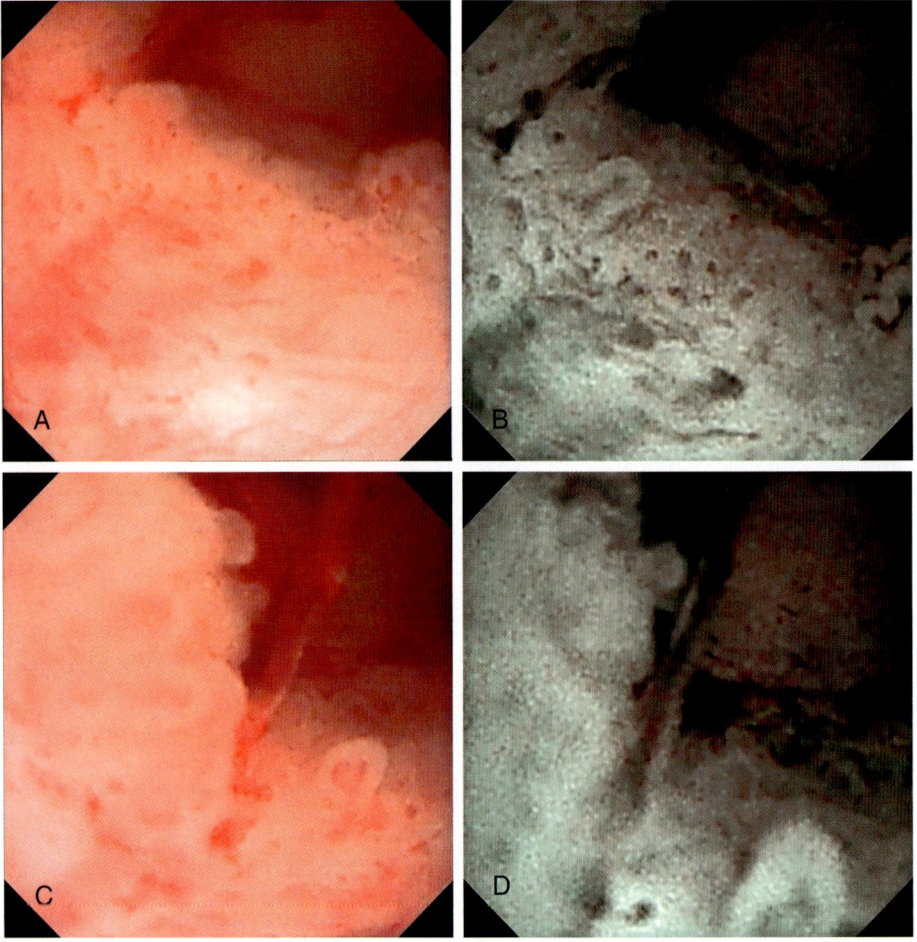

Fig. 98.4. (A) Urothelial carcinomas of the upper renal calyceal group. There are multiple carcinomas. Flexible ureteroscopes with the current digital technology provide excellent visualization of the upper urinary tract. Nevertheless, the surgeon should always scrutinize the urothelium to avoid missing sites of disease. (B) The same carcinomas as image A visualized by filters of the endoscopic system of the flexible ureteroscope. These filters could be proven useful to distinguish small tumors that could be difficult to identify in the standard image setting. (C) Sessile tumor with also some papillary morphology over its surface. (D) The same carcinoma as image C visualized by filters of the endoscopic system of the flexible ureteroscope.

by forceps or brushing are possible with URS, and these biopsies have a low false-negative rate regardless of sample size (Rojas et al., 2013).

Undergrading may occur after diagnostic biopsy, and an intensive follow-up schedule is necessary if a kidney-sparing approach is selected (Smith et al., 2011). Nevertheless, a histologic correlation of 78% to 92% between the URS biopsy specimen and the final pathologic specimen has been confirmed (Brown et al., 2007; Guarnizo et al., 2000; Keeley et al., 1997a). Histologic samples obtained by URS provide the best potential for predicting the final pathologic results. A study compared the grade and stage URS biopsy specimens of visible tumors to the surgical specimens in 42 cases (Keeley et al., 1997b). There was a 90% correlation for the low- or moderate-grade urothelial cancer specimens and 92% for the high-grade cancers. The presence of invasive cancer was successfully detected by the biopsy in 67% of cases (Keeley et al., 1997b). The visual assessment of the tumor grade during URS could be correct in 70%, and a biopsy is necessary for the staging of the upper urinary tract tumors (El-Hakim et al., 2004). URS also facilitates the selective ureteral sampling for cytology in situ (Clements et al., 2012; Ishikawa et al., 2010).

The prediction of tumor grade is accurate, but the prediction of tumor stage requires the evaluation of several parameters. According to the European guidelines, the stage assessment with the URS biopsy is notoriously difficult (Roupret et al., 2018). The URS biopsy specimens are small and usually do not include deep layers of the ureter or renal pelvis. Consequently, the precise prediction of tumor stage is difficult. Thus a more accurate prediction of the tumor stage and stratification of cases would require a combination of tumor grade, visual inspection of the tumor, radiographic studies (presence of obstruction), and urinary cytology (Clements et al., 2012; Ishikawa et al., 2010). This stratification of cases is important for decision making and the selection of radical nephroureterectomy or kidney-sparing approach for the management of UTUC (Roupret et al., 2018).

CIS of the upper urinary tract is difficult to diagnose and is hypothesized by the presence of unequivocally positive selective cytology, although the endoscopic or radiographic findings do not identify any specific lesion. The presence of ureteral CIS at the cystectomy specimen is probably the clearest diagnosis for CIS in the ureter. In a series of 40 UTUCs with localization in renal pelvis (40%), distal ureter (40%), and proximal ureter (40%), the tumor grade of the URS biopsy matched the surgical specimen in 78% of cases (Guarnizo et al., 2000). The remaining 22% the tumor grade was underestimated in URS biopsy. Lamina propria was present in the biopsy in 100% of the loop biopsies but only in 62% of the cup biopsies. In the whole population, 68% of the biopsies included the lamina propria. Ta tumors at the biopsy were upstaged to T3 stage in 45% of cases after the complete resection of the tumor (Guarnizo et al., 2000). It seems that the tumor grading may help estimating the tumor stage. Grade 3 tumor in the biopsy accurately predicts the tumor stage in more than 90% of cases (Skolarikos et al., 2003).

URS should be reserved for diagnostic uncertainty, if kidney-sparing treatment is considered, or in patients with a solitary kidney. URS could provide information regardless of obtaining biopsies or not (Roupret et al., 2018). As mentioned earlier, the tumor stage prediction requires the combination of evidence obtained by different investigations, and the decision making for a kidney-sparing approach should be based on this evidence. The surgeon should never forget that recent studies showed a higher rate of intravesical recurrence in patients (particularly in case of renal pelvic tumor) who underwent URS before RNU (Marchioni et al., 2017; Yoo et al., 2017).

Recent technologic developments in the flexible ureteroscopes and the application of novel imaging techniques have improved the visualization and diagnosis of flat tumors (Bus et al., 2015). The results of narrow band imaging are promising but require further confirmation (Abouassaly et al., 2010; Brien et al., 2010; Kata et al., 2016; Matsuoka et al., 2003). Optical coherence tomography and confocal endomicroscopy (Cellvizio) have been proposed for improved evaluation of tumor grade and/or staging. Optical coherence tomography and confocal endomicroscopy have a good correlation between the intraoperative imaging and definitive histology (Breda et al., 2018; Bus et al., 2016).

Antegrade Endoscopic Evaluation

A percutaneous approach for the diagnosis and treatment of UTUC may be necessary in some cases. Antegrade nephroscopy, ureteroscopy, and urography could be useful for visualization, biopsy, or even tumor resection. Resection of the tumor with larger caliber scopes is possible for tumor debulking in the renal pelvis (Blute et al., 1989; Matsuoka et al., 2003; Streem et al., 1986). According to EAU guidelines, the percutaneous management could be considered for low-risk UTUC in renal pelvis. Low-risk tumors inaccessible or difficult to manage with flexible ureteroscopy could be treated by percutaneous access (Roupret et al., 2018). The percutaneous approach is being abandoned because of the use of improved flexible ureteroscopes. Nevertheless, tumor cell implantation in the retroperitoneum and the nephrostomy tube tract should always be considered by the surgeon selecting this approach (Huang et al., 1995; Tomera et al., 1982).

Radiologic Imaging

Computed tomographic (CT) urography has the highest diagnostic accuracy of the available imaging techniques (Ito et al., 2013). The sensitivity of CT urography for UTUC is 0.67 to 1.0 and specificity is 0.93 to 0.99 (Cowan et al., 2007). CT is easier to perform and requires less labor than the traditional intravenous pyelography. There have been concerns regarding missing small urinary defects (<5 mm) between the slices of the traditional CT scan. The three-dimensional reconstruction of the upper tract has been shown to be equal to the intravenous pyelography in imaging the renal pelvis and ureters (McTavish et al., 2002). Rapid acquisition of thin sections allows high-resolution isotropic images that can be viewed in multiple planes to assist with diagnosis without loss of resolution (Roupret et al., 2018). Nevertheless, CT urography exposes the patient to higher doses of radiation in comparison with the intravenous pyelography.

Findings that are suggestive of upper urinary tract tumor are radiolucent filling defects, obstruction, or incomplete filling of a part of the upper tract and inability to visualize the collecting system. Filling defects could be found in 50% to 75% of cases (Fein and McClennan, 1986; Murphy et al., 1981). Differential diagnosis of filling defects includes blood clot, stones, overlying bowel gas, external compression, sloughed papilla, and fungus ball. The presence of calcification in renal ultrasonography or CT without contrast could distinguish stones. Urothelial cancers have an average density of 46 Hounsfield units (HU) and range between 10 and 70 HU (Lantz and Hattery, 1984). The average density of a radiolucent uric acid stone is 100 HU with a range of 80 to 250 HU. Measurements of the HUs in a CT could be useful in differentiating two common causes of radiolucent filling defects on excretory or retrograde urography. It is not clear if hydronephrosis or nonvisualization of the tumor could be an indicator of higher stage for renal pelvic or ureteral tumors. No visualization of the renal pelvis was observed in only 20% of the pelvic tumors (McCarron et al., 1983). No visualization was observed in 37% to 45% of the ureteral tumors; 60% of these cases were invasive (McCarron et al., 1983). The lack of visualization of the renal pelvis or ureter has not been correlated to the tumor stage by at least two studies (Anderstrom et al., 1989; Batata and Grabstald, 1976). On the contrary, hydronephrosis with or without an associated filling defect was linked to invasive ureteral tumors in up to 80% of cases (Cho et al., 2007; McCarron et al., 1983). Advanced disease and poor oncologic outcome has been associated with hydronephrosis (Hurel et al., 2015; Messer et al., 2013). Epithelial "flat lesions" without mass effect or urothelial thickening are generally not visible with CT (Roupret et al., 2018). Enlarged lymph nodes are highly predictive of metastases in upper urinary tract tumors (Verhoest et al., 2011). For staging purposes, CT provides information on the extent of invasion, mass or masses outside the collecting system, and the presence of lymph node or distant metastases (Milestone et al., 1990). CT has a poor sensitivity in assessing the invasion of the small lesions. In a study by Scolieri et al. (2000), the CT predicted accurately the TNM stage in 60% of the patients and understaged 16% and overstaged 24%. The CT could also determine poor functioning areas of a kidney such as obstructed areas based on the detection of urine (with contrast) excretion (Kenney and Stanley, 1987).

Retrograde urography could be useful for the evaluation of radiolucent, noncalcified lesions and incompletely filled or obstructed renal infundibula or calyces. These cases could be also investigated with URS with or without biopsy. Retrograde urography has an accuracy of 75% for the diagnosis of upper tract tumor and remains an option for the detection of UTUCs (Ito et al., 2011; Murphy et al., 1981; Rouprét et al., 2018). Some have suggested that ultrasonography has sensitivity equal to that of urography in evaluating patients with painless gross hematuria for upper tract malignant disease (Data et al., 2002; Yip et al., 1999).

Magnetic resonance (MR) urography is indicated in patients to whom the radiation or iodinated contrast media are contraindicated and cannot undergo CT urography (Matsuoka et al., 2003; Takahashi et al., 2010). The sensitivity of MR urography is 0.75 after contrast injection for tumors smaller than 2 cm (Matsuoka et al., 2003; Takahashi et al., 2010). Gadolinium-based contrast media for MR urography should be limited in patients with severe renal impairment (<30 mL/min creatinine clearance). These contrasts have a risk of nephrogenic systemic fibrosis. CT urography is generally preferred to MR urography for diagnosing and staging UTUC (Rouprét et al., 2018).

Evaluation of the contralateral kidney is important not only because of possible bilateral presence of the disease but also because it allows a determination of the functionality of the contralateral kidney. At times, a split-function renal scan may be helpful in determining the contribution of the "diseased" and the presumed "normal" kidney to the patient's overall renal function.

Cytology and Tumor Markers

Urine cytology could be used for the diagnosis of upper urinary tract tumors. Nevertheless, the sensitivity of voided urine (or bladder wash) cytology remains low and is related to the grade of the tumor. The sensitivity of cytology has been estimated at about 20% for grade 1, 45% for grade 2, and 75% for grade 3 tumors (Konety and Getzenberg, 2001; Murphy and Soloway, 1982). The interpretation of an abnormal voided cytology requires caution because the cytology does not provide any information on the site of origin of the malignant cells. Urine collection or washing of the ureter with a ureteral catheter could provide more accurate cytologic results. Cytology is less sensitive for UTUC in comparison with the bladder tumors and is advised to be performed in situ in the renal collecting system (Messer et al., 2011). Nevertheless, false-negative or false-positive results may range between 22% and 35% (Zincke et al., 1976). Saline washings increase the cell yield and improve the results of cytologic evaluation. Brush biopsy through a retrograde catheter or ureteroscope is related to better accuracy. These techniques could increase the sensitivity of urine cytology in the range of 90% (Blute et al., 1989; Streem et al., 1986). Brush biopsies have been associated with complications such as massive hemorrhage and preformation of the urinary tract (Blute et al., 1981). Cytologic specimens should be obtained before the instillation of any contrast agent. Especially, ionic, high osmolarity contrast agents may deteriorate the cytologic specimens (Messer et al., 2013; Terris, 2004).

The sensitivity of fluorescence in situ hybridization (FISH) for molecular abnormalities characteristic of UTUCs is similarly high to bladder cancer. The most appropriate population for FISH are the patients with low-grade recurrent disease under surveillance and kidney-sparing therapy for UTUCs (Chen and Grasso, 2008; Johannes et al., 2010). As a result, FISH is not routinely used for the surveillance of UTUCs (Chen and Grasso, 2008; Johannes et al., 2010).

STAGING AND CLASSIFICATION

Natural History

Recurrence

Poor prognosis is common in UTUCs. A study from the 1970s reported that metastatic disease is present in up to 19% of patients at diagnosis

> **KEY POINTS: DIAGNOSIS**
> - Localized disease is characterized by hematuria, dysuria, and flank pain.
> - Advanced disease is characterized by flank or abdominal mass, weight loss, anorexia, and bone pain.
> - Cystoscopy should always be performed.
> - Flexible ureteroscopy with biopsy is a key approach for diagnosis.
> - Computed tomography urography has the highest diagnostic accuracy.
> - Urine collection or washing of the ureter with a ureteral catheter could provide the most accurate cytologic results.

(Akaza et al., 1970). In recent years, multicenter studies showed that cancer-specific outcomes of matched cohorts have similar frequency between the upper and lower tract urothelial cancers despite the more invasive and poorly differentiated nature of UTUCs (Catto et al., 2007; Moussa et al., 2010). When patients with UTUC and bladder cancer were respectively treated with the nephroureterectomy and radical cystectomy, the prognosis for recurrence was related to the location of the tumor and stage. The UTUC had a worse prognosis in comparison with bladder cancer in pT4 disease. On the contrary, bladder cancer patients had worse prognosis in the group of non–muscle-invasive cancer, whereas the pT2 and pT3 diseases did not exhibit any statistical difference in terms of recurrence (Rink et al., 2012). The differences in the non–muscle-invasive stage may be attributed to the presence of aggressive features (high-grade disease), which are treated with transurethral resection with or without intravesical instillations for bladder cancer, whereas the UTUC cases are treated with radical nephroureterectomy because of the lack of efficient staging methods. Thus patients with bladder cancer may already harbor features of aggressive disease such as lymphovascular disease, persistent disease at transurethral invasion, and failure to respond to intravesical therapy. In the case of the pT4 cohort, patients with pT4a disease have prostatic stromal invasion, which can be still treated by radical cystoprostatectomy with curative intent (Green et al., 2013).

Involvement of the Ureter or Renal Collecting System

Ureteral tumors are in 70% of the UTUC cases in the distal ureter, 25% in the mid-ureter, and 5% in the upper ureter (Anderstrom et al., 1989). This phenomenon could be attributed to the downstream implantation of cancer cells, and this dictates the radical treatment by complete excision of the whole ureter. Synchronous or metachronous bilateral disease has an incidence of 1.6% to 6.0% of sporadic UTUC (Babaian and Johnson, 1980; Kang et al., 2003; Murphy et al., 1981). The location of the UTUC at presentation is a prognostic factor in some studies (Ouzzane et al., 2011; Yafi et al., 2012). When the effect of tumor stage is adjusted, patients with ureteral and/or multifocal tumors seem to have a worse prognosis than those with renal pelvic tumors (Chromecki et al., 2012; Ouzzane et al., 2011; Williams et al., 2013; Yafi et al., 2012).

Synchronous and Asynchronous Localizations

Upper Tract Recurrence After Bladder Cancer. The risk for UTUC after the treatment of bladder cancer has been reported by several large series (Canales et al., 2006; Mullerad et al., 2004; Oldbring et al., 1989; Rabbani et al., 2001; Solsona et al., 1997; Sved et al., 2004; Tran et al., 2008; Wright et al., 2009). Upper tract recurrence after bladder cancer treatment has an incidence of 2% to 6% and is diagnosed later with a median time to recurrence more than 3 years (Reddy and Kader, 2018). These rates have significant fluctuation when traditional series are considered (Herr et al., 1996; Solsona et al., 1997). In most of the traditional series, the recurrence rate ranges between 2% and 4% with an interval to recurrence ranging from 17 to 170 months, but there are also series with rates up to 25%. This discrepancy in numbers could be attributed to patient selection criteria, tumor grading, and stage and dysplastic tumors included in these series. Risk factors for upper tract recurrence are the presence of distal ureteral tumor, multifocal or recurrent urothelial carcinoma, non–muscle-invasive bladder cancer, and the presence of carcinoma in situ. A recurrence rate of only 0.8% at 15 years was observed in patients without any of these factors. Patients with more than 3 of these factors had 13.5% risk of recurrence in the same period (Volkmer et al., 2009). These recurrences are diagnosed after the onset of symptoms in more than 50% of cases and at advanced stage in 70%. Primary detection is done by cytology and upper urinary tract imaging in 7% and 29.6% of cases, respectively (Picozzi et al., 2012). Symptoms include flank pain and hematuria. The prognosis is poor: 18% to 33% of the patients have metastatic lesion at diagnosis (Huguet, 2013).

Data from the SEER database from 91,245 patients with bladder cancer showed that 657 (0.7%) developed UTUC over a median follow-up period of 4.1 years. The relative risk of recurrence in the upper urinary tract was stable over long-term follow-up. Upper tract surveillance should be rigorous over extended time periods (Rabbani et al., 2001). According to several investigations, recurrences are more frequent in patients with CIS than in patients with papillary urothelial cancers and in patients treated with cystectomy for CIS rather than for invasive cancer (Canales et al., 2006; Slaton et al., 1999; Solsona et al., 1997). Upper tract recurrence was more likely to occur in patients with T1 stage than those with Ta, patients with high-grade bladder disease, and when the lesions were located at the bladder trigone or periureteral sites. The pathologic evaluation showed that the recurrence was more likely to be superficial (Ta, T1, Tis) and to involve only the distal ureter (Wright et al., 2009). On the contrary, an earlier study observed that Ta, T1, and Tis bladder cancer treated with bacille Calmette-Guérin (BCG) was associated with 21% recurrence in the upper urinary tract after a median period of 7.3 years. Most of these patients had invasive tumors at diagnosis, and 38.8% of them died from UTUC (Herr et al., 1996).

The largest meta-analysis available included more than 13,000 patients from 27 studies. All these patients underwent cystectomy for bladder cancer. The overall prevalence of UTUC after cystectomy ranged from 0.75% to 6.4%. Recurrence was observed between 2.4 to 164 months in an advanced stage or metastatic state in 64.6% and 35.6% of cases, respectively. Patients with G1 tumor had 8 times greater probability for UTUC compared with those with G2 disease. G1 cases had 10 times higher probability than G3 cases. Patients with CIS had a twice-higher probability for UTUC than those with invasive disease. Multifocality increases the risk of recurrence 3 times. Positive ureteral or urethral margin and history of UTUC increase the risk 7 times. The negative node status increases the risk eightfold. The type of urinary diversion did not influence the recurrence rate. Patients with continent diversion had more favorable disease, and consequently a selection bias was introduced to this subgroup of patients. The follow-up schedule varied among studies and there was no specific protocol for the early detection of UTUC. Symptoms usually motivated the diagnostic evaluation for UTUC. The authors proposed the elimination of cytology and excretory urography for the follow-up of these patients. Computed tomography should be used instead (Picozzi et al., 2012).

The presence of ureteral reflux and bladder cancer located close to a ureteral orifice has been shown to predispose to UTUC (Herr et al., 1992; Hudson and Herr, 1995; Zincke et al., 1984). Delayed recurrence is more frequent in the ureter in comparison with the renal pelvis and happens earlier (at 40 vs. 67 months). Patients treated by cystectomy for disease refractory to BCG and patients with CIS of the bladder treated by BCG are associated with 30% incidence of UTUC. In these cases and in all cases of high-risk bladder cancer, annual evaluation of the upper tract is advisable (Herr et al., 1996).

Bladder Recurrence After Upper Tract Tumors. Patients with UTUC have a significant risk for recurrence of the disease in the bladder. The estimated risk is based on several reports and varies between 15% and 75% within 5 years of the development of the UTUC (Anderstrom et al., 1989; Hisataki et al., 2000; Huben et al., 1988; Kakizoe et al., 1980; Kang et al., 2003; Miyake et al., 2000). The higher incidence of metachronous bladder cancers in comparison with metachronous UTUC after bladder cancer has resulted in the proposal of several theories, which include downstream seeding, longer exposure time to carcinogens in the bladder, and greater number of urothelial cells in the bladder that are subject to random carcinogenic events. The most widely accepted theory is the downstream seeding, which is further supported by the fact that the bladder tumor recurrences after UTUC are monoclonal (Junker et al., 2005) and by the pattern of recurrence after nephroureterectomy. Bladder recurrence usually takes place within 2 years after the treatment of UTUC and is located at the site of bladder trauma after the ureterectomy (Kang et al., 2003). The high incidence of recurrences of UTUC in the bladder dictates the need for scheduled follow-up of all patients diagnosed with UTUC.

Specific gene mutations have been proposed for cases of rapidly recurrent high-grade cancers (Habuchi et al., 1993; Harris and Neal, 1992; Lunec et al., 1992). UTUC multifocality has been related to higher bladder tumor incidence (Matsui et al., 2005). Low-grade UTUCs tend to have a less rapid recurrence in the bladder, and microsatellite studies have showed that there is discordance between the upper tract tumors and the metachronous bladder tumor in 46% of cases (Takahashi et al., 2000), supporting a field effect (Takahashi et al., 2001). Increased UTUC stage at nephroureterectomy correlated to a higher risk for bladder recurrence (Hisataki et al., 2000, Matsui et al., 2005, Terakawa et al., 2008). In a multivariate analysis of a multi-institutional study, the presence of a bladder tumor before UTUC was the only independent risk factor for bladder recurrence after radical nephroureterectomy. Another study correlated only the grade of the UTUC with the pathologic findings of the metachronous bladder tumor (Novara et al., 2009).

A meta-analysis identified significant predictors for bladder recurrence after nephroureterectomy (Seisen et al., 2015). Three major categories were proposed by the authors:
1. Patient-specific factors: male gender, previous bladder cancer, smoking, and preoperative chronic kidney disease
2. Tumor-specific factors: positive preoperative urinary cytology, ureteral location, multifocality, invasive pT stage, and necrosis
3. Treatment-specific factors: laparoscopic approach, extravesical bladder cuff removal, and positive surgical margins (Roupret et al., 2018; Seisen et al., 2015)

The diagnostic ureteroscopy has been related to a higher risk of bladder recurrence after radical nephroureterectomy, especially when the UTUC is in the renal pelvis (Marchioni et al., 2017; Yoo et al., 2017).

Carcinoma in Situ. The presence of CIS increases the incidence of bilateral and multifocal disease. Bilateral disease has an overall incidence of 3% to 5% of UTUC cases. The presence of CIS increases this incidence to 25% (Herr et al., 1996). Patients with CIS have higher risk for subsequent panurothelial disease because there is a high probability for multifocal disease. Conservative management should be considered when feasible, and follow-up investigation should include bladder, upper urinary tract, and urethra.

Metastatic Potential of Upper Urinary Tract Carcinoma

Dissemination of Disease. UTUCs have significant spread potential. The tumors could be spread via direct invasion to the renal parenchyma or the surrounding structures. Lymphatic and hematogenous dissemination is also possible. Epithelial spread by seeding or direct extension could also take place. High-grade tumors have a propensity to invasive expansion, which could result in non–organ-confined disease (>pT2). The non–organ-confined disease is the most significant predictor of the development of metastases (95%), followed by vascular invasion (83%) and lymphatic invasion (77%) (Davis et al., 1987; Margulis et al., 2009).

Lymphatic. The lymphatic spread of UTUC is directly associated with the depth of invasion of the tumor. The lymphatic spread is also related to the location of the tumor. Tumors in the renal pelvis and upper or lower two-thirds of the ureter may spread to the renal hilar, para-aortic, paracaval, interaortocaval, and ipsilateral common iliac and pelvic lymph nodes (Batata and Grabstald, 1976; Kondo et al., 2010).

Hematogenous. Liver, lung, and bones are the common sites of hematogenous spread of UTUC (Batata et al., 1975; Brown et al., 2006). Direct extension of renal pelvic UTUC to the renal vein and vena cava is very rare (Geiger et al., 1986; Jitsukawa et al., 1985).

Epithelial. The epithelial spread of urothelial carcinomas results in synchronous and metachronous tumors. The epithelial spread of the tumor with urinary seeding and/or intraepithelial migration is explained by the monoclonal theory (Harris and Neal, 1992). According to this theory, multiple tumors are originating from single genetically modified neoplastic cells, and the spread could occur in antegrade (more common) or retrograde fashion. The higher incidence of bladder recurrence could be related to the antegrade seeding. This explanation was based on the high recurrence rates in patients who underwent incomplete ureterectomy or in whom the ureteral stump was left in situ after nephrectomy (Johnson and Babaian, 1979). The "field effect" proposes that the urothelium has a propensity to diffusely form unrelated de novo tumors caused by a mutagenic environment. This theory could explain the phenomenon that some multifocal cancers have been noted to derive from different clones (Hafner et al., 2002). The idea of molecular evolution of a single clone is possible; current evidence suggests that the urothelial clones can develop monoclonally through epithelial intraluminal dissemination as well as development of cancer over a "field."

Panurothelial Disease. The definition of panurothelial disease is the involvement of bladder and two extravesical sites. The involvement of bladder and both ureters in a female patient represents panurothelial disease. In the case of male patients, this definition could include the bladder along with one or both upper urinary tracts and/or the prostatic urethra. The treatment of panurothelial disease and its outcomes remains unclear because the disease is uncommon and current evidence is based on retrospective studies.

In a series of 35 patients, the highest risk for panurothelial disease was observed in the patients with high-risk superficial multifocal bladder tumors and those with CIS (Solsona et al., 2002). Cystectomy was performed for high-grade or invasive disease. The noninfiltrating tumors of the upper tract were managed conservatively with local resection, whereas more aggressive tumors led to radical excision. Unfortunately, patients with panurothelial disease represent a clinical dilemma because only the removal of the whole urinary tract would allow the cure of the disease. In another study, 35 patients with bladder and bilateral upper urinary tract urothelial carcinomas were followed for an average time of 95 months (Nguyen et al., 2014). The authors divided the population into patients with primary pathology in the bladder (n = 18) and those with primary pathology in the upper urinary tract (n = 17). There was no statistically significant difference in the oncologic outcomes between the two groups. The authors observed the transition from low-grade disease to multifocal high-grade disease, tumor invasion, and progression in 8 patients. Four patients with initial presentation of low-grade multifocal disease progressed to high-grade tumors, metastases, and death. There was a similar distribution of men and women. Almost half of the patients did not have smoking history. Genetic factors may have played a role in these patients. Most of the patients with this transition of the disease aggressiveness had a history of another malignancy or a family history of cancer.

Recently, a retrospective study evaluated 64 patients who initially underwent cystectomy and radical nephroureterectomy for metachronous UTUC (Li et al., 2017). The median time from radical cystectomy to radical nephroureterectomy was 2.7 years. After the radical nephroureterectomy, the pathology showed 39% locally advanced disease (pT3/pT4) and 11% positive node status. After radical cystectomy, the respective figures were 17% and 6%. Median survival after nephroureterectomy was 3.1 years. The lymph node involvement on radical nephroureterectomy was significantly associated with worse overall mortality. The renal function is diminished after these procedures, and eventually none of the patients was eligible for cisplatin-based chemotherapy.

Patients with panurothelial disease are a complicated population with significant therapeutic dilemmas, and current literature does not provide enough evidence for establishing a management algorithm. The role of systematic disease is not established. Cystectomy is indicated for patients with multifocal high-grade disease. Close surveillance of the upper tract is also mandatory. The total removal of the genitourinary system would have been an option for younger patients with early recognition of disease progression to prevent metastases and death.

> **KEY POINTS: STAGING AND CLASSIFICATION**
>
> - Ureteral tumors are in the distal ureter (70% of cases), mid-ureter (25% of cases), and upper ureter (5% of cases). Bilateral disease is found in in 3% to 5% of cases.
> - Prognosis for recurrence after radical nephroureterectomy is related to the location of the tumor and stage.
> - The recurrence rate is 2% to 4% with an interval of 17 to 170 months.
> - Bladder recurrence is 15% to 75% within 5 years.
> - CIS involves a higher incidence of bilateral and multifocal disease.
> - Disease spread is typically direct expansion of the tumor to lymphatics and bloodstream.

PROGNOSIS

TNM Classification

UTUC has a similar classification and morphology with the bladder carcinoma (Roupret et al., 2018). Noninvasive papillary tumors (papillary urothelial tumors of low malignant potential and low- and high-grade papillary UC) (Soukup et al., 2017), flat lesions (CIS), and invasive carcinoma can be distinguished. Nonurothelial differentiation (i.e., histologic variants) is associated with an adverse risk factor (Roupret et al., 2018).

The TNM classification and staging system is the most commonly used and is shown in Table 98.1 (Brierley, 2017). The regional lymph nodes (LNs) for pelvic and upper ureteral tumors are the hilar and retroperitoneal LNs. For the mid- and distal ureteral tumors the respective LNs are the intrapelvic LNs. The laterality of the LNs does not affect N classification. The renal pelvic subclassification (pT3) provides discrimination between the microscopic infiltration of the renal parenchyma, which is represented as pT3a, and the macroscopic infiltration or invasion of the peripelvic adipose tissue, which is represented as pT3b (Park et al., 2014; Rink et al., 2012; Roscigno et al., 2012). The American Joint Committee on Cancer (AJCC) staging system could also be used. The differences and similarities of these two staging systems are presented in Table 98.2.

Histologic Grading

The 1973 World Health Organization (WHO) classification was used for tumor grading for several decades. The tumors were graded as G1 to G3 (Roupret et al., 2018). The 2004/2016 WHO classification distinguishes between noninvasive tumors: papillary urothelial neoplasia of low malignant potential and low- and high-grade carcinomas based on histologic characteristics (low grade vs. high grade). The current EAU guidelines are based on the 2004/2016 WHO classification (Roupret et al., 2018).

Prognostic Factors

Preoperative Factors

Age-Sex-Ethnicity. Age is one of the most important demographic predictors of survival in UTUC (Kim et al., 2017a and 2017b). Decreased cancer-specific survival has been reported in patients of older age at the time of radical nephroureterectomy. Older age represents an independent factor for decreased survival (Lughezzani et al., 2012; Matsuoka et al., 2003; Park et al., 2014; Shariat et al.,

TABLE 98.1 Tumor Node Metastasis (TNM) Classification for Upper Urinary Tract Carcinoma

T: PRIMARY TUMOR

TX	Primary tumor cannot be assessed
T0	No evidence if primary tumor
Ta	Noninvasive papillary carcinoma
Tis	Carcinoma in situ
T1	Tumor invades subepithelial connective tissue
T2	Tumor invades muscularis
T3	Renal pelvis: tumor invades beyond muscularis into peripelvic fat or renal parenchyma
	Ureter: tumor invades beyond muscularis into perinephric fat
T4	Tumor invades adjacent organs or through the kidney into perinephric fat

N: REGIONAL LYMPH NODES

NX	Regional lymph nodes cannot be assessed
N0	No regional lymph nodes metastasis
N1	Metastasis in a single lymph node 2 cm or less in the greatest diameter
N2	Metastasis in a single lymph node more than 2 cm in the greatest diameter

M: DISTANT METASTASIS

M0	No distant metastasis
M1	Distant metastasis

TABLE 98.2 AJCC Staging System in Conjunction With the TNM System

AJCC STAGING SYSTEM	TNM CLASSIFICATION SYSTEM
0	T0
I	Ta, Tis, T1, N0, M0
II	T2, N0, M0
III	T3, N0, M0
IV	T4 or T, N+, M+

AJCC, American Joint Committee on Cancer; *TNM,* tumor node metastasis.

2010). Nevertheless, radical nephroureterectomy could be curative for elderly patients and is an inadequate indicator of outcome (Chromecki et al., 2011; Shariat et al., 2010). Thus age alone should not prevent a potentially curable approach. Gender is no longer considered an independent prognostic factor influencing UTUC mortality (Fernández et al., 2009; Lughezzani et al., 2012; Matsuoka et al., 2003).

Controversial results have been presented in the literature regarding the impact of race on the outcome of UTUC treatment. No difference in outcome among races was reported by a multicenter study (Matsumoto et al., 2011; Rouprêt et al., 2018). On the contrary, population-based studies showed a worse outcome for African-American patients than other ethnicities. Differences at presentation in risk factors, disease characteristics, and predictors of adverse oncologic outcomes have been noted between Chinese and American patients (risk factor, disease characteristics, and predictors of adverse oncologic outcomes) (Singla et al., 2017). The comparison of Japanese and European patients revealed no differences in survival (Matsumoto et al., 2011).

Tobacco Consumption. There is a close association between tobacco consumption and prognosis because cessation of smoking improves cancer control (Rouprêt et al., 2018). Being a smoker at diagnosis increases the risk for disease recurrence and mortality after radical nephroureterectomy (Rink et al., 2012; Simsir et al., 2011) and recurrence of the urothelial cancer in the bladder (Xylinas et al., 2014).

Tumor Location. Some studies proposed the initial location of the UTUC as a prognostic factor (Ouzzane et al., 2011; Yafi et al., 2012). Patients with ureteral and/or multifocal tumors seemed to have a worse prognosis than renal pelvic tumors when the stage was adjusted (Chromecki et al., 2012; Lughezzani et al., 2012; Ouzzane et al., 2011; Williams et al., 2013; Yafi et al., 2012).

Surgical Delay. When an invasive UTUC is diagnosed, the delay of the treatment may increase the risk of disease progression. It is advisable to perform radical nephroureterectomy within 12 weeks, if possible, from the diagnosis and decision for the treatment (Gadzinski et al., 2012; Sundi et al., 2012; Waldert et al., 2010).

Other. Cancer-specific survival after radical nephroureterectomy is correlated with the American Society of Anesthesiologists (ASA) score (Berod et al., 2012). ASA score is also correlated to poor performance status after radical surgery (Carrion et al., 2016). Obesity and higher body mass index has a negative impact on the cancer-specific outcomes in UTUCs (Ehdaie et al., 2011). The pretreatment-derived neutrophil-lymphocyte ratio seems to be related to higher cancer-specific mortality (Dalpiaz et al., 2014).

Postoperative Factors

Tumor Stage and Grade. The primary recognized prognostic factors are tumor stage and grade (Clements et al., 2012; Kim et al., 2017a,b; Lughezzani et al., 2012; Mbeutcha et al., 2017; Petrelli et al., 2017). UTUCs that invade the muscle wall usually have a very poor prognosis. The 5-year specific survival is less than 50% for pT2/pT3 stage and less than 10% for pT4 stage (Abouassaly et al., 2010; Jeldres et al., 2010; Lughezzani et al., 2012). The main prognostic factors are presented in Fig. 98.5.

The decision making for UTUC is based on the histologic characteristics and biology of the tumor. The benign papillomas have an excellent course regardless of the extent of treatment (Batata and Grabstald, 1976; Bloom et al., 1970). The existence of low-grade papillomas of low-grade malignant potential (PUNLMP) in the bladder remains an issue of debate (Cheng et al., 1999, 2000; Oyasu, 2000). The WHO 2004/2016 classification has reassigned this histologic type from Grade 1 of the 1973 WHO classification to low-grade carcinomas (Babjuk et al., 2017). Thus PUNLMP are treated the same way as low-grade disease. Differences between upper tract papillomas and bladder papillomas are not clearly defined and require further investigation.

Papillary tumors have been suggested to have better outcomes than sessile lesions (Fritsche et al., 2012; Remzi et al., 2009). The majority of the renal pelvis tumors are papillary (85%), whereas the sessile tumors represent 15%. These figures are like those of bladder cancer. Nonetheless, 50% of tumors are papillary and 80% sessile in the T1 and T2 stages, respectively (Cummings, 1980; Williams, 1991). As a result, the invasive tumors of the renal pelvis represent 50% to 60% of cases, which contrasts the noninvasive nature of most bladder cancers. Moreover, 55% to 75% of the ureteral tumors are low grade and low stage, but invasive tumors are more commonly encountered in the ureter in comparison with the bladder (Anderstrom et al., 1989; Williams, 1991). Sessile growth pattern is a strong prognosticator for worse outcome (Fritsche et al., 2012; Remzi et al., 2009).

Renal pelvis tumors are encountered slightly more frequently than ureteral tumors (Batata and Grabstald, 1976; Maulard-Durdux et al., 1996). The incidence of ureteral tumors in the distal, middle, and proximal segments is 70%, 25%, and 5% of cases, respectively (Anderstrom et al., 1989; Babaian and Johnson, 1980; Williams, 1991). When conservative treatment has taken place, the recurrence is usually distributed in an antegrade fashion in 33% to 55% of cases, and recurrence proximal to the initial site is uncommon (Babaian and Johnson, 1980; Cummings, 1980; Johnson and Babaian, 1979; Mazeman, 1976; McCarron et al., 1983). UTUC is associated with a high rate of ipsilateral recurrence, which is probably related to the multifocal field carcinogenesis and the downstream seeding.

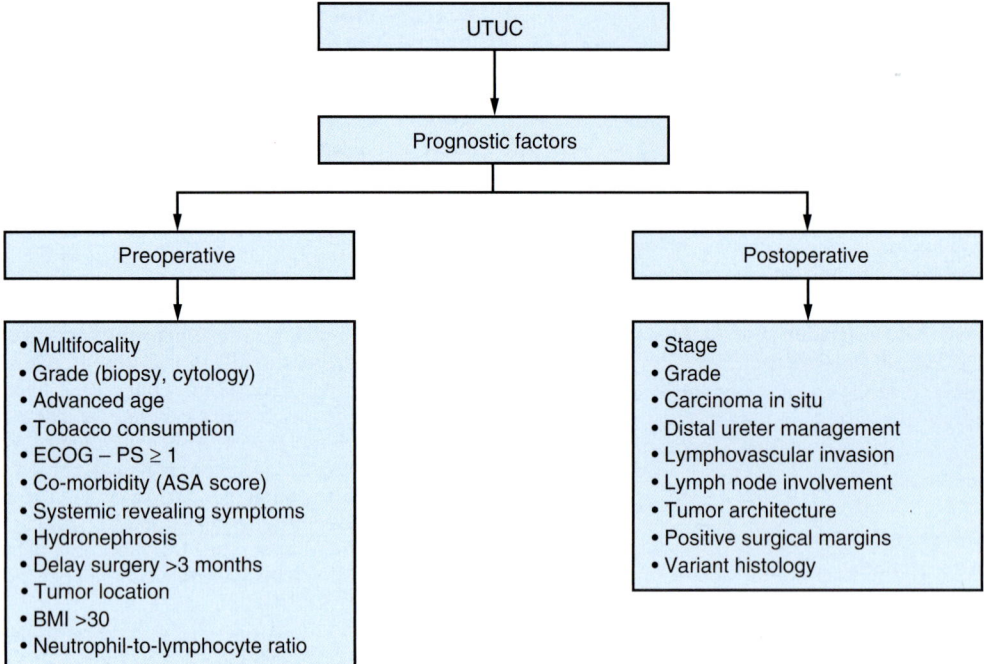

Fig. 98.5. Upper urinary tract urothelial carcinoma (UTUC): prognostic factors. *ASA*, American Society of Anesthesiologists; *BMI*, body mass index; *ECOG – PS*, Eastern Cooperative Oncology Group Performance Status. (Modified from Rouprêt M, Babjuk M, Compérat E, et al: European Association of Urology Guidelines on Upper Urinary Tract Urothelial Carcinoma: 2017 Update, *Eur Urol* 73[1]:111–122, 2018.)

Areas of atypia, dysplasia, and CIS are observed in 60% to 95% of the nephroureterectomy specimens for renal pelvis tumors (Harris and Neal, 1992; Heney et al., 1981; Johansson et al., 1976; Kakizoe et al., 1980; McCarron et al., 1983; Melamed and Reuter, 1993). Concomitant CIS in organ-confined UTUC and a history of bladder CIS are associated with a higher risk of recurrence and cancer-specific mortality (Redrow et al., 2017; Wheat et al., 2012).

Tumor size has not been established as a prognostic criterion. Still, tumors larger than 3 to 4 cm may be related to worse survival and a higher risk of bladder recurrence (Cho et al., 2007; Simone et al., 2009). Extensive tumor necrosis (>10% of the tumor area) is an independent prognostic predictor in patients who undergo radical nephroureterectomy (Seitz et al., 2010; Zigeuner et al., 2010). Extensive necrosis seems to correlate with aggressive clinicopathologic features such advanced stage, high grade, lymph node invasion, presence of CIS, sessile architecture, and lymph node metastases (Zigeuner et al., 2010). Controversial evidence has been reported regarding the presence of tumor necrosis and the decreased recurrence-free and cancer-specific survival (Seitz et al., 2010; Simone et al., 2009; Zigeuner et al., 2010).

Metachronous bilateral UTUCs have been reported to be a rare event and represent only 3.1% of the UTUC cases. These cases are related to increased age and short survival time after the diagnosis (Holmäng and Johansson, 2004). Recurrence in the bladder after UTUC confers a multifocal risk that should affect decision making for treatment, while it presents another expression for field carcinogenesis. CIS involves the distal ureter in 7% to 25% of the patients undergoing cystectomy (Herr et al., 1998; Melamed and Reuter, 1993; Solsona et al., 1997). History of bladder tumor is present in 15% to 50% of the UTUCs (Babaian and Johnson, 1980; Batata and Grabstald, 1976). Recurrence of the urothelial cancer in the upper urinary tract after the treatment of a bladder tumor takes place in 2% to 4% of the bladder cancer cases with a mean interval of 70 months (Herr et al., 1996; Melamed and Reuter, 1993; Oldbring et al., 1989; Shinka et al., 1988). In the patients after cystectomy, recurrence is 3% to 9% (Mufti et al., 1988; Zincke and Neves, 1984).

UTUC associated with environmental exposure (aristolochic acid nephropathy, which includes Balkan and Chinese herbal nephropathy, arsenic endemic regions), analgesic abuse, and Lynch syndrome has a higher tendency to multiple and bilateral recurrences than sporadic tumors (Hubosky et al., 2013; Johansson and Wahlqvist, 1979; Mahoney et al., 1977; Markovic, 1972; Melamed and Reuter, 1993; Petkovic, 1972; Stewart et al., 1999; Tan et al., 2008). Balkan nephropathy is commonly related to low-grade tumors. Nevertheless, these cases may also be related to renal insufficiency, which undermines the role of the conservative treatment. The degree of scarring of renal papillae seen in phenacetin abuse has been correlated in a dose-dependent manner with the risk of high tumor grade and progression. Moreover, the development of squamous carcinoma of the renal pelvis has been reported in calcified renal papillae after analgesic abuse (Stewart et al., 1999).

Tumor stage remains the single most important factor for the oncologic outcome of the UTUC patients (Anderstrom et al., 1989; Babaian and Johnson, 1980; Batata et al., 1975; Bloom et al., 1970; Cummings, 1980; Guinan et al., 1992; McCarron et al., 1983; Terrell et al., 1995). UTUCs spread through the lymphatic and hematogenous routes and by direct extension into surrounding structures. Most metastases develop in the first 2 to 3 years after surgery (Brown et al., 2006). The common metastatic sites are the lungs, liver, bones, and regional lymph nodes. The thin muscle layer of the renal pelvis and ureter could allow for an earlier involvement of surrounding tissue in comparison to the bladder cancer (Cummings, 1980; Richie, 1988). The renal parenchyma may serve as a barrier to the distant spread of renal pelvis tumors of T3 stage, whereas the periureteral spread is related to a high risk for dissemination of the disease along the periureteral vascular and lymphatic supply.

Improved survival of patients with stage T3 renal pelvis tumors versus ureteral tumors has been reported by several investigators (Batata and Grabstald, 1976; Guinan et al., 1992; Park et al., 2004). This observation was also reported from a series of 611 patients treated at 97 hospitals (Guinan et al., 1992). The 5-year survival rates for patients with stage T3 tumors of the renal pelvis and ureter were 54% and 24%, respectively. In a multivariate analysis, patients with ureteral tumors had a higher local and distant failure rate than did those with renal pelvis tumors of the same stage and grade (Park et al., 2004). Some have proposed subclassification of renal pelvis tumors into pT3a for infiltration of the renal parenchyma and pT3b for invasion of peripelvic adipose tissue, because the patients with pT3b have an increased risk of recurrence (Roscigno et al., 2012). Several studies showed that the presence of hydronephrosis is a valuable and independent predictive factor for advanced disease stage and survival in UTUC patients (Brien et al., 2010; Cho et al., 2007; Ito et al., 2011; Ng et al., 2011).

Lymph Node Involvement. Lymph node metastases and extranodal extension are powerful predictors of survival outcomes in UTUC (Fajkovic et al., 2012). Positive regional LNs are an independent factor for poor survival prognosis (Brown et al., 2006; Hall et al., 1998; Margulis et al., 2009). Optimal tumor staging is achieved by lymph node dissection at the time of radical nephroureterectomy (Lughezzani et al., 2010). Depending on the stage and grade of the tumor, up to 40% of patients appear to harbor lymphatic metastases. In a study of patients who underwent lymphadenectomy at the time of radical nephrectomy, lymph node density of 30% or more was associated with poor clinical outcomes (Bolenz et al., 2009). Its curative role is debated.

Lymphovascular Invasion. Lymphovascular invasion (LVI) is observed in approximately 20% of UTUCs and represents an independent predictor of survival (Kikuchi et al., 2009; Novara et al., 2010). LVI status should be identified and specifically reported in the pathologic reports of all UTUC specimens (Godfrey et al., 2012; Kikuchi et al., 2009). LVI is not identified on URS biopsy specimens and serves only as a prognostic factor after surgical resection. In a multicenter study including 1453 patients who underwent radical nephroureterectomy, the multivariate analysis showed that LVI was an independent predictor of disease recurrence and survival for patients with negative lymph nodes or unknown nodal status. LVI was not an independent predictor of outcome for lymph node–positive patients (Kikuchi et al., 2009).

Surgical Margins

The presence of positive soft tissue surgical margin after radical nephroureterectomy has been established as a significant factor for developing disease recurrence. When the stage is greater than 2, pathologists should investigate for and report positive margins at the level of ureteral transection, bladder cuff, and around the tumor (Colin et al., 2012).

Molecular Markers

The characterization of genetic pathways leading to UTUC is ongoing. Bladder cancer and UTUC share similarities but also disparities on a genetic and epigenetic level, which render these two cancers as divergent entities. There have been studies investigating the prognostic impact of molecular markers. These markers include cell adhesion (E-cadherin and CD24) (Favaretto et al., 2017), cell differentiation (Snail and human epidermal growth factor receptor [EGFR] HER-2) (Soria et al., 2017), angiogenesis (hypoxia inducible factor 1α and metalloproteinases), cell proliferation (Ki-67), epithelial-mesenchymal transition (Snail), mitosis (Aurora A), apoptosis (Bcl-2 and survivin), vascular invasion (RON), and c-met protein (MET) (Lughezzani et al., 2012; Scarpini et al., 2012). Microsatellite instability (MSI) has been proposed as an independent molecular prognostic marker (Roupret, 2005). MSI typing could facilitate the detection of germline mutations and hereditary cancers (Roupret et al., 2008). In addition, there is a prognostic value of PD-1 and PDL-1 expression in patients with high-grade UTUC (Krabbe et al., 2017). UTUC is a cancer with low incidence, and any molecular studies are retrospective, although most of them have a small sample size. Current evidence is sufficient for the introduction of any of the markers in the daily clinical practice. Nonetheless, some markers show promise for the future.

Microsatellite instability and hypermethylation are emerging as key differences between upper and lower tract urothelial tumors. Nevertheless, it has been reported that several gene foci on chromosome 9 are mutated in 50% of UTUC cases (Rigola et al., 2001). Comparative genomic hybridization showed concordance between tumors of the renal pelvis and bladder in the losses at 2q, 8p, 9q, 11p, 13q, 17p, and 18q, and gains at 1q, 6p, 8q, and 17q chromosomes (Rigola et al., 2001). Similar gene expression was observed between renal pelvic and bladder tumors. Cytogenetic alterations such as +1p36, +6p22, +7, +8q22, −9p21, +11q, −13q, +17,+19q13, and +20q were noted (Zhang et al., 2010).

Patients with HNPCC (Lynch syndrome) show genomic alterations in DNA mismatch repair genes (Amira et al., 2003). Microsatellite instability has been related to an inverted growth pattern of cancer. In the latter cases, the microsatellite instability had a sensitivity and specificity of 82% and probably could be considered a marker for inverted growth in UTUCs (Hartmann et al., 2003). A urine-based assay testing for a total panel of 77 markers for microsatellite instability was evaluated in 30 patients. The assay detected 83.3% of cases of a UTUC (Ho et al., 2008). Testing for microsatellite instability on resected tumor and normal tissues to screen for Lynch syndrome is a well-established tool for colon cancer. This approach could be considered for patients with UTUC meeting criteria suggestive of Lynch syndrome (Audenet et al., 2012).

Cell Cycle Markers. The TP53 nuclear protein staining of cytology specimens obtained during ureteroscopy were correlated to the presence of UTUC. In a study, 28 out of 36 patients with TP53-positive specimens had evidence of urothelial carcinoma. In the serial evaluation of these patients, 80% of the remaining patients had confirmed UTUC. All 14 TP53-negative specimens were obtained from patients who did not have a sign of concurrent malignant disease on ureteroscopy (Keeley et al., 1997a). Decreased TP53 immunoreactivity and TP53 overexpression in UTUCs have been associated with advanced tumor stage and poor prognosis. When the stage and grade were considered in the multivariate analysis, no such correlation was confirmed (Zigeuner et al., 2004).

CDKN1B (formerly known as p27), a cyclin-dependent kinase inhibitor, has been proposed to predict the prognosis of UTUCs. Low levels of CDKN1B staining were indicating a worse disease-specific survival (Kamai et al., 2000).

Apoptosis. Expression of Bcl-2 and survivin correlates with advanced cancers, and levels of survivin are associated with disease-specific survival (Jeong et al., 2009).

Cell Migration and Invasion. Expression of E-cadherin and matrix metalloproteinases (MMPs) was related to poor prognosis (Inoue et al., 2002). There is a correlation between the immunohistochemistry of MMPs and the pT stage and disease-specific survival (Miyata et al., 2004).

Angiogenesis. Angiogenesis is essential for tumor cell growth. Hypoxia-inducible factor-1α (HIF-1α) is a transcription factor that plays an important role in cellular hypoxia adaptation. Positive HIF-1α expression was found in two-thirds of patients with UTUC and was absent in the cases of normal urothelium. The expression of HIF-1α was significantly associated with high T stage, nodal stage, grade, and cancer-specific survival (HR = 2.23; $P = 0.004$) (Ke et al., 2008).

Cell Proliferation. Overexpression of Ki-67 has been associated with progression, decreased disease-specific survival (Jeon et al., 2010), and development of metachronous tumors (Joung et al., 2008). Epidermal growth factor receptor (EGFR) was related to stage, grade, and squamous differentiation of UTUC. Overexpression and immunoreactivity of nuclear factor-κB (NF-κB) predicts disease-specific survival and overall survival. HER2 overexpression is rare in UTUC and was related to higher stage and grade.

Cell Differentiation. Uroplakin III expression is associated with lower stage and grade. Cancer-specific survival is significantly better when uroplakin III is expressed. On multivariate analysis it outperformed stage and lymph node status as a predictor of survival (Ohtsuka et al., 2006). Snail contributes to the epithelial-mesenchymal transition in cell differentiation. Strong Snail staining is observed in invasive UTUC. It is associated with stage, grade, and LVI. It is a predictor of recurrence and disease-specific survival (Kosaka et al., 2010). In situ hybridization of telomerase mRNA component hTR is positive in 98.4% of UTUCs. hTR score is increased with stage and may be associated with disease-free and overall survival (Nakanishi et al., 1999).

Mitosis. Aurora-A regulates spindle assembly during mitosis. Its overexpression was related to the presence of vascular invasion and recurrence (Scarpini et al., 2012).

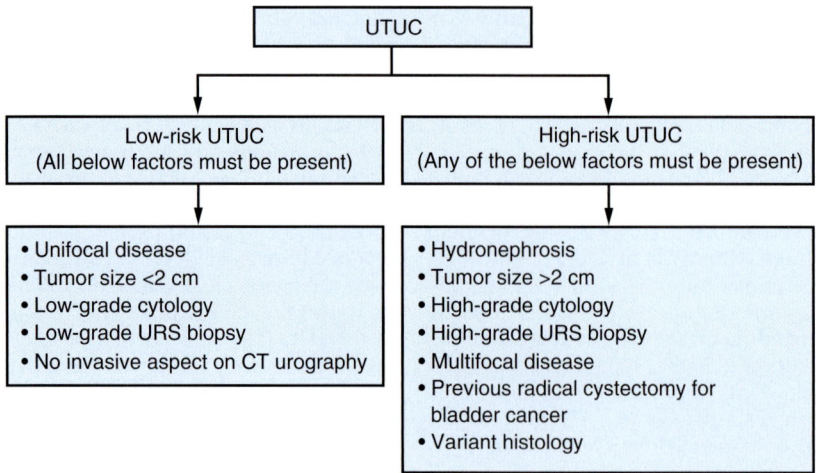

Fig. 98.6. Risk stratification of upper urinary tract urothelial carcinoma (UTUC). *CT*, Computed tomography; *URS*, ureteroscopy. (Modified from Rouprêt M, Babjuk M, Compérat E, et al: European Association of Urology Guidelines on Upper Urinary Tract Urothelial Carcinoma: 2017 Update, *Eur Urol* 73[1]:111–122, 2018.)

The roles of members of the MET proto-oncogene family of tyrosine kinases, c-MET and RON, have been investigated in UTUC (Comperat et al., 2008). c-MET overexpression correlated with vascular invasion and a worse clinical outcome. The overexpression of RON did not correlate with the outcome of UTUC.

Abnormal expression of cyclooxygenase-2 (COX-2) has been observed in various human cancers and in bladder urothelial cancer. Abnormal expression of COX-2 in stromal cells of UTUCs was associated with high tumor stage and grade and poor prognosis (Kang et al., 2008).

Other Markers

Ploidy-flow cytometry was used for providing information on tumor ploidy. The survival of patients with UTUC was correlated with tumor aneuploidy. In a study from the 1980s, tumor aneuploidy was correlated to poor 5- and 10-year survival rates of 25% and 0, respectively (Blute et al., 1988).

Efforts have been made during recent years for the development of rapid urine tests for the detection of urothelial malignant neoplasms. These rapid urine tests have been extensively studied for bladder cancer. The knowledge of their use in UTUCs remains limited. Urinary levels of NMP22 is a nuclear matrix protein–based marker. Patients with UTUC have elevated urinary levels of NMP22 (Carpinito et al., 1996). This investigation seems to have higher sensitivity for detecting the presence of UTUC but lower specificity in comparison with cytology.

The cytogenetic detection of molecular abnormalities by fluorescent in situ hybridization (FISH) has been investigated in 16 UTUC cases. Urine FISH was reported to have a sensitivity of 87.5% and a specificity of 80% for detection of UTUCs (Akkad et al., 2007). The cytology was compared with UroVysion, which is a multitarget FISH system, in 50 patients. The overall sensitivity/specificity of cytology was 20.8%/97.4% in comparison with 100%/89.5% of FISH (Mian et al., 2010). In a study including 285 patients with hematuria and negative cytology, 11 (3.9%) patients had positive FISH, of which 9 (81.8%) had UTUC. None of the patients with negative FISH was diagnosed with UTUC. The specificity and sensitivity were 99.3% and 100%, respectively (Huang et al., 2012). One study compared the analysis of fibrinogen-fibrin degradation products (AuraTek FDP) with the bladder tumor antigen (BTA) test and urine cytology. The accuracy of the FDP test was 83% compared with 62% for BTA and 59% for cytology (Siemens et al., 2003).

Predictive Tools

Accurate predictive tools are rare for UTUC. For preoperative decision making, there are two models in the preoperative setting. The one is helpful in predicting lymph node involvement of locally advanced cancer that could guide the decision to perform an LND and to decide on the extent of LND at the time of radical nephroureterectomy (Margulis et al., 2010). The other facilitates the selection of the cases with non–organ-confined UTUC to undergo radical nephroureterectomy (Favaretto et al., 2012). Five nomograms predict the survival rates postoperatively. The prediction is based on standard pathologic features (Cha et al., 2012; Ku et al., 2013; Roupret et al., 2013; Seisen et al., 2014; Yates et al., 2012). One of these nomograms is based on only four variables and was reported to have high prognostic accuracy and risk stratification for patients with high-grade urothelial carcinoma of the upper urinary tract after extirpative surgery (Krabbe et al., 2017). Further clinical research would establish one of these nomograms in the clinical practice.

Risk Stratification

Tumor stage is difficult to assert based on the clinical criteria. The UTUC cases could be stratified between low- and high-risk tumors to distinguish the cases that are more appropriate for kidney-sparing treatment rather than radical surgery (Roupret, 2014; Seisen et al., 2015; Fig. 98.6).

> **KEY POINTS: PROGNOSTIC FACTORS**
> - Use the TNM classification and staging system.
> - Use the 2004/2016 WHO grading classification.
> - Age alone should not prevent a curable approach.
> - Ureteral and/or multifocal tumors have a worse prognosis than renal pelvic tumors.
> - Muscle invasive tumors have a poor prognosis.
> - Positive regional LNs have a poor survival prognosis.
> - Lymphovascular invasion is a predictor of disease recurrence and survival.

REFERENCES

The complete reference list is available online at ExpertConsult.com.

99
Surgical Management of Upper Urinary Tract Urothelial Tumors

Thomas W. Jarret, MD, Surena F. Matin, MD, and Armine K. Smith, MD

DIAGNOSIS

Ureteroscopic Evaluation and Biopsy

Although the diagnosis can be made in obvious cases with CT urogram, cystoscopy, and a positive urinary cytology (Potrezke et al., 2016), technical advances achieved in the realm of endoscopic equipment have made flexible and rigid ureteroscopy a key part of the evaluation (and treatment) of upper urinary tract tumors. **Diagnostic accuracy can be improved from approximately 75% with excretory or retrograde urography alone to 85% to 90% when it is combined with ureteroscopy** (Blute et al., 1989; Streem et al., 1986). Although pyelovenous and pyelolymphatic migration has been reported with ureteroscopy, this phenomenon appears to be uncommon and should not preclude its use (Guo et al., 2017; Lim et al., 1993). Generally the tumor is biopsied and the treatment is contingent on the patient factors along with the biopsy results. Occasionally, the tumor is biopsied and treated in the same setting. Percutaneous access to the renal pelvis and antegrade ureteroscopy may be required for diagnosis or treatment; examples include patients with urinary diversion. These techniques are described in more detail in later sections.

In addition to biopsy, ureteroscopy allows direct tumor visualization of areas that may have not been seen on imaging and provides information that may assist with treatment planning. **Preoperative ureteroscopy has clear benefits when there is a question of diagnosis and/or if conservative management is being considered.**

Because of the small size and shallow depth of ureteroscopic biopsy specimens, a precise correlation with eventual tumor stage is difficult. Therefore, in predicting the tumor stage, a combination of the radiographic studies, the visualized appearance of the tumor, and the tumor grade provides the surgeon with the best estimation for risk stratification.

TREATMENT ALGORITHM

The gold standard therapy for treatment of upper tract urothelial carcinoma (UTUC) is nephroureterectomy with a cuff of bladder, provided there is a normal contralateral kidney. The European Association of Urology (EAU) devised a risk-adapted protocol for kidney-sparing management (Box 99.1; Rouprét, 2018).

All patients with low-risk disease should be considered for kidney-sparing treatment irrespective of the contralateral kidney because of the lower morbidity of the procedures without compromising oncologic outcomes. Kidney-sparing surgery can also be considered in select patients with higher-risk situations such as (1) serious renal insufficiency, (2) solitary kidney, (3) bilateral tumors, and/or (4) poor surgical candidate. Certainly the treatment chosen must not significantly compromise oncologic outcomes. The risks of cancer control must be weighed against the preservation of renal function. In situations of high-grade disease, segmental resection should be considered over endoscopic management, which can only reliably treat surface tumors (Seisen, 2016).

SURGICAL MANAGEMENT

The treatment of upper tract urothelial tumors has undergone significant changes. **The relatively low frequency of these lesions and paucity of prospective randomized trials do not permit absolute conclusions about treatment impact on outcomes.** In the past, treatment recommendations were based, at least in part, on practical limitations in follow-up and detection of local disease recurrence. Technologic improvements in imaging and, most important, direct endoscopic visualization of all levels of the urinary tract allow earlier and more accurate initial diagnosis and treatment and improved follow-up. Treatment may be based primarily on the risk the tumor poses and on the efficacy of a specific treatment rather than on other considerations. The specific indications and techniques for each form of treatment (open vs. laparoscopic radical nephroureterectomy; open vs. retrograde endoscopic vs. percutaneous renal-sparing tumor ablation) are addressed later in this chapter. However, the following introductory considerations apply. The least invasive treatment necessary for safe control of the tumor is preferred, but never at the risk of compromising oncologic control. UTUC is unforgiving to surgical indiscretions, which usually cannot be salvaged by other modalities. Most upper tract urothelial tumors are not large or bulky. Thus laparoscopic surgery is ideal, at least for the renal portion of radical nephroureterectomy when the tumor warrants removal of the entire renal unit. A variety of approaches with various combinations of laparoscopic and open techniques are employed for distal ureterectomy. Select low-grade noninvasive upper tract tumors can be managed initially by ablative renal-sparing surgery. Retrograde ureteroscopy and ureteropyeloscopy are preferred when tumor size, number, and access allow complete tumor ablation. Percutaneous antegrade tumor ablation is chosen when the anatomy and the tumor do not allow complete ablation through a retrograde approach.

Radical Nephroureterectomy

Indications

Radical nephroureterectomy with excision of a bladder cuff is the gold standard for large, high-grade, suspected invasive tumors of the renal pelvis and proximal ureter (Babaian and Johnson, 1980; Batata and Grabstald, 1976; Cummings, 1980; McCarron et al., 1983; Messing and Catalona, 1998; Murphy et al., 1981; Nocks et al., 1982; Richie, 1988; Skinner, 1978; Williams, 1991). Radical surgery also retains a role in treatment of low-grade, noninvasive tumors of the renal pelvis and upper ureter when they are large, multifocal, or rapidly recurring despite maximal efforts at conservative surgery.

Techniques

Open Radical Nephrectomy. The choice among a variety of surgical approaches to open radical nephroureterectomy is dictated primarily by the surgeon's experience and patient's body habitus. Nephroureterectomy is one of the few multi-quadrant operations that urologists perform with a variety of approaches. The patient may be positioned

BOX 99.1 Risk-Adapted Protocol for Kidney-Sparing Management

HIGH-RISK UTUC
Clinical factors
- Hydronephrosis
- High grade
- Tumor >1 cm
- Invasive features on imaging
- Multifocal disease
- Failed endoscopic treatment

Clinical factors
- Smoking
- Previous bladder UCC and/or cystectomy

LOW-RISK UTUC
Clinical factors
- Low-grade biopsy
- Low-grade cytology
- Tumor <1 cm
- No invasive features on imaging
- Unifocal disease
- Compliant patient

UCC, Urothelial cell carcinoma; *UTUC*, upper tract urothelial cancer.
Modified from Rouprêt M, Babjuk M, Compérat E, et al.: European Association of Urology Guidelines on Upper Urinary Tract Urothelial Carcinoma: 2017 Update. *Eur Urol* 73:111–122, 2018.

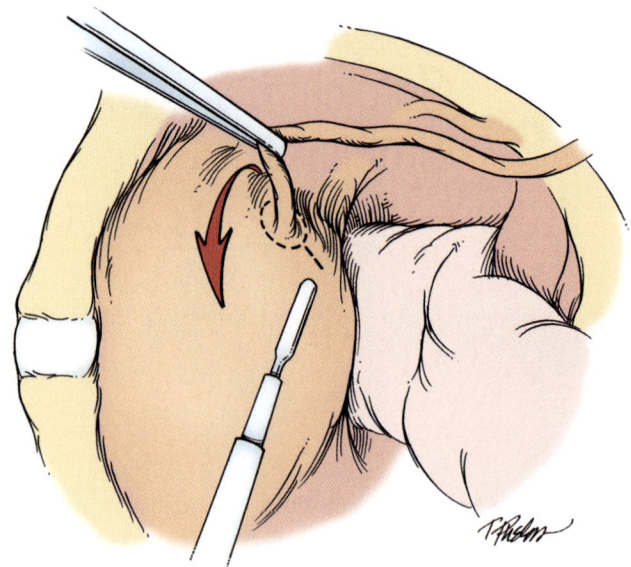

Fig. 99.2. Complete distal ureterectomy by extravesical approach. Traction is placed, everting the orifice outside the bladder. Care must be taken to ensure complete removal and to avoid injury to the contralateral ureteral orifice.

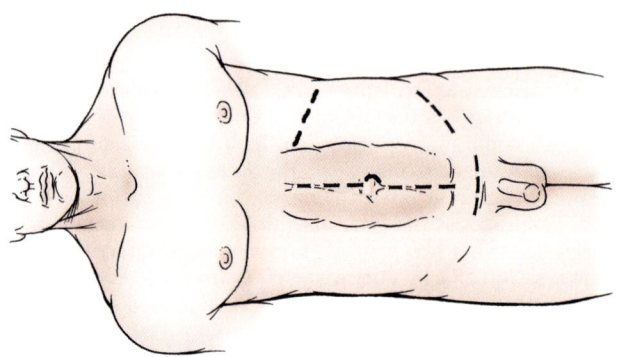

Fig. 99.1. Choice of incision for radical nephroureterectomy (midline, subcostal, flank, or thoracoabdominal) is dictated by the surgeon's preference and experience. Unless a midline incision is used, an additional Gibson, low midline, or Pfannenstiel incision is necessary for bladder cuff removal.

supine or in modified flank position. In male patients the genitalia are included in the surgical field so that the bladder catheter may be accessed during the procedure. The midline approach gives the most optimal exposure to the retroperitoneal lymph nodes and bladder. This incision, however, may be limiting in exposure of the upper pole of the left kidney, especially in obese patients. Other incisions are flank, subcostal, and thoracoabdominal. The choice of these incisions necessitates using an additional Gibson, midline, or Pfannenstiel incision for bladder cuff removal (Fig. 99.1). After the white line of Toldt is incised, the ipsilateral colon is mobilized to expose the Gerota fascia. Ideally, the hilum is controlled before excessive manipulation of the kidney and ureter. The renal hilum is exposed, reflecting the duodenum medially on the right side. For left-sided tumors, care should be taken to avoid injury to the pancreatic tail and spleen. The renal artery and vein are secured and divided in a standard manner. The variety of options for ligating the vessels is used, including suture ligature, ties, and a combination of ties with clips and stapling devices using an endovascular load. The ureter is typically ligated at this time to prevent migration of tumor fragments into the bladder. The entire kidney is mobilized, taking care to stay outside of Gerota fascia. Attachments between liver and kidney on the right side and splenorenal ligament on the left side are incised, allowing mobility of the kidney. Adrenalectomy does not aid the oncologic control of UTUC, unless its direct involvement is suspected by preoperative imaging or intraoperative examination. Thus as a routine, concomitant adrenalectomy is unnecessary.

Management of Distal Ureter and Bladder Cuff. Complete removal of the distal ureter and bladder cuff offers superior oncologic outcomes to incomplete resection. In addition, an adequate cystoscopic surveillance of a residual distal ureter stump after nephroureterectomy is almost impossible, contributing to high rates of local recurrence. **Therefore the entire distal ureter, including the intramural portion and the ureteral orifice, must be removed.** The kidney and proximal ureter may be kept in continuity with the distal segment; however, the bulk of the attached kidney makes its manipulation difficult, and, apart from helping the pathologist with specimen orientation, this technique is not necessary as long as the distal ureter is divided in the controlled manner between ties or clips at a location that is free of gross tumor. There are at least five different techniques described for distal ureterectomy, and most of these apply to open and laparoscopic surgery.

Traditional Open Distal Ureterectomy. Using a Gibson, low midline or Pfannestiel incision, bladder cuff removal is performed by extravesical (Fig. 99.2), transvesical (Fig. 99.3), or combined approach. Either of these methods is acceptable, provided that the whole ureter, including the intramural portion and mucosa of ureteral orifice, is removed with the surgeon's visual confirmation of complete resection. For the extravesical approach, the distal ureter is freed toward the bladder to the point of the intramural ureter. Gentle traction on the ureter and full bladder may aid in this step and for adequate access to the entire intramural ureter, the lateral pedicle of the bladder (obliterated artery, superior, middle, and inferior vesical arteries) may be ligated and divided. Care must be taken to avoid uncontrolled entry to urinary tract. A cuff of bladder is removed en bloc with the ureter by applying a clamp to bladder wall and excising the full intramural portion of the ureter, taking care to stay away from the contralateral ureteral orifice. In the transvesical approach, anterior cystotomy is made, and intravesical dissection of ureter is performed, including a traditional 1-cm mucosal cuff around the orifice. A wider margin can be taken if a gross tumor is seen protruding from the orifice, and if an invasive intramural tumor is suspected, an en bloc partial cystectomy may be required to ensure negative margins. Cystotomy defects are closed in two layers with interrupted or running absorbable sutures: the first layer should incorporate mucosa, and the second layer should include detrusor muscle and adventitia. A Foley catheter is placed and maintained for 5 to 7 days, and a suction drain is left in the perivesical space.

Transvesical Ligation and Detachment Technique. This technique mimics the open bladder cuff removal. Before nephrectomy portion, the patient is placed in low lithotomy position, the cystoscope is passed into the bladder and kept in place, and the bladder is filled. One or two 5-mm trocars are placed intravesically from the suprapubic area. An Endoloop is placed around the ureteral orifice, and a ureteral catheter is advanced into the ureter through the Endoloop. Using a Collins knife, the surgeon incises the bladder cuff, and this incision is carried into the extravesical space (Fig. 99.4). Retraction is provided by the grasper through the one of the trochars. Once the ureter is freed, the Endoloop is cinched around the ureter as the catheter is removed. This creates a "closed" urothelium with subsequent en bloc removal of specimen, and extravasation of fluid from the bladder is minimized by continuous suction from the second intravesical trocar. There has been excellent clinical success reported with this technique (Gill et al., 1999), but the learning curve is difficult, and repositioning of the patient for nephrectomy portion is required. Patients with distal ureteral tumors, disease in the bladder, or prior pelvic radiation are not candidates for this technique.

Transurethral Resection of the Ureteral Orifice. This approach is also referred to as a "pluck" technique and can be used in patients with proximal tumors and absence of bladder disease (Abercrombie et al., 1988; Palou et al., 1995). With the patient in the lithotomy position, the resectoscope is inserted into the bladder, and aggressive resection of ureteral orifice and intramural ureter is performed down to perivesical fat (Fig. 99.5). This facilitates the plucking of the distal ureter during the nephrectomy portion of the procedure. Even though equivalent oncologic outcomes were reported in limited studies

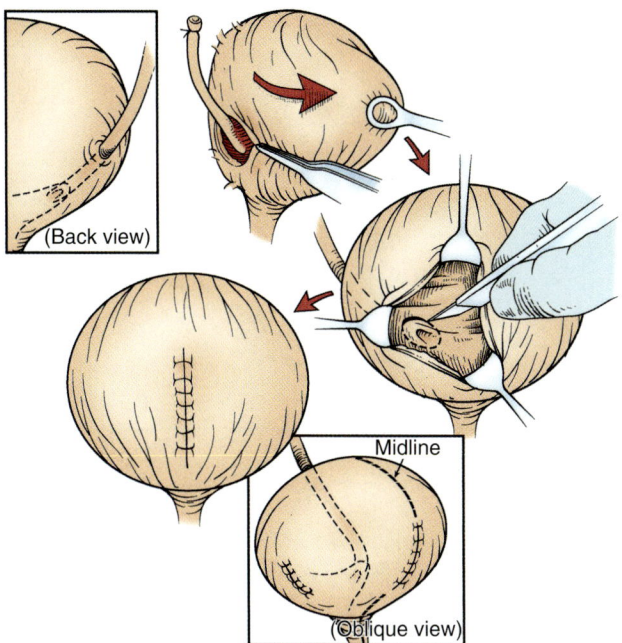

Fig. 99.3. Complete distal ureterectomy with bladder cuff is performed by combined extravesical and transvesical dissection.

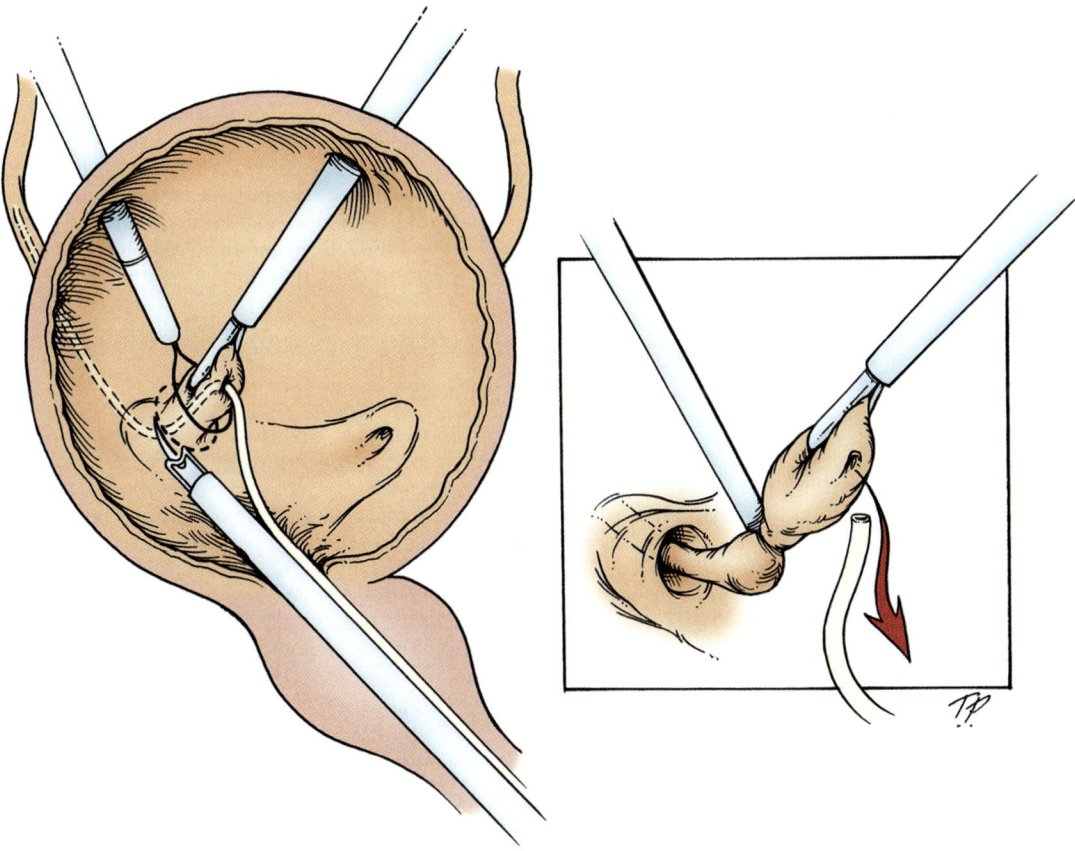

Fig. 99.4. A ureteral catheter is placed, and two laparoscopic ports are placed transvesically. The ureteral orifice is tented up; a loop is placed around the orifice to occlude the opening and to place traction on the ureter. A Collins knife then facilitates the dissection to the extravesical space.

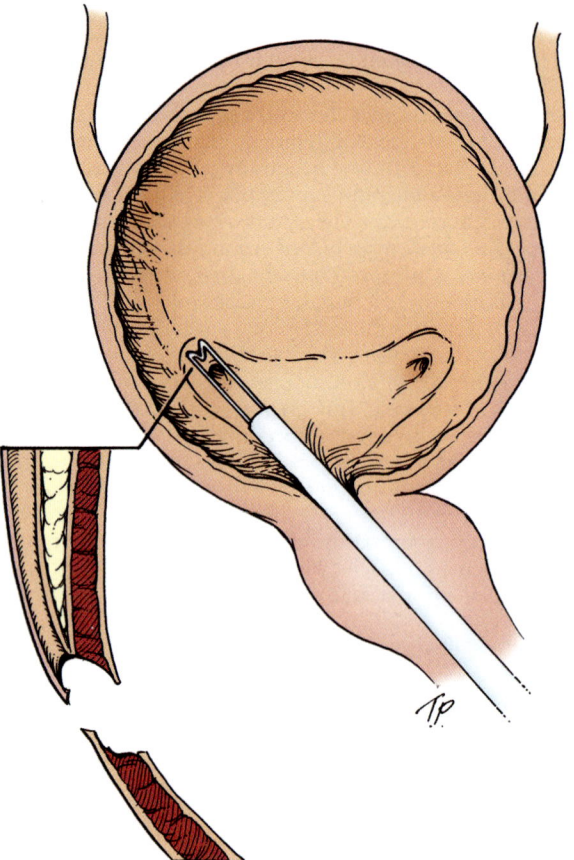

Fig. 99.5. The entire orifice and intramural ureter are resected transurethrally until the extravesical fat is seen. This portion is usually done at the beginning but can be done at the end of the procedure.

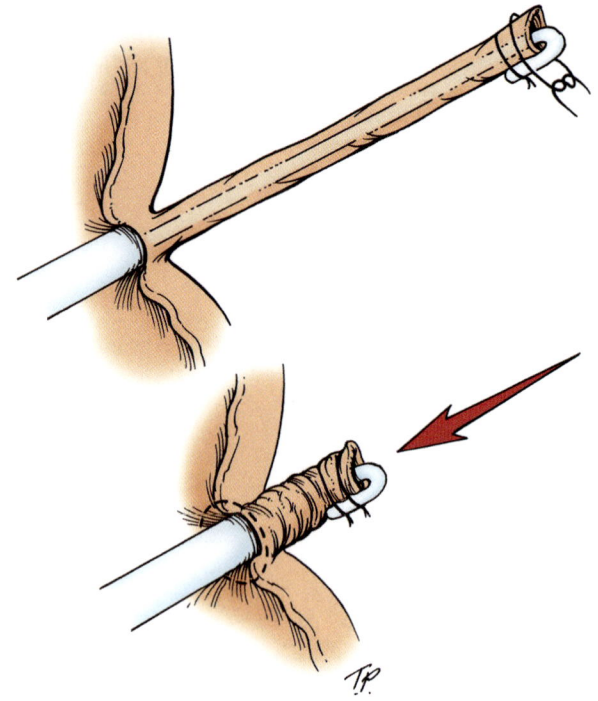

Fig. 99.6. With the intussusception technique, a ureteral catheter is placed at the beginning of the case. After nephrectomy the ureter is divided and the catheter is secured to the distal portion of the ureter. The patient is moved to the lithotomy position, and the ureter is intussuscepted into the bladder with retrograde traction. A resectoscope is used to excise the attached orifice.

(Walton et al., 2009), concerns about tumor seeding of extravesical space and the potential of leaving an incompletely resected ureter caused this technique to be largely abandoned (Arango et al., 1997; Jones and Moisey, 1993).

Intussusception (Stripping) Technique. This technique was initially described in 1953, and several modifications have been described since then (Angulo et al., 1998; Clayman et al., 1983; McDonald, 1953; Roth et al., 1996). It is contraindicated in the presence of ureteral tumors. At the beginning of the procedure, a ureteral catheter is placed in the ureter, and nephrectomy is carried out as usual. The distal ureter is isolated extravesically, and a tie is placed around it, securing the catheter to the ureter (Fig. 99.6). After the nephrectomy portion is completed, the ureter is transected between ties, and the bladder cuff is incised cystoscopically using a Collins knife. Pulling on the ureteral catheter everts the distal ureter inside the bladder. The intussuscepted ureter is then removed by traction out of the urethra. The edges of the bladder mucosa can be fulgurated. The concerns with this technique include exposure of bladder urothelium to ureteral mucosa with extensive manipulation of ureter and the potential for incomplete intramural ureter excision. In addition, the failure rate of 18.7% has been described, in which there was disruption of the ureter during manipulation and the need for an additional surgical incision (Giovansili et al., 2004).

Total Laparoscopic Technique. This approach is attractive to many because it avoids incision into the urinary tract, and in experienced hands the operative time is reduced. Initially, cystoscopy may be performed and the ureteral orifice cauterized, which may be preceded by placement of a ureteral catheter and incision of intramural tunnel at the 12 o'clock position. The nephrectomy portion is performed as usual, and the distal ureter is traced to the detrusor muscle. The ureteral dissection is carried down to the bladder. The detrusor muscle is split and the ureter retracted in antegrade direction. The endovascular stapler is then used to place a staple line as distally as possible. The fulguration mark helps serve as an identifier of bladder cuff (Fig. 99.7). The concerns with this technique include the potential for leaving ureter mucosa within the staple line and inability for the pathologist to evaluate the distal margin because of the presence of staples. Laparoscopic stapling has been associated with a higher risk of positive margins, which in this disease is associated with significantly reduced survival (Matin and Gill, 2005; Steinberg and Matin, 2004). Contraindications include the presence of distal ureteral tumors.

Laparoscopic Radical Nephroureterectomy

Indications

The indications for laparoscopic nephroureterectomy are the same as those for open nephroureterectomy. Exceptions may include large bulky tumors with involvement of adjacent structures or those in which extended lymph node dissections may be considered. Laparoscopic nephroureterectomy can be performed by transperitoneal, retroperitoneal, hand-assisted (Ni et al., 2012), and robotic approaches. **The laparoscopic approach generally shows a significant decrease in morbidity compared with an open surgical approach for appropriately selected patients.** All laparoscopic techniques involve two distinct portions of the procedure: nephrectomy/proximal ureterectomy and excision of the distal ureter with intact specimen extraction for accurate staging. Management of the distal ureter was described previously in the chapter. Several factors must be considered with laparoscopic nephroureterectomy, including the risk of tumor seeding from the ureter and the bladder. For these reasons, removal of an intact specimen is desirable. The incision should be strategically placed for extraction of the specimen and dissection of the distal ureter. Because an incision is necessary regardless of the approach chosen, some techniques for avoidance of a second incision for the distal ureter described previously have less utility.

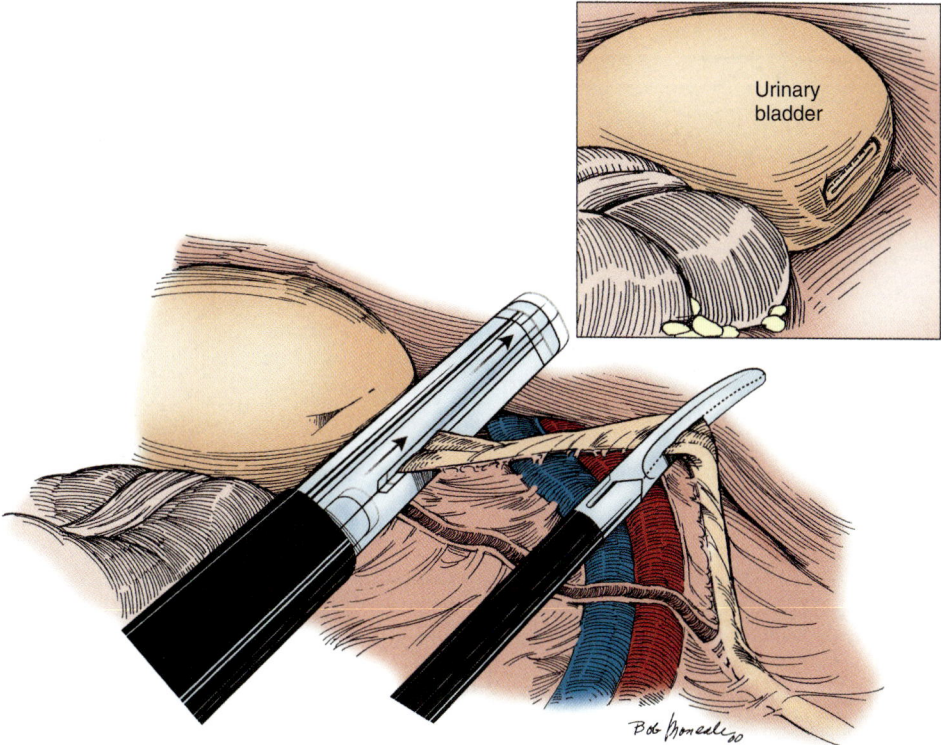

Fig. 99.7. The ureter is dissected extravesically to the ureteral orifice. Lateral traction is placed on the ureter, everting the orifice, and the endovascular stapling device is placed at the distal margin, providing simultaneous ligation and division of the distal ureter at the level of the bladder. A cystoscope can be placed to ensure that the entire ureter is removed.

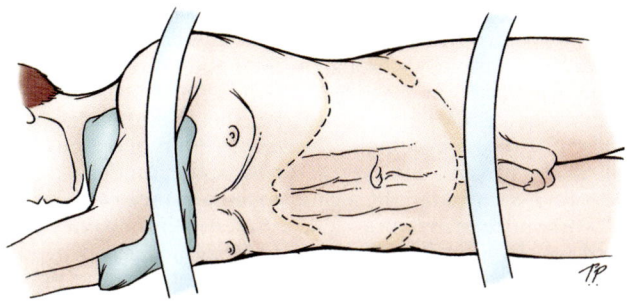

Fig. 99.8. The patient is positioned on the table in a modified lateral decubitus position with the ipsilateral flank rotated up 15 degrees. The patient is secured to the table at the chest, waist, and lower extremity. This setup allows the patient to be moved to the full flank or supine position with simple rotation of the operating table. (From Jarrett TW: Laparoscopic nephroureterectomy. In Bishoff JT, Kavoussi LR, editors: *Atlas of laparoscopic retroperitoneal surgery,* Philadelphia, 2000, Saunders, p 105.)

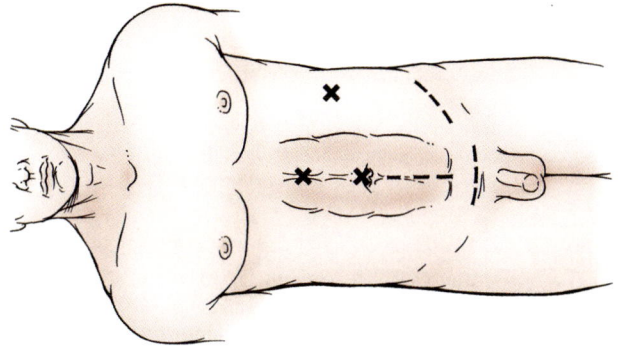

Fig. 99.9. Port configuration for laparoscopic-assisted nephroureterectomy. Three ports are typically used for the kidney and upper ureteral dissection. A fourth midline port between the umbilicus and symphysis can be placed, if needed, for further ureteral dissection. The incision is then strategically placed to allow the distal ureteral dissection and specimen removal. The choice of incision largely depends on patient factors and level of dissection reached during the laparoscopic portion of the procedure. A low abdominal (midline or Pfannenstiel) incision is favored if the dissection is below the iliac vessels. A Gibson-type incision will give exposure of the more proximal ureter, if necessary.

Technique

Transperitoneal Laparoscopic Nephroureterectomy
Laparoscopic Removal of Kidney Down to Mid-Ureter. The patient is placed supine with the ipsilateral hip and shoulder rotated approximately 20 degrees (Fig. 99.8). The patient is secured to the table and can be easily moved from the flank position (nephrectomy portion) to the modified supine position (open portion) by rotating the operative table. The ipsilateral flank and urethra are prepared and draped, and a Foley catheter is placed before insufflation of the abdomen. The abdomen is insufflated, and three or four trocars are placed as outlined in Fig. 99.9, with the first usually being the lateral trocar. Subsequent trocars are placed under direct vision. With this configuration, the camera is kept at the umbilicus for the entire procedure. The upper midline and lateral trocars are used by the surgeon for the dissection of the kidney and the proximal half of the ureter. The lower midline and lateral trocars are used for the dissection of the distal ureter. A 3-mm trocar just below the xiphoid can be helpful in retracting the spleen and liver for left- and right-sided lesions, respectively. The exception is with obese patients, when shifting of the trocars may be necessary to provide optimal visualization (Fig. 99.10). If a hand-assist approach is chosen, the hand port site should be placed so that it can be used for the dissection of the distal ureter and open bladder cuff as indicated. The table is rotated so that the patient is in the flank position. The peritoneum is incised

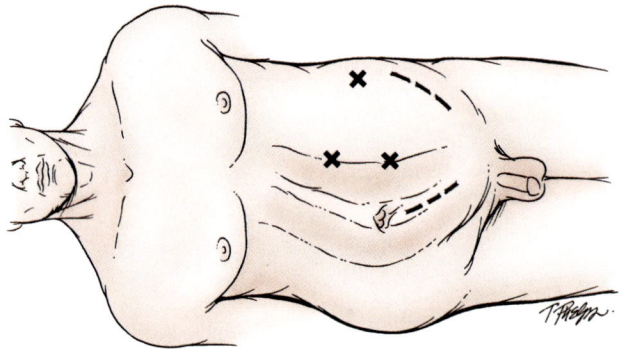

Fig. 99.10. For obese patients undergoing laparoscopic-assisted nephroureterectomy, the trocars are shifted laterally to accommodate the increased distance from the kidney.

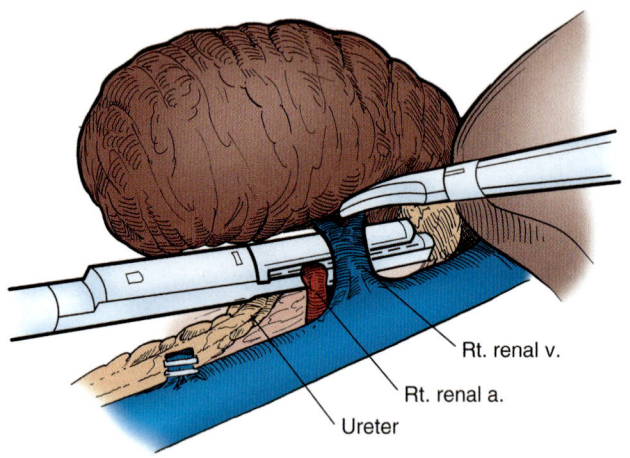

Fig. 99.11. The vessels of the renal hilum are carefully dissected, and the endovascular stapling device, with a vascular load, is used to simultaneously ligate and divide the vessels in a controlled environment. (From Jarrett TW: Laparoscopic nephroureterectomy. In Bishoff JT, Kavoussi LR, editors: *Atlas of laparoscopic retroperitoneal surgery*, Philadelphia, 2000, Saunders, p 112.)

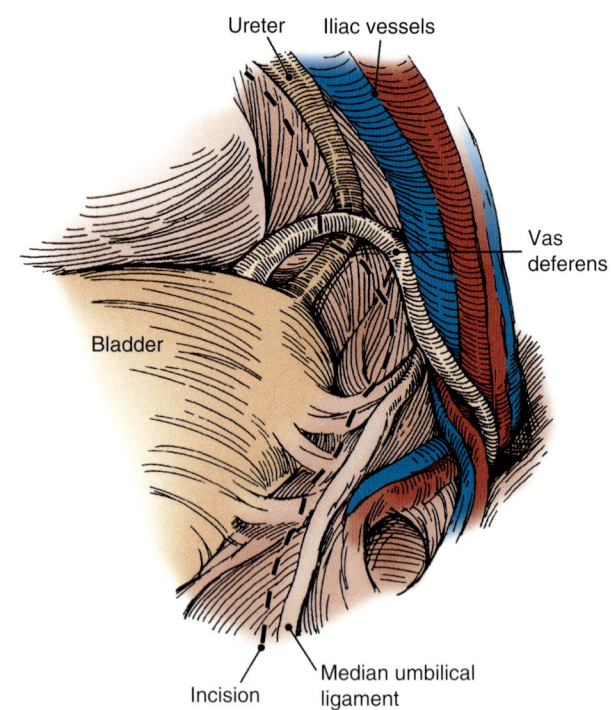

Fig. 99.12. The peritoneal incision is continued below the iliac vessels medial to the median umbilical ligament and lateral to the bladder. The vas deferens is divided between clips in the male patient. In the female patient the round ligament is divided, giving full exposure of the distal ureter to the bladder.

along the white line of Toldt from the level of the iliac vessels to the hepatic flexure on the right and to the splenic flexure on the left. The colon is moved medially by releasing the renocolic ligaments while leaving the lateral attachments of the Gerota fascia in place to prevent the kidney from "flopping" medially. The colon mesentery should be mobilized medial to the great vessels to facilitate dissection of the ureter, renal hilum, and local lymph nodes as needed.

Proximal Ureteronephrectomy. The proximal ureter is identified, just medial to the lower pole of the kidney, and dissected toward the renal pelvis, avoiding skeletonization and maintaining copious periureteral fat if any tumor is located in this area. If an invasive ureteral lesion is suspected, the dissection should include a wide margin of tissue. The renal hilum is identified, and its vessels are exposed with a combination of blunt and sharp dissection. The artery is ligated and divided by use of a stapling device with a vascular load or multiple clips. The renal vein is then divided in a similar fashion (Fig. 99.11). With vascular control ensured, most prefer to ligate the ureter with a clip as previously described, and the kidney is dissected free outside the Gerota fascia. Similar as described for open nephroureterectomy, the adrenal gland does not have to be removed routinely. The ureteral dissection is continued distally, keeping in mind that the ureteral blood supply is generally anteromedially located in the proximal third, medially located in the middle third, and laterally located in the distal third. Dissection of the lower half may require placement of the fourth trocar. In the area of primary disease, surrounding tissue should be left to provide an adequate tumor margin. The ureteral dissection is continued as far as is technically feasible. If the distal limits of the dissection are below the level of the iliac vessels, the remainder of the procedure can easily be completed through a lower abdominal incision. The specimen is placed in the pelvis, and the renal bed is inspected meticulously for bleeding. At this time, the 10-mm port sites may be closed before proceeding to the open portion of the case.

Open Distal Ureterectomy With Excision of Bladder Cuff. The patient is now moved to the supine position, which can usually be done without re-preparation, and a low midline Pfannenstiel or Gibson incision is made. The choice of incision largely depends on the tumor location, the body habitus of the patient, and the most caudal level of ureteral dissection attained during the laparoscopic portion. The Gibson incision is preferable when the distal ureter cannot be freed laparoscopically to the level of the iliac vessels.

Dissection of the Distal Ureter. To consider a total laparoscopic procedure or to minimize the open distal portion, the ureteral dissection must continue to the level of the bladder. The patient is placed in the Trendelenburg position to move the bowel contents out of the pelvis. The peritoneal incision is extended from the level of the iliac vessels into the pelvis lateral to the bladder and medial to the medial umbilical ligament (Fig. 99.12). The vas deferens in male patients or the round ligament in female patients is clipped and divided if exposure is limited. The ureter can now be traced between the bladder and the medial umbilical ligament down to its origin at the bladder. Optimal exposure of the entire intramural ureter is gained by division of the lateral pedicle of the bladder, allowing medial rotation of the bladder, exposing the entire length of the ureter. The bladder cuff may be dissected extravesically, freeing the ureter from the surrounding detrusor muscle, or alternatively, opening the bladder immediately around the ureteral orifice allows direct visual confirmation for complete resection of the bladder cuff. Yet another alternative during a complete extravesical approach is flexible cystoscopy in confirming complete ureterectomy and patency of the contralateral ureteral orifice. The techniques for open distal ureterectomy and bladder cuff excision are described in the section on open techniques.

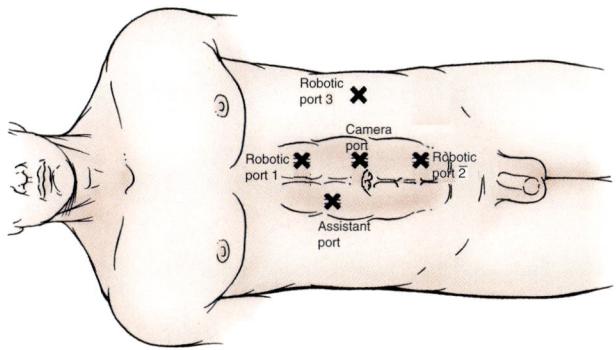

Fig. 99.13. Port configuration for robot-assisted laparoscopic nephroureterectomy. For nephrectomy and upper ureterectomy portion, the retraction instrument is placed in port 3, and for distal ureterectomy with bladder cuff removal, the retraction instrument is moved to port 1 and the left arm to port 3.

Robot-Assisted Laparoscopic Nephroureterectomy. With the increased use of robots in urologic surgery, robot-assisted nephroureterectomy has become a feasible alternative to more traditional open or laparoscopic technique. The availability of da Vinci Xi system with longer instruments and improved range of motion with less arm clashing has allowed performance of the surgery without the need to re-dock the robot or reposition the patient for distal ureterectomy portion. Proper port positioning is paramount to the success of this technique (Fig. 99.13). The 12-mm camera port is placed at the level of umbilicus, lateral to rectus sheath, followed by placement of cephalad (port #1) and caudad (port #2) 8-mm robotic ports, both of which are positioned 7 to 8 cm away from the camera port on the same line. The third robotic port (port #3) is placed about 5 cm cranial to iliac crest, close to the anterior axillary line. The assistant port is placed in the midline in or around the umbilicus. Docking the robot, the left arm is placed in port #1, right arm in port #2, and the fourth arm is placed in port #3 and used for retraction. Once the nephrectomy portion is completed, the retraction instrument is moved to port #1 and left arm to port #3 for distal ureter and bladder cuff dissection. For extravesical dissection of the ureter, the distended bladder is helpful in tracing the ureterovesical junction. Once the distal ureter is dissected out of the detrusor, the bladder can be emptied. Placement of stay sutures medial and lateral to the incision site of ureterovesical junction aids in subsequent reconstruction of bladder. Bladder should be closed in two layers (Hemal et al., 2011). For the Xi system the robotic trocars position should be modified to a straight diagonal line starting with cephalad port at midline and the rest of the ports placed caudally and toward the iliac crest at 8-cm increments. The camera port is initially placed in the second port from the top and moved to the third port for the bladder cuff portion of the surgery.

Results

The first laparoscopic nephroureterectomy was performed in 1991 by Clayman et al. Since that time the technical aspects and safety of laparoscopic procedures have been well established. There are multiple reviews and published series of laparoscopic nephroureterectomy with varying techniques (Bariol et al., 2004; Hsueh et al., 2004; Jarrett et al., 2001; Matin and Gill, 2005; Ni et al., 2012; Rai et al., 2012; Stifleman et al., 2001; Wolf et al., 2005). Each varies with regard to approach (transperitoneal vs. retroperitoneal), management of the distal ureter by open removal, transurethral resection, and total laparoscopic management. As with other laparoscopic renal procedures, there is no clear-cut benefit of any one approach with regard to morbidity, cosmesis, or return to activity.

All, however, show a benefit with regard to morbidity compared with open surgery. The efficacy of laparoscopic nephroureterectomy is being established for cancer control. With intermediate and long-term follow-up, cancer-related outcomes appear comparable with those of the open counterpart (McNeill et al., 2000). El Fettouh et al. (2002), in a multi-institutional study with 116 patients, showed the local and bladder recurrence rates to be 2% and 24%, respectively. The rate of distant metastasis was 9%, and positive margins were seen in 4.5% of cases. Berger et al. (2008) showed a 5-year cancer-specific survival of 80%, 70%, 68%, 60%, and 0 for stage Ta/Tis, T1, T2, T3, and T4 lesions, respectively. Schatteman et al., (2007) similarly showed cancer-specific survival rates of 100%, 86%, 100%, 77%, and 0 for stage Ta, T1, Tis, T3, and T4 lesions. In both studies there was a worsening prognosis with increasing tumor stage. Long-term data are available from Muntener et al. (2007a), who studied 37 patients with follow-up of 60 to 148 months. In this study, 11 patients had disease progression and died 7 to 59 months after the operation. Tumor stage was the only factor significantly associated with disease recurrence. Ni et al. (2012) compared open with laparoscopic outcomes in a larger review of comparative studies. Although the results were not statistically significant, the study showed that laparoscopic surgery had a higher 5-year cancer-specific survival and lower bladder and overall recurrence rate compared with open surgery. With appropriate patient selection, a laparoscopic approach offers reliable safety and oncologic efficacy with the advantage of lower morbidity for well-selected patients. In the only surgical randomized controlled trial comparing laparoscopic and open extirpative surgery, Simone et al. (2009) showed no difference in metastasis-free and cancer-specific survival in patients with organ-confined disease. However, in this study, patients with high-grade disease or at least pT3 stage benefited from open nephroureterectomy.

Local recurrence and port-site seeding are major concerns. There have been a few reported instances of port-site seeding involving UTUC. Two of these cases were discovered after simple nephrectomy for presumed benign disease in which the principles of surgical oncology were inadvertently not followed (Ahmed et al., 1998; Otani et al., 1999). All were for high-grade disease. Muntener et al. (2007b) reported a single case of local recurrence among 166 cases. In this instance there was obvious violation of the ipsilateral urinary tract, noted perioperatively. Although the potential for seeding exists, it seems to be decreasing and does not appear any higher than that for the open surgical counterpart as long as good surgical principles are followed.

In summary, there does not appear to be a significant difference between laparoscopic and open nephroureterectomy when the principles of surgical oncology are followed. Management of the bladder cuff still has shown variability and a tendency toward higher recurrences with minimally invasive approaches. Lymphadenectomy can be performed laparoscopically and should be used based on the clinical situation. Even extended lymph node dissections can be considered in those with advanced laparoscopic skills.

Lymphadenectomy

There is still controversy surrounding the lymphadenectomy for UTUC. For renal pelvis and proximal or mid-ureteral tumors it most commonly includes the ipsilateral renal hilar nodes and the adjacent para-aortic or paracaval nodes, and pelvic nodes for distal ureteral tumors (Abe et al., 2008; Babaian and Johnson, 1980; Batata et al., 1975; Batata and Grabstald, 1976; Brausi et al., 2007, Cummings, 1980; Grabstald et al., 1971; Heney et al., 1981; Johansson and Wahlquist, 1979; Kondo et al., 2007; McCarron et al., 1983; Messing and Catalona, 1998; Richie, 1988; Skinner, 1978; Williams, 1991). This dissection adds little time or morbidity to the surgery. Kondo and Tanabe (2012) proposed an extended lymphadenectomy template based on the location of the tumor (Fig. 99.14). For tumors of renal pelvis this includes ipsilateral hilar, paracaval, retrocaval, and interaortocaval nodes up to the level of inferior mesenteric artery for right-sided tumors, and ipsilateral hilar and para-aortic up to the level of inferior mesenteric artery for left-sided tumors. For tumors of the upper two-thirds of the ureter (above crossing of inferior mesenteric artery to the common iliac artery), the template is similar, but the distal border of dissection is extended to the level of aortic bifurcation. For tumors of the lower one-third of the ureter, these include ipsilateral obturator, internal, external and common iliac, and presacral packets. A recent mapping study looked at the pattern

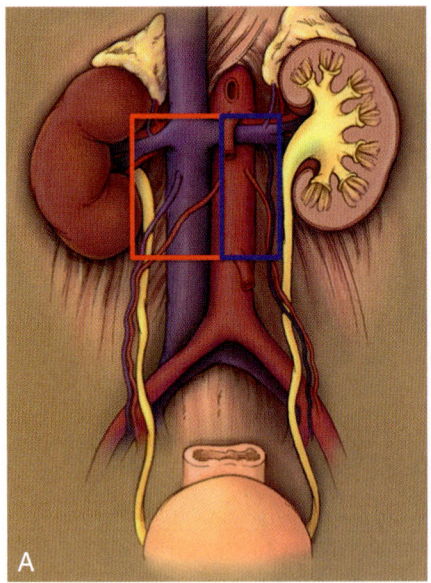 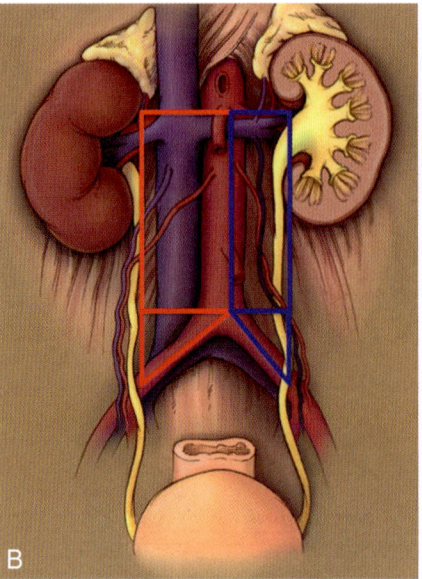 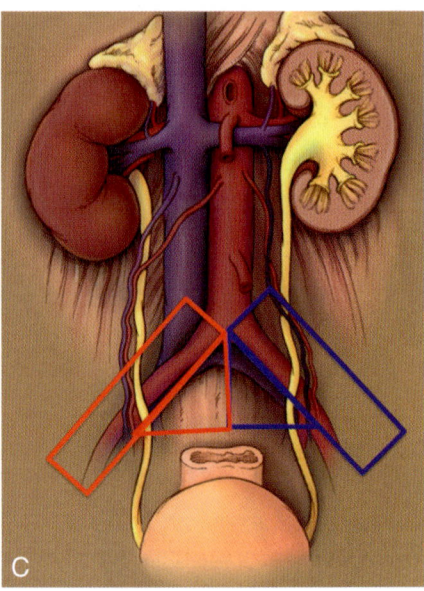

Fig. 99.14. (A) In addition to ipsilateral hilar nodes, the extended lymphadenectomy template for tumors of the renal pelvis includes paracaval, retrocaval, and interaortocaval lymph nodes for right-sided, and para-aortic lymph nodes for left-sided tumors. The inferior mesenteric artery marks the inferior boundary of the template. (B) For tumors of the upper two-thirds of the ureter, this template is extended to the level of bifurcation of aorta. (C) The extended lymphadenectomy template for tumors in the distal ureter includes ipsilateral common, external and internal iliac, obturator, and presacral nodes.

of spread to lymph nodes based on the location and side of the primary tumor (Matin et al., 2015). For right-sided tumors of the renal pelvis and proximal ureter, lymphadenectomy of the hilar, paracaval, and retrocaval nodes captured 82.9% of metastases, and adding interaortocaval dissection increased this number to 95.8%. For left-sided tumors, dissection of hilar and para-aortic nodes captured 86.9% of metastases, and addition of interaortocaval nodes increased that number to 90.2%. Data for mid-ureteral and distal ureteral tumors were less conclusive.

The analysis of the UTUC literature is complicated by a lack of uniformity in templates for lymphadenectomy and the inconsistent pattern of spread, especially for mid-ureteral and distal ureteral tumors. Lymph node involvement is reported in 12% to 25% of patients, although it increases with advanced stage and grade. The reported numbers are 0 to 3% in pTa/pTis, 0 to 6.3% in pT1, 0 to 40% in pT2, 19% to 47% in pT3, and 20% to 100% in pT4. However, the median number of nodes removed and boundaries of lymphadenectomy varied widely in these studies (Weight and Gettman, 2011). Multiple series of lymphadenectomy at the time of nephroureterectomy (Abe et al., 2010; Burger et al., 2011; Lughezzani et al., 2010; Roscigno et al., 2008, 2009; Secin et al., 2007) confirm than oncologic outcomes for patients with pN0 are better than pNx and worse for pN+ compared with pNx groups. The importance of the number of lymph nodes removed was addressed by Roscigno et al. (2009), reporting that removal of 8 or more nodes increased the chance of finding positive LNs by 49% and improved disease-specific survival for those with greater than pT1 disease. A 2017 study by Zareba et al. confirmed that an increase in lymph node yield was an independent predictor of overall survival. In another recent study from a single institution (Lenis et al., 2018), the type of surgical approach (open vs. robotic) did not appear to compromise the nodal yield. Kondo et al. (2010) stressed the importance of the dissection template over the nodal counts for survival difference. For patients with muscle invasive tumors of renal pelvis, template lymphadenectomy was an independent predictor of overall survival in multivariate analysis (Kondo et al., 2014a). Several other studies explored the effects of lymphadenectomy on survival, suggesting a potential therapeutic benefit (Brausi et al., 2007; Kondo et al., 2007, 2014b). The latter study also addressed the perioperative complications, citing 13% overall complication rate for renal pelvis disease and 15% for ureteral disease, including 5.2% incidence of lymphatic or chylous leak. These numbers were in line with other studies for open and laparoscopic surgery (Abe et al., 2015; Mitropoulos et al., 2017).

In summary, although prospective studies are needed to assess the role and optimal extent of lymphadenectomy in UTUC, emerging data validate its importance in the treatment of this cancer. It is safe and beneficial for accurate staging and appears to have prognostic and therapeutic value in patients with invasive disease (T2-T4), especially in the setting of tumors of renal pelvis and proximal ureter.

Results

Multiple series reported on strong correlation of outcome with tumor stage and grade. Recently, additional prognostic factors, such as tumor architecture, presence of carcinoma in situ (CIS), lymphovascular invasion, and lymph node positivity, were shown to correlate to oncologic outcomes (Cha et al., 2012; Margulis et al., 2009).

Complete ureterectomy with bowel cuff excision should accompany nephroureterectomy for UTUC. The risk of tumor recurrence in a remaining ureteral stump is 30% to 75% (Babaian and Johnson, 1980; Bloom et al., 1970; Johansson and Wahlquist, 1979; Kakizoe et al., 1980; McCarron et al., 1983; Mullen and Kovacs, 1980; Strong et al., 1976). Techniques such as simple extravesical dissection and tenting up of the ureter result in an incomplete removal of the distal ureter (Strong et al., 1976). Smith et al. (2009) presented data on a single-center experience comparing oncologic outcomes following variations in technique of distal ureterectomy. The techniques were divided into definitive, which included any approach that resulted in excision of distal ureter with bladder mucosal cuff, and nondefinitive, which included detachment of the ureter at or above the level of detrusor. **Nondefinitive management of the distal ureter was associated with a higher rate of local and distal recurrence and inferior disease-specific and overall survival.** Complete ureterectomy with a bowel cuff should also be performed in the setting of a renal unit draining into a urinary diversion. Tumor recurrence rates up to 37.5% have been reported when ureteroenteric anastomosis was not removed (Mufti et al., 1988).

Multiple series recommend radical nephroureterectomy as a treatment that provides optimal oncologic control (Batata et al., 1975; Johansson and Wahlquist, 1979; McCarron et al., 1983; Murphy et al., 1980; Zungri et al., 1990). Margulis et al. (2009) conducted a retrospective review of 1363 patients from 12 tertiary care centers worldwide who underwent radical nephroureterectomy with curative intent. Although the data for open and laparoscopic cases were pooled together, the majority (77%) had open nephroureterectomy. The pT stage was evenly distributed between Ta, T1, T2, and T3, but less than 5% of patients had each T0, Tcis, or T4. Two-thirds of patients had high-grade tumors, and 28% had concomitant CIS. Around 10% of patients had lymph node positivity, and 16% received perioperative chemotherapy. Disease recurrence was observed in 28% of patients at a median of 10.4 months. During a median follow-up of 37.2 months, 30% of patients died, and 61% of deaths were attributable to their disease. In summary, radical nephroureterectomy provides reasonable oncologic control, with outcomes largely dependent on clinicopathological characteristics. It is warranted for patients with high-grade invasive organ confined or locally advanced disease (stage T1–4, N0–2, M0). **Comparative data of extirpative vs. conservative management are lacking because the population of the patients who undergo these surgeries is very diverse. Treatment decisions in patients with compromised renal function must balance the potential curative effect of radical surgery to the morbidity associated with dialysis.**

Segmental Ureteral Resection

For purposes of this section, segmental ureterectomy primarily indicates distal ureterectomy with ureteral reimplant. True segmental resection of the proximal ureter with primary uretero-ureterostomy is rarely indicated but is discussed in the technical portions of this chapter, as is total ureterectomy requiring ileal ureter replacement or autotransplantation. Several studies have compared results of nephroureterectomy with segmental ureteral resection, but because these are all retrospective and selection for these patients are very different, there is significant selection bias and the quality of the data remains poor. Segmental resection performed to preserve renal function in patients with compromised renal function must not compromise oncologic efficacy for the sake of avoiding the morbidity associated with dialysis. It is critical to evaluate the entire upper tract above the tumor with ureteroscopy to ensure there is no multifocality. In addition, if high-grade disease is present, many practitioners also do an ipsilateral pelvic lymph node dissection. Advantages to a segmental ureterectomy are the ability to preserve renal function while also providing a pathological specimen that can inform the need and extent of adjuvant therapy.

Open Segmental Ureterectomy

Ureteroureterostomy
Indications. Segmental ureterectomy is indicated for tumors of the proximal ureter or mid-ureter that are not able to be removed endoscopically or for high-grade or invasive tumors when preservation of the renal unit is necessary. Achieving a clear margin and still being able to mobilize enough well-vascularized ureter to perform a tension-free anastomosis is paramount to the success of this procedure and the major limiting challenge. It is a rare and narrowly indicated procedure for when there is only a small tumor without any multifocality elsewhere, and not endoscopically manageable.

Technique. The patient is positioned in full or modified flank position. A flank incision from the tip of the 12th rib provides access to the proximal ureter or mid-ureter. With use of an extraperitoneal approach, the ureter is identified, mobilized, and secured with vessel loops. The tumor is palpated, and the ureter is ligated 1 to 2 cm above and below the suspected tumor margin (Fig. 99.15). This location can be also verified by preoperative cross-sectional imaging. The diseased ureter is excised and clear margins ascertained by frozen pathology. After regional lymphadenectomy is performed, both ends of the ureter are spatulated and anastomosed with an interrupted 4-0 Vicryl suture. The success of reconstruction depends on preservation of the blood supply to the ureter and adequate mobilization of the ureteral edges to achieve a tension-free anastomosis. If a large segment of ureter is excised, mobilization and descensus of kidney may be performed to provide additional length to the proximal ureter. A ureteral stent is placed before completion of the anastomosis. Placement of a drain is up to the surgeon's preference. For laparoscopic or robotic approaches, the patient is also in flank position and the trocar placement is similar as to a pyeloplasty or nephrectomy. Extreme care is taken to follow oncologic principles to ensure nonviolation of tumor and obtain negative margins.

Distal Ureterectomy and Direct Neocystostomy or Ureteroneocystostomy With a Bladder Psoas Muscle Hitch or a Boari Flap. The distal ureterectomy is performed as described in the prior section, with the exception that the entire distal ureter and bladder cuff must be excised, and the posterior cystotomy at the bladder cuff site is closed in two layers. For laparoscopic or robotic approaches, the patient is placed in dorsolithotomy or supine and in Trendelenburg position, similar to an approach for prostatectomy. The ureter is mobilized to achieve a tension-free anastomosis and spatulated. Ureterovesical anastomosis may be performed using an extravesical or intravesical approach. Whether to perform a refluxing or nonrefluxing anastomosis remains a matter of debate. The benefits of a nonrefluxing anastomosis include a limit of infection to the lower tract and the theoretic possibility of avoiding seeding of the upper tract. A refluxing anastomosis may make surveillance of the upper tracts easier. If an extravesical approach is desired, bladder detrusor muscle is incised, exposing the mucosa. A mucosal slit is performed at the distal aspect of this incision. An anastomosis is performed using continuous or interrupted 3-0 polyglactin or polydioxanone sutures through the full thickness of the ureter and bladder mucosa. At the distal portion of the anastomosis, two of these sutures are passed through the full thickness wall of the bladder to anchor the ureter and prevent sliding out of the tunnel. The bladder detrusor is then closed on the top of the ureter with interrupted absorbable sutures, such as 2-0 polyglactin, to achieve a nonrefluxing mechanism. A ureteral stent may be placed before completion of the anastomosis.

For the intravesical technique, an anterior cystotomy is made. An incision is made at the posterolateral wall of the bladder and a 2- to 3-cm submucosal tunnel is fashioned. The ureter is brought through this tunnel. After the ureter is spatulated, the anastomosis is performed with interrupted absorbable sutures.

If a long segment of distal ureter is excised and a tension-free anastomosis cannot be achieved by simple ureteroneocystostomy, an additional 5 cm in length can be gained by using a psoas hitch of the bladder. The bladder is mobilized anteriorly and laterally, and in women the round ligament is divided. The contralateral superior vesical artery and entire lateral pedicle can also be divided to gain further mobility. The ipsilateral dome of the bladder is sutured to the psoas tendon using several interrupted sutures. Care should be taken to avoid injury or entrapment of the nerve (Lenis et al., 2018). The ureterovesical anastomosis is then completed in a tension-free manner. If additional length is desired, a Boari flap can help gain another 10 to 15 cm in length and in some cases may be able to reach all the way to renal pelvis (Fig. 99.16). If a Boari flap is planned, it is advisable to obtain a preoperative cystogram to assess bladder capacity, because a small-capacity bladder, especially if radiated, is a contraindication to this technique. A U-shaped bladder wall flap or, if a longer segment is desired, an L-shaped segment, is developed. To ensure a good blood supply to the flap, the base of the flap should be at least 2 cm greater than the apex. To achieve adequate width of the tubularized segment, the width of the flap should be at least three times the diameter of the ureter. The tip of the flap is secured to the psoas muscle using interrupted absorbable suture, and the spatulated ureter is anastomosed to the flap in the end-to-end fashion. The flap is then tubularized and closed with two layers of absorbable sutures. A ureteral catheter is placed before closure of the flap. After all of these techniques, it is advisable to use a suction drain in the retroperitoneum and 5- to 7-day Foley drainage of the bladder. After extensive reconstruction, a cystogram should precede Foley removal.

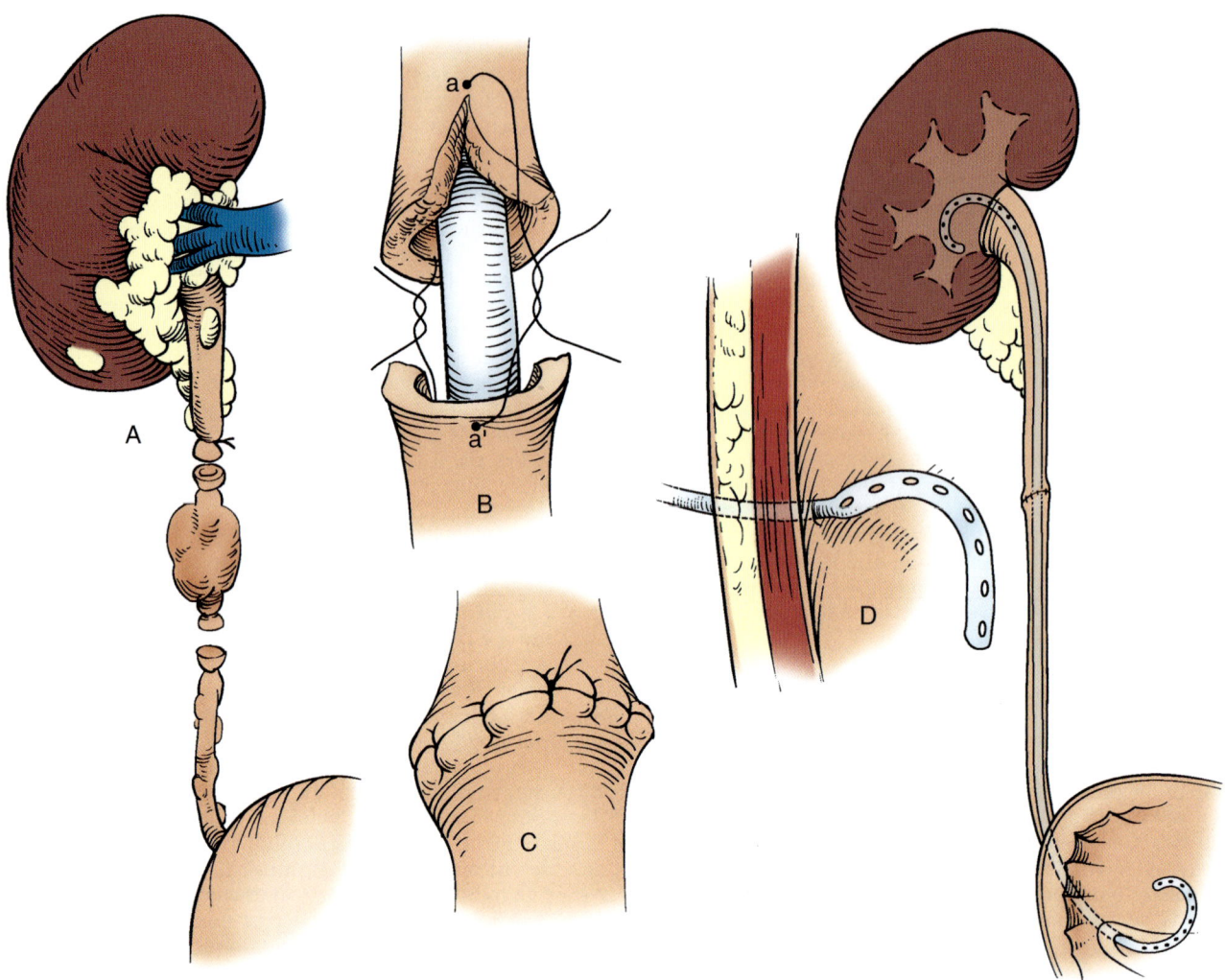

Fig. 99.15. (A) Segmental ureterectomy between ties for a large, invasive tumor of the mid-ureter. (B and C) Ureteroureterostomy of spatulated ends of the ureter. The repair is performed over an internal stent. (D) Completed repair with closed-suction drain in retroperitoneal space.

Ileal Ureteral Replacement

When a long segment of ureter is diseased, a segment of ileum can be used to reconstruct the urinary system. The appendix has also been used for segmental ureteral substitution (Goldwasser et al., 1994). Through a midline intraperitoneal incision, 20 to 25 cm of ileum is harvested at least 15 cm away from the ileocecal valve. Bowel continuity is re-established using a stapled anastomosis. With a running absorbable suture, the ileal segment is anastomosed to the renal pelvis proximally in an end-to-end fashion and an isoperistaltic direction. If the proximal portion of the ureter is healthy, the ileal segment can be anastomosed to it in an end-to-side fashion. A ureteral stent is placed before completion of the anastomosis. Distally, the segment is anastomosed to the posterior wall of the bladder in an end-to-side manner through an intravesical approach. This anastomosis is done in two layers. A suction drain is positioned in the retroperitoneum close to anastomotic sites. Optimal drainage is important for proper healing, so a large Foley catheter is inserted in the bladder and left for at least 1 week or longer postoperatively. It may have to be irrigated frequently. A nephrostomy tube may be used to drain the kidney. Before removal of the tubes, a cystogram and nephrostogram are obtained.

In skilled hands, renal autotransplantation is a feasible alternative to ileal replacement. Another approach that may help avoid ileal reconstruction involves mobilization of the kidney with subsequent nephropexy of the Gerota fascia to the cut edge of the peritoneum, placing traction in the caudal direction (Fig. 99.17). It may add up to 8 to 10 cm of length on the left side because of a longer left renal vein. This approach has been used laparoscopically, avoiding the need for a second flank incision (Sutherland et al., 2011).

Laparoscopic or Robotic Distal Ureterectomy and Reimplantation

Various laparoscopic techniques for distal ureterectomy and reimplantation have been reported. The robotic approach may assist with the reconstruction portion of the procedure. The indications are the same as those for the open counterpart, and the techniques are reserved for low-risk distal tumors. The distal ureter is dissected down to the ureteral orifice, and the proximal end is anastomosed to the bladder using standard techniques. The early reports are encouraging, but strict adherence to oncologic principles must be followed.

Results

In the past, some authors recommended radical nephroureterectomy for all patients with upper tract urothelial tumors (Skinner, 1978). Others suggested segmental ureterectomy only for patients with low-grade, noninvasive tumors of the distal ureter (Babaian et al.,

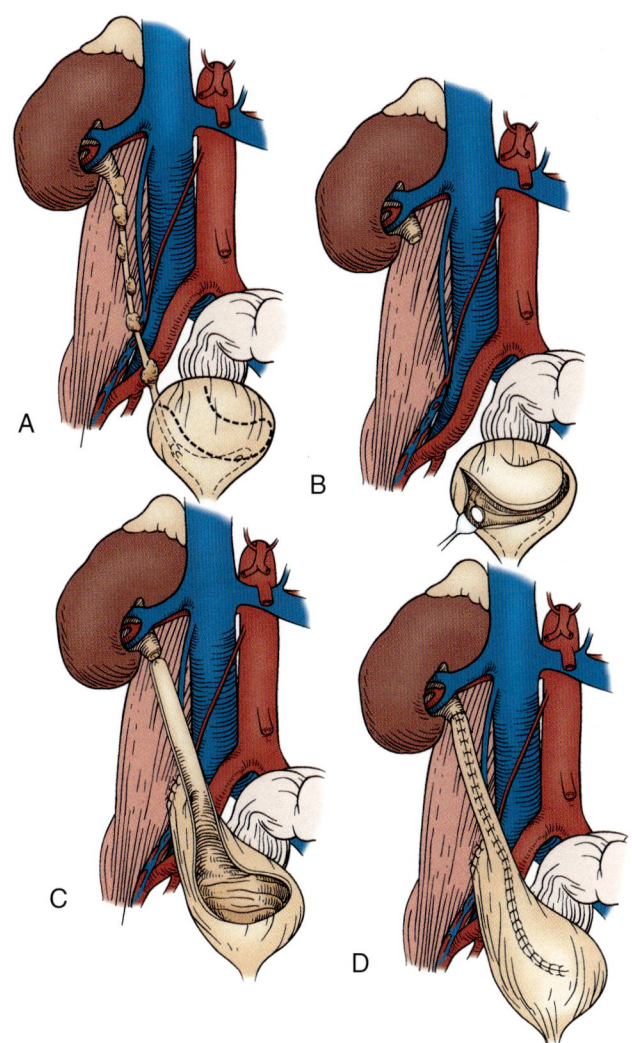

Fig. 99.16. (A) Subtotal ureterectomy required for nephron sparing in a patient with multiple diffuse ureteral tumors. (B) A spiral flap is fashioned from the anterior bladder wall. (C) The psoas hitch plus Boari flap reaches the remaining proximal ureter. (D) Completed anastomosis and bladder closure.

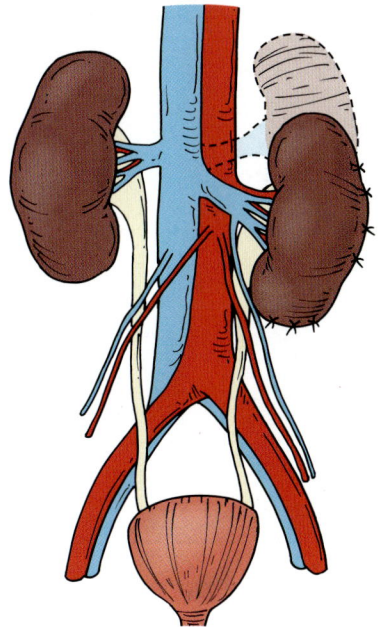

Fig. 99.17. Mobilization of the kidney with subsequent nephropexy of Gerota fascia to cut the edge of the peritoneum, placing traction in the caudal direction, may add up to 10 cm of length on the left side.

TABLE 99.1 Literature Review of Overall Survival of Patients With Upper Tract Urothelial Tumors (Renal Pelvis or Ureter) by Stage and Grade

	5-YEAR SURVIVAL (%)
TUMOR GRADE	
1–2	40–87
3–4	0–33
TNM STAGE	
Ta, T1, Tcis	60–90
T2	43–75
T3	16–33
T4	0–5
N+	0–4
M+	0

TNM, Tumor node metastasis.

1980). Most ureteral cancers occur in the distal ureter, followed by mid-ureter and proximal ureter (Vaughn et al., 2009). Most studies show similar oncologic outcomes as nephroureterectomy with properly selected patients. The outcome of patients with UTUC of the ureter strongly correlates with tumor stage and grade regardless of the extent of surgical treatment (Table 99.1). A single-center study evaluating the prognostic factors in urothelial tumors of the ureter showed an 80% 10-year progression-free survival and 10% ipsilateral tumor recurrence (Lehmann et al., 2007), although the majority of these patients had non–muscle-invasive disease. Overall, 145 patients were evaluated, and 51 underwent segmental ureterectomy. When adjusted for clinicopathological characteristics, the outcomes were similar for patients who underwent nephroureterectomy versus segmental ureterectomy. The mean follow-up in this study was 96 months. Leitenberger et al. (1996) reported their experience with organ-sparing surgery for ureter cancer. Out of 40 patients, 13 underwent extirpative nephron-sparing surgery, and recurrence was observed in 4 patients, all of whom had invasive disease. Anderstrom et al. (1989) reported no tumor-related deaths and only 1 recurrence among 21 patients treated with segmental ureterectomy for low-grade, noninvasive ureteral tumors who were observed for a median of 83 months. McCarron et al. (1983) reported 5-year survival of 64% for patients with stage Ta tumors treated by either segmental ureterectomy or endoscopic tumor ablation. In the same series, 5-year tumor-free survival rates were 66% and 50% for stage T1 and T2 tumors, respectively, treated with segmental or distal ureterectomy. In the series by Grabstald et al. (1971), disease-specific survival rates were 64% and 100% for stage Ta to T1 and stage T2 disease, respectively. All deaths were from unrelated causes. In contrast, for patients with stage T3 disease, cancer-specific survival was only 7% and the rate of death caused by tumor was 87%. A recent Surveillance, Epidemiology, and End Results database review of 2044 patients with a mean follow-up of 30 months showed no difference in 5-year cancer-specific mortality in segmental ureterectomy versus nephroureterectomy, adjusted for pathological stage (Jeldres et al., 2010). A more recent single institution comparison of 112 patients with ureteral cancer treated either by radical nephroureterectomy or segmental ureterectomy found no significant differences in bladder, local, or distant recurrence and no difference in survival outcomes after a mean follow-up of 44 and 48 months (Hung et al., 2014).

The risk of ipsilateral recurrence after conservative treatment of ureteral tumors is 33% to 55% (Babaian et al., 1980; Johnson

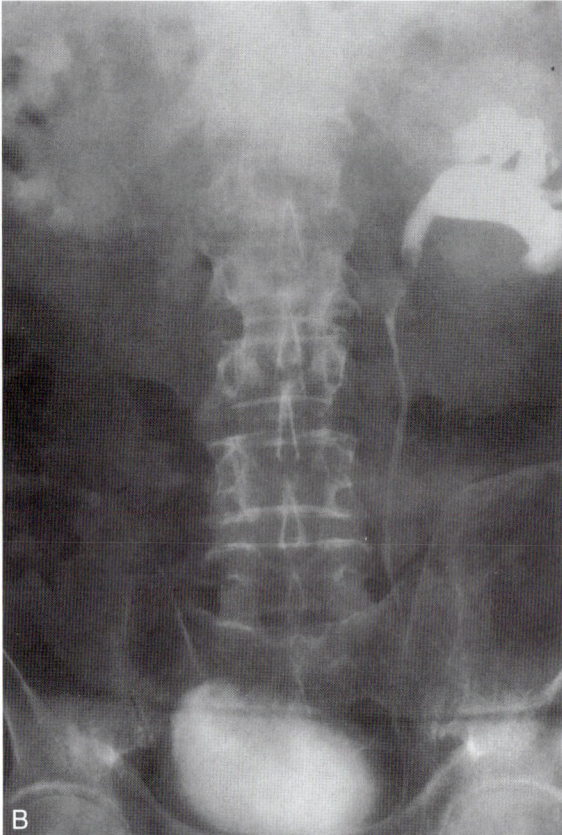

Fig. 99.18. Patient with synchronous bilateral tumors. (A) Right renal cell carcinoma that required radical nephrectomy. (B) Left proximal ureteral tumor that required combined ureteroscopic and antegrade percutaneous ablation.

et al., 1979; Mazeman, 1976; McCarron et al., 1983; Williams, 1991). Most recurrences are distal to the original lesion, but proximal recurrences are also seen (Strong et al., 1976). The risk for recurrence and the need for follow-up are lifelong (Herr, 1998), because late recurrence can be seen (Grossman, 1978). These historical studies also reflect results of when ureteroscopic evaluation was much more limited. If patients have a thorough ureteroscopic evaluation and are properly selected for ureterectomy, the results are probably more favorable (Hung et al., 2014). Segmental ureterectomy is offered for low-grade, non–muscle-invasive disease of the proximal ureter or mid-ureter that is not amenable to complete ablation by endoscopic means because of tumor size or multiplicity. Distal ureterectomy and neocystostomy may be offered for low-grade, low-stage, or in select cases, high-grade, locally invasive tumors of the distal ureter when renal preservation is necessary. As mentioned previously, in the presence of high-grade disease, consideration should also be given for lymphadenectomy.

ENDOUROLOGIC MANAGEMENT

Basic Attributes

Hugh Hampton Young described the first endoscopic evaluation of the upper urinary tract in 1912. Subsequent advances in technology allow us to reach all parts of the urinary tract with minimal morbidity through antegrade and retrograde approaches. Diagnosis and treatment of UTUC have become possible with these improvements because tumor biopsy and ablation by various energy sources are possible even through the smallest instruments. In addition, miniaturization has made follow-up surveillance of the upper tract more practical with the use of smaller ureteroscopes, which usually do not require previous stenting, or with active dilation of the distal ureter.

Tumors of the upper urinary tract can be approached in a retrograde or antegrade fashion. The approach chosen depends largely on the tumor location and size. In general, a retrograde ureteroscopic approach is used for low-volume ureteral and renal tumors. An antegrade percutaneous approach is preferred for

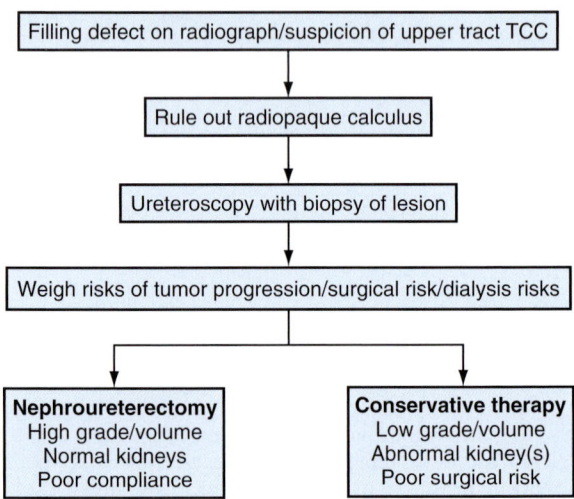

Fig. 99.19. Algorithm for endoscopic approach to upper tract transitional cell carcinoma (TCC).

larger tumors of the upper ureter or kidney and for those that cannot be adequately manipulated in a retrograde approach because of location (e.g., lower pole calyx) or previous urinary diversion. In cases with multifocal involvement, combined antegrade and retrograde approaches can be considered (Fig. 99.18).

The basic principles for treatment of UTUC are similar to those for the bladder counterpart (Fig. 99.19). The tumor is sampled and ablated by electrocautery or laser energy sources. Tumor grading is a valuable tool when considering a patient for endoscopic treatment. Almås et al. (2016) showed results indicating that endoscopic treatment of UTUC is safe and feasible for verified low-grade disease whereas its use for high-grade tumors has poor results. A staged procedure should be considered for high-volume disease or disease that is thought to represent high pathological grade or stage. In such cases, when subsequent nephroureterectomy most likely will be necessary for cure, only biopsy and partial ablation are performed to minimize the risks of perforation or major complications. Endoscopic management is completed only after the pathological examination shows that the patient is an acceptable candidate for continued minimally invasive endoscopic management. If the pathological process is unresectable, of high grade, or invasive, the patient should proceed immediately to nephroureterectomy. Segmental resection can be considered in cases of solitary kidney or significant renal insufficiency provided he or she is medically fit. Patients who undergo renal-sparing therapy must be committed to a lifetime of follow-up with radiographs and endoscopy.

Retrograde Ureteroscopic

Ureteroscopy and Ureteropyeloscopy

The ureteroscopic approach to tumors was first described by Goodman in 1984 and is generally favored for ureteral and smaller renal tumors. With the advent of small-diameter rigid and flexible ureteroscopes, tumor location is less of a limiting factor than it used to be. **The advantage of a ureteroscopic approach is lower morbidity than that of the percutaneous and open surgical counterparts, with the maintenance of a closed system. With a closed system, nonurothelial surfaces are not exposed to the possibility of tumor seeding.**

The major disadvantages of a retrograde approach are related to the smaller instruments required. Smaller endoscopes have a smaller field of view and working channel. This limits the size of tumor that can be approached in a retrograde fashion. In addition, some portions of the upper urinary tract, such as the lower pole calyces, cannot be reliably reached with working instruments. Smaller instruments limit the ability to remove large tumors and to obtain deep specimens for reliable staging. In addition, retrograde ureteroscopy is difficult in patients with prior urinary diversion.

Technique and Instrumentation. A wide variety of ureteroscopic instruments are available, each with its own distinct advantages and disadvantages. In general, rigid ureteroscopes are used primarily for the distal and mid-ureter. Access to the upper ureter and kidney with rigid endoscopy is unreliable, especially in the male patient. Larger, rigid ureteroscopes provide better visualization because of their larger field of view and better irrigation. Smaller rigid ureteroscopes (8 Fr) generally do not require active dilation of the ureteral orifice (Fig. 99.20A). Newer-generation, flexible ureteropyeloscopes are available in sizes smaller than 8 Fr to allow simple and reliable passage to most portions of the urinary tract (Abdel-Razzak and Bagley, 1993; Chen and Bagley, 2000; Chen et al., 2000; Grasso and Bagley, 1994). These are generally preferred in the upper ureter and kidney, where the rigid ureteroscope cannot be reliably passed. **Flexible ureteroscopes, however, have technical limitations, such as a small working channel, that limit irrigant flow and the diameter of working instruments. Further limitations of flexible ureteroscopy include reduced access to certain areas of the kidney, such as the lower pole, where the infundibulopelvic angle may limit passage of the scope, and prior urinary diversion** (Fig. 99.20B).

Endoscopic Evaluation and Collection of Urine Cytology Specimen. Cystoscopy is performed and the bladder inspected for concomitant bladder disease. The ureteral orifice is identified and inspected for lateralizing hematuria. A small-diameter (6.9 or 7.5 Fr) ureteroscope is passed directly into the ureteral orifice, and the distal ureter is inspected for any trauma from a previously placed guidewire or dilation. A guidewire is then placed through the ureteroscope and up the ureter to the level of the renal pelvis under fluoroscopic guidance. The flexible ureteroscope is used to visualize the remaining urothelium. All lesions are mapped. **When a lesion or suspicious area is seen, a normal saline washing of the area is performed before biopsy or intervention** (Bian et al., 1995). If the ureter does not accept the smaller ureteroscope, active dilation of the ureter is necessary.

There are no recommendations regarding the use of ureteral access sheaths. They provide the advantage of allowing for a low pressure system and allow for repeated access to the ureter. Larger specimens can be removed with less theoretical risk of downstream seeding because the lower ureter is bypassed during removal. The downside is the need for additional dilation of the ureteral orifice and the need for postprocedure stenting.

Tumor Confined to the Intramural Ureter

A second type of case is tumor in the intramural ureter. When a tumor protrudes from the ureteral orifice, complete ureteroscopic

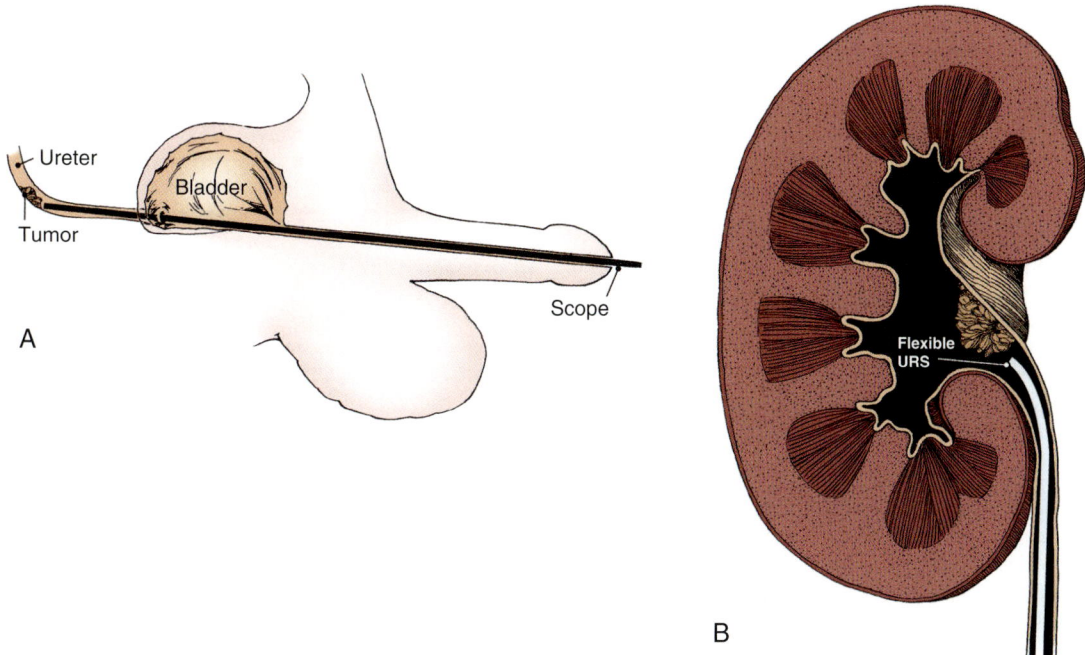

Fig. 99.20. (A) Rigid ureteroscopic approach. (B) Flexible ureteroscopic approach. *URS*, Ureteroscope.

ablation of the tumor or aggressive transurethral resection of the entire most distal ureter can be done with acceptable results (Palou et al., 2000).

Biopsy and Definitive Treatment. Three general approaches can be used for tumor ablation: bulk excision with ablation of the base, resection of the tumor to its base, and diagnostic biopsy followed by ablation with electrocautery or laser energy sources. Regardless of technique used, special attention to biopsy specimens is necessary. Specimens are frequently minute and should be placed in fixative at once and are specially labeled for either histologic or cytologic evaluation (Tawfiek et al., 1997).

Ureteroscopic Techniques. The tumor is debulked by use of either biopsy forceps or a flat wire basket engaged adjacent to the tumor (Fig. 99.21A). Next, the tumor base is treated with either electrocautery or laser energy sources. This technique is especially useful for low-grade papillary tumor on a narrow stalk. The specimen is sent for pathological evaluation.

Alternatively, a ureteroscopic resectoscope is used to remove the tumor (Fig. 99.21B). Only the intraluminal tumor is resected, and no attempt is made to resect deep (beyond the lamina propria). Extra care is necessary in the mid-ureter and upper ureter, where the wall is thin and prone to perforation. With larger volume disease of the distal ureter, Jarrett et al. (1995a) described extensive dilation of the ureter followed by resection with a long standard resectoscope. **The tumor is adequately sampled with forceps and sent to the pathology laboratory for diagnostic evaluation. The tumor bulk is then ablated to its base with laser or electrosurgical energy** (Fig. 99.21C and D). Multiple biopsy specimens are often required when small, flexible 3-Fr biopsy forceps are used. Electrocautery delivered through a small Bugbee electrode (2 or 3 Fr) can be used to fulgurate tumors. However, the variable depth of penetration can make its use in the ureter dangerous, and circumferential fulguration should be avoided because of the high risk of stricture formation. More recently, laser energy with either neodymium:yttrium-aluminum-garnet (Nd:YAG) (Carson, 1991; Schilling et al., 1986; Schmeller and Hofstetter, 1989; Smith et al., 1984) or holmium:YAG (Ho:YAG) (Bagley and Erhard, 1995; Matsuoka et al., 2003; Razvi et al., 1995; Suoka et al., 2003) sources has been popular. Each has characteristic advantages (Fig. 99.22) and can be delivered through small, flexible fibers (200 or 365 μm) that fit through small, flexible ureteroscopes without significant alteration of irrigant flow or scope deflection. The holmium:YAG laser is well suited for use in the ureter. The tissue penetration is less than 0.5 mm, which allows tumor ablation with excellent hemostasis and minimal risk of full-thickness injury to the ureter. Its shallow penetration may, however, make its use cumbersome with larger tumors, especially in the renal pelvis. Settings most commonly used for the holmium:YAG laser are energy of 0.6 to 1 J with frequency of 10 Hz. The Nd:YAG laser has a tissue penetration of up to 5 to 6 mm, depending on laser settings and duration of treatment. In contrast to the holmium:YAG laser, which ablates tumor, the Nd:YAG laser works by coagulative necrosis with subsequent sloughing of the necrotic tumor. The safety margin is significantly lower and can limit its use in the ureter, where the ureteral wall is thin. Settings most commonly used for the Nd:YAG laser are 15 W for 2 seconds for ablation of tumor and 5 to 10 W for 2 seconds for coagulation.

A ureteral stent is placed for a variable duration to aid with the healing process. Large tumors usually require multiple treatment sessions during several months.

Results

There are no published series of randomized controlled trials comparing endoscopic therapy and nephroureterectomy, and all are case series (level 4 evidence). Multiple series have shown the safety and efficacy of ureteroscopic treatment of UTUC (Cutress et al., 2012; Daneshmand et al., 2003; Gadzinski et al., 2010; Krambeck et al., 2007; Lucas et al., 2008; Thompson et al., 2008). See Table 99.2 for a summary of the largest current series. In a literature review of 736 patients (Cutress et al., 2012), the overall recurrence rates for upper tract was 53%, and the risk of bladder recurrence was 34%. Disease progression was present in 15% with 9% recurring with metastatic disease. The failure rate of ureteroscopic therapy was 24% with 19% undergoing subsequent nephroureterectomy. There was, however, considerable bias for favorable tumor characteristics (unifocal, low grade, and small tumor size). As with any urothelial cancer, the most important prognostic indicator for tumor recurrence was grade. Cutress et al. (2012) showed the upper tract recurrence rate for grades 1, 2, and 3 lesions to be 52%, 54%, and 76%, respectively. The upper tract recurrence rate and disease-free survival were worse with higher-grade tumors.

The literature shows the long-term feasibility of the ureteroscopic approach, but concerns over the high rate of ipsilateral recurrences remain. Daneshmand et al. (2003) reported a large number of recurrences with an overall ipsilateral recurrence rate of 90% with three to four recurrences per patient. Cutress et al. (2012) reported 5-year recurrence-free survival of 13% to 54% in the largest series. This is important in considering patients with a normal contralateral kidney. Patients must be counseled in the need for lifetime follow-up and possible treatment of ipsilateral recurrence.

Complications were uncommon and usually related to the patient's comorbidities. Complications specific to ureteroscopic therapy were 14% (Cutress et al., 2012) and included ureteral perforation, which can be managed with indwelling ureteral stent; ureteral stricture occurred in 11%. The complication rates seemed to have dropped in more contemporary series, most likely related to smaller endoscopes, improved laser energy sources, and refinements in endoscopic techniques.

Two major concerns of the ureteroscopic approach are the accuracy of ureteroscopic biopsies and the limitations of biopsies, especially with regard to staging. Retrospective reviews of patients who underwent ureteroscopic biopsy followed by nephroureterectomy found the accuracy of ureteroscopic diagnosis to be 89% to 94% and the pathological grading to match the open surgical technique in 70% to 92% (Guarnizo et al., 2000; Keeley et al., 1997a; Smith et al., 2011). From prior studies, we know that there is a good correlation between grade of lesion and stage (Chasko et al., 1981; Heney et al., 1981). This holds true for the ureteroscopic approach (Keeley et al., 1997b) because 87% of patients with grade 1 or grade 2 tumors had noninvasive disease (stage Ta or T1), whereas 67% of patients with grade 3 tumors had invasive disease (stage T2 or T3). This information supports the notion that tumor grade is the most important prognostic factor and, although stage cannot be directly assessed, noninvasive disease can be expected in most cases of low-grade tumor.

A final concern is whether ureteroscopy promotes progression or spread of disease to other urothelial surfaces or metastatic sites. There have been reports of increased tumor appearance in refluxing ureters of patients with bladder tumors (de Torres Mateos et al., 1987) and in the ipsilateral urinary tract and bladder of patients after ureteroscopic treatment. However, Kulp and Bagley (1994) reported on 13 patients who underwent multiple ureteroscopic treatments followed by nephroureterectomy; they found no unusual propagation of cancer in the specimens. Concerns that ureteroscopy may promote metastatic spread were raised by Lim et al. (1993), who found tumor cells in renal lymphatics after ureteroscopy. However, Hendin et al. (1999) reported no increased risk of metastatic disease in a group of patients who underwent ureteroscopy before nephroureterectomy compared with a group undergoing nephroureterectomy alone.

Antegrade Nephroureteroscopic

The percutaneous approach was first described by Tomera et al. in 1982 and is generally favored for larger tumors located proximally in the renal pelvis or proximal ureter. **The main advantage of the percutaneous approach is the ability to use larger instruments that can remove a large volume of tumor** in any portion of the renal collecting system. The EAU recommends against endoscopic therapy for tumors greater than 1 cm (Rouprêt et al., 2018); however, multiple reports have shown successful treatment of larger tumors (Cutress et al., 2012). Because deeper biopsy specimens are obtained, tumor

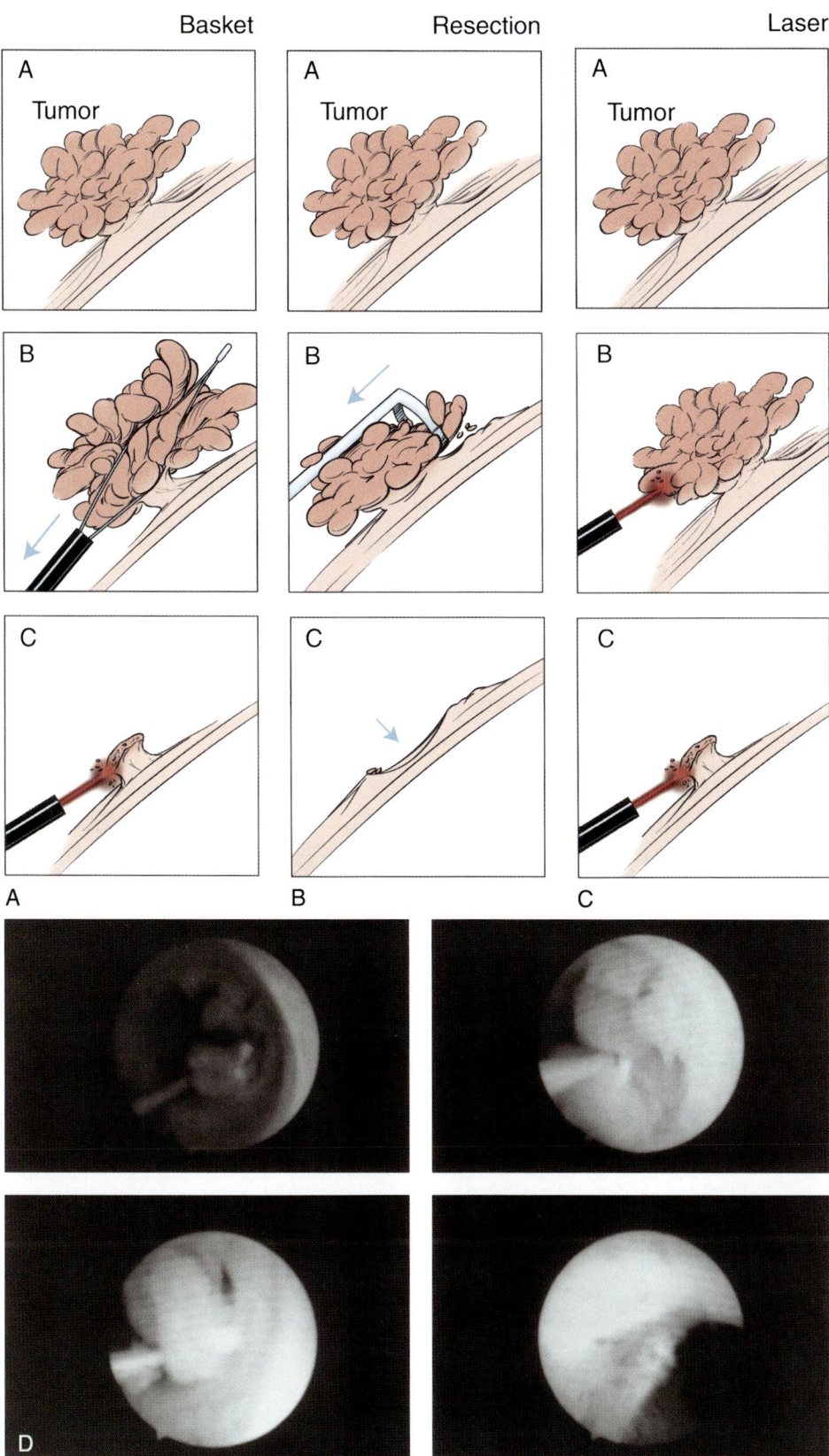

Fig. 99.21. Techniques for ureteroscopic treatment of ureteral and renal tumors. (A) The tumor is identified and removed piecemeal by grasping forceps to its base. (B) Alternatively, a flat wire basket can be deployed alongside the tumor. The tumor is engaged and removed, with care taken not to avulse the adjacent ureter. With either of these techniques, the base is treated with electrocautery or a laser energy source. (C) The tumor is identified and removed by a ureteroscopic resectoscope. The technique differs from the technique for bladder tumors in that only intraluminal tumor is resected. No attempt is made to resect deep, as with a bladder tumor. The scope is not arching deep into the tissue. (D) The tumor is sampled for diagnostic purposes. The bulk of the tumor is then ablated with electrosurgical or laser energy. In general, laser energy is preferred because it has more reliable delivery of energy and depth of penetration. The two most commonly used energy sources are holmium:yttrium-aluminum-garnet and neodymium:yttrium-aluminum-garnet.

TABLE 99.2 Ureteroscopic Management

STUDY	NUMBER OF PATIENTS	FOLLOW-UP (mo)	UPPER TRACT RECURRENCE (%)	BLADDER RECURRENCE (%)	NEPHROURETERECTOMY RATE (%)	DISEASE PROGRESSION (%)	FAILED MANAGEMENT (%)	COMPLICATIONS (%)
Martinez-Piñeiro et al., 1996	54	31	23	ND	10	ND	28	23
Daneshmand et al., 2003	30	31	90	23	13	20	47	17
Johnson et al., 2005	35	52	68	ND	3	0	3	9
Gadzinski et al., 2010	34	18	31	15	ND	15	ND	9
Pak et al., 2009	57	53	90	ND	19	7	19	ND
Thompson et al., 2008	83	55	55	45	33	14	33	
Cutress et al., 2012	73	54	69	43	19	19	30	16

ND, Not disclosed.
Modified from Cutress ML, Stewart GD, Zakikhani P, et al.: Ureteroscopic and percutaneous management of upper tract urothelial carcinoma (UTUC): systematic review. BJU Int 110:614–628, 2012.

staging as well as grading is usually possible. In addition, a percutaneous approach may avoid the limitations of flexible ureteroscopy, especially in complicated calyceal systems or areas difficult to access, such as the lower pole calyx or the upper urinary tract of patients with urinary diversion. With a percutaneous approach, the established nephrostomy tract can be maintained for immediate postoperative nephroscopy and administration of topical adjuvant therapy.

The main disadvantages are the increased morbidity compared with ureteroscopy and the potential for tumor seeding outside the urinary tract. Establishment of the nephrostomy tract has inherent risks, and the procedure usually requires inpatient admission. Distinct risks related to a percutaneous approach are loss of urothelial integrity and exposure of nonurothelial surfaces to tumor cells. This open system provides the possibility of tumor implantation in the nephrostomy tract.

Technique and Instrumentation

Establishment of the Nephrostomy Tract. Cystoscopy is performed, and an open-ended ureteral catheter is positioned in the pelvis. Contrast material is injected to define the calyceal anatomy, and a percutaneous nephrostomy tract is established through the desired calyx (Fig. 99.23). If the patient is in the prone split-leg position, a flexible ureteroscope can be passed to the desired area and renal access obtained under direct and fluoroscopic guidance. Tumors in peripheral calyces are best approached with direct puncture distal to the tumor (Fig. 99.24), avoiding trauma to or direct puncture into the tumor. Disease in the renal pelvis and upper ureter is best approached through an upper or middle pole access to allow scope maneuvering through the collecting system and down the ureteropelvic junction. The tract is dilated by either sequential (Amplatz) or balloon

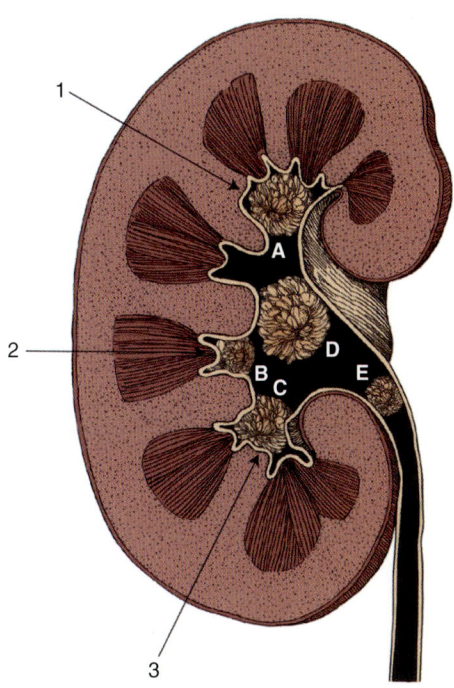

Fig. 99.23. Nephrostomy tract puncture site. Position of the nephrostomy is imperative for successful percutaneous resection of transitional cell carcinoma of the renal collecting system and upper ureter and requires careful preoperative evaluation of radiographs for tumor location. Tumors in peripheral calyces (A to C) are best approached by direct puncture as far distally in the calyx as possible. Tumors in the renal pelvis (D) and upper ureter (E) are best approached by puncture to an upper (1) or middle (2) calyx, which allows the scope to be maneuvered in the renal pelvis and down the ureter. Tumors in the lower calyx are approached by lower calyx puncture (3).

Ho:YAG
  Minimal penetration (<0.5 mm)
  Efficient ablation of tumor
  Precise cutting
  Setting 0.6–1.2 joules/8–10 Hz

Nd:YAG
  Deep penetration (5–6 mm)
  Excellent hemostasis
  Tumor ablation by coagulative necrosis
  Settings: 20–30 watts

Fig. 99.22. Characteristics of holmium:yttrium-aluminum-garnet (Ho:YAG) and neodymium:yttrium-aluminum-garnet (Nd:YAG) laser energy sources.

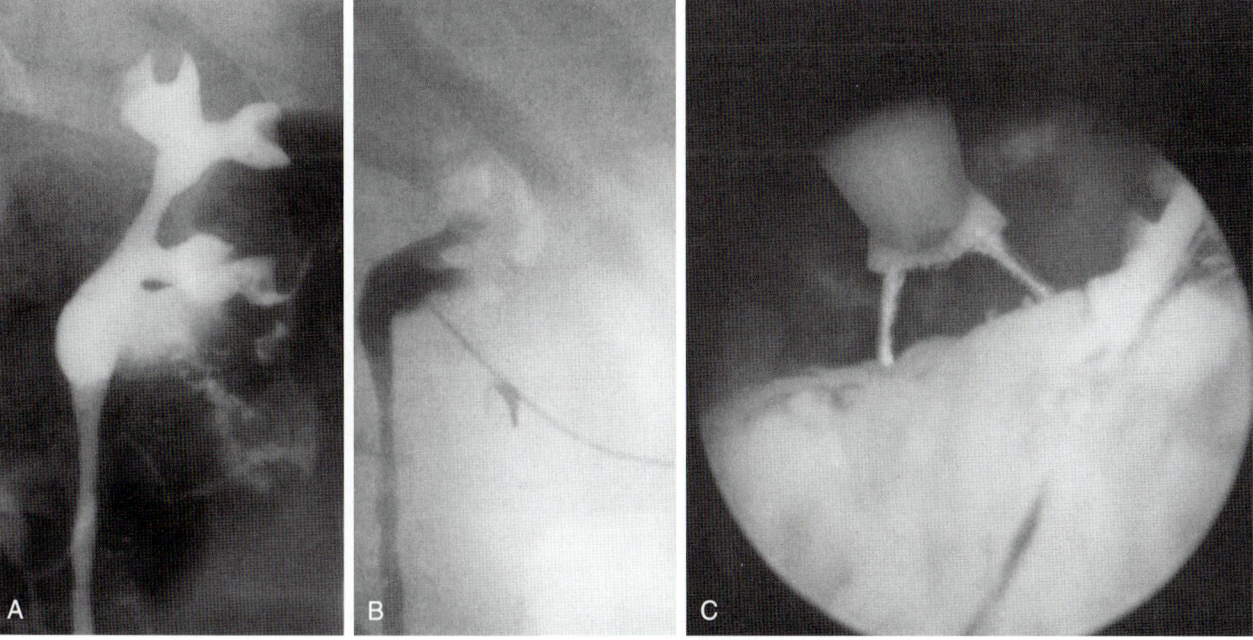

Fig. 99.24. (A) Retrograde pyelogram of a man with transitional cell carcinoma of the lower calyx in a solitary kidney. (B) Access distal in the calyx allows a clear view of the tumor. (C) Subsequent resection.

dilation to accommodate a 30-Fr sheath. Correct positioning of the nephrostomy tract is crucial to the success of the procedure and should be done by the urologist or by the radiologist after direct consultation with the operating surgeon. Some practitioners prefer to perform this in two stages, with establishment of a tract first and allowing this to mature over 1 to 2 weeks, followed by tract dilation and treatment. Alternatively, if only a diagnostic procedure must be performed, such as evaluation of a positive cytology after cystectomy and diversion, the initial smaller nephrostomy tract may be used to introduce a flexible ureteroscope. Otherwise, a nephroscope is inserted, and the ureteral catheter is grasped, brought out the tract, and exchanged for a stiff guidewire, thus providing antegrade and retrograde control. Complete nephroscopy is performed with rigid and flexible endoscopes when necessary. Any suspicion of upper ureteral involvement warrants antegrade ureteroscopy.

Biopsy and Definitive Therapy. **After identification, the tumors are removed by one of the following three techniques.** In the first technique, which uses a cold-cup biopsy forceps through a standard nephroscope, the bulk of the tumor is grasped by forceps and removed in piecemeal fashion until the base is reached (Fig. 99.25A). A separate biopsy of the base is performed for staging purposes, and the base is cauterized with a Bugbee electrode and

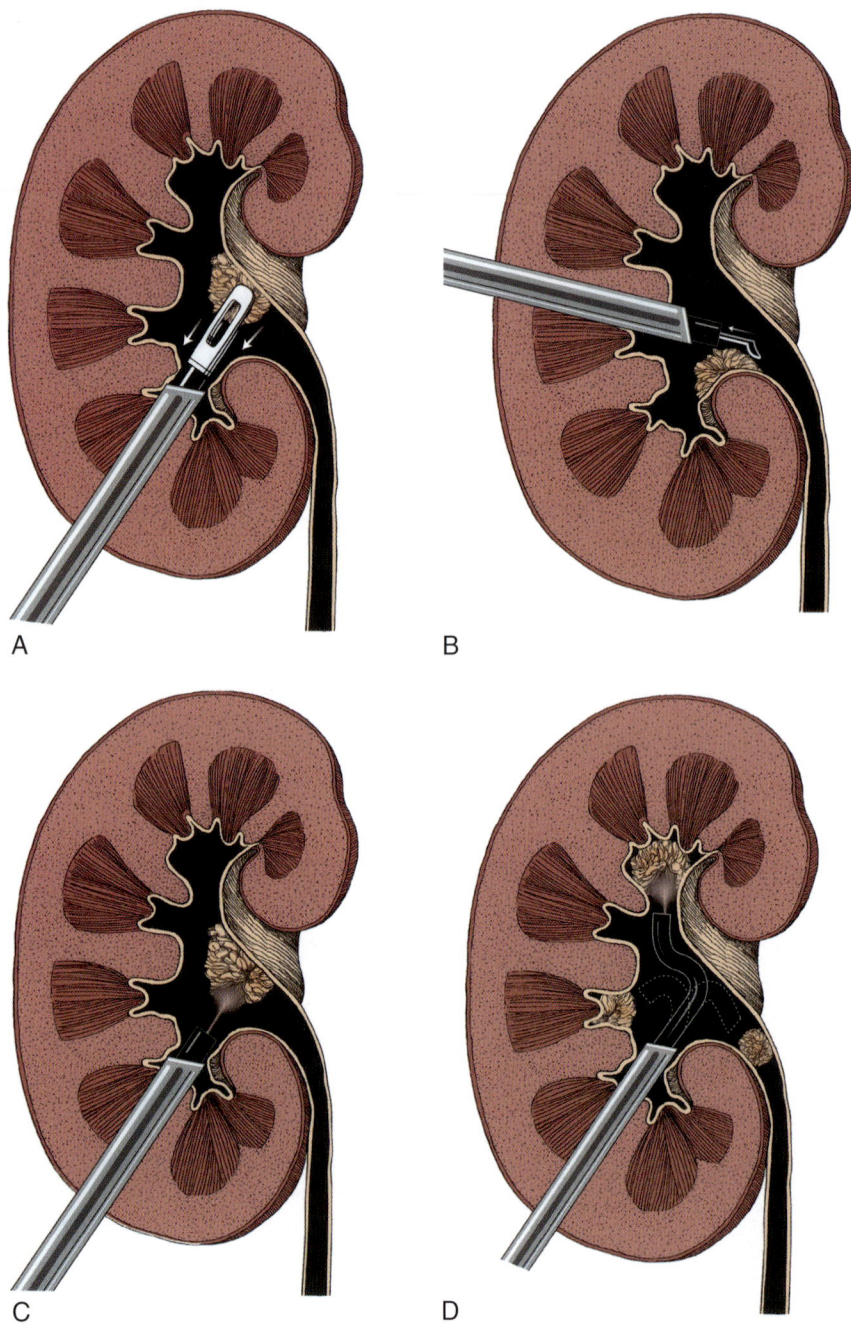

Fig. 99.25. Techniques for percutaneous removal of transitional cell carcinoma of the renal collecting system. (A) The tumor is identified and debulked by forceps to its base. The base is sampled and sent separately for evaluation. This technique works well for papillary tumors on a narrow stalk. Broad-based tumors may cause excessive bleeding and are best approached with resection or laser therapy. (B) With use of a standard resectoscope, the tumor is identified and resected to its base. Special care should be taken to avoid resection into major renal vasculature. The tumor is identified, sampled for diagnostic purposes, and treated by holmium or neodymium laser sources. This can be done through a standard nephroscope (C) or with a flexible cystoscope (D).

cautery. Low-grade papillary lesions on a thin stalk are easily treated in this manner with minimal bleeding.

Alternatively, a cutting loop from a standard resectoscope or bipolar resectocope is used to remove the tumor to its base (see Fig. 99.25B). A monopolar resection does carry the risk of absorption of large volumes of hypo-osmotic irrigant, and thus bipolar resection may be preferred. Once again, the base should be resected and sent separately for staging purposes. This approach is more effective for larger, broad-based tumors for which simple debulking to a stalk is not possible.

For the third technique, which uses flexible or rigid endoscopes, the tumor is sampled and treated with a holmium:YAG or Nd:YAG laser at 25 to 30 W (Fig. 99.25C and D). Tissue may also be obtained with a small snare used for gastrointestinal polyps.

Regardless of approach, a nephrostomy tube is left in place. This access can be used for second-look follow-up nephroscopy to ensure complete tumor removal (Fig. 99.26). Nephroureterectomy is indicated if the pathological examination shows high-grade or invasive disease.

Second-Look Nephroscopy. Follow-up nephroscopy is performed 4 to 14 days later to allow adequate healing. The tumor resection site is identified, and any residual tumor is removed. If no tumor is identified, the base should be sampled and treated by cautery or the Nd:YAG laser (15 to 20 W and 3-second exposures). The nephrostomy tube can be removed several days later if all tumors have been removed. If the patient is being considered for adjuvant topical therapy, a small, 8-Fr nephrostomy tube is left to provide access for instillations. Some authors advocate third-look nephroscopy before removal of the nephrostomy tube (Jarrett et al., 1995b).

Results

As with the ureteroscopic approach, there are no randomized controlled trials and only limited contemporary case series (Table 99.3) with adequate numbers and follow-up from which to draw reasonable conclusions (Goel et al., 2003; Palou et al., 2004; Rastinehad et al., 2009; Rouprel et al., 2007). In the longest series to date, Motamedinia et al. (2015) had an average follow-up of 76.9 months and had 87% for imperative conditions and 90% for elective conditions. In a literature review of 288 patients, Cutress et al. (2012) found an overall recurrence rate of upper tract recurrence rate of 26% and a bladder recurrence rate of 31%. Failed endoscopic management occurred in 32% with a nephroureterectomy rate of 22%. Disease progression occurred in 17% with 6% advancing to metastatic disease. As expected, tumor grade strongly predicted outcomes. Cutress et al. (2012) showed the upper tract recurrence rate for grades 1, 2, and 3 lesions to be 23%, 30%, and 40%, respectively. Lee et al. (1999) reviewed their 13-year experience with percutaneous management, comparing 50 patients who underwent percutaneous management with 60 patients who underwent nephroureterectomy and found no significant difference in overall survival. As expected, patients with low-grade disease did well regardless of modality and patients with high-grade disease did poorly regardless of treatment option.

Most would agree from the literature that percutaneous management is acceptable in patients with low-grade (grade 1) disease regardless of the status of the contralateral kidney, provided the patient is committed to lifelong endoscopic follow-up. Patients with high-grade or grade 3 disease do poorly regardless of modality chosen but should probably undergo nephroureterectomy to maximize cancer therapy (provided they are medically fit). The largest area of controversy surrounds the use of percutaneous management for patients with grade 2 disease and a normal contralateral kidney. With more invasive lesions, the potential for disease progression and metastatic disease is significant and nephroureterectomy should be considered. Interestingly, there appears to be a lower rate of upper tract recurrence with a percutaneous approach when compared with the ureteroscopic approach. Cutress et al. (2012) showed a 52% upper tract recurrence compared with 37% for ureteroscopy when comparing pooled data.

Complications from percutaneous management of tumors are similar to those for benign renal processes and include bleeding, systemic absorption of hypo-osmotic irrigation (with monopolar resection), perforation of the collecting system, and secondary ureteropelvic junction obstruction. Cutress showed the overall complication rate to be 27%; transfusion, dialysis, and renal failure were the most significant. Complications increase in number and severity with higher tumor grade (Jarrett et al., 1995a). This finding

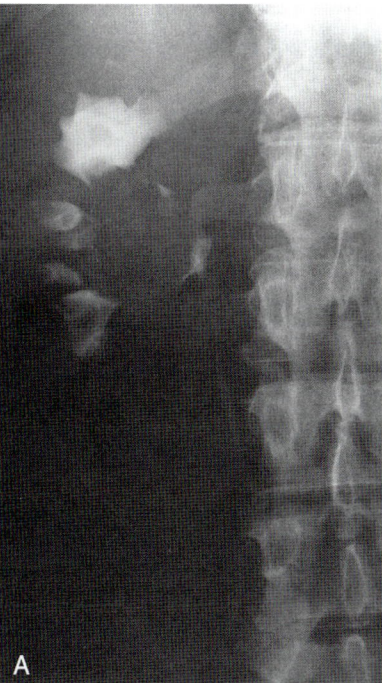
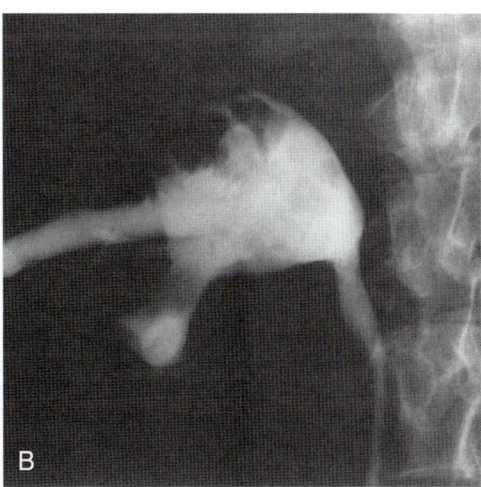
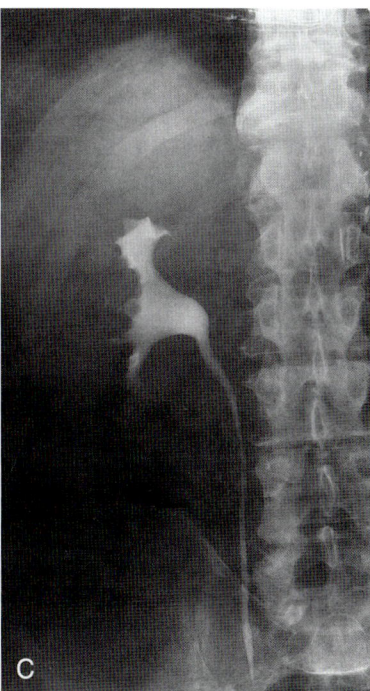

Fig. 99.26. (A) A 65-year-old man with a solitary kidney and a 5-cm renal pelvis tumor. (B) Nephrostogram after patient underwent staged resection. (C) Three-month follow-up retrograde pyelogram after completed resection. The patient showed grade 1 transitional cell carcinoma without invasion to submucosa.

TABLE 99.3 Percutaneous Management

STUDY	NUMBER OF PATIENTS (%)	FOLLOW-UP (mo)	UPPER TRACT RECURRENCE (%)	BLADDER RECURRENCE	NEPHROURETERECTOMY RATE (%)	DISEASE PROGRESSION (%)	FAILED MANAGEMENT (%)	COMPLICATIONS (%)
Jarrett et al., 1995b	36	55	33	ND	42	16	33	25
Patel et al., 1996	26	45	35	42	19	8	23	27
Goel et al., 2003	20	64	65	15	50	35	50	20
Palou et al., 2004	34	51	44	ND	26	ND	—	6
Roupret et al., 2007	24	62	13	17	21	17	—	10
Rastinehad et al., 2009	89	61	33	ND	13	20	—	ND

ND, Not disclosed.
Modified from Cutress ML, Stewart GD, Zakikhani P, et al.: Ureteroscopic and percutaneous management of upper tract urothelial carcinoma (UTUC): systematic review. BJU Int 110:614–628, 2012.

is probably due to the more extensive pathological process and treatments necessary to eradicate the tumor. Unlike ureteroscopic resection, the percutaneous method can stage tumors and, as expected, stage increases with tumor grade.

A major concern of the percutaneous approach is the potential seeding of nonurothelial surfaces with tumor cells. There have been limited reports of nephrostomy tract infiltration with high-grade tumors. Schwartzmann et al. (2017) reported on their only instance and summarized 7 additional case reports. All were high-grade tumors with 5 of urothelial and 3 of squamous histology. Cutress et al. (2012), however, only showed a 0.3% overall rate of tumor seeding in a large review of the percutaneous approach. Tract seeding is a possibility but appears to be an uncommon event.

Consideration for Urinary Diversions

With cases of prior urinary diversion, identification of the ureteroenteric anastomosis is difficult and may require antegrade percutaneous passage of a guidewire down the ureter before endoscopy. For conduits and neobladders, a trial with flexible endoscopy into the diversion and identification of the ureteroenteric anastomosis is reasonable. Knowledge of the type of anastomosis is essential. For conduits, knowledge location of the ureters (i.e., Wallace vs. Bricker) is essential to location of the ureters. Similarly with a neobladder, identification is also possible provided the pouch anatomy is known (i.e., Studer). Identification of the ureters is usually not possible with a catheterizable continent urinary diversion. With all types of diversion, if the ureters are not identifiable, antegrade passage of a wire into the pouch may be necessary by the urologist or with the assistance of interventional radiology. The wire can be retrieved from the diversion, and the ureteroscope can be passed in a retrograde fashion. The nephrostomy tract does not have to be fully dilated in this setting. Wagner et al. (2008) described their experience with endoscopic monitoring of patients with ureteral carcinoma in situ (CIS) after radical cystectomy. If this is not possible, then dilation of the tract and antegrade uretero-nephroscopy may be necessary.

Management of Positive Upper Tract Urinary Cytology and Carcinoma in situ

Evaluation

An unequivocal positive voiding urinary cytology usually indicates the presence of urothelial carcinoma. Most cases are from a bladder source; however, extravesical sites may be involved, including the upper urinary tracts and the prostatic urethra in men. Often the diagnosis is difficult because of the limitations of radiographic evaluation of upper tracts and the complexity of upper tract endoscopy compared with the bladder. In addition, the interpretation of minute pathological specimens of the upper urinary tract makes precise histologic diagnosis and staging difficult. Fig. 99.27 outlines the algorithm for management of a positive urinary cytology as described by Schwalb et al. (1994). The cytology must be repeated to confirm the findings. The next step involves radiographic evaluation of the upper tracts, usually with CT urography and a complete bladder evaluation including bladder biopsies and tumor resection if tumor is present. If the bladder evaluation was positive for urothelial carcinoma, the initial treatment at that point is to treat the bladder with either intravesical therapy and/or tumor resection and follow the voided urinary cytologies. If these remain positive despite a negative bladder evaluation or after successful treatment of the bladder, then one should proceed to evaluating extravesical sites and consider repeat bladder evaluation at the same time. Evaluation of extravesical sites should include selective cytologies from each upper urinary tract, ensuring noncontamination of the specimen from the bladder or urethra, retrograde pyelograms (if not evaluated or visualized on CT urogram), as well as resection of a representative specimen of the prostatic urethra in men. Ureteroscopy can also be done at this time to allow for direct visualization of the upper urinary tracts, or done once the positive cytology is lateralized.

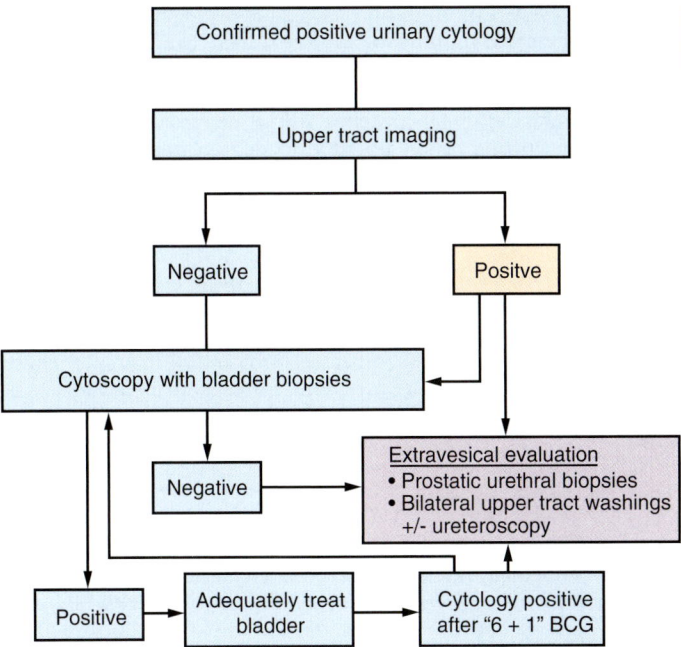

Fig. 99.27. Algorithm for management of a positive urinary cytology.

Carcinoma in situ of the Upper Urinary Tracts

The diagnosis of isolated CIS of the upper urinary tracts is a difficult one because of the inability to evaluate the urothelium of the upper tracts with adequate tissue samples. **In most cases the diagnosis is one of exclusion, wherein there is a persistent positive selective cytology in the absence of any ureteroscopic and radiographic findings** (Redrow et al., 2016). This is to be distinguished from cases in which CIS is coexistent with a high-grade papillary UTUC, in which case radical and possibly multimodal treatment is indicated, as the presence of CIS in addition to papillary tumors is associated with significantly worse recurrence-free and cancer-specific survival (Otto, 2011; Wheat, 2012). Treatment for isolated upper tract CIS is not well established: radical nephroureterectomy was performed in the past for a unilateral cytologic abnormality of the upper tract (Gittes, 1980; McCarron et al., 1983; Messing et al., 1998; Williams, 1991). This practice may not be recommended in the modern era. Upper tract cytology has the same limitations in specificity as bladder cytology. Furthermore, properly collected upper tract samples are of limited volume and cell count compared with bladder washings. Any source of inflammation, such as urinary infection or calculus, may produce a false-positive result. A subsequent cytologic abnormality from the contralateral side during follow-up is not rare in cases of true-positive results from early CIS (Khan et al., 1979; Murphy et al., 1974). There is one large series and many small series of topical therapy of the upper tract with immune therapy and chemotherapy via retrograde and antegrade approaches with variable response rates. Patients with CIS appear to do equally as well as their bladder counterparts in these limited, retrospective studies (Giannarini et al., 2011; Redrow et al., 2016) (see the section on topical therapy for results of topical therapy for upper tract CIS). Placement of a nephrostomy tube seems to be the more reliable delivery system; alternatively, a weekly cystoscopy can be performed and a ureteral catheter placed in the upper calyx (Metcalfe et al., 2017). Most would not intervene initially with surgical intervention in the absence of any histologic, radiographic, or endoscopic finding because of the limitations of cytology alone with false-positive results and the high risk for bilateral disease in the future. In addition, segmental resection is usually not effective in addressing the problem because of the field-effect nature of the disease. Nephroureterectomy is, however, indicated with radiographic or endoscopic confirmation that the patient has more than just surface disease. Frequent-interval re-evaluation with urinalysis, bladder and possible selective cytology, cystoscopy every 3 months, and retrograde pyelography or ureteropyeloscopy every 6 months are indicated for 1 to 2 years.

Another scenario is CIS of ureteral margins during radical cystectomy. There is controversy over the proper management of this finding, which definitely confers a risk of disease progression but may require a long follow-up time to demonstrate a recurrence. However, many do not progress, and when they do, recurrences may not be isolated to the distal ureteral margin. Wagner et al. (2008) studied a select group with serial endoscopy and found that recurrences were found at the site of the margin and at other sites. Herr et al. (1996) showed that many did not show any tumor at the margin site but did show a high risk of overall disease progression to death from metastatic disease. Whalen et al. (2015) performed 590 intraoperative ureteral frozen sections in 241 patients. These were positive in 12.9% of cases, and conversion to negative was accomplished in 82%. The authors showed that conversion from positive to negative was associated with improved survival.

Expectant Management

There is very little information on the role of active surveillance. UTUC was originally not thought to be amenable to active surveillance because of the risks of disease progression especially with high-risk disease, flank pain, chronic hematuria, and urinary tract obstruction. Some recent studies have shown that this approach can be considered in selected cases. Syed et al. (2018) reported on a group of patients diagnosed with UTUC but not treated and found a marked decrease overall survival in the untreated group (1.9 vs. 7.8). Thus for patients with a very short life expectancy, this approach may be chosen.

Adjuvant Topical Therapy

Adjuvant Intravesical Topical Chemotherapy After Nephroureterectomy to Decrease Bladder Recurrence. Patients with upper urinary tract tumors have a 30% to 50% risk for development of bladder cancer after nephroureterectomy (Hisataki et al., 2000; Ito et al., 2013; Kakizoe et al., 1980; Kang et al., 2003; O'Brien et al., 2011). Most recurrences in the bladder are likely a result of seeding and occur within 2 years (Catto et al., 2006; Kang et al., 2003; Takahashi et al., 2001). Data already exist showing the efficacy of mitomycin-C, and most recently, gemcitabine (Messing et al., 2017) to reduce post-transurethral resection of bladder tumor (TURBT) recurrences. Two randomized controlled studies have definitively shown a decreased risk of recurrence with use of a single postoperative dose of topical chemotherapy after nephroureterectomy. O'Brien et al. (2011) first showed that a single intravesical dose of mitomycin-C was able to reduce the risk of bladder tumor from 28% in the control arm to 16% in the mitomycin arm within the first year after nephroureterectomy. In that study, mitomycin was given at variable times and biopsy confirmation of bladder recurrence was not required. Another randomized prospective study by Ito et al. (2013) using a single dose of intravesical pirarubicin showed reduction of bladder recurrence at 2 years from 42% in the control arm to 17% in the pirarubicin arm. In the Ito et al. study, treatment was given consistently within 5 days and biopsy confirmation of disease was required. Interestingly, given the differences in study design and different drugs used, the results of both studies are remarkably similar at the 1-year mark. Finally and most importantly, both studies consistently showed a very low rate of adverse effects and good tolerance in patients. **Perioperative single-dose intravesical chemotherapy should now be considered as a standard of care for prevention of bladder cancer after nephroureterectomy.**

Technique

Within 3 to 7 days after nephroureterectomy and with the catheter still in place from surgery, patients undergo cystogram to confirm absence of leakage from the site of bladder cuff resection. If the scan is negative, a single dose of mitomycin, gemcitabine, or other proven chemotherapeutic is instilled into the bladder, and the catheter is clamped, allowing a dwell time of at least 1 and up to 2 hours. Patients should be instructed to arrive for treatment relatively dehydrated, and in the case of mitomycin, have been alkalinized with oral sodium bicarbonate starting the day prior (1 to 1.5 g sodium bicarbonate at night and in the morning on treatment day). Some of the authors have made two changes to the protocol as described in prior studies. Given the newer data on the efficacy of gemcitabine after TURBT (Messing et al., 2017), especially because of its efficacy for low- and high-grade disease, some have switched to the use of this compound instead of mitomycin. In addition, it does not require urinary alkalinization for optimized efficacy. Another major change has been to instill the gemcitabine *at the time of nephroureterectomy*. The rationale for this change is the following: (1) it does not require the patient to return for cystogram and an additional clinic visit; (2) it allows for possible earlier removal of the urinary catheter after surgery and before discharge; (3) it would preclude situations when leakage at the site of the bladder cuff would result in treatment being canceled; and (4) it is given, theoretically, at the most effective time period when seeding is thought to occur. In cases of intraoperative chemotherapy instillation, the following steps are taken. A 2- or 3-way urinary catheter is placed either on the sterile field or sterilely off the field, and the bladder is drained, after which the chemotherapy can be administered intravesically before the surgery is started. A clamp is placed on the outflow (also on inflow if using a 3-way catheter; we do this when the catheter is placed off the sterile field to allow the nursing circulator to easily irrigate the bladder using attached irrigation tubing). The anesthesia team is requested to minimize intravenous fluid administration because the bladder will be clamped for 1 to 2 hours. After surgery has started, once the ureter is clipped below the level of the tumor and after at least 1 and up to 2 hours of dwell time, the circulator can remove the clamp(s) and drain the bladder. By the time surgical dissection reaches the distal ureter and bladder cuff, the bladder has been fully drained of the chemotherapy. In addition, the use of the 3-way catheter allows additional bladder irrigation to wash out any possible residual chemotherapy, and after closure of the cystotomy, confirmation of a watertight closure of the cystotomy site.

After Organ-Sparing Therapy

Any procedure short of extirpative surgery has a higher local recurrence because of the established risk of ipsilateral recurrence. Several approaches are available to minimize these risks and that consist of reliable instillation of immunotherapeutic or chemotherapeutic agents to the upper tract.

Instillation Therapy. Instillation therapy is used in two settings for treatment of UTUC, namely as primary treatment for CIS, and as adjuvant therapy after endoscopic or organ-sparing therapy. Delivery of the agents presents an additional challenge and can be accomplished in several ways. Accepted, reliable techniques include antegrade instillation through a nephrostomy tube (Fig. 99.28) and retrograde instillation directly via a ureteral catheter. Attempting to induce reflux in a patient using an indwelling ureteral stent or by iatrogenically created vesicoureteral reflux appears to be an unreliable method of effective drug administration to the upper tracts and is not recommended. Patel and Fuchs (1998) described a technique of outpatient instillation through a ureteral catheter placed suprapubically, but given the concern over tumor implantation, this technique is not recommended. Regardless of the technique chosen, administration to the upper urinary tract should be done under low pressure and in the absence of active infection to minimize the risk of bacterial sepsis or systemic absorption of the agent.

Results

The same agents used to treat urothelial carcinoma of the bladder are used to treat tumors of the upper urinary tract. Most historical studies are small, retrospective, uncontrolled series of patients undergoing therapy with **thiotepa** (Elliott et al., 1996; Patel et al., 1996), **mitomycin** (Cornu et al., 2010; Cutress et al., 2012), **and bacille Calmette-Guérin (BCG)** (Palou et al., 2004). See Table 99.4 for a summary.

TABLE 99.4 Adjuvant Upper Tract Instillation

AGENT	NO. OF PATIENTS	MEAN FOLLOW-UP (mo)	COMPLICATIONS (%)	BENEFIT SHOWN
THIOTEPA				
Elliot et al., 1996	4	60	ND	Benefit not evaluated
Patel et al., 1996	1	1	1 death from sepsis	No benefit
MMC				
Keeley et al., 1997a	19	30	10	Safety, no definite benefit
Martínez-Piñeiro et al, 1996	41	31	3 deaths from systemic absorption	14% recurrence compared with 25% without MMC
Cornu et al., 2010	35	24	9	Benefit not evaluated
Cutress et al., 2012	73	63	18	No benefit
BCG				
Clark et al., 1999	17	21	ND	No benefit
Palou et al., 2004	34	51	6	No benefit
Giannarini et al., 2011	22	42	201 deaths from sepsis	No benefit
Rastinehad et al., 2009	89	61	2 deaths from sepsis	No benefit

BCG, Bacille Calmette-Guérin; *MMC*, mitomycin C; *ND*, not disclosed.
Modified from Cutress ML, Stewart GD, Zakikhani P, et al.: Ureteroscopic and percutaneous management of upper tract urothelial carcinoma (UTUC): systematic review. *BJU Int* 110:614–628, 2012.

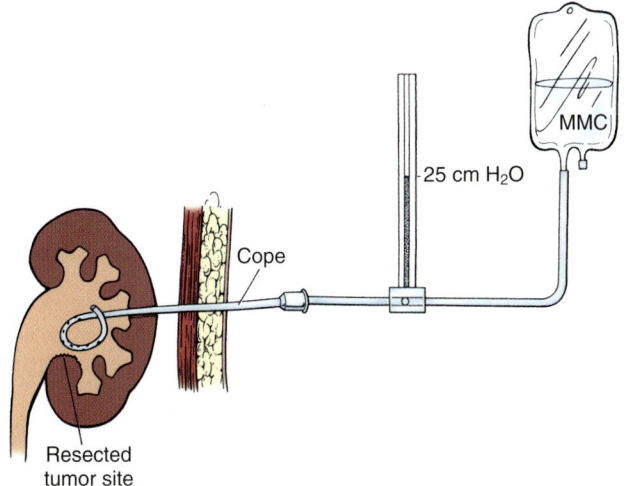

Fig. 99.28. Setup for administration of topical immunotherapy or chemotherapy to the upper urinary tract through a previously placed nephrostomy tube. Therapy is instilled by gravity with a mechanism that prevents excessive intrarenal pressures. High pressures have been linked to complications of systemic absorption and bacterial sepsis. *MMC*, Mitomycin C.

Gemcitabine has been used intravesically as an alternative to BCG with fewer side effects. We may see a larger role in the upper urinary tract. Although the cumulative experience appears encouraging, definitive conclusions are not easily reached. Possible reasons for this include (1) insufficient numbers to show clinical significance because of the relative rarity of the disease; (2) tumors of the upper urinary tract, which have a tumor biology different from that of their bladder counterparts; and (3) a nonstandardized and possibly inadequate delivery system that, unlike in the bladder, does not allow uniform delivery of the agent with adequate dwell time to enable a clinical response.

The largest experience is from use of BCG via a nephrostomy tube for primary treatment of CIS, and in this setting favorable responses are seen. In a recent update of this experience with 55 patients, a 57% 5-year recurrence-free survival was seen; on the other hand, patients treated in an adjuvant fashion after endoscopic ablation of papillary tumors had inferior results (Giannarini et al., 2011).

The greatest experience with chemotherapy is with the use of mitomycin C, but because of the smaller numbers of patients and variable selection criteria, no definite conclusions can be reached, with the exception that mitomycin is very well tolerated and has a very low adverse event profile (Audenet et al., 2013). A recent single-institutional experience with use of mitomycin-c given as induction and maintenance therapy via nephrostomy tube or weekly cystoscopically placed ureteral catheter in 27 patients showed 60% recurrence-free, 80% progression-free, and 76% nephroureterectomy-free survival at a median follow-up of 19 months (range 7–92) (Metcalfe, 2016).

In the study with intrarenal perfusion of BCG, despite initial return of cytology results to normal, 50% of patients (5 of 10) developed disease recurrence after a mean follow-up of 50.9 months, and all of these had cancer-specific mortality (Hayashida et al., 2004). The initial results regarding response are encouraging; however, the recurrences with possible disease progression should not give the clinician optimism for long-term cure. Although removal of a renal unit for CIS alone is not urged, patients need to be followed vigilantly for disease progression.

One of the most promising avenues that may radically change the paradigm for how low-grade UTUC is endoscopically managed is undergoing clinical trial evaluation at the time of this writing. The Optimized DeLivery of Mitomycin for Primary UTUC Study (Olympus) is the first sponsored trial specifically for UTUC (https://clinicaltrials.gov/NCT02793128). The study is a phase 3, prospective, open-label, single-arm trial designed to assess the efficacy, safety, and tolerability of treatment with MitoGel. This compound is a unique reverse-polymer hydrogel admixed with mitomycin, which transitions from a viscous liquid to a gel when warmed to body temperature and subsequently dissolves at a constant rate in urine over the course of several hours, delivering mitomycin at a higher concentration and longer time period than conventional methods. The study is designed for low-grade, low-volume tumors. Although the study is ongoing and results are not yet available, the results of its use in the compassionate use setting were presented by Lin et al. (2017). Of 22 patients, 18 of whom had low-grade disease, 16 (73%) completed 6 weekly treatments and 9 (41% of total population, 59% of those who completed treatment) had a complete response. **If found effective, well-tolerated, and approved, Mitogel therapy will significantly change the endoscopic management of low-grade UTUC by providing a viable therapy for not only primary topical chemoablation but also adjuvant therapy.**

The most common complications of instillation therapy are bacterial sepsis and development of strictures. To minimize infections, patients must be evaluated for active infection before each treatment, and only a low-pressure delivery system should be used. Stricture formation may be related to prior endoscopy, ureteral catheter placement, or the agent used, or a combination of all these factors (Aboumarzouk et al., 2013; Metcalfe et al., 2017). Agent-specific complications of the various therapies include ramifications of systemic absorption of the agent Bellman et al. (1994) such as described upper urinary tract complications of percutaneous BCG instillation. Granulomatous involvement of the kidney in the absence of systemic signs of BCG infection was most commonly seen. Mukamel et al., (1991) saw an inordinate decrease in renal function for patients receiving BCG who had vesicoureteral reflux.

Systemic Chemotherapy. The use of agents for UTUC has been extrapolated from chemotherapy regimens used in bladder urothelial cancer. In 2018 significant strides were made, with presentation of 2 separate prospective trials on the use of systemic chemotherapy, one a randomized adjuvant trial, the other a nonrandomized, GFR-stratified neoadjuvant trial.

The strongest current rationale for use of neoadjuvant therapy is the high proportion of significant baseline chronic kidney disease in patients with UTUC, which worsens after nephroureterectomy, rendering patients ineligible to receive the full-dose cisplatinum-based chemotherapy postoperatively (Lane et al., 2010). There are two reports on the use of neoadjuvant therapy. The initial data came from a small series of 15 patients who received MVAC (methotrexate, vinblastine, adriamycin, and cisplatin), MEC (methotrexate, etoposide, and cisplatin), or MVEC (methotrexate, vinblastine, epirubicin, and cisplatin) regimens before nephroureterectomy (Igawa et al., 1995). All of the patients had advanced disease, with 6 having clinical T2N0M0, 4 with T3N0-1M0, and 5 with T4N0-3M0 disease. Of these patients, 13% achieved complete, and 40% partial, pathological response. The authors reported a positive correlation between pathological response and disease-specific survival. Another larger retrospective case-control study (Matin et al., 2010) of 150 high-risk UTUC patients, 43 of whom received neoadjuvant therapy with a variety of regimens (MVAC, cisplatin-gemcitabine-ifosfamide, gemcitabine-paclitaxel-doxorubicin [GTA], cisplatin-gemcitabine [GC], and others), observed a significant incidence of pathological downstaging of tumors and a 14% complete response rate. A survival update of these patients showed significant improvement in 5-year survival in those receiving neoadjuvant chemotherapy versus a matched historical cohort (94% vs. 58%, $P < 0.001$) (Porten et al., 2013). **This data informed the development of the first collaborative prospective UTUC trial in the United States. The intergroup trial EA8141 was a phase 2, nonrandomized study of neoadjuvant chemotherapy for patients at high risk of recurrence after nephroureterectomy.** Patients were stratified based on kidney function, with those having a creatinine clearance of more than 50 receiving accelerated MVAC for 4 cycles before surgery, and those with clearance of 30 to 49 receiving carboplatin and gemcitabine for 4 cycles before surgery. The study was closed in 2017 after all 30 patients were enrolled in the MVAC arm and about half as many in the Carbo/Gem arm. Results were presented at the 2018 American Urological Association meeting, with the study meeting its predefined efficacy end point of pathological 14% complete remission and 60% downstaging to less than pT1N0, and no new safety concerns in patients with creatinine clearance of more than 50. **EA8141 confirms the efficacy of the neoadjuvant approach with pathological end points, which are well-accepted surrogates for survival. Once published in the peer-reviewed literature, it will be considered as an acceptable standard of care for patients with high-risk UTUC, and especially for those anticipated to have a postoperative creatinine clearance of less than 50.**

Adjuvant therapy has been used infrequently in the treatment of UTUC, and, until very recently, most publications are based on retrospective review of institutional experience. A study of 27 patients with pT3N0M0, 16 of whom received platinum-based therapy after nephroureterectomy, reported no significant difference in recurrence-free and disease-specific survival after 40 months of follow-up (Lee et al., 2006). Another study compared the outcomes of 24 patients with pT2-3N0M0 disease who received MVAC chemotherapy after nephroureterectomy with those of a similar group of patients who did not receive adjuvant therapy. The authors did not observe a significant difference in 10-year overall survival rates. A multi-institutional retrospective review of pT3-4N0M0 and N+ patients (Hellenthal et al., 2009) who did or did not receive platinum-based chemotherapy failed to show a significant difference in the overall or disease-specific survival rates. However, in this cohort, adjuvant therapy was more commonly used in patients with higher tumor grade and stage. In contrast, Kwak et al. (2006) showed a twofold decrease in recurrence of cancer and a significant reduction in disease-specific mortality (28.1% vs. 81.8%) in the pT2-3N0M0 patient population who received platinum-based chemotherapy. A recent large, multi-institutional retrospective study of 1544 patients with pT2-4 Nany M0 having nephroureterectomy from 15 centers treated between 2000 and 2015 was reported (Necchi et al., 2018). Patients receiving adjuvant therapy (n = 312) were compared with those not receiving adjuvant (n = 1232) using propensity score matching and inverse probability of treatment weighting to analyze overall survival. The authors found no improvement in overall survival. In retrospect, all of these studies were biased in one direction or another as a result of unmeasured selection biases, as became evident when prospective data were available.

In 2018 the results of the phase III randomized trial of Peri-Operative Chemotherapy Versus Surveillance in Upper Tract Urothelial Cancer (POUT) were presented after the trial was stopped early as a result of meeting predefined efficacy criteria (Birtle et al., 2018). This study randomized patients having undergone nephroureterectomy with high risk of recurrence (pT2-4 N0-3 M0) to adjuvant chemotherapy (n = 125) versus surveillance (n = 123). Patients in the adjuvant arm received gemcitabine and cisplatin if postoperative creatinine clearance was more than 50 and gemcitabine-carboplatin if clearance was 30 to 49. At a median follow-up of 17.6 months, 2-year disease-free survival was 51% for surveillance (95% confidence interval [CI] 39, 61) and 70% for chemotherapy (95% CI 58, 79). Progression-free survival favored chemotherapy, with hazard ratio (HR) = 0.49 (95% CI 0.30, 0.79, $P = 0.003$). **The POUT trial is the largest trial completed for UTUC, and once published, will establish adjuvant chemotherapy as a standard for patients with high risk of recurrence after nephroureterectomy.** Although the POUT data establish the efficacy of adjuvant therapy overall, more detailed information is needed to determine how many patients were precluded from the trial as a result of low kidney function, and the extent of efficacy of the gemcitabine-carboplatin arm, as carboplatin in the metastatic setting has limited efficacy (see the next section). Interestingly, the 2-year disease-free survival result from POUT (70%) is inferior to the 5-year cancer-specific survival obtained from neoadjuvant chemotherapy in the Matin et al. study (90%). Although the latter was retrospective, its results are similar to those obtained from the EA8141 trial. Further studies are needed to determine whether neoadjuvant or adjuvant therapy is superior; in the meantime, the consideration of post-nephroureterectomy kidney function remains paramount in planning a treatment course for the patient.

Treatment of Lymph Node–Positive and Metastatic Disease
Chemotherapy

There are limited data on efficacy of chemotherapy in lymph node positive and metastatic UTUC. Prospective randomized trials comparing chemotherapeutic regimens for UTUC are not feasible because of the rarity of these patients. Therefore other than the two recently completed prospective trials on neoadjuvant and adjuvant chemotherapy for localized or locally advanced UTUC, the data for chemotherapy response rates are extrapolated from observations in urothelial cancer, most of which do not stratify results by original location of tumor. In a study of 184 patients accrued over three consecutive time intervals from 1986 to 2004 at MD Anderson Cancer Center, the median recurrence-free survival was 2.4 years and did not improve over time (Brown et al., 2006). The decline in renal function after

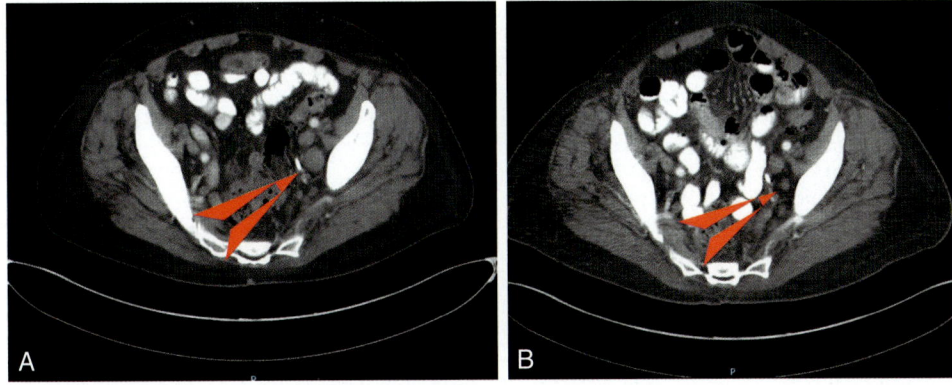

Fig. 99.29. (A) A patient with urothelial cell carcinoma of the kidney and left inguinal lymphadenopathy. (B) The patient had a sustained almost complete response at 9 weeks and 16 weeks after treatment with cabozantinib. *Red arrowhead* points to resolving adenopathy.

nephroureterectomy in these mostly elderly patients may compromise the ability to administer effective postoperative chemotherapy and is yet another reason to consider neoadjuvant chemotherapy for patients with high-risk upper tract tumors. **When there is evidence of regional lymph node metastases, initial chemotherapy should be given as the primary therapy, and surgery should be withheld until a good—ideally a complete—radiographic response is seen. Generally, two additional cycles after maximal response are given (usually a total of 6 cycles). At that time, consolidative surgery that includes lymphadenectomy can be offered, similar to the paradigm for bladder urothelial carcinoma.**

The MVAC regimen continues to have the highest response rate (Sternberg et al., 1989); however, its toxicity prohibits optimal dosage and duration in a large proportion of patients. In addition, complete responses are rare in the metastatic setting, and the duration of response is limited, with overall survival of 12 to 24 months. **A variation of standard MVAC is the dose-dense regimen, whereby all drugs are given at the same time with cell support, and this regimen has actually been shown to have a lower toxicity profile and may have better responses** (Sternberg et al., 2006). There is considerable ongoing investigation with newer agents, including paclitaxel, ifosfamide, carboplatin, gemcitabine, and vinflunine, used in various combinations and sequences (Bajorin et al., 1998; Bamias et al., 2006; Kaufman et al., 2000; Lorusso et al., 2000; Redman et al., 1998; Roth et al., 1994; Siefker-Radtke et al., 2013; Vaughn et al., 1998, 2009). Carboplatin is frequently substituted for cisplatin because of either limitations of renal function or concerns over toxicity with the latter, but the results with carboplatin remain inferior (Galsky et al., 2012). Many of these show initial overall response rates similar to the response rate to the MVAC regimen and lower toxicity. However, thus far, complete responses are rare, and there are no head-to-head comparison studies evaluating their durability or survival advantage compared with the MVAC regimen.

Results from a recent randomized phase III study comparing paclitaxel, cisplatin, and gemcitabine (PCG) versus GC in chemotherapy-naive patients with metastatic or locally advanced urothelial cancer (Bellmunt et al., 2012) showed that after a median follow-up of 4.6 years, with addition of paclitaxel, there was improvement in median overall survival (15.8 months vs. 12.7 months). The overall response rate was 55.5% with the use of PCG and 43.6 with GC, and both of the regimens were well tolerated. Of the 626 patients in this cohort, 82 had primary carcinoma of the renal pelvis or ureter; although there was no specific breakdown of the outcomes for this group of patients, on post hoc analysis the overall survival benefit was more pronounced in the group of patients with primary bladder tumors.

Another effective combination in patients with poor renal reserve is with gemcitabine, taxol, and doxorubicin (GTA). In many cases, patients can experience an improvement in kidney function after a few cycles, allowing for subsequent switching to a cisplatin regimen (Campbell et al., 2017).

There have been encouraging early results with cabozantinib, the inhibitor of MET and vascular endothelial growth factor pathways, in patients in whom previous chemotherapy has failed (Fig. 99.29). The patient accrual portion of a phase II trial is ongoing; it is hoped that this trial will provide further insight into the effects of this drug, which has shown clinical activity in multiple solid tumors.

Immunotherapy

Recently, immune modulation using a variety of checkpoint inhibitors has shown promise in the treatment of multiple malignancies, including urothelial carcinoma, and it promises to significantly change the outcomes for patients with metastatic urothelial cancer. Until now, options for patients progressing after platinum chemotherapy were poor and this was a major area of unmet need. Targeting the inhibitory surface receptor PD-1 (programmed death-1), activation of which by programmed cell death-ligand 1 (PD-L1) confers inhibition of T-cell proliferation and cytokine production, produced remarkable clinical activity in phase 1 clinical trials in metastatic urothelial carcinoma (Powles et al., 2014) with favorable side effect profile, and most importantly, infrequent renal impairment. These studies paved the way to tremendous success of new drugs approved for treatment of urothelial cancer, primarily PD-1, and PD-L1 inhibitors. UTUC patients may particularly derive a benefit from these treatments given the higher rates of microsatellite instability in UTUC than in bladder urothelial cancer, as high MSI appears to be particularly responsive to immune checkpoint inhibition. All of the following drugs are approved for patients with advanced urothelial cancer that has stopped responding or progressed after platinum chemotherapy.

Anti–PD-1 Approved Therapies. Nivolumab is a PD-1 inhibitor approved in 2017 after a phase 2 trial with median follow-up of 7 months showed objective rates of 16.1%, 28.4%, and 23.8% in those with <1%, >1%, and >5%, respectively, PD-L1 expression (not statistically significant). Grades 3 and 4 adverse events occurred in 18%, and there were 3 of 270 patients who had treatment-related death. The authors concluded that nivolumab monotherapy provided meaningful clinical benefit with an acceptable safety profile (Sharma et al., 2017). Pembrolizumab is another monoclonal antibody directed against PD-1 approved in 2017. Results of the KEYNOTE-045 study showed after a median follow-up of 27.7 months a median overall survival of 10.3 months for patients treated with pembrolizumab versus 7.3 months for those treated with chemotherapy (HR = 0.70; $P = 0.00017$). Moreover, responses appear to remain durable even after completion of therapy (Bellmunt et al., 2017). Interestingly, and similar to the nivolumab trial, patients with higher PD-L1 staining in tumor and immune cells did not appear to have substantially better survival outcomes.

Anti–PD-L1 Approved Therapies. Atezolizumab was the first PD-L1 inhibitor found to be active in urothelial cancer (Powles et al., 2014) and was approved in 2016 as first-line treatment for advanced or metastatic urothelial carcinoma ineligible for cisplatin chemotherapy. The IMvigor211 phase 3 trial showed similar objective response compared with chemotherapy (23% vs. 22%), but patients receiving atezolizumab had longer duration of response (15.9 months vs. 8.3 months), which was not statistically significant at the time, and had fewer high grade adverse events (Powles et al., 2018). Avelumab is unique in that it not only is a PD-L1 inhibitor but also acts via antibody-dependent cell-mediated toxicity, which directly lyses cells. It was approved for patients with platinum-refractory urothelial cancer, after initial results from a phase 1b trial showed an objective response from a nonrandomized clinical trial of 16.5% and a progression-free survival rate at 12 weeks of 35.6%. Adverse events occurred in 41% and 6% of patients died of treatment-related events. A subsequent pooled study of 2 cohorts (23.7% of which were UTUC patients) showed response rates of 17.6%, including 9 complete responses, and disease control rate of 41.2% (Patel et al., 2017). Durvalumab was shown in an open label phase 1/2 study in mostly previously treated urothelial cancer to have objective response rate of 17.8%, including 7 complete responses. Responses were early, durable, and were not related to expression of PD-L1 expression. Grade 3/4 treatment-related adverse events occurred in 6.8%, with 2 of 3 patients (1.6%) stopping treatment because of adverse events dying from immune-mediated events (Powles et al., 2017).

Molecular Alterations and Future of Genomic-Driven Therapy

Recent genomic studies are starting to improve our understanding of urothelial cancer in general, and specifically UTUC (Moss et al., 2017; Rouprêt et al., 2005); these show that despite phenotypic similarities, these cancers are genomically somewhat dissimilar. Microsatellite instability has been shown to be high in UTUC as compared with bladder cancer, which now has important implications for genomic-driven therapy with the approval of pembrolizumab for any solid tumor with high MSI (Le et al., 2015). In the first genomic study of UTUC, Sfakianos et al. (2015) compared tumor and germline DNA using a 300 cancer gene array. They found significant higher rate of mutations in *FGFR3* (35.6% vs. 21.6%; $P = 0.065$), *HRAS* (13.6% vs. 1.0%; $P = 0.001$), and *CDKN2B* (15.3% vs. 3.9%; $P = 0.016$) in high-grade UTUC than high-grade bladder cancer, and fewer mutations in TP53 (25.4% vs. 57.8%; $P < 0.001$) and RB1 (0 vs. 18.6%; $P < 0.001$). Mutations in chromatin-modifying genes were common, similar to bladder cancer. A second study by Moss et al. (Moss et al., 2017) reported a comprehensive genomic study of 31 UTUC samples using whole exome sequencing, RNA sequencing, and protein analysis. Of 2784 mutated genes, *FGFR3* was the most commonly mutated (74.1%), including in high-grade tumors (92% low-grade, 60% high-grade), followed by *KMT2D* (44.4%), *PIK3CA* (25.9%), and *TP53* (22.2%). Several patients had hypermutated genes, some of which were associated with deficient mismatch repair proteins associated with Lynch syndrome. APOBEC and CpG were the most common mutational signatures. RNA sequencing revealed clustering into 4 putative molecular subtypes with unique clinical behaviors, with one of the subtypes having highly upregulated expression of CTLA-4, PD-1, and PD-L1.

Relevant to these findings are the recent data showing activity of erdafitinib, a pan-FGFR inhibitor, for metastatic urothelial cancer, the first targeted agent for this indication. An ongoing phase 2 study showed a 42% response among 59 patients with metastatic urothelial cancer having specific *FGFR* mutations. The disease control rate was 73% to 74% for patients who received intermittent and continuous dosing (Loriot et al., 2018).

In summary, UTUC, like bladder cancer, is chemosensitive, but established chemotherapy regimens are toxic and lack sustained response. Unique to this population is the high rate of baseline chronic kidney disease, which worsens after nephroureterectomy. Immunotherapy with checkpoint inhibitors are starting to significantly improve the outlook for treatment-naive and platinum-refractory metastatic urothelial cancer, and the growing understanding of molecular alterations and genomic-driven therapy promises to continue expanding on this success.

Radiotherapy

There is a limited role for radiation outside treatment other than in the palliative setting. The proximity of the bowel to the upper urinary tract limits the dosing needed for effective primary therapy.

FOLLOW-UP

Issues in Assessing for Recurrence

The propensity of upper tract tumors for multifocal recurrence and metastatic spread with more dysplastic lesions makes follow-up complicated. Postoperative evaluation must routinely include evaluation of the bladder, the ipsilateral (if organ-sparing therapy was chosen) and contralateral urinary tracts, and the extraurinary sites for local and metastatic spread. A follow-up regimen is thus dependent on the time from surgery, the approach chosen (organ sparing vs. radical), and the potential for metastatic spread. Conservative recommendations for time intervals are listed in Fig. 99.30. The European Association of Urology recommendations for follow-up are much less strict, particularly for those who have radical nephroureterectomy rather than kidney-sparing treatment. Cystoscopy is recommended only at 3 and 6 months and then annually, and computed tomography every 6 to 12 months for 2 years then annually, depending on risk. After kidney-sparing management, cytology and ureteroscopy are recommended at 3, 6, 12, 18, and 24 months and annually thereafter (Rouprêt et al., 2018). The later sections detail some of the considerations and issues that address the need for individualizing follow-up care.

General Procedures

All patients should be assessed at regular intervals the first year after they are rendered tumor free by endoscopic or open surgical approaches (Keeley et al., 1997a). After the first year, this evaluation can be spaced out. This schedule is largely based on work with bladder urothelial carcinoma, showing that most tumor recurrences after bladder resection develop in the first year (Loening et al., 1980; Varkarakis et al., 1974). The upper urinary tract is more difficult to monitor, and delayed recognition of upper tract tumor recurrence may lead to disease progression and poor results (Mazeman, 1976). Evaluation should include history, physical examination, urinalysis,

---

- Physical examination, urine cytology (only for high-grade lesions), and cystoscopy
    - Every 3 months–first year
    - Every 6 months thereafter–years 2 through 3
    - Yearly–thereafter
- Contralateral imaging (IVU or retrograde pyelography)–yearly
- Ipsilateral endoscopy (patients undergoing organ-sparing therapy)–
    - Every 6 months–first several years
    - Yearly–thereafter
- Metastatic evaluation–necessary in all patients with significant risk of disease progression (i.e., high grade or invasive disease)
    - Physical examination, chest x-ray, comprehensive metabolic panel with liver enzymes
        - Every 3 months–first year
        - Every 6 months–years 2 through 3
        - Yearly–years 4 and 5
        - After 5 years–evaluation of urothelium only
    - Computed tomography or MRI of abdomen and pelvis
        - Every 6 months–years 1 and 2
        - Yearly–years 3 through 5
- Bone scan–only for elevated alkaline phosphatase level or symptoms of bone pain

Fig. 99.30. Follow-up begins after open surgery or when the patient is rendered tumor free by endoscopic management. The commencement of follow-up may be altered according to the potential for disease progression. *IVU,* Intravenous urography.

and office cystoscopy because of the high risk of bladder recurrences in patients treated conservatively and with nephroureterectomy (Mazeman, 1976). If the patient requires endoscopic evaluation of the upper urinary tract, cystoscopy can be done in conjunction with that procedure. Recent data suggest that patients treated for UTUC who do not develop a bladder recurrence in the first 6 to 12 months can have more rapid de-escalation of cystoscopic monitoring. As noted earlier, the European Association of Urology guidelines recommend a cystoscopy at 3 months and then annually (Rouprêt et al., 2018).

Urine cytology may be helpful in assessing for upper tract recurrence, especially for high-grade tumors (Murphy et al., 1981). The usefulness, however, is decreased with less dysplastic tumors (Grace et al., 1967; Sarnacki et al., 1971; Zincke et al., 1976). The same tumor markers under study for bladder urothelial carcinoma are promising for UTUC (Brown, 2000).

Specific Procedures

Bilateral disease, either synchronous or metachronous, is seen in 1% to 4% of patients (Babaian et al., 1980; Murphy et al., 1981; Petković, 1975), and thus imaging of the contralateral kidney is required on a regular basis. Yearly CT urography is usually sufficient, having replaced intravenous urography, and also can serve for metastatic surveillance. However, retrograde pyelography may be necessary if the patient is not a candidate for injection of iodinated contrast medium or if the urographic phase is not diagnostic. Magnetic resonance urography is another option for those unable to receive iodinated contrast, but patients with a creatinine clearance below 30 mg/dL may not receive gadolinium contrast because of concerns with development of nephrogenic systemic fibrosis. In these cases, MR urography with carefully performed and reformatted T2-weighted images can sometimes provide useful images. CT or ultrasonography is helpful in distinguishing stones from soft tissue densities. Further evaluation of filling defects on imaging studies usually requires ureteroscopic evaluation.

If an organ-sparing approach is chosen, the entire ipsilateral urinary tract must be assessed as well as the remainder of the urinary tract. The frequency and duration of the follow-up assessments depend largely on the grade and stage of the lesion, but they are usually every 6 months for several years and annually thereafter. Radiographic evaluation of the upper tracts alone may not be adequate because Keeley et al. (1997a) showed that 75% of early tumor recurrences were visible endoscopically and not radiographically. With tumors approached in a percutaneous fashion, early follow-up nephroscopy can be performed through the established nephrostomy tract.

In the past, the burden of repeated endoscopic evaluation of the upper urinary tracts was a major deterrent to conservative therapy. The use of smaller, 7.5-Fr flexible ureteroscopes has greatly eased the burden of follow-up because ureteroscopes can be reliably passed up the ureter without the need for dilation of the ureteral orifice or prior stenting. Others have advocated resection of the ureteral orifice to facilitate subsequent surveillance ureteroscopy in the office setting (Kerbl et al., 1993). Even though technology has somewhat facilitated follow-up, physician and patient must be committed to nephron-sparing treatment.

Metastatic Restaging

Metastatic restaging is required in all patients at significant risk for disease progression to local or distant sites and can be performed every 3 to 6 months in the first 2 years after surgery, because the majority of patients who recur with metastases do so within the first 2 to 3 years. This group includes those with high-grade or high-stage (>pT1) disease. Metastatic restaging is usually not necessary as frequently for low-grade disease when the risks of invasive and subsequent metastatic disease are negligible, and this can be done every 6 to 12 months in the first 2 years. Included in metastatic restaging is imaging of the ipsilateral renal bed for recurrence with cross-sectional imaging. Follow-up restaging includes chest radiography, liver function tests, cross-sectional body imaging, and selective use of bone scintigraphy based on symptoms or elevated serum markers. Follow-up of the upper tracts should be lifelong because of a lifetime risk of development of upper tract tumors in patients with prior bladder cancer (Herr et al., 1996).

REFERENCES

The complete reference list is available online at ExpertConsult.com.

100

Retroperitoneal Tumors

Timothy A. Masterson, MD, K. Clint Cary, MD, MPH, and Richard S. Foster, MD

OVERVIEW

The retroperitoneum (RP) is a common location for many pathologic conditions with which urologists must be familiar. Tumors within this region often involve adjacent structures including parts of the urinary tract, RP vasculature, and lymphatic circulation. Understanding the fundamental differences among a variety of tumors, both malignant and benign, that are unique to this location is important for making appropriate management decisions for patients. The origin of many tumors is primary to the RP, and for others it serves as a destination for metastatic deposits. In this chapter, we will review the anatomy of the RP, initial evaluation of the RP mass, differential diagnosis, and management strategies. Beyond this, we will discuss important perioperative management considerations, the surgical approach to the RP, and adjuvant therapies. Conditions unique to the kidneys and adrenal glands are discussed elsewhere.

ANATOMIC CONSIDERATIONS OF THE RETROPERITONEUM

Within the RP, an in-depth understanding of the anatomy is imperative. Borders include the diaphragm superiorly, inlet to the true pelvis inferiorly, insulation by the peritoneal contents anteriorly, the body wall posteriorly, and extension to the flank musculature laterally. Inclusive within the RP is the upper urinary tract (including the kidneys, renal pelvis, and proximal/middle portions of the ureter); adrenal glands; great vessels (infradiaphragmatic aorta and vena cava, common iliac vessels, lumbar branches); RP lymphatics and connective tissues (RP fat, Gerota fat, and fascia); and portions of the sensory, motor, and autonomic nervous systems (sympathetic chain of ganglia, postganglionic sympathetic and para-sympathetic nerve fibers). The close approximation of the peritoneal contents, including the second and third portions of the duodenum, ascending and descending colon, pancreas, and splenic hilum, warrant special consideration, as many of the conditions we will discuss present clinically as expansile tumors that distort and invade adjacent structures.

Specific to the right RP, tumors in the upper RP require attention not only regarding potential involvement of the kidney/ureter and adrenal gland, but more importantly the duodenum, vena cava, posterior diaphragm, and right segments of the liver. Involvement of the mesentery of the right colon can be difficult to assess on preoperative imaging, but indistinct tumor borders with loss of fat planes may raise concerns for its involvement. As for the left RP, involvement of the aorta, splenic hilum, and tail of the pancreas raise the greatest concerns. Similar to right-sided tumors, involvement of the diaphragm and mesentery of the left colon needs to be assessed. Similar to both, involvement/invasion of the posterior body wall and psoas muscle may be present. Depending on depth into the psoas muscle, trauma and/or disruption of sensory and motor nerves may be encountered. Paresthesias along the anterior and medial thigh may manifest as a result of transient or permanent injury to the genitofemoral nerve. Of greater concern, harm to the psoas muscle and femoral nerve can result in motor weakness and functional impairment with lower extremity flexion at the hip and extension from the knee.

Understanding in the preoperative setting the potential for involvement of any of these structures allows for a safer operation and better outcome. Consultation with hepatobiliary, vascular, thoracic, and/or general surgeons may be necessary to facilitate optimal care depending on the tumor location. Additionally, this will help establish appropriate expectations as to the degree of convalescence and recovery for the patient in the postoperative period.

KEY POINT

- The confines of the RP represent a specific anatomic compartment that houses or borders portions of the urinary, vascular, hepatobiliary, gastrointestinal, neurologic, and lymphatic systems. Accordingly, tumors arising within this region often involve multiple organ systems and require careful consideration/planning before intervention.

INITIAL EVALUATION OF THE RETROPERITONEAL MASS

Because of the insulation that the RP provides, tumors may grow to sizable dimensions without detection or symptoms. In a series of patients undergoing treatment for RP sarcoma, the average dimensions of tumors resected exceeded 15 cm (Fabre-Guillevin et al., 2006). Regardless of whether the mass is identified by incidental detection on routine imaging for other causes or by patient symptoms, understanding the next most appropriate steps in the evaluation is important.

Almost exclusively, computed tomography (CT) of the chest, abdomen, and pelvis represents the optimal initial imaging modality for characterizing masses occurring within the RP (National Comprehensive Cancer Network guidelines, 2018). **CT allows for detail of the lesion through demonstration of size, internal density, presence of calcifications, relation to adjacent organs, infiltration of borders, and presence of regional or distant spread. With intravenous contrast enhancement, identification of cystic changes or necrosis can be depicted.** Additionally, the use of oral contrast can aid in the assessment of duodenal, small bowel, and colonic involvement (Cohan et al., 1988; Katz et al., 2007; Tzeng et al., 2007). In the setting of fat-containing tumors, negative Hounsfield units can identify areas whose features can be pathognomonic in certain conditions such as liposarcomas, angiomyolipomas (AMLs), and myelolipomas. Limitations of CT imaging lies in the inability to discriminate histologic origin or malignant potential based on radiographic appearance alone. Magnetic resonance imaging (MRI) adds value in helping discriminate the degree of vascular involvement when central vessels are distorted, helps define the presence of cystic components or fat within masses, and provides greater resolution of internal characteristics when intravenous contrast administration cannot be provided in the setting of contrast allergy or poor renal function for enhancement during CT imaging. Positron emission tomography/computed tomography (PET/CT) increasingly has been used and plays an important role selectively in a handful of scenarios. Most notable would be assessing viability of postchemotherapy residual masses in the setting of advanced/metastatic seminoma to the RP, risk assessment and estimation of tumor grade/histologic subtypes of RP liposarcomas (Schwarzbach et al., 2001; Brenner et al., 2006), and staging and treatment adaptation in certain subtypes of lymphoma (Tateishi et al., 2010; Hutchings and Barrington, 2009).

Laboratory testing certainly plays an important role, especially in the evaluation of young male patients with a newly discovered RP mass. Serum tumor marker assessment evaluating for elevations in α-fetoprotein (AFP) and human chorionic gonadotropin (hCG) remains a critical tool in the diagnosis, prognostication, and management of germ cell tumors (GCTs). Blood cell counts can identify dyscrasias that may suggest lymphoproliferative disorders, and metabolic panels provide assessment of kidney and liver function.

The role of diagnostic sampling of tumors via fine-needle aspiration (FNA) or core-needle biopsy remains an essential tool in guiding therapy. In the era of personalized medicine, much can be learned from tissue samples as far as histologic subtype and tumor grade. Additionally, when sequencing of various therapies may be altered based on the findings on biopsy, this information becomes essential. An excellent example would be the case of RP lymphoma, in which the initial therapy is systemic chemotherapy in all circumstances and regimen based on lymphoma subtype. In the case of many sarcomas, surgical therapy was the historical mainstay of initial treatment; therefore, surgical biopsy played little role in its initial evaluation. However, as discussed later in this chapter, multimodal therapies are now often employed in the setting of high-grade tumors (von Mehren et al., 2018; Gronchi et al., 2004; Grobmyer et al., 2010). **As such, biopsy may select certain patients for neoadjuvant therapies such as chemotherapy or radiation before surgical resection.** When a biopsy is indicated, how to approach (transperitoneal vs. RP) and type of biopsy (FNA vs. core) are often dictated by clinical presentation and limitations of access. At times, open or laparoscopic biopsies can be incorporated when larger tissue samples are needed to solidify the correct diagnosis, often in advanced or unresectable situations. In general, the incremental benefit of core biopsy (typically using a 14- or 16-gauge coaxial needle) over FNA in ensuring adequate tissue for diagnostic testing and discriminatory abilities by histopathology when cellular architecture is needed has been well documented (Bennert and Abdul-Karim, 1994; Domanski, 2007). Exceptions to the benefits of biopsy include liposarcoma, a tumor in which biopsy is often nondiagnostic and notoriously limited in guiding treatment decisions (Ikoma et al., 2015).

> **KEY POINTS**
> - Many tumors of the RP grow silently over months or years, thus presenting with sizeable dimensions and adjacent organ involvement.
> - Cross-sectional imaging offers the best means of assessing size and extent of disease. Serologic testing plays an important role, specifically in GCTs.
> - FNA and/or core biopsy remain an important tool in the evaluation and management of many diseases, and its diagnostic value should be considered in the initial workup of all RP masses.

DIFFERENTIAL DIAGNOSIS

Tumors occurring in the RP need to be carefully evaluated to allow for categorization into specific groups, for which management can vary widely. These categories include both primary and metastatic tumors of germ cell/gonadal, mesodermal, neurologic, and hematologic origins. We will discuss each entity in terms of relative incidence and demographics, common clinical/radiographic/pathologic/histologic characteristics, genetic predispositions when present, and prognosis. Table 100.1 provides a comprehensive list of relevant immunohistochemical features and genetic associations of the most common entities included in the following sections.

Germ Cell/Gonadal Origins

Tumors of germ cell or gonadal origin can occur in the RP as a primary tumor or as a metastatic deposit. Although uncommon in frequency as compared with other solid tumors, the presence of a RP mass in a young male patient should immediately raise concerns of this entity. Similarly, tumors arising from the stromal elements of the testis can also find the RP as a landing zone in a similarly predictable fashion. Classified as either seminomas or nonseminomas among GCT entities versus Leydig cell, Sertoli cell, or granulosa cell tumors among the greater category of sex cord stromal tumors, each of these cancers has a distinct biologic potential that dictates specific considerations in management.

Germ Cell Tumor

Although discussed in greater detail elsewhere in this book, these remain important considerations because of their propensity to metastasize to the RP, and occasionally arise within the RP as a primary tumor. The incidence of GCTs is increasing in the population, with Hispanics representing the ethnicity with the most rapid rise (Ghazarian et al., 2017). Most commonly they are discovered as an enlarging mass in the scrotum. Within the RP, they can develop as heterogeneous, circumscribed masses along the lymphatic chains of the RP lymph nodes. CT imaging provides the best means of characterizing RP disease, and scrotal ultrasonography can aid in the detection of primary disease within the testis when present. This general category is broken down into divergent pathways of pure seminomas and nonseminomas, which includes embryonal carcinoma, yolk sac tumor, choriocarcinoma, and teratoma. Important to this classification are the clinical differences that motivate variations in management, including the distribution and rate of developing distant disease, serologic assessments, susceptibility to chemotherapy, surgery and radiation, and the risk for long-term relapse.

Seminomatous GCTs arise from the germinal epithelium of the seminiferous tubules. Occurring in the third to fifth decades of life, they represent roughly one-half of all GCT cases at presentation. Serologic testing reveals an elevated hCG in 10% to 15% of cases, corresponding to the presence of syncytiotrophoblasts in the tumor. The presence of an elevated AFP when attributable to the tumor excludes the category of pure seminoma. The tumors themselves are fleshy and tan in appearance on the cut surface. Histologically, they appear as sheets of polygonal cells with abundant clear cytoplasm that are separated into nests by fibrous septae, with a lymphocytic infiltration being present in the majority of cases. A uniform, orderly distribution of prominent nucleoli is typical, contrasting the disorganized appearance in embryonal carcinoma. Additionally, the presence of mitotic figures is numerous. Immunohistochemistry (IHC) typically reveals nuclear staining for OCT4/SALL4/NANOG and cytoplasmic staining for PLAP/CD117/D2-40. Historically, seminoma has been classified into three entities including classic type, spermatocytic, and anaplastic. Although the spermatocytic entity rarely, if ever, metastasizes, the significance of subclassification into classic versus anaplastic variants has little prognostic value. The majority of these tumors remain confined to the testis and are cured with orchiectomy; however, when metastatic they are notably chemotherapy and radiotherapy sensitive. **Pure seminomas remain one of the most curable solid tumors, even in the metastatic setting, with cure rates approaching 98%.**

Nonseminomatous GCTs includes at least one the following histologies: embryonal carcinoma, yolk sac tumor, choriocarcinoma, and teratoma. These tumors usually present in the late teens thru early thirties, although later presentations can occur. Their radiographic characteristics are similar in the testicle and RP as seminomas; however, serologic differences exist. **The production of AFP is specific for yolk sac tumor and embryonal carcinoma elements, whereas hCG can be produced by choriocarcinoma, embryonal carcinoma, and seminoma.** Depending on the components present within the tumor, variable degrees of hemorrhage, necrosis, cystic changes, and calcifications can be present. Histologically, each component within nonseminoma is distinct. Embryonal carcinoma consists of

TABLE 100.1 Immunohistochemical and Genetic Characteristics

	NOTABLE POSITIVES	NOTABLE NEGATIVE	GENETIC MARKERS
Seminoma	Nuclear: OCT4/SALL4/NANOG Cytoplasmic: PLAP/CD117/D2-40	CD30/pan-keratin	i(12p)
Nonseminoma		Inhibin/calretinin	i(12p)
Embryonal	Nuclear: OCT4/SALL4/SOX2 Cytoplasmic: CD30/pan-keratin/CK7	CD117/D2-40	
Yolk sac tumor	AFP/SALL4/glypican-3/pan-keratin	OCT4/CD30/CK7	
Choriocarcinoma	hCG/pan-keratin	OCT4/CD30	
Teratoma			
Sex cord stromal tumor			
Leydig cell tumor	Inhibin/calretinin	SALL4/PLAP	
Sertoli cell tumor	Inhibin/calretinin/β-catenin (nuclear expression)[a]	SALL4/PLAP	A subset harbor *CTNNB1* gene (β-catenin) mutations
Granulosa cell tumor	Inhibin/calretinin	SALL4/PLAP	
Liposarcoma			
Well-differentiated/de-differentiated tumor	MDM2/CDK4/S100		Ring chromosomes or amplification of 12q
Pleomorphic tumor	S100	MDM2/CDK4	
Leiomyosarcoma	SMA/desmin/H-Caldesmon	MDM2/CD117/HMB-45/DOG1	
Undifferentiated pleomorphic sarcoma (i.e., malignant fibrous histiocytoma)	Variable, positive IHC usually not helpful	Negative for markers that would indicate lineage of differentiation	
Synovial sarcoma	TLE1/CD99/EMA/pan-keratin	FLI1	t(X;18)
Solitary fibrous tumor	STAT6/CD34	Desmin/S100/DOG1	*NAB2-STAT6* gene fusion product
Extraskeletal Ewing sarcoma	CD99/FLI1	TLE1/EMA/pan-keratin	Translocations involving *EWSR1* gene, especially *FLI1-EWS* resulting in t(11;22)
Desmoplastic small round cell tumor	EMA/desmin/pan-keratin/WT1 (only the antibody directed against C-terminus of the protein)		t(11;22)(p13;q12) *WT1-EWSR1* gene fusion protein
Perivascular epitheliod cell tumor (PEComa)	Variably positive for melanocytic markers (e.g., HMB-45 and melan A) and muscle markers (e.g., SMA and desmin)		Deletions of *TSC2* gene; subset harbor *TFE3* gene rearrangements
Fibromatosis (desmoid tumor)	β-catenin (nuclear expression)		Associated with Gardner syndrome (*APC* gene); sporadic cases harbor *CTNNB1* (β-catenin) mutations
Ganglioneuroblastoma	CD56/chromogranin A/neurofilament/synaptophysin/neuron-specific enolase		LOH at 11q and 1p; *MYCN* gene amplification
Paraganglioma	Synaptophysin/chromogranin A/GATA3		Neurofibromatosis type 1 (NF-1), *SDHB* gene mutations
Neurofibroma	S100		NF-1 (multifocal and/or plexiform)
Malignant peripheral nerve sheath tumor	S100 (patchy)	H3K27me3 (~50% of malignant peripheral nerve sheath tumor)	NF-1 (if associated with neurofibroma or associated with major nerve); subset harbor *PRC2* gene inactivation
Lymphoma			
Hodgkin (classic Hodgkin lymphoma)	CD30/PAX5	CD45	
Non-Hodgkin lymphoma	Variable depending on type, usually CD45		
Plasma cell neoplasm	CD138/CD38	CD45/CD20	
Cystic lymphangioma	CD31/CD34/D2-40		
Cystic mesothelioma	Calretinin/pan-keratin		
RP cancer of unknown primary origin			

[a]60% to 70% of Sertoli cell tumors demonstrate nuclear expression of β-catenin, which is very specific for Sertoli cell tumor, however lack of nuclear expression does not exclude Sertoli cell tumor as a possibility.

polygonadal cells in clusters with varying degrees of eosinophilic cytoplasm and prominent nucleoli. Typical IHC staining patterns include OCT4, SALL4, and SOX2 in the nucleus (Cao et al., 2009; Gopalan et al., 2009; Jones et al., 2004). Cytoplasmic and cell wall staining is positive for CD30, CK7, and pan-keratin in most, with AFP positivity in up to one-third. Yolk sac tumor, in contrast, can have a variable architectural pattern and is OCT4 and CD30 negative, weakly positive for AFP, but positive for SALL4, glypican-3, and pan-keratin. Choriocarcinomas are associated with extensive hemorrhage and necrosis, and diffusely contain syncytiotrophoblasts and mononuclear trophoblasts. IHC staining is diffusely positive for hCG and pan-cytokeratin, and similarly OCT4 and CD30 negative. Lastly, teratoma is composed of random distributions from multiple germ layers, ranging from squamous/glandular epithelium, to stromal tissues with smooth muscle/bone/cartilage, to mature and immature neural tissues. Occasionally, somatic transformation of teratomatous elements into sarcomas and carcinomas can be seen. Cystic changes are common as well. IHC plays little role in the characterization of teratoma because of its unique architectural features and marbling of elements. Genetically, GCTs demonstrate the characteristic presence of chromosome 12p abnormalities in the majority of cases. Clinically, the components of embryonal carcinoma, yolk sac tumor, and choriocarcinoma are chemosensitive, similar to seminomas. However, because of the common presence of teratomatous elements, which are resistant to chemotherapy and radiotherapy, surgery often plays a more significant role in the setting of advanced disease.

The incidence of truly extragonadal GCTs in the RP remains somewhat controversial. The presence of GCT elements localized primarily to the mediastinum or RP in the absence of a testicular primary tumor occurs in 3% to 5% of all reported cases of GCT. In a multicenter collaboration evaluating 635 patients with extragonadal GCTs, 45% were localized to the RP (Bokemeyer et al., 2002). **However, when extragonadal GCTs of the RP lateralize to the left or right landing zones, over 70% of cases in one series had histologic evidence of either teratoma (20%) or necrosis/fibrosis (80%) within the ipsilateral testicle at time of orchiectomy after chemotherapy** (Brown et al., 2008). Regardless, when the presence of a GCT histology is identified serologically or pathologically to the RP, initial management is treatment with platinum-based chemotherapy. If known to be of nonseminomatous differentiation, resection of residual disease after chemotherapy is recommended in all cases (Albany and Einhorn, 2013).

Sex Cord Stromal Tumor

Sex cord stromal testicular tumors, which include Leydig, Sertoli, and granulosa cell types, compose less than 5% of all testicular neoplasms. Of the sex cord stromal tumors, Leydig cell tumors are the most common and generally occur between 30 and 60 years of age. The presence of Reinke crystals is a classic histologic finding, however, this is only present in roughly 30% of cases. Histologically, these tumors can be confused with tumors seen in congenital adrenal hyperplasia, which can be differentiated by an elevated adrenocorticotropic hormone level. Sertoli cell tumors compose less than 1% of testicular neoplasms. They are most common between 35 and 50 years of age. They can be associated with Peutz-Jeghers syndrome. They can be misinterpreted as seminomas, and therefore careful histologic assessment is important to guide therapy. A positive cytokeratin and inhibin stain with an absent PLAP stain favors Sertoli cell tumor over seminoma. Granulosa cell tumors are one of the rarest types. Two types exist: juvenile and adult. The juvenile type is benign and accounts for up to 7% of prepubertal testicular neoplasms. Most commonly, the juvenile type occurs before 6 months of age (Kao et al., 2015). Microscopically, the juvenile tumors typically show a lobular growth, punctuated by variably sized and shaped follicles. The adult type resembles that of granulosa tumors of the ovary. Twenty-five percent of patients present with infertility and gynecomastia. In general, these tumors are slow growing with limited reports of RP metastases.

Although most of these rare tumors are benign, approximately 10% will metastasize (Grem et al., 1986; Kim et al., 1985; Kratzer et al., 1997). These malignant tumors respond poorly to chemotherapy or radiotherapy. Similar to mixed GCTs, metastatic forms of sex cord stromal tumors will frequently spread to the retroperitoneum, and then to the lung. The ideal timing of surgery has been questioned because of high mortality rates for patients who develop metastasis while on surveillance, despite adequate resection. As a result, several studies have examined predictive pathologic and clinical factors to identify patients who would benefit from immediate retroperitoneal lymph node dissection (RPLND) in the clinical absence of metastatic disease to pathologically stage and hopefully prevent further nodal spread. **Although the presence of metastatic disease is the only reliable indicator of malignant phenotype, various primary tumor characteristics have been evaluated for their ability to predict aggressive behavior. These characteristics include older age, primary tumor size larger than 4 to 5 cm, necrosis, mitotic rate greater than 3 to 5 per 10 high-power fields, moderate-to-severe nuclear atypia, infiltrative tumor margins/invasion of adjacent structures, and lymphovascular invasion.** Although there are some reported cures with positive RP lymph nodes, the presence of radiologic enlarged lymph nodes is a poor prognostic sign (Mosharafa et al., 2003; Silberstein et al., 2014).

Mesodermal Origins

Tumors that arise from mesodermal origins compose the greater category of soft-tissue tumors including sarcoma and benign mesenchymal tumors. Among sarcomas, these most commonly include liposarcomas, leiomyosarcomas, malignant fibrous histiocytomas (MFHs), and, less commonly, angiosarcomas, rhabdomyosarcoma, and myxosarcomas. Tumors of the benign variety include lipomas, leiomyomas, fibromas, hemangiopericytomas, PEComas, chordomas, myelolipomas, xanthogranulomas, myxomas, and gastrointestinal stromal tumors. The following sections will discuss those entities that are more commonly associated with the RP, for which clinical decisions will be more relevant and impactful.

Soft tissue sarcomas represent approximately 1% of all solid cancers in adults, with tumors arising from the retroperitoneum in roughly 15% to 20% of those cases (Olimpiadi et al., 2015; Pisters, 2007; van Houdt et al., 2017). With as many as 50 different subtypes of sarcoma having been described, very few are likely to be discovered in the RP. With considerable overlap and varied histologic appearance, clinicopathologic characteristics and molecular diagnostics are often necessary to identify the true nature of these tumors. This requires more than ever the integration of IHC, molecular and cytogenetic characterization, as well as clinical details for the clinician and pathologist to render an accurate diagnosis.

Liposarcoma

Liposarcoma represents a malignant, locally aggressive tumor composed of adipocytes with nuclear atypia and hyperchromasia. These tumors can be classified as well-differentiated or de-differentiated, based on the presence or absence of higher-grade, nonlipogenic components within the tumor. Combined, these entities represent roughly 60% of all retroperitoneal sarcomas (Gronchi et al., 2016; Tan et al., 2016). Both typically present as painless masses, often found incidentally during a workup for other conditions or screening examinations. Growth rates of the de-differentiated tumors tend to be rapid, often drawing attention to a clinically more aggressive phenotype of liposarcoma. Radiographically, liposarcomas on CT have a low signal intensity but demonstrate mass-effect of the surrounding structures (Fig. 100.1). Areas of greater signal intensity internally within the tumor often reflect de-differentiated components (Fig. 100.2).

Histologically, well differentiated liposarcomas can be characterized into three distinct groups: adipocytic (lipoma-like), sclerosing, and inflammatory. Adipocytic tumors resemble lipomas morphologically, with hyperchromatic and atypical nuclei scantly distributed among fat lobules, often rendering core biopsies inconclusive. Sclerosing-type liposarcomas contain a hyalinized stroma intermixed with variable amounts of atypical adipocytes scattered throughout. Lastly, inflammatory-type liposarcomas have an inflammatory infiltrate interspersed among adipocytic changes. Depending on the degree

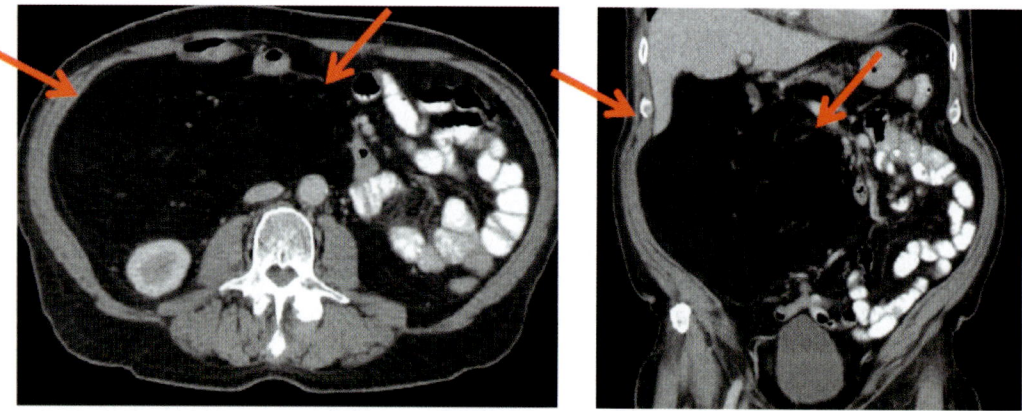

Fig. 100.1. Well-differentiated liposarcoma *(arrows)*.

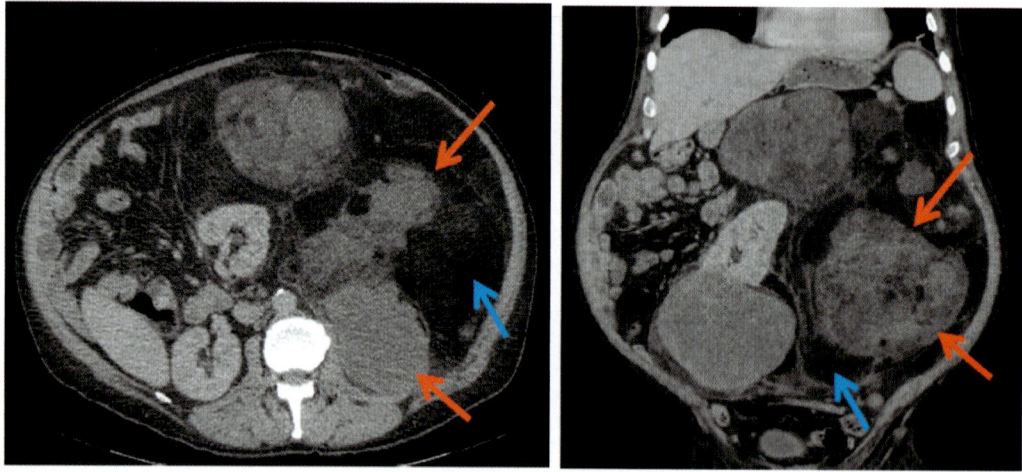

Fig. 100.2. Mixed tumor of well-differentiated *(blue arrows)* and de-differentiated liposarcoma *(red arrows)*.

of lymphoid aggregates within the tumor, these can sometimes be difficult to distinguish from a primary lymphoproliferative malignancy. **As with most cases of liposarcomas, a combination of histologic features along with clinical and anatomic presentation are often required to render the appropriate diagnosis.**

De-differentiated liposarcomas often arise from well differentiated components, therefore histologic appearance reveals atypical adipocytes surrounding regions of fleshy, nonlipogenic areas. Within these de-differentiated regions of the tumor, cells can have a mixture of patterns that appear similar to undifferentiated spindle cell sarcomas, myxoid tumors, and areas containing meningothelial and pleomorphic-like features. Not uncommonly, components of osteosarcoma, rhabdomyosarcoma, leiomyosarcoma, and small round cell morphologies can be seen within the tumor.

Cytologically, both well-differentiated and de-differentiated tumors demonstrate overexpression and/or amplification of genes localized to chromosome 12q (Sandberg, 2004), including MDM2, S100, and CDK4. Accordingly, monoclonal antibodies against these genes can be utilized through fluorescence in-situ hybridization or IHC to solidify the diagnosis of liposarcoma when suspected in otherwise limited tissue samples or in the presence of abundant stroma or inflammatory cells that obscure the diagnosis.

Prognostically, these tumors have a predilection for relapse. In well-differentiated tumors, up to 40% of tumors will recur locally (Fletcher et al., 1996; Gronchi et al., 2015b; Lucas et al., 1994; Singer et al., 2003; Tan et al., 2016; Tseng et al., 2014). Similar numbers have been reported for local relapse in de-differentiated tumors as well. However, unlike well-differentiated tumors, de-differentiated liposarcomas are associated with a higher rate of distant metastasis (up to 20% of cases) and a 5-year cancer-specific mortality of 30% (Fletcher et al., 1996; Henricks et al., 1997; Lahat et al., 2008;

Linehan et al., 2000; Tan et al., 2016; Tseng et al., 2014). The risk for local recurrence depends partly on tumor biology and surgical factors. Differing opinions with regard to the impact of surgical margin status (R0 vs. R1 resections) exist (Keung et al., 2014; Lahat et al., 2008; Neuhaus et al., 2005; Singer et al., 2003); however, most would agree that negative margins optimize outcomes for patients. Current strategies involving radical compartment resections for liposarcomas have been reported to improve local recurrence rates (Bonvalot et al., 2009; Gronchi et al., 2009, 2012, 2016; Raut et al., 2010). Average time reported for recurrent disease is roughly 2 years; therefore, long-term observation is needed (MacNeill et al., 2017). In the setting of unresectable or metastatic disease, use of anthracycline-based regimens has been associated with modest improvements in short-term survival (Jones et al., 2005). More recently, the safety and efficacy of immune checkpoint inhibitors (Pembrolizumab) was assessed in a phase II study, with objective responses seen in 2 of 10 patients (Tawbi et al., 2017).

Pleomorphic Liposarcoma

These tumors represent a very rare type of liposarcoma. They occur predominantly in adult patients, occurring more commonly in the extremities, but can be seen in the RP and along the spermatic cord (Hornick et al., 2004). They typically are fast-growing tumors, and histologically demonstrate pleomorphic lipoblasts that do *not* overexpress MDM2 or CDK4. Tissue samples often have frequent mitotic figures seen per high-power microscopic field, and can vary with the degree of spindle and epithelioid cells intermixed. These tumors can often resemble poorly differentiated carcinomas or renal cell carcinomas on needle biopsy. Ultimately, the identification of poorly differentiated lipoblasts on histologic sectioning is imperative

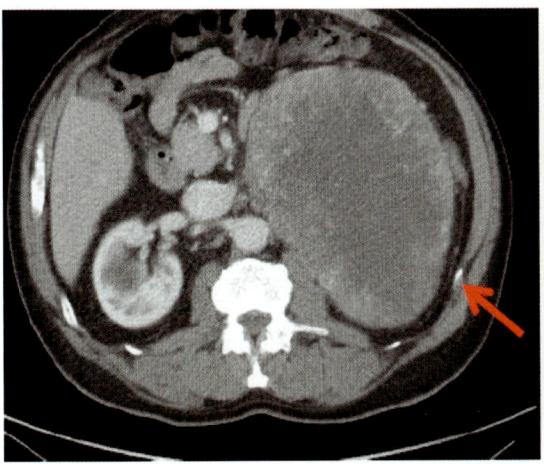 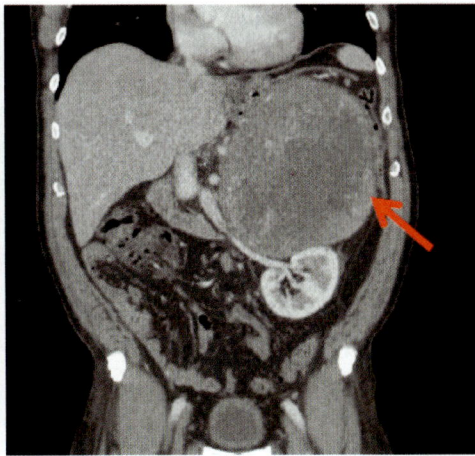

Fig. 100.3. Leiomyosarcoma *(arrows)*.

for diagnosing these tumors. These tumors progress rapidly to widespread metastatic disease, with dissemination to the lungs being most common.

Leiomyosarcoma

Malignant tumors arising from smooth muscle cells are characterized as leiomyosarcomas. These tumors represent the second most common sarcoma type within the RP, occurring in about 20% of RP sarcoma cases (Gronchi et al., 2016; Tan et al., 2016). Arising from the media of RP blood vessels, muscularis of collecting system within the urinary tract, or other smooth muscle–containing structures of the RP, these tumors can grow silently until mass-effect or obstruction presents itself, often leading to problems of venous return, urinary drainage and function, or impingement of the gastrointestinal system. In females, many RP leiomyosarcomas are of gynecologic origin. Similar to liposarcomas, many can be detected as incidental findings. **In rare circumstances, these tumors can develop in the setting of Epstein-Barr viral infections in immunosuppressed patients** (Deyrup et al., 2004; McClain et al., 1995).

Clinically, these tumors grow as homogeneous tumors that encase structures with fleshy bundles of tissue (Fig. 100.3). On occasion, necrosis or cystic areas can be seen. Cytologically, these tumors reveal fascicles of atypical smooth muscle bundles with varying amounts of nuclear atypia depending on the grade of the tumor. Although de-differentiation to other sarcoma types can be seen, this is a less common phenomenon. When a smooth muscle–containing tumor is identified, criteria have been proposed to distinguish malignant from benign entities. These parameters include location of the primary tumor (RP vs. somatic soft tissues), mitotic rate, nuclear and cellular atypia, and presence/absence of necrosis. With increasing degrees of atypia, necrosis, and mitoses, these tumors can be classified from leiomyomas, to smooth muscle tumors of low malignant potential (STUMP), to leiomyosarcomas. (Marušić and Billings, 2017). IHC plays a similarly important role in the characterization and differentiation from other soft-tissue tumors. Markers such as smooth muscle actin (SMA), desmin, and H-Caldesmon can suggest this diagnosis when staining positive, and MDM2, CD117, HMB-45, and DOG1 are typically negative.

Similar to de-differentiated liposarcomas, local and regional recurrences are common, with distant spread occurring frequently. Diagnosing these tumors on needle biopsy oftentimes underestimates the aggressiveness of disease, and an aggressive multimodal approach is often needed.

Malignant Fibrous Histiocytoma/Undifferentiated Pleomorphic Sarcoma

Tumors arising from fibroblastic and histiocyte-like cells compose the entity of malignant fibrous histiocytoma/undifferentiated pleomorphic sarcoma (MFH/UPS). Commonly occurring in the fifth and sixth decades of life, these tumors account for roughly one-fourth of soft-tissue sarcomas (Giménez Bachs et al., 2004; Ros et al., 1984; Schaefer and Fletcher, 2014). Often clinically silent, these tumors can reach large dimensions before being detected. Radiographic characteristics reveal heterogeneous soft-tissue masses caused by central necrosis, hemorrhage, and myxoid degeneration, typical of RP sarcomas (Fig. 100.4). The absence of fat within the tumor separates these tumors radiographically from liposarcomas, and rarely is there invasion of vascular structures. Peripheral nodular enhancement of a lobulated mass is common, with calcifications occurring in 10% of cases (Neville and Herts, 2004; Ros et al., 1984). Metastatic disease when present is typically to the lungs, liver, and bone. Tissue sampling is required to differentiate from other conditions, revealing spindle-shaped fibroblasts along with round histiocyte-like cells, lymphocytes, foamy cells, and giant cells. Histologic features also include a pseudoangiomatoid pattern, plasma and lymphocytic infiltrations, and a fibrous pseudocapsule (Grossman et al., 1996). Tumors most commonly stain positive for desmin, epithelial membrane antigen, CD68, and CD99 (García and Folpe, 2010). Gene translocations have been characterized in MFH/UPS tumors, resulting in the following gene fusion products: FUS/ATF1, EWSR1/ATF1, and EWSR1/CREB1 (Antonescu et al., 2007; Rossi et al., 2007; Waters et al., 2000). Among MFH/UPS, variations can exist and have been classified into distinct types: storiform-pleomorphic, myxoid, giant cell, angiomatoid, and inflammatory. The storiform-pleomorphic and myxoid tumors tend to represent high-grade sarcomas, whereas the others are often characterized as low-grade lesions. Treatment remains surgical in the absence of metastatic disease, with wide resection to achieve negative margins being associated with a risk reduction for local/distant relapse and improved survival (Yamaguchi et al., 2004). Limited data exist defining the benefits for adjuvant chemotherapy or radiotherapy in this disease. Overall 5-year survival in one series for MFH was 51% (Fabre-Guillevin et al., 2006).

Synovial Sarcoma

Although common in other locations, retroperitoneal synovial sarcomas are uncommon and occur across all age demographics (Chatzipantelis and Kafiri, 2008; Sultan et al., 2009). These mesenchymal tumors can arise from a variety of sources such as kidneys, adrenal glands, or other viscera (Fig. 100.5). Confusion can occur when arising from nerve structures, leading clinicians to suspect malignant peripheral nerve sheath tumors (Chrisinger et al., 2017). **They can grow to large sizes without symptoms within the RP, developing intratumoral calcifications that can hint at the diagnosis. Although rare, a history of prior radiation can be associated with development of these tumors** (van de Rijn et al., 1997).

The majority are encapsulated tumors, with cystic degeneration being present in many. Microscopically, they appear in a herringbone pattern with spindle cells. Mitotic activity is variable and correlates with tumor grade. They can demonstrate areas of differentiation

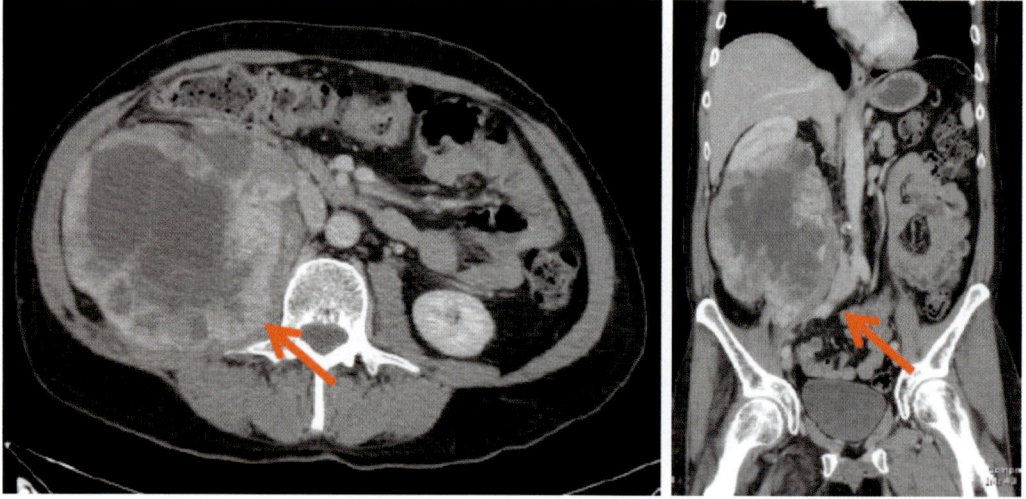

Fig. 100.4. Malignant fibrous histiocytoma *(arrows).*

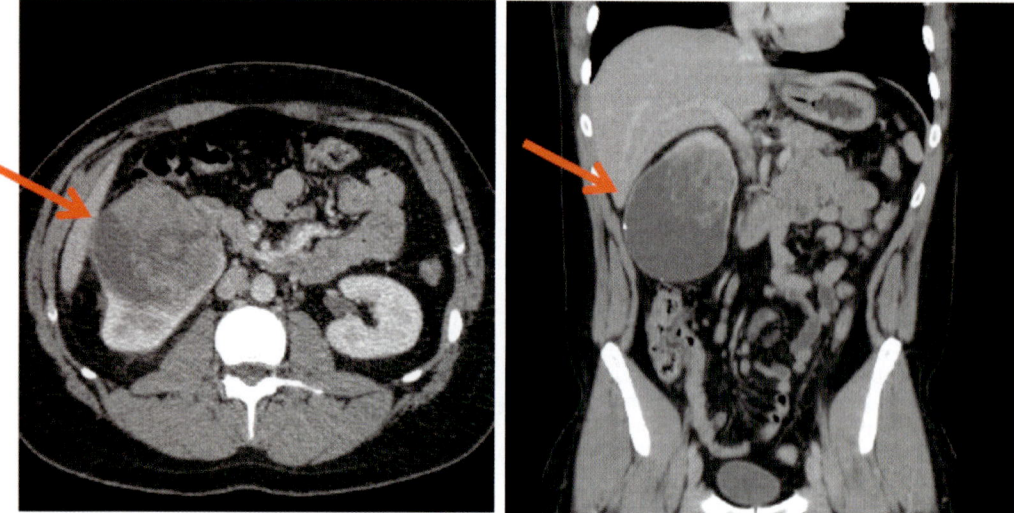

Fig. 100.5. Synovial sarcoma of the kidney *(arrows).*

into glandular, cystic, and undifferentiated round cell morphologies, rendering them often confused with other tumors. IHC testing for TLE1 is positive in 90% of cases, but is not exclusive (Terry et al., 2007). Molecular changes typical for synovial sarcomas include their translocations of X;18, which is present in the majority of cases. (Turc-Carel et al., 1986).

Outcomes are dependent on grade of tumor. Favorable characteristics include younger age at presentation and presence of diffuse calcifications (Soule, 1986).

Solitary Fibrous Tumor

Previously referred to as *hemangiopericytomas,* these fibroblastic tumors can occur throughout the body. Occurring predominantly in younger patients, they can grow to very large sizes before clinical symptoms develop (Fig. 100.6). **In rare occasions, a paraneoplastic phenomenon associated with hypoglycemia has been described, resulting from oversecretion of insulin-like growth factor (Doege-Potter Syndrome)** (Han et al., 2017).

Solitary fibrous tumors can be characterized by a "patternless" architecture, with myxoid degeneration and fatty differentiation occurring in some tumors (Demicco et al., 2012). Tumors with high mitotic indices and greater pleomorphism represent biologically more aggressive tumor behavior, with one-third of cases demonstrating these malignant features. (England et al., 1989; Demicco et al., 2017; Morimitsu et al., 2000). Unique to these tumors is near-uniform positivity for the *NAB2-STAT6* gene fusion product (Robinson et al., 2013).

Prognosis is variable, as the majority of these follow an indolent course. Unfortunately, clinico-pathologic features reflect tumor biology poorly, with a subset of cases demonstrating relatively benign features developing regional and distant metastases. Criteria have been established to further risk-stratify patients including advancing age, high mitotic rate, necrosis, and tumor size as signatures for more aggressive tumors (Demicco et al., 2017). Overtly malignant cases are associated with a poor prognosis. Overall survival rates for all cases of solitary fibrous tumor at 8 years have been reported in the 75% range for most series. (Ardoino et al., 2010; Gronchi et al., 2013, 2015a, 2016; Pasquali et al., 2016; Raut et al., 2016; Wang et al., 2014). Complete en bloc resection is standard management, noting that preservation of adjacent organs is recommended when feasible, as wide margins are not routinely needed (Pasquali et al., 2016; Trans-Atlantic RPS Working Group, 2015). **Perioperative radiotherapy can be used as an adjunct to treatment, as these tumors are radiosensitive** (Kawamura et al., 2007; Liu et al., 2014; Saynak et al., 2010).

Ewing and Ewing-Like Sarcoma

Primarily tumors of bone origin, these malignant small, round, blue tumors can rarely occur in soft tissues of the RP (Fig. 100.7). **Ewing**

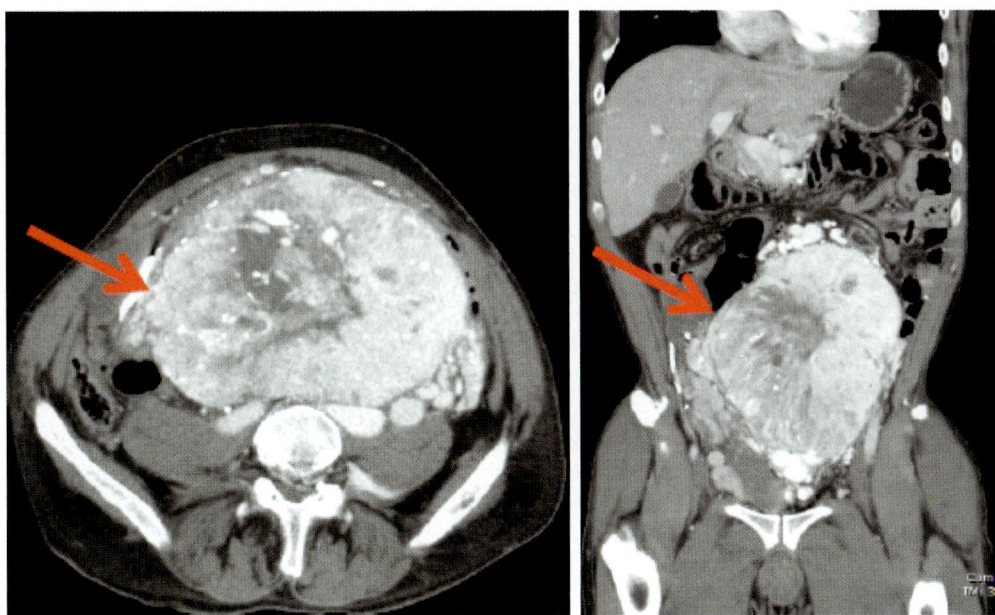

Fig. 100.6. Solitary fibrous tumor *(arrows)*.

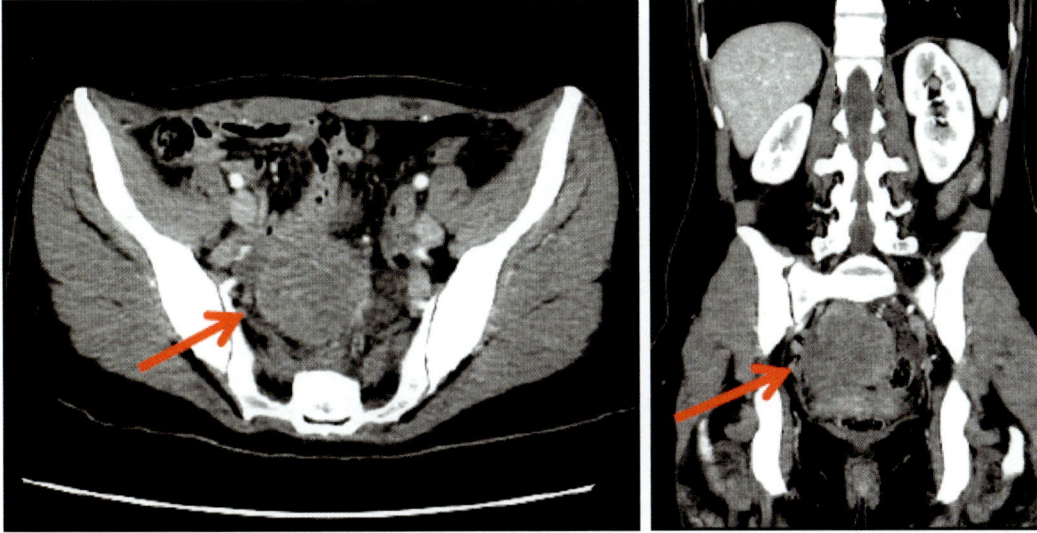

Fig. 100.7. Ewing sarcoma *(arrows)*.

sarcomas are associated with *EWSR1* translocations with the ETS transcription factor family. Typically a disease of young adult Caucasian males, neuropathic pain can be a presenting symptom when tumors develop adjacent to peripheral nerves. Unlike other sarcomas, these tumors tend to be infiltrative in their margins, rendering primary surgery alone unlikely to cure patients. Current standards recommend chemotherapy in combination for management, with cure rates exceeding 50% with multimodal therapies. Presence of larger tumor size, presence of metastatic disease, and relative absence of tumor necrosis after chemotherapy are poor prognostic features. Among Ewing-like sarcomas, the presence of the *CIC*-gene rearrangement is also considered to be associated with a poor outcome (Antonescu et al., 2017).

Desmoplastic Small Round Cell Tumors

Another translocation-associated sarcoma, these morphologically small round cell tumors are characterized by the t(11;22)(p13;q12) *WT1-EWSR1* gene fusion protein. Occurring mostly in young males, these tumors present with multifocal peritoneal implantations of tumor. Abdominal pain and distention is the most common complaint. Imaging often reveals heterogeneous enhancement of the mass with central necrosis being common (Pickhardt et al., 1999). The presence of abdominal ascites is typical, given the predilection for liver involvement. Histologic staining of the EWSR1-WT1 fusion product is diagnostic for these tumors. Prognosis is universally poor, despite multimodal therapy to address widespread disease.

Unclassified Sarcomas

These tumors with no distinct characteristics that would define a particular line of differentiation serve as a diagnosis of exclusion and occur in up to 20% of cases. This category of tumor is associated with a history of prior radiation therapy in one-fourth of patients (Gladdy et al., 2010). Typically associated with a rapid growth rate and aggressive clinical course, prognosis is universally poor. Important for these patients is to rule out the presence of de-differentiated liposarcoma through *MDM2* screening to avoid misclassification.

Perivascular Epitheliod Cell Tumor

Perivascular epitheliod cell tumor (PEComa) represents a broad range of neoplasms with perivascular epithelioid cell differentiation. This category of tumors includes renal and extrarenal angiomyolipoma (AML), extrapulmonary clear-cell sugar tumor, clear cell myomelanocytic tumor, pigmented melanotic tumor, lymphangioleiomyomatosis (LAM), and malignant PEComa (Fletcher, 2014). Accordingly, clinical presentation and behavior is quite diverse. Features associated with a malignant phenotype include large tumor size (>5 cm), high cellularity and atypia, mitotic index greater than 1/hpf, tumor necrosis, and vascular invasion. (Folpe et al., 2005). **Most PEComas are sporadic in nature, with inherited conditions such as tuberous sclerosis being responsible for the remainder.** In a distinct subset of cases, *TFE3* gene rearrangements can be identified, typically occurring in younger patients (Argani et al., 2010; Malinowska et al., 2012; Tanaka et al., 2009). Surgical management with wide local excision is indicated in tumors demonstrating adverse features, as PEComas are largely chemoresistant tumors. In unresectable or metastatic cases, use of mTOR inhibitors such as temsirolimus, everolimus, rapamycin, or sirolimus has been shown to demonstrate responses and prolonged survival (Bissler et al., 2008; Curatolo and Moavero, 2012; Dickson et al., 2013; Kenerson et al., 2007; Wagner et al., 2010).

Desmoid Tumor

These fibroblastic tumors are locally advanced tumors that demonstrate rapid growth and disruption of fascial planes, resulting in adjacent organ involvement leading to ureteral or bowel obstruction (Fig. 100.8). With a peak incidence in the third decade of life, these tumors are radiographically heterogeneous and difficult to differentiate from sarcomas. Histologically, they are composed of spindle-shaped cells, extracellular collagen, and myxoid matrix (Dinauer et al., 2007; Rajiah et al., 2011). Although not known for distant spread or metastasis, they recur locally in up to one-half of patients despite wide resection (Dinauer et al., 2007).

Neurogenic Origins

Tumors arising from neurogenic origins such as ganglion cells, paraganglionic tissues, and peripheral nerve sheaths compose roughly 10% of RP primary tumors. Distribution of tumors occur along sympathetic ganglia posterior to the great vessels, within the adrenal glands, or in the location of the organ of Zuckerkandl. Prognosis for these tumors tends to be much improved compared with sarcomas, with many representing benign tumors.

Tumors of Sympathetic Ganglia

Tumors arising from the sympathetic neural tissue fall within this class of retroperitoneal pathology. These include ganglioneuromas, neuroblastomas, and ganglioneuroblastomas. These tumors can arise from the adrenal medulla or along the course of the sympathetic chain of ganglia. Although most have a relatively benign course, some behave aggressively with regional and distant dissemination.

Ganglioneuromas are benign tumors arising from the nerve cells of the sympathetic ganglia. Commonly seen in the third or fourth decades, they occur equally among men and women. **When originating from the adrenal medulla, secretion of catecholamines, vasoactive intestinal peptide, or androgenic proteins can be seen** (Otal et al., 2001; Rha et al., 2003). Usually discovered incidentally, they are well circumscribed tumors radiographically, with calcifications being present in up to 30% of tumors (Rajiah et al., 2011). Prognosis is excellent with local removal.

Neuroblastomas are malignant tumors arising from primitive neuroblasts found within the adrenal medulla and sympathetic chain. These tumors occur largely within the first decade of life, with two-thirds originating from the adrenal medulla. These are heterogeneous tumors radiographically with course calcifications seen in the majority of cases. Most have evidence of metastatic disease at the time of presentation, and local invasion with encasement of adjacent organs, making local therapy challenging.

Ganglioneuroblastomas have features of both ganglioneuromas and neuroblastomas (Fig. 100.9). Also seen primarily in the pediatric population, they occur most commonly in the 2- to 4-year-old age group. However, cases in the adult population do occur between the late second to early fourth decades of life (Jrebi et al., 2014). Presenting with abdominal or back pain, these tumors often metastasize to regional lymph nodes, bone, brain, liver, and skin (Smith et al., 2013). **Staging imaging studies most useful include MRI and metaiodobenzylguanidine (MIBG) scanning to assess for bony involvement and local extent of the tumor.** Diagnosis is made on histologic assessment, which typically reveals IHC staining that is positive for CD-56, chromogranin A, neurofilament, synaptophysin, neuron-specific enolase, and LOH at 11q and 1p (Jrebi et al., 2014; Park et al., 2010). **Additionally, *n-Myc* gene amplification, when present, represents a negative prognostic feature.** Although treatment of these tumors is surgical resection when localized with or without

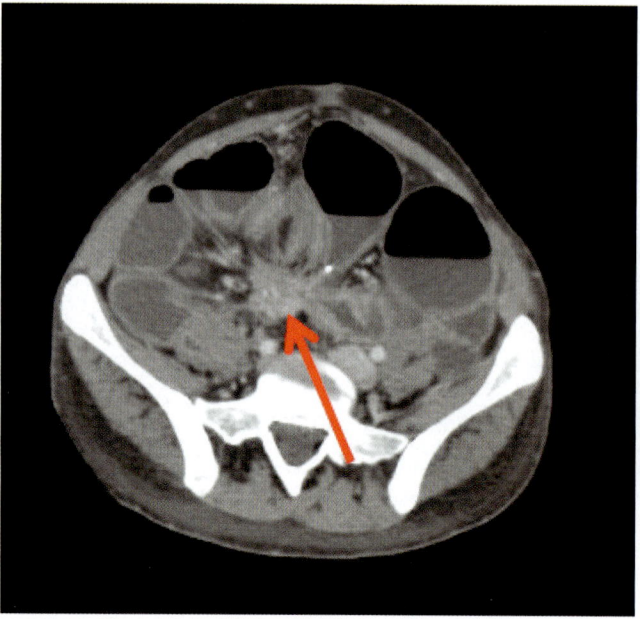
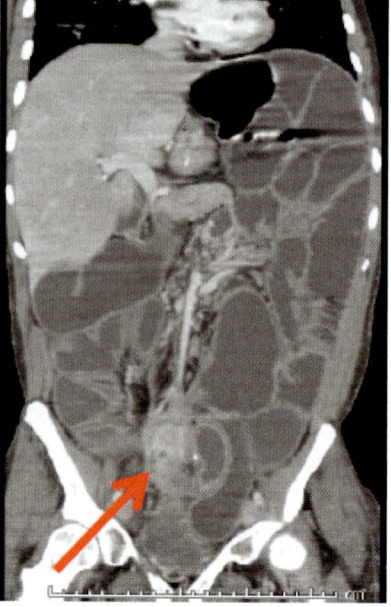

Fig. 100.8. Desmoid tumor with secondary bowel obstruction *(arrows)*.

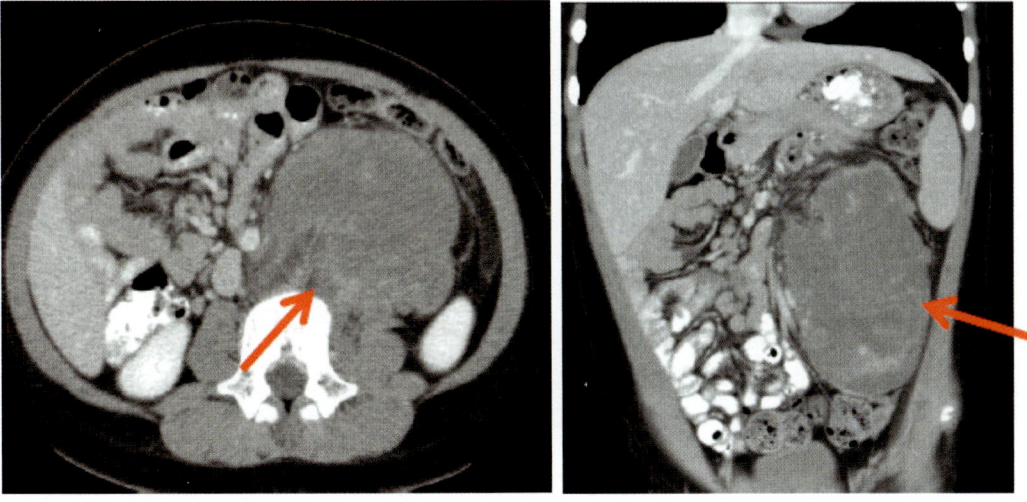

Fig. 100.9. Ganglioneuroblastoma *(arrows)*.

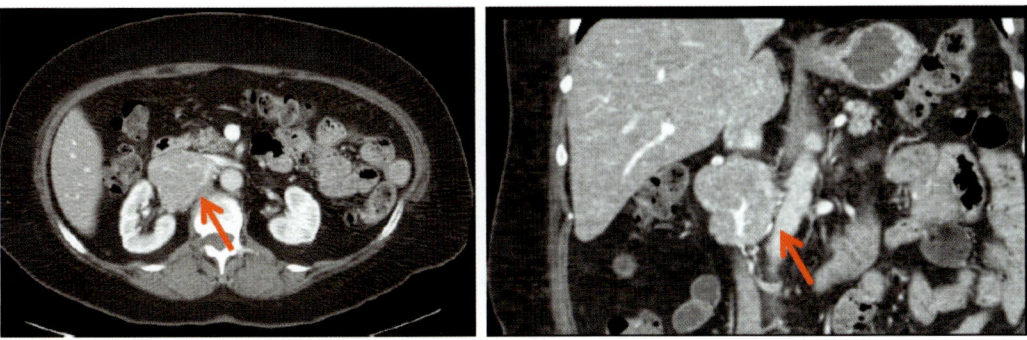

Fig. 100.10. Paraganglioma *(arrows)*.

adjuvant chemotherapy, they tend to disseminate widely. In one series, over one-half of patients at presentation had distant metastatic disease at the time of presentation (Jrebi et al., 2014). Therefore, neoadjuvant chemotherapy is recommended utilizing pediatric regimens that often include a combination of several drugs, such as cyclophosphamide, cisplatin, ifosfamide, vincristine, doxorubicin, etoposide, cis-retinoic acid, and carboplatin. Overall, prognosis is quite poor for these rare adult tumors.

Tumors of Paraganglionic System

Also derived from neural tissues found in the adrenal medulla and RP ganglia, these tumors arise from specialized neural crest cells (Neville and Herts, 2004). **When occurring from the neural crest cells found within the adrenal gland, they are referred to as pheochromocytomas. Extra-adrenal locations are classified as paragangliomas** (Rajiah et al., 2011).

Extra-adrenal paragangliomas occur most commonly in the third to fourth decades of life and are gender-neutral. Although they can occur anywhere within the RP, the most common location is within the organ of Zuckerkandl, which is located anteriorly along the aorta below the takeoff of the inferior mesenteric artery near the aortic bifurcation (Fig. 100.10). Radiographically, they demonstrate similar characteristics as pheochromocytomas, including the characteristic high–signal intensity appearance on T2-weighed MRI images (Rha et al., 2003). Also similar to pheochromocytomas, production of catecholamines is common, with elevations occurring in roughly 40% of cases (Neville and Herts, 2004; Tohme et al., 2006). Immunohistologic characteristics include a yellow-gray appearing tumor grossly, with large polygonal and pleomorphic cells that stain positive for synaptophysin and chromogranin A (Sun et al., 1998). Features of necrosis, high mitotic index, atypical nucleoli, infiltrative borders, and vascular invasion again poorly predict malignant potential, with metastases occurring in 20% to 50% of cases (Neville and Herts, 2004). Management is surgical in nature, as tumors respond poorly to other therapies. **Genetic predispositions for these tumors can be seen in patients with neurofibromatosis type 1 (NF-1; Kimura et al., 2002) and multiple endocrine neoplasia type 2a** (Gullu et al., 2005).

Tumors of Nerve Sheath Origin

Schwannomas, neurofibromas, and malignant peripheral nerve sheath tumors represent this class of tumor. Schwannomas are benign tumors arising from the Schwann cells responsible for myelinating peripheral nerves. Slow growing in nature, they typically occur in the paravertebral location, and patients present with symptoms related to nerve compression. They appear homogeneous and circumscribed on cross-sectional imaging when small, but can develop cystic degeneration and calcifications as they grow. As they arise from neural crest cells, they stain positive for S-100 on IHC. They are encapsulated tumors, and complete local resection is usually curative.

Neurofibromas are similarly benign tumors of the nerve sheath. However, they originate from nonmyelinating Schwann cells. **Commonly associated with NF-1, an autosomal dominant genetically inherited condition, sporadic tumors can also occur in the RP.** With a male predilection, these tumors occur mostly in the third to fifth decade of life (Neville and Herts, 2004). Radiographically, they are well-circumscribed with homogeneous appearance on CT. Treatment is surgical, as malignant transformation can occur in up to 20% of cases, most commonly occurring in patients with NF-1 and those exposed to radiation (Neville and Herts, 2004; Isler et al., 1996).

Malignant peripheral nerve sheath tumors are rare among soft-tissue sarcomas, representing less than 10% of cases in the RP (Deger et al., 2015; Gronchi et al., 2016; Le Guellec et al., 2016; Tan et al., 2016). Arising from cellular components of peripheral nerves along

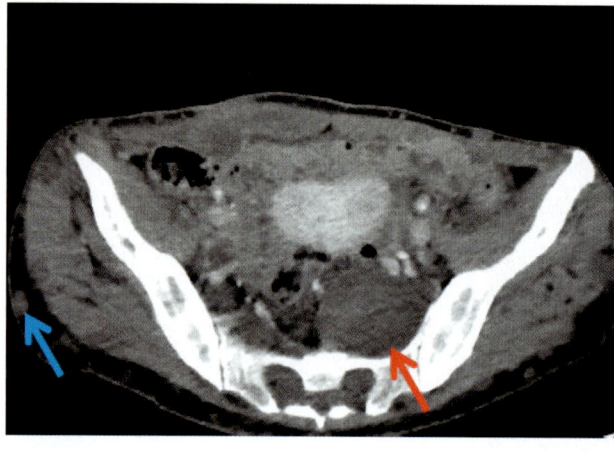
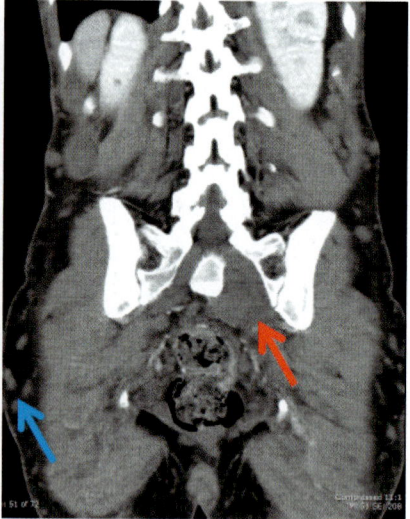

Fig. 100.11. Malignant peripheral nerve sheath tumor (red arrows) in patient with neurofibromas (indicated by blue arrows).

the sacral or lumbar nerve plexus, roughly one-half are associated with genetic predisposing conditions (most commonly NF-1), with the remainder representing sporadic tumor development (Le Guellec et al., 2016). Among sporadic cases, a history of prior radiation has been reported and is likely causative (Gladdy et al., 2010). Clinical presentations often relate to symptoms related to nerve irritation, pain, paresthesias, or paralysis (Fig. 100.11). Among patients with NF-1, discovery of these tumors often occurs in adolescence. Radiographically indistinguishable from schwannomas or neurofibromas, biopsy remains the gold standard for diagnosis.

Malignant peripheral nerve sheath tumors are similarly fleshy tumors, often associated with hemorrhage or necrosis. Microscopically, they demonstrate spindle-shaped cells with herringbone orientation. Not uncommonly, heterogeneous areas of tumor may have a benign component of neurofibromas adjacent to areas of malignant peripheral nerve sheath tumors, rendering diagnosis challenging in limited samples. Immunohistochemical staining can help with diagnosis, with roughly one-half of cases staining positive for S100, along with loss of H3K27me3 expression. A clinical history of prior radiation, NF1, or clinical/radiographic evidence of peripheral nerve origin help key in on this clinical entity.

Management remains surgical for all cases. Preoperative chemotherapy and radiation remain ineffective at eradicating disease, but both have shown to improve complete surgical resection rates (Anghileri et al., 2006). Although infiltration into adjacent structures is uncommon, extension along nerve roots can occur. Prognosis is closely associated with achieving negative margins. As these tumors arise from peripheral nerves, complete resection of those nerves is required, and loss of neurologic function is inevitable. Among malignant peripheral nerve sheath tumor patients with negative margins, 5-year survival rates approach 70%, compared with roughly 20% for those with positive margins at time of resection (Wong et al., 1998). In unresectable tumors, anthracycline-based chemotherapy and palliative radiation should be considered (Kroep et al., 2011).

Hematologic Conditions/Lymphomas of the Retroperitoneum

Hematologic conditions represent a significant number of the masses that develop within the RP. Lymphomas being the most common, other conditions such as extramedullary myeloma/plasmacytomas and other lymphoproliferative diseases can occur as well.

Lymphomas

Constituting almost one-third of primary RP tumors, lymphomas represent hematologic cancers of lymphoid tissues occurring throughout the body. They can be categorized into Hodgkin and non-Hodgkin varieties, with prognostic differences separating the two. Radiographically, lymphomas are circumscribed, confluent, commonly homogeneous masses located typically along the RP and pelvic lymph node chains (Fig. 100.12). The issue of greatest importance to the urologist is their relative similarity to other RP tumors. Hence the importance of tissue sampling with FNA and/or core needle biopsy, as these tumors rarely, if ever, warrant surgical intervention and are best managed with chemotherapy.

Plasmacytoma

The spectrum of plasma cell infiltration on one end and multiple osseous and extramedullary lesions on the other reflects the range of clinical presentations that are characterized as plasmacytoma when focal and multiple myeloma when diffuse. Although multiple myeloma represents the most common primary osseous malignancy in adults, extramedullary manifestations of the disease occur in <10% of newly diagnosed patients (Hanrahan et al., 2010; Touzeau and Moreau, 2016). Locations of disease outside of bone include the abdomen/pelvis, skin and soft tissues, and paraspinous regions (Ames et al., 2017; Usmani et al., 2012). In a comprehensive review of the literature by Ames et al., the RP was the location for extraosseous lesions in 23 of 2538 cases reported at the time of the 2017 article (Ames et al., 2017). Serologic testing during the initial evaluation is typically positive for elevated IgG levels, and serum electrophoresis can reveal the finding of an "M spike," suggestive of elevated levels of the myeloma protein, which can lead to impaired immune function, clotting, and kidney damage. Percutaneous biopsy with FNA or core-needle biopsy is often needed to diagnose. When suspected, a bone marrow aspiration and skeletal survey are recommended. Conventional radiographs for detection of bone disease have been supplanted by whole-body CT, with PET/CT imaging serving as the main imaging modality to assess response to therapy (Cavo et al., 2017; Rajkumar et al., 2014; Regelink et al., 2013). These tumors on histopathologic assessment reveal a monoclonal plasma cell infiltration of polygonal cells with homogeneous amphophilic cytoplasm and asymmetric nuclei. IHC typically reveals positivity for CD138 and Bcl-2. In the setting of isolated RP disease, case reports of complete response to wide surgical excision (Hong et al., 2009; Sharma et al., 2004), radiation, and chemotherapy have been reported (Chao et al., 2005; Chen et al., 1998; Saito et al., 2003).

Cystic Masses

Cystic masses occurring alone in the RP are rare. However, several entities that present as asymptomatic, predominantly cystic lesions can occur. Among these include cystic lymphangioma, cystic teratoma,

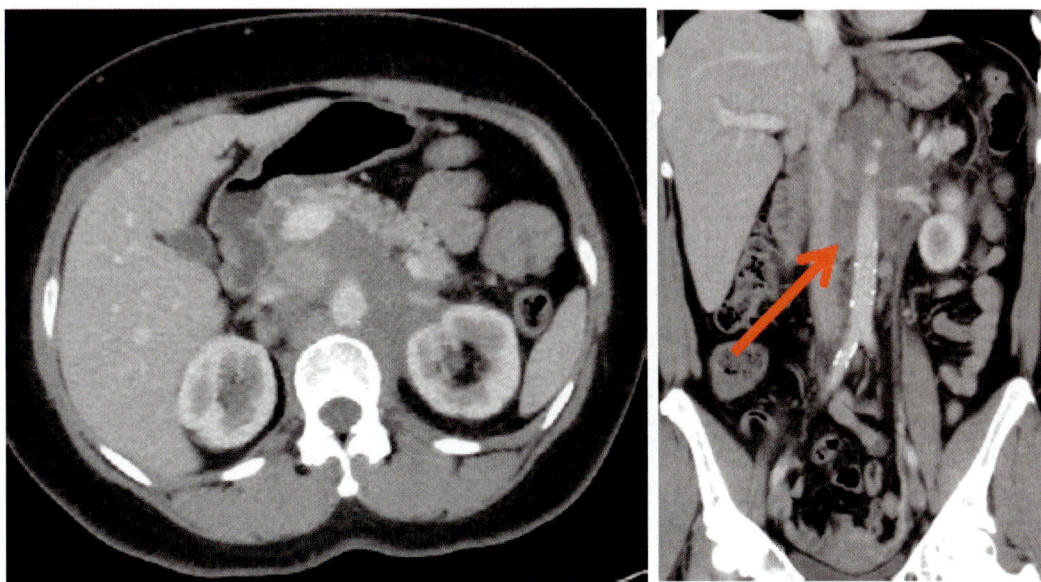

Fig. 100.12. Lymphoma *(arrows)*.

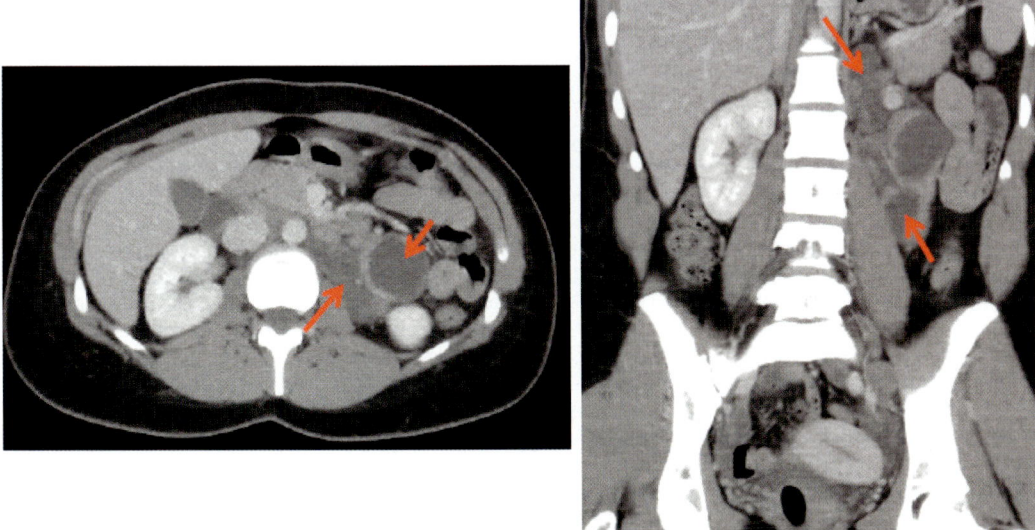

Fig. 100.13. Cystic lymphangioma *(arrows)*.

cystadenoma, cystadenocarcinoma, cystic mesothelioma, and cystic changes of solid neoplasms. Given the fact that treatment strategies vary greatly depending on the nature of the lesion, clinical diagnostics based on presentation, radiographic findings, and serologic testing are imperative. This is particularly relevant given the general cautionary recommendations against percutaneous biopsy or aspiration of lesions because of the risk for rupture and/or sampling limitations.

Cystic Lymphangioma

Arising from acquired loss or abnormal congenital communication of lymphatic ducts with upstream channels, these represent uncommon RP masses. They are seen most frequently in the pediatric population, but can present in adulthood and occur most frequently in men. (Davidson and Hartman, 1990; Munechika et al., 1987). **Resulting in progressive accumulation of cystic masses, these appear radiographically as thin-walled, multiseptated lesions, often crossing the midline into several** compartments (Fig. 100.13). Histologically, lymphangiomas can be classified into three distinct patterns (cystic, cavernous, and capillary), with the cystic type representing the most common (Casadei et al., 2003). The cystic spaces are lined with a single layer of endothelium, containing clear or milky lymphatic fluid within them. Immunohistochemical markers for lymphatic endothelium include CD31, CD34, and D2-40 (Gui et al., 2003). Treatment is complete surgical removal for symptomatic relief and exclusion of other entities. More conservative measures such as cyst aspiration or marsupialization have been abandoned because of high rates of recurrence (Surlin et al., 2011).

Mucinous Cystadenoma

Predominantly a tumor in women, these present as a unilocular cyst with homogeneous features. Although the true etiology of these lesions remains unclear, some hypothesize these represent invaginations of the peritoneal mesothelial layer resulting in cyst formation. Subsequent mucinous metaplasia develops, which can result in eventual malignant transformation in some cases (Pennell and Gusdon, 1989). Diagnostics are limited, and aspiration of fluid for cytologic analysis often provides little information. Management is complete surgical removal for histologic confirmation and treatment. On histopathology, the cyst is lined by a single layer of columnar epithelium with basal nuclei and pale cytoplasm.

Cystic Mesothelioma

Arising from the serous lining of the pleural, pericardial, or peritoneal spaces, cystic mesothelioma can occur rarely in the RP space. **Unlike malignant mesothelioma of the pleura, cystic mesothelioma is not associated with prior asbestos exposure.** Usually presenting with vague abdominal pain, they appear radiographically similar to lymphangiomas with multilocular, thin-walled cysts (Lee et al., 2009). Unlike lymphangiomas, these occur more commonly in women. Wide surgical resection is the treatment of choice, as local recurrences can occur.

Cystic Change of Solid Retroperitoneal Tumors

There remains a variety of tumors in which cystic changes can occur either arising from serous or mucinous production within the lesion, or with degenerative changes in response to treatments such as chemotherapy or radiation. A detailed history is paramount in evaluating these patients, paying particular attention to a history of prior treatment of cancer, presence of constitutional symptoms at time of presentation, and family history. In patients with a history of GCT, cystic teratoma can predominate within the RP. This is especially relevant after chemotherapy in the setting of growing tumor or late relapse. Similarly, paragangliomas can develop central areas of low attenuation on CT imaging, possibly resulting from internal hemorrhage and subsequent liquefaction (Yang et al., 2005). Other tumors demonstrating similar features include leiomyosarcomas, neurilemmomas, and gastrointestinal stromal tumors.

Retroperitoneal Cancer of Unknown Primary Origin

In the setting of a newly discovered tumor, the goal is to identify the site of origin and provide disease-specific therapy. However, when the primary origin of disease cannot be identified, determining what type of therapy to administer becomes uncertain. Cancer of an unknown primary origin presents several challenges to the treating clinician, representing up to 5% of new cancer diagnoses worldwide (Greco and Hainsworth, 1992; Levi et al., 2002; Miura et al., 1995). The median age at presentation is approximately 60 years of age, with a slight male predominance. Presenting clinically in a variety of patterns, radiographic distribution and immunohistochemical characterization through tissue biopsy samples become the mainstay of their evaluation. **Among all sites of disease, adenocarcinomas are the most common histologic subtype (50% of cases), followed by undifferentiated carcinomas (30%), squamous carcinomas (15%), and undifferentiated neoplasms** (Greco et al., 1997). In the RP, poorly differentiated carcinomas predominate, oftentimes presenting as soft-tissue masses encompassing the great vessels. Molecular and genetic analysis may reveal aberrancies of chromosomes 1 and 12, along with overexpression of Bcl-2 and p53 detected in up to one-half of patients (Bar-Eli et al., 1993; Briasoulis et al., 1998). IHC may also reveal increases of c-myc, ras, and c-erB-B2 protein expression (Hainsworth et al., 2001; Pavlidis and Fizazi, 2005). **Assessment for isochromosome i(12)p when assessing young male patients may identify patients with RP primary GCTs** (Abbruzzese et al., 1993; Bell et al., 1989). Additionally, serologic testing of tumor markers including AFP/B-hCG in young males and PSA in older men should be incorporated into the clinical workup. Despite several advances in immunohistochemical and genetic characterizations, less than 20% of cases historically will have a primary origin of disease identified. Completion of the workup includes whole-body imaging to stage and aid in identification of a primary tumor. Although CT imaging has been the mainstay of initial radiographic assessment, PET/CT scans have come into prominence to help in the workup of these lesions (Lassen et al., 1999; Rades et al., 2001).

Initial therapies are based on grouping or classifications according to the histologic characterizations and radiographic distribution. For tumors predominantly localized to the central/midline RP, especially when tissue analysis reveals i(12)p positivity, platinum-based combination chemotherapy is recommended. Response rates are reported in up to 50% of patients, with complete radiographic response rates occurring in 15% to 25% of cases (Greco et al., 1986; van der Gaast et al., 1990). Among those with poorly differentiated neuroendocrine carcinomas of the RP, again platinum-based regimens are recommended (Greco and Hainsworth, 1997; Pavlidis et al., 2003). Lastly, for those rare cases in which a cancer of unknown primary origin presents as a single, small, localized metastasis, considerations for local therapy with surgical extirpation and/or focused radiotherapy can be considered (Pavlidis et al., 2003).

Future horizons in this set of difficult-to-characterize tumors include gene expression profiles and whole-genome-based analysis. These technologies will hopefully provide a greater ability to characterize these tumors accurately according to the tissue of origin and individualize therapies with greater efficacy.

> **KEY POINT**
>
> - A multitude of histologic entities can exist within the RT that present with an infiltrative or expanding mass. Using a multidisciplinary approach with radiographic staging, consideration for pretreatment biopsy when indicated, specialized serologic and immunohistochemical characterization, and multimodal therapy including surgery, systemic therapies, and radiotherapy are pivotal for optimizing outcomes.

SURGICAL MANAGEMENT OF THE RETROPERITONEAL TUMOR

Preoperative Considerations

We do not recommend bowel preparation or dietary modifications before RP surgery. For GCTs, serum tumor markers should be checked within 7 to 10 days of surgery. Increased quantities of blood products should be considered for patients requiring more complex resections. **Preoperative sperm banking should be offered to patients who desire future paternity if retroperitoneal masses are in the path of the postganglionic sympathetic nerve fibers.** It is important for the urologist to have a medical oncology partner who possesses the clinical ability to assess bleomycin toxicity, to limit the dose when necessary, and to obtain pulmonary function testing when appropriate before sending the patient to surgery to minimize risk for postoperative acute respiratory distress syndrome. Additionally, the surgeon should ensure that the anesthesia provider is aware of any prior receipt of bleomycin and that he or she is familiar and comfortable with management of these patients. Specifically, low fraction of inspired oxygen (FiO_2) and conservative intraoperative fluid resuscitation are important in minimizing the risk for postoperative lung toxicity (Donat and Levy, 1998; Goldiner et al., 1978). Preoperative CT of the abdomen and pelvis should be thoroughly reviewed at initial consultation and immediately before surgery. A current CT scan of the chest is also required in patients with a history of pulmonary masses, planned concurrent resection of thoracic disease, or other radiographic/serologic evidence of disease progression. We prefer that preoperative imaging be performed within 6 weeks of the surgery date. **Careful inspection of imaging can usually prevent unplanned intraoperative consultations of other surgical specialists.** Preoperative identification of total inferior vena cava (IVC) thrombosis is important because the operation is made simpler by resection of the IVC (Beck and Lalka, 1998). Patients with incomplete occlusion requiring IVC resection may require reconstruction with a cadaveric allograft.

Surgical Technique

An orogastric tube is sufficient for intraoperative gastric decompression. Nasogastric tubes are generally reserved for patients with duodenal involvement that requires resection/repair, or high-volume retroperitoneal masses that require complete mobilization of the mesentery and placement of the bowels on the patient's chest for the duration of the surgery. The patient is placed in the supine

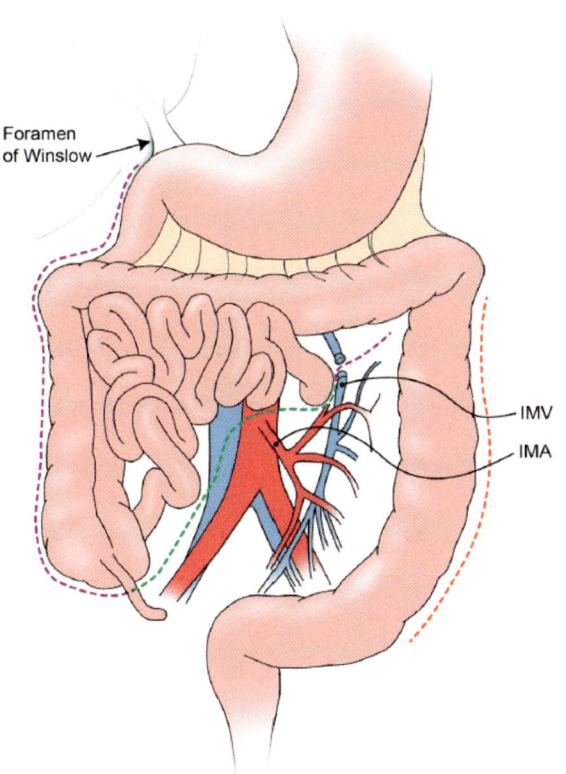

Fig. 100.14. Exposure of the retroperitoneum. *IMA*, Inferior mesenteric artery; *IMV*, inferior mesenteric vein. (Image courtesy of Indiana University School of Medicine, 2014.)

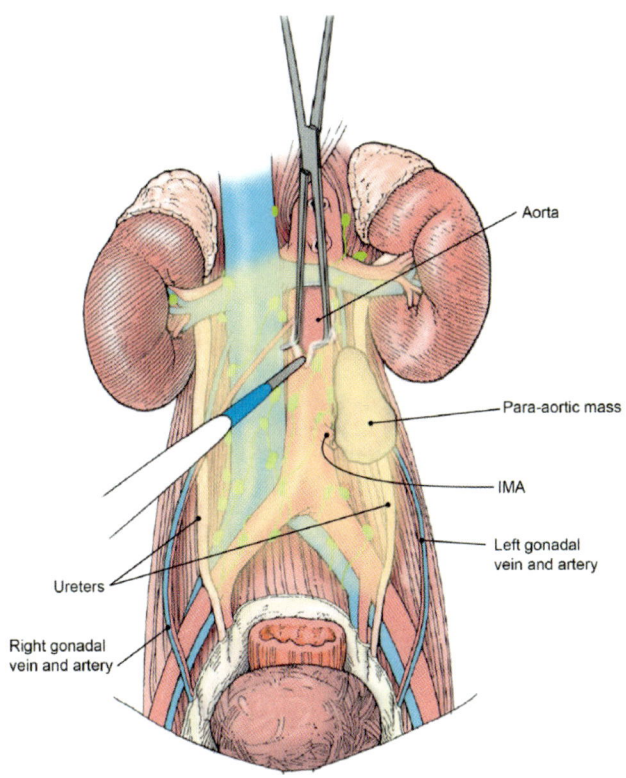

Fig. 100.15. The split-and-roll technique. *IMA*, Inferior mesenteric artery.

position, and a ventral midline incision is made. When the peritoneal cavity is entered, a thorough inspection of abdominal viscera is performed. The falciform ligament is identified, ligated, and divided to minimize the risk for hepatic retraction injury. A self-retaining retractor is then placed.

Exposure of the Retroperitoneum

For smaller paracaval and interaortocaval masses, the root of the mesentery is opened from the inferior tip of the cecum to the medial aspect of the inferior mesenteric vein (Fig. 100.14, *green dotted line*). In the case of large right RP, interaortocaval, and/or paracaval masses, the mesenteric incision can be continued around the inferior portion of the cecum to the right white line of Toldt and up to the foramen of Winslow to permit placement of the bowels on the chest (see Fig. 100.14, *green and purple line*). In the case of larger left RP and para-aortic masses, the inferior mesenteric vein is often ligated and divided to improve exposure of the left retroperitoneum. Alternatively, in the case of a small-volume disease in the left RP, the mass and/or para-aortic lymphatics can be approached through the left white line of Toldt (see Fig. 100.14, *red dotted line*).

The plane between the mesentery and the retroperitoneal fat is developed by identifying the gonadal vein and developing the plane along its anterior surface. The duodenum is dissected off of the IVC and left renal vein. Before placing retractors in this region, the superior mesenteric artery must be identified (usually by palpation). The blades of the retractors should then be placed on either side of the superior mesenteric artery.

Approach to the Retroperitoneum

Split-and-Roll Technique. Central within the RP are the vena cava and aorta. Accordingly, the surgical technique to manage any RP mass requires a thoughtful approach to exposing these structures. The large lymphatics coursing over the left renal vein should be ligated and divided. When the chosen template includes splitting over both great vessels, we prefer to perform the split on the aorta first rather than the IVC to avoid precaval right-sided accessory lower pole renal arteries. The advantage of performing the IVC split first is that the right-sided postganglionic sympathetic nerve fibers can be identified and traced to the superior hypogastric plexus, minimizing risk for injury during the aortic split. The split is started at the 12 o'clock position of the aorta, immediately inferior to the left renal vein (Fig. 100.15), and continued caudally, taking care to identify prospectively the inferior mesenteric artery and (1) preserve it in cases of a right RP procedure or (2) doubly ligate and divide this structure to expose the left para-aortic region in cases of a bilateral RP dissection. If a nerve-sparing technique is to be performed, the split should be stopped at the inferior mesenteric artery, and postganglionic sympathetic fibers should be identified before proceeding caudally.

Left Para-Aortic Region. As mentioned previously, the left RP can be approached laterally through the left white line of Toldt or medially through the mesenteric root depending on the distribution of disease. The left gonadal vein is doubly ligated and divided where it crosses the left ureter. The ureter is swept laterally and placed behind a retractor to minimize the risk for subsequent injury. The split is continued down the 12 o'clock position of the aorta and left common iliac artery until the left ureter is reached. The lymphatic tissue is rolled laterally off of the aorta and left common iliac artery. The three left-sided lumbar arteries located between the renal hilum and aortic bifurcation are identified, doubly ligated, and divided.

The mass and surrounding lymphatics are rolled inferiorly off of the left renal vein. The left gonadal and lumbar vein (when present) are doubly ligated and divided where they drain into the left renal vein. The lateral aspect of the packet is dissected off of the lower pole of the kidney and ureter.

The caudal extent of the packet is rolled superiorly off of the posterior body wall. The left genitofemoral nerve and sympathetic trunk should be identified and preserved when possible. The lumbar veins and body wall ends of the divided lumbar arteries should be identified and controlled. The packet is rolled up to the crus of the diaphragm. Lymphatics should be ligated as they course through the crus and into the retrocrural region. When the para-aortic resection is complete, tension on the ureteral retractor should be released to prevent prolonged ischemia.

Interaortocaval Region. If a right-sided nerve-sparing technique is to be performed, the IVC split and roll is performed next. Otherwise, the medial side of the aorta can be controlled first. The IVC split is performed from the renal hilum to the crossover of the right common iliac artery, where it is continued inferolaterally until the right ureter is reached. The right gonadal vein is doubly ligated and divided at the IVC. The lymphatic tissue is rolled medially off of the IVC. The nerves are visible, running obliquely along the lateral edge of the packet as it is peeled off the medial border of the IVC. The lumbar veins located between the renal hilum and the common iliac veins are identified, doubly ligated, and divided. In contrast with the lumbar arteries, the number and positions of the veins are unpredictable. When the medial aspect of the IVC has been controlled, lymphatic tissue is rolled laterally off of the IVC, and any lumbar veins encountered are ligated and divided. Before harvesting the interaortocaval mass, the right gonadal vein is ligated and divided where it crosses the right ureter. The ureter is placed behind a retractor to keep it out of the field of dissection.

Lymphatic tissue is rolled medially off of the aorta. The medial three lumbar arteries are identified, ligated, and divided. The interaortocaval mass and lymphatic tissue are harvested off of the anterior spinous ligament. The right sympathetic trunk is encountered at the right lateral border of the interaortocaval packet and should be preserved when possible. As the tumor is rolled off of the anterior spinous ligament, the cut ends of the lumbar vessels should be controlled as they enter and exit the body wall. The superior aspect of the packet is rolled inferiorly off of the renal vessels exposing the crus of the diaphragm. Taking care to avoid injury to the renal artery, the lymphatics coursing into the retrocrural region must be ligated to prevent postoperative lymph leak and chylous ascites.

Right Paracaval Region. The right paracaval lymphatics tend to be the smallest of the three major lymph node packets because the right kidney and ureter are located very close to the lateral border of the IVC. Masses in this location can be approached similarly to those in the interaortocaval region. The lymphatic tissue is rolled laterally and superiorly off of the right common iliac artery until the crossover of the right ureter is reached. The tissue is rolled superiorly off of the psoas fascia, taking care to preserve the right sympathetic trunk and the genitofemoral nerve. This roll is continued superiorly toward the right renal hilum and crus of the diaphragm. This packet often tapers to nothing and crosses under the IVC before the actual renal hilum is reached.

Surgical Modifications

Template Considerations for Management of Metastatic Germ Cell Tumors

Primary Retroperitoneal Lymph Node Dissection. In the 1970s and 1980s, the development of curative cisplatin-based chemotherapeutic regimens (Einhorn and Donohue, 1977), elucidation of distinct lymphatic spread for right-sided versus left-sided testicular tumors (Donohue et al., 1982; Ray et al., 1974; Weissbach and Boedefeld, 1987), and description of surgical techniques to preserve the postganglionic sympathetic nerve fibers involved in seminal emission and antegrade ejaculation (Colleselli et al., 1990; Donohue et al., 1990; Jewett et al., 1988) significantly altered management of the retroperitoneum in patients with testicular GCT. In 1974, Ray et al. presented a series of 283 patients undergoing RPLND at Memorial Sloan Kettering Cancer Center (MSKCC) from 1944 to 1971. Dissections were predominantly infrahilar and evolved from a full bilateral dissection to a "modified bilateral" dissection as the primary landing zones of right-sided versus left-sided primaries became apparent. These modified bilateral templates were very similar to modified unilateral templates with the exception that lymphatic tissue below the inferior mesenteric artery (IMA) was routinely resected. The detailed description of distinct templates based on the laterality of the testicular primary was the first of its kind and set the stage for further refinement.

Donohue et al. (1982) published a pathologic lymph node mapping study performed at Indiana University on 104 patients found to have pathologically positive nodes (pN+) at primary RPLND. Full bilateral dissections to include bilateral suprahilar dissections were performed on every patient. **Investigators found that left-sided tumors were most likely to metastasize to the left para-aortic lymph nodes, whereas right-sided tumors were most likely to metastasize to interaortocaval and precaval regions. Spread to contralateral retroperitoneum and suprahilar regions was rare but increased with tumor bulk.** Metastasis to the interiliac region was rare. This study confirmed the relatively predictable pattern of the lymphatic spread of testicular GCTs and provided strong pathologic evidence for the use of "modified bilateral" templates proposed by Ray et al. (1974) in patients with low-stage retroperitoneal disease. Omission of the contralateral retroperitoneum and interiliac regions resulted in the preservation of antegrade ejaculation in most patients. Omission of suprahilar regions decreased the risk for postoperative chylous ascites, renovascular injuries, and pancreatic complications.

In 1987, Weissbach and Boedefeld reported a multi-institutional retrospective review of 214 patients with nonbulky pathologic stage II disease (Weissbach and Boedefeld, 1987). The authors recommended a more reduced left-sided template including the para-aortic and upper preaortic nodes. The authors also proposed that a frozen section be sent from the primary landing zone; if the section was positive, a full bilateral infrahilar RPLND should be performed.

The end result of these template studies has been a more efficient, less morbid, and maximally effective RPLND. There is still significant debate among experts regarding the ideal extent of surgical templates. Most experts agree that suprahilar/retrocrural and interiliac resections can safely be omitted from the standard RPLND template. However, controversy exists regarding the need to resect the contralateral retroperitoneal lymphatic tissue. The boundaries of the modified unilateral templates and a full bilateral template are demonstrated in Fig. 100.16.

Eggener et al. (2007) reviewed a series of 500 patients undergoing primary RPLND for clinical stage I or IIA testicular cancer at MSKCC. Bilateral infrahilar dissection was usually performed. The authors analyzed the 191 patients (38%) with pathologic stage II disease for the anatomic distribution of positive-node packets and applied five modified templates to these results. They reported that 3% to 23% of patients with pathologically positive nodes were found to have disease outside of the modified unilateral template, depending on which one was applied. Extratemplate disease was seen more commonly with right-sided than left-sided tumors. Given these results, the authors recommended full bilateral infrahilar nerve–sparing RPLND for patients with clinical stage I or IIA testicular cancer.

To date, no prospective or retrospective studies have compared the modified unilateral templates with the full bilateral templates. Cancer-specific and overall survival approach 100% in all published series. Expanding the templates cannot be expected to improve either of these outcomes. The question is whether performance of a full bilateral infrahilar RPLND would prevent retroperitoneal relapses that would occur after a properly performed modified unilateral template. When comparing series from centers that use the modified unilateral templates with series from centers that use the bilateral infrahilar templates, outcomes are very similar (Table 100.2) (Donohue et al., 1993; Hermans et al., 2000; Nicolai et al., 2004; Stephenson et al., 2005). Although the MSKCC series reported an increased proportion of patients being cured by surgery alone, patients with pN2 disease routinely receive adjuvant postoperative chemotherapy at that center (Stephenson et al., 2005). In the first Indiana study, most of the node-positive patients were randomly assigned to observation versus adjuvant chemotherapy on protocol (Donohue et al., 1993). In the more recent Indiana study, pN1 patients and most pN2 patients were observed with chemotherapy reserved for patients who experienced recurrence and pN3 patients (Hermans et al., 2000).

The appropriate boundaries of the primary RPLND template are controversial. Use of the templates recommended in the studies by Ray, Donohue, Weissbach, and Eggener and their colleagues will

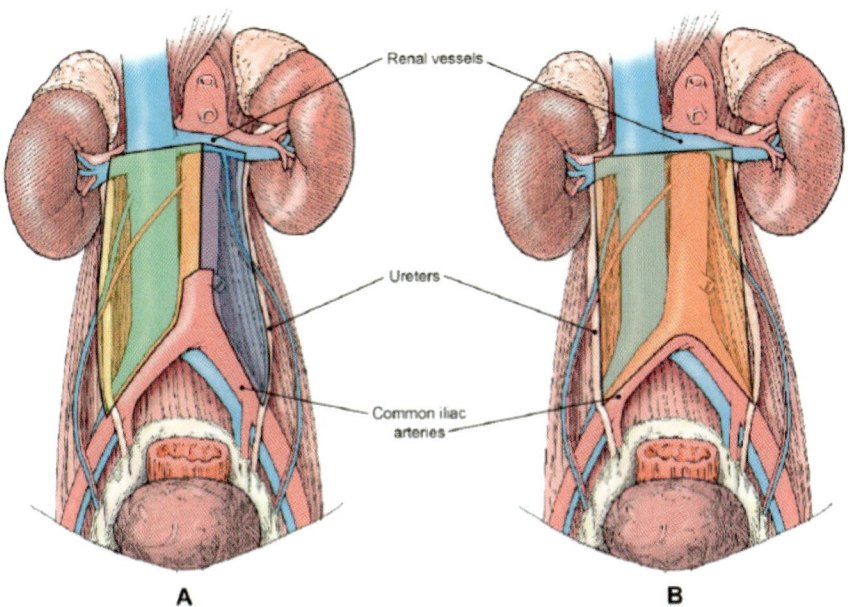

Fig. 100.16. Template modifications in retroperitoneal lymph node dissection templates. (A) Modified unilateral templates—right-sided shaded in yellow, left-sided shaded in purple. (B) Modified bilateral template—shaded area. (Image courtesy of Indiana University School of Medicine, 2014.)

TABLE 100.2 Selected Primary Retroperitoneal Lymph Node Dissection Series

STUDY	NO. OF PATIENTS	NO. pN+ (%)	RECURRENCE RATE FOR pN0 (%)	RECURRENCE RATE FOR pN+ MANAGED WITH RPLND ALONE (%)	FOLLOW-UP (YEARS)	CSS (%)
Donohue et al., 1993	378	112 (29.6)	31 (12)	22 (34)	6.2	99.2
Hermans et al., 2000	292	66 (22.4)	23 (10.2)	7 (22.6)	3.8	100
Nicolai et al., 2004	322	60 (20)	NR	NR	7.2	98.8
Stephenson et al., 2005	308	91 (29.5)	NR (7)	NR (34)	4.9	99.7

CSS, Cancer-specific survival; *RPLND*, retroperitoneal lymph node dissection.

undoubtedly result in excellent survival outcomes. The question of which template offers greatest balance of oncologic control and minimization of morbidity remains unanswered.

Postchemotherapy Retroperitoneal Lymph Node Dissection. Donohue et al. first reported their experience performing consolidative RPLND after cisplatin-based chemotherapy in 1982. Most tumors containing teratoma and/or viable malignancy were located in their respective primary landing zones. However, given the frequent contralateral crossover in the setting of bulky disease and the inability to obtain reliable confirmation of histology intraoperatively, the authors stressed the importance of the PC-RPLND being "as complete as possible" (Donohue et al., 1982). The standard PC-RPLND became resection of all macroscopic disease along with a full bilateral infrahilar dissection. This approach provides excellent local control of the RP, but is associated with significant morbidity including anejaculation in patients in whom a nerve-sparing technique is not possible.

Several groups investigated whether modified unilateral templates can safely be applied to appropriately selected patients in the postchemotherapy setting (Beck et al., 2007; Carver et al., 2007; Ehrlich et al., 2006; Heidenreich et al., 2009; Herr, 1997; Rabbani et al., 1998; Steiner et al., 2008; Wood et al., 1992). When bilateral dissections were performed, rates of disease outside the unilateral template are reported to range from 18% to 32% (Carver et al., 2007). However, rates of disease outside of the unilateral template and outside of macroscopic disease ranged from 2% to 18.6%. Variability in these percentages is likely a function of patient selection and the specific template used. Safe use of the unilateral modified templates in the postchemotherapy setting relies on selection of the correct template and appropriate patient selection. Patients meeting the following criteria may be considered for modified unilateral template PC-RPLND according to data emerging from centers performing the following surgeries:

- Well-defined lesion measuring 5 cm or less confined to the primary landing zone of the primary tumor on imaging before and after chemotherapy
- Normal postchemotherapy serum tumor markers
- International Germ Cell Cancer Collaborative Group (IGCCCG) good/intermediate risk

Use of these selection criteria has resulted in in-field retroperitoneal recurrence rates of 0% to 1%, antegrade ejaculation rates of 85% to 99%, and cancer-specific survival of 98% to 100% at postoperative follow-up times of 2.6 to 10 years (Cho et al., 2017; Heidenreich et al., 2009; Steiner et al., 2008). Although these data are encouraging with regard to the use of the modified unilateral templates in PC-RPLND, the standard of care for patients requiring postchemotherapy resection remains resection of all macroscopic disease and a full bilateral infrahilar template RPLND. To date, there have been no prospective studies comparing outcomes in patients undergoing bilateral versus modified unilateral template PC-RPLND. If unilateral modified templates are to be used at PC-RPLND, strict adherence to the above-listed selection criteria is important.

Nerve-Sparing RPLND. The anatomy of the four postganglionic efferent sympathetic fibers (L1 to L4) involved in antegrade ejaculation

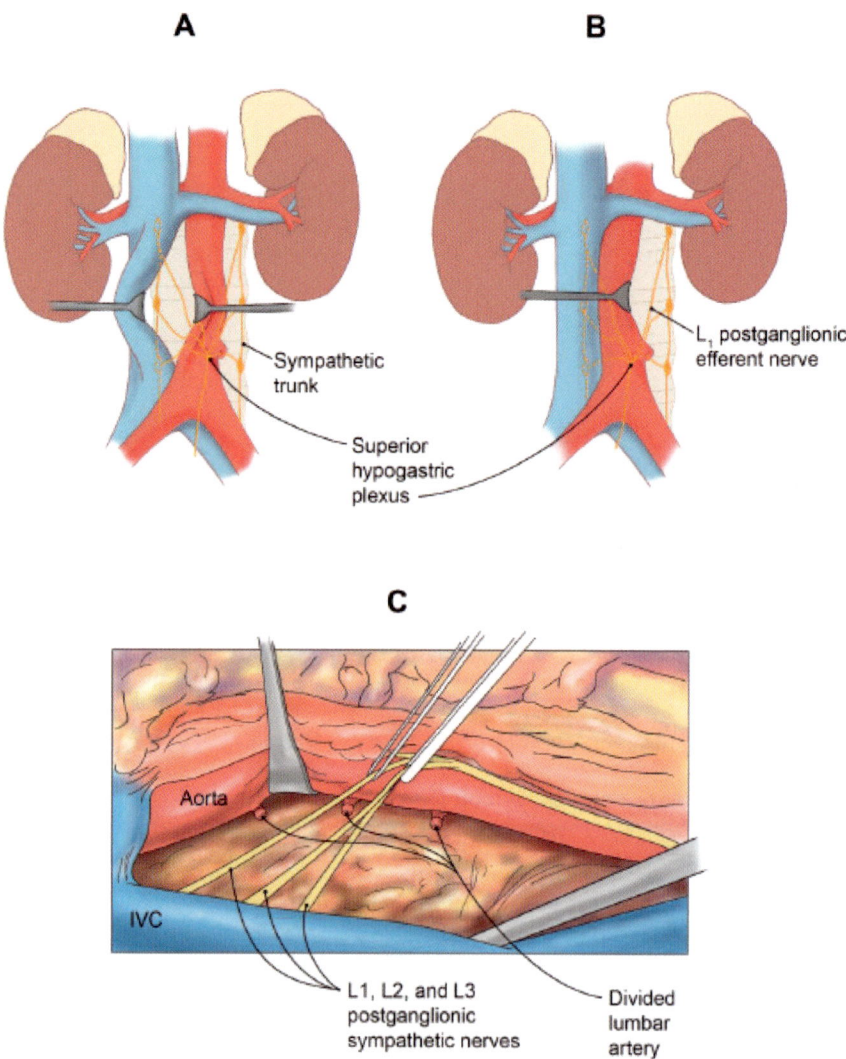

Fig. 100.17. Nerve-sparing for ejaculatory function preservation. (A) Location of right-sided postganglionic sympathetic nerves. (B) Location of left-sided postganglionic sympathetic nerves. (C) Right-sided nerve-sparing technique with ligated lumbar arteries. *IVC*, Inferior vena cava. (Image courtesy of Indiana University School of Medicine, 2014.)

demonstrates significant variability from patient to patient. The L2 and L3 fibers are usually fused. Although the L2 to L4 fibers tend to take a more anterior course along the aorta and common iliac vessels, the L1 fiber takes a more shallow, caudal, and oblique course, exiting the sympathetic trunk near the level of the ipsilateral renal hilum Fig. 100.17.

The left-sided postganglionic sympathetic nerves are first identified as they course along the lateral border of the aorta and left common iliac artery and onto the anterior surface of these vessels immediately caudal to the IMA (see Fig. 100.17). A Kittner sponge can be used to sweep the fatty connective tissue gently away revealing the shiny off-white nerve fibers running obliquely over the aorta and joining the contralateral postganglionic fibers in the superior hypogastric plexus. Fibers can be tagged with vessel loops to provide continued gentle traction as they are dissected to their origins at the sympathetic trunk. Alternatively, the left sympathetic trunk can be identified first distal to the level of the IMA and traced cranially until the postganglionic fibers are sequentially encountered.

The right-sided postganglionic nerve fibers are best identified as the precaval and interaortocaval lymphatic tissue is rolled medially off of the IVC. The postganglionic fibers can be seen coursing obliquely in an anterior and inferior direction toward the superior hypogastric plexus. These can be cleared of overlying tissue using a Kittner sponge. As described previously, the individual fibers should be encircled with vessel loops to place them on traction as they are traced down to their origins in the right sympathetic trunk.

When the nerve fibers have been dissected free for the entirety of their courses through the RPLND template, the lymphatic packets around the fibers should be dissected. The specimen must be sequentially passed through the web of postganglionic fibers as it is released from the body wall. Care must be taken to avoid injuring the fibers during specimen harvest and obtaining hemostasis. The nerve fibers often exit the sympathetic trunks in close proximity to the lumbar vessels, which puts them at particular risk for collateral injury if lumbar bleeding is encountered. Patients who undergo bilateral nerve-sparing or unilateral nerve-sparing with contralateral complete resection may experience an anejaculatory period postoperatively. This likely results from neuropraxia.

Auxiliary Procedures

The following discussion of auxiliary procedures applies to advanced-stage tumor of the RP because these procedures are rarely, if ever, required during treatment of smaller-volume disease. The most common auxiliary procedure is a nephrectomy, followed by vascular reconstruction or resection. As the volume of retroperitoneal disease increases, so does the likelihood of requiring resection of adjacent organs and/or structures.

Nephrectomy. Nephrectomy at the time of PC-RPLND is the most commonly performed auxiliary procedure for GCTs. The incidence of nephrectomy at PC-RPLND ranges from 5% to 31% (Cary et al., 2013; Djaladat et al., 2012; Nash et al, 1998; Stephenson et al., 2006). **In the setting of sarcomas, the reported incidence of the nephrectomy in 1007 patients with primary RP sarcoma is upward of 55%** (Gronchi et al., 2016).

Recognition of preoperative risk factors associated with nephrectomy at the time of RP surgery is vital for surgical planning and patient counseling. Nephrectomy is usually needed in high-risk settings such as salvage RPLND, desperation RPLND, resection of late relapse, or reoperative RPLND. Additional risk factors include retroperitoneal mass size and location of primary tumor (i.e., left vs. right testicle for GCTs). In the Indiana University study, men who had an RP mass size greater than 10 cm had a ninefold increase in odds of nephrectomy compared with men who had retroperitoneal mass less than 2 cm. Left-sided primary tumors with left para-aortic retroperitoneal masses had significantly increased odds of nephrectomy compared with right-sided tumors (odds ratio 5.44, P <.0001) (Cary et al., 2013).

It is important to consider postoperative renal function after nephrectomy because these patients may require postoperative adjuvant chemotherapy. Studies from Indiana University and MSKCC reported a decline in renal function after nephrectomy (Nash et al., 1998; Stephenson et al., 2006). However, this decreased renal function neither resulted in the need for renal replacement therapy nor compromised subsequent adjuvant or salvage chemotherapy when necessary. Despite changes in renal function, most patients can tolerate subsequent chemotherapy if needed and avoid renal replacement therapy. However, progression to chronic kidney disease is largely dependent on age and preoperative GFR.

Vascular Reconstruction
Aortic Replacement

In some cases, RP tumor encasement of the aorta requires en bloc aortic resection with reconstruction to remove the RP mass adequately. When this clinical situation occurs, it is crucial to alert additional surgical teams (i.e., vascular surgery) preoperatively to ensure successful clinical outcomes. It is ideal to anticipate the need for aortic replacement preoperatively to allow proper patient counseling and time to coordinate between surgical services. An aortic tube graft is most commonly used for reconstruction; however, an aortobi-iliac graft may be used depending on the extent of tumor involvement.

Several studies evaluated the indications for aortic resection and its morbidity. In 2001, Beck et al. reported 15 patients who underwent aortic replacement during PC-RPLND. Over a 30-year span involving more than 1200 patients, approximately 1% required this procedure. Two-thirds of these patients had received at least one course of salvage chemotherapy and/or had elevated serum tumor markers at the time of surgery. The indication for aortic replacement in these patients was tumor fixation to the aorta, with en bloc resection of the aorta deemed necessary for complete tumor removal. At a median follow-up of 34 months, 33% of these patients were disease-free. Given the chemoresistant nature of the disease and bulky tumor burden surrounding the aorta in most of these patients with advanced GCT and sarcoma, aortic resection is a worthwhile undertaking and may provide a therapeutic benefit in a significant proportion of patients.

When the decision for aortic resection has been made, the principles of the operation do not change substantially. The IVC should be dissected away from the mass and aorta using the split-and-roll technique with division of lumbar veins. The left ureter should be freed from the retroperitoneal mass. If the tumor does not encroach on the left renal hilum, this is also dissected free. The vascular surgery team assists with this dissection to ensure adequate length of the aorta cranial and caudal to the tumor, which allows for proximal and distal vascular control and ease of graft anastomoses. The aorta is cross-clamped and resected en bloc with the retroperitoneal mass. Lumbar arteries are divided during this process. Before cross-clamping, the patient is usually administered intravenous heparin to minimize the risk for arterial thrombosis. The graft is sewn into place using standard vascular surgery principles.

Vena Caval Resection

Most cases requiring IVC resection have bulky stage disease. The incidence of IVC resection reported in the literature for GCTs range from 5% to 10% (Beck and Lalka, 1998; Nash et al., 1998; Winter et al., 2012). In 1991, Donohue et al. reported on 40 patients who underwent IVC resection without reconstruction. In this study, the three indications for caval resection were necessity for tumor clearance (38%), vena caval scar occlusion (14%), and vena caval tumor thrombus (48%). The decision for en bloc caval resection was justified by the adverse nodal pathology, which included active cancer in 63% and teratoma in 31% of the specimens. For patients with lower-extremity edema and imaging concerning for IVC compression/occlusion, venacavography, ultrasonography, or magnetic resonance imaging is helpful to assess for flow through the IVC and guide intraoperative decision making.

Routine reconstruction of the vena cava after resection is not required. Data on 65 infrarenal IVC resections without reconstruction by Beck and Lalka (1998) support this approach. This study evaluated the long-term sequelae of IVC resection using a survey developed by an international consensus conference on chronic venous disease held by the American Venous Forum (Beebe et al., 1996). The median follow-up for these patients was 89 months. Of patients, 75% had a disability score of 0 to 1 (none or mild disability). Only one patient had the highest possible disability score. Although these patients are at higher risk for chylous ascites and other periprocedural complications (Baniel et al, 1993), long-term venous congestion seems to be less of an issue; this is particularly true if there is complete occlusion with development of collateral circulation present preoperatively. Slow progressive retroperitoneal tumor growth with accompanying desmoplastic reaction to chemotherapy likely results in a gradual occlusion of caval blood flow allowing for adequate development of venous collateral circulation. The development of this collateral venous return likely results in less morbidity from caval resection in patients with testicular cancer compared with patients with acute IVC occlusion.

In the sarcoma population, caval resection with or without reconstruction is well described as well. The necessity of this mirrors the indications in GCTs with the ultimate goal of obtaining negative margins. Different techniques have been described for vena caval reconstruction (e.g., Dacron, PTFE, homografts) in the sarcoma population. Late morbidity of vena caval reconstruction in this group with a prosthesis results in graft thrombosis in 10% to 40% of cases (Fiore et al, 2012; Quinones-Baldrich et al, 2012).

Tumor Thrombectomy

Intraluminal thrombi occur infrequently in GCTs and sarcoma, but has been reported most commonly in the vena cava. Additional locations are reported in the renal vein and least commonly in the aorta. The largest published series of this phenomenon comes from the Indiana group. Johnston et al. (2013) reported on 89 patients with 98 intraluminal thrombi. Seventy-three percent of these occurred in the vena cava and were managed with either cavectomy, partial cavectomy, or thrombectomy. Of the renal vein thrombi, 90% were managed with nephrectomy. The histology of these resected thrombi was bland thrombus in 32%, necrosis in 23%, teratoma in 29%, and residual cancer in 16%.

Complications
Ejaculatory Function

Early studies on ejaculatory outcomes after modified unilateral template RPLND without nerve-sparing technique reported postoperative antegrade ejaculation in 75% to 87% of patients (Fossa et al, 1985; Pizzocaro et al, 1985; Weissbach et al, 1985) However, in a more recent series, Beck et al. (2010) reported preservation of antegrade ejaculation in 97% of men undergoing modified unilateral template dissection without ipsilateral nerve–sparing technique. Additionally, 99.2% of men undergoing modified unilateral template dissection with ipsilateral nerve sparing maintained antegrade ejaculation in this series. These superior outcomes likely reflect improved understanding of the anatomy of postganglionic sympathetic nerve fibers allowing for the avoidance of damage to contralateral fibers caudal to the IMA.

Nerve-sparing RPLND results in preservation of antegrade ejaculation in 90% to 100% of patients (Beck et al., 2010; Donohue et al., 1990; Heidenreich et al., 2003; Jewett and Torbey, 1988). Although Jewett and Torbey reported temporary postoperative anejaculation in most patients, Donohue observed no such anejaculatory period (Donohue et al., 1993; Jewett and Torbey, 1988). In the study by Jewett and Torbey, bilateral template RPLND was performed in all patients, whereas ipsilateral nerve–sparing and modified unilateral template dissections were performed in most patients in the study by Donohue (Donohue et al., 1993; Jewett and Torbey, 1988). Neuropraxia likely accounted for the temporary anejaculation reported by Jewett and Torbey (1988).

Vascular

Retroperitoneal tumors requiring major vascular resection have a modest increase in vascular morbidity. In a recent series of 65 patients who required vena caval reconstruction, the incidence of perioperative thrombosis was 22%, including 9% with deep venous thrombosis and 12% with pulmonary embolus (Hicks et al, 2016).

Venous thromboembolism (VTE) rates reported after primary RPLND and PC-RPLND for GCTs are consistently low; this is likely the result of a young, otherwise healthy patient population. The rate of pulmonary embolism after primary RPLND has been reported to be less than 1% (Baniel et al., 1994; Heidenreich et al., 2003; Subramanian et al., 2010). After PC-RPLND, the rates range from 0.1% to 3.1% (Baniel et al., 1995; Subramanian et al., 2010). The incidence of deep venous thrombosis is more difficult to determine because these cases are not consistently reported in the literature and are likely most often asymptomatic. Reported rates range from 0% to 1% in primary RPLND and PC-RPLND (Heidenreich et al., 2003; Subramanian et al., 2010).

Lymphatic

Lymphocele. The incidence of subclinical lymphocele after RPLND is unknown. However, it is thought that lymphoceles are relatively common and clinically insignificant in most cases. Symptomatic retroperitoneal lymphoceles are extremely rare, with reported rates ranging from 0% to 1.7% (Baniel et al., 1994, 1995; Heidenreich et al., 2003; Subramanian et al., 2010). Symptoms can be related to ureteral compression, displacement of abdominal viscera (if very large), or secondary infection. CT scan demonstrates a thin-walled cystic lesion in the resection bed. Air within the lymphocele and/or rim enhancement should raise concern for an infection. Meticulous attention to ligation of large-caliber lymphatics during resection likely decreases the risk for developing a symptomatic lymphocele. Treatment of symptomatic and/or infected lymphoceles includes percutaneous drainage with systemic antibiotics reserved for infected lymphoceles. Additionally, in the setting of infected lymphocele, one should consider leaving an indwelling drain rather than simple percutaneous aspiration.

Chylous Ascites. Chylous ascites refers to the accumulation of chylomicron-containing lymphatic fluid in the peritoneal cavity. Chylous ascites has been reported to occur in 0.2% to 2.1% of patients undergoing primary RPLND and 2% to 7% of patients undergoing PC-RPLND (Baniel et al., 1994, 1995; Evans et al., 2006; Heidenreich et al., 2003; Subramanian et al., 2010). Patients typically present with complaints of increasing abdominal fullness, anorexia, nausea, vomiting, abdominal pain, and dyspnea. Patients often have a fluid wave on abdominal examination, which can help distinguish ascites from an ileus. Additionally, accumulated peritoneal fluid results in significant weight gain. Fluid has a milky color if paracentesis is performed. **Chylous ascites is alkaline, stains positive for Sudan black, and demonstrates a triglyceride concentration greater than that of serum. However, these tests are usually unnecessary because clinical examination and/or gross inspection of aspirating fluid should be enough to confirm the diagnosis.**

Suprahilar resections are thought to carry a higher risk for chylous ascites because of disruption of the cisterna chyli and its contributing lymphatics. The cisterna chyli is located at the level of the L1-L2 vertebral bodies, medial to the posterior surface of the aorta in the retrocrural space. The association of IVC resection and chylous ascites is thought to be related to increased venous pressure below the level of the IVC producing increased capillary leak and ultimately third-spacing of lymphatic fluid into the retroperitoneum (Baniel et al., 1993). In a review of the MD Anderson Cancer Center experience, Evans et al. (2006) found an increased number of preoperative cycles of chemotherapy, increased estimated blood loss, and longer operative time to be associated with development of chylous ascites.

We recommend a graduated approach to the management of chylous ascites. In general, patients with symptomatic chylous ascites should first be managed with paracentesis. Although an indwelling drain can be left, we recommend simple paracentesis with consideration of low-fat/medium-chain triglyceride diet and intramuscular octreotide. If ascites reaccumulates, an indwelling drain should be placed. If these dietary modifications have already been instituted, patients should be given nothing by mouth, and total parenteral nutrition should be initiated. Although the use of octreotide in the setting of chylous ascites has not been studied in the urologic literature, it has demonstrated efficacy in minimizing chylous leaks after hepaticopancreaticobiliary surgery (Shapiro et al., 1996; Kuboki et al., 2013). Persistent high-volume chylous drainage (>100 mL/24 hr) despite these modifications is exceedingly rare. When it does occur, options include continued observation with conservative management, placement of a peritoneovenous (LeVeen) shunt, or surgical exploration with attempted ligation of the lymphatic leak. The latter two options should be reserved as last resorts. Peritoneovenous shunts have been reported to be associated with a significant incidence of occlusion and/or malfunction often requiring revision after placement, sepsis, and potentially fat embolization (Evans et al., 2006). Regardless of treatment modality that ultimately results in resolution of chylous ascites, consideration should be given to a continued low-fat diet with medium-chain triglycerides for 1 to 3 months after resolution of lymph leak.

Neurologic

In the Indiana PC-RPLND review, no cases of paraplegia were noted. Seven cases of peripheral nerve injury were reported (Baniel et al., 1995). All of these cases were secondary to patient positioning and potentially retractor placement (femoral neuropraxia). Careful attention to appropriate patient positioning by the surgical and anesthesia teams is important in minimizing peripheral nerve damage. In a review of 268 patients undergoing postchemotherapy resection of mediastinal disease for testicular or primary retroperitoneal GCT, Kesler et al. (2003) reported 6 patients (2.2%) with paraplegia. Patients with bulky mediastinal and retroperitoneal disease are at an increased risk for developing paraplegia. The likelihood of neurologic complications increases with the scale of para-aortic resection.

Approximately 5% of patients with primary retroperitoneal sarcomas will require major lumbar nerve resections (Mullen and van Houdt, 2018). This most commonly results from the sarcoma arising from the nerve root itself. The most commonly affected nerves are the femoral and obturator nerves. There are also several sensory nerves that can be affected, such as the genitofemoral, ilioinguinal, and so forth. The femoral nerve is the most functionally important nerve of this group affecting ipsilateral knee extension requiring a hinged knee brace in severe cases.

Postoperative Care

Surgical drains are not routinely placed. However, large-volume retroperitoneal, retrocrural, or duodenal resections may require a drain. We leave a Penrose drain for large-volume resections, given the propensity of postoperative abdominal third spacing. This drain is typically removed after the patient has resumed a regular diet and drainage remains serous and less than 100 mL for 24 hours.

In the absence of bowel repair/anastomoses, patients are given sips of ice chips on the evening of surgery. On postoperative day 1, patients are advanced to unlimited clear liquids, and they are encouraged to spend most of the day in a chair and ambulating. If patients tolerate clear liquids, they are advanced to a regular diet and transitioned off of intravenous pain medications on postoperative day 2. Patients are typically discharged between postoperative days 2 and 5 depending on how quickly they are able to tolerate a regular diet. Patients undergoing larger resections tend to have longer inpatient stays.

> **KEY POINT**
> - Surgical preparation and management of the RP mass requires careful consideration of all potential risks and obstacles, need for a thoughtful approach to surgical exposure and mobilization of the mass, preparation in advance and coordination of consultation for the possibility of auxiliary procedures when indicated, and a keen understanding of the short- and long-term complications that come along with RP surgery.

DISEASE-SPECIFIC NEOADJUVANT AND ADJUVANT THERAPIES

Radiation

The use of multimodal therapy has increased among cancer management strategies over time. Among RP tumors, focusing mostly on sarcoma-based treatments, the use of radiation as an adjunct to surgical extirpation has become more prevalent over time with the goal of reducing local recurrences. Extrapolating from experiences in extremity soft-tissue sarcomas, the incorporation of perioperative radiotherapy in RP soft-tissue sarcoma has demonstrated improvements in survival outcomes (Nussbaum et al., 2016). However, long-term data on associated toxicities and impact on recurrence patterns requires more investigation. Controversies as to the timing of radiation, overall radiotherapy dose, and overall distribution continue to evolve. In one of the first prospective clinical trials using perioperative radiotherapy in RP sarcoma, 35 patients were randomized to receive either intraoperative (20 Gy)/postoperative (35–40 Gy) combination radiotherapy versus postoperative (50–55 Gy) radiotherapy alone (control group) (Sindelar et al., 1993). Local control with regard to locoregional relapse was higher in the intraoperative group (40% vs. 80%), and overall survival was similar (45 vs. 52 months). However, radiation-related toxicities were significant in both groups, with disabling radiation enteritis occurring more often in the control group (50% vs. 13%) and radiation-related peripheral neuropathy more frequent in the intraoperative cohort (60% vs. 5%). Interestingly, use of adjunctive chemotherapy offered no perceivable benefit with a regimen of cyclophosphamide, adriamycin, and methotrexate. The use of low-dose brachytherapy has been assessed in a phase I/II trial as an adjunct to preoperative radiotherapy, but severe toxicity was reported and the trial was closed accordingly (Jones et al., 2002). Two prospective trials hoping to compare preoperative radiotherapy to surgery alone have been initiated (NCT00091351 & NCT1344018), but results are still awaited.

In the absence of robust prospective data, large observational studies have been performed that offer some insight into the value of perioperative radiotherapy. In a case-control, propensity score-matched cohort study involving more than 9000 patients included in the National Cancer Database, the use of preoperative (563 patients), postoperative (2215 patients), and no-radiotherapy (6290 patients) was compared (Nussbaum et al., 2016). Results demonstrated a survival advantage for the use of any radiotherapy in the management of RP sarcoma patients (hazard ratio [HR] = 0.70 for preoperative; HR = 0.78 for postoperative). Similar assessment of survival benefits using postoperative radiotherapy using the Surveillance, Epidemiology, and End Results (SEER) database have been published with disparate results. Bates et al. (2018) assessed outcomes from 1973 to 2010 among 480 patients with RP sarcoma; 30% received adjuvant radiotherapy with a survival advantage at 3 years (HR = 0.79, P = 0.023). Conversely, in a larger cohort from the SEER database (1535 patients), Tseng et al. (2011) reported on 5-year overall survival and disease-specific survival outcomes. No differences were seen among those receiving or not receiving adjuvant radiotherapy, with the exception of those being treated for malignant fibrous histiocytoma. **Limitations for all of these retrospective studies include the inability to assess local control rates, toxicity-related differences, variations in radiotherapy dose administered, timing of treatment, or control for differences in patient selection.** Others have attempted to identify thresholds for radiation-related toxicity based on dose administered. Rates of late complications associated with 50–60 Gy range from 5% at 10 years up to 40% at 3.5 years, largely related to bowel-associated toxicity (Ballo et al., 2007; Bishop et al., 2015; Gilbeau et al., 2002; Le Péchoux et al., 2013; Pezner et al., 2011; Zlotecki et al., 2005). Most of the toxicity is attributable to the use of adjuvant radiotherapy, with preoperative radiotherapy having fewer issues reported.

Overall, the optimal role of perioperative radiotherapy in the setting of RP sarcoma remains uncertain. Although the incorporation of radiotherapy seems to improve local control rates, this comes at the expense of greater toxicity, particularly when used in the postoperative setting, with marginal improvements in overall survival. If radiotherapy is to be considered, its use in the preoperative setting seems to have the most promise. Results from the prospective European Organization for Research and Treatment of Cancer-STBSG trial are being eagerly awaited to clarify the benefits and risks associated with preoperative therapy. Intraoperative electron beam or brachytherapy as adjuncts to surgical resection remain investigational and warrant further assessment in the setting of a clinical trial.

Chemotherapy and Systemic Therapies

Outside of platinum-based chemotherapy used in the management of metastatic GCTs, data supporting the use of systemic therapies in localized RP sarcomas are limited. The majority of RP sarcomas identified largely represent chemotherapy-resistant entities, such as liposarcomas and leiomyosarcomas. However, there remain certain histologic subtypes for which chemotherapy represents the primary modality of treatment (i.e., lymphomas); therefore, the importance of accurate characterization of the primary tumor remains pivotal. In the absence of metastatic disease, the question at time of diagnosis is whether neoadjuvant systemic therapy impacts the risk for distant spread, improves resectability, and reduces positive surgical margins.

Although prospective studies enrolling large numbers of patients are lacking, several retrospective analyses have been published in soft-tissue sarcoma. However, heterogeneity of RP tumor subtypes limits their impact. **Table 100.3 summarizes the relative response rates of the various RP sarcoma subtypes as reported in the literature.** Overall, selective tumors have demonstrated responses to systemic therapies. Most notable examples include myxoid liposarcomas, synovial sarcomas, and Ewing sarcoma. Although standard use of neoadjuvant chemotherapy is recommended only in Ewing sarcoma based on response rates in extremity locations, its role among other entities remains uncertain. In the setting of a resectable tumor, the benefits of neoadjuvant chemotherapy remain uncertain. For tumors in which resectability is a concern or if regional or distant spread is documented, then multimodal therapy including induction chemotherapy should be considered. In RP tumors for which minimal response to chemotherapy has been recorded (i.e., well-differentiated liposarcoma, leiomyosarcoma), resection of local, regional, and/or systemic disease when feasible can be recommended in select cases. Otherwise, enrollment into clinical trials serves as the only alternative option for these patients. Some early successes have been reported with targeted therapies, particularly with MDM2 and CDK4 inhibitors in liposarcomas (Constantinidou et al., 2012; Dickson et al., 2013,

TABLE 100.3 Chemotherapy Trials in Sarcoma

	NUMBER OF PATIENTS	PRIMARY RP LOCATION (%)	INTENT FOR CT	REGIMEN USED	RESPONSE RATES	R0 RESECTION	COMMENTS
RETROPERITONEAL SARCOMA NOS							
Miura et al., 2015	8653	100%	NAC: 11% None: 89%	NR	NAC (yes/no) OS 40 vs. 52 months	40.3%	Poorer survival outcomes demonstrated with use of CT
Bremjit et al., 2014	132	100%	NAC: 21% None: 79%	NR	No improvement in OS with NAC (HR = 1.6)	48%	No reported benefit with preoperative CT or radiation in survival outcomes
Gronchi et al., 2016	1007	100%	NAC: 15% Adjuvant: 3% None: 82%	NR	No improvement in OS with NAC (HR = 1.17)	95% (R0/R1 reported together)	No reported benefit with preoperative CT or radiation in survival outcomes
Movva et al., 2015	16,370	22%	Metastatic: 100%	NR	82.7 vs. 51.3 months (CT vs. not), HR = 0.85	NA	Stratified by histology, CT improved survival only for undifferentiated pleomorphic sarcoma
LIPOSARCOMA							
Jones et al., 2005	88	43%	Metastatic: 100%	Variable (Doxy/Ifos)	Well-differentiated 0% De-differentiated 25% Myxoid 48%	NA	Myxoid liposarcoma represents a CT-sensitive tumor relative to well-differentiated and de-differentiated liposarcomas
Italiano et al., 2012	208	77.5%	Metastatic: 100%	Antracycline-based regimen (85%)	1% CR 11% PR 48% stable disease 39% no response	NA	No notable differences between well-differentiated vs. de-differentiated in response
MYXOID LIPOSARCOMA							
Katz et al., 2012	37	4%	NAC: 70% Metastatic: 30%	Doxy/Ifos	0% CR 38% PR 62% Stable	80%	All patients with R0 resection also received preoperative XRT
SYNOVIAL SARCOMA							
Wu et al., 2017	89		NAC: 84%		NAC >> Adj		
Chakiba et al., 2014	65	42%	NAC: 69%				
Vlenterie et al., 2016	313	17%	Metastatic: 100%		Improved PFS (6.3 vs. 3.7 months) for SS vs. other histology		Demonstrated improved response in SS
MALIGNANT PERIPHERAL NERVE SHEATH TUMOR							
Hirbe et al., 2017	5	1 patient	NAC	Ifosphamide Epirubicin	80% response in tumor	100%	Limited data to only one patient receiving NAC

CT, Chemotherapy; HR, hazard ratio; NA, not applicable; NAC, neoadjuvant chemotherapy; NOS, not otherwise specified; NR, not reported; OS, overall survival; RP, retroperitoneal; SS, synovial sarcoma; XRT, x-ray therapy.

2016; Ray-Coquard et al., 2012), tyrosine kinase inhibitors in refractory soft-tissue sarcomas (Mahmood et al., 2011; Nakayama et al., 2016; van der Graaf et al., 2012), and immune-modulating therapies (Tseng et al., 2015).

> **KEY POINTS**
>
> - Adjuvant and neoadjuvant therapies will continue to be expanded and incorporated as part of the multimodal approach to cancer treatment.
> - No disease process has exemplified this more than the management approach for testicular cancer patients.
> - In sarcoma, the heterogeneity across the spectrum of histologic entities and their biologic differences in response to radiation and systemic therapies restrict one's ability to make sweeping recommendations as to the timing and sequencing of different therapies.
> - Accordingly, using a multidisciplinary team to explore all available options to ensure optimal management of the RP mass offers patients the greatest chance of a favorable outcome.

CONCLUSIONS

The evaluation, diagnostics, and therapeutic management strategies of the RP mass requires careful initial consideration. Although many entities discovered are managed with surgical excision, some follow divergent therapies that warrant accurate characterization up front to facilitate these decisions. For metastatic GCT, clinical pathways have been standardized, and referral to experienced centers for coordination of care is recommended. Similar recommendations exist for the presence of RP sarcomas, given their uncommon nature, variable clinical behavior, and need for multidisciplinary care. Multimodal therapy can be considered, but limited data exist regarding the role and impact of neoadjuvant or adjuvant therapies with chemotherapy or radiation in RP sarcoma treatment. Given that the majority of lesions occurring in the RP ultimately require surgical intervention, having an in-depth familiarity of these clinical entities, their radiographic and histologic features, and perioperative needs is essential for the optimization of care for these patients.

REFERENCES

The complete reference list is available online at ExpertConsult.com.

101 Open Surgery of the Kidney

Aria F. Olumi, MD, and Michael L. Blute, MD

HISTORICAL PERSPECTIVE

Kidney-related diseases have significantly helped our understanding of the normal physiology of the kidney. As a result of better understanding of the pathophysiology and anatomic structures of the kidney, surgical approaches to management of renally related disease have evolved. From the first successful nephrectomy in 1869 for management of ureterovaginal fistula to the first radical nephrectomy, renal vasculature and caval reconstructions and advances made in retroperitoneal and transabdominal approaches for renal surgery have all stemmed from improved understanding of the surgical anatomy of the kidney and its surrounding structures. Therefore, for appropriate decision making in the perioperative period, detailed knowledge of the renal anatomy is paramount. Renal anatomy has been discussed in detail in the anatomy chapters of this book, and it will not be repeated here. The reader is referred to those chapters for review and understanding of the important surgical anatomic landmarks necessary for renal surgery.

PREOPERATIVE EVALUATION AND PREPARATION

Before any renal surgery, a global assessment of the patient's renal function is important. Routinely, preoperative urinalysis, urine culture, and serum creatinine (SCr) and hemoglobin are evaluated. Patients with locally advanced or metastatic disease should be screened for hepatic dysfunction (Stauffer syndrome) and any associated coagulopathy. Renal function can be evaluated by estimating the **glomerular filtration rate (GFR) using the Modification of Diet in Renal Disease Study equation** (Levey et al., 1999):

$$\text{GFR (mL/min/1.73 m}^2\text{)} = 186 \times (\text{SCr})^{-1.154} \times (\text{Age})^{-0.203} \times (0.742 \text{ if female}) \times (1.212 \text{ if African-American})$$

Those in good health with two normally functioning kidneys are at low risk for requiring postoperative dialysis following open renal surgery; however, patients with GFR less than 60 mL/min or significant proteinuria are at increased risk for requiring dialysis. As a result, perioperative consultation with a nephrologist can be most useful in optimizing a patient's renal function pre- and postoperatively.

Assessment of cardiac and pulmonary status is important before any surgery, but because of the potential for significant cardiopulmonary compromise resulting from intraoperative positioning, potential for blood loss, and possible fluid shifts, particular care needs to be taken to maximize cardiopulmonary function preoperatively (Fleisher et al., 2007a, 2007b).

In the modern era, cross-sectional imaging is a necessary step before any renal surgery (Bradley et al., 2011). Computed tomography (CT) and/or magnetic resonance imaging (MRI) studies are useful for proper surgical planning and assessment of renal parenchyma, renal pelvis and ureter, and renal vasculature (Fig. 101.1) (Derweesh et al., 2003; Herts, 2005).

Renal artery embolization (RAE) has been employed for palliation of inoperable renal tumors to control bleeding for large locally advanced renal tumors (eFig. 101.2) (Klimberg et al., 1985). In addition, RAE has been utilized to aid in surgical dissection of large renal tumors (Wszolek et al, 2008). Possible benefits of RAE before nephrectomy include shrinkage of an arterialized tumor thrombus to ease surgical removal, reduced blood loss, facilitation of dissection as a result of tissue plane edema, and ability to ligate the renal vein before the renal artery. However, because postinfarction syndrome, which includes flank pain, nausea, and fever, occurs in approximately three-fourths of patients, RAE is not utilized by all surgeons, and in some retrospective series RAE is associated with high blood loss, possibly secondary to the increased edema associated with the infarcted renal tissue (Schwartz et al., 2007).

Surgical site infection can be minimized by following the American Urological Association's guidelines (Wolf et al., 2008). A single dose of cefazolin or clindamycin for patients undergoing renal surgery with negative urine culture is prescribed. Any active urinary tract infection should be treated preoperatively.

Prophylactic Measures

Mechanical bowel preparation is not indicated for open renal surgery unless there is concern about intestinal involvement of a pathologic process or iatrogenic intestinal trauma is likely because of multiple prior abdominal surgeries, with likely requirement of extensive lysis of adhesions. When bowel preparation is utilized, potential adverse effects need to be considered, including chronic renal deficiency, particularly in older adults (Heher et al., 2008). For renal surgeries that may require long postoperative care and management in the intensive care unit, prophylaxis with proton pump inhibitors or sucralfate has been shown to reduce gastric stress ulcers (Bredenoord et al., 2013).

Although there is little evidence to support the use of thromboembolic prophylaxis for renal surgery, extrapolation from other similar surgeries suggests that routine use of intermittent pneumatic compression devices is useful to reduce the risk for postoperative deep venous thrombosis. The American College of Chest Physicians advises pharmacologic therapy once the bleeding risk has diminished (Geerts et al., 2008). The American Urological Association recommends use of mechanical prophylaxis in all patients undergoing open surgery and consideration of pharmacologic prophylaxis in patients with elevated risk for deep venous thrombosis.

For cigarette smokers who are anticipating elective open renal surgery, if time permits, a 4- to 6-week preoperative smoking cessation program has been shown to reduce postoperative complications. Other strategies to reduce postoperative respiratory complications include the use of incentive spirometry in high-risk patients or simply deep breathing exercises in low-risk individuals (Overend et al., 2001).

Surgical Instruments

Self-retaining retractors (Omni-Tract, Omni-Tract Surgical, St. Paul, MN; Bookwalter, Codman & Shurtleff, Raynham, MA; or Balfour, Sklar Surgical Instruments, West Chester, PA), long genitourinary surgical instruments, bulldog and/or Satinsky vascular pedicle clamps, surgical clips, and a suction drain are common instruments available and used for most open renal surgeries.

SURGICAL APPROACHES

Adequate exposure is the hallmark of effective open renal surgery. Anatomic knowledge and consideration of adjacent visceral organs

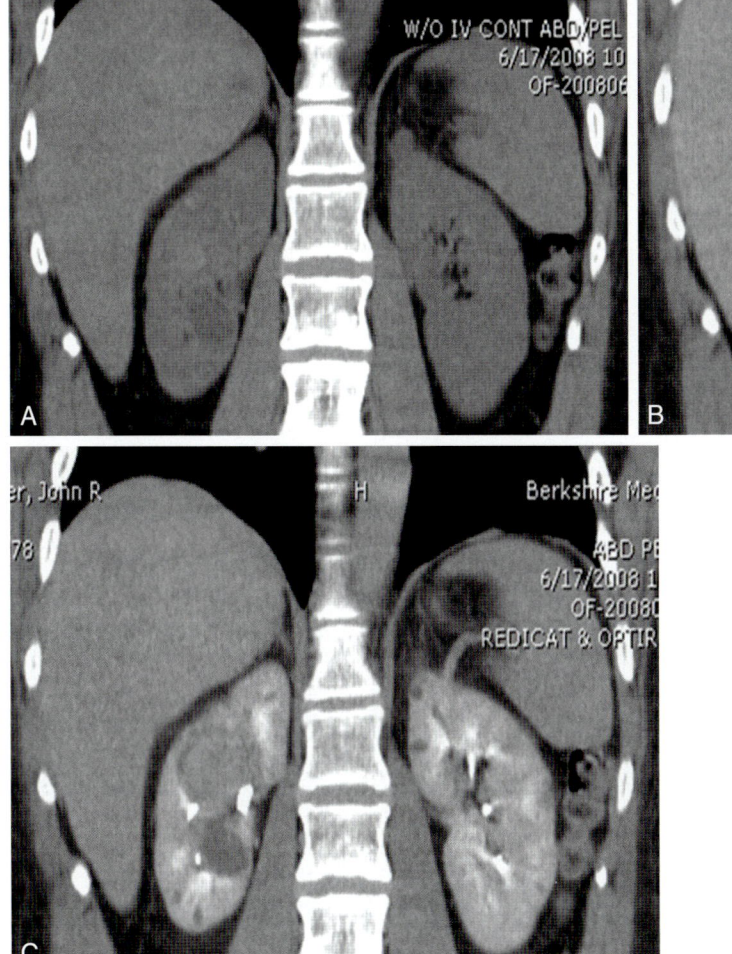

Fig. 101.1. (A) Preoperative computed tomography imaging demonstrates a large (4-cm) hilar lesion during a noncontrast film in a patient with a history of von Hippel-Lindau disease. (B) Contrast administration demonstrates enhancement of a large intrarenal mass and nearby simple cyst. (C) Delayed images depict close proximity to collecting system.

during the surgical approach are critical for safe surgical management. For right kidney surgery, the liver, colon, and duodenum serve as critical landmark structures, and for left kidney surgery, the spleen, tail of the pancreas, and colon need to be heeded. Proper incision and exposure minimize the amount of required retraction and minimize the likelihood of retractor-related injuries. The ideal surgical approach is tailored not only to the operation being performed but also to the anatomy as defined on preoperative imaging, previous surgical history, body habitus, and presence of limiting factors such as kyphoscoliosis or pulmonary disease (Wotkowicz and Libertino, 2007).

Flank Approaches

For a flank incision, with the patient in the lateral decubitus position, the table is flexed between the iliac crest and costal margin. With the kidney bar raised, the structures of the retroperitoneum are better exposed; however, care needs to be taken to avoid injury to a previously repaired contralateral kidney.

Flank approaches may not be ideal in patients with preexisting cardiopulmonary deficits because exaggerated lateral decubitus positioning may compromise pulmonary function and venous return to the heart. In patients with severe kyphosis, the flank approach may not allow proper exposure of the retroperitoneum and may lead to unanticipated pressure on the flank and vertebral bones.

Therefore, the surgeon needs to be familiar with other approaches and tailor the incision for each individual case.

Subcostal Flank Approach

The subcostal approach provides excellent exposure to the proximal ureter and renal parenchyma. It is well suited for approaches to the lower renal pole, ureteropelvic junction, and proximal ureter. However, access to the renal hilum is poor, making the subcostal approach somewhat limiting for management of large renal masses. In addition, it is not an ideal approach for partial nephrectomy because excellent exposure and access to the renal hilum are required (Fig. 101.3).

After induction of anesthesia, insertion of an endotracheal tube, and introduction of a Foley catheter into the urinary bladder to monitor urine output, the patient is placed in the lateral decubitus position. The head is supported to avoid excess flexion at the cervical spine. A kidney bar can be employed if necessary; the tip of the 12th rib should be positioned over the kidney bar (eFig. 101.4). The patient's back is supported by a rolled blanket or surgical beanbag. To preserve stability and prevent forward roll, the dependent leg is flexed at the hip and knee, and the top leg is kept straight. A pillow is placed between the knees. An axillary roll is deployed just caudal to the axilla to prevent compression or injury of the axillary neurovascular bundle. Other pressure points, including the upper foot,

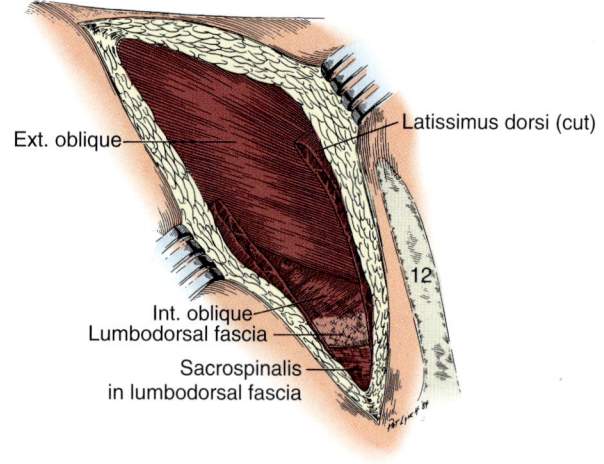

Fig. 101.3. Left subcostal incision. The latissimus dorsi muscle has been divided to expose the lumbodorsal fascia and the posterior aspects of the abdominal muscles.

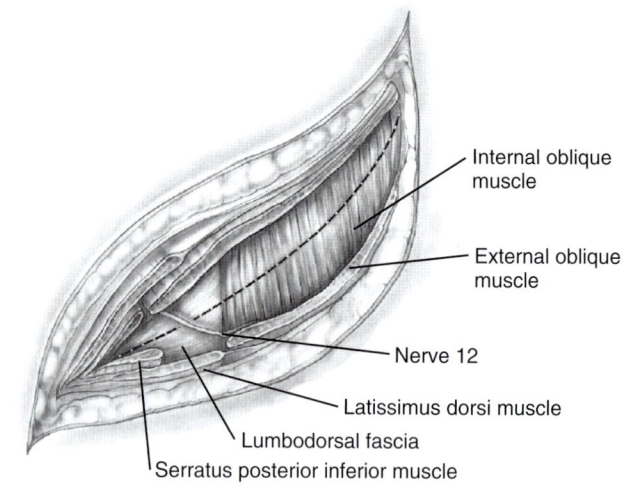

Fig. 101.6. Dissection through flank muscles. (From Libertino JA, ed. *Reconstructive urologic surgery*. 3rd ed. Philadelphia, PA: Mosby; 1998.)

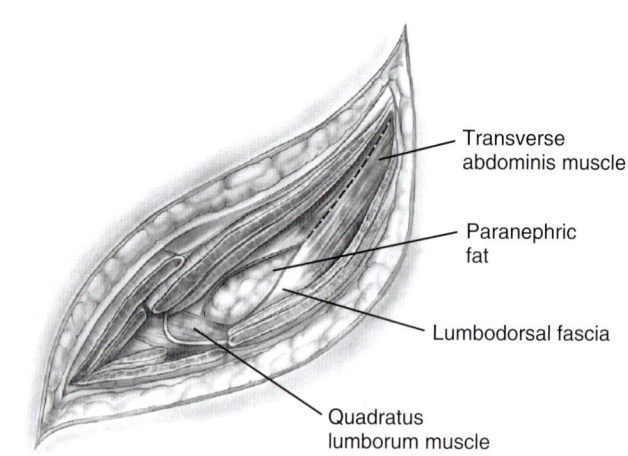

Fig. 101.7. Opening lumbodorsal fascia to gain entrance to retroperitoneum. (From Libertino JA, ed. *Reconstructive urologic surgery*. 3rd ed. Philadelphia, PA: Mosby; 1998.)

are padded with foam. The nondependent arm should be placed on a padded Mayo stand so that the arm is horizontal with slight forward rotation at the shoulder. The bed is flexed until the flank muscles are under stretch. The bed is placed in the Trendelenburg position so that the flank is rendered parallel to the floor. The patient is secured to the mobile part of the operating table with 2-inch-wide adhesive tape, which fixes the patient in place while allowing adjustment of flexion.

After sterile preparation and draping, the skin incision begins at the costovertebral angle, approximately at the lateral border of the sacrospinalis muscle just inferior to the 12th rib. The incision is made a fingerbreadth below and parallel to the 12th rib and is carried onto the anterior abdominal wall. In an attempt to avoid the subcostal nerve, the incision can be curved gently downward at the midaxillary line. If needed, the incision can be extended caudally or medially to the lateral border of the rectus abdominis.

The incision is carried sharply through the subcutaneous tissue, exposing the fascia of the latissimus dorsi and external oblique muscles. Electrocautery is used to incise the muscles in the line of the incision, starting with the latissimus dorsi posteriorly (eFig. 101.5). The posterior inferior serratus muscles, which insert into the lower four ribs, are also encountered in the posterior portion of the wound and transected. In the anterior aspect of the wound, the external oblique muscle is divided. These maneuvers expose the fused lumbodorsal fascia, which gives rise to the internal oblique and transversus abdominis muscles. The lumbodorsal fascia and internal oblique muscle are divided (Fig. 101.6). By using two fingers inserted into an opening created in the lumbodorsal fascia at the tip of the 12th rib, the peritoneum is swept medially as the transversus abdominis is split digitally. The subcostal nerve should be identified between the internal oblique and transversus abdominis muscles and spared (Figs. 101.7 and 101.8).

To maximize exposure in the posterior aspect of the incision, one may incise the posterior angle of the lumbodorsal fascia, exposing the sacrospinalis and quadratus lumborum muscles. Dividing the costovertebral ligament permits superior retraction of the 12th rib if enhanced exposure is deemed necessary. A Bookwalter flank retractor is used for exposure.

Supracostal Flank Approach

The supracostal flank incision (above the 11th or 12th rib) is favored by many open renal surgeons. An extraperitoneal, extrapleural approach can potentially minimize postoperative complications and lead to a more rapid recovery. Turner Warwick (1965), who popularized the approach, believed that the supracostal approach provides maximal posterior exposure, simplifies wound closure, and is less morbid than a transcostal incision requiring rib resection. More recently, an 8-cm modified mini-flank supra–11th rib incision has been described as a safe, effective approach to radical or partial nephrectomy for renal cortical tumors (Diblasio et al., 2006).

The level of the incision is determined by the patient's anatomy, the location of the lesion, and the planned procedure. Positioning is similar to that described for the subcostal flank approach.

A skin incision at the superior aspect of the 11th or 12th rib is made, beginning at the lateral border of the sacrospinalis muscle and continuing to the lateral border of the ipsilateral rectus abdominis muscle. The incision is carried through the subcutaneous tissue. The latissimus dorsi and posterior inferior serratus muscles are transected in the posterior aspect of the wound, revealing the intercostal muscles.

The external and internal oblique muscles are divided. The lumbodorsal fascia is opened at the tip of the rib to avoid both peritoneum and pleura. Moving medially, the transversus abdominis muscle is divided carefully while sweeping the peritoneum medially and inferiorly. The diaphragm is exposed by transection of the transversalis muscle. The pleura is identified between the divided transversus abdominis muscle and the diaphragm and can be mobilized superiorly.

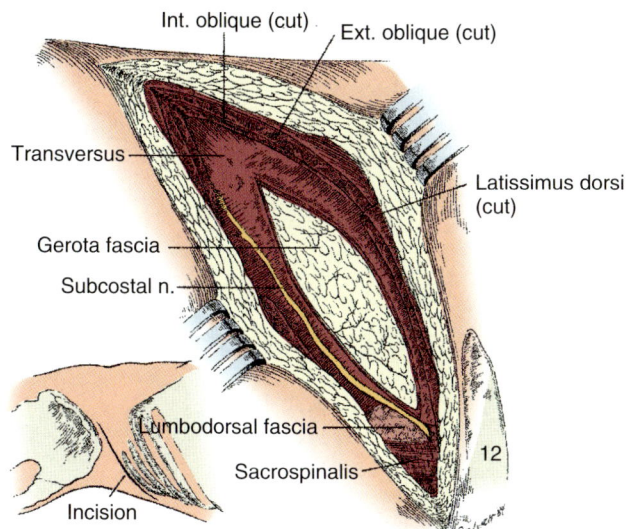

Fig. 101.8. The lumbodorsal fascia and transverse abdominal muscle have been divided to expose the Gerota fascia. The subcostal nerve and vessels pierce the lumbodorsal fascia posteriorly and course forward on the transverse abdominal muscle.

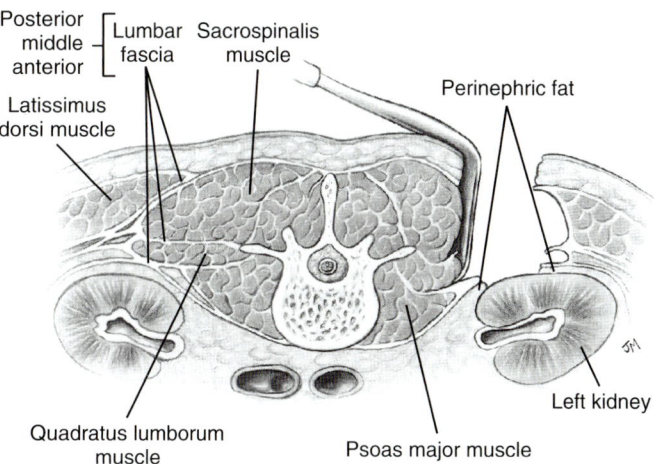

Fig. 101.10. Cross-sectional view of Gil-Vernet approach. (From Libertino JA, ed. *Reconstructive urologic surgery*. 3rd ed. Philadelphia, PA: Mosby; 1998.)

The lateral aspect of the sacrospinalis is identified and is either incised or retracted to permit access to the neck of the rib and its attachments. Division of the intercostal muscles should start at the most distal aspect of the rib and proceed toward the spine. The corresponding intercostal nerve is identified and spared. To avoid the neurovascular bundle, the intercostal muscles are divided in close proximity to the superior aspect of the rib. The plane between the chest wall and pleura is developed by entering the investing fascia surrounding the intercostal nerve, which allows an extrapleural dissection (eFig. 101.9). The slips of the diaphragm attached to the inferior ribs are transected.

Dorsal Lumbotomy Approach

This approach is typically reserved for pediatric patients and for thin adults requiring bilateral nephrectomy. The advantage to this approach is low morbidity because no muscle is transected. The main disadvantage is lack of exposure, particularly to the renal hilum and its vessels, making this approach very challenging, particularly for obese and muscular individuals and patients with high-riding enlarged kidneys (Andaloro and Lilien, 1975; Gardiner et al., 1979; Novick, 1980).

The patient is first anesthetized and intubated in the supine position. The patient is then rolled into the prone position (ventral decubitus/ventral recumbent position) with the help of several operating room personnel, and the operating table is flexed approximately 10 degrees. The arms may be tucked inward or positioned and supported cranially in an overhead swimming position. To protect the face and endotracheal tube, a C-shaped face support or doughnut-shaped foam pad may be used. The head can be rotated sideways or face downward. Eyes and ears are appropriately padded. To avoid axillary plexus injury, the humerus should not be forced into the axilla. The elbow should be flexed approximately 90 degrees and padded to prevent ulnar nerve injury. The knees should be padded and, to avoid pressure injury to the toes, the ankles should be supported and raised so that the toes do not touch the operating table. If necessary, the breasts should be displaced medially and cranially. Women who are pregnant or lactating, have breast implants, are obese, or have enlarged breasts are at risk for trauma to their breasts. The penis and scrotum should not be compressed by the body weight. In cases in which there are bowel/urinary abdominal stomas, extreme care should be taken to avoid excess pressure on these structures. In such cases, longitudinal torso frames/rolls should be used to minimize pressure from the anterior chest/abdominal structures.

The prone position may be poorly tolerated by older adults, patients with cervical spine pathology, patients with unstable chest walls following trauma, and patients with a known thoracic outlet syndrome. From a cardiovascular standpoint, the thoracic outlet syndrome (resulting from an anomalous cervical rib or some other anatomic reason) can occur particularly when the arms are located in the swimmer's position and the head is turned to one side. Because of increased pressure on the sternum, unanticipated pressure may be generated on the mediastinum, reducing coronary blood flow. Hemodynamically, the central venous pressure may rise, resulting in venous engorgement and potentially increased bleeding. From a respiratory standpoint, an increased amount of work is required to breathe when prone, an endotracheal tube can be displaced accidentally, and the risk for venous air embolism from central lines is increased. From a neurologic standpoint, rotation of the head can modify the cerebral blood flow and place the patient at risk for cerebral ischemia.

The dorsal lumbotomy approach is an anatomic approach to the kidney, with incision of fascial planes rather than muscle (Fig. 101.10). A vertical skin incision is made from the inferior border of the 12th rib to the iliac crest, in line with the lateral border of the sacrospinalis muscle. The subcutaneous tissues are divided, exposing the latissimus dorsi muscle. The aponeurosis of the latissimus dorsi is separated from the posterior layer of the lumbodorsal fascia where it overlies the sacrospinalis muscle. The posterior layer of the lumbodorsal fascia, a strong fascial covering, is incised, which allows the sacrospinalis muscle to be retracted medially. The costovertebral ligament is divided, which permits superolateral retraction of the 12th rib, which improves access superiorly. The fused middle and anterior layers of the lumbodorsal fascia are divided, permitting the quadratus lumborum muscle to be retracted medially. The ilioinguinal nerve should be identified and spared. Entry into the paranephric space is achieved by incising the transversalis fascia. Division of the perinephric fascia reveals the kidney.

Thoracoabdominal Approach

The thoracoabdominal approach (Fig. 101.11) is ideal for the management of large renal masses, suprarenal or upper pole masses, renal tumors with venous extension, and tumors involving adjacent structures.

The patient is positioned in a semioblique manner as described earlier for the flank approaches, with a rolled blanket or beanbag supporting the flank. The legs are positioned similarly to the traditional flank position. The pelvis is rotated to a more horizontal position than for the flank incisions, at an angle of approximately 45 degrees.

The level of the incision is determined by the nature of the tumor, including size and relationship to surrounding structures. Depending

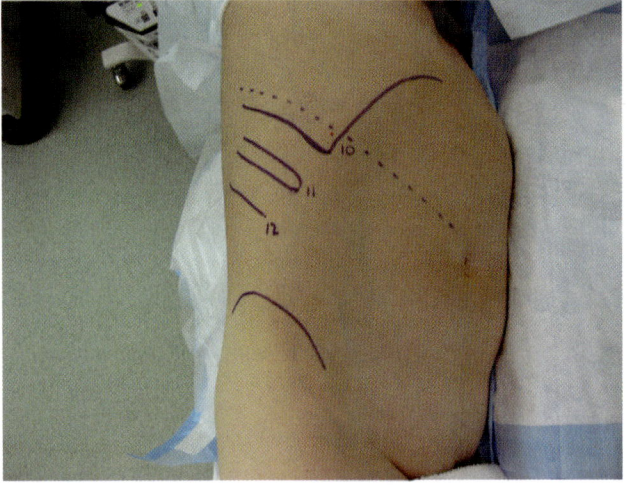

Fig. 101.11. Thoracoabdominal incision at the supra–10th rib border with the patient in the lateral decubitus position.

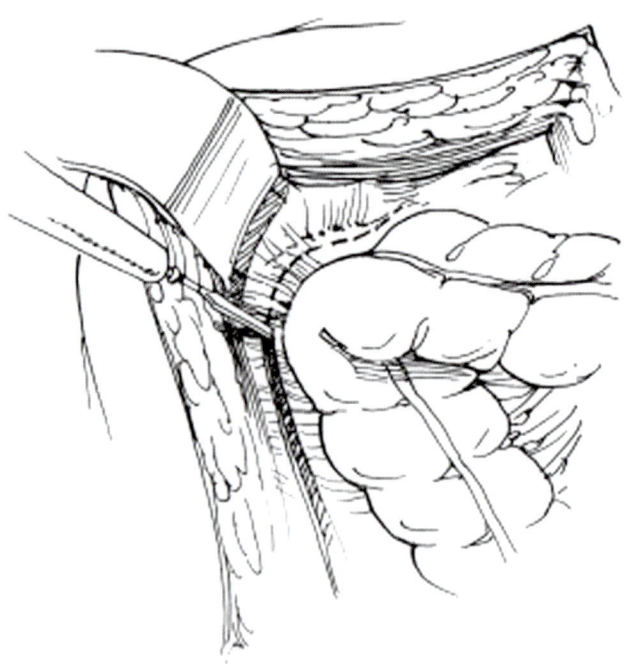

Fig. 101.14. The white line of Toldt is incised from the hepatic flexure to the common iliac artery, and the ascending colon is reflected medially. (From Smith JA Jr, Howards SS, Preminger GM, eds. *Hinman's atlas of urologic surgery.* 3rd ed. Philadelphia, PA: Saunders; 2012.)

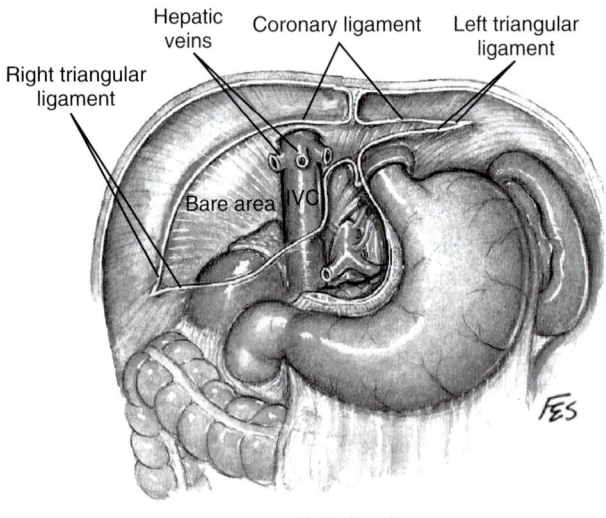

Fig. 101.12. Relationship of the liver and triangular and coronary ligaments to the inferior vena cava *(IVC)*. (© The Lahey Clinic.)

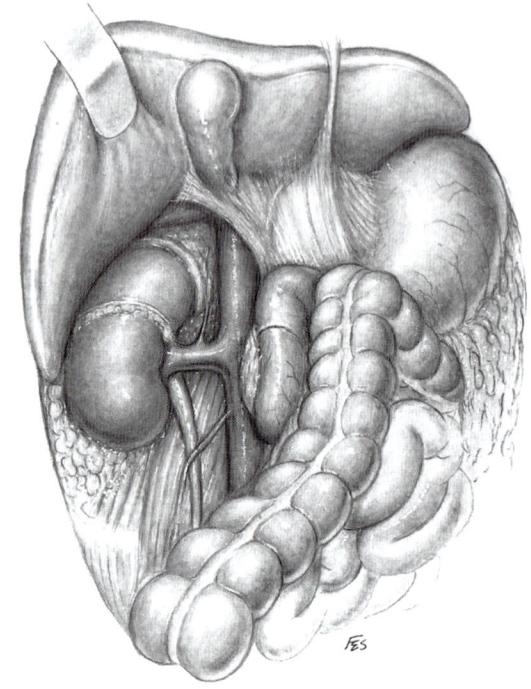

Fig. 101.16. Access to the vena cava can be achieved using the Langenbeck maneuver whereby the right triangular and coronary ligaments of the liver are divided, permitting the right lobe of the liver to be rotated medially and cephalad, exposing the retrohepatic inferior vena cava up to the diaphragms. (© The Lahey Clinic.)

on the location of the tumor, access is gained through the 8th, 9th, 10th, or 11th intercostal space. The skin incision begins at the lateral aspect of the sacrospinalis muscle over the 10th or 11th rib and can travel as far as the contralateral rectus abdominis muscle or caudally toward the symphysis pubis.

The internal oblique and transversus abdominis muscles are transected. The underlying peritoneum is opened, and the peritoneal cavity and chest are entered. Staying close to the superior border of the rib, the intercostal muscles are divided, which exposes the underlying pleura and diaphragm. The pleura is opened sharply, taking care to avoid the lung. The costovertebral ligament is divided. The diaphragm is opened from its thoracic surface. Starting anteriorly and proceeding posteriorly, the diaphragm is opened in a curvilinear fashion staying about two fingerbreadths from the chest wall to avoid injuring the more central phrenic nerve.

The liver or spleen is gently retracted upward. Additional hepatic mobility can be obtained by dividing the coronary ligament and the right triangular ligament of the liver (Fig. 101.12, eFig. 101.13; Video 101.1). For right-sided tumors, the kidney and great vessels are approached by mobilizing the colon medially and kocherizing the duodenum (Fig. 101.14 and eFig. 101.15, Fig. 101.16). For left-sided tumors, the colon and the tail of the pancreas are mobilized (eFig. 101.17, Fig. 101.18).

Anterior Approaches

Anterior Midline Approach

An anterior midline incision is the incision of choice for management of renal trauma because it permits exploration for associated intraperitoneal injuries. It can also be employed for renovascular surgery,

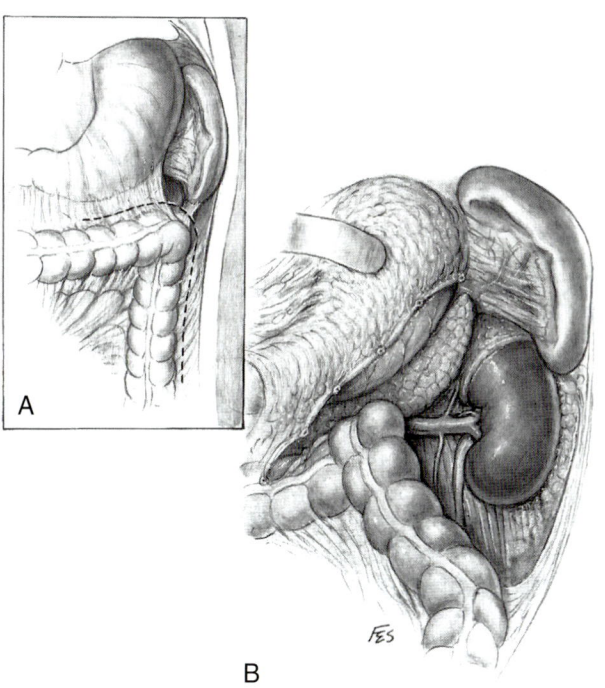

Fig. 101.18. (A) The left gastrocolic, phrenocolic, and lateral peritoneal attachments are divided. (B) The stomach, pancreas, and spleen are gently retracted upward without mobilizing the kidney. (© The Lahey Clinic.)

for reconstructive procedures, including ileal ureteral replacement, and for bilateral renal procedures.

With the patient in the supine position, a midline skin incision is carried out between the xiphoid process and the symphysis pubis. After dividing the subcutaneous tissues with electrocautery, the linea alba is sharply incised to expose the underlying preperitoneal fat and peritoneum. The peritoneum is grasped with two smooth forceps and incised. The ligamentum teres should be divided and suture-ligated.

Control of the renal pedicle can be obtained directly through the posterior parietal peritoneum or by medial reflection of the colon. On the left, the approach involves a vertical incision in the posterior peritoneum below the ligament of Treitz. This space contains the anterior surface of the aorta, the crossing left renal vein, and often the inferior mesenteric vein (IMV) and gonadal vessels. The superior mesenteric artery (SMA) should be on the anterior surface of the aorta and is usually 1 to 2 cm cephalad to the left renal vein. Gentle dissection along the hilum at this level provides good vascular control. A second approach to the left renal hilum is through the lesser sac. In this approach, the gastrocolic omentum is divided and entered. The transverse colon can then be retracted inferiorly. The peritoneum below the pancreas can be incised. The vessels are identified. This permits access to the renal pedicle both anteriorly and posteriorly. The artery can be isolated posteriorly and the venous system identified and controlled anteriorly.

Similarly, the right kidney can be reached directly by incision of the hepatic flexure and the Kocher maneuver to free the duodenum and reflect it medially. Further incision along the white line of Toldt frees the colon, permitting exposure of the anterior Gerota fascia. After the duodenum is reflected, the anterior surface of the vena cava is exposed. Care is taken not to injure the pancreas, gonadal vein, adrenal vein, or accessory renal vessels. The main renal vein is mobilized. Posterior to the renal vein along its superior margin lies the renal artery (eFig. 101.19), which normally runs a retrocaval course. The renal artery can be isolated here or between the vena cava and aorta when greater length is required.

Anterior Subcostal Approach

For the anterior subcostal approach, the patient is placed in the supine position. Some surgeons choose to place a rolled blanket under the lumbar spine to facilitate exposure with hyperlordosis. However, **excessive hyperlordosis can lead to excessive unwanted tension on the great vessels, minimizing blood flow. Also, excessive hyperlordosis may lead to postoperative lower back pain. In patients with spinal stenosis, hyperlordosis is not recommended.** In the supine position, the arms can be tucked at the side or abducted at 90 degrees while supported on arm pads. The elbows should be well protected with adequate padding to avoid ulnar nerve injury.

The supine position can cause several important problems; therefore care should be taken to avoid complications from positioning. The pressure points (occiput, dorsal torso, sacrum, dorsal legs, and heels) should be well padded. From a cardiovascular perspective, supine positioning can result in supine hypotension (aortocaval syndrome) if excess adiposity or abdominal masses compress the great vessels. From a musculoskeletal perspective, low back pain is frequent, particularly in patients with scoliotic and kyphotic spine deformities. Artificial hip and knee joints may also be placed under stress.

Chevron Incision (Bilateral Anterior Subcostal Approach)

The chevron incision, which is composed of bilateral anterior subcostal incisions, is ideal for renovascular surgery and radical nephrectomy with inferior vena cava (IVC) tumor thrombectomy. Exposure of the renal pedicles and great vessels is outstanding. The incision starts at the tip of the 11th rib, extends approximately two fingerbreadths below and parallel to the costal margin, curves superiorly in the midline, travels parallel to the contralateral costal margin, and terminates at the tip of the contralateral 11th rib.

SURGERY FOR BENIGN DISEASES

Simple Nephrectomy

Simple nephrectomy—removal of the kidney within the Gerota fascia—is used to manage nonmalignant diseases of the kidney (eFig. 101.20). Indications for simple nephrectomy include durable nonfunction or poor function of a kidney as a result of obstruction, infection, trauma, stones, nephrosclerosis, vesicoureteral reflux, polycystic kidney, or congenital dysplasia. Simple nephrectomy of a functional kidney may be employed to relieve intractable symptoms or associated problems, such as bleeding, pain, hypertension, or persistent infection.

Using one of the incisions described earlier, typically a flank incision, access to the retroperitoneal cavity is obtained. A self-retaining retractor (Finochietto, Bookwalter, or Omni-Tract retractor) is used to expose the visceral organs. The posterior layer of the renal fascia is bluntly dissected from the muscles of the posterior abdominal wall. The anterior layer of renal fascia is dissected from the colonic mesentery and peritoneum, leaving a fascial compartment in which the kidney, adrenal gland, and perirenal fat lie. The renal fascia is incised, and the perirenal fat is separated from the kidney using a combination of blunt dissection and electrocautery. Improper entry into the subrenal capsule must be avoided as this can lead to additional bleeding and difficulty in identifying the appropriate surgical planes. The surgeon must beware of aberrant vessels, typically found near the poles and in areas resistant to blunt dissection. In cases in which posterior dissection is difficult because of adherence of the kidney to the psoas muscle, inclusion of the psoas fascia in the dissection may be helpful and necessary. In cases of a large hydronephrotic kidney, in which exposure can be difficult, puncture and aspiration of the renal pelvic contents may decompress and aid mobilization of the kidney. Next, the adrenal gland is dissected from the upper pole of the kidney by maintaining the dissection plane directly on the renal capsule. The superior attachments of the kidney to the spleen, pancreas, and liver are freed to allow safe caudal retraction of the kidney.

Next, the lower pole of the kidney is mobilized and the ureter isolated, and the gonadal vein, usually found adjacent to the ureter, is identified. Care should be taken to mobilize the gonadal vein medially to avoid traction injury and avulsion of the vein. Once the

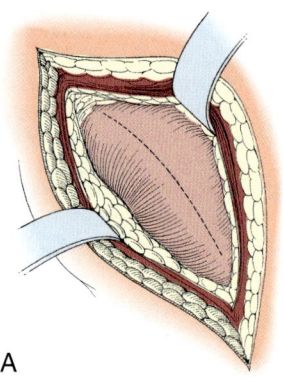 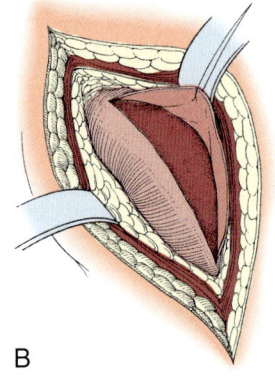 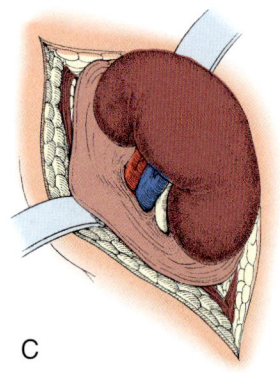 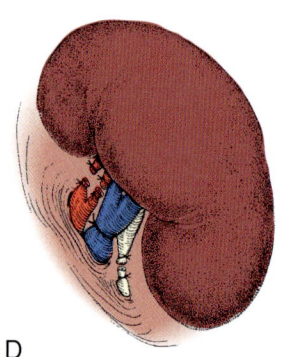

Fig. 101.21. (A to D) Technique of subcapsular nephrectomy.

inferior pole is mobilized, the ureter can be divided in between surgical clips or 2-0 silk ties. Division of the ureter provides access to the posterior part of the kidney and better exposure of the renal hilar structures. From a caudocranial approach, the renal vein is usually identified after division of the ureter. Combination of blunt and sharp dissections will allow identification of the renal artery posterior to the renal vein (Fig. 101.21).

Partial Nephrectomy for Benign Disease

Partial nephrectomy, in addition to its common utilization for treatment of small-sized renal cancer, can sometime be used for benign diseases. Some clinical scenarios in which partial nephrectomy may be indicated in benign diseases include hydronephrosis with parenchymal atrophy, atrophic pyelonephritis in a duplicated kidney, infected calyceal diverticulum, segmental traumatic renal injury with irreversible damage, and removal of benign renal tumors (angiomyolipoma or oncocytoma).

Partial nephrectomy for benign disease entities can be approached by excision of the renal capsule from the diseased site. The excised renal capsule can be successfully used for renorrhaphy (Fig. 101.22). Further details and techniques of partial nephrectomy are described in the Partial Nephrectomy for Malignant Disease section later in this chapter.

Open Nephrostomy

With the advancement in percutaneous nephrostomy tube placements, open surgical insertion of nephrostomy tubes is rare. However, when percutaneous nephrostomy tube placement is not technically feasible and endoscopic placement of a ureteral stent is not an option, open surgical placement of a nephrostomy tube can be a lifesaving procedure (eFig. 101.23).

Through a retroperitoneal flank incision, the Gerota fascia is identified and incised. The kidney is mobilized within the Gerota fascia to expose the posterior surface, and the ureter is identified inferiorly. The ureter is followed superiorly to identify the renal pelvis. The renal pelvis is incised after placement of two 2-0 absorbable Vicryl (Ethicon, Cincinnati, OH) holding sutures away from the ureteropelvic junction. Using a hooked scalpel or sharp tenotomy scissors, a 2-cm incision is made parallel to the long axis of the kidney between the holding sutures. Next, a stone forceps is passed through the pyelotomy incision into the lower pole calyx. The tip of the forceps is aimed at the convex border of the kidney, because a nephrostomy on the anterior or posterior surface of the kidney has a higher risk for hemorrhage from damage to intrarenal vessels. While pressure is applied with the forceps, the tip of the forceps is palpated at the convex border of the kidney. A radial capsulotomy is made over the tip of the forceps. The tract through the parenchyma is widened. From the exterior surface of the kidney, a Malecot catheter with a threaded 0 silk suture at the tip is guided through the renal parenchyma; the tip is placed in the renal pelvis, and the guiding 0 silk suture is removed. The Malecot catheter is secured to the renal capsule using a 3-0 absorbable purse-string suture, the pyelotomy is closed with 4-0 Vicryl sutures, and then the holding sutures are removed. The distal end of the Malecot catheter is externalized through a stab incision from the anterior flank, avoiding kinking of the tube to ensure proper drainage. The Malecot catheter is secured to the skin externally using a drain stitch (2-0 silk or 3-0 nylon). A Penrose drain or Jackson-Pratt drain (Cardinal Health, Dublin, OH) is placed in the perinephric area, and the flank incision is closed.

Extracorporeal Renal Surgery

Extracorporeal renal surgery (ECRS) with autotransplantation is an operative technique that is rarely used in contemporary urologic practice because open in situ renal exposure with vascular clamping and hypothermia provides excellent access to the kidney for nearly all forms of renal surgery. The advantages of ECRS are better exposure and illumination, a bloodless surgical field, the ability to protect the kidney from prolonged ischemia, and the opportunity to use an operating microscope (Husberg et al., 1975; Ota et al., 1967; Putnam et al., 1975). Currently, ECRS is reserved for reconstruction of complex renal pathologies in cases of a solitary kidney, when percutaneous approaches are not appropriate or possible, and when routine in situ operative exposure is inadequate (Fig. 101.24). Additionally, ECRS is used when addressing anatomic problems in a donated kidney that is destined for allogeneic transplantation. Specific indications for which ECRS may be a valid option are as follows:

Renovascular diseases
- Prolonged ischemia (>45 minutes) is anticipated
- Segmental renal artery disease
- Multivessel disease
- Arteriovenous malformations refractory to embolization
- Large intrarenal arterial aneurysms

Renal transplantation
- Repair of vascular anomaly
- Repair of collecting system anomaly

Malignancy in solitary kidney
- Large, central mass encroaching on the renal pedicle
- Large, central renal pelvic tumor
- Multiple subcortical neoplasms

Preoperative Considerations

Thorough abdominal imaging studies (CT scan and/or magnetic resonance angiogram) should be obtained to fully evaluate the renal parenchyma, collecting system, and vasculature. In select cases, digital subtraction arteriography may be used to evaluate the vascular anatomy.

Chapter 101 Open Surgery of the Kidney 2255

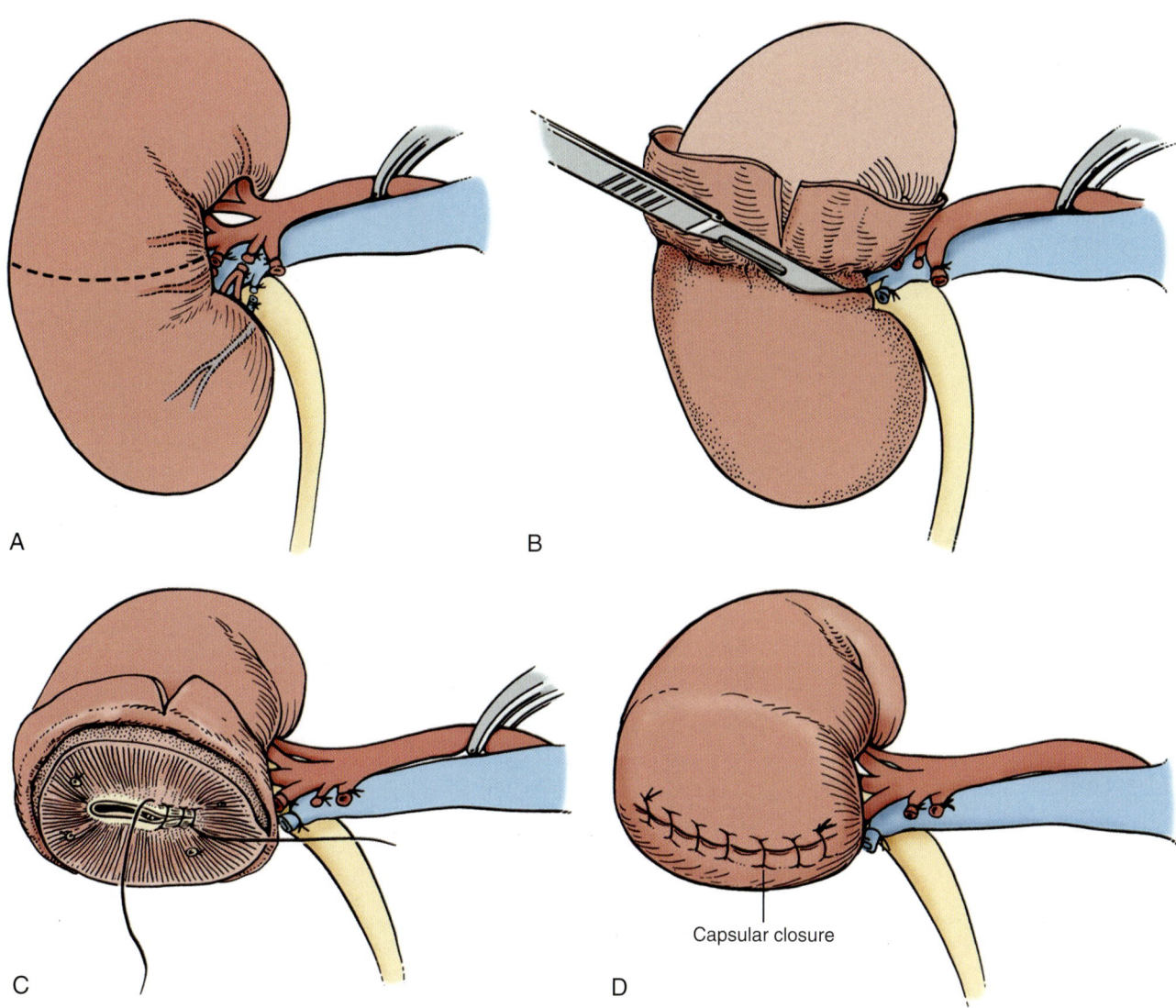

Fig. 101.22. (A to D) Technique of transverse renal resection for a benign disorder. The renal capsule from the diseased parenchyma is preserved and used to cover the transected renal surface.

The patient's renal function is assessed by serum creatinine level. Strong consideration should be given to obtaining a preoperative nephrology consultation to help maximize renal function preoperatively and to make necessary preparations in case of hemodialysis postoperatively.

A seated operative bench should be available with ice slush, renal transplant preservation solution (e.g., Euro-Collins or UW solution), and microvascular instruments.

Surgical Procedure

Because access to both the retroperitoneum and iliac fossa (for autotransplantation) is required, a number of different single- or double-incision approaches are possible. Following incision and abdominal exploration, the kidney is exposed as for a living related donor nephrectomy. When the kidney is mobilized and the only remaining attachments are the ureter, renal vein, and renal artery, 12.5 g of mannitol and 20 mg of furosemide are rapidly infused intravenously. The ureter is ligated as far distally as possible and transected, preserving as much periureteral tissue as possible. Although the ureter can be preserved intact, we do not favor this approach because it limits positioning the autotransplanted kidney in the opposite iliac fossa, and the long length of ureter is prone to ischemia and kinking, leading to obstruction. Vascular clamps are applied to each renal vessel directly where they exit the aorta and IVC (a C-shaped clamp is useful to gain length on the right renal vein), and the renal vessels are transected directly on the clamps.

Immediately after dividing the renal vessels, the kidney is placed on the workbench in a pan of ice slush covered with a towel. The kidney is flushed intra-arterially by gravity flow with renal preservation solution at 6° C. Flushing the kidney should continue until it is cooled and the renal effluent is clear (∼500 to 1000 mL). The kidney is kept in the ice slush basin during the procedure to maintain hypothermia.

For renovascular disease, the vasculature of the renal hilum is dissected and vascular repair is done. For neoplasms, the Gerota fascia and the perirenal fat are removed and partial nephrectomy is undertaken. After reconstruction of the renal vasculature or the nephrectomy parenchymal defect is achieved, the renal artery and vein are flushed independently with preservation solution to assess for potential sites of bleeding. Retrograde flushing of the ureter is done to assess for collecting system leaks, which should be repaired if identified.

The kidney may be transplanted into either lower quadrant. The kidney is transferred to the iliac fossa, and the renal vein is anastomosed to the external iliac vein. The renal artery anastomosis can be achieved by either end-to-end anastomosis to the hypogastric artery or end-to-side anastomosis with the external iliac artery. During

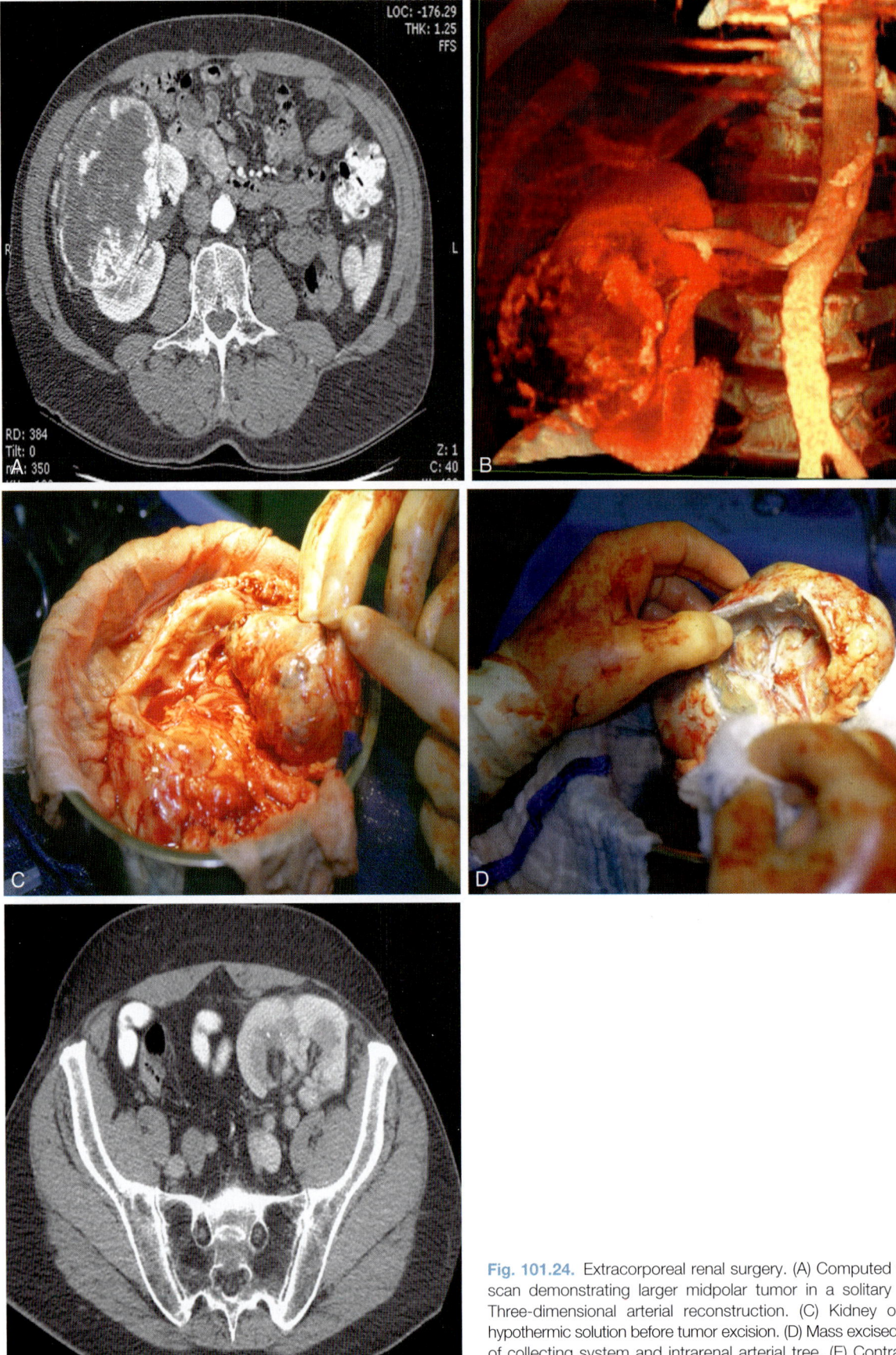

Fig. 101.24. Extracorporeal renal surgery. (A) Computed tomography (CT) scan demonstrating larger midpolar tumor in a solitary right kidney. (B) Three-dimensional arterial reconstruction. (C) Kidney on back table in hypothermic solution before tumor excision. (D) Mass excised with preservation of collecting system and intrarenal arterial tree. (E) Contrast-enhanced CT scan 4 years later demonstrating no evidence of recurrence.

the anastomosis, the vessels should be irrigated with heparin solution (10,000 units of heparin in 100 mL of normal saline), and the surgeon should consider injecting 10 mg of verapamil into the renal artery following the anastomosis to help vasodilation. The ureter is implanted into the dome of the bladder with a tension-free anastomosis. Before completion of the ureteral anastomosis, a ureteral stent is placed. Finally, a closed suction drain is placed.

SURGERY FOR MALIGNANCY
Radical Nephrectomy

Radical nephrectomy refers to complete removal of the kidney outside the Gerota fascia together with the ipsilateral adrenal gland and complete regional lymphadenectomy from the crus of the diaphragm to the aortic bifurcation, as described by Robson et al. (1969) for management of renal malignancy. Today, the adrenal gland is typically spared when technically possible because removal of the adrenal gland, when not involved by tumor, has not been shown to improve survival of patients with renal cancer. Extensive lymphadenectomy is only done in select cases when it is strongly felt that it may contribute to improved patient survival without adding complications to the patient's recovery.

Radical nephrectomy is reserved for renal tumors that are not amenable to partial nephrectomy. Indications for radical nephrectomy include tumors in nonfunctional kidneys, large tumors replacing the majority of renal parenchyma, tumors associated with detectable regional lymphadenopathy, or tumors associated with renal vein thrombus.

All renal tumors suspicious of malignancy should be staged with abdominopelvic CT or MRI and chest imaging with chest radiograph or chest CT (Fig. 101.25) (Bradley et al., 2011; Chen and Uzzo, 2011). If any sign of metastatic disease is present, a bone scan and head CT should also be obtained. The cross-sectional imaging should be closely evaluated for tumor thrombus, enlarged retroperitoneal nodes, and any embryologic abnormalities of the renal collecting system and vasculature.

Before surgery, percutaneous renal biopsy can be considered in patients with another malignancy to evaluate for potential metastatic disease, to evaluate for the possibility of lymphoma in cases of infiltrative-appearing renal masses on imaging studies and solid masses that will be managed nonoperatively with percutaneous modalities (radiofrequency or cryotherapy), or in nonoperative cases when the histology may dictate the type of systemic therapy (Pandharipande et al., 2010; Psutka et al., 2013;Volpe et al., 2007). In cases of bilateral renal tumors, percutaneous renal biopsy should be considered to guide management (Blute et al., 2000).

At times, preoperative angioembolization is undertaken for the kidney with a large renal mass and regional lymphadenopathy (Schwartz et al., 2007). Potentially, angioembolization can reduce the amount of intraoperative blood loss and provide the ability to ligate the renal vein before the renal artery, which may be necessary as a result of extensive hilar lymphadenopathy. Angioembolization may also reduce the size of the primary tumor, thereby technically improving the feasibility of nephrectomy. Disadvantages of angioembolization include postinfarction painful syndrome, risk for tumor lysis syndrome, risk for embolization of tumor thrombi, and risk for vascular trauma.

Ipsilateral adrenalectomy should be considered in large upper pole tumors when the surgical plane between the kidney and adrenal gland may be compromised. Otherwise, routine adrenalectomy is not required because the overall incidence of adrenal metastasis is less than 5%. Because preoperative CT and MRI may miss 20% to 25% of adrenal metastases, one must consider clinical indicators of adrenal involvement to guide surgical practice (Siemer et al., 2004). Typically, adrenalectomy is indicated when there is diffuse involvement by tumor, large tumor size (>10 cm), extrarenal tumor extension, tumor thrombus, lymphadenopathy and regional metastasis, or an adrenal mass on imaging.

Regional lymphadenectomy is not required in every radical nephrectomy because the overall incidence of lymph node disease is about 5%. Regional lymphadenectomy should be considered in patients who may have a reasonable chance of benefiting from the added surgery. Blute et al. and Crispen et al. discussed the probability of regional nodal involvement (Blute et al, 2004a; Crispen et al., 2011). Indications for regional lymphadenectomy include enlarged lymph nodes on imaging, cytoreductive surgery for metastatic disease, tumor size greater than 10 cm, nuclear grade 3 or greater, sarcomatoid histology, presence of tumor necrosis on imaging, extrarenal tumor extension, and tumor thrombus and direct tumoral invasion of adjacent organs.

In cases of adjacent organ involvement (colon and/or spleen), preoperative planning for splenectomy and/or partial colectomy is important (Blute et al., 2004a). Because of the presence of its bilaminar capsule, the liver is not usually directly invaded by renal tumors despite preoperative imaging studies that may suggest extension of right-sided renal tumors to the liver. However, in rare circumstances when a right-sided renal tumor does directly invade into the liver, appropriate preoperative surgical planning is essential.

Surgical Procedure

The most commonly used incisions for radical nephrectomy are subcostal flank incisions, which are described earlier in this chapter. In brief, for a subcostal approach, the patient is placed in a modified lateral decubitus position. After incising through the skin and muscular layers, a Balfour, Bookwalter, or Omni-Tract retractor is placed, and, for a right-sided approach, the liver and gallbladder are

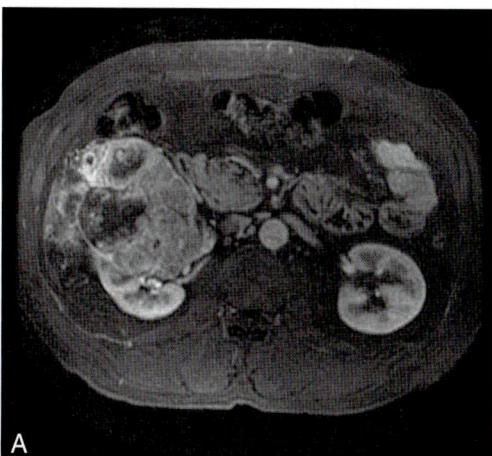 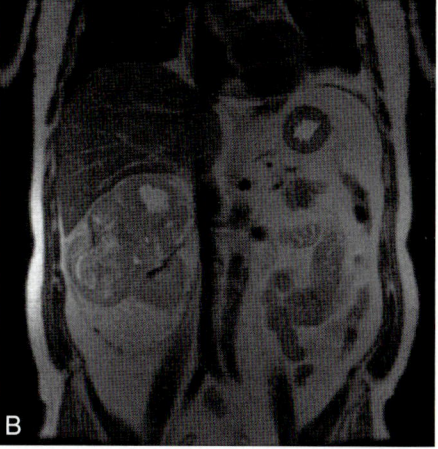

Fig. 101.25. Axial (A) and coronal (B) magnetic resonance images of a right-sided renal mass.

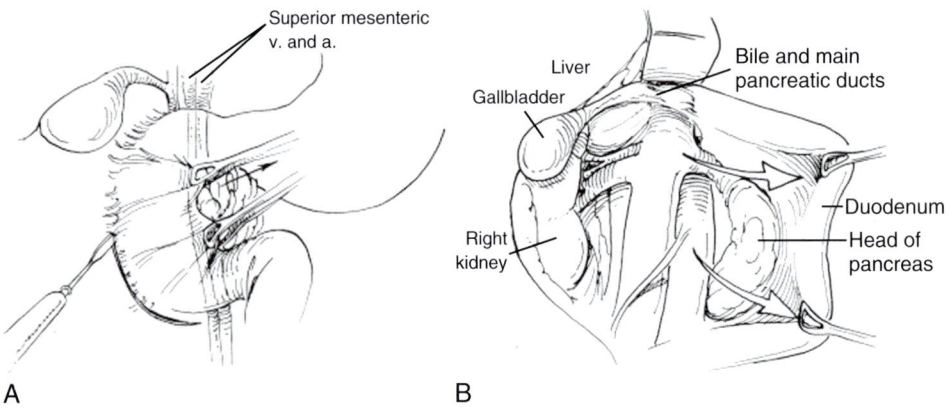

Fig. 101.26. (A and B) Kocher maneuver. (From Smith JA Jr, Howards SS, Preminger GM, eds. *Hinman's atlas of urologic surgery.* 3rd ed. Philadelphia, PA: Saunders; 2012.)

packed away superiorly. When additional mobilization of the liver is required, the avascular right triangular ligament is incised. The posterior parietal peritoneum on the white line of Toldt is incised from the pelvis (region of the iliac artery) to the right upper quadrant (region of hepatic flexure). The anterior pararenal space is developed by dissecting in the plane between the anterior renal fascia and the mesentery of the ascending colon. With large inflammatory masses, the anterior pararenal space may be difficult to develop. It is important to avoid injury to the ascending mesocolon because injury to the right colic and ileocolic arteries may devitalize this segment of colon. It is important to resect the renal fascia in its entirety for the best chance of surgical cure and to avoid intra-abdominal tumor spillage.

After mobilizing the hepatic flexure of the colon using sharp and blunt dissection, the second part of the duodenum is mobilized medially using the Kocher maneuver (Fig. 101.26). With medially located tumors, mobilization of the duodenum should be performed with extreme care to avoid injury.

After mobilization of the duodenum, the IVC is identified posteriorly. Dissection anterior to the IVC will enable identification of the renal vein and gonadal vein (on the right side). Placement of a vessel loop will enable gentle traction of the renal vein. The renal vein is palpated for any tumor thrombus. Next the renal artery is identified posterior to the renal vein. If identification of the renal artery is difficult, attention is turned to the lower pole of the kidney to identify the ureter and gonadal vein. If technically feasible, the gonadal vein is spared. However, often because of the large size of the renal tumor, the gonadal vein cannot be safely left intact without the risk for avulsion from the IVC (right side) or left renal vein. With ligation of the ureter, the kidney is lifted from a posterior to an anterior position to aid in identification of the renal artery posterior to the kidney.

Another option for identifying the right renal artery in difficult hilar dissections is to dissect in the interaortocaval region at its takeoff from the aorta (Fig. 101.27). The right renal artery can be ligated with a 0 silk suture or in emergent cases with a surgical clip. With the renal artery controlled, the right kidney and tumor will decrease in size and engorgement, easing the dissection of the kidney at the hilum and the remaining sites. The right renal vein, which should now be flaccid, is examined for any tumor thrombus and subsequently doubly ligated with a 0 silk tie and 2-0 silk suture ligature and divided. Identification of the renal artery should be technically much easier lateral to the IVC, which can now be doubly ligated and divided. Attention should be given to the lumbar veins, which enter the IVC (eFig. 101.28). If avulsed, bleeding should be controlled with suture ligatures and not surgical clips because surgical clips do not provide adequate hemostasis for the lumbar veins. These veins can retract, thereby exacerbating the degree of retroperitoneal bleeding, which will be difficult to access and control.

For left radical nephrectomy, after incision of the white line of Toldt from the splenic flexure to the common iliac artery, the descending

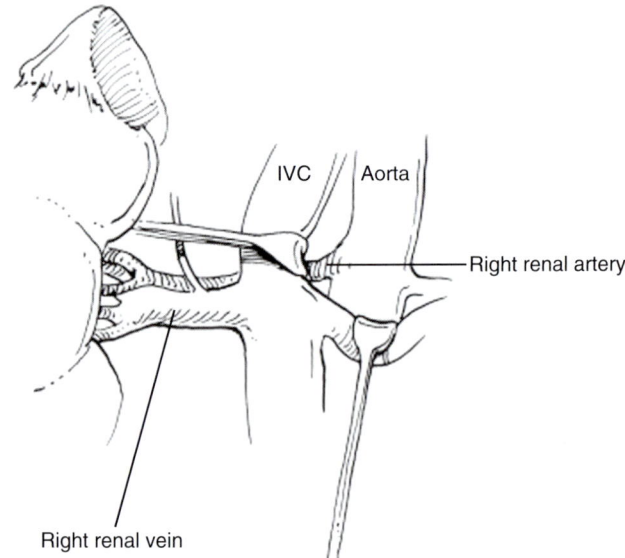

Fig. 101.27. The anteromedial surface of the inferior vena cava *(IVC)* can be used as a guide to identify the short right renal vein. The right renal artery is usually located deep to the right renal vein and is sometimes easier to identify in the interaortocaval groove. (From Smith JA Jr, Howards SS, Preminger GM, eds. *Hinman's atlas of urologic surgery.* 3rd ed. Philadelphia, PA: Saunders; 2012.)

colon is reflected medially. The renocolic ligament is divided, and extreme care is taken to avoid injury to the tail of the pancreas. The left renal vein is identified using the anterior surface of the aorta as a guide. The left renal artery is usually located cranial and posterior to the left renal vein. After further mobilization of the lower pole of the kidney, the left ureter and the left gonadal vein are identified. The left gonadal vein can be traced to its insertion to help identify the left renal vein. Depending on the size and location of the tumor, the surgeon determines whether the left gonadal vein should be left intact or tied off and transected to help with mobilization of the kidney. The ureter is divided, and the inferior and posterior surface of the kidney is mobilized to identify the left renal artery. Once the left renal artery and vein are identified, the renal artery is ligated with two right-angle clamps and divided. Preferably, the proximal end of the renal artery is clamped with two right-angle clamps and the distal end with one right-angle clamp. The renal artery is divided using a fine scalpel. The proximal end is ligated with a 0 silk suture and further secured with a 2-0 silk suture ligature; the distal end is tied with a 0 silk tie. With the renal artery secured and divided, the renal vein is secured and divided in a similar fashion.

At times, the renal artery and vein cannot be separated individually because of significant hilar lymphadenopathy. Then, a whole-pedicle clamp technique may be utilized to control the hilar vessels (eFig. 101.29). Although the risk for arteriovenous fistula may be associated with en bloc ligation of the whole renal pedicle (Lacombe, 1985), some small clinical series have not found any evidence of such fistulas in patients undergoing nephrectomy who have been managed with en bloc stapling of the renal hilum (Chung et al, 2013; Ou et al, 2008). The vascular pedicle is bluntly dissected until the pedicle has a 2- to 3-cm diameter. Long curved vascular clamps (e.g., Satinsky clamps) or renal pedicle clamps (e.g., Crawford, Young, Mayo) are used to clamp the renal artery and vein together. The pedicle is pinched, and the first clamp is placed at the lowermost aspect of the pedicle to ensure adequate length for ligation of the pedicle and that the clamp extends far enough beyond the structures within the pedicle to engage the suture. A second clamp is placed above and adjacent to the first under direct vision. A third clamp is placed on the pedicle near the renal parenchyma. The pedicle is divided between the second and the third clamps, leaving vascular stumps protruding. A 0 silk suture is looped below the lower clamp to tie off. It is prudent to tie the pedicle twice and also use suture ligature to minimize the risk with silk ties, which may slip off the vascular pedicle. Various other techniques can be utilized for controlling the vascular pedicles (Figs. 101.30 and 101.31).

In the emergent condition of loss of control of the renal hilar vascular pedicle, it is important to stay calm. The surgeon must inform the anesthesiologist and all operating room personnel of major bleeding and request aggressive hydration and availability of blood products. Compression can be applied using a fingertip or sponge stick to achieve hemostasis as best as possible so that the rest of the operating room staff can prepare. Compression can also be applied on the IVC and/or aorta to control bleeding. Two Yankauer suction tubes can be used to clear the surgical wound. Vascular occlusion clamps are used to clamp and ligate actively bleeding vessels. Clamping should not be done blindly; rather, one should suction, pack, retract, and dissect to get better exposure. If the bleeding is occurring from the renal artery, the surgeon can compress the aorta above the renal artery, clamp the arterial stump with a vascular clamp, and repair the defect with two layered running vascular sutures. If the bleeding is occurring from the IVC because of an avulsed or lacerated renal

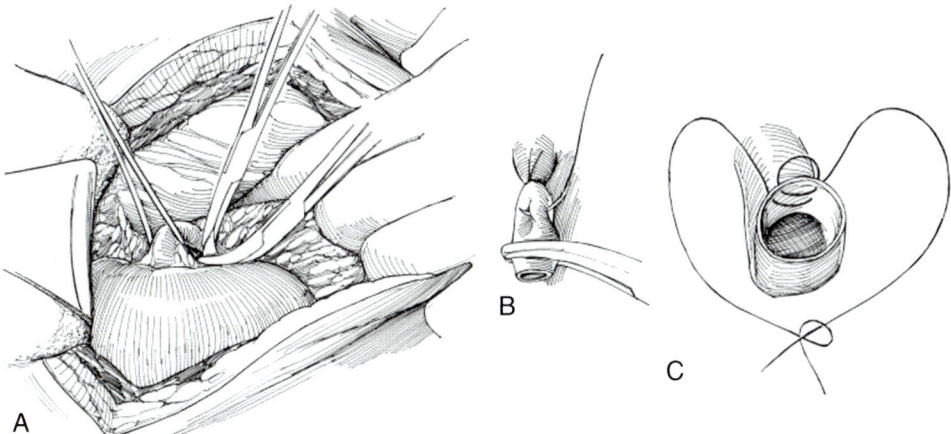

Fig. 101.30. (A to C) "Cut first, ligate second" method for securing the renal hilum. (From Smith JA Jr, Howards SS, Preminger GM, eds. *Hinman's atlas of urologic surgery*. 3rd ed. Philadelphia, PA: Saunders; 2012.)

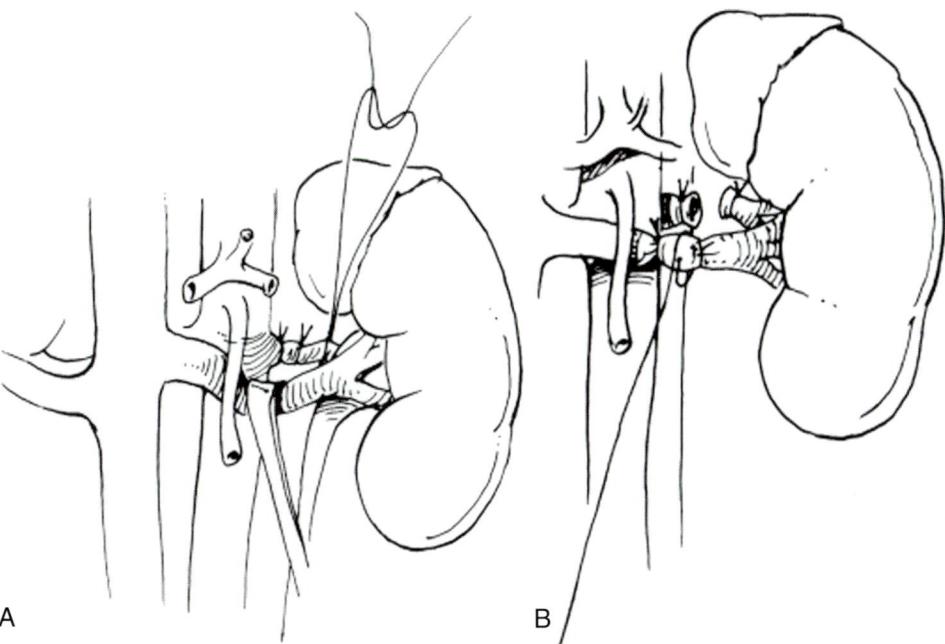

Fig. 101.31. (A and B) "Ligate first, cut second" method for securing the renal hilum. (From Smith JA Jr, Howards SS, Preminger GM, eds. *Hinman's atlas of urologic surgery*. 3rd ed. Philadelphia, PA: Saunders; 2012.)

vein, or avulsed gonadal or lumbar vein, a finger can be placed on the hole until the hole can be grasped with an Allis clamp (Scanlan International, St. Paul, MN). Pulling up on the clamp will normally stop the bleeding, allowing the defect to be visualized for repair.

For repair, polypropylene (Prolene) sutures (Ethicon, Cincinnati, OH)—typically 30 inch or 36 inch (75 cm or 90 cm)—are used; 3-0 or 4-0 sutures can be used for IVC or aortic repairs, and 4-0 or 5-0 sutures can be used for renal vessel repairs. We recommend using double-armed sutures with tapered needles—$\frac{3}{8}$-circle BB (17 mm) for arterial repair (they are less likely to fracture a calcific arterial plaque) and $\frac{1}{2}$-circle RB-1 (17 mm) or SH (26 mm) for venous repair.

Regional Lymphadenectomy for Renal Cancer

The role of regional lymphadenectomy for renal cell carcinoma (RCC) has remained controversial. Multiple retrospective studies have suggested a possible benefit to regional lymphadenectomy for carefully selected patients (Blute et al., 2004a; Crispen et al., 2011; Capitanio et al., 2013; Kim et al, 2004; Lam et al., 2004, 2006; Sun et al., 2014). A prospective randomized trial that was carried out by the European Organization for Research and Treatment of Cancer included 772 patients. Patients were randomly assigned to two groups—one that underwent regional lymphadenectomy and one that did not. Although no overall survival benefit was shown for patients who underwent regional lymphadenectomy for management of RCC, the study included a high percentage of patients with localized small and low-stage tumors who may not have benefited from lymphadenectomy at all (Blom et al., 2009).

For right-sided renal masses when lymphadenectomy is considered, the paracaval, precaval, retrocaval, and interaortocaval nodes from the right crus of the diaphragm to the bifurcation of the IVC are sampled (Fig. 101.32). A right-angle clamp and electrocautery are used to split the lymphatic tissue from the anterior surface of the IVC. The lymphatic tissue is cleared cranially from the right crus of the diaphragm (located 3 to 4 cm above the right renal vein) and caudally until the bifurcation of the IVC. The right gonadal vein is ligated at its insertion into the IVC with a 2-0 silk suture, to avoid avulsion of the vein. Next the lymphatic tissue is cleared off the lateral aspect of the IVC (paracaval nodes). The IVC is gently elevated with a vein retractor to expose the lumbar branches. The lumbar veins (typically four or five branches on either side of the IVC) are carefully ligated with 3-0 silk ties and transected. The lymphatic trunks located above the renal vein are ligated with surgical clips. Care to adequately ligate the lymphatic trunks is essential because large quantities of lymph and chyle drain through the cisterna chyli and thoracic duct, and failure to appropriately control them can result in chylous ascites (eFig. 101.33). Once the lumbar veins are secured and the superior aspect of the lymphatic trunk above the renal vein is secured, the assistant rolls the IVC medially with gentle pressure using two sponge sticks. Next the lymphatic tissue is cleared off the retrocaval region. The nodal tissue overlying the anterior surface of the aorta is then split and divided to the superior border of the left renal vein. Division of the nodal packet is followed to the medial border of the IVC, and the aortocaval nodal packet is cleared to the level of the common iliac vessels.

For left-sided renal masses, the lymphatic tissue on the anteromedial surface of the aorta is clipped and divided, and then rolled laterally (Fig. 101.34). The split is continued cranially along the aorta to the level of the SMA and caudally past the inferior mesenteric artery (IMA) to the bifurcation of the aorta. Although the IMA and the celiac trunk have to be preserved, the IMA can be tied and divided in case of involved lymphadenopathy. Once the lymphatics are dissected off the anterior and lateral surface of the aorta, the assistant gently elevates the aorta on either side to expose, secure, and divide the lumbar arteries. Once the lumbar arteries are properly secured, the aorta is rolled medially and the tissue between the anterior longitudinal vertebral ligament and the aorta (retroaortic lymph nodes) is resected. The interaortocaval nodes are resected only if they are palpable or visualized on preoperative imaging, or if there is extensive nodal involvement around the aorta.

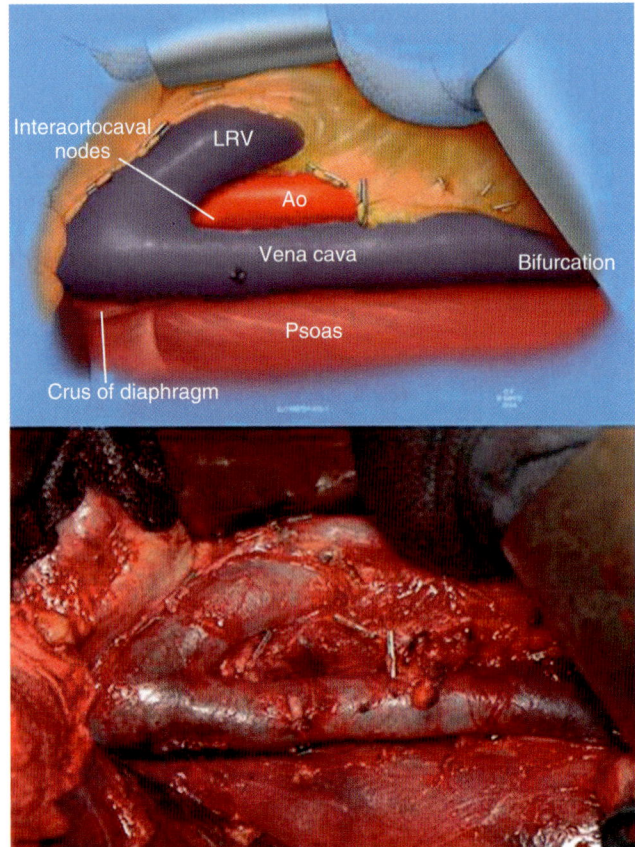

Fig. 101.32. Extended lymphadenectomy for right-sided renal masses. *Ao*, aorta; *LRV*, left renal vein.

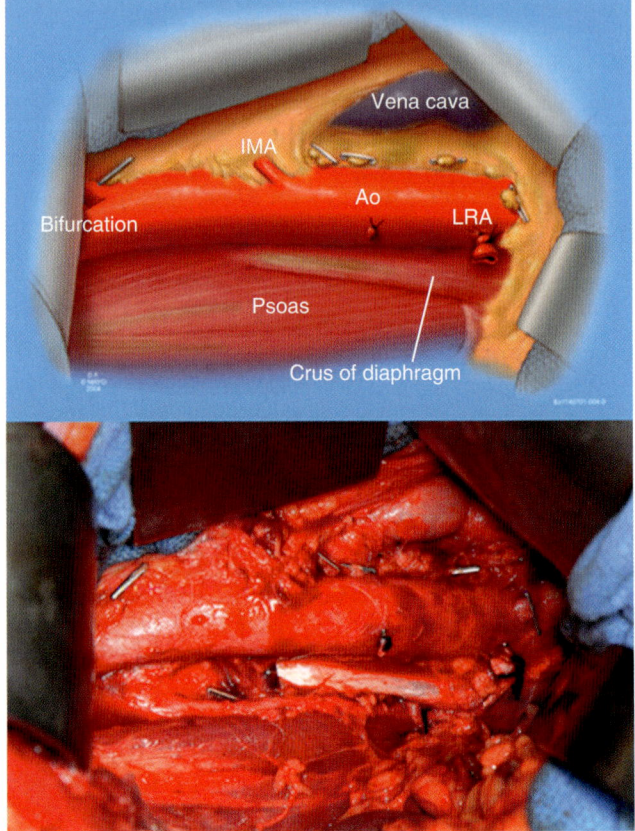

Fig. 101.34. Extended lymphadenectomy for left-sided renal masses. *Ao*, Aorta; *IMA*, inferior mesenteric artery; *LRA*, left renal artery.

Wound Closure

Once the surgical procedure is completed, the surgeon should investigate for hemostasis and evaluate adjacent organs for any signs of injury. The diaphragm and pleura are tissues that can be inadvertently injured secondary to retraction during radical open renal surgery. To test for pleural injury, the retroperitoneum is filled to the level of the flank incision with saline. The anesthesiologist then inflates the lungs with high inspiratory volumes. Bubbling of saline irrigation in the retroperitoneum with deep inspiration would suggest a pneumothorax. In case of a small pleural injury, the pleural cavity can be closed with running nonabsorbable sutures. Before complete closure of the pleura, the tip of a 14-Fr red rubber catheter is placed in the pleural cavity. The end of the catheter is placed in a saline-filled bowl. The anesthesiologist provides a deep inspiratory breath to evacuate any air from the pleural cavity through the red rubber catheter and into the saline bowl. Once the air is evacuated from the pleural cavity as evidenced by bubbles in the saline bowl, the red rubber catheter is removed and the assistant cinches the pleural incision tight for an airtight closure. A postoperative chest radiograph is essential to assess for any significant pneumothorax, even in cases when pneumothorax is not suspected.

The fascial layers are approximated typically in two layers—the transversus abdominis and internal oblique fasciae are approximated together, and the external oblique fascia is approximated as a separate layer. A 1:1 mixture of bupivacaine (0.5%) and lidocaine (1%) solutions is injected into the wound for pain control. The subcutaneous tissue is approximated using 3-0 absorbable sutures. The skin is approximated with skin staples or a subcuticular 4-0 poliglecaprone 25 (Monocryl) suture (Ethicon, Cincinnati, OH).

Intra- and Postoperative Complications

Damage During Suprahilar and Retrocrural Lymphadenectomy. Dissecting the lymphatic tissue located above the left renal vein (suprahilar and retrocrural nodes) in the interaortocaval space should be undertaken with great caution and care because the duodenum, pancreas, SMA, celiac trunk, superior mesenteric autonomic plexus, and cisterna chyli can all be easily damaged in this area with serious sequelae. In general, we consider dissecting this area if the nodes are noticeably palpable or enlarged on preoperative imaging.

Injury to the Vasculature of the Gut. During radical nephrectomy, a number of important gastrointestinal blood vessels may be encountered that have become involved by tumor, resulting in iatrogenic injury. The IMA provides the blood supply to the distal transverse, descending, and sigmoid colon. It can be safely ligated as long as the marginal artery of the colon (marginal artery of Drummond, arch of Riolan) is patent and can supply blood from the SMA to the left colonic arcades. The SMA provides the blood supply to the entire small bowel and to the cecum and ascending and transverse colon, whereas the celiac trunk feeds the esophagus, stomach, pancreas, liver, spleen, and part of the duodenum. Ligation of either the SMA or the celiac trunk is a catastrophic event that occurs predominantly with left-sided nephrectomy and that must be rapidly reversed if the patient is to survive. A vascular surgeon should be immediately called to the operating room and the vessel in question should be repaired.

The IMV is found in the mesentery of the descending colon, immediately lateral to the ligament of Treitz. It is a useful landmark for mobilization of the right colon and small bowel mesentery to access the retroperitoneum, because the posterior peritoneum is incised immediately medial to the IMV. The IMV can be safely ligated during surgery without consequence.

In contrast, the superior mesenteric vein (SMV) should not be ligated unless that is the only surgical option. It runs in the root of the small bowel mesentery and joins the splenic vein and IMV to form the portal vein. Repair of an SMV laceration is done by first clipping the small venous branches entering the SMV and then isolating the injury with atraumatic vascular clamps. Venorrhaphy using 6-0 Prolene is usually adequate to repair the vein. If the vein has been ligated and transected, serious bowel edema and venous engorgement will result, which can impair venous return through the portal venous system. The net result is the development of systemic hypotension/splanchnic hypertension syndrome, which is characterized by venous thrombosis, bowel ischemia, and necrosis. If possible, a ligated SMV should be reanastomosed primarily or repaired using autologous venous grafting. Gore-Tex vascular grafts (W. L. Gore & Associates, Flagstaff, AZ) should only be used when autologous veins are not available because the thrombosis rate is high. The abdomen should not be closed primarily in cases of SMV injury because abdominal compartment syndrome will occur.

Injury to the Liver and Spleen. Small hepatic injuries (capsular tears and minor lacerations) can usually be managed effectively with argon beam coagulation or electrocautery. Fibrin glue and topical hemostatic meshes (e.g., Surgicel Absorbable Hemostat, Ethicon, Cincinnati, OH) are useful adjuncts. More serious splenic injuries can be managed with splenorrhaphy or splenectomy. Minor hepatic lacerations can be repaired using the same basic principles as for partial nephrectomy closure, with a synthetic absorbable suture on a ½-circle tapered needle and Nu-Knit pledgets (Ethicon, Cincinnati, OH), as described in the Enucleation for Small Cortical Tumors section later in this chapter.

Injury to the Duodenum. Most intramural hematomas of the duodenum are managed expectantly. However, if the hematoma is large and narrowing the duodenal lumen, incision of the serosa and muscularis (but not the mucosa) can be performed to drain the hematoma and achieve hemostasis. The defect should be closed in one layer with interrupted 3-0 silk sutures. The involved segment may initially appear nonviable; however, no resection should be performed because the initial perception is false. Consultation with a general surgeon or gastrointestinal surgeon can be very helpful.

Minor electrocautery or laceration injuries should be managed with careful debridement of the nonviable tissue and closure in two layers, the mucosal layer with continuous 4-0 chromic or Vicryl suture on a ½-circle tapered needle, and the serosa and muscularis layer with a 3-0 silk interrupted suture on a ½-circle tapered needle. An omental flap is placed over the injury, and a closed suction drain is inserted.

Injury to the Pancreas. The first step in management of pancreatic injury is a thorough inspection of the organ. Superficial lacerations and contusions can usually be managed by applying fibrin glue and inserting a closed suction drain. The drain is monitored for an alkaline pH and lipase/amylase levels to determine whether a pancreatic fistula is developing. If the injury to the pancreas is deep and/or involves the pancreatic duct, consultation with a gastrointestinal surgeon is essential for appropriate repair and management.

Pulmonary Complications. Large postoperative pleural effusions can be managed with aspiration initially, followed by chest tube drainage if necessary.

Partial Nephrectomy for Malignant Disease

When technically feasible, partial nephrectomy is the preferred method of choice for managing most renal masses to preserve maximum renal function (Fig. 101.35). Although in the past partial nephrectomy was reserved for specific conditions (bilateral tumors, tumor in a solitary kidney, patient at high risk for future renal failure) and small tumors less than 4 cm in diameter (Novick et al., 1991), indications for partial nephrectomy have considerably widened to include most renal masses that can be safely and completely removed independent of their size (Blute and Inman, 2012; Blute et al., 2003; Gill et al., 2007).

Relative contraindications to partial nephrectomy include the following:

Technical issues
- Cold ischemia time greater than 45 minutes (consider extracorporeal approach)
- Less than 20% of global nephron mass retained

Cancer-related issues
- Diffuse encasement of renal pedicle by tumor
- Diffuse invasion of central collecting system

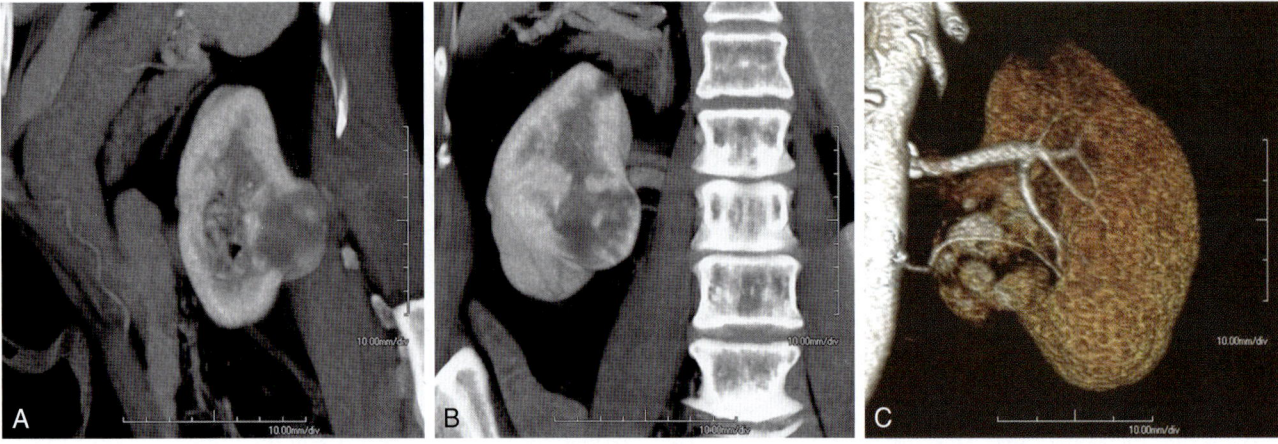

Fig. 101.35. (A) Contrast-enhanced computed tomography scan demonstrating right renal mass. (B) Three-dimensional reconstruction demonstrates a large intrarenal component to the mass. (C) Arterial reconstruction shows lower pole renal artery in close proximity to the renal mass.

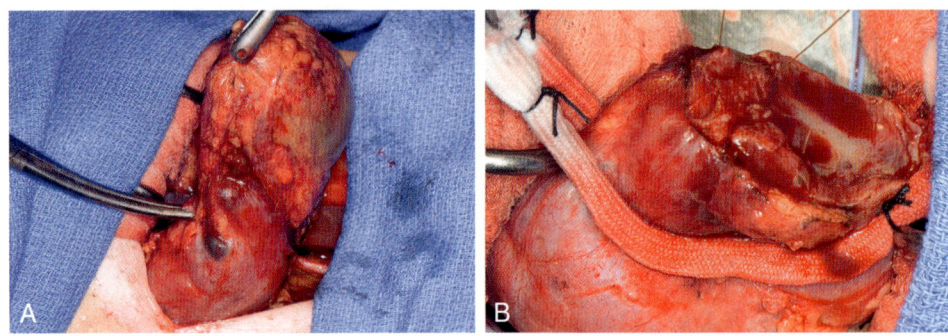

Fig. 101.36. (A and B) Partial nephrectomy for a large polar tumor using a Satinsky clamp on the renal parenchyma for ischemia.

- Tumor thrombus involving major renal veins
- Adjacent organ invasion (stage cT4)
- Regional lymphadenopathy (stage cTxN1)

Preoperative Considerations

In addition to the preoperative considerations for radical nephrectomy, there are additional concepts to consider related to partial nephrectomy.

Hyperfiltration Injury. When a significant portion of renal parenchyma is removed, the renal blood flow is delivered to a smaller number of nephrons, which can lead to increased glomerular capillary perfusion pressure that results in an increased single-nephron glomerular filtration rate called *hyperfiltration* (Goldfarb, 1995; Steckler et al., 1990). Over decades, the hyperfiltration can injure the remaining nephrons, resulting in focal segmental glomerulosclerosis and the clinical manifestations of proteinuria and progressive renal failure. Hyperfiltration injury is most common when the total nephron mass of both kidneys is reduced by more than 80%.

Renal Ischemia and Hypothermia. To minimize blood loss and allow for adequate surgical visibility, it is often necessary to employ vascular compression during partial nephrectomy. Options include manual compression, a renal compression clamp (Kaufmann clamp), selective clamping of the renal artery, and en bloc clamping of the entire renal pedicle. Manual and clamp compression of renal parenchyma is preferable because vascular clamping is associated with a higher incidence of renal complications (Fig. 101.36). It is unclear whether leaving the renal vein unclamped for retrograde renal perfusion offers any tangible benefit. Attempting to limit warm ischemia to 20 minutes and cold ischemia to 35 minutes helps maintain renal function (Thompson et al., 2007).

Adequate renal hypothermia (core renal temperature of 20° C) takes at least 15 minutes to achieve if the kidney is packed with ice slush. To help prevent acute postoperative renal failure, intravenous mannitol (12.5 g) and furosemide (20 mg) should be infused about 15 minutes before renal artery clamping (Hanley and Davidson, 1981; Tiggeler et al., 1985). Although evidence supporting this practice is somewhat limited, both drugs are quite safe as long as the patient is well hydrated (Novick et al., 1991).

Enucleation and Surgical Margin. Simple tumor enucleation can be safely conducted in small renal tumors while preserving a small rim of normal tissue and a negative surgical margin (Carini et al., 2006).

Multifocality and Tumor Size. The incidence of multifocality is approximately 2% for clear cell and chromophobe RCC and 10% for papillary RCC (Fig. 101.37). Multifocal tumors are also more common as the primary tumor size increases (Blute et al., 2003). Careful inspection of the entire renal surface should be done at the time of partial nephrectomy to ensure that intraoperative findings corroborate preoperative imaging studies. If additional unanticipated renal mass(es) are encountered intraoperatively, partial nephrectomy is still the treatment of choice for multifocal tumors as long as they can be safely resected with clear surgical margins.

Hereditary Renal Malignancy. Hereditary renal tumors are usually multifocal and bilateral, with high likelihood of recurrence. Except for patients with hereditary leiomyomatosis and RCC who should be aggressively treated with wide excision, most patients with hereditary syndromes can be safely observed with little chance of metastasis until the renal tumors reach 3 cm in size (Maher et al., 1991; Seizinger, 1991; Richards et al., 1993). When partial nephrectomy is performed, the perirenal fat and renal fascia should be preserved. The entire renal surface should be visualized, and all visible tumors should be resected. Intraoperative ultrasound can be

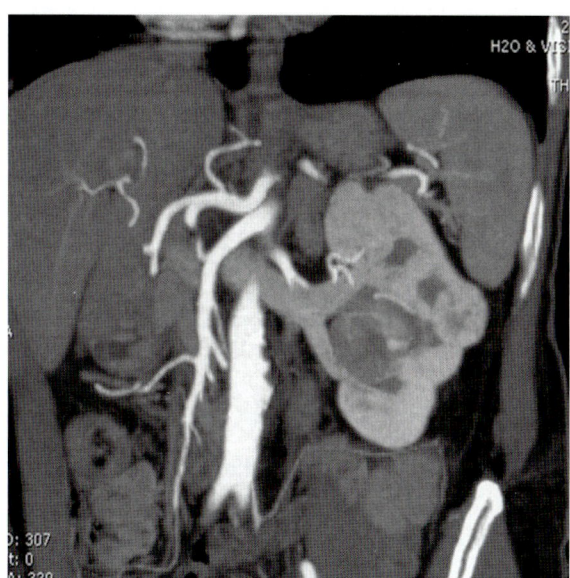

Fig. 101.37. Three-dimensional computed tomography reconstruction demonstrating a hilar tumor and peripheral tumor.

used to identify any subcortical tumors that could also be resected (eFig. 101.38). Hypothermia is advisable to minimize injury to the renal parenchyma.

Enucleation for Small Cortical Tumors

The surgeon should ensure that renal cooling is available, even though ischemia time seldom exceeds 30 minutes. Two cylinder-shaped cigarette-like bolsters are prepared by rolling Nu-Knit Absorbable Hemostat and tying each end with absorbable sutures. Two pledgets are prepared by folding Nu-Knit into a double-layer strip 5 to 10 cm wide and 1 cm long. We prefer Nu-Knit because it is absorbable and it maintains its integrity without immediate shrinkage when wet. In addition, it has excellent tensile strength when sutured.

The kidney is exposed using either the anterior subcostal or flank approach as described earlier. The entire surface of the kidney is freed of perirenal fat, with the exception of the perirenal fat overlying the tumor. While removing the perirenal fat, special care should be taken to avoid injury to the ureter, particularly for lower pole tumors. Intravenous mannitol and furosemide are administered and the renal pedicle is exposed sufficiently to allow safe application of a vascular clamp if necessary. Vessel loops are placed around the renal vein and artery individually.

The renal cortex surrounding the tumor is marked circumferentially using electrocautery. The plane outside the tumor pseudocapsule and within the normal parenchyma is identified and bluntly dissected with small closed Metzenbaum scissors. For enucleation of small lesions, renal occlusion is usually not necessary. However, if there is excessive bleeding that hampers proper visualization of the resection margin, then manual compression of the kidney or clamping of the renal pedicle can help. When small vessels within the kidney are encountered, they are divided sharply with scissors. The tumor is excised, and the margins are examined for gross evidence of a positive surgical margin; the deep margin of the excised tumor is assessed by frozen-section analysis. Small bleeding vessels in the renal parenchyma are controlled with 4-0 absorbable figure-of-eight sutures on a tapered needle or by coagulation with an argon beam coagulator or bipolar electrocautery. The integrity of the collecting system is verified by checking for injury and repairing with absorbable suture if necessary (Fig. 101.39).

A Nu-Knit pledget that was prepared earlier is placed along each border of the excised renal parenchyma and in the bottom of the excised parenchyma (Fig. 101.40). The defect is closed with 2-0 absorbable horizontal mattress sutures on a long ½-circle tapered needle. The suture is placed through the pledget and about 1 to 2 cm into the renal parenchyma to prevent capsular and parenchymal tearing. The pledgets allow even distribution of tension along the renal capsule, reducing the likelihood of tearing the capsule. If clamping was used, the pedicle is unclamped and inspection is done for bleeding, ischemia, or urine leakage of the kidney and for adjacent organ trauma.

The perirenal fat and renal fascia are replaced around the kidney. A closed suction drain in the pararenal space is placed to monitor for bleeding and urine leaks. The closed suction drain is removed after 2 to 5 days when the output is minimal. A Foley catheter is used to monitor the urine output. Unless there is a large renal collecting system defect, a ureteral stent is not typically required.

Wedge Resection for Large Cortical Tumors

For large tumors, intravenous mannitol and furosemide are administered, and then the renal artery is clamped with a vascular bulldog clamp. Based on the surgeon's preference, when partial nephrectomy is being performed for larger tumor sizes or lesions that are close to the renal hilum, the renal vein may also be clamped after clamping the renal artery to provide better hemostasis during partial nephrectomy (Fig. 101.41). A plastic bag or sheet is placed around the kidney and filled with ice slush. The kidney is allowed to cool to 20° C (approximately 15 minutes).

The renal capsule is circumferentially incised 5 to 10 mm peripheral to the tumor with electrocautery. Using a combination of blunt and sharp dissection with Metzenbaum scissors, the tumor is excised with a small rim of normal parenchyma. The specimen is inspected for visible tumor at the resection margin, then submitted for frozen-section analysis.

Bleeding vessels are controlled with figure-of-eight sutures or with argon beam or bipolar electrocautery. The deep resection margin of the kidney must be inspected for any residual tumor or any sign of collecting system injury. If there is any doubt about collecting system injury, 10 to 20 mL of diluted indigo carmine is injected into the renal pelvis while occluding the ureter to assess for leaks. The collecting system is closed with a 4-0 absorbable suture on a tapered needle.

The renal parenchymal defect is reconstructed using Nu-Knit bolsters and pledgets as described earlier. Fibrin glue is applied to the renal parenchymal defect. Finally, the renal vessels are unclamped—if the renal vein and the renal artery is clamped, the renal vein is unclamped first, followed by unclamping the renal artery.

Segmental Nephrectomy for Large Polar Tumors

Intravenous mannitol and furosemide are administered, and the renal pedicle is completely dissected, including the segmental branches (Fig. 101.42, eFig. 101.43). A bulldog clamp is applied to the apical segmental artery (or basilar segmental artery for lower pole tumors), and the line of ischemia is observed. The avascular line can be further demarcated by injecting 5 mL of indigo carmine directly into the clamped artery (eFig. 101.44). The line of ischemia is the optimal site for transection of the kidney and should be lightly marked with electrocautery. The apical segmental artery is ligated, then the renal pedicle is clamped en bloc with a curved Satinsky clamp. A plastic bag or sheet is placed around the kidney and filled with ice slush to cool the kidney to 20° C (approximately 15 minutes). The renal capsule is incised along the line of ischemia with electrocautery. Using blunt dissection, the pole of the kidney is excised (Fig. 101.45). Bleeding vessels are controlled, working expeditiously and accurately. The clamp is released to check for uncontrolled bleeders. If hemostasis is adequate, collecting system repair is begun; otherwise the pedicle is reclamped and vascular control resumed.

The collecting system is inspected for injury. If the defect in the collecting system is large, a guidewire is inserted into the defect and manually guided into the ureter and bladder. A 6-Fr double-J ureteral stent is inserted over the guidewire with the proximal coil in the renal pelvis. The collecting system is closed with a running 4-0 absorbable noncutting suture.

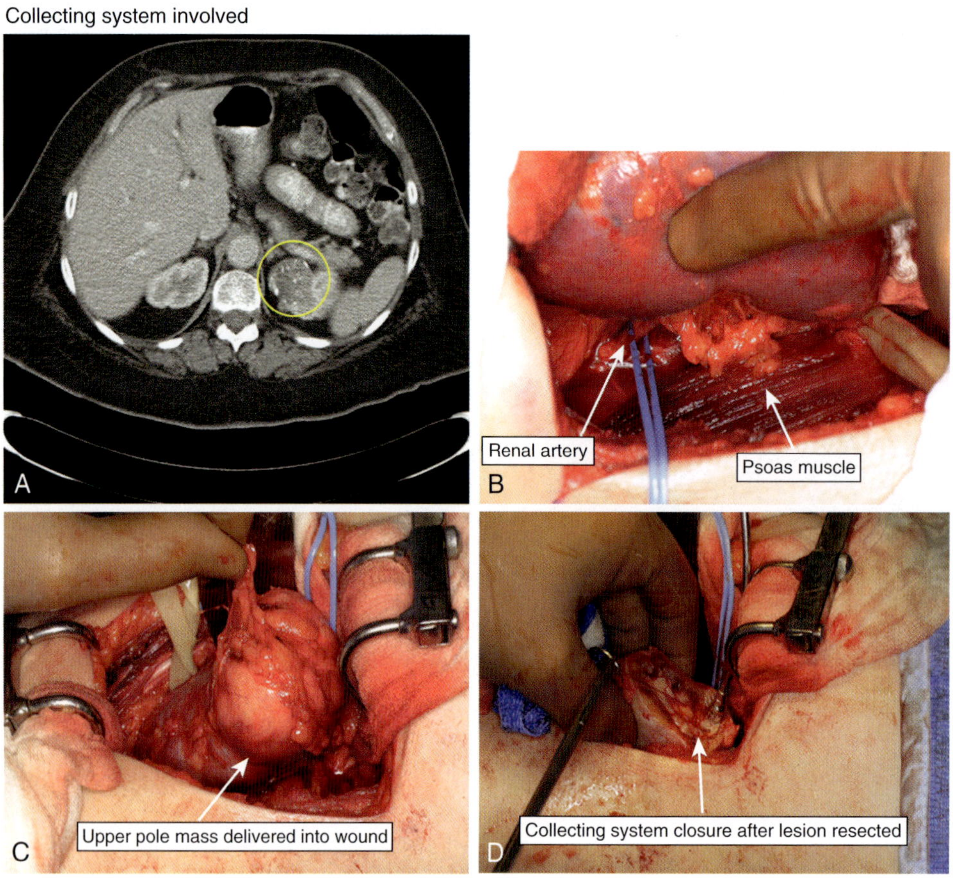

2264 PART XI Neoplasms of the Upper Urinary Tract

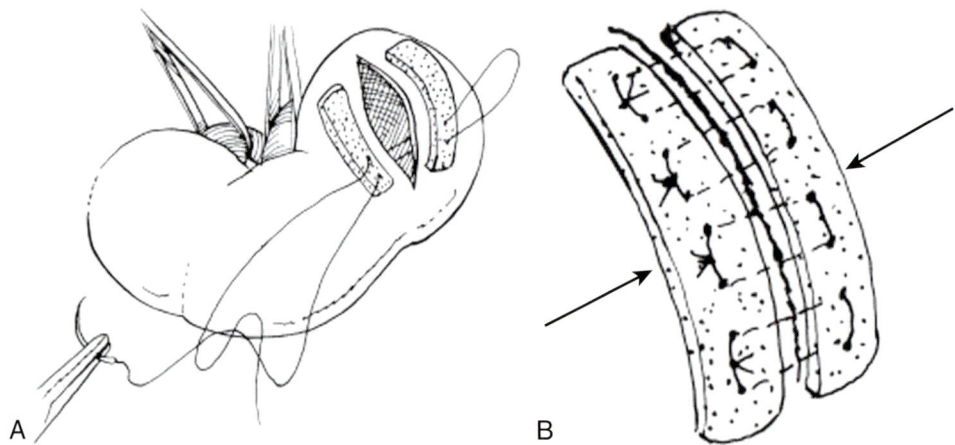

Fig. 101.39. (A) Renal tumor involving the collecting system demonstrated on computed tomography scan. (B) Securing the renal artery. (C) Identifying the upper pole mass. (D) Repair of the collecting system after lesion is resected.

Fig. 101.40. (A and B) A Nu-Knit pledget is placed along each border of the crater, and a Nu-Knit bolster is placed into the bottom of the crater (not required if the defect is very small). The defect is closed with a 2-0 absorbable horizontal mattress suture. (From Smith JA Jr, Howards SS, Preminger GM, eds. *Hinman's atlas of urologic surgery.* 3rd ed. Philadelphia, PA: Saunders; 2012.)

The renal capsule is closed using Nu-Knit pledgets and horizontal mattress sutures as described earlier. Because the defect is large, we use a larger needle (e.g., XLH, GS-27) for segmental polar nephrectomies and heminephrectomies than for enucleation and wedge resections. Nephropexy should be considered if the kidney is quite mobile; however, injury to retroperitoneal nerves overlying the psoas and quadratus lumborum muscles must be avoided (eFig. 101.46). The kidney is covered with perirenal fat and renal fascia, and a closed suction drain is placed to monitor output postoperatively. The indwelling Foley catheter is removed when the patient is mobile and stable. Depending on the output of the closed suction drain, it can be removed 5 to 10 days postoperatively. If a ureteral stent is used, it should not be removed for 4 to 6 weeks postoperatively. After removal of the indwelling Foley catheter, if the output of the closed suction drain is increased, the transurethral indwelling Foley catheter is reinserted to reduce the intrapelvic urine pressure, which should minimize the output from the closed suction drain.

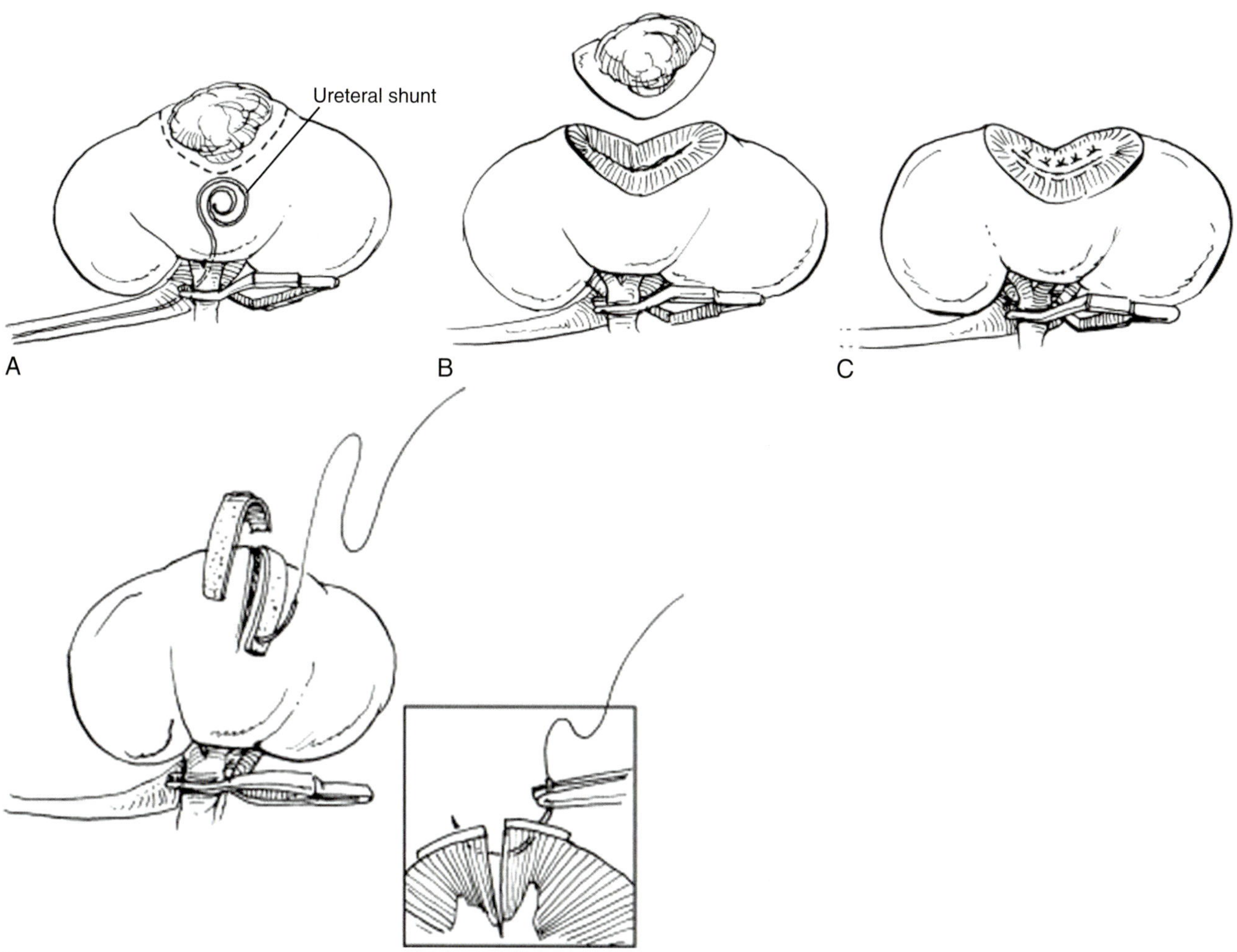

Fig. 101.41. (A) The renal capsule is circumferentially incised 5 to 10 mm peripheral to the tumor with electrocautery. (B) A combination of blunt and sharp dissection with Metzenbaum scissors is used to excise the tumor with a small rim of normal parenchyma. (C) Bleeding vessels are controlled, and the collecting system is closed. (D) The defect is reconstructed using Nu-Knit bolsters and pledgets. (From Smith JA Jr, Howards SS, Preminger GM, eds. *Hinman's atlas of urologic surgery*. 3rd ed. Philadelphia, PA: Saunders; 2012.)

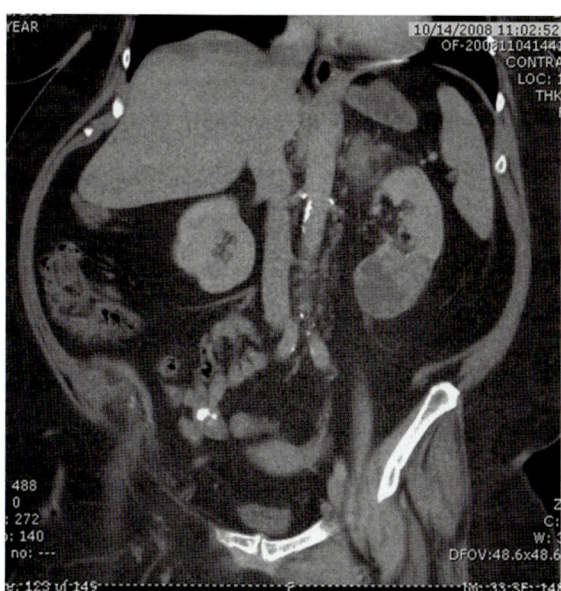

Fig. 101.42. Left renal mass in the lower pole on computed tomography scan.

Complications Associated With Partial Nephrectomy

Urinary Fistulae. Partial nephrectomies that involve incision of the collecting system, because of the size and location of the tumor, increase the possibility of urinary leakage. Most urinary fistulae present themselves in about 1 week postoperatively. Therefore, in cases of deep renal resections, it is advisable to keep the closed suction abdominal drain in place for 7 to 10 days. If a urinary fistula is suspected, the diagnosis is confirmed by checking the effluent for creatinine, which will be present at a level manyfold higher than the serum creatinine level. Alternatively, an intravenous ampule of indigo carmine, when injected and collected in the closed suction drain, can also confirm the diagnosis.

If a closed suction drain is not present and a urinary fistula is suspected, a urinary collection in the retroperitoneum can become symptomatic. Abdominal imaging is used to confirm the diagnosis. The treatment of urinary fistulae requires three tubes: (1) a retroperitoneal closed suction drain to collect the urinoma, (2) a double-J ureteral stent that is placed after retrograde pyelography, and (3) a Foley catheter to keep the entire collecting system at low pressure. Most fistulas resolve within 4 to 6 weeks with conservative management, and reoperation is rarely required.

Postoperative Bleeding. Delayed bleeding can occur following partial nephrectomy, particularly in patients who require postoperative anticoagulation therapy. If a drain is in place, initial management is

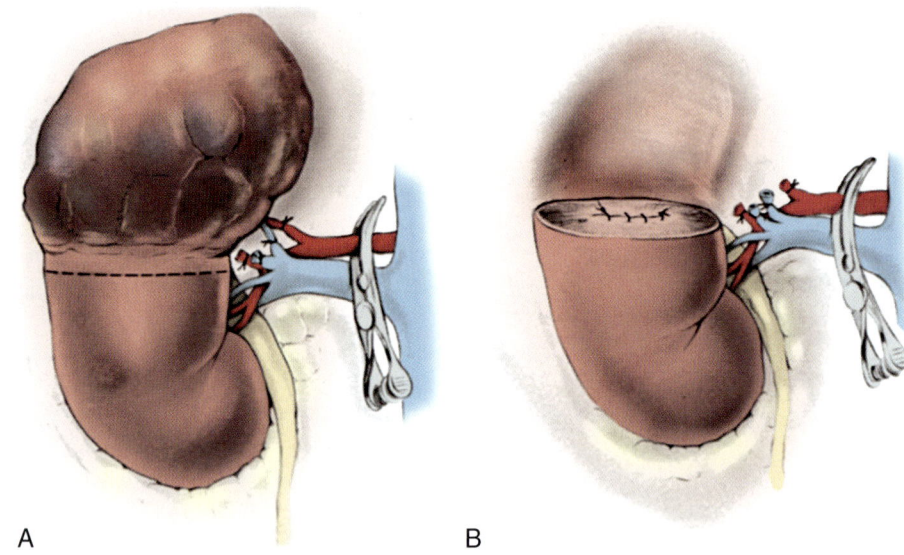

Fig. 101.45. (A and B) Technique of transverse resection for a tumor involving the upper half of the kidney. (From Novick AC: Partial nephrectomy for renal cell carcinoma. *Urol Clin North Am* 14:419, 1987.)

conservative and consists of bed rest, hydration, close clinical monitoring, and serial evaluations of blood counts. In situations in which more than 1 to 2 units of transfused blood products are required, renal angioembolization should be attempted. Usually, bleeding segmental and subsegmental arteries can be selectively embolized and the kidney salvaged without need for complete nephrectomy. Life-threatening hemorrhage can also occur and require complete angioinfarction of the kidney or reoperative exploration.

Renal Insufficiency. Acute renal failure may follow partial nephrectomy in a solitary kidney, related to large size of the tumor, excessive removal of renal parenchyma, and prolonged ischemic time. Obstruction of the collecting system, drug toxicity, vascular thrombosis, and vascular disruption are other causes that should be considered. Although most cases of postoperative renal insufficiency are mild and temporary, some cases require hemodialysis for electrolyte and fluid management. Hyperfiltration injury can also cause a gradual decrease in renal function over time, typically associated with proteinuria.

Vena Caval Thrombectomy

Tumor thrombus within the venous drainage system of the kidney can occur with many retroperitoneal tumors. In children, Wilms tumor, clear cell sarcoma of the kidney, adrenocortical carcinoma, and neuroblastoma can all be associated with IVC thrombi. In adults, urothelial carcinoma of the renal pelvis, lymphoma, retroperitoneal sarcoma, adrenocortical carcinoma, pheochromocytoma, and angiomyolipoma are all potential sources of an IVC thrombus. RCC is the most common cause associated with IVC tumor thrombus, accounting for 18% of all tumors that have venous thrombi (Blute et al., 2004b). The two components associated with IVC thrombi are tumor thrombus (tumor cells contained within bland thrombus) and bland thrombus (blood coagulum without tumor cells). Venous drainage is hampered by venous thrombus encouraging formation of bland thrombus. Distinction between these two forms of venous thrombus is critical and forms the basis of operative management for IVC thrombi.

Management of a tumor with an associated IVC thrombus can be technically challenging. In the case of RCC with venous thrombus, 10% have associated positive regional lymph nodes, 25% have associated metastases, and 50% have perirenal fat invasion. Usually, IVC thrombectomy is accompanied by radical nephrectomy and regional lymph node dissection.

Preoperative Considerations

Pulmonary Embolism, Anticoagulation, and IVC Filters. Patients with renal tumors are at increased risk for pulmonary embolism as a result of malignancy-associated hypercoagulability and venous thrombus embolization. We suggest anticoagulation with intravenous or low-molecular-weight heparin to be started as soon as tumor thrombus is detected. Although evidence supporting the use of preoperative anticoagulation is limited, several potential benefits include reduced risk for pulmonary embolism, tumor thrombus shrinkage, and bland thrombus shrinkage and/or prevention. Temporary suprarenal IVC filters are also an option for patients with level 0, I, and II tumor thrombi. However, because of the risk for contralateral renal and hepatic vein thrombosis, the risk for provoking embolization, and the impediment that these devices can pose to future IVC thrombectomy, we do not recommend use of suprarenal IVC filters. Given the risk for intraoperative thrombus detachment and the possibility of interval thrombus growth in the period immediately preceding surgery, we recommend the use of transesophageal echocardiography (TEE) for level II to IV thrombi.

Preoperative angioembolization can be considered because tumor thrombi have an independent blood supply arising from the renal artery and/or aorta in one-third of cases. Angiographic infarction of the blood supply to the tumor thrombus can help shrink a large thrombus to a more manageable size, potentially avoiding the need for bypass or extensive mobilization of the liver. Angioembolization can be considered when caval thrombi appear to invade the IVC, when the thrombus invades the intrahepatic or suprahepatic veins and cannot be excised, when the thrombus is associated with a bleeding kidney, and when deep hypothermic arrest is planned because the patency of the coronary arteries can be simultaneously assessed. The optimal timing for angioembolization is unknown, but it is usually performed 1 day before surgery at most centers. There is a potential risk for causing iatrogenic pulmonary embolization of the tumor thrombus when angiography is performed; however, this risk appears to be minimal. We seldom use angioembolization, but it is associated with ischemia-related flank pain and tumor lysis syndrome.

Urologists who do not routinely handle the IVC and aorta should consult a vascular surgeon for level II and III thrombi to aid in vena caval control and reconstruction. Consultation with a cardiothoracic surgeon preoperatively for all level III and IV

thrombi is essential because access to the mediastinal compartment for vascular bypass and thrombus removal may be required. Involvement of a cardiologist or cardiac anesthesiologist is essential for level II to IV thrombi to allow for intraoperative TEE.

Tumor Thrombus Level. Traditionally, IVC thrombi have been defined and managed according to the cranial extent of the tumor thrombus (Fig. 101.47). MRI provides excellent overall assessment of the level of tumor thrombus involvement; however, reconstructed CT angiograms can also produce excellent images to determine the level of the tumor thrombus. Assessment of the bland thrombus, a grouping system that complements the traditional tumor thrombus levels, can help with intraoperative decision making (Tables 101.1 and 101.2). The key addition of this grouping system is the consideration of the location and extent of bland thrombus and its impact on IVC management (Fig. 101.48).

Level I Vena Caval Thrombectomy: Right-Sided Tumor

Usually, level I thrombi are partially occlusive, are nonadherent, and do not require extensive IVC dissection or any form of bypass. Some groups mobilize the kidney after the thrombectomy is complete, to minimize the risk for embolization, while others mobilize the kidney first followed by thrombectomy.

Using an anterior midline, anterior subcostal, or modified flank incision, access is gained to the kidney as previously described. The great vessels and the renal hilum are exposed. Using care not to manipulate the renal vein or IVC too much, the renal artery is identified in the interaortocaval region and secured with a 0 silk ligature or a large clip. Ligating the renal artery early will help reduce the blood flow to the kidney and minimize the amount of potential blood loss. The kidney is mobilized outside the renal fascia, and the IVC is dissected above the right renal vein. The left renal vein, suprarenal IVC, and infrarenal IVC are identified and secured with vessel loops. To help with temporary ligation of these vessels, 3- to 6-inch portions of an 18-Fr red rubber catheter are passed through the vessel loop and used as Rummel tourniquets (eFig. 101.49). Although this degree of vascular control may not be necessary for all level I thrombi, it is prudent to have adequate vascular control if there is any doubt about the extension of the level of thrombus. Starting cranially, the IVC is gently pinched closed, and then the Rummel tourniquets are applied so that the infrarenal IVC, left renal vein, and suprarenal IVC are closed in that order. The IVC is milked with the left hand toward the ostium of the right renal vein. A C-shaped Satinsky vascular clamp is placed around the ostium of the right renal vein partially occluding the IVC (Fig. 101.50), ensuring that the thrombus is located within the jaws of the clamp before complete closure. The IVC is palpated for evidence of any other thrombus. Suction and two sponge sticks (to compress the IVC if necessary) are readied, and laparotomy sponges are placed around the renal vein to collect any spillage of tumor thrombus after opening of the renal vein. The renal ostium is circumferentially incised using a scalpel or fine-tipped Metzenbaum or Potts scissors. At least one-half of the width of the IVC must be maintained for proper closure.

The thrombus is extracted by gentle downward traction on the renal vein. A gauze is wrapped around the renal vein stump and

TABLE 101.1 Traditional Staging and Management of Inferior Vena Caval Thrombi

THROMBUS LEVEL	INCIDENCE RATE IN RCC	PROPORTION OF THROMBI	CRANIAL EXTENT OF THROMBUS	MANAGEMENT OF TUMOR THROMBUS
0	12%	65%	Confined to renal vein	Radical nephrectomy
I	2%	10%	Within 2 cm of renal vein ostium	IVC milking, partial IVC occlusion, ostial cavotomy
II	3%	15%	Below hepatic veins	Complete IVC mobilization/control, infrahepatic cavotomy
III	1%	5%	Between hepatic veins and diaphragm	Complete occlusion: suprahepatic IVC clamping, infrahepatic cavotomy
Partial occlusion: venovenous bypass, infrahepatic cavotomy
IV	1%	5%	Above diaphragm	Deep hypothermic arrest, infrahepatic cavotomy, right atriotomy

IVC, Inferior vena cava; *RCC,* renal cell carcinoma.
Data from Blute ML, Leibovich BC, Lohse CM, et al. The Mayo Clinic experience with surgical management, complications and outcome for patients with renal cell carcinoma and venous tumour thrombus. *BJU Int* 94:33–41, 2004.

TABLE 101.2 The Mayo Clinic Thrombus Grouping System for Inferior Vena Caval Thrombi

MAYO THROMBUS GROUP	INCIDENCE RATE IN RCC	PROPORTION OF THROMBI	ASSOCIATED BLAND THROMBUS	ADDITIONAL IVC MANAGEMENT
A	17%	90%	None	None
B	<1%	1%	At or below common iliac veins	Infrarenal IVC filter (e.g., Greenfield)
C	1%	5%	Infrarenal IVC, separate from tumor thrombus	Infrarenal IVC interruption with vena caval clip
D	0.5%	4%	Infrarenal IVC, mixed with tumor thrombus	Infrarenal IVC resection

IVC, Inferior vena cava; *RCC,* renal cell carcinoma.
Data from Blute ML, Leibovich BC, Lohse CM, et al. The Mayo Clinic experience with surgical management, complications and outcome for patients with renal cell carcinoma and venous tumour thrombus. *BJU Int* 94:33–41, 2004.

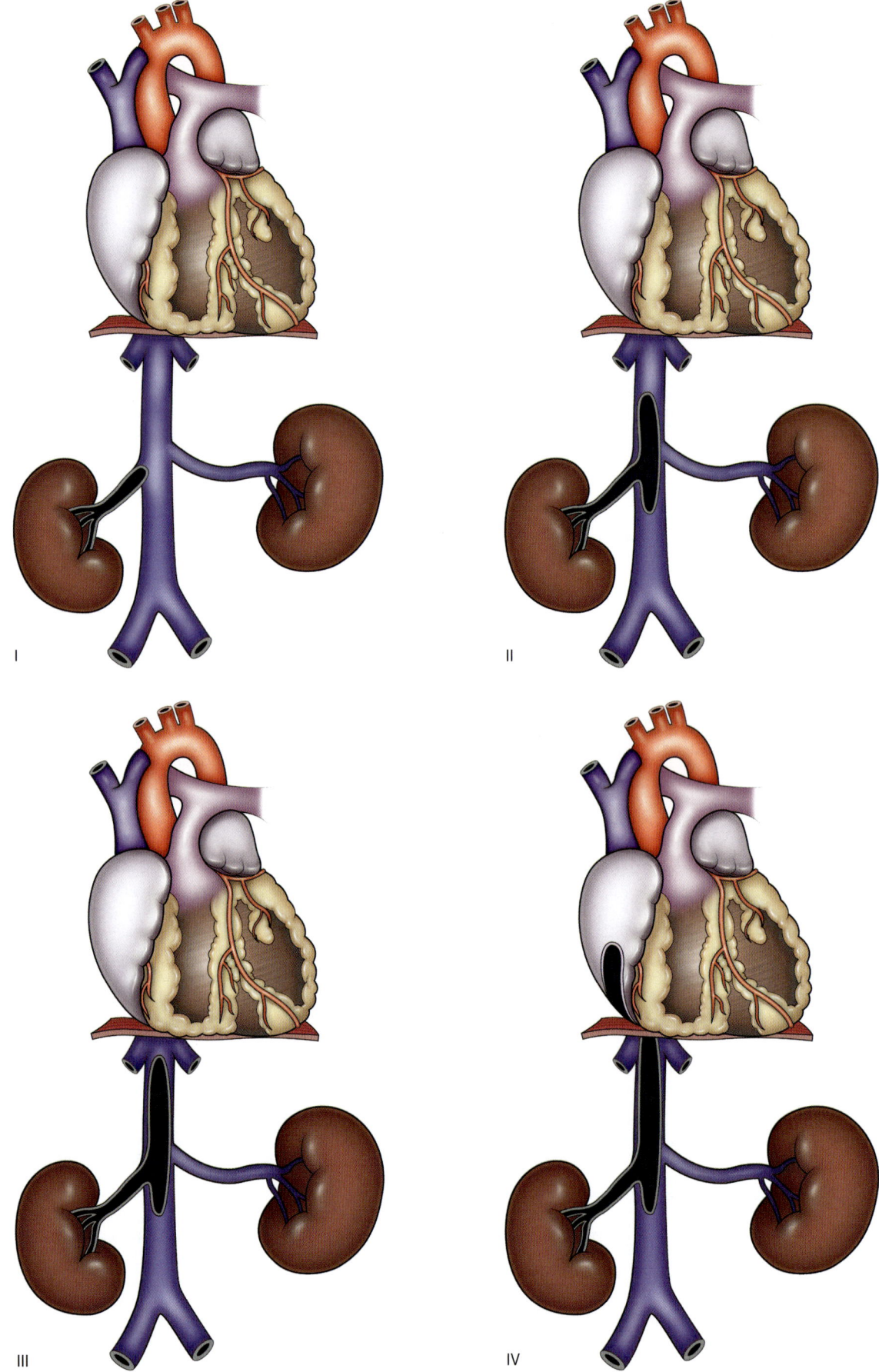

Fig. 101.47. (I to IV) Classification of venous tumor thrombus extension. (From Wang GJ, Carpenter JP, Fairman RM, et al. Single-center experience of caval thrombectomy in patients with renal cell carcinoma with tumor thrombus extension into the inferior vena cava. *Vasc Endovasc Surg* 42:335–40, 2008.)

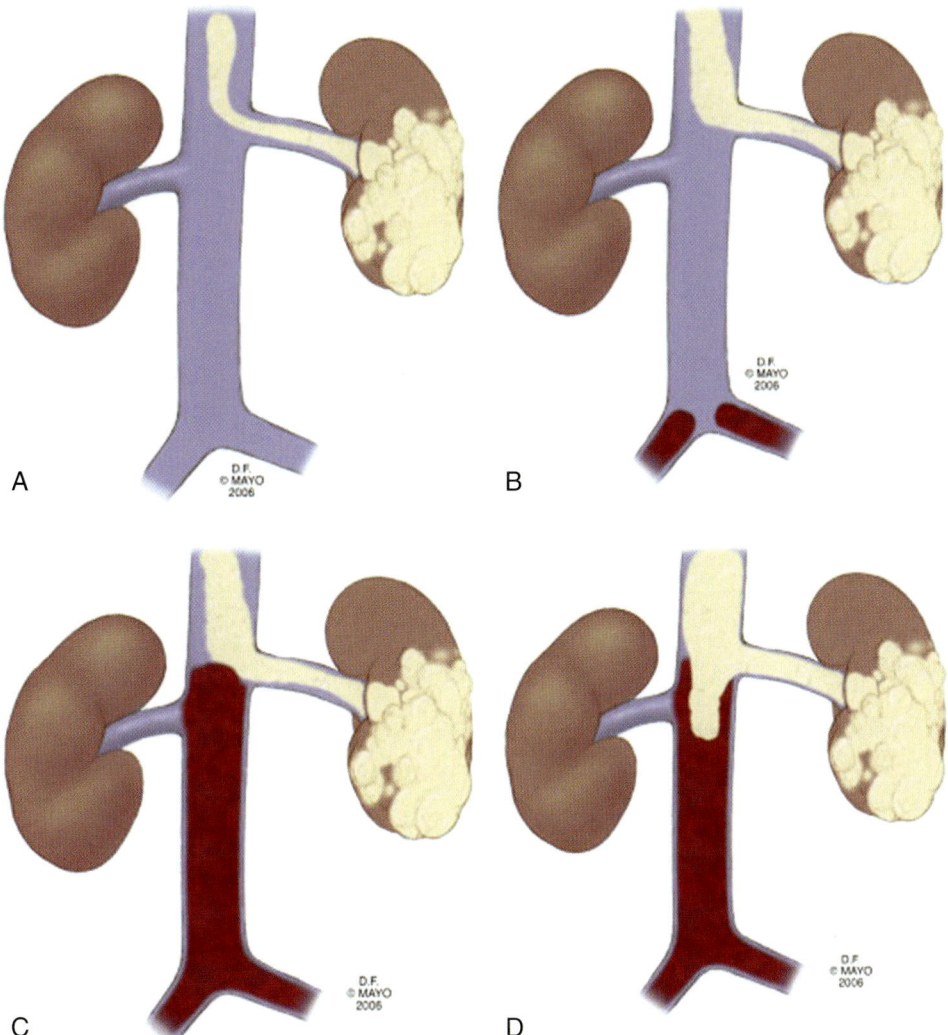

Fig. 101.48. (A to D) Mayo Clinic classification scheme for IVC interruption based on degree of venous occlusion and bland thrombus. (From Blute ML, Boorjian SA, Leibovich BC, et al. Results of inferior vena caval interruption by Greenfield filter, ligation or resection during radical nephrectomy and tumor thrombectomy. *J Urol* 178:440-5, 2007. Reprinted with permission of Mayo Foundation for Medical Education and Research. All rights reserved.)

secured with a silk ligature to prevent tumor spillage (Fig. 101.51). The medial attachments of the kidney are dissected, ligating the renal artery again before division.

The IVC is inspected for evidence of residual thrombus, irrigating its lumen with heparinized saline solution (100 units/mL) for improved visualization. The IVC defect is closed with a running closure using a 4-0 Prolene suture on a BB vascular needle (Fig. 101.52). Before tying the knot, the anesthesiologist should apply positive airway pressure, pinch the infrarenal IVC closed, and then release the Satinsky clamp. The surgeon should allow 5 to 10 mL of blood to escape from the caval defect to flush out any residual thrombus fragments and debris before pulling the suture tight and tying the closure. A right regional lymphadenectomy is performed, irrigating the wound copiously with sterile water. The surgeon may consider placement of a closed suction catheter to monitor for bleeding.

Level II Vena Caval Thrombectomy: Left-Sided Tumor

Exposure for a tumor thrombus associated with a left-sided tumor is more difficult because the IVC is best accessed from the right retroperitoneum. Both the right and the left colon must be mobilized to get adequate exposure. The anterior midline and chevron incisions provide the best access for left-sided tumors associated with tumor thrombi in the IVC.

After a subcostal chevron incision is made, the left colon is mobilized and the left anterior pararenal space is developed. The left renal artery is then identified and ligated near its origin close to the aorta. The adrenal, lumbar, and gonadal branches of the left renal vein are ligated and divided. These branches are often dilated and friable and occasionally contain thrombi. The kidney is mobilized outside the renal fascia, and the ureter is divided.

The right colon and small bowel are mobilized, the Kocher maneuver is performed, and the right anterior space is developed and the great vessels are exposed. The IVC is carefully dissected to its bifurcation, ligating the right gonadal vein on its anterior surface. Vascular control is obtained sequentially in the following order: (1) the ipsilateral (left) renal artery is ligated, (2) the infrarenal IVC is clamped, (3) the contralateral (right) renal vein is clamped, (4) the suprarenal IVC is clamped, and (5) accessory hepatic veins are ligated to the caudate lobe (this is an optional maneuver to gain 2 to 3 cm of extra infrahepatic IVC exposure) (eFig. 101.53). Optionally, one can clamp the contralateral renal artery to prevent renal engorgement while the venous outflow is temporarily clamped. This is more of an issue for left-sided tumors because the right kidney does not have significant venous collateralization to shunt blood when the right renal vein is clamped. While obtaining vascular control, one must be very gentle to avoid dislodging the thrombus. The lumbar veins are ligated and divided as required. Before clamping,

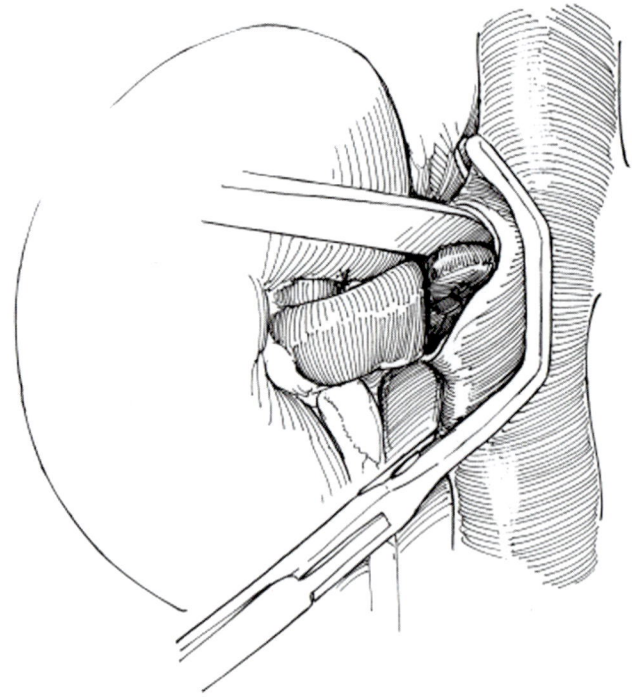

Fig. 101.50. Right-sided level I tumor thrombus. A C-shaped Satinsky vascular clamp is placed around the ostium of the right renal vein, partially occluding the inferior vena cava. (From Smith JA Jr, Howards SS, Preminger GM, eds. *Hinman's atlas of urologic surgery*. 3rd ed. Philadelphia, PA: Saunders; 2012.)

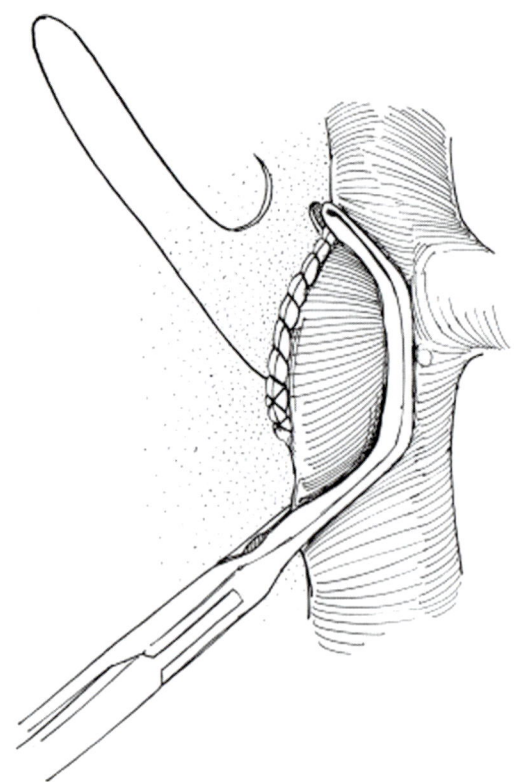

Fig. 101.52. Right-sided level I tumor thrombus. Closing the inferior vena cava defect. (From Smith JA Jr, Howards SS, Preminger GM, eds. *Hinman's atlas of urologic surgery*. 3rd ed. Philadelphia, PA: Saunders; 2012.)

The renal vein ostium is circumferentially excised, and the incision is extended superiorly onto the anterior surface of the IVC using Potts scissors (Fig. 101.54). A Penfield dissector is used to carefully extract the tumor thrombus from the IVC. Lumbar veins can be a source of troublesome bleeding at this stage and should be ligated or sutured as needed. The gross tumor thrombus and kidney are removed en bloc. The IVC is flushed with heparinized saline solution, and the intima is inspected for signs of caval invasion. Any suspicious areas should be biopsied or resected. The IVC lumen can be safely narrowed to about 50% of its preoperative size without requiring special measures. The caval defect is closed with a running 4-0 Prolene suture. Before tying the knot, the infrarenal clamp is released and 5 to 10 mL of blood is allowed to seep from the cavotomy to clear the IVC of air and debris. After tying the suture, the contralateral renal clamp is released followed by the suprarenal IVC clamp. Regional lymphadenectomy is performed, consideration is given to leaving a closed suction drain, and the wound is irrigated and the incision closed.

Level III-IV Vena Caval Thrombectomy: Intra-Abdominal Approach

Intrahepatic tumor thrombi are very challenging cases to treat. The operating room should be set up for possible cardiopulmonary bypass (CPB), including deep hypothermic arrest. Intraoperative TEE should be available to measure the cranial extent of the thrombus and to monitor the thrombus for fracture and embolization (Fig. 101.55). Cardiac function is evaluated with TEE so that the anesthesiologist can appropriately manage the patient's hemodynamics.

The key decision for level III thrombi is whether to attempt an intra-abdominal thrombus extraction with complete hepatic mobilization or use a combined intrathoracic/intra-abdominal approach with bypass. This decision can only be made intraoperatively, after the renal artery is ligated, the liver is mobilized, and the IVC is exposed and evaluated. If the IVC can be clamped below the hepatic veins, this is preferable because the venous return from the liver is significant. As a rule of thumb, patents with free-floating partially occlusive

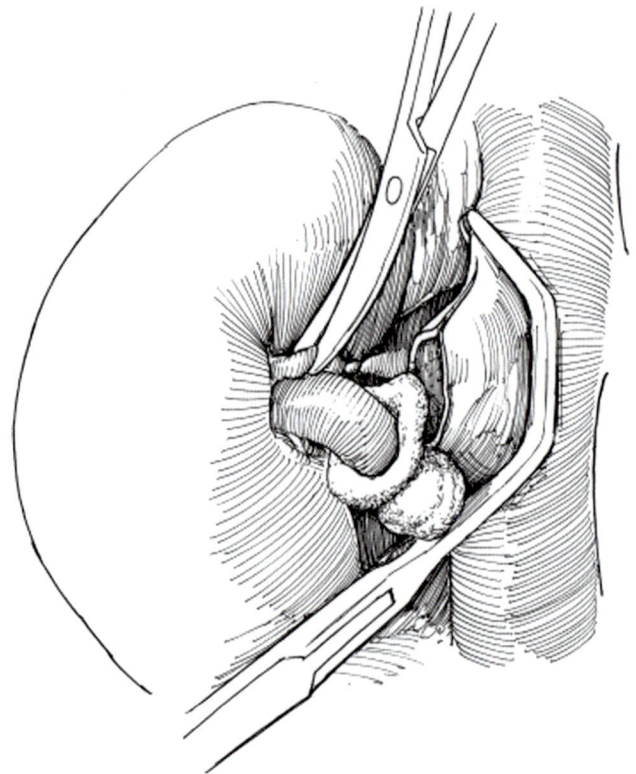

Fig. 101.51. Right-sided level I tumor thrombus. Preventing tumor spillage. (From Smith JA Jr, Howards SS, Preminger GM, eds. *Hinman's atlas of urologic surgery*. 3rd ed. Philadelphia, PA: Saunders; 2012.)

some may use 0.5 mg/kg of intravenous heparin to prevent clamp-related thrombotic complications. Our experience has been that bleeding, not clotting, is the principal problem encountered with vena caval thrombectomy, and we do not routinely heparinize our patients.

Chapter 101 Open Surgery of the Kidney 2271

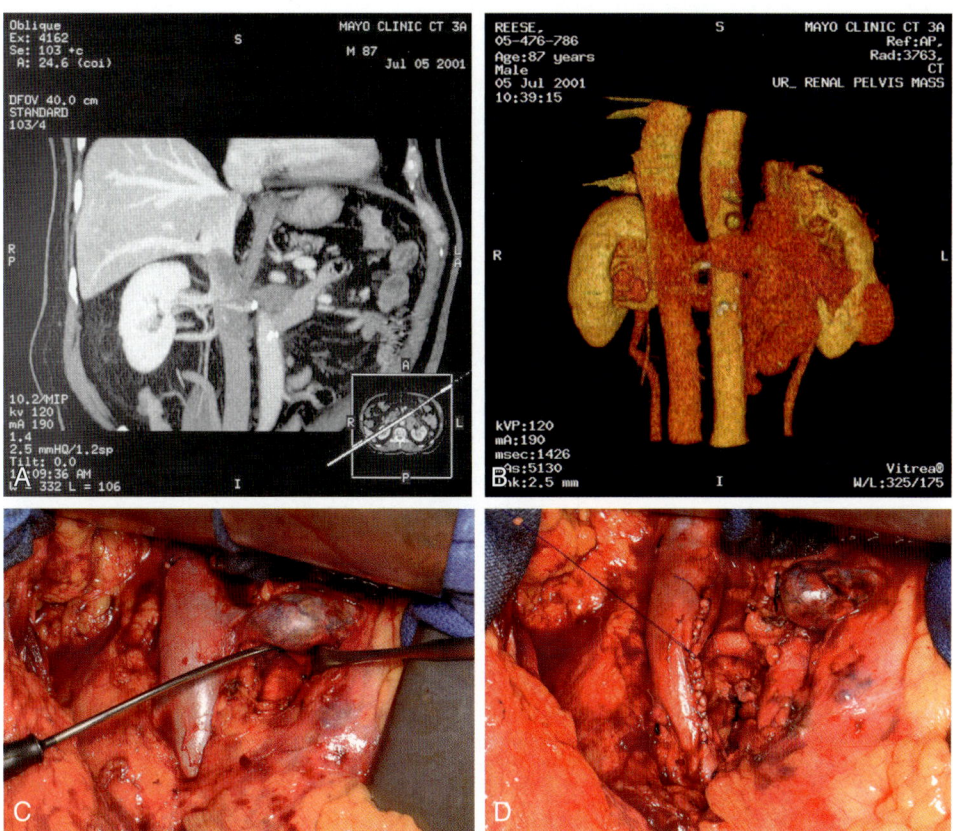

Fig. 101.54. Coronal computed tomography scan (A) and three-dimensional reconstruction (B) of a level II left-sided tumor thrombus. (C) Securing vascular control. (D) Repair of inferior vena caval defect.

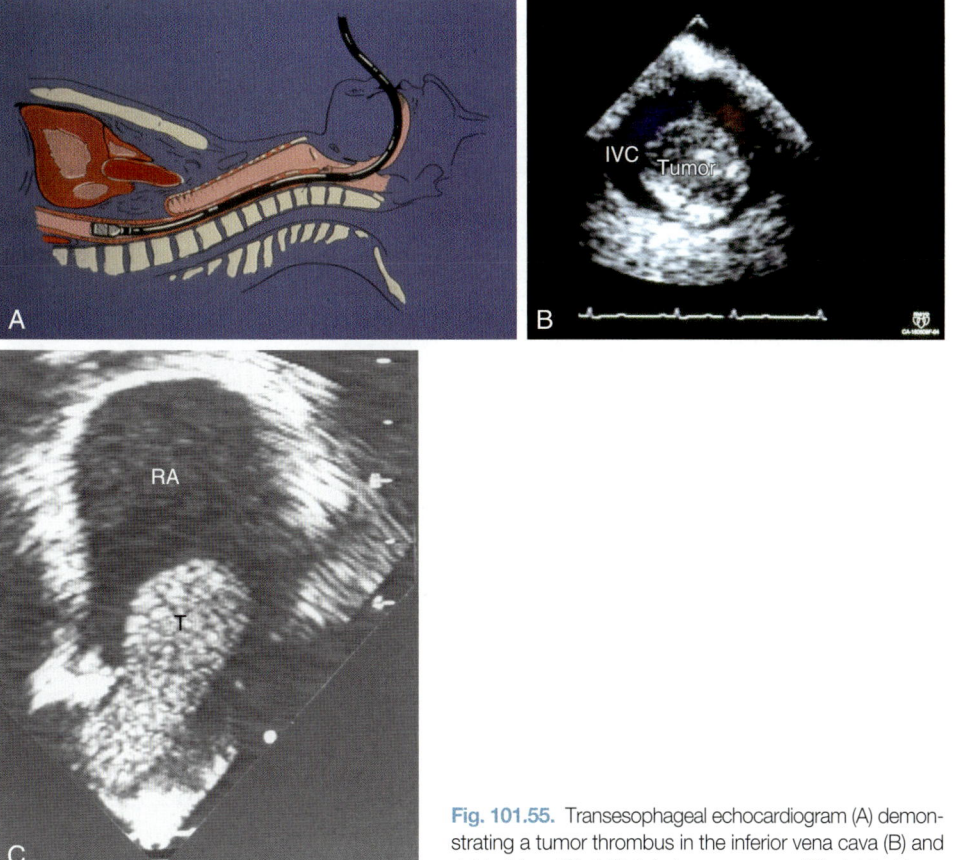

Fig. 101.55. Transesophageal echocardiogram (A) demonstrating a tumor thrombus in the inferior vena cava (B) and right atrium (C). *IVC,* Inferior vena cava; *RA,* right atrium.

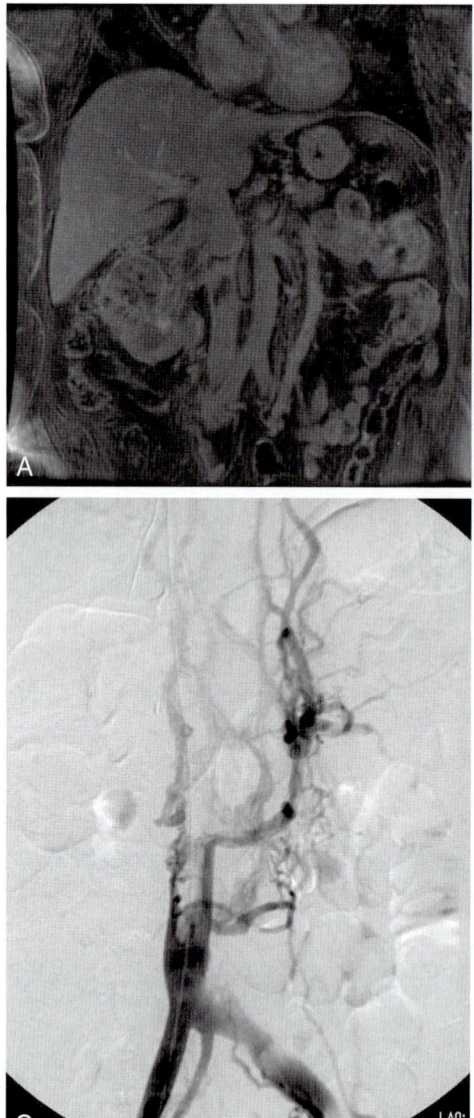
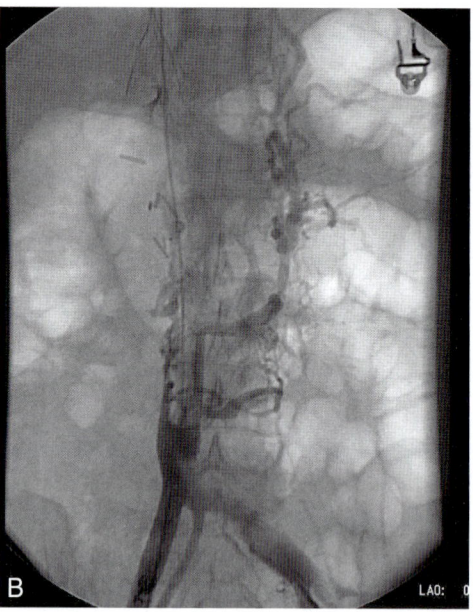

Fig. 101.56. Renal cell carcinoma tumor thrombus causing complete inferior vena caval occlusion with extensive collateralization to the azygous system demonstrated on computed tomography scan (A) and angiogram (B and C).

thrombi will not tolerate suprahepatic clamping very well and should probably undergo bypass. Contrarily, patients with completely occlusive thrombi will typically have developed extensive collateral venous drainage networks and therefore tolerate clamping much better (Fig. 101.56). Occasionally, a level IV thrombus can be milked into the abdomen through a small diaphragmatic incision and treated intra-abdominally. It is crucial that IVC control not compromise the operation because bleeding and hypotension can lead to an incomplete tumor resection, a result that is universally fatal. Techniques of bypass are discussed in a later section.

We prefer the anterior midline incision for level III and IV thrombi; however, a chevron incision with added sternotomy can also be used. The right kidney and great vessels are exposed as described for a level I thrombus, and the right renal artery is ligated in the interaortocaval area. The infrahepatic IVC is gently dissected. The infrarenal IVC and left renal vein are isolated, and Rummel tourniquets are placed around them.

The liver is mobilized by ligating and dividing the ligamentum teres, the remnant of the obliterated left umbilical vein that is located at the lower free border of the falciform ligament. The falciform ligament is divided with electrocautery up to the upper border of the liver, where it branches into the coronary ligament on the right and the left triangular ligament on the left (see Fig. 101.12). The superior layer of the coronary ligament is divided with scissors or electrocautery, taking care not to injure the liver or the IVC, which is located just behind the ligament in the bare area of the liver. Division of the superior layer of the coronary ligament continues along the right border of the liver until it forms the right triangular ligament (the fused superior and inferior layers of the coronary ligament), which should also be divided. Mobilization of the right lobe of the liver is completed by dividing the inferior layer of the coronary ligament, the attachment that ties the liver to the diaphragm, upward toward the IVC.

The left triangular ligament is divided anteriorly, and hepatic mobilization is completed by dividing the posterior aspects of the left triangular ligament toward the IVC. The right lobe of the liver can now be safely and gently rotated toward the midline so that the IVC can be evaluated on the posterior surface of the liver (Fig. 101.57). For tumors of the left kidney, it may be necessary to divide the diaphragmatic attachments of the spleen so that it can be rotated toward the midline with the pancreas without being traumatized.

The plane between the posterior surface of the liver and the anterior surface of the IVC is developed. The help of a hepatic surgeon with this portion of the procedure should be considered. This plane contains venous branches from the liver that are divided into upper and lower groups. The most important group is the upper group that contains the right, middle, and left hepatic veins, the principal outflow from the liver, and therefore cannot be divided. Tumor thrombus can extend into these veins, and they must be carefully inspected and cleared of any thrombus during thrombectomy. Obstruction of these

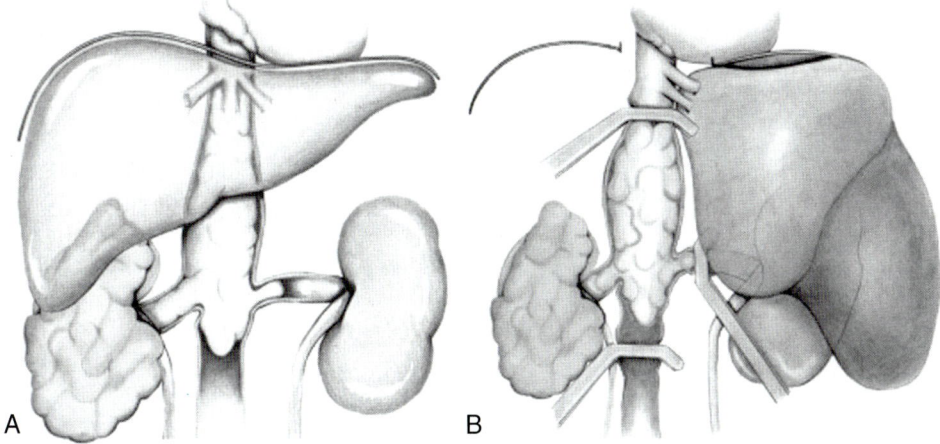

Fig. 101.57. (A and B) Mobilizing the liver to expose the inferior vena cava for management of tumor thrombus. (From Ciancio G, Livingstone AS, Soloway M. Surgical management of renal cell carcinoma with tumor thrombus in the renal and inferior vena cava: the University of Miami experience in using liver transplantation techniques. *Eur Urol* 51:988–95, 2007.)

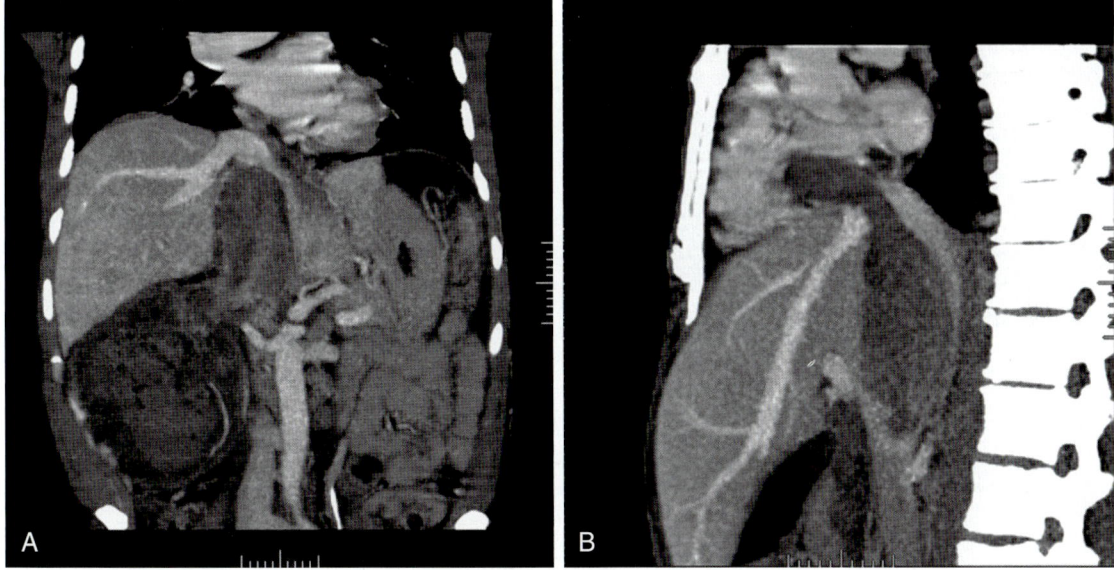

Fig. 101.59. (A) Coronal magnetic resonance image demonstrates tumor extending to the level of the diaphragm. (B) Sagittal magnetic resonance reconstruction demonstrates thrombus that extends farther into the right atrium. The patient would eventually require cardiopulmonary bypass and deep hypothermic circulatory arrest.

three veins leads to the Budd-Chiari syndrome. The lower group of hepatic veins (the accessory hepatic veins) drain blood principally from the caudate lobe (with a small contribution from the right lobe) and can be safely divided. The accessory hepatic veins are ligated with 2-0 silk, and the plane between the IVC and the liver is developed. Additionally, the lumbar veins are ligated with 2-0 silk, and the plane between the IVC and the posterior abdominal wall is developed. The IVC should now be fully mobilized.

A window is created in the lesser omentum, and the porta hepatis (also called the *portal triad* or *hepatic pedicle*), which contains the portal vein, common hepatic artery, and common bile duct, is encircled with a Rummel tourniquet. Clamping the porta hepatis (the Pringle maneuver) is necessary to prevent massive blood loss if the IVC is clamped above the major hepatic veins (eFig. 101.58). Clamping the IVC above and below the hepatic veins while performing the Pringle maneuver is called *total hepatic vascular occlusion*. If the IVC is clamped below the major hepatic veins and the accessory hepatic veins are ligated, the Pringle maneuver may not be necessary.

Under normothermic conditions, the porta hepatis can be clamped for up to 60 minutes, although a clamping time of 20 minutes or less is preferred because ischemic hepatic injury and portal vein thrombosis can ensue. Another complication of the Pringle maneuver is splenic engorgement and rupture as a result of backup of venous drainage from the splenic vein, which normally empties into the portal vein.

The resectability of the tumor and thrombus is determined using TEE and a thorough intraoperative assessment of the anatomy. If the thrombus is below the hepatic veins or can be milked below these veins, it is usually safe to proceed without bypass. If the thrombus involves the hepatic veins or extends above the liver, bypass is often required (Fig. 101.59). The IVC is occluded above the liver and thrombus, and the patient's hemodynamic response is observed over 2 to 5 minutes. Clamping the suprahepatic IVC results in a 60% reduction in cardiac preload, an 80% increase in peripheral vascular resistance, a 50% increase in heart rate, a 40% drop in cardiac output, and a 10% to 20% drop in mean arterial blood pressure. If the cardiac output drops more than 50% or the mean arterial blood pressure drops more than 30%, the patient will not tolerate suprahepatic IVC clamping. Options for managing this situation include bypass (our preference) and clamping of the supraceliac aorta. If the IVC clamping trial is tolerated and the thrombus can be removed in less than 30 minutes, it is safe to proceed with the intra-abdominal procedure.

In sequence, the infrarenal IVC, the contralateral (left) renal vein, the porta hepatis, and the suprahepatic IVC are clamped. For left-sided tumors, the right renal artery should be clamped before the right renal vein because there is no good collateral venous drainage for the right kidney. The ostium of the right renal vein is circumferentially incised, and the incision is extended upward toward the intrahepatic IVC. The incision should be large enough to permit extraction of all of the tumor thrombus and careful inspection of the intima of the IVC. The thrombus and kidney are excised (Fig. 101.60). With the help of a Penfield dissector, the IVC is cleared of adherent thrombus. A Fogarty balloon catheter (Edwards Lifesciences Corporation, Irvine, CA) or 20-Fr Foley catheter can be used as an embolectomy catheter if the thrombus is out of reach. If involved with tumor that cannot be scraped away, the IVC should be completely or partially resected and reconstructed (see the Patching, Replacing, and Interrupting the Inferior Vena Cava section later in this chapter). During deep hypothermic arrest, a cystoscope can be used to inspect the hepatic veins and suprahepatic IVC, which allows for a smaller caval incision. The IVC is closed as described for level II thrombus. The hepatic ligaments are tacked back into place to prevent torsion of the liver. A regional lymphadenectomy is performed, and a closed suction drain is inserted.

Level III-IV Vena Caval Thrombectomy: Combined Intra-Abdominal and Intrathoracic Approach

Level III thrombi that cannot be removed intra-abdominally and most level IV thrombi are managed with a combined intra-abdominal and intrathoracic approach. Thoracoabdominal, chevron laparotomy with sternotomy, and anterior midline laparotomy with sternotomy incisions can be used to provide access to the chest and abdomen (eFig. 101.61). We prefer the anterior midline laparotomy with sternotomy. A cardiothoracic surgeon needs to participate with the planned operation.

The abdominal portion of the case is identical to the intra-abdominal approach described earlier. Once the abdominal phase is completed, the cardiothoracic surgeon is called to the operating room and a median sternotomy is performed. The pericardium is opened, and the right heart is exposed. Often, mobilization of the liver and IVC is easier once the sternotomy is completed (Fig. 101.62).

The blood supply is bypassed using one of the techniques described in the following sections. Once on bypass, the ostium of the renal vein is circumferentially excised, the incision is extended cranially on the IVC, and the thrombus is extracted. A right atriotomy is usually performed to help remove the suprahepatic thrombus. The atrium and IVC are then closed. The patient is taken off bypass and

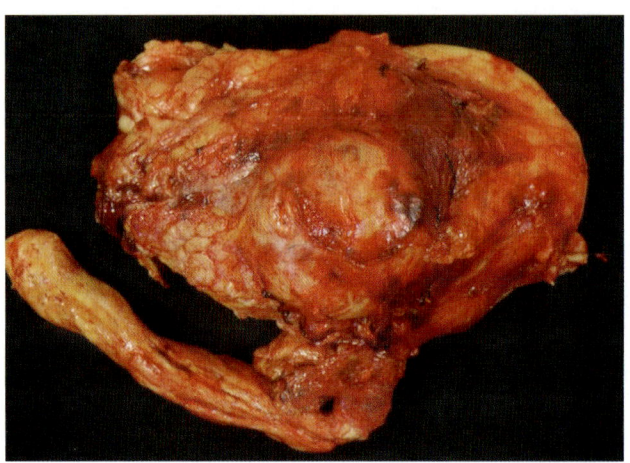

Fig. 101.60. Resected renal mass and intact inferior vena caval thrombus.

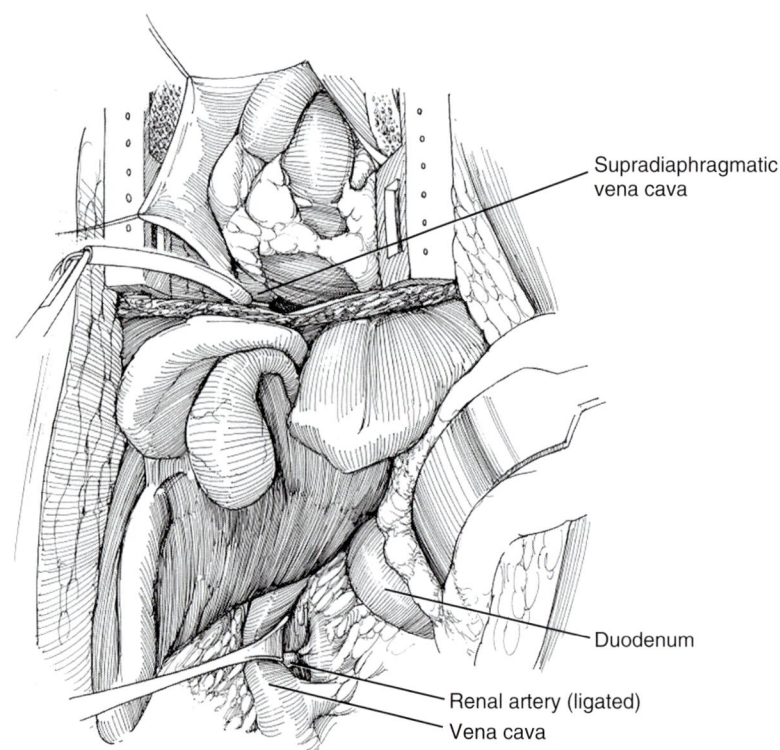

Fig. 101.62. Median sternotomy with pericardium opened exposing the right heart. (From Smith JA Jr, Howards SS, Preminger GM, eds. *Hinman's atlas of urologic surgery*. 3rd ed. Philadelphia, PA: Saunders; 2012.)

thoracotomy tubes, and closed suction abdominal drains are placed. The hepatic ligaments are tacked back into place to prevent torsion of the liver, and regional lymphadenectomy is performed.

Bypass Techniques for Inferior Vena Caval Surgery

The requirement of bypass significantly complicates and prolongs IVC thrombectomy. However, bypass is often critical to performing the procedure safely and completely and should be used whenever required. Bypass should be considered in patients in whom the IVC cross-clamping trial causes significant hypotension, and in patients in whom there is preoperative cardiac or hepatic dysfunction, contralateral renal dysfunction, or portal venous hypertension, and when there is major intraoperative bleeding that is difficult to control.

Venovenous Bypass. This is the least invasive bypass technique for IVC thrombi and involves shunting the venous blood from below the renal veins to the venous return of the heart with the aid of a pump. Venovenous bypass (VVB) can be done without opening the chest, which is a key advantage that it has over traditional CPB. Two main options are available for infrarenal cannulation: a percutaneous approach through the femoral vein or a direct intraoperative approach through the IVC just above its bifurcation. When cannulating the IVC, it is important to position the tip of the cannula as far from the tumor thrombus as possible to avoid dislodging it, which can cause a massive pulmonary embolism, and to avoid aspirating and recirculating tumor cells. Several options are available for delivering the shunted blood back to the heart: a percutaneous approach via the internal jugular vein, a cutdown approach to the brachial/axillary vein, and a direct intraoperative approach through the right atrium. One advantage of VVB is that full heparinization is not required, which may help minimize postoperative bleeding problems. However, a key disadvantage is that the blood flow to the intercostal and lumbar arteries and the intercostal and lumbar veins is not interrupted during VVB, a problem that can lead to major bleeding once the cavotomy is performed to extract the thrombus. VVB should not be used when atrial thrombi cannot be completely milked into the IVC, when there is extensive bland thrombus in the iliac veins or infrarenal IVC, or when there is preexisting Budd-Chiari syndrome.

For percutaneous VVB, immediately following intubation, the anesthesiologist should insert an 8- to 18-Fr heparin-bonded arterial cannula into the internal jugular vein using the Seldinger technique (Fig. 101.63). A 6-cm, 18-gauge hollow needle is inserted into the femoral vein, a guidewire is placed, the tract is dilated, and a 14- to 20-Fr heparin-bonded arterial cannula is advanced into the common iliac vein. Both cannulae are connected to a perfusion pump using heparin-bonded tubing. The portal vein can also be cannulated with a 20-Fr cannula and its venous flow returned to the pump, although this is usually not necessary. The incision is performed, and the kidney and IVC are dissected. Once all the vessels are clamped, the perfusion pump is started and the thrombectomy is performed under pump, ligating any troublesome lumbar and intercostal veins. Once thrombectomy and IVC repair are complete, the vessels are unclamped in the same order they were clamped.

For open VVB, the kidney and IVC are dissected, the liver is mobilized, and a sternotomy is performed (eFig. 101.64). A 20-Fr cannula is inserted into the infrarenal IVC well away from the tumor thrombus, and then a 14- to 20-Fr cannula is inserted into the auricle of the right atrium. The infrarenal IVC, renal vein, porta hepatis, and suprarenal IVC are clamped, and then bypass is started. Thrombectomy is performed as quickly as possible.

Cardiopulmonary Bypass With and Without Deep Hypothermic Arrest. CPB can be performed with or without deep hypothermic arrest (Fig. 101.65). CPB with hypothermic arrest involves stopping the heart and starting bypass, cooling the patient to 16° C to 18° C, and draining all of the blood from the patient. Although very invasive, CPB with hypothermic arrest offers several benefits. First, it can be used in cases in which the thrombus cannot be milked below an intrapericardial IVC clamp. Second, there is no need to clamp the aorta or porta hepatis or to ligate as many lumbar and hepatic veins because blood flow to these structures is no longer present. However, all vessels that have been traumatized or transected

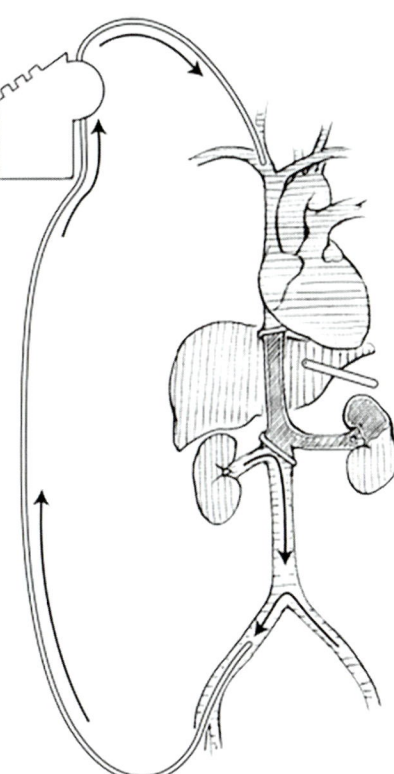

Fig. 101.63. Percutaneous venovenous bypass. (From Smith JA Jr, Howards SS, Preminger GM, eds. *Hinman's atlas of urologic surgery*. 3rd ed. Philadelphia, PA: Saunders; 2012.)

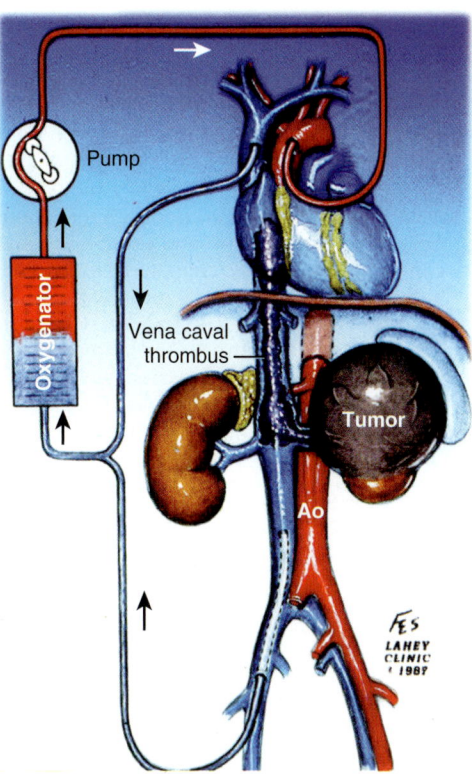

Fig. 101.65. Traditional median sternotomy approach with cannulation of the aortic arch, superior vena cava, and right femoral vein for cardiopulmonary bypass. *Ao,* Aorta. (© The Lahey Clinic.)

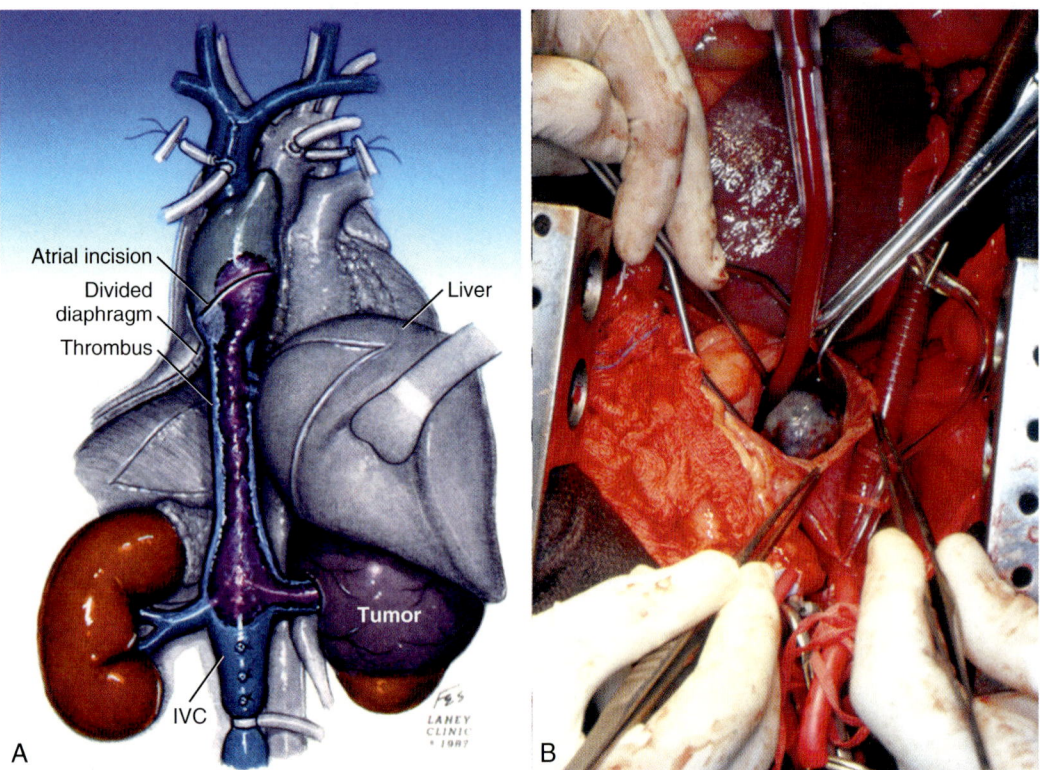

Fig. 101.66. (A and B) Tumor thrombus extension into the right atrium is removed using a traditional median sternotomy approach and an atriotomy for retrieval of the thrombus. *IVC,* Inferior vena cava. (A, © The Lahey Clinic; B, from Wotkowicz C, Libertino JA, Sorcini A, et al. Management of renal cell carcinoma with vena cava and atrial thrombus: minimal access vs. median sternotomy with circulatory arrest. *BJU Int* 98:289–97, 2006.)

must be controlled because they will bleed once the patient is taken off bypass. Third, the absence of active blood flow allows for complete inspection of the IVC and hepatic veins, thereby aiding in achieving a complete thrombectomy. Fourth, the risk for embolization during thrombectomy is lower. Fifth, the surgeon is allowed up to 60 minutes to perform thrombectomy (although <40 minutes is certainly a better target), whereas IVC clamping without bypass is only tolerated for about 30 minutes.

For CPB with deep hypothermia, the kidney and IVC are dissected and the liver is mobilized. The cardiothoracic surgeon performs the sternotomy, opens the pericardium, and exposes the heart and its vessels. Heparin-bonded cannulae are placed in the infrarenal IVC and the right atrium to collect venous blood, and a cannula is placed into the aortic arch for outflow. The patient is heparinized, and bypass is started. The aorta is clamped, and cardioplegia solution is administered. The temperature of the recirculated blood is dropped to 10° C to 14° C, and the patient is cooled for 15 to 30 minutes until a core temperature of 16° C to 18° C is reached. Intraoperative electroencephalography should be performed to determine when the brain has been adequately cooled. When sufficient cooling has been achieved, the perfusion pump is stopped and 95% of the patient's blood volume is drained into the pump reservoir. Tumor thrombectomy should be performed as quickly as possible, taking great care to ligate all potential bleeders (Fig. 101.66 and eFig. 101.67). If the patient has known coronary artery disease, coronary artery bypass can be performed at the same time. If the resection is taking longer than anticipated, the surgeon should consider allowing a 10-mL/kg/min trickle of blood to flow to the organs or using retrograde cerebral perfusion.

Once the IVC and right atrium are repaired, warm blood is reinfused from the pump reservoir and CPB is restarted. Hemostasis is performed while the patient warms to 37° C over the next 30 to 45 minutes. Once the heart has restarted pumping, bypass is stopped, the cannulae are removed, and protamine sulfate is administered.

Coagulopathy is common, and fresh frozen plasma, platelets, and packed red blood cells should be available to administer. Thoracostomy tubes and closed suction abdominal drains are inserted.

Patching, Replacing, and Interrupting the Inferior Vena Cava

Patch Cavoplasty. If the IVC is expected to be less than 50% of its original size, a patch cavoplasty is necessary to prevent IVC stenosis and thrombosis-related events (Fig. 101.68). Autologous and bovine pericardium, polytetrafluoroethylene (PTFE), collagen-impregnated Dacron (DuPont, Wilmington, DE), and autologous saphenous vein are materials that can be used for patch cavoplasty.

The patch is sized to a bit larger dimension than the caval defect, typically configured to an oval shape. A double-armed 5-0 Prolene suture on a BB needle is used to sew the patch in place. Small and regular suture bites will assure a tight closure. Intraluminal inversion of the edges of the patch should be avoided to prevent excess thrombogenesis. Some surgeons prefer tacking both apices of the defect first and then running a strand of suture from each apex to the midpoint between the apices, which requires four knots. Alternatively, the graft can be parachuted into position and sewn into place circumferentially, requiring only one knot. Minimal manipulation of the patch is helpful to prevent inadvertent damage to the patch and caval edge. Liberal use of heparinized saline solution can help with visualization. Before final closure of the cava, the caudal IVC clamp should be released and 5 to 10 mL of venous blood allowed to escape from the cavotomy, providing for removal of air, debris, and clot before unclamping the cranial caval clamp.

Vena Caval Replacement. In situations in which a circumferential section of IVC has been removed or if a vena cava defect is too large for simple patching, vena caval replacement is necessary (Fig. 101.69). Typically, we use PTFE grafts to replace the IVC, although others have described spiraled saphenous vein, superficial femoral vein, and tubularized pericardium as options (Helfand et al., 2011;

heparin is administered. The IVC is clamped, and the affected portion is excised. The cranial IVC-patch anastomosis is completed first. Subsequently, the graft is clamped followed by releasing the cranial IVC clamp to test the upper IVC-patch anastomosis. Next the graft is sized and cut to fit the IVC defect and the caudal IVC-patch anastomosis is completed. Before closure of the lower IVC anastomosis, the graft is unclamped and 5 to 10 mL of blood is allowed to escape from the graft through the cavotomy. The graft is then reclamped and the infrarenal IVC is unclamped, and 5 to 10 mL of blood is allowed to escape from the infrarenal IVC. Closure of the anastomosis is completed by tying the final knot, and the IVC is unclamped. The graft is wrapped with omentum or retroperitoneal fat, and then the hepatic ligaments are reapproximated to prevent torsion of the IVC graft.

Postoperatively, low-dose intravenous heparin or a reduced dosage of low-molecular-weight heparin is given. Once the patient's bowel function has recovered, lifelong oral warfarin is used with a target international normalized ratio of 2 to 3.

Inferior Vena Cava Filtration and Permanent Interruption for Bland Thrombus

Occasionally, a patient with an infrarenal bland thrombus requires management at the time of tumor thrombectomy. For bland thrombus that is limited to the pelvic veins, intraoperative placement of an infrarenal vena caval filter is indicated. When the bland thrombus diffusely involves the infrarenal IVC, the optimal management is permanent interruption of the IVC. Necessary intraoperative care is required to preserve the collateral lumbar venous drainage because these vessels provide a "release valve" for the impaired caval blood flow. When the infrarenal IVC is occluded with bland thrombus that is distinct and separate from the tumor thrombus, the best form of management is usually permanent interruption without resection because attempts at complete removal of diffuse organized bland thrombus are almost always unsuccessful and often result in vascular injury. Options for permanent interruption of the IVC include serrated vena caval clips (e.g., Adams-DeWeese clip, Moretz clip), cross-stapling with a vascular GIA stapler (Covidien Ltd., Mansfield, MA), suture plication, and suture ligation. Serrated vena caval clips and vascular staplers offer the advantage of easy application, while serrated vena caval clips allow partial blood flow through the IVC.

When the bland thrombus in the infrarenal IVC is admixed with tumor thrombus that has undergone retrograde growth, segmental resection of the IVC with permanent interruption of the IVC will maximize the chance of cure. Because it is not possible to accurately dissect tumor thrombus from bland thrombus and assure complete resection of tumor, resection of the IVC below the level of the contralateral renal vein ostium is recommended. Resection should be as close to the renal vein ostium as possible to prevent turbulent and thrombogenic flow in the upper stump. In addition, maximal preservation of the lumbar veins in the lower stump is important to ensure good collateral drainage.

Perioperative Complications

Air Embolism. Air embolism to the right heart and pulmonary arteries is a serious and potentially lethal complication associated with caval thrombectomy. Risk for air embolism can be significantly reduced by releasing the caudal IVC clamp first and allowing air and some blood (5 to 10 mL) to escape from the IVC repair site before removing the cranial clamp.

Acute Pulmonary Embolism. Tumor and bland thrombus can embolize during and after surgery. Minimizing intraoperative manipulation of the kidney and IVC before vascular control helps reduce the likelihood of acute thrombotic pulmonary embolism. Early preoperative or intraoperative placement of a Greenfield filter (Boston Scientific, Natick, MA) in a patient with pelvic bland thrombus can also help reduce the risk for pulmonary embolism. If respiratory distress is encountered during surgery, strong consideration should be given to prompt thoracotomy, pulmonary arteriotomy, and extraction of the thrombus.

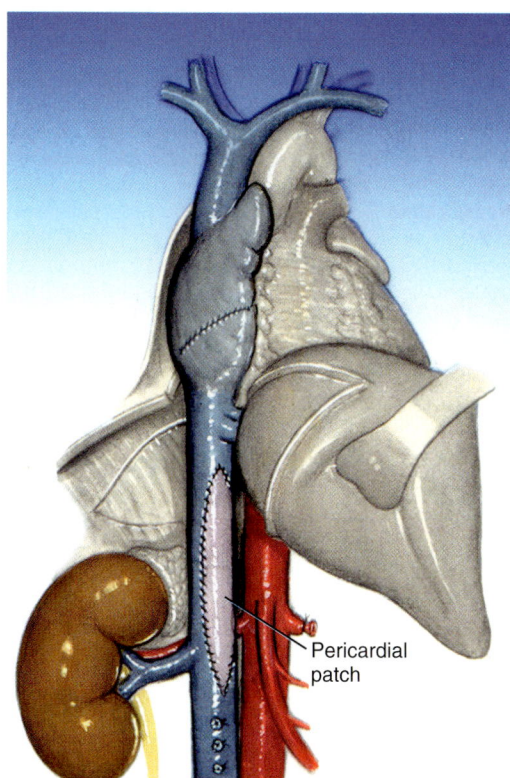

Fig. 101.68. Vena caval reconstruction using a pericardial patch graft.

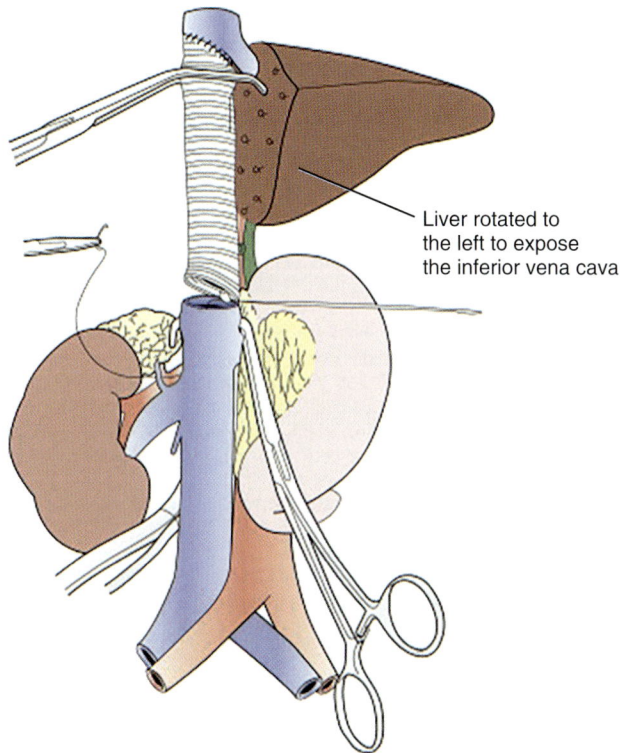

Fig. 101.69. Vena caval replacement with polytetrafluoroethylene graft. (From Bower TC, Nagorney DM, Toomey BJ, et al. Vena cava replacement for malignant disease: is there a role? *Ann Vasc Surg* 7:51–62, 1993.)

Hyams et al., 2011; Pulitano et al., 2013; Quinones-Baldrich et al., 2012). Typically a graft size of 16 to 20 mm in diameter is required. The large diameter of the graft reduces the risk for thrombosis.

The liver is mobilized, and the IVC is exposed completely. Vascular bypass is used if clinically indicated, and 5000 units of intravenous

Massive Hemorrhage. Major bleeding can occur during and after the surgery. If uncontrolled major bleeding occurs in a patient who is not on bypass, the surgeon should consider clamping the aorta above the celiac trunk or initiating deep hypothermic CPB. However, CPB can also lead to major coagulopathy, potentially worsening the degree of hemorrhage. Fresh frozen plasma, platelets, and red blood cells should be transfused liberally as indicated. Using a Cell Saver (Haemonetics Corporation, Braintree, MA) is not recommended for oncologic surgery because tumor cells can be disseminated.

Hepatic Dysfunction. Temporary hepatic dysfunction, characterized by elevated transaminases and alkaline phosphatase, is common in patients with levels III and IV thrombi that require suprahepatic IVC clamping and/or bypass. Minimizing clamping of the porta hepatis as much as possible can reduce hepatic ischemia and thereby the degree of postoperative hepatic dysfunction. Liver enzymes typically peak 2 to 3 days postoperatively and slowly resolve thereafter.

Organ Ischemia. Cardiac ischemia is most common in patients undergoing suprahepatic IVC clamping without bypass. Patients with poor preoperative cardiac function are probably best managed with CPB. Renal and intestinal ischemia can also result during thrombectomy, requiring close postoperative monitoring.

Videos 101.2, 101.3, and 101.4 show procedures related to this chapter.

KEY POINTS

- The origin of the right renal artery is posterior to the left renal vein and the IVC. During a difficult right radical nephrectomy, the right renal artery may be more accessible posterior and medial to the IVC, near the site of origin from the aorta.
- Although the right gonadal and adrenal veins drain into the IVC, the drainage of the left gonadal and left adrenal veins is different as they drain into the left renal vein.
- Simple nephrectomy, removal of the kidney within the Gerota fascia, is used for management of benign renal entities.
- The key elements of radical nephrectomy are early ligation of the renal artery and vein and removal of the kidney outside of the Gerota fascia. When technically feasible, the ipsilateral adrenal gland should be spared.
- For left radical nephrectomy, particularly for upper pole renal masses, identification of the left renal artery from the posterior approach is recommended to avoid inadvertent ligation of the SMA, which is on the anterior surface of the aorta 1 to 2 cm cephalad to the left renal vein.
- Regional lymphadenectomy extending from the crus of the diaphragm to the aortic bifurcation is employed in select cases of advanced local disease and when technically feasible.
- The impact of lymphadenectomy on progression-free and overall survival is controversial.
- To maintain the maximum number of functioning nephrons, partial nephrectomy is the treatment of choice for stage T1 renal tumors when technically feasible, even in the absence of identifiable renal insufficiency.
- The goal of partial nephrectomy is complete excision of the tumor with negative surgical margins and maximal preservation of benign adjacent parenchyma. Various techniques have been used, including enucleation, polar segmental nephrectomy, transverse resection, wedge resection, and extracorporeal partial nephrectomy with renal autotransplantation.
- In patients with known IVC tumor thrombus, intraoperative TEE should be utilized after the patient is anesthetized and intubated to appropriately assess the distal extent of the tumor thrombus before initiating the surgical procedure.
- When performing right radical nephrectomy with tumor thrombectomy, the suprarenal IVC can be resected, but only if the left renal vein has been ligated distal to its venous tributaries (i.e., gonadal, lumbar, and adrenal veins).
- Given the lack of venous tributaries on the right side, the suprarenal IVC should not be resected for a left-sided tumor unless one provides alternative venous drainage for the right kidney with autotransplantation or a saphenous vein graft to the splenic, portal, or inferior mesenteric vein.
- Alternatives to CPB may include venovenous bypass and extensive liver mobilization.
- When reconstructing the IVC, the lumen can be safely narrowed by half and closed primarily. To maintain the lumen in larger resections, the cava can be reconstructed with a pericardial graft or PTFE.

SUGGESTED READINGS

Blom JH, van Poppel H, Marechal JM, et al: Radical nephrectomy with and without lymph-node dissection: final results of European Organization for Research and Treatment of Cancer (EORTC) randomized phase 3 trial 30881, *Eur Urol* 55:28–34, 2009.

Blute ML, Amling CL, Bryant SC, et al: Management and extended outcome of patients with synchronous bilateral solid renal neoplasms in the absence of von Hippel-Lindau disease, *Mayo Clin Proc* 75:1020–1026, 2000.

Blute ML, Leibovich BC, Cheville JC, et al: A protocol for performing extended lymph node dissection using primary tumor pathological features for patients treated with radical nephrectomy for clear cell renal cell carcinoma, *J Urol* 172:465–469, 2004a.

Blute ML, Leibovich BC, Lohse CM, et al: The Mayo Clinic experience with surgical management, complications and outcome for patients with renal cell carcinoma and venous tumour thrombus, *BJU Int* 94:33–41, 2004b.

Crawford ED, Skinner DG: Intercostal nerve block with thoracoabdominal and flank incisions, *Urology* 19:25–28, 1982.

Gill IS, Kavoussi LR, Lane BR, et al: Comparison of 1,800 laparoscopic and open partial nephrectomies for single renal tumors, *J Urol* 178:41–46, 2007.

Hanley MJ, Davidson K: Prior mannitol and furosemide infusion in a model of ischemic acute renal failure, *Am J Physiol* 241:F556–F564, 1981.

Novick AC, Gephardt G, Guz B, et al: Long-term follow-up after partial removal of a solitary kidney, *N Engl J Med* 325:1058–1062, 1991.

Novick AC, Jackson CL, Straffon RA: The role of renal autotransplantation in complex urological reconstruction, *J Urol* 143:452–457, 1990.

Psutka SP, Feldman AS, McDougal WS, et al: Long-term oncologic outcomes after radiofrequency ablation for T1 renal cell carcinoma, *Eur Urol* 63:486–492, 2013.

Schwartz MJ, Smith EB, Trost DW, et al: Renal artery embolization: clinical indications and experience from over 100 cases, *BJU Int* 99:881–886, 2007.

Siemer S, Lehmann J, Kamradt J, et al: Adrenal metastases in 1635 patients with renal cell carcinoma: outcome and indication for adrenalectomy, *J Urol* 171:2155–2159, discussion 2159, 2004.

Stormont TJ, Bilhartz DL, Zincke H: Pitfalls of "bench surgery" and autotransplantation of renal cell carcinoma, *Mayo Clin Proc* 67:621–628, 1992.

Volpe A, Kachura JR, Geddie WR, et al: Techniques, safety and accuracy of sampling of renal tumors by fine needle aspiration and core biopsy, *J Urol* 178:379–386, 2007.

Zincke H, Sen SE: Experience with extracorporeal surgery and autotransplantation for renal cell and transitional cell cancer of the kidney, *J Urol* 140:25–27, 1988.

REFERENCES

The complete reference list is available online at ExpertConsult.com.

102 Laparoscopic and Robotic Surgery of the Kidney

Daniel M. Moreira, MD, MHS, and Louis R. Kavoussi, MD, MBA

The first laparoscopic nephrectomy was described by Ralph Clayman and colleagues at Washington University in St. Louis in 1991. Subsequently, minimally invasive techniques have been applied to all surgical renal pathology. Expanding surgical experience has shown equivalent long-term outcomes and improved recovery compared with open surgery. The introduction of "robotic" technology has led to a widespread adoption of minimally invasive renal surgery; laparoscopic radical nephrectomy has become the most common approach for renal tumors not amenable to partial nephrectomy (Kerbl et al., 2011). **Multiple studies have demonstrated that minimally invasive renal surgery provides less incisional pain, shorter convalescence, and better cosmesis compared with open surgery** (Gill et al., 2007; Lane et al., 2008; Tan et al., 2011). This chapter discusses indications, present techniques, and results and outlines potential complications of laparoscopy and robotic-assisted laparoscopic surgery as applied to the kidney.

PATIENT EVALUATION AND PREPARATION

Patient selection and preparation for laparoscopic and robotic renal surgery follow the same principles of general laparoscopic surgery and comparable open renal surgery, which are discussed in Chapters 9 and 101, respectively. **Relevant history and physical exam are important to identify potential issues that could arise during surgery.** For example, body habitus should be taken into consideration when positioning the patient on the surgical table and obtaining access. Prior abdominal and/or retroperitoneal surgery may influence trocar placement and surgical approach (e.g., transperitoneal vs. extraperitoneal access) (Cadeddu et al., 1999; Chen et al., 1998).

Anesthetic Considerations for Laparoscopy

Laparoscopic renal surgery requires general anesthesia. **The patient's pulmonary and cardiac function must tolerate this approach; the pneumoperitoneum can compromise ventilation and venous return.** For example, patients with severe chronic pulmonary disease may not be able to compensate for the pneumoperitoneum-induced hypercarbia. In these cases, lower insufflation pressures, use of helium insufflation, or conversion to open surgery may be required (Whalley and Berrigan, 2000).

Considerations in Obese Patients

Although not a contraindication to laparoscopic or robotic surgery, obesity frequently poses a challenge to the surgical team. **Difficulties include the distorted or hidden anatomy resulting from the excess adipose tissue, limited range of trocar and instrument motion, need for longer instruments, and higher pneumoperitoneum pressures.** These challenges may translate into higher complication rates and conversion to open surgery (Mendoza et al., 1996).

Considerations in Elderly Patients

The benefits of minimally invasive renal surgery have been demonstrated in all patient groups irrespective of age. **Some of the minimally invasive renal surgery benefits are particularly advantageous in the elderly population, including reduced postoperative pain and minimization of narcotic use leading to early mobilization** (Salami et al., 2013).

SURGICAL APPROACHES AND OBTAINING ACCESS

The minimally invasive approaches to renal surgery can be broadly divided into categories: transperitoneal, retroperitoneal, hand-assisted, robotic, laparoendoscopic single-site surgery (LESS), and natural orifice transluminal endoscopic surgery (NOTES). Although each approach has specific situational advantages, data from randomized clinical trials and retrospective studies suggest these approaches have comparable outcomes with only potential cosmetic differences. **Thus the choice of surgical approach should be based on availability of resources, surgeon's experience, and patient as well as disease characteristics.**

Transperitoneal Approach

This is the most traditional and widely used surgical approach. Its advantages include the largest working space, familiar anatomic landmarks, and several options for trocar and instrument placement.

Patient Positioning and Trocar Placement

After intravenous access, anesthesia induction, endotracheal intubation, bladder catheter, sequential compression stockings, and orogastric tube placement, the patient is placed in the modified flank position (from 30- to 45-degree flank up). If desired, table flexion to increase the distance between the ribs and iliac crest may facilitate trocar placement. All pressure points should be carefully padded and the patient secured to the table to allow lateral tilting of the table (Fig. 102.1). Arms may be secured on pillows or arm rest. The operating room is configured to maximize the use of space and allow all members of the surgical team to view the procedure (Fig. 102.2). The entire abdomen and flank are included in the field of skin preparation and draping, in case conversion to open surgery is required. After pneumoperitoneum is achieved, three to five trocars are placed (Fig. 102.3). A wide variety of trocar configurations are effective for renal surgery. The following is a guide for trocar placement, and adaptations may be required on a case-by-case basis.

A 10-mm camera port is inserted at the umbilicus, and a 5- or 10-mm trocar is placed in the midline about 2 cm below the xiphoid process. A 12-mm trocar is inserted in the anterior axillary line at the level of the umbilicus. This trocar is used for instrumentation and the passage of sutures, clamps, or staplers. In short patients, the 12-mm trocar may be placed in the midline, halfway between the umbilicus and pubis. In obese patients, all trocar sites are laterally shifted (see Fig. 102.3). Additional trocars may be placed for the use of retractors to assist visualization or exposure (Fig. 102.4), including a low midline 10- or 12-mm trocar for colon retraction and a 5-mm subxiphoid for liver retraction.

Retroperitoneal Approach

This approach resembles the open surgical technique in which the peritoneal cavity is not violated. It may be preferred for select cases

2279

of partial nephrectomy, pyeloplasty, cyst marsupialization, or renal biopsies. Moreover, this may be preferred especially in instances of extensive intraperitoneal adhesions. **In appropriately selected partial nephrectomy cases such as those with posterior tumors, the retroperitoneal approach may be faster and equally safe compared with the transperitoneal approach** (Fan et al., 2013). **The main limitations of the retroperitoneal approach include the following: limited working space leading to limited distance between trocars and decreased triangulation; less familiar anatomic landmarks; and surgical dissection being much closer to the lens, which may cause frequent smudging of the image.**

Patient Positioning and Trocar Placement

The patient is placed in a full flank position. Table flexion is used to increase the distance between the ribs and iliac crest to facilitate trocar placement. An axillary roll is placed to protect the lower arm. All pressure points should be carefully padded and the patient secured to the table to allow lateral tilting of the table. Arms may be secured on pillows or an arm rest. A trocar transverse incision

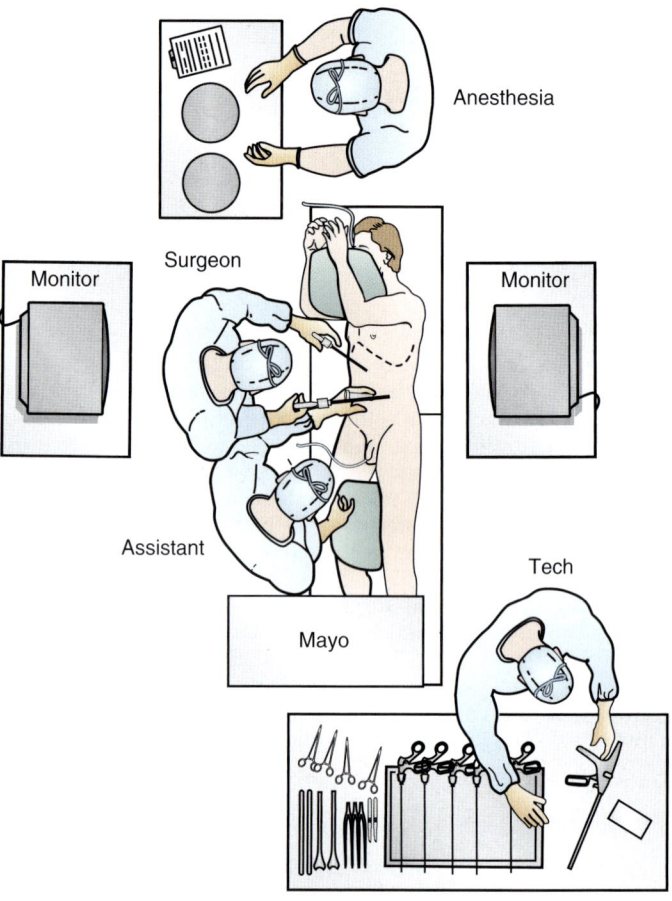

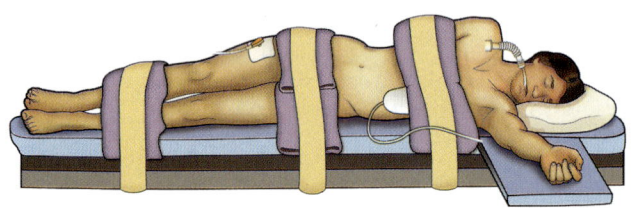

Fig. 102.1. The patient is placed in a modified flank position with the operative side tilted up 30 to 45 degrees using a gel roll or a rolled blanket supporting the back. The lower arm is placed on a padded arm rest, and the other arm is flexed at the elbow and rested over the chest. Wide cloth or silk tape is used to secure the patient to the operating table to allow for table rotation during the surgery.

Fig. 102.2. The operating room configured for left nephrectomy. Two monitors allow the assistant to follow the procedure. The scrub technician (tech) is positioned to easily assist with instrument passage and exchange.

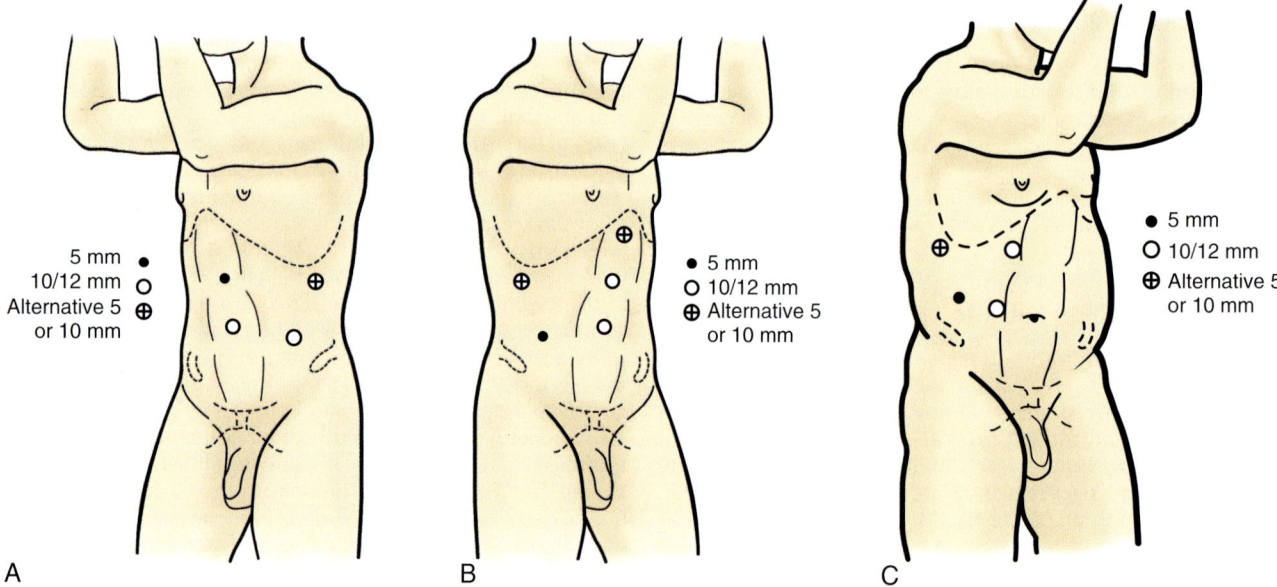

Fig. 102.3. Trocar sites for left-sided (A) and right-sided (B) procedures. A 12-mm trocar is placed lateral to the rectus at the level of the umbilicus, a second 10-mm trocar is placed at the umbilicus, and a 5-mm trocar is inserted in the midline between the umbilicus and the xiphoid process. (C) In obese patients, all trocars are shifted laterally. Optional accessory subcostal, subxiphoid, and low midline trocar positions, which may be helpful for retraction, are also shown.

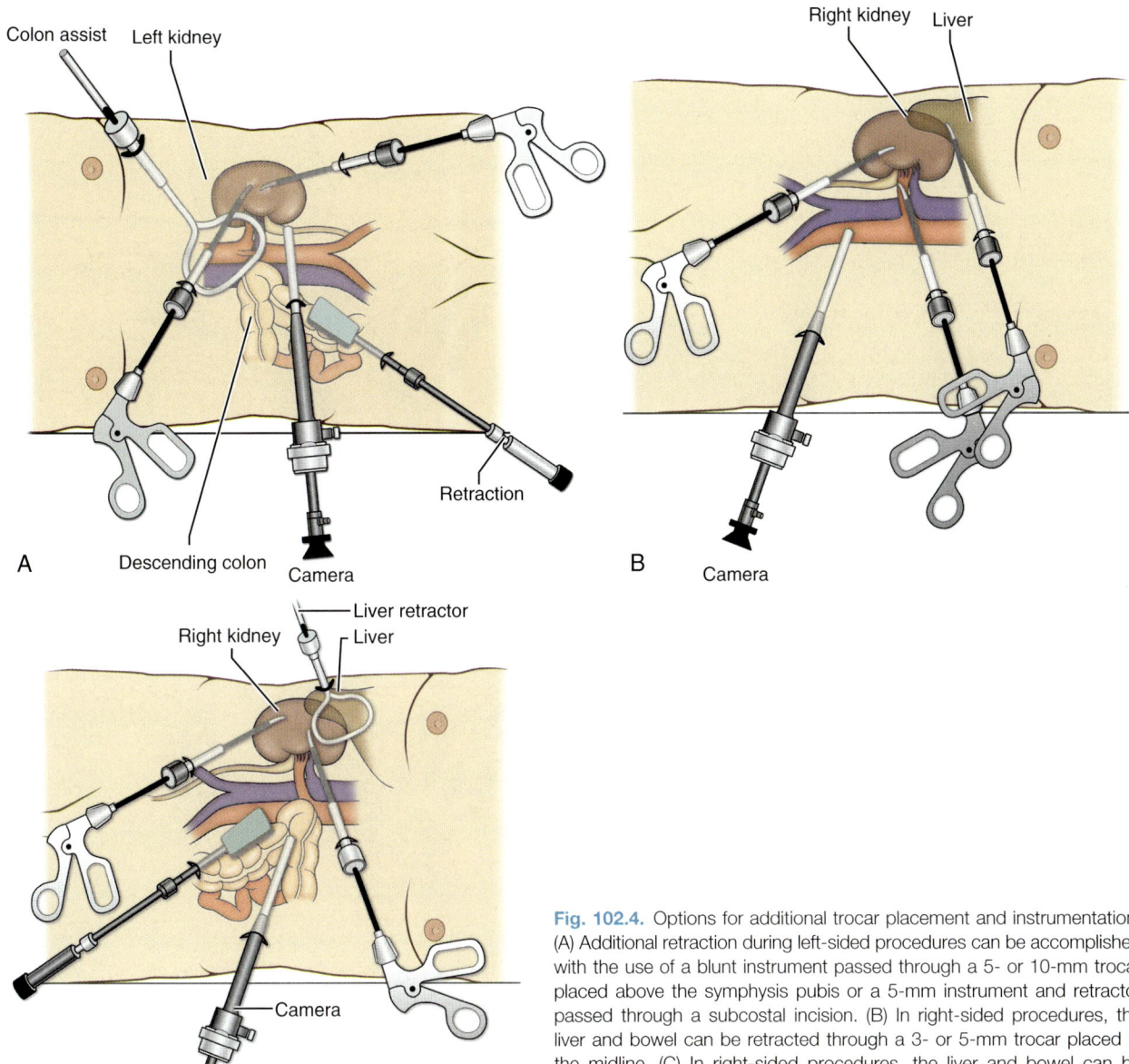

Fig. 102.4. Options for additional trocar placement and instrumentation. (A) Additional retraction during left-sided procedures can be accomplished with the use of a blunt instrument passed through a 5- or 10-mm trocar placed above the symphysis pubis or a 5-mm instrument and retractor passed through a subcostal incision. (B) In right-sided procedures, the liver and bowel can be retracted through a 3- or 5-mm trocar placed in the midline. (C) In right-sided procedures, the liver and bowel can be retracted through a 5-mm trocar with a 5-mm instrument. An optional 10-mm lower midline trocar may also be placed for retraction, freeing the two other working hands for dissection.

is made in the posterior axillary line, halfway between the tip of the 12th rib and the iliac crest (Fig. 102.5A). After the lumbodorsal fascia is divided and the retroperitoneum is entered, a working space is developed using blunt dissection with the laparoscope through a visual obturator or the finger. When manual dissection is used, a finger is placed in the space between the psoas muscle and the kidney (Fig. 102.5B). A balloon dilator is introduced in the cavity and distended with gas or fluid. This displaces the adjacent fat and peritoneum to create a suitable working space (Fig. 102.5C). A simple balloon can be constructed using two fingers of a size 8 or 9 glove (Gaur, 1992). A blunt tip trocar (US Surgical, Norwalk, CT) is then passed through the incision, and the trocar cuff is expanded and cinched to the skin to prevent gas leakage (Fig. 102.5D). Care must be taken to place the balloon completely in the retroperitoneum to avoid dilating the muscle and causing postoperative flank hernia. Alternatively, a 0-degree lens and visual obturator through the initial incision can be used to enter the retroperitoneal space (Fig. 102.6A). The appearance of the characteristic yellow retroperitoneal fat confirms the correct trocar placement. Insufflation is initiated, and blunt dissection using the laparoscope or a laparoscope with a working channel is performed to further develop the working space (Fig. 103.6B). Caution must be taken to avoid entering too anteriorly, which may cause inadvertent peritoneal violation or colon injury, or too posteriorly, which may result in bleeding from the quadratus lumborum or psoas muscles. Once the working space is fully established, the anatomic structures should be identified for orientation and additional trocar placement. Typically, a 5-mm trocar is placed just off the tip of the 12th rib, and a 12-mm trocar is placed posteriorly and superiorly relative to the camera port, both under laparoscopic visualization (see Fig. 103.5A). In cases in which the retroperitoneal approach does not allow the safe completion of the procedure, an initial retroperitoneal access can be expanded to a transperitoneal approach by opening the peritoneum under direct vision.

Hand-Assisted Laparoscopy

The hand-assisted approach combines some of the benefits of pure laparoscopy, such as improved visualization and smaller incisions, with the advantages of open surgery, including the use

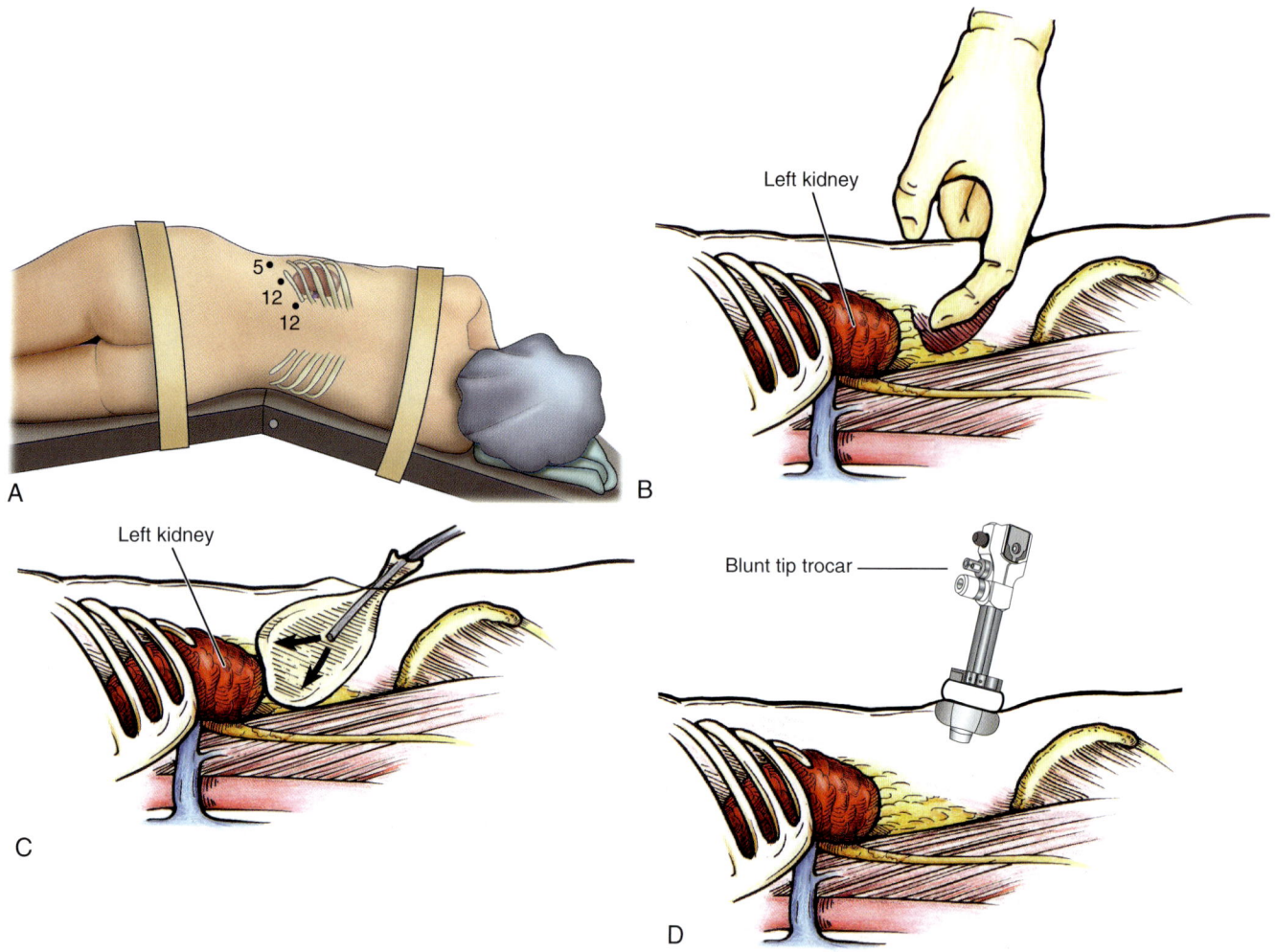

Fig. 102.5. Trocar placement for retroperitoneal kidney surgery. (A) With the patient in the full lateral position, the hips flexed, and the kidney rest elevated, a 15-mm incision is made 2 cm below the tip of the 12th rib, between the rib and the anterior superior iliac spine. (B) The index finger is inserted through the incision and used for blunt dissection to create a hole from the skin through the muscle into the retroperitoneal space. If the finger is in the correct position, the surgeon should feel the smooth surface of psoas muscle and the lower pole of the kidney covered by Gerota fascia. (C) To quickly create the working space, insert a balloon created from the finger of a size 8 or 9 glove, secured with silk suture over a simple red rubber catheter. The balloon is then filled with 600 to 800 mL of saline. (D) A blunt tip trocar (US Surgical, Norwalk, CT) is used to seal the trocar site. Because of its low profile, it will not obstruct the view or take up useful space in the retroperitoneum. The balloon and collar configuration eliminates the need for sutures and allows 360-degree rotation.

of the surgeon's hand for dissection, retraction, and hemostasis, while maintaining tactile feedback. In addition, the same incision, large enough for the hand, is also used to extract the surgical specimen. This approach is attractive for the novice laparoscopic surgeon particularly and in cases of significant scarring around the kidney, when difficult dissection is anticipated. Hand assistance may also be used in the event of an emergency, such as bleeding, by extending a trocar site and placing a hand port to assist in vascular control and repair.

Patient Positioning and Trocar Placement

The patient is posited for a transperitoneal approach (see earlier). First, the hand port incision is made through the skin and fascia and into the peritoneal cavity. The hand port location depends on the operative side, patient's body habitus, surgeon's handedness, and personal preferences (Figs. 102.7 and 102.8). The incision should not be too large given this may cause leakage of gas and difficulty to maintain an adequate pneumoperitoneal pressure. After the hand port is placed, the pneumoperitoneum is established, and additional trocars are placed under direct laparoscopic visualization. Care must be taken in the port placement to avoid the hand getting in the way of the laparoscope or other instruments. The surgeon should be aware of the increased pressure in the arm (from 30 to 100 mm Hg), which may cause tingling, numbness, and pain in the hand and forearm (Monga et al., 2004; Ost et al., 2006).

Robotic-Assisted Laparoscopy

The robotic approach allows surgeons with limited laparoscopic skills to perform minimally invasive reconstructive renal surgery. It has the advantages of a three-dimensional view of the surgical field, greater degree of instrument motion, elimination of tremor, ergonomic position, and the ability to scale motions. The robotic kidney surgery can be done transperitoneally or retroperitoneally via multiple or single-site ports.

Chapter 102 Laparoscopic and Robotic Surgery of the Kidney 2283

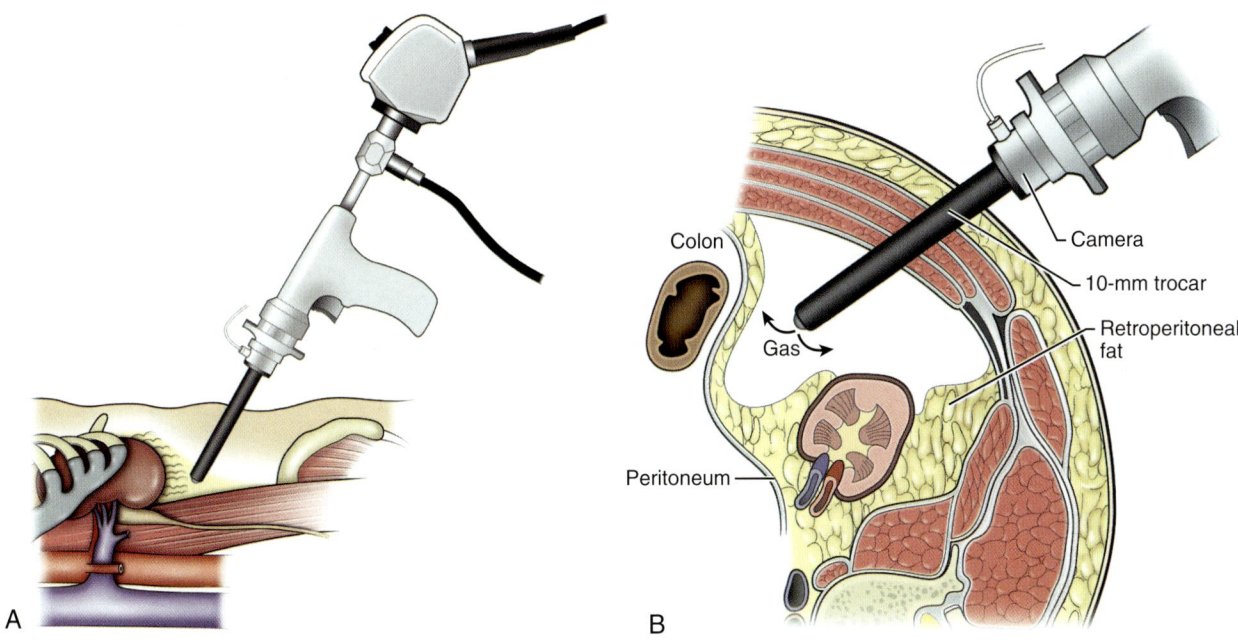

Fig. 102.6. (A) Standing behind the patient, the surgeon initially develops a space bluntly between the psoas muscle and the kidney using the visual obturator with the 0-degree laparoscope through it. (B) Together, they are used to bluntly push the peritoneum medially, creating a working space large enough to allow placement of additional trocars.

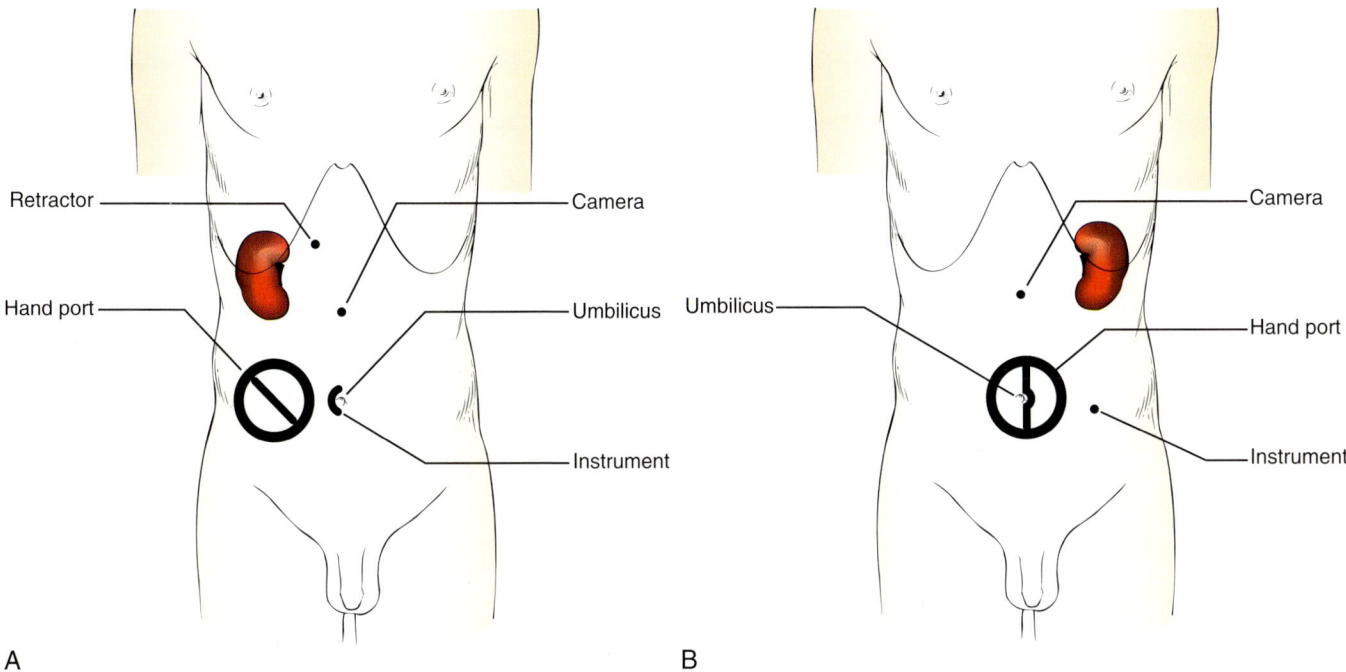

Fig. 102.7. Port placement for a right-handed surgeon for hand assistance. (A) For a right-sided kidney, the hand-assisted device is placed in the right lower quadrant for insertion of the left hand, and dissection is performed with instruments in the right hand placed through an umbilical trocar. The camera is placed several centimeters above the umbilicus in the midline. On the right side, retraction of the liver is usually necessary to allow visualization and dissection of the renal hilum. A liver or bowel retractor can be placed through a subcostal trocar to assist with visualization or irrigation and aspiration. (B) For the left kidney, the hand-assisted device and left hand are placed though a periumbilical incision, and dissection is performed with the right hand using an instrument placed in the subcostal margin just medial to the nipple. The camera is placed several centimeters lateral to the edge of the actual hand-assisted device (not the edge of the incision). Additional assistance can be delivered through the most lateral trocar site.

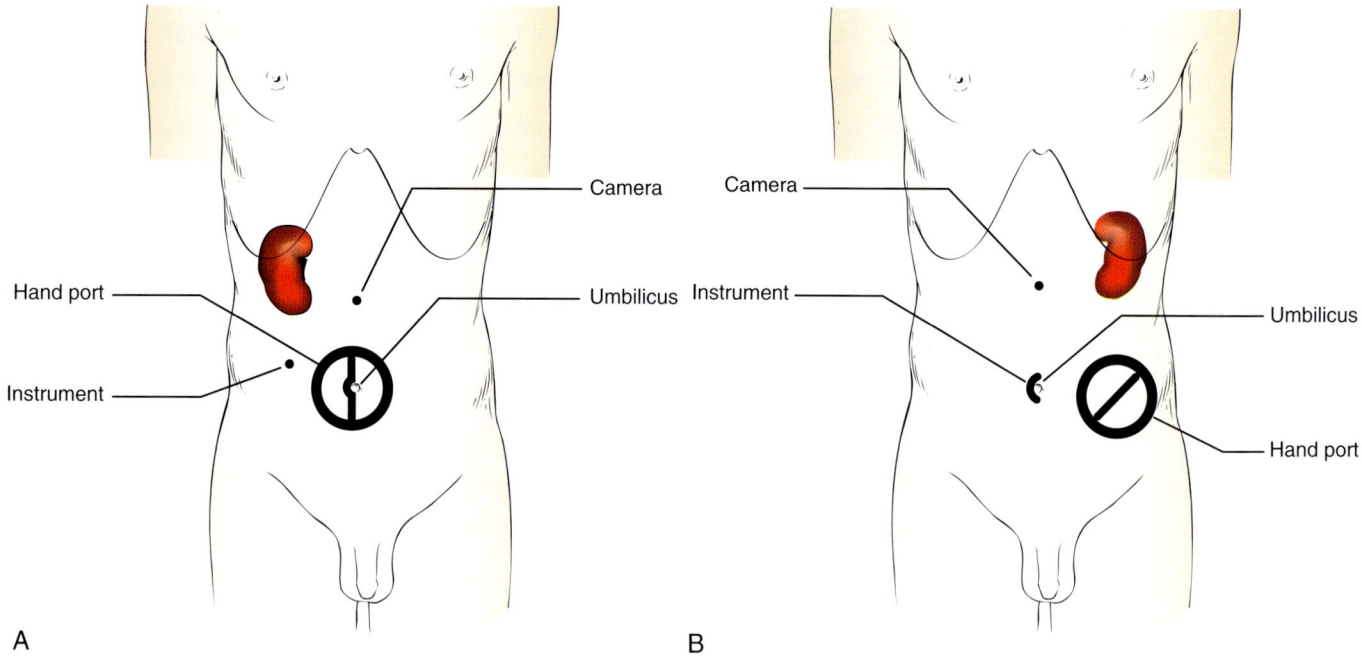

Fig. 102.8. Port placement for a left-handed surgeon for hand assistance. (A) When operating on the right kidney, a left-handed surgeon places the hand-assisted port in the periumbilical location for insertion of the right hand. The working port for the left hand is placed lateral to the rectus muscle, in line with or just inferior to the level of the umbilicus. The camera is placed through a lateral trocar in the anterior axillary line. Additional assistance with retraction of the liver can be accomplished through a subcostal trocar. (B) For a left-handed surgeon operating on the left kidney, the hand-assisted port is placed in the left lower quadrant for insertion of the right hand. The left hand works with the instrument passed through an umbilical trocar, and the camera is placed midway between the umbilicus and the xiphoid process. Additional assistance with retraction or aspiration can be accomplished through a fourth trocar placed at the subcostal margin.

Patient Positioning and Trocar Placement

Patient positioning depends on the surgical approach (transperitoneal or retroperitoneal), number of robotic arms used, and tumor location (in cases of partial nephrectomy) (Fig. 102.9). In most cases, the patient is positioned in the flank position with or without table flexion and secure to the table as previously described. In a three-arm configuration, the camera port is placed in the periumbilical area and two robotic trocars in the anterior axillary line, one above the iliac crest and a second one subcostal. A 12-mm assistant trocar is inserted in the low midline to allow passage of sutures, clamps, stapler devices, suction, or retraction. An additional 5- or 12-mm subxiphoid trocar may be used, if necessary (Fig. 102.10A). In a four-arm configuration an additional robotic trocar is placed in the lower quadrant (Fig. 102.10B). Attention must be paid to avoid robotic arm collision, especially in short patients. Lateral port placement shift may be required in obese patients.

Laparoendoscopic Single-Site Surgery and Natural Orifice Transluminal Endoscopic Surgery

LESS consolidates all laparoscopic ports in a single skin incision (Box et al., 2008). NOTES uses one or more patent natural orifices of the body for access. These approaches have evolved with the goal of further improving cosmesis and reducing postoperative pain. Virtually all renal procedures have now been performed via LESS, whereas the experience with pure NOTES is limited to a small number of procedures (Autorino et al., 2010; Kaouk et al., 2010). However, hybrid NOTES with standard laparoscopic approaches, using the vagina as an access and extraction site during nephrectomy, have been reported by several authors (Alcaraz et al., 2011; Branco et al., 2008; Gill et al., 2002; Xue et al., 2015).

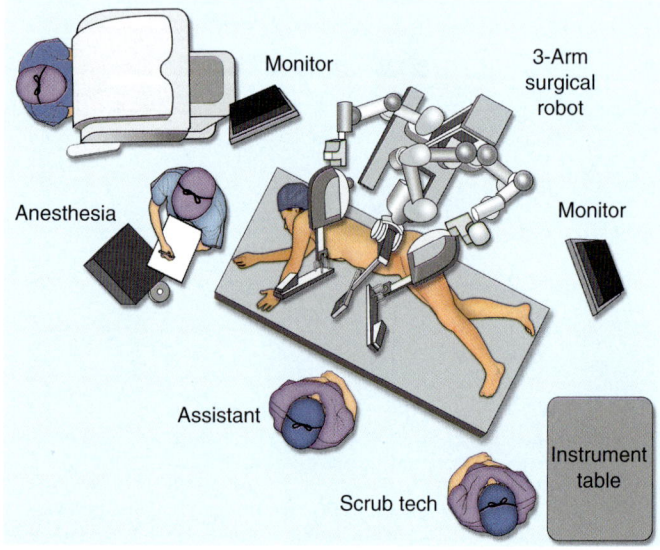

Fig. 102.9. Operating room configured for left-sided robotic-assisted laparoscopic partial nephrectomy.

Patient Positioning and Trocar Placement

A variety of accepted LESS methods of positioning and trocar use have been described and are currently used. Most approaches involve the placement of a multichannel access in the umbilicus or below the waistline to minimize visible scars. Modified flank and full flank

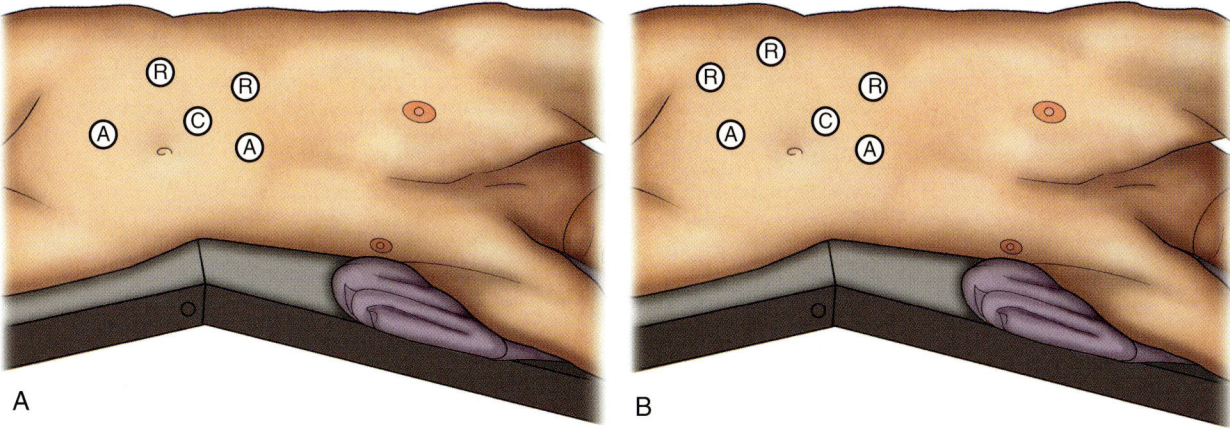

Fig. 102.10. Trocar placement for robotic-assisted laparoscopic renal surgery. (A) Three-arm system configuration. (B) Four-arm system configuration. *A*, Assistant trocar; *C*, camera port; *R*, robotic trocar.

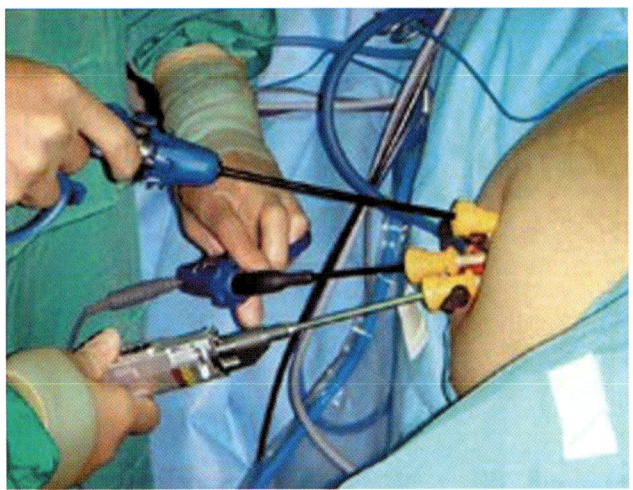

Fig. 102.11. Laparoendoscopic single-site surgery performed using three low-profile trocars inserted through a single small extraction incision. A flexible laparoscope and flexible instrumentation may be used. (From Tracy CR, Raman JD, Cadeddu JA, et al.: Laparoendoscopic single-site surgery in urology: where have we been and where are we heading? *Nat Clin Pract Urol* 5:561–568, 2008.)

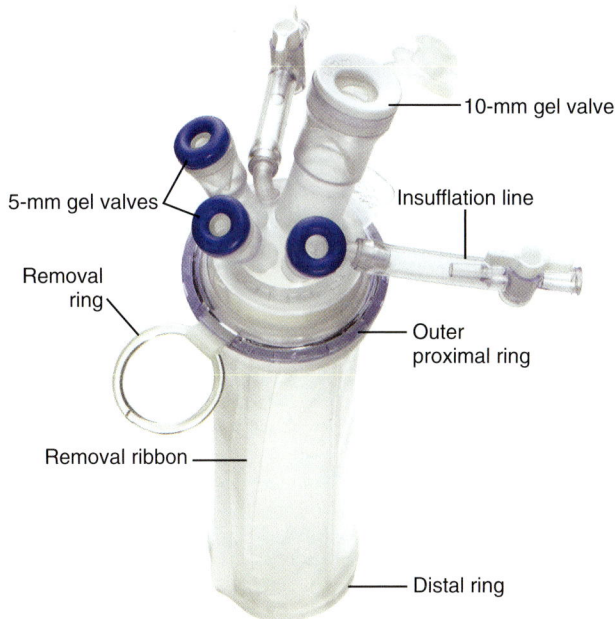

Fig. 102.12. Purpose-specific device for laparoendoscopic single-site surgery. The TriPort system (Advanced Surgical Concepts, Bray, Ireland) allows for passage of multiple instruments through a single incision.

positions have been described, mirroring positioning for standard transperitoneal or retroperitoneal laparoscopic kidney surgery, respectively. After the pneumoperitoneum is established, multiple traditional low-profile trocars close together within a single, small extraction incision (Fig. 102.11) or a purpose-specific access device (Fig. 102.12) are placed. Conventional laparoscopic instrumentation can be used; however, flexible or articulated instruments provide extra degrees of motion. Moreover, a single-site surgical version of the daVinci device has been developed. Characteristics of various single-site access options are described in Table 102.1. **LESS approaches can be technically challenging, largely because of the limited triangulation afforded by the clustering of instruments entering the intracorporal working space.**

SIMPLE NEPHRECTOMY

Laparoscopic simple nephrectomy is indicated in the treatment of many benign renal diseases, including chronic pyelonephritis, obstructive or reflux nephropathy, renal tuberculosis, multicystic dysplastic kidney, renovascular hypertension, acquired renal cystic disease in dialysis patients, nephrosclerosis, symptomatic autosomal dominant polycystic kidney disease (ADPKD), and post–kidney transplantation hypertension (Gupta and Gautam, 2005). Chronic refractory pyelonephritis, including xanthogranulomatous pyelonephritis, can be managed laparoscopically; however, these conditions are usually associated with dense perinephric adhesions, loss of tissue planes, and a higher risk for complication and conversion to open surgery (Gupta et al., 1997). In some cases, the use of hand assistance or subcapsular nephrectomy technique may be needed to safely complete the procedure.

Procedure

Reflection of the Colon

For right and left transperitoneal renal surgery, the colon should be reflected medially. For a left nephrectomy, an incision of the peritoneum at the level of the line of Toldt is carried from below the lower pole of the kidney inferiorly to above the upper pole

TABLE 102.1 Access Options for Laparoendoscopic Single-Site Surgery (LESS)

ACCESS TYPE	DESCRIPTION
Keyhole	Use of three closely approximated periumbilical trocars placed side by side in a single skin incision or three separate incisions. No additional purpose-built device required. Typically used with articulating camera and specialized instrumentation. Insufflation through one of the trocars.
TriPort +/TriPort 15/QuadPort + (Advanced Surgical Concepts, Bray, Ireland)	Open or closed access, may be used with multiple incision sizes, typically 2.5- to 5-cm fascial incision. Anchored by inner (intra-abdominal) and outer rings drawn together with cylindric sleeve. Three-port (one 12-mm and two 5-mm) and four-port (two 12-mm and two 5-mm) configurations available. Insufflation through valve housing.
Uni-X (Pnavel Systems, Cleveland, OH)	Open access technique, requires 2-cm fascial incision. Anchored with preplaced fascial sutures. Single port encompassing three 5-mm access ports. Typically used with articulating camera and specialized instrumentation. Insufflation through valve housing.
GelPort/GelPoint (Applied Medical, Rancho Santa Margarita, CA)	Open access technique, requires 2.5- to 5-cm fascial incision. Anchored by inner and outer rings drawn together with cylindric sleeve. Can accommodate all trocar sizes. May allow for wider spacing of trocars. Insufflation through trocar placed through device.
AirSeal (SurgiQuest, Milford, CT)	Various trocar sizes up to 27 mm, oval-shaped trocar accommodating multiple instruments. High-velocity CO_2 recycling system to maintain pneumoperitoneum pressures without mechanical valve.
SILS (Covidien, Mansfield, MA)	Single biconcave piece of foam with a valve for insufflation and three holes to accommodate trocars (three 5-mm low-profile trocars or two 5-mm trocars and one 10- to 12-mm trocar). Inserted via open Hasson technique through minimum 2-cm fascial incision with the aid of a Péan clamp.
SPIDER (TransEnterix, Morrisville, NC)	Single-access device allowing for the use of flexible instruments passed through articulating instrument delivery tubes. Additional working channels allow for use of conventional laparoscopic instruments as well.
Homemade port (using Applied Medical [Rancho Santa Margarita, CA] wound retractor)	Similar to GelPoint trocar using a wound retractor from the same company in addition to a sterile surgical glove. Surgical glove secured to the wound retractor using suture or sterile rubber bands. Trocars can be passed through each of the fingers of the surgical glove portion of the access device.
OCTO Port (DalimSurgNET, Seoul, Korea)	Available in two base sizes requiring fascial incisions ranging from 1.5 to 5 cm. Uses a wound retractor and multiple attachments allowing for up to four ports.
Single Site Laparoscopy (SSL) Access System (Ethicon Endo-Surgery, Somerville, NJ)	Similar to other access devices in using a wound retractor base with an attachment cap. Integrates channels (two 5-mm instruments and a 10- to 12-mm instrument) with no trocar components protruding above the low-profile cap that can rotate. Placed through 2- to 4-cm fascial openings and able to traverse abdominal wall thickness up to 7 cm.

superiorly lateral to the spleen (Fig. 102.13). Care must be taken to avoid injury to the diaphragm. The inferior limit is extended as needed to obtain adequate reflection of the colon. Dissection of the lateral attachments of the kidney should be avoided at this time given these will prevent the kidney from rolling over and obscuring the hilum. The lienocolic ligament should be incised to allow the spleen to fall medially along with the pancreas and the colon (see Fig. 102.13). The thin colorenal attachments are incised and the colon is medially retracted (Fig. 102.14). Identification of the plane between the mesenteric fat, which has brighter yellow hue, and the pale yellow retroperitoneal or Gerota fat is key for a proper dissection and to avoid making an incision in the mesocolon or Gerota fascia. If the mesocolon is accidentally opened, it should be repaired to prevent the development of an internal hernia (Regan et al., 2003). A paddle retractor may be placed through an additional lower midline trocar to aid in retracting the colon, pancreas, and spleen medially (see Fig. 102.4A).

For a right nephrectomy, a liver retractor inserted through an anterior axillary line or high midline port may be needed to expose the upper pole of the kidney (see Fig. 102.4B and C). After the peritoneal incision as described earlier, medial traction on the colon reveals colorenal attachments that must be divided to complete the colon reflection. Care must be taken to avoid thermal injury to the duodenum. Again, a low midline retractor may be helpful for visualization. Lateral dissection of the duodenum (Kocher maneuver) may be required to fully expose the medial aspect of the kidney and the connective tissue overlying the renal hilum and inferior vena cava (IVC) (Fig. 102.15). This should be done without electrocautery adjacent to the duodenum.

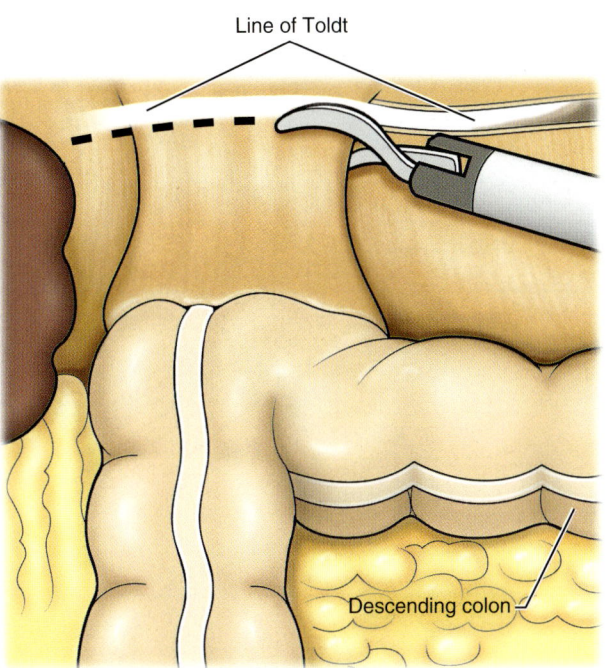

Fig. 102.13. Incision of the white line of Toldt with endoshears, bipolar cautery, or ultrasonic energy allows reflection of the colon. Continuing superiorly allows incision of the lienocolic ligament, facilitating reflection of the spleen, pancreas, and colon.

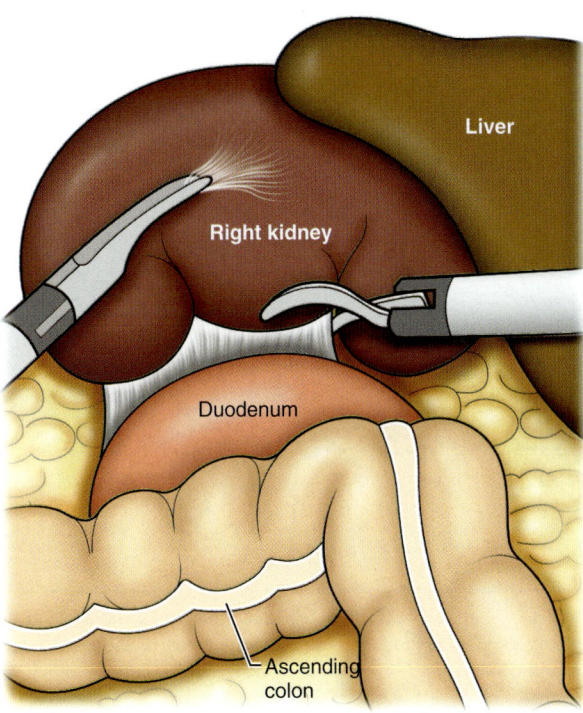

Fig. 102.15. On the right side, the colon is reflected, and a Kocher maneuver may be performed to completely expose the kidney and the renal hilum.

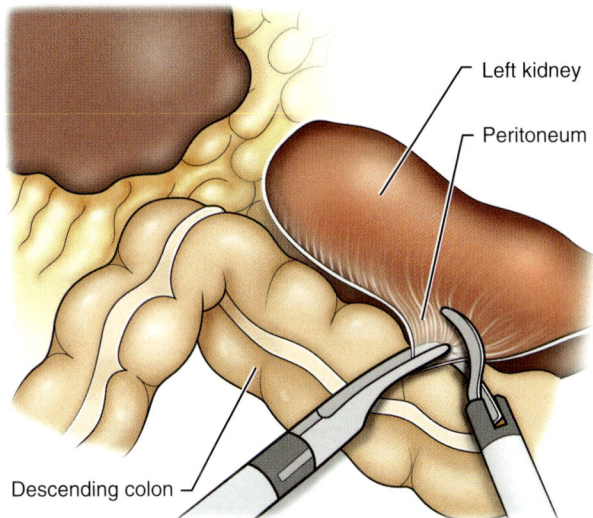

Fig. 102.14. Medial traction on the colon helps identify additional colorenal attachments and assists in differentiating the undersurface of the large bowel mesentery. Care must be taken at this step to avoid creating a mesenteric window.

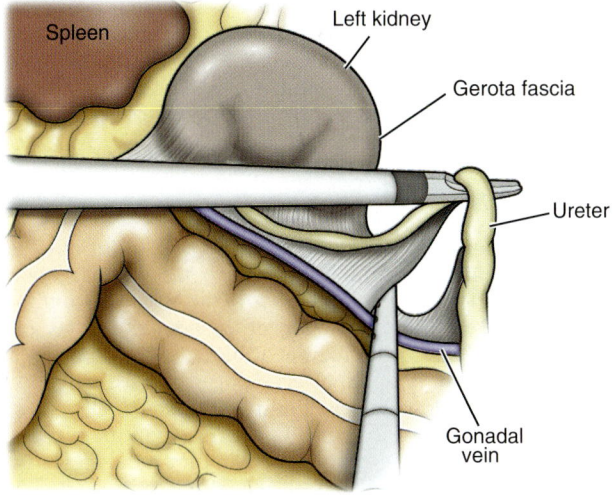

Fig. 102.16. A curved dissector, in the left hand, is placed beneath the ureter and used to provide anterolateral elevation. On the right side the angle of insertion from the gonadal vein to the vena cava can be a source of significant bleeding if torn during elevation.

Dissection of the Ureter

Once the colon is medially reflected, the psoas muscle and tendon should be identified inferior to the lower pole of the kidney. Following the psoas medially, the gonadal vessels are usually encountered first, and the ureter is usually located just posterior to these vessels. Ureteral peristalsis can help differentiate the ureter from adjacent vascular structures. Once identified, the ureter is elevated, the gonadal vessels are swept medially, and the dissection is carried up proximally to the lower pole of the kidney. The ureter is not divided at this time, because it can be used to help elevate the kidney (Fig. 102.16). The tissue posterior to the ureter and lower pole of the kidney is swept anteriorly to further expose the anterior surface of the psoas muscle. Care should be taken to stay above the psoas fascia to minimize injury to cutaneous nerves, which would result in postoperative thigh numbness.

Identification of the Renal Hilum

Safe dissection of the renal hilum requires adequate exposure by medial retraction of the colon and small bowel by gravity or the lower midline retractor, as well as anterior-lateral retraction of the kidney by lifting it out of the renal fossa (Fig. 102.17). The hilar dissection is facilitated by keeping the hilum on traction with firm

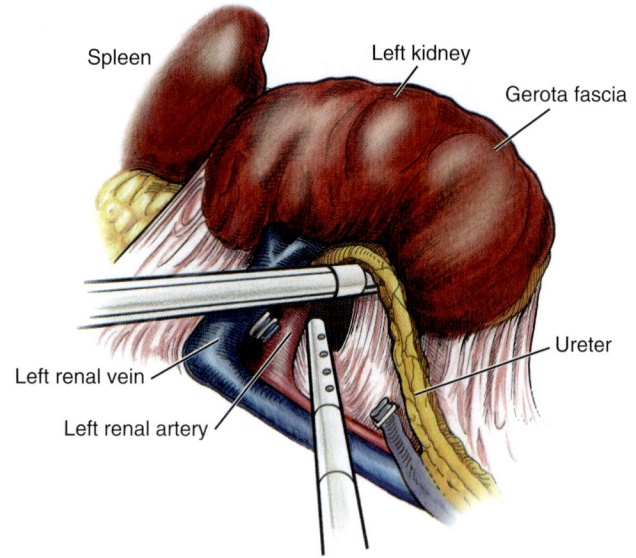

Fig. 102.17. The lower pole of the kidney and ureter are firmly retracted anterolaterally, placing the hilum on stretch. The left gonadal vein has been ligated and divided.

anterior-lateral retraction of the kidney. This can be accomplished by gently placing the lateral grasper under the ureter and kidney until it abuts the abdominal sidewall. Care must be taken to avoid placing the grasper into the renal parenchyma. With the ureter and lower pole of the kidney elevated, vessels entering the renal hilum can be identified and bluntly dissected. A gentle, layer-by-layer dissection is performed until the renal vein is identified. Gonadal, lumbar, and accessory venous branches can be clipped and divided as needed. Clips should not be placed in the anticipated staple line to prevent stapler misfire.

Securing the Renal Blood Vessels

Once the hilum is exposed and kept under traction, the renal artery should be identified typically posterior to the vein. Preoperative imaging is usually helpful to identify the location and number of renal vessels. Meticulous dissection of the vein and artery can be accomplished with a combination of blunt and sharp dissection using irrigator-aspirator tip, hook electrode, scissors, or laparoscopic forceps. With an endoscopic vascular stapler, first the artery is ligated and divided, then the vein (Fig. 102.18). It is important to ensure that the stapler covers the entire vessel. En bloc renal hilar vascular staple ligation appears to be a safe alternative to individual vessel ligation (Lai and Rais-Bahrami, 2017). In some cases, additional clips may be needed for complete hemostasis. Plastic clips alone are contraindicated for the ligation of the renal artery because of reports of fatal cases of clip failure (Hsi et al., 2007).

Dissection of the Upper Pole

After the hilar vessels are divided, the dissection continues posteriorly and superiorly to the upper pole. The adrenal gland is preserved by carrying the dissection on to the upper pole of the kidney (Fig. 102.19). This can be accomplished by incising the Gerota fascia anteriorly, just above the hilum. The perinephric fat is then gently peeled off circumferentially above the upper pole of the kidney. The ureter is then clipped and divided, and the lateral attachments of the kidney are divided. This allows the kidney to be rotated anteriorly above the liver (on the right) or spleen (on the left) to facilitate incision of the uppermost attachments under direct vision. In cases of extreme fibrosis, a subcapsular nephrectomy can be performed once the artery and vein have been controlled (Moore et al., 1998). Care should be taken to avoid a diaphragmatic injury.

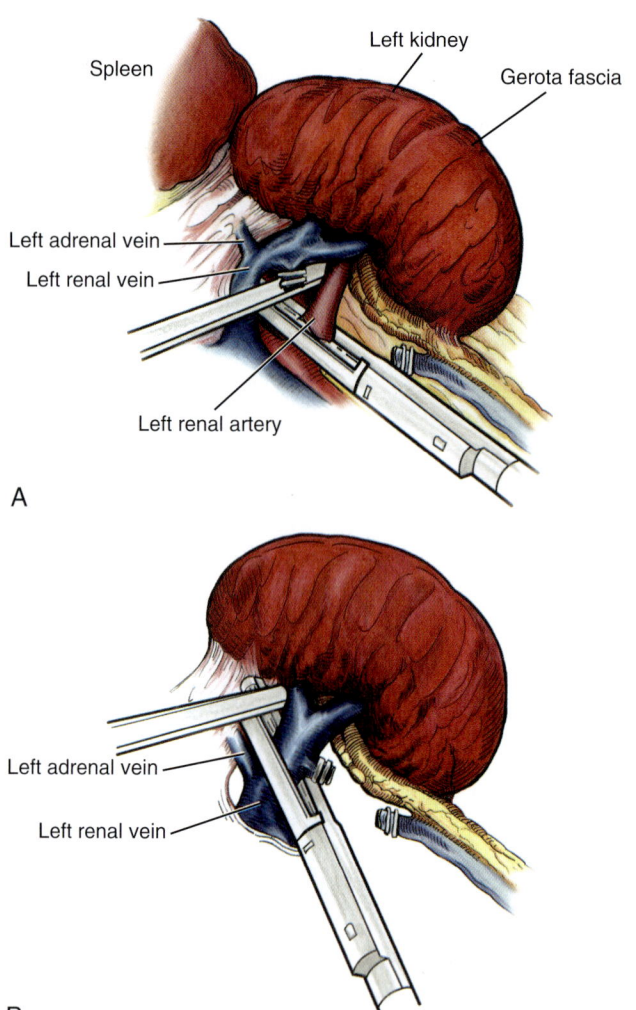

Fig. 102.18. (A) First, the renal artery is stapled using an endovascular gastrointestinal anastomosis (GIA) stapler. (B) The renal vein is secured lateral to the adrenal vein with the GIA stapler. If clips are used on the gonadal or adrenal vessels, the surgeon must be careful to exclude them from the jaws of the stapler.

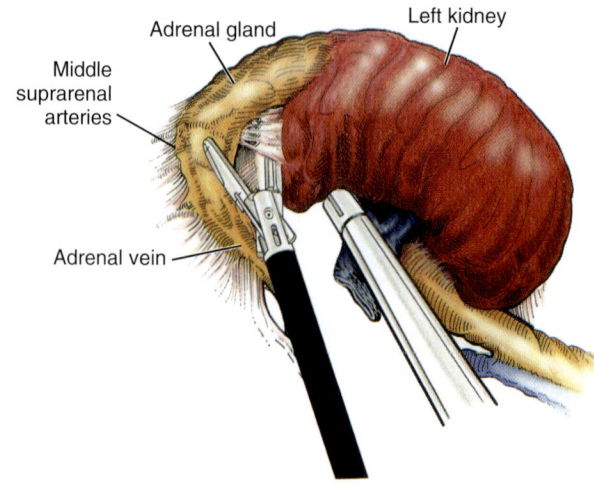

Fig. 102.19. The adrenal gland can be preserved during simple nephrectomy or radical nephrectomy as indicated by dissecting it from the superior pole of the kidney.

Organ Entrapment and Extraction

The kidney can be removed intact or piecemeal after morcellation. The specimen is placed in an extraction bag and removed intact through an extended trocar site or Pfannenstiel incision (Fig. 102.20). Morcellation can be accomplished using ring forceps and Kocher clamp (Fig. 102.21) or using a purpose-built morcellator system.

Postoperative Management

The orogastric tube is removed at the end of the procedure. Diet can be resumed as tolerated, and the Foley catheter can be removed once the patient is comfortably ambulating. Unrestricted activity can usually be resumed as tolerated. Heavy lifting should be deferred for 4 to 6 weeks in those cases with an extraction incision.

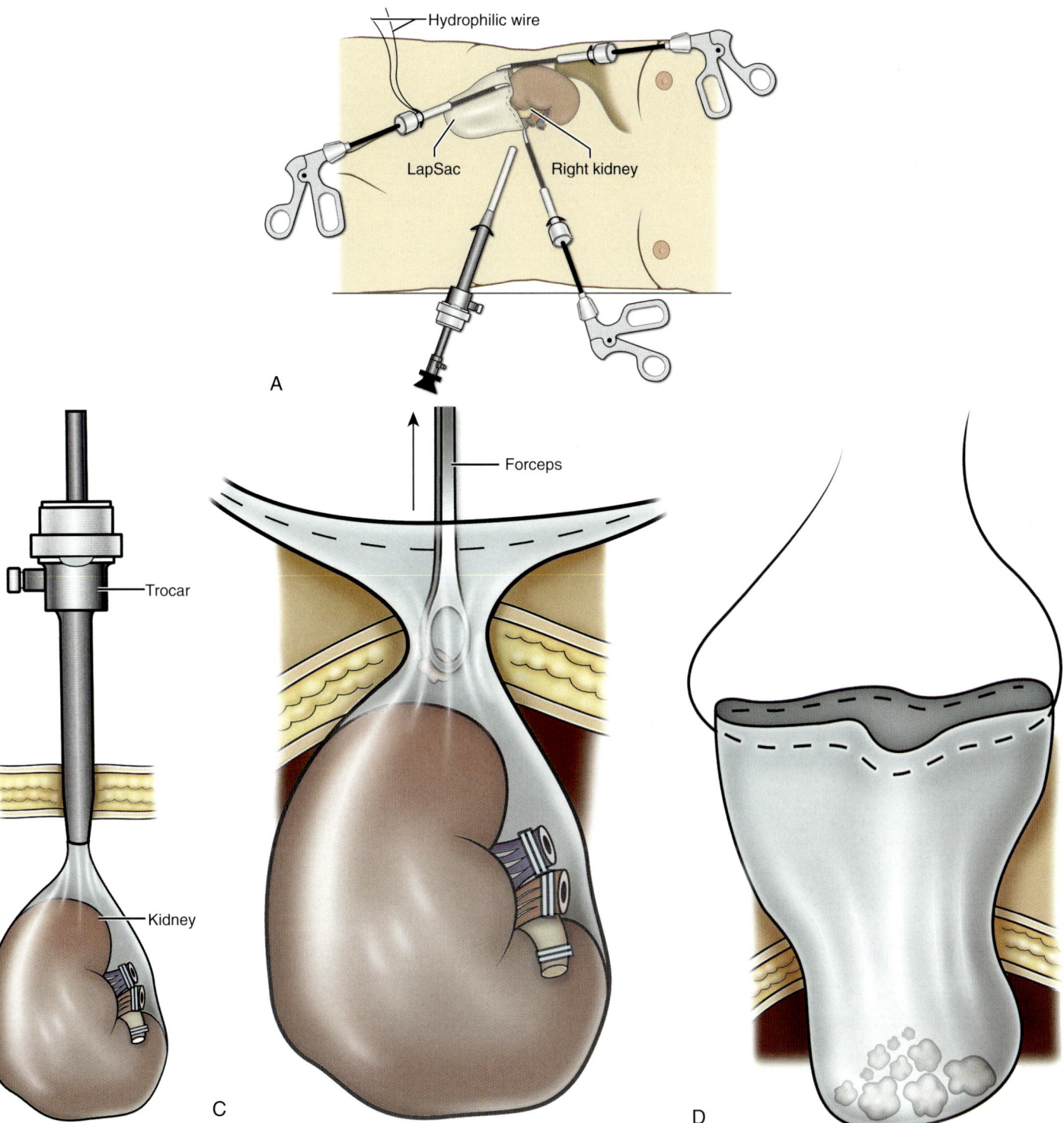

Fig. 102.20. Removal of the intact specimen. (A) The camera is moved to the lateral port site and an Endo Catch device (Covidien, Dublin, Ireland) is placed through the umbilical trocar site to entrap the specimen. (B) Alternatively, the specimen may be extracted through a Pfannenstiel incision. To accomplish this, the Endo Catch device is brought in through a separate 10-mm suprapubic incision. (C) The trocar is then removed, bringing the Endo Catch device with it through the trocar site, and the suture is cut and clamped. (D) A 4- to 6-cm incision is made including one of the trocar sites. The surgeon's finger protects the specimen and underlying structures from injury.

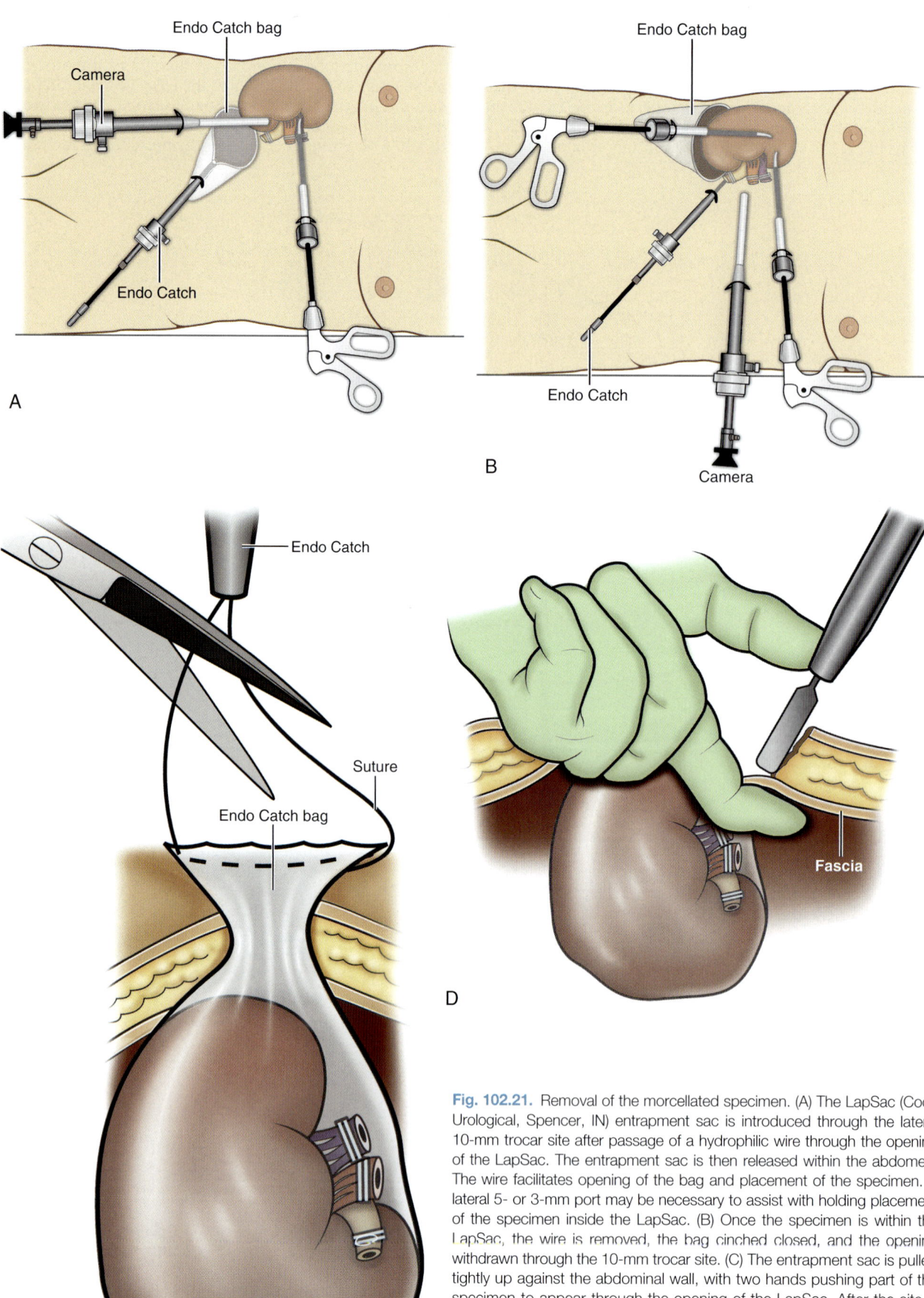

Fig. 102.21. Removal of the morcellated specimen. (A) The LapSac (Cook Urological, Spencer, IN) entrapment sac is introduced through the lateral 10-mm trocar site after passage of a hydrophilic wire through the opening of the LapSac. The entrapment sac is then released within the abdomen. The wire facilitates opening of the bag and placement of the specimen. A lateral 5- or 3-mm port may be necessary to assist with holding placement of the specimen inside the LapSac. (B) Once the specimen is within the LapSac, the wire is removed, the bag cinched closed, and the opening withdrawn through the 10-mm trocar site. (C) The entrapment sac is pulled tightly up against the abdominal wall, with two hands pushing part of the specimen to appear through the opening of the LapSac. After the site is carefully draped, manual morcellation with ring forceps or a Kelly clamp can be used. (D) The entrapment sac is removed once the remaining specimen fragments are small enough to be extracted through the trocar site. Only the tissue visible from the opening is grasped. Blind passes into the bag may injure surrounding bowel segments.

Results

The postoperative results of laparoscopic nephrectomy are comparable with those of open surgery, with less pain, less blood loss, shorter hospital stay, quicker return to normal activity, and comparable complication rates (Dunn et al., 2000; Fornara et al. 2001; Wolf et al., 2001). In spite of the higher operating room and supply costs associated with the laparoscopic approach, laparoscopic nephrectomy is cost effective compared with open surgery because of short operating times and brief lengths of stay (Lotan et al., 2002).

SURGERY FOR RENAL CYSTIC DISEASE

Although common, renal cysts rarely require surgical intervention. **Indications for operative treatment include cyst-associated pain, infection, obstruction, or concerns for malignancy.** The evaluation of renal cysts is discussed in Chapter 96. Symptomatic benign cysts can be initially managed with percutaneous needle aspiration. A sclerosing agent may be used to potentially reduce the risk of recurrence (Rane, 2004; Fig. 102.22). Caution should be taken to avoid extravasation of these agents into the collecting system because of the risk of fibrosis. Benign cysts not amenable to percutaneous treatment can be managed with cyst decortication, marsupialization, or unroofing (Okeke et al., 2003). Multiple and bilateral cysts can be treated in the same operation (Roberts et al., 2001). Laparoscopic cyst decortication has been shown to be an effective treatment for cyst-related pain in individuals with ADPKD. In cases of end-stage renal disease, bilateral synchronous laparoscopic nephrectomy may be performed in patients with enlarged, symptomatic, or infected kidneys. Renal cysts suspicious to harbor malignancy can be explored, biopsied, and treated laparoscopically with cryoablation, enucleation, or partial or radical nephrectomy (Wehle and Grabstald, 1986).

Procedure

The kidney is mobilized as previously described. After Gerota fascia is incised and the renal capsule exposed, the cyst is identified. Intraoperative ultrasound can be used to assist in locating the cyst. Hilar control is usually not required. Dissection of the cyst wall from surrounding structures is done before draining the cyst's contents. The wall of the cyst can be grasped and excised, cutting along the junction between the cyst wall and the renal parenchyma (Fig. 102.23). Lesions suspicious for malignancy can be biopsied. The cyst wall may be fulgurated with either electrocautery or argon beam coagulator. Care should be taken when ablating the surface, because inadvertent or occult entry into the collecting system can easily occur. Packing with hemostatic agents or suturing may be necessary. In cases in which the collecting system is entered, it is recommended to leave a drain (Fig. 102.24). If malignancy is noted, extirpative surgery or cryoablation may be used to treat the remainder of the lesion or kidney.

Results

Laparoscopic management of symptomatic renal cysts is highly effective. Retrospective studies suggest a greater than 90% postoperative

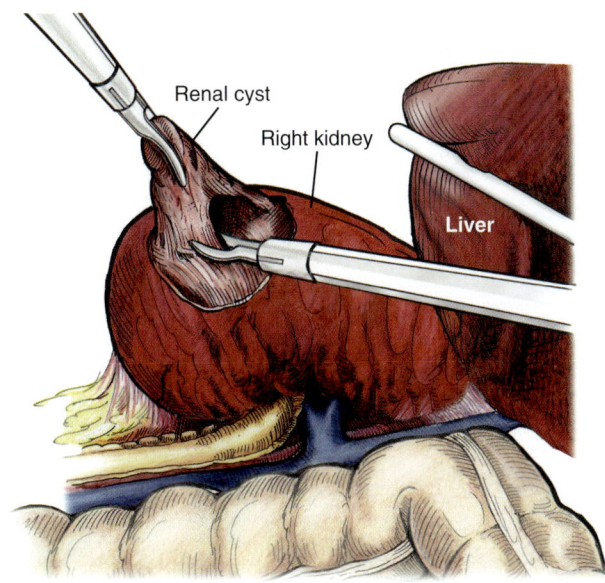

Fig. 102.23. The cyst fluid is aspirated with a laparoscopic aspiration needle. After decompression of the cyst, the wall can easily be grasped and manipulated. The cyst is elevated with a grasper and scissors or ultrasonic shears to circumferentially excise the cyst wall. The edge of the cyst is carefully inspected, and biopsies are performed using the 5-mm laparoscopic biopsy forceps as needed.

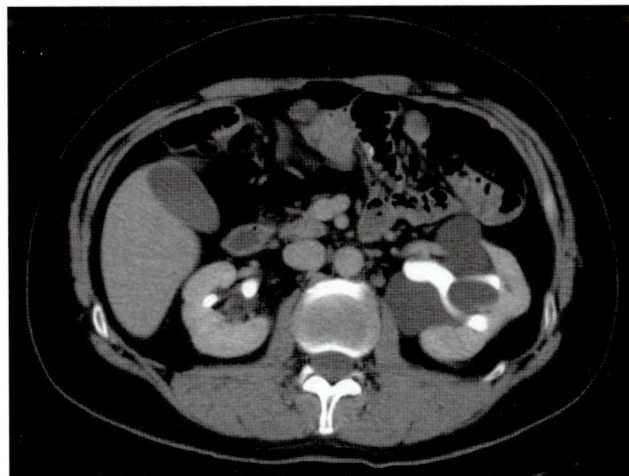

Fig. 102.22. Axial computed tomography scan in delayed phase after intravenous contrast administration, demonstrating peripelvic cysts in a patient with left flank pain.

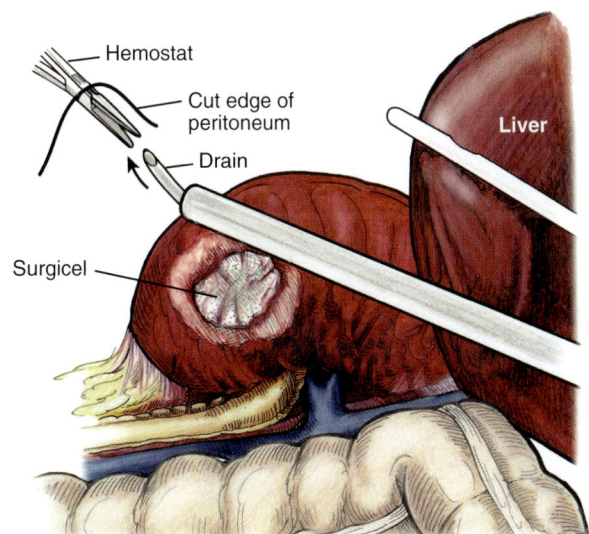

Fig. 102.24. Drain placement after renal cyst excision. If the collecting system has been entered, it is closed and a drain placed. To insert the drain, a hemostat is passed through a small stab incision in the side and advanced into the abdominal cavity under direct vision. A drain is placed through a trocar site and advanced toward the open hemostat using the trocar to direct the drain. The colon is brought back over the kidney and attached to the sidewall to "reperitonealize" the kidney and drain.

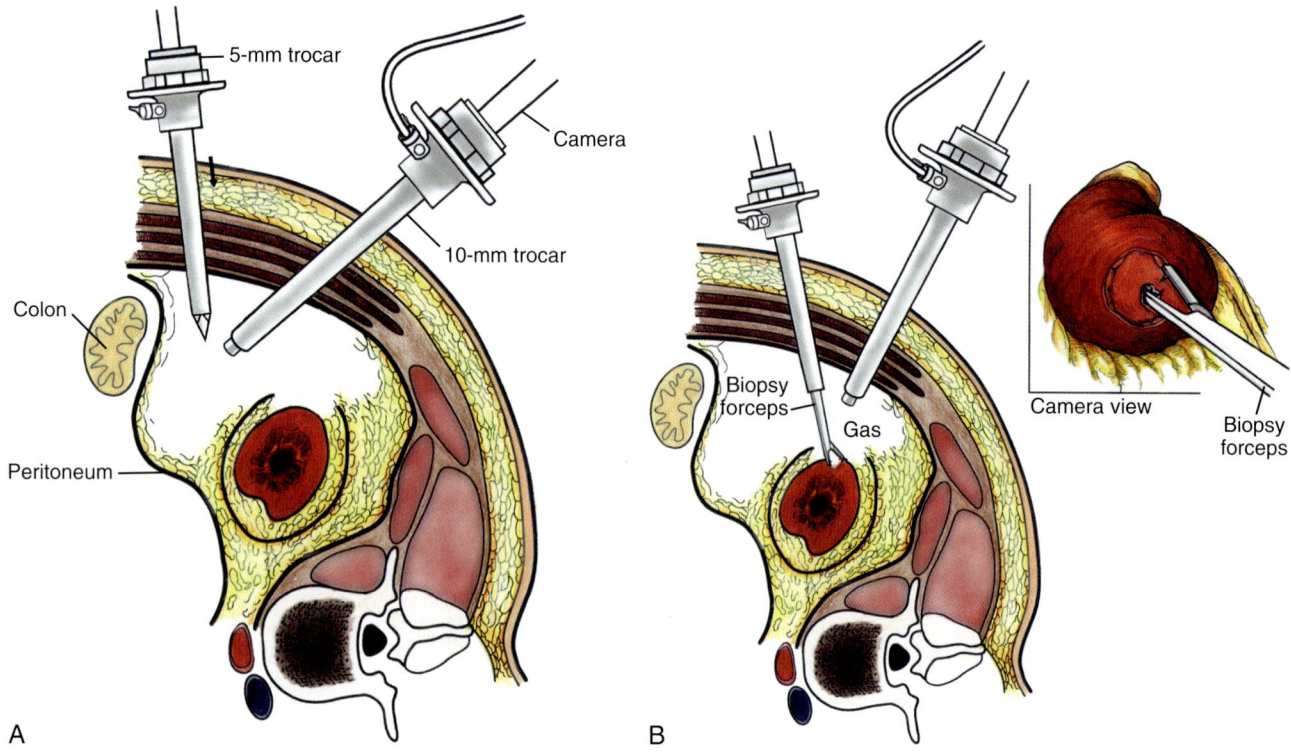

Fig. 102.25. (A) After establishment of a working space, a 5-mm trocar is placed under direct vision. The working instruments are passed through this port. The camera can be used to assist with dissection and is frequently cleaned to maintain adequate visualization. (B) Gerota fascia is opened with the use of the scissors. With 5-mm two-tooth laparoscopic biopsy forceps, two or three samples are taken from the lower pole of the kidney.

symptom improvement (Atug et al., 2006; Lee et al., 2003; Thwaini et al., 2007). In a series of 45 laparoscopic cyst decortications, the mean operative time was 89 minutes, mean estimated blood loss 85 mL, and a major complication was observed in only 1 case requiring conversion to open surgery as a result of bleeding. A total of 95% of patients achieved radiographic resolution of the cyst, and 91% were pain free after a median follow-up of 39 months (Thwaini et al., 2007).

RENAL BIOPSY FOR MEDICAL RENAL DISEASE

Renal biopsy plays a central role in the diagnosis and management of patients with hematuria and proteinuria of glomerular origin and/or unexplained renal failure. **Although renal biopsy is typically done percutaneously under CT or ultrasound guidance, there are circumstances in which a laparoscopic biopsy may be preferred, including failed previous attempts at percutaneous biopsy, renal anatomic abnormalities, bleeding diathesis, morbid obesity, multiple renal cysts, or a solitary kidney.**

Procedure

The patient is positioned, and access is obtained based on the chosen technique as previously described. Although LESS approaches have been described (Micali et al., 2014), a two-port retroperitoneal technique is typically preferred. A 10-mm trocar is placed above the iliac crest in the posterior axillary line, and a 5-mm trocar is placed at the same level at the anterior axillary line. Blunt dissection is used to open Gerota fascia to expose the lower pole of the kidney. The use of a balloon dilator can help develop the working space. Ultrasound can facilitate the localization of the kidney in cases of abundant retroperitoneal and perinephric adipose tissue. A 5-mm biopsy forceps is used to take samples of the cortical parenchyma (Fig. 102.25). Alternatively, an 18-gauge Trucut needle can be used for deeper tissue sampling. This can be passed percutaneously under visual guidance. Electrocautery or an argon beam coagulator is used to achieve hemostasis (Gimenez et al., 1998).

Results

The largest laparoscopic renal biopsy series including 74 patients showed a mean operative time of 123 minutes and mean estimated blood loss of 76 mL. Nearly 60% and 75% of the patients were discharged within 24 and 48 hours, respectively, with the remainder staying longer as a result of preexisting medical conditions. The most common complication was bleeding in 3 cases, followed by nonrenal tissue biopsy in 2 cases and inability to obtain a specimen in 2 cases. A series of 14 LESS renal biopsies showed a mean operative time of 53 minutes, estimated blood loss less than 50 mL, and hospital stay less than 24 hours in all cases. Patients did not require additional analgesia postoperatively, and no complications were observed (Micali et al., 2014).

NEPHROPEXY

Nephropexy is the surgical fixation of a mobile (ptotic) kidney. Anatomically, nephroptosis is defined as a significant descent (>5 cm or two vertebral bodies on an intravenous urography) of the kidney as the patient moves from supine to erect (Fig. 102.26; Srirangam et al., 2009). Nephropexy is usually indicated in cases of nephroptosis associated with pain (longer than 3 months duration), evidence of restricted blood flow, and/or urinary drainage on intravenous urography, nuclear medicine scan, or color Doppler imaging.

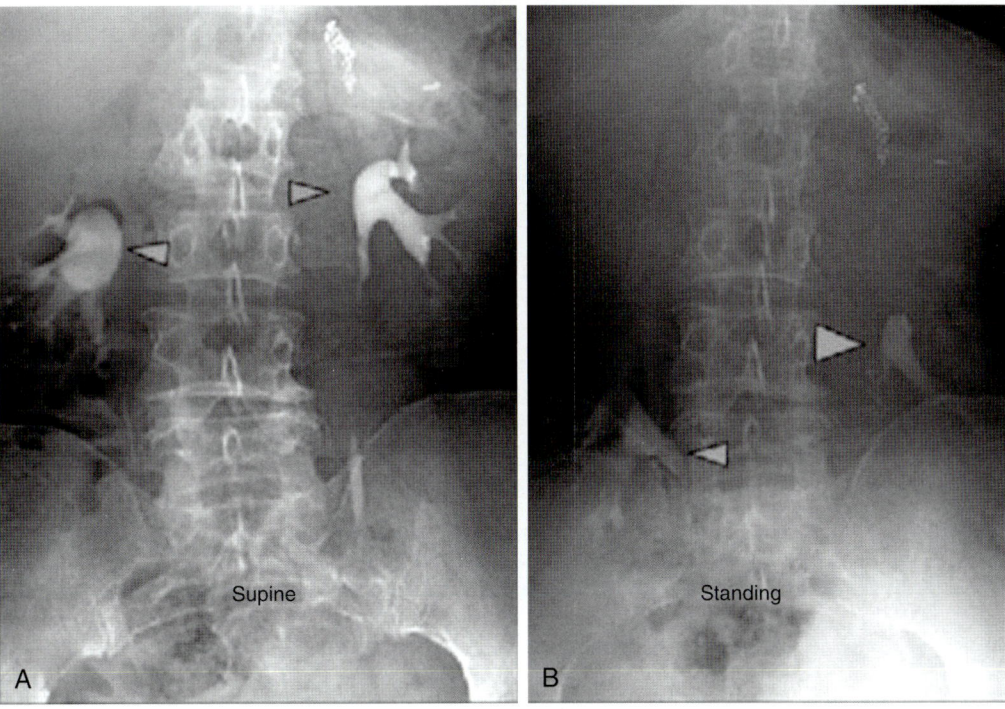

Fig. 102.26. Intravenous pyelogram demonstrating bilateral ptotic kidneys in the supine (A) and standing (B) positions. (From El-Moula MG, Izaki H, Kishimoto T, et al.: Laparoscopic nephropexy. *J Laparoendosc Adv Surg Tech A* 18:230–236, 2008.)

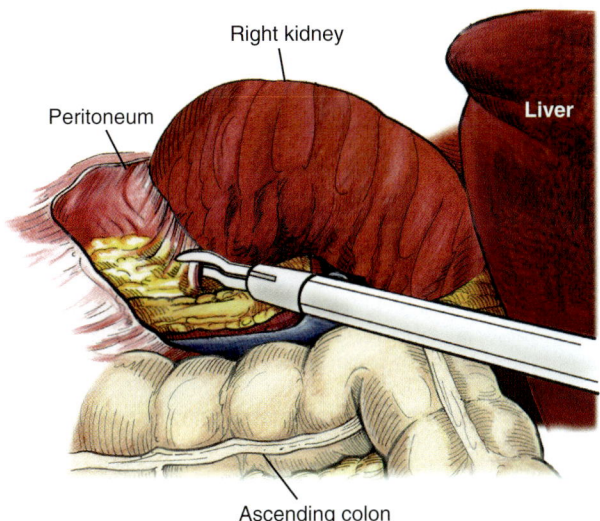

Fig. 102.27. The kidney is stripped of overlying Gerota fascia down to the surface of the renal capsule. All remaining attachments are divided, allowing full mobility for repositioning.

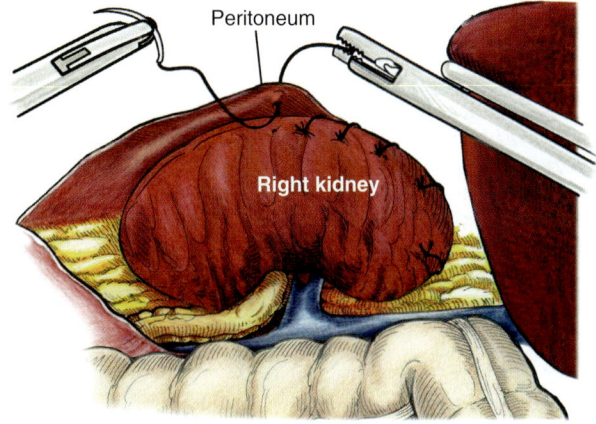

Fig. 102.28. Nephropexy. Once the kidney is free of lateral and posterior attachments, multiple 2-0 sutures are placed into the capsule and the lateral edge of the fascia overlying the abdominal wall. Sutures may also be placed between the anterior renal capsule and the parietal peritoneum for additional support.

Procedure

Dissection is performed to mobilize the entire affected kidney and expose the underlying psoas and quadratus lumborum fascia (Fig. 102.27). Renal fixation can be accomplished either by suture fixation or with use of foreign material, such as mesh or tissue adhesive. For suture fixation, interrupted nonabsorbable sutures securing the lateral edge of the renal capsule to the underlying muscle fascia are placed starting at the upper pole moving down to the lower pole (Fig. 102.28). Additional sutures between the anterior renal capsule and the parietal peritoneum can be placed for additional support. Alternatively, a tension-free tape or mesh can be used to trap the kidney against the dorsal abdominal wall. In this technique, after the kidney is mobilized, the needle attached to the tape is directed below the lower pole and pushed through the abdominal wall. The tape is guided just over the lateral margin of the kidney and pushed through the abdominal wall, so the kidney is trapped by the tape. The sling is tightened until the kidney is securely fixed to the dorsal abdominal wall (Hubner et al., 2004).

Results

Retrospective series of laparoscopic nephropexy suggest a 90% to 100% pain improvement, 80% to 95% resolution of the 5-cm

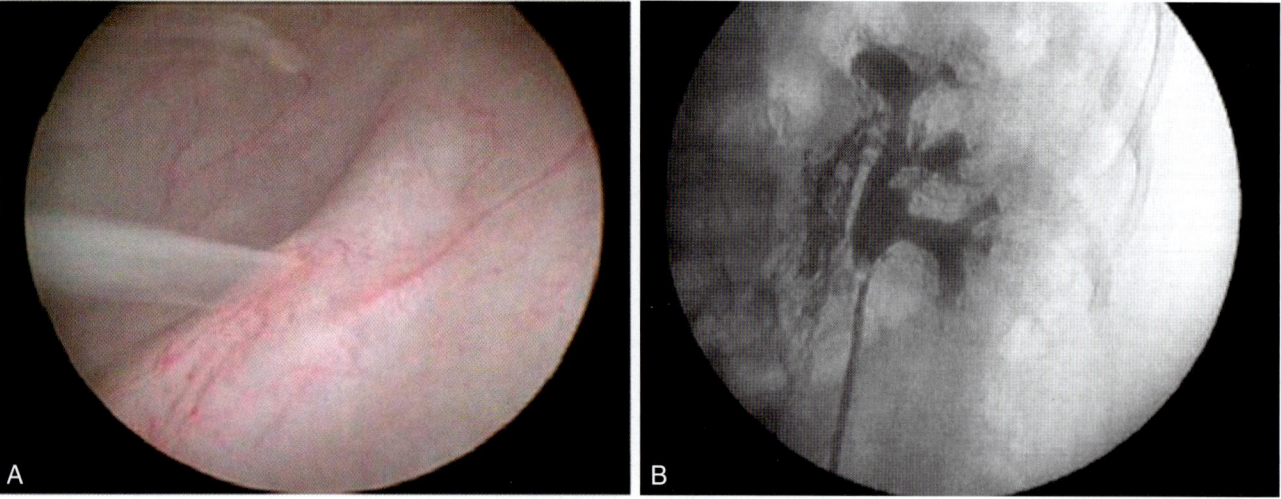

Fig. 102.29. Chyluria. (A) Cystoscopy demonstrating milky white efflux from the left ureteral orifice. (B) Retrograde pyelogram demonstrating lymphorenal fistula. (From Eisner BH, Tanrikut C, Dahl DM: Chyluria secondary to lymphorenal fistula. *Kidney Int* 76:126, 2009.)

renal descent, and 90% improvement in renal function measured by nuclear medicine scan (Elashry et al., 1995; Fornara et al., 1997; Plas et al., 2001). In a series of 48 laparoscopic nephropexies, the median estimate blood loss was 50 mL, mean operative time was 95 minutes, and there were no major complications (Gozen et al., 2008). Nearly 90% of patients were satisfied and would undergo the operation again.

CALYCEAL DIVERTICULECTOMY

Several laparoscopic techniques to treat calyceal diverticula have been described, including unroofing, excision, ablation, and obliteration of the diverticulum as well as partial nephrectomy. **Indications for operative intervention include chronic pain, recurrent urinary tract infection, gross hematuria, and decline in renal function** (Waingankar et al., 2014). The modern principles of treatment include the removal of stones and widening of the infundibular drainage to prevent urinary stasis or complete ablation of the diverticula cavity.

Procedure

The kidney is dissected as previously described. After Gerota fascia is incised and the renal capsule exposed, there is usually a divot noted on the parenchyma overlying the diverticulum. The overlying parenchyma is incised with electrocautery revealing the diverticula cavity. Hilar control is usually not required unless a partial excision of the kidney is planned. Intraoperative ultrasound and/or injection of dye via a preoperatively placed externalized ureteral catheter can be used to assist in locating the diverticulum as well as os. Stones should be removed with a grasper and placed in an extraction bag. The diverticulum cavity is obliterated with argon beam coagulation or monopolar cautery. The infundibulum in communication with the collecting system may be closed with suture. Perirenal fat may be placed into the defect to further decrease the likelihood of recurrence. A drain is usually left in place after closure of the collecting system defect.

Results

Although only small series and case reports of laparoscopic calyceal diverticulectomy are available, authors have reported excellent results with this treatment modality, including 50% to 100% pain resolution, and 90% to 100% stone-free rate. In an analysis of 31 cases, only 1 complication (urinary leak) was observed (Gonzalez et al., 2011). In a series of 6 minimally invasive calyceal diverticulectomies, the mean operative time was 162 minutes, mean estimated blood loss was 150 mL, and mean hospital stay was 2 days (Taylor and Thiel, 2015).

NEPHROLYSIS

Nephrolysis consists of the renal mobilization with skeletonization of the hilar vessels and upper ureter with ligation of the lymphatic channels. It is indicated in select cases of loin pain hematuria syndrome and chyluria. There are very limited data on nephrolysis for the management of loin pain hematuria syndrome. Nephrolysis is an effective treatment for severe refractory chyluria, where there is lymphatic rupture and/or fistulous connections into the pyelocaliceal system (Fig. 102.29).

Procedure and Results

Traditionally, the affected kidney is fully mobilized, ensuring complete lymphatic dissociation. A recent study suggests the dissection of the upper pole may be safely omitted in cases of chyluria (Zhang et al., 2016). The use of an omental wrap around the hilum has been described and may provide an additional barrier against recurrence of chyluria (Dalela et al., 2004). In a series of 59 laparoscopic nephrolysis for chyluria, the mean operative time was 79 minutes, estimated blood loss was 49 mL, and only 1 patient developed disease recurrence (Zhang et al., 2012).

RADICAL NEPHRECTOMY

The indications for minimally invasive radical nephrectomy are similar to those for open surgery. Renal tumors as large as 25 cm have been successfully removed laparoscopically. Complex kidney cancers such as those involving the IVC, lymph nodes, and adjacent or distant organs may also be managed using minimally invasive techniques (Berger et al., 2009; Rabets et al., 2004; Simmons et al., 2007; Steinnerd et al., 2007).

Transperitoneal

Procedure

The patient is positioned and trocars are placed for transperitoneal access as described earlier in the chapter. Additional trocars or a

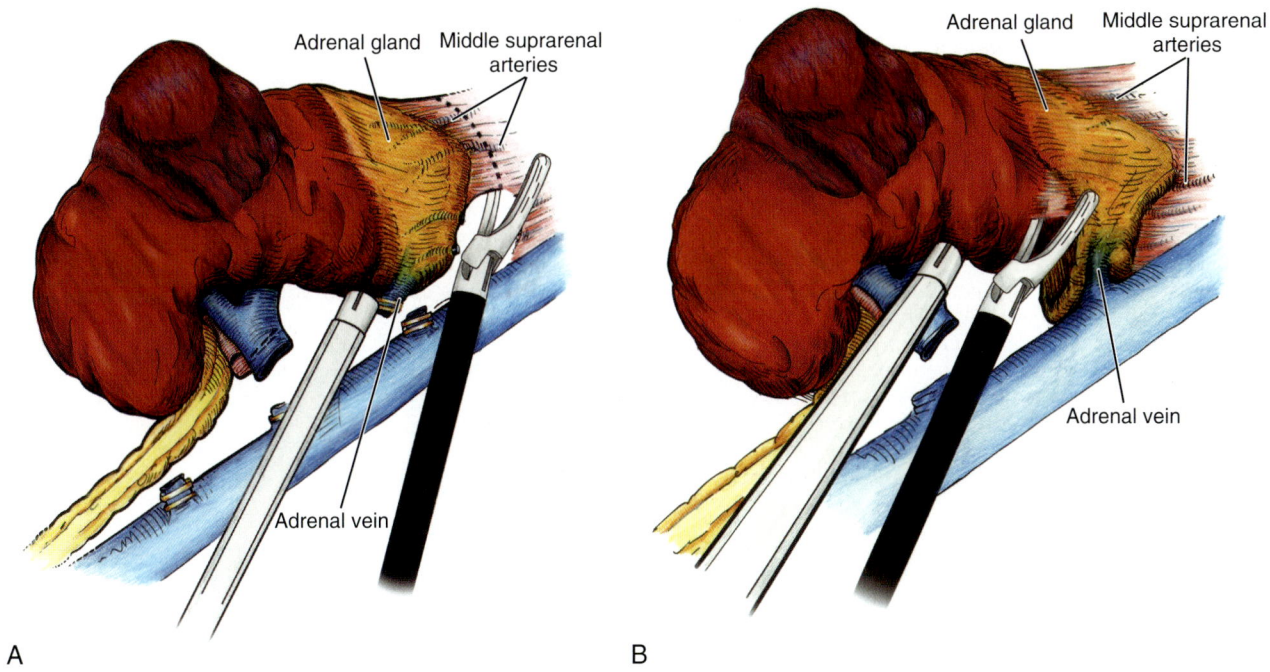

Fig. 102.30. (A) Inclusion of the adrenal gland during right laparoscopic radical nephrectomy can be readily accomplished using ultrasonic or bipolar shears to control the multiple arterial branches to the adrenal gland. Inferior retraction of the specimen facilitates exposure of this surgical plane. (B) Adrenal-sparing, right radical nephrectomy. Use of a blunt instrument above the hilum to put anterior and inferior traction on the kidney helps to expose the correct plane and place the connective tissue on stretch. Ultrasonic or bipolar shears are again useful to avoid any bleeding that may be encountered in this plane.

hand port are placed as needed, especially in cases of larger tumors, IVC involvement, or adjacent organ invasion. Laparoscopic radical nephrectomy is essentially identical to laparoscopic simple nephrectomy except that the Gerota fascia and fat are left intact during dissection. When indicated, the adrenal gland can be removed en bloc with the kidney (Fig. 102.30A). This can be accomplished by ligating the renal vein medial to the take-off of the adrenal vein. For adrenal-sparing nephrectomy, the fascia is opened over the upper medial aspect of the kidney (Fig. 102.30B). Regional lymph nodes may be removed, and a full hilar or retroperitoneal dissection can be carried out if deemed necessary. Excision of part of the adjacent organs, such as the diaphragm, pancreas, liver, spleen, and bowel, can be accomplished if needed (Molina et al., 2004; O'Malley et al., 2009).

Results

Laparoscopic radical nephrectomy offers minimally invasive advantages with similar long-term oncologic outcomes compared with open surgery (Campbell et al., 2017; EAU Guidelines: http://uroweb.org/guideline/renal-cell-carcinoma/). **Laparoscopic radical nephrectomy is associated with shorter hospital stay, time to start oral intake, and convalescence time; less estimated blood loss, lower blood transfusion rate, fewer analgesic requirements, and improved cosmesis compared with the open approach** (Fornara et al., 2001; Rassweiler et al., 1998; Tan et al., 2011; Wolf et al., 2001). A systematic review and meta-analysis of 37 prospective and retrospective studies comparing laparoscopic to open radical nephrectomy showed the laparoscopic approach was associated with a 29% lower risk of postoperative complications (Liu et al., 2017). There were no significant differences in cancer-specific mortality, tumor recurrence, or intraoperative complications. A large multi-institutional study including 1555 patients comparing laparoscopic with open radical nephrectomy demonstrated equivalent 5-year overall (laparoscopic: 93.5% vs. open: 89.8%) and recurrence-free (laparoscopic: 94.0% vs. open: 92.8%) survival rates (Jeon et al., 2011). Similar results were observed in studies with long-term follow-up in which the 10-year recurrence-free, cancer-specific, and overall survivals were 94%, 97%, and 76% for laparoscopic nephrectomy compared with 87%, 86%, and 58% for open surgery, respectively (Permpongkosol et al., 2005). Similarly, a study of laparoscopic nephrectomy for renal cell carcinoma followed for 10 years or more showed a 10-year recurrence-free, cancer-specific, and overall survival of 86%, 92%, and 65%, respectively (Berger et al., 2009).

Retroperitoneal

Procedure

The patient is positioned, and trocars are placed for retroperitoneal access as previously described. After identification of the psoas muscle and tendon, the retroperitoneal space anterior to the muscle is developed. Medial dissection in this plane will reveal the ureter. Elevation of the ureter allows the visualization and subsequent elevation of the lower pole of the kidney. This places the renal vessels on stretch, facilitating their dissection. The arterial pulsation may be indirectly visualized through overlying connective tissue. A gentle layer-by-layer dissection allows the renal vessels to come more directly into view. Use of the right-angle dissector allows the artery and vein to be circumferentially freed from the surrounding tissue, and the endovascular stapler or clips are used to divide the artery and vein sequentially. During surgery on the left kidney, a lumbar vein typically requires dissection, ligation, and division to allow direct access to the renal hilum. Once the renal hilum is ligated, the posterior dissection is carried in a cephalad direction to the upper pole followed by dissection of the lateral and anterior aspects of the kidney. Continuous identification of anatomic landmarks is key to avoid disorientation.

Results

Retroperitoneal radical nephrectomy has comparable complication rates, analgesic requirements, hospital course, convalescence, and oncologic outcomes compared with transperitoneal surgery. Three randomized clinical trials compared pure transperitoneal with retroperitoneal laparoscopic nephrectomy. In the first study with 40 patients, no significant differences in estimated blood loss, operative time, complication rates, and hospital stay were noted (Nambirajan et al., 2004). A second study including 52 transperitoneal and 50 retroperitoneal radical nephrectomies found no significant difference in estimated blood loss, narcotic use, hospital stay, or complication rate (Desai et al., 2005). However, retroperitoneal surgery was associated with shorter operative time (150 vs. 207 minutes). A third study including 62 patients found retroperitoneal nephrectomy was associated with shorter operative time (120 vs. 140 minutes), lower pain scores, lower analgesic requirements, shorter convalescence, and lower complication rate (13% vs. 6%) (Garg et al., 2014). A meta-analysis of 12 studies comparing the two approaches showed the retroperitoneal was associated with shorter operative time, and lower intraoperative complication rate (Fan et al., 2013). No significant differences in time to oral intake, postoperative analgesic requirement, postoperative complications, blood transfusion, or oncologic outcomes were observed.

Hand-Assisted

Procedure

Patient positioning, hand port, and trocar placement are done as described earlier in the chapter. The steps in hand-assisted laparoscopic nephrectomy are similar to those of standard laparoscopic surgery, but the nondominant hand is used throughout for retraction and blunt dissection. The line of Toldt is incised while the hand retracts the colon medially (Fig. 102.31). The surgeon's hand and fingers may be used to simultaneously place lateral traction on the kidney and medial traction on the bowel, helping to demonstrate the plane posterior to the mesocolon and anterior to the Gerota fascia. On the left side, the hand may also be used to retract the spleen and pancreas medially while dividing the lienorenal attachments. On the right, the hand is used to retract the liver anteriorly to expose the upper pole. After the colon is mobilized, the psoas muscle is identified, and the ureter is elevated. On the left, the gonadal vein is typically elevated in the packet along with the ureter while, on the right, the gonadal vein is reflected medially. With the ureter elevated, the hand can bluntly dissect and elevate the entire kidney off the psoas muscle, and the ureter is then followed to the renal hilum. The fingers are then used to place anterolateral traction on the kidney, while the thumb pushes the bowel and mesentery medially to expose the hilum. Once the renal vessels are sufficiently skeletonized, the endovascular stapler or clips are used to ligate and divide the artery and vein (Fig. 102.32). The lateral and superior attachments may then be divided, using a LigaSure device or Harmonic scalpel (Ethicon), while the hand keeps them on traction. The hand should

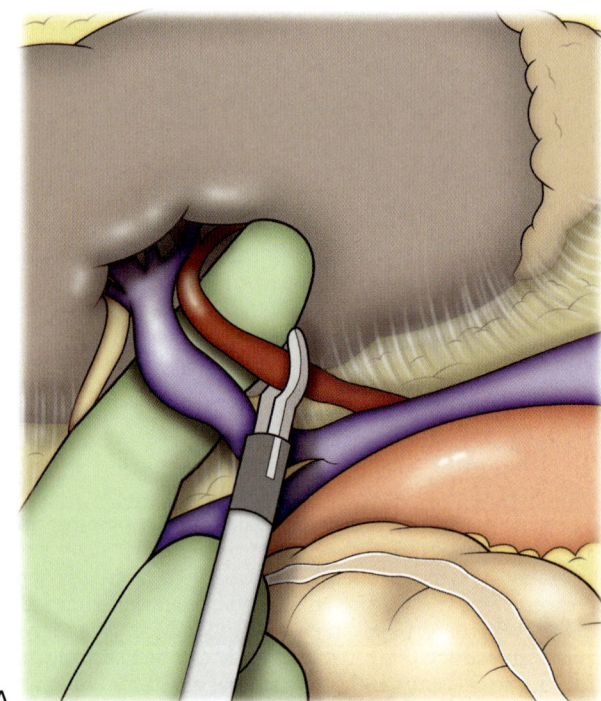

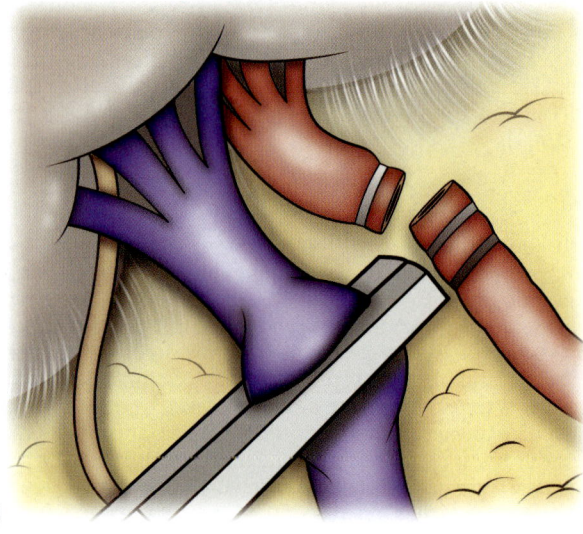

Fig. 102.32. (A) With the renal hilum on stretch and the bowel retracted medially to expose the vessels, the fingers can be used to palpate the renal artery and guide a stapler or clip applier to secure and divide the artery. (B) Once the artery is divided, the renal vein is freed circumferentially and divided with an endovascular stapler.

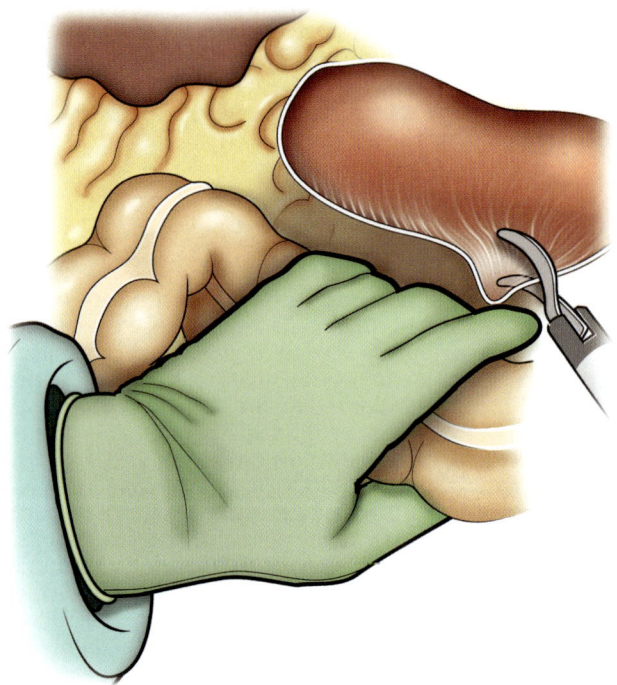

Fig. 102.31. The nondominant hand is used to retract the colon medially and to dissect tissue planes, while the dominant hand uses endoscopic scissors to divide colon attachments.

not be used to bluntly dissect the adrenal gland free from the upper pole because this typically results in bleeding. A rolled laparotomy sponge placed through the hand port at the beginning of the procedure may assist with retraction and hemostasis. The previously made hand-port incision allows rapid removal of sponge and the specimen. However, because hand-port metastases have been reported, it is recommended to place the specimen in a removal device before extraction (Chen et al., 2003). At the conclusion of the procedure, the hand-port incision is irrigated and closed.

Results

Hand-assisted laparoscopic radical nephrectomy offers recovery, morbidity, and cost that are comparable with those of pure laparoscopy surgery. A study of 22 hand-assisted and 16 standard laparoscopic radical nephrectomies found comparable operative times and no difference in the complication rate, hospital costs or stay, return to activity, or overall pain score (Nelson and Wolf, 2002). In two separate studies the rate of wound-related complications such as wound infection and incisional hernia was slightly higher in hand-assisted approach compared with pure laparoscopy (Nadler et al., 2006; Okeke et al., 2002). Oncologic outcomes seem comparable with the ones achieved with pure laparoscopy or open surgery (Chung et al., 2007; Gabr et al., 2009; Kawauchi et al., 2007). A study of 147 standard and 108 hand-assisted laparoscopic radical nephrectomies found comparable operative times and conversion to open surgery and complication rates (Gabr et al., 2009). After a median follow-up of 35 months, recurrence-free, cancer-specific, and overall survivals were similar between surgical techniques.

Special Considerations

Large Tumors

Although renal masses larger than 7 cm pose a surgical challenge, minimally invasive techniques have been shown to be a feasible and safe treatment option in most cases of large renal masses (Luciani et al., 2013; Stewart et al., 2012). A study of 200 laparoscopic radical nephrectomies for tumors larger than 7 cm showed a conversion rate to open surgery of 5% and complication rate of 20% (Pierorazio et al., 2012). **Because of the bulk of the tumor, the working space can be reduced and normal anatomic landmarks distorted, potentially leading to disorientation.** In some cases, the hilum may be obscured by large perihilar collateral vascularity or the kidney may fall over the hilum. Continuous intraoperative reference to preoperative imaging as well as use of intraoperative ultrasonography is helpful. It may be beneficial to use a hand port or additional trocars to assist in the lateral distraction of the kidney and allow for more widely distributed retraction of the kidney.

En Bloc Hilar Vessel Stapling

In spite of previous concerns of arteriovenous fistula formation in cases of en bloc hilar vessel stapling, this approach has been shown to be a safe alternative. A meta-analysis of 595 cases of en bloc stapling followed for an average of 2 years did not reveal any cases of arteriovenous fistula. Moreover, en bloc stapling was associated with almost identical complication rates and a significant reduction in operative time by an average of 43 minutes (Lai and Rais-Bahrami, 2017).

Tumor Seeding and Port-Site Recurrence

Tumor seeding is a rare complication of laparoscopic renal surgery. In a multi-institutional survey including nearly 11,000 laparoscopic urologic surgeries for cancer, tumor seeding was observed in 13 cases (0.1%), of which 10 were port-site recurrences (Micali et al., 2004). In another study of 1098 laparoscopic urologic procedures for malignancy, two port-site recurrences (0.18%) were identified (Rassweiler et al., 2003). Tumor aggressiveness, patient immune status, local wound factors, surgical technique, and tumor spillage are potential factors associated with tumor seeding. **Pneumoperitoneum, aerosolization of tumor cells, insufflation gas type, and laparoscopic wound closure techniques have been studied and have been shown to be noncontributory** (Halpin et al., 2005). Sound surgical technique avoiding tumor spillage and careful tumor extraction with the assistance of an impermeable retrieval bag are recommended to minimize the risk of tumor seeding.

Specimen Extraction

Specimen extraction can be accomplished by removing it intact or after morcellation. Although morcellation can achieve smaller extraction incisions with better cosmesis, and potentially shorter recovery, it is surrounded by controversy because of concerns of inadequate pathological evaluation and the risk of tumor seeding. A study of 57 laparoscopic nephrectomies in which 23 specimens were removed intact and 33 after morcellation found the mean incision length for morcellated specimens was 1.2 cm compared with 7.1 cm in the intact extraction group (Hernandez et al., 2003). No significant differences in operative time, pain, or hospital stay were observed. In a multi-institutional study of 188 radical nephrectomies in which specimens were removed after morcellation, one port site recurrence was identified (Wu et al., 2009). The authors concluded intracorporal mechanical morcellation after radical nephrectomy is a safe and effective way of specimen extraction. A study of 9 pathological evaluations before and after ex vivo morcellation showed morcellation did not affect the of histologic diagnosis, grade, or stage (Landman et al., 2000). Only tumor size was not assessable after morcellation. Conversely, in a study of 23 renal specimens after morcellation, tumor size, renal capsule involvement, and renal vein involvement could not be adequately evaluated for renal cell carcinoma and invasion could not be properly assessed for urothelial carcinoma of the renal pelvis (Rabban et al., 2001). Thus morcellation can be used in select cases, but it is not considered standard of care. **If the specimen is to be morcellated, the surgeon should strictly adhere to proper technique including the use of a purpose-built sac, adequate draping, and change of gowns, gloves, and instruments after morcellation.** The LapSac (Cook Urological, Spencer, IN) has been shown to be impermeable to bacteria and tumor cells, even after its use for morcellation (Urban et al., 1993). The sac is prepared by passing a moistened hydrophilic wire alternating through every third hole in the sac, which is then rolled from the bottom up and passed through a 12-mm trocar site. The trocar is replaced, leaving the wire and drawstrings outside the trocar. Graspers are used to place the specimen in the sac, which is held open by the wire, and the wire is removed (Wakabayashi et al., 2003). The drawstrings are grasped and brought through the periumbilical incision along with the neck of the sac, which is held tightly against the abdomen. Enlarging the trocar site by 1 cm allows small amounts of tissue to protrude through the mouth of the sac. The morcellation process is performed with a ring forceps, working with alternating bites on the protruding tissue. Deep passes with the forceps should be avoided to prevent unintentional incorporation of bowel into the forceps. Pneumoperitoneum and direct laparoscopic visualization should also be maintained during the process to allow monitoring of the sac intracorporeally to avoid injury to structures resting against the sac or sac perforation.

Lymphadenectomy

Routine retroperitoneal lymphadenectomy at the time of nephrectomy remains controversial. Although the removal of retroperitoneal lymph nodes allows for better disease staging and prognostication, the oncologic benefit of this procedure remains unclear (Blom et al., 2009; Gershman et al., 2017). Moreover, there is no consensus on the extent of node dissection to be performed. A study of 50 laparoscopic radical nephrectomies alone and 50 laparoscopic nephrectomies with lymphadenectomy showed that 10% of the cases had positive nodes (Chapman et al., 2008). Estimated blood loss, length of hospitalization, and complication rates were similar between groups. These results suggest that minimally invasive lymphadenectomy is feasible

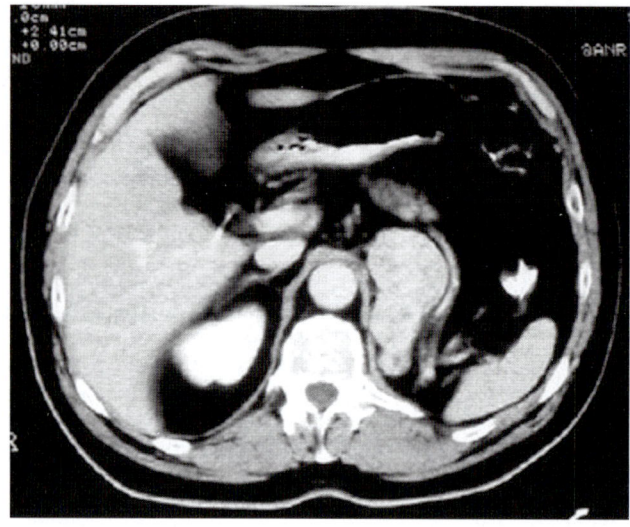

Fig. 102.33. Renal fossa recurrence. (From Nóbrega de Jesus CM, Silva Casafus FA, et al.: Surgical treatment of renal cell carcinoma recurrence at the renal fossa following radical nephrectomy. *Sao Paulo Med J* 126:194–196, 2008.)

and a safe procedure. However, currently only 6% of the laparoscopic nephrectomies are accompanied by lymphadenectomy (Filson et al., 2012). For right-sided tumors, lymphadenectomy involved sampling the paracaval, precaval, retrocaval, and interaortocaval nodes from the crus of the diaphragm to the bifurcation of the IVC. For left renal masses, the paraaortic and preaortic nodes are sampled from the crus of the diaphragm to the bifurcation of the aorta; the interaortocaval nodes are removed when suspicious for malignant involvement.

Local Recurrence

Isolated local recurrence is defined as recurrence in the ipsilateral retroperitoneal lymph nodes, renal fossa, or adrenal gland without evidence of distant metastasis (Fig. 102.33). Its incidence after radical nephrectomy is approximately 2% (Itano et al., 2000; Margulis et al., 2009). A study of 54 isolated local recurrence treated with open resection showed median recurrence-free and cancer-specific survival rates of 11 and 61 months, respectively (Margulis et al., 2009). Given its rarity, only a few series of cases of minimally invasive excision of isolated local recurrence after nephrectomy have been published. A series of 5 patients (1 open conversion resulting from IVC invasion) undergoing hand-assisted excision of isolated local recurrence showed cancer-specific and disease-free survival rates were 60% and 20%, respectively, after a mean follow-up of 43 months (Bandi et al., 2008). The robotic approach has also been described to manage isolated local recurrence (Gilbert and Abaza, 2015).

Renal Vein and Caval Tumor Thrombus

With the evolution of minimally invasive techniques and increasing surgical experience, laparoscopic surgery is now used to manage complex renal tumors, including those associated with renal vein and caval thrombus (Abaza et al., 2016; Desai et al., 2003). In a study of 37 laparoscopic radical nephrectomies for renal masses with renal vein thrombus, the median estimated blood loss was 200 mL, median length of hospital stay was 3 days, and complication rate was 14% (Guzzo et al., 2009). **The authors concluded laparoscopic radical nephrectomy in the setting of renal vein thrombus is feasible but complex and requires significant laparoscopic skills.** Management of renal vein thrombus usually involves complete laparoscopic mobilization of the kidney and ligation of the renal artery followed by use of a laparoscopic DeBakey, vessel loop, or hand-assistance to "milk" the tumor thrombus back toward the kidney. This allows either the endovascular stapler to be deployed on the renal vein excluding the thrombus, or a laparoscopic Satinsky clamp to be placed to isolate a cuff of the IVC so that the cuff may be excised to allow intact specimen extraction without tumor at the margin. In cases in which a cuff of the IVC is excised en bloc with the renal vein stump, the cavotomy may be oversewn using Prolene suture mirroring the open procedure. Intraoperative ultrasonography can aid in assessing the location and extent of the thrombus (Hsu et al., 2003). A tangential clamping of the IVC using a laparoscopic Satinsky clamp can be used to manage short caval thrombi. Long caval thrombi require circumferential dissection of the IVC above and below the thrombus to allow the placement of Rommel tourniquets or vascular clamps. The contralateral renal vein should also be controlled and lumbar veins ligated as needed. The IVC is open after the blood flow is interrupted. The thrombus is excised, and the IVC is closed using Prolene sutures and flushed with heparinized saline before reestablishing blood flow. A study of robotic-assisted radical nephrectomy in 30 level II and 2 level III IVC thrombus cases showed a need for IVC cross-clamping in 24 cases, and 1 case required synthetic patch cavoplasty (Abaza et al., 2016). Mean operative time was 292 minutes, mean blood loss was 400 mL, with no conversions to open surgery or aborted procedures. Three patients required transfusions and no Clavien grades III through V complications were observed. **The authors concluded robotic nephrectomy in the setting of IVC thrombus is feasible in selected patients. Given the complexity of the procedure and potential for catastrophic complications, these should be performed by experienced surgeons.**

Cytoreductive Nephrectomy

Cytoreductive nephrectomy has been shown to provide survival benefits in metastatic renal cell carcinoma. A study of 22 laparoscopic and 42 open cytoreductive nephrectomies showed shorter length of stay (2.3 vs. 6.1 days), less estimated blood loss (300 vs. 1,200 mL), and shorter interval from surgery to the initiation of systemic therapy (36 vs. 61 days) in the laparoscopic group, but the overall survival at 1 year was similar between groups (61% vs. 65%) (Rabets et al., 2004). Similar results have been reported in separate studies (Eisenberg et al., 2006; Matin et al., 2006; Nunez Bragayrac et al. 2016), although the shorter interval to systemic therapy has not been consistently observed.

Surgical Salvage After Failed Ablative Therapies

Several studies have shown the feasibility of the minimally invasive nephrectomy in the management after failed ablative therapies (Breda et al., 2010; Kowalczyk et al., 2009; Nguyen et al., 2008). However, the surgery can be technically challenging as a result of perinephric fibrosis causing loss of tissue planes around the lesion. A report of 10 patients undergoing salvage surgery showed that laparoscopic nephrectomy was only possible in four patients, and the remainder required either open partial or radical nephrectomy (Nguyen et al., 2008).

PARTIAL NEPHRECTOMY

Partial nephrectomy is increasingly used for the management of renal masses. The preservation of renal function with reduced morbidity and equivalent oncologic outcomes led to a paradigm shift away from radical nephrectomy. The minimally invasive approach has emerged as a management option that reduces operative time, blood loss, and hospital stay (Gill et al., 2007; Lane and Gill, 2010).

Indications

The first laparoscopic partial nephrectomy was reported in 1993 by Winfield et al., with the retroperitoneal approach introduced 1 year later (Gill et al., 1994). Initially, laparoscopic partial nephrectomy (Video 102.1) was used in the management of small exophytic renal masses (clinical stage T1a) (Fig. 102.34). With increasing experience, the indications of minimally invasive partial nephrectomy have

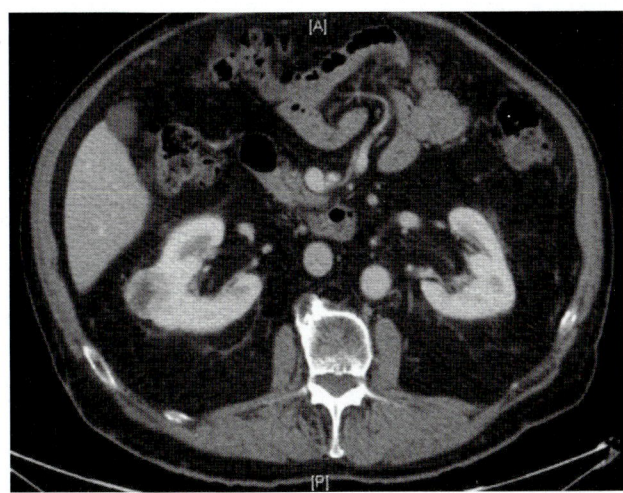

Fig. 102.34. Computed tomography scan with intravenous contrast demonstrating a partially exophytic mid-pole clinical T1a lesion in the right kidney.

expanded to include large and complex renal tumors. Tumor complexity can be characterized using RENAL nephrometry score, which takes into consideration tumor Radius, Exophytic/endophytic appearance, Nearness to the collecting system, Anterior/posterior position, and Location relative to the polar line (Kutikov and Uzzo, 2009). Anatomic complexity measured by RENAL nephrometry has been shown to correlate with risk of complications, warm ischemia time, operative time, hospital stay, estimated blood loss, and risk of recurrence after surgery (Hayn et al., 2011; Nagahara et al., 2016; Watts et al., 2017).

Clinical Stage T1b and Greater Tumors

With the increasing experience of minimally invasive nephron-sparing surgery for the management of small renal masses and advances in laparoscopic techniques, select larger renal masses can be treated with minimally invasive partial nephrectomy. Although there are no randomized clinical trials comparing partial with radical nephrectomy in the management of large renal masses, retrospective studies have shown feasibility and safety of nephron-sparing surgery for large renal tumors. A study of 35 laparoscopic partial and 75 radical nephrectomies for tumors larger than 4 cm (clinical stage pT1b or greater) showed similar negative margin rates, overall and cancer-specific and disease-free survival between groups (Simmons et al., 2009). A 2-stage worsening in chronic kidney disease stage occurred in 12% vs. 0 of the radical and partial nephrectomy groups. A similar study found longer operative times and higher estimated blood loss in the laparoscopic partial nephrectomy group, but the rate of complications and oncologic outcomes was similar between laparoscopic partial and radical nephrectomies (Deklaj et al., 2010). Radical nephrectomy was associated with a nearly 30% decline in estimated glomerular filtration rate compared with only 12% in the partial nephrectomy group. **These studies suggest with adequate laparoscopic experience and appropriate patient selection, the perioperative outcomes of laparoscopic partial nephrectomy for clinical T1b tumors appear comparable with those achieved by radical nephrectomy.** A multi-institutional study of robotic partial nephrectomy for the treatment of 1358 T1a, 379 T1b, and 41 T2a renal masses showed comparable complication rates, negative surgical margins, length of stay, and renal function decline across all three groups (Delto et al., 2018). However, larger tumors were associated with increased operative (T1a: 160, T1b: 190, and T2a: 224 minutes) and ischemia time (T1a: 15, T1b: 18, and T2a: 20 minutes), increased estimated blood loss (T1a: 100, T1b: 150, and T2a: 200 mL), and higher risk of recurrence at 1 year (T1a: 1%, T1b: 0, and T2a: 8%). A study of 133 open, 57 laparoscopic, and 95 robot-assisted partial nephrectomies for the management of pT1b renal tumors showed comparable perioperative complications, negative surgical margins, and ischemia time across all three surgical approaches (Porpiglia et al., 2016). Shah et al. (2016) looked at 1250 partial nephrectomies and found a 27% rate of upstaging in patients with clinical t1b compared with 4.4% in patients with clinical t1a disease. Furthermore, 33% of these recurred. Coupling this with the fact that medical renal disease is much different than surgically induced renal disease, caution should be taken in applying partial nephrectomy to larger tumors and indications for sparing parenchyma should be well defined.

Laparoscopic Heminephrectomy

Heminephrectomy involves the excision of 30% or more of the renal parenchyma. Specific technical considerations include deeper parenchymal resection, transection of large intraparenchymal blood vessels with potential need for clipping or suturing, and intentional entry into the pelvicalyceal system, in some cases, requiring surgical repair. A study of 41 laparoscopic heminephrectomies compared with 41 matched partial nephrectomies showed similar estimated blood loss, operative time, hospital stay, overall complication rate, and postoperative serum creatinine (Finelli et al., 2005). Heminephrectomy was associated with larger parenchymal resections, pelvicalyceal system repair, and longer warm ischemia time (39 vs. 33 minutes). Similar findings have been reported by other authors (Sobey et al., 2012).

Central and Hilar Tumors

Central tumors are defined as those abutting or invading the central renal sinus fat and/or the collecting system. These tumors deeply infiltrate the renal parenchyma, and their excision frequently requires intraoperative ultrasound guidance, intentional entry into and potentially suture-repair of the pelvicalyceal system along with complex parenchymal reconstruction, all within the time constraints of renal ischemia. A study of 154 central and 209 peripheral tumors undergoing laparoscopic partial nephrectomy showed comparable estimated blood loss, complication rates, surgical margins, and postoperative creatinine levels. Central tumors were associated with longer warm ischemia time (33.5 vs. 30 minutes), operative time (3.5 vs. 3.0 hours), and hospital stay (67 vs. 60 hours) (Frank et al., 2006). A similar analysis of laparoscopic partial nephrectomy for 53 central and 159 peripheral tumors showed similar estimated blood loss, operative time, and complication rates (Nadu et al., 2009). Central tumors were associated with longer warm ischemia time (37 vs. 28 minutes), lower conversion rate to open surgery (1% vs 6%), and less positive surgical margins (0 vs. 5%). **Hilar tumors are defined as tumors located in the renal hilum in direct contact with the renal artery and/or vein.** Preoperative three-dimensional reconstruction of triphasic spiral CT assists surgical planning by detailing the number, interrelationship, anatomic course, and position of the renal vessels in relation to the tumor (Gill et al., 2005). A study of 43 hilar tumors treated with laparoscopic partial nephrectomy found no significant differences in any perioperative parameter investigated, including warm ischemia time, surgical margins, and postoperative renal functional outcomes at 6 months' follow-up (George et al., 2014). **These authors conclude minimally invasive partial nephrectomy for central and hilar tumors can be performed safely by an experienced surgeon with perioperative outcomes comparable with those of peripheral tumors.**

Tumor in a Solitary Kidney

Partial nephrectomy in a solitary kidney poses a challenge regardless of the surgical approach. A multi-institutional study of 74 patients undergoing robotic partial nephrectomy for renal mass in a solitary kidney showed a mean warm ischemia time of 15.5 minutes, 24% 3-month complication rate, 95% negative surgical margins, and only one conversion to radical nephrectomy (Arora et al., 2018). These results are comparable with previous reports of partial nephrectomy in solitary kidneys (Reynolds et al., 2017; Zargar, et al. 2014). **These authors concluded that minimally invasive partial nephrectomy for management of tumors in a solitary kidney is safe and offered** reliable preservation of renal function and comparable outcomes with open surgery.

Multiple Tumors

Nephron-sparing surgery is an attractive treatment option for multifocal ipsilateral tumors because of the potential for contralateral recurrence. In a matched analysis of 33 patients undergoing partial nephrectomy for multiple tumors, resection of multiple tumors was associated with long operative time and hospitalization with comparable blood loss, complication rates, and renal functional outcomes (Abreu et al., 2013). Bilateral laparoscopic partial nephrectomies can be performed in a staged or single-setting fashion. In a study of 13 cases of bilateral renal masses, 11 (85%) were successfully treated in a single setting (Reisiger et al., 2005). The authors concluded that bilateral single-setting surgery is feasible and should only be performed in select cases when the primary procedure has been completed expeditiously and without complications.

Repeat Partial Nephrectomy

Repeat renal surgery can pose a technical challenge and result in higher blood loss and complication rates compared with first-time renal surgery. Studies of patients with hereditary kidney cancers showed repeat laparoscopic and robotic partial nephrectomy to be safe and feasible in select cases (Johnson et al., 2008). A study of 26 repeat robotic partial nephrectomies showed significantly higher estimated blood loss and longer hospitalization and a trend toward higher complication rates in the repeat surgery group with similar renal functional outcomes (Watson et al., 2016).

Other Indications

Minimally invasive partial nephrectomy has been performed in multiple clinical scenarios including in combination with adrenalectomy for upper pole tumor (Ramani et al., 2003), in patients with renal artery disease (Steinberg et al., 2003), tumors in congenitally anomalous kidney, such as horseshoe kidney (Tsivian et al., 2007), obese patients (Romero et al., 2008), and hereditary renal cell carcinoma (Watson et al., 2016). Although each of these scenarios poses different challenges, the minimally invasive partial nephrectomy in most clinical settings should realistically be able to safely remove the tumor while sparing normal renal parenchyma, minimizing ischemia and operative times, and minimizing postoperative complications.

Procedure

The primary goal of partial nephrectomy is complete tumor excision with negative margins and adequate hemostasis while paying attention to warm ischemia time. Successful minimally invasive partial nephrectomy requires an in-depth understanding of three-dimensional (3D) renal anatomy, real-time intraoperative appreciation of visual anatomic cues, and precise and efficient intracorporal suturing.

Transperitoneal Laparoscopic Partial Nephrectomy

The advantages of the transperitoneal approach include a large working space, familiar landmarks, greater versatility of instrument angles, and technical ease of suturing. The initial portion of the procedure is performed as previously described for transperitoneal access to the kidney.

Retroperitoneal Laparoscopic Partial Nephrectomy

The advantages of the retroperitoneal approach include no need for bowel mobilization and a more direct access to the posterior aspect of kidney and the renal hilum at the cost of a smaller working space and less familiar landmarks. After the retroperitoneum is entered and the working space established as previously described, the psoas muscle should be identified, and the kidney may be lifted anteriorly off the psoas muscle to allow visualization of the arterial pulsation.

The dissection of the renal hilum can then proceed to facilitate bulldog clamp placement when deemed necessary. A meta-analysis of 8 retrospective studies comparing transperitoneal to retroperitoneal laparoscopic partial nephrectomy indicated the retroperitoneal approach was associated with shorter operative time, lower estimated blood loss, and a shorter length of hospital stay (Ren et al., 2014). Complication rates and conversion to open surgery were comparable between the two approaches. A study comparing 100 transperitoneal and 63 retroperitoneal laparoscopic partial nephrectomies found that 77% of the posterior tumors were managed via retroperitoneal approach, whereas 97% of the anterior tumors were managed with transperitoneal surgery (Ng et al., 2005). The retroperitoneal approach was associated with smaller lesions, less pyelocaliceal system repair, shorter operative time, shorter warm ischemia time, and a shorter length of hospital stay. The choice of transperitoneal or retroperitoneal approach mainly relies on tumor location and the surgeon's preference. Other factors that may influence the decision include tumor size, number of tumors, number of arteries supplying the kidney, amount of visceral fat surrounding the kidney, and prior abdominal surgeries.

Robotic-Assisted Laparoscopic Partial Nephrectomy

Robotics have facilitated the diffusion of minimally invasive partial nephrectomy by reducing difficulty of intracorporal tumor resection and suturing, resulting in a shorter learning curve for individuals not skilled in pure laparoscopic techniques (Alameddine et al., 2018; Pierorazio et al., 2011). A meta-analysis of 23 nonrandomized studies of beginning laparoscopic surgeons comparing robotic with laparoscopic partial nephrectomy found the robotic-assisted approach was associated with a lower rate of conversion to open surgery and radical nephrectomy, shorter warm ischemia time, smaller changes in estimated glomerular filtration rate, and shorter length of hospital stay (Choi et al., 2015). Complication rate, operative time, estimated blood loss, and surgical margins were comparable between groups. Although robotic-assisted retroperitoneal laparoscopic partial nephrectomy techniques have been described, the transperitoneal approach is the one most commonly used (Ludwig et al., 2017). The initial portion of the procedure is performed as previously described for robotic-assisted laparoscopy. The beginning of the case can be done with conventional laparoscopy and the robot docked at any time, usually for tumor resection and renorrhaphy, or the robotic assistance can be used throughout the case, starting immediately after trocar insertion. Depending on the technique and instrumentation used, the responsibilities of the bedside assistant may include aiding in clamping the renal hilum, providing suction and retraction to maintain a clean operative field, delivery and cutting of sutures, clip placement, and the operation of the intraoperative ultrasound.

Tumor Localization and Excision

Once the initial dissection is complete, tumor localization can be achieved by directed inspection of the kidney and intraoperative ultrasonography, which can estimate tumor size and depth (Fig. 102.35). The Gerota fascia is entered away from the lesion to expose the renal capsule. In some cases in which the adherent fat is not easily dissecting off the renal capsule, a subcapsular dissection to visually identify the borders of the tumor before resection may be needed (Davidiuk et al., 2014). Using the monopolar scissors, the capsule is scored circumferentially around the tumor (Fig. 102.36), and the hilum is clamped (Fig. 102.37). The scored line may be incised using cold scissors (Fig. 102.38), and with the assistance of a grasper or suction device to provide countertraction and a clear operative field, the tumor excision is completed. Tumor excision can be accomplished with (standard partial nephrectomy) or without a rim of normal parenchyma (tumor enucleation). Standard partial nephrectomy and tumor enucleation seem to have comparable surgical margins and perioperative outcomes (Blackwell et al., 2017; Longo et al., 2014; Minervini et al. 2011; Takagi et al., 2017). A retrospective review of 982 standard partial nephrectomies and 537 tumor enucleations found comparable progression-free and cancer-specific survivals

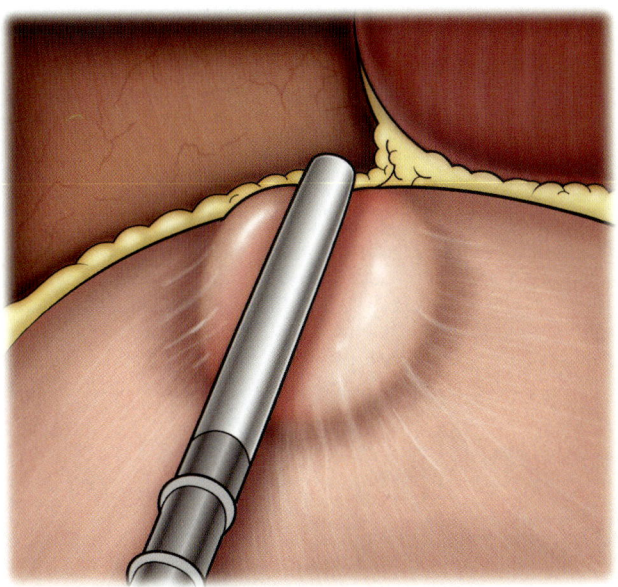

Fig. 102.35. Intraoperative ultrasonography is used to confirm location, width, and depth of the tumor.

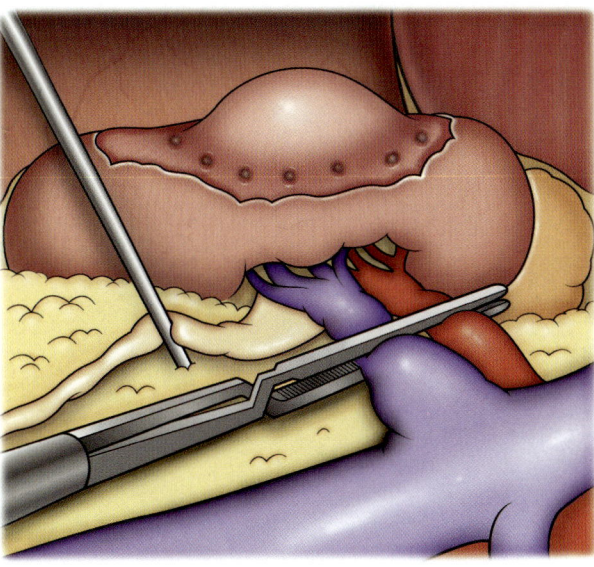

Fig. 102.37. Once the margin around the tumor has been scored, the hilum is clamped en bloc using a laparoscopic Satinsky clamp, or the artery and vein are clamped separately using bulldog clamps.

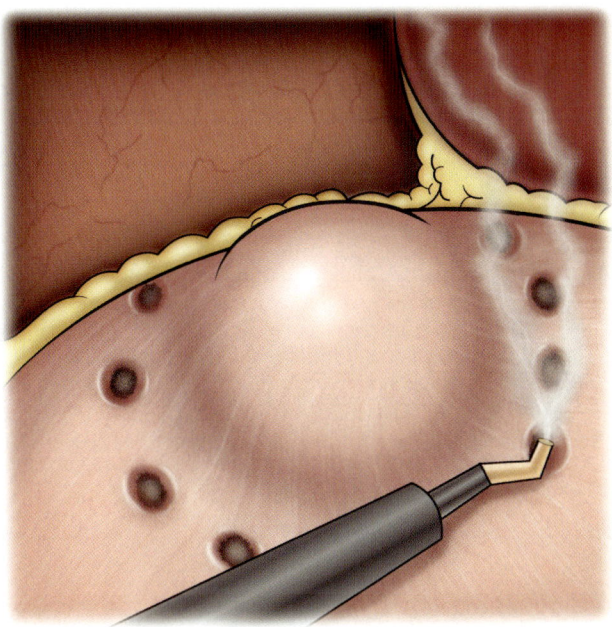

Fig. 102.36. After the Gerota fascia is cleared to expose the lesion and the renal capsule, with use of monopolar scissors or hook cautery, the capsule is scored circumferentially around the tumor.

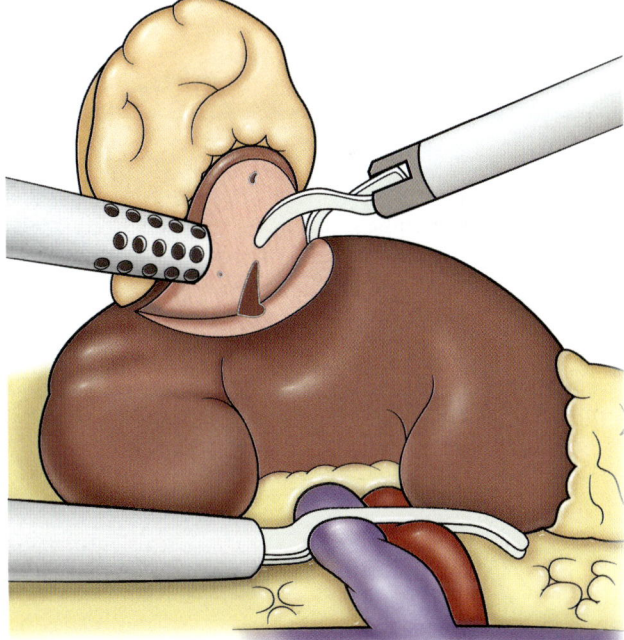

Fig. 102.38. The scored margin around the tumor is incised using cold shears with the renal hilum clamped. The suction-irrigator provides countertraction and helps to maintain a clear operative field and adequate margin of normal renal tissue.

in the two groups after a 10-year follow-up (Minervini et al., 2011). Tumor enucleation should be considered in patients with familial renal cell carcinoma, multifocal disease, or severe renal dysfunction to optimize parenchymal mass preservation (Campbell et al., 2017). After complete excision, the tumor should be placed in a bag for later extraction.

Hemostasis

Suture renorrhaphy is the most reliable technique to achieve hemostasis of the partial nephrectomy bed (Fig. 102.39). This can be accomplished with or without adjunctive hemostatic or sealing agents, or a Surgicel bolster (Johnson and Johnson, New Brunswick, NJ).

A popular renorrhaphy technique involves the use of locking clips applied to the suture, which are then slid toward the renal capsule to keep the renal parenchyma under tension (Benway et al., 2009). Barbed suture run in a horizontal mattress is the authors' preferred choice. This eliminates the need for knot tying. In addition, suturing or clip ligation of individual vessels may be required to control large vessels in the nephrectomy bed. During extrication, surgical clips may also be used to ligate any visualized vessels while coming across the surface of the parenchyma. A number of tissue sealants are available and used based on surgeon preference: gelatin matrix thrombin sealant (Floseal; Baxter, Deerfield, IL), fibrin glue (Tisseel;

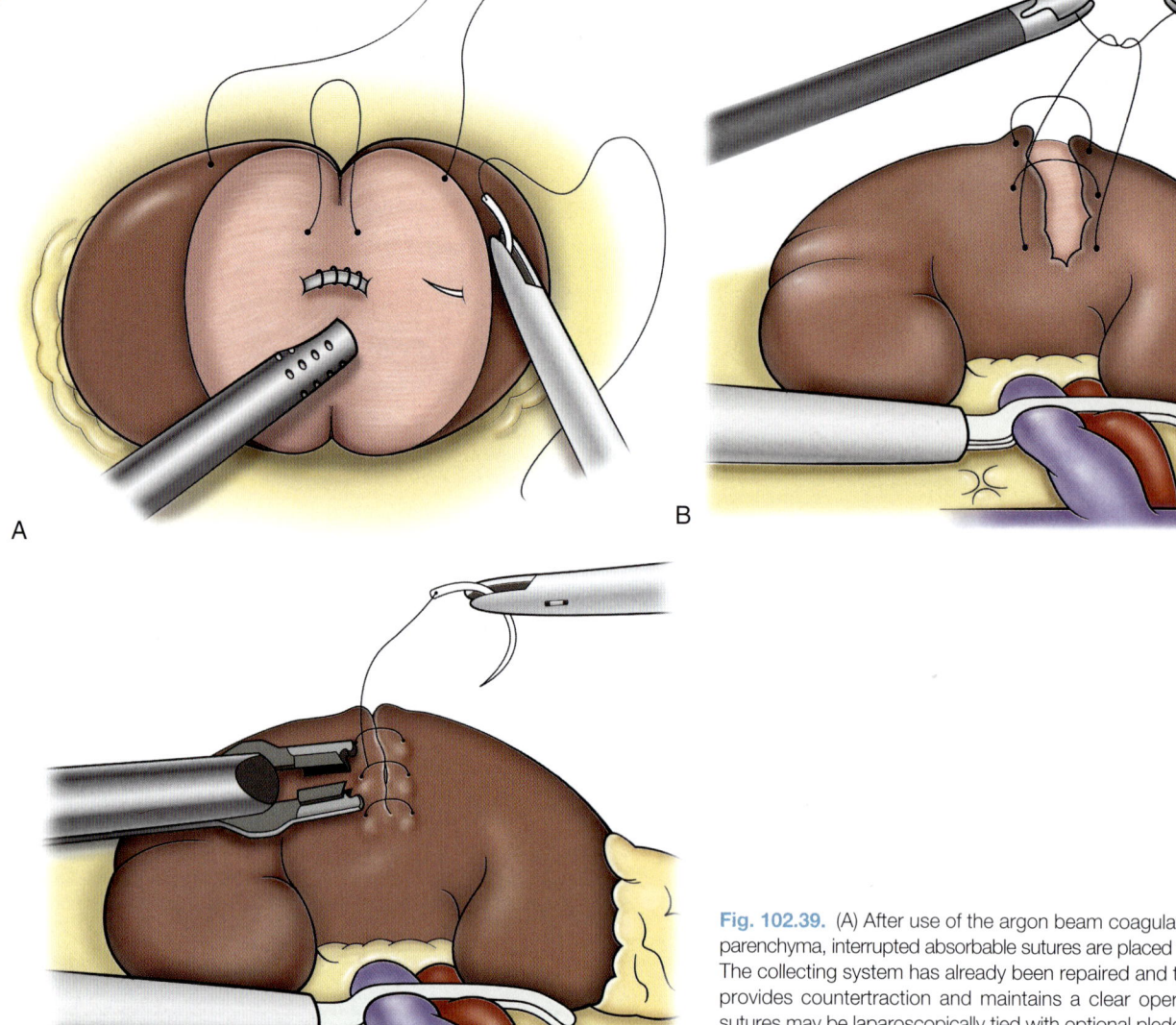

Fig. 102.39. (A) After use of the argon beam coagulator on the exposed parenchyma, interrupted absorbable sutures are placed for the renorrhaphy. The collecting system has already been repaired and the suction-irrigator provides countertraction and maintains a clear operative field. (B) The sutures may be laparoscopically tied with optional pledgets to help prevent capsular tearing during closure. (C) Alternatively, sutures with preplaced Lapra-Ty clips (Ethicon, Cincinnati, OH) at the tail are used and secured with an additional Lapra-Ty clip after the needle is passed and tension on the closure is adjusted.

Baxter), fibrin sealant (Evicel; Ethicon, Somerville, NJ), polyethylene glycol hydrogel (Coseal; Baxter), cyanoacrylate glue (Dermabond; Ethicon), and BioGlue (CryoLife; Atlanta, GA). No study published has clearly demonstrated a clear benefit of any of these agents.

Collecting System Repair

Incision and resection of the pelvicalyceal system may be needed during an excision of tumors abutting or invading the collecting system. It is estimated that in 60% of the laparoscopic partial nephrectomies the pelvicalyceal system is violated. Risk factors for pelvicalyceal system violation include larger tumor sizes, endophytic lesions, and solid tumors (Meeks et al., 2008; Shikanov et al., 2009; Zorn et al., 2007). Suture repair of the pelvicalyceal system can be done with running 3-0 or 4-0 polyglactin (Fig. 102.40). Alternatively, the renal parenchyma and capsule can be closed over the defect without primary pelvicalyceal system repair. In either case, a drain should be placed to reduce the risk of perinephric urinoma. Several nonrandomized studies comparing suture repair of the pelvicalyceal system versus no repair showed increased in mean operative time and was ischemia time in the repair group without any differences in postoperative renal function or complication rates including urinary fistula (Desai et al., 2003; Williams et al., 2017; Zorn et al., 2007).

Renal Hypothermia

Several minimally invasive renal hypothermia techniques that have been described in the literature include surface cooling with ice slush, instillation of cold saline via retrograde ureteral catheter, and intra-arterial cold perfusion (Gill et al., 2003; Kijvikai et al., 2010; Landman et al., 2003). Although these techniques are feasible, their effects on preserving renal function have not been established (Arai et al., 2011; Abe et al., 2012; Ramirez et al., 2016). Moreover, most tumors subjected to partial nephrectomy do not require an inordinately extended period of warm ischemia for resection and reconstruction. Hypothermic techniques may be considered in cases of a solitary kidney or significant renal insufficiency, depending on surgeon preference, tumor complexity, and anticipated long ischemia time.

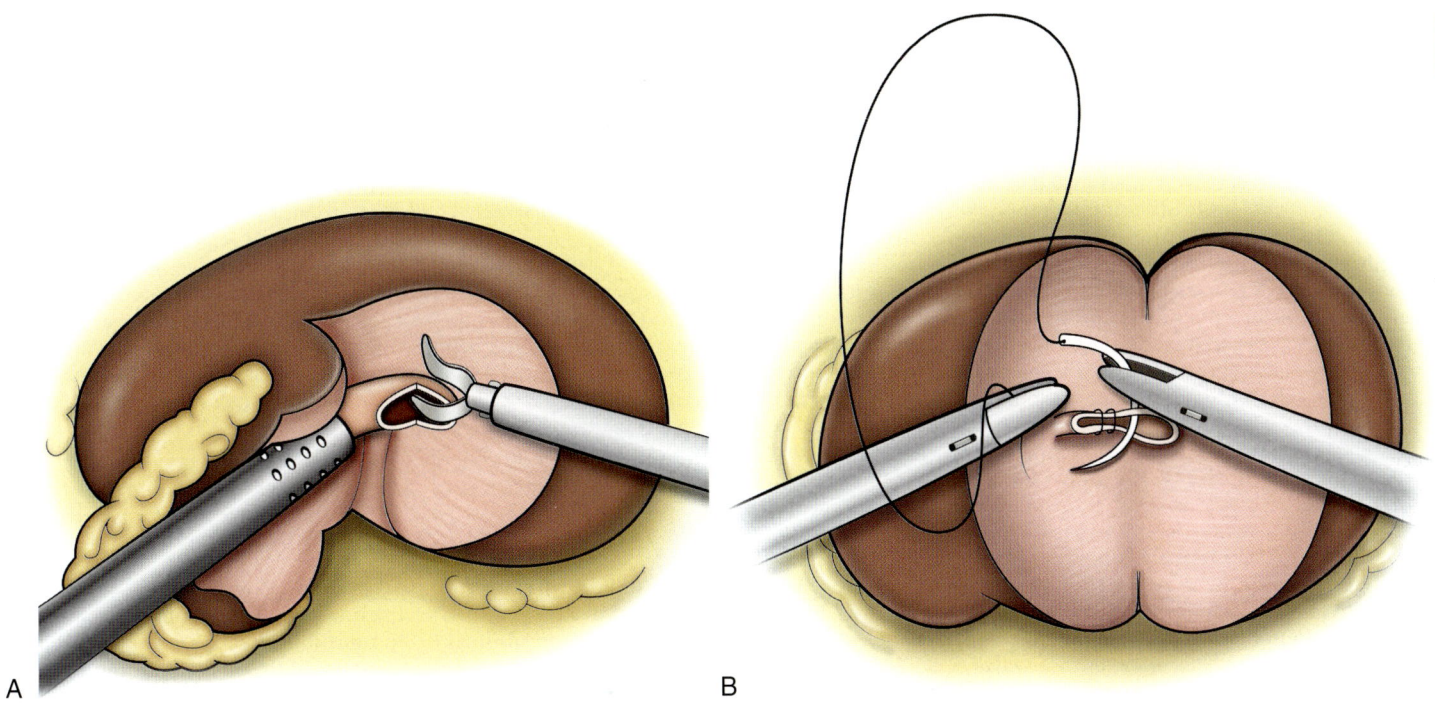

Fig. 102.40. (A) When deep resection is required, the collecting system will often be transected. With occlusion of the renal vessels, these defects can easily be identified and closed using absorbable sutures. The cut edge of the collecting system is identified with the tip of the needle and elevated. (B) An interrupted figure-of-eight suture or running suture is used to completely close the collecting system. The integrity of the repair can be determined by intravenous indigo carmine administration or retrograde instillation, if a ureteral catheter was placed at the beginning of the case. Care must be taken not to destroy the suture, if argon beam coagulation of the parenchyma surface will be performed.

Warm Ischemia and Hilar Control

Hilar control can be accomplished by using bulldog clamps on the renal artery with or without venous clamping, or a laparoscopic Satinsky clamp for en bloc hilar clamping. In a case-control study of patients undergoing laparoscopic partial nephrectomy with artery-only clamping (N = 25) versus combined clamping of the artery and vein (N = 53), artery-only clamping was associated with lower postoperative creatine rise, whereas both techniques had comparable estimated blood loss, warm ischemia time, and complication rates (Gong et al., 2008). Traditionally, the entire tumor excision and renorrhaphy is done while the hilum is clamped. The limit of safe renal warm ischemia time has historically been 30 minutes. However, there are conflicting data suggesting that up to 90 minutes may be reasonably safe, whereas other studies suggest every minute of warm ischemia counts toward worse renal damage (Orvieto et al., 2005; Thompson et al., 2010). Modifications of the surgical technique to accomplish shorter ischemia times have been described, including early unclamping, before the completion of the renorrhaphy (Nguyen and Gill, 2008). A study of 430 laparoscopic partial nephrectomies comparing early unclamping to the conventional technique found early unclamping to be associated with shorter warm ischemia time and comparable estimated blood loss and complication rates (Peyronnet et al., 2014). A similar study with 70 patients found early hilar unclamping was associated with improved postoperative renal function (Campbell et al., 2017).

Off-Clamp Partial Nephrectomy. Select tumors, especially small, exophytic, and noninfiltrating lesions, can be excised without hilar clamping (Novak et al., 2012). Even larger, deeper, central, or hilar tumors, which may require more substantial dissection and reconstruction, can be safely excised off-clamp with adequate experience (Kreshover et al., 2013; Simone et al., 2013). A meta-analysis of 10 studies including 728 off-clamp and 1267 on-clamp partial nephrectomies found that off-clamp surgery had a higher blood transfusion rate but lower overall postoperative complication rate, lower positive margin rate, and better preservation of renal function than the on-clamp approach (Liu et al., 2014). Similarly, a retrospective review of 289 on-clamp and 150 off-clamp laparoscopic partial nephrectomies found the off-clamp technique to be associated with lower reduction in estimated glomerular filtration rate (GFR) immediately postoperatively and at 6 months, slightly lower complication rates, and increased estimated blood loss (George et al., 2013). Other perioperative outcomes were comparable between groups. A 5-year follow-up study of the same cohort found no differences in GFR beyond the early postoperative period (Shah et al., 2016). A similar study including only partial nephrectomy in solitary kidneys found the off-clamp technique to be associated with improved estimated GFR in the early and late postoperative periods (Wszolek et al., 2011).

Selective Arterial Clamping. Selective arterial clamping techniques by interrupting single or multiple arterial branches supplying the area of the tumor without causing global renal ischemia have been described (Patil and Gill, 2011). The theoretic advantages of this approach include a relatively bloodless field for tumor resection, without compromising blood flow to the entire kidney. A retrospective study of 121 partial nephrectomies comparing selective arterial clamping with hilar clamping found selective clamping to be associated with improved postoperative renal function, longer operative times, higher transfusion rates, and comparable perioperative complication rates and length of hospital stay (Desai et al., 2014). The use of duplex ultrasound and near-infrared fluorescence imaging can facilitate selective arterial clamping during partial nephrectomy (Borofsky et al., 2013; Rao et al., 2013).

Parenchymal Compression. Another alternative to hilar clamping is the compression of renal parenchyma that can be accomplished by hand compression (in hand-assisted surgery) or by using a laparoscopic clamp. Reports using these techniques have demonstrated their feasibility and safety in selected cases, especially in cases of peripherally located tumors (Simon et al., 2009; Verhoest et al., 2007).

Results

The feasibility, safety, and effectiveness of minimally invasive partial nephrectomy have been demonstrated by several authors (Gill et al., 2010; Lane and Gill, 2010; Permpongkosol et al., 2006; Saika et al., 2003). **Studies comparing laparoscopic and open partial nephrectomy with radical nephrectomy suggest that nephron-sparing surgery is associated with equivalent oncologic outcomes in properly selected patients and improved overall survival, likely resulting from reduced rates of renal insufficiency and cardiovascular morbidity** (Huang et al., 2006; Thompson et al., 2008). However, the only randomized trial comparing open partial with open radical nephrectomy found nephron-sparing surgery was associated with slightly worse overall survival and comparable progression-free survival (Van Poppel et al., 2011). The authors acknowledge that their findings contradict those of prior retrospective studies and encourage a minimally invasive nephron-sparing approach when feasible. **A multitude of observational studies compared laparoscopic with open partial nephrectomy showing consistent results, including shorter operative time, lower estimated blood loss, and shorter hospital stay in patients treated with laparoscopy** (Abdelhafez et al., 2017; Gill et al., 2007; Gong et al., 2008; Marszalek et al., 2009). In a study including 771 laparoscopic and 1028 open partial nephrectomies for clinical T1 renal masses, the laparoscopic approach was associated with lower shorter operative time, decreased estimated blood loss, shorter hospital stay and comparable intraoperative complications (1.8% vs. 1%), positive surgical margins (1.6% vs. 1%), and 3-year oncologic and functional outcomes (Gill et al., 2007). Laparoscopy was also associated with slightly higher overall postoperative complications (25% vs. 19%) and longer warm ischemia time (30 vs. 20 minutes).

Comparative series of laparoscopic and open partial nephrectomy have shown the two approaches have similar long-term oncologic outcomes (Springer et al., 2013). A study of 200 laparoscopic and 200 open partial nephrectomies for clinical T1 renal masses matched for age, sex, and tumor size found comparable 5-year local recurrence-free survival (laparoscopic: 97% vs. open 98%), metastasis-free survival (laparoscopic: 99% vs open: 96%), and overall survival (laparoscopic: 96% vs. open: 85%) (Marszalek et al., 2009). The 10-year oncologic outcomes were evaluated in a larger study including 625 laparoscopic and 916 open partial nephrectomies for clinical stage T1 renal tumors (Lane et al., 2013). Subjects in the open nephrectomy groups had significantly larger tumors, more malignant tumors, and worse baseline renal function. At 5 years, both surgical approaches had comparable recurrence-free survival in the pT1a (laparoscopic: 98% vs. open: 97%) and pT1b (laparoscopic: 93% vs. open: 93%) subgroups. At 10 years, the overall survival for laparoscopic and open approaches were 78% and 72%, respectively. The recurrence rate in the open partial nephrectomy cohort was higher likely because of inherent differences between the cohorts. On multivariable analysis, predictors of metastasis included larger tumor size, absolute indication, and comorbidity but not surgical approach. **The authors concluded that laparoscopic and open partial nephrectomy provide equivalent long-term overall and recurrence-free survival for pT1 tumors.**

Multiple authors compared robot-assisted partial nephrectomy with open nephrectomy showing similar benefits of the robot-assisted approach, including less estimated blood loss, shorter hospital stay, and lower complications rates with comparable warm ischemia times and positive margin rates (Ficarra et al., 2014; Kara et al., 2016; Oh et al., 2016; Wang et al., 2017). Two meta-analyses, one including 8 retrospective studies and 3418 surgeries and another including 16 studies and 3024 surgeries, comparing robot-assisted to open partial nephrectomy demonstrated that the robot-assisted approach was associated with a lower rate of perioperative complications, less estimated blood loss, and shorter length of hospital stay with comparable conversion to radical nephrectomy, warm ischemia time, estimated GFR changes, margin status, and overall cost (Shen et al., 2016; Wu et al., 2014).

Positive Surgical Margins

Complete tumor excision with negative surgical margins should always be the goal in any oncologic procedure. Unfortunately, positive margins are observed in 0 to 7% of the minimally invasive partial nephrectomy series (Borghesi et al., 2013; Shah et al., 2016; Tabayoyong et al., 2015). Several studies failed to demonstrate worse oncologic outcomes among patients with positive surgical margins (Kang et al., 2016; Permpongkosol et al., 2006; Sutherland et al., 2002). Indeed, a study of 1390 partial nephrectomies with a positive margin rate of 5.5% showed 93% disease-free survival at 10 years regardless of margins status (Yossepowitch et al., 2008). More recently, a multi-institutional review of 1240 partial nephrectomies with a positive margins rate of 7.8% showed a twofold increase in the risk of recurrence among all patients and a 7.5-fold increase among high-risk tumors (pT2-3 or nuclear grade 3–4) (Shah et al., 2016). The increased risk of recurrence was not observed among low-risk tumors.

LAPAROSCOPIC ABLATIVE TECHNIQUES

Renal ablative treatments use extremes of temperature to cause apoptosis in cancer cells. **Their primary goals are complete tumor destruction with minimal or no morbidity. Compared with partial nephrectomy, the potential advantages of thermal ablation include less blood loss, short operative time, decreased need for dissection, and fewer complications** (Long et al., 2017). Thermal ablation can be administered percutaneously or laparoscopically. The percutaneous approach is preferred for treatment of small renal masses because of its lower morbidity. **However, the laparoscopic approach offers certain advantages such as direct tumor visualization, mobilization of the kidney, and dissection and retraction of surrounding structures** (Zargar et al., 2015). Although thermal ablation can be used to treat most small renal masses, most common indications include lesions in patients with significant comorbidities, solitary kidney, and hereditary renal cell carcinoma. Multiple energy-delivery systems have been described including cryoablation, radiofrequency ablation (RFA), and microwave therapy. Cryoablation and RFA are the most widely used and studied thermal ablation techniques and are discussed in the next sections.

Cryoablation

Transperitoneal or retroperitoneal approaches can be used for laparoscopic cryoablation, depending on tumor location. The kidney is dissected as previously described, Gerota fascia is incised, and the tumor is exposed. The fat overlying the tumor may be excised. Biopsy samples of the tumor may also be taken with a 14- or 18-gauge biopsy needle for histopathologic diagnosis. Cryoprobes may be placed percutaneously and maneuvered into the tumor using direct visualization and laparoscopic ultrasonography guidance. The number of and spacing between probes are dictated by probe-specific ablative shape and diameter and tumor size. Probes are typically arranged parallel to each another in a triangular or quadrangular configuration ensuring cryolesion overlap. The tip of the probes should be advanced just beyond the deepest margin of the tumor. The progress of the iceball formation may be monitored in real time using intraoperative ultrasonography, and the iceball should extend approximately 0.5 to 1 cm beyond the edge of the tumor. Because the progress of the iceball cannot be abruptly stopped, caution should be exercised to avoid contact of the iceball with the renal collecting system, ureter, renal vasculature, or adjacent organs. After two consecutive freeze-thaw cycles are completed, the probes are removed with a gentle twisting motion. If any bleeding occurs, it can usually be controlled by applying pressure or, if necessary, hemostatic agents such as fibrin glue or Floseal (Schiffman et al., 2014).

Radiofrequency Ablation

RFA can also be delivered laparoscopically via the transperitoneal or retroperitoneal approaches. After the kidney is dissected, Gerota fascia is open and the tumor exposed, the RFA probe is introduced into the tumor, and the tines are deployed to a diameter that ensures ablation of the tumor and a 1-cm margin of normal renal tissue. The diameter of the ablation zone varies according to the length, diameter, surface area, and temperature of the electrode. Thermal damage occurs through frictional heating resulting from ionic oscillation by a monopolar or bipolar high-frequency alternating current, which can induce temperatures between 60° and 100°C throughout the tumor (Gervais et al., 2005; Goldberg et al., 2000). Temperatures above 105°C should be avoided to prevent tissue vaporization. Unfortunately, there is no current imaging technique that effectively monitors the progress of RFA lesions intraoperatively, and most of the treatment is based on direct temperature measurement or measurement of electrical impedance.

Results

Laparoscopic thermal ablation is an effective treatment for small renal masses. A retrospective review of 167 tumors treated with laparoscopic cryoablation, with a medium tumor size of 2.4 cm, showed a recurrence-free and overall survival of 79% and 86% at 5 years (Kim et al., 2014). Similarly, a study of 79 patients with 111 small renal masses undergoing laparoscopic RFA, with median tumor size of 2.2 cm and mean follow-up of 59 months, demonstrated a recurrence-free survival of 93.3% (Ramirez et al., 2014). Larger tumor size, endophytic lesions, and hilar location are associated with higher treatment failure rates (Tsivian et al., 2010). Indeed, a study of 31 patients with renal masses from 4 to 7 cm in diameter treated with percutaneous and laparoscopic cryoablation showed a recurrence-free survival of nearly 70% at 2 years compared with 100% among those treated with partial nephrectomy (Caputo et al., 2017). In a meta-analysis of 788 patients treated with laparoscopic and 687 with percutaneous cryoablation, laparoscopic cryoablation had less incomplete ablation and higher cancer-specific survival, whereas the percutaneous group had shorter hospital stays and lower costs (Aboumarzouk et al., 2018). There are no direct comparisons between laparoscopic cryoablation and RFA. A meta-analysis comparing percutaneous and laparoscopic cryoablation with RFA showed similar efficacy and complication rates (El Dib et al., 2012). However, a review of 47 studies including predominantly laparoscopic cryoablation and percutaneous RFA demonstrated fewer retreatments (8.5% vs. 1.3%), improved local tumor control, and lower risk of metastatic progression in the cryoablation group (Kunkle and Uzzo, 2008). There are no randomized trials comparing thermal ablation with other treatment modalities, including partial nephrectomy. A meta-analysis of 13 observational studies comparing laparoscopic cryoablation with laparoscopic partial nephrectomy for the treatment of small renal tumors showed laparoscopic cryoablation had better perioperative outcomes (operative times, estimated blood loss, length of stay, and complication rates) but higher local and metastatic tumor progression (Klatte et al., 2014). Another meta-analysis including 99 studies and 6471 tumors demonstrated increased local progression rates in the cryoablation and RFA groups compared with partial nephrectomy, with similar metastatic progression rates (Kunkle et al., 2008). Conversely, a study of 1424 small renal masses showed comparable recurrence-free survival between laparoscopic partial nephrectomy and percutaneous ablation. Metastases-free survival was superior for partial nephrectomy and percutaneous cryoablation compared with RFA (Thompson et al., 2015).

Complications

Laparoscopic renal ablation is generally well tolerated. A review of 148 laparoscopic cryoablations showed an overall complication rate of 15.5%, with 3.1% considered major complications. The risk factors for complications included larger tumor size, preexisting heart disease, and female gender (Laguna et al., 2009). Similarly, a series of 139 laparoscopic cryoablations and 133 RFAs showed an overall complication rate of 11%, with 1.8% classified as major and 9.2% as minor. Major complications included significant hemorrhage, ileus, ureteropelvic junction obstruction requiring nephrectomy, urinoma, conversion to open surgery, and death. The most common complication was pain or paresthesia at the ablation probe insertion site (Johnson et al., 2004). A meta-analysis including 457 laparoscopic ablations did not find any significant difference in complication rates between cryoablation and RFA (El Dib et al., 2012). Likewise, an analysis of 118 patients undergoing laparoscopic cryoablation or laparoscopic partial nephrectomy for tumor in a solitary kidney revealed comparable complication rates (Bhindi et al., 2018).

LAPAROENDOSCOPIC SINGLE-SITE SURGERY OF THE KIDNEY

LESS approaches have been successfully used in a wide range of renal procedures, including pyeloplasty, simple nephrectomy, donor nephrectomy, radical nephrectomy, nephroureterectomy, partial nephrectomy, renal cyst decortication, and renal cryoablation.

Renal Laparoendoscopic Single-Site Surgery

The surgical techniques used in LESS are similar to the ones of the conventional laparoscopy, usually following the same steps described previously for conventional laparoscopy. However, adaptations of the surgical equipment and techniques to overcome the limited triangulation and the clustering of instruments is frequently needed. For example, the use of flexible scopes and articulating instruments may facilitate the dissection (Fig. 102.41). In addition, the use of offset optics, custom hand piece, and instruments and scopes of variable length may help prevent instrument collision. In a multi-institutional review of 1076 urologic LESS procedures, an additional port was used in 23% (Kaouk et al., 2011). The overall conversion rate was 21%, with 20% of the cases converted to conventional laparoscopy and 1% to open surgery. Peri- and intraoperative complication rates were 9.5% and 3%, respectively. In a randomized trial comparing upper urinary tract LESS with laparoscopy including 60 patients found similar operative time, estimated blood loss, complication rate, and hospital stay between the two approaches (Abdel-Karim et al., 2017). However, LESS was associated with fewer analgesic requirements. A meta-analysis of 3 randomized clinical trials including 179 patients comparing

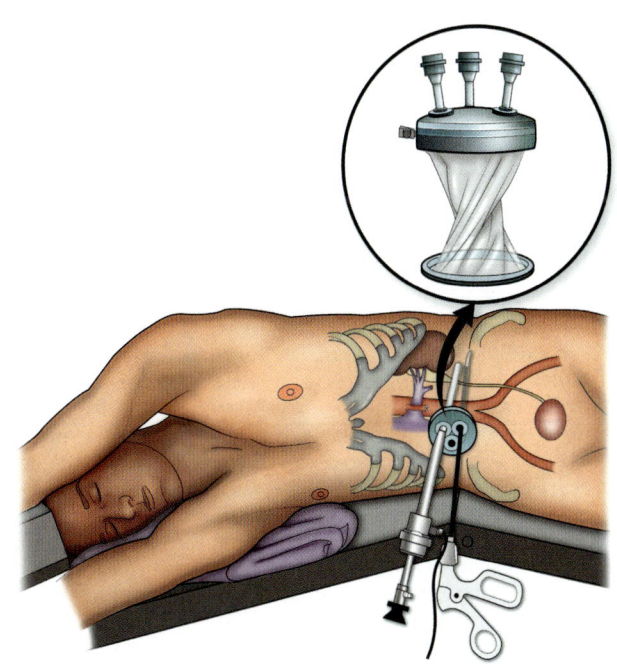

Fig. 102.41. Laparoendoscopic single-site surgery donor nephrectomy using a purpose-specific device with multichannel instrument access. A 2-mm instrument is also used to aid in retraction, hilar dissection, and extraction.

LESS donor nephrectomy with conventional laparoscopic nephrectomy found no difference in hospital stay, time to return to normal activities, blood transfusions, conversion rates, or total analgesic requirement (Gupta et al., 2016). LESS was associated with lower postoperative pain scores. A retrospective study of 141 patients comparing LESS with conventional laparoscopic nephrectomy for renal mass found comparable perioperative outcomes and disease-free and overall survivals (Antonelli et al., 2013). **Thus the main advantages of LESS over conventional laparoscopy include improved pain and cosmesis without compromising perioperative or long-term outcomes.**

Robotic Laparoendoscopic Single-Site Surgery

Robotic laparoendoscopic single-site (R-LESS) surgery has the potential to minimize the morbidity of multiport approaches while overcoming some of the technical challenges of LESS. In a retrospective study of 89 conventional robotic partial nephrectomy and 78 R-LESS partial nephrectomies, R-LESS was associated with longer operative time, longer warm ischemia time, and greater decline in estimated GFR (Komninos et al., 2014). Hospital stay, estimated blood loss, surgical margins, and perioperative complication rates were comparable between the two approaches. In another study of 80 conventional robotic partial nephrectomies and 79 R-LESS partial nephrectomies, R-LESS was associated with longer operative time and warm ischemia, lower postoperative pain scores, similar surgical margins, postoperative renal function, and perioperative complication rates (Shin et al., 2014). **Thus, similar to LESS, the main advantages of R-LESS are reduced pain and improved cosmesis. However, increased technical challenges result in longer operative times.** New robotic platforms to overcome these technical challenges are being assessed.

COMPLICATIONS FF LAPAROSCOPIC RENAL SURGERY

Complications are deviations from the normal postoperative course. Knowledge of each procedure and its potential pitfalls is key for preventing adverse events. Patient education about the potential risks of surgery is also essential. A study of 16,869 laparoscopic renal surgeries revealed an overall complication rate of 14.7% with 3.5% intraoperative and 12.1% postoperative complications. Most commonly reported intraoperative complications were bleeding (1.7%); bowel (0.3%), spleen (0.3%), and liver (0.1%) injuries; and pneumothorax (0.3%). Postoperative complications included bleeding (1.6%), wound infection (1.4%), pneumonia (1.2%), and prolonged ileus (1.1%). Reported complication rates were higher after partial nephrectomy (18.6%) compared with radical nephrectomy (15.4%) and simple nephrectomy (11.0%) (Henderson et al., 2016). Surgical approach may also correlate with complications. In a meta-analysis including 2240 partial nephrectomies, although the risk of complications was similar between robotic and laparoscopic approaches, robotic partial nephrectomy was associated with a nearly 50% lower risk of conversion to open surgery (Choi et al., 2015). Several patient-level factors including obesity and other comorbidities and prior abdominal surgery are associated with a higher complication risk (Zaid et al., 2017). Advanced age does not seem to be a major risk factor for complications. Several studies showed comparable morbidity of laparoscopic renal surgery in young and elderly patients (Thomas et al., 2009; Varkarakis et al., 2004). Although previous surgery is not a contraindication to laparoscopic renal surgery, it requires special consideration given the resulting intra-abdominal adhesions and increased possibility of bowel injury during insufflation, trocar placement, or dissection. Placement of the Veress needle and initial trocar away from previous scars and surgical fields, open trocar placement, or retroperitoneal approach may be needed to minimize access injuries and avoid adhesions (Hasson, 1971). Disease-related factors such as large tumors, and centrally located renal lesions also correlate with a higher complication rate (Simhan et al., 2011). Indeed, in a retrospective review of 482 laparoscopic nephrectomies most of the conversions to open surgery occurred in cases of infectious cause such as chronic pyelonephritis (Rassweiler et al., 1998). Finally, surgeon-related factors such as surgical experience also play a role. A multi-institutional study of 185 laparoscopic nephrectomies showed that 70% of the complications occurred during the first 20 cases at each institution. A learning curve of approximately 20 laparoscopic nephrectomy cases is also supported by other reports (Fahlenkamp et al., 1999; Keeley and Tolley, 1998; Rassweiler et al., 1998). In a series of laparoscopic partial nephrectomies, the complication rate continued to decrease even after 750 cases, implying a longer learning curve for more complex procedures (Gill et al., 2010). **When complications occur, early recognition and appropriate intervention can often minimize their morbid consequences.** Laparoscopic renal surgeries share several potential risks with traditional open approaches. However, there are differences in the type and presentation of these complications. All situations are individual, and unique problems may arise and require innovative actions.

Vascular Complications

Vascular injuries are the most common complication of urologic laparoscopic surgery (Fahlenkamp et al., 1999; Permpongkosol et al., 2007). **Major vascular injuries during laparoscopic surgery are rare, with an incidence of less than 1 in 1000** (Simforoosh et al., 2014). Although intraoperative vascular injuries can occur at any step of the procedure, most of the life-threatening vascular complications occur during the access phase of laparoscopy, including insertion of a Veress needle or the first trocar, or during the dissection of the renal hilum. Direct injury to the aorta, IVC, renal artery, or vein as well as their branches can result in significant bleeding, quickly leading to hemodynamic instability. Injuries to the renal hilum usually occur when structures are not fully identified before transection, during hilar dissection with a sharp instrument, or when the stapler does not completely cover the vessel or misfires (Meraney et al., 2002). If an arterial injury is identified, adequate hemostasis can be achieved with the use of clips, sutures, cautery, or vascular stapler depending on the location, size, and nature of the injury as well as surrounding structures. A hand may be placed in a lower abdominal midline incision to hold pressure if bleeding is brisk. In this manner, laparoscopic suturing or conversion to open surgery can be done in a controlled manner. Mild to moderate venous bleeding can frequently be controlled by applying direct pressure with a gauze for several minutes. Dissection may continue with the gauze in place. If a hole is visible, placement of a clip or suture may be attempted once a grasper has controlled the bleeding. Blind clip placement or suturing can lead to a worsening of the situation and additional complications.

Cases of inadvertent ligation of important vascular structures have been reported, including IVC, aorta, contralateral renal vessels, and inferior mesenteric vessels. Most of these injuries occurred during retroperitoneal procedures and unfortunately most were only diagnosed postoperatively (McAllister et al. 2004; Simforoosh et al., 2014). Equipment malfunction can also result in bleeding. Most reported cases of hemostatic device failure in laparoscopic renal surgery are related to vascular staplers (63%), nonlocking titanium clips (33%), and locking clips (4%) (Hsi et al., 2007). Most stapler failures are missing or malformed staple line, stapler locking up, or partial or no cutting. Clip failures include jamming or difficulty feeding clips, inability to close clips, and clip dislodgement, especially with locking clips (Hsi et al., 2009). A review of vascular stapler malfunction showed blood loss from 200 to 1200 mL and 20% conversion to open surgery (Chan et al., 2000). A 2% mortality rate was associated with hemostatic device failure (Hsi et al., 2007). Preventable causes of stapler malfunction include stapling over clips or incomplete transection resulting from incorrect placement. **Proper anatomic orientation, identification of vascular structures, and meticulous surgical dissection are important to prevent vascular complications.** At the end of surgery, the abdominal cavity should be inspected for bleeding. Reducing the intraperitoneal insufflation pressures may unmask occult venous bleeding. **Common areas of postoperative bleeding include the bed of the dissection, adrenal** gland, mesentery, gonadal vessels, and ureteral stump. Postoperative hemorrhage can occur after laparoscopic renal surgery. Hypotension associated with tachycardia and decreasing hematocrit suggest postoperative bleeding. CT scanning may be appropriate in identifying the site of bleeding. Only a small fraction require surgical intervention because most cases respond to conservative measures. For hemorrhage originating from the renal artery, most cases can be successfully managed with angiography and embolization (Jeon et al., 2016). Gross hematuria after partial nephrectomy may indicate the renal artery pseudoaneurysm. Pseudoaneurysm occurs in 2% after partial nephrectomy. Most patients present within 30 days after surgery with gross hematuria. Almost all patients with renal artery pseudoaneurysm can be successfully treated with angiography and embolization (Jain et al., 2013).

Although the risk of deep vein thrombosis (DVT) after laparoscopic renal surgery is low (Montgomery and Wolf, 2005), the decision on when and how to use prophylaxis for DVT must be based on the patient's stratification risks. Several prophylactic methods have been proposed, including unfractioned heparin, fractioned heparin, low-molecular-weight heparin, sequential compressive stocking devices (SCDs), and combination therapy, but the optimal prophylaxis is still controversial. For low-risk patients, SCDs are usually the recommended option, whereas high-risk individuals may require pharmacologic prophylaxis (Forrest et al., 2009).

Urinary Complications

Persistent urine leakage is a potential complication of any renal surgery in which the pelvicalyceal system is violated. The reported incidence of urinary leak after partial nephrectomy varies from 0.8% to 10% after laparoscopic and robotic partial nephrectomy, but it is occasionally seen after cyst or tumor ablation (Meeks et al., 2008; Potretzke et al., 2016). Factors associated with urinary leak include large tumor size, hilar location, pelvicalyceal repair, prolonged operative, and warm ischemia time. Most cases of urinary leak require no intervention other than percutaneous drainage. When conservative management fails or there is evidence of distal obstruction, additional intervention may be required, such as ureteral stenting and bladder decompression (Kundu et al., 2010).

Visceral and Bowel Complications

One of the most significant complications of laparoscopic surgery is unrecognized bowel injury (Fig. 102.42), which has a mortality rate of about 3%. The incidence of bowel injury in the urologic literature varies from 0.1% to 0.8% (Bishoff et al., 1999; Schwartz et al., 2010). Bowel injuries can occur at any point during the procedure, including access in 32% of the cases. The most common cause of unrecognized injury is the use of thermal energy adjacent to the bowel, responsible for nearly 50% of the cases. When recognized intraoperatively, superficial thermal injuries may be oversewn with 3-0 silk suture to imbricate the affected area. In addition, given only a small portion of the laparoscopic instrument is in the visual field, injuries can occur out of the surgeon's view during introduction or retraction of instruments. The presentation of unrecognized bowel injury after laparoscopic surgery is variable but typically includes persistent and increased trocar site pain at the site closest to the bowel injury without significant erythema or purulent drainage. Thermal injuries usually present later than nonthermal bowel injuries. Patients may develop abdominal distention, nausea, diarrhea, anorexia, low-grade fever, persistent bowel sounds, and low or normal white blood cell count. The patient's condition can rapidly deteriorate to hemodynamic instability and death if the injury is not recognized and appropriately treated (Bishoff et al., 1999).

CT with oral contrast is the initial diagnostic modality of choice (Cadeddu et al., 1997), and open exploration is usually required to evacuate bowel spillage and perform the necessary repair. In rare cases, when a controlled fistula develops, conservative management with bowel rest and parenteral nutrition may be used, but this may take several months to resolve. When reflecting the colon, the surgeon

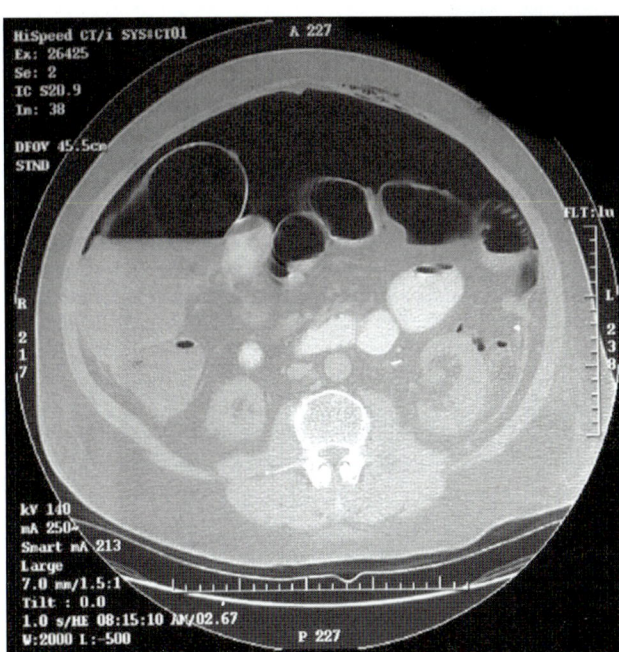

Fig. 102.42. Computed tomography (CT) scan taken 9 days after partial nephrectomy when the patient visited the clinic for routine follow-up complaining of distention and worsening abdominal pain for the previous 3 days, low-grade fever, leukopenia, and pain out of proportion at a single trocar site. CT shows dilated loops of large bowel and significant amounts of free air. Exploration revealed a small perforation in the cecum.

must take care to avoid making a hole in the mesentery, especially on the left side. Any mesenteric defects should be closed because of the possibility of bowel herniation (Regan et al., 2003). During closure of the mesentery, care should be taken to avoid compromising the vascular supply to the colon. The incidence of splenic and pancreatic injury during laparoscopic left renal surgery varies from 0 to 0.5% (Canby-Hagino et al., 2000; Varkarakis et al., 2004). Splenic injuries are most commonly caused by vigorous traction on splenic ligaments. Most cases of splenic bleeding can be controlled with argon beam coagulation and topical hemostatic agents; however, some cases require splenectomy (Biggs et al., 2005; Canby-Hagino et al., 2000). Injuries to the pancreas may be insidious, and careful inspection at the end of surgery is advisable. Capsular pancreatic injuries can be managed by closing the defect with nonabsorbable suture and/or drain placement. Deeper injuries can cause pancreatic leak and usually require formal repair or isolation of the segment with a stapler (Varkarakis et al., 2004). Intraoperative general surgery consultation is advisable. Injury to the liver or gallbladder can occur during right renal surgery. Most liver injuries can be managed with topical hemostatic therapy and argon beam coagulation. Gallbladder injuries are best managed by cholecystectomy.

Other Complications

Diaphragmatic injuries can occur during the upper pole renal dissection on either side. Most significant diaphragmatic injuries with resulting pneumothorax are immediately recognized because of a sudden increase in peak airway pressures, and the patient becomes difficult to ventilate. Immediate treatment is needed to prevent tension pneumothorax. These injuries can be repaired by suturing the hole in the diaphragm while a central line catheter is placed into the ipsilateral anterior second intercostal space and placed to a water seal. A chest radiograph should be obtained at the end of the procedure to ensure the pneumothorax is resolved and the catheter can be safely removed. When significant pneumothorax persists, a chest tube insertion is advisable (Aron et al., 2007; Del Pizzo et al., 2003). The incidence of unrecognized pneumothorax after laparoscopic nephrectomy is approximately 0.3%, and routine postoperative chest radiograph for asymptomatic patients with low suspicion for diaphragmatic injury is not recommended (Simon et al., 2005). Neuromuscular injuries occur in 2.7% of laparoscopic urologic surgeries and include abdominal wall neuralgia, motor and sensory deficit, rhabdomyolysis, orchialgia, and others. Most of these are caused by direct surgical trauma or the anatomic stress of positioning. Although most of these complications occur with similar frequency compared with open surgery, the risk of rhabdomyolysis may be increased with the laparoscopic approach. Shorter operative times and positioning patients in a partial rather than full flank position may reduce the incidence of rhabdomyolysis (Wolf et al., 2000). Thigh paresthesias may be avoided by preserving the psoas fascia during posterior renal dissection. Additional reported complications associated with minimally invasive renal surgery include incisional hernia, prolonged ileus, pulmonary embolus, and pneumonia.

MINIMALLY INVASIVE RENAL SURGERY IN UROLOGIC PRACTICE

Since its inception, the adoption of minimally invasive renal surgery has progressively increased. Data from Surveillance, Epidemiology and End Results-Medicare indicate laparoscopic nephrectomy use increased from 1.5% in 1995 to 45% in 2005 (Filson et al., 2011). Similarly, the use of laparoscopic partial nephrectomy for small renal masses increased from 15% in 2004 to 22% in 2009 (Banegas et al., 2016). More recently with the introduction of robotic technology, the use of robotic radical nephrectomy has increased from 1.5% to 27% from 2003 to 2015 (Jeong et al., 2017). This was accompanied by a decrease in laparoscopic radical nephrectomies, which raised some concerns regarding cost effectiveness because robot radical nephrectomy was associated with higher costs but similar outcomes compared with laparoscopic surgery (Yang et al. 2014). Data from the National Cancer Database indicate an increase in the use of robotic partial nephrectomy from 41% in 2010 to 63% in 2013 (Alameddine et al., 2018). Although the adoption of minimally invasive techniques in renal surgery is increasing, this has been occurring at slow pace. A complex array of reasons may account for this observation, including the differential incidence of kidney and prostate cancer, marketing of robotics, referral patterns, and consumer demand (Richstone and Kavoussi, 2008).

SUMMARY

Minimally invasive surgery is the preferred treatment approach for many renal diseases. **Patients have undoubtedly gained from the benefits of minimally invasive surgery: less perioperative morbidity without sacrificing therapeutic outcomes.** As surgical tools continue to evolve, even more minimally invasive options may become more pervasive and potentially offer additional benefits to patients.

KEY POINTS: LAPAROSCOPIC AND ROBOTIC SURGERY OF THE KIDNEY

- Minimally invasive renal surgery provides less incisional pain, shorter convalescence, and better cosmesis compared with open surgery with comparable efficacy and long-term outcomes.
- The indications for minimally invasive renal surgery are generally similar to those for open renal surgery.
- The basic principles of oncologic surgery including complete tumor excision with negative margins associated with maximization of renal parenchyma preservation when feasible should be followed when using minimally invasive approaches to treat renal tumors.
- Familiarity with the anatomic landmarks, surgical techniques, instrumentation, and knowledge of each procedure and its potential pitfalls are key for successful minimally invasive surgery.

SUGGESTED READINGS

AUA guidelines on Renal Mass and Localized Renal Cancer. Available from: http://www.auanet.org/guidelines/renal-mass-and-localized-renal-cancer-new-(2017).

Berger A, Brandina R, Atalla MA, et al: Laparoscopic radical nephrectomy for renal cell carcinoma: oncological outcomes at 10 years or more, *J Urol* 182(5):2172–2176, 2009.

Blom JH, van Poppel H, Marechal JM, et al: Radical nephrectomy with and without lymph-node dissection: final results of European Organization for Research and Treatment of Cancer (EORTC) randomized phase 3 trial 30881, *Eur Urol* 55(1):28–34, 2009.

Choi JE, You JH, Kim DK, et al: Comparison of perioperative outcomes between robotic and laparoscopic partial nephrectomy: a systematic review and meta-analysis, *Eur Urol* 67(5):891–901, 2015.

EAU guidelines on Renal Cell Carcinoma. Available from: http://uroweb.org/guideline/renal-cell-carcinoma/.

Fahlenkamp D, Rassweiler J, Fornara P, et al: Complications of laparoscopic procedures in urology: experience with 2,407 procedures at 4 German centers, *J Urol* 162(3 Pt 1):765–770, discussion 770–761, 1999.

Gill IS, Kavoussi LR, Lane BR, et al: Comparison of 1,800 laparoscopic and open partial nephrectomies for single renal tumors, *J Urol* 178(1):41–46, 2007.

Kaouk JH, Autorino R, Kim FJ, et al: Laparoendoscopic single-site surgery in urology: worldwide multi-institutional analysis of 1076 cases, *Eur Urol* 60(5):998–1005, 2011.

Permpongkosol S, Link RE, Su LM, et al: Complications of 2,775 urological laparoscopic procedures: 1993 to 2005, *J Urol* 177(2):580–585, 2007.

Shah PH, Moreira DM, Okhunov Z, et al: Positive surgical margins increase risk of recurrence after partial nephrectomy for high risk renal tumors, *J Urol* 196(2):327–334, 2016.

REFERENCES

The complete reference list is available online at ExpertConsult.com.

103 Nonsurgical Focal Therapy for Renal Tumors

Chad R. Tracy, MD, and Jeffrey A. Cadeddu, MD

The incidence of localized renal cell carcinoma (RCC) is rising as a result of the increasing use of cross-sectional imaging. Along with the increasing incidence in the diagnosis of renal masses, there has been a parallel down-staging of newly detected renal masses such that more than 70% are small and organ confined (clinical stage T1) (Chen and Uzzo, 2011; Volpe et al., 2004). The overall result is a paradigm shift in management over the last decade, with an increasing focus on minimally invasive treatment and nephron-sparing surgery. Accordingly, in addition to cancer-specific survival (CSS), emphasis is now placed on preservation of renal function and avoidance of treatment-related morbidity in the management of early stage RCC. Therefore the 2017 American Urological Association (AUA) guidelines for the management of clinical stage 1 renal masses recommends nephron-sparing surgery as standard of care, with consideration of ablative therapies as valid alternatives for patients with cT1a tumors less than 3 cm in diameter or for those with substantial comorbidities (Campbell et al., 2017).

Partial nephrectomy is the gold standard for the treatment of small renal tumors because it provides comparable oncologic outcomes (>95% CSS) compared with radical nephrectomy and is associated with improved preservation of renal function, superior cardiac outcomes, and improved overall survival (Huang et al., 2009; Pierorazio et al., 2016; Zini et al., 2009). However, irrespective of an open or laparoscopic/robotic surgical approach, nephron-sparing surgery is underused because of the comparative risks and attendant technical demands associated with the procedure (Abouassaly et al., 2009). Recent Surveillance, Epidemiology, and End Results (SEER) data found that partial nephrectomy use is increasing, yet many patients with localized renal tumors still undergo radical nephrectomy (Smaldone et al., 2012). Thus, to increase the number of patients offered nephron-sparing surgery and broaden the minimally invasive treatment options available to patients with small renal tumors, energy-based systems, including cryoablation (CA) and radiofrequency ablation (RFA), were introduced in the 1990s.

Focal ablative therapies offer several advantages compared with extirpative surgery. First, these modalities are less technically demanding than open, laparoscopic, or robotic partial nephrectomy, because renorrhaphy and hilar dissection are not obligatory. Consequently, renal tumor ablation is associated with shorter convalescence and fewer complications than extirpative surgery (Desai et al., 2005; Pierorazio et al., 2016). Equally important, several studies clearly demonstrated minimal impact on postablation renal function, with comparable or better postoperative renal function found when compared with that of partial nephrectomy (Bhindi et al., 2017; Lucas et al., 2008; Raman et al., 2008b; Ross et al., 2017; Woldu et al., 2015). Finally, all of the ablation modalities offer treatment versatility because they can be deployed in open, laparoscopic, or percutaneous procedures. Given these advantages, well-recognized indications for CA and RFA include patients with small renal tumors who are either poor surgical candidates or at risk for renal insufficiency, including patients with solitary kidneys, bilateral renal tumors, and hereditary syndromes such as von Hippel-Lindau disease. However, because of the excellent long-term published results, there is now growing experience with the treatment of the sporadic small renal tumors in healthy patients (Stern et al., 2009). Together with more robust operator experience and improved patient selection, renal CA and RFA technologies are now a viable treatment alternative for small renal tumors, in particular for those patients presenting with cT1a tumors less than 3 cm in diameter (2017 AUA guidelines). Experience with less mature (microwave ablation [MWA]) or novel technologies (irreversible electroporation [IRE] and stereotactic radiotherapy) are promising and hint at an expanding repertoire of minimally invasive modalities for renal tumor management in the near future.

CRYOABLATION

Background and Mode of Action

CA, or cryotherapy, is the practice of using extreme cold temperatures to treat a wide variety of pathological conditions. The use of cold therapy in medicine can be traced to the early Egyptians, who used cold to treat inflammatory conditions as early as 2500 BCE. However, CA was not used with a goal of tissue destruction until the mid-1800s, when an English physician, Dr. James Arnott, described using a combination of ice and salt to obtain temperatures (−18°C to −24°C) sufficient to treat breast, cervical, and skin cancers (Arnott, 1850). Over the course of the ensuing decades, multiple investigators described the use of cooled gases for treatment of various skin conditions, beginning with liquified air (−190°C), followed by solidified carbon dioxide (−78.5°C), liquid oxygen (−182.9°C), and then eventually liquid nitrogen (−196°C) (Freiman and Bouganim, 2005). In 1963 Cooper and Lee developed the first modern cryoprobe using pressurized liquid nitrogen passed through a three-channel probe (one inflow and two outflow) to achieve controlled temperatures of −196°C (Cooper, 1963). This revolutionary probe opened the possibility of treating less accessible areas rather than relegating cryotherapy solely to superficial areas such as the skin.

Although Cooper's design allowed for intra-abdominal treatment of large volumes, its use was limited by an inability to control or monitor the extent of the cryolesion. Without the availability of intraoperative imaging to visualize the expanding frozen tissue or "iceball," physicians were forced to rely on physical examination to monitor treatment, such as digital rectal examination during prostate cryotherapy, which often led to excessive ablation and irreparable collateral damage (Weber and Lee, 2005). In the mid-1980s, Onik et al. (1984, 1985) discovered that the cryogenic ice-tissue interface was highly echogenic on ultrasonography, which allowed for real-time guidance for treating intra-abdominal malignancies. Further animal studies confirmed a close correlation between the sonographically visible iceball and the zone of cell death, providing a reliable and reproducible method of targeting and destroying tumors without attendant collateral damage (Campbell et al., 1998; Steed et al., 1997; Weber et al., 1998).

After nitrogen-based cryoprobes and ultrasound guidance, the next significant breakthrough in the use of CA came with the development of argon gas–based probes, which rely on the Joule-Thomson principle (low temperatures are achieved by the rapid expansion of high-pressure, inert gas) to generate temperatures of −185.7°C within the target tissues. In addition to providing a reliable target temperature, argon-based systems are more efficient than nitrogen-based probes, with target temperatures reached faster and with a steeper internal thermal gradient (Rewcastle et al., 1999). The majority of commercially available CA units now employ argon gas–based systems (CryoHit, Galil Medical, Plymouth Meeting, PA; CryoCare, CryoCare CS, Endocare, Irvine, CA; SeedNet, Oncura, Philadelphia, PA).

2309

Tissue destruction during CA occurs during the freezing and thawing processes. Rapid freezing in the area closest to the cryoprobe forms ice crystals within the intracellular space that cause direct cellular injury through mechanical trauma to plasma membranes and organelles, leading to subsequent cell death mediated by ischemia and apoptosis (Baust and Gage, 2005; Hoffmann and Bischof, 2002; Ishiguro and Rubinsky, 1994; Mazur, 1977). As the freezing process expands further from the cryoprobe, the cooling process is slower, which encourages extracellular ice crystals to form, leading to a depletion of extracellular water and an osmotic gradient that causes further intracellular damage through dehydration and membrane rupture. During the thawing phase, extracellular osmolarity decreases as ice crystals melt, which leads to cellular edema and further disruption of cell membranes resulting from the rapid influx of water back into cells (Erinjeri and Clark, 2010). In addition to direct cellular damage, injury to blood vessel endothelium during the freezing process results in platelet activation, vascular thrombosis, and tissue ischemia (Kahlenberg et al., 1998; Rupp et al., 2002; Weber et al., 1997). The summative pathological consequence of treatment is coagulative necrosis, cellular apoptosis, and eventual fibrosis and scar formation.

Treatment Temperature

Tissue destruction during CA requires a certain threshold temperature, which is unique to the cell type and cellular environment of the target tissue. Whereas normal renal parenchyma is typically destroyed at $-19.4°C$, small animal models of CA indicate that temperatures as low as $-50°C$ may be necessary to guarantee complete cellular death of cancerous tissue because of its more fibrous nature (Chosy et al., 1998; Gage and Baust, 1998; Larson et al., 2000). **Therefore the preferred target tissue temperature during CA is at or below $-40°C$.** Importantly, the temperature of the progressing iceball is not uniform, with temperatures increasing the further the distance from the cryoprobe. Campbell et al. (1998) measured intrarenal temperatures during CA and referenced these to the leading edge of the ice-tissue interface. At the edge of the iceball, the temperature was measured at $0°C$, correlating with the onset of the freezing process, whereas temperatures consistently below $-20°C$ were not reached until 3.1 mm inside. Based on these findings, most authors advocate creating an iceball treatment zone that is at least 5 to 10 mm beyond the edge of the target lesion. Alternatively, small temperature probes may be positioned around the tumor periphery to ensure that adequate treatment temperatures ($-40°C$) are achieved (Rukstalis et al., 2001), which may be especially important for complex tumors or more challenging anatomy (Vernez et al., 2017). Depending on the size of the lesion and the type and size of probe used, reaching the appropriate target temperature within the entire mass may require the use of multiple cryoprobes (Breen et al., 2013). In addition, freezing is subject to the "heat sink" phenomenon, in which large blood vessels adjacent to the tumor may dissipate ice formation and require more extreme temperatures or longer periods of cooling (see the section on radiofrequency ablation and heat sink).

Freeze-Thaw Cycles

In vivo animal studies initially demonstrated adequate cell kill in normal tissue employing a single freeze-thaw cycle (Weber et al., 1997). However, further studies on implanted tumor cells in mice, then in dogs, found that multiple freeze-thaw cycles promoted a larger and more adequate area of liquefactive necrosis, improving subsequent cure rates (Neel et al., 1971; Woolley et al., 2002). **Therefore, in treatment of renal malignancies, the current recommendation is to perform a double freeze-thaw cycle to ensure complete cellular death.** The thawing process is also instrumental in cellular death and may be performed in a passive or active manner. Passive thawing, which relies on the iceball melting without any intervention after the cessation of argon gas through the cryoprobe, is more time consuming than active thawing, in which helium gas (rather than argon) is forced through the cryoprobe, creating a warming effect secondary to the Joule-Thomson principle. Although clearly more efficient, there are conflicting data on whether an active thaw is as effective as a passive thaw, leading to variation in practice patterns between centers (Klossner et al., 2007; Woolley et al., 2002). Some authors advocate a passive thaw between cycles and an active thaw at the end of treatment so that post-treatment bleeding may be more rapidly addressed (White and Kaouk, 2012).

Duration of Treatment

The duration of treatment to produce complete cellular death in humans is unknown. Auge et al. (2006) performed a prospective study in nine female farm pigs with CA performed for 5, 10, or 15 minutes. Although all lesions demonstrated complete cellular necrosis 5 mm from the probe, only animals treated for 10 or 15 minutes had necrosis extending 10 mm or more beyond the probes. Furthermore, animals treated for only 5 minutes had excessive bleeding, whereas those treated for 15 minutes had an increased risk for tumor fracture and subsequent hemorrhage. **Based on these findings, most contemporary series use a freeze cycle of 8 to 10 minutes** (Breen et al., 2013; Kim et al., 2013).

> **KEY POINTS: CRYOABLATION**
> - CA employs argon gas–based systems to achieve treatment temperatures of less than $-40°C$ through the Joule-Thomson principle.
> - CA of renal tumors should be performed under real-time imaging, with the treatment area approximately 5 to 10 mm beyond the margin of the tumor.
> - A double freeze-thaw cycle, each 8 to 10 minutes in duration, is currently the standard of care during renal tumor CA.

RADIOFREQUENCY ABLATION

Background and Mode of Action

RFA is the use of radiofrequency energy to heat tissue to the point of cellular death. RFA uses monopolar alternating electric current that is delivered directly into the target tissue at a frequency of 450 to 1200 kHz, leading to vibration of ions within tissue and resulting in molecular friction and heat production. Increasing temperature within the target tissue leads to cellular protein denaturation and cell membrane disintegration (Hsu et al., 2000; Tracy et al., 2010). Importantly, heat is not directly supplied by the probe, but rather by the agitation of ions within the tissue (Cosman et al., 1984). Study of the effect of radiofrequency energy dates back more than 100 years to 1891 when d'Arsonval described the ability of radiofrequency waves to heat living tissue. Without a clear understanding of the technology and an inability to effectively control the energy, the use of radiofrequency energy in surgery did not become more mainstream until 1928, when Cushing and Bovie developed the electrocautery knife. Using radiofrequency energy, they described an ability to cauterize or cut tissue, ushering in the development of the modern-day electrocautery probe, which desiccates tissue at the point of contact when alternating current passes through the patient and then dissipates to a remotely placed grounding pad on the patient's lower extremities.

In 1990 two individual groups of researchers simultaneously reported the development of probes that could be used for percutaneous ablation (McGahan et al., 1990; Rossi et al., 1990). These probes consisted of a layer of insulation down to an exposed metal tip, which allowed for percutaneous passage of the needle to deeper target tissues. Using these needles, the amount of tissue destruction could be controlled along the central axis of the lesion by adjusting the length of the exposed, uninsulated portion of the needle. Although effective in ablating along the long axis of the lesion, these initial probes were limited in their ability to create circumferential tissue damage, preventing their use in lesions greater than 1.5 cm. Further refinements using these initial designs led to the development of modern RFA generators and probes, which are capable of treating larger and more complex lesions.

Variations in Radiofrequency Ablation Equipment

RFA can be performed with either a temperature-based or impedance-based monitoring system. Temperature-based systems work by measuring tissue temperatures at the tip of the electrode and are based on achieving a specific temperature for a given period. These systems accurately measure the temperature of the tissue at the electrode tip; however, they do not measure the temperature of the surrounding parenchyma. Alternatively, impedance-based systems measure the tissue impedance (resistance to alternating current) at the electrode tip and are based on achieving a predetermined impedance level at the tissue-probe interface that indicates complete tissue desiccation and thereby ablation. **There are no explicit clinical data that support the superiority of impedance or temperature-based systems.**

The original ablation probes, which were designed as single-electrode monopolar probes controlled by varying the exposed uninsulated tip, were capable of treating tumors no greater than 2 cm (McGahan et al., 1993). Therefore the treatment of larger tumors or the acquisition of an adequate tumor margin often required additional probes or treatment of overlapping regions. To achieve a larger overall treatment volume, LeVeen (1997) introduced an insulated monopolar probe (Boston Scientific, Natick, MA) with 12 deployable tines that function as radiofrequency antennas for the wider dispersion of current. These tines are deployed in an umbrella shape to create a spherical lesion. When high impedance is encountered at one prong, current is redirected to areas of lower impedance. The similar starburst–shaped RITA device (AngioDynamics, Queensbury, NY) uses thermistors embedded in five of the nine electrical tines to modulate energy based on the aggregate average temperature of the electrodes. An alternative monopolar system, by Covidien (Boulder, CO) uses an impedance-based system composed of a single 17-gauge ("cool tip") electrode that is cooled internally with chilled saline to prevent charring of tissue adjacent to the probe. A direct comparison of these systems in the porcine liver demonstrated larger zones of ablation with the "cool tip" systems, more spheric ablation volumes with the 12-tine electrodes, and better reproducibility with the 9-tine electrodes (Pereira et al., 2004). Clinical validation studies have suggested more complete necrosis, better lesion accuracy, and superior treatment outcomes with multitine electrodes (Curley et al., 2000; Rehman et al., 2004; Rossi et al., 1998).

Another major classification in RFA technology is the differentiation between "dry" and "wet" RFA. As tissue desiccation increases in the target lesion, the charring effect (carbonization) on tissue leads to increased impedance and resistance to the alternating current of the electrode, limiting the size of the ablation zone with a single electrode to less than 4 cm. "Wet" RFA probes deliver a constant saline infusion into the tissue and in proximity to the probe to lower the temperature at the probe tip, thus mitigating the charring effect and corresponding premature rise in impedance, allowing for larger zones of ablation (Collyer et al., 2001; Goldberg et al., 1996; Lorentzen et al., 1997; Pereira et al., 2004). In addition, interstitial hypertonic saline infusion forms a virtual "liquid electrode" beyond the metal electrode so that the total electrode surface area is augmented (Ni et al., 1999). **Although lesions tend to be larger using "wet" RFA, there is less control of the exact size of ablation, which may lead to overtreatment of the target zone and disruption of adjacent normal parenchyma** (Frich et al., 2005).

Radiofrequency energy also can be delivered through bipolar electrodes. These devices generate current between two separate electrodes (one active and one negative), within the target tissue. The purported advantage of bipolar energy is that significantly higher temperatures are induced compared with those of monopolar devices (Nakada et al., 2003). In addition, heat is generated not only at the active probe but also adjacent to the ground needle and between the two electrodes (McGahan et al., 1996), resulting in a focus of coagulation necrosis that is larger than with a conventional monopolar electrode. The use of two separate electrodes, however, produces an elliptical area of coagulation necrosis rather than spherical; because most renal tumors are spherical, this technology has not been widely adapted for RFA of renal masses. In addition, clinical studies have revealed that the bipolar probes are less accurate than monopolar-based probes, with a wider variability in desired and actual target size (Rathke et al., 2014).

Treatment Temperature

The ability of RFA to ablate the target tissue relies on power delivered to the probe, the maximum temperature obtained, and the duration of the ablation (McGahan and Dodd, 2001). As stated, alternating radiofrequency current creates cellular agitation and, as a result of electrical impedance of the tissue, local heating. Provided that electrical impedance remains low, an expanding sphere of tissue damage emanates outward from the treatment probe. If current is administered too rapidly, charring occurs, which dessicates the tissue at the probe-tissue interface. This may lead to increased electrical impedance, blocking energy transfer and halting the heating process (Djavan et al., 2000; Finelli et al., 2003). To prevent this phenomenon, which may lead to incomplete or nonuniform ablation, temperatures during RFA are generally kept at or below 105°C. It is also important to reach a minimum target temperature at which cellular death occurs. In in vitro studies using human prostate tissue, Bhowmick et al. (2004a, 2004b) achieved irreversible cell injury when benign and malignant cell lines were heated to 45°C for 60 minutes, 55°C for 5 minutes, and 70°C for 1 minute. Similarly, Walsh et al. (2007) found that even short exposures at temperatures higher than 70°C are lethal to human RCC in vitro. **To maximize cellular death without carbonization, modern temperature-based generators are programmed to reach a target temperature of 90°C to 105°C, and ablation should not be considered successful unless a minimum of 70°C is uniformly reached during the treatment cycle.** Impedance-based systems are typically started at 40 to 80 W and increased at 10 W/min to a maximum of 130 to 200 W until an impedance of 200 to 500 ohms is reached.

The ability of the thermal technology to reach its target temperature within the tissue depends not only on the probe itself and the energy delivered but also on the surrounding treatment environment (Goldberg et al., 2000). In particular, **when the target zone is highly vascularized or is adjacent to large vessels, thermal energy is preferentially dispersed to the comparatively cooler blood within these vessels. This heat sink effect may therefore spare tumor cells in proximity to large blood vessels and lead to treatment failures.** Temporary renal ischemia during RFA experimentally increases the size of the initial treatment lesion and shortens the time to reach target temperature (Corwin et al., 2001). However, hilar occlusion is not currently recommended because of the risk for arterial thrombosis and ischemia-reperfusion injury to normal parenchyma. To prevent complications of vascular clamping, some authors advocate selective arterial embolization when performing RFA (Hall et al., 2000). The authors have successfully employed this approach for a few central or large (>4 cm) tumors to reduce the circulatory heat sink.

Although most studies show cellular death with a single RFA treatment, studies in animals using CA have demonstrated improved cell death with multiple cycles. Therefore, when employing a temperature-based system, we typically recommend using two separate RFA cycles separated by a minimum 30-second cool-down period (Park et al., 2006a).

Intraoperative Monitoring

Although it is possible to visualize placement of the RFA probe using ultrasonography, magnetic resonance imaging (MRI), or CT guidance, there is currently no reliable manner to evaluate the zone of treatment radiographically (Rendon et al., 2001; Renshaw, 2004). In contrast to CA, in which the expanding iceball indicates the zone of treatment, the RFA treatment zone is determined solely by the probe choice, accurate placement, and measurement of electrical impedance or temperature. An alternative method, which also may be used with CA, is to place nonconducting temperature probes around the periphery of the tumor or at the deep margin to measure real-time treatment temperatures independent of the RFA device. Using this method, Carey and Leveillee (2007) demonstrated 100% clinical success in treating tumors up to 5 cm in diameter. Experimental imaging modalities, including real-time contrast-enhanced ultrasonography (Chen et al., 2013; Johnson et al., 2005), magnetic resonance thermometry (Ertürk et al., 2016), and magnetic resonance elastography (Li et al., 2013), have shown some promise experimentally but have not been properly evaluated in the clinical setting. The successful ablation of a renal lesion with RFA therefore is highly dependent on precise probe placement, and outcome is typically determined only by feedback from the generator, thermal probes, and the absence of contrast enhancement during percutaneous axial image-guided RFA.

> **KEY POINTS: RADIOFREQUENCY ABLATION**
>
> - Transfer of radiofrequency energy generates ionic friction and agitation within tissue that results in heating. When temperatures exceed 70°C for 1 minute or more, irreversible coagulative necrosis and tissue desiccation occur.
> - Treatment may be either temperature-based or impedance-based.
> - Real-time monitoring of ablation depends on measurement of electrical impedance and temperature rather than visual or radiographic cues.

SURGICAL TECHNIQUE

Transperitoneal and Retroperitoneal Laparoscopic Renal Cryoablation and Radiofrequency Ablation

See Chapter 61 for these modalities.

Percutaneous Renal Cryoablation and Radiofrequency Ablation (See Video 103.1)

Depending on treating physician preference, percutaneous tumor ablation is performed under either conscious sedation with local anesthesia or general endotracheal anesthesia on an outpatient basis or with 23-hour observation. General endotracheal anesthesia enables control of respiration during probe placement and tumor biopsy that may translate into more accurate targeting and improved overall outcomes (Gupta et al., 2009). Conversely, conscious sedation minimizes the morbidity and time of the procedure. After administration of intravenous prophylactic antibiotics, the patient is positioned in either a prone or modified flank position on the CT gantry, with the choice of position largely dictated by the tumor location. CT guidance is by far the preferred and most common targeting technique, although ultrasound and magnetic resonance guidance also have been reported (Dong et al., 2016; vanOostenbrugge et al., 2017).

A noncontrast CT image is obtained first to confirm tumor size and position in the prone or lateral position, and a contrast-enhanced CT image is then often obtained to better delineate the tumor. A radiographic grid placed on the patient's skin can help localize placement of the needle. A 20-gauge "finder needle" or access sheath may be inserted under CT guidance near the expected location of the tumor, with position confirmed through repeated imaging. Using this finder needle as a guide, the ablation probe(s) is then positioned to treat the tumor. The number of probes and the duration of treatment are determined based on lesion size in accordance with the manufacturer's recommendations. Serial imaging is used to confirm the placement of all treatment probes/tines. Before a thermal ablation is scheduled, needle biopsy confirming malignancy is strongly recommended to confirm the need for treatment and dictate follow-up (Campbell et al., 2017). However, if a tumor biopsy has not been performed preprocedure, an 18-gauge core biopsy needle should be obtained and sent for permanent section before the initiation of therapy. Importantly, the treatment probes should be placed into the tumor before the biopsy is obtained because perinephric hematoma formation may obscure visualization of the tumor. Probe and biopsy needle positioning and adjustments are performed with breath holding to standardize the position of the mobile kidney with each sequential pass of the needle.

Monitoring of treatment efficacy during CA employs imaging of the ablation zone. **Although each cryoprobe tip reaches temperatures of −140°C to −190°C, there is a steep temperature gradient that falls to 0°C at the edge of the iceball.** Temperatures of less than −20°C are achieved at a distance of 3.1 mm inside the edge of the iceball (Campbell et al., 1998). **Because tumor cell death is reliably achieved at target temperatures of −40°C (Campbell et al., 1998), the iceball should propagate 5 to 10 mm beyond the tumor margin to ensure complete treatment.** The iceball appears as a distinct hypodense zone on CT imaging (Fig. 103.1). As previously mentioned in the section on mechanism of action, two freeze-thaw cycles are performed to obtain more complete tissue necrosis (Woolley et al., 2002). Unlike RFA, with which lesions are typically treated for a predetermined period, there is no standard duration for a freeze cycle as long as the intended ablation zone size is attained. Ten minutes is commonly used during the initial cycle, and the second cycle is generally shorter (6 to 8 minutes) based on animal evidence demonstrating inadequate necrosis at 5 minutes and increased tissue fracture at 15 minutes. Thus 10-minute freeze cycles represent an optimal compromise with adequate tumor necrosis and fewer complications (Auge et al., 2006). Each freeze cycle is followed by either an active (helium-based) or passive thaw. Although there is conflicting evidence regarding an active versus passive thaw, some authors suggest an active thaw during at least the second thaw cycle to decrease operative time and allow the surgeon to more rapidly address post-treatment bleeding (White and Kaouk, 2012). After the second cycle thaw, the probe is gently twisted, and, if there is no resistance, it is removed atraumatically. A contrast-enhanced CT is repeated after treatment to assess completeness of ablation and rule out complications.

Monitoring of treatment efficacy during RFA employs measurement of tissue temperature or impedance, using either single multitined probes (with incorporated thermistors) or multiple single-shaft probes that measure tissue impedance as the end point. At our institutions, a 14-gauge Starburst XL (AngioDynamics, Queensbury, NY) **RFA probe is deployed, and its position is adjusted to ensure complete lesion coverage plus a peritumoral margin of at least 5 mm** (Fig. 103.2). To limit radiation exposure to the patient, confirmatory scans should be limited to 3 to 4 3-mm images centered around the target lesion at a lower current than standard helical imaging (70 mA vs. 150 mA) (Tracy et al., 2015). Ablation cycles of 5, 7, and 8 minutes at a target temperature of 105°C are then delivered for tine deployments of less than 2 cm, 2 to 3 cm, and 3 to 4 cm, respectively. After a 30-second cool-down, a second cycle of similar duration is performed. During the initial and secondary cool-down cycles, the passive tissue temperature in each quadrant should be at least 70°C, confirming the absence of a large heat sink. Contrast-enhanced helical CT is repeated after treatment to assess completeness of ablation and rule out complications. If inadequately treated areas are identified, the radiofrequency probe is repositioned and the treatment is repeated in a similar fashion. Depending on the manufacturer, the probe tract is ablated during probe withdrawal. For ablation of larger lesions, some authors have described the use of nonconducting temperature probes placed at the peripheral and deep margins of the tumor for active temperature monitoring (Carey and Leveillee, 2007). Rather than multitined probes, multiple individual probes also can be used in overlapping ablations (Karam et al., 2011). Patients who undergo percutaneous CA or RFA under general anesthesia or conscious sedation are discharged in a same-day fashion, whereas those with significant comorbidities or complication typically are admitted overnight.

TREATMENT SUCCESS AND FOLLOW-UP PROTOCOL AFTER TUMOR ABLATION

Interpretation of treatment success after renal tumor ablation had been a controversial subject, but with maturing experience and

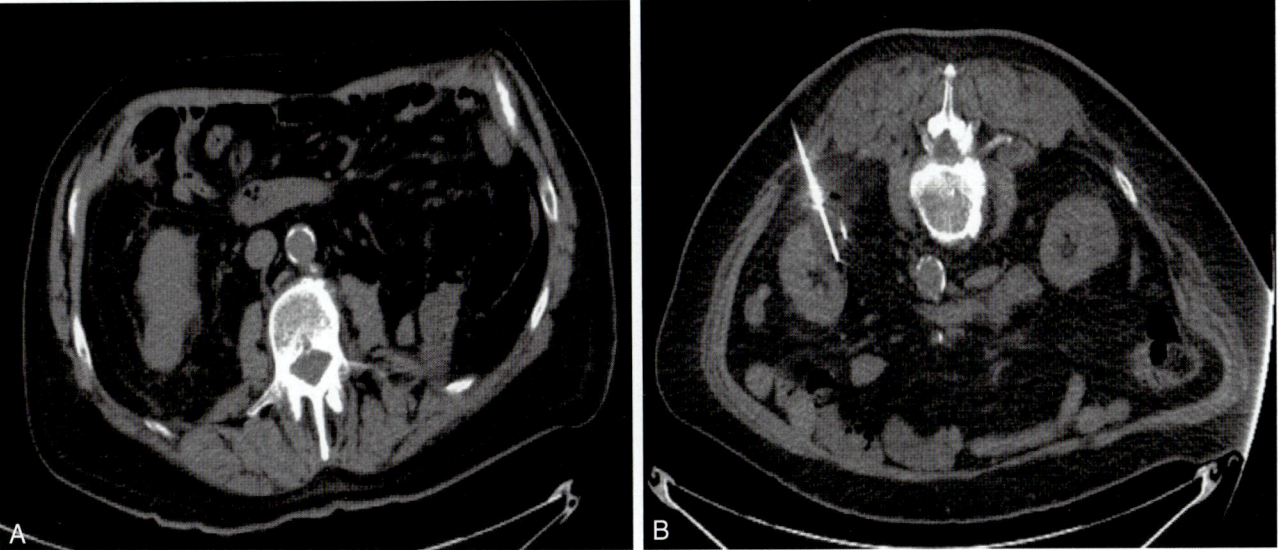

Fig. 103.1. Percutaneous cryoablation. (A) Preoperative imaging demonstrates a 2.6-cm exophytic renal cell carcinoma on the posterior aspect of the right kidney. (B) Intraoperative image during percutaneous ablations shows low attenuation area corresponding to the iceball. (Courtesy Ardeshir Rastinehad, MD, Department of Urology, North Shore–Long Island Jewish Health system.)

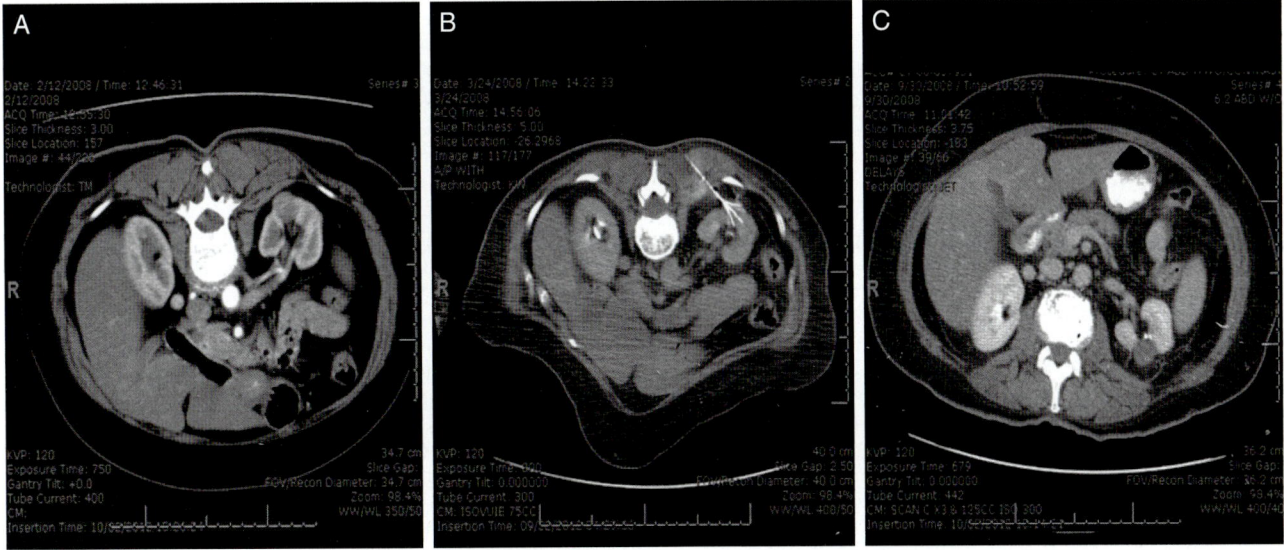

Fig. 103.2. Radiofrequency ablation (RFA) probe positioning and postablation findings. (A) Posterior left renal tumor before ablation. (B) RFA probe positioned. (C) Six months after ablation imaging with characteristic periablation halo sign.

standardization of follow-up protocols, **radiographic cross-sectional imaging is the accepted measure of treatment efficacy** (Donat et al., 2013; Matin et al., 2006). Routine postablative biopsy is not recommended because the interpretation of biopsy findings after ablation is highly contentious and unresolved. When enhancement and involution are incongruent or recurrence is suspected, multisite-directed core biopsies are appropriate.

Radiographic Interpretation of Success

No pathological margins are rendered with in situ ablation; therefore imaging characteristics serve as a surrogate marker of treatment efficacy. In general, the **complete loss of contrast enhancement on follow-up CT or MRI is considered evidence of thorough tissue destruction and attendant treatment success** (Matsumoto et al., 2004; McAchran et al., 2005). At most centers, the first postablation CT or MRI image is obtained at 6 to 12 weeks. **If persistent enhancement is identified in any portion of the treated lesion on initial imaging, it is classified as an incomplete ablation and repeat ablation is scheduled** (Fig. 103.3). Conversely, if a lesion demonstrates an initial complete loss of contrast enhancement and later demonstrates enlargement of the lesion and/or contrast enhancement, this is considered local tumor recurrence or progression (Matin, 2010).

In addition to contrast-related characteristics, lesions that undergo CA or RFA demonstrate characteristic but strikingly different appearances on follow-up imaging. **The majority of lesions treated with CA demonstrate a greater than 50% reduction in size in the first year after treatment** (Deane and Clayman, 2006; Kawamoto et al., 2009). This contraction is due to cellular breakdown and phagocytosis. Conversely, **lesions treated with RFA often demonstrate minimal postablative contraction and a have a distinctive fibrotic halo or circular demarcation around the treatment zone when performed percutaneously** (see Fig. 103.2C), representing a foreign-body giant

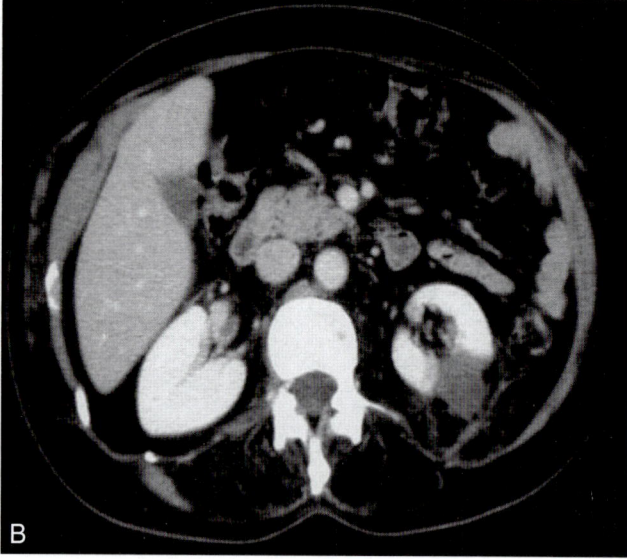

Fig. 103.3. Incomplete ablation with radiofrequency ablation. (A) Six-week follow-up computed tomography scan shows contrast enhancement of a left renal cell carcinoma indicative of an incomplete ablation *(arrowheads)*. (B) After repeat ablation, the tumor shows no further enhancement on subsequent 6-week follow-up.

cell fibrotic response (Park et al., 2006b). **Enlargement of a lesion, regardless of the treatment modality or the enhancement characteristics, should be considered a tumor recurrence,** and biopsy and/or treatment (observation vs. repeat ablation vs. extirpative surgery) should be strongly considered.

Recommended Radiographic Follow-Up Protocol

The AUA guidelines for the follow-up of an ablated renal tumor recommend that **CT or MRI with and without intravenous contrast should be performed at 3 to 6 months after ablation and then annually thereafter for 5 years** (Donat et al., 2013). There are no available data suggesting the superiority of MRI or CT in routine follow-up. Ultrasonography should not be routinely employed to evaluate lesions after ablation unless specific protocols are in place for contrast-enhanced ultrasonography.

Role of Preablation and Postablation Biopsy

To establish a diagnosis and provide uniformity and improved outcomes-based data, the AUA Small Renal Mass and the Follow-up for Clinically Localized Renal Neoplasms Guidelines Panels recommend that tumor biopsy be universally performed before ablation (Campbell et al., 2017; Donat et al., 2013). The diagnostic accuracy in specimen interpretation is high (Schmidbauer et al., 2008) and will help define the frequency of postablation follow-up. Conversely, one of the chief criticisms of in situ renal ablation has been the inability to render definitive pathological evidence of treatment success. Efficacy with ablative technologies is therefore predicated solely on indirect radiographic interpretation, as previously discussed. The role of a routine postablation biopsy has yielded conflicting data on its utility given questions surrounding the oncologic accuracy of the histologic interpretation, inherent sampling error, and poor correlation with long-term oncologic results (Klingler et al., 2007; Lin et al., 2004; Matlaga et al., 2002; Raman et al., 2008a; Weight et al., 2008). Considering the dual limitations of imaging studies and biopsy findings, **a multi-institutional study on the incidence and patterns of recurrence after energy ablative therapy concluded that radiographic detection of residual or recurrent disease is the current state of the art when performed correctly** (Matin, 2010).

> **KEY POINTS: FOLLOW-UP AFTER TUMOR ABLATION**
>
> - Complete loss of contrast enhancement on follow-up CT or MRI is considered evidence of complete tissue destruction and treatment success.
> - The majority of lesions treated with CA demonstrate a greater than 50% reduction in size in the first year after treatment. Lesions treated with RFA demonstrate minimal postablative contraction and a have a distinctive fibrotic halo or circular demarcation around the treatment zone. Enlargement of a lesion, regardless of the treatment modality or the enhancement characteristics, should be construed as an ominous sign of local tumor recurrence.
> - The AUA Guidelines Panel recommends that a pretreatment tumor biopsy be universally performed before ablation.
> - The same Guidelines Panel recommends that a CT or MRI scan with intravenous contrast should be performed at 3 and 6 months after ablation and then annually thereafter for 5 years.

ONCOLOGIC OUTCOMES

Several confounding variables in the literature complicate the interpretation and comparison of oncologic success after thermal ablation, including small cohort sizes, short follow-up, inclusion of patients with benign masses, lack of preablation biopsy, inclusion of patients with confounding features for RCC recurrence such as hereditary cancer syndromes, use of various (and evolving) technologies, and variable definitions of recurrence. Fortunately, as the ablative literature continues to mature, the quality of evidence has continued to improve, with the majority of series now controlling for most of these variables. Tables 103.1 and 103.2 summarize RCC-specific outcomes for RFA and CA, respectively, in select series with intermediate- to long-term follow-up. Although a direct comparison between ablation and partial nephrectomy is limited by patient, tumor, and surgeon selection biases, as well as inconsistent definitions of postablation recurrence, **data suggest that progression-free survival and disease-specific survival are similar for energy ablative therapy and extirpative**

TABLE 103.1 Intermediate-Term to Long-Term Outcomes After Radiofrequency Ablation of Biopsy-Proved Renal Cell Carcinoma

AUTHOR	NO. PATIENTS (NO. TUMORS)	FOLLOW-UP (yr) (RANGE)	TUMOR SIZE (cm) (RANGE)	TECHNIQUE	% LOCAL RECURRENCE-FREE SURVIVAL	% METASTATIC RECURRENCE	% OVERALL DISEASE-FREE SURVIVAL	% CANCER-SPECIFIC SURVIVAL	% OVERALL SURVIVAL
Psutka et al., 2013	185 (185)	Median 6.43 (0.5–13.4)	Median 3 (1–6.5)	Perc	5-yr: 95.2	5-yr MFS 99.4	5-yr DFS 87.6	5-yr CSS 99.4	5-yr OS 73.3
Tracy et al., 2010	160 (179)	Mean 2.25 (0.13–7.5)	Mean 2.4 (1.0–5.4)	Perc and Lap	5-yr: 90	5-yr MFS 95	—	5-yr CSS 99	5-yr OS 85[a]
Zagoria et al., 2011	41 (48)	Median 4.67 (IQR 3–5.3)	Median 2.6 (0.7–8.2)	Perc	5-yr: 88	5-yr MFS 93	5-yr DFS 83[b]	1/41 (2.4) died of RCC	5-yr OS 66
Olweny et al., 2012	37 (37)	Median 6.5 (IQR 5.8–7.1)	Median 2.1 (IQR 1.8–2.8)	Perc and Lap	5-yr: 91.7	5-yr MFS 97.2	5-yr DFS 89	5-yr CSS 97.2	5-yr OS 97.2
Levinson et al., 2008	18 (18)	Mean 4.8 (3.4–6.7)	Mean 2.1 (1–4)	Perc	5-yr: 79.9	5-yr MFS 100	5-yr DFS 79.9	5-yr CSS 100	5-yr OS 58.3
Wah et al., 2014	165 (200)	Mean 3.8 (0.2–8)	Mean 2.9 (1–5.6)	Perc	5-yr: 93.5	5-yr MFS 87.7	—	5-yr CSS 97.9	5-yr OS 75.8
Atwell et al., 2013	222 (256)	Mean 2.8 (1.2–4.1)	Mean 1.9 (0.6–3)	Perc	5-yr: 98.1	5 yr: 98.1[c]	—	5 yr: 98.7[c]	—

[a]Overall survival for entire cohort, including 22% with nondiagnostic or benign histology.
[b]No recurrences observed in patients with tumors less than 4 cm in size.
[c]Patients with no history of RCC.
CSS, Cancer-specific survival; DFS, disease-free survival; IQR, interquartile range; Lap, laparoscopic; MFS, metastasis-free survival; OS, overall survival; Perc, percutaneous; RCC, renal cell carcinoma.

TABLE 103.2 Intermediate-Term to Long-Term Outcomes After Cryoablation for Biopsy-Proved Renal Cell Carcinoma

AUTHOR	NO. PATIENTS (NO. TUMORS)	FOLLOW UP (yr) (RANGE)	TUMOR SIZE (cm) (RANGE)	APPROACH	% LOCAL RECURRENCE-FREE SURVIVAL	% METASTATIC RECURRENCE	% OVERALL DISEASE-FREE SURVIVAL	% CANCER-SPECIFIC SURVIVAL	% OVERALL SURVIVAL
Caputo et al., 2015	100	Mean 8.2	Mean 2.4 (0.5–5.2)	Lap	97	—	10-yr DFS 86.5	10-yr CSS 92.6	10-yr OS 53.8
Guazzoni et al., 2010	44	Mean 5.1	Median 2.14 (0.5–4)	Lap	93.2[a]	95.5 MFS	—	5-yr CSS 100	5-yr OS 93.2
Johnson et al., 2014	67	Mean 8.2	Mean 2.3 (0.86–7)	Lap	91.4	98.6	10-yr DFS 86.5	10-yr CSS 98.2	10-yr OS 70.7
Nielsen et al., 2017	514	Median (IQR) 3 (1.2–4.7)	Median (IQR) 2.5 (2.0–3.0)	Lap	93.8	—	10-yr DFS 80	10-yr 99	10-yr OS 64.4
Tanagho et al., 2012	35	Mean 6.3 (SD 3.3)	Mean 2.5 (SD 0.98)	Lap	6-yr LRFS 80	6-yr MFS 100	6-yr DFS 80	6-yr CSS 100	6-yr OS 76.2

[a]Although these patients received salvage therapy by radiofrequency ablation or radical nephrectomy, the authors did not include them in their analysis of recurrences.
CSS, Cancer-specific survival; DFS, disease-free survival; IQR, interquartile range; Lap, laparoscopic; LRFS, local recurrence-free survival; MFS, metastasis-free survival; OS, overall survival; RFS, recurrence-free survival.

therapy in the intermediate term, exceeding 90% in each case. In a head-to-head comparison of RFA and partial nephrectomy in patients with sporadic unilateral T1a RCC, 5-year actual local recurrence-free survival (LRFS), overall disease-free survival (DFS), and progression-free survival were statistically similar between cohorts when including patients who may have required a second ablation for incomplete primary treatment (Olweny et al., 2012). Similarly, a separate comparison of TA (CA and RFA) to partial nephrectomy showed no difference in recurrence-free survival (RFS) among the varying modalities at 3 years of follow-up (Thompson et al., 2015).

Altogether, intermediate and long term results of CA and RFA demonstrate the durability of ablation for the treatment of small cortical neoplasms, allowing for expanding indications. **The AUA guidelines now recommend that physicians consider thermal ablation as an alternative approach for the management of cT1a renal masses less than 3 cm in diameter** (Campbell et al., 2017), with an understanding that tumor recurrence or persistence may be more likely and that repeat ablation may be required.

Local Recurrence-Free Survival

The definition of local recurrence-free survival is likely the most contested point with regard to comparing CA, RFA, and partial nephrectomy. In addition to varying time points for defining success ranging from days to months, surgical approach may confound initial success rates. In particular, compared with partial nephrectomy and cryotherapy, which has been generally reported in the literature using either an open or laparoscopic technique, the majority of RFA cases are performed percutaneously. Because percutaneous treatments are considered to be easily repeatable, physicians performing the procedure may be less aggressive with their initial treatment compared with those approaching a malignancy in an open or laparoscopic fashion. Surgeons performing percutaneous ablation therefore may be more accepting of persistent disease on short-term follow-up, presuming that the tumor may be completely ablated with a second, minimally invasive procedure. Indeed, several studies have demonstrated similar recurrence-free survival rates between CA and RFA when taking into account the percutaneous versus laparoscopic approach (Matin et al., 2006; Permpongkosol et al., 2006; Zargar et al., 2015).

Local recurrence is most often defined as any evidence of residual disease remaining in the treated kidney after the primary ablation procedure. Using this definition, **the 2009 AUA Guidelines Panel examined 10 studies of CA and 10 studies of RFA and determined a local recurrence-free survival of 90.6% (83.8% to 94.7%) for CA and 87.0% (83.2% to 90%) for RFA** (Campbell et al., 2017). **When compared with alternative extirpative treatments, the 2017 AUA guidelines recognized that CA and RFA demonstrated significantly higher rates of local recurrence but no significant difference in local recurrence-free survival when considering repeat ablation.** Importantly, in a more recent meta-analysis, El Dib et al. (2012) reviewed 31 case series (20 CA, 11 RFA) and found no difference in the clinical efficacy (89% vs. 90%) between CA and RFA, respectively.

Several recent meta-analysis have investigated the risk for local tumor recurrence after TA compared with extirpative surgery. In an analysis of 147 studies on the management of localized renal masses, Pierorazio et al. (2016) found that at a median of 60 months in the extirpative cohorts and 48.6 months in thermal ablation cohorts, there was an increased local recurrence-free survival (LRFS) with partial nephrectomy compared with TA (98.9% vs. 93%). However, this difference became insignificant when considering the LRFS after a subsequent salvage ablative procedure, which increased the efficacy of TA to 97% to 100%. Likewise, Katsanos et al. (2014) found that in 587 patients with small renal tumors who underwent TA versus nephrectomy, there was no meaningful difference in local recurrence rate (3.6% vs. 3.6%) at 5 years. A cohort study using data from the SEER registry found that patients undergoing nephron-sparing surgery had a 5-year disease-specific survival that was incrementally improved (1.7%) over ablation (Whitson et al., 2012), although there was no significant difference in the risk for death when comparing the two treatments. Interestingly, the authors noted that the difference in disease-specific survival between nephron-sparing surgery and ablation has decreased over time, possibly indicating improved outcomes from ablative procedures as a result of increased experience, improved patient selection, and technical modifications.

In addition to surgical factors and their influence on outcomes after ablative procedures, long-term follow-up data suggest that **tumor size is a significant indicator of ablation success.** Best et al. (2012) found that in patients undergoing RFA, the 5-year overall local recurrence-free survival in 108 biopsy-proved RCCs was 95% for those with tumors smaller than 3 cm but only 78% for those with tumors 3 cm or larger ($P = 0.002$). This was similar to a subsequent study by Psutka et al. (2013), which demonstrated a 5-year LRFS and overall disease-free survival after RFA of 96.1% and 91.5% with tumors smaller than 4 cm (T1a) compared with 91.9% and 74.5% in tumors larger than 4 cm (T1b). Tanagho et al. (2012) demonstrated a 6-year overall disease-free survival of 80% after CA, with tumor size 2.6 cm or greater the only predictor of oncologic failure on multivariate analysis. Expanding on this observation, a more recent publication by Caputo et al. (2017) evaluated their experience treating T1b tumors (>4 and <7 cm) with CA vs. partial nephrectomy and found a 23% recurrence rate with CA compared with PN despite a modest overall tumor size in the CA and PN cohorts (4.3 cm vs. 4.6 cm, $P = 0.07$).

Metastatic Recurrence-Free Survival

Metastatic recurrence-free survival is generally defined as any disease present in the body other than in the treated kidney or associated renal fossa after primary treatment. Based on this definition, **recent meta-analyses have found no difference in metastasis-free survival when comparing extirpative surgery and TA** (Katsanos et al., 2014; Pierorazio et al., 2016).

As seen in Tables 103.1 and 103.2, multiple centers have reported on their intermediate- to long-term outcomes, including multiple series with more than 5 years of follow-up for RFA (Best et al., 2012; Olweny et al., 2012; Psutka et al., 2013; Tracy et al., 2010; Zagoria et al., 2011) and CA (Aron et al., 2010; Tanagho et al., 2012). Although the presence of confounding factors precludes meaningful comparisons among these studies, **these data seem to support the fact that outcomes for ablative procedures are durable beyond 5 years and up to 10 years.**

Cancer-Specific Survival

The AUA meta-analysis published in 2009 evaluated the risk for dying from RCC after CA or RFA and concluded that **CSS was 95.2% (89.2% to 97.9%) with CA and 98.1% (95.2% to 99.2%) with RFA with no significant difference in CSS between CA and RFA.** Although selection bias and short duration of follow-up may confound these results, more recent publications reporting on long-term outcomes have verified a CSS ranging from 80% to 100% at up to 10 years for CA (Caputo et al., 2017; Tanagho et al., 2012; Zargar et al., 2015) and approximately 98% for RFA (Olweny et al., 2012; Psutka et al., 2013; Zagoria et al., 2011). **Recent meta-analyses have found no difference in CSS when comparing extirpative surgery and TA** (Katsanos et al., 2014; Pierorazio et al., 2016).

Overall Survival

Patients undergoing ablative procedures tend to be older and have more comorbidities than those undergoing extirpative surgery (Campbell et al., 2017). Thus the mean overall survival rate after ablative procedures is typically 75% to 85% at 5 years, decreasing to 54% to 64% at 10 years (Caputo et al., 2015; Nielsen et al, 2017; Psutka et al., 2013; Tracy et al., 2010).

Cryoablation Versus Radiofrequency Ablation

No data directly compare percutaneous and laparoscopic CA to its respective RFA counterparts. Beyond issues of ill-defined radiologic and pathological end points, there is considerable variability in patient selection, tumor size and location, technique, and approach (laparoscopic vs. percutaneous), as well as inherent bias for a particular ablative modality.

Two large single-institution studies with significant experience with CA and RFA have reported comparable oncologic outcomes, impact on renal function, and complication rates. In 2006 Hegarty et al. compared outcomes in a somewhat disparate cohort of 164 laparoscopic CA procedures and 82 percutaneous RFA procedures. Although there was no significant difference in tumor size between the two groups, the RFA cohort contained more patients with central tumors and tumors in solitary kidneys, which likely accounted for the higher radiographic evidence of disease persistence or recurrence noted in patients who underwent percutaneous RFA (11% vs. 2% for laparoscopic CA). Importantly, there was no significant impact on renal function with either modality, and the short-term CSS for CA and RFA were comparable at 98% and 100%, respectively. More recently, Atwell et al. (2013) reported their single-institution contemporary outcomes comparing percutaneous ablation using either RFA or CA. Overall, in their experience with 445 tumors 3 cm or smaller over a 10-year period (256 RFA, 189 CA), the local tumor recurrence rate was 3.2% for RFA at a mean of 2.8 years and 2.8% for CA at a mean of 0.9 year. In patients with biopsy-proved RCC, there was no difference in local recurrence-free survival at 1 (100% vs. 97.3%), 3 (98.1% vs. 90.6%), and 5 years (98.1% vs. 90.6%), when comparing RFA and CA, respectively.

Ultimately, the result of multiple meta-analyses offers the most insight into the comparative oncologic merit and potential limitations of CA and RFA (Campbell et al., 2017; El Dib et al., 2012; Kunkle and Uzzo, 2008). **It appears that there is no significant difference in the risk for local tumor recurrence, disease progression/metastasis, CSS, and overall survival between CA and RFA, leading more recent studies to combine the two modalities into one category when comparing outcomes with extirpative procedures** (Pierorazio et al., 2016). Currently, RFA and CA are recognized options for patients who elect thermal ablation (Campbell et al., 2017), **with choice of therapy type dependent on institutional preference as well as tumor characteristics.**

Laparoscopic Versus Percutaneous Renal Tumor Ablation

One limitation when comparing series of renal tumor ablation to each other is the variability in technique. The assumption that the success of a laparoscopic and percutaneous ablation is comparable remains debatable. Indeed, until recently the vast majority of published CA series were approached laparoscopically, whereas more than 95% of RFA procedures were performed percutaneously. Zargar et al. (2015) retrospectively compared 275 patients undergoing laparoscopic cryoablation (LCA) to 137 undergoing percutaneous cryoablation (PCA) at their institution. Despite an increase in tumor complexity in the percutaneous cohort, the authors found no difference in 5-year recurrence-free survival (RFS) for LCA vs. PCA (79% vs. 80%) at a median of 4.4 and 3.1 years, respectively. Likewise there was no difference in incomplete treatment (6.9% vs. 6.6%) or local recurrence based on approach for LCA versus PCA (13.1% vs. 14.6%). Similarly, Leveillee et al. (2013) reported their experience with laparoscopic and percutaneous RFA in 274 patients with 292 tumors. The radiographic recurrence rate for either approach was only 4%. **Given morbidity and cost advantages, the percutaneous approach for thermal ablation is preferred** (Campbell et al., 2017). Similar studies comparing laparoscopic and percutaneous tumor ablation have confirmed these findings for RFA and CA (Derweesh et al., 2008; Hinshaw et al., 2008; Hui et al., 2008; O'Malley et al., 2006).

COMPLICATIONS

A meta-analysis comparing urologic and nonurologic complications after CA, RFA, and alternative extirpative approaches (Campbell et al., 2017) revealed that **the incidence of major urologic complications with renal CA and RFA was 4.9% (range 3.3% to 7.4%) and 6.0% (4.3% to 8.2%), respectively. Major nonurologic problems occurred in 5% (3.5% to 7.2%) of patients undergoing CA and** 4.5% (3.2% to 6.2%) of those undergoing RFA. **The risk for major urologic complications was lower with ablative techniques than with either laparoscopic or open partial nephrectomy. There was no significant difference in urologic complications with CA versus RFA.** Likewise, the more recent meta-analysis by Katsanos et al. (2014) also showed significantly fewer overall and major complications with TA compared with nephrectomy (7.4% vs. 11.1% and 2.3% vs. 5%, respectively).

The majority of complications that occur with renal ablation are minor, with major complications occurring in approximately 2% of cases (Katsanos et al., 2014). However, up to 20% of complications may require hospital readmission, procedural intervention, or transfusion (Johnson et al., 2004). **Laparoscopic ablation tends to have a higher rate of complications than percutaneous ablation, with an estimated one-third of laparoscopic ablation complications occurring as a result of laparoscopic technique** (Johnson et al., 2004). Complications decrease significantly, regardless of surgical approach, with increasing operative experience.

Several authors have attempted to objectively determine the risk for complications using patient and tumor characteristics. Using the findings of prior studies on extirpative surgery for renal malignancy that demonstrated that the RENAL nephrometry score (Kutikov and Uzzo, 2009) can predict surgeon preference and postoperative complications (Canter et al., 2011; Rosevear et al., 2012), most authors have now started to include this variable in their outcomes. In a retrospective review of 77 laparoscopic CAs performed at three high-volume centers, Okhunov et al. (2012) reported their complication rates based on low (4 to 6), moderate (7 to 19), or high (10 to 12) nephrometry scores. Overall, their cohort had a complication rate of 19.5%, including 9.5% with major complications. There was a significant association with tumor complexity and complications, with no complications in the low complexity cohort compared with 35% and 100% of those with moderate or high nephrometry scores, respectively. Similarly, Schmit et al. (2013) reported their extensive experience with 679 percutaneous tumor ablations, stratifying patients by renal complexity based on nephrometry score to predict outcomes and complications of percutaneous ablation (CA and RFA). In their series, 5.6% of patients developed major complications, including 7.8% of CAs and 2.7% of RFAs. Patients with complications had a higher mean nephrometry score than those who did not experience complications (8.1 vs. 6.8), and patients with high-complexity tumors (nephrometry score 10 to 12) had a 14.3% risk for major complications. Although there was a clear difference between complications with regard to ablative technology (CA vs. RFA), the results were difficult to compare because the authors typically performed CA on larger, more complex lesions and RFA on more exophytic and smaller lesions. Seidman et al. (2013) evaluated their experience with percutaneous and laparoscopic RFA and identified an overall complication rate of 7.5%, with a major complication rate of 2%, neither of which were predicted based on nephrometry complexity. Importantly, mean tumor complexity was less than 8 for all of the cohorts, which likely limited the ability to discern among risk categories. Accordingly, the

> **KEY POINTS: ONCOLOGIC OUTCOMES**
>
> - The interpretation of oncologic outcomes after renal tumor ablation is subject to confounding variables such as the inclusion of nonmalignant tumors.
> - When compared with alternative extirpative treatments, CA and RFA demonstrate significantly higher rates of local recurrence, albeit they can be salvaged with repeat ablation or surgery.
> - There is no apparent significant difference in metastatic recurrence-free survival when comparing RFA and CA to each other or against extirpative treatments.
> - Any discussion of oncologic efficacy regarding ablative technologies must focus on long-term markers of success, such as metastasis-free survival, CSS, renal function preservation, and quality-of-life outcomes.

authors subsequently suggested a modification to the scoring system, where the R score was modified to 1 if less than 3 cm, 2 if 3 to 4 cm, or 3 if greater than 4 cm. Using this scoring system, they were able to accurately predict initial treatment failure and DFS at 3 years (Gahan et al., 2015).

In addition to tumor factors, various patient factors also influence the risk of complications as well as success of ablation. In the multi-institutional EuRECA study, which evaluated 808 patients undergoing laparoscopic CA across eight European institutions, 16.6% of patients had a complication, 3.2% of which were considered major. Although nephrometry score was not included, multivariable analysis showed that an American Society of Anesthesiology (ASA) score of more than 3 was associated with a threefold increased risk of overall complications (Nielsen et al., 2017).

Historically, the most common complication after renal tumor ablation was pain or paresthesia at the percutaneous probe insertion site, occurring in up to 8% of patients (Farrell et al., 2003b). However, current generation cryoprobes are thermally insulated along the shaft, which has led to a decrease in freezer burns as were seen with prior generations. The active portion of the RFA probe is only along the most distal aspect. However, with RFA, to prevent inadvertent nerve damage, tract ablation should be performed only long enough to remove the probe from the kidney and surrounding the Gerota fascia. Electrical skin burns after RFA, which may occur at the site of the grounding pads, should be incredibly rare and can be avoided by placing the pads at the exact same level on the patient's posterior thigh (McDougal et al., 2005). Because energy returning to the generator travels in the shortest arc, the pads should be placed perpendicular to the long axis of the thigh to increase surface area for energy dissipation.

Currently, **the most common perioperative complication from percutaneous ablation is intraoperative or postoperative hemorrhage**, which may occur in up to 11% to 27% of patients undergoing ablative renal procedures (Finley et al., 2008), with transfusion rates of 3.2% (2% to 4.9%) with CA and 2.4% (1.4% to 4%) with RFA (Campbell et al., 2017). As experience matures, the risk of postoperative blood transfusion continues to decline with more recent series reporting rates between 0 and 2% (Nielsen et al., 2017; Okhunov et al., 2017). **The primary risk factor for hemorrhage is the use of multiple probes for treatment of larger renal masses** (Okhunov et al., 2017). **To decrease the risk for tumor fracture during CA, probes should be given adequate time to thaw because premature removal increases the risk for tumor fracture and hemorrhage. Bleeding during needle placement may be controlled by initiating the ablation, especially with the coagulative nature of RFA.** Bleeding during laparoscopic ablation can be managed with the use of hemostatic agents combined with direct pressure. If bleeding continues after ablation, consideration should be given to selective angioembolization. As with any percutaneous needle placement, percutaneous ablation risks damage to the abdominal wall vasculature, and thus care should be taken to avoid intercostal arteries. When injury does occur, it is typically visualized during the procedure with routine imaging. The expanding hematoma may be observed with serial imaging (if rapidly expanding) or serial hematocrit levels (if stable), with only the rare case requiring angiographic embolization.

Complications from damage to surrounding intra-abdominal organs can be minimized through appropriate patient selection, preoperative planning, and good surgical technique. Cross-sectional preoperative imaging is essential to determine if a tumor should be managed with a laparoscopic or percutaneous approach. For patients in whom there may be a concern regarding adjacent organs, additional imaging can be obtained with the patient in various positions to plan an appropriate needle path. Patients with anterior tumors, tumors close to the collecting system, or without a suitable access tract on preoperative imaging should be scheduled for laparoscopic ablation or have consideration for displacement of organs using intraprocedural hydrodissection. **Ideal patients for percutaneous treatment are those with posterior or lateral tumors, those with tumors located more than 0.5 cm from the ureteropelvic junction or renal pelvis, and those with tumors at least 1 cm from surrounding bowel.**

Urothelial damage may manifest as minor hematuria, hematuria with significant clots, or urinary tract obstruction. Patients with hematuria should be managed conservatively, unless they present with significant hemorrhage, at which time they can be managed with selective angioembolization. There have been several reports of urinary fistula or collecting system injury after RFA as well as CA (Brown and Bhayani, 2007; Gervais et al., 2005a, 2005b; Janzen et al., 2005). **Permanent urothelial damage may manifest as either calyceal obstruction or ureteral obstruction if damage occurs at the ureteropelvic junction or distally** (Johnson et al., 2003). In extreme cases, damage to the urinary tract may result in perirenal urinoma formation or cutaneous urinary fistula. Patients with ureteral obstruction or urine leakage from the collecting system may be managed conservatively or with insertion of an indwelling ureteral stent (Fig. 103.4). Patients with significant urinoma accumulation should have a percutaneous drain placed.

Injury to the pleural cavity resulting in pneumothorax or hemothorax can occur if probes are placed above the twelfth rib to treat upper pole lesions. These complications are typically recognized either during the procedure as breathing difficulties or with percutaneous access on routine imaging during tumor treatment. If a simple pneumothorax is identified, it may be treated by aspiration using a small needle inserted into the pleural space at the conclusion of the case. In the absence of a large or persistent pneumothorax, placement of a chest tube should be performed sparingly. Postoperatively, chest pain or shortness of breath should trigger suspicion of pneumothorax and prompt performance of an upright chest radiograph.

Colon injury after renal mass ablation is exceedingly rare and should be largely preventable with appropriate surgical technique. During percutaneous access, tumors within close proximity to bowel may be dissected free from the treatment area by injecting saline to hydrodissect tissues and develop a safe working space around the tumor (Clark et al., 2006; Farrell et al., 2003a; Lee et al., 2006; Fig. 103.5). However, reproducibility and surgeon familiarity with the patient's anatomy may make these lesions more suitable for the laparoscopic approach by which the bowel can be safely removed from the operative field. Patients with colon damage should be managed along with a general surgical consultation. Patients with a controlled colon-nephric fistula should be initially managed with placement of a ureteral stent, whereas those with a persistent fistula or with colon-cutaneous fistulas may require surgical diversion or a trial of total peripheral nutrition (Vanderbrink et al., 2007). Patients with frank colon perforation and signs of peritonitis should be managed with prompt surgical exploration.

When posterior tumors are treated percutaneously, damage to the nerves running along the posterior abdominal wall can lead to self-limiting neuralgia or neuroapraxias (Baker et al., 2007; Lee et al., 2006). This complication can be avoided by positioning the patient so that the tumor falls away from the body wall or by hydrodissecting the plane between kidney and body wall (Lee et al., 2006). For patients with multiple posterior tumors or with limited perinephric fat between the kidney and body wall, strong consideration should be given to the laparoscopic approach in which the kidney can be physically relocated away from the body wall.

Postoperative infection after tumor ablation, in the absence of a large hematoma or urinoma, is exceedingly rare but may be lethal (Schmit et al., 2013). Patients at risk for infection are those with chronic colonization of the urinary tract (e.g., ileal conduit) or active infection at the time of procedure (Bandi et al., 2007; Brown and Bhayani, 2007). When infectious complications do occur, they typically manifest from 1 to 6 months later as a chronic drainage or retroperitoneal abscess. Patients at risk for urinary tract infection (UTI) should be screened by urine culture and treated appropriately before their ablation procedure. Whereas we routinely administer perioperative prophylactic antibiotics at the time of the surgery, some authors suggest broad-spectrum coverage 2 days before and 2 weeks after surgery for patients at high risk for infection (Wah et al., 2008).

NEW ABLATION MODALITIES

High-Intensity Focused Ultrasonography

As an acoustic wave is propagated through tissue, a portion of its energy is absorbed and converted into heat (Madersbacher et al.,

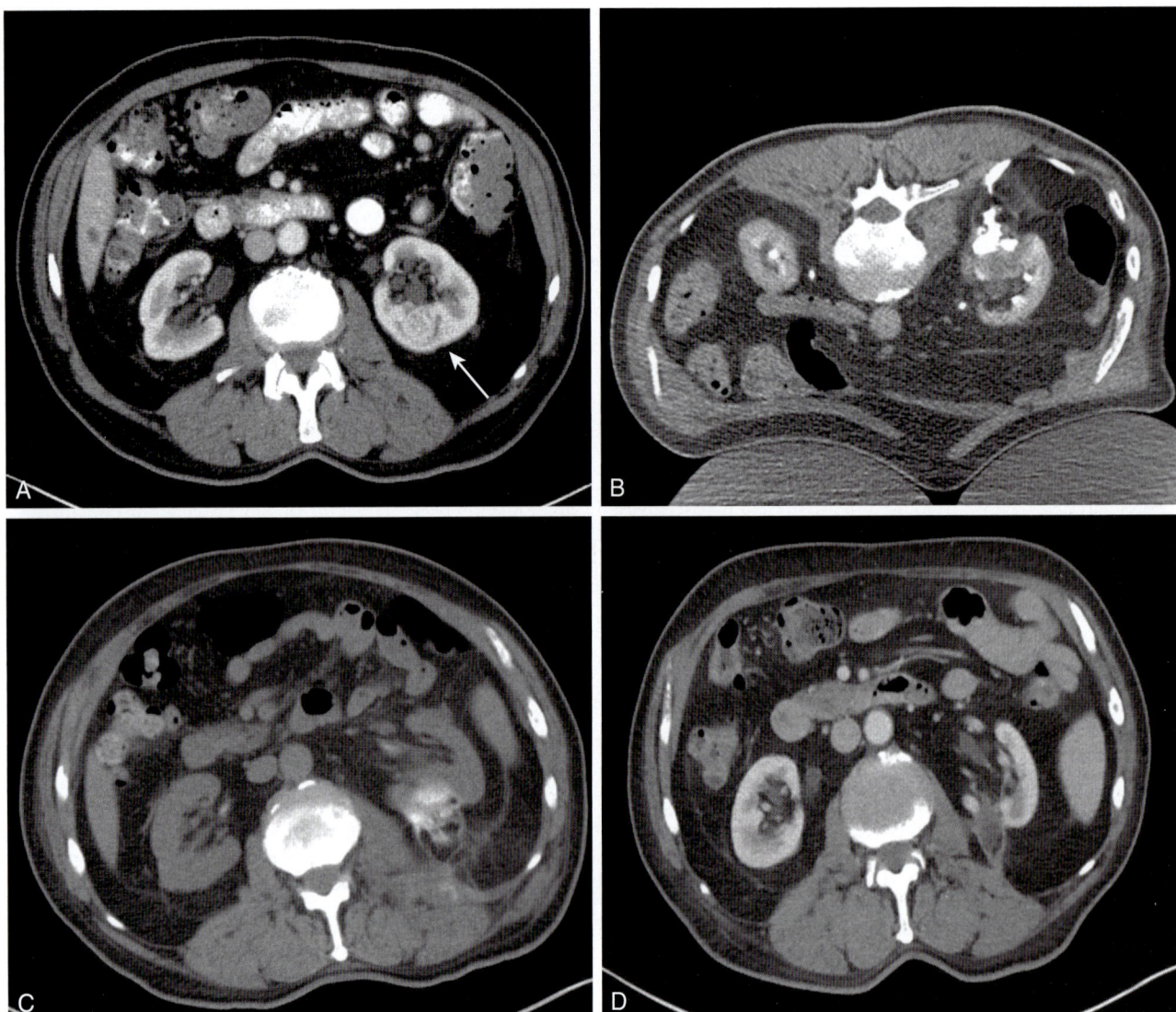

Fig. 103.4. Urine leak after percutaneous radiofrequency ablation (RFA). (A) Preoperative imaging shows 2.5-cm endophytic left renal mass (arrow). (B) Immediate postoperative image after ablation shows urinary extravasation at the site of RFA. (C) Postoperative day 1 computed tomography (CT) image shows no change in the fluid collection. (D) Three-year follow-up CT shows involution of the treated area with postoperative halo.

KEY POINTS: COMPLICATIONS AFTER TUMOR ABLATION

- The risk for major urologic complications is lower with ablative techniques (~5%) than with either laparoscopic or open partial nephrectomy. There is no significant difference in urologic complications between CA and RFA.
- For CA, postoperative hemorrhage is the most commonly cited major adverse risk.
- Bleeding is less common with RFA than CA and may be ideally suited for those at risk for postoperative hemorrhage.
- The risk for complications with CA may be predicted by tumor complexity.
- Commonly cited minor complications with CA and RFA include pain and paresthesia at the probe insertion site, UTIs, damage to surrounding structures, and self-limited hematuria.

1995; Vricella et al., 2009). When the ultrasound waves are focused with an appropriately shaped transducer, the temperature at the focal point can exceed the threshold for cell death, while adjacent tissue is spared. At sufficiently high intensities (>3500 W/cm^3), cavitation and microbubble formation occur that yield extremely high temperatures and a mechanically disrupting "shock wave" effect similar to that seen with extracorporeal shock wave lithotripsy (Kieran et al., 2007). Termed high-intensity focused ultrasound (HIFU), it is a unique thermal ablation technology in that it can be administered in an entirely noninvasive, extracorporeal fashion minimizing or eliminating the risk for tumor seeding, hemorrhage, or urinary extravasation.

HIFU employs a transducer used for treatment and monitoring. Under real-time guidance, the HIFU beam is focused on the treatment zone and a defined area is ablated. The transducer is then refocused to ablate overlapping volumes and "paint" a larger overall volume of tissue. Treatment times can be lengthy, with a mean reported duration of nearly 5.5 hours (1.5 to 9 hours) (Häcker et al., 2006; Köhrmann et al., 2002; Marberger et al., 2005). A myriad of

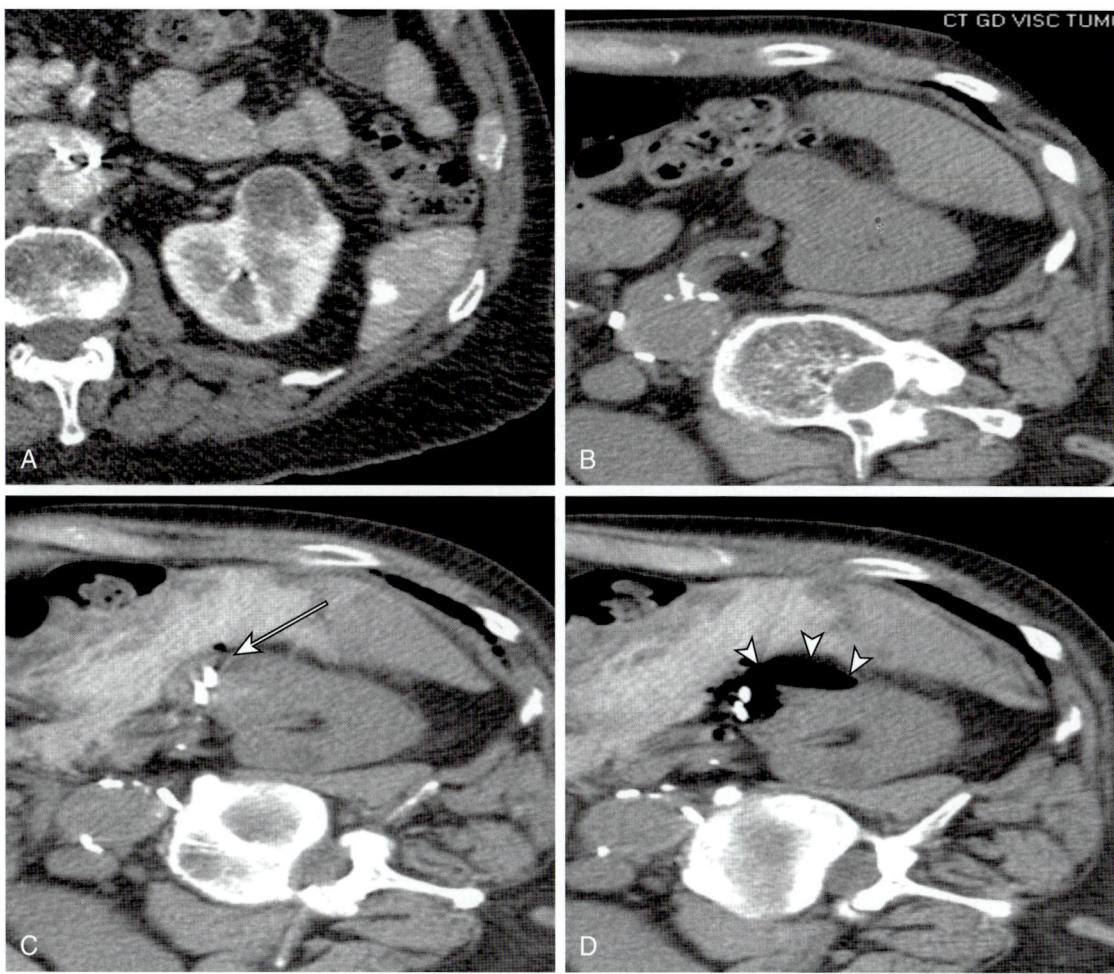

Fig. 103.5. Intraoperative hydrodissection for anterior tumor. (A) Preoperative imaging shows a 3-cm anterior renal mass. (B) Intraoperative imaging demonstrates large bowel anterior to the lesion. (C) D5 + contrast is injected percutaneously to hydrodissect bowel and create a window for placement of two cryoprobes *(arrow)*. (D) Iceball is demonstrated by hypodense lesion adjacent to the cryoprobes *(arrowheads)*. (Courtesy Fred Lee Jr, MD, University of Wisconsin.)

parameters, including focal length, type of transducer employed, and type of treatment system have been investigated and are beyond the scope of this chapter.

Although early clinical trials have established the feasibility of transcutaneous HIFU, based on the data available and the existing clinical hurdles, it should be considered only investigational at this time. Two important ablate-and-resect studies have noted incomplete treatment in all specimens, highlighting the challenge of accurate targeting (Marberger et al., 2005; Vallancien et al., 1993). Ritchie et al. (2010) reported a very limited experience with transcutaneous HIFU ablation and subsequent intermediate-term radiographic follow-up. MRI 2 weeks after treatment suggested viable tumor in 8 of 15 treated tumors. Of 14 patients with at least 6 months' follow-up, 10 appeared to have tumor involution with loss of enhancement and shrinkage (mean follow-up 36 months). Purported explanations for these collective incomplete treatments have included poor targeting secondary to respiratory movement and acoustic interference (acoustic shadowing, reverberation, and refraction) and lack of effective intraoperative monitoring of treatment progress. To circumvent these issues, laparoscopic HIFU has been investigated, and although results are favorable, its viability as a treatment modality is questionable because it would compete with established laparoscopic CA and RFA techniques (Klingler et al., 2008). **In summary, outcomes with renal HIFU have stagnated and proved inferior to alternative ablative technologies, and its use in this regard should be considered investigational.**

Radiation Therapy

Historically, radiation therapy was considered ineffective in the treatment of RCC. It remains unclear whether poor outcomes with conventional external-beam linear accelerator radiation systems were due to an inherent resistance to radiation or to limitations with radiation delivery (Camphausen and Coia, 2008). There are many technical challenges associated with treatment of kidney tumors, including limited radiation tolerance of the normal parenchyma, significant scatter with attendant damage to the surrounding tissues, and difficulty of target localization.

Stereotactic body radiation therapy (SBRT) is a "treatment method to deliver a high dose of radiation to the target, using either a single dose or a small number of fractions with a high degree of precision within the body" (Potters et al., 2010). As opposed to conventional radiation delivery techniques, modern stereotactic treatment systems employ three-dimensional coordinates to target and compensate for respiratory movement and radiation scatter by automatically tracking, detecting, and correcting for tumor and/or organ movement without interrupting the treatment or repositioning the patient. This tracking system is image guided and dependent on a constant reference point (e.g., fiducial marker) that is continually recognized by the linear accelerator. High-dose radiation beams move in real time with the respiratory cycle and are therefore extremely accurate (Ponsky et al., 2007). Not only is radiation scatter minimized but also higher doses may be applied in a focal manner that effectively ablates masses in the kidney without compromising overall renal function. Ponsky et al. (2003) first evaluated stereotactic radiosurgery in the porcine kidney using the CyberKnife (Accuray, Palo Alto, CA) treatment system. Treatment doses between 24 to 40 Gy resulted in complete necrosis in the treatment zone with no collateral damage to adjacent tissue. Building on this initial animal experience, Ponsky et al. (2007) subsequently performed a phase I study on three human patients with a mean renal tumor size of 2 cm. A total of 16 Gy was administered in a fractionated fashion. Patients were followed for 8 weeks, after which a partial nephrectomy was performed. No adverse events or radiation toxicities were noted. Histopathology demonstrated residual RCC in two patients and no evidence of viable tumor in the remaining patient.

Svedman et al. (2006) performed a retrospective study evaluating the efficacy and safety of stereotactic radiosurgery in the management of inoperable or metastatic primary RCC. Thirty patients with 82 lesions underwent treatment with varied dose/fractionation schedules. At a median follow-up of 52 months, complete response was noted in 21% of patients, with another 58% demonstrating a partial/stable response.

A critical and systematic review of SBRT for primary RCC recently identified 10 studies consisting of 126 patients treated with between one and six fractions (Siva et al., 2012). The most common treatment regimen was 40 Gy over five fractions. Median or mean follow-up ranged from 9 to 57 months. Local control was defined only radiologically and was estimated at 94% at 2 years. The weighted rate of grade 3 or higher adverse effects was only 3.8%; the most common was radiation dermatitis and enteritis.

Most recently, Sun et al. (2016) clarified the expected radiographic appearance of RCC ablated with SBRT using a fixed body frame rather than fiducial markers. They treated 41 renal tumors (all but 8 biopsy-confirmed carcinomas) with SBRT (21–48 Gy over 3 treatments) with a mean follow-up of 1.5 years. Unlike thermal ablation wherein successful treatment is characterized by complete loss of enhancement and gradual involution of the mass, it appears that the early 1-year response to SBRT is unique and may be clinically challenging to interpret. There was no statistical change in tumor enhancement during follow-up, and 75% were stable in size (though previously growing), 20% demonstrated a partial response, and a complete response occurred in only 1 patient. No tumor was biopsied during follow-up. Staehler et al. (2016) reported a success rate of 98% at 2 years with a convenient single treatment (25 Gy) for 45 tumors all less than 4 cm in diameter.

Certainly, the responsiveness of RCC to stereotactic radiosurgery in the aforementioned trials argues against its radioresistant reputation. **Presently its use should be considered experimental because there is no consensus for dose fractionation, technique (with or without fiducial markers), or appropriate criteria for imaging interpretation. With improved treatment protocols and well-designed prospective trials, SABR ultimately may play a significant role in the treatment of RCC.**

Microwave Ablation

Microwave ablation (MWA) delivers energy through semiflexible probes that are inserted directly into the target lesion and functions in a similar fashion to RFA. Medical applications of microwave energy operate in the 900-MHz to 2.45-GHz range of the electromagnetic spectrum and create rapid water ion oscillation in the tissue and frictional heat. The degree of tissue penetration and heat produced is related to the water content of the target tissue, which can be more difficult to predict in the heterogeneous kidney parenchyma environment (Moore et al., 2010; Rehman et al., 2004). MWA is capable of achieving treatment temperatures (>60°C) with greater rapidity than RFA and is not limited by tissue charring and desiccation as experienced with RFA. These qualities may translate into more efficient treatment times and may make MWA less susceptible to the heat sink phenomenon (Cornelis et al., 2017; Liang and Wang, 2007).

MWA technology was initially designed for the percutaneous treatment of liver tumors and has enjoyed considerable success in this capacity. Its use in the management of renal tumors remains immature. Clark et al. (2007) performed a phase I study in which 10 patients underwent MWA of suspected RCC at the time of radical nephrectomy. When examined pathologically, lesions as large as 5.7 cm × 4.7 cm × 3.8 cm were achieved with complete and uniform tissue necrosis. Following the initial data, MWA has continued to expand in the clinical realm. Although there was initially some concern for high treatment failures (Castle et al., 2011), more contemporary series have reported a success rate greater than 90% for pT1a and pT1b tumors (Lin et al., 2014; Wells et al., 2016). The only direct comparison of MWA to partial nephrectomy reported comparable 3-year recurrence-free survival of 90% and 97%, respectively (Guan et al., 2012). Although there are several theoretical advantages of MWA over CA and RFA, there are insufficient follow-up data and further study is required (Cornelis et al., 2017).

At this point, MWA offers considerable promise as an alternative thermal ablative technology. However, larger prospective studies with longer follow-up are necessary to better understand the optimal tumor characteristics, risks, and morbidity.

Irreversible Electroporation

Irreversible electroporation (IRE), is a novel nonthermal method for ablation of living tissue that potentially offers advantages over RFA and CA. Electroporation is a process whereby an electric field applied across cells generates nanoscale pores within cellular membranes that can be either reversible or lethally irreversible depending on the magnitude of voltage applied. IRE is produced through a series of electrical pulses delivered by a single (bipolar) or multiple (monopolar) electrodes. With appropriate modulation it is able to ablate a substantial and reproducible amount of tissue by increasing cell membrane permeability that ultimately leads to cell death (Edd et al., 2006). The result is a nonthermal effect that preserves the extracellular matrix, tissue scaffolding, ductal structures, and large blood vessels (Deodhar et al., 2011; Edd et al., 2006).

Because of the potential to avoid the shortcomings of thermal ablation, there is a great deal of interest in applying IRE to ablation of renal tumors. Although IRE has been shown to be effective in ablating liver and prostate tissue, these results cannot be readily extrapolated to the kidney, which is substantially different given the vigorous arterial blood supply, complex collecting system, and presence of urinary solutes in varying concentrations. The efficacy of IRE ablation of renal parenchyma was first described by Tracy et al. (2011). When IRE bipolar and monopolar electrodes (Angiodynamics, Queensbury, NY) were used to perform laparoscopic ablations on porcine kidneys, histopathological evaluation revealed absence of cellular viability immediately after IRE treatment that evolved to diffuse cellular necrosis by 7 days and chronic inflammation, cellular contraction, and fibrosis by day 14. In addition to its effect on the parenchyma, IRE appeared to provide some urothelial sparing with initial ulceration followed by signs of early repair and viability. Other authors subsequently confirmed these findings using image-guided percutaneous placement of IRE electrodes (Deodhar et al., 2011).

There is very limited clinical experience with percutaneous IRE. In a series of five patients Diehl et al. (2016) demonstrated the safety of IRE in treating SRM in solitary kidneys, although oncologic outcomes were not reported. Most recently, Canvasser et al. (2017) reported on 36 tumors in 35 patients who underwent IRE. Mean tumor size was 2.0 cm with a median R.E.N.A.L nephrometry score of 5. No major (Clavien grade II or higher) intraoperative or postoperative complications occurred and initial treatment success rate was 92%. The 2-year actuarial local recurrence-free survival was 78% for patients with biopsy-confirmed RCC, 85% with biopsy-confirmed or a history of RCC, and 89% for the intent-to-treat cohort.

In summary, the experience with IRE ablation of renal tumors is very limited, and its use in this regard should be considered investigational.

Targeted Embolization and Ablation

Because of the heat sink phenomenon with RFA, highly vascular central lesions or lesions positioned adjacent to the renal hilum are often inadequately ablated. Studies estimate treatment failures to be as high as 40%. In an attempt to address conductive heat loss, investigators have performed selective arterial embolization before CA and RFA (Gebauer et al., 2007; Mahnken et al., 2009; Moynagh et al., 2015; Yamakado et al., 2006). Theoretically, selective embolization should allow for more homogeneous heating and improved tissue necrosis. **Clinical reports are sporadic and anecdotal. Therefore the use of targeted angioembolization before RFA remains investigational.**

KEY POINTS: NEW ABLATION TECHNOLOGIES

- Although there are a number of promising ablation modalities on the horizon, the majority of these should be considered investigational.
- The most promising future ablation modalities appear to be stereotactic radiosurgery, microwave thermotherapy, and IRE. However, significant study is required to further determine their potential benefits compared with the well-established methods of CA and RFA.

CONCLUSION

Once considered experimental and appropriate only for patients with significant comorbidities, CA and RFA are currently considered viable alternatives to extirpative management of cT1a renal carcinoma. In situ ablation confers less treatment-related morbidity than either open or laparoscopic partial nephrectomy and offers comparable renal function preservation compared with partial nephrectomy. CA and RFA are technically less challenging than other nephron-sparing approaches, although learning curves exist for patient selection, tumor targeting, probe deployment, and generator use. Results from recent meta-analyses demonstrate modestly inferior local tumor control compared with partial and radical nephrectomy, but with equivalent cancer-specific and overall survival when salvage ablation is considered. No prospective literature currently exists that addresses the superiority of CA or RFA. Ultimately, the decision to treat a small renal mass with an ablative technology should take into account tumor-related characteristics, patient demographics and comorbidities, and the values and desires of the patient.

SUGGESTED READINGS

Atwell TD, Schmit GD, Boorjian SA, et al: Percutaneous ablation of renal masses measuring 3.0 cm and smaller: comparative local control and complications after radiofrequency ablation and cryoablation, *AJR Am J Roentgenol* 200:461–466, 2013.

Best SL, Park S, Yaacoub RF, et al: Long-term outcomes of renal tumor radiofrequency ablation stratified by tumor diameter: size matters, *J Urol* 187:1183, 2012.

Carraway WA, Raman JD, Cadeddu JA: Current status of renal radiofrequency ablation, *Curr Opin Urol* 19:143–147, 2009.

Davenport MS, Caoili EM, Cohan RH, et al: MRI and CT characteristics of successfully ablated renal masses: imaging surveillance after radiofrequency ablation, *AJR Am J Roentgenol* 192:1571–1578, 2009.

Karam JA, Ahrar K, Matin SF: Ablation of kidney tumors, *Surg Oncol Clin N Am* 20:341–353, 2011.

Kunkle DA, Egleston BL, Uzzo RG: Excise, ablate or observe: the small renal mass dilemma—a meta-analysis and review, *J Urol* 179:1227–1234, 2008.

Miller DC, Saigal CS, Banerjee M, et al: Diffusion of surgical innovation among patients with kidney cancer, *Cancer* 112:1708–1717, 2008.

Novick AC, Campbell SC, Belldegrun A, et al: *Guideline for management of the clinical stage 1 renal mass*, 2009 (website). Available from: http://www.auanet.org/content/guidelines-and-quality-care/clinical-guidelines/main-reports/renalmass09.pdf.

Ponsky LE, Crownover RL, Rosen MJ, et al: Initial evaluation of Cyberknife technology for extracorporeal renal tissue ablation, *Urology* 61:498–501, 2003.

Weight CJ, Kaouk JH, Hegarty NJ, et al: Correlation of radiographic imaging and histopathology following cryoablation and radio frequency ablation for renal tumors, *J Urol* 179:1277–1281, 2008.

REFERENCES

The complete reference list is available online at ExpertConsult.com.

104 Treatment of Advanced Renal Cell Carcinoma

Ramaprasad Srinivasan, MD, PhD, and W. Marston Linehan, MD

Renal cell carcinoma (RCC) is a term that includes a variety of cancers arising in the kidney and encompasses several histologically, biologically, and clinically distinct entities (Linehan et al., 2007, 2009). An estimated 65,340 new cases of cancer arising in the kidney or renal pelvis were diagnosed in 2018 in the United States (Siegel et al., 2018). **Approximately one-third of all patients with newly diagnosed RCC are seen initially with synchronous metastatic disease, and an additional 20% to 40% of patients with clinically localized disease at diagnosis eventually develop metastases** (Bukowski et al., 1997; Rabinovitch et al., 1994; Skinner et al., 1971). Metastatic RCC is almost always fatal, with 10-year survival rates of less than 5% (Bukowski et al., 1997; Motzer et al., 1999, 2000; Motzer and Russo, 2000; Negrier et al., 2002); patients with metastatic disease account for the majority of deaths (approximately 13,860 a year in the United States) related to RCC (Siegel et al., 2018).

Advances in our understanding of the genetic and molecular changes underlying the individual subtypes of RCC have led to the development of novel agents designed to reverse or modulate aberrant pathways contributing to renal oncogenesis. Over the past decade, these "targeted" therapeutic strategies have become an integral component in the management of metastatic clear cell kidney cancer. However, surgery, irradiation, and cytokine therapy remain appropriate choices in the management of selected patients with advanced clear cell RCC. More recently, the recognition that agents modulating T-cell function may have activity against a variety of solid tumors, including RCC, has reinvigorated interest in immunotherapy strategies; the efficacy of several immune "checkpoint" inhibitors in clear cell RCC has been clearly demonstrated in the front-line setting and in patients who have progressed on therapy directed against the vascular endothelial growth factor (VEGF) axis. Although the optimal management of patients with advanced clear cell RCC remains to be determined, the standard of care is evolving rapidly, with emerging data from a variety of strategies, including dual immune checkpoint inhibition and combinations of agents targeting the PD1/PDL1 interaction and those targeting VEGF or VEGF receptors beginning to demonstrate superiority over previously accepted standards. Last, the advent of techniques that allow comprehensive interrogation of the cancer genome has allowed identification of hitherto unrecognized alterations affecting diverse cellular functions, including carbohydrate and amino acid metabolism as well as chromatin remodeling in clear cell RCC. Although the precise contribution of these changes to the genesis and progression of kidney cancer remains to be determined, it is likely that a better understanding of these pathways will spawn additional strategies to combat what remains a largely incurable group of malignancies.

Although agents effective in clear cell RCC are often used in patients with other subtypes of RCC, there is scant evidence from prospective studies to justify their utility in non–clear cell RCC variants. Elucidation of aberrant oncogenic pathways in papillary, chromophobe, and other variants of RCC has paved the way for evaluation of targeted therapeutic approaches in these histologic subtypes (Linehan, 2009; Ricketts et al., 2016).

PROGNOSTIC FACTORS

Patients with metastatic RCC generally have a poor prognosis: the majority succumb to their disease. Ten-year survival in patients diagnosed with metastatic disease was estimated to be less than 5% in the era of cytokine therapy and is unlikely to change significantly with targeted therapy. It is hoped that newer immunotherapeutic strategies may be associated with a higher proportion of complete and/or durable responders, but longer follow-up of patients treated with these emerging strategies is required to better quantify long-term benefit. However, **several clinical features, such as a long time interval between initial diagnosis and appearance of metastatic disease and presence of fewer sites of metastatic disease, have been associated with better outcome. Conversely, poor performance status and the presence of lymph node and/or liver metastases have long been recognized to be associated with shorter survival.**

Investigators at the Memorial Sloan Kettering Cancer Center evaluated a variety of clinical and laboratory parameters in 670 patients enrolled on various clinical trials of chemotherapy or cytokine therapy (most treated with interferon-α) in an effort to identify those pretreatment factors that were able to best predict outcome (Motzer et al., 1999). **In a multivariate analysis, a poor performance status (Karnofsky score <80), an elevated serum lactate dehydrogenase (LDH) level (>1.5 times upper limit of normal), a low hemoglobin (less than the lower limit of normal), an elevated corrected calcium concentration (>10 g/dL), and lack of prior nephrectomy were independent predictors of a poor outcome (Table 104.1). Patients could be stratified into three distinct prognostic groups based on these five poor prognostic factors (Table 104.2). The overall survival (OS) times in patients with no adverse factors (favorable-risk group), one to two risk factors (intermediate-risk group), and more than three risk factors (poor-risk group) were 20 months, 10 months, and 4 months, respectively** (Fig. 104.1; Motzer et al., 1999). Subsequently, the same group identified poor performance status, high serum calcium, low hemoglobin, elevated LDH, and a short time interval from initial diagnosis to initiation of systemic therapy (<1 year) as factors that could best predict a poor outcome in 463 patients receiving interferon-based therapy in the first-line setting (Motzer et al., 2002). This prognostic model was found to be predictive of survival in an independent data set derived from patients treated at the Cleveland Clinic, providing independent, external validation of the proposed model (Mekhail et al., 2005). Similar prognostic schemes have also been proposed by the Groupe Français d'Immunotherapie, by the International Kidney Cancer Working Group, and by investigators from the University of California, Los Angeles (Manola et al., 2011; Negrier et al., 2002; Tsui et al., 2000).

Modifications of these prognostic schemes as well as identification of reliable molecular markers are under investigation as suitable predictors of response to and survival after therapy with newer targeted agents against VEGF and mammalian target of rapamycin (mTOR) pathway components (Choueiri et al., 2007, 2008; Motzer et al., 2008). The most comprehensive effort to define prognostic factors in patients undergoing therapy with VEGF-pathway antagonists was undertaken by the International Metastatic Renal Cell Carcinoma Database Consortium (IMDC). **Using data from a group of 645 patients treated with first-line VEGF-targeted agents at several US and Canadian centers, the IMDC investigators confirmed the prognostic relevance of several components of the Memorial Sloan Kettering Cancer Center model (performance status, hypercalcemia, anemia, and time from diagnosis to treatment); in addition, neutrophilia and thrombocytosis were identified as additional, independent predictors of poor outcome. Patients were divided into three risk categories based on the number of adverse prognostic factors associated with their disease** (Heng et al., 2009).

TABLE 104.1 Adverse Prognostic Factors in 670 Patients Treated With Chemotherapy or Immunotherapy at the Memorial Sloan Kettering Cancer Center

- Karnofsky performance score < 80%
- Elevated lactate dehydrogenase (>1.5 times upper limit of normal)
- Low hemoglobin (<lower limit of normal)
- Elevated corrected calcium (>10 mg/dL)
- Absence of prior nephrectomy

TABLE 104.2 Risk Stratification Based on Adverse Prognostic Factors in 670 Patients Treated With Chemotherapy or Immunotherapy at the Memorial Sloan Kettering Cancer Center

RISK GROUP	NO. OF ADVERSE PROGNOSTIC FACTORS	MEDIAN OVERALL SURVIVAL
Good	0	20 months
Intermediate	1–2	10 months
Poor	3–5	4 months

Data from Motzer RJ, Mazumdar M, Bacik J, et al.: Survival and prognostic stratification of 670 patients with advanced renal cell carcinoma. *J Clin Oncol* 17:2530–2540, 1999.

TABLE 104.3 Adverse Prognostic Factors in 849 Patients Treated With First-Line VEGF-Targeted Therapy

- Karnofsky performance score <80%
- Neutrophilia (>upper limit of normal)
- Low hemoglobin (<lower limit of normal)
- Elevated corrected calcium (>upper limit of normal)
- Thrombocytosis (>upper limit of normal)
- <1 yr from diagnosis to VEGF-targeted therapy

TABLE 104.4 Risk Stratification Based on Adverse Prognostic Factors in 849 Patients Treated With First-Line VEGF-Targeted Therapy

RISK GROUP	NO. OF ADVERSE PROGNOSTIC FACTORS	MEDIAN OVERALL SURVIVAL
Good	0	43.2 months
Intermediate	1–2	22.5 months
Poor	3–6	7.8 months

Data from Heng DY, Xie W, Regan MM, et al.: External validation and comparison with other models of the International Metastatic Renal-Cell Carcinoma Database Consortium prognostic model: a population-based study. *Lancet Oncol* 14(2):141–148, 2013.

This model was validated by the same group in an independent cohort of 849 patients and shown to be comparable with other prognostic models such as the MSKCC model. In their updated analysis, median OS was 43.2 months in patients with no risk factors, 22.5 months in those with 1 or 2 risk factors, and 7.8 months in those with 3 or more risk factors (Fig. 104.1B and Tables 104.3 and

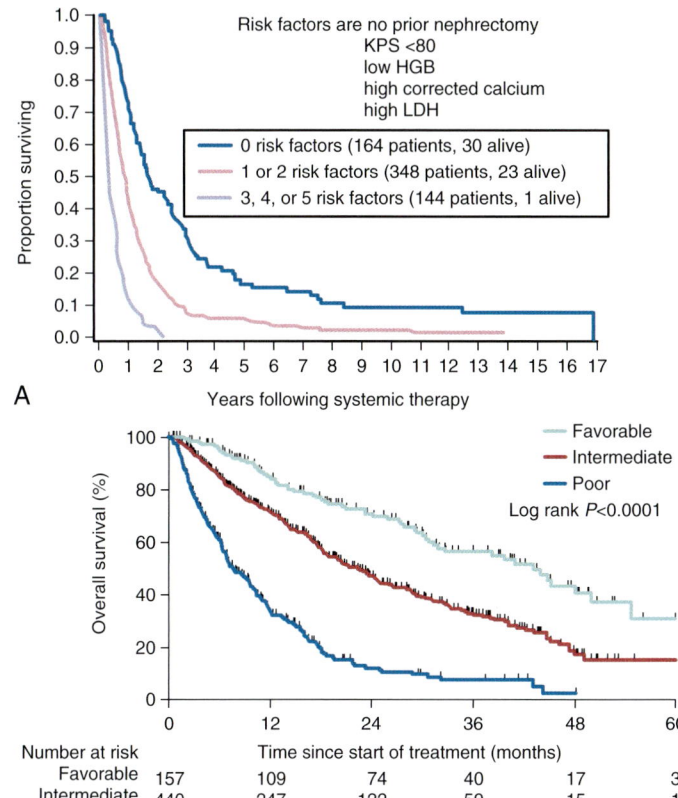

Fig. 104.1. (A) Survival analysis stratified according to risk group in 670 patients treated with chemotherapy or immunotherapy at the Memorial Sloan Kettering Cancer Center (*n* = 656; 14 patients missing one or more of the five risk factors were excluded). *HGB*, hemoglobin; *KPS*, Karnofsky performance score; *LDH*, lactate dehydrogenase. (Data from Motzer RJ, Mazumdar M, Bacik J, et al.: Survival and prognostic stratification of 670 patients with advanced renal cell carcinoma. *J Clin Oncol* 17:2530–2540, 1999.) (B) Survival analysis stratified according to risk group in 849 patients treated with first-line VEGF-targeted therapy. (IMDC Prognostic Criteria; data from Heng D, Xie W, Regan M, et al.: External validation and comparison with other models of the International Metastatic Renal Cell-Carcinoma Database Consortium prognostic model: a population-based study. Lancet Oncol 14[2]:141–148, 2013.)

104.4; Heng et al., 2013). Validated prognostic models are used in clinical practice to help make appropriate management decisions as well as in the design and interpretation of clinical trials.

SURGICAL MANAGEMENT OF METASTATIC RENAL CELL CARCINOMA

Debulking or Cytoreductive Nephrectomy in Patients With Metastatic Renal Cell Carcinoma

The role of cytoreductive nephrectomy preceding systemic therapy has been extensively studied in the era of cytokine therapy. The impetus for exploring this approach in metastatic RCC came from the perception that bulky tumors may inhibit key components of the immune system critical for combating cancer, and from observations suggesting that removal of large primary tumors may provide clinical benefit. To support this practice, early proponents of cytoreductive nephrectomy had cited (1) the rare but well-described occurrence of spontaneous regression of metastatic lesions after nephrectomy (Bloom, 1973; Marcus et al., 1993; Middleton, 1980; Snow and Schellhammer, 1982); (2) preclinical data suggesting that large primary tumors may inhibit T-cell function (Bukowski et al., 1998; Kudoh et al., 1997; Ling et al., 1998; Uzzo et al., 1999a,b); and (3) the inability of systemic agents, particularly cytokines, to induce meaningful responses in primary renal tumors in most patients (Rackley et al., 1994; Sella et al., 1993; Wagner et al., 1999). However, the risk of perioperative morbidity and mortality and the inability of a significant proportion of patients undergoing nephrectomy to subsequently receive systemic therapy clearly underlined the need for unequivocal evidence of clinical benefit as well as the ability to identify patients likely to benefit from this approach.

Nephrectomy as the sole therapeutic intervention in the context of metastatic disease is unlikely to alter outcome, as suggested by small retrospective analyses (deKernion et al., 1978). However, several retrospective studies have demonstrated the feasibility of a combined modality approach in which nephrectomy is followed by cytokine therapy, with some suggesting that this approach may favorably affect response and survival. Investigators from the National Cancer Institute (NCI) reported their experience in 195 patients undergoing nephrectomy followed by high-dose interleukin-2 (IL-2) therapy between the years 1985 and 1996 (Walther et al., 1997). An overall response rate of 18% (including a complete response rate of 4%) after IL-2 therapy was observed in this study. A notable finding that emerged from this study was that, although the majority of patients underwent successful resection of the primary tumor, only 107/195 (55%) went on to receive IL-2 therapy. Rapid postoperative disease progression and perioperative surgical and medical morbidity were the most common factors preventing delivery of systemic therapy, suggesting that careful patient selection may play an important role in the successful application of this combined modality approach.

The impact of patient and/or disease characteristics on outcome was further highlighted by a retrospective study addressing this issue. In a 1995 series by Bennet et al. of 30 patients, including several patients with unfavorable performance status (Eastern Cooperative Oncology Group [ECOG] 2) and multiple metastatic sites including patients with brain or liver metastases, only 7 (23%) were able to proceed with IL-2 after nephrectomy. Conversely, in a series that included only patients with favorable clinical/prognostic factors (e.g., good performance status, minimal comorbidity, no liver or brain metastases), the majority of patients were able to proceed to systemic therapy after nephrectomy, with high response rates (35% to 40%) and OS (median 20 to 22 months) after cytokine-based treatment (Fallick et al., 1997; Figlin et al., 1997). More recently, in a population based analysis of more than 5000 patients with metastatic kidney cancer identified in the Surveillance, Epidemiology, and End Results database, cytoreductive nephrectomy appeared to be associated with a better OS and cancer-specific survival (Zini et al., 2009). **Although these retrospective analyses and small single-arm prospective studies confirmed the feasibility of a tandem surgical/systemic therapy approach, their major contribution was in laying the foundation for controlled, prospective studies to determine if outcomes with systemic therapy could be improved by prior nephrectomy.**

The most compelling evidence in support of cytoreductive nephrectomy is provided by two randomized phase III studies conducted by the Southwest Oncology Group (SWOG) and the European Organization for Research and Treatment of Cancer (EORTC). The larger of the two studies, SWOG 8949, randomized 241 patients with metastatic RCC to receive interferon-α-2b either as initial therapy or after cytoreductive nephrectomy (Flanigan et al., 2001). Salient eligibility criteria included a histologic diagnosis of kidney cancer (all histologic subtypes were allowed); good performance status (ECOG 0 or 1); presence of a resectable primary renal tumor; no prior chemotherapy, irradiation, or immunotherapy; and adequate organ function. **Although there were no significant differences in the response rates to interferon observed in the two study arms, OS was improved in the surgery plus interferon arm (median 11.1 vs. 8.1 months for interferon alone, $P = 0.05$)** (Fig. 104.2). These data were recapitulated in a smaller EORTC trial (a total of 85 patients randomized to interferon alone or interferon after nephrectomy) that used a similar design and reported a survival advantage favoring the surgery plus interferon arm (median OS 17 vs. 7 months, $P = 0.03$) (Mickisch et al., 2001). A combined analysis of both trials revealed data that were consistent with those reported in the individual trials (Flanigan et al., 2004). **These data supported the use of cytoreductive nephrectomy in carefully selected patients with metastatic RCC who are likely candidates for subsequent cytokine therapy** (data summarized in Table 104.5). Although some patients with non–clear cell histologic subtypes of RCC were included in the aforementioned trials, the role of nephrectomy before systemic therapy in these patients is unclear.

Since the advent of VEGFR-targeted therapy, cytoreductive nephrectomy had remained the practice, based largely on data generated in the era of cytokine therapy and supported by retrospective series and outcome analysis from a national cancer database. Several retrospective series suggest that patients with metastatic clear cell RCC benefited from undergoing cytoreductive nephrectomy before initiation of systemic therapy with tyrosine kinase inhibitors

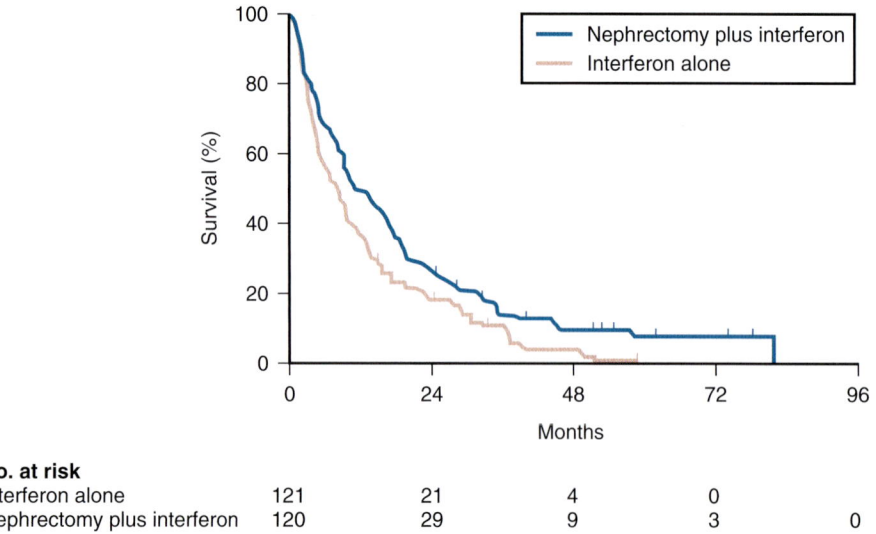

Fig. 104.2. Actuarial survival among 241 patients with metastatic renal cell carcinoma randomized to either interferon-α alone or interferon-α after cytoreductive nephrectomy. (Modified from Flanigan RC et al.: Nephrectomy followed by interferon alfa-2b compared with interferon alfa-2b alone for metastatic renal-cell cancer. *N Engl J Med* 345:1655–1659, 2001.)

TABLE 104.5 Summary of Outcome in Randomized Studies of Interferon-α Alone or Interferon-α After Cytoreductive Nephrectomy in Patients With Metastatic Kidney Cancer

STUDY	TOTAL	IFN	Nx Plus IFN	IFN	Nx Plus IFN	P	IFN	Nx Plus IFN	P
	NO. OF ELIGIBLE PATIENTS			**RESPONSE RATE AFTER IFN (%)**			**MEDIAN OVERALL SURVIVAL (MO)**		
Flanigan et al., 2001	241	121	120	3.6	3.3	NS	8.1	11.1	.05
Mickisch et al., 2001	83	42	41	12	19	.38	7	17	.03
Flanigan et al., 2004	331	163	161	5.7	6.9	.60	7.8	13.6	.002

IFN, Interferon-α; *Nx*, cytoreductive nephrectomy.

targeting VEGFR. In one early series of 314 patients who had received VEGF-pathway antagonists, 201 underwent prior cytoreductive surgery, and the remainder (n = 113) proceeded to systemic therapy without surgical debulking of their primary tumor. In a univariate analysis, cytoreductive surgery was associated with a more favorable outcome (median OS 19.8 vs 9.4 months, HR 0.44; 95% CI 0.32–0.59; $P < 0.01$), a difference that persisted after adjusting for confounding prognostic/risk factors (HR 0.68; 95% CI 0.46–0.99; $P = 0.04$) (Choueiri et al., 2011). Data from the National Cancer Database also suggested that cytoreductive nephrectomy was used more frequently at academic centers and associated with a survival advantage (Hanna et al., 2016). Although these data were subject to the inherent bias associated with analyses of this nature, they nonetheless provided some justification for clinicians who continued the practice of cytoreductive nephrectomy in the era of targeted systemic therapy.

The French Association of Urology and Urogenital Tumors Study Group undertook the CARMENA study (Cancer du Rein Metastatique Nephrectomie et Antiangiogéniques) in a bid to provide more definitive, prospective data to address this issue (Mejean et al., 2018). A total of 576 patients with metastatic clear cell RCC were randomized equally to one of two arms: cytoreductive nephrectomy followed by sunitinib or sunitinib alone. The primary objective was to ascertain the noninferiority of sunitinib alone, with OS as the primary end point. The study was hampered by low accrual, with only 450 patients accrued at 79 centers across Europe over 9 years, leading to premature closure of the trial. With a median follow-up of 50.9 months, the OS in the nephrectomy arm was 13.9 months (95% CI 11.8–18.3) versus 18.4 months in the sunitinib arm (95% CI 14.7–23.0; HR 0.89; 95% CI 0.76–1.10), leading the authors to conclude that sunitinib alone was not inferior to cytoreductive nephrectomy followed by sunitinib in patients with intermediate or poor prognosis (Fig. 104.3).

To evaluate the impact of these data on clinical practice, several aspects of this study merit further attention. First, almost 45% of the patients randomized were characterized as having poor prognosis by MSKCC criteria, a group that is typically not offered cytoreductive nephrectomy. Consequently, approximately 25% of patients assigned to the nephrectomy arm did not receive the intended treatment, including 7% who did not undergo nephrectomy and 18% who did not receive sunitinib after a nephrectomy. Conversely, 17% of patients who received sunitinib as initial therapy underwent a subsequent cytoreductive nephrectomy. When the survival analysis was limited to patients who received the intended treatment, it was no longer clear that sunitinib alone was non-inferior (upper limit of 95% CI crossed the preset boundary for non-inferiority). Second, a population most likely to benefit from cytoreductive nephrectomy may have been underrepresented because investigators screening patients were allowed to exclude patients with low metastatic burden at their discretion. Third, the study was stopped prematurely with far fewer events than originally planned, reducing statistical power. In fact, a planned interim analysis at the time the study halted further accrual failed to meet statistical parameters for stopping the study early, and the outcome may have been different had the study been allowed to meet the original accrual goal. Although findings from this study reiterate that patients with poor prognosis are not likely to benefit

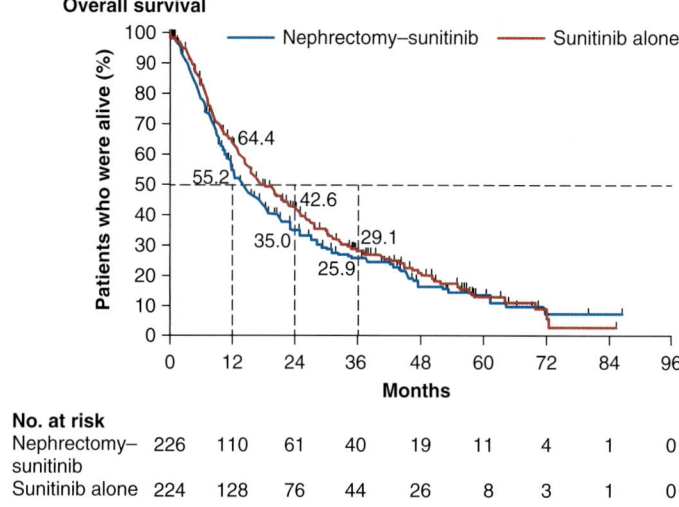

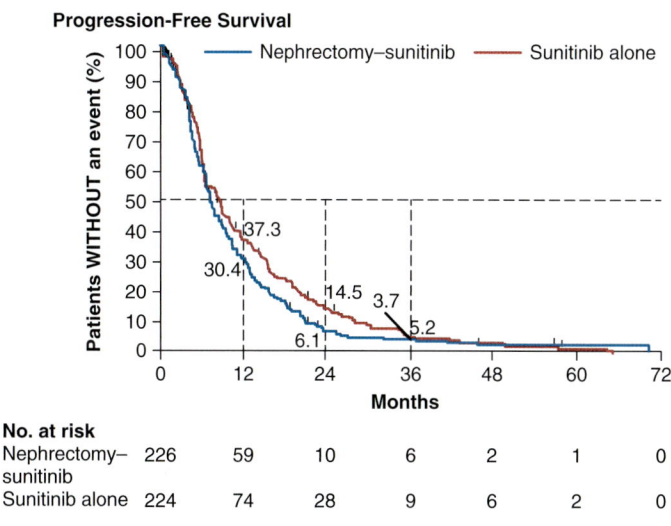

Fig. 104.3. Kaplan-Meier Curves for Overall Survival (A) and Progression Free Survival (B) among 450 patients with metastatic clear cell cancer treated with either sunitinib alone or sunitinib following cytoreductive nephrectomy. (Mejean et al., *N Engl J Med* 379:417-427, 2018.)

from cytoreductive nephrectomy, the impact of these data on current clinical practice (i.e., the use of cytoreductive surgery in appropriately selected patients with low metastatic burden and other favorable features) remains uncertain. Furthermore, the relevance of data from the CARMENA study in the current era also requires careful consideration, because sunitinib is no longer the standard initial therapy in most newly diagnosed patients.

> **KEY POINTS: CYTOREDUCTIVE NEPHRECTOMY IN METASTATIC RENAL CELL CARCINOMA**
>
> - Two randomized studies have demonstrated improved survival in carefully selected metastatic RCC patients undergoing cytoreductive nephrectomy followed by cytokine therapy (interferon-α) compared with those receiving cytokine therapy alone.
> - Several patient and/or disease characteristics appear to influence outcome; for example, patients with poor performance status, medical comorbidity, rapidly progressive disease, and presence of brain metastases are unlikely to benefit from this approach.
> - Although several retrospective studies suggested that cytoreductive nephrectomy may be of benefit in the era of VEGFR-targeted therapy, a randomized study failed to demonstrate an advantage in patients with intermediate and poor prognoses. These data, however, do not specifically address the utility of nephrectomy in patients with relatively low metastatic burden and other favorable features who may benefit from this approach.

Resection of Metastases

Most patients with metastatic RCC will not achieve a cure or long-term disease remission with currently available systemic agents. However, resection of limited metastatic disease has been reported by several groups to be associated with long disease-free intervals and OS in some patients. Metastasectomy has not been evaluated systematically in a prospective, randomized fashion, and the favorable outcome ascribed to resection in patients with solitary metastatic disease may reflect patient selection bias, inherent differences in tumor biology, and natural history or other confounding factors.

Most studies detailing outcome after metastasectomy are retrospective series. In most series, isolated pulmonary metastases were the lesions most commonly amenable to resection with curative intent. The OS of patients undergoing complete resection of limited metastatic disease is impressive, with reported median 5-year survival rates of 35% to 50% in many series (Friedel et al., 1999; Kierney et al., 1994; Middleton, 1967; Murthy et al., 2005; O'Dea et al., 1978; Pogrebniak et al., 1992; Russo et al., 2007; Skinner et al., 1971; Tolia and Whitmore, 1975). The larger of these studies have also attempted to identify patients most likely to benefit from this approach. In a series of 278 patients with recurrent RCC treated at the Memorial Sloan Kettering Cancer Center, 211 were reported to have undergone either complete (141 patients) or incomplete (70 patients) resection of recurrent tumor from a variety of metastatic sites (Kavolius et al., 1998). In this series, complete or "curative" resection was associated with a longer OS (44% 5-year survival vs. 14% in patients undergoing incomplete resection); multivariate analysis also identified the presence of a solitary metastatic lesion, age younger than 60 years, and a disease-free interval of more than 1 year as favorable prognostic indicators. In addition, some studies have suggested that pulmonary metastases, smaller tumor size (<4 cm in one series), and metachronous lesions are predictors of better outcome after metastasectomy (Friedel et al., 1999; Murthy et al., 2005; Piltz et al., 2002). In a retrospective single institution study of 125 patients who had one or more metastatic lesions surgically removed, Alt et al. (2011) confirmed that patients who underwent complete metastatectomy had improved outcomes; furthermore, complete metastasectomy appeared to be feasible and predictive of improved cancer-specific survival even in patients with multiple metastatic lesions. Although not supported by convincing evidence of survival benefit from prospective studies, resection of isolated metastatic lesions is a reasonable and widely employed practice in well-selected patients with RCC.

> **KEY POINTS: METASTASECTOMY**
>
> - Resection of isolated metastatic lesions is appropriate in selected patients.
> - Several retrospective studies have suggested that patients undergoing complete resection of isolated metastatic foci may experience long disease-free intervals with median overall survival rates of 35% to 50% in some reports.
> - Several factors are associated with an improved outcome after metastasectomy, including complete resection, presence of solitary metastatic lesions, age younger than 60 years, smaller tumor size, presence of pulmonary metastases, and development of metachronous metastatic disease.
> - There are no prospective, randomized studies demonstrating a favorable outcome with metastasectomy. It is therefore possible that the favorable outcome after resection of limited metastatic disease may be a reflection of patient selection bias, differences in tumor biology and natural history, or other confounding factors not related to resection.

Palliative Surgery

Cytoreductive nephrectomy can be performed with palliative intent in patients with intractable pain, hematuria, constitutional symptoms, or a variety of paraneoplastic manifestations such as hypercalcemia, erythrocytosis, secondary thrombocytosis, or hypertension. Symptoms such as pain and laboratory abnormalities including hypercalcemia can often be effectively managed medically, whereas symptoms such as hematuria may be amenable to alternative treatment approaches (e.g., angioembolization). Furthermore, resection of the primary renal tumor does not always result in clinical benefit; for instance, in one series, only a little more than half the patients (7/12) with hypercalcemia experienced clinically meaningful reductions in serum calcium levels (Walther et al., 1997). Cytoreductive nephrectomy with palliative intent is therefore performed relatively infrequently but is appropriate in some patients.

Resection of metastases to alleviate pain or to forestall potentially life-threatening or debilitating complications is often indicated in a variety of situations. Patients who may benefit from noncurative resection of metastatic lesions include those with solitary brain metastases, metastatic lesions in weight-bearing bones or joints, or vertebral metastatic lesions with impending spinal cord or radicular compromise (Kollender et al., 2000; Sheehan et al., 2003; Sundaresan et al., 1986). Surgical resection is often combined with radiation and/or systemic therapy in many of the aforementioned situations.

It is our current practice to offer cytoreductive nephrectomy to well-selected patients with metastatic clear cell RCC.

> **KEY POINTS: PALLIATIVE SURGERY IN ADVANCED RENAL CELL CARCINOMA**
>
> - In some patients with advanced RCC, cytoreductive nephrectomy may help alleviate symptoms related to the primary tumor (e.g., intractable pain, hematuria) or paraneoplastic manifestations.
> - However, nonsurgical options are often effective in palliating symptoms associated with RCC; cytoreductive nephrectomy is hence infrequently performed with purely palliative intent.
> - Resection of metastatic lesions (often in combination with radiation or systemic therapy) is sometimes performed for relief of symptoms or to prevent life-threatening or disabling sequelae.

IMMUNOLOGIC APPROACHES IN THE MANAGEMENT OF ADVANCED CLEAR CELL RENAL CELL CARCINOMA

The host immune system has long been believed to play an important role in the causation and control of renal cell cancer. A report detailing spontaneous regression of metastatic lesions after radical nephrectomy provides perhaps the earliest evidence implicating the immune system in the regulation of kidney cancer. The phenomenon of spontaneous regression, thought to represent T- or B-cell mediated antitumor immunity, has sparked great enthusiasm over the years and generated several reports describing this phenomenon (Braren et al., 1974; Edwards et al., 1996; Kavoussi et al., 1986; Marcus et al., 1993; Middleton, Jr., 1980; Robson, 1982; Silber et al., 1975; Snow and Schellhammer, 1982). Although rare **(it is estimated that the true incidence of spontaneous regression is less than 1%)** and often transient, the presumed immunologic mechanisms underlying this event have nonetheless played an important part in the development of immunotherapeutic approaches in kidney cancer. The presence of immune cells, notably cytotoxic T lymphocytes, in resected tumors and the identification of tumor-associated antigens that can serve as human leukocyte antigen (HLA)-restricted targets on tumor cells for T cell–mediated cytotoxicity have also kindled interest in immune-based strategies in renal cell cancer (Ada, 1999; Boon et al., 1997; Finke et al., 1994; Rosenberg, 1999; Takahashi et al., 2008). Early clinical studies explored the efficacy of agents believed to act as nonspecific stimulators of the host immune system, such as cytokines, with or without adoptive cellular therapy. More recently, investigators have evaluated a variety of novel approaches, including allogeneic immunotherapy, vaccines, and modulators of T-cell function. Most immunotherapy strategies have been directed at clear cell RCC, and the utility of these approaches in non–clear cell variants remains to be explored.

Interferons

The interferons are a group of proteins with diverse biologic functions, including immunomodulatory properties. Interferon-α was one of the earliest cytokines to be evaluated for activity in RCC. Initial trials with interferon used leukocyte-derived interferon. The subsequent availability of recombinant interferon-α in the early to mid-1980s allowed investigators to evaluate higher doses of this cytokine in a series of phase II trials. **Initial trials demonstrated overall response rates of 16% to 26% in patients treated with interferon-α, and several subsequent trials have confirmed the activity of this agent, with response rates generally in the 10% to 15% range** (deKernion et al., 1983; Figlin et al., 1988; Minasian et al., 1993; Motzer et al., 2002; Muss et al., 1987; Quesada, 1989; Quesada et al., 1983, 1985; Rosenberg et al., 1987; Umeda and Niijima, 1986). **The limited long-term survival data available suggest that durable complete responses with this agent are relatively rare (<2%).** A variety of dosing schedules and routes have been evaluated to determine the optimal interferon regimen; no single mode of administration or dosing schedule has so far demonstrated superiority over others (Kirkwood et al., 1985; Minasian et al., 1993; Muss et al., 1987; Umeda and Niijima, 1986). Similarly, the addition of chemotherapy or other cytokines to interferon-α has failed to improve the outcomes seen with single-agent therapy (Ellerhorst et al., 1997; Negrier et al., 2000a,b; Ravaud et al., 1994, 1998; Rosenberg et al., 1989; Sella et al., 1992; Tourani et al., 1998, 2003).

Several prospective, randomized trials evaluating the efficacy of interferon-α have demonstrated a modest but statistically significant improvement in outcome after treatment with this agent. A randomized phase III study that assigned 335 patients to receive either interferon-α or medroxyprogesterone demonstrated a higher response rate (14% vs. 2%) and OS (median 8.5 vs. 6 months, hazard ratio 0.72, $P = 0.017$), favoring the interferon arm of the study (Medical Research Council Renal Cancer, 1999). A second study randomized 160 patients with metastatic RCC to receive vinblastine alone or in combination with interferon-α; a higher response rate (16% vs. 2.5%) and improved OS (median 16 vs. 9 months, $P = 0.0049$) with the addition of interferon was observed in this study (Table 104.6; Pyrhonen et al., 1999). Two additional randomized studies suggested that vinblastine is unlikely to have contributed significantly to the activity of this combination by showing that survival was not improved with the addition of vinblastine to interferon-α (Fossa et al., 1992; Neidhart et al., 1991). Last, a meta-analysis of randomized trials of interferon against a variety of agents suggested that interferon-based therapy conferred a survival advantage (Coppin et al., 2005). **Despite its relatively modest activity, based on the just-described data and relative ease of administration compared with IL-2, interferon was commonly the agent of choice in the initial treatment of metastatic RCC until the advent of VEGF pathway antagonists.**

Interleukin-2

Clinical trials in the early 1980s initially identified IL-2 as an active agent in RCC, with some IL-2–based regimens leading to objective response rates in excess of 30% (Rosenberg et al., 1989, 1993). In a subsequent report detailing 255 patients treated on a series of phase II trials at the NCI, a more modest overall response rate of 15% (37/255 patients) was noted (Fyfe et al., 1996). **Several trials conducted by the NCI and the Cytokine Working Group as well as meta-analyses of published data have consistently demonstrated response rates in the range of 15% to 20%** (Dutcher et al., 1997; Fisher et al., 1988; Lotze et al., 1986; Rosenberg et al., 1987, 1989, 1993). **More importantly, 7% to 9% of patients receiving high-dose IL-2 are reported to have achieved complete regression of all metastatic tumors, with the majority of complete responders (>80%) demonstrating no evidence of disease recurrence on long-term follow-up** (Fisher et al., 1997, 2000; Rosenberg et al., 1998). There have also been reports of long-term disease-free remission in partial

TABLE 104.6 Summary of Results From Selected Randomized Trials of Interferon-α in Metastatic Renal Cell Carcinoma

STUDY	AGENT(S)	PHASE	NO. OF PATIENTS TOTAL (RANDOMIZED)	OVERALL RESPONSE RATE (%)	OVERALL SURVIVAL MEDIAN (mo)	P
Medical Research Council, 1999	IFN vs. MPA	III	335 (167 vs. 168)	13 vs. 7	8.5 vs. 6.0	<0.01
Pyrhonen et al., 1999	IFN + vinblastine vs. vinblastine	III	160 (79 vs. 81)	16 vs. 2.5	15.8 vs. 8.8	<0.01
Neidhart et al., 1991	IFN vs. IFN + vinblastine	III	165 (82 vs. 83)	13 vs. 13	NA	NS
Fossa et al., 1992	IFN vs. IFN + vinblastine	III	178 (87 vs. 91)	11 vs. 24	12 vs. 12	NS

IFN, Interferon; *MPA*, medroxyprogesterone acetate; *NA*, not available; *NS*, not significant.

responders whose limited disease burden after IL-2 therapy rendered them amenable to resection of localized metastases. **High-dose IL-2 was approved by the US Food and Drug Administration (FDA) for the treatment of metastatic kidney cancer in 1992, based largely on its ability to induce durable complete responses in some patients.**

The initial studies with IL-2 were conducted using an intravenous bolus regimen with doses of 600,000 or 720,000 IU/kg administered every 8 hours as tolerated to a maximum of 15 doses. A major limitation of this dosing regimen is the considerable associated toxicity that has limited its widespread use. Vascular leak syndrome, and the resulting hypotension, third-space fluid retention, respiratory compromise, and multiorgan damage are some of the more problematic concomitants of IL-2 therapy and led to an unacceptably high treatment-related mortality rate (2% to 5%) in early studies with this agent (Kammula et al., 1998; Rosenberg et al., 1987). Subsequently, careful patient selection, intensive monitoring schemes, and early interventions with IV fluids, vasopressors, and antibiotics have significantly reduced mortality associated with IL-2 (Kammula et al., 1998). However, the significant morbidity and expense associated with delivering bolus high-dose IL-2 have led several investigators to explore alternative regimens aimed at reducing toxicity without compromising efficacy. Numerous single-arm phase II studies have evaluated a variety of alternative regimens, including daily subcutaneous administration and continuous intravenous infusion (Atkins et al., 2001; Escudier et al., 1994a,b, 1995; Negrier et al., 2000, 2005, 2008). Many of these studies have reported overall response rates of 10% to 30%, suggesting comparable efficacy with high-dose bolus administration based on data from historical controls. However, two randomized studies have demonstrated that, although well tolerated, lower-dose regimens are associated with lower overall response rates, as well with fewer durable, complete responses (Table 104.7; McDermott et al., 2005; Yang et al., 2003). **Based on these data, we only recommend high-dose IL-2 regimens in patients being considered for cytokine therapy.**

Attempts to enhance the efficacy of IL-2 therapy have led investigators to explore combination therapy with other cytokines, cytotoxic chemotherapy, and adoptive cellular immunotherapy. Early experience with combination cytokine therapy was promising: one study reported a 31% overall response rate in patients treated with high-dose bolus IL-2 and interferon (Rosenberg et al., 1989). However, subsequent studies have indicated that this combination is more toxic and no more effective than IL-2 alone (Bukowski et al., 1997; Dutcher et al., 1997; Ravaud et al., 1994; Tourani et al., 1998, 2003). A multicenter, randomized phase III study compared the efficacy of intermediate-dose IL-2 administered by continuous intravenous infusion with interferon-α or the combination in 425 patients with metastatic clear cell RCC (Negrier et al., 1998). **Although the combination of IL-2 and interferon resulted in a higher response rate (18.6%) and 1-year event-free survival (EFS; 20%) compared with IL-2 (overall response rate 6.5%, 1-year EFS 15%) or interferon (overall response rate 7.5%, 1-year EFS 12%) alone, there was no significant difference in survival between the groups.** Combination therapy also resulted in higher toxicity than either agent given alone. Regimens combining IL-2 and cytotoxic chemotherapy (particularly 5-fluorouracil [5-FU]) have been the subject of numerous studies. Unfortunately, reports of high response rates in initial studies (49% in a study using IL-2, interferon, and 5-FU) could not be reproduced in later studies (Atzpodien et al., 1993; Dutcher et al., 2000; Ellerhorst et al., 1997; Negrier et al., 2000). Similarly, despite the promise of preclinical and early clinical studies, the addition of ex vivo expanded tumor-infiltrating lymphocytes or lymphokine-activated killer cells to high-dose IL-2 has not reliably demonstrated improved clinical benefit, and these approaches have been largely abandoned (Figlin et al., 1999; Law et al., 1995; Rosenberg et al., 1993).

Given the considerable toxicity associated with high-dose IL-2 and the relatively small proportion of patients who derive benefit from this therapy, identification of predictors of response and long-term outcome has received considerable attention. The predictive value of a variety of histologic, clinical, laboratory, and molecular parameters has been studied. **Patients with clear cell RCC appear most likely to benefit from IL-2 therapy,** although the exceedingly small number of patients with non–clear cell histologies typically enrolled in studies of IL-2 makes it difficult to draw definitive conclusions about efficacy in this subgroup of patients. **Patient performance status, number of metastatic sites, site of metastases, prior nephrectomy, and time from nephrectomy to systemic therapy are some of the factors that may affect outcome.** In one study, patients with more than one site of metastasis, those with metastatic disease within 1 year of diagnosis, and those with liver metastases had the worst outcome, with a median survival of 6 months (Negrier et al., 2002). Overexpression of carbonic anhydrase IX (CAIX or G250) has been observed in a retrospective analysis to be associated with a higher probability of response to IL-2 (Atkins et al., 2005); however, a prospective trial of 120 advanced kidney cancer patients designed to evaluate the impact of prespecified "good-risk" clinical features or biomarkers (i.e., CAIX) on outcome revealed that CAIX expression was not predictive of response (McDermott et al., 2015). **The role of cytokine therapy in the current management of kidney cancer has changed with the availability of novel inhibitors of VEGF and mTOR pathways, as well as immune checkpoint inhibitors**

TABLE 104.7 Summary of Results From Selected Randomized Trials of Interleukin-2 in Metastatic Renal Cell Carcinoma

STUDY	TREATMENT ARMS	NO. OF PATIENTS	DOSE, ROUTE, AND SCHEDULE	RESPONSE ORR	P	OVERALL SURVIVAL MEDIAN (mo)	P
Négrier et al., 1998	IL-2	138	18 × 10⁶ IU/m²/d × 5 days, CIV	6.5		12	
	IFN	147	18 × 10⁶ IU three times a week, SC	7.5		13	0.55
	IL-2 + IFN	140	18 × 10⁶ IU/m²/d × 5 days, CIV + 6 × 10⁶ IU three times a week, SC	18.6	0.01	17	
Yang et al., 2003b	IL-2	156	720,000 U/kg every 8 hours × 5 days, IV bolus	21		NA	
	IL-2	150	72,000 U/kg every 8 hours × 5 days, IV bolus	13	0.048	NA	0.41
	IL-2	94	250,000 U/d × 5 days, SC, week 1; 125,000 U/d × 5 days, SC, weeks 2 to 6	10	0.033	NA	0.38
McDermott et al., 2005	IL-2	96	600,000 U/kg every 8 hours × 5 days, IV bolus	23		17	
	IL-2 + IFN	96	5 × 10⁶ IU/m² every 8 hours × 3, then 5 × 10⁶ IU/m²/d × 5 days/week, SC + 5 × 10⁶ IU three times a week, SC	10	0.018	13	0.21

CIV, Continuous intravenous infusion; *IFN*, interferon-α; *IL-2*, interleukin-2; *IV*, intravenous; *NA*, not available; *ORR*, overall response rate; *SC*, subcutaneous.

with activity in clear cell RCC. Single-agent interferon, once the standard in many institutions, is no longer used in the treatment of clear cell RCC. However, given the inability of newer targeted agents to induce durable responses, high-dose intravenous IL-2 remains a reasonable option in most carefully selected patients with metastatic clear cell RCC.

Allogeneic Hematopoietic Stem Cell Transplantation

Allogeneic hematopoietic stem cell transplantation allows the replacement of host or recipient immune and hematopoietic systems with those of a healthy, HLA-compatible donor. The therapeutic potential of hematopoietic stem cell transplantation lies largely in the ability of the transplanted donor graft to generate an allogeneic antitumor immune response known as the graft-versus-tumor effect. This approach has been used successfully with curative intent in a variety of hematologic malignancies (Thomas et al., 1977; Weiden et al., 1979, 1981). The ability of a variety of immune-based approaches to induce remissions in patients with RCC and evidence suggesting that the host immune system in these patients may be compromised and/or tolerant to tumor cells have led several investigators to evaluate allogeneic hematopoietic stem cell transplantation in kidney cancer.

The approach was initially studied by investigators at the National Heart, Lung and Blood Institute exploring the efficacy of reduced intensity hematopoietic stem cell transplantation in patients with treatment-refractory metastatic RCC. Eligible patients underwent reduced intensity conditioning with cyclophosphamide (120 mg/kg) and fludarabine (125 mg/m^2) followed by infusion of a granulocyte colony-stimulating factor–mobilized peripheral blood stem cell graft from a 5/6 or 6/6 HLA-matched sibling donor. The initial experience with hematopoietic stem cell transplantation in metastatic RCC was published by Childs et al. (2000). Ten of the first 19 patients treated with this transplant approach had tumor shrinkage, including 3 who had a complete response and 7 who had a partial response. As more recently reported, 74 patients have undergone hematopoietic stem cell transplantation for RCC at the National Institutes of Health. Of these, 73 patients have demonstrated durable engraftment, achieving 100% donor T cell chimerism by day 100 post-transplant. Twenty-nine of 74 (39%) patients have had a disease response, including 7 complete (9%) and 22 partial responders (30%) (Takahashi et al., 2008). In one responder, T cells recognizing an endogenous retroviral element (HERV-E) were identified and believed to mediate antitumor responses. Preliminary data suggest that disease response after hematopoietic stem cell transplantation is a clinically meaningful phenomenon because regression of metastatic RCC appears to be associated with a trend toward improved survival. Survival in nonresponders has been less than 6 months, in contrast to those achieving a partial response who survived a median 2.5 years post-transplant. Several durable responses have been noted, and the first patient who underwent a transplant remains in complete remission more than 10 years after the procedure.

Hematopoietic stem cell transplantation is associated with a variety of adverse events typically associated with conditioning chemotherapy (e.g., pancytopenia), a variety of opportunistic infections, and graft-versus-host disease (GVHD). Eight patients in the aforementioned series died of transplant-related causes (transplant-related mortality of 11%), most because of GVHD and its attendant infectious complications. Several other trials have since confirmed the efficacy of this approach in RCC (Table 104.8; Artz et al., 2005; Barkholt et al., 2006; Bregni et al., 2002; Rini et al., 2001, 2002). However, a Cancer and Leukemia Group B (CALGB) intergroup trial evaluating the feasibility of performing hematopoietic stem cell transplantation for metastatic RCC in a multi-institutional setting in the United States reported no responses in 22 patients undergoing hematopoietic stem cell transplantation from an HLA-matched sibling donor after cyclophosphamide/fludarabine–based conditioning (Rini et al., 2006). Median OS was only 5½ months, with most patients dying of disease progression (median time to progression of 3 months). Inclusion of a number of patients with multiple adverse prognostic factors, sparing use of donor lymphocyte infusions (only 2/22 patients received donor lymphocyte infusions despite disease progression in the majority), and inclusion of patients with non–clear cell histology are some of the factors that may account for the poor outcome observed in this trial. This trial clearly highlights the importance of appropriate patient selection and the need for identifying prognostic factors likely to predict for a favorable outcome. In a European multicenter study of 106 patients undergoing transplantation, chronic GVHD, good performance status (Karnofsky score = 80), administration of donor lymphocyte infusions, and fewer than three sites of metastatic disease were identified as factors favorably affecting survival (Barkholt et al., 2006). Given the high morbidity and mortality with this approach, careful patient selection is of great importance. With the advent of agents targeting the VEGF pathway and immune checkpoint inhibitors, **hematopoietic stem cell transplantation is no longer being explored as a viable therapeutic approach in RCC. However, the recognition that specific RCC-associated antigens may serve as targets for cytotoxic T cell responses provides the basis for exploring antigen-specific adoptive cellular therapy approaches.**

Immune "Checkpoint" Inhibitors

The host immune response to tumors is a highly complex process that is regulated at multiple levels. The interplay between multiple stimulatory and inhibitory processes determines the nature and extent of the antitumor response generated by the host immune system. Over the last few years, it has become increasingly evident that

TABLE 104.8 Summary of Results From Selected Trials of Allogeneic Hematopoietic Stem Cell Transplantation in Metastatic Renal Cell Carcinoma

STUDIES	CONDITIONING AGENTS	GVHD PROPHYLAXIS	aGVHD (II–IV)	cGVHD	TRM	RESPONSE (PR OR CR)
Childs et al., 2000; Takahashi et al., 2008	Cy + Flu	CSP (First 25 patients) CSP + MMF (subsequent patients)	55%	21%	11%	39%
Artz et al., 2005; Rini et al., 2001, 2002	Cy + Flu	Tacro + MMF	22%	39%	14%	22%
Bregni et al., 2002	Cy + Flu + Thiotepa	CSP + MTX	86%	71%	0%	57%
Barkholt et al., 2006	Multiple fludarabine-based regimens	CSP ± MMF or MTX	40%	33%	16%	32%
Rini et al., 2006	Flu + Cy	Tacro + MTX	32%	23%	9%	0%

aGVHD, Acute graft-versus-host disease; *ATG*, antithymocyte globulin; *cGVHD*, chronic graft-versus-host disease; *CR*, complete response; *CSP*, cyclosporine; *Cy*, cyclophosphamide; *GVHD*, graft-versus-host disease; *MMF*, mycophenolate mofetil; *MTX*, methotrexate; *PR*, partial response; *Tacro*, tacrolimus; *TRM*, treatment-related mortality.

several inhibitory receptors on effector immune cells such as CD8+ T-lymphocytes play a key role in tightly regulating the immune response to tumors; furthermore, antitumor responses can be downregulated by activation of T cell receptors such as cytotoxic T-lymphocyte–associated antigen (CTLA-4) and those mediating programmed cell death (PD-1).

Pharmacologic targeting of immune checkpoints such as CTLA-4 and the PD-1 axis has been successfully explored in many solid tumors, including RCC. A single-arm phase II study of ipilimumab, a monoclonal antibody targeting CTLA-4, demonstrated activity in patients with clear cell activity, including in some who had previously progressed after IL-2 therapy (Yang et al., 2007). The most notable side effects associated with this agent included autoimmune events such as enteritis and hypophysitis. Although autoimmune adverse events were highly predictive of response, they were sufficiently severe (grade 3–4 in up to one-third of the patients), dampening enthusiasm for further development of this agent in RCC.

More recently, PD-1 and its ligands (PD-L1, PD-L2) have attracted attention as potential antitumor targets. Although PD-1 is expressed on CD+ T cells, PD-L1 and PD-L2 are expressed on the surface of tumor cells, macrophages, and other cells; patients whose tumors contain PD-1–positive tumor-infiltrating lymphocytes (TIL) are more likely to have larger tumors, higher-grade tumors, advanced-stage RCC, and sarcomatoid differentiation than patients without PD-1–positive TILs (Thompson et al., 2007). Engagement of PD-1 on T cells by its ligand leads to downregulation of antigen-driven immune responses (Fife et al., 2009; Sznol and Chen, 2013).

A number of antibodies targeting the PD-1/PD-L1 checkpoint have been evaluated clinically with several approved for use in a variety of malignancies by the FDA. In a large phase I study with multiple expansion cohorts, patients with advanced melanoma, non–small-cell lung cancer, castration-resistant prostate cancer, colorectal cancer, or renal cancer were treated with nivolumab (anti-PD-1 antibody) (Topalian et al., 2012). A total of 33 RCC patients were enrolled, and 9 patients (27%) had an objective response. Despite the fairly short follow-up, several durable responses were evident, with 5 patients demonstrating a response lasting 1 year or more. Furthermore, stable disease lasting 24 weeks or more was seen in an additional 9 patients (27%). Interestingly, pretreatment tumor specimens from 42 patients (5 RCC) were analyzed for PD-L1 expression on the surface of tumor cells. None of the 17 patients with PD-L1 negative tumors experienced a response, whereas 9/25 (36%) with PD-L1 expression had an objective response, suggesting that PD-L1 expression should be further evaluated as a predictive biomarker. As anticipated, several patients experienced adverse events of possible autoimmune cause, including diarrhea, hypophysitis, and vitiligo.

A second phase I, dose-escalating study evaluating inhibition of the PD-1 checkpoint was conducted with BMS-936559, a PD-L1 specific monoclonal antibody, in patients with advanced solid tumors (Brahmer et al., 2012). Out of 75 patients, 17 had RCC. Two out of 17 RCC patients (12%) had an objective response, lasting 4 and 17 months, respectively. Seven additional patients (41%) had stable disease lasting at least 24 weeks.

Based on the encouraging data from early phase studies, nivolumab has been evaluated in large randomized phase III studies in treatment-naive patients with metastatic clear cell RCC and in those who have progressed on prior therapy targeting the VEGF/VEGFR axis. The first of these studies (CheckMate 025), enrolled 821 patients with advanced RCC with a clear cell component who had progressed on treatment with one or two antiangiogenic agents (Motzer et al., 2015). Patients were randomized to receive either 3 mg/kg of nivolumab every 2 weeks or 10 mg of everolimus daily. The primary end point of the study was overall survival, whereas secondary objectives included evaluation of progression-free survival (PFS), overall response rate, and safety. Although the PFS was not different between the two arms [4.6 months (95% CI 3.7–5.4) with nivolumab and 4.4 months (95% CI 3.7–5.5) with everolimus (hazard ratio, 0.88; 95% CI 0.75–1.03; P = 0.11)], nivolumab was associated with a higher response rate (25% vs. 5%; odds ratio 5.98; 95% CI 3.68–9.72; P < 0.001) and improved OS. **The median OS was 25 months (95% CI 21.8–not estimable) for nivolumab and 19.6 months (95% CI 17.6–23.1) for everolimus (HR 0.73; 98.5% CI 0.57–0.93; P = 0.002) (Fig. 104.4). Nivolumab was generally well tolerated, with 19% of the patients experiencing a grade 3 to 4 adverse event compared with 37% in patients treated with everolimus.** The adverse event profile was consistent with that seen in other studies of similar checkpoint inhibitors and included a variety of autoimmune phenomena and fatigue. **Based on these data, nivolumab as a single agent is a reasonable option in patients who have progressed on prior therapy with inhibitors of the VEGF axis. These data also provided the impetus for evaluating PD-1/PD-L1 checkpoint inhibitors in the front-line setting, largely in combination with other immune checkpoint inhibitors and antagonists of the VEGF axis.**

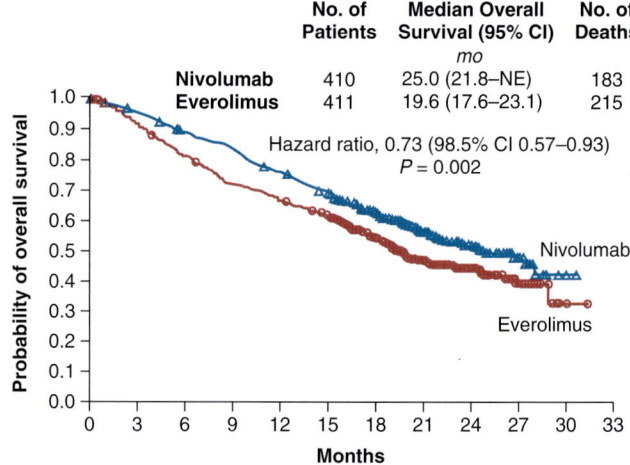

Fig. 104.4. Kaplan-Meier estimates of overall survival in 821 previously treated patients with metastatic clear cell renal cell cancer receiving either nivolumab or everolimus. (Motzer RJ, Escudier B, McDermott D, et al.: Nivolumab versus everolimus in advanced renal-cell carcinoma. *N Engl J Med* 373:1803–1813, 2015.)

MOLECULAR BASIS FOR TARGETED APPROACHES IN CLEAR CELL RENAL CELL CARCINOMA

The development of antagonists of the VEGF pathway in the treatment of clear cell RCC is an often-cited paradigm in the evolution of rational targeted therapeutic strategies and represents a logical progression from identification of an oncogenic cellular pathway to rational drug design and structured clinical evaluation. The earliest clues to the central role played by VEGF in renal oncogenesis came from studies attempting to identify the genetic basis of the von Hippel-Lindau familial kidney cancer syndrome. **In the early 1990s, investigators at the National Cancer Institute studying families with von-Hippel-Lindau disease used genetic linkage analysis to identify germline mutations or deletions in the *VHL* gene as the basis for this disease** (Latif et al., 1993). Individuals carrying germline *VHL* mutations are at increased risk for developing tumors in multiple organs, including bilateral, multifocal clear cell kidney cancer. **The *VHL* gene is a classic tumor suppressor gene, with inactivation of the normal *VHL* allele in affected tissues by a somatic "second hit" required for tumor formation.**

The *VHL* gene resides on the short arm of chromosome 3 and encodes the VHL protein, which can be synthesized as two alternatively spliced variants (Gnarra et al., 1996; Iliopoulos et al., 1998; Latif et al., 1993; Linehan, 2003). One of the better understood functions of the VHL protein is its association with elongins B and C and CUL2 to form a protein complex that tags certain cellular proteins for delivery to and degradation by the ubiquitin system (Duan et al., 1995; Kaelin, 2004; Linehan, 2003; Pause et al., 1997; Stebbins et al., 1999). Proteins targeted for ubiquitin-mediated degradation include the α subunits of a group of transcriptionally active proteins known as hypoxia-inducible factors (HIFs) (Cockman et al., 2000; Iliopoulos et al., 1996; Ivan et al., 2001; Jaakkola et al., 2001; Maxwell et al., 1999; Ohh et al., 2000; Pause et al., 1997). In cells with intact VHL function, HIF levels are controlled primarily by ambient oxygen tension. In normoxic conditions, hydroxylation of key proline residues on HIF promotes its association with the VHL/elongin/CUL complex and subsequent degradation; conversely, hypoxia impedes prolyl hydroxylation of HIF and its subsequent degradation, leading to intracellular accumulation of HIF α subunits. **Mutations in *VHL* interfere with its binding to either HIF or elongin/CUL2 and promote HIF accumulation even under normoxia. HIF accumulation, in turn, leads to the upregulation of a variety of proangiogenic** and growth factors, including VEGF, platelet-derived growth factor (PDGF), transforming growth factor-α, Glut-1, and erythropoietin, which are believed to play critical roles in the development and progression of clear cell RCC (Fig. 104.5; Duan et al., 1995; Iliopoulos et al., 1996; Kaelin, 2004; Linehan et al., 2007). Although originally identified as a germline defect in von Hippel-Lindau families, evidence of somatic *VHL* inactivation by mutation or promoter hypermethylation has been observed in a high proportion of sporadic clear cell tumors (91% in one series) (Gnarra et al., 1996; Herman et al., 1994; Nickerson et al., 2008; Zhuang et al., 1996a,b). The recognition of VHL loss as a central event in renal oncogenesis has paved the way for the development of novel agents targeting components of this pathway in the management of metastatic clear cell RCC.

TARGETED MOLECULAR AGENTS IN CLEAR CELL RENAL CELL CARCINOMA

Antagonists of the Vascular Endothelial Growth Factor Pathway

Bevacizumab

Bevacizumab, a humanized monoclonal antibody against VEGF-A, was the first VEGF pathway antagonist used in clinical trials to test the hypothesis that modulation of aberrantly expressed components of the VHL pathway would be associated with clinical activity in clear cell RCC. In a three-arm phase II study, patients with metastatic clear cell RCC whose disease had progressed after prior cytokine therapy were randomized to receive either one of two dose levels of bevacizumab (10 mg/kg or 3 mg/kg administered every 2 weeks intravenously) or placebo (Table 104.9; Yang et al., 2003). **An interim efficacy analysis performed after 116 patients (of a planned 240 patients) were enrolled in the study demonstrated a significantly longer PFS in patients assigned to 10 mg/kg bevacizumab compared with those receiving placebo (4.8 vs 2.5 months, $P < 0.001$).** There was no corresponding improvement in OS, although the crossover design used in this trial (patients progressing on placebo were allowed to cross over to the bevacizumab arm) may have influenced this outcome. The overall response rate in patients receiving bevacizumab was modest (objective response rate of 10%, all in patients assigned to the 10-mg/kg dose). The agent was well tolerated; bleeding, hypertension, fatigue, and proteinuria were some of the more common adverse events reported. Single-agent bevacizumab has not been compared with either cytokines (often used in first-line treatment before the advent of VEGF pathway antagonists) or other VEGF pathway antagonists such as sunitinib in prospective trials.

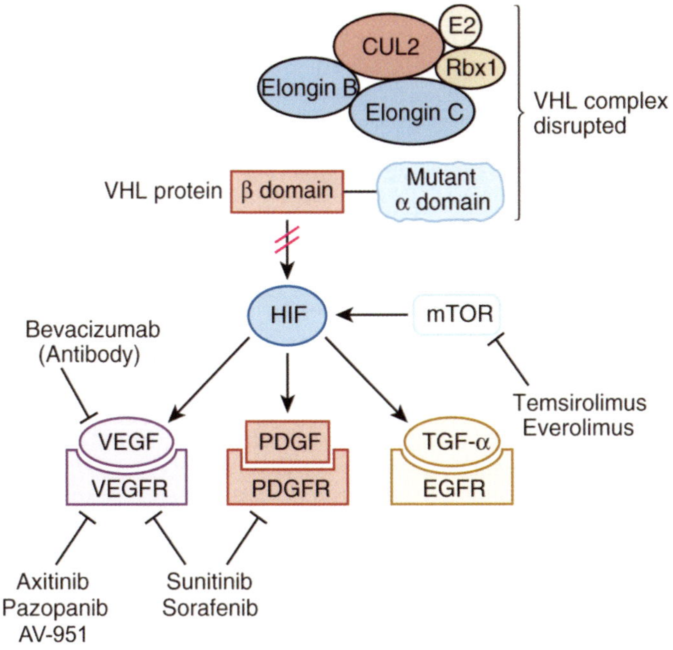

Fig. 104.5. Targeting the VHL pathway in clear cell renal cell carcinoma. Loss of VHL activity leads to accumulation of HIF and several proangiogenic and growth factors that can serve as targets for anticancer drugs. HIF can also be upregulated by mTOR, which promotes HIF translation. (Modified from Linehan WM, Bratslavsky G, Pinto PA, et al.: Molecular diagnosis and therapy of kidney cancer. *Annu Rev Med* 61:329–343, 2010.)

TABLE 104.9 Summary of Selected Studies of Bevacizumab-Based Regimens in Metastatic Renal Cell Carcinoma

STUDY	AGENT(S)	PHASE	STUDY POPULATION	NO. OF PATIENTS	OVERALL RESPONSE RATE (RECIST)	MEDIAN PFS (MO)	MEDIAN OS (MO)
Yang et al., 2003a	Bev (10 mg/kg) vs. Bev (3 mg/kg) vs. placebo	Randomized, 3-arm phase II	Cytokine-refractory clear cell	116	10% vs. 0 vs. 0	4.8 vs. 3.0 vs. 2.5	
Escudier et al., 2007b	Bev + IFN-α vs. IFN-α	Randomized phase III	Previously untreated clear cell	649	31% vs. 13%	10.2 vs. 5.4	NR vs. 19.8
Rini et al., 2008a	Bev + IFN-α vs. IFN-α	Randomized phase III	Previously untreated clear cell	732	26% vs. 13%	8.5 vs. 5.2	NA
Bukowski et al., 2007	Bev + Erlotinib vs. Bev	Randomized phase II	Previously untreated clear cell	104	14% vs. 13%	9.9 vs. 8.5	20 vs. NR

Bev, Bevacizumab; *IFN-α*, interferon-α; *NA*, not available; *NR*, not reached; *OS*, overall survival; *PFS*, progression-free survival.

Several strategies for improving the efficacy of bevacizumab have been explored, including combination with cytokines (interferon-α) and other targeted agents (e.g., erlotinib, a small molecule inhibitor of epidermal growth factor receptor tyrosine kinase activity). A single-arm phase II study of bevacizumab plus erlotinib showed promising activity with an overall response rate of 25% (higher than would be expected with bevacizumab alone based on historical data) and median PFS of 11 months (Hainsworth et al., 2005). However, a subsequent randomized phase II study failed to demonstrate the superiority of this combination (median PFS 9.9 months) over bevacizumab alone (median PFS 8.5 months, $P = 0.58$) in patients with advanced clear cell RCC (Bukowski et al., 2007). Two large randomized phase III studies have compared the combination of bevacizumab and interferon-α to interferon-α alone (see Table 104.9). In a Cancer and Leukemia Group B study (CALGB 90206) of 752 patients with previously untreated metastatic clear cell RCC randomized to one of two treatment arms, a higher response rate (25.5% vs. 13.1%, $P < 0.0001$) and PFS (8.5 months vs. 5.2 months, $P < 0.0001$) were observed in patients assigned to bevacizumab plus interferon-α compared with those receiving interferon-α alone (Rini et al., 2008). A multicenter European trial (AVOREN) with a similar design also reported similar results with PFS (10.2 vs. 5.4 months, $P = 0.0001$) and objective response rate (31% vs. 13%) favoring the combination arm (Escudier et al., 2007). Updated survival data from both trials were recently reported, demonstrating no improvement in OS associated with the addition of bevacizumab to interferon (Escudier et al., 2010; Rini et al., 2010).

Although neither study permitted crossover of patients assigned to interferon-α at progression, a significant number of patients (>60%) subsequently received anticancer therapy off protocol, potentially confounding OS analysis. Both trials reported a higher incidence of some grade 3 adverse events, such as hypertension, fatigue, anorexia, and asthenia in patients receiving combination therapy. The CALGB and Avoren trials were large, well-designed, and well-conducted multicenter studies that suggest that the addition of bevacizumab to interferon may be associated with clinical benefit (i.e., improvement in PFS). However, these trials did not include an arm with bevacizumab alone (because insufficient evidence of single-agent activity at the time these trials were designed to justify a bevacizumab-only arm), making it difficult to determine if inclusion of interferon in this regimen, with its attendant toxicities, adds meaningful clinical benefit. Interestingly, the median PFS observed in the combination arm of the CALGB trial (8½ months) is similar to that observed with bevacizumab alone in a phase II trial of previously untreated patients with clear cell RCC (Bukowski et al., 2007). Last, bevacizumab (either alone or in combination with interferon) has not been compared prospectively with VEGF receptor (VEGFR) antagonists such as sunitinib or pazopanib. Bevacizumab was not widely used as a single agent in the initial therapy for metastatic clear cell RCC but is being explored in combination studies with other agents, including inhibitors of the PD-1/PD-L1 checkpoint, because of its favorable toxicity profile. Ongoing and future trials may help determine the best use of this agent in the overall management of patients with clear cell RCC.

Sorafenib

Sorafenib is an oral receptor kinase inhibitor with activity against VEGFR2, PDGF receptor-β, and raf-1. A phase II trial using a randomized discontinuation design provided initial evidence that sorafenib is active in RCC (see Table 104.10; Ratain et al., 2006). Subsequently, a global, multicenter, placebo-controlled randomized phase III trial with 903 patients (the TARGET study) was undertaken to evaluate the efficacy of sorafenib in patients with metastatic RCC who had previously received cytokine therapy (Escudier et al., 2007). This trial echoed the results seen in the phase II trial, with patients randomized to receive sorafenib experiencing a longer PFS (median 5.5 months) versus those receiving placebo (2.8 months, $P < 0.01$) at a planned interim analysis. Mature survival data from this trial were subsequently presented and demonstrated no significant difference in OS between the two groups (17.8 months for sorafenib vs. 15.3 months with placebo, $P = 0.146$) in an intent-to-treat analysis (Escudier et al., 2009). The side effect profile of sorafenib is comparable to that of other agents in this class and includes hypertension, fatigue, rash, hand-foot syndrome, and diarrhea. The efficacy of sorafenib in the first-line setting was investigated in a randomized phase II study that assigned 189 previously untreated patients with metastatic clear cell RCC to receive either sorafenib or interferon-α (Escudier et al., 2009). Although patients receiving sorafenib had a higher likelihood of achieving tumor regression (68% vs. 39%), PFS in the two groups was nearly identical (median 5.7 months for sorafenib vs. 5.6 months for interferon, $P = NS$) (Table 104.10). Although sorafenib is FDA-approved for the treatment of advanced kidney cancer, it is infrequently, if ever, used in the management of these patients in view of the plethora of more effective treatment options available.

Sunitinib

Sunitinib is an oral VEGFR kinase inhibitor widely used until recently in the initial treatment of metastatic clear cell RCC. It is a potent inhibitor of VEGFR2, PDGFR-β, c-KIT, and fms-like tyrosine kinase-3. As with sorafenib, simultaneous targeting of VEGF and PDGF pathways by this agent is likely to act synergistically in inhibiting tumor angiogenesis, by directly disrupting VEGF-mediated vascular endothelial development and proliferation and

TABLE 104.10 Summary of Selected Studies of Sorafenib in Metastatic Renal Cell Carcinoma

STUDIES	AGENT(S)	PHASE	STUDY POPULATION	NO. OF PATIENTS	OVERALL RESPONSE RATE (RECIST)	MEDIAN PFS (MO)	MEDIAN OS (MO)
Ratain et al., 2006	Sorafenib vs. placebo	Phase II randomized discontinuation	Treatment-refractory, all histologic subtypes	202		6 vs. 1.5	NA
Escudier et al., 2007a, 2009a	Sorafenib vs. placebo	Randomized phase III	Cytokine-refractory clear cell	903	10% vs. 2%	5.5 vs. 2.8	17.8 vs. 15.2
Escudier et al., 2009b	Sorafenib vs. IFN-α	Randomized phase II	Previously untreated clear cell	189	5% vs. 9%	5.7 vs. 5.6	NA

IFN-α, Interferon-α; *NA,* not available; *NR,* not reached; *OS,* overall survival; *PFS,* progression-free survival.

TABLE 104.11 Summary of Selected Studies of Sunitinib in Metastatic Renal Cell Carcinoma

STUDIES	AGENT(S)	PHASE	STUDY POPULATION	NO. OF PATIENTS	OVERALL RESPONSE RATE (RECIST)	MEDIAN PFS (MO)	MEDIAN OS (MO)
Motzer et al., 2007, 2009	Sunitinib vs. IFN-α	Randomized phase III	Previously untreated clear cell	750	31% vs. 6%	11 vs. 5	26.4 vs. 21.08
Motzer et al., 2006a	Sunitinib	Single-arm phase II	Cytokine-refractory clear cell	63	40%	8.7	NA
Motzer et al., 2006b	Sunitinib	Single-arm phase II	Cytokine-refractory clear cell	106	44%	8.1	NA

NA, Not available; OS, overall survival; PFS, progression-free survival.

by interfering with vascular pericyte function, which is dependent on the integrity of PDGF signaling. Initial evaluation of sunitinib was undertaken with two single-arm open-label phase II trials in patients with metastatic RCC, most of whom had previously received cytokine therapy (Motzer et al., 2006a,b). Sunitinib was administered orally at a dose of 50 mg/d during the first 4 weeks of a 6-week cycle on both trials (Table 104.11). Remarkably high overall response rates (30% to 40%) with a median PFS of more than 8½ months were observed in these trials, leading to the approval of this agent for treatment of advanced RCC by the FDA.

A landmark phase III randomized trial comparing sunitinib with interferon-α as first-line therapy in patients with metastatic clear cell RCC further demonstrated the activity of sunitinib in this patient population (Motzer et al., 2007). In this study, 750 patients were randomized to receive either sunitinib or interferon-α. **An interim analysis based on independent, third-party radiologic assessment demonstrated a significantly superior PFS (median 11 months vs. 5 months, $P = 0.001$) and overall response rate (31% vs. 6%, $P = 0.001$) favoring the sunitinib arm** (Fig. 104.6). Gastrointestinal events, particularly diarrhea, dermatologic manifestations such as rash and hand-foot syndrome, constitutional symptoms such as fatigue and asthenia, and hypertension were the most commonly adverse events associated with sunitinib, whereas bone marrow suppression and hypothyroidism were other notable side effects. Sunitinib also performed better than interferon in a quality-of-life assessment conducted as part of the study. Mature survival data from this study were subsequently reported and demonstrated a clear trend toward superior OS in the sunitinib study arm based on an intent-to-treat analysis (median OS 26.4 vs. 21.8 months, $P = 0.051$) (Motzer et al., 2009). Based on these data, sunitinib was widely used in the initial management of metastatic clear cell RCC patients in the United States. **However, recent studies have demonstrated the superiority of PD-1/PD-L1 checkpoint inhibitor–based combinations over sunitinib in the first-line setting, particularly in patients with intermediate and poor prognosis RCC. Currently, sunitinib is largely used in the treatment of good prognosis patients or those unable to receive checkpoint inhibitor-based therapy.**

Pazopanib

Agents such as sunitinib and sorafenib have activity against a wide array of targets, some of which may not be relevant in clear cell RCC. Although these agents are relatively well tolerated when compared with conventional cytotoxic chemotherapy, dose reductions and termination of treatment resulting from toxicity are not infrequently warranted in patients receiving these drugs. A variety of newer agents with selective activity against the VEGFR family were evaluated as a possible means of diminishing the side effects associated with therapy without compromising efficacy (Table 104.12). One agent in this class, pazopanib, is a potent inhibitor of the VEGF receptors but retains activity against PDGFR. Pazopanib was evaluated in a randomized, double-blind, placebo-controlled phase III trial in patients with metastatic clear cell RCC who had received no or one prior cytokine-based therapy (Sternberg et al., 2010). **In the 435 patients randomized (2:1) to receive either pazopanib or placebo, PFS (median 9.4 months vs. 4.2 months, $P = 0.0000001$) and response rates (30% vs. 3%) clearly favored the pazopanib study arm. Pazopanib was associated with superior outcomes in the treatment-naive ($N = 233$; median PFS 11.1 vs. 2.8 months; HR 0.40; 95% CI 0.27–0.60; $P < 0.0001$), and the cytokine-pretreated subpopulations ($N = 202$; median PFS, 7.4 vs. 4.2 months; HR 0.54; 95% CI 0.35–0.84; $P < 0.001$). Furthermore, reported toxicities were mild, with very few grade 3 and 4 adverse events encountered.** However, mature survival data from this trial demonstrated OS was not significantly better in the pazopanib arm compared with placebo (median OS 22.9 vs. 20.5 months, respectively; hazard ratio [HR] = 0.91; 95% confidence interval [CI], 0.71–1.16; one-sided $P = 0.224$) (Sternberg et al., 2013).

The efficacy and/or tolerability of pazopanib and sunitinib were subsequently compared in at least two studies. In a recently published multicenter phase III randomized trial (COMPARZ) of 1110 patients with previously untreated metastatic clear cell kidney cancer comparing the efficacy and safety of the two agents, patients were randomized to receive either pazopanib 800 mg once daily ($N = 557$) or a standard sunitinib regimen (50 mg once daily for 4 weeks followed by 2 weeks with no treatment, $N = 553$) (Motzer et al., 2013). The primary end point was PFS, and the study was powered to evaluate non-inferiority of pazopanib versus sunitinib. Secondary end points included OS, quality of life, and safety. Median PFS in patients treated with pazopanib was 8.4 months compared with 9.5 for sunitinib. Based on predefined criteria, PFS with pazopanib was determined to be noninferior to sunitinib (HR 1.05; 95% CI 0.90–1.22). Overall survival was comparable in the two groups with a median OS of 28.4 months in the pazopanib group versus 29.3 months in the sunitinib group (HR 0.91; 95% CI 0.76–1.08). However, differences were noted in the adverse event profile and patient tolerability between the two groups. Patients treated with sunitinib had a higher incidence of fatigue (63% vs. 55%), thrombocytopenia (78% vs. 41%), and hand-foot syndrome (50% vs. 29%), whereas increased levels of alanine aminotransferase were more common in the pazopanib group (60% vs. 43%). Quality-of-life assessments related to fatigue or soreness in the mouth, throat, and hands or feet during the first 6 months of treatment favored pazopanib.

Results from a second, smaller study evaluating patient preference between pazopanib and sunitinib (PISCES) also demonstrated that pazopanib was generally better tolerated (Escudier et al., 2014). One hundred and sixty eight previously untreated patients with metastatic clear cell RCC were randomized to receive pazopanib for 10 weeks followed by a 2-week washout and then sunitinib for 10 weeks (on a 4 week on/2 week off schedule) or vice versa. After completing 22 weeks of therapy, the patients were asked to complete a questionnaire assessing which agent they preferred. Pazopanib was preferred by 70% of the patients, although sunitinib was preferred by 22% of the patients (8% had no specific preference between the agents). **Based on these data, pazopanib is a reasonable alternative to sunitinib in those cases in which the latter would be a suitable therapeutic**

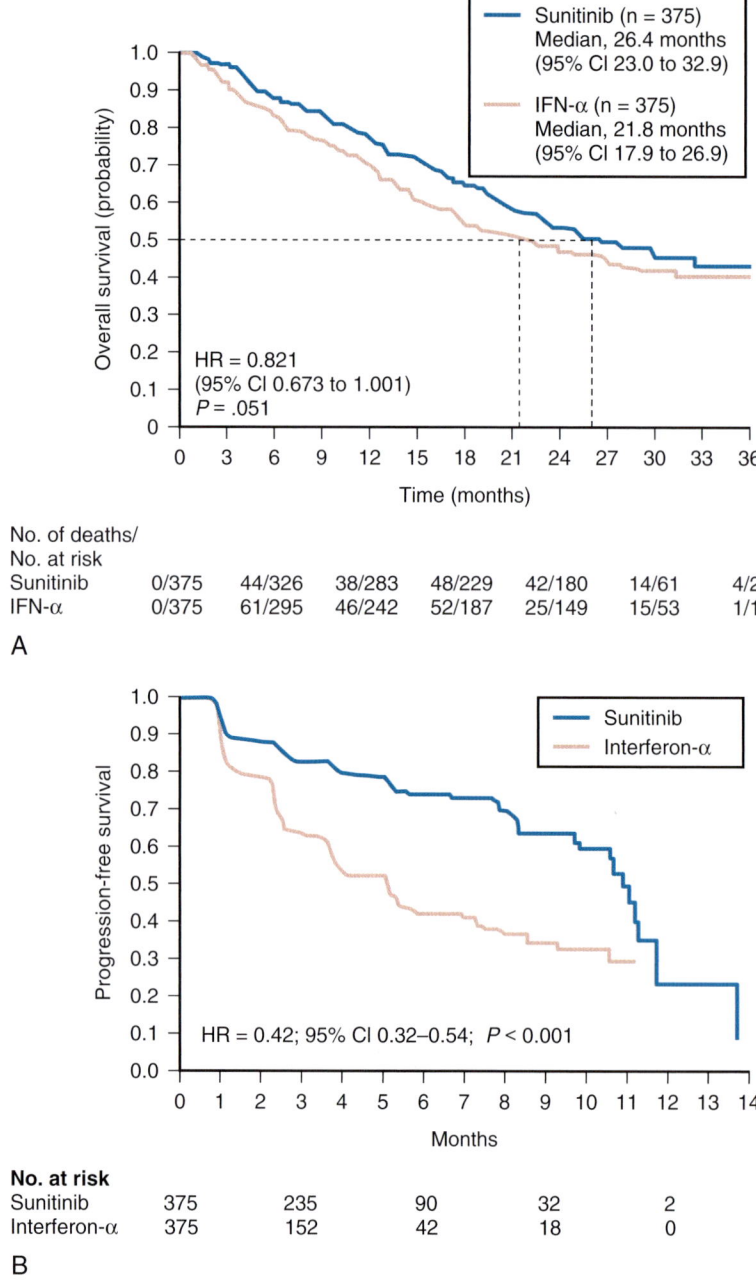

Fig. 104.6. Kaplan-Meier analysis of overall survival (A) and progression-free survival (B) in 750 previously untreated patients with metastatic renal cell carcinoma receiving either sunitinib or interferon-α. (Data from Motzer RJ, Hutson TE, Tomczak P, et al.: Overall survival and updated results for sunitinib compared with interferon alfa in patients with metastatic renal cell carcinoma. *J Clin Oncol* 27:3584–3590, 2009; and Motzer RJ, Hutson TE, Tomczak P, et al.: Sunitinib versus interferon alfa in metastatic renal-cell carcinoma. *N Engl J Med* 356:115–124, 2007.)

option. Although pazopanib appears to be better tolerated than sunitinib by the majority of patients, it appears to be associated with an increased incidence of hepatotoxicity and must be used with caution in patients at risk for this complication. At least some patients found sunitinib more tolerable than pazopanib. With the advent of effective combination therapies containing immune checkpoint inhibitors, the role of single-agent pazopanib is limited, particularly in the first-line setting, largely to good-risk patients.

Axitinib

Axitinib is a highly selective oral small molecule tyrosine kinase inhibitor of VEGFR1, VEGFR2, and VEGFR3. In a phase II trial of axitinib in 52 patients with advanced kidney cancer, an overall response rate of 44%, including two complete responses (4%), and a median time to progression of 15.7 months were reported (Rixe et al., 2007). Most patients treated on this study displayed some degree of tumor shrinkage, and many had been pretreated with either IL-2 or interferon. Diarrhea, fatigue, and hypertension were the most commonly encountered grade 3 and 4 events and were amenable to medical management in most patients. Axtinib was the subject of a phase III trial that compared its efficacy to that of sorafenib (a first-generation VEGFR and RAF inhibitor) in the second-line setting (Motzer et al., 2013; Rini et al., 2011; see Table 104.12). **In this study, 723 patients with clear cell RCC who progressed on one first-line therapy containing sunitinib, bevacizumab, temsirolimus,**

TABLE 104.12 Summary of Selected Studies of Selective VEGFR Antagonists in Metastatic Renal Cell Carcinoma

STUDY	AGENT(S)	PHASE	STUDY POPULATION	NO. OF PATIENTS	OVERALL RESPONSE RATE (RECIST)	MEDIAN PFS (MO)	MEDIAN OS (MO)
Sternberg et al., 2010 Sternberg et al., 2013	Pazopanib vs. placebo	Randomized phase III	Metastatic clear cell RCC patients with 0-1 prior cytokine therapy	435	30% vs. 3%	9.2 vs. 4.2	22.9 vs. 20.5
Motzer et al., 2013	Tivozanib vs. Sorafenib	Randomized phase III	Metastatic clear cell RCC; 0-1 prior therapies	517	33% vs. 23%	11.9 vs. 9.1	28.8 vs. 29.3
Rini et al., 2011; Motzer et al., 2013	Axitinib vs. Sorafenib	Randomized phase III	Second-line clear cell RCC	723	19% vs. 9%	6.7 vs. 4.7	20.1 vs 19.2
Motzer et al., 2013	Pazopanib vs. Sunitinib	Randomized phase III	Previously untreated clear cell RCC	1110	31% vs. 25%	10.5 vs. 10.2	28.4 vs 29.3

NA, Not available; *OS*, overall survival; *PFS*, progression-free survival; *RCC*, renal cell carcinoma.

or cytokines were randomized to receive axitinib (starting dose of 5 mg PO BID, N = 361) or sorafenib (400 mg PO BID, N = 362). Patients on the axitinib arm were allowed to receive higher doses (up to 10 mg PO twice daily) if lower dose levels were well tolerated; there was no dose-escalation in the sorafenib arm. Median progression-free survival (PFS), as measured by response criteria in solid tumors (RECIST), was 6.7 months in the axitinib arm compared with 4.7 months in the sorafenib arm (HR 0.665; 95% CI 0.544–0.812; $P < 0.0001$). The benefit from axitinib was most pronounced in patients who had previously received cytokines (median PFS 12.1 months for axitinib vs 6.5 months for sorafenib; HR 0.464; 95% CI 0.318–0.676; $P < 0.0001$). Patients previously treated with a VEGF pathway antagonist also appeared to benefit, although the improvement in PFS was modest. For instance, in patients who had received sunitinib in the first-line setting, median PFS was 4 to 8 months with axitinib and 3 to 4 months with sorafenib (HR 0.741; 95% CI 0.573–0.958; $P = 0.0107$). OS in the two arms was comparable with a median OS of 20.1 months with axitinib (95% CI 16.7–23.4) and 19.2 months (17.5–22.3) with sorafenib (HR 0.969; 95% CI 0.800–1.174; one-sided $P = 0.3744$). **Based on the improved PFS compared with sorafenib in the AXIS trial, axitinib was approved by the FDA for use in the second-line setting in patients with advanced RCC.** Axitinib is also being explored in combination with PD-1 or PD-L1 inhibitors, with available data suggesting that these regimens are well tolerated and highly effective.

Newer VEGFR-Based Targeted Therapy Strategies

Attempts to improve on outcomes associated with conventional angiogenesis inhibitors such as sunitinib and pazopanib have led to the development of agents that target VEGFR and other specific pathways believed to play a role in clear cell RCC. This has led to the development and successful clinical evaluation of strategies targeting Met and related pathways as well as those targeting FGFR.

Cabozantinib

Despite advances in our ability to target the VEGF pathway in a clinically meaningful manner, most patients with clear cell RCC eventually progress and die from their disease. Identifying mechanisms mediating primary and acquired or adaptive resistance to VEGF pathway inhibition is an area of active investigation. The Met pathway appears to be important in clear cell RCC, with preclinical models suggesting that HIF-mediated overexpression of Met may engender resistance to agents targeting the VEGF axis (Koochekpour et al., 1999). Moreover, Met and a related kinase, Axl, are overexpressed in clear cell RCC and appear to portend worse prognosis. Cabozantinib is a multityrosine kinase inhibitor with activity against VEGFR, Met, and Axl. After demonstration of activity in a single-arm phase II study in clear cell RCC patients who had received multiple prior lines of therapy, cabozantinib was evaluated in a randomized phase III study (METEOR) (Choueiri et al., 2015, 2016). A total of 658 clear cell RCC patients who had received prior therapy with VEGF or VEGFR-targeted therapy were randomized to receive either cabozantinib (60 mg PO every day) or everolimus (10 mg PO every day). Cabozantinib was associated with a higher response rate (21% with cabozantinib vs. 5% with everolimus; $P < 0.001$), and superior PFS (median PFS 7.4 months with cabozantinib vs. 3.8 months with everolimus; HR 0.58; 95% CI 0.45–0.75; $P < 0.001$). A subsequent analysis, after 430 deaths (198 for cabozantinib and 232 for everolimus), showed that cabozantinib was also associated with better OS (median OS was 21.4 months with cabozantinib and 17.1 months with everolimus; HR 0.70; 95% CI 0.58–0.85; $P = 0.0002$) (Fig. 104.7). Although cabozantinib therapy was associated with significant toxicity (60% of patients required a dose reduction, mostly because of fatigue, diarrhea, or palmar plantar erythrodysesthesia), most patients were managed with dose reductions, with only 10% requiring permanent discontinuation because of toxicity. **These data established cabozantinib as a reasonable option in patients who had received a prior angiogenesis inhibitor.**

Subsequent attempts to ascertain the efficacy of cabozantinib in the front-line setting led to a randomized phase II study (CABOSUN); 157 patients with intermediate or poor-risk clear cell RCC (based on IMDC criteria) were randomized to receive either sunitinib or cabozantinib at standard doses (Choueiri et al., 2017; Table 104.13). Treatment with cabozantinib was associated with a significant improvement in the primary end point, PFS (median PFS 8.2 vs. 5.6 months with sunitinib; adjusted HR 0.66; 95% CI 0.46–0.95; one-sided $P = 0.012$). Cabozantinib was also associated with a better ORR (46% [95% CI 34–57] vs. 18%; 95% CI 10–28] for sunitinib) (Fig. 104.8). **Based on these data, the FDA expanded the approval of cabozantinib to include patients with untreated advanced RCC.**

Lenvatinib

Activation of alternative means of promoting and supporting angiogenesis in the face of VEGF inhibition has emerged as a possible

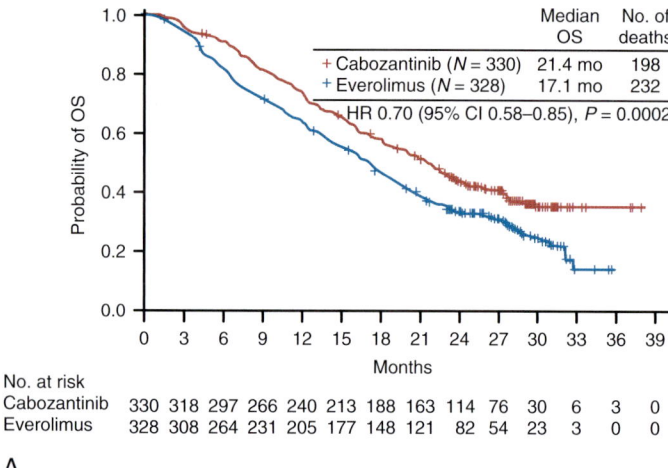

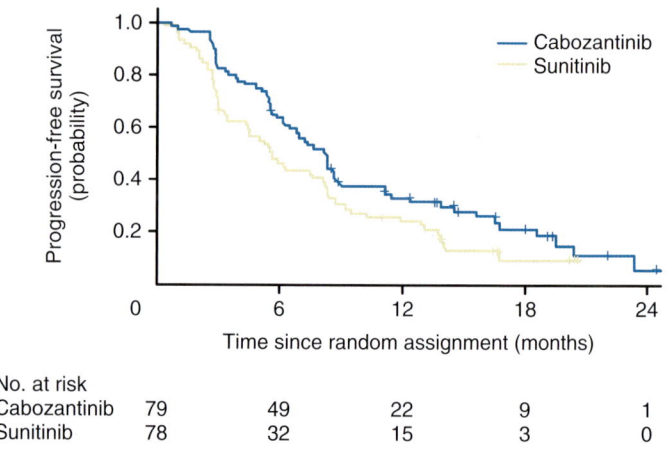

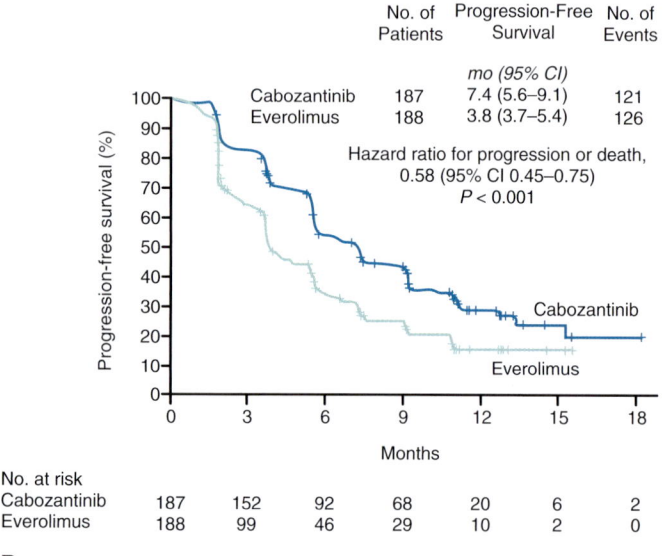

Fig. 104.7. Kaplan-Meier estimates of (A) overall survival (OS) and (B) progression-free survival in 658 patients with metastatic clear cell RCC receiving either cabozantinib or everolimus. (Modified from Motzer RJ, Escudier B, Powles T, et al.: Long-term follow-up of overall survival for cabozantanib versus everolimus in advanced renal cell carcinoma. *Br J Cancer* 118:1176–1178, 2018 and Choueiri TK, Escudier B, Powles T, et al.: Cabozantinib versus everolimus in advanced renal-cell carcinoma. *N Engl J Med* 373:1814–1823, 2015.)

Fig. 104.8. Kaplan Meier estimate of progression-free survival in 157 previously untreated patients with metastatic clear cell renal cell carcinoma receiving either sunitinib or cabozantinib. (Choueiri TK, Halabi S, Sanford BL, et al.: Cabozantinib versus sunitinib as initial targeted therapy for patients with metastatic renal cell carcinoma of poor or intermediate risk: the Alliance A031203 CABOSUN trial. *J Clin Oncol* 35[6]:591–597.)

Lenvatinib is a newer multikinase inhibitor of VEGFR1, VEGFR2, and VEGFR3, with **additional** inhibitory activity against fibroblast growth factor receptors (FGFR1, FGFR2, FGFR3, and FGFR4), PDGFRα, RET, and KIT. In a three-arm randomized phase II study of 153 patients with clear cell RCC who had progressed on prior VEGF-targeted therapy, lenvatinib (24 mg/d) was compared with everolimus (10 mg/d) alone or with a combination of lenvatinib (18 mg/d) plus everolimus (5 mg/d) (Motzer et al., 2015) (see Table 104.13). The combination of lenvatinib and everolimus significantly prolonged PFS compared with everolimus alone (median 14.6 months [95% CI 5.9–20.1] vs. 5.5 months [3.5–7.1]; HR 0.40; 95% CI 0.24–0.68; $P = 0.0005$); single-agent lenvatinib also significantly prolonged PFS compared with everolimus alone (HR 0.61; 95% CI 0.38–0.98; $P = 0.048$). However, there was no significant difference in outcome between the combination and lenvatinib alone (median PFS 7.4 months [95% CI 5.6–10.2]; HR 0.66; 95% CI 0.39–1.10; $P = 0.12$). Although these data should be confirmed in a larger study, they formed the basis for approval of the combination of lenvatinib and everolimus in patients who had progressed on prior anti-angiogenesis therapy. This combination is the subject of an ongoing randomized phase III study in previously untreated patients with clear cell RCC and is being compared to sunitinib and a combination of lenvatinib and pembrolizumab.

Inhibitors of the Mammalian Target of Rapamycin

mTOR is a key intracellular protein that is a component of several signaling cascades including those mediating the effects of some growth factors. **It appears to play a role in regulating translation and stability of HIF-1α, and preclinical models have suggested that growth inhibition occurring in response to mTOR inhibitors correlates with a block in HIF-1α translation** (Hudson et al., 2002; Thomas et al., 2006). Two analogues of sirolimus, **temsirolimus** and **everolimus,** have been clinically evaluated with demonstrable activity in RCC.

A phase II trial of **temsirolimus** evaluated three different doses (25 mg, 75 mg, and 250 mg per week administered intravenously) in 111 patients assigned randomly to one of the dose levels (see Table 104.13). The overall response rate observed on this trial was modest (7%, including one patient with a complete response), and the median PFS was 15 months (Atkins et al., 2004). Responses and PFS appeared to be independent of temsirolimus dose. An exploratory subgroup analysis based on stratification of patients according to MSKCC risk groups revealed that patients in the poor-risk group had a longer median OS compared with historical controls receiving

contributor to resistance in preclinical models. FGF receptors (FGFR1 and FGFR2) have been proposed as important mediators of resistance after effective VEGF pathway inhibition in some models (Korc and Friesel, 2009; Welti et al., 2011). A randomized phase II study evaluated the use of sunitinib and nintedanib, a small angiokinase inhibitor with activity against VEGFR-1-3, PDGFR-α/β, FGFR-1-3, RET, and Flt3 and found modest activity and no discernible advantage to nintedanib (Eisen et al., 2015). A subsequent phase III study with dovitinib, an oral inhibitor of VEGFR, PDGFR, and FGFR also dampened enthusiasm for further evaluating this class of drugs as a single agent in RCC. In this open-label randomized phase III trial, 570 patients with clear cell RCC who had received one prior VEGF and one prior mTOR therapy were randomized 1 : 1 to dovitinib or sorafenib with PFS as the primary end point (Motzer et al., 2014). PFS was comparable, with a median of 3.7 and 3.6 months (HR 0.86; 95% CI 0.72–1.94, $P = 0.063$) in the dovitinib and sorafenib arms, respectively. Median OS (HR 0.96; 95% CI 0.75–1.22; $P = 0.357$) was also similar (11.1 and 11 months in the dovitinib and sorafenib arms, respectively).

TABLE 104.13 Summary of Selected Studies of Newer Targeted Multikinase Inhibitors in Metastatic Renal Cell Carcinoma

STUDY	AGENT(S)	PHASE	STUDY POPULATION	NO. OF PATIENTS	OVERALL RESPONSE RATE (RECIST)	MEDIAN PFS (MO)	MEDIAN OS (MO)
METEOR (Choueiri et al., 2015; Motzer et al., 2018)	Cabozantinib vs. Everolimus	Randomized phase III	Metastatic clear cell RCC patients who had progressed on anti-VEGFR therapy	658	31% vs. 5%	7.4 vs. 3.8	21.4 vs. 17.1
CABOSUN Choueiri et al., 2017	Cabozantinib vs. Sunitinib	Randomized phase II	Untreated intermediate or poor risk metastatic clear cell RCC	157	33% vs. 12%	8.2 vs 5.6	NA
Everolimus with or without Lenvatinib (Motzer et al., 2015)	Lenvatinb plus Everolimus vs. Everolimus	Randomized phase II	Metastatic clear cell RCC patients who had progressed on anti-VEGFR therapy	101	43% vs. 6%	14.1. vs. 5.5	

RCC, Renal cell carcinoma.

interferon-α (8.2 vs. 4.9 months). Based on this observation, a three-arm randomized phase III trial of 626 patients with three or more predefined poor-risk features was undertaken (Hudes et al., 2007). Patients with previously untreated metastatic kidney cancer of all histologic subtypes were eligible and randomized to receive temsirolimus alone (25 mg intravenously every week), interferon-α alone (up to 18 million units subcutaneously three times a week), or temsirolimus (15 mg intravenously every week) plus interferon-α (6 million units subcutaneously three times a week). PFS was superior in both temsirolimus-containing arms compared with interferon alone (median 3.8 months vs. 1.9 months). **Importantly, the trial also demonstrated a significantly higher OS in the temsirolimus arm compared with the interferon-only arm (median OS 10.9 vs. 7.3 months, $P = 0.008$)**, whereas the addition of temsirolimus did not appear to significantly alter OS compared with interferon alone (median OS 8.4 vs. 7.3 months, $P = 0.70$) (Fig. 104.9). Temsirolimus was fairly well tolerated, and most common adverse events such as mucositis, fatigue, rash, hyperglycemia, hypophosphatemia, hypercholesterolemia, and pulmonary complications were amenable to medical and/or supportive measures. **Based on these data, temsirolimus was approved by the FDA for the treatment of patients with metastatic RCC, and the agent is a reasonable front-line choice in patients presenting with poor-risk features. However, its utility as well as relative efficacy in this patient population compared with immune checkpoint inhibitor therapy has not been evaluated.**

Everolimus is an orally bioavailable inhibitor of mTOR. It was the subject of a phase III trial in patients with metastatic clear cell RCC whose disease had progressed after therapy with sunitinib, sorafenib, or both (Motzer et al., 2008). Patients were randomized to receive either everolimus, 10 mg once daily ($n = 272$), or placebo ($n = 138$) (Table 104.14). **The trial was stopped after an interim analysis demonstrated superior PFS in the everolimus arm (median 4 months) compared with the placebo arm (median 1.9 months)** (Fig. 104.10). At the time of this analysis, median survival had not been reached in the everolimus group and was 8.8 months for the placebo group; OS was not significantly different in the two groups. **Everolimus has been supplanted by other agents including nivolumab, and cabozantinib in the post-front-line setting.** However, it is a reasonable option when used in combination with lenvatinib.

Combination and Sequential Therapy With Agents Targeting the VHL Pathway

Combinations of two or more classes of agents with activity centered on different components of the VHL pathway provide an attractive strategy that may increase efficacy as well as eliminating potential mechanisms of resistance. **A major limitation of this approach is the overlapping toxicity profile of several drugs, necessitating significant dose reductions of individual drugs** (Feldman et al., 2009; Patel et al., 2009). Several combinations of mTOR and VEGF-pathway antagonists have been evaluated in phase I trials. In general, combinations of first generation VEGFR inhibitors such as sunitinib, with an mTOR inhibitor are associated with significant toxicity discouraging their evaluation in phase 2/3 studies (Hainsworth et al., 2013; Patel et al., 2009). However, bevacizumab-based combinations appear to be better tolerated and have been evaluated in several trials.

The activity of bevacizumab in combination with everolimus was evaluated in a phase II trial of metastatic clear cell RCC patients ($n = 80$); both treatment-naive patients ($n = 50$) and patients who had previously received sunitinib and/or sorafenib were eligible (Hainsworth et al., 2010). Median PFS in the treatment-naive and previously treated populations was 9.1 and 7.1 months, respectively. The combination was further evaluated in a phase III trial (RECORD-2), which compared its efficacy with that of bevacizumab plus interferon-α (Ravaud et al., 2015). This study demonstrated similar median PFS, OS, and safety profiles in both groups, which suggests no additional advantage to replacing interferon-α with everolimus in combination with bevacizumab. The INTORACT trial compared the combination of either temsirolimus or interferon-α to bevacizumab (Rini et al., 2014): 791 patients with previously untreated metastatic clear cell RCC were randomized to one of the aforementioned groups; the primary end point of the trial was PFS. There was no significant difference between the temsirolimus and interferon-α groups in median PFS (9.1 months vs. 9.3 months, HR 1.1; 95% CI 0.9–1.3; $P = 0.80$), OS (25.8 months vs. 25.5 months, HR 1.0; 95% CI 0.9–1.3; $P = 0.6$) or objective response rates (27.0% vs. 27.4%, RR 1.0; 95% CI 0.8–1.3; $P = 1.0$). The combination of temsirolimus plus

TABLE 104.14 Summary of Selected Studies of mTOR Inhibitors in Metastatic Renal Cell Carcinoma

STUDY	AGENT(S)	PHASE	STUDY POPULATION	NO. OF PATIENTS	OVERALL RESPONSE RATE (RECIST)	MEDIAN PFS (MO)	MEDIAN OS (MO)
Hudes et al., 2007	Tem vs. IFN-α vs. tem/IFN-α	Randomized phase III	Poor prognosis, previously untreated, all histologic subtypes	626	8.6% vs. 4.8% vs. 8.1%	5.5 vs. 3.1 vs. 4.7	10.9 vs. 7.3 vs. 8.4
Motzer et al., 2008b	Everolimus vs. placebo	Randomized phase III	Clear cell RCC refractory to VEGF-targeted therapy	410	1% vs. 0	4.0 vs. 1.9	NR vs. 8.8

IFN-α, Interferon-α; NR, not reached; OS, overall survival; PFS, progression-free survival; RCC, renal cell carcinoma; tem, temsirolimus.

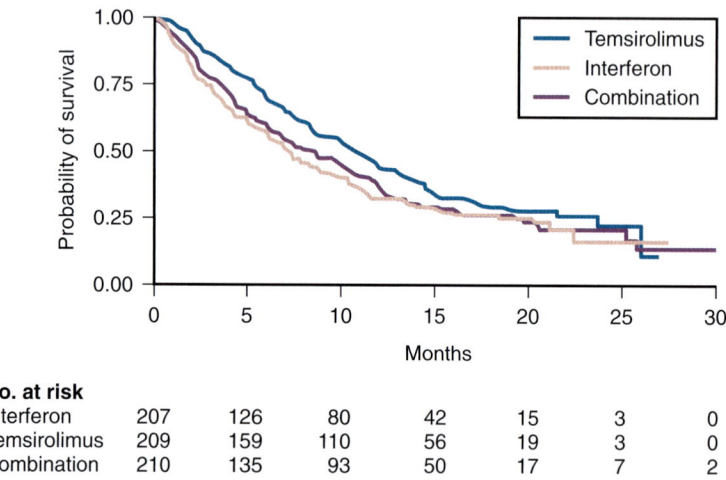

Fig. 104.9. Kaplan-Meier estimates of overall survival in 626 metastatic renal cell carcinoma patients with adverse prognostic features randomized to receive temsirolimus alone, interferon-α alone, or combination therapy. (From Hudes G, Carducci M, Tomczak P, et al.: Temsirolimus, interferon alfa, or both for advanced renal-cell carcinoma. N Engl J Med 356:2271–2281, 2007.)

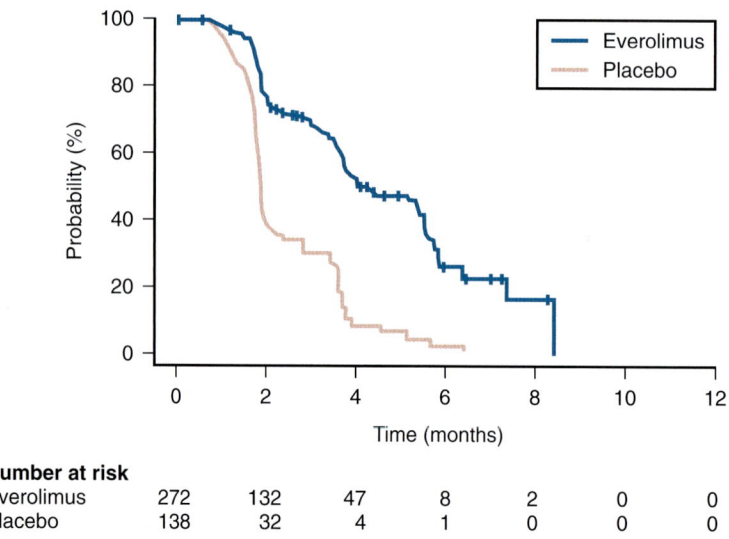

Fig. 104.10. Kaplan-Meier estimates of progression-free survival in 410 patients with metastatic renal cell carcinoma randomized to everolimus or placebo. (From Motzer RJ et al.: Efficacy of everolimus in advanced renal cell carcinoma: a double-blind, randomised, placebo-controlled phase III trial. Lancet 372:449–456, 2008b.)

bevacizumab, however, appeared to be better tolerated, with superior symptom scores, as assessed by the validated Functional Assessment of Cancer Therapy-Kidney Symptom Index (FKSI)-15 and FKSI-Disease Related Symptoms, without a significant difference in global health outcomes. Based on these studies, **combinations of bevacizumab with a mTOR inhibitor do not appear to offer additional activity compared with previously established standard of care options in the first-line setting and are unlikely to be evaluated against newer standards.**

IMMUNE "CHECKPOINT" INHIBITOR–BASED COMBINATION STRATEGIES

Although the advent of inhibitors of PD1/PD-L1 has led to improved outcomes in patients with advanced clear cell RCC, a significant proportion of patients do not appear to benefit from these agents. In addition, complete responses, a potential surrogate for long-term disease-free interval, occur in less than 10% of patients treated with nivolumab or other checkpoint inhibitors given as a single agent. Consequently, there has been significant interest in evaluating combination strategies using inhibitors of the PD1/PD-L1 interaction in a bid to improve outcomes.

Cytotoxic T-lymphocyte associated protein 4 (CTLA-4) is a CD28 homolog expressed on T cells. Binding of B7 costimulatory molecules to CTLA-4 suppresses antigen-dependent T cell stimulation, and inhibitors of this interaction have demonstrable clinical activity in advanced cancer, including melanoma and RCC. Ipilimumab, a CTLA-4 inhibitor, is FDA-approved in melanoma, and the combination of PD-1/CTLA-4 blockade appears to be synergistic in the treatment of metastatic melanoma but is associated with significant toxicity. Consequently, a phase I study evaluating various doses of nivolumab and ipilimumab in combination was conducted in patients with advanced RCC (CheckMate 016) and led to the identification of nivolumab 3 mg/kg every 3 weeks and ipilimumab 1 mg/kg every 3 weeks for 4 doses as the combination associated with the most acceptable level of adverse events (<40% grade 3–4 adverse events, compared with more than 60% grade 3–4 events in regimens containing higher doses of ipilimumab) (Hammers et al., 2017).

This regimen was subsequently studied in previously untreated patients with metastatic clear cell RCC (CheckMate 214) in a phase III study with sunitinib as the comparator (Motzer et al., 2018). A total of 1096 patients were randomized 1:1 to receive either sunitinib or nivolumab plus ipilimumab. Of these, 847 patients were classified as having intermediate or poor risk based on IMDC prognostic criteria and constituted the population that was the subject of the primary end point analysis; OS, PFS, and overall response rate were the co-primary end points. With a median follow-up of 25.6 months, the combination of nivolumab and ipilimumab was determined to be superior to sunitinib. The median OS was not reached with nivolumab plus ipilimumab versus 26.0 months with sunitinib (HR for death, 0.63; $P < 0.001$), while the objective response rate was 42% versus 27% ($P < 0.001$) with a complete response rate of 9% versus 1% (Fig. 104.11). The median PFS was 11.6 months and 8.4 months, respectively (HR for disease progression or death, 0.82; $P = 0.03$, not significant per the prespecified 0.009 threshold). As anticipated, a significant proportion of patients treated with the combination experienced grade 3 to 4 adverse events (46%); immune-related side effects requiring high-dose glucocorticoid therapy were seen in 35% of patients, and 22% of patients had their treatment permanently discontinued because of toxicity. A total of 249 patients with good prognostic features were also treated on this study; these patients tended to have better outcomes with sunitinib compared with the immunotherapy combination. In a study of patient-reported outcomes of patients with advanced renal cell carcinoma treated with nivolumab plus ipilimumab versus sunitinib (CheckMate 214), Cella et al. (2019) found that nivolumab plus ipilimumab leads to fewer symptoms and better HRQoL than sunitinib in patients with intermediate- or poor-risk disease. **Based on these data, the combination of nivolumab plus ipilimumab is now considered a reasonable standard of care option in the front-line therapy of patients with intermediate or poor-risk clear cell RCC.**

The addition of agents targeting the VEGF axis to immune checkpoint blockade is another strategy that is under investigation. In addition to the single agent activity of both classes of agents, there is ample preclinical evidence to suggest synergistic antitumor effect when VEGF pathway antagonists are combined with inhibitors of the PD1/PD-L1 interaction. Several studies suggest that VEGF-pathway inhibitors have an immunomodulatory effect. Sunitinib appears to decrease regulatory T cells, and sunitinib and sorafenib downregulate the function of suppressive tumor-associated macrophages, thereby enhancing an antitumor immune response (Ko et al., 2010; Lin et al., 2013; Porta et al., 2011). Although early studies combining nivolumab (2 mg/kg IV) and sunitinib (50 mg, 4 weeks on, 2 weeks off) or pazopanib (800 mg daily) in previously treated metastatic RCC demonstrated notable antitumor activity with an ORR of 52% in the sunitinib arm and 45% in the pazopanib arm, the associated toxicity was considered prohibitive (Amin et al., 2018).

Subsequent studies sought to mitigate the potential risk of combination therapy by using newer, more specific VEGF pathway antagonists. A number of these combinations are deemed safe and are the subject of phase III studies in untreated metastatic clear cell RCC patients. Pembrolizumab (an anti-PD1 antibody) and avelumab (an antibody directed against PD-L1) have been studied in combination with axitinib, demonstrating high response rates and manageable toxicity in phase I/II studies. Data from a phase III randomized study of avelumab and axitinib have been reported and demonstrate the superiority of this combination compared with sunitinib (JAVELIN Renal 101 Study) in 882 patients with previously untreated RCC, including 560 who had positive staining for PD-L1; specifically, the combination arm was associated with a higher PFS (13.8 vs. 7.2 months; HR 0.61; $P < 0.0001$) and overall response rate (55.2% [95% CI 49.9–61.2] vs. 25.5% [95% CI 20.6–30.9]) in the PD-L1 + population (Choueiri et al., 2017). Although grade 3 or greater toxicity was encountered in more than 70% of patients in both arms, the rate of permanent treatment discontinuation was much higher in the combination arm (22% vs. 13%). Similarly, the combination of bevacizumab and atezolizumab, another anti PD-L1 antibody, was also shown to be associated with a superior PFS compared with sunitinib in a randomized phase III study in previously untreated patients with metastatic RCC whose tumors expressed PD-L1 (Motzer et al., 2018). Other studies of similar design, including a phase III study comparing sunitinib against a combination of pembrolizumab and axitinib are ongoing. **Although mature overall survival data from these studies are not yet available, combinations of agents targeting the PD1 and VEGF axis appear to be associated with a better PFS and higher response rate compared with front-line VEGFR-targeted therapy. Although these combinations have not been compared directly to dual PD1/CTLA4 blockade, they appear to have at least comparable efficacy and a more favorable toxicity profile and are on the cusp of regulatory approval in the front-line setting.**

OTHER TREATMENT OPTIONS IN PATIENTS WITH CLEAR CELL RENAL CELL CARCINOMA

Chemotherapy

Conventional cytotoxic chemotherapy has been largely ineffective in the management of clear cell RCC. Numerous chemotherapeutic agents including 5-FU, platinum compounds, gemcitabine, vinblastine, and bleomycin have been evaluated as single agents in this disease but have failed to demonstrate clinically meaningful activity; a wide array of combination chemotherapy regimens have fared little better (Amato, 2000; Haas et al., 1976; Hahn et al., 1977; Mertens et al., 1993, 1994; Rini et al., 2000, 2005; Stadler et al., 2006; Zaniboni et al., 1989). **Comprehensive meta-analyses of chemotherapy trials in RCC indicate the overall response rate is 5.5% to 6.0%** (Yagoda et al., 1995). Although the mechanisms underlying this profound chemoresistance have not been fully elucidated, overexpression of the multidrug resistance gene *(MDR)* has been proposed as one possible culprit (Fojo et al., 1987). However, the addition of MDR inhibitors such as toremifene, cyclosporine, and verapamil to conventional

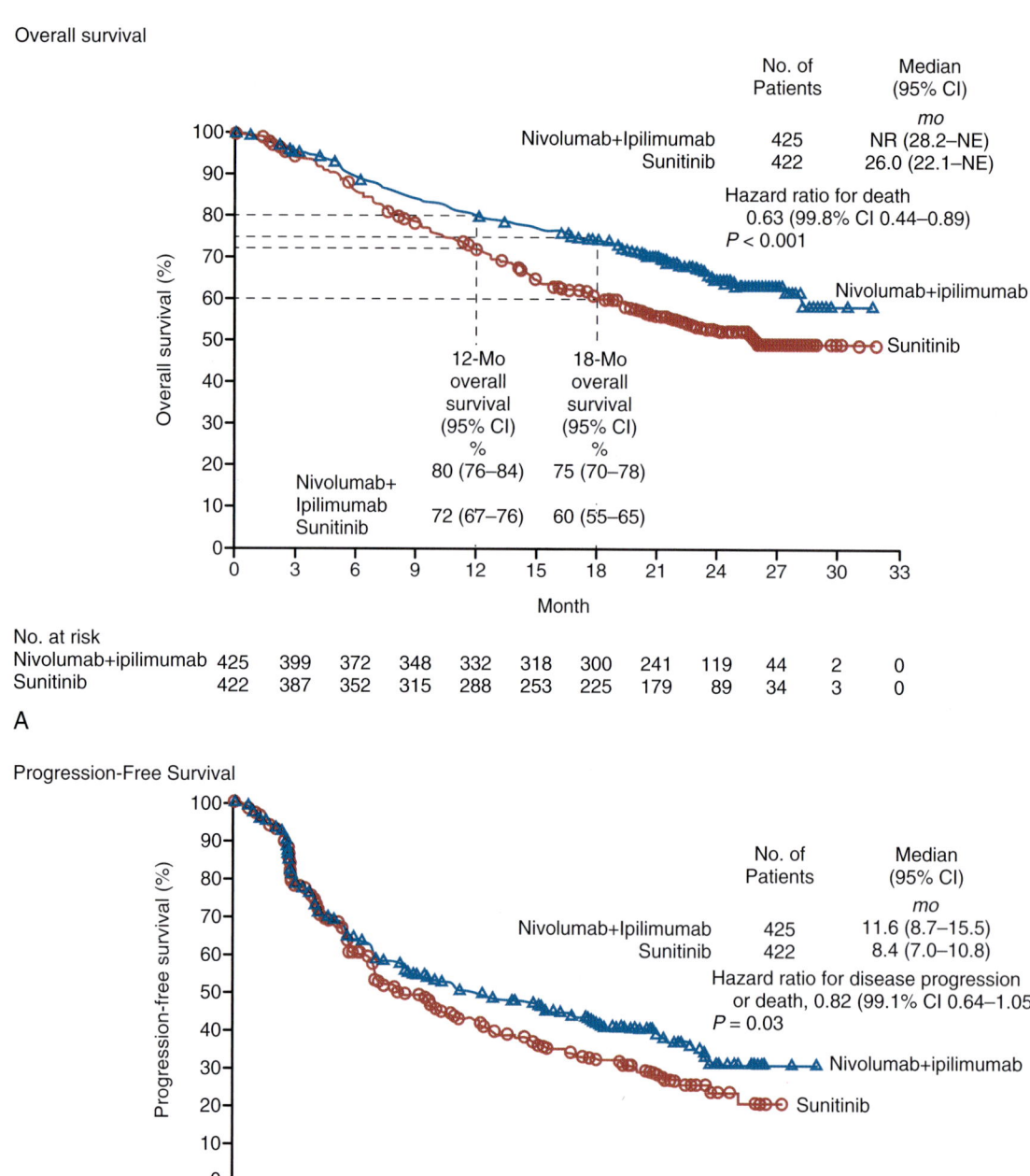

Fig. 104.11. Kaplan Meier analysis of overall survival (Panel A) and progression free survival (Panel B) in 847 patients with previously untreated intermediate or poor risk metastatic clear cell renal cell carcinoma receiving either nivolumab plus ipilimumab or sunitinib. (Motzer Tannir NM, McDermott DF, et al.: Nivolumab plus ipilimumab versus sunitinib in advanced renal-cell carcinoma. *N Engl J Med* 378:1277–1290, 2018.)

chemotherapeutic agents has failed to improve their efficacy, suggesting that other, as yet unrecognized, factors may be at play (Braybrooke et al., 2000). **Cytotoxic chemotherapy has no role in the current management of most patients with clear cell RCC.** One situation in which chemotherapy may bear further investigation is in patients whose tumors demonstrate a sarcomatoid component; a small case series has suggested promising activity for gemcitabine-based chemotherapy in this setting, prompting further study of this approach (Nanus et al., 2004).

Hormonal Therapy

Hormonal therapy had been the subject of trials in RCC in the 1970s and 1980s, preceding the advent of cytokines. These studies were prompted by the lack of effective therapies for kidney cancer and by the belief that a male preponderance (kidney cancer occurs approximately twice as frequently in males) implied a hormonal basis for this malignancy. Hormonal agents such as medroxyprogesterone have been noted to induce tumor regressions in a small minority of patients, but overall response rates are too low (approximately 2%) to have meaningful clinical impact in most patients (Braybrooke et al., 2000; Harris, 1983; Medical Research Council Renal Cancer, 1999; Schomburg et al., 1993). **Progestational and other hormonal agents have no role in the current management of renal cell cancer.**

SYSTEMIC THERAPY FOR NON–CLEAR CELL VARIANTS OF RENAL CELL CARCINOMA

Non–clear cell subtypes of kidney cancer are relatively rare (constituting approximately 15% to 25% of all kidney cancer) and have been the subject of few prospective studies. Given the unavailability of agents of proven efficacy in papillary, chromophobe, and other rare histologic subtypes, patients with non–clear cell renal tumors often receive agents with activity in clear cell RCC.

VEGFR inhibitors active in clear cell RCC have only modest efficacy in papillary RCC. Sorafenib and sunitinib were shown to have minimal activity in retrospective studies of papillary RCC patients (Choueiri et al., 2008). Prospective phase II trials with sunitinib have demonstrated that this agent is associated with low response rates (5% to 10%) in papillary RCC. The Southwest Oncology Group reported an 11% overall response rate with erlotinib, an oral EGFR inhibitor, in 52 patients with metastatic papillary RCC with a 6-month PFS of only 29%.

An exploratory subgroup analysis of patients enrolled in large randomized phase III study evaluating the efficacy of temsirolimus versus interferon in "poor prognosis" patients suggests that mTOR inhibitors may have activity in some non–clear cell variants. Approximately 20% of the patients enrolled in this trial had non–clear cell histologies (predominantly papillary RCC). The outcome of 37 patients with non–clear cell RCC treated with temsirolimus (OS and PFS) was found to be better than that of 36 patients receiving interferon in this subgroup analysis. Although these data suggest that temsirolimus may have activity in some non–clear cell variants, these conclusions are limited by the fact that this is a subgroup analysis (Dutcher et al., 2009). Everolimus was evaluated in a relatively large open-labeled, multicenter phase II clinical trial evaluating as a first-line agent in patients with metastatic papillary RCC (RAPTOR) (Escudier et al., 2016). At the time of a preliminary intent-to-treat analysis ($n = 83$), median PFS was 3.7 months (95% CI 2.4–5.5), whereas median OS was 21 months (95% CI 15.4–28) by independent radiology review. Common grade 3 or 4 adverse events included asthenia (10.6%), fatigue (5.4%), and anemia (5.4%). Around 27.2% of the patients discontinued treatment because of adverse events. A second phase II trial of everolimus in patients with metastatic non–clear cell RCC was recently published. Of the 49 patients enrolled, 29 (59%) had papillary RCC (Koh et al., 2013); 23 patients (47%) had prior anti-VEGF therapy. Partial response was noted in 5/49 (10%), stable disease in 25 (51%), and disease progression in 16 (32.7%) of the patients. Interestingly, 2 out of 5 patients with objective response to everolimus had chromophobe RCC, whereas 2 had pRCC and 1 had an unclassified RCC variant. The median PFS in this study was 5.2 months, and patients with chromophobe RCC had a trend toward longer PFS compared with other nccRCC patients ($P = 0.084$). Based on the two foregoing trials, everolimus appears to have modest activity in patients with papillary/non–clear cell RCC.

At least two phase II randomized studies have compared the activity of sunitinib and everolimus in patients with non–clear cell RCC. As was seen with single agent studies, both agents were associated with modest response rates and PFS (Armstrong et al., 2016; Tannir et al., 2016). Although neither agent was clearly superior, there was a trend toward better outcome with sunitinib.

Recent advances in our understanding of the genetic and molecular alterations underlying several RCC subtypes have begun to lead to a more rational and individualized approach to their management. As with clear cell RCC, hereditary forms of papillary and chromophobe RCC hold the key to the identification of critical molecular events leading to these tumors in familial and sporadic settings (Linehan, 2003, 2009). Hereditary papillary renal cancer (HPRC) is a familial condition characterized by the predisposition of affected individuals to develop bilateral, multifocal papillary type I RCC. **HPRC is characterized by the presence of activating germline mutations in the tyrosine kinase domain of the proto-oncogene *MET*, which is located on chromosome 7; this is usually accompanied by nonrandom duplication of the chromosome containing the mutated allele in the tumors** (Linehan, 2003, 2009; Schmidt et al., 1997, 1998, 1999, 2004; Zhuang et al., 1998). MET is a cell surface receptor that is normally activated on binding its ligand, hepatocyte growth factor (HGF) but is rendered constitutionally active in the presence of mutations in the kinase domain of this protein (Bottaro et al., 1991; Dharmawardana et al., 2004; Giubellino et al., 2009; Peruzzi and Bottaro, 2006). The HGF/MET pathway is involved in regulating a variety of biologic functions, including cell growth, proliferation, and motility (Fig. 104.12) (Giubellino et al., 2009; Jeffers et al., 1998). Somatic MET alterations have been noted in a proportion of patients with sporadic papillary RCC, with activating mutations identified in approximately 13% of papillary tumors in one series. Trisomy 7 (*HGF* and *MET* are located on chromosome 7) has been described in more than two-thirds of papillary tumors and may represent an alternative mechanism contributing to activation of the MET pathway in these tumors (Henke and Erbersdobler, 2002; Kovacs et al., 1991).

The realization that MET activation may play an important role in some forms of papillary RCC has led to the evaluation of foretinib, a novel tyrosine kinase inhibitor with activity against MET and VEGFR2 in this RCC subtype. Two dosing regimens were evaluated in sequential patient cohorts: (1) an intermittent dosing regimen of 240 mg of foretinib given days 1 to 5 of every 14-day cycle ($n = 37$), and (2) a continuous daily dosing regimen of 80 mg/day ($n = 37$). The primary end point was ORR based on response evaluation criteria in solid tumors (RECIST). An ORR of 13.5% with a median PFS of 9.3 months was reported in the entire study population. A subgroup analysis was undertaken to determine if MET pathway activation was associated with treatment outcome. The presence of a germline *MET* mutation was associated with a high likelihood of response, with 5 of 10 patients (50%) demonstrating a PR in this group compared with 5 of 57 responders (9%) in the absence of germline alterations. The side effect profile for foretinib appeared similar to that of other anti-VEGFR agents; hypertension was the most commonly reported AE. Although the primary end point of ORR greater than 25% was not met, **foretinib has activity in pRCC, notably in the germline *MET* mutation cohort, indicating that MET inhibition may be a viable treatment option for a subset of patients with pRCC.** More selective inhibitors of Met, including savolitinib and crizotinib, which lack significant activity against the VEGF receptors, have also been evaluated in phase II studies; data from these studies appear to confirm the notion that inhibitors of Met may have activity against tumors that have Met activation (Choueiri et al., 2017; Schoffski et al., 2017). At least two ongoing randomized studies are evaluating the efficacy of Met inhibitors compared with sunitinib, in patients with advanced papillary RCC.

A second form of hereditary pRCC is associated with alterations in the *fumarate hydratase* gene (*FH*), which encodes a tricarboxylic acid cycle enzyme that catalyzes the conversion of fumarate to malate. Germline *FH* mutations are seen in patients with hereditary leiomyomatosis and renal cell cancer (HLRCC), a condition associated with a highly aggressive variant of type II pRCC (Linehan et al., 2013; Ricketts et al., 2016; Shuch et al., 2013). It has long been recognized that accumulation of fumarate resulting from FH inactivation leads to a VHL-independent upregulation of intracellular HIF and transcriptional activation of downstream proangiogenic and growth factors (Isaacs et al., 2005). Loss of FH activity promotes a metabolic shift in these tumors, characterized by disruption of the Krebs cycle and a consequent reliance on aerobic glycolysis to satisfy cellular bioenergetic requirements.

Investigators at the National Cancer Institute have recently attempted to therapeutically exploit the exquisite sensitivity of this variant of papillary RCC to glucose deprivation (Yang et al., 2010). They hypothesized that a combination of bevacizumab, a monoclonal antibody to VEGF and erlotinib (inhibitor of EFGR

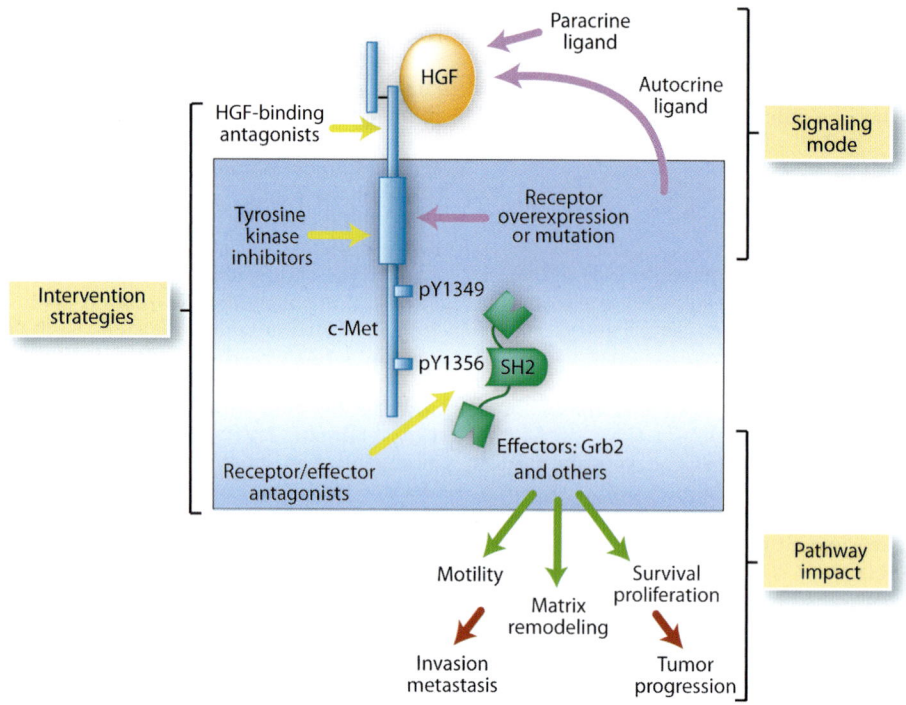

Fig. 104.12. MET oncogenic signaling pathway. Important downstream biochemical and biologic consequences of MET activation (by HGF binding or by constitutive activation of the receptor tyrosine kinase activity by mutation) are represented. The MET ligand (HGF), MET tyrosine kinase activity, and downstream effectors (such as Grb-2) are potential targets for drugs in tumors with aberrant pathway activation. (From Peruzzi B, Bottaro DP: Targeting the c-Met signaling pathway in cancer. *Clin Cancer Res* 12:3657–3660, 2006.)

kinase activity) would severely constrain glucose delivery to the tumor microenvironment and disrupt critical cellular processes. The combination of bevacizumab and erlotinib is currently being evaluated in patients with metastatic papillary RCC and interim data from his trial were recently presented (Srinivasan et al., 2014). This interim analysis included the first 41 individuals enrolled, of whom 21 had sporadic papillary RCC and 20 had HLRCC-associated kidney cancer. Sixteen patients had received at least one prior systemic therapy regimen. The overall RECIST response rate was 46% (19/41) in the entire cohort with a median PFS of 12.8 months; partial responses were seen in 13 out of 20 (65%) individuals with HLRCC and 6 out of 20 (29%) individuals with sporadic pRCC. After a median follow-up of 10.7 months, median PFS was 10.5 months (95% CI 7.4–18.6 months). Although these results are promising and suggest that the combination of bevacizumab and erlotinib is highly active in some forms of papillary RCC, further follow-up is required to clearly define the efficacy of this regimen in this population.

Cytotoxic chemotherapy has been used with modest success in collecting duct carcinoma, a rare kidney cancer variant with similarities to urothelial malignancies. In a series of 23 patients with metastatic collecting duct carcinoma, a response rate of 26% (including one complete response) was reported with a regimen comprising gemcitabine and carboplatin. Median PFS (7.1 months) and OS (10.5 months) were modest (Oudard et al., 2007).

In summary, there is no standard approach of proven efficacy for most patients with non–clear cell RCC, although some promising approaches are being evaluated. Enrollment in suitable trials should be considered for all patients with non–clear cell RCC.

SUGGESTED READINGS

Atkins MB, Dutcher J, Weiss G, et al: Kidney cancer: the Cytokine Working Group experience (1986-2001): part I. IL-2-based clinical trials, *Med Oncol* 18:197–207, 2001.

Choueiri TK, Escudier B, Powles T, et al: Cabozantinib versus everolimus in advanced renal-cell carcinoma, *N Engl J Med* 373:1814–1823, 2015.

Choueiri TK, Escudier B, Powles T, et al: Cabozantinib versus everolimus in advanced renal cell carcinoma (METEOR): final results from a randomised, open-label, phase 3 trial, *Lancet Oncol* 17:917–927, 2016.

Choueiri TK, Halabi S, Sanford BL, et al: Cabozantinib versus sunitinib as initial targeted therapy for patients with metastatic renal cell carcinoma of poor or intermediate risk: the Alliance A031203 CABOSUN Trial, *J Clin Oncol* 35:591–597, 2017.

Flanigan RC, Salmon SE, Blumenstein BA, et al: Nephrectomy followed by interferon alfa-2b compared with interferon alfa-2b alone for metastatic renal-cell cancer, *New Engl J Med* 345:1655–1659, 2001.

Fyfe GA, Fisher RI, Rosenberg SA, et al: Long-term response data for 255 patients with metastatic renal cell carcinoma treated with high-dose recombinant interleukin-2 therapy, *J Clin Oncol* 14:2410–2411, 1996.

Heng DY, Xie W, Regan MM, et al: External validation and comparison with other models of the International Metastatic Renal-Cell Carcinoma Database Consortium prognostic model: a population-based study, *Lancet Oncol* 14:141–148, 2013.

Hudes G, Carducci M, Tomczak P, et al: Temsirolimus, interferon alfa, or both for advanced renal-cell carcinoma, *New Engl J Med* 356:2271–2281, 2007.

Mejean A, Ravaud A, Thezenas S, et al: Sunitinib alone or after nephrectomy in metastatic renal-cell carcinoma, *N Engl J Med* 379:417–427, 2018.

Motzer RJ, Hutson TE, Tomczak P, et al: Sunitinib versus interferon alfa in metastatic renal-cell carcinoma, *New Engl J Med* 356:115–124, 2007.

Motzer RJ, Mazumdar M, Bacik J, et al: Survival and prognostic stratification of 670 patients with advanced renal cell carcinoma, *J Clin Oncol* 17:2530–2540, 1999.

Motzer RJ, Escudier B, McDermott DF, et al: Nivolumab versus everolimus in advanced renal-cell carcinoma, *N Engl J Med* 373:1803–1813, 2015.

Motzer RJ, Tannir NM, McDermott DF, et al: Nivolumab plus ipilimumab versus sunitinib in advanced renal-cell carcinoma, *N Engl J Med* 378:1277–1290, 2018.

REFERENCES

The complete reference list is available online at ExpertConsult.com.

INDEX

Page numbers followed by "*f*" indicate figures, "*t*" indicate tables, "*b*" indicate boxes, and "*e*" indicate online content.

A

AAST. *see* American Association for Surgery of Trauma
Abdomen
  clinical staging of, TGCTs and, 1689, 1689*f*
  exiting of
    after laparoscopic and robotic surgery, 218-219
    complications related to, 230
  hostile, 463
Abdominal aorta, 1669, 1669.e1*f*, 1671*f*, 1672*t*
Abdominal distention, 383, 387*b*
Abdominal incisions, in urologic surgery, 135-136
  Gibson incision, 135-136, 138*f*
  midline incision, 135, 136*f*-137*f*
  Pfannestiel incision, 135, 138*f*
Abdominal leak point pressure (ALPP)
  measurement of, 2561-2562, 2562*f*
  for sling procedure, 2833
Abdominal mesh removal, 2887
Abdominal obesity, 1418-1419
Abdominal paravaginal repair, for pelvic organ prolapse, 2780*t*, 2787, 2788*f*
Abdominal pressure, increased, urinary incontinence during, 2516
Abdominal sacrocolpopexy, for apical pelvic organ prolapse repair, 2798-2809
  complications of, 2804, 2806*t*
  cost of, 2809
  laparoscopic
    comparison with, 2806, 2807*t*
    versus robotic-assisted, 2806-2809, 2808*t*
    versus robotic-assisted colpopexy, 2809
    technique for, 2802*f*-2803*f*, 2803-2804
  learning curve in, 2809
  open, technique for, 2798-2800, 2800*f*-2801*f*
  results of, 2804-2806, 2805*t*
  robotic-assisted laparoscopic, 2800-2803, 2801*f*-2803*f*
Abdominal sacrohysteropexy, 2822-2823, 2824*f*
Abdominal surgery, operative team placement for
  retroperitoneal procedures, 207, 207*f*
  transperitoneal procedures, 206, 206*f*, 206.e1*f*
  complication of, 223*t*
Abdominal testis, surgical management of, 967-968
  Fowler-Stephens orchidopexy, 967-968
  laparoscopic orchidopexy, 967-968
  open transabdominal orchidopexy, 967
Abdominal wall
  closure of, for classic bladder exstrophy, 545-548, 546*f*-548*f*
  defects, in bladder exstrophy, 533
  lower
    inguinal canal, 2445-2447, 2448*f*
    internal surface of, 2447-2448, 2448*f*
    musculature of, 2444-2445, 2447*f*-2448*f*
    skin and subcutaneous fascia, 2444, 2446*f*
  posterior, 1658-1665
    flank muscles of, 1658-1665, 1662*f*-1664*f*, 1664*t*
  in prune-belly syndrome, 585-586, 586*f*-587*f*
  reconstruction of, for prune-belly syndrome, 594-595

Abdominal wall defects, 410
Abdominal wall related complications, after robot-assisted cystectomy, 3272
Abdominoperineal resection (APR), LUTD after, 2620-2621
Abdominoscrotal hydroceles, 889, 892-893
Abiraterone, 3677-3678, 3677*f*, 3693-3695, 3694*f*
Ablation
  adjuvants to, 3638
  approach of, 3624
  brachytherapy, 3632-3638
  cryotherapy, 3624-3628, 3625*f*, 3627*t*
  follow up, 3638
  high-intensity focused ultrasonography, 3628, 3629*t*-3630*t*, 3631*f*-3632*f*
  irreversible electroporation, 3628-3632, 3635*f*, 3636*t*
  laser, 3628, 3633*f*, 3634*t*, 3635*f*
  other modalities, 3638
  types, 3624, 3624*f*
  vascular-targeted photodynamic therapy, 3632, 3637*t*
Ablative therapy
  adrenal surgery, 2424-2425
  failure of, laparoscopic radical nephrectomy after, 2298
  laparoscopic ablation *versus*, 2318
  laparoscopic kidney, 2304-2305
  for renal tumors, 2309, 2322
    new modalities of, 2319-2323, 2323*b*
Abnormal adrenal function disorders, 2383-2384
Absorbable gelatin matrix agents, 147
Absorbable stapling techniques, for cutaneous continent urinary diversion, 3227-3228
  right colon pouch, 3228, 3229*f*
  stapled sigmoid reservoir, 3228, 3230*f*
  W-stapled reservoir, 3228-3229, 3231*f*
Absorbable sutures, 149-150
Absorbed dose, 28
Absorbent products
  for bladder emptying/storage failure, 2904
  for urinary incontinence, in geriatric patients, 2920.e6
Absorption, of ultrasound waves, 71, 72*f*
Absorptive hypercalciuria (AH), 2019
ACC. *see* Adrenal cortical carcinoma
Access needles, 169-170, 170*f*
Accreditation, for ultrasonography, 89-90
Acellular human dermis, allograft slings and, 2834-2835
^{11}C-acetate positron emission tomography scan, 3662, 3662*f*
Acetazolamide, in stone formation, 2033
Acetylcholine (ACh)
  in bladder function, 2474-2475
  botulinum toxins and, 2512, 2720.e3
  for detrusor underactivity, 2660-2661
  mechanism of action of, 2681
  in ureteral function, 1887
Acid-base balance, filtrate transport, 1911-1912, 1912*f*, 1912*b*
Acid-base metabolic, pneumoperitoneum effects on, 222
Acid-base physiology, 461

Acidosis
  after augmentation cystoplasty, 698
  requiring treatment, with intestinal anastomoses, 3180*t*
Acontractile detrusor, 2521, 2565
Acoustical shadow, 71, 71*f*
Acquired curvatures of penis, 1837-1838
Acquired diverticula, 525
Acquired immunodeficiency syndrome (AIDS), lower urinary tract dysfunction and, 2625
Acquired renal cystic diseases (ARCD), 772-774, 774*b*
  clinical features of, 772
  etiology of, 772
  evaluation of, 773
  histopathology of, 772-773, 773*f*
  treatment of, 773-774
Acquired renal scars, 499-500
Acquired scarring, pathophysiology of, 500-501, 500*f*-501*f*
  age, 500
  bacterial virulence, 500
  host susceptibility and response, 500
  hypertension, 501
  papillary anatomy, 500
  renal failure and somatic growth, 501
  renal growth, 501
Acrosome, 1442.e1
ACTH-dependent Cushing syndrome, 2361, 2361*f*
  Cushing disease, 2361
  ectopic ACTH syndrome, 2361, 2362*f*, 2362*t*, 2366
  treatment of, 2365-2366, 2366*f*
ACTH-independent bilateral macronodular adrenal hyperplasia, 2362
ACTH-independent Cushing syndrome, 2362, 2366-2367
Actin, in thin filaments, 2471
Actinomyosin cross-bridge cycling, 2472-2473, 2472*f*, 2473*f*
Action potentials
  of smooth muscles, of bladder, 2473-2474, 2474*f*
  of ureteral muscle cells, 1879-1881, 1879*f*-1880*f*
Active surveillance
  barriers to, of prostate cancer
    economics, 3546
    nomenclature, 3546
  complementary roles of focal therapy and, 3620
  of prostate cancer, 3537-3547, 3539*b*
    barriers to, 3545-3546
    management of men on, 3541-3542
    outcomes of, 3540-3542, 3540*t*, 3540*b*
    patient selection in, 3540-3541, 3541*t*
    research questions in, 3546-3547
    watchful waiting, 3541
  for RCC, 2173, 2173*t*
Activin, 1390, 1391*f*
Activities of daily living (ADLs), of geriatric urology patient, 2909
Activity product ratio, 2010
Acupuncture, for PE, 1572.e3
Acute adenolymphangitis (ADL), as filariasis clinical manifestation, 1329
Acute chest syndrome, 451

Acute disseminated encephalomyelitis (ADEM), lower urinary tract dysfunction and, 2625-2626
Acute epididymitis, 1202-1223
Acute focal or multifocal bacterial nephritis, 1171.e1, 1171.e1f
Acute interstitial nephritis (AIN), AKI caused by, 1925, 1925t
Acute kidney injury (AKI), 1921-1927, 1927b
　in children, 353-354, 353t, 353b-354b
　　prerenal, 353-354
　definition of, 1921, 1922t
　differential diagnosis of, 1925-1926, 1926t
　epidemiology and classification of, 1922
　　postrenal, 1923
　　prerenal, 1922-1923
　management of, 1926-1927, 1927t
　staging of, 1922t
Acute orchitis, 1218-1219
Acute post-streptococcal glomerulonephritis, 346
Acute pyelonephritis, 1168-1171, 1168f-1169f, 1170t
Acute renal injury, fractional excretion of sodium for, 777
Acute schistosomiasis, 1324
Acute scrotum, 893-899, 893b
　epididymitis, 898-899
　MRI, 414
　pain causes of, 899, 899b
　spermatic cord torsion, 893-897
　torsion of appendix testis and epididymis, 897-898, 898f
　ultrasonography of, 410-411, 411f-412f, 412b
Acute transverse myelitis, lower urinary tract dysfunction with, 2617
Acute tubular necrosis, resulting from ischemic injury, 1923
Acute upper respiratory tract infection (URTI), 450
Acute urinary retention (AUR)
　age and, 3337, 3337f
　with benign prostatic hyperplasia, 3336-3339, 3337f-3339f, 3337t-3338t, 3400-3401, 3400t
　epidemiology
　　of analytical, 3337-3339
　　of descriptive, 3336, 3337t
　lower urinary tract symptoms with, 3337-3338, 3338t
　management of, 3400-3401, 3401f
　prevention with medical therapy, 3401, 3401b
　prostate volume in, 3338-3339, 3338f-3339f
　serum PSA in, 3338-3339, 3338f-3339f
　urodynamic parameters of, 3338, 3338f
AD. see Atopic dermatitis
Adalimumab, for BPS/IC oral therapy, 1243
Adaptive immune system, 1334-1336, 1335f
ADEM. see Acute disseminated encephalomyelitis
Adenine, 1346.e1, 1346.e2f
Adenocarcinoma
　of bladder, 3090, 3090f
　　in pediatric patients, 1118
　of nonurothelial malignant lesions, 2189
　of rete testis, 1708
　of Skene gland, urethral diverticula differentiated from, 2986, 2986f
Adenomas
　as benign lesions, 2362, 2389-2391, 2390f, 2391b
　metanephric, 2128-2129, 2129f, 2129b
　papillary, of kidney, 2128, 2128b
　prostatic, enucleation of
　　retropubic simple prostatectomy for, 3451-3452, 3451f-3452f
　　in robot-assisted laparoscopic simple prostatectomy, 3455
　　suprapubic prostatectomy for, 3453, 3453f
Adenomatoid tumors, of testicular adnexa, 1709

Adenosine, and ED, 1499
Adenosine triphosphate (ATP), urothelium release of, 2469
Adenylyl cyclase pathway, in ED, 1498
ADHD. see Attention-deficit/hyperactivity disorder
Adherence, 428-429
Adhesins, 428-429
Adjuvant androgen deprivation
　with radiation therapy, for locally advanced prostate cancer, 3653-3654
　with radical prostatectomy, for locally advanced prostate cancer, 3652
Adjuvant chemotherapy
　for muscle-invasive bladder cancer, 3120-3125
　randomized trials of, 3121-3123, 3121t
　for penile cancer, 1798-1800
Adjuvant intravesical topical chemotherapy, after nephroureterectomy, 2220
Adjuvant radiation therapy
　after radical prostatectomy, for locally advanced prostate cancer, 3650-3652, 3651t
　for biochemical recurrence after radical prostatectomy, salvage radiation therapy versus, 3664-3665
Adjuvant therapy, in lymph node metastatic prostate cancer, 3684
Adjuvant topical therapy, for UTUC, 2220
ADL. see Acute adenolymphangitis
ADLs. see Activities of daily living
ADPKD. see Autosomal dominant polycystic kidney disease
Adrenal adenomas
　as benign lesions, 2362, 2393-2394, 2393f, 2394b
　MRI and, 51-52
Adrenal cancer, in nuclear medicine, 43
Adrenal cortex, physiology of, 2356-2357, 2357f, 2357t-2358t
Adrenal cortical carcinoma (ACC)
　malignant lesions, 2362, 2384-2388, 2384f, 2385t, 2386f, 2386b, 2387t, 2388b
　MRI and, 52
　pediatric, 2388
　surgery, 2408-2409, 2408b-2409b
Adrenal cyst, as benign lesion, 2393-2394, 2393f, 2394b
Adrenal disorders, 2354-2404
　of abnormal adrenal function, 2383-2384
　anatomy and, 2355f, 2356, 2356b
　benign lesions, 2389-2394
　　adenoma, 2362, 2389-2391, 2390f, 2391b
　　adrenal cyst, 2393-2394, 2393f, 2394b
　　ganglioneuromas, 2392-2393, 2393b
　　myelolipoma, 2392, 2392f, 2392b
　　oncocytoma, 2391, 2392b
　　pheochromocytoma. see Pheochromocytoma
　of decreased adrenal function, 2380-2383, 2383b
　　clinical characteristics, 2381-2382, 2382t
　　diagnostic tests, 2382
　　overview and epidemiology, 2380-2381
　　pathophysiology, 2381, 2381f
　　prognosis, 2383
　　treatment, 2382-2383, 2383t
　embryology and, 2354-2356, 2356b
　histology and, 2355f, 2356
　historical background, 2354
　of increased adrenal function, 2360-2380
　　Cushing syndrome. see Cushing syndrome
　　pheochromocytoma. see Pheochromocytoma
　　primary aldosteronism. see Primary aldosteronism
　malignant lesions, 2384-2388
　　adrenal cortical carcinoma, 2384-2388, 2384f, 2385t, 2386f, 2386b, 2387t, 2388b

Adrenal disorders (Continued)
　malignant pheochromocytomas, 2373, 2375, 2389
　metastases, 2388-2389, 2389f, 2390b
　neuroblastoma. see Neuroblastoma
　pheochromocytomas, 2373, 2375, 2389
　physiology and, 2356-2360, 2360b
　　adrenal cortex, 2356-2357, 2357f, 2357t-2358t
　　adrenal medulla, 2358-2360, 2358f, 2359t-2360t
Adrenal glands, 2345-2354, 2346f, 2353b
　anatomic relationships in, 2345
　anatomy, 2355f, 2356, 2356b, 2405-2406
　embryology, 2345-2351, 2351f, 2354-2356, 2356b
　histology, 2351-2352, 2351f, 2355f, 2356
　nerves, 2345, 2350f
　physiology, 2356-2360, 2360b
　　adrenal cortex, 2356-2357, 2357f, 2357t-2358t
　　adrenal medulla, 2358-2360, 2358f, 2359t-2360t
　radiology, 2352-2353, 2352f
　surgical landmarks, 2345, 2347f-2348f
　vasculature, 2345, 2348f-2349f, 2355f, 2356, 2405-2406, 2406f
Adrenal incidentalomas
　adrenal surgery for, 2409b
　evaluation of, 2394, 2394t
Adrenal lesions, 54, 57t
Adrenal magnetic resonance imaging, 51-54
Adrenal medulla, physiology of, 2358-2360, 2358f, 2359t-2360t
Adrenal sex steroid hypersecretion, in evaluation of adrenal masses, 2401-2402
Adrenal surgery, 2405-2426, 2426b
　ablative therapy, 2424-2425
　complications, 2423-2424, 2423b-2424b
　for Conn syndrome, 2409-2410, 2409b
　for Cushing syndrome, 2409b, 2410
　evolution of, 2405
　future of, 2425-2426
　hand-assisted, 2419
　indications, 2403, 2403f, 2404b, 2406-2407, 2406f, 2407b
　laparoendoscopic single-site, 2419-2420
　laparoscopic adrenalectomy, 2407-2409, 2407b
　　left, 2414-2415, 2415f-2416f, 2417-2418
　　outcomes, 2421-2423
　　retroperitoneal approach, 2417-2418, 2418f, 2422
　　right, 2415-2416, 2417f-2418f, 2418
　　transperitoneal approach, 2414-2417, 2415f-2417f, 2422
　natural orifice transluminal endoscopic surgery, 2421
　open adrenalectomy, 2410-2414
　　anterior transabdominal approach, 2412-2413, 2412f-2413f
　　flank retroperitoneal approach, 2410-2411, 2410f-2411f
　　left, 2412-2413, 2412f-2413f
　　outcomes, 2421-2423
　　posterior lumbodorsal approach, 2411-2412, 2411f-2412f
　　thoracoabdominal approach, 2413-2414, 2413f-2414f
　partial adrenalectomy, 2421, 2421b
　perioperative management for, 2409-2410
　for pheochromocytoma, 2409, 2409b
　preoperative and perioperative management for, 2409-2410, 2409b
　robot-assisted, 2418-2419, 2419f-2420f, 2422-2423
　surgical anatomy, 2405-2406, 2406f
Adrenal tumors
　ablative therapy for, 2424-2425
　Cushing syndrome and, 2362

Adrenal tumors (Continued)
  evaluation of, 2394-2403
    adrenal incidentalomas, 2394, 2394t
    assessment of function, 2399-2403, 2400b, 2401f, 2402t, 2403b
    biopsy, 2398-2399, 2399f, 2399b
    imaging, 2394-2398, 2396f-2397f, 2397b
    size and growth, 2397-2398, 2398f, 2398b, 2408
    surgical indications, 2403, 2403f, 2404b
α-Adrenergic agonists, 1888
  for stress urinary incontinence in women, 2714
β-Adrenergic agonists
  for stress urinary incontinence in women, 2714
  ureteral response to, 1885
Adrenergic agonists, for stress urinary incontinence, 2501
β3-Adrenergic agonists, for OAB, 2647
α1-Adrenergic antagonists, for PE, 1572.e1
α-Adrenergic antagonists, 1534
β-Adrenergic antagonists
  to facilitate bladder filling and urine storage, 2682t, 2698-2699
  with antimuscarinics, 2706
  for stress urinary incontinence in women, 2714
  ureteral response to, 1888
α-Adrenergic blockers
  and ED, 1506
  for OAB, 2647
α1-Adrenergic blockers
  adverse events with, 3369
  for benign prostatic hyperplasia, 3355-3356
  cardiovascular diseases with, 3369-3370
  classification of, 3356-3357, 3356t
  comparison of, 3367-3369, 3368t
  complications associated with, 3370-3371
  in elderly, 3370
  hemodynamic side effects of, 3369, 3369f
  intraoperative floppy iris syndrome, 3370
  nonselective, 3356
  5α-reductase inhibitors and, 3385, 3386f
  safety profile of, 3369
  selective, 3356-3357
  sexual function and, 3370
β-Adrenergic blockers, and ED, 1506
α-Adrenergic receptor antagonists, for bowel-bladder dysfunction, 657-658
Adrenergic receptors
  pharmacology of, 2500-2501, 2501b
    α-adrenergic receptors, 2500-2501, 2501f
    β-adrenergic receptors, 2500
  in ureteral function, 1888
Adrenogenital syndrome, testicular "tumor" of, 1708
α-Adrenoreceptor antagonists
  for detrusor underactivity, 2661
  to facilitate bladder emptying, 2719-2720
  to facilitate bladder filling and urine storage, 2682t, 2697-2698
  with 5α-Reductase inhibitors, 2707
ADT. see Androgen deprivation therapy
Advance TOT sling, 2887-2888
Advanced imaging, for pediatric urology, 390-391
  computed tomography, 390-391
  magnetic resonance imaging, 390
Advancement flap, laparoscopic or robotic, 3031, 3032f
Advancement procedures, for hypospadias, 918-920
  M inverted V glansplasty, 920, 922f
  meatal advancement glanuloplasty, 920, 921f
  urethral, 920, 922f
  urethromeatoplasty, 918
AdvaSeal-S, 215.e2
Aerobactin, 429
Aerobic glycolysis, 96

Afferent arterioles, 1869
Afferent neuropeptides, lower urinary tract and, 2501-2502
  endothelins, 2502
  prostanoids, 2502
  tachykinins, 2501-2502, 2501t
Afferent pathways
  in detrusor underactivity, 2653-2655, 2655f
  in lower urinary tract, 2481-2486, 2487b
    cannabinoids, 2486
    functional properties of, 2482-2483, 2483f
    modulators of, 2483-2484
    neuromodulation of, 2511
    nitric oxide in, 2484, 2484f
    pelvic organ interactions with, 2486, 2486f
    properties of, 2481
    purinergic signaling, 2484-2485, 2485f
    spinal cord pathways of, 2481-2482, 2481t, 2482f
    transient receptor potential cation channels, 2485
  in overactive bladder and detrusor overactivity, 2641-2642
AFFINITY study, 3702
AFFIRM study, 3695, 3695f
Aflibercept, 3700
African plum, for benign prostatic hyperplasia, 3398
Age
  acute urinary retention and, 3337, 3337f
  and aging, 2922b
    biology and principles of, 2905-2906
    demographics of, 2906-2908, 2907f-2908f
    detrusor muscle and, 2653, 2654f
    geriatric urology and, 2905-2923
    lower urinary system and, 2906
    lower urinary tract dysfunction and, 652, 2509-2510, 2510b, 2633
    orthotopic urinary diversion and, 3237
    physiologic, 2905-2906
    prevalence of OAB and, 2639
    renal calculi and, 2089-2090
    ureter physiology effects of, 1900, 1901f
    and urinary incontinence, 2582-2583
    urinary incontinence and conservative interventions for, 2735
    UTUC variations and, 2185
  colposuspension and, 2756
  prostate cancer diagnosis and, 3459
  renal calculi and, 2006
Age-based self-assessment pain tools, 448-449, 448f
Agency for Healthcare Research and Quality (AHRQ), 101
Agenesis, 949
Aging
  hypothalamic-pituitary-gonadal axis and, 1392
  Peyronie's disease and, 1600
β3-Agonist (Mirabegron)
  for benign prostatic hyperplasia, 3381-3393
  indication, efficacy, and safety profile of, 3381-3382
AH. see Absorptive hypercalciuria
AHRQ. see Agency for Healthcare Research and Quality
AIDS. see Acquired immunodeficiency syndrome
AIN. see Acute interstitial nephritis
Air-charged catheters, for urodynamic studies, 2558
Air embolism, vena caval thrombectomy causing, 2277
AirSeal System, 211, 211.e3f
AKI. see Acute kidney injury
Albumin, 1436
Albuminuria
  in CKD, 1928, 1928t
  in urine, during pregnancy, 283

Albuterol (Ventolin), for contrast media reaction treatment, 30-31
Alcohol
  consumption, prostate cancer and, 3465
  and ED, 1509
  use, benign prostatic hyperplasia and, 3322
Aldosterone hypersecretion, in evaluation of adrenal masses, 2401, 2401f
Aldosterone receptor antagonists, and ED, 1507
Alfuzosin
  for benign prostatic hyperplasia, 3361-3363, 3362t
  to facilitate bladder emptying, 2682t, 2720.e1
Alfuzosin, Finasteride and Combination study, 3385
Aligning catheters, for PFUIs, 1828
Alkali agents, for pediatric kidney stone disease, 869
Alkalosis, after augmentation cystoplasty, 698.e1
Allantois, 319f, 330f
Allergic dermatitis
  atopic dermatitis, 1275-1276, 1276f
  contact dermatitis, 1276-1277, 1277f
  differential diagnosis, 1275b
  erythema multiforme and Stevens-Johnson syndrome, 1277-1278, 1278f
Allergy
  contrast media and, 32
  patient history of, 8
Allogeneic hematopoietic stem cell transplantation, for RCC, 2331, 2331t
Allograft, for pubovaginal sling, 2834-2835
  outcomes of, 2841-2843, 2841t-2842t
Allopurinol
  for chronic scrotal pain syndrome, 1216
  for pediatric kidney stone disease, 870
Alpha hemolysin, 429
5-Alpha reductase inhibitors, for nocturia, 2674
Alpha/beta ratio, 3593
Alpha-blockers, for chronic scrotal pain syndrome, 1215
Alport syndrome, 347
ALPP. see Abdominal leak point pressure
Alprostadil, 1535
ALSYMPCA trial, 3704, 3705f
Alternative hormone treatments, in ED, 1530
Alternative therapies, for ED, 1537-1538
Alveolar RMS, 1111, 1112f, 1113b
Alzheimer disease, and ED, 1502
Amantadine, for delayed ejaculation, 1579
Ambiguous genitalia, 386, 998-1018, 999f, 999b
Ambulatory urodynamics, 2571-2574, 2574b
  clinical utility of, 2571-2574
  monitoring, 484-485
Amebiasis, of genitourinary tract, 1332
American Academy of Pediatrics Guidelines, for febrile urinary tract infection diagnosis and management in young children, 507, 508t
American Association for Surgery of Trauma (AAST), Organ Injury Severity Scale for Kidney, 1992t
American Joint Committee on Cancer and Union International Control Cancer (AJCC and UICC) staging systems, for penile squamous cell carcinoma, 1748-1750
American Joint Committee on Cancer (AJCC) staging system, for UTUC, 2194, 2195t
American Society of Anesthesiologists Classification and Risk, in urologic surgery, 119, 120t, 120b
American Society of Anesthesiologists Task Force Recommendation, on the prevention of peripheral neuropathies, 146t
American Urological Association (AUA)
  best practice statement
    on antibiotic, prophylaxis, 188
    on use of VTE prophylaxis, 231

American Urological Association (AUA) *(Continued)*
  Guideline for the Surgical Management of Stress Urinary Incontinence, 2875-2876
  RCC management guidelines of, 2162-2163, 2163f
  Symptom Score, 109
American Urological Association Symptom Index (AUASI), for benign prostatic hyperplasia, 3344
γ-Aminobutyric acid (GABA), 1494, 1495t
  in efferent pathways to bladder, 2488
  in inhibition of micturition, 2704
Aminoglutethimide, 3677
Aminoglycosides
  prophylaxis with, for uncomplicated urologic procedures, 1194t-1196t
  for UTIs, 1150t-1153t, 1154, 1155f
Aminopenicillins, for UTIs, 1154
Aminophylline, for ureteral relaxation, 1899
Amitriptyline (Elavil)
  for BPS/IC oral therapy, 1241-1242, 1241t
  urethral function effects of, 1903
Ammonium acid urate stones, 2066
  in renal calculi, 2032
Amniotic fluid, 404
  pulmonary development and, 716-717
Amoxicillin, for UTIs, 1151t-1153t, 1154, 1187t
Ampicillin, for UTIs, 1151t-1153t, 1154, 1170t, 1187t
Amplatz dilators, 171, 171f
Amplitude-coded color Doppler sonography, 389
Ampulla, 335
Amputation
  penile, traumatic, 3050-3051
  of penis, for penile cancer, 1752-1753
Amyloidosis
  lower urinary tract dysfunction and, 2632
  of urethra, reconstructive surgery for, 1810
Anaerobes, in urinary tract, 1133
Anal perineum, female, 2435, 2436f
Anal sphincter, 2435
Anal triangle
  female, 2434
  male, 2449-2450
Analgesia
  for pediatric patients, 447b
    children of Jehovah's Witnesses, 448
    children with asthma, 447-448
    children with spina bifida, 452
  for prostate biopsy, 3496-3497
Analgesics, UTUC risk and, 2187
Anaplastic Wilms tumor, 1100
Anastomosis, excision and primary, for transmen, 3071
Ancillary procedures, in pediatric kidney stone disease, 861
Androgen, 1390
  for benign prostatic hyperplasia, manipulation of, 3371-3379
    aromatase inhibitors for, 3377
    cetrorelix, 3377
    chlormadinone acetate, 3377
    dutasteride, 3374-3376, 3374f, 3375t, 3376f
    finasteride, 3371-3374, 3373t
    flutamide, 3376-3377
    literature interpretation for, 3371
    literature review for, 3371
    pharmacological classification for, 3371, 3372t
    rationale for, 3371
    5α-reductase inhibitors and sexual dysfunction, 3378
    selective estrogen and androgen receptor modulators, 3377
    summary for, 3379
    tolerability and safety of, 3378
    zanoterone, 3376

Androgen *(Continued)*
  lower urinary tract and, 2503
  in nuclear matrix, 3294-3295
  plasma binding proteins of, 3282f, 3284
  in prostate cancer, 3462, 3466, 3467f
  in prostate growth, 3282-3283, 3283f
    metabolism of, 3286-3287, 3286f, 3287t
    regulation of, 3285-3286, 3285f
  role in benign prostatic hyperplasia, 3306-3308, 3306f
  sources of, 3673, 3674t, 3674b
  stromal-epithelial interaction regulation by, 3287
  synthesis inhibition, 3677-3678
Androgen axis
  androgen sources in, 3673, 3674t, 3674b
  blockade mechanisms for, 3673-3678, 3679b
  response to, 3679-3680
  molecular biology of, 3672-3673, 3672f, 3673t, 3673b
Androgen-binding protein, 1396-1398
Androgen deprivation therapy (ADT), 3687
  for biochemical recurrence after radiation therapy, 3668-3670
  for biochemical recurrence after radical prostatectomy, 3665
    salvage radiation therapy with, 3663-3664
  continuous, 3683-3684
  intermittent *versus* continuous, 3684-3685
  for localized prostate cancer, immediate *versus* delayed, 3684
  for locally advanced prostate cancer, 3655-3656, 3656b
    intermittent, 3656
    quality of life, 3656
Androgen receptor (AR), 3293b
  in benign prostatic hyperplasia, 3307
  chaperonin binding, 3289
  defects of, 1013-1014
  dimerization of, 3291
  DNA-binding domain, 3289-3290
  function of, 3295b
  ligand-binding domain, 3290-3291
  modulation of, for castration-resistant prostate cancer, 3695-3696, 3695f
  nuclear localization of, 3291
  post-translational modifications of, 3291
  in prostate cancer, 3472
  in prostate growth regulation, 3288-3292, 3289f-3290f
  structure of, 3295b
  transcriptional activation domains, 3291-3292, 3291b, 3292f
Androgen receptor-associated biomarkers, 3685-3686
Androgen receptor-dependent chromatin remodeling, in prostate growth regulation, 3293-3295
Androgen receptor splice variant 7 (AR-V7), 3696
Androgen receptor splice variants, 3685
Androgen suppression, combined with radiation, 3600-3602, 3602b
  background and potential mechanisms of, 3600
  localized disease and, 3600-3602, 3601t
  locally advanced disease and, 3602
    benefit of, 3602
  optimal duration of, 3602
Andropause, 1392
Androstenedione, 3283, 3283f
Anejaculation, 1451
  causes of, 1574, 1574t
  and neurologic disorders, 1576-1577
  treatment of, 1578-1579, 1579t
Anemia
  in CKD, 355
  hormonal therapy and, 3682

Anesthesia
  acute perioperative events, 452-453
    nonspecific fever, 453
    sepsis, 452, 453b
    trauma, 452-453
    URTIs, 453
    UTI, 453
  children with asthma, 447-448
  comorbidities, 450-453
  disposal of unused narcotics, 456, 457t
  ERAS protocols, 453-455
  in geriatric urology patient, 2912
  intraoperative considerations, 453-454
    anaphylaxis, 454-455
    fluid management, 454
    malignant hyperthermia, 454-455
    pain management, 455
    preoperative antibiotics, 453-454, 454t
  for laparoscopic and robotic surgery, complications related, 228
  for laparoscopic kidney surgery, 2279
  laparoscopic procedures, 455-456
  for laparoscopic radical prostatectomy, 3568-3570
  for pediatric kidney stone disease, 861
  for pediatric patients, 447, 447b
  for percutaneous nephrolithotomy, 2104
  perioperative home, 447, 457b
  perioperative planning and postoperative considerations, 450-453, 452b
    acute upper respiratory tract infection (URTI), 450
    anaphylaxis, 454-455, 455b
    for asthma and pulmonary disease, 450
    for cardiovascular anomalies, 450-451
    chemotherapy and, 451
    congenital adrenal hyperplasia, 452
    fluid management, 454
    hematologic disorders, 451
    oncologic disorders, 451-452
    pheochromocytoma, 451-452
    for premature infants, 450
    for renal abnormalities, 451
    spina bifida, 452
  post care unit and pain management, 456
  postoperative management, 455-456
    immediate, 455-456
    inpatient, 456
    outpatient, 456
  and potential neurocognitive effects, 447
  preoperative assessment
    department of social services, 448
    diabetes and metabolic disorders, 449-450
    enteral tube feeds, 449
    fasting times, 449
    for Jehovah's witness, 448
    ketogenic diet, 449
    medication administration, 450
    NPO status, 449, 449t
    pain assessment tools, 448-449
    risk, 447-448
    setting, 448
    special, 448
  preoperative studies, 450
    chest X-ray, 450
    laboratory tests, 450
    pulmonary function testing, 450
    urine evaluation, 450
  preparation for surgery, risk, 447-448
  pubovaginal sling procedure, 2836-2837
  for retropubic radical prostatectomy, 3551-3552, 3551f
  for simple prostatectomy, 3450
  for vasectomy, 1850
Aneurysm
  as laparoscopic and robotic surgery contraindication, 204
  in penile implant, 1593, 1593f

Angioembolization
  indications for, 1072-1073
  of isolated renal segment, 1072
  for renal injuries, 1986, 1986f
Angiogenesis
  in castration-resistant prostate cancer, 3700-3701
  in RCC, 2146
  in UTUC, 2197
Angiography
  in adrenal radiology, 2353
  interventional, for priapism, 1560-1561, 1561f
  of renal artery, 179f
  renovascular hypertension, screening tests for, MRA, 1917-1918, 1918b
  for renovascular hypertension screening, 1917-1918, 1918b
Angiokeratomas of Fordyce, 1302, 1303f
Angiomyolipoma (AML), 293
  in pediatric patients, 1110, 1110f
  renal, 2125-2128, 2128b
    diagnosis of, 2125-2126, 2126f
    epidemiology of, 2125
    management of, 2126-2128, 2127f
    pathophysiology of, 2125
Angiotensin, urethral function effects of, 1902
Angiotensin II (AT2)
  renal vascular tone control by, 1913
  in tubulointerstitial fibrosis, 788
  type 1 receptor antagonists, and ED, 1507
Angiotensin receptor blockers (ARBs), AKI caused by, 1922
Angiotensin-converting enzyme (ACE), 788
Angiotensin-converting enzyme (ACE) inhibitors
  AKI caused by, 1922
  and ED, 1506-1507
Anhydrous ethanol, for prostatic injections, 3447
Animal bites, of penis, 3050
Animal models, laparoscopic training with, 232
Animal protein
  in pediatric kidney stone disease, 869
  for urinary lithiasis, 2047-2048, 2048b
Annexin A3, as prostate cancer biomarker, 3487
Anogenital distance, 305
Anorectal defects
  in bladder exstrophy, 533
  urinary fistula with, 622-623, 622f
Anorectal malformation, 386, 644-645, 650b
  pathogenesis of, 645
  presentation of, 644-645, 646f
  specific recommendations for, 645
Anorgasmia, patient history of, 6
ANP. see Atrial natriuretic peptide
Antegrade endoscopic evaluation, for UTUC, 2191
Antegrade injection, of male stress urinary incontinence, 2896-2897
Antegrade nephroureteroscopy, for UTUC, 2212-2219
  biopsy and definitive therapy in, 2216-2217, 2216f-2217f
  consideration for urinary diversions, 2219
  establishment of nephrostomy tract, 2215-2216, 2215f
  result of, 2217-2219, 2218t
  second-look nephroscopy in, 2217
Antegrade pyelography
  for genitourinary tuberculosis diagnosis, 1312-1313
  for ureterovaginal fistula, 2943
  for urinary tract obstruction, 781
Antegrade ureterography, of ureteral injuries, 1995
Antenatal urinary incontinence, 2726

Anterior approaches, for open kidney surgery, 2252-2253
  chevron incision, 2253
  midline, 2252-2253, 2253.e1f
  subcostal, 2253
Anterior colporrhaphy, for pelvic organ prolapse
  complications of, 2782-2783
  results with, 2779-2782, 2780t
  technique for, 2779, 2779f
Anterior compartment prolapse, 2587
Anterior cutaneous perforating nerves, 136f
Anterior extraperitoneal approach, to laparoscopic pyeloplasty, 1956
Anterior labial commissure, 1627.e1
Anterior pituitary, in HPG axis, 1390-1391, 1391f
Anterior-posterior renal pelvic diameter, in perinatal urology, 359-360, 360t
Anterior transabdominal approach, to open adrenalectomy, 2412-2413, 2412f-2413f
Anterior trunk, 2451t, 2452
Antiandrogens, 3674-3676, 3675f
  and ED, 1508, 1509t
  nonsteroidal, 3674-3676
  for priapism, 1553
  steroidal, 3674
  withdrawal syndrome, 3676
Antibiotic prophylaxis, in urologic surgery, 127-128, 127b
Antibiotic Prophylaxis and Recurrent Urinary Tract Infection in Children (PRIVENT) study, 516
Antibiotics
  for BPS/IC oral therapy, 1243
  for hypospadias, preoperative, 916-918
  for inguinal lymphadenectomy, 1801
  before inguinal node dissection, 1800-1801
  pediatric stone disease and, 867
  for percutaneous nephrolithotomy, 2104
  prophylaxis with, for cystourethroscopy, 188, 189t
  for prostate biopsy, 3496, 3496t
  for renal calculi, pretreatment, 2071
  urethral function effects of, 1904
  for vesicovaginal fistula surgery, 2934
Anticholinergic medication
  detrusor underactivity and, 2657
  for urinary incontinence, in geriatric patients, 2919.e1
Anticholinergic receptor blockers, for benign prostatic hyperplasia, 3389-3393, 3390t, 3392f
Anticholinergics. see also Antimuscarinic agents
  for bowel-bladder dysfunction, 657
  for enuresis, 665
Anticholinesterases, ureteral response to, 1887-1888
Anticoagulants, for vena caval thrombectomy, 2266-2267
Anticoagulated patient
  holmium laser enucleation of prostate and, 3438
  monopolar transurethral resection of prostate in, 3416
  photoselective vaporization of prostate and, 3441
Anticoagulation
  for inguinal lymphadenectomy, 1801
  before inguinal node dissection, 1801
Anticonvulsants, and ED, 1508
Antidepressants
  and ED, 1507-1508
  to facilitate bladder filling and urine storage, 2682t, 2702-2703
Antiglomerular basement membrane (Anti-GBM) disease, 347
Antihistamines
  for BPS/IC oral therapy, 1242
  for contrast media reaction treatment, 31

Antihypertensive agents
  and ED, 1506-1507, 1509t
  effect on sexual function, 1507t
Antihypertensive and Lipid-Lowering Treatment to Prevent Heart Attack Trial (ALLHAT), 3369-3370
Anti-inflammatory therapy, for chronic scrotal pain syndrome, 1215
Antimicrobial formulary, for UTIs, 1150-1155, 1150t-1151t, 1155f
Antimicrobial prophylaxis
  for common urologic procedures, 1193-1201, 1193b, 1194t-1196t, 1201t, 1201b
  for lower tract endoscopy, 1198
  for open and laparoscopic surgery, 1199-1200
  principles of, 1193-1197, 1193b, 1194t-1196t
  for shock wave lithotripsy, 1198
  special considerations, 1200-1201, 1201t
  for transurethral resection of prostate and bladder, 1198-1199
  for TRUSP biopsy, 1197-1198
  for upper tract endoscopy, 1199
  for urethral catheterization and removal, 1193b, 1194t-1196t, 1197
  for urodynamics, 1197
  for UTIs, 1130, 1162-1163
Antimicrobial selection, for uncomplicated cystitis, 1156-1157
Antimicrobial suppression, for UTIs, 1130
Antimicrobial therapy, for UTIs
  antimicrobial formulary for, 1150-1155, 1150t-1153t, 1155f
  bacterial resistance to, 1144-1146, 1145t-1146t, 1147b
  duration of, 1155
  principles of, 1149-1155, 1155f, 1155b
  prophylaxis, 1130
  selection of agents in, 1155-1157
  suppression, 1130
Antimuscarinic agents
  adverse effects of, 2683-2684
  clinical use of, 2683
  to facilitate bladder filling and urine storage, 2681-2684, 2682t, 2697b
    with 5α-reductase inhibitors, 2707
    with α-adrenoreceptor antagonists, 2704-2706
    atropine sulfate, 2684
    with β₃-adrenoreceptor agonist, 2706
    combinations of, 2706-2707
    darifenacin hydrobromide, 2684-2685
    fesoterodine fumarate, 2685-2687
    flavoxate hydrochloride, 2696
    imidafenacin, 2687
    oxybutynin chloride, 2693
    propantheline bromide, 2688
    propiverine hydrochloride, 2695-2696
    solifenacin succinate, 2688-2689
    tolterodine tartrate, 2689-2691
    trospium chloride, 2691-2692
  mechanism of action of, 2681-2682, 2681f
  for neuromuscular dysfunction of lower urinary tract, 633-634
  nocturnal polyuria and, 2668-2669
  pharmacologic properties of, 2682-2683
  for urinary incontinence
    in geriatric patients, 2920.e3
    urgency, 2544
Anti-neutrophil cytoplasmic antibodies (ANCA)-associated glomerulonephritis, 347
Antioxidant therapy, for calcium oxalate precipitation, 2020
Anti-PD-1 approved therapies, 2223
Anti-PD-L1 approved therapies, 2223-2224
Antiproliferative factor (APF), in BPS/IC etiology, 1232.e7, 1232.e8b
Antipsychotics, and ED, 1507

Antireflux procedure
    for classic bladder exstrophy, 554–556, 555f–556f
    for urinary tract reconstruction, 683–685, 685b
        with intestinal segments, 683–685
        psoas hitch for, 683, 684f
        single ureteral reimplant for, 683
        transureteroureterostomy for, 683, 683f
Antiretroviral agents
    and ED, 1509
    in stone formation, 2032–2033
Antiseptics, for cystourethroscopy, 189
Antisperm antibodies, 1398–1399
Antithrombotic therapy, in urologic surgery, 32–34, 57t
Antituberculosis drugs, 1311t, 1315–1317, 1315t–1316t
Anuria, 386, 461
Anxiety
    contrast media and, 32
    prostatitis and, 1210
Anxiolytics, and ED, 1508
Aorta, 1669, 1669.e1f, 1671f, 1672t
    in radical nephrectomy, 2258, 2258f, 2258.e1f
    reconstruction of, RPLND with, 1719
Aortic aneurysm, as laparoscopic and robotic surgery contraindication, 204
Aortic replacement, in retroperitoneal tumors, 2243
Apalutamide, 3676, 3695–3696
Aphallia, 876–877, 877f
Aphthous ulcers, 1286–1287, 1287f
Apical mesh complications, 2886–2887
Apical prolapse, 2587
Apoptosis
    after renal obstruction, 790
    as evolutionarily conserved process, 1365–1366
    in GU cancers, 1365–1367, 1367b
        alternative regulators of, 1366–1367
        extrinsic pathway, 1366.e1f–1366.e2f, 1366.e2
        global defects in, 1366–1367
        intrinsic pathway, 1366.e1, 1366.e1f
        TP53 role in, 1366
    pathway, in castration-resistant prostate cancer, 3701–3702
    regulation of, 783–784
        in benign prostatic hyperplasia, 3309
        in UTUC, 2197
Apparent diffusion coefficient maps, 63–64, 64f
Appendicovesicostomy, 708, 708f
Appendix
    for continent urinary diversions, 707–708
    in ileocecocystoplasty, 694
Appendix epididymis, 319f
Appendix testis, 319f
APR. see Abdominoperineal resection
Aprepitant, to facilitate bladder filling and urine storage, 2713.e4
Aquaporin 2 (AQP2), 793
Aquaporins (AQPs), 793
AR. see Androgen receptor
ARBs. see Angiotensin receptor blockers
ARCD. see Acquired renal cystic diseases
Arcuate arteries, 1869
Arcus tendineus fascia pelvis (ATFP), 2427, 2429f, 2438
Arcus tendineus levator ani (ATLA), 2427, 2429f
Area under the curve (AUC), 3479
Areflexia, 2565
    in detrusor underactivity, 2650
L-Arginine
    for BPS/IC oral therapy, 1241t, 1243
    for female sexual arousal disorders, 1650
Arginine vasopressin (AVP), in water regulation, 2668, 2670f

Argon beam coagulator
    for laparoscopic and robotic surgery, 215.e1
    for monopolar electrosurgery, 235
Aristolochic acid nephropathy, in UTUC, 2187
Aromatase inhibitors, for benign prostatic hyperplasia, 3377
Arousal, female sexual dysfunction and, 1637
ARPKD. see Autosomal recessive polycystic kidney disease
Arsenic, UTUC risk and, 2187
Arterial revascularization, in ED, 1537
Arterial supply, to male pelvis, 2451–2452, 2451t
Arterial system, 1807.e9
    of retroperitoneum, 1669–1672, 1669.e1f–1669.e2f, 1671f, 1671.e1f, 1672t
Arterial system, surgical anatomy of, 3548, 3549f
Arterioureteral fistulas, 1993
Arteriovenous fistulas (AVFs), renal, 737
Artifacts, of ultrasonography images, 71–73, 72f–73f
Artificial somatic-autonomic reflex pathway procedure, for neuromuscular dysfunction of lower urinary tract, 638
Artificial urinary sphincter (AUS), 2546–2547
    for bladder neck reconstruction, 687–688
        results with, 687–688
        technique for, 687.e1
    complications with, 3005–3008, 3008b
        mechanical failure, 3007
        sling, 3008
        special circumstances of, 3007–3008
        urethral atrophy, 3007
        urethral erosion, 3006–3007
        urinary retention, 3005
    evaluation of persistent incontinence after, 2997–2998
    history and development of, 2994, 2994f
    implantation technique, 3000, 3001f, 3003f
        bladder neck, 3003–3004, 3005b
        control pump placement, 3000, 3002f
        making connections, 3000, 3002f
        outcomes of, 3003t
        pressure-regulating balloon, 3000
        tandem cuff, 3000–3002, 3003f
        transcorporal, 3002, 3004f
        trans-scrotal, 3002–3003, 3003f
    infection, 3005–3006
    long-term results with, 3008, 3009b
    for neuromuscular dysfunction of lower urinary tract, 637
AR-V7. see Androgen receptor splice variant 7
As low as reasonably achievable (ALARA) principle, 78, 403, 403b
ASB. see Asymptomatic bacteriuria
Ascending route of infection, 1131
Ascent anomaly, 339, 339f
Ascites
    laparoscopic and robotic surgery causing, 231.e1
    as laparoscopic and robotic surgery contraindication, 204
Ask-Upmark kidney, 744, 744f
Aspiration
    of gastric contents, during laparoscopic and robotic surgery, 228.e1
    of testis, technique of, 1847–1848
Assisted reproduction, 1445–1452, 1445.e3, 1445.e3t
Asthma
    contrast media and, 32
    preoperative care for pediatric patients with, 447–448
Asymmetrical unit membrane (AUM), of urothelium of bladder, 2462, 2463f
Asymptomatic bacteriuria (ASB), 434–435
    in elderly, 1147–1149, 1147t
    in geriatric patients, 2920.e10–2920.e11
    in pregnancy, 1185

Atamestane, for benign prostatic hyperplasia, 3377
ATFP. see Arcus tendineus fascia pelvis
Atherosclerotic renal artery stenosis, 1930–1933
    arterial physiology, concepts in, 1930–1931, 1930f–1931f
    clinical features of, 1931–1932
    diagnostic evaluation of, 1931–1932
    hypertension in, pathophysiology of, 1930–1931
    ischemic nephropathy, pathophysiology of, 1931
    laboratory features of, 1932
    radiographic assessment of, 1932–1933
    therapeutic options for, 1933
        medical management, 1933
        procedural management, 1933
ATLA. see Arcus tendineus levator ani
Atopic dermatitis (AD), 1275–1276, 1276f
ATP. see Adenosine triphosphate
Atrial natriuretic peptide (ANP)
    in bilateral ureteral obstruction, 791–792
    renal vascular tone control by, 1913, 1913f
Atropine, ureteral response to, 1888
Atropine sulfate, to facilitate bladder filling and urine storage, 2682t, 2684
Attention Deficit Hyperactivity Disorder scale, 477
Attention-deficit/hyperactivity disorder (ADHD)
    lower urinary tract dysfunction and, 2633
    and priapism, 1545
Attenuation mechanisms, in ultrasonography, 71, 71f–72f
Attribution bias, 103–104
"Atypical suspicious for carcinoma,", 3506
AUA. see American Urological Association
AUASI. see American Urological Association Symptom Index
AUC. see Area under the curve
Audiovisual and vibratory stimulation, in ED, 1526
Augmentation cystoplasty, 2889–2890
    approach to, 701
    bladder capacity after, 2889–2890
    bladder compliance after, 697–698, 697f, 2889
    bladder level after, 2889–2890, 2890b
    capacity of, 2889
    cecocystoplasty for, 694
    complications of, 635–636, 696–701
        calculi, 699
        delayed spontaneous bladder perforation, 700–701, 700f
        metabolic, 698
        mucus, 698
        urinary tract infection, 699
    contraindications to, 2890
    detrusor overactivity and, 2889–2890
    gastrocystoplasty for, 695
    gastrointestinal effects of, 696–697
    historical perspective on, 2889
    ileocecocystoplasty for, 694, 694f–695f
    ileocystoplasty for, 692–693, 693f
    ileovesicostomy for, 702, 702b
    indications for, 2889–2890
    intestinal segment management for, 692
    native bladder management for, 692, 692f
    necessity of, 701–702
    for neuromuscular dysfunction of lower urinary tract, 635–636
    postoperative management of, 695–696
        early, 695
        late, 696
    pregnancy and, 701
    quality of life and, 702
    in renal transplantation, 1058
    results with, 696–701
    segment choice for, 701
    sigmoid cystoplasty for, 694–695, 696f
    techniques for, 2890

Augmentation cystoplasty *(Continued)*
　for urinary tract reconstruction, in pediatric patients, 691-706, 702*b*
Augmented anastomosis, for urethral stricture disease, 1821-1823, 1826*f*-1827*f*
Augmented bladders
　renal transplantation and, 1057-1058
　tumors of, in pediatric patients, 1118
Augmented valved rectum, 3209
AUM. *see* Asymmetrical unit membrane
AUR. *see* Acute urinary retention
AUS. *see* Artificial urinary sphincter
Autoaugmentation
　for augmentation cystoplasty, 703-705, 704*f*
　for neuromuscular dysfunction of lower urinary tract, 636
Autoimmunity, BPS/IC etiology and, 1232. e2-1232.e3, 1232.e3*b*
Autologous graft, for pubovaginal sling, 2834
　outcomes of, 2839-2841, 2840*t*
Autonomic dysreflexia
　lower urinary tract dysfunction with, 2614-2615
　symptoms of, 2614
　treatment of, 2614-2615
Autonomic nervous system
　and ED, 1527
　in retroperitoneum, 1674-1675, 1676*f*-1677*f*
Autonomic pathways, penile erection and, 1490, 1490*f*
Autonomy, definition of, 115
Autosomal dominant polycystic kidney disease (ADPKD), 349-350, 405, 750-755, 755*b*
　clinical features of, 752
　emerging therapeutics for, 755
　evaluation of, 753-754, 753*f*-754*f*
　extrarenal manifestations of, 752-753
　genetics of, 750-751
　histopathology of, 753, 753*f*
　pathogenesis of, 751-752
　prognosis of, 754-755
　renal cell carcinoma association with, 753
　renal cell carcinoma in, 2158
　treatment of, 754-755
Autosomal recessive polycystic kidney disease (ARPKD), 349, 405, 746-749, 751*b*
　clinical features of, 748
　evaluation of, 748-749, 749*f*-750*f*
　genetics of, 748
　histopathology of, 748, 748*f*
　treatment of, 749
Autotransplantation
　ureteral injuries, upper, 1997
　for ureteral stricture disease, 1975
AVFs. *see* Arteriovenous fistulas
Avitene Microfibrillar Collagen Hemostat, 215. e2
AVP. *see* Arginine vasopressin
Avulsion
　injury, ureteral, with ureteroscopy, 2002
　in ureteroscopic stone management, 2109
Axial flaps, for urethral and penile reconstruction, 1807, 1807*f*-1808*f*
Axial resolution, of ultrasonography images, 70, 70*f*
Axitinib, for RCC, 2179*t*-2180*t*, 2336-2337, 2337*t*
Azathioprine derivatives, for BPS/IC oral therapy, 1241*t*, 1243
Azoospermia, 1445.e1
Azotemia, with benign prostatic hyperplasia, 3336
Aztreonam, for UTIs, 1151*t*-1153*t*, 1154-1155

B

Bacille Calmette-Guérin (BCG)
　in bladder cancer, 1333, 1334*f*, 1338-1339, 1339*f*

Bacille Calmette-Guérin (BCG) *(Continued)*
　for non-muscle-invasive bladder cancer, 3099-3100
　　carcinoma treatment in situ with, 3100
　　contraindications to, 3102*b*
　　mechanism of action of, 3100
　　prophylaxis to prevent recurrence, 3100-3101
　　residual tumor treatment, 3100
　　toxicity management of, 3102*b*
Baclofen
　drug delivery of, 2720.e2
　to facilitate bladder emptying, 2720.e2-2720. e3
　to facilitate bladder filling and urine storage, 2682*t*, 2704
　for priapism, 1553-1554
Bacteremia, 427, 428*f*
　UTIs and, 1182-1187, 1184*b*
Bacteria
　cell wall components, in septic shock, 1183
　mesh complication with, 2878
　urease production by, 2030-2031, 2031*t*
　in urine, 23, 24*f*
　urothelial cancer and, 3099
Bacterial adherence, 1134-1135
Bacterial adhesins, 1134
Bacterial fimbriae, 428-429
Bacterial nephritis, 435, 435*f*
Bacterial persistence, in recurrent UTIs, 1160-1161
Bacterial "relapse," renal infection from, 1177.e1
Bacterial resistance, to UTI antimicrobial therapy, 1144-1146, 1145*t*-1146*t*, 1147*b*
Bacterial type 1 (mannose-sensitive) pili, 1134
Bacterial vaginosis, 1271-1272, 1272*t*
Bacteriology, sepsis and, 1184
Bacteriuria
　after augmentation cystoplasty, 699
　catheter-associated, 1190, 1191*b*
　in elderly, 1188-1190, 1190*b*
　　asymptomatic, 1147-1149, 1147*t*, 1147*b*-1149*b*
　　diagnosis, 1188-1189
　　epidemiology, 1188
　　management, 1189-1190, 1189*t*
　　pathogenesis, 1188
　　screening for, 1188
　in pregnancy, 1184-1185, 1188*b*
　　anatomic and physiologic changes and, 1185-1186, 1185*t*, 1186*f*
　　complications of, 1186-1187
　　management of, 1186-1187, 1187*t*
　　pathogenesis, 1185
　UTIs and, 1129, 1159
Bacteroides fragilis, infection after mid-urethral sling surgery, 2870-2871
Baden-Walker classification, of PFDs, 2529-2530
Baden-Walker Halfway Scoring System, 2588
Balanitis
　infection, 1288
　pseudoepitheliomatous, keratotic, and micaceous, 1299-1300, 1300*f*
　urethral reconstructive surgery for, 1811
　Zoon, 1302, 1303*f*
Balanitis xerotica obliterans (BXO), 875-876, 876*f*, 939, 940*f*
Balanoposthitis, 1288, 1289*f*
Ballistic lithotripsy, 2111-2112, 2112*f*
Balloon catheters, 173
Balloon dilation
　for achieving extraperitoneal access and developing extraperitoneal space, 209, 210*f*
　for ureteral stricture disease
　　antegrade, 1967-1968
　　results with, 1968
　　retrograde, 1966-1967, 1967*f*-1968*f*
　for ureteroenteric strictures, 1977

Balloon dilators, 171-172, 171*f*-172*f*
Balloon incision, cautery wire, for ureteroenteric strictures, 1977
Barotrauma, during laparoscopic and robotic surgery, 225
Barrier function, of urothelium of bladder, 2467-2468, 2468*f*
Barrington nucleus, 2493
Bartter syndrome, 349, 2019
Basal cell carcinoma (BCC)
　as neoplastic condition, 1297-1298, 1300*f*
　of penis, 1772
Basal cells
　epididymis, 1374-1375, 1403-1404
　of prostate, 3278, 3278*f*
Base excision repair (BER), 1351.e1, 1351.e1*f*
Baseline urinary function, localized prostate cancer and, 3524
Bashful bladder
　detrusor underactivity and, 2659
　lower urinary tract dysfunction and, 2628-2629
Basic Laparoscopic Urologic Surgery (BLUS), 471
"Bayesian" problem, 3543
BBD. *see* Bladder and bowel dysfunction
BCC. *see* Basal cell carcinoma
BCG. *see* Bacille Calmette-Guérin
BCI. *see* Bladder contractility index
BCR. *see* Bulbocavernosus reflex
BD. *see* Behçet disease
BDL. *see* Biomarker Development Laboratory
Beckwith-Wiedemann syndrome (BWS), genomic alterations in, 1098, 1354*t*
Behavior, norms of, masculinity and, 1416
Behavioral modification, for bowel-bladder dysfunction, 656
Behavioral therapy (BT)
　for enuresis, 663, 664*f*
　for OAB, 2647
　for urinary incontinence, in geriatric patient, 2920.e3
Behavioral training
　levels of evidence and recommendations for, 2722.e1*b*, 2722.e4*b*
　with urge suppression, 2727-2729, 2728*f*
Behavioral treatment programs, for urinary incontinence, 2722-2738, 2738*b*
　adherence to, 2734-2735
　assessment for, 2722-2723, 2723.e1*f*-2723. e2*f*, 2724*f*
　bladder training, 2728*f*, 2730-2732, 2730.e1*t*
　common, 2722, 2723*f*
　conditions benefitting from, 2722.e1*t*
　indications for, 2722
　levels of evidence and recommendations for, 2722.e1*b*, 2722.e4*b*
　lifestyle modifications as, 2722, 2722.e1*b*
　models of delivery, 2737-2738, 2737.e1*f*
　patient education for, 2723
　for pelvic floor dysfunction, 2732-2735
　pelvic floor muscle electrical stimulation, 2729-2730
　pelvic floor muscle training for. *see* Pelvic floor muscle training
　for prevention, 2735-2736
　role of biofeedback in, 2727.e1*f*, 2729
　vaginal and urethral mechanical devices, 2736-2737
Behçet disease (BD), 1286-1287, 1287*f*
Bell-shaped curve, 480
Beneficence, definition of, 115
Benign bounce phenomenon, brachytherapy and, 3608
Benign cutaneous diseases, of external genitalia, of male genitalia
　angiokeratomas of Fordyce, 1302, 1303*f*
　ectopic sebaceous glands, 1303*f*, 1304
　median raphe cysts, 1304

Benign cutaneous diseases, of external genitalia, of male genitalia (Continued)
  pearly penile papules, 1302, 1303f
  sclerosing lymphangitis, 1302–1304
  Zoon balanitis, 1302, 1303f
Benign disease, bladder surgery for, 3010–3047
  anatomy of, 3010
  bladder stones, 3043–3046
  diverticulectomy, 3010–3019, 3011f, 3011b, 3046b–3047b
  enterocystoplasty, 3034–3038
  foreign-body removal, 3043–3046
  partial cystectomy, 3038–3043
  psoas hitch and Boari flap, 3026–3034
  surgical considerations of, 3010
  urachal surgery, 3038–3043
  ureteral reimplantation, 3019–3026
Benign idiopathic urethrorrhagia, 401
Benign joint hypermobility syndrome, lower urinary tract dysfunction and, 2633
Benign lesions, adrenal, 2389–2394
  adenoma, 2362, 2389–2391, 2390f, 2391b
  adrenal cyst, 2393–2394, 2393f, 2394b
  ganglioneuromas, 2392–2393, 2393b
  myelolipoma, 2392, 2392f, 2392b
  oncocytoma, 2391, 2392b
  pheochromocytoma. see Pheochromocytoma
Benign multilocular cyst, 765–766, 765f, 766b, 767f
Benign oncocytomas, 98
Benign prostatic hyperplasia (BPH), 3063, 3305–3342
  acute urinary retention with, 3400–3401, 3400t
    as complication of, 3336–3339, 3337f–3339f, 3337t–3338t
  α1-adrenergic blockers for, 3355–3356
    adverse events with, 3369
    alfuzosin, 3361–3363, 3362t
    anticholinergic receptor blockers with, 3389–3393, 3390t, 3392f
    cardiovascular diseases with, 3369–3370
    classification of, 3356–3357, 3356t
    comparison of, 3367–3369, 3368t
    complications associated with, 3370–3371
    doxazosin for, 3359–3361, 3360t–3361t
    in elderly, 3370
    hemodynamic side effects of, 3369, 3369f
    hypertension with, 3369–3370
    intraoperative floppy iris syndrome, 3370
    literature review for, 3357–3367
    naftopidil, 3365–3367, 3367t
    nonselective, 3356
    phosphodiesterase type 5 inhibitors with, 3393, 3394t
    rationale for, 3355–3356, 3355f
    safety profile of, 3369
    selective, 3356–3357
    sexual function and, 3370
    silodosin, 3365, 3365f, 3366t
    summary for, 3371
    tamsulosin, 3363–3365, 3363f, 3364t
    terazosin for, 3357–3359, 3357t–3358t, 3359f
  α-adrenergic receptors in, 2500
  β3-agonist (Mirabegron) for, 3381–3393
    indication, efficacy, and safety profile, 3381–3382
    phosphodiesterase type 5 inhibitors, 3382
  alcohol use and, 3322
  anatomic features of, 3313–3314, 3313f–3314f
  androgen manipulation for, 3371–3379
    aromatase inhibitors for, 3377
    cetrorelix, 3377
    chlormadinone acetate, 3377
    dutasteride, 3374–3376, 3374f, 3375t, 3376f
    finasteride, 3371–3374, 3373t
    flutamide, 3376–3377
    literature interpretation for, 3371
    literature review for, 3371

Benign prostatic hyperplasia (BPH) (Continued)
    pharmacological classification for, 3371, 3372t
    rationale for, 3371
    5α-reductase inhibitors and sexual dysfunction, 3378
    selective estrogen and androgen receptor modulators, 3377
    summary for, 3379
    tolerability and safety of, 3378
    zanoterone, 3376
  anticholinergic receptor blockers for
    α-adrenergic blockers with, 3389–3393, 3390t, 3392f
    β3-agonists, 3393
  autopsy prevalence of, 3317, 3317f
  bladder obstruction in
    measures of, 3320
    response to, 3315–3316
  body mass index and, 3324, 3325t
  clinical prevalence of, 3317, 3318f
  combination therapy for, 3385
    α-adrenergic blockers and 5α-reductase inhibitors, 3385, 3386f
    Combination of Avodart and Tamsulosin Study, 3386–3389, 3389f, 3389t
    Medical Therapy of Prostatic Symptoms Trial, 3385–3386, 3387f–3388f, 3387t
  complications of, 3335–3339
    acute urinary retention with, as complication of, 3336–3339, 3337f–3339f, 3337t–3338t
    bladder decompensation, 3335
    bladder stones, 3335
    hematuria, 3336
    mortality, 3335
    upper urinary tract deterioration and azotemia, 3336
    urinary incontinence, 3335
    urinary tract infections, 3336
  cystourethrogram for, 3348
  cystourethroscopy for, 3348
  diagnostic evaluation of, 3343–3351, 3351b
  diet and, 3324, 3325t
  epidemiology of, 3316–3335, 3341b
    analytical studies, 3320–3327
    definitions for, 3316–3317
    descriptive studies for, 3317–3320
    parameter correlations, 3324–3327, 3326f–3327f, 3327t
  etiology of, 3305–3313, 3316b
    androgen receptors in, 3307
    androgen role in, 3306–3308, 3306t
    cytokines, 3311, 3312f
    dihydrotestosterone in, 3307–3308, 3308f
    estrogen role in, 3308–3309, 3308t
    familial factors in, 3311–3312, 3311t
    genetic factors in, 3311–3312, 3311t
    growth factors, 3309–3310, 3310f
    hyperplasia, 3305–3306
    inflammatory pathways in, 3311, 3312f
    programmed cell death regulation, 3309
    prolactin, 3313
    signaling pathways in, 3310–3311
    steroid 5α-reductase in, 3307–3308, 3308f
    stromal-epithelial interaction, 3309
  filling cystometry for, 3347
  frequency-volume charts and bladder diaries of, 3344–3345
  future directions for, 3401–3402, 3402f
  health-related quality of life and, 3319
  histologic features of, 3314–3315, 3314f
  histologic prevalence of, 3317, 3317f
  hypertension and, 3322
  imaging for, 3347
  instrumental investigations of, 3346–3351
  laboratory tests of, 3345–3346
  liver cirrhosis and, 3322
  lower urinary tract function and, 2528
  in lower urinary tract symptoms, 3305, 3306f

Benign prostatic hyperplasia (BPH) (Continued)
    management of lower urinary tract symptoms caused by, 3351–3371
      conservative, 3351, 3352f–3353f
      lifestyle and dietary modifications, 3351–3353
      watchful waiting, 3351
    medical history for, 3343
    medications and, 3324
      effects of, 3404
    metabolic syndrome and, 3324, 3325t
    muscarinic receptor antagonists for, 3379–3381
      efficacy of, 3379–3381, 3380t
      rationale and indication for, 3379, 3379t
      summary for, 3381
      tolerability and safety profile of, 3381
    natural history of, 3316–3335
    obesity and, 3324, 3325t
    pathology of, 3313–3315
    pathophysiology of, 3313–3316, 3313f
    phosphodiesterase type 5 inhibitors for, 3382, 3382f, 3383t–3384t, 3385f
      α1-adrenergic blockers with, 3393, 3394t
    physical activity and, 3324, 3325t
    physical examination for, 3344
    phytotherapy for, 3393–3399
      current role of, 3395
      extract composition of, 3394, 3394t–3395t
      Hypoxis rooperi (South African star grass), 3398
      lycopene, 3398–3399
      mechanism of action, 3394–3395, 3395t
      origin of agents for, 3394, 3394t
      Pygeum africanum (African plum), 3398
      Serenoa repens (saw palmetto berry), 3395–3398, 3396f, 3397t
      summary for, 3399
    postvoid residual volume for, 3346
    pressure-flow study for, 3347
    prostate and bladder imaging for, 3348
    prostate size and, 3320, 3320f, 3404
    prostate-specific antigen in, 3345
    religion and, 3320–3321
    serum creatinine measurement for, 3345–3346
    sexual activity and, 3322, 3322f, 3323t
    smoking and, 3324
    smooth muscle in, 3315, 3315f
    socioeconomic factors in, 3321, 3321t
    surgery for, 3321, 3339–3340, 3340f
    surgical treatment for, 3403–3404
    symptom of
      assessment of, 3343–3344
      severity and frequency of, 3317–3319, 3319f
    untreated, natural history of, 3327–3328
      baseline symptom severity in, 3331–3332
      clinical parameters of, 3328, 3328t
      disease progression in, 3332, 3332f–3333f, 3334t
      longitudinal population-based studies, 3333–3335, 3334f, 3334t–3335t
      outcomes of interest with, 3328, 3328t
      perception of improvement, 3328
      placebo control groups in, 3331, 3331t
      placebo/sham effect in, 3331–3332
      sham control groups in, 3331
      study methods for, 3328–3335, 3329t
      watchful waiting studies for, 3329–3330, 3330f, 3330t
    upper-tract imaging for, 3347–3348
    upper urinary tract in, deterioration of, 3336
    urinalysis for, 3345
    urodynamics for, 3347
    uroflowmetry for, 3346–3347, 3346f
    vasectomy and, 3322, 3322f, 3323t
Benign prostatic obstruction (BPO), bladder outlet obstruction and, 2566

Benign renal tumors, 2121-2132. see also Renal cysts
　angiomyolipoma, 2125-2128, 2126f-2127f, 2128b
　cystic nephroma, 2129-2130, 2129f
　diagnosis of, 2121
　leiomyoma, 2131, 2131f, 2131b
　metanephric adenoma, 2128-2129, 2129f, 2129b
　mixed epithelial and stromal, 2130, 2130f, 2130b
　mixed mesenchymal and epithelial, 2129-2130, 2129f
　oncocytoma, 2123-2125, 2124f, 2125b
　other, 2131-2132, 2132b
　papillary adenoma, of kidney, 2128, 2128b
Benign urethral tumors, 1776
　FEPs, 1776
　hemangiomas, 1776
　leiomyomas, 1776
Benzodiazepines, to facilitate bladder emptying, 2720.e2
BER. see Base excision repair
Berger disease, 17
Beta-blockers, contrast media and, 32
Bethanechol (Urecholine)
　administration of, 2717
　for detrusor underactivity, 2660-2661
　efficacy of, 2718
　to facilitate bladder emptying, 2716-2717
　side effects of, 2718
　supersensitivity test, 2565
　ureteral response to, 1887
Bevacizumab, 1358, 3700
　for RCC, 2146, 2333-2334, 2333t
BEZ235, 3700
BF. see Biofeedback
Bicalutamide, 3675
Bicarbonate reabsorption, in neonate, 342
Bicycle riding, long-distance, penile implants and, 1596, 1597f
Bifid pelvis, 737, 738f
Bifid scrotum, 886, 887f
Bifid ureters, 820-821
BII. see BPH Impact Index
Bilateral anterior subcostal approach, for open kidney surgery, 2253
Bilateral renal agenesis (BRA), 714-717
　amniotic fluid production and, 716-717
　diagnosis of, 717
　gross pathologic description of, 715, 716f
　incidence of, 714
　mammalian kidney organogenesis in, 714-715
　phenotypic features associated with, 715-716, 717f
　postnatal radiographic evaluation of, 717
　prognosis of, 717
　renal embryology and possible etiology of, 714
Bilateral vanishing testes syndrome, 1005-1006
Bilirubin, in urine, 20
Binary survival outcomes, 104-105
Biochemical evaluation, of pheochromocytoma, 2376, 2377f, 2377t
Biochemical recurrence
　after radiation therapy, 3665-3670
　　androgen deprivation therapy after, 3668-3670
　　biopsy, 3666
　　imaging for, 3666-3667
　　natural history, 3666
　　prostate-specific antigen bounce, 3666
　　prostate-specific antigen recurrence, 3665-3666
　　salvage brachytherapy, 3668
　　salvage cryotherapy, 3667-3668, 3669t
　　salvage high-intensity focused ultrasound, 3668
　　salvage radical prostatectomy, 3667, 3667t

Biochemical recurrence (Continued)
　after radical prostatectomy, 3659-3665
　　adjuvant radiation therapy, 3664-3665
　　androgen deprivation therapy, 3665
　　androgen deprivation therapy with salvage radiation therapy for, 3663-3664
　　definition of, 3659
　　imaging of, 3661-3662, 3662f
　　natural history of, 3660-3661
　　prediction of, 3659-3660, 3660t
　　salvage radiation therapy dose response, 3663
　　salvage radiation therapy for, 3662-3663
　　ultrasensitive prostate-specific antigen for, 3661
　　whole-pelvis versus prostatic bed radiation therapy, 3664, 3664f-3665f
　of prostate cancer, management strategies for, 3659-3670, 3670b
Bioethics, 115
Biofeedback (BF)
　for bowel-bladder dysfunction, 656-657
　for genito-pelvic pain-penetration disorder, 1653
　with PFMT, 2727.e1f, 2729, 2729f, 2729.e1f-2729.e2f
Biofilm, 434
　formation, 430, 434
BioGlue, 215.e2
Biologic grafts, for posterior compartment repair, 2829
Biologic therapies, for neuroblastoma, 1095-1096
Biologically active agents, 148
Biomarker Development Laboratory (BDL), 3478-3479
Biomarker Reference Laboratories (BRL), 3478-3479
Biomarkers
　for non-muscle-invasive bladder cancer, 3109, 3109f
　for penile cancer, 1759, 1759t
　telomerase activity as, 1364
　for testicular tumors, in pediatric patients, 1122, 1122f
Biopsy
　bladder, for RMS, 1113
　prostate, after radiotherapy for biochemical recurrence, 3666
　renal
　　laparoscopic, 2292, 2292f
　　ultrasound guidance of, 79-80
　　for renal tumor ablation, 2314
　　in retrograde ureteroscopic, 2212
　testis, 1454-1456
　　aspiration, percutaneous, 1455
　　complications of, 1456
　　indications of, 1454-1455
　　open testis biopsy: microsurgical technique for, 1455, 1456f
　　percutaneous, 1455
　in transurethral resection of bladder tumor, for non-muscle-invasive bladder cancer, 3096
Biopsy-based lesion identification, for focal therapy for prostate cancer, 3621
Biosyn suture, 149
Biothesiometry, 1527
Bipolar electrocautery, 466
Bipolar electrosurgical devices, 237
　for laparoscopic and robotic surgery, 214
Bipolar resectoscope, 172
Bipolar transurethral resection of the prostate (B-TURP), 3418-3420
　complications with, 3419
　　intraoperative, 3419
　　perioperative, 3419
　　postoperative, 3419
　concept for, 3418-3419

Bipolar transurethral resection of the prostate (B-TURP) (Continued)
　conclusion for, 3419-3420
　outcomes with, 3419
　　comparative studies, 3419
　　single-cohort studies, 3419
　technique for, 3419
Birmingham Reflux Study (Birmingham Reflux Study Group 1987), 515
Birt-Hogg-Dubé (BHD) syndrome, genomic alterations in, 1354t, 1358, 2142t, 2144-2145
BISF-W. see Brief Index of Sexual Function for Women
Bisphosphonates, for castration-resistant prostate cancer, 3703-3704
Bites, animal and human, penile, 3050
Bladder, 315f, 324f
　afferent pathways in, 2481-2486, 2487b
　　cannabinoids, 2486
　　in detrusor underactivity, 2653-2655, 2655f
　　functional properties of, 2482-2483, 2483f
　　modulators of, 2483-2484
　　nitric oxide in, 2484, 2484f
　　pelvic organ interactions with, 2486, 2486f
　　properties of, 2481
　　purinergic signaling, 2484-2485, 2485f
　　spinal cord pathways of, 2481-2482, 2481t, 2482f
　　transient receptor potential cation channels, 2485
　aging and, 2509-2510
　anatomy of, 2461-2513, 2462f, 3010
　　lamina propria of, 2462-2463
　　smooth muscle of, 2465, 2465f
　　stroma of, 2463
　　urothelium of, 2461-2462, 2462f-2463f. see also Urothelium, of bladder
　　vasculature of, 2462-2463, 2464f
　capacity of
　　nocturnal, 661-662
　　pharmacologic therapy to increase, 2679-2700
　　reconstruction and, 681-682
　cells, receptivity in UTIs, 1136-1137, 1137f
　changes, during pregnancy, 1185
　closure of, for classic bladder exstrophy, 545-548, 546f-548f
　contractility of
　　bladder emptying and, 2716-2718
　　pharmacologic therapy to inhibit, 2679-2700
　contraction of
　　muscarinic receptors and, 2679-2681
　　normal, in voiding, 2515-2516
　decompensation, in benign prostatic hyperplasia, 3335
　defects in, in bladder exstrophy, 535-537, 536f-537f
　defunctionalized, lower urinary tract dysfunction and, 2632-2633
　development of, 329-333, 333b
　dynamics of, 681-682
　dysfunction of, 680-681
　　with posterior urethral valves, 616-619
　efferent pathways to, 2487-2493, 2487f
　　adrenergic, 2488
　　in detrusor underactivity, 2653, 2655f
　　glutamate in, 2488, 2489f
　　glycine and γ-aminobutyric acid in, 2488
　　purinergic, 2488-2489
　　reflex circuitry, 2489-2493, 2490f
　　serotonin in, 2488-2489
　　terminal nerve fibers, 2487-2488
　　transmitters in, 2488, 2490b, 2491f-2492f, 2491t

Bladder (Continued)
    emptying failure of, 2903-2904, 2903b-2904b
        absorbent products for, 2904
        catheterization for, 2900-2902, 2900f
        external collecting devices for, 2903-2904
        intravesical pressure increases for, 2902-2903
    emptying of
        benign prostatic hyperplasia and, 3354-3355
        failure of, 2518-2519
        reconstruction and, 682
        therapy to facilitate, 2520b
        urodynamic studies of, 2564-2566
    estrogens and, 2503
    filling of. see also Continence
        abnormalities of, 2516-2519, 2516b-2517b, 2518t
        bladder response during, 2514-2515
        mechanics of, 2478-2479
        outlet response to, 2515
        smooth muscles in, 2478
        urodynamic studies of, 2552t-2553t, 2559
    in genitourinary tuberculosis, 1309
    glycosaminoglycan layer, 1232.e5-1232.e7, 1232.e7b
    high-pressure, spinal cord injury with, host defense mechanisms in UTIs and, 1140
    injuries of, 3054-3057, 3055b-3056b
        clinical signs and symptoms of, 3056
        complications with, 3057
        diagnosis of, 3055-3056
        etiology of, 3054-3055
        with holmium laser enucleation of prostate, 3438
        management of, 3056-3057, 3056.e1f
        outcomes with, 3057
        radiographic imaging of, 3055-3056, 3055f
    male
        circulation of, 2456
        innervation of, 2456
        relationship with, 2448f
        trigone, 2455-2456, 2456f
        ureterovesical junction of, 2455-2456, 2456f
    mesh perforation of, in midurethral sling, 2868-2870, 2868f, 2869t, 2870b
    natural defenses of, 1138-1139
    necrosis of, with transurethral vaporization of prostate, 3426
    neoplasia in, 1360-1361
    neural tube defects and, early intervention for, 628, 628f
    obstruction of
        response to, 3315-3316
        RMS causing, 1113
    overactive. see Overactive bladder
    paralytic, 2522
    perforation of
        after augmentation cystoplasty, 700-701, 700f
        in transurethral resection of bladder tumor, 3135, 3135f
    pharmacology of, 2497-2503
        adrenergic mechanisms, 2500-2501, 2501f, 2501b
        muscarinic mechanisms, 2497-2500, 2499t, 2500b
        sex steroids, 2502-2503
    physical examination for, 10, 10f-11f
    in prune-belly syndrome, 582-583, 584f
    pudendal nerve stimulation and, 2511
        inhibitory and excitatory frequencies for, 2511
    reconstruction of, 690-691
        after RMS treatment, 1116
    regeneration of, for augmentation cystoplasty, 706

Bladder (Continued)
    sensation of
        altered, filling/storage failure due to, 2517-2518
        detrusor underactivity and, 2659
        terminology for, 2581
    sensory input of, pharmacologic therapy to decrease, 2679-2700
    smooth muscle of, 1185, 2465, 2465f
    storage failure of, 2517-2518, 2903-2904, 2904b
        absorbent products for, 2904
        augmentation cystoplasty for, 2889-2890
        external collecting devices for, 2903-2904
    storage function of
        after retropubic suspension surgery, 2770
        pharmacologic therapy to facilitate, 2679-2716
        urinary incontinence and, 2581
        urodynamic studies of, 2552t-2553t, 2559
    suburothelial interstitial cells of, 2470, 2470f
    surgical considerations of, 3010
    transabdominal pelvic ultrasonography, 80-81, 80f-81f
    transurethral resection of, 1198-1199
    trigone of, 2455-2456, 2456f
    tumors of. see Bladder tumors
    underactive, 2506-2507, 2650
        parasympathomimetics for, 2660-2661
        pediatric, 660
    unstable, 2637
    UPEC persistence in, 1136-1137, 1138f
    urothelium of, genetic alterations in, 1360-1361
    voiding of. see also Micturition
        bashful bladder, 2628-2629
        mechanics of, 2479
Bladder advancement flap, laparoscopic or robotic, 3031, 3033f
Bladder and bowel dysfunction (BBD), 397-399, 495
    conservative management of, 656
    neuromodulation for, 658, 659t
    in pediatric patients, 654
    pharmacotherapy for, 657-658
    treatment for, 655-656
    urotherapy for, 655-656
Bladder anomalies, in children, 518-527
    acquired, 525-526, 527b
        inflammatory, 526
        noninflammatory, 525-526
    congenital, 518-525, 523b
        embryology of urinary bladder, 518
        normal and abnormal antenatal sonographic findings of bladder, 518-525
Bladder augmentation, pharmacologic therapy in, to facilitate bladder filling and urine storage, 2718
Bladder calculi
    after renal transplantation, 2117
    bladder outlet obstruction with bladder lithiasis, 2115-2116
    etiopathogenesis of, 2114-2115
    lithotripsy
        for EHL, 241
        pneumatic, 244.e4
    medical management of, 2066-2067
    in patients with spinal cord injury, 2116-2117
    in urinary diversions and augmented bladder, 2116
Bladder cancer
    BCG in, 1333, 1334f, 1338-1339, 1339f
    bladder diverticula with, 2969-2971, 3011
    chronic inflammation role in, 1336-1338, 1337f-1338f
    diminished bladder capacity and, 2671
    DNA methylation in, 1349
        CDH1 and RASSF1A genes, 1350
        hypermethylation, 1350
        hypomethylation, 1350
        INK4A gene, 1350

Bladder cancer (Continued)
    genomic alterations in, 1358-1360
        alterations in normal and benign urothelium, 1360-1361
        detection and surveillance using, 1361
        before neoplasia, 1360-1361
    in geriatric patients, 2920.e12-2920.e13
    hereditary, 3076
    immune checkpoint blockade in, 1342
    immunotherapy for, 1333
    long-term indwelling catheterization and, 2616
    metastatic
        chemotherapy for, 3127t
        FDA-approved agents and future directions for, 3130
        first-line, immune checkpoint inhibitor therapy, 3130
        immune checkpoint inhibitor therapy, 3129-3130
        management of, 3112-3132, 3131b
        multiagent, second-line chemotherapy for, 3129
        randomized trials in, 3127-3128, 3127t
        second-line, immune checkpoint inhibitor therapy, 3130
        second-line chemotherapy for, 3128, 3128t
        single agent, second-line chemotherapy for, 3128-3129, 3129t
        targeted therapy for, 3130-3131
    minimally invasive, 3144
    as non-AIDS-defining urologic malignancy, 1268
    in nuclear medicine, 43
    screening for, molecular genetics-based assays for, 1361
    UTUC after, 2192-2193
Bladder cancer, pediatric
    in augmented bladders, 1118
    carcinoma, 1118
    TCC, 1117-1118
    urachal carcinoma, 1118
Bladder coil, 174f
Bladder compliance (C), 2478
    after augmentation cystoplasty, 697-698, 697f
    impaired, urodynamic studies of, 2560-2561, 2560f-2561f
Bladder contractility index (BCI), 2567, 2567f, 2659
Bladder cooling reflex, 2485
Bladder cuff
    management, 2200
    open distal ureterectomy with excision of, 2204
Bladder diary, 3
    for behavioral treatment programs, 2723, 2724f
    for benign prostatic hyperplasia (BPH), 3344-3345
    Questionnaire-Based Voiding Diary, 2723, 2723.e1f-2723.e2f
    for urinary incontinence, male, 2541, 2541f
Bladder diverticula, 509-510, 509.e1f, 2964-2972, 2965f-2966f
    associated conditions, 2969-2971
        bladder outlet obstruction, 2969
        endoscopic examination, 2969, 2970f
        ipsilateral vesicoureteral reflux, 2971
        malignancy, 2969-2971
    classification of, 2964-2965
    diagnosis of, 2965-2969, 2971b
        evaluation of, 2965-2967, 2966f
        imaging of, 2965f, 2967, 2968f-2969f
        presentation of, 2965-2967, 2966f
        urodynamics of, 2967-2969
    etiology of, 2964-2965
    malignancy, 3011
    management of, 2971-2972, 2972b, 2973f
        endoscopic, 2972
        indications for intervention, 2972
        observation and nonsurgical, 2972

Bladder diverticula *(Continued)*
  nonsurgical management of, 2972
  pathophysiology of, 2964-2965
  surgical management of, laparoscopic and robotic diverticulectomy, 2972
  techniques for repair, complication with, 2991, 2991f
Bladder diverticulectomy, 3010-3019, 3011f, 3011b, 3046b-3047b
  complications of, 3018-3019
  evaluation of, 3011-3012, 3012f
  laparoscopic and robotic techniques, 3015-3018, 3016f-3017f
  outcomes of, 3018-3019
  postoperative care of, 3018-3019
  surgical indications, 3011-3012, 3012f
  surgical technique of, 3012-3018, 3012f
Bladder duplication, 521-522, 521f
Bladder dysfunction, after pediatric renal transplantation, 1063
Bladder epithelial grafts, 1806
Bladder exstrophy, 330, 379-380, 381f
  recommendations for, 379-380
Bladder filling, ureteral function effects of, 1893
Bladder function
  localized prostate cancer and, 3524
  in prune-belly syndrome, 596-600
Bladder functional assessment, for ureteral anomalies, 806
Bladder health promotion research, for LUTS prevention, 2735-2736
Bladder hemangiomas, 525
Bladder imaging, for benign prostatic hyperplasia, 3348
Bladder infections, 1166b
  complicated, 1158-1159, 1158f, 1158t
  emphysematous cystitis, 1158-1159
  recurrent UTIs, 1159-1166, 1160t, 1160b
    bacterial persistence, 1160-1161
    cranberry, 1163-1164, 1164f
    D-mannose, 1166
    estrogen, 1164-1165, 1164f
    immunoactive prophylaxis, 1166
    low-dose continuous prophylaxis for, 1162-1163
    management, 1161-1166, 1161f
    methenamine, 1165-1166, 1165t
    non-antibiotic management, 1163
    probiotics, 1165
  uncomplicated cystitis, 1155-1158
    antimicrobial selection for, 1156-1157
    clinical presentation, 1156
    follow-up, 1157-1158
    laboratory diagnosis, 1156
    management, 1156-1157, 1157f
    risk factors, 1156b
  unresolved UTIs, 1159, 1159b
Bladder injury
  complications of seminal vesicle surgery, 1863
  and intraoperative consultation, 299-300, 303b
    diagnosis/recognition, 300
    incidence, 299, 299t
    management, 300
    mechanisms, 299-300, 300t
  during laparoscopic and robotic surgery, 230.e1
  perforation/extrusion and, 2882-2883, 2882f
Bladder mobilization, for ureteral reimplantation, 3021, 3021f
Bladder mucosa, in vesicovaginal fistula repair, 2940, 2941f
Bladder neck, 1807.e4f, 1807.e8
  division of, 690
  in laparoscopic radical prostatectomy
    identification and transection of, 3573, 3573f
    reconstruction of, 3577

Bladder neck *(Continued)*
  mesh perforation/extrusion at, 2883, 2883b, 2884f-2885f
  in neuromuscular dysfunction of lower urinary tract, 637
  in retropubic radical prostatectomy
    division of, 3559-3560, 3560f-3561f
    reconstruction and anastomosis of, 3560-3562, 3561f-3562f
Bladder neck closure
  in classic bladder exstrophy
    failure of, 563-564, 564b
    outcomes and results of, 558-559, 559t, 559b, 560f
  for vesicoureteral reflux, 2615
Bladder neck contracture
  after photoselective vaporization of prostate, 3441
  after retropubic radical prostatectomy, 3564
  with bipolar transurethral resection of prostate, 3419
  with holmium laser enucleation of prostate, 3438
  with monopolar transurethral resection of prostate, 3417
Bladder neck dysfunction, 2519
  lower urinary tract dysfunction and, 2627-2628
  videourodynamics for, 2570, 2570f
Bladder neck reconstruction
  artificial urinary sphincter for, 687-688
  bladder neck division for, 690
  bulking agents for, 687
  fascial sling for, 686-687
  Pippi Salle procedure for, 690, 691f
  urethral lengthening for, 688-690, 689f
  in urinary tract reconstruction, 685-690, 690b
  Young-Dees-Leadbetter repair for, 685-686
Bladder neck slings, for neuromuscular dysfunction of lower urinary tract, 637
Bladder neck stenosis, after transurethral microwave therapy, 3430
Bladder neck stricture, in robotic prostatectomy, 3580
Bladder outlet
  closure of, 2898, 2899f
  overactivity of, emptying/voiding failure from, 2519
  response of, to filling, 2515
  storage failure at, 2890-2898, 2898b
    adjustable continence therapy, 2895, 2895f
    adverse events of, 2893
    bladder outlet closure, 2898, 2898b, 2899f
    cell-based therapy, 2895-2898
    complications of, 2895
    human studies, 2896
    injectable agents for male stress urinary incontinence, 2896-2897
    injection techniques of, 2891-2893, 2892f
    outcomes of, 2895
    patient selection, indications, and contraindications, 2891
    periprocedure care of, 2893
    urethral bulking agents, 2890-2895
  surgery of, for detrusor underactivity, 2662-2663
  underactivity of
    emptying/voiding failure from, 2518-2519
    filling/storage failure from, 2518
  ureteroceles and, 806-807, 807f-808f
Bladder outlet obstruction (BOO)
  after pubovaginal sling procedure, 2845-2848, 2848b
    surgical management of, 2846-2848, 2847t
  in benign prostatic hyperplasia, medical treatment and, 3354
  with bladder diverticula, 2964-2965
  detrusor underactivity and, 2655-2656, 2657b

Bladder outlet obstruction (BOO) *(Continued)*
  emptying/voiding failure from, 2519
  in geriatric patients, 2920.e7
  mechanisms of, 2505-2506, 2506b
  in mesh complication, 2880
  nocturia and, 2671-2673
  urodynamic studies of
    in men, 2566-2567, 2567f
    in women, 2567-2568
  videourodynamic studies of
    in women, 2570, 2570f
    in women, lower urinary tract dysfunction and, 2628
Bladder output relation (BOR), 2566, 2566f
Bladder pain syndrome (BPS), 2517-2518
  female sexual dysfunction and, 1657
  overactive bladder distinguished from, 2637, 2638f
  terminology for, 2637
Bladder pain syndrome and interstitial cystitis (BPS/IC), 1224-1250
  definition of, 1224, 1225f-1226f, 1226b
  diagnosis of, 1225b, 1233, 1234t, 1235f, 1236b, 1239b
    markers in, 1238
    potassium chloride test, 1238-1239
  epidemiology of
    associated disorders, 1230-1231, 1230t, 1231f, 1231b
    natural history, 1228-1229, 1230b
    prevalence, 1226, 1227t-1228t, 1229b
  etiology of, 1231-1232, 1232f, 1232.e11b
    animal models, 1232.e1
    antiproliferative factor, 1232.e7, 1232.e8b
    autoimmunity and inflammation, 1232.e2-1232.e3, 1232.e3b
    bladder glycosaminoglycan layer and epithelial permeability, 1232.e5-1232.e7, 1232.e7b
    genetics, 1232.e10
    infection, 1232.e1-1232.e2
    mast cells and histamine, 1232.e4-1232.e5, 1232.e5b
    neurobiology, 1232.e7-1232.e9, 1232.e9b
    nitric oxide metabolism, 1232.e9
    other potential causes, 1232.e10-1232.e11
    pelvic organ cross-sensitization, 1232.e9, 1232.e9b
    urine abnormalities, 1232.e9-1232.e10
  historical perspective of, 1224-1225, 1225b
  mechanisms of, 2507-2509, 2509b
  nomenclature, 1224
  pathology, 1232-1235, 1233b
  surgical therapy for, 1247-1248, 1249b
    historical procedures, 1247-1248
    for Hunner lesion, 1248
    hydrodistention, 1247
    major procedures, 1248
    surgical considerations, 1247
  taxonomy, 1224, 1225f
  treatment of, 1239b
    conservative therapies, 1239-1240
    diet, 1240-1241, 1240b
    intravesical therapies, 1241t, 1244-1247, 1245b
    neuromodulation, 1246-1247, 1247b
    oral therapies, 1241-1244, 1241t, 1244b
    surgical therapy, 1247-1248, 1249b
  urgency, 1225-1226, 1226f, 1226b
  urine studies
    biopsy, 1236-1238, 1237f
    clinical assessment and research, 1235.e1, 1235.e1b
    office cystoscopy, 1236, 1237f
    urodynamic evaluation, 1235-1236
    voiding diary, 1235
Bladder recurrence, UTUC after, 2193
Bladder retraining, types of, 3352

Bladder RMS, 1111
  biopsy of, 1113
  epidemiology and syndromic associations of, 1111
  imaging evaluation of, 1113-1114
  pathology and molecular biology of, 1111-1113, 1112f, 1113b
  presenting symptoms and examination of, 1113-1117, 1113t, 1113b
  staging and COG risk group assignment of, 1113-1114, 1114t
  treatment of, 1115b
    COG multimodal approaches to, 1114-1115
    European Cooperative Group approaches to, 1115
    evolution of multimodal, 1114
    late effects of, 1116-1117
    outcomes of, 1116
    surgical reconstruction, 1116
    for very young children, 1116
Bladder spasm, 932
Bladder sphincter function, effects of sex reassignment surgery on, 3062-3063
Bladder stones, 243.e1, 244.e3-244.e4, 3043-3046
  with benign prostatic hyperplasia, 3335
  complications of, 3046
  endourologic approach to, 2115, 2116f
  evaluation of, 3043-3044
  laparoscopic and robotic technique, 3044-3045, 3045f-3046f
  management of, 2115
    medical, 2115
  open surgery for, 2115
  open technique of, 3044, 3045f
  percutaneous, 3045-3046
  postoperative care of, 3046
  presentation of, 2115
  surgical indication of, 3043-3044
  surgical technique of, 3044-3046
Bladder surgery, for genitourinary tuberculosis treatment, 1317-1318
Bladder training
  evidence for, 2730
  for urinary incontinence, 2722.e2b-2722.e4b, 2728f, 2730, 2730.e1t
Bladder tumor antigen (BTA) assay, of bladder tumor, 3079-3081
Bladder tumors, 3073-3090, 3078b
  benign, 3010-3047
    anatomy of, 3010
    bladder stones, 3043-3046
    diverticulectomy, 3010-3019, 3011f, 3011b, 3046b-3047b
    enterocystoplasty, 3034-3038
    foreign-body removal, 3043-3046
    partial cystectomy, 3038-3043
    psoas hitch and Boari flap, 3026-3034
    surgical considerations of, 3010
    urachal surgery, 3038-3043
    ureteral reimplantation, 3019-3026
  benign, pediatric, 1119
  nonurothelial malignancy, 3089-3090, 3089f
    prostatic urethral cancer, 3084
    sarcomas. see Sarcomas, of bladder
  during pregnancy, and urologic malignancy, 293
Bladder urinary diversion, rectal, 3209-3211
  augmented valved rectum, 3209
  folded rectosigmoid bladder, 3209
  hemi-Kock pouch procedures with valved rectum, 3209-3210
  Mainz II pouch, 3210-3211
  sigma-rectum pouch, 3210-3211
  T pouch procedures with valved rectum, 3209-3210, 3210f
Bladder wall
  collagen of, 2463-2464
  elastin of, 2464
  matrix of, 2464
  stroma of, 2463

Bladder wall thickness (BWT), 3348
Blake drains, 148
Bland thrombus, IVC filtration and permanent interruption for, 2277
Bleeding
  after midurethral sling, 2874
  during anterior colporrhaphy, 2782
  complication of scrotal surgery, 1855
  in monopolar transurethral resection of prostate, 3415
  with prostate biopsy, 3499
  at the sheath site, 226-227, 227f
Bleomycin, for penile cancer, 1771
Bleomycin-etoposide-cisplatin (BEP), for seminomas, 1705
Blind access, 169
Blind trocar placement, complications related to, 225-226
α-Blockade, for pheochromocytoma, 2378, 2379f
β-Blockade, for pheochromocytoma, 2378, 2379f
α-Blockers
  for nocturia, 2674
  transurethral microwave therapy versus, 3429
Blockers of inhibition, to facilitate bladder emptying, 2719
Blood-based biomarkers, for prostate cancer, 3480-3485
Blood-epididymis barrier, 1404
Blood/hematuria, 16
  differential diagnosis and evaluation of, 16
Blood loss/transfusion, in robotic prostatectomy, 3580
Blood pressure, anesthesia-related changes in, during laparoscopic and robotic surgery, 228.e1
Blood products
  transfusions, preoperative considerations for, for laparoscopic and robotic surgery, 204
  for urologic surgery, 147-148
Blood-testis barrier, 1373, 1398-1399, 1399f
Blood tests, for male urinary incontinence, 2543
"BLUE stent,", 834-835, 834f
Blunt dissection instrumentation, for laparoscopic and robotic surgery, 218
Blunt trauma
  renal, 1982
    imaging of, 1984
    nonoperative management of, 1986-1987
    renal artery thrombosis with, 1990
  ureteral, 1992, 1992t
    diagnosis of, 1992-1993
BLUS. see Basic Laparoscopic Urologic Surgery
BMI. see Body mass index
Boari flap, 3026-3034
  with bladder advancement flap, 3031
  complications with, 3032
  evaluation for, 3026
  laparoendoscopic single-site, 3031
  laparoscopic or robotic, 3030-3031, 3030f-3031f
  for lower ureteral injuries, 1999, 2000f
  with mega-Boari flap, 3033f
  outcomes with, 3033-3034
  postoperative care of, 3032
  surgical indication for, 3026
  surgical technique for, 3027-3028, 3028f
  with ureteroneocystostomy, 1973
Body habitus, hormonal therapy and, 3681
Body mass index (BMI)
  benign prostatic hyperplasia and, 3324, 3325t
  in bladder tumor, 3076
  male SUI and, 2540-2541
  prostate cancer and, 3465, 3465f
  urinary incontinence and, 2582
Body weight, renal calculi and, 2027-2028
Bone mineralization, renal regulation of, 1914, 1914f
Bone morphogenic protein-7 (BMP-7), in tubulointerstitial fibrosis, 787

Bone scan, for localized prostate cancer, 3527
Bone scan index, 3679
Bone-anchored porcine single-incision sling, 2843
Bone-anchored sling, history and development of, 2994
Bony pelvis
  female, 2427, 2428f
  male, 2444
BOO. see Bladder outlet obstruction
BOR. see Bladder output relation
Bors-Comarr classification, of voiding dysfunction, 2522-2523, 2523b
Bosniak category IV lesions, 770
Bosniak classification, for renal cystic lesions, 2122, 2122f, 2122t, 2137, 2137t
Botox, for chronic scrotal pain syndrome, 1221
Bottleneck technique, 1845, 1847f
Botulinum toxin (BoNT). see also OnabotulinumtoxinA
  adverse effects of, 2709
  for bowel-bladder dysfunction, 658
  clinical use of, 2708
  for detrusor underactivity, 2662
  efficacy of, 2709
  to facilitate bladder emptying, 2720.e3
  to facilitate bladder filling and urine storage, 2682t, 2707-2709
  mechanism of action of, 2707-2709
  for neuromuscular dysfunction of lower urinary tract, 634-635
  for OAB, 2647
  for Parkinson disease, 2606
  for prostatic injections, 3447
Botulinum-A toxin, for PE, 1572.e3
Bowel cleansing, before inguinal node dissection, 1801
Bowel disorders, normal versus abnormal, 667, 668t
Bowel dysfunction, in geriatric patients, 2920.e9
Bowel entrapment, during laparoscopic and robotic surgery, 230
Bowel function
  localized prostate cancer and, 3525
  urinary incontinence and, 2734
Bowel injury, 275-281, 276f
  duodenal and pancreatic injuries, during nephrectomy, 277, 277f
  during laparoscopic and robotic surgery, 228f, 229
  laparoscopic kidney surgery causing, 2307, 2307f
  lymphoceles, 280-281, 281f
  management, 278
  mechanism of, 276-277
  port site hernia, 278, 278f-279f
  rectal injury, 277-278
  in robotic prostatectomy, 3580
  venous thromboembolism, 278-280, 279t-280t
Bowel insufflation, during laparoscopic and robotic surgery, 224
Bowel interposition, for ureteral injuries, upper, 1998, 1998f
Bowel mobilization, in transurethral resection of bladder tumor, 3137, 3137f
Bowel obstruction, 3272
  with intestinal anastomoses, 3180-3181, 3180t, 3181f
Bowel preparation
  preoperative, for laparoscopic and robotic surgery, 204
  for urinary tract reconstruction, 682
  in urologic surgery, 124-125
Bowel resection, orthoptic urinary diversion and, 3238-3239
Bowen disease, of penis, 1742, 1742.e1f
Bowenoid papulosis
  as neoplastic condition, 1296, 1298f
  of penis, 1742
BP. see Bullous pemphigoid

BPH. *see* Benign prostatic hyperplasia
BPH Impact Index (BII), 110*t*
   for benign prostatic hyperplasia, 3344
BPO. *see* Benign prostatic obstruction
BPS. *see* Bladder pain syndrome
BPS/IC. *see* Bladder pain syndrome and interstitial cystitis
BRA. *see* Bilateral renal agenesis
Brachytherapy, 3632–3638
   benign bounce phenomenon and, 3608
   combined with external irradiation, 3613–3615
   external beam radiation therapy *versus*, 3612–3613, 3614*t*
   outcomes for, 3612
   for penile cancer, 1765–1767, 1767*f*–1768*f*
   for prostate cancer, 3591, 3596–3600, 3600*b*
     combined with external irradiation, 3599–3600
     high-dose-rate, 3598–3599
     low-dose-rate, technique and trends of, 3596, 3597*f*
     patient selection for, 3599
     permanent implant quality assessment, 3597–3598, 3597*f*, 3598*t*
     transrectal ultrasound-guided, 3591–3592, 3592*f*
Bradley classification, of voiding dysfunction, 2524
Brain circuits, in detrusor underactivity, 2653, 2655*f*
Brain metastases, of TGCTs, 1706–1707, 1707*b*
Brain tumor
   lower urinary tract dysfunction with, 2604
   neurogenic bladder with, 648
Brainstem
   bladder modulatory mechanisms of, 2493–2494, 2495*f*
     neurotransmitters and modulators within, 2495–2496
     neuromuscular lower urinary tract dysfunction at and above, 2602–2607
Brainstem stroke, lower urinary tract dysfunction with, 2603
Branchio-oto-renal syndrome, 336–337
Bricker anastomosis, 3187, 3187*f*
Brief Index of Sexual Function for Women (BISF-W), 112, 112*t*
Brindley system, 2741–2742
Bristol Female Lower Urinary Tract Symptoms (BFLUTS) Questionnaire, 110
Bristol Stool Scale, 473–474, 474*f*, 667–668, 668*f*
BRL. *see* Biomarker Reference Laboratories
Broad ligament, 2430, 2431*f*
Brödel-type orientation, 162, 163*f*
Brushite calculi, surgical management of, 2076
   stone fragility and, 2077.e1
Brushite stone formers, 2011–2012, 2013*f*
Brushite stones, surgical management of, method selection for, 2077.e2
BT. *see* Behavioral therapy
B-TURP. *see* Bipolar transurethral resection of the prostate
Buccal mucosa, in complex penile reconstruction, 946
Bulbar urethra, 1807.e8
Bulbocavernosus reflex (BCR), in pelvic floor disorders, 2530
Bulbospongiosus, 2435
Bulbourethral artery, 1383
Bulbourethral glands, 1383
Bulbous urethra, 1383, 1383*f*, 1807.e2*f*, 1807.e4*f*
Bullous pemphigoid (BP), 1284–1285, 1285*f*
Bumetanide, in stone formation, 2033
Bupropion
   for female sexual arousal disorders, 1650
   for female sexual interest disorder, 1645

Burch colposuspension, 2763–2766, 2766*b*
   Marshall-Marchetti-Krantz procedure *versus*, 2773
   paravaginal repair *versus*, 2766
   prophylactic colposuspension, 2765
   pubovaginal sling *versus*, 2771, 2772*f*
   reoperative surgery, 2765–2766
   results with, 2763–2765
   suspensions in, configuration of, 2758
   technique for, 2763, 2764*f*
   urethral elevation in, 2758
Buried penis, 394, 877–878, 878*f*–879*f*
Burns, of penis, 3053
Buschke-Löwenstein tumor, 1742.e1*f*, 1742.e3
Buspirone, for female sexual interest disorder, 1645
BWS. *see* Beckwith-Wiedemann syndrome
BWT. *see* Bladder wall thickness
BXO. *see* Balanitis xerotica obliterans
Byars flap procedure, 927, 931*f*
Bypass techniques, for vena caval thrombectomy, 2275–2276, 2275*f*–2276*f*, 2275.e1*f*, 2276.e1*f*

C

C3 complement, in prostatic secretions, 3298*t*, 3302
CA. *see* Cryoablation
Cabazitaxel, 3692–3693, 3693*f*
Cabozantinib, 3701
   for RCC, 2337, 2338*f*
C-acetate PET/CT, 43
Cadaveric fascia lata
   allograft slings and, 2834–2835
   for pelvic organ prolapse reconstructive surgery, 2781*t*–2782*t*, 2786, 2786*f*
Cadaveric models, laparoscopic training with, 232
Cadherins, in prostate growth regulation, 3288
Caffeine reduction
   for OAB, 2647
   for urinary incontinence, 2733
CAH. *see* Congenital adrenal hyperplasia
Caiman 5 vessel-sealing system, 214.e1*f*
Cake or lump kidney, 728*f*–729*f*, 729
Calcifying nanoparticles (CNPs), 2011
Calcitonin gene-related peptide (CGRP)
   and ED, 1499
   in ureteral function, 1887
Calcium
   filtrate transport, 1911, 1912*f*
   metabolism of, 2015–2016
   in pediatric kidney stone disease, 869
   in prostate cancer, 3463–3465
   PTH and, 1914, 1914*f*, 2016
   sensitization to, 2472–2473
   in smooth muscle contraction, 2472–2473, 2472*b*, 2473*f*, 2475–2476, 2476*f*
   in ureter physiology
     excitation-contraction coupling and, 1884–1885
     as second messengers, 1885–1887, 1885*f*–1886*f*
   vitamin D and, 1914, 2015
Calcium antagonists
   to facilitate bladder filling and urine storage, 2682*t*, 2696–2697
   urethral function effects of, 1903
Calcium apatite, 2011
Calcium-based calculi in, 2048–2049, 2049*b*
   dietary, 2049
Calcium channel blockers (CCBs)
   and ED, 1507
   for pheochromocytoma, 2379–2380, 2379*f*
   ureteral function effects of, 1900
Calcium channels, in detrusor muscle, 2474–2475, 2475*f*
Calcium hydroxylapatite (Coaptite), for female urinary incontinence, 2894–2895

Calcium-induced calcium release (CICR), 2476
Calcium oxalate stones
   of crystal formation, 2010
   formation of, 2008
   formers of, 2011–2012
   homogeneous nucleation, 2011
   Randall plaques and, 2011, 2012*f*–2013*f*, 2018
   surgical management of, 2076
   stone fragility and, 2077.e2
Calcium stones, in renal calculi, 2018–2026
   hypercalciuria, 2018–2020
   hyperoxaluria, 2020–2023, 2021*f*–2022*f*
   hyperuricosuria, 2023–2024, 2024*f*
   hypocitraturia, 2024
   hypomagnesiuria, 2026
Calculi
   after augmentation cystoplasty, 699
   HIV and, 1266
Caldesmon (CaD), 2472, 2473*f*
Calicovesicostomy, for ureteropelvic junction obstruction, laparoscopic, 1960
Calyceal diverticula
   percutaneous nephrolithotomy and, 2105, 2105*f*
   renal calculi with, 2034
     surgical management of, 2077–2078, 2077.e1*f*
Calyceal diverticulectomy, laparoscopic, 2294
Calyceal diverticulum, 737–738, 739*f*, 774, 774*f*
Calyceal fornix, 161, 162*f*
Calyces, 1865.e1*f*
   hydrocalycosis, 738
   megacalycosis, 738–739, 740*f*
   renal, 1869, 1869.e1*f*
   normal urothelium of, 2188
Cameras, for laparoscopic and robotic surgery, 213
Camey II orthotopic substitute, 3243, 3243*f*
cAMP. *see* Cyclic adenosine monophosphate
Camper fascia, 2444, 2446*f*
Cancer
   chronic inflammation in GU cancers, 1336, 1338*b*
     bladder cancer, 1336–1338, 1337*f*–1338*f*
     kidney cancer, 1338
     prostate cancer, 1338
   female urethral, 1782–1785, 1785*b*
   fertility preservation in, 1452
   immunologic response to, 1333–1345, 1336*b*
     adaptive immune system, 1334–1336, 1335*f*
     immune editing hypothesis, 1336, 1337*f*
     innate immune system, 1333–1334, 1334*f*–1335*f*, 1334*t*–1335*t*
   immunotherapy for, 1333–1345, 1341*b*, 1343*b*
     BCG in bladder cancer, 1333–1334, 1334*f*, 1338–1339, 1339*f*
     cancer vaccines, 1339–1340, 1340*f*–1341*f*
     combination, 1343–1345, 1345*f*
     immune checkpoint blockade, 1342, 1342*f*
   male urethral, 1776–1782, 1782*b*
   surgery, 2959–2960
   of testis, 1440
   with urinary intestinal diversion, 3203–3204
   vaccines for, 1339–1340, 1340*f*
     for genitourinary tumors, 1341–1342, 1342*f*
     for kidney cancer, 1340–1341
     for prostate cancer, 1341, 1341*f*
CancerSEEK test, 3485
Candida albicans, 445
Candidal intertrigo, 1293–1294, 1294*f*
Candidiasis, 1272, 1272*t*
Cannabinoids
   in bladder afferent pathway, 2486
   in ED, 1495, 1495*t*
   to facilitate bladder filling and urine storage, 2713.e2–2713.e3

Cantwell-Ransley procedure, for classic bladder exstrophy repair, modified, 551–552, 552f–553f
Capacitive coupling, 237
Capillary hemangioma, 1304–1306
Capio suture capturing device, for sacrospinous ligament fixation, 2795
Caprini risk assessment model, 279t
Caprosyn suture, 149
Capsaicin
  to facilitate bladder filling and urine storage, 2682t, 2709
  intravesical, 2709.e1
  for prostate cancer, 3544
  ureteral response to, 1889
Capsular invasion, 3507
Capsular penetration, 3507
Capsular perforations
  with bipolar transurethral resection of prostate, 3419
  with holmium laser enucleation of prostate, 3438
  with transurethral incision of prostate, 3435
  with transurethral vaporization of prostate, 3425–3426
Capsular polysaccharides, 429
Carbamylcholine (Carbachol), ureteral response to, 1887
Carbon dioxide (CO), as insufflant choice, 241
Carbon monoxide (CO)
  in ED, 1498
  renal vascular tone control by, 1913
Carbon-11 (11C), 91
Carbon-coated zirconium beads (Durasphere), for female urinary incontinence, 2894
Carbonic anhydrase inhibitors, in stone formation, 2033
Carbonic anhydrase IX (CA-IX, MN-9), 98, 2136
Carboplatin
  for NSGCTs, 1697
  for penile cancer, 1771
  for seminomas, 1704, 1704t
Carcinoid tumors, of kidney, 2181t, 2183
Carcinoma in situ (CIS)
  of penis, 1742
  of upper urinary tracts, 2219–2220
  UTUC association with, 2193
Cardiac abnormalities, contrast media and, 32
Cardiac arrest, anesthesia-related, during laparoscopic and robotic surgery, 228.e1
Cardiac arrhythmias
  anesthesia-related, during laparoscopic and robotic surgery, 228.e1
  pneumoperitoneum causing, 221
Cardiac glycosides, urethral function effects of, 1903–1904
Cardiac ischemia, during vena caval thrombectomy, 2278
Cardinal ligament, 2429–2430, 2431f
Cardinal veins, retrocaval ureter and, 1963, 1966b
Cardiopulmonary bypass (CPB), for vena caval thrombectomy, 2275–2276, 2275f–2276f, 2276.e1f
Cardiovascular disease (CVD)
  α-blocker therapy in patients with, 3369–3370
  and ED, 1504
  erectile dysfunction and, 1425–1426, 1426b
  prostatitis and, 1210
  renal calculi and, 2008–2009
Cardiovascular morbidity/mortality, hormonal therapy and, 3681
Cardiovascular system
  abnormalities of, with cloacal exstrophy, 575
  pneumoperitoneum effects on, 220–221
  Wilms tumor treatment effects on, 1108
Carnitine, for PD, 1611, 1616t
Carter-Thomason needle-point suture passer, 219, 219f

Caruncle, urethral, urethral diverticula differentiated from, 2987, 2987f
Casale continent catheterizable stoma, 711, 712f
Caspases, in GU cancers, 1365–1366
Castration-resistant prostate cancer
  anaplastic phenotype, 3705
  assessment of, 3687–3689
  bisphosphonates for, 3703–3704
  clinical considerations for, 3687–3690, 3690b
  cytotoxic chemotherapy for, 3690–3693, 3694b
    chemotherapeutic agents as, 3690–3693
    evaluation of treatment efficacy, 3690
    platinum agents as, 3693
  epidural cord compression in, 3702
  immunotherapy for, 3697–3699, 3699b
    immune checkpoint blockade as, 3698
    pembrolizumab, 3698–3699
    ProstVac-VF, 3698
    sipuleucel-T, 3697–3698, 3697f
  metastatic, 3689–3690
  neuroendocrine subtype, 3704–3705
  nonmetastatic, 3689
  novel hormonal therapies for, 3693–3696, 3696b
    androgen receptor modulation as, 3695–3696, 3695f
    AR-V7 as, 3696
    CYP17 inhibition as, 3693–3695, 3694f
  palliative management of, 3702–3704, 3705b
    bone-targeted approaches as, 3703–3704
    pain and spinal cord compression as, 3702, 3703t
  prognostic considerations for, 3687–3689, 3688f
  radiopharmaceuticals for, 3704
  RANK ligand inhibitors for, 3704
  targeted treatments for, 3699–3702, 3702b
    angiogenesis, 3700–3701
    apoptosis pathway in, 3701–3702
    DNA repair, 3702
    MET signaling, 3701
    PI3K/Akt/mTOR pathway in, 3699–3700
  treatment for, 3687–3706
Casts, in urine, 23, 23f–24f
Catch bonds, 1135
Catecholamine hypersecretion, in evaluation of adrenal masses, 2402–2403, 2402t
Catecholamine synthesis blockade, for pheochromocytoma, 2378–2379, 2379f
Catecholamine testing, for pheochromocytoma, 2377
Catecholamines, adrenal medulla physiology and, 2358–2360, 2359t–2360t
Category I cysts, 769
Category II cysts, 769
Category III cysts, 769–770
Catheter-associated bacteriuria, UTIs and, 1190, 1191b
Catheter-associated UTI (CAUTI), 433
Catheter placement, for urodynamics, 2535
Catheterization
  anatomic considerations in, 152
  for bladder emptying failure, 2900–2902, 2900f
  continuous, 2901–2902
  of children, urethral, 153
  difficult, 156–158
  history of, 152
  lower urinary tract, 152–159
    technique of, 152–155
  in men, urethral, 153
  preparation for, 152–153
  suprapubic, 155–156
  ureteral, 1197
  urethral, antimicrobial prophylaxis for urologic procedures and, 1197
  in women, urethral, 153
Catheterized urine specimens, in urine collection, 1141

Catheters
  air-charged, for urodynamic studies, 2558
  condom, 155
  diagnostic, 154–155, 155f
  double-lumen, 154
  drain, 155
  hematuria, 154, 154f
  indwelling, in geriatric patients, 2919
  knotting and balloon malfunction, 159
  long-term, bladder cancer and, 2616
  single-lumen, 154
  sizing, 153–154, 154t
  types of, 153–155
  water-filled, for urodynamic studies, 2558
Cation transport, urinary tract obstruction and, 794
Cauda equina, 2619
Cauda equina syndrome, 2620
Cauterization, energy modalities for, 235–241
  electrosurgery, 235–241, 236f
  ultrasound instrumentation, 237–238
Cautery wire balloon incision, for ureteroenteric strictures, 1977
CAUTI. see Catheter-associated UTI
CAVD. see Congenital absence of vas deferens
Caveolae, in ED, 1499
Cavernosal nerves, 1378
Cavernosal veins, 1807.e5f
Cavernosogram, of penis, 1386, 1387f
Cavernous smooth muscle content test, 1525
Cavitation mechanism, in ultrasonography, 77
Cavoplasty, for IVC, 2276, 2277f
CBCL. see Child Behavior Checklist
CBE. see Classic bladder exstrophy
CCBs. see Calcium channel blockers
C-choline and F-fluorocholine, 43
CCI. see Charlson Comorbidity Index
CCSK. see Clear cell sarcoma of kidney
CDC. see Centers for Disease Control and Prevention
CDH1 gene, in bladder cancer, 1350
CDKIs. see Cyclin-dependent kinase inhibitors
CDKN1B, in UTUC, 2197
Cecil-Culp repair, for hypospadias fistula, 947f
Cecocystoplasty, 694
Cecum, proximal, 3211
Celecoxib, urethral function effects of, 1903
Cell adhesion molecules, in prostate growth regulation, 3287–3288, 3288b
Cell-based therapy, of male stress urinary incontinence, 2897
Cell cycle deregulation, in GU cancers, 1347–1348, 1349b
  CDKIs, 1347.e1, 1347.e1f
  cell cycle entry, 1347.e1
  cell cycle progression through S phase, 1347.e2
  cyclin-dependent kinases and cyclins, 1347.e1, 1347.e1f
  G_1/S checkpoint, 1347.e2
  G2M checkpoint, 1347.e2–1347.e3
  mitosis, 1347.e2
  mitotic arrest and spindle assembly checkpoint, 1347.e3
  RB1, 1347.e1, 1347.e1f
  S phase arrest, 1347.e2
  TP53, 1347.e2, 1347.e2f, 1348
Cell cycle markers, in UTUC, 2197
Cell cycle progression, in prostate cancer, 3543
Cell differentiation, in UTUC, 2197
Cell migration and invasion, in UTUC, 2197
Cell proliferation, in UTUC, 2197
Cells, in urine, 21–23, 21f–23f
CellSearch system, 3484–3485, 3485f
Cellular proliferation, 305
Cellules, 2967
Cellulitis, 1288–1289, 1290f
  genital skin loss and, 3053
Centers for Disease Control and Prevention (CDC), 1251

Central defect, in pelvic floor support mechanism, 2597-2598
Central perineal tendon, 1807.e10
Central venous pressure, pneumoperitoneum effects on, 221
Cephalad renal ectopia, 724-725, 726f
Cephalexin, for UTIs, 1170t
Cephalosporins
  prophylaxis with, for uncomplicated urologic procedures, 1194t-1196t
  for UTIs, 1151t-1153t, 1154, 1187t
Cerebellar ataxia, lower urinary tract dysfunction with, 2604
Cerebral palsy (CP)
  lower urinary tract dysfunction with, 2604-2605
  pathogenesis of, 647-648
  presentation of, 647, 650b
  specific recommendations of, 648
Cerebrovascular accident (CVA), lower urinary tract dysfunction and, 2602-2603
Cerebrovascular disease, lower urinary tract dysfunction and, 2602-2603
Cernilton, 3399
  for diminished bladder, 2674
Cervical atresia, 984-985, 985f
Cervical myelopathy, lower urinary tract dysfunction with, 2617
Cervical RMS, in pediatric patients, 1120
Cervix, 325, 325f
  anatomy of, 2436
Cesarean delivery, urinary incontinence and, 2583
Cetrorelix, for benign prostatic hyperplasia, 3377
CEVC. see Clinical Epidemiological Validation Center
CGA. see Comprehensive geriatric assessment
cGMP. see Cyclic guanosine monophosphate
CGRP. see Calcitonin gene-related peptide
Chancroid, 1255t, 1259-1260, 1259f
Chaperone-usher pathway (CUP), 428-429
Chaperonin, androgen receptor binding of, 3289
Charlson Combined Comorbidity Index, 107-108
Charlson Comorbidity Index (CCI), 2909, 3522
Checkpoint inhibition, in GU cancers, 1367-1368, 1368b
Chemical exposure, in workplace, 1416
Chemodenervation, for urinary incontinence, in geriatric patients, 2920.e5
Chemokines, 1333-1334, 1335f, 1335t
Chemotherapy
  for bladder tumor, 3077
  for castration-resistant prostate cancer, 3690-3693
    cabazitaxel, 3692-3693, 3693f
    docetaxel, 3690-3692, 3691f-3692f
    mitoxantrone, 3690, 3693f
  for metastatic bladder cancer, 3125
    second-line, 3128, 3128t
  for metastatic RCC, 2341-2342
  for muscle-invasive bladder cancer, 3121-3123, 3121t
    randomized trials in, 3127-3128, 3127t
  for neuroblastoma, 1093f, 1095
  at PC-RPLND, 1727
  for penile cancer, 1769-1771, 1772b
    adjuvant, 1771
    combination, 1770-1771
    single-agent, 1769-1770
    surgical consolidation after, 1771
  with radiation therapy, for locally advanced prostate cancer, 3654-3655
  for RCC, resistance to, 2145
  for retroperitoneal tumors, 2245-2247, 2246t
  for TGCTs
    with brain metastases, 1706-1707, 1707b
    NSGCTs, 1695

Chemotherapy (Continued)
    post-salvage, 1701
    relapsed tumors, 1700
    residual mass management after, 1698-1700, 1698t-1699t
    seminomas, 1704, 1704t
    toxicity of, 1707
  for UTUC, 2222-2223, 2223f
  for Wilms tumor, 1100, 1102f
Chest, imaging of, for TGCTs, 1690
Chest X-ray, 450
Chevron and subcostal incision, kidney and retroperitoneum approaches, 137-138, 139f
Chevron incision, for open kidney surgery, 2253
Chief complaint, in patient history, 1
Child Behavior Checklist (CBCL), 477, 654
Childbearing women, prevention of urinary incontinence and, 2735
Childhood diseases, and male infertility, 1432-1434
Children
  fundamentals of
    MRI in, 412-413
    sonography in, 404
  ionizing radiation in, 403
  megaureter in, 849-852, 852b
    cutaneous ureterostomy for, 850-851, 850f
    definition of, 849
    definitive reconstruction for, 850-851, 850f
    dilatation and stenting for, 852
    etiology, occurrence, and presentation of, 849
    excisional tapering for, 851-852, 851f
    Kalicinski plication technique for, 851, 851f
    outcomes with, 852
    remodeling for, 837f-839f, 851
    Starr plication technique for, 851, 851f
    surgical indications for, 849-850
    surgical management of, 850-852, 850f-851f
    ureteral polyps with, 835-836
    ureteral strictures with, 835
  surgery of ureter in, 826-852
  ureteropelvic junction obstruction in, 826-836
    associated anomalies, 826
    clinical presentation of, 826, 827f
    complications with, 832f, 835, 835f
    definition of, 826
    dismembered pyeloplasty, 828, 828f-830f
    endoscopic approach to, 830
    flank approach to, 829
    laparoscopic pyeloplasty for, 830-834, 833f-834f
    lower pole, 826, 827f
    minimally invasive techniques for, 830-835
    nondismembered pyeloplasty for, 828-829, 829f-831f
    outcomes with, 835
    posterior lumbotomy for, 829, 832f
    secondary, 826
    surgical approach to, 829
    surgical indications for, 826-827
    surgical repair of, 827-828
  urethral catheterization of, 153
  UTI in, 426
    diagnosis of, 426b
  vesicoureteral reflux in, 836-846, 836b
    clinical presentation of, 836
    Cohen Cross-Trigonal technique for, 840, 841f
    complications of ureteral reimplantation for, 844-846
    definition of, 836
    early complications of, 844-846
    endoscopic treatment of, 846-849
    extravesical procedures for, 840-842, 842f-843f

Children (Continued)
    Glenn-Anderson technique for, 840, 840f
    incision for, 836, 837f-839f
    intravesical procedures for, 836-840
    long-term complications of, 846
    minimally invasive procedures for, 842-844
    Politano-Leadbetter technique for, 837f-839f, 840
    postoperative evaluation of, 844
    reoperative reimplantation for, 846
    robotic-assisted laparoscopic ureteral reimplantation- extravesical for, 844, 845f
    surgical management of, 836
Children's Oncology Group (COG)
  staging systems and risk group assignments of
    for bladder RMS, 1113-1114, 1114t
    for testicular tumors, 1122, 1122t
  treatment recommendations of, bladder RMS approaches, 1114-1115
Chills, patient history of, 7
Chlamydia
  as fastidious organism in UTIs, 1133
  as nongonococcal urethritis, 1253
  prostatitis microbiology and, 1205-1206
Chloride absorption, after augmentation cystoplasty, 698
Chlormadinone acetate, for benign prostatic hyperplasia, 3377
Chloroquine derivatives, for BPS/IC oral therapy, 1241t, 1243
Cholecalciferol (vitamin D3), 1914
Cholesterol, testosterone synthesis from, 1395-1396
Choline PET/CT, 43
Cholinergic agonists, ureteral response to, 1887
Chondroitin sulfate, in crystal formation, 2014
"Choosing Wisely" campaign, 3527
"Chop-fmru,", 413
Chordee
  in classic bladder exstrophy repair, 551
  without hypospadias, 1836
Choriocarcinoma
  histology of, 1683-1684, 1683f
  spread of, 1706
Chromatin remodeling
  androgen receptor-dependent, 3293-3295
  in prostate cancer, 3470
Chromogranin A testing, for pheochromocytoma, 2377
Chromophobe RCC, pathology of, 2149t-2151t, 2152-2153, 2154f
Chromosomal abnormalities
  in GU cancers, 1351-1352, 1362b
    bladder cancer, 1358-1360
    bladder RMS, 1111-1113
    CNAs, 1354, 1354t-1355t
    gross abnormalities, 1351, 1352b
    neuroblastoma, 1087
    prostate cancer, 1352-1353, 1354t
    renal cancer, 1353, 1354t, 1355f, 1358
    testicular cancer, 1121, 1353, 1361-1362
    Wilms tumor, 1096-1099, 1097t, 1354t
  male reproductive physiology and, age-related, 1401-1402
Chromosomal instability
  telomerase reversal of, 1364
  telomeres and, 1362
Chromosomal recombination, 1401
Chromosomal sex, 990, 991f, 991b
Chromosome abnormalities, association with pathologic stage of prostate cancer, 3642t
Chromosomes, basics of, 1346.e4
Chronic bacterial prostatitis
  evaluation of, 1211-1214, 1214b
    assessment, 1211, 1212f
    history, 1211
    laboratory/office studies, 1213-1214, 1214b

Chronic bacterial prostatitis *(Continued)*
    physical examination, 1211–1213, 1213f
    review of symptoms, 1211
  histopathology, 1205–1207, 1207b
  symptoms, 1209–1211
    anxiety and depression, 1210
    association with other medical diseases, 1210
    multidisciplinary approach, 1209–1210
    phenotypic approach to symptoms and symptom clustering, 1210–1211, 1210f
    prevalence, 1209
    severity, 1210
    sexual dysfunction, 1210
  treatment of, 1214–1218, 1218b
    Cochrane review, 1218
    conservative, 1216
    minimally invasive therapies, 1216–1217
    pharmacologic, 1214–1216
    prostate-specific, 1217
    summary and approach, 1218
Chronic constipation, pelvic organ prolapse and, 2591
Chronic diarrhea, ammonium acid urate stones from, 2032
Chronic epididymitis, 1202–1223
  nonmedical therapy for, 1221
  nonradical surgical treatments, 1221
  surgical therapy, 1221–1222
Chronic flank pain, genitourinary trauma and, 1078
Chronic inflammation
  in cancer immune response, 1336, 1338b
    bladder cancer, 1336–1338, 1337f–1338f
    kidney cancer, 1338
    prostate cancer, 1338
  UTUC risk and, 2187
Chronic kidney disease (CKD), 1927–1934, 1934b
  bone disease, 355
  in children, 354–355, 354t, 355b
  definition of, 1927, 1928f, 1928t
  genitourinary trauma and, 1078
  renal calculi and, 2009
Chronic Kidney Disease Epidemiology Collaboration (CKD-EPI) equation, 777, 1905
Chronic pelvic pain syndrome (CPPS)
  epidemiology, 1202
  evaluation of, 1211–1214, 1214b
    assessment, 1211, 1212f
    history, 1211
    laboratory/office studies, 1213–1214, 1214b
    physical examination, 1211–1213, 1213f
    review of symptoms, 1211
  historical perspective, 1202
  symptoms in, 1209–1211
    anxiety and depression, 1210
    association with other medical diseases, 1210
    multidisciplinary approach, 1209–1210
    phenotypic approach to symptoms and symptom clustering, 1210–1211, 1210f
    prevalence, 1209
    severity, 1210
    sexual dysfunction, 1210
  treatment of, 1214–1218, 1218b
    Cochrane review, 1218
    conservative, 1216
    minimally invasive therapies, 1216–1217
    pharmacologic, 1214–1216
    prostate-specific, 1217
    summary and approach, 1218
Chronic pyelonephritis, 1176–1177, 1177f
Chronic renal failure, and ED, 1511
Chronic scrotal pain
  complication of scrotal surgery, 1855
  surgical management of, 1853–1855, 1854f
Chronic scrotal pain syndrome, 1219–1220, 1222b
  nonmedical therapy for, 1221

Chronic scrotal pain syndrome *(Continued)*
  nonradical surgical treatments, 1221
  surgical therapy, 1221–1222, 1223f
Chylous ascites
  after RPLND, 1731, 2244
  laparoscopic and robotic surgery causing, 231.e1
Chyluria
  as filariasis clinical manifestation, 1330
  nephrolysis for, 2294, 2294f
CIC. see Clean intermittent catheterization
CICR. see Calcium-induced calcium release
Cidofovir, for condylomata acuminata, 1742.e3
CIQ-FLUTS. see International Consultation on Incontinence Questionnaire Female Lower Urinary Symptoms
Circle nephrostomy tube, 174f
Circulating tumor cells (CTCs), as prostate cancer biomarkers, 3484–3485, 3485f
Circulating tumor DNA, as prostate cancer biomarkers, 3484–3485, 3485f
Circumcision, 393, 872–876, 873b
  complications of, 873–874, 874f, 876b
    urethral reconstructive surgery and, 1811–1812
  female, 987–988, 988f
  penile cancer management with, 1752–1753
  for penile carcinoma, prevention of, 1743
  for posterior urethral valves, 615
  for prune-belly syndrome, 593
Circumferential compression mechanism, of stone fragmentation, 2096–2097
CIS. see Carcinoma in situ
Cisapride, to facilitate bladder emptying, 2718
Cisplatin
  for penile cancer, 1770
  for TGCTs, toxicity of, 1707
Citrate
  in crystal formation, 2014, 2024
  in pediatric kidney stone disease, 869
Citric acid, in prostatic secretions, 3295
Citrus juices, for hypocitraturia, 2053–2054
CJD. see Creutzfeldt-Jakob prion disease
CKD. see Chronic kidney disease
Classic bladder exstrophy (CBE), 290–291
  abdominal wall defects in, 533
  anatomic considerations in, 531–537
  anorectal defects in, 533
  antireflux procedure for, 554–556, 555f–556f
  chordee in, 551
  complete repair for, 544, 544f
    continence outcomes with, 560
    technical aspects of, 550, 550f
  continence procedure for, 554–556, 555f–556f
  continence with, 565
  continent urinary diversion for, 564–565, 565b
  epispadias repair for, 550–551
    failure of, 564
  evaluation of, at birth, 539–542, 539f, 539b
  female genital defect in, 534–535, 535f
  fertility, 290–291
  genital anatomy, 290
  immobilization techniques for, complications of, 542–543, 543t, 543b
  Kelly repair for, 544
    continence outcomes with, 561
    technical aspects of, 549–550, 549f
  long-term adjustment issues with, 567–568, 568b
  male genital defect in, 533–534, 533f–534f
  management of, at birth, 539–542, 539f
  Mitchell repair for, 544, 544f
    continence outcomes with, 560
    technical aspects of, 550, 550f
  mode of delivery, 291
  modern staged repair of exstrophy, 545
    bladder, posterior urethral, and abdominal wall closure for, 545–548, 546f–548f

Classic bladder exstrophy (CBE) *(Continued)*
    combined bladder closure and epispadias repair, 548
    management after, 548–549
  osteotomy for, 540–542, 541f–542f
    complications of, 542–543
  outcomes and results of modern initial repair, 556–559
    bladder neck repair, 558–559, 559t, 559b, 560f
    epispadias repair, 557–558
    initial closure, 557
  pelvic bone defects in, 531–532, 531f
  pelvic floor defects in, 532, 532f
  penile reconstruction for, 551–552, 552f–553f
  penile skin closure for, 552–554
  pregnancy, 291
  reconstruction failures and complications, 561–565
    epispadias repair, 564
    failed bladder neck repair, 563–564, 564b
    failed closure, 561–563, 561f–562f, 561t, 563b
  Schrott-Erlangen approach to, 545
    continence outcomes with, 560
  spinal defects in, 531–532
  surgical options in newborn with, 543–545
    Mainz repair, 545
  surgical reconstruction of, 538–556
    alternative, 564–565
    female exstrophy, 554
    patient selection for, 540
    postoperative care, 556
    postoperative problems, 554
    small exstrophy bladder unsuitable for newborn closure, 540
  ureterosigmoidostomy for, 564
  urethral reconstruction for, 564
  urinary defects in, 535–537, 536f–537f
Classic Wilms tumor, 1100, 1100f
Classical Cushing syndrome, 2363, 2363f, 2364t
Clavien-Dindo scale, 260–261, 261t
Clavien-Dindo System of Classifying Complications, 105–106, 106t
Clean intermittent catheterization (CIC)
  for bladder emptying failure, 2901
  for bowel-bladder dysfunction, 657
  for renal transplantation, 1057
  for urinary tract infections, 625
Cleansing enema, for prostate biopsy, 3496
Clear cell RCC
  chemotherapy, 2341–2342
  familial form of, 1354t, 1358, 2141–2143, 2143t, 2144f
  hormonal therapy, 2342–2343
  immunologic approaches to, 2329–2332
    allogeneic hematopoietic stem cell transplantation, 2331, 2331t
    IL-2, 2329–2331, 2330t
    immune checkpoint inhibitors, 2331–2332, 2332f
    interferons, 2329, 2329t
  pathology of, 2149t–2151t, 2151–2152, 2152f
  targeted molecular therapies for
    basis of, 2332–2333, 2333f
    combination and sequential therapy with, 2339–2341
    immune "checkpoint" inhibitor-based combination strategies, 2341, 2342f
    mTOR pathway inhibitors, 2326–2327, 2338–2339, 2340f, 2340t
    other, 2341–2343
    VEGFR-based, 2326–2327, 2333–2337, 2333t–2335t, 2336f, 2337t
Clear cell sarcoma of kidney (CCSK), in pediatric patients, 1108–1109
Clenbuterol, for stress urinary incontinence in women, 2714
Climate, renal calculi and, 2007
Clindamycin, prophylaxis with, for uncomplicated urologic procedures, 1194t–1196t

Clinic, in transitional urology, 1047
Clinical Epidemiological Validation Center (CEVC), 3478-3479
Clinical question, in urodynamic studies, 2551-2552
Clinical target volume (CTV), 3590
Clinical trials, for locally advanced prostate cancer, 3657, 3657t-3658t
Clipping devices, for laparoscopic and robotic surgery, 216-217, 217f
Clitoral complex, 1627.e2-1627.e4, 1627.e3f
Clitoris, 1627.e1, 2435, 2436f-2437f
  disorders of, 975, 977b
    diminutive clitoris, 975, 976f
    hypertrophied clitoris, 975, 975f
Clitorodynia, sexual pain and, 1651-1652
Clitoroplasty, initial management, timing, and principles for, 1026, 1026f, 1028f-1029f
Cloaca, 330f
Cloacal anomalies, 1019-1042
  classification of, 1019-1025
  evaluation of, 1021
    history and physical examination for, 1021-1022, 1022f
    radiographic and endoscopic evaluation of, 1024-1025, 1025f
Cloacal exstrophy, 380, 381t, 573-576
  anatomic considerations for, 574-575
  cardiovascular abnormalities with, 575
  evaluation of, at birth, 576, 576b
  failed, 579
  gender assignment for, 576-577, 577f
  genitourinary abnormalities with, 575
  intestinal tract abnormalities with, 575
  long-term adjustment issues with, 567-568, 568b
  long-term issues in, 580, 580b
  management of, at birth, 576, 577b
  neurospinal abnormalities with, 574-575, 574f
  prenatal diagnosis of, 576
  pulmonary abnormalities with, 575
  sexuality with, male concerns, 566
  skeletal system abnormalities with, 575
  surgical reconstruction of, 576-580
    immediate, 577-578
  urinary continence creation in, 579-580
  urinary tract reconstruction of, 578-579
    modern staged, 578, 578t
    osteotomy role in, 578-579
    single-stage, 579
  variants of, 575f, 576
Cloacal malformation, 380-382
Clonidine
  to facilitate bladder emptying, 2720
  suppression testing, for pheochromocytoma, 2377
Clorpactin, for BPS/IC treatment, 1244.e1
Closed access techniques
  for achieving transperitoneal access and establishing pneumoperitoneum, 207-209
  complications related to, 224
"Closing zipper," in hypospadias, 905
Cloudy urine, cause of, 14
CLPP. see Cough leak point pressure
Clusterin, 3701
c-MET gene, 2143-2144
  in UTUC, 2198
CMG. see Cystometrogram
CMN. see Congenital mesoblastic nephroma
CNAs. see Copy number alterations
CNF. see Congenital nephrotic syndrome of Finnish type
CNPs. see Calcifying nanoparticles
CNS. see Congenital nephrotic syndrome
Coaxial introducer, 170
Cobb-Ragde needles, in pubovaginal sling placement, 2838-2839

Cocaine, ureteral response to, 1888
Cockcroft-Gault formula, 1905
Coffee, UTUC risk and, 2186
COG. see Children's Oncology Group
Cognition, of geriatric urology patient, 2910, 2911f
Cognitive function, hormonal therapy and, 3681
Cognitive/mental fusion, 3622
Cohen Cross-Trigonal technique, for vesicoureteral reflux in children, 840, 841f
Coherence, 238
Coital alignment technique, for female orgasmic disorder, 1647
Coital incontinence, 2540
Colchicine, for PD, 1611, 1616t
Collagen
  of bladder wall, 2463-2464
  of male stress urinary incontinence, 2897
  of urethra, 2468
Collagen disorders, and PD, 1602
Collagenase Clostridium histolyticum, for PD, 1613, 1617t
Collecting duct RCC
  pathology of, 2149t-2151t, 2154
  systemic therapy for, 2344
Collecting system, 161-162, 162f
  injury, 179
  of kidney, 336
  obstruction, 182
  radiologic anatomy of, 1872-1873
Collecting system repair, laparoscopic repair of, 2302, 2303f
Colles fascia, 1807.e9-1807.e10, 2444, 2446f
Collimator, 91
Collings knives, 172
Colon
  pseudo-obstruction of, 3181
  reflection of, for simple nephrectomy, 2285-2286, 2287f
  selection, 3162
  for urinary diversion
    preparation for, 3160-3161, 3161f
    selection of, 3161
Colon conduit, 3196-3197, 3196f, 3198t
Colon isolation, in robot-assisted intracorporeal continent cutaneous diversion, 3269, 3269f
Colon mobilization, in robot-assisted intracorporeal continent cutaneous diversion, 3269, 3269f
Colon pouches
  creation, in robot-assisted intracorporeal continent cutaneous diversion, 3269
  right
    with intussuscepted terminal ileum, 3219-3220
    for orthoptic urinary diversion, 3246
Color Doppler ultrasonography, 73, 388
  transrectal, for prostate biopsy, 3500-3501, 3500f-3502f
  for urinary tract obstruction, 778
Color flow with spectral display ultrasonography, 73-74
Colpexin sphere, 2726, 2726f, 2726.e1f
Colpocleisis, for apical pelvic organ prolapse repair, 2809-2814, 2920.e10
  partial
    results with, 2812-2814
    technique for, 2811-2812, 2811f
  total
    results with, 2812
    technique for, 2812, 2813f
Colpoperineorrhaphy, posterior, 2825
Colpopexy and Urinary Reduction Efforts (CARE) trial, 2535-2536

Colporrhaphy
  anterior
    complications of, 2782-2783
    results with, 2779-2782, 2780t
    technique for, 2779, 2779f
  posterior, 2825-2829, 2825f
    perineorrhaphy, technique for, 2827-2829
    results with, 2827-2829, 2828t
    site specific, technique for, 2826-2827, 2826f-2827f
Colposuspension
  Burch. see Burch colposuspension
  definition of, 2757
  laparoscopic, 2759
  open retropubic, 2757
  prophylactic, 2765
  tension-free vaginal tape procedure compared with, 2773-2774
Columns of Bertin, 1866
Combination ballistic and ultrasonic devices, 2112-2113
Combination of Avodart and Tamsulosin (CombAT) Study, 3386-3389, 3389f, 3389t
Combination therapies, in ED, 1537-1538
Combined intracavernosal injection and stimulation, in ED, 1521
Combined intra-extravesical approach, for bladder diverticula, 3015, 3015f
Comet tail artifact, 74f
Commensal bacteria, 427-428
Common excretory duct, 328
Common iliac arteries, 1873.e1f, 1874
Common iliac lymphadenectomy, 3152, 3153f-3154f
Common penile artery, 1807.e5f, 1807.e9
Common Terminology Criteria for Adverse Events (CTCAE), 105, 106t
Communicating hydrocele, 889
  epidemiology and pathogenesis of, 889
Comorbidity, definition of, 107-108
Comparative Effectiveness Analysis of Surgery and Radiation (CEASAR) study, 3532
Compensatory renal growth, with urinary tract obstruction, 794-795
Complete repair, for classic bladder exstrophy, 544, 544f
  continence outcomes with, 560
  technical aspects of, 550, 550f
Complex cystic masses, 50
Complex stones, percutaneous nephrolithotomy and, 2106
Complexed prostate-specific antigen, in prostate cancer, 3518
Compliance number, 2560-2561
Compound calyx, 161
Comprehensive geriatric assessment (CGA), 2913
Compressive dressings and stockings, for inguinal lymphadenectomy, 1801
Computed tomography (CT), 45-51, 46f-48f, 51b, 416-418
  of adrenal glands, 2352, 2352f
  in adrenal mass evaluation, 2395-2396, 2396f
  after orthoptic urinary diversion, 3235, 3235f
  for biochemical recurrence after radical prostatectomy, 3662
  of bladder diverticula, 2967, 2968f
  of bladder injuries, 3055f
  of bladder RMS, 1113
  of bladder/urethra, 418
  for calculus disease, 418
  for cysts/masses, 416
  fundamentals of, 416
  infection and, 418, 418f
  for inguinal node dissection, 1792
  of IVC tumor thrombus, 2175, 2175f
  of kidney, 1868f

Computed tomography (CT) (Continued)
  for kidney preoperative evaluation, 2248, 2249f
  for localized prostate cancer, 3527
  of male pelvis, 2458, 2458f–2459f
  of matrix stones, 2076, 2076f
  of neuroblastoma, 1089
  obstruction of kidney/ureter, 416
  for pediatric genitourinary trauma, 1066
  of pediatric stone disease, 854
  radiation exposure with, 780
  of RCC, 2159–2160, 2160f
  renal, 390–391
  of renal angiomyolipoma, 2125–2126, 2126f
  of renal calculi, pretreatment assessment, 2071
  of renal injuries, 1984–1985, 1984f–1985f
  of renal lymphoma, 2182, 2182t
  of renal tumor ablation, 2313, 2314f
  for renal tumor evaluation, 2134–2135, 2136f–2137f
  for renovascular hypertension screening, 1917–1918, 1918b
  of retrocaval ureter, 1963, 1965f
  of retroperitoneal fibrosis, 1979, 1979f
  scrotum/testes/internal genitalia, 418
  of seminal vesicles and ejaculatory ducts, 1378
  trauma and, 418
  of ureteral injuries, 1995, 1995f
  of ureteropelvic junction obstruction, 1943, 1944f–1945f
  for ureterovaginal fistula, 2945f
  of urinary lithiasis, 2037–2038, 2037f, 2037t
  of urinary tract obstruction, 779–780
  for UTIs, 1144, 1168, 1169f, 1178–1179, 1179f
  of UTUC, 2193
Computed tomography angiography (CTA), of kidneys, 1869.e2f
Concealed penis, 394
Concentration product (C_p), 2009
Concentration product ratio (CPR), 2010
"Concerning a New Kind of Ray,", 3587
Condom catheters, 155, 156f, 2920.e6
Conduction velocity, ureteral, 1883
Condyloma acuminatum, 988
Condylomata acuminata, malignant transformation of, 1742.e2
Congenital absence of vas deferens (CAVD), 903
Congenital adrenal hyperplasia (CAH), 311, 380–382, 1007–1010, 1007f–1008f, 1007b, 1438, 2383–2384
  lower urinary tract dysfunction and, 2633
  postnatal treatment of, 382
  prenatal treatment of, 382
Congenital anomalies, genitourinary trauma and, 1075–1076
Congenital bilateral absence of the vas deferens, 1450
Congenital bladder diverticulum, 3011
Congenital cryptorchidism, 949, 953–954
Congenital curvature of penis, 1836–1837
Congenital defects versus acquired scar, 498–499
Congenital disorders, and delayed ejaculation, 1575
Congenital diverticula, 522
  urethral, reconstructive surgery for, 1810
Congenital megacystis, 376–377, 519–521, 519f, 520t
Congenital mesoblastic nephroma (CMN), in pediatric patients, 1109
Congenital nephrosis, 756
Congenital nephrotic syndrome (CNS), 345
Congenital nephrotic syndrome of Finnish type (CNF), 756
Congenital neurogenic bladder, diagnostic evaluation and follow-up of, 631, 631f, 632t
Congenital penile curvature, 914, 917f
Congenital penile nevi, 883, 883f
Congenital strictures, 1815

Congenital unilateral absence of the vas deferens, 1449–1450
Congenital urethral fistula, 883, 883f
Conn syndrome, adrenal surgery for, 2409–2410, 2409b
Connexin 43, 2476–2477, 2477f
Conservative therapies, for BPS/IC treatment, 1239–1240
Constipation. see Defecation disorders
Constitutional symptoms, patient history of, 7
Consultation, intraoperative, 296–304, 298b
Contact dermatitis, 1276–1277, 1277f
Content validity, 109
Contextual features, definition of, 116
CONTILIFE, 111t
Continence
  during abdominal pressure increases, 2516
  after creation of neobladder, 3272–3273, 3272t
  after orthoptic urinary diversion, 3251–3254, 3252t–3253t, 3254b
  bladder expansion in, 2593, 2593b
  bladder outlet in, 2593–2595
  in cloacal exstrophy, 579–580
  estrogens and, 2713
  lower urinary tract neural control in, 2593
  in male epispadias, 569–570, 570t
  mechanisms of, 2593–2595
    development of, 329–333
  medical diagnoses and, 2527
  physiotherapy, role of, in laparoscopic radical prostatectomy, 3579
  procedure, for classic bladder exstrophy, 554–556, 555f–556f
  promotion and advocacy for, 2920.e9
  reflex circuitry controlling, 2489–2493, 2490f
    somatic to visceral reflexes, 2492
    sphincter to bladder reflexes, 2490f, 2491–2492, 2492f
    storage phase, 2490–2491, 2490f–2491f, 2491t
  sphincteric mechanisms in, 2593–2595
    female, 2594–2595, 2595b
    male, 2594, 2594f, 2595b
Continent catheterizable channels, for bladder emptying failure, 2898–2900, 2899f
Continent catheterizable stoma, 292
Continent catheterizing pouches, 3211–3226, 3212f
  continent ileal reservoir, 3213–3215, 3214f
  double T pouch, 3215, 3216f–3217f
  gastric pouch, 3225–3226, 3225f–3226f
  general care, 3213
  general procedural methodology, 3212–3213
  Indiana pouch, 3220–3224, 3222f–3223f
  Mainz pouch I, 3215–3219, 3218f–3221f
  Penn pouch, 3224–3225, 3224f
  right colon pouches with intussuscepted terminal ileum, 3219–3220
Continent ileal reservoir, 3213–3215, 3214f
Continent urinary diversions, 191, 3208–3226
  catheterizable stoma for, 706–711
  for classic bladder exstrophy, 564–565, 565b
  considerations for, 706
  continent vesicostomy, 710–711
  cutaneous, 3206–3232, 3231b
    absorbable stapling techniques in, 3227–3228
    comments on, 3208
    continent catheterizing pouches, 3211–3226, 3212f
    cystectomy for, 3206–3208, 3207f
    general considerations of, 3206
    operative technique variations for, 3227–3229
    patient preparation of, 3206
    patient selection of, 3206
    postoperative care of, 3208
    quality-of-life assessments, 3226–3227
    rectal bladder urinary diversion, 3209–3211

Continent urinary diversions (Continued)
  flap valves for, 707–709
  hydraulic valves for, 710
  ileocecal valve for, 709–710
  mechanisms for, 706–711, 707f
  Mitrofanoff principle for, 707–709
  nipple valves for, 707
  for pediatric patients, 706–713, 711b
    considerations to, 706
    results with, 709
    technique for, 708–709, 708f
  ureterosigmoidostomy for, 706–707
Continent vesicostomy, 710–711
Continuous incontinence, patient history of, 5
Continuous occlusion test, 2659
Continuous positive airway pressure (CPAP)
  for nocturnal polyuria, 2669
  for obstructive sleep apnea, 2920.e8
Continuous urinary incontinence, 2540, 2581
Continuous wave lasers, 238
Contractile activity, of ureters, 1883–1887, 1883f
  calcium and excitation-contraction coupling, 1884–1885
  proteins, 1883–1884, 1883f–1884f
  second messengers in, 1885–1887, 1885f–1886f
  urothelial effects on, 1885
Contractile (motor) function, in overactive bladder, 2640
Contractile proteins
  of smooth muscles, 2470–2472, 2471f–2473f
  of ureters, 1883–1884, 1883f–1884f
Contractile tissue, epididymal, 1403f, 1404
Contralateral internal ring, 892, 892f
Contrast agents, in ultrasonography, 76–77
Contrast media, 29–35, 35b
  adverse reactions, 29–34, 30t
  allergic-like reactions, 30
  considerations, 32–34
  contrast reactions, treatment of, 30–31
  delayed contrast reactions, 32
  magnetic resonance imaging contrast agents, 34–35
  premedication, 31–32, 31b
Contrast nephropathy, 1923–1924
Contusion, ureteral, 1996
Convective radiofrequency water vapor thermal therapy, 3421–3422
  complications of, 3422
  conclusion for, 3422
  outcomes with, 3422
    comparative studies, 3422
    single-cohort studies, 3422
  technique for, 3421–3422, 3421f–3422f
Conventional radiation, 3587
Conventional radiography, 28, 29f, 29b, 415
  intravenous pyelography, 415
  plain abdominal radiography, 415
  retrograde pyelography, 415
Convergent validity, 109
Cooper ligament, 2444, 2447f–2448f
Cope catheter, 173, 173f
Cope retention mechanism, 173
Copy number alterations (CNAs), in GU cancers, 1354, 1354t–1355t
Cordonnier and Nesbit techniques, in urinary diversion, 3187
Corpora amylacea, 1203
Corpora cavernosa, 1383–1384
  anatomy of, 1807.e1f–1807.e2f
Corporal perforation, 1589–1591, 1590f
Corpus cavernosum electromyography, and single potential analysis of cavernous electrical activity, 1527
Corpus spongiosum, 1383–1384
  anatomy of, 1807.e1f–1807.e3f, 1807.e6f–1807.e7f
Cortical defects, vesicoureteral reflux, 498–501, 500b
  acquired renal scars, 499–500

Cortical defects, vesicoureteral reflux *(Continued)*
 congenital defects *versus* acquired scar, 498-499
 pathophysiology of acquired scarring, 500-501, 500f-501f
 reflux-associated renal dysplasia, 499, 499f, 499t, 499.e1f
Cortical microcystic disease, 756-757
Cortical renal scan with DMSA, 440
Cortical sex cords, 319f
Corticobasal degeneration, lower urinary tract dysfunction and, 2631
Corticosteroids
 in genitourinary tuberculosis medical therapy, 1316-1317
 and nephrotic syndrome, 345, 348b
Corticotropin-releasing factor (CRF), 2495-2496
Cortisol hypersecretion, testing for, 2399-2401
Corynebacterial infection, as cutaneous disease of external genitalia, 1292-1293, 1293f
CoSeal, 215.e2
COU-AA-301 study, 3694, 3694f
Cough leak point pressure (CLPP), 2562
Council catheters, 153, 173f
Cowden syndrome, 2142t, 2145
COX-2 inhibitors
 to facilitate bladder filling and urine storage, 2703
 urethral function effects of, 1903
 for urinary tract obstruction, 795
CP. *see* Cerebral palsy
CPAP. *see* Continuous positive airway pressure
CPB. *see* Cardiopulmonary bypass
CPDN. *see* Cystic partially differentiated nephroblastoma
CPPS. *see* Chronic pelvic pain syndrome
CPR. *see* Concentration product ratio
Cranial suspensory ligament (CSL), 318-320
Creatinine
 GFR and, 777, 1905, 1906f
 serum
  for benign prostatic hyperplasia, 3345-3346
  measurement, in AKI, 1921, 1922t
Creatinine clearance (CrCl), GFR estimation with, 1905
Credé maneuver, 2902
Creep, ureteral, 1891
Cremasteric artery, 1370-1371, 1372f, 1375, 1393
Cremasteric muscle, 1394f
Creutzfeldt-Jakob prion disease (CJD), allografts and, 2835
CRF. *see* Corticotropin-releasing factor
Criterion validity, 109
Crossed renal ectopia, 727-728, 727f-728f, 731b
Cross-organ sensitization, 2486, 2508
Cross-sectional imaging, of pheochromocytoma, 2375
Cryoablation (CA)
 for locally advanced prostate cancer, 3655
 for renal tumors, 2309-2310, 2310b
  background and mode of action, 2309-2310
  complications of, 2318-2319, 2320f-2321f, 2320b
  duration, 2310
  follow-up for, 2312-2314, 2314b
  freeze-thaw cycles, 2310
  laparoscopic, 2304
  oncologic outcomes of, 2314-2318, 2315t-2316t, 2318b
  percutaneous, 2312, 2313f, 2318
  RFA *versus*, 2317-2318
  success of, 2313-2314, 2314f
  treatment temperature, 2310

Cryotherapy, 3624-3628, 3625f, 3627t
Cryptorchidism, 321, 322f-323f, 413f, 949, 972b, 1432-1433, 1440, 1449
 acquired, 949, 954
 adjuvant hormonal therapy for, 965
 associated pathology of, 961-964
  epididymis anomalies with, 962-963, 962f
  gubernacular anomalies with, 962-963
  processus vaginalis anomalies with, 962-963
  testicular anomalies with, 963-964
  testicular maldevelopment, 961-964
 cancer risk and, 1680
 congenital, 949, 953-954
 definitions for, 949
 diagnosis of, 958-964
  nonpalpable testes, 959-961, 960f
  palpable testes, 958-959, 959f
 diagnostic laparoscopy for, 960-961
 epidemiology of, 953-954
 etiology, diagnosis and management of, 949-958
 examination in, 958, 958f
 genetic susceptibility to, 954-955
 hormonal defects of, 950f, 956-957
 hormonal evaluation of, 960
 human chorionic gonadotropin for, 964-965
 imaging of, 960
 luteinizing hormone-releasing hormone for, 964-965
 management of, 959f, 964
 medical management of, 964-965
 MRI of, 415
 pathogenesis of, 954-958
 prognosis for, 968-972
 surgical management of, 965-968
  abdominal testis, 967-968
  palpable testis, 966-967
 syndromic, 957-958
 testicular cancer and, 970-972
 testicular embryology and, 949-953
 testicular hormone production for, 950-951, 950f
 ultrasonography of, 412, 412b
Crystallization
 inhibitors and promoters of, 2014-2015
 in urine, 2009
Crystals
 aggregation of, 2011
 homogeneous nucleation of, 2011
 oxidative stress and, 2013-2014
 retention of, 2011
 scanning electron micrographs of, 2041, 2042f
 in urine, 23, 24f
CSL. *see* Cranial suspensory ligament
CT. *see* Computed tomography
CT urogram (CTU), for genitourinary tuberculosis diagnosis, 1312, 1313f
CTA. *see* Computed tomography angiography
CTCAE. *see* Common Terminology Criteria for Adverse Events
"CTC-Chip,", 3485
CTCL. *see* Cutaneous T-cell lymphoma
CTCs. *see* Circulating tumor cells
CTLA-4. *see* Cytotoxic T-lymphocyte antigen-4
CTV. *see* Clinical target volume
Culp-DeWeerd spiral flap, for ureteropelvic junction obstruction, 1960-1961, 1961f
CUP. *see* Chaperone-usher pathway
Curriculum, for men's health center, 1427
Curvatures of penis, 394, 880-881, 881f
 correction of, 306-310, 311f
 reconstructive surgery for, 1836-1838, 1838b
  acquired, 1837-1838
  congenital, 1836-1837
Cushing disease, 2361

Cushing syndrome, 2360-2367, 2367b
 ACTH-dependent, 2361, 2361f
  Cushing disease, 2361
  ectopic ACTH syndrome, 2361, 2362f, 2362t, 2366
  treatment of, 2365-2366, 2366f
 ACTH-independent, 2362, 2366-2367
  bilateral macronodular adrenal hyperplasia, 2362
 adrenal surgery for, 2409b, 2410
 adrenal tumors and, 2362
 clinical characteristics, 2363-2364
  classical, 2363, 2363f, 2364t
  subclinical Cushing syndrome, 2363-2364
 diagnostic tests, 2364-2365, 2365f, 2365b, 2400, 2400b
 epidemiology of, 2360
 exogenous, 2361, 2365
 increased adrenal function in, 2360-2367, 2361f-2363f, 2362t, 2364t, 2365f-2366f, 2365b, 2367b, 2400b
 overview of, 2360-2361
 pathophysiology of, 2360-2362, 2361f-2362f, 2362t
 primary pigmented nodular adrenocortical disease, 2362
 prognosis, 2367
 treatment, 2365-2367, 2409b, 2410
Cutaneous artery, 136f
Cutaneous continent urinary diversion, 3206-3232, 3231b
 absorbable stapling techniques in, 3227-3228
  right colon pouch, 3228, 3229f
  stapled sigmoid reservoir, 3228, 3230f
  W-stapled reservoir, 3228-3229, 3231f
 comments on, 3208
 continent catheterizing pouches, 3211-3226, 3212f
  continent ileal reservoir, 3213-3215, 3214f
  double T pouch, 3215, 3216f-3217f
  gastric pouch, 3225-3226, 3225f-3226f
  general care, 3213
  general procedural methodology, 3212-3213
  Indiana pouch, 3220-3224, 3222f-3223f
  Mainz pouch I, 3215-3219, 3218f-3221f
  Penn pouch, 3224-3225, 3224f
  right colon pouches with intussuscepted terminal ileum, 3219-3220
 cystectomy for, 3206-3208, 3207f
 general considerations of, 3206
 operative technique variations for, 3227-3229
  conduit conversion to continent reservoir, 3227
  minimally invasive, 3227
 patient preparation of, 3206
 patient selection of, 3206
 postoperative care of, 3208
 quality-of-life assessments, 3226-3227
 rectal bladder urinary diversion, 3209-3211
  augmented valved rectum, 3209
  folded rectosigmoid bladder, 3209
  hemi-Kock pouch procedures with valved rectum, 3209-3210
  Mainz II pouch, 3210-3211
  sigma-rectum pouch, 3210-3211
  T pouch procedures with valved rectum, 3209-3210, 3210f
Cutaneous diseases, of external genitalia, 1273-1306, 1306b
 allergic dermatitis
  atopic dermatitis, 1275-1276, 1276f
  contact dermatitis, 1276-1277, 1277f
  differential diagnosis, 1275b
  erythema multiforme and Stevens-Johnson syndrome, 1277-1278, 1278f

Cutaneous diseases, of external genitalia (*Continued*)
  basic dermatology, 1273, 1274f, 1274t
  benign, of male genitalia
    angiokeratomas of Fordyce, 1302, 1303f
    ectopic sebaceous glands, 1303f, 1304
    median raphe cysts, 1304
    pearly penile papules, 1302, 1303f
    sclerosing lymphangitis, 1302–1304
    Zoon balanitis, 1302, 1303f
  common miscellaneous
    capillary hemangioma, 1304–1306
    dermatofibroma, 1304, 1305f
    epidermoid cyst, 1304, 1305f
    lentigo simplex, 1304, 1305f
    mole, 1304, 1305f
    neurofibroma, 1304, 1305f
    seborrheic keratosis, 1304, 1305f
    skin tag, 1304
    vitiligo, 1305f, 1306
  dermatologic therapy, 1273–1275, 1275f
  infections and infestations
    balanitis, 1288
    balanoposthitis, 1288, 1289f
    candidal intertrigo, 1293–1294, 1294f
    cellulitis, 1288–1289, 1290f
    corynebacterial infection (trichomycosis axillaris and erythrasma), 1292–1293, 1293f
    dermatophyte infection, 1294–1295, 1295f
    ecthyma gangrenosum, 1293, 1294f
    erysipelas, 1288–1289
    folliculitis, 1290–1291, 1291f
    Fournier gangrene, 1289–1290, 1290f
    furunculosis, 1291, 1291f
    genital bite wounds, 1293, 1294f
    hidradenitis suppurativa, 1291–1292, 1292f
    infestation, 1295–1296, 1296f–1297f
    STDs, 1288, 1289f
  neoplastic conditions
    basal cell carcinoma, 1297–1298, 1300f
    bowenoid papulosis, 1296, 1298f
    cutaneous T-cell lymphoma, 1302, 1302f
    extramammary Paget disease, 1301–1302, 1301f
    Kaposi sarcoma, 1298–1299, 1300f
    melanoma, 1300–1301
    pseudoepitheliomatous, keratotic, and micaceous balanitis, 1299–1300, 1300f
    squamous cell carcinoma, 1296, 1299f
    squamous cell carcinoma in situ, 1296, 1298f
    verrucous carcinoma (Buschke-Lowenstein tumor), 1296–1297, 1299f
  noninfectious genital ulcers, 1286–1288, 1286b
    aphthous ulcers and Behçet disease, 1286–1287, 1287f
    pyoderma gangrenosum, 1287–1288, 1288f
    traumatic causes, 1288, 1288f
  papulosquamous disorders, 1278–1283, 1278b
    fixed drug eruption, 1282, 1283f
    lichen nitidus, 1281
    lichen planus, 1280–1281, 1281f
    lichen sclerosus, 1281–1282, 1282f
    psoriasis, 1278–1279, 1279f
    reactive arthritis, 1279–1280, 1280f
    seborrheic dermatitis, 1282–1283
  vesicobullous disorders, 1283–1286, 1284b
    bullous pemphigoid, 1284–1285, 1285f
    dermatitis herpetiformis, 1285
    Hailey-Hailey disease, 1285–1286, 1286f
    linear IgA bullous dermatosis, 1285, 1285f
    pemphigus vulgaris, 1284, 1284f
Cutaneous fistulae, 2962
Cutaneous horn, of penis, 1742.e1, 1742.e1f
Cutaneous lesions, penile premalignant, 1742
  Buschke-Löwenstein tumor, 1742.e1f, 1742.e3
  non-human papillomavirus-related, 1742.e1–1742.e2
  virus-related, 1742.e2–1742.e3, 1743b

Cutaneous T-cell lymphoma (CTCL), as neoplastic condition, 1302, 1302f
"Cut-to-the-light" procedure, 3059
CVA. *see* Cerebrovascular accident
CVD. *see* Cardiovascular disease
CxBladder, of bladder tumor, 3081
CyberWand, 245
Cyclic adenosine monophosphate (cAMP), in ureteral contractions, 1885
Cyclic guanosine monophosphate (cGMP), in ureteral contractions, 1885
Cyclic guanosine monophosphate-signaling pathway, 1497–1499
Cyclin D2, 3616
Cyclin-dependent kinase inhibitors (CDKIs), in GU cancers, 1347.e1, 1347.e1f
Cyclin-dependent kinases, in GU cancers, 1347.e1, 1347.e1f
Cyclins, in GU cancers, 1347.e1, 1347.e1f
Cyclooxygenase (COX) inhibitors
  to facilitate bladder filling and urine storage, 2703
  urethral function effects of, 1903
Cyclooxygenase-2 (COX-2), in UTUC, 2198
Cyclosporine, for BPS/IC oral therapy, 1241t, 1242–1243
CYP17 inhibition, 3693–3695, 3694f
Cyproheptadine, for delayed ejaculation, 1579
Cyproterone acetate, 3674
Cystadenomas, of testicular adnexa, 1709
Cystatin C, GFR estimation with, 1905
Cystectomy
  for cutaneous continent urinary diversion, 3206–3208, 3207f
  for non-muscle-invasive bladder cancer, 3106–3107, 3107b
  oncologic outcomes following, radical, 3118–3119
  partial, 3038–3043
    evaluation for, 3038–3040
    extraperitoneal approach to, 3040–3041
    open, 3040
    outcomes with, 3042–3043
    surgical indications for, 3038–3040
    surgical technique for, 3040–3041
    transperitoneal approach to, 3041–3042, 3042f–3043f
  with pelvic lymph node dissection, radical
    anatomic extent of, 3115–3116
    bilateral, 3115
    density of, 3117
    distal urethra management, 3118
    extracapsular nodal extension, 3117
    intraoperative decision making, 3117–3118
    intraoperative frozen sections of ureter, 3117–3118
    managing female urethra in, 3118
    for muscle-invasive bladder cancer, 3114–3119
    number removed in, 3125
    oncologic outcomes following, 3118–3119, 3118t
Cystic and solid renal masses, CT and, 48–50, 50f, 52f
Cystic dysplasia of rete testis, 899
Cystic fibrosis transmembrane conductance regulator, 1450
  mutation assessment, for male infertility, 1443
Cystic lymphangioma, retroperitoneal tumors and, 2237, 2237f
Cystic masses, retroperitoneal tumors and, 2236–2237
Cystic mesothelioma, retroperitoneal tumors and, 2238
Cystic nephroma, 765–766, 765f, 766b, 767f, 2129–2130, 2129f
Cystic partially differentiated nephroblastoma (CPDN), in pediatric patients, 1109
Cystic renal disease, 339, 349–350

Cystine stones, in renal calculi, 2029–2030, 2029f
Cystinuria, 859, 2029, 2060–2068, 2063b
  ammonium acid urate stones, 2066
  bladder calculi, medical management of, 2066–2067
  clinical considerations of, 2060–2061
  compliance and quality of life, 2062–2063
  conservative strategies of, 2061
  drug-containing calculi, 2065–2066, 2066t
  follow-up of, 2062
  infection calculi, 2063–2065, 2063f, 2064t, 2065b
  medical therapy for, 2061–2062
  metabolic stone formation, 2066
  miscellaneous and drug-induced stones, 2065, 2065b
Cystitis
  definition of, 1129
  diminished bladder capacity and, 2671
  mechanosensitive afferent sensitization with, 2508
  spinal cord chemical changes with, 2507
  with spinal cord injury, 2467
Cystitis cystica, 526
  of bladder, 3082, 3082f
Cystitis glandularis, of bladder, 3082, 3082f
Cystocele, 2526, 2587, 2589f
Cystography
  after modern staged repair of exstrophy, 548–549
  of bladder injuries, 3055f–3056f
Cystolithotripsy
  EHL for, 241.e2
  laser, 244.e4
Cystometrogram (CMG), in urodynamic studies, 2556, 2557f
Cystometry, in urodynamic studies, 2556, 2557f
Cystoplasty
  reduction, for prune-belly syndrome, 592
  sigmoid, 694–695, 696f
Cystoscopy, 156, 2443, 2443f
  after modern staged repair of exstrophy, 548–549
  antimicrobial prophylaxis for, 1198
  of bladder tumor, 3078–3079
  in diagnostic of hematuria, 250–251
  for genitourinary tuberculosis diagnosis, 1313–1314, 1314f
  for non-muscle-invasive bladder cancer, 3096
    surveillance, 3108
  for partial cystectomy, 3038
  for pelvic floor disorder assessment, 2534
  in pubovaginal sling placement and fixation, 2838–2839
  in retropubic midurethral sling, 2853
  for sphincteric urinary incontinence, 2996–2997, 2997f
  for transurethral resection of bladder tumor, 3133
  for urothelial cancer, 3091
  for UTUC, 2190
Cystourethoscopy, 26, 26t
Cystourethrogram
  for benign prostatic hyperplasia, 3348
  for striated sphincter dyssynergia, 2611f
Cystourethroscopy
  for benign prostatic hyperplasia, 3348
  equipment for, 186–187, 186t, 188f–189f, 188t
  indications for, 185–186, 186t, 191b
  patient preparation for, 187–190, 189t
  special circumstances in
    continent urinary diversions, 191
    suprapubic cystostomy, 190–191
  technique for, 190, 190f
  for urethral diverticula, 2982, 2982f
Cysts
  of Gartner duct, urethral diverticula differentiated from, 2986, 2986f

Cysts (Continued)
  of prostate, on transrectal ultrasonography, 3493, 3493f
  of scrotal wall, excision of, 1844
  simple, 766–770, 770b
    classification of, 768–770, 769b, 770f
    clinical features of, 766
    evaluation of, 768, 768f–769f
    histopathology of, 766–768
    prognosis of, 770, 770f
    treatment of, 770, 770f
  of Skene gland, urethral diverticula differentiated from, 2974, 2986f
  vestibular, 976–977, 977f
Cytochrome P450 oxidoreductase deficiency, 1011
Cytokine regulation, 788
Cytokines, 1333–1334, 1335f, 1335t
  in benign prostatic hyperplasia, 3311, 3312f
  septic shock and, 1183
  in tubulointerstitial fibrosis, 787–788
Cytoreductive androgen deprivation therapy (ADT), for localized prostate cancer, 3524
Cytoreductive nephrectomy
  laparoscopic, 2298
  for metastatic RCC, 2325–2328, 2326f–2327f, 2327t, 2328b
Cytosine, 1346.e1, 1346.e2f
Cytosolic free calcium, 1495
Cytotoxic T-lymphocyte antigen-4 (CTLA-4), 2146

D

da Vinci robotic platform, 467
da Vinci Robotic System, 211, 212.e2f
  instrumentation for, 218, 218f
  virtual reality training for, 231.e2, 233.e1f
da Vinci Surgical System, 2822–2823
DA-8031, for PE, 1572.e2
Danish Prostatic Symptom Score (DAN-PSS), 110t, 3344
DAN-PSS. see Danish Prostatic Symptom Score
Dantrolene, to facilitate bladder emptying, 2720.e3
Dapoxetine, and PE, 1571
Darifenacin hydrobromide, to facilitate bladder filling and urine storage, 2682t, 2684–2685
Darkfield examination, syphilis test, 1258
Dartos pouch procedure, 1855
Data Management and Coordinating Center (DMCC), 3478–3479
Davis and Trattner Diagnostic Foley catheters, 154
Daytime urinary incontinence, bladder dysfunction and, 655–660, 660b
DBD. see Diabetes-induced bladder dysfunction
DDR. see DNA damage response
De novo detrusor overactivity, as complication of anterior colporrhaphy, 2782
Debulking nephrectomy, for metastatic RCC, 2325–2328, 2326f–2327f, 2327t, 2328b
Decipher assay, 3488
Decipher biopsy test, 3542–3543
Decipher test, 3521
Decision making, in intraoperative consultation, 296–297, 297f
Decreased adrenal function disorders, 2380–2383, 2383b
  clinical characteristics, 2381–2382, 2382t
  diagnostic tests, 2382
  overview and epidemiology, 2380–2381
  pathophysiology, 2381, 2381f
  prognosis, 2383
  treatment, 2382–2383, 2383t
De-differentiated liposarcomas, in retroperitoneum, 2230
Deep brain stimulation, for Parkinson disease, 2606
Deep perineal space, 1807.e10

Deep venous thrombosis (DVT)
  after laparoscopic and robotic surgery, 231
  after retropubic radical prostatectomy, 3563
  prophylaxis, after laparoscopic radical prostatectomy, 3579
Defecation disorders, 667–679, 667b
  classification of, 667–671, 668t
  disimpaction for, 672
  epidemiology of, 667–671, 668t
  evaluation of, 667–669, 668.e1f, 669t, 671b
  imaging studies of, 669–671, 669f–670f, 669.e1f, 670.e1f
  large bowel/rectum washout for, 672
  maintenance therapy for, 672–673
  management of, 671–678, 671f, 673b, 679b
  nonpharmacologic interventions, 671–673
  prognosis of, 673
  surgical management of, 673–678, 673f
    enema regimen for, 677–678, 678f
    operative technique for, 674–677, 675f–677f
    outcomes with, 678, 678f, 678t
    patient selection and preparation for, 674
  urinary tract and, 667, 668f
Deferential artery, 1370–1371, 1372f, 1375, 1393, 1394f
Definitive perineostomy, for transmen, 3072, 3072f
Deflazacort, for ureteral stone passage, 1900
Defunctionalized bladder, lower urinary tract dysfunction and, 2632–2633
Dehydroepiandrosterone (DHEA), 3281, 3283f
Delayed contrast reactions, in contrast media, 32
Delayed ejaculation, 1572–1579, 1579b
  causes of, 1574, 1574t
  and congenital disorders, 1575
  and endocrinopathy, 1575
  epidemiology of, 1574
  evaluation of, 1577–1578, 1577t, 1578f
  iatrogenic causes of, 1575
  and infective disorders, 1575
  and neurologic disorders, 1576–1577
  psychological, 1574–1575
  terminology and definition of, 1573–1574
  treatment of, 1578–1579
    pelvic cancers, 1575–1576
    pharmacotherapy, 1578–1579, 1579t
    psychological strategies, 1578
Delayed orchiectomy, 1712
Delayed spontaneous bladder perforation, after augmentation cystoplasty, 700–701, 700f
Delayed voiding, 2732
Delirium, 2914
Delivery
  sphincter function and, 2596
  urinary incontinence and, 2583
Dementia, lower urinary tract dysfunction with, 2603–2604
Dénes technique, 595, 598f–600f
Denosumab, 3704
Dent disease, 349
Depression
  in geriatric urology patient, 2910
  prostatitis and, 1210
Dermal grafts, for urethral and penile reconstruction, 1805–1806
Dermatitis herpetiformis, 1285
Dermatofibroma, 1304, 1305f
Dermatophyte infection, 1294–1295, 1295f
Dermoid cysts, testicular, 1708
Derogatis Interview for Sexual Functioning (DISF), 112, 112t
Desmoid tumor, retroperitoneal tumors and, 2234, 2234f
Desmopressin (DDAVP)
  in children, 2711
  efficacy of, 2712
  for enuresis, 664

Desmopressin (DDAVP) (Continued)
  to facilitate bladder filling and urine storage, 2682t, 2710–2712
  gender and, 2712
  for nocturia, 2672t, 2920.e8–2920.e9
  for nocturnal enuresis, 2712
  for nocturnal polyuria, 2669–2670, 2673t
  in nocturnal polyuria, 2713b
Desperation RPLND, 1728, 1728t
Desperation surgery, for NSGCTs, 1701
Detection bias, 105
Detrusor contractility, impaired, in detrusor underactivity, 2650
Detrusor contraction assessment
  duration, 2659
  speed, 2659
  strength, 2657–2659, 2658f
Detrusor failure, in detrusor underactivity, 2650
Detrusor hyperactivity with impaired contractility (DHIC), 2651
  in geriatric patients, 2919.e2
Detrusor hyperreflexia, 2637
Detrusor leak point pressure (DLPP), 485–486
  urodynamic studies of, 2561f, 2562
Detrusor muscle, 2465, 2465f
  acontractile, 2521, 2565
  actinomyosin cross-bridge cycling, 2472–2473, 2472b, 2473f
  action potentials of, 2473–2474, 2474f
  aging and, 2509–2510, 2653, 2654f
  areflexia of, 2521
    after CVA, 2602
    after traumatic brain injury, 2604
    with cerebellar ataxia, 2604
    with lumbar disk protrusion, 2619–2620
    with MS, 2608
    with Parkinson disease, 2605–2606
    urodynamic classification of, 2521–2522, 2522b
  calcium signaling in, 2475–2476, 2476f
  contractile proteins, 2470–2472, 2471f–2473f
  contraction of
    electrical stimulation and, 2729
    muscarinic receptors and, 2680
  electrical response propagation, 2476–2477, 2477f
  excitation-contraction coupling in, 2474–2475, 2475f
  interstitial cells of, 2477–2478, 2478f
  involuntary contractions of, 2559
  membrane electrical properties of, 2473–2474, 2474f
  motor sensory network in, 2479–2480, 2479f
  normal function of, 2564
  overactivity, neurogenic, 2521–2522
Detrusor overactivity (DO), 496, 2833
  afferent mechanisms in, 2642
  after CVA, 2602
  benign prostatic hyperplasia and, 3355
  with brain tumor, 2604
  with cerebellar ataxia, 2604
  herpesvirus infection and, 2621–2622
  hypothesis of, 2642
  idiopathic, 2560
  interstitial cells and, 2477–2478, 2478f
  with MS, 2608
  neurogenic, 2560
  neuromodulation for, rationale for, 2510, 2510f
  nocturnal, 2671
  with Parkinson disease, 2605
  pharmacologic therapy for, 2682t
    antimuscarinic agents, 2681
  spinal cord injury and, 2504–2505, 2505b
  stress-induced, urodynamic studies of, 2563, 2563f
  with suprasacral spinal cord injury, 2610
  test induced, 2560
  with traumatic brain injury, 2604

Detrusor overactivity (DO) *(Continued)*
  urodynamic studies of, 2560–2561, 2560f–2561f
  vasculature in, 2463
Detrusor overactivity incontinence (DOI), 2543, 2581
  cough-induced, 2543
Detrusor sphincter dyssynergia (DSD), 2521
  with autonomic dysreflexia, 2614
  lower urinary tract dysfunction and, 2627
  with Parkinson disease, 2605
  urinary incontinence and, 2595–2596
Detrusor underactivity (DUA), 2521, 2565, 2650
  definition of, 2650, 2651f, 2652b
  diagnosis of, 2657–2659, 2658t, 2659b
    ambulatory urodynamics, 2659
    bladder sensation, 2659
    detrusor contraction duration, 2659
    detrusor contraction speed, 2659
    detrusor contraction strength, 2657–2659, 2658f
  epidemiology of, 2650–2652, 2652t, 2653f
  etiopathogenesis of, 2653–2657, 2654f–2655f, 2657b
    bladder outlet obstruction, 2655–2656, 2657b
    diabetes mellitus, 2656–2657, 2657b
    myogenic factors, 2653
    neurogenic factors, 2653–2655
    neurologic disease or injury, 2657, 2657b
    specific factors, 2655–2657, 2656b
  in geriatric patients, 2919.e2
  management of, 2659–2663, 2660f, 2663b
    bladder outlet surgery for, 2662–2663
    botulinum toxin, 2662
    conservative, 2660
    electrical stimulation, 2661–2662
    initial assessment for, 2656b, 2660
    pharmacotherapies for, 2660–2661
    reconstructive surgery for, 2663
    urinary diversion for, 2663
  prevalence of, 2652t
  regenerative medicine for, 2663
  symptoms of, 2650, 2651f, 2652b
  terminology for, 2650, 2652b
  treatment of, 2719b
Detrusor wall thickness (DWT), 3348
Developmental disorders, and male infertility, 1449–1450
Dexamethasone sodium sulfate, for contrast media, 32
Dextroamphetamine, for BPS/IC oral therapy, 1243
DGN. *see* Dorsal genital nerve
DHEA. *see* Dehydroepiandrosterone
DHIC. *see* Detrusor hyperactivity with impaired contractility
DHT. *see* Dihydrotestosterone
Diabetes-induced bladder dysfunction (DBD), 2656–2657
Diabetes insipidus, 2678
Diabetes mellitus
  detrusor underactivity and, 2656–2657, 2657b
  ED and, 1510, 1510t–1511t
  hormonal therapy and, 3681
  host defense mechanisms in UTIs and, 1139
  hyperoxaluria and, 2059–2060
  low urine pH and, 2027–2028
  lower urinary tract dysfunction and, 2622–2624, 2624b
  Peyronie's disease and, 1600, 1601f
  renal calculi and, 2008
  ureteral function effects of, 1900
Diabetic cystopathy, 2623, 2656–2657
Diacylglycerol (DG), in ureteral contractions, 1885
Diagnosis, of UTIs, 1141–1143, 1141b, 1142.e1t, 1143f

Diagnostic and Statistical Manual of Mental Disorders (DSM-5), and premature ejaculation, 1567
Diagnostic catheters, 154–155, 155f
Diagnostic evaluation, in ED, 1517–1519, 1528b
  cardiovascular risk assessment tools for, 1519
  laboratory tests, 1519
  medical history, 1518
  physical examination for, 1519
  psychosocial history, 1519
  questionnaires and sexual function symptom scores, 1519, 1520f
  sexual history, 1518, 1518t
Dialysis, in renal transplantation, 1058
Diameter, of ureters, 1891
Diaphragm, anatomy of, 2448–2449, 2449f
DIAPPERS acronym, 2526t, 2539
Diarrhea, with bowel preparation, 3165, 3166t
Diclofenac, urethral function effects of, 1903
Diet
  after laparoscopic radical prostatectomy, 3579
  benign prostatic hyperplasia and, 3324, 3325t
  bladder cancer and, 3077–3078
  for BPS/IC treatment, 1240–1241, 1240b
  and exercise, for metabolic syndrome, 1422
  prostate cancer and, 3464–3465, 3544
  urinary incontinence and, 2586
Dietary calcium, 2049
Dietary hyperoxaluria, 2023
Dietary supplements, bladder cancer and, 3078
Differentiation, in urinary tract obstruction, 784–786, 785f
Diffuse mesangial sclerosis (DMS), 756
Diffuse pelvic floor hypertonicity, 2881
Diffusion-weighted imaging (DWI), 61, 63–64, 64f
Diffusion-weighted imaging magnetic resonance imaging (DWI-MRI), for biochemical recurrence after radiotherapy, 3666–3667
Digital palpation, for PFM function assessment, 2723
Digital rectal examination (DRE)
  for pelvic floor disorders, 2530
  physical examination for, 11–12
  for prostate cancer, 3515
    tumor extent prediction with, 3519
  for simple prostatectomy, 3450
Digital ureteroscopes, 195, 195f, 196t
  care and sterilization of, 195–197
Digoxin, and ED, 1508–1509
Dihydrotestosterone (DHT), 1391, 3371
  in benign prostatic hyperplasia, 3307–3308, 3308f
  epididymal function and, 1406
  in prostate, 3280–3281, 3282t
    cancer, 3466, 3467f
  in vas deferens, 1407
Dihydroxyadenine stones, in renal calculi, 2031–2032
1,25-Dihydroxycholecalciferol (Calcitriol), 1914
  in calcium metabolism, 2015
Dilated bladder, 519–521
Dilation devices, for ureteroscopy, 197
Dilators and insertion, for genito-pelvic pain-penetration disorder, 1653
Dimercaptosuccinic acid (DMSA), 92, 796
Dimerization, of androgen receptors, 3291
Dimethyl sulfoxide (DMSO), 1244
  to facilitate bladder filling and urine storage, 2703–2704
Diminished bladder capacity
  causes of, 2671
  management of, 2671–2674, 2675t–2677t
  nocturia and, 2667, 2668t, 2671–2674
  nocturnal polyuria and, 2674–2678
Diminutive clitoris, 975, 976f
Diode lasers, 240
Diphallia, 877, 877f
Dipsogenic polydipsia, 2678

Dipstick test, 15
Dipstick urinalysis, 479
Direct cutaneous artery, 136f
Direct neocystostomy, 2207, 2209f
Direct visualization, 459
Directed masturbation, for female orgasmic disorder, 1647
Disc kidney, 728f, 729
Disease-specific mortality, 103–104
DISF. *see* Derogatis Interview for Sexual Functioning
Disimpaction, 672
Disk disease, lower urinary tract dysfunction with, 2619–2620
Disk prolapse, lower urinary tract dysfunction with, 2619
Dismembered pyeloplasty, 1952–1953
  indications for, 1952–1953
  technique of, 1953, 1953f–1954f
  for ureteropelvic junction obstruction, 1945–1946, 1953f–1954f
    in children, 828, 828f–830f
  results of, 1957–1958, 1959t
Disorders of sex development (DSD), 990–1018, 1449
  ambiguous genitalia, 998–1018, 999f, 999b
  of gonadal differentiation and development, 1000–1007
    46,XX males, 1000–1001
    bilateral vanishing testes syndrome, 1005–1006
    embryonic testicular regression, 1005–1006
    Klinefelter syndrome and variants, 1000
    syndromes of gonadal dysgenesis, 1001–1005
    ovotesticular, 999f, 1006–1007
    testicular tumors associated with, 1122–1124, 1123t
  46,XX, 1007–1011
    congenital adrenal hyperplasia, 1007–1010, 1007f–1008f, 1007b
    secondary to maternal androgens and progestins and maternal tumors, 1010–1011
  46,XY, 1011–1017
    androgen receptor and postreceptor defects, 1013–1014
    Leydig cell aplasia, 1011
    Mayer-Rokitansky-Küster-Hauser syndrome, 1017
    persistent Müllerian duct syndrome, 1016–1017, 1016f
    5α-reductase deficiency, 1014–1016, 1015f
    testosterone biosynthesis disorders, 1011–1013
Disorders of sexual differentiation, 908
Disposable probes, 245
Disruptive Behavior Disorders Rating instrument, 477
Dissection, energy modalities
  for electrosurgery, 235–241, 236f
  ultrasound instrumentation, 237–238
Dissemination of disease, of UTUC, 2193
Dissertatio de Arthritide: Mantissa Schematica: De Acupunctura, 2749
Distal hypospadias, repair of, 918
Distal renal tubular acidosis
  type 1, 2025–2026, 2025f
    causes of, 2055b
    chronic diarrheal states, 2055–2056
  type 4, 2026
Distal ureter
  stone localization and, 2086, 2086t
  surgery of, 3010
Distal ureterectomy
  with bladder psoas muscle hitch/Boari flap, 2207, 2209f
  laparoscopic or robotic, reimplantation and, 2208, 2209t
Distal vagina, 980, 1627, 1627.e1
Distraction injuries, urethral, ED with, 3059

Diuresis
　postobstructive, 796
　ureteral function effects of, 1893
Diuretic renal scintigraphy, 419-423, 419f-424f
Diuretic renography, 390
　for UPJO and reflux differentiation, 1943
　for ureteropelvic junction obstruction, 1944, 1946f
　for urinary tract obstruction, 779
Diuretic scintigraphy, 41-42, 41f-42f
Diuretics
　and ED, 1506
　for pediatric kidney stone disease, 869
Divergent validity, 109
Diverticulectomy
　bladder, 3010-3019, 3011f, 3011b, 3046b-3047b
　　complications of, 3018-3019
　　evaluation of, 3011-3012, 3012f
　　laparoscopic and robotic techniques, 3015-3018, 3016f-3017f
　　outcomes of, 3018-3019
　　postoperative care of, 3018-3019
　　surgical indications, 3011-3012, 3012f
　　surgical technique of, 3012-3018, 3012f
　bladder outlet, 2971-2972
　calyceal, 2294
　laparoscopic, 3012-3013
　urethral, 2989b, 2991-2992, 2991t
DLPP. see Detrusor leak point pressure
DMCC. see Data Management and Coordinating Center
DMS. see Diffuse mesangial sclerosis
DMSA. see Dimercaptosuccinic acid
DMSA renal cortical scintigraphy, 418
DMSO. see Dimethyl sulfoxide
DNA
　basics of, 1346.e1-1346.e4, 1346.e2f
　damage and repair of, 1350-1351, 1351b
　　DSB repair, 1351.e1f-1351.e2f, 1351.e2
　　mechanisms, 1351.e1, 1351.e1f
DNA-binding domain, of androgen receptors, 3289-3290
DNA damage response (DDR), 1350-1351
DNA hypermethylation, in prostate cancer, 3470
DNA methylation, 1348-1350, 1350b
　in bladder cancer, 1349
　in prostate cancer, 1349
DO. see Detrusor overactivity
Docetaxel
　for castration-resistant prostate cancer, 3690-3692, 3691f-3692f
　cisplatin, and 5-fluorouracil (TPF), for penile cancer, 1770
　for non-muscle-invasive bladder cancer, 3105
Documentation
　in intraoperative consultation, 297-298
　　surgical time out, 298, 298t
　ultrasonography, 76, 77f
DOI. see Detrusor overactivity incontinence
Domestic station, patient history of, 9
Donabedian, Avedis, 101
Donabedian model, 101
Dopamine
　agonists, for female sexual arousal disorders, 1650
　in ED, 1494, 1495t
　in ejaculatory response, 1564
　in PD, 2605
Dopaminergic agonists, 1534
Doppler ultrasound, 73-74
　for urinary tract obstruction, 778
Dorsal artery, of penis, 1385f, 1387f, 1807.e5f
Dorsal genital nerve (DGN), electrical stimulation of, 2752
Dorsal lithotomy, 467f
Dorsal lumbotomy
　approach, for open kidney surgery, 2251, 2251f
　urologic surgery, 141-142, 141f-142f

Dorsal nerve
　conduction velocity, 1527
　of penis, 1386
Dorsal plication, 912, 912f
Dorsal rhizotomy, 2741-2742
　clinical results of, 2743, 2744t
　effect of, 2742-2743
　goal of, 2742-2743
　patient selection for, 2742
　post-stimulus voiding in, technique of, 2742
　stimulator of, 2741-2742, 2742f
　surgical implantation technique of, 2742-2743, 2743f
Dorsal segmental artery, 136f
Dorsal shortening technique, 912-913, 915f
Dorsal vein, of penis, 1384-1385, 1807.e5f
Dorsal vein complex (DVC)
　division of, in retropubic radical prostatectomy, 3553-3554, 3554f
　ligation of
　　in laparoscopic radical prostatectomy, 3572-3573, 3573f
　　in retropubic radical prostatectomy, 3553-3556, 3553f
Dose-volume histogram (DVH), 3587-3588, 3588f
Double dye test, for ureterovaginal fistula, 2943
Double T pouch, 3215, 3216f-3217f
Double-lumen catheters, 154
Double-strand breaks (DSBs), repair of, 1351.e1f-1351.e2f, 1351.e2
Dovitinib, for RCC, 2337-2338
Down training, 2732
Doxazosin
　for benign prostatic hyperplasia, 3359-3361, 3360t-3361t
　for diminished bladder, 2674, 2675t-2677t
　to facilitate bladder emptying, 2720.e1
　to facilitate bladder filling and urine storage, 2682t
　ureteral response to, 1888
Doxepin, to facilitate bladder filling and urine storage, 2702
Doxorubicin (Adriamycin), for non-muscle invasive bladder cancer, 3103-3104
Doyen rib stripper, 140
Drain catheters, 155
Drainage, renal, for urinary tract obstruction, 795
DRE. see Digital rectal examination
Dribble-Stop, 2546
Dromedary hump, 1865
Drug-containing calculi, 2065-2066, 2066t
Drug-induced erectile dysfunction, 1506-1509
Drug-resistant tuberculosis, 1318
Drug toxicity, AKI caused by, 1924-1925, 1924t
Drugs
　lower urinary tract function and, 2528, 2528t
　renal calculi induced by, 2032
　transport of, prostatic secretions and, 3303-3304, 3304b
Dry matrix agents, 147
DSBs. see Double-strand breaks
DSD. see Disorders of sex development
DSM-5. see Diagnostic and Statistical Manual of Mental Disorders
DSNB. see Dynamic sentinel node biopsy
DUA. see Detrusor underactivity
Dual-modality lithotripters, 244-246, 245f, 246b
　LithoClast Ultra, 244-245
Dual-source CT (DSCT), 45
Ductuli efferentes, 1393
Ductus (vas) deferens, physiology of, 1406-1407, 1408b
　absorption and secretion and, 1407
　cytoarchitecture, 1406
　functions of, 1406
　gross architecture, 1406
　sperm transport and, 1406-1407

Duke Activity Status Index, 120, 121t
Duloxetine
　to facilitate bladder filling and urine storage, 2682t, 2702-2703
　for stress urinary incontinence, 2504, 2546
　　in men, 2716
　　in women, 2715-2716
Duodenum, 1668, 1668.e2f, 1669f-1670f
　injury of, during radical nephrectomy, 2261
Duplex Doppler ultrasonography, 388
　or renovascular hypertension screening, 1917-1918, 1918b
Duplex kidney, genitourinary trauma and, 1076
Duplex ultrasonography, in ED, 1521-1523, 1522f
Duplicated collecting system, ureteral calculi with, surgical management of, 2087
Duplicated urethra, 310
Duplication anomaly, 333
Dutasteride, for benign prostatic hyperplasia, 3374-3376, 3374f, 3375t, 3376f
DVC. see Dorsal vein complex
DVH. see Dose-volume histogram
DVISS. see Dysfunctional Voiding and Incontinence Scoring System
DVSS. see Dysfunctional Voiding Symptom Score
DVT. see Deep venous thrombosis
DWI. see Diffusion-weighted imaging
DWI-MRI. see Diffusion-weighted imaging magnetic resonance imaging
DWT. see Detrusor wall thickness
Dye testing, for pelvic floor disorders, 2533
Dynamic contrast-enhanced magnetic resonance imaging, 64, 65f
Dynamic dosimetry, 3598
Dynamic infusion cavernosometry and cavernosography, in ED, 1523, 1523f-1524f
Dynamic pressure perfusion studies, for ureteropelvic junction obstruction, 1944-1945
Dynamic renal imaging, 92-93
　with Technetium-99m Mercaptoacetyltriglycine (^{99}mTc-MAG3), 92-93, 94f
Dynamic sentinel node biopsy (DSNB)
　of inguinal nodes, for penile cancer, 1760-1761
　for penile cancer, 1793
Dysfunctional elimination syndrome, 432
Dysfunctional voiding, 2568-2569
Dysfunctional Voiding and Incontinence Scoring System (DVISS), 476
Dysfunctional Voiding Symptom Score (DVSS), 476, 653
Dyslipidemia, 1419
Dyspareunia
　female sexual dysfunction and, 1637
　genito-pelvic pain-penetration disorder and, 1652
Dysplastic lesion, of upper tract urothelium, 2188
Dysuria
　after photoselective vaporization of prostate, 3440
　after transurethral needle ablation of prostate, 3433
　patient history of, 3-4
　of urethral diverticula, 2980

E

Early detection research network (EDRN), 3478
Eastern Cooperative Oncology Group (ECOG) Scale, 107, 107t
Echelon Flex, 216, 216f
Echinococcosis, of genitourinary tract, 1332
Economics
　of metabolic evaluation of urinary lithiasis, 2044-2045, 2045b

Economics (*Continued*)
  prostate cancer and, 3546
  of ureteral calculi surgical management, 2088.e1
ECRS. *see* Extracorporeal renal surgery
Ecthyma gangrenosum, 1293, 1294*f*
Ectoderm, 305
Ectodermal ingrowth theory, 905
Ectopic ACTH syndrome, 2361, 2362*f*, 2362*t*, 2366
Ectopic corticotropin-releasing hormone, 2361–2362
Ectopic kidney, 177
  genitourinary trauma and, 1076, 1077*f*
Ectopic scrotum, 886–887, 888*f*
Ectopic sebaceous glands, 1303*f*, 1304
Ectopic ureter, 333, 798
  anatomic description of, 798*b*, 799*f*
  ureterostomy for, 819
Ectopic ureteral insertion, 977, 978*f*
ED. *see* Erectile dysfunction
EDCs. *see* Endocrine-disrupting chemicals
Edging artifact, in ultrasonography, 72, 73*f*
EDRN. *see* Early detection research network
Education
  for female orgasmic disorder, 1647
  for genito-pelvic pain-penetration disorder, 1653
EEC. *see* Exstrophy-epispadias complex
Effective dose, 28
Efferent pathways, to bladder, 2487–2493, 2487*f*
  adrenergic, 2488
  in detrusor underactivity, 2653, 2655*f*
  glutamate in, 2488, 2489*f*
  glycine and γ-aminobutyric acid in, 2488
  purinergic, 2488–2489
  reflex circuitry, 2489–2493, 2490*f*
  serotonin in, 2488–2489
  terminal nerve fibers, 2487–2488
  transmitters in, 2488, 2490*b*, 2491*f*–2492*f*, 2491*t*
"Eggplant deformity," with penile fracture, 3048, 3048.e1*f*
EHL. *see* Electrohydraulic lithotripsy
Ehlers-Danlos syndrome, lower urinary tract dysfunction and, 2631
Ehrlich technique, 595
Eight edition TNM penile staging system, 1748–1750, 1750*t*
Ejaculation
  delayed, 1572–1579, 1579*b*
    causes of, 1574, 1574*t*
    and congenital disorders, 1575
    and endocrinopathy, 1575
    epidemiology of, 1574
    evaluation of, 1577–1578, 1577*t*, 1578*f*
    iatrogenic causes of, 1575
    and infective disorders, 1575
    and neurologic disorders, 1576–1577
    pharmacotherapy, 1578–1579, 1579*t*
    psychological, 1574–1575
    psychological strategies, 1578
    terminology and definition of, 1573–1574
    treatment of, 1578–1579
    and treatment of pelvic cancers, 1575–1576
  disorders, α₁-blocker therapy associated with, 3370
  failure, patient history of, 6
  premature, 1564–1572, 1572*b*
    and assessment of erectile function, 1570
    causes of, 1568–1569
    classification of, 1564–1565
    definition of, 1565–1567, 1565.e1, 1566*t*
    and determination of intravaginal ejaculation latency time, 1569
    diagnosis of, 1569
    evaluation of, 1569
    patient-reported outcome measures, 1569–1570
    physical examination of, 1570, 1570*f*
    prevalence of, 1567–1568, 1567*f*
    treatment of, 1570–1572

Ejaculatory anhedonia, 1580
Ejaculatory ductal obstruction, 1450–1451
  delayed ejaculation and, 1575
Ejaculatory ducts, 315*f*, 1407, 1408*f*, 1408*b*
  anatomy of, 1454
Ejaculatory dysfunction
  after monopolar transurethral resection of prostate, 3418
  after retroperitoneal tumors management, 2243–2244
  after RPLND, 1729–1730
  after transurethral microwave therapy, 3430
  after transurethral needle ablation of prostate, 3433
  in male infertility, 1450–1451
Elastin, of bladder wall, 2464
Elderly
  α1-adrenergic blockers in, 3370
  bacteriuria in, 1188–1190, 1190*b*
    asymptomatic, 1147–1149, 1147*t*, 1147*b*–1149*b*
    diagnosis, 1188–1189
    epidemiology, 1188
    management, 1189–1190, 1189*t*
    pathogenesis, 1188
    screening for, 1188
  for laparoscopic kidney surgery, 2279
  mid-urethral sling outcomes in, 2862–2863, 2863*b*
  mistreatment of, 2921–2922
  sexual health in, 2920–2921
  in urologic surgery, 121–122
Electrical activity, of ureters
  action potentials, 1879–1881, 1879*f*–1880*f*
  pacemaker potentials and pacemaker activity, 1881–1882, 1882*f*
  propagation, 1882–1883
  resting potential, 1878–1879, 1879*f*, 1881, 1881*b*
Electrical stimulation, 2739–2755, 2755*b*
  constant *versus* intermittent, 2754–2755
  current and future perspectives for, 2743–2746
  for detrusor underactivity, 2661–2662
  for genito-pelvic pain-penetration disorder, 1653
  history of, 2739–2740
  levels of evidence and recommendations for, 2722.e2*b*–2722.e4*b*
  neurophysiology of, 2740–2741, 2741*f*
  of pelvic floor muscle, 2729–2730
  rechargeable neurostimulator of, 2755
  sacral anterior root stimulation, 2741–2742, 2742*f*
  sacral dorsal rhizotomy, 2741–2742, 2742*f*
    clinical results of, 2743, 2744*t*
    goal and effect of, 2742–2743
    patient selection in, 2742
    surgical implantation technique of, 2742–2743, 2743*f*
  techniques of, 2747–2754
    dorsal genital nerve, 2752
    intravesical, 2747–2748
    percutaneous tibial nerve, 2748–2751, 2749*f*
    pudendal nerve, 2751–2752
    sacral nerve, 2752–2754
    transcutaneous, 2748
  types of, 2729
  working mechanism of, 2746–2747, 2746*f*–2747*f*
Electrocardiogram, 450
Electrohydraulic (spark gap) generator, 2094, 2095*f*
Electrohydraulic lithotripsy (EHL), 197, 241*f*, 241*b*, 2109–2110, 2110*f*
  for bladder stones, 241
  chemical stone composition and, 241
  physics and mechanism of action of, 241
  tissue effects, 243
  ureteroscopy with, 243.e1

Electrolyte abnormalities
  in CKD, 355
  with urinary intestinal diversion, 3199–3201, 3199*t*, 3200*f*
Electromagnetic generator, 2094, 2095*f*
Electromotive drug administration (EMDA), 1614, 1617*t*
Electromyography (EMG)
  for PFM function assessment, 2723
  in urodynamic studies, 2557, 2559
  for urodynamics, 2535
Electrostimulation, for neuromuscular dysfunction of lower urinary tract, 637
Electrosurgery
  devices for laparoscopic and robotic surgery, 214
  safety of, 236–237
  tissue dissection and cauterization with, 235–237, 236*f*
Electrotonic spread, in ureteral cells, 1882
Elephantiasis, as filariasis clinical manifestation, 1330, 1330*f*
11p15 locus, in Wilms tumor, 1097*t*, 1098
Elocalcitol, to facilitate bladder filling and urine storage, 2713.e1
EM. *see* Erythema multiforme
Embolization
  before kidney surgery, 2248, 2248.e1*f*
  of prostate, 3445–3446
  for renal injuries, 1986, 1986*f*
  for renal tumors, targeted, 2323
Embolotherapy, 903, 903.e1*f*
Embryology, 799–800, 801*b*
  of exstrophy-epispadias complex, 530, 530*f*
  of female genitalia, 973–974, 974*f*, 974*b*
  of neuroblastoma, 1087–1088
  of prune-belly syndrome, 581
  of supernumerary kidney, 721
  of testis, 949–953
  of thoracic kidney, 725–726
  of unilateral renal agenesis, 718, 719*f*
  of vagina, 973–974, 974*f*, 974*b*
Embryonal carcinoma (EC), histology of, 1682–1683, 1683*f*
Embryonal RMS, 1111, 1112*f*, 1113*b*
Embryonic testicular regression, 1005–1006
EMDA. *see* Electromotive drug administration
Emergency situations, 118
EMG. *see* Electromyography
Emphysema, subcutaneous, during laparoscopic and robotic surgery, 225
Emphysematous cystitis, 1158–1159
Emphysematous pyelonephritis, 1171–1172, 1171*f*
Empirical treatment, in male infertility, 1452
EMT. *see* Epithelial-mesenchymal transition
En bloc hilar vessel stapling, in laparoscopic radical nephrectomy, 2297
Encephalitis, and ED, 1502
Endo Close, 219
Endo Stitch, 215
EndoAvitene, 215.e2
Endocarditis, antimicrobial prophylaxis for uncomplicated urologic procedures and, 1200
Endocrine, concepts of, basic, for HPG axis, 1390, 1391*f*
Endocrine-disrupting chemicals (EDCs), cryptorchidism and, 949
Endocrine evaluation, and male infertility, 1436–1438
Endocrinology, of prostate, 3280–3295, 3281*f*
  adrenal androgens, 3282–3283, 3283*f*
  androgen-binding proteins in plasma, 3282*f*, 3284
  androgen production by testes, 3281–3282, 3282*f*–3283*f*, 3282*t*
  estrogens in male, 3282*t*, 3283–3284
End-of-life care, 2922
Endometriosis, of bladder, 3039, 3040*f*

Endopelvic fascia, 2850
  incision of, in retropubic radical prostatectomy, 3552, 3552f
Endopyeloplasty, percutaneous, for ureteropelvic junction obstruction, 1949
Endopyelotomy, for ureteropelvic junction obstruction, 191–192
Endoscopic incision (direct vision internal urethrotomy), for transmen, 3071
Endoscopic inguinal lymphadenectomy, for penile cancer, 1794
Endoscopic surgery, 145
  complications of, of seminal vesicle surgery, 1863
Endoscopy, 185–202
  of bladder diverticula, 2969, 2970f
    management of, 2972
  of cloacal anomalies, 1024–1025, 1025f
  equipment and video-endoscopic systems for, 185, 186f–187f
  female pelvis anatomy for, 2443, 2443f, 2443b
  in genitourinary tuberculosis treatment, 1317
  history of, 185
  kidney anatomy for, 1865.e2f
  for male urinary incontinence, 2543
  of ureteral anomalies, 799f–800f, 808, 808f–809f
  of urogenital sinus abnormalities, 1023f–1024f
Endothelial dysfunction, 1420
Endothelins (ETs)
  lower urinary tract and, 2502
  renal vascular tone control by, 1913
  urethral function effects of, 1903–1904
Endothelium, ED and, 1506
Endoureterotomy, for ureteral stricture disease, 1968–1969
  antegrade approach to, 1969
  combined retrograde and antegrade approach, 1969
  results with, 1969
  retrograde ureteroscopic approach to, 1968–1969, 1969f
Endourologic management
  of upper tract urothelial cancer, 2210–2224
    antegrade nephroureteroscopic, 2212–2219, 2215f–2217f, 2218t
    basic attributes, 2210–2211, 2210f
    lymph node-positive and metastatic disease treatment, 2222–2224, 2223f
    positive upper tract urinary cytology and carcinoma in situ management, 2219–2222, 2219f, 2221f, 2221t
    retrograde ureteroscopic, 2211–2212, 2211f, 2213f, 2214t, 2215f
  for ureteral stricture disease, 1966–1969, 1971b
  for ureteroenteric anastomotic stricture, 1977, 1978f
  for ureteropelvic junction obstruction, 1947, 1952b
Endourology, rise of, 2069.e2–2069.e3
Endovascular stents, for renovascular injuries, 1990
EndoWrist instruments, 218, 218f
End-stage renal disease (ESRD)
  in children, 355–357
  in CKD, 1929–1930
  neural tube defects and, early intervention for, 629
Enema
  cleansing, for prostate biopsy, 3496
  for defecation disorders, 677–678, 678f
Energetic harmony, 2749
Energy modalities in urologic surgery, for tissue dissection and cauterization
  electrosurgery, 235–241, 236f
  ultrasound instrumentation, 237–238

Enhanced recovery after surgery (ERAS), 453–455, 3165–3169, 3167t–3168t, 3170t–3174t
Enteral nutrition, 122
Enteral tube feeds, 449
Enteric hyperoxaluria, 2022–2023, 2022f, 2056
  medical therapy for, 2057
Enterobiasis, of genitourinary tract, 1332
Enterocele, 2526, 2587, 2589f
Enterococcus, 442
Enterocystoplasty, 3034–3038
  complications with, 3036–3038
  evaluation for, 3034–3035
  laparoscopic and robotic techniques, 3036, 3037f
  outcomes with, 3037–3038
  postoperative care of, 3036–3038
  seromuscular, 705–706, 705f
  surgical indication of, 3034–3035
  surgical technique for, 3035–3036, 3035f
Enucleation, for small renal tumors, 2263, 2264f
Enuresis
  alarm for, 663–664
  alternative therapies for, 665
  background on, 660–661
  behavioral therapy for, 663, 664f
  combination therapy for, 665
  epidemiology of, 661, 661f
  evaluation of, 662–663
  genetics of, 661
  natural history of, 661, 661f
  nocturnal, 2539, 2581
  pathophysiology of, 661–662, 662f
  patient history of, 6
  pediatric, 660–665, 665b
  pharmacotherapy for, 664
  terminology for, 660–661
  treatment of, 663–664, 2547
Enuresis risoria, 658–660
Environmental factors, UTUC variations and, 2186–2188
Environmental pollution, bladder cancer and, 3077
Enzalutamide, 3676, 3695–3696, 3695f
Eosinophilic cystitis, 526, 526f
EP. *see* Etoposide-cisplatin
EPD. *see* Extramammary Paget disease
Ephedrine
  in stone formation, 2033
  surgical management of, 2077.e2–2077.e3
  for stress urinary incontinence in women, 2714
Epidemiology of Lower Urinary Tract Symptoms (EpiLUTS) II, 2734
Epidermal growth factor receptor (EGFR) therapy, for metastatic bladder cancer, 3131
Epidermoid cysts, 1123, 1304, 1305f
  testicular, 1708
Epididymal appendix, 391–392, 392f
Epididymal cysts, 903
Epididymal tumor excision, 1850
Epididymal/vasal injury, complication of scrotal surgery, 1856
Epididymectomy, 1853
  for chronic scrotal pain syndrome, 1222
Epididymis, 319f, 1850
  acute, 1853
  anatomy of, 1376b
    arterial supply, 1375
    blood supply of, 1454, 1454t
    gross structure, 1374, 1374f–1375f
    innervation in, 1403
    lymphatic supply, 1375
    microanatomic architecture, 1374–1375
    nerve supply, 1375
    vascular and lymph supply, 1402–1403
    venous drainage, 1375

Epididymis *(Continued)*
  anomalies of, 903
    cryptorchidism and, 962–963, 962f
    appendix, torsion of, 897–898
  chronic, 1853
  in genitourinary tuberculosis, 1309
  HIV and, 1266
  imaging of
    magnetic resonance imaging, 1376
    ultrasound, 1375–1376, 1376f
  palpable abnormalities of, 1853
  physiology of, 1402–1406, 1406b
    cytoarchitecture, 1403–1404
    gross architecture in, 1402–1403, 1403f
    regulation of, 1405–1406
Epididymitis, 898–899
  after photoselective vaporization of prostate, 3441
  as STD, 1255
Epididymo-orchitis, 392, 410–411
Epidural cord compression, in castration-resistant prostate cancer, 3702, 3703t
Epigenetic anomalies, and male infertility, 1446
Epigenetic changes, male reproductive physiology and, age-related, 1402
Epigenetic events, in prostate cancer, 3470
Epigenetic modifications, as prostate cancer biomarkers, 3487–3489
Epispadias, 568–572, 572b, 1449
  female, 570–572, 571f–572f
    associated anomalies, 571
    operative techniques for, 571, 573f
    surgical objectives for, 571
    surgical results for, 571–572
  male, 568–570, 568f
    associated anomalies, 568–569
    genital reconstruction in, 569
    surgical management of, 569–570
    urethral reconstruction in, 569
    urinary continence in, 569–570, 570t
  repair of, 550–551
    failure of, 564
    outcomes and results with, 557–558
Epithelial cell receptivity, in UTIs
  bladder cells, 1136–1137, 1137f
  vaginal cells, 1135–1136, 1135f
  variation in, 1136
Epithelial-mesenchymal transition (EMT), 789
Epithelial metaplasia, of bladder, 3081
Epithelial permeability, bladder glycosaminoglycan layer and, 1232.e5–1232.e7, 1232.e7b
Epithelial spread, of UTUC, 2194
Epithelial stem cells, of prostate, 3278f, 3279
Epithelium, epididymal, 1403–1404, 1403f
EPO. *see* Erythropoietin
Epoöphoron, 319f
Epstein criteria, of localized prostate cancer, 3526–3527
EQUIL 2, 2010
ERAS. *see* Enhanced recovery after surgery
Erbium:YAG (Er:YAG) laser lithotripsy, basic physics of, 244
Erectile bodies, of penis, 1807.e6f–1807.e7f
Erectile dysfunction (ED), 1425–1426
  after laparoscopic radical prostatectomy, 3579
  after photoselective vaporization of prostate, 3442
  after retropubic radical prostatectomy, 3564
  after robotic radical prostatectomy, 3582–3583, 3582f
  arteriogenic, 1504–1505
  cardiovascular disease and, 1425–1426, 1426b
  causes of
    arteriogenic, 1505
    cavernous (venogenic), 1505t
    drug-induced, 1506–1509

Erectile dysfunction (ED) *(Continued)*
classification of, 1502b
corporal structural defects and, 1505-1506
endocrinologic, 1503-1504
epidemiology of, 1513-1514
evaluation and management of, 1513-1538
diagnostic evaluation, 1517-1519, 1518f
historical perspective, 1513, 1514t
management principles, 1515-1517, 1515t, 1516f
public health significance, 1513-1514
specialized evaluation and testing, 1519-1529, 1521t
treatment considerations, 1529-1538
HIV and, 1267
hormonal therapy and, 3681
intraoperative troubleshooting, 1588-1591, 1592b
crural crossover, 1589-1591, 1590f
fibrotic corpora, 1588-1589, 1589f
metabolic syndrome and, 1422
neurogenic, 1502-1503
pathophysiology of, 1500-1512, 1512b
incidence and epidemiology of, 1500-1512
patient history of, 6, 8t
and PD, 1600-1601
perspectives on, 1512
postoperative complications of, 1591-1596, 1596b
cylinder aneurysm as, 1593, 1593f
cylinder erosion as, 1594, 1595f
cylinder extrusion as, 1593-1594, 1594f-1595f
infection as, 1591-1593, 1592f, 1593b
penile necrosis after implant placement, 1595-1596, 1595f
visceral erosion of the reservoir, 1594-1595, 1595f
preoperative preparation for, 1583-1584
device placement for, 1585-1588, 1585f-1587f, 1588b
incision for, 1584-1585, 1585f
reservoir placement, 1586-1588, 1587f-1588f
primary, 1511-1512
prostate cancer and, 3606
psychogenic, 1501-1502
risk factors for, 1501, 1502f
surgery for, 1582-1598
device placement for, 1585-1588, 1585f-1587f
incision for, 1584-1585, 1585f
informed consent for, 1582-1583, 1584b
patient and partner satisfaction for, 1597-1598
postoperative care for, 1596-1597
in special situations, 1596
types of implants for, 1582, 1583f
with transurethral vaporization of prostate, 3426
with urethral distraction injury, 3060
vascular, 1505
Erectile Dysfunction Inventory of Treatment Satisfaction, 111
Erectile prosthesis, testicular implants and, 3069, 3070f
Erector spinae, 1658, 1662f-1665f, 1664t
Ergot alkaloids, with RPF, 1978
Erlotinib, for RCC, 2343-2344
Erosion, in penile implant, 1594, 1595f
Erysipelas, 1288-1289
Erythema multiforme (EM), 1277-1278, 1278f
Erythromycin, in pregnancy, 1187t
Erythroplasia of Queyrat, 1742
Erythropoiesis, renal regulation of, 1914
Erythropoietin (EPO), 1914
Escherichia coli, 428, 429f
ESRD. *see* End-stage renal disease
Established urinary incontinence, in geriatric patients, 2919
Estradiol, 1391, 1434, 1437

Estrogens, 1390, 1394
benign prostatic hyperplasia role of, 3308-3309, 3308t
bladder and, 2503
continence mechanism and, 2713
to facilitate bladder filling and urine storage, 2682t
and female sexual response, 1627.e5
in male, 3282t, 3283-3284
for overactive bladder, 2709-2710
in prostate cancer, 3462-3463
for stress urinary incontinence in women, 2713-2714
supplementation of, for vesicovaginal fistula surgery, 2934
urethra and, 2503
for urgency urinary incontinence, 2709-2710
for UTIs, 1164-1165, 1164f
ESWL. *see* Extracorporeal shock wave lithotripsy
ESWT. *see* Extracorporeal shock wave therapy
Ethics, 115-118
medical, 115-116
Ethnicity
renal calculi and, 2006
urinary incontinence and, 2583-2585
Etoposide-cisplatin (EP), for seminomas, 1705
ETs. *see* Endothelins
ETS family gene fusions, 3469
European Cooperative Groups, bladder RMS treatment approaches of, 1115
Everolimus, for RCC, 2337, 2338f
Evicel, 215.e2
Ewing sarcoma, retroperitoneal tumors and, 2232-2233, 2233f
Ewing-like sarcoma, retroperitoneal tumors and, 2232-2233, 2233f
Excisional tapering, for megaureter in children, 851-852, 851f
Excitation-contraction coupling
in detrusor muscle, 2474-2475, 2475f
in ureters, 1884-1885
Excretory urography
ureter anatomy on, 1873-1874
of ureteropelvic junction obstruction, 1943, 1944f
of urinary tract obstruction, 780
Excurrent ducts, of testis, 1454
Exercise, for prostate cancer, 3543-3544
Exercise-induced hematuria, 18
Exogenous Cushing syndrome, 2361, 2365
Expressed prostatic secretions, 24, 25f
Exstrophy
in perinatal urology, 379-382
in transitional urology, 1049-1050
female with, 1051-1052
long-term reconstructive outcomes, 1049
urologic, 1049-1050
Exstrophy-epispadias complex (EEC), 528-580, 529f, 531b
adolescents with, 565
adults with, 565
embryology of, 530, 530f
fertility with
female patient, 567
male patient, 566
historical aspects of, 528
incidence of, 528-530
inheritance of, 528-530
long-term adjustment issues with, 567-568, 568b
prenatal diagnosis of, 538, 538b
pseudoexstrophy, 537
quality of life with, 567
sexuality with
female concerns, 566-567
male concerns, 565-566
split symphysis variant of, 538
variants of, 537-538, 538f
Extended-core biopsy techniques, 3497, 3498f

Extended pelvic lymphadenectomy
common iliac, 3152, 3153f-3154f
external iliac, 3148-3149, 3151f
hypogastric, 3149-3152, 3153f
obturator, 3149, 3152f
presacral, 3152, 3154f
Extended sentinel lymph node dissection, for penile cancer, 1760
Extensively drug-resistant tuberculosis, 1318
External beam hypofractionation, outcomes for, 3611-3612, 3611t, 3612b, 3613t
External-beam radiation therapy, for penile cancer, 1765, 1766f
External beam radiation treatment, for prostate cancer, 3593-3596, 3596b
brachytherapy *versus*, 3612-3613, 3614t
fractionation, 3593
heavy particle beams/proton therapy, 3594-3596, 3594f, 3595t
high dose rate as a boost with, 3599
outcomes for, 3609-3610, 3610t
radiobiologic basis for hypofractionation, 3593, 3593t
stereotactic body radiation therapy, 3593-3594
tumor control after, 3611b
External collecting devices, 2903-2904
External compression (Credé), 2902
External genitalia, 312b
male, development of, 1392, 1392f
External iliac lymphadenectomy, 3148-3149, 3151f
External irradiation, brachytherapy combined with, 3599-3600
External sphincter
damage, orthoptic urinary diversion and, 3238
male sphincteric mechanisms and, 2594
urodynamic studies of, 2568-2569
Extracellular matrix, in obstructive nephropathy, 788-790
Extracorporeal renal surgery (ECRS), 2254-2257, 2256f
preoperative considerations for, 2254-2255
surgical procedure for, 2255-2257
Extracorporeal shock wave lithotripsy (ESWL), 2094-2103, 2103b, 2115
adjuncts to improve, 2102, 2102b
bioeffects of, 2097-2100
acute renal injury as, 2098-2099, 2098f-2099f, 2099b
chronic renal injury as, 2099-2100, 2099t
extrarenal damage as, 2097-2098, 2097f
combination of ultrasonography and fluoroscopy for, 2095
fluoroscopy for, 2094-2095
future direction in, 2102-2103, 2103f
generator types for, 2094
electrohydraulic (spark gap), 2094, 2095f
electromagnetic, 2094, 2095f
piezoelectric, 2094, 2096f
imaging systems for, 2094-2095
methods and physical principles, 2094-2097
optimization of, 2100-2102, 2100b, 2101f, 2102b
stone fragmentation in, 2095-2097, 2096f
tissue injury from, 2100
ultrasonography for, 2095
Extracorporeal shock wave therapy (ESWT), and PD, 1614, 1617t
Extraction, in laser lithotripsy, 2111
Extragenital skin harvest, for hypospadias, 945
Extramammary Paget disease (EPD), as neoplastic condition, 1301-1302, 1301f
Extraperitoneal approach
anterior, to laparoscopic pyeloplasty, 1956
operative team placement for, 211
Extrapituitary endocrine modulators, 1448
Extraprostatic extension, 3507, 3511
Extratesticular endocrine dysfunction, male infertility and, 1448-1449

Extravaginal spermatic cord torsion, 897, 897f
Extravasation of contrast material, contrast media and, 32
Extrinsic apoptotic pathway, 1366.e1f–1366.e2f, 1366.e2
Extrusion, in penile implant, 1593–1594, 1594f–1595f
Eyeball UDS, 2534
Eye-of-the-needle technique, 166–167, 167f

F

F antigens, 428–429
FAAH. *see* Fatty acid amide hydrolase
Fabry disease, 1302, 1303f
Facility setup, for urodynamic studies, 2552–2553
Factors, additional, in urodynamic studies, 2554
Failed epispadias repair, reconstructive surgery for, 1813
Failed hypospadias repair, reconstructive surgery for, 1812–1813
Fallopian tubes
   anatomy of, 2436–2437
   for continent urinary diversions, 709
Falls, nocturia and, 2666
Familial benign prostatic hyperplasia, 3311–3312, 3311t
Familial hypomagnesemia with hypercalciuria and nephrocalcinosis (FHHNC), 2019
Familial hypoplastic glomerulocystic kidney disease, 756–757
Familial papillary RCC, molecular genetics of, 1354t, 1358
Familial RCC, 2141–2145, 2142t–2143t, 2144f
   treatment of, 2173–2174, 2174f
Familial Wilms tumor, 1098
Family history, 9
   prostate cancer and, 3542
Fanconi syndrome, 348
Fascia lata, 2834
   harvest of, 2837
Fasciae
   of anterior abdominal wall, 2429f
   of lower abdominal wall, 2444, 2446f
   pelvic
      female, 2427, 2429f
      male, 2448f, 2449, 2452f
   of perineum and perineal body, 2449, 2450f
Fascial closure
   after laparoscopic and robotic surgery, 218–219
   techniques, 150–151
Fascial sling
   for bladder neck reconstruction, 686–687
   results with, 686–687
   technique for, 686
FAST. *see* Focused assessment with sonography for trauma
Fast spin-echo (FSE), 412–413
Fast-twitch fibers, of urethral striated muscle, 2466
Fatty acid amide hydrolase (FAAH), 2713.e2
Febrile child, 426
Fecal diversion, for radiation fistula, 2956
Fecal impaction, transient urinary incontinence and, 2919.e1
Fecal incontinence (FI)
   in geriatric patients, 2920.e9
   ultrasound for, 2439, 2440f
Female circumcision, 987–988, 988f
Female external genitalia, 2435–2436, 2436f–2437f
   abnormalities of
      acquired, 986–988
      cervical atresia, 984–985, 985f
      clitoris, 975, 977b
      congenital, 975–986
      lateral fusion, 985–986
      management of, 973–989

Female external genitalia *(Continued)*
      structural, 974
      vagina, 978–986, 982b
      vertical fusion, 979–981
      vestibule, 975–977, 977b
   acquired disorders of, 986–988, 988b
      condyloma acuminatum, 988
      female circumcision, 987–988, 988f
      labial adhesions, 986–987, 987f
   defect of, in bladder exstrophy, 534–535, 535f
   development of, 307f, 310–311, 311f–313f
   embryology of, 973–974, 974f, 974b
   evaluation and classification of, 974, 975f
Female genital-pelvic pain dysfunction, 1636
Female orgasmic disorder, 1646, 1648b
   assessment for, 1646–1647
   with desire and arousal problem, 1647–1648
   medical treatment for, 1647–1648
   medication-induced, 1648
   psychosocial treatment for, 1647
   sexual enhancement products, 1647
Female pelvis
   anatomy of, 2427–2443, 2439b
      anal perineum of, 2435
      bony pelvis, 2427, 2428f
      external genitalia of, 2435–2436, 2436f–2437f
      fascia of, 2427, 2429f
      innervation of, 2433–2434
      ligaments of, 2428–2430, 2430f–2432f
      lymphatic drainage of, 2433, 2434f
      muscles of pelvic floor, 2430–2432, 2432f
      organ support of, 2438, 2438f
      organs of, 2436–2438, 2437f
      perineum of, 2434–2435, 2435f
      peritoneum of, 2427, 2429f
      urethra, 2438–2439, 2439f, 2465–2466, 2466f
      vasculature of, 2432–2433, 2433f
   endoscopic anatomy of, 2443, 2443f, 2443b
   radiographic anatomy of, 2439–2443
      fluoroscopy, 2442–2443, 2442f
      magnetic resonance imaging, 2440–2442, 2440f–2442f
      ultrasound, 2439, 2440f
Female persistent genital arousal disorders, 1650, 1650t
   psychosocial characterization and etiologic factors, 1650
   treatment targets for, 1650
Female radical cystectomy, 3155–3157, 3157f–3158f
Female reproductive system, pediatric tumors of, 1121b
   cervical or uterine RMS, 1120
   ovarian, 1120–1121
   vaginal RMS, 1119–1120, 1119f
   vulvar RMS, 1119
Female reproductive tract, development of, 324–327, 324f–325f
Female sexual arousal disorders, 1648–1649, 1651b
   interview assessment for, 1649, 1649t
   pharmacotherapy for, 1649–1650
      hormonal therapy, 1649–1650
      nonhormonal therapy, 1650
   potential treatments for, 1649
Female sexual arousal dysfunction, 1636
Female sexual dysfunction
   epidemiology of, 1636–1637, 1637b
   lower urinary tract dysfunction and, 1654–1655, 1657b
      clinical signs and investigations for, 1655
      epidemiology of, 1654
      etiology and classification of, 1654–1655
      links and treatments, 1655–1657
      self-image/body image connected to, 1657
      sexual lifestyle and communication and, 1654–1655, 1654t

Female Sexual Function Inventory (FSFI), 112, 112t
Female sexual interest-arousal disorders, 1635–1636
Female sexual interest disorder, 1640–1648, 1646b
   definition of, 1640–1641
   evaluation of, 1641–1643, 1642t–1643t
   pathophysiology of, 1641, 1641f
   treatment for, 1643, 1644f
      medical, 1643–1646
      psychological, 1643
Female sexual organs, anatomy and physiology of, 1627, 1627b
Female sexual response
   hormonal regulators of, 1627.e5–1627.e6
   neurogenic mediators of, 1627.e5
Female stress urinary incontinence, use of injectable agents for, 2890–2891
Female urethra, 152
   catheterization of, 153
Female urethral cancer, 1782–1785, 1785b
   anatomy and pathology of, 1782–1785, 1783f
   epidemiology, etiology, and clinical presentation of, 1782
   evaluation and staging of, 1783
   prognosis of, 1783–1784
   recurrence after cystectomy, 1787–1789, 1789b
   treatment of, 1784–1785
Females, with exstrophy, 1051–1052
   fertility, 1051
   pregnancy and delivery, 1051–1052
   procedentia repair, 1051
   reconstruction of genitalia, 1051
   sexual function, 1051
Female-to-male transexuals. *see* Transmen
Female-to-male transgender, reconstructive surgery for, 1841–1842, 1842b
Femoral nerve, 2453t
Fenretinide, for neuroblastoma, 1096
FEPs. *see* Fibroepithelial polyps
Fertility
   after RPLND, 1729
   with cryptorchidism, 969–970
   with exstrophy-epispadias complex
      female patient, 567
      male patient, 566
   in prune-belly syndrome, 600
   RMS treatment effects on, 1116–1117
   sperm, 1405, 1405f
   urologic surgery and, 288
   Wilms tumor treatment effects on, 1108
Fesoterodine
   for diminished bladder, 2674, 2675t–2677t
   to facilitate bladder filling and urine storage, 2682t, 2685–2687
   for urinary incontinence, in geriatric patients, 2920.e4
Fetal cystoscopy, in urinary tract dilation, 364–365
Fetal magnetic resonance imaging, 358, 359f
Fetal myelomeningocele closure, outcomes for, 382
α-Fetoprotein (AFP), in pediatric patients, 1122, 1122f
Fetus, fundamentals of, 404
   MRI in, 412–413
Fever
   evaluation and management of, 426–433, 427f
   patient history of, 7
   UTI diagnosis and, 1143
^{18}F-FACBC, 99
F-FDG PET/CT, 43
FFP. *see* Fresh frozen plasma
FG. *see* Fournier gangrene
FGF. *see* Fibroblast growth factors

FH gene, systemic therapy targeting, 2343
FHHNC. *see* Familial hypomagnesemia with hypercalciuria and nephrocalcinosis
FI. *see* Fecal incontinence
Fibrin-based glue, for laparoscopic and robotic surgery, 215.e2
Fibrin sealants, 148
Fibroblast growth factor receptor therapy, for metastatic bladder cancer, 3131
Fibroblast growth factors (FGF), in prostate development, 3276
Fibroblasts, in tubulointerstitial fibrosis, 782f, 789
Fibrocystin, 748
Fibroepithelial polyps (FEPs), 526
　of ureter, 821–822, 821f–822f
　of urethra, 1776
Fibrosis
　mechanisms of, 788–790
　in obstructive nephropathy, 788–790
　PC-RPLND findings of, survival outcomes associated with, 1726, 1727t
　pelvic, as laparoscopic and robotic surgery contraindication, 203
Fibrotic corpora, 1588–1589, 1589f
Fibrotic gene expression, and PD, 1606
Fibrous dysplasia, 1933–1934, 1934f
Filariasis, of genitourinary tract, 1328–1331, 1332b
　diagnosis, 1330
　epidemiology, 1328–1329
　organisms, 1328, 1328f
　pathology and clinical manifestations, 1329–1330, 1329f–1330f
　prevention and control, 1331
　treatment, 1330–1331
Filling cystometry, for benign prostatic hyperplasia, 3347
Filtrate transport, 1906–1913
　acid-base balance, 1911–1912, 1912f, 1912b
　calcium, 1911, 1912f
　potassium, 1909–1910, 1910b
　sodium, 1906–1909, 1907f–1910f, 1909b
　solutes, 1912–1913
　water, 1910–1911, 1911f, 1911b
Fimbria, 319f, 324f
Finasteride
　for benign prostatic hyperplasia, 3371–3374, 3373t
　for diminished bladder, 2674, 2675t–2677t
Fine-needle aspiration cytology, for penile cancer, 1760
FIRSTANA trial, 3693
First-morning void, 2667
FISH. *see* Fluorescence in situ hybridization
Fistula obstruction, 3272
Fistulae
　classification of, 2930–2931, 2931f
　complex, of posterior urethra, 1835–1836, 1836b
　cutaneous, 2962
　with intestinal anastomoses, 3179–3180
　other urinary, 2962, 2962b
　radiation, 2960–2962
　　chemotherapy of, 2961–2962
　　combination therapies of, 2962
　　diversion procedures for, 2961
　　interpositional grafts for, 2961
　　management approaches for, 2961
　　recommendations for, 2961
　　repair techniques for, 2961
　urethral, 883, 883f
　urethrocutaneous, 935–937, 936f–937f
　urinary tract, 2924–2963, 2924b
　　after renal preservation surgery, 2962
　　after renal transplantation, 2962
　　general considerations of, 2924
　　management of, 2925b
　　other, 2962, 2962b
　　surgical repair of, 2925b

Fistulae *(Continued)*
　urocutaneous, 2962
　uroenteric, 2952–2953
　　pyeloenteric, 2953–2955, 2953f
　　vesicoenteric, 2953t
　urogynecologic, 2946
　　ureterovaginal, 2942, 2942b
　　urethrovaginal, 2947–2951
　　vesicouterine, 2946–2947, 2947b
　　vesicovaginal, 2924–2926
　urovascular, 2958
　　pyelovascular, 2958
　　renovascular, 2958
　　ureterovascular, 2958–2959
Fixed drug eruption, as papulosquamous disorder, 1282, 1283f
Fixed particle growth theory, 2011
FLA. *see* Focal laser ablation
Flank approaches
　for open kidney surgery, 2249–2251
　　subcostal, 2249–2250, 2249.e1f, 2250f–2251f, 2250.e1f
　　supracostal, 2250–2251, 2251.e1f
　to ureteropelvic junction obstruction in children, 829
Flank incision, kidney and retroperitoneum approaches, 138–140
　12th rib supracostal and 11th rib transcostal, 140, 140f
　true flank incision, 139–140, 140f
Flank muscles, of posterior abdominal wall, 1658, 1662f–1664f, 1664t
Flank pain, 400
　UTI diagnosis and, 1143
Flank retroperitoneal approach, in open adrenalectomy, 2410–2411, 2410f–2411f
Flap urethroplasty, for transmen, 3071
Flaps
　for continent urinary diversions, 707–709. *see also* specific flaps
　for penile transplantation, 1838–1842, 1840f, 1842b
　for ureteropelvic junction obstruction, 1960–1962
　　Culp-DeWeerd spiral flap, 1960–1961, 1961f
　　Foley Y-V plasty, 1960, 1960f
　　intubated ureterotomy, 1961–1962, 1963f
　　salvage procedures, 1963
　　Scardino-Prince vertical flap, 1961, 1962f
　for urethral and penile reconstruction, 1807, 1807f
　　axial, 1807, 1807f–1808f
　　island, 1807
　　peninsular, 1807
　　random, 1807, 1807f
　for urethral stricture disease, 1823–1827, 1824f–1825f
Flavoxate hydrochloride, to facilitate bladder filling and urine storage, 2682t, 2696
Flexible cystourethroscopes, 186–187, 189t
Flexible laser lithotripsy, 244.e4
Flexible lithotripters, 2109–2111
Flexible ureteroscopes, 194f–195f, 195, 196t
　care and sterilization of, 195–197, 197f
　technique, 201
Flibanserin, for female sexual interest disorder, 1645–1646
Flip-flap technique (Mathieu), 924, 924f
FloSeal, 148, 215.e2
　for renal trauma, 1990, 1990f
FLS. *see* Fundamentals of Laparoscopic Surgery
Fluid intake, for pediatric kidney stone disease, 868–869
Fluids
　bladder cancer and, 3077
　intake of, renal calculi and, 2009
　management of, 2732–2733
　　evidence for, 2733
　　excessive, 2732–2733
　　inadequate, 2733
　　timing of, 2733

Fluorescence in situ hybridization (FISH), of bladder tumor, 3079
Fluorine-18 (^{18}F), 91
(^{18}F)fluoro-D-glucose (18F-FDG), 96, 97f, 100b
　for bladder cancer, 97
　for kidney cancer, 97–98
　for penile cancer, 100
　for prostate cancer, 98–100
　for testis cancer, 100
Fluoroquinolones
　prophylaxis with
　　for cystourethroscopy, 189
　　for uncomplicated urologic procedures, 1194t–1196t
　for UTIs, 1151t–1153t, 1153–1154, 1156, 1187t
Fluoroscopic-guided access, 166–169, 166f–167f
Fluoroscopic imaging, for urodynamics, 2535
Fluoroscopy, 389
　of female pelvis, 2442–2443, 2442f
　of male pelvis, 2457–2458
　of pediatric stone disease, 861
　ureteroscopy, 199
5-Fluorouracil
　for condylomata acuminata, 1742.e3
　for penile cancer, 1770
Flurbiprofen, to facilitate bladder filling and urine storage, 2682t, 2703
Flush stoma, 3182–3183
Flutamide
　for benign prostatic hyperplasia, 3376–3377
　for prostate cancer, 3674
Focal ablative therapy, for locally advanced prostate cancer, 3655
　cryoablation, 3655
　high-intensity focused ultrasound, 3655
Focal extraprostatic extension, 3511
Focal laser ablation (FLA), 3628, 3633f, 3634t, 3635f
Focal segmental glomerulosclerosis (FSGS), 345
Focal therapy, for prostate cancer, 3616–3639, 3639b
　ablation patterns and current technologies of, 3624–3638
　　ablation approach, 3624
　　ablation types, 3624, 3624f
　　adjuvants to, 3638
　　brachytherapy, 3632–3638
　　cryotherapy, 3624–3628, 3625f, 3627t
　　follow up, 3638
　　high-intensity focused ultrasonography, 3628, 3629t–3630t, 3631f–3632f
　　irreversible electroporation, 3628–3632, 3635f, 3636t
　　laser, 3628, 3633f, 3634t, 3635f
　　other modalities, 3638
　　vascular-targeted photodynamic therapy, 3632, 3637t
　advanced imaging techniques in, 3621–3622
　　MRI-targeted/fusion biopsy, 3622
　　multiparametric magnetic resonance imaging, 3621–3622
　biologic basis for, 3616–3620
　　multifocality of, *versus* index lesion hypothesis, 3617–3620, 3619t, 3620f
　　using cancer grade as indication of aggressiveness, 3616–3617, 3617f
　clinical applications of, 3620
　　complementary roles and active surveillance, 3620
　　index lesion treatment, 3620
　concepts of, 3616
　future research for, 3638–3639
　historical perspective of, 3616
　patient selection for, 3620–3621
　　biopsy-based lesion identification, 3621
　promising imaging modalities of, 3622–3624
　　contemporary patient selection criteria, 3622–3624, 3623t
　　multiparametric ultrasonography, 3622
　　positron emission tomography, 3622

Focused assessment with sonography for trauma (FAST), of upper urinary tract, 1066
Focused ultrasound, for renal tumor ablation, 2319-2321
Folded rectosigmoid bladder, 3209
Foley catheters, 173, 484
Foley Y-V plasty, for ureteropelvic junction obstruction, 1960, 1960f
Follicle cells, 319f
Follicle-stimulating hormone (FSH), 1390, 1391f, 1437
Folliculitis, 1290-1291, 1291f
Foods, bladder cancer and, 3078
Force-length relations, of ureters, 1890, 1890f
Force-velocity relations, of ureters, 1890-1891, 1891f
Foregut, 318f
Foreign-body removal, bladder, 3043-3046
  complications of, 3046
  evaluation of, 3043-3044
  laparoscopic and robotic technique, 3044-3045, 3045f-3046f
  open technique of, 3044, 3045f
  percutaneous, 3045-3046
  postoperative care of, 3046
  surgical indication of, 3043-3044
  surgical technique of, 3044-3046
Formation product (K_f), 2009
46,XX DSD, 1007-1011
46,XX males, 1000-1001
46,XY complete, 998t, 1004-1005, 1005f
46,XY DSD, 1011-1017
Fosfomycin, for UTIs, 1151t-1153t, 1153
Fosfomycin trometamol, for UTIs, 1156
Fossa navicularis, 1383, 1383f-1384f, 1807.e2f, 1807.e4f, 1807.e8
Four-Box framework, 116, 117t
Fourchette, 1627.e2
Fournier gangrene (FG), 1289-1290, 1290f
  genital skin loss and, 3053
Four-principles framework, 115
Four-way catheter, 154f
Fowler syndrome, 2629, 2720.e3
Fowler-Stephens orchidopexy, 967-968
fPSA. see Free prostate-specific antigen
12-Fr Cope nephrostomy tube, 181, 181f
Fractional excretion of sodium (FENa), urinary tract obstruction and, 777
Fractionation, in radiation therapy, 3593
Fracture
  of penis, 3048-3049, 3048.e1f, 3049f-3050f, 3049.e1f
  of testis, 3051-3053
Fragmentation, in laser lithotripsy, 2111
Frailty, 2913-2914, 2913f
  definition of, 108
Frank hematuria, 247
Frasier syndrome, 998t, 1004
Free crystal particle growth, 2011
Free graft urethroplasty, for transmen, 3071
Free prostate-specific antigen (fPSA), 3481-3482, 3481t, 3482f, 3517-3518
  isoforms, 3483-3484, 3483f
Free water loss, 341-342
Frequency-volume chart, 2666
  for benign prostatic hyperplasia, 3344-3345
  nocturia classification with, 2667, 2668t
Frequently-relapsing nephrotic syndrome (FRNS), 345
Fresh frozen plasma (FFP), transfusion with, 147
Fresh prostatic cancer tissues, genomic research on, 3586
FRNS. see Frequently-relapsing nephrotic syndrome
Fructose, in prostatic secretions, 3295-3296
FSE. see Fast spin-echo
FSFI. see Female Sexual Function Inventory
FSGS. see Focal segmental glomerulosclerosis

FSH. see Follicle-stimulating hormone
Fuhrman's classification system, for RCC, 2148, 2148t
Full-thickness skin grafts, for urethral and penile reconstruction, 1805, 1806f
Functional acute kidney injury, in children, 353
Functional capacity, 120
Functional imaging
  in adrenal mass evaluation, 2396-2397
  of pheochromocytoma, 2375-2376, 2376f
Functional incidental training, in toileting programs, 2730.e1t
Functional incontinence, patient history of, 6
Functional phase, of dynamic renal imaging, 93
Functional profile length, 2563
Functional status
  assessment of, 107
  definition of, 106-107
Fundamentals of Laparoscopic Surgery (FLS), 471
Funguria, 445
Funiculoepididymitis, as filariasis clinical manifestation, 1329
Furosemide
  for nocturnal polyuria, 2673t
  in stone formation, 2033
Furunculosis, 1291, 1291f
Fusion anomalies, genitourinary trauma and, 1076, 1077f
Future business plan, for men's health center, 1427

G

G_1/S checkpoint, deregulation of, in GU cancers, 1347.e2
G2M checkpoint, deregulation of, 1347.e2-1347.e3
Gabapentin, to facilitate bladder filling and urine storage, 2713.e3
^{67}Ga-citrate, 96
Gadolinium, for contrast media, 34
Gadolinium-based contrast media (GBCM), contrast media and, 32-33
Galdakao-modified supine position, 165
Gallium-68 (^{68}Ga), 91, 92t
Ganglioneuroblastomas, in retroperitoneum, 2234, 2235f
Ganglioneuroma
  as benign lesion, 2392-2393, 2393b
  in retroperitoneum, 2234
GAP. see Glans approximation procedure
^{68}Ga-PSMA PET scans, 3667
Gardasil, 1262
Gartner duct cysts, 319f, 977, 977f
  urethral diverticula differentiated from, 2986, 2986f
GAS. see Gender-affirmation surgery
Gas embolism
  during laparoscopic and robotic surgery, 224-225
  vena caval thrombectomy causing, 2277
Gasless laparoscopic transperitoneal approach, 2416-2417, 2417f
Gastric contents, aspiration of, during laparoscopic and robotic surgery, 228.e1
Gastric pouch, for cutaneous continent urinary diversion, 3225-3226, 3225f-3226f
Gastrocystoplasty, 695
Gastroenterologic changes, with aging, 2906
Gastrointestinal cystoplasty, alternatives to, 702-706, 706b
  autoaugmentation, 703-705, 704f
  bladder regeneration, 706
  seromuscular enterocystoplasty, 705-706, 705f
  ureterocystoplasty, 703, 703f
Gastrointestinal injury
  during laparoscopic and robotic surgery, 225-226

Gastrointestinal injury (Continued)
  laparoscopic kidney surgery causing, 2307, 2307f
  during radical nephrectomy, 2261
Gastrointestinal tract
  abnormalities of, with cloacal exstrophy, 575
  after augmentation cystoplasty, 696-697
  in prune-belly syndrome, 587-588, 587f
Gastrointestinal viscera, in retroperitoneum, 1668-1669, 1668.e2f, 1669f-1670f, 1674b
Gastroparesis, lower urinary tract dysfunction and, 2630
GBCM. see Gadolinium-based contrast media
GBS. see Guillain-Barré syndrome
GC. see Genomic classifier
GCTs. see Germ cell tumors
GD. see Gender dysphoria
GEARS. see Global Evaluative Assessment of Robotic Skills
GelPort, 212, 212f
Gemcitabine, for non-muscle-invasive bladder cancer, 3105
Gender
  assignment of
    for cloacal exstrophy, 576-577, 577f
    in newborn, 1000
  desmopressin and, 2712
  lower urinary tract dysfunction and, 652
  renal calculi and, 2005-2006
  UTUC variations and, 2185
Gender-affirmation surgery (GAS), 3062
Gender dysphoria (GD), 3062
Gender identity, 3062
  role, and orientation, 996-997
Gender nonconforming youths, urologic issues in, 3062
Gender reassignment surgery (GRS), 3062
Gene amplification, androgen receptor and, 3685-3686
Gene fusions, in prostate cancer, 3468-3470
  as biomarkers for, 3486
Gene rearrangements
  in prostate cancer, 1352-1353, 1354t
  in renal cancer, 1353, 1354t
  in testicular cancer, 1353
General anesthesia
  for laparoscopic and robotic surgery, complications related to, 228
  in urologic surgery, 132
General appearance, physical examination for, 9-10
Genes
  oncogenes, 1346-1347, 1347b
  structure of, 1346.e4
  tumor suppressor, 1346-1347, 1347f, 1347b
Genetic factors, in pelvic organ prolapse, 2591
Genetic mutations, male reproductive physiology and, age-related, 1402
Genetic predisposition, UTUC variations and, 2185, 2186f
Genetic syndromes, male infertility and, 1445-1446
Genetic testing, for evaluation of pediatric stone disease, 351
Genetics
  of autosomal dominant polycystic kidney disease, 750-751
  of autosomal recessive polycystic kidney disease, 748
  of benign prostatic hyperplasia, 3311-3312, 3311t
  of bladder tumor, 3076
  in BPS/IC etiology, 1232.e10
  of clear cell RCC, 2141-2143, 2143t, 2144f
  of enuresis, 661
  of hernia and hydroceles, 889
  of juvenile nephronophthisis, 755
  of lower urinary tract function, 2528
  of neuroblastoma, 1096-1099

Genetics (Continued)
  overview of, 741
  of prune-belly syndrome, 581
  of tuberous sclerosis complex, 757, 759f
Genital bite wounds, 1293, 1294f
Genital burns, 3054
Genital lymphedema, 884-885
Genital Perception Score (GPS), 942-943
Genital ridges, 318f
Genital ulcers
  noninfectious, 1286-1288, 1286b
    aphthous ulcers and Behçet disease, 1286-1287, 1287f
    pyoderma gangrenosum, 1287-1288, 1288f
    traumatic causes, 1288, 1288f
  STDs, 1255-1261, 1255t
    chancroid, 1255t, 1259-1260, 1259f
    diagnosis of, 1256
    granuloma inguinale, 1260
    herpes, 1255t
    HPV, 1261, 1262f
    lymphogranuloma, 1255t, 1260-1261, 1260f
    Molluscum contagiosum, 1261, 1261f
    pediculosis pubis, 1271
    presentation of, 1256, 1256f
    scabies, 1271
    syphilis, 1255t, 1257, 1257f-1258f, 1257t
    treatment of, 1256-1257, 1256t
    vaginitis, 1271-1272, 1272t
Genitalia
  ambiguous, 998-1018, 999f, 999b
  external, development of, 305-310, 307f-310f, 312f
  masculinization of, 305
Genitalia of female, external, 395-398
  bladder and bowel dysfunction, 397-398
  development of, 307f, 310-311, 311f-313f
  foreign body, 398
  hymenal disorders, 395, 396f
  hymenal skin tags, 395
  interlabial masses, 395
  labial adhesions, 395, 396f
  paraurethral cyst, 395, 397f
  prolapsing ureterocele, 395, 397f
  urethral prolapse, 395, 397f
  vaginal discharge, 397
  vaginal rhabdomyosarcoma, 397
Genitalia of male, external, 391-395
  abnormal penile orientation, 394
    hypospadias, 394
    parameatal urethral cyst, 394
    penile curvature, 394
    penile torsion, 394
    priapism, 394-395
  penile conditions, 393-395
    buried penis, 394
    circumcision, 393
    concealed penis, 394
    foreskin, 393
    inconspicuous penis, 394
    paraphimosis, 393
    phimosis, 393
    smegma pearl, 393-394
    smegmoma, 393-394, 393f
    webbed penis, 394
  scrotal conditions, 391-393
    epididymo-orchitis, 392
    hernia, 392
    hydrocele, 392
    scrotal and testicular pain, 391
    scrotal mass, 392
    testicular torsion, 391
    testicular tumor, 392-393
    torsion of testicular, 391-392
    undescended testicle, 391
    varicocele, 392
Genitocerebral evoked potential, 1527
Genitofemoral nerve, 1372-1373, 2447f-2448f, 2453, 2453t
Genitography, 390

Genito-pelvic pain-penetration disorder, 1636, 1651-1653, 1653b
  clinical presentation of, 1652, 1652f
  clitoris and clitorodynia, 1651-1652
  pain and sex, 1651
  provoked vestibulodynia, 1651
  treatment for, 1653
Genitourinary malignancies, 1940-1941, 1941b
  bladder cancer, 1941
  molecular imaging of, 96-100
  prostate cancer, 1941
  renal cell carcinoma, 1940-1941, 1940f
Genitourinary problem index (GUPI), 1211, 1212f
Genitourinary region, pediatric, 391-402
  external
    of female, 395-398
    of male, 391-395
    sexual abuse, 398, 400
  urinary tract, 398-402
    infection of, 398-399, 402b
    pyelonephritis, 398-399
    urinary incontinence, 399-400
    vesicoureteral reflux, 399
Genitourinary surgery, genito-pelvic pain-penetration disorder and, 1652-1653
Genitourinary tract
  abnormalities of, with cloacal exstrophy, 575
  embryology of, 305-340, 306f-307f
    external genitalia, development of, 305-310, 307f-310f
    female external genitalia, 307f, 310-311, 311f-313f
    gonads, development of, 317-322, 318f
    human seminal vesicle, development of, 317
    kidneys, 333-340, 333f-334f, 339b
    Müllerian structures, 322-329, 323f, 327b
    ureter, development of, 329-333, 332f, 332t
Genitourinary trauma
  genitourinary malignancies, 2920
  in geriatric patients, 2920.e11
Genitourinary tuberculosis (GUTB), 1307-1319
  clinical manifestations and pathologic features of, 1308-1309
    bladder, 1309
    epididymis, vas deferens, testes, and scrotum, 1309
    kidney, 1308-1309
    prostate and seminal vesicles, 1309
    ureter, 1309
    urethra and penis, 1309
  development of, 1308
  diagnosis of, 1309-1314
    culture, 1310
    histopathology, 1310
    nucleic acid amplification tests, 1310
    radiography, 1311-1313, 1311f-1313f
    screening tests, 1310-1311
  management, in special situations, 1318-1319
  relapse, 1318
  transmission and host immune response, 1307-1308
  treatment of, 1315-1318
    medical therapy, 1311t, 1315-1317, 1315t-1316t
    surgical therapy, 1317-1318
Genome, GU cancer alterations in, 1351-1362, 1362b
  bladder cancer, 1358-1360
  bladder RMS, 1111-1113
  CNAs, 1354, 1354t-1355t
  gross chromosomal abnormalities, 1351-1352, 1352b
  prostate cancer, 1352-1353, 1354t, 1355f
  renal cancer, 1353, 1354t, 1358
  testicular cancer, 1121, 1353, 1361-1362
  Wilms tumor, 1096-1099, 1097f, 1354t
Genomic assessment, in male infertility, 1442-1443

Genomic classifier (GC), of prostate cancer, 3542-3543
Genomic expression profiles, as prostate cancer biomarkers, 3488
Genomic predictors, hormonal therapy and, 3680
Genomic prostate score (GPS), 3543
Genomic sequence assessment, for male infertility, 1443
Genomic tests, for localized prostate cancer, 3529
Geography
  renal calculi and, 2006-2007, 2007f
  in transitional urology, 1047
Geriatric patients, in urinary incontinence, 2917-2920
  absorbent products for, 2920.e6
  behavioral therapies for, 2920.e3
  clinical evaluation of, 2920
  costs of, 2918
  established, 2919
  history for, 2920.e1
  laboratory testing for, 2920.e2
  negative impacts of, 2918-2919
  pharmacotherapies for, 2920.e3-2920.e4
  physical examination for, 2920.e1
  PVR assessment, 2920.e1
  risk factors of, 2918
  surgical therapies for, 2920.e4-2920.e6
  transient, 2919
  treatment of, 2920
  urine containment for, 2920.e6
  urodynamic studies for, 2920.e2
  voiding diaries, 2920.e1-2920.e2
Geriatric syndromes, 2913-2917
  asymptomatic bacteriuria, 2920.e10-2920.e11
  bladder outlet obstruction, 2920.e7
  delirium, 2914
  falls, 2915
  fecal incontinence, 2920.e9
  frailty, 2913-2914, 2913f
  genitourinary malignancies, 2920
  genitourinary trauma, 2920.e11
  hematuria, 2920.e11
  medication optimization, 2915-2917, 2916t-2917t
  neurogenic bladder, 2920.e7-2920.e8
  nocturia, 2920.e8-2920.e9
  pelvic organ prolapse, 2920.e9-2920.e10
  polypharmacy, 2915-2917
  pressure ulcers, 2915
  underactive bladder, 2920.e7-2920.e8
  urinary incontinence, 2917-2920
  urinary retention, 2920.e7-2920.e8
  urinary tract infections, 2920.e10-2920.e11
Geriatric urology patient
  care coordination of, 2921
  clinical evaluation of, 2908-2922, 2909f
    activities of daily living, 2909
    cognition of, 2910, 2911f
    comprehensive geriatric assessment, 2913
    depression in, 2910
    functional assessment, 2909-2910
    instrumental activities of daily living, 2909
    mobility of, 2909-2910
  discharge planning for, 2921
  end-of-life care, 2922
  palliative care of, 2922
  surgical risk and medical optimization in, 2911-2913, 2911b-2912b
    anesthesia, 2912
    prehabilitation, 2912-2913
Germ cell neoplasia in situ, 1692-1693, 1693b
Germ cell tumors (GCTs)
  in female pediatric patients, 1120
  retroperitoneal tumors and, 2227-2229
Germ cell/gonadal origins, retroperitoneal tumors and, 2227
Germ cells
  in spermatogenesis, 1396, 1399, 1401
  of testis, 1398, 1398f

Gerota fascia, 1667-1668, 1667f-1668f, 1668b, 1865-1866, 1865.e4f
GETUG-16 trial, 3663-3664
GFR. see Glomerular filtration rate
Giant condyloma acuminatum, of penis, 1742.e1f, 1742.e3
Gibson incision, of abdomen, 135-136, 138f
Giggle incontinence, 658-660, 2540
Gitelman syndrome, 349
Glans approximation procedure (GAP), 907f, 920-921
Glans dehiscence, 937, 938f
Glans meatus and penile shaft (GMS) score, 907-908, 908f
Glans penis, 1383-1384
Glanular adhesions, of penis, 874-875, 874f
Glanular urethra, 305
Gleason grading system, 3507-3508, 3508f, 3509b, 3510-3511
Gleason scoring system, of localized prostate cancer, 3526
Glenn-Anderson technique, for vesicoureteral reflux in children, 840, 840f
Glial-derived neurotrophic factor (Gdnf)/RET, vesicoureteral reflux and, 491.e1
Global Action Plan Prostate Cancer Active Surveillance (GAP3), 3545
Global Evaluative Assessment of Robotic Skills (GEARS), 470
Global Objective Assessment of Laparoscopy (GOALS), 470
Global polyuria, 2667, 2668t
Glomerular capillary tuft, 335-336
Glomerular disease, 258-259
  in children, 344-348, 344b
    nephrotic syndrome, 344-345
Glomerular filtration rate (GFR), 341, 1905-1914
  aging and, 2905
  in AKI, 1921, 1922t
  clinical assessment of, 1905, 1906f
  determinants of, 1905
  developmental changes in, 342
  filtrate transport, 1906-1913
  nephron anatomy, 1906, 1906f-1907f, 1907b
  preoperative evaluation of, 2248
  renal hormone effects, 1913-1914
  urinary tract obstruction and
    in bilateral ureteral obstruction, 791-792
    renal blood flow and, 791
    renal vascular resistance and, 791
    in unilateral ureteral obstruction, 791
Glomerular hematuria, 16-17, 16t, 17f
Glomerulonephritis, 345-346
  in CKD, 1929
Glomerulosclerosis, with urinary tract obstruction, 781, 782f
Glucocorticoid-induced hypercalcemia, 2020
Glucocorticoids
  in adrenal cortex physiology, 2357, 2358t
  hypercalcemia induced by, 2020
Glucose
  homeostasis, 2665-2666
  in urine, 19-20
Glucosuria, 479
Glue, for laparoscopic and robotic surgery, 215.e2
Glutamate, in efferent pathways to bladder, 2488, 2489f
Glutaraldehyde cross-linked (GAX) bovine collagen (Contigen), for female urinary incontinence, 2893-2894, 2894f
Gluteal compartment syndrome, 262
Glycine, in efferent pathways to bladder, 2488
Glycosaminoglycans
  for BPS/IC treatment, 1244-1245
  in crystal formation, 2014
  in crystal matrix, 2015
  layer, of bladder urothelium, 2467-2468

GnRH. see Gonadotropin-releasing hormone
GnRH analogues, for priapism, 1553
GOALS. see Global Objective Assessment of Laparoscopy
Goldman's cardiac risk index, 120t
Gonadal descent, 318-322
Gonadal dysfunction, opioid abuse and, 1426-1427
Gonadal dysgenesis, 1001-1005
  mixed, 998t, 1002-1004, 1003f, 1003b, 1004t
  partial, 1004
  46,XX "pure,", 998t, 1002
  46,XY complete, 998t, 1004-1005, 1005f
Gonadal stage of differentiation, 993-994, 994f, 994b
Gonadal stromal tumors, in male pediatric patients, 1124, 1124f
Gonadal veins, 1672-1673
  dissection of, for RPLND, 1716
Gonadoblastomas, 1708
Gonadotropin-releasing hormone (GnRH), 1390, 1391f, 1391t
Gonadotropin-releasing hormone (GnRH) antagonists, to facilitate bladder filling and urine storage, 2713.e3
Gonads, development of, 317-322, 318f, 321f-322f, 322b
Goniometer, 912
Gonocytes, 951, 1399
Goodpasture syndrome, 347
GPS. see Genital Perception Score
Grading systems, in perinatal urology, 358-361
Graduated introducer, 170
Grafts
  for pelvic organ prolapse reconstructive surgery, 2776
    anterior compartment, 2783, 2785f
    biologics versus mesh, 2787
    cadaveric fascia, 2781t-2782t, 2786, 2786f
    polypropylene mesh, 2781t-2782t, 2783-2786, 2786f
    porcine dermis, 2781t-2782t, 2786-2787, 2787f
    posterior compartment, 2829
  for pubovaginal sling, 2834-2835
    harvest for, 2837, 2837f
  for renal transplantation, 1058, 1058.e2f
  for urethral and penile reconstruction, 1805-1807, 1806f
    dermal, 1805-1806
    full-thickness skin, 1805, 1806f
    oral mucosa, 1806, 1806f
    split-thickness skin, 1805
    vein, 1806
  for urethral stricture disease, 1821f-1823f
Granuloma inguinale, 1260
Granulomatous disease
  hypercalcemia in, 2020
  hypercalciuria in, 2050
Granulomatous orchitis, 1219
Granulomatous prostatitis, histopathology, 1203
Granulosa cell tumors, of testis, 1708
Grasping instrumentation, for laparoscopic and robotic surgery, 218
Gray-scale ultrasound, 73
Greater omentum, in vesicovaginal fistula repair, 2940
Groin pain, 2880
  in mesh complication, 2881-2882
Gross hematuria, 252-253, 400-401
Gross tumor volume (GTV), 3590
Growth
  impairment, and chronic kidney disease, 354-355
  in prune-belly syndrome, 600
  regulation, in urinary tract obstruction, 783-784

Growth factors
  in benign prostatic hyperplasia, 3309-3310, 3310f
  in tubulointerstitial fibrosis, 787-788
GRS. see Gender reassignment surgery
Grynfeltt lumbar triangle, 169
GTV. see Gross tumor volume
Guaifenesin, in stone formation, 2033
  surgical management of, 2077.e2-2077.e3
Guanine, 1346.e1, 1346.e2f
Guanylyl cyclase pathway, in ED, 1498
Guarding reflex, in bladder filling, 2515
Gubernacular anomalies, cryptorchidism and, 962-963
Gubernaculum
  anomalies of, cryptorchidism and, 962-963
  development of, testis descent and, 951-952, 952f
Guidewires, 170
  for ureteroscopy, 197
Guillain-Barré syndrome (GBS), lower urinary tract dysfunction with, 2624
Gunshot wounds
  penile, 3049-3050
  renal, 1982
    nonoperative management of, 1986-1987
  ureteral, 1995-1996
    diagnosis of, 1995-1996
GUPI. see Genitourinary problem index
Gut, 324f
GUTB. see Genitourinary tuberculosis
Gynecologic history, pelvic floor disorders and, 2527-2528
Gynecologic laparoscopy, ureteral injuries after, 1993
Gynecomastia, hormonal therapy and, 3681-3682

H
Habit training, 2730.e1t, 2731
Hailey-Hailey disease, 1285-1286, 1286f
Hald-Bradley classification, of voiding dysfunction, 2523-2524, 2523b
HALN. see Hand-assisted laparoscopic nephrectomy
Haloperidol, for delirium, 2914
Hammock anastomosis, in urinary diversion, 3189
Hammock hypothesis, of urinary incontinence, 2466, 2518, 2596, 2597b
Hand-assist devices, for laparoscopic and robotic surgery, 212, 212f
Hand-assisted adrenal surgery, 2419
Hand-assisted laparoscopic nephrectomy (HALN), 2296-2297, 2296f
Hand-assisted laparoscopy, for kidney, 2281-2282, 2283f
Hand port access, for transperitoneal access, 209
Harmonic Scalpel, 466, 466f
Harmonic scanning ultrasound, 74, 75f
Hasson technique, 271-272, 464
  for achieving extraperitoneal access and developing extraperitoneal space, 209-210, 210f
  for achieving transperitoneal access and establishing pneumoperitoneum, 209, 209f
  complications related to, 224
Hautmann pouch, for orthoptic urinary diversion, 3245, 3246f
Hawthorne effect, 484-485
Hayflick "limit," aging and, 2905
HBOT. see Hyperbaric oxygen therapy
hCG. see Human chorionic gonadotropin
HDCT. see High-dose chemotherapy
HDRB. see High-dose rate brachytherapy
Headache, orgasmic, 1580-1581
Health, norms of, masculinity and, 1416
Health care, global implications for, 2907-2908

Health issues, in geriatric patients, 2920.e13
Health policy, in ED, 1514, 1515b
Health-related quality of life (HRQoL), 108
　benign prostatic hyperplasia and, 3319
　pelvic floor disorders and, 2532t–2533t
Health services, outcomes research and, 101
Heart, 318f
　in prune-belly syndrome, 586
Heart and Estrogen/Progestin Replacement Study (HERS), 2710
Heart disease, nocturia and, 2665
Heart rate variability and sympathetic skin response test, 1527
Heavy particle beams, 3594–3596, 3594f, 3595t
Hedgehog signaling pathway, in prostate development, 3276
Heineke-Mikulicz principle, of urethromeatoplasty, 918, 921f
Heineke-Mikulicz procedure, for lower ureteral injuries, 1999
Heineke-Mikulicz urethroplasty, urethral reconstruction and, 3071
Helium, as insufflant choice, 220
Hemangiomas
　congenital, 888
　renal, 2131–2132
　subcutaneous, 888
　urethral, 1776
　　reconstructive surgery for, 1808
Hemangiopericytomas, in retroperitoneum, 2232, 2233f
Hematogenous route of infection, 1131.e1
Hematogenous spread, of UTUC, 2194
Hematologic dyscrasias, priapism and, 1542, 1542b
Hematoma
　after midurethral sling, 2874
　postoperative, complication of scrotal surgery, 1855
　urinoma compared with, 1988
Hematopoietic stem cell transplantation, for RCC, 2331, 2331t
Hematospermia
　patient history of, 6–7
　prostate biopsy and, 3499
Hematuria, 1936
　after transurethral microwave therapy, 3430
　with benign prostatic hyperplasia, 3336
　in children, 342–343, 343b
　　cause of, 342b, 343
　classification of, 247
　CT and, 50–51
　evaluation of, 247–259
　　for urothelial cancer, 3078
　in geriatric patients, 2920.e11
　gross, 252–253, 386–387, 386t
　hemorrhagic cystitis, 253–255, 253b, 255b
　management of, 247–259
　microscopic, 247–250, 250b
　patient history of, 3
　in pregnant, 283–284
　prostatic origin, 255–257, 256f, 257b
　in renal injuries, 1982–1983
　timing of, 247
　upper tract imaging in diagnostic evaluation of, 248t, 251
　upper urinary tract, 258–259, 258b–259b
　in ureteral injuries, 1995
　urethral bleeding, 257–258, 258b
　urinary biomarkers, 248t, 252
　urine cytology for, 248t, 252
　UTUC causing, 2189–2190
Hematuria catheter, 154, 154f
Hematuria-dysuria syndrome, after augmentation cystoplasty, 698.e1
Hemi-Kock pouch
　for orthoptic urinary diversion, 3243–3244, 3244f
　procedure for with valved rectum, 3209–3210
Heminephrectomy, laparoscopic, 2299

Hemodynamics
　changes in, with urinary tract obstruction, 791–792, 793b
　during laparoscopic and robotic surgery, approach and patient position effects on, 222
Hemoglobinopathies, 451
Hem-o-Lock clips, 216–217, 217f, 217b, 467
Hemolysin, 429
Hemolytic uremic syndrome (HUS), 347–348
Hemorrhage
　with holmium laser enucleation of prostate, 3438
　with intestinal anastomoses, 3181
　laparoscopic kidney surgery causing, 2306–2307
　with monopolar transurethral resection of prostate, 3417
　partial nephrectomy causing, 2265–2266
　with percutaneous antegrade endopyelotomy, 1949
　tray, for laparoscopic surgery, 226b
　during vena caval thrombectomy, 2278
Hemorrhagic cystitis, 253–255, 253b, 255b, 526
　management of, 254–255, 254f
Hemostasis
　instrumentation, for laparoscopic and robotic surgery, 214–215, 218
　for monopolar transurethral resection of prostate, 3410–3415
Henoch-Schönlein purpura (HSP), 346–347, 899
Heparin
　for vena caval thrombectomy, 2266
　VTE prophylaxis with for laparoscopic and robotic surgery, 231
Heparin sulfate, in crystal formation, 2014
Hepatic cysts, 752
Hepatic dysfunction, during vena caval thrombectomy, 2278
Hepatic function, aging and, 2906
Hepatic resections, RPLND with, 1719–1720
Hepatitis, allografts and, 2835
Hepatitis B, STDs and, 1268–1269, 1269t
Hepatitis C, STDs and, 1270
Hepatobiliary evaluation, 121
Hepatorenal ligament, 1865
Hereditary hypophosphatemic rickets with hypercalciuria (HHRH), 2019
Hereditary leiomyomatosis and RCC (HLRCC) syndrome, 1358, 2142t, 2144
　systemic therapy for, 2343
Hereditary nonpolyposis colorectal cancer, genomic alterations in, 1354t
Hereditary papillary RCC (HPRCC) syndrome
　genomic alterations in, 1354t, 1358, 2142t, 2143–2144
　systemic therapy for, 2343–2344, 2344f
Hereditary pheochromocytoma, 2373, 2374t, 2375, 2380
Hereditary prostate cancer (HPC), genomic alterations in, 1354–1355, 1354t, 1355f
Hereditary renal malignancy, in partial nephrectomy, 2262–2263
Hereditary spastic paraplegia (HSP), lower urinary tract dysfunction and, 2624–2625
Herlyn-Werner-Wunderlich syndrome, 985–986, 986f
Hernia, 392, 888–893, 892b
　after laparoscopic and robotic surgery, 231
　definitions for, 888, 889f
　diagnosis of, 889–890
　embryology of, 888–889
　epidemiology and pathogenesis of, 889
　genetics of, 889
　with intestinal anastomoses, 3180t
　as laparoscopic and robotic surgery contraindication, 204
　physical examination of, 890, 890f
　radiologic imaging of, 890, 890f
Herpes, genital ulcers, 1255t

Herpesvirus infection, lower urinary tract dysfunction with, 2621–2622
HERS. see Heart and Estrogen/Progestin Replacement Study
HGPIN. see High-grade prostatic intraepithelial neoplasia
HHRH. see Hereditary hypophosphatemic rickets with hypercalciuria
Hidden incision endoscopic surgery (HIdES), 458, 459f
HIdES. see Hidden incision endoscopic surgery
Hidradenitis suppurativa (HS), 1291–1292, 1292f
HIFU. see High-intensity focused ultrasound ablation
High-dose chemotherapy (HDCT), for NSGCTs, 1697–1698
High-dose rate brachytherapy (HDRB), 1767, 3668
　for prostate cancer, 3598–3599
　　as boost with external beam radiation therapy, 3599
　　monotherapy, 3599
High-dose-rate monotherapy, 3599
High-energy linear accelerators, 3587
High-grade prostatic intraepithelial neoplasia (HGPIN), 3506, 3507f
High-intensity focused ultrasonography, 3628, 3629t–3630t, 3631f–3632f
　for locally advanced prostate cancer, 3655
High-intensity focused ultrasound ablation (HIFU), for renal tumor ablation, 2319–2321
High-pressure bladder, spinal cord injury with, host defense mechanisms in UTIs and, 1140
Hillier, Thomas, 160
Hindgut, 318f
Hinge region, of urothelium of bladder, 2462, 2463f
Hippocratic oath, 115, 116b
Histamine
　in BPS/IC etiology, 1232.e4, 1232.e5b
　urethral function effects of, 1901–1902
Histamine antagonists, urethral function effects of, 1901–1902
Histamine H_2 receptor antagonists, and ED, 1509
Histology, adrenal, 2351–2352, 2351f, 2355f, 2356
Histone post-translational modifications, in prostate cancer, 3470
History. see Patient history
History of present illness, 1–7
HIV. see Human immunodeficiency virus
H-line measurement, 2441–2442, 2442f
HO. see Hyperbaric oxygen
Hodson-type kidney, 162, 163f, 164
HoLEP. see Holmium laser enucleation of prostate
Holmium laser
　for bladder mesh perforation, 2868–2869
　use of, 168–169
Holmium laser enucleation of prostate (HoLEP), 3436
　in anticoagulated patient, 3438
　complications with, 3438
　　intraoperative, 3438
　　perioperative, 3438
　　postoperative, 3438
　conclusion for, 3438
　introduction and concept for, 3436
　open prostatectomy versus, 3437
　outcomes with, 3437–3438
　　comparative series, 3437–3438
　　single-cohort series, 3437
　technique for, 3436
　　intraoperative, 3436
　　postoperative, 3436
　　preoperative, 3436
　thulium laser versus, 3442–3443
　transurethral resection of prostate versus, 3437

Holmium:YAG (Ho:YAG) laser, 240, 245b
　basic physics of, 244
Homeobox gene, 317
Homogeneous nucleation, 2011
HOPE. see Hypospadias Objective Penile Evaluation
Hormonal evaluation, and ED, 1527-1529
Hormonal therapy
　for benign prostatic hyperplasia, 3371
　for ED, 1529
　for metastatic RCC, 2342-2343
　for priapism, 1553
　for prostate cancer, 3671-3686
　　androgen axis molecular biology and, 3672-3673, 3672f, 3673t, 3673b
　　androgen blockade mechanisms, 3673-3678, 3679b
　　androgen blockade response in, 3679-3680
　　androgen synthesis inhibition, 3677-3678
　　anemia, 3682
　　antiandrogens, 3674-3676, 3675f
　　body habitus changes with, 3681
　　cardiovascular morbidity and mortality, 3681
　　with chemotherapy, 3683
　　clinical follow-up on, 3679-3682, 3680b
　　cognitive function and, 3681
　　combination therapy, 3682-3683, 3683b
　　combined androgen blockade, 3682
　　complications of, 3680-3682, 3682b
　　diabetes and, 3681
　　gynecomastia, 3681
　　historical overview of, 3671-3672
　　hot flashes, 3680-3681
　　metabolic syndrome and, 3681
　　osteoporosis and, 3680
　　with radiation therapy, 3682
　　with radical prostatectomy, 3682
　　sexual dysfunction and, 3681
　　timing of, 3683-3686
　urinary incontinence and, 2585
Hormones
　for female orgasmic disorder, 1648
　for female sexual interest disorder, 1643-1645
　of HPG axis
　　anterior pituitary, 1390-1391, 1391f
　　hypothalamus, 1390, 1391f
　　testis, 953, 1391-1392, 1391f
　laparoscopic and robotic surgery effects on, 222
　renal
　　bone mineral regulation by, 1914, 1914f
　　erythropoiesis regulation by, 1914
　　red blood cell production, 1914
　　vasoconstriction, 1913
　　vasodilation, 1913
Horseshoe kidneys, 177, 177f, 731-733, 733b, 1869.e2f
　anomalies of, 731-732, 732f
　description for, 731
　diagnosis and radiographic appearance of, 732, 732f
　incidence of, 731
　percutaneous nephrolithotomy and, 2105-2106
　prognosis of, 732-733
　renal calculi and, 2034
　　surgical management of, 2078-2081, 2079f
　symptoms of, 732
HOSE. see Hypospadias Objective Scoring Evaluation
Host defense mechanisms, alterations in, in UTI pathogenesis, 1139-1140
　diabetes mellitus, 1139
　HIV, 1140
　obstruction, 1139
　pregnancy, 1140
　RPN, 1139-1140, 1139b

Host defense mechanisms, alterations in, in UTI pathogenesis (Continued)
　spinal cord injury with high-pressure bladders, 1140
　underlying disease, 1139
　vesicoureteral reflux, 1139
Hostile Abdomen Index Scoring Table, 463t
Hot flashes, hormonal therapy and, 3680-3681
Hounsfield units, 46-48
24-hour voiding frequency, 3345
Hox homeobox genes, 317
HPC. see Hereditary prostate cancer
HPV. see Human papillomavirus
HRQoL. see Health-related quality of life
HS. see Hidradenitis suppurativa
HSP. see Henoch-Schönlein purpura
HTN. see Hypertension
Human bites, of penis, 3050
Human chorionic gonadotropin (hCG), in TGCTs, 1686
Human herpesvirus 8, penis, tumors of, 1742.e5
Human immunodeficiency virus (HIV)
　allografts and, 2835
　circumcision protection against, 1812
　genitourinary tuberculosis management and, 1318
　host defense mechanisms in UTIs and, 1140
　occupational exposure to, 1264-1265
　penis tumors related to, 1742.e5
　as STD, 1264-1268
　　diagnosis, 1264
　　erectile dysfunction and, 1267
　　interactions with other STDs, 1257, 1264-1268
　　Kaposi sarcoma, 1267-1268
　　male circumcision, 1264
　　malignancy, 1267
　　nephrolithiasis, 1266
　　non-AIDS-defining urologic malignancies, 1268
　　nonulcerating skin infections and, 1265
　　postexposure prophylaxis, 1264-1265
　　pre-exposure prophylaxis, 1265
　　prostatitis and, 1266
　　renal dysfunction and, 1266-1267
　　renal infections, 1266
　　testis, epididymis, seminal vesicles and, 1266
　　urologic manifestations of, 1265-1268, 1265f
　　UTI and, 1265-1266
　　voiding dysfunction and, 1267
　vaccine, 1262-1263
Human kallikrein 2 (hK2)
　as prostate cancer biomarkers, 3484
　in prostate cancer diagnosis, 3518
　in prostatic secretions, 3298, 3298t
Human kallikrein 11 (hK11), in prostatic secretions, 3298t, 3299
Human kallikrein 14 (KLK14), in prostatic secretions, 3298t, 3299
Human kallikrein L1, in prostatic secretions, 3298-3299, 3298t
Human papillomavirus (HPV)
　as genital ulcers, 1261, 1262f
　penis tumors and
　　carcinoma, 1743-1744
　　premalignant lesions, 1742
Human prostate, 311-317, 313f-316f, 315t, 317t, 317b
Human seminal vesicle, development of, 317
Hunner lesion, surgery for, 1248
HUS. see Hemolytic uremic syndrome
Hutch diverticula, bladder, 3011
Hydraulic valves, for continent urinary diversions, 710
Hydrocalycosis, 738

Hydrocele, 392, 1394
　as filariasis clinical manifestation, 1329-1330, 1330f
　recurrence, complication of scrotal surgery, 1856
Hydrocelectomy, 1845
Hydroceles, 888-893, 892b
　abdominoscrotal, 889, 892-893
　communicating, 889
　definitions for, 889, 889f
　diagnosis of, 889-890
　embryology of, 888-889
　genetics of, 889
　noncommunicating, 889
　physical examination of, 890, 890f
　radiologic imaging of, 890, 890f
　scrotal, 889
　of spermatic cord, 889
　surgical repair of, 891
Hydrocephalus, normal-pressure
　lower urinary tract dysfunction with, 2604
　transient urinary incontinence and, 2919.e1
Hydrodistention, for BPS/IC treatment, 1247
Hydrogen ions, transport of, urinary tract obstruction and, 793-794
Hydrogen sulfide, in ED, 1498
Hydronephrosis
　after pediatric renal transplantation, 1062-1063, 1063f
　Color Doppler ultrasonography for, 778
　versus cystic renal diseases, 404, 404f, 408f
　infected, 1174
　neonatal diagnosis of, 1943
　prevalence of, 776
　retroperitoneal fibrosis with, 1978
　urinary tract obstruction and, 776-777
　UTUC with, 2196-2197
Hydrothorax, 180
Hydroureter, urinary tract obstruction and, 776
Hydroureteronephrosis of pregnancy, 1900
25-Hydroxycholecalciferol (Calcidiol), 1914
17α-Hydroxylase deficiency, 1012
3β-Hydroxysteroid dehydrogenase deficiency, 1011-1012
17β-Hydroxysteroid oxidoreductase deficiency, 1012-1013
Hymen, imperforate, 327, 328f, 978-979, 979f
Hymen vaginae, 1627.e2
Hymenal disorders, 395
　imperforate hymen, 395
Hymenal skin tags, 395, 978-979, 979f
Hyperbaric oxygen (HO), 945
Hyperbaric oxygen therapy (HBOT), 255
Hypercalcemia
　glucocorticoid-induced, 2020
　in granulomatous disease, 2020
　malignancy-associated, 2020
　in RCC, 2156
　in sarcoidosis, 2020
Hypercalcemic-induced hypercalciuria, 2020
Hypercalciuria, 350, 857-858, 858t, 2050-2053
　absorptive, 2019
　calcium stone formation associated with, 2018-2020
　calcium supplementation, 2050-2051
　clinical considerations of, 2050
　conservative strategies for, 2051
　hypercalcemic-induced, 2020
　idiopathic, 2050, 2051b
　medical therapy for, 2051-2053, 2053b
　renal, 2019-2020
　resorptive, 2020, 2050, 2050b
　in sarcoidosis and granulomatous disease, 2050
Hypercapnia, 461
Hyperfiltration injury, in partial nephrectomy, 2262
Hyperkalemia, 353
Hyperlipidemia, and ED, 1504

Hypermobile glans penis, 1591, 1591f
Hypermobility, in stress urinary incontinence, 2757, 2834
Hypernatremia, 353
Hyperoxaluria, 350, 858, 858t, 2056-2060, 2057b
　calcium stone formation, 2020-2023, 2021f-2022f, 2057-2058
　causes of, 2021
　clinical considerations of, 2056
　conservative strategies for, 2056-2057, 2057b
　diabetes, obesity, and metabolic syndrome, 2059-2060
　dietary, 2023
　enteric, 2022-2023, 2056
　hypomagnesuric calcium nephrolithiasis, 2058t
　idiopathic, 2023
　medical therapy for, 2057
　primary, 2021-2022, 2021f, 2056-2057
　uric acid stones, 2058-2059
Hyperparathyroidism, primary, with resorptive hypercalciuria, 2020
Hyperprolactinemia treatments, 1530-1532
Hypertension (HTN), 1419-1420
　after renal injury, 1992
　benign prostatic hyperplasia and, 3322
　　with α1-adrenergic blockers, 3369-3370
　in children, 351-353, 352b
　and ED, 1504-1505
　genitourinary trauma and, 1077-1078
　nocturia and, 2665
　in RCC, 2156
　renal calculi and, 2008
　with renovascular injuries, 1990
　staging of, 351-352
　with urinary tract obstruction, 794
Hypertensive emergency, 351-352
Hyperthyroidism
　contrast media and, 32
　lower urinary tract dysfunction and, 2630
Hypertrophied clitoris, 975, 975f
Hyperuricemia, and ED, 1511
Hyperuricosuria, 858t, 859
　in calcium stone formation, 2023-2024
　in uric acid stone formation, 2029
Hyperuricosuric calcium oxalate nephrolithiasis, 2057-2058
Hypoactive sexual desire dysfunction, 1636
Hypocitraturia, 858-859, 2053-2056, 2054b, 2055f
　calcium stone formation associated with, 2024
　clinical considerations of, 2053
　conservative strategies for, 2053-2054
　distal renal tubular acidosis (type 1) in, 2055-2056, 2055f
　medical therapy for, 2054
　thiazide-induced hypocitraturia, 2056
Hypofractionation, radiobiologic basis for, 3593, 3593t
Hypogastric artery, 2432, 2433f, 2452
Hypogastric lymphadenectomy, 3149-3152, 3153f
Hypogastric plexus, 2434
Hypogonadism, 1430
　and ED, 1504
　and PD, 1602
Hypogonadotropic hypogonadism, 1447-1448
Hypohedonic orgasm, 1636
Hypokalemic metabolic alkalosis, 349
Hypomagnesiuria, in calcium stone formation, 2026
Hypomagnesuric calcium nephrolithiasis, 2058, 2058t
Hypomethylation, in bladder cancer, 1350
Hyponatremia, 353
　with desmopressin, 2711
　as effect of desmopressin, 2670
Hypoplastic glomerulocystic disease, 756-757

Hypospadias, 306, 310f, 394, 905-948, 1449
　advancement procedures for, 918-920
　　M inverted V glansplasty, 920, 922f
　　meatal advancement glanuloplasty, 920, 921f
　　urethral, 920, 922f
　　urethromeatoplasty, 918
　anatomic imaging of, 941
　assessment and management for
　　intraoperative, 911, 911b
　　preoperative, 932-934
　complications of, 934-941
　　balanitis xerotica obliterans, 939, 940f
　　glans dehiscence, 937, 938f
　　meatal stenosis, 937-938
　　recurrent penile curvature, 939-941, 940f
　　skin, 941
　　urethral diverticulum, 938-939, 939f
　　urethral stricture, 938
　　urethrocutaneous fistula, 935-937, 936f-937f
　diagnosis of, 905-908, 907f
　disorders of sexual differentiation in, 908
　embryology of, 905, 905b, 906f
　etiology of, 908-909, 909b
　improving outcomes for, 941
　outcome assessment for, 942-943
　outcomes after, 941-947
　　sexual function, 942
　　urinary stream, 942
　patient-reported outcomes in, 942-943
　postoperative management for, 932-934
　　dressing, 918, 920f
　　medications, 932
　　urinary diversion, 932
　preoperative androgen stimulation for, 910-911
　proximal, 925-932, 925b, 948f
　pudendal nerve block for, 911
　reoperations for, 943-947, 945b, 948b
　　buccal mucosa, 946
　　dorsal inlay graft, 934f, 946
　　tubularized, incised plate procedure, 916-918, 922-924
　repair of, failure of, reconstructive surgery for, 1812-1813
　surgical assessment for, 909-918
　surgical repair for
　　Byars flaps, 927, 931f
　　comments on, 932, 932b, 935f
　　distal, 918
　　general considerations of, 916-918, 918b, 919f
　　graft or flap, 932, 934f
　　one-stage, 925-926
　　preputial flaps, 926f, 938-939
　　proximal, 925-932, 925b
　　scrotoplasty, 941
　　technical aspects of, 925-926, 926f
　　two-stage, 926-927
　　two-stage with free graft, 927, 929f
　　two-stage with pedicle flap, 927-932, 931f
　in transitional urology, 1049
　tubularization techniques for, 920-941
　　flip-flap technique, 924, 924f
　　glans approximation procedure, 907f, 920-921
　　island onlay flap procedure, 924-925, 926f
　　slitlike adjusted Mathieu procedure for, 924, 925f
　　Thiersch Duplay repair, 921-922, 923f
　urethral plate formation for, 905
　urethroplasty for
　　algorithm for, 912f, 914
　　complications with, 936t
　　distal tubularized incised plate, 923f
　　hair-bearing skin, 918
　　proximal tubularized incised plate, 928f
　ventral penile curvature and, 911-914, 916b
　　artificial erection for, 911-912

Hypospadias (Continued)
　　dorsal shortening technique for, 912-913, 915f
　　goniometer for, 912
　　significance of, 911
　　ventral corporal lengthening procedures for, 913, 915f-916f
Hypospadias Objective Penile Evaluation (HOPE), 942-943, 943t, 944f
Hypospadias Objective Scoring Evaluation (HOSE), 942-943
Hypothalamic-pituitary-adrenal axis physiology, normal, 2360-2361, 2361f
Hypothalamic-pituitary-gonadal (HPG) axis, 1390-1402, 1393b
　aging and, 1392
　basic endocrine concepts for, 1390, 1391f
　components of, 1390-1392
　　anterior pituitary, 1390-1391, 1391f
　　hypothalamus, 1390, 1391f
　　testis, 1391-1392, 1391f
　development of, 1392, 1392f
　and ED, 1503
Hypothalamus
　in HPG axis, 1390, 1391f
　micturition control by, 2496
Hypothermia
　anesthesia-related, during laparoscopic and robotic surgery, 228.e1
　for laparoscopic partial nephrectomy, 2302
　for partial nephrectomy, 2262
　in urologic surgery, 125, 145
Hypothermic arrest, for vena caval thrombectomy, 2275-2276
Hypoxia-induced factor-1α (HIF-1α), 3700
Hypoxis rooperi (South African star grass), for benign prostatic hyperplasia, 3398
Hysterectomy, 3063-3064
　laparoscopic, ureteral injuries after, 1993
　lower urinary tract dysfunction after, 2621
　pelvic organ prolapse and, 2591
　vaginal, with McCall culdoplasty technique, 2814-2815, 2815f
Hysteresis, ureteral, 1890, 1890f
Hysteropexy, 2815-2823
　minimally invasive sacrohysteropexy, 2822-2823, 2824t
　minimally invasive uterosacral, 2820-2822, 2821t
　open abdominal sacrohysteropexy, 2822-2823, 2824t
　sacrospinous, 2817-2820
　transvaginal uterosacral ligament, 2817, 2819t

I
IADLs. see Instrumental activities of daily living
Iatrogenic factors, in UTUC etiology, 2187-2188
Iatrogenic fistulae, 2926-2942, 2927f
Iatrogenic priapism
　ADHD and, 1545
　intracavernous injections for, 1544-1545
Iatrogenic urethral strictures, 1815
IBS. see Irritable bowel syndrome
Ibuprofen, 932-934
ICAs. see Intracranial aneurysms
Ice-water test, 2485, 2505
ICI. see International Consultation on Incontinence
ICIQ. see International Consultation on Incontinence Questionnaire
ICIQ-BD. see International Consultation on Incontinence Questionnaire Bladder Diary
ICIQ-MLUTS. see International Consultation on Incontinence Questionnaire Male Lower Urinary Tract Symptoms
ICIQ-Nocturia Quality of Life Question (ICIQ-Nqol), 110t
ICIQ-UI-SF. see International Consultation on Incontinence Questionnaire Urinary Incontinence Short Form
ICS. see International Continence Society

ICSmale Questionnaire, 110t
IDC-P. *see* Intraductal carcinoma of the prostate
IDCs. *see* Involuntary detrusor contractions
Idiopathic detrusor overactivity (IDO), 2504
　resiniferatoxin in, 2709.e1
Idiopathic hypercalciuria, 2018
Idiopathic hyperoxaluria, 2023
Idiopathic hypocitraturic calcium nephrolithiasis, 2054
Idiopathic scrotal edema, 899
Idiopathic strictures, 1815
IDO. *see* Idiopathic detrusor overactivity
IFIS. *see* Intraoperative floppy iris syndrome
IFNs. *see* Interferons
Ifosfamide, for NSGCTs, 1697
IGCCCG. *see* International Germ Cell Cancer Collaborative Group
IGFs. *see* Insulin-like growth factors
IGRAs. *see* Interferon-gamma release assays
IIEF. *see* International Index of Erectile Function
IIQ. *see* Incontinence Impact Questionnaire
Ileal conduit, 3193-3196, 3194f-3195f, 3195t
　in minimally invasive urinary diversion, 3261-3262
Ileal neobladder, for orthoptic urinary diversion, 3245, 3246f
Ileal reservoirs
　continent, 3213-3215, 3214f
　for orthoptic urinary diversion, 3243
Ileal ureteral replacement, 2208, 2209f
Ileal ureteral substitution
　minimally invasive, for ureteral stricture disease, 1973-1975
　for ureteral stricture disease, 1973-1975, 1974f
Ileal vesicostomy, 3197-3198
Ileocecal conduit, colon conduit and, 3196, 3198t
Ileocecal valve
　for continent urinary diversions, 709-710
　in ileocecocystoplasty, 694
　imbricating, in robot-assisted intracorporeal continent cutaneous diversion, 3269
Ileocecocystoplasty, 694, 694f-695f
Ileocolic anastomosis, in robot-assisted intracorporeal continent cutaneous diversion, 3269, 3269f
Ileocystoplasty, 692-693, 693f
Ileostomy bowel diversions, ammonium acid urate stones from, 2032
Ileovesicostomy, 702, 702b
Ileum
　selection, 3162
　tapering of, in robot-assisted intracorporeal continent cutaneous diversion, 3269
Ileus, after RPLND, 1731
Iliac aneurysm, as laparoscopic and robotic surgery contraindication, 204
Iliac arteries, 2451-2452, 2451t
Iliac crests, 2428f
Iliac lymph nodes, 2433
Iliac spines, 2428f, 2445f
Iliac veins, 2452
Iliacus, 1658, 1662f-1665f, 1664t
Iliococcygeus muscle, 2430-2432, 2432f
Iliococcygeus suspension, for apical pelvic organ prolapse repair, 2797-2798, 2799f
Iliohypogastric nerve, 2447f-2448f, 2453, 2453t
Ilioinguinal nerve, 2447f-2448f, 2453, 2453t
Illicit drug use, patient history of, 9
ILND. *see* Inguinal lymphadenectomy
IMA. *see* Inferior mesenteric artery
Image guidance, to prostate cancer, 3589
Image-guided radiation therapy, for prostate cancer, 3589-3590, 3591f-3592f
Image storage, ultrasonography, 76, 77f
Imaging
　in adrenal mass evaluation, 2394-2398, 2396f-2397f, 2397b

Imaging (*Continued*)
　for benign prostatic hyperplasia, 3347
　for male urinary incontinence, 2543
　for pediatric urology, 388-391
　　prenatal ultrasonography, 389
　　renal bladder ultrasound, 388-389
　　ultrasonography, 388-389
　of pheochromocytoma, 2375, 2376f
　techniques, for UTIs, 1143-1144, 1144b
　　CT and MRI, 1144
　　indications, 1144b
　　radionuclide studies, 1144.e1
　　ultrasonography, 1144
　　voiding cystourethrogram, 1144
Imidafenacin, to facilitate bladder filling and urine storage, 2682, 2682t
Imipramine (Tofranil)
　to facilitate bladder filling and urine storage, 2682t, 2702
　for nocturnal polyuria, 2668, 2673t
　for stress urinary incontinence in women, 2714-2715
　ureteral response to, 1888
Imiquimod cream, for condylomata acuminata, 1742.e3
Immune checkpoint blockade, 1342, 1342f
　in bladder cancer, 1342
　in kidney cancer, 1343
　in prostate cancer, 1343
Immune editing hypothesis, 1336, 1337f
Immune response, pathogen recognition, 1138-1139
ImmunoCyt, of bladder tumor, 3081
Immunoglobulin A (IgA) nephropathy, 346
Immunoglobulins, in prostatic secretions, 3298t, 3302
Immunologic effects, of laparoscopic and robotic surgery, 223
Immunologic function, aging and, 2906
Immunology, immune response in GU cancers, 1333-1345, 1336b
　adaptive immune system, 1334-1336, 1335f
　immune editing hypothesis, 1336, 1337f
　inflammation effects in, 1336, 1337f-1338f, 1338b
　innate immune system, 1333-1334, 1334f-1335f, 1334t-1335t
Immunomodulator drugs, for BPS/IC oral therapy, 1241t, 1242-1243
Immunosuppressed patients, penile implants for, 1596
Immunosuppression, in end stage renal disease, 357
Immunotherapy
　for castration-resistant prostate cancer, 3697-3699, 3699b
　for GU cancers, 1333-1345, 1341b, 1343b
　　BCG in bladder cancer, 1333, 1334f, 1338-1339, 1339f
　　cancer vaccines, 1339-1340, 1340f-1341f
　　combination, 1343-1345, 1345f
　　immune checkpoint blockade, 1342, 1342f
　for non-muscle-invasive bladder cancer, 3099-3103, 3103b
　　Bacille Calmette-Guérin, 3099-3100
　　interferon, 3102-3103
　　investigational, 3103
　for UTUC, 2223-2224
IMPACT study, 3697, 3697f
Impedance, in ultrasonography, 71, 71f
Imperforate hymen, 395, 396f, 978-979, 979f
Implants, for ED, 1582
　inflatable, 1582, 1583f
　semirigid rods, 1582, 1583f, 1584t
IMT. *see* Inflammatory myofibroblastic tumor
IMV. *see* Inferior mesenteric vein
In vitro fertilization, 1428, 1445.e3
Incidental urolithiasis, 402

Incidentalomas, adrenal
　adrenal surgery for, 2409b
　evaluation of, 2394, 2394t
Incision instrumentation, for laparoscopic and robotic surgery, 214-215
Incisional hernia, after laparoscopic and robotic surgery, 231
Inclusion cysts, 882-883, 882f
Inconspicuous penis, 394, 872t, 877-879, 879f
Incontinence Impact Questionnaire (IIQ), 110, 111t
Incontinence Quality of Life Instrument (I-QOL), 111t
Incontinence Symptom Index (ISI-P), 477
Incontinent urinary diversion, for neuromuscular dysfunction of lower urinary tract, 636-637
Increased through transmission, in ultrasonography, 72, 72f
Index lesion hypothesis, multifocality of prostate cancer *versus*, 3617-3620, 3619t, 3620f
Index of Premature Ejaculation (IPE), 112t
Indiana pouch, 3220-3224, 3222f-3223f
Indigo carmine, toxicity of, 1994
Indinavir sulfate (Crixivan), in stone formation, 2032-2033
Indirect inguinal hernia, 889
Indirect medical risk factors, in bladder tumor, 3077
Indium-111 (^{111}In), 91, 92t
　capromab pendetide scanning, for biochemical recurrence after radical prostatectomy, 3661
Indomethacin
　to facilitate bladder filling and urine storage, 2682t, 2703
　urethral function effects of, 1902
Induction process, 785-786, 786f
Indwelling catheters, for urinary incontinence, in geriatric patients, 2920.e5
Indwelling orthopedic hardware, antimicrobial prophylaxis for uncomplicated urologic procedures and, 1201
Infected hydronephrosis and pyonephrosis, 1174, 1174f
Infection
　after midurethral sling, 2870-2871
　after prostate biopsy, 3499
　with artificial urinary sphincter, 3005-3006
　in BPS/IC etiology, 1232.e1-1232.e2
　complicated, 1129, 1130b
　complication of scrotal surgery, 1856
　from cutaneous diseases of external genitalia
　　balanitis, 1288
　　balanoposthitis, 1288, 1289f
　　candidal intertrigo, 1293-1294, 1294f
　　cellulitis, 1288-1289, 1290f
　　corynebacterial infection (trichomycosis axillaris and erythrasma), 1292-1293, 1293f
　　dermatophyte infection, 1294-1295, 1295f
　　ecthyma gangrenosum, 1293, 1294f
　　erysipelas, 1288-1289
　　folliculitis, 1290-1291, 1291f
　　Fournier gangrene, 1289-1290, 1290f
　　furunculosis, 1291, 1291f
　　genital bite wounds, 1293, 1294f
　　hidradenitis suppurativa, 1291-1292, 1292f
　　infestation, 1295-1296, 1296f
　　STDs, 1288, 1289f
　host factors increasing risk of, 1193b
　and inflammation, and male infertility, 1432
　with intestinal anastomoses, 3180
　penile implant and, 1591-1593, 1592f, 1593b
　with percutaneous antegrade endopyelotomy, 1949
　preoperative care for pediatric patients with, 447-448

Infection (Continued)
  prostate cancer and, 3461, 3462f
  prostatitis and, 1207
  renal transplantation and, 1056-1057, 1061
  ureteral anomalies and, 801-802
  ureteral function effects of, 1899
  with urinary intestinal diversion, 3198-3205, 3205b
  UTUC risk and, 2187
Infection calculi, 2063-2065, 2063f, 2064t, 2065b
Infection stones, 2030-2031
  bacteriology of, 2030-2031, 2031t
  epidemiology of, 2031
  pathogenesis of, 2030, 2030f
Infectious granulomatous nephritis
  malacoplakia, 1179-1181, 1180f
  renal echinococcosis, 1181.e1, 1181.e2f
  XGP, 1177-1179, 1178f-1179f
Infective disorders, and delayed ejaculation, 1575
Inferior epigastric artery, 136f
Inferior mesenteric artery (IMA), in radical nephrectomy, 2261
Inferior mesenteric vein (IMV), in radical nephrectomy, 2261
Inferior vena cava (IVC)
  filtration and permanent interruption of, 2277
  patching, replacing, and interrupting of, 2276-2277, 2277f
  in radical nephrectomy, 2258, 2258f, 2258.e1f
  RCC involvement of, 2174-2176, 2175f-2176f, 2298
  resection of, RPLND with, 1718-1719
  in retroperitoneum, 1672
Inferior vesical artery, 1380, 1380f
Infertility
  ligation with resulting, complication of scrotal surgery, 1856
  male, 1428-1452
    abdominal, imaging of, 1444, 1445f
    assisted reproduction, 1445-1452, 1445.e3, 1445.e3t
    causes of, 1446-1447
    and childhood diseases, 1432-1434
    and chromosomal numerical disorders, 1445-1446
    cranial, imaging of, 1444-1445, 1445f
    developmental disorders and, 1449-1450
    diagnoses and therapies for, 1445, 1452b
    and ejaculatory dysfunction, 1450-1451
    epidemiology of, 1428
    epigenetic anomalies and, 1446
    and extratesticular endocrine dysfunction, 1448-1449
    and genetic syndromes, 1445-1446
    and genetics, 1433
    and genomic assessment, 1442-1443
    history of, 1428-1434, 1429t, 1434b
    and hypogonadotropic hypogonadism, 1447-1448
    imaging of, 1443-1445, 1445b
    and infections and inflammation, 1432
    laboratory evaluation of, 1436-1443, 1443b
    and microductal obstruction, 1447, 1447f
    and pediatric surgery, 1432
    physical examination of, 1434-1436, 1436b
    and pituitary dysfunction, 1447-1448
    and spermatogenic dysfunction, 1446
    and steroidogenic dysfunction, 1447
    structural chromosomal anomalies and, 1446
    and structural sperm abnormalities, 1451-1452
    testicular dysgenesis hypothesis, and childhood diseases, 1433

Infertility (Continued)
    testis histopathology and, 1445, 1445.e1f-1445.e2f, 1445.e2b
    vasography for, 1444
    venography for, 1444
  TGCT and, 1690
Infestation, as cutaneous disease of external genitalia, 1295-1296, 1296f-1297f
Infibulation, 987-988, 988f
Inflammation
  in BPS/IC etiology, 1232.e2-1232.e3, 1232.e3b
  in cancer immune response, 1336, 1338b
  pathways of, in benign prostatic hyperplasia, 3311, 3312f
  prostate cancer and, 3461, 3462f
  prostatitis and, 1207
  triggers for, 3477b
Inflammatory bowel disease, ammonium acid urate stones from, 2032
Inflammatory cell infiltration, in tubulointerstitial fibrosis, 787
Inflammatory myofibroblastic tumor (IMT), in pediatric patients, 1119
Inflammatory strictures, 1815
Informed consent, 115-118
  elements of, 117-118
  for erectile dysfunction, surgery for, 1582-1583, 1584b
  exception to, requirement, 118
    emergency situations, 118
    patients without decision-making capacity, 118
    pediatric patients, 118
  history of, 116-117
  quality of, 118
Infraumbilical, 135
Infundibulopelvic stenosis, 739-740, 740f
Inguinal canal, anatomy of, 2445-2447, 2448f
Inguinal hernia
  epidemiology and pathogenesis of, 889
  female, 988
  surgical repair of, 890-891
    complications with, 891
    laparoscopic, 891-892
    scrotal approach to, 891
    standard, 891
Inguinal incisions, in urologic surgery, 140-141
  inguinal ligament, incision above, 140-141, 141f
  and pelvic lymphadenectomy, in penile cancer, 141, 141f
Inguinal ligament, incision above, 140-141, 141f
Inguinal lymph nodes, 1386
  anatomy of, 1790, 1791f
Inguinal lymphadenectomy (ILND), 1753-1756
  in clinically negative groins
    DSNB, 1760-1761
    laparoscopic and robotic ILND, 1761
    modified complete ILND, 1761
    sentinel lymph node biopsy, 1760
    superficial inguinal node dissection, 1761
  complications of, 1801-1802
  indications for
    expectant management of, 1759-1760, 1760t
    modified procedures, 1760-1762
    traditional procedures, 1761-1762
    watchful waiting, 1759
  palpable adenopathy in selection for, 1753-1756
  for penile cancer
    immediate versus delayed, 1756
    indications for modified procedures, 1760-1762
    indications for traditional procedures, 1761-1762
    indications for watchful waiting, 1759
    molecular prognostic markers for, 1759, 1759t

Inguinal lymphadenectomy (ILND) (Continued)
    morbidity versus benefit, 1756-1757, 1756t, 1757f
    palpable adenopathy in selection for, 1753-1756
    prognostic significance of metastatic disease, 1753, 1754t-1755t
    tumor histology in selection for, 1757-1759, 1758t
  postoperative care after, 1801
    antibiotics for, 1801
    anticoagulation for, 1801
    bed rest in, 1801
    compressive dressings and stockings for, 1801
    dietary considerations of, 1801
    drainage, 1801
    prognostic significance of metastatic disease, 1753, 1754t-1755t
Inguinal node dissection, 1790-1803, 1803b
  anatomic considerations for
    inguinal anatomy, 1790-1791, 1791f
    penile lymphatics, 1790
    urethral lymphatics, 1790
  endoscopic anatomy of, 1791
  follow-up after, 1802-1803, 1802t
  imaging evaluation of, 1791-1792
  oncologic control after, 1802, 1802t
  patient before surgery, preparation of, 1800-1801
    antibiotics, 1800-1801
    anticoagulation, 1801
    bowel cleansing, 1801
  for penile cancer, 1792, 1792b
    nonpalpable inguinal adenopathy, 1792-1796
    palpable inguinal adenopathy or positive inguinal lymph nodes, 1796-1800
    surgical management of, 1792
Inguinal nodes
  palpable adenopathy in selection for, 1753-1756
  penile cancer metastasis to
    imaging studies for, 1747-1748
    risk-based management for, 1762-1765, 1763f-1764f
    treatment of, for penile cancer, 1753-1765, 1762b
  palpable adenopathy in selection for, 1753-1756
  prognostic significance of metastatic disease, 1753, 1754t-1755t
Inguinal orchiopexy, 966-967
Inherited genetic markers, as prostate cancer biomarkers, 3488-3489
Inhibin, 1390, 1391f
Inhibitors, of crystal formation, 2014-2015
Injection therapy
  for bladder neck reconstruction, 687
  for female stress urinary, in geriatric patients, 2920.e5
  for prostate, 3446-3447
Injuries, of bladder, 3054-3057, 3055b-3056b
INK4A gene (p16), in bladder cancer, 1350
Innate immune system, 1333-1334, 1334f-1335f, 1334t
  cytokines and chemokines, 1333-1334, 1335f, 1335t
Innervation
  of bladder, 2456
  of labium majus, 2436
  motor nerve, of bladder smooth muscle, 2465, 2465f, 2480, 2480f
  of pelvis
    female, 2433-2434
    male, 2447f-2448f, 2453, 2453f, 2453t, 2454b
  of vagina, 2438
Innominate bones, 2444

Inositol 1,4,5-trisphosphate (IP3), in ureteral contractions, 1885
In-oxine, 96
Insemination, intrauterine, 1445.e3
Insensible urinary incontinence (IUI), 2540, 2581
  overactive bladder and, 2637
  pathophysiology of, 2597
INSS. see International Neuroblastoma Staging System
Instillation therapy, 2220, 2221f
Institutional support, in transitional urology, 1045
Instrument development, 108
Instrumental activities of daily living (IADLs), of geriatric urology patient, 2909
Instrumentation, for visualization, 213, 213.e1f
Insufflant, for laparoscopic and robotic surgery, 220
Insufflation, for laparoscopic and robotic surgery, complications related to, 224-225
Insulin resistance, low urine pH and, 2027-2028
Insulin-like growth factor-3, 1392
Insulin-like growth factors (IGFs)
  in compensatory renal growth, 794-795
  in prostate cancer, 3463
Integral theory, 2596, 2597b, 2831
Integrated endoscopy systems, for laparoscopic surgery, 205-206, 205.e1f
Intensity-modulated radiation therapy, for prostate cancer, 3588-3589, 3589f, 3589t
Interaortocaval lymph nodes, 1372
Inter-α-trypsin, in crystal formation, 2015
Intercellular communication, penile erection and, 1500
Interference, of ultrasound waves, 71, 71f
Interferon alfa-2b (IFNs), for PD, 1612-1613, 1617t
Interferon-gamma release assays (IGRAs), for genitourinary tuberculosis, 1311
Interferons (IFNs)
  for clear cell RCC, 2329, 2329t
  for condylomata acuminata, 1742.e3
  for metastatic RCC, 2326, 2326f, 2327t
  for non-muscle-invasive bladder cancer, 3102-3103
  for RCC, 2178-2179
Interlabial masses, 395, 398b
Interleukin-2 (IL-2), for metastatic RCC, 2326, 2329-2331, 2330t
Interleukin-18 (IL-18), in tubulointerstitial fibrosis, 788
Interleukins, 1334, 1335f, 1335t
Interlobar arteries, 1869
Interlobular arteries, of kidney, 1869, 1870.e1f
Interlobular veins, of kidney, 1869-1870
Intermediate cells, of prostate, 3278f, 3279
Intermediate junctions, ureteral, 1877, 1883
Intermediate stratum, 2427, 2429f
Intermittent testicular torsion, 1855
Internal genitalia, male, development of, 1392, 1392f
Internal iliac arteries, 1873.e1f, 1874
Internal iliac lymph nodes, 1381
Internal iliac veins, 1381, 1874
Internal pudendal artery, 1381, 1807.e4f
Internal spermatic artery, 1393, 1394f
Internal sphincter
  male sphincteric mechanisms and, 2594
  urodynamic studies of, 2569
Internal urethrotomy, for urethral stricture disease, 1818
International Association for the Study of Pain, 448
International Classification of Vesicoureteral Reflux, 498t

International Consultation on Incontinence (ICI)
  Oxford guidelines
    for behavior therapy, 2722.e4b
    to facilitate bladder filling and urine storage, 2681t
  pelvic floor disorder questionnaires, 2531, 2532t-2533t
International Consultation on Incontinence Modular Questionnaire-male LUTS (ICIQ-MLUTS), 3344
International Consultation on Incontinence Questionnaire (ICIQ), 111t
International Consultation on Incontinence Questionnaire Bladder Diary (ICIQ-BD), 2541, 2541f
International Consultation on Incontinence Questionnaire Female Lower Urinary Symptoms (ICIQ-FLUTS), 111t
International Consultation on Incontinence Questionnaire Male Lower Urinary Tract Symptoms (ICIQ-MLUTS), 2541, 2541.e1f-2541.e2f
International Consultation on Incontinence Questionnaire Urinary Incontinence Short Form (ICIQ-UI-SF), 2541, 2542f
International Continence Society (ICS)
  classification of voiding dysfunction, 2517, 2521b
  nocturia definition of, 2664
  transient incontinence causes, 2525, 2526t
International Germ Cell Cancer Collaborative Group (IGCCCG), risk classification for advanced GCTs, 1690, 1691t
International Index of Erectile Function (IIEF), 112t
International Neuroblastoma Staging System (INSS), 1090t-1091t, 1091
International Prostate Symptom Score (IPSS), 4t-5t, 109, 110t
  for benign prostatic hyperplasia, 3344
  for male urinary incontinence, 2541
  for nocturia, 2664
  for pelvic floor disorders, 2531
International Reflux Study in Children, 515
International Society for Sexual Medicine, and Premature ejaculation, 1565-1567
  rationales for, 1567.e1-1567.e2
International Society of Urological Pathology, Gleason grading system, 3511
Interpolar calyx, 166
Interposition material, in urethrovaginal fistulae, 2951
Interrupted-shaped curve, 480
Interstitial cells
  bladder outlet obstruction and, 2506
  of detrusor muscle, 2477-2478, 2478f
Interstitial cystitis, female sexual dysfunction and, 1657
Interstitium, of testis, 1394-1396
  in testosterone synthesis, 1394
Interventional angiography, for priapism, 1560-1561, 1561f
Intestinal anastomoses, in urinary intestinal diversion, 3169-3184, 3184b
  abdominal stomas with, 3182-3183
  complications of, 3183-3184, 3186t
    flush, 3182-3183
    loop end ileostomy, 3183, 3183f
    nipple (rosebud), 3182, 3182f-3183f
  with biofragmentable ring, 3179
  complications of, 3179-3181
    bowel obstruction, 3180-3181, 3180t, 3181f
    fistulas, 3179-3180
    hemorrhage, 3181
    infection, 3180
    intestinal stenosis, 3181, 3181f
    pseudo-obstruction, 3181
    sepsis, 3180

Intestinal anastomoses, in urinary intestinal diversion (Continued)
    complications of isolated intestinal segment, 3181-3182
      intestinal stricture, 3181
      segment elongation, 3181-3182, 3182f
    compression, 3179
    laparoscopic and robotic, 3178-3179, 3178f-3179f
    stapled, 3176-3178
      ileal-ileal, 3177-3178, 3178f
      ileocolonic end-to-end, 3176, 3176f
      ileocolonic with circular device, 3177, 3177f
    types of, 3174-3176
      end-to-side ileocolic, 3175-3176, 3176f
      ileocolonic end-to-end, 3176, 3176f
      single-layer suture, 3175, 3175f
      two-layer suture, 3174-3175, 3175f
Intestinal antireflux valves, in urinary intestinal diversion, 3189-3191
    intussuscepted ileal valve, 3190-3191, 3191f
    intussuscepted ileocecal valve, 3189-3190, 3191f
    nipple valve, 3191, 3192f
Intestinal motility
    pneumoperitoneum effects on, 222
    urinary intestinal diversion and, 3203
Intestinal neobladders, pharmacologic therapy in, to facilitate bladder filling and urine storage, 2712-2713
Intestinal segments
    for antireflux procedure, 683-685
    in augmentation cystoplasty, 692
      effects of, 696-697
    neuromechanical aspects of, 3204-3205
    used in urinary diversion, minimally invasive, 3268
Intestinal stenosis, with intestinal anastomoses, 3181, 3181f
Intestinal stricture, with intestinal anastomoses, 3181
Intestinal tract abnormalities, with cloacal exstrophy, 575
Intimal fibroplasia, 1916, 1916f
Intra-abdominal pressure, for laparoscopic and robotic surgery, 220-221
Intra-abdominal vessels, injury of, during laparoscopic and robotic surgery, 226
Intracavernosal injection, in ED, 1534-1535, 1535f
Intracorporeal lithotripsy, 2109-2113
    ballistic lithotripsy, 2111-2112, 2112f
    combination ballistic and ultrasonic devices in, 2112-2113
    commonly used, 242t
    electrohydraulic lithotripsy, 2109-2110, 2110f
    laser lithotripsy, 2110-2111
    pneumatic, 243b
      basic physics of, 243
      for percutaneous nephrolithotomy, 243.e1
      tissue effects of, 243
      ureteroscopy with, 243.e1
    ultrasonic lithotripsy, 2112, 2112f
Intracorporeal neobladder, in minimally invasive urinary diversion, 3262-3273, 3263t
Intracranial aneurysms (ICAs), 752
Intradetrusor therapies, for BPS/IC treatment, 1245-1246
Intraductal carcinoma of the prostate (IDC-P), 3506
Intralabial masses, in female, 386
Intraluminal lithotripsy, ureteroscopic devices for, 197
    retropulsion prevention devices for, 198, 198f
    stone retrieval devices, 198
    ureteral access sheaths for, 199, 199f, 199t
Intramural ureter, tumor confined to, 2211-2212, 2213f, 2215f

Intraoperative consultation, 296-304, 298b
  bladder injury, 299-300, 303b
  decision making, 296-297, 297f
  documentation, 297-298
  ethical considerations, 296
    patient-physician relationship, 296
  placental cases, 303-304
  renal injury, 302-303
  ureteral injury, 300-302
  urethral injury, 298-299
Intraoperative floppy iris syndrome (IFIS), α1-adrenergic blockers and, 3370
Intraoperative management, in urologic surgery, 125-134
  anesthetic considerations, 130-132
  antibiotic prophylaxis, 127-128, 127b
  pain management, 134
  patient management, 125
  patient positioning, 126-127, 126b, 128b
  patient safety, 126
  skin preparation, 132-133
  transfusion considerations, 133
  venous thromboembolic prophylaxis, 128-130, 129t-131t, 131b
Intraoperative obturator nerve injury, 262
Intraoperative planning, 3596
Intraoperative urethral injury, 2883
Intraoperative vascular complications, 269-270
Intraperitoneal urine leak, in robotic prostatectomy, 3580
Intraprostatically injected drugs, to facilitate bladder filling and urine storage, 2713.e2-2713.e3
Intrarenal schwannoma, 2132
Intrarenal vasculature, 162-164, 163f
Intrascrotal pain, surgical management of, 1853-1855
Intratesticular varicocele, 901-902
Intratubular germ cell neoplasia (ITGCN), 1680
Intraurethral valve-pump, for women with impaired detrusor contractility, 2902-2903
Intrauterine insemination, 1445.e3, 1445.e3t
Intravaginal devices, for urinary incontinence, 2736-2737, 2736.e1f, 2737f, 2737.e1f
Intravaginal slingplasty, 2831, 2851
Intravascular volume management, for pheochromocytoma, 2379f, 2380
Intravenous general anesthesia, 132
Intravenous pyelography, 415, 806, 807f
  of ureteral injuries, 1995-1996, 1996f
Intravenous urography (IVU), 35, 36f
  for genitourinary tuberculosis diagnosis, 1312, 1312f-1313f
  for ureterovaginal fistula, 2929, 2944f
  for vesicovaginal fistula, 2929
Intravesical approach, for bladder diverticula, 3013-3015, 3013f-3014f
Intravesical chemotherapy, for non-muscle invasive bladder cancer, 3103-3105, 3104t, 3105b
  combination therapy, 3105
  doxorubicin, 3103-3104
  mitomycin C, 3104-3105
  novel agents, 3103
  to prevent implantation, 3103-3105
  thiotepa, 3103
  valrubicin, 3104
Intravesical electrotherapy (IVE), for detrusor underactivity, 2661-2662
Intravesical pressure, increasing
  external compression for, 2902-2903
    to facilitate bladder emptying, 2716-2718
    to facilitate bladder emptying, 2902-2903
  intraurethral valve-pump for women with impaired detrusor contractility, 2902-2903
  reflex contraction promotion or initiation, 2902
  stimulated myoplasty, 2903
Intravesical prostatic protrusion (IPP), 3348
Intravesical stimulation, 2747-2748

Intravesical therapies, for BPS/IC treatment, 1241t, 1244-1247, 1245b
  Clorpactin, 1244.e1
  DMSO, 1244
  glycosaminoglycans, 1244-1245
  intradetrusor therapies, 1245-1246
  silver nitrate, 1244.e1
Intrinsic apoptotic pathway, 1366.e1, 1366.e1f
Intrinsic kidney injury, 1923
Intrinsic renal disease, AKI due to, 1923
Intrinsic sphincter dysfunction, 2518
Intrinsic sphincteric deficiency (ISD), 2518
  causes of, 2595-2596
  midurethral sling for, outcomes of, 2859-2860
  quantification of, 2562
  sling procedure and, 2834
  stress urinary incontinence and, 2597, 2757
  urinary incontinence and, 2595-2596
Introitus, 1627.e1
Intubated ureterotomy, for ureteropelvic junction obstruction, 1961-1962, 1963f
Intussuscepted ileal valve, 3190-3191, 3191f
Intussuscepted ileocecal valve, 3189-3190, 3191f
Inverse treatment planning, 3588
Inverted papilloma, of bladder, 3081
Involuntary detrusor contractions (IDCs), 2560
Iodinated intravenous contrast agents, 292
Iodine-123 (^{123}I), 91
Iodine-124 (^{124}I), 91
Ion channels
  in detrusor muscle, 2474, 2474f
  in ED, 1499
Ionic transport, across bladder urothelium, 2469
Ionizing radiation, technique of, 403, 403b
IPE. see Index of Premature Ejaculation
Ipilimumab, 2146
  for RCC, 2332
IPP. see Intravesical prostatic protrusion
Ipsilateral vesicoureteral reflux, bladder diverticula with, 2971
IPSS. see International Prostate Symptom Score
I-QOL. see Incontinence Quality of Life Instrument
IRE. see Irreversible electroporation
Irinotecan, for penile cancer, 1770
Irreversible electroporation (IRE), 3628-3632, 3635f, 3636f
  for renal tumors, 2322
Irritable bowel syndrome (IBS), cross-organ sensitization in, 2486
Irritative lower urinary tract symptoms, patient history of, 3
Isaacs syndrome, lower urinary tract dysfunction and, 2630
Ischemic nephropathy, 1915, 1921-1935
Ischemic priapism, 1539, 1540f
  epidemiology and pathophysiology of, 1541-1545, 1543f
  penile implants in, 1596
Ischial spine, 2427, 2428f
Ischiococcygeus muscle, 2432f, 2434
Ischiorectal fossa, 2435
ISD. see Intrinsic sphincteric deficiency
ISI-P. see Incontinence Symptom Index
Island flaps, for urethral and penile reconstruction, 1807
Island onlay flap procedure (OIF), 924-925, 926f
Isoproterenol, ureteral response to, 1885, 1888
Isovolumetric pressure, 2659
ITGCN. see Intratubular germ cell neoplasia
IUI. see Insensible urinary incontinence
IV pyelography (IVP)
  of renal injuries, 1985, 1995-1996, 1996f
  for renal tumor evaluation, 2134
IVC. see Inferior vena cava
IVC filters, for vena caval thrombectomy, 2266-2267

IVE. see Intravesical electrotherapy
IVU. see Intravenous urography

J

Jaboulay (Winkelman) technique, 1845, 1847f
Jackson-Pratt drains, 148
Jehovah's Witnesses
  anesthesia preoperative considerations for, 448
  blood transfusion and, 133
Jejunal conduit, 3195-3196, 3196t
Jejunum, selection, 3162
JESS. see Joint Expert Speciation System
Joint Expert Speciation System (JESS), 2010
Justice, definition of, 115
Juvenile granulosa cell tumors, 1120-1121
Juvenile nephronophthisis, 747t, 755-756, 756f, 756b
  clinical features of, 755-756
  evaluation of, 756, 756f
  genetics of, 755
  treatment of, 756
Juvenile xanthogranuloma, 883
Juxtaglomerular cell tumor, 2132

K

K antigens, 429
Kalicinski plication technique, for megaureter in children, 851, 851f
Kaposi sarcoma (KS)
  HIV and, 1267-1268, 1298-1299, 1300f
  as neoplastic condition, 1298-1299, 1300f
  of penis, 1742.e5
Karnofsky Performance Scale (KPS), 107, 107t
Karyotype, for male infertility, 1442
Kaye nephrostomy tamponade balloon, 178f
KDIGO. see Kidney Disease: Improving Global Outcomes
Kegel's exercises, 2833
Kelly repair, for classic bladder exstrophy, 544
  continence outcomes with, 561
  technical aspects of, 549-550, 549f
Ketoconazole, 3677
Ketogenic diet, 449
Ketones, in urine, 19-20
Ketorolac, for urinary tract obstruction, 795
Kidney, 324f, 333-340, 333f-334f, 339b
  deterioration of, in urinary intestinal diversion, 3192-3193, 3193b
  early events in, 334
  molecular mechanisms of, 336
Kidney and retroperitoneum anterior approaches, 136-138, 138f, 139t
  Chevron and subcostal incision, 137-138, 139f
  thoracoabdominal incision, 136-137
Kidney cancer
  in geriatric patients, 2920.e13
  in nuclear medicine, 42
Kidney Disease: Improving Global Outcomes (KDIGO)
  AKI definition by, 1921, 1922t
  CKD classification by, 1927, 1928f
Kidney disease, nocturia and, 2665
Kidney infections, 1181b
  infectious granulomatous nephritis malacoplakia, 1179-1181, 1180f
  renal echinococcosis, 1181.e1, 1181.e2f
  XGP, 1177-1179, 1178f-1179f
  renal infection (bacterial nephritis), 1166-1181
    acute focal or multifocal bacterial nephritis, 1171.e1, 1171.e1f
    for acute pyelonephritis, 1168-1171, 1168f-1169f, 1170t
    bacterial "relapse,", 1177.e1
    chronic pyelonephritis, 1176-1177, 1177f
    emphysematous pyelonephritis, 1171-1172, 1171f
    infected hydronephrosis and pyonephrosis, 1174, 1174f

Kidney infections (Continued)
    pathology, 1166-1168, 1167f-1168f
    perinephric abscess, 1174-1176, 1175f
    renal abscess, 1172-1174, 1172f-1173f
Kidney surgery, 2248-2278, 2278b
  approaches used in, 2248-2253
    anterior, 2252-2253, 2253.e1f
    dorsal lumbotomy, 2251, 2251f
    flank, 2249-2251, 2249.e1f, 2250f-2251f, 2250.e1f, 2251.e1f
    thoracoabdominal, 2251-2252, 2252f-2253f, 2252.e1f
  for benign diseases, 2253-2257
    extracorporeal renal surgery, 2254-2257, 2256f
    open nephrectomy, 2254, 2254.e1f
    partial nephrectomy, 2254, 2255f
    simple nephrectomy, 2253-2254, 2253.e2f, 2254f
  historical perspective, 2248
  for malignancy, 2257-2278
    partial nephrectomy, 2261-2266, 2262f-2266f, 2263.e1f-2263.e2f, 2264.e1f
    radical nephrectomy, 2257-2261, 2257f-2260f, 2258.e1f, 2259.e1f, 2260.e1f
    vena caval thrombectomy. see Vena caval thrombectomy
  preoperative evaluation and preparation for, 2248, 2248.e1f, 2249f
  prophylactic measures, 2248
  surgical instruments, 2248
Kidneys, 1865-1872, 1868b
  AAST Organ Injury Severity Scale for, 1992t
  anatomy of, 1865-1876
    congenital anomalies in, 1869, 1869.e1f-1869.e2f
    gross and microscopic, 1866-1868, 1866.e1f-1866.e2f, 1867f
    innervation, 1872, 1872.e1f
    lymphatic drainage, 1870-1871, 1870.e1f
    radiologic, 1868-1869, 1868f, 1868.e1f, 1869b, 1869.e1f-1869.e2f
    surface anatomy and relationships, 1865-1866, 1865.e1f-1865.e4f, 1866f
    vasculature, 1869-1870, 1869.e2f-1869.e3f, 1870f-1871f, 1871b
  anatomy of, changes during pregnancy, 1185-1186, 1185t
  Ask-Upmark, 744, 744f
  cake or lump, 728f
  calcium absorption in, 2016
  collecting system of, 794
  cystic disease of, 741-775
  developing, pathological changes in, with urinary tract obstruction, 781-786
  disc, 728f
  drainage of, for urinary tract obstruction, 795
  ectopic
    inferior, 729
    superior, 728f, 729-731
  functional imaging of, 91-96
    ^{99}TC-MAG3 and ^{99m}TC-DTPA for, 92-93
    dosing and pharmacokinetics in, 92
    image acquisition and interpretation in, 92-93
    patient preparation for, 92
    relevant renal physiology of, 91-92
    Technetium-99m diethyltriaminepentaacetic acid (^{99m}TC-DTPA) for, 92
    Technetium-99m dimercaptosuccinic acid (^{99m}TC-DMSA) for, 92
    Technetium-99m mercaptoacetyltriglycine (^{99m}TC-MAG3) for, 92
  in genitourinary tuberculosis, 1308-1309
  growth regulation of, 783, 783t-784t
  horseshoe, 731-733, 733b
  localization, in UTI diagnosis, 1142.e1t, 1143
  L-shaped, 728f

Kidneys (Continued)
  mature, pathological changes in, with urinary tract obstruction, 781, 782f
  organoneogenesis of
    molecular mechanisms of, 721
    new advances in, 714-715
  physical examination for, 10-12, 10f
  in prune-belly syndrome, 581, 582f
  sigmoid, 728f
  size of, with spina bifida, 629
  solitary, upper urinary tract calculi and, 2089
  supernumerary, 721-722, 722f-723f
  thoracic, 725-727, 726f
  urine egress from, in urinary tract obstruction, 794
Kidney-ureter-bladder (KUB) radiograph, kidney anatomy, 1868
King's Health Questionnaire, 111t
Kinins, urethral function effects of, 1902
Kisspeptin protein, 1392
Klinefelter syndrome and variants, 1000
Klippel-Trénaunay-Weber syndrome, 888
"The Knack, 2725, 2725.e1t
Kocher maneuver, for radical nephrectomy, 2258, 2258f
Kock ileal reservoir, for orthoptic urinary diversion, 3243-3244, 3244f
Kock pouch, 3213-3215, 3214f
KPS. see Karnofsky Performance Scale
KS. see Kaposi sarcoma
KUL-7211, ureteral response to, 1888-1889

L

LABD. see Linear IgA bullous dermatosis
Labia majora, 1627.e1, 2435, 2436f-2437f
Labia minora, 1627.e1
Labial adhesions, 395, 396f, 986-987, 987f
Labioplasty, initial management, timing, and principles for, 1026, 1026f, 1028f-1029f
Labor, vesicovaginal fistulae with, 2925
Lactate dehydrogenase (LDH)
  in prostatic secretions, 3302
  in TGCTs, 1686
Lamina propria, 2462-2463
Laminectomy, LUT function and, 2620
Laparoendoscopic single-site surgery (LESS), 458, 466, 2419-2420
  access devices for, 212
  Boari flap, 3031
  instrumentation for, 218
  for kidney surgery
    clinical experience of, 2305-2306, 2305f
    robotic, 2306
    surgical approaches and access for, 2284-2285, 2285f, 2286t
  pyeloplasty, for ureteropelvic junction obstruction, 1956-1957, 1957f
Laparoscopes, for laparoscopic and robotic surgery, 213, 213.e1f
Laparoscopic adrenalectomy, 2407-2409, 2407b
  left, 2414-2415, 2415f-2416f, 2417-2418
  outcomes, 2421-2423
  retroperitoneal approach, 2417-2418, 2418f, 2422
  right, 2415-2416, 2417f-2418f, 2418
  transperitoneal approach, 2414-2417, 2415f-2417f, 2422
Laparoscopic and robotic surgery, in children
  acid-base physiology during, 461
  advantages in postoperative pain control after, 459
  approach to, 465, 465b
    retroperitoneal, 465
    transperitoneal, 465
    vesicoscopic, 465
  cardiovascular changes during, 460
  comparative effectiveness of access technique for, 465

Laparoscopic and robotic surgery, in children (Continued)
  equipment and instrumentation for, 465-467, 468b
    clips, 467
    hemostatic devices, 466
    laparoscopic ports, 465-466
    robotic-assisted surgery, 467
    single-site surgery, 466
    staplers, 466
    suture assistance, 467
  intracranial pressure during, 461
  learning curves for, 460
  minimally invasive surgery, 458-460
  open access for, 464, 464f
  pneumoperitoneum during
    physiology of, 460-461, 462b
    stress response to, 461
  principles of, 458-472
  pulmonary changes during, 460-461
  renal physiology during, 461
  Veress needle access for, 463, 464f
  visual obturator access for, 464-465
Laparoscopic calicovesicostomy, for ureteropelvic junction obstruction, 1960
Laparoscopic carts, 205, 205.e1f
Laparoscopic colposuspension, 2759
Laparoscopic dismembered tubularized flap pyeloplasty, for ureteropelvic junction obstruction, 1960
Laparoscopic heminephrectomy, 2299
Laparoscopic hysterectomy, ureteral injuries after, 1993
Laparoscopic ILND, for penile cancer, 1761
Laparoscopic kidney surgery, 2279-2308, 2308b
  ablative techniques, 2304-2305, 2318
  biopsy for medical renal disease, 2292, 2292f
  calyceal diverticulectomy, 2294
  complications of, 2306-2308, 2307f
  laparoendoscopic single-site surgery
    clinical experience of, 2305-2306, 2305f
    robotic, 2306
    surgical approaches and access for, 2284-2285, 2285f, 2286t
  nephrolysis, 2294, 2294f
  nephropexy, 2292-2294, 2293f
    procedure for, 2293f
    results of, 2293-2294
  partial nephrectomy. see Laparoscopic partial nephrectomy
  patient evaluation and preparation for, 2279
  radical nephrectomy. see Laparoscopic radical nephrectomy
  for renal cystic disease, 2291-2292, 2291f
    procedure for, 2291, 2291f
    results of, 2291-2292
  simple nephrectomy, 2285-2291
    dissection of ureter, 2287, 2287f
    identification of renal hilum, 2287-2288, 2288f
    organ entrapment and extraction, 2289, 2289f-2290f
    postoperative management for, 2289
    reflection of colon, 2285-2286, 2287f
    results of, 2291
    securing of renal blood vessels, 2288, 2288f
    upper pole dissection, 2288, 2288f
  surgical approaches and access for, 2279-2285
    hand-assisted laparoscopy, 2281-2282, 2283f
    laparoendoscopic single-site surgery and natural orifice transluminal endoscopic surgery, 2284-2285, 2285f, 2286t
    retroperitoneal, 2279-2281, 2282f
    robotic-assisted laparoscopy, 2282-2284, 2284f-2285f
    transperitoneal, 2279, 2280f-2281f

Laparoscopic live-donor nephrectomy, 270
Laparoscopic partial nephrectomy (LPN), 2298-2304
  indications for, 2298-2300, 2299f
    central and hilar tumors, 2299
    clinical stage T1b and greater tumors, 2299
    laparoscopic heminephrectomy, 2299
    multiple tumor management, 2300
    repeat, 2300
    tumors in solitary kidneys, 2299-2300
  positive surgical margins in, 2304
  procedure for, 2300-2304
    collecting system repair, 2302, 2303f
    hemostasis, 2301-2302, 2302f
    renal hypothermia, 2302
    retroperitoneal approach, 2300
    robotic-assisted, 2300
    transperitoneal approach, 2300
    tumor localization and excision, 2300-2301, 2301f
    warm ischemia and hilar control, 2303-2304
  results of, 2304
Laparoscopic Prostatectomy Robot Open (LAPPRO) study, 3581
Laparoscopic pyelolithotomy, for pediatric kidney stone disease, 868-870
Laparoscopic pyeloplasty
  technique of, 832-834, 833f
  for ureteropelvic junction obstruction
    anterior extraperitoneal approach to, 1956
    in children, 830-834, 833f-834f
    with concomitant pyelolithotomy, 1958-1960
    dismembered tubularized flap for, 1960
    indications and contraindications for, 1955
    results of, 1957-1958, 1959t
    retroperitoneal approach to, 1956
    robotic-assisted, 1956, 1957f
    single-site surgery approach, 1956-1957
    techniques for, 1955-1957
    transmesenteric modification of transperitoneal approach to, 1956
    transperitoneal approach to, 1955-1956, 1955f
    vascular transposition for, 1956
Laparoscopic radical nephrectomy (LRN), 2294-2298
  hand-assisted, 2296-2297, 2296f
  retroperitoneal approach to, 2295-2296
  special considerations for, 2297-2298
    cytoreductive nephrectomy, 2298
    en bloc hilar vessel stapling, 2297
    large tumors, 2297
    local recurrence, 2298, 2298f
    lymphadenectomy, 2297-2298
    port-site recurrence, 2297
    renal vein and caval tumor thrombus, 2298
    specimen extraction, 2297
    surgical salvage after failed ablative therapies, 2298
    tumor seeding, 2297
  transperitoneal approach to, 2294-2295, 2295f
Laparoscopic radical nephroureterectomy, for UTUC, 2202-2205
  indications of, 2202
  results of, 2205
  robot-assisted, 2205, 2205f
  transperitoneal laparoscopic nephroureterectomy, 2203-2204, 2203f-2204f
Laparoscopic radical prostatectomy (LRP)
  abdominal access in, 3570, 3571f
  anesthesia for, 3568-3570
  apical dissection, 3576-3577, 3577f
  bladder neck in, identification and transection of, 3573, 3573f
  bladder neck reconstruction, 3577
  blood loss/transfusion with, 3580
  bowel preparation for, 3567

Laparoscopic radical prostatectomy (LRP) (Continued)
  contraindications for, 3566-3567
  deep dorsal venous complex litigation in, 3572-3573, 3573f
  evolution of, 3566
  extraperitoneal approach to, 3570-3571, 3571f
    transperitoneal approach versus, 3571
  hospital stay with, 3581
  indications for, 3566-3567
  informed consent for, 3567-3568
  instrumentation for, 3567, 3568b, 3570b
  insufflation in, 3570, 3571f
  intraoperative inspection of prostate, 3577
  neurovascular bundle preservation in, 3575-3576, 3575f-3576f
  operating room personnel for, 3568, 3569f
  outcomes with, functional, 3581-3583
  pain management, 3578-3579
  patient positioning for, 3568, 3569f
  patient selection for, 3566-3567, 3570b
  postoperative complications of, 3580-3581
  postoperative management for, 3578-3580
  preoperative preparation for, 3567-3570, 3570b
  prostate and rectum plane development in, 3574-3575, 3574f
  prostatic pedicle control in, 3575, 3575f
  return to normal activity, 3579
  robotic-assisted versus, 3570
  role of continence physiotherapy in, 3579
  seminal vesicle dissection in, 3573-3574, 3574f
  space of Retzius development for, 3571-3572, 3572f
  specimens
    delivery in, 3578
    entrapment in, 3577
  technique of, 3578b
  transperitoneal approach to, 3570
    extraperitoneal approach versus, 3571
  trocar placement in, 3570, 3571f
  vasa deferentia dissection in, 3573-3574, 3574f
  vesicourethral anastomosis, 3577-3578, 3578f
  posterior support of, 3577, 3578f
Laparoscopic removal, of kidney down to mid-ureter, 2203-2204, 2203f-2204f
Laparoscopic retroperitoneal lymph node dissection, for testicular tumors, 1734-1741, 1741b
  bilateral, 1738
  complications of, 1739-1740, 1739t
  duplication of, 1735
  postoperative care after, 1738-1739
  prospective nerve-sparing techniques for, 1739
  rationale and evolution of, 1734
  results and current status of, 1740-1741, 1740t
  staging, 1734-1735
  surgical technique for, 1735-1738
    approach for, 1735
    left-sided dissection, 1736-1738
    patient positioning and port placement for, 1735-1736, 1735f-1736f
    right-sided dissection, 1736, 1736f
Laparoscopic retropubic suspension surgery, 2768-2769, 2769b
Laparoscopic sacrocolpopexy, for apical pelvic organ prolapse repair, 2802f-2803f, 2803-2804
Laparoscopic surgery, 145
  access technology for hand-assist devices, 212, 212f
    trocars, 211, 211f
  common urologic procedures, antimicrobial prophylaxis for, 1199-1200

Laparoscopic surgery (Continued)
  complications and troubleshooting, 223-231, 232b
    anesthesia-related, 228
    early postoperative, 230-231
    equipment-related, 223-224
    exit-related, 230
    late postoperative, 231
    during learning curve, 223
    pneumoperitoneum-related, 224
    of seminal vesicle surgery, 1864
  equipment placement for, 205-207, 205.e1f
  instrumentation used in
    for da Vinci Robotic System, 218, 218f
    for grasping and blunt dissection, 218
    for incising and hemostasis, 214-215
    for LESS, 218
    for morcellation, 218
    for NOTES, 218
    for port site closure, 219
    for retraction, 218
    for specimen entrapment, 217-218, 217f
    for stapling and clipping, 216-217, 216f
    surgical pharmaceuticals, 215
    for suturing and tissue anastomosis, 215-216, 215.e2f
    for visualization, 213, 213.e1f
  operative team placement for
    retroperitoneal upper abdominal procedures, 207, 207f
    transperitoneal upper abdominal procedures, 206, 206f
  for partial nephrectomy, 811-813, 814f
  physiologic considerations in, 223b
    hemodynamic effects related to approach and patient position, 222
    hormonal and metabolic effects during surgery, 222-223
    immunologic effects, 223
    insufflant choice, 220
    pneumoperitoneum pressure choice, 220
  preoperative preparation for, 204b
    blood products, 204
    bowel preparation, 204
    operating room setup, 205, 205b
    patient positioning, 205f
    patient selection and contraindications, 203-204
    prophylaxis, 205
  procedure for, 219b
    abdomen exit, 218-219
    achieving extraperitoneal access and developing extraperitoneal space, 210-211
    achieving retroperitoneal access and developing retroperitoneal space, 209-210
    achieving transperitoneal access and establishing pneumoperitoneum, 209
    hand-assist device placement, 212
    initial incision, 207
    port removal and fascial closure, 218-219
    port site closure, 219
    skin closure, 219
    trocar placement, 212-213
  training and practicing for, 231-233
    equipment for, 232
    formal programs for, 233
  ureteral injuries with, 1993
Laparoscopic training boxes, 232, 232f, 232.e1f
Laparoscopic ureterocalicostomy, for ureteropelvic junction obstruction, 1958
Laparoscopic ureterolysis, for retroperitoneal fibrosis, 1980
Laparoscopic ureteroneocystostomy, for ureteral stricture disease, 1972, 1972f
  with Boari flap, 1973
  with psoas hitch, 1972-1973
Laparoscopic ureteroureterostomy, for ureteral stricture disease, 1972

Lapides classification, of voiding dysfunction, 2522-2523, 2522b
Lapides Diagnostic Foley catheter, 154
Lapra-Ty clips, 215, 215f
Laser ablation, for penile cancer, 1752
Laser cystolithotripsy, 244.e4
Laser instrumentation
    for laparoscopic and robotic surgery, 214
    for tissue dissection and cauterization
        CO2 laser, 241
        delivery systems for, 238-241
        diode laser, 240
        Ho:YAG laser, 240
        KTP laser, 239
        LBO laser, 239-240
        light-tissue interaction, 238-239
        Nd:YAG laser, 239
        pulsed and continuous wave lasers, 238
        soft tissue applications, 238-241
        Thu:YAG laser, 240-241
Laser lithotripsy, 2110-2111
    Ho:YAG and Er:YAG, basic physics of, 244
Laser treatments, for benign prostatic hyperplasia, 3435-3438, 3443b
    safety for, 3435-3436
Lasers, for urethral stricture disease, 1818-1828
Late-night salivary cortisol, in evaluation of adrenal masses, 2400
Late relapse RPLND, 1728t, 1729
Latent pacemakers, ureteral, 1882
Latent stress incontinence, 2563
Latent syphilis, 1257-1258
Lateral cutaneous nerve, 136f
Lateral decubitus position, 146
Lateral defect, in pelvic floor support mechanism, 2597-2598
Lateral fusion abnormalities, 985-986, 985f
    inguinal hernias, 988
    rhabdomyosarcoma, 986, 986f
    uterus and cervix duplication, 985-986, 986f
Lateral plexuses, 2452
Lateral resolution, of ultrasonography images, 70, 70f
Lax suspensory ligament, penile implants and, 1596, 1596f
Laxative abuse, ammonium acid urate stones from, 2032
LDH. see Lactate dehydrogenase
Le Duc technique, in urinary diversion, 3189, 3189f
Leadbetter and Clarke technique, in urinary diversion, 3185, 3185f, 3186t
Lead-time bias, 102, 103f
Leak point pressures, urodynamic studies of, 2561-2563
    abdominal, 2561, 2562f
    detrusor, 2561f, 2562
Left adrenalectomy
    laparoscopic, 2414-2415, 2415f-2416f, 2417-2418
    open, 2412-2413, 2412f-2413f
Leiomyoma
    bladder, 3038, 3039f
    renal, 2131, 2131f, 2131b
    of urethra, 1776
Leiomyosarcoma
    of kidney, 2181
    retroperitoneal tumors and, 2231, 2231f
Length-time bias, 103, 103f
Lentigo simplex, 1304, 1305f
Lenvatinib, for RCC, 2337-2338
Leptin, 1392
    in prostate cancer, 3463
Lesion
    measurable, 104
    target, 104-105
LESS. see Laparoendoscopic single-site surgery
Leucine aminopeptidase, in prostatic secretions, 3302

Leukemia
    of kidney, 2181-2183, 2182t
    testicular metastases of, 1124-1125, 1709
Leukocyte esterase, 437
    in urine, 20-21, 20f
Leukoplakia, of bladder, 3082
Levator ani muscle, 2430-2432, 2432f
    complex, 2597
Levator plate, 2430-2432, 2432f
Leydig cell aplasia, 1011
Leydig cell tumors, 1124, 1124f, 1707-1708
Leydig cells, 305, 1370
    testis cytoarchitecture and, 1394
    testosterone production by, 3280-3281
    testosterone synthesis in, 1394
        control of, 1395-1396
LGPIN. see Low-grade prostatic intraepithelial neoplasia
LGV. see Lymphogranuloma venereum
LH. see Luteinizing hormone
Libido, loss of
    hormonal therapy and, 3681
    patient history of, 6
Lichen nitidus (LN), as papulosquamous disorder, 1281
Lichen planus (LP), as papulosquamous disorder, 1280-1281, 1281f
Lichen sclerosus (LS)
    male, 1742.e1-1742.e2
        reconstructive surgery for, 1808-1810, 1809f
    as papulosquamous disorder, 1281-1282, 1282f
Lichen sclerosus et atrophicus, in male, circumcision and, 875, 876f
Lidocaine, for cystourethroscopy, 189-190
Lifestyle modifications
    for ED, 1529
    for urinary incontinence, 2732-2734
        bowel function, 2734
        caffeine reduction, 2733
        dietary irritants, 2733-2734
        fluid management, 2732-2733
        levels of evidence and recommendations, 2722.e1b
        obesity and weight reduction, 2734
Ligaments, of female pelvis, 2428-2430, 2430f-2432f
Ligand-binding domain, of androgen receptors, 3290-3291
LigaSure device, 466
LigaSure vessel-sealing system, 214
Ligation, of ureter, 2000-2001, 2001f
Light-tissue interaction, 238-239, 239f
Likelihood ratio (LR), 3479-3480
Likert scales, 108-109
Linea alba, 2444, 2447f-2448f
Linear IgA bullous dermatosis (LABD), 1285, 1285f
Linear-quadratic formula, 3593
Lipomeningocele, 639-641, 642b
    pathogenesis of, 639-641, 641f
    presentation of, 639, 639t, 640f-641f
    recommendations for, 641, 642f
Lipopolysaccharide (LPS), 1138
Liposarcoma
    of kidney, 2181
    retroperitoneal tumors and, 2229-2230, 2230f
    of testicular adnexa, 1709
Lipotoxicity, 2028-2029
Lithium triborate (LBO) laser, 239-240
LithoClast Ultra, 244-245
Lithotomy position, 146
Lithotripsy
    dual-modality, 244-246, 245f
    holmium:YAG and Erbium: YAG laser, 244

Lithotripsy (Continued)
    intracorporeal, 2109-2113
        ballistic lithotripsy, 2111-2112, 2112f
        combination ballistic and ultrasonic devices in, 2112-2113
        electrohydraulic lithotripsy, 2109-2110, 2110f
        laser lithotripsy, 2110-2111
        ultrasonic lithotripsy, 2112, 2112f
    pneumatic, 243, 243b
        basic physics of, 243
        tissue effects, 243
    ultrasonic, 243, 244b
        basic physics of, 243
        tissue effects of, 243
Live animal models, laparoscopic training with, 232
Liver cirrhosis, benign prostatic hyperplasia and, 3322
Liver injury, during radical nephrectomy, 2261
LN. see Lichen nitidus
Localization, in UTI diagnosis, 1142.e1t, 1143
Localized prostate cancer
    active management strategies for, 3522-3536
    androgen deprivation therapy for, 3683-3684
    host evaluation of, 3522-3529
        bladder function, 3524
        bowel function and other conditions affecting treatment choice, 3525
        longevity assessment and competing risks for mortality, 3522-3524, 3523f
        patient preference and biases, 3525
        sexual function, 3524-3525
    patient counseling of, 3532-3535, 3532f
        observation versus active treatment, 3532-3534, 3533t-3534t
        partial gland versus whole gland treatment, 3534-3535
        surgery versus radiation versus whole-gland ablation, 3535
        treatment delivery type, 3535
    risk assessment of, 3525-3529
        Epstein criteria, 3526-3527
        genomic tests for risk stratification, 3529
        Gleason scoring and grade groups, 3526
        low, intermediate, and high risk definition, 3525-3526, 3526t
        nomograms for prediction of stage, 3527-3528
        prostate magnetic resonance imaging in, 3528-3529
        staging, 3527
        stratification nomograms, 3528, 3528f
        tools for risk stratification, 3525
    treatment selection of, 3529-3532
        comparative population-based studies, 3529-3531, 3530f
        functional outcomes, 3531-3532
        oncologic outcomes, 3529-3532
Locally advanced prostate cancer
    androgen deprivation for, 3655-3656, 3656b
        intermittent, 3656
        quality of life, 3656
    clinical trials for, 3657, 3657t-3658t
    contemporary risk assessment for, 3640-3641, 3640b
    definition of, 3640-3643
    focal ablative therapy for, 3655
        cryoablation, 3655
        high-intensity focused ultrasound, 3655
    imaging modalities for, 3641-3642, 3641f-3642f
    immediate versus delayed ADT in, 3684
    incidence trends of, 3643-3644, 3643b
    management of delayed sequelae, 3657
    natural history of, 3644-3645, 3645f, 3645t
    novel markers for, 3642-3643, 3642t

Locally advanced prostate cancer *(Continued)*
  radiation therapy for, 3652–3655, 3653*t*
    adjuvant androgen deprivation with, 3653–3654
    chemotherapy with, 3654–3655
    neoadjuvant androgen deprivation with, 3652–3653, 3654*b*
  radical prostatectomy for, 3645–3652, 3648*b*
    adjuvant androgen deprivation with, 3652
    adjuvant radiation therapy, 3650–3652, 3651*t*, 3652*b*
    for clinical stage T3, 3645–3652, 3646*t*
    neoadjuvant androgen deprivation, 3648–3649, 3648*t*–3649*t*
    neoadjuvant chemotherapy and chemotherapy-hormonal therapy, 3649–3650, 3650*t*
    outcomes of, 3646–3647, 3647*f*
    pathologic findings in, 3643, 3643*t*
  treatment, 3640–3658
  trends of, 3643–3644, 3643*b*, 3644*f*
LOCM. *see* Low-osmolality contrast media
Loop diuretics, in stone formation, 2033
  surgical management of, 2077.e3
Loop end ileostomy, 3183, 3183*f*
Loopography, 38, 39*f*
Lord plication, 1845, 1847*f*
Lost stone, in ureteroscopic stone management, 2109
Low-dose continuous prophylaxis, for recurrent UTIs, 1162–1163
Low-dose rate brachytherapy, 1765–1767
  for prostate cancer, 3596, 3597*f*
Lower extremity compartment syndrome, 262, 263*f*
Lower motor neuron (LMN) lesion, voiding dysfunction after, 2522, 2523*b*
Lower pole renal calculi, surgical management of, 2081–2084, 2081*f*, 2082*t*, 2083*f*
Lower tract endoscopy
  antimicrobial prophylaxis for, 1198
  cystoscopy, antimicrobial prophylaxis for, 1198
Lower tract urinary complications, 267–269
  bladder injuries, 267
  urine leaks, after radical prostatectomy, 267–269, 268*f*–269*f*
Lower urinary system, aging and, 2906
Lower urinary tract, assessment of, 503–505
  cystographic imaging, 503–504, 504*f*
  cystoscopy and the positioning of the instillation of contrast cystogram, 504–505
Lower urinary tract (LUT)
  afferent pathways in, 2481–2486, 2487*b*
    cannabinoids, 2486
    functional properties of, 2482–2483, 2483*f*
    modulators of, 2483–2484
    nitric oxide in, 2484, 2484*f*
    pelvic organ interactions with, 2486, 2486*f*
    properties of, 2481
    purinergic signaling, 2484–2485, 2485*f*
    spinal cord pathways of, 2481–2482, 2481*t*, 2482*f*
    transient receptor potential cation channels, 2485
  anatomy of, 2461, 2462*f*
    bladder. *see* Bladder, anatomy of
    urethra. *see* Urethra, anatomy of
  efferent pathways of, 2487–2493, 2487*f*, 2489*f*–2492*f*, 2490*b*, 2491*t*
  electrical stimulation of, techniques of, 2747–2754
    dorsal genital nerve, 2752
    intravesical, 2747–2748
    percutaneous tibial nerve, 2748–2751, 2749*f*
    pudendal nerve, 2751–2752
    sacral nerve, 2752–2754
    transcutaneous, 2748

Lower urinary tract (LUT) *(Continued)*
  function of, 2679
    mechanisms underlying two phases of, 2514
    normal, 2514–2516
    sensory aspects of, 2516
    two-phase concept of, 2514–2516
  neural control of, 2480–2497, 2593
    parasympathetic pathways, 2480, 2480*f*
    peripheral nervous system, 2480–2497, 2480*f*
    somatic pathways, 2480*f*–2481*f*, 2481
    supraspinal pathways, 2493–2497, 2495*f*–2496*f*
    sympathetic pathways, 2480, 2480*f*
  overview of, 2580
  pharmacology of, 2497–2503
    adrenergic mechanisms, 2500–2501, 2501*f*, 2501*b*
    afferent neuropeptides, 2501–2502, 2501*t*
    muscarinic mechanisms, 2497–2500, 2499*t*, 2500*b*
    sex steroids, 2502–2503
    urethral tone in women, 2501
  posterior urethral valves and, 603–604, 605*f*–606*f*
  supraspinal pathways in, 2493–2497
    additional regions in, 2496–2497
    bladder modulatory mechanisms, 2493–2494, 2495*f*
    brain-bladder control model, 2497, 2498*f*
    central circuitry regulation of, 2494–2495
    cerebral control of voiding, 2496
    human brain imaging studies in, 2496, 2496*f*
    modulators in, 2495–2496
    neurotransmitters in, 2495–2496
    pontine micturition center, 2493–2494, 2495*f*
  transabdominal pelvic ultrasonography of, 80–81, 80*f*, 82*f*
  trauma and, 2527
Lower urinary tract calculi, 2114–2120, 2120*b*
  bladder calculi
    after renal transplantation, 2117
    bladder outlet obstruction with bladder lithiasis, 2115–2116
    etiopathogenesis of, 2114–2115
    in patients with spinal cord injury, 2116–2117
    in urinary diversions and augmented bladder, 2116
  bladder stones
    endourologic approach to, 2115, 2116*f*
    management of, 2115
    open surgery for, 2115
    presentation of, 2115
  history of, 2114
  in special situations, 2115–2117
  unusual, 2118–2120
    preputial calculi, 2118–2119
    prostatic calculi, 2119–2120, 2119*f*
  urethral calculi, 2117–2120
    clinical presentation and evaluation of, 2117–2118
    pathogenesis and composition of, 2117
    primary, 2117
    treatment of, 2118, 2119*f*
Lower urinary tract catheterization, 152–159, 159*b*
  complications of, 158–159
    erosion, 159
    iatrogenic trauma, 159
    infection, 158–159, 159*b*
    malignancy, 159
    stricture, 159
  contraindications of, 152
  diagnostic, 152
  difficulty with, 156–158, 158*f*
    abnormal anatomy, 157–158
    artificial urinary sphincter, 158

Lower urinary tract catheterization *(Continued)*
    bladder neck reconstruction, 158
    bladder replacement, 157
    continent urinary reservoir, 157–158
    obesity, 157
    posterior urethral valves, 157
    prostatic obstruction, 156–157
    reconstruction of, 157
    urethral stricture, 157
    urethral trauma, 157
    urinary conduit, 158
  indications for, 152, 155*b*
  technique of, 152–155
  therapeutic, 152
  types of, 153–155
Lower urinary tract complications, 1939–1940
  benign prostatic hyperplasia, 1939
  transplant, small bladder after, 1939
  urine incontinence, 1939–1940
  voiding dysfunction, 1939
Lower urinary tract dysfunction (LUTD), 2503–2512. *see also* Urinary incontinence; Voiding dysfunction
  aging and, 2509–2510, 2510*b*
  bladder outlet obstruction, 2505–2506, 2506*b*
  bladder pain syndrome and interstitial cystitis, 2507–2509, 2509*b*
  bowel dysfunction, 654
  bowel function, 473–474
  in children, 473–488
  clinical aids, 474–475
  clinical evaluation of, 473–479
  detrusor underactivity and, 2651–2652
  evaluation strategies for specific, 486–488
    anorectal malformations, 487
    cerebral palsy, 487
    non-neurogenic, 486–487
    pelvic tumors, 487
    posterior urethral valves, 487
    sacral agenesis, 487
    spinal cord injury, 487
    spinal dysraphism, 487
    transverse myelitis, 488
  and female sexual dysfunction, 1654–1655, 1657*b*
    clinical signs and investigations for, 1655
    epidemiology of, 1654
    etiology and classification of, 1654–1655
    links and treatments, 1655–1657
    self-image/body image connected to, 1657
    sexual lifestyle and communication and, 1654–1655, 1654*t*
  future research for, 2512–2513
  genitourinary malignancies, 2920
  history of, 473–477, 479*b*
  idiopathic detrusor overactivity, 2504
  infections, 475–476
  laboratory testing, 479–480
    additional, 479–480
    urinalysis, 479, 480*b*
    urine culture, 479
  neurologic diseases and
    acute disseminated encephalomyelitis, 2625–2626
    AIDS, 2625
    hereditary spastic paraplegia, 2624–2625
    Lyme disease, 2624
    reflex sympathetic dystrophy, 2626
    schistosomal myelopathy, 2626
    syringomyelia, 2626
    systemic lupus erythematosus, 2626
    tropical spastic paraparesis, 2625
    tuberculosis, 2626–2627
  neurologic function, 476
  neuromodulation, 2510–2512
    to inhibit OAB, rationale for, 2511, 2511*f*
    inhibitory and excitatory stimulation frequencies, 2511
    onabotulinumtoxinA, 2512
    pudendal nerve stimulation, 2511
    sacral, mechanism of action, 2510

Lower urinary tract dysfunction (LUTD) (Continued)
  somatic afferents activation, in foot, 2511-2512
  for voiding, rationale for, 2510, 2510f
  nocturia, 2505
  overactive bladder, 2504
  pathophysiology and classification of, 2514-2524
  pediatric, 652
    clinical significance of, 652
    comorbidities with, 653-654, 655b
    epidemiology of, 652, 655b
    giggle incontinence, 658-660
    pollakiuria, 660
    quality-of-life and, 652-653, 655b
    self-esteem and, 652-653
    terminology of, 654-655
    underactive bladder, 660
    urinary incontinence and, 655-660, 660b
    vaginal reflux, 660
  physical examination, 477-479, 479b
    abdominal, 478
    of female, 479
    genital, 478-479
    of male, 479
    neurologic examination, 477-478, 478f, 478t
    vital signs, 477
  psychological associations with, 654
  signs and symptoms of, 2580
  spinal cord injury and neurogenic detrusor overactivity, 2504-2505
  storage symptoms of, 473
  stress urinary incontinence, 2504
  terminology of, 2580-2581, 2581t
  urinary tract infections and, 653
  urodynamic evaluation, 480-486, 486b
    formal, 483-486
    frequency, 486
    interpretation of studies, 485-486
    noninvasive testing, 480-483, 483b
    patch electromyography, 483
    in pediatric setting, 485
    pelvic ultrasonography, 482-483, 482f
    unique considerations in pediatric, 484-485
    uroflowmetry, 480-481
    video, 485
  validated questionnaires, 476-477
  vesicoureteral reflux and, 653-654
  voiding symptoms of, 473, 474f
Lower urinary tract obstruction, 375-377, 376f-377f, 384
  congenital megacystis, 376-377
  posterior urethral valve, 375, 377f
  prune belly syndrome/megalourethra, 375
  recommendations for, 377, 377f
  urethral stenosis/atresia, 376
Lower urinary tract symptoms (LUTS), 109
  with acute urinary retention, 3337-3338, 3338t
  aging and, 2643
  benign prostatic hyperplasia in, 3305, 3306f
  bias associated with trials on medical treatment of, 3355
    adverse events, 3355
    sample size, 3355
  classification of, 2540t
  clinical end points of, 3354
  clinical indications for, 3354
  in detrusor underactivity, 2650, 2651f
  drugs used in treatment of, 2682t, 2708b
  management of, 3351-3371, 3353b
    conservative, 3351, 3352f-3353f
    lifestyle and dietary modifications, 3351-3353
    watchful waiting, 3351

Lower urinary tract symptoms (LUTS) (Continued)
  medical therapy of, 3353-3354
    impact and trends of, 3354
  metabolic syndrome and, 1421
  outcome measures for, 3354-3355
  with Parkinson disease, 2605
  patient history of, 3-6, 4t-5t
  practical flowchart for evaluation of patients with, 3349-3351, 3349f-3350f
  prevalence of, 2650, 2681
  prognosis of patients receiving medical treatment for, 3399-3400, 3399b
  questionnaires for, 2532t-2533t
  related to overactive bladder, 2638-2639
  result of, 2681
  review of literature on currently approved α_1-blockers for treatment of, 3357-3367
    alfuzosin, 3361-3363, 3362f
    doxazosin, 3359-3361, 3360t-3361t
    naftopidil, 3365-3367, 3367t
    silodosin, 3365, 3365f, 3366t
    tamsulosin, 3363-3365, 3363f, 3364t
    terazosin, 3357-3359, 3357t-3358t, 3359f
  symptoms of, 3354
  terminology of, 2580-2581, 2581t
  urodynamic observations of, 2580
  urodynamic studies of, 2550-2579
    evidence-based review of, 2574-2578
  videourodynamics for, 2570, 2571f
Low-grade prostatic intraepithelial neoplasia (LGPIN), 3506
Low-osmolality contrast media (LOCM), 30
Lowsley retractor, 156
LP. see Lichen planus
LPN. see Laparoscopic partial nephrectomy
LPS. see Lipopolysaccharide
LR. see Likelihood ratio
LRN. see Laparoscopic radical nephrectomy
LRP. see Laparoscopic radical prostatectomy
LS. see Lichen sclerosus
L-shaped kidney, 728f, 729
Lumbar notch, 169, 170f
Lumbar vein, 1869-1870
Lumbodorsal fascia, in retroperitoneum, 1665-1666, 1666f, 1666.e1f
Lumbosacral plexus, 1675-1676, 1675.e1f, 1677f-1678f, 1679t, 2447f-2448f, 2453, 2453f, 2453t
Lumbosacral trunk, 2453t
Luminal epithelial cells, 3278, 3278f
Lungs
  development of, amniotic fluid and, 716-717
  in prune-belly syndrome, 586-587
LUT. see Lower urinary tract
LUTD. see Lower urinary tract dysfunction
Luteinizing hormone (LH), 1390, 1391f, 1395-1396, 1429, 1437
Luteinizing hormone receptor abnormality, 1011
Luteinizing hormone-releasing hormone agonists, 3676
Luteinizing hormone-releasing hormone antagonists, 3676-3677
LUTS. see Lower urinary tract symptoms
LVI. see Lymphovascular invasion
17,20-Lyase deficiency, 1012
Lycopene, for benign prostatic hyperplasia, 3398-3399
Lyme disease, lower urinary tract dysfunction and, 2624
Lymph node metastases, 3511
Lymph node-positive, treatment of, 2222-2224, 2223f
Lymph nodes
  counts, RPLND outcomes and, 1729
  iliac, 2433
  number of identified, 3116-3117, 3116f

Lymphadenectomy
  common iliac, 3152, 3153f-3154f
  external iliac, 3148-3149, 3151f
  hypogastric, 3149-3152, 3153f
  inguinal
    antibiotics for, 1801
    anticoagulation for, 1801
    bed rest in, 1801
    complications of, 1801-1802
    compressive dressings and stockings for, 1801
    dietary considerations of, 1801
    drainage, 1801
    postoperative care after, 1801
  laparoscopic radical nephrectomy with, 2297-2298
  obturator, 3149, 3152f
  patient positioning and port placement for, 1736, 1737f-1738f
  presacral, 3152, 3154f
  for RCC, 2177, 2177f, 2260, 2260f, 2260.e1f
  in retropubic radical prostatectomy, 3551-3552, 3551f
  for UTUC, 2205-2207, 2206f
Lymphangiomas, renal, 2132
Lymphatic complications, after RPLND, 2244
Lymphatic drainage
  of bladder, 2456
  of kidneys, 1870-1871, 1870.e1f
  of pelvis
    female, 2433, 2434f
    male, 2452-2453
  of retroperitoneum, 1674, 1675f
  of ureters, 1870-1871, 1870.e1f
  of uterus, 2436-2437
  of vulva, 2436
Lymphatic spread
  of infection, 1131.e1
  of UTUC, 2193-2194
Lymphedema
  as filariasis clinical manifestation, 1329
  genital, 884-885
Lymphocele, 280-281, 280t, 281f, 1938-1939
  after RPLND, 1731, 2244
  diagnosis of, 1939
  laparoscopic and robotic surgery causing, 231.e1
  treatment of, 1939
Lymphogranuloma venereum (LGV), 1255t, 1260-1261, 1260f
Lymphoma
  of kidney, 2181-2183, 2182t
  prostatic, 3513
  retroperitoneal tumors and, 2236, 2237f
  testicular metastases of, 1124-1125, 1709
Lymphovascular invasion (LVI), UTUC with, 2197

M

M inverted V glansplasty (MIV), 920, 922f
M region, 2493
MACE. see Malone antegrade continence enema
Machado-Joseph (MJ) disease, lower urinary tract dysfunction and, 2632
Macrohematuria, 247
Magnesium
  in calcium stone formation, 2017
  in crystal formation, 2014
  metabolism of, 2016
  transport of, urinary tract obstruction and, 794
Magnetic resonance angiography (MRA), for renovascular hypertension screening, 1917-1918, 1918b
Magnetic resonance fusion-guided prostate biopsy, 66-67

Magnetic resonance imaging (MRI), 51–67, 61t, 67b, 390, 412–415
　of acute scrotum, 414
　adrenal, 51–54
　of adrenal glands, 2352
　for adrenal mass evaluation, 2395–2396
　for biochemical recurrence after radical prostatectomy, 3662
　of bladder RMS, 1113
　of bladder/urethra, 414
　cranial, 1444–1445, 1445f
　of cyst/masses/stones, 413–414
　for differences of sex development, 415
　and ED, 1528
　of epididymis, 1375–1376
　of female pelvis, 2440–2442, 2440f–2442f
　fundamentals of, 412–413
　for genitourinary tuberculosis diagnosis, 1313
　for infection, 414
　for inguinal node dissection, 1792
　of IVC tumor thrombus, 2175
　of kidney/ureter, 413–414, 1866.e2f
　　hydronephrosis, 413
　for locally advanced prostate cancer, 3641, 3641f
　of male pelvis, 2458–2460, 2459f–2460f
　with nanotechnology, for inguinal node dissection, 1792
　for neuroblastoma, 1089, 1089f–1090f
　for other congenital malformations, 414
　for pelvic organ prolapse, 2589f, 2597
　of penis, 1386, 1388f
　of posterior urethral valves, 607, 608f
　in pregnant, 284
　of prostate, 61–63, 1380–1381, 1381f
　　for localized prostate cancer, 3527–3529
　for prostate cancer, 3542–3543, 3543b
　protocol of, 412–413
　for radiation therapy for prostate cancer, 3590–3591
　renal, 390
　of renal calculi, pretreatment assessment, 2071
　for renal tumor ablation, 2313, 2314f
　for renal tumor evaluation, 2135, 2138f
　for retroperitoneal fibrosis, 1979, 1979f
　for sedation in child, 413
　of seminal vesicles and ejaculatory ducts, 1378, 1378f
　of testis, 1373–1374
　for TGCTs, 1686
　for undescended testis, 415
　for ureteral anomalies, 805, 805f–806f
　for urethral diverticula, 2983, 2985f
Magnetic resonance imaging-targeted/fusion biopsy, for prostate cancer, 3622
Magnetic resonance spectroscopic imaging (MRSI), for biochemical recurrence after radiotherapy, 3666
Magnetic resonance spectroscopy, 64
Magnetic resonance urography (MRU), 412–413
　for urinary tract obstruction, 780
MAGPI. see Meatal advancement glanuloplasty
Mainz II pouch, 3210–3211
Mainz III, for orthoptic urinary diversion, 3246, 3248f
Mainz pouch I, 3215–3219, 3218f–3221f
Mainz repair, for classic bladder exstrophy, 545
Major vascular reconstruction, RPLND with, 1718–1719, 1719f
Malacoplakia, 1179–1181, 1180f
Male, 1050–1051
　fertility, 1051
　　penile concerns and management, 1050, 1050f
　　sexual function, 1050–1051
Male apical dissection, 3155
Male climacteric, 1392

Male external genitalia, 871.e1t, 871.e2f
　anomalies of, 871–886
　　acute scrotum, 893–899
　　epididymal and vasal, 903
　　hernia, 888–893
　　hydrocele, 888–893
　　penile, 871–886
　　scrotal, 886–888
　　varicocele, 899–903
　　vascular lesions of, 888
　benign cutaneous diseases of
　　angiokeratomas of Fordyce, 1302, 1303f
　　ectopic sebaceous glands, 1303f, 1304
　　median raphe cysts, 1304
　　pearly penile papules, 1302, 1303f
　　sclerosing lymphangitis, 1302–1304
　　Zoon balanitis, 1302, 1303f
　defect of, in bladder exstrophy, 533–534, 533f–534f
　embryology of, 871
　injuries of, 3048–3054, 3054b
　management of abnormalities of, 871–904
　normal, 871
　penile reconstruction of, 3054
　skin loss from, 3053–3054, 3053f–3054f
　surgical repair of, 890–892
　ultrasonography of, 871, 871.e2f
Male infertility, 1428–1452
　assisted reproduction, 1445–1452, 1445.e3, 1445.e3t
　causes of, 1446–1447
　and childhood diseases, 1432–1434
　　testicular dysgenesis hypothesis, 1433
　and chromosomal numerical disorders, 1445–1446
　developmental disorders and, 1449–1450
　diagnoses and therapies for, 1445, 1452b
　and ejaculatory dysfunction, 1450–1451
　epidemiology of, 1428
　epigenetic anomalies and, 1446
　and extratesticular endocrine dysfunction, 1448–1449
　and genetic syndromes, 1445–1446
　and genetics, 1433
　and genomic assessment, 1442–1443
　history of, 1428–1434, 1429t, 1434b
　and hypogonadotropic hypogonadism, 1447–1448
　imaging of, 1443–1445, 1445b
　　abdominal, 1444, 1445f
　　cranial, 1444–1445, 1445f
　and infections and inflammation, 1432
　laboratory evaluation of, 1436–1443, 1443b
　and microductal obstruction, 1447, 1447f
　and pediatric surgery, 1432
　physical examination of, 1434–1436, 1436b
　and pituitary dysfunction, 1447–1448
　and spermatogenic dysfunction, 1446
　and steroidogenic dysfunction, 1447
　structural chromosomal anomalies and, 1446
　and structural sperm abnormalities, 1451–1452
　surgical management of, 1453–1484
　　electroejaculation, 1472
　　orchiopexy in adults, 1483–1484, 1483f
　　sperm retrieval techniques, 1472–1476
　　surgery of epididymis, 1467–1471, 1468f–1469f, 1468t
　　surgical anatomy in, 1453–1454
　　testis biopsy, 1454–1456
　　transurethral resection of ejaculatory ducts, 1471–1472, 1472f
　　varicocelectomy, 1476–1483, 1476f, 1476t
　　vasography, 1457–1460, 1457f–1459f
　　vasovasostomy, 1460–1467, 1461f–1462f, 1463t
　testis histopathology and, 1445, 1445.e1f–1445.e2f, 1445.e2b
　vasography for, 1444
　venography for, 1444

Male lichen sclerosus, 1742.e1–1742.e2
Male lumpectomy, 3616
Male menopause, 1392
Male mesh slings, 2887–2888, 2887b–2888b, 2888f
Male orgasm and ejaculation, disorders of, 1564–1581
　anatomy and physiology of ejaculatory response, 1564, 1565f
　delayed ejaculation, anejaculation, and anorgasmia, 1572–1579
　painful ejaculation, 1581
　postorgasmic illness syndrome, 1581
　premature ejaculation, 1564–1572
　retrograde ejaculation, 1579
Male Overactive Bladder in Veterans (MOTIVE) study, 2727
Male pelvis
　anatomy of, 2444–2460, 2449b
　　arterial supply, 2451–2452, 2451t
　　bladder, 2448f, 2455, 2456f
　　bony pelvis of, 2444
　　innervation of, 2447f–2448f, 2453, 2453f, 2453t, 2454b
　　lower abdominal wall, 2444–2448, 2445f–2448f
　　lymphatics, 2452–2453
　　musculature of, 2448–2449, 2449f
　　pelvic fascia of, 2449, 2452f
　　pelvic ureter, 2456, 2456f
　　perineum, 2450f–2451f, 2451b
　　perineum and perineal body fasciae, 2449–2450, 2450f–2451f
　　rectum, 2450f, 2454, 2455f
　　soft tissues of, 2448–2449, 2449f
　　urethra, 2465, 2465f
　　vasculature of, 2451–2452, 2451t
　　venous supply, 2452
　　viscera, 2454–2456, 2457b
　endoscopic anatomy of, 2456–2457, 2457f, 2460b
　　CT, 2458, 2458f–2459f
　　magnetic resonance imaging, 2458–2460, 2460f
　　radiographs and fluoroscopy, 2457–2458
Male reproductive system
　pediatric tumors of, paratesticular RMS, 1126–1127, 1127b
　physiology of, 1390–1410
　　ductus (vas) deferens, 1406–1407
　　seminal vesicle and ejaculatory ducts, 1407–1408
　　testis, 1392–1394, 1393f–1394f
Male reproductive system anatomy
　epididymis, 1374, 1374f–1376f, 1376b
　penis, 1383–1386, 1387b, 1807, 1807.e1f–1807.e7f
　prostate, 1378–1381, 1379f–1381f, 1381b
　scrotum, 1387–1389, 1388f, 1389b
　seminal vesicles and ejaculatory ducts, 1377–1378, 1378f, 1378b
　testis, 1370–1374, 1371f–1373f, 1374b
　urethra, 1381–1383, 1381f–1384f, 1384b, 1807, 1807.e1f–1807.e7f, 2465, 2465f
　vas deferens, 1376–1377, 1376f–1377f, 1377b
Male stress incontinence, 3009
Male stress urinary incontinence, injectable agents for, 2896–2897
　after urinary diversion, 2897–2898
　injection techniques, 2896–2897
Male urethra, 152
　catheterization of, 153
Male urethral cancer, 1776–1782, 1782b
　anterior, 1777–1781
　carcinoma of penile urethra, 1778–1780, 1779f–1780f
　epidemiology, etiology, and clinical presentation of, 1776–1777
　evaluation and staging of, 1777, 1778f, 1778t
　pathology of, 1777, 1777f, 1777t

Male urethral cancer *(Continued)*
  posterior, 1781–1782, 1782t
  recurrence after cystectomy, 1786t, 1789b
  treatment of, 1778, 1779t
Malecot catheters, 155, 155f, 173, 174f
Male-to-female transexuals. *see* Transwomen
Malignancy, PC-RPLND findings of, survival outcomes associated with, 1726–1727, 1727t
Malignancy-associated hypercalcemia, 2020
Malignant fibrous histiocytoma/undifferentiated pleomorphic sarcoma, retroperitoneal tumors and, 2231, 2232f
Malignant lesions
  adrenal, 2384–2388
    adrenal cortical carcinoma, 2384–2388, 2384f, 2385t, 2386f, 2386b, 2387t, 2388b
    malignant pheochromocytomas, 2373, 2375, 2389
    metastases, 2388–2389, 2389f, 2390b
    neuroblastoma. *see* Neuroblastoma
  of bladder, 3083–3084, 3083f–3084f
Malignant peripheral nerve sheath tumors, in retroperitoneum, 2235–2236
Malignant pheochromocytomas, 2373, 2375, 2389
Malone antegrade continence enema (MACE), 673, 674f–675f, 678t
Malrotation, of kidney, 1869, 1869.e1f
Mammalian target of rapamycin (mTOR)
  inhibitors, for metastatic RCC, 2326–2327, 2338–2339, 2340f, 2340t
  in RCC, 2145, 2145t
Management principles, of ED
  cardiac risk assessment, 1516–1517, 1517f
  early detection, 1515, 1515t
  follow-up care, 1517
  goal-directed management, 1516
  role of partner interview, 1516
  shared decision making and treatment planning, 1515–1516
  specialist referral, 1517
  step-care approach, 1516
Manchester procedure, in uterine sparing, 2816–2817, 2819t
Mannose-sensitive adhesin, 429
Manometry, for PFM activity measurement, 2729
Manual dexterity, orthoptic urinary diversion and, 3238
Manual dilation, for achieving retroperitoneal access and developing retroperitoneal space, 210
Manual therapy, for genito-pelvic pain-penetration disorder, 1653
Margins, 3511
Marionette stitch, for minimally invasive urinary diversion, 3261–3262, 3261f
Marshall-Marchetti-Krantz (MMK) procedure, 2762–2763, 2763b
  Burch colposuspension *versus*, 2773
  results with, 2762–2763
  technique for, 2762, 2762f
Martius flap
  in urethrovaginal fistulae, 2950
  in vesicovaginal fistula repair, 2940, 2949f
Martius labial fat pad graft, 2866–2868
Masked hypertension, 352
Mast cells, in BPS/IC etiology, 1232.e4–1232.e5, 1232.e5b
Mastectomy, 3063–3064
Maternal anemia, from bacteriuria in pregnancy, 1186.e1
Maternal-fetal ultrasound, 358, 359f
Matrix
  of bladder wall, 2464
  renal calculi and, 2015

Matrix GLA protein (MGP), in crystal formation, 2015
Matrix stones
  composition of, 2076–2077, 2076f
  imaging of, 2076, 2076f
  in renal calculi, 2032
Matrix substance A, 2015
Maturation arrest, 1445.e1, 1445.e2f
Maximum birth weight, pelvic organ prolapse and, 2591
Maximum urethral closure pressure (MUCP), 2563, 2757
  for sling procedure, 2831, 2833
Maximum urethral pressure (MUP), 2563
Maximum voided volume (MVV), 2667
Mayer-Rokitansky-Küster-Hauser syndrome (MRKH), 720, 1017
McCall culdoplasty technique, vaginal hysterectomy with, 2814–2815, 2815f
MCDK. *see* Multicystic dysplastic kidney
McGuire's technique, for pubovaginal sling, modified, 2834
MCKD. *see* Medullary cystic kidney disease
MDSC. *see* Microsurgical denervation of the spermatic cord
Meatal advancement glanuloplasty (MAGPI), 920, 921f
Meatal retrusion, 938
Meatal stenosis, 875, 875f, 937–938
  urethral, reconstructive surgery for, 1811
Meatotomy, urethral reconstruction and, 3071
Mechanical assistants, for laparoscopic and robotic surgery, 218.e2
Mechanical bowel preparation, in urologic surgery, 125
Mechanical index (MI), in ultrasonography, 78
Mechanical injury, during laparoscopic and robotic surgery, 229
Mechanical properties, of ureters, 1890–1891
  force-length relations, 1890, 1890f
  force-velocity relations, 1890–1891, 1891f
  pressure-length-diameter relations, 1891
Mechanical reliability, repair for, 1597, 1597f
Medial fibroplasia, 1915, 1915f
Medial hyperplasia, 1916
Median raphe cysts, 882, 882f, 1304
Median umbilical ligament, 330–333
Medical conditions
  in bladder tumor, 3076–3077
  urinary incontinence and, 2586
Medical devices, in ED, 1536–1537
Medical ethics, 115–116, 118b
  in clinical practice, 115–116
  four-principles of, 115
  history of, 115
Medical expulsive therapy (MET), for ureteral calculi
  in megaureter, 2087
  stone localization and, 2085
Medical history, adrenal surgery and, 2407–2408
Medical indications, 116
Medical management, in schistosomiasis treatment, 1326–1327
Medical therapy
  for adrenal cortical carcinoma, 2387–2388
  for genitourinary tuberculosis treatment, 1311t, 1315–1317, 1315t–1316t
Medical Therapy of Prostatic Symptoms (MTOPS) Trial, 3385–3386, 3387f–3388f, 3387t
Medication change, for ED, 1529
Medication optimization, in geriatric patient, 2915–2917, 2916t–2917t
Medication-related stones
  in renal calculi, 2032–2033
  surgical management of, 2077.e2–2077.e3

Medications
  benign prostatic hyperplasia and, 3324
  patient history of, 7–8
  transient urinary incontinence and, 2919.e1
Medullary cystic kidney disease (MCKD), 747t, 755–756, 756f, 756b
  clinical features of, 755–756
  evaluation of, 756, 756f
  genetics of, 755
  treatment of, 756
Medullary sex cord, 319f
Medullary sponge kidney (MSK), 771–772, 771f, 772b
  clinical features of, 771
  diagnosis of, 771
  histopathology of, 771
  prognosis of, 771–772
  renal calculi and, 2034–2035
  treatment of, 771–772
Megacalycosis, 738–739, 740f
Megacystis microcolon intestinal hypoperistalsis syndrome (MMIHS), 520–521
Megacystis-megaureter association, 510
Megaureter
  in children, 849–852, 852b
    cutaneous ureterostomy for, 850–851, 850f
    definition of, 849
    definitive reconstruction for, 850–851, 850f
    dilatation and stenting for, 852
    etiology, occurrence, and presentation of, 849
    excisional tapering for, 851–852, 851f
    Kalicinski plication technique for, 851, 851f
    outcomes with, 852
    remodeling for, 837f–839f, 851
    Starr plication technique for, 851, 851f
    surgical indications for, 849–850
    surgical management of, 850–852, 850f–851f
    ureteral polyps with, 835–836
    ureteral strictures with, 835
  ureteral calculi in, surgical management of, 2087
  ureterovesical junction obstruction, 374–375
  recommendations for, 374–375
Meiosis, testis germ cells and, 1400–1401, 1401t
Melanocortin-receptor agonists, 1534
Melanocortins, in ED, 1494, 1495t
Melanoma, as neoplastic condition, 1300–1301
Melatonin, 1392
MELD score, in assessment of perioperative mortality, 121
Membrane potential, of smooth muscles, of bladder, 2473–2474, 2474f
Membranoproliferative glomerulonephritis (MPGN), 346
Membranous glomerulonephritis (MGN), with RPF, 1978
Membranous nephropathy (MN), 345
Membranous urethra, 1382, 1382f–1383f, 1807.e4f, 1807.e8
Memorial Sloan-Kettering Cancer Center (MSKCC) penile rehabilitation program, 3579
MEN. *see* Multiple endocrine neoplasia
Menopause
  genito-pelvic pain-penetration disorder and, 1652
  pelvic organ prolapse and, 2591
Men's health, integrated, 1411–1427
  cardiovascular risk, and testosterone therapy, 1424–1425, 1425b
  health centers for, 1427
  mental health and opioid abuse in men, 1426–1427, 1427b
  metabolic syndrome and, 1417–1424, 1424b

Men's health, integrated *(Continued)*
  rationale for, 1411–1417, 1417b
    gender longevity gap, 1411, 1412t–1415t, 1415f
    global men's health movement, 1417
    health and wellness gap by gender, 1411, 1415t
    poorer health of men, explanation of, 1411–1416
    targets and effective interventions, 1416–1417
Mental illness, in men, 1426
Mepartricin, for chronic scrotal pain syndrome, 1216
Meperidine (Demerol), urethral function effects of, 1902
Mesenchymal condensation, 3275–3276
Mesenchymal-epithelial conversion, 338
Mesenchymal tumors, of prostate, 3512
Mesenteric blood flow, pneumoperitoneum effects on, 222
Mesh complications, 2877–2888, 2878b
  among three slings, 2880–2887
  apical, 2886–2887
    exposure, treatment of, 2886–2887, 2886f
  male, 2887–2888, 2887b–2888b, 2888f
  materials for, 2877
  in midurethral sling, 2877
    bladder, perforation of, 2868–2870, 2868f, 2869t, 2870b
    contraction of, 2877
    exposure of, 2864–2866, 2864f, 2865t, 2866b, 2877, 2878f
    extrusion of, 2877
    perforation of, 2877, 2879f
    prominence of, 2877
    risk factors for, 2879–2880
    for stress urinary incontinence, 2879
    urethra, perforation of, 2866–2868, 2867t, 2870b
  prolapse, treatment of, 2885
  and properties, 2877–2878
  surgical removal, 2885–2886, 2886b
  surrounding, 2877
  transvaginal (anterior and posterior wall), 2883–2885
Mesoderm, 305
Mesodermal origins, retroperitoneal tumors and, 2229
Mesonephric duct, 324f
  degenerating, 319f
  ureteral development from, 1877
Mesonephric tubules, 319f, 324f
Mesonephros, 324f, 334–335, 334f
Mesotheliomas, of testicular adnexa, 1709
Mesovarium, 2437–2438
MESTs. *see* Mixed epithelial and stromal tumors
MET. *see* Medical expulsive therapy
MET gene, systemic therapy targeting, 2343, 2344f
MET signaling, in castration-resistant prostate cancer, 3701
Metabolic changes, with aging, 2906
Metabolic syndrome (MetS)
  benign prostatic hyperplasia and, 3324, 3325t
  bladder cancer, 1421
  definition of, 1417–1418, 1417f, 1418t
  and ED, 1510–1511
  hormonal therapy and, 3681
  hyperoxaluria and, 2059–2060
  novel strategy for, 1422
    diet and exercise, 1422
    metformin, 1422
    statins, 1422
    testosterone therapy, 1422
  physiology of, 1418–1420, 1419f
    abdominal obesity, 1418–1419
    dietary factors, 1420
    dyslipidemia, 1419
    endothelial dysfunction, 1420
    genetics, 1420

Metabolic syndrome (MetS) *(Continued)*
    glucocorticoid and stress-response mediators, 1420
    hypercoagulable state, 1420
    hypertension, 1419–1420
    insulin resistance, 1419
    obstructive sleep apnea, 1420
  prevalence and predictors of, 1418
  renal calculi and, 2008
  sleep duration and, 2665–2666
  urologic disorders and, 1420–1422
    bladder cancer, 1421
    erectile dysfunction, 1422
    low testosterone and erectile dysfunction, 1422
    lower urinary tract symptoms, 1421
    overactive bladder, 1421
    prostate cancer, 1421–1422
    renal insufficiency, 1420
    renal stones, 1420–1421
    tumor, 1421
Metabolomics, for prostate cancer biomarkers, 3479
Metanephric adenofibroma, in pediatric patients, 1109
Metanephric adenoma, of kidney, 2128–2129, 2129f, 2129b
Metanephric mesenchyme, ureteric bud outgrowth, 336–338, 337f
Metanephrine testing, for pheochromocytoma, 2377, 2377f
Metanephros, 335–336, 335f
Metaplastic lesion, of upper tract urothelium, 2188
Metastasectomy, in advanced RCC, 2328, 2328b
Metastasis
  adrenal disorder, 2388–2389, 2389f, 2390b
  after renal tumor ablation, 2317
  MRI and, 53–54
  neuroblastoma with, 1089
  of penile cancer
    primary tumor histology in prediction of, 1757–1759, 1758t
    prognostic significance of, 1753, 1754t–1755t
    risk-based management for, 1762–1765, 1763f–1764f
  from prostate, castration-resistant, 3689–3690
  renal, 2181t, 2183
  testicular, 1124, 1709
Metastatic bladder cancer
  chemotherapy for, 3127t
  FDA-approved agents and future directions, 3130
  immune checkpoint inhibitor therapy, 3129–3130
    first-line, 3130
    second-line, 3130
  management of, 3112–3132, 3131b
  randomized trials in, 3127–3128, 3127t
  second-line chemotherapy for, 3128, 3128t
    multiagent, 3129
    single agent, 3128–3129, 3129t
  targeted therapy for, 3130–3131
Metastatic disease, treatment of, 2222–2224, 2223f
Metastatic potential, of UTUC, 2193–2194
Metastatic prostate cancer, castration-sensitive, phase III clinical trials for, 3678t
Metastatic RCC, 2177
  treatment of, 2325–2328
    advanced, immunologic approaches, 2329–2332, 2329t–2331t, 2332f
    chemotherapy, 2341–2342
    debulking or cytoreductive nephrectomy, 2325–2328, 2326f–2327f, 2327t, 2328b
    hormonal therapy, 2342–2343
    palliative surgery, 2328, 2328b
    prognostic factors and, 2324–2325, 2325f, 2325t

Metastatic RCC *(Continued)*
    resection of metastases, 2328, 2328b
    systemic therapy for non–clear cell variants, 2343–2344, 2344f
    targeted molecular agents in, 2324, 2333–2341, 2333t–2335t, 2336f, 2337t
Metastatic restaging, in UTUC, 2225
Metformin, 449
  and gadolinium, contrast media and, 34
  and iodinated contrast, contrast media and, 33–34
  for metabolic syndrome, 1422
  for prostate cancer, 3545
  in prostate cancer prevention, 3475
Methacholine (Mecholyl), ureteral response to, 1887
Methenamine, for UTIs, 1165–1166, 1165t
Methotrexate
  for BPS/IC oral therapy, 1241t, 1243
  for penile cancer, 1770
Methoxamine, for stress urinary incontinence in women, 2714
α-Methylacyl coenzyme A racemase (AMACR) gene, as prostate cancer biomarker, 3487
Methylene blue
  for pelvic floor disorder testing, 2533
  toxicity of, 1994
  ureteral response to, 1886
Methylprednisolone sodium succinate, for contrast media, 32
Methysergide (Sansert), with RPF, 1978
Meticulous padding, 164–165, 165f
Metoclopramide, to facilitate bladder emptying, 2718
Metoidioplasty, 3068–3069
Metronidazole, prophylaxis with, for uncomplicated urologic procedures, 1194t–1196t
MetS. *see* Metabolic syndrome
Meyers scale, 473–474, 474f
MGN. *see* Membranous glomerulonephritis
MGP. *see* Matrix GLA protein
MHCs. *see* Myosin heavy chains
MI. *see* Mechanical index
Mic-Key button, for bladder emptying, 711
Microbiology, TB, 1307
Microbiome, in GU cancers, 1368–1369, 1369b
Microductal aplasia, 1449–1450
Microductal obstruction, 1447, 1447f
Microfibrillar collagen (Avitene), 147
Microhematuria, 401
Microlithiasis, testicular, in pediatric patients, 1124–1125
Micromotions, 2642
Micronutrients, for prostate cancer, 3544
Micropapillary urothelial carcinoma (MPUC), 3088
Micropenis, 872t, 879–880, 880f, 880.e1b, 881b
Microphthalmia-associated transcription factor-associated cancer syndrome, 2145
Microporous polysaccharide spheres (Arista), 147
MicroRNA (miRNA), as prostate cancer biomarker, 3487
Microsatellite instability, in UTUC, 2197
Microscopic hematuria, 247–250, 250b, 252b, 479
  American Urologic Association (AUA) guideline panel define, 247
  causes of, 247, 248b, 249t
  criteria for diagnosis of, 247, 248t
  cystoscopy in diagnostic evaluation of, 250–251
  guideline-based evaluation of, 250–252, 251f
  natural history, in patients with negative evaluation, 252
  requirement for, 247
  screening for, 250
  selection of patient, for evaluation of, 247–250, 248t
  symptomatic, 252

Microsurgical denervation of the spermatic cord (MDSC), 1853-1855, 1854f-1855f
Microsurgical epididymal sperm aspiration, in sperm retrieval, 1473-1474, 1473f-1474f
Microwave ablation (MWA), for renal tumors, 2322
Micturating cystourethrogram, 415-416
Micturition
  brainstem modulatory mechanisms of, 2493-2494, 2495f
  cerebral control of, 2496
  charts, 3344
  mechanics of, 2479
  neuromodulation for, rationale for, 2510, 2510f
  nitric oxide and, 2484
  physiology of, 2564, 2564f
  pontine micturition center in, 2493-2494, 2495f
  reflex circuitry controlling, 2489-2493, 2490f
    emptying phase, 2490f, 2491t, 2492
    urethra to bladder reflexes, 2492-2493, 2492f-2494f
Micturition cycle, 2516
  abnormalities of, 2600
  bladder emptying/voiding in
    failure of, pathophysiology of, 2516
    urodynamic studies of, 2564-2566
  bladder filling/storage in
    failure of, pathophysiology of, 2516
    urodynamic studies of, 2552t-2553t, 2559
  phases of, mechanisms underlying, 2514
Micturitional urethral pressure profile (MUPP), 2567
Midline incision, of abdomen, 135, 136f-137f
Midodrine, for stress urinary incontinence in women, 2714
Mid-ureter, stone localization and, 2086t
Midurethral sling (MUS), 2849-2851
  age of, 2831-2832
  anatomy of, 2850, 2851b
  complications of, 2863-2866, 2864.e1t-2864.e2t
    bleeding after, 2874
    infection and pain after, 2870-2871
    management of SUI after, 2874
    mesh exposure in, 2864-2866, 2864f, 2865t, 2866b
    mesh perforation of bladder, 2868-2870, 2868f, 2869t, 2870b
    mesh perforation of urethra, 2866-2868, 2867t, 2870b
    regulatory and legal issues related to, 2874-2876
    serious, 2874
    sexual dysfunction after, 2873
    trocar injury to urinary tract, 2866-2873
    urethral perforation during placement, 2866-2868, 2866f, 2867t
    voiding dysfunction after, 2871-2873, 2872t, 2873b
  evolution of, 2830-2831
  materials for, 2851, 2851b
  mechanics of, 2849-2850, 2851b
  mesh complications of, 2877
    among three slings, 2880-2887
    contraction of, 2877
    exposure of, 2877, 2878f
    extrusion of, 2877
    perforation of, 2877, 2879f
    prominence of, 2877
    risk factors for, 2879-2880
    for stress urinary incontinence, 2879
  operative procedures for, 2851-2863
    anesthesia for, 2851-2854
    patient counseling for, 2851
    positioning for, 2851-2854
    preparation for, 2851-2854

Midurethral sling (MUS) (Continued)
  outcomes of
    for elderly women, 2862-2863, 2863b
    for intrinsic sphincteric deficiency, 2859-2860
    for mixed urinary incontinence, 2858-2859
    for obese patients, 2863, 2863b
    for pelvic organ prolapse, 2861-2862
    for predominantly SUI, 2854
    for recurrent SUI, 2860-2861, 2861b
  retropubic
    anatomy of, 2850
    complications of, 2863-2866
    outcomes for, 2854-2856, 2855t
    removal of, 2870
    surgical approach to, 2851-2853, 2852f-2853f
  retropubic, complications of, 2880
  single-incision
    anatomy of, 2851
    complications of, 2863-2866, 2879
    outcomes for, 2857-2858
    surgical approach to, 2854, 2855f
  for stress urinary incontinence, 2879
  transobturator
    anatomy of, 2850-2851
    complications of, 2863-2866
    inside-out, surgical approach for, 2853-2854, 2854f
    outcomes for, 2856-2857, 2857t
    outside-in, surgical approach for, 2853
Mild androgen insensitivity syndrome, 1014
Milnacipran hydrochloride, to facilitate bladder filling and urine storage, 2702
Mindfulness, for female orgasmic disorder, 1647
Mineral metabolism, 2017b
Mineralocorticoids, in adrenal histology, 2356, 2357t
Mini balloon button, for bladder emptying, 711
Mini Mental State Examination (MMSE), 2910
Mini-Cog, 2910, 2911f
Minimally invasive and endoscopic management of benign prostatic hyperplasia, 3403-3448
  defining outcomes for, 3405-3407
    comparing to other treatments, 3407, 3408t
    response rates, 3405-3407
    secondary procedures, 3407
  epidemiology of, 3403-3404, 3404b
  failed, failing, and future directions for, 3443-3447
    aquablation (aquabeam), 3444-3445, 3445f
    prostate embolization, 3445-3446
    prostate stents, 3443-3444
    prostatic injections, 3446-3447
    Temporary Implantable Nitinol Device, 3444
  increasing age and, 3404
  laser treatments, 3435-3438
    safety for, 3435-3436
  marketshare, 3403-3404, 3404b
  non-laser options for, 3409-3443, 3422b, 3435b
  presurgical factors for, 3407-3409, 3409b
    antibiotic coverage for, 3409
    histologic specimen for, 3409
    matching treatment with patient, 3409
    treatment indications, 3407-3409
  workup for, 3404-3405, 3405f-3406f
Minimally invasive ileal ureteral substitution, for ureteral stricture disease, 1973-1975, 1974f
Minimally invasive pelvic lymph node dissection, 3584-3586
  complications of, 3585-3586, 3586b
  future of, 3586
  indications for, 3584
  surgical technique of, 3584-3585, 3585f

Minimally invasive surgery (MIS)
  access, 463-465, 465b
    comparative effectiveness of, 465
    open, 464, 464f
    Veress needle, 463, 464f
    visual obturator, 464-465
  additional benefit of, 459
  advantages and disadvantages of, 458-459, 459f, 459t, 460b
  approach to, 465, 465b
    retroperitoneal, 465
    transperitoneal, 465
    vesicoscopic, 465
  assessment, 470
  complications of, 468-469, 469b
    incisional hernia, 468-469, 469f
    pulmonary air embolus, 469
    vascular injury, 468, 469f
    visceral injury, 468
  cost of, 460
  drawbacks of, 460
  learning curves, 472
  length-of-stay benefits for selected, 458-459, 459t
  patient selection for, 462-463, 463b
  pediatric urologic procedures, 462t
  simulation training and evaluation of, 469-472, 470f-471f, 472b
  skills acquisition, stages of, 470t
  training, 470
  in urologic practice, 2308
  warm-up, 471-472
Minimally invasive urinary diversion, 3258-3273
  anatomic considerations in
    men, 3260-3261, 3260f
    women, 3261
  complications of, 3270, 3271t
  Florin: Florence robotic intracorporeal neobladder, 3267
    configuration and setup, 3267, 3267f
    uretero-neobladder anastomosis, 3267
  functional outcomes with, 3272-3273
  future direction for, 3273
  hospital stay for, 3259
  ileal conduit, 3261-3262
    bowel restoration, 3262
    bowel segment isolation, 3262
    bowel selection for, 3261
    left ureter transfer for, 3261
    marionette stitch, 3261-3262, 3261f
    pre-stoma preparation, 3262, 3262b
    ureteroileal anastomosis, 3262
  intracorporeal versus extracorporeal, 3273
  learning curve for, 3270
  modified Studer neobladder: Karolinska Institute Technique, 3263t, 3264-3265
    bowel detubularization, 3264
    closure of neobladder, 3265
    configuration and setup, 3264, 3264f
    neobladder creation, 3264
    neobladder-urethral anastomosis, 3264
    uretero-neobladder anastomosis, 3264
  modified Studer neobladder: The USC Institute of Urology Technique, 3265
    configuration and setup, 3265, 3265f
    neobladder-urethral anastomosis and cross-folding of pouch, 3265
    rotation of pouch, 3265
    uretero-neobladder anastomosis, 3265
  modified "W" Hautmann neobladder: The Roswell Park Comprehensive Cancer Center Technique, 3267-3269
    configuration and setup, 3267-3268, 3268f
    neobladder creation, 3268
    uretero-neobladder anastomosis, 3268-3269

Minimally invasive urinary diversion (Continued)
  modified Y neobladder: The Clinique Saint-Augustin Technique, 3266
    configuration and setup, 3266, 3266f
    neobladder creation, 3266
    uretero-neobladder anastomosis, 3266
  operative time for, 3270
  outcomes with, 3270
  Padua neobladder, 3266-3267
    configuration and setup, 3266-3267, 3267f
    uretero-neobladder anastomosis, 3267
  patient position for, 3259-3260, 3259f, 3260b
  patient selection for, 3258
  port placement for, 3259-3260, 3259f, 3260b
  postoperative care for, 3269-3270
  preoperative care for, 3259, 3259b
  pyramid neobladder: The University College London Hospital technique, 3265-3266
    configuration and setup, 3265, 3266f
    formation of, 3265-3266
    uretero-neobladder anastomosis, 3266
  surgeon choice in, 3258-3259
Mi-Prostate Score (MiPS), 3486
MiPS. see Mi-Prostate Score
Mirabegron, 2500, 2544
  adverse effects of, 2700
  for benign prostatic hyperplasia, 3381-3393
  for diminished bladder, 2674, 2675t-2677t
  efficacy of, 2699-2700
  to facilitate bladder filling and urine storage, 2682t, 2699-2700
  with antimuscarinics, 2706
  indication, efficacy, and safety profile of, 3381-3382
  for OAB, 2647
  pharmacokinetics of, 2699
  tolerability of, 2700
  for urinary incontinence, in geriatric patients, 2920.e4
MIS. see Minimally invasive surgery
Mismatch repair (MMR), 1351.e1, 1351.e1f
Misoprostol, for BPS/IC oral therapy, 1241t, 1243
Mitchell repair, for classic bladder exstrophy, 544, 544f
  continence outcomes with, 560
  technical aspects of, 550, 550f
Mitomycin C (MMC), for non-muscle-invasive bladder cancer, 3104-3105
Mitosis
  deregulation of, in GU cancers, 1347.e2
  in UTUC, 2197-2198
Mitotic arrest, deregulation of, 1347.e3
Mitoxantrone, 3690, 3693f
Mitrofanoff principle, for continent urinary diversions, 707-709
MIV. see M inverted V glansplasty
Mixed epithelial and stromal tumors (MESTs), of kidney, 2130, 2130f, 2130b
Mixed fiber mesh, for anterior compartment repair, 2781t-2782t
Mixed gonadal dysgenesis, 998t, 1002-1004, 1003f, 1003b, 1004t
Mixed mesenchymal and epithelial tumors, renal, 2129-2130, 2129f
Mixed urinary incontinence (MUI)
  definition of, 2539, 2581
  midurethral sling for, outcomes of, 2858-2859
  overactive bladder and, 2637
  patient history of, 5
  pubovaginal sling for, outcomes of, 2844-2845
  treatment of, 2547
MK2206, 3700
MLCs. see Myosin light chains
M-line measurement, 2441-2442, 2442f
MMC. see Mitomycin C

MMIHS. see Megacystis microcolon intestinal hypoperistalsis syndrome
MMR. see Mismatch repair
MMSE. see Mini Mental State Examination
MN. see Membranous nephropathy
Modafinil, for PE, 1572.e2-1572.e3
Modern staged reconstruction, of cloacal exstrophy, 578, 578t
Modern staged repair of exstrophy (MRSE), 545
  bladder, posterior urethral, and abdominal wall closure for, 545-548, 546f-548f
  combined bladder closure and epispadias repair, 548
  management after, 548-549, 549b
Modified Cantwell-Ransley repair, for classic bladder exstrophy, 551-552, 552f-553f
Modified cardiac risk index, 120t
Modified complete ILND, for penile cancer, 1761
Modified inguinal lymph node dissection, for penile cancer, 1794
Modified supine positioning, 467f
Modified Young-Dees-Leadbetter bladder neck reconstruction, 555f-556f
Modulators, within brainstem networks, 2495-2496
Mohs micrographic surgery, for penile cancer, 1752
Mole, 1304, 1305f
Molecular genetics of GU cancers, 1346-1369, 1346.e1-1346.e4
  apoptosis, 1365-1367, 1367b
    extrinsic pathway of, 1366.e1f-1366.e2f, 1366.e2
    intrinsic pathway of, 1366.e1, 1366.e1f
  basic concepts for
    chromosomes and gene structure, 1346.e4
    DNA, 1346.e1-1346.e4, 1346.e2f
    protein synthesis, 1346.e3-1346.e4, 1346.e3f-1346.e4f
    transcription, 1346.e3, 1346.e3f
  cell cycle deregulation, 1347-1348, 1349b
    CDKIs, 1347.e1, 1347.e1f
    cell cycle entry, 1347.e1
    cell cycle progression through S phase, 1347.e2
    cyclin-dependent kinases and cyclins, 1347.e1, 1347.e1f
    G₁/S checkpoint, 1347.e2
    G2M checkpoint, 1347.e2-1347.e3
    mitosis, 1347.e2
    mitotic arrest and spindle assembly checkpoint, 1347.e3
    RB1, 1347.e1, 1347.e1f
    S phase arrest, 1347.e2
    TP53, 1347.e2, 1347.e2f, 1348
  checkpoint inhibition, 1367-1368, 1368b
  DNA damage and repair, 1350-1351, 1351b
    DSB repair, 1351.e1f-1351.e2f, 1351.e2
    mechanisms, 1351.e1, 1351.e1f
  DNA methylation, 1348-1350, 1350b
  genomic alterations, 1351-1362, 1362b
    in bladder cancer, 1358-1360
    bladder RMS, 1111-1113
    CNAs, 1354, 1354t-1355t
    gross chromosomal abnormalities, 1351-1352, 1352b
    in prostate cancer, 1352-1353, 1354t, 1355f
    in renal cancer, 1353, 1354t, 1358
    in testicular cancer, 1121, 1353, 1361-1362
    in Wilms tumor, 1096-1099, 1097t, 1354t
  microbiome, 1368-1369, 1369b
  oncogenes, 1346-1347, 1347b
  stem cells, 1367, 1368b
  telomerase, 1362-1365, 1363f, 1365b
    chromosome stabilizing activity of, 1364
    as potential diagnostic marker, 1364
    therapies based on, 1365

Molecular genetics of GU cancers (Continued)
  telomeres, 1362-1365, 1365b
    cancers and premalignant lesions with short, 1363-1364
    chromosomal instability and, 1362
    prostate cancer prognosis using, 1364-1365
    as tumor suppressive mechanism, 1363, 1363f
  terminology for, 1346.e1b-1346.e2b
  tumor suppressor genes, 1346-1347, 1347f, 1347b
Molecular imaging, 91
Molecular oxygen, penile erection and, 1500
Molluscum contagiosum, 1261, 1261f
Monfort technique, 595, 596f-597f
Monopolar electrocautery, 466
Monopolar electrosurgery
  argon beam coagulator, 215.e1
  devices for, 237
  in laparoscopic and robotic surgery, 214
  generator settings for, 235-236
  physics of, 235, 236f
  safety of, 236-237
Monopolar thermal energy, 468
Monopolar transurethral resection of the prostate (M-TURP), 3409-3418
  in anticoagulated patient, 3416
  complications of, 3416-3418
    intraoperative, 3416-3417
    perioperative, 3416-3417
    postoperative, 3417-3418
  conclusion for, 3418
  outcomes with, 3416
  technique for, 3410-3416
    intraoperative, 3410-3415, 3411f-3414f, 3414f-3415f
    postoperative, 3415-3416
    preoperative, 3410
Monosymptomatic enuresis (MSE), 660
Mons pubis, 1627.e1, 2435, 2436f-2437f
Montelukast, for BPS/IC oral therapy, 1241t, 1242
Monti procedure, for ureteral injury, upper, 1998
Morbid obesity, in urologic surgery, 122
Morcellation instrumentation, for laparoscopic and robotic surgery, 218
Morphine, urethral function effects of, 1902
Mortality
  after RPLND, 1731
  with benign prostatic hyperplasia, 3335
  definition of, 102
  early, nocturia and, 2664-2666
  in locally advanced prostate cancer, 3644, 3645f
  prostate cancer, rates of, 3457, 3458f
    global, 3458-3459
    screening effect of, 3459-3460
  rate, 102
Motility, sperm, 1404-1405, 1405f
Motor nerve innervation, in detrusor muscle, 2465, 2465f, 2480, 2480f
Motor paralytic bladder, 2522
MPGN. see Membranoproliferative glomerulonephritis
MPUC. see Micropapillary urothelial carcinoma
MRA. see Magnetic resonance angiography
MRI. see Magnetic resonance imaging
MRKH. see Mayer-Rokitansky-Küster-Hauser syndrome
MRSE. see Modern staged repair of exstrophy
MRSI. see Magnetic resonance spectroscopic imaging
MRU. see Magnetic resonance urography
MS. see Multiple sclerosis
MSA. see Multiple system atrophy
MSE. see Monosymptomatic enuresis
MSK. see Medullary sponge kidney
⁹⁹mTc hexamethylpropyleneamine oxine (⁹⁹mTc-HMPAO), 96

mTOR. see Mammalian target of rapamycin
M-TURP. see Monopolar transurethral resection of the prostate
Mucinous cystadenoma, retroperitoneal tumors and, 2237
Mucosal glands, 315f
Mucosal plexus, 2463
MUCP. see Maximum urethral closure pressure
Mucus, after augmentation cystoplasty, 698
MUI. see Mixed urinary incontinence
Müllerian Aplasia, 980-981, 981f
Müllerian duct, 324f
Müllerian-inhibiting substance (MIS), 317-318, 1392, 1392f
Müllerian tubercle, 324, 776
Multichannel UDS, 2536, 2565f
Multicystic dysplastic kidney (MCDK), 339-340, 349, 350b, 377-378, 378f, 401, 405, 762-765, 762f, 765b
   clinical features of, 762
   duplex anomaly, recommendation of, 379, 381f
   duplication anomalies/ureterocele/ectopic ureter, 378-379, 379f-380f
   etiology of, 762
   evaluation of, 763, 763f-764f
   histopathology of, 762-763, 763f
   prognosis of, 763-765
   recommendations for, 378
   treatment of, 763-765
Multidetector computed tomography urography (CTU), for urinary tract obstruction, 779-780
Multidisciplinary approach, to pelvic pain study, 1209-1210
Multidisciplinary team, in transitional urology, 1045
Multidrug-resistant tuberculosis, 1318
Multimodal physical therapy, for genito-pelvic pain-penetration disorder, 1653
Multiparametric magnetic resonance imaging, 66, 66f-67f, 66t
   of prostate, 3502-3504, 3502t-3503t, 3502b, 3504f
   for prostate cancer, 3621-3622
Multiparametric ultrasonography, 77f
   prostate, 3502
   for prostate cancer, 3622
Multiple endocrine neoplasia (MEN), genomic alterations in, 1354t-1355t
Multiple malformation syndromes with renal cysts, 747t, 757-761
   tuberous sclerosis complex, 757-759
   von Hippel-Landau disease, 759-761
Multiple sclerosis (MS)
   cause of, 2607
   lower urinary tract dysfunction and, 2607-2608
   overview of, 2607
   treatment for, 2608
Multiple system atrophy (MSA), lower urinary tract dysfunction with, 2606-2607, 2607b
MUP. see Maximum urethral pressure
MUPP. see Micturitional urethral pressure profile
MUS. see Midurethral sling
Muscarinic receptor antagonists, for benign prostatic hyperplasia, 3379-3381
   efficacy of, 3379-3381, 3380t
   rationale and indication for, 3379, 3379t
   summary for, 3381
   tolerability and safety profile of, 3381
Muscarinic receptors
   in bladder function, 2470
      contraction, 2679-2681
   distribution of, 2680t
   pharmacology of, 2497-2500, 2499t, 2500b
      for detrusor underactivity, 2661
   selectivity of, 2499

Muscle-invasive bladder cancer
   adjuvant chemoradiation for, 3122
   adjuvant chemotherapy for, 3120-3125
      randomized trials of, 3121-3123, 3121t
   bladder preservation with, 3122-3123
      partial cystectomy, 3124-3125
      radiation monotherapy, 3124
      radical transurethral resection, 3124
      single modality treatment for, 3124-3125
      trimodal therapy for, 3123, 3123t
      trimodality therapy for, 3123-3124
   clinical presentation of, 3112-3114
   clinical staging for, 3112-3113, 3113t
   diagnosis of, 3112-3114
   grossly positive nodes and, 3117
   histology of, 3112
   management of, 3112-3132, 3131b
   natural history of, 3112
   neoadjuvant chemotherapy for, 3119-3120, 3120t
   pathologic staging for, 3113-3114, 3114t
   prognostic nomograms for, 3125-3127, 3126f
   radical cystectomy and pelvic lymph node dissection for, 3114-3119
Muscles
   of abdominal wall, lower, 2444-2448, 2447f-2448f
   of pelvic floor
      female, 2430-2432, 2432f
      male, 2449, 2449f
   in prune-belly syndrome, 587, 600
Musculocutaneous artery, 136f
Mutation, androgen receptor and, 3685-3686
Mutations (SPOP, FOXA1, IDH1), tumors defined by, 3470-3472, 3470f
MVV. see Maximum voided volume
MWA. see Microwave ablation
Myasthenia gravis
   contrast media and, 32
   lower urinary tract dysfunction and, 2630
Mycobacterium tuberculosis, 1133
Mycophenolate mofetil (CellCept), for BPS/IC oral therapy, 1243
Mycoplasma genitalium, 1253-1254
Myelodysplasia
   early intervention in, 628
   renal dysfunction in, 629
   sexuality and, 629-630
Myelolipoma
   as benign lesions, 2392, 2392f, 2392b
   MRI and, 52-53, 53f-56f, 58f
Myelomeningocele
   closure, prenatal counseling for prenatal surgery for, 362
   lower urinary tract dysfunction with, 2617
   prenatal closure of, 625
   presentation of, 625f
   urologic surgery and, 288-290
Myofibroblasts, 2470, 2470f
   and PD, 1605
Myogenic hypothesis, 2642
Myoplasty
   for bladder emptying, 2903
   stimulated, 2903
Myosin, in thick filaments, 2471, 2471f
Myosin heavy chains (MHCs), 2471, 2471f
Myosin light chains (MLCs), 2471
Myotonic dystrophy, lower urinary tract dysfunction and, 2631

N
NAATs. see Nucleic acid amplification tests
Naftopidil
   for benign prostatic hyperplasia, 3365-3367, 3367t
   to facilitate bladder filling and urine storage, 2682t
   for ureteral stone passage, 1900
Naloxone, to facilitate bladder emptying, 2719

Narcotic considerations, patient history of, 2-3
Narrow band imaging (NBI), for non-muscle invasive bladder cancer, 3097-3098
NASA TLX. see National Aeronautics and Space Administration Task Load Index assessment
National Aeronautics and Space Administration Task Load Index assessment (NASA TLX), 471
National Institutes for Clinical Excellence Guidelines, 507
Natriuretic peptides, in ED, 1498
Natural orifice transluminal endoscopic surgery (NOTES), 2421
   instrumentation for, 218
   for kidney surgery, 2284-2285, 2285f, 2286t
NBCi. see Nocturnal bladder capacity index
NBI. see Narrow band imaging
NCCT. see Noncontrast computed tomography
NDO. see Neurogenic detrusor overactivity; Nocturnal detrusor overactivity
Nd:YAG. see Neodymium:yttrium-aluminum-garnet
Near-infrared spectroscopy (NIRS), for benign prostatic hyperplasia, 3349
Necrosis
   PC-RPLND findings of, survival outcomes associated with, 1726
   penile, implant for, 1595-1596, 1595f
Needle biopsy
   for prostate adenocarcinoma, 3509-3510, 3510b
   for prostate cancer, 3519-3520
Needle drivers, for laparoscopic and robotic surgery, 215, 215.e3f
Needle suspension repair, retropubic suspension surgery *versus*, 2771
Negative feedback, in HPG axis, 1390, 1391f
Neoadjuvant androgen deprivation
   with radiation therapy, for locally advanced prostate cancer, 3652-3653, 3654b
   with radical prostatectomy, for locally advanced prostate cancer, 3648-3649, 3648t-3649t
Neoadjuvant chemotherapy, for muscle-invasive bladder cancer, 3119-3120, 3120t
Neoadjuvant chemotherapy-hormonal therapy, with radical prostatectomy, for locally advanced prostate cancer, 3649-3650, 3650t
Neobladder-urethral anastomosis
   maneuvers facilitating, 3268-3269
   for minimally invasive urinary diversion, 3264
Neodymium:yttrium-aluminum-garnet (Nd:YAG), 239
Neonatal urologic emergencies, 382-383
Neonates
   hydronephrosis diagnosis in, 1943
   with UPJO, 1943
Neoplasia, of bladder, 1360-1361
Neoplastic conditions, of cutaneous diseases of external genitalia
   basal cell carcinoma, 1297-1298, 1300f
   bowenoid papulosis, 1296, 1298f
   cutaneous T-cell lymphoma, 1302, 1302f
   extramammary Paget disease, 1301-1302, 1301f
   Kaposi sarcoma, 1298-1299, 1300f
   melanoma, 1300-1301
   pseudoepitheliomatous, keratotic, and micaceous balanitis, 1299-1300, 1300f
   squamous cell carcinoma, 1296, 1299f
   squamous cell carcinoma in situ, 1296, 1298f
   verrucous carcinoma, 1296-1297, 1299f
Neostigmine, ureteral response to, 1887-1888
Nephrectomy, 444
   for genitourinary tuberculosis treatment, 1317
   history of, 2133

Nephrectomy (Continued)
  for metastatic RCC, 2325-2328, 2326f-2327f, 2327t, 2328b
  open, technique of, 2254, 2254.e1f
  renal bleeding and, 1988-1989
  in renal transplantation, 1058
  for renal trauma
    partial, 1989-1990, 1989f
    total, 1991
  for retroperitoneal tumors, 2243
  RPLND with, 1718, 1718t
  segmental, for large polar tumors, 2263-2264, 2263.e1f-2263.e2f, 2264.e1f, 2265f
  for ureteral anomalies
    laparoscopic partial, 811-813, 814f
    open partial, 811, 812f-814f
    upper pole partial, 811-813, 812f, 814b
  for ureteral injuries, upper, 1998
  for ureteropelvic junction obstruction, 1946-1947
Nephric ducts, formation of, 336
Nephroblastomatosis, 1101, 1101f
Nephrocalcin
  in crystal formation, 2014
  in crystal matrix, 2015
Nephrogenic adenoma, 526
  of bladder, 3082
    in pediatric patients, 1119
Nephrogenic rests, 1100-1101, 1101f
Nephrogenic systemic fibrosis (NSF), 773
  contrast media and, 34-35
Nephrolithiasis, 400, 1939. see also Urinary lithiasis
  child with, 854-856, 855f-856f
  HIV and, 1266
  treatment of, 1939
Nephrolithotomy
  percutaneous, 243.e1, 244.e3
    for bladder stones, 244.e3-244.e4
    ShockPulse-SE, 245-246
  for ureteropelvic junction obstruction, percutaneous antegrade endopyelotomy simultaneous with, 1949
Nephrolysis, laparoscopic, 2294, 2294f
Nephron, 1866-1868, 1867f
  anatomy, 1906, 1906f-1907f, 1907b
  hydrogen ion transport in, urinary tract obstruction and, 793
  sodium transport in, urinary tract obstruction and, 793
Nephronophthisis, 350
Nephron-sparing surgery, for RCC, 2173-2174, 2174f
Nephropathy, aristolochic acid, 2196
Nephropexy, laparoscopic, 2292-2294, 2293f
  procedure for, 2293f
  results of, 2293-2294
Nephropleural fistula, 180
Nephrostomy tract, establishment of, in antegrade nephroureteroscopic, for UTUC, 2215-2216, 2215f
Nephrostomy tube, for pediatric genitourinary trauma, 1072
Nephrotic syndrome, in children, 344-345
Nephroureteral stent, 173, 174f, 176b
Nephroureterectomy
  for posterior urethral valves, 615
  radical, 2199-2202
    distal ureter and bladder cuff management, 2200
    indications of, 2199
    laparoscopic, 2202-2205
    open, 2199-2200, 2200f
    total laparoscopic technique in, 2202, 2203f
    traditional open distal ureterectomy in, 2200-2201, 2200f-2201f
    transurethral resection of ureteral orifice, 2201-2202, 2202f

Nephroureterectomy (Continued)
    transvesical ligation and detachment technique in, 2201, 2201f
  robot-assisted, 2205, 2205f
  transperitoneal, 2203-2204, 2203f-2204f
NER. see Nucleotide excision repair
Nerve growth factor (NGF)
  in bladder outlet obstruction, 2506
  in bladder pain syndrome and interstitial cystitis, 2508
  in detrusor overactivity, 2505
  in overactive bladder, 2504
Nerve injury, during laparoscopic and robotic surgery, 230
Nerve sheath tumors, retroperitoneal tumors and, 2235-2236, 2236f
Nerves, adrenal, 2345, 2350f
Nerve-sparing RPLND, 2241-2242, 2242f
Nervous system
  of lower urinary tract, peripheral nervous system, 2480-2497, 2480f
  of retroperitoneum, 1674-1679
    autonomic nervous system, 1674-1675, 1676f-1677f
    somatic nervous system, 1675-1679, 1675.e1f, 1677f-1678f, 1679t
  in ureteral function
    parasympathetic, 1887-1888
    purinergic, 1889-1890
    sensory innervation and peptidergic agents, 1889
    sympathetic, 1888-1889
Nested variant, of urothelial cancer, 3088
Neural injury, in robotic prostatectomy, 3580
Neural tube defects (NTD), 624-631, 626b
  early intervention for, 628-629, 629b
  epidemiology of, 624
  findings with, 626-628
  pathogenesis of, 624, 626t
  perinatal concerns with, 625
  postnatal management of
    congenital neurogenic bladder, 631, 631f, 632t
    initial, 626
    neurogenic bowel dysfunction, 631
  prenatal closure of, bladder function after, 625
  prevention of, 290
  risk factors for, 624
  upper urinary tract deterioration with, 626-628, 627f
Neurobiology, in BPS/IC etiology, 1232.e7-1232.e9, 1232.e9b
Neuroblastoma, 1087-1096, 1096b, 2388
  clinical presentation and pattern of spread of, 1088-1089, 1089f
  diagnosis of
    imaging, 1089, 1089f-1090f
    laboratory evaluation, 1089
    screening, 1089-1090
    staging, 1090-1091, 1090t-1091t
  epidemiology and genetics of, 1087
  pathology of, 1088, 1088f-1089f
  prognosis of, 1091-1092
    biologic variables affecting, 1092
    clinical variables affecting, 1091-1092
  in retroperitoneum, 2234
  spontaneous regression of, 1087-1088
  treatment of
    biologic therapies, 1095-1096
    chemotherapy, 1093f, 1095
    radiotherapy, 1096
    spinal cord decompression, 1096
    surgery, 1092-1095, 1093f
Neuroendocrine cells, of prostate, 3278f, 3279
Neurofibroma, 1304, 1305f
  in retroperitoneum, 2235
Neurogenic acontractile detrusor, 2565

Neurogenic bladder
  autonomous, 2522
  with CNS tumors, 648
  diminished bladder capacity and, 2671
  reflex, 2522
  renal transplantation and, 1057-1058
  sensory, 2522
  uninhibited, 2522
Neurogenic bladder dysfunction, 2964
Neurogenic bowel dysfunction, management of, with spina bifida, 631
Neurogenic detrusor overactivity (NDO), 2521
  capsaicin for, 2709.e1
  detrusor underactivity and, 2521
  resiniferatoxin in, 2709.e1
  urinary incontinence and, 2595
Neurogenic lower urinary tract dysfunction (NLUTD)
  urodynamic studies, evidence-based review of, 2577-2578
  videourodynamics for, 2569-2570
Neurogenic origins, retroperitoneal tumors and, 2234
Neuroimaging, in ED, 1526
Neurologic complications, after RPLND, 1731, 2244
Neurologic conditions, pelvic floor disorders and, 2527
Neurologic disease
  detrusor underactivity and, 2657, 2657b
  prostatitis and, 1210
Neurologic examination
  for pelvic floor disorders, 2530
  physical examination for, 12, 12f
Neuromodulation. see also Electrical stimulation
  for bowel-bladder dysfunction, 658, 659t
  for BPS/IC treatment, 1246-1247, 1247b
  for chronic scrotal pain syndrome, 1221
  for lower urinary tract dysfunction, 2510-2512
    to inhibit OAB, rationale for, 2511, 2511f
    inhibitory and excitatory stimulation frequencies, 2511
    onabotulinumtoxinA, 2512
    pudendal nerve stimulation, 2511
    somatic afferents activation, in foot, 2511-2512
    for voiding, rationale for, 2510, 2510f
  for neuromuscular dysfunction of lower urinary tract, 637-638
  sacral, mechanism of action, 2510
  for urinary incontinence, in geriatric patients, 2920.e5
Neuromuscular complication, in urologic surgery, 261-262
Neuromuscular dysfunction of lower urinary tract, 624-651, 2600-2636. see also Voiding dysfunction
  acquired immunodeficiency syndrome and, 2625
  acute disseminated encephalomyelitis and, 2625-2626
  aging and, 2633
  amyloidosis, 2632
  amyotrophic lateral sclerosis and, 2624
  attention-deficit/hyperactivity disorder, 2633
  bashful bladder, 2628-2629
  benign joint hypermobility syndrome, 2633
  bladder neck dysfunction, 2627-2628
  bladder outlet obstruction in women, 2628
  in children
    anorectal malformation, 644-645
    causes of, 624, 625t
    management principles for, 632-638, 632t-633t, 633b
    medical management for, 633-634, 633t, 638b
    neuromodulation for, 637-638
    renal function assessment with, 629-631
    surgical management of, 635-638, 638b

Neuromuscular dysfunction of lower urinary tract (Continued)
vesicoureteral reflux in, 638–639, 638f, 639b
congenital adrenal hyperplasia, 2633
corticobasal degeneration, 2631
defunctionalized bladder, 2632–2633
detrusor sphincter dyssynergia and, 2627
distal to spinal cord, 2619–2624
childbirth, 2621
diabetes mellitus, 2622–2624, 2624b
disk disease, 2619–2620
Guillain-Barré syndrome, 2624
herpesvirus infection, 2621–2622
hysterectomy, 2621
radical pelvic surgery, 2620–2621
spinal stenosis, 2620
dysfunctional voiding, 2627
Ehlers-Danlos syndrome, 2631
Fowler syndrome, 2629
gastroparesis, 2630
hereditary spastic paraplegia and, 2624–2625
hyperthyroidism, 2630
Isaacs syndrome, 2630
Lyme disease and, 2624
Machado-Joseph disease, 2632
myasthenia gravis, 2630
myotonic dystrophy, 2631
neuroplasticity and, 2600–2602
at or above brainstem, 2602–2607
brain tumor, 2604
brainstem stroke, 2603
cerebellar ataxia, 2604
cerebral palsy, 2604–2605
cerebrovascular disease, 2602–2603
dementia, 2603–2604
multiple system atrophy, 2606–2607, 2607b
normal-pressure hydrocephalus, 2604
Parkinson disease, 2605–2606
progressive supranuclear palsy, 2607
traumatic brain injury, 2604
patterns of, 2600–2602, 2601t
radiation, 2632
reflex sympathetic dystrophy and, 2626
sacrococcygeal teratoma, 2631
schistosomal myelopathy and, 2626
schizophrenia, 2630
spinal cord involvement in, 2607–2619
acute transverse myelitis, 2617
autonomic dysreflexia, 2614–2615
bladder cancer and, 2616
cervical myelopathy, 2617
follow-up for, 2616–2617
multiple sclerosis, 2607–2608
neurologic and urodynamic correlation, 2612–2614
neurospinal dysraphism, 2617–2619
pernicious anemia, 2619
poliomyelitis, 2619
sacral injury, 2611–2612, 2613f, 2613b
spinal cord injury, 2609–2617, 2609b
spinal shock, 2610
subacute combined degeneration, 2619
suprasacral injury, 2610–2611, 2611f–2612f, 2612b
tabes dorsalis, 2619
urinary tract infection, 2615
vesicoureteral reflux, 2615
in women, 2615–2616
syringomyelia and, 2626
systemic lupus erythematosus and, 2626
systemic sclerosis, 2631
treatment of, 2634–2635, 2634b
tropical spastic paraparesis and, 2625
tuberculosis and, 2626–2627
urinary retention, postoperative, 2629–2630
Wernicke encephalopathy, 2631
Williams-Beuren syndrome, 2631–2632

Neuroplasticity, in lower urinary tract dysfunction, 2600–2602
Neurospinal abnormalities, with cloacal exstrophy, 574–575, 574f
Neurospinal dysraphism, lower urinary tract dysfunction with, 2617–2619
Neurotransmitters, within brainstem networks, 2495–2496
Neurovascular bundle (NVB)
injury, complications of seminal vesicle surgery, 1864
preservation of, in laparoscopic radical prostatectomy, 3575–3576, 3575f–3576f
in retropubic radical prostatectomy, 3555–3556
high anterior release of, at apex, 3557–3558, 3558f–3559f
identification of, 3556–3558
preservation of, 3556–3557, 3556f–3557f
wide excision of, 3558, 3559f
Neutrons, 3594
NGF. see Nerve growth factor
NHCT. see Noncontrast helical computed tomography
Nicardipine, for PD, 1612, 1617t
Nicotinic agonists, ureteral response to, 1887
Nifedipine
for BPS/IC oral therapy, 1241t, 1243
for ureteral relaxation, 1900
Nighttime, definition of, 2666
Nilutamide, 3675–3676
Nintedanib, for RCC, 2337–2338
Nipple (rosebud) stoma, 3182, 3182f–3183f
Nipple valve, 3191, 3192f
for continent urinary diversions, 707
NIRS. see Near-infrared spectroscopy
Nitric oxide (NO)
bladder afferent pathway and, 2484, 2484f
in ED, 1494, 1495t, 1497–1498
to facilitate bladder emptying, 2720.e1
metabolism of, in BPS/IC etiology, 1232.e9
and PD, 1605
renal vascular tone control by, 1913
ureteral response to, 1886, 1886f
urothelium release of, 2469
Nitrite, 437
Nitrite tests, in urine, 20–21, 20f
Nitrofurantoin, 441
for UTIs, 1150–1153, 1151t–1153t, 1156, 1163, 1187t
Nitrous oxide, as insufflant choice, 220
NK1-receptor antagonists, to facilitate bladder filling and urine storage, 2713.e4
Nkx3.1, 3276
NLUTD. see Neurogenic lower urinary tract dysfunction
NMIBC. see Non-muscle-invasive bladder cancer
NO. see Nitric oxide
No drainage tube, 176
Nocturia, 2581, 2664–2678, 3345
behavioral therapy with urge suppression for, 2727
bladder capacity and, 2667, 2668t, 2671–2674
classification of, 2667, 2668t, 2669f
definition of, 2664, 2665t
degree of bother of, 2664
drug effects causing, 2671b
evaluation of, 2666–2667, 2667b, 2678b
in geriatric patients, 2920.e8–2920.e9
mechanisms of, 2505
mortality, early and, 2664–2666
nocturnal polyuria and, 662, 2667–2668, 2668t
overactive bladder and, 2637
polyuria and, 2667–2668, 2668t
prevalence of, 2461, 2664
rationale for evaluation and management of, 2664–2666, 2666b

Nocturia (Continued)
societal costs of, 2666
treatment algorithm for, 2669f
Nocturia Quality of Life (N-QoL) score, 2669
Nocturnal bladder capacity index (NBCi), 2667
Nocturnal detrusor overactivity (NDO), 2671
Nocturnal enuresis, 2539, 2581
desmopressin for, 2712
treatment of, 2547
Nocturnal polyuria
diminished bladder capacity and, 2674–2678
epidemiology and causes of, 2667–2668, 2670f
management of, 2668–2671, 2673t
nocturia and, 662, 2667–2668, 2668t
with obstructive sleep apnea, 2668
Nocturnal polyuria index (NPi), 2667
Nocturnal urine volume (NUV), 2667
Node-positive disease, outcomes of prostatectomy for, 3647–3648
Nonabsorbable sutures, 150
Non-AIDS-defining urologic malignancies, 1268
Nonatherosclerotic renal artery diseases, 1933–1934
Noncommunicating hydroceles, epidemiology and pathogenesis of, 889
Noncontrast computed tomography (NCCT), of urinary calculi, 2037, 2037f
Noncontrast helical computed tomography (NHCT), for urinary tract obstruction, 779
Nondilated or absent bladder, 518–519
bladder agenesis, 518–519
bladder hypoplasia, 519
cloacal and bladder exstrophy, 519
Nondismembered pyeloplasty, for ureteropelvic junction obstruction in children, 828–829, 829f–831f
Nonfilarial parasitic infections, of genitourinary tract
amebiasis, 1332
echinococcosis, 1332
enterobiasis, 1332
trichomoniasis, 1332
Nonfocal extraprostatic extension, 3511
Nonglomerular hematuria, 17–18
Nongonococcal urethritis, 1253, 1254f
Chlamydia, 1253
Mycoplasma genitalium, 1253–1254
recurrent and persistent, 1254
Trichomatis vaginalis, 1254
Noninfectious genital ulcers, 1286–1288, 1286b
aphthous ulcers and Behçet disease, 1286–1287, 1287f
pyoderma gangrenosum, 1287–1288, 1288f
traumatic causes, 1288, 1288f
Nonionizing radiation, technique of, 403, 403b
Nonmaleficence, definition of, 115
Nonmonosymptomatic enuresis, 660
Non-muscle-invasive bladder cancer (NMIBC), 3075
Bacille Calmette-Guérin for, 3099–3100
carcinoma treatment in situ with, 3100
contraindications to, 3102b
mechanism of action of, 3100
prophylaxis to prevent recurrence, 3100–3101
residual tumor treatment, 3100
toxicity management of, 3102b
biology of, 3092–3094
early cystectomy for, 3106–3107, 3107b
endoscopic surgical management of, 3094–3098, 3099b
confocal laser endomicroscopy for, 3097–3098
fluorescence cystoscopy for, 3097–3098, 3098f
laser resection for, 3097
narrow band imaging for, 3097–3098
office-based, 3097

Non-muscle-invasive bladder cancer (NMIBC) (Continued)
    optical coherent tomography for, 3097–3098
    immunotherapy for, 3099–3103, 3103b
        Bacille Calmette-Guérin, 3099–3100
        interferon, 3102–3103
        investigational, 3103
    intravesical chemotherapy for, 3103–3105, 3104t, 3105b
        combination therapy, 3105
        doxorubicin, 3103–3104
        mitomycin C, 3104–3105
        novel agents, 3103
        to prevent implantation, 3103–3105
        to prevent tumor implantation, 3100b
        thiotepa, 3103
        valrubicin, 3104
    intravesical immunotherapy for, 3099–3103
        Bacille Calmette-Guérin, 3099–3100
    intravesical therapy of, 3098–3105
    management strategies for, 3091–3111
    pathology of, 3092t, 3094b
        characteristics by stage, 3094, 3094t
    perioperative intravesical therapy for, 3098–3099
    prevention of
        secondary, 3110
        surveillance for, 3107–3110, 3108t, 3111b
    refractory high-grade disease, 3105–3107
        alternative options for, 3106
        management of, 3106, 3107b
    surveillance for, 3108–3109
        cystoscopic, 3108–3109
        extravesical, 3110
        tumor markers, 3109–3110, 3109f
        urine cytology, 3109
    transurethral resection for
        complications of, 3096
        repeat, 3096–3097
Non-rapid eye movement (NREM), 2665
Nonrefluxing ureteral reimplantation, 3021–3022, 3022–3025, 3022f–3024f
Nonselective α₁-blockers, 3356
Nonseminoma germ cell tumors (NSGCTs), 2227–2229
    chemotherapy for, 1695, 1696t, 1697
    clinical stage I tumors, 1693–1696, 1694t
        retroperitoneal lymph node dissection, 1694–1695, 1695t
        risk assessment, 1693
        surveillance, 1693–1694, 1694t
        treatment selection for, 1695–1696
    clinical stage IIA and IIB, 1696–1697
    clinical stage IIC and III tumors, 1697–1700
    clinical stage IS, 1696
    genomic alterations in, 1361
    relapse after, 1701–1702
    residual mass management after, 1698–1700, 1698t–1699t
    treatment of, 1692, 1692b, 1702b
Nonstaghorn renal calculi, 2069–2070
    stone burden of
        between 1 and 2 cm, 2073–2074, 2073f
        greater than 2 cm, 2074
        up to 1 cm, 2072–2073, 2072b
Nonsteroidal antiandrogens, 3674–3676
Nonsteroidal anti-inflammatory drugs (NSAIDs)
    RI and, 778
    for urinary tract obstruction, 795
Nonsurgical focal therapy, of renal tumors, 2309–2323
    complications, 2318–2319, 2320f–2321f, 2320b
    cryoablation, 2309–2310, 2310b. see also Cryoablation (CA), for renal tumors
    new ablation modalities, 2319–2323, 2323b
    oncologic outcomes, 2314–2318, 2315t–2316t, 2318b
    radiofrequency ablation, 2310–2312, 2312b
    surgical technique, 2312

Nonsurgical focal therapy, of renal tumors (Continued)
    treatment success and follow-up protocol after tumor ablation, 2312–2314, 2314b
Nontreponemal syphilis tests, 1258
Nontuberculous mycobacteria, 1133
Nonulcerating skin infections, HIV and, 1265
Nonurothelial malignant lesions, 2189
    adenocarcinoma, 2189
    other, 2189
    squamous cell carcinoma, 2189
Norephedrine, for stress urinary incontinence in women, 2714
Norepinephrine
    in ED, 1494, 1495t
    renal vascular tone control by, 1913
    ureteral response to, 1888
Normal compliance, 2560–2561
Normal detrusor function, 2565
Normal-pressure hydrocephalus, lower urinary tract dysfunction with, 2604
Normal scrotal position, 949
Normocomplementemic glomerulonephritis, 346–348
Normothermia, definition of, 145
North American and International Finasteride trial, 3372
Nosocomial UTIs, 433
NOTES. see Natural orifice transluminal endoscopic surgery
Novel markers, for locally advanced prostate cancer, 3642–3643, 3642t
NPi. see Nocturnal polyuria index
NPO guidelines, 449, 449t
    enteral tube feeds, 449
    ketogenic diet, 449
    special, 449
NR0B1 gene, 992f, 992t, 993
NR5A1 gene, 992–993, 992f, 992t
NREM. see Non-rapid eye movement
NS-398, urethral function effects of, 1903
NSAIDs. see Nonsteroidal anti-inflammatory drugs
NSF. see Nephrogenic systemic fibrosis
NSGCTs. see Nonseminoma germ cell tumors
NTD. see Neural tube defects
Nuclear cystography, 389–390
Nuclear imaging, 806, 806f
Nuclear localization, of androgen receptors, 3291
Nuclear matrix, androgens in, 3294–3295
Nuclear medicine
    basic principles of, 91–100
    imaging agents in, 91
    in urologic oncology, 42–44
Nuclear renography, for urinary tract obstruction, 779
Nuclear scintigraphy, 40–44, 44b
Nucleation, 2011
Nucleic acid amplification tests (NAATs), for genitourinary tuberculosis, 1310
Nucleotide excision repair (NER), 1351.e1, 1351.e1f
Nucleotides, 1346.e1, 1346.e2f
Numeric pain rating scale, 448f
Nurses' Health Study, 2710
Nursing Home Setting, urinary incontinence in, 2919–2920
Nutcracker syndrome, 1869–1870
Nutrition, urinary intestinal diversion and, 3203
Nutritional status, in urologic surgery, 122–123
NUV. see Nocturnal urine volume
NVB. see Neurovascular bundle
NX-1207, to facilitate bladder filling and urine storage, 2713.e2

O

OAB. see Overactive bladder
Obesity, 1418–1419
    abdominal, 1418–1419
    benign prostatic hyperplasia and, 3324, 3325t

Obesity (Continued)
    and ED, 1504
    hyperoxaluria and, 2059–2060
    as laparoscopic and robotic surgery contraindication, 203
    laparoscopic kidney surgery and, 2279
    midurethral sling outcomes with, 2863, 2863b
    morbid, percutaneous nephrolithotomy and, 2106–2107
    orthotopic urinary diversion and, 3238
    prostate cancer and, 3465, 3465f, 3544
    in retropubic suspension surgery, 2756
    upper urinary tract calculi and, 2089
    urinary incontinence and, 2585–2586, 2734
Objective structured assessment of technical skills (OSATS) tool, 470
Obstetric fistulae, 2925–2926, 2926f
Obstetric history, pelvic floor disorders and, 2527–2528
Obstructed hemivagina and ipsilateral renal agenesis (OHVIRA) syndrome, 327, 328f
Obstructed labor injury complex, 2925
Obstruction
    bladder
        response to, 3315–3316
        RMS causing, 1113
    of seminal vesicles and ejaculatory ducts, 1407
    ureteropelvic junction. see Ureteropelvic junction obstruction
    urinary tract. see Urinary tract obstruction
    in UTI host defense mechanisms, 1139
Obstructive sleep apnea (OSA), 1420
    metabolic syndrome and, 1420
    nocturnal polyuria with, 2668
    treatment of, 2920.e8
ObTape, 2851
Obturator internus, 2448–2449, 2449f
Obturator lymph node, 1380
Obturator lymphadenectomy, 3149, 3152f
Obturator nerve, 2453t
OBTX. see OnabotulinumtoxinA
Occult spinal dysraphism, 389
"Occult" stress urinary incontinence, 2591–2592
Occupation
    patient history of, 9
    renal calculi and, 2007–2008
Occupational exposures, UTUC risk and, 2186
Occupational risk, in bladder tumor, 3076, 3076t
Odd-skipped related 1 (Osr1), vesicoureteral reflux and, 491.e1
ODS. see Output display standard
Off-clamp partial nephrectomy, 2303
Ogilvie syndrome, with intestinal anastomoses, 3181
Olaparib, 3702
Older women, prevention of urinary incontinence and, 2735
Oligohydramnios, prenatal sonogram for, 409f
Oligomeganephronia, 742–744, 743f
Oliguria, 386, 461
Omental herniation, 468–469
OnabotulinumtoxinA (OBTX), 286
    to facilitate bladder filling and urine storage, 2707–2708
    neuromodulation with, 2512
    in surgical management of voiding dysfunction, 2848
    for UUI, 2546
Oncocytoma, 2391, 2392b
    renal, 2123–2125, 2125b
        epidemiology and etiology of, 2123
        evaluation of, 2124
        management of, 2124–2125
        pathophysiology of, 2123–2124, 2124f
Oncogenes, 1346–1347, 1347b
Oncologic fistulae, 2959

Oncology
  chronic inflammation in GU cancers, 1336, 1338b
    bladder cancer, 1336-1338, 1337f-1338f
    kidney cancer, 1338
    prostate cancer, 1338
  immunologic response in GU cancers, 1333-1345, 1336b
    adaptive immune system, 1334-1336, 1335f
    immune editing hypothesis, 1336, 1337f
    innate immune system, 1333-1334, 1334f-1335f, 1334t-1335t
  immunotherapy for GU cancers, 1333-1345, 1341b, 1343b
    BCG in bladder cancer, 1333, 1334f, 1338-1339, 1339f
    cancer vaccines, 1339-1340, 1340f-1341f
    combination, 1343-1345, 1345f
    immune checkpoint blockade, 1342, 1342f
  molecular genetics in. see Molecular genetics
  pediatric. see Pediatric oncology
Oncotype DX Prostate Cancer Test, 3488, 3521
One-kidney, one-clip model, of renovascular hypertension, 1917, 1918f
One-port catheters, 153
On-table intravenous pyelography, for pediatric genitourinary trauma, 1073-1074
Open access techniques
  for achieving extraperitoneal access and developing extraperitoneal space, 210-211
  for achieving retroperitoneal access and developing retroperitoneal space, 209-210
  for achieving transperitoneal access and establishing pneumoperitoneum, 209, 209f
  complications related to, 224
Open adrenalectomy, 2410-2414
  anterior transabdominal approach, 2412-2413, 2412f-2413f
  flank retroperitoneal approach, 2410-2411, 2410f-2411f
  left, 2412-2413, 2412f-2413f
  outcomes, 2421-2423
  posterior lumbodorsal approach, 2411-2412, 2411f-2412f
  thoracoabdominal approach, 2413-2414, 2413f-2414f
Open cystotomy, 156, 156f
Open distal ureterectomy with excision of bladder cuff, 2204
Open flank incision, 459f
Open nephrectomy, technique of, for benign diseases, 2254, 2254.e1f
Open prostatectomy, robotic prostatectomy versus, 3532
Open radical prostatectomy, 3548-3565
Open reconstruction, for urethral stricture disease, 1819-1828
Open segmental ureterectomy, 2207, 2208f-2209f
Open simple prostatectomy, 3450
  incision for, 3450
  patient positioning for, 3450
  space of Retzius development for, 3450
Open surgery, common urologic procedures, antimicrobial prophylaxis for, 1199-1200
Open transabdominal orchidopexy, 967
Operating room setup, for laparoscopic and robotic surgery, 205, 205b
Operative nerve injury, 262
Operative team placement, for laparoscopic and robotic surgery
  retroperitoneal upper abdominal procedures, 207, 207f
  transperitoneal upper abdominal procedures, 206f, 206.e1f
Opiates, and ED, 1509

Opioid-receptor antagonists, to facilitate bladder emptying, 2719
Opioids
  abuse, in men, 1426
  and ED, 1494-1495, 1495t
  for urinary tract obstruction, 795
Oral mucosa grafts, for urethral and penile reconstruction, 1806, 1806f
Oral therapies, for BPS/IC treatment, 1241-1244, 1241t, 1244b
Orchalgia, 1219-1220
  nonmedical therapy for, 1221
  nonradical surgical treatments, 1221
  surgical therapy, 1221-1222
Orchidopexy
  Fowler-Stephens, 967-968
  laparoscopic, 967-968
  open transabdominal, 967
  for prune-belly syndrome, 593-594
  transscrotal, 967, 967f
Orchiectomy, 3674
  castration-resistant prostate cancer and, 3688
  for chronic scrotal pain syndrome, 1222
  delayed, 1712
  evaluation after, 1712
  partial. see Partial orchiectomy
  radical. see Radical orchiectomy
  simple, 1848
    technique of, 1848, 1849f
  for TGCTs, 1686
Orchiopexy, in adults, 1483-1484, 1483f
Orchitis, 1440
  acute, 1202-1223
Orciprenaline, ureteral response to, 1888
Organ Injury Severity Scale for Kidney, of AAST, 1992t
Organ ischemia, during vena caval thrombectomy, 2278
Organ preservation, in penile cancer management, 1751
Organ transplantation. see Transplantation
Organomegaly, as laparoscopic and robotic surgery contraindication, 204
Organ-sparing therapy, UTUC after, 2220
Orgasm, female sexual dysfunction and, 1637
Orgasmic headache, 1580-1581
Orteronel, 3695
Orthophosphate, for hypercalciuria, 2052-2053
Orthostatic proteinuria, 343-344
Orthotopic Mainz pouch, for orthotopic urinary diversion, 3246, 3248f
Orthotopic neobladder, 3178
Orthotopic urinary diversion, 3233-3257
  basic principles of, 3234-3235, 3235b
  bladder substitution in
    bowel segment selection for, 3241-3249, 3242b
    reflux prevention in, 3241-3242, 3242b
  complications of, 3249-3257
  continence mechanism in, 3239, 3241b
  continence preservation in
    anterior apical dissection in male patient, 3239-3240
    urethra preservation in female patient, 3240-3241, 3240f
  follow-up for, 3255, 3255b
  general perioperative management for, 3242-3243
  history of, 3233-3234, 3234f, 3234b
  oncologic factors for, 3235-3237, 3237b
    locally advanced tumor stage, 3237
    urethral recurrence risk in men, 3235-3236
    urethral recurrence risk in women, 3236
  patient selection for, 3235-3239, 3235f
    patient-related factors, 3237-3239, 3239b
  quality of life after, 3255-3257, 3256t, 3257b
  results with, 3249-3257
    continence in, 3251-3254, 3252t-3253t, 3254b
    urinary retention with, 3254, 3254b

Orthotopic urinary diversion (Continued)
  surgical techniques for, 3243-3246
    Camey II, 3243, 3243f
    colon and ileocolic pouches, 3246-3248
    ileal neobladder, 3245, 3246f
    ileal reservoirs, 3243
    Kock ileal reservoir, 3243-3244, 3244f
    minimally invasive, 3248-3249
    orthotopic Mainz pouch, 3246, 3248f
    Padua pouch, 3248, 3250f
    right colon pouch, 3246
    serous-lined extramural tunnel, 3244-3245, 3245f
    sigmoid pouch, 3248, 3249f
    Studer pouch, 3245, 3247f
    T pouch modification, 3245-3246, 3247f
OSA. see Obstructive sleep apnea
Osmolality, 15
Osmotic effect, of urothelium of bladder, 2467
Osteogenic sarcoma, of kidney, 2181
Osteomalacia, with urinary intestinal diversion, 3201-3202
Osteopontin, in crystal formation, 2011, 2014-2015
Osteoporosis, hormonal therapy and, 3680
Osteotomy
  for classic bladder exstrophy, 540-542, 541f-542f
  complications of, 542-543
  in urinary tract reconstruction, of cloacal exstrophy, 578-579, 579f
Ouabain, urethral function effects of, 1903
Outcomes research, 101
  binary survival, 104-105
  definition of, 101
  disease progression, 104-105
  disease-specific mortality in, 103-104
  health services and, 101
  health-related quality of life, 112-113. see also Health-related quality of life
  measure, 101-102
  overall mortality in, 102-103
  proxy endpoints, 104
  recurrence, 104-105
  sexual dysfunction, 110-112
  short-term, 105-108
Outflow resistance, 682
Output display standard (ODS), in ultrasonography, 78
Ovarian formation, 318
Ovarian tumors, in pediatric patients, 1120
Ovariectomy, 3063-3064
Ovaries
  anatomy of, 324f, 2437-2438
  function of, 995
  ligament of, 321
Overactive bladder (OAB), 1421, 2637-2649, 2915
  afferent mechanisms in, 2641-2642
  after retropubic suspension surgery, 2770
  clinical assessment of, 2643-2646, 2646b
    advanced evaluation, 2645-2646, 2645f-2646f
    initial evaluation, 2643-2645, 2644t
    laboratory examination, 2645
    physical examination, 2645
  costs of, 2640
  definitions for, 2637, 2638f, 2638t, 2639b
  detrusor overactivity with, 2640
  economics of, 2638-2640
  epidemiology of, 2638-2640, 2639t
  estrogens for, 2709-2710, 2713-2714
  etiology of, 2643, 2643b
  female sexual dysfunction and, 1655-1656
  health burden of, 2639-2640
  incidence and progression of, 2639
  management of, 2646-2649, 2649b
    approach, 2647-2649, 2648f
    first-line therapy, 2646-2647

Overactive bladder (OAB) *(Continued)*
    fourth-line therapy, 2647
    second-line therapy, 2647
    third-line therapy, 2647
  mechanisms of, 2504, 2713.e4b
  metabolic syndrome and, 1421
  neuromodulation for, 2510
    rationale for, 2511, 2511f
  nocturnal bladder capacity and, 661–662
  pathophysiology of, 2517, 2640–2643, 2640f–2641f, 2643b
  pelvic organ prolapse and, 2591
  pharmacologic therapy for, 2682t, 2704b
    antimuscarinic agents, 2681, 2681f
  prevalence of, 2591, 2638–2639
  questionnaires for, 2532t–2533t
  sacral nerve stimulation for, 2752–2753
  terminology for, 2637, 2638f, 2638t, 2639b
    bladder pain syndrome distinguished from, 2637, 2638f
    mixed symptoms incorporating urinary urgency, 2637, 2638f
  urgency urinary incontinence with, 2539
Overactive Bladder Questionnaire (OAB-Q), 111t
Overflow incontinence, patient history of, 5–6
Overflow proteinuria, 18
Overnight low-dose dexamethasone suppression test, in evaluation of adrenal masses, 2400
Overnight water deprivation test (OWDT), 2678
Ovotesticular disorder of sexual development, 322, 323f, 999f, 1006–1007
OWDT. *see* Overnight water deprivation test
Oxalate
  in calcium stone formation, 2020
  foods containing, 2057b
  metabolism of, 2016–2017
Oxalobacter formigenes, 2017
Oxford guidelines
  for behavior therapy, 2722.e4b
  to facilitate bladder filling and urine storage, 2681t
Oxidative stress, stone disease and, 2013–2014
Oxidized regenerated cellulose agents, 147
Oxybutynin, 2498, 2499t, 3381
  for urinary incontinence, 657
Oxybutynin chloride
  effects on cognition of, 2695
  extended release, 2693–2694
  to facilitate bladder filling and urine storage, 2682, 2682t
    with α-adrenoreceptor antagonists, 2705
    with other antimuscarinics, 2693
  immediate-release, 2693
  intravesical administration of, 2695
  rectal administration of, 2695
  topical gel, 2694
  transdermal, 2694
Oxygen free radicals and oxidative stress, and PD, 1605
Oxytocin
  in ED, 1494, 1495t
  for female orgasmic disorder, 1648
  for female sexual arousal disorders, 1650
Oxytocin antagonists, for PE, 1572.e2

P

P (mannose-resistant) pili, 429, 1134–1135
p16. *see* INK4A gene
Pacemaker activity, 1881–1882, 1882f
Pacemaker potentials, 1881–1882, 1882f
Packed red blood cells, for urologic surgery, 147
Paclitaxel, for non–muscle-invasive bladder cancer, 3105
Paclitaxel, ifosfamide, and cisplatin (TIP)
  for NSGCTs, 1700
  for penile cancer, 1770
Pad tests
  for male urinary incontinence, 2541–2543
  for pelvic floor disorders, 2531–2533
  use of, 109–110

PADAM. *see* Partial androgen deficiency in aging male
Padua pouch, for orthotopic urinary diversion, 3248, 3250f
Pagano technique, in urinary diversion, 3186–3187, 3187f
Pain
  after laparoscopic and robotic surgery, 230–231
  after midurethral sling, 2870–2871
  in castration-resistant prostate cancer, 3702, 3703t
  definition of, 448
  intensity of, 448f
  management of. *see also* Analgesia
    after laparoscopic radical prostatectomy, 3578–3579
  in urinary tract obstruction, 795
  patient history of, 2–3
  ureteral anomalies and, 802
Painful orgasm, 1636
Paired box gene 2 *(PAX2)*, vesicoureteral reflux and, 491.e1
Palliative care, 2922
Palliative surgery, for metastatic RCC, 2328, 2328b
Palpable testis, surgical management of, 966–967
  inguinal orchiopexy, 966–967
  transscrotal orchidopexy, 967, 967f
Pampiniform plexus, 1372, 1372f–1373f, 1393
Pancreas, 1668, 1668.e2f, 1669f–1670f
Pancreatic injury
  during laparoscopic and robotic surgery, 230.e1
  during radical nephrectomy, 2261
Panurothelial disease, UTUC, 2194
Papaverine, 1535
Papillary adenoma, of kidney, 2128, 2128b
Papillary necrosis, hematuria and, 18
Papillary RCC
  molecular genetics of, 1354t, 1358
  pathology of, 2149t–2151t, 2152, 2153f
Papillary urothelial neoplasm of low malignant potential (PUNLMP), 3083–3084, 3083f, 3092
Papilloma
  of bladder, 3081, 3081f
  of upper urinary tract, 2188
Papulosquamous disorders, 1278–1283, 1278b
  fixed drug eruption, 1282, 1283f
  lichen nitidus, 1281
  lichen planus, 1280–1281, 1281f
  lichen sclerosus, 1281–1282, 1282f
  psoriasis, 1278–1279, 1279f
  reactive arthritis, 1279–1280, 1280f
  seborrheic dermatitis, 1282–1283
Paracolpium, 2438
Paradoxical incontinence. *see* Overflow incontinence
Paraganglioma
  of adrenal gland, 2235, 2235f
  of bladder, 3038–3039, 3039f
Paraganglionic system tumors, retroperitoneal tumors and, 2235, 2235f
Parameatal urethral cyst, 394, 882, 882f
Parametrium, 2438
Paraneoplastic syndromes, in RCC, 2156
Paranephric fat, 1865–1866
Parapelvic cyst, 775, 775f
Paraphimosis, 393, 871–872, 872f
Paraphimosis, urethral reconstructive surgery for, 1811
Pararenal space, anterior, 1668, 1668.e1f–1668.e2f
Parasites, in urine, 24, 25f
Parasitic infections, of genitourinary tract, 1319–1332
  filariasis, 1328–1331, 1332b
    diagnosis, 1330
    epidemiology, 1328–1329

Parasitic infections, of genitourinary tract *(Continued)*
    organisms, 1328, 1328f
    pathology and clinical manifestations, 1329–1330, 1329f–1330f
    prevention and control, 1331
    treatment, 1330–1331
  nonfilarial
    amebiasis, 1332
    echinococcosis, 1332
    enterobiasis, 1332
    trichomoniasis, 1332. *see also* Trichomoniasis
  schistosomiasis, 1319–1328, 1328b
    biology and life cycle, 1319, 1320f–1321f
    clinical manifestations, 1324
    diagnosis, 1325–1326, 1325f–1326f
    epidemiology, 1319–1321
    history, 1319
    pathogenesis and pathology, 1321–1324, 1321f, 1323f
    prevention and control, 1327–1328
    prognosis, 1327
    treatment, 1326–1327
Parasympathetic blocking agents, ureteral response to, 1888
Parasympathetic decentralization, LUTD and, 2620–2621
Parasympathetic nervous system
  in retroperitoneum, 1675
  in ureteral function, 1887–1888
Parasympathetic pathways, of lower urinary tract, 2480, 2480f
Parasympathetic transmission, in neural control of LUT, 2593
Parasympathomimetics
  for detrusor underactivity, 2660–2661
  to facilitate bladder emptying, 2716–2718
Paratesticular cancer, RMS in pediatric patients, 1126–1127, 1127b
  outcomes of, 1126–1127
  presentation and staging of, 1126
  RPLND role in, 1126
  treatment of, 1126
Parathyroid hormone (PTH)
  in calcium metabolism, 2016
  in renal hypercalciuria, 2019
  renal regulation of, 1914, 1914f
  in resorptive hypercalciuria, 2020
Paraureteral congenital diverticula, 522, 522f
Paraureteral diverticula, 525
Paraurethral cysts, 394f, 395, 397f, 976–977, 977f
Paravaginal repair procedures
  for female incontinence, 2766–2767, 2767b
    Burch colposuspension *versus*, 2773
    results with, 2766–2767
    suspensions in, configuration of, 2758
    technique for, 2766, 2767f
    tissue approximation in, 2759
    urethral elevation in, 2758
  for pelvic organ prolapse
    abdominal, 2779, 2780t
    vaginal, 2780t, 2783, 2784f–2785f
Parenchymal compression, for laparoscopic partial nephrectomy, 2303–2304
Parental counseling for fetal intervention, 362
Parity, urinary incontinence and, 2583
Parkinson disease (PD)
  detrusor underactivity and, 2657
  diagnosis of, 2605
  in ED, 1502
  lower urinary tract dysfunction with, 2605–2606
  pathophysiology of, 2605
  treatment for, 2605
Paroxetine hydrochloride, to facilitate bladder filling and urine storage, 2702
Partial adrenalectomy, 2421, 2421b
Partial androgen deficiency in aging male (PADAM), 1392

Partial colpocleisis, for apical pelvic organ prolapse repair
  results with, 2812-2814
  technique for, 2811-2812, 2811f-2812f
Partial cystectomy, 3038-3043
  evaluation for, 3038-3040
  extraperitoneal approach to, 3040-3041
  for muscle-invasive bladder cancer, 3124-3125
  open, 3040
  outcomes with, 3042-3043
  surgical indications for, 3038-3040
  surgical technique for, 3040-3041
  transperitoneal approach to, 3041-3042, 3042f-3043f
  with transurethral resection of bladder tumor, 3143, 3144f
Partial gonadal dysgenesis, 1004
Partial nephrectomy (PN)
  for benign diseases, 2254, 2255f
  laparoscopic. see Laparoscopic partial nephrectomy
  for malignancy, 2261-2266, 2262f
    complications of, 2265-2266
    enucleation for small cortical tumors, 2263, 2264f
    preoperative considerations for, 2262-2263, 2262f-2263f, 2263.e1f
    segmental nephrectomy for large polar tumors, 2263-2264, 2263.e1f-2263.e2f, 2264.e1f, 2265f
    wedge resection for large cortical tumors, 2263, 2265f
  for RCC, local recurrence after, 2164-2169, 2165b, 2167t, 2169f
  for renal injuries, 1989-1990, 1989f
  for Wilms tumor, 1107-1108
Partial orchiectomy, 1712
  technique for, 1712
  for TGCT, 1686-1688
Partial prostate ablation, 3624
Partial scrotectomy, 1844-1845, 1846f
Partial transection, for lower ureteral injuries, 1999
Partial ureteral obstruction (PUO), hemodynamic changes with, 792
Partial urogenital mobilization (PUM), 1033-1034, 1034f-1036f
Partin tables, 3527-3528
Past surgical history, 7
Patch cavoplasty, for IVC, 2276, 2277f
Patch electromyography, 483
Patent urachus, 523-525, 524f
Pathogenesis
  of bacteriuria in pregnancy, 1185
  UTI, 1131-1140, 1140b
    alterations in host defense mechanisms, 1139-1140
    bacterial virulence factors, 1133-1134
    early events in UPEC pathogenesis, 1134-1135, 1134f
    epithelial cell receptivity, 1135-1137
    fastidious organisms, 1133
    natural defenses of urinary tract against, 1137-1139
    phase variation of bacterial pili in vivo, 1135.e1, 1135.e1f
    routes of infection, 1131
    urinary pathogens, 1132, 1133f
Patient. see Geriatric patients; Pediatric patients
Patient biases, of localized prostate cancer, 3525
Patient counseling, of localized prostate cancer, 3532-3535, 3532f
Patient decision making, 118, 118f
Patient growth, after augmentation cystoplasty, 698
Patient history, 1-9
  chief complaint, 1
  medical history, 7-9

Patient history (Continued)
  overview, 1
  physical examination, 9-12
  of present illness, 1-7
  special populations, 12-13
Patient positioning, 205
  for laparoscopic and robotic surgery, 205f
    hemodynamic effects related to, 222
  for laparoscopic kidney surgery, 2279-2285
    hand-assisted laparoscopy, 2281-2282, 2283f
    laparoendoscopic single-site surgery and natural orifice transluminal endoscopic surgery, 2284-2285, 2285f, 2286t
    retroperitoneal, 2279-2281, 2282f
    robotic-assisted laparoscopy, 2282-2284, 2284f-2285f
    transperitoneal, 2279, 2280f-2281f
  for laparoscopic radical prostatectomy, 3568, 3569f
  for open simple prostatectomy, 3450
  for prostate biopsy, 3497
  for robot-assisted laparoscopic simple prostatectomy, 3454
Patient preparation
  for cystourethroscopy, 187-190, 189t
  for surgery. see Preoperative care
  for ureteroscopy, 199-200
  for urodynamic studies, 2552
Patient safety, in ultrasonography, 77-78
Patient selection
  for brachytherapy, 3599
  for focal therapy for prostate cancer, 3620-3621
  for prostate cancer, 3540-3541
Patient-physician relationship, in intraoperative consultation, 296
Patient-reported outcome measures, for male urinary incontinence, 2541, 2541.e1f-2541.e2f, 2542f
Patient-reported outcomes, 108-113, 110t, 476
  methods of assessing, 108-109
  selecting an appropriate, 477
  tools for use in females with sexual dysfunction, 112t
  tools for use in men with sexual dysfunction, 112t
  tools for use primarily in women with urinary incontinence, 111t
Pazopanib, for RCC, 2179t-2180t, 2335-2336
PBR. see Peripheral benzodiazepine receptor
PBS. see Prune-belly syndrome
PCA3. see Prostate cancer antigen 3
PCI. see Protein C inhibitor
PCN. see Percutaneous nephrostomy
PCPT. see Prostate Cancer Prevention Trial
PCr. see Plasma creatinine
PC-RPLND. see Postchemotherapy retroperitoneal lymph node dissection
PCS. see Post-chemotherapy surgery
PD-1. see Programmed death-1
PDE5-I. see Phosphodiesterase type 5 inhibitors
PDT. see Photodynamic therapy
Pearly penile papules, 1302, 1303f
Pectus excavatum, 587f, 600
Pediatric ACC, 2388
Pediatric catheters, size of, 153t
Pediatric genitourinary trauma, 1065-1086
  assessment of
    computed tomography for, 1066
    focused assessment with sonography for trauma, 1066
    renal trauma grading system for, 1066-1072, 1067f-1069f, 1067t, 1069t
    renal ultrasonography for, 1066
  bladder injuries, 1080-1083, 1080t, 1083b
    imaging of, 1080
    management, 1080-1081
    pelvic fracture of, 1080
    presentation of, 1080

Pediatric genitourinary trauma (Continued)
  blunt versus penetrating, 1069
  genital injury in, 1083-1086, 1086b
  indications for renal imaging for, 1065, 1066t
  management of, 1069-1070
    angioembolization of isolated renal segment, 1072
    chronic flank pain, 1078
    chronic kidney disease, 1078
    congenital anomalies and renal injuries, 1075-1076
    control of renal vasculature, 1074
    early repeat imaging, 1070
    follow-up and activities with solitary kidney, 1078
    follow-up and long-term issues, 1076, 1078b
    fusion anomalies and ectopic kidney, 1076, 1077f
    hypertension, 1077-1078
    late repeat imaging and assessment of renal function, 1077
    nephrostomy tube, 1072
    nonoperative, 1070, 1073b
    on-table intravenous pyelography or ultrasonography, 1073-1074
    operative, 1073-1078, 1076b
    percutaneous drain, 1071-1072, 1072f
    persistent urine leak, 1070, 1071f
    reconstruction versus nephrectomy, 1074
    renal arterial laceration, 1074
    renal arterial occlusion, 1074
    renal exploration, 1073
    renal exploration with repair of urine leak, 1072
    renal pelvis rupture, 1075
    ureteral stent, 1071
    ureteropelvic junction disruption, 1074-1075, 1075f
    ureteropelvic junction obstruction, 1076, 1076f
  penile, 1083-1084, 1083t
  persistent or delayed bleeding of, 1072-1073
  scrotal, 1084, 1084t, 1085f
  ureteral, 1078-1079, 1080b
    American Association for Surgery of Trauma Classification, 1079, 1079t
    distal ureteral injury surgical repair, 1079
    epidemiology of, 1078
    follow-up imaging, 1079
    imaging findings of, 1079
    lengthy ureteral injuries, 1079
    management of, 1079
    presentation of, 1078-1079
    proximal or mid-ureteral injury surgical repair, 1079
  urethral, 1081-1083, 1081t, 1083b
    evaluation of, 1081
    in females, 1083
    management of, 1081-1083, 1082f
  vaginal, 1084-1086, 1085t
Pediatric kidney stone disease
  conservative management of, 865b
  evaluation of, 854-856, 859b
  extrarenal manifestations of, 853-859, 854b
  goals of therapy for, 860-861
  laparoscopic and robotic-assisted pyelolithotomy for, 868-870
  management of, 853-870, 854f
  medical expulsion therapy for, 859-860
  medical history in, 856-857
  medications for, 869-870
  metabolic investigations in, 856-857, 857t
  percutaneous nephrolithotomy, 865-868, 866t, 868b
    complications, 868
    planning for, 867
    technique for, 867-868, 867f-868f

Pediatric kidney stone disease (Continued)
  physical examination for, 856-857
  secondary prevention for, 868-869
  shock wave lithotripsy for, 864-865, 865b
    limitations and concerns with, 865
    stone size, location, and composition, 864-865
    technique for, 865
  surgical management of, 860, 860t
  ureteroscopic management of, 861-863, 864b
    equipment for, 863, 863f
    indications for, 861, 862t
    limitations and complications of, 864
    technique for, 863-864, 863f
  urinary metabolic abnormalities of, 857-858
    cystinuria, 859
    hypercalciuria, 857-858, 858t
    hyperoxaluria, 858, 858t
    hyperuricosuria, 858t, 859
    hypocitraturia, 858-859
    primary hyperoxaluria, 858
    secondary hyperoxaluria, 858-859
Pediatric nephrology, urologic aspects of, 341-357
  acute kidney injury, 353-354, 353t, 353b-354b
  chronic kidney disease, 354-355, 354t, 355b
  cystic renal disease, 349-350
  end-stage renal disease, 355-357
  fluid and electrolyte homeostasis, 341-342
  glomerular disease, 344-348, 344b
  hematuria, 342-343, 343b
  hypertension, 351-353, 352b
  proteinuria, 343-344, 344b
  renal function, 341-342
  tubulopathies, 348-349
  urolithiasis, medical management, 350-351, 351b
Pediatric oncology, 1087-1127
  adrenal tumors, neuroblastoma. see Neuroblastoma
  bladder tumors
    adenocarcinoma and squamous cell carcinoma, 1118
    in augmented bladders, 1118
    benign, 1119
    RMS. see Bladder RMS
    TCC, 1117-1118
    urachal carcinoma, 1118
  female genital tract tumors, 1121b
    cervical or uterine RMS, 1120
    ovarian, 1120-1121
    vaginal RMS, 1119-1120, 1119f
    vulvar RMS, 1119
  male reproductive tumors
    paratesticular RMS, 1126-1127, 1127b
    testicular. see Testicular tumors
  renal tumors
    angiomyolipoma, 1110, 1110f
    CCSK, 1108-1109
    CMN, 1109
    CPDN, 1109
    metanephric adenofibroma, 1109
    RCC, 1109-1110
    RTK, 1109
    solitary multilocular cyst nephroma, 1109
    Wilms tumor. see Wilms tumor
Pediatric patients
  bladder and bowel dysfunction. see Bladder and bowel dysfunction
  bladder anomalies in. see Bladder anomalies, in children
  imaging of. see specific imaging modalities
  kidneys of, 1065
  lower urinary tract dysfunction in, 652
    clinical significance of, 652
    comorbidities with, 653-654, 655b
    enuresis. see Enuresis
    epidemiology of, 652, 655b
    giggle incontinence, 658-660
    pollakiuria, 660

Pediatric patients (Continued)
    quality-of-life and, 652-653, 655b
    self-esteem and, 652-653
    terminology of, 654-655
    underactive bladder, 660
    urinary incontinence and, 655-660, 660b
    vaginal reflux, 660
  neuromuscular dysfunction of lower urinary tract in. see Neuromuscular dysfunction of lower urinary tract, in children
  transitional urology for. see Transitional urology
  ureteral anomalies in. see Ureteral anomalies
  urinary tract reconstruction in
    antireflux, 683-685, 685b
    augmentation cystoplasty for, 691-706, 702b. see also Augmentation cystoplasty
    bladder neck reconstruction, 685-690, 690b
    continent urinary diversions, 706-713, 711b. see also Continent urinary diversions
    patient evaluation for, 681-682, 683b
    patient preparation for, 682-683, 683b
    summary for, 713
    urodynamics for, 681-682
Pediatric Penile Perception Score (PPS), 942-943, 942f
Pediatric renal transplantation, 1054-1064
  bladder preparation for
    capacity, 1056, 1056f
    clean intermittent catheterization, 1057
    general issues, 1054-1055
    hypertonicity, 1055-1056
    infections, 1056-1057
  complications with, 1060-1064, 1061t, 1064b
    bladder dysfunction, 1063
    hydronephrosis, 1062-1063, 1063f
    infection, 1061
    obstruction, 1062-1063, 1062f-1063f
    reflux, 1062, 1062f
    stones, 1063-1064
    urine leaks, 1060-1061, 1061f, 1061.e1f
  cutaneous stomas for, 1058
  defunctionalized bladder, 1057-1058
    augmentation decision, 1057-1058
    neuropathic, 1057
    non-neuropathic, 1057
  native kidney management, 1059, 1059.e4f-1059.e5f
    nephrectomy with, 1059
  pretransplant assessment for, 1054, 1054b, 1055f
  pretransplant preparation for, 1054-1059, 1057b
  reconstruction strategies for, 1058-1059, 1059b
    dialysis issues, 1058
    enterocystoplasty, 1058-1059, 1058.e1f
    graft placement, 1058, 1058.e2f
    native nephrectomy, 1059, 1059.e2f-1059.e4f
    timing of, 1058
  ureteral anastomosis, 1060, 1060b, 1060.e1f-1060.e4f
  ureteral stenting, 1060
Pediatric sepsis, 452
Pediatric Urinary Incontinence Quality of Life Score (PinQ), 476-477, 653
Pediatric urogenital imaging, 403-425
  computed tomography for, 416-418
  conventional radiography for, 415
  DMSA renal cortical scintigraphy, 418
  magnetic resonance imaging for, 412-415
  technique of, 403
    ionizing, 403, 403b
    nonionizing, 403, 403b
  ultrasonography for, 404-412
  voiding cystourethrography (VCUG), 415-416
Pediatric urology, 395b
  advanced imaging for, 390-391
    computed tomography, 390-391
    magnetic resonance imaging, 390

Pediatric urology (Continued)
  flank pain in, 400
  imaging for, 388-391
    prenatal ultrasonography, 389
    renal bladder ultrasound, 388-389
    ultrasonography, 388-389
  overview of, 388
  presentations by genitourinary region, 391-402
  renal scintigraphy for, 390
    diuretic renography, 390
    renal cortical scintigraphy, 390
  triage of common, 389t
  urodynamic testing, 390
  voiding cystourethrogram, 389-390
    fluoroscopy, 389
    genitography, 390
    nuclear cystography, 389-390
Pedicle effect, 468
Pediculosis pubis
  infestation, 1295-1296, 1296f
  as STD, 1271
PEKMB. see Pseudoepitheliomatous, keratotic, and micaceous balanitis
Pelvic abscesses, after mid-urethral sling surgery, 2870
Pelvic arterial ischemia, detrusor inactivity and, 2657
Pelvic autonomic plexus, 2453-2454, 2454f-2455f
Pelvic bone defects, in bladder exstrophy, 531-532, 531f
Pelvic cystic lesion, and distended bladder, 385
Pelvic drain, after laparoscopic radical prostatectomy, 3579
Pelvic examination
  in female, physical examination for, 12
  for PFDs, 2528
Pelvic fascia
  female, 2427, 2429f
  male, 2449, 2452f
  surgical anatomy of, 3549-3550, 3550f
Pelvic fibrosis, as laparoscopic and robotic surgery contraindication, 203
Pelvic floor
  defects in
    in bladder exstrophy, 532, 532f
    prostatitis and, 1208, 1208f
  female, 2427, 2428f
    muscles of, 2430-2432, 2432f
  genitourinary malignancies, 2920
  support mechanism of, 2597-2598, 2598f
Pelvic floor disorders (PFDs)
  diagnostic evaluation of, 2525-2528
    benign prostatic hyperplasia, 2528
    general considerations for, 2525-2526, 2526t, 2526b, 2527f
    genetics and, 2528
    history for, 2526, 2528b
    history of present illness, 2527
    male incontinence, 2528
    medications and, 2528, 2528t
    past medical and surgical history, 2527-2528
  impact of, 2525
  management of, 2537-2538
    for incontinence, 2537
    for pelvic prolapse, 2537-2538
  physical examination for, 2528-2530, 2529f-2530f, 2529t-2530t, 2530b
  supplemental evaluation of, 2530-2537, 2531t, 2533b
    cystoscopy, 2534
    dye testing, 2533
    magnetic resonance imaging, 2536-2537
    pad tests, 2531-2533
    postvoid residual, 2534
    quality of life instruments for, 2531, 2532t-2533t
    questionnaires for, 2531, 2532t-2533t
    radiographic imaging, 2536

Pelvic floor disorders (PFDs) (Continued)
　　ultrasonography, 2536
　　urinalysis, 2534
　　urodynamics, 2534-2536, 2536b
　　voiding diaries for, 2530
　symptom quantification instruments for, 2531
　terminology of, 2526t
Pelvic floor muscle (PFM)
　assessment of, for PFMT, 2723-2725
　contraction of, to prevent stress incontinence, 2540, 2725
　dysfunction of, behavioral training for, 2732-2735
　electrical stimulation of, 2729-2730
　female, 2430-2432, 2432f
　for SUI, 2540
　teaching control of, 2725
Pelvic floor muscle exercise (PFME), for urinary incontinence, in geriatric patients, 2919.e2
Pelvic floor muscle training (PFMT), 2723-2727
　assessment of PFMF, 2723-2725
　biofeedback for, 2729, 2729f, 2729.e1f-2729.e2f
　evidence for, 2725-2726
　exercise regimens for, 2725, 2725.e1t
　handout for, 2725.e1t
　levels of evidence and recommendations for, 2722.e1b-2722.e4b
　as nonsurgical treatment option, 2833
　for prevention of stress incontinence, 2725
　teaching of, 2725
　vaginal cones for, 2726, 2726.e1f
Pelvic floor physiotherapy
　for chronic scrotal pain syndrome, 1221
　for detrusor underactivity, 2660
Pelvic fracture, bladder injuries with, 3057
Pelvic fracture urethral injuries (PFUIs), 1828-1834
　evaluation of, 1829
　postoperative management of, 1832-1834, 1834f
　repair of, 1829-1832, 1830f-1833f
Pelvic inlet, female, 2427, 2428f
Pelvic lymphadenectomy (PLND)
　extended
　　common iliac, 3152, 3153f-3154f
　　external iliac, 3148-3149, 3151f
　　hypogastric, 3149-3152, 3153f
　　obturator, 3149, 3152f
　　presacral, 3152, 3154f
　in laparoscopic radical prostatectomy, 3577
　for penile cancer, 1761-1762
　for prostate cancer staging, 3521
　radical cystectomy with
　　anatomic extent of, 3115-3116
　　bilateral, 3115
　　density of, 3117
　　distal urethra management, 3118
　　extracapsular nodal extension, 3117
　　intraoperative decision making, 3117-3118
　　intraoperative frozen sections of ureter, 3117-3118
　　managing female urethra in, 3118
　　for muscle-invasive bladder cancer, 3114-3119
　　number of lymph nodes identified, 3116-3117, 3116f
　　oncologic outcomes following, 3118-3119, 3118t
　　prostatic urothelial carcinoma and, 3118
　　with transurethral resection of bladder tumor, 3137-3138, 3138f-3139f
Pelvic muscle electromyography (EMG), 2557
Pelvic muscle training device, 2727f
Pelvic nerve afferents, 2481-2482, 2481t, 2482f
Pelvic node dissection, in robotic prostatectomy, 3580-3581
Pelvic organ cross-sensitization, in BPS/IC etiology, 1232.e9, 1232.e9b

Pelvic organ prolapse (POP). see also Pelvic floor disorders
　classification of, 2526, 2527f, 2587-2589, 2589b
　　systems for, 2529-2530, 2529f, 2530t
　conditions associated with, 2592b
　consequences of, 2592-2593, 2592b
　definition of, 2587-2589, 2589b
　epidemiology of, 2590-2591, 2591b
　female sexual dysfunction and, 1656-1657
　financial impact of, 2593
　in geriatric patients, 2920.e9-2920.e10
　history of, 2528
　imaging of, 2441-2442, 2442f
　incidence of, 2590
　midurethral sling outcomes for, 2861-2862
　pathophysiology of, 2598-2599, 2599b
　physical examination of, 2588-2589, 2588f-2589f
　prevalence of, 2590
　on quality of life, 2592-2593
　questionnaires for, 2532t-2533t
　reconstructive surgery for, 2776-2829
　　in anterior compartment, 2778-2790, 2790b
　　　abdominal paravaginal repair, 2780t-2782t, 2787, 2788f
　　　anterior colporrhaphy, 2778-2783, 2779f, 2780t
　　　with cadaveric fascia, 2781t-2782t, 2786, 2786f
　　　with grafts, 2783, 2785f
　　　with polypropylene mesh, 2781t-2782t, 2783-2786, 2786f
　　　with porcine dermis, 2781t-2782t, 2786-2787, 2787f
　　　with sling, 2788-2790, 2789f
　　　vaginal paravaginal repair, 2780t, 2783, 2784f-2785f
　　in apical compartment, 2790-2809
　　　abdominal sacrocolpopexy, 2798-2809, 2800f-2801f
　　　colpocleisis, 2809-2814. see also Colpocleisis, for apical pelvic organ prolapse repair
　　　comparison of procedures of, 2809-2823
　　　hysteropexy, 2815-2823
　　　iliococcygeus suspension, 2797-2798, 2799f
　　　sacrospinous ligament fixation, 2793-2797. see also Sacrospinous ligament fixation (SSLF), for pelvic organ prolapse repair
　　　uterine prolapse, 2814
　　　uterine sparing, 2815-2823
　　　uterosacral ligament suspension, 2790-2793
　　　vaginal hysterectomy with McCall culdoplasty technique, 2814-2815, 2815f
　　in apical vaginal compartment
　　　colpocleisis. see Colpocleisis, for apical pelvic organ prolapse repair
　　　sacrospinous ligament fixation. see Sacrospinous ligament fixation
　　approach to, 2778t
　　mesh for, 2776-2778, 2778t
　　　complications from, 2787
　　in posterior compartment, 2823-2829, 2829b
　　　interposition graft repairs of, 2829
　　　posterior colporrhaphy, 2825-2829, 2825f
　　preoperative counseling for, 2776, 2777b
　　preparation for, 2776, 2777b
　risk factors for, 2590-2591
　social impact of, 2592
　societal costs of, 2592
　symptoms of, 2587-2588
　urinary incontinence and, 2591-2592, 2592b

Pelvic Organ Prolapse Quantification (POPQ), 2529-2530, 2529f, 2530t, 2588, 2589f
Pelvic organs, female, 2436-2438, 2437f
Pelvic pain, 2988
　in mesh complication, 2881
Pelvic plexus, for retropubic radical prostatectomy, 3548, 3549f
Pelvic plexus injury, LUTD after, 2620-2621
Pelvic resections, RPLND with, 1720
Pelvic sidewalls, female, 2430, 2432f
Pelvic surgery, 645-647
　medical diagnoses and, 2528
　operative team placement for, transperitoneal and extraperitoneal procedures, 207, 208f
　pathogenesis for, 647
　presentation for, 645-647
　specific recommendations for, 647
Pelvic ultrasonography, 482-483, 482f
　bladder wall thickness, 482, 483f
　postvoid residual, 482
　rectal diameter, 482
　transabdominal. see Transabdominal pelvic ultrasonography
　urinary debris, 482
Pelvicalyceal system, anatomy of, 1872-1873, 1872f
　endoscopic, 1875-1876, 1875b, 1875.e1f
Pelvis
　clinical staging of, TGCTs and, 1689, 1689f
　female. see Female pelvis
　male. see Male pelvis
Pembrolizumab, for microsatellite instability-high cancers, 3698-3699
Pemphigus vulgaris, 1284, 1284f
Pendulous urethra. see Penile urethra
Penectomy, for penile cancer, 1752
Penetrating trauma
　bladder, 3055
　penile, 3049-3051
　renal, 1982
　　imaging of, 1984
　　nonoperative management of, 1987
　scrotal, 3051
　ureteral, 1992, 1992t
　　diagnosis of, 1992-1993
Penile angiography, 1523, 1524f
Penile anomalies, 871-886
　abnormal number, 876-877
　　aphallia, 876-877, 877f
　　diphallia, 877, 877f
　abnormal orientation, 880-882
　　curvature, 880-881, 881f
　accessory urethral openings, 883-884
　　congenital urethral fistula, 883, 883f
　　urethral duplication, 883-884, 884f
　genital lymphedema, 884-885
　inconspicuous penis, 872t, 877-879, 879f
　　buried penis, 877-878, 878f-879f
　　webbed penis, 878-879, 879f
　masses, 882-883
　　congenital penile nevi, 883, 883f
　　inclusion cysts, 882-883, 882f
　　juvenile xanthogranuloma, 883
　　median raphe cysts, 882, 882f
　　parameatal urethral cyst, 882, 882f
　micropenis, 872t, 879-880, 880f, 880.e1b, 881b
　penoscrotal transposition, 885-886, 886f
　prepuce, 871-876
　　circumcision, 872-876
　　phimosis and paraphimosis, 871-872, 872f
　priapism, 885, 885b
　torsion, 881-882, 881f
Penile blood flow, historical and investigational studies of, 1523-1525
Penile brachial pressure index, 1523

Penile cancer
  chemotherapy for, 1769–1771, 1772b
    adjuvant, 1771
    combination, 1770–1771, 1770t
    single-agent, 1769–1770
    surgical consolidation after, 1771
  inguinal lymph node dissection for. see
      Inguinal lymphadenectomy
  as non-AIDS-defining urologic malignancy, 1268
  nonpalpable inguinal adenopathy, 1792–1796, 1792b
    dynamic sentinel lymph node biopsy, 1793
    endoscopic inguinal lymphadenectomy, 1794
    follow-up, 1793
    modified inguinal lymph node dissection, 1794
    robotic inguinal lymphadenectomy, 1794
    sentinel lymph node biopsy, 1792–1793
    superficial inguinal lymph node dissection, 1793–1794
    surgical technique, 1794–1796, 1795f, 1797f–1798f
    technique of, 1793
  nonsquamous neoplasms, 1771–1775, 1775b
    adenosquamous carcinoma, 1774
    basal cell carcinoma, 1772
    extramammary Paget disease, 1774
    lymphoreticular malignant neoplasm, 1774
    melanoma, 1772, 1773f
    metastases, 1774–1775
    sarcomas, 1772–1774
  palpable inguinal adenopathy or positive inguinal lymph nodes, 1796–1800
    adjuvant chemotherapy, 1798–1800
    curative purposes, surgery for, 1796
    palliative purposes, surgery for, 1800
    radical inguinal lymph node dissection, 1796–1798, 1799f–1800f
  radiation therapy for, 1765–1769, 1769b
    adverse effects of, 1767–1768
    inguinal areas, 1768–1769, 1769f
    primary lesion, 1765–1768
  risk-based management of inguinal region in, 1762–1765, 1763f–1764f
    bulky adenopathy and fixed nodal metastasis, 1765
    high-risk patients, 1762–1765
    low- to intermediate-risk patients, 1762
    very low-risk patients, 1762
  surgical management of, 1753t, 1753b, 1792
    amputation, 1752–1753
Penile elephantiasis, as filariasis clinical manifestation, 1330
Penile erection, 1485–1512. see also Erectile dysfunction
  physiology of, 1485–1500, 1490b, 1495b
    functional anatomy of, 1485–1487, 1486f–1488f, 1486t
    hemodynamics and mechanism of erection and detumescence, 1487–1489, 1489f, 1490t
    historical context of, 1485
    neuroanatomy and neurophysiology of, 1489–1495, 1490f, 1491t–1492t
    smooth muscle, 1495–1500, 1496f–1497f, 1500b, 1501f
Penile imaging, in priapism, 1549–1550, 1550f, 1550b
Penile incisions, in urologic surgery, 143–144, 143f
Penile magnetic resonance imaging, 1524
Penile near infrared spectrophotometry, 1524–1525
Penile pain, patient history of, 2
Penile plethysmography, 1524
Penile prosthesis
  for Peyronie's disease
    indications for, 1624
    techniques for, 1624–1625, 1625t
  surgery, 1537

Penile rehabilitation, role of, in laparoscopic radical prostatectomy, 3579
Penile revascularization surgery, 1537
Penile thermal sensory testing, 1527
Penile torsion, 394
Penile traction, and PD, 1614–1615, 1617t
Penile transplantation, 1838–1842, 1840f, 1842b
  after trauma, 1841
Penile tumescence and rigidity monitoring, 1525–1526, 1525f
Penile urethra, 1383, 1383f, 1807.e4f, 1807.e8
  carcinoma of, 1780–1781, 1781f
Peninsular flaps, for urethral and penile reconstruction, 1807
Penis
  amputation of
    for penile cancer, 1752–1753
    traumatic, 3050–3051
  anatomy of, 1387b, 1485–1487, 1486t, 1807.e8–1807.e9, 1807.e10b
    arterial supply, 1384–1385, 1386f, 1807.e5f
    arteries, 1487, 1487f
    blood supply, 1807.e8–1807.e9
    corpora cavernosa, corpus spongiosum, and glans penis, 1485–1486
    lymphatics, 1386, 1807.e9
    nerve supply, 1386, 1387f, 1807.e9
    reconstructive surgery and, 1807, 1807.e1f–1807.e7f
    sphincteric, 1807.e8
    structure, 1383–1384, 1385f–1386f
    urethral, 1807.e8
    venous drainage, 1385, 1487, 1488f, 1807.e5f
  curvatures of. see Curvatures of penis
  in genitourinary tuberculosis, 1309
  imaging of
    cavernosogram, 1386, 1387f
    Doppler ultrasound, 1386, 1387f
    magnetic resonance imaging, 1386, 1388f
  injuries and trauma of, 3048–3051
    amputation, 3050–3051
    animal and human bites, 3050
    burns, 3053
    with circumcision, 874f, 875
    fracture, 3048–3049, 3048.e1f, 3049f–3050f, 3049.e1f
    gunshot wounds, 3049–3050
    microvascular, 3050
    penetrating, 3049–3051
    strangulation, 3051
    total reconstruction after, 1841
    zipper, 3051
  length of, 871, 872t
  nerve supply of, 305–306
  neuroanatomy and neurophysiology of
    neurotransmitters and, 1492–1495, 1495t
    spinal centers and peripheral pathways, 1489–1491, 1490f, 1491t
    supraspinal pathways and centers, 1491–1492, 1491t–1493t
  physical examination for, 10–11
  physiology of
    corpora cavernosa, 1488–1489, 1489f
    corpus spongiosum and glans penis, 1489, 1490t
  preservation of, in penile cancer management, 1751
  reattachment of, 3051b
  reconstructive surgery of, 1804–1842, 1805b, 1813b, 3054
    for amyloidosis, 1810
    anatomy of, 1807, 1807.e1f–1807.e7f
    balanitis xerotica obliterans, 939, 940f
    for balanitis xerotica obliterans, 939, 940f
    for circumcision complications, 1811–1812
    in classic bladder exstrophy, 551–552, 552f–553f
    for curvatures of penis, 1836–1838, 1838b
    for failed epispadias repair, 1813

Penis (Continued)
    for failed hypospadias repair, 1812–1813
    for female-to-male transgender, 1841–1842, 1842b
    for fistulae of posterior urethra, 1835–1836, 1836b
    for glans dehiscence, 937, 938f
    for LS, 1808–1810, 1809f
    in male epispadias, 569
    for meatal stenosis, 937–938, 1811
    for paraphimosis, balanitis, and phimosis, 1811
    penile transplantation, 1838–1842, 1840f, 1842b
    for PFUIs, 1828–1834, 1830f–1834f
    principles of, 1804–1807, 1806f–1807f, 1808b
    for recurrent penile curvature, 939–941, 940f
    for urethral diverticulum, 938–939, 939f, 1810–1811
    for urethral stricture, 938, 1814–1828, 1814f, 1828b
    for urethrocutaneous fistula, 935–937, 936f–937f, 1810
    for vesicourethral distraction defects, 1834b, 1835, 1836b
  skin complications of, 874
  tumors of, 1742–1775
    malignant. see Penile cancer
    premalignant cutaneous lesions, 1742
      Buschke-Löwenstein tumor (giant condyloma acuminatum), 1742.e1f, 1742.e3
      carcinoma in situ (penile intraepithelial neoplasia), 1742
      non-human papillomavirus-related, 1742.e1–1742.e2
      virus-related, 1742.e2–1742.e3, 1743b
    squamous cell carcinoma, 1743–1751. see also Squamous cell carcinoma
    surgical management of, 1751–1753, 1753t, 1753b
      circumcision and limited excision strategies, 1752–1753
      contemporary penile amputation, 1752–1753
      laser ablation, 1752
      Mohs micrographic surgery, 1752
      organ preservation, 1751
  ultrasonography of, 85–88, 86f
Penn pouch, 3224–3225, 3224f
Penoscrotal transposition, 886f
Penrose drains, 148
Pentosan polysulfate, for chronic scrotal pain syndrome, 1216
Pentoxifylline, for PD, 1611, 1616t
Peptide hormones, of reproductive axis, 1390, 1391f
Peptidergic agents, in ureteral function, 1889
PERC Mentor, 176, 177f
Percutaneous antegrade endopyelotomy, for ureteropelvic junction obstruction, 1947
  complications with, 1949
  indications and contraindications for, 1947, 1947f
  patient preparation for, 1947
  postoperative care for, 1948
  results with, 1949
  technique of, 1947–1948
Percutaneous drain, for pediatric genitourinary trauma, 1071–1072, 1072f
Percutaneous endopyeloplasty, for ureteropelvic junction obstruction, 1949
Percutaneous epididymal sperm aspiration, in sperm retrieval, 1474, 1474f
Percutaneous nephrolithotomy (PCNL), 243.e1, 2103–2107, 2105b
  anesthesia for, 2104
  antibiotics for, 2104
  calyceal diverticula and, 2105, 2105f

Percutaneous nephrolithotomy (PCNL) (Continued)
clinical use of, 246
complications of, 2107
CyberWand, 245
horseshoe kidney and, 2105–2106
laser fragmentation, 244.e3
morbid obesity and, 2089, 2106–2107
old age and frailty and, 2089–2090
patient preparation, 2103–2104
pediatric, 865–868, 866t, 868b
  complications, 868
  planning for, 867
  technique for, 867–868, 867f–868f
prior renal surgery and, 2090
for renal calculi
  in calyceal diverticula, 2078
  in horseshoe kidneys, 2080
  lower pole calculi, 2081, 2081f, 2082t, 2083f
  in renal ectopia, 2080, 2081f
  stone composition and, 2076, 2076f
  stone localization and, 2075
renal function and, 2088–2089
renal transplants and, 2091
ShockPulse-SE, 245–246
solitary kidney and, 2089
spinal deformity or limb contractures and, 2090
for staghorn calculi, 2074
staghorn calculi or complex stones and, 2106
stone burden and
  between 1 and 2 cm, 2073
  greater than 2 cm, 2074
  up to 1 cm, 2072–2073
stone removal in, 2104–2105
tissue effects, 246
transplantation and pelvic kidneys and, 2106, 2106f
uncorrected coagulopathy and, 2090
for ureteral calculi
  duplicated collecting system and, 2087
  in megaureter, 2087
  outcome of, 2091–2093
  stone composition and, 2087
  stone localization and, 2085–2086, 2086t
urinary diversion and, 2091
urinary tract infection and, 2088
Percutaneous nephrostomy drains, 288
Percutaneous nerve evaluation test, for sacral neuromodulation, 2754
Percutaneous posterior tibial nerve stimulation (PTNS), for UUI, 2546
Percutaneous procedures, antimicrobial prophylaxis for, 1199
Percutaneous pyelolithotomy, 160
Percutaneous renal access and drainage, 160–182
anatomic considerations of, 160–164
  collecting system, 161–162, 162f
  intrarenal vasculature, 162–164, 163f
  perirenal anatomy, 160–161, 161f
  renal parenchyma, 161–162
anesthetic considerations for, 165
complications, 178–182, 182b
  acute hemorrhage, 178
  death, 182
  delayed hemorrhage, 178–179
  fever and sepsis, 181
  loss of renal function, 182
  metabolic and physiologic, 181
  neuromusculoskeletal, 181–182
  pleural injury, 180–181
  venous thromboembolism, 182
  visceral injury, 179–180
history of, 160
image guidance for puncture, 166–169

Percutaneous renal access and drainage (Continued)
indications of, 160
  diagnostic studies, 160
  percutaneous renal surgery, 160
  simple drainage, 160
  therapeutic instillations, 160
obtaining, 169b
postprocedural drainage, 173–176
  general considerations of, 174–175
special situations, 177–178
  horseshoe kidney, 177
surgical technique, 164–176
  advanced guidance techniques, 169–172
  antimicrobial prophylaxis, 164
  choice of calyx for access, 165
  diagnostic imaging, 164
  interpolar calyx, 166
  lower pole calyx, 166
  management of anticoagulation, 164
  obtaining access, 164
  patient positioning, 164
  prone position, 164–165, 165f
  supine position, 165
  upper pole calyx, 165–166, 166f
training for, 176
Percutaneous renal tumor ablation, 2312, 2313f, 2318
Percutaneous Shunting in Lower Urinary Tract Obstruction (PLUTO) trial, 364
Percutaneous stone removal, 2069.e2
Percutaneous surgery, 243.e2
Percutaneous tibial nerve stimulation (PTNS), 2748–2751, 2749f
  clinical results of, 2749–2750
  compared with other treatments, 2750
  history of, 2749
  implantable, 2750–2751, 2751f
  prognostic factors for, 2750
  technique of, 2749, 2750f
Perforating artery, 136f
Perforation
  of bladder, in transurethral resection of bladder tumor, 3135f
  with monopolar transurethral resection of prostate, 3417
  ureteral, ureteroscopic, 2002
  in ureteroscopic stone management, 2108
Perfusion phase, 92–93
Perfusion studies, for UPJO, 1944–1945
Perinatal neuroblastoma, surgical treatment of, 1093
Perinatal testicular torsion, 897, 897f
Perinatal urology, 358–387
  congenital adrenal hyperplasia, 382, 383f
  exstrophy, 379–382
  grading systems, 358–361
  key conditions, 372–375
  kidney anomalies, 377–379
  lower urinary tract obstruction, 375–377, 376f–377f
  perinatal urgencies/emergencies, 382–387
  postnatal evaluation and management, 366–370, 367b, 370b
    imaging, 367–370
    magnetic resonance urography, 369–370
    renal scintigraphy, 367–369, 369f–370f
    renal ultrasound/resolution of urinary tract dilation, 367, 368f
    voiding cystourethrogram, 367
  postnatal urinary tract dilation, management recommendations for, 370–372
  prenatal imaging, 358, 358b
  prenatal multidisciplinary consultations, 361–362, 362b
  urinary tract dilation, 362–366
  urogenital sinus, 382, 382b, 383f

Perineal body, 1807.e10, 2434
  fasciae of, 2449, 2450f–2451f
  female sexual organs, 1627.e2
Perineal bone-anchored slings, 2887
Perineal incisions, in urologic surgery, 144
Perineal membrane, 2434
Perineal pain, after transurethral needle ablation of prostate, 3433
Perineal ultrasonography, of penis and male urethra, 85, 87f
Perineal urethrostomy, for urethral stricture disease, 1827–1828
Perineorrhaphy, posterior colporrhaphy with, for pelvic organ prolapse repair, 2827–2829
Perinephric abscess
  after renal injury, 1992
  as renal infection, 1174–1176, 1175f
Perinephric fat, 1865
Perineum
  fasciae of, 2449, 2450f–2451f
  female, 2434–2435, 2435f
    Fournier gangrene and, 1289–1290, 1290f
  male, 2450f–2451f, 2451b
    anatomy of, 1807.e9–1807.e10, 1807.e10b
Perineural invasion, 3512
Perioperative intravesical therapy, for non–muscle-invasive bladder cancer, 3098–3099
Peripheral benzodiazepine receptor (PBR), 1394–1395
Peripheral (or modified-peripheral) loading, 3596
Peripheral nervous system, of lower urinary tract, 2480–2497, 2480f
  afferent pathways in, 2481–2486, 2481t, 2482f–2486f, 2487b
  efferent pathways to, 2487–2493, 2487f, 2489f–2492f, 2490b, 2491t
  parasympathetic pathways, 2480, 2480f
  somatic pathways, 2480f–2481f, 2481
  supraspinal pathways, 2493–2497, 2495f–2496f
  sympathetic pathways, 2480, 2480f
Peripheral neuropathy, 146
Periprostatic plexus, 1380
Perirenal anatomy, 160–161, 161f
Peristalsis, of ureters
  cellular, 1877
  contractile activity, 1883–1887, 1883f–1886f
  development of, 1877–1878, 1878f
  drug effects on, 1901–1903
  electrical activity, 1878–1883, 1879f–1880f
  mechanical properties, 1890–1891, 1890f–1891f
  nervous system function in, 1887–1890
  urine transport, 1891–1894, 1892f–1893f
Peritoneal dialysis, in children, 356, 357b
Peritoneal flap, for vesicovaginal fistula repair, 2940, 2940f
Peritoneum
  female, 2427, 2429f
  male, 2448f, 2449
Peritubular tissue, 1398, 1398f
Periureteral fascia, 1865
Periurethral abscess, 1182, 1182b
Periurethral bulking agents
  as alternative treatment for slings, 2833
  for neuromuscular dysfunction of lower urinary tract, 637
  urethral diverticula differentiated from, 2987
Periurethral glands, 2439
  urethral diverticula and, 2976
Periurethral region, natural defenses of, 1137
Periurethral technique, injection, 2892
Perivascular epithelioid cell tumor, retroperitoneal tumors and, 2234
Permeability, of urothelium of bladder, 2461–2462, 2467, 2468f
Pernicious anemia, lower urinary tract dysfunction with, 2619

Persistent genital arousal disorder, 1636
Persistent Müllerian duct syndrome (PMDS), 322, 323f, 1016-1017, 1016f
Persistent penile erection, with monopolar transurethral resection of prostate, 3417
Pessaries
  continence, 2736, 2736f, 2736.e1f
  for pelvic organ prolapse, 2920.e9-2920.e10
PET. see Positron emission tomography
Peyronie's disease (PD)
  and aging, 1600
  and collagen disorders, 1602
  and combination therapy, 1615
  curvatures of penis associated with, 1837-1838
  and diabetes, 1600, 1601f
  diagnosis and management of, 1599-1626
    epidemiology, 1599-1602, 1602b
    etiology, 1604-1606, 1606b
    evaluation of patient, 1607-1609, 1607f-1609f, 1609b
    general considerations with, 1599, 1600b
    natural history of, 1599
    nonsurgical treatment, 1610-1616, 1616b
    penile anatomy, 1602-1604, 1603f-1604f
    surgical, 1616-1625
    symptoms, 1606-1607
    treatment protocols, 1609-1610
  and electromotive drug administration, 1614
  erectile dysfunction and, 1600-1601
  etiology of, 1604-1606, 1606b
  and extracorporeal shock wave therapy, 1614
  and fibrotic gene expression, 1606
  and hypogonadism, 1602
  and impact of wound healing, 1603-1604
  incidence of, 1599-1600
  intralesional injections for, 1612-1613, 1617t
  oral medications for, 1610-1612, 1616t
  and penile traction, 1614-1615
  and psychological aspects, 1601-1602
  and radiation therapy, 1615-1616
  and radical prostatectomy, 1602
  and role of myofibroblasts, 1605
  and role of nitric oxide, 1605
  and role of oxygen free radicals and oxidative stress, 1605
  and role of transforming growth factor-β1, 1605-1606
  surgical management of, 1616-1625, 1626b
    indications, 1616-1618, 1618b, 1619t
    penile prosthesis, 1624-1625
    tunica lengthening procedures, 1621-1624
    tunical shortening procedures, 1618-1621, 1620f-1621f, 1622t
  topical drug application for, 1613-1614
  and vacuum therapy, 1615
Pezzer tube, 155, 155f
Pfannenstiel incision, of abdomen, 135, 138f
PFDs. see Pelvic floor disorders
P fimbriae, 431
PFM. see Pelvic floor muscle
PFME. see Pelvic floor muscle exercise
PFMT. see Pelvic floor muscle training
PFUIs. see Pelvic fracture urethral injuries
PG. see Pyoderma gangrenosum
PGI-I. see Post-operative Patient Global Impression of Improvement
pH, of urine, 15-16
  low
    in calcium stone formation, 2024-2025
    in uric acid stone formation, 2027-2029, 2028f
Phallic urethra, 3068, 3069f
Phalloplasty, 3068
Pharmacologic therapy
  in ED, 1532-1536, 1533b, 1538b
    future directions for, 1538
    intracavernosal injection, 1534-1535, 1535f
    intraurethral suppositories, 1535-1536
    oral, 1532-1534
    transdermal/topical, 1536

Pharmacologic therapy (Continued)
  to facilitate bladder emptying, 2716-2720
    by bladder contractility, 2716-2718
    by decreasing outlet resistance, 2719-2720, 2720b
    by increasing intravesical pressure, 2716-2718
  to facilitate bladder filling and urine storage, 2679-2716, 2682t
    α-adrenoreceptor antagonists, 2682t, 2697-2698
    β-adrenoreceptor antagonists, 2682t, 2698-2699
    antidepressants, 2682t, 2702-2703
    antimuscarinic agents, 2681-2684, 2682t, 2697b. see also Antimuscarinic agents, to facilitate bladder filling and urine storage
    in augmented or intestinal neobladders, 2712-2713
    botulinum toxins, 2682t, 2707-2709
    cannabinoids, 2713.e2-2713.e3
    centrally acting drugs, 2713.e3-2713.e4
    combinations for, 2704-2707
    cyclooxygenase inhibitors, 2682t, 2703
    desmopressin for, 2710-2712
    dimethyl sulfoxide, 2703-2704
    estrogens for, 2709-2710, 2713-2714
    future possibilities of, 2713
    gabapentin, 2713.e3
    gonadotropin-releasing hormone antagonists, 2713.e3
    guidelines for, 2681t
    by increasing outlet resistance, 2713-2716
    by inhibiting bladder contractility, 2679-2700
    intraprostatically injected drugs, 2713.e2-2713.e3
    membrane channel activity, 2682t, 2696-2697
    mirabegron, 2699-2700
    muscarinic receptors in, 2679-2681, 2680t
    NK$_1$-receptor antagonists, 2713.e4
    phosphodiesterase inhibitors, 2682t, 2700-2702
    prostanoid-receptor agonists and antagonists, 2713.e1-2713.e2
    toxins, 2707-2709
    tramadol, 2713.e3-2713.e4
    transient receptor potential channel antagonists, 2713.e1
    vanilloids for, 2709
    vitamin D$_3$-receptor analogues, 2713.e1
  for hypospadias, 945
  for lower urinary tract, 2497-2503
    adrenergic mechanisms, 2500-2501, 2501f, 2501b
    afferent neuropeptides, 2501-2502, 2501t
    muscarinic mechanisms, 2497-2500, 2499t, 2500b
    sex steroids, 2502-2503
    urethral tone in women, 2501
Phenazopyridine, for pelvic floor disorder testing, 2533
Phenotypic gender development, 1390
Phenotypic sexual differentiation, 995-996, 995f-997f
Phenoxybenzamine
  to facilitate bladder emptying, 2720.e1
  ureteral response to, 1888
Phentolamine (Regitine), 1535
  ureteral response to, 1888
Phenylephrine
  in priapism, 1551
  ureteral response to, 1888
Phenylpropanolamine (PPA), for stress urinary incontinence in women, 2714
Pheochromocytoma, 451-452
  clinical characteristics, 2373-2375, 2375t
  contrast media and, 32

Pheochromocytoma (Continued)
  diagnostic tests, 2375-2378, 2376f-2378f, 2377t, 2402, 2402t
  hereditary, 2373, 2374t, 2375, 2380
  increased adrenal function in, 2373-2380, 2373f, 2374t-2375t, 2376f-2379f, 2377t
  malignant, 2373, 2375, 2380
  MRI and, 54
  overview and epidemiology, 2373, 2373f
  pathophysiology, 2373
  prognosis, 2380
  surgery, 2409, 2409b
  treatment, 2378, 2379f, 2409, 2409b
Phimosis, 393, 871-872, 872f
  urethral reconstructive surgery for, 1811
Phosphate
  in crystal formation, 2014
  transport of, urinary tract obstruction and, 794
Phosphatidylinositol 3-kinase (PI3K) pathway, in prostate cancer, 3469
Phosphaturia, in urine, 14
Phosphodiesterase
  in ED, 1498-1499
  for PE, 1572
Phosphodiesterase inhibitors
  for BPS/IC oral therapy, 1243
  to facilitate bladder filling and urine storage, 2682t, 2700-2702
Phosphodiesterase type 5 inhibitors (PDE5-I)
  for benign prostatic hyperplasia, 3382, 3393, 3394t
  for chronic scrotal pain syndrome, 1216
  for ED, 1532-1534, 1532t
  for female orgasmic disorder, 1648
  for female sexual arousal disorders, 1650
  for PD, 1611-1612
  for priapism, 1554
  rationale and efficacy of, 3382-3385, 3382f, 3383t-3384t, 3385f
Phosphorus, metabolism of, 2016
Phosphorylcholine, in prostatic secretions, 3296
Photodynamic therapy (PDT), for refractory high-grade non-muscle-invasive bladder cancer, 3106
Photon, 238
Photoselective vaporization of prostate (PVP), 3438-3442
  in anticoagulated patients, 3441
  complications with, 3441-3442
    intraoperative, 3441
    perioperative, 3441
    postoperative, 3441-3442
  concept and introduction for, 3438-3439
  conclusion for, 3442
  outcomes with, 3440-3441
    comparative studies, 3440-3441
    single-cohort studies, 3440
  technique for, 3439-3440
    intraoperative, 3439
    postoperative, 3439-3440
    preoperative, 3439
Phototherapy, for chronic scrotal pain syndrome, 1216
Physical activity, benign prostatic hyperplasia and, 3324, 3325t
Physical examination, 1434-1436, 1436b
  bladder, 10, 10f-11f
  of male reproductive system, 1435-1436
    phallus, examination of, 1436
    prostate and seminal vesicles, 1436
    scrotum, examination of, 1435
    spermatic cord, examination of, 1435-1436
    testis and epididymis, examination of, 1435, 1435f
  penis, 10-11
  scrotum, 11, 11f
  in urinalysis, 14
Physiologic hydronephrosis, of pregnancy, 284
Physostigmine, ureteral response to, 1887-1888

Phytotherapy
    for benign prostatic hyperplasia, 3393-3399
        current role of, 3395
        extract composition of, 3394, 3394t-3395t
        mechanism of action, 3394-3395, 3395t
        origin of agents for, 3394, 3394t
PI3K/Akt/mTOR pathway, in castration-resistant prostate cancer, 3699-3700
PIA. see Proliferative inflammatory atrophy
Piezoelectric generator, 2094, 2096f
Pigment-related kidney injury, 1924
Pigtail drains, 148
Pili, 428-429
    bacterial type 1 (mannose-sensitive), 1134
    classification of, 429
    P (mannose-resistant), 1134-1135
PIN. see Prostatic intraepithelial neoplasia
Pioglitazone, bladder cancer and, 3077
Pippi Salle procedure, for bladder neck reconstruction, 690, 691f
PIRADS. see Prostate Image Reporting and Data System
Pituitary tumors, 1448
Pivmecillinam, for UTIs, 1155-1156
PIVOT, 3530-3531
Placenta accreta, 294, 303
Placental abnormality, urologic management of, 294-295, 295b
Plain abdominal radiography, 35-36, 36f-37f, 415
Planning target volume (PTV), 3590
Plaques, of urothelium of bladder, 2462
Plasma creatinine (PCr), GFR estimation with, 1905, 1906f
Plasma free metanephrines, in evaluation of adrenal masses, 2402, 2402t
Plasma markers, GFR estimation with, 1905, 1906f
Plasmacytoma, retroperitoneal tumors and, 2236
Plateau-shaped curve, 480
Platelet transfusion, 147
Platinum agents, 3693
Pleomorphic liposarcoma, retroperitoneal tumors and, 2230-2231
PLESS. see Proscar Long-Term Efficacy and Safety Study
PLISSIT Model, for female sexual function, 1628-1629, 1628t-1629t
PLND. see Pelvic lymphadenectomy
Ploidy-flow cytometry, in UTUC, 2198
PNET. see Primitive neuroectodermal tumor
Pneumatic compression stockings, VTE prophylaxis with, for laparoscopic and robotic surgery, 231
Pneumatic lithotripsy, 243, 243b
    basic physics, 243
    tissue effects of, 243
Pneumaturia, patient history of, 7
Pneumomediastinum, during laparoscopic and robotic surgery, 225
Pneumopericardium, during laparoscopic and robotic surgery, 225
Pneumoperitoneum
    for laparoscopic and robotic surgery
        acid-base metabolic effects of, 222
        cardiovascular effects of, 220-221
        complications related to, 224
        mesenteric blood flow and intestinal motility effects of, 222
        pressure of, 220
        renal effects of, 221
        respiratory effects of, 221
    physiology of, 460-461, 462b
    stress response to, 461
Pneumothorax, during laparoscopic and robotic surgery, 225
Podophyllin, for condylomata acuminata, 1742.e3

Poiseuille's law, 932, 935f
Polaris Loop stent, 176f
Pole calyx
    lower, 166, 166.e1f
    upper, 165-166, 166f, 166.e1f
Poliomyelitis, lower urinary tract dysfunction with, 2619
Politano-Leadbetter technique, for vesicoureteral reflux in children, 837f-839f, 840
Political support, in transitional urology, 1045
Pollakiuria, 660
Poly-ADP-ribose polymerase (PARP) inhibitors, 3702
Polyamide (Nylon), 150
Polyamines, in prostatic secretions, 3296
Polyanion macromolecules, in crystal formation, 2014
Polycythemia, in RCC, 2156
Polydioxanone suture, 150
Polyductin, 748
Polyester (Mersilene), 150
Polyglactin 910 suture, 149-150
Polyglactin mesh, for anterior compartment repair, 2781t-2782t
Polyglyconate (Maxon) suture, 150
Polyorchidism, 963
Polypharmacy, 2915-2917
Polypropylene (Prolene), 150
Polypropylene mesh, for pelvic organ prolapse reconstructive surgery, 2781t-2782t, 2783-2786, 2786f
Polyuria
    etiology of, 2678
    management of, 2678
    nocturia and, 2667, 2668t, 2678
    transient urinary incontinence and, 2919.e1
Pontine micturition center, 2493-2494, 2495f
Pontine tegmentum, 2493
POPQ. see Pelvic Organ Prolapse Quantification
Population trends, aging and, 2906-2907
Porcine dermis, anterior repair with, for pelvic organ prolapse reconstructive surgery, 2781t-2782t, 2786-2787, 2787f
Porcine origin, of xenograft sling material, 2835
Port removal, after laparoscopic and robotic surgery, 218-219
Port site closure, after laparoscopic and robotic surgery, 219
Port-site hernias, 468-469
Port-site recurrence, of renal malignancy, 2297
Positional complication, in urologic surgery, 261-262
Positional nerve injury, in urologic surgery, 261-262
Positioning. see Patient positioning
Position-related neuropathy, 146
Positive upper tract urinary cytology, 2219-2222, 2219f
Positron emission tomography (PET), 42
    for biochemical recurrence after radical prostatectomy, 3662, 3662f
    degree of radiotracer of, 91
    degree of visual conspicuity of, 91
    for inguinal node dissection, 1792
    physical characteristics of, 92t
    principles of, 91
    for prostate cancer, 3622
    radionuclides in, 91
Positron emission tomography magnetic resonance imaging, 44, 45t
Postchemotherapy retroperitoneal lymph node dissection (PC-RPLND), 2241
    adjuvant chemotherapy at, 1727
    auxiliary procedures for, 1717-1720, 1721b
    hepatic resection, 1719-1720
    major vascular reconstruction, 1718-1719, 1719f
    nephrectomy, 1718, 1718t

Postchemotherapy retroperitoneal lymph node dissection (PC-RPLND) (Continued)
    pelvic resection, 1720
    supradiaphragmatic disease, management of, 1720
    clinical complete remission to induction chemotherapy, 1721-1722, 1722t
    in high-risk populations
        desperation RPLND, 1728, 1728t
        late relapse RPLND, 1728t, 1729
        reoperative RPLND, 1728t, 1729
        salvage RPLND, 1727-1728, 1728t
    histologic findings at, survival outcomes and, 1726-1727, 1727t, 1727b
Post-chemotherapy surgery (PCS)
    for NSGCTs, 1698-1700, 1698t-1699t
    for seminomas, 1705-1706
Postcoital syndrome, 1636
Postcontrast acute kidney injury, contrast media and, 32-33
Posterior colpoperineorrhaphy, 2825
Posterior colporrhaphy, for pelvic organ prolapse repair, 2825-2829, 2825f
    perineorrhaphy, technique for, 2827-2829
    results with, 2827-2829, 2828t
    site specific, 2826-2827, 2826f-2827f
Posterior compartment prolapse, 2587
Posterior labial commissure, 1627.e1
Posterior lumbodorsal approach, to open adrenalectomy, 2411-2412, 2411f-2412f
Posterior lumbosacral incision, in urologic surgery, 141-142, 141f-142f
Posterior lumbotomy, for ureteropelvic junction obstruction in children, 829, 832f
Posterior pararenal space, 1666-1667, 1667f
Posterior pedicle dissection, ureteral control and, 3152-3157, 3155f-3156f
Posterior urethral valves, 375, 377f, 1053, 1053b
    sexual function and fertility, 1053
Posterolateral and multiple congenital diverticula, 522, 523f
Postexposure prophylaxis, for HIV treatment, 1264-1265
Posthysterectomy vesicovaginal fistulae, 2926-2927
Postmicturition leakage or dribble, 2540
    treatment of, 2547
Postnatal detection, incidental, of ureteral anomalies, 801
Postobstructive diuresis, 796
Postoperative care
    for laparoscopic simple nephrectomy, 2289
    for RPLND, 1717
Postoperative complications, adrenal surgery, 2424, 2424b
Postoperative management, for pheochromocytoma, 2380
Post-operative Patient Global Impression of Improvement (PGI-I), 2531
Postoperative urinary retention, lower urinary tract dysfunction and, 2629-2630
Postorgasmic illness syndrome (POIS), 1564, 1581, 1581.e1b, 1636
Postpartum, urinary incontinence and, PFMT for, 2726
Post-prostatectomy, vesicourethral region, 2993
Postprostatectomy incontinence (PPI), 2596
    PFMT for, 2726
Postrenal kidney injury, 1923
Post-SSRI sexual dysfunction, 1580
Post-translational modifications, of androgen, 3291
Post-void dribbling, for transmen, 3072
Postvoid residual (PVR), 482
    measurement in urinary incontinence, in men, 2543
    pelvic floor disorders and, 2534
    for sling procedure, 2832
    urinary flow rate with, 2565

Postvoid residual (PVR) (Continued)
    in urinary incontinence, in geriatric patients, 2920.e1
    in urodynamic studies, 2556
Postvoid residual volume, in benign prostatic hyperplasia, 3346
Potaba, for PD, 1610, 1616t
Potassium
    filtrate transport, 1909-1910, 1910b
    in kidney, of neonate, 342, 342b
    transport of, urinary tract obstruction and, 794
Potassium channel openers
    to facilitate bladder filling and urine storage, 2682t, 2697
    urethral function effects of, 1903
Potassium channels, in detrusor muscle, 2474, 2474f
Potassium chloride test, for BPS/IC diagnosis, 1238-1239
Potassium titanyl phosphate (KTP) laser, 239
Pouch calculi, with intestinal anastomoses, 3180t
Pouch of Douglas, 2427-2428
Power Doppler ultrasonography, 74
    transrectal, for prostate biopsy, 3500-3501, 3500f-3502f
PPNAD. see Primary pigmented nodular adrenocortical disease
Practice accreditation, for ultrasonography, 89-90
Prazosin
    to facilitate bladder filling and urine storage, 2682t, 2720.e1
    ureteral response to, 1888
Precalyceal canalicular ectasia, 771
Precipitancy, 2919.e2
PRECISION trial, 3503-3504
Precoital pseudoephedrine, for delayed ejaculation, 1579
Precursor malignant lesions, of bladder, 3082-3083, 3083f
Pre-exposure prophylaxis, for HIV, 1265
Pregnancy
    augmentation cystoplasty and, 701
    bacteriuria in, 1184-1185, 1188b
        anatomic and physiologic changes and, 1185-1186, 1185t, 1186f
        complications of, 1186-1187
        management of, 1186-1187, 1187t
        pathogenesis, 1185
        renal insufficiency and, 1187.e1
    classic bladder exstrophy, 290-291
    with congenital urologic conditions, 288-291, 291b
        fertility, 288
        mode of delivery, 289-290
        myelomeningocele, 288-290
    considerations for imaging in, 284-285
    functional and anatomic urologic concerns during, 291-292
        continent catheterizable stoma, 292
        intermittent catheterization, 291
        urinary diversion, 291-292
        urinary tract infection and urinary diversion, 292
    genitourinary tuberculosis management during, 1318
    host defense mechanisms in UTIs and, 1140
    as laparoscopic and robotic surgery contraindication, 204
    neural tube defects, prevention of, 290
    PFMT during, 2726
    physiologic changes during, 282-284
        cardiovascular, 282
        hematologic, 282-283
        hematuria, 283-284
        renal and urinary tract, 283
        respiratory, 282
        urine chemistries during, 283

Pregnancy (Continued)
    physiologic hydronephrosis of, 284
    reflux and, 510-511, 511b
    renal calculi in, 2035
    RMS treatment effects on, 1116-1117
    surgical management of, 285
    ureter physiology effects of, 1900-1901
    urinary incontinence and, 2583
        conservative interventions for, 2735
    urinary tract infections in, management of, 293-294
    urolithiasis in, 286-288, 288b
    urologic considerations in, 282-295
    urologic malignancy during, 292-293
    urologic medication administration during, 285-286
    in urologic surgery, 122
    Wilms tumor treatment effects on, 1108
Premature ejaculation, 1564-1572, 1572b
    and assessment of erectile function, 1570
    causes of, 1568-1569
        acquired premature ejaculation, 1568
        comorbid erectile dysfunction, 1568
        hyperthyroidism and, 1568-1569
        lifelong premature ejaculation, 1568
        prostate disease, 1568
        sexual performance anxiety, psychological or relationship problems and, 1568
    classification of, 1564-1565
    definition of, 1565-1567, 1565.e1, 1566t
    and determination of intravaginal ejaculation latency time, 1569
    diagnosis of, 1569
    evaluation of, 1569
        medical history in, 1569, 1569t
    patient history of, 6
    patient-reported outcome measures, 1569-1570
        index of premature ejaculation, 1570.e1
        premature ejaculation diagnostic tool, 1570.e1
        premature ejaculation profile, 1570.e1
    physical examination of, 1570, 1570f
    prevalence of, 1567-1568, 1567f
    treatment of, 1570-1572
        pharmacologic, 1571-1572, 1573t
        psychosexual therapy, 1571
Prematurity, from bacteriuria in pregnancy, 1186
Prenatal detection, of ureteral anomalies, 801
Prenatal hydronephrosis, 401
Prenatal imaging, and perinatal urology, 358, 358b
Prenatal mortality, from bacteriuria in pregnancy, 1186
Prenatal multidisciplinary consultations, 361-362, 362b
Prenatal ultrasonography, for pediatric urology, 389
Prenatal urinary tract dilation, etiology of, 372, 372t
Preoperative cardiovascular evaluation, 119-120
    clinical markers, 120
    functional capacity, 120
    surgery-specific cardiac risk, 120
Preoperative care
    for adrenal surgery, 2409-2410, 2409b
    evaluation
        for kidney surgery, 2248, 2248.e1f, 2249f
        for laparoscopic kidney surgery, 2279
    for laparoscopic and robotic surgery
        blood products, 204
        bowel preparation, 204
        operating room setup, 205, 205b
        patient positioning, 205, 205f
        patient selection and contraindications, 203-204
        prophylaxis, 205
    for minimally invasive urinary diversion, 3259, 3259b
    preparation for surgery
        for kidney surgery, 2248, 2248.e1f, 2249f
        for laparoscopic kidney surgery, 2279

Preoperative evaluation, 119
Preoperative management, for pheochromocytoma, 2378-2380
Preoperative multiparametric magnetic resonance imaging, use of, 3567
Preputial calculi, 2118-2119
Prerenal kidney injury, 353-354, 1922-1923
Presacral lymphadenectomy, 3152, 3154f
Prespermatogonia, 951
Pressure effects, for laparoscopic and robotic surgery, 221t
Pressure transmission theory, 2597b
Pressure ulcers, 2915
Pressure-flow study
    for benign prostatic hyperplasia, 3347
    in urodynamic studies, 2557
Presurgical testing, 119
    American Society of Anesthesiologists Classification and Risk, 119, 120t, 120b
Preureteral iliac artery, 824
Preureteral vena cava, 822-824, 823f, 824b
PREVAIL study, 3696
Prevesical space, 2427, 2429f, 2850
PRF. see Retroperitoneal fibrosis
Priapism, 394-395, 885, 885b, 1539-1563
    causes of, 1542b
    classifying, 1539
    definition of, 1539, 1540b
    epidemiology and pathophysiology
        in children, 1546
        etiology of ischemic priapism (veno-occlusive, low-flow), 1541-1545, 1543f
        etiology of nonischemic (arterial, high-flow), 1546, 1546f
        etiology of stuttering (intermittent), 1545-1546, 1545b
    epidemiology of, 1540-1546
    evaluation and diagnosis of, 1547-1550
        history of, 1547, 1548f, 1548b
        laboratory testing in, 1548-1549, 1549f, 1549t
        penile imaging in, 1549-1550, 1550f, 1550b
        physical examination for, 1548, 1549t
    historical perspectives of, 1539-1540
    interventional angiography, 1560-1561, 1561f
    ischemic, 1539, 1540f
        penile implants in, 1596
    medical treatments for, 1550-1554, 1552b, 1554b
        ischemic priapism, 1550-1552, 1551f, 1552b
        stuttering, 1553-1554
    molecular basis of, 1547
    nonischemic priapism, 1539, 1541f
    sickle cell disease and, 1544, 1547b
    stuttering priapism, 1539
    surgical management of arterial, 1561, 1562f-1563f, 1562b
    surgical management of ischemic, 1554-1560, 1558b
        immediate implantation of penile prosthesis, 1558-1560, 1560f, 1560b
        shunting, 1554-1558, 1555f-1559f, 1556b
Primary aldosteronism
    clinical characteristics, 2368
    diagnostic tests, 2368-2372, 2369b-2370b, 2370f-2371f
    increased adrenal function in, 2367-2372, 2367f-2368f, 2369b-2370b, 2370f-2371f, 2372b
    overview and epidemiology, 2367
    pathophysiology, 2367-2368, 2367f-2368f
    treatment and prognosis, 2372, 2409b
Primary ciliary dyskinesia, 1452
Primary cutaneous lesions, 1273, 1274t
Primary erectile dysfunction, causes of micropenis, 1511
    vascular abnormalities, 1511-1512
Primary hyperoxaluria, 858, 2056-2057
    medical therapy for, 2057

Primary hyperoxalurias (PHs), 350, 2021–2022, 2021f
Primary nephrotic syndrome, in children, 344
Primary pigmented nodular adrenocortical disease (PPNAD), 2362
Primary syphilis, 1255t, 1257, 1257f–1258f
Primary urethral calculi, 2117
Primary vestibulodynia, 1651
Primitive neuroectodermal tumor (PNET), of kidney, 2181t, 2183
Primordial germ cells, 318f
Principal cells, epididymis, 1374–1375, 1403–1404
Pringle maneuver, in vena caval thrombectomy, 2273, 2273.e1f
Prior surgery, as laparoscopic and robotic surgery contraindication, 203
Probiotics, for UTIs, 1165
Processus vaginalis, 318–320
　cryptorchidism and, 962–963
Procidentia repair, 1051
Programmed cell death. see Apoptosis
Programmed death-1 (PD-1), 2146
Progression, disease, 104–105
Progressive renal dysfunction, urinary tract obstruction and, 776, 777f
Projected isovolumetric pressure (PIP), 2658, 2658f
Prolactin, 1391, 1391f
　in benign prostatic hyperplasia, 3313
　in ED, 1494, 1495t
Prolapsed ureterocele, 395, 397f, 977, 978f
Prolaris test, 3488, 3521
Proliferative inflammatory atrophy (PIA), prostate cancer and, 3461
Promoters, of crystal formation, 2014–2015
Prompted voiding, 2730.e1t, 2731–2732
Prone position, 164–165, 165f
　modifications to, 165
Prone position for percutaneous nephroscopy, 146–147
Pronephros, 334–335, 334f
Propagation, electrical, in ureteral cells, 1882–1883
Propantheline bromide, to facilitate bladder filling and urine storage, 2682t, 2688
Prophylactic antibiotics, for UTI, 371–372
Prophylactic colposuspension, 2765
Prophylactic pelvic nodal treatment, for prostate cancer, 3602–3603, 3603b
Propiverine hydrochloride, to facilitate bladder filling and urine storage, 2682t, 2695–2696
　with α-adrenoreceptor antagonists, 2704
Propranolol (Inderal), ureteral response to, 1888
Proscar Long-Term Efficacy and Safety Study (PLESS), 3332, 3372–3373
PROSELICA trial, 3692–3693
Prospective European Doxazosin and Combination Therapy (PREDICT) study, 3385
PROSPER study, 3696
Prospermatogonia, 951
Prostaglandins (PGs)
　to facilitate bladder emptying, 2718–2719
　for female sexual arousal disorders, 1650
　in prostatic secretions, 3296
　urethral function effects of, 1902–1903
　urothelium release of, 2469–2470
Prostanoid-receptor agonists and antagonists, to facilitate bladder filling and urine storage, 2713.e1–2713.e2
Prostanoids
　for detrusor underactivity, 2661
　lower urinary tract and, 2502

Prostate
　anatomy of, 1381b
　　arterial supply, 1380, 1380f
　　gross structure, 1378–1379, 1379f
　　lymphatic drainage, 1380
　　microanatomic architecture, 1379–1380
　　nerve supply, 1380
　　ultrasonographic, 3490, 3491f–3492f
　　venous drainage, 1380
　cell types of, 3277t, 3278–3279, 3278f, 3279b
　　basal cells, 3278, 3278f
　　epithelial stem cells, 3278f, 3279
　　intermediate cells, 3278f, 3279
　　luminal epithelial, 3278
　　neuroendocrine cells, 3278f, 3279
　development of, 311–317, 313f–316f, 315t, 317t, 317b, 3274–3280, 3277t, 3278b
　　budding induction, 3274–3276
　　budding of, 3274, 3275f
　　cytodifferentiation, 3274
　　epithelial budding, 3276
　　fibroblast growth factors, 3276
　　hedgehog signaling pathway, 3276
　　molecular features of, 3274–3277
　　Nkx3.1 and Sox9, 3276
　　regional differentiation, 3274
　　transforming growth factor-β superfamily, 3276–3277
　　Wnt signaling pathway, 3276
　　zonal and lobar anatomy, 3277, 3277t
　endocrine control of growth of, 3280–3295, 3281f, 3284b
　　adrenal androgens, 3282–3283, 3283f
　　androgen production by testes, 3281–3282, 3282f–3283f, 3282t
　　androgen-binding proteins in plasma, 3282f, 3284
　　estrogens in male, 3282t, 3283–3284
　fate of, in transwomen, 3063
　in genitourinary tuberculosis, 1309
　growth regulation of
　　androgen action at cellular level, 3285–3286, 3285f
　　androgen metabolism in, 3286–3287, 3286f, 3287f
　　androgen receptor in, 3288–3292, 3289f–3290f
　　androgen receptor-dependent chromatin remodeling, 3293–3295
　　cell adhesion molecules, 3287–3288, 3288b
　　at molecular level, 3288–3292
　　protein growth factors in, 3284–3285, 3284f
　　5α-reductase metabolism in, 3286–3287, 3286f, 3287t
　　steroid receptors, 3288–3292
　　steroids in, 3284–3285, 3284f
　　stromal-epithelial interactions, 3287
　localization studies, 1143
　MRI of, T2-weighted, 1380–1381, 1381f
　in prune-belly syndrome, 583–584, 584f
　secretions of. see Prostatic secretions
　size of, benign prostatic hyperplasia and, 3320, 3320f, 3404
　stents for, 3443–3444
　stroma of, 3280
　tissue matrix of, 3280
　transabdominal pelvic ultrasonography of, 80–81, 82f
　transrectal ultrasound of, 88–89, 89f, 1380, 1380f, 3493, 3493f. see also Transrectal ultrasonography, of prostate
　transurethral resection of, 1198–1199
　volume of
　　in acute urinary retention, 3338–3339, 3338f–3339f
　　transurethral microwave therapy and, 3426

Prostate adenocarcinoma, 3506–3512
　Gleason grading of, 3507–3509, 3508f, 3509b
　location of, 3507
　needle biopsy of, 3509–3510, 3510b
　radical prostatectomy specimens for, 3510–3512
　spread of, 3507
　staging classification for, 3506–3507
　subtypes of, 3512–3513
　　malignant tumors, 3513
　　mesenchymal, 3512
　　urothelial carcinoma, 3512–3513
　transurethral resection specimens for, 3510
　treatment effect and, 3512
　volume of, 3507
Prostate biopsy, 3494–3500, 3504b
　for adenocarcinoma, 3509–3510, 3510b
　advanced techniques for, 3500–3504
　after radiotherapy, for biochemical recurrence, 3666
　analgesia for, 3496–3497
　antibiotic prophylaxis for, 3496, 3496t
　bleeding with, 3499
　cleansing enema for, 3496
　complications of, 3499–3500
　contraindications to, 3495
　extended-core techniques, 3497, 3498f
　indications for, 3494–3495, 3495b
　infections after, 3499
　investigational techniques for, 3500–3504
　needle, 3519–3520
　patient positioning for, 3497
　patient preparation for, 3495–3497
　postradiation therapy, 3608
　　imaging and sampling error, 3609
　　interpretation of, 3608–3609, 3609b
　　timing of, 3608–3609
　PSA triggers for, 3516–3517
　repeat, 3497–3498
　risks of, 3499–3500
　saturation, 3497–3498
　sextant, 3497
　transperineal, 3498–3499
　transrectal techniques, 3497–3498
　transurethral, 3499
Prostate cancer, 1421–1422, 3063
　abiraterone for, 3677–3678, 3677f
　adenocarcinoma. see Prostate adenocarcinoma
　African-Americans versus Caucasians, 3472, 3472f
　aminoglutethimide for, 3677
　androgen receptor in, 3472
　androgens, influence of, 3462, 3466, 3467f
　bicalutamide for, 3675
　biomarkers for, 3478–3489, 3489b, 3542–3543
　　annexin A3, 3487
　　blood-based, 3480–3485
　　cell cycle progression, 3543
　　circulating tumor cells, 3484–3485, 3485f
　　development of, 3478–3479
　　epigenetic modifications, 3487–3489
　　gene fusions, 3486
　　genomic classifier, 3542–3543
　　genomic expression profiles, 3488
　　genomic prostate score, 3543
　　human kallikrein 2, 3484
　　inherited genetic markers, 3488–3489
　　metabolomics, 3479
　　α-methylacyl coenzyme A racemase gene, 3487
　　microRNA, 3487
　　performance assessment, 3479–3480
　　prostate cancer antigen 3, 3485–3486, 3485f
　　prostate-specific membrane antigen, 3484
　　tissue-based, 3487–3489
　　urine-based, 3485–3487

Prostate cancer (Continued)
    The Cancer Genome Atlas and, 3467-3468, 3469f
    castration-resistant. see Castration-resistant prostate cancer
    chemoprevention of, 3473, 3477b
        metformin, 3475
        pharmacologic agents for, 3473-3475
        Prostate Cancer Prevention Trial on, 3473-3475, 3474f
        rationale for, 3470f, 3473
        5α-reductase inhibitors for, 3473-3475
        Reduction by Dutasteride of Prostate Cancer Events Trial, 3475
        selenium, 3476, 3476f
        soy, 3476
        statins, 3475
        toremifene citrate, 3475
        tumorigenesis model for, 3472-3473
        vitamin E, 3476, 3476f
    chronic inflammation role in, 1338
    and delayed ejaculation, 1575-1576
    diagnosis of, 3514-3518, 3521b
        age at, 3459
        digital rectal examination for, 3515
        prostate cancer gene 3, 3518
        prostate-specific antigen for, 3515-3517
        stage at, 3459
    DNA methylation in, 1349
    DNA repair defects and, 3472
    enzalutamide for, 3676
    epidemiology of, 3457-3460, 3477b
        molecular, 3461-3462, 3477b
    epigenetic changes in, 3470-3472, 3471f
    etiology of, 3465-3473, 3477b
    flutamide for, 3674
    focal therapy for. see Focal therapy, for prostate cancer
    gene fusions in, 3468-3470
    genomic alterations in
        gene rearrangements, 1352-1353, 1354t
        HPC, 1354-1355, 1354t, 1355f
        sporadic prostate cancer, 1355-1358
    in geriatric patients, 2920.e12
    hereditary. see Hereditary prostate cancer
    hormonal therapy for. see Hormonal therapy, for prostate cancer
    immune checkpoint blockade in, 1343
    incidence of, 3457, 3458f, 3458t
        global, 3458-3459
        screening effect of, 3459-3460
    ketoconazole for, 3677
    lifestyle management of, 3543-3544
        diet, 3544
        exercise, 3543-3544
        micronutrients, 3544
        smoking cessation, 3543
        weight control, 3544
    localized. see Localized prostate cancer
    locally advanced. see Locally advanced prostate cancer
    magnetic resonance imaging of, 3542-3543, 3543b
    management strategies for biochemical recurrence of, 3659-3670
    metabolic syndrome and, 1421-1422
    molecular genetics of, 3465-3473, 3477b
    mortality rates of, 3457, 3458f
        global, 3458-3459
        screening effect of, 3459-3460
    mutations (SPOP, FOXA1, IDH1) in, 3470-3472, 3470f
    natural history of, 3537-3539
        molecular genetics of Gleason pattern 3 versus patterns 4 and 5, 3538-3539, 3538t
    nilutamide for, 3675-3676
    as non-AIDS-defining urologic malignancies, 1268
    in nuclear medicine, 43
    overdiagnosis and overtreatment of, 3537

Prostate cancer (Continued)
    pharmacologic intervention of, 3544-3545
    phosphatidylinositol 3-kinase pathway, 3469
    prognostic value of telomere length for, 1364-1365
    prostate-specific antigen. see Prostate-specific antigen
    psychological aspects of, 3543
    racial differences and, 3457-3458
    RB1 in, 1348
    risk factors for, 3460-3465, 3542
        alcohol consumption, 3465
        androgens, 3462
        calcium, 3463-3465
        diet, 3464-3465
        estrogens, 3462-3463
        familial, 3460-3461, 3460t, 3461f, 3477b
        family history, 3542
        genetic, 3460-3461, 3460t, 3461f, 3477b
        infection, 3461, 3462f, 3477b
        inflammation, 3461, 3462f, 3477b
        insulin-like growth factor axis, 3463
        leptin, 3463
        monitoring, 3542
        obesity, 3465, 3465f
        race, 3542
        sexual activity, 3463-3464
        sexually transmitted disease, 3463-3464
        smoking, 3464
        vasectomy, 3464
        vitamin D, 3463-3465
        vitamin D receptor, 3463-3465
    screening for, 3514-3515
        general concepts of, 3514
        randomized trials for, 3514
        specialty group recommendations for, 3514-3515
    SPOP mutations in, 3470-3472
    sporadic, 1355-1358
    staging of, 3518-3521, 3521b
        classifications for, 3519, 3519t
        clinical versus pathologic, 3518-3519
        combined pretreatment parameters in, 3520
        general concepts of, 3518-3519
        imaging for, 3520
        molecular, 3520-3521
        needle biopsy, 3519-3520
        pelvic lymphadenectomy, 3521
        tumor extent prediction, 3519
    stem cells in, 3466, 3468f
    summary for, 3545
    tissue-based genomics of, 3543
    TP53 gene in, 3469
    tumor initiation and progression in, somatic mutations associated with, 3466-3467, 3469f
    vaccines for, 1341, 1341f
Prostate cancer antigen 3 (PCA3), as prostate cancer biomarker, 3485-3486, 3485f, 3518
Prostate cancer imaging
    imaging studies with metastatic, 100f
    PET radiotracers for, 99t
Prostate Cancer Intervention versus Observation Trial (PIVOT), 3539
Prostate Cancer Outcomes Study, 3531
Prostate Cancer Prevention Trial (PCPT), 3473-3475, 3474f
Prostate D90, 3597
Prostate embolization, 3445-3446
Prostate HistoScanning, 3501-3502
Prostate Image Reporting and Data System (PIRADS), 3502, 3502t-3503t, 3502b, 3622
Prostate imaging, for benign prostatic hyperplasia, 3348
Prostate Intervention Versus Observation Trial (PIVOT), 3620
Prostate stem cell antigen (PSCA), in prostatic secretions, 3298t, 3300-3301

Prostate surgery
    lower urinary tract function and, 2528
    orthotopic urinary diversion and, 3238-3239
Prostate Testing for Cancer and Treatment (ProtecT), 3531
Prostate V100, 3597
Prostatectomy
    holmium laser enucleation of prostate versus, 3437
    radical. see Radical prostatectomy
    simple, 3449-3456, 3456b
        anesthesia for, 3450
        complications with, 3455
        contraindications for, 3450
        indications for, 3449-3450
        open, 3450
        operating day preparation for, 3450
        postoperative management for, 3454-3455
        preoperative evaluation for, 3450
        retropubic, 3450-3452, 3451f-3452f
        robotic-assisted laparoscopic, 3454-3455
        summary for, 3455-3456
        suprapubic, 3452-3454, 3452f-3454f
        surgical technique for, 3450-3454
    SUI following, 2546
    urinary incontinence and, conservative interventions for, 2735
Prostate-specific antigen (PSA), 25, 3679, 3688
    in acute urinary retention, 3338-3339, 3338f-3339f
    in benign prostatic hyperplasia, 3345
    in biochemical recurrence
        after radiation therapy, 3665-3666
        after radical prostatectomy, 3661
    free, 3481-3482, 3481t, 3482f
    isoforms of, 3483-3484, 3483f
    measurement of, for urine incontinence, 2543
    in prostate cancer, 3515-3517
        as biomarker, 3480-3484, 3480f-3481f
        biopsy triggers, 3516-3517
        clinical use for, 3516, 3516t
        complex, 3518
        derivatives and molecular forms of, 3517-3518
        factors influencing, 3515-3516
        free, 3517-3518
        isoforms, 3518
        multiplex tests, 3518
        tumor extent prediction with, 3519
        velocity of, 3517
        volume-based parameters of, 3517
    in prostatic secretions, 3297, 3298t
        derivatives of, 3297-3298, 3298t
    radiation therapy and, 3606-3607
        doubling time, 3607-3608
        failure and, 3606-3607
        nadir value significance, 3607-3608
        neoadjuvant hormones, 3608
        time to nadir of, 3607
Prostate-specific membrane antigen (PSMA), 99, 3622
    as prostate cancer biomarker, 3484
    in prostatic secretions, 3298t, 3300
Prostate-specific protein 94 (PSP-94), in prostatic secretions, 3298t, 3301-3302
Prostate-specific transglutaminases, in prostatic secretions, 3298t, 3299-3303
Prostatic abscess, histopathology, 1205, 1205f
Prostatic acid phosphatase, in prostatic secretions, 3298t, 3301
Prostatic calculi, 2119-2120, 2119f
    clinical presentation of, 2119
    etiopathogenesis and composition of, 2119
    evaluation and management of, 2119-2120
Prostatic epithelial squamous metaplasia, 316
Prostatic injections, 3446-3447
Prostatic intraepithelial neoplasia (PIN), 3506, 3507f, 3513b
    high-grade, 3506, 3507f
    low-grade, 3506

Index I-65

Prostatic lymphoma, 3513
Prostatic neoplasia, pathology of, 3506-3513
Prostatic obstruction, 156-157
Prostatic pain, patient history of, 2
Prostatic secretions, 3295-3304
  drug transport and, 3303-3304, 3304b
  nonpeptide components of, 3295-3297
    citric acid, 3295
    fructose, 3295-3296
    phosphorylcholine, 3296
    polyamines, 3296
    prostaglandins, 3296
    zinc, 3296-3297
  proteins in, 3297-3303, 3298t-3299t, 3299b
    C3 complement, 3302
    human kallikrein 2, 3298
    human kallikrein 11, 3299
    human kallikrein 14, 3299
    human kallikrein L1, 3298-3299
    immunoglobulins, 3302
    lactate dehydrogenase, 3302
    leucine aminopeptidase, 3302
    prostate stem cell antigen, 3300-3301
    prostate-specific antigen, 3297
    prostate-specific antigen derivatives, 3297-3298
    prostate-specific membrane antigen, 3300
    prostate-specific protein 94, 3301-3302
    prostate-specific transglutaminases, 3299-3303
    prostatic acid phosphatase, 3301
    protein C inhibitor, 3302
    semenogelins I and II, 3300
    seminal vesicle secretory proteins, 3303
    transferrin, 3302
    zinc α_2-glycoprotein, 3302-3303
Prostatic urethra, 1382, 1382f, 1807.e4f, 1807.e8
Prostatic urethral lift (PUL), 3420-3421, 3420f
  complications of, 3421
  conclusion for, 3421
  outcomes with, 3420-3421
    comparative studies, 3421
    single-cohort studies, 3420-3421
Prostatic utricle, 1382
Prostatitis, 1202-1223
  chronic bacterial, 1205-1207, 1207b. see also Chronic bacterial prostatitis
  current classification, 1202, 1205b
  epidemiology, 1202
  etiology, 1207-1209, 1209b
    abnormal sensory processing, 1209
    endocrine abnormalities, 1208
    genetics, 1208-1209
    infection, 1207
    inflammation, 1207
    neurologic causes, 1207-1208
    pelvic floor dysfunction, 1208, 1208f
    psychosocial factors, 1208
  granulomatous, 1203
  histopathology, 1202-1203, 1203f
  historical perspective, 1202
  HIV and, 1266
  microbiology, 1204
  prostatic abscess, 1205, 1205f
  in transwomen, 3063
ProstVac-VF, 1341, 1341f, 3698
Protein C inhibitor (PCI), in prostatic secretions, 3302
Protein kinase G (PKG), in ED, 1498
Protein malnutrition, and chronic kidney disease, 354
Protein synthesis, basics of, 1346.e3-1346.e4, 1346.e3f-1346.e4f
Proteins
  androgen-binding, in plasma, 3282f, 3284
  of bladder urothelium
    tight junction, 2467, 2468f
    uroplakins, 2462

Proteins (Continued)
    connexin 43, 2476-2477, 2477f
    contractile, of smooth muscles, 2470-2472, 2471f-2473f
    RhoA, 2473, 2473f
Proteinuria, 15t, 18-19, 19f
  in children, 343-344, 344b
  in urine, during pregnancy, 283
Proteolytic balance, dysregulation of, 782f, 789
Proton beams, 3594-3595
Proton therapy, 3594-3596, 3594f, 3595t
Provoked vestibulodynia, genito-pelvic pain-penetration disorder, 1651
Proximal renal tubular acidosis, 348, 2026
Proximal ureter, stone localization and, 2085-2086, 2086t
Proximal ureteronephrectomy, 2204, 2204f
Proxy endpoints, 104
Prune-belly syndrome (PBS), 375, 410f, 581-601
  adult presentation of, 590
  clinical features of, 581-588, 583b, 588b
    abdominal wall defect, 585-586, 586f-587f
    bladder, 582-583, 584f
    cardiac anomalies, 586
    extragenitourinary abnormalities, 585-588, 585t
    gastrointestinal abnormalities, 587-588, 587f
    genitourinary anomalies, 581-585
    kidneys, 581, 582f
    oral abnormalities, 588
    orthopedic abnormalities, 588, 588f
    prostate, 583-584, 584f
    pulmonary anomalies, 586-587
    sex organs, 583-584
    testes, 584-585, 585f
    ureters, 581-582, 582f-583f
    urethra, anterior, 584, 585f
  description of, 581
  embryology of, 581
  evaluation of, 590-595
  female syndrome, 590
  genetics of, 581
  incidence of, 581
  incomplete, 590
  long-term outlook with, 595-600, 600b
  management of, 590-595, 591b
  neonatal presentation of, 589
  prenatal, diagnosis and management of, 588-589, 589f
  presentation of, 588-590
  spectrum of, 589-590, 589t
  surgical management of, 591-595, 595b
    abdominal wall reconstruction, 594-595
    cutaneous vesicostomy, 592, 592f
    Dénes technique, 595, 598f-600f
    Ehrlich technique, 595
    Furness technique, 595
    internal urethrotomy, 592
    Monfort technique, 595, 596f-597f
    orchidopexy, 593-594, 594f
    Randolph technique, 595
    reduction cystoplasty, 592
    supravesical urinary diversion, 591-592
    ureteral reconstruction, 592
    urethral reconstruction, 592-593, 593f
PRX302, 3447
  to facilitate bladder filling and urine storage, 2713.e2
PSA. see Prostate-specific antigen
PSCA. see Prostate stem cell antigen
Pseudoaneurysm, 274-275
Pseudoepitheliomatous, keratotic, and micaceous balanitis (PEKMB), 1299-1300, 1300f, 1742.e1
Pseudoexstrophy, 537
Pseudoincontinence, patient history of, 5
Pseudomembranous enterocolitis, with bowel preparation, 3165, 3166t

Pseudomonas aeruginosa, 442
Pseudo-obstruction of colon, with intestinal anastomoses, 3181
Pseudoureterocele, 801
PSMA. see Prostate-specific membrane antigen
Psoas, 1658, 1662f-1665f, 1664t
Psoas hitch, 3026-3034
  evaluation for, 3026
  laparoscopic and robotic technique of, 3028-3029, 3029f
  for lower ureteral injuries, 1998-1999, 1999f
  surgical indication for, 3026
  surgical technique for, 3026-3027, 3027f
  with ureteroneocystostomy, 1973
  for urinary tract reconstruction, 683, 684f
Psoas syndrome, 262
Psoriasis, as papulosquamous disorder, 1278-1279, 1279f
Psychological evaluation, in ED, 1526
Psychological Impact of Erectile Dysfunction (PIED) scale, 112t
Psychological screening, 477
Psychometric analysis, 108
Psychophysiologic evaluation, in ED, 1525-1526
Psychosexual development, 996-997, 997b
Psychosexual therapy, for ED, 1529
Psychotropic medication, and ED, 1507-1508, 1509t
PTH. see Parathyroid hormone
PTNS. see Percutaneous tibial nerve stimulation
Puberty, 1392
Pubic lice. see Pediculosis pubis
Pubic rami, 2427
Pubic tubercles, 2428f
Public health notification, from USFDA Center for Devices and Radiological Health, 2777
Pubococcygeal line (PCL), 2537
Pubococcygeus muscle, 2430-2432, 2432f
Puboprostatic ligaments, division of, in retropubic radical prostatectomy, 3552, 3552f
Pubovaginal sling (PVS), 2833-2835
  allograft
    materials for, 2834-2835
    outcomes of, 2841-2843, 2841t-2842t
  anatomy for, 2834
  autologous graft
    materials for, 2834
    outcomes of, 2839-2841, 2840t
  complications of, 2848-2849, 2849b
    nonurologic, 2849
    perforation and exposure, 2848-2849
  evolution of, 2830
  materials for, 2834-2835, 2836b
  mechanics of, 2834
  operative procedure for, 2836-2839, 2839b
    anesthesia for, 2836-2837
    counseling, 2836
    graft harvest for, 2837, 2837f
    patient positioning for, 2836-2837
    postoperative care for, 2839
    preparation for, 2836-2837
    sling placement and fixation in, 2838-2839, 2838f-2839f
    vaginal dissection for, 2837-2838, 2838f
  outcomes of, 2839-2844, 2845b
    for mixed urinary incontinence, 2844-2845
    for urethral reconstruction, 2845
  retropubic suspension surgery versus, 2771-2773, 2772f
  synthetic prosthetic
    materials for, 2835, 2836t
    outcomes of, 2843
  voiding dysfunction after, 2845-2848, 2848b
    surgical management of, 2846-2848, 2847t
  xenograft
    materials for, 2835
    outcomes of, 2843-2844, 2844t

Pubovesical ligaments, 2429-2430, 2438
Pudendal arteries, 1807.e4f
    preservation of, in retropubic radical prostatectomy, 3552, 3552f
Pudendal nerve, 2434
    stimulation of, 2511, 2751-2752
        inhibitory and excitatory stimulation frequencies, 2511
Pulmonary abnormalities, with cloacal exstrophy, 575
Pulmonary complications
    after RPLND, 1730
    of radical nephrectomy, 2261-2266
Pulmonary embolism
    after laparoscopic and robotic surgery, 231
    after retropubic radical prostatectomy, 3563
    vena caval thrombectomy and, 2266-2267, 2277
Pulmonary evaluation, 120-121
Pulmonary hypoplasia, with posterior urethral valves, 610-611, 610f
Pulsed radiofrequency, for chronic scrotal pain syndrome, 1221
Pulsed wave lasers, 238
PUM. see Partial urogenital mobilization
PUNLMP. see Papillary urothelial neoplasm of low malignant potential
PUO. see Partial ureteral obstruction
Purinergic nervous system, in ureteral function, 1889-1890
Purinergic signaling
    in bladder afferent pathway, 2484-2485, 2485f
    in bladder pain syndrome and interstitial cystitis, 2508
PVP. see Photoselective vaporization of prostate
PVR. see Postvoid residual
PVS. see Pubovaginal sling
Pyeloenteric fistulae, 2953-2955, 2953f-2954f
Pyelogenic cyst, 774, 774f
Pyelography
    antegrade. see Antegrade pyelography
    intravenous. see Intravenous pyelography
    for pediatric genitourinary trauma, 1073-1074
    retrograde. see Retrograde pyelography
Pyelolithotomy, laparoscopic pyeloplasty with, for ureteropelvic junction obstruction with, 1958-1960
Pyelolymphatic backflow, 38
Pyelonephritis, 398-400, 1129
    acute, 1168-1171, 1168f-1169f, 1170t
    chronic, 1176-1177, 1177f
    emphysematous, 1171-1172, 1171f
    with ureterointestinal anastomoses in urinary intestinal diversion, 3180t, 3192
    XGP, 1177-1179, 1178f-1179f
Pyeloplasty, 836b
    with concomitant pyelolithotomy, 1958-1960
    dismembered. see Dismembered pyeloplasty
    laparoscopic. see Laparoscopic pyeloplasty
    laparoscopic dismembered tubularized flap, 1960
    nondismembered. see Nondismembered pyeloplasty
    open surgery, 1953
    for prune-belly syndrome, 592
    results of, 1957-1958, 1959t
    salvage procedures for, 1963
Pyelopyelostomy, for retrocaval ureter, 1963, 1965f
Pyelosinus backflow, 38
Pyelotubular backflow, 38
Pyeloureterostomy, for ureteral anomalies, 816-817, 817b
Pyelovascular fistulae, 2958
Pygeum africanum (African plum)
    for benign prostatic hyperplasia, 3398
    for nocturia, 2674
Pyoderma gangrenosum (PG), 1287-1288, 1288f
Pyonephrosis, 435
    infected, 1174, 1174f

Pyridium, for pelvic floor disorder testing, 2533
Pyridoxine, for pediatric kidney stone disease, 870
Pyrophosphate, in crystal formation, 2014
Pyuria, 14, 426, 1129

Q
Qmax, 480-481, 481t
QOL-MED, 112t
Q-tip test, for urethral mobility, 2529
Quadratic fixation
    mechanisms of action of, 2995, 2995f
    mechanisms of continence of, 2995
Quadratus lumborum, 1658, 1662f-1665f, 1664t
Quadruple ureters, 821
Quality of care, definition of, 101
Quality of life. see also Health-related quality of life
    after androgen deprivation therapy, 3656
    after orthotopic urinary diversion, 3255-3257, 3256t, 3257b
    augmentation cystoplasty and, 702
    with cutaneous continent urinary diversion, 3226-3227
    cystinuria and, 2062-2063
    definition of, 116
    with exstrophy-epispadias complex, 567
    lower urinary tract dysfunction and, in pediatric patients, 652-653, 655b
    nocturia and, 2664
    with posterior urethral valves, 620, 623b
    in prune-belly syndrome, 595
Quality-of-life questionnaires
    for male urinary incontinence, 2541, 2541.e1f-2541.e2f, 2542f
    for pelvic floor disorders, 2531, 2532t-2533t
Quercetin, for BPS/IC oral therapy, 1241t, 1243
Questionnaire-Based Voiding Diary (QVD), 2723, 2723.e1f-2723.e2f
Quick flicks, 2730
Quiescent intracellular reservoir (QIR), 429
QVD. see Questionnaire-Based Voiding Diary

R
RAA. see Renal artery aneurysm
Race
    pelvic organ prolapse and, 2591
    urinary incontinence and, 2583-2585
    UTUC variations and, 2185
Race, prostate cancer and, 3457-3458, 3542
Rad, 28
Radiation
    for adrenal cortical carcinoma, 2387
    bladder cancer and, 3077
    in pediatric kidney stone disease, 861
    for retroperitoneal tumors, 2245
Radiation exposure, 28
    with CT, 780
    lower urinary tract dysfunction and, 2632
    medical diagnoses and, 2527
Radiation fistulae, 2959-2962
    chemotherapy of, 2961-2962
    combination therapies of, 2962
    diversion procedures for, 2961
    interpositional grafts for, 2961
    management approaches for, 2961
    recommendations for, 2961
    repair techniques for, 2961
Radiation therapy
    adjuvant. see Adjuvant radiation therapy
    after partial orchiectomy, 1712
    biochemical recurrence after. see Biochemical recurrence, after radiation therapy
    brachytherapy. see Brachytherapy
    definitive, 3665-3666
    external beam. see External beam radiation treatment

Radiation therapy (Continued)
    for locally advanced prostate cancer, 3652-3655, 3653t
        adjuvant androgen deprivation with, 3653-3654
        chemotherapy with, 3654-3655
        neoadjuvant androgen deprivation with, 3652-3653, 3654b
    for muscle-invasive bladder cancer, 3122
    for neuroblastoma, 1096
    in non-muscle-invasive bladder cancer, 3106
    for PD, 1615-1616, 1617t
    for penile cancer, 1765-1769, 1769b
        adverse effects of, 1767-1768
        inguinal areas, 1768-1769, 1769f
        primary lesion, 1765-1768
    for prostate cancer, 3587-3615
        androgen suppression combined with, 3600-3602, 3602b
            background and potential mechanisms of, 3600
            localized disease and, 3600-3602, 3601t
            locally advanced disease and, 3602
            optimal duration of, 3602
        CT-based treatment planning and three-dimensional conformal radiotherapy, 3587-3588, 3588f
        evaluating response to, 3606-3609, 3609b
        high-energy linear accelerators, 3587
        in high-risk or locally advanced disease, 3611
        historical perspective on, 3587-3592, 3592b
        hormonal therapy with, 3682
        image-guided radiation therapy and treatment margins, 3589-3590, 3591f-3592f
        intensity-modulated radiation therapy, 3588-3589, 3589f, 3589t
        multiparametric magnetic resonance imaging in, 3590-3591
        postradiation therapy biopsy, 3608
            imaging and sampling error, 3609
            interpretation of, 3608-3609, 3609b
            timing of, 3608-3609
        prostate-specific antigen and, 3606-3607
            doubling time, 3607-3608
            failure and, 3606-3607
            nadir value significance, 3607-3608
            neoadjuvant hormones, 3608
            time to nadir of, 3607
        role of prophylactic pelvic nodal treatment, 3602-3603, 3603b
        technological advances of, 3587-3592, 3592b
        transrectal ultrasound-guided brachytherapy, 3591-3592, 3592f
        treatment morbidity and quality-of-life outcomes of, 3603-3606, 3604t-3605t, 3606b
            erectile dysfunction and management, 3606
            rectal toxicity and management, 3603-3604
            rectal-sparing strategies, 3604, 3604f
            urinary toxicity and management, 3604-3606
    for renal tumor ablation, 2321-2322
    salvage. see Salvage radiation therapy
    for seminomas, 1702-1703, 1703t
    stereotactic body, 3593-3594
    for TGCTs, 1692
    in uroradiology, 28-29, 29t
        radiation protection, 28-29
        relative radiation levels, 28, 29t
Radiation Therapy Oncology Group (RTOG), 3594
Radical cystectomy
    continence preservation in
        anterior apical dissection in male patient, 3239-3240, 3241b
        urethra preservation in female patient, 3240-3241, 3240f

Radical cystectomy (Continued)
  history of, 3133
  indications for, 3144
  oncologic outcomes of, 3118–3119, 3133
  with pelvic lymph node dissection
    anatomic extent of, 3115–3116
    bilateral, 3115
    density of, 3117
    distal urethra management, 3118
    extracapsular nodal extension, 3117
    intraoperative decision making, 3117–3118
    intraoperative frozen sections of ureter, 3117–3118
    managing female urethra in, 3118
    for muscle-invasive bladder cancer, 3114–3119
    number removed in, 3125
    oncologic outcomes following, 3118–3119, 3118t
  robotic. see Robotic radical cystectomy
  with transurethral resection of bladder tumor
    female, 3141–3143, 3142f–3143f
    male, 3138–3141, 3139f–3141f
Radical inguinal lymph node dissection, for penile cancer, 1796–1798, 1799f–1800f
Radical nephrectomy
  laparoscopic. see Laparoscopic radical nephrectomy
  for malignancy, 2257–2261, 2257f
    complications of, 2261
    regional lymphadenectomy with, 2260, 2260f, 2260.e1f
    surgical procedure for, 2257–2260, 2258f–2259f, 2258.e1f, 2259.e1f
    wound closure for, 2261
  for RCC, local recurrence after, 2164–2165, 2165–2166, 2165b, 2166f, 2167t, 2168f
Radical nephroureterectomy, for UTUC, 2199–2202
  distal ureter and bladder cuff management, 2200
  indications of, 2199
  laparoscopic, 2202–2205
  open, 2199–2200, 2200f
  total laparoscopic technique in, 2202, 2203f
  traditional open distal ureterectomy in, 2200–2201, 2200f–2201f
  transurethral resection of ureteral orifice, 2201–2202, 2202f
  transvesical ligation and detachment technique in, 2201, 2201f
Radical orchiectomy, 1711
  technique for, 1711–1712
  for TGCTs, 1686
Radical pelvic irradiation, localized prostate cancer and, 3525
Radical prostatectomy
  biochemical recurrence after, 3659–3665. see also Biochemical recurrence, after radical prostatectomy
  for locally advanced prostate cancer, 3645–3652, 3648b
    adjuvant androgen deprivation with, 3652
    adjuvant radiation therapy, 3650–3652, 3651t, 3652b
    for clinical stage T3, 3645–3652, 3646t
    neoadjuvant androgen deprivation, 3648–3649, 3648t–3649t
    neoadjuvant chemotherapy and chemotherapy-hormonal therapy, 3649–3650, 3650t
    outcomes of, 3646–3647, 3647f
    pathologic findings with, 3643, 3643t
    and PD, 1602
  for prostate adenocarcinoma, 3510–3512
  for prostate cancer, hormonal therapy with, 3682
  retropubic. see Retropubic radical prostatectomy

Radical prostatectomy (Continued)
  salvage. see Salvage radical prostatectomy
  urinary incontinence after
    prevalence of, 2587
    risk factors for, 2587
    sphincteric function and, 2596
Radiofrequency ablation (RFA)
  for RCC, 2171
  for renal tumors, 2310–2312, 2312b
    background and mode of action, 2310–2312
    CA versus, 2317–2318
    complications of, 2318–2319, 2320f–2321f, 2320b
    equipment variations, 2311
    follow-up for, 2312–2314, 2314b
    intraoperative monitoring, 2311–2312
    laparoscopic, 2304–2305
    oncologic outcomes of, 2314–2318, 2315t–2316t, 2318b
    percutaneous, 2312, 2313f, 2318
    treatment temperature, 2311
Radiography
  of bladder injuries, 3055–3056
  of cloacal anomalies, 1024–1025
  of defecation disorders, 669–670, 669f–670f
  for genitourinary tuberculosis, 1311–1313, 1311f–1313f
  intravenous urography. see Intravenous urography
  loopography. see Loopography
  of male pelvis, 2457–2458
  of neuroblastoma, 1089
  retrograde pyelography. see Retrograde pyelography
  retrograde urethrography. see Retrograde urethrography
  static cystography. see Static cystography
  for ureteropelvic junction obstruction, 1943, 1944f
  of urethral diverticula, 2982–2983, 2983f–2984f
  of urinary lithiasis, 2038
  of urogenital sinus abnormalities, 1023–1024
  voiding cystourethrogram. see Voiding cystourethrogram
Radioisotopic penography, 1524
Radiologic imaging
  of pediatric urology, 388
  for UTUC, 2191–2192
Radionuclide cystography, 423, 424f–425f
Radionuclide renal scan, for posterior urethral valves, 608
Radionuclide studies, for UTIs, 1144.e1
Radionuclide testicular scanning, 423
Radiopharmaceuticals
  for castration-resistant prostate cancer, 3704
  for nuclear imaging of kidneys, 96b
Radiotherapy and Androgen Deprivation in Combination after Local Surgery (RADICALS), 3663–3664
Radiotracers, 91
Radium-223, for castration-resistant prostate cancer, 3704
RAE. see Renal artery embolization
RaLPN. see Robotic-assisted laparoscopic partial nephrectomy
RALRP. see Robotic-assisted laparoscopic radical prostatectomy
Randall plaques, 2011, 2012f–2013f, 2018
Randolph technique, 595
Random flaps, for urethral and penile reconstruction, 1807, 1807f
Randomized Intervention for Management of Vesicoureteral Reflux (RIVUR) study, 515–516
RANK ligand inhibitors, for castration-resistant prostate cancer, 3704
Rapid eye movement (REM), 2665

RAS. see Renal artery stenosis
RASSF1A gene, in bladder cancer, 1349
RAVES (Radiotherapy-Adjuvant Versus Early Salvage) trial, 3664–3665
RAZOR trial, of robotic cystectomy, 3144
RBF. see Renal blood flow
RCC. see Renal cell carcinoma
RCCT. see Renal concentrating capacity test
Reactive arthritis
  as papulosquamous disorder, 1279–1280, 1280f
  urethral involvement in, reconstructive surgery for, 1808
    for reactive arthritis, 1808
    for urethral hemangioma process, 1808
Real-time CT fluoroscopy, 45
Real-time elastography (RTE), 74, 75f
  of scrotum, 84
Real-time or ultrasound dosimetry, 3598
Reanastomosis, for urethral stricture disease, 1819–1820, 1819f–1820f
Reboxetine, for delayed ejaculation, 1579
Reconstructive surgery
  after bladder RMS treatment, 1116
  for cloacal anomalies, 1037–1041, 1040b
    definitive, 1039–1041, 1039f
    gastrointestinal tract decompression for, 1038
    genitourinary tract decompression for, 1038–1039, 1038f
    initial management, timing, and principles for, 1037–1038
    obstructive urinary repair, 1039
    results of, 1040–1041, 1041t
  for detrusor underactivity, 2663
  for disorders of sex development and urogenital sinus
    current operative techniques for, 1028–1034, 1029f
    high vaginal confluence: with or without clitoral hypertrophy, 1030–1033, 1031f–1033f
    initial management, timing, and principles, 1025–1028, 1026f
    low vaginal confluence: clitoral hypertrophy, 1028–1030, 1030f, 1030b
    results of, 1034–1037
    total and partial urogenital mobilization, 1033–1034, 1034f–1036f
  microvascular, 3050
  penile and urethral, 1804–1842, 1805b, 1813b
    for amyloidosis, 1810
    anatomy of, 1807, 1807.e1f–1807.e7f
    for balanitis xerotica obliterans, 939, 940f
    for circumcision complications, 1811–1812
    in classic bladder exstrophy, 551–552, 552f–553f
    for curvatures of penis, 1836–1838, 1838b
    for failed epispadias repair, 1813
    for failed hypospadias repair, 1812–1813
    female-to-male transgender, 1841–1842, 1842b
    for fistulae of posterior urethra, 1835–1836, 1836b
    for glans dehiscence, 937, 938f
    for LS, 1808–1810, 1809f
    in male epispadias, 569
    for meatal stenosis, 937–938, 1811
    for paraphimosis, balanitis, and phimosis, 1811
    penile transplantation, 1838–1842, 1840f, 1842b
    for PFUIs, 1828–1834, 1830f–1834f
    principles of, 1804–1807, 1806f–1807f, 1808b
    for reactive arthritis, 1808
    for recurrent penile curvature, 939–941, 940f

Reconstructive surgery (Continued)
  for urethral diverticulum, 938–939, 939f, 1810–1811
  for urethral hemangioma process, 1808
  for urethral stricture, 938, 1814–1828, 1814f, 1828b
  for urethrocutaneous fistula, 935–937, 936f–937f, 1810
  for vesicourethral distraction defects, 1834f, 1835, 1836b
Rectal bladder urinary diversion, 3209–3211
  augmented valved rectum, 3209
  folded rectosigmoid bladder, 3209
  hemi-Kock pouch procedures with valved rectum, 3209–3210
  Mainz II pouch, 3210–3211
  sigma-rectum pouch, 3210–3211
  T pouch procedures with valved rectum, 3209–3210, 3210f
Rectal carcinoma, and delayed ejaculation, 1576
Rectal fascia, 2427, 2429f
Rectal injury
  bowel injury and, 277–278
  complications of seminal vesicle surgery, 1864
Rectal mucosal grafts, 1807
Rectal toxicity, prostate cancer and, 3603–3604
Rectocele, 2526, 2587
  repair of, 2825
Rectourethral fistulae (RUF), 2955–2958, 2956f, 2958b
Rectouterine pouch, 2427–2428, 2429f
Rectovaginal space, 2427, 2429f
Rectovesical pouch, bladder, 3010
Rectum, anatomy of, 2449, 2450f, 2454, 2455f
Rectus abdominis, 136f, 2447, 2447f–2448f
Rectus muscle flap, in urethrovaginal fistulae, 2950
Rectus sheath, 2444, 2447f–2448f
Recurrent cryptorchidism, 949
Recurrent infection, in bladder tumor, 3077
Recurrent penile curvature, 913f–914f, 939–941, 940f
Recurrent stenosis, after urethral injury, 3060
Recurrent uric acid stone formation, ammonium acid urate stones from, 2032
Recurrent UTIs, 1159–1166, 1160t, 1160b
  ammonium acid urate stones from, 2032
  bacterial persistence and, 1160–1161
  cranberry, 1163–1164, 1164f
  D-mannose, 1166
  estrogen, 1164–1165, 1164f
  immunoactive prophylaxis, 1166
  low-dose continuous prophylaxis for, 1162–1163
  management, 1161–1166, 1161f
  methenamine, 1165t, 1166
  non-antibiotic management, 1163
  probiotics, 1165
REDUCE. see Reduction by Dutasteride of Prostate Cancer Events
5α-Reductase
  in benign prostatic hyperplasia, 3307–3308, 3308f
  prostate metabolism, 3286–3287, 3286f, 3287t
5α-Reductase deficiency, 1014–1016, 1015f
5α-Reductase inhibitors
  α-adrenergic blockers and, 3385, 3386f
  for benign prostatic hyperplasia, 3378
  for chemoprevention of prostate cancer, 3473–3475
  for chronic scrotal pain syndrome, 1215
  to facilitate bladder filling and urine storage
    with α-adrenoreceptor antagonists, 2707
    with antimuscarinic agents, 2707
  for priapism, 1553
  prostate-specific antigen and, 3515
5α-Reductase-specific antibodies (5ARIs), in prostate cancer, 3544

Reduction by Dutasteride of Clinical Progression Events in Expectant Management of Prostate Cancer (REDEEM) study, 3544
Reduction by Dutasteride of Prostate Cancer Events (REDUCE), 3475
Re-entry catheter, 173, 174f
Reflection, of ultrasound waves, 71, 71f
Reflex circuitry
  controlling continence, 2489–2493, 2490f
    somatic to visceral reflexes, 2492
    sphincter to bladder reflexes, 2490f, 2491–2492, 2492f
    storage phase, 2490–2491, 2490f–2491f, 2491t
  controlling micturition, 2489–2493, 2490f
    emptying phase, 2490f, 2491t, 2492
    urethra to bladder reflexes, 2492–2493, 2492f–2494f
Reflex contraction, promotion or initiation of, 2902
Reflex sympathetic dystrophy (RSD), lower urinary tract dysfunction and, 2626
Reflux nephropathy, 742
Reflux-associated renal dysplasia, 499, 499f, 499t, 499.e1f
Refluxing ureteral reimplantation, 3023–3026, 3023f
Refractory urinary storage symptoms, after urethrolysis, 2848
Regional anesthesia, in urologic surgery, 131–132
Regions of interest (ROI), 3587–3588
Regitine. see Phentolamine
Reiter syndrome. see Reactive arthritis
Relapse, tumors
  NSGCTs, 1700–1702
  seminomas, 1706
Relative jet frequency (RJF), 778
Relative saturation ratio (RSR), 2010
Reliability, definition of, 109
Religion, benign prostatic hyperplasia and, 3320–3321
REM. see Rapid eye movement
Renal abscess, 1172–1174, 1172f–1173f
Renal agenesis, 741–742
  unilateral. see Unilateral renal agenesis
Renal anomalies, 510
Renal arterial clamping, for laparoscopic partial nephrectomy, 2303
Renal arterial laceration, for pediatric genitourinary trauma, 1074
Renal arterial occlusion, for pediatric genitourinary trauma, 1074
Renal arteries, 1671–1672
  occlusion of. see Ischemic nephropathy; Renovascular hypertension
  in radical nephrectomy, 2258, 2258f, 2258.e1f
  in simple nephrectomy, 2288, 2288f
Renal arteriovenous fistula, 737
Renal artery aneurysm (RAA), 736–737
Renal artery embolization (RAE), before kidney surgery, 2248, 2248.e1f
Renal artery stenosis (RAS)
  diagnosis of, 1916–1918, 1917f–1918f, 1918b
  incidence and etiology of, 1914b
  management of, 1918–1919
    medical therapy, 1918
    percutaneous intervention, 1918–1919, 1919f
    surgical, 1919, 1920b
  pathophysiology of, 1915–1916, 1915f–1916f, 1915t, 1916b
    one-kidney, one-clip model of, 1917, 1918f
    two-kidney, one-clip model of, 1917, 1917f
  in renovascular hypertension, 1915
  screening tests for
    angiography, 1917–1918, 1918b
    CT, 1917–1918, 1918b
    duplex Doppler ultrasonography, 1917–1918, 1918b
    MRA, 1917–1918, 1918b

Renal artery thrombosis (RAT), 387
Renal bladder ultrasound, for pediatric urology, 388–389
Renal bleeding
  nephrectomy and, 1988–1989
  with renal injury, 1991
Renal blood flow (RBF), 1905, 1906b
  aging and, 2905
  urinary tract obstruction and
    in bilateral ureteral obstruction, 791–792
    GFR and, 791
    renal vascular resistance and, 791
    in unilateral ureteral obstruction, 791
Renal calculi, 2069.e1, 2084b
  ammonium acid urate stones in, 2032
  anatomic predisposition to, 2033–2035
    caliceal diverticula, 2034
    horseshoe kidneys, 2034
    medullary sponge kidney, 2034–2035
    ureteropelvic junction obstruction, 2034
  calcium stones in, 2018–2026
    hypercalciuria, 2018–2020
    hyperoxaluria, 2020–2023, 2021f–2022f
    hyperuricosuria, 2023–2024, 2024f
    hypocitraturia, 2024
    hypomagnesiuria, 2026
  classification of, 2017–2018, 2017t–2018t
  clinical factors of, 2088–2091, 2091b
    duration, 2091
    morbid obesity and, 2089
    old age and frailty, 2089–2090
    prior renal surgery, 2090
    renal function, 2088–2089
    renal transplants, 2091
    solitary kidney, 2089
    spinal deformity or limb contractures, 2090
    uncorrected coagulopathy, 2090
    urinary diversion, 2091
    urinary tract infection and, 2088
  composition of, treatment decision based on, 2076
  cystine stones in, 2029–2030, 2029f
  dihydroxyadenine stones in, 2031–2032
  epidemiology of, 2005–2009, 2009b
    age, 2006
    cardiovascular disease, 2008–2009
    chronic kidney disease, 2009
    climate, 2007
    gender, 2005–2006
    geography, 2006–2007, 2007f
    obesity, diabetes, and metabolic syndrome, 2008
    occupation, 2007–2008
    race and ethnicity, 2006
    water intake, 2009
  infection stones in, 2030–2031
    bacteriology of, 2030–2031, 2031t
    epidemiology of, 2031
    pathogenesis of, 2030, 2030f
  matrix stones in, 2032
  medication-related stones in, 2032–2033
  mineral metabolism and, 2015–2017, 2017b
    calcium, 2015–2016
    magnesium, 2016
    oxalate, 2016–2017
    phosphorus, 2016
  natural history of, 2069–2070
  nonmedical management of, 2069–2093
    anatomic factors in, 2077–2084
    in calyceal diverticula, 2077–2078, 2077.e1f
    factors affecting, 2070b
    imaging for, 2071
    laboratory tests for, 2071
    lower pole calculi, 2081–2084, 2081f, 2082t, 2083f
    medical history for, 2071
    pretreatment assessment for, 2070–2071
    in renal ectopia, 2080–2081, 2081f
    stone burden and treatment decision, 2072–2074, 2072b, 2073f
    stone composition and, 2076

Renal calculi *(Continued)*
 stone localization and, 2075–2076
 treatment algorithm for, 2069, 2070f
 in ureteropelvic junction obstruction, 2077
 nonstaghorn. *see* Nonstaghorn renal calculi
 pathophysiology of, 2017–2035, 2035b
 physicochemistry of, 2009–2015, 2015b
  inhibitors and promoters, 2014–2015
  matrix of, 2015
  nucleation and crystal growth, 2010–2014, 2012f–2013f
  saturation state in, 2009–2010, 2010f–2011f
 in pregnancy, 2035
 staghorn. *see* Staghorn calculi
 technical factors of, 2088
 uric acid stones in, 2026–2029, 2027f–2028f
  hyperuricosuria, 2029
  low urinary volume, 2029
  low urine pH, 2027–2029, 2028f
 with urinary intestinal diversion, 3180t, 3195–3196
 in urinary tract obstruction, 778
 xanthine stones in, 2031–2032
Renal calyces, 1869, 1869.e1f
Renal cell carcinoma (RCC)
 autosomal dominant polycystic kidney disease association with, 753, 2158
 clear cell type, 55
 clinical associations of, 2156–2158
 clinical presentation of, 2155–2156, 2156t, 2156b
 etiology of, 2140–2141, 2141b
 familial, 2141–2145, 2142t–2143t, 2144f
  treatment of, 2173–2174, 2174f
 historical considerations for, 2133
 incidence of, 2138–2140
 metastatic. *see* Metastatic RCC
 as non-AIDS-defining urologic malignancy, 1268
 pathology of, 2148–2155, 2148t–2151t, 2153b
  chromophobe RCC, 2149t–2151t, 2152–2153, 2154f
  classification systems, 2149–2151, 2149t–2151t
  clear cell RCC, 2149t–2151t, 2151–2152, 2152f
  collecting duct RCC, 2149t–2151t, 2154
  papillary RCC, 2149t–2151t, 2152, 2153f
  renal medullary RCC, 2149t–2151t, 2154–2155
  sarcomatoid and rhabdoid differentiation, 2149t–2151t, 2155, 2155f
  unclassified, 2149t–2151t, 2155
 in pediatric patients, 1109–1110
 prognosis of, 2160–2162, 2161t
 screening for, 2156–2158, 2157t
 staging of, 2158–2160, 2158t–2159t, 2160f, 2160b
 treatment of advanced, 2325–2328
  chemotherapy, 2341–2342
  debulking or cytoreductive nephrectomy, 2325–2328, 2326f–2327f, 2327t, 2328b
  hormonal therapy, 2342–2343
  palliative surgery, 2328, 2328b
  prognostic factors and, 2324–2325, 2325f, 2325t
  resection of metastases, 2328, 2328b
  systemic therapy for non–clear cell variants, 2343–2344, 2344f
  targeted molecular agents in, 2324, 2333–2341, 2333t–2335t, 2336f, 2337t
 treatment of localized, 2162–2174
  active surveillance, 2173, 2173t
  AUA guidelines for, 2162–2163, 2163f
  nephron-sparing surgery in, 2173–2174, 2174f
  partial nephrectomy, 2164–2169, 2165b, 2167t, 2169f

Renal cell carcinoma (RCC) *(Continued)*
  radical nephrectomy, 2164–2165, 2165–2166, 2165b, 2166f, 2167t, 2168f
  risk stratification and renal mass biopsy, 2163–2164, 2164f, 2164b
  thermal ablative therapies, 2171–2173, 2171f, 2172t
  tumor enucleation, 2170–2171, 2170f
 treatment of locally advanced, 2174–2180, 2174f
  adjuvant therapy, 2178–2180, 2178b
  IVC involvement, 2174–2176, 2175f–2176f, 2298. *see also* Vena caval thrombectomy
  local recurrence, 2178, 2178b
  locally invasive, 2176–2177
  lymph node dissection, 2177–2178, 2177f, 2177t, 2260, 2260f, 2260.e1f
 with tuberous sclerosis complex, 758
 tumor biology clinical implications in, 2145–2148
  angiogenesis and targeted pathways, 2146, 2148
  cancer genome research, 2146–2148
  immunobiology and immune tolerance, 2145–2146, 2147f
  resistance to cytotoxic therapy, 2145, 2145t
Renal clearance, 1905
Renal concentrating capacity test (RCCT), 2678
Renal cortex, 1866, 1866.e1f
Renal cortical scintigraphy, 390
Renal cystic diseases, 745–746, 746f
 acquired. *see* Acquired renal cystic diseases
 benign multilocular cyst, 765–766, 765f, 766b, 767f
 classification of, 745–746, 745b
 congenital nephrosis, 756
 familial hypoplastic glomerulocystic kidney disease, 756–757
 inheritable, 745b, 746
 medullary, 747t, 755–756, 756f, 756b
 medullary sponge kidney, 771–772, 771f, 772b
 multicystic dysplastic kidney, 762–765, 762f, 765b
 multiple malformation syndromes, 747t, 762b
 polycystic, 751t
  autosomal dominant, 750–755, 755b
  autosomal recessive, 746–749, 751b
Renal cysts, 401–402, 405, 2121–2123, 2123b
 epidemiology, etiology, and pathophysiology of, 2121
 evaluation of, 2122, 2122f, 2122t
 laparoscopic surgery for, 2291–2292, 2291f
  procedure for, 2291, 2291f
  results of, 2291–2292
 management options of, 2123, 2123f
 multiple malformation syndromes with. *see* Multiple malformation syndromes with renal cysts
 natural history of, 2121–2122
 papillary adenoma, of kidney, 2128, 2128b
Renal descensus, for ureteral stricture disease, 1973
Renal drainage, for urinary tract obstruction, 795
Renal dysfunction, HIV and, 1266–1267
Renal dysplasia, 741–742, 741b
 definition of, 741, 742f
 etiology of, 741–742, 742f–743f
Renal echinococcosis, 1181.e1, 1181.e2f
Renal ectopia, 1869, 1869.e1f
 cephalad, 724–725, 726f
 crossed, 727–728, 728f, 731b
 simple, 724f–725f
Renal exploration
 for pediatric genitourinary trauma, 1073
 for renal injuries, 1988–1989, 1988f

Renal (Gerota) fascia, 1865
Renal function
 after RCC surgery, 2164–2169, 2165b, 2167t, 2169f
 aging and, 2905
 orthotopic urinary diversion and, 3237–3238
 in posterior urethral valves, 619, 620b
 in prune-belly syndrome, 595–596
 upper urinary tract calculi and, 2088–2089
Renal functional assessment
 for benign prostatic hyperplasia, 3345–3346
 for ureteral anomalies, 806, 806f
Renal hilum, 1865, 1869
 identification of, for simple nephrectomy, 2287–2288, 2288f
Renal hypercalciuria, 2019–2020
Renal hypodysplasia, 742–745, 745b
Renal hypoplasia, 742–745, 745b
Renal infection (bacterial nephritis), 1166–1177
 acute focal or multifocal bacterial nephritis, 1171.e1, 1171.e1f
 for acute pyelonephritis, 1168–1171, 1168f–1169f, 1170t
 bacterial "relapse,", 1177.e1
 chronic pyelonephritis, 1176–1177, 1177f
 emphysematous pyelonephritis, 1171–1172, 1171f
 HIV and, 1266
 infected hydronephrosis and pyonephrosis, 1174, 1174f
 pathology, 1166–1168, 1167f–1168f
 perinephric abscess, 1174–1176, 1175f
 renal abscess, 1172–1174, 1172f–1173f
Renal injuries, 1982–1992, 1992b
 angioembolization for, 1986, 1986f
 classification of, 1983–1986, 1983f, 1983t
 damage control for, 1991
 genitourinary trauma and, 1075–1076
 hematuria in, 1982–1983
 history for, 1982–1983
 imaging of
  CT, 1984–1985, 1984f–1985f
  indications for, 1984, 1984f
  IVP, 1985
 in intraoperative consultation, 302–303
  diagnosis/recognition, 302–303
  incidence, 302
  management, 303
  mechanisms, 302
 nonoperative management of, 1986–1988, 1987f
 operative management of, 1988–1991
  complications with, 1991–1992
  indications for, 1991
  partial nephrectomy, 1989–1990, 1989f
  renal exploration for, 1988–1989, 1988f
  renal reconstruction, 1989–1991, 1989f–1990f
  renorrhaphy, 1989, 1989f
  for renovascular injuries, 1990–1991, 1990f–1991f
  total nephrectomy, 1991
 pediatric, 1065
 presentation of, 1982–1983
 renal trauma grading system for, 1066–1072, 1067f–1069f, 1067t, 1069t
Renal insufficiency, 1921–1935
 bacteriuria in pregnancy and, 1187.e1
 metabolic syndrome and, 1420
 partial nephrectomy causing, 2266
Renal ischemia. *see also* Ischemic nephropathy; Renovascular hypertension
 for laparoscopic partial nephrectomy, 2303–2304
 for partial nephrectomy, 2262, 2262f
Renal magnetic resonance imaging, 55–67, 59f–60f

Renal malignancies, 2133-2184, 2134t
  chronic inflammation role in, 1336
  classification of, 2133-2134, 2137t
  genomic alterations in, 1353, 1354t, 1358
  hereditary. see Hereditary leiomyomatosis and RCC syndrome; Hereditary papillary RCC syndrome
  historical considerations for, 2133
  immune checkpoint blockade in, 1343
  lymphoma and leukemia, 2181-2183, 2182t
  metastases, 2181t, 2183
  other, 2181t, 2183-2184
  port-site recurrence of, 2297
  radiographic evaluation of, 2134-2138, 2135t, 2136f
    CT, 2134-2135, 2136f, 2174f
    for cystic lesions, 2137-2138, 2139f-2140f
    MRI, 2135, 2138f
    ultrasonography, 2135
  RCC, 2138-2162. see also Renal cell carcinoma
  sarcomas, 2180-2181, 2181t, 2182f
  surgical techniques for. see Kidney surgery
  vaccines for, 1339-1340
Renal medulla, 1866, 1866.e1f-1866.e2f, 1867f
Renal medullary RCC, pathology of, 2149t-2151t, 2154-2155
Renal morphogenesis, 341
Renal osteodystrophy, 355
Renal pain, patient history of, 2
Renal papilla, 1866, 1866.e1f-1866.e2f
Renal papillary necrosis (RPN), host defense mechanisms in UTIs and, 1139-1140, 1139b
Renal parenchyma, 161-162
  radiologic anatomy of, 1868-1869, 1868f, 1868.e1f, 1869f, 1869.e1f-1869.e2f
Renal pelvic perforation, 179, 180f
Renal pelvis
  normal upper tract urothelium, 2188
  physiology of, 1877-1904
  rupture of, for pediatric genitourinary trauma, 1075
  urothelial neoplasms, 2188-2189
Renal physiology, 1905-1920
  hormonal, renal hormone effects, 1913-1914, 1913f-1914f, 1914b
  vascular
    blood flow. see Renal blood flow
    glomerular filtration. see Glomerular filtration rate
Renal preservation surgery, urinary leak after, 2962
Renal rotation, anomalies of, 733-735, 735b
  description for, 733
  diagnosis of, 734, 735f
  dorsal position in, 733
  incidence of, 733
  lateral position in, 733-735
  prognosis of, 735
  symptoms of, 734
  ventral position in, 733
  ventromedial position in, 733
Renal scintigraphy, 367-369, 369f-370f, 390
  diuretic renography, 390
  renal cortical scintigraphy, 390
Renal sinus, 1865
  cyst of, 775, 775f
Renal stones, 406
  metabolic syndrome and, 1420-1421
Renal threshold, 19-20
Renal transplantation
  evaluation, 94-95
  genitourinary tuberculosis management and, 1318-1319
  pediatric. see Pediatric renal transplantation
  in posterior urethral valves, 619-620
  urinary leak after, 2962

Renal transplantation (Continued)
  urologic complications of, 1936-1941
    genitourinary malignancies, 1940-1941, 1941b
      bladder cancer, 1941
      prostate cancer, 1941
      renal cell carcinoma, 1940-1941, 1940f
    hematuria, 1936
    lower urinary tract complications, 1939-1940
      benign prostatic hyperplasia, 1939
      transplant, small bladder after, 1939
      urine incontinence, 1939-1940
      voiding dysfunction, 1939
    lymphocele, 1938-1939
    nephrolithiasis, 1939
    ureteral leak, 1937, 1937b
    ureteral stent management, 1936, 1936b
    ureteral structure, 1937-1938, 1937t, 1938b
    vesicoureteral reflux, 1938
Renal trauma. see Renal injuries
Renal tubular acidosis (RTA)
  in calcium stone formation, 2025-2026, 2025f
  type 1 (distal), 2025-2026, 2025f
  type 2 (proximal), 2026
  type 4 (distal), 2026
Renal tubular disorders, 348, 349b
Renal tubules
  apoptosis in, 790
  urinary tract obstruction and, 791
Renal tumors, 402
  benign, 2121-2132. see also Renal cysts
    angiomyolipoma, 2125-2128, 2126f-2127f, 2128b
    cystic nephroma, 2129-2130, 2129f
    diagnosis of, 2121
    leiomyoma, 2131, 2131f, 2131b
    metanephric adenoma, 2128-2129, 2129f, 2129b
    mixed epithelial and stromal, 2130, 2130f, 2130b
    mixed mesenchymal and epithelial, 2129-2130, 2129f
    oncocytoma, 2123-2125, 2124f, 2125b
    other, 2131-2132, 2132f, 2132b
    papillary adenoma, of kidney, 2128, 2128b
  imaging and clinical risk stratification of, 2133-2134, 2135t
  malignant. see Renal malignancies
  nonsurgical focal therapy of, 2309-2323
    complications, 2318-2319, 2320f-2321f, 2320b
    cryoablation, 2309-2310, 2310b. see also Cryoablation (CA), for renal tumors
    new ablation modalities, 2319-2323, 2323b
    oncologic outcomes, 2314-2318, 2315t-2316t, 2318b
    radiofrequency ablation, 2310-2312, 2312b
    surgical technique, 2312
    treatment success and follow-up protocol after tumor ablation, 2312-2314, 2314b
  pediatric
    angiomyolipoma, 1110, 1110f
    CCSK, 1108-1109
    CMN, 1109
    CPDN, 1109
    metanephric adenofibroma, 1109
    neuroblastoma. see Neuroblastoma
    RCC, 1109-1110
    RTK, 1109
    solitary multilocular cyst nephroma, 1109
    Wilms tumor. see Wilms tumor
  radiologic evaluation of, 2134-2138, 2135t, 2136f
    CT, 2134-2135, 2136f, 2174f
    for cystic lesions, 2137-2138, 2139f-2140f
    MRI, 2135, 2138f
    ultrasonography, 2135
  surgical techniques for. see Kidney surgery

Renal ultrasonography
  for acute pyelonephritis, 1168
  indications for, 78
  limitations of, 80
  normal findings in, 78-79, 79f
  procedural applications of, 79-80
  technique of, 78
Renal vascular development, 338-340
Renal vascular hypertension, evaluation of, 94
Renal vasculature
  anomalies of, 735-736, 737b
    aberrant, accessory, or multiple vessels, 735-736, 736f
    renal arteriovenous fistula, 737
    renal artery aneurysm, 736-737
  hormonal, renal hormone effects, 1913-1914, 1913f-1914f, 1914b
Renal vein thrombosis, AKI caused by, 1925
Renal vein tumor thrombus, laparoscopic radical nephrectomy for, 2298
Renal veins, 1673, 1869-1870
  in radical nephrectomy, 2258, 2258f, 2258.e1f
  in simple nephrectomy, 2288, 2288f
Renal/abdominal solid masses, 405-406
Renin-angiotensin system (RAS), erectile dysfunction and, 1493
Reninoma, 2132
Renography
  diuretic. see Diuretic renography
  normal curve of, 779
  nuclear, for urinary tract obstruction, 779
  in transitional urology, 1048
Renomedullary interstitial cell tumors, 2132
Renorrhaphy, for renal injuries, 1989, 1989f
Renovascular fistulae, 2958
Renovascular hypertension, 1915-1919
  diagnosis of, 1916-1918, 1917f-1918f, 1918b
  incidence and etiology of, 1914b
  management of, 1918-1919
    medical therapy, 1918
    percutaneous intervention, 1918-1919, 1919f
    surgical, 1919, 1920b
  pathophysiology of, 1915-1916, 1915f-1916f, 1915t, 1916b
    one-kidney, one-clip model of, 1917, 1918f
    two-kidney, one-clip model of, 1917, 1917f
  screening tests for
    angiography, 1917-1918, 1918b
    CT, 1917-1918, 1918b
    duplex Doppler ultrasonography, 1917-1918, 1918b
    MRA, 1917-1918, 1918b
Renovascular injuries, operative management of, 1990-1991, 1990f-1991f
Reoperative RPLND, 1728t, 1729
Replantation, of penis, 3050-3051
Reports, ultrasonography, 76-77
Reproductive system
  female. see Female reproductive system
  male. see Male reproductive system
Residual tumor, after treatment
  NSGCTs with, 1698-1700, 1698t-1699t
  seminomas with, 1705-1706
Resiniferatoxin, 2485
  to facilitate bladder filling and urine storage, 2682t, 2709
  in idiopathic detrusor overactivity, 2709.e1
  in neurogenic detrusor overactivity, 2709.e1
  urgency and, 2709.e1
Resistance, to chemotherapy, RCC with, 2145, 2145t
Resolution, of ultrasonography images, 70-71, 70f
Resorptive hypercalciuria, 2020
Respiratory system
  aging and, 2906
  pneumoperitoneum effects on, 221
Response Evaluation Criteria In Solid Tumors (RECIST), 104, 105t

Resting membrane potential (RMP), of ureteral muscle cells, 1878-1879, 1879f, 1881, 1881b
Restriction point, RB1 and, 1347.e1, 1347.e1f
Rete testis, 1393
  adenocarcinoma of, 1708
  cystic dysplasia of, 899
Retention sutures, 151
Retinoblastoma susceptibility protein (RB1), in GU cancers, 1347.e1, 1347.e1f
13-cis-Retinoic acid, for neuroblastoma, 1095-1096
Retractile testis, 949, 1855
Retraction instrumentation, for laparoscopic and robotic surgery, 218
Retrocaval ureter
  etiology and diagnosis of, 1963, 1965f, 1966b
  operative intervention for, 1963-1965, 1965f
    laparoscopic surgical intervention, 1963-1965
Retrocrural disease, resection of, 1720, 1721f
Retrograde ejaculation, 1451
  after transurethral needle ablation of prostate, 3433
  with holmium laser enucleation of prostate, 3438
  with transurethral incision of prostate, 3435
  treatment of, 1579, 1580f
Retrograde injection, of male stress urinary incontinence, 2896, 2897f
Retrograde intrarenal surgery. *see* Ureterorenoscopy
Retrograde pyelography, 36-38, 415
  complications, 38, 38f
  for genitourinary tuberculosis diagnosis, 1312-1313
  indications, 37
  limitations, 37
  technique, 36-37, 37f
  of urinary tract obstruction, 780-781
Retrograde renal access drainage, 182-184, 184b
  guide wire placement of, 183, 183f
  history, 182
  indications, 182
  stent placement of, 183, 183f
  stent tolerance, 184
  stent varieties of, 183-184
    design, 183-184, 184f
    materials, 183
  surgical technique of, 182-183
Retrograde ureterography, of ureteral injuries, 1995
Retrograde ureteroscopic endopyelotomy, for ureteropelvic junction obstruction, 1949-1950
  complications of, 1950
  indications and contraindications for, 1950
  other, 1950
  results with, 1950
  technique for, 1950, 1951f-1952f
Retrograde ureteroscopic endoureterotomy, for ureteral stricture disease, 1968-1969, 1969f
  antegrade approach combined with, 1969
Retrograde urethrography, 38, 39f
Retroiliac ureter, 824
Retroperitoneal approach, 832
  to laparoscopic adrenalectomy, 2417-2418, 2418f, 2422
  for laparoscopic and robotic surgery, 1956
    operative team placement for, 207, 207f
  to laparoscopic kidney surgery, 2279-2281, 2282f
  to laparoscopic partial nephrectomy, 2300
Retroperitoneal cancer of unknown primary origin, retroperitoneal tumors and, 2238

Retroperitoneal fibrosis (RPF), 1981b
  evaluation of, 1978-1979
  management of
    initial, 1979
    medical, 1979-1980
    surgical, 1980, 1981f
  presentation and etiology of, 1977-1978
Retroperitoneal incision, for renal exploration, 1988, 1988f
Retroperitoneal lymph node dissection (RPLND), 1713-1717, 1713f, 2240-2241, 2241f, 2241t
  auxiliary procedures for, 1717-1720, 1721b
    hepatic resection, 1719-1720
    major vascular reconstruction, 1718-1719, 1719f
    nephrectomy, 1718, 1718t
    pelvic resection, 1720
    supradiaphragmatic disease, management of, 1720
  complications of, 1730-1731, 1730t
    chylous ascites, 1731
    ileus, 1731
    lymphocele, 1731
    mortality, 1731
    neurologic, 1731
    pulmonary, 1730
    VTE, 1731
  high-risk
    desperation, 1728, 1728t
    late relapse, 1728t, 1729
    reoperative, 1728t, 1729
    salvage, 1727-1728, 1728t
  laparoscopic. *see* Laparoscopic retroperitoneal lymph node dissection
  management of clinical complete remission to induction chemotherapy, 1721-1722, 1722t
  for NSGCTs, 1694-1695, 1695t
  outcomes and functional considerations of
    fertility, 1729-1730
    lymph node counts, 1729
  in paratesticular RMS, 1126
  preoperative planning for, 1713-1714
  robotic. *see* Robotic-assisted retroperitoneal lymph node dissection
  surgical technique for, 1714-1717
    closure and postoperative care, 1717
    gonadal vein dissection, 1716
    interaortocaval packet, 1715-1716, 1716f
    left para-aortic packet, 1714-1715
    nerve sparing, 1716-1717, 1717f
    retroperitoneum exposure, 1714, 1714f
    right paracaval packet, 1716
    split and roll technique, 1714, 1715f
  template use in, 1722-1723, 1723f, 1723t
  TGCT staging with, 1689-1690
  in unique situations, 1731-1733, 1733b
    for seminoma, 1731-1732
    for sex cord stromal tumors, 1732-1733
Retroperitoneal tumors (RPTs), 2226-2247
  anatomic considerations of retroperitoneum, 2226, 2226b
  differential diagnosis of, 2227-2238, 2228t, 2238b
    cystic change of solid retroperitoneal tumors, 2238
    cystic lymphangioma, 2237, 2237f
    cystic masses, 2236-2237
    cystic mesothelioma, 2238
    desmoid tumor, 2234, 2234f
    Ewing and Ewing-like sarcoma, 2232-2233, 2233f
    germ cell tumor, 2227-2229
    germ cell/gonadal origins, 2227
    hematologic conditions/lymphomas of retroperitoneum, 2236
    leiomyosarcoma, 2231, 2231f
    liposarcoma, 2229-2230, 2230f

Retroperitoneal tumors (RPTs) *(Continued)*
  lymphomas, 2236, 2237f
  malignant fibrous histiocytoma/undifferentiated pleomorphic sarcoma, 2231, 2232f
  mesodermal origins, 2229
  mucinous cystadenoma, 2237
  nerve sheath tumors, 2235-2236, 2236f
  neurogenic origins, 2234
  paraganglionic system tumors, 2235, 2235f
  perivascular epithelioid cell tumor, 2234
  plasmacytoma, 2236
  pleomorphic liposarcoma, 2230-2231
  retroperitoneal cancer of unknown primary origin, 2238
  sex cord stromal tumor, 2229
  solitary fibrous tumor, 2232, 2233f
  sympathetic ganglia tumors, 2234-2235, 2235f
  synovial sarcoma, 2231-2232, 2232f
  unclassified sarcomas, 2233
  disease-specific neoadjuvant and adjuvant therapies for, 2245-2247, 2246t, 2247b
  initial evaluation of, 2226-2227, 2227b
  surgical management of, 2238-2245, 2245b
    auxiliary procedures for, 2242-2243
    complications of, 2243-2244
    modifications for, 2240-2243
    postoperative care in, 2244-2245
    preoperative considerations, 2238
    technique for, 2238-2240
    template considerations for management of metastatic germ cell tumors, 2240-2242, 2241f, 2241t
    vascular reconstruction in, 2243
Retroperitoneum
  anatomic considerations of, 2226, 2226b
  anatomy of, 1658-1679, 1659f-1661f, 1659t, 1661b, 1666b
    10th, 11th, and 12th ribs, 1658-1665, 1658.e1f, 1665f
    arterial system, 1669-1672, 1669.e1f-1669.e2f, 1671f, 1671.e1f, 1672t
    body surface landmarks, 1658, 1662f
    fasciae and spaces, 1666-1668, 1666.e1f, 1667f-1668f, 1668b, 1674b
    gastrointestinal viscera, 1668-1669, 1668.e2f, 1669f-1670f, 1674b
    lumbodorsal fascia, 1665-1666, 1666f, 1666.e1f
    lymphatic system, 1674, 1675f
    nervous structures, 1674-1679, 1679b
    posterior abdominal wall, 1658, 1662f-1664f, 1664t
    psoas, iliacus, quadratus lumborum, and erector spinae, 1658, 1662f-1665f, 1664t
    spine, 1658, 1658.e1f
    vasculature, 1669-1674
    venous system, 1672-1674, 1672.e1f
  approach to, 2239-2240
  exposure of, 2239, 2239f
  exposure of, for RPLND, 1714, 1714f
  interaortocaval region in, 2240
  left para-aortic region in, 2239-2240
  right paracaval region in, 2240
  split-and-roll technique for, 2239, 2239f
Retropubic mid-urethral slings
  anatomy of, 2850
  complications of, 2863-2866
  outcomes for, 2854-2856, 2855t
  surgical approach to, 2851-2853, 2852f-2853f
Retropubic radical prostatectomy (RRP)
  accessory pudendal artery preservation in, 3552, 3552f
  anesthesia for, 3551-3552, 3551f
  bladder neck division, 3559-3560, 3560f-3561f

Retropubic radical prostatectomy (RRP) (Continued)
  bladder neck reconstruction and anastomosis, 3560–3562, 3561f–3562f
  complications with, 3563–3564
    bladder neck contracture, 3564
    erectile dysfunction, 3564
    intraoperative, 3563
    postoperative, 3563–3564
    thromboembolic events, 3563
    urinary incontinence, 3564
  dorsal vein complex division, 3553–3554, 3554f
  dorsal vein complex ligation, 3553–3556, 3553f
  endopelvic fascia incision for, 3552, 3552f
  exposure for, 3552
  incision for, 3551–3552, 3551f
  instruments for, 3551
  lateral pedicles division in, 3558–3559, 3560f
  lymphadenectomy in, 3551–3552, 3551f
  neurovascular bundle in, 3555–3556
    high anterior release of, at apex, 3557–3558, 3558f–3559f
    identification of, 3556–3558
    preservation of, 3556–3557, 3556f–3557f
    wide excision of, 3558, 3559f
  posterior dissection in, 3558–3559, 3560f
  postoperative management for, 3562–3563
  preoperative preparation for, 3550–3551
  puboprostatic ligament division for, 3552, 3552f
  seminal vesicle excision in, 3559–3560, 3560f–3561f
  surgical anatomy of, 3548–3550, 3564b–3565b
    pelvic fascia, 3549–3550, 3550f
    pelvic plexus, 3548, 3549f
    striated urethral sphincter, 3549, 3549f–3550f
    venous and arterial, 3548, 3549f
  surgical technique for, 3550–3563
  urethra division and suture placement, 3554–3555, 3555f
Retropubic simple prostatectomy, 3450–3452
  adenoma enucleation for, 3451–3452, 3451f–3452f
  hemostatic maneuvers in, 3451, 3451f
  prostate exposure for, 3450, 3451f
Retropubic space, bladder, 3010
Retropubic suspension surgery, for incontinence in women, 2756–2775
  comparisons with, 2771–2774
    anterior repair, 2771, 2771b
    needle suspension, 2771, 2771b
    pubovaginal sling, 2771–2773, 2772f, 2773b
    between techniques, 2773
    tension-free vaginal tape procedure, 2773–2774, 2774b
  complications of, 2769–2771, 2771b
    bladder overactivity, 2770
    postoperative voiding difficulty, 2770
    vaginal prolapse, 2770–2771
  hypermobility in, 2757
  indications for, 2759–2761, 2760f
  intrinsic sphincter deficiency contribution, 2757
    issues of, 2759
  key points for, 2775b
  laparoscopic, 2768–2769, 2769b
  outcomes, assessment for
    cure, definition of, 2759
    follow-up, duration of, 2759
    patient's *versus* physician's perspective, 2759
  potential contraindications for, 2760
  surgical procedures for, 2756–2757, 2757–2759, 2757b
    Burch colposuspension, 2757–2758, 2758f. see also Burch colposuspension

Retropubic suspension surgery, for incontinence in women (Continued)
    Marshall-Marchetti-Krantz procedure, 2757–2758, 2758f. see also Marshall-Marchetti-Krantz procedure
    paravaginal defect repair, 2757–2758, 2758f. see also Paravaginal repair
    vagino-obturator shelf repair, 2757–2758, 2758f. see also Vagino-obturator shelf repair
  technical issues for, 2761–2762
    bladder drainage for, 2761
    dissection for, 2761
    drains for, 2762
    suture material for, 2761
  technique, choice of, 2757–2759
  therapeutic options for, 2756–2757, 2757b
  use of synthetic mesh in, 2774
  vaginal surgery *versus*, 2760–2761, 2761b
Retropulsion prevention devices, for ureteroscopic intraluminal lithotripsy, 198, 198f
Retrorectal space, 2427, 2429f
Reverberation artifact, in ultrasonography, 73, 73f–74f
Review of systems, patient history of, 9
RFA. see Radiofrequency ablation
Rhabdoid differentiation, 2149t–2151t, 2155, 2155f
Rhabdoid tumor of kidney (RTK), in pediatric patients, 1109
Rhabdomyolysis, after laparoscopic and robotic surgery, 231
Rhabdomyosarcoma (RMS), 986, 986f
  bladder. see Bladder RMS
  cervical or uterine, in pediatric patients, 1120
  paratesticular, in pediatric patients, 1126–1127, 1127b
  perineal, 1127, 1127f
  of prostate, 3512
  of testicular adnexa, 1709
  vaginal, in pediatric patients, 1119–1120, 1119f
  vulvar, in pediatric patients, 1119
Rhabdosphincter, 2467
  male sphincteric mechanisms and, 2594
Rho kinase signaling pathway, 1495, 1497f
RhoA, 2473, 2473f
Rhythmic suprapubic manual pressure, 2902
Ribs, in retroperitoneum, 1658–1665, 1658.e1f, 1665f
Right adrenalectomy
  laparoscopic, 2415–2416, 2417f–2418f, 2418
  open, 2413, 2413f
Right colon pouches
  with intussuscepted terminal ileum, 3219–3220
  operative technique variations for, 3228, 3229f
Rigid cystourethroscopes, 186, 188f–189f, 188t
Rigid lithotripters, 2111–2112
Rigid metal dilators, 171, 171f
RIVUR study. see Randomized Intervention for Management of Vesicoureteral Reflux (RIVUR) study
RJF. see Relative jet frequency
R-LESS. see Robotic laparoscopic single-site surgery
RMS. see Rhabdomyosarcoma
RNA
  in transcription, 1346.e3, 1346.e3f
  in translation, 1346.e3, 1346.e3f–1346.e4f
Robot-assisted adrenalectomy, 2418–2419, 2419f–2420f, 2422–2423
Robot-assisted approach, incorporation of, in minimally invasive urinary diversion, 3258, 3258b
Robot-assisted intracorporeal continent cutaneous diversion, 3269–3270, 3269f, 3270b

Robotic inguinal lymphadenectomy, for penile cancer, 1761, 1794
  background of, 1794
  surgical technique for, 1761
Robotic laparoscopic single-site surgery (R-LESS), for kidney surgery, 2306
Robotic machine failure, in robotic prostatectomy, 3580
Robotic partial nephrectomy, 811–813, 814f
Robotic port site incisions, 459f
Robotic prostatectomy, open prostatectomy *versus*, 3532
Robotic radical cystectomy, 3143–3157, 3159b
  anterior vascular pedicle dissection, 3148, 3149f–3150f
  extended pelvic lymphadenectomy, 3148–3152
  instrumentation of, 3146, 3146t
  lateral space of Retzius, 3148, 3149f–3150f
  patient positioning of, 3145, 3145f
  patient selection of, 3144–3145
  port and assistant placement of, 3145–3146, 3145f
  posterior dissection of, 3146, 3146t, 3147f–3148f
  reoperation after, 3270–3273
  sigmoid release of, 3146, 3146t, 3147f
  ureteral control and posterior pedicle dissection, 3152–3157, 3155f–3156f
Robotic surgery, 203
  access technology for
    hand-assist devices, 212
    LESS devices, 212, 212.e2f
    trocars, 211, 211f, 212.e2f
  complications and troubleshooting in, 223–231, 232b
    anesthesia-related, 228
    early postoperative, 230–231
    equipment-related, 223–231
    exit-related, 230
    late postoperative, 231
    during learning curve, 223
    pneumoperitoneum-related, 224
    seminal vesicle surgery, 1864
  equipment placement for, 205–207, 205.e1f
  instrumentation used in
    abdomen exit, 218–219
    for da Vinci Robotic System, 218, 218f
    for grasping and blunt dissection, 218
    for incising and hemostasis, 215–216, 215.e3f
    for LESS, 218
    for morcellation, 218
    for NOTES, 218
    for port site closure, 219
    for retraction, 218
    for specimen entrapment, 217–218, 217f
    for stapling and clipping, 216–217
    surgical pharmaceuticals, 215
    for suturing and tissue anastomosis, 215–216
  operative team placement for
    retroperitoneal upper abdominal procedures, 207, 207f
    transperitoneal and extraperitoneal pelvic procedures, 207
    transperitoneal upper abdominal procedures, 206.e1f, 207.e1f
  physiologic considerations in, 223b
    hemodynamic effects related to approach and patient position, 222
    hormonal and metabolic effects during surgery, 222–223
    immunologic effects, 223
    insufflant choice, 220
    pneumoperitoneum pressure choice, 220
  preoperative preparation for, 204b
    blood products, 204
    bowel preparation, 204
    operating room setup, 205, 205b
    patient positioning, 205, 205f

Robotic surgery (Continued)
    patient selection and contraindications, 203-204
    prophylaxis, 205
    procedure for, 219b
        abdomen exit, 218-219
        hand-assist device placement, 212
        port removal and fascial closure, 218-219
        port site closure, 219
        pre-incision checklist, 207
        skin closure, 219
        trocar placement, 212-213
    training and practicing for, 231-233, 233b
        equipment for, 232
        formal programs for, 233
    ureteral injuries with, 1993
Robotic systems, 206, 206.e1f
Robotic-assisted laparoscopic partial nephrectomy (RaLPN), 2300
Robotic-assisted laparoscopic radical prostatectomy (RALRP)
    complications of, 3580, 3583b
    evolution of, 3566
    outcomes of, 3579-3580, 3583b
        oncologic, 3583
    pure laparoscopic versus, 3570
    quality-of-life outcomes after, 3581
    technique of, 3578b
Robotic-assisted laparoscopic sacrocolpopexy, for apical pelvic organ prolapse repair, 2800-2803, 2801f-2803f
Robotic-assisted laparoscopic simple prostatectomy, 3454-3455
    abdominal access, insufflation, and trocar placement for, 3454-3455
    adenoma enucleation in, 3455
    adenoma extraction and closure for, 3455
    bladder neck incision for, 3455
    hemostasis and vesicourethral anastomosis, 3455
    patient positioning for, 3454
    space of Retzius development for, 3455
Robotic-assisted laparoscopic surgery
    bladder diverticulectomy. see Bladder diverticulectomy
    Boari flap. see Boari flap
    for kidney, 2282-2284, 2284f-2285f
    pyelolithotomy, for pediatric kidney stone disease, 868-870
    pyeloplasty, for ureteropelvic junction obstruction, 1956
    pyelopyelostomy, for retrocaval ureter, 1963
    ureteral reimplantation. see Ureteral reimplantation
    ureteroureterostomy, for ureteral stricture disease, 1972
    for vesicovaginal fistula. see Vesicovaginal fistula
Robotic-assisted pyeloplasty, 832
    techniques of, 832-834, 833f
Robotic-assisted retroperitoneal lymph node dissection, 1734-1741, 1741b
    complications of, 1739-1740, 1739t
    postoperative care for, 1738-1739
    prospective nerve-sparing techniques for, 1739
    rationale and evolution of, 1734
    results and current status for, 1740-1741
    surgical technique for, 1735-1738
        port placement and technique, 1738, 1738f
        preoperative patient preparation and technical considerations for, 1735
Roentgen, Wilhelm Conrad, 3587
Rolipram, for ureteral relaxation, 1899
Rome IV criteria, for functional constipation in children, 474, 474t, 475f
RON, in UTUC, 2198
Rosebud stoma, 3182, 3182f-3183f
Round ligament, 2430, 2431f

RPLND. see Retroperitoneal lymph node dissection
RPTs. see Retroperitoneal tumors
RRP. see Retropubic radical prostatectomy
RSD. see Reflex sympathetic dystrophy
RSPO1 gene, 992f, 992t, 993
RSR. see Relative saturation ratio
RTA. see Renal tubular acidosis
RTE. see Real-time elastography
RTK. see Rhabdoid tumor of kidney
RUF. see Rectourethral fistulae

S
S phase, deregulation of progression through, in GU cancers, 1347.e1
S phase arrest, deregulation of, in GU cancers, 1347.e2
Saccules, 2967
SACD. see Subacute combined degeneration
Sacral agenesis, 487, 641-644, 644b
    pathogenesis of, 642-643
    presentation of, 641-642, 643f-644f
    specific recommendations for, 643-644
Sacral arteries, 2451-2452, 2451t
Sacral dorsal rhizotomy, 2741-2742, 2742f
    clinical results of, 2743, 2744t
    goal and effect of, 2742-2743
    patient selection in, 2742
    surgical implantation technique of, 2742-2743, 2743f
Sacral evoked response: bulbocavernosus reflex latency, 1527
Sacral nerve stimulation (SNS), 2510, 2752-2754
    current indications for, 2752
    implantation procedure for, 2753-2754
        percutaneous nerve evaluation test, 2754
        staged implant procedure, 2754, 2754f
    indications for, 2753, 2753f
    for nonobstructive chronic underactive bladder, 2753
    for OAB with or without urinary continence, 2752-2753
    outcomes for, 2752
    patient selection for, 2753-2754
Sacral neuromodulation (SNM), 2739
    for detrusor underactivity, 2662
    for neuromuscular dysfunction of lower urinary tract, 637-638
    for OAB, 2647
    for UUI, 2546
Sacral plexus, 2433
    neuromodulation of, 2510
Sacral spinal cord injury
    lower urinary tract dysfunction with, 2611-2612, 2613f
    management with, 2613b
Sacrococcygeal teratoma, lower urinary tract dysfunction and, 2631
Sacrocolpopexy, abdominal, for apical pelvic organ prolapse repair, 2798-2809
    complications of, 2804, 2806t
    cost of, 2809
    laparoscopic
        comparison with, 2806, 2807t
        versus robotic-assisted, 2806-2809, 2808t
        versus robotic-assisted colpopexy, 2809
        technique for, 2802f-2803f, 2803-2804
    learning curve in, 2809
    open, technique for, 2798-2800, 2800f-2801f
    results of, 2804-2806, 2805t
    robotic-assisted laparoscopic, 2800-2803, 2801f-2803f, 2810t-2811t
Sacrohysteropexy
    minimally invasive, 2822-2823, 2824t
    open abdominal, 2822-2823, 2824t
    results with, 2823
Sacroiliac ligaments, 2428-2429
Sacrospinous ligament colposuspension, 2433

Sacrospinous ligament fixation (SSLF), for pelvic organ prolapse repair, 2793-2797
    complications with, 2797
    results of, 2795-2797, 2796t-2797t
    surgical anatomy for, 2794-2795, 2795f
    technique for, 2795, 2796f
Sacrospinous ligaments, 2428-2429
Sacrotuberous ligaments, 2428-2429
Sacrum, 2427, 2428f, 2444
Salbutamol, to facilitate bladder filling and urine storage, 2682t
Saline drop test examination, for bowel injury, 276
Salvage brachytherapy, for biochemical recurrence after radiation therapy, 3668
Salvage cryotherapy, for biochemical recurrence after radiation therapy, 3667-3668, 3669t
Salvage high-intensity focused ultrasound, for biochemical recurrence after radiation therapy, 3668
Salvage radiation therapy, for biochemical recurrence after radical prostatectomy, 3662-3663
    adjuvant radiation therapy versus, 3664-3665
    androgen deprivation therapy (ADT), 3663-3664
    dose response, 3663
    whole-pelvis versus prostatic bed radiation therapy, 3664, 3664f-3665f
Salvage radical prostatectomy, for biochemical recurrence after radiation therapy, 3667, 3667t
Salvage robotic-assisted radical prostatectomy, 3583-3584
    technique of, 3584
Salvage RPLND, 1727-1728, 1728t
Sansert. see Methysergide
Saphenous hiatus, 1791
Sarcoidosis
    hypercalcemia in, 2020
    hypercalciuria in, 2050
Sarcomas
    of bladder
        adenocarcinoma, 3090, 3090f
        small cell carcinoma, 3089, 3089f
        squamous cell cancer, 3089-3090, 3089f
        urachal adenocarcinoma, 3090, 3090b
    of kidney, 2180-2181, 2181t, 2182f
    of prostate, 3512
    of testicular adnexa, 1709
Sarcomatoid differentiation, in RCC, 2149t-2151t, 2155, 2155f
Saw palmetto berry, for benign prostatic hyperplasia, 3395-3398, 3396f, 3397t
Scabies
    infestation, 1295-1296, 1297f
    as STD, 1271
Scalpels, for laparoscopic and robotic surgery, 214
Scandinavian Prostate Cancer Group Study Number 4 (SPCG-4), 3529-3530, 3539
Scanning electron microscope (SEM)
    of bladder blood vessels, 2464f
    of urothelium, 2462, 2463f
Scardino-Prince vertical flap, for ureteropelvic junction obstruction, 1961, 1962f
Scarpa fascia, 2444, 2446f
Scattering, of ultrasound waves, 71, 71f
SCC. see Squamous cell carcinoma
SCCis. see Squamous cell carcinoma in situ
SCD. see Sickle cell disease
Scheduled voiding regimens. see Toileting programs
Schistosomal myelopathy, lower urinary tract dysfunction and, 2626
Schistosomiasis
    in bladder tumor, 3077
    of genitourinary tract, 1319-1328, 1328b
        biology and life cycle, 1319, 1320f-1321f

Schistosomiasis (Continued)
    diagnosis, 1325–1326, 1325f–1326f
    epidemiology, 1319–1321, 1321–1324, 1321f, 1323f
    history, 1319
    prevention and control, 1327–1328
    prognosis, 1327
    treatment, 1326–1327
        surgical management in, 1327
Schizophrenia, lower urinary tract dysfunction and, 2630
Schrott-Erlangen approach, for classic bladder exstrophy, 545
    continence outcomes with, 560
Schwannomas
    intrarenal, 2132
    in retroperitoneum, 2235
SCI. see Spinal cord injury
Sciatic nerve injury, 261–262
Scintillation crystal, 91
Scissors, for laparoscopic and robotic surgery, 214
Scleroderma, lower urinary tract dysfunction and, 2631
Sclerosing lymphangitis, 1302–1304
Sclerotherapy, 903, 903.e1f, 1845–1847, 1848t
Screening tests, for genitourinary tuberculosis, 1310–1311
Scrotal agenesis, 887, 887.e1f
Scrotal anomalies, 886–888
    bifid scrotum, 886, 887f
    ectopic scrotum, 886–887, 888f
    scrotal agenesis, 887, 887.e1f
    scrotal hypoplasia, 887
    scrotoschisis, 887–888, 888.e1f
Scrotal elephantiasis, as filariasis clinical manifestation, 1330, 1330f
Scrotal engulfment, 885–886, 886f
Scrotal hydrocele, 889
Scrotal incision, in urologic surgery, 142–143
Scrotal mass, 392
    in neonate, 387, 387t
Scrotal pain, patient history of, 2
Scrotal reconstruction, 3054, 3054.e1f
Scrotal ultrasonography, for pediatric urology, 389
Scrotal wall, 1843
Scrotectomy, 1844–1845, 1846f
Scrotoplasty, 941, 3068
Scrotum, 1843
    access into, 1844
    acute. see Acute scrotum
    anatomy of, 1389b, 1843, 1844f
        arterial supply, 1387–1389
        gross structure, 1387–1389, 1388f
        lymphatic drainage, 1389
        nerve supply, 1389
        venous drainage, 1389
    in genitourinary tuberculosis, 1309
    penetrating injuries to, 3051
    physical examination for, 11, 11f
    surgeries of, 1843–1864
        approaches to, 1844, 1850b, 1855b
        complications of, 1855–1856
        innervation, 1843
        preoperative considerations of, 1843–1844
        reconstruction, 1845, 1847f
        vasectomy. see Vasectomy
    ultrasonography of, 81–84, 1373
        for GCTs, 1685–1686, 1685f
        indications for, 82
        normal findings in, 82–83, 83f–85f
        procedural applications of, 83
        sonoelastography, 84
        technique of, 82
SCSTs. see Sex cord-stromal tumors
SDHRCC. see Succinate dehydrogenase RCC
Sealants, for laparoscopic and robotic surgery, 215.e2

Seborrheic dermatitis (SD), as papulosquamous disorder, 1282–1283
Seborrheic keratosis, 1304, 1305f
Second malignancies
    after bladder RMS treatment, 1117
    after Wilms tumor treatment, 1108
Second messengers, in ureteral contractions, 1885–1887, 1885f–1886f
Secondary cryptorchidism, 949
Secondary cutaneous lesions, 1273, 1274t
Secondary hyperoxaluria, 858–859
Secondary paraureteral diverticula, 525
Secondary syphilis, 1257, 1258f
Secondary therapy, receipt of, 105
Secondary vestibulodynia, 1651
Second-look nephroscopy, in antegrade nephroureteroscopic, for UTUC, 2217
Sedation, 484
Segmental hypoplasia, 744, 744f
Segmental nephrectomy, for large renal tumors, 2263–2264, 2263.e1f–2263.e2f, 2264.e1f, 2265f
Segmental pyelonephritis, 388–389
Segmental ureteral resection, for UTUC, 2207–2210
    ileal ureteral replacement, 2208, 2209f
    laparoscopic or robotic distal ureterectomy and reimplantation, 2208, 2209t
    open segmental ureterectomy, 2207, 2208f–2209f
    results of, 2208–2210
SELECT. see Selenium and Vitamin E Cancer Prevention Trial
Selective α_1-blockers, 3356–3357
Selective androgen receptor modulators, for benign prostatic hyperplasia, 3377
Selective estrogen receptor modulators (SERMs), for benign prostatic hyperplasia, 3377
Selective serotonin reuptake inhibitors, and PE, 1571–1572
Selective tissue estrogenic activity regulator, for female sexual arousal disorders, 1649–1650
SelectMDx test, 3486
Selenium, in prostate cancer prevention, 3476, 3476f
Selenium and Vitamin E Cancer Prevention Trial (SELECT), 3476, 3476f
Self-care practices, for bowel function, 2734
Self-catheterization, orthotopic urinary diversion and, 3238
Self-styled dilators, for achieving extraperitoneal access and developing extraperitoneal space, 210
SEM. see Scanning electron microscope
Semen
    coagulation and liquefaction of, 3303, 3304b
    density of, 896–897
    evaluation of, in male infertility, 1438–1442
        acrosome reaction, 1442
        bulk semen parameters, 1438–1440, 1438t
        comet assay, 1441–1442
        computer-assisted semen analysis, 1440.e2
        denatured sperm DNA assays, 1442
        pyospermia assays, 1440–1441
        reactive oxygen species, 1442
        secondary semen assays, 1440–1441
        semen volume, 1439
        sperm density, 1439
        sperm DNA integrity assays, 1441
        sperm fluorescence in situ hybridization, 1442
        sperm morphology, 1439–1440
        sperm motility, 1439
        sperm mucus interaction, 1442
        sperm ovum interaction, 1442
        sperm ultrastructural assessment, 1442
        sperm vitality, 1440
        tertiary and investigational sperm assays, 1441–1442
        TUNEL assay, 1441, 1441f

Semenogelins I and II, in prostatic secretions, 3298t, 3300
Seminal vesicle and ejaculatory ducts, physiology of, 1407–1408, 1408b
    gross architecture and cytoarchitecture, 1407
    unit function, 1407
Seminal vesicle cysts (SVCs), management of, 1862–1863
Seminal vesicle invasion, 3511
Seminal vesicle secretory proteins, in prostatic secretions of, 3303
Seminal vesicles
    anatomy of, 1378b, 1856, 1856f–1858f
        arterial supply, 1377
        gross structure, 1377
        lymphatic drainage, 1378
        microanatomic architecture, 1377
        nerve supply, 1378
        venous drainage, 1378
    development of, 3280
    dissection of, in laparoscopic radical prostatectomy, 3573–3574, 3574f
    embryology of, 1856, 1856f–1858f
    in genitourinary tuberculosis, 1309
    HIV and, 1266
    imaging
        CT, 1378
        MRI, 1378, 1378f
        transrectal ultrasound, 1378
    in retropubic radical prostatectomy, excision of, 3559–3560, 3560f–3561f
    surgeries of, 1843–1864, 1863b
        anterior approach to, 1856–1857, 1859f–1861f
        complications of, 1863–1864
        perineal approach to, 1857
        posterior approach to, 1857–1862, 1862f
        preoperative considerations of, 1843–1844
        scrotal wall procedures, 1844–1845
        testis, 1845–1850
        transrectal ultrasound-guided aspiration, 1863
        transurethral endoscopic treatments, 1863
        tumor excision, 1863
Seminiferous epithelium, 1445.e1, 1445.e2f
Seminiferous tubules, 1370, 1371f, 1373, 1393, 1393f, 1396–1398
Seminomas, 1680, 1702–1706, 1706b
    genomic alterations in, 1353, 1361
    histology of, 1682, 1683f
    treatment of, 1692, 1692b
        clinical stage I tumors, 1702–1704
        clinical stage IIA and IIB tumors, 1704–1705
        clinical stage IIC and III tumors, 1705–1706
        relapsed tumors, 1706
    treatment of, RPLND, 1731–1732
Seminomatous GCTs, 2227
Semirigid ureteroscopes, 192, 192f, 193t
    care and sterilization of, 195–197
    technique for, 199–201, 201f
Senior-Loken syndrome, 756
Sensate focus, for female orgasmic disorder, 1647
Sensation, bladder
    altered, filling/storage failure due to, 2517–2518
    detrusor underactivity and, 2659
    terminology for, 2581
Sensorineural deafness, 347
Sensor-transducer function, of bladder urothelium, 2469–2470
Sensory innervation, in ureteral function, 1889
Sensory nerve (afferent) signaling, in overactive bladder, 2640
Sentinel lymph node biopsy
    of inguinal nodes, for penile cancer, 1760
    for penile cancer, 1792–1793
Sepsis
    with intestinal anastomoses, 3180
    UTIs and, 1182–1187, 1183b–1184b

Septic shock, UTIs and, 1182–1187, 1184b
Serenoa repens (saw palmetto berry), for benign prostatic hyperplasia, 3395–3398, 3396f, 3397t
Serlopitant, to facilitate bladder filling and urine storage, 2713.e4
Serology, syphilis tests, 1258
Seromuscular enterocystoplasty, 705–706, 705f
Serotonin (5-HT)
  in ED, 1494, 1495t
  in efferent pathways to bladder, 2488–2489
  in ejaculatory response, 1564
  urethral function effects of, 1902
Serotonin-noradrenaline uptake inhibitors, for stress urinary incontinence in women, 2714–2716
Serotonin-receptor effectors, 1534
Serous-lined extramural tunnel, for orthotopic urinary diversion, 3244–3245, 3245f
Sertoli cell tumors, 1124, 1708
Sertoli cell-only syndrome, 1445.e1, 1445.e1f
Sertoli cells, 1392, 1437
  testis physiology and, 1396–1398, 1397f
Serum gonadotropin measurements, 1528
Serum laboratory studies, in urine, 25
Serum prolactin measurement, 1528
Serum testosterone measurements, 1527–1528
Serum tests, for UTIs, 438
Serum thyroid function tests, 1528–1529
Severe bilateral urinary tract dilation, considerations for, 371
Sex cord-stromal tumors (SCSTs), 1707–1708
  retroperitoneal tumors and, 2229
  treatment of, RPLND, 1732–1733
Sex determination, 1392
Sex hormone-binding globulin, 1434, 1436–1437, 1437b
Sex reassignment surgery (SRS), 3062
Sex steroids, lower urinary tract and, 2502–2503
Sextant biopsy, of prostate, 3497
Sexual activity
  benign prostatic hyperplasia and, 3322, 3322f, 3323t
  prostate cancer and, 3463–3464
Sexual development, 990–997
  disorders of. *see* Disorders of sex development
  gender identity, role, and orientation, 996–997
  gonadal function, 994–995, 994b
    ovary, 995
    testis, 994, 995f
  gonadal stage of differentiation, 993–994, 994f, 994b
  normal genotypic development, 990–993
    additional genes in, 991–993, 992f, 992t
    chromosomal sex, 990, 991f, 991b
    SRY, 990, 991f–992f
  normal phenotypic development, 993–994
  phenotypic, 995–996, 995f–997f
  psychosexual development, 996–997, 997b
Sexual dysfunction. *see also* Erectile dysfunction
  after mid-urethral slings, 2873
  after transurethral needle ablation of prostate, 3433
  benign prostatic hyperplasia and, 3378
  of female
    arousal dysfunction, 1636
    definitions of, 1635, 1637b
    DSM-5 definitions of, 1635–1636, 1635t
    epidemiology, 1636–1637, 1637b
    female sexual interest-arousal disorder, 1635–1636
    genital-pelvic pain dysfunction, 1636
    genito-pelvic pain-penetration disorder, 1636
    hypoactive sexual desire dysfunction, 1636
    hypohedonic orgasm, 1636
    orgasmic disorder, 1636
    painful orgasm, 1636

Sexual dysfunction *(Continued)*
  persistent genital arousal disorder, 1636
  postcoital syndrome, 1636
  sexual arousal dysfunction, 1636
  hormonal therapy and, 3681
  patient history of, 6
  prostatitis and, 1210
Sexual function
  α1-adrenergic blockers and, 3370
  of female
    evaluation of sexual wellness, 1627–1637
    female sexual physiology, 1627.e4
    female sexual response, 1627.e4–1627.e5, 1627.e4f
    international consultation on sexual medicine, 1636
    mental aspects of sexual response, 1627.e6
    physiologic measures of, 1634, 1634t
    PLISSIT model for, 1628–1629, 1628t–1629t
    in special populations, 1637–1640, 1640b
      fertility in transgender people, 1638–1639
      gender dysphoria and hormonal treatment, 1638, 1639t
      in LGBTQ, 1637–1638, 1638t
      malignancies in female transgender patients, 1639–1640
      sexuality and disability, 1640
  localized prostate cancer and, 3524–3525
  pelvic organ prolapse and, 2593
  in prune-belly syndrome, 600
  transurethral microwave therapy and, 3430
Sexual health, in elderly, 2920–2921
Sexual Health Inventory for Men (SHIM), 112t
Sexual history, and male infertility, 1433–1434
Sexual intercourse, penile fracture with, 3048
Sexual maturation, 1390
Sexual Quality of Life for Men (SQOL-M), 112t
Sexual relations, patient history of, 9
Sexual wellness in women, evaluation of, 1627–1637, 1635b
  history, 1627–1629, 1628t–1630t
  laboratory tests for, 1633–1634
  partner, 1629
  physical examination in, 1629–1633, 1632f–1633f
  questionnaires for, 1629, 1630t–1632t
Sexuality
  with exstrophy-epispadias complex
    female concerns, 566–567
    male concerns, 565–566
  neural tube defects and, 629–631
Sexually transmitted diseases (STDs), 1251–1272, 1272b
  CDC screening recommendations for, 1251–1252
  cutaneous infections and infestations from, 1288, 1289f
  epidemiology of, 1251–1252, 1252t
  epididymitis, 1255
  genital ulcers, 1255–1261, 1255t
    chancroid, 1255t, 1259–1260, 1259f
    diagnosis of, 1256
    granuloma inguinale, 1260
    herpes, 1255t
    HPV, 1261, 1262f
    lymphogranuloma, 1255t, 1260–1261, 1260f
    Molluscum contagiosum, 1261, 1261f
    pediculosis pubis, 1271
    presentation of, 1256, 1256f
    scabies, 1271
    syphilis, 1255t, 1257, 1257f–1258f, 1257t
    treatment of, 1256–1257, 1256t
    vaginitis, 1271–1272, 1272t
  gonococcal infections, 1252

Sexually transmitted diseases (STDs) *(Continued)*
  HIV, 1264–1268
    diagnosis, 1264
    erectile dysfunction and, 1267
    interactions with other STDs, 1257, 1264–1268
    Kaposi sarcoma, 1267–1268
    male circumcision, 1264
    malignancy, 1267
    nephrolithiasis, 1266
    non-AIDS-defining urologic malignancies, 1268
    nonulcerating skin infections and, 1265
    postexposure prophylaxis, 1264–1265
    pre-exposure prophylaxis, 1265
    prostatitis and, 1266
    renal dysfunction and, 1266–1267
    renal infections, 1266
    testis, epididymis, seminal vesicles and, 1266
    urologic manifestations of, 1265–1268, 1265f
    UTI and, 1265–1266
    voiding dysfunction and, 1267
  nongonococcal urethritis, 1253, 1254f
    chlamydia, 1253
    Mycoplasma genitalium, 1253–1254
    recurrent and persistent, 1254
    Trichomonas vaginalis, 1254
  prostate cancer and, 3463–3464
  reportable, 1252
  urethritis, 1252–1254
  viral hepatitis and, 1268–1271, 1269t
  Zika virus, 1263–1264
Shared decision making, in localized prostate cancer, 3525
Sharp dissectors, for laparoscopic and robotic surgery, 214
Shear stress mechanism, of stone fragmentation, 2097
Shear wave elastography (SWE), 74, 76f
Shock wave lithotripsy (SWL), 2094–2103, 2103b
  adjuncts to improve, 2102, 2102b
  attenuation values and, 2077.e2
  bioeffects of, 2097–2100
    acute renal injury as, 2098–2099, 2098f–2099f, 2099b
    chronic renal injury as, 2099–2100, 2099t
    extrarenal damage as, 2097–2098, 2097f
  combination of ultrasonography and fluoroscopy for, 2095
  contraindications to, 2072b
  extracorporeal, 2069.e2–2069.e3
  factors negatively affecting success of, 2072b
  fluoroscopy for, 2094–2095
  future direction in, 2102–2103, 2103f
  generator types for, 2094
    electrohydraulic (spark gap), 2094, 2095f
    electromagnetic, 2094, 2095f
    piezoelectric, 2094, 2096f
  imaging systems for, 2094–2095
  methods and physical principles, 2094–2097
  morbid obesity and, 2089
  old age and frailty and, 2089–2090
  optimization of, 2100–2102, 2100b, 2101f, 2102b
  pediatric, 864–865, 865b
    limitations and concerns with, 865
    stone size, location, and composition, 864–865
    technique for, 865
  prior renal surgery and, 2090
  for renal calculi
    in calyceal diverticula, 2078
    in horseshoe kidneys, 2079
    lower pole calculi, 2081, 2081f, 2082t, 2083f
    in renal ectopia, 2081
    stone composition and, 2076, 2076f
    stone localization and, 2075

Shock wave lithotripsy (SWL) (Continued)
  renal function and, 2088-2089
  renal transplants and, 2091
  solitary kidney and, 2089
  spinal deformity or limb contractures and, 2090
  for staghorn calculi, 2074
  stone burden and
    between 1 to 2 cm, 2073
    greater than 2 cm, 2074
    up to 1 cm, 2072
  stone fragmentation in, 2095-2097, 2096f
  tissue injury from, 2100
  ultrasonography for, 2095
  uncorrected coagulopathy and, 2090
  for ureteral calculi
    duplicated collecting system and, 2087
    in megaureter, 2087
    outcome of, 2091
    stone burden and, 2087
    stone composition and, 2087
    stone localization and, 2085-2086, 2086t
    with ureteral stricture or stenosis, 2087-2088
  urinary diversion and, 2091
  urinary tract infection and, 2088
ShockPulse-SE, 245-246
Short bowel, urinary intestinal diversion and, 3203
Short Screening Instrument for Psychological Problems in Enuresis (SSIPPE), 477
Shunting, for ischemic priapism, 1554-1558, 1555f-1559f, 1556b
Shy-Drager syndrome, lower urinary tract dysfunction with, 2606
Sickle cell disease (SCD), 451
  and priapism, 1544, 1547b
Sickle cell trait and disease, contrast media and, 32
Siderophore aerobactin, 429
Sigma-rectum pouch, 3210-3211
Sigmoid colon, colon conduit and, 3196, 3197f, 3198t
Sigmoid cystoplasty, 694-695, 696f
Sigmoid kidney, 728f, 729
Sigmoid pouch, for orthotopic urinary diversion, 3248, 3249f
Signal transduction cascade, 429, 430f
Signal transmission, in urodynamic studies, 2558
Sildenafil (Viagra)
  to facilitate bladder filling and urine storage, 2682t, 2701
  for ureteral relaxation, 1899
Silicate stones, 2033
Silicone catheters, 152
Silicone microimplants (Macroplastique), 2894, 2894f
  for female urinary incontinence, 2894
  of male stress urinary incontinence, 2897
Silk suture, 150-151
Silodosin
  for benign prostatic hyperplasia, 3365, 3365f, 3366t
  to facilitate bladder emptying, 2720.e1
  to facilitate bladder filling and urine storage, 2682t
  ureteral response to, 1888
SILS Port, 212.e1, 212.e1f
Silver nitrate, for BPS/IC treatment, 1244.e1
Simple cysts, 766-770, 770b
  classification of, 768-770, 769b, 770f
  clinical features of, 766
  evaluation of, 768, 768f-769f
  histopathology of, 766-768
  prognosis of, 770, 770f
  treatment of, 770, 770f
Simple nephrectomy
  laparoscopic, 2285-2291
    dissection of ureter, 2287, 2287f

Simple nephrectomy (Continued)
    identification of renal hilum, 2287-2288, 2288f
    organ entrapment and extraction, 2289, 2289f-2290f
    postoperative management for, 2289
    reflection of colon, 2285-2286, 2287f
    results of, 2291
    securing of renal blood vessels, 2288, 2288f
    upper pole dissection, 2288, 2288f
  open, 2253-2254, 2253.e2f, 2254f
Simple orchiectomy, 1848
  technique of, 1848, 1849f
Simple prostatectomy, nocturia and, 2671-2673
Simple renal ectopia, anomalies of, 723-724, 724f-725f
  description for, 723-724
  diagnosis of, 724
  incidence of, 723
  prognosis of, 724
Sims-Huhner test, 1442.e2
Simulation, 3587-3588
Single-incision mid-urethral slings
  anatomy of, 2851
  complications of, 2863-2866
  outcomes for, 2857-2858
  surgical approach to, 2854, 2855f
Single-lumen catheters, 154
Single-photon emission computed tomography (SPECT), 91, 440
Single photon imaging
  physical characteristics of, 92t
  principles of, 91
  three-dimensional images in, 91
Sinovaginal bulbs, 325-326, 776
Sipuleucel-T, 1341, 3697-3698, 3697f
Skeletal muscle, smooth muscles compared with, 2471t
Skeletal system abnormalities, with cloacal exstrophy, 575
Skene gland, cysts of, urethral diverticula differentiated from, 2974, 2986f
Skin, of external genitalia, loss of, 3053-3054, 3053f-3054f
Skin bridge, of penis, 874-875, 874f
Skin closure, 150-151
  after laparoscopic and robotic surgery, 219
Skin tag, 1304
Skin tags
  hymenal, 978-979, 979f
SLE. see Systemic lupus erythematosus
Sleep
  enuresis and, 662
  nocturia effect on, 2664-2665
  states of, 2665
Sleep efficiency, definition of, 2664-2665
Sleep latency, definition of, 2664-2665
Slings, 2830-2876
  alternative treatment options to, 2833
  evolution of, 2830-2831, 2832b
  mid-urethral. see Midurethral sling
  for pelvic organ prolapse, anterior compartment, 2788-2790, 2789f
  preoperative assessment for, 2832-2833, 2833b
  pubovaginal. see Pubovaginal sling
  for urinary incontinence, in geriatric patients, 2920.e5
Slitlike adjusted Mathieu (SLAM) procedure, 924, 925f
Slow-twitch fibers
  male sphincteric mechanisms and, 2594
  of urethral striated muscle, 2467
Slow-wave sleep (SWS), glucose homeostasis and, 2665-2666
SMA. see Superior mesenteric artery
Small bowel, for urinary diversion, 3160
Small bowel anastomosis
  tunneled, 3188
  in urinary diversion, 3187-3189
    Bricker anastomosis, 3187, 3187f

Small bowel anastomosis (Continued)
    Hammock anastomosis, 3189
    Le Duc technique, 3189, 3189f
    split-nipple technique, 3188-3189, 3188f
    tunneled, 3188, 3188f
    ureteral dipping technique, 3189
    ureteral-small bowel, 3189, 3190f
    Wallace technique, 3187-3188, 3188f
Small cell carcinoma
  of bladder, 3089, 3089f
  of kidney, 2181t, 2183
Small cell neuroendocrine prostate cancer, 3693
Smegma pearl, 393-394
Smegmoma, 393-394, 393f
Smoking
  benign prostatic hyperplasia and, 3324
  in bladder tumor, 3076
  and ED, 1509
  penile cancer and, 1744
  prostate cancer and, 3464, 3543
  urinary incontinence and, 2586
  UTUC risk and, 2186
Smooth muscles
  in benign prostatic hyperplasia, 3315, 3315f
  of bladder, 2465, 2465f
    actinomyosin cross-bridge cycling, 2472-2473, 2472b, 2473f
    action potentials of, 2473-2474, 2474f
    calcium signaling in, 2475-2476, 2476f
    contractile proteins, 2470-2472, 2471f-2473f
    electrical response propagation, 2476-2477, 2477f
    excitation-contraction coupling in, 2474-2475, 2475f
    during filling, 2478
    interstitial cells of, 2477-2478, 2478f
    membrane electrical properties of, 2473-2474, 2474f
    motor sensory network in, 2479-2480, 2479f
    physiology of, 2470-2478, 2478b
    during voiding, 2479
  of penis, physiology of, 1495-1500
    cytosolic calcium, and calcium sensitization pathway, 1495
    intracavernous tissue architecture and erectile response, 1500, 1501t
    modulation of antitumescence pathways by protumescence pathways, 1496-1500
    molecular pathways that directly modulate intracellular free calcium and, 1495
    molecular pathways that indirectly modulate intracellular free calcium and, 1495-1496
  skeletal muscle compared with, 2471t
  of urethral sphincter, 2467
    CVA and, 2603
Smooth sphincter, decreasing outlet resistance at, to facilitate bladder emptying, 2719-2720
Smooth sphincter dyssynergia, 2521-2522
  with autonomic dysreflexia, 2614
SMV. see Superior mesenteric vein
SNM. see Sacral neuromodulation
SNS. see Sacral nerve stimulation
Social history, 8-9
Social Security Administration (SSA), 102
Society for Fetal Urology classification, 404, 405f
Society for Fetal Urology grading system, 360-361, 360f
Socioeconomic factors, in benign prostatic hyperplasia, 3321, 3321t
Sodium
  filtrate transport, 1906-1909, 1907f-1910f, 1909b
  fractional excretion of, urinary tract obstruction and, 777
  hypercalciuria and, 2051
  in kidney, of neonate, 342, 342b

Sodium (Continued)
  in pediatric kidney stone disease, 869
  transport of, urinary tract obstruction and, 793
Sodium cellulose phosphate, for hypercalciuria, 2053
Sodium pentosan polysulfate, for BPS/IC oral therapy, 1242
Soft tissue sarcomas, in retroperitoneum, 2229
Solid retroperitoneal tumors, cystic change of, retroperitoneal tumors and, 2238
Solid/cystic renal masses, 384-385
Solifenacin
  for diminished bladder, 2668-2669, 2675t-2677t
  to facilitate bladder filling and urine storage, 2682, 2682t
  with β-adrenoreceptor antagonists, 2700
Solitary fibrous tumor
  of kidney, 2132
  retroperitoneal tumors and, 2232, 2233f
Solitary multilocular cyst nephroma, in pediatric patients, 1109
Solubility product, 2009-2010, 2010f
Solutes, filtrate transport, 1912-1913
Somatic nervous system
  and ED, 1527
  in retroperitoneum, 1675-1679, 1675.e1f, 1677f-1678f, 1679t
Somatic pathways
  of lower urinary tract, 2480f-2481f, 2481
  penile erection and, 1490-1491
Sonic Hedgehog protein, ED and, 1506
Sonoelastography
  limitations of, 84, 85f
  mode of, 74-75
  of scrotum, 84
Sonography, 403, 405b
  prenatal, 404, 407f
Sorafenib, 1358
  for RCC, 2179t-2180t, 2334, 2334t
South African star grass, for benign prostatic hyperplasia, 3398
Southwest Oncology Group (SWOG), 3691, 3692f
SOX9 gene, 992f, 992t, 993, 3276
Soy, in prostate cancer prevention, 3476
Space of Retzius, 2850
  development of
    for laparoscopic radical prostatectomy, 3571-3572, 3572f
    of open simple prostatectomy, 3450
    of robot-assisted laparoscopic simple prostatectomy, 3455
Spall fracture mechanism, of stone fragmentation, 2095-2096
Spallation, of stone fragmentation, 2095-2096
SPARTAN trial, 3696
Spatial compounding ultrasonography, 74
Specialist nurse, in transitional urology, 1046-1047
Specific gravity, of urine, 15
Specimen collection, for urinalysis, 14
Specimen entrapment instrumentation, for laparoscopic and robotic surgery, 217-218, 217f
Speckling, in ultrasonography, 71, 72f
SPECT. see Single-photon emission computed tomography
Sperm cryopreservation, for TGCT patients, 1690
Sperm granuloma, complication of scrotal surgery, 1856
Sperm production, age-related decrease in, 1392
Sperm retrieval
  in anejaculation, 1580
  surgical techniques for, 1472-1476, 1473t
    microsurgical epididymal sperm aspiration, 1473-1474, 1473f-1474f

Sperm retrieval (Continued)
    percutaneous epididymal sperm aspiration, 1474, 1474f
    postmortem, 1476
    testicular sperm extraction, 1474-1475, 1474f-1475f, 1475t
Spermatic cord, 1393
Spermatic cord dissection, patient positioning and port placement for, 1736, 1736f, 1738
Spermatic cord torsion, 893-897
  acute intravaginal, 893-894
    clinical presentation of, 894
    diagnostic studies of, 894, 895f
    management and surgical treatment of, 894-896, 896f
    predisposing factors for, 893-894
    prognosis for, 896-897
  extravaginal, 897, 897f
  intermittent intravaginal, 897
Spermatic vessel ligation, for prune-belly syndrome, 594
Spermatids, 1398, 1398f
Spermatoceles, excision of, 1850
Spermatocytes, 1396, 1397f-1398f, 1400-1401
Spermatocytic tumors, histology of, 1682
Spermatogenesis, 1399-1402
  cycle of, 1399, 1399f
  genetics of, 1401
    paternal age and, 1401-1402, 1402b
  germ cells in, 1396, 1401
  meiosis, 1401
  Sertoli cells in, 1396, 1401
  spermiogenesis, 1401
  testis stem cell migration, 1399
  testis stem cell proliferation, 1400
  testis stem cell renewal, 1400, 1400f
Spermatogonia, 1396
Spermatotoxicity, 1429-1432
  medications and
    antibiotics, 1430
    antihypertensives, 1430
    anti-inflammatory agents, 1431
    antipsychotics, 1430
    cytotoxic chemotherapeutics, 1430-1431
    endocrine modulators, 1429
    environmental toxicants, 1431
    opioids, 1430
    phosphodiesterase V inhibitors, 1431
    radiation, 1431-1432
    recreational drugs, 1430
    thermal toxicity, 1431
Spermatozoa, 1408-1410, 1409f, 1410b
  epididymal function and, 1404-1406
    maturation, 1404-1405
    storage of, 1404
    transport of, 1404
  maturation of
    biochemical changes, 1405
    fertility, 1405, 1405f
    motility, 1404-1405, 1405f
  production. see Spermatogenesis
  vas deferens function and, 1406-1407
Sphincteric urinary incontinence
  cause of, 2993
  classification of, 2993-2998
  diagnosis of, 2995-2998
  etiology of, 2993-2998
  evaluation of, 2995-2998, 2996f, 2998b
    cystoscopy for, 2996-2997, 2997f
    history for, 2995
    laboratory of, 2996
    patient-reported measures, 2995-2996
    physical examination for, 2996
    urodynamics for, 2997
  history and development of devices, 2993-2994, 2994f
  implantation device technique, 3000-3005
    artificial urinary sphincter, 3000, 3001f, 3003f

Sphincteric urinary incontinence (Continued)
    four-arm sling, 3005, 3005b
    operative preparation of, 3000
    transobturator bulbourethral sling, 3005, 3006f
  improving quality of evidence, 3009
  indications for surgery, 2998-2999, 2999b
  innovations and emerging concepts in device design, 2994-2995
  mechanisms of continence with surgical devices, 2995
  pathophysiology of, 2993-2998
  training paradigms of, 3009
Spina bifida (SB)
  kidney size with, 629
  lower urinary tract dysfunction with, 2617
  neuropathic bladder, 1052-1053
    changes in function and continence, 1052
    preparation for pregnancy, 1052-1053
    renal and urologic concerns, 1052
    sex and sexuality, 1052
Spinal cord
  abnormalities of, with cloacal exstrophy, 574-575
  cystitis and, chemical changes with, 2507
  neuromuscular lower urinary tract dysfunction involvement of, 2607-2619
  segment numbering for, 2609
Spinal cord compression, neuroblastoma causing, 1096
Spinal cord injury (SCI)
  bladder calculi in patients with, 2116-2117
  cystitis with, 2467
  and delayed ejaculation, 1576-1577, 1576t
  epidemiology of, 2609, 2609b
  general concepts of, 2609, 2609b
  with high-pressure bladders, host defense mechanisms in UTIs and, 1140
  lower urinary tract dysfunction with, 2609-2617, 2609b
    autonomic dysreflexia, 2614-2615
    bladder cancer and, 2616
    follow-up for, 2616-2617
    neurologic and urodynamic correlation, 2612-2614
    sacral, 2611-2612, 2613f, 2613b
    spinal shock, 2610
    suprasacral, 2610-2611, 2611f-2612f, 2612b
    urinary tract infection, 2615
    vesicoureteral reflux, 2615
    in women, 2615-2616
  morbidity of, 2609, 2609b
  neurogenic detrusor overactivity and, 2504-2505
  traumatic, 648-649, 650b
    pathogenesis of, 648
    presentation of, 648, 648f
    specific recommendations for, 649
  urothelium and, 2467
Spinal cord pathways, in lower urinary tract, 2481-2482, 2481t, 2482f
Spinal defects, in bladder exstrophy, 531-532
Spinal dysraphism, 487
  lower urinary tract dysfunction with, 2617-2619
  occult, 644, 645t
Spinal shock, lower urinary tract dysfunction with, 2610
Spinal stenosis, lower urinary tract dysfunction with, 2620
Spinal ultrasound, 389
Spindle assembly checkpoint, deregulation of, 1347.e3
Spine, anatomy of, in retroperitoneum, 1658, 1658.e1f
Splenic injury
  during laparoscopic and robotic surgery, 230.e1
  during radical nephrectomy, 2261

Splenogonadal fusion, 963, 963f
Splenorenal ligament, 1865
Split onlay skin flap (SOS) hypospadias repair technique, 946f
Split symphysis variant of exstrophy-epispadias complex, 538
Split-and-roll technique, for RPLND, 2239, 2239f
Split-nipple technique, in urinary diversion, 3188-3189, 3188f
Split-thickness skin grafts, for urethral and penile reconstruction, 1805
SPOP mutations, in prostate cancer, 3470-3472
Sporadic glomerulocystic kidney disease (GCKD), 772
Sporadic prostate cancer, 1355-1358
Spread-out Bragg peak, 3594, 3594f
Squamous cell carcinoma (SCC)
  of bladder, 3089-3090, 3089f
    in pediatric patients, 1118
  as neoplastic condition, 1296, 1299f
  of penis, 1743-1751
    biopsy for, 1746, 1747b
    delay in, 1745
    diagnosis of, 1745-1751
    differential diagnosis of, 1751
    etiology of, 1743-1744, 1745b
    examination for, 1745-1746
    histologic features of, 1746, 1747b
    invasive, 1743
    invasive carcinoma, 1743
    laboratory studies of, 1746-1747
    natural history of, 1745, 1746b
    presentation of, 1745, 1746b
    prevention of, 1744, 1745b
    radiologic studies of, 1747-1748, 1748b
    signs of, 1745
    staging of, 1748-1751, 1748t-1749t, 1750f, 1751t, 1751b
    symptoms of, 1745
  of upper urinary tract, 2189
Squamous cell carcinoma in situ (SCCis), as neoplastic condition, 1296, 1298f
Squeezing-splitting mechanism, of stone fragmentation, 2096-2097
SRY gene, 990, 991f-992f, 1392
SSIGN score. see Stage, Size, Grade and Necrosis (SSIGN) score
SSIPPE. see Short Screening Instrument for Psychological Problems in Enuresis
SSIs. see Surgical site infections
SSLF. see Sacrospinous ligament fixation
Stab wounds
  renal, 1982
    nonoperative management of, 1986-1987
  ureteral, 1995-1996
    diagnosis of, 1995-1996
Staccato-shaped curve, 480
Stage, Size, Grade and Necrosis (SSIGN) score, 2162
Staged implant procedure, for sacral neuromodulation, 2754
Staged tubularized autograft (STAG) repair, 927, 930f
Staghorn calculi, 2070, 2070f
  epidemiology of, 2031
  percutaneous nephrolithotomy and, 2106
  surgical treatment selection for, 2074-2075
Stamey incontinence grading system, 2893t
Stamey needles, in pubovaginal sling placement, 2838-2839
Standardized uptake value (SUV), 91
Stapled sigmoid reservoir, for cutaneous continent urinary diversion, 3228, 3230f
Staplers, 466
Stapling devices, for laparoscopic and robotic surgery, 216, 216f
StAR. see Steroid acute regulatory protein
Starr plication technique, for megaureter in children, 851, 851f

States of saturation, renal calculi and, 2009-2010, 2010f-2011f
Static cystography, 39, 40f
Statins
  and ED, 1509
  for metabolic syndrome, 1422
  for prostate cancer, 3544-3545
  in prostate cancer prevention, 3475
Stauffer syndrome, 2156
STDs. see Sexually transmitted diseases
Stem cell transplantation, for RCC, 2331, 2331t
Stem cells
  in GU cancers, 1367, 1368b
  in prostate cancer, 3466, 3468f
  testis
    migration of, 1399
    proliferation of, 1400
    renewal of, 1400, 1400f
Stenosis, urethral, reconstructive surgery for, 1811
Stents
  endovascular, for renovascular injuries, 1990
  for prostate, 3443-3444
  ureteral. see Ureteral stents
    for ureteroenteric strictures, 1977
    for ureteropelvic junction obstruction, 834-835
    in percutaneous antegrade endopyelotomy, 1948
  for urethral stricture disease, 1818-1819
Stepper, 3592
Stereotactic body radiation therapy, 3593-3594
Sterilization, of ureteroscopes, 195-197
Steroid acute regulatory protein (StAR), 1394-1395
  deficiency of, 1011
Steroid hormones, of male reproductive system, 1390, 1391f
Steroid-dependent nephrotic syndrome (SDNS), 345
Steroidogenic dysfunction, 1447
Steroid-resistant nephrotic syndrome (SRNS), 345
Steroids
  for retroperitoneal fibrosis, 1980
  sex, lower urinary tract and, 2502-2503
Steroid-sensitive nephrotic syndrome (SSNS), and nephrotic syndrome, 345
Stevens-Johnson syndrome, 1277-1278, 1278f
Stimulated myoplasty, 2903
Stoma
  for intestinal anastomoses in urinary intestinal diversion, 3161f
  complications of, 3180t
  flush, 3182-3183
  loop end ileostomy, 3183, 3183f
  nipple (rosebud), 3182, 3182f-3183f
  in minimally invasive urinary diversion, preparation of, 3262, 3262b
Stomach
  selection, 3162
  for urinary diversion, 3160
Stone breakage mechanism, of stone fragmentation, 2097
Stone clearance, 861
Stone composition, after shock wave lithotripsy, 865
Stone disease. see Calculi
Stone fragility, 2077.e1-2077.e2
Stone location, after shock wave lithotripsy, 865
Stone removal
  laparoscopic and robotic, 2113
  in percutaneous nephrolithotomy, 2104-2105
Stone retrieval devices, for ureteroscopic, intraluminal lithotripsy, 198
Stone size, after shock wave lithotripsy, 864-865
Stones. see Calculi
Stop test, 2659
"Straddle fractures," urethral injuries with, 3057, 3057.e1f
Straight ureteral catheter, 166.e1f

Streak gonad, 321-322, 323f
Stress Incontinence Surgical Treatment Efficacy Trial (SISTEr), 2840-2841
Stress relaxation, ureteral, 1885, 1885f
Stress strategies, 2725, 2725.e1t
Stress urinary incontinence (SUI)
  adrenergic agonists for, 2501
  with bipolar transurethral resection of prostate, 3419
  BMI and, 2540-2541
  cause of, 2834
  definition of, 2539, 2581
  estrogens for, 2713-2714
  female
    algorithm for management of, 2760f
    drugs used for treatment of, 2713-2716
    urodynamic studies, evidence-based review in, 2574-2576
    use of injectable agents for, 2890-2891
  genuine, 2518
  hypermobility in, 2757, 2834
  male
    drugs used for treatment for, 2716
    injectable agents for, 2896-2897
      after urinary diversion, 2897-2898
      injection techniques, 2896-2897
  mechanisms of, 2504
  occult, urodynamic studies of, 2563
  pathophysiology of, 2517, 2596-2597, 2597b
    intrinsic sphincteric deficiency in, 2597, 2757, 2834, 2859-2860
    urethral support and, loss of, 2596-2597, 2596f
  patient history of, 4
  pelvic floor muscle training for, 2540, 2723
  recurrent, midurethral sling outcomes for, 2860-2861, 2861b
  treatment for
    choice of, 2757
    in men, 2546-2547, 2546t, 2547b
    midurethral sling. see Midurethral sling
    pharmacologic, 2683t, 2713, 2717b
    pubovaginal sling for. see Pubovaginal sling
    surgical, 2574
  urethral collagen and, 2467
  urethral slings for, 2831
Striated muscles, of urethral sphincter, 2466-2467
  fiber types of, 2466-2467
Striated sphincter, decreasing outlet resistance at, to facilitate bladder emptying, 2720
Striated sphincter dyssynergia, 2521-2522
  after CVA, 2603
  baclofen for, 2720.e2-2720.e3
  with cerebellar ataxia, 2604
  cystourethrogram of, 2611f
  with MS, 2608
  with suprasacral spinal cord injury, 2610
  with traumatic brain injury, 2604
Striated urethral sphincter, surgical anatomy of, 3549, 3549f-3550f
Strickler technique, in urinary diversion, 3186, 3186t, 3187f
Stricture
  ureteral. see Ureteral strictures
  with ureterointestinal anastomoses, in urinary intestinal diversion, 3192
  in ureteroscopic stone management, 2108
  urethral. see Urethral strictures
Stroke
  and ED, 1502
  lower urinary tract dysfunction and, 2602-2603
Stroma
  of bladder wall, 2463
  of prostate, 3280
  of urethra, 2468
Stromal-epithelial interactions
  in benign prostatic hyperplasia, 3309
  in prostate growth, 3287

Structural chromosomal anomalies, male infertility and, 1446
Structural sperm abnormalities, in male infertility, 1451-1452
Structure, definition of, 101
Studer neobladder, modified, for minimally invasive urinary diversion, 3263t, 3264-3265
Studer pouch, for orthotopic urinary diversion, 3245, 3247f
Subacute combined degeneration (SACD), lower urinary tract dysfunction and, 2619
Subclinical Cushing syndrome, 2363-2364
Subclinical filariasis, 1329
Subcostal artery, 136f
Subcostal flank approach, for open kidney surgery, 2249-2250, 2249.e1f, 2250f-2251f, 2250.e1f
Subcutaneous emphysema, during laparoscopic and robotic surgery, 225
Subcutaneous tissue expansion, for hypospadias, 945
Subepithelial plexus, 2463
Submucosal stone, in ureteroscopic stone management, 2109
Substance P, in ureteral function, 1889
Suburethral hammock, 2831
Suburethral slings, 2830
Suburothelial interstitial cells, 2470, 2470f
Succinate dehydrogenase RCC (SDHRCC), 2142t, 2144
Sudeck's point, 3161
SUI. see Stress urinary incontinence
Sunitinib, 3700
    for RCC, 2179t-2180t, 2334-2335, 2335t, 2336f
Superficial bladder cancer. see Non-muscle-invasive bladder cancer
Superficial fascia, 136f
Superficial inguinal lymph node dissection, for penile cancer, 1761, 1793-1794
Superficial perineal space, 1807.e10
Superior ectopic kidney, 728f, 729-731
    anomalies of, 729-730, 730f
    diagnosis of, 730-731
    prognosis of, 731
    symptoms of, 730, 730f
Superior lumbar triangle, 169
Superior mesenteric artery (SMA), 1869-1870
    in radical nephrectomy, 2261
Superior mesenteric vein (SMV), in radical nephrectomy, 2261
Superior vesical artery, 1377
Supernumerary kidney, 721-722, 722f-723f
Supernumerary renal arteries, 1869
Supine hypotensive syndrome, in pregnant, 282
Supine position, 146, 165
    modifications to, 165
Suplatast tosilate, for BPS/IC oral therapy, 1241t, 1243
Supracostal flank approach, for open kidney surgery, 2250-2251, 2251.e1f
Supradiaphragmatic tumors, testicular tumors with, 1720
Suprapubic aspiration, 437
    in urine collection, 1141
Suprapubic catheterization, 155-156
    techniques of, 156
        placement with a guidewire and Seldinger technique, 156
Suprapubic cystostomy, 190-191
    for posterior urethral injury, 3058, 3058f
Suprapubic simple prostatectomy, 3452-3454
    adenoma enucleation for, 3453, 3453f
    closure for, 3453-3454, 3454f
    hemostatic maneuvers for, 3452f, 3453
    prostate exposure for, 3452-3453, 3452f

Suprasacral spinal cord injury
    lower urinary tract dysfunction with, 2610-2611, 2611f-2612f
    management with, 2612b
Supraspinal pathways, in lower urinary tract, 2493-2497
    additional regions in, 2496-2497
    bladder modulatory mechanisms, 2493-2494, 2495f
    brain-bladder control model, 2497, 2498f
    central circuitry regulation of, 2494-2495
    cerebral control of voiding, 2496
    human brain imaging studies in, 2496, 2496f
    modulators in, 2495-2496
    neurotransmitters in, 2495-2496
    pontine micturition center, 2493-2494, 2495f
Supravesical urinary diversion, for prune-belly syndrome, 591-592
Surface electrode electromyography (sEMG), for PFM activity measurement, 2729
Surgery
    adrenal. see Adrenal surgery
    in ED, 1537
    for genito-pelvic pain-penetration disorder, 1653, 1653.e1f
    for hypospadias
        Byars flap, 927, 931f
        distal, 918
        general considerations of, 916-918, 918b
        graft or flap, 932, 934f
        one-stage, 925-926
        preputial flaps, 926f, 938-939
        proximal, 925-932, 925b
        scrotoplasty, 941
        technical aspects of, 925-926, 926f
        two-stage, 926-927
        two-stage, with free graft, 927, 929f
        two-stage, with pedicle flap, 927-932, 931f
    kidney. see Kidney surgery
    for Peyronie's disease (PD), 1616-1625, 1626b
        indications, 1610f, 1616-1618, 1618b, 1619t
        penile prosthesis, 1624-1625
        tunica lengthening procedures, 1621-1624
        tunical shortening procedures, 1618-1621, 1620f-1621f, 1622f
    postoperative care for. see Postoperative care
    preoperative care for. see Preoperative care
    preparation for, 123-125
        antithrombotic therapy, 32-34
        bowel preparation, 124-125
        medication management, 32
Surgery-specific cardiac risk, 120
Surgical antimicrobial prophylaxis, in pediatric kidney stone disease, 861
Surgical castration, 3371
Surgical history, adrenal surgery and, 2407-2408
Surgical landmarks, of adrenal glands, 2345, 2347f-2348f, 2405-2406, 2406f
Surgical mesh removal, 2885-2886, 2886b
Surgical neurotomy, cryoablation, and neuromodulation, of dorsal penile nerve, 1572.e3
Surgical outcomes, assessment of, 101-114
Surgical pharmaceuticals, for laparoscopic and robotic surgery, 215
Surgical site infections (SSIs), 453-454
    risk of, 145
Surgical wounds
    classification of, 1201t
    of radical nephrectomy, closure of, 2261
Surgiflo, 148
Surveillance
    active, for RCC, 2173, 2173t
    for NSGCTs, 1693-1694, 1694t
    for penile cancer, 1757
    for seminomas, 1703-1704, 1703t

Suturing instrumentation, for laparoscopic and robotic surgery, 215-216, 216f
SWE. see Shear wave elastography
Swedish Reflux Study, 515
SWL. see Shock wave lithotripsy
Swyer syndrome, 998t, 1004-1005, 1005f
Sympathetic ganglia tumors, retroperitoneal tumors and, 2234-2235, 2235f
Sympathetic nervous system
    in retroperitoneum, 1675
    in ureteral function, 1888-1889
Sympathetic pathways, of lower urinary tract, 2480, 2480f
Sympathetic transmission, in neural control of LUT, 2593
Sympathomimetic agents, for neuromuscular dysfunction of lower urinary tract, 634, 634f
Symptom Impact Index (SII), 111t
Symptom Severity Index (SSI), 111t
Symptomatic microscopic hematuria, 252
Symptoms Management After Reducing Therapy (SMART) trial, 3389
Syndrome of complete androgen insensitivity, 1013-1014
Syndrome of partial androgen resistance, 1014
Syndromic cryptorchidism, 957-958
SYNERGY study, 3702
Synovial sarcoma, retroperitoneal tumors and, 2231-2232, 2232f
Synthetic mesh, for posterior compartment repair, 2829
Synthetic prosthetic materials, for pubovaginal sling, 2835, 2836t
    outcomes of, 2843
Syphilis
    diagnosis, 1258-1259
    as genital ulcers, 1255t, 1257, 1257f-1258f, 1257t
    treatment, 1259, 1259t
Syringomyelia, lower urinary tract dysfunction and, 2626
Systemic chemotherapy, for UTUC, 2222
Systemic lupus erythematosus (SLE), lower urinary tract dysfunction and, 2626
Systemic sclerosis, lower urinary tract dysfunction and, 2631
Systemic therapies, for retroperitoneal tumors, 2245-2247

T

T pouch
    for orthotopic urinary diversion, 3245-3246, 3247f
    with valved rectum, 3209-3210, 3210f
T2-weighted imaging, 63, 63f
Tabes dorsalis, lower urinary tract dysfunction with, 2619
Tachykinins
    lower urinary tract and, 2501-2502, 2501t
    in ureteral function, 1889
Tadalafil
    for benign prostatic hyperplasia, 3385
    to facilitate bladder filling and urine storage, 2682t, 2701
    for ureteral relaxation, 1899
    for urinary incontinence, 2544-2546
Tamm-Horsfall protein
    in crystal formation, 2014
    in crystal matrix, 2015
Tamoxifen, for PD, 1611, 1616t
Tamsulosin
    for benign prostatic hyperplasia, 3363-3365, 3363f, 3364t
    for detrusor underactivity, 2661
    for diminished bladder capacity, 2675t-2677t
    to facilitate bladder emptying, 2720.e1
    to facilitate bladder filling and urine storage, 2682t
    with antimuscarinic agent, 2704

Tamsulosin (Continued)
  for nocturia, 2671–2673
  ureteral response to, 1888
Tanner classification, 871, 872t
"Taqaandan," penile fracture with, 3048
Targeted angioembolization, for renal tumors, 2323
Targeted molecular therapies, for advanced RCC
  basis of, 2332–2333, 2333f
  combination and sequential therapy with, 2339–2341
  immune "checkpoint" inhibitor-based combination strategies, 2341, 2342f
  mTOR pathway inhibitors, 2326–2327, 2338–2339, 2340f, 2340t
  VEGFR-based, 2326–2327, 2333–2337, 2333t–2335t, 2336f, 2337f
Tasquinimod, 3700–3701
TAX 327 study, 3691, 3691f
TCC. see Transitional cell carcinoma
99mTc-DMSA. see Technetium-99m dimercaptosuccinic acid
99mTC-DTPA. see TECHNETIUM-99M-DIETHYLENETRIAMINE PENTAACETIC ACID
99mTc-MAG3. see Technetium-99m-mercaptoacetyl triglycine
TCS. see Tethered cord syndrome
99mTc-sestamibi, 98, 98f
Tea, UTUC risk and, 2186
Technetium-99m (99mTc), 91, 92t
Technetium-99m dimercaptosuccinic acid (99mTc-DMSA), 92, 96b
  for imaging infections of kidney, 96
  renal cortical imaging with, 95–96
Technetium-99m-diethylenetriamine pentaacetic acid (99mTc-DTPA), 41, 92, 96b
  dynamic renal scintigraphy with, 94–95
  scintigraphy, 94–95
Technetium-99m-mercaptoacetyl triglycine (99mTc-MAG3), 41, 41f, 92, 94f, 96b
  additional applications of, 94–95
  dynamic renal imaging with, 92–93
  dynamic renal scintigraphy with, 94–95
  renogram, 95f
Telomerase, in GU cancers, 1362–1365, 1363f, 1365b
  chromosome stabilizing activity of, 1364
  as potential diagnostic marker, 1364
  therapies based on, 1365
Telomere shortening, 2905
Telomeres, in GU cancers, 1362–1365, 1365b
  cancers and premalignant lesions with short, 1363–1364
  chromosomal instability and, 1362
  prostate cancer prognosis using, 1364–1365
  as tumor suppressive mechanism, 1363, 1363f
Temperature, epididymal function and, 1406
Temporal lobe epilepsy, and ED, 1502
Temsirolimus (Torisel), 2148
  for RCC, 2338–2339, 2339t–2340t, 2340f
Tension-free vaginal tape (TVT) procedure
  colposuspension compared with, 2773–2774
  evolution of, 2831
Teratomas, 1122
  histology of, 1683f, 1684
  PC-RPLND findings of, survival outcomes associated with, 1726, 1727t
Terazosin
  for autonomic dysreflexia, 2615
  for benign prostatic hyperplasia, 3357–3359, 3357t–3358t, 3359f
  for diminished bladder, 2674, 2675t–2677t
  to facilitate bladder emptying, 2682t, 2720.e1
Terbutaline, to facilitate bladder filling and urine storage, 2682t, 2714
Terminal ileum, right colon pouches with intussuscepted, 3219–3220
Tertiary or late syphilis, 1258
Testicular adnexa, tumors of, 1709

Testicular anomalies, cryptorchidism and, 963–964
Testicular artery, 1370–1371, 1372f–1373f, 1375
Testicular cancer. see also Paratesticular cancer
  and delayed ejaculation, 1576
  genomic alterations in, 1361–1362
    gene rearrangements, 1353
  in geriatric patients, 2920.e13
  non–germ cell, 1707–1709
    adenocarcinoma of rete testis, 1708
    dermoid and epidermoid cysts, 1708
    secondary metastases, 1709
    sex cord-stromal tumors, 1707–1708
  in nuclear medicine, 43–44, 44f
  pediatric, 1121–1125, 1125b
    biomarkers for, 1122, 1122f
    epidemiology of, 1121
    gonadal stromal tumors, 1124, 1124f
    leukemia and lymphoma metastases, 1124–1125
    management algorithms for, 1125, 1125f
    microlithiasis, 1124–1125
    pathogenesis and molecular biology of, 1121
    presentation of, 1121–1122
    sexual development disorders associated with, 1122–1124, 1123t
    staging of, 1122, 1122t
    testis-sparing surgery technique for, 1125
    ultrasonography of, 1122
  staging of, 1687t–1688t
Testicular dysgenesis syndrome (TDS), 909, 955–956
Testicular fixation, with suture, 1855
Testicular formation, 317–318, 319f, 320t
Testicular germ cell tumors (TGCTs), 1680–1707, 1681t, 1684b, 1688b
  clinical staging of, 1687t–1688t, 1689–1690, 1691b
    chest imaging and, 1690
    imaging studies, 1689
    prognostic classification of advanced germ cell tumor, 1690, 1691t
    serum tumor markers in, 1690
    sperm cryopreservation, 1690
  diagnosis delay, 1685
  diagnostic testing and initial management of, 1685–1688
    contralateral testis biopsy, 1688
    partial orchiectomy, 1686–1688
    radical inguinal orchiectomy, 1686
    scrotal ultrasound, 1685–1686, 1685f
    serum tumor markers, 1686
    for suspected extragonadal GCTs, 1688
  differential diagnosis of, 1685
  epidemiology of, 1680
  genomic alterations in, 1122t, 1361
  histologic classification of, 1682–1684
    choriocarcinoma, 1683–1684, 1683f
    EC, 1682–1683, 1683f
    germ cell tumor neoplasia in situ, 1682
    seminoma, 1682, 1683f
    spermatocytic tumor, 1682
    teratoma, 1683f, 1684
    YSTs, 1683f, 1684
  initial presentation of, 1684–1685
  pathogenesis and biology of, 1681–1682
  physical examination for, 1685
  risk factors for, 1680–1681
  signs and symptoms of, 1684–1685
  suspected, 1688
  treatment of, 1691–1693
    brain metastases, 1706–1707, 1707b
    NSGCTs, 1692, 1692b
    relapse after, 1700–1702
    residual mass management after, 1698–1700, 1698f–1699f
    seminomas, 1692, 1692b
    sequelae of, 1707, 1707b
    therapeutic principles, 1691–1692
Testicular hypotrophy, 900–901

Testicular injury
  complications with, 3053
  diagnosis of, 3051–3052, 3052f
  etiology of, 3051
  management of, 3052–3053, 3052f
  outcome of, 3053
Testicular maldevelopment, cryptorchidism and, 961–964
Testicular microlithiasis, 971–972, 971f
  in pediatric patients, 1124–1125
Testicular prosthesis placement, 1848–1850, 1849f
Testicular retraction, 949
Testicular rupture, 899
Testicular sperm extraction, 1474–1475, 1474f–1475f, 1475t
Testicular torsion, 387, 391–392, 392f, 1432
  perinatal, 897, 897f
Testicular tumors, 392–393
  laparoscopic retroperitoneal lymph node dissection, 1734–1741, 1741b
    bilateral, 1738
    complications of, 1739–1740, 1739t
    duplication of, 1735
    postoperative care after, 1738–1739
    prospective nerve-sparing techniques for, 1739
    rationale and evolution of, 1734
    results and current status of, 1740–1741, 1740f
    staging, 1734–1735
    surgical technique for, 1735–1738
  malignant. see Testicular cancer
  management of, 1711–1712
  as non–AIDS-defining urologic malignancies, 1268
  robotic-assisted retroperitoneal lymph node dissection, 1734–1741, 1741b
    complications of, 1739–1740, 1739t
    postoperative care for, 1738–1739
    prospective nerve-sparing techniques for, 1739
    rationale and evolution of, 1734
    results and current status for, 1740–1741
    surgical technique for, 1735–1738
  surgery of, 1711–1733, 1712b
    delayed orchiectomy, 1712
    evaluation after, 1712
    in high-risk populations, 1727–1729, 1728t, 1729b
    histologic findings and survival outcomes of, 1726–1727, 1727t, 1727b
    history, and physical examination, ultrasonography, and preorchiectomy evaluation, 1711–1712
    outcomes, functional considerations, and complications of, 1729–1731, 1732b
    for seminoma, 1731–1732
    for sex cord stromal tumors, 1732–1733
    surgical decision making for, 1721–1726, 1726b
      adjuvant chemotherapy for primary RPLND, 1724–1726
      in cases of clinical complete remission to induction chemotherapy, 1721–1722, 1722t
      template use in PC-RPLND, 1723–1724, 1724f, 1725t
      template use in primary RLND, 1722–1723, 1723f, 1723t
Testis
  anatomy of, 1374b
    arterial supply to, 1370–1371, 1372f, 1393
    blood supply of, 1453–1454, 1454t
    gross structure, 1370, 1371f
    lymphatic supply, 1372, 1373f
    microanatomic architecture, 1370, 1371f
    nerve supply, 1372–1373
    venous drainage, 1372, 1372f–1373f
  androgen production by, 3281–3282, 3282f–3283f, 3282t

Testis *(Continued)*
  anomalies of, cryptorchidism and, 963-964
  appendix, torsion of, 897-898, 898f
  descent of
    gubernacular development and, 951-952, 952f
    regulation of, 952-953
  differentiation of, 949-950
  embryology of, 949-953
  function of, 994, 995f
  in genitourinary tuberculosis, 1309
  HIV and, 1266
  hormones of, 950-951, 1391-1392, 1391f
  imaging of
    magnetic resonance imaging, 1373-1374
    scanning electron micrograph, 1393f
    ultrasound, 1373, 1373f-1374f
  inflammation of. *see* Orchitis
  injuries of, 3051-3053
  magnetic resonance imaging, 1373-1374
  neoplasms of, 1680-1710, 1681t
  physiology of, 1392-1394, 1402b
    cytoarchitecture, 1394-1399, 1395f-1396f
    gross architecture in, 1392-1394, 1393f-1394f
    in HPG axis, 1391-1392, 1391f
  in prune-belly syndrome, 584-585, 585f
  ultrasonography of, 82, 1373, 1373f-1374f
    indications for, 82
    normal findings in, 78f, 82-83, 83f-84f
    procedural applications of, 83
    sonoelastography, 84
  undescended. *see* Cryptorchidism
  vanishing, 959-960, 960f
Testis stem cell
  migration of, 1399
  proliferation of, 1400
  renewal of, 1400, 1400f
Testis-sparing surgery
  for pediatric tumors, 1125
  for TGCT, 1686-1688
Testosterone
  aging effects on, 1392
  biosynthesis disorders of, 1011-1013
  cycles of, 1396, 1396f
  epididymal function and, 1406
  for female sexual arousal disorders, 1649-1650
  for female sexual response, 1627.e5-1627.e6
  in HPG axis, 1391
  lower urinary tract and, 2503
  in prostate cancer, 3466, 3467f
  sources of, 3673
  synthesis of, 1394-1395, 3280-3281, 3283f
    control of, 1395-1396
Testosterone therapy, 1529-1532, 1531t
  buccal, 1530
  cardiovascular risk of, 1424-1425
  intramuscular, 1530
  for metabolic syndrome, 1422
  oral, 1530
  subcutaneous, 1530
  transdermal, 1530
Tethered cord syndrome (TCS), lower urinary tract dysfunction with, 2618
TGCTs. *see* Testicular germ cell tumors
The Cancer Genome Atlas (TGCA), 3467-3468, 3469f
Theophylline, for ureteral relaxation, 1899
Thermal ablative therapies, for RCC, 2171-2173, 2171f, 2172t
"Thermal dose,", 3426
Thermal index (TI), in ultrasonography, 78
Thermodynamic solubility product (K_{sp}), 2009
Thiazide-induced hypocitraturia, 2056
Thiazides
  for hypercalciuria, 2051-2052, 2052t
  in stone formation, 2033
Thick filaments, 2471, 2471f

Thiersch Duplay (TD) repair, 921-922, 923f
Thigh pain, in mesh complication, 2881
Thin filaments, 2470-2471
Thiol-containing agents, for pediatric kidney stone disease, 869-870
Thiotepa, for non-muscle-invasive bladder cancer, 3103
Thoracic kidney, 725-727, 726f
  anomalies of, 726
  description for, 726
  diagnosis of, 726, 726f
  embryology of, 725-726
  incidence of, 725
  prognosis of, 727
  symptoms of, 726
Thoracoabdominal approach
  for kidney surgery, 2251-2252, 2252f-2253f, 2252.e1f
  to open adrenalectomy, 2413-2414, 2413f-2414f
Thoracoabdominal incision, kidney and retroperitoneum approaches, 136-137
Thoracostomy, 181
Three-dimensional conformal radiotherapy, for prostate cancer, 3587-3588, 3588f
Three-dimensional laparoscopic systems, 213
Three-dimensional scanning, in ultrasonography, 75, 77f
Three-port catheters, 153
Thrombectomy, vena caval, 2266-2278, 2278b
  bypass techniques for, 2275-2276, 2275f-2276f, 2275.e1f, 2276.e1f
  IVC filtration and permanent interruption for bland thrombus, 2277
  level I, right-sided tumor technique, 2267-2269, 2267.e1f, 2269.e1f, 2270f
  level II, left-sided tumor technique, 2269-2270, 2269.e1f, 2271f
  level III-IV
    combined intra-abdominal and intrathoracic approach, 2274-2275, 2274f, 2274.e1f
    intra-abdominal approach technique, 2270-2274, 2271f-2274f, 2273.e1f
  patching, replacing, and interrupting of IVC in, 2276-2277, 2277f
  perioperative complications, 2277-2278
  preoperative considerations for, 2266-2267, 2267t, 2268f-2269f
Thromboembolic events, after retropubic radical prostatectomy, 3563
Thulium laser, 3442-3443
  complications with, 3443
    intraoperative, 3443
    perioperative, 3443
    postoperative, 3443
  concept and introduction for, 3442
  conclusion for, 3443
  holmium laser enucleation of prostate *versus*, 3442-3443
  outcomes with, 3442-3443
    comparative series, 3442-3443
    single-cohort series, 3442
  technique for, 3442
  transurethral resection of prostate *versus*, 3442
Thulium:YAG (Thu:YAG) laser, 240-241
Thymine, 1346.e1, 1346.e2f
Tibial nerve stimulation, for OAB, 2647
Tight junction (TJ) proteins, in bladder urothelium, 2467, 2468f
Time activity curve (TAC), 92-93, 93f
Timed Up and Go (TUG) test, 2910
Timed voiding, 2730.e1t, 2731
Tisseel VH Fibrin Sealant, 215.e2
Tissue adhesives (Bioglue), 148
Tissue anastomosis instrumentation, for laparoscopic and robotic surgery, 215-216
Tissue banking, genomic research on, 3586
Tissue matrix, of prostate, 3280

Tissue transfer, principles of, 1805
Tissue-based biomarkers, 3487-3489
Tissue-based genomics, caveats of, 3543
TMP. *see* Trimethoprim
TMP-SMX. *see* Trimethoprim-sulfamethoxazole
TNF-α. *see* Tumor necrosis factor-α
TNM staging. *see* Tumor, nodes, and metastases (TNM) staging
Tofranil. *see* Imipramine
Toileting programs
  bladder training, 2728f, 2730, 2730.e1t
  caregiver-administered, challenges of, 2732.e1
  delayed voiding, 2732
  habit training, 2730.e1t, 2731
  prompted voiding, 2730.e1t, 2731-2732
  timed voiding, 2730.e1t, 2731
  understanding, 2730.e1
  for urinary incontinence, 2730-2731
Tolterodine, 2498, 2499t
  for diminished bladder, 2674, 2675t-2677t
  to facilitate bladder filling and urine storage, 2682, 2682t
    with α-adrenoreceptor antagonists, 2697-2698
    with other antimuscarinics, 2685
Tonsil clamps, in pubovaginal sling placement, 2838-2839
TOOKAD Soluble, 3632
Top-down approach (TDA), 439
Topical local anesthetics, for PE, 1572
Topical therapy, for genito-pelvic pain-penetration disorder, 1653
Topical thrombin agents, 148
Topiramate, in stone formation, 2033
Toremifene citrate, in prostate cancer prevention, 3475
Torisel. *see* Temsirolimus
Toronto group, 3540
Torsion of appendix testis and epididymis, 897-898
Torulopsis glabrata, 445
Total colpocleisis, for apical pelvic organ prolapse repair
  results with, 2812
  technique for, 2812, 2813f
Total laparoscopic technique, in nephroureterectomy, for UTUC, 2202, 2203f
Total nephrectomy, for renal injuries, 1991
Total parenteral nutrition (TPN), 122
Total scrotectomy, 1844-1845, 1846f
Total urogenital mobilization (TUM), 1033-1034, 1034f-1036f
Tower-shaped curve, 480
Toxins, to facilitate bladder filling and urine storage, 2682t, 2707-2709, 2709b
  botulinum toxins, 2707-2709
  capsaicin, 2709
  resiniferatoxin, 2709
TP53
  in apoptosis, 1366
  in GU cancers, 1347.e2, 1347.e2f, 1348
  in prostate cancer, 3469
  in Wilms tumor, 1098
TPE. *see* Tropical pulmonary eosinophilia
Tract dilation, 170-172
Tract sealants, 176
Traditional open distal ureterectomy, in UTUC, 2200-2201, 2200f-2201f
Tramadol
  to facilitate bladder filling and urine storage, 2713.e3-2713.e4
  for PE, 1572.e1
Trans Tasman Radiation Oncology Group (TROG), 3600-3602
Transabdominal pelvic ultrasonography
  indications for, 80
  limitations of, 81
  normal findings in, 80-81, 80f, 82f

Transabdominal pelvic ultrasonography (Continued)
  procedural applications of, 81
  technique of, 80
Transcolonic technique of Goodwin, in urinary diversion, 3185-3186, 3186f
Transcription, basics of, 1346.e3, 1346.e3f
Transcriptional activation domains, of androgen receptors, 3291-3292, 3291b, 3292f
Transcutaneous electrostimulation, 2748
  sacral dermatome, 2748
  tibial nerve, 2748
Transducers, in urodynamic studies, 2558
Transection, of ureter, delayed recognition, 2001-2002
Transepithelial resistance (TER), 2467
Transferrin, in prostatic secretions, 3298t, 3302
Transforming growth factor-β superfamily, in prostate development, 3276-3277
Transforming growth factor-β1 (TGF-β1)
  and PD, 1605-1606
  in tubulointerstitial fibrosis, 787
Transfusion protocol, massive, 147
Transgender. see also Transmen; Transwomen
  female-to-male, 1841-1842, 1842b
  special urologic considerations in, 3062-3072, 3072b
  early postoperative care of, 3069-3070
Transient receptor potential (TRP) channels
  antagonists of, to facilitate bladder filling and urine storage, 2713.e1
  in bladder afferent pathway, 2485
Transient urinary incontinence
  in geriatric patients, 2919.e1
  with holmium laser enucleation of prostate, 3438
Transient urinary tract dilation, 372-373, 373f
Transitional cell carcinoma (TCC). see also Urothelial cancer
  pediatric, 1117-1118, 1123-1124, 1124f
  upper tract and lower tract magnetic resonance imaging for, 61, 62f
Transitional urology, 1043-1053
  barriers to, 1045-1047
    expanding numbers and management of service long-term, 1046
    importance of specialist nurses, 1046-1047
    institutional, 1045-1046
    patients, 1046
    professional, 1046
  clinical delivery to, 1047
    geography, 1047
  clinical practice:major diagnosis of, 1047-1050, 1050b
    blood tests, 1049
    exstrophy, 1049-1050
    flow rates, 1048
    functional assessment of reconstructed urinary tract, 1047-1048
    hypospadias, 1049
    renography, 1048
    ultrasonography, 1048-1049
    video-urodynamics, 1048, 1048f
  definitions for, 1043-1045
    failure of transition, 1044
    models for transition, 1044-1045
    transfer, 1044
    transition, 1043-1045, 1044t
  patient population to, 1045
  patient/parent preparation for, 1047, 1047b
  setting up a service of, 1045
    institutional and political support, 1045
    multidisciplinary team, 1045
    training, 1045
Translation, basics of, 1346.e3, 1346.e3f-1346.e4f
Transmen
  transurethral catheterization in, 3070
  urethral complications in, 3070-3071
  urologic issues in, 3063-3069
    diagnosis of, 3063

Transmen (Continued)
  genitoperineal transformation, 3066-3068
  metoidioplasty, 3068-3069
  phallic urethra, 3068
  phalloplasty, 3068
  preoperative care of, 3063
  removal of female anatomic structures, 3063-3066
  scrotoplasty, 3068
  sex reassignment surgery, 3063
  testicular implants and erectile prosthesis, 3069, 3070f
Transmural cystotomy, nonrefluxing ureteral reimplantation and, 3021-3022
Transneuronal tracing, 2494-2495
Transobturator AdVance sling, long-term results with, 3008
Transobturator bulbourethral slings
  implantation technique for, 3005
  outcomes with, 3003t
Transobturator mid-urethral slings
  anatomy of, 2850-2851
  complications of, 2863-2866
  outcomes for, 2856-2857, 2857t
  surgical approach for
    inside-out, 2853-2854, 2854f
    outside-in, 2853
Transobturator slings
  history and development of, 2994
  mechanisms of continence, 2995
Transperineal prostate biopsy, 3498-3499
Transperineal ultrasound, 85, 87f-88f
Transperitoneal approach
  to laparoscopic adrenalectomy, 2414-2417, 2415f-2417f, 2422
  to laparoscopic kidney surgery, 2279, 2280f-2281f
  to laparoscopic partial nephrectomy, 2300
  to laparoscopic radical nephrectomy, 2294-2295, 2295f
  robot-assisted, 2418-2419, 2419f-2420f
Transperitoneal laparoscopic nephroureterectomy, 2203-2204, 2203f-2204f
Transplant kidney, 177-178
Transplantation
  hematopoietic stem cell, for RCC, 2331, 2331t
  percutaneous nephrolithotomy and, 2106, 2106f
  renal. see Renal transplantation
Transport, of sperm
  by epididymis, 1404
  by vas deferens, 1406-1407
Transrectal prostate biopsy, 3497-3498
Transrectal ultrasonography (TRUS), 1444
  of locally advanced prostate cancer, 3641, 3641f
  of prostate, 88-89, 89f, 1380, 1380f, 3490
    after treatment, 3493-3494
    anatomy of, 3490, 3491f-3492f
    cancer, 3493, 3493f
    color Doppler, 3500-3501, 3500f-3502f
    cystic lesions, 3493, 3493f
    elastography, 3501, 3502f
    gray-scale, 3490-3494, 3494b
    investigational techniques for, 3501-3504
    machine setting for, 3491
    other malignancies and, 3494
    power Doppler, 3500-3501, 3500f-3502f
    probe manipulation in, 3491-3492, 3492f
    Prostate HistoScanning, 3501-3502
    techniques for, 3491-3492
    volume calculations in, 3492-3493
  of seminal vesicles and ejaculatory ducts, 1378
Transrectal ultrasound-guided aspiration, 1863
Transrectal ultrasound-guided brachytherapy, for prostate cancer, 3591-3592, 3592f
Transrectal ultrasound-guided prostate (TRUSP) biopsy, antimicrobial prophylaxis, 1197-1198

Transscrotal orchidopexy, 967, 967f
Transumbilical approach, 464
Transureteroureterostomy (TUU)
  for midureteral injuries, 1998
  for urinary tract reconstruction, 683, 683f
  for vesicoureteral reflux, 2615
Transurethral endoscopic treatments, 1863
Transurethral incision (TUI), for ureteroceles, 817-819, 818f-819f, 819b
  reflux outcomes after, 819
Transurethral incision of prostate (TUIP), 3434-3435
  complications with, 3435
    intraoperative, 3435
    perioperative, 3435
    postoperative, 3435
  introduction and concept of, 3434
  outcomes with, 3434-3435
    comparative studies, 3434-3435
    single-cohort studies, 3434
  summary for, 3435
  technique for, 3434, 3434f
  transurethral resection of prostate versus, 3434-3435
Transurethral microwave therapy (TUMT), 3426-3430
  α-blocker versus, 3429
  complications with, 3430
    intraoperative, 3430
    perioperative, 3430
    postoperative, 3430
  conclusion for, 3430
  contraindications to, 3427-3428
  introduction and concept of, 3426, 3427f
  mechanism of action of, 3426-3427
    morphology changes, 3427
    nerve degeneration/sensory changes, 3426-3427
  outcomes with, 3428-3430
    comparative studies for, 3429
    prediction of, 3428
    single-cohort studies, 3428-3429
  sham versus, 3429
  technique for, 3427-3428
    intraoperative, 3428, 3428f
    postoperative, 3428
    preoperative, 3427-3428, 3428f
  transurethral resection of prostate versus, 3429-3430
Transurethral needle ablation (TUNA), 3430-3434
  complications with, 3433
    intraoperative, 3433
    perioperative, 3433
    postoperative, 3433
  conclusion for, 3433-3434
  introduction and concept of, 3430-3431, 3431f
  other minimally invasive surgical techniques versus, 3433
  outcomes with, 3432-3433
    comparative studies, 3433
    single-cohort studies, 3432-3433
  technique for, 3431-3432
    intraoperative, 3431-3432, 3432f
    postoperative, 3432
    preoperative, 3431
  transurethral resection of prostate versus, 3433
Transurethral prostate biopsy, 3499
Transurethral resection (TUR), 1454
  of diverticular neck, for bladder diverticula, 2972
  of ureteral orifice, in UTUC, 2201-2202, 2202f
Transurethral resection of bladder tumor (TURBT), 3133-3135, 3134f, 3159b
  bladder perforation with, 3135, 3135f
  challenges with, 3134-3135
  cystoscopy for, 3133
  goal of, 3134
  history of, 3133

Transurethral resection of bladder tumor (TURBT) *(Continued)*
  of muscle-invasive bladder cancer, radical, 3124
  of non-muscle-invasive bladder cancer, 3096-3097
    complications of, 3096
    repeat, 3096-3097
  partial cystectomy with, 3143, 3144f
  patient preparation for, 3135-3136
  pelvic lymphadenectomy with, 3137-3138, 3138f-3139f
  physical examination and, 3113
  physical examination of, 3133
  postoperative care for, 3157
  radical cystectomy
    female, 3141-3143, 3142f-3143f
    male, 3138-3141, 3139f-3141f
  surgical technique for, 3136-3137, 3136f-3137f
Transurethral resection of ejaculatory ducts (TURED), 1454, 1471-1472
  complications of, 1471-1472
    epididymitis, 1471
    reflux, 1471
    retrograde ejaculation, 1471-1472
  diagnosis for, 1471
  results for, 1472
  technique for, 1471, 1472f
Transurethral resection of prostate (TURP)
  for adenocarcinoma, 3510
  bipolar. *see* Bipolar transurethral resection of the prostate
  holmium laser enucleation of prostate *versus*, 3437
  for localized prostate cancer, 3524
  monopolar. *see* Monopolar transurethral resection of the prostate
  for nocturia, 2671-2673
  thulium laser *versus*, 3442
  transurethral incision of prostate *versus*, 3434-3435
  transurethral microwave therapy *versus*, 3429-3430
  transurethral needle ablation of prostate *versus*, 3433
  urinary incontinence after, risk factors for, 2587
Transurethral technique, injection, 2892-2893, 2893f
Transurethral vaporization of prostate (TUVP), 3422-3426
  comparative studies for, 3425
    bipolar studies, 3425
    monopolar studies, 3425
  complications of, 3425-3426
    intraoperative, 3425-3426
    perioperative, 3425-3426
    postoperative, 3426
  conclusion for, 3426
  electrode for, 3423, 3423f
  introduction and concept of, 3422-3424, 3423f
  outcomes with, 3424-3425
    animal/in vitro studies, 3424
    single-cohort studies, 3424-3425
  technique for, 3424
    intraoperative, 3424
    postoperative, 3424
    preoperative, 3424
Transvaginal uterosacral ligament hysteropexy, 2817, 2819t
Transversalis fascia, 1666-1667, 1667f, 2427, 2429f, 2447f-2448f
Transverse colon, colon conduit and, 3196
Transverse myelitis, 649-650, 650b
  pathogenesis of, 650
  presentation of, 649-650, 650f
  specific recommendations for, 650

Transverse preputial island flap (TPIF), 925, 927f
Transverse testicular ectopia (TTE), 963-964
Transverse vaginal septum, 327, 979-980, 979f-980f
Transverse vesical fold, bladder, 3010
Transversus abdominis, 136f
Transvesical ligation and detachment technique, in nephroureterectomy, in UTUC, 2201, 2201f
Transwomen
  fate of prostate in, 3063
  urologic issues in, 3062-3063
  vaginoplasty in, 3062
Trauma
  of external genitalia, 3048-3054, 3054b
    genital skin loss, 3053-3054, 3053f-3054f
    penile reconstructions, 3054
    penis, 874f, 875, 3048-3049, 3048.e1f, 3049f-3050f, 3049.e1f
  genital and lower urinary tract, 3048-3061, 3061b
  LUT function and, 2527
  noninfectious genital ulcers caused by, 1288, 1288f
  renal. *see* Renal injuries
  spinal cord. *see* Spinal cord injury
  testis, 3051-3053
  ureteral. *see* Ureteral injuries
Traumatic brain injury, lower urinary tract dysfunction with, 2604
Traumatic urethral strictures, 1815
Treatment margins, for prostate cancer, 3589-3590, 3591f-3592f
Trendelenburg position, 146-147, 460-461
Treponemal syphilis tests, 1258-1259
Triamterene
  in stone formation, 2033
  in stone formation, surgical management of, 2077.e3
Triangulation, 218.e3, 218.e3f
  technique, 167, 168f
Trichloroacetic acid, for condylomata acuminata, 1742.e3
Trichomonas vaginalis, 1254
Trichomoniasis, 1272, 1272t
  of genitourinary tract, 1332
Tricyclic antidepressants (TCAs)
  for BPS/IC oral therapy, 1241t, 1242
  for enuresis, 664-665
  to facilitate bladder filling and urine storage, 2702
  and PE, 1571-1572
Trigone of bladder, 2455-2456, 2456f
  formation of, 328-329, 331f
Trimethoprim (TMP), for UTIs, 1156, 1187t
Trimethoprim-sulfamethoxazole (TMP-SMX)
  prophylaxis with
    for common urologic procedures, 1156, 1162, 1170t, 1194t-1196t
    for cystourethroscopy, 189
  for UTIs, 1153
TriPort, 212.e1, 212.e1f
Trocars
  for laparoscopic and robotic access, 211, 211f, 211.e2f
  complications related to placement of, 225-226
  for laparoscopic kidney surgery, 2279-2285
    hand-assisted laparoscopy, 2282, 2283f
    laparoendoscopic single-site surgery and natural orifice transluminal endoscopic surgery, 2284-2285, 2285f, 2286t
    retroperitoneal, 2280-2281, 2282f
    robotic-assisted laparoscopy, 2282-2284, 2284f-2285f
    transperitoneal, 2279, 2280f-2281f
  in midurethral sling, injury to urinary tract with, 2866-2873

TROPIC study, 3692, 3693f
Tropical pulmonary eosinophilia (TPE), as filariasis clinical manifestation, 1330
Tropical spastic paraparesis, lower urinary tract dysfunction and, 2625
Tropomyosin (TM), 2472, 2473f
Trospium chloride
  for diminished bladder, 2674, 2675t-2677t
  to facilitate bladder filling and urine storage, 2682t, 2683
  with other antimuscarinics, 2691-2692
TRP channels. *see* Transient receptor potential (TRP) channels
TRPA1, 2485
TRPM8, 2485
TRPV4, 2485
True flank incision, 139-140, 140f
TRUS. *see* Transrectal ultrasonography
TRUSP biopsy. *see* Transrectal ultrasound-guided prostate (TRUSP) biopsy
TSC. *see* Tuberous sclerosis complex
Tubeless percutaneous procedure, 175-176
Tubercular epididymitis, 1221
Tuberculin skin test (TST), 1310
Tuberculosis (TB), 1307-1332, 1319b
  drug-resistant, 1318
  epidemiology, 1307
  genitourinary. *see* Genitourinary tuberculosis
  history, 1307
  lower urinary tract dysfunction and, 2626-2627
  microbiology, 1307
  relapse, 1318
Tuberous sclerosis complex (TSC), 757-759, 757f-758f, 2125, 2142t, 2145
  clinical features of, 757-758
  genetics of, 757, 759f
  radiographic evaluation of, 758-759, 758f
  renal cell carcinoma in, 758, 2157-2158
  treatment of, 759
Tubular function, 341-342
  developmental changes in, 342
Tubular proteinuria, 18
Tubularization techniques, for hypospadias, 920-941
  flip-flap, 924, 924f
  glans approximation procedure, 907f, 920-921
  island onlay flap procedure, 924-925, 926f
  slitlike adjusted Mathieu procedure for, 924, 925f
  Thiersch Duplay repair, 921-922, 923f
Tubularized incised plate urethroplasty
  distal, 923f
  proximal, 928f
  for reoperation, 916-918, 922-924, 923f
Tubulogenesis, 338
Tubulointerstitial fibrosis, 786-790, 790b
Tubulopathies, 348-349
TUI. *see* Transurethral incision
TUIP. *see* Transurethral incision of prostate
TUM. *see* Total urogenital mobilization
Tumor, nodes, and metastases (TNM) staging, 3084, 3085t, 3086f
  for RCC, 2158-2159, 2159t
  of urethral cancer, 1777, 1778f, 1778t
  for UTUC, 2194, 2195t, 2198b
Tumor enucleation, for RCC, 2170-2171, 2170f
Tumor lysis syndrome (TLS), 1924
Tumor necrosis factor-α (TNF-α), in tubulointerstitial fibrosis, 787
Tumor suppressor genes, 1346-1347, 1347f, 1347b
Tumor syndromes, 1354, 1354t
  in prostate cancer, 1354-1355, 1354t, 1355f
  in renal cancer, 1354t, 1358
Tumor thrombectomy, in retroperitoneal tumors, 2243
Tumor volume, 3511

Tumorigenesis model, for prostate cancer, 3472-3473
Tumors. *see also* Malignancy; Oncology; *specific tumors*
　formation of, augmentation cystoplasty and, 699-700
　renal, metabolic syndrome and, 1421
TUMT. *see* Transurethral microwave therapy
TUNA. *see* Transurethral needle ablation
Tunica albuginea, 317, 1370, 1371f, 1374f, 1392-1393, 1599
　anatomy of, 1486-1487, 1486f
　in penile fracture, 3048
Tunica lengthening
　graft materials for, 1622-1623
　grafting surgical technique for, 1623-1624
　postoperative management for, 1624
Tunica vaginalis grafts, 1807
Tunical shortening, procedures for, 1618-1621, 1620f-1621f, 1622t
TUR. *see* Transurethral resection
TURBT. *see* Transurethral resection of bladder tumor
TURED. *see* Transurethral resection of ejaculatory ducts
Turner syndrome, 1001-1002, 1001f-1002f, 1002b
TURP. *see* Transurethral resection of prostate
TUU. *see* Transureteroureterostomy
TUVP. *see* Transurethral vaporization of prostate
TVT procedure. *see* Tension-free vaginal tape (TVT) procedure
Two-kidney, one-clip model, of renovascular hypertension, 1917, 1917f
Two-port catheters, 153
Two-stage urethroplasty, for transmen, 3071
Tyramine, ureteral response to, 1888
Tyrosine kinase inhibitors, for RCC, 2167-2168

U
UA. *see* Urinalysis
UCLA Integrated Staging System (UISS), for RCC, 2162
UCSF and the Cancer of the Prostate Risk Assessment (CAPRA) score, 3528
UDS. *see* Urodynamic studies
UISS. *see* UCLA Integrated Staging System
Ulaanbaatar repair, 927-932, 933f
Ulcers. *see* Genital ulcers
Ulnar nerve injury, 261-262
Ultrafiltration, in end stage renal disease, 356
Ultrasensitive prostate-specific antigen (uPSA), for biochemical recurrence after radical prostatectomy, 3661
Ultrasonic lithotripsy, 243, 244b, 2112, 2112f
　basic physics of, 243
　tissue effects of, 243
Ultrasonography, 68-90, 90b, 391b, 404-412
　abdominal wall defects, 410
　of adrenal glands, 2352
　in adrenal mass evaluation, 2395
　bladder tumors, 408-409
　bladder/urethra, 408-412, 409f-410f
　　obstruction of, 408
　clinical urologic
　　penis and male urethra, 85-88, 86f
　　renal, 78-80, 79f
　　scrotum, 81-84, 83f-85f
　　transabdominal pelvic, 80-81, 80f-82f
　　TRUS of prostate, 88-89, 89f
　contrast agents in, 76-77
　for cysts/masses/stones, 405-406, 406b, 407f, 411-412
　　abdominal solid, 405-406
　　renal, 405
　　renal stones, 406
　　ureteral stones, 406
　of defecation disorders, 669-670, 670f, 670.e1f
　for differences of sex development, 412
　documentation and image storage in, 76, 77f

Ultrasonography *(Continued)*
　Doppler. *see* Doppler ultrasound
　of epididymis, 1375-1376, 1376f
　of exstrophy-epispadias complex, 538, 539f
　of female pelvis, 2439, 2440f
　with fine-needle aspiration cytology, for inguinal node dissection, 1791-1792
　fundamental of, in fetus and child, 404
　history of, 68, 69f
　infection and, 406-407, 408b, 409
　of kidney/ureter, 404-407, 1868, 1868.e1f
　of male external genitalia, 871, 871.e2f
　midline pelvic cysts, 408-409
　modes of
　　Doppler, 73-74
　　gray-scale, 73
　　harmonic scanning, 74, 75f
　　sonoelastography, 74-75
　　spatial compounding, 74
　　three-dimensional scanning, 75, 77f
　noncontrast voiding, 406-407
　obstruction, of kidney/ureter, 404-405, 405b
　　dilated ureters, 404
　　functional interpretation of, 404-405
　　hydronephrosis *versus* cystic renal diseases, 404
　of other congenital malformation, 407, 410
　patient safety in, 77-78
　pediatric
　　genitourinary trauma, 1073-1074
　　stone disease, 854-856, 855f
　　urology, 388-389
　of penile fracture, 3048-3049, 3049f
　of penis, 1386, 1387f
　for PFM function assessment, 2723
　physical principles of, 68-73, 69f
　　artifacts, 71-73, 72f
　　attenuation mechanisms, 71, 71f-72f
　　image generation, 70, 70f
　　resolution, 70-71, 70f
　of posterior urethral valves, 607, 607f
　practice accreditation for, 89-90
　in pregnant, 284
　prenatal, 389
　renal bladder, 388-389
　for renal calculi, 778-779
　　pretreatment assessment, 2071
　for renal tumor evaluation, 2135
　for renovascular hypertension screening, 1917-1918, 1918b
　scrotal, 389, 1373, 1443-1444, 1444f
　　for GCTs, 1685-1686, 1685f
　of testis, 1373, 1373f-1374f
　　injury to, 3052, 3052f
　in transitional urology, 1048-1049
　transrectal. *see* Transrectal ultrasonography
　for trauma, 407, 408b
　　scrotum, acute, 410-411, 411f-412f, 412b
　of undescended testis, 412, 412b
　of ureteral anomalies, 803-805, 804f-805f
　ureteral anomalies, imaging interpretation of, 804f, 806
　for ureteral calculi, 778-779
　for ureteropelvic junction obstruction, 1943
　urethral, 1384f
　of urethral diverticula, 2983
　of urinary lithiasis, 2038, 2038f-2039f
　for urinary tract obstruction, 778-781
　for UTIs, 1144, 1168, 1169f
　Wilms tumor screening with, 1098-1099, 1099f
Ultrasound instrumentation
　for laparoscopic and robotic surgery, 214-215
　for tissue dissection and cauterization, 237-238
Ultrasound-guided access, 169, 169f
Umbrella cells, 2461-2462, 2463f, 2467
UMN bladder, in Bors-Comarr classification system, 2523
Unclassified RCC, 2149t-2151t, 2155

Unclassified sarcomas, retroperitoneal tumors and, 2233
Uncomplicated cystitis, 1155-1158
　antimicrobial selection for, 1156-1157
　clinical presentation, 1156
　follow-up, 1157-1158
　laboratory diagnosis, 1156
　management, 1156-1157, 1157f
　risk factors, 1156b
Underactive bladder. *see* Bladder, underactive
Underactive detrusor. *see* Detrusor underactivity (DUA)
Undescended testis, 391, 949-972. *see also* Cryptorchidism
Unilateral levator hypertonicity, 2881
Unilateral renal agenesis (URA), 717-721
　anomalies of other organ systems and, 720
　associations with, 718
　current concepts regarding prognosis in adults with, 720-721
　diagnosis of, 720
　embryology of, 718, 719f
　genitourinary and adrenal anomalies with, 718-719
　　in female, 719-720
　　in male, 719
　incidence of, 718
　prognosis of, 720
　special considerations in, 720
Unilateral renal cystic disease, 770
Unilateral ureteral obstruction (UUO)
　hemodynamic changes with, 791, 791f
　renal recovery after, 795
　tubular function with, 792-793
Unresolved UTIs, 1159, 1159b
Unstable bladder, 2637
Up training, 2732
UPEC. *see* Uropathogenic *E. coli*
UPJ. *see* Ureteropelvic junction
UPP. *see* Urethral pressure profile
Upper abdominal surgery, operative team placement for
　retroperitoneal procedures, 207, 207f
　transperitoneal procedures, 206, 206f, 206.e1f
Upper motor neuron (UMN) lesion, voiding dysfunction after, 2522, 2523f
Upper respiratory infections (URIs), perioperative care for pediatric patients with, 447-448
Upper tract endoscopy
　antimicrobial prophylaxis for, 1199
　equipment for, 192-199, 192f, 193t, 195f, 196t, 199f, 199t
　indications for, 191-192
　percutaneous procedures, antimicrobial prophylaxis for, 1199
　technique, 199-201, 201f
　ureteroscopy, antimicrobial prophylaxis for, 1199
Upper tract urothelial cancer (UTUC), 2185-2199
　diagnosis of, 2189-2192, 2192b, 2199
　　cystoscopy for, 2190
　　uretero-renoscopic evaluation for, 2190-2191, 2190f
　　ureteroscopic evaluation and biopsy for, 2199
　endourologic management of, 2210-2224
　　antegrade nephroureteroscopic, 2212-2219, 2215f-2217f, 2218t
　　basic attributes, 2210-2211, 2210f
　　lymph node-positive and metastatic disease treatment, 2222-2224, 2223f
　　positive upper tract urinary cytology and carcinoma in situ management, 2219-2222, 2219f, 2221f, 2221t
　　retrograde ureteroscopic, 2211-2212, 2211f, 2213f, 2214t, 2215f
　epidemiology of, 2185, 2185b
　　incidence of, 2185
　　mortality rate of, 2185
　　variations by gender, race, and age, 2185

Upper tract urothelial cancer (UTUC) (Continued)
  follow-up in, 2224–2225, 2224f
  histopathology of, 2188–2189, 2189b
    micropapillary variant of, 2188
    normal upper tract urothelium, 2188
    urothelial carcinoma, 2188, 2189f
  natural history of, 2192–2194
    panurothelial disease, 2194
  prognosis of, 2194–2198
    histologic grading of, 2194
    postoperative factors, 2195–2197
    preoperative factors, 2194–2195
    surgical margins, 2197–2198
  prognostic factors of
    age-sex-ethnicity, 2194–2195
    lymph node involvement, 2197
    lymphovascular invasion, 2197
    molecular markers, 2197–2198
    predictive tools, 2198
    risk stratification, 2198, 2198f
    surgical delay, 2195
    tobacco consumption, 2195
    tumor location, 2195
    tumor stage and grade, 2195–2197, 2196f
  risk factors of, 2185–2188, 2188b
    environmental factors, 2186–2188
    genetic predisposition, 2185, 2186f
  staging of, 2192–2194, 2194b
  surgical management of, 2199–2210
    distal ureter and bladder cuff management, 2200
    ileal ureteral replacement, 2208, 2209f
    intussusception (stripping) technique in, 2202, 2202f
    laparoscopic or robotic distal ureterectomy and reimplantation, 2208, 2209t
    laparoscopic radical nephroureterectomy, 2202–2205
    lymphadenectomy, 2205–2207, 2206f
    open radical nephrectomy in, 2199–2200, 2200f
    open segmental ureterectomy, 2207, 2208f–2209f
    robot-assisted laparoscopic nephroureterectomy, 2205, 2205f
    segmental ureteral resection, 2207–2210
    total laparoscopic technique in, 2202, 2203f
    traditional open distal ureterectomy in, 2200–2201, 2200f–2201f
    transperitoneal laparoscopic nephroureterectomy, 2203–2204, 2203f–2204f
    transurethral resection of ureteral orifice, 2201–2202, 2202f
    transvesical ligation and detachment technique in, 2201, 2201f
    treatment algorithm for, 2199, 2200b
  ureter compared with collecting system, 2192
Upper urinary tract
  anomalies of, 714–740
    collecting system. see Upper urinary tract collecting system, anomalies of
    renal vasculature. see Renal vasculature, anomalies of
    rotation of, 733–735, 735b
  anomalies of ascent of, 722–727, 727b
    cephalad renal ectopia, 724–725
    simple renal ectopia, 722–724
    thoracic kidney, 725–727
  anomalies of form and fusion of, 727–733
    cake or lump kidney, 728f–729f, 729
    crossed renal ectopia, 727–728, 727f–728f, 731b
    disc kidney, 728f, 729
    horseshoe kidney, 731–733
    inferior ectopic kidney, 729
    L-shaped kidney, 728f, 729

Upper urinary tract (Continued)
    sigmoid kidney, 728f, 729
    superior ectopic kidney, 728f, 729–731
  anomalies of number of, 714–722, 722b, 734t
    bilateral renal agenesis. see Bilateral renal agenesis
    supernumerary kidney, 721–722
    unilateral renal agenesis. see Unilateral renal agenesis
  assessment of, 505–507
    controversies in usage of invasive investigations, 506
    rationale for serial assessment of upper tracts, 505
    renal scintigraphy, 505–506, 506f
    renal scintigraphy and the top-down approach, 506–507
    renal sonography, 505
  defects in, in bladder exstrophy, 535–537
  deterioration of
    with benign prostatic hyperplasia, 3336
    early intervention for, 628
    with neural tube defects, 626–628, 627f
  dysfunction of, 680
  posterior urethral valves and, 604–605, 606f
  urothelium of, abnormal, 2188
Upper urinary tract bleeding, 258b–259b
  lateralizing essential hematuria evaluation of, 259
  vascular condition affecting, 259
Upper urinary tract calculi, 2094–2113
  extracorporeal shock wave lithotripsy, 2094–2103, 2103b
    bioeffects of, 2097–2100
    future direction in, 2102–2103, 2103f
    methods and physical principles, 2094–2097
    techniques to optimize outcome of, 2100–2102, 2100b, 2101f, 2102b
  intracorporeal lithotripsy for, 2109–2113
    ballistic lithotripsy, 2111–2112, 2112f
    combination ballistic and ultrasonic devices in, 2112–2113
    electrohydraulic lithotripsy, 2109–2110, 2110f
    laser lithotripsy, 2110–2111
    ultrasonic lithotripsy, 2112, 2112f
  nonmedical management of, 2069–2093
  percutaneous nephrolithotomy for, 2103–2107, 2105b
    anesthesia for, 2104
    antibiotics for, 2104
    calyceal diverticula and, 2105, 2105f
    complications of, 2107
    horseshoe kidney and, 2105–2106
    morbid obesity and, 2106–2107
    patient preparation, 2103–2104
    staghorn calculi or complex stones and, 2106
    stone removal in, 2104–2105
    transplantation and pelvic kidneys and, 2106, 2106f
  ureteroscopic stone management, 2107–2109
    avulsion in, 2109
    perforation in, 2108
    stricture in, 2108
    submucosal stone and lost stone in, 2109
Upper urinary tract collecting system, anomalies of, 737–740, 740b
  bifid pelvis, 737, 738f
  calyceal diverticulum, 737–738, 739f
  hydrocalycosis, 738
  infundibulopelvic stenosis, 739–740, 740f
  megacalycosis, 738–739, 740f
Upper urinary tract drainage, fundamentals of, 160–184

Upper urinary tract obstruction, 383–384, 384f
  evaluation of, 1942
  management of, 1942–1981
  retrocaval ureter. see Retrocaval ureter
  retroperitoneal fibrosis. see Retroperitoneal fibrosis
  ureteroenteric anastomotic stricture. see Ureteroenteric anastomotic stricture
  ureteropelvic junction obstruction. see Ureteropelvic junction obstruction
Upper urinary tract tumors, benign
  others, 2189
  papillomas, 2188
  von Brunn nests, 2188
Upper-tract imaging, for benign prostatic hyperplasia, 3347–3348
Urachal abnormalities, of bladder, 3039–3040, 3041f
Urachal adenocarcinoma, of bladder, 3090, 3090b
Urachal anomalies, 330–333, 522–525, 524f, 525b
Urachal carcinoma, in pediatric patients, 1118
Urachal cyst, 525
Urachal diverticulum, 525
Urachal sinus, 525
Urachus
  anatomy of, 2448f, 2455
  surgery of, 3038–3043
    complications with, 3042
    evaluation for, 3038–3040
    laparoscopic and robotic techniques, 3043f
    outcomes with, 3042–3043
    postoperative care of, 3042
    surgical indications for, 3038–3040
    surgical technique for, 3041
Uracil, 1346.e1, 1346.e2f
UraTape, 2851
Ureaplasma infection, 1253
Urease, bacteria production by, 2030–2031, 2031t
Uresta, 2736–2737, 2737f
Ureter, 324f
  access of, for ureteroscopy, 200, 200f
  anatomy of, 1865–1876, 1872f, 1873.e1f
    arteries, veins, and lymphatic drainage of, 1873.e1f, 1874, 1874b
    cellular, 1877
    endoscopic, 1875–1876, 1875b, 1875.e1f
    microscopic, 1875, 1875.e1f
    nerve supply of, 1874
    pelvic, 2456, 2456f
    radiologic, 1873–1874, 1874b
  aperistaltic segment of, 1942, 1943f
  development of, 329–333, 332f, 332t
  dissection of, for simple nephrectomy, 2287, 2287f
  distal
    dissection of, 2204, 2204f
    management, 2200
  in genitourinary tuberculosis, 1309
  herniation of, 824
  muscle-invasive bladder cancer involvement, 3119–3120, 3120t
  normal urothelium of, 2188
  pharmacology, 1877–1904
  physiology of, 1877–1904
    cellular, 1877
    contractile activity, 1883–1887, 1883f–1886f
    development of, 1877–1878, 1878f
    drug effects on, 1901–1903
    electrical activity, 1878–1883, 1879f–1880f
    mechanical properties, 1890–1891, 1890f–1891f
    nervous system function, 1887–1890
    urine transport, 1891–1894, 1892f–1893f
  in prune-belly syndrome, 581–582, 582f–583f
  in renal transplantation, 1060

Ureter (Continued)
  vascular anomalies involving, 822-824
  vascular obstruction of, 824
Ureteral access sheaths, for ureteroscopy, 199, 199f, 199t
Ureteral anomalies, 798-825, 822b
  anatomic assessment of, 803
  classification and anatomic description of, 798-801
    ectopic ureter, 798, 798b, 799f
    ureterocele, 798-799, 799f, 800b
  clinical management of, 808-820
    fetal, 810
    general, 810
    goals for, 808-809, 811b
    historical perspective on, 809-810
    neonatal, 810
    observational, 810-811
    summary for, 819-820, 819f, 820t
  clinical presentation of, 801-802, 802b
  ectopic ureter. see Ectopic ureter
  embryology and etiology of, 799-800, 801b
  endoscopic evaluation of, 799f-800f, 808, 808f-809f
  evaluation of, 802-808, 809b
    magnetic resonance imaging, 805, 805f-806f
    physical examination, 803, 803f-804f
    ultrasonography, 803-805, 804f-805f
  functional assessment of, 805-807
    bladder, 806
    renal, 806, 806f
    voiding cystourethrogram for, 805
  general patterns of, 798
  imaging of, 801
  incontinence and, 802
  infection and, 801-802
  late presentation of, 802
  lower tract reconstruction for, 813-816
  nonurgent management of, 810
  of number, 820-821
  pain and, 802
  of position, 822-824
  prolapse of, 802, 803f
  pyeloureterostomy for, 816-817, 817b
    laparoscopic, 817, 817f
  total reconstruction for, 811
  upper pole partial nephrectomy for, 811-813, 812f, 814b
    complications with, 813
    laparoscopic, 811-813, 814f
    open, 811, 812f-814f
    outcomes with, 813
  ureteral clipping of, 813
  ureteral-trigonal-renal development and, 800-801
  ureteroceles. see Ureteroceles
  ureteroureterostomy for, 816-817, 817f, 817b
    laparoscopic, 817, 817f
    open, 816-817
  urgent management of, 810
Ureteral calculi, 2069.e1
  clinical factors of, 2088-2091, 2091b
    duration, 2091
    morbid obesity and, 2089
    old age and frailty, 2089-2090
    prior renal surgery, 2090
    renal function, 2088-2089
    renal transplants, 2091
    solitary kidney, 2089
    spinal deformity or limb contractures, 2090
    uncorrected coagulopathy, 2090
    urinary diversion, 2091
    urinary tract infection and, 2088
  residual fragments, assessment and fate of, 2091-2093, 2093b
  spontaneous passage of, 2085, 2085t
  surgical management of, 2084-2093, 2084b, 2088b
    anatomic factors, 2087-2088
    duplicated collecting system and, 2087

Ureteral calculi (Continued)
    megaureter and, 2087
    natural history of, 2084-2085
    pretreatment assessment for, 2085
    stone burden in, 2087
    stone composition and, 2087
    stone factors for, 2085-2087
    stone location in, 2085-2087, 2086t
    treatment algorithm, 2084f
    ureteral stricture or stenosis, 2087-2088
  technical factors of, 2088
  ureteral function effects of, 1899-1900
  in urinary tract obstruction, 778-779
Ureteral catheterization, UTI diagnosis and, 1142.e1t, 1143
Ureteral development, 313f, 327, 329f
Ureteral dipping technique, in urinary diversion, 3189
Ureteral duplication, 508-509, 508.e1f
Ureteral function
  age effects on, 1900, 1901f
  effect of calculi and stents on, 1899-1900
  effect of diabetes on, 1900
  effect of infection on, 1899
  effects of obstruction on, 1894-1898, 1894f-1897f
    physiologic methodologies for, 1897-1898, 1898f
  pathologic processes affecting, 1894-1900, 1894f-1899f, 1901f
  pregnancy effects on, 1900-1901
  vesicoureteral reflux and, 1898-1899, 1899f
Ureteral injuries, 264-267, 1992-2002
  cause of, 1992-1995
  complications of seminal vesicle surgery, 1864
  diagnosis of, 1995-1996
    hematuria, 1995
    intraoperative recognition, 1995
  external trauma, 1992-1993, 1992t
    contusion, 1996
    management for, 1996-1999
  imaging of, 1995-1996
    antegrade ureterography, 1995
    computed tomography, 1995, 1995f
    intravenous pyelography, 1995-1996, 1996f
    retrograde ureterography, 1995
  incidence and anatomic landmarks, 264-265
  in intraoperative consultation, 300-302
    diagnosis/recognition, 300-301
    grade 1 and 2 injury, 301-302
    grade 3 to 5 distal ureteral injury, 302
    grade 3 to 5 mid-and proximal ureteral injury, 302
    grade 5 injury, 302
    incidence, 300, 300t
    management, 301
    mechanisms, 300, 301t
    principles of repair, 301
    ureteral catheters, 302
    ureteroscopic avulsion injury, 302
  intraoperative management, 265, 266f
  key points of, 2002f-2003f, 2002b
  during laparoscopic and robotic surgery, 230.e1
  lower, 1998-1999
    Boari flap for, 1999, 2000f
    partial transection for, 1999
    psoas bladder hitch for, 1998-1999, 1999f
    ureteroneocystostomy for, 1998
  management of, 1996-2002, 1996f
    damage control, 1999
    general principles of, 1996, 1997f
  mechanisms of, 265
  midureteral, 1998
  with monopolar transurethral resection of prostate, 3417
  presentation of unrecognized, 265-266
  in robotic prostatectomy, 3580
  strictures, 267

Ureteral injuries (Continued)
  surgical, 1993-1994, 1999-2002
    avoidance and detection of, 1993-1994, 1994f
    delayed recognition of, 2001-2002
    immediate recognition of, 2001
    ligation, 2000-2001, 2001f
    robotic and laparoscopic, 1993
    tenuous ureteral blood supply, 1994
    timing of repair of, 1999-2002
    with vascular surgery, 1993
  upper, 1996-1998
    autotransplantation for, 1997
    bowel interposition for, 1998, 1998f
    monitoring after repair, 1998
    nephrectomy for, 1998
    ureterocalicostomy for, 1997
    ureteroureterostomy for, 1996-1997, 1997f
  ureteroscopic, 1994-1995, 2002
    avulsion, 2002
    perforation, 2002
  ureterovaginal fistula, 266-267
Ureteral leak, 1937, 1937b
  diagnosis of, 1937
  treatment of, 1937
Ureteral mobilization, for ureteral reimplantation, 3020-3021, 3021f
Ureteral obstruction
  partial, hemodynamic changes with, 792
  ureteral stenting for, 795
Ureteral pain, patient history of, 2
Ureteral polyps, with megaureter in children, 835-836
Ureteral reconstruction, for prune-belly syndrome, 592
Ureteral reimplantation, 3019-3026
  complications with, 3025
  evaluation of, 3019, 3019f-3020f
  laparoscopic and robotic techniques of, 3023-3024, 3024f
  nonrefluxing, 3021-3022, 3022-3025, 3022f-3024f
  outcomes of, 3025-3026
  postoperative care of, 3025
  refluxing, 3023-3026, 3023f
  surgical indications of, 3019, 3019f-3020f
  surgical technique for, 3020-3021
Ureteral stents
  management of, 1936, 1936b
    diagnosis and treatment of, 1936, 1937f
    prevention of, 1936
    retained, 1936
    timing of, 1936
  for pediatric genitourinary trauma, 1071
  for ureteral obstruction, 795
  for ureterovaginal fistula, 2945, 2945f
Ureteral stones, 406
Ureteral strictures, 1937-1938, 1937t, 1938b
  autotransplantation for, 1975
  balloon dilation for
    antegrade, 1967-1968
    results with, 1968
    retrograde, 1966-1967, 1967f-1968f
  buccal mucosa grafting, 1975
  diagnosis of, 1937-1938
  diagnostic studies of, 1966
  endoureterotomy for, 1968-1969
    antegrade approach to, 1969
    combined retrograde and antegrade approach, 1969
    results with, 1969
    retrograde ureteroscopic approach to, 1968-1969, 1969f
  etiology of, 1965-1966, 1966b
  intervention for
    endourologic, 1966-1969, 1967f-1970f
    indications for, 1966
    surgical, 1969-1975, 1970t, 1976b
  management algorithm for, 1969f
  with megaureter in children, 835
  minimally invasive ileal ureteral substitution for, 1973-1975, 1974f

Ureteral strictures *(Continued)*
  psoas hitch, 1972–1973
  renal descensus for, 1973
  transureteroureterostomy for, 1973
  treatment of, 1938, 1938f
  ureteral stent placement for, 1966
  ureteroneocystostomy for, 1972
  ureteroscopy for, 191–192
  ureteroureterostomy for, 1970–1972
    open approach, 1970–1972, 1971f
    postoperative care, 1972
Ureteral surgery, for genitourinary tuberculosis treatment, 1317–1318
Ureteral tapering, 1897–1898
Ureteral tumors, benign
  other, 2189
  papilloma, 2188
  von Brunn nests, 2188
Ureteric bud branching, 335f, 337–338
Ureteric fistulae, 2942–2946, 2946b
  diagnosis of, 2943–2946, 2943f, 2945f
  etiology of, 2942–2943, 2942b
  management of, 2943–2946, 2943f, 2945f
  presentation of, 2942–2943
Ureterocalicostomy
  for ureteral injuries, upper, 1997
  for ureteropelvic junction obstruction
    laparoscopic and robotic-assisted, 1958
    for UPJ reconstruction, 1962, 1964f
Ureteroceles, 333, 798–825. *see also* Ureteral anomalies
  anatomic description of, 798–799, 799f
  bladder outlet and, 806–807, 807f–808f
  excision of, and common-sheath reimplantation, 813–816, 815f–816f, 817b
  prolapsed, 802, 803f, 977, 978f
  transurethral incision for, 817–819, 818f–819f, 819b
  reflux outcomes after, 819
  voiding dysfunction and, 820
Ureterocolonic anastomosis
  in robot-assisted intracorporeal continent cutaneous diversion, 3269
  in urinary diversion, 3185–3187
    complications of, 3191–3192
      stricture, 3192
      urinary fistula, 3191–3192
    Cordonnier and Nesbit techniques, 3187
    intestinal antireflux valves, 3189–3191
      intussuscepted ileal valve, 3189–3190, 3191f
      intussuscepted ileocecal valve, 3189–3190, 3191f
    Leadbetter and Clarke technique, 3185, 3185f
    Pagano technique, 3186–3187, 3187f
    Strickler technique, 3186, 3186t, 3187f
    transcolonic technique of Goodwin, 3185–3186, 3186f
Ureterocystoneostomy, for prune-belly syndrome, 592
Ureterocystoplasty, 703, 703f
Ureteroenteric anastomotic stricture, 1977b
  evaluation of, 1976
  incidence and etiology of, 1975–1976
  intervention for
    endourologic, 1976–1977, 1978f
    initial management and, 1976–1977
Uretero-enteric strictures, 3272
Ureteroileal anastomosis, for minimally invasive urinary diversion, 3262
Ureterointestinal anastomosis, for urinary diversion, 3184–3192
  complications of, pyelonephritis, 3180t
  intestinal antireflux valves, nipple valve, 3191, 3192f

Ureterointestinal anastomosis, for urinary diversion *(Continued)*
  small bowel anastomoses, 3187–3189
    Bricker anastomosis, 3187, 3187f
    Hammock anastomosis, 3189
    Le Duc technique, 3189, 3189f
    split-nipple technique, 3188–3189, 3188f
    tunneled, 3188, 3188f
    ureteral dipping technique, 3189
    ureteral-small bowel, 3189, 3190f
    Wallace technique, 3187–3188, 3188f
  ureterocolonic anastomoses, 3185–3187
    Cordonnier and Nesbit techniques, 3187
    Leadbetter and Clarke technique, 3185, 3185f
    Pagano technique, 3186–3187, 3187f
    Strickler technique, 3186, 3186t, 3187f
    transcolonic technique of Goodwin, 3185–3186, 3186f
    ureterocolonic anastomoses, 3185–3187
Ureterolysis, for retroperitoneal fibrosis, outcomes of, 1980
Ureteroneocystostomy
  with a bladder psoas muscle hitch or Boari flap, 2207, 2209f
  for ureteral stricture disease, 1972
Ureteronephrectomy, proximal, 2204, 2204f
Ureteropelvic junction (UPJ)
  disruption of, for pediatric genitourinary trauma, 1074–1075, 1075f
  flap procedures of, 1960–1962
    Culp-DeWeerd spiral flap, 1960–1961, 1961f
    Foley Y-V plasty, 1960, 1960f
    intubated ureterotomy, 1961–1962, 1963f
    Scardino-Prince vertical flap, 1961, 1962f
    ureterocalicostomy for, 1962, 1964f
  injury of, 1992–1993
  surgical exposure to, 1953, 1953f–1954f
  urine transport and, 1891, 1892f
Ureteropelvic junction obstruction (UPJO), 400, 507–508, 509f, 1942–1963, 1952b
  acquired, 1943
  calicovesicostomy for, laparoscopic, 1960
  congenital, 1942, 1943f
  diagnosis of, 1942
  dismembered pyeloplasty, 1952–1953
  flap procedures for, 1960–1962
    Culp-DeWeerd spiral flap, 1960–1961, 1961f
    Foley Y-V plasty, 1960, 1960f
    intubated ureterotomy, 1961–1962, 1963f
    salvage procedures, 1963
    Scardino-Prince vertical flap, 1961, 1962f
    ureterocalicostomy for, 1962, 1964f
  genitourinary trauma and, 1076, 1076f
  interventions for, 1947
    endourologic management of, 1947, 1952b
    historical notes on, 1951–1952
    indications for, 1945–1963
    management of complications for, 1963
    nephrectomy for, 1946–1947
    operative, 1951–1953
    options for, 1947–1950
    postoperative care for, 1963
  intrinsic, 1942
  nephrolithotomy for, percutaneous antegrade endopyelotomy simultaneous with, 1949
  pathogenesis of, 1942–1943, 1943f
  patient presentation and diagnostic studies for, 1943–1945, 1944f–1946f
  pattern of dilation, 373–374
    recommendations for, 373–374
  in pediatric patients, 826–852
    associated anomalies, 826
    clinical presentation of, 826, 827f
    complications with, 832f, 835, 835f
    definition of, 826
    dismembered pyeloplasty, 828, 828f–830f

Ureteropelvic junction obstruction (UPJO) *(Continued)*
  endoscopic approach to, 830
  flank approach to, 829
  laparoscopic pyeloplasty for, 830–834, 833f–834f
  lower pole, 826, 827f
  minimally invasive techniques for, 830–835
  nondismembered pyeloplasty for, 828–829, 829f–831f
  outcomes with, 835
  posterior lumbotomy for, 829, 832f
  secondary, 826
  surgical approach to, 829
  surgical indications for, 826–827
  surgical repair of, 827–828
  percutaneous antegrade endopyelotomy for, 1947, 1947f–1948f
  nephrolithotomy simultaneous with, 1949
  percutaneous endopyelotomy for, 1949
  postoperative care and complications, 1957
  pyeloplasty for
    dismembered, 1945–1946, 1953f–1954f
    laparoscopic and robotic intervention, 1953–1955, 1960b
    laparoscopic dismembered tubularized flap, 1960
    open surgery, 1953
    with pyelolithotomy, 1958–1960
    salvage procedures for, 1963
  renal calculi with, surgical management of, 2077
  results of, 1957–1958, 1959t
    minimally invasive approaches, 1957–1958
    open approach, 1957
  retrograde ureteroscopic endopyelotomy for, 1949–1950, 1951f–1952f
  surgical approaches to, 1953–1958
  ureterocalicostomy for, laparoscopic and robotic-assisted, 1958
  ureteroscopy for, 191–192
Ureteropelvic surgery, for genitourinary tuberculosis treatment, 1317–1318
Ureteroplasty, for prune-belly syndrome, 592
Ureteropyeloscopy, 2211, 2211f
Ureterorenoscopy (URS), 2069.e2
  morbid obesity and, 2089
  old age and frailty and, 2089–2090
  prior renal surgery and, 2090
  for renal calculi
    in calyceal diverticula, 2078
    in horseshoe kidneys, 2079
    in renal ectopia, 2081
    stone composition and, 2076, 2076f
    stone localization and, 2075
  renal function and, 2088–2089
  solitary kidney and, 2089
  spinal deformity or limb contractures and, 2090
  stone burden and
    between 1 and 2 cm, 2073
    greater than 2 cm, 2074
    up to 1 cm, 2072
  uncorrected coagulopathy and, 2090
  for ureteral calculi, 2087–2088
    duplicated collecting system and, 2087
    in megaureter, 2087
    outcome of, 2091–2093
    stone burden and, 2087
    stone composition and, 2087
    stone localization and, 2085–2086, 2086t
  urinary diversion and, 2091
  urinary tract infection and, 2088
Ureteroscopic endoureterotomy, retrograde, for ureteral stricture disease, 1968–1969, 1969f
Ureteroscopic stone management, 2107–2109
  avulsion in, 2109
  perforation in, 2108
  stricture in, 2108
  submucosal stone and lost stone in, 2109

Ureteroscopic-assisted fluoroscopic access, 168-169, 168f
Ureteroscopy, 202b, 2211, 2211f
　antimicrobial prophylaxis for, 1199
　common supplies for, 200t
　dual-modality lithotripters, 244-246
　EHL with, 243.e1
　equipment for, 192, 192f, 193t, 195f, 196t, 198f-199f, 199t
　flexible, 244.e2
　fragmentation, 243.e2
　for genitourinary tuberculosis diagnosis, 1313-1314, 1314f
　indications for, 191-192
　intracorporeal lithotripters used in, 244.e4f
　laser fragmentation, 244.e2
　technique, 199-201, 201f
　ultrasonic lithotripsy, 243.e2
　ureteral injuries with, 1994-1995, 2002
　　avulsion, 2002
　　perforation, 2002
Ureterosigmoidostomy
　for classic bladder exstrophy, 564
　for continent urinary diversions, 706-707
　history of, 3233
　tumor formation and, 699
Ureterostomy
　cutaneous, for megaureter in children, 850-851, 850f
　for ectopic ureter, 819
Ureterotomy, intubated, for ureteropelvic junction obstruction, 1961-1962, 1963f
Ureteroureterostomy, 2207, 2208f
　laparoscopic, 817
　open, 816-817
　for ureteral anomalies, 816-817, 817f, 817b
　for ureteral injuries, upper, 1996-1997, 1997f
　for ureteral stricture disease, 1970-1972
　　laparoscopic or robotic approach, 1972
　　open approach, 1970-1972, 1971f
　　postoperative care, 1972
Ureterovaginal fistula (UVF), 266-267, 2942, 2942b
Ureterovascular fistulae, 2958-2959
Ureterovesical junction (UVJ), 1873, 1877, 2455-2456, 2456f
　with epispadias, 569
　physiology of, 1891, 1892f
Ureters
　bifid, 820-821
　quadruple, 821
　triplication of, 821
Urethra, 315f
　α-adrenergic receptors in, 2500-2501, 2501f
　anatomy of, 2461, 2462f
　　common to both genders, 2466
　　female, 2438-2439, 2439f, 2465-2466, 2466f, 2974-2975, 2974f, 3010
　　male, 1381-1383, 1381f-1384f, 1384b, 1807.e2f, 1807.e4f, 2465, 2465f
　　tone, 2468-2469
　caruncle of, urethral diverticula differentiated from, 2987, 2987f
　closure of, for classic bladder exstrophy, 545-548, 546f-548f
　distraction injuries of, 1807.e2f
　division of, in retropubic radical prostatectomy, 3554-3555, 3555f
　duplication of, 310, 883-884, 884f
　estrogens and, 2503
　female, 152, 1627.e2
　　in orthotopic urinary diversion, 3240-3241, 3240f
　　radical cystectomy and, 3118
　function of
　　during filling/storage, 2521
　　during voiding, 2521
　in genitourinary tuberculosis, 1309
　　treatment, 1318
　hypermobility of, filling/storage failure due to, 2518

Urethra (Continued)
　instability of, filling/storage failure due to, 2518
　localization studies, 1143
　male, 152
　　anatomy of, 1381-1383, 1381f-1384f, 1384b, 1807.e2f, 1807.e4f, 2465, 2465f
　　ultrasonography of, 85-88, 86f, 1384f
　mesh perforation/extrusion at, 2883, 2883b, 2884f-2885f
　　in midurethral sling, 2866-2868, 2867t, 2870b
　mobility of, Q-tip test for, 2529
　necrosis of, with transurethral vaporization of prostate, 3426
　prolapse of, urethral diverticula differentiated from, 2986-2987
　in prune-belly syndrome, 584, 585f
　reconstructive surgery of, 1804-1842, 1805b, 1813b
　　for amyloidosis, 1810
　　anatomy of, 1807, 1807.e1f-1807.e7f
　　for balanitis xerotica obliterans, 939, 940f
　　for circumcision complications, 1811-1812
　　for curvatures of penis, 1836-1838, 1838b
　　for failed epispadias repair, 1813
　　for failed hypospadias repair, 1812-1813
　　for female-to-male transgender, 1841-1842, 1842f
　　for glans dehiscence, 937, 938f
　　for LS, 1808-1810, 1809f
　　for meatal stenosis, 937-938, 1811
　　for paraphimosis, balanitis, and phimosis, 1811
　　penile transplantation, 1838-1842, 1840f, 1842b
　　for PFUIs, 1828-1834, 1830f-1834f
　　principles of, 1804-1807, 1806f-1807f, 1808b
　　for reactive arthritis, 1808
　　for recurrent penile curvature, 939-941, 940f
　　for urethral diverticulum, 938-939, 939f, 1810-1811
　　for urethral hemangioma process, 1808
　　for urethral stricture, 938, 1814-1828, 1814f, 1828b
　　for urethrocutaneous fistula, 935-937, 936f-937f, 1810
　　for vesicourethral distraction defects, 1834b, 1835, 1836b
　stroma of, 2468
　support mechanisms, stress urinary incontinence and, 2596-2597, 2596f
　tone of, in women, 2501
Urethra Resistance Factor (URA), 2566
Urethral advancement procedure, 920, 922f
Urethral atresia, 620-621, 621f
Urethral atrophy, with artificial urinary sphincter, 3007
Urethral bleeding, 257-258
Urethral calculi, 2117-2120
　clinical presentation and evaluation of, 2117-2118
　pathogenesis and composition of, 2117
　primary, 2117
　treatment of, 2118
Urethral cancer
　female, 1782-1785, 1785b
　　anatomy and pathology of, 1782-1785, 1783f
　　epidemiology, etiology, and clinical presentation of, 1782
　　evaluation and staging of, 1783
　　prognosis of, 1783-1784
　　recurrence after cystectomy, 1787-1789, 1789b
　　treatment of, 1784-1785
　male, 1776-1782, 1782b
　　anterior, 1777-1781

Urethral cancer (Continued)
　　carcinoma of penile urethra, 1778-1780, 1779f-1780f
　　epidemiology, etiology, and clinical presentation of, 1776-1777
　　evaluation and staging of, 1777, 1778f, 1778t
　　pathology of, 1777, 1777f, 1777t
　　posterior, 1781-1782, 1782t
　　recurrence after cystectomy, 1785-1787, 1786t, 1789b
　　treatment of, 1778, 1779t
Urethral caruncle, 2920.e10
Urethral catheterization
　after laparoscopic radical prostatectomy, 3579
　antimicrobial prophylaxis for urologic procedures and, 1193b, 1194t-1196t, 1197
Urethral closure pressure profile (UCP), 2563
Urethral compressor, 2438-2439
Urethral dilation
　in mesh complication, 2880
　for neuromuscular dysfunction of lower urinary tract, 637
　as surgical technique
　　for detrusor underactivity, 2663
　　for urethral stricture disease, 1817-1818
　for transmen, 3071
Urethral discharge, patient history of, 7
Urethral diverticula (UD), 2966f, 2975-2992
　anatomy and histology of, 2977, 2978f, 2978t-2980t
　classification of, 2987
　differential diagnosis of, 2983-2987
　　Gartner duct abnormalities, 2986, 2986f
　　periurethral bulking agents, 2987
　　Skene gland abnormalities, 2984-2986, 2986f
　　urethral caruncle, 2987
　　urethral mucosal prolapse, 2986-2987
　　vaginal leiomyoma, 2983-2984, 2985f
　　vaginal wall cysts, 2986, 2986f
　etiology of, 2975-2976, 2975f
　evaluation and diagnosis of, 2981-2982
　　cystourethroscopy, 2982, 2982f
　　history and physical examination, 2981-2982, 2981f
　　urine studies, 2982
　　urodynamics, 2982
　female, 2972-2975, 2974f, 2987b
　imaging of, 2982-2987, 2983f
　management of, 2992b
　pathophysiology of, 2975-2976, 2975f
　presentation of, 2980-2981, 2981b
　prevalence of, 2976-2977
　reconstructive surgery for, 1810-1811
　stress urinary incontinence and, 2988-2992, 2988f
　surgical repair of, 2987-2988
　　alternative techniques for, 2989
　　indications for, 2987-2988
　urethral calculi within, 2977, 2977f
　urethral diverticulectomy for
　　complications of, 2991, 2991f, 2991t
　　excision and reconstruction, 2989, 2989b
　　persistence of symptoms following, 2991-2992
　　postoperative care for, 2991
　　preoperative preparation for, 2989
　　procedure for, 2989-2991, 2990f
　　techniques for, 2989-2992, 2989b
Urethral diverticulectomy, 2989b, 2991-2992, 2991t
Urethral diverticulum, 938-939, 939f
Urethral duplication, 621-622, 621f-622f
Urethral erosion, with artificial urinary sphincter, 3006-3007
Urethral fistula, for transmen, 3070
Urethral hair growth, for transmen, 3072
Urethral hemangioma, reconstructive surgery for, 1808

Urethral injection therapy, for female stress urinary incontinence, 2893
Urethral injury, 3057-3061
　anterior, 3060-3061, 3060.e1f
　　initial management of, 3060
　　delayed reconstruction of, 3060-3061
　　posterior, 3059, 3059f
　distraction, ED with, 3059
　gunshot wounds, 3049-3050
　initial, primary realignment for, 3058-3059, 3058f
　and intraoperative consultation, 298-299
　　diagnosis, 299
　　incidence, 298
　　management, 299
　　mechanisms, 298-299
　with penile fracture, 3048
　posterior, 3057-3060
　　diagnosis of, 3057, 3057f
　　endoscopic treatment, 3059
　　etiology of, 3057, 3057.e1f
　　immediate open, 3056
　　initial management of, 3057-3059
　　suprapubic cystostomy, 3057-3058
　　surgical reconstruction, 3059-3060
　　urethrography for, 3057, 3058f
Urethral instability, filling/storage failure due to, 2518
Urethral lengthening
　for bladder neck reconstruction, 688-690
　results with, 689-690
　technique for, 688-689, 689f
Urethral meatus, 1807.e8
　location of, 907, 907f-908f
Urethral obstruction, after pediatric renal transplantation, 1062-1063, 1062f-1063f
Urethral orifice, 1627.e2
Urethral polyp, 976, 976f
Urethral pressure, during bladder filling, 2515
Urethral pressure profile (UPP)
　micturitional, 2567
　in urodynamic studies, 2557
Urethral pressure profilometry
　urodynamic studies of, 2563-2564, 2564f
Urethral prolapse, 395, 397f, 975-976, 976f
Urethral reconstruction
　in classic bladder exstrophy, 564
　in male epispadias, 569
　for prune-belly syndrome, 592-593, 593f
　pubovaginal sling for, outcomes of, 2845
　for transmen, 3071-3072
Urethral region, natural defenses of, 1137
Urethral slings, stress urinary incontinence and, 2831
Urethral sphincter
　coordination of, urodynamic studies of, 2568-2569, 2569f-2570f
　CVA and, 2603
　deficiency of, intrinsic, 2518
　　quantification of, 2562
　development of, 2466
　disk disease and, 2620
　dynamics of, 682
　female, 2465-2466, 2466f
　male, 2465f
　mechanisms of, urinary incontinence and, 2596-2597, 2596f
　micturition and, 2494
　neurospinal dysraphism and, 2618
　obstruction of, nonrelaxing, 2521
　with Parkinson disease, 2605
　tone of, 2466
Urethral stenosis/atresia, 376
Urethral strictures, 157, 938, 1814-1828, 1814f, 1828b
　after photoselective vaporization of prostate, 3441
　after transurethral microwave therapy, 3430
　anatomic considerations for, 1814

Urethral strictures (Continued)
　with bipolar transurethral resection of prostate, 3419
　decision making, 1817
　diagnosis and evaluation of, 1815-1817, 1816f-1817f
　etiology of, 1814-1815
　with holmium laser enucleation of prostate, 3438
　with monopolar transurethral resection of prostate, 3417-3418
　orthotopic urinary diversion and, 3238
　prior pelvic radiation and, 3238
　for transmen, 3070-3071, 3071f
　treatment, 1817-1818, 1828b
　　augmented anastomosis, 1821-1823, 1826f-1827f
　　dilation, 1817-1818
　　excision and reanastomosis, 1819-1820, 1819f-1820f
　　flap onlay, 1823-1827, 1824f-1825f
　　graft onlay, 1821f-1823f
　　internal urethrotomy, 1818
　　lasers, 1818-1828
　　open reconstruction, 1819-1828
　　perineal urethrostomy, 1827-1828
　　vessel-sparing technique, 1820, 1820f-1821f
Urethral tumors, 1776-1789
　benign, 1776
　　FEPs, 1776
　　hemangiomas, 1776
　　leiomyomas, 1776
　malignant. see Urethral cancer
Urethral valves
　anterior, 620
　posterior, 602-623
　　antenatal management of, 608-610, 610b
　　bladder dysfunction with, 616-619
　　circumcision for, 615
　　clinical presentation of, 608-611
　　delayed presentation of, 611
　　description of, 602, 603f
　　diagnosis of, 607-608, 608b
　　epidemiology of, 602-603, 603b
　　initial management of, 608-611
　　laboratory studies for, 608
　　lower urinary tract and, 603-604, 605f-606f
　　nephroureterectomy, 615
　　pathophysiology of, 603-606, 604t, 606b
　　postnatal management of, 610-611, 611b
　　pulmonary hypoplasia with, 610-611, 610f
　　quality of life with, 620, 623b
　　radionuclide renal scan for, 608
　　renal function prognostic indicators in, 619, 620b
　　surgical intervention for, 611-615, 615b
　　transplantation in, 619-620
　　ultrasonography of, 607, 607f
　　upper tract diversion, 613-614, 615f
　　upper urinary tract and, 604-605, 606f
　　urinomas with, 611, 611f
　　valve ablation for, 611-615, 612f
　　valve bladder syndrome with, 617-619, 617f-618f
　　vesicostomy for, 612-613, 613f-614f
　　vesicoureteral reflux and dysplasia, 606, 606b, 607f
　　vesicoureteral reflux in, 615-616, 619b
　　voiding cystourethrography for, 608, 609f
Urethrectomy
　after cutaneous diversion, 1787, 1788f
　after orthotopic diversion, 1787
Urethritis, 258, 436. see also Nongonococcal urethritis
　in differential diagnosis, 1140-1141
　as STD, 1252-1254

Urethrocutaneous fistula, 935-937, 936f-937f
　reconstructive surgery for, 1810
Urethrography, for posterior urethral injury, 3057, 3058f
Urethrolysis, for voiding dysfunction after pubovaginal sling, 2846, 2847t
Urethromeatoplasty, 918
Urethroplasty
　algorithm for, 912f, 914
　complications of, 934-941, 936t
　　balanitis xerotica obliterans, 939, 940f
　　glans dehiscence, 937, 938f
　　meatal stenosis, 937-938
　　recurrent penile curvature, 939-941, 940f
　　skin, 941
　　urethral diverticulum, 938-939, 939f
　　urethral stricture, 938
　　urethrocutaneous fistula, 935-937, 936f-937f
　genitoperineal transformation, 3066-3068
　hair-bearing skin for, 918
　outcome assessment for, 942-943
　for posterior urethral injury, 3059, 3059.e1f
　tubularized incised plate
　　distal, 923f
　　proximal, 928f
Urethrorrhagia, 622
Urethroscopy, for posterior urethral injury, 3057
Urethrostomy, perineal, for urethral stricture disease, 1827-1828
Urethrotomy, internal, for prune-belly syndrome, 592
Urethrovaginal fistulae, 2868, 2947-2951, 2953b
　diagnosis of, 2948-2950, 2949f-2950f
　etiology of, 2947-2948
　presentation of, 2947-2948, 2948f-2949f
　treatment of, 2950-2951
　　abdominal approach for, 2951
　　complications, 2951
　　follow-up, 2951
　　labial flaps, 2950-2951
　　neourethra, 2950-2951
　　operative technique for, 2951, 2952f
　　posterior approach for, 2951
　　vaginal approach for, 2950
　　vaginal flaps, 2950-2951
Urge suppression, behavioral training with, 2727-2729, 2728f
Urge-Incontinence Impact Questionnaire (U-IIQ), 111t
Urgency urinary incontinence (UUI)
　behavioral therapy with urge suppression for, 2727-2729, 2728f
　definition of, 2539, 2581, 2637, 2638f
　estrogens for, 2709-2710, 2711b
　in mesh complication, 2880
　patient history of, 4-5
　percutaneous tibial nerve stimulation for, 2750
　treatment of, 2544-2546, 2547b
Urge-Urinary Distress Inventory (U-UDI), 111t
Uric acid
　in calcium stone formation, 2023-2024
　in uric acid stone formation, 2026-2029, 2027f-2028f
Uric acid stones, 2058-2059, 2060b
　clinical considerations of, 2058-2059
　diagnosis of, 2060
　low urine pH, 2059, 2059f
　prevention of
　　conservative, 2060
　　medical treatment for, 2060
　in renal calculi, 2026-2029, 2027f-2028f
　hyperuricosuria, 2029
　low urinary volume, 2029
　low urine pH, 2027-2029, 2028f
Uricase, 2026

Urinalysis (UA), 14, 437
  for benign prostatic hyperplasia, 3345
  color of, 14, 15t
  for pelvic floor disorder assessment, 2534
  physical and gross examination, 14
  for RCC, 2157
  for renal calculi, pretreatment assessment, 2070-2071
  specimen collection of, 14
  for sphincteric urinary incontinence, 2995
  turbidity, 14
  for urinary incontinence, in men, 2541
  for urinary tract obstruction, 777
  for UTI diagnosis, 1142
Urinary acidification
  in neonate, 342
  urinary tract obstruction and, 793-794
Urinary ascites, 384
Urinary bladder, surgery of, 3010
Urinary catheters, falls and, 2915
Urinary complications, 262-263
Urinary continence
  after robotic radical prostatectomy, 3581-3582, 3581f-3582f
  physiology of, 2593-2595
Urinary dipstick, sensitivity of, 16
Urinary diversion
  in antegrade nephroureteroscopic, for UTUC, 2219
  cutaneous continent. see Cutaneous continent urinary diversion
  for detrusor underactivity, 2663
  for hypospadias postoperative management, 932
  minimally invasive. see Minimally invasive urinary diversion
  for neuromuscular dysfunction of lower urinary tract, 636-637
  orthotopic. see Orthotopic urinary diversion
  for posterior urethral valves, 613-614, 615f
  for urinary incontinence, in geriatric patients, 2920.e5
Urinary fistula
  with anorectal malformation, 622-623, 622f
  partial nephrectomy causing, 2265
  with ureterointestinal anastomoses in urinary intestinal diversion, 3186t, 3191-3192
Urinary flow rate, with postvoid residual, 2565
Urinary fractionated metanephrines, in evaluation of adrenal masses, 2402-2403, 2402t
Urinary free cortisol (UFC) evaluation, in evaluation of adrenal masses, 2400-2401
Urinary hesitancy, 4
Urinary incontinence (UI), 109-110, 399-400, 1083, 2580-2599. see also Pelvic floor disorders
  after retropubic radical prostatectomy, 3564
  aging and, 2582-2583
  anogenital herpes and, 2622
  associated with chronic retention, 2540
  with benign prostatic hyperplasia, 3335
  with brain tumor, 2604
  causes of, 2526
  classification of, 2580
  coital, 2540
  conservative management of, 2722-2738
    adherence to, 2734-2735
    assessment for, 2722-2723
    behavioral training with urge suppression, 2727-2729, 2728f
    biofeedback for, 2727.e1f, 2729, 2729f, 2729.e1f-2729.e2f
    bladder training, 2728f, 2730-2732, 2730.e1t
    indications for, 2722
    lifestyle modifications, 2722, 2722.e1b
    patient education for, 2723
    for pelvic floor dysfunction, 2732-2735
    pelvic floor muscle electrical stimulation, 2729-2730

Urinary incontinence (UI) (Continued)
    pelvic floor muscle training for. see Pelvic floor muscle training
    for prevention, 2735-2736
    toileting programs for, 2730-2731, 2730.e1t
  continuous, 2540, 2581
  CVA and, 2602
  daytime. see Bladder and bowel dysfunction
  definition of, 2539, 2580
  diagnosis of, 2526
  diet and, 2586
  epidemiology of, 2581-2582
  female
    retropubic suspension surgery for. see Retropubic suspension surgery
    urethra and, 2466
    use of injectable agents for, 2890-2891, 2891t
  female sexual dysfunction and, 1655-1656
  general comments on, 2581-2582
  in geriatric patients, 2917-2920
    absorbent products for, 2920.e6
    behavioral therapies for, 2920.e3
    clinical evaluation of, 2920
    costs of, 2918
    established, 2919
    history for, 2920.e1
    laboratory testing for, 2920.e2
    negative impacts of, 2918-2919
    pharmacotherapies for, 2920.e3-2920.e4
    physical examination for, 2920.e1
    PVR assessment, 2920.e1
    risk factors of, 2918
    surgical therapies for, 2920.e4-2920.e6
    transient, 2919
    treatment of, 2920
    urine containment for, 2920.e6
    urodynamic studies for, 2920.e2
    voiding diaries, 2920.e1-2920.e2
  giggle, 2540
  hammock hypothesis of, 2466, 2518, 2596, 2597b
  herpesvirus infection and, 2621-2622
  hormonal therapy and, 2585
  incidence of, 2582, 2582b
  insensible, 2540
  lower urinary tract dysfunction and, 655-660, 660b
  male, 2539-2549, 2539b
    cause of, 2993
    classification of, 2993-2998
    diagnosis of, 2995-2998
    epidemiology of, 2587
    etiology of, 2993-2998
    evaluation of, 2540-2544, 2544b, 2995-2998, 2996f, 2998b
    first-line investigations for, 2540-2544
    history and development of devices, 2993-2994, 2994f
    history for, 2540
    implantation device technique, 3000-3005
    improving quality of evidence, 3009
    incidence of, 2587
    indications for surgery, 2998-2999, 2999b
    innovations and emerging concepts in device design, 2994-2995
    management of, 2544-2547, 2545f, 2548f-2549f
    mechanisms of continence with surgical devices, 2995
    pathophysiology of, 2993-2998
    physical examination for, 2540
    prevalence of, 2587
    principal methods in, 2544
    remission rates of, 2587
    risk factors for, 2587
    sphincteric, 2993-3009. see also Sphincteric urinary incontinence
    training paradigms of, 3009

Urinary incontinence (UI) (Continued)
    mechanical devices for, 2736-2737
      intravaginal, 2736-2737, 2736.e1f, 2737f, 2737.e1f
    medical conditions and, 2586
    mixed, 2539, 2581
      treatment of, 2547
    neurospinal dysraphism and, 2618
    nocturnal enuresis, 2539, 2581
      treatment of, 2547
    in nursing home setting, 2919-2920
    obesity and, 2585-2586
    pathophysiology of, 2595-2596
      bladder storage and, 2595
      sphincteric function, 2595-2596
    patient history of, 4-6, 8t
    pelvic organ prolapse and, 2591-2592, 2592b
    physiology of, 2593-2595
    postmicturition leakage or dribble, 2540
      treatment of, 2547
    postpartum, PFMT for, 2726
    pregnancy and, 2583
    prevalence of
      in adult women, 2581-2582, 2583f
      urinary urge incontinence, 2585f
      worldwide, 2584f
    questionnaires for, 2532t-2533t, 2582
    race and ethnicity and, 2583-2585
    radiation therapy and, 3606
    remission of, 2582, 2582b
    risk factors for, 2582-2586, 2586b
    signs and symptoms of, 2580
    smoking and, 2586
    social impact of, 2592, 2592b
    societal costs of, 2592, 2592b
    stress. see Stress urinary incontinence (SUI)
    terminology of, 2580-2581, 2581t
    types of, 2539-2540
    ureteral anomalies and, 802
    urethral diverticula and, 2982
    urgency, 2539, 2581, 2637, 2638f
      treatment of, 2544-2546
    urodynamic observations of, 2580
    in women, 2581-2582
Urinary intestinal diversion
  bowel preparation for, 3162-3169, 3169b
    antibiotic, 3164-3165, 3164t-3165t
    diarrhea and pseudomembranous enterocolitis with, 3165, 3166t
    mechanical, 3163-3164, 3163t
  complications of, urinary fistula, 3186t, 3191-3192
  conduit urinary diversion types, 3193-3198, 3198b
    colon conduit, 3196-3197, 3196f, 3198t
    ileal conduit, 3193-3196, 3194f-3195f, 3195t
    ileal vesicostomy, 3197-3198
    jejunal conduit, 3195-3196, 3196t
    management of, 3195f, 3198
  intestinal anastomoses for. see Intestinal anastomoses, in urinary intestinal diversion
  intestinal segments in, 3160-3205
  metabolic problems of, 3198-3205, 3205b
    altered sensorium, 3201
    cancer, 3203-3204
    drug absorption abnormalities, 3201
    electrolyte abnormalities, 3199-3201, 3199t, 3200f
    growth and development, 3202
    infection, 3202
    intestinal motility, 3203
    nutritional problems, 3203
    osteomalacia, 3201-3202
    short bowel, 3203
    stones, 3202

Urinary intestinal diversion *(Continued)*
  neuromechanical aspects of intestinal segments in, 3204-3205
    motor activity, 3204-3205, 3204f
    volume-pressure considerations, 3204, 3204f
  postoperative recovery of, 3162-3169, 3169b
  renal deterioration in, 3180t, 3192-3193, 3193b
  selection for, 3161-3162, 3162b
  surgical anatomy for, 3160-3161, 3161b
    of colon, 3160-3161, 3161f
    of small bowel, 3160
    of stomach, 3160
  ureterointestinal anastomoses, 3184-3192. *see also* Ureterointestinal anastomosis, for urinary diversion
Urinary lithiasis. *see also* Renal calculi
  calcium-based calculi in, 2048-2049, 2049b
    dietary, 2049
  classification of, 2046-2048
    animal protein for, 2047-2048, 2048b
    fluid recommendation for, 2047
    general recommendation for, 2047-2048
  cystinuria in, 2060-2068, 2063b
    ammonium acid urate stones, 2066
    bladder calculi, medical management of, 2066-2067
    clinical considerations of, 2060-2061
    compliance and quality of life, 2062-2063
    conservative strategies of, 2061
    drug-containing calculi, 2065-2066, 2066t
    follow-up of, 2062
    infection calculi, 2063-2065, 2063f, 2064t, 2065b
    medical therapy for, 2061-2062
    metabolic stone formation, 2066
    miscellaneous and drug-induced stones, 2065, 2065b
  distal renal tubular acidosis (type 1) in, 2055-2056, 2055f
    causes of, 2055b
    chronic diarrheal states, 2055-2056
  epidemiology and morbidity from, 2036, 2036b
  evaluation of, 2036-2068
  hypercalciuria in, 2050-2053
    calcium supplementation, 2050-2051
    clinical considerations of, 2050
    conservative strategies for, 2051
    idiopathic, 2051b
    medical therapy for, 2051-2053, 2053b
    resorptive, 2050, 2050b
    in sarcoidosis and granulomatous disease, 2050
  hyperoxaluria, 2056-2060, 2057b
    calcium stone formation, 2057-2058
    clinical considerations of, 2056
    conservative strategies for, 2056-2057, 2057b
    diabetes, obesity, and metabolic syndrome, 2059-2060
    enteric, 2056
    hypomagnesuric calcium nephrolithiasis, 2058t
    medical therapy for, 2057
    primary, 2056-2057
    uric acid stones, 2058-2059
  hypocitraturia in, 2053-2056, 2054b, 2055f
    clinical considerations of, 2053
    conservative strategies for, 2053-2054
    distal renal tubular acidosis (type 1) in, 2055-2056, 2055f
    medical therapy for, 2054
    thiazide-induced hypocitraturia, 2056
  imaging for, 2036-2039, 2039b
    computed tomography, 2037-2038, 2037f, 2037t
    modalities, 2038-2039

Urinary lithiasis *(Continued)*
    radiography, 2038
    ultrasound, 2038, 2039f
  medical management of, 2036-2068
    follow-up considerations in, 2067-2068, 2067f
  metabolic evaluation for, 2039-2045
    24-hour urine collection, 2043-2044, 2044f
    economics of, 2044-2045, 2045b
    of first-time stone former, 2039
    for high-risk and recurrent stone formers, 2042-2043, 2043b
    of high-risk stone former, 2040b, 2043b
    in newly diagnosed stone formers, 2040-2041, 2040b-2041b, 2041t, 2042f
    patient selection for, 2040b
    stone analysis in, 2045-2046, 2045t, 2046f, 2046b
Urinary markers, 25-26
  for urothelial cancer, 3109
Urinary metabolic abnormalities, of pediatric kidney stone disease, 857-858
  cystinuria, 859
  hypercalciuria, 857-858, 858t
  hyperoxaluria, 858, 858t
  hyperuricosuria, 858t, 859
  hypocitraturia, 858-859
  primary hyperoxaluria, 858
  secondary hyperoxaluria, 858-859
Urinary oxalate, 2010
Urinary prothrombin fragment 1 (F1), in crystal formation, 2015
Urinary retention, 384, 385f, 2980
  after CVA, 2602
  after monopolar transurethral resection of prostate, 3418
  after orthotopic urinary diversion, 3254, 3254b
  with artificial urinary sphincter, 3005
  with botulinum toxins, 2709
  with brain tumor, 2604
  detrusor underactivity and, 2657
  in geriatric patients, 2920.e7-2920.e8
  with herpesvirus infections, 2621-2622
  lower urinary tract dysfunction and, 2629
  neuromodulation for, 2510
  postoperative, lower urinary tract dysfunction and, 2629-2630
  risk factors for, 2880
  with spinal cord injury, 648-649
  with spinal shock, 2610
  with subacute combined degeneration, 2619-2620
  with transurethral incision of prostate, 3435
Urinary sediment, in urinalysis, 21
Urinary sheaths, 2920.e6
Urinary sphincter, artificial
  complications with, 3005-3008, 3008b
  evaluation of persistent incontinence after, 2997-2998
  history and development of, 2994, 2994f
  implantation technique, 3000, 3001f, 3003f
  infection, 3005-3006
  long-term results with, 3008, 3009b
Urinary storage symptoms
  after monopolar transurethral resection of prostate, 3418
  after photoselective vaporization of prostate, 3441
Urinary toxicity, prostate cancer and, 3604-3606
Urinary tract
  anaerobes in, 1133
  anatomic and physiologic changes during pregnancy, 1185-1186
  defecation disorders and, 667, 668f
  defects in, in bladder exstrophy, 535-537

Urinary tract *(Continued)*
  dysfunction of, 680-681
  fistulae of. *see* Fistulae
  functional, 680-681
    active voiding phase, 680
    passive storage phase, 680
  functional assessment of, 1047-1048
  lower. *see* Lower urinary tract
  natural defenses against UTIs, 1137-1139
    bladder, 1138-1139
    periurethral and urethral region, 1137
    urine, 1137
  trocar injury to, in midurethral sling, 2866-2873
  upper. *see* Upper urinary tract
Urinary tract dilation, 358, 362-366
  fetal cystoscopy, 364-365
  grading system, 361, 361f, 362b
  lower urinary tract obstruction, prenatal intervention for, 362-364, 363t, 365f-366f
  P1 (lower risk), 370, 371b
  P2 (intermediate risk), 370-371
  P3 (high risk), 371
  prenatal management, 362-366
  risk stratification and management for prenatal urinary tract dilation, 362, 363f-364f
  vesicoamniotic shunt placement *versus* fetal cystoscopy, 365-366, 367f
Urinary tract imaging, 28-67, 91-100
  conventional radiography, 28
  infection imaging, 96
  radiation management, in uroradiology, 28-29
Urinary tract infections (UTIs), 371-372, 372f, 372b, 398-399, 402b, 475-476, 1129-1201
  adherence in, 428-429
  after augmentation cystoplasty, 699
  after mid-urethral sling surgery, 2873-2874
  after photoselective vaporization of prostate, 3441
  antimicrobial prophylaxis for common urologic procedures and, 1193-1201, 1193b, 1194t-1196t, 1201t, 1201b
    for lower tract endoscopy, 1198
    for open and laparoscopic surgery, 1199-1200
    principles of, 1193-1197, 1193b, 1194t-1196t
    for shock wave lithotripsy, 1198
    special considerations, 1200-1201, 1201t
    for transurethral resection of prostate and bladder, 1198-1199
    for TRUSP biopsy, 1197-1198
    for upper tract endoscopy, 1199
    for urethral catheterization and removal, 1193b, 1194t-1196t, 1197
    for urodynamics, 1197
  antimicrobial therapy for
    agent selection in, 1155-1157, 1186-1187, 1187t
    antimicrobial formulary for, 1150-1155, 1150t-1153t, 1155f
    bacterial resistance to, 1144-1146, 1145t-1146t, 1147b
    duration of, 1155
    principles of, 1149-1155, 1155f, 1155b
    prophylaxis, 1130, 1162-1163
    suppression, 1130
  bacteremia and, 1182-1187, 1184b
  bacterial factors of, 430b
  bacteriuria in elderly, 1188-1190, 1190b
    asymptomatic, 1147-1149, 1147t, 1147b-1149b
    diagnosis, 1188-1189
    epidemiology, 1188
    management, 1189-1190, 1189t
    pathogenesis, 1188
    screening for, 1188

Urinary tract infections (UTIs) (Continued)
  bacteriuria in pregnancy, 1184–1185, 1188b
    anatomic and physiologic changes and, 1185–1186, 1185t, 1186f
    complications of, 1186–1187
    management of, 1186–1187, 1187t
    pathogenesis, 1185
    renal insufficiency and, 1187.e1
  with benign prostatic hyperplasia, 3336
  bladder infections, 1155–1166
  catheter-associated bacteriuria, 1190, 1191b
  clean intermittent catheterization and, 625
  definitions of, 426, 1129–1131, 1130f, 1131b
  Escherichia coli causing, 428, 429f
  evaluation, 1140–1143, 1140b, 1143b
    diagnosis, 1141–1143, 1141b, 1142.e1t, 1143f
    symptoms and signs, 1140–1141
  Fournier gangrene, 1182, 1182b
  genitourinary malignancies, 2920
  in geriatric patients, 2920.e10–2920.e11
  HIV and, 1265–1266
  imaging techniques, 1143–1144, 1144b
    CT, 1144, 1168
    indications, 1144b
    MRI, 1144
    radionuclide studies, 1144.e1
    ultrasonography, 1144, 1168, 1168f
    voiding cystourethrogram, 1144
  incidence and epidemiology, 1131, 1131b, 1132f
  kidney infections. *see* Kidney infections
  management of, during pregnancy, 293–294
  pathogenesis, 426–430, 1131–1140, 1140b
    alterations in host defense mechanisms, 1139–1140
    bacterial virulence factors, 1133–1134
    early events in UPEC pathogenesis, 1134–1135, 1134f
    epithelial cell receptivity, 1135–1137
    fastidious organisms, 1133
    natural defenses of urinary tract against, 1137–1139
    phase variation of bacterial pili in vivo, 1135.e1, 1135.e1f
    routes of infection, 1131
    urinary pathogens, 1132, 1133f
  in pediatric patients, 426–446, 653
    antibiotics for, 434
    bacterial factors leading to, 427–428
    classification of, 433–435, 435b
      acute renal abscess, 435
      asymptomatic bacteriuria, 434–435
      bacterial nephritis, 435, 435f
      pyonephrosis, 435
    complicated, 433
    diagnosis of, 426b, 435–440, 438b
      catheter insertion for, 436–437
      computed tomography, 440
      laboratories for, 436–438, 438b
      magnetic resonance imaging, 440
      physical examination, 436
      radiographic imaging for, 438–440, 439t, 440b
      serum tests for, 438
      symptoms of, 435–436, 438b
      ^{99m}Tc-Dimercaptosuccinic acid, 440
      ultrasound for, 439
      urinalysis for, 437
      urine collection methods for, 436–437
      urine culture, 437–438
      urine dipstick tests, 437
      urine microscopic examination, 437
      voiding cystourethrogram, 439–440
    host risk factors leading to, 430–433, 433b
      age, 430
      anatomic abnormalities, 432
      bladder and bowel dysfunction, 432, 443–444
      circumcision, 431

Urinary tract infections (UTIs) (Continued)
    fecal and perineal bacterial colonization, 431–432
    gender, 430
    genetics, 431
    iatrogenic factors, 433
    immune status, 433
    neurogenic bladder, 432–433
    race, 430–431
    sexual activity, 432
    vesicoureteral reflux, 432
  management of, 440–442
    after, 442–444
    antibiotic duration for, 441
    antibiotic selection, 441–442, 441t–442t
    antibiotic treatment for, 440–441
    inpatient, 441
    outpatient, 441
    prophylactic antibiotics, 443
    vesicoureteral reflux, 444
  nosocomial, 433
  pathogenesis of, 426–430
  recurrent, 434
  sequelae of, 444–445, 445b
    long-term, 444–445
    renal scarring, 444
    xanthogranulomatous pyelonephritis (XGP), 444
  uncommon, 445
    funguria, 445
    viral cystitis, 445
  uncomplicated, 433
  upper, 433–434
periurethral abscess, 1182, 1182b
recurrent, 434
renal calculi and, 2088
in renal transplantation, 1059
risk factors, 1156b
sepsis and, 1182–1187, 1183b–1184b
septic shock and, 1182–1187, 1184b
sexual activity and, 432
with spinal cord injury, 2615
  management of, 1191–1192, 1192b
symptoms of, 435–436, 438b
transient urinary incontinence and, 2919.e1
typical, 427
uncomplicated, 428f
unresolved, 1159, 1159b
urethritis and, 436
virulence factors of, 428
Urinary tract injury, during laparoscopic and robotic surgery, 230.e1
Urinary tract obstruction
  cation transport and, 794
  clinical impact of, 794–795, 794b
  clinical presentation in, 776
    children, 776
  compensatory renal growth with, 794–795
  congenital
    antegrade pyelography for, 781
    retrograde pyelography for, 780–781
    Whitaker test for, 780
  definition of, 776–777
  diagnostic imaging for, 778–781, 781b
    computed tomography, 779–780
    excretory urography, 780
    magnetic resonance urography, 780
    nuclear renography, 779
    ultrasonography, 778–779
  emerging therapeutic options for, 790
  hemodynamic changes with, 791–792, 793b
    bilateral ureteral obstruction, 791–792, 792f
    glomerular filtration and, 791
    partial ureteral obstruction, 792
    renal blood flow, 791–792
    renal vascular resistance, 791–792
    unilateral ureteral obstruction, 791, 791f
  hydrogen ion transport and, 793–794
  hypertension with, 794

Urinary tract obstruction (Continued)
  laboratory studies for, 777–778
    biomarkers of, 778
    fractional excretion of sodium, 777
    renal function assessment, 777–778
    urinalysis, 777
  pathological changes of, 781–786
  pathophysiology of, 776–797
  postobstructive diuresis after, 796
  prevalence of, 776
  progressive renal dysfunction and, 776, 777f
  renal recovery after, 795–796
  sodium transport and, 793
  treatment of, 795–796, 797b
    pain management, 795
    renal drainage, 795
    surgical intervention for, 796
  tubular function effects of, 792–794
  tubulointerstitial fibrosis with, 786–790, 790b
  urinary acidification and, 793–794
  urinary concentration ability with, 793
  urine egress from kidney in, 794
  Whitaker test for, 780
Urinary tract reconstruction
  for cloacal exstrophy, 578–579
    modern staged, 578, 578t
    osteotomy role in, 578–579, 579f
    single-stage, 579
  in pediatric patients
    antireflux, 683–685, 685b
    augmentation cystoplasty for, 691–706, 702b. *see also* Augmentation cystoplasty
    bladder neck reconstruction, 685–690, 690b
    continent urinary diversions, 706–713, 711b. *see also* Continent urinary diversions
    patient evaluation for, 681–682, 683b
    patient preparation for, 682–683, 683b
    summary for, 713
    urodynamics for, 681–682
Urinary tract trauma, upper, 1982–2004
Urinary urgency
  with holmium laser enucleation of prostate, 3438
  patient history of, 3–4
Urine
  abnormalities, in BPS/IC etiology, 1232.e9–1232.e10
  acidification of, urinary tract obstruction and, 793–794
  analysis. *see* Urinalysis
  chemical examination of, 15–27, 25b–27b
    additional serum studies, 26
    bacteria, 23, 24f
    Berger disease, 17
    bilirubin and urobilinogen, 20
    blood/hematuria, 16
    casts, 23, 23f–24f
    cells, 21–23, 21f–23f
    crystals, 23, 24f
    CT and MRI, 27
    cystometrography and multichannel urodynamic studies, 26–27
    cystourethroscopy, 26
    expressed prostatic secretions, 24, 25f
    glomerular hematuria, 16–17, 16t, 17f
    glucose and ketones, 19–20
    intravenous pyelogram, and plain radiographs, 27
    leukocyte esterase and nitrite tests, 20–21, 20f
    microscopy technique, 21
    nonglomerular hematuria, 17–18
    office diagnostic procedures, 26
    parasites, 24, 25f
    pH, 15–16
    prostate-specific antigen, 25
    proteinuria, 15t, 18–19
    radiologic imaging, 27
    serum laboratory studies, 25
    specific gravity and osmolality, 15

Urine *(Continued)*
　ultrasonography, 27
　urinary markers, 25–26
　urinary sediment, 21
　uroflowmetry and ultrasound, for postvoid residual, 26
　yeast, 22f, 23
　concentration of, with urinary tract obstruction, 793
　crystallization in, 2009
　culture, for UTI diagnosis, 1142–1143, 1143f
　egress from kidney, in urinary tract obstruction, 794
　natural defenses of, 1137
　pH, low
　　in calcium stone formation, 2024–2025
　　in uric acid stone formation, 2027–2029, 2028f
　physical and gross examination of, 14
　volume of, low, in uric acid stone formation, 2029
Urine containment, for urinary incontinence, in geriatric patients, 2920.e6
Urine culture, 437–438
　reconstruction and, 682
Urine cytology
　of bladder tumor, 3079, 3079f, 3080t
　endoscopic evaluation and collection of, 2211
　for non–muscle-invasive bladder cancer surveillance, 3109
　for UTUC diagnosis, 2192
Urine dipstick tests, 437
Urine flow rate, male urinary incontinence and, 2543
Urine leaks
　after partial nephrectomy, 263–264
　after upper tract urologic surgery, 263–264
　indications for intervention for, 1071
　with intestinal anastomoses, 3180t
　management, 263–264, 264f–265f
　persistent, 1070
　renal exploration with repair of, 1072
　risk factors and diagnosis, 263, 264f
Urine microscopic examination, 437
Urine transport, 1891–1894
　bladder filling and neurogenic vesical dysfunction effects on, 1893
　diuresis effects, 1893
　ureteropelvic junction, physiology of, 1891, 1892f
　ureterovesical junction, physiology of, 1893–1894
　urinary bolus propulsion in, 1892–1893, 1893f
Urine-based biomarkers, 3485–3487
Urinoma
　hematoma compared with, 1988
　for pediatric genitourinary trauma, 1071, 1071f
　with posterior urethral valves, 611, 611f
Urobilinogen, in urine, 20
Urocutaneous fistulae, 2962
Urodynamic catheters, 155
Urodynamic observations, of urinary incontinence, 2580
Urodynamic stress incontinence (USI), 2543
Urodynamic stress test, 2562
Urodynamic studies (UDS), 2550–2579
　of acute urinary retention, 3338, 3338f
　after radical pelvic surgery, 2620–2621
　ambulatory, 2571–2574
　　clinical utility of, 2571–2574
　analysis and interpretation in, 2559–2569, 2569b
　antimicrobial prophylaxis for, 1197
　for benign prostatic hyperplasia, 3347
　of bladder diverticula, 2967
　clinical applications of, evidence-based, 2574–2578
　　guidelines, 2574

Urodynamic studies (UDS) *(Continued)*
　in lower urinary tract symptoms, 2576–2577
　in neurogenic lower urinary tract dysfunction, 2577–2578
　in stress incontinence in women, 2574–2576
　in clinical practice, 2550–2551, 2551b
　components of, 2556–2557, 2557f
　conduction of, 2551–2554
　cystometrogram in, 2556, 2557f
　definition of, 2550
　of detrusor underactivity, 2650, 2651f
　electromyography in, 2557, 2559
　equipment for, 2557–2559, 2559b
　eyeball, 2534
　of filling and storage phase, 2552t–2553t, 2559
　　detrusor overactivity and impaired compliance, 2560–2561, 2560f–2561f
　　leak point pressures, 2561–2563, 2562f–2563f
　　normal, 2559–2560, 2559f
　　occult stress incontinence, 2563
　　stress-induced detrusor overactivity, 2563, 2563f
　　urethral pressure profilometry, 2563–2564, 2564f
　guidelines for, 2550
　key points of, 2578b
　for male urinary incontinence, 2543–2544
　of MS, 2607
　multichannel, 2536, 2565f
　neurologic injury and, 2612–2614
　in overactive bladder, 2645
　Parkinson disease and, 2605
　for pelvic floor disorders assessment, 2534–2536, 2536b
　postvoid residual in, 2556
　preparation for, 2551–2554, 2554b–2556b
　pressure-flow studies in, 2557
　room for, 2552–2553
　rules for, 2551
　signal transmission and transducers for, 2558
　of sphincteric urinary incontinence, 2997
　terminology for, 2554b–2556b
　of urethral diverticula, 2982
　urethral pressure profile in, 2557
　of urinary incontinence, in geriatric patients, 2920.e2
　for urinary tract reconstruction, in pediatric patients, 681–682
　uroflowmetry in, 2556, 2557f, 2558–2559
　video. *see* Videourodynamics
　of voiding and emptying phase, 2564–2566
　　bladder outlet obstruction in men, 2566–2567, 2567f
　　bladder outlet obstruction in women, 2567–2568
　　normal, 2564–2565, 2564f–2565f
　　sphincter coordination, 2568–2569, 2569f–2570f
　　voiding pressure-flow studies, 2565–2566, 2566f
　of voiding dysfunction, functional classification and, 2551
Urodynamic systems, 2557–2558
Urodynamic testing
　setup, 480–486, 480f
　in urine, 26
Uroenteric fistulae, 2952–2953
　pyeloenteric, 2953–2955, 2953f
　urethrovaginal. *see* Urethrovaginal fistulae
　vesicoenteric, 2953t. *see also* Vesicoenteric fistulae
Uroflow, 942
Uroflowmetry
　for benign prostatic hyperplasia, 3346–3347, 3346f

Uroflowmetry *(Continued)*
　test equipment, 480–481, 480f–481f
　in urodynamic studies, 2556, 2557f, 2558–2559
Urogenital Distress Inventory, 110, 111t
Urogenital hiatus, 2434
Urogenital imaging, pediatric, 403–425
　computed tomography for, 416–418
　conventional radiography, 415
　DMSA renal cortical scintigraphy, 418
　magnetic resonance imaging for, 412–415
　technique of, 403
　　ionizing, 403, 403b
　　nonionizing, 403, 403b
　ultrasonography for, 404–412
Urogenital sinus, 380–382
　abnormalities of, 1019b
　　classification of, 1019–1025, 1020f–1021f
　　evaluation of, 1019–1021, 1022b
　　history and physical examination for, 1021–1022
　　outcomes of reconstruction, 1037b
　　radiographic and endoscopic evaluation of, 1023–1025, 1023f–1024f
　　urogenital mobilization, 1036b
　formation of, 320t, 328, 330f–331f
　surgical reconstruction of. *see* Reconstructive surgery, for disorders of sex development and urogenital sinus
Urogenital triangle
　female, 2434
　male, 2450, 2451f
Urogynecologic fistulae, 2946
　ureterovaginal, 2942, 2942b
　urethrovaginal, 2947–2951
　vesicouterine, 2946–2947, 2947b
　vesicovaginal, 2924–2926
Urolithiasis
　CT and, 48, 49f
　lithotripsy for. *see* Lithotripsy
　medical management, 350–351, 351b
　in pregnancy, 286–288, 288b
　　etiology, 286
　　evaluation, 286–288
　ureteroscopy for, 191
Urologic cancer, in geriatric patients, 2920.e13
Urologic considerations, in pregnancy, 282–295
Urologic disorders, and metabolic syndrome, 1420–1422
　bladder cancer, 1421
　low testosterone and erectile dysfunction, 1422
　lower urinary tract symptoms, 1421
　overactive bladder, 1421
　prostate cancer, 1421–1422
　renal insufficiency, 1420
　renal stones, 1420–1421
　tumor, 1421
Urologic evaluation of child, 388–402
Urologic malignancy, during pregnancy, 292–293
　angiomyolipoma, 293
　bladder tumors, 293
　renal tumors, 292–293
Urologic oncology, nuclear medicine in, 42–44
Urologic patient, evaluation of, 1–27, 13b, 27b
Urologic surgeon, 145
Urologic surgery
　adverse events during, 145
　blood products for, 147–148
　　biologically active agents, 148
　　component therapy, 147
　　dry matrix agents, 147
　　hemostatic agents, 147
　　massive transfusion protocol, 147
　　packed red blood cells, 147
　complications of, 260–281, 281b
　　bowel injury, 275–281, 276f
　　classification of, 260–261

Urologic surgery (Continued)
　　Clavien-Dindo scale, 260-261, 261t
　　lower tract urinary, 267-269
　　neuromuscular, 261-262
　　physiologic, 261
　　positional, 261-262
　　ureteral injury, 264-267
　　urinary, 262-263
　　urine leaks, after upper tract urologic surgery, 263-264
　　vascular, 269-275, 270f
　drains during, 148
　　Blake, 148
　　Jackson-Pratt, 148
　　Penrose, 148
　　pigtail, 148
　hypothermia during, 145
　incision closure for, 148-151
　　fascial closure techniques, 150-151
　　retention sutures, 151
　　skin closure, 150-151
　lithotomy position during, 146
　patient environment during, 145-147
　patient positioning in, 146-147
　patient safety during, 145
　patient temperature during, 145
　physiologic complication in, 261
　preventable injuries during, 145
　principles of, 119-151, 134b, 144b, 151b
　　abdominal incisions, 135-136
　　flank incision, 138-140
　　hepatobiliary evaluation, 121
　　incisions for specific surgeries, 141-144
　　inguinal incisions, 140-141
　　intraoperative management, 125-134
　　kidney and retroperitoneum anterior approaches, 136-138, 138f, 139t
　　preoperative evaluation, 119
　　preparation, 123-125
　　presurgical testing, 119
　　pulmonary evaluation, 120-121
　　special populations, 121-123
　skin preparation in, 145
　suture material for, 148-151, 149t
　　absorbable, 149-150
　　Biosyn, 149
　　Caprosyn, 149
　　nonabsorbable, 150
　　plain gut and chronic gut, 149
　　poliglecaprone, 149
　　polyamide (Nylon), 150
　　polydioxanone, 150
　　polyester (Mersilene), 150
　　polyglactin 910, 149-150
　　polyglyconate, 150
　　polypropylene (Prolene), 150
　　silk, 150-151
Urology
　assessing surgical complications in, 105-106, 106t
　　pain in, 108
　　risk of, 106-108
　commonly assessed short-term outcomes in, 105-108
　conceptual framework for assessing the effectiveness of treatment and improving care in, 101-102
　geriatric syndromes and, 2913-2917
　　asymptomatic bacteriuria, 2920.e10-2920.e11
　　bladder outlet obstruction, 2920.e7
　　delirium, 2914
　　falls, 2915
　　fecal incontinence, 2920.e9
　　frailty, 2913-2914, 2913f
　　genitourinary malignancies, 2920
　　genitourinary trauma, 2920.e11
　　hematuria, 2920.e11
　　medication optimization, 2915-2917, 2916t-2917t
　　neurogenic bladder, 2920.e7-2920.e8

Urology (Continued)
　　nocturia, 2920.e8-2920.e9
　　pelvic organ prolapse, 2920.e9-2920.e10
　　polypharmacy, 2915-2917
　　pressure ulcers, 2915
　　underactive bladder, 2920.e7-2920.e8
　　urinary incontinence, 2917-2920
　　urinary retention, 2920.e7-2920.e8
　　urinary tract infections, 2920.e10-2920.e11
　health care costs, 114, 114b
　health-related quality of life in, 112-113, 113t
　long-term disease outcomes commonly assessed in, 102-105
　outcomes of interest in, 113-114
　patient satisfaction, 113
　patient-reported outcomes in, 108-113
　specific symptom scales, 109-113
UroLume stent, for urethral stricture disease, 1819
Uropathogenic bacteria, 427-428, 430f
Uropathogenic E. coli (UPEC), 1132
　pathogenesis, early events in, 1134-1135, 1134f
　persistence, in bladder, 1136-1137, 1138f
Uroplakin III, vesicoureteral reflux and, 491.e1
Uroplakins, of bladder urothelium, 2462
Uropontin, in crystal formation, 2014-2015
Uroradiology, radiation management in, 28-29, 29t
Uroselectivity, 2680-2681
Urothelial cancer. see also Bladder tumors
　detection of, 3078-3081, 3081b, 3092
　direct extension of, 3084
　with divergent differentiation, of urothelial cancer, 3088-3089
　economic impact of, 3075
　epidemiology of, 3073-3075, 3074f-3075f
　　gender, racial, and age differences, 3073-3075
　　incidence of, 3073
　　mortality of, 3073
　　prevalence of, 3073
　histologic variants of, 3087-3090, 3088b
　　clear cell, 3087-3088
　　micropapillary, 3088, 3088f
　　nested variant, 3088, 3089f
　　plasmacytoid, 3088
　　sarcomatoid, 3088
　pathological grading of, 3092, 3092f-3093f
　pathological staging of, 3091-3092
　pathology of, 3076t, 3081-3087, 3091-3094, 3092t
　　cystitis cystica, 3082, 3082f
　　cystitis glandularis, 3082, 3082f
　　epithelial metaplasia, 3081
　　inverted papilloma, 3081
　　leukoplakia, 3082
　　malignant lesions, 3083-3084, 3083f-3084f
　　molecular biology of, 3084-3087, 3087f
　　nephrogenic adenoma, 3082
　　papilloma, 3081, 3081f-3082f
　　precursor malignant lesions, 3082-3083, 3083f
　　staging, 3084, 3085t-3086t, 3086f
　prevention of, 3107-3110, 3108t
　of prostate, 3512-3513
　recurrence, 3118
　risk factors of, 3075-3078
Urothelial cell carcinoma, genomic alterations in, 1359
Urothelial malignant lesions, of upper tract urothelium, 2188
Urothelium
　of bladder, 2461-2462, 2462f-2463f
　　asymmetrical unit membrane (AUM), 2462, 2463f
　　barrier function of, 2467-2468, 2468f
　　glycosaminoglycan layer of, 2467-2468
　　hinge region of, 2462, 2463f
　　ionic transport of, 2469

Urothelium (Continued)
　　permeability of, 2461-2462, 2467, 2468f
　　physiology of, 2467-2470, 2470b
　　plaques of, 2462
　　sensor-transducer function of, 2469-2470
　　suburothelial interstitial cells, 2470, 2470f
　　umbrella cells, 2461-2462, 2463f, 2467
　genetic alterations in, 1358-1359
　idiopathic OAB and, 2504
　of upper urinary tract, normal, 2188
　of ureters, contractile activity and, 1885
Urothelium-based hypothesis, 2642
Urothelium-derived inhibitory factors, 2470
Urotherapy, for bowel-bladder dysfunction, 655-656
Urovascular fistulae, 2958, 2959b
　pyelovascular, 2958
　renovascular, 2958
　ureterovascular, 2958-2959
USI. see Urodynamic stress incontinence
Uterine artery, 2432, 2433f, 2436
Uterine body, anatomy of, 2436
Uterine procidentia, 2526
Uterine prolapse, 2814
　exstrophy-epispadias complex and, 567
　hysteropexy, 2815-2823
　　minimally invasive sacrohysteropexy, 2822-2823, 2824t
　　minimally invasive uterosacral, 2820-2822, 2821t
　　open abdominal sacrohysteropexy, 2822-2823, 2824t
　　sacrospinous, 2817-2820
　　transvaginal uterosacral ligament, 2817, 2819t
　uterine sparing and, 2815-2823, 2816t
Uterine RMS, in pediatric patients, 1120
Uterine tube, 324-325, 324f-325f
Uterosacral fold, 2427-2428, 2429f
Uterosacral hysteropexy, minimally invasive, 2820-2822, 2821t
Uterosacral ligament, 2429-2430, 2431f
　surgical anatomy of, 2789f, 2790, 2791f
Uterosacral ligament suspension, for apical vaginal vault prolapse repair, 2790-2793
　abdominal approach to, 2791, 2793f
　high suspension, 2790-2791, 2792f
　results of, 2792-2793, 2794t
Uterovaginal canal, 324f
Uterus
　anatomy of, 2436
　imaging of, 2440-2441, 2441f-2442f
　round ligament of, 321
Uterus corpus, 325, 325f
Uterus didelphys, 327
UTIs. see Urinary tract infections
Utricle, 315f
UTUC. see Upper tract urothelial cancer
UUI. see Urgency urinary incontinence
UVF. see Ureterovaginal fistula
UVJ. see Ureterovesical junction

V

Vaccination, for GU cancers, 1339-1340, 1340f
　genitourinary tumors, 1341-1342, 1342f
　kidney cancer, 1340-1341
　prostate cancer, 1341
Vacuum therapy, and PD, 1615, 1617t
Vagina, 325-327, 326f-327f
　anatomy of, 2438
　disorders of, 978-986, 982b
　　associated findings, 981-982
　　hymenal skin tags, 978-979, 979f
　　imperforate hymen, 978-979, 979f
　　transverse vaginal septum, 979-980, 979f-980f
　　vaginal agenesis, 980-981, 981f
　　vaginal atresia, 980
　　vertical fusion, 979-981

Vagina (Continued)
  embryology of, 973-974, 974f, 974b
  leiomyoma of, urethral diverticula differentiated from, 2983-2984, 2985f
Vaginal agenesis, 327, 980-981, 981f
Vaginal atresia, 980
Vaginal birth, urinary incontinence and, 2583
Vaginal cells, receptivity of, in UTIs, 1135-1136, 1135f
Vaginal cones
  for pelvic floor muscle training, 2722.e2b-2722.e4b, 2726, 2726.e1f
  for urinary incontinence, in geriatric patient, 2920.e3
Vaginal delivery, for congenital urologic conditions, 290
Vaginal discharge, 397
Vaginal hysterectomy, for uterine prolapse, 2814
Vaginal mesh
  exposure
    after mid-urethral sling surgery, 2864, 2864f
    complications from, 2880, 2881f
  removal, complications from, 2882, 2882b
Vaginal pain, in mesh complication, 2881
Vaginal paravaginal repair, for pelvic organ prolapse, 2780t, 2783, 2784f-2785f
Vaginal prolapse, after retropubic suspension surgery, 2770-2771
Vaginal pull-down maneuver, 974, 975f
Vaginal reflux, pediatric, 660
Vaginal replacement surgery, 982-984, 985b
  intestinal neovagina creation for, 983-984, 983f-984f
  skin neovagina creation for, 982-983, 982f
Vaginal rhabdomyosarcoma, 397
Vaginal RMS, in pediatric patients, 1119-1120, 1119f
Vaginal wall cysts, urethral diverticula differentiated from, 2986, 2986f
Vaginectomy, 3064-3066, 3064f-3068f
Vaginismus, female sexual dysfunction and, 1637
Vaginitis, 1140, 1271-1272, 1272t
Vagino-obturator shelf (VOS) repair, 2767-2768
  results with, 2768
  suspensions in, configuration of, 2758
  technique for, 2767-2768, 2767f
  tissue approximation in, 2759
  urethral elevation in, 2758
Vaginoplasty, 3062
  initial management, timing, and principles for, 1026, 1026f, 1028f-1029f
Valid surrogate end point, 104
Validated questionnaires, 476-477
Validity, definition of, 109
Valrubicin, for non-muscle-invasive bladder cancer, 3104
Valsalva leak point pressure (VLPP), 2562, 2597
Valsalva maneuver, 2902
Valve bladder syndrome, 617-619, 617f-618f
Vancomycin
  prophylaxis with, for uncomplicated urologic procedures, 1194t-1196t
  for UTIs, 1150t-1151t
Vanilloids, to facilitate bladder filling and urine storage, 2709
Vanillylmandelic acid testing, for pheochromocytoma, 2377
Vanishing testis, 959-960, 960f
Vardenafil (Levitra)
  to facilitate bladder filling and urine storage, 2682t, 2701
  for ureteral relaxation, 1899
Varicocele, 899-903, 900b, 1440, 1450
  associated pathologic processes, 900-901
  diagnosis and classification of, 900, 900t
  epidemiology of, 899-900
  hormonal function, 901

Varicocele (Continued)
  intratesticular, 901-902
  pathogenesis of, 899-900
  sclerotherapy or embolotherapy for, 903, 903.e1f
  semen quality in, 901
  surgical repair of, 902, 902t
  testicular histology, 901
  treatment for, 902-903
  varicocelectomy for
    retroperitoneal or laparoscopic, 902-903, 903f
    subinguinal or inguinal microsurgical, 902
Varicocelectomy, 1855
  complications of, 1482
    hydrocele, 1482
    testicular artery injury, 1482
    varicocele recurrence, 1482
  laparoscopic, 902-903, 903f, 1477
  microsurgical inguinal and subinguinal operations for, 1477-1481
    anesthesia for, 1477
    approaches for, 1478, 1478f-1479f, 1478t
    delivery of testis, 1478t, 1480-1481, 1481f
    dissection of cord, 1479-1480, 1479f-1481f
  radiographic occlusion technique for, 1481-1482
  results for, 1482-1483
  retroperitoneal, 902-903, 903f, 1476-1477, 1476f
  scrotal operations for, 1476
  subinguinal or inguinal microsurgical, 902
Vas deferens, 1850-1853
  anatomy of, 1377b
    arterial supply, 1377
    gross structure, 1376, 1376f-1377f
    lymphatic drainage, 1377
    microanatomic architecture, 1376-1377
    nerve supply, 1377
    venous drainage, 1377
  anomalies of, 903
  blood supply of, 1454, 1454t
  dissection of, in laparoscopic radical prostatectomy, 3573-3574, 3574f
  in genitourinary tuberculosis, 1309
  imaging of
    transrectal ultrasound, 1444.e3
    vasogram, 1377
Vas isolation, methods of, 1850
Vascular anomaly, 338-339
Vascular changes, with aging, 2906
Vascular complications, after RPLND, 2244
Vascular complications, of urologic surgery, 269-275
  access technique, comparison of, 271-272
  diagnosis of, 274-275, 275f
  epigastric vessels, injury of, 272
  injury, mechanisms of, 271
  major vessels, injury of, 272-273, 273f
  management, 270, 270f
    intraoperative vascular complications, 269-270
  postoperative vascular complications, 274
  stapler malfunction, 273-274, 274f
  vascular incidents, management of, 272, 272f
  vascular injury, during abdominal access, 271
Vascular endothelial growth factor (VEGF)
  inhibitors of
    for metastatic bladder cancer, 3130-3131
    for metastatic RCC, 2326-2327, 2333-2337, 2333t-2335t, 2336f, 2337t
  in RCC, 2146
Vascular evaluation, in ED, 1521-1523
Vascular injury
  during abdominal access, 271
  during laparoscopic and robotic surgery, 229-230

Vascular injury (Continued)
  laparoscopic kidney surgery causing, 2306-2307
  during radical nephrectomy, 2261
Vascular invasion, 3512
Vascular malformations, 888, 888f
Vascular reconstruction, RPLND with, 1718-1719, 1719f
Vascular surgery, ureteral injuries with, 1993
Vascular transposition, for laparoscopic pyeloplasty, 1956
Vascular-targeted photodynamic (VTP) therapy, 3632, 3637t
Vasculature
  adrenal, 2345, 2348f-2349f, 2355f, 2356, 2405-2406, 2406f
  of bladder, 2455, 2456f, 2462-2463, 2464f
  of epididymis, 1375
  of pelvis
    female, 2432-2433, 2433f
    male, 2451-2452, 2451t
  of penis, 1807.e4f
  of prostate, 1380, 1380f
  renal, 1869-1870
  of scrotum, 1843
  of testis, 1370-1371, 1372f
  of urethra, 2438-2439, 2439f
  of uterus, 2436
  of vagina, 2438
Vasectomy, 1440, 1850-1853, 1853b
  conventional technique for, 1850-1851
  failure, complication of scrotal surgery, 1856
  minimally invasive, 1851, 1851f
  no-scalpel technique for, 1851-1853, 1852f
  prostate cancer and, 3464
  reversal, 1853
Vasoactive drugs, for PE, 1572.e2
Vasoactive intestinal polypeptide, 1535
Vasoconstriction, renal hormone effects, 1913
Vasodilation, renal hormone effects, 1913
Vasoepididymostomy, 1467-1471
  indications for, 1468
  intussusception, 1469-1470, 1470f
  long-term follow-up evaluation and results, 1471
  techniques for, and microsurgical end-to-side, 1468-1469, 1468f-1469f, 1468t
  varicocelectomy and, 1470
Vasoepididymostomy, for chronic scrotal pain syndrome, 1221
Vasogram, of vas deferens, 1377
Vasography, 1457-1460
  complications of, 1458-1459
    hematoma, 1459
    injury to vasal blood supply, 1459
    sperm granuloma, 1459
    stricture, 1458-1459
  fine-needle, 1459-1460
  in male, 1444
  techniques, and interpretation of findings, 1457-1458, 1457f-1459f
  transrectal and seminal vesiculography, 1459-1460
Vasopressin, renal vascular tone control by, 1913
Vasovasostomy, 1460-1467
  and anastomosis in convoluted, 1465-1466, 1466f
  anastomotic techniques for, 1463-1464
  anesthesia for, 1460
  for chronic scrotal pain syndrome, 1221
  crossed, 1466
    technique for, 1466, 1466f
  long-term follow-up evaluation for, 1467
  and microsurgical multilayer microdot method, 1464-1465, 1464f-1465f
  and multiple vasal obstructions, 1462
  postoperative complications of, 1467
  postoperative management for, 1467

Vasovasostomy (Continued)
    preoperative evaluation for, 1460
        laboratory tests, 1460
        physical examination, 1460
    preparation of vasa, 1461, 1461f–1462f
    set-up for, 1464
    surgical approaches for
        inguinal, 1460–1461
        scrotal, 1460, 1461f
    and transposition of testis, 1466, 1467f
    and varicocelectomy, 1462–1463
    and vasoepididymostomy, 1461–1462, 1463t
    wound closure, 1466–1467
VCUG. see Voiding cystourethrogram
VDR. see Vitamin D receptor
VEGF. see Vascular endothelial growth factor
Vein grafts, for urethral and penile reconstruction, 1806
Velocity of sound, 70f
Vena caval replacement, 2276–2277, 2277f
Vena caval resection, in retroperitoneal tumors, 2243
Vena caval thrombectomy, 2266–2278, 2278b
    bypass techniques for, 2275–2276, 2275f–2276f, 2275.e1f, 2276.e1f
    IVC filtration and permanent interruption for bland thrombus, 2277
    level I, right-sided tumor technique, 2267–2269, 2267.e1f, 2269.e1f, 2270f
    level II, left-sided tumor technique, 2269–2270, 2269.e1f, 2271f
    level III-IV
        combined intra-abdominal and intrathoracic approach, 2274–2275, 2274f, 2274.e1f
        intra-abdominal approach technique, 2270–2274, 2271f–2274f, 2273.e1f
    patching, replacing, and interrupting of IVC in, 2276–2277, 2277f
    perioperative complications, 2277–2278
    preoperative considerations for, 2266–2267, 2267t, 2268f–2269f
Veneficus, 427–428
Venereal warts. see Condylomata acuminata
Venography, 1444, 1444.e1
Venous drainage, 1807.e8–1807.e9
Venous flow, pneumoperitoneum effects on, 220–221
Venous gas embolism, 181
Venous reconstruction, in ED, 1537
Venous supply, to male pelvis, 2452
Venous system
    of retroperitoneum, 1672–1674, 1672.e1f
    surgical anatomy of, 3548, 3549f
Venous thromboembolism (VTE), 278–280, 279t–280t
    after RPLND, 1731
    prophylaxis for, in urologic surgery, 128–130, 129t–131t, 131b
Venous tumor thrombus
    laparoscopic radical nephrectomy for, 2298
    in RCC, 2160
    surgery for. see Vena caval thrombectomy
Venovenous bypass (VVB), for vena caval thrombectomy, 2275, 2275f, 2275.e1f
Ventral corporal lengthening procedures, 913, 915f–916f
Ventral penile curvature, 911–914, 916b
    artificial erection for, 911–912
    assessment and management of, 911–914
    dorsal shortening technique for, 912–913, 915f
    goniometer for, 912
    significance of, 911
    ventral corporal lengthening procedures for, 913, 915f–916f
Ventriculoperitoneal (VP) shunts, 461
Verapamil, for PD, 1612, 1617t

Veress needle, 463, 464f
    for achieving transperitoneal access and establishing pneumoperitoneum, 207–209
    complications related to, 224
    vascular injury, 469f
Verrucous carcinoma (Buschke-Lowenstein tumor)
    as neoplastic condition, 1296–1297, 1299f
    of penis, 1742.e1
Vertebral column abnormalities, with cloacal exstrophy, 575
Vertical fusion, abnormalities of, 979–981
Verumontanum, 315f, 1382, 1382f–1383f
Vesicle pain, patient history of, 2
Vesicoamniotic shunt placement versus fetal cystoscopy, 365–366, 367f
Vesicobullous disorders, 1283–1286, 1284b
    bullous pemphigoid, 1284–1285, 1285f
    dermatitis herpetiformis, 1285
    Hailey-Hailey disease, 1285–1286, 1286f
    linear IgA bullous dermatosis, 1285, 1285f
    pemphigus vulgaris, 1284, 1284f
Vesicoenteric fistulae, 2953t, 2955b
    etiology of, 2952–2953, 2953t
    presentation of, 2952–2953, 2953t
Vesicopelvic ligament, 2429–2430
Vesicostomy
    continent, 710–711
    cutaneous, 690–691
        for posterior urethral valves, 612–613, 613f–614f
        for prune-belly syndrome, 592, 592f
Vesicoureteral reflux (VUR), 330, 374, 374f–375f, 399, 489–517, 836–846, 836b, 1139, 1938
    after pediatric renal transplantation, 1062, 1062f
    assessment of, 95
    associated anomalies and conditions, 507–511
        bladder diverticula, 509–510, 509.e1f
        megacystis-megaureter association, 510
        other anomalies, 510
        pregnancy and reflux, 510–511, 511b
        renal anomalies, 510
        ureteral duplication, 508–509, 508.e1f
        ureteropelvic junction obstruction, 507–508, 509f
    causes of, 495–497
        clinical correlates, 496–497, 497f
        primary reflux, 495
        secondary reflux, 495–496, 496f
    clinical presentation of, 836
    Cohen Cross-Trigonal technique for, 840, 841f
    complications of ureteral reimplantation for, 844–846
        contralateral reflux, 844
        obstruction, 844–846
        persistent reflux, 844
    controversies in usage of invasive investigations, 507
        American Academy of Pediatrics Guidelines for febrile urinary tract infection diagnosis and management in young children, 507, 508t
        National Institutes for Clinical Excellence Guidelines, 507
    cortical defects, 498–501, 500b
        acquired renal scars, 499–500
        congenital defects versus acquired scar, 498–499
        pathophysiology of acquired scarring, 500–501, 500f–501f
        reflux-associated renal dysplasia, 499, 499f, 499t, 499.e1f
    defecation disorders and, 667, 667.e1f
    definition of, 836
    demographics, 489–490, 490b
        age, 490, 490t
        prevalence, 489

Vesicoureteral reflux (VUR) (Continued)
        race, 490
        reflux in the fetus, 490
        sex, 489–490
    diagnosis and evaluation of, 501–503, 502b, 1938
        confirmation of urinary tract infection, 501–502
        evaluating urinary tract infection, 502–503, 503f
    early complications of, 844–846
    embryology of ureterovesical junction, 493
    endoscopic treatment of, 846–849
        follow-up for, 847–848
        injection technique, 846–847, 847f
        materials used for, 848
        recurrence after, 848–849
    with epispadias, 569
    extravesical procedures for, 840–842, 842f–843f
    functional anatomy of the antireflux mechanism, 493–495, 494f, 494t, 495b
    Glenn-Anderson technique for, 840, 840f
    grading of, 497–498, 498f, 498t
    historical perspective, 489
    incision for, 836, 837f–839f
    inheritance and genetics, 490–492, 492b
        genes involved, 491–492, 492f–493f
        sibling reflux, 490–491
    intravesical procedures for, 836–840
        ureter mobilization, 836–840, 837f–839f
    long-term complications of, 846
        obstruction, 846
        recurrent or persistent reflux, 846
    lower urinary tract, assessment of, 503–505
        cystographic imaging, 503–504, 504f
        cystoscopy and the positioning of the instillation of contrast cystogram, 504–505
    minimally invasive procedures for, 842–844
    natural history and management, 511–517, 516b
        antibiotic controversies and potential new approaches, 514–515
        individualizing patient care, 516–517, 517f
        landmark studies, 515–516
        medical management: continuous antibiotic prophylaxis, 513–514, 513t
        principles, 512–513
        resolution by age, 512, 512f
        resolution by grade, 511
        spontaneous resolution, 511
    neural tube defects and, early intervention for, 628
    in neuromuscular dysfunction of lower urinary tract, 638–639, 638f, 639b
    in pediatric patients, 653–654
    Politano-Leadbetter technique for, 837f–839f, 840
    with posterior urethral valves, 615–616, 619b
    postoperative evaluation of, 844
    recommendations for, 374
    reoperative reimplantation for, 846
    robotic-assisted laparoscopic ureteral reimplantation- extravesical for, 844, 845f
    surgical management of, 836
    treatment of, 1938
    upper urinary tract, assessment of, 505–507
        controversies in usage of invasive investigations, 506
        rationale for serial assessment of upper tracts, 505
        renal scintigraphy, 505–506, 506f
        renal scintigraphy and the top-down approach, 506–507
        renal sonography, 505
    ureteral function relation with, 1898–1899, 1899f
    ureteropelvic junction obstruction with, 1943
    urinary tract dysfunction with, 2615

Vesicoureteral reflux (VUR) (Continued)
　urinary tract infection and, 497, 497b
　Valsalva maneuver and, 2902
Vesicoureteral reflux and dysplasia (VURD), posterior urethral valves and, 606, 606b, 607f
Vesicourethral distraction defects, 1834b, 1835, 1836b
Vesicouterine fistulae, 2946-2947, 2947b
　diagnosis of, 2946-2947, 2946f-2947f
　etiology of, 2946
　management of, 2946-2947
　presentation of, 2946
Vesicouterine pouch, 2427-2428, 2429f
　bladder, 3010
Vesicovaginal fistula (VVF), 2924-2926, 2925f, 2925b, 2942b
　abdominal techniques for, 2937
　　suprapubic intraperitoneal or extraperitoneal, 2937, 2937f-2938f
　　transvesical, 2937
　　vaginal versus, 2933-2934, 2933t
　adjuvant procedures in repair of, 2939-2942
　　greater omentum, 2940
　　Martius flap, 2939-2940, 2939f
　　other flap and graft techniques, 2940, 2941f
　　peritoneal flap, 2940, 2940f
　causes of, 2927b
　conservative and minimally invasive therapy for, 2931-2932, 2932f
　etiology of, 2925, 2925f, 2925b
　history of, 2929
　intraoperative risk factors for, 2927-2930
　　cystoscopy for, 2929, 2929f
　　diagnosis of, 2928
　　evaluation of, 2928
　　imaging for, 2929, 2930f-2931f
　　physical examination of, 2928-2929, 2928f
　　presentation of, 2928
　　urine studies for, 2929-2930
　laparoscopic approaches to, 2937-2939, 2939t
　　transabdominal transvesical, 2940
　posthysterectomy, 2926-2927
　prevalence of, 2925
　robotic approaches to, 2937-2939
　surgery for
　　abdominal versus vaginal approach, 2932-2933, 2933-2934, 2933t
　　adjuvant flaps or grafts, 2934
　　antibiotics, 2934
　　estrogen supplementation, 2934
　　excision versus no excision, 2934
　　immediate versus delayed, 2933
　　indications for, 2934-2935
　　outcomes of, 2942
　　postoperative drainage, 2934
　　preoperative counseling for, 2934-2935
　treatment for, 2931-2942
　urinary diversion and, 2940-2942
　vaginal techniques for, 2935-2937
　　abdominal versus, 2933-2934, 2933t
　　complications with, 2936-2937
　　other transvaginal techniques, 2937
　　vaginal flap or flap-splitting technique, 2935-2936, 2935f-2936f
Vesicovaginal space, 2427, 2429f
Vesiculodeferential artery, 1377
Vessel-sparing technique, for urethral stricture disease, 1820, 1820f-1821f
Vestibular cysts, 976-977, 977f
Vestibule, 1627.e1
　disorders of, 975-977, 977b
　　ectopic ureteral insertion, 977, 978f
　　prolapsed ureterocele, 977, 978f
　　urethral polyp, 976, 976f
　　urethral prolapse, 975-976, 976f
　　vestibular cysts, 976-977, 977f

Veterans Affairs Cooperative Study, 3385
VHL. see von Hippel-Lindau disease
VHL gene, 2141-2143, 2143t, 2144f, 2332-2333, 2333f
Viagra. see Sildenafil
Vicryl suture, 149-150
Video-endoscopic systems, 185, 186f-187f
Videourodynamics (VUDS), 1048, 1048f, 2569-2571, 2571b, 2572f
　for benign prostatic hyperplasia, 3347
　for bladder neck dysfunction, 2570, 2570f
　for BOO diagnosis in women, 2570, 2570f
　for LUTS in men, 2570, 2571f
　methods of, 2570
　for neuropathic voiding dysfunction, 2573f
　for pelvic floor disorders, 2535
　for voiding phase dysfunction, 2570
Vinblastine-ifosfamide-cisplatin (VeIP), for NSGCTs, 1697
Vincristine, for penile cancer, 1771
Viral hepatitis, STDs and, 1268-1271, 1269t
Virchow triad, in pregnancy, 283
Virtual reality trainers, for laparoscopic and robotic surgery, 232-233
Virtue Quadratic male sling, 2887
Virulent bacteria, 427-428
Virus-related tumors, of penis, 1742.e2-1742.e3, 1743b
　Bowenoid papulosis, 1742.e2
　HPV, 1742.e5
　Kaposi sarcoma, 1742.e5
Visceral injury
　during laparoscopic and robotic surgery, 224
　laparoscopic kidney surgery causing, 2307, 2307f
Visible hematuria, 247
Visual estimation targeting (VET), 3622
Visual obturator access, 464-465
Vital signs, 9
Vitamin D
　in absorptive hypercalciuria, 2019
　in calcium metabolism, 2015
　in prostate cancer, 3463-3465
　renal regulation of, 1914, 1914f
Vitamin D receptor (VDR), 2019
　in prostate cancer, 3463-3465
Vitamin D$_3$-receptor analogues, to facilitate bladder filling and urine storage, 2713.e1
Vitamin E
　for PD, 1611, 1616t
　in prostate cancer prevention, 3476, 3476f
Vitiligo, 1305f, 1306
VLPP. see Valsalva leak point pressure
Voided urine specimens, in urine collection, 1141
Voiding. see also Micturition
　bashful bladder, 2628-2629
　with normal bladder contraction, 2515-2516
　therapy to facilitate, 2520b
Voiding cystourethrogram (VCUG), 39-40, 40f, 367, 389-390, 404-405, 406f, 414f, 415-416
　bladder, 3011
　of bladder diverticula, 2965f
　for bladder/urethra, 415-416
　　cysts/masses, 415
　　infection, 415
　　obstruction of, 415, 416f
　for differences of sex development, 416, 417f
　fluoroscopy, 389
　fundamentals of, 415
　genitography, 390
　of kidney/ureter, 415
　　cysts/masses, 415
　　infection, 415
　　obstruction of, 415
　nuclear cystography, 389-390
　of posterior urethral valves, 608, 609f
　for scrotum/testes/internal genitalia, 416

Voiding cystourethrogram (VCUG) (Continued)
　trauma and, 415-416, 417f
　for ureteral anomalies, 805
　for vesicovaginal fistula, 2929, 2930f
Voiding diaries, 476f
　for PFDs evaluation, 2531
　for urinary incontinence, in geriatric patients, 2920.e1-2920.e2
Voiding dysfunction
　after mid-urethral sling, 2871-2873, 2872t, 2873b
　　management of, 2871-2873
　after pubovaginal sling procedure, 2845-2848, 2848b
　　surgical management of, 2846-2848, 2847t
　behavioral treatment for, 2732
　benign prostatic hyperplasia in, 3305, 3306f
　classification of
　　functional, 2551
　classification systems of, 2519-2524
　　Bors-Comarr, 2522-2523, 2523b
　　Bradley, 2524
　　functional, 2516b-2517b, 2518t, 2519b-2521b, 2520-2521
　　Hald-Bradley, 2523-2524, 2523b
　　International Continence Society, 2517, 2521b
　　Lapides, 2522-2523, 2522b
　　urodynamic, 2521-2522, 2522b
　electrical stimulation in, 2746-2747, 2746f-2747f
　HIV and, 1267
　lower urinary tract dysfunction and, 2627
　neurogenic, 2967
　neuropathic
　　patterns of, 2600-2602
　　videourodynamics for, 2573f
　postoperative, after retropubic suspension surgery, 2770
　ureterocele and, 820
　urodynamic studies of, functional classification, 2551
　videourodynamics for, 2570
von Brunn nests, of upper urinary tract, 2188
von Hippel-Lindau disease (VHL), 759-761
　classification of, 760, 760t
　clinical features of, 760
　etiology of, 760
　evaluation of, 761
　histopathology of, 760-761
　screening for, 761, 761t
　targeted molecular therapies for
　　basis of, 2332-2333, 2333f
　　combination and sequential therapy with, 2339-2341
　　mTOR pathway inhibitors, 2326-2327, 2338-2339, 2340f, 2340t
　　VEGFR-based, 2326-2327, 2333-2337, 2333t-2335t, 2336f, 2337t
　treatment of, 761
von Hippel-Lindau syndrome
　genomic alterations in, 1354t, 1358, 2141-2143, 2143t, 2144f
　RCC screening for, 2158
　treatment of RCC in, 2173-2174, 2174f
VOS repair. see Vagino-obturator shelf (VOS) repair
VTE. see Venous thromboembolism
VUDS. see Videourodynamics
Vulva, 1627.e1-1627.e2, 1627.e1f, 2436, 2436f-2437f
Vulvar RMS, in pediatric patients, 1119
VUR. see Vesicoureteral reflux
VVB. see Venovenous bypass
VVF. see Vesicovaginal fistula

W

Wallace technique, in urinary diversion, 3187-3188, 3188f

Warburg effect, 96
WAS. see Water avoidance stress
Watchful waiting. see also Surveillance
  for benign prostatic hyperplasia, studies on, 3329–3330, 3330f, 3330t
  for lower urinary tract symptoms, 3351
  for prostate cancer, 3541
Water
  filtrate transport, 1910–1911, 1911f, 1911b
  intake of, renal calculi and, 2009
  urothelium permeability to, 2467
Water avoidance stress (WAS), bladder pain syndrome and interstitial cystitis and, 2508
Water imbalance, diabetes insipidus, 2678
Water-filled catheters, for urodynamic studies, 2558
Watts factor (WF), 2658
Wavelength, 70f
WBS. see Williams-Beuren syndrome
Webbed penis, 394, 878–879, 879f
Wedge resection, for large renal tumors, 2263, 2265f
Weight control, for prostate cancer, 3544
Weight loss, for OAB, 2647
Weight reduction, for urinary incontinence, 2734
Well differentiated liposarcomas, in retroperitoneum, 2229–2230
Wernicke encephalopathy, lower urinary tract dysfunction and, 2631
WHI. see Women's Health Initiative
Whitaker test, 160
  for urinary tract obstruction, 780
White blood cell, priapism and, 1542
White coat hypertension, 352
White line of Toldt, 1866
Whole-body bone scan, 42
Williams-Beuren syndrome (WBS), lower urinary tract dysfunction and, 2631–2632
Wilms tumor, 402, 1096–1110, 1110b, 2181t, 2183
  biology and genetics of, 1096–1099, 1097t, 1354t
  epidemiology of, 1096

Wilms tumor (Continued)
  pathology of, 1099–1101
    after preoperative chemotherapy, 1100
    anaplasia, 1100
    favorable histology, 1100, 1100f
    nephrogenic rests, 1100–1101, 1101f
  preoperative evaluation of, 1101–1103, 1103t
  screening for, 1098–1099, 1099f, 1099t
  treatment of
    chemotherapy, 1106–1108, 1107f
    late effects of, 1108–1110
    partial nephrectomy, 1107–1108
    surgical considerations of, 1103–1104, 1105f
Window technique, 1845
Wisconsin Stone Quality of Life (WiSQoL) questionnaire, 175
Wnt signaling pathway, 3276
WNT4 gene, 992f, 992t, 993
Wolffian duct (WD), 324f, 334–335, 714
Women's Health Initiative (WHI), 2710
Wong-Baker FACES, 448f
World Health Organization, RCC classification system of, 2148t
Wound. see also Surgical wounds
  genital bite, 1293, 1294f
Wound dressing, 151
Wound healing, and PD, 1603–1604
Wound infections. see also Surgical site infections
  after laparoscopic and robotic surgery, 231
W-stapled reservoir, for cutaneous continent urinary diversion, 3228–3229, 3231f
WT1 gene, 991–992, 992f, 992t, 1097, 1097t
WTX gene, 1097–1098, 1097t

X
Xanthine stones
  in renal calculi, 2031–2032
  surgical management of, 2077.e3
Xanthogranulomatous pyelonephritis (XGP), 444, 1177–1179, 1178f–1179f
Xenograft, for pubovaginal sling, 2835
  outcomes of, 2843–2844, 2844t
XGP. see Xanthogranulomatous pyelonephritis

Y
Y chromosome microdeletion testing, for male infertility, 1442–1443
Yang-Monti technique, 709, 710f
Yeast, in urine, 22f, 23
Yellowfins stirrups, 3580
Yerba mate, UTUC risk and, 2186
Yoga, for female orgasmic disorder, 1647
Yolk sac, 318f
Yolk sac tumors (YSTs)
  in female pediatric patients, 1120
  testicular
    histology of, 1683f, 1684
    in pediatric patients, 1123–1124, 1124f
Young-Dees-Leadbetter bladder neck reconstruction, 685–686
  modified, 555f–556f
  results with, 685–686
  technique for, 685
YSTs. see Yolk sac tumors

Z
Zanoterone, for benign prostatic hyperplasia, 3376
Zika virus, STD and, 1264–1268
Zinc, in prostatic secretions, 3296–3297
Zinc α$_2$-glycoprotein, in prostatic secretions, 3302–3303
Zipper injuries, to penis, 3051
Zoledronate, 3703
Zona fasciculata, in adrenal cortex physiology, 2357, 2357f, 2358t
Zona glomerulosa, in adrenal cortex physiology, 2356–2357
Zona reticularis, in adrenal cortex physiology, 2357
Zonal anatomy, prostate, 1379f–1380f, 1380–1381
Zonisamide, in stone formation, 2033